18th Edition

Handbook of Pediatrics

Gerald B. Merenstein
David W. Kaplan
Adam A. Rosenb

a LANGE medical .

18th Edition

Handbook of Pediatrics

GERALD B. MERENSTEIN, MD, FAAP
Professor and Vice Chair
Department of Pediatrics
University of Colorado Health Sciences Center:
The Children's Hospital
Denver, Colorado

DAVID W. KAPLAN, MD, MPH
Professor
Head, Adolescent Medicine
Department of Pediatrics
University of Colorado Health Sciences Center:
The Children's Hospital
Denver, Colorado

ADAM A. ROSENBERG, MD
Associate Professor
Department of Pediatrics
University of Colorado Health Sciences Center:
The Children's Hospital
Denver, Colorado

APPLETON & LANGE
Stamford, Connecticut

97 98 99 00 / 10 9 8 7 6 5 4 3 2 1

Prentice Hall International (UK) Limited, *London*
Prentice Hall of Australia Pty. Limited, *Sydney*
Prentice Hall Canada, Inc., *Toronto*
Prentice Hall Hispanoamericana, S.A., *Mexico*
Prentice Hall of India Private Limited, *New Delhi*
Prentice Hall of Japan, Inc., *Tokyo*
Simon & Schuster Asia Pte. Ltd., *Singapore*
Editora Prentice Hall do Brasil Ltda., *Rio de Janeiro*
Prentice Hall, *Upper Saddle River, New Jersey*

ISBN 0-8385-3625-5
ISBN 0440-1921

Acquisitions Editor: Shelley Reinhardt
Production Editor: Christine Langan
Senior Art Manager: Eve Siegel

PRINTED IN THE UNITED STATES OF AMERICA

Table of Contents

The Authors

Steven H. Abman, MD
Professor, Pediatric Pulmonary Medicine, University of Colorado School of Medicine/The Children's Hospital, Denver.

Mark J. Abzug, MD
Associate Professor, Department of Pediatrics, Pediatric Infectious Diseases, University of Colorado Health Sciences Center/The Children's Hospital, Denver.

Peter W. Aldoretta, MD, FAAP
Neonatologist, Woman's Hospital, Baton Rouge, Louisiana.

Marsha S. Anderson, MD
Fellow, Department of Infectious Disease, The Children's Hospital, University of Colorado, Denver.

F. Keith Battan, MD
Assistant Professor, Department of Pediatrics, University of Colorado School of Medicine; Associate Director, Emergency Services, Denver Children's Hospital, Denver.

Stephen Berman, MD
Professor of Pediatrics, University of Colorado School of Medicine/The Children's Hospital, Denver.

Holly U. Biffl, MD
Chief Resident, The Children's Hospital, Denver.

David Burgess, MD
Associate Professor, Department of Pediatrics, University of Colorado School of Medicine, Denver.

H. Peter Chase, MD
Professor of Pediatrics; Clinical Director, Barbara Davis Center for Childhood Diabetes, University of Colorado School of Medicine, Denver.

Richard C. Dart, MD
Director, Rocky Mountain Poison and Drug Center, Denver, Colorado.

Jeffrey I. Dolgan, PhD
Assistant Clinical Professor, Psychiatry, University of Colorado Health Sciences Center; Associate Clinical Professor, Psychology, Denver University, Denver.

Robert E. Eilert, MD
Clinical Professor of Orthopaedic Surgery, University of Colorado Health Sciences Center, Denver; Chairman, Department of Orthopaedic Surgery, The Children's Hospital, Denver.

Stewart Gabel, MD
Chairman, Department of Psychiatry and Behavioral Sciences, The Children's Hospital, Denver; Associate Professor of Psychiatry and Pediatrics, University of Colorado Health Sciences Center, Denver.

Benjamin A. Gitterman, MD
Associate Professor of Pediatrics & Health Care Sciences, George Washington University Medical Center; Director, General Pediatric Ambulatory Center, Children's National Medical Center, Washington, DC.

Ronald W. Gotlin, MD
Professor of Pediatrics, University of Colorado Health Sciences Center/The Children's Hospital, Denver.

K. Michael Hambidge, MD, ScD
Professor, Pediatrics; Director, Center for Human Nutrition, University of Colorado Health Sciences Center/The Children's Hospital, Denver.

Taru Hays, MD
Professor of Pediatrics, University of Colorado Health Sciences Center/The Children's Hospital, Denver.

Rebecca A. Hea, PsyD
Outpatient Clinical Coordinator, Denver Children's Home, Denver, Colorado.

Roxann M. Headley, MD
Assistant Professor of Pediatrics, University of Colorado School of Medicine; Medical Director, Primary Care Clinics at The Children's Hospital, Denver.

D. Dunbar Ivy, MD
Assistant Professor of Pediatrics, Section of Pediatric Cardiology, University of Colorado Health Sciences Center/The Children's Hospital, Denver.

Joanne Solliday Janas, MD
Pediatric Neurologist, Child Neurology Associates, Atlanta, Georgia.

Alan K. Kamada, PharmD
Assistant Professor, Clinical Pharmacology Division, Department of Pediatrics, National Jewish Center for Immunology and Respiratory Medicine, Denver; Adjoint Assistant Professor, Department of Pharmacy Practice, School of Pharmacy, University of Colorado Health Sciences Center, Denver.

David W. Kaplan, MD, MPH
Professor of Pediatrics; Chief, Section of Adolescent Medicine, University of Colorado Health Sciences Center/The Children's Hospital, Denver.

Kevin Kirchner, MD
Private Practice Physician, Georgia Pediatric Pulmonology Associates, PC, Scottish Rite Children's Medical Center, Atlanta, Georgia.

Nancy F. Krebs, MD
Assistant Professor, Department of Pediatrics, Section of Nutrition; Associate Director, University of Colorado Center for Human Nutrition, University of Colorado Center for Human Nutrition, University of Colorado Health Sciences Center/The Children's Hospital, Denver.

Carol A. Ledwith, MD
Assistant Professor of Pediatrics, University of Colorado Health Sciences Center/The Children's Hospital, Denver.

Gary M. Lum, MD
Professor of Pediatrics and Medicine; Chief, Pediatric Renal Section, Department of Pediatrics, University of Colorado School of Medicine, University of Colorado Health Sciences Center/The Children's Hospital, Denver.

Kathleen A. Mammel, MD
Assistant Professor of Pediatrics, University of Colorado Health Sciences Center/The Children's Hospital, Denver.

Thomas J. McIntee, MD
Pediatrician, Rice Clinic Pediatrics, Stevens Point, Wisconsin.

Sandra J. Meech, MD
Fellow in Pediatric Hematology/Oncology, University of Colorado Health Sciences Center/The Children's Hospital, Denver.

Gerald B. Merenstein, MD
Professor, Department of Pediatrics, University of Colorado Health Sciences Center/The Children's Hospital, Denver.

Joseph G. Morelli, MD
Associate Professor of Dermatology and Pediatrics, University of Colorado School of Medicine, University of Colorado Health Sciences Center, Denver.

John W. Ogle, MD
Associate Professor of Pediatrics, University of Colorado School of Medicine, Denver; Director, Pediatric Service, Denver General Hospital, Denver.

David S. Pearlman, MD
Clinical Professor of Pediatrics, University of Colorado School of Medicine, Denver.

Mark G. Roback, MD
Assistant Professor of Pediatrics, University of Colorado Health Sciences Center/The Children's Hospital, Denver.

Adam A. Rosenberg, MD
Associate Professor, Department of Pediatrics, University of Colorado Health Sciences Center/The Children's Hospital, Denver.

Barry H. Rumack, MD
Clinical Professor of Pediatrics, University of Colorado Health Sciences Center, Denver.

Robert A. Sargent, MD, FAAP, FACS, FAAO
Associate Clinical Professor of Ophthalmology. University of Colorado Health Sciences Center/The Children's Hospital, Denver.

Michael S. Schaffer, MD
Associate Professor of Pediatrics, Section of Cardiology, University of Colorado School of Medicine; Director, Pediatric Electrophysiology, The Children's Hospital, Denver.

Barton D. Schmitt, MD
Professor of Pediatrics, University of Colorado School of Medicine; Director, General Pediatric Consultative Services, The Children's Hospital, Denver.

Alan R. Seay, MD
Professor of Pediatrics and Neurology; Head, Division of Neurology, University of Colorado Health Sciences Center/The Children's Hospital, Denver.

Elizabeth M. Shaffer, MD
Associate Professor of Pediatrics, University of Colorado Health Sciences Center/The Children's Hospital, Denver.

Judith M. Sondheimer, MD
Professor of Pediatrics; Chief, Section of Gastroenterology, Hepatology, and Nutrition, University of Colorado Health Sciences Center/The Children's Hospital, Denver.

Steven B. Spedale, MD
Medical Director of Neonatology, Woman's Hospital; Clinical Assistant Professor of Pediatrics, Tulane University School of Medicine, Baton Rouge, Louisiana.

Linda C. Stork, MD
Associate Professor, Department of Pediatrics, Section of Hematology and Oncology, University of Colorado School of Medicine, University of Colorado Health Sciences Center/The Children's Hospital, Denver.

Eva Sujansky, MD
Associate Professor of Pediatrics and Biochemistry, Biophysics, and Genetics; Co-Director, Division of Genetic Services, University of Colorado Health Sciences Center/The Children's Hospital, Denver.

Stanley J. Szefler, MD
Professor of Pediatrics and Pharmacology, University of Colorado Health Sciences Center; Director of Clinical Pharmacology, National Jewish Center for Immunology & Respiratory Medicine, Denver.

Suzanne M. Tanner, MD
Assistant Professor, Departments of Orthopedics and Pediatrics, CU Sports Medicine Center, Denver.

Elaine Van Gundy, MD
Assistant Professor, Creighton University, School of Medicine, Omaha, Nebraska.

William L. Weston, MD
Professor and Chairman, Department of Dermatology; Professor of Pediatrics, University of Colorado School of Medicine, Denver.

NOTICE

Not all of the drugs mentioned in this book have been approved by the FDA for use in infants or in children younger than age 6 or age 12. Such drugs should not be used if effective alternatives are available; they may be used if no effective alternatives are available or if the known risk of toxicity of alternative drugs or the risk of nontreatment is outweighed by the probable advantages of treatment.

Because of the possibility of an error in the article or book from which a particular drug dosage is obtained, or an error appearing in the text of this book, our readers are urged to consult appropriate references, including the manufacturer's package insert, especially when prescribing new drugs or those with which they are not adequately familiar.

—The Authors

Preface

Handbook of Pediatrics offers a convenient, up-to-date source of practical information on the care of children from infancy through adolescence. Focusing on the **clinical** aspects of pediatric care, the eighteenth edition covers a range of topics, including growth and development of the healthy child, ambulatory care, preventive medicine, and diagnosis and management of common pediatric disorders. Pertinent physiologic and pharmacologic principles support the clinical information.

Audience

Handbook of Pediatrics serves the needs of all health professionals involved in the day-to-day care of pediatric patients. **Medical, nursing and physician assistant students, and pediatric and family medicine residents** working in the ambulatory care or hospital setting will appreciate the concise description of diseases and the accessibility of information. **Practicing physicians, nurses, nurse practitioners, and physician assistants,** particularly those in primary care, will find the Handbook a ready and useful reference for a broad spectrum of information; included are chapters on dermatology, cardiology, gastroenterology, and other relevant pediatric subspecialties.

New to This Edition

The eighteenth edition of *Handbook of Pediatrics* continues to reflect the original intent of Dr. Silver and colleagues to provide an up-to-date digest of pediatric information. The team of editors and contributors has continued to revise, reorganize, and update the book to enhance its usefulness in today's practice. The editors continue to strive to present as much information as possible in the form of tables and figures for ready access to information, while assuring appropriate physiologic principles are presented. Many chapters have important revisions, including extensive changes in these:

- Behavioral, Psychosocial, & Psychiatric Pediatrics
- Infectious Diseases: Viral
- Infectious Diseases: Bacterial, Parasitic, & Fungal
- Pediatric Procedures

Continuing Features

- Normal values of blood chemistry, urine, bone marrow, peripheral blood, feces, sweat, and cerebrospinal fluid.
- Description of the most commonly used laboratory tests.
- Extensive pediatric antibiotic formulary.
- Extensive general pediatric drug formulary.

Acknowledgments

We wish to thank the authors who contributed to this edition and the editors and authors who worked on previous editions. We are especially appreciative of the support provided by our Lange editors.

We wish to express our gratitude to our readers throughout the world who have provided us with helpful suggestions. Comments and suggestions for future editions can be sent to us in care of Appleton & Lange, 107 Elm Street, PO Box 120041, Stamford, CT 06912-0041.

Gerald B. Merenstein
David W. Kaplan
Adam A. Rosenberg

Denver, Colorado
December 1996

Pediatric History & Physical Examination | 1

Benjamin A. Gitterman, MD

HISTORY

For many pediatric problems, the history is the most important factor in arriving at a correct diagnosis. The physician's interaction with the patient and the parents during history-taking is also the first stage in the psychotherapeutic management of the patient. Keep in mind that socioeconomic, cultural, and educational factors may influence the caregiver-patient communication process; you should therefore provide assurance of confidentiality as part of the process.

The outline in Table 1–1 should be modified and adapted as appropriate for the age of the child and the reason for the consultation.

Source of History & Reason for Referral

The history and reason for the consultation should be obtained from the parent or whoever is responsible for the care of the child. You can also obtain much valuable information from the child. Interview adolescents in private whenever possible; they may be uncomfortable discussing sensitive information in the presence of their parents.

Identifying Information

The clinician should obtain the following basic information about the child: name, address, and telephone number; sex; date and place of birth; race, religion, and nationality; source of referral; parents' names, occupations, and home or business telephone numbers.

Chief Complaint (CC)

Make a brief record of the patient's or informant's own account of the presenting complaint and its duration.

Table 1–1. Taking a pediatric history.

Source of history and reason for referral	Operations
Identifying information	Accidents and injuries
Chief complaint	Medications
History of present illness	Family history
Birth history	Personal history
Development	Social history
Nutrition	Habits
Illnesses	Review of systems
Immunizations and tests	

History of Present Illness (HPI)

The HPI should include the following inquiries or observations:

1. When was the patient last entirely well?
2. How and when did the condition begin?
3. Progress of disease; order and date of onset of new symptoms.
4. Specific symptoms and physical signs that may have developed.
5. Pertinent negative data obtained by direct questioning.
6. Aggravating and alleviating factors.
7. Significant medical attention and medications or home therapies given, and over what period of time.
8. In acute infections, statement of type and degree of exposure, and interval since exposure.
9. For the well child, factors of significance and general condition since last visit.
10. Examiner's opinion of the informant's reliability.

Birth History

A. Antenatal: Obtain basic information regarding the mother's health during pregnancy, including prenatal care, diet, infections (eg, rubella) and other illnesses, vomiting, bleeding, preeclampsia-eclampsia and other complications. Ask about Rh typing and serologic tests, pelvimetry, medications, x-ray procedures, amniocentesis.

B. Natal: Note the duration of pregnancy, kind and duration of labor, type of delivery, sedation and anesthesia (if known), birth weight, state of infant at birth, resuscitation required, onset of respiration, first cry, special procedures.

C. Neonatal: Ask about the child's Apgar score, color (cyanosis, pallor, jaundice), and cry; and about any twitching, excessive mucus, paralysis, convulsions, fever, hemorrhage, congenital abnormalities, or birth injuries. Also note presence of any rashes as well as any difficulties in sucking or feeding. Record the length of hospital stay and the child's discharge weight.

Development

1. Milestones: record the child's age when he or she first raised head, rolled over, sat alone, pulled up, walked with help, walked alone, talked (meaningful words, sentences). A standardized developmental screening test (eg, Denver II) should be used if possible (Chapter 2).
2. Urinary continence during night; during day.
3. Control of defecation.
4. Comparison of development with that of siblings and parents.
5. Any period of failure to grow or unusual growth.
6. School grade, quality of work.

Nutrition

A. Breast or Formula Feeding: Record the type of feeding, duration, major formula changes, time of weaning, difficulties.

B. Supplements: Note the addition of vitamins (type, amount, duration), iron, or fluoride to the child's diet.

C. Solid Foods: Ask when solid foods were introduced, how taken, types, unusual family dietary habits (eg, vegetarian), balancing of food groups.

D. Appetite: Record the child's food likes and dislikes, idiosyncrasies, allergies, general attitude to eating.

Illnesses

A. Hospitalizations: Record dates and reasons (accidents, poisoning, other emergencies, tests, etc) for hospitalizations.

B. Infections: Note the child's age at onset, type of infection, number and severity of episodes.

C. Contagious Diseases: Record the child's age at exposure to the following infectious diseases: measles, rubella, chickenpox, mumps, pertussis, diphtheria, scarlet fever. Note presence and severity of any complications.

D. Other Serious Noninfectious Illnesses: Obtain information about such illnesses as neoplastic diseases and genetic disorders.

Immunizations & Tests

Indicate child's age at immunization, type and number of immunizations, boosters, reactions, if any.

A. Inoculations: Diphtheria, tetanus, pertussis, measles, rubella, mumps, *Haemophilus influenzae*, hepatitis B, others.

B. Oral Immunizations: Poliomyelitis.

C. Serum Injections: Passive immunizations.

D. Tests: Tuberculin, serology, anemia, lead, sickle cell, others.

Surgery

Record type of surgery, child's age, complications, if any; reasons for operation; child's apparent response.

Accidents & Injuries

Obtain information about the nature and severity of injuries and sequelae, if any.

Medications

Inquire about type of medications (eg, cold remedies, aspirin, laxatives, analgesics); long-term use; any allergies to medications.

Family History

1. Note basic information about child's parents (age and health conditions). If the child does not live with his or her birth parents, record the legal guardian's relationship to the child.
2. Obtain basic information about the child's siblings, if any (age[s], condition of health, significant previous illnesses and problems). Note child's birth order within sibship.
3. Obtain information about mother's childbearing history (stillbirths, miscarriages, abortions); also (if relevant) note age at death and cause of death of members of immediate family.
4. Inquire about the presence of the following conditions in family members: tuberculosis, allergies, blood dyscrasias, mental or nervous diseases, diabetes, cardiovascular diseases, kidney diseases, hypertension, rheumatic fever, neoplastic diseases, congenital abnormalities, convulsive disorders, other hereditary conditions.
5. Record observations about the health of the child's extrafamilial contacts (baby-sitters, day-care personnel and other caregivers, schoolmates, etc).

Personal History

A. Social Behavior & Interests: The clinician should obtain basic information about the child's interpersonal development, with such questions as the following.

1. How does he or she relate to others (eg, independent, clinging, negativistic, aggressive, submissive, shy, extraverted)?
2. Is there age-appropriate separation from parents?
3. Does the child have hobbies and similar interests that involve interacting with others?
4. Is he or she easy or difficult to get along with?
5. How is the child similar to or different from siblings?

B. School Progress: Ask about the child's preschool activities (child care, Head Start, nursery school, etc); for older children, record basic information about academic performance, special aptitudes or problems, reactions to school.

Social History

A. Family Structure: Record information about adults in the home and their relationship to child; stability of family structure; sources of income; description of home (size, number of rooms, living conditions, sleeping facilities), type of neighborhood, access to play facilities. If parents work outside the home, identify the child's caregivers and their relation to the child. If family's primary language is other than English, note language(s) spoken at home.

B. Family Support Systems: Ask about the presence of relatives nearby or close friends to provide support and give parents "time off."

C. Child Care: Obtain information about child care arrangements (eg, baby-sitter, nanny, day-care center, child care co-op) and the parents' satisfaction with these arrangements.

D. School: Record information about the type and location of school (public, parochial, boarding, other private), students per classroom, child's and parents' satisfaction with school.

E. Insurance: Record the type of health coverage, if any.

Environmental History

A. Indoor Air Pollution: Note whether child's health appears to be affected by house dust, mold, animal dander, fumes from disinfectants or other chemicals, ventilation problems, "sick building syndrome."

B. Pesticides & Lawn Care Products: Ask parents about accessibility of these products and security of household storage; proper washing of fresh fruits and vegetables.

C. Lead: Inquire about the presence of lead-based paints on household woodwork/furnishings or lead-glazed pottery in the household.

D. Playground Hazards: For older children, note location(s) of play areas, local traffic conditions, adult supervision, sturdiness of play equipment.

E. Arts & Crafts Hazards: For older children and adolescents, note activities involving use of potentially hazardous objects, substances, or equipment:

1. Sharp or penetrating objects (eg, knives, needles, scissors, leather punches, saws, nails, tacks, staple guns)
2. Inhalants and petroleum distillates (glue, paint, turpentine and other thinners, kerosene, wood polish, aerosol products)
3. Small objects that could be swallowed or aspirated (beads, pins, small buttons)
4. Flammable, toxic, or explosive substances or materials (eg, helium, etching acid, paint remover, kerosene, photograph developer, bleach)
5. Electrically operated craft equipment (eg, lathes, pottery wheels and kilns, sewing machines, electric saws, airbrushes, paint sprayers)

F. Electromagnetic Hazards: Ask parents about accessibility or secure storage of electrical devices and tools; accessibility of electrical outlets; condition and placement of extension cords, multiple plugs, multiple outlets; use of electrical equipment (eg, shavers, hair dryers, space heaters) in bathrooms or near other sources of water.

Personal Habits

A. Sleeping: The examiner should note the duration of the child's sleep, as well as such disturbances as snoring, restlessness, dreaming, nightmares.

B. Recreation: Note basic information about the child's exercise and play habits, favorite sports, etc.

C. Elimination: Briefly describe the patterns and age-appropriateness of the child's urinary and bowel habits.

D. Behavioral Concerns: Note problematic behaviors (including familial patterns) such as excessive bed-wetting, masturbation, thumb-sucking, nail-biting, breath-holding, temper tantrums, tics, nervousness, undue thirst, others. The examiner should also include school problems (learning or perceptual disorders, school phobia, etc).

E. Adolescent Habits: For teenagers, note the presence of smoking, alcohol or substance abuse; eating or exercise disorders, abuse of steroids; sexual activity, use of birth control, knowledge regarding sexually transmitted diseases; involvement in gangs, use of guns and other weapons. Questions about these matters need not be asked immediately but should be routine if appropriate to the patient's age.

F. Dental Hygiene: Note the child's self-care habits (brushing, flossing), and date of most recent preventive check.

G. Safety: Ask parents or caregivers about the use of infant- or child-restraining devices in automobiles, use of bicycle helmets, teaching basic traffic safety; careful storage of medicines and toxic substances, covering of electrical outlets, as well as other (age-appropriate) safety measures.

H. Family Modeling of Health Habits: The examiner should record information about family behaviors regarding smoking, alcohol consumption, exercise, safety, diet, hygiene, responsible use of medications.

Review of Systems

A. General Review: Record any unusual weight gains or losses, fatigue, fevers, growth patterns, recent behavioral changes.

B. Skin: Check for rashes, lumps, itching, dryness, color changes, changes in hair or nails, easy bruising.

C. Eyes: Record vision, date of last eye examination, use of glasses or contact lenses, pain, redness, excessive tearing, double vision, lazy eye.

D. Ears, Nose, & Throat: Note the presence of frequent colds, sore throats, sneezing, stuffy nose, nasal discharge or postnasal drip, mouth breathing, snoring, otitis, adenitis, allergies; note hearing acuity.

E. Dental: Record child's age at eruption of deciduous and permanent teeth; note presence of bleeding gums, pyorrhea, condition of teeth, other concerns.

F. Cardiorespiratory System: Record the frequency and nature of any disturbances; note the presence of dyspnea, chest pain, cough, sputum, wheezing, history of pneumonia, cyanosis, syncope, tachycardia.

G. Gastrointestinal System: Note the existence of any swallowing problems, spitting, vomiting, diarrhea, constipation, type of stool, abdominal pain or discomfort, jaundice, changes in bowel movements, blood in stool.

H. Genitourinary System: Note the presence of enuresis, dysuria, frequency, polyuria, pyuria, hematuria, character of urine stream, vaginal itching or discharge; note menstrual history, bladder control, abnormalities of genitalia, bruising or evidence of trauma.

I. Neuromuscular System: Inquire about headache, nervousness, dizziness, tingling, convulsions, habit spasms, ataxia, muscle or joint pains, postural deformities, exercise tolerance, gait. Screen the child for scoliosis.

J. Endocrine System: Check for disturbances of growth, excessive fluid intake, polyphagia, goiter, thyroid disease, age at onset of pubertal changes.

PHYSICAL EXAMINATION

Every child should have a complete systematic examination at regular intervals (Table 1–2). The examination should not be restricted to those portions of the body considered to be involved in the presenting complaint.

Approaching the Child

Adequate time should be allowed for the child and the examiner to become acquainted. The child should be treated as an individual whose feelings and sensibilities are well developed, and the examiner's conduct should be appropriate to the child's age. A friendly manner, quiet voice, and slow, easy approach will help to facilitate the examination. If the physician is not able to establish a friendly relationship but feels that it is important to proceed with the examination, this should be done in an orderly, systematic manner in the hope that the child will then accept the necessary procedures.

The examiner's hands should be washed in warm water and should be warm before the examination begins.

Table 1–2. The physical examination.

Vital signs	Neck
General appearance	Thorax
Skin	Lungs
Lymph nodes	Heart
Head	Abdomen
Face	Male and female genitalia
Eyes	Rectum and anus
Nose	Extremities
Mouth	Spine and back
Throat	Neurologic examination
Ears	Developmental assessment

Observing the Child

Although very young children may not be able to speak, an observant and receptive examiner can obtain much information. The total evaluation of the child should include impressions obtained from the time the child enters the room; assessment should not be based solely on the period during which the patient is on the examining table. This is also the best time to assess interactions between parent and child; the examiner's impressions of all these considerations should be recorded at the time of the examination.

In general, one can obtain more information by careful inspection than by any other method of examination.

Holding the Child for Examination

Most segments of the examination can be performed while the child is held in the parent's lap or over the parent's shoulder. Certain parts of the examination can sometimes be done more easily with the child prone or held against the parent so that the examiner is out of the child's direct line of sight.

Removing the Child's Clothing

The child's clothes should be removed gradually to prevent chilling and to minimize resistance if he or she is shy. To save time and to avoid creating unpleasant associations with the caregiver in the child's mind, suggest that the parent undress the child and take his or her temperature. The considerable degree of modesty that some children exhibit should be respected.

Sequence of Examination

In most cases, it is best to begin the examination of the young child in an area that is least likely to be associated with pain or discomfort. The ears and throat usually should be examined last. The examiner should develop a regular sequence of examination that can be adapted to each child as required by special circumstances.

Painful Procedures

Before performing a disagreeable, painful, or upsetting examination, the examiner should tell the child (1) what is likely to happen and how the child can help; (2) that the examination is necessary; and (3) that it will be performed as rapidly and as painlessly as possible. Do not tell a child falsehoods, such as that a painful procedure "won't hurt at all."

Vital Signs

Record the child's temperature, pulse rate, and respiratory rate (TPR); blood pressure (Chapter 16); weight; and height. Weight should be recorded at each visit; height should be determined at regular intervals. The child's height, weight, and head circumference should be plotted on standardized growth curves and the approximate percentiles recorded. Multiple measurements at intervals are more valuable than one-time measurements, since the former give information regarding growth patterns. Blood pressure should be compared with standard percentiles.

General Appearance

The examiner should ask whether the child's overall appearance is healthy or not, as well as note the degree of prostration (if present); degree of cooperation; state of comfort, nutrition, and consciousness; abnormalities; gait, posture, and coordination; estimate of intelligence; reactions to parents, physician, and examination; nature of cry and degree of activity; facies and facial expressions.

Skin

The child's skin should be examined with regard to color (cyanosis, jaundice, pallor, erythema), texture, eruptions, hydration, edema, hemorrhagic manifestations, scars, dilated vessels and direction of blood flow, hemangiomas, café-au-lait areas and nevi, mongolian spots, pigmentation, turgor, elasticity, subcutaneous nodules, sensitivity, hair distribution, character, desquamation, and capillary refill.

Practical notes:

1. Loss of turgor, especially of the calf muscles and skin over the abdomen, is evidence of dehydration.
2. The soles and palms are often bluish and cold in early infancy; this finding is of no significance.
3. The degree of anemia cannot be reliably determined by inspection, since pallor (even in the newborn) may be normal and not due to anemia.
4. To demonstrate pitting edema in a child, the examiner may need to exert prolonged pressure.
5. A few small pigmented nevi are commonly found, particularly in older children.
6. Spider nevi occur in about one-sixth of children under age 5 years and almost one-half of older children.

7. Mongolian spots (large, flat, black or blue-black areas) are frequently present over the lower back and buttocks; they have no pathologic significance. They occur most commonly in children from Native American, African American, or Asian families.
8. Cyanosis will not be evident unless at least 5 gm of reduced hemoglobin is present; therefore, it develops less readily in an anemic child.
9. Carotenemia is usually most prominent over the palms and soles and around the nose but often spares the conjunctivae.
10. Striae and wrinkling may indicate rapid weight gain or loss.

Lymph Nodes

The examiner should note the location, size, sensitivity, mobility, and consistency of the lymph nodes. One should routinely attempt to palpate the suboccipital, preauricular, anterior cervical, posterior cervical, submaxillary, sublingual, axillary, epitrochlear, and inguinal nodes.

Practical notes:

1. Enlargement of the lymph nodes occurs much more readily in children than in adults.
2. Small inguinal lymph nodes are palpable in almost all healthy young children. Small, mobile, nontender shotty nodes are commonly found as residua of previous infection.

Head

The examiner should note size, shape, circumference, asymmetry, cephalhematoma, bossae, craniotabes, control, molding, bruits, fontanelles (size, tension, number, abnormally late or early closure), sutures, dilated veins, scalp, hair (texture, distribution, parasites), face, transillumination.

Practical notes:

1. Measure the child's head at its greatest circumference; this is usually at the mid-forehead anteriorly and around the most prominent portion of the occiput posteriorly. The ratio of head circumference to circumference of the chest or abdomen is usually of little value.
2. Fontanelle tension is best determined with the child quiet and sitting upright.
3. Slight pulsations over the anterior fontanelle may occur in normal infants.

4. Although bruits may be heard over the temporal areas in normal children, the possibility of an existing abnormality should be ruled out.
5. Craniotabes may be found in normal newborn infants (especially premature infants) and during the first 2–4 months of life.
6. A positive Macewen sign ("cracked pot" sound when the skull is percussed with one finger) may be present in normal infants as long as the fontanelle is open.
7. Transillumination of the skull can be performed by means of a flashlight with a sponge rubber collar so that it fits tightly when held against the child's head.

Face

The examiner should check for symmetry, paralysis, distance between nose and mouth, depth of nasolabial folds, bridge of nose, distribution of hair, size of mandible, swellings, hypertelorism, Chvostek's sign, and tenderness over sinuses.

Eyes

Look for the presence of photophobia; visual acuity; muscular control and conjugate gaze; nystagmus; Mongolian slant; Brushfield's spots; epicanthic folds; lacrimation; discharge; lids; exophthalmos or enophthalmos; the condition of the conjunctivae; pupillary size, shape, reaction to light and accommodation; color of iris; media (corneal opacities, cataracts); fundi; visual fields (in older children).

Practical notes:

1. Newborn infants will usually open their eyes if placed prone, supported with one hand on the abdomen, and lifted over the examiner's head.
2. Occasionally, one pupil will appear larger than the other. This is normal, and occurs only in bright or subdued light.
3. Examination of the fundi should be part of every complete physical examination.
4. Dilation of the pupils may be necessary for adequate visualization of the eyes.
5. A mild degree of strabismus may be present during the first 6 months of life but should be considered abnormal after that time.
6. To test for strabismus in a very young or uncooperative child, note where a distant source of light is reflected from the surface of the eyes; the reflection should be present on corresponding portions of each eye.

7. Small areas of capillary dilatation are commonly seen on the eyelids of normal newborn infants.
8. Most infants produce visible tears during the first few days of life.

Nose

The clinician should examine the exterior, shape, mucosa, patency, discharge, bleeding, pressure over sinuses, flaring of nostrils, and septum.

Mouth

Note the condition of the child's lips (thinness, downturning, fissures, color, cleft); teeth (number, position, caries, mottling, discoloration, notching, malocclusion or misalignment); mucosa (color, redness of Stensen's duct, enanthems, Bohn's nodules, Epstein's pearls); also, the gums, palate, tongue, uvula, mouth breathing, geographic tongue (usually normal).

Practical note: If the tongue can be extended as far as the alveolar ridge, there will be no interference with nursing or speaking. Frenectomy is not a preventive measure for being tongue-tied.

Throat

The examiner should observe the tonsils (size, inflammation, exudate, crypts, inflammation of the anterior pillars), epiglottis, mucosa, hypertrophic lymphoid tissue, postnasal drip, voice (hoarseness, stridor, grunting, type of cry, speech).

Practical notes:

1. Before examining a child's throat, the clinician should examine the mouth. To help the child overcome fear of the instruments, allow him or her to handle the tongue blade, nasal speculum, and flashlight. Then ask the child to stick out his or her tongue and say "Ah," louder and louder. In some cases, this maneuver may allow an adequate examination of the throat. In others, a cooperative child may be asked to "pant like a puppy;" while the child is breathing in this way, the physician can apply the tongue blade firmly to the rear of the tongue. Gagging need not be elicited to obtain a satisfactory examination. In still other cases, you may prefer to examine one side of the child's tongue at a time, pushing the base of the tongue first to one side and then to the other. This may be less unpleasant for the child and is less apt to cause gagging.

2. Young children may have to be restrained to adequately examine the throat. Eliciting a gag reflex may be necessary if the oropharynx is to be visualized.
3. A small child's head may be restrained satisfactorily with the parent's help. Have the parent place his or her hands at the level of the child's elbows, while holding his or her arms firmly against the sides of the child's head.
4. A child who can sit up can be held on the parent's lap, with the back against the parent's chest. The child's left hand is held in the parent's left, the right hand in the right, and the hands are placed against the child's groin or lower thighs to prevent slipping. If you are examining the throat in natural light, ask the parent to face the light. If you are using artificial light and a head mirror, place the light behind the parent. In either case, use one hand to hold the child's head in position and the other to manipulate the tongue blade.
5. Young children seldom complain of sore throat even in the presence of significant infection of the pharynx and tonsils. Therefore, the throat should receive thorough examination whether or not the child complains of discomfort.

Ears

The examiner should check the pinnas (position, size), canals, tympanic membranes (landmarks, mobility, perforation, inflammation, discharge), mastoid tenderness and swelling, hearing.

Practical notes:

1. A hearing test is an important part of the physical examination of every infant and child. If a parent says that the child does not hear well, this must be investigated until disproved.
2. The ears of all sick children should be examined whether or not the child complains of earache.
3. When examining the ears, you may find it helpful to place the speculum just within the canal, remove it and place it gently in the other ear, remove it again, and proceed in this way, advancing from one ear to the other gradually until a satisfactory examination is completed.
4. In examining the ears, use as large a speculum as possible and insert it no further than necessary, to avoid both discomfort and pushing wax in front of the speculum so that it obscures the field. Balance the otoscope in your hand by holding the handle at the end

nearest the speculum. Position one finger against the child's head to prevent injury resulting from sudden movement.

5. Pneumatic insufflation to test mobility of the tympanic membrane should always be included in the examination.
6. The child may be restrained most easily if he or she is lying prone.
7. Low-set ears are present in a number of congenital syndromes, including several associated with mental retardation. The ears may be considered low-set if they lie below a line drawn from the lateral angle of the eye to the external occipital protuberance.
8. Congenital anomalies of the urinary tract are frequently associated with abnormalities of the pinnas.
9. To examine the ears of an infant, you will usually need to draw the auricle backward and downward; in older children, draw the external ear backward and upward.

Neck

Note the position of the child's neck (torticollis, opisthotonos, inability to support head, mobility): also check swelling, thyroid (size, contour, bruit, isthmus, nodules, tenderness), lymph nodes, veins, position of trachea, sternocleidomastoid (swelling, shortening), webbing, edema, auscultation, movement, tonic neck reflex.

Practical note: In the older child, the size and shape of the thyroid gland may be more clearly defined if the gland is palpated from behind.

Thorax

The clinician should observe thoracic shape and symmetry, veins, retractions and pulsations, beading; the presence of Harrison's groove, flaring of ribs, pigeon breast, funnel shape; the size and position of nipples, breasts, length of sternum, intercostal and substernal retraction, asymmetry, scapulae, clavicles; the presence of scoliosis.

Practical note: In normal children, one breast usually begins to develop before the other during puberty. Tenderness of the breast is relatively common in both sexes. Gynecomastia is not unusual in pubescent boys.

Lungs

Check for type of breathing, dyspnea, prolongation of expiration, cough, fremitus, flatness or dullness to percussion, rales, wheezing; check expansion, resonance, quality of breath and voice sounds.

Practical notes:

1. Breath sounds in infants and children normally are more intense and more localized in the bronchi, and expiration is more prolonged than in adults.
2. Most of the young child's respiratory movement is produced by abdominal movement; there is very little intercostal motion.
3. If the stethoscope is placed over the child's mouth and the sounds heard by this route are subtracted from the sounds heard through the chest wall, the difference usually represents the amount produced intrathoracically.

Heart

The clinician should note the location and intensity of apex beat, precordial bulging, pulsation of vessels, thrills, size, shape, auscultation (rate, rhythm, force, quality of sounds—compare with pulse with respect to rate and rhythm; friction rub—variation with pressure), murmurs (location, position in cycle, intensity, pitch, effect of change of position, transmission, effect of exercise) (Chapter 16).

Practical notes:

1. Many children normally have sinus dysrhythmia. The child should be asked to take a deep breath to determine its effect on the rhythm.
2. Extrasystoles are not uncommon in childhood.
3. The heart should be examined with the child in different positions: erect, recumbent, and turned to the left.

Abdomen

Check the child's abdomen with regard to size and contour, visible peristalsis, respiratory movements, veins (distension, direction of flow), umbilicus, hernia, musculature, tenderness and rigidity, rebound tenderness, tympany, shifting dullness, pulsation, palpable organs or masses (size, shape, position, mobility), fluid wave, reflexes, femoral pulsations, bowel sounds.

Practical notes:

1. The abdomen may be examined with the child prone in the parent's lap, held over the shoulder, or seated on the examining table facing away from the doctor. These positions may be particularly helpful whenever you must palpate a tender or rigid abdomen or an

abdominal mass. In the infant, the examination may be aided by having the child suck at a "sugar tip" or a bottle.
2. Light palpation, especially of the spleen, will often yield more information than deep palpation.
3. Umbilical hernias are common during the first 2 years of life. They usually disappear spontaneously.

Male Genitalia

The examiner should note circumcision, meatal opening, hypospadias, phimosis, adherent foreskin, size of testes, cryptorchidism, scrotum, hydrocele, hernia, pubertal changes. Tanner stage (I–V; Chapter 9, Figure 9–2) should be noted.

Practical notes:

1. In examining a suspected case of cryptorchidism, palpate for the testicles before the child has fully undressed or become chilled or had the cremasteric reflex stimulated. In some cases, you may find it helpful to examine the child while he is in a warm bath. A boy can also be examined while sitting in a chair holding his knees with his heels on the seat; the increased intra-abdominal pressure may push the testes into the scrotum.
2. To examine for cryptorchidism, start above the inguinal canal and work downward to prevent pushing the testes up into the canal or abdomen.
3. The penis of an obese boy may be so obscured by fat as to appear abnormally small. If this fat is pushed back, the penis is usually found to be of normal size.

Female Genitalia

In girls, the clinician should observe the vagina (imperforate, discharge, adhesions), size of vaginal opening (in prepubertal children), clitoral hypertrophy, pubertal changes. Tanner stage should be noted (I–V; Chapter 9, Figure 9–2).

Practical note: Digital or speculum examination is rarely indicated before puberty, excepting cases of rape, suspected sexual abuse, or other trauma to the genitals.

Rectum & Anus

Check for the presence of irritation, fissures, prolapse, imperforate anus. Note muscle tone, character of stool, masses, tenderness, sensation.

Practical note: Perform rectal examinations with your little finger (inserted slowly). Examine the stool on glove finger (gross, microscopic, culture guaiac) as indicated.

Extremities

A. General: Note the presence of deformities, hemiatrophy, bowleg (common in infancy), knock-knee (common at age 2–3 years), paralysis, asymmetry, edema; note temperature, posture, gait, and stance.

B. Joints: Check for swelling, redness, pain, limitations, tenderness, motion, rheumatic nodules, carrying angle of elbows, tibial torsion.

C. Hands & Feet: Note the presence of extra digits, clubbing, simian lines, curvature of little fingers, nail deformities, splinter hemorrhages, flatfeet (feet commonly appear flat during first 2 years of life); abnormalities of feet; dermatoglyphics; width of thumbs and big toes; syndactyly; length of various segments; dimpling of dorsa; temperature.

D. Peripheral Vessels: The examiner should observe the presence, absence, or diminution of arterial pulses.

Practical note: Normal femoral arterial pulsations during the newborn period do not definitively exclude coarctation.

Spine & Back

Check the child's overall posture; curvatures; rigidity; webbed neck; spina bifida; pilonidal dimple or cyst; tufts of hair; mobility; mongolian spots; tenderness over spine, pelvis, and kidneys.

Neurologic Examination (after Vazuka)

A. Cerebral Function: The examiner should note the child's general behavior, level of consciousness, intelligence, emotional status, memory, orientation, illusions, hallucinations, cortical sensory interpretation, cortical motor integration, ability to understand and communicate, auditory-verbal and visual-verbal comprehension, visual recognition of objects, speech, ability to write, performance of skilled motor skills.

B. Cranial Nerves: The functioning of the cranial nerves should be evaluated as follows:

1. I (olfactory)–Identification of odors; disorders of smell.

2. II (optic)–Visual acuity, visual fields, ophthalmoscopic examination.

3. III (oculomotor), IV (trochlear), and VI (abducens)–Ocular movements, strabismus, ptosis, dilatation of pupil, nystagmus, pupillary accommodation, pupillary light reflexes.

4. V (trigeminal)–Facial sensations, corneal reflex, masseter and temporal muscle reflexes, maxillary reflex (jaw jerk).

5. VII (facial)–Wrinkling forehead, frowning, smiling, raising eyebrows, asymmetry of face, strength of eyelid muscles, taste on anterior portion of tongue.

6. VIII (vestibulocochlear)–

a. Cochlear–Hearing, lateralization, air and bone conduction, tinnitus.

b. Vestibular–Caloric tests.

7. IX (glossopharyngeal) and X (vagus)–Pharyngeal gag reflex; ability to swallow and speak clearly; sensation of mucosa of pharynx, soft palate, and tonsils; movement of pharynx, larynx, and soft palate; autonomic functions.

8. XI (accessory)–Strength of trapezius and sternocleidomastoid muscles.

9. XII (hypoglossal)–Protrusion of tongue, tremor, strength of tongue.

Practical note: Cranial nerve function can usually be evaluated by observation in young children; formal testing is not realistic in most cases.

C. Cerebellar Function: The examiner should ask the child to perform the following maneuvers: touch finger to nose and finger to examiner's finger; rapidly alternate pronation and supination of hands; run one heel down the other shin and make a requested motion with foot; stand with eyes closed, walk normally, then walk heel to toe. The examiner should also check for tremor, ataxia, general posture, arm swing when walking, nystagmus, abnormalities of muscle tone and speech.

D. Motor System: Observe muscle size, consistency, and tone; muscle contours and outlines; muscle strength; myotonic contraction; slow relaxation; symmetry of posture; fasciculations; tremor; resistance to passive movement; involuntary movement.

E. Reflexes: Check for the presence of the following reflexes:

1. Deep–Biceps, brachioradialis, triceps, patellar, and Achilles; rapidity and strength of contraction and relaxation.

2. Superficial–Abdominal, cremasteric, plantar, and gluteal.

3. Neonatal–Babinski, Landau, Moro, rooting, sucking, grasping, and tonic neck.

Developmental Assessment

Both the history of milestones and screening tests for [intellectual, motor, and psychosocial] development are integral parts of a routine physical evaluation.

Practical note: Screening devices are not diagnostic of particular problems but merely indicate a need for more specific developmental evaluation (Chapter 2).

Development & Growth | 2

David Burgess, MD

Development and growth are continuous dynamic processes occurring from conception to maturity, taking place in an orderly sequence that is similar for all persons. At any specific age, however, wide individual variations can be found among normal children; these variations reflect active responses of growing human beings to numerous hereditary and environmental factors.

Development includes maturation of organs and systems; acquisition of physical, intellectual, and interpersonal skills; ability to adapt more readily to stress; assumption of personal responsibility; and capacities for creative expression. **Growth** signifies increase in size.

DEVELOPMENTAL SCREENING & SURVEILLANCE

To provide comprehensive pediatric care, physicians and other health care providers should understand the markers of normal development at all ages, and should be particularly familiar with these criteria in young children. Systematic screening and surveillance are two approaches for monitoring of development and identification of developmental deviations.

Screening Tests

In accordance with the guidelines for health supervision developed by the American Academy of Pediatrics (AAP), a two-stage developmental screening program was devised for use in primary health care settings to detect developmental delays in infancy and the preschool years. The first stage consists of the Revised Prescreening Developmental Questionnaire (R-PDQ) (Figure 2–1) and is followed by the Denver II (the 1990 revision of the Denver Developmental Screening Test (DDST)) (Figure 2–2) as a second-stage screening for children suspected of having developmental delays.

A. First-Stage Screening: The R-PDQ is a questionnaire for parents or caregivers designed to achieve three goals:

R-PDQ age: (_____yr__11__ mo__2__ completed wks)

			For Office Use
39. Gets to Sitting Can your baby get to a sitting position without help?	(YES)	NO	(11) G M
40. Imitates Speech Sounds Write down 2 or 3 words that your baby tries to imitate with a recognizable sound (not necessarily complete words). In your judgment does (s)he try to imitate words?	YES	(NO)	((11)) L Delay
41. Bangs 2 Cubes Held in Hands Without your moving his/her hands can your baby bang together 2 small blocks? Rattles and pan lids do not count.	YES	(NO)	No Delay (12-1) FMA

Figure 2–1. Revised prescreening developmental questionnaire.

1. To educate parents about developmental issues in their children.
2. To provide systematic documentation of the developmental progress of individual children.
3. To facilitate early identification of children with developmental delays.

Administration of the R-PDQ consists of the following steps (using the age-appropriate R-PDQ form):

1. Calculation of the child's R-PDQ age.
2. Administration of the R-PDQ to the child's caregiver, who answers all appropriate questions by following available instructions.
3. Identification of delays. A **delay** is defined as an item passed by 90% of children (in the Denver II norming studies) at a younger age than that of the child being screened. A **caution** is an item passed by 75% of children in the Denver II norming sample at a younger age than the child being tested.

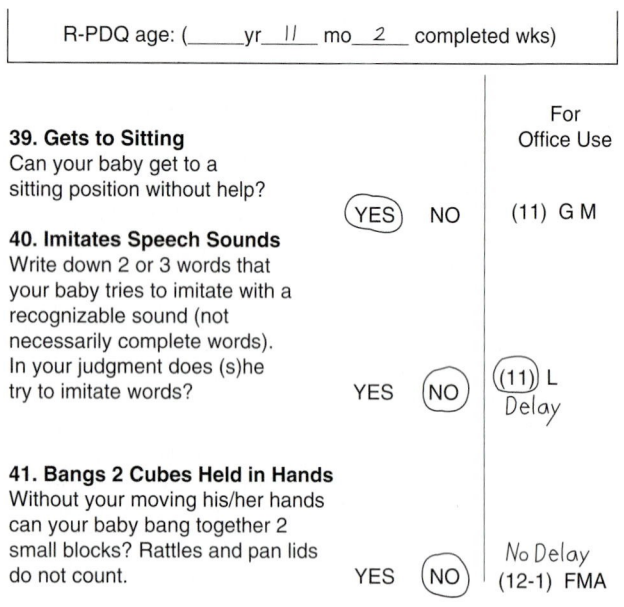

Children who have no delays on the R-PDQ are considered developmentally normal. If a child has one or more delays, the clinician should consider second-stage screening with the Denver II.

B. Second-Stage Screening: The use of the R-PDQ will identify 15–30% of the pediatric population as suspect. Children who are tentatively identified on first-stage screening should be considered for second-stage screening with the Denver II. A child who receives a suspect result on the Denver II (one or more delays as defined above, and/or two or more cautions) should be considered for further medical/developmental evaluation.

To use the Denver II effectively, individual examiners must be trained to administer and interpret the test properly. Denver II training consists of an introductory video tape, the Denver II training manual, a written proficiency test accompanied by a video test, practice testing, and administration of the Denver II for a trained observer. Completion of this training insures that the Denver II will be administered in a standardized, reliable manner. A free catalog describing the training materials, the Denver II, and the R-PDQ is available from Denver Developmental Materials, P.O. Box 6919, Denver, CO 80206-0919, (303) 355-4729.

C. Developmental Surveillance: Developmental surveillance is a concept based on skilled professional observations of a child throughout his or her history in the child health care system. Developmental surveillance includes the taking of a relevant developmental history, accurate observing, and attentive listening to parental concerns. It is a process of continuous monitoring of a child's development rather than a static record compiled at one point in time. The R-PDQ and/or the Denver II can be used to improve the accuracy of this process. Whether the clinician uses the R-PDQ/Denver II to perform systematic screening of a defined population or as part of a specific child's developmental surveillance, he or she should not interpret the results on the basis of one score but rather within the context of each child's overall assessment, including medical history, physical findings, and parental concerns.

GROWTH

General Considerations

A. Fetal Growth: The rate of fetal growth in utero is extremely rapid. During the early months, the fetal rate of gain in length is greater than the rate of gain in weight when expressed as a percentage

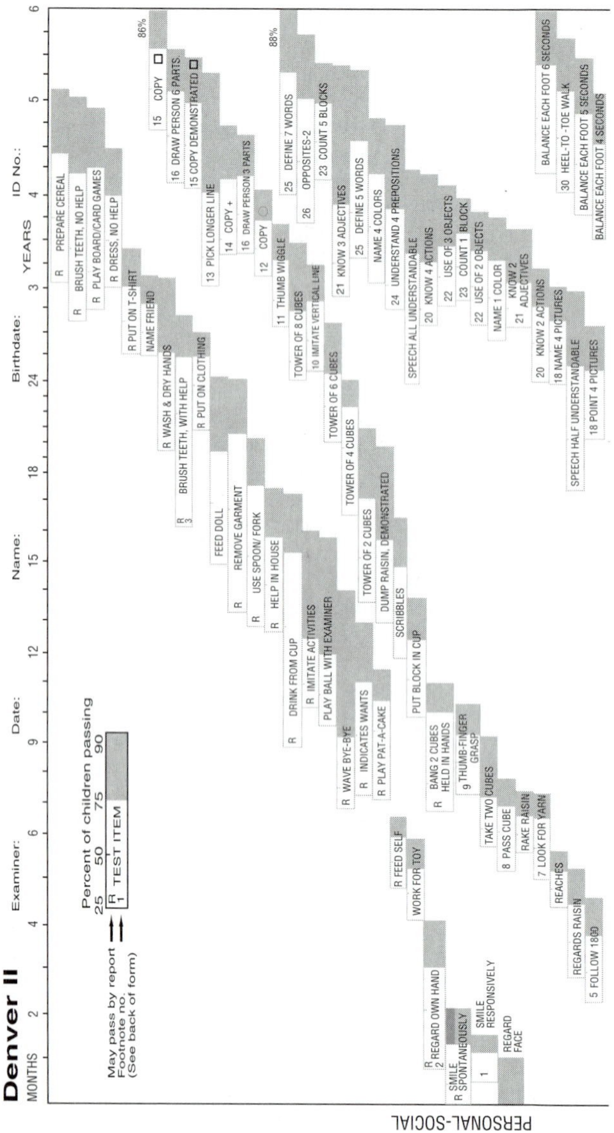
Denver II
MONTHS
Examiner:
Date:
Name:
Birthdate:
YEARS
ID No.:
May pass by report
Footnote no.
(See back of form)
Percent of children passing
25 50 75 90
R 1 TEST ITEM
PERSONAL-SOCIAL
R SMILE SPONTANEOUSLY
SMILE RESPONSIVELY
REGARD FACE
R 2 REGARD OWN HAND
WORK FOR TOY
R FEED SELF
R PLAY PAT-A-CAKE
R INDICATES WANTS
R WAVE BYE-BYE
PLAY BALL WITH EXAMINER
R IMITATE ACTIVITIES
R DRINK FROM CUP
R HELP IN HOUSE
R USE SPOON/ FORK
R REMOVE GARMENT
FEED DOLL
R PUT ON CLOTHING
R 3 BRUSH TEETH, WITH HELP
R WASH & DRY HANDS
NAME FRIEND
R PUT ON T-SHIRT
R DRESS, NO HELP
R PLAY BOARD/CARD GAMES
R BRUSH TEETH, NO HELP
R PREPARE CEREAL
5 FOLLOW 180°
REGARDS RAISIN
REACHES
7 LOOK FOR YARN
RAKE RAISIN
8 PASS CUBE
TAKE TWO CUBES
9 THUMB-FINGER GRASP
R BANG 2 CUBES HELD IN HANDS
PUT BLOCK IN CUP
SCRIBBLES
DUMP RAISIN, DEMONSTRATED
TOWER OF 2 CUBES
TOWER OF 4 CUBES
TOWER OF 6 CUBES
10 IMITATE VERTICAL LINE
TOWER OF 8 CUBES
11 THUMB WIGGLE
12 COPY
16 DRAW PERSON 3 PARTS
14 COPY +
13 PICK LONGER LINE
15 COPY DEMONSTRATED
16 DRAW PERSON 6 PARTS
15 COPY
86%
18 POINT 4 PICTURES
SPEECH HALF UNDERSTANDABLE
18 NAME 4 PICTURES
20 KNOW 2 ACTIONS
21 KNOW 2 ADJECTIVES
NAME 1 COLOR
22 USE OF 2 OBJECTS
23 COUNT 1 BLOCK
22 USE OF 3 OBJECTS
20 KNOW 4 ACTIONS
SPEECH ALL UNDERSTANDABLE
24 UNDERSTAND 4 PREPOSITIONS
NAME 4 COLORS
25 DEFINE 5 WORDS
21 KNOW 3 ADJECTIVES
23 COUNT 5 BLOCKS
26 OPPOSITES-2
25 DEFINE 7 WORDS
88%
BALANCE EACH FOOT 4 SECONDS
BALANCE EACH FOOT 5 SECONDS
30 HEEL-TO -TOE WALK
BALANCE EACH FOOT 6 SECONDS

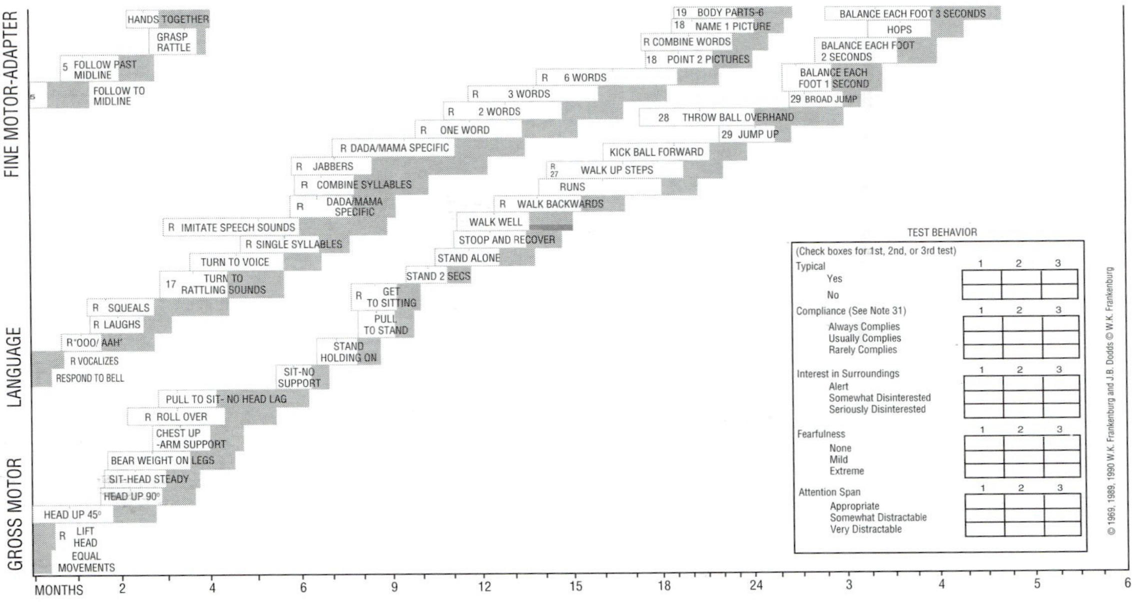

Figure 2–2. Denver II.

of the birth value. By the eighth month, the fetus has achieved 80% of its birth length and only 50% of its birth weight .

B. Height: Rate of growth is generally more important than the child's actual size. For more accurate comparisons, data should be recorded both as absolute figures and as percentiles for that particular age; the rate of growth should then be determined. Birth length doubles by approximately age 4 years and triples by age 13 years. The average child grows approximately 10 in (25 cm) in the first year of life, 5 in (12.5 cm) in the second, 3–4 in (7.5–10 cm) in the third, and approximately 2–3 in (5–7.5 cm) per year thereafter until the growth spurt of puberty.

C. Weight: Body weight is probably the best index of nutrition and growth. The average infant weighs approximately 7 lb 5 oz (3.33 kg) at birth. Within the first few days of life, the newborn loses up to 10% of the birth weight. Birth weight doubles between 4 and 5 months of age, triples by the end of the first year, and quadruples by the end of the child's second year. Between ages 2 and 9 years, the annual increment in weight averages about 5 lb (2.25 kg) per year.

D. Growth at Puberty: See Chapter 9.

E. Growth Charts: Standard growth charts are available for plotting height, weight, and head circumference longitudinally during well child care.

Specific Considerations

A. Head & Skull: At birth the head is approximately two-thirds to three-fourths of its total mature size, whereas the rest of the body is only one-fourth its adult size.

Six fontanelles (anterior, posterior, two sphenoid, and two mastoid) are usually present at birth. The anterior fontanelle normally closes between 10 and 14 months of age, but may close by 3 months or remain open until 18 months. The posterior fontanelle usually closes by 4 months, but in some children may not be palpable at birth. Cranial sutures do not ossify completely until later childhood. Growth of the skull, as determined by increasing head circumference, is a much more accurate index of brain growth than is the presence or size of fontanelles.

B. Sinuses: The maxillary and ethmoid sinuses are present at birth, but are not usually aerated for approximately 6 months. The sphenoid sinuses are not usually visible on x-ray until after the third year of life. Frontal sinuses usually become visible by x-ray between 7 and 9 years of age, but seldom before age 5.

The mastoid process at birth is relatively large and has a relatively wide communication with the middle ear. Its cellular structure gradually appears between birth and age 3 years.

C. Respiration & Heart Rate: The respiratory rate decreases steadily during childhood, averaging approximately 30 breaths per minute during the first year of life, 25 during the second year, 20 during the eighth year, and 18 by the 15th year.

The heart rate falls steadily throughout childhood, averaging about 150 beats per minute (bpm) in utero, 130 bpm at birth, 105 bpm during the second year of life, 90 bpm during the fourth year, 80 bpm during the sixth year, and 70 bpm during the tenth year.

D. Abdomen: Gas may be roentgenographically visualized in the stomach almost immediately after birth, in the ileum within 2 hours, and on average, in the rectum in 3–4 hours.

E. Muscle: At birth, muscle constitutes 25% of total body weight, as compared with 43% in the adult.

F. Ossification Centers: At birth, the average full-term infant has five ossification centers demonstrable by x-ray: distal end of femur, proximal end of tibia, calcaneus, talus, and cuboid. The clavicle is the first bone to calcify in utero, calcification beginning during the fifth fetal week.

G. Senses: At birth, the newborn infant has mature sensory receptors for pressure, pain, and temperature over the entire body surface, in the mouth, and in the external genitalia; there are also mature pain receptors in the viscera and proprioceptive receptors in muscles, joints, and tendons.

1. Taste: The ability to taste is present in the newborn infant, who is capable of distinguishing the four basic tastes.

2. Olfaction: The human infant is born with fully mature olfactory receptors.

3. Hearing: Normal infants can hear almost immediately after birth, but respond to sounds at a subcortical level.

4. Vision: About 80% of newborn infants are hyperopic. At birth, the infant demonstrates an awareness of light and dark, possesses peripheral vision, and is capable of rudimentary fixation on near objects. At 4 months of age, visual acuity is 20/300–20/200; at 10 months, 20/200; and by 2–3 years may reach 20/30–20/20.

Strabismus may be a normal finding for the first 4–6 months of life, but persistent deviation requires evaluation.

Susceptibility to amblyopia (subnormal visual acuity in one or both eyes despite correction of refractive error) is greatest during the first 2–3 years of life and lasts until full visual stability has been achieved by the age of 5–6 years. The key to successful treatment of amblyopia is early detection (Chapter 14).

H. Water Content: The water content of the body is approximately 95% by weight during early fetal life, 65–75% at birth, and 55–60% at maturity.

I. Blood: At birth, 5% of all red blood cells may be reticulocytes; this percentage drops to less than 1% after the second week of life. Nucleated red cells (up to 5% as a percentage of total number of nucleated cells) and immature lymphocytes may be present in the newborn, but disappear within the first week of life. Fetal hemoglobin accounts for 80% of total hemoglobin at birth, 70% of the total at 2 weeks, and 45% at 5 weeks; it falls to less than 10% by 20 weeks.

The leukocyte count is high at birth, rises slightly during the first 48 hours after birth, falls for the next 2–3 weeks, and then rises again. The lymphocyte count is highest during the first year of life, and then falls progressively during the remainder of childhood.

J. Urine: The average infant secretes 15–50 mL of urine per 24 hours during the first 2 days of life, 50–300 mL per day during the next week, and 400–500 mL per day by the latter half of the first year. There is subsequently a gradual increase in urinary output; children secrete 700–1500 mL per day between 8 and 14 years.

K. Tears: Tears often are not present with crying until after 1–3 months of age.

L. Teeth: Table 2–1 outlines the stages of dental growth and development.

The opinions and assertions contained in this manuscript are the private views of the authors and are not to be construed as official or as reflecting the views of the United States Departments Army or Defense.

Table 2–1. Dental growth and development.

Primary or Deciduous Teeth						
	Calcification		Eruption		Shedding	
	Begins At	**Complete At**	**Maxillary**	**Mandibular**	**Maxillary**	**Mandibular**
Central incisors	4th fetal mo	18–24 mo	6–10 mo	5–8 mo	7–8 yr	6–7 yr
Lateral incisors	5th fetal mo	18–24 mo	8–12 mo	7–10 mo	8–9 yr	7–8 yr
Cuspids	6th fetal mo	30–39 mo	16–20 mo	16–20 mo	11–12 yr	9–11 yr
First molars	5th fetal mo	24–30 mo	11–18 mo	11–18 mo	9–11 yr	10–12 yr
Second molars	6th fetal mo	36 mo	20–30 mo	20–30 mo	9–12 yr	11–13 yr

(*continued*)

Table 2–1. *(continued)*.

Secondary or Permanent Teeth				
	Calcification		Eruption[1]	
	Begins At	Complete At	Maxillary	Mandibular
Central incisors	3–4 mo	9–10 yr	7–8 yr (3)	6–7 yr (2)
Lateral incisors	Maxilla 10–12 mo Mandible 3–4 mo	10–11 yr	8–9 yr (5)	7–8 yr (4)
Cuspids	4–5 mo	12–15 yr	11–12 yr (11)	9–11 yr (6)
First premolars	18–24 mo	12–13 yr	10–11 yr (7)	10–12 yr (8)
Second premolars	24–30 mo	12–14 yr	10–12 yr (9)	11–13 yr (10)
First molars	Birth	9–10 yr	5½–7 yr (1)	5½–7 yr (1a)
Second molars	30–36 mo	14–16 yr	12–14 yr (12)	12–13 yr (12a)
Third molars	Maxilla 7–9 yr Mandible 8–10 yr	18–25 yr	17–30 yr (13)	17–30 yr (13a)

[1] Figures in parentheses indicate order of eruption. Many otherwise normal infants do not conform strictly to the stated schedule.

Ambulatory Pediatrics | 3

Roxann M. Headley, MD, & Barton D. Schmitt, MD

Health supervision visits are the key to preventive pediatrics. The visit has several purposes: responding to the parent's or child's current concerns, examining for physical abnormalities (Chapter 1), assessing growth and development (Chapter 2), presenting age-appropriate anticipatory guidance, obtaining laboratory screening tests, and administering immunizations (Chapter 6).

PARENTAL CONCERNS

The first part of each well-child visit should be directed toward dealing with the parent's current concerns. Prior to the baby's birth, a prenatal visit with the pediatrician allows expectant parents an opportunity to ask about feeding, circumcision (if the baby is male), recommended schedules for visits and immunizations, as well as office policies. First-time mothers who are breast-feeding should come in with the baby for a feeding assessment and weight check within 1 week of delivery.

A health supervision visit without parental concerns is unusual. Some mothers bring a written list of questions. In most cases, these have to do with fairly commonplace issues of weight gain, crying, sleep patterns, and the like. Many of the most predictable questions, unfortunately, have no clear-cut answers. Seasoned pediatricians usually enjoy these discussions and the satisfaction that comes with reassuring anxious parents. When an issue is identified which warrants in-depth evaluation or counseling, (eg, bereavement), it is good practice to schedule a special visit to allow more time for discussion; or the health supervision visit can be postponed and the present time used to explore the immediate problem.

PHYSICAL EXAMINATION

The physician should perform a complete physical examination at each health supervision visit. Guidelines for good practice in approaching children as patients, as well as a detailed outline for review of systems, are discussed in Chapter 1. The greatest concern is to rule out disorders that are treatable when detected early, but potentially serious when undetected. These disorders (with relevant testing procedures indicated in parentheses) include but are not limited to congenital heart disease, retinoblastoma (red fundus reflection test), strabismus (corneal light reflection test), congenital hip dislocation (Ortolani maneuver), scoliosis, coarctation of the aorta (femoral pulses), hypertension, imperforate hymen, labial adhesions, and dental caries. The examination can also be used as an opportunity for teaching, particularly when dealing with health concerns in the adolescent population (eg, self-examination of the breast or testes), activities for developmental stimulation, or perineal hygiene.

Growth Parameters

At each visit during the first three years of life, the child's height, weight and head circumference should be carefully measured and plotted. To ensure accurate weight measurements for longitudinal comparisons, infants should be undressed completely and young children should be dressed only in underpants. Recumbent length is plotted on the birth-to-36-month chart. When the child is old enough to be measured standing upright, parameters are plotted on the 2–18-year growth chart. If circumferential head growth has been steady for the first two years, routine measurement may be suspended. If a central nervous system (CNS) problem exists or develops, however, or the child manifests failure to thrive, head measurements should continue to be taken. Tracking growth velocity for each of these parameters allows the clinician to detect deviations from normal patterns of development at an early stage (eg, growth deficiency [failure to thrive]).

Blood Pressure

Blood pressure screening for low-risk children is recommended beginning at three years of age. To obtain an accurate measurement, the cuff must cover two-thirds of the child's upper arm. Interpretation of the measurement is made by consulting a table of normative pressures for the child's age (Table 3–1). Blood pressure varies with height and weight; there is also some difference between the sexes, especially in newborns and older teenagers. If the child has renal or

Table 3–1. Normative blood pressures in the pediatric population.[1]

	Age in years							
	Newborn	1	3	6	9	12	15	18
Systolic[2] (mm Hg)	76–87	105	106	111	115	121	127–129	127–136
Diastolic[2] (mm Hg)	68	68	68	70	74	77	79–82	80–84

[1] Adapted from Report of the Second Task Force on Blood Pressure Control in Children.
[2] 90th percentile values. Ranges reflect differences between the sexes with average values for males being at the high end of the range.

cardiac abnormalities, a blood pressure reading *must* be obtained at each visit, regardless of age.

Hearing & Vision

Sensory functions, specifically vision and hearing, are addressed by history taking and physical examination at each visit. Infants should be evaluated for ability to focus on an object, usually the examiner's face. An ophthalmoscopic examination of the anterior chamber checks for bleeding that may have occurred during the birth process. The presence of bilateral red reflexes rules out opacification from congenital cataracts or retinoblastoma.

Physicians should attempt office screening of vision using Allen cards or the Snellen Illiterate E chart as soon as children reach their third birthday (Chapter 14). Test each eye separately. Give credit for a line on which more than 50% of the child's answers are correct. If the child cannot follow verbal instructions, rescreen him or her in six months. Because visual acuity improves with age, results of the test should be interpreted according to the cut-off values in Table 3–2.

The corneal light reflex test may be performed at any age to screen for alignment of the eyes; a cover test allows for a functional evaluation for strabismus. The reader is referred to Chapter 14 for further details of optical testing.

In the newborn period, any infant whose history indicates that he or she is at high risk for hearing deficits should be tested. Pure tone audiometry in the office can be used for testing, beginning at three years of age. See Chapter 13 for further discussion of hearing deficits and auditory testing.

Table 3–2. Age-appropriate visual acuity.[1]

Age (yr)	Minimal Acceptable Acuity
3	20/40
4	20/30
5	20/20

[1] Refer to an ophthalmologist if minimal acuity is not met at a given age or if there is a difference in scores between eyes of two or more lines.

School Readiness Examination

Whenever a child is about to start school (preschool, kindergarten, first grade), the health care provider should screen for readiness in the following seven areas:

1. Hearing: can the child hear well enough to understand others?
2. Vision: can the child see the blackboard or recognize other objects at a distance?
3. Speech: can others understand what the child says (especially if English is not his or her first language)?
4. Social skills: is the child able to share, take turns, be part of a group?
5. Separation: is the child able to cope with brief separations from the parents (eg, with baby-sitters)?
6. Development: is the child's development age-appropriate, as measured by standardized tests (eg, the Denver II)?
7. Attention span: is it adequate for learning tasks?

ANTICIPATORY GUIDANCE

Anticipatory guidance may include age-appropriate nutritional counseling, injury prevention, behavioral counseling, suggestions for developmental stimulation, sex education, dental recommendations, and health promotion information. Special counseling is in order for adolescents (Chapter 9). A list of suggested topics to be discussed at particular ages is found in Table 3–3.

Injury Prevention

Injuries are the leading cause of death for children after the first year of life and adolescents. For young people between 15 and 24 years, injuries are responsible for more than 75% of deaths. Each year

Table 3–3. Anticipatory guidance topics.[1]

Age	Safety	Nutrition	Development	Health
Birth–2 months	Car seat Sleep on back or side Smoke detector	No solids	Stimulation	No honey Exposure to second-hand smoke Immunizations
4–6 months	Falling	If bottle-fed, iron fortified formula No bottle in bed	Rolling Sitting	Fever
9–12 months	Poisons locked up Choking on small objects Hot liquids causing burns	Finger foods Cup Spoon	Crawling, walking, "mama," "dada," pincer grasp, social games	Dental hygiene
15–18 months	Hot water <130 °F Sunscreen Drowning: tub, pail, pool Falls	Set mealtimes Self-feeding Bottle weaning	3–6 words Runs, climbs, stoops Indicates wants and needs Discipline	
2–5 years	Traffic safety Gun safety	Healthy snacks Prudent diet	Peer play Television habits	Family models of exercise, diet Handwashing
6–12 years	Helmets for bicycling, skating Seatbelts Swim lessons/water safety	Fat intake	Chores/responsibility Honesty/respect Sex education School	Smoking Drugs
13–18 years	Sports safety	Junk foods/soda pop Weight control	Responsibility at home Independence	Risk behaviors Exercise

[1] Introduction of a topic is recommended at the age listed; however, reinforcement of the topic is appropriate at later ages as well.

16 million visits to emergency departments occur as a result of pediatric injuries; more than a half million children are hospitalized; and 100,000 children under 15 years of age are left with permanent disabilities.

Injury prevention advice should be an integral part of medical care provided for all infants and children. It must be age-appropriate and specific. Passive prevention strategies should be emphasized as they are more effective than active strategies. For example, the use of child-proof cupboard latches to prevent accidental ingestion of household poisons will be more effective than instructing parents to watch their children closely.

A parent-answered questionnaire assessing home safety measures can be filled out while families are waiting for the physician. Advice can then be tailored to the family's specific situation or needs, and an office handout can be given. A model program, the Injury Prevention Program (TIPP), is available from the American Academy of Pediatrics (AAP).

Motor Vehicles: The foremost killer and crippler of children in the United States is the automobile. Safety for children includes proper restraints within the vehicle. Car safety seats are mandated by law in the United States; their consistent use could reduce fatalities and hospitalizations by at least 50%. The type of safety seat to be used depends on the child's weight or height:

1. Weight less than 20 lb: rear-facing infant seat; avoid seats with air bags.
2. Weight 20–40 lb: forward-facing toddler seat.
3. Weight 40–60 lb: shield booster seat with lap belt.
4. Weight over 60 lb: regular lap belt.
5. Height over 48 inches: adult shoulder strap with lap belt.

The leading cause of injury and death among children aged 5–9 years is the motor vehicle–pedestrian collision. When the child is a motor vehicle occupant in a crash, the case fatality rate is 1.0%; when the child is a pedestrian in a motor vehicle collision, the case-fatality rate increases 300%.

Bicycles and Motorcycles: Millions of people enjoy cycling for sport and utility, but thousands are injured and hundreds die each year unnecessarily from bicycle and motorcycle mishaps. Head trauma accounts for 75% of all bicycle-related fatalities. More than 85% of brain injuries sustained in bicycle accidents can be prevented through regular use of helmets. Safety awareness programs to increase helmet use for bicycling, in-line skating and motorcycling merit support.

Firearms: On average, 14 children and adolescents a day are killed by firearms in the United States. Injuries from firearms are higher for young people aged 15–24 years than for any other age group; black males are especially vulnerable. Some gun deaths are accidental but the majority are due to homicide or suicide. The risk of suicide in the general population, including children and adolescents, is five times greater if there is a gun in the home. Although handguns are often kept at home for protection, a gun is more likely to kill a family member or friend than an intruder. Only 0.5% of the home firearm deaths each year involve intruders. The most effective way to prevent firearm injuries is to remove guns from the home. If families insist, however, on keeping firearms in the home, they should be advised to store them in a locked container with the ammunition stored separately.

Water Accidents: Children between the ages of 1 and 3 years have the highest rate of accidental drowning. In some warm-weather states (Arizona, California, Florida) drowning deaths exceed the number of deaths due to motor vehicle or pedestrian accidents. For every death, 6 children are hospitalized; up to 10% of the survivors suffer severe brain damage. Children under 1 year of age are most likely to drown in the bathtub; children 1–4 years, most frequently in home swimming pools; and school-aged children and teens, most often in lakes or the ocean. Backyard pools should be securely fenced; parents should learn cardiopulmonary resuscitation (CPR). School-aged children should be taught to swim, but in addition should always be supervised by adults when they are in the water.

Burns: Burns are the leading cause of childhood injury-related death within the home. Burn injuries include smoke inhalation, contact burns, scalds, electrical, chemical, and ultraviolet burns. Scalds are the most common type of burn seen in pediatric practice. While the majority of scalds involve food and beverages, nearly a quarter involve tap water; thus parents should be advised to set hot water heaters lower than 130 °F. The greatest number of deaths, however, are caused by smoke inhalation. Smoke detectors can prevent 85% of the injuries and deaths caused by house fires. In addition, parents should check electrical appliances and cords for proper insulation and functioning; unused outlets should be child-proofed with plastic plugs.

Prudent Diet

By 2 years of age, a prudent diet includes diverse sources of food, encourages the intake of foods high in fiber, and limits the intake of sodium and fat. Specific nutrient guidelines are:

- carbohydrates: about 55% of total calories
- protein: about 15–20% of total calories
- total fat: < 30% of total calories
- saturated fat: < 10% of total calories
- cholesterol: < 300 mg/d.

The reader is referred to Chapter 4 for a detailed discussion of children's nutritional requirements.

LABORATORY SCREENING TESTS

A health supervision flow chart or sheet (Figure 3–1) is a helpful reminder to office personnel that certain procedures, laboratory tests, developmental evaluations, and immunizations are recommended for children of specific ages.

Newborn Screening

As part of a preventive public health program, all infants should have blood taken prior to discharge from the nursery in order to screen for inherited conditions. Although some of these diseases are rare, the burden of suffering imposed is high and the effectiveness of early intervention is generally quite good. The reader is referred to Chapter 7 for further information regarding screening of neonates.

It must be remembered that screening does not equal diagnosis. If symptoms of disease are present despite negative test results, the infant should receive further testing. If test results are positive, they must be confirmed and parental anxiety addressed.

Lead Toxicity

Developing infants and children are at special risk for the adverse affects of lead exposure. While acute or chronic high blood lead levels (> 55 μg/dL) can produce multi-organ system effects (colic, nausea, nephritis, muscle aches, encephalopathy, seizures, headache, and anemia), numerous studies have demonstrated that even children with low levels of lead (10–25 μg/dL) can have more behavior problems, more learning disabilities, and lower IQs than cohorts with levels < 10 μg/dL even after confounding variables are controlled. Furthermore, the effects persist into adulthood. The primary source of lead exposure in this country remains lead-based paint, even though its use has been banned since 1977. It is likely that environmental controls (eg, elimination of leaded gasolines and paints) and educational interventions have brought about a nationwide decline in lead levels, from a mean of 16 μg/dL in 1976 to about 5 μg/dL today. Considerable variation exists in different parts of the United States.

All children should be screened by questionnaire for possible environmental risk factors at the time of health supervision visits between the ages of 6 months and 6 years (Table 3–4). Although the questionnaire is of limited use in identifying high-risk children, it allows for the discussion of risk factors with families. If any risk factor is identified, a blood lead level should be obtained at that time. In addition, routine screening of blood lead levels should be performed on all children at 9–12 months and at 2 years of age, regardless of the presence or absence of historical risk factors. A venous sample is preferable to a capillary specimen because the latter may be falsely elevated. Blood lead levels < 10 μg/dL are acceptable. Children with confirmed blood levels > 15 μg/dL should be evaluated for iron deficiency; supplemental iron may be given prophylactically, their environment investigated, and development assessed. Chelation therapy is considered for levels > 25 μg/dL; *it is emergent for levels* ≥ 70 μg/dL. As more data are collected, low-risk communities may be identified in which routine blood lead screening would be unnecessary.

Anemia

Iron deficiency is the most common cause of anemia in young children, although the incidence has declined in recent years due in large part to the use of iron-fortified feeding formulas. Infants born prematurely, in a multiple pregnancy, or to iron-deficient mothers are at increased risk for iron deficiency. Asymptomatic iron deficiency anemia in the young child has been associated with impaired behavior and developmental deficits persisting into school age despite correction of the anemia. Therefore, screening of infants at 9 months of age is a reasonable precaution. A screening hematocrit is also recommended for pregnant teenagers because low maternal hemoglobin levels have been associated with low birthweight infants, prematurity, and high perinatal mortality.

Blood Cholesterol & Lipoproteins

Blood screening of cholesterol and lipoproteins in children should be based upon risk factors. If either parent has a cholesterol level > 240 mg/dL, the child should be screened by 2–3 years of age. If there is a history of cardiovascular disease in a parent or grandparent before 55 years of age, the child's blood should receive a complete lipoprotein analysis (fasting cholesterol, high- and low-density

Name: ______________________ Date of Birth: ______________________

Directions: Record date for all immunizations.
Record value for head circumference, height, weight, BP, and Hct.
Record N (normal) or ABN (abnormal) for all items.

	NB	2 wk	2 mo	4 mo	6 mo	9 mo	12 mo	15 mo	18 mo	2 yr	3 yr	4 yr	5 yr	6 yr	8 yr	10 yr	12 yr	14 yr	16 yr	18 yr
Today's date																				
Head circumference																				
Height (cm)																				
Weight (kg)																				
BP																				
Dental caries screen																				
DTP (Td after 6 years)[1]																				
Polio																				
Measles, mumps, rubella[2]																				
Haemophilus influenza type b																				
Hepatitis B (low-risk)																				
Varicella																				
TB test[3]																				

	NB	2 wk	2 mo	4 mo	6 mo	9 mo	12 mo	15 mo	18 mo	2 yr	3 yr	4 yr	5 yr	6 yr	8 yr	10 yr	12 yr	14 yr	16 yr	18 yr
Hearing [4]																				
Vision [5]																				
Developmental screen [6]																				
Newborn screen																				
Hct																				
Sickle cell test for black patients [8]																				
Pap smear/GC[9]																				

[1]Acellular DTP may be used for the 4th and 5th doses after 15 mo.

[2]MMR booster is given once, generally at 5 years of age or later per state guidelines.

[3]TB test yearly for high-risk groups.

[4]High-risk inquiry; nursery screen (NB)
Listens to soft sounds (2 mo)
Turns to sound (6 mo)
Audiometrics (3 yr and thereafter)

[5]Red reflex (NB or 2 wk)
Regards smiling face (2 mo)
Follows past midline (4mo)
Corneal light reflections test (6 mo)
Visual acuity (3 yr and thereafter)
Color vision once (6 yr)

[6]Informal screening should occur at all visits with formal testing (eg Denver II) at 9 mo and at regular intervals.

[7]PKU, hypothyroidism, etc (NB)
PKU retest (2 wk) if first test done before 48 hours
Perform according to state law.

[8]Perform at 2 mo of age, if not performed as newborn.

[9]Sexually active patients.

Figure 3–1. Health maintenance flow sheet.

Table 3–4. Lead exposure screening questionnaire.[1]

Does your child:

1. Live in or regularly visit a house with peeling or chipping paint built before 1960? This could include a day care center, preschool, the home of a babysitter or relative, etc.
2. Live in or regularly visit a house built before 1960 with recent, ongoing, or planned renovation or remodeling?
3. Have a brother or sister, housemate, or playmate being followed up or treated for lead poisoning (ie, blood level ≥ 15 mg/dL)?
4. Live with an adult whose job or hobby involves exposure to lead?
5. Live near an active lead smelter, battery recycling plant, or other industry likely to release lead?

[1] From the Centers for Disease Control and Prevention, Atlanta.

lipoproteins [HDLs and LDLs], and triglycerides). For all children, a prudent diet is advised as described in Chapter 4.

A table of age-appropriate lipid profiles is included in the Appendix.

Bacteriuria

At present, routine screening of asymptomatic children for bacteriuria is debated. For infant males the prevalence of asymptomatic bacteriuria is 2–4%; for early grade-school girls it is 5–6%. It has not been demonstrated that detection and treatment of asymptomatic bacteriuria effectively prevents pyelonephritis and subsequent development of renal scarring. Dipstick urinalysis, including the nitrite test for bacteriuria and the leukocyte esterase test for pyuria, is itself an inexpensive screening test. Its 20% false-positive rate, however, increases the cost by necessitating retesting or urine culture. Nevertheless, the AAP and other professional groups recommend a screening urinalysis for all children around 5 years of age.

Tuberculosis

In 1993 there were 2301 new cases of tuberculosis (TB) in children reported in the United States. This figure is part of a disturbing nationwide upward trend in the case rate since the mid-1980's. In general, persons who belong to subpopulations at risk for tuberculosis should be screened. In the pediatric population, high-risk infants, children, and adolescents include those with infectious or high-risk contacts; those who are immunosuppressed, including HIV-positive persons; those from countries with a high prevalence of TB (Asia, Pacific Islands), those with a chest radiograph suggesting disease, and those with clinical symptoms of TB. The **Mantoux test**, or **purified protein derivative (PPD)** test, is the recommended screening instrument. It can be given to children as young as 12 months of age and repeated yearly if the risk persists. The tine test is no longer recommended because, since the prevalence of infection in the United States is low, the positive predictive value of this test is quite low.

IMMUNIZATIONS

Because of the importance of immunization in children's health care, as well as providing documentation for school entry, primary care providers must keep accurate records of vaccinations and other forms of immunization. A child's immunization status can be easily monitored on a health supervision flow sheet (Figure 3–1). A copy of the record should also be given to the parents and updated by the nurse as additional immunizations or boosters are given. Details of specific immunization procedures and tests can be found in Chapter 6.

FEVER

Fever in children warrants specific discussion in that it is a symptom which frequently prompts parents to call for advice or bring children to the pediatrician's office. Evaluation of fever is therefore an important part of routine telephone or office triage. Two areas deserve special mention: (1) educating parents and office staff about fever; and (2) evaluation of fever in children under three years of age.

Definition & Measurement

A child's temperature can be measured in the mouth, the rectum, or the axillae. Rectal temperature is generally considered more reliable than oral temperature, especially in children who are mouth breathers. The following temperatures are usually indicative of fever:

- Rectal: temperature over 38 °C (100.4 °F).
- Oral: temperature over 37.5 °C (99.5 °F).
- Axillary: temperature over 37 °C (98.6 °F).

Body temperature normally fluctuates during the day; it may be a half degree *below* normal in the morning, rising to a half degree *above* normal in the evening. Mild elevations of 1–1.5 °C can be caused by exercise, excessive clothing, a hot bath or hot weather. Bottle or breast feedings may raise an infant's temperature for a half hour or more; likewise, warm food or drink can elevate an oral temperature. If any of the foregoing causes is suspected, take the temperature again in a half hour after eliminating the possible cause.

Causes

Fever is a symptom, not a disease. It occurs when (1) there is a rise in the hypothalamic set-point (caused by infection, malignancy, collagen vascular disease, some drugs, etc.); (2) the body's heat production or environmental heat exceeds heat loss mechanisms (eg, malignant hyperthermia, excessive environmental heat); or (3) heat loss mechanisms are defective (eg, ectodermal dysphasia). The vast majority of fevers at any level are caused by viral illnesses. There is, however, a direct relationship between fever magnitude and serious bacterial infection. Teething, often cited as a cause of fever in infants, does not cause fever over 38.4 °C (101 °F).

Course

Most fevers associated with viral illnesses last for 2–3 days. Fever causes no harm (eg, brain damage) when it is lower than 41.7 °C (107 °F). Fortunately, the brain's thermostat keeps untreated fevers caused by infections below 41.1 °C (106 °F). While all children run fevers on occasion, only 4% develop febrile convulsions. This type of seizure is generally harmless.

Guidelines for Evaluation

For purposes of triage, the following guidelines may be helpful:

The child should be evaluated *immediately* if:

- He or she is younger than 2 months old.
- The fever is > 40.1 °C (104 °F).
- The child is crying inconsolably or whimpering.
- The child cries when moved or otherwise touched by the parent.
- The child is difficult to awaken.
- The neck is stiff.
- Any purple spots (petechiae) are present on the skin.
- Breathing is difficult and not improved by clearing the nose.
- The child is drooling saliva and is unable to swallow.
- A convulsion has occurred.
- The child acts or looks very sick.

The child should be seen *within 24 hours* if:

- The child is 2–4 months old (unless fever occurs within 48 hours of a diphtheria-pertussis-tetanus (DPT) shot and the infant has no other serious symptoms).
- The fever is > 40 °C (104 °F) (especially if the child is under 3 years old).
- Burning or pain occurs with urination.
- The fever has been present more than 24 hours without an obvious cause or locus of infection.
- The fever went away for more than 24 hours and then returned.
- The fever has been present more than 72 hours.

Treatment

Overtreatment: "Fever phobia" is a term that describes parents' overly anxious response to the fevers that all children experience. Because of widespread misconceptions about fever (eg, the notion that low-grade fevers can cause brain damage or that untreated fevers will continue to rise), many parents overtreat low-grade fevers. Teaching parents about fever can reduce the number of telephone calls and visits to the doctor. You may find it helpful to give parents an office handout summarizing necessary information.

Acetaminophen: Children older than 2 months of age can be given acetaminophen every 4–6 hours. Acetaminophen is indicated if the fever is over 39 °C (102 °F) or the child is uncomfortable. Acetaminophen will reduce the fever by 1–2 °C within 2 hours after it is given. Acetaminophen and other antipyretics do not bring the temperature down to normal unless the fever was low-grade to begin with.

Ibuprofen: Ibuprofen is similar to acetaminophen in safety and in its ability to lower fever. One advantage of ibuprofen over acetaminophen, however, is its longer duration of action (6–8 hours versus 4–6 hours). Because the dose (10 mg/kg), strength (100 mg/5 mL), and dosing interval (6–8 hours) of liquid ibuprofen differ from those of acetaminophen, the use of ibuprofen should be reviewed carefully with parents.

Aspirin: Several studies have linked the use of aspirin during viral illnesses (especially chickenpox and influenza) to **Reye's syndrome,** which is a rare but severe complication of viral infections marked by rapid-onset liver failure and encephalopathy. Parents should therefore be advised *not* to give children aspirin for fever.

Other Treatment Measures: Children can be sponged with lukewarm water (*never* rubbing alcohol) for febrile delirium, febrile seizure, or any fever over 41.1 °C (106 °F). Ideally, acetaminophen should be given 30 minutes prior to sponging to reset the hypothalamic temperature set point, so that the sponge bath will not cause shivering. Heat stroke requires immediate cold water sponging; antipyretics are *not* beneficial. Also encourage the child to take extra fluids.

FEVER WITHOUT FOCUS

Essentials of Diagnosis

- Child less than 3 years of age with fever.
- No focal infection found on physical examination.

General Considerations

Children under the age of three years who present with a fever and no obvious source of infection present a special challenge to physicians. Both minor illnesses as well as serious bacterial infections (SBIs) (sepsis, meningitis, urinary tract infections [UTIs], pneumonia, septic arthritis/osteomyelitis, and enteritis) are common at this age.

Bacterial pathogens most commonly seen in the infant less than 2 months of age are group B streptococcus and *Escherichia coli. Streptococcus pneumoniae* and *Haemophilus influenzae* type b are more commonly encountered in older children, although the incidence of *H influenzae* type b disease has fallen dramatically since the introduction of this vaccine for infants. Other pathogens responsible for invasive disease include *Staphylococcus aureus, Salmonella* and other gram-negative organisms.

In general, the higher the fever, the greater the risk of SBIs. In infants younger than 30 days, the rate of SBIs was 4.4% for temperatures 38.1–39 °C (100–102 °F), 7.6% for 39.1–39.9 °C (102–104 °F) and 18% for temperatures ≥ 40 °C (104 °F). Several studies report the risk of occult bacteremia in children 3–36 months of age with fever without source to be in the range of 3–11%.

Management

An expert panel's review of the literature has suggested the following treatment guidelines for fever without source in infants and children less than 3 years of age:

1. Hospitalize any child who appears toxic. Serious disease may be present in an infant without fever; in fact, a newborn may be hypothermic.

2. Hospitalize newborns under 4 weeks of age. Most experts maintain that infants under a month of age should have a work-up for sepsis and be hospitalized, even though the risk of SBI if they meet the criteria for low risk is quite small. In general, hospitalized infants are placed on parenteral antibiotics pending culture results; however, they can also be kept under observation without antibiotics.

3. Identify low-risk febrile infants (1–3 months of age). The following factors are considered to indicate low risk:

- non-toxic
- previously healthy
- no bacterial focus (except otitis media) on examination
- good social situation
- white blood cell count (WBC) 5000–15,000/mm^3, < 1500 bands/mm^3. In general, the higher the WBC or the higher the absolute neutrophil count, the greater the likelihood of bacteremia. When the WBC exceeds 15,000/mm^3, the probability of bacteremia increases fivefold.
- urinalysis with < 5 WBCs/high-power field (hpf)
- if diarrhea is present, < 5 WBCs/hpf in stool.

Febrile infants who do *not* fall into these low-risk categories should be hospitalized; others should be managed as outpatients with one of two options: (1) Culture urine; reevaluate in 24 hours; (2) Culture blood, urine, and cerebrospinal fluid (CSF); administer ceftriaxone 50 mg/kg; reevaluate in 24 hours. Parenteral antibiotics are more effective than oral antibiotics. The probability of an SBI in low-risk infants is 0.2%.

4. Determine the temperature of previously healthy children 3 months–3 years of age. If the fever is < 39.0 °C (102 °F), give antipyretics and keep child under observation. If the temperature is ≥ 39.0 °C (102 °F) obtain a WBC. If the count is ≥ 15,000/mm^3, obtain a blood culture and treat with ceftriaxone 50 mg/kg. Males < 6 months of age and females < 2 years of age should also have a urine specimen for culture collected either by catheter or suprapubic tap; chest x-ray (CXR) and stool culture only if indicated by history or examination.

Follow-up

Infants and children with positive blood or CSF cultures should be admitted and treated with parental antibiotics. If the blood culture grows nonresistant *S pneumoniae* and the child is afebrile on follow-up visit, outpatient therapy with oral amoxicillin or penicillin is sufficient. Urinary tract infections (UTIs) may also be treated on an outpa-

Table 3–5. Acceptable weight gain by age.

Age (mo)	Weight gain (g/d)
Birth–3	20–30
3–6	15–20
6–9	10–15
9–12	6–11
12–18	5–8
18–24	3–7

Table 3–6. Evaluation and treatment of growth deficiency.

Initial Evaluation		Further	
History	**Examination**	**Evaluation**	**Treatment**
Birth	Growth measurements	Prospective 3-day diet record	**Standard** High-calorie diet
Feeding and nutrition	Vital signs	Laboratory tests, if indicated	Frequent monitoring (every 1–2 weeks)
Stooling and voiding	Complete examination		Education in nutrition and child development
Growth pattern	Developmental screening (eg, Denver II)		Psychosocial support of primary caretaker
Recurrent infection	Observation of child-caretaker interaction		**Adjunctive (as indicated)**
Hospitalizations			Developmental interventions
HIV risk factors			Daycare
Development			Other medical treatment
Social situation			Rarely, hospitalization
Family milieu			
Review of systems			

HIV = human immunodeficiency virus.

tient basis with oral antibiotics based upon sensitivities, if the child is afebrile.

GROWTH DEFICIENCY (FAILURE TO THRIVE)

Growth deficiency, or "failure to thrive," occurs when there is a deceleration of growth velocity resulting in crossing two major percentile lines on the growth chart, or when a height-to-weight plot is lower than the fifth percentile. Because growth is so rapid in the first 6 months of life, providers should be concerned if there is no weight gain over a 2-month period. Growth deficiency is present in about 8% of the pediatric population. Acceptable weight gain varies by age (Table 3–5).

The reader is referred to Chapter 4 for a detailed description of various patterns of growth deficiency. Evaluation and treatment of growth deficiency is provided in Table 3–6.

4 | Nutrition & Feeding

K. Michael Hambidge, MD, ScD, &
Nancy F. Krebs, MD, MS

The act of feeding is important to the young child not only because of the nutritive substances obtained from the food but also because of the emotional and psychologic benefits derived. Drinking and eating are intense experiences to an infant and can and should be sources of great satisfaction. From these experiences and from the persons who feed them, infants obtain many of their early ideas about the nature of life and people.

Parents must be made to understand that there is much individual variation in the nutritional needs and desires of infants and that differences occur in the same child at various times.

The feeding of children has become more flexible and simple as knowledge of their nutritional requirements increases; however, certain basic information and data are necessary for a practical understanding of the subject.

Neither strict adherence to a time schedule nor feeding when the infant cries is necessary for successful and satisfactory feeding. For most parents and infants, a flexible schedule with reasonable regularity is most satisfactory, but in some cases either a strict routine or complete "demand" feeding gives better results.

BREAST-FEEDING

Advantages & Contraindications

Apart from considerations of economy and convenience (temperature, asepsis, automatic adjustment in most instances to infant's needs), breast-feeding is superior to bottle-feeding for many reasons. The composition of breast milk is ideal for nearly all infants, as breast milk has specific antibacterial and antiviral activities that protect infants from gastrointestinal and respiratory disease. Breast-feeding produces less infantile allergy and is psychologically beneficial to both mother and infant.

In the past decade, breast-feeding has been reestablished as the predominant mode of feeding the young infant in the United States. Unfortunately, breast-feeding rates remain low among several subpopulations of women, including low-income, minority, and young mothers. Many mothers face unique obstacles to maintaining lactation once they return to work. Skilled use of the breast pump may help to maintain lactation in this circumstance.

Breast-feeding may be temporarily impossible for a weak, ill, or premature infant. Difficulties may also arise in an infant with a cleft palate, although in such cases breast milk may be expressed and fed in another way.

Absolute contraindications to breast-feeding (eg, galactosemia) are rare. Maternal infection with human immunodeficiency virus in developed countries and untreated tuberculosis are other contraindications.

Infants weighing less than 1500 g are likely to benefit from the addition of an infant milk fortifier to increase the density of energy, protein, calcium, and phosphorus. Some breast-fed infants with cystic fibrosis also will need a supplement.

Transmission of Drugs & Toxins in Breast Milk

Virtually all drugs consumed by the mother will appear in her breast milk to some degree, usually in homeopathic amounts. Drug excretion into milk is affected by the drug's ionization, lipid solubility, protein binding, and molecular size, as well as other factors. Effects on the infant also depend on the route of administration, the dosage, and the mother's timing in taking the drugs. Another determining factor is the drug's metabolites and its absorption in the gastrointestinal tract. It is believed that the level of drugs present in breast milk is lowest just before the mother takes medications.

Table 4–1 lists drugs and other contraindications to breast-feeding. A regional drug center should be consulted for up-to-date information on which drugs are contraindicated. When a course of therapy of a potentially hazardous drug will be brief, the mother can temporarily interrupt breast-feeding and maintain her supply by expressing and discarding her milk.

Composition of Breast Milk (Table 4–2)

Favorable features of human milk include an optimal amino acid and protein content for the normal infant; a generous but not excessive quantity of essential fatty acids; an adequate but relatively low sodium content; a low solute load compared with cow's milk; and

Table 4–1. Contraindications to breast-feeding.

Drugs
Maternal use of illicit drugs
Radioactive compounds
Antimetabolites
Lithium
Valium (diazepam)
Chloramphenicol, tetracycline
Maternal infection
Tuberculosis
Human immunodeficiency virus (in developed countries)
? hepatitis C
Infant conditions
Galactosemia

very favorable absorption of iron, calcium, and zinc, which results in the provision of adequate quantities of these nutrients to the infant fully breast-fed for 4–6 months.

Breast-fed infants do require standard neonatal prophylactic vitamin K and may require vitamin D supplements if not regularly exposed to sunlight or if maternal vitamin D status is suboptimal. Breast milk will be low in vitamin B_{12} if the mother is a strict, unsupplemented vegetarian. Maternal undernutrition is generally associated with lower breast milk supply, but with preservation of nutritional quality.

Management of Breast-Feeding

Perinatal hospital routines and follow-up pediatric care have a great impact on the successful initiation of breast-feeding. Breast-feeding is promoted by prenatal and postpartum education, frequent mother/baby contact after delivery, one-on-one advice about breast-feeding technique, demand feeding, rooming in, avoidance of bottle supplements, early follow-up after delivery, maternal confidence, family support, adequate maternity leave, and accurate advice for common problems such as sore nipples.

Before discharge, individualized assessment should identify those mother/baby pairs needing additional support. In all such cases, there should be early follow-up after discharge. The onset of copious milk secretion between the second and fourth postpartum day is a critical time in the establishment of lactation.

A. Prelactation (Colostrum) Phase: Colostrum is a yellow, alkaline breast secretion that may be produced during the last few months of pregnancy and for the first 2–4 days after delivery. It has a higher specific gravity (1.040–1.060); a higher content of protein, fat-soluble vitamins, and minerals; and a lower content of carbohydrate and fat than breast milk.

Colostrum contains secretory immunoglobulin A (IgA), leukocytes, and other immune substances that play a part in the immune defenses of the newborn. Colostrum has a natural laxative action and is an ideal starter food.

Although the milk may not "come in" until 2–4 days after delivery, prelactation nursing is very important because of the value of colostrum, the effect of the nursing stimulus to increase milk supply and lessen engorgement, and the opportunity nursing provides for the mother and infant to become accustomed to one another. While some infants nurse irregularly the first few days, others demand feeding as often as every 2 hours. Nursing is commonly limited to 5 minutes per breast per feeding the first day, 10 minutes per breast per feeding the second day, and 15 minutes or longer per breast per feeding thereafter.

There is no need for routine supplementation for the full-term, healthy infant who appears satisfied, but when the infant is persistently hungry or has an underlying condition (eg, hypoglycemia) requiring increased caloric intake, then formula may be offered after nursing until the milk comes in. Once milk is in, further supplements should not be given unless there is evidence of inadequate milk intake.

B. Lactation Phase: Forty-eight to 96 hours postpartum, the mother's breasts change from soft to firm and full as lactogenesis occurs. The infant may be fed at each hungry period, day and night, which is usually every 1.5–3 hours during the first month with longer intervals (4–5 hours) at night. The infant should nurse at the first breast for approximately 10 minutes and then be put to the other breast and allowed to suckle for up to 15 minutes (unless the nipples are sore). Feedings lasting more than 45 minutes usually are indicative of ineffective nursing or insufficient milk supply. During the early weeks of lactation, the milk supply seems to be more sensitive to negative stimuli such as maternal fatigue, anxiety, and lack of suckling. The infant will typically have frequent, somewhat loose bowel movements (often with each feeding) during this period. Dark transition stools, infrequent bowel movements, or scant volumes in the young breast-fed infant are common indicators of insufficient milk.

The **let-down reflex**, by which milk is actively ejected through

Table 4–2. Comparison of composition of milk and commercial formula (per 1000 mL).[1]

Component	Unit	Human Milk	Typical Commercial Formula	Whole Cow's Milk
Osmolality	mosm/kg water	282	290	275
Energy	kcal	67	67	61
Carbohydrate (lactose)	g	7.3	7.2	4.7
Fat	g	4.2	3.8	3.3
Minerals				
Calcium	mg	25	51	119
Chloride	mg (meq)	40 (1.1)	53 (1.5)	102 (2.9)
Copper	μg	35	41	30
Fluorine	μg	7	20	15
Iodine	μg	7	10	5
Iron	μg	40	150 (1200 w/Fe)	50
Magnesium	mg	3	4.1	13
Manganese	μg	0.4	3	2–4
Phosphorus	mg	15	39	93
Potassium	mg (meq)	58 (1.5)	78 (2)	152 (3.9)

Sodium	mg (meq)	15 (0.8)	25 (1.1)	49 (2.1)
Zinc	μg	100–300	500	300
Proteins				
Casein	mg	187	1185	2700
Lactalbumin	mg	161	52	400
Total proteins	g	0.9	1.5	3.3
Vitamins				
A (retinol equivalents)	μg (IU)	47 (155)	75 (250)	31 (126)
B_6 (pyridoxine)	μg	28	40	42
B_{12} (cyanocobalamin)	ng	26	150	357
C (ascorbic acid)	mg	4	5.5	0.9
D	μg (IU)	0.04 (1.6)	1 (40)	1 (42)
E (total tocopherols)	μg (IU)	315 (0.32)	1700 (1.7)	80 (0.08)
K	μg	0.21	3	6
Folic acid	μg	5.2	5	5
Niacin	μg	200	790	84
Pantothenic acid	μg	225	300	314
Riboflavin	μg	35	100	162
Thiamine	μg	16	65	30

[1] Adapted from various sources.

the duct system for easy access to the infant, is usually conditioned and evident by 2 weeks. The mother feels “tightening,” “stinging,” “tingling,” or “burning” circumferentially in both breasts shortly after the infant begins nursing. The nursing mother should eat a well-balanced diet with additional intake of protein, calcium, and fluids. Drinking a glass of liquid with each nursing is helpful. Additional rest, with several naps each day, should be encouraged.

“Frequency days,” or “appetite spurts,” when infants desire to nurse more often than their established routine, typically occur for several days at approximately 3 weeks, 6 weeks, 3 months, and 6 months of age. Increased frequency of nursing increases the milk supply and allows resumption of the former nursing schedule.

Problems with Breast-Feeding

A. Failure to Thrive: Some breast-fed infants fail to thrive. The most common cause of early failure to thrive is poorly managed mammary engorgement, which will rapidly decrease milk supply. Few breast-fed infants lose as much as 10% of their birth weight in the absence of breast-feeding problems. Unrelieved engorgement can result from inappropriately long intervals between feeding, improper infant suckling, a nondemanding infant, sore nipples, maternal or infant illness, nursing from only one breast, and latching difficulties. Poor maternal knowledge and lack of maternal fluids and rest can all be factors. Some infants are too sleepy to do well on an *ad libitum* regimen and, in particular, may need waking to feed at night. Primary lactation failure is rare but does occur.

Some decline in weight for age percentiles after 3 months should not necessarily be taken as an indication of inadequate nutrition, since the commonly used percentile charts have been constructed from data on infants who have been primarily formula-fed. However, if there is a decline in weight-for-length of more than 20 percentile points, solids should be introduced earlier than may otherwise be intended and formula supplement may be indicated for individual infants.

B. Breast-Feeding Jaundice: Breast-feeding jaundice is exaggerated physiologic jaundice associated with inadequate intake of breast milk, infrequent stooling, and unsatisfactory weight gain. Where possible, this condition should be managed by increasing the frequency of nursing and, if necessary, augmenting the infant’s suckling with regular breast pumping. Supplemental feedings may be necessary until adequate milk supply can be established.

C. Breast-Milk Jaundice: In a small percentage of breast-fed infants, **breast-milk jaundice** occurs as the result of an unidentified property of the milk that inhibits conjugation of bilirubin or deconjugates bile in the lumen of the small intestine. In severe cases, interruption of breast-feeding for 24–36 hours may be necessary. The mother's breast should be emptied with an electric breast pump during this period.

D. Sore Nipples: Mild nipple tenderness requires attention to proper positioning of the infant and correct latch-on. Ancillary measures include nursing for shorter periods, beginning feeds on the less sore side, air-drying the nipples after nursing, and the application of lanolin cream. Severe nipple pain and cracking usually indicate improper infant attachment. Temporary pumping, which is well tolerated, may be needed.

E. Mastitis: Maternal mastitis should be suspected when a nursing mother complains of a "flu-like" illness, with local breast tenderness. Antibiotic therapy providing coverage against beta-lactamase–producing organisms should be given for 10 days. Analgesics may be necessary, but breast-feeding should be continued. Breast pumping may be a helpful adjunctive therapy.

FORMULA FEEDING

The standard milk-based infant formulas (Table 4–3) contain heat-treated protein (at reduced concentration), lactose and minerals from cow's milk, vegetable oils, minerals, and vitamin additives. Iron-fortified formulas are recommended after 2 months. Standard formulas contain 20 kcal/oz and 0.45 g protein/oz.

As an alternative to proprietary infant formulas, use evaporated milk formula. To prepare 32 oz of formula, mix 1 can (13 oz) of whole evaporated milk, 1½ cans (19 oz) of water, and 2 tablespoons of corn syrup. To make 5 oz, mix 2 oz of evaporated milk, 3 oz of water, and 1 teaspoon of corn syrup.

Infants should be fed formula for a minimum of 6 months, or, ideally, for the entire first year of life. Low-fat and skim milk are inappropriate for use in the first year of life.

Lactose intolerance is the main indicator for a soy-based formula. Semi-elemental formulas have a wide range of uses in intestinal disease, including malabsorption syndromes, chronic diarrhea, and short-bowel syndrome. They are also used in infants who are intolerant of cow's protein and soy protein. Elemental formulas also find some applications in infancy, for example, when continuous drip feeding is indicated in infants with cystic fibrosis. Special formulas

Table 4–3. Selected normal and special infant formulas.[1]

Product	Protein Source, Amount	CHO Source, Amount	Fat Source, Amount	Indications for Use	Comments (Nutritional Adequacy)
Milk-based formulas					
Enfamil (Mead Johnson)[2]	Nonfat cow's milk, reduced mineral whey, 1.5 g/dL	Lactose, 6.9 g/dL	Coconut, soy oils, 3.8 g/dL	For full-term and premature infants with no special nutritional re-quirements	Available fortified with iron, 12 mg/L; whey: casein ratio 60:40
Similac (Ross)[2]	Nonfat cow's milk, 1.5 g/dL	Lactose, 7.2 g/dL	Coconut, soy oils, 3.6 g/dL	Same as Enfamil	Available fortified with iron, 12 mg/L
Lactofree (Mead Johnson)	Whole milk protein isolate; 1.5 g/dL	Corn syrup solids, 7.0 g/dL	Vegetable oils (palm olein, soy, coco-nut, high oleic sunflower) 3.7 g/dL	Lactose intolerance, galactosemia	Protein 2.2 g/100 kcal; Ca:P ratio 1.5:1; Iron fortified
Soy-protein formulas					
Isomil (Ross)	Soy protein isolate, 1.8 g/dL	Sucrose, corn syrup,[3] 6.8 g/dL	Coconut, soy oils, 3.7 g/dL	For infants with lac-tose intolerance or milk-protein allergy	Supplemented with iron, 12 mg/L
ProSoBee (Mead Johnson)	Soy protein isolate with added L-methionine, 2.0 g/dL	Corn syrup solids 6.6 g/dL	Soy, coconut oils, 3.5 g/dL	ISame as Isomi	Same as Isomill

Products for premature infants					
Enfamil Premature Formula (Mead Johnson)	Nonfat cow's milk, demineralized whey, 2.4 g/dL	Lactose, corn syrup solids, 7.5 g/dL	MCT[4] (coconut source), corn, coconut oils, 3.4 g/dL	For rapidly growing low-birth-weight infants	Protein, 3 g/100 kcal; Ca:P ratio, 2:1; E:PUFA ratio,[5] 2.8:1
Similac 24 Special Care (Ross)	Nonfat cow's milk, whey protein concentrate, 2.2 g/dL	Lactose, glucose polymers, 8.5 g/dL	MCT,[4] coconut, soy oils, 4.3 g/dL	Same as Enfamil Premature Formula	Protein, 2.7 g/100 kcal; E:PUFA ratio[5] 2.5:1, osmolality, 280 mosm/kg water
Neocare (Ross)	Nonfat cow's milk, whey protein concentrate, 1.9 g/dL; casein: whey 40:60	Corn syrup solids, lactose, 7.6 g/dL	LCT + MCT (soy, coconut oils), 4.1 g/dL	Post-discharged premature infant for first year of life	Protein 2.6 g/100 kcal; Ca:P ratio 1.7:1; Zn 1.2 mg/100 kcal
Partially demineralized whey formulas					
Similac PM 60/40 (Ross)	Whey, caseinate, 1.6 g/dL	Lactose, 6.8 g/dL	Coconut, soy oils, 3.7 g/dL	For newborns pre disposed to hy pocalcemia and infants with renal or heart disease	Ca:P ratio, 2:1; low phosphorus; relatively low solute load; Na = 7 meq/L E:PUFA ratio,[5] 1.0:1

(*continued*)

Table 4–3. Selected normal and special infant formulas[1] (*continued*).

Product	Protein Source, Amount	CHO Source, Amount	Fat Source, Amount	Indications for Use	Comments (Nutritional Adequacy)
Semi-elemental formulas					
Nutramigen (Mead Johnson)	Casein hydrolysate, 1.9 g/dL	Modified corn starch, corn syrup solids, 9.0 mg/dL	Corn oil, 2.6 g/dL	For infants and children intolerant of food proteins and for galactosemic patients	
Pregestamil (Mead Johnson)	Casein hydrolysate, 70% amino acids, 30% peptides, 1.9 g/dL	Corn syrup solids, dextrose 6.9 g/dL	60% MCT,[4] 20% corn oil, 20% high oleic safflower, 3.8 g/dL	For infants with malabsorption syndromes	
Alimentum (Ross)	Casein hydrolysate 1.8 g/dL	71% sucrose, 29% modified tapioca starch, 6.9 g/dL	50% MCT,[4] 40% safflower oil, 10% soy oil, 3.8 g/dL	Same as Pregestamil	
Other formulas for malabsorption syndromes					
Portagen (Mead Johnson)	Sodium caseinate, 2.3 g/dL	Sucrose, corn syrup solids, 7.7 g/dL	88% MCT[4] (coconut source), corn oil, 3.2 g/dL	For management of chyluria, intestinal lymphangiectasia	88% MCT[4] oil, low in essential fatty acids

Peptamen Jr. (Clintec)	Whey hydrolysate, peptides	Maltodextrin, starch 13.8 g/dL	50% MCT, sunflower oil, 3.8 g/dL	For children with malabsorption	Available with flavor packets
Elemental formula					
Pediatric Vivonex	Free amino acids, 2.4 g/dL	Maltodextrin, modi fied starch, 12.6 g/dL	MCT, soybean oil, 2.2 g/dL	For children with malabsorption, severe protein allergies	
Products for infants with inborn errors					
Lofenallac (Mead Johnson)	Casein hydrolysate, L-Amino acids	Corn syrup solids, modified tapioca starch	Corn oil	For infants and chil dren with phenylketonuria	*Must* be supplemented with other foods or infant formula to provide minimal phenylalanine
MSUD Diet (Mead Johnson)	L-Amino acids	Corn syrup solids, modified tapioca starch	Corn oil	For children with branched-chain ketoaciduria	Leucine-, isoleucine-, and valine-free; *must* be supplemented
Phenyl-Free (Mead Johnson)	L-Amino acids	Sucrose, corn syrup solids, modified tapioca starch	Corn and coconut oils	For children over 1 year of age with phenylketonuria	Phenylalanine-free. Permits increased supple mentation with normal foods

(*continued*)

Table 4–3. Selected normal and special infant formulas[1] (*continued*).

Product	Protein Source, Amount	CHO Source, Amount	Fat Source, Amount	Indications for Use	Comments (Nutritional Adequacy)
Products for infants with inborn errors (*continued*)					
Analog XP (Ross Laboratories)	L-Amino acids	Corn syrup solids	Peanut oil, animal fat (pork), coconut oil	For infants and children with phenylketonuria	Phenylalanine-free; must be supplemented with other milk, formula or foods.
Product 3232A (Mead Johnson)	Enzymatically treated casein	Modified tapioca starch	MCT,[4] corn oil	Protein hydrolysate formula base for use in diagnosis and nutritional management of infants with disaccharidase deficiencies	Monosaccharide- and disaccharide-free powder
Product 80056 (Mead Johnson)	None	Corn syrup solids, modified tapioca starch	Corn oil	For formulation of special diets for infants requiring specific mixtures of amino acids	Protein-free; carbohydrate, fat, vitamin, and mineral mix

[1] Committee on Nutrition, American Academy of Pediatrics: Commentary on breast feeding and infant formulas including proposed standards for formulas. Pediatrics 1976;57:278. Committee on Nutrition, American Academy of Pediatrics: Nutritional needs of low-birthweight infants. Pediatrics 1977;60:519.

[2] Ready-to-use, concentrated liquid, and powder forms.

[3] Composed of glucose, maltose, and dextrins.

[4] Medium-chain triglycerides (MCT).

[5] Ratio of vitamin E (E) to polyunsaturated fatty acids (PUFA).

are marketed for several inborn metabolic diseases and for a variety of disease states. Polycose and medium-chain triglycerides are used as formula supplements. Increasing the concentration of the formulas to provide > 24 kcal/oz is preferable if the aim is an overall increase in nutrient density.

Infants who are fed most complete proprietary infant formulas require no additional vitamin supplements. Those fed evaporated milk formula should have daily supplements of vitamins C and D. Supplemental vitamin D is recommended for breast-fed infants if consistent exposure to sunlight cannot be assured and for darkly pigmented infants. It is most conveniently given as a multivitamin liquid preparation.

"SOLID" FOODS

1. Solid foods can be introduced gradually starting at age 4–6 months. Solids should not be introduced until the infant can sit with support and show good control of the head and neck. The infant should be able to indicate a desire for food by opening the mouth and leaning forward and indicate disinterest by leaning back and turning away.

   Start with an iron-fortified cereal, preferably rice. This may be followed by pureed vegetables, fruits, strained meat, and egg yolks. Junior-type foods can be introduced at age 7–8 months.
2. There is no exact order for starting solid foods. The physiologic requirement for foods other than milk first occurs at about age 4–6 months, when a need for iron develops. When solid foods are started, they should initially be given in small amounts for several consecutive days to determine the infant's reaction and to note if any adverse response occurs. The amount should be gradually increased if the food is well tolerated.
3. Many infants can learn to take semisolid food from a small spoon by age 4 months. If the infant cannot master spoon-feeding, postpone the attempt for a few weeks; otherwise, undesirable behavior may result and may make spoon-feeding difficult for months.
4. The transition from strained to chopped foods should be gradual and may be started when the infant begins to make chewing motions.
5. Egg white, wheat, orange juice, corn, and other allergenic foods should not be given (especially when there is a family predisposition to allergy) until the child is in the latter part of the first year of life.
6. Infants should be encouraged to feed themselves with fingers or a spoon when they wish to do so, usually at around 6 months.

7. Avoid feeding nuts, popcorn, and other foods that are easily aspirated to all children under age 4 years.

NUTRIENT REQUIREMENTS

Energy requirements for infants, based on measurements of energy expenditure and energy intakes of breast-fed infants, are presented in Table 4–4. The components of energy expenditure are given in Table 4–5. There are wide individual variations in energy requirements. In general, appetite and growth provide useful guides. Protein requirements for infants are also given in Table 4-4. Infants require 43% and children 36% of their protein as essential amino acids. Cysteine, tyrosine, and taurine are considered partially essential in the premature infant.

Infants should receive 45–50% of their calories as fat until age 2 years, after which fat consumption should be reduced to < 30% of calories. At least 2% of calories should be provided as essential fatty acids of the ω6 series, and up to 1% as the ω3 series.

Medium-chain triglycerides (MCTs), energy density 7.6 kcal/g, are not essential in the normal diet but are invaluable in malabsorption syndromes. MCTs are especially useful when bile secretion is diminished or absorption and transport of long-chain fatty acids is impaired by other mechanisms. MCTs are very readily absorbed without mycelle formation and are transported via the portal circulation directly to the liver, where they undergo rapid beta-oxidation (without the need for carnitine) or ketogenesis.

Recommended dietary allowances (RDAs), which exceed the actual requirements of most individuals, can be found in the reference *Recommended Dietary Allowances*, 10th edition (National Academy Press, 1989). The utility of the RDAs is especially limited for young infants because recommendations cover a wide age range at a time when physiologic changes are occurring rapidly. It should be emphasized that the RDAs are not designed to provide guidelines for individual requirements.

NUTRIENT DEFICIENCIES AND EXCESSES

Failure to Thrive

Failure to thrive (FTT) is a term that is commonly applied to mild or moderate undernutrition. Errors in diet or feeding technique (eg, wrong dilution of formula, inadequate breast-feeding, too-small holes in bottle nipples) account for about 20% of cases of FTT. Thirty

Table 4–4. Guide to protein, energy, and fluid requirements of infants and frequency of feeds.[1]

Age (mo)[2]	0	1	2	3	4	5	6	7	8	9	10	11	12
Calories (kcal/kg/d)	120	115	105	95			90						
Protein (g/kg/day)	2.25 0–3 months			2.0 3–4 months	1.7 4–6 months					1.5 6–12 months			
Fluid	130–200 mL/kg/d (2–3 oz/lb/d)			130–165 mL/kg/d (2–2.5 oz/lb/d)						130 mL/kg/d (2 oz/lb/d)			
Number of feedings (per day)	8–12		4–5				3–4					3	
Amount (oz) per feeding	2.5–4	3.5–5	4–6	5–7	6–8	7–9							

[1] Some prepared milk formulas may be deficient in vitamins C and D and need to be supplemented with vitamins (25–50 mg of vitamin C and 400 units of vitamin D daily). Iron supplementation of formulas is recommended after 2 months.

[2] Underweight or overweight infants generally have the same food requirements as do infants of the same age with a normal weight. Undiluted whole milk or formulas of equal parts of evaporated milk and water should not be used for young infants, since their kidneys do not have a range of safety in the event of high environmental or body temperature.

Table 4–5. Approximate daily expenditure of calories during the first year of life.

Use	Amount (kcal/kg/d)
Basal metabolism	50
Thermic effect of foods	5
Caloric loss in the excreta	10
Allowance for bodily activity[1]	2–20
Growth	50 → 10
Total	120 → 90

[1] Range is for infants up to 1 month old to those 6–12 months old.

percent are secondary to organic disease, and 50% result from nutritional deprivation. Whatever the primary event, malnutrition is the final common pathway, and the pattern of impaired growth is "wasting," or a low weight-for-length percentile with the weight-age declining earlier and more severely than the length-age. The end result, if not effectively treated at an early stage, is "stunting," which is characterized by a low height-for-age percentile and relatively normal weight-for-height percentile. In the United States, stunting of nutritional origin is usually seen only after infancy, but frequently occurs before 6 months of age in less developed countries. Stunting must be distinguished from endocrinopathy and structural dystrophia. If the head circumference is severely affected, the differential diagnosis includes primary central nervous system disease, severe intrauterine growth retardation, or very severe and early FTT.

For malnourished infants, requirements can be based on ideal body weight (ie, 50th percentile weight-for-height age) or by calculating energy required for the desired "catch-up" growth (5 kcal/g new tissue). Protein requirements also increase during "catch-up" growth (0.2 g protein/g new tissue). Weight velocity during rehabilitation of wasted infants is up to 20 times normal, but in stunting does not exceed three times normal.

Marasmus & Kwashiorkor

Marasmus is the end result of severe undernutrition in which there has been successful adaptation to prolonged lack of energy and nutrients. Body weight is less than 60% median for age.

Table 4–6. Comparison of clinical and laboratory features of marasmus and kwashiorkor.

Clinical	Marasmus	Kwashiorkor
Weight loss	++++	++
Loss of muscle	++++	+
Loss of fat	++++	+
Edema	−−−	++++
Psychological impairment	++	++++
Anorexia	+	++++
Hepatomegaly	−−−	++
Associated infections	++	++++
Diarrhea	+++	+++
Skin lesions	−−−	++
Hair changes	+	++
Laboratory Features		
Anemia	+	+++
Low serum albumin, transferrin, etc	+	++++
Impaired sodium homeostasis	+	++++
Total body potassium deficiency	++	++++
Prothrombin time	Normal	Prolonged
Immune system	Depressed	Depressed

Kwashiorkor is edematous malnutrition with body weight 60–80% median for age. In kwashiorkor, hepatic protein synthesis is depressed at an early stage. Adaptation to malnutrition is poor, and a life-threatening disease develops despite the presence of some energy reserves and skeletal muscle. The etiology of this complex state of malnutrition remains controversial. Lack of protein or certain amino acids in the diet appears to be a contributory factor in at least some cases. The features of kwashiorkor and marasmus are compared in Table 4–6.

Whereas FTT can be managed with aggressive nutritional rehabilitation from the outset, great care and patience are required in the initial management of kwashiorkor. Small, frequent oral feeds should be given to avoid hypoglycemia. During the acute phase, provide only maintenance energy (95 kcal/kg/d) and protein (less than 1.5 g/kg/d), a very generous supply of potassium to replace intracellular losses, and a minimal amount of sodium (avoid intravenous sodium completely, as intracellular sodium levels and total body sodium are abnormally high). Infections must be treated aggressively. Initial progress over the first 1–2 weeks is characterized by loss of weight as the edema resolves. During the recovery phase, provide 3.5 g protein and 150–200 kcal/kg/d with abundant minerals, vitamins, and trace elements.

Obesity

Obesity is a rapidly increasing problem in the United States; weight problems are evident in up to 1 in 3 children as young as 6 years of age. Obesity results from an imbalance between energy intake and expenditure. However, it frequently involves more than simply overeating. For example, energy expenditure is probably low in preobese states and definitely low in postobese states.

For nutritional management, obtain a diet history to evaluate serving sizes, eating, and activity patterns. Focus on reducing or eliminating specific items. For example, encourage intake of skim milk, nonsugared cereals, and avoidance of high-energy snacks and high-fat foods. Even without counting calories, these measures are likely to reduce energy intake by about one-third. A reduction of 500 kcal/d will result in the loss of 1 pound of fat per week, provided the same rate of energy expenditure is maintained as weight is lost. Exercise and behavioral modification are important components of weight management. Involvement of the entire family is critical to success, since frequently the child's obesity reflects lack of structure or poor limit-setting in the home.

Essential Fatty Acids

Clinical features of ω6 deficiency include growth failure, abnormal scaliness of the skin, erythematous skin lesions, decreased capillary resistance, increased fragility of erythrocytes, thrombocytopenia, poor wound healing, and increased susceptibility to infection. Deficiency of ω3 fatty acids (linoleic) has been less clearly documented, but recent evidence shows that visual acuity is compromised by feeding premature infants formulas that lack docosohexanoic acid (22:6 ω3). Excess ω6 fatty acids may lead to an undesirable increase in the production of leukotrienes and thromboxane.

Carbohydrates

A high intake of complex carbohydrates (more than 55–60% of calories) and of fiber is a key feature of the diet now recommended for children older than 2 years. Ketosis develops with diets containing less than 10% carbohydrates.

Sucrose is currently consumed in large quantities by children and adolescents in North America in such items as soda, candy, and sweetened breakfast cereals. A high intake of sucrose predisposes to obesity and is a major risk factor for dental caries.

Vitamins, Minerals, & Micronutrients

See Table 4–7 for a discussion of nutrient sources, deficiency states, and toxicity.

INTRAVENOUS NUTRITION

Indications

The principal indication for total parenteral nutrition (TPN) is loss of ability to absorb nutrients from the gastrointestinal tract. Supplemental intravenous (IV) nutrition, which can be administered via a peripheral vein, is useful as a temporary measure in the premature neonate or the malnourished postoperative surgical patient.

Catheter Selection & Placement

The **Broviac** is the catheter of choice. Use a double-lumen catheter if required for multiple purposes. If TPN will be needed for less than one month, a Perq catheter can be inserted into a peripheral vein and advanced centrally. The tip of the central venous catheter should be located in the superior vena cava or right atrium. Check placement radiologically before using.

Complications

Because of the cost and the risk of complications, TPN should be used only with adequate indication. Complications include mechanical difficulties that result from problems with insertion; thrombosis of a major vessel; metabolic complications including TPN liver disease and bone disease; and, most commonly, septic complications.

Central catheters may be lost because of sepsis; lack of response to therapy; thrombosis; composition of the infusate (excessive concentrations of calcium and phosphorus); incompatible medications administered with the infusate; or slipping, kinking, or breaking of the catheter. Most breaks are exterior to the skin and can be repaired with kits, which must be kept readily available. Urokinase is effective in dissolving recently formed clots in the catheter.

Nutrient Requirements & Administration

Energy requirements are approximately 10% lower than those for enteral feeding. At least 60% of energy is provided as dextrose mono-

Table 4–7. Deficiency states and toxicity of vitamins and minerals.

Nutrient	Examples of Good Food Sources	Deficient States				Toxicity
		Etiology	Clinical Features	Diagnosis	Treatment	
Vitamin A	Dairy products, fortified margarine, eggs, liver, carotene (from vegetables)	Fat malabsorption, prematurity, TPN, protein–energy malnutrition, cultural (lack of vegetables)	Night blindness → xerophthalmia & Bitot's spots, keratomalacia → ulceration & perforation of cornea → prolapse of lens and iris → blindness, follicular hyperkeratosis & pruritus. ?predisposes to BPD in the premature	Serum retinol < 10 μg/dL, retinol; RBP < 0.7	Fat malabsorption: 2,500–5000 IU/d, eye changes: 50,000 IU orally or IM, preparation: aquasol A (water soluble), [0.1 mL = 5000 IU = 1.6 mg]	> 20,000 IU/d: vomiting, increased intracranial pressure; irritability, headaches, emotional lability, insomnia, dry desquamating skin, myalgia and arthralgia, abdominal pain, hepatosplenomegaly, cortical thickening of bones of hands and feet
Vitamin D	Ultraviolet light synthesis of D_3 in skin; fortified milk & formulas, fish oils	Lack of adequate sunlight coupled with low dietary intake, fat malabsorption syndromes, hydroxylation decreased by hepatic and renal disease and by P450 stimulating drugs, inborn errors of metabolism	Rickets (children), osteomalacia (adults)	Skeletal radiologic abnormalities, high alk phos and PTH, low serum P, low 25-OH D	Fat malabsorption: may need calciferol (vit D_3) 800–1200 IU/d or 25-OH D (Rocaltrol) 5–7 μg/kg/d; rickets: D_3 1600–5000 IU/d (1 mg = 8000 IU); renal disease: + 1,25 OH_2D 0.5–0.2 μg/kg/d	> 40,000 IU/d: hypercalcemia, vomiting, constipation, nephrocalcinosis

Vitamin E	Vegetable oils, wheat germ, nuts, seeds	Fat malabsorption syndromes; especially cholestatic liver disease, abetalipoproteinemia, isolated inborn error of Vitamin E metabolism, increased utilization during oxidant stress, premature infant	Decreased red cell half life may cause hemolytic anemia; progressive neurologic disorders (loss of deep tendon reflexes, loss of coordination, weakness, scoliosis, etc); ?predisposes to oxidant; injury to retina, lung, and brain in premature infant	Serum Vitamin E < 3 µg/mL < 0.8 mg Vitamin E/1 g total lipids, increased H_2O_2 induced hemolysis	Fat malabsorption: 20 mg/kg/d (< 200 mg); abetalipoproteinemia: 100–200 mg/d	25–100 mg/kg/d IM in premature infants associated with necrotizing enterocolitis and liver toxicity but probably due to polysorbate 80 solubilizer
Vitamin K	Vitamin K_1: leafy vegetables, soybean oil, fruits, seeds, cow's milk; Vitamin K_2: intestinal bacteria	Newborn (especially breast fed), fat malabsorption syndrome, anticoagulant drugs (eg, warfarin)	Hemorrhagic disease of newborn, hemorrhage into skin, GI and GU tracts, gingiva, lungs, joints, CNS	Plasma levels of PIVKA, prothrombin time	Newborn: 0.5–1.0 mg IM; children: 3–10 mg IM or IV; malabsorption: 2.5 mg $\times$ 2 weekly or 5 mg/d orally; warfarin reversal: 50–100 mg IV	

(continued)

Table 4–7. Deficiency states and toxicity of vitamins and minerals (*continued*).

Nutrient	Examples of Good Food Sources	Deficient States				Toxicity
		Etiology	Clinical Features	Diagnosis	Treatment	
Vitamin C	Fruits: citrus, strawberries, melons; vegetables: broccoli, green pepper, tomato, potato	Prematurity, no dietary fruits or vegetables	Anorexia, apathy, fever, failure-to-thrive; anemia; increased susceptibility to infections; petechiae; long bone tenderness (severe deficiency: scurvy)	Serum ascorbate < 0.2 mg/dL, low leukocyte ascorbate	Scurvy: 5–10 mg/kg/d IV or PO	Interferes with copper absorption; decreased tolerance to hypoxia; decreased oxalic acid excretion
Folic acid	Orange juice, whole grains, green leafy vegetables, legumes and meats (heat labile; easily destroyed in cooking)	Prematurity; term breast fed infants whose mothers are folate deficient; term infants fed whole cow's or goat's milk; kwashiorkor; dependence on foods cooked for long periods; malabsorption due to sprue, celiac disease; drugs including phenytoin, sulfasalazine	Megaloblastic anemia; hypersegmented neutrophils; delayed maturation of CNS in infants; maternal deficiency in 1st trimester may cause neural tube defects	Serum erythrocyte folate, urinary excretion of FIGLU	0.5–1.0 mg/d of pteroylgutamic acid (PO)	None (except masking B_{12} deficiency)

Thiamine	Whole grains, pork, legumes	Alcoholism, hemodialysis, inborn errors of metabolism; breast-fed infant of deficient mother	Beri-beri: muscle tenderness, weakness; foot/wrist drop, sensory neuropathy; cardiomyopathy → congestive heart failure → edema. Wernicke-Korsakoff Syndrome: Confusion, ataxia, ophthalmoplegia, psychosis	Erythrocyte transketolase	0.3–1 mg/d (PO)	Very low
Riboflavin	Dairy products, eggs, liver, wheat germ	Diabetes, oral contraceptive use (subclinical), phototherapy for hyperbilirubinemia in newborns on IV nutrition	Cheilosis, angular stomatitis, seborrheic dermatitis, photophobia	Erythrocyte glutathione reductase	0.4–1.0 mg/d (PO)	Very low

(*continued*)

Table 4–7. Deficiency states and toxicity of vitamins and minerals (*continued*).

Nutrient	Examples of Good Food Sources	Deficient States				Toxicity
		Etiology	Clinical Features	Diagnosis	Treatment	
Niacin	Meats, poultry, fish, legumes; *precursor:* tryptophan (sources include milk, eggs); 60 mg tryptophan equivalent to 1 mg niacin	Chronic low intake; associated with predominantly corn-based diets	Pellagra: severe diarrhea, dermatitis (aggravated by sun exposure), dementia	Urine N_1-methylniacinamide (N_1-ME) and N_1-methyl-6-pyridone-3-carboxamide; random urine N_1-ME to creatinine $\leq$ 0.5 mg/1 g creatinine suggestive of deficiency	6 mg (PO)	Relatively nontoxic; doses at 2–6 g/d associated with peripheral vasodilation, increase uric acid, hepatotoxicity, glucose intolerance
Pyridoxine	Meat, fish, poultry; broccoli; whole grains	Drug interactions: isoniazid, penicillamine, oral contraceptives; historically, heat destruction in processing of infant formula; inborn errors of metabolism; infants fed goat's milk	Seborrheic dermatitis; peripheral neuropathy, seizures, hyperoxaluria, anemia	Erythrocyte glutamic pyruvic transaminase index > 1.25; urine xanthurenic acid after tryptophan load (2–5 g)	Ratio $\geq$ 0.02 mg B_6 per gram protein ingested	Sensory neuropathy in adults associated with 2–6 g/d doses

Biotin	Organ meats, egg yolks, legumes, nuts	Ingestion of raw egg whites (binding by avidin); prolonged antibiotic therapy; inborn errors of metabolism; hemodialysis	Seborrheic dermatitis; alopecia, glossitis, pallor	Plasma biotin and urinary excretion	20 mg/d IV	Very low
Cobalamin (B_{12})	Animal foods	Poor absorption from deficient intrinsic factor secretion, gastrectomy, Crohn's disease, ileal resection; strict vegetarians	Hypersegmented neutrophils, megaloblastic anemia, posterior and lateral column demyelinization in spinal cord, paresthesias, sensory deficits, loss of deep tendon reflexes, confusion, memory defects. *Note:* Neurologic changes may be irreversible	Serum B_{12} level, serum folate, erythrocyte folate, Schilling test	30–50 μg IM; 1 mg/d IV	Low

(*continued*)

Table 4–7. Deficiency states and toxicity of vitamins and minerals (*continued*).

Nutrient	Examples of Good Food Sources	Deficient States				Toxicity
		Etiology	Clinical Features	Diagnosis	Treatment	
Carnitine	Red meats, dairy products	Infants (especially premature) who are fed implemented soy formulas or fed IV, dialysis patients, inherited defects in carnitine synthesis, organic acidemics, valproic acid	Fatty liver hypoglycemia, progressive muscle weakness, cardiomyopathy	Serum carnitine	Oral or IV carnitine, oral doses = 50–300 mg/kg/d	None recognized
Iron	Animal meats, breast milk, iron-fortified formula, iron-fortified infant cereal, whole grains, legumes (absorption enhanced with concurrent ascorbate)	Dietary deficiency, blood loss, prematurity, generalized malnutrition	Microcytic anemia, impaired cognitive development, decreased exercise tolerance, anorexia, failure-to-thrive	Complete blood count, serum ferritin, serum iron/total iron binding capacity, erythrocyte protoporphyrin	3 mg iron/kg/d; avoid accidental overdose	Acute hemorrhagic gastroenteritis, shock; acidosis; coagulation defects; coma; hepatic failure and death
Iodine	Milk, green leafy vegetables	Geochemical deficiency	Goiter, hypothyroidism, cretinism (fetus), deafness (fetus)	Thyroid function tests and urine iodine	Iodized salt or water, iodized oil orally or intravenously (2–4 mL)	Thyrotoxicosis, goiter

Zinc	Animal meats, shellfish, legumes, whole grains	Dietary deficiency; generalized malnutrition, prematurity, intravenous nutrition, diarrhea, renal disease, chelation therapy, inborn metabolic diseases	Acro orifacial skin lesions, diarrhea, alopecia, growth retardation, anorexia, immune dysfunction, impaired wound healing, personality changes, impaired taste perception	Plasma zinc $< 60\ \mu g/dL$	1 mg Zn^{++}/kg body wt/d	*Chronic:* copper deficiency, depressed HDL cholesterol; *acute:* diarrhea, vomiting, irritability, headache and lethargy
Copper	Animal meats, shellfish, nuts, whole grain, legumes, some water supplies	General malnutrition, diarrhea, prematurity, intravenous nutrition, excess zinc intake, inborn metabolic disease, chelation therapy, cow's milk diet	Anemia (microcytic unresponsive to iron), neutropenia, osteoporosis, fractures, seborrheic skin lesions, failure-to-thrive, impaired CNS function, connective tissue defects	Plasma copper, plasma ceruloplasmin, red cell superoxide dismutase	Infants: 0.2–0.6 mg Cu/d as 1% solution of copper sulfate; children < 1–2 mg Cu/d	*Chronic:* ?Cirrhosis, ?recurrent diarrhea and vomiting, ?prooxidant mediated CNS damage; *acute:* gastrointestinal disfunction, hepatic central lobular necrosis, intravascular hemolysis, renal tubular damage, cardiotoxicity

(*continued*)

Table 4–7. Deficiency states and toxicity of vitamins and minerals (*continued*).

Nutrient	Examples of Good Food Sources	Deficient States				Toxicity
		Etiology	Clinical Features	Diagnosis	Treatment	
Selenium	Animal meats, fish, whole grain, cereals	Geochemical, intravenous nutrition, low-selenium synthetic diets, premature infants, generalized malnutrition	Cardiomyopathy, skeletal myopathy, macrocytosis and hair depigmentation	Plasma selenium, whole blood selenium, hair selenium, plasma glutathione peroxidase	0.1 mg sodium selenite/d	*Chronic:* loss of hair, rough finger nails, fatigue; *acute:* vomiting and diarrhea, paresthesias and irritability
Manganese	Whole grain cereals, legumes, nuts, tea	None confirmed				Extrapyramidal central nervous system dysfunction, ?cholestatic liver damage
Calcium	Dairy products, vegetables, canned salmon/sardines	Prematurity; milk-free diet; lactating adolescent; vitamin D deficiency; diuretics	Osteoporosis/rickets, increased blood pressure	Hypocalcemia (rarely due to calcium deficiency), dietary history most useful	Calcium supplement for the very low birth weight infant, adequate intake of dairy products and calcium supplement	Primarily iatrogenic, associated with excessive infusion, infiltration

Phosphorus	Meat, fish, poultry, eggs, cow's milk, cheese, whole grains, nuts, legumes	Protein energy malnutrition, prematurity (human milk), intravenous feeding, severe burns, acidosis, phosphate binding antacids; hypophosphatemia triggered by: glucose loading, insulin, nutritional rehabilitation	Respiratory insufficiency, decreased cardiac contractility, hematologic abnormalities, osteomalacia, bone pain, behavioral changes, peripheral neuropathy, muscle weakness, myalgia	Hypophosphatemia, elevated creatine phosphokinase	Phosphate salts, skimmed milk	Neonatal tetany; if due to renal failure: hyperparathyroidism, metabolic bone disease
Magnesium	Vegetables (chlorophyll), cereals, nuts	Protein energy malnutrition, renal magnesium wasting, impaired magnesium absorption	Muscle fasciculation/tremors, muscle weakness, cardiac arrhythmias (depressed S-T & T), personality changes, neurologic abnormalities, rickets (2° to impaired calcium metabolism)	Hypomagnesemia, decrease in muscle Mg	Magnesium salts	Lethargy, respiratory arrest

(continued)

Table 4–7. Deficiency states and toxicity of vitamins and minerals (*continued*).

Nutrient	Examples of Good Food Sources	Deficient States				Toxicity
		Etiology	Clinical Features	Diagnosis	Treatment	
Sodium	*High:* many processed foods including bread, cured meats, cheese, butter, margarine; *low:* fruits, vegetables, nuts (unsalted), grains, human milk	Diarrhea, excessive sweating, cystic fibrosis	Dehydration, anorexia, vomiting, mental apathy, muscle cramps, seizures	Serum sodium (may be misleadingly low in protein energy malnutrition and in hypermetabolic states)	Oral or parenteral saline	With insufficient water → hypernatremic dehydration; with adequate water → edema; hypertension: increase in intracellular sodium impairs cellular metabolism
Potassium	Unprocessed foods (meat, fish, potatoes, beans, bananas, apricots, prunes, raisins, whole grains)	Protein energy malnutrition, any catabolic state, acidosis, diarrhea, loop diuretics	Muscle weakness, mental confusion, cardiac arrhythmias, sudden death	Hypokalemia, muscle K	High intake of potassium salt (PO) if kidney functioning	Muscle weakness, mental apathy
Chloride	Closely linked to sodium	Chloride inadvertently low in infant formulas, cystic fibrosis, severe vomiting, diarrhea, loop diuretics, Bartter's syndrome	Hypochloremic, hypokalemic alkalosis, failure-to-thrive (including impaired head growth), anorexia, lethargy, muscle weakness, vomiting	Hypochloremia: urine chloride depends on the cause of chloride depletion	Sodium/potassium chloride	

hydrate (3.4 kcal/g). Dextrose concentrations greater than 12.5% (630 mosm/kg water) cannot be administered via peripheral vein. With a central catheter, start with D10 and advance by approximately 2.5% per day as tolerance (due to decreased endogenous glucose production) increases, up to 20% or higher, if needed. The rate of advance and final concentration will depend on flow rates.

Tolerance to IV dextrose is especially limited in premature infants and hypermetabolic ICU patients. Excess administration of dextrose will cause hyperglycemia, osmotic diuresis, fatty liver, and elevated $PaCO_2$. If unexpected hyperglycemia occurs, check for uneven flow rate, sepsis, stress, pancreatitis or errors in dextrose concentration. When the infusate is discontinued either temporarily or during cyclic IV feeding, taper glucose delivery over at least 2 hours to avoid hypoglycemia. A minimum of about 5% of total calories per week should be provided as an intravenous fat emulsion (2.7% calories as essential fatty acids) to avoid risk of essential fatty acid deficiency. The potential advantages of providing up to 40% of calories as lipid include the high energy density, low osmolality, low CO_2 production, and negligible energy cost of storage. Administration of fat emulsions beyond tolerance will impair leukocyte function, cause coagulation defects, decrease pulmonary oxygen diffusion, and compete with bilirubin and drugs for albumin binding sites. Commence fat emulsion with 1 g/kg/d and, as tolerated, advance by 0.5 g/kg/d up to a maximum of 3 g/kg/d.

Provide nitrogen (1 g N = 6.25 g protein) as an amino acid solution, usually 1–3% depending on flow rate and requirements (the same as for enteral feeding). Trophamine (McGaw) may currently be the best source of nitrogen for the premature infant because of added cysteine (40 mg/g trophamine). Optimal N (g):kcal ratios are usually 1:150–300. When energy intake is low, administration of nitrogen will improve, but not correct, negative nitrogen balance. When nitrogen intake is low, provision of energy (> 70 kcal/kg/d in an infant) will improve negative nitrogen balance.

One vial (5 mL) of MVI Pediatric (Armour) meets the vitamin guidelines for term infants. Administer 2 mL (40% of a single-dose vial) per kg to premature infants. Additional supplements of vitamins A (250 μg) and E (10 mg) may be beneficial.

Mineral and trace element recommendations are given in Figure 4–1.

Ordering

See sample order form in Figure 4–1. Orders should be reviewed daily.

PEDIATRIC PARENTERAL NUTRITION (PN) ORDER FORM

Imprint Patient Plate

Weight of patient ______________kg   Central line________   Peripheral line __________   ______________

Rate ____________________

	Standard Order	Modifications To Standard Order	*Adjustments for Neonates and Premature Infants (Circle these when required and cross out corresponding items* under "standard order")
Protein (as amino acid)* ____________	g%		*Use trophamine and cysteine for patients in level II and III nurseries who have a central line or are on a day 6 of peripheral therapy.
Dextrose ______________________	g%		
Na ____________________________	30 meq/L		
K _____________________________	25 meq/L		
Cl ____________________________	20 meq/L		
Acetate ________________________	45 meq/L		
Ca (as gluconate) (10 mM Ca/L) _____	20 meq/L		
Mg (as sulfate) __________________	3 meq/L		
P _____________________________	10 meq/L		
MVI Pediatric ____________________	*5.0 mL/d		*2 mL/kg/d for patients < 2.5 kg
Zinc __________________________	*1.0 mg/L		*Zn: 400 μg/kg/d < 2 kg body weight 250 μg/kg/d others < 3 mo old

Copper ______________________ 200 μg /L

Manganese __________________ 5.0 μg/L

Chromium ___________________ 2.0 μg/L

Selenium ____________________ 20.0 μg/L

Iodide _______________________ 10 μg /L

Heparin _____________________ 1000 Units/L

Cysteine (40 mg/g trophamine)* ______ mg/L *Use only with trophamine

Pharmacy will automatically account for electrolytes provided in amino acid preparation.

Changes in Na or K to be made as: Cl only___, or Acetate only___, Cl: Acetate 1:1__, or other

Cl: Acetate ratio (specify____________________).

Date:_____________ Signature:_________________________________M.D.

Figure 4–1. Pediatric parenteral nutrition (PN) order form. (Modified from the pediatric parenteral nutrition order form of the University of Colorado Health Sciences Center Department of Pharmacy.)

Monitoring

Maintain PN flow chart at bedside or in hospital chart.

1. Weight daily; height and head circumference weekly.
2. Urine glucose, specific gravity: dipstick once each shift while changing concentrations of dextrose.
3. Blood glucose: 4 hours after starting or changing infusion rate or changing glucose concentration; then every third day.
4. Serum Na-K-Cl-CO_2-BUN: daily for 2 days after starting or changing infusion rate or changing composition of infusate; then every third day.
5. Serum Ca-Mg-P: initially, then weekly, when flow rate and composition are stabilized.
6. Total protein, albumin, bilirubin, AST, GGT, alkaline phosphatase, CBC: initially bi-weekly. Zinc and copper: initially, then monthly for chronic TPN.
7. Serum triglycerides (monitor if IV fat emulsion is used): 1 day after starting or changing quantity of fat, then weekly. (Draw level just prior to starting daily infusion of fat emulsion.)

Note: These assays will need to be performed more frequently in some patients according to their clinical status and the results of previous assays.

Fluids & Electrolytes | 5

Carol A. Ledwith, MD

Children differ from adults in their fluid and electrolyte requirements. Children have: (1) a greater percentage of total body weight that is water; (2) a higher basal metabolic rate; and (3) a higher body surface area-to weight ratio. These features lead to greater water turnover per kilogram of body weight when compared with adults. Severe dehydration is a pediatric emergency. Fluid and electrolyte therapy for children may be understood in terms of four major components: (1) rapid volume expansion to treat shock and restore perfusion; (2) continuation of deficit replacement; (3) provision of maintenance requirements; and (4) replacement of ongoing losses.

MAINTENANCE REQUIREMENTS

Calculations of water requirements are based on caloric expenditure. One mL of water is required for every Kcal burned. Electrolyte needs are based on water requirements. Electrolyte losses occur primarily through the urine with smaller amounts lost through the skin and stool. During short-term intravenous hydration, the solution must provide enough glucose to prevent ketosis and minimize protein breakdown. Table 5–1 outlines the calculation of maintenance requirements based on body weight.

Special Considerations

Maintenance requirements differ according to the clinical situation. They may need to be adjusted upward for premature and low-birth-weight infants, fever, sweating, respiratory distress, skin disease, diabetes insipidus, high-output renal failure, burns, and phototherapy.

Requirements need to be adjusted downward for syndrome of inappropriate anti-diuretic hormone secretion (SIADH), increased intracranial pressure, congestive heart failure (CHF), and oliguric renal failure.

Table 5–1. 24-hour maintenance requirements.

Water	100 mL/kg for first 10 kg 50 mL/kg for next 10 kg 20 mL/kg for each kg above 20 kg
Sodium	3 meq/100 mL H_2O = 30 meq/L
Potassium	2 meq/100 mL H_2O = 20 meq/L
Glucose	5 g/100 mL H_2O = 5% dextrose solution

Example: A 23-kg patient requires:

$$[(10 \times 100) + (10 \times 50) + (3 \times 20)] \text{ mL/24 h} = 1560 \text{ mL/24 h}$$

Therefore, appropriate maintenance solution is D_5¼ NS[1] with 20 meq/L KCl at 65 mL/h

[1]NS (Normal Saline) = 154 meq/L Na^+, ½ NS = 77 meq/L, ¼ NS = 38 meq/L.

DEHYDRATION

General Considerations

Children are at high risk for dehydration. There are many reasons for this: (1) Children have an increased incidence of gastrointestinal (GI) disease, especially gastroenteritis; (2) GI symptoms occur with many nongastrointestinal diseases; (3) children suffer relatively greater GI losses than do adults; (4) infants cannot respond to thirst independently. *All* sick children, not merely those with gastroenteritis, should be assessed for their hydration status.

History

A detailed history must be taken to determine the child's fluid intake and the exact type of fluid that he or she has been drinking. History should include frequency and amount of vomiting, diarrhea, and urine output. If a previous recent weight is known it can be extremely useful in calculating the degree of dehydration. Weight loss with an acute illness represents water loss and is the most accurate measure of the water deficit. (1 mL H_2O = 1 g). Degree and duration of fever, underlying medical conditions, and medications given must also be noted.

Clinical Assessment

Table 5–2 shows the patterns in physical findings and laboratory values with increasing levels of dehydration. In general, the most reliable signs and symptoms of dehydration in children are prolonged

Table 5–2. Estimating the severity of dehydration.[1]

Physical Signs	Mild	Moderate	Severe
Weight loss			
Infant	5%	10%	15%
Older child	3%	6%	9%
Vital signs			
Pulse	± ↑	↑	↑ ↑
Blood pressure	normal	normal	normal or ↓
Eyes	± tearing	↓ tearing ± sunken	↓ tearing sunken
Mucous membranes	± tacky	tacky/dry	parched
Skin			
Turgor	± ↓	↓	↓ ↓
Perfusion	normal	± mottled	poor/mottled
Capillary refill[2]	2–3 s	3–4 s	> 4 s
Laboratory findings			
Urine output	↓	↓ ↓	↓ ↓ ↓
Urine specific gravity	↑	↑	↑
BUN	normal	± ↑	↑
CO_2	↓	↓ ↓	↓ ↓ ↓

[1] Adapted from Barkin RM (editor): *Emergency Pediatrics,* Mosby, 1986, p 44.
[2] Normal capillary refill is < 2 seconds. Not accurate with hypoxia or a cold extremity.

capillary refill time, decreased urine output, altered mental status/decreased level of consciousness, and tachycardia. Low or falling blood pressure is a late sign of shock in the pediatric population. Children respond to hypovolemic dehydration primarily with tachycardia and are able to maintain their blood pressure even in the face of severe hypovolemia. Shock is defined by inadequate tissue perfusion and not by hypotension. Do *not* be reassured by a normal blood pressure.

Types of Dehydration

The type of dehydration is defined by the serum sodium (Na^+) concentration. **Isotonic dehydration** is defined as a loss of total body water combined with maintenance of a serum sodium of 130–150 meq/L. Isotonic dehydration is the most common form. See Tables 5–3 and 5–4 for management. **Hypertonic (hypernatremic) dehydration** is characterized by a serum sodium of > 150 meq/L in the presence of a total body water deficit. **Hypotonic (hyponatremic) dehydration** is defined as a loss of water and sodium with a serum sodium < 130 meq/L. Consult the algorithms in Tables 5–5 and 5–6

Table 5–3. Acute hypovolemic dehydration: principles of initial management.

Volume expansion for **ALL** types of dehydration
Always give bolus with isotonic fluid
(NS, LR [Lactated Ringer's]) 20 mL/kg

↓

Bedside rapid glucose check
Give bolus with glucose as indicated
D_{10}2–4 mL/kg if < 3 months
D_{25}2 mL/kg if > 3 months

↓

Obtain serum electrolytes,[1] urea nitrogen, glucose

↓

Continue to treat with isotonic fluid in 20 mL/kg boluses until perfusion is restored and patient is hemodynamically stable

↓

Calculate and begin deficit replacement (Table 5–4) when adequate tissue perfusion has been demonstrated (improved capillary refill, urine output, decrease in tachycardia, and improved mental status)

↓

If after 40 mL/kg of isotonic fluid perfusion has not been restored, consider other causes such as hemorrhagic shock, septic shock, cardiogenic shock

[1] Electrolytes = sodium (Na^+), potassium (K^+), chloride (CL^-), bicarbonate (HCO_3^-).

for management guidelines. Additional causes of hypo- and hypernatremia are listed in Table 5–7.

SPECIFIC ELECTROLYTE DISTURBANCES

1. HYPERKALEMIA

Clinical Findings

Causes of hyperkalemia include renal failure, hemolysis, rhabdomyolysis, adrenal insufficiency, tumor cell lysis during induction chemotherapy, tissue destruction seen with burns and crush injuries, and excess administrations (usually IV). *Always* document serum potassium (K^+) with a nonhemolyzed specimen.

Clinical effects of hyperkalemia include listlessness, confusion, paresthesias, peripheral vascular collapse, bradycardia, and asystole.

Table 5–4. Isotonic dehydration: management guidelines.

Procedure	Example
Calculate fluid deficit based on weight loss, if known, or based on estimated percent dehydration.	Known 10 kg previous (hydrated) weight. Now weighs 9 kg = 1 kg (1000 mL) deficit. **or** Current weight 9 kg with estimated 10% dehydration; therefore, current weight is 90% of hydrated weight 9 kg = 90% × (hydrated weight). 9/.9 = 10kg = hydrated weight. 10kg – 9kg = 1kg (1000 mL) deficit.
↓	↓
Subtract bolus fluids from total deficit	If 200 mL bolus fluids given; remaining deficit is 800 mL
↓	↓
Replace ½ of total deficit over the first 8 h, and ½ of total deficit over the next 16 h	400/8 = 50 mL/h × 8 h then 400/16 = 25 mL/h × 16 h
↓	↓
Add in maintenance fluid requirements (based on hydrated weight)	1000 mL/24h = 40 mL/h maintenance therefore; 40 + 50 = 90 mL/h × 8 h, then 40 + 25 = 65 mL/h × 16 h
↓	↓
For isotonic dehydration, appropriate electrolyte solution is same as maintenance solution.	[2]D_5¼ NS with 20 meq/L KCl.
↓	↓
Replace ongoing losses; diarrhea; nasogastric, duodenal or jejunal secretions; vomiting; urine (such as with diabetic patient).	For most accurate assessment when output is high, send fluid of concern for electrolyte concentrations and order additional solutions accordingly. Output may be calculated every 8 h and replaced mL per mL.

[1] Treat shock as in Table 5–3 with isotonic solution.

[2] K acetate rather than KCl may be used in acidotic patients. Do not add K^+ until serum potassium is documented or patient has produced urine.

Table 5–5. Hypotonic dehydration.

Seizures secondary to hyponatremia (Usually not seen with serum $Na^+ \geq 120$ meq/L)	No seizures — go directly to deficit replacement
↓	

Administer 3% NaCl intravenously over 1 h
(3% NaCl = 0.5 meq NaCl/mL)
Correct with this formula (desired Na^+ = 120 meq/L):
(Desired Na^+ – measured Na) × 0.6 × weight (kg) = meq NaCl required
General rule: 6 mL/kg of 3% NaCl raises Na^+ by 5 meq/L

Deficit Replacement

Procedure	Example
Calculate fluid deficit as in isotonic dehydration	For the 10 kg (hydrated weight) infant with 10% dehydration = 1000 mL deficit
↓	↓
Calculate Na^+ deficit with desired Na^+ 135 meq/L	For Na^+ = 115 meq/L (135 – 115) × 0.6 × 10kg = 120 meq Na^+ deficit
↓	↓
Replace ½ of total water and Na^+ deficit over the first 8 h, and ½ over the next 16 h. Add in maintenance fluid and Na^+ requirements	Water / Na Deficit 1000 mL / 120 meq Maintenance 1000 mL/24 h / 30 meq/24 h 1st 8 h: 500 mL deficit 320 mL maintenance (water) 60 meq deficit + 10 meq maintenance (Na^+) Total = 70 meq Na^+ in 820 mL water or D_5½ NS at 100 mL/h for 8 h. Then D_5½ NS at 70 mL/h for next 16 h (500 + 680 mL H_2O; 80 meq Na^+)

Table 5–5. Hypotonic dehydration (*continued*).

Note:

- If 3% NaCl given, subtract this from total Na^+ deficit
- Remember to subtract bolus fluids from total fluid deficit
- Replace ongoing losses as in isotonic dehydration
- Add potassium as indicated
- Follow Na carefully: Na^+ should correct over 24 h. Rate of rise should not exceed 2 meq/L/h
- Too rapid correction may lead to central pontine myelinolysis.

[1] Treat shock as in Table 5–3 with isotonic solution.
[2] 0.6 = volume of distribution for Na^+.

Table 5–6. Hypertonic dehydration.

Procedure	Example
Calculate fluid deficit as in isotonic dehydration	For the 10 kg infant with 10% dehydration = 1000 mL deficit
↓	↓
Replace this deficit evenly over 48 h Add maintenance fluids	1000 mL deficit + 2000 mL maintenance (48 h) = 3000 mL at 60 mL/h. Use D_5¼ NS as higher Na^+ concentration will not allow serum Na^+ to decrease (½ NS may be considered; ¾ NS and NS are **not** appropriate solutions)
↓	↓
If serum Na^+ is not correcting, may need to replace free water portion of deficit as D_5W. Formula to calculate free water deficit: 4 mL/kg free water for each meq of Na^+ that serum Na^+ exceeds 145.	If serum Na^+ = 160: (160 − 145) × 4 mL/kg × 10 kg = 600 mL (free water deficit) Replace with D_5W over 48 h at 12 mL/h. Give maintenance and remainder of total fluid deficit as D_5¼ NS.

Note:

- Goal is to lower serum Na^+ slowly (0.5 meq/L/h); follow every 2 h
- Too rapid correction may cause cerebral edema and refractory seizures
- Remember to subtract bolus fluids from total fluid deficit
- Replace ongoing losses as in isotonic dehydration
- Add potassium as indicated

[1] Treat shock as in Table 5–3 with isotonic solution.

Table 5–7. Hyponatremia and hypernatremia: classification and etiologies.

Hyponatremia
↓ total body sodium > ↓ total body water
(as in hypovolemic dehydration)
Commonly seen in infants and children with gastroenteritis who are rehydrated with water, weak tea, or other no sodium or low sodium fluids.

↑ total body sodium < ↑ total body water
(conditions associated with edema)
Congestive heart failure, renal failure, hepatic failure

normal total body sodium with ↑ total body water
SIADH, water intoxication

↓ total body sodium with normal or ↓ total body water
Seen in patients with excessive sodium losses such as in cystic fibrosis, adrenal insufficiency.

Factitious
Hyperglycemia, mannitol, hyperlipidemia

Hypernatremia
↑ total body sodium
Seen most commonly secondary to excessive sodium administration, such as through inadequately diluted powdered or concentrated formula

↓ total body water
Diabetes insipidus

↓ total body sodium < ↓ total body water
Osmotic diuretics
Gastroenteritis and dehydration with excessive sodium in oral rehydration solution

The most important clinical effects of hyperkalemia are cardiac. Electrocardiographic changes include peaked T waves, widened QRS complex, increased P-R interval, heart block, and ventricular tachycardia or fibrillation. Symptoms will often not manifest until the potassium rises above 7 meq/L. (Normal potassium ranges are higher for premature and newborn infants.) Consult the algorithm in Table 5–8 for management guidelines.

2. HYPOKALEMIA

Clinical Findings

Causes of hypokalemia include: vomiting, diarrhea, nasogastric suction, inadequate intake, diuretics, correction of metabolic acidosis,

Table 5–8. Treatment of hyperkalemia.

Serum potassium > 6 meq/L but < 7 meq/L

↓

Repeat serum potassium

↓

Continuously monitor ECG

↓

Withhold all potassium

↓

Kayexalate exchange resin 1 g/kg po or pr

↓

If serum potassium is > 7 meq/L or cardiovascular instability is present: follow algorithm as above; then proceed.

↓

Furosemide 1 mg/kg IV

↓

Calcium gluconate (10% solution) 0.5 mL/kg IV over 3 min (maximum 10 mL) (0.5 mL/kg = 50 mg/kg of 10% solution). Best emergency treatment for dysrhythmias

↓

Sodium bicarbonate 1–2 meq/kg IV. This transiently moves potassium intracellularly.

↓

Glucose 0.5 g/kg/h and insulin 1 U regular for each 3 g glucose

↓

Dialysis is indicated for refractory symptomatic hyperkalemia

↓

Treat the underlying condition

Table 5–9. Treatment of hypokalemia.

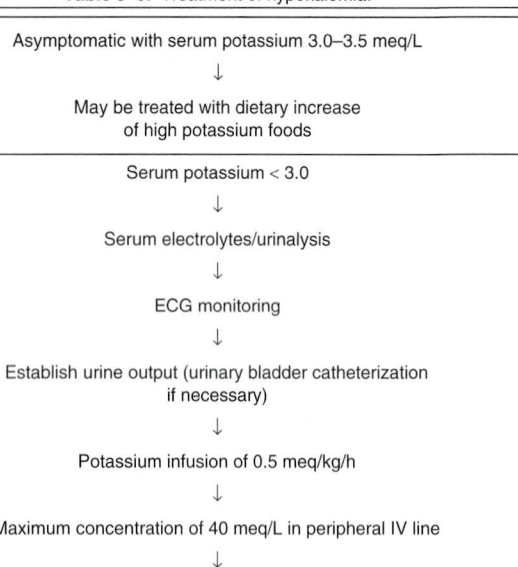

Asymptomatic with serum potassium 3.0–3.5 meq/L ↓ May be treated with dietary increase of high potassium foods
Serum potassium < 3.0 ↓ Serum electrolytes/urinalysis ↓ ECG monitoring ↓ Establish urine output (urinary bladder catheterization if necessary) ↓ Potassium infusion of 0.5 meq/kg/h ↓ Maximum concentration of 40 meq/L in peripheral IV line ↓ Recheck serum potassium after 1 meq/kg infused (2 h) ↓ Always treat the underlying cause

and renal tubular acidosis. The clinical effects include weakness, hypotonia, decreased deep tendon reflexes, and ileus. With more severe hypokalemia (serum potassium < 2.5) respiratory depression and cardiac effects may be seen. Electrocardiographic changes consistent with hypokalemia include flattened T waves, the presence of U waves, S-T segment depression, and AV block. AV block may be exacerbated if the patient is taking digitalis.

Consult the algorithm in Table 5–9 for treatment guidelines.

3. ACID-BASE DISTURBANCES

The normal pH range is 7.38–7.42. pH changes 0.15 units for every 10 meq/L change in serum bicarbonate HCO_3^- and 0.08 units for every 10 torr change in PCO_2.

Table 5–10. Causes of metabolic acidosis.

Normal anion gap	
	GI losses: diarrhea, enterostomies, fistulas
	Renal tubular acidosis
	Hyperalimentation
Increased anion gap	
	Lactic acidosis
	Diabetic ketoacidosis
	Inborn errors of metabolism
	Uremia
	Ingestions (ethanol, methanol, ethylene glycol, salicylates, paraldehyde)

Metabolic Acidosis

One of the main consequences of dehydration is acidosis. Acidosis results from inadequate tissue perfusion, decreased O_2 delivery, lactic acid and keto-acid production, increase in hydrogen ion secondary to decreased renal perfusion, or direct bicarbonate losses (eg, in diarrheal stools).

Calculation of the anion gap can help determine the cause of acidosis (Table 5–10).

$$\textbf{Anion gap} = \textbf{Na} - (\textbf{CL} + \textbf{HCO}_3^-).$$

A normal anion gap is 8–16 meq/L. An increased anion gap suggests accumulation of organic acids.

Treatment of acidosis involves identification of the underlying cause. Bicarbonate therapy is rarely indicated, although it may be considered when a metabolic acidosis with pH less than 7.0 is documented, and if adequate ventilation is established. The vast majority of lactic acidoses associated with dehydration will resolve with rehydration. The dose of bicarbonate is calculated as follows:

$$\textbf{bicarbonate dose} = \textbf{weight (kg)} \times \textbf{base deficit} \times \textbf{0.6}$$

The **base deficit** is easily obtained from the following formula:

$$\textbf{base deficit} = \textbf{desired HCO}_3^- - \textbf{the measured HCO}_3^-$$

Half the calculated dose can be given immediately with the remainder given over the next 1–2 hours.

Monitor patients carefully for hypokalemia when intravenous bicarbonate is administered.

Respiratory Acidosis

Respiratory acidosis occurs as a result of hypoventilation due to pulmonary disease or central respiratory depression. Treatment is adequate ventilation. Bicarbonate therapy is *not* indicated and will exacerbate the acidosis.

Metabolic Alkalosis

This condition results from loss of hydrogen ion (vomiting), excess intake of bicarbonate, or as compensation for excess renal loss of chloride (Cl^-) from diuretics. The underlying cause must be treated.

Respiratory Alkalosis

The presence of a respiratory alkalosis suggests hyperventilation or salicylate intoxication. Treatment involves identification of the underlying cause.

ORAL REHYDRATION THERAPY

Oral rehydration should be considered for pediatric patients with mild to moderate (3–10%) dehydration. Vomiting is *not* a contraindication to oral rehydration. Most children with a history of vomiting will succeed with oral rehydration.

Success with oral rehydration requires explicit instructions to caretakers and a committed and patient staff.

Maintenance solutions (45–50 mmol/L Na^+) [Lytren (Mead Johnson), Pedialyte (Ross), Resol (Wyeth), Ricelyte (Mead Johnson)] or rehydration solutions (75–90 mmol/L Na^+) [Rehydralyte (Ross), WHO-ORS] may be used in the initial oral rehydration phase. Glucose-based (20–25 g of glucose per liter) or rice-based oral rehydration solutions are available.

Five to 15 mL aliquots should be administered by spoon or syringe every 10–20 minutes. Volumes may be gradually increased and the interval between feeds decreased as tolerated by the patient.

Contraindications to oral rehydration include hemodynamic instability, serum $Na^+ < 120$ meq/L or > 160 meq/L, clinical suspicion of acute surgical abdomen, or concurrent conditions such as altered mental status or severe respiratory distress.

Failure of oral rehydration (persistent vomiting, inability to keep up with ongoing losses) indicates the need for intravenous hydration.

Immunization Procedures, Vaccines, Antisera, & Skin Tests | 6

John W. Ogle, MD

Active immunity to infectious diseases occurs following inoculation of bacterial, viral, and parasitic antigens, either in a live attenuated form, as inactivated whole organisms, or as portions or products of organisms. New vaccines are being developed and tested and are introduced periodically. In addition, vaccine composition, recommended schedules, and contraindications continue to change. Readers are advised to consult the recommendations of the Advisory Committee for Immunization Practices (ACIP) and the *Report of the Committee on Infectious Diseases* of the American Academy of Pediatrics (the *Red Book*) to supplement the information given in this chapter.

Passive immunity, administered in the form of intravenous gamma globulin (IVIG) or as one of several specific immune globulins or animal serum, provides temporary protection against infection or disease. Only a limited number of infectious agents are susceptible to passive antibody. In general, it is preferable to use a vaccine for a disease (if available) to provide active immunity than to provide passive protection.

PROCEDURES FOR ACTIVE IMMUNIZATION

General Principles

A. Sources of Information: *Always* consult authoritative sources before using any of the vaccines, sera, or immune globulins. Among these sources are (1) The CDC's *Morbidity and Mortality Weekly Report* (MMWR), (2) the American Academy of Pediatrics' periodic updates of the *Report of the Committee on Infectious Diseases* (the *Red Book*), (3) the manufacturer's package insert that accompanies each biologic product, and (4) the CDC's *Health Information for International Travel.* The package inserts are reasonably complete, but the recommendations may contain conflicting information (usually occasioned by legal considerations), in which case it is best to follow the advice of the CDC or the American Academy of Pediatrics.

B. Informed Consent: Providers are required to provide detailed information to parents on the risks and benefits of immunization. Providers may use brochures developed by the CDC, which are available through local health departments, or may develop and use their own materials provided they conform to the requirements of the law. Signed informed consent must be obtained prior to immunization.

C. Storage & Administration of Vaccines: Scrupulous attention should be paid to proper handling and storage of vaccines and other biologic products. The work area used for vaccine storage and preparation of injections should be separate from areas used for collection or storage of potentially contaminated patient samples, such as cultures and blood samples. Consult the package insert for specifications for each product, as instructions vary for different types of products and manufacturers.

Aseptic technique should be used in removing vaccine from a vial, preparing the injection site, and administering the vaccine. Intramuscular injections are best given to children in either the lateral thigh or, in older children, the deltoid muscle. Administration in the gluteal region can cause injury to the sciatic nerve, and therefore should be avoided. The tissue at the injection site should be compressed and the needle should be inserted in the upper lateral quadrant of the thigh with the syringe directed inferiorly at a 45-degree angle to the long axis of the leg and posteriorly at a 45-degree angle to a line parallel to the table top. Before injecting the vaccine, the syringe plunger should be pulled back; if blood appears, the needle should be withdrawn, new vaccine drawn up into a new syringe, and injected into a different site. To decrease the likelihood of local reactions to vaccines, a needle long enough to enter the muscle—2.5 cm or 1 inch—is recommended for intramuscular injections in children of all ages. When injecting an irritating material, the injection site should be rotated at subsequent inoculations and the injection site noted in the chart. Two vaccines should never be injected into the same site, and separate vaccines should never be mixed in one syringe.

D. Monitoring & Reporting Adverse Reactions: Parents should be informed of any possible adverse reactions and given specific instructions for reporting such reactions. Severe reactions require a physical assessment of the child and appropriate therapeutic intervention. The parents should be given an immunization record, which should be updated each time a vaccine is given. The National Childhood Vaccine Injury Act, which went into effect on March 21, 1988, requires health care providers to record certain information and events. The health care provider who administers the vaccine should enter into the permanent medical record the following information: date of vaccine administration; vaccine manufacturer and lot number; and the name, address, and title of the person administering the vaccine. Certain reportable adverse events after vaccination are listed in Table 6–1. Adverse events due to vaccines must be reported to the Vaccine Adverse Events Reporting System (VAERS). Forms may be requested by calling (800) 822–7967. Adverse events that must be reported are found in Table 6–1.

The National Childhood Vaccine Injury Act of 1988 provides compensation to families for certain illnesses temporally related to immunization. Compensable events are listed in Table 6–1. A panel of special masters is appointed to hear evidence and decide on compensation adjudicate claims. Compensation forms are available by calling (800) 338–2382. Claims for compensation through the National Vaccine Injury Compensation Program must be filed within 3 years of the first symptom or within 2 years after death.

E. General Precautions & Contraindications: The physician should be aware of the recommended precautions and contraindications for each vaccine. The following are general guidelines: (1) Avoid giving live vaccines to women during pregnancy. (2) Do not administer a live vaccine to any person suspected or proved to be immunodeficient (eg, a patient with a known or suspected congenital defect, a patient with an acquired immunodeficiency disease, or a patient receiving immunosuppressive therapy or corticosteroids). (3) Vaccines are generally given only to healthy children; however, minor illness, whether there is fever or not, is not a contraindication to live viral vaccine administration. DTP should not be given to children who have a febrile illness because the symptoms may be attributed to the vaccine. However, if a child has a nonfebrile upper respiratory tract infection, DTP vaccine can be administered as scheduled, to prevent multiple visits or a delay in completing the immunization schedule.

Table 6–1. Reportable events following immunizations.[1]

Vaccine/ Toxoid[2]	Adverse Event	Interval from Vaccination to Onset of Event	
		For Reporting[3]	For Compensation[4]
DTP, P, DTP/poliovirus combined	A. Anaphylaxis or anaphylactic shock	24 h	24 h
	B. Encephalopathy (or encephalitis)[5]	7 d	3 d
	C. Shock-collapse or hypotonic-hyporesponsive collapse[6]	7 d	3 d
	D. Residual seizure disorder[7]	(See footnote[7])	3 d
	E. Any acute complication or sequela (including death) of above events	No limit	Not applicable
	F. Events described as contraindications to additional doses of vaccine (see manufacturer's package insert[8])	(See package insert[8])	
Measles, mumps, and rubella; DT, Td, T	A. Anaphylaxis or anaphylactic shock	24 h	24 h
	B. Encephalopathy (or encephalitis)[5]	15 d for measles, mumps, and rubella vaccine; 7 d for DT, Td, and T	15 d for measles, mumps, and rubella vaccine; 3 d for DT, Td, and T
	C. Residual seizure disorder[7]	(See footnote[7])	15 d for measles, mumps, or rubella vaccine; 3 d for DT, Td, and T
	D. Any acute complication or sequela (including death) of above events	No limit	
	E. Events described as contraindica-	(See package insert[8])	

	tions to additional doses of vaccine (see manufacturer's package insert[8])		
OPV	A. Paralytic poliomyelitis		
	• in a nonimmunodeficient recipient	30 d	30 d
	• in an immunodeficient recipient	6 mo	6 mo
	• in a vaccine-associated community case	No limit	Not applicable
	B. Any acute complication or sequela (including death) of above events	No limit	Not applicable
	C. Events described as contraindications to additional doses of vaccine (see manufacturer's package insert[8])	(See package insert[8])	
Inactivated polio vaccine	A. Anaphylaxis or anaphylactic shock	24 h	24 h
	B. Any acute complication or sequela (including death) of above events	No limit	Not applicable
	C. Events described as contraindications to additional doses of vaccine (see manufacturer's package insert[8])	(See package insert[8])	

[1] As of December 1993. Used with permission, 1994 Red Book: Report of the Committee on Infectious Diseases, 23rd ed., American Academy of Pediatrics, Elk Grove, IL, p. 32–33.

[2] The vaccine/toxoid abbreviations, in alphabetical order, are: DT = diphtheria and tetanus toxoids; DPT = diphtheria and tetanus toxoids and pertussis vaccine (pediatric); OPV = oral poliovirus vaccine, live, trivalent; P = pertussis vaccine; T = tetanus toxoid; and Td = tetanus and diphtheria toxoids (for adult use).

(continued)

Table 6–1. Reportable events following immunizations (*continued*).[1]

[3] Adverse events that are required by *National Childhood Vaccine Injury Act of 1986* (NCVIA) to be reported to Vaccine Adverse Events Reporting System (VAERS) if their onset is within the indicated interval after vaccination.

[4] Adverse events that may be compensable under NCVIA if the onset is within this interval after vaccination.

[5] Encephalopathy means any significant acquired abnormality of, injury to, or impairment of function of, the brain. Among the frequent manifestations of encephalopathy are focal and diffuse neurologic signs, increased intracranial pressure, or changes lasting at least 6 h in level of consciousness, with or without convulsions. The neurologic signs and symptoms of encephalopathy may be temporary with complete recovery or may result in various degrees of permanent impairment. Signs and symptoms such as high-pitched and unusual screaming, persistent inconsolable crying, and bulging fontanelle are compatible with an encephalopathy, but in and of themselves are not conclusive evidence of encephalopathy. Encephalopathy can usually be documented by slow-wave activity on an electroencephalogram.

[6] Shock-collapse or hypotonic-hyporesponsive collapse may include signs and symptoms such as decrease or loss of muscle tone, paralysis (partial or complete), hemiplegia, hemiparesis, loss of color or turning pale white or blue, unresponsiveness to environmental stimuli, depression of or loss of consciousness, prolonged sleeping with difficulty being aroused, or cardiovascular or respiratory arrest.

[7] Residual seizure disorder may have occurred if no other seizure or convulsion unaccompanied by fever or accompanied by a fever of < 102 °F occurred before the first seizure or convulsion after the administration of the vaccine involved, and if, in the case of measles-, mumps-, or rubella-containing vaccines, the first seizure or convulsion occurred within 15 d after vaccination, or, in the case of any other vaccine, the first seizure or convulsion occurred within 3 d after vaccination, and, if 2 or more seizures or convulsions unaccompanied by fever or accompanied by a fever of < 102 °F occurred within 1 yr after vaccination. The terms “seizure” and “convulsion” include grand mal, petit mal, absence, myoclonic, tonic-clonic, and focal motor seizures and signs.

[8] Refer to the CONTRAINDICATION section of the manufacturer’s package insert for each vaccine/toxoid.

PRIMARY IMMUNIZATION OF CHILDREN IN THE FIRST YEAR OF LIFE

The recommended schedule of immunizations is listed in Table 6–1. Adequate protection against diphtheria, pertussis, tetanus, *Haemophilus influenzae* type b, hepatitis B, and poliomyelitis should be initiated early in infancy and carried through with the recommended "booster" doses of vaccine. A combination product containing measles, mumps, and rubella vaccines (MMR) is administered at 12–15 months of age, with a second dose recommended for school-aged children. A single dose of varicella vaccine given at 12–18 months is recommended by the American Academy of Pediatrics. By the time of school entry, the healthy child should have received all vaccines in the primary series and thereafter need only be given booster doses of the adult preparation of diphtheria-tetanus toxoid (Td) at 10-year intervals. Pertussis vaccine should not be given after 7 years of age, and no additional doses of poliovirus vaccine are required.

The following guidelines pertain to variations from the schedule shown in Figure 6–1.

(1) If a child misses any of the DTP doses, ignore the interval and proceed with completion of the schedule.
(2) If pertussis vaccine is contraindicated in a child under 7 years of age, the pediatric preparation of diphtheria-tetanus toxoid (DT) should be substituted for DTP.

IMMUNIZATION OF CHILDREN NOT IMMUNIZED IN INFANCY

The schedule for immunization of persons not immunized in infancy is shown in Table 6–2. The following guidelines should be observed:

(1) Pediatric DT is used only for children 7 years of age. Adult Td is used for primary immunization of older children and adults (Table 6–2).
(2) Live oral poliovirus vaccine (OPV) should not be given to persons over 18 years of age. Inactivated (killed, Salk) poliovirus vaccine (IVP) should be used instead. Follow the manufacturer's instructions for dosage and booster intervals.
(3) MMR can be administered to persons older than 15 months.

Recommended Ages for Administration of Currently Licensed Childhood Vaccines–August 1995

Vaccines are listed under the routinely recommended ages. Solid bars indicate range of acceptable ages for vaccination. Shaded bars indicate new recommendations or vaccines licensed since publication of the Recommended Childhood Immunization Schedule in January 1995. Hepatitis B vaccine is recommended at 11–12 years of age for children not previously vaccinated. Varicella zoster virus vaccine is recommended at 11–12 years of age for children not previously vaccinated, and who lack a reliable history of chickenpox.

Age ► Vaccine ▼	Birth	2 mo	4 mo	6 mo	12[1] mo	15 mo	18 mo	4–6 yr	11–12 yr	14–16 yr
Hepatitis B [2,3]	Hep B–1	Hep B–1								
		Hep B–2	Hep B–2	Hep B–3	Hep B–3	Hep B–3	Hep B–3		Hep B[3]	
Diphtheria, tetanus, pertussis[4]		DTP	DTP	DTP	DTP[1,4]	DTaP at 15+ m	DTaP at 15+ m	DTP or DtaP	Td	Td
H influenzae type b[5]		Hib	Hib	Hib[5]	Hib[1,5]	Hib[1,5]				
Polio		OPV	OPV	OPV	OPV	OPV	OPV	OPV		
Measles, mumps, rubella[6]					MMR[1,6]	MMR[1,6]		MMR or	[6]MMR	
Varicella zoster[7]					VZV[7]	VZV[7]	VZV[7]		VZV[7]	

[1]Vaccines recommended in the second year of life (12–15 months of age) may be given at either one or two visits.

[2]Infants born to HBsAg-negative mothers should receive 2.5 μg of Merck Sharp and Dohme (MSD) vaccine (Recombivax HB) or 10 μg of SmithKline Beecham (SKB) vaccine (Engerix-B). The second dose should be given between 1 and 4 months of age, if at least one month has elapsed since receipt of the first dose. The third dose is recommended between 6 and 18 months of age.
Infants born to HBsAg-positive mothers should receive immunoprophylaxis for hepatitis B with 0.5 mL hepatitis B immune globulin

(HBIG) within 12 hours of birth, and either 5 μg of MSD vaccine (Recombivax HB) or 10μg of SKB vaccine (Engerix-B) at a separate site. In these infants, the second dose of vaccine is recommended at 1 month of age and the third dose at 6 months of age. All pregnant women should be screened for HBsAg in an early prenatal visit.

[3]Hepatitis B vaccine is recommended for adolescents who have not previously received three doses of vaccine. The three-dose series should be initiated or completed at the 11 to 12 year old visit for persons not previously fully vaccinated. The second dose should be administered at least 1 month after the first dose, and the third dose should be administered at least 4 months after the first dose.

[4]The fourth dose of DTP may be administered as early as 12 months of age, provided at least 6 months have elapsed since DTP3. Combined DTP-Hib products may be used when these two vaccines are to be administered simultaneously. DTaP (diphtheria and tetanus toxoids and acellular pertussis vaccine) is licensed for use for the fourth and/or fifth dose of DTP vaccine in children 15 months of age or older and may be preferred for these doses in children in this age group. Td (tetanus and diphtheria toxoids, absorbed, for adult use) is recommended at 11–12 years of age if at least 5 years have elapsed since the last dose of DTP, DTP-Hib, or DT.

[5]Three *H influenzae* type b conjugate vaccines are available for use in infants: HbOC(HibTITER) (Lederle Praxis); PRP -T(ActHIB; Omni-HIB) (Pasteur Mérieux, distributed by SmithKline Beecham; Connaught); and PRP-OMP (Pedvax HIB) (Merck Sharp & Dohme). Children who have received PRP-OMP at 2 and 4 months of age do not require a dose at 6 months of age. After the primary infant Hib conjugate vaccine series is completed, any licensed Hib conjugate vaccine may be used as a booster dose at 12–15 months.

[6]The second dose of MMR vaccine should be administered *EITHER* at 4–6 years of age *OR* at 11–12 years of age, consistent with state school immunization requirements.

[7]Varicella zoster virus vaccine (VZV) is routinely recommended at 12–18 months of age. Children who have not been vaccinated previously and who lack a reliable history of chickenpox should be vaccinated by 13 years of age. VZV can be administered to susceptible children any time after 12 months of age. Children under 13 years of age should receive a single 0.5 mL dose; persons 13 years of age and older should receive two 0.5 doses 4–8 weeks apart.

Figure 6–1. Recommended childhood immunization schedule, United States, January–June 1996.

Table 6–2. Recommended immunization schedule for normal children not immunized in the first year of life.[1]

Recommended Time/Age	Immunizations[4]	Comments
		YOUNGER THAN 7 YEARS
First visit	DTP, OPV, MMR	MMR if child ≥ 15 months old; tuberculin testing may be done at same time.
	HbCV[3]	For children aged 15–59 months, can be given simultaneously with DTP and other vaccines (at separate sites).[4]
Interval after first visit		
2 months	DTP, OPV (HbCV)[5]	Second and third dose of HbCV is indicated only in children whose first dose was received when younger than 15 months.
4 months	DTP (HbCV)	Third dose of OPV is not indicated in the USA but is desirable in other geographic areas where polio is endemic.
10–16 months	DTP, (DTaP)[6] OPV	OPV is not necessary if third dose was given earlier.
4–6 years (at or before school entry)	DTP (DTaP),[6] OPV (MMR)[5]	DTP is not necessary if the fourth dose was given after the fourth birthday; OPV is not necessary if the third dose was given after the fourth birthday.
11–12 years	MMR	At entry to middle school or junior high.
10 years later	Td	Repeat every 10 years throughout life.

7 YEARS AND OLDER[7,6]

First visit	Td, OPV, MMR[9]	
Interval after first visit		
2 months	Td, OPV	
8–14 months	Td, OPV	
11–12 years	MMR	Repeat every 10 years throughout life.
10 years later	Td	At entry to middle school or junior high.

[1] Reproduced with permission from: Immunization. In: *Current Pediatric Diagnosis and Treatment,* 12th ed, Norwalk, CT: Appleton & Lange; 1995, p. 235.

[2] Abbreviations are explained in Table 6–1.

[3] See *Haemophilus influenzae* vaccination section.

[4] The initial 3 doses of DTP can be given at 1- to 2-month intervals; hence, for the child in whom immunization is initiated at age 15 months or older, one visit could be eliminated by giving DTP, OPV, and MMR and HBV at the first visit; DTP and HbCV at the second visit (1 month later); and DTP, HBV, and OPV at the third visit (2 months after the first visit). Subsequent doses of DTP and OPV 10–16 months after the first visit are still indicated. HbCV, MMR, DTP, and HBV can be given simultaneously at separate sites if failure of the patient to return for future immunizations is a concern.

[5] Please see section on hepatitis B vaccine for discussion of recommendations by the AAP and ACIP.

[6] DTaP is recommended only if 3 prior doses of DTP have been administered.

[7] The ACIP recommends MMR at this time.

[8] If person is $\geq$ 18 years old, routine poliovirus vaccination is not indicated in the USA.

[9] Minimal interval between doses of MMR is 1 month.

(4) *Haemophilus influenzae* b conjugate vaccine should be given to all children between the ages of 2 months and 5 years. Only those children at high risk (eg, splenectomized children, or children with sickle cell disease or immunodeficiency) should receive the vaccine after the fifth birthday if they have never received it before.

IMMUNIZATIONS FOR ALL CHILDREN

Diphtheria

Immunization against diphtheria is effected by administration of toxoid to stimulate antitoxin production. Levels of antitoxin are related to immunity against disease.

A. Diphtheria-Tetanus-Pertussis (DTP): This vaccine is used routinely in infants and children. It combines diphtheria and tetanus toxoids with a suspension of killed *Bordetella pertussis* organisms. Three doses of 0.5 mL each are given intramuscularly at 2-month intervals; the first dose is usually given when the infant is 2 months of age (Figure 6–1). Booster doses may be given 6–12 months after the third DTP dose. The fifth dose of DTP is given between 4 and 6 years of age. Thereafter, the pertussis component of the vaccine is not used. DTP and live virus vaccines may be given at the same time. If pertussis is prevalent in the community, immunization may be started as early as 2 weeks of age and doses may be given 4 weeks apart. Reduced or split doses of vaccine may not be efficacious and are not recommended. Premature infants should be appropriately immunized according to the schedule given in Table 6–2. Altered dosages or schedules should not be used, with the exception that administration of OPV should be delayed, in hospitalized newborns, until hospital discharge.

B. Diphtheria-Tetanus-Acellular Pertussis (DTaP): Acellular pertussis vaccine combined with diphtheria and tetanus toxoids may be substituted for DTP at the fourth and fifth doses only. Acellular vaccines contain some or all of the following antigens: pertussis toxin, filamentous hemagglutinins, agglutinogens, and pertactin. Several different acellular vaccines were developed and used in Japan with estimated vaccine efficacy of 90%. Recent trials conducted abroad suggest these vaccines offer variable, but significant, protection against severe pertussis.

DTaP is licensed only as the fourth or fifth dose for children previously immunized with 3 doses of DTP. DTaP is administered intramuscularly in a dose of 0.5 mL.

C. Diphtheria-Tetanus (DT) (Pediatric): This preparation contains full amounts of diphtheria and tetanus toxoids and is used in children for whom pertussis vaccine is contraindicated. Three doses of 0.5 mL each are given intramuscularly at 4–8 week intervals, with a booster injection 6–12 months later. DT toxoid should not be given to anyone older than 7 years.

D. Diphtheria-Tetanus (Td) (Adult): This preparation contains less diphtheria toxoid than does the DT preparation and should be used for booster doses in older children and adults. The dose is 0.5 mL intramuscularly, given at the intervals shown in Table 6–2.

E. Diphtheria (D): This toxoid is used only when combined preparations are contraindicated.

Pertussis

Immunization with suspensions of phase I *Bordetella pertussis* prepared as vaccine can effectively reduce the risk of clinical pertussis. Infants are immunized with DTP; children over 7 years of age do not receive the pertussis component. Common adverse effects of pertussis vaccine include redness, pain or swelling at vaccination site, fever, drowsiness, fretfulness, anorexia, and vomiting. These reactions occur shortly after the vaccine and subside within 24–48 hours; however, the tendency of these reactions to occur increases with subsequent doses of the vaccine. Children who experience these reactions should receive additional doses of the vaccine as scheduled; the administration of acetaminophen (15 mg/kg per dose) given at the time of vaccination and every 4 hours for three doses may decrease side effects to the pertussis vaccine.

More serious adverse reactions, including encephalopathy, have been reported after pertussis vaccine, but experts disagree whether the vaccine causes the reactions. None of the reported reactions are unique to pertussis vaccine, as all the reactions also occur in young children who have not received pertussis vaccine. Nonetheless, future administration of pertussis vaccine is contraindicated in children who have any of the following reactions: encephalopathy within 7 days; convulsion, with or without fever, within 3 days; persistent inconsolable screaming or crying for 3 or more hours within 48 hours; collapse or shock-like state within 48 hours; unexplained temperature of 40.5° C (104.9° F) or higher within 48 hours; and an immediate severe or anaphylactic allergic reaction.

Children with a progressive neurologic disorder who have a developmental delay or neurologic findings should have pertussis immunization delayed. The evolution of neurologic signs and symptoms caused by the underlying disorder may be blamed on the pertussis component. These conditions include infantile spasms, tuberous sclerosis, and metabolic and neurodegenerative diseases. The decision to defer pertussis immunization should be reassessed at each visit based on the neurologic status of the child and the risk of contracting pertussis in the community. Infants and children with well-controlled seizures may be vaccinated with pertussis, however, the risk of a seizure post-immunization is increased compared to children without a history of seizures. The clinician must weigh the likelihood of seizures compared to the risk of pertussis. The risk of contracting pertussis is increased in children who may travel to areas where pertussis is endemic and in children in day-care centers, special clinics, or residential care institutions. A family history of seizures, sudden infant death syndrome, or severe reaction to pertussis vaccine by a family member is not a contraindication to pertussis immunization. All families should be informed of the risks and benefits of pertussis vaccine and given advice about appropriate medical care in the event of a seizure or other adverse reactions.

Fever, local reactions, and minor systemic reactions occur in 10–33% of children following DPT vaccination. In comparison, these adverse reactions are significantly reduced following acellular pertussis vaccine. Hyperpyrexia (temperature $> 40.5°$ C), febrile seizures, persistent inconsolable crying, and hypotonic-hyporesponsive events occur uncommonly following DPT and are expected to be even more uncommon following acellular pertussis, however, data on the frequency of these events are unavailable. Severe neurologic events such as encephalopathy and prolonged seizures are rare following DTP, and no data are available on the incidence of temporal association with DTaP.

Tetanus

Tetanus toxoid is an excellent immunizing agent. Every child should receive adsorbed tetanus toxoid during infancy, usually administered in the form of DTP vaccine (see under Diphtheria, above, and Figure 6–1). Older children and adults receive Td or booster injections of purified tetanus toxoid (T) every 10 years unless wound management dictates otherwise. More frequent boosters may be accompanied by local hypersensitivity reactions.

Poliomyelitis

Live, trivalent oral poliovirus vaccine (OPV) provides effective immunity and is the choice for immunization of infants in most countries. Inactivated poliovirus vaccines (IPV) are used increasingly because of the rare cases of poliomyelitis associated with OPV.

A. Live Polio Vaccine: Attenuated strains of virus types I, II, and III are grown in cell culture. Standardized suspensions of virus are stored frozen until they are administered orally. OPV is commonly administered at 6–8 weeks and at 4 months of age. Additional doses are given at 6–18 months and at 4–6 years of age. This schedule usually ensures development of antibodies and immunity to all three types of viruses. An additional dose may be given later in life under special circumstances (eg, travel to endemic regions, an outbreak of poliomyelitis).

OPV is contraindicated in children with immunodeficiency diseases, including HIV infection. Children who have household contacts with immunodeficiency diseases, or who are immunosuppressed because of pharmacologic or radiation therapy should receive IPV because of the risk of paralytic disease following OPV. Vaccine-associated paralysis in vaccines or contacts have been reported to occur at a rate of one in 6.9 million. Parents and vaccinees should be informed of this rare adverse reaction.

B. Inactivated Polio Vaccine: Enhanced-potency inactivated polio vaccine (IPV-E) has a higher antigen content than previous IPV vaccine, and contains antigens of all three polio virus strains. IPV-E is administered in a dose of 0.5 mL subcutaneously. IPV-E is given in two doses 4–8 weeks apart with a final dose 6–12 months later. An additional dose is given at 4–6 years. The necessity for 5-year booster doses, which were recommended for IPV, has not been established for IPV-E. IPV-E is the polio vaccine of choice for patients with HIV infection or other immunodeficiencies, transplant recipients, and partially immunized adults. Family members and other close contacts of patients with impaired immunity should also receive IPV-E.

Measles

Live attenuated measles virus vaccine is grown in cell culture and given subcutaneously in combination as MMR (measles, mumps, rubella). MMR may be inactivated by heat and light, so the vaccine must be kept at 35.6–46.5° C or colder and must be protected from light.

The number of reported cases of measles in the United States decreased from 500,000 per year to a nadir of 1497 in 1983. An increase to 18,000 cases occurred in 1989, and over 27,000 cases occurred in 1990. Measles cases occur most frequently in unvaccinated preschool-aged children and previously vaccinated school-aged children. Both children in junior high school and college students have been infected during measles outbreaks in schools.

The increase in measles cases in school-aged children prompted the ACIP and American Academy of Pediatrics (AAP) to recommend a two-dose schedule for administration of MMR vaccine. The new two-dose schedule attempts to protect the estimated 5% of children who do not respond to the initial dose of MMR.

The first dose of MMR is usually given at 12–15 months of age but can be given at any age thereafter. The ACIP recommends a second dose of MMR upon entrance to kindergarten (4–6 years of age). This recommendation was made to fit into the pre-existing immunization schedule for children. In contrast, the AAP recommends the second dose of MMR at the time of entry to middle or junior high school (11–12 years of age).

State or local health departments may require the second dose of MMR at school entry. Practitioners should be familiar with current local requirements.

Colleges, technical schools, and post-high school educational programs should require students who were born after 1957 to provide documentation of two doses of measles-containing vaccine, documentation of physician-diagnosed measles disease, or laboratory evidence of measles immunity. Students who lack documentation of measles immunity should receive one dose of MMR at the time of school entry and a second dose of MMR no less than 1 month after the first dose. Similar recommendations apply to medical personnel.

During local measles outbreaks or in areas with recurrent measles transmission among preschool-aged children (a county with five cases of measles among preschool children during each of the previous 5 years, a county with a recent outbreak among unvaccinated preschool-aged children, and cities with large unvaccinated populations), monovalent measles vaccine may be recommended as early as 6 months of age or the first visit thereafter. Children vaccinated with MMR before 12 months of age should have a repeat vaccination at 12–15 months of age and a third dose at the time of entry to junior high or middle school.

During school outbreaks of measles, all children and their siblings born after January 1, 1957, who have not received 2 doses of measles-containing vaccine after 12 months of age should be revaccinated.

The "further attenuated" measles virus vaccine (Moraten strain) is the only vaccine currently available in the United States. In 5% of children, the live MMR vaccine may produce a transient rash 6–14 days after vaccination. Five to 15% of children develop a fever of 39.4° C (103° F) or higher beginning 6–14 days postvaccination and lasting 1–2 days. Children with febrile seizures may be given antipyretic prophylaxis realizing that the treatment should begin before the expected onset of fever and continued for 1 week. Postvaccine encephalitis has been reported in 1 per 3 million doses of MMR.

Contraindications to measles vaccine include pregnancy, immunodeficiency, immunosuppression, recent administration of immune globulin, and known anaphylactic reaction to materials in the vaccine (eg, eggs, neomycin).

Although immunodeficiency is a contraindication to the administration of live virus vaccines, children with pediatric HIV infection should receive MMR. Measles is a severe disease with frequent mortality in children with HIV infection. The risk of adverse reactions to MMR in children with symptomatic HIV is small, and must be weighed against the likelihood of acquiring severe measles infection.

Mumps

Mumps is usually benign, but can be accompanied by aseptic meningitis, pancreatitis, orchitis, or oophoritis. Live vaccine confers immunity.

Live attenuated mumps vaccine is a chick embryo-adapted virus that is usually given together as MMR. Mumps vaccine is dispensed as a freeze-dried powder that must be reconstituted before subcutaneous administration. (Follow manufacturer's directions for reconstitution.)

Contraindications to mumps vaccine are listed in the manufacturer's package insert and include immunodeficiency, hypersensitivity to eggs, and all contraindications to measles vaccine (listed above).

Rubella

Rubella is a benign disease in children, but infection in pregnant women and the resulting fetal infection can have catastrophic consequences. Maternal antibodies can fully protect the fetus. Live attenuated rubella vaccine (strain RA 27/3, grown in diploid cells) is recommended for all infants, usually in combination with live measles and mumps vaccines. The contraindications are the same as for measles and mumps vaccines.

Rubella vaccine may be given to prepubertal girls and to nonpregnant, susceptible women (eg, those with negative serologic test results). Such persons should be advised not to become pregnant for at least 3 months after receiving this vaccine. The vaccine strain occasionally has been isolated from placental tissues of women inadvertently vaccinated during pregnancy, but no fetal abnormalities have been definitely associated with such an occurrence. Inadvertent administration of rubella vaccine to more than 250 pregnant women has not resulted in congenital rubella syndrome. Efforts should be made to ensure that other groups, such as college students, military recruits, and postpubertal males and females, are immunized. Prenatal and antepartum screening for rubella is recommended and the vaccine should be administered to susceptible women in the immediate postpartum period prior to discharge. Protection of day care workers, school employees, and health care workers, both male and female, should be ensured either with a history of immunization or actual disease.

Adverse reactions, which may occur 5–12 days after immunization, include fever, rash, and lymphadenopathy in a small number of children. Postpubertal females may have pain in small peripheral joints 7–21 days postvaccination, but arthritis is uncommon.

Haemophilus influenzae Type b Conjugate Vaccine

Sepsis, epiglottitis, and meningitis are examples of severe infections caused by *Haemophilus influenzae* type b (HIB) in young infants. The initial vaccine directed against HIB, the PRP vaccine, was poorly immunogenic, particularly in infants less than 2 years of age. Conjugate vaccines composed of capsular polysaccharide linked to protein molecules are far more immunogenic and have been successfully used to immunize infants beginning at 2 months of age. Widespread use of conjugate vaccines has reduced the incidence of invasive HIB infections significantly. In most communities, HIB is now an uncommon pathogen.

Four different conjugate vaccines are available. PRP-D (manufactured by Connaught Laboratories) is composed of capsular polysaccharide covalently linked to diphtheria toxoid. This vaccine is indicated only for infants older than 15 months. This vaccine conferred limited protection in a study in Alaskan native infants and therefore is not licensed for infants younger than 12 months.

HBOC vaccine (manufactured by Lederle-Praxis) is composed of capsular polysaccharide directly linked to a mutant diphtheria toxoid (CRM-197). This vaccine was shown 100% protective (95% confidence interval, 68–100%) in a large study in Northern California where infants were vaccinated at 2, 4, and 6 months of age.

PRP-OMP vaccine (manufactured by Merck, Sharpe, and Dohme) is composed of capsular polysaccharide linked with a spacer molecule to an outer membrane protein of *Neisseria meningitidis*. PRP-OMP was shown effective in a large study conducted in Navajo children. Children immunized at 2 and 4 months were protected for disease with an estimated efficacy of 93% (95% confidence interval, 45–99%).

PRP-T vaccine (manufactured by Pasteur Merieux Vaccins) consists of capsular polysaccharide linked to tetanus toxoid. This vaccine is highly immunogenic in young infants.

HBOC and PRP-OMP were approved for administration on different schedules. HBOC and PRP-T are administered at 2, 4, and 6 months, with a booster dose at 15–18 months. PRP-OMP is administered at 2 and 4 months, with a third dose at 12 months. It is preferable to complete the schedule of immunization with the vaccine initially used. HBOC, PRP-OMP, PRP-T, and PRP-D are considered to be equally safe and efficacious when used in children older than 15 months.

All infants should receive immunization against HIB using HBOC, PRP-T, or PRP-OMP beginning at 2 months. The schedule for immunization is complex and is summarized in Figure 6–1 and Table 6–3. Unimmunized children older than 5 years who are at risk for invasive disease due to sickle cell anemia or asplenia should be immunized with a single dose of any of the 3 conjugate vaccines.

Table 6–3. Schedule for hib conjugate vaccine administration.[2]

Vaccine	Age at First Vaccination (months)	Primary Series	Booster
HbOC/PRP-T[1]	2–6	3 doses 2 months apart	12–15 months
	7–11	2 doses 2 months apart	12–18 months
	12–14	1 dose	2 months later
	15–59	1 dose	
PRP-OMP	2–6	2 doses 2 months apart	12–15 months
	7–11	2 doses 2 months apart	12–18 months
	12–14	1 dose	2 months later
	15–59	1 dose	
PRP-D	15–59	1 dose	

[1] DPT-HbOC may be administered by the same schedule for primary immunization as HbOC/PRP-T (when the series begins at 2–6 months of age). A booster dose of DTP or DTaP should be administered at 4–6 years of age, before kindergarten or elementary school. This booster is not necessary if the fourth vaccinating dose was administered after the fourth birthday.

[2] Used with permission from: Immunization, In: *Current Pediatric Diagnosis and Treatment*, 12th ed., Appleton & Lange, 1995, p. 245.

The dose and route for all four conjugate vaccines is 0.5 mL intramuscularly. Adverse effects are uncommon with these vaccines, consisting of fever, local reactions, or mild systemic reactions in fewer than 5% of vaccinees.

Hepatitis B Vaccine

Universal immunization against hepatitis B is now recommended for all infants. Although hepatitis B vaccination has been available since 1982, the policy of selective immunization of high risk populations has not appreciably diminished morbidity and mortality due to hepatitis B. Patients at high risk for hepatitis B often do not seek immunization. Furthermore, 40% or more of patients with hepatitis B infection lack identifiable risk factors. Universal immunization in childhood is recommended rather than immunization at an older age because of the success of childhood immunization programs, and the decreased cost of immunization during infancy. Although universal immunization is recommended, this program is both controversial and expensive, due to the high price of vaccine. Antibody levels correlate with protection against hepatitis B. Antibody is known to persist for 5–8 years following immunization in the majority of patients, and protection may be more long-lived. The longevity of protection from immunization in infancy is not known, but currently, booster doses are not recommended.

Two recombinant vaccines are currently available. Plasma derived HBsAg vaccine is no longer available. Recombivax HB (Merck, Sharpe and Dohme) containing 10 μg/mL and Engerix-B (SmithKline) containing 20 μg/mL are available for routine use, although the dosage and schedule vary with the age of the patient (Table 6–4).

All women should be tested for hepatitis B during pregnancy. Infants born to chronically infected women should receive hepatitis B immune globulin (HBIG) 0.5 mL intramuscularly and hepatitis B vaccine at a different site as soon as practical within 12 hours following birth. Infants born to HBsAg negative women should be immunized at 0–2 days, 1–2 months, and 6–18 months.

Adolescents at high risk of hepatitis B infection due to sexual activity or intravenous drug abuse should also receive immunization. Many other patient populations should be offered vaccination: hemodialysis patients, individuals likely to be exposed occupationally to blood, and caregivers of chronically infected patients. Postexposure prophylaxis following percutaneous or mucosal exposure to an HBsAg individual is also recommended.

The rate of adverse events following immunization is very low and usually limited to minor local reactions and fever (less than 5%).

Table 6–4. Recommended schedule for immunization with hepatitis B vaccine.

	Dose of Vaccine	
	Recombivax (mL)	Engerix-B[1] (mL)
Infants[2]		
Mother HBsAg-negative[3]	0.25	0.50
Mother HBsAg-positive[4]	0.50	0.50
Children[5] < 11 years	0.25	0.50
Children[5] 11–19 years	0.50	1.00
Adults[5] > 20 years	1.00	1.00
Immunosuppressed and dialysis	1.00	2.00

[1] Engerix-B also licensed on schedule of 0, 1, 2, and 12 months.
[2] All pregnant women should be screened. Infants born to HBsAg-positive women should receive 0.5 mL HBIG at birth or within 12 hours. The schedule for immunization consists of 3 doses at 0–2 days, 1–2 months, and 6–18 months.
[3] An alternative schedule (2, 4, and 6–18 months) for infants born to HBsAg-negative mothers is acceptable but not preferred. The preferred schedule is 0–2 days, 1 month, 6 months.
[4] Infants born to HBsAg-positive women should be tested at 9 months for HBsAg and anti-HBs. An additional dose of vaccine should be administered to infants who are HBsAg-negative to infants who are HBsAg-negative and anti-HBs < 10 IU.
[5] Older children not vaccinated at birth and adults are immunized at 0, 1, and 6 months.

Varicella-Zoster

Varicella zoster vaccine is a live, attenuated virus newly licensed March 17, 1995. The vaccine was developed in Japan and has been used extensively since the 1970s. The vaccine is stored lyophilized, frozen to −15° C or colder, and is stable for up to 18 months. After reconstitution, the vaccine should be used within 30 minutes. The recommended dose is 0.5 mL subcutaneously.

The American Academy of Pediatrics recommends universal immunization of children at 12–18 months of age. Children aged 18 months through 13 years should also receive one dose of vaccine if they lack a history of varicella and were not previously immunized. Children older than 13 years should also be immunized, but require two doses separated by 4–8 weeks.

Varicella vaccine is very immunogenic, as greater than 95% of recipients seroconvert after one dose. The vaccine is highly protective against severe clinical varicella. Breakthrough varicella characterized by mild rash with less than 50 lesions and little or no fever occurs in

10–15% of vaccinees. A mild vaccine-associated rash with a median of 2–5 lesions occurs in 5–10% of vaccinees. Fever is no more common in vaccinees than unvaccinated controls.

Universal immunization is controversial because of the expense of the vaccine, and because additional injections are required. Nonetheless, cost-benefit analyses demonstrate that a significant reduction in costs to families, as well as reduced morbidity, will follow widespread immunization. Currently, there is no evidence that immunity wanes after immunization. The incidence of varicella-zoster reactivation (shingles) is reduced after immunization compared to natural disease in immunocompromised children. Varicella vaccine is not currently licensed for immunocompromised patients, although data suggest children with acute lymphocytic leukemia will benefit.

IMMUNIZATION FOR CHILDREN WITH SPECIAL INDICATIONS

Cholera

For children traveling to or residing in areas where cholera is endemic (or for travel to countries that require a certificate of cholera vaccination), suspensions of killed *Vibrio cholerae* vaccine give only partial protection from disease and must be repeated at 6-month intervals. The vaccine is not recommended in the control of cholera outbreaks nor for infants less than 6 months of age. The vaccination is used primarily to satisfy the requirements of several countries for vaccination prior to travel. Newer subunit or recombinant live vaccines appear safer and more efficacious in several trials and will probably replace currently available killed vaccines. Careful attention to sanitation, including disinfection or boiling of water and thorough cooking of food, prevents transmission of cholera. Antimicrobial prophylaxis with tetracycline, trimethropim-sulfamethoxazole, erythromycin, or furazolidone will prevent infection if given within 24 hours following exposure.

Hepatitis A vaccine (Havrix) was licensed in 1995 for children or adults traveling to or living in areas with increased risk of hepatitis A. The vaccine is an inactivated virus manufactured in pediatric (age 2–18 years) and adult (age older than 18 years) formulations. Children receive 0.5 mL IM with additional doses 1 month and 6–12 months later. Adults receive 1.0 mL intramuscularly of the adult preparation with a second dose 6–12 months later.

The vaccine is highly immunogenic and estimated to be greater than 94% protective. Patients traveling or living in undeveloped countries with poor or questionable sanitation should be immunized. Children younger than 2 years should receive immune serum globulin (see Immune Globulins below).

Influenza

Epidemic influenza A or B may cause serious respiratory disease in infants or children with cardiac, pulmonary, metabolic, renal, or neurologic disease, including those with immunodeficiency and immunosuppression. Institutionalized children or those in child-care centers are at special risk. For these individuals, influenza vaccines may reduce the risk of serious illness or complications. Routine immunization is recommended *only* for children at increased risk–not for normal healthy infants and children.

The subtypes of influenza A and B to be incorporated into vaccines are selected every year, and are based on the strains expected to circulate during the next season. Viruses are grown in embryonated chicken eggs, purified, chemically inactivated, and made into "split" virus products. To avoid severe febrile reactions, *only* the split virus form of vaccine should be given to children less than 12 years old. Two doses, given 4 or more weeks apart, are required for initial immunization of children 8 years and younger. For children previously vaccinated, one dose is indicated every year. Each year, the Center for Disease Control issues recommendations for influenza vaccine usage in children. Anaphylaxis to eggs is a contraindication to immunization.

Meningococcal Meningitis

Polysaccharide vaccine-containing antigens from meningococcus groups A, C, Y, and W-135 are available. The type A polysaccharide is immunogenic in children 3 months of age and older, but the other types are poorly immunogenic in infants less than 2 years of age. Meningococcal vaccine is indicated (1) during meningococcal outbreaks, (2) if an individual plans to visit or reside in a country with endemic meningococcal disease, (3) for children with asplenia, and (4) for individuals with increased susceptibility to disease owing to absence of the terminal components of the complement cascade. The dose is 0.5 mL subcutaneously. The vaccine is well tolerated.

Plague

Killed *Yersinia pestis* vaccine may be used in children traveling in or residing in areas where plague is highly endemic, but is not recommended for routine use in plague enzootic areas of the country. The vaccine should be given in doses recommended by the manufacturer. Control of exposure to vectors and use of chemoprophylaxis for exposed individuals are necessary.

Pneumococcal Vaccine

A mixture of capsular polysaccharides from 23 types of pneumococci, including those that account for about 80% of bacteremic infections, is available. This preparation is not recommended for routine immunization. It should be considered for use in children at high risk of death from pneumococcal infection and in children over 2 years of age who suffer from sickle cell disease, asplenia, nephrosis, immunodeficiency, cerebrospinal fluid leakage, and HIV infection. Vaccination of children with recurrent otitis media is controversial, but the vaccine may be beneficial. The vaccine is well tolerated in children, but some children 2 years of age or older fail to develop adequate antibody responses. Children in high-risk groups should receive penicillin prophylaxis against life-threatening pneumococcal infections. The dose is 0.5 mL given intramuscularly or subcutaneously, and the vaccine is generally given only once. Routine revaccination is not indicated. However, some centers revaccinate children with sickle cell anemia, nephrotic syndrome, renal failure, transplant recipients, and asplenia 3–5 years after initial vaccination because of their very high risk of pneumococcal infection.

Rabies

Rabies develops following bites by rabid animals. It is almost always fatal. Because the disease is so feared, many persons receive rabies treatment after contact with an animal even when the chance may be very small that the animal was rabid.

The risk of rabies is dependent on the species of animal, the nature of the bite or exposure, and the geographic locale. Local health authorities are usually very knowledgeable regarding the risk of rabies and should be consulted prior to beginning vaccination.

Two vaccines are licensed for use in the United States. Rabies vaccine, or adsorbed (RVA), was developed and is available from Smith Kline Beecham, Philadelphia, PA. The vaccine is a cell culture-derived vaccine that is used for either preexposure or postexposure use.

Human diploid cell rabies vaccine (HDCV) is supplied in lyophilized form for either preexposure or postexposure use. Preexposure immunization requires three 1 mL doses of vaccine given intramuscularly on days 0, 7, and 21 or 28. Intradermal administration of HDCV only (RVA cannot be used) can be recommended as an alternative to intramuscular immunization. 0.1 mL of HDCV is given intradermally on days 0, 7, and 21 or 28. Postexposure vaccination in previously unimmunized individuals consists of five 1-mL intramuscular doses on days 0, 3, 7, 14, and 28. The vaccine should not be given in the buttock; the deltoid muscle is the preferred site in adults, and the anterolateral thigh should be used in children. For postexposure vaccination, 20 IU/kg of rabies immune globulin (RIG) is recommended. One half the dose is infiltrated around the wound and the remainder is given intramuscularly at a site separate from the vaccine. Persons with previous vaccination need only 1 mL of RVA given intramuscularly on days 0 and 3. Adverse reactions to RVA are similar to those to HDCV and include pain, redness, and swelling at injection site in 85–90% of vaccinees, and fever, nausea, and arthralgia in 10%. Approximately 6% of persons vaccinated with HDCV developed a serum sickness-like allergic reaction.

Tuberculosis

Bacille Calmette-Guérin (BCG) is an attenuated strain of *Mycobacterium bovis*; different substrains of the organism are produced as vaccine in different countries. These substrains exhibit marked differences in invasiveness and immunogenicity. Studies of the effectiveness of BCG vary significantly, and therefore, use of BCG is controversial. Administration of BCG is limited to individuals who have a negative tuberculin skin test and who are at very high risk of infection because of intimate and prolonged contact with persons untreated or ineffectively treated for pulmonary tuberculosis, or exposure to persons with isoniazid- or rifampin-resistant tuberculosis and who cannot be removed from the source of exposure. BCG is also recommended for infants and children who live in areas where the rate of new infections exceeds 1% per year and where usual treatment programs have failed. The manufacturer's recommendations must be followed. BCG is not recommended for health care workers. These workers should be monitored by periodic tuberculin skin testing and isoniazid therapy for skin test-positive workers. Use of BCG varies widely in different countries, depending on socioeconomic conditions and available measures for medical and public health control of active tuberculosis. Any form of immune deficiency is an absolute contraindication to the administration of BCG because of the possibility of disseminated and fatal BCG infection. The tuberculin skin test in a child injected with BCG will yield positive results, at least temporarily. The PPD should be repeated 2–3 months after immunization; immunization should be repeated if the child remains PPD negative. Immunization with BCG should not supplant isoniazid prophylaxis, which is of proved efficacy. The dose of vaccine is 0.05 mL intradermally in neonates and 0.1 mL in older individuals.

Typhoid

Immunization against *Salmonella typhi* infection is possible, but currently available vaccines are of moderate efficacy. Immunization is indicated for travelers to endemic areas, individuals with close contact to typhoid carriers such as household contacts, and laboratory workers with frequent contact with *S typhi.*

An inactivated vaccine has been available for many years and is associated with a high rate of systemic and local reactions. The dose is 0.25 mL subcutaneously for children < 10 years, and 0.5 mL subcutaneously in older children and adults. The vaccine is given twice, separated by at least 4 weeks.

An oral, live attenuated vaccine derived from *S. typhi*, Ty21a, is available for adults and children 6 years and older. The dose of oral vaccine is one capsule per day every other day for a total of four capsules. Vomiting and diarrhea are infrequent reactions following oral immunization.

Booster doses are given every 3 years when parenteral vaccine is used. The manufacturer recommends revaccination after oral vaccine in 5 years.

Yellow Fever

For children 9 months of age or older living in or visiting areas where yellow fever is endemic, a single injection of live attenuated vaccine (consisting of the 17D strain of yellow fever virus) is indicated. Infants younger than 4 months are at higher risk of encephalitis that is temporally associated with yellow fever vaccine, and should not be immunized. The vaccine is administered only by certain public health officials and may be repeated 6–8 years later. Yellow fever and cholera vaccines should be administered at least 3 weeks apart if both are required because of poor immune response to both when simultaneously administered. A valid certificate for yellow fever vaccination is required for travel to some countries.

Japanese Encephalitis

Japanese encephalitis vaccine is an inactivated virus grown in mouse brains. Travelers to rural areas of Asia endemic for the virus who plan stays of 30 days or greater should consider immunization. Information on endemic and epidemic areas and current recommendations are available from the CDC (303–221–6400). The vaccine is given as three 1.0 mL doses on days 0, 7, and 30. In children 1 to 3 years, 0.5 mL doses are given. Children younger than 1 year should not be immunized.

MATERIALS USED FOR PASSIVE IMMUNIZATION

IMMUNE GLOBULINS

Standard immune globulin (IG) is prepared from pooled plasma and contains sufficient antibodies against measles, hepatitis, and other pathogens to be used as follows:

(1) For **measles prophylaxis** in unimmunized individuals exposed to the disease, give 0.25 mL/kg IM as a single dose; the maximum dose is 15 mL. For immunocompromised susceptible individuals, the dose is 0.5 mL/kg. Prophylaxis should be given within 6 days of exposure.

(2) For **hepatitis A prophylaxis** in individuals exposed to hepatitis A virus, give 0.02 mL/kg intramuscularly. Susceptible individuals include family contacts of the index case and day care workers and children in the same classroom as the index case. If the day care setting involves children who are not yet toilet trained and HAV infection is identified in an employee or child, or if household contacts of 2 children in a day care setting contract HAV, all employees and enrolled children should receive IG. If the exposure is continuous, such as occurs in endemic areas of the world, 0.06 mL should be given and may be repeated in 5 months.

Recent studies have shown that intravenous immunoglobulin (IVIG) is more effective than intramuscular immune globulin. Several preparations of IVIG are now available for use in a number of conditions, yet its use in other conditions remains controversial. There is good evidence that IVIG is efficacious in the following conditions: primary hypogammaglobulinemia, selected cases of idiopathic thrombocytopenic purpura, Kawasaki disease, bone marrow and renal transplant recipients at risk for cytomegalovirus infections, and patients with lymphocytic leukemia.

Several special immune globulins are available: tetanus (TIG), rabies (RIG), varicella-zoster (VZIG), and hepatitis B (HBIG). Consult the product brochure, and follow the advice of the CDC and the Infectious Diseases Committee of the American Academy of Pediatrics for their use in specific situations.

SKIN TEST

Tuberculin Skin Test (Mantoux Test)

The Mantoux Test (0.1 mL of intermediate strength purified protein derivative containing 5 TU and inoculated intradermally) is read at 48–72 hours. False-negative reactions are seen in malnourished and immunocompromised patients, and in those with overwhelming disease. Temporary suppression is associated with viral infections (measles, mumps, influenza, varicella) after live virus immunization, and when corticosteroid or other immunosuppressive agents are given. A control antigen that is expected to yield a positive result in children with normal immunity should be given (tetanus, *Candida antigens*, or DT).

Tine tests consist of old tuberculin (OT) or PPD on multiple puncture metal tines. Tine tests are not recommended for screening high risk populations or patients with suspected tuberculosis due to frequent false-negative results. Positive tine tests need to be confirmed by Mantoux tests. As such, tine testing should not be used.

Mantoux testing is recommended in persons with suspected tuberculosis. Family members and other close contacts should also be tested. High-risk populations should be screened annually.

The interpretation of a Mantoux test depends on the estimated risk of tuberculosis. Usually ≥ 10 mm of induration is considered a positive reaction. In patients at high risk of tuberculosis due to contact with an active case, to chest radiograph consistent with tuberculosis, or to immunocompromise, induration of ≥ 5 mm should be considered positive.

False-positive Mantoux tests (usually 5–10 mm) are often due to nontuberculous mycobacterial infection. False-negative Mantoux tests are often due to subcutaneous injection of PPD.

Care of the Newborn | 7

Peter W. Aldoretta, MD, & Steven B. Spedale, MD

Assessment and care of the newborn can be divided into three distinct phases: antenatal evaluation, delivery room management, and postnatal care.

ANTENATAL EVALUATION

The antenatal evaluation begins with a thorough history that includes the medical history of both the mother and father, the mother's previous obstetrical history, and the history of the current pregnancy. Many of the medical problems presented by a sick neonate may be anticipated from a complete history. Particular attention should be paid to acute or chronic maternal illnesses (Table 7–1). Medications taken during pregnancy and labor, including illicit drugs, may affect the newborn's presentation and outcome (Tables 7–2 and 7–20). High-risk pregnancies should be identified early and monitored carefully for evidence of fetal compromise. Whenever possible, you should make arrangements to deliver mothers with high-risk pregnancies at perinatal centers, thus avoiding transport of a sick neonate after delivery.

DELIVERY ROOM MANAGEMENT

Transition from Fetus to Newborn

Fetal circulation is shown in Figure 7–1. In utero, oxygenated blood is delivered from the placenta to the fetus by the umbilical vein. Most of this is preferentially shunted through the right atrium into the left atrium via the foramen ovale and then into the left ventricle for distribution to the myocardium, brain, and upper body. The remaining blood in the right atrium (including superior vena cava blood) flows preferentially through the right atrium into the right ventricle and out via the main pulmonary artery. As the pulmonary vascular resistance of the fetus is higher than the systemic circulation (reflecting low pla-

Table 7–1. Maternal diseases affecting the fetus.

Maternal Disorder	Fetal or Neonatal Effects
Cholestasis	Preterm delivery
Cyanotic congenital disease	Intrauterine growth retardation (IUGR)
Diabetes mellitus (including gestational)	Large-for-gestational-age infants, hypoglycemia, hypocalcemia, immaturity
Endemic goiter	Neonatal hypothyroidism
Graves' disease	Transient neonatal thyrotoxicosis
Hyperparathyroidism	Hypocalcemia
Hypertension	Intrauterine growth retardation, stillbirth
Idiopathic thrombocytopenia	Thrombocytopenia, bleeding
Immune neutropenia	Fetal neutropenia
Infection (bacterial and viral)	See Table 7–11
Myasthenia gravis	Transient neonatal myasthenia
Obesity	Large-for-gestational-age infants, hypoglycemia
Preeclampsia-eclampsia (toxemia)	Intrauterine growth retardation, stillbirth, asphyxia
Phenylketonuria	Microcephaly, mental retardation
Renal disease	Intrauterine growth retardation, abortion
Rhesus immunization	Fetal anemia, hydrops
Sickle cell anemia	Intrauterine growth retardation
Systemic lupus erythematosus	Congenital heart block, transient rash, anemia, leukopenia, thrombocytopenia, pericardial effusion

[1] Adapted and modified from Behrman RE Shiono PH: In Fanaroff AA, Martin RJ (editors): *Neonatal-Perinatal Medicine, Diseases of the Fetus and Infant,* 5th ed. Vol 1. Mosby, 1992, p 9.

cental resistance), most of the right ventricular output is shunted across the ductus arteriosus into the aorta which supplies the lower body. Blood returns to the placenta via the umbilical arteries.

With the onset of spontaneous respirations at birth, pulmonary vascular resistance falls and pulmonary blood flow increases secondary to the uncoiling of pulmonary vessels and vasodilation as a result of increasing PaO_2. Pressures decrease in the pulmonary artery, right ventricle, and right atrium, while left atrial pressure rises because of an increase in pulmonary venous return. Systemic vascular resistance also increases owing to the removal of the placenta from the circulation. Left atrial pressure exceeds right atrial pressure, thus

Table 7–2. Maternal drug consumption and effects in the fetus and neonate.[1]

Drug Class	Effect(s)
Antipsychotics/Tranquilizers	
Benzodiazepines	May cause craniofacial defects, hypotonia, withdrawal symptoms
Meprobamate/chlordiazepoxide	Probably not teratogenic
Phenothiazines/tricyclic antidepressants	Probably not teratogenic; may cause withdrawal symptoms, urinary retention
Lithium	Increased risk of right-sided heart disease
Thalidomide	Phocomelia
Hormones	
Androgens/progestogens	Increased risk of masculinization of female fetus
Estrogens (diethylstilbestrol)	Vaginal adenosis/adenocarcinoma in adolescence
Clomiphene	Probably not teratogenic
Adrenal corticosteroids	Probably not teratogenic; may cause neonatal adrenal insufficiency
Antihypertensives	Fetal hypotension
Antimicrobials	
Sulfonamides, oxacillin, cephalothin	Competitive binding with serum bilirubin; may increase risk of hyperbilirubinemia
Tetracyclines	Staining of dentition
Aminoglycosides	Auditory nerve defects and ocular nerve damage following prenatal exposure
Streptomycin	Deafness
Nitrofurantoin	Hemolysis
Chloramphenicol	Cardiovascular collapse and "gray baby" syndrome
Quinine	Thrombocytopenia and deafness
Anticonvulsants	
Hydantoins	Fetal hydantoin syndrome; neonatal hemorrhage due to depletion of vitamin K-dependent factors
Barbiturates (phenobarbital, secobarbital)	Congenital anomalies similar to those caused by hydantoin, valproic acid, and carbamazepine
Valproic Acid	Congenital anomalies (craniofacial, cardiovascular, and neural tube)
Trimethadione	Congenital anomalies (fetal trimethadione syndrome-craniofacial, growth retardation, and cardiovascular)
Carbamazepine	Risk of myelomeningocele

(continued)

Table 7–2. Maternal drug consumption and effects in the fetus and neonate (*continued*).[1]

Drug Class	Effect(s)
Antineoplastic agents	All are teratogenic
Anticoagulants	
Warfarin	Fetal and placental hemorrhage, craniofacial and bone defects with first-trimester exposure
Antiemetics; Antihistamines	No association with malformations
Nonnarcotic Analgesics, Anti-inflammatory, Antipyretic Agents	No association with malformations except for salicylate (may increase bleeding risks, possible intrauterine closure of the ductus arteriosus)
Hypoglycemics	
Insulin	Hypoglycemia
Vitamins and iron	
Isotretinoin	Congenital anomalies (ear, cardiovascular, neural tube, thymus)
Diuretics	
Benzothiadiazides	Thrombocytopenia, altered carbohydrate metabolism and hyperbilirubinemia
Cardiovascular agents	
Propranolol	IUGR, bradycardia, and hypoglycemia
Antiarrhythmics, digitalis, glycosides, antihypertensives	Probably not teratogenic
Caffeine	Low birth-weight infants
During Labor	
Barbiturates	CNS and respiratory depression, slowed metabolism
	Depends on dose and timing of administration prior to birth. May cause CNS and respiratory depression, and bradycardia
Paracervical block	Fetal bradycardia
Spinal anesthetics	Maternal hypotension, fetal bradycardia
General anesthetics	Respiratory depression
Magnesium sulfate	Respiratory depression
Drugs of Abuse (See Table 7–20.)	

[1]Adapted and modified from Aranda JV, Hales BF, Rieder MF: In Fanaroff AA, Martin RJ (editors): *Neonatal-Perinatal Medicine, Diseases of the Fetus and Infant,* 5th ed. Vol. 1. Mosby, 1992, p 127.

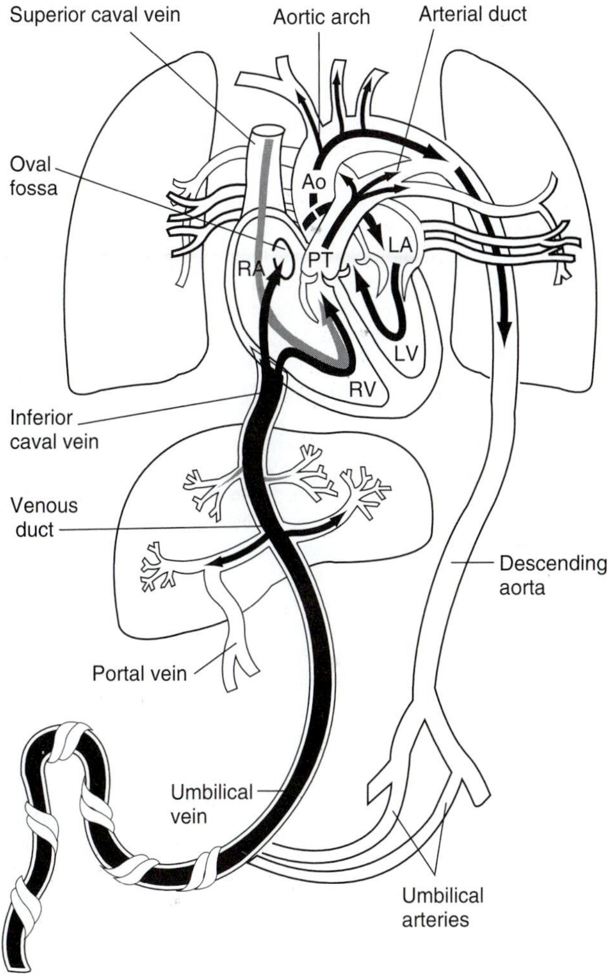

Figure 7–1. Diagram of the course of fetal circulation.

closing the foramen ovale. Systemic pressure exceeds pulmonary pressures and shunting through the ductus arteriosus is reversed. Increasing arterial oxygen tension leads to constriction of the ductus arteriosus.

Successful transition also requires that the neonate remove fetal lung fluid present prior to birth and establish adequate lung volume. As much as 30 mL of fetal lung fluid is removed during passage through the birth canal as a result of the physiologic "squeeze." Additional fluid removal via absorption by alveolar epithelial cells, as well as increases in pulmonary blood and lymphatic flows, occurs in the first few hours after vaginal delivery. Initial lung inflation may require pressures of 30–40 cm H_2O. Subsequent breaths usually require only 15–20 cm H_2O. During the first 24 hours post delivery, the infant's PaO_2 increases from about 55 torr to 90 torr.

The goal of high-risk obstetrics and neonatal resuscitation is prevention of asphyxia, a condition in which hypoxemia and metabolic acidosis are present in the fetus or newborn infant. Asphyxia may result in end-organ damage. The physiology of asphyxia is illustrated in Figure 7–2. **Primary apnea** is defined as cessation of respiration during the period following hypoxia as the heart rate and blood pressure begin to fall. In primary apnea, tactile stimulation and oxygen are sufficient to induce respirations. If asphyxia continues, however, the infant develops gasping respiration followed by **secondary** or **terminal apnea**, a period of respiratory cessation marked by continued decline in heart rate and blood pressure. Positive pressure ventilation is usually required in secondary apnea for resuscitation. This sequence may occur in utero; therefore, you should assume that an infant who is apneic at birth is in secondary apnea and proceed quickly with resuscitative efforts.

Neonatal Resuscitation

Preparation and anticipation are the keys to successful neonatal resuscitation. Personnel attending deliveries should be certified in neonatal resuscitation, demonstrated by participation in the American Heart Association and American Academy of Pediatrics Neonatal Resuscitation Course. Supplies and equipment necessary for successful resuscitation are listed in Table 7–3. The algorithm for neonatal resuscitation is presented in Figure 7–3.

Most neonates will respond to positive pressure ventilation with 100% oxygen. Neonates rarely require cardiac massage or drugs. Mechanical causes for a failed resuscitation are listed in Table 7–4. Medications for resuscitation are described in Table 7–5.

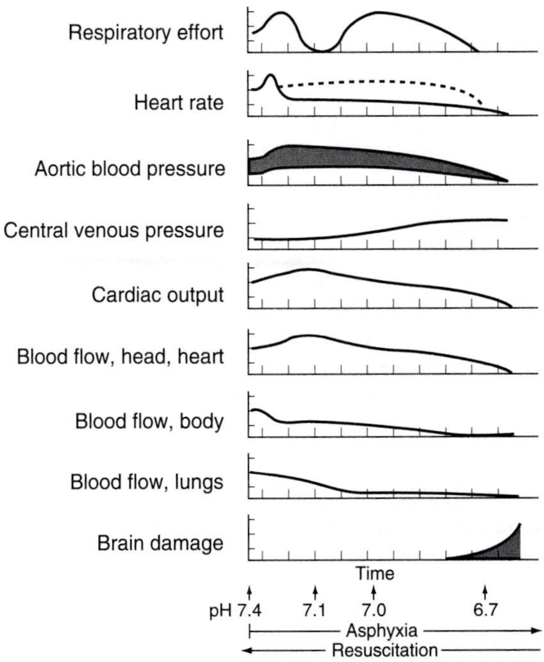

Figure 7–2. Schematic sequence of cardiopulmonary changes with asphyxia and resuscitation. (Adapted from Dawes G: *Foetal and Neonatal Physiology.* Year Book;1968.) (Reproduced with permission from Avery GB: *Neonatology: Pathophysiology and Management of the Newborn.* Lippincott;1987).

Apgar scores (Table 7–6) should be assigned at 1 and 5 minutes post delivery and every 5 minutes thereafter until 20 minutes have passed or until consecutive scores of 7 or higher are obtained. Assessment of Apgar scores should not interfere with the pace of resuscitation. A brief screening examination should be performed in the delivery room. Special emphasis should be placed on identifying dysmorphic features, adequate chest expansion and air exchange, heart tones, abdominal masses, testicular torsion, birth trauma, and skin perfusion. The umbilical cord should be checked for the number of vessels present.

Table 7–3. Equipment for neonatal resuscitation.[1]

Suction Equipment
Bulb syringe
Mechanical suction
Suction catheters: 5F, 6F, 8F, 10F
8F feeding tube and 20-mL syringe
Meconium aspirator
Bag-and-Mask Equipment
Neonatal resuscitation bag with a pressure-release valve or pressure gauge; bag must be capable of delivering oxygen 90–100%
Face masks, newborn and premature sizes (cushioned-rim masks preferred)
Oral airways, newborn and premature sizes
Oxygen with flowmeter and tubing
Intubation Equipment
Laryngoscope with straight blades, No. 0 (preterm) and No. 1 (term)
Extra bulbs and batteries for laryngoscope
Endotracheal tubes: 2.5, 3.0, 3.5, 4.0 mm
Stylet
Scissors
Gloves
Administration of Medications
(see Table 7–5)
Miscellaneous
Radiant warmer
Stethoscope
Cardiotachometer with ECG (oscilloscope desirable)
Adhesve tape, 1/2- or 3/4-inch
Syringes: 1, 3, 5, 10, 20, 50 mL
Needles: 25-, 21-, 18-gauge
Alcohol sponges
Umbilical artery catheterization tray
Umbilical tape
Umbilical catheters: 3.5F, 5F
Three-way stopcocks
Feeding tube, 5F

[1] Modified with permission from American Academy of Pediatrics, American Heart Association: *Neonatal Resuscitation*, 1994.

Indications for Endotracheal Intubation

Endotracheal intubation should be considered:

1. When the amniotic fluid is stained with meconium (below)
2. In preterm infants, especially those below 1000 grams
3. When a diaphragmatic hernia is suspected
4. When bag and mask ventilation is ineffective
5. When prolonged positive pressure ventilation is necessary

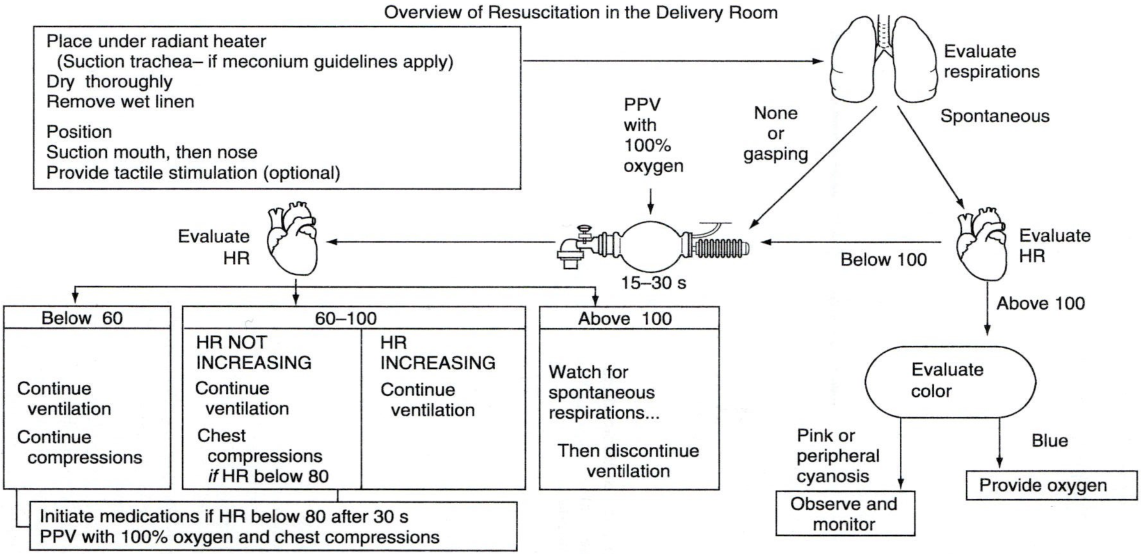

Figure 7–3. Overview of resuscitation in the delivery room. (Reproduced with permission from American Academy of Pediatrics, American Heart Association: *Neonatal Resuscitation;*1994.)

Table 7–4. Mechanical causes of failed resuscitation.[1]

Cause	Examples
Equipment failure	Malfunctioning ambu bag, oxygen not connected or running
Endotracheal tube malposition	Esophagus, right main stem bronchus
Occluded endotracheal tube	
Insufficient inflation pressure to expand lungs	Poor face/mask seal, improper position of mask on infant's face, occluded airway, inadequate inflation pressure
Space-occupying lesions in the thorax	Pneumothorax, pleural effusions, diaphragmatic hernia
Pulmonary hypoplasia	Extreme prematurity, oligohydramnios

[1] Reproduced with permission from Rosenberg AA: Neonatal adaptation. In: *Obstetrics: Normal and Problem Pregnancies,* 1st ed. Gabbe SB, Niebyl JR, Simpson JL (editors). Churchill Livingstone, 1986.

Management of Infants With Meconium-Stained Amniotic Fluid

Amniotic fluid is stained with meconium in approximately 10–20% of all deliveries; the frequency increases to over 39% in deliveries after 42 weeks' gestation. Careful monitoring of fetal well-being is required in these cases. Management of infants with meconium-stained amniotic fluid is outlined in Figure 7–4.

POSTNATAL CARE

Immediate Care of the Newborn

Place the infant in a heated crib or under a radiant warmer and maintain a stable axillary temperature between 36.3 °C and 36.9 °C. Avoid heat loss by drying the baby thoroughly and postponing the initial bath until the infant has stabilized and the temperature is normal. Assess gestational age based on maternal menstrual history and obstetric milestones, and gestational age assessment and physical examination of the neonate (Figure 7–5). Plot growth parameters (weight, length, head circumference) versus gestational age to determine if the infant is appropriate-size-for-gestational-age (AGA), small-for-gestational-age (SGA), or large-for-gestational-age (LGA) (Figure 7–6). Administer vitamin K_1 oxide (phytonadione) in a single parenteral dose of 0.5–1.0 mg within 1 hour of birth to prevent **hemor-**

rhagic disease of the newborn (HDN). Instill 1% silver nitrate, 0.5% erythromycin, or 1% tetracycline into the eyes as prophylaxis against gonococcal ophthalmia. In areas where the rate of chlamydial infection is low, silver nitrate is recommended, especially if penicillinase-producing *Neisseria gonorrhoeae* (PPNG) is present. The effectiveness of erythromycin or tetracycline in the prevention of ophthalmia caused by PPNG has not been established. No topical regimen has proven efficacy in preventing chlamydial conjunctivitis. It is recommended, however, that infants born to mothers with chlamydial cervicitis be treated with a 14-day course of oral erythromycin.

Physical Examination

All infants should have a complete physical examination within 12 hours of birth; sick infants as soon as they are stable. Term newborns have the following characteristics at birth and shortly thereafter.

A. Resting posture: Extremities are flexed and somewhat hypertonic. Positioning may reflect the infant's position in utero (eg, thighs flexed on abdomen following breech presentation). Fists are clenched. Asymmetries of skull, face, jaw, or extremities may result from intrauterine pressures.

B. Skin: Skin is usually ruddy and often mottled. Localized cyanosis of hands and feet (acrocyanosis) normally disappears after several days. Skin may appear dry and peeling in postterm newborns.

Other characteristics of the skin may include:

1. **Lanugo** (fine downy growth of hair) may be present over the shoulders and back.
2. **Vernix caseosa** (whitish or clay-colored, cheesy, greasy material) may cover the body but is usually found on the back and scalp and in the creases of term infants.
3. Facial **milia** (distended sebaceous glands producing tiny whitish papules) are especially prominent over the nose, chin, or cheeks.
4. **Mongolian spots** (benign bluish pigmentation over the lower back, buttocks, or extensor surfaces) may be found in infants of dark-skinned races.
5. Capillary hemangiomas ("flame nevi") are common over the eyelids, forehead, and neck.
6. Petechiae are sometimes present over the head, neck, and back, especially in association with nuchal cord. If petechiae are generalized, thrombocytopenia should be suspected.
7. **Miliaria**, caused by blocked sweat gland ducts, are pustules without a red base.

Table 7–5. Medications for neonatal resuscitation.[1]

Medication	Concentration to Administer	Preparation	Dosage/ Route[2]	Total Dose/Infant		Rate/Precautions	
				Weight (in kg)		**Total mL**	
Epinephrine	1:10,000	1 mL	0.1–0.3 mL/kg	1		0.1–0.3	Give rapidly
				2		0.2–0.6	May dilute with normal saline to 1–2 mL if giving
				3		0.3–0.9	
			IV or ET	4		0.4–1.2	ET
Volume expanders	Whole blood	40 mL	10 mL/kg	**Weight (in kg)**		**Total mL**	
	5% Albumin-saline			1		10	Give over 5–10 minutes
			IV	2		20	
	Normal saline		3	30			
	Ringer's lactate			4		40	
				Weight (kg)	**Total Dose**	**Total mL**	
Sodium bicarbonate	0.5 mEq/mL (4.2% solution)	20 mL or two 10-mL prefilled syringes	2 mEq/kg IV	1	2	4	Give *slowly*, over at least 2 minutes
				2	4	8	
				3	6	12	
				4	8	16	Give only if infant is being effectively ventilated

				Weight (kg)	Total Dose (mEq)	Total mL	
Naloxone hydrochloride	0.4 mg/mL	1 mL	0.1 mg/kg	1	0.1	0.25	
			(0.25 mL/kg)	2	0.2	0.50	Give rapidly
			IV, ET	3	0.3	0.75	IV, ET preferred
			IM, SQ	4	0.4	1.00	IM, SQ acceptable
	1.0 mg/mL	1 mL	0.1 mL/kg	1	0.1	0.1	
			(0.1 mL/kg)	2	0.2	0.2	
			IV, ET	3	0.3	0.3	
			IM, SQ	4	0.4	0.4	
				Weight (kg)	**Total μg/min**		
Dopamine	$\frac{6 \times \text{Weight (kg)} \times \text{Desired (μg/kg/min)}}{\text{Desired fluid (mL/h)}} =$	mg of dopamine per 100 mL of solution	Begin at 5 μg/kg/min (may increase to 20 μg/kg/min if necessary) IV	1	5–20		Give as continuous infusion using an infusion pump
				2	10–40		
				3	15–60		Monitor heart rate and blood pressure closely
				4	20–80		Seek consultation

[1] From *Textbook of Neonatal Resuscitation* © 1987, 1990, 1994 American Heart Association

[2] IM, intramuscular; ET, endotracheal; IV, intravenous; SQ, subcutaneous

Table 7–6. Apgar score for evaluating newborn infants.[1]

Sign	Score 0	1	2
A Appearance (color)	Blue; pale	Body pink; extremities blue	Completely pink
P Pulse (heart rate)	Absent	< 100	> 100
G Grimace (reflex irritability in response to stimulation of sole of foot	No response	Grimace	Cry
A Activity (muscle tone)	Limp	Some flexion of extremities	Active motion
R Respiration (respiratory effort)	Absent	Slow; irregular	Good strong cry

[1] Practical epigram of Apgar Score. (Reproduced with permission from Butterfield J, Covey M: *JAMA* 1962;**181**:353. Copyright American Medical Association.)

8. Newborns of 32 weeks' or more gestational age may perspire when too warm. The forehead is usually the first site to perspire.
9. **Erythema toxicum** is characterized by erythematous raised areas with a pustule filled with eosinophils.
10. **Pustular melanosis** is a pustular rash marked by the presence of pigment in ruptured pustules. The pustules are noninfectious but may contain neutrophils.

    The reader is referred to Chapter 12 for information regarding the management of skin disorders in neonates.

C. Head: The head of neonates is large in proportion to the rest of the body; it may exhibit considerable molding with overriding of the cranial bones. Other features may include the following:

1. **Caput succedaneum** (localized or fairly extensive ill-defined soft tissue swelling) may be present over the scalp or other presenting parts. It usually extends over a suture line.
2. Cephalhematoma (see Birth Injuries)
3. The anterior and posterior fontanelles are soft and may measure 0.6–3.6 cm in any direction. They may be small initially. A third

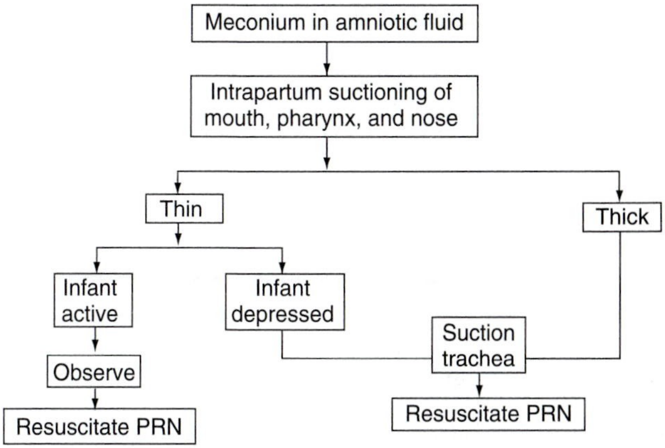

Figure 7–4. Suggested approach to meconium in the amniotic fluid. (Reproduced with permission from American Academy of Pediatrics, American Heart Association: *Neonatal Resuscitation;*1994.)

fontanelle between these two is present in approximately 6% of infants and is more likely to occur in children with various abnormalities.

4. Transillumination of a term infant's head normally produces a circle of light no greater than 1.5 cm beyond the light source.
5. **Craniotabes** (slight indentation and recoil of parietal bones, elicited by pressing lightly with the thumb) is normal in newborns.

D. Face: Unusual facies occur with many congenital syndromes. Check the neonate's face for bruising or forceps marks and facial nerve palsy. Note also:

1. **Eyes:** The irises are slate-gray except in infants of dark-skinned races. Tears may or may not be present. Most term infants look toward light sources and focus transiently on human faces. Subconjunctival, scleral, and retinal hemorrhages occur with birth trauma. The pupillary light reflex should be present. Lens opacities are abnormal. A red reflex can be seen on ophthalmoscopic examination. The infant will turn to follow a person's face more intently than other visual stimuli.
2. **Ears:** The eardrums may be difficult to visualize but have a characteristic opaque appearance and decreased mobility. Severe mal-

MATURATIONAL ASSESSMENT OF GESTATIONAL AGE (New Ballard Score)

Name__________ Date/Time of birth__________ Sex__________

Hospital No.__________ Date/Time of exam__________ Birth weight__________

Race__________ Age when examined__________ Length__________

Apgar score: 1 minute_____ 5 minutes_____ 10 minutes_____ Head circ.__________

Examiner__________

NEUROMUSCULAR MATURITY

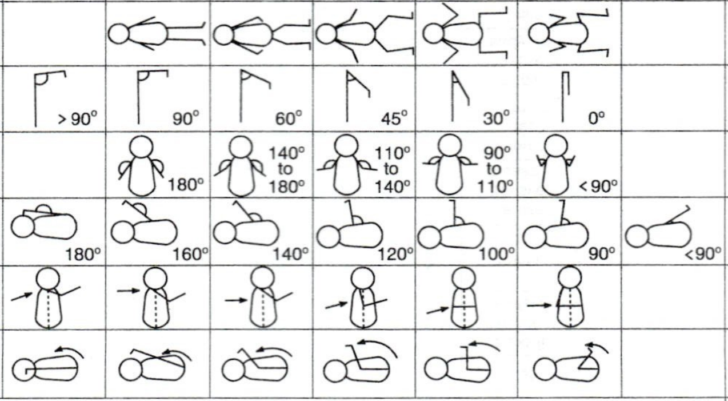

Neuromuscular maturity sign	Score -1	0	1	2	3	4	5	Record score here
Posture								
Square window (wrist)	> 90°	90°	60°	45°	30°	0°		
Arm recoil		180°	140° to 180°	110° to 140°	90° to 110°	< 90°		
Popliteal angle	180°	160°	140°	120°	100°	90°	<90°	
Scarf sign								
Heal to ear								
							Total neuromuscular maturity score	

SCORE

Neuromuscular ________

Physical ________

Total ________

Maturity rating

Score	Weeks
-10	20
-5	22
0	24
5	26
10	28
15	30
20	32
25	34
30	36
35	38
40	40
45	42
50	44

GESTATIONAL AGE

(weeks)

By dates ________

By ultrasound ________

By exam ________

PHYSICAL MATURITY

Physical maturity sign	Score							Record score here
	-1	0	1	2	3	4	5	
Sign	sticky friable transparent	gelatinous red translucent	smooth pink visible veins	superficial peeling &/or rash, few veins	cracking pale areas rare veins	parchment deep cracking no vessels	leathery cracked wrinkled	
Lanugo	none	sparse	abundant	thinning	bald areas	mostly bald		
Plantar surface	heel-toe 40-50mm:-1 <40 mm:-2	>50 m no crease	faint red marks	anterior transverse crease only	creases ant. 2/3	creases over entire sole		
Breast	imperceptible	barely perceptible	flat areola no bud	stippled areola 1-2 mm bud	raised areola 3-4 mm bud	full areola 5-10 mm bud		
Eye/ ear	lids fused loosely:-1 tightly:-2	lids open pinna flat stays folded	sl. curved pinna; soft slow recoil	well curved pinna; soft but ready recoil	formed and firm instant recoil	thick cartilage ear stiff		
Genitals (male)	scrotum flat, smooth	scrotum empty faint rugae	testes in upper canal rare rugae	testes descending few rugae	teste down good rugae	teste pendulous deep rugae		
Genitals (female)	clitoris prominent & labia flat	prominent clitoris & small labia minora	prominent clitoris & en-larging minora	majora & minora equally prominent	majora large minora small	majora cover clitoris & minora		
							Total physical maturity score	

Figure 7–5. Maturational assessment of gestational age (New Ballard Score). (Reprinted from Ballard JL, Khoury JC, Wedig K et al: New Ballard Score, expanded to include extremely premature infants. J Pediatr 1991;119:417.)

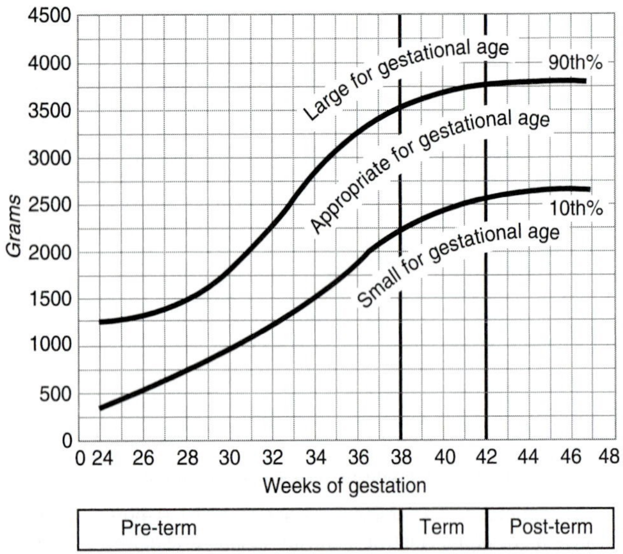

Figure 7–6. University of Colorado Medical Center classification of newborns by birth weight and gestational age. (Adapted from Battaglia FC, Lubchenco LO: J Pediatr 1967;71:159.) (Reproduced with permission from Avery GB: *Neonatology: Pathophysiology and Management of the Newborn.* Lippincott;1987.)

formation of the pinnas may be associated with abnormalities of the genitourinary tract. Ear tags should prompt the clinician to assess hearing loss and take a family history. Normal newborns respond to sounds with a startle, blink, head turning, or cry.

3. **Nose:** Newborns are preferential nosebreathers and experience respiratory distress in bilateral choanal atresia. Confirm nasal patency by passage of a nasogastric tube if you suspect obstruction.
4. **Mouth:** Small, pearl-like retention cysts at the gum margins and in the midline of the palate (Bohn's and Epstein's pearls) are common but insignificant. Natal teeth should be removed. Rule out clefts of the lip and of the hard and soft palate. Examine the size of the tongue and mandible. The tonsils are quite small. Excessive drooling occurs with esophageal atresia.
5. **Cheeks:** The cheeks are full because of sucking pads.

E. Neck: Check for webbing, sinus tracts, and masses.

F. Chest: Check for fractured clavicles. Note also:

1. **Breasts:** The breasts are palpable in most mature males and females. Their size is determined by gestational age, maternal hormones, and adequacy of nutrition.
2. **Lungs:** Neonatal breathing is abdominal and may be shallow and irregular. The rate is usually 40–60 breaths per minute, with a range of 20–100 breaths per minute. Breath sounds are harsh and bronchial. Faint rales may be heard immediately following birth but normally clear in several hours.
3. **Heart:** The rate averages 130 beats per minute (bpm), but rates from 90–180 bpm may be present for brief periods in normal infants. Sinus dysrhythmia may be present. Transient murmurs are common. Check brachial and femoral pulses to rule out coarctation of the aorta. Blood pressure is fairly constant over a wide range of gestational age and birthweight (Table 7–7). Lower blood pressures tend to be seen in sick preterm infants who suffered perinatal hypoxia, and in those requiring mechanical ventilation.

G. Abdomen: The abdomen is normally flat at birth but soon becomes more protuberant; a markedly scaphoid abdomen suggests diaphragmatic hernia. Two arteries and one vein are usually present in the umbilical cord. The liver is palpable. The tip of the spleen can be felt in 10% of newborns. Both kidneys can and should be palpated. Bowel sounds are audible shortly after birth.

H. Genitalia: Appearance in either sex depends on gestational age (Figure 7–5). Edema is common, particularly after breech delivery. Rule out ambiguous genitalia. In females, an imperforate hymen may be visible. Females may also develop a whitish discharge with or without blood. In males the prepuce is adherent to the glans of the penis. White epithelial pearls 1–2 mm in diameter may be present at the tip of the prepuce.

Table 7–7. Blood pressure at different gestational ages.[1]

Gestational age (wk)	Systolic (mm Hg)	Diastolic (mm Hg)
< 24	48–63	24–39
24–28	48–58	25–36
29–32	47–59	24–34
> 32	48–60	24–34

[1] Modified from Hegyi T et al: J Pediatr 1994;124:627.

I. Anus: Patency should be checked. An anteriorly displaced anus may be associated with stenosis (Chapter 17).

J. Skeleton: Check for skeletal abnormalities (eg, absence of bones, clubfoot, syndactyly, polydactyly). Examine for hip dislocation by attempting to dislocate the femur posteriorly and then abducting the legs to relocate the femur. Examine for extremity or clavicular fractures, palsies, and arthrogryposis (limited joint movement). Rule out myelomeningocele and other spinal deformities (eg, scoliosis).

K. Nervous system:

1. **Neurologic development** is dependent on gestational age.
2. Assess **muscle tone and strength**.
3. Assess character of **cry**.
4. **Most reflexes**, including the Moro, tonic neck, grasp, sucking, rooting, stepping, Babinski, deep tendon, abdominal, cremasteric, and Chvostek reflexes, are normally present at birth.

Routine Care of the Term Infant

A. Observation: Following stabilization, observations should be made and recorded every 8 hours. Most importantly, they should include vital signs, overall well being, voiding and stooling patterns, and feeding patterns. The normal full-term neonate passes meconium in the first 24 hours post delivery and voids within the first 12 hours. Delays beyond 48 and 24 hours, respectively, may indicate obstruction. Daily weights should be obtained; a weight loss of 5–10% over the third to fifth day may be expected.

B. Feedings: Both breast and bottle feeding can be started immediately if the infant is stable. For infants who have undergone a difficult delivery and resuscitation, feedings should be delayed until they are stable. Feedings may be initiated with breast milk or formula. Sterile water feedings are *not* necessary. The normal term infant should feed every 2–4 hours with volumes of feeding increasing from 1/2–1 ounce per feed to 1 1/2–2 ounces per feed on day 3. Breast-fed infants will also feed every 2–3 hours, increasing from 4 to 10 minutes on each side. Formula-fed babies should be given supplemental fluoride (0.25 mg/d) if they do not live in an area with a fluoridated water supply. Because of the poor passage of fluoride into human milk, breast-fed infants should receive supplemental fluoride.

C. Laboratory screening: Cord blood is used for blood typing, Rh determination, and Coombs antibody testing. Most states have mandatory screening programs for inborn errors of metabolism (eg, phenylketonuria [PKU], maple syrup urine disease, homocystinuria, galactosemia, etc) and for congenital hypothyroidism. Samples of blood for screening tests should ideally be taken after the infant has had adequate intake of milk (protein) for 24 hours.

D. Circumcision: The decision to circumcise a male infant should be made by parents after consultation with the pediatrician/obstetrician.

E. Length of hospitalization: In current practice, neonates and their mothers are routinely discharged after 24–48 hours. Nurseries should instruct parents in routine matters of newborn care with special emphasis on important signs and symptoms (eg, jaundice, lethargy, poor feeding, vomiting, and fever). Routine outpatient follow-up should be scheduled for 48–72 hours post delivery in infants discharged in less than 24 hours.

Care of the Small-for-Gestational-Age (SGA) Infant

Regardless of gestational age, the SGA infant's weight is less than the tenth percentile for that age (Figure 7–6). The infant often appears malnourished. With increasingly severe growth retardation, the infant's length and head circumference are compromised (Chapter 3). Asymmetric growth retardation (sparing of growth in length and head circumference) implies a problem occurring late in pregnancy (placental insufficiency of any etiology), whereas symmetric growth retardation (weight, length, and head circumference $< 10\%$) implies an event in early pregnancy (eg, chromosomal abnormality, drug or alcohol use, congenital viral infection).

SGA infants have a higher morbidity and mortality rate than do AGA infants. SGA infants may present with severe asphyxia in the delivery room and should be carefully examined for congenital anomalies and intrauterine infections. Approximately two-thirds of preterm SGA and one-third of term SGA infants develop **neonatal hypoglycemia** (blood glucose < 40 mg/dL). SGA infants are also more likely to develop polycythemia/hyperviscosity and feeding difficulties.

Care of the Large-for-Gestational-Age (LGA) Infant

LGA neonates have birth weights which are greater than the 90th percentile for gestational age. These infants are more likely to have birth injuries and hypoglycemia.

Infants of diabetic mothers (IDMs) are often LGA and have a characteristic macrosomic appearance with a round full facies. In addition, they are immature for gestational age with an increased incidence of respiratory distress syndrome. Other problems of the IDM include polycythemia, hypocalcemia, hyperbilirubinemia, cardiomyopathy, small left colon syndrome, and an increased incidence of congenital anomalies, including caudal regression.

Care of the Premature Infant

Initial support and resuscitation of the premature infant is the same as that for a term infant. However, he or she may need extra support owing to functional and anatomic immaturity of various organs. In the immediate postdelivery period these measures include support of respiration (mechanical ventilation and oxygen), thermoregulation (radiant warmer or isolette), and fluid intake (often increased secondary to water loss through the skin). Intravenous glucose and subsequent parenteral nutrition are often necessary. Enteral feedings via a feeding tube may be required for infants delivered prior to 36 weeks' gestation.

DISEASES OF THE NEWBORN

DISEASES OF THE RESPIRATORY SYSTEM

Apnea

A. Clinical Findings: Apneic episodes occur mainly in preterm infants. **Apnea** in neonates is defined as a respiratory pause longer than 20 seconds, or shorter if accompanied by cyanosis and bradycardia. Prematurity is the most common cause, associated with the immaturity of central respiratory regulation centers and of protective mechanisms that aid in maintaining airway patency. Apnea must be differentiated from **periodic breathing**, which is characterized by regularly occurring ventilatory cycles interrupted by short pauses *not* associated with bradycardia or color changes. The causes of apnea are listed in Table 7–8.

B. Treatment: Therapy should be directed toward the underlying cause. If apnea is due to prematurity, cutaneous stimulation may relieve mild symptoms. Frequent or severe apnea may require intubation. Ventilation or pharmacologic therapy with theophylline (loading dose 5 mg/kg; maintenance dose 1–2 mg/kg q6–12h) or caffeine (loading dose 10 mg/kg [base] or 20 mg/kg [citrate]; maintenance 2.5–5.0 mg/kg q24h). Drug levels must be followed (normal 5–10 μg/mL).

Table 7–8. Causes of apnea in infants.

1.	Temperature instability: cold or heat stress
2.	Response to passage of a feeding tube
3.	Gastroesophageal reflux
4.	Hypoxemia: pulmonary parenchymal disease
	patent ductus arteriosus
	? anemia
5.	Infection: sepsis (viral or bacterial)
	necrotizing enterocolitis
6.	Metabolic: hypoglycemia
	hyponatremia
7.	Intracranial hemorrhage
8.	Posthemorrhagic hydrocephalus
9.	Seizures
10.	Drugs (eg, morphine, maternal magnesium administration)
11.	Apnea of prematurity

C. Prognosis: In the majority of premature infants, apnea and bradycardia cease by 34–36 weeks postconception. If these symptoms persist at time of discharge, home monitoring should be considered as well as continued use of methylxanthines. Home monitoring, however, has not been effective in reducing **sudden infant death syndrome (SIDS)**.

Respiratory Distress in the Newborn

A. Clinical Findings: Respiratory distress is among the most common neonatal problems. Causes include cardiopulmonary and other abnormalities and are listed in Table 7–9. The most important clinical features include a respiratory rate greater than 60/minute with or without associated cyanosis, nasal flaring, intercostal and sternal retractions, and expiratory grunting. Most noncardiopulmonary causes can be ruled out by history, physical examination and a few simple laboratory tests (eg, glucose chemstrip, blood gas, hematocrit). The differential diagnosis of common causes of respiratory distress in term infants is presented in Table 7–10.

Hyaline Membrane Disease

A. Clinical Findings: Premature infants represent the largest population of infants with respiratory distress. The most common cause is **hyaline membrane disease (HMD)** or deficiency of surfactant. Surfactant deficiency results in poor lung compliance and atelectasis. Diagnosis is based on gestational age of infant, clinical presenta-

Table 7 9. Respiratory distress in the newborn.[1]

Non-cardiopulmonary	Cardiovascular	Pulmonary
Hypo- or hyperthermia	Left-sided outflow tract obstruction	Upper airway
Hypoglycemia	Hypoplastic left heart	obstruction
Polycythemia	Aortic stenosis	Choanal atresia
Metabolic acidosis	Coarctation of the aorta	Vocal cord paralysis
Drug intoxications; withdrawal	Cyanotic lesions	Lingual thyroid
CNS insult	Transposition of the great vessels	Laryngomalacia
Asphyxia	Total anomalous pulmonary venous return	Meconium aspiration
Hemorrhage	Tricuspid atresia	Amniotic fluid aspiration
Neuromuscular disease	Right-sided outflow obstruction	Transient tachypnea
Phrenic nerve injury		Pneumonia
Skeletal abnormalities		Pulmonary hypoplasia
Asphyxiating thoracic dystrophy		Hyaline membrane disease
		Pneumothorax, pleural effusions
		Mass Lesions
		Lobar emphysema
		Cystic adenomatoid malformation

CNS = central nervous system

[1]Reproduced with permission from Rosenberg AA: Neonatal adaptation. In *Obstetrics: Normal and Problem Pregnancies,* 1st ed. Gabbe SB, Niebyl JR, Simpson JL (editors). Churchill Livingstone, 1986.

Table 7–10. Common causes of respiratory distress in the term infant.

Condition	Presentation	Diagnosis	Course
Delayed absorption of amniotic fluid (TTN)	slightly preterm infant or term infant delivered by C-section. Tachypnea, cyanosis, grunting, retractions soon after birth	CXR-hyperexpansion, perihilar streaking, interlobar fluid	usually require < 40% FiO_2; resolves 12–72 hours
Amniotic fluid aspiration	tachypnea, cyanosis, grunting, retractions soon after birth	CXR-hyperexpanded; patchy infiltrates	protracted course of 4–7 days; may require supplemental O_2 30–60%
Meconium aspiration	as for amniotic fluid aspiration; barrel chest, fetal distress	CXR-hyperexpansion, course irregular infiltrates	resolves 4–7 days, may require high FiO_2. At risk for PPHN and air leaks.
Pneumonia	Onset of respiratory symptoms within 6–12 hrs of birth, history of prolonged rupture of membranes, ± chorio-amnionitis, associated shock, absolute neutropenia on CBC	CXR-variable-can mimic TTN, aspiration syndromes, HMD	variable; mortality rate
Pneumothorax	tachypnea, shifted heart sounds, cyanosis,	CXR; transillumination	usually resolve within 24–48h. Rarely requires drainage. FiO_2 requirement usually < 40%

CBC = complete blood count; CXR = chest x-ray; HMD = hyaline membrane disease; PPHN = persistent pulmonary hypertension of the newborn; TTN = transient tachypnea of newborn

tion and chest x-ray (CXR). The incidence of HMD is 5% at 35–36 weeks but rises to 65% at 29–30 weeks. On CXR, the lung fields classically have a "ground glass" appearance with normal to small lung volumes and evidence of atelectasis as shown by the appearance of air bronchograms.

B. Treatment: The overall goal of therapy is to maintain a PaO_2 60–70 mm Hg with a normal pH and $PaCO_2$ (35–45 mm Hg). Respiratory assessment includes arterial blood gas sampling and noninvasive monitoring with pulse oximetry, transcutaneous O_2 and CO_2 monitoring. Arterial access through either a peripheral or umbilical artery catheter may be needed if the infants require a FiO_2 above 0.40. The need for intubation is present if the infant is unable to maintain a $PaO_2 > 60$ and $PaCO_2 < 50$ mm Hg in $FIO_2 > 0.60$. Infants born after 30 weeks' gestation may benefit from a trial of continuous positive airway pressure (CPAP) alone.

The availability of exogenous surfactant replacement has dramatically changed the management of HMD. Commercially available surfactant preparations include bovine and porcine lung extracts as well as a synthetic surfactant (Exosurf). Each of these compounds has demonstrated the ability to decrease mortality from HMD, especially in the very immature infant (23–26 weeks). In addition, ventilator settings and oxygen requirements are lower over the first few days of life, and the incidence of air leak complications is decreased. Some studies have shown a significant cost savings for infants treated with surfactants. A consistent decrease in the incidence of other complications of prematurity such as necrotizing enterocolitis (NEC), patent ductus arteriosus (PDA), intracranial hemorrhage, or chronic lung disease has not occurred.

The administration of corticosteroids to the mother at least 24 hours prior to delivery has been shown to cause a significant decrease in the incidence of HMD in preterm infants.

C. Prognosis: Mortality from HMD is less than 10% for infants greater than 28 weeks' gestation, and increases in more immature infants. The major long-term sequela is the development of chronic lung disease in 20% of the survivors.

DISEASES OF THE CARDIOVASCULAR SYSTEM

Cardiovascular causes of respiratory distress in the neonatal period can be divided into two groups: those associated with structural heart disease (present with cyanosis or congestive heart failure) and those associated with shunting through fetal pathways and a structurally normal heart.

Structural Heart Disease

A. Clinical Findings: Examples of cyanotic lesions are transposition of the great vessels, total anomalous pulmonary venous return, tricuspid atresia, certain types of truncus arteriosus, and right heart obstruction (pulmonary/tricuspid atresia). Cyanosis presents early and may not be associated with any respiratory distress. Over time, however, many infants will develop respiratory symptoms due to increased pulmonary blood flow or secondary to metabolic acidosis from hypoxia. Diagnostic aids include failure of an infant's PaO_2 to increase significantly when placed in 100% oxygen (all lesions), decreased pulmonary lung markings on CXR (right heart obstruction), and left-sided forces predominating on electrocardiography (tricuspid atresia). Diagnosis can be confirmed with echocardiography.

Infants presenting with congestive heart failure (CHF) usually have some form of left outflow obstruction (aortic stenosis, aortic atresia, coarctation). Infants with obstructive lesions do well until the patent ductus arteriosus, which previously had provided for most or all of the systemic flow, closes (1–2 d). At this time heart failure and metabolic acidosis develop. Diagnostic aids include abnormal pulses on physical exam. CXR shows a large heart with pulmonary edema. Arterial blood gases (ABGs) are remarkable for profound metabolic acidosis. Lesions involving left-to-right shunting (VSD) do well until the pulmonary vascular resistance drops (3–4 wk) and shunting becomes significant leading to heart failure.

B. Treatment: Infants presenting with any structural lesion may require basic stabilization. Specific therapy includes infusion of prostaglandin E_1, 0.025–0.1 μg/kg/min to maintain ductal patency. In some cyanotic lesions, this will improve pulmonary blood flow and PaO_2 by allowing shunting through the ductus to the pulmonary artery. In left-sided outflow tract obstruction, systemic blood flow is duct-dependent, so this will improve systemic perfusion and resolve the baby's acidosis. Further specific therapies are covered in Chapter 16.

C. Prognosis: Prognoses for structural heart lesions depend on the type and severity of the lesion; they are reviewed in Chapter 16.

Shunting Through Fetal Pathways

I. Patent Ductus Arteriosus (PDA)

A. Clinical Findings: This is the most frequent cardiovascular disorder seen in the preterm infant. Presentation may occur as early as day 1–2 in small prematures, but most often becomes clinically significant on days 3–7 as the infant is recovering from HMD. As pulmonary vascular resistance falls below systemic resistance there is increasing left-to-right shunting; this initially results in the characteristic physical findings (hyperdynamic precordium, increased peripheral pulses, widened pulse pressure, systolic murmur). If untreated it may progress to CHF and pulmonary edema. Respiratory support may need to be increased. Echocardiogram is confirmatory.

B. Treatment: PDA may require surgical as well as medical management. Indomethacin (0.2 mg/kg IV per dose) every 12–24 hours for 3 doses results in ductal closure in approximately two-thirds of the cases. If the ductus reopens, a second trial may be undertaken. If this fails, surgical ligation is indicated. A major side effect of indomethacin is a transient oliguria, which can be treated with fluid restriction until the urine output improves. Contraindications include hyperkalemia, creatinine >2 mg/dL, or marked thrombocytopenia (platelet count $< 50{,}000/\text{mm}^3$).

II. Persistent Pulmonary Hypertension of the Newborn (PPHN)

A. Clinical Findings: Most often seen in full- or post-term infants, PPHN represents a failure of the pulmonary vasculature to move from the intrauterine state of high resistance and low flow to the normal postnatal low resistance, high-flow state. The increased pulmonary vascular resistance may be *reversible*, secondary to increased pulmonary vasoreactivity, or less commonly may be *irreversible*, resulting from an anatomically abnormal pulmonary vascular bed with decreased cross-sectional diameter (eg, pulmonary hypoplasia secondary to congenital diaphragmatic hernia or oligohydramnios sequence). Reversible pulmonary hypertension can result from a variety of insults and disorders; these include perinatal asphyxia, meconium aspiration, sepsis, pneumonia, HMD, chronic intrauterine hypoxia, polycythemia, and hypothermia. The clinical syndrome is characterized by (1) early-onset respiratory distress (frequently from birth); (2) hypoxemia out of proportion to CXR findings; (3) minimal improvement in PaO_2 with 100% oxygen; (4) marked lability of oxygenation; (5) right-to-left shunting through a PDA or foramen ovale, occasionally producing significant differences in pre- and postductal oxygen saturations; (6) single, increased S_2 on auscultation; (7) ± myocardial depression with hypotension. Echocardiogram can help with the diagnosis by demonstrating right-to-left shunting or tricuspid or pulmonary regurgitation.

B. Treatment: Therapy for PPHN includes supportive treatment for associated disorders (antibiotics for sepsis and pneumonia, fluid and electrolyte management for renal failure, etc). Specific therapies are primarily directed at raising systemic pressure above pulmonary pressure in order to prevent right-to-left shunting and reverse hypoxemia. These include (1) oxygen and mechanical ventilation (oxygen is a pulmonary vasodilator; adequate lung inflation helps to mechanically decrease pulmonary resistance); (2) colloid infusions (10–30 mL/kg) to improve systemic pressure; (3) systemic vasopressors to aid compromised cardiac function (dopamine 5–20 μg/kg/min and/or dobutamine 5–20 μg/kg/min); and (4) alkalosis to raise pH to 7.55–7.65 (achieved with hyperventilation and/or administration of sodium bicarbonate).

High-frequency ventilation devices (both jet ventilation and oscillatory ventilation) have proven useful in the management of selected cases of PPHN. Studies evaluating high-frequency ventilation as rescue therapy in PPHN refractory to conventional ventilation have demonstrated improved oxygenation and carbon dioxide elimination with no apparent increase in morbidity. Nitric oxide has been recently identified as a potent endogenous vasodilator and can be used without risk of systemic hypotension; it is rapidly metabolized, and when given in inhaled form acts as a selective pulmonary vasodilator. It is currently undergoing studies for efficacy in PPHN and has shown promising results.

As a highly invasive treatment with tremendous potential for morbidity, **extracorporeal membrane oxygenation (ECMO)** remains a therapy of last resort for infants with PPHN. In ECMO, blood is removed for exogenous oxygenation and returned through a continuous circuit allowing a period of lung rest for infants with potentially reversible disease. In venoarterial ECMO, blood is removed from the right side of the circulation through an internal jugular cannula and oxygenated blood returned through a cannula in the common carotid artery. In venovenous ECMO, blood is both removed from and returned to the right side of the circulation with either a two-catheter system or a single double-lumen catheter in the right atrium. Both entail the significant risk of prolonged heparinization, but venovenous ECMO avoids the need for unilateral carotid artery ligation. Only venoarterial ECMO provides the added benefit of supporting systemic blood flow, however, which may be important in infants with significant myocardial dysfunction.

C. Prognosis: Mortality rates with PPHN will vary widely depending upon severity and the nature of associated disorders. Major morbidities include neurologic deficits (both motor and cognitive) which may be severe in up to 20%, hearing loss, and chronic lung disease.

BIRTH INJURIES

Birth injuries occur during both labor and delivery. Risk factors include macrosomia, cephalopelvic disproportion, prematurity, dystocia, prolonged labor, and abnormal presentation.

Soft tissue injuries consisting of petechiae, erythema, and ecchymoses are common. They usually involve the presenting part of the infant and most often require no treatment. Note that petechiae away from the presenting part may represent signs of an underlying hemorrhagic disorder.

Cephalhematoma is a subperiosteal collection of blood caused by localized trauma; it is present in 0.4–2.5% of live births. Cephalhematoma presents as a swelling on day 1 that does not cross suture lines. Most commonly the swelling overlies the parietal bone. Rarely there can be enough bleeding to cause shock or anemia. Subgaleal bleeds occur beneath the scalp and are not restricted by sutures. This type of injury is rare, but can result in significant blood loss. Subdural and subarachnoid bleeds may also result from a traumatic delivery.

The most common fracture resulting from birth trauma involves the clavicle. This type of fracture may be clinically palpable or suspect in an infant who does not move an upper extremity. Therapy is usually not necessary; healing occurs with good callus formation in 7–10 days. The most common long bone fracture involves the humerus.

Nerve injuries most often involve the brachial plexus or facial nerves. Three types of brachial plexus injuries may require attention: (1) **Duchenne-Erb:** upper arm paralysis resulting from damage to the fifth and sixth cervical nerves; (2) **Klumpke's** (lower arm): damage to the eight cervical and first thoracic nerves; and (3) entire arm. Treatment involves physical therapy to prevent contractures. Most infants will recover good arm function, although 15% will suffer significant handicap. Phrenic nerve injuries (brachial plexus injuries) can also occur during deliveries in which the infant's neck is severely stretched. Brachial plexus damage is associated with 80–90% of phrenic injuries. The clinical presentation of a phrenic nerve injury includes tachypnea and cyanosis. Facial nerve injuries occur at the point where the nerve emerges from the stylomastoid foramen. Unilateral facial muscle weakness will be seen with complete resolution over several days in most cases.

NEONATAL HYPERBILIRUBINEMIA

Bilirubin Metabolism

Bilirubin in the neonate is derived from breakdown of circulating red blood cells (RBCs) (75%) and ineffective erythropoiesis and tissue heme proteins (25%). Heme is converted to unconjugated (lipid-soluble) bilirubin in the reticuloendothelial system and is transported by albumin to the liver. In the liver it is conjugated with glucuronic acid in a reaction catalyzed by glucuronyl transferase. The conjugated bilirubin (water-soluble) is secreted into the biliary tree for excretion via the gastrointestinal (GI) tract. The enzyme B-glucuronidase is present in the small bowel and hydrolyzes some of the conjugated bilirubin. This unconjugated bilirubin can then be reabsorbed into the circulation, adding to the total load of unconjugated bilirubin (enterohepatic circulation).

Physiologic Hyperbilirubinemia (Physiologic Jaundice)

This is a transient hyperbilirubinemia in the first week post delivery seen in most newborns (average 5–7 mg/dL). It is secondary to low levels of glucuronyl transferase and increased bilirubin load from an increased RBC volume with decreased survival, increased ineffective erythropoiesis, and enterohepatic circulation. Clinically, physiologic jaundice should (1) *not* present on day 1; (2) total bilirubin should rise by less than 5 mg/dL/d peaking at less than 12.9 mg/dL on days 3–4 (term infant) and 15 mg/dL on days 5–7 (preterm infant); (3) the conjugated fraction should be less than 2 mg/dL; and (4) jaundice should persist no longer than one week in the term infant and two weeks in the preterm infant.

Nonphysiologic Hyperbilirubinemia

If the diagnostic criteria for physiologic jaundice are not met, the cause of the jaundice must be investigated. Appropriate laboratory tests at this time include complete blood count (CBC), platelets, reticulocyte count, Coombs' test, and peripheral blood smear. Causes include:

A. Overproduction of bilirubin

1. Increased rate of hemolysis (increased unconjugated bilirubin and reticulocyte count).

a. Positive Coombs': Rh incompatibility, ABO incompatibility, other blood group sensitization.

b. Negative Coombs': RBC membrane defects (spherocytosis, elliptocytosis, pyknocytosis, stomatocytosis) and RBC enzyme defects (glucose-6-phosphate deficiency, pyruvate kinase deficiency, hexokinase deficiency).

2. Nonhemolytic causes (increased unconjugated bilirubin, normal reticulocyte count).

a. Extravascular hematoma: Cephalhematoma, bruising, CNS hemorrhage.

b. Polycythemia

c. Exaggerated enterohepatic circulation: GI obstruction, ileus.

B. Decreased rate of conjugation (increased unconjugated bilirubin, normal reticulocyte count)

1. Physiologic jaundice

2. Crigler-Najjar (type I glucuronyltransferase deficiency, autosomal recessive)

3. Type II glucuronyltransferase deficiency, autosomal dominant

4. Breast milk jaundice

C. Abnormalities of excretion or reabsorption (increased conjugated and unconjugated bilirubin, Coombs' negative, normal reticulocyte count)

1. Hepatitis (viral, bacterial, parasitic, toxic)

2. Metabolic (galactosemia, glycogen storage disease, cystic fibrosis, hypothyroidism)

3. Biliary atresia

4. Choledochal cyst

5. Obstruction of the ampulla of Vater

6. Sepsis

Bilirubin Toxicity

The importance of monitoring serum bilirubin is to prevent **kernicterus** (staining of the basal ganglia and hippocampus). Kernicterus occurs when unconjugated bilirubin enters nerve cells and produces cell death. Mortality is high. Clinical symptoms include lethargy, refusal to feed, high-pitched cry, hypertonicity, opisthotonos, seizures, and apnea. Sequelae include athetoid cerebral palsy, high-frequency hearing loss, paralysis of upward gaze, and dental dysplasia. The risk of kernicterus in a given infant is not well-defined for either term or premature infants. The only group in which a specific bilirubin level (20 mg/dL) has been associated with an increased risk of kernicterus is infants with Rh hemolytic disease. This observation was extended to the clinical management of all neonates, although no definitive data existed for these infants. The risk is likely negligible for term infants without hemolytic disease, even at levels > 25 mg/dL. Significant data for premature infants are not available. The clinician must rely on individualized clinical evaluation, including assessment of jaundice in light of prematurity.

Treatment

Two modalities are in use today for treatment of hyperbilirubinemia. In phototherapy, unconjugated bilirubin in the skin is converted to a water-soluble photoisomer and excreted in the bile and urine. The infant's eyes should be shielded and fluid administration should be increased to compensate for evaporative losses. Other side effects are loose stools, skin rashes, and problems with thermoregulation.

Guidelines for phototherapy are outlined in Table 7–11. In very immature babies, many centers institute prophylactic phototherapy. When phototherapy is not sufficient to bring about a significant decrease in serum bilirubin; or if the bilirubin level is at or approaching toxic ranges, double-volume exchange transfusions are used. As discussed above, it is difficult to specify a precise bilirubin level at which exchange transfusions should be performed. Well term infants are probably safe with levels as high as 25–30 mg/dL. In healthy preterm infants of more than 32 weeks, a level of 20 mg/dL can be used, whereas sick infants in this age range are usually exchanged at lower levels (15–18 mg/dL). In infants of less than 32 weeks, exchange transfusions are performed for levels of 12–15 mg/dL in most settings.

In addition, exchange transfusions are also used for other indications in the care of erythroblastic infants (Rh sensitization). A partial isovolemic exchange done with packed red cells (35 mL/kg) corrects the anemia and adjusts blood volume. An early double-volume exchange with whole blood will remove the sensitized cells in order to decrease the number of subsequent exchange transfusions to remove bilirubin. Indications for early double-volume exchange are cord hematocrit < 40% or bilirubin > 6.0 mg/dL.

Specific Causes of Hyperbilirubinemia

A. Breast milk jaundice: Breast milk jaundice is an unconjugated hyperbilirubinemia that peaks late (usually by days 6–14). The infant is well, and bilirubin levels are approximately 12–20 mg/dL. Breast milk jaundice can be distinguished from other causes by a prompt reduction in bilirubin upon substituting formula feeds for 1–2 days. This entity is to be distinguished from jaundice in the breast-fed infant during the first week post delivery. Breast-fed infants, when

Table 7–11. Management of hyperbilirubinemia in the healthy term newborn.[1]

	TSB Level, mg/dL (μmol/L)			
Age in hours	Consider phototherapy[2]	Phototherapy	Exchange transfusion if intensive phototherapy fails[3]	Exchange transfusion and intensive phototherapy
≤ 24[4]	...	...	...	...
25–48	≥12 (170)	≥15 (260)	≥20 (340)	≥25 (430)
49–72	≥15 (260)	≥18 (310)	≥25 (430)	≥30 (510)
> 72	≥17 (290)	≥20 (430)	≥25 (430)	≥30 (510)

[1] Modified from American Academy of Pediatrics. *Pracice Parameter: Management of Hyperbilirubinemia n the Healthy Term Newborn.* 1994.

[2] Phototherapy at these TSB levels is a clinical option, meaning that the intervention is available and may be used on the basis of individual clinical judgment.

[3] Intensive phototherapy should produce a decline of TSB of 1–2 mg/dl within 4–6 hours. The TSB level should continue to fall and remain below the threshold level for exchange transfusion. If this fall does not occur, it is considered a failure of phototherapy.

[4] Term infants who are clinically jaundiced at ≤ 24 hours old are not considered healthy and require further evaluation. Generally a bilirubin ≥ 10 on day 1 indicates phototherapy.

TSB = total serum bilirubin.

compared to formula-fed infants, have higher bilirubin levels due to decreased intake over the first several days of life. The treatment is not cessation of breast feeding, but increased frequency of feedings or provision of feeding supplements.

B. ABO incompatibility: ABO incompatibility is an indirect hyperbilirubinemia secondary to destruction of neonatal RBCs by maternal immunoglobulin G (IgG) which crosses the placenta into the fetal circulation (mother O, infant A or B). The infants may have both isolated anemia or jaundice, or neither. Since the amount of circulating IgG antibody varies, it is not possible to predict the severity of the process from one pregnancy to another.

C. Erythroblastosis: Erythroblastosis is caused by isoimmunization to Rh antigens (D, C, E, d, c, or e), Kell, Duffy, Lutheran, or Kidd. Most commonly, D antigen is involved. Fetal blood may enter the maternal circulation as an initiating event. The problem worsens with subsequent pregnancies. Clinically, some infants are more affected than others. The more severely affected infants will have **hydrops** (pleural effusions, ascites) secondary to intrauterine high output failure from anemia and hypoproteinemia. Less severe cases are characterized by hepatosplenomegaly, anemia, or jaundice. Administration of Rhogam (anti-D) to Rh-negative mothers can prevent most cases of erythroblastosis.

D. Extravascular hemorrhage: Extravascular hemorrhage within the body (eg, cephalhematoma, bruising, CNS hemorrhage) may result in an unconjugated hyperbilirubinemia secondary to a extra bilirubin load for the liver. The bilirubin/jaundice usually peaks at 3–4 days of age.

E. Gastrointestinal tract obstruction: GI tract obstruction (functional or structural) can result in unconjugated hyperbilirubinemia due to enhanced enterohepatic circulation of bilirubin.

INFECTION OF THE NEWBORN

A. Clinical Findings: There are three major routes of perinatal infection: (1) blood-borne transplacental infection of the fetus (eg, CMV, rubella, syphilis); (2) ascending infection with disruption of the barrier provided by the amniotic membranes (eg, bacterial infection after ruptured membranes); and (3) infection via passage through an infected birth canal or exposure to infected blood at delivery (eg, herpes simplex, hepatitis B infections).

Early-onset bacterial infections are related to perinatal risk factors and usually present on the first day post delivery. Symptoms include respiratory distress (most common), poor perfusion, and hypotension. Late-onset disease is more subtle and may present with poor feeding, lethargy, hypotonia, temperature instability, altered perfusion, new or increased oxygen requirement, and apnea. Laboratory findings may include an abnormal CBC (decreased total count, neutropenia, increased immature/mature neutrophil ratio, thrombocytopenia); hyperglycemia; elevated C-reactive protein (CRP); and an unexplained metabolic acidosis. Serum latex agglutination may be helpful in the diagnosis of Group B streptococcus. Urine latex agglutinations are also used but have a high incidence of false positives. Definitive diagnosis is made from positive blood and cerebrospinal fluid (CSF) cultures. Signs suggestive of congenital viral infection include small size for gestational age (symmetrical growth retardation), petechiae, jaundice, and hepatosplenomegaly. Specific neonatal infections are reviewed in Table 7–12.

B. Treatment: Guidelines for evaluation and management of term infants are listed in Table 7–13. Keep in mind that respiratory distress in a preterm neonate may also be evidence of infection. Preterm infants have a five-fold risk for infection compared to term infants. Blood cultures should be taken from all premature infants with respiratory distress. Empiric antibiotics should be given for 48–72 hours until cultures are negative. Infants with strong clinical signs of sepsis should have their CSF examined. Intravenous gamma globulin (500–750 mg/kg) may be given to infants with known or clinically suspect infections.

C. Prognosis: The prognosis for neonatal infection depends on the specific agent and type of infection.

DISORDERS OF THE GASTROINTESTINAL SYSTEM

Tracheoesophageal Fistula/Esophageal Atresia

A. Clinical Findings: Tracheoesophageal fistula (TEF) and esophageal atresia consist of a blind esophageal pouch with a fistulous connection between either the proximal or distal esophagus and airway. There is often a maternal history of polyhydramnios and infant history of copious secretions, choking, cyanosis and respiratory distress. CXR following placement of a nasogastric tube will show the tube in the blind proximal pouch. If a TEF is present to the distal esophagus, gas will be present in the abdomen.

B. Treatment: Surgery provides the definitive therapy. It may be staged if initial reanastomosis of esophageal ends is not possible. A gastrostomy may also be performed until reanastomosis heals. Prior to surgery, the goal is to minimize aspiration of gastric fluid through the fistula into the lungs. The infant should be supported with IV fluids and glucose, elevation of the head of the bed, and placement of a nasogastric tube in the proximal pouch attached to continuous suction.

C. Prognosis: Prognosis is determined primarily by the presence or absence of associated anomalies (vertebral, cardiac, limb, and anal).

Obstructive Lesions

A. Clinical Findings: Obstructive lesions are classified as high or low based on their location with respect to the ligament of Treitz. Clinical findings suggestive of high obstruction include a maternal history of polyhydramnios and early onset of emesis, often bilious (Table 7–14).

Distal obstructions present with increasing intolerance of feeds, abdominal distension and decreased or absent stooling. Imperforate anus should be ruled out early as it is often missed on cursory examination. Other causes of distal obstruction include meconium ileus, Hirschsprung's disease, meconium plug, small left colon, and ileal and colonic atresia. Plain films will show gaseous distension with air through a considerable portion of the bowel and air fluid levels. Meconium ileus or plug and small left colon are diagnosed by contrast enema. Contrast enema and rectal biopsy are used to diagnose Hirschsprung's disease (Chapter 17).

B. Treatment: Definitive treatment is surgical, with the exception of meconium plug and small left colon. Prior to surgery, infants should be treated with nasogastric suction and administration of IV fluids.

C. Prognosis: Most lesions carry a good prognosis. Ten percent of infants with meconium plug will have cystic fibrosis (CF), while all infants with meconium ileus will have CF. Imperforate anus is associated with other anomalies (vertebral, renal, cardiac, limb). Duodenal atresia is associated with trisomy 21. Otherwise, most of these infants do well after surgical repair.

Abdominal Wall Defects

Omphaloceles are formed by incomplete closure of the anterior abdominal wall after the return of midgut to the abdominal cavity.

Table 7–12. Characteristics of specific neonatal infections.

Infection	Etiologies	Clinical Tips	Treatment
Bacterial sepsis	GBS, Gram-negative enteric (*E coli*), *S aureus, L monocytogenes, Enterococcus, S epidermidis*	Early onset: shock, pneumonia; late onset: meningitis, local infection. Maternal diarrhea may be associated with listeria. *S epidermidis* is increased with indwelling lines	Ampicillin plus aminoglycoside or third-generation cephalosporin. Vancomycin for *S epidermidis*. Duration of therapy 10–14 d
Fungal sepsis	*C albicans*	High-risk group; VLBW infants with indwelling lines	Amphotericin B, flucytosine
Meningitis	GBS, gram-negative enterics, viral (enterovirus)	High-risk group; infants with bacterial sepsis	Appropriate antibiotics for 21 d
Pneumonia	Bacterial, viral (CMV, RSV, adenovirus, influenza, parainfluenza), *Ureaplasma, Mycoplasma, Chlamydia*	Infection in utero or upon passage through birth canal. Older neonates: look for new onset respiratory distress or an increase in FiO_2 on ventilator settings in infants receiving respiratory support	Specific therapy when known. Ventilatory support as needed
Urinary tract infection	Gram-negative enterics	Uncommon early-onset infection; usually associated with GU anomalies. Obtain urine culture by aspiration or catheterization	Treat 10–14 d. Evaluate for GU anomalies
Osteomyelitis	GBS, *S aureus*	Uncommon in neonates. Usually late-onset disease	See chapter 21
Otitis	Usual bacterial agents, gram-negatives	Gram-negatives more common in long-term patients. Seen with increased incidence in infants with prolonged endotracheal intubation	Appropriate antibiotics
Omphalitis	Group A strep, *S aureus,* gram-negatives	Some degree of purulent material at the base of cord is common. Diagnosis requires erythema, edema of surrounding soft tissues.	Broad-spectrum antibiotics

Congenital viral infection	CMV	Most common transmitted in utero virus. Clinical disease: SGA, hepatosplenomegaly, petechiae, thrombocytopenia, increased conjugated bilirubin. Mortality 20% with symptomatic CMV, sequelae in 90% of survivors and 5–15% asymptomatic infants. Sequelae: hearing loss, mental retardation, delayed motor development, chorioretinitis, optic atrophy, seizures, language delay, learning disabilities. Fetal/neonatal infection increased with primary maternal infection. Diagnosis: Viral cultures (blood, CSF, urine, throat, placenta, amniotic fluid)	Ganciclovir, CMV immune globulin
	Rubella	80% of fetal infection during 1st trimester. Clinical syndrome: adenopathy, bone radiolucencies, encephalitis, cardiac defects, cataracts, retinopathy, IUGR, hepatosplenomegaly, thrombocytopenia, purpura. Sequelae: mental retardation, hearing loss. Diagnosis: Compare infant and maternal IgG; specific IgM in infant. Cultures of pharyngeal secretions	Supportive therapy. Prevention: Prenatal immunization for mother
	Varicella	Congenital infection (1st/2nd trimester) rare. Findings: limb hypoplasia, cutaneous scars, microcephaly, cortical atrophy, cataracts, chorioretinitis. Perinatal exposure (5 days before to 2 days after delivery) causes severe-fatal disseminated varicella. Diagnosis: Rise in maternal IgG. IgM in infant. Culture vesicles	Prevention: VZIG to baby in perinatal period. Can treat illness with acyclovir

(*continued*)

Table 7–12. Characteristics of specific neonatal infections (*continued*).

Infection	Etiologies	Clinical Tips	Treatment
	Parvovirus B19 (Erythema infectiosum, Fifth Disease)	Most often manifested as mild systemic symptoms, fever, distinctive rash. Infection during pregnancy can cause fetal hydrops and death	Supportive
Parasitic	Toxoplasmosis (*Toxoplasma gondii*)	Congenital infection (1st/2nd trimester). 40% children infected (15% severe clinical damage). Exposure to cat feces, raw meat. Sequelae: IUGR, chorioretinitis, seizures, jaundice, hydrocephalus, microcephaly, hepatosplenomegaly, adenopathy, cataracts, thrombocytopenia, pneumonia. Diagnosis: IgG serologies in mother. IgM in infants	Can potentially treat known cases transplacentally by treating mother
Perinatal acquired	Herpes simplex	Usually acquired through passage birth canal. Primary maternal infection carries higher risk to infant. reactivated disease. Risk likely low to infant with reactivated disease. Local/disseminated disease (onset 5–14 days). 70% may present with local skin or oral vesicles. Progression of disease common. Disseminated: pneumonia, shock, hepatitis. CNS (onset 14–28 days). Lethargy, instability, seizures. Diagnosis: Viral cultures	Acyclovir prevents progres sion of local disease. Decreases mortality with disseminated and CNS disease
	Hepatitis B	Screen mothers with HbsAg. Clinical illness rare at birth. Exposed infants at risk to be chronic carriers	Maternal HbsAg positive-HBIG at birth followed by vaccination. Vaccine now recommended for all newborns

	Enterovirus	Late summer/fall: maternal illness (fever, diarrhea, rash) in week prior to delivery. Infant: fever, rash, diarrhea, lethargy. May be more severe with meningoencephalitis, myocarditis, hepatitis, pneumonia, shock DIC. Diagnosis: Viral cultures (rectal, CSF, blood)	No therapy. Prognosis good except for disseminated disease
	Human immunodeficiency virus (HIV)	Clinical features: IUGR, microcephaly, prominent forehead, flattened nasal bridge, prominence of eyes, blue sclera, hypertelorism, long philtrum, patulous lips. May be transplacental or perinatal. Majority of infected infants present < 2 yrs	Prenatal therapy of mother with AZT decreases transmission to fetus
Other congenital dseases	Syphilis (*T pallidum*)	Transplancental infection. Symptoms: mucocutaneous lesions, lymphadenopathy, hepatitis, bony changes, hydrops. Diagnosis: Darkfield identification of organism. Presumptive: rising serologies (VDRL); FTA-IgM. CSF exam	IV/IM PCN 10–14 days
	Tuberculosis	Congenital form rare (mother with hematogenous spread). Women with pulmonary form infect infant after delivery	Mother with positive skin and neg CXR: treat mother with INH and follow infant with skin tests. Mother with active disease requires separation from infant until mother no longer contagious. Follow with skin tests

(*continued*)

Table 7–12. Characteristics of specific neonatal infections (*continued*).

Infection	Etiologies	Clinical Tips	Treatment
Conjunctivitis	*Neisseria gonorrhoeae*	Onset 3–7 days. Gram-negative intracellular diplococci on Gram's stain	Ceftriaxone or Cefotaxime
	Chlamydia	Onset 5 days to several wks. Congestion, edema, and discharge	PO erythromycin

CMV = cytomegalovirus; CNS = central nervous system; CSF = cerebrospinal fluid; CXR = chest x-ray; DIC = disseminated intravascular coagulation; FTA = fluorescent treponemal antibody; GBS = Group B streptococcus; GU = genitourinary; INH = isoniazid; IUGR = intra-uterine gestational retardation; RSV = respiratory syncytial virus; SGA = small for gestational age; VDRL = venereal disease research laboratory test; VLBW = very low birth weight; VZIG = varicella zoster immune globulin.

Table 7–13. Management of bacterial infection in the term infant.

Risk Factor	Clinical Signs[1]	Evaluation and Treatment
12–18 h rupture of membranes	None	Observation
> 12–18 h rupture of membranes; chorioamnionitis ± maternal antibiotics	None	CBC, CSF and blood cultures, 48–72 hr broad-spectrum antibiotics
None or any of the above	Present	CBC, CSF and blood culture, ± urine culture, broad-spectrum antibiotics[2]

CBC = complete blood count; CSF = cerebrospinal fluid.

[1] In any infant without signs consistent with infection, it is reasonable simply to observe without treatment, provided close observation is possible.

[2] Any infant, irrespective of age of presentation, who appears infected by clinical criteria should have a CSF examination. Urine culture is indicated in the evaluation of infants who were initially well and develop symptoms after 2–3 days in the nursery.

The defect is usually covered by a sac, with the umbilical cord inserted into the center of the defect. The size of the defect varies but may contain intestine, stomach, liver, and spleen. There is a high incidence of associated anomalies including cardiac, other gastrointestinal, and chromosomal anomalies. Acute therapy includes covering the defect with sterile warm saline dressings to prevent fluid loss, nasogastric decompression, IV fluids and glucose. Definitive therapy is surgery.

Gastroschisis is a defect in the anterior abdominal wall lateral to the umbilicus. There is no covering sac, and herniated viscera are lim-

Table 7–14. High intestinal obstruction in the neonate.

Lesion	Clinical Tips
Duodenal atresia	Non-bilious emesis. Abdominal x-ray will show double bubble (stomach/dilated duodenum). May be associated with trisomy 21.
Malrotation with volvulus	Bilious emesis. Abdominal x-ray often needs to be supplemented with contrast studies for diagnosis (contrast enema looking for location of caecum or upper GI study). PROMPT surgical repair necessary to prevent ischemic damage from torsion of intestine and superior mesenteric artery.
High jejunal atresia	Bilious emesis. Diagnosis confirmed with upper GI.

ited to the intestines. The underlying cause may be an infarct to the abdominal wall. Other than intestinal atresia, associated anomalies are uncommon. Acute therapy is the same as for omphalocele. Definitive therapy is surgical.

Diaphragmatic Hernia

Diaphragmatic hernia is a herniation of abdominal organs into the hemithorax, usually the left, and is caused by a defect in the posterior lateral diaphragm. Infants present in the delivery room with respiratory distress, cyanosis, decreased breath sounds on the side of the hernia, and shift of the mediastinum to the opposite side of the hernia. Definitive repair is surgical but infants often require extensive resuscitation including intubation and nasogastric decompression. Postoperative course is often complicated by PPHN.

Acquired Conditions

Necrotizing enterocolitis (NEC) is the most commonly seen acquired GI emergency in the newborn period, usually affecting premature infants. The pathogenesis is multifactorial and is related to previous ischemic episodes, bacterial or viral infection, and immunologic immaturity of the premature GI tract.

A. Clinical Findings: The primary presenting sign is abdominal distension with or without associated vomiting, increased gastric residua, heme positive stool, abdominal tenderness, temperature instability, increased apnea and bradycardia, decreased urine output, and poor perfusion. CBC may show increased WBC with bandemia and decreased platelets. Diagnosis is confirmed by the presence of pneumatosis intestinalis (air in bowel wall on x-ray).

B. Treatment: Surgery is required if evidence of necrotic bowel (perforation with free air on x-ray, fixed dilated loop on serial films, abdominal wall cellulitis, progressive deterioration) is present. Otherwise, medical management consisting of nasogastric decompression, IV fluids (TPN), bowel rest (NPO), and systemic antibiotics is usually sufficient in 75% of cases. Infants should not be refed until the disease is resolved, examination of the abdomen is normal, and x-ray reveals resolution of pneumatosis. Resolution usually takes 10–14 days.

C. Prognosis: The mortality rate is 10%. Long-term prognosis is usually good in cases that respond to medical management. Complications include stricture at 6–8 weeks after initial onset. Long-term surgical prognosis depends on the amount of intestine lost. Infants with resultant short gut often require prolonged hospitalization.

DISEASES OF THE BLOOD/HEMATOPOIETIC SYSTEM

Bleeding Disorders

A. Clinical Findings: Bleeding in newborns may result from physiologic deficiencies of coagulation factors (inherited or acquired), influences of maternal disease or drugs, immaturity of blood vessels, vulnerability to birth trauma, and other conditions associated with bleeding (eg, sepsis and asphyxia). The common neonatal bleeding disorders are disseminated intravascular coagulation (DIC), hemorrhagic disease of the newborn (HDN) due to vitamin K deficiency, platelet disorders including thrombocytopenia, and inherited deficiencies of coagulation factors. The differential diagnosis of bleeding in neonates is presented in Table 7–15. Conditions associated with DIC are presented in Table 7–16 and the differential diagnosis of thrombocytopenia (platelet count < 150,000) in Table 7–17.

B. Treatment: Treatment for DIC includes replacement of depleted coagulation factors and identification of the underlying cause. HDN is treated with Vitamin K 1 mg IM or IV. Thrombocytopenia is treated by 10 mL/kg of platelets. Indication for transfusion in the term infant is clinical bleeding or a total count lower than 10,000–20,000/μL. In the preterm infant at risk for intraventricular hemorrhage, transfusion is indicated for counts lower than 40–50,000/μL. Isoimmune thrombocytopenia requires transfusion of maternal platelets. Infants born to mothers with ITP may benefit from intravenous immunoglobulin and corticosteroids.

Anemia

A. Clinical Findings: Anemia can be caused by hemorrhage, hemolysis, or failure of RBC production. Evaluation of anemia includes: (1) clinical assessment for signs of acute blood loss; and (2) laboratory evaluation consisting of CBC, peripheral smear, reticulocyte count, and direct and indirect Coombs' tests. Anemia in the first 24–48 hours of life is due to hemorrhage or hemolysis. Kleihauer-Betke on maternal blood should be performed when a fetomaternal bleed is suspected.

Hemorrhage can occur in utero (fetoplacental, fetomaternal, twin-twin); perinatally (cord rupture, placenta previa, placental incision at C-section); or internally (intracranial, rupture of liver or spleen). Infants with chronic blood loss (eg, fetomaternal) will be pale at birth but will compensate without signs of volume loss. Initial hematocrit will be low. Acute bleeding will present with hypovolemia (tachycardia, poor perfusion, hypotension) and a normal or low initial

Table 7–15. Clinical and laboratory approach to the differential diagnosis of bleeding in the neonate.[1]

Laboratory Investigations			
Platelets	Prothrombin Time	Partial Thromboplastin Time	Possible Diagnosis
Sick Neonates			
Decreased	Increased	Increased	Disseminated intravascular coagulation
Decreased	Normal	Normal	Platelet-consumption (infection, necrotizing enterocolitis, renal-vein thrombosis)
Normal	Increased	Increased	Liver disease, heparinization
Normal	Normal	Normal	Altered vascular integrity (eg, extreme prematurity, severe hypoxia and acidosis, hyperosmolality)
Healthy Neonates			
Decreased	Normal	Normal	Immune thrombocytopenia, occult infection or thrombosis, bone marrow hypoplasia (rare), leukemia (rare)
Normal	Increased	Increased	Hemorrhagic disease of newborn (vitamin K deficiency)
Normal	Normal	Increased	Hereditary clotting factor deficiencies
Normal	Normal	Normal	Bleeding due to local factors (trauma, anatomic abnormalities), qualitative platelet abnormalities (rare), factor XIII deficiency (rare): disrupted vessel from anatomical lesion (eg, ulcer, hemangioma), swallowed maternal blood

[1]Modified from Pramanik AK: Bleeding disorders in neonates. Pediatr Rev 1992;13:5.

Table 7–16. Clinical conditions in the sick bleeding neonate associated with disseminated intravascular coagulation.[1]

Obstetric Complications	Neonatal Infections	Miscellaneous Conditions
Abruptio placentae	Bacterial (gram-positive and gram-negative organisms)	Respiratory distress syndrome (severe)
Preeclampsia and eclampsia	Toxoplasmosis	Severe erythroblastosis fetalis
Dead twin fetus	Syphilis	Giant hemangioma
Fetal distress	Rubella	Renal-vein thrombosis
Amniotic fluid embolism	Cytomegalovirus	Severe hypoxia and acidosis
Complicated breech extraction	Herpes, hepatitis	Prolonged indwelling vascular catheter
	Other viral infections	

[1]Modified from Pramanik AK: Bleeding disorders in neonates. Pediatr Rev 1992;13:5.

Table 7–17. Differential diagnosis of neonatal thrombocytopenia.

Disorder	Clinical Tips
Immune	
passively acquired antibody (ITP, SLE, drug-induced)	proper history, maternal thrombocytopenia
isoimmune sensitization to PLA-1 antigen	positive antiplatelet antibodies in baby's serum, sustained rise in platelets by transfusion of mother's platelets
Infections	
bacterial	sick infants with other signs consistent with infections
congenital viral infections	
Syndromes	
absent radii	
Fanconi's anemia	congenital anomalies, also associated with pancytopenia
DIC	sick infants, abnormalities of clotting factors
Giant hemangioma	
Thrombosis	infants with hyperviscous blood, vascular catheters
high-risk infant with RDS, pulmonary hypertension, etc.	isolated decrease in platelets is not uncommon in sick infants even in the absence of DIC

DIC = disseminated intravascular coagulation; ITP = idiopathic thrombocytopenic purpura; RDS = respiratory distress syndrome; SLE = systemic lupus erythematosus.

hematocrit. Hemolysis is caused by blood group incompatibility, enzyme/membrane abnormalities, infection, and DIC.

B. Treatment: Acute treatment is provision of volume (10–20 mL/kg) as 5% albumin, normal saline (NS), or with whole blood to restore normovolemia. Later treatment with packed red cells is indicated for symptomatic anemia.

Anemia in the Premature Infant

Anemia of prematurity is due to decreased erythropoietin production in response to a low red cell m procedures in sick neonates. Symptoms include poor feeding, lethargy, tachycardia, poor weight gain, and apnea. Transfusion may be indicated if an infant is symptomatic (usually occurs with a hematocrit < 25%). Recent studies of exogenous erythropoietin (Epoetin alfa) [250 IU/kg SC three times per week] administration suggest that this treatment may decrease but not obviate the need for transfusions in premature infants. Adequate supplemental iron must be given as well (4–8 mg/kg/d).

Supplemental iron should be started in premature infants at 2 months of age to prevent iron deficiency anemia.

Polycythemia

A. Clinical Findings: Polycythemia occurs in 2–5% of live births. Causes include twin-twin transfusion, maternal-fetal transfusion, intrapartum transfusion from the placenta associated with fetal distress, and chronic intrauterine hypoxia. The consequence is hyperviscosity which decreases effective perfusion of capillary beds in the microcirculation. Clinical consequences can affect any organ system; they are summarized in Table 7–18. Venous hematocrits > 70% at less than 12 hours of age and 65% after 12 hours of age should be considered indicative of hyperviscosity.

B. Treatment: Treatment with partial exchange transfusion is recommended for symptomatic infants; treatment of asymptomatic infants based on the hematocrit alone is controversial. Albumin (5%) is transfused over a constant rate through a peripheral IV while blood is removed through an umbilical venous line. The exchange volume can be calculated from the following equation, when the desired hematocrit is 50–55% and blood volume is 80 mL/kg.

$$\frac{\text{Peripheral venous Hct} - \text{Desired Hct}}{\text{Peripheral venous Hct}} \times \text{blood volume/kg} \times \text{body weight}$$

Table 7–18. Organ-related symptoms of hyperviscosity.

Central nervous system	Irritability, jitteriness, seizures, lethargy
Cardiopulmonary	Respiratory distress secondary to congestive heart failure or persistent pulmonary hypertension
Gastrointestinal	Vomiting, heme-positive stools, distension, NEC
Renal	Decreased urine output, renal vein thrombosis
Metabolic	Hypoglycemia
Hematologic	Hyperbilirubinemia, thrombocytopenia

NEC = necrotizing enterocolitis.

C. Prognosis: Follow-up studies at 1–2 years have revealed that infants with hyperviscosity have more frequent motor problems, more neurologic abnormalities, and delayed speech development. At 7 years of age, some subtle findings persist. Whether this outcome can be improved by treatment is unclear.

METABOLIC DISORDERS

Hypoglycemia

Hypoglycemia in neonates is defined as blood glucose lower than 40 mg/dL. Although glucose concentration normally decreases in all infants during the postpartum period, most term babies have stable glucose concentrations (50–80 mg/dL) by 3 hrs post delivery. Two high-risk groups for hypoglycemia are infants of diabetic mothers (IDMs) and infants with intrauterine growth retardation (IUGR).

In IDMs, hypoglycemia develops because of an imbalance in insulin-glucagon secretion due to hyperinsulinemia from islet cell hyperplasia. These infants are macrosomic because other sites grow abnormally in utero secondary to an increased flow of nutrients. They may also have asymmetric septal cardiac hypertrophy, small left colon, hypercoagulability, and polycythemia. As these infants are immature for gestational age, there is an increased risk for HMD, hypocalcemia, and hyperbilirubinemia. IDMs are also at increased risk for congenital anomalies likely related to first-trimester glucose control.

Intrauterine growth-retarded infants have appropriate endocrine control but low carbohydrate stores in the form of glycogen. Other causes of hypoglycemia include other disorders with increased islet cell hyperplasia (Beckwith-Wiedemann, nesidioblastosis, erythroblas-

Table 17–19. Hypoglycemia: Suggested therapeutic regimens.

Screening Test	Presence of Symptoms	Action
Test strip 20–40 mg/dL	None	Confirm with blood glucose; if the infant is alert and vigorous, feed; follow frequent test strips. If the baby continues after 1 or 2 feeds to have test strips < 40 mg/dL, provide intravenous glucose at 6 mg/g/min.
Test strip < 40 mg/dL	Present	Confirm with blood glucose; provide bolus (2 cc/kg) of $D_{10}W$ followed by an infusion of 6 mg/kg/min.
Test strip < 20 mg/dL	±	Confirm with blood glucose; provide bolus (2 mL/kg) of $D_{10}W$ followed by an infusion of 6 mg/kg/min. If IV access cannot be obtained immediately, an umbilical venous line should be utilized.

tosis fetalis); inborn errors (leucine sensitivity, glycogen storage diseases, galactosemia); and endocrine disorders (panhypopituitarism). Hypoglycemia may also be associated with birth asphyxia and sepsis.

A. Clinical Findings: Symptoms may be nonspecific and include lethargy, irritability, poor feeding, and regurgitation. More severe symptoms include cardiorespiratory distress, apnea and seizures. Catecholamine-related symptoms may be present, such as pallor, sweating, cold extremities and increased heart rate. Hypoglycemia may be detected by commercially available test strips, although these may be unreliable with glucose levels lower than 40 mg/dL. All low glucose levels should be supplemented by direct measurement with a glucose analyzer.

B. Treatment: A treatment regimen is outlined in Table 7–19.

C. Prognosis: Prompt treatment improves prognosis. CNS sequelae occur with hypoglycemic seizures.

Hypocalcemia

Hypocalcemia is defined as a total serum concentration lower than 7 mg/dL (equivalent to calcium activity of 3.5 meq/L). Early-onset hypocalcemia (day 1–2) is seen in IDMs and cases of sepsis, asphyxia, prematurity and maternal hyperparathyroidism. Late-onset hypocalcemia (1–2 weeks of age) is seen in infants receiving modified cow's milk with high phosphorus content.

A. Clinical Findings: Clinical signs include a high-pitched cry, jitteriness, tremulousness, and seizures.

B. Treatment: Calcium gluconate (0.5–1 g/kg/d) may be given orally (45–90 mg/kg elemental calcium). It is administered IV for symptomatic hypocalcemia. Cautious IV use is necessary to prevent the right atrial calcium concentration rising too quickly causing bradycardia. Close observation for tissue infiltrates is important. The dosage is 10% calcium gluconate as a 1–2 mL/kg bolus over 10–20 minutes followed by a continuous infusion of 0.5–1 gm/kg/d. Do not add calcium salts to IV solutions with sodium bicarbonate as they will precipitate.

C. Prognosis: Prognosis is good.

INFANTS OF MOTHERS WITH DRUG ABUSE

Drug abuse continues to be a serious problem across the United States. A full maternal history of drug consumption is often difficult to obtain but must be pursued. Withdrawal symptoms in neonates are common with many drugs, narcotics and alcohol being most prominent. Treatment protocols are outlined in Table 7–20.

RENAL DISORDERS

Renal function is dependent on postconceptional age. Normal renal function and test values are presented in Table 7–21. Normal urine output is 1–3 mL/kg/hr.

The most common disorders seen in newborns are (1) renal failure, (2) renal vein thrombosis (RVT), and (3) congenital anomalies.

Renal Failure

A. Clinical Findings: Renal failure is often seen following an asphyxial episode, hypovolemia, or sepsis. Two phases are present: (1) anuria/oliguria (first 2–3 days) associated with hematuria, proteinuria, and increased creatinine; and (2) polyuria with increased urine losses of sodium and bicarbonate.

B. Treatment: The initial step is fluid resuscitation if necessary followed by fluid restriction equal to insensible water losses (40–60 mL/kg/d) plus urine losses. The infant must be monitored for hyperkalemia in the presence of oliguria/anuria. During the polyuric phase, infants should be allowed to diurese if they are fluid-overloaded, provided that water, salt, and acid-base balance are carefully followed.

Table 7–20. Drugs commonly abused during pregnancy.

Drug	Clinical Tips	Treatment and Prognosis
Narcotics (heroin, methadone, propoxyphene, codeine)	Heroin/methadone withdrawal similar with methadone having longer duration. Early-onset 1–2 d, although methadone withdrawal may be delayed. Symptoms: irritability, hyperactivity, tremors, high-pitched cry, excessive hunger, salivation, sweating, sneezing, yawning, nasal stuffiness, tachypnea, diarrhea, and seizures.	Supportive care (quiet environment, swaddling) usually sufficient. Medical control: phenobarbital (loading dose 15–20 mg/kg load with maintenance dose 5 mg/kg divided BID) Valium, paregoric. Prognosis good but mortality can occur in severe cases. Increased incidence of sudden infant death syndrome
Ethanol	Fetal/newborn effects proportional to amount consumed. Effects: IUGR, dysmorphic features (short palpebral fissures, microcephaly), cardiac and joint anomalies; withdrawal similar to narcotics.	Treat as in narcotic withdrawal. Postnatal growth may be slow, mental retardation, hyperactivity in severe cases
Nicotine	IUGR	Education of mother important
Cocaine	Abruptio placentae and CNS infarct to infant may occur secondary to vasoconstrictive properties of drug. Increased incidence of GU anomalies.	Screen infant for metabolites with suspected maternal history. Close observation, no specific therapy

BID = bis in die (twice daily); CNS = central nervous system; GU = genitourinary; IUGR = intra-uterine growth retardation

Table 7–21. Summary of neonatal renal function.

Function	Premature	Full-term	2 wk	8 wk	1 yr
Glomerular filtration (mL/min/1.73 m^2)	13–58	15–60	50	63–80	120
Concentrating ability (mOsm/L)	480	800	900	1200	1400
Urine volume (mL/24 h)	24–72/kg	15–60/kg	250–400	250–400	500–600
Tests	**Gestational Age**				
Creatinine (mg/dL)	< 28 wk	29–32 wk	33–36 wk	36–42 wk	
0–2 d	1.2	1.1	1.1	0.8	
28 d	0.7	0.6	0.45	0.3	

Renal Vein Thrombosis (RVT)

RVT is seen most frequently in IDMs and infants with dehydration and polycythemia. Clinically, it may be suspected on the basis of new renal mass (usually unilateral), hematuria, and proteinuria. Anuria may be present if RVT is bilateral. Diagnosis can be confirmed with renal ultrasonography. Treatment involves correction of the predisposing condition and heparinization. Systemic hypertension has been noted in some infants.

Congenital Anomalies

Abdominal masses in the newborn are most frequently due to renal enlargement: multicystic/dysplastic kidney and hydronephrosis. Anomalies might also be suspected on basis of maternal history of oligohydramnios which can be associated with renal agenesis or posterior urethral valves. Diagnosis in most cases is aided by renal ultrasonography.

BRAIN & NEUROLOGIC DISORDERS

Hypoxic Ischemic Encephalopathy

Hypoxic ischemic encephalopathy (HIE) occurs in both preterm and term infants. It is often associated with intraventricular hemorrhage in the preterm infant.

A. Clinical Findings: Infants with evidence of fetal distress before and during labor are at risk for HIE. Clinical features include: (1) birth to 12 hours: decreased level of consciousness, hypotonia, decreased spontaneous movement, periodic breathing or apnea, possible seizures; (2) 12–24 hours: seizures, apnea, jitteriness, weakness; (3) over 24 hrs: decreased level of consciousness, progressive apnea, onset of brain stem dysfunction, hypotonia, poor feeding.

The severity and duration of clinical signs correlate with the severity of insult. Other helpful diagnostic tools include electroencephalography, computed tomography (CT scan), evoked potentials, and magnetic resonance imaging (MRI).

B. Treatment: The mainstay of therapy is to provide adequate oxygen to the injured brain with normal PaO_2 and blood pressure. Fluids may be modestly restricted, glucose normalized, and anticonvulsants given for seizures.

C. Prognosis: The best predictor of outcome is the severity of clinical encephalopathy; severe symptoms are correlated with a 75% chance of death and 100% rate of neurologic sequelae. The major sequelae in survivors are cerebral palsy and mental retardation.

Intracranial Bleeding

A. Subdural hemorrhage: Subdural bleeding is usually related to birth trauma and occurs in three locations (tentorial laceration, falx laceration, rupture of superficial cerebral veins). The major complication in the first two types is extension of bleeding infratentorially, causing brain stem compression requiring immediate surgical drainage. Bleeds in the third location are the most common and may be asymptomatic or cause seizures on days 2–3. Diagnosis can be confirmed with CT scan or MRI. The prognosis is poor for bleeding in the first two locations; 75% of infants with bleeding of the third type have normal follow-up.

B. Subarachnoid hemorrhage: Subarachnoid bleeding is the most common type of hemorrhage. In premature infants, it is associated with germinal matrix bleed and in term infants with birth trauma. The most common presentation is with seizures and irritability on the second day post delivery. Diagnosis is aided by CT scan and lumbar puncture. The prognosis is good.

C. Periventricular/intraventricular hemorrhage: Intraventricular hemorrhage is seen almost exclusively in premature infants. The incidence is 25–35% in infants less than 31 weeks and weighing less than 1500 grams. Other risk factors include birth asphyxia, severe respiratory distress and pneumothorax. Bleeding is most commonly seen in the subependymal germinal matrix but may extend into the ventricular cavity. Primary parenchymal hemorrhages can be seen as well. Fifty percent of bleeds occur by 24 hours of age and the vast majority by 4 days. Clinically, these bleeds range from asymptomatic to rapid-catastrophic presentations (coma, hypoventilation, acidosis, shock, drop in hematocrit). Diagnosis is made by real-time ultrasonography. The grading system is as follows:

- Grade I: germinal matrix bleed only
- Grade II: intraventricular bleed without enlargement of the ventricles
- Grade III: intraventricular bleed with enlargement of the ventricles
- Grade IV: any of the above plus intracerebral hemorrhage.

The majority of bleeds that occur (> 60%) are small (Grades I and II). Routine screening is at 4–7 days in infants less than 31 weeks or any sick infant between 31 and 35 weeks. Follow-up for grades I/II should be done at 2 weeks of age; for grades III/IV within one week of initial screen. Further follow-ups are dictated by progression of ventricular enlargement. The clinician should also seek evidence of periventricular leukomalacia (cystic changes in periventricular white matter) which is usually evident by 1 month of age.

1. Treatment: Initial treatment should be based on the infant's status. The more severely affected may require volume resuscitation, transfusion, and increased ventilatory support. If progressive post-hemorrhagic hydrocephalus develops, it can be controlled by decreasing CSF production (Lasix 1 mg/kg/d plus Diamox, increasing doses from 25–100 mg/kg/d) or by removal of CSF with daily lumbar puncture.

2. Prognosis: There is no mortality with grade I/II bleeds, while grades III/IV carry a 10–20% mortality risk. Ventriculomegaly is rare with grade I, but is found in 54–87% of cases in grades II–IV. Long-term neurologic risk in grades I/II is no different from that for other premature infants who experience no bleeding. With grades III/IV, severe sequelae occur in 20–25%, mild in 35%. The major long-term sequelae include hydrocephalus, cerebral palsy, and mental retardation.

Seizures

Organized tonic-clonic seizures in infants are rare due to incomplete cortical organization and a preponderance of inhibitory synapses. The most common type of seizure is characterized by a constellation of findings including horizontal deviation of eyes with blinking or fluttering; sucking, smacking, or drooling; swimming, rowing or paddling movements; and apneic spells. The clinician may also see strictly tonic or multifocal clonic episodes. The differential diagnosis of neonatal seizures is outlined in Table 7–22.

Table 7–22. Differential diagnosis of neonatal seizures.

Diagnosis	Comment
Hypoxic-ischemic encephalopathy	Most common etiology (60%); onset first 24 h
Intracranial hemorrhage	Up to 15% of cases: PVH/IVH, subdural, or subarachnoid bleeds
Infection	12% of cases
Hypoglycemia	SGA, IDM
Hypocalcemia, hypomagnesemia	Low-birth-weight infant, IDMs
Hyponatremia	Rare, seen with SIADH
Disorders of amino and organic acid metabolism, hyperammonemia	Associated acidosis, altered level of consciousness
Pyridoxine dependency	Seizures refractory to routine therapy; cessation of seizures after administration of pyridoxine
Developmental defects	Other anomalies, chromosomal syndromes
Drug withdrawal	—
No cause found	10% of cases

IDM = infant of diabetic mother; PVH/IVH = periventricular hemorrhage/intraventricular hemorrhage; SGA = small for gestational age; SIADH = syndrome of inappropriate secretion of antidiuretic hormone

A. Treatment: Supportive therapy to assure adequate ventilation and perfusion should be provided. Hypoglycemia should be promptly treated; other therapy is directed towards specific underlying causes. Phenobarbital (20 mg/kg as a loading dose with supplemental doses of 5 mg/kg/d up to 40 mg/kg) can be given. If seizures persist, therapy with dilantin, sodium valproate,and lorazepam may be tried. A trial of pyridoxine for refractory seizures is indicated.

B. Prognosis: Prognosis is related to the cause of the seizures; the more difficult to control, the worse the prognosis. Seizures due to hypoglycemia and CNS infection, some inborn errors of metabolism and developmental defects also have a high rate of poor outcome.

REFERENCES

American Academy of Pediatrics/American Heart Association. *Textbook of Neonatal Resuscitation*, 1994.

American Academy of Pediatrics/American College of Obstetricians and Gynecologists. *Guidelines for Perinatal Care.* 3rd ed, 1992.

Avery GB, Fletcher MA, MacDonald MG (editors): *Neonatology: Pathophysiology and Management of the Newborn*, 4th ed. Lippincott, 1994.

Battaglia FC, Meschia G: *An Introduction to Fetal Physiology.* Academic Press, 1988.

Briggs GG, Freeman RK, Yaffe SJ: *Drugs in Pregnancy and Lactation*, 4th ed. Williams & Wilkins, 1994.

Creasy RK, Resnik R (editors): *Maternal-Fetal Medicine: Principles and Practice,* 3rd ed. Saunders, 1994.

Fanaroff AA, Martin RJ (editors): *Neonatal-Perinatal Medicine, Diseases of the Fetus and Infant,* 5th ed. Mosby, 1992.

Goldsmith JP, Karotkin EH (editors): *Assisted Ventilation of the Neonate,* 2nd ed. Saunders, 1988.

Jones KL (editor): *Smith's Recognizable Patterns of Human Malformation,* 4th ed. Saunders, 1988.

Klaus MH, Fanaroff AA (editors): *Care of the High-Risk Neonate,* 3rd ed. Saunders, 1986.

Remington JS, Klein JO (editors): *Infectious Diseases of the Fetus and Newborn Infant,* 2nd ed. Saunders, 1983.

Volpe JJ (editor): *Neurology of the Newborn,* 2nd ed. Saunders, 1987.

8 | Behavioral, Psychosocial, & Psychiatric Pediatrics

Stewart Gabel, MD, Jeffrey I. Dolgan, PhD, &
Rebecca A. Hea, PsyD

ASSESSMENT

This section discusses assessment procedures for emotional and behavioral disorders relevant to pediatric practice. Parents often feel less threatened taking their children to the pediatrician than to a psychologist or psychiatrist for behavioral or emotional symptoms because they are apprehensive about the social stigma attached to mental health concerns. When parents bring a child for an office visit, the pediatrician must consider several important lines of development: physical development, gross and fine motor skills, language, and psychosocial maturation. Physical development, motor skills, and some other developmental landmarks may be more readily assessed because they concern tangible parameters (eg, height and weight). Psychosocial issues are typically less clear-cut and are therefore more difficult to assess. For instance, children may have temper tantrums because they are in physical pain, are emotionally abused at home, or are normal toddlers for whom tantrums are age-appropriate behavior.

To obtain relevant information about the existence and nature of a significant behavior problem, the pediatrician must interview both child and family, as well as take an overall family history (Table 8–1).

THE ASSESSMENT INTERVIEW

Interviewing the Parents

Begin your assessment by asking parents if they have any current concerns about the child's behavior or development. Address major

Table 8–1. Outline for pediatric psychosocial assessment interview.

PART I. The Child

A. Presenting Problem

1. Brief description of problem: its nature, onset, duration or frequency, setting, severity, triggers or precipitating events
2. Presentation for evaluation
   a. timing
   b. family's previous use of mental health resources, if any
   c. referral source, if any
3. Family's previous approaches to problem
   a. family's general approach to problem-solving
   b. family's disciplinary style, methods, and delegation of authority
   c. child's attitude toward problem and response(s) to previous interventions

B. Child's History

1. Medical
   a. history of prenatal, perinatal, or subsequent problems, if any
   b. hospitalizations, if any; note reason, duration, and nature of tests or treatment
   c. neurologic problems or deficits, if any
   d. history of routine childhood illnesses and immunizations
   e. current physical problems, if any
   f. record of current medications, if any
2. Developmental
   a. review general developmental landmarks: gross motor, fine motor, language, personal, and social skills. Note delays, if any
   b. comparison of child's developmental pattern with sibs
3. Psychosocial
   a. review general points and any difficulties in developmental transitions: weaning, autonomy issues, feeding, toilet training, locomotion, school entry, etc
   b. note history of problem habits (eg, thumb-sucking, head banging), if any
   c. factors which may influence child's psychosocial development, if any (eg, moves, family crises, family's racial, religious, or ethnic identity)

C. Child's Present Psychosocial Functioning

1. Other problems, if any; note brief description and treatment history
2. Brief description of child's general temperament, personality traits and relational style
   a. child's popularity with others
   b. child's relational preferences in family, school, other activities
      (1) child's preferred companions
      (2) general extraversion or introversion
   c. child's moods, ways of handling emotions, communication patterns

(*continued*)

Table 8–1. Outline for pediatric psychosocial assessment interview (*continued*).

C. Child's Present Psychosocial Functioning (*continued*)

3. School
   a. type of school: public, private, parochial, boarding, Montessori, experimental, specialized, etc
   b. child's special educational needs, if any
   c. child's general attitude toward school; note history of school avoidance or school refusal, if any
   d. child's general level of achievement
4. Extracurricular activities and interests
   a. note child's areas of interest (music, art, sports, etc)
   b. enjoyment of "solo" activities
   c. participation in clubs or groups connected to areas of interest

PART II. Family and Community

A. Parents/Caregivers

1. Note ages, occupations, interests, etc; if child is being reared by relatives other than birth parents (eg, grandparents), note relationship to child and date of adoption or assumption of responsibility for child
2. Marital history
   a. date of marriage; dates of birth or adoption of children
   b. note previous marriages of either partner, if any; in cases of separation and divorce, note
      (1) child's contacts with birth parent(s)
      (2) custodial parent's present marital status or relationships
      (3) child's attitude toward custodial parent's relationship, if any
3. If the family is non-traditional in structure, describe briefly (eg, common-law marriage, same-sex partnership, commune, etc); note child's attitude toward situation
4. Parents' general relational style or interactional patterns
   a. attitudes toward discipline
   b. understanding of child development
5. Family stressors, if any (eg, illness, unemployment, rapid succession of pregnancies, substance abuse, etc)

B. Siblings

1. Note ages, sex, individual characteristics and problems
   a. locate child's birth order within sibship
   b. note degree of relationship to child (eg, full or half-sibling)
2. Note child's interactions with sibs, both positive and negative
   a. areas of recurrent conflict or stress
   b. parents' handling of sibling issues
      (1) general disciplinary style
      (2) problems with favoritism or scapegoating
3. If child is an only child:
   a. note child's attitudes or feeling about having no sibs

Table 8–1. Outline for pediatric psychosocial assessment interview.

C. Other Relatives
1. List ages, sex, relationship to child
2. Degree of involvement with child
   a. geographical location
   b. financial or other assistance to child
   c. reactions or response (if any) to child's presenting problem
3. Child's attitude toward relatives
4. Note child's problems with relatives, if any (eg, incest)

D. Home and Community
1. Features of family's home and neighborhood
   a. type, size, and condition of house or apartment
   b. location: rural, small town, suburb, inner city, etc
   c. environmental stressors, if any (degree of privacy; traffic patterns; closeness to airport or other source of noise; crime or violence, etc)
   d. relationship (if any) between child's problem and family's location or housing
2. Family's participation in community groups
   a. church, synagogue, or other religious group
   b. civic or political groups
   c. cultural activities (museums, orchestras, etc)
   d. effects (if any) of child's problem on family's participation in these activities

PART III. Clinician's Observations
In this section, the clinician should note:
1. Overall impression of child and child's problem
2. Any significant discrepancies:
   a. between different parents' or caregivers' accounts of child's history, problem, or characteristics
   b. between parents'/caregivers' accounts and medical or other written records (eg, case notes from previous therapists)
   c. between parents' statement of problem and clinician's own impression and observations

issues first. You may have to provide the parents with background information so that they can determine whether or not their child's behavior is developmentally appropriate. Develop a good working alliance with the family so that the parent or child being interviewed will feel comfortable in disclosing information.

Parents will provide you with a great deal of information in *what* they convey and *how* they convey it. Conversational style as well as content may help you understand the family's dynamics and their impact on the child's functioning.

Interviewing the Child

Effective child interviews depend on good rapport between the clinician and the child. You can foster rapport by using age-appropriate language and sitting at the child's eye level. One way to create a relaxed atmosphere for younger children is to sit on the floor or at a small table and engage the child in play before questions are asked. It is best not to stand or loom over the child in such a way as to make him or her uncomfortable; children are keenly aware of the difference in size between adults and themselves. When you begin your interview, ask the child about family, friends, school, teachers and other important adults, and personal interests. As you engage the child in conversation about these subjects, make a running assessment of the child's language, thought processes, mood, behavior, and interpersonal style, as noted below. Standard texts will help you interpret your observations in these areas.

Family History

Obtaining a family history of psychiatric illness may be helpful in determining if a specific condition is present in a child or adolescent. This is particularly important with disorders that have a strong genetic component (eg, bipolar disorder). In the course of history taking, you may also uncover useful information about the family's attitudes toward mental health problems or mental health care providers.

MENTAL STATUS EXAMINATION (MSE)

A mental status assessment should cover the following areas:

- child's appearance and behavior: grooming, personal hygiene, physical size and proportion (may indicate malnutrition), relatedness, activity level
- motor movements: smooth or jerky; posture and gait; abnormal movements, such as tics
- perceptual disturbances: hallucinations (visual, aural, olfactory); disturbances of tactile perception
- mood and affect: depressed, flat, manic, anxious, agitated, relaxed, limited range
- thought rate and pattern (inferred from speech): logical or illogical; coherent or disconnected; easy to follow, pressured, rapid, tangential

- thought content: peculiar or morbid preoccupations or themes; suspiciousness; age-inappropriate subject matter; delusional thinking
- cognitive functioning and orientation

In some situations, you may need to conduct a more thorough MSE. For younger children, use simple questions appropriate to their age; with respect to time, their knowledge of day or night rather than the exact hour is sufficient. Ask some general information questions in order to determine the child's fund of knowledge and his or her basic verbal and relational skills (eg, "Who is the President? Where does he live?"). To assess immediate memory, you can recite a short series of numbers and ask the child to repeat them. To assess short-term memory, list three unrelated items (eg, "baseball, frog, and teapot"). The child is asked to repeat these items and asked to list them again 3–5 minutes later, while the interview continues. Long-term memory can be determined by asking about the contents of the child's dinner last night or about recent events at home or school that you can verify from other sources.

Abstraction and detection of essential similarities are also included in the cognitive portion of the mental status exam. Common questions include "What do a fly and a tree have in common?" and for younger children, "How are a ball and wheel the same?" Adolescents can be asked to explain the meaning of a common proverb, such as "Don't cry over spilled milk." Another brief mental screen involves the performance of calculations. Young children can be asked to count to 10, and then count backward to one. You can ask latency-aged children to count backward from 30 by threes. Adolescents can start with 100 and count backward by sevens.

PHYSICAL EXAMINATION

You should note possible physical causes for emotional symptoms as well as their psychosocial dimension. A complete physical examination should be performed to rule out organic factors. Numerous medical disorders (eg, hyperthyroidism) have behavioral manifestations (eg, hyperactivity). In other cases, undiagnosed physical problems (eg, nearsightedness) may affect the child's school performance or social adjustment (eg, inability to see the blackboard or recognize friends).

COMMON PSYCHOSOCIAL PROBLEMS

This section provides a concise discussion of common behavioral and psychosocial issues in younger children. Problems that present more frequently during adolescence (eg, runaway behavior and suicide) are discussed in Chapter 9.

CHILD ABUSE AND NEGLECT

Child abuse and neglect is a major nationwide problem. Available data suggest that 2–2.5% of children in the United States are abused or neglected annually. The rise in reported cases over the past decade is a function of improved recognition and assessment of abused children by professionals, mandatory reporting statutes, expanded definitions of abuse and neglect, and broad-based changes in the social structure of the family.

Assessment of Abuse and Neglect

Pediatricians are not the only professionals who may become aware of abuse in a family; other physicians, psychologists, dentists, school nurses, teachers, and clergy may also notice problems. You may wish to contact the American Academy of Pediatrics for further information, including a list of experts in child abuse available for consultation.

When confronted with a case of abuse, keep the following priorities in mind:

1. **Immediate treatment**: Physical injuries and sexually transmitted diseases must be treated at once. In cases of neglect or failure to thrive, the children must be placed in settings or facilities that offer proper feeding and nutrition.
2. **Assessment of child's safety**: Evaluate the child's physical and social environment for potential re-injury or repeated abuse. Rely on your hospital's Child Protection Team for help in evaluation, management, or disposition of abuse cases.
3. **Reporting**: Complete your jurisdiction's mandated reporting procedure as soon as possible after treating the child. Maintain appropriate communication with child protective services and law enforcement agencies.

A. Behavioral Characteristics of Abused Children: Child maltreatment includes physical, sexual, and emotional abuse. In evaluating the appearance and behavior of a given child, you should note any "red flags" that may signal maltreatment.

Abused children commonly exhibit behavior that is regressive or runs to extremes. They may be unusually shy and fearful around adults or aggressive and disrespectful of adults. They may reject friendly overtures or act "love-hungry." Their behavior may swing rapidly from one extreme to the other or may exhibit sudden mood changes.

Abused children often present as self-absorbed, withdrawn, or "spaced-out." They may have problems in school because they cannot focus on the tasks at hand. In extreme cases the child may manifest dissociative symptoms (eg, "feeling unreal"). Older children may engage in self-cutting, self-mutilation, or other forms of intentional self-harm.

In some instances, abused children behave in a parentified manner; that is, they act as their parents' caretakers and often assume responsibilities within the family that are age-inappropriate. An example would be a 9-year-old who is expected to do the family cooking and laundry, supervise younger siblings, and serve as a parent's confidante about adult problems.

B. Characteristics of Abusive Parents: When you interview a child's parents, be alert for indicators of abusive attitudes and behaviors. As you engage the parents in conversation, note their general attitudes toward authority, responsibility, and caregiving. Abusive parents frequently exhibit resentment of authority figures and reluctance to assume responsibility for their behavior. They may be evasive or distrustful in answering routine questions or may be hostile toward you or other personnel. They may present as immature or dependent, seeking someone to take care of them or to take the blame for their problems. They may express age-inappropriate expectations of children (eg, expecting a 6-month-old to be toilet-trained) or show ignorance of normal developmental patterns. Some abusive parents subscribe to a harsh and authoritarian philosophy of child-rearing and may show little affection toward children or express concerns about "spoiling" them.

In some cases, you may need to assess the parents for signs of alcohol or substance abuse. Although addiction to mood-altering chemicals does not *cause* child abuse, it reinforces the immaturity, denial, and poor social skills that often characterize abusive parents.

C. Historical Factors: As you take the family's medical and social history, note the presence of any of the following signs: a history of failure to keep medical appointments or refusal of diagnostic studies; a pattern of taking the child to a variety of different providers within a short period of time; evidence of social isolation (absence of extended family ties, community involvement, or friendship networks); unreliable or discrepant accounts of the child's medical history; reiterated expressions of hostility toward the child or inappropriate reactions to the seriousness of the child's condition. It may be useful to note a family history of multiple stressors (eg, unemployment, chronic illness, rapid succession of pregnancies) to help assess the degree of risk for child abuse. Note also that the risk may vary for different children within the same family; a child who requires a disproportionate share of the family's resources because of special medical or educational needs may be singled out for maltreatment.

Types of Abuse

A. Physical Abuse: Physical abuse or nonaccidental trauma is bodily harm done to children by a caretaker or trusted adults. It may involve the use of a weapon; hitting or striking the child with an object; burning or scalding the child; forced feeding or forced ingestion of nonfood items (eg, fecal matter); confinement (eg, in closets or storage areas) or bondage; and sleep deprivation. You should be aware of the following external indicators of physical abuse: age-inappropriate injuries (eg, leg fractures in a 3-month-old infant); bruises or wounds in unusual locations on the child's body (eg, the inner thigh); patterned bruises or welts; lacerations of the mouth or dental evidence of forced feeding; stocking or glove distribution of burn or scald marks; a series of bruises or injuries in different stages of healing in the same area of the child's body. In some cases the child's medical history will indicate repeated hospitalizations or treatments for the same injury (eg, the child is reported to have broken the same arm four times in a 2-year period).

Radiologic and laboratory findings may also be suggestive of physical abuse. You should note any of the following: metaphyseal "corner" or "bucket handle" fractures of the long bones in infants; spiral fractures of the long bones in pre-ambulatory infants; multiple fractures of the ribs or long bones; computed tomographic or magnetic resonance imaging findings of subdural hemorrhage in infants; or ultrasonographic evidence of abdominal injury.

B. Neglect: Neglect is a form of abuse that is often overlooked because the consequences of care withheld, including medical care, are harder to assess and not always physically demonstrable.

1. Malnutrition and Failure to Thrive– The absence of subcutaneous fat in cheeks, buttocks, and extremities, and the appearance of "deprivation dwarfism" in older children are common findings in some cases of neglect. The child may also have a depressed appearance and manner. See Chapter 4 for information about nutritional requirements and treatment of undernourished children.

2. Munchausen by Proxy Syndrome– Munchausen by proxy syndrome is a factitious disorder in which a parent creates symptoms of illness in a child to satisfy a disturbed need to assume the patient role. Children suffering from this syndrome may present with dehydration or electrolyte imbalance caused by induced vomiting or diarrhea.

C. Emotional Abuse: While all forms of abuse create emotional suffering in children, it is also possible for parents to abuse children emotionally without physical or sexual contact. Some experts consider emotional abuse the most common form of maltreatment. It may include verbal abuse of various types, ranging from shaming, humiliating, and teasing to cursing, intimidating, or terrorizing the child. It may also include emotional abuse such as killing a child's pet in front of him or her, refusing to speak to or interact with the child, or threatening to abandon the child.

Emotional abuse may not be evident from physical workups but is often suggested by the child's behavior. Such behaviors as extreme timidity or aggressiveness, mistrustfulness, or intense fear of rejection may be signs of emotional abuse. Many emotionally abused children present with clinical depression.

D. Sexual Abuse: Sexual abuse of children is a complex phenomenon that may or may not involve physical contact. In cases of completed intercourse, the child may present with a sexually transmitted disease, a genital discharge or infection, or injury to the oral, genital, or anal areas. In some cases, the child may complain of pain when urinating or defecating. Sexual abuse may, however, also involve touching or fondling short of intercourse; using the child for pornographic pictures; forcing the child to stimulate the adult, etc. In these instances, the child may respond to the abuse with a variety of diffuse symptoms, ranging from depression, gastrointestinal complaints, and sleep disturbances to age-inappropriate interest in or knowledge of sexual matters; exhibitionism; and compulsive masturbation.

If you suspect that a child may have been sexually abused, you may wish to consult a specialist trained in interviewing children. If there is *any* possibility that the child might have to appear in court, forensic considerations require avoidance of leading questions and other language that may be interpreted as influencing the child's answers.

Treatment and Prevention

After treatment of medical emergencies, placement of malnourished children, and assessment of the child's environment, long-term follow-up of abused children should include preventive measures. These fall into two primary categories: intervention and education. High-risk families may benefit from home visitors who are trained public health nurses and paraprofessionals. Family members can be given the number of the local hotline for stressed parents; these lines are staffed by persons who can help caregivers regain control of themselves before they abuse the child. In addition, many cities have support groups for abusive parents. *Keep a list of hotline numbers and support groups in your office and update it regularly.* Many abused children and their families will require psychotherapeutic and family treatment.

Educational measures include anticipatory instruction for parents regarding children's developmental patterns and age-appropriate expectations, as well as information about proper nutrition, hygiene, and household safety. You may find it helpful to make up office handouts with this information for parents to take with them. Keep in mind that many abusive parents are afraid to ask questions of authority figures; if you can convey that you are open to questions about childrearing, they may welcome the opportunity to discuss their problems with parenting.

SLEEP DIFFICULTIES

Bedtime refusal is a common pediatric behavioral presentation. It may take a variety of forms, from inundating the parents with questions, requests for water, or other delaying tactics to outright refusal to go to bed or remain in the bedroom. A psychoeducational approach pointing out to parents that these are manipulative behaviors is often helpful. In other instances, the parents may need to monitor the child's activities prior to bedtime, to make sure that he or she is not being overstimulated by television shows, games, or play. Establishing a bedtime ritual that is patterned and predictable may help the child to quiet down and feel secure before going to sleep.

Parents may need to check the child's bedroom to see that it is dark or dimly lit, quiet, and a comfortable temperature. Families who live in urban areas with a high level of traffic and other noise may have children kept awake by environmental stimuli.

In a few cases, the child's diet or prescribed medication may need assessment. Some children drink large quantities of soft drinks containing caffeine. Others may be taking medications that have a stimulant side effect.

See the section on sleep disorders below for information on the differential diagnosis and management of *disordered* sleep.

ENURESIS

Children may have problems with bladder control for a variety of reasons. Table 8–2 lists possible causes for enuresis. Enuresis may be a symptom of regression in a child who is upset by changes in the family (eg, birth of new sibling or parental separation), moving, or other emotional stressors. Enuresis that does not arise from medically or surgically treatable causes may respond to behavioral modification approaches. These methods typically encourage children to get up to urinate during the night, urinate less frequently during the day, and

Table 8–2. Causes of enuresis.[1]

Nonpathologic causes (97%)
Small functional bladder capacity
Inability to delay micturition urge
Nighttime polyuria because anti-diuretic hormone (ADH) levels fail to rise at night
Nighttime polyuria because child drinks too much in the evening
Child does not wake up when bladder feels full
Disease states (3%)
Medically treatable
Urinary tract infection
Diabetes insipidus
Diabetes mellitus
Fecal impaction or constipation
Surgically treatable
Ectopic ureter
Lower urinary tract obstruction
Neurogenic bladder
Bladder calculus or foreign body
Sleep apnea secondary to large adenoids

[1] From Schmitt BD: Nocturnal enuresis: Finding the treatment that fits the child. *Contemp Pediatr* September, 1990, p 72.

drink more in the morning and early afternoon. Children benefit from discouragement of evening fluids and the establishment of a morning routine for wet pajamas and wet bedding, and also benefit from receiving a positive response to dry nights. Some parents find wet bedding alarms to be helpful. Medications to control enuresis appear to be effective only as long as the child continues to take them; they do not "cure" the problem.

PSYCHIATRIC DISORDERS

This third section describes the most common psychiatric disorders or syndromes that are seen in pediatric practice. The following information is based on the *Diagnostic and Statistical Manual, Fourth edition*, or DSM-IV, published by the American Psychiatric Association (1994). More detailed information about any of the disorders discussed below can be found in DSM-IV.

MENTAL RETARDATION

Mental retardation is not itself an emotional disturbance; however, it is commonly associated with a number of behavioral and emotional symptoms, including poor impulse control, low self-esteem, self-inflicted harm, and depression. Causes include a complex array of physical and psychosocial factors; 30–40% of cases seen in clinical settings have no clear etiology. Medical conditions to be ruled out include inborn errors of metabolism (eg, Tay-Sachs disease); abnormalities in genes (eg, tuberous sclerosis) or chromosomes (eg, Down's syndrome, fragile X syndrome); perinatal difficulties (toxins in utero, fetal alcohol syndrome, hypoxia, infection, prematurity, fetal malnutrition); and certain childhood infections (meningitis, lead encephalopathy).

Physical examination and laboratory findings are not specific to mental retardation; abnormalities reflect the associated or underlying condition.

Diagnostic Characteristics

Mental retardation is defined as significant subaverage general intellectual functioning (ie, an IQ of ~ 70 or below). It involves concurrent deficits or impairments in adaptive functioning. Its onset occurs before 18 years of age.

Associated Features

The prevalence in the general pediatric population is ~ 1%. Mental retardation is classified according to four degrees of severity:

1. **Mild**: IQ 50–55 to approximately 70 (about 85% of people with mental retardation)
2. **Moderate**: IQ 35–40 to 50–55 (about 10% of the retarded)
3. **Severe**: IQ 20–25 to 35–40 (about 3–4% of the retarded)
4. **Profound**: IQ < 20 (about 1–2% of the retarded)

Increased severity of mental retardation is associated with increased likelihood of other neurologic or medical disorders (eg, seizures). Lower socioeconomic groups tend to be overrepresented in cases of retardation without determinate biological causality, but the degree of retardation tends to be milder.

It is important to distinguish mental retardation from learning or communication disorders. The former are characterized by impairment in a specific area of development, such as reading. In pervasive developmental disorders, *qualitative* impairments occur in a number of developmental areas (eg, social interaction) regardless of the level of intellectual ability. Mental retardation and pervasive developmental disorders, such as autism, may occur together, however. The patient's course may be variable, although mental retardation is often lifelong.

Treatment

Treatment of mental retardation is based on a multidimensional evaluation of the child's functioning.

1. **Special education** is required for the child's intellectual deficits. An individualized educational plan should be developed for each student by school personnel in consultation with parents.
2. **Speech therapy, physical therapy or occupational therapy** may also be useful adjunctive treatments for associated problems such as visual motor deficits.
3. **Medical treatment for underlying conditions** such as hypothyroidism.
4. **Alleviation of psychosocial factors** (eg, isolation or lack of stimulation).
5. **Appropriate psychopharmacologic treatment** of associated mental disorders. Psychostimulants may be prescribed for associ-

ated attention-deficit/hyperactivity disorder. You may wish to consult a child psychiatrist for detailed information about pharmacotherapy for specific behavior problems.

6. **Supportive psychotherapy** for children and adolescents with milder degrees of mental retardation. This modality may include problem-solving approaches. Family behavior management and supportive approaches for parents may also be helpful.
7. **Treatment of parental reactions** to the child's condition (eg, grief, anger, or shame) and the ongoing difficulties imposed on other family members. Effective treatment may include supportive psychotherapy or family systems approaches.

LEARNING DISORDERS

Diagnostic Characteristics

Learning disorders, also called **learning disabilities** or **academic skill disorders**, are deemed to be present when a child's achievement on standardized tests of reading, mathematics, or written expression falls substantially below predicted performance based on age, schooling, and level of intelligence. Learning disorders also interfere with academic achievement in the classroom.

Classification

Learning disorders include reading disorder (also known as dyslexia), mathematics disorder, and disorder of written expression.

A. Reading Disorder: This type of learning disorder should be suspected when the child's reading achievement, as measured by standardized tests of reading accuracy or comprehension, is substantially below expectations based on chronologic age, IQ, and education. Most children with reading disorders are male. It is estimated that 4% of school-aged children are affected. Genetic factors probably contribute.

B. Mathematics Disorder: This disorder is likely to be present when mathematical ability, as measured by standardized tests, is substantially below expectations based on chronologic age, IQ, and education. About 1% of school-age children are thought to be affected.

C. Disorder of Written Expression: This disorder should be suspected when writing skills, as measured by standardized tests (or functional assessment of writing skills), are substantially below expectations based on age, IQ, and education and when significant interference with academic achievement is present.

Associated Features

Prevalence estimates for learning disorders range from 2% to 10%. These disorders may be associated with numerous behavioral and emotional problems, including low self-esteem and poor social skills. Children and adolescents with conduct disorder, oppositional defiant disorder and attention-deficit/hyperactivity disorder (A-D/HD) have an increased likelihood of associated learning disorders. Language delays and other developmental problems may be more common in this population. Genetic susceptibility and certain neurologic or medical conditions (eg, fetal alcohol syndrome, fragile X syndrome) may also be associated with learning disorders. The differential diagnosis includes lack of opportunity to acquire academic skills, poor teaching, inadequate schooling, and physical causes (impaired vision or hearing). Mental retardation is diagnosed when there is a sufficiently severe general impairment in intellectual functioning.

Treatment

1. **Educational intervention** is the primary line of treatment for learning disorders. An individualized educational program should be developed by school personnel in consultation with parents.
2. **Associated or causative medical disorders** should be treated if possible (eg, lead intoxication).
3. **Concurrent behavioral and emotional problems** may be treated with psychotherapy or pharmacotherapy, depending on the problem. Treatment for A-D/HD is usually helpful for classroom behavior and performance. Recent studies suggest that longer-term academic gains occur when A-D/HD is treated appropriately.
4. There is no widely recognized **pharmacologic intervention** for learning disorders themselves.
5. **Supportive or psychoeducational interventions** may be helpful for children and parents in dealing with emotional reactions to the learning disorder (eg, poor self-esteem or guilt).

COMMUNICATION DISORDERS

Several disorders in the pediatric population are characterized by communication difficulties. These include expressive language disorder, mixed receptive-expressive language disorder, phonological disorder, and stuttering.

Expressive Language Disorder

A. Diagnostic Characteristics: Expressive language disorder may be suspected when the child's scores on standardized measures of expressive language development are below scores on measures of nonverbal intellectual capacity and receptive language development. Symptoms include limited vocabulary, limited amount of speech, difficulty acquiring new words, word-finding errors, and slow rate of language development.

B. Associated Features: The disorder is present in 3–5% of school-aged children; it is more common in males. It must be differentiated from acquired aphasia associated with neurologic conditions. Expressive language disorder is commonly associated with other developmental, learning, and psychiatric disorders.

C. Treatment: Treatment of expressive language disorder usually necessitates speech and language therapy, special education measures for any associated learning difficulties, and psychological/psychiatric treatment for associated emotional or behavioral problems.

Mixed Receptive-Expressive Language Disorder

A. Diagnostic Characteristics: In this disorder, the child's scores on measures of both receptive and expressive language development are below those obtained on measures of nonverbal intellectual capacity. Symptoms include those of expressive language disorder (above) as well as impairment in receptive language development (difficulty understanding words, sentences, or types of words).

B. Associated Features: As with expressive language disorder, this mixed form is more common in males. It is thought to affect up to 3% of school-aged children. Other developmental, learning, and psychiatric disorders are commonly associated with this communication disorder.

C. Treatment: Treatment follows the same guidelines as for expressive language disorder.

Phonological Disorder (Developmental Articulation Disorder)

A. Diagnostic Characteristics: In this disorder, the child fails to use age-appropriate and developmentally expected speech sounds. Phonological disorder includes errors in sound production (articulation), use, representation, or organization. Substitutions of one sound for another are common.

B. Associated Features: Phonological disorder is more common in males. Approximately 2–3% of 6- to 7-year-old children present with moderate to severe symptoms.

C. Treatment: Treatment of phonological disorder includes speech therapy, an examination to rule out hearing impairment, and specific treatment for such impairment or other causal and associated factors.

Stuttering

A. Diagnostic Characteristics: Stuttering includes disturbances in the normal fluency and time patterning of speech. It is marked by frequent occurrences of one or more of the following: sound and syllable repetitions, sound prolongations, interjections, or broken words.

B. Associated Features: Stuttering may be associated with other communication disorders. It is more common in males and occurs in 1% of prepubertal children. The age of peak onset is about 5 years; almost all cases occur before age 10. Most children with stuttering recover.

C. Treatment: Speech therapy (and language therapy if needed) is the treatment of choice for stuttering.

PERVASIVE DEVELOPMENTAL DISORDERS

Pervasive developmental disorders are characterized by severe and pervasive impairment in several areas of development, including reciprocal social interaction and communication skills. Children with these disorders often display stereotypic behavior, interests, and activities. The qualitative impairments are distinctly deviant relative to the child's developmental level or mental age. These disorders usually manifest in the first years of life and are often associated with some degree of mental retardation. They may be associated with various medical conditions and chromosomal abnormalities.

Autistic Disorder

A. Diagnostic Characteristics: Autistic disorder is characterized by qualitative impairment in the child's social interaction, as exemplified by marked impairment in the use of nonverbal behaviors (eg, eye contact); failure to develop peer relationships appropriate to developmental level; and lack of social or emotional reciprocity. Qualitative impairments in communication are exemplified by delay in or lack of development of spoken language; stereotyped or repetitive speech; lack of varied make-believe play or social imitative play. The onset of autistic disorder is usually before age 3.

B. Associated Features: Mental retardation occurs in about 75% of cases of autistic disorder, generally with an uneven profile of cognitive skills. A variety of problematic, odd, or unusual behaviors may be present, such as hyperactivity, hypersensitivity to sensory stimuli, odd eating or sleeping patterns, or self-injurious behavior. Causes may include neurologic or other medical conditions (eg, encephalitis, tuberous sclerosis, fetal anoxia, or maternal rubella). Seizures may develop in 25% of cases, usually in adolescence. Males are more likely to develop autistic disorder than females.

C. Treatment: The treatment of autistic disorder usually requires a number of different therapeutic modalities.

1. Evaluate the child for any underlying or associated medical/neurological condition (eg, tuberous sclerosis). Give anticonvulsant medication for associated seizures.

2. Special education classes to address social, learning, or behavioral difficulties are important. If possible, the child should attend such classes at specialized centers for the treatment of children with autistic disorder.

3. Neuroleptic medications may be prescribed for symptomatic improvement of a variety of inappropriate behaviors.

4. Psychostimulants may be prescribed for associated behavioral problems such as hyperactivity.

5. Family intervention for behavior management and support may be helpful.

ATTENTION-DEFICIT/HYPERACTIVITY DISORDER (A-D/HD)

A. Diagnostic Characteristics: A-D/HD is marked by a persistent, long-standing pattern of inattention or hyperactivity and impulsivity that is more frequent and severe than usually observed in children at a comparable level of development. Its usual onset is before age 7. Diagnosis requires evidence of impairment in at least two settings (eg, home and school). There must also be evidence of interference with developmentally appropriate social, academic, or occupational functioning. **Inattention** is manifested by symptoms such as failure to give close attention to details, making careless mistakes, difficulty sustaining attention in tasks or play, not following through on instructions, failure to complete schoolwork, difficulty organizing tasks, avoidance of tasks requiring sustained mental effort, and being easily distracted or forgetful. **Hyperactivity** is manifested by symptoms such as fidgetiness, inability to remain seated in school, difficulty playing or participating in activities quietly, running about in inappropriate situations or being "always on the go." **Impulsivity** is manifested by blurting out answers before questions have been completed, difficulty waiting in line, and interrupting or intruding on others.

B. Associated Features: A-D/HD may be associated with low frustration tolerance, temper outbursts, mood lability, lowered morale, and poor self-esteem. It is often concurrent with other learning disorders and psychiatric diagnoses (eg, oppositional defiant disorder or conduct disorder). The child's academic achievement is often compromised. A small percentage of cases may be caused by neurologic or medical conditions such as encephalitis. The male-to-female ratio for A-D/HD is 4–9:1. The disorder occurs in 3–5% of school-aged children. It is usually first diagnosed in the elementary school years, but symptoms typically appear earlier. The symptoms commonly, though not invariably, diminish in adolescence or adulthood. There is an increased risk for alcohol/substance abuse and antisocial behavior in adult life in those who have associated conduct disorder.

C. Treatment:

1. Behavioral and Cognitive-Behavioral Therapy– Behavioral therapy for A-D/HD emphasizes the use of clear rewards and consequences for particular behaviors. Cognitive-behavioral treatment emphasizes cognitive strategies (eg, listening before forming conclusions or rehearsing alternatives prior to action) that may help the child curb maladaptive or impulsive behaviors. These treatment modalities may be sufficient in milder cases of A-D/HD but usually must be combined with medication in more severe cases.

2. Pharmacotherapy–

a. Psychostimulants are the mainstay of pharmacologic treatment for A-D/HD. About two-thirds of children diagnosed with the disorder will respond to these agents. The three psychostimulants most widely used are methylphenidate (Ritalin), dextroamphetamine sulfate (Dexedrine), and magnesium pemoline (Cylert). There are no demonstrated differences in efficacy among these three stimulants. Because of their shorter half-lives, methylphenidate and dextroamphetamine are given two or more times per day, whereas pemoline is given only once. Longer-acting forms of dextroamphetamine and methylphenidate (sustained-release) are now available.

Methylphenidate is the single most widely used psychostimulant in the treatment of A-DH/D. Its onset of action usually is within ½ hour, allowing for very rapid evaluation of efficacy at a given dose. Half-life is about 3–4 hours, necessitating a lunch-time dose for most school children. The sustained-release form allows once-daily dosing but is not directly comparable in efficacy to methylphenidate tablets. In general, the sustained-release form has a slower onset of action, a longer duration of action, and a lower peak blood level. In some cases, the sustained-release form and regular methylphenidate tablets can be combined to achieve both rapid onset and sustained action.

Dosages vary for children receiving psychostimulants. At higher dosages, cognitive blunting and impaired learning may occur. The usual dosage for methylphenidate is about 0.3 mg/kg/dose or slightly higer, up to a Food and Drug Administration (FDA)-approved dosage of 60 mg/d. Dextroamphetamine dosage is usually about one-half that of methylphenidate, up to an FDA-approved dosage of 40 mg/d. The dosage of magnesium pemoline is not converted directly to that of the other stimulants and varies from about 18.75 mg/d to 112.5 mg/d.

There is a rebound effect with short-acting psychostimulants; children sometimes become more active, inattentive, and impulsive as the most recent dosage "wears off." The rebound effect typically occurs in late afternoon, when the child returns home. Parents who see only the rebound behavior may complain that the medication is ineffective or worsens the situation. The child's teacher may need to be consulted about the medication's effect during the school day. Rebound effects can often be managed by giving a smaller dosage (eg, one-half of the last dosage) in late afternoon, which allows for a more gradual tapering of medication effects on behavior without interfering with sleep.

The side effects of psychostimulants are usually mild and can be managed by lowered dosage, discontinuation, or slower upward titration. Common side effects include insomnia, abdominal pain, decreased appetite, and irritability. Height and weight gain may be decreased (growth suppression) in children treated with psychostimulants. This effect is usually more pronounced for weight than for height and is completely reversible in preadolescents when the medication is withdrawn. The complete reversibility of this effect for adolescents is not certain. The growth suppressant effect of psychostimulants is related in part to dosage level; reduction often alleviates the problem. Drug holidays (eg, weekends, school vacation) may be helpful.

Another side effect of psychostimulant usage is the development of tics, which may progress in some children to Tourette's disorder (below). Psychostimulants do not appear to cause Tourette's disorder in nonsusceptible children; however, by precipitating tics in susceptible youth, psychostimulants may lead to earlier emergence of the disorder. In general, a personal or family history of tics is a contraindication to the use of psychostimulants. Since about 25% of children with Tourette's disorder have A-D/HD, however, they may receive psychostimulants as well as such agents as haloperidol or clonidine, which suppress tics.

Ongoing evaluation of medication efficacy is important. In addition to direct discussions with teachers, parents, and children themselves, the use of various behavior rating scales (eg, Conners scales) by parents and teachers can be helpful.

b. Other medications for children unresponsive to or intolerant of psychostimulants include clonidine and desipramine.

(1) Clonidine is an alpha-adrenergic agonist that has been used successfully in children with A-D/HD and is thought to be particularly helpful in those children with coexistent oppositional defiant disorder, conduct disorder, or aggressivity. The dosage of clonidine usually ranges from about 3 to 6 μg/kg/d in three to four divided doses. Dosing often begins at 0.05 mg/d and is gradually increased by 0.05 mg/d every 3 days or so, depending of the side effects and efficacy in reducing target symptoms. Sedation, hypotension, and depression may be significant side effects associated with clonidine. If sedation occurs, holding the dosage temporarily or reducing the current dosage for a brief period may be helpful. Monitoring of symptoms related to decreased blood pressure (eg, lightheadedness) and actual blood pressure recording should be performed during clonidine treatment. If clonidine is to be withdrawn, this should be done gradually since rebound hypertension may occur. A clonidine skin patch (transdermal system) also is available and is sometimes preferred by patients and their families. It is usually easier to begin with the oral dosage, however, and to switch to the transdermal system after treatment response has occurred. There is significant variability between the oral and transdermal routes in terms of dosage required, however, making it necessary to sometimes modify the dosage in switching to the transdermal system. Skin irritation may be a problem with the transdermal system, and return to oral clonidine is sometimes required.

(2) Desipramine is a tricyclic antidepressant that has been used effectively in treating symptoms of A-D/HD in children. For some clinicians, it had been the drug of choice in children with A-D/HD who did not respond to psychostimulants until recent reports became available of sudden death occurring in a small number of children treated with desipramine. Tricyclic antidepressants are known to have a number of cardiac effects, including increases in heart rate, PR interval, and QRS interval. Whether these cases of sudden death were caused by the use of desipramine has not been definitely determined. Nonetheless, it is advised that pediatricians wishing to prescribe desipramine for the treatment of A-D/HD seek additional child and adolescent psychiatric and cardiology consultation.

3. Adjunctive Treatment Modalities–Children diagnosed with A-D/HD usually require evaluation of associated learning problems and individualized educational plans. Supportive counseling and psychoeducational intervention for the child's family may also be helpful.

CONDUCT DISORDER

A. Diagnostic Characteristics: Conduct disorder is a repetitive, persistent pattern of behavior that violates the basic rights of others or major age-appropriate societal norms or rules. Behaviors fall into four groups: **aggressive** (eg, causes or threatens physical harm to others), **nonaggressive** (eg, causes property loss or damage), **deceitfulness or theft,** and **serious violation of rules** (eg, running away from home, truancy from school). The disorder usually presents in a variety of settings, including home, school, or community. Typical behaviors include bullying, threatening others, initiating physical fights, physical cruelty to animals, stealing, fire setting, destruction of others' property, breaking into someone else's house, running away, etc.

B. Associated Features: The onset of conduct disorder may be either in childhood or adolescence; early onset is more likely in males, is more often associated with aggression, and carries a poorer prognosis. Early sexual activity, alcohol and drug use, development of antisocial personality disorder, and criminality are more common in persons diagnosed with conduct disorder. This subpopulation also attempts suicide more frequently than the general population. Academic achievement is often low; conduct disorder frequently coexists with A-D/HD and learning disorders. Predisposing factors include harsh or inconsistent parenting, abuse, lack of supervision, and association with a delinquent peer group. Conduct disorder is present in 6–16% of males and 2–9% females. Most cases improve as the youth grows older, but a sizable minority manifest adult antisocial personality disorder. Conduct disorder appears to have both genetic and environmental causes.

C. Treatment: Treatment of conduct disorder often includes therapy directed at concurrent disorders.

1. Evaluate and treat associated psychiatric disorders, such as A-D/HD or depression. About 75% of children with severe conduct disorder also have A-D/HD; assessment for this specific disorder is especially important.

2. Evaluate and treat associated learning disorders. Many youth with conduct disorder are in the low-average range intellectually. Individualized educational plans should be developed to address academic and social deficiencies.

3. Behavior therapy and cognitive-behavior therapy may be helpful.

4. Pharmacotherapy may be indicated for conduct disorder as well as for A-D/HD. Some children are helped by medications such as lithium carbonate or carbamazepine to reduce aggressive behavior or mood instability. Severely disturbed youth sometimes benefit from neuroleptic agents such as haloperidol. Pediatricians should consult a specialist in child and adolescent psychiatry before prescribing these medications.

5. Therapy may be required for other family members, as many children with conduct disorder have been neglected, abused, or reared by parents with alcohol or substance abuse/dependence problems or depression. Referral to social service agencies may be needed.

OPPOSITIONAL DEFIANT DISORDER

A. Diagnostic Characteristics: Oppositional defiant disorder is defined as a recurrent pattern of negativistic, defiant, disobedient, or hostile behavior toward authority figures. It includes such behaviors as loss of temper, arguing with adults, and intentional frustration of others, without the more serious violations of social norms and legal codes that characterize conduct disorder. oppositional defiant disorder may manifest only in the home.

B. Associated Features: This disorder may be associated with A-D/HD and learning disorders. It appears to be more common in males before puberty; however, the postpubertal gender ratio is nearly equal. Oppositional defiant disorder occurs in about 2–16% of children and adolescents. In some cases, it is a precursor of conduct disorder.

C. Treatment: Treatment plans may vary according to symptom severity and associated disorders. Milder cases may respond to individual therapy or family therapy; more severe cases may require interventions similar to those for conduct disorder. Associated disorders should receive specific treatment.

PICA

A. Diagnostic Characteristics: Pica involves the persistent eating of non-nutritive substances in a developmentally inappropriate pattern. Paint, plaster, string, hair, animal droppings, sand, insects, leaves, or clay may all be ingested. Food aversion is not characteristic of pica.

B. Associated Features: Pica is frequently associated with mental retardation. It may in turn cause medical conditions such as lead intoxication or intestinal obstruction. Poverty and lack of parental supervision are risk factors.

C. Treatment: Treatment of pica may include medical intervention as indicated for secondary consequences. In addition, the child's environment may require evaluation for adequacy of supervision and stimulation, or risk factors such as lead-based paint.

TOURETTE'S DISORDER

A. Diagnostic Characteristics: Tourette's disorder is characterized by both multiple motor and one or more vocal tics many times during the day, nearly every day, or intermittently throughout a period of more than 1 year. Onset is usually during childhood or early adolescence. The prevalence is 4–5 individuals per 10,000; the disorder is more common in males. Tourette's disorder is chronic but may have occasional remissions and relapses.

B. Associated Features: Tourette's disorder requires careful differential diagnosis; motor tics must be distinguished from abnormal movements accompanying other conditions, such as choreiform movements in Huntington's disease or stereotypic movements in autistic disorder. The anatomic location, severity, and frequency of the tics vary over time. Tourette's disorder may be associated with obsessive-compulsive disorder (OCD), A-D/HD, and learning disorders. There may be concurrent depression or other psychiatric disturbances related to social embarrassment.

C. Treatment: Treatment of Tourette's disorder usually involves a multimodal approach.

1. Medications for concurrent disorders (eg, A-D/HD or OCD) are often indicated but should be prescribed after consultation with or in conjunction with a child and adolescent psychiatrist or pediatric neurologist versed in the evaluation and treatment of children with Tourette's disorder.

Neuroleptics (haloperidol, pimozide) and clonidine are the mainstays of treatment for the tics themselves. Neuroleptics may be more effective than clonidine but are associated with side effects that often reduce compliance. Short-term side effects include tremor, rigidity, and bradykinesia. Long-term side effects include tardive dyskinesia, a potentially irreversible movement disorder.

Clonidine may be useful for the tics and is often prescribed when the child suffers from concurrent A-D/HD. At times, psychostimulants are given with neuroleptics or clonidine to treat A-D/HD in a child with Tourette's disorder.

Newer selective serotonin reuptake inhibitors (SSRIs) (eg, fluoxetine) and the tricyclic antidepressant clomipramine (which also inhibits serotonin reuptake) have been found effective in decreasing symptoms of OCD. They have been given to children with Tourette's disorder who have obsessive-compulsive symptoms.

2. Educational evaluation and remediation as indicated. Special educational classes and an individualized treatment plan may be helpful.

3. Individual and family treatment/support for the secondary consequences (social rejection, ridicule, embarrassment) associated with the disorder.

SEPARATION ANXIETY DISORDER

A. Diagnostic Characteristics: Separation anxiety disorder is marked by the child's excessive anxiety about separation from the home or from those with whom he or she is attached. The anxiety is more intense than expected for the child's developmental level and is not connected to recent trauma. Symptoms may include recurrent distress when separation from home is anticipated; persistent worry about loss of or harm befalling major attachment figures; school refusal; or reluctance to go to sleep or be at home alone. There may be associated sleep disturbances, such as nightmares involving themes of separation or loss. Physical symptoms (eg, headaches or nausea) may be present when the child anticipates separation.

B. Associated Features: Children with separation anxiety disorder tend to come from close-knit families, although excessive demands from the child may produce family conflict. School refusal may result in academic and social difficulties. Depression is frequently associated with separation anxiety disorder. The prevalence of separation anxiety disorder is about 4% in children and young adolescents. It appears to be more frequent in females. Children diagnosed with separation anxiety disorder are at increased risk in later life for panic disorder with agoraphobia.

C. Treatment:

1. Many children with separation anxiety disorder present with somatic complaints prior to feared separation. A medical evaluation to rule out organic illness may be reassuring to parents and child. A supportive attitude toward the family is important.

2. Individual therapy with a strong behavioral component may be helpful. The child's return to school is usually a major goal.

3. When necessary, the parents should be educated regarding developmentally appropriate separation and independence. If the child is receiving behavioral therapy, parents should be involved in the program.

4. Medication may be useful in severe or less tractable cases. Behavioral and family intervention should be tried first. Imipramine has been used with varying success; however, its usefulness is limited by concerns about cardiac toxicity and side effects (dry mouth and blurred vision). Clonazepam, a high-potency benzodiazepine, may be beneficial. Concerns about addiction and withdrawal symptoms on discontinuation require caution prior to use and make psychiatric consultation important.

GENERALIZED ANXIETY DISORDER (GAD)

A. Diagnostic Characteristics: Children with generalized anxiety disorder (GAD) manifest excessive worry and anxiety about numerous events or activities, often in the context of performance-related activities (academic examinations, athletic contests). The anxiety is difficult to control and is often accompanied by restlessness, fatigue, difficulties in concentration, irritability, muscle tension, sleep disturbances, or gastrointestinal complaints.

B. Associated Features: Intensity, duration, or frequency of the anxiety is out of proportion to the likelihood the feared event will happen. Associated somatic symptoms are common. Worry about catastrophic events such as earthquakes or nuclear war may occur. Children diagnosed with GAD may also manifest perfectionist or approval-seeking tendencies.

C. Treatment:

1. As with separation anxiety disorder, somatic symptoms may require medical evaluation to rule out organic causes.

2. Individual psychotherapy with parent counseling may be useful. Assessment of family characteristics (eg, excessively high standards or competitiveness) is indicated; likewise, history taking is indicated to screen for recent events that may be implicated in the child's anxiety. Pediatricians should keep in mind that children may react with much greater anxiety than adults to some situations (eg, parent's hospitalization for minor surgery).

3. Medication as adjunctive therapy may be considered, as in separation anxiety disorder, discussed earlier. Because GAD is often long-term and associated with family characteristics, caution is advised in the use of medications. A trial of psychotherapy with family intervention is usually warranted before medication is prescribed.

SUBSTANCE-RELATED DISORDERS

Substance abuse presents more frequently in adolescents than in younger children. This topic is discussed in detail in Chapter 9.

MOOD DISORDERS

Mood disorders fall into two general categories: depression and mania. Mania may occur by itself, in combination with depression, or in a cyclical pattern with depression. **Bipolar disorder** refers to mood disorders involving one or more manic or hypomanic episodes. Less severe but more chronic periods of depressed mood are sometimes termed **dysthymic disorder,** which is associated with some but not all of the symptoms of a major depressive episode.

Major Depressive Episode

A. Diagnostic Characteristics: Depression in children is marked by depressed mood (feeling "down," sad, hopeless), irritability, or anhedonia. Diagnosis of a major depressive episode in children requires at least 2 weeks of depressed mood and associated symptoms. These symptoms may include appetite and weight changes, insomnia or hypersomnia, psychomotor agitation or retardation, fatigue, or feelings of worthlessness or inappropriate guilt. The child's ability to think or concentrate may be diminished. There may be recurrent thoughts of death or suicide.

B. Associated Features: It is important to rule out other causes, such as organic factors or normal grief.

Diagnostic instruments for the assessment of depression in children are available. The initial presentation of a major depressive episode may include physical symptoms, behavior problems (including substance abuse), or associated conduct disorder. There is a high risk of suicide. Sleep electroencephalographic abnormalities are common, including prolonged sleep latency. Several neurotransmitters, such as serotonin, have been implicated in severe depressive disorders. Untreated episodes usually last 6 months or longer, followed for most by return to premorbid level of functioning. In prepubertal children, males and females are equally affected; in adolescence, females are diagnosed with major depression more frequently than males. First episodes commonly follow a severe psychosocial stressor.

C. Treatment:

1. As with anxiety disorders, possible physical causes should be ruled out. Discussion of unexplained somatic symptoms may allow further exploration of potentially problematic areas, such as psychosocial and family stressors, academic difficulties, peer difficulties, and alcohol- and substance-related problems.

2. Psychotherapy for both child and family should be considered prior to medication, depending on the severity of the episode, need for hospitalization, or suicidal ideation. Appropriate mental health consultation is important.

3. Pharmacotherapy should not be the only treatment modality used in most cases of major depressive episode in children but should be used in conjunction with psychotherapy. Several types of agents have been tried. **Tricyclic antidepressants,** while effective in adults, have not been shown to be effective overall in major depressive episodes in children and adolescents. Individual children or adolescents may benefit, however. Side effects, such as blurred vision and dry mouth, may be problematic. The potential for cardiac toxicity is a concern. Some antidepressants may trigger episodes of mania in susceptible individuals; close observation is important. Newer SSRIs such as fluoxetine and sertraline have been given to children but have not been widely studied in the pediatric population.

POST-TRAUMATIC STRESS DISORDER (PTSD)

A. Diagnostic Characteristics: PTSD is characterized by exposure to a traumatic event in which the person has experienced, witnessed, or was confronted with an event(s) that involved actual or threatened death or serious injury, or threat to the physical integrity of self or others. The response to the event involves intense fear, helplessness, or horror. PTSD includes symptoms of numbing, intrusive re-experiencing of the event, and symptoms of increased arousal (difficulty falling asleep, irritability, hypervigilance, and exaggerated startle response). A child suffering from PTSD may seek to avoid cues or situations that resemble or symbolize the traumatic event. Repetitive play expressing themes or aspects of the trauma may be exhibited. Other associated symptoms include feelings of detachment or estrangement from others, restricted range of affect, and a sense of foreshortened future (in children, expecting to die young or refusing to plan for future education or careers).

B. Associated Features: PTSD in children may result from childhood sexual or physical abuse or domestic violence. Symptoms of PTSD typically begin within 3 months of the precipitating event, although delays in onset are not unusual.

C. Treatment: In addition to individual psychotherapy, family counseling may be helpful. If the child was involved in a group or collective trauma (eg, plane crash, natural disaster, explosion), he or she may benefit from therapy groups formed for survivors of large-scale traumas. Medication for PTSD has not been well studied in children. In adults, symptom-specific medications such as antidepressants have been used. Clonidine and SSRIs have also been tried. Pediatricians should consult specialists in child psychiatry before prescribing medications for PTSD.

EATING DISORDERS

Eating disorders present more often in adolescents than in younger children and are discussed in Chapter 9.

SLEEP DISORDERS

Sleep disorders are common in pediatric practice; they include nightmare disorder, sleep terror disorder, and sleepwalking disorder. Consult Chapter 20 for information about neurologic disorders and sleep disturbances.

Nightmare Disorder

A. Diagnostic Characteristics: In nightmare disorder, the child experiences repeated awakenings from sleep with detailed recall of extended and extremely frightening dreams that usually involve threats to survival, security, or self-esteem. The child exhibits rapid re-orientation and alertness on awakening. The nightmares occur almost exclusively during rapid eye movement (REM) sleep, most commonly during the second half of the night. The sleep disturbance causes significant distress or impairment in daytime functioning.

B. Associated Features: Nightmares are common in childhood and do not necessarily signify a mental disorder. If the frequency is high or impairment significant, consider associated psychiatric disorder. Nightmare disorder must be differentiated from sleep terror disorder, which usually occurs in the first third of the night, begins during non-REM (NREM) sleep, and is associated with no dream recall or only single images without storylike quality.

C. Treatment: In general, supportive or psychoeducational counseling for the child and parents is sufficient. In cases of high frequency or significant dysfunction, evaluation for psychosocial stressors and emotional or behavioral difficulties is warranted.

Sleep Terror Disorder

A. Diagnostic Characteristics: Sleep terror disorder is characterized by recurrent episodes of abrupt awakening from sleep, usually during the first third of the major sleep episode. These episodes begin with a panicky scream. There may be yelling, screaming, and crying. Intense fear and signs of autonomic arousal (tachycardia, tachypnea, diaphoresis) occur. The child is relatively unresponsive to comforting from others. There is no detailed dream recall, and the child is amnestic for the episode.

B. Associated Features: Sleep deprivation, fatigue, and physical or emotional stress increase the likelihood of this disorder. It is more common in males; age of onset is usually 4–12 years, with spontaneous resolution during adolescence. Sleep terror disorder is not usually associated with other mental disorders.

C. Treatment: Treatment is usually supportive and psychoeducational and should include the establishment of a regular sleep schedule for the child. In severe cases, short-term or intermittent use of a benzodiazepine may be helpful. Imipramine has also been used.

Sleepwalking Disorder

A. Diagnostic Characteristics: Sleepwalking disorder is characterized by repeated episodes of rising from bed during sleep and walking about. The sleepwalking usually occurs during the first third of a major sleep episode. The child is relatively unresponsive to others, is awakened with great difficulty, and is amnestic for the episode on awakening.

B. Associated Features: Sleepwalking disorder may be associated with injuries caused by falls; it may also be associated with sleep terror disorder. It is usually not associated with other mental disorders. Sleepwalking episodes typically begin during NREM sleep; heart and respiratory rate may increase at the beginning of the episode. Ten percent to 30% of children have at least one episode of sleepwalking. The prevalence of repeated episodes and impairment is much lower. Onset is usually between 4 and 8 years of age. Sleepwalking disorder generally resolves spontaneously during adolescence.

C. Treatment: Treatment is usually supportive and psychoeducational. In addition to the establishment of a regular sleep schedule, the child's safety should be ensured by appropriate attention to environmental hazards. Medication is seldom indicated. Benzodiazepines and imipramine have been used.

9 | Adolescence

David W. Kaplan, MD, MPH, &
Kathleen A. Mammel, MD

Adolescence is a unique period of rapid physical, emotional, cognitive, and social growth and development bridging childhood and adult life. Generally, adolescence "begins" at age 11–12 years and ends between ages 18 and 21.

The developmental passage from childhood to adulthood encompasses:

1. Completion of puberty and somatic growth.
2. Development of social, emotional, and cognitive skills–moving from concrete to abstract thinking.
3. Establishment of an independent identity and separation from the family.
4. Preparation for a career or vocation.

DEMOGRAPHY

In the United States in 1995, 18.0 million adolescents were between the ages of 15 and 19 years; 17.9 million were 20–24 years of age. The adolescent/young adult population—15–24 years—comprises 13.7% of the US population.

MORTALITY

The three leading causes of mortality in the adolescent population aged 15–19 years in 1992 were unintentional injuries (43.3% –78% of all unintentional injuries were caused by motor vehicle crashes), suicides (12.8%), and homicides (22.9%). During the past 20 years, fatalities due to motor vehicle crashes, suicide, and homicide have increased between 300 and 400%. The major threats of death for the adolescent population are due to societal and environmental rather than organic factors.

MORBIDITY

Major morbidity during adolescence is primarily psychosocial: unintended pregnancy, sexually transmitted diseases, substance abuse, smoking, truancy and quitting school, depression, running away from home, physical violence, and juvenile delinquency. Early identification of teenagers at risk for these problems is important not only to prevent immediate complications but also to prevent future associated problems. High-risk behavior in one aspect of life is often associated with or may lead to problems in another area (Figure 9–1).

Some of the early indicators of an adolescent at high risk include:

1. Decline in academic performance.
2. Excessive school absences; cutting class.
3. Frequent or persistent psychosomatic complaints.
4. Changes in sleeping or eating habits.
5. Difficulty concentrating; persistent boredom.
6. Signs or symptoms of depression, extreme stress, or anxiety.
7. Withdrawal from friends or family or change to a new peer group.
8. Radical personality changes, or unusually severe violent or rebellious behavior.
9. Parent-adolescent conflict.
10. Sexual acting-out.
11. Conflict with the law.
12. Expressions of suicidal or homicidal thoughts; preoccupation with themes of death.
13. Substance abuse.
14. Running away from home.

DELIVERY OF HEALTH SERVICES

How, where, why, and when adolescents seek health care depends on a number of factors: ability to pay for care, distance, transportation, accessibility of services, time out of school, and privacy. Teenagers concerned about pregnancy or contraception, symptoms of a sexually transmitted disease or depression, or problems with substance abuse are often reluctant to confide in their parents for fear of

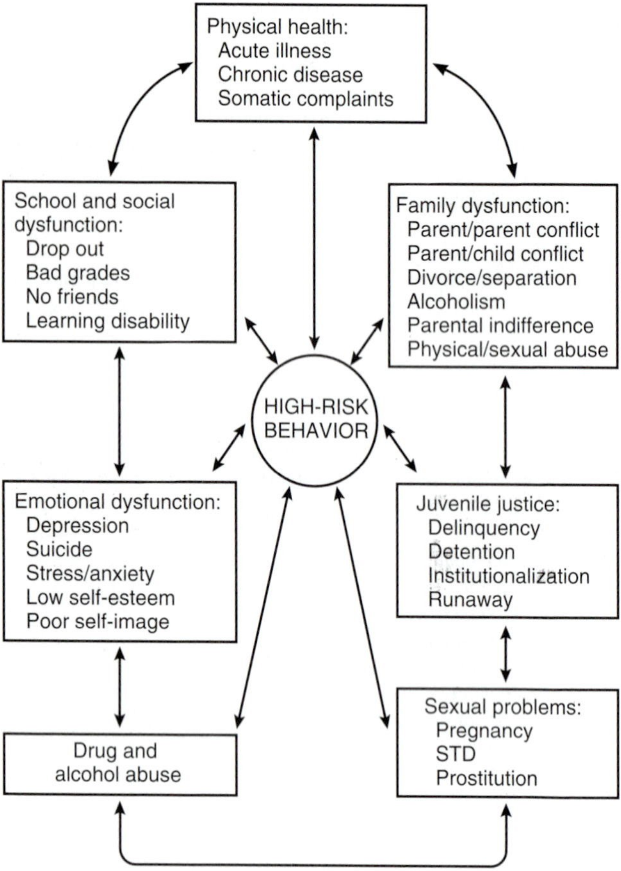

Figure 9–1. Interrelationships of high-risk adolescent behaviors.

disappointing them and being punished. For the physician, establishing a trusting and confidential relationship is basic to meeting an adolescent patient's health-care needs. If the patient senses the physician may disclose information about a confidential problem to parents or guardians, the patient may lie or withhold information essential to proper diagnosis and treatment.

RELATING TO THE ADOLESCENT PATIENT

The manner in which the physician initially approaches the adolescent may determine the success or failure of the visit. The physician should act in a simple and honest fashion, without an authoritarian or excessively "professional" attitude. Because many young adolescents have fragile self-esteem, clinicians must be careful not to overpower and intimidate the patient. In communicating with an adolescent, be especially sensitive to the young person's developmental level; recognize that physical appearance and chronological age may be misleading as measures of cognitive development.

CONFIDENTIALITY

It is helpful at the beginning of the visit to talk with the adolescent and his or her parents about expectations. The issue of confidentiality should be addressed straightforwardly; tell the parents you will meet first with the teenager alone, and then with all three of them. Adequate time must be spent with both the patient and parent(s), or important information may be missed. At the beginning of the interview with the patient, you may find it useful to say something like "I am likely to ask you some personal questions. This is not because I am trying to snoop into your private life, but because these matters may be important to your health. I want to assure you that I will keep our conversation confidential, just between the two of us. If there is something I think we should discuss with your parents, I will ask your permission first. The only exception would be a life-threatening problem."

THE INTERVIEW

The course of the interview during the first few minutes of the visit often determines the absence or establishment of a trusting relationship. Spending a few minutes getting to know the patient is time well invested.

History taking should include an assessment of progress in psychodevelopmental tasks as well as personal behaviors that are potentially detrimental to the patient's health (eg, smoking). The review of systems should include questions about:

1. Nutrition: Number and balance of meals; calcium, iron, cholesterol intake.
2. Sleep: Number of hours; problems with insomnia, hypersomnia, or frequent wakening.
3. Safety measures: proper and regular use of automobile seat belts, bicycle or motorcycle helmets, protective athletic gear.
4. Self-care: Maintenance of proper dental hygiene and physical exercise; knowledge of testicular or breast self-examination.
5. Family relationships: Quality of the adolescent's relationships with parents/caregivers, siblings, relatives.
6. Peers: Same-sex best friend or buddy, boy/girl friend, involvement in group activities.
7. School: Attendance, grades, extracurricular activities.
8. Educational and vocational interests: College, career, short- and long-term vocational plans.
9. Tobacco: Use of cigarettes, snuff, chewing tobacco.
10. Substance abuse: Frequency, extent, and history of alcohol or drug use.
11. Sexuality: Sexual orientation and activity, contraceptive use, pregnancies, history of sexually transmitted disease, number of sexual partners, risk for infection with human immunodeficiency virus (HIV).
12. Psychological health: Signs of depression, anxiety, or excessive stress.

The physician's personal attention and interest may be a new experience for the teenager who has probably experienced medical care only when accompanied by parents or caregivers. The teenager should leave the visit with a sense of having his or her "own physician."

THE PHYSICAL EXAMINATION

During early adolescence, many teenagers may be quite shy and modest, especially if examined by a physician of the opposite sex. The examiner should address shyness directly as it can usually be allayed by verbal acknowledgment of the uneasiness, explanation of the purposes of the examination, and discussion of the findings during the examination. A pictorial chart of sexual development (Figure 9–2) is extremely useful for showing patients their current stage of development and the changes they can expect in the future.

GROWTH AND DEVELOPMENT

PHYSICAL GROWTH

Pediatricians should understand the physical changes of puberty because they are often implicated in the differential diagnosis of adolescents' medical problems, and because they have wide-ranging effects on adolescents' psychosocial adjustment and maturation. Pubertal growth and physical development result from activation in late childhood of the hypothalamic-pituitary-gonadal axis. Before the onset of puberty, pituitary and gonadal hormones remain at very low levels. With the onset of puberty, the inhibition of gonadotropin-releasing hormone (GnRH) in the hypothalamus is removed, thus allowing pulsatile production and release of the gonadotropins, luteinizing hormone (LH) and follicle-stimulating hormone (FSH). In early to middle adolescence, there is an increase in pulse frequency and amplitude of LH and FSH secretion, which stimulates the gonads to produce sex steroids (estrogen or testosterone). In the female, FSH stimulates ovarian maturation, granulosa cell function, and estradiol secretion. LH is important in ovulation of the mature ovum and is also involved in corpus luteum formation and progesterone secretion. Initially, estradiol has an inhibitory effect on the release of LH and FSH. Eventually, estradiol becomes stimulatory and the secretions of LH and FSH become cyclic. There is a progressive increase in estradiol that results in maturation of the female genital tract and development of the breasts.

In the male, LH stimulates the interstitial cells of the testes, which produce testosterone. FSH stimulates the production of spermatocytes in the presence of testosterone. The testes also produce inhibin, which is a Sertoli-cell protein that inhibits the secretion of FSH. During puberty, circulating testosterone increases more than 20-fold. Levels of testosterone correlate with the physical stages of puberty and the degree of skeletal maturation.

Tanner's scale of sexual maturation is useful clinically to categorize genital development. Tanner staging includes age ranges of normal development and specific descriptions for each stage of pubic hair growth, penis and testes development in boys, and breast maturation in girls. The chronologic development of this process with reference to each Tanner stage is shown in Figures 9–2 A and B.

The pubertal growth spurt usually takes 2–4 years. It begins nearly 2 years earlier in girls than in boys, but lasts longer in boys.

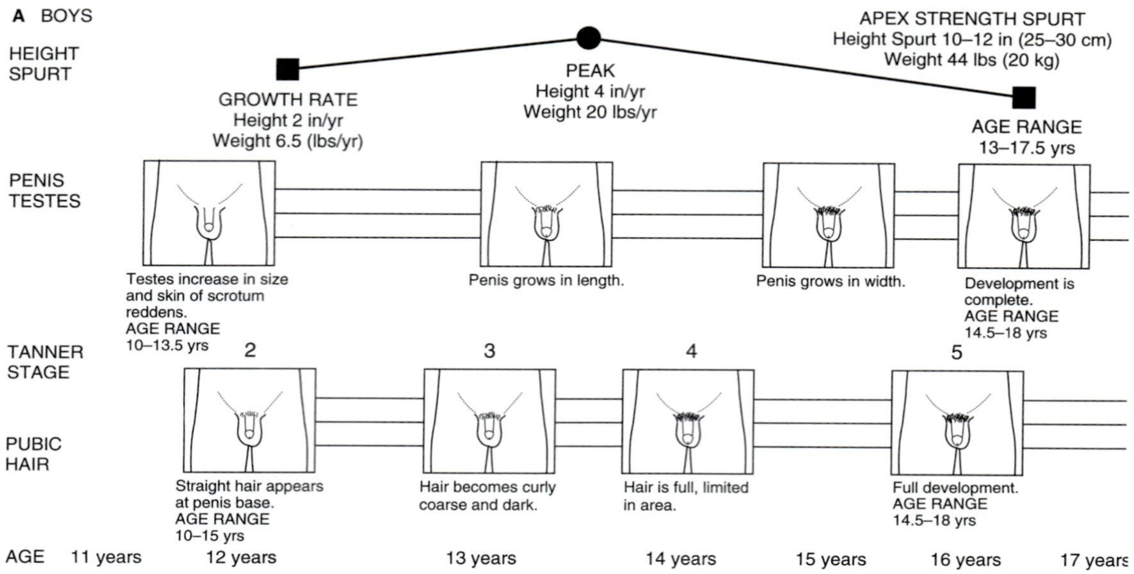
A BOYS
HEIGHT SPURT
GROWTH RATE
Height 2 in/yr
Weight 6.5 (lbs/yr)
PEAK
Height 4 in/yr
Weight 20 lbs/yr
APEX STRENGTH SPURT
Height Spurt 10–12 in (25–30 cm)
Weight 44 lbs (20 kg)
AGE RANGE
13–17.5 yrs
PENIS TESTES
Testes increase in size and skin of scrotum reddens.
AGE RANGE
10–13.5 yrs
Penis grows in length.
Penis grows in width.
Development is complete.
AGE RANGE
14.5–18 yrs
TANNER STAGE
2
3
4
5
PUBIC HAIR
Straight hair appears at penis base.
AGE RANGE
10–15 yrs
Hair becomes curly coarse and dark.
Hair is full, limited in area.
Full development.
AGE RANGE
14.5–18 yrs
AGE
11 years
12 years
13 years
14 years
15 years
16 years
17 years

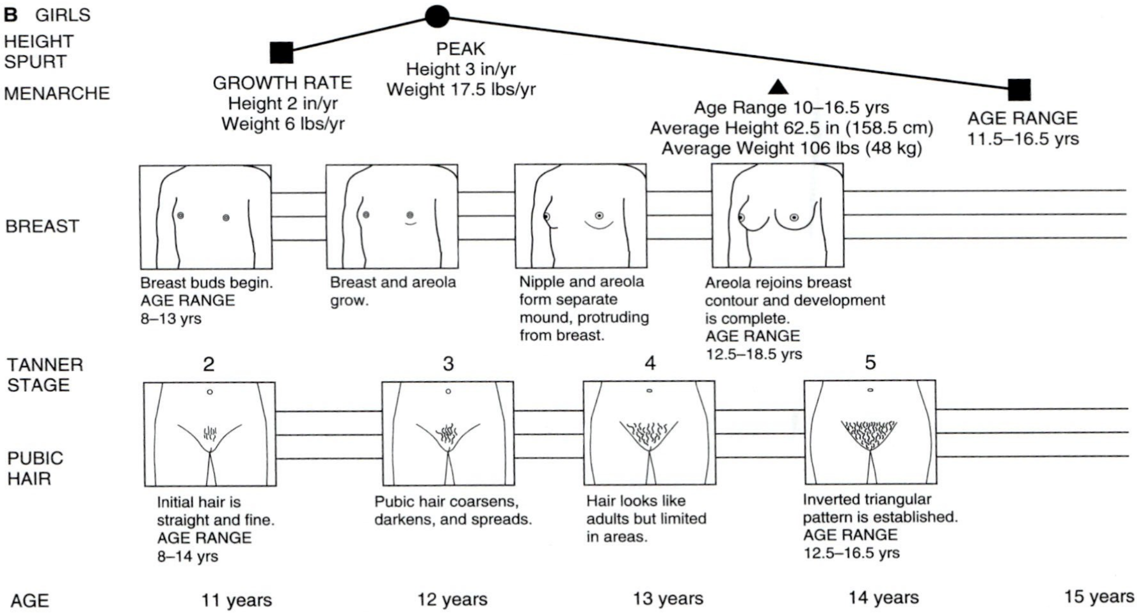

Figure 9–2. (A) Adolescent male sexual maturation and growth. **(B)** Adolescent female sexual maturation and growth. (Adapted from Tanner JM: *Growth at Adolescence.* Blackwell;1962.)

Girls reach their peak height velocity (PHV) between 11.5 and 12 years of age, and boys at ages 13.5–14 years. Linear growth at peak velocity is 9.5 + 1.5 cm per year for boys and 8.3 + 1.2 cm per year for girls. During adolescence, a teenager's weight doubles, and height increases by 15–20%. In the United States, the average age of menarche is 12¾ years. However, menarche may be delayed until age 16 or begin as early as age 10. The first conspicuous sign of puberty in girls is development of breast buds between the ages of 8 and 11 years. The first sign of puberty in the male, usually between the ages of 10 and 12, is thinning of the scrotum and testicular growth.

PSYCHOSOCIAL DEVELOPMENT

Adolescents are struggling to find out who they are, what they want to do with their lives, and what their personal strengths and weaknesses are. These questions arise primarily because teenagers are in the process of establishing their own identity. Adolescence is a period of progressive individuation and separation from the family. Because of the rapid physical, emotional, cognitive, and social growth that occurs during adolescence, it is useful to divide the period into three phases of development. **Early adolescence** occurs roughly between ages 10 and 13; **middle adolescence** between ages 14 and 16; and **late adolescence,** at age 17 and older.

Early Adolescence

Early adolescence (ages 10–13) is characterized by rapid growth and the development of secondary sex characteristics. Young adolescents are often preoccupied with the changes taking place in their bodies. Because of these rapid transformations, body image, self-concept, and self-esteem fluctuate dramatically. Young adolescents may worry intensely about how their growth and development deviates from their friends' patterns, especially with regard to short stature in boys and delayed breast development or delayed menarche in girls. As the young teenager becomes more independent, and family ties loosen, allegiance shifts from parents to peers, who become much more important. Young teenagers still think concretely and cannot easily conceptualize the future. They may have vague professional goals, or aspirations limited to current peer group interests, such as becoming a lead singer in a rock group or an athletic superstar.

Middle Adolescence

During middle adolescence (14–16 years), with the rapid pubertal growth of early adolescence leveling off, teenagers begin to adjust physically and become more comfortable with their "new" bodies. Intense emotions and wide mood swings are typical of this age group. Cognitively, as teenagers move from concrete thinking to formal operations, they develop greater competence with abstract thought. With this new mental power comes a sense of omnipotence and a belief that the world can be changed merely by thinking about it (sometimes called "magical thinking"). Sexually active teenagers may believe they don't need to use contraception because they "can't get pregnant—it won't happen to me." Other adolescents may drive recklessly, or drive under the influence of mood-altering substances. In an effort to establish their own identity, teens relate to other people, including peers, in narcissistic ways; experimenting with different images or dress styles is quite common. Peers usually determine the standards for identification, behavior, activities, and fashion; and provide emotional support, intimacy, empathy, and the sharing of guilt and anxiety, during adolescent struggles for autonomy.

Late Adolescence

Late adolescents (17 years and older) are less self-centered and begin to demonstrate care for others; these teenagers often seek involvement in volunteer activities. Social relationships shift from the peer group to the individual. Dating becomes much more intimate. The older adolescent strives for greater independence from the family. The ability to think abstractly allows older adolescents to delay immediate gratification and plan ahead in terms of future education, activities, and careers. With regard to morals, older adolescents may have very rigid concepts of right and wrong. Late adolescence is typically a period of idealism.

BEHAVIORAL AND PSYCHOLOGIC HEALTH

Adolescents with emotional disorders often present with somatic symptoms that do not appear to have biologic causes (eg, abdominal pain, headaches, dizziness/syncope, fatigue, sleep problems, and chest pain). The emotional basis of such a complaint may be varied: somatoform disorder, depression, or stress and anxiety.

PSYCHOPHYSIOLOGIC SYMPTOMS AND CONVERSION REACTIONS

The most common somatoform disorders during adolescence are conversion reactions. A **conversion reaction** is a psychophysiologic process in which painful emotions, especially anxiety, depression, and guilt, are communicated through a physical symptom. The symptom may appear at times of stress such as parental conflict or divorce, serious illness in a family member, or moving and a change of school. Psychophysiologic symptoms result when anxiety activates the autonomic nervous system, resulting in tachycardia, hyperventilation, and vasoconstriction. The degree to which the conversion symptom lessens anxiety, depression, or the unpleasant feeling is referred to as **primary gain.** Conversion symptoms not only diminish unpleasant feelings but also benefit the adolescent by removing him or her from conflict or an uncomfortable situation. This benefit is referred to as **secondary gain.** Specific symptoms may be based on existing or previous illness (eg, pseudoseizures in adolescents with a history of epilepsy). Adolescents with conversion symptoms tend to have overprotective parents and to become increasingly dependent on their parents as the symptoms become the major focus of both the parent's and adolescent's life.

Diagnosis & Treatment

In cases of suspected conversion reaction, the patient's history and physical findings are usually inconsistent with anatomic and physiologic concepts. It is critical from the outset that the physician emphasize to the patient and his or her family that both physical and emotional causes for the symptom need to be understood. The relationship between physical causes of emotional pain and emotional causes of physical pain should be explained. The patient should come to understand that the symptom may persist, and that at least a short-term goal is to help them continue normal daily activities in school and with friends. Medication is rarely helpful in relieving or resolving conversion symptoms. Discussion of the symptom itself should be kept to a minimum; however, the physician should be supportive and avoid suggesting that the pain is imaginary. As the parents gain further insight into the symptom's origin, they will become less indulgent of the patient's complaints, facilitating the resumption of normal activities. If management is successful, the adolescent will acquire increased coping skills and become more independent, with decreasing secondary gain.

If the symptom continues to interfere with daily activities, school attendance, participation in extracurricular activities, or involvement with peers, and the patient and parents believe that no progress is being made, psychologic referral is indicated.

DEPRESSION

Presentation

Moderate or severe depression may present during adolescence in a variety of ways. It may be similar to presentation in adults, with vegetative signs such as "blue" moods nearly every day, crying spells or inability to cry, discouragement, irritability, sense of emptiness and meaninglessness, negative expectations of self and the environment, low self-esteem, isolation, helplessness, marked anhedonia, significant weight loss or weight gain, insomnia or hypersomnia, fatigue or loss of energy, and diminished ability to reason or concentrate. However, it is not unusual for a serious depression to be masked because the teenager does not exhibit outward severe feelings of sadness. He or she may present instead with recurrent or persistent psychosomatic complaints, such as abdominal pain, chest pain, headache, lethargy, appetite disturbances, dizziness and syncope, or other nonspecific symptoms. Other behavioral manifestations of a masked depression may include school truancy, running away from home, defiance of authorities, self-destructive behavior, drug and alcohol abuse, sexual acting-out, and vandalism or other delinquent acts.

Diagnosis

A complete history and physical examination should be performed, including a careful review of the patient's medical and psychosocial history. The family history should be explored for psychiatric problems.

The teenager should be questioned directly about any specific symptoms of depression (as noted above), expression of suicidal thoughts, or preoccupation with themes of death. The history should include an assessment of the patient's school performance, change in work or other outside activities, family transitions (eg, divorce), or death of a close relative. The teenager may have withdrawn from friends or family, or begun to associate with a new group of friends. Is there a history of drug and alcohol abuse, conflict with the law, sexual acting-out, running away from home, unusual severe violent or rebellious behavior, or radical personality change?

Because a number of physical disorders can mimic, cause, or exacerbate major depression, adolescents presenting with significant depressive symptoms deserve a thorough medical evaluation to rule out any contributing or underlying medical illness. Commonly prescribed medications in this age group, such as birth control pills and anticonvulsants, may be responsible for depressive symptoms, as may illicit drugs such as marijuana, phencyclidine, amphetamines, and cocaine.

The majority of physical disorders presenting with depressive symptoms are usually evident by history of present illness, past medical history, and physical examination. However, some routine laboratory studies are indicated, including a complete blood count (CBC), sedimentation rate, urinalysis, electrolytes, blood urea nitrogen (BUN), calcium, T_4 and TSH, serology, and liver enzymes.

The risk of depression appears to be greatest in families with a history of depression of early onset and chronicity.

Treatment

The primary care physician may be able to counsel adolescents and parents if an underlying depression is mild or seems to be the result of an acute identifiable personal loss or frustration, and if the patient is not contemplating suicide or appears to be at risk for other life-threatening behaviors. If there is evidence of a long-standing depressive disorder, suicidal thoughts, or psychotic ideation; or if the physician does not feel competent to counsel or have an interest in counseling the patient, a psychologic referral should be made.

ADOLESCENT SUICIDE

In the United States in 1992 there were 4693 suicides in persons aged 15–24. In the 15- to 19-year-old age group, males had a rate 400% higher than females, and white males had the highest rate. The ratio of attempted to completed suicides is estimated to be 50:1 to 100:1, and is three times higher in females than in males. Among completed suicides, deaths due to firearms are the number one cause for both males and females, accounting for more than 60% of the suicide deaths.

Acute depressive reactions (transient grief responses) to the loss of a close family member or friend through death or separation may last for weeks or even months. If an adolescent is unable to work through the grief and becomes increasingly depressed, is unable to function at school or socially, has sleep and appetite disturbances, and feelings of hopelessness and helplessness, the magnitude of the depression fulfills the diagnostic criteria of major depression; the teenager should be considered to be at increased risk for suicide. As discussed in the preceding section, symptoms of depression during adolescence may be masked.

Another group of suicidal adolescents includes angry teenagers who feel ineffective and want to have an impact on their environment. They may be only mildly depressed and may not have a long-standing wish to die. Teenagers in this group—usually females—may "try out" or "gesture" suicide as a form of revenge or to gain attention by frightening or worrying another person.

The last group of adolescents at risk for suicide comprises teenagers with a serious thought disorder, such as acute schizophrenia or a psychotic depressive disorder.

Diagnosis

In teenagers at risk, the physician must determine the extent of the patient's depression and the degree of risk in adolescents with a history of self-inflicted harm. The evaluation should include interviews with both the teenager and his or her family. The history should include the medical, social, emotional, and academic background, as described above. When seeing depressed patients, the physician should always inquire about thoughts of suicide with such questions as the following: "Are things ever so bad that life doesn't seem worth living?" "Have you thought of taking your life?" If the patient mentions suicidal ideation, you can assess the immediacy of risk by determining whether the patient has a concrete, feasible plan. Although the patients who are at greatest risk have a concrete plan that can be carried out in the near future, especially if they have rehearsed the scenario, the physician should not dismiss potential risks of suicide in adolescents who do not describe a specific means or setting. The physician should pay attention to "gut feelings." There may be subtle nonverbal signs that the patient is at greater risk than is apparent on the surface.

Management

Primary care physicians are often in a unique position to identify adolescents at risk for suicide, in that many teenagers who attempt suicide seek medical attention within a few weeks prior to the attempt. These visits often involve vague somatic complaints or subtle signs of depression. If there is evidence of depression, the physician must assess its severity and the degree of suicidal risk. The physician should always obtain emergency psychologic consultation for any teenager who is severely depressed, psychotic, or acutely suicidal. It is the psychologist's or psychiatrist's responsibility to assess the seriousness of suicidal ideation and decide whether hospitalization or outpatient treatment is appropriate.

SUBSTANCE ABUSE

Substance abuse is a serious problem in a society that promotes quick fixes for complex problems. In 1993, a national survey of high-school seniors reported that 51.0% had used alcohol and 15.5% smoked marijuana in the past 30 days; 6.1% reported that they had tried cocaine.

Risk Factors

The causes of substance abuse are multifactorial, including personality characteristics, genetic influences, peer pressure, parental examples, and cultural influences.

Children whose parents exemplify healthy attitudes toward drugs and provide consistent authoritative discipline involving warmth and discussion of problems; those whose peers do not use drugs; those who understand the consequences of substance abuse; and those who consider good health and achievement to be important are relatively protected from substance abuse.

Stages of Substance Involvement and Abuse

Chemical dependency is the result of a gradual process of habituation. Macdonald has suggested five stages of substance abuse which are outlined in Table 9–1. Progression through these stages may occur at a variable rate, and not every user will progress to stage 4. However, the earlier in life that substance abuse begins, the greater the risk for development of chemical dependency.

Substances Abused

Although tobacco and alcohol are considered "gateway" drugs for young persons experimenting with substance use, many teenagers also use marijuana during adolescence. See Table 9–2 for drugs commonly abused by teenagers and their effects. Anabolic steroid users are more likely to use multiple drugs and engage in the use of injected drugs.

Diagnosis

History taking is the key to accurate differential diagnosis of substance abuse; a history obtained in a nonjudgmental manner may be highly informative. In an adolescent who has progressed to advanced stages of involvement, however, denial may lead to minimization of use. Significant diagnostic clues include episodes of acute drug abuse (eg, accidental or intentional overdosing); deteriorating academic or athletic performance; personality changes (mood swings, lack of motivation); worsening family relationships; change of peer groups; trouble with the law; or persistent regular drug use despite parental or medical intervention. When substance abuse is suspected or established in an adolescent, an assessment of the adolescent's involvement with the drug (age at onset, drugs used, duration and frequency of use, attitude toward use); involvement with a drug-using peer group or subculture; family structure; and psychologic profile (any preexisting psychiatric, developmental, or educational difficulties) will assist in decisions regarding appropriate management. Information should also be obtained from the parents, who may suspect substance abuse or may be in denial and thereby enabling the adolescent.

Physical examination may provide few clues apart from needle marks or weight loss and malnutrition. In some cases, sexually transmitted diseases are associated with drug abuse in that the teenager may be exchanging sex for drugs or engaging in unsafe sex under the influence of drugs. Laboratory tests are usually helpful only with acute intoxication, when a blood alcohol and urine toxin screen should be obtained. When it is known that one chemical has been used at the time of acute intoxication, a drug screen should be obtained to look for other substances because of the possibility of multiple drug abuse (cross-addiction) or adulteration or misrepresentation of material. Drug testing apart from an episode of acute intoxication or a drug-free maintenance program is generally of little help and may endanger the patient-physician relationship.

Management

Prevention and early intervention during the stage of experimental use is most effective. Management depends on the stage of the adolescent's involvement (Table 9–1).

EATING DISORDERS

Prevalence rates for eating disorders among adolescents have risen steadily over the past four decades. Of 15- to 19-year-old females,

Table 9–1. Stages of substance abuse.[1]

Stage	Drugs	Sources	Frequency	Feelings	Behavior	Treatment
Stage 0 Curiosity	None	Available—but not used	—	Curious	Risk-taking Desire for acceptance	Optimal time Anticipatory guidance to develop good coping skills and strong self-esteem Clear family guidelines on drug and alcohol use Drug education
Stage 1 Experimentation	Tobacco Alcohol Marijuana	House supply Friends Siblings	Weekend use for recreational purposes	Excitement Pleasure Few consequences Learns how easy it is to feel good	Lying Little change	Drug education Attention to societal messages, reduce supply Strict, loving rules at home Drug-free alternative activities established
Stage 2 Regular use	As above, plus hashish or hash oil, tranquilizers, sedatives, amphetamines	Buying	Progresses to mid-week use Purpose is to get high	Excitement followed by guilt	Mood swings Faltering school performance Truancy Changing peer groups Changing style of dress	Drug-free self-help groups (Alcoholics or Narcotics Anonymous) Family involvement Psychiatric counseling unhelpful unless family therapy and after-care provided

Stage 3 Psychologic or chemical dependency	As above, plus stimulants, hallucinogens	Selling to support their habit Possibly stealing or prostitution in exchange for drugs	Daily	Euphoric highs followed by depression, shame, guilt, and perhaps suicidal thoughts	Pathological lying School failure Family fights Involvement with the law over curfew, truancy, vandalism, shoplifting, or driving under the influence, breaking and entering, violence	Inpatient or foster-care programs that require family involvement and provide after-care
Stage 4 Using drugs to feel "normal"	As above; any available drug, including opiates	Any way possible	All day	Euphoria rare and harder to achieve Chronic depression	Drifters with repeated failures and psychologic symptoms of paranoia and aggression Overdosing, black-outs, amnesia occur regularly Chronic cough, fatigue, malnutrition	Inpatient or foster-care programs that require family involvement and provide after-care

[1]Reproduced with permission, from Macdonald DI: *Drugs, Drinking, and Adolescents.* Year Book, 1984. © 1984 Year Book Medical Publishers, Inc.

Table 9–2. Subjective, objective, and adverse effects of commonly abused drugs.

Drug	Street Name	Subjective Effects	Objective Effects	Adverse/Overdose Reactions
Cannabis Marijuana Hashish Hash oil THC	Pot Grass Weed Mary Jane Hash Tea Reefer Joint	Sedation Tranquilization Mild hallucination or pleasurable change in perception	Tachycardia Conjunctival irritation Impaired abstract thinking, reading comprehension, verbal ability, short-term memory, counting, color discrimination Impaired driving ability	Acute anxiety Serious reaction uncommon unless adulterated with hallucinogens
Alcohol	Booze	Stimulation as blood level rises Subsequent sedation, release of inhibitions	Slurred speech Ataxia Impaired driving performance	Poor judgment Impaired cognitive and motor abilities Emotional changes Respiratory depression Decrease in temperature Coma, shock, death
CNS Stimulants Cocaine Amphetamines	Cocaine Coke Snow Dust Amphetamines Uppers Speed Meth Bennies Dexies	Euphoric effects: exhilaration, calmness, sense of power; omnipotence and unlimited energy in high doses Perception of decrease in appetite, thirst, fatigue Dysphoria or "wired" irritability after euphoric phase	Local anesthetic Sympathomimetic: mydriasis, hypertension, tachycardia, tachypnea, temperature elevation, tremor, agitation	Anxiety Elevated temperature Seizures Respiratory arrest Arrhythmia Death Hallucinations and paranoia

CNS Depressants Group I Sedatives Tranquilizers	Downers Quaaludes, Ludes Blues, Bluebirds Reds, Red devils Yellows, Yellow jackets	Relaxation Facilitation of social behavior With higher doses, loss of inhibitions, sedation, drowsiness	Nystagmus on lateral gaze Slurred speech, ataxia Impulsiveness	Coma Death
CNS Depressants Group II Nitrous oxide Toluene Trichlorethylene Methanol Acetone Gasoline Fluorinated hydrocarbons		Sedation Heightened visual imagery Hallucination Euphoria	Drowsiness Rhinitis, bronchitis Odor of inhalant on breath Metabolic abnormalities	Coma is rare Idiosyncratic reaction to fluorinated hydrocarbons resulting in sudden death by cardiac arrhythmia
Nitrites Amyl nitrite Isobutyl nitrite	Rush Locker room Poppers Bolt	Sudden, transient, pleasurable tingling Headache Pounding heart	Tachycardia Hypotension	Exacerbation of preexisting cardiac disease, syncope Elevated intraocular pressure Coma, rarely sudden death Methemoglobinemia
Hallucinogens Group I Lysergic acid diethylamide Mescaline Psilocybin	Acid LSD Peyote Button Mesc Mushrooms	Vivid sensory stimulation and distortion Introspection Awareness of drug-induced state	Dizziness, nausea Paresthesias Sympathomimetic effects Varying mental status as changes from hallucinating to coherent recountings	Idiosyncratic "bad trips" or panic reactions with terrifying hallucinations that may last from hours to more than a day

(*continued*)

Table 9–2. Subjective, objective, and adverse effects of commonly abused drugs (*continued*).

Drug	Street Name	Subjective Effects	Objective Effects	Adverse/Overdose Reactions
Hallucinogens Group II Phencyclidine	PCP Angel dust	Low doses (1–5 mg) produce floating euphoria or numbness Doses of 5–15 mg cause confusion, agitation, impairment of communication, and distorted body perception Higher doses may cause psychotic reactions lasting from days to months	Sympathomimetic effects Drooling Rotatory nystagmus Decreased response to pain Combative and aggressive or silent and withdrawn	Muscle rigidity, opisthotonos, seizures, coma Toxic psychosis (rotatory nystagmus and fever may be the only signs to differentiate from non-toxic psychosis) Hypertensive crises with CNS hemorrhage and death
Opiates Heroin Morphine Meperidine Propoxyphene Methadone Codeine	Dope H Horse Smack Meth	With IV use a sudden "rush" and sensation similar to orgasm With other routes, euphoria, drowsiness, decreased appetite and libido Nausea, vomiting, and dizziness may occur in novices	Oriented but indifferent Slurred speech, unsteady gait Slowed heart and respiratory rates Pinpoint pupils Needle tracks in IV users	CNS and respiratory depression responsive to naloxone (Narcan) Pulmonary edema 24–36 hours after use, not responsive to naloxone Death

0.48 have anorexia nervosa. In the 1980's, 1–5% of teenage girls met strict criteria for bulimia nervosa. Many more teenagers who do not meet full criteria in the *Diagnostic and Statistical Manual, Fourth Edition* (DSM-IV) for eating disorders (Table 9–3) need medical and psychiatric intervention nonetheless.

Presentation and Diagnosis

Some eating disorder patients present with fatigue, abdominal pain, nausea, fainting spells, hair loss, amenorrhea, or at the urging of a school nurse or coach. Bulimics, however, may present on their own initiative and may feel relieved to have someone who knows their secret.

A diagnosis of anorexia nervosa or bulimia nervosa is largely based on history and meeting specific diagnostic criteria (Table 9–3); however, a low threshold of suspicion is advised so that subclinical cases will not be missed. An adequate history will include the presenting symptoms; weight history, including the patient's desired weight; dietary intake, unusual eating behaviors, or avoided foods; history of any compensatory behaviors such as vomiting, excessive exercise, or use of diet pills, diuretics, emetics, or laxatives; and menstrual history

Table 9–3. Diagnostic criteria for eating disorders.[1]

Anorexia nervosa

Weight loss or failure to gain weight during growth such that weight is 15% below that expected for age and height.

Fear of weight gain or fatness despite being underweight.

Disturbed body image—feels all or part of the body is fat even when severely underweight, or self-evaluation overly influenced by body image.

For postmenarchal females, interruption of menstrual cycles for at least 3 months.

Bulimia nervosa

Repeated binge eating (excessive number of calories in short period of time accompanied by the perception that one lacks control over eating).

Recurrent compensatory behaviors to prevent weight gain (self-induced emesis; use of laxatives, diuretics, or emetics; excessive exercise, or severely restricted intake).

The binge eating and compensatory behaviors both occur at a frequency of at least twice a week for 3 months or more.

Self-evaluation is overly influenced by body image.

Not occurring exclusively as part of anorexia nervosa.

[1] Modified and reproduced from American Psychiatric Association: *Diagnostic and Statistical Manual of Mental Disorders,* 4th ed. APA Press, Washington, DC, 1994.

for irregular cycles, secondary amenorrhea, or delay in a perfectionistic drive in anorexics or impulsiveness in bulimics (eg, substance abuse or sexual promiscuity) or to family dysfunction. Review of systems should focus on symptoms of possible complications of the above behaviors (eg, dental problems) and on symptoms of other diseases in the differential diagnosis.

Physical Findings

Findings on physical examination are often normal, but they do not rule out the diagnosis of an eating disorder. The anorexic's weight will quantitate the actual loss; however, bulimics are usually of normal weight or within 10 pounds (under or over) of normal weight. The vital signs of the anorexic may indicate hypothermia, bradycardia, or hypotension. Other findings in anorexia include dry skin, presence of fine, downy lanugo hair on the body or more pigmented body hair, limpness and loss of shine in scalp hair, excoriation over the sacral spine from excessive situps, prominent ribs, atrophied breasts, scaphoid abdomen, palpable hard stool in the rectal vault, cold extremities, squaring off of the convergence of the thighs, or edema of the extremities. In patients with self-induced emesis there may be loss of tooth enamel, particularly on the posterior aspect of the front teeth, or calluses on the dorsum of the fingers.

Laboratory Findings

The goal of laboratory tests is the exclusion of other diagnoses and assessment of the patient's status. Most laboratory studies will not show changes until late in the course of the disease. A CBC is useful to assess nutritional status. A sedimentation rate will help rule out other disorders such as inflammatory bowel disease (IBD) or collagen vascular disease. Electrolyte tests may detect the presence of hypochloremic alkalosis and hypokalemia from vomiting or the metabolic acidosis of laxative abuse. Serum total protein and albumin are usually normal until late. Prealbumin, transferrin, or C_3 complement levels can help assess the degree of malnutrition. Bone densitometry should be done at baseline for severely malnourished teens, especially those with a prolonged history or delayed growth. Serum calcium, phosphorus, and magnesium should be followed closely during refeeding as these elements may quickly become depleted. Other laboratory studies, such as thyroid function tests, x-rays, electrocardiography, upper gastrointestinal series, or computed tomography of the head need be done only as indicated by the presentation.

Differential Diagnosis

The list of causes of weight loss is extensive. Such causes as malignancy, collagen vascular disease, diabetes mellitus, hyperthyroidism, malabsorptive syndromes, IBD, or chronic renal, pulmonary, or cardiac disease warrant consideration in the suspected anorexic. However, with these disorders there may be weight loss but there is no associated disturbance of body image or fear of obesity. Keep in mind also that a number of psychiatric disturbances, including depression, may be associated with loss of appetite and weight. Some unusual central nervous system disorders may present like bulimia, but again there is no distorted body image or overconcern with body shape or weight.

Although early studies of eating disorders suggested that the great majority of patients are female, more recent findings indicate that the number of males with eating disorders is rising. Thus the pediatrician should not exclude these disorders from the differential diagnosis on the basis of sex.

Complications

Eating disorders can result in severe consequences to nearly every system of the body, including electrolyte and acid-base disturbances; depressed gonadotropins; altered thyroid tests; menstrual irregularities; dysrhythmias; congestive heart failure; osteopenia and osteoporosis; disturbed thermoregulation; cortical atrophy of the brain; constipation; gastric dilatation, delayed emptying, and rupture; and bone marrow suppression.

Management

Patients of either sex will need reassurance that the clinician understands their struggle, aims to restore them to health, won't let them become fat, and will help them to regain control. The parents need to understand that eating disorders are symptoms of underlying issues, often a family problem; that the family is very important to resolution of the disorder; and that treatment requires mental health intervention.

Restoration of the nutritional and physiologic state is an early goal of treatment. An individualized contract can be drawn up and signed by the patient that addresses such issues as long-term weight goals, rate of weight gain, amount of exercise, frequency of visits and of laboratory workups, minimal weight signaling need for hospitalization, and consequences of failed weight goals.

In most cases, the patient's increased intake will be adequate to replace nutrient deficits and to gain weight. In extremely malnour-

Table 9–4. Indications for hospitalization of an adolescent with an eating disorder.

Medical
Weight < 75% of ideal body weight
Severe metabolic disturbance
Heart rate < 40 beats/min
Temperature < 36 °C
Systolic blood pressure < 70 mm Hg
Serum K+ < 2.5 meq/L despite oral K+ replacement
Severe dehydration
Cardiac dysrhythmia
Arrested growth and development
Acute food refusal
Severe binging and purging
Failure to respond to outpatient treatment
Psychiatric
Severe depression or risk of suicide
Psychotic symptoms
Family crisis (eg, death or divorce)
Failure to comply with a therapeutic contract, or inadequate response to outpatient treatment

ished and noncompliant hospitalized patients, nasogastric tube feedings or hyperalimentation may initially be necessary. Hospitalization may become necessary for medical or psychiatric reasons (Table 9–4).

Prognosis

It appears that 40–60% of significantly ill anorexics make a good physical and psychosocial recovery, and that 75% improve in weight. The mortality rate ranges from 0–19% and is at least 5% in those receiving therapy. As few as 40–50% of treated bulimics are considered cured, and there is a greater likelihood of serious medical complications, risk of suicide, and death than for anorexics without bulimic behavior.

EXOGENOUS OBESITY

Background

If a child enters adolescence obese, the odds are 4:1 against later achievement of normal weight; but if a child leaves adolescence obese, the odds are 28:1 against later normal weight. The associated medical risks of obesity include pediatric and adult hypertension, elevated triglyceride levels, cerebrovascular accidents, diabetes mellitus, gallbladder disease, slipped capital femoral epiphyses, degenerative arthritis, and pregnancy complications. The psychosocial hazards of obesity tend to be the greatest consequence for adolescents, who may experience alienation, distorted peer relations, poor self-esteem, guilt, depression, or distortions of body image.

Diagnosis

The history should include onset of obesity, eating and exercise habits, amount of time spent in sedentary activities (eg, television watching or computer games), food allergies, previous successful or unsuccessful attempts at weight loss, and family history of obesity. In addition, one needs to assess the patient's readiness to lose weight. A complete physical examination should be performed. Height, weight, and body mass index (BMI) should be plotted; a BMI above the 85th percentile is considered at risk of overweight and above the 95th percentile is overweight. Triceps skinfold (TSF) thickness is the most practical way to measure obesity in children and teenagers, but reproducibility is inconsistent. A TSF of more than one standard deviation above the mean (85th percentile) or weight of 20% over ideal body weight defines obesity. Laboratory evaluation should include CBC, urinalysis, and cholesterol level. Endocrine causes such as hypothyroidism or Cushing's disease can usually be excluded on the basis of history and physical examination, but in some cases exclusion of these may require additional studies.

Management

An age-appropriate behavior modification program incorporating good dietary counseling and exercise is optimal (Table 9–5).

SCHOOL FAILURE

When children graduate from grade school to middle school or junior high school, they encounter a significant increase in the content, amount, and complexity of course work. Academic failure presenting at adolescence has a broad differential diagnosis: (1) limited intellectual abilities; (2) specific learning disabilities; (3) depression or emotional problems; (4) physical causes (eg, poor eyesight or hearing); (5) missed attendance secondary to chronic disease (eg, asthma,

Table 9–5. Program components for weight-control interventions.[1]

Component	Specific Aspects
Physical activity	
Cardiovascular fitness	a. Frequency: 3–4 ×/week
High calorie equivalent	b. Intensity: 50–60% maximal ability (55–65% max heart rate)
	c. Duration: 15 min at start, building to 30–40 min
	d. Mode: use of large-muscle activity such as walk/jog, swim, or cycle
	e. Interest: encourage a wide variety of recreational activities
	f. Enjoyment: focus on the fun of movement and the enjoyment of being physically active
Nutrition education	
	a. Teach critical aspects of quality nutrition, ie, food groups, serving requirements, and variety
	b. Develop understanding of calorie balance: calories in vs calories out
	c. Alert children to pressures of media advertising
	d. Instruct on role of snacks and ideas for "good" snacking
	e. Assist children on balancing fast-food eating and calorie intake
	f. Teach children to reduce intake of high-calorie, low-nutrition treats
Behavior modification	
Change eating habits	a. Identify cues that affect eating, eg, location of meals, size of plates, food in easy-to-see places
Increase habitual physical activity	b. Identify behavior that negatively affects weight control: speed of eating, habitual second portions, high-calorie food choices, "pickiness"
	c. Contract for increased levels of activity using record cards or activity contracts
	d. Develop strategies for more functional activity, such as walking to school, taking stairs, sitting rather than lying
	e. Develop interest in a variety of recreational areas: tennis, dance, skating, etc
	f. Identify cues that lead to inactivity: frequent TV watching, lying down after school or meals, friends who do not like active play

[1] Reproduced with permission, from Ward DS, Bar-Or O: Role of the physician and physical education teacher in the treatment of obesity at school. Pediatrician 1986;13:44.

rheumatic fever) or neurologic dysfunction; (6) problems with concentration, sometimes caused by family crises (eg, divorce, death of a parent); (7) attention deficit/hyperactivity disorder (ADHD); (8) lack of motivation; (9) difficulties learning English as a second language; or (10) problems with substance abuse. Each of these possible causes must be explored in depth.

Diagnosis

A thorough history, physical examination, appropriate laboratory studies, and educational and psychologic testing should be performed. The clinician should obtain a detailed medical history with specific inquiries about chronic disease or any sensory deficits. A large number of school days missed in combination with a parental response that the student was "too sick to go to school," suggests school avoidance. A history of attention deficit disorder or stimulant medication use in the past may be an indication of ongoing problems with concentration. Educational records, including previous intelligence and achievement tests, provide important background information. The student's emotional history may reveal past episodes of counseling for depression or other significant psychiatric problems. Conflict in the family due to factors such as divorce or alcoholism may distract the adolescent from academic responsibilities. There may be a family history of school problems in other siblings or family members, or the family may be immigrants still in the process of adjusting to the United States. In some instances, information about the school itself may be relevant: the school may be troubled by gang warfare or other urban problems, or there may be a "poor fit" between the student and the school (eg, a student accustomed to experimental programs is sent to a military academy).

Treatment

Management must be individualized to address specific needs, foster strengths, and implement a feasible program. With specific learning disabilities (eg, dyslexia) an individual prescription for regular and special educational courses, teachers, and extracurricular activities is advised. Psychological counseling is helpful for students who need to work on coping skills, self-esteem, and social adjustment. If there is a history of hyperactivity or attention deficit disorder, with poor ability to concentrate, a trial of psychostimulant medication may be useful. If the teenager appears to be depressed or gives evidence of other serious emotional problems, further psychologic evaluation should be recommended.

BREAST DISORDERS

A breast examination should become part of the routine physical examination in females as soon as breast budding occurs. Breast examination begins with inspection for symmetry and Tanner stage (Figure 9–2). Asymmetry is usually a normal variation but may be due to unilateral breast hypoplasia or amastia, absence of the pectoralis major muscle, or virginal hypertrophy.

BREAST MASSES

Most breast masses in adolescents are benign; however, approximately 150 cases of adenocarcinoma are reported each year in the United States in women under 25 years of age. Fibroadenomas account for 90% of breast lumps in teenagers seen in referral clinics, with the remaining 10% being cysts. In practice, cysts may account for as many as 50% of breast masses in adolescents, but they are readily diagnosed and many resolve spontaneously. Suspicious lesions should be referred to a surgeon immediately (Table 9–6).

GALACTORRHEA

In teenagers, **galactorrhea**, or inappropriate nipple discharge, is most often a benign condition; however, a careful history and work-up are necessary. Galactorrhea is associated with numerous prescription and illicit drugs, (Table 9–7), as well as with a number of central nervous system (CNS), endocrine, or chest-wall disorders (Table 9–8).

Evaluation

If there is no history of pregnancy or drug use, TSH and prolactin levels should be obtained. An elevated TSH confirms the diagnosis of hypothyroidism. An elevated prolactin and normal TSH, often accompanied by amenorrhea, suggest a hypothalamic or pituitary tumor; computed tomography is then indicated. When the prolactin level is normal, unusual causes such as adrenal, renal, or ovarian tumors should be considered. For those with a negative work-up and persistent galactorrhea, careful follow-up is required. In many cases, symptoms resolve spontaneously without a diagnosis.

Treatment

Treatment of galactorrhea depends on the underlying cause. Prolactinomas may be surgically removed or suppressed with bromocriptine. Bromocriptine may also be beneficial in some amenorrheic females with normal prolactin levels.

GYNECOMASTIA

Gynecomastia is a common concern of male adolescents, in the majority of whom (60–70%) transient subareolar breast tissue develops during Tanner stages II and III. Proposed etiologies include testosterone-estrogen imbalance, increased prolactin level, and abnormal serum binding protein levels.

Clinical Findings

In type I idiopathic gynecomastia, the adolescent presents with a unilateral (20% bilateral), tender, firm mass beneath the areola. More generalized breast enlargement is classified as type II. Pseudogynecomastia refers to excessive fat tissue or prominent pectoralis muscles.

Differential Diagnosis

Gynecomastia may be drug-induced (Table 9–7) or related to any one of a host of disorders (Table 9–9).

Treatment

If gynecomastia is idiopathic, reassure the patient that the process is both common and benign. Resolution may take several months to 2 years. Pharmacotherapeutic agents, such as dihydrotestosterone heptanoate, danazol, clomiphene, and tamoxifen, have been used with variable results. Surgery is reserved for adolescents with significant psychologic trauma or severe breast enlargement.

GYNECOLOGIC DISORDERS & ISSUES

MENSTRUAL PHYSIOLOGY

The menstrual cycle is divided into three phases: follicular, ovulatory, and luteal. Hypothalamic, pituitary, and ovarian hormones

Table 9–6. Breast lesions.

Type	Clinical Findings	Progression	Treatment
Fibroadenoma	Rubbery, well-demarcated, nontender mass, usually in upper outer quadrant. Most < 5 cm; 25% will be multiple or recurrent.	Slow-growing, quiescent after teen years.	Follow for 2–3 menstrual cycles. If no change, ultrasound differentiates solid tumor from cyst. Solid tumors should be referred for excisional biopsy.
Cysts	Tender, spongy masses, often multiple. Increased symptoms premenstrually.	About half of cysts spontaneously regress over 2–3 menstrual cycles.	Persistent cysts may be drained by needle aspiration. Refer suspicious lesions to breast surgeon.
Fibrocystic breasts	Cyclical tenderness and nodularity bilaterally, most common in third and fourth decades, but seen in adolescence.	Increase and diminish under cyclical influence of estrogen–progesterone balance.	Reassurance. Oral contraceptives reduce the risk of fibrocystic breasts. Some women report decreased symptoms after vitamin E treatment or when methylxanthines are limited in the diet, but recent studies have not proven this.
Breast abscess	Unilateral brest pain with overlying inflammatory changes, breast mass palpable late in course. Often due to *Staphylococcus aureus.*	Infection may extend deeper than suspected on exam.	Surgical incision and drainage when fluctuant. Oral antibiotics (dicloxacillin or cephalosporin) for 2–4 weeks.
Adenocarcinoma	Hard, nonmobile, well-circumscribed, painless mass.	Generally indolent course.	Refer for surgical treatment.
Cystosarcoma phylloides	Firm, rubbery, tender, warm, cystic; associated with skin necrosis.	May suddenly enlarge. Most often benign; rarely metastasizes.	Surgical removal is indicated.

Giant juvenile fibroadenoma	Remarkably large fibroadenoma with overlying dilated superficial veins.	Benign.	Requires excision to prevent breast atrophy for cosmetic reasons.
Intraductal papilloma	Cylindrical tumor arising from epithelium duct; often subareolar but may be in periphery in adolescents; associated nipple discharge.	Most are benign.	Requires excision for cytologic diagnosis.
Fat necrosis	Localized inflammatory process in one breast; follows trauma in half of cases.	Subsequent scarring may be confused with malignancy.	Biopsy if suspicious in scarring stage.
Virginal or juvenile hypertrophy	Massive enlargement of both, or less often one, breasts, attributed to end-organ hypersensitivity to normal hormone levels around menarche.	Benign. May cause embarrassment.	Cosmetic reduction may be done at a later date.

Table 9–7. Drugs associated with breast symptoms (galactorrhea, gynecomastia, pain, mass).[1]

Street drugs (illicit or abused)
Marijuana
Opiates
Amphetamines
Meprobamate
Hormones or related drugs
Oral contraceptives
Estrogens
Tamoxifen
Bromocriptine withdrawal
Methyltestosterone
Human chorionic gonadotropin
Chemotherapeutic agents
Vincristine
Busulfan
Prescription medications
Antidepressants
Benzodiazepines
Butyrophenones
Cimetidine
Digoxin
Isoniazid
Methyldopa
Phenothiazines & derivatives
Reserpine
Spironolactone

[1] Modified and reproduced with permission, from Beach RK: Routine breast exams: A chance to reassure, guide, and protect. Contemp Pediatr 1987;Oct:70.

work in concert through a complex system of positive and negative feedback to bring about monthly ovulation (Figure 9–3) and, if fertilization does not occur, menstruation.

MENSTRUAL DISORDERS

Amenorrhea

Amenorrhea is the absence of expected menses. It may result from anatomic abnormalities, chromosomal deviations, or physiologic delay (Table 9–10).

Table 9–8. Causes of galactorrhea.[1]

1. Hypothalamic disorders
Functional
Postpartum
Without pregnancy
Pathologic
Infiltrative
Sarcoid
Histiocytosis X
Hypothalamic tumors
Section of pituitary stalk
2. Drug therapy
Tranquilizers
Tricyclic antidepressants
Methyldopa
Rauwolfia alkaloids
Oral contraceptives
Estrogens
3. Neoplasms
Pituitary tumors
Prolactin secretion only
Prolactin and ACTH secretion (Cushing's disease)
Growth hormone secretion with or without prolactin secretion (acromegaly)
Ectopic prolactin-secreting tumors
4. Hypothyroidism
5. Neurogenic stimulation
Breast stimulation
Chest-wall lesions (herpes zoster, thoracotomy)

[1] Reproduced with permission, from Fraser WM, Blackard WG: Medical conditions that affect the breast and lactation. Clin Obstet Gynecol 1975;18:51.

Primary amenorrhea refers to delay in menarche such that there are no menstrual periods or secondary sex characteristics by 14 years of age or no menses in the presence of secondary sex characteristics by 16 years of age. **Secondary amenorrhea** is defined as the absence of menses for at least three cycles after regular cycles have been established. In some instances, evaluation should begin immediately, without waiting for the specified age or duration of lapsed periods (eg, in suspected pregnancy, short stature with the stigmata of Turner's syndrome, or an anatomic defect).

A. Evaluation for Primary Amenorrhea: The history should include information about the onset of puberty, the age at menarche for other female relatives, the patient's level of exercise, and a com-

Table 9–9. Disorders associated with gynecomastia.[1]

Klinefelter's syndrome
Traumatic paraplegia
Male pseudohermaphroditism
Testicular feminization syndrome
Reifenstein's syndrome
17-ketosteroid reductase deficiency
Endocrine tumors (seminoma, Leydig cell tumor, teratoma, feminizing adrenal tumor, hepatoma, leukemia, hemophilia, bronchogenic carcinoma, leprosy, etc)
Hypothyroidism
Hyperthyroidism
Cirrhosis
Herpes zoster
Friedreich's ataxia

[1] Reproduced with permission, from McAnarney ER, Greydanus DE: Adolescence. In: *Current Pediatric Diagnosis and Treatment,* 9th ed. Kempe CH, Silver HK, O'Brien D, et al (eds). Appleton and Lange, 1987.

prehensive psychosocial history. The clinician should perform a careful physical examination, keeping in mind that estrogen is responsible for breast development; maturation of the external genitalia, vagina, and uterus; and menstruation. If the pelvic examination reveals normal female external genitalia and pelvic organs, a vaginal smear for estrogen influence or a progesterone challenge may be performed (Figure 9–4).

If signs of virilization are present (Figure 9–5), testosterone and dehydroepiandrosterone sulfate (DHEAS) levels will separate polycystic ovary syndrome (PCOS) from adrenal causes of virilization and amenorrhea. PCOS is a spectrum of disorders not necessarily accompanied by the classic symptoms of obesity, hirsutism, oligomenorrhea, and infertility. Because of insufficient FSH, androstenedione cannot be converted to estradiol in the ovarian follicle, resulting in anovulation and excessive androgen production.

Figure 9–3. Physiology of the normal ovulatory menstrual cycle: gonadotropin secretion, ovarian hormone production, follicular maturation, and endometrial changes during one cycle. FSH = follicle-stimulating hormone; LH = luteinizing hormone. (Modified and reproduced with permission from Emans SJH, Goldstein DP: *Pediatrics & Adolescent Gynecology,* 2nd ed. Little, Brown;1982.)

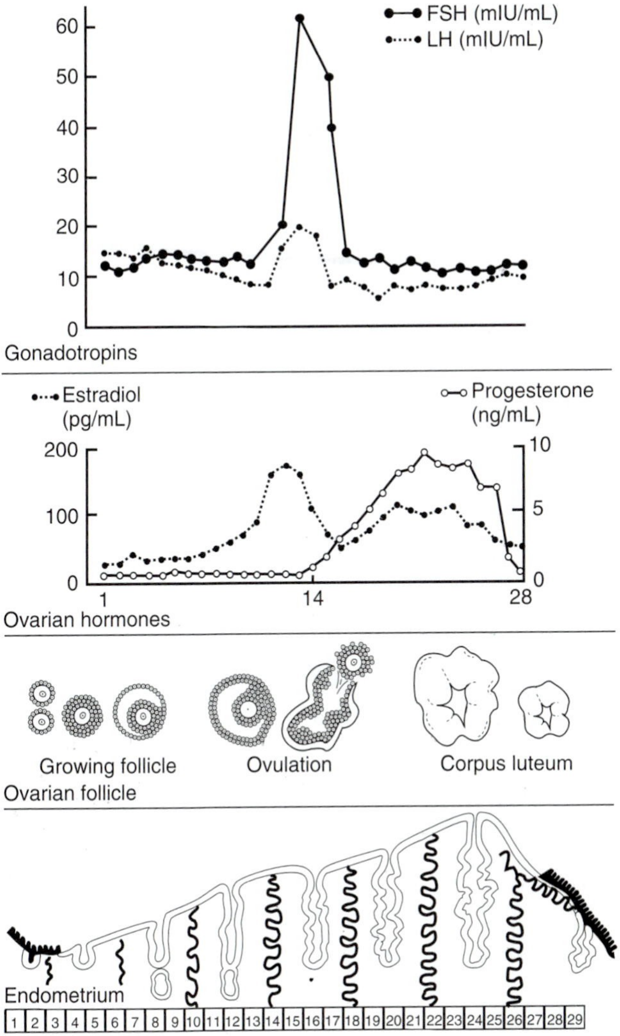

FSH (mIU/mL)
LH (mIU/mL)
60
50
40
30
20
10
0
Gonadotropins
Estradiol (pg/mL)
Progesterone (ng/mL)
200
100
0
10
5
0
1
14
28
Ovarian hormones
Growing follicle
Ovulation
Corpus luteum
Ovarian follicle
Endometrium
1 2 3 4 5 6 7 8 9 10 11 12 13 14 15 16 17 18 19 20 21 22 23 24 25 26 27 28 29

Table 9–10. Causes of amenorrhea.

Hypothalamic—Pituitary Axis
Hypothalamic repression
- Emotional stress
- Depression
- Chronic disease
- Weight loss; severe dieting
- Obesity
- Strenuous athletics
- Drugs (post-BCP, phenothiazines)

CNS lesion
- Pituitary lesion—adenoma, prolatinoma
- Craniopharyngioma and other brain stem or parasellar tumors
- Head injury with hypothalamic contusion
- Infiltrative process (sarcoidosis)
- Vascular disease (hypothalamic vasculitis)

Congenital conditions[1]
- Kallman's syndrome

Ovaries
Gonadal dysgenesis[1]
- Turner's syndrome (XO)
- Mosaic (XX/XO)

Injury to ovary
- Autoimmune disease (may include thyroid, adrenal, islet cells)
- Infection (mumps, oophoritis)
- Toxins (alkylating chemotherapeutic agents)
- Irradiation
- Trauma, torsion (rare)

Polycystic ovary syndrome (Stein-Leventhal) (virilization may be present)

Ovarian failure
- Premature menopause—may result from causes of ovarian injury above
- Resistant ovary
- Variant of gonadal dysgenesis (mosaic)

Uterovaginal Outflow Tract
Müllerian dysgenesis[1]
- Congenital deformity or absence of uterus, fallopian tubes, or vagina

Imperforate hymen, transverse vaginal septum, vaginal agenesis, agenesis of the cervix[1]

Testicular feminization (absent uterus)[1]

Uterine lining defect
- Asherman's syndrome (intrauterine synechiae postcurettage or endometritis)
- TB, brucellosis

Defect in Hormone Synthesis/Action (virilization may be present)
Adrenal hyperplasia[1]
Cushing's syndrome
Adrenal tumor
Ovarian tumor (rare)
Drugs (steroids, ACTH)

[1] Indicates condition usually presenting as primary amenorrhea.

If physical examination reveals the absence of a uterus (Figure 9–5), a karyotype should be performed to differentiate testicular feminization from Müllerian duct defect, since the management of each differs.

B. Evaluation and Management of Secondary Amenorrhea: Secondary amenorrhea results when there is unopposed estrogen stimulation, maintaining the endometrium in the proliferative phase. The most common causes are pregnancy, stress, and polycystic ovary syndrome (Figure 9–6). The history should focus on issues of stress, weight change, strenuous exercise, sexual activity, and contraceptive use. Review of systems should include questions about headaches, visual changes, and galactorrhea. Physical examination should include a careful funduscopic examination, visual fields, palpation of the thyroid, measurement of blood pressure and heart rate, compression of the areola to check for galactorrhea, and a search for signs of excessive levels of androgen such as hirsutism, clitoromegaly, severe acne, or ovarian enlargement.

The first laboratory study obtained is a pregnancy test, even if the patient denies sexual activity. If the test result is negative, a vaginal smear for estrogen or progesterone challenge should be done to determine whether the patient has an estrogen-primed uterus that will respond with bleeding upon withdrawal of the drug.

Dysmenorrhea

Dysmenorrhea is the most common gynecologic complaint of adolescent girls, with an incidence of about 60%. Dysmenorrhea can be divided into primary and secondary types on the basis of whether there is any underlying pelvic pathology. **Primary spasmodic dysmenorrhea** accounts for 80% of adolescent dysmenorrhea and most often affects women under 25 years of age. **Secondary dysmenorrhea** is most often due to sexually transmitted infection, endometriosis, congenital anomalies, or a complication of pregnancy (Table 9–11).

Dysfunctional Uterine Bleeding

Dysfunctional uterine bleeding (DUB) may be referred to as hypermenorrhea or polymenorrhea. It results when an endometrium that has proliferated under unopposed estrogen stimulation finally begins to slough incompletely, causing irregular, painless bleeding. The unopposed estrogen stimulation occurs during anovulatory cycles, common in younger adolescents who have not been menstruating for long; but it also occurs in older adolescents during times of stress or illness.

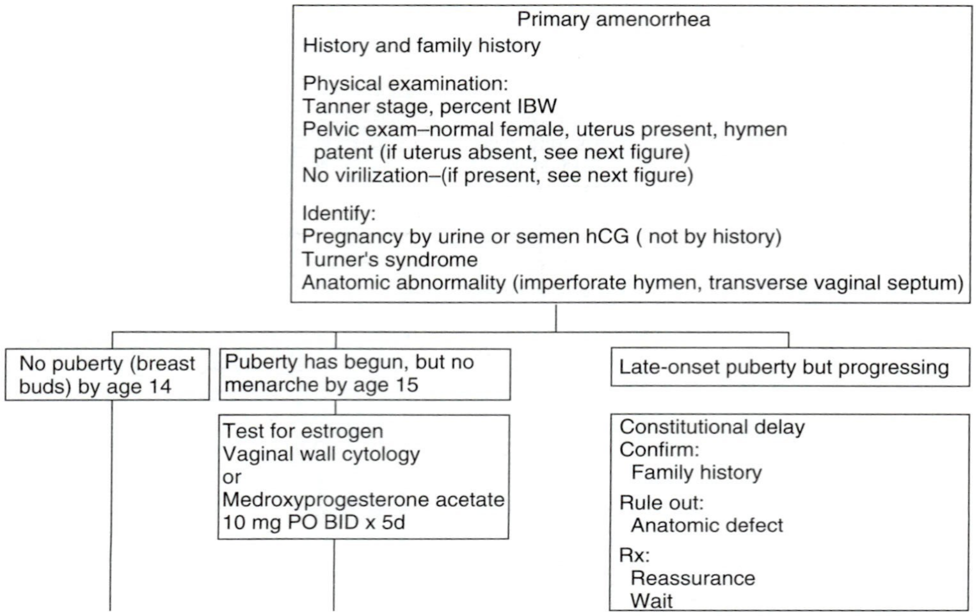
Primary amenorrhea
History and family history
Physical examination:
Tanner stage, percent IBW
Pelvic exam–normal female, uterus present, hymen patent (if uterus absent, see next figure)
No virilization–(if present, see next figure)
Identify:
Pregnancy by urine or semen hCG (not by history)
Turner's syndrome
Anatomic abnormality (imperforate hymen, transverse vaginal septum)
No puberty (breast buds) by age 14
Puberty has begun, but no menarche by age 15
Late-onset puberty but progressing
Test for estrogen
Vaginal wall cytology
or
Medroxyprogesterone acetate 10 mg PO BID x 5d
Constitutional delay
Confirm:
Family history
Rule out:
Anatomic defect
Rx:
Reassurance
Wait

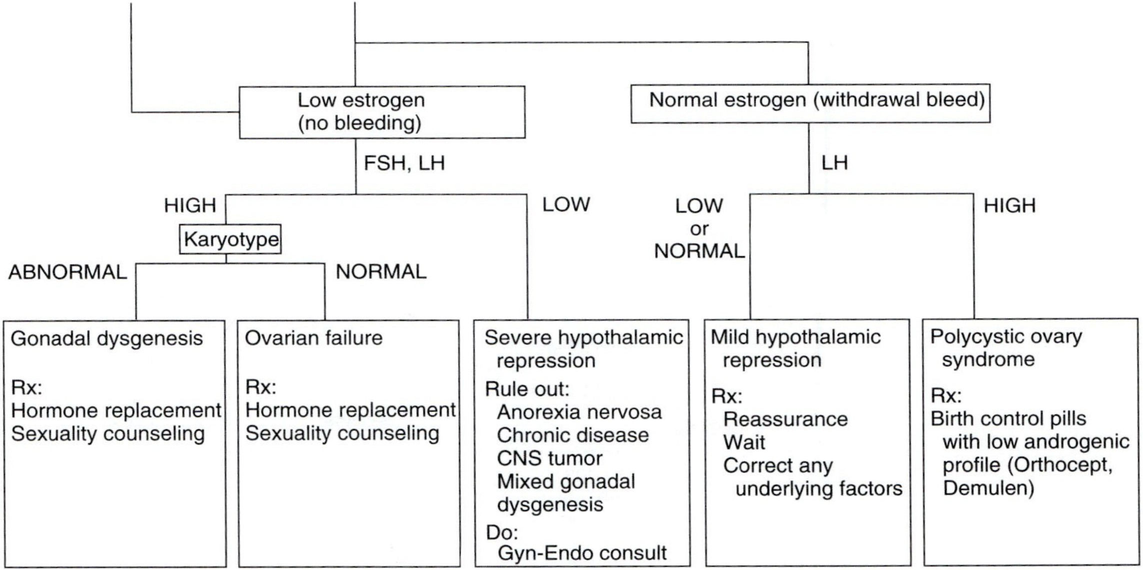

Figure 9–4. Evaluation of primary amenorrhea in a normal female. (Modified from Roberta K. Beach, MD.)

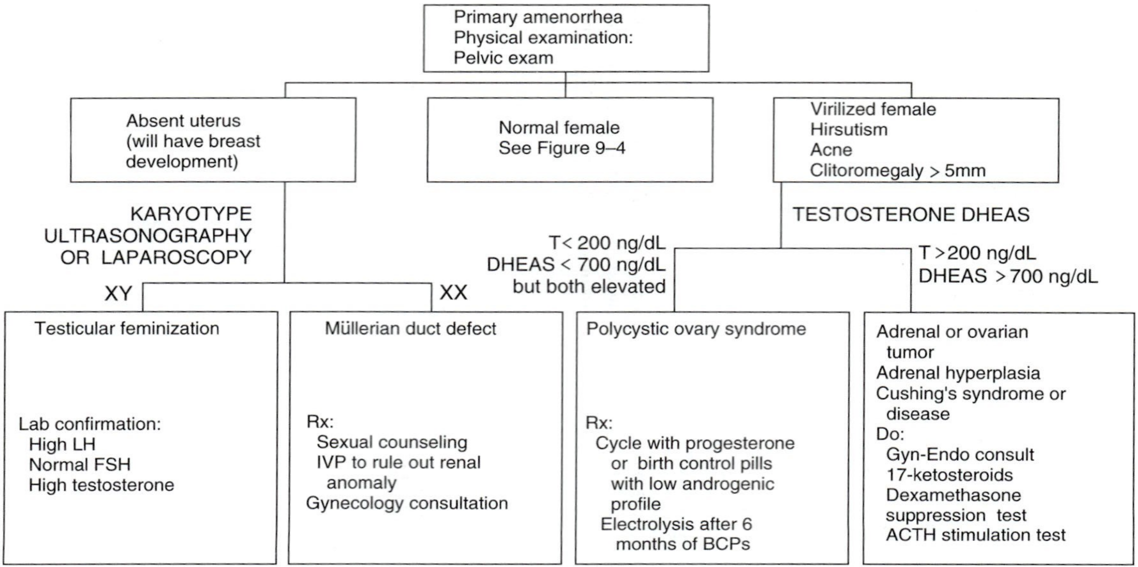

Figure 9–5. Evaluation of primary amenorrhea in a female without a uterus or with virilization. (Modified from Roberta K. Beach, MD.)

A. Findings: Typically, the adolescent will present with a history of several years of regular cycles; she then begins to have menses every 2 weeks, or complains of having bleeding for 2–3 weeks after 2–3 months of amenorrhea. A history of painless, irregular periods at intervals of less than 3 weeks may also be elicited. Bleeding for longer than 10 days should be considered abnormal. Dysfunctional uterine bleeding must be considered a diagnosis of exclusion (Table 9–12).

B. Management: A pregnancy test and pelvic examination with appropriate cultures should be performed in sexually active patients. A CBC with platelets should also be obtained. Additional coagulation studies should be done if the patient presents with severe bleeding or within 1 year of menarche. Hormonal studies may be performed based on the history and physical findings. Management depends on the severity of the problem (Table 9–13).

Severe dysfunctional bleeding requires hospitalization if the patient presents with low hemoglobin levels, orthostatic symptoms, and heavy vaginal bleeding. Hemodynamic instability should be treated with fluids and blood transfusions as needed. Premarin, 25 mg intravenously, may be given for its hemostatic effect (Table 9–13). Gynecologic consult should be obtained.

Mittelschmerz

Mittelschmerz refers to the pain caused by spillage of fluid from the ruptured follicular cyst at the time of ovulation, irritating the peritoneum. The patient presents with a history of midcycle, unilateral dull or aching abdominal pain lasting a few minutes or as long as 8 hours. Rarely this pain mimics the acute abdominal findings of appendicitis, torsion or rupture of an ovarian cyst, or ectopic pregnancy, in which case laparoscopy may be necessary. The patient should be reassured and treated symptomatically.

Ovarian Cysts

Functional cysts account for 20–50% of ovarian masses in adolescents and are a variation of the normal physiologic process. They may be asymptomatic or may cause menstrual irregularity, constipation, or urinary frequency. Functional cysts, unless large, rarely cause abdominal pain. However, torsion or hemorrhage of an ovarian cyst may present as an acute or subacute abdomen. **Follicular cysts** account for most ovarian cysts; they are usually 4 cm or smaller in diameter and resolve spontaneously. **Lutein cysts** occur less commonly, and may be 5–10 cm in diameter. The patient should be referred to a

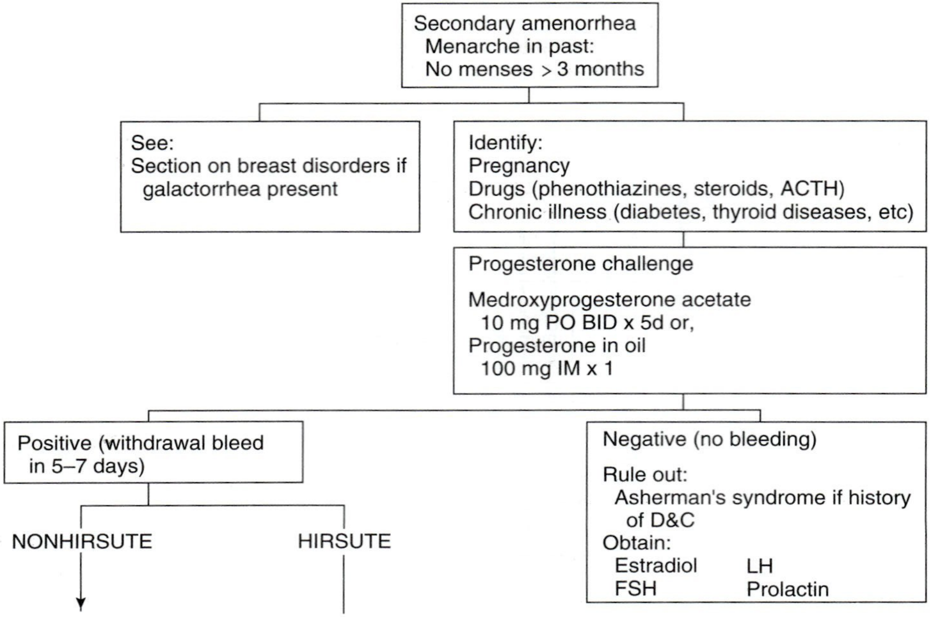
Secondary amenorrhea
Menarche in past:
No menses > 3 months
See:
Section on breast disorders if galactorrhea present
Identify:
Pregnancy
Drugs (phenothiazines, steroids, ACTH)
Chronic illness (diabetes, thyroid diseases, etc)
Progesterone challenge
Medroxyprogesterone acetate
10 mg PO BID x 5d or,
Progesterone in oil
100 mg IM x 1
Positive (withdrawal bleed in 5–7 days)
NONHIRSUTE
HIRSUTE
Negative (no bleeding)
Rule out:
Asherman's syndrome if history of D&C
Obtain:
Estradiol
LH
FSH
Prolactin

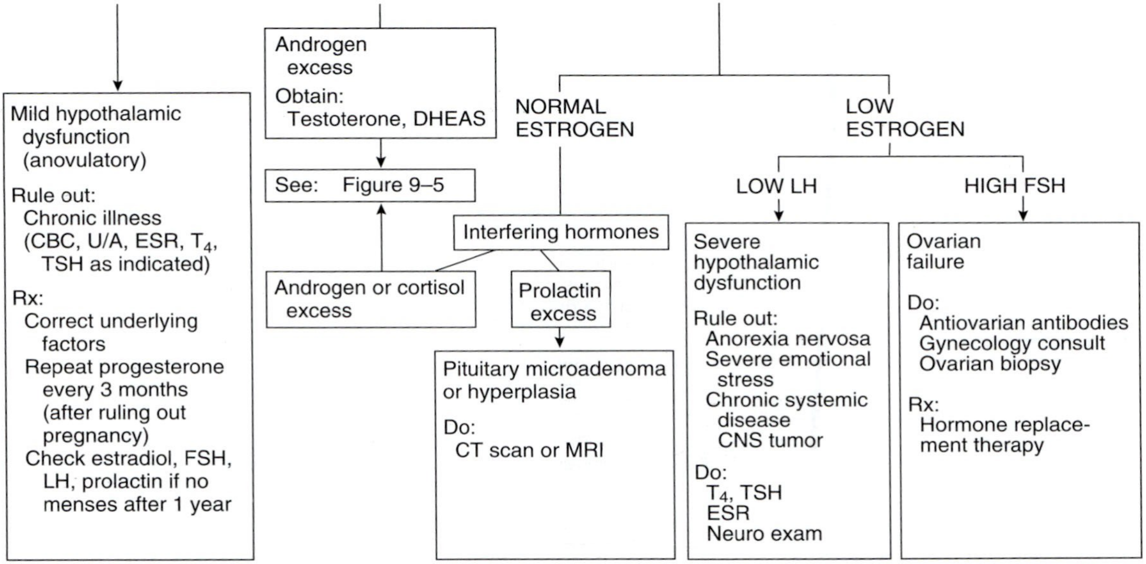

Figure 9–6. Evaluation of secondary amenorrhea. (Modified from Mammel KA: Secondary amenorrhea. In: Berman S, ed. *Pediatric Decision Making*, 3rd ed. Decker;1995.)

Table 9–11. Dysmenorrhea in the adolescent.

Primary Dysmenorrhea—no pelvic pathology

	Etiology	Onset and Duration	Symptoms	Pelvic Exam	Treatment
Primary spasmodic	Excessive amount of prostaglandin $F2_{\alpha}$, which attaches to myometrium causing uterine contractions, hypoxia, and ischemia. Also, directly sensitizes pain receptors.	Begins with onset of flow or just prior and lasts 1–2 days Does not start until 6–18 months after menarche, when cycles become ovulatory.	Lower abdominal cramps radiating to lower back and thighs. Associated nausea, vomiting, diarrhea, and urinary frequency also due to excess prostaglandins.	Normal. May wait to examine if never sexually active and history is consistent with primary spasmodic dysmenorrhea.	Mild: heating pad, warm baths, nonprescription analgesics. Moderate–severe: prostaglandin inhibitors at onset of flow or pain. Oral contraceptives for sexually active patients.
Psychogenic	May have history of sexual abuse or may have difficulty adjusting to womanhood. May have secondary gain from school or work avoidance.	Starts at menarche. Pain begins with anticipation of menses and lasts throughout flow.	Abdominal cramps.	Normal.	Educate regarding normal menstrual function. Reassure that pain does not indicate pathology. Relaxation techniques and biofeedback. Counseling to understand under lying issues.

Secondary Dysmenorrhea—underlying pathology present. (Always perform pelvic exam if secondary dysmenorrhea suspected or patient is sexually active. Gonorrhea culture, test for chlamydia, CBC, and ESR should be obtained.)

Infection	Most often due to a sexually transmitted disease such as chlamydia or gonorrhea.	Recent onset of pelvic cramps.	Pelvic cramps, excessive bleeding, intermenstrual spotting or vaginal discharge.	Mucopurulent or purulent discharge from cervical os, cervical friability, cervical motion tenderness, adnexal tenderness, pos-	Appropriate antibiotics.

				itive culture for STD.	
Endometriosis	Aberrant implants of endometrial tissue in pelvis or abdomen; may result from reflux.	Generally starts more than 2 years after menarche.	Pelvic pain, may occur intermenstrually.	Two-thirds are tender on exam, especially during late luteal phase.	Hormonal suppression by oral contraceptives or danazol. Surgery may be necessary for extensive disease.
Complication of pregnancy	Spontaneous abortion, ectopic pregnancy.	Acute onset.	Pelvic cramps associated with a delay in menses.	Positive hCG, enlarged uterus or adnexal mass.	Immediate gynecologic consult.
Congenital anomalies	Transverse vaginal septum, septate uterus, or cervical stenosis.	Onset at menarche.	Pelvic cramps.	Underlying congenital anomaly may be apparent. May require exam under anesthesia.	Gynecologic consult for ultrasound, hysteroscopy, or laparoscopy.
IUD	Increased uterine contractions, or increased risk for pelvic infection.	Onset after placement of IUD or acutely if due to infection.	Pelvic cramps, heavy menstrual bleeding, may have vaginal discharge.	Normal, or see infection above.	Prostaglandin inhibitors or mefenamic acid may be drug of choice because it also reduces flow. Give appropriate antibiotics and consider removal of IUD if infection is present.
Pelvic adhesions	Previous abdominal surgery or pelvic inflammatory disease.	Delayed onset after surgery or PID.	Abdominal pain, may or may not be associated with menstrual cycles; posible alteration in bowel pattern.	Variable.	Surgery.

Table 9–12. Differential diagnosis of dysfunctional uterine bleeding in adolescents.

Pelvic inflammatory disease or cervicitis
Complication of pregnancy: ectopic pregnancy, threatened abortion, incomplete abortion, missed abortion
Breakthrough bleeding on oral contraceptives
Blood dyscrasias: iron deficiency, thrombocytopenia, coagulopathy, von Willebrand's disease, leukemia
Endocrine disorders: hypothyroidism, hyperthyroidism, diabetes mellitus, adrenal disease, hyperprolactinemia
Trauma
Foreign body
Uterine, vaginal, ovarian abnormalities: carcinoma, fibroids, adenosis from DES, premature menopause

gynecologist for laparoscopy if she is premenarchal; the cyst has a solid component or is larger than 5 cm on ultrasonography; there are symptoms or signs suggestive of hemorrhage or torsion; or the cyst fails to regress after 2–3 menstrual cycles.

CONTRACEPTION

Sexually active adolescent females wait an average of 1 year after first intercourse before seeking contraception. One-half of teen pregnancies in the United States, however, occur in the first 6 months of initiating sexual intercourse. Sexuality, contraception, and pregnancy prevention are areas with which the pediatrician has become familiar out of necessity.

Counseling Teenagers About Contraception

Adolescents may have poorly formed skills for making decisions of any kind and often benefit from a decision-making framework that can be applied to a variety of situations, particularly those involving peer pressure. By talking with teenagers about their alternatives to sexual intercourse and the implications of coitus (unintended pregnancy; sexually transmitted diseases; possible emotional trauma; and effects on education, career, income, and responsibilities if a pregnancy occurs), the physician can help them to make better-informed decisions before they find themselves in a dilemma.

Abstinence is the most commonly used method of birth control. It is prudent, however, to encourage adolescents to learn about and

Table 9–13. Management of dysfunctional uterine bleeding[1] (DUB).[2]

	Mild	Moderate	Severe
Characteristics	Hct > 33% or Hgb > 11 g/dL	Hct 27–33% or Hgb 9–11 g/dL	Hct < 27% or Hgb < 9 g/dL (or dropping)
Acute treatment	Menstrual calendar Iron supplementation Consider OCPs if patient is sexually active and desires contraception (standard once-daily dose)	*Begin:* OCPs (1/35) cycle 4 pills/day × 4 days 3 pills/day × 4 days 2 pills/day × 13–19 days withdrawal bleeding × 7 days	Blood transfusion, PRN *Consider:* Conjugated estrogens, 25 mg IV q 4–6 h × 24 h until bleeding stops; antiemetic *Begin:* OCPs (1/35) cycle 4 pills/day × 4 days 3 pills/day × 4 days 2 pills/day × 13–19 days withdrawal bleeding × 7 days
Long-term treatment	*Monitor:* Iron status (Hgb/Hct) *Follow-up* in 2 months	*Next:* OCPs (1/35)[3] cycle for 3 months. Begin OCPs the Sunday after withdrawal bleeding begins. Length of use dependent on resolution of anemia. Iron supplementation. *Monitor:* Iron status *Follow-up* within 2–3 weeks and every 3 months	*Next:* OCPs (1/50)[4] cycle for 3 months. Begin OCPs the Sunday after withdrawal bleeding begins. Length of use dependent on resolution of anemia. Iron supplementation. *Monitor:* Iron status *Follow-up* within 2–3 weeks and every 3 months

[1] Reproduced with permission, from Blythe M: Common menstrual problems, Part 3: Abnormal uterine bleeding. Adolescent Health Update 1992;4:1.

[2] DX = Prolonged painless menses (≥ 8 days); heavy flow (> 6 tampons/pads per day); short cycles (≤ 21 days); no other etiology found.

[3] Triphasic OCP is acceptable.

[4] Use pill with 50 mcg of ethinyl estradiol for first 3 months, then 30–35 mcg monophasic or triphasic pill.

use contraception at the time they do begin to engage in sexual intercourse. Thorough counseling about expected side effects improves compliance. Adolescents should understand the menstrual cycle and be taught either that there is no "safe" period or that ovulation occurs 2 weeks before the next menstrual period and may be difficult to predict. Since teenagers frequently have irregular cycles and engage in spontaneous and unplanned coitus, they will not find the rhythm or calendar method effective. Adolescents also need to be informed that withdrawal (coitus interruptus) is not a reliable method of contraception (Table 9–14).

A. Birth Control Pills: Before beginning oral contraceptives, a careful menstrual history, medical history, and family medical history should be taken. In addition, baseline weight and blood pressure should be established, breast and pelvic examination should be performed, and specimens for urinalysis, Papanicolaou (Pap) smear, gonorrhea culture, and chlamydia culture or antigen-detection test obtained.

If there are no contraindications (Table 9–15), the patient may begin her first pack of pills with her next menstrual period. A triphasic or a low-dose combined oral contraceptive is used for teenagers without contraindications to the use of estrogen. It is always wise to use 28-day packs with adolescents rather than 21-day packs to reduce the chance of missed pills. The patient should be instructed on the use of her type of pills, as well as possible risks and side effects and their warning signs. She should use a back-up method such as condoms and foam for the first 2 weeks to assure protection. A follow-up visit in 1 month and every 2–3 months thereafter for the first year may improve compliance, as teenagers often discontinue birth control pills for nonmedical reasons or because of minor side effects.

A different type of combined oral contraceptive should be tried if the patient has a persistent minor side effect for more than the first 2 or 3 months. Adjustments should be made on the basis of hormonal effects. Changes are most often made for persistent breakthrough bleeding not related to missed pills.

B. Injectable Hormonal Contraceptives: The depot form of medroxyprogesterone acetate (DMPA) has rapidly gained popularity among teenagers since it was approved by the Federal Drug Administration (FDA) as a contraceptive in 1992. DMPA is given as a 150-mg deep intramuscular injection into the gluteal or deltoid muscle every 12 weeks with a 2-week grace period. The first injection should be given within the first 5 days of the menstrual cycle to provide immediate protection. Advantages of DMPA include a failure rate of less than

0.3%, long-acting protection, minimal compliance issues, no interference with intercourse, and lack of estrogen-related side effects. Some teenagers consider its 50% rate of amenorrhea at 1 year of use a desirable side effect. Other side effects include unpredictable menstrual patterns, possible weight gain or mood changes, and a potential for diminished bone density, which remains under investigation.

The levonorgestrel subdermal implant (Norplant), which is inserted under the skin of the upper arm, became available in the United States in 1991. Its ease of use, lack of compliance issues, less than 1% failure rate, and 5-year protection make the subdermal implant an ideal method for teenagers who can tolerate its associated menstrual irregularities.

PREGNANCY

There are more than 1 million pregnancies among teenagers in the United States each year. Of these, about 40% are terminated by abortion, 13% end in miscarriage, and 47% are carried to term. About 45% of 15-to-19-year-old females are sexually active; more than one-third of these become pregnant within 2 years of beginning sexual intercourse. More than 80% of these pregnancies are unintended, and about 60% of pregnancies in women younger than 20 years occur out of wedlock.

Young maternal age and associated maternal risk factors have been linked to adverse neonatal outcome, including higher rates of low-birth-weight babies (< 2500 g) and neonatal mortality. The psychosocial consequences for the adolescent mother and her infant are extensive.

Presentation

An adolescent may present with delayed or missed menses or may even request a pregnancy test, but often will present with an unrelated concern (hidden agenda) or a vague somatic complaint. Clinicians need to have a low threshold for suspecting pregnancy. If there is *any* suspicion, a urine pregnancy test should be performed.

Diagnosis

History, as above, and physical examination may assist in making the diagnosis of pregnancy. Bluish coloring and softening of the cervix may be noted on speculum examination. The uterine fundus may be palpable on abdominal examination if sufficient time has

Table 9–14. Commonly used contraceptives in the United States.

Method	Action	Failure Rate[1]	Side Effects	Benefits	Comments
Condoms	Barrier, spermicidal action of nonoxynol-9 in some	12	None	Protect against STD	Require no medical visit or prescription
Spermicides	Spermicidal action	21	Local irritation	Non-oxynol 9 is bactericidal and viricidal	
Sponges	Barriers, spermicidal	18–28	Possible risk of toxic shock syndrome		Higher failure rates in parous than nulliparous women. Withdrawn from market 1995
Combined oral contraceptives	1) Suppress ovulation 2) Thicken cervical mucus and make sperm penetration difficult 3) Atrophy of endometrium diminishes chance of implantation	0.1	Risk of thromboembolism, MI, stroke, hypertension, hepatoma, death exists but rare in teenagers	Improve dysmenorrhea and acne Protect against PID, ovarian and endometrial cancer, benign breast masses Decrease menstrual blood loss	May be method of choice for adolescents who have unplanned intercourse. Serious risks increase after age 30, especially in smokers. See Table 9–16 for contraindications
Mini pill	1) Thickens cervical mucus 2) Causes atrophy of endometrium 3) Ovulation suppressed in only 15–40% of cycles	0.5	Less predictable menstrual patterns		May be used in patients who should avoid exogenous estrogens

Depo-Provera	1) Suppresses ovulation 2) Thickens cervical mucus 3) Causes atrophy of endometrium.	0.3	Unpredictable menstrual patterns, moderate weight gain, mood changes, potential decrease in bone density	↓ sickling and Hgb in SS disease. May ↓ seizures in some epileptics.	50% become amenorrheic by 1 year of use.
Subdermal progestin implant (Norplant)	1) Thickens cervical mucus 2) Causes atrophy of endometrium 3) Suppresses LH surge	0.04[2]	Irregular bleeding, mood changes, hair loss, pigmentation change at insertion site	No temporal relationship to sexual activity	Emphasize need for annual check-ups despite 5-year duration. Contraindicated in those with active liver disease, acute thromboembolic disorder, undiagnosed genital bleeding, pregnancy
IUD	Prevents implantation through local inflammatory response and local production of prostaglandins	3	STDs, PID and its sequelae, heavy menstrual flow, dysmenorrhea	No temporal relationship to sexual activity	Not the method of choice for teens who have multiple partners and their childbearing years ahead of them, given STD risk
Diaphragm	Barrier Spermicidal action of contraceptive gel used in conjunction	18	None		Must be comfortable inserting and checking fit

[1] Among typical couples who initiate use of a method, the percentage who experience an accidental pregnancy during the first year if they do not stop use for any other reason.
[2] Rate increases to 1.1% by end of fifth year.

Table 9–15. Contraindications to combined birth control pills.[1]

Absolute contraindications
History of thrombophlebitis, thromboembolic disorder, cerebrovascular disorder, ischemic heart disease
Known or suspected carcinoma of the breast or estrogen-dependent neoplasia
Known or suspected pregnancy
History of benign or malignant liver tumor
Undiagnosed abnormal vaginal bleeding
Strong relative contraindications
Severe vascular or migraine headaches
Hypertension
Diabetes
Active gallbladder dsease
Mononucleosis, acute phase
Sickle cell disease or sickle C disease
Upcoming major surgery
Long leg cast or major injury to lower leg
Known impaired liver function at present time
Completion of term pregnancy within past 10–14 days

[1] Modified and reproduced with permission, from *Contraceptive Technology 1988–1989,* 14th revised ed. Breedlove B, Judy B, Martin N (eds). Irvington Publishers, Inc., 1988.

lapsed. If uterine size on bimanual examination does not correspond to dates, one must consider ectopic pregnancy, incomplete or missed abortion, twin gestation, or inaccurate dates. Laboratory tests for human chorionic gonadotropin (hCG) are simple to perform and usually establish the diagnosis.

Special Issues in Management

When an adolescent presents for pregnancy testing, it is wise to discuss her hopes and plans before performing the test. If she wants to conceive and the test is negative, further counseling into the implications of teen pregnancy and parenthood should be undertaken. For those who do not wish to be pregnant, this is a good time to begin contraception.

If the adolescent is pregnant, discuss her support systems and her options with her. Many teenagers need help in involving their parents. Since teenagers are often ambivalent about their plans and may have a high level of denial, it is prudent to follow up with her in 1 week to be certain that a decision has been made and to assist her into prenatal care if she has chosen to maintain the pregnancy.

It has been shown that maternal age in and of itself is not responsible for low birth weight and poor fetal outcome, but that low maternal prepregnancy weight, poor weight gain, delay in prenatal care, low socioeconomic status, and black race are contributing factors. The poor nutritional status of some teenagers as well as their erratic eating patterns; habits of smoking, drinking, or substance abuse; and high prevalence of sexually transmitted diseases also contributes to the problem. Teenagers are also at greater risk of toxemia of pregnancy, iron deficiency anemia, cephalopelvic disproportion, prolonged labor, premature labor, and maternal death. Early prenatal care and good nutrition can make a difference with a number of these potential complications.

Because of the high risk of a second unintended pregnancy within the next 2 years, postpartum contraceptive counseling and follow-up is imperative.

VULVOVAGINITIS

Vaginitis has two main causes: pathogens or indigenous flora after a change in milieu of the vagina. Monilial vulvovaginitis and bacterial vaginosis (formerly referred to as *Gardnerella, Haemophilus*, or nonspecific vaginitis) may be found in sexually nonactive patients; they are examples of indigenous flora that may cause infection. Bacterial vaginosis is more prevalent in those who are sexually active. In sexually active patients, trichomonal infections or cervicitis from sexually transmitted pathogens must be considered. (See section on sexually transmitted diseases [STDs]). For this reason, sexually active patients or those suspected to be victims of sexual abuse should have appropriate specimens taken for STDs even if yeast or bacterial vaginosis is identified (Table 9–16).

SEXUALLY TRANSMITTED DISEASES AND PELVIC INFLAMMATORY DISEASE

STDs

The 15- to 25-year-old age group has the highest incidence of sexually transmitted diseases (STDs) because of multiple sexual partners, lack of use of barrier methods of contraception, and delay in seeking treatment.

Chlamydia trachomatis, an obligate intracellular body half the

Table 9–16. Vulvovaginitis.

	Causes	Description	Tests	Treatment
Physiologic leukorrhea	Physiologic	Clear, white, nonodorous discharge beginning around menarche.	Wet prep may show few squamous epithelial cells and < 5 PMN/hpf.	Reassure patient that this is normal.
Monilial vulvovaginitis	*Candida* (yeast)	Thick, white, adherent, cheesy discharge; erythematous mucosa; associated pruritus.	Leukocytes on wet prep. Budding yeast or mycelia on KOH prep. Slides may be negative.	Treat on basis of exam if slides negative. Nystatin, clotrimazole, or terconazole vaginal creams or suppositories for 3–7 nightly doses.
Bacterial vaginosis	Indigenous vaginal flora: *gardnerella, bacteroides, peptococcus,* lactobacilli	Thin, homogenous, gray-white discharge adherent to vaginal wall; diffuse vaginal erythema; malodorous.	Whiff test (KOH drop added to smear of discharge) results in fishy odor. Abundance of clue cells (stippled vaginal epithelial cells) on wet prep.	Metronidazole 500 mg orally twice a day for 7 days. Ampicillin 500 mg orally four times daily for 7 days is alternative during pregnancy.
Sexually transmitted diseases (see next section)	See next section	Cervix may appear inflamed, friable, ulcerated, or normal.	Wet prep, gonorrhea culture, *chlamydia* culture or antigen detection should be performed.	See next section.
Foreign body vaginitis	Retained tampons most common cause.	Extremely malodorous purulent discharge.	Speculum exam to visualize.	Remove foreign body. Antibiotics are generally not necessary.
Allergic or contact vaginitis	Bubble baths, feminine hygiene sprays, vaginal contraceptives	Erythematous vaginal mucosa.	Rule out sexually transmitted diseases.	Discontinue use of offending agent.

size of the gonococcus, is the most common cause of STDs, with 2–3 million new cases per year in the United States; peak incidence is in the 15- to 20-year-old age group. One-quarter to one-half of those infected are asymptomatic; one-quarter to one-half are coinfected with gonorrhea. *Chlamydia* accounts for 20–30% of the 170,000 cases of pelvic inflammatory disease (PID) each year and is responsible for more than 60% of PID cases in women under 20 years old (Table 9–17).

Neisseria gonorrhoeae is the second most common cause of STD, with peak incidence in the 15- to 25-year-old age group. Of all cases, 5–25% are associated with another STD, and more than 50% of those infected are asymptomatic (Table 9–17).

In view of the prevalence of STDs in the adolescent population and the reluctance of teenagers to discuss them, the clinician needs to ask adolescents routinely about sexual activity, number of partners, and STD symptoms when they present for regular physical examinations or sexually related symptoms (dysuria, penile or vaginal discharge, genital lesion, or abdominal pain). As females are frequently asymptomatic, the clinician should obtain a wet preparation, gonorrhea culture, and test for chlamydia at the time of the annual Pap smear in sexually active females. Although males are usually symptomatic, a significant number of those with chlamydia are asymptomatic. Males with gonorrhea may find their symptoms resolve, and thus fail to seek treatment. If leukocyte esterase is positive on a urinalysis of the first 10 cc voided, further tests for STDs can be undertaken in asymptomatic males.

When an STD is diagnosed, the adolescent and his or her partner(s) should be treated simultaneously with the appropriate antibiotic regimen (Tables 9–18, 9–19, 9–20, and 9–21). Serology will need to be followed in the case of syphilis. It is essential to emphasize abstinence until both partners complete treatment to avoid reinfection or spread, and to advise use of barrier methods of contraception to prevent future infections. Possible complications and the implications of recurrent infections with regard to fertility and ectopic pregnancy should also be discussed. Adolescents should also be made aware of the possibility of transmission of an STD to the fetus. They should be followed closely because poor compliance with treatment is common in this age group.

PELVIC INFLAMMATORY DISEASE (PID)

Acute PID, or salpingitis, is the most common serious infection occurring in young women (Table 9–17). The adolescent age group

Table 9–17. Urethritis, cervicitis, and pelvic inflammatory disease.

	Agents	Symptoms	Physical Findings	Laboratory Findings	Complications
Urethritis	*Chlamydia* Gonorrhea *Ureaplasma* *Mycoplasma* *Trichomonas*	Dysuria Urethral discharge May be asymptomatic	Exam may be normal. Clear, white, or purulent penile discharge. (May occur in females, often in association with cervicitis.)	U/A: Moderate WBCs without bacteriuria Gram's stain: PMNs, may show gram-negative intracellular diplococci if due to gonorrhea. Gonorrhea culture: may be positive. *Chlamydia* culture or antigen detection test: may be positive.	Nontender penile edema Prostatitis Epididymitis Orchitis
Cervicitis	*Chlamydia* Gonorrhea Herpes *Trichomonas*	Asymptomatic Possible vaginal discharge or dysuria	Cervix may appear normal, or may have erythema, petechiae, irregular raised surface, friability, or ulcerations. Mucopurulent or purulent cervical discharge.	Wet prep: > 10 WBCs/hpf if due to gonorrhea or chlamydia. Gonorrhea culture: may be positive. *Chlamydia* culture or antigen detection test: may be positive Trichomonads may be seen on wet prep	Pelvic inflammatory disease Infection of Bartholin glands
PID	*Chlamydia* Gonorrhea Normal vaginal aerobic and anaerobic flora may be secondary invaders	Abdominal pain may be minimal Vaginal discharge in 75% Excessive menstrual bleeding or intermenstrual spotting in 40% Fever in 40% Dysuria in 15%	Lower abdominal tenderness. Uterine, adnexal, or cervical motion tenderness. Abnormal cervical discharge in half.	May have elevated WBC, ESR, but may be normal. Cervical culture for gonorrhea or chlamydia may be positive.	Tubovarian abscess Fitz-Hugh-Curtis syndrome Tubal occlusion Infertility Ectopic pregnancy Chronic abdominal pain

Table 9–18. Treatment of urethritis or cervicitis in adolescents.[1]

	Drug of Choice	Alternatives
Gonorrhea	Ceftriaxone 125–250 mg IM once, followed by treatment for *Chlamydia,* below	Cefixime 400 mg orally once; or ciprofloxacin[2] 500 mg orally once; or ofloxacin[2] 400 mg orally once; or spectinomycin 2 g IM once, plus treatment for *Chlamydia*
Chlamydia trachomatis	Doxycycline[3] 100 mg orally bid for 7 days or azithromycin[3,4] 1 g orally once	Erythromycin 500 mg orally 4 times daily for 7 days or ofloxacin[2] 300 mg orally 2 times daily for 7 days

[1] Modified and reproduced with permission, from Treatment of sexually transmitted diseases. *Med Lett Drugs Ther* 1994;36:1.
[2] Quinolones, such as ciprofloxacin, are contraindicated during pregnancy and in children 16 years of age or younger.
[3] Contraindicated during pregnancy.
[4] Not tested in patients under 16 years of age.

has the highest rate of PID, with an annual rate of 1.5% in females 15–19 years old. Risk factors for PID include sexual activity, multiple partners (5 times greater risk than for one partner), age lower than 25, presence of an IUD (2–4 times greater risk than for nonusers), nulliparous status, previous episodes of PID (2 times greater risk), history of uncomplicated STD, and prior induced abortion.

The diagnosis of PID is not straightforward; hence, the following guidelines have been suggested. The three major criteria of lower abdominal pain and tenderness, cervical motion tenderness, and adnexal tenderness must be present. In addition, one of the following minor criteria must be present: temperature higher than 38°C; leukocytosis higher than 10,500 WBC/mm^3; culdocentesis yielding peritoneal fluid containing WBCs and bacteria; inflammatory mass noted on pelvic examination or ultrasonography; elevated ESR; cervical Gram's stain suggestive of gonorrhea or positive chlamydia antigen detection test; or more than 5 WBCs per oil-immersion field on Gram's stain of endocervical discharge.

The differential diagnosis of PID includes acute appendicitis, mesenteric lymphadenitis, cholecystitis, ectopic pregnancy, intrauterine pregnancy, ovarian cyst or tumor, endometriosis, urinary tract infection, and renal calculus.

If there is the slightest suspicion of PID the patient should be

Table 9–19. Treatment of pelvic inflammatory disease.[1]

	Drug of Choice	Dosage	Alternatives
Hospitalized patients	Cefoxitin or cefotetan either one plus doxycycline followed by doxycycline[2]	2 g IV every 6 hours 2 g IV every 12 hours 100 mg IV every 12 hours until improved 100 mg orally twice daily to complete 14 days	Clindamycin 900 mg IV every 8 hours plus gentamicin 2 mg/kg IV once followed by gentamicin 1.5 mg/kg IV every 8 hours until improved followed by doxycycline[2] 100 mg orally twice daily to complete 14 days
Outpatients	Cefoxitin plus probenecid or ceftriaxone either one followed by doxycycline[2]	2 g IM once 1 g orally once 250 mg IM once 100 mg orally twice daily for 14 days	Ofloxacin[2,3] 450 mg orally 4 times daily for 14 days, plus clindamycin 450 mg orally 4 times daily for 14 days or metronidazole 500 mg orally 2 times daily for 14 days

[1] Modified and reproduced with permission, from Treatment of sexually transmitted diseases. *Med Lett Drugs Ther* 1994;36:1.
[2] Contraindicated during pregnancy.
[3] Not tested in patients under 16 years of age.

treated with appropriate antibiotics while cultures are pending (Table 9–19). The patient should be hospitalized if she exhibits serious fever or toxicity, is unable to tolerate oral medication and fluids, has not responded to outpatient therapy or is unlikely to comply with it, is a younger adolescent, or is seriously ill with an unclear diagnosis.

GENITAL LESIONS

Condylomata acuminata, or genital warts, are caused by human papilloma virus (HPV). Warts typically occur at the site of minute skin trauma on the external genitalia but may be present on the cervix and indiscernible to the unaided eye. It is now accepted that HPV is the most important causal agent in the development of cervical in-

Table 9–20. Diagnosis and treatment of genital lesions.

Lesion	Agent	Clinical Findings	Treatment
Condylomata acuminata (genital warts)	Human papilloma virus	Verrucous skin lesion most often occurring on the glans penis or corona in males and posterior introitus in females.	Apply 20–25% podophyllin in tincture of benzoin to wart after applying petroleum jelly to normal skin. Wash off in 4 hours. Do not use on vaginal or anal mucosa, or during pregnancy. Refer for colposcopy if HPV effects are noted on Pap smear. (Additional treatments: liquid nitrogen, laser, 5-FU, surgical excision, trichloroacetic acid, interferon.)
Herpes	Herpes simplex virus (HSV-2 in 80–95% and HSV-1 in remainder)	Cluster of painful papules which progress to vesicles, pustules, ulcers, and crusts. Systemic symptoms with primary episode. Prodromal tingling with recurrences.	Acyclovir 400 mg orally 3 times a day for 7–10 days (primary) or 5 days (recurrence). May shorten duration of eruptions. Institute with prodromal symptoms.
Syphilis	*Treponema pallidum*		Penicillin G benzathine 2.4 million units IM once OR doxycycline 100 mg orally twice daily for 14 days OR Erythromycin 500 mg orally 4 times a day for 14 days.
Primary		Painless, clean ulcer with an erythematous, indurated border (chancre) which is positive on darkfield exam.	
Secondary		Broad-based, flat, mucoid lesions (condylomata lata) on the genitals.	

Table 9–21. Diagnosis and treatment of sexually transmitted parasites.

	Symptoms	Clinical Findings	Treatment
Trichomoniasis	Asymptomatic or pruritic vaginal discharge in females or clear penile discharge in males.	Copious frothy vaginal discharge. Motile flagellated trichomonad seen on wet prep of vaginal discharge or spun urinalysis	Metronidazole[1] 2 g orally once or 500 mg orally 2 times a day for 7 days.
Pediculosis pubis (crab lice)	Pruritic rash.	Lice and opalescent nits found anchored to pubic hairs.	Lindane or pyrethrin is applied to pubic hair and surrounding skin, worked into a lather for 4–10 minutes, and rinsed off. Nits are combed out. Fomites and linens need to be washed in hot water. Treat close contacts.
Scabies	Pruritic rash of groin, thighs, or abdomen.	Scabetic burrows and erythematous, maculopapular scaliness and tendency to impetignize.	Permethrin 5% (Elimite cream) is applied from head to soles, left on for 8–14 hours, then showered off. Fomites & close contacts must be treated.

[1]Metronidazole is generally contraindicated during the first trimester of pregnancy. Clotrimazole 100 mg intravaginally at bedtime for 7 days is a less effective alternative which may be used during pregnancy.

traepithelial neoplasia and invasive cervical cancers and appears to be associated with penile cancer (Table 9–20).

Herpes Simplex Virus

The primary episode of genital herpes is generally more symptomatic and prolonged than recurrences and is characterized by such systemic symptoms as fever, headache, malaise, myalgias, and a cluster of painful papules that progress to vesicles, pustules, ulcers, and finally crusts (Table 9–20). Fifty percent of new cases may be asymptomatic.

Syphilis

The primary stage of syphilis typically presents with a painless chancre. Diagnosis is made by immediate darkfield examination of a microscope slide that has been pressed to the base of the lesion with a drop of saline added. VDRL can be done for further investigation, but results may be negative early in the course of the disease. The chancre may be self-limited. After a latency period of 4–6 weeks, the disease may resurface in its secondary stage, characterized by a diffuse, nonpruritic, maculopapular rash that includes the palms and soles, mucous patches on the mucosal surfaces, generalized lymphadenopathy, constitutional symptoms, and the presence of condylomata on the genitals. At this stage, diagnosis is established by VDRL. The tertiary stage is divided into early latent and late benign and may manifest cardiovascular and CNS complications. These include dissection of the ascending aorta, seizures, stroke, optic atrophy, and tabes dorsalis. All stages may be treated with penicillin. The VDRL should be repeated 3, 6, and 12 months after treatment.

TRICHOMONAS AND ARTHROPODS

See Table 9–21.

HUMAN IMMUNODEFICIENCY VIRUS

AIDS results from infection with the human immunodeficiency virus (HIV), which is transmitted in blood and semen, and potentially other body fluids, through sexual and needle contact.

As of 1992, only 0.39% of AIDS cases in the United States were reported in 13- to 19-year-olds. A multicenter seroprevalence study of

HIV in adolescents in 24 cities in the United States in 1990–1992 found the median clinic-specific prevalence to be 0.2% for adolescent medicine clinics, 0.3% for correctional facilities, 0.5% in STD clinics, and 1.1% in homeless youth centers; however, rates ranged from 0–17% at specific settings. Although the male/female ratio of AIDS in the adult population is 9:1, in adolescents it is 4:1. While 87% of AIDS cases among adults are attributable to males having sex with males, injectable drug use, or both, in the 13- to 19-year-old group only 41% are attributed to these causes. Fourteen percent of adolescent AIDS is due to heterosexual transmission, compared with 6% of all cases. Among adolescent females with AIDS, heterosexual contact is the most common risk factor. Adolescents are at significant potential risk because of their propensity for multiple sexual partners and their limited use of barrier contraceptives, as well as the use of drugs by some. A large number of infected young adults 20–29 years old acquired HIV infection as adolescents.

Preventive measures need to be taken to ensure that adolescents have the necessary knowledge to protect themselves from HIV in current and future relationships and to eliminate AIDS-related hysteria. They need to be instructed in risk factors for HIV, modes of transmission, means of protection, and availability of confidential testing. The safer sex practices promoted as a result of AIDS can reduce the rate of all kinds of STDs if heeded. Adolescence is an ideal time to promote these practices, as it is a time when intimate relationships are beginning and decisions about sexual activity become important.

Infectious Diseases: Viral | 10

Mark J. Abzug, MD

VIRAL DISEASES

ROSEOLA INFANTUM/HUMAN HERPESVIRUS 6 (Exanthem Subitum)

Roseola infantum is an acute febrile disease of infants and young children characterized by fever followed by a faint rash. The incubation period is estimated to be approximately 9 days. Human herpesvirus 6 (HHV-6) has been identified as the causative agent of roseola and other less distinct febrile illnesses in infancy and early childhood.

Clinical Findings (Table 10–1)

A. Symptoms & Signs:

1. Roseola–Onset is sudden, with sustained or spiking fever as high as 41.1 °C (106 °F). Fever persists for 1–5 days (average, 3 days), falls by crisis, and then may be subnormal for a few hours just before the rash appears. The rash, which appears when the temperature returns to normal, is faintly erythematous, maculopapular, and principally confined to the trunk. Other physical findings may include mild pharyngitis, enlargement of the postoccipital nodes, and irritability.

2. Other Manifestations–HHV-6 is a frequent cause of febrile illness with or without rash in the first 2 years of life. This virus may also produce illness in immunocompromised patients, including febrile episodes, encephalitis, bone marrow suppression, hepatitis, and pneumonitis. Rare cases of disseminated infections have been reported.

B. Laboratory Findings: Findings include progressive leukopenia to 3000–5000 white cells, with a relative lymphocytosis as high as 90%.

Table 10–1. Diagnostic features of some acute exanthems.

Disease	Prodromal Signs & Symptoms	Nature of Eruption	Other Diagnostic Features	Laboratory Findings
Chickenpox (varicella)	0–1 d of fever, anorexia, headache	Rapid evolution of macules to papules, vesicles, crusts; vesicles extremely fragile; all stages simultaneously present in successive outcroppings; lesions superficial; distribution centripetal	Lesions on scalp and mucous membranes	Fluorescent antibody stain and viral culture of lesions
Drug eruption	Occasionally fever	Maculopapular rash resembling rubella; rarely papulovesicular		Eosinophilia
Enterovirus infection	1–2 d of fever, malaise	Maculopapular rash resembling rubella; rarely papulovesicular or petechial	Aseptic meningitis	Virus isolation from stool or CSF
Erythema infectiosum	No prodrome. Usually in epidemics	Red, flushed cheeks; circumoral pallor, maculopapules on extremities	"Slapped face" appearance	WBC normal; serology
Exanthema subitum	3–4 d of high fever	As fever falls by crisis, pink maculopapules appear on chest and trunk; fade in 1–3 d		WBC low; serology

Infectious mononucleosis	Fever, adenopathy, sore throat	Maculopapular rash resembling rubella, rarely papulovesicular; distribution scattered, asymmetrical	Splenomegaly, tonsillar exudate	Atypical lymphs in blood smears; slide heterophil agglutination test and specific serology
Meningococcemia	Hours of fever, vomiting	Maculopapules, petechiae, purpura	Meningeal signs, toxicity, shock	WBC high. Bacterial cultures of blood and CSF
Rocky Mountain spotted fever	3–4 d of fever, chills, severe headache	Maculopapules, petechiae; distribution centrifugal	History of tick bite	Serology
Rubella (German measles)	Little or no prodrome	Maculopapular, pink; begins on head and neck, spreads downward, fades in 3 d. No desquamation	Lymphadenopathy, postauricular or occipital	WBC normal or low; serology
Rubeola (measles)	3–4 d of fever, coryza, conjunctivitis, cough	Maculopapular, brick-red; begins on head and neck; spreads downward. In 5–6 d, rash is brownish, desquamating	Koplik's spots on buccal mucosa	WBC low. Virus isolation in cell culture; serology
Scarlet fever	½–2 d of malaise, sore throat, fever, vomiting	Generalized, punctate, red; prominent on neck, in axillae, groin, skin folds; circumoral pallor; fine desquamation involves hands and feet	Strawberry tongue, exudative tonsillitis	Group A hemolytic streptococci cultures from throat; rise in antistreptolysin O titer

CSF = cerebrospinal fluid; WBC = white blood cell count.

Complications

Seizures are the principal complication. They may be the first sign of illness and are usually associated with a rapidly rising temperature. Encephalitis also can occur (Chapter 20).

Treatment

A. Specific Measures: None available.

B. General Measures: Antipyretics and tepid sponge baths may be used to minimize discomfort and risk of febrile seizures.

Prognosis

The prognosis for full recovery is excellent.

MEASLES
(Rubeola)

Measles is a highly communicable disease; the highest incidence is between 2 and 14 years of age. The incubation period is 8–14 days, the majority of cases occurring 10 days after exposure.

Clinical Findings (Table 10–1)

A. Symptoms & Signs:

1. Prodrome–Fever is usually the first sign and persists throughout the prodrome. It ranges from 38.3–40 °C (101–104 °F), tends to be higher just before the rash appears, and may be lower after the rash erupts. Sore throat, nasal discharge, and dry, barking cough are common prodromal signs. Nonpurulent conjunctivitis appears toward the end of the prodrome and is accompanied by photophobia. Lymphadenopathy of the posterior cervical lymph nodes may occur. The causative virus is easily transmitted via nose and throat secretions during the prodromal period (3–5 days).

Koplik's spots are fine white spots on a faint erythematous base that appear first on the buccal mucosa opposite the molar teeth. The spots may spread over the entire inside of the mouth by the third or fourth day of the prodrome. They usually disappear as the exanthem becomes well established.

2. Rash–Rash appears on about the fifth day of disease. The pink, blotchy, irregular, macular erythema darkens and coalesces into larger red patches of varying size and shape. The rash first appears on the face and behind the ears, then spreads to the chest, abdomen, and extremities. It lasts 4–7 days and may be accompanied by mild itching. A fine brawny desquamation of the face and trunk may follow, lasting 2–3 days; light brown pigmentation may then appear.

B. Laboratory Findings: Leukopenia is present during the prodrome and early stages of the rash. There is usually a sharp rise in the white cell count (WBC) with the onset of any bacterial complication. In the absence of complications, the WBC slowly rises to normal as the rash fades.

Complications

A. Bacterial Infection:

1. Otitis Media–Ear infection may appear toward the end of the prodrome or during the course of the rash (Chapter 13).

2. Tracheobronchitis–There may be secondary bacterial involvement in addition to inflammation caused by rubeola. This infection is usually accompanied by a more productive cough.

3. Bronchopneumonia–While rubeola virus often causes a specific pneumonitis, secondary bacterial invasion is a relatively common complication.

B. Encephalitis: Encephalitis (Chapter 20) occurs in about 1 of 1000 cases; there is no relation to severity of measles. The first sign may be increasing lethargy or seizures. Lumbar puncture shows 0–200 cells, mostly lymphocytes. Subacute sclerosing panencephalitis (SSPE) is a late degenerative central nervous system (CNS) complication that results from persistent infection.

C. Hemorrhagic Measles: This rare form of the disease has a high mortality rate and is characterized by generalized bleeding and purpura.

D. Tuberculosis: Active pulmonary tuberculosis may be aggravated by measles.

Treatment

A. Specific Measures: Vitamin A should be considered for children with complications of measles, immunodeficiency, or clinical evidence of (or epidemiologic risk factors for) vitamin A deficiency.

B. General Measures: Measures include isolation for 4 days from onset of rash and supportive therapies.

C. Treatment of Complications: Bacterial complications should be treated with appropriate antibacterial agents. For treatment of patients with encephalitis, see Chapter 20.

Prophylaxis

Live measles virus vaccine should be given at 12–15 months of age, or at any age thereafter in susceptible persons (Chapter 6). Recommendations call for a second vaccination, either at the time of school entry (around 5 years of age) or at the time of middle/junior high school entry (around seventh grade). Measles vaccine may be given between 6 and 12 months of age in high-risk areas. Measles vaccine is contraindicated in immunocompromised children, except for HIV-infected patients. Measles vaccine given within 72 hours of measles exposure may be effective as postexposure prophylaxis. Standard immune globulin can prevent the disease in exposed susceptible persons if it is administered within 6 days of exposure. The dose is 0.25 mL/kg (0.5 mL/kg in immunocompromised children). One of these methods of postexposure prophylaxis is recommended for exposed infants younger than 12 months.

Prognosis

In uncomplicated cases or patients with bacterial complications, the prognosis is excellent. In patients with encephalitis, the prognosis is guarded; the incidence of permanent sequelae is high.

RUBELLA
(German Measles)

Rubella is a mild febrile virus infection that frequently occurs in epidemics. It is probably transmitted by droplets. The incubation period is 12–21 days (average, 16 days).

Clinical Findings (Table 10–1)

A. Symptoms & Signs:

1. Typical Rubella–The prodrome, if present, lasts only a few days and is characterized by slight malaise, occasional tender postauricular and occipital lymph nodes, and no catarrhal symptoms. Rash may be the first sign of disease and consists of faint, fine, discrete, erythematous maculopapules, which may coalesce, appearing first on the face and spreading rapidly over the trunk and extremities. The rash generally disappears by the third day. Fever rarely exceeds 38.3 °C (101 °F) and usually lasts less than 2 days.

2. Rubella Without Rash–Rubella sine eruption occurs as a febrile lymphadenopathy that may persist for a week or more. During epidemics, this syndrome may represent over 40% of cases with infection.

3. Congenital Rubella–This syndrome usually involves infants whose mothers contracted rubella in the first trimester of pregnancy. The majority of these infants show growth retardation, microcephaly, hepatosplenomegaly, and purpura, in addition to mental deficiency and congenital defects of the heart, eye, and ear. Marked thrombocytopenia and radiographic metaphysitis are common findings. Rubella virus is easily isolated from such patients, and they must be considered to be highly contagious. A late-onset congenital rubella syndrome has been reported, with minimal signs at birth and acute onset of severe clinical disease after 3–6 months.

B. Laboratory Findings: Transient leukopenia is usually noted.

Complications

If a woman contracts rubella during the first month of pregnancy, there is a 50% chance of fetal abnormality. By the third month of pregnancy, the risk of abnormalities decreases to less than 10%.

Encephalitis and thrombocytopenic purpura are rare. Polyarthritis occurs in 25% of cases in patients older than 16 years.

Treatment

A. Specific Measures: None available.

B. General Measures: Isolation is required for 7 days after the onset of rash. Infants with congenital rubella may be contagious for more than 1 year. Symptomatic measures are rarely necessary.

C. Treatment of Complications: For treatment of encephalitis and purpura, see Chapters 19 and 20 respectively.

Prophylaxis

Live rubella vaccine is normally administered in combination with measles and mumps vaccine at 12–15 months of age. It should be given along with the second recommended dose of measles vaccine (Chapter 6). Live rubella vaccine can be administered at any age after 12 months in susceptible persons. Adolescents and young adults with no history of immunization should be identified and vaccinated. A history of disease is unreliable and should not be used to determine the need for vaccination. Females of childbearing age should avoid pregnancy for 3 months after vaccination, although surveillance data suggest that no cases of congenital rubella syndrome have occurred in the offspring of women inadvertently given live rubella vaccine shortly before or within 3 months of conception. Rubella vaccine is contraindicated in immunocompromised patients, except those with HIV infection.

Standard immune globulin is *not* reliable in preventing infection in pregnant women exposed to rubella virus infection and is therefore not routinely recommended. Rubella serology should be measured immediately after exposure. If findings are negative (susceptible), measurement should be repeated at 3 and 6 weeks, to document occurrence of maternal infection. *All pregnant women regardless of immune status should be cautioned against exposure to any person with an illness that suggests rubella.*

Prognosis

The prognosis in patients with acquired infection is excellent. In patients with congenital disease, the prognosis is universally poor. A progressive degenerative panencephalitis has been reported. Late manifestations of brain damage such as behavior problems, increasing mental retardation, and minimal brain dysfunction (Chapter 8) may occur.

ERYTHEMA INFECTIOSUM (Fifth Disease & Parvovirus B19)

Erythema infectiosum is a mild, minimally febrile contagious disease usually occurring in family or institutional epidemics. The incubation period is estimated to be 4–14 days. Human parvovirus B19 has been demonstrated to be the causative agent.

Clinical Findings (Table 10–1)

A. Symptoms & Signs: There is usually no prodrome. The initial symptom is rash, which appears first on the cheeks and ears as red coalescent macules that are warm and slightly raised. Circumoral pallor is marked, leading to a "slapped cheek" appearance. This eruption fades within 4 days, followed 1 day later by a lacy, reticulated maculopapular erythematous rash that appears on the extensor surfaces of the extremities and spreads over 2–3 days to the flexor surfaces and trunk. The rash lasts 3–7 days but may recur over 1–3 weeks in response to environmental changes. Children are no longer infectious by the time they have developed a rash. Pruritus, headache, and arthralgia are occasional additional symptoms.

B. Laboratory Findings: The WBC is normal.

Complications

Human parvovirus has been implicated in arthritis syndromes, particularly in adults, and is the cause of aplastic crises in patients with chronic hemolytic disorders. Intrauterine parvovirus infection may produce hydrops and fetal death. Infection in immunocompromised patients may lead to chronic infection and anemia.

Treatment

Treatment is not indicated in uncomplicated cases. Patients with hemolytic conditions may require transfusions. Intrauterine transfusion has been suggested for fetal infections. Intravenous immune globulin may be effective in immunodeficient patients with chronic infection.

Prophylaxis

Advise pregnant women to avoid exposure to a known outbreak of erythema infectiosum. Should exposure occur, acute serology (immunoglobulin G [IgG] and immunoglobulin M [IgM]) can be measured; if findings are negative (susceptible), the IgG and IgM titers can be rechecked in 3 or more weeks to document whether maternal infection has occurred. Pregnant women with known infection may be followed with serum alpha-fetoprotein levels and frequent ultrasonography for the earliest detection of fetal hydrops.

Prognosis

Prognosis of uncomplicated erythema infectiosum and aplastic crises, if adequately supported by transfusion therapy, is excellent. It appears that most though not all intrauterine infections that produce hydrops will result in fetal loss.

VARICELLA (Chickenpox) & HERPES ZOSTER (Shingles)

Varicella is an extremely communicable acute disease caused by the varicella zoster virus. It is spread by respiratory droplets or by direct contact with freshly infected vesicles. Varicella is communicable from 1–2 days before until 6 days after appearance of the rash. The incubation period is 10–21 days (average, 15 days).

With rare exceptions, post-infection immunity to varicella is lifelong, although persons with a history of varicella may later develop herpes zoster.

Clinical Findings (Table 10–1)

A. Symptoms & Signs:

1. Prodrome–The prodrome is usually not apparent; there may be slight malaise and fever for 24 hours.

2. Rash–Usually, the first sign of varicella is a rash. Lesions tend to appear in crops (2–4 crops in 2–6 days). All stages and sizes may be present at the same time and in the same vicinity. Lesions occur first on the scalp and mucous surfaces; then on the body. They are numerous over the chest, back, and shoulders; less numerous on the extremities; and seldom seen on the palms and soles. Successive stages include macules, papules, vesicles on erythematous bases, and pustules or scabs.

3. Pruritus–Pruritus is minimal at first but may become severe in lesions in the pustular stage.

4. Fever–Fever may occur during the first few days of rash, but systemic symptoms are usually minimal.

5. Herpes Zoster–Herpes zoster (shingles) occurs in persons who have had varicella but is rarely seen in very young children. There may be pain in the area of the rash before the vesicles erupt. Lesions resemble those of varicella but are confined to dermatomal distributions. The most common site is the chest, but lesions may also follow the distribution of the trigeminal nerve root. The vesicles are usually dry and beginning to heal by the fourth or fifth day.

B. Laboratory Findings: Leukopenia occurs early. The WBC may rise with extensive secondary infection of vesicles.

Complications

Secondary infection of vesicles is a common complication of varicella. Encephalitis, nephritis, hepatitis, arthritis, glomerulonephritis, thrombocytopenia, and **Reye's syndrome** (Chapter 3) occur rarely. Severe disease with visceral involvement (including pneumonia) occurs in some immunocompromised individuals and in some normal adults and newborns. Congenital infection with cicatricial skin lesions and neurologic and eye abnormalities occasionally results from infection during the first or early second trimester of pregnancy.

Treatment

A. Specific Measures: Intravenous acyclovir is generally reserved for complicated cases (eg, immunocompromised patients or those with disseminated visceral involvement). Oral acyclovir, which reduces the duration and extent of skin lesions and fever, may be beneficial in children with underlying disease or otherwise at increased risk of severe disease, including being older than 12 years of age.

B. General Measures: Pruritus may be relieved by local application of calamine lotion or mild topical anesthetic ointments, or by administration of systemic antihistamines. Salicylates should be avoided because of increased risk of Reye's syndrome.

C. Treatment of Complications: Treat secondary infection with antibiotics active against group A streptococcus and *Staphylococcus aureus*. For general treatment measures in patients with encephalitis, see Chapter 20.

Prophylaxis

Varicella zoster immune globulin (VZIG) may prevent or modify the course of progressive disease in susceptible immunodeficient persons exposed to the virus. For maximal benefit, VZIG should be administered within 96 hours of exposure. Protection with VZIG is also recommended for susceptible pregnant women, for neonates whose mothers develop chickenpox between 5 days before and 2 days after delivery, and for premature neonates exposed postnatally. Live attenuated varicella virus vaccine is recommended for children ≥ 12 months of age without a prior history of chickenpox. Two doses 1–2 months apart are required for children older than 13 years. Vaccination is not approved for immunocompromised children, although several clinical trials in select populations are under way. Vaccination is also contraindicated in pregnant women and should not be given to patients receiving salicylate therapy.

Prognosis

In uncomplicated disease, the prognosis is excellent. Scarring is not uncommon. Encephalitis may lead to significant neurologic sequelae in some patients. Severe illness and death may occur in immunodeficient patients or neonates with disseminated disease. Congenital disease may result in long-term extremity, neurologic, or ocular abnormalities. In patients with herpes zoster, pain along the nerve root may persist for several months.

MUMPS
(Epidemic Parotitis)

Mumps is an acute viral disease that commonly affects the salivary glands, chiefly the parotid gland (about 60% of cases), and frequently the central nervous system. It is uncommon in children younger than 3 years and adults older than 40. Mumps spreads directly by the respiratory route. It is communicable from 2 days before the appearance of symptoms to the disappearance of salivary gland swelling. The incubation period is usually 12–24 days (average, 16–18 days).

Clinical Findings (Table 10–1)

A. Symptoms & Signs:

1. Gland Involvement–A prodrome of 1–2 days may precede salivary gland involvement. It is characterized by fever, malaise, and pain in or behind the ear on chewing or swallowing. Tender swelling and brawny edema of the parotid gland are common. Submaxillary and sublingual glands may be involved also or in the absence of parotid gland involvement. Pain is referred to the ear and is aggravated by chewing, swallowing, opening the mouth, and sometimes by ingestion of sour substances. Tenderness persists for 1–3 days; swelling is present for 7–10 days. The skin over the gland is normal. Openings of ducts of the involved gland and especially the papilla of **Stensen's duct** (opposite the upper second molar) may be puffy and red. Fever may be absent or as high as 40 °C (104 °F). Malaise, anorexia, and headache may be present.

2. "Inapparent" Mumps Infection–This infection has a short course, with fever lasting 1–5 days without apparent salivary gland involvement.

3. Central Nervous System Involvement–Mumps encephalitis may precede, accompany, or follow inflammation of the salivary glands. It may also occur without such involvement. Mumps meningitis is heralded by the sudden onset of meningeal irritation. Headache, vomiting, stiff neck and back, and lethargy are characteristic. Fever recurs or increases, up to 41.1 °C (106 °F). Symptoms seldom last more than 5 days. Transient paresis may suggest poliomyelitis. Asymptomatic CNS inflammation with pleocytosis may be found in over 50% of mumps cases.

4. Other Organ Involvement–Mastitis, arthritis, and thyroiditis may occur. Other organs may be involved, including the following:

a. Testicles & Ovaries–These organs are usually involved during or after adolescence; however, orchitis can occur in childhood. Orchitis may occur in the absence of distinctive salivary gland involvement.

b. Pancreas–Pancreatic involvement is marked by a sudden onset of pain in the mid- or upper abdomen, with vomiting, prostration, and usually, fever.

c. Kidney–Nephritis is rare and mild, with complete recovery in most cases.

d. Ear–Deafness occasionally occurs and may be permanent.

B. Laboratory Findings: The WBC usually shows leukopenia and relative lymphocytosis.

Complications

Paresis of the facial nerve has been reported. Serious sequelae of CNS involvement are rare. Testicular involvement (usually unilateral) may produce atrophy, but sterility is rare.

Treatment

A. Specific Measures: None available.

B. General Measures: Measures include bed rest, isolation of the patient until the salivary swelling is gone, local application of cold or heat to swollen salivary glands, analgesics, washing mouth with fat-free broth or saline solution, and avoidance of highly flavored or acidic foods and drinks.

C. Treatment of Complications:

1. CNS Involvement–Treatment is symptomatic for mild encephalitis. Lumbar puncture may be useful in reducing headache.

2. Orchitis–Suspension of the scrotum in a sling or suspensory, application of ice packs, and use of analgesics may be indicated. Anesthetic infiltration around the spermatic cord at the external inguinal ring may produce dramatic relief.

3. Pancreatitis & Oophoritis–Treatment is symptomatic only.

Prophylaxis

Live mumps virus vaccine is usually given in combination with measles and rubella vaccine at 12–15 months of age. It may be administered to any preadolescent or adolescent with a negative history for vaccine (Chapter 6), but should not be given to pregnant females. A second dose of vaccine is recommended (with measles and rubella vaccine) at school entry or at entry into middle school/junior high school. There is no effective passive protection for mumps exposure.

Prognosis

The prognosis is excellent even with extensive organ system involvement. Sterility very rarely results from orchitis in the postadolescent male. Death may occasionally result from encephalitis.

ENTEROVIRUS INFECTION (Coxsackieviruses, Echoviruses, & Other Nonpolio Enteroviruses)

Enteroviruses are responsible for a large variety of illnesses that occur during epidemics in the summer and fall. They are spread by the enteric-oral route, possibly by the respiratory route; incubation periods are usually 3–6 days.

Clinical Findings (Table 10–1)

A. "Summer Grippe": An acute, brief, febrile illness lasting 1–4 days without other specific signs or symptoms.

B. Exanthematous Disease: A febrile illness associated with a macular, maculopapular, or petechial rash on the face, trunk, and extremities. The illness may be accompanied by pharyngitis or gastrointestinal (GI) symptoms. Frequently caused by echovirus strains.

C. Herpangina: A febrile illness lasting 1–4 days associated with pharyngitis, including hyperemia of the anterior tonsillar pillars and vesicles in the posterior oropharynx. Usually associated with Coxsackie A viruses.

D. Hand-Foot-Mouth Syndrome: Also caused by Coxsackie A viruses; a papulovesicular eruption is present on the oropharynx, hand or foot, and often buttocks.

E. Aseptic Meningitis: Caused by both Coxsackie viruses and echoviruses, this self-limited febrile illness is accompanied by headache, nausea, vomiting, meningismus, and sometimes rashes. Spinal fluid may show a pleocytosis, usually less than 500/mL, and usually mononuclear cells, although these findings are variable. Paralytic disease occasionally occurs with some viral strains. Chronic meningoencephalitis may occur in patients with humoral immunodeficiency.

F. Pleurodynia (Bornholm Disease): Fever is accompanied by dyspnea, pleuritic chest pain, and often abdominal pain. Pleurodynia is usually caused by Coxsackie B viruses, and tends to occur in older children and adults.

G. Myocarditis & Pericarditis: Enteroviruses, especially Coxsackie B viruses, are a major cause of viral myocarditis. They may occasionally lead to sudden cardiac death or chronic heart failure.

H. Neonatal Infection: Infected neonates may have variable combinations of sepsis, meningoencephalitis, myocarditis (caused by Coxsackie B viruses), hepatitis (caused by echoviruses), and pneumonia. Epidemics in newborn nurseries have been reported.

I. Conjunctivitis: Specific serotypes have been implicated in acute (epidemic) hemorrhagic conjunctivitis.

J. Upper Respiratory Tract Infection

K. Gastroenteritis: Seen most often in young infants.

Treatment

No specific therapies are available. Immune globulin may be beneficial for infections in immunodeficient hosts and perhaps in some neonatal infections.

Prophylaxis

Careful and thorough hand washing can minimize spread of infection.

Prognosis

Prognosis is generally excellent. Paresis, when present, is usually transient. Myocarditis will occasionally lead to chronic heart failure or death. Severe neonatal disease has a high mortality rate.

VIRAL HEPATITIS

Several causal agents are presently recognized, with distinct morphologic and antigenic characteristics.

Hepatitis A virus (HAV) is transmitted by the fecal-oral route and by contaminated food or water. Day care centers have been identified as important sites of HAV transmission. The incubation period is 15–50 days (average, 25–30 days).

Hepatitis B virus (HBV) is transmitted via blood, mucous secretions, and open wounds. Transmission may occur either from acutely infected patients or from chronically infected carriers. Perinatal transmission typically involves a mother who is hepatitis B surface antigen (HBsAg) positive, especially if she is also hepatitis B e antigen (HBeAg) positive. The incubation period of hepatitis B is 45–160 days (average, 120 days).

Hepatitis delta (D) virus is a helper virus that leads to accelerated acute or chronic hepatitis, but only in the presence of coinfection with HBV. It is transmitted via the same routes as HBV; however, perinatal transmission is unusual. The incubation period is approximately 14–56 days.

Hepatitis C virus (HCV) is the major etiologic agent of parenterally-acquired non-A, non-B hepatitis. It is transmitted by blood;

it is probably also sexually transmitted and can be acquired perinatally. A significant number of infected individuals have no identified risk factor. The incubation period is 14–168 days (average, 49–63 days).

Hepatitis E virus (HEV) is an enterically transmitted agent of hepatitis that has caused outbreaks in Asia, Africa, and Central America. It has an incubation period of 15–60 days (average, 40 days).

Clinical Findings

A. Symptoms & Signs:

1. Hepatitis A–This form is most often asymptomatic or mild and nonspecific in infants and young children. The virus may produce acute clinical hepatitis with fever, jaundice, anorexia, nausea and vomiting, abdominal pain, and hepatomegaly; it generally resolves within 2–4 weeks. Fulminant hepatitis rarely occurs. Chronic infection does not occur.

2. Hepatitis B–This virus may also produce asymptomatic or mild anicteric illness in children. The hepatitis tends to be subacute; fever, jaundice, anorexia, nausea, malaise, and tender liver enlargement may be accompanied by rash or arthralgias/arthritis. Fulminant hepatitis, chronic hepatitis, or chronic asymptomatic viral carriage may occur.

3. Hepatitis Delta–May co-infect patients, or aggravate acute or chronic disease in patients with hepatitis B infection.

4. Hepatitis C–This virus may produce asymptomatic infection or an insidious mild illness marked by jaundice and malaise. Symptoms and transaminase values may fluctuate. Chronic infection and chronic hepatitis are frequent occurrences. Fulminant hepatitis may also occur.

5. Hepatitis E–Produces acute illness characterized by jaundice, malaise, fever, abdominal pain, and arthralgia. Chronic infection is not described. Fulminant infection may occur, particularly in pregnant women.

B. Laboratory Findings: Elevations in hepatic transaminases associated with elevated bilirubin levels are frequent findings. Specific serologic markers are available to diagnose infections by HAV, HBV, hepatitis delta, and HCV.

Complications

Complications of acute severe hepatitis include hemorrhage, encephalopathy, ascites, renal failure, and hepatic necrosis. Chronic or recurring hepatitis can occur after acute infection with hepatitis B, delta, or hepatitis C virus; it may proceed to cirrhosis. Infection with HBV (especially perinatal infection) or HCV may lead to chronic viral carriage, which is associated with an increased risk of cirrhosis and hepatocellular carcinoma.

Treatment

A. Specific Measures: Interferon may be useful for some cases of chronic hepatitis caused by HBV or HCV.

B. General Measures: Attention to dietary needs (including vitamins), and treatment of complications (eg, coagulopathy or encephalopathy).

Prophylaxis

Standard immune globulin can prevent overt disease from HAV infection but may not prevent infection. A dose of 0.02 mL/kg given within 2 weeks of exposure is recommended for sexual, familial, and day care contacts. Travelers to endemic regions should receive 0.02 mL/kg for visits up to 3 months; 0.06 mL/kg every 5 months is recommended for longer stays. **Inactivated hepatitis A vaccine** is recommended for individuals at significant risk, including residents of and travelers to endemic areas, and persons exposed to HAV.

Hepatitis B immune globulin (HBIG) is effective in preventing hepatitis B infection in susceptible persons exposed to the blood of an infected person. Exposure may occur via needle pricks, mucosal surfaces, sexual activity, and some household contacts. HBIG is given in a dose of 0.06 mL/kg as soon as possible after exposure (but within 14 days); the hepatitis B vaccine series should also be initiated. Perinatal exposure requires administration of 0.5 mL of HBIG as soon after birth as possible, preferably in the delivery room but within 12–48 hours, as well as initiation of hepatitis B vaccine (see below).

Recombinant inactivated hepatitis B vaccine is effective in the prevention of hepatitis B. The vaccine regimen consists of three doses administered intramuscularly. The first dose is followed in 1 month by the second and in 6 months by the third. Alternative regimens are available. In addition to administration following blood or perinatal exposure, vaccination (and HBIG) is recommended for some household and sexual contacts of persons with hepatitis B as well as for other high-risk groups. Vaccination is now recommended as a universal precaution for newborns; it should also be given to nonimmunized adolescents when feasible. Following the neonatal vaccine series given for perinatal exposure, serum anti-HBs antibody and hepatitis B surface antigen should be measured 1–3 months after the last immunization. If the antibody titer and surface antigen are negative, additional vaccine doses should be administered and anti-HBs should be remeasured. If the surface antigen is positive, perform follow-up testing to determine whether chronic carriage has occurred. Prophylaxis with immune globulin for exposure to blood from a patient with hepatitis C infection is unlikely to be effective.

Prognosis

Hepatitis A is usually a self-limited disease. In the absence of acute hepatic failure, the prognosis is good. Severe acute hepatitis or chronic progressive or recurrent liver disease may result from hepatitis B and hepatitis C infections, and may lead to cirrhosis. Hepatitis E may occasionally produce fatal disease, particularly in pregnant women.

HERPES SIMPLEX INFECTIONS

Herpes simplex virus typically produces a subclinical or clinical primary infection, followed by latent persistence of the virus in a sensory ganglion. Recurrences are triggered by fever, trauma, or other stress. Herpes simplex virus type 1 (HSV-1) occurs principally around the mouth and produces lesions on the face and upper part of the body; it is commonly transmitted by saliva or respiratory droplets. Herpes simplex virus type 2 (HSV-2) occurs principally on the genitals and the lower parts of the body and is often a sexually transmitted disease (STD). HSV-2 is the type more commonly implicated in neonatal herpes infection. The incubation period of genital HSV-2 infection is approximately 2–14 days.

Clinical Findings

A. Symptoms & Signs:

1. Acute Herpetic Gingivostomatitis–This is a typical primary infection of young children, with extensive vesicles and ulcers on the gums, palate, and buccal mucosa. Pain, bleeding, and fever are common. Herpetic gingivostomatitis is self-limited and heals in 1–2 weeks. Primary oral infection is often subclinical.

2. Recurrent "Cold Sores"–These findings are most common at the mucocutaneous junctions of the lips or nose. They recur at the same site in a given person, with the virus latent in the trigeminal ganglion between recurrences. Individual vesicles develop 36–60 hours after being triggered (eg, by sunburn), persist for 2–4 days, and then rupture, leaving an ulcer that crusts and heals without scarring.

3. Whitlow–This is a vesicular paronychia caused by primary or secondary infection of a finger with HSV.

4. Genital Herpes–Vesicles and ulceration occur on the genitalia, with significant surrounding inflammation. Recurrent lesions occur at the same site (penis, vulva, cervix), liberating virus and serving as a source of infection during sexual contact.

Primary episodes may be severe, while recurrent lesions may be associated with minimal inflammation and symptoms.

5. Keratoconjunctivitis–This may be a primary or recurrent infection, usually caused by HSV-1. Recurrent lesions often take the form of dendritic lesions or ulcers of the corneal epithelium. The corneal stroma may be involved, leading to opacity and impairment of vision or blindness.

6. Eczema Herpeticum–This herpetic infection consists of vesicular lesions concentrated in areas of eczematous dermatitis. Unless the child is immunodeficient, these widespread lesions usually heal.

7. Encephalitis–This may be a primary or a recurrent infection; findings include headache, fever, sensory impairment, seizures, or signs pointing to a lesion of the temporal lobe (eg, aphasia, behavioral disorders, psychomotor convulsions). Necrotizing encephalitis is often fatal in untreated patients. Brain biopsy permits virus isolation; cerebrospinal fluid (CSF) findings are often negative, but viral DNA in CSF is frequently detectable by polymerase chain reaction. HSV-1 may also be responsible for 2–5% of cases of viral aseptic meningitis, which has an almost universally favorable outcome.

8. Neonatal Herpes–This is a primary perinatal infection transmitted from asymptomatically shed virus or lesions on the mother's genitalia. Manifestations include cutaneous and oral vesicles; keratoconjunctivitis and chorioretinitis; meningoencephalitis; or multisystem disease affecting the liver, lungs, and other organs. Disease usually occurs in the first month of life. Congenital disease apparent at birth also occurs.

9. Infection in Immunocompromised Hosts–Herpes simplex may produce disseminated mucocutaneous or visceral disease. Pneumonia, hepatitis, or encephalitis may occur.

B. Laboratory Findings: Scrapings from ulcerations on the base of vesicles show multinucleated giant cells in Giemsa-stained smears or positive antigen testing. Swabs or aspirates from early lesions (first to fourth days) inoculated into cell cultures permit growth of the virus in 1–3 days.

Treatment

Several drugs can inhibit herpes simplex virus replication. Idoxuridine, vidarabine, and trifluridine ophthalmic preparations, applied topically for herpetic keratitis, and local debridement will greatly accelerate corneal healing. These treatments will not, however, affect the rate of recurrence. In neonates, intravenous acyclovir must be used in addition to topical treatment of herpes keratitis.

Intravenous acyclovir is indicated for the treatment of neonatal HSV infection, HSV disease in immunocompromised hosts, HSV encephalitis, severe eczema herpeticum, and severe primary genital herpes infection.

Oral acyclovir may be used for treatment or prophylaxis of genital herpes and for treatment or prophylaxis of HSV infections in immunocompromised patients.

Antiviral resistance has been observed in immunocompromised patients after prolonged treatment with acyclovir. Foscarnet is a suitable alternative.

Prophylaxis

Susceptible individuals should avoid contact with open lesions. Transmission of genital herpes may be minimized by the use of condoms. Caesarean section may prevent some neonatal infections when the mother has active genital lesions at the time of delivery. Cultures obtained from at-risk mothers and babies at the time of delivery or 24–48 hours afterward may be useful in guiding management.

Prognosis

In most cases of mucocutaneous disease, the prognosis is excellent. In patients with CNS involvement and in newborns or other compromised hosts with systemic disease, the prognosis is guarded.

INFECTIOUS MONONUCLEOSIS (Epstein-Barr Virus)

Infectious mononucleosis is the prototype disease caused by Epstein-Barr (EB) virus, although EB virus produces a range of illnesses from asymptomatic infection to severe progressive disease. Infectious mononucleosis may occur at any age; it is rare in infancy and most common in later childhood and the early adult years. Intimate personal contact is required for transmission. The incubation period ranges from approximately 30 to 50 days.

Clinical Findings

A. Symptoms & Signs: Mononucleosis is usually marked by gradual onset of malaise and fever. A sore throat becomes apparent and sometimes becomes severe, with swelling of the neck and a membrane on the tonsils and pharynx. There is generalized lymphadenopathy, especially of the cervical nodes. The liver and spleen are characteristically enlarged, usually after the first week of symptoms. A morbilliform, scarlatiniform, or petechial rash may appear.

B. Laboratory Findings: A leukocytosis develops very early, with a predominant lymphocytosis, including large immature vacuolated lymphocytes. A rising titer of heterophil agglutinins usually appears in the serum by the second week; a slide agglutination test demonstrates the same antibody and can be used for diagnostic purposes. In uncertain cases, an EB virus serology panel can determine the timing of EB virus infection.

Complications

A secondary infection in the throat with group A streptococcus is the most common complication. Myocarditis, encephalitis, meningitis, Guillain-Barré syndrome, thrombocytopenia, hemolytic anemia, and agranulocytosis have been reported. Rupture of the spleen may occur from trauma to the abdomen. EB virus infection in immunodeficient patients, including transplant recipients, may produce disseminated infection or B-cell lymphomas. EB virus also causes African Burkitt's lymphoma and nasopharyngeal carcinoma, and is the incriminated agent in some cases of hemophagocytic syndrome.

Treatment

A. Specific Measures: Antiviral therapy with acyclovir has been used in immunocompromised patients. Reduction of immune suppression has been useful in some transplant patients.

B. General Measures: Pharyngitis complicated by group A streptococci should be treated with penicillin (Chapter 11). Steroids may be useful for severe tonsillar swelling that threatens airway patency. Contact sports and trauma should be avoided during acute illness and convalescence.

Prognosis

Infectious mononucleosis usually runs its course in 10–20 days. The prognosis is excellent in most cases. Rupture of the spleen is a serious complication requiring surgical intervention.

CYTOMEGALOVIRUS DISEASE

Cytomegalovirus (CMV) is the cause of severe congenital infection as well as milder acquired infections. Routes of transmission include transplacental transmission, cervical contact during birth, breast milk, contact with saliva or urine, and blood transfusion or tissue transplantation. While most infections are asymptomatic, certain clinical entities may result.

Clinical Findings

A. Symptoms & Signs:

1. Congenital Cytomegalic Inclusion Disease–A minority of congenitally infected infants show evidence of this severe illness. Most infants with severe disease are infected as a result of a primary maternal infection during pregnancy. Findings include intrauterine growth retardation (IUGR), jaundice shortly after birth, hepatosplenomegaly, purpura, pneumonitis, and encephalitis. Laboratory findings include thrombocytopenia, erythroblastosis, hyperbilirubinemia, and marked lymphocytosis. Sequelae include intracranial calcifications, microcephaly, mental retardation, and chorioretinitis. The prognosis is poor. Fortunately, the majority of congenital infections cause only mild symptoms (eg, hearing loss, mild developmental delay) or are asymptomatic.

2. Acute Acquired Disease–This form of CMV infection resembles infectious mononucleosis. There is a sudden onset of fever, malaise, joint pain, and myalgia. Pharyngitis is minimal, and respiratory symptoms are absent. Lymphadenopathy is generalized. The liver shows enlargement and often slight tenderness. Laboratory findings include the hematologic picture of mononucleosis as well as hyperbilirubinemia. Heterophil antibody does not appear.

3. Generalized Systemic Disease–This form occurs in immunosuppressed persons, especially following organ transplant procedures, and in patients with human immunodeficiency virus (HIV) infection. Manifestations include pneumonitis, hepatitis, colitis, chorioretinitis, encephalitis, and leukopenia, often with a lymphocytosis. Generalized disease is occasionally fatal. Transplant patients who acquire primary infection are at especially high risk of serious disease.

B. Laboratory Findings: CMV infection may be diagnosed by virus culture of urine, saliva, leukocytes, or other secretions and tissues. Serologic tests are also available.

Treatment

Ganciclovir and foscarnet are available for the treatment of severe CMV-associated disease. CMV immune globulin may be synergistic with ganciclovir in bone marrow transplant patients with CMV pneumonia. Ganciclovir-resistant CMV in immunocompromised patients may respond to foscarnet.

Prophylaxis

Careful hand washing is the most effective way of preventing infection. Attempts should be made to avoid CMV-contaminated transfusions to high-risk groups (eg, premature newborns or immunosuppressed patients) by freezing blood in glycerol, filtering out white blood cells, or using blood from seronegative donors. Infection or illness with CMV in immunocompromised patients may be reduced with prophylactic regimens consisting of acyclovir, ganciclovir, or (CMV) immune globulin. CMV vaccines are being developed.

Prognosis

Ninety percent of survivors of the congenital cytomegalic inclusion disease are neurologically impaired, with microcephaly, mental retardation, or hearing loss. Up to 10–15% of asymptomatic congenitally infected neonates will develop hearing loss or mild developmental delay. Acquired infection may be severe in immunocompromised hosts.

INFLUENZA

Influenza is an acute systemic viral disease that usually occurs in epidemics. It is caused by a distinct class of virus with three main serotypes (A, B, and C) based on ribonucleoproteins. Subclassification of each type is based on the surface proteins hemagglutinin and neuraminidase. The incubation period is 1–3 days.

Clinical Findings

Onset of influenza is abrupt, with sudden fever rising to 39.4–40 °C (103–104 °F), extreme malaise, myalgia, headache, a dry, nonproductive cough, and nasal congestion. Small infants may exhibit only fever, cough, and marked irritability. Physical findings are minimal; they may include nasal congestion, pharyngitis, and myositis.

Complications

Primary complications are rare but may include pneumonia, croup, myocarditis, and encephalopathy. Secondary complications include pneumonia and otitis media. The bacterial agent most often responsible is *S aureus*. Reye's syndrome (Chapter 3) is a rare complication of influenza B infection.

Treatment

Amantadine and rimantadine reduce symptoms of influenza A if begun early in the illness. Treatment for 2–5 days is recommended for children with severe disease and in those at high risk for severe infection.

Give acetaminophen for antipyresis; avoid salicylates because of the risk of Reye's syndrome.

Prophylaxis

Immunization against influenza is recommended as annual prophylaxis for high-risk children and their close contacts. Children at risk include persons with chronic cardiopulmonary disease, immunocompromised patients, children with hemoglobinopathies, those with chronic metabolic or renal diseases, and those on chronic aspirin therapy.

Chemoprophylaxis with amantadine or rimantadine (against influenza A) is an alternative modality during an identified community outbreak.

Prognosis

The prognosis of influenza is good in normal hosts. The course of illness may be severe in those with underlying diseases, especially persons with preexistent cardiopulmonary disease and those who develop such primary complications as myocarditis or secondary bacterial superinfections (eg, pneumonia).

ACQUIRED IMMUNODEFICIENCY SYNDROME (AIDS)

AIDS is caused by human immunodeficiency virus (HIV), a human retrovirus that infects the helper-inducer subset of T cells as well as other cells and tissues.

Adults and older children at risk include intravenous drug abusers, recipients of infected blood or blood products, and persons with infected sex partners (homosexual or heterosexual). New pediatric HIV infections most commonly (> 80%) occur in offspring of parents infected with HIV, whether or not either parent is symptomatic. Approximately 20% of infants of HIV antibody-positive mothers will be infected. The relative importance of transplacental infection versus intrapartum infection is not known.

Clinical Findings

A. Symptoms & Signs: Common findings in pediatric AIDS include failure to thrive, lymphadenopathy, hepatosplenomegaly, persistent thrush, recurrent bacterial infections, diarrhea, parotitis, and lymphoid interstitial pneumonitis. Opportunistic infections occur, including *Pneumocystis carinii* pneumonia, cryptosporidiosis, CMV infection, cryptococcal meningitis, tuberculosis, and *Mycobacterium avium-intracellulare* infection. Cardiomyopathy, hepatitis, retinitis, or nephropathy may develop. Developmental delay and encephalopathy are frequent.

B. Laboratory Findings: Frequent features of AIDS include hypergammaglobulinemia, thrombocytopenia, lymphopenia, and decreased T4 (helper) lymphocytes. Diagnosis is generally made in older children and adults via serum ELISA and Western blot assays for IgG antibody. Diagnosis is more difficult in the first 18 months of life because of the presence of passively acquired maternal antibodies. Diagnostic modalities useful in this age group include viral culture, polymerase chain reaction, and p24 antigen detection.

Complications

The course of HIV infection in children is quite variable. Some infants with HIV infection have a rapidly progressive illness in the first 2 years of life, with *P carinii* pneumonia, encephalopathy, recurrent bacterial infections, failure to thrive, and frequently death. Other children have more benign illness, with minimal symptoms during early childhood.

Treatment

Zidovudine (azidothymidine or AZT), didanosine (ddI), zalcitabine (dideoxycitidine or ddC), and other reverse transcriptase inhibitors have in vitro activity against HIV and are effective in treating symptomatic patients. Studies currently in progress are addressing the utility of early treatment of mildly symptomatic children and defining optional combinations of antiviral agents. Intravenous immune globulin may benefit some patients with recurrent bacterial infections. Treatment of typical bacterial and opportunistic infections is important in the total care of AIDS patients.

Prophylaxis (usually with trimethoprim-sulfamethoxazole) against *P carinii* pneumonia is instituted according to age-dependent thresholds in the T4 lymphocyte count and may be given to all indeterminate and HIV-infected infants younger than 1 year. Immunizations for the HIV-infected child should include DPT, inactivated poliovirus, *Haemophilus influenzae* B, and measles/mumps/rubella. Children older than 2 years should also receive pneumococcal vaccine. Annual immunization against influenza is also recommended, particularly in symptomatic children.

A regimen consisting of oral zidovudine during pregnancy followed by intravenous AZT during delivery and oral AZT for neonates for 6 weeks has been demonstrated to reduce significantly the rate of vertical transmission of HIV infection. This approach is recommended for pregnant women identified with HIV infection.

Prognosis

Children infected with HIV represent a spectrum of prognoses ranging from rapid death to survival for many years from the time of diagnosis. While most HIV infections are presumed to progress eventually to symptomatic illness, persons with prolonged asymptomatic infection or prolonged survival have been described. Poor prognostic factors include symptoms in the first year, *Pneumocystis* pneumonia, encephalopathy, and severe wasting.

POLIOMYELITIS

Poliomyelitis is an acute viral infection of the spinal cord and brain stem. In its severe form, it leads to neuron destruction and irreversible muscular paralysis. The paralytic forms have a mortality rate of 10%. This disease is very rare in countries with widespread immunization.

The disease is caused by poliovirus serotypes 1, 2, and 3, which are enteroviruses. They are transmitted by the fecal-oral route and possibly by the respiratory route. The incubation period is 3–6 days for abortive poliomyelitis and 7–21 days for paralytic disease.

Clinical Findings

A. Symptoms & Signs: Poliovirus infection may be asymptomatic or produce a nonspecific febrile illness (abortive poliomyelitis). Other forms of infection include:

1. Nonparalytic Poliomyelitis–Symptoms and signs are those of a febrile aseptic meningitis.

2. Paralytic Poliomyelitis (Spinal Type)–Paralysis may occur without obvious antecedent illness, especially in infants. Paralysis usually begins and progresses during the febrile stage of the illness. Tremor upon sustained effort may be present before weakness occurs. Muscle tightness and pain on stretching may simulate paralysis. The CSF white cell count may be normal in 10–15% of cases.

3. Bulbar Polioencephalitis–This infection is a paralytic poliomyelitis that includes involvement of the cranial nerves and brain stem. Significant lower spinal involvement may be absent. Any cranial nerve may be affected; however, swallowing difficulties predominate. Polioencephalitis is the term used in cases of impairment of cerebral function.

4. Respiratory Difficulty in Poliomyelitis–Respiratory difficulty may occur with paralysis of intercostal muscles. Manifestations include anxiety, increased respiratory rate, and reluctance to vocalize. Paralyses of the diaphragm, which are easily overlooked, are usually associated with intercostal paralysis. Damage to the medullary respiratory center may also occur, sometimes with severe symptoms of irregular, shallow, and spasmodic breathing. Obstruction of the pharynx or trachea, caused by aspiration of saliva secondary to pharyngeal or palatal paralysis, may also occur.

B. Laboratory Findings: Poliovirus can be grown from stool and throat specimens; it is rarely recovered from CSF. Serology can demonstrate seroconversion.

Treatment

A. Specific Measures: None available.

B. General Measures: Many patients with mild forms of poliomyelitis can be cared for at home. Special facilities and trained professional personnel are required for seriously ill patients.

Bed rest is indicated. Hot packs and soaks, bed boards, foot boards, and splints may be used. Physiotherapy is the most important single factor in recovery.

C. Treatment of Respiratory Difficulties: Intercostal or diaphragm paralysis requires artificial ventilation. A tank respirator, chest respirator (cuirass), or a positive-pressure ventilator may be used. Tracheostomy may be required in patients with paralysis of muscles of swallowing, weakness of muscles of respiration, or bulbar poliomyelitis.

Prophylaxis

The paralytic consequences of infection with poliomyelitis virus can be avoided by prophylactic use of live oral (or inactive/intramuscular) vaccine (Chapter 6). The vaccine should be administered to infants and children according to the routine schedule.

Oral live attenuated vaccine has a very small risk of causing paralytic poliomyelitis; this risk is increased in immunocompromised hosts. Therefore, inactivated intramuscular vaccine should be used in persons with immune deficiency and those who are in close contact with immunocompromised hosts. The inactivated vaccine is also the preferred vaccine for adults, as they have a slightly higher risk of developing vaccine-associated paralytic poliomyelitis than do children. Adults who are at increased risk for exposure to poliovirus (eg, travelers to or residents of areas with endemic or epidemic disease) are candidates for immunization.

Prognosis

The prognosis with paralytic polio is guarded, although muscle function may improve within the first 2 years after infection. In the bulbar form, prognosis is good if complications are overcome. Patients with polioencephalitis usually have a poor prognosis for survival. If the respiratory center is severely involved, the prognosis is poor.

RESPIRATORY SYNCYTIAL VIRUS

Respiratory syncytial virus (RSV) is the most frequent cause of viral lower respiratory tract infection in infants. The incubation period ranges between 2 and 8 days. Annual epidemics in winter and early spring typically occur in temperate climates.

Clinical Findings

A. Symptoms & Signs: RSV causes upper respiratory infection, bronchiolitis or pneumonia. Symptoms include fever, anorexia, lethargy, tachypnea, cough, and respiratory distress. Patients may have nasal flaring, retractions, rales, rhonchi, or wheezes. Apnea may be a presenting manifestation.

B. Laboratory Findings: Chest radiographs may show hyperexpansion, atelectasis, or scattered infiltrates. Blood gas or oximetry may reveal hypoxemia. Diagnosis can be made by viral isolation from nasopharyngeal secretions or rapid antigen detection (ELISA, immunofluorescence).

Complications

RSV infections in young infants may produce severe apnea or progressive pulmonary infection. Children at particular risk include premature babies, infants with congenital heart disease or chronic pulmonary disease (including bronchopulmonary dysplasia), and immunodeficient patients.

Treatment

Most infants with RSV require only supportive care. Oxygen is used for hypoxemia; mechanical ventilation may be required for significant apnea or pulmonary involvement. Ribavirin is an antiviral agent that may be delivered via aerosol to infants with RSV disease; it is generally reserved for patients with severe disease or those in high-risk groups. Studies of new methods of passive and active immunization hold promise. RSVIVIG may be beneficial in preventing RSV disease in infants with chronic lung disease.

Prognosis

The prognosis varies with the degree of illness and the presence of underlying risk factors. The majority of patients recover fully, although some may exhibit reactive airway diseases in later childhood.

PARAINFLUENZA VIRUS

Parainfluenza viruses are RNA viruses with four subtypes that frequently cause pediatric respiratory infections. They are the most frequent cause of croup. Transmitted by direct personal contact and by nasopharyngeal secretions, they have an incubation period of 2–6 days.

Clinical Findings

A. Symptoms & Signs: Parainfluenza viruses may cause croup, upper respiratory tract infections and lower respiratory tract disease.

1. Croup–Parainfluenza virus 1 is responsible for most croup in autumn; parainfluenza 2 is sometimes implicated. Parainfluenza 3 tends to predominate in spring and summer. Affected toddlers and young children develop stridor, barking cough, and respiratory distress, usually with upper respiratory symptoms and low-grade fever.

2. Lower Respiratory Infections–Parainfluenza viruses may cause pneumonia and bronchiolitis in infants and young children. Severe persistent infection can occur in immunocompromised children.

B. Laboratory Findings: Diagnosis may be made by viral isolation from or detection of viral antigen in respiratory secretions. Less commonly, the diagnosis is made by acute and convalescent serologic evaluation.

Treatment

Treatment is generally supportive, including mist, oxygen, and a non-invasive environment (particularly for croup). Patients with croup often have clinical improvement with aerosolized epinephrine (short-lived) and with dexamethasone. Severe croup or lower respiratory disease occasionally requires intubation and mechanical ventilation. Ribavirin aerosol has been used for some immunodeficient patients with progressive or chronic pneumonia.

Prognosis

The prognosis is good for those with mild to moderate illness. Patients with severe disease and immunocompromised persons may have long-term morbidity.

ADENOVIRUSES

Adenoviruses consist of 47 serotypes that are responsible for a wide range of respiratory and gastrointestinal illnesses. Adenovirus-associated respiratory illness peaks in the winter and spring, and institutional epidemics (particularly among military recruits) may occur at those times. Adenoviruses are spread via respiratory contact and fecal-oral contamination; the incubation period is 2–14 days.

Clinical Findings

A. Symptoms & Signs: Respiratory manifestations include nonspecific upper respiratory infection, conjunctivitis, keratoconjunctivitis, pharyngitis, pharyngoconjunctival fever, croup, pertussis-like illness, bronchiolitis, and pneumonia. Adenovirus infections may occasionally be associated with meningoencephalitis. Other illnesses caused by adenoviruses include gastroenteritis and hemorrhagic cystitis.

B. Laboratory Findings: Respiratory adenoviruses may be isolated from cultures of conjunctivae, pharynx, or stool. Enteric adenoviruses are more easily detected by electron microscopy of stool or by antigen detection. Diagnosis of recent infection may also be made serologically.

Treatment

Treatment is supportive, including oxygen and mechanical ventilation as needed for pneumonia and fluid therapy for gastroenteritis.

Prophylaxis

Live adenovirus vaccines against several serotypes are available for military personnel.

Prognosis

Prognosis is generally good, although severe pneumonia may cause significant morbidity or mortality in immunocompromised patients and neonates.

HANTAVIRUSES

Hantaviruses, classified as Bunyaviruses, cause hemorrhagic fever with renal syndrome (Korean hemorrhagic fever and nephropathia epidemica, caused by Hantaan virus and Puumala virus respectively); and hantavirus pulmonary syndrome (Muerte Canyon virus and other strains). The hemorrhagic fever syndromes have been described primarily in Asia and Europe, while the pulmonary syndrome, first described in 1993, has been observed in North America. Hantavirus pulmonary syndrome has been observed in adolescents and adults, but not young children. The causative agents infect rodents and small mammals; humans acquire the viruses by contact (especially via aerosol inhalation) with infected secretions and excreta.

Clinical Findings

A. Symptoms & Signs: Hantavirus pulmonary syndrome is characterized by fever and flu-like illness, progressing to noncardiogenic pulmonary edema, respiratory failure, and shock.

B. Laboratory Findings: Suggestive findings include hemoconcentration, hypoalbuminemia, thrombocytopenia, leukocytosis, hypoxemia, and pulmonary edema. Confirmatory diagnosis can be made by detection of IgM antibody, or by detection of virus in tissue by polymerase chain reaction or immunohistochemistry.

Treatment

Intensive care, including respiratory and fluid management, is necessary for hantavirus pulmonary syndrome. The efficacy of ribavirin is under investigation.

Prophylaxis

Prophylactic measures are primarily environmental. Elimination of rodent reservoirs and reduction of direct contact with rodents and their excreta is advised.

Prognosis

Significant mortality has been described with hantavirus pulmonary syndrome, but patients who recover appear to be free of residua.

ROTAVIRUS

Rotaviruses are RNA viruses associated with diarrheal illness. They are the most frequent cause of gastroenteritis worldwide.

Clinical Findings

A. Symptoms & Signs: Vomiting, watery diarrhea, and mild fever are frequent. Cough and rhinorrhea may also be present. Severe infection, particularly in infants, may induce dehydration and acidosis.

B. Laboratory Findings: Serum electrolytes may reflect dehydration or acidosis. Diagnosis may be made by detection of viral antigens in stool via ELISA or latex agglutination, or by visualization of virus in stool with electron microscopy.

Treatment

A. Specific Measures: None available. Oral immune globulin may be helpful for prolonged infection in immunocompromised patients.

B. General Measures: Fluid therapy, oral or parenteral, is essential to prevent and treat dehydration.

Prophylaxis

Thorough hand washing and good hygiene are the major preventive measures. Live attenuated oral vaccines are being developed.

Prognosis

Prognosis is good if hydration is maintained. Some patients with severe diarrhea may suffer from malabsorption for a period after the acute enteritis subsides. Death is usually caused by severe dehydration or electrolyte imbalance.

Infectious Diseases: Bacterial, Parasitic, & Fungal | 11

Mark J. Abzug, MD

BACTERIAL DISEASES

STREPTOCOCCAL DISEASES

Various disease states directly or indirectly ascribed to streptococci are very important in pediatric populations. These illnesses are spread by respiratory secretions.

Etiology

Streptococci are gram-positive and characteristically appear in chains. They may be classified as follows:

A. β-Hemolytic Streptococci: Groups A, B, and D are the principal pathogens. Group A infections most commonly occur in children and adults; group B may cause severe disease in infants, pregnant women, and the elderly.

B. Non–β-Hemolytic Streptococci: These commonly exhibit alpha hemolysis or no hemolysis on blood agar culture. Viridans streptococci and some group D streptococci are included in this category.

C. Peptostreptococci: These are anaerobic, produce variable hemolysis, are found in the pharynx and intestinal tract, and are sometimes pathogenic.

Clinical Findings

A. Symptoms & Signs: Streptococci produce a variety of clinical diseases. Certain entities show a definite concentration in specific age groups.

1. Infection in Neonates–Neonatal infections are principally caused by group B streptococci, especially type III. There are two clinical syndromes—early onset and late onset. In the **early onset syndrome** (in infants younger than 7 days of age), infection is acquired from the maternal vagina. Early onset disease frequently includes apnea, shock, pneumonia, sepsis, and meningitis. Mortality is high. The **late-onset syndrome** affects infants between 1 week and 4 months of age and may result from person-to-person transmission. Meningitis, cellulitis, bacteremia, septic arthritis, and osteomyelitis are common manifestations.

2. Infection in Young Children (< 3 Years Old)–Group A streptococcal infection is insidious with mild constitutional symptoms, mucopurulent nasal discharge, and suppurative complications (otitis media, lymphadenitis). Exudative tonsillitis is uncommon, and sore throat is apparently absent. Rheumatic fever, nephritis, and scarlet fever rarely occur in association with this form of the disease.

3. Infection in Older Children–The onset of Group A streptococcal infection is usually sudden, with temperature over 39 °C (102.2 °F). The throat is moderately sore and beefy red, with edema of anterior pillars and palatal petechiae. Exudative tonsillitis, with a white-yellow membrane, is relatively frequent. Anterior cervical lymph nodes are large and tender. Scarlet fever consists of streptococcal pharyngitis plus a rash due to host susceptibility to erythrogenic toxin. The rash appears 12–48 hours after onset of fever; it begins in areas of warmth and pressure, spreads rapidly to involve the entire body below the chin, and reaches its maximum in 1–2 days (Table 10–1). It is characterized by a diffuse erythema of the skin, with sandpaper-like texture. The rash fades on pressure and does not involve the circumoral region. Transverse lines that do *not* fade on pressure are found at the elbow (Pastia's sign). The exanthem is usually followed by desquamation beginning in the second week with peeling of the fingertips. The tongue may be coated but then desquamates and becomes beefy red.

4. Skin Infection–In streptococcal disease of the skin, streptococci may enter the skin and subcutaneous tissues through abrasions or wounds and may produce impetigo; erysipelas, a superficially spreading infection with edema and erythema; or cellulitis. Wound infection with streptococci may result in "surgical scarlet fever" when the organism produces erythrogenic toxin in a patient lacking antibody to toxin.

B. Laboratory Findings: The white blood cell count (WBC) is usually elevated in patients with uncomplicated group A streptococcal upper respiratory tract infection (URI); it may go to 20,000/μL or higher in patients with suppurative complications. An anti-group A streptococcal antibody screen (Streptozyme) will usually become positive; antistreptolysin titers will rise above 150 U in the course of

Group A streptococcal infection. A documented rise (or fall) in titer is a more reliable measure of recent streptococcal infection. Throat culture is generally positive for group A streptococci and is the diagnostic method of choice. Positive rapid antigen tests correlate well with culture results. Negative test results should be confirmed by culture, since rapid tests may fail to detect small numbers of streptococci.

Neonatal group B streptococcal infection may be identified by positive culture of blood, cerebrospinal fluid, or other involved body site or by positive latex agglutination of serum or cerebrospinal fluid (CSF) for group B streptococcal antigen.

Complications

A wide variety of clinical conditions may result from the presence of streptococci in the patient's upper respiratory tract, skin, or blood.

A. Otitis Media: (Chapter 13)

B. Adenitis: Usually cervical.

C. Septicemia: Most common in compromised hosts or the very young. A toxic-shock-like syndrome with shock and multiorgan dysfunction may also occur.

D. Pneumonia: Pneumonia may be severe and is frequently complicated by empyema.

E. "Metastatic Foci:" These include meningitis, septic arthritis, osteomyelitis, and omphalitis (neonates).

F. Vaginitis & Perianal Cellulitis

G. Nonsuppurative Complications: These include rheumatic fever (Chapter 16) and acute glomerulonephritis (Chapter 18).

Treatment

A. Specific Measures:

1. Group B Streptococcal Infections–Parenteral penicillin or ampicillin is the therapy of choice. Combination therapy with an aminoglycoside is recommended until clinical stabilization and improvement have been observed. Treatment is ordinarily administered for 10–14 days (14–21 days for meningitis).

2. Group A Streptococcal Infections–Oral penicillin V for 10 days or intramuscular benzathine penicillin are recommended for uncomplicated group A streptococcal infections. Alternatives for penicillin-allergic patients include erythromycin, cephalosporins, and clindamycin. Some clinicians also recommend these antibiotics in cases of failure of penicillin therapy. Severe infections should be treated with parenteral antibiotics. Prompt therapy for group A streptococcal infections will prevent acute rheumatic fever in most cases. Resistance of group A streptococcus to erythromycin does occur, but resistance to penicillin has not been documented.

3. Group A Streptococcal Carriers–These do not usually require antibiotic therapy unless there is a personal or family history of acute rheumatic fever. However, illnesses accompanied by a positive throat culture require a course of antibiotic treatment.

Prophylaxis

Antibiotic prophylaxis against group A streptococcal infection with penicillin or sulfisoxazole is indicated to prevent recurrent disease in persons with a history of rheumatic fever.

For group B streptococcal infections the following are recommended:

1. Prepartum vaginal and anal cultures to identify group B streptococcal carriage.
2. Intrapartum treatment (with ampicillin or penicillin G) of carriers with risk factors (eg, preterm labor, fever, multiple births, premature or prolonged rupture of membranes, and previous infant with group B streptococcal infection).

Prognosis

The prognosis for the patient with uncomplicated group A streptococcal infection is excellent when penicillin is given. Uncomplicated cases of older childhood-type infection subside in 4–5 days with or without specific treatment, but treatment is recommended for all children to prevent nonsuppurative complications. Cases of group A streptococcal sepsis, visceral infection, or toxic-shock-like illness may have considerable morbidity; some prove fatal. The prognosis for neonates with group B streptococcal infection varies with the severity of infection. The prognosis for patients with severe sepsis, pneumonia, or meningitis is guarded.

PNEUMOCOCCAL DISEASES

Streptococcus pneumoniae is a gram-positive diplococcus with 84 serotypes based on specific capsular polysaccharides. Types 6, 14, 18, 19, and 23 are more likely to cause disease in children than in adults. The disease is spread by respiratory droplets.

Clinical Findings

A. Symptoms & Signs:

1. Otitis Media & Sinusitis: (Chapter 13)

2. Bacteremia–*S pneumoniae* is the most frequent cause of bacteremia in children over 1 month of age. Fever without localizing signs may be the only presenting finding of occult pneumococcal bacteremia.

3. Pneumonia–Pneumonia is usually peribronchial in the child under 6 years of age. Typical lobar pneumonia occurs more commonly in older children.

4. Meningitis

5. Peritonitis–Most likely to occur in patients with chronic glomerulonephritis and nephrosis.

B. Laboratory Findings: Leukocytosis is the rule in pneumococcal infection. Blood cultures should be done when pneumonia, meningitis, or peritonitis is suspected; Gram's stain and culture of material from the infection site should be obtained when possible. Rapid tests such as latex agglutination may also be helpful, but keep in mind that they tend to be insensitive.

Complications

Localized pneumococcal infection may result from bacteremia or respiratory spread; infected sites may include joints, pericardium, pleural space, and bone.

Treatment

Penicillin is the drug of choice for susceptible isolates. In cases of penicillin allergy, patients may be treated with oral erythromycin, trimethoprim-sulfamethoxazole, clindamycin, or cephalexin. Severe infections should be treated parenterally. Resistance of *S pneumoniae* to penicillin and cephalosporins is increasing. Antibiotic susceptibility testing should be performed on all isolates from normally sterile sites. Treatment for resistant isolates (especially if *full* resistance is observed) should be undertaken with vancomycin; a third-generation cephalosporin (eg, cefotaxime or ceftriaxone); rifampin; or chloramphenicol.

Prophylaxis

Polyvalent polysaccharide vaccine is available and contains antigens of 23 different types of pneumococci, which account for more than 90% of strains producing bacteremic disease in adults and children. Experience in the pediatric population is limited; however, the vaccine is ineffective in children younger than 2 years of age. It is recommended for children older than 2 years in the following high-risk categories: children with functional (sickle cell disease), congenital, or surgical asplenia; nephrotic syndrome or chronic renal failure; cerebrospinal leaks; antibody-deficient states (response is not ensured in this group, but some children may respond); acquired immune deficiency states; and human immunodeficiency virus (HIV) infection. Revaccination after 3–5 years should be considered for children in high-risk groups. Development of protein-conjugated pneumococcal polysaccharide vaccines is in progress.

Antibiotic prophylaxis is recommended by many practitioners to prevent pneumococcal infections in patients with anatomic or functional asplenia (including sickle cell disease). Parents and patients should be advised that vaccine and antibiotics may not prevent all infections and that they should report for medical care immediately if there is any febrile illness. Physicians seeing such children should treat them for potential bacteremia.

STAPHYLOCOCCAL DISEASES

Staphylococci are gram-positive organisms. *S aureus,* which is coagulase-producing, is the most common pathogen. Coagulase-negative staphylococci, including *S epidermidis,* occasionally also cause invasive disease, particularly in compromised hosts and in patients with indwelling foreign bodies (eg, catheters).

Staphylococci are common in the environment and are normally found in humans in the nose and on the skin.

Clinical Findings

A. Symptoms & Signs:

1. *Staphylocccus aureus*–

a. Superficial Infection–Pyoderma/impetigo is the most common type of infection with this organism. Furuncles are discussed in Chapter 13; folliculitis and carbuncles are discussed in Chapter 12.

b. Deep Infection–Osteomyelitis or septic arthritis can occur following bloodstream spread from a local inoculation or a superficial infection. Pneumonia may occur, especially after a viral infection (eg, influenza); it tends to be severe and is usually associated with an empyema. Septicemia, with focal abscesses in the chest, abdomen, and brain, may occur.

c. Toxin Disease–Food poisoning (Table 11–1) may result from production of enterotoxin in contaminated foods, usually gravies or custards. Onset is abrupt, with vomiting, prostration, and diarrhea within 4 hours of ingestion. Staphylococcal scalded skin syndrome is an exfoliative skin disease caused by an exotoxin that occurs in infants colonized by *S aureus*. Toxic shock syndrome, also caused by an exotoxin, may result from staphylococcal infection in surgical wounds, in the vagina during menstruation and with the use of tampons, in localized abscesses, and in fulminant staphylococcal sepsis. Onset is sudden with fever, vomiting, diarrhea, and hypotension, followed by a generalized desquamating erythroderma.

2. Coagulase-Negative Staphylococci–

a. Bacteremia–Bacteremia with coagulase-negative staphylococci occurs in immunocompromised patients, including premature infants and immunosuppressed patients. Bacteremia with these organisms frequently occurs as a consequence of indwelling vascular catheters.

b. Other Foreign Body Infections–Coagulase-negative staphylococci are frequently the causative organisms of infections affecting ventriculoperitoneal shunts, peritoneal dialysis catheters, and other indwelling foreign bodies.

c. Urinary Tract Infections–*S saprophyticus* is a cause of urinary tract infections (UTIs), mostly in adolescents and adults.

B. Laboratory Findings: Leukocytosis occurs in patients with deep infection. Culture of the blood yields positive results in many cases of deep infection. Gram's stain and culture of pus from sites of local infection easily demonstrate the organism's sites.

Treatment

Most *S aureus* are resistant to penicillin and require treatment with penicillinase-resistant penicillins (eg, nafcillin or oxacillin). Alternative agents include first-generation cephalosporins, clindamycin, or vancomycin. Vancomycin is the drug of choice for methicillin-resistant *S aureus* (infrequent) and methicillin-resistant coagulase-negative staphylococci (frequent). Deep infections may require several weeks of antibiotic therapy. Abscesses generally need to be drained; foreign bodies may need to be removed. Treatment of staphylococcal toxic shock syndrome includes fluids and other supportive care, antibiotics, removal of foreign bodies (eg, tampons), and drainage of infected foci.

Table 11–1. Gastrointestinal bacterial & protozoal pathogens.

Organism	Organism Description	Epidemiology	Disease Manifestations	Laboratory Findings	Treatment	Prophylaxis
Campylobacter jejuni fetus	Comma-shaped, gram-negative rods	Fecal-oral transmission; acquisition from infected poultry, pets, farm animals, contaminated foods	*C jejuni:* Gastroenteritis, colitis, reactive arthritis, seizures, abdominal pain, Guillain-Barré syndrome *C fetus:* neonatal sepsis; sepsis in compromised hosts	Motile rods in stool wet mount; positive culture of stool (*C jejuni*) or blood (*C fetus*)	Erythromycin and fluoroquinolones shorten duration of illness and excretion of *C jejuni*	Hygiene, proper cooking of meat and pasteurization of milk
Clostridium difficile	Anaerobic gram-negative bacillus	Found in soil, hospital environment. Transmitted fecal-orally. High rate of asymptomatic colonization in neonates and young infants. Disease frequently follows antibiotic use	Pseudomembranous colitis, antibiotic-associated diarrhea, asymptomatic colonization	Stool WBCs, blood; toxin detection (ELISA or cell culture). Plaques and pseudomembranes on endoscopy	Discontinue antibiotics. Oral vancomycin, oral or IV metronidazole, or oral bacitracin	Hygiene; limit antibiotic use
Cryptosporidium parvum	Coccidian protozoan	Fecal-oral transmission and acquisition via contaminated water	Watery diarrhea, abdominal pain, anorexia. Chronic in immunocompromised; occasional dissemination in immunocompromised	Oocytes in stool or intestinal biopsy	Hydration and nourishment in normal hosts; treatment regimens in immunocompromised under investigation	Hygiene and sanitation

Entamoeba histolytica	Protozoan transmitted as cysts which produce invasive trophozoites	Fecal-oral transmission and acquisition from contaminated food or drink	Gastroenteritis, dysentery, abdominal pain, liver abscess, metastatic abscesses	Trophozoites or cysts in stool or rectal biopsy; serology for invasive disease	Asymptomatic: luminal amebicide (iodoquinol, diloxanide furoate, paromomycin); Mild-severe colitis or extraintestinal disease: tissue amebicide (metronidazole) and luminal amebicide	Hygiene, sanitation
Escherichia coli enteropathogenic (EPEC) enterotoxigenic (ETEC) enteroinvasive (EIEC) enterohemorrhagic (EHEC; 0157:H7)	Gram-negative bacillus	Fecal-oral transmission and acquisition from contaminated food, milk, or water	EPEC: diarrhea, dehydration, failure to thrive ETEC: diarrhea including traveler's diarrhea EIEC: dysentery EHEC: diarrhea, hemorrhagic colitis, hemolytic-uremic syndrome	Positive stool culture with serotyping or in vitro analysis. Lack of sorbitol fermentation to screen for EHEC strains	Hydration; EPEC: nonabsorbable antibiotic, trimethoprim-sulfamethoxazole, ampicillin ETEC: trimethoprim-sulfamethoxazole, ciprofloxacin, doxycycline EIEC: ampicillin, trimethoprim-sulfamethoxazole EHEC: role of antibiotic treatment unclear	Hygiene; food and water precautions during foreign travel and empiric antibiotic treatment for traveler's diarrhea
Giardia lamblia	Flagellated protozoan, transmitted as cysts	Fecal-oral transmission and acquisition via contaminated water	Chronic diarrhea, cramping, flatulence, steatorrhea, failure to thrive, malabsorption	Trophozoites or cysts in stool, duodenal aspiration, or biopsy	Furazolidone, metronidazole, quinacrine, paromomycin. Rehydration and nutritional support	Hygiene and sanitation; boil water from streams; filter municipal water

(*continued*)

Table 11–1. Gastrointestinal bacterial & protozoal pathogens (*continued*).

Organism	Organism Description	Epidemiology	Disease Manifestations	Laboratory Findings	Treatment	Prophylaxis
Helicobacter pylori	Gram-negative spiral bacillus	Fecal-oral transmission? Increasing acquisition with age	Asymptomatic chronic gastritis, duodenal and gastric ulceration, increased risk of gastric adenocarcinoma or lymphoma	Histologic staining, culture, urease production, urea breath test, serology	Combination therapy including amoxicillin, tetracycline, metronidazole, and/or bismuth	Disinfection of endoscopes
Salmonella choleraesuis enteritidis typhi	Gram-negative bacillus	Fecal-oral transmission and acquisition from contaminated foods, poultry, eggs, and pet turtles	Gastroenteritis, bacteremia, localized infections (osteomyelitis, meningitis, pneumonia, peritonitis, enteric fever). Complications: dehydration, hemorrhage, perforation	Leukopenia (enteric fever); leukocytosis (gastroenteritis). Stool WBCs; positive cultures from stool, blood, bone marrow, involved site	Ampicillin, amoxicillin, chloramphenicol, trimethoprim-sulfamethoxazole, ceftriaxone, cefotaxime, fluoroquinolones (depending on susceptibilities) for enteric fever, bacteremia, invasive disease, or gastroenteritis in patients at high risk for invasive disease (< 3 months of age, immunocompromised, hemoglobinopathy, severe colitis). Antibiotic	Sanitation. Typhoid vaccine for travelers to endemic regions

					treatment may promote prolonged carriage and is not used for uncomplicated illness. Corticosteroids for severe enteric fever	
Shigella boydii dysenteriae flexneri sonnei	Gram-negative bacillus	Fecal-oral trans mission and acquisition from contaminated water and foods. Flies may serve as vectors	Gastroenteritis, bacillary dysentery, encephalopathy. Complications: dehydration, seizures, hemolytic uremic syndrome, Reiter's syndrome	Leukocytosis; stool WBCs; positive culture from stool, rarely blood	Trimethoprim-sulfamethoxazole, ampicillin, tetracycline, chloramphenicol, ceftriaxone, cefotaxime, fluoroquinolones (depending on susceptibilities); hydration	Sanitation and hygiene
Vibrio cholerae	Gram-negative, curved, flagellated rod	Transmission via contaminated food, water, or shellfish	Profuse watery diarrhea, vomiting, shock	Darkfield microscopy of stools; positive culture of stool; positive serology	Tetracycline, doxycycline, trimethoprim-sulfamethoxazole, furazolidone, erythromycin, fluoroqunolones. Rehydration	Hygiene and adequate cooking of foods and boiling of water; antibiotic treatment for contacts; vaccine has limited efficacy

(*continued*)

Table 11–1. Gastrointestinal bacterial & protozoal pathogens (*continued*).

Organism	Organism Description	Epidemiology	Disease Manifestations	Laboratory Findings	Treatment	Prophylaxis
Yersinia enterocolitica	Gram-negative bacillus	Acquired from contaminated food (swine), milk, or water; animal contact; transfusion; fecal-oral transmission. Associated with cooler climates; increased incidence in winter. Bacteremia associated with iron storage syndromes	Enterocolitis, pseudoappendicitis, abscesses, bacteremia, disseminated infection; post-infectious reactive arthritis, erythema nodosum	Stool WBCs, blood; cold enrichment culture	Aminoglycosides, cefotaxime, trimethoprim-sulfamethoxazole, tetracycline	Avoid ingestion of uncooked meat, unpasteurized milk, and contaminated water

ELISA = enzyme-linked immunosorbent assay; WBC = white blood cell count.

Prophylaxis

For prophylaxis of recurrent furunculosis, see Chapter 13. Prevent food poisoning by adequate refrigeration and sanitation. Cleanliness and antiseptic measures can control excessive spread from draining lesions. Hand washing is always an important control measure.

Prognosis

In the typical case of superficial infection with adequate treatment, the prognosis is excellent. In deep infections with sepsis, pneumonia, brain abscess, or other localization, the prognosis is guarded. Patients with osteomyelitis have an excellent prognosis if they are treated promptly.

HAEMOPHILUS INFLUENZAE B DISEASES

Haemophilus influenzae B used to be the cause of most cases of bacterial meningitis in pediatrics. The organism is an encapsulated gram-negative pleomorphic rod. It usually infects infants and children younger than 6 years of age. Its incidence has decreased as a result of immunization.

Clinical Findings

A. Symptoms & Signs: ***H influenzae B*** causes a wide spectrum of disease, including meningitis, pneumonia, empyema, bacteremia, epiglottitis, cellulitis (buccal, periorbital, or other), septic arthritis, osteomyelitis, pericarditis, and uvulitis. More than one of these processes may coexist. Patients usually present with fever and irritability and then go on to have specific localizing findings depending on the site of infection.

B. Laboratory Findings: Leukocytosis with a shift to the left is frequently present. A Gram's stain of fluid obtained from the infection site is frequently positive; latex agglutination of such fluid or urine is frequently positive. The organism can be cultured on chocolate agar from blood or from fluid or swabs obtained from the site of localization.

Treatment

A. Specific Measures: Useful parenteral antibiotics for *H influenzae B* include ampicillin, cefotaxime, ceftriaxone, cefuroxime, and chloramphenicol. Antibiotic susceptibility testing will guide the choice; ampicillin resistance is common (up to 40%), and chloramphenicol resistance is occasional. Parenteral therapy is usually administered initially; oral agents may be used to complete a course of therapy for nonmeningitic disease after improvement with parenteral therapy.

B. General Measures: Intensive support may be needed for severely ill patients, including those with meningitis, sepsis, pneumonia, pericarditis, and epiglottitis. Patients with epiglottitis require emergent tracheal intubation to assure an adequate airway. Patients with pericarditis, empyema, and arthritis usually benefit from aspiration or drainage of infected fluid.

Prophylaxis

Rifampin (20 mg/kg/d qd for 4 days; adult dose (600 mg/d) is recommended for children who develop *H influenzae B* disease and for their household contacts. In addition, many experts recommend similar prophylaxis of day care and nursery school contacts of index patients, particularly if there are incompletely vaccinated or unvaccinated attendees younger than 2 years of age. (Prophylaxis is indicated for children both vaccinated and unvaccinated against *H influenzae B*.) Children exposed to *H influenzae B* in whom a febrile illness develops should receive medical attention.

Immunization against *H influenzae B* disease is currently recommended for children, beginning in infancy with a vaccine that conjugates *H influenzae B* capsular polysaccharide to a protein carrier. All children younger than 60 months should receive the vaccine series; children older than 60 months who are in high-risk groups (eg, those with asplenia, sickle cell disease, or malignancy) should receive a conjugate vaccine. Children who have had invasive *H influenzae B* disease prior to the age of 24 months should be vaccinated with a conjugate vaccine; those with invasive disease after 24 months do not require vaccination.

Prognosis

Patients with mild to moderate disease who receive prompt therapy usually have a good prognosis. Patients with severe infections, including sepsis, pericarditis, meningitis, and epiglottitis, have a more guarded outcome, particularly if there is a delay in therapy.

MENINGOCOCCAL DISEASES

Neisseria meningitidis is a gram-negative diplococcus that is a common pathogen in children as well as adults.

Clinical Findings

A. Symptoms & Signs: Septicemia, or meningococcemia, presents with fever, irritability, lethargy, and often a maculopapular or petechial rash. In severe cases, hypotension, disseminated intravascular coagulation (DIC), and coma may occur (Waterhouse-Friderichsen syndrome). Meningococcal meningitis may also occur with or without the signs of meningococcemia. Other meningococcal infections include bacteremia, pericarditis, arthritis, and pneumonia, alone or in combination. Chronic meningococcemia is a form of bacteremia that persists for more than 1 week and is associated with fever, rash, and arthralgia.

B. Laboratory Findings: Leukocytosis with a left shift is common; thrombocytopenia is present in severe meningococcemia.

The diagnosis may be made by Gram's stain and culture of blood, CSF, joint fluid, or petechial aspirate. Latex agglutination of urine, serum, or CSF may be positive, although sensitivity is lacking.

Treatment

A. Specific Measures: The antibiotic of choice is penicillin G or ampicillin (except when resistance is reported). Alternatives include chloramphenicol, cefotaxime, and ceftriaxone.

B. General Measures: Intensive supportive care may be required for patients with meningococcemia or meningitis, particularly if shock and coagulopathy are present.

Prophylaxis

Prophylaxis is recommended for contacts of a patient with meningococcal disease (eg, household, day care, and nursery persons) as well as any others who have had contact with the index patient's oral secretions. Medical personnel involved with resuscitation or airway care should receive prophylaxis. The drug of choice for prophylaxis is rifampin (10 mg/kg q12h for 2 days; adult dose 600 mg q12h); sulfisoxazole, ceftriaxone, and ciprofloxacin are alternative choices. Contacts in whom a febrile illness develops should receive medical attention.

Meningococcal vaccine is a quadrivalent polysaccharide vaccine. It is recommended for children 2 years of age and older in high-risk groups for meningococcal disease (eg, asplenic children or those with a deficiency of terminal complement). The vaccine should also be given to persons traveling to regions with hyperendemic or epidemic disease and to aid in interrupting outbreaks.

Prognosis

Patients with isolated focal disease who receive prompt therapy have a good prognosis. Patients with overwhelming meningococcemia have a guarded prognosis; features suggestive of a poor prognosis include hypotension, leukopenia, purpura, and absence of meningitis.

PERTUSSIS
(Whooping Cough)

Bordetella pertussis is a gram-negative bacillus. Transmission occurs by droplets during the catarrhal and paroxysmal stages of whooping cough. Pertussis is communicable from 1 week before to 3 weeks after onset of paroxysms. The incubation period is 7–10 days. A pertussis-like syndrome may be caused by *B parapertussis, Chlamydia trachomatis,* or several other respiratory tract viruses.

Clinical Findings

A. Symptoms & Signs: Insidious onset of symptoms of a mild URI occurs, with rhinitis, sneezing, lacrimation, slight fever, and irritating cough (catarrhal stage). Within 2 weeks, the cough becomes paroxysmal; a repeated series of many coughs during one expiration is followed by a sudden deep inspiration with a characteristic crowing sound, or "whoop." Eating often precipitates paroxysms, which may then cause vomiting. Tenacious mucus may also be coughed and vomited. The paroxysmal stage lasts 2–6 weeks, but a habit of coughing may continue for many weeks (convalescent stage). Typical paroxysms and "whoops" may not be present in young infants or older children and adults.

B. Laboratory Findings: The WBC may be very high, with predominant lymphocytosis. Cultures are best obtained by nasopharyngeal swab or washings. Results are generally positive during the catarrhal stage and the first week or two of the paroxysmal stage. The fluorescent antibody test performed on nasal secretions may give a rapid diagnosis but has variable sensitivity and specificity.

Complications

Pneumonia accounts for most of the deaths caused by pertussis. Atelectasis, emphysema, and bronchiectasis are other pulmonary complications. Neurologic complications include seizures, apnea, and encephalopathy.

Treatment

A. Specific Measures: Erythromycin will quickly eradicate organisms and reduce the possibility of transmission. It will *not* influence the course of the clinical disease unless begun during the catarrhal stage. Corticosteroids and albuterol may be beneficial in reducing coughing paroxysms.

B. General Measures:

1. Respiration–Because of anoxic periods during paroxysms, infants may require constant attendance and such measures as insertion of an airway, mechanical ventilation, and suctioning of the oropharynx. Oxygen should be administered to infants who have significant desaturation during paroxysms. Bacterial superinfections of the respiratory tract require specific antimicrobial treatment.

2. Parenteral Fluids–Severe paroxysms may prevent adequate intake of fluids and necessitate parenteral therapy.

3. Feedings–Frequent small feedings are less likely to cause vomiting. Thick feedings are often retained better than more fluid ones. If post-tussive vomiting occurs during or immediately after a feeding, the child should be fed again. Paroxysms are less likely to occur at this time.

Prophylaxis

For recommendations concerning active immunization in early infancy, consult Table 6–3. Exposed household, day care, and other close contacts of a pertussis patient should receive a 14–day course of erythromycin.

Prognosis

Disease in infants younger than 1 year of age may be severe and is sometimes accompanied by a poor prognosis (especially if complications have occurred). The prognosis is good in patients older than 1 year and in those with uncomplicated infection.

DIPHTHERIA

Diphtheria is an acute febrile infection, usually of the throat, and is most common during the winter in temperate zones. With active immunization in early childhood, the disease is now rare in the United States.

Diphtheria is caused by a gram-positive, pleomorphic rod, *Corynebacterium diphtheriae.* The disease is transmitted by droplets from the respiratory tracts of carriers or patients. The incubation period is 1–7 days (average, 3 days).

Clinical Findings

A. Symptoms and Signs:

1. Pharyngeal–Findings include mild sore throat, moderate fever to 38.5 °C (101.2–102.2 °F), rapid pulse, severe prostration, and exudate. A membrane forms in the throat and spreads from the tonsils to the anterior pillars and uvula. It is typically dirty gray or gray–green when fully developed but may be white early in the course. The edges of the membrane are slightly elevated; bleeding results if it is scraped off. (This procedure is contraindicated as it hastens absorption of toxin.)

2. Nasal–Nasal discharge is a potent source of spread of infection to others, and serosanguineous nasal discharge may excoriate the patient's upper lip. A membrane may be visible on turbinates; constitutional manifestations are slight.

3. Laryngeal–*Findings of laryngeal involvement are the most serious* and include hoarseness or aphonia, croupy cough, fever up to 39.5–40.0 °C (103–104 °F), marked prostration, cyanosis, difficulty in breathing, and, eventually, respiratory obstruction. Brawny edema of the neck may occur, and membrane formation may be visible in the pharynx.

4. Cutaneous, Vaginal, & Wound–Findings include ulcerative lesions with membrane formation. The lesions are persistent and often anesthetic.

B. Laboratory Findings: The WBC is normal, or there may be a slight leukocytosis. A smear of exudate stained with methylene blue shows rods with midpolar bars. Cultures on Loëffler's medium yield positive results.

Complications

A. Myocarditis: Myocarditis is a direct result of toxin. Clinical diagnosis is discussed in Chapter 16. Electrocardiography shows T-wave changes and partial or complete atrioventricular block.

B. Neuritis: Neuritis is usually a late development. Both sensory loss and motor paralyses develop rapidly once neuritis becomes apparent. Complete recovery is usual.

1. Pharyngeal & Palatal Muscles–These are the earliest muscles to become involved. Manifestations include nasal voice, dysphagia, and nasal regurgitation of fluids. Vocal cord paralysis may occur.

2. Extrinsic Eye Muscles–Diplopia and strabismus are manifestations.

3. Skeletal Muscles–Involvement of the legs and arms may end in quadriplegia.

C. Bronchopneumonia

D. Proteinuria: Proteinuria usually clears as the temperature returns to normal, but nephritis may occur.

E. Thrombocytopenia

Treatment

A. Specific Measures: The following measures apply to the treatment of all types of diphtheria.

1. Antitoxin–Diphtheria antitoxin in sufficient dosage *must be given promptly*. The longer the time between onset of disease and administration of antitoxin, the higher the mortality. Give antitoxin if disease is considered possible from clinical manifestations; do *not* wait for culture results. The dosage is 20,000–100,000 U for patients of any age, depending on the site, severity, and duration of the disease. *Always* test for horse serum sensitivity before administration (Chapter 6); the preferred route is intravenous.

2. Antibiotics–Erythromycin (best) or penicillin G for 14 days should be used in treatment and to shorten the carrier state.

3. Toxoid–Diphtheria may not confer immunity. Patients recovered from diphtheria should receive a full primary course of immunization (Chapter 6).

B. General Measures: Parenteral fluids and monitoring of the patient's airway are important elements of supportive care. Special measures for the treatment of patients with laryngeal diphtheria include avoidance of sedation, suction of the larynx as necessary, tracheal intubation or tracheostomy for respiratory obstruction, and humidity.

C. Treatment of Complications:

1. Myocarditis–Treat with oxygen, antiarrhythmics, and blood pressure support as indicated.

2. Neuritis–Dysphagia may necessitate the use of an indwelling nasogastric tube. Intercostal paralysis may necessitate the use of a mechanical ventilator.

Prophylaxis

Prophylactic measures include active immunization in early childhood (Table 6–3), culture of and antibiotic treatment of close contacts, and booster immunization of contacts.

Prognosis

The prognosis is always guarded, varying with the day of disease on which antitoxin treatment is given. After 6 days without treatment, mortality is almost 50%. Myocarditis within the first 10 days is an ominous sign.

TETANUS

Tetanus is an acute disease characterized by painful muscular contractions. The causative organism, *Clostridium tetani,* is an anaerobic, spore-forming, gram-positive organism that produces a very powerful neurotoxin which acts on motor nerve end-plates and anterior horn cells of the spinal cord and brain stem. Bacilli and spores are widely distributed in soil and dust and are present in the feces of animals and humans. Infection is most often acquired by contamination of a puncture wound or, in the newborn, the umbilical cord.

Clinical Findings

A. Symptoms & Signs: The incubation period varies from 3 days to 3 weeks, depending upon the size of the inoculum and the rapidity of its growth. Onset may be marked by spasm and cramplike pain in the muscles of the back and abdomen or about the site of inoculation, together with restlessness, irritability, difficulty in swallowing, and sometimes convulsions. A gradual increase in muscular tension occurs in the next 48 hours, with stiff neck, positive Kernig's sign, tightness of masseters, anxious facies, and stiffness of the arms and legs. Facial expression is modified by inability to open the mouth (trismus). Swallowing is difficult. Recurring tetanic spasms occur and last 5–10 seconds; they are characterized by agonizing pain, stiffening of the body, retraction of the head, opisthotonos, and clenching of the jaws or hands. Fever is usually low-grade but rarely may be as high as 40 °C (104 °F). Auditory or tactile stimuli may trigger convulsions. Severe spasms may occur for 1 week or longer and then gradually subside. Local tetanus, with muscle spasms limited to the area around the initial wound, may also occur.

B. Laboratory Findings: CSF shows a slight increase in pressure, with a normal cell count. Anaerobic culture of excised necrotic tissue may yield positive results; however, the diagnosis is usually made on clinical presentation.

Treatment

A. Specific Measures:

1. **Tetanus immune globulin (TIG)** is preferred in a single dose of 3000–6000 U, part delivered intramuscularly and part infiltrated locally around the wound. If human TIG is not available, give tetanus antitoxin (equine), 50,000–100,000 U intravenously, after testing for horse serum sensitivity. The value of antitoxin treatment is questionable in mild cases and when treatment is delayed for several days after the appearance of symptoms.
2. Surgical exploration of the wound, with excision of necrotic tissue and cleaning and drainage, is indicated to eliminate a local source of infection.
3. Give parenteral penicillin or tetracycline for 10–14 days.

B. General Measures:

1. Keep the patient in a quiet, dark room; minimize handling.
2. Give sedation as indicated; benzodiazepines and barbiturates are useful.
3. Gentle aspiration of secretions in the nasopharynx should be performed as required.
4. Oxygen and intravenous fluids should be given as required.
5. Airway maintenance may necessitate tracheal intubation or tracheostomy.

Prophylaxis

Active immunization with a booster every 10 years will prevent tetanus in children and adults.

Adequate debridement of wounds is one of the most important preventive measures. In addition, administration of tetanus toxoid, TIG, or both may be indicated depending on the type of wound and the patient's immunization status (Table 11–2).

Prognosis

The mortality rate in infants is 70%; in other age groups, mortality rates range from 10–60%.

BOTULISM

Classification

Three clinical syndromes caused by the neuromuscular paralytic effects of the neurotoxins produced by *Clostridium botulinum* are recognized:

Table 11–2. Guide to tetanus prophylaxis in routine wound management.[1]

History of Adsorbed Tetanus Toxoid (doses)	Clean, Minor Wounds		All Other Wounds[2]	
	Td[3]	**TIG**	**Td[3]**	**TIG**
Unknown or < 3	Yes	No	Yes	Yes
≥ 3[4]	No[5]	No	No[6]	No

DTP = diphtheria (toxoid)-tetanus (toxoid)-pertussis (vaccine); DTaP = diphtheria (toxoid)-tetanus (toxoid)-acellular pertussis (vaccine); Td = adult-type tetanus and diphtheria toxoids; TIG = tetanus immune globulin.

[1] Modified and reproduced with permission.

[2] Such as, but not limited to, wounds contaminated with dirt, feces, soil, and saliva; puncture wounds; avulsions; and wounds resulting from missiles, crushing, burns, and frostbite.

[3] For children < 7 years old; DTP or DTaP (if ≥ 3 doses of DTP have been previously given) is preferred to tetanus toxoid alone; if pertussis vaccine is contraindicated, DT is given. For persons ≥ 7 years of age, Td is preferred to tetanus toxoid alone.

[4] If only 3 doses of fluid toxoid have been received, then a fourth dose of toxoid, preferably an adsorbed toxoid, should be given.

[5] Yes, if > 10 years since last dose.

[6] Yes, if > 5 years since last dose. (More frequent boosters are not needed and can accentuate side effects.)

A. Endogenous Toxin Syndrome: Infant botulism is the result of colonization of the infant's intestinal tract with *C botulinum.* Contaminated honey and corn syrups have been implicated in some cases. Toxin is produced in the infant bowel and absorbed to produce symptoms.

B. Exogenous Toxin Syndrome: Poisoning from food contaminated by botulinum toxin may occur if the food has been improperly processed or canned.

C. Wound Infection: Botulism may result from growth of *C botulinum* and toxin production in a colonized wound.

Clinical Findings

A. Symptoms & Signs:

1. Endogenous Toxin Syndrome–Onset of infant botulism occurs within the first 6 months of life. Manifestations include apathy, weakness, constipation, floppiness, sudden apnea, and ocular palsies.

2. Exogenous Toxin Syndrome–Sudden onset of food poisoning occurs 12–36 hours after ingestion of contaminated food. Double vision, nystagmus, dry mouth, and dysphagia may occur. There may be progressive descending motor paralysis with no sensory impairment or meningeal signs.

3. Wound Infection–Onset is 4–14 days after injury. Symptoms are similar to those found in patients with exogenous toxin syndrome.

B. Laboratory Findings: All possible food sources should be sampled for culture when exogenous botulism is suspected. Exogenous toxin can be demonstrated in the wound, vomitus, serum, stool, or implicated food. In infant disease, endogenous toxin may be found in the stool or serum. The organism can sometimes be cultured from the infant's feces. Other laboratory findings are usually normal. CSF findings are normal. Electromyography shows characteristic findings.

Treatment

A. Specific Measures: Equine antitoxin should be given for food-borne and wound botulism after testing for hypersensitivity. Endogenous disease in the infant does not require antitoxin. Antibiotic therapy (penicillin) is recommended only for wound botulism.

B. General Measures: Tracheal intubation or tracheostomy may be necessary to remove pooled secretions. Mechanical ventilation may be required if respiratory musculature is severely affected. Tube feeding may be necessary with prolonged paralysis. In infant disease, the possibility of sudden death resulting from respiratory arrest dictates constant and careful observation. The use of aminoglycoside antibiotics may exacerbate symptoms.

Prophylaxis

The best prophylaxis for exogenous disease is to ensure proper food preservation (eg, use of a pressure cooker to kill *C botulinum* spores in home-canned foodstuffs). Honey should not be given to small infants.

Prognosis

The mortality rate in exogenous disease is 20–50%. In endogenous disease, most infants recover after an illness that may last several weeks to months.

TUBERCULOSIS

Tuberculosis, caused by the acid-fast bacillus *Mycobacterium tuberculosis,* is a cause of significant morbidity and mortality worldwide. High-risk groups include persons in developing regions, and, in the United States, minority groups (especially in urban areas) and homeless or institutionalized persons. Tuberculosis is currently linked to HIV infection, as individuals with impaired cellular immunity are at risk of severe disease.

Transmission occurs via droplets from the respiratory tract of patients with active pulmonary tuberculosis. Transplacental infection or acquisition from infected amniotic fluid occasionally occurs. The incubation period to skin test reactivity is 2–10 weeks, although disease may not result for many years or may never result. The risk of disease is greatest in the 2 years following infection.

Clinical Findings

A. Symptoms & Signs:

1. Primary Infection–Initial pulmonary infection may be asymptomatic; or may produce symptomatic pulmonary disease, lymphadenopathy, or metastatic disease (eg, meningitis, mastoiditis, osteomyelitis, arthritis, cutaneous infection, renal disease, or miliary tuberculosis). Meningeal, bony, and miliary disease are relatively more common in children.

2. Reactivation–Latent infection may reactivate years after the primary infection, generally in the lung but also in the kidney and other organs.

B. Laboratory Findings: The diagnosis is made on the basis of clinical findings and typical radiographic findings, in combination with identification and isolation of *M tuberculosis* in body fluids or tissues. Skin testing by the **Mantoux (intradermal) technique** often provides supportive evidence of the diagnosis when isolation of the causative organism is not possible. Interpretation of the Mantoux test varies with the risk status of the patient. Skin testing may be negative in the presence of infection in immunocompromised patients, in patients in the early phase of infection, and in infants younger than 6 months of age.

Complications

The most dreaded complication is tuberculous meningitis, which may be progressive, causing increased intracranial pressure, severe neurologic sequelae, and possibly death.

Other complications include central nervous system (CNS) tuberculoma, pericarditis, ocular tuberculosis, and gastrointestinal (GI) infection.

Treatment

A. Specific Measures: Tuberculous therapy uses prolonged, multiple drug protocols to eradicate the slow-growing organisms and limit the emergence of resistant organisms. Currently recommended regimens use 6-to-12-month treatment courses of two to four drugs, depending on the extent of disease. Uncomplicated pulmonary infection may be treated with a 6-month regimen of isoniazid, rifampin, and pyrazinamide (the latter for the first 2 months). Severe extrapulmonary disease, such as bone/joint, meningeal, and miliary infection, is treated for up to 12 months, with four drugs given during the first 2 months (eg, isoniazid, rifampin, pyrazinamide, and streptomycin), followed by administration of isoniazid and rifampin if the isolate is fully susceptible.

Treatment of tuberculosis must be guided by in vitro susceptibility testing. Drug-resistant tuberculosis is usually treated with multiple drugs for prolonged courses (12–18 months).

Immunocompromised patients such as those with HIV infection are generally treated with more than two drugs (at least initially) for prolonged courses. Congenital disease is generally treated with more than two drugs for 12 months.

B. General Measures: Corticosteroids are considered adjunctive treatment for tuberculous meningitis, pleural effusions, pericarditis, miliary disease, and obstructive endobronchial disease.

Prophylaxis

Regular (annual) tuberculin test screening is recommended in such high-risk populations as minority groups, underprivileged populations, families with members who have immigrated from high-risk countries, communities with high rates of tuberculosis, and individuals in contact with known cases of tuberculosis. Periodic screening is appropriate in lower-risk groups.

Isoniazid prophylaxis is indicated for all individuals younger than 35 years of age with a positive skin test and no evidence of disease; a 9-month course is recommended for normal children.

Isoniazid is also given to contacts of a patient with active tuberculosis. If a skin test 2–3 months later is negative, prophylaxis is discontinued; if it is positive, prophylaxis is continued for a total of 9 months. If contact involves a patient with isoniazid-resistant tuberculosis, rifampin may be substituted.

Bacillus Calmette-Guérin (BCG) vaccine, consisting of live attenuated strains of *M bovis,* is used worldwide. BCG is indicated in the United States in situations in which repeated exposure to tuberculosis is anticipated and is not otherwise preventable. The vaccine is contraindicated in immunodeficient persons.

GONORRHEA

Neisseria gonorrhoeae is a gram-negative, coffee bean–shaped diplococcus usually found both intracellularly and extracellularly in purulent exudate. Neonatal infection may be acquired during delivery by direct contact with infected discharge in the mother's vagina. In childhood, infection may be acquired during sexual abuse, by contact with infected vaginal or urethral discharge or, very rarely, from household exposure.

Clinical Findings

A. Symptoms & Signs: For gonococcal conjunctivitis of the newborn, see Chapter 14. Urethritis with purulent discharge may occur in males, and gonorrheal vulvovaginitis may occur in prepubertal females. Although the vaginal mucosa in adults is resistant to gonococcal infection, both the vagina and the vulva are readily infected before puberty, most commonly from birth to 5 years of age. The infection can be spread by contact with contaminated articles (in rare cases) or infected children or adults. It is manifested by itching and burning of the vulva and vagina. The genital mucosa are red and edematous, and there is a profuse yellow purulent discharge. Acute salpingitis (pelvic inflammatory disease) may develop suddenly after several weeks or months of inapparent infection; however, this is more common in postpubertal females. Perihepatitis in conjunction with salpingitis is characterized by right upper abdominal tenderness and, occasionally, abnormal results of liver function tests. Pharyngitis and proctitis are occasional manifestations of gonococcal disease.

B. Laboratory Findings: A smear of purulent exudate may show intracellular organisms. Cultures on Thayer-Martin medium or other suitable media should be carried out for any suspected case. All isolates from children should be confirmed by a reference laboratory because of the medicolegal implications of positive results.

Complications

Complications of conjunctivitis include corneal ulceration and opacity. Vaginitis may be associated with spread to regional organs or with bacteremia, purulent arthritis, or skin lesions. Skin lesions have an erythematous base, with central hemorrhage. They later become necrotic and vesicular. Nonpurulent polyarthritis also may occur, with low-grade fever, pain and swelling of joints, and redness and tenderness over the wrist, ankle, knee, finger, foot, and other joints of the extremities. Tenosynovitis is also common.

Treatment

A. Specific Measures: Because of increasing resistance, penicillins and tetracyclines are no longer recommended for gonococcal infections. Recommended options include ceftriaxone, cefotaxime, cefixime, spectinomycin, and ofloxacin. Local resistance patterns as well as susceptibilities of individual isolates should be used to guide therapy. The dosage and duration of therapy vary with the site of infection.

B. General Measures:

1. Neonates with gonococcal infection should be hospitalized. In addition to parenteral antibiotics, frequent irrigation of the eyes is crucial.
2. Anticipatory therapy of potential copathogens, for example *Chlamydia trachomatis,* is important for any patient with gonorrhea. In addition, serologic testing for syphilis should be performed.
3. Children who have gonococcal infections should be evaluated for possible sexual abuse.
4. Children and adolescents with gonococcal infections should be considered for screening for HIV and for hepatitis B immunization.

Prophylaxis

For prophylaxis of conjunctivitis, see Chapter 14. Pregnant women should undergo routine screening for gonorrhea. In addition, pregnant women with vaginitis should be examined and cultured prior to delivery, with appropriate treatment of the neonate if maternal cultures are positive. Examination, culturing, and treatment of sexual partners of any person with gonorrhea must be carried out. (Asymptomatic vaginal or urethral infection is common.)

Prognosis

The prognosis is excellent with prompt treatment. Untreated conjunctivitis may result in corneal scarring. Salpingitis as a result of spread from the vagina may be asymptomatic and chronic and may lead to sterility.

TULAREMIA

The causative agent of tularemia is *Francisella tularensis,* a gram-negative coccobacillus. The infection is transmitted through (1) direct contact with the blood of an infected rabbit, ground squirrel, or (more rarely) any one of many species of wild or domestic mammals; (2) through bites of infected ticks or mosquitoes; (3) through ingestion of improperly cooked meat from wild mammals, usually rabbits; or (4) from drinking contaminated water. The incubation period is 1–21 days (average, 3–5 days).

Clinical Findings

A. Symptoms & Signs: Onset is sudden, with fever to 40–40.5 °C (104–105 °F), vomiting, chills in older children, and seizures (rarely) in infected infants. Cutaneous eruptions of various types occur in about 10% of children. The clinical picture depends on the portal of entry.

1. Ulceroglandular–The lesion on the extremity where the bacteria enter the skin is at first papular but rapidly breaks down and becomes a punched-out ulcer. It is accompanied by enlargement and tenderness of regional lymph nodes and sometimes by nodules along the course of the lymphatics. Without therapy, suppuration of the lymph nodes frequently occurs. In some cases, there is lymphadenopathy but no detectable primary lesion (glandular type).

2. Oropharyngeal–Ulceration and formation of a membrane on the pharynx and tonsils are accompanied by enlargement of the cervical lymph nodes.

3. Oculoglandular–Infection is acquired when infectious material is rubbed into the eye. Findings include acute conjunctivitis with edema; photophobia; itching and pain in the eye; swelling of the upper lid, which may show scattered small yellow nodules; and enlargement of lymph glands in the neck, axilla, and scalp.

4. Typhoidal–The organism's point of entry cannot be determined, and the symptoms are systemic.

5. Pneumonic

B. Laboratory Findings: The WBC may be normal, or there may be a slight leukocytosis. Serology shows a positive rising titer, beginning around 7 days from onset. Culture of blood and material (on special media) from other sites of infection may be positive; an indirect fluorescent antibody stain can also be done on potentially infected tissues or exudates.

Treatment

Streptomycin or gentamicin are the drugs of choice. Tetracyclines or chloramphenicol may be used as alternatives; they are, however, associated with a greater chance of relapse.

Prophylaxis

Prophylactic measures include proper handling and cooking of meat from wild mammals, wearing rubber gloves when handling potentially infected animals, using extreme care in handling laboratory materials, and minimizing the chances of tick and mosquito bites. A live attenuated vaccine is recommended for persons with repeated exposures.

Prognosis

The mortality rate in patients with untreated ulceroglandular tularemia is 5%; in patients with the pneumonic type, it is 30%. Early chemotherapy eliminates fatalities.

PLAGUE

Plague is a disease primarily of rats and other small rodents. It is transmitted to humans by a variety of rodent fleas, as well as by direct contact with infected rodents, rabbits, and domestic animals (especially cats). The pneumonic form of the disease may be transmitted by droplet inhalation.

The causative agent is *Yersinia pestis,* a gram-negative, bipolar-staining, pleomorphic bacillus.

Clinical Findings

A. Symptoms & Signs: The incubation period is 2–6 days. Plague has three clinical syndromes:

1. Bubonic Plague–Onset is sudden, with chills, fever to 40 °C (104 °F), vomiting, and lethargy. There is tender, firm enlargement of the inguinal, axillary, and cervical lymph nodes (buboes) by the third day. Meningismus, seizures, and delirium may occur.

2. Pneumonic Plague–Findings are as above but with the absence of buboes and onset of cough on the first day. The patient may expectorate mucoid or thin, blood-tinged or bright-red sputum. Clinical signs of pneumonia may be absent at first.

3. Fulminant (Septicemic) Plague–Onset is as above but with overwhelming bloodstream invasion prior to nodal enlargement or pneumonia.

B. Laboratory Findings: Leukocytosis appears early, with counts as high as 50,000/μL (mostly polymorphonuclear leukocytes). Early blood cultures show positive results. Organisms can be cultured from lymph node contents, sputum, and sometimes from CSF. *Y pestis* may also be identified in stains of blood smears, lymph node aspirates, CSF, or sputum. Serologic testing may also indicate the occurrence of recent infection.

Treatment

A. Specific Measures: Streptomycin is the drug of choice. Tetracycline, chloramphenicol, or sulfonamides may be used as alternative agents. Chloramphenicol should be included in the therapy of meningitis.

B. General Measures: Strict isolation of patients with pneumonic plague and disinfection of all secretions are mandatory.

Prophylaxis

Periodic surveys of rodents and their ectoparasites in endemic areas will provide guidelines for extensive rodent and flea control measures. Total eradication of plague from wild rodents in an endemic area is rarely possible. Active immunization in endemic areas and for those with occupational exposure may be indicated (Chapter 6). Antibiotic prophylaxis with tetracycline or a sulfonamide may provide protection for those exposed to plague infection, especially by the respiratory route.

Prognosis

If treatment can be started early enough in the disease, the prognosis is excellent. Delay in treatment may result in death from fulminant disease. Without treatment, the prognosis is poor.

BRUCELLOSIS
(Undulant Fever, Malta Fever)

Brucellosis is caused by one of four strains of gram-negative brucellae: *Brucella abortus, B melitensis, B canis,* and *B suis*). Although these varieties are most commonly found in cattle, goats, dogs, and hogs respectively, they have also been isolated in other species of animals. The incubation period ranges from a few days to several weeks.

Transmission is by direct contact with diseased animals or their tissues or with unpasteurized milk or cheese from diseased cows and goats.

Clinical Findings

A. Symptoms & Signs: In acute brucellosis, onset is gradual and insidious, with fever and weight loss. Fever may at first be low-grade and present in the evening only, but in the course of days or weeks it may reach 40 °C (104 °F) and exhibit a wave-like character over a period of 2–4 days. Chronic brucellosis is manifested by low-grade fever, sweats, malaise, arthralgia, depression, hepatomegaly, splenomegaly, and leukopenia.

B. Laboratory Findings: The WBC is usually normal to low, with relative or absolute lymphocytosis. Brucellae can be recovered from blood, bone marrow, urine, and local abscesses, usually with difficulty and requiring long incubation in special medium. An agglutination titer > 1:160 or a rising titer will support the diagnosis. A prozone phenomenon in which the agglutination occurs in high dilutions but not in low ones is common. Serologic tests may give a cross-reaction with tularemia, yersinia, and cholera.

Complications

Complications include endocarditis, pneumonia, meningoencephalitis, and osteomyelitis.

Treatment

Tetracyclines are the drugs of choice. Continue treatment for a minimum of 4–6 weeks. In severe illness, add streptomycin, gentamicin, or rifampin, alone or in combination. Trimethoprim-sulfamethoxazole may be used in lieu of tetracycline in young children.

Prophylaxis

Milk and milk products should be pasteurized.

Prognosis

In patients with acute infection, the prognosis is good with adequate treatment. In patients with chronic infection, response to treatment may be poor, although the disease is usually not fatal.

MYCOPLASMA PNEUMONIAE INFECTIONS

Mycoplasmas are free-living organisms without cell walls. The common clinical diseases caused by *Mycoplasma pneumoniae* are pneumonia and tracheobronchitis, which are most frequent in persons 5–18 years of age and especially in young adults. The incubation period is 2–3 weeks.

Clinical Findings

A. Symptoms & Signs: Mycoplasmic diseases have a gradual onset, with moderate fever, malaise, and sore throat. Nonproductive cough occurs after 3–5 days; it becomes persistent and sometimes paroxysmal, resembling pertussis. Other findings include abdominal pain, vomiting, nausea, and dry rales occasionally accompanied by friction rub.

B. Laboratory Findings: The WBC is normal early in the disease but later may show leukocytosis. Autohemagglutinins for type O human erythrocytes (cold agglutinins) usually appear after the first 10 days of disease. Complement fixation and other antibody tests are useful, particularly when a four-fold rise in titer is demonstrated. Mycoplasma may be grown on special media and will indicate either current or recent infection.

C. Imaging: X-ray findings are those of pneumonitis, with infiltrates developing around the hilum and gradually spreading. Pleural effusion may be apparent.

Complications

Otitis media or bullous myringitis is common in younger individuals. CNS disease, hemolytic anemia, exanthems, Stevens-Johnson syndrome, and arthritis have all been reported. Severe respiratory disease may be seen in immunocompromised hosts, in children with sickle cell disease, and in children with trisomy 21.

Treatment

Erythromycin in young children or tetracycline in those older than 9 years of age is the drug of choice (Chapter 31). Therapy does not affect the rate of transmission.

Prognosis

With adequate treatment, the prognosis is excellent.

CHLAMYDIAL INFECTIONS

The species of the genus *Chlamydia* are obligate intracellular bacteria, classified as *C trachomatis, C psittaci,* and *C pneumoniae* (TWAR agent). These agents cause several diseases in humans.

Clinical Findings

A. Symptoms & Signs:

1. Inclusion Conjunctivitis & Trachoma–Neonatal inclusion conjunctivitis (inclusion blennorrhea) and trachoma are caused by *C trachomatis.* Neonatal infection is acquired during passage through the cervix and causes a purulent conjunctivitis within the first few weeks after birth. This conjunctivitis usually heals without scarring. Trachoma is a chronic keratoconjunctivitis that may cause scarring and blindness.

2. Pneumonitis–Neonatal pneumonitis, also a result of *C trachomatis* infection acquired during birth, is characterized by onset during early infancy, with progressive tachypnea, staccato cough, cyanosis, and vomiting. It is an afebrile illness. Chest x-ray shows bilateral infiltrates.

3. Lymphogranuloma Venereum–Infection is caused by particular strains of *C trachomatis* acquired via sexual contact. Inguinal nodes in the male and perirectal nodes in the female become infected, enlarge, and suppurate. Clinical presentations include buboes in males and proctitis in females or homosexual males.

4. Urethritis & Cervicitis–Caused by *C trachomatis,* these infections are clinically similar to gonococcal disease and may be mistaken for resistant gonococcal infection. Chlamydial infection of these structures may be asymptomatic and persistent.

5. Psittacosis–Caused by *C psittaci*, psittacosis (ornithosis) is acquired by contact with parrots, parakeets, pigeons, chickens, ducks, and other wild birds. There is a sudden onset of fever, chills, and nonproductive cough, with clinical signs of pneumonia or bronchiolitis (Chapter 15). Multisystem involvement rarely occurs.

6. *Chlamydia pneumoniae*–A febrile respiratory illness consisting of pharyngitis, fever, cough, cervical adenopathy, and pneumonia is caused by this agent, which is antigenically distinct from *C trachomatis* and *C psittaci.*

B. Laboratory Findings: Chlamydiae can be cultured, with difficulty, on special media. Testing is available for *C trachomatis, C pneumoniae,* and *C psittaci.* Characteristic inclusion bodies are found on Giemsa-stained smears of discharge in neonatal conjunctivitis and trachoma. Fluorescent antibody staining and enzyme-linked immunoassay tests are widely available for diagnosing *C trachomatis* infections, and DNA detection tests are available. Culture, not rapid detection techniques, is the appropriate diagnostic method for genital specimens from children under evaluation for possible sexual abuse.

Serologic tests are diagnostic in lymphogranuloma venereum, psittacosis, and *C pneumoniae* agent infection.

Complications

Neonatal inclusion conjunctivitis (rarely) and trachoma (relatively commonly) may produce corneal scarring and vision problems if untreated. Untreated lymphogranuloma venereum in boys may produce extensive scarring around draining inguinal nodes; in girls, perirectal scarring may cause rectal stricture. Untreated urethritis in boys may cause chronic discharge and dysuria persisting for many weeks. Untreated cervicitis in girls may cause salpingitis with resultant scarring and sterility. Untreated neonatal chlamydial pneumonia may produce chronic illness.

Treatment

A. Specific Measures:

1. Inclusion Conjunctivitis–Therapy with oral erythromycin for 14 days (Chapter 14) is the recommended treatment. Sulfonamides are an acceptable alternative. Topical therapy does not eradicate nasopharyngeal carriage.

2. Trachoma–Give oral doxycycline or erythromycin in addition to local antibiotic treatment. Continue therapy for 40 days.

3. Pneumonitis–Treat with oral erythromycin or a sulfonamide for 14 days.

4. Lymphogranuloma Venereum–Give tetracycline, azithromycin, a sulfonamide, or erythromycin for 3–6 weeks (Chapter 31).

5. Urethritis & Cervicitis–Oral doxycycline, azithromycin, or erythromycin may reduce symptoms but will not always eradicate the organisms. Amoxicillin or sulfisoxazole may be used during pregnancy, but are less effective.

6. Psittacosis–Give oral tetracyclines or erythromycin (Chapter 31).

7. *C pneumoniae*–Erythromycin and tetracycline are the drugs of choice.

Prophylaxis

Topical erythromycin, tetracycline, or silver nitrate do not reliably prevent neonatal chlamydial conjunctivitis. Identification and treatment of pregnant women who are infected may prevent neonatal conjunctivitis and pneumonia. Mothers (and their sexual partners) of infected infants and sexual partners of patients with identified or probable chlamydial infections should be evaluated and treated.

Prognosis

With early diagnosis and treatment of chlamydial infections, complications are minimal and the prognosis excellent.

KAWASAKI DISEASE
(Mucocutaneous Lymph Node Syndrome)

Kawasaki disease is a vasculitic illness of unknown etiology. It occurs primarily in children younger than 8 years of age.

Clinical Findings

A. Symptoms & Signs: Onset is abrupt, with fever as high as 40 °C (104 °F) and a diffuse rash over the body. The lips are very red, and the tongue has a bright "strawberry" appearance. The patient's conjunctivae, palms, and soles are red and swollen. The cervical lymph nodes are often enlarged. Fever usually subsides in 1–3 weeks. There is a characteristic peeling of the skin, beginning with the fingertips and toenails. Associated symptoms or findings may include carditis, arthralgia, pyuria, gallbladder hydrops, and aseptic meningitis. Young infants may not show the full range of clinical findings.

B. Laboratory Findings: Leukocytosis, elevated sedimentation rate, and sterile pyuria are common. The platelet count generally rises as the illness progresses.

Echocardiographic and electrocardiographic evaluations are critical both at diagnosis and during follow-up.

Complications

Complications include carditis, arthritis, dilation or aneurysms of coronary arteries, and aneurysms in other large arteries.

Treatment

Intravenous gamma globulin reduces the acute inflammatory signs of Kawasaki disease and also appears to reduce the frequency of coronary artery dilation and aneurysm. Aspirin is generally given in high anti-inflammatory doses during the acute phase of illness, followed by lower antiplatelet doses during the subacute and convalescent phases.

Prognosis

Patients with coronary artery involvement are at risk of coronary thrombosis, myocardial infarction, and sudden death. Mild coronary vessel dilation often regresses over weeks or months.

BACTERIAL INFECTIONS OF THE CENTRAL NERVOUS SYSTEM

GENERAL CONSIDERATIONS IN MENINGITIS

The most frequent causative agents are group B streptococcus and gram-negative enterics in neonates and *Streptococcus pneumoniae, Neisseria meningitidis, and Haemophilus influenzae B,* in infants and children (Table 11–3).

Symptoms & Signs

A. "Meningeal" Signs: These include stiffness of the neck (inability to touch the chin to the chest), stiffness of the back (inability to sit up normally), a positive **Kernig's sign** (inability to extend the knee when the leg is flexed anteriorly at the hip), and a positive **Brudzinski's sign** (bending the head forward produces flexure movements of the lower extremity).

B. Increased Intracranial Pressure: Findings include bulging fontanelles in small infants and irritability, headache (may be intermittent), projectile vomiting (or vomiting may be absent), diplopia, "choking" of the optic disks, slowing of the pulse, irregular respirations, and increase in blood pressure.

C. Change in Sensorium: Such changes range from mild lethargy to coma.

D. Seizures: Seizures are usually generalized and are more common in infants.

E. Fever: Onset of high- or low-grade fever may be sudden or insidious, or there may be a marked change in pattern during a minor illness.

F. Shock: Shock may appear in the course of many types of CNS infection.

G. Other: In children younger than 18 months, irritability, persistent crying, poor feeding, diarrhea, or vomiting may be the *only* symptoms. Fever may be absent or low-grade in neonates and young infants, and meningeal signs may not be found. Therefore, the index of suspicion must be higher for infants.

Examination of Cerebrospinal Fluid (CSF)

When CNS infection is suspected, lumbar puncture and examination of CSF must be performed to establish the diagnosis. Gross examination, cell count, chemistries, and microscopic examination for bacteria may all be performed immediately after lumbar puncture. Latex agglutination and counterimmunoelectrophoresis are rapid diagnostic tests that may be used to identify capsular antigens of meningococci, pneumococci, *Haemophilus influenzae,* or group B streptococcus in CSF, although their yield is usually not better than that of a Gram's stain in a child who has not been pretreated with antibiotics.

Differential Diagnosis

Bacterial meningitis must be differentiated from other types of CNS infection and disease (eg, granulomatous meningitis associated with tuberculosis, coccidioidomycosis, cryptococcosis, and syphilis) and from viral meningoencephalitis.

Partially treated bacterial meningitis may present with similar clinical and laboratory findings as aseptic meningitis.

A purulent infectious process in close proximity to the central nervous system may introduce white cells or protein into the cerebrospinal fluid. Parameningeal infections include brain abscess, osteomyelitis of the skull or vertebrae, epidural abscess, or mastoiditis.

Meningismus may occur in such infections as pneumonia, shigellosis, salmonellosis, otitis media, and meningeal invasion by neoplastic cells. In the latter instance, there may be not only increased numbers of cells in the spinal fluid but also a lowered glucose level.

Complications

CNS infection may produce fatality rates of up to 20% and long-term sequelae in up to 30% of survivors. Complications include hydrocephalus, especially in infants (uncommon since the advent of specific therapy); subdural accumulation of fluid, especially in a patient younger than 2 years; deafness; paresis; mental retardation; focal epilepsy; and neurodevelopmental residua. Persistent fever may be due to intracranial abscess, lateral sinus thrombosis, mastoiditis, drug reaction, continued sepsis, secondary infection, phlebitis, or simply to persistent meningeal inflammation.

Treatment

A. Emergency Measures: Treat shock, hypoglycemia, and hypoxemia; avoid overhydration and aggravation of brain edema. Institute measures for treatment of increased intracranial pressure if appropriate.

B. Specific Measures:

1. Infection With Known Organism–Treat with antibiotics appropriate for the causative organism.

Table 11–3. Bacterial meningitis: specific agents.

Organism	Epidemiology	Clinical Findings	Laboratory Findings	Complications	Treatment	Prophylaxis
Gram-negative enterics (*Citrobacter diversus*, *Enterobacter* species, *Escherichia coli*, *Klebsiella pneumoniae*, *Pseudomonas aeruginosa*)	Increased risk in premature neonates or other compromised hosts; may be associated with UTI, foreign body, other focus of infection, break in skin or mucosal integrity	Usually acute onset, with systemic illness	Gram's stain of CSF may reveal gram-negative rods. Cultures of CSF and often blood are positive	Tends to have severe course, with resultant morbidity. Brain abscess may occur	Cefotaxime, ceftazidime, trimethoprim-sulfamethoxazole and/or an aminoglycoside, depending on susceptibilities	—
Group B streptococcus	Neonates; increased risk with prematurity, prolonged rupture of membranes, maternal infection	May present as early onset or late onset disease. Findings may be nonspecific	Gram's stain of CSF may show gram-positive cocci in chains; CSF and blood cultures usually positive. Latex agglutination frequently positive (urine, CSF, serum)	Long-term sequelae may include intellectual impairment, motor deficits, hearing loss, seizures	Penicillin G, or ampicillin; an aminoglycoside may be added for possible synergy	Intrapartum antibiotic prophylaxis of high-risk women carrying group B streptococcus is recommended

Haemophilus influenzae B	Previously most frequent cause of pediatric meningitis (now decreased because of immunization); most frequent under 5 yr, especially < 2 yr	May be of rapid or insidious onset; frequently follows URI. May have associated foci of infection, eg, arthritis, cellulitis	Gram's stain of CSF may show gram-negative pleomorphic rods. CSF culture and often blood culture positive. Latex agglutination may be positive in CSF, serum, or urine	Persistent or recurrent fevers; secondary sites of infection (arthritis, pericarditis; subdural effusions or empyemas). Long-term morbidity, especially hearing loss, may ensue	Ampicillin, cefotaxime, ceftriaxone, chloramphenicol depending on susceptibilities. Ampicillin resistance ranges from 25% to 50%. Dexamethasone should be considered to reduce hearing loss and/or neurologic sequelae	Rifampin prophylaxis of contacts; *Haemophilus influenzae B* vaccine
Listeria monocytogenes	Neonates; patients with defective cell-mediated immunity	May present as early onset or late onset disease in neonates. May be associated with maternal illness	Gram's stain of CSF shows gram-positive rods. Cultures of CSF and blood usually positive	May have long-term morbidity if severe and/or treatment delayed	Ampicillin, plus an aminoglycoside initially	Maternal avoidance of foods implicated in listeriosis outbreaks; treat maternal infections when identified
Mycobacterium tuberculosis	Infected contact can usually be identfied; patient often in high-risk geographic or ethnic group	Onset may be gradual; encephalopathic symptoms may predominate. Tuberculous pneumonia often but not invariably present	Positive tuberculin skin test; moderate CSF pleocytosis with low CSF glucose and elevated protein. Acid-fast bacilli may be identified in or grown from CSF or detected with DNA probes	Long-term sequelae may develop as for other bacterial meningitides	Prolonged antituberculous therapy with isoniazid, rifampin, and initially, usually a third and fourth drug (pyrazinamide, streptomycin, or ethambutol) depending on susceptibilities. Corticosteroids should also be considered	Prophylactic administration of isoniazid to contacts of active tuberculosis and to skin-test positive patients. Use of BCG in rare circumstances in the United States

(*continued*)

Table 11–3. Bacterial meningitis: specific agents (*continued*).

Organism	Epidemiology	Clinical Findings	Laboratory Findings	Complications	Treatment	Prophylaxis
Neisseria meningitidis	Most frequent in infants and young children. Increased risk in patients with terminal complement deficiency	Morbilliform, petechial, or purpuric rash frequent. May present with shock	Gram's stain of CSF may show gram-negative diplococci. Organism may be grown from CSF, blood, and petechial lesions. Latex agglutination test may be helpful, though lacks sensitivity	Secondary sites of infection may occur. DIC, myocarditis, pericarditis, Waterhouse-Friderichsen syndrome, shock, long-term morbidity, including hearing loss	Penicillin G, ampicillin, cefotaxime, ceftriaxone, chloramphenicol. Rarely penicillin-resistant. Dexamethasone should be considered to reduce hearing loss and/or neurologic sequelae	Rifampin prophylaxis of close contacts (sulfisoxazole, ceftriaxone, and ciprofloxacin are alternatives); vaccination of children in high-risk groups
Streptococcus pneumoniae	Increased risk in children with deficiencies of humoral immunity or splenic function; common cause of posttraumatic meningitis	Frequently follows URI or other infection (otitis, sinusitis, pneumonia)	Gram's stain of CSF may show gram-positive diplococci. Organism often isolated from CSF and/or blood. Latex agglutination may be positive in CSF, serum, or urine	Secondary sites of infection may occur. Long-term morbidity is common, including hearing loss, seizures, motor deficits, and intellectual impairment	Penicillin G or ampicillin. If strain is not fully susceptible to penicillin, alternatives include vancomycin, rifampin, cefotaxime, ceftriaxone, chloramphenicol. Dexamethasone should be considered to reduce hearing loss and/or neurologic sequelae	Antibiotic prophylaxis for asplenic and sickle cell patients; pneumococcal vaccine for high-risk groups

BCG = Bacillus Calmette-Guérin; CSF = cerebrospinal fluid; DIC = disseminated intravascular coagulation; URI = upper respiratory tract infection; UTI = urinary tract infection.

2. Suspected Infection With Unidentified Bacterial Organism–Obtain all diagnostic material before instituting antimicrobial therapy, if possible. Meningitis of unknown cause in premature infants and infants younger than 1 month should be treated with ampicillin plus cefotaxime or ampicillin plus gentamicin. Children older than 1 month should be given cefotaxime or ceftriaxone in combination with ampicillin, in the first 3 months of life. After 3 months of age, empiric treatment with cefotaxime or ceftriaxone is appropriate. Additional empiric treatment of penicillin/cephalosporin-resistant *S pneumoniae* (eg, with vancomycin, rifampin, or both) should be provided in most cases outside the immediate neonatal period, pending culture and susceptibility testing.

3. Corticosteroids–Dexamethasone has been shown in some studies to reduce hearing loss and some neurologic sequelae of bacterial meningitis (particularly when caused by *Haemophilus influenzae B*). When given, it should be started with (or before) the administration of antibiotics. Studies in neonates have not been performed as of this writing.

BRAIN ABSCESS

Brain abscess is usually caused by one of the common pyogenic bacteria: streptococci, oral anaerobes, pneumococci, staphylococci, or gram negatives. The source of infection is often a septic focus elsewhere in the body (eg, oropharyngeal infection, sinusitis, otitis media, pneumonia, osteomyelitis, subacute infective endocarditis, furuncles). After skull fracture, organisms may enter through the paranasal sinuses or middle ear. Patients with right-to-left cardiopulmonary shunts are at increased risk of brain abscess.

Clinical Findings

A. Symptoms & Signs: Findings may be few and diagnosis difficult. Onset is gradual, with fever, vomiting, and lethargy sometimes proceeding to coma. Increased intracranial pressure may be present, manifested by bulging fontanelles (infants) or papilledema (older children). Neurologic signs related to special areas of the brain may be present, and focal seizures may occur. A history of infection elsewhere in the body should be sought.

B. Laboratory Findings: Leukocytosis, elevated sedimentation rate, and CSF changes may occur.

C. Imaging: Cranial sutures may be widened. Computed tomography, magnetic resonance imaging, radionuclide brain scanning, and arteriography may suggest a specific diagnosis and location.

Treatment

A. Specific Measures: Surgical aspiration and drainage are usually indicated for diagnosis and treatment. Identification of the pathogen will allow specific antibiotic therapy. Until the agent is identified, broad-spectrum antimicrobial therapy should be initiated (eg, combinations of penicillin, nafcillin, vancomycin, chloramphenicol, cefotaxime, or metronidazole, as dictated by particular circumstances).

B. General Measures: Give anticonvulsants for seizures. Treat increased intracranial pressure, if present.

Prognosis

When appropriate treatment is initiated early, the prognosis is good. For extensive disease or when therapy is delayed, the prognosis is guarded. Brain damage may occur, with resultant cortical deficits.

SPIROCHETAL DISEASES

SYPHILIS

Syphilis is caused by *Treponema pallidum.* Congenital syphilis is transmitted transplacentally or at delivery. If the mother has been infected recently, the disease is almost always transmitted to the infant. The longer the interval between infection of the mother and conception, the greater the likelihood that the infant will be free of disease. Intrauterine infection may produce intrauterine death or congenital syphilis.

Syphilis may be acquired in childhood or adolescence by contact of an abrasion or laceration with infectious secretions, by contact with infected nipples, by kissing infectious lesions, or by sexual contact (including sexual abuse).

Clinical Findings

A. Symptoms & Signs: Childhood syphilis may occur in early or late congenital forms or follow the same patterns as adult disease.

1. Early Congenital Syphilis–Signs generally appear before the sixth week of life. The more severe the infection, the earlier the onset. Rhinitis, or "snuffles"—a profuse, persistent, mucopurulent nasal discharge—is usually the first symptom. The discharge may be blood-tinged. Skin rash follows onset of rhinitis and appears as a maculopapular or morbilliform eruption, heaviest on the child's back, buttocks, and backs of thighs. Bullous lesions on the hands and feet are suggestive. Other findings include bleeding ulcerations and fissures of mucous membranes of the mouth, anus, and contiguous areas; anemia, with erythroblasts often present in large numbers; osteochondritis or periostitis (or both), with pseudoparalysis, pathologic fractures, and a characteristic x-ray appearance of increased density, widening of the epiphyseal line, and scattered areas of decreased density; hepatomegaly and splenomegaly (jaundice may be prominent); pneumonia; and chorioretinitis, with eventual atrophy.

2. Late Congenital Syphilis–Symptoms do not usually occur until after the second year of life. There may be maldevelopment of bones of the nose ("saddle nose") and legs ("saber shins"). Neurosyphilis may occur, with clinical evidence of meningitis, paresis, tabes, or a slowly developing hydrocephalus. Deciduous teeth are normal. Permanent dentition may include Hutchinson's teeth, in which the upper central incisors have a characteristic V-shaped notch in a peg-shaped tooth. The first permanent molars may have multiple cusps ("mulberry molars"). Other findings include rhagades, or scars around the mouth and nose; interstitial keratitis, usually occurring in children between 6 and 12 years of age; and conjunctivitis, which gradually infiltrates deeply into the cornea and produces opacity.

3. Acquired Syphilis–Symptoms in children are similar to those in adults, with three stages: (1) mucocutaneous ulcerative lesions; (2) rash; and (3) tertiary syphilis with its cardiovascular or neurologic changes.

B. Laboratory Findings: Darkfield microscopic examination of scrapings from mucocutaneous lesions and nasal discharge may show treponemal spirochetes.

Serologic tests for syphilis include nontreponemal tests (Venereal Disease Research Laboratory [VDRL]; rapid plasma reagin [RPR]; automated reagin test [ART]) and treponemal tests (fluorescent treponemal antibody absorption [FTA-ABS]; microhemagglutination, *Treponema pallidum* [MHA-TP]; *Treponema pallidum* immobilization [TPI]). The nontreponemal tests are useful for screening; positive tests need to be confirmed with specific treponemal tests. Nontreponemal tests should be followed after therapy; a declining titer correlates with successful treatment, whereas a persistent elevated titer suggests ongoing infection. Nontreponemal tests usually become nonreactive within 1–2 years of adequate therapy, whereas treponemal tests remain positive indefinitely.

Diagnosis of congenital syphilis is based on clinical findings as well as serologic tests. Positive nontreponemal and treponemal tests on neonatal serum may reflect neonatal or maternal infection (even a satisfactorily treated maternal infection). In some cases, the only way to confirm neonatal infection is to follow the neonate's nontreponemal titer; a rising titer over the first few months suggests active infection.

Children with suspected congenital syphilis or acquired syphilis of > 1 year's duration should have their CSF analyzed. Increases in protein or cell count or a positive nontreponemal test (VDRL) result on CSF suggests neurologic involvement.

C. Imaging: Findings are characteristic in congenital syphilis. All of the long bones may be affected. Changes are apparent early in the disease. The epiphyseal line shows increased density, with decreased density proximal to it. In severe cases, destructive lesions occur near the ends of the long bones. Periostitis appears as a widening of the shaft of the long bones, with eventual calcification and distortion of the normal curvature.

Treatment

A. Specific Measures:

1. Congenital Syphilis–Give aqueous penicillin G intravenously for 10–14 days or procaine penicillin G intramuscularly for 10 days.

Therapy should be provided for neonates with clinical syphilis and for newborns whose mothers had syphilis during pregnancy but were untreated, had inadequate treatment, had unknown treatment, had non-penicillin treatment, did not have a four-fold decrease in nontreponemal antibody titer, or had treatment during the last 4 weeks of pregnancy.

Infants who are asymptomatic and are born to mothers who received appropriate treatment for syphilis during pregnancy do not need therapy; their nontreponemal test titer should be followed monthly until negative. Treatment should be provided, however, if the titer is not negative by 6 months or if follow-up cannot be assured.

2. Acquired Syphilis–Give intramuscular benzathine penicillin G once for disease of < 1 year's duration. Infection of > 1 year's duration should be treated once a week for 3 weeks.

3. Penicillin Sensitivity–In persons allergic to penicillin, give tetracycline or erythromycin for 14 days. Penicillin should be used whenever safely possible during pregnancy.

B. Complications of Specific Therapy: The Jarisch-Herxheimer reaction, with fever associated with the sudden destruction of spirochetes, occurs within the first 24 hours of treatment and subsides within the next 24 hours.

C. Follow-up Treatment: Nontreponemal serologic tests should be performed at intervals of 3 months for at least 1 year. Retreatment should be considered if titers do not fall to the negative range. For those with initially abnormal cerebrospinal fluid, CSF examinations should be performed at 6-month intervals for at least 2 years or until normal. Retreatment should be considered if abnormal CSF findings are still present by 2 years of age.

Prophylaxis

All pregnant women should be screened for syphilis at least once, early in pregnancy. High-risk patients should be screened a second time late in pregnancy. If syphilis is diagnosed early in pregnancy, treatment may be completed before delivery. The chances of preventing the disease in the newborn are excellent even if the mother is not treated until the seventh or eighth month of pregnancy.

Sexual contacts of patients identified as having syphilis should be tested and treated.

Prognosis

Rapid treatment of infants with early congenital syphilis or of older patients with early acquired disease usually results in cure as well as normal growth and development. In children with late congenital syphilis, the prognosis for cure of the spirochetal infection is good, but pathologic changes in the bones, nervous system, and eyes will remain throughout life.

LEPTOSPIROSIS

Leptospirosis is an acute febrile disease caused by *Leptospira* serovariants of *L interrogans.* The most common species (or serovariants) implicated are *L canicola, L icterohaemorrhagiae,* and *L pomona.* The infection is transmitted through ingestion of food or water contaminated with the urine of reservoir animals (dogs, rats, cattle, swine). Ingestion may occur while bathing in contaminated water. Contact with carcasses and rat bites also transmit infection. The incubation period is 7–13 days.

Clinical Findings

A. Symptoms & Signs: Onset is abrupt, with fever to 39.5–40.5 °C (103–105 °F). Pharyngitis, cervical lymphadenopathy, and conjunctivitis accompany the first phase of the disease, which lasts 3–5 days and is followed by subsidence of fever and symptoms. The second phase of the disease appears after 2 or 3 days, with recurrence of fever and the onset of joint pain, vomiting, headache, and often a rash, which is morbilliform and sometimes purpuric. Meningitis and (more rarely) uveitis may develop at this phase of the disease.

B. Laboratory Findings: The WBC usually is markedly elevated (as high as 50,000 μL), sometimes with immature forms. Cerebrospinal fluid may show 100–200 cells/μL. Leptospirae may occasionally be seen on darkfield examination, silver stain, or fluorescent antibody stain of blood, urine, or CSF. The organism can be cultured (on special media) from these body fluids. Serum bilirubin levels may be elevated, and the aspartate aminotransferase (AST) [serum glutamic-oxaloacetic transaminase, or SGOT] level may be abnormal. The diagnosis is most often made serologically; antibody is detectable after the first 7 days of disease.

Complications

Renal involvement, with hematuria, proteinuria, and oliguria, occurs in about 50% of cases. Myositis and jaundice, with an enlarged and tender liver, are also common. Symptomatic meningitis may become apparent in the second phase of the disease. Myocarditis may infrequently occur.

Treatment

A. Specific Measures: Administer procaine penicillin G intravenously for 7 days. In patients with penicillin sensitivity, give doxycycline.

B. Complications of Specific Therapy: The Jarisch-Herxheimer reaction may occur, as in the treatment of syphilis.

Prophylaxis

Preventive measures include rodent control, protective clothing for occupational exposures, and prophylactic doxycycline.

Prognosis

In the absence of renal or hepatic involvement, recovery is complete after 10–21 days. With severe kidney and liver involvement, the mortality rate may be as high as 30%.

RELAPSING FEVER

Relapsing fever is endemic in many parts of the world, especially mountainous areas. Causative organisms include *Borrelia recurrentis, B hermsii,* and related *Borrelia* species. The reservoirs are rodents, other small mammals, and humans with relapsing fever. Transmission to humans occurs by lice or ticks and occasionally by contact with the blood of infected rodents.

Clinical Findings

A. Symptoms & Signs: After an incubation period of 2–14 days, onset is abrupt, with fever, chills, tachycardia, nausea, vomiting, headache, hepatosplenomegaly, arthralgia, and cough. Usually within the first 2 days, a macular or morbilliform rash appears over the trunk and extremities. Petechiae may also appear. Without treatment, the fever falls by crisis in 3–10 days. Relapse characteristically occurs at intervals of 1–2 weeks, with relapses becoming progressively shorter and milder. As many as 10 such episodes may occur in the absence of treatment.

B. Laboratory Findings: Diagnosis is based on the clinical course and the observation of spirochetes in the peripheral blood by darkfield examination or by use of Wright's stain, Giemsa stain, or acridine orange stain on thick smears or buffy coat smears. Aids to diagnosis include inoculation of blood in mice, proteus OX-K agglutinin serology, and direct serology.

Complications

Complications include meningitis, iridocyclitis, epistaxis, myocarditis, and intrauterine infection, which can lead to abortion or neonatal disease.

Treatment

Treatment with penicillin, tetracyclines, erythromycin, or chloramphenicol is successful. As with syphilis and leptospirosis, the Jarisch-Herxheimer reaction may occur in the first 24 hours of treatment.

Prophylaxis

Minimizing contact with lice and ticks by good hygiene, appropriate clothing, and insect repellents is appropriate.

Prognosis

Prognosis is good except in debilitated patients.

LYME DISEASE

Lyme disease, caused by the spirochete *Borrelia burgdorferi,* is a multisystem disorder that is prevalent in the United States (upper Atlantic Coast, Midwest, West Coast), Europe, and Australia. The major vectors are ticks, particularly *Ixodes* ticks.

Clinical Findings

A. Symptoms & Signs: An annular erythematous skin lesion—**erythema chronicum migrans**—develops in most patients at the site of a tick bite; the incubation period is 3–32 days. More extensive rashes, conjunctivitis, fever, malaise, arthralgia, or meningitis may also develop. Weeks to months later, involvement of several organ systems may occur: neurologic (Bell's palsy, cranial or peripheral neuritis, meningitis), cardiac (conduction block, myocarditis), or joint (chronic arthritis). These later findings may develop without the prior appearance of erythema chronicum migrans. There are anecdotal reports of apparent intrauterine infection with adverse pregnancy outcome.

B. Laboratory Findings: The most widely available diagnostic test is enzyme-linked immunosorbent assay (ELISA) serology. Antibody may not be detectable for several weeks following onset of infection, and sensitivity and specificity may be lacking. Western blot testing may improve sensitivity and specificity. Antibodies may not develop in patients treated early in the disease. Culture is not routinely available and lacks sensitivity.

Treatment

A. Specific Measures: Oral doxycycline, amoxicillin, penicillin V, cefuroxime, or erythromycin for 10–30 days are recommended for early disease (erythema chronicum migrans). High-dose intravenous ceftriaxone or penicillin G for 14–21 days is recommended for the later stages of Lyme disease.

B. General Measures: Nonsteroidal anti-inflammatory agents (NSAIDs) may be useful for patients with arthritis.

Prophylaxis

The major preventive measure is avoidance of tick exposure, for example, by wearing protective clothing in endemic areas, by using tick repellents, and by removing ticks promptly. Antibiotic prophylaxis following tick bites is not recommended in most circumstances.

Prognosis

Patients treated early in the infection usually have a favorable course; patients with delayed therapy may have more chronic courses.

RICKETTSIAL DISEASES

The **rickettsiae** are very small intracellular bacteria that irregularly stain gram-negative. They are divided immunologically into distinct groups and subgroups. Although most groups stimulate the production in humans of agglutinins against strains of *Proteus vulgaris,* the determination of complement-fixing antibodies is a more accurate and acceptable serologic testing method (Table 11–4). The major causative agent of cat-scratch disease has been identified as *Bartonella henselae* (formerly *Rochalimaea henselae*), a gram-negative rickettsia.

PROTOZOAL DISEASES

MALARIA

Malaria is an acute or chronic febrile disease caused by one of four types of plasmodia: *Plasmodium vivax, P malariae, P falciparum,* and *P ovale.* Transmission occurs through the bite of the female *Anopheles* mosquito, in which the sexual cycle of the parasite occurs. Transmission via transfusion and congenital infection is less common. The asexual cycle occurs in humans. Infection is widespread in the tropics and subtropics. The incubation period ranges from 6–30 days; relapses may occur with *P vivax* and *P ovale* infection.

Clinical Findings

A. Symptoms & Signs: Sudden onset of paroxysms of fever to 39.5–40.5 °C (103–105 °F) may be accompanied by seizures in the very young. Chills are sometimes present, last at least 2–4 hours, and are followed by sweating. In young children, paroxysms may be continuous or recur irregularly. In older children, paroxysmal recurrence varies with type of infection: 48 hours for *P vivax, P falciparum,* and *P ovale*; and 72 hours for *P malariae.* Diarrhea and vomiting are frequent; splenomegaly is usually present. Hemolysis may lead to clini-

Table 11–4. Rickettsial diseases: epidemiology and clinical manifestations.

Disease	Agent	Natural Host	Vector	Geographic Prevalence
Epidemiology				
Cat-scratch disease	*Bartonella henselae*	Cats, other animals	—	Worldwide
Ehrlichiosis	*Ehrlichia chaffeensis*	Humans	Tick	Southeast, South Central, western United States
Endemic typhus	*Rickettsia typhi*	Rats	Rat flea	Worldwide, including southern and southeastern United States
Epidemic typhus	*Rickettsia prowazekii*	Humans	Body louse	Africa, Asia, Europe, Central and South America
Q fever	*Coxiella burnetii*	Farm and wild animals (including sheep, goats, cows, cats)	—	Worldwide
Rickettsialpox	*Rickettsia akari*	House mice	Mouse mite	Africa, Asia, United States
Rocky Mountain spotted fever	*Rickettsia rickettsii*	Ticks, small animals, dogs	Tick	North and South America, including southern and eastern United States and upper Rocky Mountain states

Disease	Clinical Findings	Complications	Treatment	Prophylaxis
Cat-scratch disease	Fever, malaise, papular lesions at inoculation site, regional lymphadenitis. Generally self-limiting within a few months.	Encephalopathy, osteomyelitis, hepatitis, thrombocytopenia, conjunctivitis, erythema nodosum	Symptomatic; needle aspiration; antibiotics (eg, gentamicin, trimethoprim-sulfamethoxazole) for systemic disease	—
Ehrlichiosis	Fever, chills, myalgia, headache, arthralgia, vomiting, + rash	Pneumonitis, renal failure, encephalopathy	Tetracycline; chloramphenicol	Minimize tick exposure
Endemic typhus	Fever, headache, myalgia, macular rash	Unusual	Doxycycline; chloramphenicol	Insecticides; rat control
Epidemic typhus	Nausea, vomiting, fever, headache, maculopapular hemorrhagic rash	Encephalopathy, myocarditis, renal failure, bacterial pneumonia; relapse (Brill-Zinsser disease)	Tetracycline; chloramphenicol; pediculocides	Delousing
Q fever	Fever, malaise, headache, cough, weakness, hepatosplenomegaly	Pneumonia, endocarditis, hepatitis	Doxycycline; chloramphenicol	Reduce animal exposure; pasteurize milk
Rickettsialpox	Papulovesicular rash, fever, headache, myalgia, photophobia; eschar and lymphadenopathy at site of mite bite	Rare	Tetracycline; chloramphenicol	Insecticides; rodent control
Rocky Mountain spotted fever	Fever, maculopapular hemorrhagic rash, headache, myalgia, nausea, vomiting, conjunctivitis	Shock, disseminated intravascular coagulation, multisystem failure	Chloramphenicol; tetracycline; supportive care	Minimize tick exposure

cal jaundice and pallor. The child may be asymptomatic or have mild manifestations of illness between paroxysms. In infants, infection—including congenital infection—may cause lethargy, irritability, anorexia, and other findings suggestive of sepsis.

B. Laboratory Findings: There is rapid onset of anemia; serum bilirubin levels are increased. Thin and thick blood smears and bone marrow smears show parasites.

Complications

"Blackwater fever" is rare in childhood. It is usually associated with *P falciparum* infection and is characterized by hemoglobinuria and shock-like state. Coagulopathy, encephalopathy, and multiorgan failure may also result from *P falciparum* infection. Nephrosis may complicate chronic *P malariae* infection.

Treatment

A. Specific Measures: Treatment is dictated in part by the malarial species involved and the region in which infection was contracted.

1. Chloroquine–Chloroquine phosphate (Aralen), given once daily orally for 3 days, is the drug of choice for *P vivax, P ovale, P malariae,* and nonresistant *P falciparum* infections.

If oral therapy is not possible, give intravenous quinine dihydrochloride or quinidine gluconate and begin oral chloroquine as soon as possible.

2. Quinine, Pyrimethamine, & Sulfadiazine–Oral quinine sulfate (3–7 days) and tetracycline (7 days), clindamycin (3 days), or pyrimethamine-sulfadoxine (1 dose) should be used for *P falciparum* infections acquired in areas of known chloroquine resistance. Alternatives are mefloquine hydrochloride and quinidine gluconate for patients who cannot tolerate oral medication.

3. Primaquine Phosphate–Administer this agent with chloroquine to prevent relapses in patients with *P vivax* and *P ovale* infections. Give orally once daily for 14 days. Patients should be screened for glucose-6-phosphate dehydrogenase (G6PD) deficiency before primaquine is begun.

B. General Measures: Fluid therapy is most important. Urge oral intake and, if not satisfactory, give parenteral fluids. Control high fever. Treat anemia with iron.

Prophylaxis

Pregnant women from nonendemic areas should be discouraged from traveling to malarial areas. Although chloroquine can be given safely in standard prophylactic doses during pregnancy, other antimicrobials may be fetotoxic.

Since true prophylaxis (prevention of infection by the destruction of sporozoites) is unavailable for travelers to endemic areas, a drug is given that suppresses schizogony and clinical symptoms. The most commonly used suppressive drug is chloroquine, given orally each week, beginning 1 week before travel to an endemic area and continued for 4 weeks after return. Travelers to areas where *P ovale* and *P vivax* are endemic may also be given primaquine phosphate for 14 days after departure from the endemic region to prevent relapses. Be sure to rule out G6PD deficiency before beginning primaquine.

Falciparum malaria resistant to chloroquine is widespread in Southeast Asia, Indonesia, some islands of the South Pacific (including the Philippines and Papua New Guinea), and South America; it has been documented in the Indian subcontinent, East Africa, and parts of Panama. Chemoprophylaxis with chloroquine is not always effective in these areas. Chemoprophylaxis of travelers to areas with chloroquine-resistance is recommended with weekly mefloquine beginning 1 week before travel through 4 weeks after return. Alternatives when mefloquine is contraindicated include chloroquine prophylaxis (with or without proguanil) in combination with pyrimethamine-sulfadoxine (Fansidar); use for presumptive treatment of a febrile illness (while medical care is sought) and prophylaxis with doxycycline.

Caution: Pyrimethamine-sulfadoxine is contraindicated in patients with a history of sulfonamide or pyrimethamine intolerance, in pregnant women (at term), and in infants younger than 2 months. Severe, sometimes fatal, cutaneous reactions (such as Stevens-Johnson syndrome) have occurred; if any mucocutaneous signs or symptoms develop, *stop the drug immediately*.

Mefloquine is not recommended in the first trimester of pregnancy but may be considered later in pregnancy when satisfactory alternatives are unavailable. Mefloquine is also not recommended in patients with epilepsy or psychiatric disorders, in patients taking beta-blockers, or in young children. Since most malarial vectors are night biters, mosquito nets and chemical repellents in sleeping quarters are important preventive measures. While chemoprophylaxis and environmental engineering or chemical control of mosquito populations are currently the most feasible mass preventive measures, biologic control of mosquitoes and malarial vaccines are under investigation.

Persons who have traveled to areas endemic for malaria should seek medical care if they develop fever after return from their travel—even if they have taken prophylactic medication.

Prognosis

In most cases, the prognosis is excellent with proper therapy. In small infants, in the presence of malnutrition or chronic debilitating disease or with severe *P falciparum* disease, the prognosis is more guarded.

TRICHOMONIASIS

Trichomoniasis is caused by *Trichomonas vaginalis,* a flagellate protozoon. Infection is usually spread by sexual intercourse, often by an asymptomatic male carrier.

Clinical Findings

A. Symptoms & Signs: The symptoms are vaginitis and cervicitis with itching and a frothy discharge that is usually yellow–green with a characteristic "fishy" odor. Other symptoms may include abdominal pain and dysuria. Males may have urethritis or prostatitis. Trichomoniasis is very uncommon in patients before menarche. Infection is often asymptomatic.

B. Laboratory Findings: The diagnosis is usually made by visualization of the organism in a wet mount of vaginal secretions. Culture and serology are available but usually unnecessary.

Treatment

Treatment with oral metronidazole is most effective. The sexual partner should be treated concomitantly. Metronidazole should not be used in the first trimester of pregnancy; instead, clotrimazole may be used to reduce symptoms.

Prognosis

The prognosis for patients with vaginal trichomoniasis is excellent although reinfection or relapse may occur.

TOXOPLASMOSIS

Toxoplasma gondii, an obligate intracellular parasite, is found worldwide in humans and in many species of animals. The parasite is a coccidian of cats, the definitive host. Human infection occurs by ingestion of oocysts from cat feces, by ingestion of cysts in raw or undercooked meat, by transplacental transmission, or, rarely, by direct inoculation of trophozoites, as in blood transfusion.

Clinical Findings

A. Symptoms & Signs:

1. Congenital Toxoplasmosis–Congenital transmission usually occurs as a result of acute infection *during* pregnancy and may occur in any trimester. Infection has been detected in up to 1% of women during pregnancy; about 45% of women who acquire the primary infection during pregnancy and who are not treated will give birth to congenitally infected infants. Signs of congenital toxoplasmosis are present at birth in 10% of infected infants. The others may develop symptoms in the first months of life. Symptoms and signs of congenital toxoplasmosis include microcephaly, hydrocephalus, seizures, mental retardation, hepatosplenomegaly, jaundice, thrombocytopenia, pneumonitis, rash, fever, chorioretinitis, and cerebral calcification. Chorioretinitis is usually a late sequela of congenital infection, with symptoms first noted in the second or third decade of life.

2. Toxoplasmosis in the Immunocompromised Host–Toxoplasmosis may present as a disseminated disease, particularly in patients given immunosuppressive drugs; in patients with HIV infection; or in patients with lymphoreticular, hematologic, or other malignant diseases. Encephalitis and focal brain abscesses are the most common manifestations; pneumonitis and myocarditis may also occur.

3. Acquired Toxoplasmosis–

a. Fever, pharyngitis, and lymphadenopathy resembling infectious mononucleosis may occur, but with a more prolonged course (sometimes 2–6 months) and with intermittent exacerbations.

b. There may be febrile disease without symptoms or signs of specific organ system involvement. A transient morbilliform rash may appear. A prolonged and recurrent course is not uncommon.

c. Chorioretinitis, with acute onset in children or young adults, may be recurrent and prolonged (almost pathognomonic of toxoplasmosis).

B. Laboratory Findings: The WBC and differential count may resemble those of infectious mononucleosis (Chapter 10) or may be entirely normal. Various serologic tests are available to measure immunoglobulin G (IgG), immunoglobulin M (IgM), and immunoglobulin A (IgA) antibodies. A seroconversion or four-fold rise in IgG titer, a very high single IgG titer, or a positive IgM test will confirm the clinical diagnosis. To diagnose congenital infection, analyze maternal and neonatal sera simultaneously for IgG and IgM. A positive neonatal IgM (or IgA) or a very high or rising IgG level suggests the diagnosis of cong can be diagnosed occasionally by histologic examination of tissue or by detection of organisms, antigen, or DNA in bone marrow aspirates, CSF sediment, sputum, blood, and other tissue and body fluids. Only isolation from body fluids confirms acute infection; isolation from tissue may represent chronic infection.

Skull x-rays or computed tomographic scans of the head show intracranial calcifications in recovered congenital infection.

Treatment

Treatment is indicated in immunocompromised patients, in pregnant women with acute infection, in congenitally infected infants with or without symptoms, and in patients with acquired disease whose symptoms persist for > 2 weeks or who have active chorioretinitis.

A. Specific Measures:

1. Pyrimethamine, Folinic Acid, & Sulfadiazine–Treatment includes a combination of pyrimethamine, folinic acid (calcium leucovorin), and sulfadiazine. Duration of therapy is determined by the severity of illness; treatment is usually administered for one to several months. Pyrimethamine should not be used during the first trimester of pregnancy because it is teratogenic in animals. Alternatives include spiramycin and clindamycin.

2. Prednisone–For patients with chorioretinitis or CNS disease, prednisone may be used if disease is progressive or threatens the macula.

Prophylaxis in Pregnant Women

Pregnant women who are seropositive or who do not know their toxoplasmotic status should take measures to prevent infection: (1) Avoid contact with or wear gloves when handling potentially contaminated materials (eg, cat litter boxes) and wear gloves when gardening; (2) avoid eating raw or undercooked meat; (3) wash hands thoroughly after handling raw meat; (4) wash fruits and vegetables before consumption. These same precautions apply to the nonpregnant population, especially those who are immunosuppressed.

Prognosis

Most children with congenital toxoplasmosis who are asymptomatic or have only mild abnormalities in the first year of life will subsequently develop such sequelae as ophthalmologic and neurologic abnormalities. Early therapy appears to reduce the incidence of later sequelae. Children born with clinical evidence of congenital toxoplasmosis generally have severe long-term handicaps.

PNEUMOCYSTIS PNEUMONIA

Pneumocystis is an interstitial pneumonitis occurring in immunocompromised infants and children (eg, when receiving corticosteroids or cytotoxic drugs for neoplasms or transplantations, from inborn or acquired immunodeficiency, or related to malnutrition or prematurity). It has emerged as a major problem in patients with HIV infection. The causative organism, *P carinii,* has not been classified definitively, although it is commonly believed to be either a fungus related to the yeasts or a sporozoon. The organism occurs in many animal species. The roles of human–human and animal–human transmission are still unknown.

Clinical Findings

X-rays show an interstitial pneumonitis; physical signs may include tachypnea, dyspnea, cough, and fever. Onset may be acute and fulminant or subacute and gradual. Hypoxemia is characteristically present. The diagnosis may be established by lung biopsy, by demonstration of the organism in bronchoscopic brush biopsy specimens or washes, or in induced sputum specimens. Elevated serum lactate dehydrogenase is frequently seen in HIV-infected patients with *P carinii* pneumonia.

Treatment

A. Specific Measures: Trimethoprim-sulfamethoxazole is the treatment of choice and is given intravenously or orally. Parenteral pentamidine isoethionate is also an effective therapy, but it can have significant toxicities. New therapeutic regimens include atovaquone, clindamycin plus primaquine, and trimetrexate. Corticosteroids are an efficacious adjunctive therapy in HIV-infected patients with *P carinii* pneumonia.

B. General Measures: Oxygen and mechanical ventilation (if needed) are important supportive measures. The cause of impaired immunity should be eliminated if known and if possible.

Prophylaxis

Trimethoprim-sulfamethoxazole in subtherapeutic doses prevents infection in patients at risk if administered throughout the period of increased susceptibility. Other potentially useful prophylactic regimens include aerosolized pentamidine, intravenous pentamidine, oral pyrimethamine-sulfadoxine (Fansidar), dapsone, and dapsone-pyrimethamine.

Prophylaxis is provided to HIV-infected patients at high risk for *P carinii* pneumonia, including (1) patients with prior episodes; (2) patients with a low CD4 cell count (according to age-specific criteria in children and $< 200/mm^3$ or $< 20\%$ of lymphocytes in adolescents and adults); and (3) all HIV-infected children younger than 1 year.

METAZOAL DISEASES

Metazoal diseases are outlined in Table 11–5.

MYCOTIC INFECTIONS

Many of the systemic mycoses share a number of characteristics. Infection of humans occurs through inhalation of free-living fungal spores, which are present in the dust or soil in endemic areas. Primary pulmonary infections are usually mild or asymptomatic, and most infections have a tendency to heal, mainly through cellular immune mechanisms. Specific skin test results become positive after primary infection and remain positive throughout life. In a few specifically predisposed persons, the disease progresses after primary infection (immediately or after a latent period) and may disseminate and involve many organs—and may be fatal. Dissemination may occur years after primary infection if the person is subsequently immunosuppressed by disease (eg, lymphoma) or drugs.

SYSTEMIC MYCOSES

Systemic mycoses are outlined in Table 11–6.

CANDIDIASIS

Candida albicans and other *Candida* species are found in the normal flora of human mucous membranes, especially in the respira-

Table 11–5. Diseases caused by helminths.

Agent	Geographic Prevalence	Definitive Host (Mature Worms)	Intermediate Host (Larval Stages)	Route of Human Infection	Directly Communicable Human-to-Human	Eggs in Human Feces	Stage of Parasite Causing Disease	Pathology	Diagnostic Tests	Specific Treatment
Ancylostoma braziliense, A caninum (cat and dog hookworm)	Southern United States	Cats, dogs	Humans	Invasion of larvae in soil through skin	No	No	Larva	Cutaneous larva migrans, with serpiginous skin eruption at site of entry	Clinical diagnosis	Self-limited; freezing, thiabendazole, albendazole
Ancylostoma duodenale, Necator americanus (hookworm)	Tropics and subtropics, Europe, Asia	Humans	—	Larvae in soil enter through skin	Yes	Yes	Larva in skin and lungs; adult in bowel	Dermatitis and pneumonitis in larval stage; anemia, melena, anorexia from adult worm in bowel	Detection of ova in stool	Mebendazole, pyrantel pamoate
Ascaris lumbricoides (roundworm)	Tropics and areas with poor sanitation	Humans	—	Ingestion of eggs in soil	Yes (via soil)	Yes	Larva in lungs; adult in bowel	Pneumonitis in larval stage; adult worm may cause intestinal obstruction, abdominal pain, peritonitis	Detection of ova or adult worms in stool	Pyrantel pamoate, mebendazole, albendazole
Diphyllobothrium latum (fish tapeworm)	Worldwide	Humans, other mammals	Copepods, fish	Ingestion of fish containing larval worms	No	Yes	Adult	Vitamin B_{12} deficiency; intestinal irritation; anemia	Identification of ova or proglottids in stool	Niclosamide, praziquantel

(*continued*)

Table 11–5. Diseases caused by helminths (*continued*).

Agent	Geographic Prevalence	Definitive Host (Mature Worms)	Intermediate Host (Larval Stages)	Route of Human Infection	Directly Communicable Human-to-Human	Eggs in Human Feces	Stage of Parasite Causing Disease	Pathology	Diagnostic Tests	Specific Treatment
Dipylidium caninum (dog tapeworm)	Worldwide	Dogs, cats, humans	Fleas	Ingestion of fleas containing larval worms	No	Yes	Adult	Intestinal irritation	Identification of ova in stool	Niclosamide, praziquantel
Echinococcus granulosus (unilocular hydatid cyst)	Scattered foci worldwide	Dogs, wolves	Domestic and wild herbivores (including sheep), humans	Ingestion of worm eggs from canine feces	No	No	Larva (hydatid)	Circumscribed unilocular cysts in lung, liver, other viscera	History, radiographs, serology, biopsies	Surgical removal, albendazole, mebendazole
Echinococcus multilocularis (alveolar hydatid cyst)	Northern hemisphere	Foxes, dogs	Field rodents, humans	Ingestion of worm eggs from canine feces	No	No	Larva (hydatid)	Invasive multilocular cysts in liver	History, radiographs, biopsies, serology	Surgical removal, albendazole, mebendazole
Enterobius vermicularis (pinworm)	Worldwide	Humans	—	Ingestion of eggs on clothing, in food, in dust, etc	Yes	Yes	Adult female	Anal irritation and itching; vaginal inflammation; abdominal pain	Scotch tape exam under microscope	Pyrantel pamoate, mebendazole, albendazole

Hymenolepsis nana (dwarf tapeworm)	Worldwide in warm climates	Humans, rodents	Humans, rodents	Ingestion of worm eggs from human feces or infected insects	Yes	Yes	Adult	Intestinal irritation	Detection of ova in stool	Niclosamide, praziquantel
Schistosoma mansoni, S japonicum, S haematobium (blood flukes)	*S mansoni*—tropics *S japonicum*—Far East, Southeast Asia *S haematobium*—Africa, Asia	Humans	Snails	Invasion of skin by cercariae in bodies of fresh water	No	Yes (*S mansoni* and *S japonicum*) (*S haematobium* in urine)	Adult	Maturation in veins draining intestines (*S mansoni, S japonicum*) or bladder (*S haematobium*) producing enteritis, hepatomegaly, portal hypertension, or hematuria and urinary symptoms	Demonstration of eggs in stool or urine, tissue biopsies, serology	Praziquantel, oxamniquine (*S mansoni*), metrifonate (*S haematobium*), surgical removal
Strongyloides stercoralis (thread worms)	Tropics and subtropics	Humans, dogs, cats	—	Larvae enter through skin	Yes	Rare	Larva and adult	Pneumonitis and intestinal irritation, disseminated disease in immunocompromised host	Identification of larvae in stool or duodenal aspirate; serology	Thiabendazole, ivermectin
Taenia saginata (beef tapeworm)	Africa, Central and South America, Europe, Asia	Humans	Cattle	Ingestion of beef containing larval worms	No	Yes	Adult	Intestinal irritation with nausea, diarrhea	Identification of ova or proglottids in stool, serology	Niclosamide, praziquantel

(*continued*)

Table 11–5. Diseases caused by helminths (*continued*).

Agent	Geographic Prevalence	Definitive Host (Mature Worms)	Intermediate Host (Larval Stages)	Route of Human Infection	Directly Communicable Human-to-Human	Eggs in Human Feces	Stage of Parasite Causing Disease	Pathology	Diagnostic Tests	Specific Treatment
Taenia solium (pork tapeworm)	Africa, Asia, Central and South America, Europe	Humans	Hogs	Ingestion of pork containing larval worms	Yes	Yes	Adult	Intestinal irritation with nausea, diarrhea	Identification of ova or proglottids in stool, serology	Niclosamide, praziquantel
			Humans	Ingestion of worm eggs from human feces	No	No	Larva (cysticercus)	Cysticercosis with lesions in muscles, brain, viscera, eyes. Seizures common	Muscle or brain biopsy; computed tomography scan of head; serology	Surgical removal, praziquantel, albendazole, corticosteroids
Toxocara canis, *T cati* (dog and cat roundworm)	North America, Europe	Dogs, cats	Humans	Ingestion of worm eggs in soil	No	No	Larva	Visceral larva migrans with fever, systemic symptoms, and infection of eyes, lung, heart, brain, liver	Eosinophilia, organ biopsy, serology	Thiabendazole, diethylcarbamazine, albendazole, corticosteroids. Corticosteroid injection and surgery for ocular disease

Trichinella spiralis (trichina worm)	Worldwide	Hogs, bears, rats	Hogs, bears, rats, humans	Ingestion of larvae in meat	No	No	Larva in muscle, heart, and brain	Encystment of larvae in tissue (especially muscle) causes necrosis and inflammation. Symptoms produced include diarrhea, myalgia, fever, periorbital edema, urticaria, headache, myocardial failure	Eosinophilia, serology, muscle biopsy, examination of suspect meat	Mebendazole, thiabendazole, corticosteroids
Trichuris trichiura (whipworm)	Worldwide	Humans	—	Ingestion of eggs in soil	Yes (via soil)	Yes	Adult	Adult worm in mucosa of colon usually produces no reactions or symptoms. Abdominal pain, colitis, and rectal prolapse may occur in severe infections	Identification of ova in stool	Mebendazole, albendazole

(*continued*)

Table 11–5. Diseases caused by helminths (*continued*).

Agent	Geographic Prevalence	Definitive Host (Mature Worms)	Intermediate Host (Larval Stages)	Route of Human Infection	Directly Communicable Human-to-Human	Eggs in Human Feces	Stage of Parasite Causing Disease	Pathology	Diagnostic Tests	Specific Treatment
Wuchereria bancrofti, Brugia malayi, B timori (filaria)	Tropics, subtropics	Humans	Humans, mosquitoes	Bite by infected mosquito	No	No	Adult	Inflammation or obstruction of lymphatics, producing lymphadenopathy, lymphangitis, edema of extremities and genitalia	Demonstration of microfilariae in blood, tissue biopsies, serology	Diethylcarbamazine citrate, ivermectin, corticosteroids, surgical removal, treatment of superinfections

Table 11–6. Systemic mycoses.

Disease	Organism	Geographic Prevalence/ Environmental Source	Primary Infection	Disseminated Disease	Laboratory Findings	Treatment
Aspergillosis	*Aspergillus fumigatus, Flavus niger*	Worldwide/Soil, vegetable matter	Allergic bronchopulmonary disease; episodic fever, wheezing, fleeting infiltrates. Fungus balls in prior pulmonary cavities	Sinusitis; pulmonary infection; bone abdominal viscera, CNS involvement	Positive smears and cultures. Allergic bronchopulmonary aspergillosis; elevated IgE and eosinopils, positive precipitins to *Aspergillus*, airway colonization	Amphotericin B ± flucytosine or rifampin; itraconazole. Surgical excision. Corticosteroids for allergic bronchopulmonary disease
Blastomycosis (North American)	*Blastomyces dermatitidis*	Central and southeastern United States, Central and South America/ Soil	Cutaneous ulcerating papule and abscesses. Pulmonary densities, empyema, and lymph node enlargement	Cough, fever, cutaneous lesions; brain abscesses; abdominal viscera, bone, muscle involvement	Positive smears, cultures, and antibody	Amphotericin B; ketoconazole; itraconazole
Coccidioidomycosis	*Coccidioides immitis*	Southwestern United States, Mexico, Central and South America/Soil	Asymptomatic or fever, headache, myalgias, arthralgias, rash, URI, bronchitis, ± pulmonary cavity	Pneumonia, empyema, osteomyelitis, soft tissue infection, abdominal visceral involvement, meningitis	Elevated ESR, WBC, CXR densities and enlarged nodes. Positive antibody, smears and cultures	Primary infection: therapy generally not required. Disseminated disease: Amphotericin B; ketoconazole; fluconazole (especially meningitis); itraconazole. Surgical excision; CSF shunting

(*continued*)

Table 11–6. Systemic mycoses (*continued*).

Disease	Organism	Geographic Prevalence/ Environmental Source	Primary Infection	Disseminated Disease	Laboratory Findings	Treatment
Cryptococcosis	*Cryptococcus neoformans*	Worldwide/Soil, bird feces	Asymptomatic or influenza-like. Pulmonary consolidation	Meningitis, bone or skin lesions, lymphadenopathy	CSF inflammation, positive CSF antigen, India ink smear, culture	Primary infection: generally does not require treatment. Disseminated disease: amphotericin B, with flucytosine; fluconazole
Histoplasmosis	*Histoplasma capsulatum*	Central and southern United States/Dust, soils, bird and bat feces	Asymptomatic or influenza-like. Also, pneumonitis, fever, cough, chest pain, and enlarged nodes, liver, spleen	Fever, anemia, adenopathy, hepatomegaly, splenomegaly, pneumonitis, bone lesions, cutaneous granulomas. Chronic pulmonary histoplasmosis may occur	Leukopenia, anemia, elevated ESR. Positive smears (bone marrow and other tissues), cultures, and antibody. CXR consolidations ± calcifications	Primary infection: generally not required. Disseminated disease: amphotericin B, ketoconazole; itrazonazole; fluconazole (meningitis); surgical excision
Paracoccidioidomycosis (South American Blastomycosis)	*Paracoccidioides brasiliensis*	Central and South America/Soil	Skin and mucous membrane granulomatous lesions	Spread to lymph nodes, gut, lungs, other viscera	Positive smears, cultures, and antibody	Ketoconazole; miconazole; amphotericin B; itraconazole
Sporotrichosis	*Sporothrix schenckii*	Worldwide/Plant matter	Subcutaneous nodules and ulcers, with spread along lymphatics	Spread to bones, joints, lungs, brain uncommon	Positive smears and cultures from lesions (drainage or biopsy)	Itraconazole; potassium iodide; amphotericin B

CNS = central nervous system; CSF = cerebrospinal fluid; CXR = chest x-ray; ESR = erythrocyte sedimentation rate; IgE = immunoglobulin E; URI = upper respiratory tract infection.

tory, gastrointestinal, and female genital tracts. In these locations, *Candida* may proliferate and produce local lesions; also, *Candida* may disseminate from these locations.

Clinical Findings

A. Symptoms & Signs: Moist, warm, eroded skin in intertriginous areas, the diaper area, or nails is subject to acute and chronic surface infection. Mucous membranes of the mouth (thrush) and vagina (vaginitis) are made more susceptible to overgrowth of *Candida* by use of antimicrobial agents that suppress normal flora or by use of corticosteroids. Rarely, *Candida* invades tissues or the bloodstream—for example, in patients with indwelling catheters, immunodeficiency, leukemia, parenteral drug abuse, or prematurity—and may cause progressive systemic disease, including pneumonia, endocarditis, meningitis, renal lesions, and involvement of other organs.

B. Laboratory Findings: Diagnosis is based on visualization of yeast and pseudohyphae in material from lesions or infected tissues or on culture of *Candida* from blood, CSF, urine, or involved organs.

Treatment

Treatment consists of keeping local lesions dry and applying topical nystatin, clotrimazole, gentian violet, miconazole, amphotericin B, or other antifungal agents. Ketoconazole and fluconazole have proved effective in many cases of esophageal candidiasis and chronic mucocutaneous disease. Intravenous treatment with amphotericin B is the approach of choice for systemic infections. Oral flucytosine is added for synergy in severe infections. Therapy is usually prolonged (weeks to months; precise duration is highly individual and varies according to the patient's immune status and *Candida* species). Fluconazole is useful for esophagitis, refractory thrush, candidemia, and some cases of disseminated disease.

Prognosis

The prognosis is good for patients with local lesions but guarded for those with systemic dissemination.

12 | Skin

Joseph G. Morelli, MD, &
William L. Weston, MD

Differential diagnosis in dermatology is based on the external appearance of the skin lesion. It is therefore important to identify the color, texture, or other features of a lesion with completeness and precision. Identification of a skin lesion begins with noting its **primary** appearance; then **secondary** changes; **color; configuration;** and **distribution**.

TERMINOLOGY

Primary Lesions (First Appearance of Lesion)

A. Macule: A **macule** is any circumscribed color change in the skin that is even with the skin surface. Examples: white (vitiligo), brown (café-au-lait spot), or purple (petechia) macules.

B. Papule: Papules are solid, elevated lesions smaller than 1 cm in diameter with pointed, rounded, or flat tops. Examples: acne, warts, small lesions of psoriasis.

C. Plaque: A solid, circumscribed area greater than 1 cm in diameter, usually flat-topped. Example: psoriasis.

D. Vesicle: A circumscribed, elevated lesion less than 1 cm in diameter and containing clear serous fluid. Example: blisters of herpes simplex.

E. Bulla: A circumscribed, elevated lesion greater than 1 cm in diameter and containing clear serous fluid. Examples: bullous erythema multiforme; pemphigus.

F. Nodule: A **nodule** is a deep-seated mass with indistinct borders elevating the overlying epidermis. Examples: tumors, granuloma annulare. If a nodule moves with the skin on palpation, it is **intradermal**; if the skin moves over the nodule, it is **subcutaneous**.

G. Wheal: A circumscribed, flat-topped, firm elevation of skin resulting from tense edema of the papillary dermis. Example: urticaria.

Secondary Changes in Lesions

A. Pustule: A vesicle containing a purulent exudate. Examples: acne, folliculitis, chickenpox.

B. Scales: Dry thin plates of keratinized epidermal cells (stratum corneum). Examples: psoriasis, ichthyosis, dandruff.

C. Lichenification: Dry leathery thickening of the skin with deep and exaggerated skin lines and a shiny surface resulting from chronic rubbing of the skin. Example: atopic dermatitis.

D. Erosion & Oozing: Lesion consists of a moist, circumscribed, slightly depressed area representing a blister base with the roof of the blister removed. Examples: burns, impetigo. Most oral blisters present as erosions.

E. Crust: Dried exudate of plasma on the surface of the skin following acute dermatitis. Example: poison ivy.

F. Fissure: A linear split in the skin extending through the epidermis into the dermis. Example: angular cheilitis.

G. Scar: A flat, raised, or depressed area of fibrotic replacement of dermis or subcutaneous tissue. Examples: acne scar, burn scar, postsurgical scar.

H. Atrophy: Depression of the skin surface due to thinning of one or more layers of skin.

Color

A lesion should be described as red, yellow, brown, tan, or blue. Particular attention should be given to the blanching of red or brown lesions (eg, petechiae).

Configuration

Clues to diagnosis may be obtained from the characteristic morphologic arrangement of primary or secondary lesions.

A. Annular (circular): Annular nodules represent granuloma annulare; annular papules are more apt to be caused by dermatophyte infections.

B. Linear (straight line): Linear papules represent lichen striatus; linear vesicles, incontinentia pigmenti; linear papules with burrow, scabies.

C. Grouped: Grouped vesicles occur in herpes simplex or zoster.

Distribution

It is useful to note whether the eruption is generalized, acral (hands, feet, buttocks, or face), or localized to a specific skin region.

Description of Skin Lesions

Skin lesions are described in reverse order from that of their identification. One begins with distribution, followed by configuration, color, secondary changes, and then primary lesion; eg, guttate psoriasis could be described as generalized discrete, red, scaly papules.

DISORDERS OF THE SKIN IN NEWBORNS

No treatment is *required* for any of these transient disorders, although treatment may be given as noted below.

Milia

Milia (multiple white papules 1 mm in diameter scattered over the forehead, nose, and cheeks) are present in up to 40% of newborn infants. Histologically, milia represent superficial epidermal cysts filled with keratinous material associated with the developing pilosebaceous follicle. Their intraoral counterparts are called **Epstein's pearls** and are even more common than facial milia. All these cystic structures rupture spontaneously and exfoliate their contents.

Sebaceous Gland Hyperplasia

Prominent yellow macules at the opening of each pilosebaceous follicle, distributed predominantly over the nose, represent overgrowth of sebaceous glands in response to the same androgenic stimulation that occurs in adolescence.

Acne Neonatorum

Open and closed comedones, erythematous papules, and pustules identical in appearance to adolescent acne may occur over the forehead, cheeks, and chin of neonates. The lesions may be present at birth but usually do not appear until 3–4 weeks of age. Spontaneous resolution occurs over a period of 6 months to a year. Rarely, neonatal acne may be a manifestation of a virilizing syndrome.

Harlequin Color Change

A cutaneous vascular phenomenon unique to neonates occurs when the infant (particularly one of low birth weight) is placed on one side. The dependent half develops an erythematous flush with a sharp demarcation at the midline, and the upper half of the body becomes pale. The color changes usually subside within a few seconds after the infant is placed supine but may persist for as long as 20 minutes.

Mottling

A lacelike pattern of dilated cutaneous vessels appears over the extremities and often on the trunk of neonates exposed to lowered room temperature. This feature is transient and usually disappears completely upon rewarming.

Erythema Toxicum

Up to 50% of term infants develop **erythema toxicum**. Usually at 24–48 hours of age, blotchy erythematous macules 2–3 cm in diameter appear, most prominently on the chest but also on the back, face, and extremities. The macules are occasionally present at birth, and rarely have their onset after 4–5 days of life. The lesions vary in number from 2–3, up to as many as 100. Incidence is much higher in term infants than in premature ones. The macular erythema may fade within 24–48 hours or may progress to urticarial wheals in the center of the macules or, in 10% of cases, pustules. Examination of a Wright-stained smear of the lesion will reveal numerous eosinophils. This may be accompanied by peripheral blood eosinophilia of up to 20%. All the lesions fade and disappear by 5–7 days. A similar eruption in black newborns has a neutrophilic predominance and results in hyperpigmentation.

Sucking Blisters

Bullae, either intact or in the form of an erosion representing a blister base without inflammatory borders, may occur over the forearms, wrists, thumbs, or upper lip of neonates. The blisters presumably result from vigorous sucking in utero. They resolve without complications.

Miliaria (Heat Rash)

Obstruction of the eccrine sweat ducts occurs often in neonates; it produces one of two clinical pictures depending upon the level of obstruction. **Miliaria crystallina** is characterized by tiny (1–2 mm) superficial grouped vesicles without erythema over intertriginous areas and adjacent skin (eg, neck and upper chest). Obstruction occurs in the stratum corneum portion of the eccrine duct. More commonly, obstruction of the eccrine duct deeper in the epidermis results in erythematous grouped papuls in the same areas and is called **miliaria rubra**. Rarely, the papules may progress to pustules. Heat and high humidity predispose to eccrine duct pore closure. Removal to a cooler environment is the treatment of choice.

Subcutaneous Fat Necrosis

Reddish or purple, sharply circumscribed, firm nodules occurring over the cheeks, buttocks, arms, and thighs and occurring between day 1 and day 7 in infants represent subcutaneous fat necrosis. Cold injury is thought to play an important role. These lesions resolve spontaneously over a period of weeks, although like all instances of fat necrosis they may calcify.

BIRTHMARKS

Birthmarks may involve an overgrowth of one or more of any of the normal components of skin: pigment cells, blood vessels, lymph vessels, etc. A **nevus** is a hamartoma of highly differentiated cells that retain their normal function.

1. PIGMENT CELL BIRTHMARKS

Mongolian Spot

A blue-black macule found over the lumbosacral area in 90% of Native American, black, and Oriental infants is called a **mongolian spot**. These spots are occasionally noted over the shoulders and back and may extend over the buttocks. Histologically, they consist of spindle-shaped pigment cells located deep within the dermis. The lesions fade somewhat with time, but some traces may persist into adult life.

Café-au-Lait Spot

A café-au-lait spot is a light brown oval macule (dark brown on black skin) that may be found anywhere on the body. Ten percent of white and 22% of black children have café-au-lait spots greater than 1.5 cm in their longest diameter. These lesions persist throughout life and may increase in number with age. The presence of 6 or more café-au-lait macules greater than 1.5 cm in their longest diameter may be suggestive of neurofibromatosis. Patients with **Albright's syndrome** also have increased numbers of café-au-lait macules.

Congenital Melanocytic Nevus

An irregular dark brown to black plaque represents a **pigmented nevus**. Nevi over 10 cm in diameter are classified as **giant congenital pigmented nevi**. Often the lesions are of such size as to cover the entire trunk ("bathing suit" nevi). Transformation to melanoma has been reported in as many as 10% of cases in some series, although the true incidence is probably somewhat lower. Malignant change prior to puberty is rare for small congenital melanocytic nevi, but can occur at birth or at any time in giant nevi.

2. VASCULAR BIRTHMARKS

Vascular Malformations

Vascular malformations can be divided into two types: those that are orange or light red (**salmon patch**) and those that are dark red or bluish red (**port wine stain**).

A. Salmon Patch: Salmon patches are light red macules found over the nape of the neck, upper eyelids, and glabella. Fifty percent of infants have such lesions over their necks. Eyelid lesions fade completely within 3–6 months; some but not all glabellar lesions fade by age 5 to 6. Those on the nape of the neck usually persist into adult life.

B. Port Wine Stain: Port wine stains are dark red or purple macules appearing in any location on the body. A port wine stain covering a large portion of the face, including the first and second branches of the trigeminal nerve, may be suggestive of **Sturge-Weber syndrome**, which is characterized by seizures, mental retardation, glaucoma, and hemiplegia. Most infants with unilateral port wine stains do *not* have Sturge-Weber syndrome.

Similarly, a port wine stain over an extremity may be associated with hypertrophy of the soft tissue and bone in that extremity (**Klippel-Trenaunay-Weber syndrome**).

Treatment of port wine stains consists of a vascular-specific pulsed dye laser. Infants as young as 2 weeks of age have been successfully treated.

Hemangioma

Only 20% of hemangiomas are present at birth; the others arise within the first 2–6 weeks of life. Hemangiomas present as either hypopigmented macules, fine telangiectasias, or red papules. Superficial hemangiomas remain bright red, whereas deep hemangiomas become pulpy blue nodules. Most hemangiomas contain both a superficial and deep component (mixed). Histologically, these are benign tumors of endothelial cells. Hemangiomas grow rapidly for the first year of life and then begin to involute spontaneously. Fifty percent resolve spontaneously by age 5; 70% by age 7; 90% by age 9; and the rest remain unresolved.

After resolution, hemangiomas leave redundant skin, hyperpigmentation, telangiectasia, and fibrofatty deposits. The most common complication is ulceration and secondary bacterial infection. Treatment of noninfected ulceration can be done with the pulsed dye laser. Infected lesions require oral antibiotics.

Major complications include: (1) thrombocytopenia due to platelet trapping within the lesion (**Kasabach-Merritt syndrome**); (2) airway obstruction (hemangiomas of the head and neck are often associated with subglottic hemangiomas); (3) visual obstruction (with resulting amblyopia); and (4) cardiac decompensation (high output failure). In these instances, the treatment of choice is prednisone, 1–2 mg/kg orally daily or every other day for 4–6 weeks. Interferon α-2a has been used to treat hemangiomas unresponsive to prednisone.

Lymphangioma

Lymphangiomas are malformations of lymphatic vessels and not tumors of lymphatic endothelium. Deep lymphangiomas are rubbery, skin-colored nodules commonly occurring in the parotid area (cystic hygroma). Superficial lymphangiomas are clear. They often result in grotesque enlargement of soft tissue.

Surgical excision is the only treatment presently available, although the results are not satisfactory. The large size of the defects is associated with severe scarring and frequent recurrences.

3. EPIDERMAL BIRTHMARKS

Epidermal Nevi

Linear or groups of linear, warty, papular, unilateral lesions represent overgrowth of epidermis. These areas may range from dirty yellow to brown, or may be darkly pigmented. The histologic features of the lesions include thickening of the epidermis and elongation of the rete ridges and hyperkeratosis.

If desired, surgical excision is the treatment of choice.

Nevus Comedonicus

The lesion known as **nevus comedonicus** consists of linear groups of widely dilated follicular openings plugged with keratin, giving the appearance of localized noninflammatory acne. The treatment of choice is surgical removal. If surgery is not feasible, topical retinoic acid is helpful.

Nevus Sebaceus

The **nevus sebaceus** of Jadassohn is a hamartoma of sebaceous glands and underlying apocrine glands that is diagnosed by the appearance at birth of a yellowish hairless smooth plaque in the scalp or on the face.

Histologically, nevus sebaceus represents an overabundance of sebaceous glands without hair follicles. At puberty, with androgenic stimulation, the sebaceous cells in the nevus divide, expanding their cellular volume, and synthesize sebum, resulting in a warty mass.

Because 15% of these lesions become basal cell carcinomas after puberty, excision before puberty is recommended.

4. CONNECTIVE TISSUE BIRTHMARKS

Connective tissue nevi are smooth skin-colored papules 1–10 mm in diameter grouped on the trunk. Histologically, connective tissue nevi show thickened, abundant collagen bundles with or without associated increases of elastic tissue. Large connective tissue nevi (**shagreen patches**) are associated with tuberous sclerosis, but most individuals with connective tissue nevi do not have tuberous sclerosis.

These nevi remain throughout life; no treatment is necessary.

HEREDITARY SKIN DISORDERS

The Ichthyoses

Ichthyosis is a term applied to several heritable diseases characterized by excessive scaling of the skin. The nomenclature of this group of diseases is confusing. Major categories are listed in Table 12–1. X-linked ichthyosis is related to cholesterol sulfatase deficiency.

Scaling can be treated with hydroxy acids (eg, 5% pyruvic, citric, lactic, or salicylic acid) in petrolatum applied once or twice daily. Restoring water to the skin is also very helpful.

Epidermolysis Bullosa

The diagnostic feature of this group of diseases is the formation of hemorrhagic blisters in response to even slight trauma. Epidermolyses can be divided into scarring and nonscarring types (Table 12–2).

Treatment usually consists of systemic antibiotics for infection and protective dressings of petrolatum or zinc oxide.

Incontinentia Pigmenti

Linear blisters in the newborn represent **incontinentia pigmenti**. The blisters are replaced by hypertrophic, linear, warty bands within

Table 12–1. Four major types of ichthyosis.[1]

Name	Age at Onset	Clinical Features	Histology	Inheritance
Ichthyosis with normal epidermal turnover				
Ichthyosis vulgaris	Childhood	Fine scales, deep palmar and plantar markings	Decreased to absent granular layer, hyperkeratosis	Autosomal dominant
X-linked ichthyosis	Birth	Palms and soles spared; thick scales that darken with age; corneal opacities in patients and carrier mothers	Hyperkeratosis	X-linked
Ichthyosis with increased epidermal turnover				
Epidermolytic hyperkeratosis	Birth	Verrucous, yellow scales in flexural areas and palms and soles	Hyperkeratosis, vacuolated reticular spaces in epidermis	Autosomal dominant
Lamellar ichthyosis	Birth; collodion baby	Erythroderma, ectropion, large coarse scales; thickened palms and soles	Hyperkeratosis, many mitotic figures	Autosomal recessive

[1] Reproduced, with permission, from Frost P, Weinstein GD; Ichthyosiform dermatoses. In: *Dermatology in General Medicine.* Fitzpatrick TB (editor). McGraw-Hill, 1971.

Table 12–2. Types of epidermolysis bullosa.

Name	Age at Onset	Clinical Features	Histology	Inheritance
Nonscarring types				
Epidermolysis bullosa simplex	Birth	Hemorrhagic blisters over the lower legs; cooling prevents blisters	Disintegration of basal cells	Autosomal dominant
Recurrent bullous eruption of the hands and feet (Weber-Cockayne syndrome)	First few years of life	Blisters brought out by walking	Cytolysis of suprabasal cells; keratotic cells	Autosomal dominant
Junctional bullous epimatosis (Herlitz disease)	Birth	Erosions on legs, oral mucosa; severe perioral involvement	Separation between plasma membrane of basal cells and PAS-positive basal lamina	Autosomal recessive
Scarring types				
Epidermolysis bullosa dystrophica, dominant	Infancy	Numerous blisters on hands and feet; milia formation	Separation of PAS-positive basal lamina; anchoring fibrils lost	Autosomal dominant
Epidermolysis bullosa dystrophica, recessive	Birth	Repeated episodes of blistering, secondary infection and scarring—"mitten hands and feet"	Separation below PAS-positive basal lamina; anchoring fibrils lost	Autosomal recessive

PAS = periodic acid-Schiff stain.

several months, followed by swirling brown areas of hyperpigmentation. Most cases are thought to be X-linked dominant, lethal in male children. Mental retardation and seizures have been reported in as many as 30% of cases in one series, but the true incidence is probably much lower.

COMMON SKIN DISEASES IN INFANTS, CHILDREN, & ADOLESCENTS

ACNE

Clinical Findings

The common forms of acne in pediatric patients occur in two age groups: neonates and adolescents. Neonatal acne is a response to maternal androgen, first appearing at 4–6 weeks of age and lasting until 4–6 months. It is characterized by inflammatory papules with all lesions in the same stage at the same time. The lesions appear primarily on the face, upper chest, and back, in a distribution similar to that seen in adolescent acne. It has been hypothesized but not proved that infants who have severe neonatal acne will develop severe adolescent acne.

The onset of adolescent acne is between ages 8 and 10 in 40% of children. Early lesions are usually limited to the face and are primarily closed **comedones** (whiteheads; see below). Eventually, 85% of adolescents will devlop some form of acne.

Acne occurs in sebaceous follicles, which, unlike hair follicles, have large, abundant sebaceous glands and usually lack hair. They are located primarily on the face, upper chest, back, and penis. Obstruction of the follicle opening produces the clinical lesion of acne. If the obstruction occurs at the follicular mouth, the lesion is characterized by a wide, patulous opening filled with a plug of stratum corneum cells. This is the **open comedo**, or blackhead. Open comedones are the predominant lesion seen in early adolescent acne. The black color does not result from dirt but from the oxidation of material within the stratum corneum cellular plug. Open comedones do not often progress to inflammatory lesions. **Closed comedones,** or whiteheads, are caused by obstruction just beneath the follicular opening in the neck of the sebaceous follicle, which produces a cystic swelling of the follicular duct directly beneath the epidermis. The stratum corneum continues to accumulate within the cystic cavity. The resultant lesion is an enlarging sphere just beneath the skin surface. Most authorities believe that closed comedones are precursors of inflammatory acne. If open or closed comedones are the predominant lesions on the skin in adolescent acne, it is called **comedonal acne**.

In typical adolescent acne, several different types of lesions are present simultaneously (eg, open and closed comedones and inflammatory lesions such as papules, pustules, and cysts). Inflammatory lesions may also rarely occur as interconnecting, draining sinus tracts. Adolescents with cystic acne require prompt medical attention, since ruptured cysts and sinus tracts result in severe scar formation. New acne scars are highly vascular and have a reddish or purplish hue. Such scars return to normal skin color after several years. Acne scars may be depressed beneath the skin level, raised, or flat to the skin. In adolescents with a tendency toward keloid formation, keloidal scars can occur following acne lesions, particularly over the sternal area.

Treatment

A. Topical Keratolytic Agents: Two classes of potent keratolytic agents are available: retinoic acid and benzoyl peroxide gel. These have been found to be the most efficacious agents in the treatment of acne. Either agent may be used once daily, or the combination of retinoic acid cream applied to acne-bearing areas of the skin once daily in the evening and a benzoyl peroxide gel applied once daily in the morning may be used. This regime will control 80–85% of cases of adolescent acne.

B. Topical Antibiotics: Topical antibiotics are less effective than systemic antibiotics and at best are equivalent in potency to 250 mg of tetracycline orally once a day. One percent clindamycin phosphate solution is the most efficacious of all topical antibiotics; 1.5% and 2% topical erythromycin solutions are effective; while 1% topical tetracycline solution is minimally effective.

C. Systemic Antibiotics: Antibiotics that are concentrated in sebum, such as tetracycline and erythromycin, are very effective in inflammatory acne. The usual dose is 0.5–1 g taken once or twice daily on an empty stomach (NPO 1 hour before or after the medication). Tetracycline or erythromycin should be continued for 2–3 months until the acne lesions are suppressed.

D. Oral Retinoids: An oral retinoid, 13-*cis*-retinoic acid (isotretinoin; Accutane), offers the most efficacious treatment of severe cystic acne. The precise mechanism of its action is unknown, but decreased sebum production, decreased follicular obstruction, decreased skin bacteria, and general antiinflammatory activities have been described. The initial dosage is 40 mg once or twice daily. This drug is not effective in comedonal acne or other mild forms of acne. Side effects include dryness and scaliness of the skin, dry lips, and, occasionally, dry eyes and dry nose. Up to 10% of patients experience mild, reversible hair loss. Elevated liver enzymes and blood lipids have been described. Isotretinoin is teratogenic. Use in young women of childbearing age is not recommended.

E. Other Acne Treatments: There is no convincing evidence that dietary management, mild drying agents, abrasive scrubs, oral vitamin A, ultraviolet light, cryotherapy, or incision and drainage have any beneficial effects in the management of acne.

F. Avoidance of Cosmetics & Hair Spray: Acne can be aggravated by a variety of external factors that result in further obstruction of partially occluded sebaceous follicles. Discontinuing the use of oil-based cosmetics, face creams, and hair sprays may alleviate the comedonal component of acne within 6–8 weeks.

Patient Education & Follow-up Visits

It is important to explain the mechanism of acne and the treatment plan to adolescent patients. Time should be set aside at the first visit to answer the patient's questions. Explain that there will not be much improvement for 6–8 weeks. Establish guidelines for ideal control, and explain that the best the patient might achieve is one or two new pimples a month. A written education sheet is most useful.

BACTERIAL INFECTIONS OF THE SKIN

Impetigo

Erosions covered by honey-colored crusts are diagnostic of impetigo. Staphylococci and group A streptococci are important pathogens in this disease, which histologically consists of superficial invasion of bacteria into the upper epidermis, forming a subcorneal pustule.

Although topical antibiotics may effect a clinical cure, parenteral penicillin or oral penicillin for 10 days is necessary to eradicate streptococci. The risk of nephrogenic strains varies considerably from area to area, but active treatment of patients and contacts with systemic penicillin will significantly reduce the incidence of acute glomerulonephritis in endemic areas. Dicloxacillin or other antistaphylococcal antibiotics are used when staphylococcal infection is suspected.

Ecthyma

Ecthyma is a firm, dry crust, surrounded by erythema, that exudes purulent material. It represents deep invasion by the streptococcus through the epidermis to the superficial dermis.

Cellulitis

Cellulitis is characterized by erythematous, hot, tender, ill-defined plaques accompanied by regional lymphadenopathy. Histologically, this disorder represents invasion of microorganisms into the lower dermis and sometimes beyond, with obstruction of local lymphatics. *Haemophilus influenzae, Streptococcus pneumoniae,* and *S pyogenes* are the most common offending organisms.

Septicemia is common, and treatment with the appropriate systemic antibiotic is indicated.

Folliculitis

A pustule at the follicular opening represents **folliculitis**. If the pustule occurs at eccrine sweat orifices, it is correctly called **poritis**. Staphylococci and streptococci are the most frequent causative pathogens.

Treatment consists of measures to remove follicular obstruction: either cool wet compresses for 24 hours or keratolytics (eg, those used for acne), as well as systemic antibiotics.

Abscess

An abscess occurs deep in the skin, at the bottom of a follicle or an apocrine gland, and is diagnosed as an erythematous, firm, acutely tender nodule with ill-defined borders. Staphylococci are the most common causative organisms.

Treatment consists of incision, drainage, and administration of systemic antibiotics.

Scalded Skin Syndrome

This entity consists of the sudden onset of bright red, acutely painful skin, most obvious periorally, periorbitally, and in the flexural areas of the neck, the axillae, the popliteal and antecubital areas, and groin. The slightest pressure on the skin results in severe pain and separation of the epidermis, leaving a glistening layer (the stratum granulosum of the epidermis) beneath. **Scalded skin syndrome** is caused by a circulating toxin (exfoliation) elaborated by group II staphylococci (Chapter 11).

In all the forms of this entity, the causative staphylococci may not be isolated from the skin but rather from the nasopharynx, an abscess, blood culture, etc.

Treatment consists of systemic administration of antistaphylococcal drugs (eg, dicloxacillin, 25–50 mg/kg/d orally; or methicillin, 200–300 mg/kg/d intravenously).

Bullous Impetigo

All impetigo is bullous, with blisters forming just beneath the stratum corneum. **Bullous impetigo,** however, is characterized by a border filled with clear fluid in addition to the usual erosion covered by a honey-colored crust. Staphylococci may be isolated from the lesions, and systemic signs of circulating exfoliation are absent. **Bullous varicella** is a disorder that represents bullous impetigo in varicella lesions.

Treatment with dicloxacillin, 25–50 mg/kg/d orally for 5–6 days, is effective. Application of cool compresses to debride crusts is a helpful symptomatic measure.

FUNGAL INFECTIONS OF THE SKIN

1. DERMATOPHYTE INFECTIONS

Essentials of Diagnosis

- Red, scaly, round lesions.
- Hair loss with or without scaling in tinea capitis.

General Considerations

Dermatophytes become attached to the superficial layer of the epidermis, nails, and hair, where they proliferate. They grow mainly within the stratum corneum and do not invade the lower epidermis or dermis. Dermatitis is caused by release of toxins from the dermatophytes, especially those whose natural hosts are animals or soil (eg, *Microsporum canis* and *Trichophyton verrucosum*. Fungal infection should be suspected with any red and scaly lesion.

Specific Diagnoses

A. Tinea Capitis (Ringworm): Thickened, broken-off hairs with erythema and scaling of underlying scalp are distinguishing features (Table 12–3). Pustule formation and a boggy fluctuant mass on the scalp occur in *M canis* and *T tonsurans* infections. The mass, called a **kerion**, represents an exaggerated host response to the organ-

Table 12–3. Clinical features of tinea capitis.

Most Common Organisms	Clinical Appearance	Microscopic Appearance in KOH
Trichophyton tonsurans (60%)	Hairs broken off 2–3 mm from follicle; "black dot"; no fluorescence	Hyphae and spores within hair
Microsporum canis (39%)	Thickened broken-off hairs that fluoresce yellow-green with Wood's lamp[1]	Small spores outside of hair; hyphae within hair
Microsporum audouini (1%)	Thickened, broken-off hairs that fluoresce yellow-green with Wood's lamp[1]	Small spores outside of hair; hyphae within hair

[1] Select fluorescent hairs for examination in KOH and culture.

ism. Fungal culture should be performed in all cases of suspected tinea capitis.

B. Tinea Corporis: Tinea corporis presents either as annular marginated papules with a thin scale and clear center or as an annular confluent dermatitis. The most common organisms are *T mentagrophytes* and *M canis*. The diagnosis is made by scraping thin scales from the border of the lesion, dissolving them in 20% potassium hydroxide (KOH), and examining the preparation for hyphae.

C. Tinea Cruris ("Jock Itch"): Symmetric, sharply marginated lesions in inguinal areas are seen with tinea cruris. The most common causative organisms are *T rubrum, T mentagrophytes*, and *Epidermophyton floccosum*. Scrapings taken from the border of the lesion should be examined for dermatophytes under the microscope with 20% KOH.

D. Tinea Pedis ("Athlete's Foot"): The diagnosis of tinea pedis in a prepubertal child must always be regarded with skepticism; atopic feet or contact dermatitis is a more likely diagnosis in this age group. Tinea pedis is seen most commonly in postpubertal males with blisters on the instep of the foot. Fissuring between the toes is occasionally seen. Microscopic examination of thin scales or the undersurface of the blister roof confirms the diagnosis.

E. Tinea Unguium (Onychomycosis): Loosening of the nail plate from the nail bed (onycholysis), producing a yellow discoloration, is the first sign of fungal invasion of the nails. Thickening of the distal nail plate then occurs, followed by scaling and a crumbly appearance of the entire nail plate surface. *T rubrum* and *T mentagrophytes* are the most common causes. The diagnosis is confirmed by KOH examination. Usually one or two nails are involved. If every nail is involved, psoriasis or lichen planus is a more likely diagnosis than fungal infection.

Treatment

Treatment of dermatophytosis is quite simple: If hair or nails are involved, griseofulvin is the systemic treatment of choice. Topical antifungal agents do not enter hair or nails in sufficient concentrations to clear the infection. The absorption of griseofulvin from the gastrointestinal tract is enhanced by a fatty meal; thus, whole milk or ice cream taken with the medication increases absorption. The dosage of griseofulvin is 20 mg/kg/d. With hair infections, the hair should be cultured every 4 weeks and treatment should be continued 6–8 weeks following the first negative culture; in nail infections, for a minimum of 3 months. Griseofulvin is supplied in capsules (250 mg) or as a suspension (125 mg/5 mL). It has few side effects, and has been used successfully even in neonates.

Tinea corporis, tinea pedis, and tinea cruris can be treated effectively with topical medication after careful inspection to make certain that the hair and nails are not involved. Treatment with an imidazole antifungal agent, applied twice daily for 3–4 weeks, is recommended.

2. TINEA VERSICOLOR

Tinea versicolor is a superficial infection caused by *Pityrosporon orbiculare* (also called *Malassezia furfur*), a yeastlike fungus. It typically causes polycyclic connected hypopigmented macules and very fine scales in areas of sun-induced pigmentation. In winter, the polycyclic macules appear reddish–brown.

Treatment consists of application of selenium sulfide (Selsun), full-strength suspension. Selenium sulfide should be applied to the whole body and left on overnight. Treatment can be repeated again in a week and then monthly thereafter. The topical agent tends to be somewhat irritating, and the patient should be warned about this side effect.

3. *CANDIDA ALBICANS* INFECTIONS

In addition to being a frequent invader in diaper dermatitis, *Candida albicans* may also infect the oral mucosa, where it appears as thick white patches with an erythematous base (**thrush**); the angles of the mouth, where it causes fissures and white exudate (**perleche**); and the cuticular region of the fingers, where thickening of the cuticle, dull red erythema, and distortion of growth of the nail plate suggest the diagnosis of **candidal paronychia**. *C albicans* is able to penetrate the stratum corneum layer and locally activate the complement system.

Nystatin (Mycostatin) is the drug of first choice for *C albicans* infections. It is supplied as an ointment or a cream, as an oral suspension, and as vaginal tablets. In diaper dermatitis, the cream form can be applied every 3–4 hours. In oral thrush, the suspension should be applied directly to the mucosa with the finger or a cotton-tipped applicator, since nystatin is not absorbed and acts topically. In candidal paronychia, nystatin is applied over the area, covered with an occlusive plastic wrapping, and left on ovrnight after the application is made airtight.

Imidazole creams are effective alternatives.

VIRAL INFECTIONS OF THE SKIN

Herpes Simplex

Grouped vesicles or grouped erosions suggest herpes simplex. Microscopic findings of epidermal giant cells after scraping the vesicle base with a No. 15 blade, smearing on a slide, and staining with Wright's stain (**Tzanck smear**) suggest herpes simplex or varicella zoster. Rapid immunofluorescence tests are also available. In infants, lesions due to herpes simplex type 1 are seen on the gingiva and lips, periorbitally, or on the thumb in thumb suckers. Recurrent erosions in the mouth are usually aphthous stomatitis (Chapter 13) rather than recurrent herpes simplex. Herpes simplex type 2 is seen on the genitalia and in the mouth in adolescents. Cutaneous dissemination of herpes simplex occurs in patients with atopic dermatitis (eczema herpeticum, Kaposi's varicelliform eruption).

In severe disseminated infection, oral acyclovir may be helpful.

Varicella Zoster

Grouped vesicles in a dermatome on the trunk or face suggest herpes zoster. Zoster in children may not be painful and usually has a mild course. In patients with compromised host resistance, the appearance of an erythematous border around the vesicles is a good prognostic sign. Conversely, large bullae without a tendency to crusting imply a poor host response to a virus.

Varicella appears in crops, and many different stages of lesions are present at the same time. Itching is usually the symptom, and cool baths as frequently as necessary are sufficient to relieve symptoms. In immunosuppressed children, intravenous or oral acyclovir should be considered.

Varicella, zoster, and herpes simplex lesions undergo the same progression of changes: papule, vesicle, pustule, crust, slightly depressed scar.

Virus-Induced Tumors

A. Molluscum Contagiosum: Molluscum contagiosum consists of umbilicated white or whitish-yellow papules found in groups on the genitalia or trunk. They are common in sexually active adolescents as well as in infants and preschool children. Molluscum contagiosum is a poxvirus that induces the epidermis to proliferate, forming a pale papule.

Removal of the lesion with a sharp curet is curative. Other therapies include liquid nitrogen, topical salicylic acid, podophyllin, or cantharidin.

B. Warts: Warts are skin-colored papules with irregular, rough (verrucous) surfaces. They are intraepidermal tumors caused by infection with human papilloma virus. This DNA virus induces the epidermal cells to proliferate, thus resulting in the warty growth. The different forms of warts are caused by distinct strains of papilloma viruses.

There is no ideal therapy for warts, and some types of therapy should be avoided because the recurrence rate of warts is high. Flat warts generally require no treatment. A good response to 0.05% tretinoin (Retin-A) cream, applied once daily for 3–4 weeks, has been reported.

The best treatment for the solitary common ("vulgaris") wart is cryotherapy, ie freezing it with liquid nitrogen. Liquid nitrogen is applied by drip until the wart turns completely white and stays white for 20–25 seconds. Small plantar warts usually need not be treated. Large and painful ones are treated most effectively by applying 40% salicylic acid plaster cut with a scissors to fit the lesion. The sticky brown side of the plaster is placed against the lesion, taped on securely with adhesive tape, and left on for 5 days. The plaster is then removed, and the white necrotic warty tissue can be gently rubbed off and a new salicylic acid plaster applied. This procedure is repeated every 5 days, and the patient is seen every 4 weeks.

Sharp scalpel excision, electrosurgery, laser surgery, and radiotherapy should be avoided, since the resulting scar often becomes a more difficult problem than the wart itself. In addition, the wart may recur in the area of the scar.

Condylomata acuminata (genital warts) are best treated with 25% podophyllum resin (podophyllin) in alcohol. This should be painted on the lesions and then washed off after 4 hours. Retreatment in 7–10 days may be necessary. A condyloma not on the vulvar mucous membrane but on the adjacent skin should be treated as a common wart and frozen.

For isolated warts and periungual warts, cantharidin (Cantharone) is effective and painless in children. It causes a blister and sometimes is difficult to control. An undesirable complication is the appearance of warts along the margins of the cantharidin blister. Cantharidin is applied to the skin, allowed to dry, and covered with occlusive tape (eg, Blenderm) for 24 hours.

No wart therapy is immediate and definitive, and recurrences are reported in 20–30% of cases even with the best care.

HUMAN IMMUNODEFICIENCY VIRUS (HIV) INFECTIONS

The onset of skin lesions in perinatally acquired AIDS is 4 months; it is 11 months in transfusion-acquired AIDS. Persistent oral candidiasis and recalcitrant candidal diaper rash are the most frequent cutaneous manifestations of infantile HIV infection. Severe herpetic gingivostomatitis, herpes zoster, and molluscum contagiosum are also seen, as are recurrent staphylococcal pyodermas, tinea of the face, and onychomycosis. A generalized dermatitis with seborrheic features is extremely common. In general, persistent, recurrent or extensive skin infections are suggestive of AIDS.

INSECT INFESTATIONS (Zoonoses)

Essentials of Diagnosis

- Discrete red papules, nodules, and S-shaped burrow on skin.
- Hand and foot involvement common.

Scabies

Scabies is suggested by the appearance of linear burrows about the wrists, ankles, finger webs, areolae, anterior axillary folds, genitalia, or face (in infants). Often, there are excoriations, honey-colored crusts, and pustules from secondary infection. Identification of the female mite or her eggs and feces is necessary to confirm the diagnosis. Slice off an unscratched papule or burrow with a No. 15 blade and examine it microscopically in immersion oil to confirm the diagnosis. In a child who scratches frequently, scrape under the fingernails. Examine the parent(s) for unscratched burrows.

Lindane (gamma benzene hexachloride 1%; Kwell) is an excellent scabicide. However, since lindane is concentrated in the central nervous system, and CNS toxicity from systemic absorption in infants has been reported, the following restricted use of this agent is recommended: (1) For adults and older children, one treatment of lindane lotion or cream applied to the entire body and left on for 4 hours, followed by a shower, is sufficient; (2) Infants tend to have more organisms and many more lesions; they may require retreatment in 7–10 days. All family members should be treated for scabies simultaneously. Elimite (permethrin) may be substituted for lindane in infants.

Pediculoses (Louse Infestations)

Excoriated papules and pustules with a history of severe itching at night suggest infestation with the human body louse. This louse may be discovered in the seams of underwear but not on the body. In the scalp hair, the gelatinous nits of the louse adhere tightly to the hair shaft. The pubic louse ("crabs") may be found crawling among pubic hairs, or blue-black macules may be found dispersed through the pubic region (**maculae ceruleae**). The pubic louse is sometimes seen in the eyelashes of newborns.

Lindane (gamma benzene hexachloride; Kwell) has been the treatment of choice. Since this agent is concentrated in the central nervous system and CNS toxicity from systemic absorption in infants has been reported, the following modification in its use is recommended: For head lice, a shampoo preparation is left on the scalp for 5 minutes and rinsed out thoroughly. The hair is then combed with a fine-tooth comb to remove nits. This treatment may be repeated in 7 days. Lindane cream or lotion applied to the body for 4 hours may be necessary for body lice, but washing the clothing in boiling water followed by ironing the seams with a hot iron usually eliminates the organisms. Elimite (permethrin) is also efficacious for lice.

Lindane cream or lotion applied to the pubic area for 24 hours is sufficient to treat pediculosis pubis. It may be repeated in 4–5 days.

Papular Urticaria

Papular urticaria is characterized by grouped erythematous papules surrounded by an urticarial flare and distributed over the shoulder, upper arms, and buttocks in infants. These lesions represent delayed hypersensitivity reactions to stinging or biting insects and can be reproduced by patch testing with the offending insect. Dog and cat fleas are the usual offenders. Less commonly, mosquitoes, lice, scabies, and bird or grass mites are involved. Sensitivity is transient, lasting 4–6 months.

The logical therapy is environmental, ie removal of the offending insect. Topical corticosteroids and oral antihistamines will control symptoms.

DERMATITIS
(Eczema)

Essentials of Diagnosis

- Red skin with disruption of skin surface.
- Vesicles, crusting, or lichenification may be present.

Atopic Dermatitis

Atopic dermatitis is not a clearly defined clinical entity but rather a general term for chronic superficial inflammation of the skin that can be applied to a heterogeneous group of patients. Many (not all) patients go through three clinical phases. In the first (infantile eczema), the dermatitis begins on the cheeks and scalp and frequently expresses itself as oval patches on the trunk, later involving the extensor surfaces of the extremities. The usual age at onset is 2–3 months; this phase ends at 18 months–2 years. Only one-third of all infants with atopic eczema progress to the second phase (childhood or flexural eczema), in which the dermatitis primarily affects the antecubital and popliteal fossae, the neck, the wrist, and sometimes the hands or feet. This phase lasts from age 2 years to adolescence. Some children will have involvement of the soles of their feet only, with cracking, redness, and pain (so-called "atopic feet"). Only a third of children with typical flexural eczema will progress to adolescent eczema, which is usually manifested by dermatitis only on the hands. Atopic dermatitis is quite unusual after age 30.

Atopic dermatitis has no known cause, and despite the high incidence of asthma and hay fever in these patients (39%) and their families (70%), evidence for allergy beyond this hereditary association is limited to testimonials. The evidence for food and inhalant allergens as causes of atopic dermatitis is not specific.

A few patients with atopic dermatitis have immunodeficiency with recurrent pyodermas, unusual susceptibility to herpes simplex and vaccinia virus, hyperimmunoglobulinemia E, defective neutrophil and monocyte chemotaxis, and impaired T-lymphocyte function.

A faulty epidermal barrier may predispose th patient with atopic dermatitis to itchy skin. Inability to hold water within the stratum corneum results in rapid evaporation of water, shrinking of the stratum corneum, and cracks in the epidermal barrier. Such skin forms an ineffective barrier to the entry of various irritants; indeed, it may be clinically useful to regard atopic dermatitis as a primary irritant contact dermatitis and simply tell patients that they have sensitive or hyperirritable skin. Chronic atopic dermatitis is frequently secondarily infected with *Staphylococcus aureus* or *Streptococcus pyogenes*.

A. Treatment of Acute Stages: Application of wet dressings and topical corticosteroids is the treatment of choice for acute, weeping atopic eczema. The topical steroid is applied 4 times daily and covered with wet dressings. Systemic antibiotics chosen on the basis of appropriate skin cultures may be necessary, since lesions in the acute stages are often secondarily infected with *S aureus* or streptococci.

B. Treatment of Chronic Stages: Treatment is aimed at avoiding irritants and restoring water to the skin. No harsh soaps or shampoos should be used, and the patient should avoid woolen or synthetic clothing, or any fabric with a rough surface. Restoring water to the skin is important in atopic dermatitis. This can be accomplished by two daily "drip-dry" baths, less than 5 minutes each, after which lubricating oils or ointments are applied. Moisturel is a useful lubricant. Plain petrolatum and lards are often too greasy and may cause considerable sweat retention. Liberal use of Cetaphil lotion as a soap substitute 3 or 5 times a day is also satisfactory as a means of lubrication. A bedroom humidifier is often helpful. Topical corticosteroids should be limited to the less potent ones. There is never any reason to use high-potency corticosteroids in atopic dermatitis. In superinfected atopic dermatitis, a course of systemic antibiotics for 10–14 days (erythromycin, 40 mg/kg/d; dicloxacillin, 50 mg/kg/d) is necessary.

Treatment failures in chronic atopic dermatitis are most often due to patient noncompliance. This is a frustrating disease for parent and child.

Nummular Eczema

Nummular eczema is characterized by numerous symmetrically distributed nummular (coin-shaped) patches of dermatitis, principally on the extremities. These patches may be acute, oozing, and crusted; or dry and scaling. The disease lasts 9 months to 2 years. The differential diagnosis should include tinea corporis and atopic dermatitis.

The same topical measures should be used as for atopic dermatitis, though treatment is often more difficult. The reasons for resistance to treatment are presently unknown.

Primary Irritant Contact Dermatitis (Diaper Dermatitis)

In general, a contact dermatitis can be classified under one of two categories: primary irritant or allergic eczematous. **Primary irritant** dermatitis develops within a few hours of exposure to the offending substance, reaches peak severity at 24 hours, and then disappears. **Allergic eczematous** contact dermatitis (see below) has a delayed onset of 18 hours, peaks at 48–72 hours, and often lasts as long as 2–3 weeks, even if exposure to the antigen is discontinued.

Diaper dermatitis, the most common form of primary irritant contact dermatitis seen in pediatric practice, is due to prolonged contact of the skin with urine and feces, which contain irritating chemicals (eg, urea and intestinal enzymes). The diagnosis of diaper dermatitis is based on the appearance of erythema and thickening of the skin in the perineal area and a history of skin contact with urine or feces. In 80% of cases of diaper dermatitis lasting more than 4 days, the affected area is colonized with *Candida albicans* even before the classic signs of a beefy red, sharply marginated dermatitis with satellite lesions appear.

Treatment consists of frequent diaper changes. Because rubber or plastic pants serve as occlusive dressings, preventing the evaporation of the irritant and enhancing its penetration into the skin, they should be avoided as much as possible. Air drying of the child's skin after cleansing is useful. Streptococcal infection should be included in the differential diagnosis.

Treatment of long-standing diaper dermatitis should include application of nystatin (Mycostatin) or an imidazole cream with each diaper change.

Lichen Simplex Chronicus (Localized Neurodermatitis)

Lichen simplex chronicus is a sharply circumscribed single patch of lichenification. When patients rub or scratch the affected area to relieve itching, the morphologic skin changes known as lichenification result.

The thickened lesions are treated with topical corticosteroids. Because the epidermal barrier has thickened, penetration of topical corticosteroids is poor. Penetration of the steroid can be enhanced in several ways. Airtight occlusion with plastic dressings (eg, Saran Wrap) overnight over topical corticosteroids is useful. Alternately, flurandrenolide (Cordran) tape impregnated with corticosteroids will penetrate the lesion. Covering the lesion will also prevent scratching the area.

Allergic Eczematous Contact Dermatitis (Poison Ivy Dermatitis)

Children often present with acute dermatitis with blister formation, oozing, and crusting. The blisters are often linear, with acute onset. Plants (especially poison ivy, poison sumac, and poison oak) cause most cases of allergic contact dermatitis in children; some is caused by wearing watches or costume jewelry made from base metal containing nickel. Allergic contact dermatitis has all the features of delayed type (T-lymphocyte-mediated) hypersensitivity. Although many substances may cause such a reaction, nickel sulfate (metals), potassium dichromate, and neomycin are the most common causes. The true incidence of allergic contact dermatitis in children is not known.

Treatment of contact dermatitis in localized areas is with topical corticosteroids. In severe generalized involvement, prednisone can be given, 1–2 mg/kg/d orally for 14–21 days.

Dry Skin (Asteatotic Eczema, Xerosis)

Newborns and older children who live in arid climates are susceptible to dry skin, characterized by large cracked scales with erythematous borders. The stratum corneum is dependent upon environmental humidity for its water; when the environmental humidity falls below 30% the stratum corneum loses water, shrinks, and cracks. These cracks in the epidermal barrier allow irritating substances to enter the skin, predisposing to dermatitis.

Treatment of xerosis consists of increasing the water content of the skin's immediate external environment. House humidifiers are very useful. Two 5-minute baths a day with immediate application of oil; or ointments (petrolatum, Aquaphor) applied after the bath will allow the skin to retain water. Frequent soaping of the skin impairs its water-holding capacity and exposes it to alkaline irritation. Frequent use of emollients (eg, Moisturel, Cetaphil, Eucerin, Lubriderm) should be a major part of therapy.

Keratosis Pilaris

Follicular papules containing a white inspissated scale characterize **keratosis pilaris**. Individual lesions are discrete and may be red. They are prominent on the extensor surfaces of the upper arms and thighs and on the buttocks and cheeks. In severe cases, the lesions may be generalized. Such lesions are seen frequently in children with dry skin and have also been associated with atopic dermatitis and ichthyosis vulgaris.

Treatment is with keratolytics such as topical lactic acid or retinoic acid cream followed by skin hydration.

Pityriasis Alba

White, scaly macular areas with indistinct borders are seen over extensor surfaces of extremities and on the cheeks in children. Sun tanning exaggerates these lesions. Histologic examination reveals a mild dermatitis. These lesions may be confused with tinea versicolor.

There is no satisfactory treatment; however, the patient's parents should be reassured that pityriasis alba is a benign disease that clears up without therapy.

COMMON SKIN TUMORS

Skin tumors can be grouped into two major categories. If the skin moves with the nodule on lateral palpation, the tumor is **intradermal**; if the skin moves over the nodule, it is **subcutaneous**. Table 12–4 lists common skin tumors according to these categories.

Granuloma Annulare

Circles or semicircles of nontender intradermal nodules found over the lower legs and ankles, the dorsum of the hands and wrists, and the trunk, in that order, suggest **granuloma annulare**. Histologically, the disease appears as a central area of tissue death (necrobiosis) surrounded by macrophages and lymphocytes.

Table 12–4. Common skin tumors.

Intradermal	**Intradermal (cont'd)**
Granuloma annulare	Lymphangioma
Dermatofibroma	Hemangioma
Epidermal inclusion cyst	Hair and sweat gland hamartomas
Neurofibroma	**Subcutaneous**
Neuroma	Lipoma
Leiomyoma	Rheumatoid nodule
Pylomatrixoma	Osteoma
Melanocytic nevus	
Pyogenic granuloma	

No treatment is necessary. Lesions resolve spontaneously within 1–2 years.

Pyogenic Granuloma

A rapidly growing dark red papule with an ulcerated and crusted surface appearing 1–2 weeks after trauma to the skin suggests **pyogenic granuloma**. Histologically, this represents excessive new vessel formation with or without inflammation (granulation tissue). Technically, the papule is neither pyogenic nor granulomatous but should be regarded as an abnormal healing response.

Vascular-specific pulsed dye laser or shave excision with electrocautery are the treatments of choice.

Epidermal Inclusion Cysts

Epidermal inclusion cysts are smooth, dome-shaped nodules in the skin that may grow to 2 cm in diameter. In infants they may be found about the eyes, and in older children and adolescents on the chest, back, and scalp. They are the most common superficial lumps in children.

Treatment, if desired, is surgical excision.

Keloids

Keloids are scars raised above the skin surface with many radial projections of scar tissue. They continue to enlarge over several years. They are often found on the face, earlobes, neck, chest, and back. Keloids show no racial predilection. Treatment includes intralesional injection with triamcinolone acetonide, 20 mg/mL, or excision and injection with glucocorticosteroids.

PAPULOSQUAMOUS ERUPTIONS

Pityriasis Rosea

Erythematous papules that coalesce to form oval plaques preceded by a large oval plaque with central clearing and a scaly border (the herald patch) establish the diagnosis of **pityriasis rosea**. The herald patch has the appearance of ringworm and is often treated as such. It appears 1–30 days before the onset of the generalized papular eruption. The oval plaques are parallel in their long axis and follow Langer's lines of skin cleavage. In whites, the lesions are primarily on the trunk. In blacks, lesions are primarily on the extremities. This disease is common in school-age children and adolescents, and is presumed to be viral in origin. It lasts about 6 weeks and may be pruritic for the first 7–10 days. The major differential diagnosis is secondary syphilis, and a Venereal Disease Research Laboratory (VDRL) test should be performed if syphilis is suspected. A chronic variant of this disease may last 2–3 years; it is called **chronic parapsoriasis** or **pityriasis lichenoides chronicus**. Five consecutive daily doses of erythema-producing ultraviolet (UVB) light will decrease the pruritus and the extent of the eruption. Exposing the skin to sunlight until a mild sunburn occurs (slight redness) will hasten the disappearance of lesions. Ordinarily, no treatment is necessary.

Psoriasis

Psoriasis is characterized by erythematous papules covered by thick white scales. Guttate (droplike) psoriasis is a common form in children that often follows an episode of streptococcal pharyngitis by 2–3 weeks. The sudden onset of small (3–8 mm) papules, seen predominantly over the trunk and quickly covered with thick white scales, is characteristic of guttate psoriasis. Chronic psoriasis is marked by thick, large (5–10 cm), scaly plaques over the elbows, knees, scalp, and other sites of trauma. Pinpoint pits in the nail plate are seen as well as yellow discoloration of the nail plate resulting from onycholysis. Thickening of all 20 fingernails and toenails is an uncommon feature. The sacral and seborrheic areas are commonly involved. Psoriasis has no known cause. It demonstrates active proliferation of epidermal cells with a turnover period of 3–4 days, in contrast to 28 days for normal skin. These rapidly proliferating epidermal cells produce excessive stratum corneum, giving rise to thick opaque scales. Papulosquamous eruptions that present problems of differential diagnosis are listed in Table 12–5.

All therapy for psoriasis is aimed at diminishing epidermal

Table 12–5. Papulosquamous eruptions in children.

Psoriasis	Pityriasis rubra pilaris
Pityriasis rosea	Tinea corporis
Secondary syphilis	Dermatomyositis
Lichen planus	Lupus erythematosus
Chronic papapsoriasis	

turnover time. Sunlight or artificial ultraviolet light (UVL) alone will produce some improvement. Coal tar enhances the effect of UVL and hastens the disappearance of psoriatic lesions. Bathing or shampooing with a product containing tar (eg, Balnetar) at night, followed by UVL the next day, may be sufficient in mild cases. In more severe psoriasis, 2% crude coal tar in petrolatum should be applied after the bath. The newer tar gels (Estargel, Psorigel) do not cause staining and are most efficacious. They are applied twice daily for 6–8 weeks.

Crude coal tar therapy is messy and stains bed clothes, and patients may prefer to use topical corticosteroids. Penetration of topical corticosteroids through the enlarged epidermal barrier in psoriasis requires the use of more potent preparations (eg, fluocinonide [Lidex] 0.05%, or triamcinolone [Aristocort, Kenalog], 0.05%, 4 times daily).

Anthralin therapy is also useful for localized psoriasis. Anthralin is applied to the skin for a short period (eg, 20 minutes once daily) and is then washed off with a neutral soap (eg, Dove). A 6-week course of treatment is recommended.

Scalp care using a tar shampoo (Polytar, Zetar, many others) requires leaving the shampoo on for 5 minutes, washing it off, and then shampooing with commercial shampoo to remove scales. It may be necessary to shampoo daily until scaling is reduced.

More severe cases of psoriasis are best referred to a dermatologist.

Lichen Planus

Lichen planus consists of pruritic, light purple, flat-topped, multi-sided papules, predominantly on the lower legs, penis, wrist, and arms. A white lacy pattern may be seen in the buccal mucosa. Pruritus may be severe.

If pruritus is mild, no treatment is necessary, and the disease will resolve in 6–12 months. With severe pruritus, a trial of antihistamines (eg, diphenhydramine, 5 mg/kg/d, or hydroxyzine, 2 mg/kg/d orally) is warranted. Rapid relief of pruritus and disappearance of the lesions can be achieved by administering prednisone, 1 mg/kg/d orally for 3–4 weeks.

HAIR LOSS
(Alopecia)

Hair loss in children (Table 12–6) imposes great emotional stress on the parent and physician—often more so than on the child. A 60% hair loss in a single area is necessary before hair loss can be detected clinically. Examination should begin with the scalp to determine if there are color changes or infiltrative changes. Hairs should be examined microscopically for breaking and structural defects and to see if growing or resting hairs are being shed. Placing removed hairs in mounting fluid (Permount) facilitates examination. Three disorders account for most cases of hair loss in children: (1) **alopecia areata;** (2) **tinea capitis;** and (3) **trichotillomania.** Tinea capitis may be distinguished from alopecia by fluorescence of infected hairs under Wood's light. **Trichotillomania** represents habitual voluntary pulling out of the hair secondary to emotional distress; the patient may be unaware of the habit. In trichotillomania, the patches of hair loss are irregular, often unilateral (on the same side as the patient's dominant hand), and contain growing hairs. Treatment depends on identification and resolution of the underlying emotional problem.

Table 12–6. Causes of hair loss in children.[1]

Hair loss with scalp changes
Nodules and tumors
Nevus sebaceus
Epidermal nevus
Thickening
Linear scleroderma (morphea) (en coup de sabre)
Burn
Atrophy
Lupus erythematosus
Lichen planus
Hair loss with hair shaft defects (hair fails to grow out enough to require haircuts)
Monilethrix—alternating bands of thin and thick areas
Trichorrhexis nodosa—nodules with fragmented hair
Trichorrhexis invaginata (bamboo hair)—intussusception of one hair into another
Pili torti—hair twisted 180 degrees, brittle
Pili annulati—alternating bands of light and dark pigmentation

[1] Price VH: Office diagnosis of hair shaft defects. *Cutis* 1975;**15**:231.

REACTIVE ERYTHEMAS

Erythema Multiforme

Erythema multiforme begins with fixed papules for 7–10 days that develop a dark center and then evolve into lesions with central blisters and characteristic target lesions (iris lesions) with concentric circles of color change. Primary injury is to endothelial cells, with later destruction of epidermal basal cells and blister formation. Erythema multiforme has sometimes been diagnosed in severe mucous membrane involvement. **Stevens-Johnson syndrome**, or **erythema multiforme major**, is the usual term for severe involvement of conjunctiva, oral cavity, and genital mucosa.

Many causes are suspected, particularly herpes simplex virus, drugs, and mycoplasma infections. Recurrent erythema multiforme is usually associated with reactivation of herpes simplex virus. Stevens-Johnson syndrome is more likely to be associated with drug reactions, especially to nonsteroidals (NSAIDs), anticonvulsants, and sulfonamides. In the mild form, spontaneous healing occurs in 10–14 days; however, Stevens-Johnson syndrome may last 6–8 weeks if untreated.

Treatment is symptomatic in uncomplicated erythema multiforme. Removal of offending drugs is an obvious necessary measure. Oral antihistamines such as hydroxyzine, 2 mg/kg/d orally, are useful. Cool compresses and wet dressings will relieve pruritus.

Erythema Nodosum

Erythema nodosum consists of painful erythematous nodules on the anterior lower legs. In streptococcal infections, coccidioidomycosis, histoplasmosis, and tuberculosis, the onset of erythema nodosum parallels the appearance of cell-mediated immunity. Streptococcal infections and birth control pills are the most common causes of this panniculitis in the United States.

Treatment consists of removal of the offending drug or eradication of infection. NSAIDs may be helpful.

Drug Eruptions (Dermatitis Medicamentosa)

Prescription medications may produce urticarial, morbilliform, scarlatiniform, or bullous skin eruptions. Urticaria may appear within minutes after drug administration, but most reactions begin 7–14 days after the drug is first given. Drugs commonly implicated in skin reactions are listed in Table 12–7.

Table 12–7. Common skin reactions associated with frequently used drugs.

Drug	Common Reactions
Aspirin	Urticaria rarely; purpuric eruptions.
Anti-infective agents Erythromycin	Urticaria.
Griseofulvin	Exanthematous eruptions; rarely, cold urticaria or photodermatitis.
Penicillin and synthetic penicillins	Serum sickness, urticaria, exanthematous eruptions, anaphylactic shock. Ampicillin causes a high incidence of exanthematous eruption in patients with infectious mononucleosis.
Streptomycin	Exanthematous eruptions, urticaria, stomatitis.
Sulfonamides	Urticaria, erythema multiforme, exanthematous eruptions, Stevens-Johnson syndrome, photodermatitis.
Tetracycline	Exanthematous eruptions, urticaria; rarely, bullous eruptions. Demeclocycline (Declomycin) can cause phototoxic reactions.
Antihistamines	Exanthematous eruptions, urticaria, photodermatitis.
Barbiturates	Maculopapular eruptions, urticaria, erythema multiforme, Stevens-Johnson syndrome, bullous eruptions.
Chlorothiazides	Exanthematous eruptions, urticaria, photodermatitis, hemosiderosis of the lower extremities, leading to development of petechiae with resultant pigmentation (Schamberg's phenomenon).
Cortisone and derivatives	Acneiform drug reactions on trunk—pustular, purpuric eruptions.
Insulin	Urticaria, erythema at injection site.
Iodides (cough syrups, antiasthma preparations)	Acneiform pustules over trunk, granulomatous reaction.
Phenytoin	Exanthematous eruptions usually in first 3 weeks of treatment; gingival hyperplasia, hypertrichosis; pseudolymphoma syndrome.

NAIL DISORDERS

Nail biting and *Candida paronychia* infection are the two most common causes of nail disorders. **Onychomycosis** (fungal infection of the nails) is uncommon. Nail pitting is associated with psoriasis and alopecia areata.

MISCELLANEOUS SKIN DISORDERS ENCOUNTERED IN PEDIATRIC PRACTICE

Aphthous Stomatitis

Recurrent erosions on the gums, lips, tongue, palate, and buccal mucosa are often confused with herpes simplex. A smear of the base of such a lesion stained with Wright's stain will aid in ruling out herpes simplex by the absence of epithelial giant cells. A culture for herpes simplex is also useful in this difficult differential diagnosis problem. The reader is referred to Chapter 13 for details of treatment.

Morphea (Linear Scleroderma)

Morphea is characterized by the appearance anywhere on the body of well-circumscribed, shiny, white, firmly adherent skin. It is particularly cosmetically deforming on the face. A light purple border is indicative of an early lesion or continuing activity. Skin biopsy reveals replacement of subcutaneous fat with thickened collagen fibers. The lesions tend to burn themselves out in 3–5 years. It may be difficult to differentiate morphea from **lichen sclerosis et atrophicus**, which has similar white patches that occur primarily on the upper back and genitalia. Histopathologic differentiation is often necessary but may be difficult.

No treatments have been proven effective in altering the course of either morphea or lichen sclerosis et atrophicus.

CUTANEOUS SIGNS OF SYSTEMIC DISEASE

Cutaneous signs of systemic disease in infants and children are outlined in Table 12–8.

Table 12–8. Cutaneous signs of systemic disease in infants and children.

Sign	Disease
Acnelike erythematous papules in mid-face and white ash-leaf macules on trunk, shiny thickened patch on back, subungual fibromas	Tuberous sclerosis
Pruritic blisters on buttocks, elbows, knees, and scapula	Dermatitis herpetiformis (celiac disease)
Café-au-lait macules	Neurofibromatosis, Albright's disease
"Chicken skin"—yellow rows of soft papules with wrinkled valleys in between in neck, axillae, groin	Pseudoxanthoma elasticum
"Dirty" neck and axillae (hyperpigmented, velvety flexural papules)	Acanthosis nigricans and obesity (endocrinopathies)
Eczematous erosions around the mouth, eyes, perineum, fingers, and toes; alopecia and diarrhea	Acrodermatitis enteropathica (zinc deficiency)
Erythematous isolated papules on elbows, knees, buttocks, face	Papular acrodermatitis (viral infection, rarely Hepatitis B)
Erythematous truncal macules with central pallor	Juvenile rheumatoid arthritis
Erythematous flat-topped papules over knuckles	Dermatomyositis
Hemorrhagic (1–2 mm) macules on lips, tongue, palms (epistaxis, gastrointestinal bleeding)	Hereditary hemorrhagic telangiectasia (Osler–Weber–Rendu syndrome)

(*continued*)

Table 12–8. Cutaneous signs of systemic disease in infants and children (*continued*).

Sign	Disease
Hyperpigmentation in palmar creases, knuckles, scars, buccal mucosa, linea alba, scrotum	Addison's disease
Linear or oval vesicles on hands or feet, erosions on soft palate, tonsillar pillars	Hand, foot, and mouth syndrome (Coxsackie A16 and others)
Palpable purpura	Vasculitis
Pigmented macules on oral mucosa	Peutz–Jeghers disease (benign small intestinal polyps)
Purpuric lakes	Purpura fulminans—disseminated intravascular coagulation
Purpuric pustules on hands and feet	Gonococcemia
Purpuric (petechiae) seborrheic dermatitis	Histiocytosis X
Epidermal inclusion cysts (multiple) on face and trunk	Gardner's syndrome (premalignant polyps of colon and rectum)
Stretchy skin; healing with large purple scars	Ehlers–Danlos syndrome
Tight, hard skin, telangiectases, hypo- and hyperpigmentation	Scleroderma
Ulcers with undermined, liquefying borders	Pyoderma gangrenosum (ulcerative colitis, regional enteritis, rheumatoid arthritis)
Vitiligo (completely depigmented macules with hyperpigmented borders)	Pernicious anemia, Hashimoto's thyroiditis, Addison's disease, diabetes mellitus
Yellow papules (lower eyelids, joints, palms)	Xanthomas, hyperlipidemias

Ear, Nose, & Throat | 13

Stephen Berman, MD

DISEASES OF THE EAR

INFECTIONS OF THE EAR

Infections of the ear represent a spectrum of diseases involving the structures of the outer ear (otitis externa), middle ear (otitis media), mastoid (mastoiditis), and inner ear (labyrinthitis).

OTITIS EXTERNA

General Considerations

Otitis externa is an inflammation of the skin lining the ear canals. The most common cause is accumulation of water in the ear, often from swimming or frequent showering, leading to maceration and desquamation of the lining. Swimming pools are more problematic than lakes because chlorine kills normal ear flora. Other causes of otitis externa are trauma to the ear canal from using cotton-tipped applicators or poorly fitted ear plugs; contact dermatitis due to hair sprays, perfumes, or self-administered ear drops; and chronic drainage from a perforated tympanic membrane. Infections are often caused by *Staphylococcus aureus* or *Pseudomonas aeruginosa.*

Clinical Findings

Otitis externa is marked by pain and itching in the ear, especially with chewing or pressure on the tragus. Movement of the pinna or tragus causes considerable pain. Drainage may be minimal. The ear canal may be grossly swollen, and the patient may resist any attempt to insert an ear speculum. Debris is noticeable in the canal. It is often impossible to visualize the tympanic membrane. Hearing is normal unless complete occlusion has occurred.

Treatment

Topical treatment usually suffices. The crucial initial step is removal of the desquamated epithelium and moist cerumen. This debris can be irrigated or suctioned out using warm Burow's solution (one packet of Domeboro Powder to 250 mL tap water) or normal saline (NS). Once the ear canal is open, instill antibiotic-corticosteroid ear drops bid–qid. The corticosteroid is necessary to reduce inflammation. Oral antibiotics are indicated if there are any signs of invasiveness (eg, fever, auricular cellulitis, or tender postauricular lymph nodes). Prescribe an antistaphylococcal antibiotic while awaiting culture results. Systemic antibiotics alone without topical treatment may not clear up otitis externa. Analgesics (sometimes codeine) may be required temporarily. During the acute phase the patient should avoid swimming. Cotton earplugs are *not* helpful and may prolong the infection. Schedule a follow-up visit in 1 week to document an intact tympanic membrane. Children predisposed to otitis externa should instill 2–3 drops of a 1:1 solution of white vinegar and 70% ethyl alcohol into their ears before and after swimming to prevent this infection.

OTITIS MEDIA

Classification & Clinical Findings

Otitis media, an inflammation of the middle ear, is associated with an **effusion** (a collection of fluid) in the middle ear space or **otorrhea** (a discharge from the ear through a perforation in the tympanic membrane or ventilating tube). Otitis media can be further classified into **acute** otitis media, otitis media with **effusion** (residual or persistent), **unresponsive** otitis media, **recurrent** otitis media, otitis media **with complications**, and **chronic suppurative** otitis media.

Acute otitis media (AOM) is commonly defined as inflammation of the middle ear presenting with rapid onset of symptoms such as otalgia, fever, irritability, anorexia, or vomiting. Otoscopic findings include decreased tympanic membrane mobility, a bulging contour with impaired visibility of the ossicular landmarks, yellow or red color, exudate on the membrane, or bullae. In AOM symptoms are nonspecific and often result from an associated viral upper respiratory infection. Therefore, the case definition of acute otitis media may be based on otoscopic findings of inflammation regardless of other symptoms. Approximately one-third of cases with otoscopic signs of inflammation and decreased mobility do *not* present with fever, pain, or irritability.

Otitis media with effusion is defined as an asymptomatic middle ear effusion, sometimes associated with a "plugged ear" feeling. Findings suggestive of otitis media with effusion include visualization of air fluid levels, serous middle ear fluid, and diminished membrane mobility when the membrane is translucent. The presence of an effusion is associated with a mild to moderate conductive hearing impairment 15 dB or higher. Otitis media with effusion can also be associated with negative middle ear pressure, suggested by prominence of the lateral process, a more horizontal orientation of the malleus, and better mobility with negative compared to positive pressure.

Otitis media with residual effusion is characterized by the presence of an asymptomatic effusion without otoscopic signs of inflammation from 3–16 weeks following the diagnosis of acute otitis. After 16 weeks this condition can be considered **otitis media with persistent effusion**.

Both AOM and otitis media with effusion can be associated with decreased tympanic membrane mobility, a flat type B tympanogram and a conductive hearing loss. The distinguishing characteristics are the presence of symptoms and inflammation of the membrane. In an asymptomatic patient, it is difficult to distinguish AOM from otitis media with effusion when the membrane appears opaque, thickened, and scarred. However, bacterial pathogens can be isolated frequently from effusions in these cases with opaque membranes regardless of whether the fluid is purulent, serous, or mucoid.

Unresponsive AOM is characterized by clinical signs and symptoms associated with otoscopic findings of inflammation that continue beyond 48 hours of therapy.

Recurrent AOM can be defined as three new acute otitis media episodes within 6 months or four episodes during 1 year.

Otitis media with complications involves damage to the middle ear structures (eg, tympanosclerosis, retraction pockets, adhesions, ossicular erosion, cholesteatoma, and perforations) as well as other infratemporal and intracranial complications. **Tympanosclerosis** is caused by chronic inflammation or trauma that produces granulation tissue, hyalinization, and calcification. The appearance of a small defect in the posterior superior area of the pars tensa or in the pars flaccida suggests a **retraction pocket**. Retraction pockets occur when chronic inflammation and negative pressure in the middle ear space produce atrophy and atelectasis of the tympanic membrane. Continued inflammation can cause adhesions between the retraction pocket and the ossicles. This condition, referred to as **adhesive otitis**, predisposes to formation of a **cholesteatoma** or fixation and erosion of the ossicles. Erosion of the ossicles results from osteitis and compromise of the blood supply. Ossicular discontinuity produces a severe hearing loss with a 25–50 dB threshold. A tympanogram with very high compliance indicates ossicular discontinuity. The presence of a greasy-looking mass or debris seen in a retraction pocket or perforation suggests cholesteatoma regardless of the presence of discharge. When a perforation is present, the condition is usually painless. If no infection is present, the middle ear cavity is seen to contain thickened, inflamed mucosa. If superimposed infection is present, serous or purulent drainage will be seen, and the middle ear cavity may contain granulation tissue or even polyps. A conductive hearing loss will usually be present depending on the size of the perforation. *The site of perforation is important.* Central perforations do not usually encourage formation of cholesteatomata. Peripheral perforations, especially in the pars flaccida, may allow development of a cholesteatoma because the epithelial tissue adjacent to the perforation may invade it.

Chronic suppurative otitis media is defined as otorrhea persisting beyond 6 weeks.

MICROBIOLOGY

The most common bacterial pathogens in AOM are *S pneumoniae* and *H influenzae*, the same bacterial pathogens most frequently associated with sinusitis and pneumonia. Additional bacterial pathogens include *Moraxella catarrhalis, Streptococcus pyogenes, Staphylococcus aureus*, gram-negative enteric organisms and anaerobes. The microbiologic causes of AOM in early infancy differ from those in later life. The risk of gram-negative enteric infection is especially high in infants who are under 6 weeks of age and have been or are hospitalized in a neonatal intensive care nursery. In normal infants seen during the first 3 months of life, AOM is caused by *S aureus* and *Chlamydia trachomatis*, as well as by *S pneumoniae, H influenzae,* and *M catarrhalis.*

Aspirates of residual and persistent middle ear effusions often harbor pathogenic organisms. The most common pathogens isolated from these effusions are *H influenzae, S pneumoniae, M catarrhalis*, and *S pyogenes*. Most strains of *H influenzae* and *M catarrhalis* are β-lactamase-positive. The role of *S epidermidis* and diphtheroids is unclear.

Chronic suppurative otitis media is often caused by resistant organisms, especially *Pseudomonas*, anaerobes, and gram-negative enteric organisms. Consider performing a purified protein derivative (PPD) test to identify tuberculosis.

Recently, resistant *S pneumoniae* is emerging as a more frequent pathogen in acute and unresponsive otitis as well as in persistent effusions and chronic suppurative otitis, especially in cases with ventilating tubes. The problem of resistant strains of *S pneumoniae* is worrisome. Children with these pathogens are often younger than 18 months and have more unresponsive infections. Prior recent antibiotic treatment appears to increase the risk of the pathogen being a resistant form of *S pneumoniae*.

The relationship between viral and bacterial infections remains controversial. Since viruses have been isolated as the single agent in only 6% of middle ear aspirates with AOM, it appears that viruses promote bacterial superinfection by impairing eustachian tube function, altering nasopharyngeal bacterial growth, as well as by impairing the host's defenses.

DIAGNOSIS

Pneumatic Otoscopy

Acute otitis media is commonly over-diagnosed in clinical settings. Errors are related to professional and parental predilections for treating sick children with antibiotics, the tendency to diagnose AOM without removing enough cerumen to visualize the membrane adequately, and the mistaken belief that a red membrane with normal mobility establishes the diagnosis. A red membrane can be caused by a viral upper respiratory infection (URI), the child's crying, or efforts to remove cerumen. To assess mobility of the tympanic membrane, use a pneumatic otoscope with a rubber suction bulb and tube. When you squeeze the rubber bulb, the tympanic membrane will flap briskly if no fluid is present (normal finding). If fluid is present in the middle ear space, the mobility of the tympanic membrane will be diminished.

Cerumen Removal

Cerumen often prevents adequate visualization of the tympanic membrane. Impacted cerumen can also cause itching, pain, hearing loss, or otitis externa. Parents should be advised that earwax protects the ear in that it contains lysozymes and immunoglobulins that curtail infection, and will come out by itself. They should therefore never put anything into the ear canal to remove the ear wax.

All procedures to remove cerumen with a curet require immobilization to prevent injury to the ear canal. The physician should remove cerumen under direct vision through the operating head of an otoscope. Irrigation can also be used to remove cerumen. Very hard cerumen may adhere to the wall of the ear canal and cause pain or bleeding if you attempt to remove it with a curet. This type of wax can be softened with Cerumenex or a few drops of detergent before irrigation is attempted. After 20 minutes, irrigation with a soft bulb syringe can be started with water warmed to 35–38 °C to prevent vertigo. A commercial water-jet tooth cleaner (eg, Water Pik) is also an excellent device for removing cerumen, but it is important to set it at low power (2 or less) to prevent damage to an intact tympanic membrane. A perforated tympanic membrane is a contraindication to any form of irrigation.

Tympanometry

Tympanometry can be used to confirm otoscopic findings and identify effusions. It should not replace pneumatic otoscopy as it does not identify inflammation. Tympanometry utilizes an electroacoustic impedance bridge to measure tympanic membrane compliance and display it in graphic form. Compliance is determined at specific air pressures (from +200 to –400 mm H_2O air pressure) created in the hermetically sealed external ear canal. The existing middle ear pressure can be measured by determining the ear canal pressure at which the tympanic membrane is most compliant. Because total visualization of the tympanic membrane is not necessary, tympanometry does not require removal of cerumen unless the canal is completely blocked.

Tympanograms can be classified into three major patterns, as shown in Figure 13–1. The type A pattern, characterized by maximum compliance at normal atmospheric pressure (0 mm H_2O air pressure), indicates a normal tympanic membrane, good auditory tube function, and absence of effusion. The type B pattern identifies a nonmobile tympanic membrane, which may be associated with middle ear effusion, perforation, patent ventilation tubes, or excessive and hard-packed cerumen. The type C pattern indicates an intact mobile tympanic membrane with poor auditory tube function and excessive negative pressure (> -150 mm H_2O air pressure) in the middle ear. Middle ear effusion is present in about 20% of patients with a type C pattern.

TREATMENT

An algorithm for treatment of otitis media in children is presented in Figure 13–2.

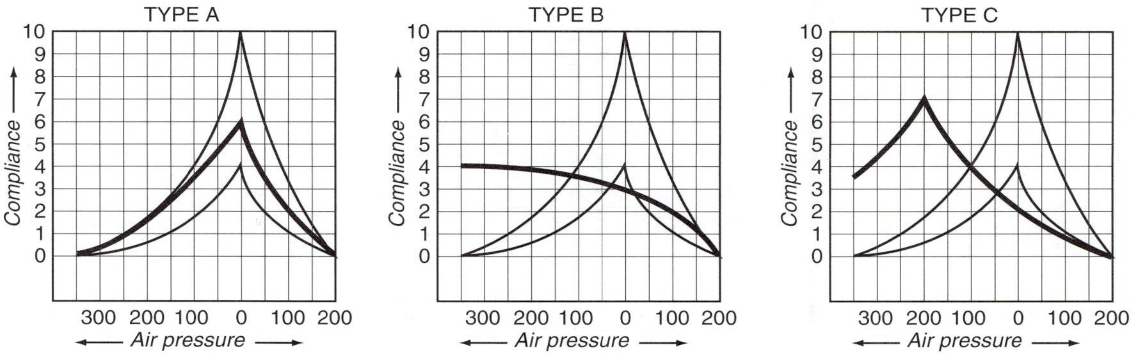

Figure 13–1. Type A tympanograms are characterized by maximum compliance at normal atmospheric pressure (0 mm H_2O air pressure). Type B tympanograms show little or no change in compliance of the tympanic membrane as air pressure in the external ear canal is varied. Type C tympanograms show near-normal compliance with significant negative middle ear pressures (typically more severe than –150 mm H_2O). (Reproduced with permission from Northern JL: Advanced techniques for measuring middle ear function. Pediatrics 1987;61:761.)

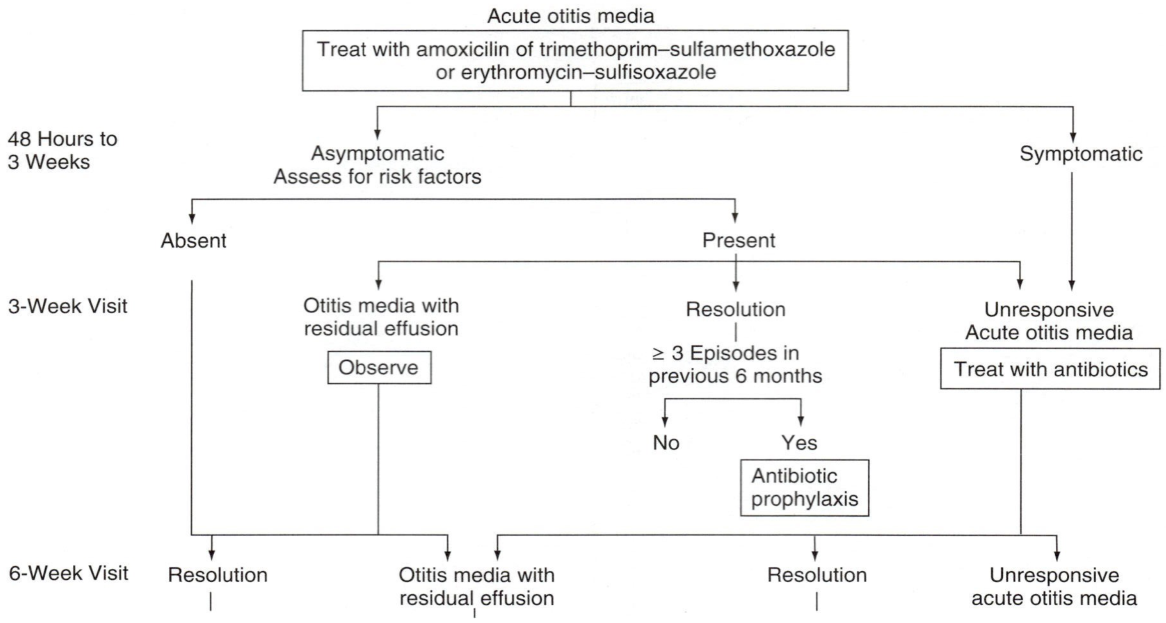
Acute otitis media
Treat with amoxicilin of trimethoprim–sulfamethoxazole or erythromycin–sulfisoxazole
48 Hours to 3 Weeks
Asymptomatic
Assess for risk factors
Symptomatic
Absent
Present
3-Week Visit
Otitis media with residual effusion
Observe
Resolution
≥ 3 Episodes in previous 6 months
No
Yes
Antibiotic prophylaxis
Unresponsive
Acute otitis media
Treat with antibiotics
6-Week Visit
Resolution
Otitis media with residual effusion
Resolution
Unresponsive acute otitis media

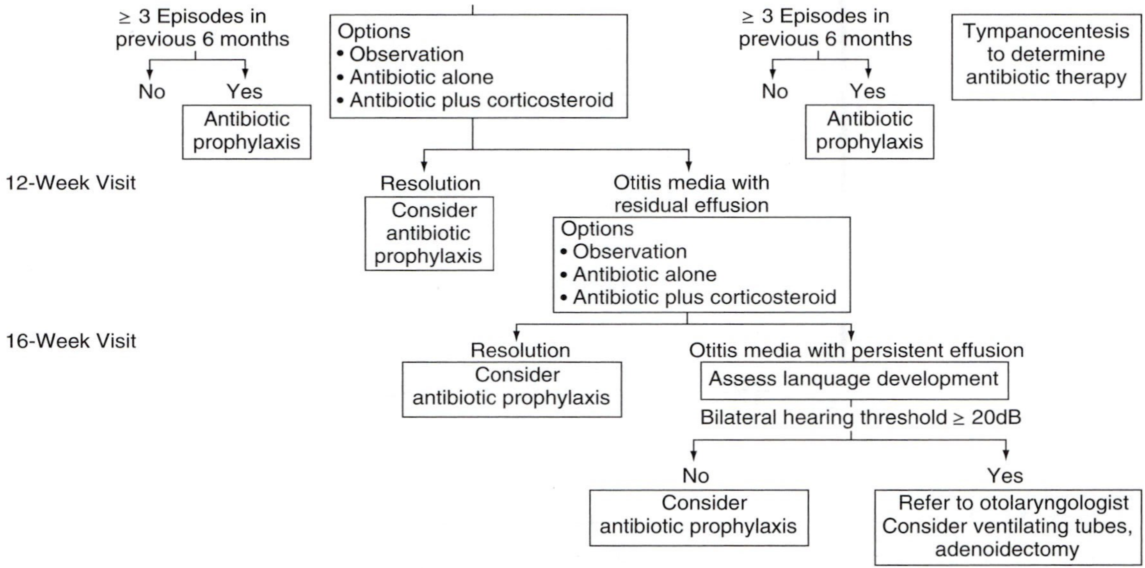

Figure 13–2. An algorithm for the diagnosis and management of otitis media in children. Risk factors for the failure of treatment are an age of less than 15 months, a history of recurrent otitis media in the patient or a sibling, and antibiotic treatment of otitis media within the previous month.

Table 13–1. Antibiotic therapy for acute otitis media with effusion in children.

Antibiotic	Dosage	Product Availability
Amoxicillin	10–15 mg/kg/dose tid (bid for prophylaxis)	Liquid: 125 and 500 mg/5 mL Caps: 250, 500 mg Chewables: 125, 250 mg
Amoxicillin/clavulanate (Augmentin)	10–15 mg/kg/dose tid	Liquid: 125, 250 mg/5 mL Chewables: 125, 250 mg Tabs: 250, 500 mg
Cefaclor (Ceclor)	10 mg/kg/dose tid	Liquid: 125, 250 mg/5 mL Caps: 250, 500 mg
Cefixime (Suprax)	8 mg/kg/day as single dose or divided bid	Liquid: 100 mg/5 mL Tabs: 200, 400 mg
Erythromycin	10 mg/kg/dose bid for prophylaxis	Liquid: 200 ml 400 mg/5 mL Chewables: 200 mg Tabs/caps: 250, 500 mg
Erythromycin/sulfisoxazole (Pediazole)	10 mg (E)/kg/dose qid	Liquid: 100 mg (E), 600 mg (S)/5 mL
Prednisone or prednisolone	0.5–1 mg/kg/dose bid	Tabs: 5, 10, 20 mg Syrup: 1 mg/1 mL
Sulfisoxazole (Gantrisin)	30–40 mg/kg/dose bid for prophylaxis	Liquid: 500 mg/5 mL Tabs: 500 mg
Trimethoprim/sulfamethoxazole (Bactrim, Septra)	5 mg (T)/kg/dose bid or 0.5 mg/kg/dose bid	Liquid: 40 (T) mg/5 mL Tabs: 80, 160 mg T:S = 1:5 ratio

T = trimethoprim component; E = erythromycin component; S = sulfisoxazole component.

Antibiotic Treatment of Acute Otitis Media

First-line antibiotics for AOM are amoxicillin, trimethoprim-sulfamethoxazole, and erythromycin plus sulfisoxazole (Table 13–1). In most cases, third-generation cephalosporins, amoxicillin plus clavulanate, or clarithromycin should *not* be used as first- or second-line antibiotics in a normal child who is not allergic to amoxicillin or sulfa containing antibiotics.

The optimal duration of therapy is variable; 5–7 days appears to be as effective as 10–14 days. If the physician is concerned about an associated bacteremia or compliance, the patient can be treated with an intramuscular injection of ceftriaxone or CR Bicillin. Procaine penicillin is similar to amoxicillin in its coverage of *H influenzae*. Antihistamines with or without decongestants are ineffective in the prevention or treatment of otitis media.

Pain Management in Acute Otitis Media

Children with pain related to AOM may get relief from acetaminophen, ibuprofen, or topical therapy with auralgan. When pain is severe, tympanocentesis results in prompt relief.

Follow-up Visits

Optimal timing for follow-up visits depends on the child's response to therapy. Reassess children when symptoms of AOM continue beyond 48 hours or recur prior to the next scheduled visit. A follow-up visit for children who become asymptomatic should be scheduled for 3–6 weeks later. Follow-up visits for children with risk factors for treatment failure should be scheduled for 3 weeks after initiation of therapy. Risk factors include age less than 15 months, a prior history of recurrent otitis media, or history of antibiotic treatment of otitis media within the preceding month. Follow-up visits for asymptomatic children without risk factors may be scheduled for 6 weeks after initiation of treatment.

Antibiotic Therapy of Unresponsive Acute Otitis Media

About 10% of children will have unresponsive AOM after 48 hours of initial antibiotic therapy. Treat unresponsive AOM in a child who has been treated initially with amoxicillin with trimethoprim-sulfamethoxazole or erythromycin plus sulfisoxazole, and vice versa (Table 13–1). The sequential administration of these antibiotics provides excellent coverage for most middle ear pathogens. Unfortunately, third-generation cephalosporins and amoxicillin plus clavulanate offer minimal advantage in covering highly resistant pneumococcal organisms. These more expensive antibiotics are chiefly useful as second-line therapy for children who are allergic to antibiotics. If the child is allergic to amoxicillin but not to cephalosporins, use a third-generation cephalosporin or clarithromycin to treat AOM that has not responded to erythromycin plus sulfisoxazole or trimethoprim-sulfisoxazole. If the child is allergic to an antibiotic containing sulfa, give amoxicillin plus clavulanate, a third-generation cephalosporin or clarithromycin when the otitis has not responded to amoxicillin. If unresponsive AOM persists after a second course of antibiotics, consider a myringotomy or tympanocentesis in order to isolate the pathogen and drain the effusion.

Tympanocentesis or Myringotomy

Tympanocentesis is performed by placing a needle through the tympanic membrane and aspirating the middle ear fluid. **Myringotomy** involves an incision of the drum with a myringotomy knife in order to drain the fluid. Indications for tympanocentesis or myringotomy are: (1) acute otitis media in a hospitalized newborn, because the pathogens may be gram-negative; (2) AOM in a patient with compromised resistance, because the organism may be unusual; (3) painful bullae of the tympanic membrane; (4) a complete workup for presumed sepsis or meningitis; (5) unresponsive otitis media despite courses of two different antibiotics; and (6) acute mastoiditis.

Management of Recurrent Otitis

The decision to administer antibiotic prophylaxis to children who have experienced three documented episodes of AOM in a 6-month period should be individualized and the risks and benefits reviewed with the parents. Antibiotic prophylaxis is as effective as ventilating tubes in preventing new otitis episodes (Table 13–1). Neither intervention, however, appears to make a major clinical difference compared to a placebo. Antibiotic prophylaxis is marginally effective in reducing the frequency of otitis episodes. The increased risk of acquiring resistant *S pneumoniae* while on continuous prophylaxis is unclear. Administration of antibiotic therapy at the onset of upper respiratory infection (URI) symptoms rather than daily continuous therapy also decreases otitis episodes, and may have less of an effect on colonization with resistant *S pneumoniae*.

Another approach to prevention of recurrent otitis is active immunization. Clinical trials of the newly developed conjugate pneumococcal vaccine to prevent AOM episodes are currently underway. Consider immunizing children with recurrent otitis with influenza vaccine and immunizing children older than 2 years with the 23-valent pneumococcal vaccine (pneumovax).

Management of Otitis Media With Residual & Persistent Effusions

The main reason to treat otitis media with effusion is the negative impact of prolonged conductive hearing impairment on language development and academic functioning. While the available data document a causal relationship between severe congenital or acquired hearing loss (usually sensorineural) and language development, the data fail to establish a causal relationship between conductive hearing loss associated with otitis media and subsequent hearing-related development. Data from several studies on the impact of conductive hearing impairment related to otitis report conflicting results.

Management options for otitis media with residual effusion present for 6 weeks to 4 months include observation, antibiotics alone, and a combination of antibiotic and corticosteroid therapy. If combination therapy is selected, a corticosteroid (prednisone) can be given for 7 days combined with an antibiotic (trimethoprim-sulfamethoxazole or an alternative) for 14–21 days. Children without a history of varicella who have been exposed in the preceding month should not receive prednisone because of the potential risk of disseminated disease if they are receiving a corticosteroid. The side effects of prednisone are similar to those noted in treating asthmatic episodes with short steroid courses: increased appetite, fluid retention, occasional vomiting, and in rare cases marked behavior changes. If the patient clears the persistent middle ear effusion unilaterally or bilaterally, follow him or her monthly. Consider administering low-dose intermittent antibiotic prophylaxis with amoxicillin 20 mg/kg/day either bid or qd, or sulfisoxazole 75 mg/kg/day either bid or qd for 3 months to prevent a recurrence of otitis media.

Ventilating tubes should be considered after otitis media with effusion has persisted for at least 4 months and is accompanied by a documented bilateral hearing impairment of 20 dB or greater. The timing should be individualized depending on the child's developmental and behavioral status as well as parental preference. Studies have established that children with otitis media with persistent effusion have a higher incidence of abnormalities such as cholesteatoma, adhesive otitis, retraction pockets, membrane atrophy, or persistent membrane perforations compared to children without a history of persistent effusion.

The main reason for surgery in the management of these children is to restore normal hearing in order to promote language development and reduce the risk of secondary learning or behavior problems. Surgical options include ventilating tubes or adenoidectomy. Adenoidectomy cannot be recommended for children under 4 years of age, however, because no data are currently available on its efficacy at this age. Adenoidectomy for otitis media without signs of upper airway obstruction is usually considered a second-line surgical intervention when a child has developed complications from the ventilating tubes or requires multiple tube reinsertions.

Management of Otitis Media With Perforation

Most perforations seen with AOM heal within 2 weeks. When perforations fail to heal after 3–6 months a surgical repair may be needed. Repair of the defect in the tympanic membrane is rarely successful during the period when children have frequent colds and recurrent auditory tube dysfunction. Tympanoplasty is usually deferred until age 9–12. The perforated eardrum can be repaired earlier if the other ear remains free of infection and effusion for a year. Swimming should be discouraged unless it is very important to the patient, in which case it can be continued using custom-fitted ear molds plus a bathing cap for girls or a scuba cap for boys. Instruct the patient to avoid diving, jumping into the water, and swimming underwater.

Management of Chronic Suppurative Otitis Media

The successful treatment of chronic suppurative otitis usually requires parenteral therapy with an antibiotic that covers *Pseudomonas* or anaerobes. The role of oral quinolone antibiotics effective against *Pseudomonas* for outpatient management is unclear because of possible side effects on growing cartilage in children. When a cholesteatoma is present, medical therapy is not effective. If the discharge does not respond to 2 weeks of aggressive therapy, suspect mastoiditis or cholesteatoma. Serious central nervous system (CNS) complications such as extradural abscess, subdural abscess, brain abscess, meningitis, labyrinthitis, or lateral sinus thrombophlebitis can occur with extension of this process. Therefore, patients with facial palsy, vertigo, or other CNS signs should be referred immediately to an otolaryngologist.

MASTOIDITIS

General Considerations

Infection of the mastoid antrum and air cells may be associated with an episode of AOM. Mastoiditis is unusual before age 2, when air cells begin to develop. The most common causative agents are *S pyogenes, S pneumoniae,* and *S aureus. H influenzae* causes mastoiditis much less frequently than might be expected. Other causative agents include *Pseudomonas, Mycobacterium,* enteropathic gram-negative rods, and *M catarrhalis.* Anaerobic organisms appear to play a role in chronic mastoiditis; however, there are no data on how frequently they cause acute mastoiditis.

Clinical Findings

The principal complaints are usually postauricular pain and fever. On examination, the mastoid area is often red and swollen. In the late stage, it may be fluctuant. The earliest finding is severe tenderness upon mastoid percussion. AOM is almost always present. Late findings in mastoiditis are a pinna that is pushed forward by postauricular swelling and an ear canal that is narrowed in the posterior superior wall because of pressure from the mastoid abscess. In infants less than 1 year of age, the swelling occurs superior to the ear and pushes the pinna downward rather than outward. In the acute phase, there is diffuse inflammatory clouding of the mastoid cells as in every case of AOM. Later there is evidence of bony destruction and resorption of the mastoid air cells. The best method to determine the extent of disease is by computed tomography.

Complications

Meningitis appears in as many as 9% of cases of acute mastoiditis, and should be suspected when a child has high fever, stiff neck, severe headache, or other meningeal signs. A lumbar puncture should be performed to diagnose this condition. Brain abscess occurs in 2% of cases and may be associated with persistent headache, recurring fever, or changes in sensorium.

Treatment

The patient must be hospitalized, because this disorder represents osteitis. Before therapy is initiated, tympanocentesis or myringotomy should be performed in order to obtain material for culture and to relieve pressure in the middle ear-mastoid space.

The initial management of uncomplicated acute mastoiditis includes intravenous antibiotic therapy. Results of Gram's stain smears taken during tympanocentesis may assist in the choice of antibiotics. Reasonable initial therapy is ceftriaxone with nafcillin or clindamycin. Indications for immediate surgery include evidence of a major complication such as meningitis, brain abscess, cavernous sinus thrombosis, acute suppurative labyrinthitis, or facial palsy. Some otolaryngologists consider the destruction of septal bone (osteitis) and resorption of the mastoid air cells an indication for surgery as well. Oral antibiotics should be continued for 4–6 weeks after the patient is discharged. The prognosis is good if treatment is started early and continued until the process is inactive.

ACUTE TRAUMA TO THE MIDDLE EAR

Head injuries, a blow to the ear canal, sudden impact with water, blast injuries, or the insertion of pointed instruments into the ear canal can lead to perforation of the tympanic membrane or hematoma of the middle ear. As many as 50% of serious penetrating wounds of the tympanic membrane are due to parental use of cotton-tipped swabs.

Treatment of middle ear hematomas chiefly consists of watchful waiting. Prophylactic antibiotics are not necessary unless signs of superimposed infection appear. The prognosis for unimpaired hearing depends upon associated dislocations or fractures of the ossicles. The patient should be followed with audiometrics until hearing has returned to normal.

Traumatic perforations of the tympanic membrane often do not heal spontaneously and should be referred to an otolaryngologist. Perforations caused by a foreign body must be attended to immediately, whereas those due to impact can be seen within 24 hours. Early debridement and placement of a graft virtually ensure closure.

FOREIGN BODY IN EAR CANAL

Children insert a wide variety of small objects into their ears. If the object is large, wedged in the canal, or difficult to remove with available instruments, refer the patient to an otolaryngologist rather than risk damage to the ear canal followed by edema that will require removal of the object under anesthesia.

Insects in the ear can be killed with an alcohol solution; caregivers can be advised to use spirits. With inanimate objects, make an initial attempt at removal by straightening the child's ear canal. This can be done by pulling on the pinna and gently shaking the child's head. The patient should be immobilized on a papoose board with the head firmly grasped by an assistant. If the object is smooth (eg, a bead), you can insert a cotton-tipped applicator with warmed dental wax or collodion and place it against the object for 1–2 minutes, after which time you can remove it. An object with an irregular surface can sometimes be removed with bayonet forceps. A steel object (eg, a ball bearing) can sometimes be removed with a magnetic probe. A right-angled hook can sometimes be inserted past the object and then withdrawn, pushing the object ahead of it.

DETECTION & MANAGEMENT OF HEARING DEFICITS

Hearing deficits are classified as conductive, sensorineural, or mixed. **Conductive** hearing loss results from a blockage of the transmission of sound waves from the external auditory canal to the inner ear. It is characterized by normal bone conduction and reduced air conduction hearing. In children, conductive losses are most often caused by middle ear effusion. **Sensorineural** hearing loss occurs when the auditory nerve or cochlear hair cells are damaged. **Mixed** hearing loss is characterized by components of both conductive and sensorineural loss. The criteria for normal hearing levels in children are lower than those in adults, since children are in the process of learning language. In children, a hearing loss of 15–30 dB is considered mild, 31–50 dB moderate, 51–80 dB severe, and 81–100 dB profound.

Conductive Hearing Loss

By far the greatest cause of conductive hearing loss during childhood is otitis media and its sequelae. Other causes include atresia, stenosis, or collapse of the ear canal; furuncle, cerumen, or foreign body in the ear; aural discharge; bony growths; otitis externa; perichondritis; middle ear anomalies (eg, stapes fixation, ossicular malformation); and cleft palate.

The average hearing loss due to middle ear effusion (whether serous, purulent, or mucoid) is 27–31 dB, the equivalent of a mild hearing loss. This loss may be intermittent in nature and may occur in one or both ears.

The American Academy of Pediatrics recommends that hearing be assessed and language development skills be monitored in children who have frequent episodes of AOM or middle ear effusion persisting longer than 3 months. The effects of hearing loss may be insidious and not discernible until the child attains the explosive phase of expressive language development (16–24 months). Therefore, the optimal times for screening very young children are 18 and 24 months. The Early Language Milestone (ELM) scale is an acceptable tool for language screening at these ages. Children 3, 4, and 5 years of age should also be screened for language delays. To mitigate the development of a communication disorder, the physician should inform the parents of a child with middle ear disease that his or her hearing may not be normal. The parents should be instructed to (1) turn off sources of background noise (eg, televisions, radios, dishwashers) when speaking to the child; (2) focus on the child's face and gain his or her direct attention before speaking; (3) speak slightly louder than usual. In addition, the child's teachers should be advised to assign him or her a seat in the front of any classroom.

Sensorineural Hearing Loss

Sensorineural hearing loss arises from lesions in the cochlear structures of the inner ear or in the neural fibers of the auditory nerve (cranial nerve VIII). Most sensorineural losses in children are congenital, with an incidence of 1:750 live births. Causes include perinatal infections, problems of prematurity, and various hereditary deafness syndromes. In some hereditary diseases (eg, **Alport's syndrome**), hearing loss is progressive and becomes apparent later in childhood. The incidence of acquired sensorineural loss in children has decreased since the advent of effective immunization programs against rubella and mumps, and the control of erythroblastosis fetalis with Rh_0(D) immune globulin. Meningitis remains the most common cause of acquired hearing loss, with deafness occurring in about 10% of children with bacterial meningitis.

In the past, the effect of unilateral deafness on school performance was thought to be insignificant. More recent studies indicate, however, that more than one-third of affected children fail one or more grades in school. Preferential classroom seating for these children is not sufficient; they should be referred to a specialist for full evaluation of their hearing deficits.

Acquisition of language skills is more severely affected by bilateral than unilateral sensorineural hearing loss. The earlier the deafness, the graver the consequences for language development. The earlier the detection and treatment of sensorineural loss (by sound amplification and language habilitation), the better the chances of a good outcome. For example, detection of deafness in a 3-month-old infant and treatment by 4 months of age will result in an optimal outcome. Unfortunately, an average of 2–3 years elapses between recognition of hearing loss and institution of treatment. The alert physician can eliminate this delay by screening children for hearing deficits.

DISEASES OF THE NOSE & PARANASAL SINUSES

ACUTE VIRAL RHINITIS
(Common Cold)

The common cold is the most frequent infectious disease encountered in the pediatric population. The incidence is higher in early childhood than in any other period of life. Children under age 5 may have 6–12 colds a year. Upper respiratory infections (URIs) may be caused by over 200 different viruses, including rhinovirus, coronavirus, adenovirus, influenza virus, parainfluenza virus, respiratory syncytial virus, and coxsackievirus (Chapter 10).

Clinical Findings

The patient usually experiences a sudden onset of clear or mucoid rhinorrhea, nasal congestion, and fever. Mild sore throat and cough are frequently associated. Although the fever is usually low-grade in older children, in the first 5 or 6 years of life it can be as high as 40.6 °C without superinfection. The nose, throat, and tympanic membrane may appear red and inflamed.

Use the following guidelines when screening children with colds for elective surgery: Surgery is usually postponed if fever or cough is present. Surgery can proceed if the child has only a runny nose, sore throat, or ear infection. If anesthesia will not require intubation, surgery can be permitted even if the child has a cough, provided that findings on chest film are normal.

Treatment

Treatment for colds is largely symptomatic. Acetaminophen is helpful for fever, sore throat, or muscle aches. A stuffy, congested nose can be treated with normal saline nose drops (mix ¼ tsp table salt with 6 oz. of water), 3 drops in each nostril. After several minutes, a suction bulb can be used to remove the secretions of infants too young to blow their noses. If this procedure fails after several attempts and the stuffy nose still interferes with feeding or sleep, consider long-acting xylometazoline (Otrivin) or oxymetazoline (Afrin) 0.05% nose drops. Drops should be used only when the nose is congested. Discontinue drops after 5 days to prevent rebound chemical rhinitis. Antihistamines are *not* effective in relieving cold symptoms. In rhinoviral colds, increased levels of histamine are not observed. Antibiotics do not prevent superinfection and should not be used. Codeine and dextromethorphan should be discouraged as they do not alleviate the symptoms of acute cough. Parents should be instructed that fast breathing or difficult breathing with retraction are signs of a lower respiratory infection such as bronchiolitis or pneumonia.

SINUSITIS

1. ACUTE SINUSITIS

General Considerations

The maxillary and ethmoidal sinuses are most commonly involved when mucociliary clearance and drainage are impaired by a

URI or allergic rhinitis. The ethmoidal sinus is the only sinus significantly developed at birth. The maxillary sinus is rudimentary at birth and visible on x-ray film by 6 months. The frontal sinus is not visible until 3–9 years of age. Clinical ethmoiditis does not usually occur until 6 months of age. About half of cases occur between 1 and 5 years of age, during which time the most common presenting sign is periorbital cellulitis. Maxillary sinusitis is seen clinically after 1 year of age. An uncommon cause of maxillary sinusitis is extension of a periapical abscess of an upper molar. Frontal sinusitis is unusual before 10 years of age.

The pathogens that cause acute sinusitis are usually *S pneumoniae, H influenzae* (nontypable), *M catarrhalis,* and β-hemolytic streptococci. Rarely, anaerobic bacterial infections can cause fulminant frontal sinusitis. Viruses can be isolated in 10% of sinus aspirates, but their pathogenic role is unclear.

Clinical Findings

Acute sinusitis in children may present either gradually or suddenly. In gradual presentations nasal discharge or postnasal drip and daytime cough persist longer than 10 days. In addition a low-grade fever is often present together with malodorous breath or intermittent, painless morning periorbital swelling. Older patients may complain of a headache, a sense of facial fullness, or facial pain overlying the involved sinus. With the more sudden toxic presentation the patient presents with a high fever and more severe pain or periorbital inflammation. Ethmoiditis causes retro-orbital pain; maxillary sinusitis causes upper molar or zygomatic pain; and frontal sinusitis causes pain above the eyebrow.

Physical examination reveals injected nasal mucosa, usually associated with mucopurulent discharge. Occasionally there is percussion tenderness overlying the sinusitis. In ethmoiditis, the tenderness is elicited by pressing medially on the inner canthus of the eye. Tenderness of the eyeball may also be present. Maxillary sinusitis reveals percussion tenderness on the maxillary bone. Frontal sinusitis reveals percussion tenderness with upward pressure on the floor of the supraorbital ridge. Periorbital swelling or mild discoloration may be present. Examination should identify exudative tonsillitis, a nasal foreign body, or dental caries and poor dental hygiene. Transillumination of the sinuses is difficult to perform and not very helpful unless it is grossly asymmetric.

In most acute cases, radiographs are not needed. Positive findings in children over one year include opacification of the involved sinuses, air-fluid levels, or mucosal thickening greater than 5 mm. Findings consistent with sinusitis may be found in asymptomatic patients with colds or nasal allergies. Many clinicians believe that CT scans rather than standard sinus radiographs should be obtained. Radiographic studies are indicated mainly in children with (1) facial swelling of unknown cause; (2) acute sinusitis unresponsive to 48 hours of therapy; (3) persistent or recurrent sinusitis; and (4) chronic asthma.

Complications

The most frequent complication of paranasal sinusitis is preseptal periorbital cellulitis secondary to ethmoiditis. Less frequently, orbital cellulitis or abscess develops. These are associated with decreased extraocular movement, proptosis, edema, and altered visual acuity. The most common complication of frontal sinusitis is osteitis of the frontal bone, called **Pott's puffy tumor**. Additional serious intracranial complications include cavernous sinus thrombosis, subdural empyema, brain abscess, and meningitis. The most common maxillary complication is cellulitis of the cheek. Rarely, osteomyelitis of the maxilla can develop.

Treatment

Oral Antibiotics: Treat acute sinusitis with oral antibiotics for 10 days. Continue antibiotic treatment for another week if the patient has improved but is not totally asymptomatic. The usual agent is amoxicillin, 15 mg/kg, tid. In areas where β-lactamase-positive pathogens are common or when the patient is allergic to penicillin, use trimethoprim-sulfamethoxazole, 5 mg/kg/dose bid, or erythromycin plus sulfamethoxazole, 10 mg/kg/dose qid. Additional possibilities include third-generation cephalosporins, amoxicillin-clavulanate, or clarithromycin. Failure to improve after 48 hours suggests a resistant organism or potential complication and is an indication to admit for parenteral therapy.

Topical and Oral Decongestants and Antihistamines: Topical decongestants and oral combinations are frequently used in acute sinusitis to promote drainage. Their effectiveness has not been evaluated, and concern has been raised about potential adverse effects related to impaired ciliary function, decreased blood flow to the mucosa, and reduced diffusion of antibiotic into the sinuses. Patients with underlying allergic rhinitis may benefit from intranasal cromolyn or corticosteroid nasal spray. Vasoconstrictor nose drops and sprays are all associated with rebound edema if used for more than 5–7 days.

Treatment of Complications: Patients with evidence of invasive infection or any CNS complications should be hospitalized immediately. Intravenous therapy with nafcillin or clindamycin, plus a third-generation cephalosporin (eg, cefotaxime) should be initiated while awaiting culture results.

Pain Management: Patients will often need acetaminophen or even codeine in order to sleep until the obstructed sinus has drained. Application of ice over the sinus may help to relieve pain.

Surgery: External drainage: in complicated cases admitted to the hospital, an otolaryngologist should always be consulted. Sinus aspiration is often helpful. For sinus intraorbital or intracranial complications, external drainage of the abscess is as important as antibiotic therapy.

2. RECURRENT OR CHRONIC SINUSITIS

Chronic or frequent episodes of sinusitis occur in a small group of patients. The most common cause is allergic rhinitis. Rarely cases result from pressure against the ostia by a septal deviation, nasal malformation, polyp, or foreign body. In cases of chronic or recurrent pyogenic pansinusitis, poor host resistance (eg, an immune defect, Kartagener's syndrome, or cystic fibrosis) must be ruled out by immunoglobulin studies, cilia studies, and a sweat chloride test. Anaerobic and staphylococcal organisms are often responsible for chronic sinusitis. If allergies and diving do not offer a sufficient explanation for the problem, the patient should be referred to an otolaryngologist for complete evaluation. Functional endoscopic sinus surgery is being employed to manage patients with recurrent or persistent sinusitis. No data are available comparing the outcome of surgical intervention with antibiotic management. There are large variations in use of this procedure by otolaryngologists especially for younger patients.

Choanal Atresia

Choanal atresia occurs bilaterally in 25% of affected children and unilaterally in 75%. Bilateral cases can cause severe respiratory distress, even apnea at birth if the child is an absolute nasal breather. Both types eventually present with a chronic nasal discharge because the normal sinus and nasal secretions can escape only anteriorly. A No. 8 soft rubber catheter should be passed through the nose and visualized in the oropharynx. If this procedure cannot be performed, a diagnosis of choanal atresia should be confirmed by radiographic study.

An oral airway should be placed immediately if the infant has bilateral choanal atresia. A dentist can fashion a comfortable temporary airway until mouth breathing is established. Feeding by syringe or medicine dropper is preferable. An otolaryngologist should decide on the optimal timing for definitive surgery, but it is usually 1 year of age.

3. RECURRENT RHINITIS IN THE OLDER CHILD

Recurrent rhinitis in older children is a frequent problem in pediatric office practice. Parents may complain that their child has "one cold after another" or "is always sick." Although the frustration is genuine, the differential diagnosis is rather simple. Approximately two-thirds of these children have recurrent colds, and another one-third have allergic rhinitis.

Allergic Rhinitis

The onset of "hay fever" is usually after 2 years of age (after the child has had adequate exposure to allergens). There is no fever or contagion among close contacts. The attacks include frequent sneezing, rubbing of the nose, and a profuse clear discharge. The nasal turbinates are swollen. The nasal smear contains over 20% eosinophils. (Nasal eosinophilia may be normal during the first 3 months of life.) Nasal secretions should be collected only when the patient is symptomatic. Between attacks or after receiving antihistamines, the eosinophil smear may be falsely negative.

Oral decongestants and antihistamines should be tried until the optimal drug and dosage are found. Avoidance of allergens (especially pet dander and tobacco smoke) should be encouraged with the help of environmental controls. If symptoms persist, treatment with cromolyn or corticosteroid nasal sprays should be considered.

A full discussion of allergic rhinitis is presented in Chapter 30.

Chemical Rhinitis

Prolonged use of vasoconstrictor nose drops beyond 7 days results in a rebound reaction and secondary nasal congestion (rhinitis medicamentosa). Discontinue the offending nose drops.

Vasomotor Rhinitis

Some children react to sudden changes in environmental temperature with prolonged congestion and rhinorrhea. Air pollution (especially tobacco smoke) may be a factor. Oral decongestants can be used periodically to give symptomatic relief.

EPISTAXIS

The human nose is a very vascular structure. In most cases, epistaxis results from mild trauma to the anterior portion of the nasal septum (**Kiesselbach's area**) caused by vigorous nose rubbing, blowing, or picking. Fewer than 5% of children with recurrent epistaxis have a bleeding disorder. Examination of Kiesselbach's area usually reveals a red, raw surface with fresh clots or old crusts. Look for telangiectasia, hemangiomas, or varicosities.

Most patients do not need a hematologic workup, but bleeding tests are indicated with any of the following: (1) family history of a bleeding disorder; (2) a history of easy bleeding; (3) spontaneous bleeding at other sites; (4) bleeding that lasts for over 30 minutes or will not clot with direct pressure; (5) onset before age 2; or (6) a drop in the hematocrit due to epistaxis. High blood pressure may also predispose to prolonged nosebleeds.

A nasopharyngeal angiofibroma may present with epistaxis with bleeding confined to the back of the throat. Lateral soft tissue films of the nasopharynx are diagnostic.

Treatment

The following approach can be used in the office or given as phone advice: Have the patient sit up and lean forward so as not to swallow blood. Pinch the nose, maintaining pressure over the bleeding site for 10 minutes by the clock. If bleeding continues, pressure is not being applied to the right spot, and should be relocated. If these maneuvers are not effective, remove clots by suction or by having the child blow the nose. The bleeding site should be visualized. A small piece of gelatin sponge (Gelfoam) or topical thrombin can be inserted over the bleeding site.

Friability of nasal vessels can be decreased with daily application of petrolatum ointment by cotton-tipped applicator. Apply the lubricant daily until 5 days have passed without a nosebleed, then weekly for 1 month; resume only if nosebleeds recur. In a very dry environment, humidification of the patient's room may be helpful. Instruct the patient to avoid aspirin and vigorous nose blowing.

NASAL FURUNCLE

A **furuncle** is an infected hair follicle in the anterior nares. Hair plucking or nose picking can provide a route of entry. The most common causative organism is *S aureus*. The diagnosis is made by finding an exquisitely tender, firm, red lump in the anterior naris. Treatment includes dicloxacillin or cephalexin orally for 5 days to prevent spread. The lesion should be gently incised and drained as soon as it points, usually with a needle. Topical bacitracin ointment may be of additional value. Since this lesion is in the drainage area of the cavernous sinus, the patient should be followed closely until healing is complete. Parents should be advised never to pick or squeeze a furuncle in this location, nor should the physician. Associated cellulitis or spread requires hospitalization for administration of intravenous antibiotics.

NASAL SEPTUM SUBLUXATION

Rarely newborn infants have subluxation of the quadrangular cartilage of the septum. The tip of the nose deviates to one side, and the inferior septal border deviates to the other. There is also leaning of the columella and instability of the nasal tip. This disorder must be distinguished from the more common transient flattening of the nose caused by the birth process.

NASAL FRACTURE

Most blows to the nose result in swelling and hematoma without fracture. Persistent nosebleed after trauma, crepitus or instability of the bones in the nasal bridge, and marked deviation of the nose to one side indicate fracture. Septal injury, however, can be ruled out only by careful intranasal examination. Patients with suspected fractures should be referred to an otolaryngologist for definitive treatment. Resetting of nasal fractures can be postponed up to 1 week without causing difficulty.

NASAL SEPTUM HEMATOMA

After trauma to the nose, it is essential to examine the interior with a nasal speculum. Hematoma of the nasal septum imposes considerable risk of pressure necrosis and resorption of the cartilage, leading to septal perforation or a saddle-back nose in adulthood. Diagnosis of hematoma is confirmed by the abrupt onset of nasal obstruction following trauma and the presence of a widened nasal septum. The normal nasal septum is 2–4 mm thick.

Treatment consists of prompt referral to an otolaryngologist for evacuation of the hematoma and packing of the nose.

FOREIGN BODIES IN THE NOSE

Foreign bodies may be removed from the nose by several maneuvers, including vigorous nose blowing if the child is old enough. If the object is round (eg, beads), collodion on a cotton-tipped applicator can be placed against it and left there for 1–2 minutes, after which it will usually be dry enough to remove the object. Irregular objects can sometimes be grasped with a bayonet forceps. If there is room to maneuver past the object, a right-angled hook can be inserted and withdrawn, pushing the object ahead of it. If these techniques are not successful and there is some space between the object and the side of the nose, a lubricated No. 8 Bardex Foley catheter can be inserted. When the balloon is past the object, it can be inflated and then used to extract the object.

Tilt the child's head over a large basin and flush the noninvolved nostril rapidly with normal saline from a nasal bulb syringe. The fluid will wash around to the involved side, in most cases forcing the object out. Closing the uninvolved nostril and placing one's mouth over the patient's mouth to administer a sudden blast of air will also force out the foreign body if sufficient pressure is exerted. If the object seems inaccessible, is wedged in, or is quite large, refer the patient to an otolaryngologist.

THE THROAT

ACUTE STOMATITIS

Recurrent Aphthous Stomatitis ("Canker Sore")

The main finding is single (2–3 at most) small (3–10 mm) ulcers on the insides of the lips and elsewhere in the mouth. There is usually no associated fever or cervical adenopathy. The ulcers are very painful and last 1–2 weeks. They may recur numerous times throughout the patient's life. The cause is unknown, though an allergic or autoimmune basis is suspected.

Treatment consists of coating the lesions with topical antacids or sucralfate qid. Topical corticosteroids, either in a dental paste (eg, triamcinolone acetonide 0.1% [Kenalog in Orabase]) or in a mouthwash administered four times a day are also helpful. Pain can be managed symptomatically by a bland diet; instructing patients to avoid salty or acid foods; switching infants from a bottle to a cup; and giving 2% viscous lidocaine prior to meals with acetaminophen or even codeine at bedtime. Do not give lidocaine to children too young to expectorate it.

Herpes Simplex Gingivostomatitis

Approximately 1% of children develop multiple (10 or more) small (1–3 mm) ulcers of the buccal mucosa, anterior pillars, inner lips, tongue, and especially the gingiva on their first exposure to the herpes simplex virus. The lesions are often associated with fever, tender cervical nodes, and generalized inflammation of the mouth. Patients are commonly under 3 years of age. This disorder lasts 7–10 days. Severe dysphagia interferes with eating and drinking. Treatment is symptomatic as described for recurrent aphthous stomatitis (above), with the exception that corticosteroids are contraindicated because they may encourage spread of the infection. Early in the course consider prescribing acyclovir suspension (200 mg/5 mL), 10 mg/kg/dose tid for 7 days. Follow the patient closely. Dehydration occasionally ensues despite liberal offerings of cold fluids, in which case the patient must be hospitalized for intravenous rehydration. Herpetic laryngotracheitis is a rare complication. See also Chapter 10.

Thrush

Oral candidiasis mainly affects bottle-fed infants and occasionally older children in a debilitated state. *Candida albicans* is a saprophyte that is normally not invasive unless the mouth is abraded. The use of broad-spectrum antibiotics may be a contributing factor. Symptoms include soreness of the mouth and refusal of feedings. Lesions consist of white curd-like plaques predominantly on the buccal mucosa. These plaques cannot be washed away after a water feeding.

Specific treatment consists of use of nystatin (Mycostatin) oral suspension, 1 mL qid for 1 week. This should be preceded by removal of any large plaques with a moistened cotton-tipped applicator or piece of gauze.

Traumatic Oral Ulcers

Ulcers are a nonspecific response of the oral mucosa to trauma. Mechanical trauma most commonly occurs on the buccal mucosa secondary to accidental biting. Thermal trauma (eg, from very hot foods) can also cause ulcerative lesions. Chemical ulcers can be produced by mucosal contact with aspirin, caustics, etc. Oral ulcers can also occur with leukemia or on a recurrent basis with cyclic neutropenia. These lesions usually need no treatment. The pain subsides in 2–3 days.

ACUTE VIRAL PHARYNGITIS & TONSILLITIS

Over 90% of cases of sore throat and fever in children are due to viral infections. Most children develop associated rhinorrhea and mild cough; in fact, they are simply having a cold. Findings seldom give any clue to the particular viral agent; however, six types of viral pharyngitis are sufficiently distinctive to warrant descriptions of specific causes.

Infectious Mononucleosis: The findings are an exudative tonsillitis, generalized cervical adenitis, and fever, most commonly in teenagers. A palpable spleen or axillary adenopathy adds weight to the diagnosis. The presence of > 20% atypical lymphocytes on a peripheral blood smear or a positive mononucleosis spot test (Monospot) confirms the diagnosis, although the Monospot is frequently negative in children under 5 years old. This diagnosis is often not considered until a patient with a presumptive diagnosis of streptococcal pharyngitis has failed to respond to 48 hours of treatment with penicillin.

Herpangina: Herpangina ulcers, 2–3 mm in size, are found on the anterior pillars and sometimes on the soft palate and uvula. There are no ulcers in the anterior mouth, as there are in herpes simplex. Herpangina is caused by several members of the coxsackie A group of viruses. A patient can have up to five bouts of herpangina in a lifetime.

Lymphonodular Pharyngitis: The classic finding is small, yellow-white nodules in the same distribution as the small ulcers in herpangina. In this condition, which is caused by coxsackievirus A10, the nodules do not ulcerate.

Hand-Foot-and-Mouth Disease: This entity is caused by coxsackieviruses A5, A10, and A16. Ulcers occur on the tongue and oral mucosa. Vesicles, which usually do not ulcerate, are found on the palms, soles, and interdigital areas. See also Chapter 10.

Pharyngoconjunctival Fever: This disorder is caused by an adenovirus. Exudative tonsillitis, conjunctivitis, and fever are the main findings.

Rubeola: The prodrome of measles looks like any nonspecific viral respiratory infection until one closely examines the buccal mucosa and the inner aspects of the lower lip. Small white specks the size of salt granules on an erythematous base (Koplik's spots) found at these sites are pathognomonic of early measles. See also Chapter 10.

Treatment

The treatment of acute viral pharyngitis is strictly symptomatic. Older children can gargle with warm saline solution or antacid solution (eg, Mylanta). Younger children can suck on hard candy (especially butterscotch). Analgesics and antipyretics are sometimes helpful. Antibiotics are *not* helpful.

ACUTE STREPTOCOCCAL PHARYNGITIS & TONSILLITIS

Approximately 10% of children with sore throat and fever have a streptococcal infection. Untreated streptococcal pharyngitis can result in acute rheumatic fever, glomerulonephritis, and suppurative complications (eg, cervical adenitis, peritonsillar abscess, otitis media, cellulitis, and septicemia). Vesicles and ulcers are suggestive of viral infection, whereas cervical adenitis, petechiae, a beefy-red uvula, and a tonsillar exudate are suggestive of streptococcal infection. A definitive diagnosis necessitates obtaining a throat culture or a rapid identification test. Rapid identification tests are very specific but lack sensitivity; a positive test indicates infection but a negative result requires confirmation with culture. Treat cases of suspected or proven *S pyogenes* infection with a 10-day course of oral penicillin V potassium or cephalosporin (eg, cephalexin) or an intramuscular injection of penicillin G benzathine. Use erythromycin for patients allergic to penicillin. Treatment failure after 10 days of penicillin V administered three times daily varies from 6% to 23%. Causes of treatment failure include unrecognized carriers, poor compliance, reacquisition of a different strain, inactivation of penicillin by β-lactamase, or the development of tolerance by *S pyogenes*. Approximately 5% of *S pyogenes* are resistant to erythromycin. Remember that trimethoprim-sulfamethoxazole is not an effective antibiotic for this pathogen. Children should receive 24 hours of therapy prior to returning to school.

If the child has a history of recurrent streptococcal infection, one must document the presence of *S pyogenes* in an asymptomatic patient following a course of therapy. If compliance or the antibiotic dosage was questionable, treat with intramuscular penicillin; otherwise, treat with an antibiotic effective against β-lactamase-producing organisms (amoxicillin plus clavulanate, a cephalosporin, or erythromycin). If this therapy fails to eradicate the organism, consider a course of clindamycin for 10 days. In general, the carrier state is harmless, not contagious, and self-limited (2–6 months). An attempt to eradicate the carrier state is warranted only if the patient or another family member has frequent streptococcal infections or when a family member or patient has a history of rheumatic fever or glomerulonephritis. Also consider treatment for carriers who live in closed or semiclosed community settings. If the patient has had three or more documented infections within 6 months, consider instituting daily penicillin prophylaxis during the winter. Refer patients for tonsillectomy only if they continue to have frequent episodes despite antibiotic prophylaxis or when persistently enlarged tonsils cause chronic upper airway obstruction.

Other rare causes of acute nonviral pharyngitis are *Corynebacterium diphtheriae, Neisseria gonorrhoeae,* group C streptococci, meningococci, *Chlamydia, Francisella tularensis,* and *Mycoplasma pneumoniae.*

RECURRENT PHARYNGITIS

School-age children are occasionally brought to a physician with a complaint of recurrent or persistent sore throat. Fever and other systemic manifestations are usually absent. This problem has three common causes: mouth breathing, postnasal drip, and school phobia.

Mouth breathing leads to dryness and irritation of the throat, especially in areas of low humidity. Occasionally, children will even complain that their lips are stuck to their teeth upon awakening. The causes of mouth breathing should be investigated. Symptomatic treatment consists of good hydration and environmental humidification.

Postnasal drip due to chronic sinusitis can lead to continuous throat irritation. Examination reveals mucopurulent secretions descending from the nasopharynx after the patient sniffs. The irritation is largely due to repeated clearing of the throat.

Children with **school avoidance problems** are brought in repeatedly for sore throats, but physical examination reveals a normal oropharynx and tonsillar area. The diagnosis is made by asking the parent if the problem has been interfering with the child's school attendance. An affirmative answer confirms the diagnosis.

PERITONSILLAR CELLULITIS OR ABSCESS (Quinsy)

Tonsillar infection occasionally penetrates the tonsillar capsule, spreads to the surrounding tissues, and causes peritonsillar cellulitis. If untreated, necrosis occurs and a tonsillar abscess forms. This can occur at any age. The most common cause is β-hemolytic streptococci. Other pathogens are group D streptococci, α-hemolytic streptococci, *S pneumoniae,* and anaerobes.

The patient complains of a severe sore throat even before the physical findings become marked. A high fever is usually present. The process is almost always unilateral. The tonsil bulges medially, and the anterior pillar is prominent. The soft palate and uvula on the involved side are edematous and displaced medially toward the uninvolved side. In severe cases, there is trismus, dysphagia, and, finally, drooling. The quality of the voice is severely impaired by the fixation of the soft palate. On palpation, the tonsil is firm and exquisitely tender. A serious complication of inadequately treated peritonsillar abscess is a lateral pharyngeal abscess. This leads to fullness and tenderness of the lateral neck, as well as torticollis. Without intervention, the abscess eventually threatens life by airway obstruction or carotid artery erosion.

Aggressive treatment in early cases of peritonsillar cellulitis will usually abort the process and prevent suppuration. The treatment of choice is home parenteral therapy or procaine penicillin by daily injection plus oral penicillin qid in high doses. Consider adding clindamycin for better coverage of β-lactamase-producing anaerobes if the rapid streptococcal test is negative. Daily follow-up is critical to detect possible abscess. If the initial swelling is marked, fluctuation or a neck mass develops, the patient appears toxic, or symptoms fail to respond to 48 hours of antibiotics, the patient should be hospitalized for intravenous penicillin or clindamycin. Consult an otolaryngologist. Incision and drainage under general anesthesia should be considered in children who fail to respond to IV antibiotics. Recurrent peritonsillar abscesses are so uncommon (7%) that routine tonsillectomy for a single bout is not indicated. Hospitalized patients can be discharged on oral antibiotics when fever has been resolved for 24 hours and they can swallow easily.

RETROPHARYNGEAL ABSCESS

Retropharyngeal nodes drain the adenoids, nasopharynx, and paranasal sinuses and can become infected. The most common causes are β-hemolytic streptococci and *S aureus.* If this pyogenic adenitis is not treated, a retropharyngeal abscess forms. The process occurs most commonly during the first 2 years of life. Beyond this age, retropharyngeal abscess usually results from superinfection of a penetrating injury of the posterior wall of the oropharynx.

The diagnosis should be strongly suspected in an infant with fever, respiratory symptoms, and neck hyperextension. Findings also include dysphagia, drooling, dyspnea, and gurgling respirations, which are due to impingement by the abscess. Prominent swelling on one side of the posterior pharyngeal wall confirms the diagnosis. Swelling usually stops at the midline because a medial raphe divides the prevertebral space. Lateral neck soft tissue films show the retropharyngeal space to be wider than the C4 vertebral body.

Retropharyngeal abscess is a surgical emergency requiring immediate hospitalization. A surgeon should incise and drain the abscess under general anesthesia to prevent its extension. The patient's head should be kept down during incision to prevent aspiration of purulent material. Intravenous hydration and antibiotics should be instituted before surgery. A semisynthetic penicillin and clindamycin are the drugs of choice pending the results of stained smear examination and culture.

LUDWIG'S ANGINA

Ludwig's angina is a rapidly progressive cellulitis of the submandibular space, which extends from the mucous membrane of the tongue to the muscular and fascial attachments of the hyoid bone. The initiating factor in over half of cases is dental disease, including abscesses and extraction. Some patients have a history of lacerations and injuries to the floor of the mouth. Group A streptococci are the most common organisms identified, but other pathogens have been recovered.

The presenting symptoms of Ludwig's angina are fever and tender swelling of the floor of the mouth. The tongue can become enlarged as well as tender and erythematous. Upward displacement of the tongue may cause dysphagia and drooling. Laboratory evaluation includes blood cultures and hypopharyngeal aspiration to identify the specific pathogen.

Treatment consists of high doses of intravenous clindamycin or ampicillin and nafcillin pending the results of cultures and sensitivity tests. Since the most common cause of death in Ludwig's angina is sudden airway obstruction, the patient must be followed closely and intubation provided for any progressive respiratory distress. Consult an otolaryngologist to identify any abscess and assess the benefit of incision and drainage.

ACUTE CERVICAL ADENITIS

General Considerations

Local infections of the ear, nose, and throat can spread to the regional node and cause a secondary inflammation there. The most commonly involved node is the jugulodigastric, which drains the tonsillar area. Cervical adenitis is most prevalent among preschool children.

The classic presentation involves a large, unilateral, solitary, tender node. About 70% of cases are caused by β-hemolytic streptococci, 20% by staphylococci, and the remainder by viruses. *H influenzae* or anaerobes have rarely been reported as the cause. Surgeons report a higher incidence of staphylococcal infection, but they see a greater proportion of atypical cases that have failed to respond to penicillin therapy and thus require incision and drainage.

The most common site of invasion is from an inflamed pharynx or tonsils. Other entry sites for pyogenic adenitis are periapical dental abscess (usually producing a submandibular adenitis), facial impetigo (infected cuts or bug bites), infected acne, and otitis externa (usually producing a preauricular adenitis).

Early treatment with antibiotics prevents many cases of pyogenic adenitis from progressing to suppuration. Once fluctuation occurs, however, antibiotic therapy alone is insufficient. When fluctuation or pointing is present and the PPD skin test is negative, needle aspiration may promote resolution and avoid the need for surgery. If not, a surgeon should incise and drain the abscess. This can be done as an office procedure or in an ambulatory surgery unit. Hospitalization is required only if the patient is toxic, dehydrated, dysphagic, dyspneic, or less than 6 months of age. The causes of chronic cervical adenopathy include infection and malignancy.

Cat-Scratch Fever

Cat-scratch fever is caused by a pleomorphic gram-negative bacillus called *Afipia felis*; it accounts for over 70% of cases of chronic cervical adenopathy. The diagnosis is aided by the finding of a primary papule in approximately 60% of cases. In over 90% of cases, cat scratches are visible or there is a history of contact with cats. The node is usually mildly tender. The cat-scratch skin test is helpful and relatively safe. The disease can be treated orally with rifampin (87% efficacy), ciprofloxacin (84% efficacy), or trimethoprim-sulfamethoxazole (58% efficacy). Intramuscular gentamicin is an acceptable alternative (about 73% efficacy).

Atypical Mycobacterial Infection

Cervical lymphadenitis can be caused by nontuberculous or atypical mycobacteria. The adenitis is often indolent, developing over a prolonged period of time without systemic involvement or much local pain. Atypical mycobacterial infections are often associated with PPD skin reactions smaller than 10 mm. A positive PPD can cause confusion regarding the possibility of tuberculosis. Fluctuant cervical nodes should be aspirated for Gram's stain and culture. While treatment usually involves surgical excision, a course of clarithromycin or rifampin may also be tried.

Cervical Node Tumors

Malignant tumors usually are not suspected unless the adenopathy persists despite treatment. Classically, the nodes are painless, nontender, and firm or hard in consistency. Tumors may occur in a single node, in unilateral multiple nodes in a chain, in bilateral cervical nodes, or as generalized adenopathy. Cancers that may present in the neck include Hodgkin's disease, lymphosarcoma, fibrosarcoma, thyroid cancer, leukemia, and cancers with an occult primary in the nasopharynx (eg, rhabdomyosarcoma). A benign tumor that presents as enlarged cervical nodes is sinus histiocytosis.

Imitators of Adenitis

Several structures in the neck can become infected and resemble an inflamed node. The first three are congenital and are listed in order of frequency.

Thyroglossal Duct Cyst: When superinfected, this congenital malformation can become acutely swollen. Helpful findings are the fact that it is in the midline, located between the hyoid bone and suprasternal notch, and moves upward when the patient sticks out the tongue or swallows. Occasionally, the cyst develops a sinus tract and opening just lateral to the midline.

Branchial Cleft Cyst: When superinfected, this can become a tender mass 3–5 cm in diameter. Aids to diagnosis are the fact that the mass is located along the anterior border of the sternocleidomastoid muscle and is smooth and fluctuant. Occasionally, a branchial cleft cyst is attached to the overlying skin by a small dimple or draining sinus tract.

Cystic Hygroma: Most of these lymphatic cysts are located in the posterior triangle just above the clavicle. The mass is soft and compressible and can be transilluminated. Over 60% of cystic hygromas are noted at birth, and the remainder usually present by 2 years of age. If they become large enough, they can compromise swallowing and breathing.

Mumps: The most common pitfall in differential diagnosis of cervical adenopathy is to mistake mumps for adenitis. A swollen parotid crosses the angle of the jaw, is associated with preauricular percussion tenderness, is bilateral in 70% of cases, and there is frequently a history of exposure to mumps without mumps immunization. Submandibular mumps can present a diagnostic dilemma.

Ranula: This sublingual retention cyst can be mistaken for a submental node.

Sternocleidomastoid Muscle Hematoma: This cervical mass is noted in infants 2–4 weeks of age. On close examination, the hematoma is found to be an immovable part of the muscle body. An associated torticollis usually confirms the diagnosis.

SNORING, MOUTH BREATHING, & UPPER AIRWAY OBSTRUCTION

Parents sometimes bring children to the office with complaints about snoring or mouth-breathing at night. Audiotapes may help to document the severity of a child's snoring; however, they cannot provide accurate documentation of episodes of upper airway obstruction.

Differential Diagnosis

Snoring or mouth-breathing in children may result from several different causes.

Large Adenoids: Large adenoids can be suspected if the soft palate is depressed or has limited elevation, the patient's speech is hyponasal in quality, or the tonsils are unusually large. The adenoids can be assessed by mirror examination, endoscopy, or radiographic studies.

Nasal Obstruction: With the child's mouth covered, test each nostril separately for patency. One or both nostrils may be too severely occluded for adequate air exchange. Even when the nasal passages are not completely occluded, the patient may prefer to breathe through the mouth for comfort. With complete obstruction, a constant nasal discharge ensues because the normal sinus and nasal secretions can escape only anteriorly.

Nasal Polyps: Polyps appear as glistening, grayish–pink, jelly-like masses just inside the anterior nares; they occur singly or in clusters. They are characteristic of cystic fibrosis and severe allergic rhinitis. Do not mistake the turbinates for polyps.

Other Causes: Persistent mouth breathing may be due to obstruction by a nasopharyngeal tumor, a meningocele, or an encephalocele herniated into the nasal cavity. If unilateral nasal obstruction and epistaxis are frequent, juvenile angiofibroma should be suspected.

Diagnosis

A lateral neck radiograph or fiberoptic nasopharyngoscopy will assess the relative size of the adenoids. When episodes of hypopnea/obstructive apnea, failure to thrive, or clinical signs of cardiac disease are present, a chest radiograph and electrocardiogram should be obtained initially. Children with severe snoring may also develop obstructive sleep apnea or hypopnea which can be identified by a sleep study polysomnogram. **Obstructive apnea** is defined as periodic cessation of air flow for longer than 5 seconds associated with respiratory effort or bradycardia, or oxygen desaturation or termination with gasping and agitated arousal. **Hypopnea** is defined as loud snoring during sleep with periods of reduced airflow for 10 seconds or longer associated with oxygen desaturation or arousal. A sleep study polysomnogram measures heart rate, oxygen saturation, oronasal airflow, chest wall movement, carbon dioxide, electrocardiogram, and electroencephalogram waves. Absent oronasal airflow with the presence of chest wall movement, oxygen desaturation, or bradycardia indicates obstruction sleep apnea.

Treatment

Consider treating patients older than 5 years of age who have enlarged adenoids or nasal obstruction with mild or intermittent obstructive symptoms with aqueous nasal beclomethasone, 1 spray in each nostril twice daily for 4–16 weeks. This treatment appears to reduce adenoidal hypertrophy and nasal airway obstructive symptoms. Immunize children without a history of varicella to prevent more serious infection if an exposure occurs while on nasal steroids. Consider adenoidectomy with or without tonsillectomy in more severely affected children.

TONSILLECTOMY & ADENOIDECTOMY (T & A)

Indications for tonsillectomy with or without adenoidectomy include pulmonary conditions (eg, chronic hypoxia related to upper airway obstruction or hypopnea/obstructive sleep apnea); orofacial conditions (eg, mandibular growth abnormalities, dental malocclusion, and swallowing disorders); speech abnormalities; and persistent or recurrent infections.

Chronic hypoxia related to upper airway obstruction can present with signs of right heart failure (**cor pulmonale**) or pulmonary hypertension. Obstructive sleep apnea presents with loud snoring during sleep, with periods of 6–10-second respiratory pauses terminating in gasping and agitated arousal. In young children sleep apnea should not be confused with restless sleep patterns, trained night feeders, and trained night crying. There is no consensus on the infectious criteria for tonsillectomy. Reasonable indications are four or more documented *S pyogenes* infections per year; documented *S pyogenes* carrier resistant to medical therapy; or six or more tonsillitis episodes per year or five or more per year for 2 years.

Adenoidectomy

The adenoids, located in the nasopharynx, are a component of the **Waldeyer ring** of lymphoid tissue with the palantive and lingual tonsils. Enlargement of the adenoids with or without infection can obstruct the upper airway, alter normal orofacial growth, and interfere with speech, swallowing, or the functioning of the eustachian tube. Most children with prolonged mouth breathing eventually develop dental malocclusion and a so-called adenoidal facies. The face is pinched and the maxilla narrowed because the molding pressures of the orbicularis oris and buccinator muscles are unopposed by the tongue. The role of adenoidal hypertrophy or chronic infection in the pathogenesis of sinusitis is unclear. Indications for adenoidectomy with or without tonsillectomy include pulmonary conditions such as chronic hypoxia related to upper airway obstruction or hypopnea/obstructive sleep apnea; orofacial conditions such as mandibular growth abnormalities, dental malocclusion, and swallowing disorders; speech abnormalities, and persistent middle ear effusion. Children with suspected velopharyngeal insufficiency (eg, cleft palate) should not have an adenoidectomy except when there is a life-threatening obstruction.

Complications of Tonsillectomy & Adenoidectomy

The mortality rate associated with combined tonsillectomy and adenoidectomy varies from 0.004–0.006% and the rate of hemorrhage has been reported to vary from 0.49–4%. Some children with previously normal speech develop hypernasal speech. The emotional hazards of hospitalization and surgery in a child under 5 years of age have been well documented. The role of tonsils in immunologic response and disease prevention is still debated.

Contraindications to Tonsillectomy & Adenoidectomy

Short Palate: Adenoids should not be removed in a child with a cleft palate, submucous cleft palate, or bifid uvula, because of the risk of aggravating velopharyngeal incompetence and causing hypernasal speech and nasal regurgitation.

Bleeding Disorder: If a chronic bleeding disorder is present, it must be diagnosed and compensated for before a T & A.

Acute Tonsillitis: T & A should be postponed until an acute tonsillitis is resolved to prevent superinfection of the wound.

DISORDERS OF THE LIPS

Labial Sucking Tubercle

A small baby may present with a small callus in the mid-upper lip. It usually is asymptomatic and disappears after cup feeding is initiated.

Cheilitis

Dry, cracked, scaling lips are usually due to sun or wind exposure. Contact dermatitis from mouthpieces of woodwind or brass instruments has also been reported. Licking the lips accentuates the process, and the patient should be warned of this connection. Liberal use of lip balms gives excellent results.

DISORDERS OF THE TONGUE

Geographic Tongue (Benign Migratory Glossitis)

This condition of unknown cause is marked by circular or elliptical smooth areas on the tongue, devoid of papillae and surrounded by a narrow ring of hyperkeratosis. The pattern may change from day to day. The lesions are painless and may last months to years. This puzzling disorder is benign, uncommon after age 6, and requires no treatment.

Fissured Tongue (Scrotal Tongue)

This condition is marked by numerous irregular fissures on the dorsum of the tongue. It occurs in approximately 1% of the general population and is usually a dominant trait. It is also frequently seen in children with trisomy 21 and other retarded patients who have the habit of chewing on a protruded tongue.

Coated Tongue (Furry Tongue)

The tongue normally becomes coated if mastication is impaired and the patient is on a liquid or soft diet. Mouth breathing, fever, or dehydration can accentuate the process.

Macroglossia

Tongue hypertrophy and protrusion may be a clue to **Beckwith-Wiedemann syndrome**, glycogen storage disease, cretinism, **Hurler's syndrome**, lymphangioma, or hemangioma. In trisomy 21, the normal-sized tongue protrudes because the oral cavity is small.

SALIVARY GLAND DISORDERS

Epidemic Parotitis (Mumps)

Readers are referred to Chapter 10 for a discussion of the clinical findings and treatment of mumps.

Suppurative Parotitis

Pyogenic parotitis is an unusual clinical disorder found chiefly in newborns and debilitated older patients. The parotid gland is swollen, tender, and often reddened. The diagnosis is made by expression of purulent material from Stensen's duct. The material should be smeared and cultured. Fever and leukocytosis may be present.

Treatment includes hospitalization with administration of intravenous nafcillin. The most common causative organism is *S aureus*.

Recurrent Idiopathic Parotitis

Some children experience repeated episodes of parotid swelling that last 1–2 weeks and then resolve spontaneously. There is usually mild pain and often no fever. The process is most often unilateral, a fact that argues against an autoimmune process as the underlying cause and suggests some sort of obstructive process. Serum amylase is normal, which speaks against a diagnosis of viral parotitis, which may occur with mumps, parainfluenza, and other viral infections. As many as ten episodes may occur from age 2 on; the number may be reduced by antibiotic prophylaxis. The problem usually resolves spontaneously at puberty.

Treatment includes analgesics for pain. A 4-day course of corticosteroids is recommended if given early in an attack. A second episode of parotid swelling without fever is an indication for referral to an otolaryngologist for a sialogram to rule out calculus of Stensen's duct. The usual finding is sialectasis. The sialogram usually improves as the recurrence rate diminishes.

Parotid Tumors

Mixed tumors, hemangiomas, and leukemia can present in the parotid gland as hard or persistent masses. The patient should be referred to a surgeon.

Ranula

A **ranula** is a retention cyst in a sublingual salivary gland. It is found on the floor of the mouth to one side of the lingual frenulum. Ranulae have been described as resembling a frog's belly, because they are thin-walled and contain a clear bluish fluid. Referral to an otolaryngologist for excision of the cyst and associated sublingual gland is the treatment of choice.

CONGENITAL ORAL MALFORMATIONS

Tongue-Tie

The tightness of the lingual frenulum varies greatly among normal people. A short frenulum prevents both protrusion and elevation of the tongue. A puckering of the midline of the tongue occurs with tongue movement. The condition in no way interferes with the ability to nurse. It is unlikely that it interferes with the ability to speak, because even children with ankyloglossia have normal speech.

Treatment consists of reassurance. Although there is no evidence to support it, clipping of the frenulum is sometimes recommended if the tongue does not protrude beyond the teeth or gums. If this degree of tongue-tie is associated with impairment of rapid articulation, the patient should be referred to an otolaryngologist for correction. Casual frenulum clipping can result in significant bleeding from a cut lingual artery or injury to the orifices of Wharton's duct.

Bifid Uvula & Submucous Cleft Palate

A bifid uvula is present in 3% of healthy children. There is, however, a close association (as high as 75%) between this and submucous cleft palate. The latter can be diagnosed by noting a translucent zone in the middle of the soft palate. Palpation of the hard palate reveals absence of the posterior bony portion. Affected children have a 40% risk of developing persistent middle ear effusion. They also are at risk of incomplete closure of the palate, resulting in hypernasal speech. During feeding, some of these infants experience nasal regurgitation of food. Children with either of these symptoms should be referred for repair to a plastic surgeon associated with a cleft palate clinic.

14 | Eye

Robert Sargent, MD

The most important role a pediatrician plays in the ophthalmologic care of children is assurance of normal visual development. Children's central visual acuity sharpens until they are 8–9 years of age; they should then attain 20/20 vision. It is not uncommon for children to have a condition that interferes with normal visual development.

VISION SCREENING

Vision screening should be performed as soon as a child can respond verbally to an examiner's questions. Verbal responsiveness sufficient for visual screening occurs around 3–4 years of age, although some children can give feedback as early as 2–3 years. In children too young to respond to screening charts, a skilled pediatrician can sense poor fixation by one eye by alternately covering each eye. **Amblyopia,** the absence of normal vision in one eye in the presence of a normal eyeball and optic nerve, requires the earliest possible detection to assure optimal treatment.

Clinicians can screen preschoolers (ages 3–5 years) for visual problems using vision screening charts and cards. Below 4 years of age, a child is most easily tested by asking the names of common objects (eg, an airplane, duck, hand, horse, telephone, umbrella) as found in the Allen Picture Test. By the age of 4 or 5, most children can be tested with the Snellen letter "E" Test. In the "E-Game," children are asked to point their finger in the direction in which the lines of the letter E point. To eliminate confusion as to which item a child is to view, a particular letter can be blocked off. Most of the eye charts are designed for a distance of 20 feet from the child, for which we use the nomenclature 20/20 as the normal visual acuity. However, a 10-foot distance using a smaller chart creates fewer distractions and is more convenient in many settings.

A more consistent testing modality for 4–5 year old preschoolers is to ask the child to identify the letters H, O, T, and V (Figure 14–1). The child holds four cards, each depicting one of these four letters. The examiner points to one of the four letters on the wall chart and the child holds up or points to the card with the letter identical to the letter on the chart.

DEVELOPMENTAL VISION PROBLEMS

AMBLYOPIA

Amblyopia is an abnormality of the central nervous system (CNS), in which the visual perceptual cortical cells of the occiput are not stimulated in the early years of life. As a result, the sensory portion of the brain that subserves the unused eye never learns to perceive a visual image crisply. Cellular maturation of the occipital cortex progresses until approximately 8–9 years of age. If one eye does not function fully during these formative years, it will never "see" normally for the remainder of the person's lifetime. Amblyopia occurs in approximately 2–3% of the population.

Etiology

A. Strabismus: Strabismus is a Greek word meaning "bent." It refers to crooked eyes, whether the deviated eye is up, down, in, or out. A crooked eye is the commonest cause of amblyopia and occurs in 2–3% of the United States population.

Epicanthal skin folds which cover the white sclera nasally are common in the young child, and an infant may appear to have crossed eyes when indeed the eyes are aligned correctly.

B. Anisometropia: Anisometropia means "not the same refraction." For example, in a child with anisometropia, one eye may not require a corrective lens, while the other eye is considerably out of focus (eg, nearsighted, farsighted, or astigmatic). The brain receives clear retinal images from the normal eye, while the unfocused eye sends a blurry image to the brain. The poorly focused eye eventually becomes amblyopic. The condition is difficult to detect without early preschool vision screening. A skilled pediatrician can sense poor fixation in one eye based on occlusion of the better eye, and resistance of the child to fixate with the poor eye. The diagnosis of anisometropia is made by an ophthalmologist by means of cycloplegic retinoscopy.

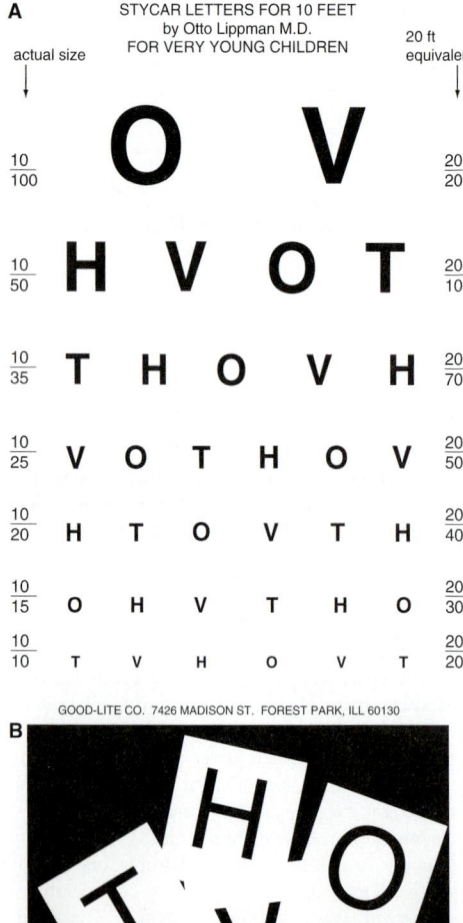

Figure 14–1. Vision testing for preschool children. To perform this test, the clinician points to a letter on this wall chart (**A**). The child is asked to point to the corresponding letter on these cards (**B**, which may be placed in the child's lap or hands.

C. Ocular Pathology That Interferes With Normal Vision:

1. Congenital cataract
2. Corneal opacities
3. Optic nerve hypoplasia
4. Vitreous hemorrhage
5. Chronic ocular inflammation
6. Unilateral trauma or surgery during the early years of life.
7. Persistent hyperplastic primary vitreous (PHPV).

Organic pathology is particularly devastating to normal visual development. One should never wait and observe these patients, but rather should refer them to an ophthalmologist who is comfortable evaluating young children.

Diagnosis

A. Pre-verbal Children: Cover testing is used for detecting crooked eyes in pre-verbal children. This is an evaluation of shifting movements of each eye when the eyes are alternately covered (Figure 14–2). If no movement occurs, there is no misalignment of the visual axes, and therefore no strabismus is present. This test is difficult to perform in young infants. The corneal light reflex from a penlight can aid in the diagnosis. The reflections should be central, or even somewhat nasal, on each side. The presence of a nasal corneal reflex is physiologic.

B. Verbal Children: Several different visual screening tests are used, depending on the child's age.

1. Three-year-olds: Allen picture cards.

2. Four- to five-year-olds: HOTV or "Tumbling E" game (Figure 14–1).

3. Six years and older: Linear alphabet.

Vision responses in children vary significantly due to differences in intellectual ability and attentiveness. If no success is obtained with a given type of test, use a simpler testing method. A *difference* of one to two lines suggests amblyopia. However, *both* eyes responding at 20/40 or 20/50 does not indicate amblyopia. Amblyopia is a *unilateral* disease process in which one eye functions less well than the other. Whenever a primary care physician suspects that a child in the early years of life has poor vision in one eye, the patient should be referred to an ophthalmologist.

Treatment

A. Patching: This is by far the most important therapy for amblyopia. It must be undertaken promptly in the early years of life, and

A

B

C

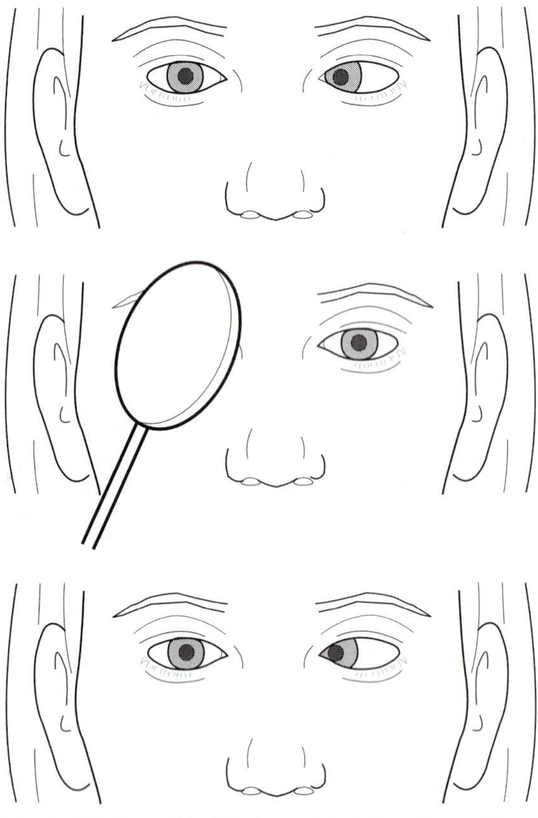

Figure 14–2. (A) The girl in this figure has left esotropia. The occluder is placed over her better, right eye (B), thereby forcing her to look out of her left eye. When the paddle is removed from the right eye, the fixation shifts back to the dominant right eye (C). Cover-uncover testing here indicates some level of amblyopia in the left eye. The clinician can estimate the degree of amblyopia by examining the fixation of the left eye when the paddle is on the right eye, and how quickly the right eye regains fixation while the left eye shifts back toward the nose. In older children, one can perform a Snellen acuity test.

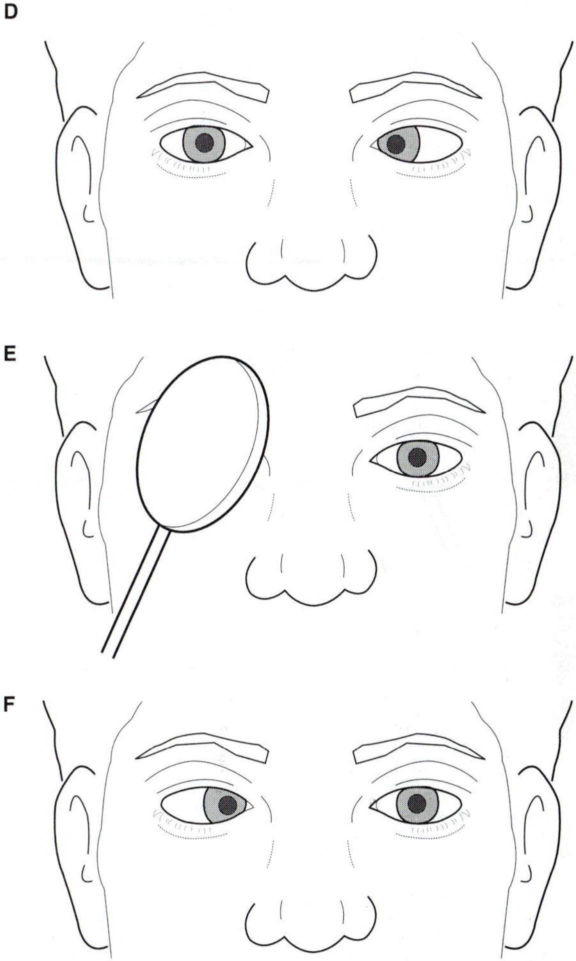

Figure 14–2. (D) The boy in this figure also has left esotropia. The right eye is covered (E), forcing him to use his left eye for fixation. When the paddle is removed (F), the child maintains fixation with the left eye, indicating good vision in the left eye. There is no amblyopia in this example.

in selected cases continued on a part-time basis until the child is 8–9 years of age.

B. Corrective Lenses: In some cases an amblyopic eye is sufficiently out of focus (referred to as anisometropia) that wearing corrective eyeglasses helps to improve visual acuity.

C. Ophthalmic Atropine: Children who resist visual occlusion (eg, by pulling off eye patches) may be helped to use the amblyopic eye by blurring the focus in the good eye. This can be done by administering ophthalmic atropine, which is an anticholinergic agent and paralyzes visual focusing. Thus, in order for the child to focus on close objects, he or she will need to use the amblyopic eye.

STRABISMUS

Strabismus is a significant problem in the pediatric population for three reasons:

1. Amblyopia is the most common and serious sequela of strabismus. The first 8–9 years of life provide the only opportunity for human eyes to develop 20/20 visual acuity. All patients with strabismus should be referred to an ophthalmologist for evaluation of possible amblyopia and patching therapy.
2. Strabismus may lead to significant secondary psychological trauma, affecting a child's self-confidence and self-esteem.
3. Strabismus may indicate the presence of neurologic, ocular, or systemic pathology. Any neurologic condition affecting the third, fourth or sixth cranial nerves can lead to strabismus. Medical diseases include diabetic neuropathy, myasthenia gravis, metastatic lesions, amyloid depositions within the muscles, and other neurologic and metabolic conditions. An eye with poor vision in early infancy usually becomes esotropic. One should suspect several possible intraocular conditions when there is a persistent unilateral esotropia. These diagnoses would include retinoblastoma, chorioretinal scars from congenital viral infections, optic nerve hypoplasia, and congenital cataracts.

Development of Ocular Alignment

The following timetable may be a useful guide in evaluating the vision of preverbal infants:

A. 0–2 Months: Dysconjugate random eye movements. Strabismus is common, particularly exotropia.

B. 2–3 Months: Child is inattentive but displays intact eye fixation and following, best noted by parent.

C. 4–5 Months: Eyes at this stage should be straight and fixating well. Generally one waits until 6 months of age before undertaking strabismus correction.

Types of Strabismus

A. Esotropia: Esotropia refers to crossed eyes (Figure 14–3A).

1. Congenital esotropia is characterized by a large angle deviation, early infantile onset, and occasional vertical strabismus. There are two types of vertical strabismus. The first is dissociated vertical deviation in which an eye floats up with inattentiveness. The second type is overacting inferior oblique muscles. Inferior oblique muscles

A

B

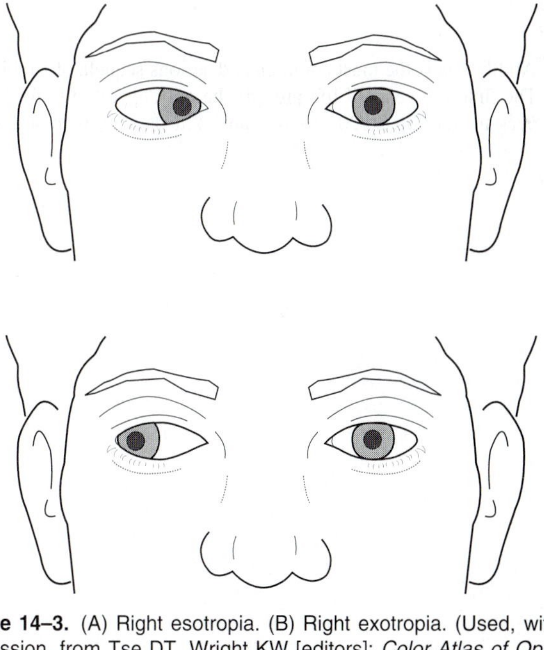

Figure 14–3. (A) Right esotropia. (B) Right exotropia. (Used, with permission, from Tse DT, Wright KW [editors]: *Color Atlas of Ophthalmic Surgery*. Lippincott, 1992.)

elevate the eye(s) when the eye(s) is turned toward the nose. Thus, when these muscles overact, one sees the eye(s) shoot upward toward the brow when the eye(s) is turned inward. Latent nystagmus is seen with congenital esotropia. Most congenital esotropes require surgery for correction of the deviation.

2. Acquired esotropia is seen in individuals who have decompensation of fusional control (eg, a CNS insult from a serious head injury or febrile illness). Diplopia is the immediate result. Children learn to suppress the diplopic image very soon; it is therefore desirable to correct an acquired esotropia without delay in order to avoid sensory suppression.

3. Accommodative esotropia results from significant farsightedness (hyperopia) in which the act of focusing to see clearly induces accommodative convergence. It usually develops between 2 and 4 years of age. Accommodative esotropia is frequently associated with amblyopia, in contrast to congenital esotropia. Treatment involves corrective lenses.

4. Intermittent, non-accommodative esotropia is not a usual categorization of esotropia; however, it represents a type of deviation whose treatment involves no glasses and no surgery. The child has straight eyes most of the time and crosses the eyes only under conditions of fatigue, illness, or stress. Therefore, the child is developing good binocular fusion and depth perception. Over a period of months or years, the fusional control can decompensate, resulting in crossed eyes for the majority of the time. When this occurs, eye muscle surgery is indicated. Ophthalmologists differ in opinion as to when to intervene surgically.

5. Duane's syndrome involves a congenitally tight medial rectus muscle that does not allow the eye to move outward. It simulates a sixth-nerve palsy on that side.

B. Exotropia: Exotropia is a condition of diverging visual axes (Figure 14–3B). It usually begins as an intermittent condition in which one eye or the other floats outward with fatigue, anxiety, or illness. Over a period of time the frequency of divergence increases because the suppression becomes better and denser. Children with intermittent exotropia tend to squint their eyelids in bright sunlight. Correction of the exotropia eliminates the squinting.

When exotropia presents later in childhood or in adult life, diplopia may result. Absence of diplopia usually indicates early-onset exotropia. The definitive treatment for exotropia is eye muscle surgery. Temporary measures include eye muscle exercises, or the use of glasses that induce accommodation (which in turn compel accommodative convergence that may control the exotropia). These therapy modalities are, however, difficult to enforce in young children.

C. Vertical Strabismus: Vertical strabismus is much less common than horizontal deviations, and is associated with diplopia, or a compensatory face turn or head tilt. Face turning and head tilting can also be seen with torticollis, congenital jerk nystagmus, and eye muscle restrictions and palsies. The condition in which an eye is depressed is called **hypotropia**, and the condition in which an eye is elevated is called **hypertropia**. Causes of vertical strabismus include congenital superior oblique palsy, Brown's syndrome (a congenitally tight superior oblique tendon), adhesion syndromes from eye muscle surgery, and fibrosis anomalies. Treatment almost always involves eye muscle surgery or prism glasses.

Treatment

The purpose of straightening a child's eyes, whether by surgery or glasses, is to allow for development of binocular fusion and depth perception. If the eyes are straight some binocular fusion may develop. If deviation is not corrected, the child is compelled either to see double or to suppress the image from the deviated eye. If the eyes are fairly straight at distance fixation, but are crossed when focusing up close, bifocal glasses are sometimes indicated for excessive convergence. This type of esotropia usually improves by adolescence.

EYE TRAUMA

EPIDEMIOLOGY

A. Preschool Children: Eye trauma in this age group may be caused by accidental bumping into hard objects (eg, table corners or chair posts). Of particular danger to toddlers are the metallic prongs that hold items for sale in department stores, supermarkets and drug stores. These are usually placed at the eyeball level of small children.

B. Elementary School Age: The most common form of injury in children between ages 6 and 12 years results from objects thrown or shot at the eye (eg, rocks, sticks, mud, snowballs, pop guns, arrows, and darts), although a direct blow to the eye from a hand or fist may also occur.

C. Adolescence: Most eye injuries in this age group are connected with sports equipment (eg, balls, bats, hockey pucks) or "shop" courses (eg, accidents from wood chips, metal splinters, broken glass, etc.), or fights. Males suffer eye injuries far more frequently than females. When a child loses an eye or has severely compromised vision, protective lenses should be used for the remaining eye.

TYPES OF EYE TRAUMA

Injuries of the eye can be divided into four broad categories:

1. Blunt contusion and dislocation of ocular tissues.
2. Laceration of the cornea and sclera with or without prolapse of intraocular contents.
3. Corneal abrasion and foreign body of the cornea.
4. Chemical burns.

Blunt Injuries

A. Categories: Blunt injuries to the eyes may be categorized as follows:

1. Subconjunctival hemorrhage: This is harmless but worrisome to parents because of the blood-red appearance of the bulbar conjunctiva.

2. Hyphema: A **hyphema** is a hemorrhage in the anterior chamber due to injury to the capillaries of the iris tissue. The amount of blood can vary from a microscopic level to complete filling of the anterior chamber. The major concern is failure of blood resorption and the development of secondary glaucoma. Re-bleeds occur most frequently on the third to fifth day post injury. In the past these children were hospitalized, but the majority of children with hyphema are now treated at home with eye rest. Treatment is primarily limitation of eye movement. Watching television is an excellent method to reduce eye movement, in contrast to performing activities that increase eye movement, such as watching a game of Ping-Pong or tennis (the eye jerks back and forth, following the ball).

3. Fracture of orbital floor between the socket and maxillary sinus: This type of injury can incarcerate the orbital contents and inferior rectus muscle below, leading to scarring and hypotropia. Usually diplopia is due to muscle contusion and will resolve in 1–2 weeks. True incarceration and restriction requires surgical intervention.

4. Disruption of the attachment of the peripheral iris to the ciliary body: This damages the outflow trabecular meshwork, which interferes with drainage of aqueous humor into the canal of Schlemm. Secondary glaucoma can occur.

5. Cataracts: These can result from blunt injuries, but are more common from lacerating injuries.

6. Dislocated lens: This type of injury interrupts clear vision and is of particular concern in children who might develop amblyopia.

7. Retinal or vitreous hemorrhage

8. Detached retina

9. Macular edema and hemorrhage

10. Choroidal rupture: This results in severe visual loss. Injuries to the posterior segment of the eye are more serious than are surface contusions and abrasions.

B. Treatment of Blunt Injuries: The pediatrician should obtain a visual acuity and refer when vision is not normal. Most cases resolve without problems and are manifest by nothing more than bruised eyelids ("shiners").

Lacerating Injuries

Lacerating injuries are ocular emergencies and require ophthalmic surgery.

A. Clinical Manifestations

1. Possible history of foreign body penetrating the globe.
2. Pain.
3. Red eye.
4. Poor vision.
5. Flat appearance to anterior chamber due to loss of aqueous humor.
6. Irregular pupil because of incarceration of the pupil edge or peripheral iris within the lacerated area.
7. Possible cataract.
8. Black or pigmented opacity on the white part of the eye indicating protrusion of uvea through scleral laceration.
9. Intravitreal or retinal foreign body.

B. Treatment

1. Obtain a visual acuity, if possible.
2. Patch or shield the eye for protection of an opened eyeball.
3. Give systemic antibiotics to get a blood level for protection of the posterior segment of the eye. Infection can occur rapidly throughout the eye (endophthalmitis), which can lead to loss of the eye itself.

4. Refer patient to an ophthalmologist.
5. Instruct patient to refrain from eating (NPO) for eventual anesthesia and surgical repair.
6. Transport patient to hospital emergency room or ophthalmologist's office.

Corneal Abrasion or Foreign Body

A. Signs & Symptoms

1. Severe localized pain.
2. Tearing.
3. Blepharospasm (squeezing eyelids).
4. Reactive conjunctival hyperemia.
5. Decreased visual acuity from the injury or copious tearing.

B. Diagnosis: Sometimes a careful history will distinguish a foreign body in the eye from a surface scratch. Inspect the upper and lower cul-de-sacs between the eye and eyelids for a foreign body. The lower lid is easy to examine, but flipping the upper lid is an art, particularly in children. The easiest way to rotate the upper lid is to use a cotton applicator as a fulcrum, and then to hold the lashes and make one decisive flip-of-the-lid. This allows examination of the tarsal plate superiorly. If a foreign body is observed, it can usually be removed with a cotton applicator.If a foreign body is not visible, you can apply fluorescein solution to the lower fornix (the crevice between the everted lower lid and the eye) in order to stain the corneal surface. Use the blue light and a +10 diopter lens of the ophthalmoscope. If a scratch is observed, it can be treated with antibiotic ointment and a tight patch. If the pain is severe, a cycloplegic dilating drop (eg, Cyclogel or homatropine) gives relief because it paralyzes the ciliary spasm contributing to the child's pain. Sometimes a patch is necessary when a foreign body is removed from the upper or lower lids, because the object may have scratched the cornea prior to its removal. Topical anesthetic drops should *not* be used, because they mask the pain.

If a foreign body *is* observed upon the cornea, instill a drop of topical anesthetic. The foreign body can be removed with the beveled edge of a 25-gauge needle, applied tangentially toward the eye. *Never* use a sharp object directed toward the eye, because a child who thrusts forward could inadvertently suffer a perforating injury from the sharp object.

C. Treatment: A tight patch over the scratched eye is important because it prevents blinking, thus minimizing pain. Prevention of blinking also allows for more rapid reepithelialization of the corneal surface. Two eye patches are placed upon the child's eye, one folded in half and the other flat upon the closed eyelid. Tape is applied from the forehead to the cheek in such a manner that the lower cheek is drawn upward before the tape is adhered to the face. When the lower cheek drops downward it flattens out the tape over the patch, applying greater pressure upon the eyeball. Additional tapes are placed nasally and temporally. Tincture of benzoin may be useful in making the skin surface sticky to improve tape adhesion.

The patch can be kept on for 24–48 hours, and then removed. Most corneal abrasions heal in this period. If there is any question about the status of the eye or vision, the child should return for a follow-up visual acuity measurement.

Chemical Injuries

Chemical injuries can be dangerous depending on the material that enters the eyes. **Alkali burns** soak into the corneal and ocular tissues leading to cellular necrosis and eventual corneal opacification. The loss of conjunctival goblet cells leads to a dry eye and a poor prognosis, even with corneal transplantation. An alkali burn may appear white and non-painful initially, but is followed by corneal ulceration and opacity.

Acid burns (eg, citric acid from grapefruit juice) produce immediate pain, irritation, tearing and conjunctival hyperemia. Apart from mechanical or chemical abrasion to the corneal surface, however, no serious injury usually ensues. In such cases irrigation of the eye suffices.

Organic solvents in the eye cause no serious injury to the globe but **mydriasis** (dilation of the pupil) may persist for weeks to months afterwards.

Thermal burns to the eye usually singe the lashes but do not cause serious pathology. If the eye perchance is exposed to a flash of heat (eg, from an explosion), a corneal abrasion results; administer topical antibiotics during management of the facial skin burn. In these situations, do *not* apply a tight patch to loose, edematous, or sloughing skin tissue.

OCULAR INFLAMMATORY DISEASES

CONJUNCTIVITIS

Conjunctivitis is inflammation of the mucosal lining of the eye; its hallmark is a red or pink eye due to vasodilatation. Secretions can be watery, mucoid or purulent. Symptoms of conjunctivitis include burning, stinging, itching, pain, or the sensation of sand, grit, or a foreign body in the eye.

Differential Diagnosis

Conjunctivitis may result from a number of different causes.

A. **Allergy**
B. **Infection:**
   1. **Bacterial**
   2. **Viral**
   3. **Fungal**
C. **Trauma**
D. **Foreign Body**
E. **Dry Eyes**
F. **Chemical Irritation**
G. **Secondary to Other Disease:**
   1. **Keratitis**
   2. **Uveitis**
   3. **Glaucoma**
   4. **Corneal Abrasion**

ALLERGIC CONJUNCTIVITIS

Allergic conjunctivitis is typically itchy and often seasonal. The discharge tends to be watery and the condition bilateral. Diagnosis can be aided by conjunctival scrapings that show eosinophils.

Treatment

A. Decongestant-antihistamine ophthalmic preparations are safest to use both to reduce the redness and give some relief as an astringent.

B. Steroids can be used for treating particularly itchy eyes. Always use fluorescein staining of the cornea to rule out dendritic keratitis as seen with herpes simplex keratitis. Steroids are contraindicated with herpes.

C. Cromolyn sodium and lodoxamide tromethamine (Alomide) are used to inhibit mast cell degranulation and are particularly helpful in treating vernal conjunctivitis that occurs around May and June. These agents should be used in patients unresponsive to steroids.

D. Environmental modification (ie, avoidance of offending allergens). An allergy work-up is usually not helpful unless the problem is chronic and recurrent.

BACTERIAL CONJUNCTIVITIS

Bacterial conjunctivitis is more often unilateral than bilateral, and is associated with pain, mucopurulent discharge and a beefy red conjunctival injection. The most common causative pathogens are *Haemophilus influenzae, Streptococcus pneumoniae, Staphylococcus aureus,* and other gram-positive organisms.

Treatment

Treatment includes antibiotic drops or ointment. If antibiotic drops are used, they should be administered every 2–4 hours while the patient is awake, and continued for at least 48 hours after signs and symptoms have disappeared. Frequent application is necessary because tearing rapidly dilutes and eliminates antibiotic solutions from the eye. Antibiotic ointments can be used less frequently, every 4–6 waking hours; however, blurring of vision may be annoying to older children. Because spread of infection is common, topical therapy may include both eyes. A number of different antibiotic preparations can be used, including topical 10% sulfacetamide or neomycin-polymyxin-bacitracin. Other options include gentamicin, tobramycin, and erythromycin. Neomycin and gentamicin ophthalmic preparations can cause an allergic reaction.

VIRAL CONJUNCTIVITIS

Viral conjunctivitis is a common complaint. It is usually bilateral and is associated with a profuse watery discharge, generalized hyperemia, and nonspecific ocular irritation, burning, or itching. The diagnostic clues for viral conjunctivitis are preauricular lymphadenopathy and associated sore throat or fever. Decongestant eye drops may help relieve the symptoms and reduce the ocular injection.

CHLAMYDIAL CONJUNCTIVITIS

Chlamydial conjunctivitis is the commonest form of infectious ophthalmia neonatorum. It is a bilateral condition with hyperacute bulbar injection with extensive mucoid discharge. The diagnosis can be made by Giemsa stain of the conjunctival scrapings or more easily with immunofluorescent monoclonal antibody stains.

Treatment of *Chlamydia* includes giving topical erythromycin or tetracycline antibiotic. Because of the association with chlamydial pneumonia, oral erythromycin for 2 weeks should supplement topical tetracycline medication.

HERPES SIMPLEX KERATOCONJUNCTIVITIS

Herpes simplex is the most serious viral pathogen affecting the eye. The DNA virus resides in conjunctival and lacrimal tissues, and can cause recurrent infections in susceptible individuals. The virus invades the corneal epithelium producing a typical dendritic pattern. Use of an ophthalmoscope with +10 magnification, blue light, and fluorescein staining will visualize the dendritic pattern. Sometimes a slit lamp is necessary for magnification. As with other viral conjunctivitis, preauricular lymphadenopathy is common. Vesicles on the lid margin and a history of stomatitis are often present.

The patient should be referred to an ophthalmologist, because blindness may result from this disease. The blindness is caused by an allergic antibody response to the viral antigen resulting in corneal opacification.

Treatment

The initial treatment of primary herpes simplex keratitis consists of application of topical antiviral agents. Either idoxuridine (IDU) ointment 0.5% or vidarabine (Vira-A) in a 3% ointment should be instilled five times a day, or trifluridine (Viroptic) in a 1% solution may be used every 2 hours (maximum dose, nine drops per day). Treatment should be continued until the lesions have cleared, although no longer than 10–12 days.

MEASLES

Rubeola typically causes a keratitis with photophobia as a bothersome side effect. The disease is self-limited and no specific ophthalmic treatment is necessary.

CHICKEN POX

Varicella infrequently involves the eyes, but may inflame any part of the anterior segment of the eye. Lesions most commonly involve the conjunctival surface, appearing as white blister-like domes of 1–2 mm with surrounding dilated capillaries. The lesions are asymptomatic, and clear as the varicella resolves. Occasionally there is crusting on the lid margin which may lead to mechanical abrasion of the cornea. In these cases, the firm crust should be removed and sterile eye ointment applied to the eye to minimize corneal irritation.

MOLLUSCUM CONTAGIOSUM

Molluscum contagiosum is a viral disease characterized by 1–2 mm solid umbilicated lesions located near the lid margin. Virus particles are released into the eye and cause a chronic conjunctivitis. Treatment involves debridement of the umbilicated tissue by pricking the central part of the pearl-like elevation with a sterile pin or needle. The central content is curetted, or treated with cryotherapy.

OPHTHALMIA NEONATORUM

Ophthalmia neonatorum is a conjunctivitis occurring in the first month of life. The most common cause is *Chlamydia* infection, but the most serious pathogen is *Neisseria gonorrhoeae*. The differential diagnosis also includes a spectrum of organisms that can infect the infant's eye from the vaginal canal during delivery, or from nosocomial infections in the hospital setting. Topical 1% silver nitrate, 0.5% erythromycin, and 1% tetracycline are considered equally effective for prophylaxis of ocular gonorrheal infection in newborn infants. The effectiveness of erythromycin and tetracycline in preventing penicillinase-producing *N gonorrhoeae* has not been established. No topical regimen has proven efficacy in preventing chlamydial conjunctivitis.

Treatment

Gonorrhea requires aggressive treatment with systemic antibiotics. Besides *Corynebacterium diphtheriae,* the gonococcus is the only organism that can penetrate intact corneal epithelium. Once the pathogen enters the eye the disease progresses rapidly to endophthalmitis and blindness. Neonates, older infants and children with gonococcal ophthalmia should be hospitalized and evaluated for disseminated gonococcal infection. Gonococcal ophthalmia should be treated for 7 days with ceftriaxone, 25–50 mg/kg/d IV or IM in a single dose, or cefotaxime 25–50 mg/kg/d IV or IM every 12 h. Infants should receive eye irrigations with buffered saline solutions until the discharge has cleared. Because of the frequency of concurrent infection with *Chlamydia trachomatis,* the mother and infant should also be tested for chlamydial infection.

Chlamydial conjunctivitis (and pneumonia) in young infants are treated with oral erythromycin (50 mg/kg/d in four divided doses) for 14 days. Topical treatment of conjunctivitis is ineffective and unnecessary.

ORBITAL CELLULITIS

Orbital cellulitis is characterized by a pink, violaceous swelling of the lid margins. There are two types: preseptal cellulitis and orbital or retrobulbar cellulitis. Both are due to upper respiratory tract infection extending from the sinuses to the periocular region.

Preseptal Cellulitis

A. Clinical Manifestations: The more common lesion, preseptal cellulitis is an inflammation anteriorly but is devoid of ocular involvement. The eye is usually white, moves easily, and is not proptotic. It is called preseptal cellulitis because the inflammation resides anterior to a fibrous septum connecting the lid margin to the orbital rim. The septum prevents extension of lid margin disease to the posterior orbital region.

B. Etiology: Preseptal cellulitis may be caused by:

1. Sinusitis with local extension.
2. Local lid disease (eg, sties or infected chalazia).
3. Lid trauma with secondary infection, occasionally with suppuration and abscess formation. In preseptal cellulitis, there is *no* proptosis, limitation of eye movement, myositic pain on eye movement, chemosis, papilledema, or compromised vision. Extension of preseptal cellulitis to the brain is rare.

In children younger than 3 years, preseptal cellulitis is far more common than orbital involvement. The most common causative pathogen is *H influenzae*, although its prevalence is reduced today because of influenza immunization. In older children, gram-positive agents are more frequent.

C. Treatment: Periorbital or preseptal cellulitis is treated by aggressive intramuscular and oral antibiotics.

Orbital or Retrobulbar Cellulitis

Orbital or retrobulbar cellulitis is a medical emergency because the focus of the infection lies between the eye and the brain. The disease can spread posteriorly to the cavernous sinus or anteriorly into the eye, resulting in vision loss.

A. Mechanism of Action: Bacterial ethmoid sinusitis extends through the thin medial bony wall into the orbital region and into the retrobulbar veins. Because these veins do not have valves, the disease can spread in a retrograde direction, creating lid margin swelling characteristic of preseptal cellulitis.

B. Clinical Manifestations:

1. Proptosis: Swelling behind the eye makes the eye appear to bulge outward. Be careful to distinguish between swollen lids per se and true exophthalmos. The easiest way to determine the difference clinically is to look over the child's forehead to see if the globe has a more anterior corneal protrusion on the involved side.

2. Myositic pain and limitation of eye movement.

3. Diplopia on side gaze due to inability to move the eye.

4. Chemosis–Chemosis refers to swelling of the conjunctiva with or without redness of the eye.

5. Venous dilatation and tortuousity of the retinal vascular tree on ophthalmoscopic examination.

6. Papilledema

7. Compromise of vision

8. Evidence of sinusitis provided by computed tomography or magnetic resonance imaging.

C. Differential Diagnosis:

1. Orbital Pseudotumor–This is a disease of unknown origin involving swelling of the soft tissue and extraocular muscles in the orbit. It is uncommon in children and is a diagnosis of exclusion when acute inflammatory disease does not respond to antibiotics. Unlike infectious orbital cellulitis, the white cell count and differential are normal; the sedimentation rate is frequently elevated. Orbital pseudotumors respond to high doses of oral steroids.

2. Rhabdomyosarcoma–Orbital involvement leads to rapid progression of lid swelling, pinkness, proptosis, and immobility of the eye. Rhabdomyosarcoma is usually asymptomatic. Diagnosis requires a biopsy. Treatment involves chemotherapy.

3. Neuroblastoma: Although metastasis can spread to the orbit, the more common finding is that of bilateral periorbital ecchymosis with minimal swelling. This is a classical sign of neuroblastoma.

4. Leukemia & Lymphoma–Either disease can have a rapid inflammatory course in the orbital region, thereby mimicking infectious orbital cellulitis.

5. Other Tumors–

1. Neurofibroma
2. Glioma of the optic nerve
3. Dermoid cysts
4. Lymphangioma
5. Hemangioma
6. Wilms' tumor

All of these tumors tend not to have the rapid course of infectious orbital cellulitis but must be considered in the differential diagnosis of exophthalmos.

STY (HORDEOLUM)

A **sty** is an acute inflammation of the oil-secreting glands in the lid margin. Sties are common occurrences in children because they tend to rub their eyes frequently, introducing gram-positive organisms. *S aureus* is the most common offending organism. Some patients have a predilection for recurrent oil gland infections, just as acne tends to afflict some teenagers more than others.

The usual presentation is one of a painful pink mass near the lid margin which occasionally spreads into an adjacent cellulitis or encapsulates into abscess. The oil gland orifice is frequently obstructed, but pressure or moist heat therapy can rupture the lesion allowing drainage of pus. Sties have no serious sequelae.

Treatment

Treatment involves hot soaks and topical antibiotic medication, 3–4 times a day. A useful approach with children is to have them watch television with a warm moist wash cloth applied to the affected lid. The wash cloth should be rewarmed periodically. Most topical antibiotics are effective in treating the infection. Ointments last longer, and can be easier to apply. On the other hand, eye drops do not blur the vision, and do not lead to a greasy-appearing lid margin.

CHALAZION

A **chalazion** is a lipogranulomatous tumor arising from the oil secreting glands within the tarsal plate (the collagenous connective tissue condensation that forms the structural support of the eyelids). Chalazia are the sequelae of chronic lid gland inflammation. The healing process leads to granulomas that incorporate lipid material from the infected ductules. They can become secondarily infected and present with a tender pink nodule on the lid. The diagnosis can be confusing between an acute sty versus a secondarily infected chalazion. The treatment is the same for both: hot soaks and topical antibiotic medications.

Uninfected chalazia are benign lumps that may present externally on the skin side, or internally on the tarsal conjunctiva. These chalazia usually require surgical excision.

An infected chalazion may last weeks to months, especially if untreated. Excision in a child requires general anesthesia. To avoid surgical excision under anesthesia, hot soaks and antibiotics should be continued for 2–3 months for resolution of the lesion. Most chalazia in children eventually clear with conservative medical treatment.

UVEITIS

Iritis is a specific term for inflammation of the anterior segment of the eye, whereas **uveitis** is a generic term for inflammation of any portion of the uveal tract. Acute iritis in children is rare and is usually associated with juvenile rheumatoid arthritis (JRA). Diagnosis of iritis requires a slit lamp examination. A work-up for JRA should be undertaken in children when iritis is diagnosed. The disease is usually unilateral and treated with steroids.

PARS PLANITIS

The anatomical structure between the anterior iris and the posterior choroid is called the **pars plana**. Inflammation of the pars plana or peripheral retinal area is infrequent, but can cause blindness. Early detection of patients with poor vision, eye pain, and secondary conjunctivitis requires evaluation by an ophthalmologist. Vision below 20/40 requires retrobulbar injection of Depo-Medrol under general anesthesia. The treatment protocol for this disease usually involves injections every two weeks for six occasions when visual acuity does not improve beyond 20/40. As long as the macular cones are not damaged, the disease usually is self-limited, but may be interrupted by chronic, recurrent inflammatory episodes over a number of years.

OBSTRUCTED NASOLACRIMAL DUCTS
(Blocked Tear Ducts)

Blocked tear ducts are the commonest cause of tearing or mucoid discharge in the neonatal period and the first year of life. The condition is commonly confused with conjunctivitis because of the mucoid discharge from the eye. The most serious condition in the differential diagnosis is congenital glaucoma.

Seven percent of newborns are born with blocked tear ducts, but in most cases, the ducts clear spontaneously. The obstruction is caused by residual epithelial membranes in the tear duct passageway.

Clinical Manifestations

1. Watery or mucoid discharge.
2. White eyeballs.
3. Crusting on lashes.
4. Adherent lid margins, particularly in the morning.
5. Reddening and maceration of skin from chronic wetness.
6. Secondary infection.
7. Clumping of lashes instead of normal feathering.
8. Tears dripping down the cheek.
9. Eye rubbing from tear crust or skin irritation.

Most blocked tear ducts are not completely occluded. On days with little lacrimation, the partial opening drains tears from the eye into the nose. But when more tears are formed secondary to irritants, rubbing, allergies, etc, the partial tear duct opening is not large enough to allow passage of tears. The tears backlog into the eye, giving a wet or mucoid appearance.

Treatment

A. Watchful Waiting: If the eyes are merely watery without redness caused by secondary infection, one can choose to wait as long as 1 year to allow the condition to resolve spontaneously.

B. Massage of Lacrimal Sac: Downward pressure upon the lacrimal sac can be applied to push mucus through the nasolacrimal duct and break any membranes blocking the way. However, studies are not conclusive that massage is beneficial.

C. Antibiotics: Antibiotic agents should be reserved for conditions involving inflammation of the bulbar conjunctiva. Tearing or mucus secretion usually recurs after resolution of the secondary infection.

D. Probing and Irrigation: This is a procedure that involves breaking of the membranes with a probe, followed by saline or water irrigation of the nasal cavity (Figure 14–4).

Most tear duct obstructions resolve spontaneously by 1 year of age. Therefore, if a child has a watery eye but does not require repetitive attention or lid margin cleansing, one can wait a full year before attempting the probing and irrigation procedure.

If a child has recurrent infection or has significant discharge throughout the day, the obstruction can be treated by probing and irrigation at any time during the first year of life. Most pediatric ophthalmologists are comfortable with performing this procedure in the office.

Prognosis

Most cases of blocked tear ducts are successfully treated with one or two courses of probing and irrigation. If these are unsuccessful, further procedures may be required. Children with Down's syndrome are particularly susceptible to failure with this procedure because of anatomical anomalies.

CONGENITAL CATARACT

A **cataract** is an opacity of the lens. Congenital cataracts are far more serious than lens opacities in adults, because dense amblyopia can result when the condition is not treated. Unilateral cataract leads to strabismus, while bilateral cataracts cause irreversible **nystagmus** (involuntary oscillation of the eyeball). A neonate with dense opacities fails to receive visual stimulation of the central nervous system. This in turn interferes with the normal sensorimotor reflexes that maintain straight and steady eyes. Permanent deterioration of vision can occur in the space of a few weeks or months.

Differential Diagnosis

A. Idiopathic

B. Familial Autosomal Dominant Heredity

C. Ophthalmologic Conditions:

1. Posterior lenticonus.

2. Microphthalmia.

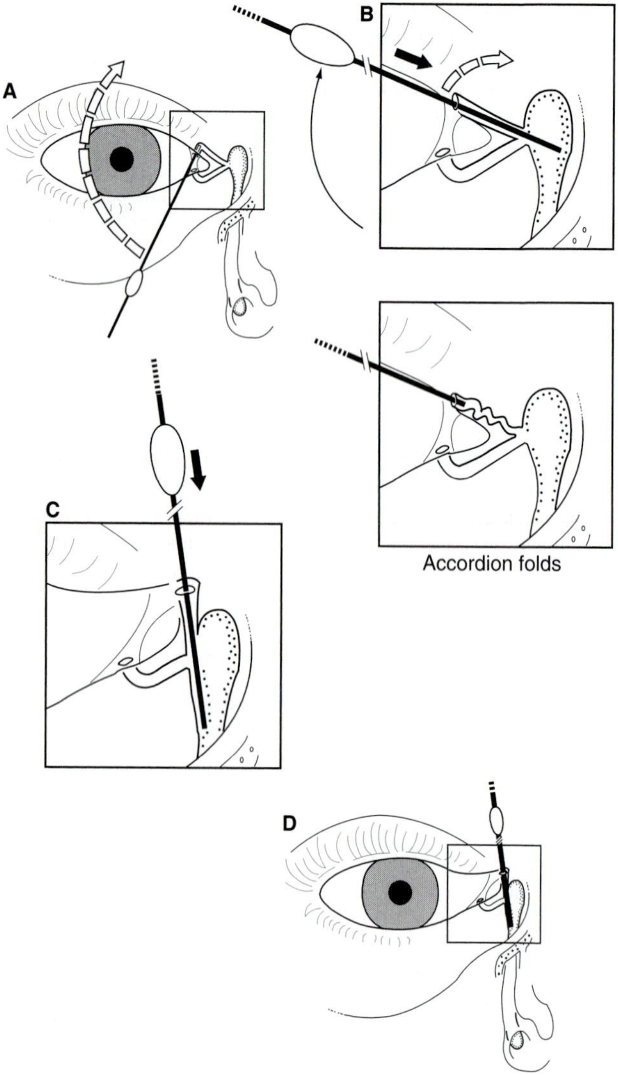
A
B
Accordion folds
C
D

3. **Aniridia.**
4. **Congenital intrauterine infections (eg, rubella).**
5. **Persistent hyperplastic primary vitreous (PHPV).**

D. **Metabolic Abnormalities:**
1. **Hyperglycemia.**
2. **Hypoglycemia.**
3. **Hypocalcemia.**
4. **Galactosemia.**

E. **Systemic Syndromes:**
1. **Lowe's syndrome.**
2. **Down's syndrome.**
3. **Hallerman-Streiff syndrome.**

Diagnosis

Diagnosis of congenital cataract is based on the following findings:

A. White pupil (leukocoria) due to opacity of the lens.

B. Unilateral strabismus, particularly esotropia, secondary to poor vision.

C. Lack of Red Reflex: This may be difficult to evaluate in a black infant because of the dense melanin pigmentation of the retina. These infants may need pupil dilatation for evaluation.

D. Clinical evidence of blindness (eg, poor fixation).

Treatment

If a congenital cataract is suspected either in the neonate or an older infant, the patient should be referred immediately to a pediatric ophthalmologist. The nature of the cataract dictates whether surgical intervention is necessary. For example, small dot-like anterior polar cataracts almost never interfere with vision, nor do trace remnants of the hyaloid system behind the lens. On the other hand, diffuse or

Figure 14–4. (A) The punctum is dilated and the Bowman probe is inserted. (B) The probe is passed through the canaliculus to the lacrimal sac. The sac is adjacent to the bony nasal wall. (C) The probe is turned inferiorly and passed through the nasolacrimal duct. This tear duct is a bony passage that connects the eye to the nose. (D) The probe is pushed into the nasal cavity, and its presence is confirmed by metal-to-metal contact with a probe that enters the nostril. (Used, with permission, from Tse DT, Wright KW [editors]: *Color Atlas of Ophthalmic Surgery.* Lippincott, 1992.)

dense cataracts require extraction of the lens. Follow-up requires frequent changes of contact lenses or eyeglass prescriptions, and careful monitoring of the child's vision for signs of amblyopia.

Children with small cataracts do not require surgical removal but the cataracts may progress with time. These children must be followed by an ophthalmologist. Lensectomy is usually considered when acuity falls below 20/70. If the child is older than 2–3 years, the eye has grown sufficiently that an intraocular lens (IOL) can be inserted. This is a new procedure in children, and is presently being investigated. An IOL obviates the need for contact lenses and puts the child's eye into optical focus immediately.

CONGENITAL GLAUCOMA

Glaucoma is a disease of high intraocular pressure associated with visual loss. The elevated pressure compresses the capillaries at the optic nerve causing ischemic damage to the neural axons connecting the optic nerve to the brain. Glaucoma in infants and children is very different from the insidious disease seen in the older adult population.

Mechanisms of Action

A. Primary Glaucoma: A congenital membrane between the iris and cornea obstructs the outflow of aqueous humor into the trabecula and canal of Schlemm.

B. Secondary Glaucomas: Mechanisms include

1. Angle closure as seen with retinopathy of prematurity, microphthalmos, persistent hyperplastic primary vitreous (PHPV)

2. Blood from trauma to the eye

3. Cellular and fibrin debris of uveitis

4. Abnormal trabecular cellular function as seen in various syndromes such as neurofibromatosis, aniridia, and Sturge-Weber syndrome.

Clinical Manifestations

A. Tearing and watering in the first year of life. This condition can mimic blocked tear ducts. Blocked tear ducts are usually associated with a mucoid discharge, while congenital glaucoma is associated with watery lacrimation.

B. Irritability

C. Squeezing eyelids (blepharospasm)

D. Severe photophobia

These findings precede clinical signs such as haziness and enlargement of the cornea.

Differential Diagnosis of Cloudy Corneas

A. Congenital Glaucoma

B. Anterior Segment Dysgenesis

C. Congenital Rubella Syndrome

D. Interstitial keratitis, particularly when caused by syphilis and tuberculosis.

E. Congenital Hereditary Endothelial Dystrophy

F. Birth trauma from forceps injury to the cornea.

Treatment

Primary congenital glaucoma usually requires surgical intervention involving incision of the membrane obstructing aqueous humor outflow. Frequently the affected eye has become enlarged prior to surgery and then becomes nearsighted. After surgery it will require care for amblyopia.

PTOSIS OF THE EYELID
(Blepharoptosis)

Congenital **ptosis** (drooping of the upper eyelid) involves muscular dystrophy of the levator palpebrae muscle. Histopathologically, the tissue lacks striated muscle fibers. Congenital ptosis occurs sporadically and usually has no familial pattern. It may be unilateral or bilateral. The droopiness is more severe later in the day with fatigue and loss of neuromuscular control. The child sometimes has to lift the chin to allow for visualization.

Differential Diagnosis

A. Congenital Muscular Dystrophy: The commonest form of congenital ptosis.

B. Horner's syndrome with sympathetic enervation.

C. Congenital fibrosis syndrome involving fibrotic extraocular muscles of the eye, as well as droopiness of the eyelids.

D. Third nerve palsies, congenital or acquired.

E. Myasthenia Gravis

F. Chronic Progressive External Ophthalmoplegia

G. Perinatal trauma caused by forceps injury to the levator muscle.

H. Mechanical Factors: large dermoid cysts, hemangiomas, and neurofibromas.

Clinical Features

A. Marcus-Gunn Jaw Winking Anomaly: During chewing or eating, occasional anomalous winking and jaw twitching occurs because of misdirected cranial nerve innervation.

B. Anisometropic Amblyopia: The droopy lid sits on the cornea and distorts the shape of the eyeball, producing astigmatism and eventual amblyopia. Ophthalmologists should rule out anisometropic amblyopia by performing a cycloplegic refraction in young children and repeating this procedure in the early years of life.

Treatment

Usual treatment involves surgery of the eyelid. The choice of technique depends on the amount of ptosis and the degree of levator muscle function. Surgery is usually performed when the child is 3–4 years of age. The exception to this rule would include infants or toddlers who raise their heads excessively in order to see.

Prognosis

Surgery for this condition has intrinsic but unavoidable complications. Most eyelids post surgery will not close completely and the lid will lag when the child gazes downward. Ointments are sometimes necessary to keep the eye moist, especially in the post-operative period.

RETINOBLASTOMA

Retinoblastoma is a rare malignancy of primitive retinal cells, usually seen in the first few years of life. There are two major types: (1) a sporadic unilateral condition caused by retinal cell mutations; and (2) a hereditary autosomal dominant form that is usually bilateral and involves germinal cell mutations. In general the hereditary forms are seen earlier, during the first year of life, while the sporadic form might first present after several years. The tumor can grow posteriorly through the optic nerve to the CNS and beyond. Most cases are detectable and treatable.

Clinical Manifestations

All neonates should be checked for red reflex, even if the examination requires a dilating drop. To examine for a red reflex, a light is shined into the eye; when light is reflected back from the retina, the red (or orange) reflex occurs. It is this phenomenon that accounts for a photographic image showing an orange pupil instead of a black pupil; the flash is reflected back from the photographic subject's retina. In persons with dark pigmentation, however, it is difficult to see a red reflex, hence the need for administering a dilating drop. Clinicians should note any of the following signs:

1. White pupil (leukocoria).
2. Strabismus.
3. Glaucoma.
4. Spontaneous hemorrhage (hyphema).
5. A solid white or yellow retinal mass that extends anteriorly into the vitreous cavity.

Treatment

Treatment of retinoblastoma includes preventive as well as therapeutic measures.

A. Genetic counseling, particularly in bilateral cases with multifocal tumors, or cases with known family history of retinoblastoma.

B. Radiation directed at the lesion. It is important to avoid the development of cataracts and retinal neovascular proliferation from the radiation.

C. Enucleation, in cases of huge tumors that are unlikely to respond to radiation, and likely to metastasize by direct extension.

D. Photocoagulation

E. Cryoapplication

F. Radon Plaque Application to posterior lesions.

G. Chemotherapy for extraocular extension.

H. Involvement of a team of specialists, including oncologists, therapeutic radiologists, pediatric and retinal ophthalmologists, and geneticists.

RETINOPATHY OF PREMATURITY

Retinopathy of prematurity (ROP) is a vascular disease of the retina seen in premature infants of less than 31 weeks' gestation, particularly in those who receive high amounts of oxygen. Vascularization of the peripheral retina is a normal process which occurs between the fourth month of pregnancy to two weeks after birth. All premature neonates undergo some degree of vessel proliferation; most do not develop pathologic changes.

ROP involves vessel proliferation into the vitreous cavity, with associated bleeding, scarring, and ultimately complete retinal detachment and blindness. The mechanism is not known precisely, but it is thought that a vasoproliferative substance is released in the peripheral avascular retina that leads to abnormal vessel growth. The end result is a cicatricial replacement of both retinal and vitreous tissue.

Clinical Manifestations

The ophthalmologist usually examines the neonate 6–8 weeks after birth, when pathologic changes may be evident. The following table summarizes the five stages of ROP development.

A. Stage I: Demarcation line or border dividing the vascular from the avascular retina.

B. Stage II: Ridge; line of previous stage acquires volume and rises above the surface retina to become a ridge.

C. Stage III: Ridge with extraretinal fibrovascular proliferation.

D. Stage IV: Subtotal retinal detachment.

E. Stage V: Total retinal detachment.

Clinically, older children present with the following findings:

1. Full recovery of central and peripheral vision.
2. Partial visual incapacity, usually loss of central acuity due to distortion of the cones in the macula area.
3. Cicatricial traction of the vessels and preretinal tissue drawn laterally, as can noted on ophthalmoscopy.
4. Severe myopia.
5. Anisometropia.
6. Mild bilateral microphthalmos.
7. Deep upper lid sulcus (indentation between the eyelid sitting upon the globe and the upper bony orbital rim).
8. Secondary glaucoma.
9. Retinal detachment.
10. Complete scarring behind the lens, called retrolental fibroplasia (RLF).

Treatment

Treatment of ROP includes the following steps and modalities:

A. Neonatal screening by ophthalmologists 6 weeks after birth.

B. Prevention, if possible, by minimization of the use of supplemental oxygen. Long-term usage is more deleterious than short, high bursts of oxygen therapy.

C. Cryoapplication to peripheral avascular retina in selected cases.

D. Vitamin E therapy: Vitamin E is an antioxidant that might retard vessel proliferation. This treatment is still under evaluation.

E. Retinal detachment surgery, when indicated.

F. Follow-up ophthalmologic examinations in selected cases.

EYELID DERMOIDS

Dermoids are benign encapsulated tumors of the eyelid, usually presenting as soft, nontender, movable masses on the outer aspect of the eyelid. They are formed during the fusion of the orbital bones, which in the early embryologic stages, incorporate ectodermal material that would otherwise differentiate into skin-like tissue; thus the term "dermoid." Sebaceous secretions and hairs can be seen inside the capsule. If the capsule is thin, the cheesy yellow contents can emerge upon traumatic impact and cause a local cellulitis.

Treatment of dermoids involves surgical excision at some time in the early years of life. Psychologically it is easier to remove these when the child is younger than 2–3 years.

HEMANGIOMA

Hemangiomas are benign capillary tumors that present as a flat pink discoloration of the skin, or as an elevated encapsulated bluish mass. A bulky hemangioma of the upper lid can close the pupil and visual axis resulting in amblyopia.

When the hemangioma has a moderate component of connective tissue there is a mottling of the red vascular tissue with gray areas giving a strawberry appearance to its surface. If the venous channels are prominent, and the tumor is subcutaneous, the hemangioma may present as a blue mass within the lid region. Characteristic of all these presentations is that of enlargement upon crying and breath holding. Hemangiomas may not be present at birth but may appear in the first 3–12 months of life. After that stage the tumor usually regresses spontaneously without treatment.

Because of the cosmetic blemish, parents and physicians may be tempted to treat these lesions early on. Most treatments, however, result in greater disfigurement and scarring. Attempts at therapy have included surgical excision, radiation, and steroids given either orally or through local injection. The best treatment in most cases is benign neglect.

When the tumor is large, intralesional steroid injections are necessary. These should be given by ophthalmologists familiar with the specific steroids and dosages.

ANISOCORIA

Anisocoria (unequal pupil size) is a common finding in the general population, presenting in early infancy. Almost all cases of anisocoria referred to pediatric ophthalmologists are benign congenital lesions that have no CNS implications. Anisocoria is a result of insufficient sympathetic innervation to the iris dilating muscle fibers. The counter-balancing parasympathetic innervation to the pupil results in miosis. The defect is in the eye with the smaller pupil, not the eye with the dilated one.

Parents sometimes indicate that the difference in pupil size is more noticeable in a dark or poorly lit room, while the pupils constrict fully in bright sunlight. From a practical point of view this has no effect upon vision at all. Only in severe cases is there a cosmetic problem. The condition is less visible with age, presumably because sympathetic innervation finally does develop.

BLINKING

During childhood, blinking is almost always a functional, unconscious tic. There is often a forced component to the closure of the eyelids, atypical of the normal orbicularis closure which takes place every 5 seconds. Associated with blinking is that of "eyes rolling up." **Hemifacial spasm** is a rare medical condition associated with blepharospasm. **Tourette's syndrome** (Chapter 8) is a known neurologic entity. Seizures may be associated with lid twitches. In preverbal toddlers, blinking can occur when vision is blurry or diplopic. Children with external ocular irritation may blink.

Respiratory Tract | 15

Kevin Kirchner, MD, & Steven H. Abman, MD

ACUTE RESPIRATORY EMERGENCIES

ACUTE RESPIRATORY FAILURE (ARF)

Acute respiratory failure (ARF) is the inability of the respiratory system to provide sufficient PaO_2 or remove enough CO_2 to meet the body's metabolic needs, because of the presence of either severe lung or airway disease, or inadequate respiratory effort. In the pediatric population, cardiopulmonary arrests are more commonly caused by respiratory problems than by primary cardiac abnormalities. Several anatomic and physiologic factors (eg, smaller airway diameters, easy fatigability of the diaphragm and other respiratory muscles, high chest wall compliance, and decreased intra-alveolar connections [pores of Kohn]) make young children more vulnerable than adults to ARF. ARF occurs in a wide variety of clinical settings (including all the disorders discussed in this chapter), and presents with variable physical findings depending on the precise cause and physiologic response.

In general, early recognition of the high risk of ARF in various clinical settings is important, in order to anticipate difficulties and initiate appropriate therapy prior to cardiopulmonary arrest (Tables 15–1, 15–2, and 15–3). Physicians may often fail to recognize the clinical severity of respiratory insufficiency without arterial blood gas measurements of arterial oxygen tension (PaO_2), carbon dioxide tension ($PaCO_2$), and pH. Although pulse oximetry and transcutaneous PO_2 monitoring are helpful in the noninvasive demonstration of serial changes in oxygenation, measurements of arterial blood gas tensions are necessary for a full assessment of acid-base balance and ventilation. $PaCO_2$ is a direct reflection of alveolar ventilation; as $PaCO_2$ rises, effective ventilation decreases proportionately. Determination of pH will help to differentiate the relative contributions of respiratory and metabolic causes of acidemia or alkalemia. A change in $PaCO_2$ of

Table 15–1. Systematic approach to acute respiratory failure.

1. Anticipate high-risk clinical setting for early monitoring and intervention prior to cardiopulmonary arrest.
2. Assessment of respiratory distress prior to arrest:
   A. *Physical examination:* mentation, cyanosis, apnea, respiratory rate, severity of distress (use of accessory muscles, grunting, retractions, paradoxical respiratory effort, breath sounds, response to oxygen administration).
   B. *Laboratory examination:* chest x-ray, monitoring with pulse oximeter and serial arterial blood gas studies.
3. Therapy dependent on clinical setting, severity of clinical findings: Intubation, ventilation, pharmacologic therapy, chest postural drainage, etc.
4. Initiate basic CPR with arrest:
   A. Airway patent? Head tilt/ chin tilt or jaw thrust; oropharyngeal/nasopharyngeal airway, endotracheal tube; cricothyrotomy.
   B. Adequacy of oxygenation? Supplemental oxygen (100%) by nasal cannula, head hood, or face mask.
   C. Adequacy of ventilation? Self-inflating bag-ventilation by face mask or through endotracheal tube.
   D. Circulation? Chest compressions if cardiac activity ineffective or absent; vascular access for fluid, drug administration; arterial and/or central venous access for monitoring.

CPR = cardiopulmonary resuscitation.

10 torr will cause a change in arterial pH of 0.08 units in the opposite direction. Similarly, a change in HCO_3 of 10 meq/L will cause a change in pH of 0.15 units. The clinical approach to the patient with ARF begins with the same "ABC" assessments used in CPR training: **a**irway, **b**reathing (effort), and **c**irculation, with further monitoring and therapeutic interventions dependent upon the severity of distress.

Table 15–2. General indications for intubation with acute respiratory failure.

Cardiopulmonary arrest, severe shock
Apnea (frequent or prolonged episodes)
Rising $PaCO_2$ (especially if >50 mm Hg, with changes in mentation, fatigue, or in face of marked respiratory effort)
Falling PaO_2 despite supplemental oxygen therapy (especially if < 60 mm Hg while breathing high fraction of inspired oxygen (FiO_2)
Marked lethargy, fatigue, encephalopathy, coma
Loss of gag reflex, inability to protect airway
Severe upper airway obstruction

Table 15–3. Age-dependent changes in pediatric sizes of endotracheal tubes, laryngoscope blades, tracheostomy tubes, and chest tubes.

Age/Weight	Internal Diameter of Endotracheal Tube (mm)	Size of Laryngoscope Blade for Intubation	Tracheostomy Size (Shiley)	Chest Tube Size (French)
Premature				
1000 g	2.5	Miller 0		10
1000–2500 g	3.0	Miller 0	Neonatal 00	10–14
Newborn–6 mo	3.0–3.5	Miller 1	Neonatal 0 Pediatric 1	12–18
6 mo–1 yr	3.5–4.0	Miller 1	Pediatric 1–2	14–20
1–2 yr	4.0–5.0	Miller 1	Pediatric 3	14–24
2–6 yr	$\frac{\text{Age (yr)} + 16}{4}$	Miller 1–2	Pediatric 3, 4	20–32
6–12 yr	Same as above	Miller/Macintosh 2	Pediatric 4	28–38
> 12 yr	Same as above	Miller/Macintosh 3	Pediatric 6	

ADULT RESPIRATORY DISTRESS SYNDROME (ARDS)/PULMONARY EDEMA

Adult respiratory distress syndrome (ARDS) is a clinical entity characterized by the progressive development of respiratory failure associated with acute lung injury due to indirect (septic or hemorrhagic shock, head trauma, burn injury, pancreatitis, others) or direct (smoke or chemical inhalation, pneumonia, aspiration, emboli) causes. Its pathophysiologic hallmark is the presence of nonhydrostatic, or permeability, edema owing to injury to the alveolar-capillary network. Nonhydrostatic edema is in contrast to the pulmonary edema secondary to elevated pulmonary venous pressures more typical of congestive heart failure (CHF).

Clinical Findings

ARDS typically progresses from tachypnea, cyanosis, and retractions to ARF within 6–48 hours of an acute catastrophic event. Although the rate of progression and the severity of illness vary, early chest x-rays (CXRs) often appear normal. However, serial studies will reveal patchy alveolar infiltrates, air bronchograms, and loss of lung volume. Diminished breath sounds and rales are typical auscultatory findings. Although initially responsive to supplemental oxygen, hypoxemia often progresses because of severe ventilation-perfusion mismatch, requiring mechanical ventilation with high mean airway pressures. Physiologically, lung compliance is low, and pulmonary artery wedge pressure [PAWP] (as measured with a pulmonary artery catheter) is normal.

Treatment

Therapy is currently supportive only. Along with treating the underlying disorder, early recognition of high-risk patients allows initiation of appropriate monitoring for progressive respiratory distress, thus decreasing the risk for sudden cardiopulmonary arrest. Monitoring generally includes a systemic arterial line for frequent arterial blood gas and continuous blood pressure measurements. Pulse oximetry provides continuous assessments of oxygenation. Assessment of fluid status often requires the placement of a Foley catheter. Dependable peripheral and central venous lines provide access for administration of blood products, fluids, and medications, and for assessing volume status. In some cases, placement of a pulmonary artery catheter will allow essential measurements of cardiac output, pulmonary artery and wedge pressures, and mixed venous oxygen tension and saturation. The overall goal of therapy is to maximize tissue oxygen delivery, which is determined by the arterial oxygen content and the cardiac index. Treatment typically includes maintaining the hematocrit above 40%, cardiac index over 4.5 L/min, and oxygen saturation above 90–92%. Volume ventilators are required to ensure delivery of sufficient tidal volume in the face of changing respiratory compliance. High levels of mean airway pressure and peak end-expiratory pressures are often necessary to correct the hypoxemia. Steroids have *not* been shown to improve the clinical course or outcome of ARDS.

Prognosis

Mortality rates of 50–60% are commonly reported for ARDS, with death often due to multiple organ-system failure associated with secondary infection and progressive respiratory failure. Some patients require prolonged ventilator support and develop chronic lung disease. Most survivors, however, appear to have few sequelae at follow-up.

ACUTE AIRWAY OBSTRUCTION

The most common causes of acute airway obstruction in children include aspiration of foreign bodies; viral croup; epiglottitis; bacterial tracheitis; peritonsillar abscess; and marked adenoidal or tonsillar hypertrophy due to infection, allergy, or trauma (most commonly postextubation).

1. FOREIGN BODY OBSTRUCTION OF THE UPPER AND LOWER AIRWAY

Foreign body aspiration contributes significantly to the morbidity and mortality of early childhood, with over 3000 deaths from this cause occurring each year. Children between 6 months and 4 years are at greatest risk.

Clinical Findings

A. Symptoms & Signs: Upper airway obstruction presents as the acute onset of cyanosis and choking, with drooling, cough, and stridor (if partial); or inability to vocalize or cough (if complete). If untreated, progressive cyanosis, loss of consciousness, seizures, and cardiopulmonary arrest follow. Onset is abrupt, usually preceded in small children by a history of running with food, a small toy, or other object in the mouth. Poor household "childproofing" or allowing older siblings to feed younger children age-inappropriate food are common findings. Lower respiratory tract obstruction generally presents with the abrupt onset of cough, wheezing, or respiratory distress. These signs may decrease or disappear over time, however, and if left untreated may lead to bronchiectasis. Lower respiratory tract obstruction should be suspected in any child with chronic cough or recurrent "pneumonias." Physical examination may reveal asymmetric breath sounds or localized wheezing or rales.

B. Laboratory Findings: *Foreign body obstruction is generally a medical emergency without the need for laboratory studies.* If obstruction is incomplete, a lateral neck x-ray may be helpful, although it generally does not replace visualization. When lower respiratory tract foreign body aspiration is suspected, inspiratory and forced expiratory (manual abdominal compression) CXRs should be obtained. The initial CXR may show asymmetric hyperinflation or atelectasis. A positive force expiratory film will show mediastinal shift away from the side of the obstruction.

Treatment

Emergency treatment of partial upper airway obstruction caused by a foreign body includes allowing the child to use his or her own cough reflex to extrude the object. Acute intervention in infants less than 1 year old includes placing the child in a face-down position over the rescuer's arm, with the head positioned below the trunk. Four measured back blows are delivered rapidly between the scapulae. If the airway is still obstructed, roll the infant over, and deliver four chest compressions as performed in CPR. Repeat this sequence until the obstruction is cleared. Blind probing of the airway to attempt to dislodge the foreign body is discouraged. If you can visualize the foreign body, you can attempt careful removal with the fingers or available instruments (eg, Magill forceps). The abdominal thrust technique (**Heimlich maneuver**) is recommended in older children.

Lower respiratory tract foreign body aspiration requires rigid bronchoscopy for removal, followed by beta-adrenergic nebulization and chest physiotherapy treatments in children with persistent symptoms.

2. INFECTIOUS CAUSES OF UPPER AIRWAY OBSTRUCTION

Several infectious agents can cause acute onset of upper airway obstruction. Although a number of these have distinctive clinical presentations, the overlap of clinical findings must be appreciated (Table 15–4). For example, viral croup may present with high fever and marked distress, as more typically seen with epiglottitis. Upper airway obstruction from a foreign body must be considered in the differential diagnosis (see above).

STATUS ASTHMATICUS

See Chapter 26, Allergic Diseases.

PLEURAL EFFUSIONS AND EMPYEMA

Pleural effusions in pediatrics are most often **parapneumonic**; that is, they are associated with a concomitant bacterial, mycoplasmal, viral, fungal, or mycobacterial lung infection. However, effusions are also associated with nephritis or nephrosis, cirrhosis, ascites, liver abscess, CHF, collagen vascular disease, pancreatitis, drug-induced lung injury, malignancy, and other causes. Clinical findings are dependent upon the underlying condition and the size of the effusion. Cough and dyspnea are common, with a secondary rise in fever often heralding the development of pleural effusion. Breath sounds are decreased or tubular in quality, with dullness to percussion over the involved area. CXR may show mediastinal shift; lateral decubitus or chest ultrasonography may help demonstrate the presence or absence of fluid loculation and the amount of fluid present. Thoracentesis provides helpful fluid samples for diagnostic and often therapeutic benefit. Studies should include pH determination (obtained in a small heparinized syringe, placed immediately on ice); stains and cultures for aerobic, anaerobic, and acid-fast organisms; cell count and differential; determination of glucose, lactate dehydrogenase (LDH), protein, and amylase; cytologic examination. Serum samples from simultaneously drawn blood should be sent for protein, glucose, amylase, and LDH. These tests help to differentiate transudate from exudate and may aid in providing a specific diagnosis for the source of the effusion and the potential need for early chest tube drainage. Chest tube drainage should be performed in the presence of a complicated parapneumonic empyema with pH < 7.15, LDH > 1000, protein > 4.5 g/dL, and/or glucose < 40 mg/dL; see Table 15–5.

Table 15–4. Infectious causes of upper airway obstruction.

Disease	Clinical Signs	Age	Season	Causes	Diagnosis and Therapy
Croup	Stridor, barking cough, mild fever, hoarseness, URI, worse at night	6 mo–3 yr	Late fall–winter	Parainfluenza (other viruses)	Cool mist, racemic epinephrine (IPPB), ± brief steroid use
Epiglottitis	Abrupt onset, toxic, anxious, high fever, drooling, dysphagia, rare cough	3–7 yr	None	*H influenzae B*	Direct visualization,[1] nasotracheal intubation, IV antibiotics, ICU admit
Retropharyngeal abscess	Acute pharyngitis, high fever, toxic, dysphagia, hyperextension of head, drooling	Variable	None	Group A strep, *S aureus*, anaerobic bacteria	Visualization,[1] lateral neck x-rays, IV antibiotics, surgery
Bacterial tracheitis	Crouplike illness, high fever, toxic	< 6 yr	Late fall–winter	*S aureus*	Visualization,[1] lateral neck x-ray, racemic epinephrine, IV antibiotics

IPPB = intermittent positive pressure breathing; URI = upper respiratory infection.

[1] Visualization should be performed by experienced personnel under controlled settings (usually in the PICU or under general anesthesia). The use of lateral neck x-rays are often helpful, but do not replace direct visualization, and should not be obtained without the patient being observed by a physician capable of managing the airway in case of an abrupt obstruction.

Table 15–5. Pleural effusions: transudate or exudate?

Type	White Blood Cell Count	Protein (g/dL)	Ratio, Pleural Fluid:Serum Protein	Ratio, Pleural Fluid:Serum LDH	Glucose	pH
1. **Transudate** (CHF, nephrosis, cirrhosis)	< 1000 (mononuclear)	< 1	< 0.5	< 0.6	= serum	> 7.40
2. **Exudate** (parapneumonic, inflammatory, collagen vascular diseases, etc)						
A. Uncomplicated	10,000	1.4–6.1	> 0.5	> 0.6	= serum	> 7.30
B. Complicated[1]	20,000 (PMNs)	> 4.5	> 0.5	> 0.6	< 40 g/dL	< 7.10

CHF = congestive heart failure; LDH = lactic dehydrogenase; PMNs = polymorphonuclear leukocytes (neutrophils).

[1] "Complicated" parapneumonic effusions are believed to require early chest tube drainage for an improved clinical response and minimization of potential sequelae.

APPARENT LIFE-THREATENING EPISODES (ALTE)

Marked controversy exists regarding the clinical management of infants with apnea or ALTE. As suggested by the long list of potential causes of ALTE or apnea (Table 15–6), these children are a heterogeneous group. Typically, infants with an ALTE present with an acute episode of apnea (central or obstructive) with or without cyanosis or pallor, changes in muscle tone, or choking and gagging. The episode is considered life-threatening by the observer, with resuscitative efforts usually initiated. Whether some children in fact represent aborted or "near-miss" sudden infant death syndrome (SIDS) is not known; however, there are reports of subsequent sudden death in such infants. Clinical evaluation includes obtaining a clear description of the event to determine whether the episode was associated with being

Table 15–6. Causes of apparent life-threatening episodes (ALTE).

Infectious
Viral (RSV, other respiratory pathogens)
Bacterial sepsis (Group B Streptococcus, pertussis, others)
Gastrointestinal
Reflux
Aspiration
Respiratory
Airway anomalies
Infection
Neurologic/Metabolic
Seizure
Central hypoventilation
Infection
Leigh's syndrome
Tumor
Carnitine deficiency
Medium-chain acyl dehydrogenase deficiency
CNS hemorrhage, stroke
Cardiac/Vascular
Cardiomyopathy
Endocardial fibroelastosis
Arrhythmia
Malformations
Pulmonary hypertension, A-V malformation
Nonaccidental Trauma
Unknown
(Apnea of infancy)

A-V = arterio-venous; CNS = central nervous system; RSV = respiratory syncytial virus.

awake or asleep, with feedings, with crying, or with signs of acute infection. Critical data include the duration of the episode, resuscitative efforts, and the infant's subsequent responses. A more complete history of developmental delays, neurologic abnormalities, signs of chronic disease, or nonaccidental trauma or neglect (eg, Munchausen by proxy syndrome [Chapter 8]) are helpful. Physical examination may help direct the laboratory evaluation, which includes sleep studies to assess respiratory pattern and oxygenation (oximetry), CXR, electrocardiography, barium swallow, esophageal pH study, air laryngotracheogram, electroencephalography, determination of serum electrolytes and hematocrit. A thorough psychosocial assessment is also an important part of the evaluation. Therapy is directed toward the identified cause. Indications for the use and duration of home apnea monitoring and respiratory stimulants, including caffeine, doxapram, and theophylline, remain controversial.

SUDDEN INFANT DEATH SYNDROME (SIDS)

SIDS, or "crib death," is a tragic but common cause of infant mortality, with an estimated frequency of 1–2 per 1000 births. Although the cause of SIDS is unknown, it generally occurs in children between 1 and 6 months of age (peak incidence: 2 months), with most deaths occurring between midnight and 8 AM. Mild upper respiratory tract infection (URI) symptoms may be present, but the role of infection is unknown. Risk factors include low birth weight; adolescent, drug-addicted, or nicotine-abusing mothers; and a family history of previous SIDS deaths. Recent epidemiologic studies suggest that infants who sleep in the prone position are at increased risk for SIDS compared to those who sleep supine or on their side. Diagnosis of SIDS is based on the clinical setting and a postmortem examination that rules out other causes of death; it may include such findings as intrathoracic petechiae, mild respiratory tract congestion, brain stem gliosis, and extramedullary hematopoiesis.

ACUTE BRONCHIOLITIS

Bronchiolitis is one of the most common causes of acute hospitalizations in young infants, especially during the winter. Although respiratory syncytial virus (RSV) is the most common cause, other agents include parainfluenza, influenza, adenovirus, *Mycoplasma*, and *Chlamydia*.

Clinical Findings

A. Symptoms & Signs: The usual course of RSV-bronchiolitis is 1–2 days of fever, rhinorrhea, and cough, followed by tachypnea, wheezing, and retractions. Some young infants, especially preterm newborns, may present with apnea and few auscultatory findings, but may later develop rales, rhonchi, and wheezing. Otitis media and superimposed bacterial pneumonia (especially pneumococcal) may develop.

B. Laboratory Findings: CXR findings include hyperinflation with mild interstitial infiltrates or segmental atelectasis. The peripheral white blood cell count (WBC) may be normal or show a mild lymphocytosis.

Treatment

Although most children infected with RSV are readily managed as outpatients, hospitalization is frequently required for those younger than 2 years. Indications for admission include hypoxemia in room air, apnea, moderate tachypnea with feeding difficulties, or marked respiratory distress. Admission is more frequent in children with underlying chronic cardiopulmonary disorders, such as congenital heart disease, bronchopulmonary dysplasia, or cystic fibrosis (CF). Arterial blood gas assessments (ABGs) or noninvasive measurements of oxygenation should be used to assess oxygen requirements and the response to therapy. Supportive therapy includes supplemental oxygen, intravenous hydration, beta-adrenergic nebulization, theophylline, or steroids. Mechanical ventilation may be required in infants with apnea or marked distress. Ribavirin therapy may be helpful for some children with coexistent cardiopulmonary disease or immunodeficiency. Its efficacy, however, remains unproven. RSV-Ig has recently been approved for prevention of infection in some high-risk populations (eg, premature infants with chronic lung disease).

Prognosis

Whereas acute outcomes are generally excellent, children with pulmonary hypertension, bronchopulmonary dysplasia, or CF may have prolonged courses with high morbidity and mortality. In addition, recurrent episodes of wheezing may follow acute infection in almost half of hospitalized patients, suggesting either a predisposition to acute bronchiolitis or an important role in the pathogenesis of chronic reactive airway disease.

CHRONIC RESPIRATORY DISORDERS

General Considerations

Diagnostic evaluation of children with chronic respiratory disease can be approached in a staged work-up, which includes consideration of age at onset of symptoms, predominant clinical respiratory signs, and related findings (Table 15–7). Because of the wide diversity of causal factors, the pace of evaluation should be based on the sever-

Table 15–7. Work-up of chronic lung disease.[1]

Initial Laboratory Studies

1. Review previous course, lab data, and radiologic studies.
2. Obtain: Chest x-ray (PA and lateral)
   - CBC with differential
   - Sweat test (pilocarpine iontophoresis)
   - Skin testing (TB, coccidioidomycosis, histoplasmosis, etc, depending on history)
   - Pulmonary function testing (if age-appropriate)
   - Sputum or nasal washings for culture

Follow-up ("Second Stage") Studies

1. More extensive pulmonary function testing (response to bronchodilator, exercise, or methacholine challenge).
2. Additional imaging studies:
   - Air laryngotracheogram
   - Barium swallow
   - Chest CT or ultrasound
3. Serologic studies.
4. Screening immunologic testing (serum immunoglobulin levels, including IgE and IgG subclasses, antistreptolysin, isohemagglutinin, and titers assessing response to past immunizations, T cell subsets, HIV status, etc).

"Third Stage" Studies

1. Flexible or rigid laryngoscopy/bronchoscopy (with or without bronchoalveolar lavage, brush sampling, biopsy, or bronchography).
2. More specialized immunologic or serologic testing.
3. Esophageal pH monitoring.
4. Cardiac catheterization, angiography.
5. Lung biopsy.

CBC = complete blood cell count; CT = computed tomography; HIV = human immunodeficiency virus; IgE = immunoglobulin E; IgG = immunoglobulin G; PA = posteroanterior; TB = tuberculosis.

[1] Reproduced, with permission, from Taussig LM, Lemen RJ: Chronic obstructive lung disease. In: *Advances in Pediatrics.* Year Book, 1979.

ity or rate of progression of clinical findings. In addition, since normal, healthy children often have 10–12 respiratory infections during infancy, physicians should carefully distinguish between a history of several different infections in a thriving child and chronic lung disorders with intermittent exacerbations superimposed on persistent respiratory signs. Evaluations should also determine the role, if any, of exposure to environmental factors (eg, household tobacco smoke, gas heat and stoves, wood-burning stoves, or air pollution from nearby factories, highways, etc).

ASTHMA

See Chapter 26, Allergic Diseases.

BRONCHOPULMONARY DYSPLASIA (BPD)

Bronchopulmonary dysplasia (BPD) is a clinical entity defined by the following criteria: (1) acute respiratory distress in the first week of life (mostly in preterm infants with hyaline membrane disease [HMD]); (2) past or present treatment with mechanical ventilation and oxygen therapy; (3) persistent signs of chronic respiratory distress, including physical signs, CXR findings, and oxygen requirement after the first month of life. Immaturity, oxygen toxicity, barotrauma, and inflammation are considered to be the major risk factors for developing BPD. Its precise definition and cause remain controversial. Iatrogenic and anatomical factors such as excessive fluid administration, patent ductus arteriosus (PDA), pulmonary interstitial emphysema, pneumothorax, infection, and inflammatory stimuli appear to play important roles in its pathogenesis and pathophysiology.

Clinical Course & Treatment

The clinical course of BPD varies widely, ranging from patients with mild oxygen requirements who improve steadily over a few months to more severely affected children who require chronic tracheostomy and mechanical ventilation. Airway hyperreactivity is common in infants with BPD, leading to frequent treatment with beta-adrenergic agonists (eg, terbutaline, albuterol [Salbutamol], and metaproterenol), theophylline, steroids and cromolyn sodium. Part of the rationale for using steroids is to decrease lung inflammation and enhance responsiveness to the nebulized bronchodilators. Recurrent atelectasis, tracheomalacia, subglottic stenosis, and other structural airway problems frequently contribute to the severity of the underlying BPD. Recurrent pulmonary edema, perhaps owing to increased vascular permeability, pulmonary hypertension, left ventricular dysfunction, or fluid overload, leads to the frequent use of long-term diuretic therapy, including administration of furosemide, hydrochlorothiazide, and spironolactone (Aldactone). Severe volume contraction, hypokalemia, hyponatremia, and alkalosis are common side effects of diuretics. To minimize the development or progression of pulmonary hypertension, infants with BPD are carefully monitored with serial pulse oximeter and blood gas tension measurements to maintain PaO_2 or O_2 saturations above 55–60 torr or 92%, respectively. Serial ECG and echocardiography studies monitor the development of right ventricular hypertrophy (**cor pulmonale**) and left ventricular hypertrophy. In addition to the cardiopulmonary abnormalities of BPD, clinical management requires close monitoring of the child's growth, nutrition, metabolic status, development, neurologic status, and related problems (eg, psychosocial adjustment).

Prognosis

Although mortality is high for advanced (Stage 4) BPD, the long-term outlook is generally favorable for most infants with the condition. More time and further study, however, are needed to determine more precisely the long-term impact of such sequelae as persistent airway hyperreactivity (asthma), exercise intolerance, and perhaps abnormal lung growth.

CYSTIC FIBROSIS (CF)

Cystic fibrosis (CF) is the most common lethal genetic disease (autosomal recessive) occurring in white children, with an estimated incidence of 1:2500 births. Although CF is found in black (1:17,000) and Asian children (1:100,000), it occurs far less frequently than in whites. Genetic studies have demonstrated that the CF gene is located on the long arm of chromosome 7 (7q31). Deletion of phenylalanine at the 508 position (delta F508) accounts for most CF mutations (70–80%). The absence of this amino acid results in an abnormal protein called the **CF transmembrane conductance regulator** (CFTR). The CFTR may have several cellular functions, but appears to be a chloride channel. This defect is believed to cause the characteristic abnormalities in sweat electrolytes and accumulation of secretions in the

Table 15–8. Presenting signs of patients with cystic fibrosis.

1. **Respiratory**
   Chronic cough, wheezing
   Persistent atelectasis
   "Recurrent pneumonia"
   Staphylococcal pneumonia
   Pseudomonas aeruginosa pneumonia, sinusitis, or bronchitis
   Clubbing
   Bronchiectasis
   Nasal polyps
   Hemoptysis
2. **Gastrointestinal/nutritional**
   Meconium ileus or plug syndrome
   Small bowel atresia
   Meconium peritonitis
   Direct hyperbilirubinemia
   Unexplained hepatomegaly, cirrhosis
   Failure to thrive
   Steatorrhea
   Chronic diarrhea
   Rectal prolapse
   Bowel obstruction
   Hypoalbuminemia
   Vitamin A, E, or K deficiency
3. **Other**
   Family history of CF
   Aspermia
   Skin "tastes salty"
   Metabolic alkalosis
   Hypoelectrolytemia
   Heat stroke, exhaustion
   Elevated intracranial pressure (vitamin A deficit)
   Intracranial hemorrhage (vitamin K deficit)

lung, pancreas, intestine, liver, and other sites, which subsequently cause multiple organ dysfunction. The clinical manifestations of CF are diverse; children with the disease may present with a wide variety of clinical abnormalities (Table 15–8). As 90% of children with CF have pancreatic insufficiency, many present with severe failure to thrive, steatorrhea, and malabsorption. These signs may present with or without respiratory disease in young infants. Diagnosis of CF is primarily based on elevated sweat chloride levels as detected by pilocarpine iontophoresis. The leading cause of morbidity and mortality, however, is progressive respiratory failure due to chronic endobronchial infection and inflammation. *Pseudomonas aeruginosa*, es-

Table 15–9. General clinical management of CF.

1. **General:** Frequent clinical assessments, every 2–4 months (depending on age, disease severity); extensive history and physical, especially growth parameters, respiratory and GI systems; psychosocial issues related to chronic disease.
2. **Nutrition:** Pancreatic enzyme supplements; caloric supplements; vitamin supplements (especially vitamin E, often A, D, and K); monitoring liver function and nutritional indices (including trace elements, protein and vitamin levels, glycosylated hemoglobin).
3. **Respiratory:** Physiotherapy (conventional, autogenic drainage, "flutter valve," PEP treatments); monitoring of oxygenation (pulse oximeter); chest x-ray; pulmonary function testing, including exercise studies; ECG; influenza vaccine (fall); Medications: aerosolized bronchodilators (if responsiveness proven), DNase therapy, cromolyn, steroids, antibiotics (oral, IV, or aerosolized; generally directed against *S aureus, P aeruginosa*).
4. **Promising interventions currently under investigation:** Amiloride; IV gammaglobulin therapy; protease inhibitors; anti-*Pseudomonas* vaccines; gene therapy

CF = cystic fibrosis; ECG = electrocardiography; GI = gastrointestinal; PEP = positive expiratory pressure.

pecially in its mucoid form, is the major bacterial pathogen associated with CF; *Staphylococcus aureus* and nontypable *Haemophilus influenzae* are other common isolates. Although clinical courses are variable, recurrent hospitalizations for respiratory exacerbations and gastrointestinal and nutritional problems are common. Prognosis has improved over the past decade but is variable; the current median age of survival is 29 years. Management approach to CF is presented in Table 15–9.

RECURRENT ASPIRATION

Although a history of breathing difficulties that occur during or shortly after a feeding, awake apnea, or vomiting can be elicited in patients with chronic aspiration, some patients present with recurrent wheezing, "recurrent pneumonia," or chronic cough, in the absence of such a history. Disorders associated with recurrent aspiration include abnormal sucking or swallowing owing to neuromuscular immaturity, brain injury, or other primary neurologic and muscle abnormalities; structural lesions of the mouth, tongue, pharynx, or jaw; esophageal dysfunction owing to vascular ring, severe reflux, achalasia, hiatal hernia, or other causes; or aspiration owing to tracheoesophageal fistula or cleft. CXR findings of migratory asymmetric infiltrates are suggestive of recurrent aspiration. Barium swallow, esophageal pH studies, and the presence of significant numbers of lipid-laden alveolar macrophages in tracheal aspirates or bronchial washings may help confirm the diagnosis. Medical management with thickened feeds, positional changes, or gastric motility agents and H_2 blockers often improves symptoms in patients with esophageal dysfunction. The decision to undergo surgical (fundoplication) intervention depends upon the severity and frequency of aspiration, as well as on its underlying cause.

INTERSTITIAL LUNG DISEASES

Pediatric interstitial lung diseases include a diverse group of clinical disorders (Table 15–10), which can be characterized by persistent inflammation and edema of the lung interstitium, alveoli, and bronchiolar walls. These developments may lead to mild dysfunction or cause progressive pulmonary fibrosis.

The clinical presentation is highly variable, but generally tachypnea is the earliest manifestation, with cough, dyspnea, retractions, and cyanosis often found. Weight loss, clubbing, hemoptysis, chest pain, and other signs may be present. Often respiratory symptoms develop insidiously. Fine rales and diminished breath sounds are heard on chest auscultation. CXR findings are highly variable, with diffuse reticular, reticulonodular, or nodular infiltrates present. Peribronchial cuffing, hilar adenopathy, and other abnormalities are present depending on the underlying cause. Pulmonary function tests often indicate a restrictive pattern, with low lung volumes and compliance and a widened gradient of alveolar-arterial oxygen tensions, especially with exercise. Diagnostic assessments include bronchoalveolar lavage and lung biopsy. Treatment and prognosis depend on the specific abnormality.

BRONCHIECTASIS

Bronchiectasis generally refers to chronic, irreversible airway injury that leads to fixed dilatation. It is most commonly caused by recurrent lower respiratory tract infections, often in association with a primary chronic disease. The latter include CF, immunodeficiencies, immotile cilia syndrome, anatomic airway obstruction, congenital deficiency of bronchial cartilage, foreign body, chronic aspiration pneu-

Table 15–10. Causes of pediatric interstitial lung disease.

Infectious
- Viral (CMV, HIV, RSV, adenovirus, influenza, parainfluenza, measles, EBV, varicella)
- *Mycoplasma*
- Protozoal (*Pneumocystis carinii*)
- Mycobacterial
- Fungal
- Bacterial (*Haemophilus influenzae, Legionella, Bordetella pertussis*)

Postinfectious
- Bronchiolitis obliterans

Inhalational
- Inorganic dusts (silica, asbestos, talcum powder)
- Organic dusts (hypersensitivity pneumonitis)
- Fumes (sulfuric acid, hydrochloric acid)
- Gases (chlorine, nitrogen dioxide, ammonia)
- Aerosols

Drug-induced
- Cytotoxic (cyclophosphamide, BCNU, CCNU, methotrexate, azathioprine, vinblastine, bleomycin, cytosine arabinoside)
- Others (nitrofurantoin, penicillamine, gold salts)

Radiation

Neoplastic
- Leukemia
- Lymphoma
- Histiocytosis

Lymphoproliferative disorders
- Pseudotumor
- Others

Metabolic
- Cystic fibrosis
- Lipidoses
- Storage disorders

Idiopathic interstitial fibrosis

Associated with collagen vascular disease, systemic vasculitis

Associated with neurocutaneous syndromes

Sarcoidosis

Pulmonary hemosiderosis

Pulmonary alveolar proteinosis

Pulmonary infiltrates with eosinophilia

Cardiac failure

Renal disease

BCNU = carmustine; CCNU = lomustine; CMV = cytomegalovirus; EBV = Epstein-Barr virus; HIV = human immunodeficiency virus; RSV = respiratory syncytial virus.

monitis, or sequelae of severe acute infections (including such agents as *Mycobacterium tuberculosis, Bordetella pertussis*, adenovirus, measles, *H influenzae*, or *S aureus*). Bronchiectasis can be classified as cylindric, varicose, or saccular, depending on its radiologic, bronchographic, or histologic appearance. **Cylindric** lesions manifest slight but uniform dilatation of the larger bronchi. **Varicose** bronchiectasis is marked by irregular dilatation and constriction of bronchi. The **saccular** form is described as having a progressively larger bronchial diameter, with gross destruction of more peripheral airways.

Clinical Findings

A. Symptoms & Signs: In 80–95% of patients with bronchiectasis, a chronic suppurative cough is present, which is generally worse in the early morning or with exercise. Purulent sputum production, hemoptysis, wheezing, and severe sinusitis may also be present. Auscultation frequently reveals localized wheezing or moist rales over the bronchiectatic lung. Digital clubbing may be present.

B. Laboratory Findings: Although CXR findings are often insensitive and not specific for the presence of bronchiectasis, the typical appearance of "tram lines," increased localized bronchovascular markings, or cystic changes may be found. The left lower lobe, right middle lobe, and lingula are the most common sites. Chest CT scanning may be helpful to confirm the presence of bronchiectasis, as well as to evaluate the rest of the lung for diffuse lesions. Bronchography can be performed in centers with personnel experienced in this technique if surgical removal is under consideration. Diagnostic evaluation depends on the clinical setting, but typically includes a sweat test; immunologic work-up; purified protein derivative (PPD) skin test, sputum cultures and stains for bacteria, fungi, and mycobacteria; barium swallow and esophageal pH study; CBC; and bronchoscopy.

Treatment

In addition to therapy specific to an underlying primary disease, aggressive chest physiotherapy after beta-adrenergic nebulization therapy is undertaken for at least 2–4 weeks. Antibiotics (based on culture results) are often given to children with bronchiectasis. Indications for surgical resection include the presence of localized disease producing severe symptoms or pulmonary hemorrhage. In the presence of diffuse lung involvement, surgery is generally not indicated.

HEMOPTYSIS, PULMONARY HEMORRHAGE, & HEMOSIDEROSIS

Acute pulmonary hemorrhage can occur with or without overt hemoptysis, and is usually accompanied by alveolar infiltrates on CXR. Hemosiderin-laden macrophages are found within the sputum and tracheal and gastric aspirates. Many cases are secondary to infection (bacterial, mycobacterial, parasitic, viral, or fungal); lung abscess; bronchiectasis (CF, immune deficiency); foreign body; coagulopathy; elevated pulmonary venous pressure (CHF); structural lesions (arteriovenous fistula, telangiectasia, sequestration, bronchogenic cyst); lung contusion; tumor; pulmonary embolus; or collagen-vascular diseases (lupus, Wegener's granulomatosis, rheumatoid arthritis, polyarteritis nodosa, Schönlein-Henoch purpura, Goodpasture's syndrome, others). **Idiopathic pulmonary hemosiderosis** refers to the accumulation of hemosiderin in the lung (alveolar macrophage). It may be related to cow's milk allergy (**Heiner's syndrome**).

Clinical findings are often nonspecific, and include cough, tachypnea, retractions, hemoptysis, poor growth, and fatigue. Some patients may present with massive hemoptysis. Auscultation reveals decreased breath sounds, wheezing, or rales. The presence of iron-deficiency anemia and hematuria should be sought. CXR findings are variable; fluffy alveolar or interstitial infiltrates may be transient, with or without atelectasis and mediastinal adenopathy. Pulmonary function testing generally reveals restrictive impairment with low lung volumes and poor compliance. Diagnostic evaluation depends upon the patient's age and associated signs (eg, serum precipitins to cow's milk proteins in infants and young children). Treatment and prognosis are dependent on the underlying etiology. Steroids or cytotoxic agents are frequently used.

CONGENITAL STRUCTURAL LESIONS

Congenital extrathoracic respiratory abnormalities cause inspiratory stridor or poor air movement despite increased respiratory effort from birth or within the first months of life. Congenital causes of airway obstruction that present in early infancy include choanal atresia; macroglossia; micrognathia (**Pierre Robin syndrome**); laryngeal atresia, cleft, web, stenosis, or cyst; subglottal hemangioma; and others. Laryngomalacia is one of the most common causes, accounting for perhaps more than half the cases. The epiglottis or arytenoid cartilages collapse into the airway during inspiration, causing laryngeal stridor. Diagnosis is readily made by flexible laryngoscopy. Although tracheostomy may be required, most children resolve their stridor within the first 2 years of life.

Congenital intrathoracic lesions are diverse and have variable clinical presentations, ranging from severe neonatal respiratory distress to mild chronic cough in older adolescents.

Tracheomalacia

Tracheomalacia consists of dynamic collapse of the trachea, often associated with other conditions, such as vascular rings, tracheoesophageal fistula (TEF), BPD, and others. It may be primary. Diagnosis can be made by air laryngotracheogram or flexible bronchoscopy.

Most children with primary tracheomalacia do not require intervention as the cartilage stiffens with growth. Nebulized ipratropium may improve the stability of the airway malacia in some patients. Occasionally, patients with tracheomalacia associated with other conditions may require surgical intervention (aortopexy, tracheostomy, tracheal reconstructive surgery).

Vascular Rings

The clinical signs of vascular rings or slings vary considerably, depending on the type of lesion and the severity of compression of central airways or the esophagus. Most commonly, stridor, wheezing, or obstructive apnea are the initial presenting signs within the first months of life. Some children may have a more delayed presentation after long-term therapy for presumed asthma. The most common type of vascular abnormality is a double aortic arch, in which the persistence of left- and right-sided embryologic fourth aortic arches leads to esophageal and tracheal compression. Aberrant innominate artery, right aortic arch with aberrant left subclavian and left ligamentum arteriosum, and pulmonary sling (distal take-off of the left pulmonary artery) are other common vascular anomalies. Laboratory evaluation includes a CXR, with particular attention to the side of the aortic arch and its tracheal caliber. Barium swallow may reveal persistent indentation of the esophagus, suggesting an aortic arch anomaly (posterior esophageal compression); a pulmonary vascular sling; or an aberrant subclavian artery (anterior esophageal compression). A normal barium esophagogram is found with aberrant innominate artery compression; however, anterior tracheal compression about 2 centimeters above the carina may be noted on lateral chest film in these patients. Further evaluation generally includes bronchoscopy to assess tracheal or bronchial compression, and, often, angiography or magnetic resonance imaging to define the anatomy more precisely. Surgical intervention is required for children with significant airway obstruction. Tracheomalacia may persist at the site of compression following surgery.

Mediastinal Masses

Mediastinal masses present with stridor, wheezing, chronic cough, or as incidental findings on CXRs obtained for other purposes. The differential diagnosis is dependent upon the mediastinal compartment in which the mass is located (Table 15–11). Although some mediastinal lesions are congenital, others develop later in childhood. Work-up includes barium swallow, chest CT scan, bronchoscopy, or exploratory thoracotomy. Skin testing for mycobacterial disease with related controls should be performed as well.

Tracheoesophageal Fistulas (TEF)

Tracheoesophageal fistulas are caused by the failure of septation of the esophagus and trachea. Distal TEF with esophageal atresia is the most common type (90%), and includes a proximal esophagus that

Table 15–11. Mediastinal masses.

Compartment	Cause
Superior	Cystic hygroma Hemangioma Thymic tumors Teratoma
Anterior	Thymoma Thymic hyperplasia Thymic cyst Teratoma Intrathoracic thyroid Lymphoma Pericardial cyst
Posterior	Neurogenic tumors Neurenteric anomaly Anterior meningocele Bronchogenic cyst
Middle	Lymphoma Lymphadenopathy Bronchogenic cyst Pericardial cyst Cardiac tumors Anomalies of the great vessels

ends in a blind pouch, with the distal esophagus connected to the trachea. Clinically, TEF may be associated with polyhydramnios, and with congenital abnormalities (35%), such as vertebral anomalies, imperforate anus, congenital heart disease, and genitourinary lesions. Cough, choking, and respiratory distress present shortly after birth. Lung injury can occur from gastric secretions entering the airway. Diagnosis is suggested by attempts to pass an esophageal catheter. A CXR will confirm the position of the nasogastric tube curled in the proximal esophagus. Treatment includes suctioning secretions from the esophageal pouch to prevent aspiration until definite surgical repair in the newborn period. Tracheomalacia often persists as a clinical problem after surgical repair. Late complications include leakage at the anastomosis site, mediastinitis, esophageal stricture, diaphragm paralysis, hiatal hernia, poor esophageal motility, and recurrent fistulas.

Pulmonary Hypoplasia

Pulmonary agenesis or **hypoplasia** represents incomplete lung development, generally reflecting an intrauterine interruption or alteration of the normal sequence of embryologic events. It may be associated with other congenital anomalies. Lungs are considered hypoplastic when their size is decreased as assessed by weight (ratio of lung to body weight is below 0.015 in premature infants less than 28 weeks' gestation, or 0.012 in older newborns). Causes include the presence of an intrathoracic mass resulting in the lack of space for lung growth (eg, diaphragmatic hernia, fetal hydrops, extralobar sequestration, thoracic neuroblastoma); decreased size of the thoracic cage (eg, asphyxiating thoracic dystrophy, achondrogenesis); decreased fetal breathing movements or diaphragmatic elevation (eventration, phrenic nerve agenesis, fetal ascites, abdominal masses); oligohydramnios (urinary outflow tract obstruction, polycystic kidneys, prolonged amniotic fluid leak); trisomies 13, 18 and 21; severe musculoskeletal disorders (arthrogryposis, osteogenesis imperfecta); and cardiac lesions (Ebstein's anomaly, pulmonic stenosis, hypoplastic right heart, scimitar syndrome). Clinical presentation is highly variable, and is related to the severity of hypoplasia as well as to associated abnormalities. Some newborns present with spontaneous pneumothorax, perinatal stress, and persistent pulmonary hypertension. Children with milder degrees of hypoplasia may present with tachypnea and related chronic respiratory signs. CXR findings include variable degrees of volume loss with a small hemithorax and mediastinal shift. Ventilation-perfusion scans, angiography, and bronchoscopy are often helpful with the clinical evaluation. Outcome is dependent on the severity of hypoplasia or related clinical problems.

Pulmonary Sequestrations

Pulmonary sequestrations are localized masses of pulmonary parenchyma that may be anatomically separate from the lung. **Extralobar** sequestrations have a distinct pleural investment and **intralobar** are located within the lung pleura. An extralobar sequestration receives its blood supply from the systemic circulation, pulmonary vessels, or both, and rarely communicates with the stomach or esophagus. The arterial supply to intralobar lesions comes from the aorta or systemic branches. Intralobar lesions are often found in lower lobes (98%), are rarely associated with congenital lesions (less than 2% versus 50% with extralobar), are rarely seen in the newborn period (unlike extralobar), and may represent acquired lesions (ie, postinfectious). Clinically, sequestrations can present as chronic cough, wheezing, recurrent pneumonias, or hemoptysis. Treatment is surgical resection.

Congenital Lobar Emphysema

This condition usually presents in the newborn period as severe respiratory distress, or during the first year of life as progressive respiratory impairment. Rarely, there is a delayed diagnosis because of mild or intermittent symptoms in older children. CXR shows overdistension of the affected lobe, with wide separation of bronchovascular markings, collapse of adjacent lung, shift of the mediastinum away from the affected side, and a depressed diaphragm on the affected side. Diagnostic studies often include fluoroscopy, ventilation-perfusion scans, chest CT scanning, angiography, and exploratory thoracotomy. Bronchoscopy may be helpful to examine whether extrinsic or intrinsic compression of the bronchus is present. The differential diagnosis includes pneumothorax, pneumatocele, atelectasis with compensatory hyperinflation secondary to ball-valve mechanism, and cystic adenomatoid malformations. Management usually involves surgical resection.

Cystic Adenomatoid Malformations (CAM)

These are unilateral hamartomatous lesions that generally present with marked respiratory distress within the first days of life. This type of lesion accounts for 95% of cases of congenital cystic lung disease. CAMs are gland-like ("adenomatoid") in appearance, and have intercommunicating cysts of various sizes. Classification of the three types of CAM is based on the size of the cysts. **Type 1** CAMs have large cysts; they are the most common (75%), and have the best prognosis for survival (98%). **Type 2** lesions consist of smaller cysts, and are often associated with other congenital anomalies (renal, cardiac, intestinal), leading to a lower (40%) rate of survival. **Type 3** CAMs present as bulky, firm masses, and have a 50% survival rate. Treatment is by surgical resection.

Bronchogenic Cysts

Bronchogenic cysts are middle mediastinal masses of variable sizes, usually located near the carina and major bronchi. These cysts usually do not communicate with the airway, and can present with acute respiratory distress and chronic cough and wheezing, or may be incidental findings on CXR. Chest CT scan or ultrasonography can differentiate solid from cystic mediastinal mass. Treatment requires surgical excision.

Pulmonary Lymphangiectasia

This is a rare and usually fatal disorder that presents as acute or persistent respiratory distress in the newborn period. It may be accompanied by generalized lymphangiectasis, **Noonan's syndrome**, asplenia, cardiovascular lesions (especially total anomalous pulmonary venous return), chylothorax, or renal malformations. CXR findings include a "ground glass" appearance, prominent interstitial markings, and hyperinflation. Therapy is largely supportive. Prognosis is poor, with most deaths occurring within the first months of life. There are isolated reports of its diagnosis and survival later in childhood.

Heart | 16

*D. Dunbar Ivy, MD, Elizabeth M. Shaffer, MD, &
Michael S. Schaffer, MD*

Cardiovascular disease in children is a significant cause of worldwide morbidity and mortality. Congenital heart defects are a major cause of these illnesses, while acquired heart diseases also play an important role. In addition, the precursors of adult heart disease begin in childhood and their prevention needs to be addressed as early as possible.

DIAGNOSTIC EVALUATION

History

Information about the perinatal period, including prenatal exposure to potential teratogens and the birth history, provides clues to particular types of heart disease. The timing of events such as neonatal distress, cyanosis, and the appearance of murmurs is helpful in differential diagnosis. Symptoms suggestive of congestive heart failure (eg, feeding difficulties and diaphoresis) are important and must be looked for. Family history is crucial in neonates because some forms of congenital heart disease are hereditary and may not be apparent at the initial evaluation of a child (Table 16–1).

Physical Examination

Cardiac examination is done in stages including inspection, palpation, and auscultation. The clinician begins the examination with a general inspection of the patient noting peripheral perfusion, color, attitude, and dysmorphic features. Vital signs, including four limb blood pressures, are imperative. Growth parameters must be assessed. The chest should be inspected for signs of dyssymmetry. Cardiac palpation and auscultation should be done with the patient in various positions (standing, sitting, and supine) because physical findings may be position-dependent (eg, the click in mitral valve prolapse). The examiner should auscultate each of the following areas: right upper sternal bor-

Table 16–1. Genetic and environmental associations.

A. CHROMOSOMAL ABNORMALITIES	
Autosomal	
Trisomy 13	VSD, PDA, dextrocardia
Trisomy 18	VSD, PDA, PS
Trisomy 21	Endocardial cushion defect, VSD, ASD
Pericentric inversion of chromosome 8	TOF, DORV, PDA
Sex Chromosome	
XO (Turner's)	Coarctation of the aorta, AS, ASD
XXXXY	PDA, ASD
Fragile X	Aortic root dilatation, MVP
B. GENE ABNORMALITIES	
Autosomal Recessive	
Ellis–van Crevald	ASD, single atrium
Friedreich's ataxia	Cardiomyopathy
Glycogen storage disease, type II	Cardiomyopathy
Jervell–Lange–Nielson	Prolonged QT interval
Hurler	Coronary artery disease, AI, MR, conduction defects
Seckel	VSD, PDA
Smith–Lemli–Opitz	VSD, PDA
Autosomal Dominant	
Ehlers–Danlos	Rupture of the large blood vessels
Holt–Oram	ASD, VSD
Marfan's	Great artery aneurysm, AI, MR
Neurofibromatosis	PS, coarctation of the aorta
Osler–Weber–Rendu	Pulmonary AV fistulas
Romano–Ward	Prolonged QT interval
Tuberous sclerosis	Myocardial rhabdomyoma, aortic aneurysm
Ullrich–Noonan	PS, ASD, IHSS
X-Linked Recessive (X-R) and X-Linked Dominant (X-D)	
Hunter (X-R)	Coronary artery disease, valve disease
Duchenne's muscular dystrophy (X-D)	Cardiomyopathy

Table 16–1. Genetic and environmental associations (*continued*).

C. TERATOGENS	
Alcohol	VSD, PDA, ASD
Phenytoin	PS, AS, coarctation of the aorta, PDA
Trimethadione	TGA, TOF, HLHS
Lithium	Ebstein's anomaly, TGA, ASD
Thalidomide	TOF, VSD, ASD, truncus arteriosus
Rubella	PPS, PDA, VSD, ASD
Maternal DM	ASH, TGA, VSD, coarctation of the aorta
Maternal phenylketonuria	TOF, VSD, ASD
Maternal SLE	Complete heart block

AI, aortic insufficiency; AS, aortic stenosis; ASD, atrial septal defect; ASH, asymmetric septal hypertrophy; AV, arteriovenous; DORV, double outlet right ventricle; HLHS, hypoplastic left heart syndrome; IHSS, idiopathic hypertrophic subaortic stenosis; MR, mitral regurgitation; MVP, mitral valve prolapse; PDA, patent ductus arteriosus; PPS, peripheral pulmonic stenosis; PS, pulmonary stenosis; SLE, systemic lupus erythematosus; TGA, transposition of the great arteries; TOF, tetralogy of Fallot; VSD, ventricular septal defect.

der and neck (aortic area); left upper sternal border and back (pulmonic area); left lower sternal border (tricuspid area); and left axilla (mitral area). The right arm and lower extremity arterial pulses must be palpated noting any discrepancy in caliber or timing. Palpation of the chest includes locating the point of maximal impulse and noting its intensity. Frequently, right ventricular preponderance is present in patients with right-sided cardiac pathology. Thrills may be present and should be noted. Auscultation must be performed in an orderly fashion. Each component of the cardiac cycle (ie, first heart sound, second heart sound, systole and diastole) must be evaluated. When characterizing murmurs, be sure to describe the timing of the murmur along with its location, intensity, and quality.

LABORATORY INVESTIGATION

Electrocardiography

An **electrocardiogram (ECG)** is a graphic representation of myocardial electric activity: the **P wave** represents atrial depolarization, the **QRS wave** represents ventricular depolarization, and the **T wave** represents ventricular repolarization. The QRS wave is a sum-

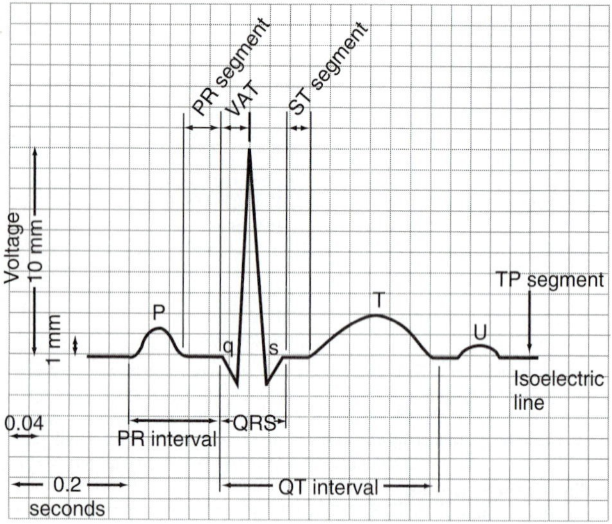

RAE: P > 2.5 mm in any lead; peaked

LAE: P > 0.08 sec; terminal deep inversion V_3R, V_1 notched

RVH: RV_1	0–24 h	> 20 mm	
	1–7 d	> 29 mm	
	1 wk–16 yr	> 20 mm	
SV_6	0–7 d	> 14 mm	
	8–30 d	> 10 mm	
	1–6 mo	> 7 mm	
	0.5–16 yr	> 5 mm	

LVH: SV_1	0–1 d	> 28 mm
	1d–1 yr	> 19 mm
	1–16 yr	> 25 mm
RV_6	0–6 m	> 16 mm
	6–12 m	> 19 mm
	1–16 yr	> 21 mm

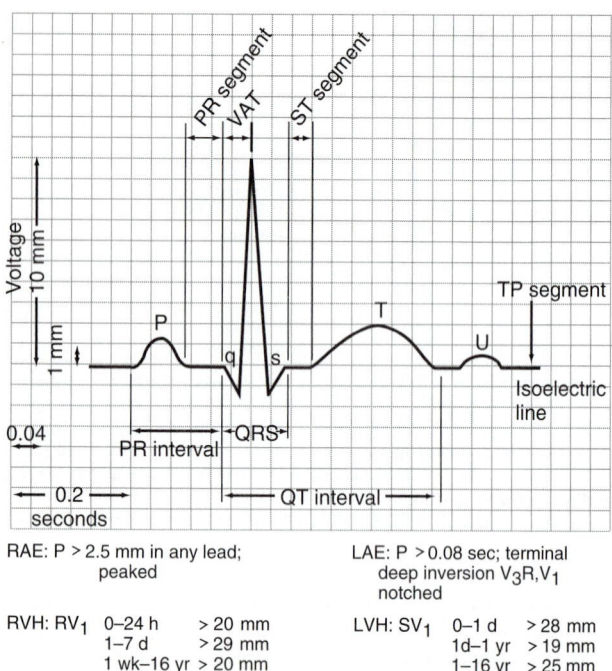

Figure 16–1. The pediatric electrocardiogram. LAE = left atrial enlargement; LVH = left ventricular hypertrophy; RAE = right atrial enlargement; RVH = right ventricular hypertrophy; VAT = ventricular activation time.

mation of both left and right ventricular activity. Throughout childhood, the heart continues to mature with a shift from right to left ventricular predominance. Thus, normal electrocardiographic criteria are dependent on the age of the subject (Figure 16–1). Increased myocardial muscle mass creates an imbalance of forces and is depicted as ventricular hypertrophy. In the presence of hypoplastic chambers, the balance of forces will be shifted and represented as hypertrophy of the opposite ventricle (eg, right ventricular hypertrophy in hypoplastic left heart syndrome).

Chest Radiography

The chest x-ray (CXR) is critical for evaluating heart size and pulmonary blood flow. The cardiothoracic ratio is increased in neonates, with 0.55 being the upper limit of normal in neonates and 0.5 the maximum in normal older children. The presence of increased and enlarged pulmonary arteries or the paucity of pulmonary vascular markings suggests increased or decreased pulmonary blood flow, respectively (Figure 16–2).

Echocardiography

Echocardiography is used extensively in evaluation and follow-up of pediatric patients with cardiac pathology. Two-dimensional imaging can supply anatomic details while Doppler studies provide pressure and flow data (Figure 16–2).

Cardiac Catheterization

Cardiac catheterization is rapidly evolving from a diagnostic tool to a technique of therapeutic intervention. Anatomic definition and intracardiac pressures are evaluated via catheterization when noninvasive means fail to elicit necessary information.

Balloon dilation valvuloplasty has become the treatment of choice for stenotic valves and post-neonatal coarctation of the aorta. Catheter occlusion of patent ductus arteriosus (PDA), atrial septal defect (ASD), systemic collaterals, and surgically placed shunts are available at some centers.

Many pediatric patients with dysrhythmias are routinely evaluated by intracardiac electrophysiologic studies to determine the mechanism of their dysrhythmias and potential therapies. Transcatheter ablation of accessory pathways can now be performed in the electrophysiologic laboratory and obviate the need for surgery.

CONGESTIVE HEART FAILURE

Congestive heart failure (CHF) is a clinical syndrome in which the heart cannot generate sufficient output to supply the needs of the body. CHF results from one of four circumstances: 1) dysfunctional myocardial tissue (eg, myocarditis or cardiomyopathy); 2) congenital cardiac malformations that decrease systemic perfusion (eg, critical

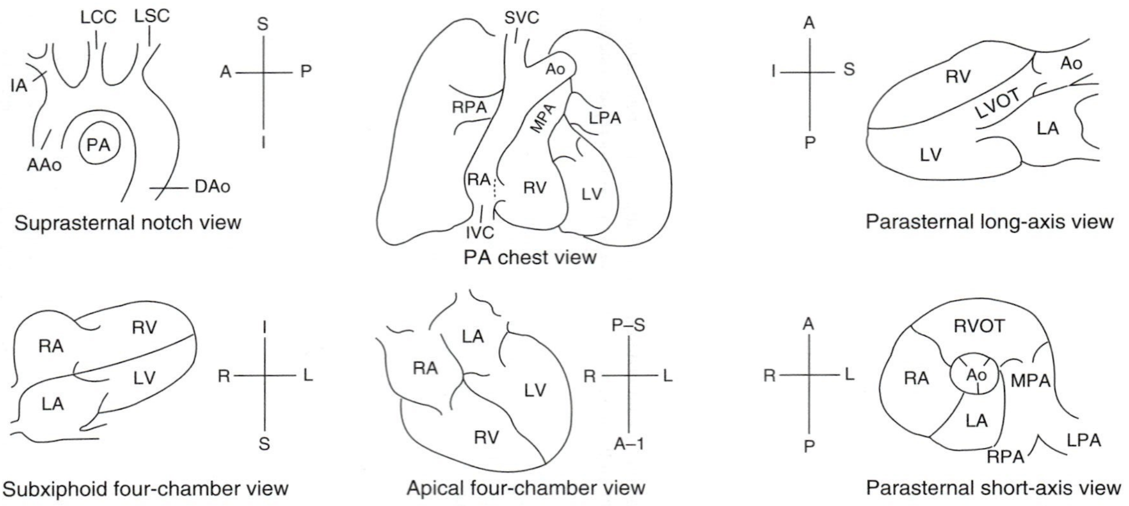

Figure 16–2. Standard chest x-ray and echocardiographic views. A = anterior; AAo = ascending aorta; Ao = aorta; DAo = descending aorta; I = inferior; IA = innominate artery; IVC = inferior vena cava; L = left; LA = left atrium; LCC = left common carotid artery; LPA = left pulmonary artery; LSC = left subclavian artery; LV = left ventricle; LVOT = left ventricular outflow tract; MPA = main pulmonary artery; P = posterior; PA = pulmonary artery; R = right; RA = right atrium; RPA = right pulmonary artery; RV = right ventricle; RVOT = right ventricular outflow tract; S = superior; SVC = superior vena cava.

aortic stenosis or large left-to-right shunts with pulmonary overcirculation); 3) normal cardiovascular systems confronted by abnormal demands (eg, thyrotoxicosis or severe anemia); and 4) dysrhythmias that fail to produce an adequate cardiac output.

Clinical Findings

Tachycardia, tachypnea, gallop rhythm, and hepatomegaly are characteristic clinical findings in CHF. Despite the numerous underlying mechanisms, findings are surprisingly similar in all cases. Additional clinical findings include diaphoresis, jugular venous distension, peripheral edema (periorbital edema in infants), cardiomegaly and, in advanced cases, cyanosis.

Treatment

Treatment of CHF should be directed at the underlying cause; however, nonspecific treatment will generally improve the patient's condition.

1. **Oxygen** should be administered unless a large left-to-right shunt is present even in the absence of cyanosis as it will increase systemic oxygen delivery and also reduce reactive pulmonary vasoconstriction.
2. **Digitalization** will improve myocardial contractility and increase cardiac output while producing diuresis.
3. **Diuretics** decrease preload and reduce pulmonary edema.
4. **Afterload reduction**, in cases of left ventricular dysfunction, will decrease systemic vascular resistance and increase cardiac output. For medication dosages, consult Table 16–2.

HYPERCYANOTIC SPELLS

Hypercyanotic or **tetralogy spells** are sudden episodes of increasing irritability, tachypnea, and intense cyanosis that may progress to syncope and seizures. They may last from minutes to hours and are frequently seen in patients with tetralogy of Fallot, tricuspid atresia, or any cardiac anomaly with reduced pulmonary blood flow and unobstructed intracardiac communication. Tetralogy spells are caused by 1) infundibular hypercontractility; 2) decreased systemic vascular resistance; or 3) decreased systemic venous return.

Hypercyanotic spells are a medical emergency. Treatment is directed at correcting the underlying problem. Frequently, soothing the

Table 16–2. Commonly used medications.

Drug	Route	Dose	Onset	Mechanisms of Action	Precautions/ Complications
Antidysrhythmics					
Adenosine	IV	Rapid IV bolus 75–100 μg/kg; if no response, 50–300 μg/kg. Maximum dose = 12 mg. Dose may be repeated once if no effect	Seconds	Purinergic agonist	Contraindicated in patients with second- or third-degree AV block, atrial fibrillation flutter and sick sinus syndrome
Atropine	IV	0.01–0.03 mg/kg/dose q4–6h. Maximum dose 0.4 mg/dose	Seconds	Parasympathetic blockade	Tachycardia
Bretylium tosylate	IV	5 mg/kg, then 1–2 mg/min	Minutes	Inhibits norepinephrine release	Hypotension
Digoxin therapeutic level: 0.6–2.0 ng/mL	PO	TDD ½, ¼, ¼ q6–8h Premature: 20–40 μg/kg Newborn–2 yr: 50 μg/kg > 2 yr: 40 μg/kg Maintenance: ¼ TDD divided bid	1–2 h	CHF: contractility Dysrhythmia: atrial conduction, AV node refractoriness	Anorexia, nausea, vomiting, headache, diarrhea, excitement, disorientation, abdominal pain, bradycardia, atrial fibrillation, ventricular tachycardia
	IV	75–80% PO dose	15–60 min		
	IM	75–80% PO dose	5–15 min		
Flecainide	PO	2–6 mg/kg/d in 2–3 divided doses	2–3h	Fast sodium channel blockade (class IC)	Contraindicated in patients with second- or third-degree AV block, bifascicular or fascicular block, sick sinus syndrome and myocardial depression. May be proarrhythmic
Lidocaine therapeutic level: 2–5 μg/mL	IV	1.0 mg/kg, then 30–50 μg/kg/min	15–90 sec	Local anesthetic. Decreases myocardial irritability	Dysrhythmia

Phenytoin therapeutic level: 10–20 μg/mL	PO	2–5 mg/kg/d, divided q8–12h	2–4h	Elevates fibrillation threshold	Bradycardia, hypotension with rapid IV infusion, blood dyscrasias, gingival hyperplasia
	IV	3–5 mg/kg loading dose	5–10 min		
Procainamide therapeutic level: 4–10 μg/mL	PO	40–60 mg/kg/d divided q6–8h	30–60 min	Slows myocardial conduction and prolongs repolarization	Hypotension, blood dyscrasias, lupuslike syndrome, acquired long QT syndrome, GI upset
	IV	10–20 mg/kg/dose	1–5 min		
Propranolol	PO	0.5–1.0 mg/kg/dose q6h	30 min	Beta blockade	Decreased cardiac output, bradycardia, hypoglycemia, asthma
	IV	0.01–0.1 mg/kg/dose q6–8h	2–5 min		
Quinidine gluconate therapeutic level: 1–6 μg/mL	PO	10–30 mg/kg/d divided q12h	Minutes	Slows myocardial conduction and prolongs repolarization	Hypotension, blood dyscrasias, tinnitus, GI upset
Sotalol	PO	2–8 mg/kg/d q12h	2–3h	Beta blockade; has bretylium-like effect	Dizziness, worsening CHF, proarrhythmia, nausea, bronchospasm, bradycardia
Verapamil	PO	3–6 mg/kg/d divided tid	Minutes	Calcium antagonist	Exacerbates heart failure; have colloid and calcium available during rapid infusion
	IV	0.1–0.15 mg/kg over 1 min			
Antihypertensives					
Captopril	PO	1–4 mg/kg/d divided q8–12h 1/10 dose for premature infants, increasing with caution	1 h	ACE inhibitor	Hypotension, decreased renal perfusion
Diazoxide	IV	3–5 mg/kg/dose	1–2 min	Arterial vasodilator	Hypotension, hyperglycemia
Hydralazine	PO	0.75–7.0 mg/kg/d divided q6–8h	Hours to days	Arterial vasodilator	Hypotension, tachycardia, lupuslike syndrome
	IV	0.8–3.0 mg/kg/d divided q4–6h	10–30 min		
Nitroprusside	IV	0.5–6.5 μg/kg/min IV drip	Minutes	Peripheral vasodilator (arterial and venous)	Hypotension, cyanide toxicity (discontinue if thiocyanate level > 12 mg/dL)
Propranolol (see above)					

(*continued*)

Table 16–2. Commonly used medications.

Drug	Route	Dose	Onset	Mechanisms of Action	Precautions/ Complications
Diuretics					
Bumetanide	PO	0.015–0.1 mg/kg/d	30–60 min	Inhibits sodium reabsorption in the ascending loop of Henle	Hypotension, hypokalemia, hypocalcemia, hyperuricemia
	IV	Dose not established	15–30 min		
Ethacrynic acid	PO	25 mg/dose; max 2–3 mg/kg/d	30 min	Inhibits sodium reabsorption in the ascending loop of Henle and proximal and distal tubules	Hypotension, hypokalemia
	IV	1 mg/kg/dose; repeat dose not recommended	5 min		
Furosemide	PO	2 mg/kg/dose	30–60 min	Inhibits sodium reabsorption in the ascending loop of Henle	Ototoxicity in renal disease, hypocalcemia, dehydration, nephrocalcinosis in premature infants
	IV	1 mg/kg/dose	Minutes		
Hydrochlorothiazide	PO	2–3 mg/kg/d	1–2 h	Inhibits renal tubular absorption of sodium	Hyperbilirubinemia, hypokalemia, hypoglycemia, hyperuricemia
Spironolactone	PO	1–3 mg/kg/d	4–5 d	Aldosterone inhibitor	Hyperkalemia, GI distress
Ductal-related					
Indomethacin	IV	0.2 mg/kg q12h (0.1 mg/kg for 2nd and 3rd dose if infant < 48 h old)	Minutes	Prostaglandin inhibitor	GI bleeding; infection, transient renal impairment. Discontinue if urine output < 0.6 mL/kg/hr
Prostaglandin E_1	IV	0.01–0.1 μg/kg/min	Minutes	Smooth muscle relaxation, especially ductal tissue. Maintenance of systemic or pulmonary perfusion in ductal-dependent CHD	Apnea, fever, hypotension

Inotropic agents					
Amrinone lactate	IV	0.75 mg/kg bolus over 3 minutes; then 5–10 μg/kg/min	Minutes	Vasodilator; increases contractility	Hypotension, thrombocytopenia, hepatic toxicity
Digoxin (see above)					
Dobutamine	IV	2.5–20 μg/kg/min	Minutes	Beta-adrenergic	Tachydysrhythmias, ectopy, hypertension; contraindicated in hypertrophic cardiomyopathy
Dopamine	IV	2–20 μg/kg/min	Minutes	Dopaminergic; beta-adrenergic. At high doses, alpha effects predominate	Tachydysrhythmias, hypertension
Epinephrine	IV	0.1–1 μg/kg/min	Minutes	Alpha- and beta-adrenergic	Tachycardia, hypertension, headaches, nausea, vomiting
Isoproterenol	IV	0.05–1 μg/kg/min	Minutes	Beta-adrenergic	Tachycardia, ventricular entropy

ACE = angiotensin-converting enzyme; AV = atrioventricular; CHD = congenital heart disease; CHF = congestive heart failure; GI = gastrointestinal; IV = intravenous; PO = oral (per os); TDD = total digitalizing dose.

child and placing him or her in a knee-chest position will break the cycle. Oxygen should be administered. Morphine sulfate 0.1–0.2 mg/kg subcutaneously will quiet the child and reduce the tachypnea. Intravenous propranolol 0.05–0.10 mg/kg may be given in acute cases; oral propranolol 1.0–4.0 mg/kg/d may be used chronically until palliative or definitive surgery can be arranged.

CONGENITAL HEART DISEASE

Congenital heart disease (CHD) occurs in approximately 6–8:1000 live births; in the United States alone 25–35,000 children with CHD are born each year. Palliative or corrective surgery is now available for well over 90% of these children, with successful intervention dependent upon early and accurate diagnosis. When a child presents with cyanosis or CHF, the clinician should immediately begin a rapid, orderly sequence of evaluation and intervention.

ACYANOTIC HEART DISEASE

Ventricular Septal Defect (VSD)

A. General Considerations: VSD is the most common form of CHD, excluding bicuspid aortic valves. It occurs in 25% of all cases of CHD, and is more common in males than in females. It is the most common lesion found in chromosomal abnormalities.

B. Anatomy: The most common location is in the perimembranous ventricular septum. VSDs can also be found in the muscular, outlet, and inlet portions of the septum. The size ranges from pinpoint to a lesion involving most of the septum. VSDs may be singular or multiple, and are frequently associated with other cardiac defects.

C. Symptoms & Signs: Physical presentation depends largely on the size of the defect, pulmonary vascular resistance (PVR) and associated lesions. CHF may worsen as PVR falls in the first months of life. In a small- to moderate-sized defect there will be a normal P_2 and a grade II–VI/VI harsh, pansystolic murmur (PSM) at the lower left sternal border. In a large shunt without pulmonary hypertension the P_2 is normal, a grade II–III/VI PSM is heard at the lower left sternal border, a mid-diastolic flow rumble is appreciated at the apex, and CHF is present. In the presence of marked pulmonary hypertension, a right ventricular lift is present, P_2 is loud, a short systolic ejection murmur is present along the left sternal border, and the patient may be cyanotic if **Eisenmenger's syndrome** (reversal of shunt) has developed.

D. Laboratory Findings: In a small shunt, the heart size will be normal on the chest x-ray (CXR) and the electrocardiogram (ECG) will be normal. In moderate-sized defects, the CXR may show mild cardiac enlargement and increased pulmonary blood flow, and the ECG will be variable. Large defects result in marked cardiomegaly with increased pulmonary vascularity; the ECG demonstrates right ventricular hypertrophy (RVH), left ventricular hypertrophy (LVH), or both. The echocardiogram is useful in defining the position and size of the defect. Doppler echocardiography can be used to estimate the pulmonary artery systolic pressure.

E. Treatment: Small defects rarely need any surgical or medical management other than prophylaxis for subacute bacterial endocarditis (SBE). There is a significant spontaneous closure rate indirectly related to the size of the defect. Anticongestive heart failure medications are used in the presence of CHF. Surgery is recommended for patients with refractory CHF, failure to thrive in spite of adequate medical and nutritional management, repeated episodes of pneumonia, or reversible pulmonary hypertension.

Patent Ductus Arteriosus (PDA)

A. General Considerations: PDA is a common form of CHD, accounting for 12% of all cases; it occurs in 20–60% of all premature infants. Females are affected twice as often as males and there appears to be an increased incidence at higher altitudes.

B. Anatomy: The ductus arteriosus is a vessel located between the pulmonary artery and the descending aorta, found in all fetuses and generally closing shortly after birth in full-term infants.

C. Symptoms & Signs: In premature infants, depending on the size of the PDA, the precordium may be hyperactive and a variable systolic murmur may be present. The pulses are often bounding. In the older child a continuous murmur can be heard at the left upper sternal border below the clavicle, with radiation to the back. The pulses are bounding.

D. Laboratory Findings: In a small PDA the CXR and ECG are normal. Moderate to large PDAs will show LVH on the ECG with cardiomegaly and increased pulmonary markings on the CXR. If pulmonary hypertension is present the ECG will show RVH or biventricular hypertrophy. Two-dimensional and Doppler echocardiogram can demonstrate the PDA. In large shunts, the left atrium will be enlarged secondary to increased pulmonary venous return.

E. Treatment: Premature infants are urgently treated either medically (indomethacin) or surgically. In the absence of pulmonary vascular obstructive disease, effective surgical ligation or transvenous occlusion in the catheterization lab is indicated for older children.

Atrial Septal Defect (ASD)

A. General Considerations: There are three types of ASDs: ostium secundum, ostium primum, and sinus venosus. **Ostia secunda** make up 80% of ASDs and 10% of all cases of CHD, and have a 2:1 female:male ratio. **Ostia prima** comprise 2% of cases of CHD and occur approximately equally among males and females. Five percent of ASDs are made up of **sinus venosus** defects.

B. Anatomy: Ostium secundum defects involve the area around the fossa ovalis. Ostium primum anomalies result from deficiencies in the atrial septum primum during the embryonic period and are associated with mitral valve clefts. The sinus venosus defect is located posteriorly to the fossa ovalis adjacent to the SVC orifice; this defect is often associated with partial anomalous pulmonary venous return of the right upper pulmonary veins.

C. Symptoms & Signs: In general, there is a right ventricular heave and the S_2 is widely split and fixed. A grade II/VI systolic ejection murmur is heard at the left upper sternal border, followed by a mid-diastolic flow rumble in the tricuspid valve region.

D. Laboratory Findings: CXR demonstrates cardiomegaly with increased pulmonary markings. The ECG shows RVH with an rsR′ in V1. Left axis deviation (LAD) and RVH with an rsR′ in V1 is seen in ostium primum defects. The echocardiogram reveals a dilated right atrium and right ventricle plus paradoxical septal motion. The defect itself can be visualized in the atrial septum with intracardiac shunt flow detected by Doppler studies.

E. Treatment: Spontaneous closure of ASDs has been reported, although it is not as common as in VSDs. Anticongestive medications are used for CHF. Where there is a large left-to-right shunt, CHF, or pulmonary congestion, surgical closure is recommended. Transvenous closure in the catheterization lab with an occluding device is now an alternative to surgical closure in some medical centers.

Atrioventricular Septal Defect

A. General Considerations: This disorder, common in Down's syndrome, is found in approximately 4% of patients with CHD. Males and females are affected equally. Pulmonary hypertension and irreversible pulmonary vascular obstructive disease are major risks.

B. Anatomy: In complete atrioventricular septal defect, there is a large AV septal defect and a common AV valve that arises from both the right and left atria. The partial form has an ostium primum ASD and an abnormal mitral valve with mitral regurgitation.

C. Symptoms & Signs: In the neonatal period the murmur may be inaudible and P_2 will be loud. A nonspecific systolic murmur along with a mid-diastolic flow rumble at the apex is usually heard in later infancy.

D. Laboratory Findings: CXR demonstrates cardiomegaly and increased pulmonary vascular markings. The ECG will show LAD with RVH, LVH, or both. Fifty percent of cases will have first-degree heart block. Echocardiography is useful in assessing the AV valve structures and the atrial and ventricular septal defects.

E. Treatment: Anticongestive medication is used to control CHF. Surgery is performed prior to the development of irreversible pulmonary vascular disease, usually before 6–12 months.

Aortic Stenosis (AS)

A. General Considerations: AS accounts for 5% of cases of CHD, with a 2:1 male predominance. AS can be classified as valvular, subvalvular, or supravalvular. Supravalvular AS is associated with **William's syndrome** (elfin facies and hypercalcemia of infancy).

B. Anatomy: In valvular AS, the valve is usually bicuspid and the leaflets are dysplastic and thickened, with decreased mobility. In severe cases the annulus itself is frequently hypoplastic.

C. Symptoms & Signs: Infants may present with CHF and weak pulses; older children are usually asymptomatic. A systolic ejection click will be heard at the apex and a grade II–VI/VI systolic ejection murmur will be heard at the upper right sternal border with radiation to the carotids. In moderate to severe disease a thrill is often palpable at the suprasternal notch and the base. The click is absent in subvalvular and supravalvular disease. Subaortic stenosis is frequently associated with aortic regurgitation.

D. Laboratory Findings: The CXR shows a normal heart size and a dilated aortic root. The ECG is similar to coarctation of the aorta (CoA) with RVH in infancy and LVH in older children. Echocardiography demonstrates the abnormal aortic valve and the left ventricular outflow tract abnormalities. Doppler flow studies can estimate the pressure gradient precisely.

E. Treatment: Balloon valvuloplasty is the initial procedure of choice for most cases of valvular AS. Surgical intervention is usually required for cases of subvalvular or supravalvular AS. Indications for intervention are symptoms, a pressure gradient greater than 60 mm Hg, an abnormal blood pressure response to exercise, or electrocardiographic evidence of myocardial strain.

Coarctation of the Aorta (CoA)

A. General Considerations: CoA accounts for 6% of cases of CHD, with a 1.7:1 male predominance. CoA is commonly seen in association with **Turner's syndrome**.

B. Anatomy: CoA is defined as a constriction of the aorta typically in the region adjacent to the ductus arteriosus (juxtaductal). It may involve a discrete narrowing or a long segment. Bicuspid aortic valves are associated findings in 50% of cases. The **CoA syndrome** consists of coarctation, PDA, tubular hypoplasia of the aortic isthmus, and VSD; and is frequently complicated by CHF.

C. Symptoms & Signs: Hypertension and decreased femoral pulses with a brachial-femoral pulse lag herald the diagnosis. In neonates the decreased femoral pulses can be masked in the presence of a large PDA. Severe CoA can present in the first weeks of life with CHF and absent femoral pulses.

D. Laboratory Findings: CXR shows cardiomegaly with pulmonary venous congestion in infants with CHF. The ECG will show RVH (LV hypoplasia). In older children the CXR may be normal, or show rib notching or poststenotic dilatation of the aorta. LVH is seen on the ECG. Echocardiography indicates a dilated right ventricle and possibly a hypoplastic left ventricle during infancy. The aortic arch and coarctation site can be visualized; in addition, aortic Doppler studies will demonstrate the disturbed arterial flow.

E. Treatment: Infants with CHF require stabilization and urgent surgery. In neonates, administration of PGE_1 (0.025–0.1 μg/kg/min) to reopen the ductus arteriosus will improve systemic perfusion and resolve acidosis. Several surgical options are currently available with excellent results. Recoarctation may occur. Balloon angioplasty in the catheterization laboratory is highly successful at relieving the obstruction in recoarctation and post-neonatal coarctation.

Hypoplastic Left Heart Syndrome (HLHS)

A. General Considerations: HLHS occurs in 1.5% of patients with CHD, with a male predominance. Without surgery it is virtually 100% fatal.

B. Anatomy: Anatomical defects include aortic and mitral atresia with small left ventricular cavity.

C. Symptoms & Signs: Patients usually present in the first week of life with CHF and weak pulses. There is a single S_2. A pulmonary ejection click is associated with a nonspecific systolic ejection murmur at the left sternal border.

D. Laboratory Findings: CXR shows cardiomegaly and interstitial pulmonary edema. The ECG shows RVH with absence of left-sided forces. There is frequently an absent Q wave in V_6. Echocardiography demonstrates the hypoplastic left ventricle and aorta.

E. Treatment: The outlook for this group of patients has changed drastically in recent years. With the advent of neonatal cardiac transplant and complex surgical repairs (**Norwood procedure**), several options are available for this lethal lesion. Currently, neonatal cardiac transplant has a two-year survival rate of 75%. Preliminary results of long-term morbidity and mortality studies are encouraging.

Pulmonary Stenosis (PS)

A. General Considerations: PS occurs in 10% of cases of CHD, with a male predominance.

B. Anatomy: The valve is conical or dome-shaped and is formed by fusion of the valve leaflets. Twenty percent of autopsied PS cases show bicuspid valves; 10–15% of cases have dysplastic valves.

C. Symptoms & Signs: In mild to moderate PS the P_2 is soft and there is a systolic ejection click. The click is followed by a grade I–III/VI systolic ejection murmur at the left upper sternal border radiating to the back. In severe PS, P_2 becomes silent and the murmur becomes longer and louder, and peaks later in systole. In severe PS, cyanosis may be the presenting sign as early as the neonatal period.

D. Laboratory Findings: The CXR in mild PS shows a normal-sized heart and dilatation of the main pulmonary artery. The degree of pulmonary artery dilatation does not correlate with the severity of the stenosis. The ECG is normal. In moderate to severe pulmonary stenosis, the ECG shows RVH and RVH with strain in critical PS. Echocardiography demonstrates the abnormal pulmonary valve and associated degree of right ventricular hypertrophy. Doppler echocardiography defines the transvalvular gradient precisely.

E. Treatment: Transcatheter balloon valvuloplasty is the recommended procedure for moderate and severe cases. It is now being performed in small infants, thus avoiding the high risks of neonatal surgery.

CYANOTIC HEART DISEASE

Cyanotic heart disease characterizes children who have right-to-left shunts and are *usually,* but not always, cyanotic. Cyanosis is determined by the presence of at least 4–5 grams of unsaturated hemoglobin in the capillary bed. On the basis of this definition, a child with a cyanotic heart lesion with anemia may not appear cyanotic. It is also important to remember that cyanotic infants may appear ashen in color rather than blue. Evaluation of cyanotic infants is outlined in Figure 16–3.

Tetralogy of Fallot (TOF)

A. General Considerations: TOF is the most common form of cyanotic cardiac malformation, accounting for 10–15% of all cases of CHD. There is a slight predominance of males over females.

B. Anatomy: TOF consists of infundibular PS, a large unrestrictive VSD, an aorta overriding the VSD, and RVH. Associated anomalies may include a right aortic arch in 25% of cases, an ASD in 15%, absent pulmonary valve, pulmonary atresia, atrioventricular septal defect, and a left superior vena cava to the coronary sinus.

C. Symptoms & Signs: Depending on the degree of right-to-left shunting, the patient may either be acyanotic (ie, pink tetralogy) or cyanotic. The degree of right ventricular outflow tract obstruction largely determines the degree of cyanosis. Auscultation reveals a single S_2 and a grade I–III/VI systolic ejection murmur at the mid- to high left sternal border. During a hypercyanotic episode the murmur diminishes in intensity and the patient becomes more cyanotic and irritable.

D. Laboratory Findings: The ECG commonly shows right axis deviation and RVH. CXR reveals a normal or small heart, often with the apex upturned, and a narrow mediastinum. The pulmonary markings are normal to decreased. The aortic arch is right-sided in approximately 25% of cases. Echocardiography demonstrates the overriding aorta, VSD, pulmonary infundibular stenosis, and the hypertrophied right ventricle. Arterial blood gas analysis demonstrates a normal pH and $Paco_2$ at rest, with a variable degree of hypoxemia.

E. Treatment: Beta blockade may prevent hypercyanotic spells. Surgical palliation is provided with creation of a systemic artery to pulmonary artery anastomosis to increase pulmonary blood flow (**Blalock-Taussig shunt**). Later, total correction is completed.

Transposition of the Great Arteries (TGA)

A. General Considerations: TGA is the second most common cyanotic heart lesion and accounts for 5–7% of all cases of CHD. There is a 3:1 male predominance.

B. Anatomy: In TGA, the aorta arises from the right ventricle and the pulmonary artery arises from the left ventricle. Associated anomalies may include a VSD (30–35%), PS and VSD (10%), PS alone (5%), or CoA (5%).

C. Symptoms & Signs: Infants with TGA are cyanotic at birth and generally appear comfortable and well developed. The first heart sound is normal; S_2 is single. The systolic murmur of PS or VSD is heard when those associated lesions are present.

D. Laboratory Findings: The ECG may be entirely normal or show right-axis deviation and RVH. In the first few days of life, the CXR can be normal or show the diagnostic triad of an oval or egg-shaped cardiac silhouette, a narrow mediastinum, and increased pulmonary markings. The echocardiogram will demonstrate the aorta arising from the right ventricle and the pulmonary artery from the left ventricle. Associated anomalies such as VSD and PS can be ascertained. Arterial blood gas analysis shows PaO_2 rarely higher than 35 mm Hg, with little or no response to supplemental oxygen and a normal $Paco_2$.

E. Treatment: Medical treatment includes starting the infant on PGE_1. At the time of cardiac catheterization, a balloon atrial septostomy is performed to enlarge an ASD and improve systemic and venous mixing. A supravalvular arterial switch with coronary artery relocation may be performed in the first 2 weeks of life. In cases not suitable for arterial switching, an atrial switch rerouting the systemic and pulmonary venous return may be performed.

Total Anomalous Pulmonary Venous Return (TAPVR)

A. General Considerations: TAPVR describes a group of disorders in which no pulmonary venous return enters directly into the left atrium. This heart lesion accounts for 2% of cases of CHD and is seen equally in males and females except when the veins enter the portal system, in which case there is an approximate 3:1 male predominance.

B. Anatomy: The pulmonary veins generally form a confluence and then enter the heart (1) via the vertical vein into the left innominate vein; (2) directly into the coronary sinus, the right atrium, or the

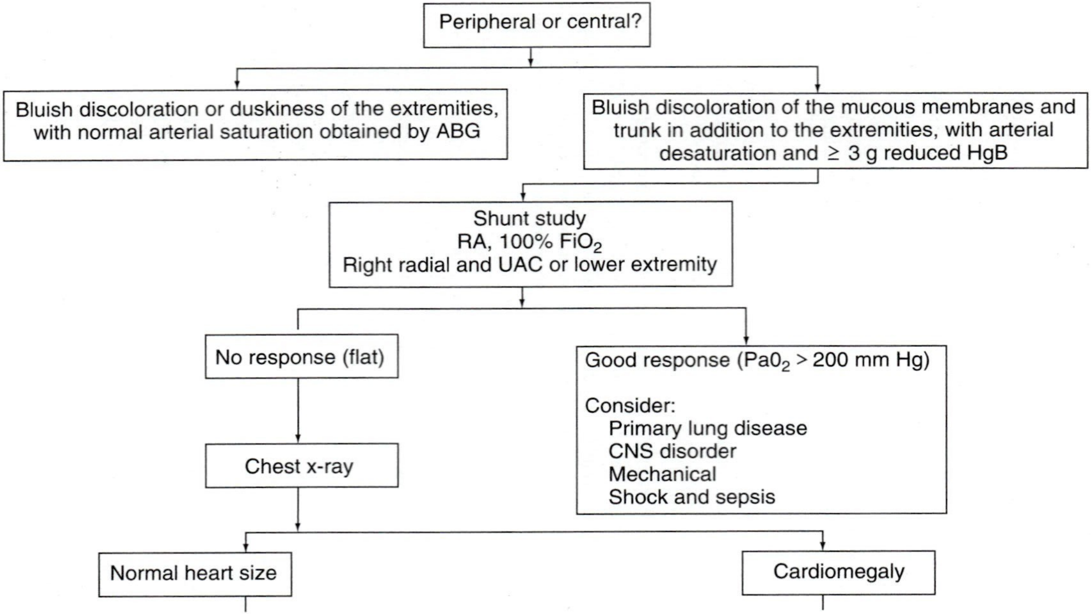
Peripheral or central?
Bluish discoloration or duskiness of the extremities, with normal arterial saturation obtained by ABG
Bluish discoloration of the mucous membranes and trunk in addition to the extremities, with arterial desaturation and ≥ 3 g reduced HgB
Shunt study
RA, 100% FiO_2
Right radial and UAC or lower extremity
No response (flat)
Good response ($Pa0_2$ > 200 mm Hg)
Consider:
Primary lung disease
CNS disorder
Mechanical
Shock and sepsis
Chest x-ray
Normal heart size
Cardiomegaly

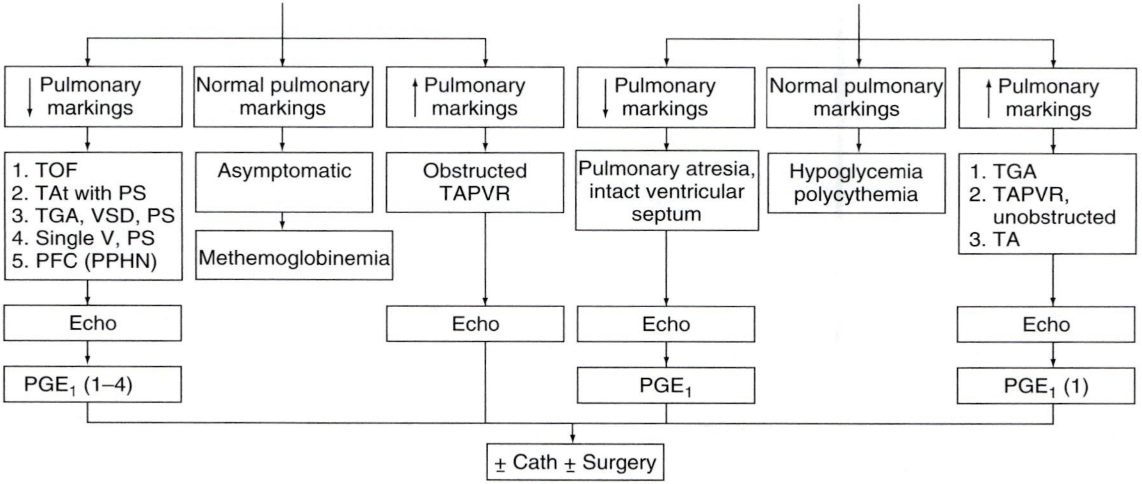

Figure 16–3. Evaluation of the cyanotic neonate. ABG = arterial blood gas; CNS = central nervous system; CoA = coarctation of the aorta; FIO_2 = % inspired oxygen; PFC = persistent fetal circulation; PGE_1 = prostaglandin; PPHN = persistent pulmonary hypertension of the newborn; PS = pulmonary stenosis; RA = room air; TAt = tricuspid atresia; TA = truncus arteriosus; TAPVR = total anomalous pulmonary venous return; TGA = transposition of the great arteries; TOF = tetralogy of Fallot; UAC = umbilical artery catheter; V = ventricle; VSD = ventricular septal defect.

right superior vena cava; or (3) across the diaphragm and into the inferior vena cava or the portal system. They may or may not be obstructed.

C. Symptoms & Signs: Patients without pulmonary venous obstruction are usually mildly cyanotic and asymptomatic at birth; CHF develops later. A right ventricular heave may be present. S_1 is loud, followed by a widely split S_2 and usually an S_3 at the apex. A grade II/VI systolic ejection murmur is usually, but not always, heard in the pulmonic region, with a mid-diastolic flow rumble in the tricuspid valve region. Patients with obstruction to pulmonary venous return usually develop signs and symptoms within 24 hours of birth, including respiratory distress, feeding problems, and cardiac failure. They are cyanotic. S_1 is normal and S_2 splits with an increased P_2. A murmur may be barely audible.

D. Laboratory Findings: In *unobstructed* TAPVR, the ECG shows right-axis deviation, right atrial enlargement (RAE), and RVH. The CXR will demonstrate increased pulmonary flow, an enlarged right heart, and occasionally a "snowman" figure when the return is supracardiac. Echocardiography shows an enlarged right atrium and ventricle. The anomalous pulmonary veins can usually be demonstrated. With *obstructed* pulmonary venous return the ECG will show RVH. The CXR reveals a normal heart size and diffuse interstitial edema. The echocardiogram shows a large right ventricle; Doppler flow studies will demonstrate the pulmonary venous obstruction.

E. Treatment: Surgical correction with reanastomosis of the pulmonary veins to the left atrium is mandatory in early infancy and is emergent when the veins are obstructed.

Tricuspid Atresia

A. General Considerations: This lesion occurs in 2% of cases of CHD and is slightly more common in males.

B. Anatomy: There is complete atresia of the tricuspid valve; therefore, no direct communication between the right atrium and the right ventricle. The right ventricle has varying degrees of hypoplasia. There is a mandatory ASD. The great vessels may be normally related or transposed; a VSD may or may not be present. The pulmonary valve may be normal, stenotic, or atretic.

C. Symptoms & Signs: The infants are cyanotic at birth. S_1 is normal; S_2 is single. A grade I–III/VI harsh systolic ejection murmur is heard along the lower left sternal border and there may be CHF when the pulmonary blood flow is increased.

D. Laboratory Findings: The ECG shows LAD, RAE, and LVH. CXR reveals a slightly to markedly enlarged heart with variable pulmonary artery markings, depending on the associated lesions. The echocardiogram demonstrates the absence of the tricuspid valve and the right ventricular hypoplasia. The relationship of the great vessels can be determined, and the status of the pulmonary valve and ventricular septum identified.

E. Treatment: A balloon atrial septostomy is performed in the catheterization lab to allow unobstructed flow to the left heart. For those patients with high pulmonary blood flow, anticongestives are utilized followed by an atriopulmonary anastomosis (**Fontan procedure**) at a later date. Pulmonary artery banding may be required to protect the pulmonary vascular bed prior to the Fontan repair. Low pulmonary blood flow indicates the need for a systemic-to-pulmonary shunt followed later by the Fontan procedure.

Pulmonary Atresia, Intact Ventricular Septum

A. General Considerations: Pulmonary atresia with an intact ventricular septum accounts for approximately 1% of cases of CHD.

B. Anatomy: The pulmonary valve does not form and the right ventricle is either small with a hypertrophied wall or of relatively normal size. The ventricular septum is intact. The tricuspid valve shows varying degrees of hypoplasia. Fistulous communication between the right ventricle and coronary arteries may occur.

C. Symptoms & Signs: Infants with this condition are cyanotic from birth. S_1 is normal and S_2 is single. A grade I–II/VI continuous murmur (PDA) may be heard at the left upper sternal border, likewise a grade I–III/VI harsh pansystolic murmur at the left lower sternal border (tricuspid regurgitation).

D. Laboratory Findings: The ECG shows a normal axis, RAE, and LVH. CXR reveals a large heart with decreased pulmonary blood flow. Echocardiography shows the atretic pulmonary valve plus an intact ventricular septum. The size of the right ventricular cavity determines treatment and can be ascertained as well as the presence and degree of tricuspid regurgitation.

E. Treatment: Prostaglandins are used to keep the ductus arteriosus open while awaiting intervention. If the right ventricle is small, a systemic-to-pulmonary shunt procedure is done and a balloon atrial septostomy is performed. If the right ventricle is of adequate size, a pulmonary valvulotomy is performed. Right ventricular outflow tract reconstruction is performed at a later date if necessary. In cases of severely hypoplastic right ventricle with right ventricular dependent coronary artery blood flow, a cardiac transplantation may be performed.

Truncus Arteriosus

A. General Considerations: Approximately 0.7% of children with CHD have truncus arteriosus, which is equally distributed between males and females. **DiGeorge's syndrome** (Chapter 24) with thymic aplasia is frequently present.

B. Anatomy: One large vessel giving rise to the aorta, pulmonary artery, and coronary arteries arises from the heart. It overrides a VSD. The truncal valve may be stenotic or incompetent. A right aortic arch is common.

C. Symptoms & Signs: When there is unobstructed pulmonary blood flow the child presents with CHF. If there is decreased flow to the lungs the infant will be cyanotic. S_1 and S_2 are loud, and a systolic ejection click is present. A grade II–IV/VI systolic ejection murmur is heard at the left lower sternal border. A diastolic decrescendo murmur of truncal valve insufficiency may be audible.

D. Laboratory Findings: ECG usually demonstrates right ventricular or biventricular hypertrophy and ST-T wave depression. CXR reveals a large boot-shaped heart with absence of the pulmonary artery segment, often a right aortic arch, and variable pulmonary markings. Echocardiography identifies the single truncal root and the large VSD.

E. Treatment: Anticongestive medications are needed for patients with high pulmonary blood flow. Early total correction is performed by closing the VSD to include the truncal root. The pulmonary arteries are detached from the root and then reanastomosed to the right ventricle, with or without an interposed conduit.

ACQUIRED HEART DISEASE

Acquired heart disease includes infectious, immunologic, and metabolic involvement of the endocardium, myocardium, or pericardium. It presents frequently in all age groups as a life-threatening situation.

ACUTE RHEUMATIC FEVER (ARF)

Rheumatic fever is discussed in Chapter 27, Collagen Diseases. The reader is also referred to Adnan D, Taubert K, Ferrieri P: Treatment of acute streptococcal pharyngitis and prevention of rheumatic fever. Pediatrics 1995;96:758.

KAWASAKI DISEASE

A. General Considerations: Kawasaki disease, or mucocutaneous lymph node syndrome, is an inflammatory disorder of unknown etiology (Chapter 11). It is characterized by multisystem involvement, most notably the heart. Eighty percent of cases involve children less than 4 years of age, with a 1.5:1 male-to-female ratio. Asians are affected more frequently than blacks, who are affected more frequently than whites.

B. Symptoms & Signs: As with acute rheumatic fever, the physical findings depend on the particular criteria present. Five criteria are required for the diagnosis.

1. Fever: Present longer than 5 days; unresponsive to antibiotics.

2. Mucous membrane involvement: Cracked, fissured lips and tongue ("strawberry tongue").

3. Nonpurulent conjunctivitis

4. Polymorphous rash: Typically involves the trunk and extremities.

5. Lymphadenopathy

6. Digital swelling and desquamation

Examination of the cardiovascular system may reveal findings consistent with myocarditis, pericarditis, and peripheral arteritis.

C. Laboratory Findings: The white blood cell count (WBC), erythrocyte sedimentation rate (ESR), and C-reactive protein value (CRP) will be elevated, as will the platelet count. A normochromic anemia can be present, as can a sterile pyuria. The ECG often shows a prolonged PR interval, ST-T wave changes, and low voltage. CXR may show cardiomegaly. Echocardiography is a vital diagnostic tool in Kawasaki disease since 20% of patients will develop coronary artery aneurysms or dilatation without treatment. Five percent of patients will develop aneurysms despite treatment. A pericardial effusion may be present.

D. Treatment: Current therapy includes aspirin and intravenous gamma globulin (IVIG). Serial ECGs and echocardiograms should be obtained since Kawasaki disease has acute and chronic phases; some findings, most notably coronary involvement, may not be present on initial examination. The reader is also referred to Adnan D, Taubert K, Gerber M: Diagnosis and therapy of Kawasaki disease in children. Circulation 1993;87:1776.

ENDOCARDITIS

A. General Considerations: Infective endocarditis is an infection of the endocardium in patients with structural heart disease or in immunocompromised hosts. Common associated cardiovascular conditions include prosthetic valves, Blalock-Taussig shunts, PDA, VSD, and bicuspid aortic valves. Infective endocarditis is rarely seen in a normal population. The most common causative organisms include *Streptococcus viridans* and *Staphylococcus aureus* along with fungi.

B. Symptoms & Signs: The patient may have a history of persistent fever and weight loss. Physical examination will be positive for changing murmurs and splenomegaly (70%), petechiae, and peripheral embolic phenomena.

C. Laboratory Findings: The ESR and WBC are often elevated and the urine can be heme positive. Blood cultures are usually positive. Cardiomegaly will be present on CXR and heart block will be seen on ECG when the aortic annulus is involved. Echocardiography will identify large endocardial vegetations, but may be normal.

D. Treatment: Appropriate antibiotics should be administered for both culture-positive and culture-negative endocarditis. Treatment for CHF and valve replacement may be necessary.

E. Prophylaxis: Many children with congenital or acquired heart disease are at increased risk for infective endocarditis; therefore, prophylactic treatment is recommended. Prophylaxis is recommended at times when there is a known increased risk for bacteremia, such as with certain dental or surgical procedures. Antibiotics are given around the time of the procedure in sufficient doses to assure adequate antibiotic concentrations in the serum during and after the procedure. Children with valve dysfunction who take chronic penicillin for secondary prevention of rheumatic fever require infective endocarditis prophylaxis with an alternative regimen because of potentially resistant oral pathogens. Children with repaired VSDs, ASDs, and PDAs who do not have cardiac residua require endocarditis prophylaxis for 6 months following surgery. Infective endocarditis prophylaxis is not recommended for children with functional murmurs or isolated secundum atrial septal defect. For specific indications and dosing regimens, consult American Heart Association recommendations (JAMA 1990; 264:2919).

MYOCARDITIS

A. General Considerations: In a majority of cases the cause is unknown. Viral etiologies are common and include Coxsackie A & B viruses, rubella, cytomegalovirus, mumps, adenovirus, and herpes viruses.

B. Symptoms & Signs: In the newborn period the onset is rapid with CHF and vascular collapse. Mitral and tricuspid regurgitation may also be present. Onset is more insidious in older children.

C. Laboratory Findings: The WBC is variable; both bacterial and viral cultures are usually negative. CXR will show cardiomegaly with moderate to marked venous congestion and possibly pneumonia. Decreased voltage, ST-T wave changes, and dysrhythmias may be seen on the ECG. Decreased contractility and dilation of the heart are seen by echocardiography.

D. Treatment: CHF is treated with digitalis, diuretics, and afterload reduction. Care is taken with digitalization, using two-thirds the total dose owing to an increased risk of toxicity. Treatment with steroids and IVIG is controversial.

PERICARDITIS

A. General Considerations: Pericarditis may be nonpurulent, secondary to rheumatic fever, viral infection, collagen vascular disease, and uremia; or purulent, caused by *Haemophilus influenzae, S aureus,* and *Streptococcus pneumoniae*. It is rarely an isolated event. Tamponade may occur and may lead to rapid deterioration and death.

B. Symptoms & Signs: Fever is present along with retrosternal chest pain. Dyspnea and grunting respirations may be present in infants. There may be jugular venous distension (JVD) and pulsus paradoxus. Cardiac examination may reveal muffled heart sounds and a pericardial friction rub.

C. Laboratory Findings: In nonpurulent pericarditis, the WBC and ESR may be elevated with negative blood cultures. In purulent pericarditis the blood culture is positive and the WBC and ESR may be elevated. In the presence of an effusion, the cardiac silhouette has a "water-bottle" shape. ST-T wave elevation can be seen on the ECG. Echocardiography can document the presence of a pericardial effusion and evidence of purulent loculation.

D. Treatment: Aspirin and other anti-inflammatory agents are used for nonpurulent pericarditis. Antibiotics and pericardiectomy are indicated in purulent pericarditis. Cardiac tamponade requires an emergent pericardiocentesis.

DYSRHYTHMIAS

Recognition and management of cardiac dysrhythmias in childhood is growing rapidly. This improvement is due partly to increased awareness secondary to the availability of advanced technology in cardiac monitoring equipment (eg, continuous heart rate monitoring in intensive care units and the 24-hour Holter monitor). Also, there is a true increase in the incidence and prevalence of dysrhythmias as more patients are surviving open heart surgery; dysrhythmias are frequently seen in these survivors. Understanding the basic underlying mechanism of dysrhythmias helps in establishing a workable approach to diagnosis and treatment. Common dysrhythmias in the pediatric population are illustrated in Figure 16–4.

SINUS DYSRHYTHMIAS

Sinus Arrhythmia

Sinus rhythm with a variable heart rate. This is a normal variant with an increase in rate with inspiration and a decrease with expiration. No treatment is required.

Sinus Bradycardia

Sinus heart rate less than the lower limits of normal for age (60 bpm in newborns, 40 bpm in older children). This may be a normal finding in athletes and in persons at rest. Other causes include sick sinus syndrome, hypertension, and central nervous system (CNS) abnormalities. Asymptomatic patients need only to be watched, while treatment should be directed at correcting the underlying cause.

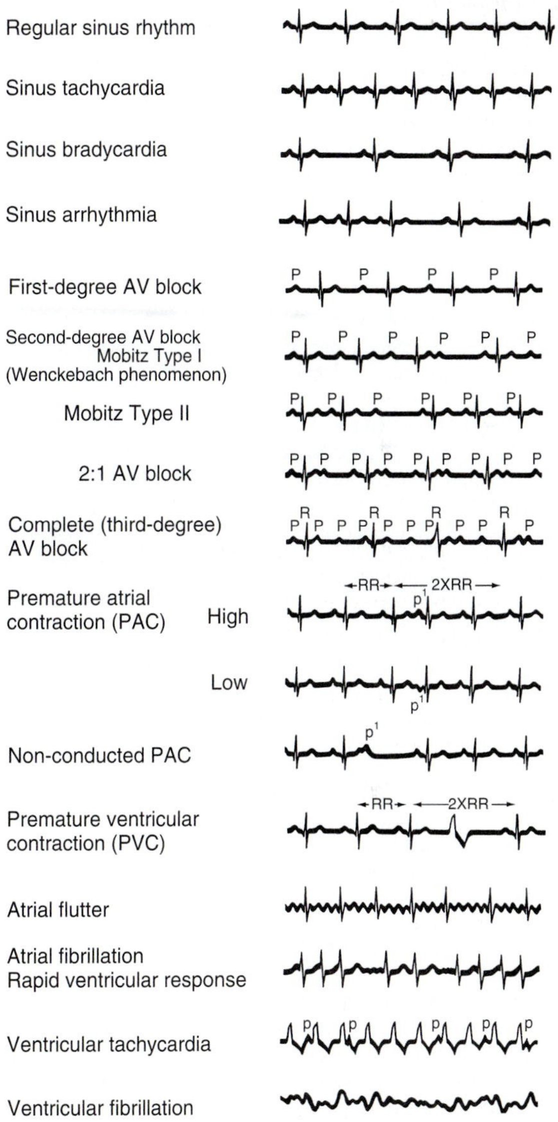

Figure 16–4. Common dysrhythmias in pediatric electrocardiograms.

Sinus Tachycardia

Sinus heart rate greater than the upper limits of normal for age (220 bpm in newborns, 190 bpm in older children). This is found in fever, anemia, hypovolemia, and CHF. Treatment should be directed at the underlying cause.

CONDUCTION ABNORMALITIES

First-Degree Heart Block

Prolonged PR interval that is greater than the upper limits of normal for age. No treatment is required.

Second-Degree Heart Block

Mobitz Type I (Wenckebach) is progressive lengthening of the PR interval until a nonconducted P wave occurs. Mobitz Type II has a consistent PR interval with an occasional nonconducted P wave. Type I may be seen in normal persons, while Type II implies advanced conduction system disease. Type I seldom requires treatment, while Type II may need temporary or permanent pacing.

Third-Degree Heart Block (Complete AV Block)

This condition may be congenital or acquired after cardiac surgery, myocarditis, or drug ingestion. Seventy-five percent of patients with congenital third-degree block *without structural heart disease* have mothers with systemic lupus erythematosus (SLE).

Treatment of acute complete block includes isoproterenol or temporary pacing. Long-term treatment requires a permanent pacemaker if the patient is symptomatic, has exercise intolerance, or has a sleeping heart rate less than 40.

PREMATURE DEPOLARIZATIONS

Premature Atrial Contraction (PAC)

Premature atrial depolarizations (P waves) that may or may not be conducted through the AV node. PACs are usually idiopathic (normal variant) but may be secondary to hypokalemia, hypoxia, hypoglycemia, atrial enlargement, or digitalis toxicity. No treatment is required unless supraventricular tachycardia (SVT) is present.

Premature Junctional Contraction (PJC)

Premature QRS waves of normal morphology not preceded by a P wave. The beats originate in the AV nodal region and have the same significance as PACs.

Premature Ventricular Contraction (PVC)

Premature QRS complex with a prolonged duration and a morphology different from the preceding normal QRS complex. It is not preceded by a P wave. PVCs may be found in a normal heart or may be secondary to hypokalemia, hypocalcemia, cardiomyopathy, or myocarditis. In asymptomatic patients with no underlying heart disease, no treatment is necessary. Treatment should be directed at correcting the underlying cause. Suppression with antidysrhythmic agents should be initiated in a hospital setting.

TACHYDYSRHYTHMIAS

Supraventricular Tachycardia (SVT) (Figure 16–5)

Atrial Flutter

Saw-tooth configuration of atrial flutter waves with atrial rates varying from 300 to 600. There may be variable AV node conduction. This rhythm is seen in right or left atrial enlargements, sick sinus syndrome, hypokalemia, hypoxia, hypoglycemia, atrial septal aneurysm, and following cardiac surgery. Acute treatment includes DC cardioversion, overdrive atrial pacing, and intravenous digitalis or procainamide.

Atrial Fibrillation

Rapid irregularly-irregular atrial rate with irregular QRS rhythm. It is rare in children but can occur in right and left atrial enlargement, hypokalemia, hypoxia, hypoglycemia, hyperthyroidism, and following atrial surgery. Acute treatment includes DC cardioversion and intravenous digitalis.

Ventricular Tachycardia

Three or more consecutive PVCs at rates of greater than 120. The PVCs may be unifocal and multifocal. The ventricular origin of the tachycardia is substantiated by the presence of fusion beats. Ventricular tachycardia can be seen in myocarditis, cardiomyopathy, digitalis toxicity, long QT syndrome, hypertrophic cardiomyopathy,

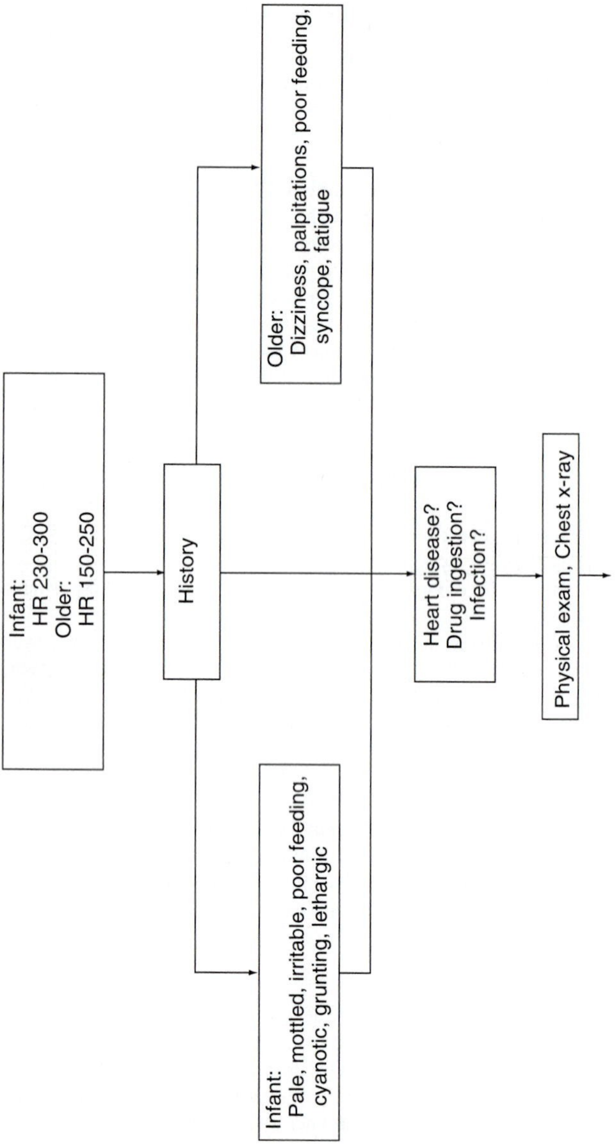
Infant:
HR 230-300
Older:
HR 150-250
History
Older:
Dizziness, palpitations, poor feeding,
syncope, fatigue
Infant:
Pale, mottled, irritable, poor feeding,
cyanotic, grunting, lethargic
Heart disease?
Drug ingestion?
Infection?
Physical exam, Chest x-ray

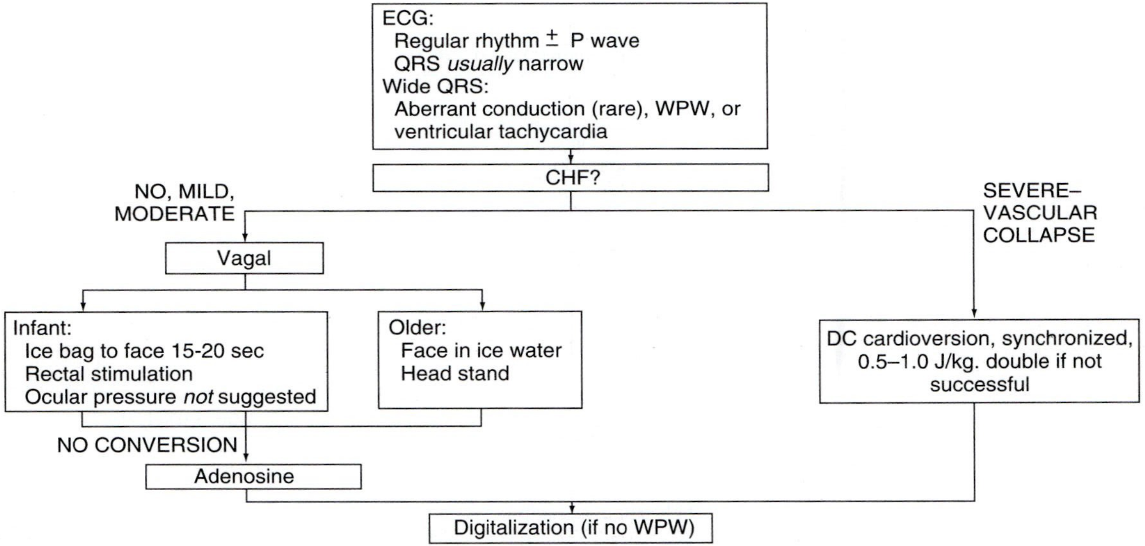

Figure 16–5. Evaluation and treatment of the child with supraventricular tachycardia. CHF = congestive heart failure; CXR = chest x-ray; DC = direct current; ECG = electrocardiogram; HR = heart rate; WPW = Wolff-Parkinson-White syndrome.

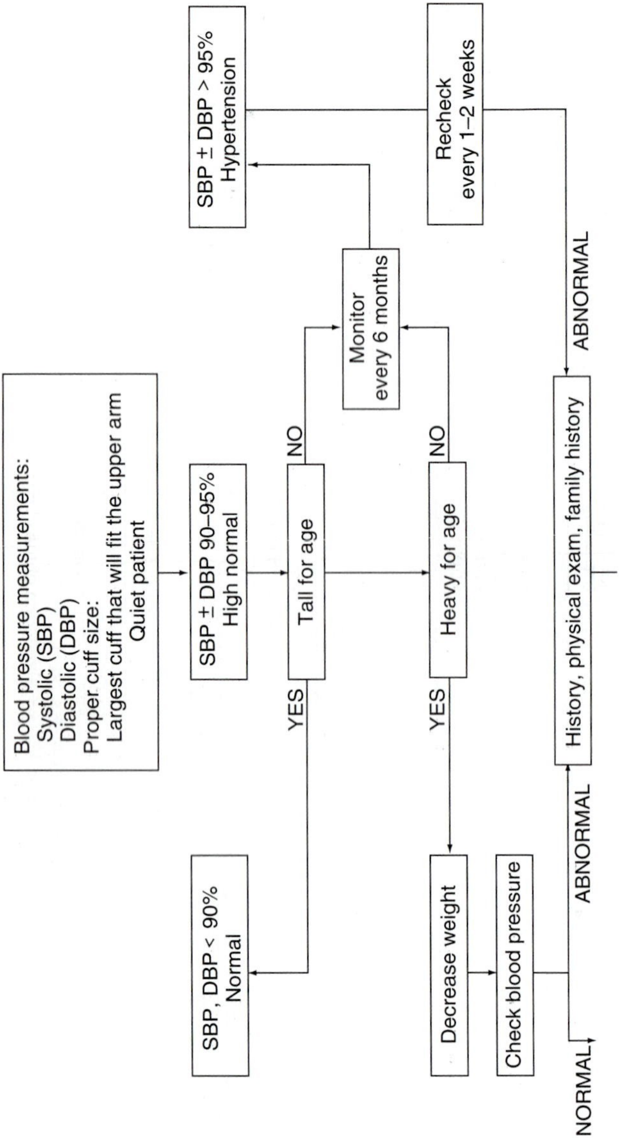
Blood pressure measurements:
Systolic (SBP)
Diastolic (DBP)
Proper cuff size:
Largest cuff that will fit the upper arm
Quiet patient
SBP ± DBP 90–95%
High normal
Tall for age
YES
NO
Heavy for age
YES
NO
Monitor every 6 months
SBP ± DBP > 95%
Hypertension
Recheck every 1–2 weeks
SBP, DBP < 90%
Normal
Decrease weight
Check blood pressure
NORMAL
ABNORMAL
ABNORMAL
History, physical exam, family history

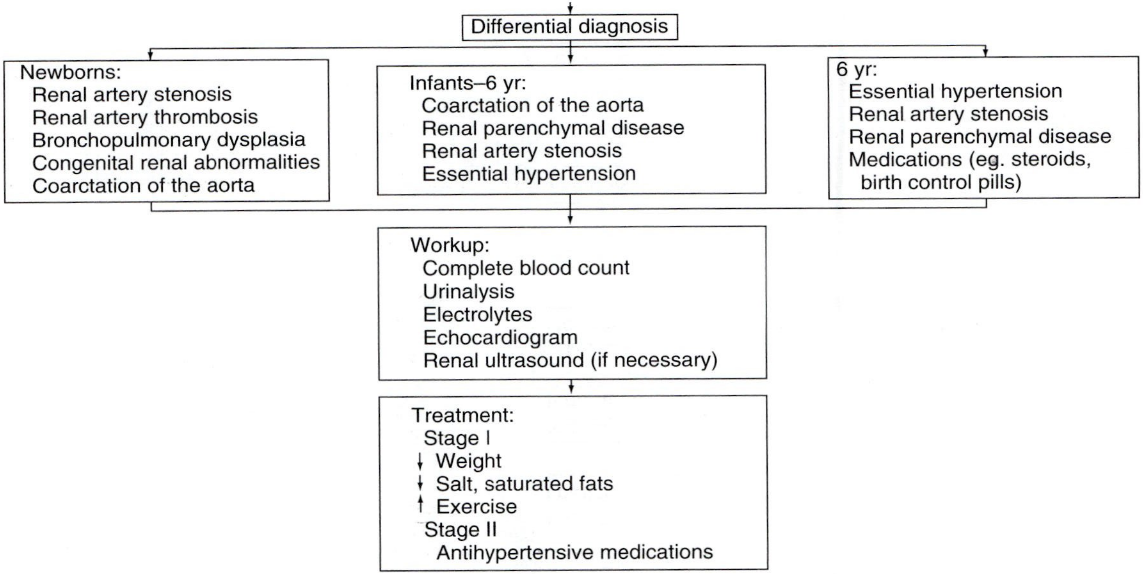
Differential diagnosis
Newborns:
Renal artery stenosis
Renal artery thrombosis
Bronchopulmonary dysplasia
Congenital renal abnormalities
Coarctation of the aorta
Infants–6 yr:
Coarctation of the aorta
Renal parenchymal disease
Renal artery stenosis
Essential hypertension
6 yr:
Essential hypertension
Renal artery stenosis
Renal parenchymal disease
Medications (eg. steroids, birth control pills)
Workup:
Complete blood count
Urinalysis
Electrolytes
Echocardiogram
Renal ultrasound (if necessary)
Treatment:
Stage I
↓ Weight
↓ Salt, saturated fats
↑ Exercise
Stage II
Antihypertensive medications

Figure 16–6. Evaluation of the child with hypertension.

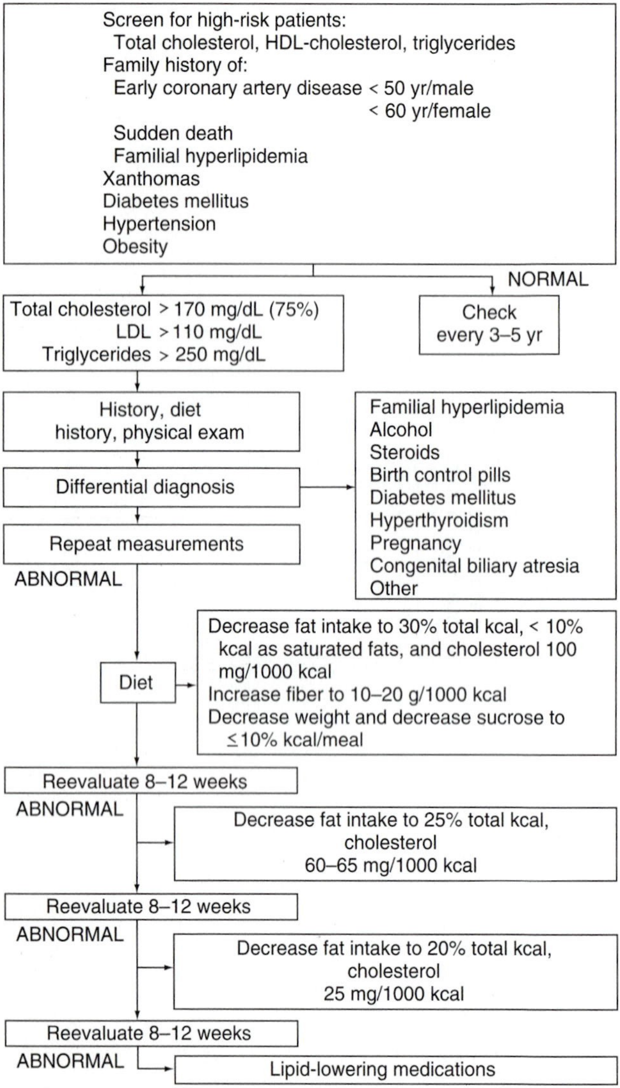
Screen for high-risk patients:
Total cholesterol, HDL-cholesterol, triglycerides
Family history of:
Early coronary artery disease < 50 yr/male
< 60 yr/female
Sudden death
Familial hyperlipidemia
Xanthomas
Diabetes mellitus
Hypertension
Obesity
NORMAL
Total cholesterol > 170 mg/dL (75%)
LDL > 110 mg/dL
Triglycerides > 250 mg/dL
Check every 3–5 yr
History, diet history, physical exam
Differential diagnosis
Familial hyperlipidemia
Alcohol
Steroids
Birth control pills
Diabetes mellitus
Hyperthyroidism
Pregnancy
Congenital biliary atresia
Other
Repeat measurements
ABNORMAL
Diet
Decrease fat intake to 30% total kcal, < 10% kcal as saturated fats, and cholesterol 100 mg/1000 kcal
Increase fiber to 10–20 g/1000 kcal
Decrease weight and decrease sucrose to ≤10% kcal/meal
Reevaluate 8–12 weeks
ABNORMAL
Decrease fat intake to 25% total kcal, cholesterol 60–65 mg/1000 kcal
Reevaluate 8–12 weeks
ABNORMAL
Decrease fat intake to 20% total kcal, cholesterol 25 mg/1000 kcal
Reevaluate 8–12 weeks
ABNORMAL
Lipid-lowering medications

myocardial tumors, and following cardiac surgery. Treatment includes DC cardioversion when the patient is hemodynamically unstable. Antidysrhythmic agents are used t suppress recurrences and must be initiated in a hospital setting.

PREVENTIVE CARDIOLOGY

Hypertension (Figure 16–6) and hyperlipidemia (Figure 16–7) are well recognized as risk factors for atherosclerotic heart disease. Long-range population-based studies have shown elevations of these risk factors to persist from childhood throughout adolescence and adulthood. Screening and intervention programs are now being offered in most pediatric centers.

Figure 16–7. Screening and evaluation of the child with hyperlipidemia. HDL = high-density lipoproteins; Hx = history; LDL = low-density lipoproteins; PE = physical examination.

17 | Gastrointestinal Tract

Judith M. Sondheimer, MD

COMMON SYMPTOMS & SIGNS

RECURRENT ABDOMINAL PAIN

Recurrent abdominal pain of childhood is characterized by at least three episodes of abdominal pain in a 3-month period in a child whose physical examination is normal. It affects 10–15% of children between 4 and 12 years of age. Recurrent abdominal pain may be severe, is sometimes associated with pallor and emesis (30%), and frequently interferes with school attendance. Fewer than 10% have organic disease. The incidence of organic disease increases in children under 3 years and in the presence of symptoms such as diarrhea, weight loss, dysuria, fever, or neurologic symptoms. The pain varies in intensity, duration, and location. The presence of nocturnal pain does *not* rule out the diagnosis. Headache, constipation, and limb pains are common findings. Emotional stress related to family or school may be found in 30–50% of patients. Laboratory evaluatproportion to the apparent degree of pain.

VOMITING

Vomiting is a non-specific symptom of many childhood diseases. Organic disease must be considered if vomiting is protracted or severe. Bilious emesis must be investigated. Causes and characteristics of vomiting are listed in Table 17–1.

RECTAL BLEEDING

See Table 17–2.

Table 17–1. Causes and characteristics of vomiting.

Cause	Emesis	Other Characteristics
Gastric Outlet Obstruction:		
Pyloric stenosis	Forceful emesis, gastric contents.	4–12 wk infant; alkalosis, weight loss, palpable mass (see Pyloric Stenosis section).
Gastric web duplication, annular pancreas	Emesis of variable force, usually gastric contents.	Presents at any age; x-ray diagnosis.
Duodenal stenosis/ atresia	Emesis of variable force depending upon severity of obstruction; usually gastric contents.	Duodenal atresia presents at birth; common in Down's syndrome.
Intestinal Obstruction:		
Malrotation with mesenteric bands	Bilious.	May be associated with intestinal volvulus.
Volvulus	See Malrotation section.	See Malrotation section.
Intussusception	See Intussusception section.	See Intussusception section.
Superior mesenteric artery syndrome	Emesis of variable force; may be bilious.	Associated with sudden weight loss; often follows body casting after scoliosis repair; x-ray shows obstruction of transverse duodenum.
Peptic Disease:		
Gastric, duodenal ulcer, gastritis, esophagitis	Emesis is especially common in young infants; may contain bright red or dark blood.	Pain, irritability; weight loss in small infants; endoscopy most accurate diagnostic test.
Motility:		
Hypokalemia	Distension, ileus and emesis.	Generalized weakness.
Hypercalcemia, hypermagnesemia	Emesis, constipation.	

(*continued*)

Table 17–1. Causes and characteristics of vomiting (*continued*).

Cause	Emesis	Other Characteristics
Pseudo-obstruction	Distension, ileus, bilious emesis.	Cause unknown; may be present at birth or present later; sometimes familial; may spare segments.
Drugs:		
Aspirin, alcohol, theophylline	Gastric contents; may contain gross blood.	History of ingestion but not necessarily overdose.
Erythromycin	Gastric contents.	Gastric motor stimulant.
Opiates	Gastric contents.	Stimulation of medullary vomiting center.
Infections:		
Gastroenteritis	Usually precedes diarrhea.	Mediated by toxin or secondary to ileus.
UTI and obstructive uropathy	Usually gastric contents, sometimes bilious.	Common in infants; probably centrally mediated.
Otitis media	Usually gastric.	Common in infancy; probably centrally mediated.
Pneumonia, pertussis bronchiolitis	Usually gastric.	Post-tussive
Central Nervous System:		
Meningitis, tumor, pseudotumor; vascular anomalies	Usually gastric; often upon change of position.	Stimulation of medullary vomiting center.
Metabolic:		
Galactosemia, fructosemia, hyperammonemia, congenital adrenal hyperplasia, organic acidemia, phenylketonuria	Usually gastric, occasionally bilious.	Sick infant; often associated with acidosis, liver function abnormalities, hypoglycemia. Seek specific diagnostic indicators for these diseases.
Gastroesophageal Reflux:		
	Gastric contents; variable force; often postprandial.	Most common under 6 months.

UTI = urinary tract infection.

Table 17–2. Common causes of gross rectal bleeding in infants and children.[1]

Kind of Blood	Diagnosis	Comments
Melena	Nasal or pharyngeal bleeding.	Possible if blood loss is large and rapid.
	Peptic disease.	
	Esophageal varices.	Look for physical signs of portal hypertension.
	Upper GI tract vascular anomalies.	
	Swallowed maternal blood.	Occurs during delivery or from mastitis in nursing mother.
Maroon or brick red	Meckel's diverticulum.	Painless bleeding, healthy infant.
	Small bowel vascular anomalies.	Painless; if large enough volume blood may be bright red.
	Small bowel polyps, lymphoma.	Rare. Usually present with obstructive symptoms.
Bright red	Colitis–IBD or infectious.	Usually small volume associated with diarrhea and pain.
	Polyps–juvenile, adenomatous.	Usually small volume, no diarrhea or pain.
	Fissure.	After defecation, associated with constipation and anal pain.
	Intussusception.	Preceded by diarrhea, vomiting, abdominal pain alternating with lethargy. "Currant jelly stool" with blood and mucus. Abdominal mass may be present.
	Foreign body.	
	Allergy.	In young infants, small volume, associated with diarrhea. May be related to milk and soy protein. Can occur in breast-fed infants.

GI = gastrointestinal; IBD = inflammatory bowel disease.

[1] This table does not include disorders causing occult rectal blood loss.

DIARRHEA

Diarrhea (defined as > 20 mL of stool/kg/d) is a common symptom in children. When it occurs acutely, it is usually infectious. See Table 11–1 (pages 316–320) for causes and treatment of bacterial, viral, and parasitic diseases causing diarrhea. The physician should consider diarrhea seriously because of the risk of dehydration, especially in young infants.

The following information should be routinely obtained:

1. Duration, frequency, and description (consistency and color) of diarrheal stools.
2. Incidence and character of vomiting.
3. Incidence, volume, and frequency of voiding; dehydration will decrease the volume and frequency of urination.
4. Estimate of weight loss. In the infant or young child, weighing at the onset of diarrhea will provide an index with which subsequent weights can be compared.
5. Possible infectious disease contact(s).

Examine the abdomen for tenderness and abnormal masses. Examine rectally for further localization and to obtain stool for microscopic examination and culture. See Table 17–3 for differential diagnosis of chronic diarrhea.

TREATMENT MEASURES FOR DIARRHEA

General Considerations

Fluid loss amounting to more than 5% of body weight must be replaced. Dehydration is often accompanied by metabolic acidosis (decreased serum HCO_3) and sometimes by hyper- or hyponatremia, depending upon the concentration of electrolyte in the stool. The potassium content of stool may be as high as 30–40 meq/L, and the dehydrated infant may be depleted of intracellular potassium with normal serum potassium. Serum electrolytes should be checked in any child with more than 5% dehydration.

Treatment

A. Parenteral Fluid Therapy: Parenteral fluid is indicated: (1) if vomiting or weakness prevents oral therapy; (2) if the patient is hypotensive; or (3) if surgical procedures are contemplated (see Chapter 4).

B. Oral Rehydration:

1. Replacement of Fluid Deficit: Commercially available oral solutions for replacement of fluid deficits from viral gastroenteritis usually contain 75 meq Na/L, 20 meq K/L, 65 meq Cl/L, 30 meq citrate or bicarbonate/L, and 25 g dextrose/L. Fluid deficit is calculated by comparing weights or by physical signs. Replacement fluids should be administered by mouth over 12–24 hours.

2. Ongoing Fluid Needs: Commercially available oral solutions for maintenance during acute viral enteritis contain slightly less sodium (45 meq/L) and chloride (35 meq/L) than replacement solution. The calorie content of these solutions is only 100 kcal/L; they should not be used as the patient's sole intake for more than 48 hours.

3. Return to Normal Caloric Intake: This should be rapid in uncomplicated viral gastroenteritis. Intestinal lactase levels may be depressed for 7–14 days, and a lactose-free formula is advisable. Gastric retention and diminished bile salt secretion may temporarily decrease fatty food tolerance.

4. Symptomatic Therapy: Anti-diarrheal medications for viral gastroenteritis are rarely indicated and may complicate fluid management. Diphenoxylate with atropine (Lomotil) should not be used in any infant under 3 years. Kaolin and pectin preparations are ineffective.

CONSTIPATION

Normal frequency of defecation in children ranges from three stools per day to 1 per week. Stooling frequency in infants is higher, but some normally defecate only 2–3 times per week. If stools are unusually hard or large, if pain or excessive straining occurs with defecation, if stool frequency is less than once per week, if impaction of the rectum with fecal leakage develops or if abdominal distension, emesis, or failure to thrive occur, symptomatic treatment and assessment of possible organic causes is indicated.

Etiology

See Table 17–4.

Treatment

A. Disimpaction: If the impacted stool is soft, disimpaction can be accomplished with laxatives such as extract of senna fruit or milk

Table 17–3. Chronic diarrhea: guide to differential diagnosis.

Cause	Age	Type of Diarrhea	Associated Features
Disease:			
Bacterial infections	Any age	Mucoid bloody stool.	Rarely chronic except in immunocompromised hosts; *Salmonella* and *Yersinia* most likely.
Viral infection	Any age	Watery.	Rarely chronic except in immunocompromised hosts; CMV, adenovirus, rotovirus.
Parasitic infestation	Any age	Depends on organism.	Amoeba, *Glardia, Cryptosporidium.*
Dietary Factors:			
Overfeeding–especially starches	<6 m	Watery.	Colicky behavior without weight loss.
Protein allergy	<2 m	Watery ± malabsorption of fat; at times blood and mucus.	Colic, emesis, anemia, hypoproteinemia.
Acrodermatitis enteropathica	<12 m	Voluminous with steatorrhea.	Malnutrition, skin rash; low serum Zn; usually genetic; sometimes secondary to severe dietary Zn deficiency.
Primary bile acid malabsorption	<1 m	Voluminous with steatorrhea.	Malnutrition; defective ileal transport of bile acids.
Irritable colon/chronic nonspecific diarrhea	6–36 m	Watery, frequent, with mucus, undigested food; no steatorrhea.	Healthy child; often starts with bout of gastro-enteritis.
Toxic diarrhea (antibiotics, cancer chemotherapy, radiation)	Any age	Loose; sometimes steatorrhea, occult blood or pus.	Vomiting; anorexia.
Functional tumors (neuro-blastoma, carcinoid, pan-creatic cholera, Zollinger-Ellison syndrome)	Any age	Secretory diarrhea, watery, persists when patient fasting.	Hypokalemia; other symptoms depend upon tumor.

Carbohydrate malabsorption: Sucrase–isomaltase	<6 m	Watery; low pH; reducing substance positive after acid hydrolysis; volume varies with sucrose intake.	Abdominal distension; poor growth; deficiency present in 0.8% Americans, 10% Native Alaskans.
Glucose galactose malabsorption	<1 m	Intractable diarrhea with feeding; stool pH low; watery; reducing substances present.	Poor growth; defect in glucose transport.
Genetic Deficiencies:			
Lactase	<4 yr	Watery diarrhea with lactose; low pH; reducing substances present.	Deficiency develops at about 4 years of age in 100% Asians, 80% U.S. blacks, 15% U.S. whites.
Acquired Deficiencies:			
Lactase and sucrase	Any age	Watery; low pH; reducing substances present.	Follows intestinal injury or infection.
Monosaccharide transport	<6 m	Watery; low pH; reducing substances present.	Rare; follows infection; made worse by malnutrition.
Pancreatic Disorders:			
Cystic fibrosis	<6 m	Steatorrhea; bulky, foul, pale.	Respiratory infection; poor weight gain.
Shwachman syndrome	<2 yr	Steatorrhea; bulky, foul, pale.	Neutropenia; short stature; bacterial infections; metaphyseal dysostosis.
Chronic pancreatitis	Any age	Steatorrhea; bulky, foul, pale.	Rare in children; usually associated with alcoholism.
Celiac disease	<12 m	Steatorrhea; bulky, foul, pale.	Emesis, distention, irritability, anorexia.
Intestinal lymphangiectasia	3 m	Voluminous, steatorrhea.	Lymphedema, lymphopenia, hypoalbuminemia.

(*continued*)

Table 17–3. Chronic diarrhea: guide to differential diagnosis (*continued*).

Cause	Age	Type of Diarrhea	Associated Features
Immune Defects:			
Hypogammaglobulinemia; IgA deficiency	Any age	Watery; sometimes steatorrhea.	Recurrent cutaneous and respiratory infection.
Combined immunodeficiency, AIDS, cellular defect	<1 m Any age <2 yr	Severe; watery; steatorrhea.	Stomatitis, skin rash, recurrent infection, opportunistic infection.
Genetic-Metabolic:			
Chloride-losing diarrhea	<1 m	Watery.	Alkalosis; growth failure.
Hypobetalipoproteinemia and α-betalipoproteinemia	<3 m	Profuse; steatorrhea.	Progressive neurologic symptoms; low serum cholesterol; acanthocytosis.
Wolman's disease	<1 m	Profuse; steatorrhea.	Emesis; severe growth failure; adrenal calcification; hypercholesterolemia.
Folate malabsorption	<1 m	Watery.	Anemia; stomatitis, seizures, retardation.
Anatomic:			
Blind (stagnant) loop/bacterial overgrowth	Any age	Watery; fat and carbohydrate malabsorption.	Caused by surgical adhesions, intestinal duplication, abnormal GI motility, partial obstruction.
Short bowel	Any age	Watery; malabsorption of all nutrients.	Rarely congenital, usually secondary to surgical resection.
Intestinal pseudo-obstruction	Any age	Watery; malabsorption of all nutrients.	Distension; may be acquired or congenital; diarrhea secondary to bacterial overgrowth.

Inflammatory Bowel Disease:			
Crohn's disease		See Table 17–9	
Ulcerative colitis		See Table 17–9	
Eosinophilic gastroenteritis	Any age	Watery or bloody depending upon site of disease.	Intestinal or gastric obstruction, eczema, asthma, increased blood eosinophiles.
Hirschsprung's disease with enterocolitis	<1 yr	Foul, liquid with WBC and RBC.	Abdominal distension, fever, history of constipation.
Malnutrition	<1 yr	Loose, steatorrhea, sometimes with carbohydrate malabsorption.	Becomes temporarily worse with refeeding.
Endocrine:			
Hyperthyroidism	Any age	Frequent, loose stool without malabsorption.	Other signs of hyperthyroidism.

CMV = cytomegalovirus; GI = gastrointestinal; IgA = immunoglobulin A; RBC = red blood cell; WBC = white blood cell; Zn = zinc.

Table 17–4. Constipation.

Characteristics	Agents
Infancy:	
Mechanical obstruction	Imperforate anus, anal stenosis. Intestinal obstruction.
Abnormal intestinal motility	Hirschsprung's disease: Lack of ganglion cells in the colon wall causes failure of peristalsis through affected areas. Intestinal pseudo-obstruction. Hypothyroidism, congenital or acquired. Hypokalemia, hypercalcemia, hypermagnesemia.
Somatic weakness or incoordination	Hypotoniamyopathy, acquired or congenital; cerebral palsy; sacral agenesis; spina bifida.
Pain on defecation	Anal fissure, perianal skin disease, or abscess.
Drugs	Narcotics, antihistamines, calcium salts, aluminum hydroxide antacids, vincristine.
Dehydrating conditions	Diabetes mellitus, diabetes insipidus, following acute gastroenteritis.
Childhood:[1]	
Retentive constipation	This is the most likely cause of constipation in healthy toddlers or school-age children. Boys are more commonly affected. Fecal leakage around an impaction is present in 60% of all children. Urinary tract infection or obstruction may be associated, especially in females.

[1] All of the features of constipation in infancy may present in childhood.

of magnesia (below). If impaction is large or hard, enemas may be required. Mineral oil instilled per rectum will lubricate the impaction; a subsequent hypertonic phosphate enema (Fleet) or normal saline enema (20–40 mL/kg) will stimulate evacuation. Tap water or soapy water enemas are not used because they may cause water intoxication or colitis.

B. Maintenance Therapy: Daily non-habituating lubricant or osmotic laxatives are recommended to induce easy daily defecation. See Table 17–5. Compliance with daily toileting and medication are the major determinants of long-term success.

Table 17–5. Commonly used medications in childhood constipation.

Drug	Age	Dose	Comment
Osmotic:			
Malt soup extract	Infant	5–10 mL bid	Surprisingly expensive!
Light corn syrup	Infant	5–10 mL bid	Inexpensive. Has been linked to infant botulism.
Lactulose	Infant and older	conc 10 g/15 mL 1–2 mL/kg/day in 2 doses	Results vary, depending upon resident bacteria. Anorexia is common. Expensive.
Milk of magnesia	>3 mos	1–3 mL/kg/day in 1–2 doses	May be used long term.
Lubricant:			
Mineral oil	>12 mos	1–3 mL/kg/day in 1–2 doses	Danger of lipid pneumonia if aspirated. Avoid use in vomiters. Don't mix with fatty food. Disimpact first to avoid leakage.
Docusate sodium	Infant and older	1–3 mg/kg/day in 2 doses	Not very effective in children. Taste is disliked.
Stimulant:			
Senna syrup	>1 yr	0.5–2 tsp bid	Habituation common.
Dulcolax	>5 yr	5–10 mg/day	Habituation common. Useful for disimpaction.

COLIC

Colic occurs in healthy infants. It is characterized by bouts of crying totaling more than 3 hours per day with apparent discomfort. The usual onset of colic is around 10 days of age, lasting through the third month. It is a source of great anxiety for parents whose ineffective attempts to calm the infant may exacerbate the condition. Prolonged crying may fill the child's stomach and intestines with air. This may lead to crampy pain and the expulsion of gas per rectum. Continuous sucking on a pacifier or frequent breast or bottle feeding may do the same. A vicious cycle of crying, air swallowing, and more crying may be established. Overfeeding in an effort to quiet the infant may cause gastric distension and discomfort. Paradoxically, genuine hunger may initiate this cycle. Colic occurs most often in a first-born infant during the first weeks at home. Family tension and parental anxiety may be aggravating factors.

Intestinal allergy to cow's milk protein, especially in families with a history of allergy in other members, may be associated with colic, emesis, and diarrhea.

Treatment

Careful physical examination and history are required to look for organic causes of fussiness such as otitis media; urinary infection; central nervous system (CNS) disorders (tumors, seizures, infections); intestinal disease (ulcer, esophagitis, gastritis, infection or obstruction); and, more rarely, osteomyelitis or injury secondary to child abuse.

The following therapeutic measures are sometimes helpful:

1. Supportive, sympathetic instruction of parents regarding colic and its benign nature. Rest and assistance with child care are essential to prevent parental exhaustion.
2. Regular schedule for feedings and naps to avoid chaotic routines, overfeeding, or underfeeding.
3. Low-level sound in the infant's sleeping area such as a radio or vacuum cleaner may be soothing.
4. Gentle movement in a swing or rides in the automobile.
5. Trial of milk-free diet may help an infant with true protein allergy. Avoid frequent formula changes.
6. Medications are rarely useful. Antihistamines, antispasmodics, and antacids have been used. Bentyl has been shown effective, but there is a risk of respiratory depression. The use of alcoholic beverages for sedation is not recommended.

LIVER DISEASE

The reader is referred to Chapter 10 for a discussion of infectious hepatitis.

Cholestasis of the Newborn

Many newborns have elevated total and unconjugated serum bilirubin secondary to physiologic jaundice, hemolytic disease, and sometimes hypothyroidism. If the direct reacting fraction of bilirubin (conjugated fraction) is greater than 20% of the total, cholestatic liver disease should be suspected and evaluated. Conjugated hyperbilirubinemia is *never* physiologic. The causes of conjugated hyperbilirubinemia are listed in Tables 17–6 and 17–7.

BILIARY ATRESIA

Biliary atresia is a progressive extrahepatic biliary obstruction in the newborn. The extrahepatic biliary tree is fibrotic and intensely inflamed, suggesting infection. Chronic complete biliary obstruction eventually compromises the intrahepatic biliary system and results in cirrhosis, portal hypertension, ascites, and liver insufficiency.

Clinical Findings

Cholestasis, hepatomegaly and acholic stools develop, usually after week two of life. Failure to thrive and nutritional deficiencies secondary to steatorrhea develop in the first few months of life. Neonatal hepatitis is the condition most often confused with biliary atresia. This and other causes of jaundice (Tables 17–7 and 17–8) must be ruled out.

Treatment

Laparotomy and operative cholangiogram should be performed to confirm the diagnosis. Bilioenteric drainage (portojejunostomy) procedures must be performed as soon as the diagnosis is confirmed. The condition cannot be surgically palliated after 12–16 weeks.

Course & Prognosis

The average survival with untreated biliary atresia is 18 months. Progression of hepatic fibrosis is common even after surgical palliation, although 30–50% of patients may remain anicteric. Liver transplantation may be required as hepatic fibrosis progresses.

Table 17–6. Causes of neonatal cholestasis.

Source	Associated Findings
Infection:	
Bacterial (UTI, sepsis, meningitis)	+ Bacterial cultures.
Viral-intrauterine (rubella, CMV, herpes, toxoplasmosis)	+ Cultures; infant often SGA with DIC and other abnormalities secondary to infection. Hepatomegaly and splenomegaly common.
Viral-acquired (HAV, HBV, HCV, EBV, herpes, Enterovirus)	+ Serologic tests; enterovirus associated with encephalitis; cutaneous lesions in herpes.
Idiopathic (giant cell) hepatitis	Negative cultures; giant cells on liver biopsy.
Metabolic:	
Cystic fibrosis	+ Sweat test; pale, fatty stools, large gallbladder with viscid bile.
Galactosemia	Emesis, acidosis; reducing substances in urine while taking lactose; decreased RBC gal-1-PO_4-uridyl transferase.
Alpha-1-antitrypsin deficiency	Baby may be SGA; variable degrees of hepatitis and cirrhosis at presentation; serum α-1-antitrypsin <70 mg%.
Tyrosinemia	Hypoalbuminemia, coagulopathy, and hepatitis, increased urinary succinyl acetone.
Parenteral nutrition	Gradual onset; jaundice a late finding occurring after several weeks of IV nutrition.
Extrahepatic biliary atresia, choledochal cyst	Acholic stools, firm large liver, generally healthy appearance (see pg 588).
Paucity of intrahepatic bile ducts:	
Alagille syndrome	Odd facies, growth failure. Hypogonadism. Peripheral pulmonic stenosis. Vertebral anomalies.
Nonsyndromatic bile duct paucity	Rapidly progressive liver disease.

CMV = cytomegalovirus; DIC = disseminated intravascular coagulation; EBV = Epstein-Barr virus; HAV = hepatitis A virus; HBV = hepatitis B virus; HCV = hepatitis C virus; RBC = red blood cell count; SGA = small for gestational age; UTI = urinary tract infection.

Table 17–7. Liver disease of older children.

Cause	Agents
Acute infection (see Chapter 10)	Cytomegalic inclusion virus
	Epstein-Barr virus
	Hepatitis A, hepatitis B, hepatitis C, hepatitis E
	Other systemic viral infections
	Bacterial agents include *N gonorrhoeae* (causes perihepatitis)
Fatty liver	Malnutrition
	Storage (Wolman's disease)
	Reye's syndrome
	Mitochondrial dysfunction (eg, carnitine deficiency, lactic acidemia)
Tumors (see Chapter 25)	Hepatoblastoma
	Hemangiomatosis
	Metastatic Wilms' tumor
	Neuroblastoma
	Gonadal tumor
	Leukemic infiltration
	Histiocytosis
Parasitic disease (see Chapter 11)	*E histolytica*
	Visceral larva migrans
	Schistosoma mansoni
	S japonicum
Metabolic/genetic/ storage diseases	Cystic fibrosis—fatty liver/biliary cirrhosis
	Glycogen storage disease
	Galactosemia
	Tyrosinemia
	Alpha-1-antitrypsin deficiency
	Neiman–Pick disease
	Gaucher's disease
	Amyloidosis
	Congenital hepatic fibrosis
	Wilson's disease
Chronic inflammatory disease	Autoimmune chronic active hepatitis
	Chronic active hepatitis B or C
	Sclerosing cholangitis, or chronic active hepatitis associated with inflammatory bowel disease

CHOLEDOCHAL CYST

Choledochal cyst is less common than biliary atresia. Symptoms include intermittent jaundice, fever, and a mass in the right upper quadrant. X-ray examination may show a mass on a plain film and indentation of the duodenum on an upper gastrointestinal (GI) se-

Table 17–8. Acid-peptic diseases.

Location	Etiology	Signs and Symptoms
Esophagus	GE reflux	Spitting and vomiting (infants), heartburn in older children, blood loss, aspiration, dysphagia. Infections of the esophagus mimic peptic esophagitis.
Stomach: Gastritis Gastric ulcer	Infection (CMV) Irritants (ASA, alcohol) *H pylori* infection Immunodeficiency (AIDS, cancer and transplant chemotherapy) Secondary: head injury, burn, sepsis, shock, Crohn's disease. Idiopathic	Epigastric pain, vomiting (especially in infancy), hematemesis, protein losing enteropathy. Decrease in mucosal defense and reperfusion injury are thought to be the cause of secondary gastritis/ulcer
Duodenitis & ulcer	Secondary ulcer—head injury, sepsis, shock, burn, chronic lung disease (CF), Crohn's disease. Drugs: NSAIDs, ASA *H pylori* infection Hypersecretion of acid: Zollinger-Ellison syndrome, gastrinoma	Epigastric pain, vomiting (especially in infancy), hematemesis.

AIDS = acquired immune deficiency syndrome; ASA = aminosalicylic acid; CF = cystic fibrosis; CMV = cytomegalovirus; GE = gastroesophageal; NSAIDs = non-steroidal anti-inflammatory drugs.

ries. Ultrasonography is preferred to confirm the diagnosis. The cyst should be excised. The prognosis is excellent if excision is done early. Newborns with choledochal cysts have a poorer prognosis than older children, with a course similar to that of extrahepatic biliary atresia.

PANCREATIC DISEASE

See Table 17–3.

CYSTIC FIBROSIS

In childhood, the most common cause of exocrine pancreatic insufficiency is **cystic fibrosis (CF)**. Malabsorption, present from birth in 85% of persons with CF, results from obstruction of the ductular system and progressive destruction of the exocrine pancreas. Exogenous pancreatic enzymes must be provided with meals to improve digestion of complex carbohydrate, protein, and fat. Other GI problems associated with CF include peptic ulcer, pancreatitis, cholecystitis, cholelithiasis, biliary cirrhosis, meconium ileus (in the newborn), distal ileal obstructions, and rectal prolapse.

SHWACHMAN SYNDROME

Shwachman syndrome is a rare condition of unknown etiology (probably genetic) characterized by exocrine pancreatic insufficiency (because of fatty replacement of acinar tissue), neutropenia (either cyclic or continuous), growth failure, and metaphyseal dysostosis. Recurrent bacterial infections occur in some patients. Diarrhea and malnutrition are common. Sweat test is normal.

PANCREATITIS

Pancreatitis is usually an acute viral infection in childhood. It is sometimes associated with overwhelming bacterial infection, connective tissue diseases, **Reye's syndrome** (Chapter 3), drug toxicity, hyperlipidemia, and rarely (in pediatrics) alcohol abuse. Forty percent of cases are idiopathic. Trauma may cause pancreatitis or pancreatic pseudocyst. Abdominal tenderness, high serum amylase, and enlarged pancreas on abdominal ultrasound with ascites are diagnostic findings. Hypocalcemia may occur. Hemorrhagic pancreatitis carries a very high mortality.

DISEASES OF THE ESOPHAGUS, STOMACH, & INTESTINE

PEPTIC ULCER DISEASE

See Table 17–8.

INFLAMMATORY BOWEL DISEASE

See Table 17–9.

The two major inflammatory bowel diseases (IBDs) in children are **Crohn's disease** (regional enteritis) and ulcerative colitis. A comparison of the two conditions is found in Table 17–9. The etiology of both is unknown, but aberrations of immune and inflammatory mediators are suspected. A family history of IBD is obtained in 25% of cases. Ulcerative colitis and Crohn's disease may occur in the same family, suggesting some common etiology for the two conditions.

GLUTEN ENTEROPATHY-CELIAC DISEASE

In celiac disease, intestinal villous atrophy occurs in response to glutens present in wheat, rye, barley, and oats. Malabsorption of all nutrients occurs owing to the diminished surface in the small intestine. It is thought that gliadin is bound by enterocytes in the intestine and that a local immune reaction ensues, which destroys the absorbing cells. Weight loss, fatty stools, anorexia, and irritability usually appear in the second year of life, often after an acute viral illness. Occasionally, severe diarrhea, dehydration, electrolyte deficiency, and prostration occur (**celiac crisis**).

Diagnosis rests on typical villous atrophy and plasma cell infiltrate in small intestinal biopsies. Antigliadin, reticulin, and endomysial antibodies are present. Diagnosis by trial of gluten-free diet is not recommended. Treatment is by gluten-free diet. Lactose tolerance is poor until intestinal recovery occurs. Vitamin and iron supplements may be necessary if diarrhea has been long-standing.

Full recovery is expected. The intestinal biopsy normalizes. The sensitivity to gluten is life-long. Ten percent of first-degree relatives are affected in this genetically determined disease.

DISACCHARIDASE DEFICIENCIES

Diminished activity of disaccharidase enzymes on the microvillous surface of the small intestine causes malabsorption of disaccharides and watery, acid, osmotic diarrhea upon ingestion of the offending sugar. Stools contain undigested disaccharides and their fermentation by-products. Symptoms also include nausea, vomiting, and flatulence. Disaccharidase deficiency may be primary (genetic) or secondary to bowel injury. Genetic lactase deficiency affects 30–50% of whites in the United States, 50–70% of African Americans, and nearly 100% of Asians and Native Americans over the age of 4 years. Genetic sucrase deficiency is rare except in Native Alaskans, for whom the prevalence is 10%. Disaccharide tolerance tests or breath hydrogen assay after an oral disaccharide test meal may be diagnostic. Direct measurement of enzyme levels in intestinal biopsies can be performed (Table 17–3). Avoidance of the offending sugars or enzyme supplements (lactase and sucrase) taken with disaccharide-containing foods reduces symptoms.

COW'S MILK ALLERGY

Cow's milk protein allergy is more often suspected than proved. The onset is usually in patients under 3 months of age. The symptoms are diarrhea, vomiting, and, in older children, a malabsorption syndrome compatible with small bowel injury. Early introduction of milk into the diet, especially following gastrointestinal infection, may predispose to this condition. Findings in infants include proctitis with eosinophils in rectal mucosa, blood in stool, and occasionally an atrophic small bowel lesion.

Diagnosis is confirmed by a response to elimination of cow's milk followed by recurrence of symptoms after reintroduction of milk. Cow's milk protein is strictly eliminated from the diet for 6 months to 1 year. Protein hydrolysate formulas may be substituted. Concomitant soy protein allergy is seen in up to 30% of these infants.

Cow's milk protein allergy usually resolves after 6–12 months.

ESOPHAGEAL ATRESIA WITH OR WITHOUT TRACHEOESOPHAGEAL FISTULA

Most infants with tracheoesophageal fistula (TEF) present at birth with cough, vomiting, apparent excessive salivation, and aspiration pneumonia. See Chapter 15 for management of respiratory problems connected with TEF. In 85–90% of cases, the upper esophagus ends in a blind pouch while the lower esophageal segment communicates with the lower trachea. In about 10% of cases, there is upper esophageal atresia without an associated distal tracheoesophageal fistula. Maternal polyhydramnios is common. In about 5% of cases there is an H-type fistula between an intact esophagus and trachea. These

Table 17–9. Features of Crohn's disease and ulcerative colitis.

Feature	Crohn's Disease	Ulcerative Colitis
Age at onset	10–20 yr	10–20 yr
Incidence (general population)	4–5/100,000	3–15/100,000
Relative incidence in children	2	1
Area of bowel affected	Oropharynx, esophagus, and stomach—rare Small bowel only, 25–30% Colon and anus only, 15% Ileocolitis, 40% Diffuse disease, 5%	Total colon, 90% Proctitis, 10%
Distribution	Segmental; disease-free skip areas common.	Continuous.
Pathology	Full thickness, acute and chronic inflammation; noncaseating granulomas (50%); fistulae, abscesses, strictures, and fibrosis may be present.	Superficial acute inflammation of mucosa with microscopic crypt abscess.
X-ray	Segmental lesions; thickened circular folds; cobblestone appearance of bowel wall secondary to longitudinal ulcers and transverse fissures; fixation and separation of loops; narrowed lumen "string sign"; fistulae.	Superficial colitis; loss of haustra; shortened colon and pseudopolyps (islands of normal tissue surrounded by denuded mucosa) are late findings.
Intestinal symptoms	Abdominal pain, diarrhea, perianal disease; enteroenteric/enterocutaneous fistula, abscess, anorexia	Abdominal pain, bloody diarrhea, urgency, and tenesmus.

Extraintestinal Symptoms:		
Arthritis/arthralgia	15%	9%
Fever	40–50%	40–50%
Stomatitis	9%	2%
Weight loss	90% (mean 5.7 kg)	68% (mean 4.1 kg)
Delayed growth and sexual development	30%	5–10%
Uveitis/conjunctivitis	15% (in Crohn's colitis)	4%
Sclerosing cholangitis	Rare	4%
Renal stones	6% (oxalate)	6% (urate)
Pyoderma gangrenosum	1.3%	5%
Erythema nodosum	8–15%	4%
Laboratory findings	High ESR; microcytic anemia; low serum iron and total iron binding capacity; increased fecal protein loss; low serum albumin.	High ESR; microcytic anemia, high WBC with "left shift."
Treatment	Corticosteroids, azulfidine (or mesalamine, olsalazine), metronidazole (especially for perianal disease), 6-MP, azathioprine; surgical resection as last resort.	Corticosteroids, azulfidine (or mesalamine, olsalazine), azathioprine, or 6-mercaptopurine; cyclosporine in very severe cases; colectomy for toxic megacolon, resistant symptoms, intractable pain or bleeding.

ESR = erythrocyte sedimentation rate; WBC = white blood cell count.

infants usually present later, after repeated bouts of aspiration pneumonia or choking with feedings. Thirty percent of infants with TEF have associated anomalies, usually cardiac or gastrointestinal. Imperforate anus is common. Careful barium esophagram is necessary to make the diagnosis. The H-type fistula, usually located in the lower cervical esophagus, is often tiny, and endoscopy or bronchoscopy may be necessary for diagnosis. Early diagnosis, normal birth weight, absence of lung disease, and a short distance between the proximal and distal esophageal segments improve the prognosis. The treatment is surgical. Stricture and fistula formation at the site of esophageal repair may occur. Gastroesophageal reflux (below) occurs in 75% of patients postoperatively. Esophageal peristaltic function is always abnormal.

Other causes of esophageal obstruction include vascular ring, especially double aortic arch, congenital stricture, and achalasia.

Esophageal strictures may develop after correction of TEF, ingestion of corrosive chemicals (eg, lye), or as a result of peptic esophagitis. **Globus hystericus**, or a sensation of esophageal obstruction in the absence of obstructing lesions, may be seen even in preschool children. These children often refuse food but usually have no difficulty swallowing their own secretions.

Diagnosis

The upper GI series is the most informative study when symptoms suggest esophageal obstruction. Vascular ring causes characteristic external compression of the esophageal outline. Location and length of stricture, esophageal dysmotility, and hiatal hernia are easily seen. Endoscopy adds more information regarding esophagitis.

INGUINAL HERNIA & HYDROCELE

Inguinal Hernia

A hernia is seen as an intermittent bulge lateral to the pubic tubercle; the bulge appears when the patient is crying, straining, or standing, and usually reduces spontaneously when the patient is relaxed or supine. The hernia usually contains bowel or mesentery. In females the ovary may herniate.

The incidence of hernia in the general population is 1%, and in premature infants, 5%. Males are affected most commonly (85% of cases). One-half of cases of inguinal hernia during childhood occur in infants under 6 months of age. Right-sided hernias are more frequent than left-sided (2:1). Twenty-five percent of patients have bilateral hernias; the percentage is higher in females. Elective repair of inguinal hernia is recommended; repair of the asymptomatic side is often performed in children less than 2 years of age, especially in females.

Incarceration (failure to reduce) occurs in about 10% of cases, most often in children under 1 year of age. The hernia becomes tender and erythematous. The abdomen becomes distended, with vomiting and signs of bowel obstruction. Pressure on testicular vessels in the inguinal canal by an incarcerated hernia can cause testicular infarction. Incarcerated hernia can often be reduced by gently squeezing the bowel back into the abdomen along the axis of the inguinal canal. Sedation (pentobarbital, 4 mg/kg, and meperidine, 1 mg/kg) is necessary in most cases. Reduction should not be attempted after 12 hours of incarceration because of the risk of bowel perforation. Immediate surgical repair is indicated.

Hydrocele

Hydrocele, or collection of fluid between the layers of the tunica vaginalis, is very common in newborns. Spontaneous regression by age 6 months is the rule. Frequent changes in size of the hydrocele indicates a patent processus vaginalis with communication to the peritoneal cavity. Since hernia may develop, communicating hydroceles should be repaired.

Acute hydrocele may develop about the testis or in the spermatic cord and may be difficult to differentiate from incarcerated hernia. Examination at the internal ring level, with one finger in the upper rectum and another feeling the abdomen from the outside, may aid in differentiation. Acute hydrocele presents as an oblong, firm swelling in the groin of a female infant and may be confused with a groin node. Exploration is required in doubtful cases.

GASTROESOPHAGEAL REFLUX

Gastroesophageal reflux occurs in 40% of healthy infants younger than 6 months. Postprandial spitting and vomiting are the most common symptoms. Infants are usually healthy, but aspiration pneumonia, esophagitis, esophageal stricture, and malnutrition occur if vomiting is severe. Reflux is common in physically and neurologically handicapped children, in those with severe scoliosis, and after tracheoesophageal fistula repair.

Diagnosis is based upon characteristic history, upper GI series, and esophageal pH monitoring in atypical cases.

Conservative measures often suffice in healthy infants as the condition usually resolves by 8–12 months. Infants are given small-volume, frequent feedings thickened with cereal and are kept in the prone position as much as possible. Medication includes antacids, H_2 receptor antagonists, and smooth muscle stimulants such as cisapride. In resistant cases, gastric fundoplication may be necessary.

CONGENITAL HERNIA OF THE DIAPHRAGM

The most common area of herniation is in the left posterolateral portion, the foramen of Bochdalek. Hernias in the foramen of Morgagni rarely present during the newborn period and rarely cause significant respiratory symptoms.

Clinical Findings

A. Symptoms & Signs: Cyanosis and dyspnea in a newborn infant suggest the diagnosis. Chest movements are asymmetric with dullness on the affected side. Breath sounds may be absent. The abdomen is scaphoid and feels less full than usual. The mediastinum shifts away from the affected side. There is usually hypoplasia of the lung on the affected side with pulmonary hypertension, which makes ventilatory management difficult.

B. Imaging: Chest x-ray usually shows a portion of the GI tract in the thorax and displacement of the mediastinum.

Treatment & Prognosis

Diaphragmatic hernia is a surgical emergency. The viscera must be reduced from the thorax. The diaphragm must be closed (or patched if the defect is large).

Persistent pulmonary hypertension and pulmonary hypoplasia are the commonest causes of mortality. Pulmonary vasodilators are sometimes helpful. Recently, **extracorporeal membrane oxygenation**, or ECMO (Chapter 7), and inhaled nitric oxide have been used with success in some of these infants.

Survival depends on the degree of pulmonary hypoplasia; survival rate is about 50%. Lung weights of infants who do not survive are about half those of normal infants of the same gestational age and birth weight. The morphology of the lung on the side of the hernia is immature. Long-term survivors have normal lung weights, although they may have emphysema and decreased blood flow.

PYLORIC STENOSIS

(Congenital Hypertrophic Pyloric Stenosis)

Pyloric stenosis is more apt to occur in firstborn infants and is more common in males than in females (4:1 ratio) between 3 and 12 weeks of age. Circular musculature of the pylorus is hypertrophied, causing obstruction of the lumen.

Symptoms & Signs

Emesis is mild at first but becomes progressively more projectile over 3–7 days. The vomitus does not contain bile. The infant appears hungry. Stools are small. Weight loss, dehydration, and hypochloremic alkalosis may be severe. Jaundice develops in 2–5% of cases. Gastric stasis results in gastritis and hematemesis in some cases. On examination, the infant is alert, irritable, dehydrated, and hungry. The epigastrium may be distended and the gastric outline obvious. Gastric peristalsis passing from left to right during feeding can be seen on the abdomen. An olive-shaped mass is palpable in the right upper quadrant, especially immediately after vomiting. Inguinal hernias develop in 10% of cases secondary to forceful emesis. Tetany as a result of alkalosis may occur.

Imaging

If the typical mass in the right upper quadrant is not palpable, the pyloric muscle may be demonstrated by ultrasonography. The upper GI series shows an enlarged stomach with a narrow, elongated pyloric channel and prolonged gastric retention of barium. The impression of the pyloric muscle on the antrum can be seen.

Treatment is surgical. Ramstedt pyloromyotomy divides the hypertrophied muscle bundles that obstruct the pylorus. Surgery should not be performed until rehydration and correction of alkalosis are complete. Complete relief is to be expected following surgical repair. Mortality is low.

MECONIUM ILEUS

Meconium ileus with small bowel obstruction is the presenting sign in 15% of newborn infants with CF. Lack of pancreatic trypsin causes thick meconium, which obstructs the lower 10–20 cm of ileum. The ileocecal valve and the entire colon are normal, albeit small.

Symptoms & Signs

Progressive bilious vomiting and abdominal distension occur in the first day or two of life. Firm masses within dilated bowel loops strongly suggest meconium ileus. In most cases, no meconium will have been passed per rectum.

Imaging

Marked intestinal dilatation is seen. A granular, mottled appearance to the intestinal content in the right lower abdomen is characteristic of inspissated meconium. Microcolon may be seen on barium enema. Free air in the peritoneal cavity or fluid between the loops of bowel indicates perforation. Calcification of the peritoneum is seen in antenatal perforation and meconium peritonitis.

Laboratory Findings

The sweat shows an increase in the chloride concentration (> 60 meq/L). Serum immunoreactive trypsinogen, usually elevated in newborns with CF, may be falsely normal in patients with meconium ileus, because of the severe antenatal reduction in exocrine pancreatic secretion.

Treatment & Prognosis

Provide continuous gastric suction through a nasogastric tube. Administer diatrizoate (Gastrografin) enemas but only when the infant is adequately hydrated. The hypertonic contrast medium draws water into the bowel and may "float out" the inspissated meconium. This procedure must be done under fluoroscopy by a radiologist familiar with newborn infants. Surgery is required if obstruction is not relieved. The ileum is opened and meconium removed. The portion of distal ileum containing the greatest amount of meconium may have to be resected with temporary ileostomy. There is no relationship between meconium ileus and the severity of the respiratory symptoms of CF.

CONGENITAL ATRESIA OR STENOSIS OF INTESTINES & COLON

Congenital intestinal atresia and stenosis probably result from vascular obstruction in the mesenteric vessels during fetal development. Atresia or stenosis of the duodenum is frequently associated with **Down's syndrome**.

Symptoms & Signs

Atresia of the intestinal tract or colon causes vomiting on the first day of life. Intestinal stenosis may not cause symptoms for weeks or months. The vomitus contains bile. Depending on the level of involvement, abdominal distension is present and becomes progressively worse. Peristaltic waves are often seen. Intestinal loops may be outlined on the abdominal wall.

Imaging

Upright abdominal x-ray shows air and fluid levels with dilatation of the bowel proximal to obstruction. The distal loops will be free of gas if the obstruction is complete. In partial obstruction, there may be gas without distension distal to the obstruction. Presence of free air in the abdominal cavity means that perforation has occurred. A granular, mottled appearance in the small bowel as a result of gas and meconium suggests meconium ileus.

Barium enema is an important part of the preoperative x-ray study. In low-intestinal atresia, it will often demonstrate the markedly decreased caliber of the unused portion of the GI tract—the so-called microcolon. The chief indication for barium enema is to rule out **Hirschsprung's disease** (below) and malrotation with volvulus, which can present with symptoms identical to those of intestinal atresia.

Treatment & Prognosis

Immediate resection of atretic or stenotic bowel with end-to-end anastomosis, where possible, is performed. If the infant is debilitated or if perforation has occurred, diverting intestinal enterostomy is performed with later resection with anastomosis.

The mortality rate in infants with atresia or stenosis is increased by delay in diagnosis. Postoperative hypomotility of the dilated proximal bowel may compromise enteral feedings, necessitating parenteral nutrition.

MALROTATION OF INTESTINES & COLON

Malrotation is the result of incomplete rotation of the gut and lack of attachment of the mesentery of the small intestine during intrauterine development. It may result in a volvulus of the midgut or obstruction of the second part of the duodenum by peritoneal bands. It may be associated with no symptoms.

Symptoms & Signs

If malrotation is accompanied by an intrinsic obstruction of the second portion of the duodenum (eg, atresia, stenosis), vomiting occurs within 48 hours of birth. Midgut volvulus may occur at any time but is most common in the first 3 months. In the early stages of midgut volvulus, the general condition is good. Bilious emesis is the significant symptom, followed by shock and acidosis secondary to bowel infarction. Abdominal distension may not be prominent.

Hematocrit and red blood cell counts (RBCs) are elevated owing to dehydration. Slight leukocytosis is usually present. Marked leukocytosis and metabolic acidosis suggests impending or actual gangrene of the bowel.

Imaging

Plain films of the abdomen may show dilatation of the stomach and duodenum. If the patient is stable, upper GI series or barium enema will reveal the malrotation.

Treatment & Prognosis

The goal of surgery is to relieve extrinsic compression in the duodenum by dividing the bands that bind the second and third portions to the retroperitoneum and by straightening the duodenojejunal junction. The midgut always twists in a clockwise fashion in North America; thus, the mass of bowel loops must be unwound in a counterclockwise direction. The small bowel is then placed in the right side of the abdomen and the colon to the left.

Recurrences after surgical correction are uncommon.

MECKEL'S DIVERTICULUM

Meckel's diverticulum may be asymptomatic throughout life or may be associated with any of the following: hemorrhage; Meckel's diverticulitis; perforation; intussusception, with the diverticulum as the leading point; patent omphalomesenteric duct, with a diverticulum opening at the umbilicus; and intestinal obstruction from a vestigial band connecting the diverticulum to the umbilicus. It is found in 2% of the population and is usually located in the distal ileum. A ^{99}Tc scan may identify a Meckel's diverticulum which contains gastric mucosa.

Bleeding from a Meckel's diverticulum is a result of peptic ulceration of the diverticulum itself or of adjacent intestinal mucosa.

Bleeding is massive but usually painless. Diverticula containing no gastric mucosa do not usually bleed. Foreign bodies occasionally impact in a diverticulum.

Treatment of a diverticulum which has bled is excision, either open or laparoscopically. Meckel's diverticula discovered incidentally at laparotomy may be removed, especially if they contain gastric mucosa.

The prognosis is excellent following surgery. If perforation of a gangrenous diverticulum has occurred, peritonitis may follow.

DUPLICATIONS OF THE GASTROINTESTINAL TRACT

Cysts of enteric origin may occur anywhere from the upper esophagus to the anus, usually sharing a common muscular wall with the GI tract. There may be communication between cyst and bowel lumen. The nature of the mucosal lining varies considerably and may not necessarily correspond with the level of the gastrointestinal tract to which the cyst is adjacent. There is considerable variation in the size and shape of these cysts.

A duplication may present as an asymptomatic mass, with bleeding, perforation and peritonitis, intestinal obstruction, malabsorption secondary to bacterial overgrowth. Neurenteric cysts usually arise from the proximal small bowel and extend toward the vertebral column; they are associated with hemivertebrae, or ventral or dorsal spina bifida. They may extend through the diaphragm into the chest. Hindgut duplications are often associated with doubling of the anus and the perineal structures.

Diagnosis can sometimes be made by use of radioactive technetium perchlorate to demonstrate ectopic gastric mucosa in the duplication or by computed tomography.

Treatment consists of resection of the duplication and, in most cases, of the adjacent bowel also. The prognosis is good.

INTUSSUSCEPTION

Intussusception is a common surgical emergency in early childhood. It is characterized by the telescoping of a proximal portion of the intestine into a more distal portion, resulting in impairment of the blood supply and necrosis of the involved segment of bowel. In 95% of cases, no cause of intussusception can be found, although viral infections have been implicated. The condition is most common in infants between the ages of 5 months and 1 year. In children over 4 years, there may be a leading point for intussusception such as Meckel's diverticulum, polyps, or lymphoma.

Intussusception most commonly involves the telescoping of the ileum into the colon. Bowel necrosis occurs if the incarcerated bowel loses its blood supply.

Symptoms & Signs

Recurrent paroxysmal abdominal pain in a healthy child suggests intussusception. The child typically perspires and draws up the legs. He or she may appear well or lethargic in the pain-free intervals. Vomiting frequently occurs but is not universally present. Fifteen percent of patients do *not* have pain.

There is pallor, sweating, and lassitude with each attack of pain. After 5 or more hours, dehydration and listlessness are noted. A low-grade fever is usually present as a result of dehydration and obstruction.

Palpation usually reveals a nontender, firm, sausage-shaped mass in the abdomen. Its location varies, but it frequently is in the upper midabdomen. The right lower quadrant is characteristically less full than usual. If the leading point of the intussusception has reached the rectum, it may be possible to palpate a mass by rectal examination. A "currant jelly" stool (blood and mucus clot) may be evacuated in a bowel movement.

Imaging

A plain film of the abdomen often shows absence of bowel gas in the right lower quadrant. Dilated small bowel suggests partial or complete obstruction of the small intestine. Barium enema examination outlines the intussusception, and obstruction to further progression of the barium is noted.

Treatment & Prognosis

After intravenous fluids are given, barium or air enema under fluoroscopic control will safely reduce intussusception in two-thirds of cases. Laparotomy is necessary if reduction is not accomplished. If too much pressure is employed or if the bowel wall has been weakened owing to impairment of its vascular supply, perforation can occur. Non-operative reduction (barium enema) should *not* be attempted if there are physical findings of peritonitis.

Surgical reduction is possible in most cases when non-operative treatment fails. The bowel is usually viable. If not, resection and anastomosis are performed.

With early treatment, the prognosis is excellent. Recurrence after non-operative reduction occurs in 2–5% of cases.

POLYPS OF THE INTESTINAL TRACT

See Table 17–10.

Juvenile Polyps

Benign juvenile polyps occur in children from 2–13 years. Sixty percent occur in the rectum. Painless, small-volume, bright-red rectal bleeding is the usual presenting symptom. In most cases, colonoscopic removal of juvenile polyps from the colon is possible. Occasionally, adenomatous changes develop in patients with multiple juvenile polyps. Most juvenile polyps will slough in time without complication.

HIRSCHSPRUNG'S DISEASE

In **Hirschsprung's disease**, there is failure of neuroblast migration from the neural crest to developing distal bowel, resulting in absence of ganglion cells in the submucosa and intermuscular bowel layers. The defect always involves the anorectal junction and may involve variable lengths of bowel proximally, including the small intestine. In most cases, only the rectosigmoid is involved. The disease is 4 times more common in males.

Symptoms & Signs

Obstipation, abdominal distension, and vomiting begin in the first days of life. Ninety percent of patients with aganglionosis fail to pass meconium during the first 24 hours of life. Obstipation may alternate with watery diarrhea. Complete obstruction, perforation, or acute enterocolitis may develop. Poor weight gain is common.

The abdomen is distended, often with palpable loops of bowel. Rectal examination shows no stool in the ampulla. There may be an explosive release of feces and flatus when the examining finger is withdrawn.

Diagnostic Testing

An upright abdominal x-ray may show distension of the colon with gas and feces. Air fluid levels are present. Pneumatosis may occur.

Table 17–10. GI polyposis syndromes.

Syndrome	Location[1]	Number	Histology	Associated Findings	Malignant Potential
Juvenile polyps	Colon.	Usually single.	Hyperplastic, hamartomatous.	None.	None in single polyps.
Familial juvenile polyposis[2]	Stomach, small bowel, colon.	Multiple.	Hamartomatous with focal adenomatous change.	Meckel diverticulum, malrotation, hydrocephaly, undescended testes.	10–25%.
Familial adenomatous polyposis[2]	Colon (stomach and small bowel).	Multiple.	Adenomatous.	None.	95–100%.
Peutz–Jegher syndrome[2]	Small bowel, stomach, colon.	Multiple.	Hamartomatous.	Pigmented cutaneous and oral macules; ovarian cysts and tumors; bony exostoses.	2–3%.
Gardner syndrome[2]	Colon (stomach, small bowel).	Multiple.	Adenomatous.	Cysts, tumors, and desmoids of skin and bone; other tumors.	95–100%.
Cronkhite–Canada syndrome	Stomach, colon (esophagus, small bowel).	Multiple.	Hamartomatous.	Alopecia, retinal pigmentation, onychodystrophy, hyperpigmentation.	Rare.
Turcot syndrome[3]	Colon.	Multiple.	Adenomatous.	Thyroid and brain tumors.	Possible.

GI = gastrointestinal.
[1] Parentheses indicate less common locations.
[2] Autosomal dominant.
[3] Autosomal recessive.

Barium enema should be performed *without* the usual bowel preparation. A transition between narrow distal aganglionic bowel and dilated normal bowel is seen. It may not be clearly discernible in neonates. The transitional segment is spastic, with an irregular, saw-toothed outline.

A deep rectal biopsy shows absence of ganglion cells in both Meissner's and Auerbach's plexuses. Marked hypertrophy of nerve trunks may be seen.

Rectal manometry demonstrates loss of the normal reflex relaxation of the internal anal sphincter upon rectal distension.

Treatment

Diverting colostomy or ileostomy is usually performed. Resection of the aganglionic segment, with colo- (or entero-) anal anastomosis is performed when the patient is 6 months or older.

ANORECTAL MALFORMATIONS

(Imperforate Anus)

Clinical Findings

A. Males: There is no opening where the anus should be. The intergluteal fold may be well developed, with good sphincter response to perineal stimulation. Look for a fistula along the median raphe. Watch for meconium in urine. There is a significant incidence of associated TEF. Absence of a perineal fistula means that the patient probably has a communication to the urethra and requires a diverting colostomy. In doubtful cases, this communication (fistula) can sometimes be seen on urethrogram.

B. Females: Look for a fistula in the posterior fourchette and perineum. Gentle dilation of the fistula with a sound will often relieve obstipation temporarily. A high vaginal fistula cannot be handled by dilation; the patient should have a colostomy.

C. General Findings: Since there is a high incidence of absence of kidneys and strictures of the ureteropelvic and ureterovesical structures, all infants with imperforate anus require thorough study of the urinary tract.

Treatment & Prognosis

Treatment is surgical. Perineal fistulas in males and females require only dilation during the newborn period; anoplasty can be done later. Diverting colostomy is necessary if no perineal fistula is present. Pull-through operations for patients with a high imperforate anus should be done after the age of 6 months. The best results are reported when a transcoccygeal approach is used. The results are poor if the child has myelomeningocele or a significant malformation of the lumbosacral spine.

All infants with perineal fistulas should be continent since bowel passes normally through the levators. Infants with a high proximal pouch and no perineal fistula have only a fair chance for complete rectal continence as anal musculature and levators may be absent.

APPENDICITIS

Appendicitis is the most common lesion of the intestinal tract requiring surgery in childhood. The cause is not clear, although some cases result from impaction of a fecalith in the lumen of the appendix. Pinworms may occasionally cause appendicitis.

Symptoms & Signs:

Periumbilical or generalized abdominal pain occurs. After 1–5 hours, the pain becomes localized in the right lower quadrant. Urinary pain or frequency may be present if the appendix lies near the bladder. Constipation occurs frequently, but diarrhea is only occasionally seen. Vomiting is a late symptom.

Fever is low-grade or may be absent early in the course. Very high fevers are suggestive of appendiceal perforation, with peritonitis. Localization of tenderness may be difficult, but an opinion may be formed by palpating each area and noting the voluntary guarding or involuntary spasm of the abdominal musculature. Most children tend to flex the right thigh in an effort to decrease the spasm of the psoas muscle. However, the elicitation of a positive psoas sign is of doubtful value in small children. There may be rectal tenderness, a mass consisting of peritoneal fluid, or an indurated omentum wrapped around an inflamed appendix.

Laboratory Findings

Two or three consecutive determinations of white blood cells (WBCs) will frequently show a rise in the total WBC, with an accompanying shift to the left in the neutrophilic series. A urinalysis should be performed in order to rule out infection of the kidney or bladder.

Imaging

In uncomplicated appendicitis, plain films of the abdomen may show a fecalith, scoliosis, or an abnormal gas pattern. When exudate has formed, evidence of peritoneal inflammation may cause disappearance of the properitoneal fat line along the right wall of the abdomen or obliteration of the psoas shadow.

A barium enema may be of value if the diagnosis is not clear since filling of the appendix tends to exclude the diagnosis of appendicitis. Abdominal ultrasound may show an enlarged appendix or abscess.

Differential diagnosis includes mesenteric adenitis, pyelitis, cystitis, pneumonitis (especially pneumococcal), gastroenteritis, peritonitis, constipation, Meckel's diverticulitis, and inflammatory bowel disease (especially Crohn's ileitis/ileocolitis).

Appendectomy should be performed as soon as the child has been prepared by adequate fluid and electrolyte administration. If there is doubt as to diagnosis, exploratory laparotomy or laparoscopy, with removal of the appendix and culture of peritoneal fluid, should be performed. Intravenous antibiotic therapy is indicated if peritoneal contamination has occurred.

FOREIGN BODIES IN THE GASTROINTESTINAL TRACT

The incidence of foreign bodies in the GI tract is highest in children 1–3 years of age. Foreign bodies lodged in the esophagus for more than 24 hours must be removed, usually by endoscopy. If passed into the stomach, round smooth foreign bodies (eg, beads) usually pass through the GI tract without incident.

Pointed foreign bodies (eg, straight pins, nails, screws) usually pass without incident. Remove endoscopically if the patient has pain, fever, vomiting, or local tenderness; or if the foreign body fails to pass from the stomach in several days (may be as long as 3–4 weeks for some smooth objects to pass). X-ray examination is required only if the foreign body has not passed in 4–5 days. If a sharp object remains in the same location for 4–5 days, the point may have penetrated the bowel, and endoscopic removal or surgery is then indicated.

18 | Kidney & Urinary Tract

Gary M. Lum, MD

CLINICAL FINDINGS

Clinical manifestations of diseases of the kidneys or urinary tract include symptoms that suggest (1) infection (eg, urgency; frequency; dysuria; and abdominal, suprapubic, or costovertebral angle pain); (2) urolithiasis (abdominal pain, colic); (3) voiding problems (frequency, straining, incontinence); and (4) chronic renal failure (CRF) from abnormal renal development (polyuria, enuresis, failure to thrive). Inability of the kidneys to elaborate a concentrated urine is one of the first signs of inadequate renal development. If urinary concentrating ability is the *only* renal abnormality noted, the diagnosis of diabetes insipidus must be entertained as well.

Renal inflammation (eg, glomerulonephritis) is often asymptomatic unless it produces an immediate, severe compromise in renal function. Subsequent disease progression can produce symptoms of CRF, including anorexia, nausea and vomiting, malaise and easy fatigability, and bone pain.

Renal compromise should be suspected in newborns with congenital absence of the abdominal musculature; abdominal masses; or abnormalities of the spinal cord, sacrum, perineum, or external genitalia. Renal anomalies may also be seen in association with ear deformities, aniridia, hemihypertrophy, chromosomal disorders, hepatic cysts or fibrosis, pulmonary hypoplasia, and congenital ascites. The presence of oligohydramnios and spontaneous pneumothorax should also raise the question of renal disease. With the application of prenatal ultrasonography, abnormalities of the urinary tract may be demonstrated early in pregnancy.

Findings such as hypertension; edema; skeletal deformity; pallor or anemia; hematuria; proteinuria; bacteriuria; crystalluria; acidosis; and elevations in blood urea nitrogen (BUN), creatinine, potassium, and serum phosphate may be encountered in various renal disease states.

DIAGNOSTIC STUDIES

Laboratory assessment of renal function begins with a carefully performed urinalysis. The urinary dipstick is a helpful screening tool. The detection of hematuria, leukocyturia, or bacteriuria, however, should be followed by microscopic inspection of the urinary sediment. Abnormal amounts of urinary protein should be quantitatively measured. If infection is suspected, the urine is sent for culture and sensitivity. If a reliably performed mid-stream, clean-catch urinary specimen cannot be obtained with confidence, a bladder catheterization or suprapubic bladder tap may be performed (Chapter 28). Bacterial colony counts of less than 10,000/mL or multiple flora are usually considered contaminants unless obtained by catheterization or bladder tap (provided proper technique is followed). Appropriate diagnostic work-up should follow to exclude genitourinary abnormalities or conditions predisposing to infection (eg, obstruction, reflux, foreign body, trauma, poor hygiene, or pinworm infestations).

Abnormalities or disease resulting in functional renal disturbance should be demonstrated and monitored by following serum BUN and creatinine (Cr) levels. Serum creatinine is a reflection of muscle metabolism and therefore is related to total body muscle mass. In general, the normal range in the pediatric population is from 0.3 to 0.8 mg%. Since normal renal function maintains the serum level in a steady-state equilibrium, a doubling of the serum creatinine reflects an approximate 50% reduction in renal function. Calculation of the renal creatinine clearance (CrCl) can be useful in estimating renal function; however, this measurement requires reliable collection of a timed (12–24 h) urinary specimen. Renal function can be calculated from the following equation:

$$\frac{\text{Urine Cr mg\%} \times \text{Volume mL/min}}{\text{Serum Cr mg\%}}$$

Verification of reliability can be demonstrated by determination of the creatinine index (24-h creatinine excretion in mg/kg body wt = 12–20). The difficulties encountered in obtaining such a specimen are avoided by estimating glomerular filtration rate with the serum creatinine. The following formula derives creatinine clearance:

$$\frac{0.55 \times \text{height (length) cm}}{\text{Serum Cr mg\%}}$$

BUN also reflects renal function, but it may be altered in other ways (eg, increased catabolism, low urinary flow rate). For example, although the usual BUN:creatinine ratio is 10:1, urinary obstruction typically produces a disproportionate rise in BUN.

Other biochemical markers of renal disease include acidosis, hyperkalemia, hypocalcemia, hyperphosphatemia; and, as a result of disturbed calcium and phosphate homeostasis, elevated alkaline phosphatase. Serologic data, such as immunoglobulins, serum complement, or antinuclear antibodies (ANA) are useful in work-ups of glomerulonephritis and should be obtained when clinically indicated. A normocytic, normochromic anemia is found later in renal failure, as are rickets or long-bone deformity secondary to renal osteodystrophy.

RADIOGRAPHIC STUDIES

Renal **ultrasonography (US)** is a noninvasive technique; it can provide information regarding diseases of the renal parenchyma (cysts, inflammatory or infiltrative disease) or collecting system (dilatation, obstruction) independent of renal function. In addition, clinicians can use Doppler techniques to investigate the integrity of the renal blood flow or the presence of thrombosis. A radioisotope scan such as a **DTPA (technetium-labelled diethylenetriamene pentaacetic acid)** scan is helpful in the search for unilateral disease, renovascular hypertension, and obstruction. A **DMSA (technetium-labelled 2,3-dimercaptosuccinic acid)** scan is useful for detecting renal scarring, and can demonstrate differential function. Angiography is indicated in ruling out renovascular disease when surgical or transluminal angioplasty is anticipated. A voiding cystourethrogram demonstrates ureteral reflux, while more invasive studies of the urinary tract have special indications and are obtained through urologic consultation.

RENAL BIOPSY

Percutaneous renal biopsy can provide histologic verification of suspected renal parenchymal disease, especially in cases of asymptomatic hematuria or proteinuria. The technique is also useful in serial documentation of disease progression or response to treatment, as well as in renal allografts.

RENAL MALFORMATIONS

Anatomical abnormalities such as a solitary cyst kidney or a completely cystic remnant of one kidney with a contralateral normal kidney may manifest little or no clinical symptomatology. If hypertension or infection are problems, urologic referral and removal should be considered.

Polycystic kidney disease (PKD) is progressive in nature. The infantile variant (autosomal recessive) is more likely to progress to renal failure during childhood years. In the autosomal dominant or adult type of PKD (except for instances which present with little or no function at birth), however, renal failure is usually not clinically manifested until the fourth or fifth decade, and sometimes not at all. Congenital nephrotic syndrome (microcystic disease); juvenile nephronopthisis (medullary cystic disease); tuberous sclerosis; and congenital renal hypoplasia, dysplasia, or aplasia can be clinically problematic at birth or at any time during the child's subsequent development.

Clinical & Laboratory Findings

Clinical findings relate to the degree of renal failure. Initial laboratory evaluation includes serum BUN, creatinine, electrolytes, calcium, and phosphate. Anomalous external genitalia, auricular malformations, or pulmonary problems may be associated with poor renal development. Renomegaly may be detected by abdominal exam. Hypertension is a common finding in PKD and tuberous sclerosis. Inability to concentrate urine is characteristic of congenital lesions that result in chronic renal failure. Hematuria, proteinuria, or infection may suggest the presence of these and other anatomic abnormalities. The appropriate, previously mentioned radiographic studies are employed in the evaluation.

URINARY TRACT MALFORMATIONS

Developmental abnormalities of the urinary tract, depending upon severity and interference with urinary flow, can seriously compromise renal parenchymal development and function. Antenatal US can provide information on the developing kidneys and urinary tract, thus allowing the physician to anticipate potential postnatal renal functional disturbances. Some degree of hydronephrosis is a common finding in utero, but postnatal US can easily dispel concern. In cases of justified concern, timely urologic intervention is of paramount importance to reduce further deleterious effects on remaining renal tissue.

Clinical & Laboratory Findings

Delays or abnormalities in voiding patterns may signal poor renal function or urinary tract obstruction. Abdominal masses, absence of abdominal musculature, and anomalies of the external genitalia or lower spine suggest urinary tract maldevelopment. Renal functional capacity will vary according to severity of the abnormality and its effect on renal parenchyma. Laboratory findings reveal the level of renal function, and diagnostic work-up proceeds as mentioned above.

URINARY TRACT INFECTIONS

Acute urinary tract infections (UTIs) in children may be limited to cystitis; in some cases one may also observe acute pyelonephritis. Newborns of both sexes and females of all ages seem at highest risk of developing UTIs.

These infections may be caused by a variety of organisms, particularly *Escherichia coli* and other organisms commonly found in the intestinal tract. Kidney involvement often results from ascending infection. Congenital abnormalities associated with obstruction and ureterovesical reflux may be important predisposing factors.

Clinical Findings

A. Symptoms & Signs: Symptoms may be mild or absent. Common symptoms of UTIs, however, include fever and chills, urinary urgency and frequency, incontinence, dysuria, and abdominal pain. Occasionally, the patient may complain of anorexia and nausea or vomiting. UTI symptoms may be more obvious with acute pyelonephritis. Signs of urinary tract infection include dull or sharp pain and tenderness in the kidney area or abdomen. Hypertension and evidence of chronic renal failure may be present. Jaundice may occur during early infancy.

B. Urinary Findings: Pyuria is characteristic, but it may be absent. Slight or moderate hematuria occasionally occurs. There may be slight proteinuria. Leukocytosis is usually in the range of 15,000–35,000/μL. A reliably performed mid-stream, clean-catch urine specimen is suitable for culture. If it cannot be obtained with confidence, a suprapubic bladder tap or catheterization may be performed (Chapter 28).

C. Urologic Studies: Intravenous urography and voiding cystourethrography are recommended by many investigators for all children after the initial infection. Others maintain that these procedures should be performed after the first urinary tract infection only for newborn infants, boys of all ages, and girls with symptoms suggestive of pyelonephritis; otherwise, they should be performed after second infections. Pediatric nephrology consultation is helpful; the need for a urologic evaluation depends on the nature and severity of any abnormalities noted.

Treatment

A. Specific Measures: Eradicate infection with appropriate chemotherapeutic or antibiotic therapy (Chapter 30) for 7 days. A prolonged course of urinary tract antisepsis (2–6 months or longer) may be indicated, especially for repeated infections. Repeated urinalyses at intervals of 1–2 months for at least a year is recommended.

B. General Measures: Force fluids during the acute stage. Discontinue bubble baths in girls, in that they expose the urethral orifice to irritation by soap. Avoid constipation. Look for evidence of pinworms in females; pinworm infestations are often associated with repeated episodes of cystitis. Sexual activity, including children's explorations of their own bodies as well as sexual abuse by adults, may also play a role.

C. Surgical Measures: There is no clear evidence that routine surgical correction (by either bladder neck revision, dilation, urethrotomy, or meatotomy) alters the course of recurrent UTIs to any significant degree. On the other hand, clearly obstructive lesions such as severe ureteric reflux, bladder dysfunction, or other abnormalities warrant urologic intervention.

D. Prophylactic Measures: After the infection is brought under control, a prophylactic regimen using trimethoprim sulfa is of value. If methenamine is used, the urine should be kept acid. Nalidixic acid is an effective substitute for methenamine. The dipstick nitrite test is a useful adjunct to home screening. Urine cultures should be repeated as clinically indicated or suggested by urinalysis.

HEMATURIA

The finding of abnormal numbers of red blood cells (RBCs) in the urine, especially if the patient is asymptomatic, suggests the possible presence of glomerular disease. Other nonrenal and largely symptomatic problems (eg, trauma, bleeding diathesis, infection, lithiasis, hypercalciuria, history of sickle cell disease, renal tumors, cystic diseases) should be excluded. A "decision tree" for clinical work-up is depicted in Figure 18–1. If the presentation is one of acute glomerulonephritis (GN), the differential diagnosis includes: postinfectious GN (most common), the GN of systemic lupus erythematosus (SLE), Henoch-Schönlein purpura (HSP), immunoglobulin A (IgA) nephropathy, and membranoproliferative GN (histologic types I, II, and III). Antiglomerular basement membrane (anti-GBM) disease (eg, **Goodpasture's syndrome**) and idiopathic rapidly progressive GN are rare occurrences in children. Hereditary forms of glomerulonephritis (eg, **Alport's syndrome**) do not present as acute GN.

Laboratory Findings (Figure 18–1)

Since preceding streptococcal disease is most frequently the cause of acute postinfectious forms of GN, a search for evidence of recent exposure may reveal elevations in antistreptolysin O titer; streptozyme; or both. Such data are of little relevance in nonacute GN or purely nephrotic syndrome presentations.

Other helpful laboratory data in evaluating GN include the serum complement. Complement may be found to be depressed in postinfectious GN, membranoproliferative GN, and SLE-GN. Normalization of serum complement is expected to be rapid (1–30 days) in typical poststreptococcal GN. Intermittent or persistent depression suggests chronic GN (eg, membranoproliferative GN varieties), or SLE, in which complement depression and antinative DNA elevations, hallmarks of disease activity, can be used to guide therapy.

Treatment

There is no specific therapy for typical poststreptococcal GN. Treatment is aimed at controlling hypertension and following the effect of disease on the glomerular filtration rate (GFR). Depending on the degree of associated renal failure (usually at > 50% reduction of GFR), measures can be taken to reduce protein, salt, and potassium intake; phosphate binders can be used to reduce dietary phosphate; and dialysis can be used as indicated in severe renal failure until (and if) renal recovery occurs. Such extreme measures would be instituted earlier in the more severe forms of GN, in which acute renal failure (ARF) progresses at a more rapid rate.

There are, of course, specific therapeutic measures that can be taken in the more severe or chronic forms of GN. Corticosteroids are useful in membranoproliferative GN and SLE. High dose, intravenous

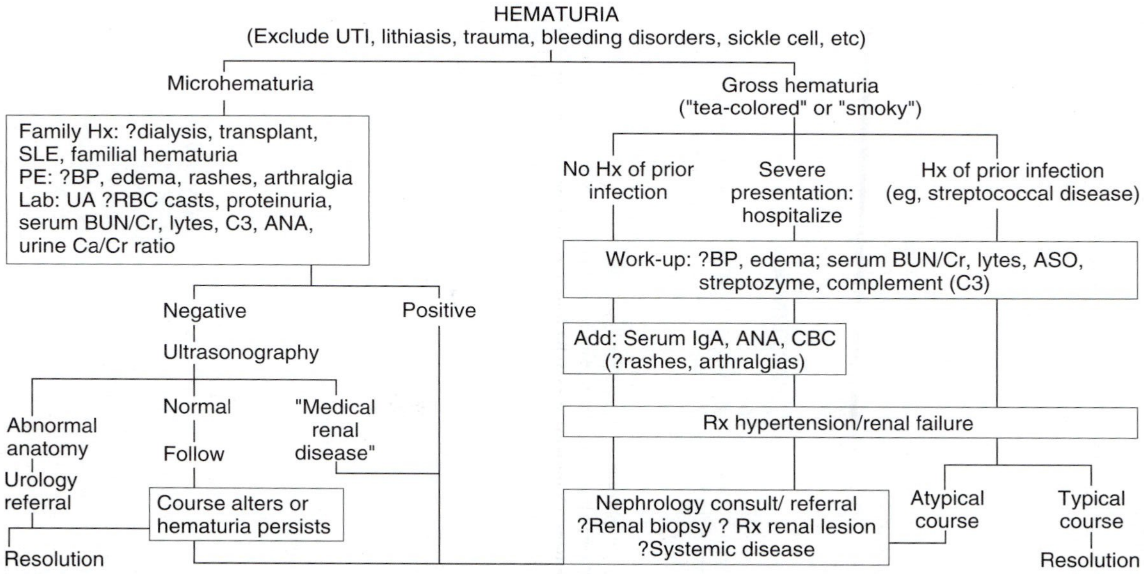

Figure 18–1. Work-up for hematuria. UTI = urinary tract infection; SLE = systemic lupus erythematosus; ANA = antinuclear antibody; ASO = antistreptolysin O titer.

corticosteroids, cytotoxic agents, anticoagulation, and plasmapheresis have been used alone and in combination with variable results in these and other GNs (eg, anti-GBM disease, rapidly progressive GN). Some cases of HSP-GN and IgA nephropathy, when severe (usually with excessive proteinuria or marked reduction in renal function) have also prompted attempts at treatment intervention, although there is no universally accepted therapy for these clinical entities. The possibility of ARF or CRF progressing toward **end-stage renal disease (ESRD)**, requiring chronic dialysis treatment or transplant, is a serious concern in all such cases.

PROTEINURIA

As in hematuria, the presence of abnormal amounts of protein in the urine suggests renal or urinary tract abnormalities. Excretion of more than 250 mg of protein in 24 hours should raise the suspicion of significant proteinuria. A urinary dipstick can estimate the amount of protein in a given specimen, but total 24-hour quantitation should be undertaken. The albumin:creatinine ratio in a spot urine specimen provides a practical screening tool. Although there is some variation with age, it is convenient to think of a ratio of less than 0.1 as normal, 0.1–1.0 as slight, 1.0–3 as moderate, and greater than 3 as heavy proteinuria; (ie, in the nephrotic range). Some children will excrete abnormal amounts of protein only while maintaining an upright posture (orthostatic or postural proteinuria). This phenomenon can be documented by measuring the protein content of urine produced during the day (upright) and comparing it with the urine formed overnight (recumbent). In such cases more than 80% of the protein lost in the urine will be demonstrated in the upright specimen. The total quantity should not exceed 1.5 g in 24 hours. The work-up is depicted in Figure 18–2.

Laboratory Findings (Figure 18–2)

Urinalysis is expected to be otherwise unrevealing in cases of isolated proteinuria (although the presence of significant quantities of RBCs suggests glomerular disease). However, as many as 20 RBCs per high-power field (no RBC casts) can be seen in the urine of children with **idiopathic nephrotic syndrome of childhood (INSC)**, in which no glomerular lesion is expected. If NS is present, lipid droplets ("Maltese crosses") can be seen in the urine with the use of Polaroid filters.

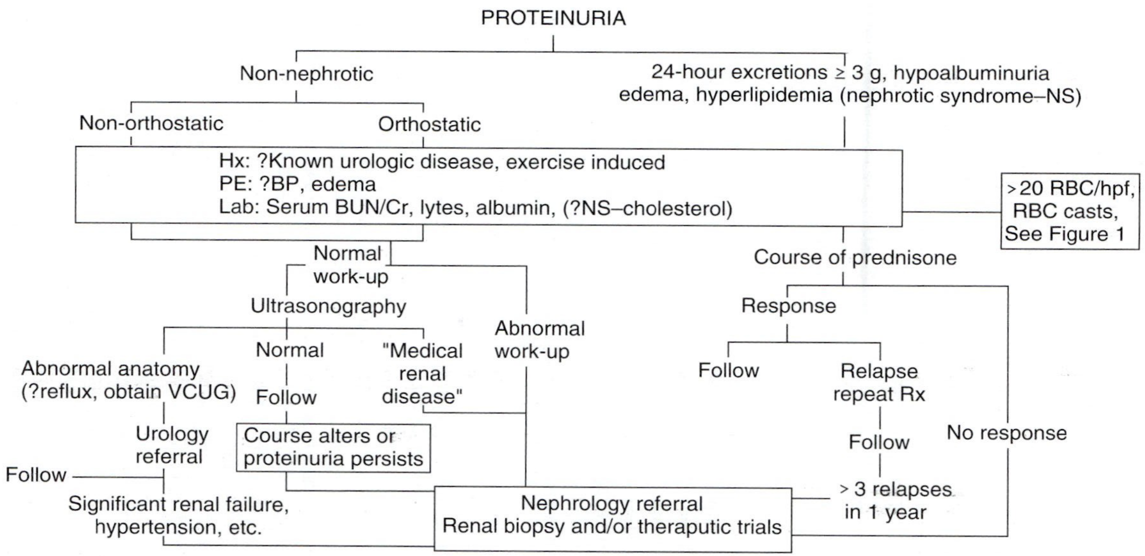

Figure 18–2. Work-up for proteinuria. BP = blood pressure; BUN/Cr = blood urea nitrogen/creatinine; Hx = history; RBC = red blood cell; hpf = high-power field; VCUG = voiding cystourethrogram.

Glomerular lesions can also produce reductions in GFR; thus, serum BUN and creatinine may be elevated. However, keep in mind that in NS, whether or not glomerular injury is responsible, circulatory volume contraction can lead to renal underperfusion ("prerenal" insufficiency) also resulting in elevations of BUN (primarily) and creatinine.

Furthermore, in NS, serum albumin will be decreased (as will measured total calcium) and serum lipids will be increased. Hyponatremia may be present. Although total body sodium is high owing to renal affinity for sodium in this state, the kidney is also avidly reabsorbing water (vasopressin) in defense of circulating volume. Factitious hyponatremia is also created by measurement of serum sodium in lipemic sera.

Treatment

The complications of NS may require immediate attention while the physician awaits the response, if any, to therapy directed at reducing or eliminating proteinuria. Restoration of life-threatening volume depletion should be accomplished with the administration of albumin. Care must be taken if hypertension is also paradoxically present. Administration of diuretics can lead to further circulating volume contraction, but can aid in mobilization of problematic edema and urine production, if administered during replenishment of serum albumin. Infections should be promptly treated. The tendency to increased intravascular thrombosis can also be a threat.

Therapy directed against specific renal lesions will first demand documentation by renal biopsy except in cases in which clinical presentations favor "minimal change" disease (INSC). If the clinical presentation strongly supports this diagnosis, corticosteroids are the treatment of choice. Approximately 85% of children with INSC respond to prednisone. A dose of 2 mg/kg of body weight (maximum 60 mg) is given as a single daily dose until the urine is protein-free (negative to trace by dipstick) for a maximum of 4 weeks. After remission has been maintained for 3–5 days, the same dose is administered every other day for 4 weeks and then is slowly tapered over another 4–6 weeks and discontinued. Of patients who do not respond to this treatment, a few will still reveal no significant histopathology on renal biopsy, but the rest will likely have either focal glomerular sclerosis (most prevalent), mesangial nephropathy, or membranous lesions. Even some initial responders may prove to be steroid-dependent or steroid-resistant with time.

When prolonged steroid exposure poses the risks associated with steroid toxicity, cytotoxic drugs such as chlorambucil and cyclophosphamide can induce longer, if not permanent, remission. They must be administered judiciously as they are not without significant side effects. Diagnostic confirmation of renal morphology with steroid resistance is again needed. Cyclosporine A is also now being used in steroid-dependent or resistant NS. Certainly the application of therapeutic trials with immunosuppressive agents requires the participation of a nephrologist.

Prognosis

INSC can be expected to resolve without sequelae. The aspects of the entity which cause the most serious concern are related to the complications of the nephrotic condition which have been previously addressed. Complications of NS are likewise of considerable concern in the other glomerular lesions capable of producing it. Of these, mesangial nephropathy has a guarded prognosis relative to progressive renal failure. On the other hand, as many as 15–20% of children with focal glomerular sclerosis develop CRF, although improved results with attempts at various treatment regimens have been reported. Corticosteroid therapy is reported to improve the prognosis of membranous nephropathy.

ACUTE RENAL FAILURE (ARF)

Renal insufficiency, or acute renal failure (ARF) may be divided for practical purposes into three sets of causes. ARF may result from (1) compromise in renal perfusion (prerenal); (2) obstruction to urinary flow (postrenal); or (3) renal parenchymal disease (renal). Examples of each of these groups are listed in Table 18–1.

Table 18–1. Causes of acute renal failure in children.

Prerenal:	Dehydration, congestive heart failure, renal arterial thrombosis, nephrotic syndrome.
Postrenal:	Urinary tract obstruction (eg, ureteropelvic and ureterovesical junctional stenoses and posterior urethral valves), urolithiasis, clot, foreign body.
Renal:	Glomerulonephritis, hemolytic uremic syndrome, systemic vasculitis, acute tubular necrosis (asphyxia, hypotension, ischemia), drugs, interstitial disease.

Clinical Findings

A. Symptoms & Signs: Depending on the degree of reduction in GFR and urine production, symptoms of ARF will range from those associated with fluid overload (eg, shortness of breath) to those of uremia (anorexia, nausea and vomiting, lethargy, etc).

Clinical signs vary from mild to severe edema, hypertension, CHF, pulmonary edema, anemia, and encephalopathy.

B. Laboratory Findings: Serum BUN and creatinine are increased in ARF and must be monitored. Serum analysis will reveal disturbances in electrolytes, most importantly potassium and bicarbonate (acidosis). Serum calcium generally decreases while phosphate increases. Anemia may be an associated finding.

Treatment

All correctable causes (usually prerenal or postrenal) should be addressed in therapy. Renal glomerular or interstitial diseases, once identified, are treated accordingly. Complications of ARF should be carefully monitored and controlled. Timely intervention with dialysis is important in reducing morbidity. Recovery is largely dependent on the nature of the renal lesion and its response to therapy.

Hemolytic uremic syndrome (HUS) is responsible for many cases of ARF in children. Management is directed at the consequences of renal failure (dialysis should be instituted in severe cases), although there have been reported improvements seen with plasma infusion or plasmapheresis in isolated cases.

Acute tubular necrosis (ATN), or vasomotor nephropathy, is the disturbance in renal function usually suspected in clinical settings in which renal ischemia or nephrotoxicity (hemoglobin, myoglobin, drugs, etc) is implicated and no other immediately identifiable cause is elucidated. Precipitating factors should be quickly identified and eliminated. Urinary indices (Table 18–2) are helpful in assessing oliguria when a distinction must be made between diminished renal perfusion and ATN. Rapid restoration of renal perfusion and induction of diuresis (furosemide, up to 5 mg/kg IV) may avert ATN or at least establish nonoliguric ATN, which by virtue of reasonable urinary output is considerably easier to manage. The treatment for this entity is otherwise largely supportive, including dialysis as indicated. Renal recovery is expected unless renal ischemia is severe enough to produce cortical necrosis, or unless metabolic toxins have caused irreversible injury. Recovery from oligoanuric ATN generally includes a nonoliguric or diuretic phase, and thus careful attention is

Table 18–2. Urinary findings in oliguria-prerenal vs ATN.

Test	Prerenal	ATN
Sodium (meq/L)	<20	>20
Fractional Na excretion[1]	<1	>1
Urine/serum creatinine	>40	<40
Osmolality (mosm/L)	>400	<400

ATN = acute tubular necrosis; Na = sodium.

[1] FENa $\frac{U/P\ Na}{U/P\ Cr} \times 100$.

directed toward preventing severe volume depletion during this period.

Overall management of prolonged ARF with oliguria includes careful attention to fluid balance. Measurement of input and output as well as daily weight is advised. Central venous pressure monitoring may be indicated. Urinary bladder catheterization may be helpful in assessing the clinical situation early in ARF.

Hypertension should be controlled with appropriate antihypertensive medications and normalization of intravascular volume. Intake of water, sodium, potassium, and phosphate should be restricted. Dietary phosphate binders (eg, calcium carbonate) should be administered as well. Reduced protein intake and adequate calories to decrease catabolism will minimize the rate of rise in serum BUN. Such restrictions can be greatly modified or eliminated with the use of dialysis.

Metabolic acidosis may be treated with bicarbonate, intravascular volume permitting. Likewise, correction of pH will aid in the intracellular movement of serum potassium; thus bicarbonate administration should be one of the first steps in treating life-threatening hyperkalemia.

Other temporizing measures to combat hyperkalemia include the infusion of dextrose and insulin. Calcium administration is cardioprotective in this situation; moreover, hypocalcemia itself may be a problem, and may be clinically manifest in tetany with correction of acidosis; alkalinization increases protein-bound calcium. Such temporizing treatment of life-threatening hyperkalemia must be followed by the removal of excess potassium with either Na-K^+ exchange resins (Kayexalate) or dialysis. Again, most, if not all, of the complexities of management and consequences of uremia may be easily handled with the institution of dialysis.

RENAL TUBULAR DEFECTS

Some renal disorders are expressed primarily, if not solely, by abnormal function of the renal tubule. The most commonly encountered abnormality of this type is isolated renal tubular acidosis (RTA). Although this is a "renal" acidosis, it is to be distinguished from the acidosis seen in CRF, which is primarily the result of decreasing renal mass. The **De Toni-Fanconi-Debré syndrome** describes a more extensively malfunctioning nephron that leads not only to renal bicarbonate losses but also to phosphaturia, glycosuria, and aminoaciduria. This abnormality is most frequently encountered in metabolic diseases (eg, cystinosis), renal developmental conditions (eg, juvenile nephronophthisis), and acquired conditions of either unknown etiology or renal toxin exposure. Some of the acquired conditions may resolve; but the usual course in untreated cystinosis, for example, is progressive CRF to end-stage disease.

The prognosis varies, however, depending on the type of isolated RTA. **Type 1 RTA** (distal tubule: hydrogen ion gradient defect/bicarbonate loss) is generally associated with more complex metabolic disorders and nephrocalcinosis. **Type 2 RTA** (proximal tubule: lowered threshold for bicarbonate reabsorption bicarbonate wasting) is most frequently encountered as a transient form in infancy, suggesting delayed renal development of normal proximal bicarbonate reclamation. If this type is an isolated tubular problem it is expected to resolve spontaneously by age 2–4 years. **Type 3 RTA** is a combination of types 1 and 2; **type 4 RTA** (deficiency in the renal physiologic effect of aldosterone) is seen primarily in adults with renal tubulo-interstitial disease.

1. RENAL TUBULAR ACIDOSIS

Clinical Findings

A. Symptoms & Signs: Failure to thrive is the most common presenting symptom of RTA. Polydypsia and polyuria may be noted. Anorexia, vomiting, constipation, and general listlessness may also be prominent features, depending on the severity of systemic acidosis and extent of urinary losses. Skeletal pain associated with rickets (usually in more severe forms of type 1 and **Fanconi's syndrome**) can also occur. There may be associated hypokalemia, producing symptomatic muscle weakness.

B. Laboratory Findings: Non-anion gap acidosis (hyperchloremic) is demonstrated with inappropriate urine pH (nonacidified).

Hypokalemia may be present, or may result from the administration of alkali therapy. Glycosuria, phosphaturia, and aminoaciduria are noted in Fanconi's syndrome. Normal urinalysis should help exclude tubulo-interstitial disease. Demonstration of normal renal architecture with ultrasonography is advisable.

Treatment

Administration of alkali is the mainstay of treating the metabolic abnormality. Sodium citrate solution (Bicitra, 1 meq each Na and HCO_3 per mL, or Polycitra, 1 meq each Na and K and 2 meq HCO_3 per mL) is commonly used. Type 1 RTA will require 1–3 meq/kg body wt/d in three divided doses. Type 2, owing to the magnitude of proximal tubular bicarbonate losses, will generally require 5–15 meq/kg/d. Fanconi's syndrome requires greater phosphate and potassium supplementation.

Course & Prognosis

Genetically transmitted or sporadic type 1 (with or without associated systemic disease) disorders resulting in nephrocalcinosis, or autoimmune diseases associated with type 1, are likely to be permanent defects. Drug-induced type 1 may resolve with discontinuation of the offending agent, as should RTA secondary to reflux nephropathy or obstruction if there is satisfactory recovery with correction of the urinary tract abnormality. Transient forms of type 2 are expected to resolve, as are those associated with drugs. Familial type 2 or that associated with Fanconi's syndrome are permanent defects.

2. NEPHROGENIC DIABETES INSIPIDUS

Another tubular disorder less frequently encountered is nephrogenic diabetes insipidus, an inherited (primarily X-linked) disorder, in which there is impaired or absent renal response to antidiuretic hormone.

Clinical Findings

A. Symptoms & Signs: Nephrogenic diabetes insipidus occurs early in infancy with irritability, failure to thrive, and poor feeding. Polyuria, polydypsia, dehydration, and rapid weight loss are remarkable, and fever may be noted.

B. Laboratory Findings: Urine output is increased and the osmolality is low, but urinalysis is otherwise unremarkable. Urinary concentration does not respond to vasopressin administration. Hypernatremia is marked (serum osmolality high) and metabolic acidosis develops with severe dehydration.

Treatment

Intake should be reduced in solutes (which obligate urinary water excretion) but appropriate in caloric content. Care must be taken to assure adequate protein intake for growth, and to avoid hyponatremia. Thiazide diuretics are useful as they decrease sodium reabsorption in the cortical diluting segment of the renal tubule, resulting in increased sodium loss, while the resulting volume contraction leads to enhanced proximal tubule absorption of fluid. A dose of 30 mg/kg of chlorthiazide per day in 3 divided doses is helpful in treating this abnormality.

Hematologic Disorders | 19

Taru Hays, MD

CHILDHOOD ANEMIAS

Anemia is a common blood disorder in children; its presentation differs from that in adults, however, in that it may be more pronounced. This is due to the fact that childhood growth patterns are associated with increased needs for blood-building substances. Furthermore, infections, which are so common in childhood, have a more profound effect on blood formation in early life than in maturity. A classification of childhood anemia based on mean corpuscular volume (MCV) is presented in Table 19–1.

PHYSIOLOGIC ANEMIA OF THE NEWBORN

A gradual drop in red cells and hemoglobin occurs normally during the first 10–12 weeks of life, owing to shortened red cell survival time, expanded intravascular volume, and improved oxygenation. The red blood cell count (RBC) is reduced to 3.5–4.5 million/μL. The hemoglobin level may reach a low of 10 g/dL in full-term infants and 7 g/dL in premature infants. This reduction is followed by a gradual increase in the number of red cells, with a correspondingly slower rise in hemoglobin level.

ANEMIA OF PREMATURITY

Although the RBC and hemoglobin levels of a premature infant are only slightly lower at birth than those of a full-term baby, the subsequent reduction that occurs is greater in premature infants. The magnitude of the drop in RBC and hemoglobin level is inversely proportionate to the infant's size. In very small infants (< 1 kg at birth), a reduction of hemoglobin to 7–8 g/dL and a reduction of red cells to

Table 19–1. Classification of anemias based on mean corpuscular volume (MCV).

Microcytic	Normocytic	Macrocytic
Iron deficiency	Hemolytic anemias	Folate deficiency
Thalassemia	Chronic disease anemia	Vitamin B_{12} deficiency
Lead poisoning	Acute blood loss	Congenital hypoplastic anemia (Diamond-Blackfan)
Pyridoxine deficiency	Anemia of infection/inflammation	Fanconi's anemia
Copper deficiency	Infiltrative process	Preleukemia
Hemoglobin E	Aplastic process	Other bone marrow failure states

2.5–3 million/μL may occur. The lowest levels are reached at about the end of the second month of life. More severe anemia occurs in premature infants than in full-term infants, because premature infants undergo a greater growth in body size and a correspondingly greater increase in blood volume. Furthermore, the total iron stores are smaller in the premature infant, since most of a newborn's iron is acquired during the last 3 months of gestation and erythropoietin production in response to anemia is lower than in the term infant.

Pallor is the principal manifestation of anemia of prematurity. The anemia generally is normochromic and normocytic early in the course of the disease and relatively hypochromic and microcytic late in the course.

The initial drop in hemoglobin level or RBC cannot be prevented by early treatment with iron. Treatment with iron along with erythropoietin injections may decrease the need for transfusions in these infants. After the second month of life, supplemental iron should be given to all preterm infants.

IRON DEFICIENCY ANEMIA

Because expansion of blood volume is part of the growth process, the need for iron in children is greater than that in adults. In the average full-term infant, the stores of iron available at birth are adequate for 3–6 months. In the premature infant, twin, or child born of a mother with severe iron deficiency, iron reserves will be expended earlier, placing these children at increased risk of developing iron deficiency anemia.

Iron deficiency anemia may result from inadequate storage, deficient intake, chronic blood loss, poor absorption and utilization of iron, or milk protein sensitivity. Iron deficiency anemia is uncommon in breast-fed infants.

Clinical Findings

A. Symptoms & Signs: Pallor may be the only early finding. Weakness, listlessness, and irritability appear later. Interference with growth may occur in cases of long-standing anemia, and delayed development (reversible) may occur in anemia of short duration. Congestive heart failure (CHF) occurs occasionally; generalized edema, rarely.

B. Laboratory Findings: In hypochromic microcytic anemia, hemoglobin and red cells are decreased. Anisocytosis and poikilocytosis may be marked. The reticulocyte count may be low, normal, or slightly elevated. The serum ferritin concentration is reduced; serum iron level is low, iron-binding capacity is increased; transferrin saturation is reduced; and the level of free erythrocyte protoporphyrin is elevated. Blood may be present in stool. Severe iron deficiency may be associated with copper deficiency, a decreased serum albumin level, thrombocytosis, and rarely thrombocytopenia.

Treatment

A. Medicinal Iron: Iron should be given as the ferrous salt. Elemental iron, 5–6 mg/kg/d in three divided doses, should be given before meals. Therapy should be continued for several months after the hemoglobin concentration returns to normal in order to build reserves of iron.

Intramuscular iron (iron dextran injection [Imferon]) should be used only when treatment with oral iron is not feasible.

B. Dietary Iron: Food contains insufficient iron for effective treatment of iron deficiency anemia. Absorption of iron from most foods is generally good; phytates (oatmeal, brown bread) may inhibit absorption. Good sources of iron include red meats; liver; dried fruits (eg, apricots, prunes, and raisins); and pinto beans. Adequate sources of iron include carrots, beans, spinach, peas, sweet potatoes, and peaches.

C. Transfusions: Transfusions of packed red cells are reserved for patients with severe symptomatic anemia in whom a rapid rise in hemoglobin concentration is desired. If evidence of heart failure is present, transfuse very slowly. Parenteral diuretics and partial exchange transfusion may be considered.

Course & Prognosis

Progressive anemia will result unless medicinal or dietary therapy is instituted and the underlying abnormality, if any, corrected. Improvement is then prompt, with a significant rise in the reticulocyte count appearing in 4–7 days and a rise in the hemoglobin concentration of approximately 0.1–0.2 g/dL/d. Simple iron deficiency anemia due to low iron intake should clear rapidly, but the presence of other deficiencies, congenital malformation, infection, or poor compliance with therapy may alter this favorable outcome.

Administration of iron, 2 mg/kg/d for full-term infants and 4 mg/kg/d for premature infants at high risk for developing iron deficiency during the first year, either in infant formulas or in a medicinal form, has been recommended to prevent iron deficiency.

ANEMIA OF CHRONIC INFECTION & INFLAMMATION

Chronic infection or inflammation is often accompanied by anemia. These conditions may inhibit iron exchange by blocking the release of catabolized iron from the red cells to the reticuloendothelial system. This form of anemia is often confused with iron deficiency anemia because the red cells may be slightly hypochromic (although they are often normal) and the reticulocyte count is low. In anemia of chronic infection, however, serum ferritin and serum iron levels are normal but total iron binding capacity is low, and the anemia does not respond to iron therapy. Anemia may be an important clue to an underlying inflammatory condition; it resolves when the primary disease process is controlled.

HYPOPLASTIC & APLASTIC ANEMIAS

Congenital hypoplastic anemia (Diamond-Blackfan anemia, a regenerative pure red blood cell anemia) is associated with decreased hemoglobin concentration and reticulocyte counts and increased MCV. Erythroid precursors are decreased or absent from the marrow. Patients usually respond well to corticosteroids; transfusions may be necessary. Skeletal malformations and short stature are common findings.

Children may develop transient erythroblastopenia, with a temporary halt in red cell production manifested by normochromic normocytic anemia, reticulocytopenia, and the absence of red cell precursors in otherwise normal bone marrow. Erythroblastopenia is usually preceded by viral or bacterial infection and can be differentiated from congenital hypoplastic anemia by the presence of normal MCV. Recovery is spontaneous without treatment, often within a few weeks.

Fanconi's anemia (hypoplastic anemia, often with pancytopenia) presenting after the age of 2 years may occur as an autosomal recessive disorder in association with abnormal pigmentation, skeletal anomalies (eg, absent, hypoplastic, or supernumerary thumb; hypoplastic or absent radius), retarded growth, hypogonadism, small head, renal anomalies (Chapter 18), microphthalmos, strabismus, and abnormalities of the genitourinary tract. Fanconi's anemia usually responds to testosterone. Bone-marrow transplantation may be considered.

Acquired aplastic anemia, characterized by pancytopenia and hypoplasia of the bone marrow, is rare in childhood. The peak incidence is 3–5 years of age. Acquired aplastic anemia may occur as a toxic reaction to drugs or chemicals (chloramphenicol, phenylbutazone, sulfonamides, solvents, insecticides), as a complication of infection, or in association with early manifestations of leukemia. Although aplastic anemia appears to be acquired in most cases, no causative agent can be identified in as many as 50% of patients (idiopathic aplastic anemia). Children with aplastic anemia present with pallor, fatigue, fever, and an increased tendency to bleed. The prognosis of aplastic anemia without treatment is extremely poor; fewer than 10% of patients recover fully within 5 years, and 50% of patients die from hemorrhage or infection within the first 6 months. Bone marrow transplant from a sibling with HLA-compatible marrow may increase survival to the 50–70% range and is presently the treatment of choice. When bone marrow transplant is not feasible, the use of immunosuppressive therapy with high-dose corticosteroids and antithymocyte globulin (ATG) may be of value in up to 50% of patients.

HEMOLYTIC ANEMIAS

GENERAL CONSIDERATIONS

Anemias associated with shortened red cell survival are known as **hemolytic anemias**. Symptoms and signs may include pallor, jaundice, and splenomegaly. Gallstones may develop after many episodes of hemolysis.

Anemia, reticulocytosis, hyperbilirubinemia, and haptoglobinemia are the hallmarks of hemolytic anemia. Urine and feces contain increased amounts of urobilinogen. With severe chronic hemolysis, erythroid hyperplasia of the bone marrow often results in widening of the marrow spaces.

Classification of Congenital Hemolytic Anemia

Congenital hemolytic anemias can be grouped into three categories:

A. Membrane Defects: Hereditary spherocytosis, hereditary elliptocytosis, hereditary stomatocytosis, pyropoikilocytosis.

B. Hemoglobinopathies: Sickle cell anemia, sickle syndromes (S-thalassemia, SC hemoglobinopathy), thalassemias, unstable hemoglobins.

C. Enzyme Defects: Glucose-6-phosphate dehydrogenase (G6PD) deficiency, pyruvate kinase deficiency, hexokinase deficiency.

Classification of Acquired Hemolytic Anemia

1. Autoimmune process.
2. Infections.
3. Toxins and drugs.
4. Thermal injury.
5. Disseminated intravascular coagulation (DIC).
6. Hemolytic-uremic syndrome.
7. Transfusion reactions.

AUTOIMMUNE HEMOLYTIC ANEMIA

In **autoimmune hemolytic anemia,** hemolysis occurs when IgG or IgM antibodies are directed against and cause damage to the red cell membranes. IgG-mediated disease is primarily an extravascular process, with hemolysis occurring in the spleen or other reticuloendothelial organs, while IgM-mediated disease is generally intravascular. The cause of anemia cannot be identified in about half of affected patients (idiopathic autoimmune hemolytic anemia). Anemia in other patients may be associated with immunoproliferative disorders (lupus erythematosus, Hodgkin's disease, and other malignant diseases); infection (especially Epstein-Barr virus, cytomegalovirus (CMV), other viral infections, and *Mycoplasma*); and chronic inflammatory conditions (ulcerative colitis).

The clinical presentation may be indolent (IgG-mediated) or fulminant (complement and IgM-mediated), with symptoms of anemia (pallor, malaise, and congestive heart failure); jaundice (common), with increased amounts of urobilinogen in the urine; and splenomegaly, which is more common with the IgG-mediated form of the disease. Laboratory findings include reticulocytosis and the presence of microspherocytes. Results of direct Coomb's tests are positive for IgG antibody in sera from patients with IgG-mediated anemia; negative for IgG antibody in sera from those with IgM-mediated anemia; and positive for complement fixation with IgM and, occasionally, with IgG.

If hemolysis is mild, treatment may not be necessary. Most patients respond to corticosteroids. Splenectomy is reserved for patients with severe hemolysis that is unresponsive to an adequate trial of corticosteroids. Other immunosuppressive therapy may be used in refractory cases. Packed red blood cell transfusion can be given for severe and profound hemolysis.

ISOIMMUNE HEMOLYTIC ANEMIA

Isoimmune hemolytic anemia is seen primarily in the newborn and is due to incompatibility with maternal Rh, ABO, or other antigens. It may also occur with transfusion reactions in patients of all ages. Findings are similar to those of autoimmune hemolytic anemia. After the source of exogenous antibody has been exhausted, the anemia is usually self-limited. Exchange transfusion may be required, especially in infants with Rh incompatibility.

HEREDITARY SPHEROCYTOSIS

Spherocytosis is an autosomal dominant disease caused by excessive destruction of abnormally shaped cells (spherocytes). The disease may be discovered during an aplastic crisis, when the reticulocyte count may be very low and the degree of anemia more profound than usual. Hyperhemolytic or aplastic crises may occur at periodic intervals.

Other members of the patient's family may have overt or subclinical disease with mild spherocytes and increased osmotic fragility of red blood cells. In a small percentage of cases, no family history can be obtained.

Findings include spherocytes, increased osmotic fragility, and reticulocytosis. Neonates may show early and exaggerated jaundice. Cholelithiasis may develop in the second or third decade.

Treatment is by splenectomy, ideally performed in patients after the age of 5 years. Until the time of splenectomy, folic acid, 1 mg/d, should be given.

Following removal of the spleen, the underlying red cell defects persist, but most patients will have a complete remission of hemolysis and anemia.

HEREDITARY ELLIPTOCYTOSIS

Hereditary elliptocytosis (ovalocytosis) is an autosomal dominant disease characterized by numerous elongated or oval cells. It is usually asymptomatic, but some patients may have mild to severe hemolysis. In the latter, splenectomy may be of value.

DEFICIENCIES OF RED CELL ENZYMES

Glucose-6-phosphate dehydrogenase (G6PD) deficiency is the most common red cell enzyme deficiency. It is inherited as an X-linked recessive trait and primarily affects males. G6PD occurs most frequently in people from Africa, the Mediterranean region, the Arabian peninsula, the Middle East, and Southeast Asia. Chronic anemia is variable, but acute episodes of severe hemolysis occur with exposure to certain drugs and foods, including primaquine, sulfonamides, aspirin, acetanilide, phenacetin, nitrofurans, synthetic vitamin K, compounds containing naphthalene, and fava beans. Approximately 15% of black males in the United States are affected by G6PD. The deficiency is less severe in blacks, and hemolysis usually occurs only with use of antimalarial agents, nitrofurans, and sulfonamides. Hemolysis is occasionally precipitated by infections. A screening test and assay are available, although the results may be normal if the reticulocyte count is high. With drug exposure, there is a rapid development of hemolytic anemia with hemoglobinuria and subsequent reticulocytosis. Blood transfusion may be required for treatment.

A number of other red cell enzyme deficiencies have been reported as causes of chronic hemolytic anemia. They are usually autosomal recessive disorders and are symptomatic only in the homozygous state. These disorders are very rare except for pyruvate kinase deficiency. Specific diagnosis is made by red cell enzyme assay. Patients with pyruvate kinase deficiency show a partial response to splenectomy. Transfusions may be needed for hemolytic or aplastic crises.

HEMOLYTIC UREMIC SYNDROME

Hemolytic uremic syndrome (HUS), occurring mainly in children between the ages of 6 months and 6 years, is characterized by (1) a sudden onset of Coomb's negative hemolytic anemia; (2) thrombocytopenia; and (3) nephropathy (with renal insufficiency, azotemia, and acute renal necrosis; see Chapter 18). Occasionally, there is central nervous system (CNS) involvement, with drowsiness and convulsions. Clinical manifestations of the syndrome are frequently preceded by diarrhea (commonly due to enterovirus infection or *Escherichia coli*) or, less often, by an upper respiratory tract infection, with an intervening symptom-free period of 1–10 days. Helmet-shaped and fragmented red cells are the hallmark of HUS. Fibrinogen and platelet deposition in the arterioles may play a very significant role in the pathophysiology of HUS.

Packed red blood cell transfusions and peritoneal dialysis are often required as supportive measures. Heparin, inhibitors of platelet function, or activators of fibrinolysin have been used in treatment, with very little effect on the course of the renal disease. Complete recovery from hematologic manifestations usually occurs, but permanent impairment of renal function is observed.

HEMOGLOBINOPATHIES

BETA-THALASSEMIA

Beta-thalassemia is a relatively common anemia that is due to an inherited defect in the synthesis of the beta chains of hemoglobin. It may occur in a severe homozygous form, characterized by pronounced changes in the blood and in various organ systems; or it may occur as a trait, with little or no anemia and no systemic changes. It is most common in Italians, Greeks, Mid-, South, and Southeast Asians. A mild beta-thalassemia gene (β^+) also occurs in blacks of African descent and may be seen in association with the sickle-cell gene.

Beta-Thalassemia Minor (Thalassemia Trait)

In the heterozygous form of β-thalassemia, evidence of mild anemia may be present. Blood smears show hypochromic microcytosis, target cells, anisocytosis, and poikilocytosis. The diagnosis may be confirmed by finding elevated levels of F or A_2 hemoglobin on hemoglobin electrophoresis. No treatment is required.

Beta-Thalassemia Major (Cooley's Anemia)

The homozygous form of β-thalassemia is a severe hypochromic microcytic anemia with hemolysis in the bone marrow that starts in the first year of life. Both parents will be carriers of the trait. Symptoms are secondary to the anemia and include pallor, characteristic facies due to widening of the skull bones, jaundice of varying degrees, and hepatosplenomegaly. Laboratory findings (Table 19–2) include hypochromic microcytic anemia, anisocytosis, poikilocytosis, basophilic stippling, and decreased fragility of the red cells, with the presence of target cells, nucleated erythrocytes, and an increased number of reticulocytes in the peripheral blood. Levels of hemoglobin F and A_2 are elevated; hemoglobin A is usually absent. Findings on x-ray include changes in the bones due to extreme marrow hyperplasia. These changes include widening of the medulla, thinning of the cortex, and coarsening of trabeculation ("hair-on-end" appearance).

Treatment

Transfusions are the only effective means of temporarily overcoming the anemia in severe cases, but they do not alter the underlying disease. Iron chelation with deferoxamine combined with hypertransfusion (maintaining hemoglobin at levels greater than 11 g/dL) are very beneficial. Chronic hypoxia and iron loading are the significant factors in the production of myocardial and hepatic damage.

Splenectomy may be necessary for a very large spleen or for evidence of hypersplenism. The risk of infection, however, in splenectomized children with thalassemia is great, and prophylactic penicillin and pneumococcal vaccine should be given. Bone marrow transplantation is the only curative treatment for thalassemia major.

ALPHA-THALASSEMIA

Alpha chains of the hemoglobin molecule are genetically determined by four genes; as a result, gene deletions can result in four degrees of α-thalassemia.

Type 1 α-thalassemia occurs primarily in Southeast Asians. The heterozygote, or 'carrier,' with two gene deletions (–/αα) also shows microcytosis, hypochromia, and mild anemia, while the homozygous state (–/–) results in hydrops fetalis and stillbirth.

Type 2 α-thalassemia is always mild. Its incidence is high in Africa, Arabia, the Middle East, and Southeast Asia. The heterozy-

Table 19–2. Summary of findings in abnormal hemoglobin diseases and thalassemia.

	Hemoglobin Type	Anemia	Splenomegaly	Pain Crises	Increased Blood Destruction	Target Cells	Sickling (Solubility) Test	Microcytosis	Hypochromia
Normal adult and child	AA (A_2* F*)	0	0	0	No	0	0	0	0
Normal newborn	AF†	0	0	0	No	0	0	0	0
Iron deficiency anemia	AA (A_2* F*)	+ to ++++	±	0	No	±	0	+ to ++++	+ to ++++
β^0-Thalassemia major	F† A_2†	++++	++++	0	Yes	++	0	++++	++++
β^0-Thalassemia minor	A (S_2† F†)	±	0 to +	0	±	+	0	++	++
β^+-Thalassemia-hemoglobin C disease	CA (F*)	+	0	0	Yes	+++	0	+	+
β^0-Thalassemia-hemoglobin E disease	EF†	+++	+++	0	Yes	++	0	+++	+++
Sickle cell trait	AS (A_2* F*)	0	0	0	No	+	+	0	0
Sickle cell anemia	SS (A_2* F†)	+++	±	+++	Yes	++	+	0	0 to +
Sickle-β^+-thalassemia	SA (A_2† F†)	+	±	+	Yes	++	+	++	++
Sickle-β^0-thalassemia	S (A_2† F†)	+++	+++	+++	Yes	++	+	++	++
Sickle-hemoglobin C disease	SC (F†)	+	++	++	Yes	+++	+	0	0
Sickle-hemoglobin D disease	SD (A_2* F†)	++	++	++	Yes	+	+	+	+

Hemoglobin C trait	AC (F*)	0	0	0	No	+++	0	0	0
Homozygous hemoglobin C disease	CC (F*)	+	0 to ++	0	Yes	++++	0	0	0
Hemoglobin D trait	AD (A_2* F*)	0	0	0	No	0	0	0	0
Hemoglobin E trait	AE (F*)	0	0	0	No	±	0	0	0
Homozygous hemoglobin E disease	EE (F†)	+	±	0	Yes	+++	0	++	0
α-Thalassemia carrier	A (A_2* F*)‡	±	0	0	0	±	0	++	+
α-Thalassemia-hemoglobin H disease	AH (A_2* F*)‡	++	++	0	++	+++	0	+++	+++
α-Thalassemia-fetal hydrops	Bart's	++++	++++	0	++	+++	0	++++	++++

* A_2 is usually < 4% and F < 2% of the total hemoglobin.
† Elevated levels.
‡ Hemoglobin Bart's is also present at birth.

gote with one gene deletion (– α/αα) is called the "silent carrier" and is clinically and hematologically normal, while the homozygote with two deletions (–α/–α) is called the "carrier" and has microcytosis, hypochromia, and mild or borderline anemia.

In the double heterozygous state for type 1 and type 2 α-thalassemia, genes are deleted (–/–α); this is known as hemoglobin H disease and occurs in Southeast Asians. It is characterized by splenomegaly and a moderate hemolytic anemia with microcytosis, hypochromia, and elevated reticulocyte count.

Diagnosis is made in the mild forms by ruling out iron deficiency (by documenting a normal serum iron or ferritin level) and β-thalassemia minor. A_2 and F hemoglobin levels are normal in α-thalassemia. Hemoglobin Bart's (γ4-globins) is present in varying degrees in all forms in the newborn infant, while hemoglobin H (β4-globins) is present in the older child with the 3-gene deletion disease.

No treatment is necessary in the mild forms. Hemoglobin H disease may require transfusions, but most patients maintain hemoglobin levels of 9–10 g/dL.

SICKLE CELL ANEMIA

Sickle cell anemia is an inherited abnormality of hemoglobin (hemoglobin S). It has a high incidence in blacks but is also common in the Arabian peninsula, Sicily, and certain parts of Greece, Turkey, and India. In hemoglobin S, the amino acid valine replaces glutamic acid at the sixth position in the beta chain. Although the sickle trait occurs in about 8% of the black population in the United States, the disease with anemia occurs in less than 1% of blacks.

Clinical Findings

A. Symptoms & Signs: Onset of clinical manifestations may be at any time during the first decade of life. Findings include "pain crises" in the long bones, dactylitis, abdominal pain, pallor, jaundice, splenomegaly (in the very young), hepatomegaly, cardiomegaly, and hemic heart murmurs. Functional asplenia occurs early in childhood due to "autosplenectomy" as a result of repeated infarctions. Patients with sickle cell anemia have an increased resistance to malarial infection; an increased susceptibility to bacterial sepsis, osteomyelitis, pneumonia, and meningitis [in particular with encapsulated organisms (eg, pneumococcus)]; and an increased risk of anesthetic complications. Enuresis and nocturia may be present. Strokes are commonly seen in young teens. During a pain crisis, the disease may mimic acute surgical abdomen or osteomyelitis. Aplastic crises may occur, with diminished red cell production superimposed on rapid destruction. In young infants, acute hemolysis and hypovolemia can be seen with splenic sequestration.

B. Laboratory Findings: Sickle-forms are seen in peripheral blood smear. Other findings include normochromic anemia, reticulocytosis, nucleated red blood cells and leukocytosis. Hyperbilirubinemia, increased excretion of urobilinogen, increased lactate dehydrogenase levels, and an abnormal hemoglobin electrophoretic pattern, with 75–100% hemoglobin S and increased amounts of fetal hemoglobin occur. There is excretion of excessive quantities of urine of low specific gravity. Severe hyponatremia may occur during a crisis. Zinc deficiency has been described and may contribute to short stature and delayed onset of puberty. Folate deficiency is also very common.

Heterozygotes (carriers of the sickle trait) may be identified by use of a screening test (Sickledex Test; sodium metabisulfite test) and hemoglobin electrophoresis. Characteristically, 25–45% hemoglobin S is found. Heterozygotes are not anemic and (except for conditions with extreme hypoxia) are asymptomatic.

Treatment

Parenteral fluid therapy, analgesics, oxygen, and transfusion for severe anemia and crises are the only consistently effective methods of treatment.

Adequate hydration of the patient at the onset of a crisis sometimes obviates the need for transfusions. Because infection exacerbates sickling of the patient's red blood cells, all infections should be treated promptly and vigorously. Sepsis and meningitis should be suspected in the febrile infant.

Folic acid, 1 mg/d, should be given. Routine administration of prophylactic penicillin for children under 5 years of age has been advocated, and pneumococcal vaccine should be given at 2 years of age.

Course & Prognosis

The course is determined by the severity of the sickling tendency and resulting hemolysis, the frequency and duration of crises, and the age of the patient. Interference with growth, nutrition, and general activity is common, although many patients lead active lives with persistent hemoglobin levels of 7–9 g/dL.

Repeated transfusions in conjunction with iron chelation using deferoxamine, designed to maintain hemoglobin levels above 11 g/dL and thus decrease bone marrow production of hemoglobin S, is recommended for patients with strokes and heart failure.

SICKLE-HEMOGLOBIN C DISEASE

Sickle-hemoglobin C disease is caused by the inheritance of hemoglobin S from one parent and hemoglobin C from the other. It occurs almost exclusively in the black population.

Clinical manifestations are similar to those of sickle cell anemia but tend to be less severe. Splenomegaly may be present and acute enlargement may occur with splenic sequestration crises. Proliferative retinopathy is common after the age of 15 years. Diagnosis is suspected by the presence of mild to moderate anemia, elevated reticulocyte counts, many target cells on blood smear, and positive results in the sickling (solubility) test. It is confirmed by hemoglobin electrophoresis.

Treatment is similar to that for sickle cell anemia and is primarily symptomatic. Patients should receive annual retinal examinations and be treated with laser therapy if retinopathy is detected.

BLEEDING DISEASES IN CHILDHOOD

GENERAL CONSIDERATIONS

Family History

A family history of easy bruising and excessive bleeding is valuable in the following disorders: (1) hemophilia (X-linked), (2) von Willebrand's disease (autosomal dominant), (3) congenital thrombocytopenia or platelet dysfunction syndromes, (4) hereditary hemorrhagic telangiectasia, and (5) deficiencies of factors II, V, VII, X, or XI (autosomal).

Physical Examination

Bleeding disorders should be considered in patients with abrupt changes in the pattern or severity of bruising and bleeding, unexplained bleeding from a circumcision, or excessive bleeding at the site of surgery.

Bruises on the extremities are found in many normal children following trauma and usually have no clinical significance. In infants and young children, petechiae can occur in the head and neck areas in association with crying, vomiting, or coughing without an underlying bleeding disorder. Mucocutaneous bleeding usually signifies an abnormality in the number or function of the platelets or a defect of the blood vessels. Hemarthrosis is uncommon except in patients with hemophilia.

Laboratory Examination

Recommended basic screening tests include platelet count, bleeding time, partial thromboplastin time (PTT), prothrombin time (PT), thrombin time, and fibrinogen level.

HEMOPHILIA

Hemophilia is an X-linked bleeding disorder transmitted by females to their male offspring. Hemophilia A (factor VIII deficiency, or classic hemophilia) accounts for 75% of cases. It occurs with an incidence of 1 per 10,000 population. Affected family members generally have equally severe disease. Hemophilia B (factor IX deficiency, or Christmas disease) is much less common. Hemophilia is divided into mild, moderate, and severe forms.

Clinical Findings

A. Symptoms & Signs: Severely affected patients are usually identified at circumcision or in the first year of life. They show signs of increased bruising and hemarthrosis (most commonly of the knees, ankles, or hips) as they begin to walk. In older patients, bleeding may occur in the large muscle groups, the genitourinary tract, or the skin. Mildly affected patients rarely have bleeding into the joints and may present with hemophilia only at the time of a surgical procedure.

B. Laboratory Findings: Consult Table 19–3. The PTT should be determined and other screening tests performed in any suspected case of hemophilia. If the PTT is prolonged, a specific-factor assay should be carried out to confirm the diagnosis.

Treatment

A. Specific Measures: The specific treatment of hemophilia consists of replacing missing clotting factors. In hemophilia A, only

Table 19–3. Differentiation by laboratory findings of coagulation defects.

Disease	Bleeding Time	Platelet Count	One-Stage Prothrombin Time	Partial Thromboplastin Time	Thrombin Time
Afibrinogenemia	N or ↑	N	↑	↑	↑
Factor II deficiency disease	V[2]	N	↑	N or ↑	N
Factor V deficiency disease	N	N	↑	↑	N
Factor VII deficiency disease	N	N	↑	N	N
Factor VIII deficiency disease	N	N	N	↑	N
Factor IX deficiency disease	N	N	N	↑	N
Factor X deficiency disease	N	N	↑	↑	N
Factor XI deficiency disease	N	N	N	↑	N
Factor XIII deficiency disease	N	N	N	N[1]	N
Thrombasthenia (Glanzmann's syndrome)	↑	N	N	N	N
Thrombocytopenia	↑	↓	N	N	N
Von Willebrand's disease	↑	N	N	↑	N

[1] Diagnosis should be suspected in a congenital bleeding state when results of all screening tests are normal. Diagnosis is confirmed by showing instability of fibrin clot in urea.
[2] Variable.

fresh frozen plasma, factor VIII concentrates, or cryoprecipitates should be used. In younger children, this can be achieved with cryoprecipitates. Older children with hemophilia A may be given factor VIII concentrates (heat-treated or recombinant). In hemophilia B, use of fresh frozen plasma or factor IX concentrate (heat-treated or recombinant) is effective. Dosage is determined by the severity of the bleeding to be treated. Adjuncts to transfusion therapy include (1) aminocaproic acid (Amicar), 100 mg/kg every 6 hours, for oral mucosal bleeding; and (2) desmopressin acetate (DDAVP, Stimate), 0.3 μg/kg given intravenously in 20 mL of saline over a 20-minute period, in mild cases of hemophilia A.

B. Special Problems:

1. Head Injuries: Head injuries can be life-threatening in severe hemophiliacs. Raise the factor level to 80–100% as soon as possible. Patients with head injuries often require repeated factor replacement initially and, if intracranial hemorrhage is documented, for several weeks.

2. Hemarthroses: In patients with bleeding into the joints or muscles, raise the factor levels to 50% every day until the pain lessens. Bed rest and a short period of immobilization (usually for no longer than 24 hours) are indicated. This is followed by a slow increase in the level of physical therapy, with an active range of motion to regain full use of the joint. Acetaminophen is usually sufficient for analgesia if the patient receives transfusion early. Aspirin should *not* be given. Subsequent therapy includes exercises (passive and then active) and prevention of ankylosis in the unphysiologic position. Repeated episodes of joint effusion may be treated by corticosteroids.

3. Sutures: If suturing is necessary, raise the factor levels to 20–40% every other day until the sutures are removed, including the day of removal.

4. Hematuria: Patients with hematuria may be treated with a short course of corticosteroids.

5. Open Wounds: In patients with bleeding from open wounds (skin, tooth socket), follow the measures outlined above, as indicated. Do *not* cauterize the wounds. Use sutures as necessary. Use pressure bandage and application of cold to accessible areas.

Prognosis

The prognosis for hemophiliacs has been much improved since the institution of home care programs of prophylactic therapy. Many of the problems of chronic joint disease have been avoided. Major problems with repeated administration of blood products include the increased risk of hepatitis, HIV infection, and the development of inhibitors (IgG antibody) to factor VIII and factor IX in 1–3% of patients. With home transfusion programs, most patients are successful in leading independent and nearly normal lifestyles.

VON WILLEBRAND'S DISEASE

Von Willebrand's disease is a mild to severe familial bleeding disorder characterized by abnormalities of the factor VIII molecule. In severe cases of classic von Willebrand's disease, the factor VIII procoagulant activity (VIIIc), the portion of the molecule that corrects the bleeding time defect and supports ristocetin-induced aggregation of platelets (VWF), and the factor VIII measured by heterologous antibodies (VWF antigen) are reduced. Variants of the disorder occur in which combinations of these portions of the factor VIII molecule are defective.

Patients with von Willebrand's disease show skin and mucous membrane bleeding (epistaxis, menorrhagia). The disorder is usually inherited as an autosomal dominant trait. Bleeding time is usually prolonged, as is the PTT, although measurements of VIIIc, VWF antigen, and VWF must be made to establish the diagnosis.

Treatment consists of infusions of fresh frozen plasma, 10–15 mL/kg; cryoprecipitate, one pack per 5 kg; or desmopressin acetate (DDAVP, Stimate), 0.3 μg/kg in 20 mL of saline, given intravenously over a 20-minute period.

Von Willebrand's disease is a lifelong condition. The prognosis is generally good with fairly minor bleeding complications.

DISSEMINATED INTRAVASCULAR COAGULATION (DIC)

Disseminated intravascular coagulation (DIC) is characterized by intravascular consumption of plasma clotting factors (factors I, II, V, and VIII) and platelets; fibrinolysis, with production of fibrin split products; widespread deposition of fibrin thrombi that produce tissue ischemia and necrosis in various organs (principally the lungs, kidneys, gastrointestinal tract, adrenals, brain, liver, pancreas, and skin); generalized hemorrhagic diathesis; microangiopathic hemolytic anemia, with fragmented, burred, and helmet-shaped erythrocytes; and shock and death. The disorder has been found in association with infections, surgical procedures, burns, neonatal conditions (especially sepsis and respiratory distress syndrome), neoplastic diseases, severe hypoxia and acidosis, other metabolic disorders, and a variety of miscellaneous causes (eg, hemangioma, transfusion reactions, drugs, HUS). Clinical manifestations of DIC depend on the systems involved. Laboratory findings include prolonged PT and PTT, increased fibrin split products, decreased levels of fibrinogen, and decreased platelet counts.

Therapy consists of treating the underlying cause (sepsis, acidosis, hypoxia) and replacing clotting factors with fresh frozen plasma, 10 mL/kg, or platelet transfusions. Indications for use of heparin include severe meningococcemia, associated large vessel thrombosis, purpura fulminans, and promyelocytic or monocytic leukemia.

THERAPEUTIC BLOOD FRACTION PRODUCTS

When therapeutic blood fractions are given, there is a risk of transmitting the hepatitis virus; this risk is greater when pooled blood fraction products are given than when single donor products are used. There appears to be an increased risk of contracting human immunodeficiency virus (HIV) with the use of factor VIII concentrates or other blood components; however, this risk is decreased by use of heat-treated concentrates and screening of donors.

Cryoprecipitates

Cryoprecipitates are a blood bank product made from fresh frozen plasma. One pack of cryoprecipitate contains 100 units.*

A dosage of one pack per 5 kg usually gives a factor VIII level of 40%. The usual level desired is 40%; however, 20% is the minimal hemostatic level.

Factor VIII Concentrate (Monoclonal; Heat-treated or Recombinant)

A. Indications: For therapy of factor VIII deficiency (hemophilia A).

B. Dosage & Administration: Reconstitute lyophilized material (stored at 4 °C) and inject by intravenous push. Dose is calculated as follows:

Units* of factor VIII
= Desired level in percent × 0.5 × Weight (kg)

Factor IX Concentrate (Monoclonal; Heat-treated or Recombinant)

A. Indications: For therapy of congenital factor IX deficiency (hemophilia B, or Christmas disease).

B. Dosage & Administration: Dosage is calculated as follows:

Units* of factor IX = Desired level in percent × Weight (kg)

PURPURAS

Purpura is defined as a disorder characterized by large, multiple, raised hematomas due to a reduced number of platelets, abnormal function of platelets, or to a defect in or abnormality of the vascular system.

Purpuras are classified by the clinical picture, the quantity and quality of platelets.

Classification of Common Purpuras

A. Quantitative defect of platelets (thrombocytopenia):

1. Idiopathic thrombocytopenic purpura.
2. Disseminated intravascular coagulation.
3. Hemolytic uremic syndrome.
4. Familial thrombocytopenia.

B. Qualitative defect of platelets (platelet dysfunction):

1. Congenital.
2. Acquired: secondary to drugs, infection, inflammation, or uremia.

C. Non-thrombocytopenic purpura:

1. Henoch-Schönlein purpura.
2. Vasculitis.
3. Vitamin C deficiency (scurvy).
4. Drugs and toxins.
5. Collagen disorders (Ehlers-Danlos syndrome, Marfan's syndrome).
6. Psychogenic purpura.

* A unit of clotting factor is the amount contained in the equivalent of 1 mL of fresh frozen plasma with 100% clotting activity.

IDIOPATHIC THROMBOCYTOPENIC PURPURA (ITP)

Idiopathic thrombocytopenic purpura (ITP) of childhood is a common bleeding disorder associated with antiplatelet antibodies. It usually occurs in patients between 2 and 10 years of age and commonly follows an infection by 2–3 weeks.

Clinical Findings

A. Symptoms & Signs: Bleeding into the skin or from the nose, gums, and urinary tract is the most common symptom of ITP. Bleeding into joints or from the bowel is uncommon. CNS bleeding occurs rarely but may be fatal. Petechiae are usually present. Splenomegaly is rare.

B. Laboratory Findings: The platelet count is decreased, and large platelets are seen. RBCs and WBCs are normal unless severe hemorrhage has occurred. Megakaryocytes in the bone marrow are normal or increased in number. Antiplatelet antibodies may be demonstrated. Coagulation studies are usually normal.

Treatment

A. Specific Measures: There is no specific treatment for ITP. Corticosteroids are useful in 60–70% of children. Indications include patients with severe thrombocytopenia with bleeding and patients at increased risk for CNS bleeding. More recently, intravenous gamma globulin has been useful in acute bleeding episodes and also in steroid-refractory thrombocytopenia. Rhogam (Anti-D immune globulin) has been useful in some patients.

B. General Measures: Pressure and application of cold packs help in arresting bleeding. Eradicate infection, if present. All medications should be given either orally or intravenously; avoid intramuscular injection. Other measures include prevention of trauma, institution or maintenance of regular diet, and avoidance of aspirin. Careful monitoring for 6–8 weeks is appropriate for many cases.

C. Surgical Measures: Splenectomy is indicated after conservative therapy has been carried out for 12 months without improvement; if the disease process is very severe, with heavy bleeding; and if the patient develops a sudden intracranial hemorrhage. Splenectomy is also indicated in adolescent girls with severe menorrhagia. The procedure should be avoided, if possible, in children under 5 years of age.

Course & Prognosis

Symptoms may continue to be evident for 2 weeks to several months, but significant improvement usually occurs within 4–6 weeks. Eighty-five percent of children with ITP will have a spontaneous and complete recovery within 6 months even without therapy, but spontaneous recovery may occur after a period of as long as 3–5 years. A few will need splenectomy.

Adolescents tend to have a more chronic course, often associated with the presence of other antibodies. ITP during adolescence may be associated with subsequent development of systemic lupus erythematosus (SLE).

ANAPHYLACTOID PURPURA

Anaphylactoid purpura (Henoch-Schönlein purpura) is a disease of unknown cause. Many patients have a history of allergic manifestations. Some cases of anaphylactoid purpura follow infections; a causal relationship with group A streptococcal infections has been suspected. The disease tends to recur, and it may persist for years.

Clinical Findings

A. Symptoms & Signs: Abdominal and joint pains are present in most children, but the pain may occur only in the abdomen (Henoch type) or only at the joints (Schönlein type). The pain may precede the development of skin lesions. Either small or large joints may be involved. The joints are painful and swollen. Ecchymoses, petechiae, or bullous hematomas may be present. The initial lesions may resemble urticaria, but these soon become hemorrhagic. They often appear first around the elbows and ankles and over the buttocks. Gastrointestinal hemorrhage is common in children. Nephritis may occur early or after the acute phase in over one-third of cases. Intussusception may develop. Associated group A β-hemolytic streptococcal infections are frequent.

B. Laboratory Findings: Platelet count is normal; thrombocytopenia is seen rarely. Eosinophilia may be present in some cases. Serum IgA levels may be elevated.

Treatment

In many cases, treatment is either unnecessary or ineffective.

A. Specific Measures: Therapy includes eradication of infection, using appropriate antibiotics, and elimination of allergens (if known). Antihistamines may be given if allergy is suspected. Anti-inflammatory agents are useful.

B. General Measures: Corticosteroids may relieve joint and abdominal symptoms; they do not appear to benefit patients with renal complications.

Course & Prognosis

The disease may vary in degree from mild to quite severe. Complete recovery eventually occurs in most cases, but recurrences are not infrequent. Nephritis occasionally persists and may become chronic.

HYPERCOAGULABILITY

Hypercoagulability describes an increased tendency toward thrombosis in patients with certain underlying conditions. Patients at risk include those with a deficiency of antithrombin III, protein C, protein S, or APC cofactor/Factor V mutations; newborns and older children with central venous catheters or prosthetic heart valves; postsurgical patients who require prolonged periods of bed rest and thus are susceptible to venous stasis; and patients with vasculitis (eg, SLE, nephritis, HUS) in which damaged endothelium provides a nidus for clot formation and occasionally for progression to a more generalized thrombotic process. Patients with antiphospholipid antibodies (eg, lupus anticoagulant or anticardiolipin antibodies) are at high risk for thrombosis.

The patient may present with pain and swelling of the involved extremity or with symptoms of a stroke. Homozygous protein C deficiency can present as purpura fulminans in neonates. The diagnosis of thrombosis is made by physical examination. Supporting laboratory findings may include decreased levels of fibrinogen, antithrombin III, protein S, or protein C; decreased platelet counts; or elevated levels of fibrin split products, monomer and dimer. However, laboratory findings may be normal even in the face of significant thrombosis. Doppler flow and venogram/arteriogram studies are more specific.

Treatment involves interruption of the triggering process. Heparinization should be instituted at once, with the goal of increasing the PTT to 1½ times that of normal. Plasma heparin level is better correlated with therapeutic heparinization, so if available heparin levels should be followed. Give a loading dose of heparin, 100 units/kg, followed by a continuous intravenous infusion of 15–20 units/kg/h. Newborn infants may require an increased dosage. Prolonged anticoagulation for 3–6 months with warfarin (Coumadin) may be indicated once the initial thrombosis is controlled. Antiplatelet agents (aspirin, sulfinpyrazone, dipyridamole) may be indicated in cases in which a prosthetic heart valve or arterial malformation is the inciting factor for thrombosis. The use of fibrinolytic agents (streptokinase, urokinase) in children is reserved for extensive and life-threatening thrombus. Local urokinase therapy is very useful in catheter-induced thrombosis.

ASPLENIA

Absence of the spleen, whether the absence is congenital, post-surgical, or functional (secondary to an underlying disease such as sickle cell anemia), places the child at significant risk for infection with encapsulated bacteria. The overall incidence of infection is 5–10%, with the mortality rate 30–50%. Those at greatest risk are children under 5 years of age and children with recent splenectomy (ie, for the first 2 years following the procedure). The classic hematologic finding is the presence of Howell-Jolly bodies on the peripheral blood smear.

Life-threatening infections are rare in older children when the spleen is removed for trauma, ITP, portal vein thrombosis, local tumors, or hereditary spherocytosis. The risk is significant in those with histiocytosis, inborn errors of metabolism, Hodgkin's disease, thalassemia, and **Wiskott-Aldrich syndrome**.

The use of prophylactic antibiotics remains controversial. Some physicians use continuous penicillin prophylaxis in the younger child, while others treat at the first sign of fever. Polyvalent pneumococcal vaccine, which protects against infection with many of the common pneumococci, should be given to all children prior to splenectomy and repeated in early childhood if given to infants under 2 years of age. Prompt therapy with antibiotics in any child with fever has been recommended.

SPLENOMEGALY

Splenomegaly is generally an indicator of systemic disease. The tip of the spleen may normally be felt in 30% of newborn infants and 5% of young children. Splenomegaly may be associated with other signs of systemic disease, particularly adenopathy, hepatomegaly, petechiae, ecchymoses, and jaundice. Less common causes of splenomegaly include acute viral infections (particularly infectious mononucleosis and cytomegalovirus); hematologic disorders (eg, congenital or acquired hemolytic anemias, red cell membrane defects, disorders of hemoglobin synthesis); metabolic diseases (eg, Gaucher's disease, Niemann-Pick disease); vascular abnormalities (eg, portal hypertension); and, rarely, cysts (eg, splenic cysts). When leukemia or other malignant neoplastic disease presents with splenomegaly, it is usually accompanied by adenopathy, pallor, and other signs of systemic illness.

Evaluation of patients with splenomegaly should include an assessment of the complete blood count (CBC), platelet count, peripheral blood smear, and reticulocyte count. Other studies may include tests for viral infection, liver-spleen scan, work-up for hemolytic anemias, and bone marrow examination for evaluation of storage diseases.

NEUTROPENIA

Neutropenia, which is defined as a total granulocyte count below 1000 μL, may result from poor release of granulocytes from the bone marrow, decreased survival of granulocytes in the circulation, or abnormalities of granulocyte production and development. Congenital forms of neutropenia include (1) cyclic neutropenia, occurring at 2- to 4-week intervals in association with mucous membrane ulcers, cervical lymphadenopathy, and stomatitis; (2) benign chronic neutropenia, which may be genetically transmitted (as a dominant or recessive trait), with manifestations of mild infection; (3) severe congenital neutropenia, transmitted as a recessive trait, with life-threatening infection in early infancy; (4) **Schwachman-Diamond syndrome**, with metaphyseal chondrodysplasia, dwarfism, pancreatic exocrine insufficiency, anemia, and thrombocytopenia; (5) cartilage-hair hypoplasia, with short limb dwarfism, abnormally fine hair, and T cell deficiencies; and (6) **Chédiak-Higashi** syndrome. Acquired neutropenias are the most common forms of childhood neutropenia and are induced by an autoimmune mechanism. Viral infections are the commonest reason for neutrophil antibodies causing both leukopenia and neutropenia. Atypical lymphocytosis and monocytosis are common associated findings. Drugs and toxins may also cause neutropenia.

Benign forms of neutropenia may not require therapy. In other forms, infections should be treated with appropriate antibiotics. Patients with fever and neutropenia associated with acute suppression of the bone marrow from cytotoxic drugs should be treated with broad-spectrum antibiotics; growth factors such as G-CSF or Gm-CSF are useful in some forms of neutropenia.

IMMUNE DEFICIENCY DISORDERS

Immune deficiency diseases are characterized by increased susceptibility to bacterial, viral, and fungal infections. Several categories are definable based upon whether the defect originates with a disturbance of antibody-producing lymphoid cells (B cells) or with thymus-derived cells that mediate cellular immunity (T cells).

Classification of Immunologic Disorders

A. Immunoglobulin deficiencies:

1. Infantile X-linked agammaglobulinemia.
2. Selective immunoglobulin deficiency (IgA deficiency and dysgammaglobulinemia).
3. Acquired hypogammaglobulinemia.
4. Transient hypogammaglobulinemia of infancy.

B. Cellular immune deficiency with "normal" immunoglobulins:

1. Thymic dysplasia (Nezelof type).
2. **DiGeorge's syndrome** (congenital absence of thymus and parathyroids; third and fourth pharyngeal pouch syndrome).

C. Combined immunoglobulin and cellular immune deficiencies:

1. **Congenital:**
   - **a.** Severe combined immunodeficiency (Swiss type agammaglobulinemia, thymic dysplasia).
   - **b.** **Wiskott-Aldrich syndrome** (dysgammaglobulinemia and progressive cellular immunity deficiency).
2. **Acquired:**
   - **a.** Lymphoid neoplasms.
   - **b.** Iatrogenic conditions (steroid or antimetabolite therapy).
   - **c.** Human immunodeficiency virus (HIV).

Clinical Findings

A. Signs & Symptoms: In patients with immunoglobulin deficiency disease, recurrent pyogenic bacterial infections predominate;

chronic otitis media, sinusitis, and bronchiectasis are especially common. In agammaglobulinemia, viral infections (eg, measles, varicella, and mumps) are weathered without incident. In individuals with cellular immunity defects, progressive vaccinia has been a frequent complication, and vaccination should be avoided. *Candida* infections are not uncommon in such patients, and unusually severe infections with CMV, herpesvirus, and *Pneumocystis* occur as well. In the acquired forms, malignant disorders of the lymphoreticular system occur with increased frequency. AIDS, which has been reported in children with hemophilia and in infants born to infected mothers (eg, IV drug abusers), is often difficult to distinguish from congenital deficiency disease.

Laboratory Findings

Diagnosis is based on results of the following studies:

1. Quantitative determination of IgG, IgM, and IgA levels.
2. Isohemagglutinin determination. These antibodies to the blood group substance belong for the most part to the IgM class. They are normally present after about 1 year of age in all individuals of blood groups A, B, and O. Therefore, their absence is presumptive evidence of IgM deficiency.
3. Absolute lymphocyte count. The count is 4000–6000/μL in normal children but reduced in patients with cellular immunity deficiency (especially in patients with severe combined immunodeficiency).
4. Examination of bone marrow for plasma cells.

Confirmatory tests include the following:

1. Results of immunization with well-characterized antigens (eg, diphtheria toxoid, tetanus toxoid) in terms of specific antibody production and plasma cell development.
2. Presence of germinal center formation, plasma cells, and small lymphocytes in a biopsy of the regional lymph node taken 1 week after antigenic stimulation.
3. Reaction to *C albicans* and mumps skin tests.
4. Induction of contact dermal hypersensitivity with dinitrochlorobenzene.
5. In vitro tests of lymphocyte function [common mitogens: phytohemagglutinin (PHA), concanavalin A (ConA), and pokeweed mitogen stimulation].

Treatment

Treatment for patients with immunoglobulin deficiency consists of replacement therapy with immune globulin, which is chiefly IgG.

Give loading dose of 200 mg/kg intravenously and then 100 mg/kg every 3 or 4 weeks. Preparations consisting solely of IgM and IgA are not yet available. Preparations suitable for intravenous use (Gamimune, Sandoglobulin) are now available.

Each individual has genetically determined differences in gamma globulins, and isoimmunization can occur as a result of giving genetically foreign gamma globulin. Since isoimmunization may have some deleterious effects, injudicious administration of immune globulin should be avoided.

Therapy of cellular immune deficiencies with bone marrow transplant is still experimental, but results are improving.

Neurologic & Muscular Disorders

20

Alan R. Seay, MD, & Joanne Janas, MD

SEIZURES

Seizure is defined as a sudden, transient disturbance of brain function manifested by involuntary motor, sensory, autonomic, or psychic phenomena. Often an alteration or loss of consciousness occurs. These alterations in neurologic function are accompanied by abnormally synchronized electrocerebral discharges. The term "epilepsy" denotes recurrent seizures that are not caused by identifiable, correctable metabolic disturbances. "Convulsion" refers to seizures that consist of generalized muscular rigidity or rhythmical jerking.

Seizures occur in approximately 2–4% of children and most childhood seizure disorders remit spontaneously. Factors that increase the probability of seizure recurrence or epilepsy when antiepileptic drugs are discontinued include the presence of preexisting neurologic deficits or mental retardation, age of onset less than 2 years, and an abnormal EEG at the time of discontinuing medication. Seizures that are difficult to control initially or that require multiple antiepileptic drugs for control are more likely to recur than seizures that are quickly suppressed by monotherapy.

Seizures and epilepsy are often classified as symptomatic (the cause is known) and idiopathic (the cause is unknown). When "idiopathic" is used to describe epilepsy, it usually implies a genetic etiology or predisposition. The younger the infant or child, the more likely the etiology for the seizure can be identified. Genetically determined epilepsy usually begins between ages 4 and 16 years. Seizures and epilepsy should not be considered idiopathic or genetic in origin until a thorough history, neurologic examination, and appropriate laboratory evaluation have excluded other possible causes.

After a specific seizure type is determined, further refinement in diagnosis results if an epileptic syndrome can be identified. An epileptic syndrome is defined by the predictable association of a certain

Table 20–1. Childhood epilepsy syndromes.

Generalized epileptic syndromes
Idiopathic
Benign familial neonatal convulsions
Primary generalized epilepsy
Juvenile myoclonic epilepsy
Childhood absence epilepsy (petit mal epilepsy)
Symptomatic
Progressive myoclonic epilepsies
West's syndrome (infantile spasms with hypsarrhythmic EEG)
Lennox-Gastaut syndrome
Localization-related epileptic syndromes
Idiopathic
Benign epilepsy of childhood with centrotemporal spikes (rolandic epilepsy)
Childhood epilepsy with occipital paroxysms
Symptomatic partial

seizure type with a specific EEG pattern in a patient with a characteristic clinical profile. The most frequently encountered childhood epilepsy syndromes are displayed in Table 20–1. The correct identification of an epileptic syndrome allows the clinician to select the most specific antiepileptic medication for the patient and helps to clarify issues related to etiology, prognosis, and genetic factors. A full discussion of these syndromes is available in numerous monographs and review articles, such as J Child Neurol 1994;9 (supplements 1 and 2).

Status epilepticus, neonatal seizures, and their therapy are discussed in other sections of this book (see Chapters 7 and 28). Table 20–2 lists the major types of childhood seizures along with their most prominent clinical manifestations and their treatment. Table 20–3 lists several of the most common antiepileptic drugs and outlines their dosages and most frequent potential side effects.

Clinical Findings

The history provides the most important information upon which to make the diagnosis of seizures or epilepsy. Some seizures, complex partial seizures for example, may be preceded by an aura, which consists of transient subjective symptoms such as numbness, tingling, visual disturbances, or a vague feeling of fear and anxiety. Patients may remember the aura, but they are amnestic for the remaining portion of the seizure. Some patients with generalized seizures experience a

Table 20–2. Common seizure types in children.

Seizure Type	Age at Onset	Clinical Manifestations	Treatment
Partial			
Simple partial (focal motor, sensory, autonomic)	Any age	No disturbance of consciousness. May involve any part of the body. May spread in fixed pattern (Jacksonian) and become generalized.	Carbamazepine, phenytoin, phenobarbital or primidone; valproic acid may be a useful adjunct.
Complex partial	Any age	Associated with impairment of consciousness. The aura may be sensation of fear, epigastric discomfort, odd smell or taste, visual or auditory hallucination. Proceeds to period of altered behavior which may be characterized by walking in a daze, facial movements such as eye blinking, lip smacking, chewing or other automatisms. If the seizure consists solely of an aura, it is classified as a partial seizure. Complex partial seizures may also generalize.	Carbamazepine, phenytoin, phenobarbital or primidone. Valproic acid may be a useful adjunct.
Generalized			
Tonic–Clonic	Any age	Loss of consciousness, ± bladder/bowel incontinence, postictal confusion.	Phenobarbital, carbamazepine, phenytoin, valproic acid, primidone.
Absence	3–15 years	Lapses of consciousness lasting about 10 seconds. Often in clusters. May see automatisms of face and hands.	Ethosuximide or valproic acid.
Myoclonic	Any age (usually 2–7 years)	Abrupt contractions of one or more muscle groups, singly or irregularly repetitive. Usually no or only brief loss of consciousness.	Valproic acid, clonazepam, ethosuximide. Imipramine is adjunct. Diazepam. Ketogenic or medium chain triglyceride diet. ACTH or corticosteroids in West's Syndrome.

Table 20–3. Common antiepileptic drugs.

Drug	Preparation	Therapeutic Plasma Concentration	Dose (Initial & Maintenance)	Laboratory Monitoring	Side Effects	Drug & Clinical Interactions
Carbamazepine (Tegretol)	Tabs: 200 mg Chewable Tabs: 100 mg Suspension: 100 mg/5 mL	6–12 μg/mL	*Under 6 yrs:* Initial: 10 mg/kg/24h PO–QD or BID or 100 mg/dose BID Increment: up to 20 mg/kg/24h *6–12 yrs:* Initial: 10 mg/kg/24h PO–QD or BID up to 100 mg/dose BID Increment: 100 mg/24h at intervals of 1 day (TID or QID) until best response Maintenance: 20–30 mg/kg/24h–PO, TID or QID **Max. dose:** 1000 mg/24h *Adolescents & Adults:* Initial: 200 mg BID Increment: 200 mg/24h at intervals of 1 day using TID or QID schedule until best response.	Baseline CBC, LFTS, electrolytes. Monitor for hematologic and hepatic toxicity.	*Acute:* Diplopia, drowsiness, vertigo, blurred vision, dry mouth, stomatitis, SIADH, dehydration, headache, diarrhea, constipation, paresthesia *Chronic:* Enzyme induction, aplastic anemia, leukopenia, hepatic enzyme elevation, nervousness	*Increased by:* INH Propxyphene Erythromycin Hepatic disease *Decreased by:* Phenobarbital Phenytoin Primidone Pregnancy

			Maintenance: 600–1200 mg/24h–TID or QID **Max.** 12–15 yr: 1000 mg/24h **Max.** Adult: 1200 mg/24h			
Clonazepam (Klonopin)	Tabs: 0.5, 1.0, 2.0 mg Suspension: 80 μg/5 mL or 0.1 mg/mL	0.013–0.072 μg/mL	*Children:* Up to 10 yr or 30 kg: Initial: 0.01–0.05 mg/kg/24h–Q8h PO Increment: 0.25–0.5 mg/24h Q3 days, up to **maximum** maintenance dose of 0.1–0.2 mg/kg/24h–Q8h *Adolescents & Adults:* Initial: 1.5 mg/24h PO–TID Increment: 0.5–1 mg/24h Q3 days **Max. dose:** 20 mg/24h		CNS depression, drowsiness and ataxia common. May cause behavioral changes and other CNS symptoms; increased bronchial secretions. GI, CV, GU and hematopoietic toxicity may occur. Use with **caution** in renal impairment.	*Increased by:* Phenytoin *Decreased by:* Phenobarbital

(*continued*)

Table 20–3. Common antiepileptic drugs (*continued*).

Drug	Preparation	Therapeutic Plasma Concentration	Dose (Initial & Maintenance)	Laboratory Monitoring	Side Effects	Drug & Clinical Interactions
Diazepam (Valium)	Tabs: 2, 5, 10 mg Oral solution: 1.5 mg/mL Injection: 5 mg/mL		*Status Epilepticus:* *Neonate:* 0.5–1.0 mg/kg/dose IV Q15–30 min × 2–3 doses *1 mo–5 yr:* 0.2–0.5 mg/kg/dose IV Q15–30 min (**max. total dose:** 5 mg) > *5 yrs:* 0.2–0.5 mg/kg/dose IV Q15–30 min (**max. total dose:** 10 mg). *Adolescents & Adults:* 5–10 mg/dose IV Q10–15 min (**max. total dose:** 30 mg)		Hypotension and respiratory depression may occur. Use with **caution** in glaucoma, shock, and depression. Give undiluted no faster than 2 mg/min. **Do not** mix with IV fluids. Not recommended for use in neonates. In status epilepticus, diazepam must be followed by long-acting anticonvulsants.	
Ethosuximide (Zarontin)	250 mg tabs 250 mg/5 mL elixir	40–100 μg/mL	*3–6 yr:* Initial: 250 mg/24h–QD–BID PO Increment: Increase 250 mg/24h every 4–7 days Maintenance: 20–40 mg/kg/24h–QD > *6 yr:* Initial: 500 mg/24h–QD–BID PO Increment: Same as above Maintenance: Same as above	Baseline CBC and LFTS. Monitor for hematologic and hepatic changes.	*Acute:* Nausea, vertigo, loss of appetite, vomiting, hiccups, headache *Chronic:* Loss of sleep, nervousness, occasional psychotic behavior, hiccups, headache, reported exacerbation of major seizures. May also see lupus-like syndrome, dystonia.	

			Adolescents & Adults: Initial: 750 mg/24h–QD Increment: Same as above Maintenance: Same as above **Max. children's dose:** 1500 mg/24h			
Lorazepam (Ativan)	Tabs: 0.5, 1, 2 mg Injection: 2, 4 mg/mL		*Status Epilepticus:* *Infants and Children:* 0.03 to 0.05 mg/kg/dose IV up to **max.** of 4 mg/dose. May repeat in 15 to 20 min. × 1. *Adolescents & Adults:* 2.5–10 mg/dose IV. May repeat in 15–20 min.		May cause respiratory depression, especially in combination with other sedatives. May also cause sedation, dizziness, mild ataxia, mood changes, rash and GI symptoms. Injectable product may be given rectally.	
Phenobarbital (Luminal)	Tabs: 8, 15, 16, 30, 32, 60, 65, 100 mg Caps: 16 mg Elixir: 15, 20 mg/5mL Injection: 30, 60, 65, 130 mg/mL	15–40μg/mL	*Children:* 10–20 mg/kg/dose IV × 1, then 5–10 mg/kg/dose Q20 min PRN **Max. total dose:** 40 mg/kg *Adolescents & Adults:* 300–800 mg IV × 1, then 120–240 mg/dose Q20 min PRN **Max. total dose:** 1–2 g *Chronic Anticonvulsant:* *Neonates:*	Baseline CBC Folate/B_{12} if anemic	IV administration may cause respiratory arrest or hypotension. **Do not exceed** push of 1 mg/kg/mn. Acute: Sedation, behavior disturbances, ataxia Chronic: Difficulty with concentration, cognitive deficit, loss of initiative, hemorrhage in newborn.	*Increased by:* Valproic acid Phenytoin Lasix Amphetamines Renal disease Hepatic disease *Decreased by:* Clonazepam Alkaline urine

(*continued*)

Table 20–3. Common antiepileptic drugs (*continued*).

Drug	Preparation	Therapeutic Plasma Concentration	Dose (Initial & Maintenance)	Laboratory Monitoring	Side Effects	Drug & Clinical Interactions
			Initial: 2–4 mg/kg/24h–QD–BID × 2w Maintenance: 5 mg/kg/24h–QD–BID *Infants:* 5–8 mg/kg/24h–QD–BID *Children:* 3–5 mg/kg/24h–QD–BID *Adolescents & Adults:* 120–250 mg/24h–QD–BID (1–3 mg/kg/24h)			
Phenytoin (Dilantin)	Chewable Tabs: 50 mg (Infatab) Prompt Caps: 30, 100 mg Extended Release Caps: 30, 100 mg Susp.: 30, 125 mg/5 mL Injection: 50 mg/mL	10–20 μg/mL	*Status Epilepticus:* 15–20 mg/kg IV **Max. dose:** 1000 mg/24h *Maintenance for Seizure Disorders:* *Infants/Children:* 4–7 mg/kg/24h–QD–BID IV or PO *Adolescents & Adults:* 300–400 mg/24h–QD–BID IV or PO	Baseline CBC, LFTS	*Acute:* Drowsiness, ataxia, diplopia, nystagmus, gastro-intestinal complaints, choreoathetosis, nausea, hypotension (after injection), Stevens-Johnson. *Chronic:* Gingival hyper-plasia, hypertrichosis, coarse facies, Dupuy-tren's contractures, folate deficiency, megaloblastic anemia, osteomalacia with	*Increased by:* Phenobarbital Valproic acid Ethosuximide Chloramphenicol Disulfiram Isoniazid Dicumarol Amphetamines Tolbutamide Chlordane Phenylbutazone Alcohol (acute) Aminosalicylic acid

				vitamin D deficiency, peripheral neuropathy, encephalopathy, cerebellar dysfunction, endocrine dysfunction (adrenal, thyroid, diabetogenesis), pseudolymphoma, immunosuppression, agranulocytosis, hemorrhage in the newborn.	Chlorpromazine Estrogens Methylphenidate Prochlorperazine Sulfaphenazole Hepatic disease *Decreased by:* Phenobarbital Carbamazepine Clonazepam Chronic ETOH Reserpine ? Theophylline Pregnancy Renal disease Mononucleosis Acute hepatitis May decrease effectiveness of OBC pills. Induces liver enzymes.
Primidone (Mysoline)	Tabs: 50, 250 mg Susp.: 250 mg/5 mL	Phenobarbital: 15–40 mg/L Mysoline: 8–12 mg/L Follow both (?)	*< 8 yrs:* Initial: 125 mg/24h QD PO Increment: 125 mg/24h weekly PO Maintenance: 10–25 mg/kg/24h–TID–QID PO *> 8 yrs–Adults:* Initial: 250 mg/24h QD PO	Metabolizes to phenobarbital, so at risk for same toxicities. *Acute:* Sedation, vertigo, nausea, unsteadiness *Chronic:* Behavior disturbances in the young, loss of libido, difficulty with concentration, hemorrhagic disease in newborn.	*Increased by:* Valproic acid Clonazepam *Decreased by:* Phenytoin

(*continued*)

Table 20–3. Common antiepileptic drugs (*continued*).

Drug	Preparation	Therapeutic Plasma Concentration	Dose (Initial & Maintenance)	Laboratory Monitoring	Side Effects	Drug & Clinical Interactions
			Increment: 250 mg/24h weekly PO Maintenance: 0.75–1.5 g/24h–TID–QID PO			
Valproic acid (Depakene)	Caps: 250 mg Syrup: 250 mg/5 mL Sprinkles: 125 mg caps		*PO:* Initial: 10–15 mg/kg/24h–QD–TID Increment: 5–10 mg/kg/24h at weekly intervals to max. of 60 mg/kg/24h Maintenance: 30–60 mg/kg/24h QD–TID *PR:* Syrup diluted 1:1 may be given PR using the same doses as those given PO.	Baseline CBC, LFTS	*Acute:* Drowsiness, gastrointestinal disturbances (nausea and vomiting) *Chronic:* Alopecia, weight gain, weight loss, tremor, ankle swelling, amenorrhea, hyperammonemia, unexplained stupor, granulocytopenia, hepatic enzyme elevation, thrombocytopenia, occasional psychosis	*Increased by:* Hepatic disease *Decreased by:* Carbamazepine Phenytoin Phenobarbital Primidone

more vague prodrome of feeling tired or having a recognizable malaise for several minutes or hours before the seizure occurs.

Proper classification of seizures and their differentiation from other types of spells depends upon an accurate and detailed account of the sequence of events leading to and during the spell. Did the patient become pale or cyanotic before he or she fell, began to jerk, or lost consciousness? Was the patient able to respond to any type of stimulation during the episode? Did the patient lose consciousness completely? Did the patient fall, become rigid, jerk rhythmically, or go limp? How long did the stiffening or jerking last? What parts of the body were involved in the stiffness or rhythmical jerking? What was the patient's behavior after the episode was over?

The proper classification of the seizures is necessary to make an accurate diagnosis, prognosis, and appropriate management decisions.

Febrile Seizures

Febrile seizures are very common, occurring in 2–3% of children. Simple febrile seizures are generalized and brief, usually lasting less than 5 minutes. They are typically triggered by infections of the ear, pharynx, or gastrointestinal tract. Febrile seizures probably reflect a genetically determined lowered seizure threshold to the stress of fever. Risk factors for the later development of non-febrile epilepsy are presented in Table 20–4. Even with these factors, the risk of epilepsy in later life is only about 15–20%. After a single febrile seizure, the probability of recurrence is estimated to be 20–40%. In general, recurrence of febrile seizures does not alter the long-term, uniformly good outlook.

After the child with a febrile seizure is examined and the history reviewed, laboratory studies including CBC, electrolytes, glucose, calcium, EEG, and brain imaging studies may be done selectively and tailored to the needs of each child. Bacterial meningitis must be excluded either by careful clinical observation or by spinal fluid examination.

Table 20–4. Febrile seizures: Risk factors for non-febrile epilepsy.

- Seizure > 15 minutes
- More than one seizure in a day
- Focal seizure
- Abnormal neurologic status preceding the seizure (eg, cerebral palsy)
- < 1 year of age
- Positive family history for epilepsy

Most neurologists elect not to use antiepileptic drugs after one or a few simple febrile seizures because of their benign nature and low risk of recurrence. Fever control with sponging and antipyretics and appropriate use of antibiotics for suspected bacterial infections constitute the major treatment approach. In addition, the family is reassured about the benign nature of simple febrile seizures. The results of an electroencephalogram are usually normal. In about 10% of patients, an EEG done within a few days of the seizure will show nonspecific occipital slowing which resolves within two weeks. In young infants, EEG results seldom aid in predicting the likelihood of future seizure recurrence, either febrile or non-febrile.

Differential Diagnosis of Seizures

Several conditions closely resemble seizures and should be considered in the differential.

A. Breath-holding Spells: These episodes occur in children between the ages of 6 months and 3 years and are precipitated by trauma, fright, anger, frustration, or emotional upset. After beginning to cry, the child holds his or her breath and then passes out. During these spells, the child may become cyanotic or pale and may have a few rhythmical clonic jerks, but consciousness is rapidly regained. Family history for similar spells is positive in about 30% of cases. The EEG is typically normal. No medical therapy is effective at preventing recurrences, and treatment is reassurance to parents about the benign nature of these spells. These spells spontaneously remit by 4 to 6 years.

B. Sleep Disturbances: Night terrors most frequently affect children between 3 and 10 years old. The episodes occur 30–90 minutes after the child falls asleep. The child begins to cry and appears fretful, agitated, and frightened. The child may be noted to have small, dilated pupils and profuse sweating. The spell lasts several minutes, then the child becomes quiet again. The child has no memory of the spell upon awakening. Results of polysomnography and EEGs are normal. No therapy is indicated. The spells spontaneously cease.

Nightmares are vivid, frightening dreams that usually occur in the early morning hours, and portions of them are remembered. Occasionally, bizarre behavior may occur during nightmares that resembles a complex partial seizure. In selected cases, an overnight EEG may help to differentiate seizures from nightmares and other sleep disturbances.

C. Migraine: Migraine attacks can result in a variety of motor and sensory deficits that resemble partial or generalized seizures. The presence and location of a throbbing headache helps to differentiate migraine attacks from seizures. Migraine episodes in general last longer than seizures and are less likely to be followed by amnesia. Family history is positive for migraine in about 65–75% of children with migraine. Propranolol, amitriptyline, and cyproheptadine are useful prophylactic agents for migraine.

Confusional migraine attacks most often affect children in late childhood and early adolescence. These attacks may occur in a child with a previous history of migraine or as the initial presentation of migraine. The child has sudden onset of delirium, confusion, agitation, and combative behavior. Throbbing headache is usually present when the child's sensorium begins to clear. Symptoms can last from 1–2 hours or occasionally as long as 20–24 hours. Resolution usually occurs after a short period of sleep. These types of spells are typically infrequent and do not require prophylactic drug therapy.

D. Syncope: Syncope is often precipitated by identifiable factors, and the patient remembers the initial symptoms of lightheadedness, dim vision, generalized weakness, and nausea. Observers notice extreme pallor and profuse sweating. The heart rate and blood pressure may be quite low. Patients regain consciousness rapidly. Occasionally, brief tonic posturing or clonic jerking occurs as a result of generalized, transient cerebral ischemia. Incontinence is rare. EEGs between attacks are normal. The family history is frequently positive for similar syncopal episodes.

E. Shuddering Spells: Shuddering or shivering attacks occur in infancy and may be the early manifestation of a familial, essential tremor. The attacks are brief, lasting several seconds, and are not associated with any impairment of consciousness. Shuddering spells may occur frequently and tend to occur as the patient awakens from sleep. EEGs are normal and the family histories frequently positive for similar spells as well as for essential tremor.

F. Gastroesophageal Reflux: Reflux of acidic gastric contents can lead to severe abdominal pain and can be accompanied by unusual posturing and movements of the head, neck and trunk. Barium swallow radiographs and gastric pH probe studies are the most frequently used and reliable tests to confirm the diagnosis.

G. Pseudoseizures: Many patients with unquestionable epileptic seizures also have non-epileptic pseudoseizures. These episodes may consist of tonic posturing, bizarre nonrhythmical jerking and thrashing movements, and impaired responsivity. The triggers for such attacks are usually obscure. In many patients, simultaneous EEG/video tape monitoring helps to clarify which spells are epileptic and which are not. A normal or non-epileptiform EEG during a spell usually confirms that a spell is a pseudoseizure.

H. Staring Spells: School teachers often make referrals for suspected seizures in youngsters who have brief staring spells. Non-epileptic inattentiveness may not be observed at home and usually does not cluster in the early morning hours as might be seen in patients with absence seizures. The child can generally be brought out of this spell by verbal or tactile stimulation. An EEG is sometimes used to reassure parents and teachers that the child is not having seizures. Long-term EEG/video tape monitoring may be needed to provide unequivocal distinction between absence seizures and brief non-epileptic staring spells.

ABNORMAL HEAD SIZE & SHAPE

Microcephaly

Microcephaly is defined as a head circumference that is 2 standard deviations or more below the mean for age and sex. The etiology may be primary (malformation, chromosomal anomaly, genetic syndrome) or secondary (infections, birth asphyxia, trauma, malnutrition, systemic disease). Microcephaly at birth indicates that the etiological process affected brain growth in utero. Babies with neonatal asphyxial brain damage will have normal head sizes at birth, but head growth rate will be slower than normal. A family history of small heads may aid in the diagnosis of familial trait microcephaly or, more rarely, autosomal dominant microcephaly. An outline of some common causes of microcephaly is provided in Table 20–5.

Microcephaly may be discovered when the child is evaluated for developmental or neurologic problems. There may be a marked backward slope of the forehead with narrowing of the bitemporal diameter. The fontanelle may be closed earlier than expected and suture lines excessively prominent.

Based on the history and clinical findings, congenital infections are evaluated by measuring serum antibody titers against CMV, HSV, toxoplasmosis, and rubella virus. The presence of organism-specific anti-IgM antibodies are the most specific diagnostic findings. The

Table 20–5. Disorders associated with microcephaly.

Genetic/Chromosomal	Trisomy 13, 18, 21
	Lissencephaly
	Rubenstein-Taybi
	Cornelia de Lange
	Familial microcephaly
Toxins	Maternal alcohol
	Antiepileptic drugs
	Maternal PKU
Infections	Congenital viral (CMV, HSV, Toxo)
	AIDS
	Bacterial meningitis
	Viral meningoencephalitis
Metabolic	Perinatal asphyxia
	Hypoglycemia
	Aminoacidopathies
Birth injury	

comparison of maternal antiviral IgG titers with the infant's antiviral IgG titers or the demonstration of rising IgG titers in the infant postnatally are important alternative ways of documenting probable congenital infections. Serum and urine organic acid screens are occasionally diagnostic. Infants born to women with untreated PKU may suffer severe microcephaly and mental retardation. Karyotyping may be considered in selected cases.

Skull films are rarely helpful in the evaluation of microcephaly. Head CT or MRI scans may aid the diagnosis by demonstrating intracranial calcifications, cerebral malformations, or cerebral atrophy.

Treatment is supportive and directed at associated motor and sensory deficits and any associated treatable condition. Catch-up growth after correction of an underlying metabolic disturbance can occur. Perhaps as many as 80% of children with microcephaly are mentally retarded to some degree.

Macrocephaly

Macrocephaly is defined as a head circumference that is 2 or more standard deviations above the mean for age and sex. A large head may be due to hydrocephalus, true megalencephaly, thickening of skull bone, or the presence of extra-axial fluid accumulations. As with microcephaly, it is important to review familial head circumferences, the onset and progression of the abnormal head size, and the child's developmental progress. A careful family history of abnormal skin pigmentation, café-au-lait spots, cutaneous tumors, or neurologic disorders that might indicate neurofibromatosis should be obtained.

A. Hydrocephalus: Hydrocephalus is characterized by increased volume of cerebrospinal fluid in association with progressive ventricular dilatation and may result from impaired reabsorption of CSF (communicating hydrocephalus) or from obstruction of CSF flow through the ventricles and into the subarachnoid space (non-communicating hydrocephalus). A wide variety of disorders, such as hemorrhage, infection, tumors, and congenital malformations can play an etiologic role in development of hydrocephalus.

Clinical features of hydrocephalus include macrocephaly and excessive head growth rate. Increased intracranial pressure causes irritability, vomiting, loss of appetite, impaired upward gaze, impaired extraocular movements, lower extremity hypertonia, and generalized hyperreflexia. Papilledema may not occur in young infants but usually is present in older children. Without treatment, hydrocephalus can result in progressive loss of vision, loss of consciousness, autonomic failure, and ultimately death.

Hydrocephalus is confirmed by head CT or MRI scans. Treatment is directed at providing an alternative outlet for CSF from the intracranial compartment, usually by ventriculoperitoneal shunting. Treatment should also be directed, if possible, at any underlying etiology.

B. Megalencephaly: A large brain may be normal or may be secondary to abnormal neuronal migration or cerebral organization. Hamartomatous proliferation of cerebral tissue is found in patients with neurocutaneous disorders, such as neurofibromatosis, tuberous sclerosis, and hypomelanosis of Ito. Large brains are also characteristic of some storage and neurometabolic disorders, for example, Alexander's disease, Canavan's disease, and the mucopolysaccharidoses.

Craniosynostosis

Craniosynostosis, or premature closure of cranial sutures, is usually a sporadic, idiopathic disorder. However, some patients have syndromes such as Apert's and Crouzon's that are inherited and are associated with characteristic abnormalities of the digits, extremities, and heart. Rarely, craniosynostosis may be associated with an underlying metabolic disturbance such as hyperthyroidism and hypophosphatasia. The most common form of craniosynostosis involves the sagittal suture and results in scaphocephaly, an elongation of the head in the anterior-to-posterior direction. Premature closure of the coronal sutures causes brachycephaly, an increase in cranial diameter from left to right. Unless multiple sutures close prematurely, intracranial volume is not compromised, and the brain's growth potential is not impaired. Neurologic functions are not affected. Surgical management of craniosynostosis is directed at preventing cosmetically unsatisfactory distortions in skull shape.

Arnold–Chiari Malformation

This malformation results from abnormal, incomplete closure of the neural tube during the first month after conception. The malformation is characterized by elongation and kinking of the brain stem and protrusion of cerebellar tonsils into the foramen magnum. This malformation is usually classified into three types.

Type I consists of elongation and displacement of the caudal end of the brain stem into the spinal canal with protrusion of the cerebellar tonsils through the foramen magnum. Minor to moderate abnormalities of the base of the skull, including basilar impression, platybasia, and small foramen magnum may be present. Type I may remain asymptomatic for years, but may cause progressive ataxia, lower cranial nerve paresis, and progressive vertigo in adolescents and adults.

Type II is the most commonly recognized variant and consists of any combination of Type I abnormalities plus a lumbosacral meningomyelocele. Hydrocephalus is present in 90% of cases. Aqueductal stenosis, hydromyelia, and syringomyelia are frequent, associated anomalies.

Type III consists of any combination of Type I or Type II abnormalities plus occipital cranium bifidum with encephalocele or cervical spinal bifida. Hydrocephalus is frequently present and is secondary to aqueductal stenosis, atresia of the fourth ventricle, or narrowing of the foramen magnum.

Dandy–Walker Malformation

Dandy–Walker malformation is characterized by vermal aplasia, cystic enlargement of the fourth ventricle, rostral displacement of the tentorium, and absence or atresia of the foramina of Magendie and Luschka. Although hydrocephalus is usually not present at birth, it often develops within the first few months of life. In those patients who develop hydrocephalus, 90% do so by 1 year of age. On physical examination, there is often a rounded protuberance or exaggeration of the occiput. In the absence of hydrocephalus and increased intracranial pressure, there may be few or no abnormal neurologic findings. An ataxic syndrome, if it develops, usually appears late, but occurs in fewer than 20% of patients. Many of the long-term neurologic deficits result directly from hydrocephalus. Diagnosis of Dandy–Walker malformation is confirmed by head CT or MRI scanning. Treatment is directed at the management of hydrocephalus.

Agenesis of the Corpus Callosum

Agenesis of the corpus callosum, once thought to be a rare cerebral malformation, has been seen frequently with modern neuroimaging techniques. Occasionally agenesis of the corpus callosum appears to be inherited in an autosomal dominant or autosomal recessive pattern. X-linked patterns have also been described. Agenesis of the corpus callosum may be found in conjunction with metabolic defects (pyruvate dehydrogenase deficiency, nonketotic hyperglycinemia). Most cases, however, are sporadic and idiopathic. Maldevelopment of the corpus callosum may be partial or complete. Many patients with agenesis of the corpus callosum have associated seizures, developmental delay, microcephaly, or mental retardation, although this malformation may be found coincidentally in normal people. In Aicardi's syndrome, agenesis of the corpus callosum is associated with infantile spasms, mental retardation, lacunar chorioretinopathy, and vertebral body abnormalities. Aicardi's syndrome is inherited in an X-linked dominant pattern.

Lissencephaly

Lissencephaly is a severe malformation of the brain characterized by an extremely smooth cortical surface with minimal development of sulci and gyri. There is primitive cytoarchitectural construction of the cerebral mantle. Pachygyria and agyria are defects in cerebral development that are closely associated with lissencephaly but which represent more restricted forms of migrational abnormalities. Patients with lissencephaly usually suffer from severe neurodevelopmental delay, microcephaly, and infantile spasms. Patients with lissencephaly frequently have additional associated malformations, dysmorphic features, or metabolic abnormalities, as in Walker-Warburg syndrome, Miller–Dieker syndrome, and Zellweger syndrome. Deletion defects of chromosome 17 have been found in some patients. It is particularly important to identify genetic syndromes so that families can be counseled appropriately regarding prognosis and recurrence risk.

DISORDERS AFFECTING MUSCLES

Progressive Spinal Muscular Atrophy

Progressive deterioration of the anterior horn cells is usually inherited in an autosomal recessive pattern and is characterized by severe progressive weakness, hypotonia, and areflexia. Muscle wasting and fasciculations are present in distal extremity, facial, and tongue muscles.

Early infantile onset and rapid progression is characteristic of Werdnig–Hoffman disease, while later onset and slow progression is typical of Kugelberg–Welander disease. Many intermediate forms are also seen. Steady progression and eventual incapacitation are common with early onset forms. Diagnosis is aided by electromyography, which provides evidence of denervation. Serum creatine kinase levels are usually normal. Molecular genetic linkage tests are now available. Muscle biopsy confirms the neurogenic nature of the illness. Therapy is supportive only. Death in later childhood results from secondary infections, pulmonary insufficiency, and congestive heart failure.

Muscular Dystrophies

The most common muscular dystrophy in childhood is Duchenne dystrophy. This X-linked recessive disorder becomes symptomatic in boys by the age of 2–3 years. Weakness is first evident in proximal muscles of the lower extremities. The child displays a waddling gait, has progressive difficulty running and walking, and soon becomes unable to stand from a sitting position without using his upper extremities to push or pull the body up. All skeletal muscles and cardiac muscle are affected by the dystrophic process. Enlargement of calf muscles occurs in 70 to 80% of patients. The serum creatine kinase level is 50 to 100-fold above normal. Abnormal EKG findings are present in 75% of patients. The diagnosis is confirmed by the presence of myopathic abnormalities on the EMG and dystrophic changes on muscle biopsy. The recent development of dystrophin staining of muscle biopsies provides the most definitive diagnostic information. No specific therapy is available. Affected boys are wheelchair confined by 12–14 years, and death occurs between 20–30 years.

Myotonic dystrophy is an autosomal dominant form of muscular dystrophy that is characterized by weakness, progressive distal muscle wasting, and inability to relax contracted muscle. When newborns and infants are symptomatic, they may display generalized hypotonia of all extremities as well as facial and tongue muscles. More than 90% of symptomatic neonates inherit the disorder from their mothers. In older patients, frontal balding, cataracts, endocrinopathies, diabetes mellitus, and immunologic disorders are common, and non-muscular manifestations, cardiac dysrrhythmias, and cardiomyopathy are frequent. Serum levels of creatine kinase are normal or only mildly elevated. The EMG demonstrates diagnostic myotonic discharges, though these findings may be absent in the neonate and very young infant. Muscle biopsy findings include excess numbers of central nuclei, ring fibers, and excessive proliferation of connective tissue. Molecular genetic testing is now available to confirm the diagnosis in suspected or atypical cases. No specific therapy is available. Painful myotonic contractions can be partially relieved by the use of phenytoin or procainamide. Prognosis is excellent for long survival, but many patients eventually require assistance to walk, and others become confined to a wheelchair.

Congenital Myopathies

Several inherited disorders of muscle structure (nemaline myopathy, central core disease, centronuclear myopathy, and myotubular myopathy) result in generalized hypotonia and non-progressive or very slowly progressive weakness in children. Many, though not all, of these disorders are symptomatic at birth or during early infancy. Typical features include facial diplegia, weak suck, poor swallow, weak cry, extraocular movement disorders, and respiratory insufficiency. Some infants with these disorders improve with age if they are given early supportive care. Serum levels of creatine kinase are normal or mildly elevated. The EMG confirms nonspecific myopathic changes. Muscle biopsy with light and electronmicroscopic studies are necessary to accurately diagnose these disorders. Specific therapy is not available.

Dermatomyositis

Generalized progressive weakness is the hallmark of dermatomyositis in childhood. Skin rashes on the face and extensor surfaces of joints are typical, but may be fleeting and absent at the time of medical evaluation. Fever, muscle pain, and muscle tenderness are not reliable signs of inflammatory myopathy. Erythrocyte sedimentation rate and serum levels of creatine kinase may be normal or moderately elevated. EMG shows nonspecific signs of a myopathic process, occasionally mixed with fibrillations. Muscle biopsy is necessary and confirms the inflammatory nature of the process. Dermatomyositis is treated with corticosteroids or other anti-inflammatory drugs. Occasionally, therapy with cytoxan, methotrexate, plasmapheresis, and intravenous gammaglobulin is beneficial. Prognosis is variable. Some patients have spontaneous resolution without therapy while other patients are refractory to all modes of therapy. Death can occur from cardiac involvement, associated gastrointestinal hemorrhage, or secondary complications of immunosuppressive therapy.

Myoneural Junction Disorders

Myasthenia gravis is uncommon in early childhood with fewer than 25% of all patients having their onset before 10 years. The disorder is characterized by generalized weakness, dysphagia, dysphonia, easy fatigability, and external ophthalmoplegia. The typical disorder that affects older children and adults is due to defective function of the post-synaptic membrane. IgG antibodies directed against acetylcholine receptors impair the ability of acetylcholine released from the presynaptic nerve terminal to attach to receptor sites in the clefts of the post-synaptic muscle membrane. Approximately 12% of infants born to mothers with this form of IgG antibody-mediated myasthenia gravis develop passively acquired, transient myasthenia gravis that spontaneously resolves in 2–6 months. These infants may be profoundly weak as neonates, but their prognosis is excellent for full recovery if they receive aggressive supportive care, including mechanical ventilation and anticholinesterase therapy. Other rare forms of non-immune mediated myasthenia have been described in neonates. These forms of congenital, persistent myasthenia gravis also produce generalized weakness.

Diagnosis of myasthenia gravis rests upon the patient's response to test doses of acetylcholinesterase inhibitors such as edrophonium and neostigmine, repetitive nerve stimulation studies, and serum levels of anti-acetylcholine receptor antibodies.

Treatment involves general support and administration of anticholinesterase medications. Pyridostigmine is the most commonly used anticholinesterase and is begun at about 5 mg per kg per day in 4–6 divided doses. The dosage is adjusted to the patient's response and to the occurrence of adverse, cholinergic side-effects. Atropine can be used to control some of the cholinergic side-effects. Cholinergic crisis occurs when the patient is overdosed with anticholinesterase medications. The patient becomes weaker and has copious salivation, excessive lacrimation, abdominal cramping, diarrhea, miosis, and hypotension. Distinguishing between a cholinergic crisis and a myasthenic crisis can usually be accomplished by giving the patient an intravenous test dose of edrophonium (0.1 mg per dose, not exceeding a total of 10 mg per dose). The patient will improve if the weakness is from worsening myasthenia, but will worsen if the weakness is the result of cholinergic crisis. Cholinergic crises are managed by discontinuing anticholinesterase medications and using atropine judiciously. In addition to anticholinesterase medications, other treatment options for myasthenia gravis include use of corticosteroids and early thymectomy. Prognosis for full recovery is excellent for infants with passively acquired, transient neonatal myasthenia gravis. The prognosis of the later onset, IgG-mediated myasthenia is generally good for improvement with therapy, and about 10–15% of young children with myasthenia eventually have spontaneous remission. For some infants with congenital, non-immune myasthenia, weakness may remain unimproved but stable while others become progressively weaker.

Infant botulism represents another disorder of myoneural junction function important in pediatrics. Typically, infants between 2 and 4 months of age ingest *Clostridium botulinum* bacteria. The neurotoxin formed by the bacteria in the child's intestinal tract is absorbed systemically, and attaches with high affinity to the membrane of the presynaptic nerve terminal. The toxin interferes with release of acetylcholine and results in weakness, hypotonia, impaired pupillary light reflexes, impaired extraocular movements, and decreased frequency of stooling. The diagnosis is confirmed by finding abnormalities on repetitive nerve stimulation tests indicative of presynaptic, myoneural junction dysfunction and by identifying botulinum toxin in stool and serum. Treatment is supportive and prognosis excellent for full recovery. Complete recovery, however, can take many months.

Other Disorders

In addition to the neuromuscular disorders described above, acute weakness and flaccidity may result from other diseases. Guillain-Barré syndrome (post-infectious polyradiculoneuritis), acute spinal cord compression, and acute transmyelitis can cause an acute clinical picture of weakness, flaccidity, and hyporeflexia. Associated clinical features such as low back pain, Babinski signs, bowel and bladder dysfunction, and sensory deficits can be used to separate these disorders diagnostically. Spinal fluid examination, nerve conduction studies, and imaging tests will provide additional diagnostic separation.

STROKE IN CHILDHOOD

Stroke is uncommon in children, occurring in 2.5–2.75 children per 100,000 per year. The onset of symptoms may be acute or subacute and may consist of hemiplegia, aphasia, vertigo, diplopia, or

Table 20–6. Conditions associated with stroke in children.

Cardiac
Cyanotic heart disease
Valvular heart disease
Cardiomyopathy
Dysrhythmias
Hematologic disorders
Polycythemia
Thrombocytopenia
Thrombocythemia
Hemoglobinopathies
Coagulopathies
Hypercoagulable states
Leukemia
Systemic vascular disorders
Carotid dissection
Vasculitis
Fibromuscular dysplasia
Diabetes
Familial hyperlipidemia
Hypertension
Homocystinuria
Mitochondrial cytopathy
Intracranial vascular anomalies
Carotid-cavernous fistula
Venous sinus and cortical vein thrombosis
Arteriovenous malformation
Arterial aneurysms
Moyamoya disease

sensory deficits. The differential diagnosis of acute onset focal or lateralized neurologic deficits should include trauma, infection, seizure, and migraine. A thorough evaluation should be done to determine the etiology of stroke so that appropriate therapy and preventive measures can be taken. Congenital cyanotic heart disease is the most common underlying systemic disorder predisposing children to stroke. A search for underlying cardiopulmonary, hematologic, systemic vascular, and intracranial vascular disorders should be undertaken (Table 20–6).

Laboratory investigations are guided by the history and physical findings. Blood studies include CBC, platelet count, sedimentation rate, ANA, electrolytes, BUN, creatinine, coagulation studies, lipid profile, and lactate levels. A urinalysis is performed, and the presence of homocystine in urine determined. An EKG and echocardiogram are indicated for all children suspected of having stroke. Head CT and MRI scans are helpful in defining the location and extent of cerebral infarctions and hemorrhages and may identify abnormal intracranial structures that are etiologically important. The development of MR angiography has drastically reduced the need for invasive, contrast angiography. EEGs frequently show nonspecific abnormalities, but rarely shed light on the cause of stroke.

Initial treatment is directed at correcting the underlying etiology if possible. In patients for whom no etiology is found, stroke recurrence is uncommon, but aspirin or other drugs that inhibit platelet aggregation may be given for several months in an attempt to reduce recurrence risks. Anticoagulation therapy is seldom used in children unless a specific coagulopathy is diagnosed. The prognosis for neurologic recovery is excellent for most children. Seizures occur in about 30% of patients at some point in their clinical course and may require antiepileptic medications.

HEADACHE

Headaches are common in children, occurring in nearly 40% of all children under 7 years of age. Migraine occurs in 2.7% of children by 7 years of age and gradually increases to 11% by 14 years. Onset of migraine by age 4 years is not uncommon. In later childhood, migraine affects twice as many girls as boys. A careful description of the headaches, associated circumstances, and associated neurologic and systemic symptoms will usually differentiate migraine from other types of headache (Table 20–7). Potential emotional problems that might trigger headaches should be identified. A careful history, together with complete general and neurologic examinations, will allow correct classification of the headache and will almost always identify those patients whose headaches are caused by an underlying systemic or progressive neurologic illness. If there is evidence of a specific intracranial condition or systemic illness, diagnostic testing and therapy should be directed at the primary disorder.

Migraine headaches usually last 2–6 hours, but many patients have both longer and shorter attacks. The frequency of headaches can vary from 1 or fewer per year to more than 1 headache a day. Between attacks the child is normal. Migraine headaches in children are commonly accompanied by loss of appetite, gastric discomfort, nausea, vomiting, light-headedness, vertigo, and photophobia. Motion sickness is prominent in about 45% of children with migraine. It is un-

Table 20–7. Features of common headaches in childhood.

Muscle contraction/tension	
	Chronic and protracted
	Diffuse squeezing or pressure sensation
	Band distribution around head
	No prodrome
	Associated anxiety and depression
	Environmental triggers prominent
Migraine	
	Acute, paroxysmal
	Unilateral or bilateral
	Temporal, retro-orbital, or frontal
	Throbbing or pulsating quality
	May have prodrome
	Positive family history (75%)
	Environmental triggers occasionally
Increased intracranial pressure/traction headache	
	Intermittent or chronic
	Progressively increasing severity or frequency through time
	Positional pain
	Diffuse pressure
	No prodrome
	Associated focal or lateralized neurologic deficits

common for children to experience or describe scotomata, visual field cuts, sensory and motor disturbances, dysphasia, or hemiplegia. Older children and adolescents may experience acute confusional episodes or subjective distortions of space, time, and body image perceptions (termed the "Alice-in-Wonderland" syndrome) as part of their migraine attack.

EEGs done during or shortly after an attack of migraine are abnormally slow or mildly dysrhythmic in up to 80% of patients, but normal between attacks. Neuroradiologic studies, such as head CT or MRI scans, are usually not indicated unless the history suggests atypical features or unless there are definite neurologic deficits.

Sleep or rest and simple analgesic therapy are the mainstays of therapy for childhood migraine. Acetaminophen or ibuprofen are usually effective and sufficient for children. For severe, persistent migraines, parenteral doses of chlorpromazine may help calm patients, relieve their nausea, allow them to fall asleep, and avoid the use of narcotics. For prophylaxis of severe or frequent migraine attacks, propranolol, amitriptyline, and cyproheptadine are useful. Calcium channel blockers, corticosteroids, and narcotics are rarely necessary for the treatment of childhood migraine. The role of sumatriptan in the management of childhood migraines has not been well defined.

ACUTE CEREBELLAR ATAXIA OF CHILDHOOD (Acute Cerebellitis)

The syndrome of acute cerebellar ataxia occurs most commonly in children 2–6 years of age. The onset is abrupt. In about 50% of cases, there is a prodromal respiratory or gastrointestinal viral-like illness or an exanthematous illness 2–3 weeks before onset. Well-known associated viral infections include varicella, rubeola, mumps, rubella, echovirus, poliovirus, infectious mononucleosis, and influenza. Bacterial infections such as scarlet fever and salmonellosis have also been implicated.

Ataxia of the trunk and extremities may be mild or so severe that the child is unable to stand or sit without support. Intention tremors may impair the child's ability to reach for objects. Hypotonia, tremor, horizontal nystagmus, and dysarthria are frequently present. The child is irritable, and vomiting is common. Signs of increased intracranial pressure are absent and the fundi are normal. Sensory and reflex examinations are normal.

Cerebrospinal fluid pressure and protein and glucose concentrations are normal. A mild lymphocytosis (up to 30 lymphocyte/mm) may be present in CSF. Attempts should be made to identify the etiologic infectious agent by appropriate virologic, bacteriologic, and immunologic studies on spinal fluid, blood, stool, throat washings, and urine. Head CT and MRI scans are normal. The EEG may show mild, diffuse, generalized background slowing, but these changes are nonspecific and the EEG rapidly returns to normal.

The syndrome of acute, parainfectious cerebellar ataxia must be differentiated from acute cerebellar ataxia due to drugs and toxins, occult neuroblastoma, and posterior fossa tumors. On occasion, acute cerebellar ataxia may be the presenting sign of acute bacterial meningitis, systemic vasculitides, trauma, or an inborn error of metabolism, such as Hartnup's and maple syrup urine disease. Acute disseminated encephalomyelitis and multiple sclerosis can cause acute ataxia in older children and adolescents.

Treatment is supportive. The use of corticosteroids is unnecessary in typical cases. Between 80 and 90% of children completely recover within 6–8 weeks. In the remainder, disorders of behavior and learning, persistent ataxia, abnormal eye movements, and speech impairment may persist for months or years, and recovery may remain incomplete.

NEURODIAGNOSTIC PROCEDURES

Electroencephalography (EEG)

EEG is most useful in evaluation of patients with seizures and patients with unexplained loss of consciousness. Activation procedures such as sleep deprivation, hyperventilation, and photic stimulation help to accentuate and provoke electrocortical, epileptiform abnormalities. Prolonged EEG recordings with or without simultaneous video taping of the patient are valuable in the diagnosis of unusual or difficult to treat seizures as well as sleep apnea, narcolepsy, and other sleep disturbances. An electrically silent EEG supports the diagnosis of death if specific clinical and technical criteria have been met.

Evoked Potentials

Cortical auditory, visual, and somatosensory evoked potentials can be recorded from the scalp overlying the temporal, occipital, and frontoparietal cortex after appropriate, repetitive stimulation of the retina, cochlea, or skin. Abnormalities indicate disturbances along sensory pathways in the peripheral or central nervous system. Since evoked potentials are largely passive examinations, requiring only that the patient remain still, they are particularly useful in the neurologic evaluation of neonates and small children, as well as patients who are unable to cooperate.

Computed Tomographic (CT) Scans

CT scans carry minimal risk and can be performed on an outpatient basis. Radiation exposure is approximately the same as that from a skull x-ray. Intravenous injection of iodinated contrast material helps to visualize structures or lesions with a high degree of vascularity. Excessive enhancement is also indicative of cerebral capillary damage and disruption of the blood-brain barrier.

Magnetic Resonance Imaging (MRI)

MRI is a noninvasive, risk-free technique that uses the magnetic properties primarily of protons in water molecules within the body to produce signals that are converted by computers into images. MRI can clearly delineate brain tumors, edema, ischemic areas, hemorrhages, hydrocephalus, vascular abnormalities, and inflammatory and infectious lesions. Sequential MRI scans are extremely useful in following the structural changes that occur in the brain and spinal cord in many neurodegenerative and metabolic disorders. Bone produces almost no image on MRI scans, making this test valuable in evaluating structures within the posterior fossa.

Head Ultrasonography

Head ultrasonography provides an excellent way to rapidly visualize the ventricles and midline brain structures in infants with open, anterior fontanelles. Ultrasound studies are used in many nurseries to screen premature neonates for intracranial hemorrhage and diagnose and follow-up periventricular ischemic injury and ventriculomegaly.

Cerebral Angiography

Angiography is useful in diagnosing cerebrovascular disorders and vascular malformations. Noninvasive CT and MRI scans together with MR angiography have eliminated the need for invasive angiography in many instances.

Sedation for Neurodiagnostic Procedures

Sedation for neuroradiologic and other neurodiagnostic procedures can be achieved with rectally administered chloral hydrate (30–60 mg/kg/dose) or parenterally administered pentobarbital (3–5 mg/kg/dose). Sedation is given at least 20 minutes before the procedure. When sedatives are administered, trained personnel and equipment should be readily available to support blood pressure and respirations in the event of an unexpected adverse reaction.

Bones & Joints | 21

Robert E. Eilert, MD

ORTHOPEDIC PROBLEMS IN THE NEWBORN

CONGENITAL AMPUTATIONS

Congenital amputations may be due to teratogens (eg, drugs or viruses), amniotic bands, or metabolic diseases (eg, diabetes in the mother) or, in rare cases, may be hereditary defects. Most are spontaneous and not genetically determined. The history of the pregnancy must be carefully reviewed for possible teratogenic factors. According to the currently accepted international classification, amputations are either terminal or longitudinal. In terminal amputation, all parts are missing distal to the level of involvement—eg, absence of the forearm, wrist, and hand in the case of a terminal below-the-elbow amputation. A longitudinal amputation consists of partial absence of structures in the extremity along one side or the other. In radial clubhand, the entire radius is absent, but the thumb may be either hypoplastic or completely absent. Complex tissue defects are nearly always associated with longitudinal amputations in that the associated nerves and muscles are usually not completely represented when a bone is absent. Bones within the axial skeleton likewise may be absent. Congenital absence of the sacrum is often associated with diabetes in the mother.

Terminal amputations are treated by means of a prosthesis, eg, to compensate for shortness of one leg. With longitudinal deficiencies, constructive surgery may be feasible with the objective of reducing deformity and stabilizing joints.

Lower extremity prostheses are best fitted at about the time of normal walking (12–15 months of age). Lower extremity prostheses are consistently well accepted, as they are necessary for balancing and walking. Upper extremity prostheses are not as well accepted. Fitting the child with a dummy type prosthesis as early as 6 months of age has the advantage of instilling an accustomed pattern of proper length and bimanual manipulation. Children fitted later than age 2 years nearly always reject upper extremity prostheses.

Children quickly learn how to function with their prostheses and can lead active lives, participating in sports with peers.

METATARSUS VARUS

Metatarsus varus is characterized by adduction of the forefoot on the hindfoot, with the heel in normal position or slightly valgus. The longitudinal arch is often creased vertically when the deformity is more rigid. The lateral border of the foot demonstrates sharp angulation at the level of the base of the fifth metatarsal, and this bone will be especially prominent. The deformity varies from flexible to rigid. Most flexible deformities are secondary to intrauterine posture and usually resolve spontaneously.

If the deformity is rigid and cannot be manipulated past the midline, splinting is appropriate to ensure the resolution of the deformity. The prognosis for this common deformity of the foot is excellent in that 85% correct by age 3–4 years with the remainder having mild problems fitting shoes.

CLUBFOOT

Classic **talipes equinovarus**, consists of three associated deformities: equinus or plantar flexion of the foot at the ankle joint, varus or inversion deformity of the heel, and forefoot varus. The incidence of talipes equinovarus is approximately 1:1000 live births. Any infant with a clubfoot should be examined carefully for associated anomalies, especially of the spine. Clubfoot tends to follow a hereditary pattern in some families or may be part of a generalized neuromuscular syndrome such as arthrogryposis or myelodysplasia.

Treatment consists manipulation of the foot to stretch the contracted tissues on the medial and posterior aspects, followed by splinting to hold the correction. When this is instituted in the nursery shortly after birth, correction is achieved much more rapidly. When treatment is delayed, the foot tends to become more rigid within a matter of days.

About half of children with clubfoot eventually need an operative procedure to lengthen the tightened structures about the foot.

A supple foot that is easily corrected by strapping and casting has a more favorable prognosis. If the foot is rigid, operative correction is indicated for normal function in walking.

DYSPLASIA OF THE HIP JOINT

In a child with dysplasia of the hip, the femoral head and the acetabulum may be in partial contact at birth. This condition is termed subluxation of the hip. A more severe defect is complete loss of contact between the femoral head and acetabulum, in which case there is frank dislocation of the hip, with the femoral head nearly always displaced laterally and superiorly due to muscle pull. At birth, there is lack of the development of both the acetabulum and the femur in cases of congenital hip dysplasia. The dysplasia becomes progressive with growth unless the dislocation is corrected. If the dislocation is corrected in the first few days or weeks of life, the dysplasia is completely reversible and a normal hip can develop. As the child becomes older and the dislocation or subluxation persists, the dysplasia will worsen to the point where it will not be completely reversible, especially after the walking age. It is important to diagnose the deformity in the nursery or, at the latest, the 6-week checkup.

Clinical Findings

The diagnosis of congenital hip dislocation in the newborn depends upon demonstrating instability of the joint by placing the infant on its back and obtaining complete relaxation by feeding with a bottle if necessary. The examiner's long finger is then placed over the greater trochanter and the thumb over the inner side of the thigh. Both hips are flexed 90 degrees and then slowly abducted from the midline. With gentle pressure, an attempt is made to lift the greater trochanter forward. A feeling of slipping as the head goes into the acetabulum is a sign of instability (Ortolani's sign). In other infants, the joint is more stable, and the deformity must be provoked by applying slight pressure with the thumb on the medial side of the thigh as the thigh is adducted, thus slipping the hip posteriorly and eliciting a jerk as the hip dislocates (Barlow's sign). The signs of instability are the most reliable criteria for diagnosing dislocation of the hip in the newborn. X-rays of the pelvis are notoriously unreliable until about 6 weeks of age.

After the first month of life, the signs of instability become less evident. Contractures begin to develop about the hip joint, causing limitation of abduction. Normally, the hip should abduct fully to 90 degrees on either side during the first few months of life. It is important that the pelvis be held level to detect asymmetry of abduction. When the hips and knees are flexed, the knees are at unequal heights, with the dislocated side lower. After the first few weeks of life, x-ray examination becomes more valuable, with lateral displacement of the femoral head being the most reliable finding. In mild cases, the only abnormality may be increased steepness of the acetabular roof, so that the acetabular angle is greater than 35 degrees.

If dysplasia of the hip has not been diagnosed during the first year of life and the child begins to walk, there will be a painless limp and a lurch to the affected side. When the child stands on the affected leg, there is a dip of the pelvis on the opposite side owing to inefficiency of the gluteus medius muscle. In children with bilateral dislocations, the loss of abduction is almost symmetric and may be deceiving. Abduction, however, is never complete, and x-ray of the pelvis is indicated in children with incomplete abduction in the first few months of life. As a child with bilateral dislocation of the hips begins to walk, she does so with a waddle. The perineum is widened as a result of lateral displacement of the hips, and there is flexion contracture as a result of posterior displacement of the hips. This flexion contracture contributes to marked lordosis, and the greater trochanters are easily palpable in their elevated position. Treatment is still possible after the child begins to walk, but the results are not nearly as effective as in children treated in the nursery.

Treatment

Dislocation or dysplasia diagnosed in the first few weeks or months of life can easily be treated by splinting, with the hip maintained in flexion and abduction. Forced abduction is contraindicated, as this often leads to avascular necrosis of the femoral head. The use of double or triple diapers is never indicated, since diapers are not adequate to obtain proper positioning of the hip. In cases of joint laxity without true dislocation, improvement will be spontaneous and diapers are excessive treatment.

Various splints to maintain flexion and abduction of the hip are available. The Pavlik harness is the most popular. Treatment of children requiring splints is best supervised by an orthopedic surgeon.

In the first 4 months of life, reduction can be obtained by simply flexing and abducting the hip; no other manipulation is usually necessary. If force is used to reduce the hip, the excessive pressure may cause avascular necrosis. In such cases, preoperative traction for 2–3 weeks may be used to relax soft tissues about the hip. Following traction in which the femur is brought down opposite the acetabulum, reduction can be easily achieved without force under general anesthesia. The child is then placed in a hipspica cast, which is used for approximately 6 months. If the reduction is not stable within a reasonable range following closed reduction, open reduction may be necessary combined with plication of the lax capsule in order to maintain reduction.

If reduction is done at an older age, operations to correct the deformities of the acetabulum and femur may be necessary during growth.

TORTICOLLIS

Wryneck deformities in infancy may be due either to injury to the sternocleidomastoid muscle during delivery or to disease affecting the cervical spine. In the case of muscular deformity, the chin is rotated to the side opposite to the affected sternocleidomastoid muscle contracture, and the head is tilted toward the side of the contracture. A mass felt in the midportion of the sternocleidomastoid muscle does not represent a true tumor but fibrous transformation within the muscle.

In mild cases, passive stretching is usually effective. If the deformity has not been corrected by passive stretching within the first year of life, surgical division of the muscle will correct it. If the deformity is left untreated, an unsightly facial asymmetry will result.

Torticollis is occasionally associated with congenital deformities of the cervical spine, and x-rays of the spine are indicated in all cases.

Acute torticollis may follow upper respiratory infection or mild trauma in children. Rotatory subluxation of the upper cervical spine should be sought by appropriate x-ray views. Traction or a cervical collar usually results in resolution of the symptoms within 1 or 2 days.

TALIPES CALCANEOVALGUS

Talipes calcaneovalgus is characterized by excessive dorsiflexion at the ankle and eversion of the foot. When present at birth, it almost always corrects spontaneously. The deformity is the reverse of classic clubfoot (talipes equinovarus) and is due to intrauterine position.

Treatment consists of passive exercises by the parents, stretching the foot into plantar flexion. In rare instances, it may be necessary to use casts to help with positioning after manipulation. Complete correction is the rule.

MUSCULOSKELETAL TRAUMA (Basic Principles of Examination & Treatment)

The force involved and the pattern of injury determine the structures which are damaged in musculoskeletal trauma. Spending the time to gain as accurate a history as possible will expedite the examination. After deciding that the rare limb threatening injury has not occurred, the next concern is whether bone and/or soft tissue have been disrupted. Once an initial visual assessment and palpation have been done, a splint should be applied to the injured part to relieve pain and prevent further damage during transportation. A fracture causes local tenderness and swelling, if not deformity. It is a rare fracture that cannot be diagnosed by looking and feeling, if the clinician is thorough and suspicious.

SOFT TISSUE TRAUMA (Sprains, Strains, & Contusions)

General information about soft tissue trauma is presented in Chapter 22. Specific entities will be discussed in greater detail in this section.

Ankle Sprains

The history will indicate that the injury was by either forceful inversion or eversion. The more common inversion injury results in tearing or injury to the lateral ligaments, whereas an eversion injury will injure the medial ligaments of the ankle. The injured ligaments may be identified by means of careful palpation for point tenderness around the ankle.

If there is more severe trauma resulting in tearing of a ligament, instability of the joint may be demonstrated by gross examination or by stress testing with x-ray documentation. Such deformity of the joint may cause persistent instability resulting from inaccurate apposition of the ligament ends during healing. If instability is evident, surgical repair of the torn ligament may be indicated.

Knee Sprains

Sprains of the collateral and cruciate ligaments are uncommon in children. These ligaments are so strong that it is more common to injure the epiphyseal growth plates, which are the weakest structures in the region of the knees of children. In adolescence, the growth plates close, and a rupture of the anterior cruciate ligament can result from a hyperextension. In such instances, the injury is apparent by anterior laxity on knee examination in extension. In most instances, operative correction is indicated.

Back Sprains

Sprains of the ligaments and muscles of the back are unusual in children but may occur as a result of violent trauma from automobile accidents or athletic injuries. A child with back pain should not be presumed to have had trauma to the spine unless the history warrants that conclusion. The reason for back pain should be carefully sought by x-ray and physical examination. Inflammation, infection, and tumors are more common causes of back pain in children than sprains.

Myositis Ossificans

Ossification within muscle occurs when there is sufficient trauma to cause a hematoma that later heals in the manner of a fracture. The injury is usually a contusion and occurs most commonly in the quadriceps of the thigh or the triceps of the arm. When such a severe injury with hematoma is recognized, it is important to splint the extremity and avoid activity. If further activity is allowed, ossification may reach spectacular proportions and resemble an osteosarcoma.

Disability is great, with local swelling and heat and extreme pain upon the slightest motion of the adjacent joint. The limb should be rested, with the knee in extension or the elbow in 90 degrees of flexion, until the local reaction has subsided. Once local heat and tenderness have decreased, gentle active exercises may be initiated. Passive stretching exercises are not indicated, because they may stimulate the ossification reaction. It is occasionally necessary to excise excessive bony tissue if it interferes with muscle function once the reaction is mature. Surgery should not be attempted before 9 months to a year after injury, because it may restart the process and lead to an even more severe reaction.

TRAUMATIC SUBLUXATIONS & DISLOCATIONS

Dislocation of a joint is always associated with severe damage to the ligaments and joint capsule. In contrast to fracture treatment, which may be safely postponed, dislocations must be reduced immediately. Dislocations can usually be reduced by gentle sustained traction. No anesthetic may be necessary immediately after the injury, because of the protective anesthesia produced by the injury. Following reduction, the joint should be splinted for transportation of the patient.

The dislocated joint should be treated by immobilization for at least 3 weeks, followed by graduated active exercises through a full range of motion. Physical therapy is usually not indicated for young children with injuries. As a matter of fact, vigorous manipulation of the joint by a therapist may be harmful. The child should be permitted to return to activity at his or her own pace.

Subluxation of the Radial Head (Nursemaid's Elbow)

Infants frequently sustain subluxation of the radial head as a result of being lifted or pulled by the hand. The child appears with the elbow fully pronated and painful. The usual complaint is that the child's elbow will not bend. X-rays are normal, but there is point tenderness over the radial head. When the elbow is placed in full supination and slowly moved from full flexion to full extension, a click may be palpated at the level of the radial head. The relief of pain is remarkable, as the child usually stops crying immediately. The elbow may be immobilized in a sling for comfort for a day.

Pulled elbow may be a clue to battering. This should be remembered during examination, especially if the problem is recurrent.

Recurrent Dislocation of the Patella

Recurrent dislocation of the patella is more common in loose-jointed individuals, especially adolescent girls. If the patella completely dislocates, it nearly always goes laterally. Pain is severe, and the patient is brought to the doctor with the knee slightly flexed, an obvious bony mass lateral to the knee joint, and a flat area over the usual location of the patella anteriorly. X-rays confirm the diagnosis. The patella may be reduced by extending the knee and placing slight pressure on the patella while gentle traction is exerted on the leg. In subluxation of the patella, the symptoms may be more subtle, and the patient may say that the knee "gives out" or "jumps out of place."

In the case of complete dislocation, the knee should be immobilized for 3–4 weeks, followed by a physical therapy program for strengthening the quadriceps muscle. Operation may be necessary to tighten the knee joint capsule if dislocation or subluxation is recurrent. In such instances, if the patella is not stabilized, repeated dislocation produces damage to the articular cartilage of the patellofemoral joint and premature degenerative arthritis.

EPIPHYSEAL SEPARATIONS & FRACTURES

Epiphyseal Separations

In children, **epiphyseal separations and fractures** are more common than ligamentous injuries because the ligaments of the joints are generally stronger than the associated growth plates. In instances where dislocation is suspected, an x-ray should be taken in order to rule out epiphyseal fracture. Films of the opposite extremity, especially around the elbow, may be valuable for comparison. Reduction of a fractured epiphysis should be done under anesthesia in order to align the growth plate with the least amount of force necessary. Fractures across the growth plate may produce bony bridges that will cause premature cessation of growth or angular deformities in the growth plate. Epiphyseal fractures around the shoulder, wrist, and fingers can usually be treated by closed reduction, but fractures of the epiphyses around the elbow often require open reduction. In the lower extremity, accurate reduction of the epiphyseal plate is necessary to prevent joint deformity if a joint surface is involved. Unfortunately, some of the most severe injuries to the epiphyseal plate occur from compression injuries, where the amount of force is not immediately apparent. If angular deformities result, corrective osteotomy can be done.

Torus Fractures

Torus fractures consist of "buckling" of the cortex as a result of minimal angular trauma. They usually occur in the distal radius or ulna. Alignment is satisfactory, and simple immobilization for 3–5 weeks is sufficient.

Greenstick Fractures

With **greenstick fractures**, there is frank disruption of the cortex on one side of the bone but no discernible cleavage plane on the opposite side. These fractures are angulated but not displaced. Reduction is achieved by straightening the arm into normal alignment, and reduction is maintained by a snugly fitting cast. It is necessary to x-ray children with greenstick fractures again in a week to 10 days to make certain that the reduction has been maintained. A slight angular deformity will be corrected by remodeling of the bone. The farther the fracture is from the growing end of the bone, the longer the time required for remodeling. The fracture can be considered healed when there are no findings of tenderness and local swelling or heat and when adequate bony callus is seen on x-ray.

Fracture of the Clavicle

Clavicular fractures are very common injuries in infants and children. They can be immobilized by a figure-of-8 dressing that retracts the shoulders and brings the clavicle to normal length. The healing callus will be apparent when the fracture has consolidated, but this unsightly lump will generally resolve over a period of months to a year.

Supracondylar Fractures of the Humerus

Supracondylar fractures tend to occur in children ages 3–6 years and are potentially dangerous because of the proximity to the brachial artery in the distal arm. They are usually associated with a significant amount of trauma, and swelling may be severe. Volkmann's ischemic contracture of muscle may occur as a result of vascular embarrassment. When severe swelling is present, the safest course is to place the arm in traction and carefully observe nerve function and the vascular supply to the hand. In these cases, the children should be hospitalized. If the blood supply is compromised, exposure of the brachial artery may be necessary, although this is rarely needed when satisfactory reduction and traction are employed. Complications associated with supracondylar fractures also include a resultant cubitus varus secondary to poor reduction. It is often difficult to ascertain adequacy of the reduction because a flexed position is necessary to maintain normal alignment. Such a "gunstock" deformity of the elbow may be somewhat unsightly but does not usually interfere with joint function.

INFECTIONS OF THE BONES & JOINTS

OSTEOMYELITIS

Osteomyelitis is an infectious process that usually begins in the spongy or medullary bone and then extends to involve compact or cortical bone. It is more common in boys than in girls or in adults of either sex. The lower extremities are most often affected, and there is commonly a history of trauma. Osteomyelitis may occur as a result of direct invasion from the outside through a penetrating wound (nail) or open fracture, but hematogenous spread of infection (eg, pyoderma or upper respiratory tract infection) from other infected areas is more common. The most common infecting organism is *Staphylococcus aureus*, which seems to have a special tendency to infect the metaphyses of growing bones. Anatomically, circulation in the long bones is such that the arterial supply to the metaphysis just below the growth plate is by end arteries, which turn sharply to end in venous sinusoids, causing a relative stasis. In the infant under 1 year of age, there is direct vascular communication with the epiphysis across the growth plate, so that direct spread may occur from the metaphysis to the epiphysis and subsequently into the joint. In the older child, the growth plate provides an effective barrier and the epiphysis is usually not involved, although the infection spreads retrograde from the metaphysis into the diaphysis and, by rupture through the cortical bone, down along the diaphysis beneath the periosteum.

Exogenous Osteomyelitis

To avoid osteomyelitis by direct extension, all wounds must be carefully examined and cleansed. Cultures of the wound made at the time of exploration and debridement may be useful if signs of inflammation and infection develop subsequently. In extensive or contaminated wounds, antibiotic coverage is indicated. Contaminated wounds should be left open and secondary closure performed 3–5 days later. If at the time of delayed closure further necrotic tissue is present, it should be excised.

If the wound is acquired outside the hospital, a synthetic penicillin is adequate for most wounds. After cultures have been read, an appropriate alternative antibiotic can be chosen if there is lingering inflammation. A tetanus toxoid booster is indicated for any questionable immunization history.

Once exogenous osteomyelitis has become established, treatment becomes more complicated, requiring extensive surgical debridement and drainage followed by careful antibiotic management (in particular for *Staphylococcus aureus*). Coverage for *Pseudomonas* should be added in cases involving nail puncture wounds. These cases require hospitalization and the use of intravenous antibiotics.

Hematogenous Osteomyelitis

Hematogenous osteomyelitis is usually caused by pyogenic bacteria; 85% of cases are due to staphylococci. Streptococci are rare causes of osteomyelitis today. Children with sickle cell anemia are especially prone to osteomyelitis caused by salmonellae.

Clinical Findings

A. Symptoms & Signs: In infants, the manifestations of osteomyelitis may be quite subtle, presenting as irritability, diarrhea, or failure to feed properly; the temperature may be normal or slightly low; and the white blood count may be normal or only slightly elevated. In older children, the manifestations are more striking, with severe local tenderness and pain, high fever, rapid pulse, and elevated white blood cell count and sedimentation rate. Osteomyelitis of a lower extremity often presents around the knee in a child 7–10 years of age. Tenderness is most marked over the metaphysis of the bone where the process has its origin.

B. Laboratory Findings: Blood cultures are often positive early. The most significant test in infancy is the aspiration of pus when suspicion arises because of lack of movement in a painful extremity. It is useful to insert a needle to the bone in the area of suspected infection and aspirate any fluid present. This fluid can be smeared and stained for organisms and cultured. Even edema fluid may be useful for determining the causative organism. The white blood cell count is usually elevated, and the sedimentation rate is high.

C. Imaging: The first manifestation to appear on x-ray is nonspecific local swelling. This is followed by elevation of the periosteum, with formation of new bone from the cambium layer of the periosteum occurring after 3–6 days. As the infection becomes chronic, areas of cortical bone are isolated by pus spreading down the medullary canal, causing rarefaction and demineralization of the bone. Such isolated pieces of cortex become ischemic and form sequestra (dead bone fragments). These x-ray findings are late, and osteomyelitis should be diagnosed clinically before significant x-ray findings are present. Bone scan is valuable in suspected cases before x-rays become positive.

Treatment

A. Specific Measures: Antibiotics should be begun intravenously as soon as the diagnosis of osteomyelitis is made. Use of methicillin, another semisynthetic penicillin, or a cephalosporin that covers penicillinase-producing *S aureus* is recommended. Gentamicin can also be given to combat gram-negative organisms until the results of cultures are available, and *Salmonella* should be covered in children with sickle cell. Antibiotics should be continued until swelling, tenderness, and local discharge have ceased and the white blood cell count and erythrocyte sedimentation rate are normal, usually a period of at least 1 month. Serial x-rays can also be used to follow bone healing. Antibiotic therapy by the intravenous route should be continued until all clinical signs are improved, including sedimentation rate. For a reliable family, oral medication may be started at that time (about 10 days), adjusting dosage by serum killing power and continued monitoring of erythrocyte sedimentation rate for at least 1 month after the ESR has returned to normal.

B. General Measures: Splinting of the limb minimizes pain and decreases spread of the infection by lymphatic channels through the soft tissue. The splint should be removed periodically to allow active use of adjacent joints and prevent stiffening and muscle atrophy. In chronic osteomyelitis, splinting may be necessary to guard against fracture of the weakened bone.

C. Surgical Measures: Aspiration of the metaphysis is a useful diagnostic measure in any case of suspected osteomyelitis. Osteomyelitis represents a collection of pus under pressure within the body. In the first 24–72 hours, it may be possible to abort osteomyelitis by the use of antibiotics alone. However, if frank pus is aspirated from the bone, surgical drainage is indicated. If the infection has not shown a dramatic response to antibiotics within 24 hours in questionable cases, surgical drainage is also indicated. It is important that all devitalized soft tissue be removed and adequate exposure of the bone obtained in order to permit free drainage. Excessive amounts of bone should not be removed when draining acute osteomyelitis, since they may not be completely replaced by the normal healing process.

In questionable cases, little damage has been done by surgical drainage, but failure to drain the pus in acute cases may lead to more severe damage.

Prognosis

When osteomyelitis is diagnosed in the early clinical stages and prompt antibiotic therapy is begun, the prognosis is excellent. If the process has been unattended for a week to 10 days, there is almost always some permanent loss of bone structure, as well as the possibility of growth abnormality.

PYOGENIC ARTHRITIS

The source of **pyogenic arthritis** varies according to the age of the child. In the infant, pyogenic arthritis often develops by spread from adjacent osteomyelitis. In the older child, it presents as an isolated infection, usually without bony involvement. In teenagers with pyogenic arthritis, an underlying systemic disease is usually the cause, eg, an obvious generalized infection or an organism that has an affinity for joints, such as the gonococcus.

In infants, the most common cause of pyogenic arthritis is *S aureus*, although gram-negative organisms may be seen. In children between 4 months and 4 years of age, *Haemophilus influenzae* is a common causative organism.

The initial effusion of the joint rapidly becomes purulent. An effusion of the joint may accompany osteomyelitis in the adjacent bone. A white blood cell count exceeding 100,000/μL in the joint fluid indicates a definite purulent infection. Generally, spread of infection is from the bone into the joint, but unattended pyogenic arthritis may also affect adjacent bone. The sedimentation rate is elevated.

Clinical Findings

A. Symptoms & Signs: In older children, the signs are striking, with fever, malaise, vomiting, and restriction of motion. In infants, pseudo-paralysis of the limb due to inflammatory neuritis may be evident. Infection of the hip joint in infants can be diagnosed if suspicion is aroused by decreased abduction of the hip in an infant who is irritable or feeding poorly. A history of umbilical catheter treatment in the newborn nursery should alert the physician to the possibility of pyogenic arthritis of the hip.

B. Imaging: Early distention of the joint capsule is nonspecific and difficult to measure by x-ray. In the infant with unrecognized pyogenic arthritis, dislocation of the joint may follow within a few days as a result of distention of the capsule by pus. Later changes include destruction of the joint space, resorption of epiphyseal cartilage, and erosion of the adjacent bone of the metaphysis.

Treatment

Diagnosis may be made by aspiration of the joint. In the hip joint, pyogenic arthritis is most easily treated by surgical drainage. In more superficial joints, such as the knee, aspiration of the joint at least twice daily may maintain adequate drainage. If fever and clinical symptoms do not subside within 24 hours after treatment is begun, open surgical drainage is indicated. Antibiotics can be specifically selected based on cultures of the aspirated pus. Before the results of cultures are available, treatment by methicillin and gentamicin will cover the usual etiologic organisms. If *H influenzae* is suspected, an extended spectrum cephalosporin (e.g., ceftriaxone) can be used.

Prognosis

The prognosis is excellent if the joint is drained early, before damage to the articular cartilage has occurred. If infection is present for more than 24 hours, there is dissolution of the proteoglycans in the articular cartilage, with subsequent arthrosis and fibrosis of the joint. Damage to the growth plate may also occur, especially within the hip joint, where the epiphyseal plate is intracapsular. This damage is usually due to interruption of blood supply producing osteonecrosis.

NONTRAUMATIC HIP PAIN OR LIMP

TRANSIENT ("TOXIC") SYNOVITIS OF THE HIP

The most common cause of limping and pain in the hip of children in the United States is **transitory synovitis**, an acute inflammatory reaction that often follows an upper respiratory infection and is generally self-limited. In questionable cases, aspiration of the hip yields only yellowish fluid, ruling out pyogenic arthritis. Generally, however, toxic synovitis of the hip is not associated with elevation of the white blood cell count or a temperature above 38.3° C (101° F). It classically affects children 3–10 years of age and is more common in boys. There is limitation of motion of the hip joint, particularly internal rotation, and x-ray changes are nonspecific, with some swelling apparent in the soft tissues around the joint.

Treatment consists of bed rest and the use of traction with slight flexion of the hip. Aspirin may shorten the course of the disease, although even with no treatment the disease usually is self-limited to a matter of days. It is important to maintain x-ray follow-up, since transient synovitis may be the precursor of avascular necrosis of the femoral head (see next section) in a small percentage of patients. X-rays can be obtained at 1 month and 3 months, or earlier if there is persistent limp or pain.

AVASCULAR NECROSIS OF THE PROXIMAL FEMUR (Legg-Calvé-Perthes Disease)

The vascular supply of bone is generally precarious, and when it is interrupted, necrosis results. In contrast to other body tissues that undergo infarction, bone removes necrotic tissue and replaces it with living bone in a process called "creeping substitution." This replacement of necrotic bone may be so complete and so perfect that a completely normal bone results. Adequacy of replacement depends upon the age of the patient, the presence or absence of associated infection, congruity of the involved joint, and other physiologic and mechanical factors.

Because of their rapid growth in relation to their blood supply, the secondary ossification centers in the epiphyses are subject to avascular necrosis. Though the pathologic and radiologic features of avascular necrosis of the epiphyses are well known, the cause is not generally agreed upon. Necrosis may follow known causes such as trauma or infection, but idiopathic lesions usually develop during periods of rapid growth of the epiphyses. Thus, the highest incidence of Legg-Calvé-Perthes disease is between 4 and 8 years of age.

Clinical Findings

A. Symptoms & Signs: Persistent pain is the most common symptom, and the patient may present with limp or limitation of motion.

B. Laboratory Findings: Laboratory findings, including studies of joint aspirates, are normal.

C. Imaging: X-ray findings correlate with the progression of the process and the extent of necrosis. The early finding is effusion of the joint associated with slight widening of the joint space and periarticular swelling. Decreased bone density in and around the joint is apparent after a few weeks. The necrotic ossification center appears more dense than the surrounding viable structures, and there is collapse or narrowing of the femoral head.

As replacement of the necrotic ossification center occurs, there is rarefaction of the bone in a patchwork fashion, producing alternating areas of rarefaction and relative density or "fragmentation" of the epiphysis.

In the hip, there may be widening of the femoral head associated with flattening. If infarction has extended across the growth plate, there will be a radiolucent lesion within the metaphysis. If the growth center of the femoral head has been damaged so that normal growth does not occur, varus deformity of the femoral neck will occur as a result of overgrowth of the greater trochanteric apophysis.

Eventually, complete replacement of the epiphysis will become apparent as new bone replaces necrotic bone. The final shape of the head will depend upon the extent of the necrosis and collapse that has occurred.

Differential Diagnosis

Differential diagnosis includes inflammatory and infectious lesions of the joints or apophyses. Transient synovitis of the hip may be distinguished from Legg-Calvé-Perthes disease by serial x-rays.

Treatment

Treatment consists simply of protection of the joint. If the joint is deeply seated within the acetabulum and normal joint motion is maintained, a reasonably good result can be expected. The hip is held in abduction and internal rotation in order to fulfill this purpose. Braces may be used. Surgery may be necessary for late deformity.

Prognosis

The prognosis for complete replacement of the necrotic femoral head in a child is excellent, but the functional result will depend upon the amount of deformity that develops during the time the softened structure exists. In Legg-Calvé-Perthes disease, the prognosis depends upon the completeness of involvement of the epiphyseal center. In general, patients with metaphyseal defects, those in whom the disease develops late in childhood, and those who have more complete involvement of the femoral head have a poorer prognosis.

EPIPHYSIOLYSIS
(Slipped Capital Femoral Epiphysis)

Epiphysiolysis is the separation of the proximal femoral epiphysis through the growth plate. The head of the femur is usually displaced medially and posteriorly relative to the neck of the femur. The condition occurs in adolescence and is more common in overweight children. Slightly over 40% of the children so affected are of the obese, hypogenital body type.

Occasionally, the condition occurs as an acute episode resulting from a fall or direct trauma to the hip. Commonly, there are vague symptoms over a protracted period of time in an otherwise healthy child who presents with pain and limp. The pain is often referred into the thigh or the medial side of the knee. It is important to examine the hip joint in any child complaining of knee pain, particularly in adolescents. The consistent finding on physical examination is limitation of internal rotation of the hip. There usually is also an associated hip flexion contracture as well as local tenderness about the hip. X-rays should be taken in both the anteroposterior and lateral planes. These must be carefully examined in early cases in order to show an abnormality where displacement of the femoral head occurs posteriorly, which is usually most easily seen on the lateral view.

Treatment is based on the same principles that govern treatment of fracture of the femoral neck in adults in that the head of the femur is fixed to the neck of the femur and the fracture line allowed to heal. Unfortunately, the severe complication of avascular necrosis occurs in 30% of these patients.

The long-term prognosis is guarded because most of these patients continue to be overweight and overstress their hip joints. Follow-up studies have shown a high incidence of premature degenerative arthritis in this group of patients. The development of avascular necrosis almost guarantees a poor prognosis, since new bone does not replace the femoral head at this late stage of skeletal growth.

About 30% of patients have bilateral involvement, and patients should be followed for slipping of the opposite side, which may occur as long as 1 or 2 years after the primary episode.

NONTRAUMATIC KNEE PAIN

OSTEOCHONDRITIS DISSECANS

In **osteochondritis dissecans**, there is a pie-shaped necrotic area of bone and cartilage adjacent to the articular surface. The fragment of bone may be broken off from the host bone and displaced into the joint as a loose body. If it remains attached, the necrotic fragment may be completely replaced by creeping substitution.

The pathologic process is precisely the same as that described above for avascular necrosing lesions of ossification centers. However, since these lesions are adjacent to articular cartilage, there may be joint damage.

The most common sites of these lesions are the knee (medial femoral condyle), the elbow joint (capitellum), and the talus (superior lateral dome).

Joint pain is the usual presenting complaint. However, local swelling or locking may be present, particularly if there is a fragment free in the joint. Laboratory studies are normal.

Treatment consists of protection of the involved area from mechanical damage. If there is a fragment free within the joint as a loose body, it must be surgically removed. For some marginal lesions, it may be worthwhile to drill the necrotic fragment in order to encourage more rapid vascular ingrowth and replacement. If large areas of a weight-bearing joint are involved, secondary degenerative arthritis may result.

FIBROUS DYSPLASIA

Dysplastic fibrous tissue replacement of the medullary canal is accompanied by the formation of metaplastic bone in fibrous dysplasia. Three forms of the disease are recognized: monostotic, polyostotic, and polyostotic with endocrine disturbances (precocious puberty in females, hyperthyroidism, and hyperadrenalism, ie, Albright's syndrome).

Clinical Findings

A. Symptoms & Signs: The lesion or lesions may be asymptomatic. Pain, if present, is probably due to pathologic fractures. In females, endocrine disturbances may be present in the polyostotic variety and associated with café au lait spots.

B. Laboratory Findings: Laboratory findings are normal unless endocrine disturbances are present, in which case there may be increased secretion of gonadotropic, thyroid, or adrenal hormones.

C. Imaging: The lesion begins centrally within the medullary canal, usually of a long bone, and expands slowly. Pathologic fracture may occur. If metaplastic bone predominates, the contents of the lesion will be of the density of bone. Marked deformity of the bone may result, and a shepherd's crook deformity of the upper femur is a classic feature of the disease. The disease is often asymmetric, and limb length disturbances may occur as a result of stimulation of epiphyseal cartilage growth.

Differential Diagnosis

The differential diagnosis may include other fibrous lesions of bone as well as destructive lesions such as bone cyst, eosinophilic granuloma, aneurysmal bone cyst, nonossifying fibroma, enchondroma, and chondromyxoid fibroma.

Treatment

If the lesion is small and asymptomatic, no treatment is needed. If the lesion is large and produces or threatens pathologic fracture, curettage and bone grafting are indicated.

Prognosis

Unless the lesions impair epiphyseal growth, the prognosis is good. Lesions tend to enlarge during the growth period but are stable during adult life. Malignant transformation is rare.

UNICAMERAL BONE CYST

Unicameral bone cyst appears in the metaphysis of a long bone, usually in the femur or humerus. It begins within the medullary canal adjacent to the epiphyseal cartilage. It probably results from some fault in enchondral ossification. The lesion is usually identified when a pathologic fracture occurs, producing pain. Laboratory findings are normal. On x-rays, the cyst is identified centrally within the medullary canal, producing expansion of the cortex and thinning over the widest portion of the cyst.

Treatment consists of curettage of the cyst if it is producing pain. The cyst may heal after a fracture and not require treatment. Curettage should be delayed if surgery would risk damage to the adjacent growth plate.

The prognosis is excellent. Some cysts will heal following pathologic fracture.

ANEURYSMAL BONE CYST

Aneurysmal bone cyst is similar to unicameral bone cyst, but it contains blood rather than clear fluid. It usually occurs in a slightly eccentric position in the long bone, expanding the cortex of the bone but not breaking the cortex, although some extraosseous mass may be produced. On x-rays, the lesion appears somewhat larger than the width of the epiphyseal cartilage, and this feature distinguishes it from unicameral bone cyst.

The aneurysmal bone cyst is filled by large vascular lakes, and the stoma of the cyst contains fibrous tissue and areas of metaplastic ossification.

The lesion may appear quite aggressive histologically, and it is important to differentiate it from osteosarcoma or hemangioma. Treatment is by curettage and bone grafting, and the prognosis is excellent.

BAKER'S CYST

Baker's cyst is a herniation of the synovium in the knee joint into the popliteal region. In children, the diagnosis may be made by aspiration of mucinous fluid, but the cyst nearly always disappears with time. Whereas Baker's cysts may be indicative of intraarticular disease in the adult, they are not associated with meniscal tears in children and rarely require excision, usually resolving spontaneously within 20 months.

FOOT DEFORMITIES

When a child begins to stand and walk, the long arch of the foot is flat with a medial bulge over the inner border of the foot. The forefeet are mildly pronated or rotated inward, with a slight valgus alignment of the knees. As the child grows and muscle power improves, the long arch is better supported and more normal relationships occur in the lower extremities.

FLATFOOT

Flatfoot is a normal condition in infants. Children presenting for examinations should be checked to determine that the heel cord is of normal length when the heel is aligned in the neutral position, allowing complete dorsiflexion and plantar flexion. As long as the foot is supple and the presence of a longitudinal arch is noted when the child is sitting in a non–weight-bearing position, the parents can be assured that a normal arch will probably develop. There is usually a familial incidence of relaxed flatfeet in children who have prolonged malalignment of the foot. In any child with a shortened heel cord or stiffness of the foot, other causes of flatfoot such as tarsal coalition or vertical talus should be ruled out by a complete orthopedic examination and x-ray.

In the child with an ordinary relaxed flatfoot, no active treatment is indicated unless there is calf or leg pain. In children who have leg pains attributable to flatfeet, a supportive shoe may relieve discomfort. An arch insert should not be prescribed unless passive correction of the arch is easily accomplished; otherwise, there will be irritation of the skin over the medial side of the foot.

CAVUS FOOT

In **cavus foot**, the deformity consists of an unusually high longitudinal arch of the foot. It may be hereditary or associated with neurologic conditions such as poliomyelitis, Charcot-Marie-Tooth disease, Friedreich's ataxia, or diastematomyelia. There is usually an associated contracture of the toe extensors, producing a claw toe deformity in which the metatarsal phalangeal joints are hyperextended and the interphalangeal joints acutely flexed. Any child presenting with cavus feet should have a careful neurologic examination including x-rays of the spine.

In painful cases, operation may be necessary to lengthen the contracted extensor and flexor tendons. Arthrodesis of the foot may be necessary later. If these feet are left untreated, they are often painful and limit walking.

The overall prognosis is much poorer than with low arch or pes planus.

CLAW TOES

In patients with **claw toes**, there is a flexion deformity of either or both interphalangeal joints, which results in the "claw." The condition is usually congenital and may be seen in association with disorders of motor weakness, such as Charcot-Marie-Tooth disease or pes cavus. Surgical correction can alleviate symptoms if the toes are painful.

BUNIONS
(Hallux Valgus)

Bunions may present in adolescence with lateral deviation of the great toe associated with a prominence over the head of first metatarsal. This deformity is painful only with shoe wear and almost always can be relieved by fitting shoes that are sufficiently wide. Surgery should be avoided in the adolescent age group, as the results are much less successful than in adult patients with the same condition.

OFFICE ORTHOPEDICS

SCOLIOSIS

The term *scoliosis* denotes lateral curvature of the spine, which is always associated with some rotation of the involved vertebrae. Scoliosis is classified by its anatomic location, in either the thoracic or lumbar spine, with rare involvement of the cervical spine. The apex of the curve is designated right or left. Thus, a right thoracic scoliosis would denote a convex leftward curve in the thoracic region, and this is the most common type of idiopathic curve. Posterior curvature of the spine (kyphosis) is normal in the thoracic area, though excessive curvature may become pathologic. Anterior curvature is called lordosis and is normal in the lumbar spine. Idiopathic scoliosis generally begins at about 8 or 10 years of age and progresses during growth. In rare instances, infantile scoliosis may be seen in children 2 years of age or less.

Idiopathic scoliosis is about 4–5 times more common in girls than in boys. The disorder is usually asymptomatic in the adolescent years, but severe curvature may lead to impairment of pulmonary function or low back pain in later years. It is important to examine the back of any adolescent during a physical examination. The examination is performed by having the patient bend forward 90 degrees with the hands joined in the midline. An abnormal finding consists of asymmetry of the height of the ribs or paravertebral muscles on one side, indicating rotation of the trunk associated with lateral curvature.

Diseases that may be associated with scoliosis include neurofibromatosis, Marfan's syndrome, cerebral palsy, muscular dystrophy, and poliomyelitis. Neurologic examination should be performed in all children with scoliosis to determine whether these disorders are present.

Five to 7% of cases of scoliosis are due to congenital vertebral anomalies such as a hemivertebral or unilateral vertebral bridge. These curves are more rigid than the more common idiopathic curve and will often increase with growth, especially during the rapid growth spurt during adolescence.

The most common type of scoliosis is so-called idiopathic scoliosis, which may be due to asymmetry of neuromuscular development. In 30% of cases, other family members are affected.

Postural compensation of the spine may lead to lateral curvature from such causes as unequal length of the lower extremities. Antalgic scoliosis may result from pressure on the spinal cord or roots by infectious processes or herniation of the nucleus pulposus. The underlying cause for painful scoliosis must be sought. The curvature will resolve as the primary problem is treated.

Clinical Findings

A. Symptoms & Signs: Scoliosis in adolescents is classically asymptomatic. It is imperative to seek the underlying cause in any case where there is pain, since in these instances the scoliosis may be secondary to some other disorder such as a bone or spinal cord tumor. Deformity of the rib cage and asymmetry of the waistline are evident with curvatures of 30 degrees or more. A lesser curvature may be detected by the forward bending test as described above.

B. Imaging: The most valuable x-rays are those taken of the entire spine in the standing position in both the anteroposterior and lateral planes. Usually, there is one primary curvature with a compensatory curvature that develops to balance the body. At times, there may be two primary curvatures, usually in the right thoracic and left lumbar regions. Any left thoracic curvature should be suspected of being secondary to neurologic or muscular disease.

Treatment

Curvatures of less than 20 degrees usually do not require treatment unless they show progression. Bracing is indicated for curvature of 20–40 degrees in a skeletally immature child. Treatment is indicated for any curvature that demonstrates progression on serial x-ray examination. Curvatures greater than 40 degrees are resistant to treatment by bracing. Thoracic curvatures greater than 60 degrees have been correlated with a poor pulmonary prognosis in adult life. Curvatures of such severity are an indication for surgical correction of the deformity and posterior spinal fusion to maintain the correction. Curvatures between 40 and 60 degrees may also require spinal fusion if they appear to be progressive, are causing decompensation of the spine, or cause unacceptable deformity.

Prognosis

Compensated small curvatures that do not progress may be well tolerated throughout life, with little deformity. The patients should be counseled regarding the genetic transmission of scoliosis and cautioned that their children should be examined at regular intervals during growth. Large thoracic curvatures greater than 60 degrees are associated with shortened life span and may progress even during adult life. Large lumbar curvatures may lead to subluxation of the vertebrae and premature arthritic degeneration of the spine, producing disabling pain in adulthood. Early detection allows for simple brace treatment. In patients so treated, the long-term prognosis is excellent and surgery is not necessary. For this reason, school screening programs for scoliosis have gained popular support in many sections of the country.

GENU VARUM & GENU VALGUM

Genu varum (bowleg) is normal from infancy through 2 years of life. The alignment then changes to **genu valgum** (knock-knee) until about 8 years of age, at which time adult alignment is attained. Criteria for referral to an orthopedist include persistent bowing beyond age 2, bowing that is increasing rather than decreasing, bowing of one leg only, and knock-knee associated with short stature.

Bracing may be appropriate, or, rarely, an osteotomy is necessary for a severe problem such as **Blount's disease** (proximal tibial epiphyseal dysplasia).

TIBIAL TORSION

The physician is often asked about "toeing in" in small children. The disorder is routinely asymptomatic. **Tibial torsion** is rotation of the leg between the knee and the ankle. Internal rotation amounts to about 20 degrees at birth but decreases to neutral rotation by 1 year of age. The deformity is sometimes accentuated by laxity of the knee ligaments, allowing excessive internal rotation of the leg in small children. In children who have a persistent internal rotation of the tibia beyond 1 year of age, it is often due to sleeping with feet turned in and can be reversed with an external rotation splint worn only at night.

FEMORAL ANTEVERSION

"Toeing in" beyond 2 or 3 years of age is usually based on **femoral anteversion**, which produces excessive internal rotation of the femur as compared with external rotation. This femoral alignment follows a natural history of progressive decrease toward neutral up to 8 years of age, with slower change to 16 years of age. Studies comparing the results of treatment with shoes or braces to the natural history have shown that little is gained by treatment. Active external rotation exercises such as ballet, skating, or bicycle riding may be worthwhile. Osteotomy for rotational correction is reserved for the rare patient who has no external rotation of hip in extension.

GANGLION

A **ganglion** is a smooth, small cystic mass connected by a pedicle to the joint capsule, usually on the dorsum of the wrist. It may also be seen in the tendon sheath over the flexor surfaces of the fingers. These ganglions can be excised if they interfere with function or cause persistent pain.

Sports Medicine | 22

Suzanne M. Tanner, MD

The pediatric sports medicine practitioner aims to prevent injuries and illness in young athletes. Since this goal is not always achievable, a second objective is to provide prompt, appropriate medical care. Practitioners treating young athletes are called upon to perform preparticipation examinations and treat sprains, strains, contusions, and overuse injuries, the most common maladies affecting active youngsters.

THE PREPARTICIPATION EXAMINATION

For many pediatricians, performing sports physical examinations is a principal source of involvement in the realm of sports medicine. The primary goal of the preparticipation evaluation is to enhance the health of athletes. It is not meant to exclude athletes from participation, but to help them participate safely. Although it is not intended as a substitute for an athlete's regular health maintenance examination, 78% of athletes view the preparticipation evaluation as their annual health examination. Careful attention to general health maintenance should therefore be included with the exam, or at another appointment.

The preparticipation examination should ideally be conducted at least 6 weeks prior to the start of practice or competition so that health disorders may be evaluated and previous injuries rehabilitated.

A complete history (Table 22–1) will identify 63–74% of problems affecting athletes. Parents should help the athlete complete the questionnaire since only 39% of histories reported by athletes agree with information given by their parents.

Important entities to detect during the preparticipation examination are listed below. Further evaluation or treatment may be recommended before the athlete is allowed to participate.

Table 22–1. Preparticipation physical evaluation.

History Date ______________

Name ______________ Sex ________ Age ________ Date of birth ______________

Grade ________ Sport ______________ ______________ ______________

Personal physician ______________ ______________ (Adress) ______________ (Physician's phone)

Explain "Yes" answers below:	Yes	No
1. Have you ever been hospitalized?	☐	☐
Have you ever had surgery?	☐	☐
2. Are you presently taking any medications or pills?	☐	☐
3. Do you hav enay allergies (medicine, bees or other stinging insects)?	☐	☐
4. Have you ever passed out during or after exercise?	☐	☐
Have you ever been dizzy during or after exercise?	☐	☐
Have you ever had chest pain during or after exercise?	☐	☐
Do you tire more quickly than your friends during exercise?	☐	☐
Have you ever had high blood pressure?	☐	☐
Have you ever been told that you have a heart murmur?	☐	☐
Have you ever had racing of your heart or skipped heartbeats?	☐	☐
Has anyone in your family died of heart problems or a sudden death before age 50?	☐	☐
5. Do you have any skin problems (itching, rashes, acne)?	☐	☐

6. Have you ever had a head injury?	☐	☐
Have you ever been knocked out or unconscious?	☐	☐
Have you ever had a seizure?	☐	☐
Have you ever had a stinger, burner or pinched nerve?	☐	☐
7. Have you ever had heat or muscle cramps?	☐	☐
Have you ever been dizzy or passed out in the heat?	☐	☐
8. Do you have trouble breathing or do you cough during or after activity?	☐	☐
9. Do you use any special equipment (pads, braces, neck rolls, mouth guard, eye guards, etc.)?	☐	☐
10. Have you had any problems with your eyes or vision?	☐	☐
Do you wear glasses or contacts or protective eye wear?	☐	☐
11. Have you ever sprained/strained, dislocated, fractured, broken or had repeated swelling or other injuries of any bones or joints?	☐	☐
☐ Head ☐ Shoulder ☐ Thigh ☐ Neck ☐ Elbow ☐ Knee ☐ Chest		
☐ Forearm ☐ Shin/calf ☐ Back ☐ Wrist ☐ Ankle ☐ Hip ☐ Hand ☐ Foot		
12. Have you had any other medical problems (infectious mononucleosis, diabetes, etc.)?	☐	☐
13. Have you had a medical problem or injury since your last evaluation?	☐	☐

14. When was your last tetanus shot? ______________________

When was your last measles immunization ______________________

15. When was your first menstrual period? ______________________

When was your last menstrual period? ______________________

What was the longest time between your periods last year? ______________________

Exercise-Induced Asthma (EIA)

EIA is common in children and adolescents. Approximately 10% of the normal population and 80–90% of asthmatics experience EIA. Only athletes with severe asthma should be deterred from participating in any sport.

Symptoms of EIA include shortness of breath, chest pain, abdominal pain, a feeling of being out of shape, and coughing after activity. Symptoms can be reduced by performing warm-up drills prior to activity and exercising in a warm, humidified environment. Sports that are well tolerated include swimming (since air is humidified), and wrestling (since bouts are of short duration).

Treatment includes inhaling a beta-2-agonist, cromolyn, or both shortly before exercise. More extensive treatment is outlined in Chapter 26.

Cardiovascular Symptoms

Careful attention to the cardiovascular system is crucial since over 95% of sudden deaths in athletes under age 30 involve the cardiovascular system. Syncope, or near syncope, may be a clue to the presence of hypertrophic cardiomyopathy, conduction abnormalities, arrhythmias, or valvular problems, such as aortic stenosis or mitral valve prolapse. Exertional chest pain may indicate congenital abnormalities of the coronary arteries or atherosclerotic disease in a child with abnormal lipid metabolism. Lung pathology or valvular problems may cause dyspnea on exertion. Palpitations or skipped beats may signify arrhythmias or conduction abnormalities, such as Wolff–Parkinson–White syndrome.

It is important to determine if family members under the age of 50 have experienced sudden cardiac death. Causes of sudden cardiac death include hypertrophic cardiomyopathy, Marfan's syndrome, and prolonged QT syndrome. These entities may have a familial component. It is also important to distinguish between dysrhythmias in a patient with a structurally sound heart and those occurring in a patient with congenital heart disease. The prognosis for the latter group is less favorable.

Repeat measurements of blood pressure, using an appropriate cuff size, should be taken if the pressure is initially elevated. As an easy rule of thumb, blood pressure greater than 125/75 for a child 10 years or younger, or a blood pressure greater than 135/85 for a child over 10 years should be further evaluated.

Children with mild hypertension may compete in all sports. Those with moderate to severe hypertension should be individually evaluated.

Skin Infections

An athlete with herpes simplex, scabies, pubic lice, molluscum contagiosum, furunculosis, carbunculosis, or impetigo may temporarily need to be disqualified from sports such as wrestling, the martial arts, swimming, or gymnastics. Infections may be spread via direct contact, swimming pools, tumbling mats, or shared towels.

Blood-Borne Pathogens

Only one case of possible transmission of human immunodeficiency virus has been reported in a sporting setting. It involved a violent collision of two soccer players resulting in profuse bleeding. One player was HIV-positive and the other individual later seroconverted. It was impossible to determine, however, whether the infection occurred from the collision or some other exposure. Since a theoretical risk of transmission of HIV exists during contact sports, voluntary avoidance of sports where blood exposure is likely is recommended for HIV-positive individuals (Table 22–2).

Transmission of hepatitis B virus has been documented in an ath-

Table 22–2. Guidelines for limiting exposure to blood-borne pathogens.

1. Athletes infected with blood-borne pathogens should be allowed to participate in all competitive sports.[1]
2. Since a hypothetical risk for transmission of a blood-borne infection does exist when there is blood-to-blood or blood-to-mucous membrane exposure, athletes who are infected with a blood-borne pathogen should be advised of risk and urged to avoid participation in "contact/collision/impact" sports.
3. Athletes with a blood-borne infection have a right to confidentiality. This includes not disclosing an individual's status to participants or staff.
4. All athletes should be informed that an athletic program is functioning under the rules cited above.
5. There is no medical or public health reason for routine or mandatory testing in sports activities.
6. Athletes and program staff should receive mandatory training on blood-borne pathogen transmission and its prevention.
7. During all athletic contests or practices, there should be strict adherence to universal precaution guidelines for preventing blood-borne infections.
8. All adolescent and young adult athletes at increased risk of hepatitis B infection should receive hepatitis B vaccine.

[1] This recommendation is subject to review if new information concerning the transmission of blood-borne pathogens becomes available.

Adapted from the American Academy of Pediatrics Committee on Sports Medicine and Fitness (1991).

Table 22–4. The 2-minute orthopedic examination.[1]

Instructions	Observations
Stand facing examiner	Acromioclavicular joints, general habitus
Look at ceiling, floor, over both shoulders; touch ears to shoulders	Cervical spine motion
Shrug shoulders (examiner resists)	Trapezius strength
Abduct shoulders 90° (examiner resists at 90°)	Deltoid strength
Full external rotation of arms	Shoulder motion
Flex and extend elbows	Elbow motion
Arms at sides, elbows 90° flexed; pronate and supinate wrists	Elbow and wrist motion
Spread fingers; make fist	Hand or finger motion and deformities
Tighten (contract) quadriceps; relax quadriceps	Symmetry and knee effusion; ankle effusion
"Duck walk" four steps (away from examiner with buttocks on heels)	Hip, knee and ankle motion
Back to examiner	Shoulder symmetry, scoliosis
Knees straight, touch toes	Scoliosis, hip motion, hamstring tightness
Raise up on toes, raise heels	Calf symmetry, leg strength

[1] Reproduced with permission from *Sports Medicine: Health Care of the Young Athlete*, 2nd ed., 1991, published by The American Academy of Pediatrics, Elk Grove Village, Illinois.

purposes by the American Academy of Pediatrics (AAP). Athletes with inadequate iron intake, especially girls participating in endurance sports, may be at risk for iron-deficiency anemia and should be screened for this disorder.

Electrocardiogram, echocardiogram, and exercise stress testing are indicated only when history and physical findings identify an individual with increased cardiovascular risks. The most common dysrhythmias in school-aged children are sinus dysrhythmias and premature atrial contractions. These are benign if the heart is structurally normal and no further work-up beyond an ECG is necessary. Athletes with structural heart disease, significant conduction defects, or cardiac symptoms should be seen by a cardiologist.

Exclusion from Sports

The AAP has classified sports based on strenuousness and probability of collision (Table 22–5). AAP guidelines for participation or exclusion from sports are listed in Table 22–6.

The physician should consider the following questions when clearing or excluding an athlete from participation:

(1) Does the problem place the athlete at increased risk of injury?
(2) Is any other participant at risk of injury because of the problem?

Table 22–5. Classification of sports by contact.[1]

Contact/ Collision	Limited Contact	Noncontact
Basketball	Baseball	Archery
Boxing*	Bicycling	Badminton
Diving	Cheerleading	Body building
Field hockey	Canoeing/kayaking (white water)	Bowling
Football	Fencing	Canoeing/kayaking (flat water)
Flag	Field	Crew/rowing
Tackle	High jump	Curling
Ice hockey	Pole vault	Dancing
Lacrosse	Floor hockey	Field
Martial arts	Gymnastics	Discus
Rodeo	Handball	Javelin
Rugby	Horseback riding	Shot put
Ski jumping	Racquetball	Golf
Soccer	Skating	Orienteering
Team handball	Ice	Power lifting
Water polo	Inline	Race walking
Wrestling	Roller	Riflery
	Skiing	Rope jumping
	Cross-country	Running
	Downhill	Sailing
	Water	Scuba diving
	Softball	Strength training
	Squash	Swimming
	Ultimate Frisbee	Table tennis
	Volleyball	Tennis
	Windsurfing/surfing	Track
		Weight lifting

* Participation not recommended.

[1] Reproduced with permission from PEDIATRICS Vol. 94 No. 5 November 1994.

Table 22–6. Medical conditions and sports participation.[1]

This table is designed to be understood by medical and nonmedical personnel. In the "Explanation" section below, "needs evaluation" means that a physician with appropriate knowledge and experience should assess the safety of a given sport for an athlete with the listed medical condition. Unless otherwise noted, this is because of the variability of the severity of the disease or of the risk of injury among the specific sports in Table 22–5, or both.

Condition	May Participate?
Atlantoaxial instability (instability of the joint between cervical vertebrae 1 and 2)	Qualified Yes
Explanation: Athlete needs evaluation to assess risk of spinal cord injury during sports participation.	
Bleeding disorder	Qualified Yes
Explanation: Athlete needs evaluation.	
Cardiovascular diseases	
Carditis (inflammation of the heart)	No
Explanation: Carditis may result in sudden death with exertion.	
Hypertension (high blood pressure)	Qualified Yes
Explanation: Those with significant essential (unexplained) hypertension should avoid weight and power lifting, body building, and strength training. Those with secondary hypertension (hypertension caused by a previously identified disease), or severe essential hypertension, need evaluation. Reference 4 defines significant and severe hypertension.	
Congenital heart disease (structural heart defects present at birth)	Qualified Yes
Explanation: Those with mild forms may participate fully; those with moderate or severe forms, or who have undergone surgery, need evaluation.	

Dysrhythmia (irregular heart rhythm)	Qualified Yes
Explanation: Athlete needs evaluation because some types require therapy or make certain sports dangerous, or both.	
Mitral valve prolapse (abnormal heart valve)	Qualified Yes
Explanation: Those with symptoms (chest pain, symptoms of possible dysrhythmia) or evidence of mitral regurgitation (leaking) on physical examination need evaluation. All others may participate fully.	
Heart murmur	Qualified Yes
Explanation: If the murmur is innocent (does not indicate heart disease), full participation is permitted. Otherwise the athlete needs evaluation (see congenital heart disease and mitral valve prolapse, above).	
Cerebral palsy	Qualified Yes
Explanation: Athlete needs evaluation.	
Diabetes mellitus	Yes
Explanation: All sports can be played with proper attention to diet, hydration, and insulin therapy. Particular attention is needed for activities that last 30 minutes or more.	
Diarrhea	Qualified No
Explanation: Unless disease is mild, no participation is permitted, because diarrhea may increase the risk of dehydration and heat illness. See "Fever" below.	
Eating disorders	
Anorexia nervosa	Qualified Yes
Bulimia nervosa	
Explanation: These patients need both medical and psychiatric assessment before participation.	

(*continued*)

Table 22–6. Medical conditions and sports participation (*continued*).

Condition	May Participate?
Eyes	
Functionally one-eyed athlete	Qualified Yes
Loss of an eye	
Detached retina	
Previous eye surgery or serious eye injury	
Explanation: A functionally one-eyed athlete has a best corrected visual acuity of <20/40 in the worse eye. These athletes would suffer significant disability if the better eye was seriously injured as would those with loss of an eye. Some athletes who have previously undergone eye surgery or had a serious eye injury may have an increased risk of injury because of weakened eye tissue. Availability of eye guards approved by the American Society for Testing Materials (ASTM) and other protective equipment may allow participation in most sports, but this must be judged on an individual basis.	
Fever	No
Explanation: Fever can increase cardiopulmonary effort, reduce maximum exercise capacity, make heat illness more likely, and increase orthostatic hypotension during exercise. Fever may rarely accompany myocarditis or other infections that may make exercise dangerous.	
Heat illness, history of	Qualified Yes
Explanation: Because of the increased likelihood of recurrence, the athlete needs individual assessment to determine the presence of predisposing conditions and to arrange a prevention strategy.	
HIV infection	Yes
Explanation: Because of the apparent minimal risk to others, all sports may be played that the state of health allows. In all athletes, skin lesions should be properly covered, and athletic personnel should use universal precautions when handling blood or body fluids with visible blood.	
Kidney: absence of one	Qualified Yes
Explanation: Athlete needs individual assessment for contact/collision and limited contact sports.	

Liver: enlarged	Qualified Yes
Explanation: If the liver is acutely enlarged, participation should be avoided because of risk of rupture. If the liver is chronically enlarged, individual assessment is needed before collision/contact or limited contact sports are played.	
Malignancy	Qualified Yes
Explanation: Athlete needs individual assessment.	
Musculoskeletal disorders	Qualified Yes
Explanation: Athlete needs individual assessment.	
Neurologic	
History of serious head or spine trauma, severe or repeated concussions, or craniotomy.	Qualified Yes
Explanation: Athlete needs individual assessment for collision/contact or limited contact sports, and also for noncontact sports if there are deficits in judgment or cognition. Recent research supports a conservative approach to management of concussion.	
Convulsive disorder, well controlled	Yes
Explanation: Risk of convulsion during participation is minimal.	
Convulsive disorder, poorly controlled	Qualified Yes
Explanation: Athlete needs individual assessment for collision/contact or limited contact sports. Avoid the following noncontact sports: archery, riflery, swimming, weight or power lifting, strength training, or sports involving heights. In these sports, occurrence of a convulsion may be a risk to self or others.	
Obesity	Qualified Yes
Explanation: Because of the risk of heat illness, obese persons need careful acclimatization and hydration.	
Organ transplant recipient	Qualified Yes
Explanation: Athlete needs individual assessment.	
Ovary: absence of one	Yes
Explanation: Risk of severe injury to the remaining ovary is minimal.	

(*continued*)

Table 22–6. Medical conditions and sports participation (*continued*).

Condition	May Participate?
Respiratory	
Pulmonary compromise including cystic fibrosis	Qualified Yes
Explanation: Athlete needs individual assessment, but generally all sports may be played if oxygenation remains satisfactory during a graded exercise test. Patients with cystic fibrosis need acclimatization and good hydration to reduce the risk of heat illness.	
Asthma	Yes
Explanation: With proper medication and education, only athletes with the most severe asthma will have to modify their participation.	
Acute upper respiratory infection	Qualified Yes
Explanation: Upper respiratory obstruction may affect pulmonary function. Athlete needs individual assessment for all but mild disease. See "Fever" above.	
Sickle cell disease	Qualified Yes
Explanation: Athlete needs individual assessment. In general, if status of the illness permits, all but high exertion, collision/contact sports may be played. Overheating, dehydration, and chilling must be avoided.	

Sickle cell trait	Yes
Explanation: It is unlikely that individuals with sickle cell trait (AS) have an increased risk of sudden death or other medical problems during athletic participation except under the most extreme conditions of heat, humidity, and possibly increased altitude.[12] These individuals, like all athletes, should be carefully conditioned, acclimatized, and hydrated to reduce any possible risk.	
Skin: boils, herpes simplex, impetigo, scabies, molluscum contagiosum	Qualified Yes
Explanation: While the patient is contagious, participation in gymnastics with mats, martial arts, wrestling, or other collision/contact or limited contact sports is not allowed. Herpes simplex virus probably is not transmitted via mats.	
Spleen, enlarged	Qualified Yes
Explanation: Patients with acutely enlarged spleens should avoid all sports because of risk of rupture. Those with chronically enlarged spleens need individual assessment before playing collision/contact or limited contact sports.	
Testicle: absent or undescended	Yes
Explanation: Certain sports may require a protective cup.	

[1] Reproduced with permission from: *Preparticipation Physical Evaluation*, a joint publication of AAFP, AAP, AMSSM, AOSSM, & AOASM, copyright 1992.

(3) Can the athlete safely participate with medication, rehabilitation, bracing, or padding?
(4) Can limited participation be allowed while treatment is being initiated?
(5) If clearance is denied for certain activities only, in what activities can the athlete safely participate?

EPIDEMIOLOGY OF SPORTS INJURIES IN THE PEDIATRIC ATHLETE

Injuries by Sport

The yearly injury incidence in all interscholastic high school sports is 27–39%. Among popular high school sports, football and wrestling are the most hazardous.

Injuries by Gender

There has been concern that sports are more dangerous for girls than boys. Injury incidence in males and females in high school and college sports, however, is generally similar. Female competitive basketball players, however, appear to have an increased risk of tears of the anterior cruciate ligament (four times greater than males).

Injuries by Age

Injury rates tend to increase by age. Teenage and college-age athletes may have a higher rate of injury than youngsters due to increased time participating in sports. At the high school and college levels, games last longer and practices are more frequent, giving the player more opportunities to become injured. In sports such as football, larger size and increased speed of players make collisions more hazardous.

Younger children are at risk for growth plate injuries.

Methods to prevent injuries are presented in Table 22–7.

SOFT TISSUE TRAUMA

Of injuries in adolescents, soft tissue injuries are by far the most common. Sprains, strains, and contusions account for 75% of all high school sports-related injuries. The knee, thigh, and ankle are the sites most commonly injured.

Table 22–7. Methods of injury prevention.[1]

Proper conditioning and acclimatization
Avoidance of training excesses
A safe environment
Resolution of previous injuries
Good supervision
Enforcement of rules concerned with safety, with continued revision as new risk factors are identified
Instruction in proper technique
Appropriate safety equipment
A careful preparticipation medical assessment
Matching of competitors by age, weight, and stage of maturation

[1] From Goldberg B, in Dyment PG (ed): *Adolescent Medicine: Sports and the Adolescent.* Hanly and Belfus, Philadelphia, Vol. 2, No. 1, Feb. 1991.

Sprain

A sprain is an injury to a ligament or joint capsule. Common sites of sprains include the lateral ankle and medial collateral ligament of the knee. Sprains are graded according to their severity (Table 22–8). Grading of sprains requires testing ligament integrity through specific tests during which stress is applied across a joint.

Strains

Strains are often called "muscle pulls." The term refers to an injury to a muscle or tendon. Common sites of strains include the shoulder and hamstrings. Grading of strains requires assessing strength, which is more subjective that grading stability for sprains (Table 22–9).

Table 22–8. Grading of sprains according to severity.[1]

Grade	Fibers Torn	Pain/Swelling	Range of Motion	Laxity
I	Less than 5%	Little	Full	None
II	5–95%	Moderate	Impaired	Noticeable
III	100%	Severe	Poor	Marked

[1] Adapted from Dyment PG (ed): *Adolescent Medicine: Sports and the Adolescent.* Hanley and Belfus, Philadelphia, Vol.2, No. 1, Feb. 1991.

Table 22–9. Grading of strains by assessing strength.[1]

Grade	Pain on Palpation or Contraction	Loss of Strength	Palpable Defect
I	Little	Little or none	–
II	Moderate	Significant	±
III	Severe	Marked	±

[1] Adapted from Dyment PG (ed): *Adolescent Medicine: Sports and the Adolescent.* Hanley and Belfus, Philadelphia, Vol. 2, No. 1, Feb. 1991.

Contusions

A contusion refers to a crushing of cells and bleeding from a direct blow. A "charley horse" refers to a contusion of the quadriceps muscles. Since muscles are more vascular than ligaments and tendons, they are prone to hematoma formation after a blow. Repetitive or severe contusions may progress to myositis ossificans, or calcification within the muscle, especially if further activity is not halted.

Treatment of Soft Tissue Injuries

Most grade I and II soft tissue injuries can be managed by the primary care physician. The aim of treatment during the first 48–72 hours following a soft tissue injury is to limit inflammation and bleeding. This promotes healing and speeds up rehabilitation. An acronym, RICE (*r*est, *i*ce, *c*ompression, and *e*levation) should guide initial management.

Rest is accomplished through cessation of activity, immobilization, and elimination or reduction of weight bearing for lower extremity injuries. These steps prevent further injury, relieve pain, and reduce inflammation. Although the length of time a body part requires rest to enhance healing varies according to the injury severity and site, rest should usually be at least 48–72 hours.

Vasoconstriction by application of cold, rather than heat, immediately after an injury decreases bleeding, inflammation, pain and spasm. The application of heat acutely after an injury may have the opposite effect. A plastic bag containing ice cubes or crushed ice can be placed over a towel on the skin. For best results, ice may be applied for 10–20 minutes, 2–4 times per day for the first 2–3 days.

The application of an elastic bandage to the injured part compresses the site and limits swelling.

Elevation is accomplished by raising the injured part on cushions or pillows. Elevation facilitates venous and lymphatic drainage.

Application of the RICE regimen alone usually limits swelling

Table 22–10. Adverse effects of NSAIDs.[1]

Gastritis
Headache
Mental status changes
Hypersensitivity
Impairment of platelet function
Impairment of renal function
Bronchospasm

[1] Adapted from Landry G, in Dyment PG (ed): *Adolescent Medicine: Sports and the Adolescent.* Hanley and Belfus, Philadelphia, Vol. 2, No. 1, Feb. 1991.

adequately for most soft tissue injuries. The role of anti-inflammatory medications in the management of soft tissue injuries is controversial due to their potential toxicity (Table 22–10).

Management of Soft Tissue Injuries After the Acute Phase

Approximately 72 hours post-injury, when swelling and pain have decreased, rehabilitation may be started. An athletic trainer or physical therapist may help design a rehabilitation program. Range of motion exercises through simple, isolated movement patterns may be performed several times per day. Once range of motion is near normal, strengthening exercises may be added. Strengthening helps the athlete to return to sports sooner and helps prevent a reinjury. Cardiovascular endurance can be maintained during rehabilitation while resting the injured part.

Return to Play

Criteria for return to play include:

- Full range of motion
- Full strength
- No swelling
- No joint instability
- No tenderness
- No pain with motion
- Ability to perform the athletic activity without limping or favoring the injured part

OVERUSE INJURIES

Today, millions of children join organized sports teams, train rigorously, and pursue sports at a young age. The reward to a young athlete may be excelling at a sport. Hours of practicing the same movement, however, may produce wear on specific body parts. Overuse, or overload, injuries refer to trauma due to repetitive microtrauma. Intrinsic and extrinsic factors may lead to overuse injuries (Table 22–11).

Examples of overuse injuries in children include the entities listed below. Treatment options are listed in Table 22–12.

Rotator Cuff Tendinitis

The rotator cuff consists of four muscles (SITS muscles, or *s*upraspinatus, *i*nfraspinatus, *t*eres minor, and *s*ubscapularis). These muscles form a tendinous cuff around the superior portion of the humerus. Children and teenagers who participate in overhead activities such as throwing, swimming, and playing volleyball may develop pain in the superior aspect of the shoulder due to inflammation of the rotator cuff.

Patellar Tendinitis (Jumper's Knee)

Jumper's knee refers to inflammation of the patellar tendon below the patella. Youngsters involved in running and jumping sports,

Table 22–11. Predisposing factors to overruse injuries.

Intrinsic Factors	Example
Leg-length inequality	May cause low back pain
Weakness	Weak quadriceps may predispose to patellofemoral (kneecap) pain
Inflexibility	Tight Achilles tendons may predispose to Sever's disease (heel pain)
Poor aerobic fitness	Poor general fitness correlates with the presence of low back pain
Growth spurt	Perhaps bones grow faster than muscles, causing inflexibility (unproven)
Extrinsic Factors	**Example**
Training errors	Suddenly increasing running mileage may lead to stress fractures
Improper technique	Deep squats while holding weights may lead to patellofemoral (kneecap) pain
Poor equipment	Shoes with poor support may lead to pain in the arch of the foot
Poor nutrition	Low calcium intake may predispose to the development of stress fractures

Table 22–12. Treatment options for overuse injuries.

Tissue	Overuse Injury	Rest	Apply Ice	NSAID[1]	Stretching	Strengthening	Shoes	Brace	Injection
Tendon	Rotation cuff tendonitis	+	+	+		Rotator cuff			+ Subacromial – Bursa injection
	Jumper's knee (patella tendonitis)	+	+	+	Quadriceps hamstrings	Quadriceps (straight leg raises)	Proper shoes	± Infrapatella strap	
Cartilage	Patellofemoral pain	+	+	+	Quadriceps hamstrings	Quadriceps (straight leg raises)	Proper shoes	± Sleeve with central patellar hole	
Bone	Stress fracture	+					Proper shoes		
	Spondylolysis	+			Hamstrings	Back and abdomen		+	
Apophysis	Osgood-Schlatter condition	+	+	+	Quadriceps hamstrings			± Infrapetella strap	
	Sever condition	+	+	+	Achilles tendon		Heel lifts Proper shoes		
Epiphyseal growth plate	Little leaguer's elbow (medial humeral epicondylitis)	+	+	+		Wrist flexor		± Elbow sleeve	

[1] NSAID = nonsteroidal anti-inflammatory drug.

such as basketball, may develop pain at the area of the patellar tendon during and after activity.

Patellofemoral Pain

Patellofemoral pain refers to discomfort around the patella. Possible sources of pain include irritation of the cartilage posterior to the patella and perhaps synovial inflammation. Predisposing conditions include weakness of the quadriceps, inflexibility of the hamstrings and quadriceps, malalignment of the extensor mechanism of the knee, and increased patellar compressive forces (running, ascending and descending stairs, full squats, and jumping).

Pain usually occurs during and after activity, ascending and descending stairs, while squatting, and after prolonged sitting. The physical examination often reveals that compression on the patella during quadriceps contraction with the knee extended is painful.

Stress Fracture

When a bone is repetitively loaded, such as while running, it may break with a load that would not normally cause it to fail if it were loaded only once. This condition is called a fatigue or stress fracture. Predisposing conditions in children include high training intensity and frequency, and perhaps poor calcium intake and hormonal imbalances associated with athletic amenorrhea.

Common sites include the fibula, metatarsal, tibia, and femoral neck. Localized pain is a presenting symptom of stress fractures. Impact, such as heel strike during running, often produces pain. The most important physical examination finding is point tenderness over bone.

Radiographs may not show evidence of a stress fracture, such as a radiolucent line or callous formation, until 7–10 days after the onset of pain. Bone scans are more sensitive.

Spondylolysis/Spondylolisthesis

These terms are derived from the Greek. *Spondylo* means vertebra, *-lysis* means crack or fracture, and *-olisthesis* means sliding down an incline. Spondylolysis is a bony defect of the pars interarticularis (a segment of the vertebrae) that usually affects the fifth lumbar vertebra. Spondylolysis may progress to spondylolisthesis, an anterior slippage of a vertebra.

In athletes, the lytic defect is thought to be due to repetitive hyperextension maneuvers, such as performing back walk-overs in gymnastics, or while high jumping.

One symptom is chronic dull aching pain of the lumbosacral spine that is exacerbated by maneuvers requiring hyperextension. Oblique radiographs of the spine are required to view the defect. A bone scan may also confirm the diagnosis.

Progression from spondylolysis to spondylolisthesis is unusual, but when slips do develop, it is often between the ages of 10 and 15 years. Approximately 90% of the slips occur at the fifth lumbar–first sacral level.

Osgood–Schlatter's Condition

Osgood–Schlatter's is not a disease, but a condition in growing, active children. It refers to traction apophysitis of the tibial tubercle. Sports requiring repetitive flexion and extension of the knee, such as basketball and soccer, are inciting factors. Physical examination reveals tenderness directly over the prominence of the tibial tubercle. Pain resolves once growth is completed, or by decreasing running, but prominence of the tibial tubercle may persist through adulthood.

Sever Condition

Sever condition can be referred to as Osgood–Schlatter's condition of the heel. A traction apophysitis at the site of attachment of the Achilles tendon to the calcaneus is the source of pain with this entity.

Little Leaguer's Elbow

The term "little leaguer's elbow" refers to all stress changes involved in pitching that occur in the skeletally immature athlete. The most common cause of elbow pain is due to distraction of the medial side of the elbow during the follow-through of a pitch. This may produce tendinitis at the site of insertion of the wrist flexor and pronator muscles to the medial epicondyle of the humerus. More serious causes of little leaguer's elbow include osteochondritis dissecans (bone fragmentation) of the capitellum and radial head due to lateral elbow compression while throwing, or separation of the medial epicondylar epiphyseal growth plate due to medial distraction forces.

Pain, tenderness and loss of extension are common findings. Radiographs may reveal osteochondritis dissecans. Comparison radiographs with the contralateral elbow may show widening of the medial epiphyseal growth plate.

Failure to protect the joint may result in the formation of loose fragments, pain, deformity, and possibly arthritis.

23 | Endocrine & Metabolic Disorders

Ronald W. Gotlin, MD, & H. Peter Chase, MD

DISTURBANCES OF GROWTH & DEVELOPMENT

SHORT STATURE

Abnormally short stature in relation to age is a common finding in childhood. In most instances, it is due to a normal variation from the average pattern of growth. The possible roles of factors such as sex, race, size of parents and other family members, intrauterine factors, nutrition, pubertal maturation, and emotional status must all be evaluated in the total assessment of the child (Table 23–1). The causes of unusually short stature can usually be differentiated on the basis of significant findings in the history, physical examination, and radiographic estimation of epiphyseal maturation ("bone age").

1. CONSTITUTIONAL DELAYED GROWTH & ADOLESCENCE

Many normal children have a delay in the onset of **epiphyseal maturation** that is considered to be "constitutional." Subsequent progress is normal. In other respects, they appear entirely normal. There is often a history of a similar pattern of growth in one of the parents or other members of the family. These children are usually short throughout childhood but reach normal adult height, although at an age later than average.

2. GROWTH HORMONE DEFICIENCY

The incidence of **growth hormone (GH) deficiency** is approximately 1:4000. More than 75% of cases are the result of a hypothalamic abnormality affecting GH releasing hormone. Approximately two-thirds of all cases involving the hypothalamus and pituitary are idiopathic (rarely familial), and the remainder are secondary to pituitary, central nervous system, or hypothalamic disease (empty sella syndrome, septooptic dysplasia, craniopharyngioma, infections, tuberculosis, sarcoidosis, toxoplasmosis, syphilis, trauma, reticuloendotheliosis, vascular anomalies, and other tumors such as gliomas). GH deficiency may be an isolated defect or may occur in combination with other pituitary hormone deficiencies.

At birth, affected infants may be small; growth retardation is evident during infancy. There may be infantile fat distribution, youthful facial features, small hands and feet, and delayed sexual maturation. Hypoglycemia and microphallus may occur. Dental development and epiphyseal maturation ("bone age") are delayed. Headaches, visual field defects, abnormal skull x-rays, and symptoms of posterior pituitary insufficiency (polyuria and polydipsia) often precede or accompany the GH deficiency in cases resulting from central nervous system disease.

GH deficiency is associated with low levels of IGF (somatomedin C) and GH in the serum; GH levels fail to rise during normal physiologic sleep in response to arginine, oral levodopa, oral clonidine, exercise, or insulin-induced hypoglycemia. Patients with hypothalamic deficiency may have a GH rise in response to growth hormone-releasing hormone. GH treatment is ineffective in this condition; treatment with recombinant IGF is effective.

Laron type dwarfism is a rare condition in which there is an inability to generate IGF_1 in response to GH. Rarely, children may have an immunoreactive GH with reduced bioactivity.

Treatment is with synthetic human growth hormone (hGH). Growth hormone-releasing hormone and growth hormone-releasing peptides may be effective in hypothalamic disease and are expected to be available soon. Protein anabolic agents (testosterone, fluoxymesterone, oxandrolone, etc) may be effective in promoting linear growth, but these drugs may cause acceleration of epiphyseal closure with decrease in eventual height.

Treatment trials employing hGH in conditions with non-hGH-dependent short stature are proceeding, and in Turner's syndrome hGH treatment is efficacious. Use of hGH for *normal* short children is controversial.

3. HYPOTHYROIDISM

See section on hypothyroidism later in this chapter under Diseases of the Thyroid.

Table 23–1. Causes of short stature.[1]

- Familial, racial, or genetic
- Constitutional short stature and delayed adolescence
- Endocrine disturbances
  - Growth hormone deficiency
    - Hereditary—gene deletion
    - Idiopathic—deficiency of growth hormone or growth hormone releasing hormone (or both) with and without associated abnormalities of midline structures of the central nervous system
    - Acquired
    - Transient—eg, psychosocial short stature
    - Organic—tumor, irradiation of the central nervous system, infection, or trauma
- Hypothyroidism
- Adrenal insufficiency
- Cushing's disease and Cushing's syndrome (including iatrogenic causes)
- Sexual precocity (androgen or estrogen excess)
- Diabetes mellitus (poorly controlled)
- Diabetes insipidus
- Hyperaldosteronism
- Inborn errors of metabolism (cont'd)
    - Sphingolipidoses (eg, Tay-Sachs disease, Niemann-Pick disease, Gaucher's disease)
    - Miscellaneous (eg, cystinosis)
  - Aminoacidemias and aminoacidurias
  - Epithelial transport disorders (eg, renal tubular acidosis, cystic fibrosis, Bartter syndrome, vasopressin-resistant diabetes insipidus, pseudohypoparathyroidism)
  - Organic acidemias and acidurias (eg, methylmalonic aciduria, orotic aciduria, maple syrup urine disease, isovaleric acidemia)
  - Metabolic anemias (eg, sickle cell disease, thalassemia, pyruvate kinase deficiency)
  - Disorders of mineral metabolism (eg, Wilson's disease, magnesium malabsorption syndrome)
  - Body defense disorders (eg, Bruton agammaglobulinemia, thymic aplasia, chronic granulomatous disease)
- Constitutional (intrinsic) diseases of bone
  - Defects of growth of tubular bones or spine (eg, achondroplasia, metatrophic dwarfism, diastrophic dwarfism, metaphyseal chondrodysplasia)

- Intrauterine growth retardation
    - Placental insufficiency
    - Intrauterine infection
    - Progeria (Hutchinson-Gilford syndrome)
    - Progeroid syndrome
        - Werner's syndrome
        - Cachectic (Cockayne's syndrome)
  - Short stature without dysmorphism
  - Short stature with dysmorphism (eg, Seckel's bird-headed dwarfism, leprechaunism, Silver's syndrome, Bloom's syndrome, Cornelia de Lange syndrome, Hallerman-Streiff syndrome)
- Inborn errors of metabolism
  - Altered metabolism of calcium or phosphorus (eg, hypophosphatemic rickets, hypophosphatasia, infantile hypercalcemia, pseudohypoparathyroidism)
  - Storage diseases
    - Mucopolysaccharidoses (eg, Hurler's syndrome, Hunter syndrome)
    - Mucolipidoses (eg, generalized gangliosidosis, fucosidosis, mannosidosis)
  - Disorganized development of cartilage and fibrous components of the skeleton (eg, multiple cartilaginous exostoses, fibrous dysplasia with skin pigmentation, precocious puberty of McCune-Albright)
  - Abnormalities of density of cortical diaphyseal structure or metaphyseal modeling (eg, osteogenesis imperfecta congenita, osteopetrosis, tubular stenosis)
- Short stature associated with chromosomal defects
  - Autosomal (eg, Down syndrome, cri du chat syndrome, trisomy 18)
  - Sex chromosomal (eg, Turner syndrome-XO, penta X, XXXY)
- Chronic systemic diseases, congenital defects, and cancers (eg, chronic infection and infestation, inflammatory bowel disease, hepatic disease, cardiovascular disease, hematologic disease, central nervous system disease, pulmonary disease, renal disease, malnutrition, collagen vascular disease)
- Psychosocial short stature (deprivation dwarfism)
- Miscellaneous syndromes (eg, arthrogryposis multiplex congenita, cerebrohepatorenal syndrome, Noonan's syndrome, Prader-Willi syndrome, Riley-Day syndrome)

---

[1] From Hathaway WE et al: *Current Pediatric Diagnosis & Treatment,* 10th ed. Appleton & Lange, 1991.

4. INTRAUTERINE GROWTH RETARDATION

Intrauterine growth retardation (IUGR) may occur in a number of disorders, including craniofacial disproportion (Table 23–1), or may occur in individuals with no accompanying significant physical abnormalities. Children with IUGR have birth weight and length below normal for gestational age. Head circumference may be normal or reduced. Thereafter, they grow parallel to but below the third percentile. Plasma GH levels are usually normal but may be elevated. There is an increased incidence of functional fasting hypoglycemia. In most instances, epiphyseal maturation ("bone age") corresponds to chronologic age or is only mildly delayed, in contrast to the more marked delay often present in children with GH and thyroid deficiency.

There is as yet no satisfactory treatment for primordial short stature, although there may be an increase in growth rate in response to pharmacologic doses of human GH or IGF_1.

5. SHORT STATURE DUE TO EMOTIONAL FACTORS

(Psychosocial Short Stature, Deprivation Dwarfism, Reversible Growth Hormone Deficiency)

Psychologic and emotional deprivation with disturbances in motor and personality development may be associated with short stature. Growth retardation in some of these children is the result of undernutrition; these children may have an increased (often voracious) appetite. In others, undernutrition does not seem to be a factor. There is a delay in epiphyseal maturation. Plasma GH and IGF_1 levels are reduced. A history of feeding problems during early infancy is common; polydipsia and polyuria are sometimes present. Emotional disturbances in the family are the rule.

Placement in a foster home or a significant change in the psychologic and emotional environment at home usually results in return to normal levels of GH and IGF_1 and improved growth, a decrease of appetite and dietary intake to more normal levels, and personality improvement. Treatment with growth-promoting agents is not indicated.

DIFFERENTIAL DIAGNOSIS OF SHORT STATURE

Short stature may accompany or be caused by a large number of conditions (see Table 23–1). When the etiologic diagnosis is not apparent from the history and physical examination, the following laboratory studies, in addition to bone age, are useful in detecting or categorizing the common causes of short stature:

1. Complete blood count (to detect chronic anemia, infection, cancer).
2. Erythrocyte sedimentation rate (often elevated in collagen vascular disease, cancer, chronic infection, inflammatory bowel disease).
3. Urinalysis and microscopic examination (occult pyelonephritis, glomerulonephritis, renal tubular disease, etc).
4. Stool examination for occult blood, parasites, and parasite ova (inflammatory bowel disease, overwhelming parasitism).
5. Serum electrolytes and phosphorus levels (mild adrenal insufficiency, renal tubular diseases, parathyroid disease, rickets, etc).
6. Blood urea nitrogen and creatinine levels (occult renal insufficiency).
7. Karyotyping (should be performed in all short girls with delayed sexual maturation with or without clinical features of Turner's syndrome).
8. Thyroid function assessment: serum free thyroxin (FT4) and thyroid-stimulating hormone (TSH) assay (short stature may be the only sign of hypothyroidism).
9. GH evaluation. Blood samples for GH determination should be obtained following 20 minutes of exercise, during normal sleep, or after administration of one of the conventional provocative agents (arginine, glucagon, levodopa, clonidine, and insulin-induced hypoglycemia). Random GH and IGF_1 determinations are of no value.

FAILURE TO THRIVE

Failure to thrive (FTT) is present when there is a perceptible declination of growth from an established pattern or when the patient's height and weight plot consistently below the third percentile. (The term is usually reserved for infants who, for various reasons, fail to gain weight.) Linear growth and head circumference may also be affected; when this occurs, the underlying condition is generally more severe. There are many reasons for failure to thrive (see below and Table 23–1), although a specific cause often cannot be established. Neglect and nonaccidental trauma may be an important cause of failure to thrive.

Classification & Etiologic Diagnosis

The diagnosis of FTT is usually apparent on the basis of the history and physical examination. In FTT, it is useful to compare the patient's chronologic age with the height age (median age for the patient's height), weight age, and head circumference. On the basis of these measurements, 3 principal patterns can be defined and will provide a starting point in the diagnostic approach.

Group 1: This group is the most common type. The head circumference is normal, and the weight is reduced out of proportion to height. In the majority of cases of FTT, undernutrition is present as a result of deficient caloric intake, malabsorption, or impaired caloric utilization.

Group 2: The head circumference is normal or enlarged for age, and the weight is only moderately reduced, usually in proportion to height. Failure to thrive is due to structural dystrophies, constitutional dwarfism, or endocrinopathies.

Group 3: Although the head circumference is normal, the weight is reduced in proportion to height, owing to a primary central nervous system deficit or intrauterine growth retardation.

An initial period of observed nutritional rehabilitation, usually in a hospital setting, is often helpful in the diagnosis. The child should be placed on a regular diet for age, and the caloric intake and weight should be carefully plotted for 1–2 weeks. During this period, evidence of lactose intolerance should be sought by checking pH and reducing substances in the stool. If stools are abnormal, the child should be placed on a lactose-free diet and further observed. Caloric intake should be increased if weight gain does not occur but intake is well tolerated. The following three patterns are often noted during the rehabilitation period. Pattern 1 is by far the most common.

Pattern 1: In this most common type, the intake is adequate and the weight gain is satisfactory, but the feeding technique is at fault. A disturbed infant-mother relationship leads to the decreased caloric intake.

Pattern 2: The intake is adequate, but there is no weight gain. If weight gain is unsatisfactory after increasing the calories to an adequate level (based on the infant's ideal weight for his or her height), malabsorption is a likely diagnosis. If malabsorption is present, it is usually necessary to differentiate pancreatic exocrine insufficiency (cystic fibrosis) from abnormalities of intestinal mucosa (celiac disease). In cystic fibrosis, growth velocity commonly declines from the time of birth, and appetite is good to voracious except during illness (eg, pneumonia). In celiac disease, growth velocity is usually not reduced until 6–12 months of age, and inadequate caloric intake may be a prominent feature.

Pattern 3: The intake is inadequate, owing to the following: (1) Sucking or swallowing difficulties due to central nervous system or neuromuscular disease or to esophageal or oropharyngeal malformations may result in inadequate intake. (2) Inability to eat large amounts is common in patients with cardiopulmonary disease or in anorexic children suffering from chronic infections, inflammatory bowel disease, and endocrine problems (eg, hypothyroidism). Patients with celiac disease often have inadequate caloric intake in addition to malabsorption. (3) Inadequate intake may be due to vomiting, spitting up, or rumination in patients with upper intestinal tract obstruction (eg, pyloric stenosis, hiatal hernia, chalasia), chronic metabolic aberrations and acidosis (eg, renal insufficiency, diabetes mellitus or insipidus, methylmalonic acidemia), congenital adrenal hyperplasia, increased intracranial pressure, or psychosocial abnormalities.

TALL STATURE

Although there are several conditions (Table 23–2) that may produce tall stature, by far the most common cause is a constitutional variation from normal. Tall stature is usually of concern only to adolescent and preadolescent girls or their parents.

On the basis of family history, previous pattern of growth, state of physiologic development, assessment of epiphyseal development

Table 23–2. Causes of tall stature.

Constitutional (familial, genetic) factors	Genetic causes
Endocrine causes	Klinefelter syndrome
Androgen deficiency (normal height as children, tall as adults)	Syndromes of XYY, XXYY (tall as adults)
Anorchidism (infection, trauma, idiopathic)	Testicular feminization
Klinefelter syndrome	Miscellaneous syndromes and entities
Androgen excess (tall as children, short as adults)	Cerebral gigantism (Soto syndrome)
Pseudosexual precocity	Diencephalic syndrome
True sexual precocity	Homocystinuria
Hyperthyroidism	Marfan's syndrome
Somatotropin excess (pituitary gigantism)	Total lipodystrophy

("bone age"), and standard growth data, the physician should make a tentative estimate of the patient's eventual height. Hormonal therapy with conjugated estrogenic substances (eg, Premarin), 5–10 mg/d orally (continuously or cyclically), has been recommended by some in cases in which the patient's predicted height is considered to be excessive. Because of known and unknown long-term effects of estrogen administration in children and variable effects of therapy, treatment with estrogen is seldom recommended and should be used with caution.

Testosterone in high doses has been used to decrease final height in excessively tall boys. The results are variable.

DIABETES INSIPIDUS

Diabetes insipidus may result from deficient secretion of vasopressin (ADH), lack of response to the kidney to ADH, or failure of osmoreceptors to respond to elevations of osmolality. Hypofuncion of the posterior lobe of the pituitary with ADH deficiency may be idiopathic or may be associated with lesions of the anterior pituitary or hypothalamus (trauma, infections, suprasellar cysts, tumors, reticuloendotheliosis, or some developmental abnormality). Congenital ADH deficiency may be transmitted as an autosomal dominant trait. In nephrogenic diabetes insipidus, a hereditary X-linked dominant disease that affects both sexes but is more severe in males, the renal tubules fail to respond normally to ADH, and no lesion of the pituitary or hypothalamus can be demonstrated (see Chapter 18).

Clinical Findings

The onset is often sudden, with polyuria, intense thirst, constipation, and evidence of dehydration. High fever, circulatory collapse, and secondary brain damage may occur in young infants on an ordinary feeding regimen. Serum osmolality may be elevated (above 305 mosm/L), but urine osmolality remains below 280 mosm/L (specific gravity approximately 1.010) even after a 7-hour test period of thirsting. Rate of growth, sexual maturation, and general body metabolism may be impaired, and hydroureter and bladder distention may develop.

Diabetes insipidus may be differentiated from psychogenic polydipsia and polyuria by permitting the normal intake of fluid for several days and then withholding water for 7 hours or until weight loss (3% or more) demonstrates adequate dehydration. With neurogenic or nephrogenic diabetes insipidus, the urine osmolality does not increase above 300 mosm/L even after the period of dehydration. Normal children and those with psychogenic polydipsia will respond to the dehydration with a urinary osmolality above 450 mosm/L. Patients with long-standing psychogenic polydipsia may be unable to concentrate urine initially, and the test may need to be repeated on several successive days. Eventually, dehydration will increase urine osmolality well above plasma osmolality. The ADH and hypertonic saline tests may be employed to distinguish between the various forms of diabetes insipidus.

Treatment

The treatment of choice for central diabetes insipidus is intranasal desmopression acetate (1-desamino-8-D-arginine vasopressin; DDAVP). Individual and temporal variations in degree of deficiency absorption and response are the rule.

The cautious use of chlorothiazide and ethacrynic acid may be of value in nephrogenic diabetes insipidus. (Levels of serum electrolytes, uric acid, and blood glucose should be checked periodically.) For nephrogenic diabetes insipidus, abundant quantities of water at short intervals and feedings containing limited electrolytes and minimal (but nutritionally adequate) amounts of protein should be administered.

SEXUAL PRECOCITY

In **sexual precocity**, the onset of secondary sexual development is earlier than anticipated by chronologic age (females less than 8 years and males less than 9 years of age), body mass, and family history. Sexual precocity is generally divided into 2 *major* types: gonadotropin releasing hormone (GnRH) dependent or true precocity, and GnRH independent pseudoprecocity. **True (complete) precocity** is the result of premature increases in gonadotropin either from stimulation of the hypothalamic-pituitary mechanism (eg, in children with no abnormality or in those with tumor, infection, trauma, etc) or, rarely, from gonadotropin-producing tumors (eg, CNS germinoma hepatoma, choriocarcinoma). **Pseudoprecocity** is initiated by nongonadotropin-producing conditions (eg, adrenal, ovarian, and testicular tumors and other lesions) or by administration of sex steroids.

A third type, **familial gonadotropin independent precocious puberty** ("testotoxicosis"), has been described in males, and is not associated with premature elevation of gonadotropin concentrations.

In the past, true sexual precocity was considered to be idiopathic in approximately 80% of girls and 50% of boys. Currently, through the use of CT and MRI imaging, small abnormalities in the region of the hypothalamus are most commonly recognized.

Sexual precocity has been arbitrarily defined as the development of secondary sex characteristics beginning before age 8 in girls and age 9 in boys. Breast development is usually the first sign in girls, but the pattern of development is variable. Height may be normal initially, but it is often increased; epiphyseal maturation ("bone age") may be even more advanced than height age, particularly in pseudoprecocious patients. Psychologic development tends to correspond to chronologic age. Ovarian luteal cysts may be present in response to gonadotropin stimulation. When sensitive assays are employed, urinary and serum gonadotropin levels are elevated for age, and adrenal androgen levels may be elevated to the pubertal range.

Adrenal lesions (see Diseases of the Adrenal Cortex, below) are the most common causes of pseudoprecocity. Gonadal tumors are uncommon causes; the granulosa cell and theca-lutein cell tumors of the ovary are the most common, are generally unilateral and of low malignant potential, and produce excessive amounts of estrogen. In almost all instances, the tumor can be palpated transabdominally or rectally, and is readily visualized by pelvic ultrasonography.

When possible, treatment is directed at the underlying cause. In the GnRH type, the treatment of choice is a GnRH agonist. These agents result in gonadotropin suppression through endocrine "down regulation." Psychologic management of the patient and family is important. Children who initially have no definable causative lesion should be examined at periodic intervals for evidence of previously occult abdominal or central nervous system lesions.

Precocious Development of the Breast (Premature Thelarche)

Precocious development of one or both breasts may occur at any age. In most cases, the onset is in the first 2 years of life; in two-thirds of these cases, breast development is obvious in the first year. The condition is not associated with other evidence of sexual maturation such as rapid growth, advanced skeletal maturation, or menstruation. It may represent unusual sensitivity of the breasts to normal amounts of circulating estrogen or a temporarily increased secretion or ingestion of estrogen. Both breasts are usually involved, and enlargement may persist for months or years; the nipples generally do not enlarge. Extensive diagnostic investigation is seldom warranted; no treatment is necessary. Puberty occurs at the normal time.

Premature Adrenarche (Premature Pubarche)

Premature development of sexual hair may occur at any age and in both sexes (more often in females than in males) and must be differentiated from adrenal hyperplasia or neoplasia exogenous androgen intake and gonadal tumors. About one-third of cases occur in organically brain-damaged children. Pubic hair usually develops first, but axillary hair is present in about half of cases when these patients are first seen. Children are of normal stature, and osseous development (bone age) is not advanced. The condition results from a premature slight increase in production of adrenal androgens. Premature adrenarche requires no treatment.

Menstruation

The age at menarche ranges from 8 to 16 years; menarche is considered delayed if it has not occurred by age 17 years or within 5 years after development of the breasts. Primary amenorrhea is the result of gonadal lesions (ie, gonadal dysgenesis) in about 60% of patients, and in such cases serum and urine gonadotropin levels are elevated. In the remaining cases of primary amenorrhea, extragonadal abnormalities are present (eg, pituitary-hypothalamic hypogonadotropinism; congenital anomalies of the tubes, uterus, or vagina; androgen excess or other endocrine imbalance; and chronic systemic disease or pelvic inflammatory disease).

Once regular periods are established, amenorrhea (ie, secondary amenorrhea; Table 23–3) during adolescence is often the result of pregnancy, strenuous physical activity, or chronic systemic disease. Secondary amenorrhea should therefore be viewed as a symptom requiring evaluation and, when possible, treatment.

GONADAL DISORDERS

Deficiency of gonadal tissue or function may result from a genetic or embryologic defect; from hormone excess or impaired blood supply affecting the fetus in utero; from inflammation and destruction following infection (eg, mumps, syphilis, tuberculosis); from trauma, irradiation, autoimmune disease, or tumor; or as a consequence of surgical castration. Secondary hypogonadism may result from pituitary insufficiency (eg, destructive lesions in or about the anterior pituitary, irradiation of the pituitary, starvation), diabetes mellitus, androgen excess (eg, congenital adrenal hyperplasia), or insufficiency of either the thyroid or adrenals.

Table 23–3. Causes of secondary amenorrhea.

I. Pregnancy.
II. Decreased ovarian function.
  A. Decreased gonadotropin level (secondary ovarian insufficiency).
    1. Due to organic and idiopathic hypothalamic disease, pituitary disease, or both.[1]
    2. Due to "functional abnormalities of the hypothalamic-pituitary axis" ("psychogenic").
    3. Due to hypothalamic-pituitary disease secondary to chronic systemic illness.
      a. Nutritional disorder (eg, anorexia nervosa).
      b. Chronic infection or systemic disease (eg, cancer, collagen vascular disease, inflammatory bowel disease).
    4. Secondary to endogenous hormones (eg, androgen excess, feminizing or masculinizing ovarian tumor).
    5. Secondary to exogenous drugs (eg, long-term contraceptive drugs, androgens, estrogens, tranquilizers).
    6. Associated with strenuous and prolonged physical activity (eg, ballet dancing, gymnastics, marathon running).
  B. Increased gonadotropin level (primary ovarian insufficiency).
    1. Due to acquired diseases (destruction of ovaries by infection or tumor, "premature menopause," radiation castration, surgical removal of ovaries).
    2. Due to ovarian agenesis and dysgenesis[1] (eg, Turner syndrome).
III. Congenital and acquired lesions of the uterine tubes and uterus, including cases of chromosomal intersex (eg, adhesions, congenital absence of the uterus, cryptomenorrhea, hysterectomy, synechia of the uterus, testicular feminization syndrome).

[1] Usually or often associated with primary amenorrhea.

CRYPTORCHIDISM

Cryptorchidism (undescended testes) is a common disorder in children. It may be unilateral or bilateral and may be classified as ectopic, total, or incomplete. About 3% of term male infants and 20% of premature male infants have undescended testes at birth. In over half of these cases, the testes will descend by the second month; by age 1 year, 80% of all undescended testes are in the scrotum. If cryptorchidism persists into adult life, failure of spermatogenesis is the rule, but testicular androgen production usually remains intact. The incidence of cancer (usually seminoma) is appreciably greater in testes that remain in the abdomen after puberty.

Cryptorchidism may merely represent delayed descent of the testes or may be due to prevention of normal descent by some mechanical lesion such as adhesions, short spermatic cord, fibrous bands, or endocrine disorders (ie, decreased gonadotropins). It is probable that many undescended testes are congenitally abnormal and that this abnormality in itself is associated with undescent.

A causal relationship between failure of spermatogenesis and an abdominal location of testes after puberty is assumed. On occasion, the apparent abnormality of abdominal testes may be reversible (even if the testes are histologically abnormal at the time they are placed in the scrotum).

Clinical Findings

In palpating the scrotum for the testes, the cremasteric reflex may be elicited, with a resultant ascent of the testes into the abdomen (pseudocryptorchidism). To prevent this ascent, the fingers should first be placed across the upper portion of the inguinal canal. Examination in a warm setting or bath is also helpful.

Treatment

The best age for medical or surgical treatment has not been determined, but early childhood is currently recommended. Some recommend surgery before age 5 years; others say during the first year. There appears to be a high incidence of azoospermia in testes operated on after age 10 years; damage to germ and Leydig cells of intraabdominal testes may occur by age 3–4 years, but the relationship of these changes to fertility is unproved. The risk of surgical injury to the testes must be weighed against the possible benefits. Surgical repair is indicated for cryptorchidism persisting beyond puberty, since the incidence of cancer is appreciably greater in glands that remain in the abdomen beyond the second decade of life.

A. Unilateral Cryptorchidism: Most cases are due to local mechanical lesions or a defective testis on the involved side. If pseudocryptorchidism has been ruled out and if descent has not occurred by age 5 years, many investigators recommend surgical exploration, with testicular biopsy and relocation by a surgeon skilled in this procedure.

B. Bilateral Cryptorchidism: The child with bilaterally undescended testes should be evaluated for sex chromosome abnormalities and genetic sex determined by chromosome analysis in the newborn period. Androgen treatment (testosterone enanthate) is indicated in the newborn male with micropenis and as replacement therapy in the male beyond the normal age of puberty who has been shown to lack functional testes.

C. Pseudocryptorchidism: Retractile testes, ie, those that are sometimes in the scrotum but not at the time of examination, generally require no treatment.

Prognosis

Following surgery, the prognosis is guarded with respect to spermatogenesis in the involved testis.

KLINEFELTER SYNDROME

Klinefelter syndrome is occasionally familial, is typically not diagnosed until the time of puberty, and is characterized by atrophic sclerosis of the seminiferous tubules, normal Leydig cells and virilization. It is often accompanied by bilateral gynecomastia, relatively long extremities (particularly legs), abnormally small testes, and azoospermia or oligospermatogenesis. Gonadotropin levels (particularly luteinizing hormone levels) are usually elevated. Testosterone levels are normal or low. Many patients have mild mental retardation and poor psychosocial skills. There is an extra X chromosome (most commonly an XXY chromosome pattern).

Klinefelter syndrome must be differentiated from other causes of primary hypogonadism, gonadotropin deficiency, and the physiologic gynecomastia that occurs in some boys at puberty.

There is no satisfactory treatment, but depot testosterone, 200–400 mg intramuscularly every 3 weeks, continued for several months, may produce positive physical and behavioral changes and reduce gynecomastia. If not, liposuction or surgical mastectomy for cosmetic purposes is indicated.

DISEASES OF THE THYROID

GOITER

Goiter is not uncommon in children and adolescents and is most commonly due to chronic lymphocytic thyroiditis (see Thyroiditis, below). It may also result from acute inflammation, iodine deficiency, infiltrative processes, neoplasms, ingestion of goitrogens, or an inborn error in thyroid metabolism (familial goiter). With the exception of hyperthyroidism (and possibly pregnancy), thyroid enlargement results from the stimulation of excess thyroid-stimulating hormone (TSH). Regardless of the cause, patients may be clinically and biochemically euthyroid, hypothyroid, or hyperthyroid.

Familial goiter results from enzymatic defects in hormonogenesis, eg, (1) iodide trapping, (2) iodide organification, (3) coupling, (4) deiodination, and (5) production of thyroglobulin and serum carrier protein. Patients with any of these defects display an autosomal recessive mode of inheritance; the organification defect may be associated with severe congenital deafness (Pendred's syndrome). The age at onset of symptoms of hypothyroidism is variable.

Substances implicated in the development of goiter include cabbage, soybeans, turnips, rutabagas, aminosalicyclic acid (PAS), resorcinol, phenylbutazone, iodides (particularly in individuals who have also received corticosteroids), and drugs that interfere with iodide trapping (eg, thiocyanates).

Clinical Findings

The clinical features and physical characteristics of patients with goiters vary depending on the cause and thyroid function tests and are seldom diagnostic.

Nodular goiter may occur during childhood. The likelihood that a nodule is malignant increases when the nodule is single, hard, or associated with paratracheal lymph node enlargement or does not concentrate radioactive iodide (see Carcinoma of the Thyroid, below).

Treatment

Remove or avoid precipitating factors if possible. With the exception of hyperthyroidism and instances where specific causes can be eliminated or corrected (eg, iodide deficiency, goitrogens). If the TSH level is elevated, treatment is with full replacement of thyroid hormone (see below). Surgery is necessary if cancer is a possibility.

Prophylaxis

Prophylaxis in endemic areas of iodine deficiency consists of the use of bread containing iodides or iodized salt (1 mg of iodine per 100 g of salt), the administration of 1–2 drops of saturated solution of potassium iodide per week, or monthly injections of depot iodide preparation. Iodination of the water supply is also a satisfactory preventive measure.

NEONATAL GOITER

Neonatal goiter may result from the transplacental passage, from mother to infant, of iodides, goitrogens, antithyroid drugs, or human-specific thyroid-stimulating immunoglobulin (TSI). The latter may occur in pregnancies in which the mother has or once had Graves' disease. The offspring may temporarily be hyperthyroid, with exophthalmos. Regardless of the cause, the goiter is usually diffuse and relatively soft but may be large and firm enough to compress the trachea, esophagus, and adjacent blood vessels. Treatment varies with the cause; iodides, antithyroid drugs, or thyroid hormone (eg, levothyroxine, 0.05 mg/d) for a few weeks may be indicated. Rarely, surgical division of the thyroid isthmus may be necessary.

HYPOTHYROIDISM

Hypothyroidism may be either congenital or acquired. Congenital hypothyroidism may be due to aplasia, hypoplasia, or maldescent of the thyroid, resulting from an embryonic defect of development; the administration of radioiodide to the mother; or, possibly, an autoimmune disease. It may be caused by defective synthesis of thyroid hormone (familial goiter; see Goiter, above). Other cases of congenital hypothyroidism may result from the maternal ingestion of medications (eg, goitrogens, propylthiouracil, methimazole, or iodides), from iodide deficiency (endemic cretinism), or, rarely, from thyroid hormone unresponsiveness. Thyroid tissue in an aberrant location is present in most patients with sporadic "athyreotic" cretinism.

Acquired (juvenile) hypothyroidism is most commonly the result of chronic lymphocytic thyroiditis (see Thyroiditis, below) but may be idiopathic or the result of surgical removal, thyrotropin deficiency (usually associated with other pituitary tropic hormone deficiencies), the ingestion of medications (eg, iodides, cobalt), or a deficiency of iodides. An ectopic thyroid gland, a relatively common cause of hypothyroidism, may maintain normal function for variable periods postnatally. Breast-feeding may mitigate severe hypothyroidism and perhaps diminish impaired neurologic development in the hypothyroid patient.

Clinical Findings

The findings depend on age at onset and the degree of deficiency.

A. Symptoms & Signs:

1. Functional Changes–Findings include decreased appetite; physical and mental sluggishness; pale, dry, coarse cool skin; decreased intestinal activity (constipation); large tongue; poor muscle tone (protuberant abdomen, umbilical hernia, lumbar lordosis); hypothermia; bradycardia; diminished sweating (variable); lateral thinning of the eye brows; carotenemia; decreased pulse pressure; hoarse voice or cry; and slow relaxation on eliciting tendon reflexes. Prolonged gestation, large size at birth, nasal obstruction and discharge, large fontanelles, hypoactivity, and persistent jaundice may also be present during the neonatal period. Even with congenital deficiency of thyroid hormone, the first findings may not appear for several days or weeks.

2. Retardation of Growth & Development–Findings include decreased growth velocity with resultant shortness of stature; infantile skeletal proportions with relatively short extremities; infantile naso-orbital configuration (flat, broad, and undeveloped bridge of nose and widely spaced eyes); retarded "bone age" and epiphyseal dysgenesis; retarded dental development and enamel hypoplasia; and large fontanelles in the neonate. Slowing of mental responsiveness and retardation of development of the brain may occur. In older children and adolescents, growth failure may be the only manifestation of hypothyroidism.

3. Sexual Precocity–Rarely, isosexual precocity may occur, resulting from elevated gonadotropin levels. Galactorrhea may be present, and menometrorrhagia has been reported in older girls. Testicular enlargement occurs rarely in boys.

4. Other Changes–Myxedema of tissues may occur. The skin may be dry, thick, scaly, and coarse, with a yellowish tinge from excessive deposition of carotene. The hair is dry, coarse, and brittle (variable) and may be excessive. Thinning of the lateral portions of the eyebrows may occur. The axillary and supraclavicular pads may be prominent. Muscular hypertrophy (Kocher, Debré-Sémélaigne syndromes) is occasionally present. Psychosis secondary to myxedema has been described. An ectopic thyroid gland may produce a mass at the base of the tongue or in the midline of the neck.

B. Laboratory Findings: Thyroxine (T_4) and thyroid-stimulating hormone (TSH) levels are the most helpful aids in diagnosing hypothyroidism. Levels of T_4 and free T_4 are reduced and TSH levels are increased in primary hypothyroidism. Serum carotene and cholesterol levels are usually elevated in hypothyroid children but may be normal in some hypothyroid infants; a rise to abnormally high levels occurs 6–8 weeks after cessation of therapy. Serum alkaline phosphatase levels and erythrocyte glucose 6-phosphate dehydrogenase activity are reduced; BUN and creatinine levels may be increased. Circulating autoantibodies to thyroid constituents may be found. Plasma GH levels and GH response to insulin-induced hypoglycemia and arginine stimulation may be subnormal.

C. Imaging: Epiphyseal development ("bone age") is delayed. The cardiac shadow may be increased. Epiphyseal dysgenesis, coxa vara, coxa plana, and vertebral anomalies may occur. The pituitary fossa may be enlarged.

Treatment

Levothyroxine sodium is a reliable synthetic agent for thyroid replacement therapy. The dose is 75–100 μg/m^2 (10–12 μg/kg in neonates). Older children, adolescents, and adults require 0.15–0.2 mg daily in one dose. In hypothyroid patients, particularly myxedematous infants, low doses (0.025–0.05 mg) should be used initially and increased weekly in small increments. The therapeutic range is evaluated by clinical response (appearance, growth, and development), sleeping pulses, and thyroid function tests (TSH and free T_4 levels). Improvement usually occurs in 1–3 weeks.

Course & Prognosis

In patients with congenital hypothyroidism, growth and motor development can be returned to normal with adequate replacement therapy. The prognosis for mental development is guarded if treatment is delayed beyond 3 months of life. In patients with acquired hypothyroidism, restoration of physical and mental function to the predisease level is variable following replacement therapy. Overtreatment with thyroid drugs may produce accelerated skeletal maturation and craniosynostosis; osteoporosis is a concern in adults.

HYPERTHYROIDISM

The clinical features of **hyperthyroidism** are the result of overproduction of thyroid hormones released in response to human thyroid stimulator immunoglobulin (TSI). The latter is an IgG antibody to thyroid receptors produced in individuals who demonstrate a reduced capacity to remove host-directed thyroid-stimulating immunoglobulins. Congenital hyperthyroidism, sometimes persisting or recurring for months or years with or without exophthalmos, may occur in infants of thyrotoxic mothers and may be associated with premature cranio synostosis, minimal brain dysfunction, advanced epiphyseal maturation, and goiter.

Hyperthyroidism (with normal T_4 levels) may result from isolated hypersecretion of triiodothyronine (T_3 toxicosis) but is uncommon during childhood.

Clinical Findings

A. Symptoms & Signs: The disease usually develops rapidly and is more common in girls (5:1), with the highest incidence between ages 12 and 14 years. The manifestations may include the following in any combination: "nervousness" (ie, restlessness, mood swings, hand tremors); palpitations and tachycardia, even during sleep, and systolic hypertension with increased pulse pressure; warm and moist skin and flushed face; exophthalmos; diffuse goiter, usually firm, with or without bruit and thrill; weakness and loss of weight in spite of polyphagia; accelerated growth and development; and poor school performance. Amenorrhea is common in adolescent girls.

B. Laboratory Findings: Levels of T_4, free T_4, and T_3 resin uptake are elevated. T3 levels may be elevated. Serum cholesterol and TSH levels are low. Circulating TSI and other antithyroid antibody levels are usually elevated and may be useful in following the course of the disease. There is moderate leukopenia and hyperglycemia. Glycosuria may be present.

Treatment

Antithyroid drugs, radioactive iodide, and surgical methods are equally capable of eliminating the manifestations of hyperthyroidism and yield approximately equal numbers of "cured" patients.

A. General Measures:

1. Restricted Physical Activity–Activity should be restricted in severe cases, in preparation for surgery or during pregnancy.

2. Diet–The diet should be high in calories, proteins, and vitamins.

3. Sedation–Large doses of barbiturates or tranquilizers may be necessary to control nervousness.

4. Sympatholytic Drugs–These drugs (eg, propranolol) decrease the peripheral conversion of T_4 to T_3 and diminish cardiovascular and some neurologic symptoms. They are also helpful in preparation for thyroid surgery.

B. Specific Measures: With medical treatment, clinical response may be noted in about 2–3 weeks, and adequate control may be achieved in 2–3 months. The thyroid gland frequently increases in size after initiation of treatment, but it usually decreases in size after 3 months.

1. Propylthiouracil–This drug blocks the hormonogenesis and release of thyroid hormone as well as the peripheral conversion of T_4 to T_3. It may be used in the initial treatment of the patient with hyperthyroidism, but if the T_4 fails to return to a normal range, surgery or RAI may be necessary, although some patients may be controlled by long-continued (> 5 years) medical therapy. Relapses occur in 25–50% of patients, and severe cases may not respond. Therapy must usually be continued at least 2–3 years with the minimum drug dosage that will produce a euthyroid state.

a. Initial Dosage–Give 100–800 mg/d in 3 or 4 divided doses 6 or 8 hours apart until results of thyroid function tests are normal and all signs and symptoms have subsided. Larger doses may be necessary.

b. Maintenance Dosage–Give 100–150 mg/d in 1–3 divided doses. The drug may be continued at higher doses until hypothyroidism has resulted, and then a supplement of oral thyroid may be added. Thyroid hormone may be necessary if the TSH concentration rises during treatment.

2. Methimazole (Tapazole)–This may be used in 1/15–1/10 the dosage of propylthiouracil. Toxic reactions are slightly more common with this drug than with the thiouracils in children.

3. Iodide–Elemental iodide is effective only transiently (1–2 weeks) and may be useful in preparation of surgery or RAI and following RAI therapy. Iodide is generally not recommended.

4. Radioactive Iodide–Radioiodide therapy is currently recommended by some either as initial treatment or if medical therapy fails. Regardless of the dose or type of radioactive iodide employed, hypothyroidism generally can be anticipated at variable periods after treatment.

5. Other Drugs–Antithyroid drugs, antibiotics, sedation, propranolol, reserpine, and guanethidine may be of value for the treatment of thyroid storm.

C. Surgical Measures: Subtotal thyroidectomy is still recommended in some centers for children, especially if close follow-up is difficult or impossible. The patient should be prepared first with bed rest, diet, propranolol, and sedation (as above) and with propylthiouracil (for 2–4 weeks). Iodide (2–10 drops daily of saturated solution of potassium iodide for 10–21 days) may be of value. Continue for 1 week after surgery.

Course & Prognosis

Medical treatment is usually effective within 2–3 years. With medical treatment alone, prolonged remissions may be expected in about one-third of cases. Hypothyroidism is likely in later life. The risk of developing leukemia or carcinoma of the thyroid after treatment with radioactive iodide has not been determined.

CARCINOMA OF THE THYROID

See also Chapter 29.

Carcinoma of the thyroid is uncommon. It is most likely to occur following irradiation of the neck and chest. Findings include goiter, neck discomfort, dysphagia, voice changes, or a nodule of the thyroid that fails to regress despite therapy with above maintenance doses of thyroid hormones for a period of 2 months. Surgical extirpation of the entire gland, with removal of all involved nodes, is the treatment of choice. Radical neck dissection is seldom necessary. Postoperatively, the patient may be allowed to become hypothyroid and a diagnostic scan with radioactive iodide may then be done; metastases, if present, can be treated with ^{131}I or removed surgically, if feasible. Subsequent thyroid replacement therapy should consist of larger than maintenance doses. Monitoring of thyroglobulin levels is useful in following the course. Patients with papillary carcinoma have a good prognosis for prolonged (> 10 years) survival.

Medullary carcinoma may be familial and associated with multiple endocrine adenomatosis, marfanoid body habitus, mucosal neuromas of the tongue and mucous membranes, and pheochromocytoma or visceral ganglioneuromas. The serum calcitonin level is elevated.

GOITROUS CRETINISM

See Familial Goiter, above.

THYROIDITIS

Acute thyroiditis produces an acute inflammatory goiter and may be due to almost any pathogenic organism (viral or bacterial) or may be nonspecific or idiopathic. Most children are euthyroid and free of symptoms, but hypothyroidism or hyperthyroidism may be present. Specific antibiotic therapy and corticosteroids may be of value.

Subacute thyroiditis (pseudotuberculosis, de Quervain's giant cell thyroiditis) is characterized by mild and transient manifestations of hypermetabolism and an enlarged, very tender, firm thyroid gland. The T_4 concentration is elevated, and ^{131}I uptake by the gland is reduced. Aspirin (mild cases) corticosteroids (severe disease), and thyroid hormone may be of value.

Chronic thyroiditis (lymphocytic or Hashimoto's struma, autoimmune thyroiditis) is common, particularly in pubertal patients ("adolescent goiter"). It may be associated with other endocrine disorders (eg, Addison's disease, type I diabetes mellitus) resulting from autoimmune damage to the organ. It is characterized by firm, nontender, diffuse or nodular, "pebbly" enlargement of the thyroid with variable activity. Occasionally, there are symptoms of mild tracheal compression. Definitive diagnosis can be made only by histologic examination; thyroid function tests, antithyroid antibody tests, and scanning studies provide varying results. Needle biopsy of the gland is often diagnostic but is not generally indicated. Treatment is with thyroid hormone in full replacement dosage when TSH levels rise. Hypothyroidism is often an end result, and lifelong treatment may be required.

DISEASES OF THE PARATHYROID GLANDS

HYPOPARATHYROIDISM

Hypoparathyroidism may be idiopathic, may result from parathyroidectomy, or may be one feature of a general autoimmune disorder associated with candidiasis, Addison's disease, pernicious anemia, diabetes mellitus, thyroiditis, ovarian failure, and alopecia. Transient hypoparathyroidism may occur in the neonate as a result of parathyroid gland immaturity; the condition is more common in the offspring of diabetic and of hyperparathyroid mothers.

Clinical Findings

A. Symptoms & Signs:

1. Tetany–Symptoms and signs include numbness, cramps and twitchings of extremities, carpopedal spasm, laryngospasm, a positive Chvostek sign (tapping of the face in front of the ear produces spasm of the facial muscles), a positive peroneal sign (tapping the fibular side of the leg over the peroneal nerve produces abduction and dorsiflexion of the foot), and a positive Trousseau sign (prolonged compression of the upper arm produces carpal spasm).

2. Prolonged Hypocalcemia–In addition to the findings listed above, prolonged hypocalcemia may be associated with growth retardation, blepharospasm and chronic conjunctivitis, cataracts, unexplained bizarre behavior, diarrhea, photophobia, irritability, loss of consciousness, convulsions, poor dentition, skin rashes, ectodermal dysplasias, fungal infections (*Candida*), "idiopathic" epilepsy, symmetric punctate calcifications of basal ganglia, and steatorrhea. Candidiasis, Addison's disease, thyroiditis, and pernicious anemia may precede or follow the hypoparathyroidism in the familial "autoimmune" form.

B. Laboratory Findings: See Table 23–4. Serum parathyroid levels are inappropriately low.

Treatment

The objective of treatment is to maintain serum calcium at a low normal level.

A. Tetany: In patients with acute or severe tetany, immediate correction of hypocalcemia is indicated. Calcium should be given intravenously and orally. Thiazide diuretics may be used to increase urinary calcium reabsorption.

B. Prolonged Hypocalcemia: For maintenance therapy in patients with hypoparathyroidism and chronic hypocalcemia, use calciferol 1,25 dihydroxycholecalciferol or dihydrotachysterol (see Chapter 38). The diet should be high in calcium, with added calcium lactate or carbonate, and should be adequate in phosphorus.

PSEUDOHYPOPARATHYROIDISM
(Albright's Brachymetacarpal Dwarfism)

Pseudohypoparathyroidism consists of a group of disorders generally having a familial X-linked dominant syndrome in which there is no lack of parathyroid hormone but a failure of response in the end organs (eg, the renal tubule). The symptoms and signs of hypocalcemia are the same as in idiopathic hypoparathyroidism. Patients with pseudohypoparathyroidism have round, full faces, stubby fingers (shortening of the first, fourth, and fifth metacarpals), mental subnormality, shortness of stature, delayed and defective dentition, and early closure of the epiphyses. X-rays may show dyschondroplastic changes in the bones of the hands, demineralization of the bones, thickening of the cortices, exostoses, and ectopic calcification of the

Table 23–4. Laboratory findings in rickets and disorders of calcium metabolism.[1]

	Metabolic Features					
	Serum Concentration				Urinary Excretion	
Condition	Ca^{2+}	P	Alk P'tase	PTH	Ca^{2+}	P
Chronic renal insufficiency	↓ (N)	↑	↑(N)	↑	↓ (N)	↓
Hypoparathyroid states	↓	↑	N		↓	↓
Malabsorption syndrome	↓ (N)	↓ (N)	↑ (N)	↑ (N)	↓	N (↑ ↓)
Rickets						
Familial hypophosphatemic vitamin D-resistant	N (↓)	↓	N	N (↑)	N	↑
Hereditary vitamin D-refractory	↓	↓ (N)	↑	↑		↑
Vitamin D-deficient	↓ (N)	↓	↑	↑	↑	↑
Transient tetany of the newborn	↓	↓ (N)	↓ (N)	↓ (N)	↓ (N)	↓ (N)

[1] Tubular reabsorption of phosphate (TRP) normally is 83–98%; the lower values are associated with higher serum levels of phosphorus. In hypoparathyroidism, TRP values vary from 40 to 70%. Low TRP values are also found in some forms of inherited renal tubular disease, eg, vitamin D-resistant rickets.

basal ganglia and subcutaneous tissues. Corneal and lenticular opacities may be present.

Treatment is with vitamin D and supplementary oral calcium lactate or carbonate.

HYPERPARATHYROIDISM

Hyperparathyroidism may be primary (occasionally familial) or secondary. Primary hyperparathyroidism may be due to adenoma or diffuse parathyroid hyperplasia. The most common causes of the secondary form are chronic renal disease (glomerulonephritis, pyelonephritis), congenital anomalies of the genitourinary tract, pseudohypoparathyroidism, and vitamin D-refractory rickets. Rarely, it may be found in osteogenesis imperfecta, cancer with bony metastases, and vitamin D-resistant rickets.

Clinical Findings

A. Symptoms & Signs:

1. Due to Hypercalcemia*–Findings include hypotonicity and weakness of muscles; chronic abdominal pain; nausea, vomiting, and poor tone of the gastrointestinal tract, with constipation; loss of weight; hyperextensibility of joints; bradycardia; and shortening of the QT interval.

2. Due to Increased Calcium and Phosphorus Excretion– Polyuria, hyposthenuria, polydipsia, and precipitation of calcium phosphate in the renal parenchyma or as urinary calculi (ie, sand or gravel) may occur.

3. Related to Changes in the Skeleton–Findings include osteitis fibrosa, absence of lamina dura around the teeth, spontaneous fractures, and a "moth-eaten" appearance of the skull.

B. Laboratory Findings: Serum calcium and parathyroid hormone, urinary phosphorus, cAMP, and hydroxyproline excretion are increased (Table 23–5).

C. Imaging: Bone changes do not usually occur in children with an adequate calcium intake. When bone changes occur, there is a generalized demineralization with a predilection for the subperiosteal cor-

* Hypercalcemia may also be secondary to immobilization, excess intake of vitamin D, sarcoidosis, milk-alkali syndrome, extensive fat necrosis of the newborn, or certain types of cancer, or it may occur as a familial disease.

Table 23–5. Laboratory findings in hypercalcemia.

Condition	Metabolic Features					Bone Pathology
	Serum Concentration			Urinary Excretion		
	Ca^{2+}	P	P'tase	Ca^{2+}	P	
Excessive vitamin D	↑	↑	N	↑	N (↑)	
Hyperparathyroidism	↑	↓	N (↑)	↑	↑	Generalized osteitis fibrosa
Hyperparathyroidism with impaired renal function	↑	N (↑)	↑	↑	↑	Generalized osteitis fibrosa
Hyperproteinemia	↑ (total) N (ionized)	N	N	N	N	
Idiopathic hypercalcemia	↑	N	N	↑	N	See text
Neoplasms of bone	N (↑)	N	N (↑)	↑	N (↑)	Bone destruction

tical bone. The distal clavicle and phalanges are usually first affected. Nephrocalcinosis is an important additional x-ray finding.

Treatment

Complete removal of tumor or subtotal removal of hyperplastic parathyroid glands is indicated. Preoperatively, fluids should be forced and the intake of calcium restricted. Postoperatively, the diet should be high in calcium, phosphorus, and vitamin D.

Treatment of secondary hyperparathyroidism (viz renal disease) is directed at the underlying disease. Decrease the intake of phosphate by use of aluminum hydroxide orally and by reduction of milk consumption.

Course & Prognosis

Although the condition may recur (particularly in patients with familial forms of hyperparathyroidism), the prognosis following subtotal parathyroidectomy or removal of an adenoma is usually quite good. The prognosis in the secondary forms depends on correction of the underlying defect. Renal function may remain abnormal.

IDIOPATHIC HYPERCALCEMIA

Idiopathic hypercalcemia (Williams's syndrome) is an uncommon disorder probably related to either excessive intake or increased sensitivity to vitamin D. The disease is characterized in its severe form by peculiar facies (receding mandible, depressed bridge of nose, relatively large mouth, prominent lips, hanging jowls, large low-set ears, "elfin" appearance), failure to thrive, mental and motor retardation, irritability, purposeless movements, constipation, hypotonia, polyuria, polydipsia, hypertension, and heart disease (especially supravalvular aortic stenosis). Generalized osteosclerosis is common, and there may be premature craniosynostosis and nephrocalcinosis with evidence of urinary tract disease. Hypercholesterolemia, azotemia, and serum vitamin A elevations may be present.

Clinical manifestations may not appear for several months. Severe disease may end in death. Mild disease may occur without the typical facies and other findings and has a good prognosis.

Treatment is by rigid restriction of dietary calcium and vitamin D and, in severely involved children, the administration of corticosteroids in high doses.

HYPOPHOSPHATASIA

Hypophosphatasia is an uncommon heritable condition characterized by rickets and a deficiency of alkaline phosphatase. The earlier the age at onset, the more severe the condition. Failure to thrive, premature loss of teeth, widening of the sutures, bulging fontanelles, convulsions, bony deformities, dwarfing, and renal lesions have been reported. Premature closure of cranial sutures may occur. Late features include osteoporosis, pseudofractures, and rachitic deformities. Signs and symptoms may be similar to those of idiopathic hypercalcemia. The serum calcium level is frequently high. The urinary hydroxyproline level is low during infancy. The plasma and urine contain phosphoethanolamine in excessive amounts. No specific treatment is available; corticosteroids may be of value.

DISEASES OF THE ADRENAL CORTEX

ADRENOCORTICAL HYPOFUNCTION
(Adrenal Crisis, Addison's Disease)

Adrenocortical hypofunction may be due to atrophy; autoimmune disease; destruction of the gland by a tumor, hemorrhage (Waterhouse-Friderichsen syndrome), or infection (eg, tuberculosis); congenital absence of the adrenal cortex; or congenital hyperplasia of the cortex associated with glucocorticoid insufficiency with or without androgen excess. It may occur as a consequence of inadequate secretion of corticotropin (ACTH) due to anterior pituitary or hypothalamic disease. Any acute illness, surgery, trauma, or exposure to excessive heat may precipitate an adrenal crisis. A temporary salt-losing disorder (possibly due to hypoaldosteronism) may occur during infancy.

Adrenogenital syndrome and associated adrenal insufficiency, congenital adrenocortical insufficiency, autoimmune adrenal insufficiency, and neoplasms are the most common causes of chronic adrenocortical insufficiency. Autoimmune Addison's disease may be associated with hypoparathyroidism, lymphocytic thyroiditis, candidiasis, pernicious anemia, ovarian failure, alopecia, and diabetes mellitus. Antiadrenal antibodies may be present.

Clinical Findings

A. Symptoms & Signs:

1. Acute Form (Adrenal Crisis)–Signs and symptoms include nausea and vomiting; diarrhea; dehydration; fever, which may be followed by hypothermia; circulatory collapse; and confusion or coma.

2. Chronic Form (Addison's Disease)–Signs and symptoms include vomiting (which becomes forceful and sometimes projectile), diarrhea, weakness, fatigue, weight loss or failure to gain weight, increased appetite for salt, dehydration, increased pigmentation (both generalized and over pressure points, scars, and mucous membranes), hypotension, and small heart size.

B. Laboratory Findings:

1. Adrenal Insufficiency–Findings suggestive of adrenal insufficiency include the following:

a. Serum sodium, chloride, and carbon dioxide levels are decreased.

b. Serum potassium and blood urea nitrogen levels are increased.

c. Urinary sodium levels are increased despite low serum sodium levels.

d. Eosinophilia and moderate neutropenia occur.

e. Fasting blood glucose levels are generally normal but may be low in crisis.

f. There is inability to excrete a water load.

2. Adrenal Cortex Function–Results of confirmatory tests to measure the functional capacity of the adrenal cortex include the following:

a. Blood cortisol, urinary free cortisol, 17-hydroxycorticosteroid levels, and ketogenic steroid excretion levels are decreased. ACTH levels are increased in primary adrenal insufficiency.

b. Blood Androstenedione and DHEA concentrations and urinary 17-ketosteroid levels are decreased except in cases due to congenital hyperplasia or tumor of the cortex. See pg 779–780.

c. Circulating eosinophil counts are elevated.

d. Corticotropin and metyrapone administration are associated with subnormal responses.

Treatment

A. Acute Form (Adrenal Crisis):

1. Treat infections with large doses of the appropriate antibiotics or other antimicrobial agents.

2. Treat hypovolemia with adequate fluid electrolyte therapy (normal saline) and p 000 (eg, isoproterenol, dopamine). Infusion of a solution of human albumin may be necessary in severe cases.

3. For replacement therapy, use the following:

a. Initially, hydrocortisone sodium succinate (Solu-Cortef), 2 mg/kg diluted in 2–10 mL of water intravenously, is given over 2–5 minutes. Following this, an infusion of normal saline and 5–10% glucose, 100 mL/kg/24 hr intravenously, is given.

b. Hydrocortisone sodium succinate, 1.5 mg/kg (12.5 mg/m^2), is given intravenously every 4–6 hours until stabilization is achieved and oral therapy tolerated.

c. Ten percent glucose in normal saline, 20 mL/kg intravenously in the first 2 hours, may be of value, particularly in infants with adrenal crisis who have congenital adrenal hyperplasia. Avoid overtreatment.

4. Fruit juices, ginger ale, milk, and soft foods should be begun as soon as possible.

B. Chronic Form (Addison's Disease): There may be variable response to different glucocorticoids in some patients. (See Table 23–6 for conversion of other corticosteroids to hydrocortisone equivalents.) Maintenance therapy following initial stabilization generally requires the use of a corticosteroid together with a liberal intake of salt and a fluorinated steroid. Children requiring prolonged adrenocorticosteroid administration should have periodic determinations of height, weight, and blood pressure (taken in the recumbent position) and assay of blood glucose, ACTH, sodium, and potassium.

1. Hydrocortisone–Dosages are as follows:

a. Physiologic replacement–

(1) Intramuscularly–0.44 mg/kg or 13–20 mg/m^2 once daily.

(2) Orally*–0.66 mg/kg in infants or 10–15 mg/m^2/d.

b. Therapeutic use–

(1) Intramuscularly–4.4 mg/kg or 130 mg/m^2 once daily.

(2) Orally*–6.6 mg/kg or 200 mg/m^2/d.

c. Therapeutic maintenance–

(1) Intramuscularly–1.3–2.2 mg/kg or 40–65 mg/m^2 once daily.

(2) Orally*–2–3.3 mg/kg or 60–100 mg/m^2/d.

d. Development of infection–If infection occurs while the patient is receiving a large dose of glucocorticoid, give about 2–3 times the physiologic maintenance dose for 3 or 4 days and then resume the larger dose.

* In 4 doses 6 hours apart (preferred) or 3 doses every 8 hours, providing approximately 50% of the total dose in the early morning.

Table 23–6. Corticosteroids.

Generic and Chemical Name	Potency per Milligram Compared With Hydrocortisone[1] Glucocorticoid Effect	Mineralocorticoid Effect
Glucocorticoids		
Hydrocortisone	1	1
Dexamethasone	30	Minimal
Fluprednisolone	13	
Methylprednisolone	5	Minimal
Prednisolone	4	Minimal
Prednisone	4	Minimal
Triamcinolone	5	Minimal
Mineralocorticoids		
Aldosterone	30	500
Fludrocortisone		15–20

[1] To convert hydrocortisone dosage to equivalent dosage in any of the other preparations listed in this table, divide by the potency factors shown.

e. Long-term maintenance–Except when used for replacement therapy (ie, in the treatment of Addison's disease and congenital adrenal hyperplasia), and in the treatment of certain malignant states, the total 2-day dose of glucocorticoid for long-term maintenance therapy may be administered as a single dose once every 48 hours. This will not diminish the therapeutic efficacy but will diminish the side effects; there may be normal growth and decreased tendency to cushingoid appearance.

2. Fludrocortisone–Give fludrocortisone, 0.05–0.2 mg daily in 2 divided doses.

3. Sodium Chloride–Give 1–3 g/d (as enteric-coated salt pills if they can be taken). Reduce the dose if edema appears.

4. Increased Dosages–Additional glucocorticoids (2–3 times the maintenance dose) may be necessary with moderate to severe acute illness, surgery, trauma, or other stress reactions after optimal glucocorticoid stabilization has been achieved.

C. Other Recommendations:

1. If corticosteroids have been administered for more than 1 month, terminate their use gradually. Abrupt withdrawal may cause a severe "rebound" of the disease or rarely produce symptoms of adrenal insufficiency.

2. Give corticosteroids to any child undergoing surgery, severe infection, or other significant stress who has received prolonged therapy with corticosteroids in the past.

3. If a child receiving maintenance doses of corticosteroids develops chickenpox, the dosage of glucocorticoids should be increased to pharmacologic levels (eg, 2 times maintenance). Corticosteroid withdrawal in these circumstances may have a fatal outcome.

4. Use of topical corticosteroids for the treatment of inflammatory skin conditions may result in absorption of significantly large amounts of corticosteroid.

D. Corticosteroids in Patients Requiring Surgery: In patients with current or previous adrenocortical insufficiency who undergo surgery, corticosteroids are given as follows:

1. Preoperatively–Give oral glucocorticoids in twice the maintenance dose 24 hours before surgery.

2. During Operation–Give hydrocortisone sodium succinate (Solu-Cortef), 1–2 mg/kg by intravenous infusion over a 6- to 12-hour period.

3. Postoperatively–Continue intravenous delivery until oral intake is resumed. Begin oral preparation as soon as possible, and give full maintenance doses daily.

ADRENOCORTICAL HYPERFUNCTION

1. CUSHING'S SYNDROME

The principal findings in **Cushing's syndrome** in children result from excessive secretion of glucocorticoid and androgenic hormones, leading to varying degrees of abnormal carbohydrate, protein, and fat metabolism and virilization. In noniatrogenic disease, there may also be overproduction of mineralocorticoids and adrenal androgens.

Cushing's syndrome is more common in females; in children under 12 years of age, noniatrogenic disease is usually due to adrenal tumor. Hemihypertrophy may be present. Cushing's syndrome is a common result of therapy with one of the corticosteroids. Rarely, it may be associated with an apparently primary adrenocortical hyperplasia or hyperplasia secondary either to basophilic adenoma of the pituitary gland or to an ectopic ACTH-producing tumor. Spontaneous remission has been reported.

Clinical Findings

A. Symptoms & Signs:

1. Due to Excessive Secretion of the Carbohydrate-regulating Hormones–"Buffalo type" adiposity, most marked on the face, neck, and trunk, may occur; a fat pad in the interscapular area is characteristic. Other findings include easy fatigability and muscle weakness, striae, plethoric facies, easy bruisability, osteoporosis, increased appetite, growth failure, hyperglycemia, psychologic disturbances, and pain in the back.

2. Due to Excessive Secretion of Androgens–Findings include an increase in the linear growth rate, hirsutism, acne, varying degrees of clitoral or penile enlargement, advanced epiphyseal maturation, and deepening of the voice. Menstrual irregularities occur in older girls.

3. Due to Excessive Production of Mineralocorticoids–Sodium retention with hypertension (rarely edema) occurs.

B. Laboratory Findings:

1. Serum chloride and potassium levels may be low.

2. Serum sodium, pH, and carbon dioxide content may be elevated.

3. Plasma and urine cortisol levels are increased, and plasma diurnal variation may not occur.

4. Excretions of urinary free cortisol, 17-ketosteroids, 17-hydroxycorticosteroids, and 17-ketogenic steroids, are generally increased; the test for free cortisol is the assay of choice. Increased secretion of ACTH occurs in patients with adrenal hyperplasia and with ACTH-secreting nonendocrine tumors but not with other adrenal tumors. Suppression of blood cortisol and 17-hydroxycorticosteroids by high doses of dexamethasone occurs with adrenal hyperplasia but not with adrenal tumors.

5. Eosinophil counts are below 50/μL.

6. Glycosuria alone or with carbohydrate intolerance and hyperglycemia may be present ("diabetic" type of glucose tolerance curve).

7. Abdominal ultrasonography, CT or MRI scanning, and radioactive cholesterol uptake studies may be helpful in localizing a tumor.

Treatment

Since almost all cases of primary adrenal hyperfunction in childhood are due to tumor, surgical removal (if possible) is indicated. Corticotropin has been recommended for preoperative and postoperative use to stimulate the nontumorous adrenal cortex, which is generally atrophied. Corticosteroids should be administered for 1 or 2 days before surgery and continued during and after operation. Supplemental potassium, normal saline solution, and fludrocortisone may be necessary.

Pituitary surgery is the treatment if choice for Cushing's disease. Irradiation or cyproheptadine may also be of value to control Cushing's disease.

Prognosis

If the tumor is malignant, the prognosis is poor. If it is benign, cure should result following proper preparation and surgery.

2. CONGENITAL ADRENAL HYPERPLASIA (CAH)

Virilization is most commonly the result of **congenital adrenal hyperplasia** or tumor; maternal androgens from endogenous and exogenous sources and tumor may also be causative in newborns.

The congenital form of adrenogenital syndrome (due to adrenal hyperplasia) is an autosomal recessive disease due to an inborn error of metabolism with a deficiency of an adrenocortical enzyme. Various types are recognized, including the following:

1. Deficiency of 21-hydroxylase (approximately 90% of cases), resulting in inability to convert 17-hydroxyprogesterone into 11-deoxycortisol. Mild forms result in androgenic changes (virilization) alone, but severe cases are associated with salt loss and electrolyte imbalance.
2. Deficiency in β-hydroxylation and a failure to convert 11-deoxycortisol to cortisol. This is associated with virilization and usually with hypertension.
3. A defect in 17-hydroxylase, with the enzyme deficiency in both the adrenals and the gonads. Hypertension, virilization, amenorrhea, and eunuchoidism may be present.
4. A partial or complete defect in β-hydroxysteroid dehydrogenase activity and a failure to convert D^5-pregnenolone to progesterone. This is associated with incomplete masculinization, hypospadias, and cryptorchidism in the male. Some degree of masculinization may occur in the female. Severe sodium loss occurs, and the infant mortality rate is high in the complete form.
5. Cholesterol desmolase deficiency with congenital lipoid adrenal hyperplasia. Clinical features are similar to those of 3β-hydroxysteroid dehydrogenase deficiency (above).

CAH in Females

In congenital hyperplasia of the adrenal cortex (pseudohermaphroditism), abnormalities of the external genitalia include an enlarged clitoris with partial to complete labial fusion and a common urogenital sinus. Growth in height is excessive and "bone age" advanced, and patients may have excessive muscularity. Pubic hair appears early, acne may be excessive, and the voice may deepen.

Pseudohermaphroditism in the female may also be produced as a result of the administration of androgens, progestins, diethylstilbestrol, and related hormones to the mother during the first trimester of pregnancy or as a result of virilizing maternal tumors. In these cases, the condition regresses after birth.

CAH in Males (Macrogenitosomia Praecox)

In males, precocious sexual development is along isosexual lines. With congenital bilateral hyperplasia of the adrenal cortex, the infant may appear normal at birth; however, during the first few months of life, the penis enlarges, the scrotum darkens, the rugae become more prominent, and acne and pubic and axillary hair appear. The testicles generally remain small, and spermatogenesis does not occur. Other symptoms and signs are similar to those of the congenital form in females. If an adrenal or testicular tumor is the cause, the tumor may be palpable or readily appreciated with ultrasonography, CT, or MRI. Rarely, an adrenal tumor in either sex produces feminization, with gynecomastia resulting in males.

Laboratory Findings

A. 21-Hydroxylase Deficiency–Blood and urine adrenal androgens and testosterone are elevated and the 17 OH progesterone level is elevated to diagnostic levels in cord and newborn blood. Aldosterone may be reduced, and excessive sodium loss occurs in salt-losing forms.

B. β-Hydroxylase Deficiency–11-Deoxycortisol (and its tetrahydro derivative), 17-hydroxycorticoid, deoxycorticosterone, 17-ketosteroid, and testosterone levels are increased.

C. 17-Hydroxylase Deficiency–17-Ketosteroid and 17-hydroxycorticoid levels are decreased; aldosterone, corticosterone, and deoxycorticosterone levels are increased.

D. β-Hydroxysteroid Dehydrogenase Deficiency–With the exception of D^5 compounds all adrenal steroid levels in the blood and urine are low.

E. Cholesterol Desmolase Deficiency–All steroid excretion is markedly decreased.

F. Tumor–Excretion of dehydroepiandrosterone may be greatly elevated.

Dexamethasone Suppression Test

If the administration of dexamethasone, 2–4 mg/d orally in 4 doses for 7 days, reduces serum and urine metabolite levels, hyperplasia rather than adenoma is the probable diagnosis.

Imaging

Genitograms using contrast material may indicate the presence of a urogenital sinus. Displacement of the kidney and calcification in the area of the adrenal may be seen on urograms or plain films of patients with tumors. Radiograph of epiphyseal maturation ("bone age") is typically advanced with 21- and 11β-hydroxylase defects after the first year of life in the untreated child.

Treatment

A. Congenital Hyperplasia of the Adrenal Cortex:

1. Hydrocortisone–Approximately 20–25 $mg/m^2/d$ orally will produce adrenal suppression and normal linear growth. Dosages of 10–25 mg/d for infants and 25–100 mg/d for older children initially are usually necessary. The drug should be given orally in divided doses several times a day, two-fifths of the total dose given as the first morning dose and two-fifths as the last dose at night. After suppression is achieved, the maintenance doses necessary to sustain control are generally 10–15 $mg/m^2/day$.

2. Mineralocorticoids–For patients with salt-losing forms of adrenogenital syndrome, therapy with fludrocortisone and sodium chloride is necessary (see pp 000–000).

3. Glucocorticoids–Glucocorticoids should be increased (by 3–4 times) during acute severe stress, surgery, or moderate infectious illnesses.

4. Surgical Measures–Recession or partial clitoridectomy is occasionally indicated in a girl with an abnormally large or sensitive clitoris but may be delayed for 1 or 2 years until the effect of therapy is determined. Surgical correction of the labial fusion and urogenital sinus may require several operations.

B. Tumor: Because the malignant lesions cannot be distinguished clinically from the benign ones, surgical removal is indicated whenever a tumor has been diagnosed. Preoperative and postoperative treatment are the same as for Cushing's syndrome due to a tumor (see Cushing's Syndrome, above).

Course & Prognosis

Untreated patients with congenital adrenal hyperplasia will show precocious virilization throughout childhood. Because of accelerated skeletal maturation, these individuals will be tall as children but short as adults. Adequate corticosteroid treatment permits normal growth and sexual maturation.

Female pseudohermaphrodites mistakenly raised as males for more than 3 years may have serious psychologic disturbances if their sex role is changed after that time.

When virilization is caused by a tumor, progression of signs and symptoms will cease after successful surgical removal; pubic hair, pigmentation, and deepening of the voice may regress or persist.

3. PRIMARY ALDOSTERONISM

Primary hyperaldosteronism may be caused by an adrenal tumor or by adrenal hyperplasia. It is characterized by paresthesias, tetany, weakness, periodic "paralysis," low serum potassium levels, hypertension, alkaline urine, proteinuria, metabolic alkalosis, carbohydrate intolerance, suppressed plasma renin activity, polyuria, and hyposthenuria that does not respond to vasopressin. The urinary aldosterone level is increased, but other steroid levels are variable. Adrenal tumors may be visualized with CT, ultrasonography, or MRI. Treatment of the tumor is by surgical removal. With hyperplasia, subtotal or total adrenalectomy is recommended if pharmacologic doses of glucocorticoid are ineffective after 2 months.

A form of secondary hyperaldosteronism occurs, possibly due to increased prostagladins, in which both renin and aldosterone levels are elevated in the absence of hypertension (Bartter's syndrome). There is associated renovascular disease with hyperplasia of the juxtaglomerular apparatus and renal electrolyte wasting.

DISEASES OF THE ADRENAL MEDULLA

PHEOCHROMOCYTOMA
(Chromaffinoma)

Pheochromocytoma is an uncommon tumor that may be located wherever there is any chromaffin tissue (eg, adrenal medulla, sympathetic ganglia, carotid body). The condition may be familial (eg, multiple endocrine adenomatosis type II), and in children the tumors are often multiple and bilateral.

Clinical Findings

Clinical manifestations of pheochromocytoma are due to excessive secretion of epinephrine or norepinephrine (or both). Attacks of anxiety and headaches should arouse suspicion. Other findings are palpitation, dizziness, weakness, nausea, vomiting, diarrhea, dilated pupils with blurring of vision, abdominal and precordial pain, rapid pulse, hypertension (usually persistent), and discomfort from heat. The symptoms may be sustained, producing all of the above findings plus papilledema, retinopathy, and cardiac enlargement.

Urine and serum catecholamine levels are increased. The 24-hour urine collection shows markedly increased urinary excretion of total catecholamines, metanephrine, and vanilmandelic acid. *Caution:* Attacks may be provoked by mechanical stimulation of the tumor or by histamine or tyramine. Results of the phentolamine (Regitine) test are positive, but the test is not specific for pheochromocytoma. Displacement of the kidney may be shown by routine x-ray. The tumor may be defined by ultrasonography, CT, or MRI of the abdomen.

Treatment

Surgical removal of the tumor is the treatment of choice, but a sudden paroxysm and death during surgery are not uncommon. The oral administration of propranolol and phentolamine preoperatively has been recommended to prevent the extreme fluctuations of blood pressure that sometimes occur during surgery. Medical treatment includes phenoxybenzamine to reduce hypertension and propranolol to lessen tachycardia and ventricular dysrhythmias.

Prognosis

Complete relief of symptoms, except those due to long-standing vascular or renal changes, is the rule after recovery. If no treatment is given, severe cardiac, renal, and cerebral damage may result.

DIABETES MELLITUS

Insulin dependent diabetes mellitus (IDDM), or type I diabetes (previously referred to as juvenile diabetes), is the primary type of diabetes occurring in people under age 40 years and is characterized by a gradual loss of insulin production. Although the majority of children in the United States no longer present in acidosis (due to the earlier diagnosis by lay and professional people), if untreated long enough acidosis will ensue.

Noninsulin-dependent diabetes mellitus (NIDDM), or type II diabetes, occurs primarily in people over 40 years of age who are overweight, but can occur in overweight teenagers and is then referred to as maturity-onset diabetes in youth (MODY). Insulin production is often elevated in NIDDM (and MODY) and the etiology is related to ineffective insulin activity. Treatment is with weight loss, exercise, oral hypoglycemic agents, and a high-fiber diet. Insulin is not initially required and acidosis is usually not a problem.

Transient diabetes may occur in the newborn and may not require insulin treatment. Similarly, the stress of illness may result in hyperglycemia and glucosuria (and even mild acetonuria) in some children. Treatment with insulin is usually not necessary. However, up to 25% of these children will have islet cell antibodies (see below) and may eventually develop type I diabetes.

Etiology

The etiology of type I diabetes is now believed to involve a genetic predisposition, environmental factors (such as viruses or chemicals), and an immunologic component. The genetic component is associated with the HLA groups DR3 and DR4 (present in 95% of Caucasian children with diabetes and 53% have DR3/DR4). In addition, the presence of aspartic acid on position 57 of the DQ beta chain of the HLA complex is considered protective of diabetes and its absence provides a marker for susceptibility. In spite of these genetic associations, there is no close family member with type I diabetes in 75% of newly diagnosed children.

It is now recognized that type I diabetes has a gradual onset and that immunologic markers (islet cell antibodies [ICA], insulin autoantibodies [IAA], and other antibodies) may be present in the sera of prediabetic children for years prior to the development of insulin dependence.

Clinical Findings

A. Symptoms & Signs:

1. Early Manifestations–The three main symptoms are thirst (polydipsia), frequent urination (polyuria) which may include nocturia or enuresis, and weight loss (or a failure to gain weight). A loss of energy is common. The presence of ketones may result in nausea and/or vomiting and, eventually, ketonemia and acidosis and a sweet-smelling breath and deep respirations (Kussmal) and, eventually, coma.

2. Chronic Complications–One-third of children with diabetes develop joint contractures, particularly of the fifth fingers. However, these are not usually disabling. Severe diabetic retinopathy and early nephropathy develop in one-third of pubertal adolescents and young adults who have had diabetes for 10–20 years. Mild retinal changes, such as microaneurysms, are much more common. The severe renal and retinal complications are more likely in patients with longitudinal poor glucose control or higher blood pressures. Use of tobacco also increases the risk. Thyroid gland enlargement is present in 20% of adolescents with diabetes, and 5% have elevated TSH levels (subclinical thyroiditis). Psychological problems also seem to be more common among adolescents with IDDM. Fortunately, stunting of growth and hepatomegaly (Mauriac's syndrome) due to chronic poor glucose control is now quite rare. Also, since it has been realized that recurrent ketoacidosis is almost always due to missed insulin shots, the incidence of this problem has been reduced greatly.

B. Laboratory Findings: Findings include glycosuria, fasting hyperglycemia (> 120 mg/dL or 6.7 mmol/L), and hyperglycemia 2 hours after a meal (> 200 mg/dL or 11.1 mmol/L). Similarly, a random blood glucose above 300 mg/dL (16.6 mmol/L) is usually indicative of diabetes. A glucose tolerance test is usually not necessary, but if done should involve giving 1.75 g/kg body weight (up to a maximum of 75 g) of glucose orally. Antibody levels (see Etiology, above) may be helpful in the borderline patient. Other findings may include ketonuria, hyperlipidemia, hemoconcentration, and ketoacidemia. The venous pH is the best test to detect the degree of acidemia. Hemoglobin A1c levels may be elevated in new, long-standing, or poorly controlled patients. Insulin levels are usually not measured, but may be elevated (as with C-peptide levels) in obese adolescents with MODY.

Treatment

A. Education: Good initial education is important in making the family feel secure and competent to handle the insulin injections, blood glucose testing, urine ketone testing, hypoglycemia, and other management that they must do. This usually requires that both parents be present for approximately 3 days (but depends on the rate of learning).

B. Insulin: Most children with moderate or large ketonuria who are not acidotic and who are not dehydrated so as to require intravenous fluid therapy are initially treated (usually as outpatients) with regular insulin IM (every 1 hour) or SQ (every 2–3 hours) at a dose of 0.1–0.2 units per kg body weight. When ketonuria diminishes, a mixture of regular insulin and long-acting insulin (usually NPH; see Table

Table 23–7. Summary of bioavailability characteristics of the insulins.

	Human Insulin Type	Onset	Peak Action	Duration
Short-acting	Regular, Actrapid, Velosulin	30–45 min	2–4 hr	5–7 hr
	Semilente, Semitard	30–60 min	4–6 hr	6–8 hr
Intermediate-acting	Lente, Lentard, Monotard	2–4 hr	8–10 hr	15–18 hr
	NPH, Insulatard, Protaphane	2–4 hr	8–10 hr	12–14 hr
Long-acting	Ultralente, Ultratard	4–5 hr	8–14 hr	15–18 hr

23–7) is started at 0.5–1.0 units per kg (total dose) per 24 hours. If ketonuria is not present at onset, usually signifying greater endogenous insulin production, the usual starting dose is 0.25 to 0.5 units per kg body weight per 24 hrs. Two-thirds of the total dose is usually given in the morning and one-third in the evening, preferably 30–60 minutes before meals. Children under age 4 years usually need only ½ to 2 units of regular insulin, children between 4 and 12 years need 1–5 units of regular insulin, and pubertal children need 5–10 units of regular insulin. The remainder of the dose is given as long-acting insulin. Dosages are usually closely monitored by phone in the first week and are titrated to home blood glucose monitoring. At puberty, the insulin dose generally increases and can reach up to 1.5 units per kg body weight per 24 hrs.

C. Diet: Five-year data are now available to show that glucose control is similar for children receiving a "sugar-restricted" diet with freedom to eat other foods to appetite, versus a specified American Diabetes Association exchange diet (originally developed for weight control and still useful if weight is a problem). If an exchange diet is used, the 24-hour caloric intake is calculated as 1000 Kcal plus an additional 100 Kcal per year of age up to 2500 Kcal. Calories are usually divided with 55% from carbohydrate, 20% from protein, and 25% from fat. Snacks are used at peak times of insulin activity or before exercise to prevent hypoglycemia (usually at 3–4 PM and sometimes at 10–11 AM), and a solid snack containing protein and fat should consistently be consumed prior to bedtime to help prevent nocturnal hypoglycemia.

D. Outpatient Management: In most children and adolescents, blood should be tested 3 times each day (in the morning, before supper, and/or at bedtime). This can be done with diagnostic paper strips (eg, Chemstrip bG Strips), which permit visual estimation of the glucose concentration when compared to a color chart, or by use of a meter (eg, The One-Touch meter manufactured by LifeScan). The desired fasting blood glucose level (or anytime there is no food intake for two or more hours), varies with the age of the child: < 5 years = 100–200 mg/dL, (< 5.5–11.1 mmol/L); 5–11 years = 80–180 mg/dL (4.4–10.0 mmol/L); and 12 years and above = 70–150 mg/dL (3.9–8.3 mmol/L). These goals take into account the greater risk for brain damage secondary to hypoglycemia and the reduced ability to recognize symptoms in the young child. In contrast, in the pubescent child, when the risk for microvascular complications is greater, lower blood glucose levels should be a goal. If the blood glucose concentration is above 240 mg/dL (13.30 mmol/L), or if the patient feels ill, urine ketone levels must also be checked. Physical examination every 3 months with particular attention to the retinas, thyroid, liver, injection sites, fingers (for blood test pricks and for contractures), and neurologic examination is recommended. The patient's understanding of the disease should be reviewed. After puberty, hemoglobin A_{1c} (glycosylated hemoglobin) levels should be determined every 3 months. With normal HbA_{1c} values up to 6.2%, children 12 years of age and older who are in good control should have values below 7.8%, children ages 5–12 years should be below 8.5%, and children under age 5 years should be between 7.5 and 9.3%. Poor control of blood glucose levels is most commonly due to inadequate insulin dosage, missed insulin injections, frequent infections, or non-compliance with diet or timing of injections.

E. Other Factors Influencing the Regulation of Diabetes:

1. Activity–Strenuous exercise tends to lower the insulin requirement. Exercise in moderation (and without significant day to day variations) is beneficial. However, patients should be cautioned against strenuous exercise unless they take extra carbohydrates beforehand or reduce the insulin dosage.

2. Infection–Any infection is serious in a diabetic patient; it completely upsets the equilibrium established by therapy, usually increasing the need for insulin. Infection may precipitate ketoacidosis. During severe infections, it is often necessary to add small doses of supplemental regular insulin every 2–4 hours until acetonuria clears. Supplements of approximately 10–20% of the total daily insulin dose are given every 3 hours as regular insulin if the patient has moderate or large ketonuria and a blood glucose level above 150 mg/dL (8.30 mmol/L). When vomiting is present without ketoacidosis, it is often best to reduce the daily insulin dose by half; regular insulin may be supplemented later if high glucose and ketone levels develop. It may also be necessary to give beverages containing sugar (eg, soda pop) to keep the blood glucose level normal if vomiting is a problem.

3. Surgery–Prior to elective surgery, the patient should be given half the usual dose of long-acting insulin in the morning; following this, 5% or 10% dextrose in water should be administered slowly intravenously before, during, and after surgery to cover the insulin. Blood glucose levels should be monitored during surgery and the early postoperative period. If blood glucose levels exceed 300 mg/dL (16.65 mmol/L), or if moderate or large levels of urine ketones appear, regular insulin may be administered as a continuous intravenous solution at the rate of 0.05 unit/kg/hr. If the patient is unable to return to oral food intake promptly, intravenous glucose and electrolytes are continued and intravenous insulin may be continued as necessary. On the day after surgery, if the patient is able to resume eating, the usual amount of long-acting insulin should be administered. As soon as possible, feedings by mouth and the usual insulin regime should be reinstituted.

4. Prevention of Hypoglycemia–Prevention of hypoglycemia is particularly important in the child under age 4 years when the brain is still developing. Hypoglycemia and posthypoglycemic hyperglycemia (Somogyi's syndrome) may be due to overdosage with insulin. This should be suspected in children receiving an insulin dosage that exceeds 1.5 units/kg/d, although the relative insulin resistance of adolescence may result in insulin doses of 1.5 units/kg/d or more during the adolescent growth spurt. All families should receive thorough education about hypoglycemia and how to manage it. Most physicians recommend the family keep glucagon (1.0 mg vials) available for emergencies (0.3 mg for children under 10 years old or 0.5 mg [SQ or IM] for older children).

DIABETIC ACIDOSIS
(Diabetic Coma)

Clinical Findings

A. Symptoms & Signs: Diabetic acidosis is characterized by marked thirst and polyuria, followed by nausea and vomiting, abdominal pain, and general malaise. Dehydration and acidosis (pH

< 7.3) develop rapidly. Respirations then become long, deep, and labored; headache, irritability, drowsiness, stupor, and (finally) coma may develop. On physical examination, the patient is irritable, drowsy, or unconscious, and there is marked dehydration. The skin and mucous membranes are usually dry, lips cherry-red, eyeballs soft, blood pressure low, pulse usually rapid and thready, hyperventilation present, temperature low, and a sweetish ("fruity") acetone breath may be detected. The abdomen may show diffuse spasm and tenderness suggestive of an acute abdominal disorder. The signs and symptoms of the precipitating cause (infection, trauma, missed injection, emotional upset, etc) will usually be found.

A syndrome of hyperosmolar nonketotic diabetic coma in children has been described. It is characterized by the presence of severe hyperglycemia, severe dehydration, and metabolic acidosis and may occur secondary to hypernatremia. The duration of illness is short. There is little or no polydipsia and polyuria, and these children are frequently insulin-resistant. In treatment, sufficient insulin (and isotonic parenteral fluid initially) should be used to normalize glucose metabolism; insulin may not be necessary when the disorder follows hypernatremia.

B. Laboratory Findings: Findings include glycosuria, ketonemia, ketonuria, and hyperglycemia. Acidosis results, and the pH may be below 7.1 (severe ketoacidosis), between 7.1 and 7.2 (moderate ketoacidosis), or between 7.2 and 7.3 (mild ketoacidosis). Serum sodium and chloride levels and the plasma carbon dioxide content are low. Serum potassium and inorganic phosphorus levels may be increased initially, but there is a major total body depletion of these elements, and levels usually decline rapidly with correction of acidosis. Total protein, hemoglobin, and blood urea nitrogen levels may be increased. Leukocytosis and increased hematocrit are often present.

Treatment

A. Objectives: Objectives are the restoration of circulation, correction of fluid and electrolyte deficit, reestablishment of normal carbohydrate metabolism, and eradication of the cause of acidosis and the hyperosmolar state.

B. Emergency Measures:

1. Hospitalize the patient if diabetic acidosis is severe. Patients with mild acidosis can be treated without hospitalization. Keep the patient warm, but avoid excessive warmth. Do not give narcotics or barbiturates.

2. Treat shock, if present, with albumin and other antishock measures (see Chapter 28).

3. Evaluate the degree of dehydration and shock by physical examination and by close inquiry to determine if there is a history of recent weight loss.

4. Obtain urine for estimation of glucose and ketone levels, specific gravity, and evidence of infection.

5. Take venous blood for measurement of pH and determination of levels of carbon dioxide, sodium chloride, potassium, glucose, inorganic phosphorus, urea nitrogen, and ketone bodies. Measurement of the blood lactic acid level may also be of value in the acidotic nonketotic patient.

6. Insulin is given as follows:

a. Intravenous insulin should not be given until the blood glucose level is known, particularly if subcutaneous injections were given previously.

b. A constant intravenous infusion of regular insulin, 0.1–0.2 unit/kg/hr, is given by use of a constant infusion pump if that method of delivery is available. One method to prepare an insulin infusion is to add regular insulin, 30 units, to 150 mL of 0.9% sodium chloride to give a dilution of 1 unit/5 mL. If 50 mL of this solution is run through the tubing prior to use, the insulin binding sites on the tubing will be saturated. A similar dose of insulin may be given intramuscularly instead of intravenously but will then need to be repeated every hour. With either route of administration, blood glucose levels should be determined hourly. Insulin may be given subcutaneously every 2–4 hours in less severely involved patients, except in markedly dehydrated patients who may have varied absorption of the drug.

7. Gastric lavage may rarely be necessary to relieve distention of the stomach and to reduce vomiting.

8. Fluids and electrolytes are given as follows:

a. First, correct extracellular dehydration, shock, anoxia, and impaired renal function with normal saline solution or, if acidosis is severe ($pH < 7.0$), a solution containing the following: sodium, 150 meq/L; chloride, 100 meq/L; and bicarbonate, 50 meq/L. Give 10–20 mL/kg over the first 1 or 2 hours of therapy. The maximum volume of fluid used for the initial reexpansion must NOT exceed 40 mL/kg (to prevent cerebral edema), and this must be considered in the 8-hour fluid totals. If shock is present, the use of albumin or other volume expander is essential.

b. Next, give 50% physiologic solution (usually without bicarbonate) at a rate calculated to restore deficits, supply maintenance amounts, and replace intercurrent losses.

c. When urine flow and circulatory efficiency are satisfactory, the blood pH level is above 7.1, and signs of hyperpnea have begun to subside (generally in 1–2 hours), replace intracellular electrolytes (potassium and phosphorus). Although serum potassium and phosphorus concentrations are usually normal or high early in acidosis, they may fall to low levels following correction of acidosis.

d. Replace the remainder of the water deficit, and when the blood glucose level falls below 250 mg/dL, 5% glucose should be added to the intravenous fluids.

C. General Measures:

1. Ascertain the precipitating cause of the acidosis, and initiate appropriate treatment.

2. Use an indwelling catheter if spontaneous voidings are not possible (rarely necessary).

3. Measure urinary acetone, blood glucose and carbon dioxide, venous pH, and serum electrolytes at frequent intervals (hourly in the first 4 hours).

4. Continuous or intermittent monitoring of the ECG is helpful to follow the effect of potassium therapy.

5. After 12–18 hours, if there is no vomiting, the remainder of the day's fluid and electrolyte requirements may be given orally in a suitable vehicle (orange juice, ginger ale, or milk). Vomiting generally subsides after ketosis has been corrected.

6. For continued fluid and electrolyte therapy, see Chapter 5.

Prognosis

With prompt and adequate therapy, the prognosis is good. The largest number of serious side effects and sequelae result from central nervous system complications. The risk of these may be minimized by attention to correction of fluid and electrolyte losses and avoidance of overzealous correction of the hyperglycemia, dehydration, or acidosis. Recurrent episodes of acidosis are due to failure to take the proper insulin, to emotional problems, to omitting insulin, or to chronic or repeated infections.

HYPOGLYCEMIA
(See also Neonatal Hypoglycemia, Chapter 7.)

Low blood glucose levels can occur when a patient with diabetes receives excessive insulin, fails to eat, or exercises too strenuously. In children who do not have diabetes, the diagnosis of hypoglycemia *should not be made* unless the blood glucose level is below 40 mg/dL; in a newborn, below 30 mg/dL. The diagnosis is unfortunately assigned frequently to children with behavioral or other problems who have never had a documented low blood glucose level.

The most common known cause of severe hypoglycemia in infants during the first year of life is inappropriate insulin secretion. During episodes of hypoglycemia, insulin levels are inappropriately elevated relative to the glucose concentration. When the pancreas is examined histologically, the islet cells may be hypertrophied in some cases; in other cases, there may be excessive numbers of islet cells, which may be arising from pancreatic ductules (nesidioblastoma). Treatment consists of avoidance of insulin stimuli (simple carbohydrates and certain amino acids viz leucine arginine). A trial of diazoxide, 10–20 mg/kg, to inhibit insulin release should be attempted. If this is unsuccessful, 80–90% pancreatomy may be indicated.

The most frequent known cause of hypoglycemia in children between 1 and 5 years of age is functional fasting ("ketotic") hypoglycemia. Functional fasting hypoglycemia is more common in males and in children who had birth weights below 2500 g, who were small for gestational age, or who have minor neurologic or behavioral disorders. There is often a history of vomiting, decreased appetite, or failure to eat during the previous 24 hours. Early morning seizures with the concurrent appearance of ketones in the urine are common in the young child. Treatment should consist of preventing excessive fasting and monitoring the urine for ketones whenever the child is ill or appears to be deviating from normal behavior patterns. If ketones are present, foods high in simple sugars should be encouraged. If the child is vomiting, parenteral glucose and fluids to prevent dehydration may be necessary.

Islet cell adenoma is the most frequent known cause of severe hypoglycemia in patients over 6 years of age. Inappropriate insulin secretion occurs and a tumor can sometimes be detected by means of intraoperative ultrasonography. Treatment is surgical removal.

There are some cases in which a cause for hypoglycemia cannot be found (group IV, idiopathic spontaneous hypoglycemia; Table 23–8). Genetic metabolic disorders (group VI) should be considered in the differential particularly when the hypoglycemia occurs in association with vomiting, seizures, feeding disorders, and physical signs of increased intracranial pressure and hepatomegaly.

Clinical Findings

A. Symptoms & Signs: Findings include weakness, hunger, irritability, faintness, sweating, changes in mood, epigastric pain, vomiting, nervousness, tachycardia, hypothermia, unsteadiness of gait,

Table 23–8. Hypoglycemia.

Classification	Clinical and Laboratory Findings	Treatment
I. Antenatal period disorders (1) Fetal malnutrition (placental (insufficiency) (2) Sepsis Offspring of diabetic mothers Erythroblastosis fetalis (3) Neonatal cold injury (4) Hypoglycemia, cardiomegaly, and pulmonary edema	Offspring of diabetic mothers and infants with erythroblastosis fetalis may have hyperinsulinemia with rebound hypoglycemia to insulinogenic stimuli; blood ratios of insulin to glucose are elevated. The other conditions listed have in common depleted hepatic glycogen and fat stores and fasting hypoglycemia.	Infusion of 10–20% glucose by peripheral vein. Frequent oral feedings. Avoidance or cautious administration of insulinogenic agents (eg, arginine, 50% dextrose) in hyperinsulinism states.
II. Hyperinsulin states (1) Islet cell hyperplasia (2) Islet cell adenoma or adenocarcinoma (3) Islet cell nesidioblastosis (4) Leucine sensitivity (5) Beckwith-Wiedemann syndrome	As a whole, this group is prone to fasting hypoglycemia and rebound hypoglycemia to insulinogenic stimuli. Diagnosis is dependent on finding of abnormally elevated insulin or proinsulin levels during the fasting state or following insulin provocation with glucose, amino acids (ie, leucine, arginine), glucagon, or tolbutamide (1–5); or finding of clinical characteristics of the EMG triad, ie, exomphalos, macroglossia, and gigantism with abdominal organomegaly (5).	(1) Avoidance of insulinogenic stimuli. (2) Catecholamines or diazoxide (or both). (3) A diet low in simple sugars and, sometimes, low in leucine. (4) Pancreatectomy.
III. Functional fasting hypoglycemia ("Ketotic hypoglycemia")	Findings include a history of low birth weight for gestational age; onset between ages 1 and 6 yr; and triad of hypoglycemia, ketosis, and blunted glycemic response to glucagon. Patients may have abnormalities in gluconeogenesis with abnormalities in hepatic handling of alanine during a fast.	Frequent feedings with diet high in carbohydrates and protein. Avoid periods of prolonged fasting.

IV. Primary neurologic disorders ("central")	Hypoglycemia is frequently observed in children with neurologic disorders of various types. No definite pattern or consistent metabolic abnormality has been demonstrated, although hyperinsulinemia has not been a feature.	Frequent feedings. Anticonvulsants when indicated.
VI. Metabolic disorders (1) Liver glycogen storage disease (2) Liver glycogen synthase deficiency (3) Fructose intolerance (4) Maple syrup urine disease (5) Deficiency of liver 1,6-diphosphatase activity	Definitive diagnosis is dependent on enzyme determination. Blunted hyperglycemia response to glucagon (1, 2, and 5), history of hypoglycemia after fructose ingestion (3), and a characteristic odor (4) are helpful for diagnosis.	(1 and 2) Frequent feedings with diet high in carbohydrates. Hyperalimentation. Portacaval diversion in severe type 1 glycogen storage disease may be indicated. (3 and 4) Rigid avoidance of offending substrate.
VII. Endocrine insufficiency syndromes (1) Hypopituitarism (2) Adrenocortical insufficiency (3) Adrenomedullary insufficiency (Broberger-Zetterström syndrome) (4) Congenital hypothyroidism (5) Glucagon deficiency	Definitive diagnosis is dependent on biochemical establishment of hormone deficiency. History of failure to thrive, growth retardation, and features of hypopituitarism (1), excessive tanning (2), and abnormal weight for gestational age (3) are helpful for diagnosis.	Replacement of deficient hormone or hormones.
VIII. Severe malnutrition states (1) Chronic diarrhea (2) Liver disease	Characteristics include fasting hypoglycemia and depleted glycogen and fat stores.	Nutritional rehabilitation.

semiconsciousness, tremors, and convulsions. Symptoms are relieved by administration of glucose. If left untreated, hypoglycemia may lead to extensive central nervous system damage; symptomatic hypoglycemia is more commonly associated with mental deterioration, disintegration of the personality, and death, but the course and prognosis are variable.

B. Laboratory Findings: (See Table 23–8.)

1. Blood glucose levels are low during an attack. There is no sharp dividing line below which a level can be regarded as abnormal, but consistent or repeated levels below 40 mg/dL, associated with signs and symptoms, should be investigated.

2. Serum insulin levels may be inappropriately elevated in hyperinsulinemic states when compared with the simultaneously obtained glucose level.

3. No single test of blood glucose regulation reliably confirms the diagnosis of hypoglycemia, and no combination of tests reliably establishes the mechanism of hypoglycemia in all children.

Treatment

Long-term treatment for specific types of hypoglycemia is outlined in Table 23–8. Acute treatment is usually necessary prior to definitive diagnosis and includes the following:

A. Glucose:

1. Infuse 10–20% dextrose via peripheral vein, at a constant rate, maintaining a blood glucose level that controls central nervous system symptoms (eg, 30 mg/dL in newborns and 40–50 mg/dL in children). If hyperinsulinemia is suspected or is a possibility, avoid bolus ("push") infusions of concentrated dextrose solutions to prevent hyperinsulinemic rebound. (Fifty percent dextrose solutions are not indicated during infancy and childhood.)

2. Instruct the patient's family to give glucose as follows if the patient is unconscious and a physician is not available: Place Insta-Glucose between the child's cheek and gums or under the tongue. If there is no response in 10 minutes, give an initial deep intramuscular injection of glucagon, usually 0.5 mL (0.5 mg). If there is no response, wait 10 more minutes and inject an additional 0.5 mL of glucagon.

3. If a diagnosis of hypoglycemia not due to hyperinsulinism or an inborn error of metabolism has been established, carbohydrates can be safely administered via any route without risk of hypoglycemic rebound.

4. If a diabetic patient is unconscious and a diagnosis of coma or insulin reaction is possible, infuse glucose (20–25%) solution, give intravenously, up to 1 mL/kg. This will overcome the insulin reaction.

B. Drugs:

1. In general, drug therapy should be employed only after a definite diagnosis (Table 23–8) is established.

2. If the cardiorespiratory status permits, catecholamines (eg, aqueous epinephrine or subcutaneous epinephrine in oil [Sus-Phrinel]) may be useful and have the unique advantage in the undiagnosed case of avoiding insulin stimulation.

3. Corticosteroids, corticotropin, and glucagon may be helpful in controlling hypoglycemia, but they may stimulate insulin production, and the action of glucagon in neonates is unpredictable. Glucagon is useful in hyperinsulin states; corticotropin and conticosteroids are occasionally successful over acute short intervals.

4. In severe chronic hyperinsulinism states, an oral preparation of diazoxide is useful. Diazoxide, a nondiuretic benzothiadiazine, may be of value in controlling chronic idiopathic hypoglycemia and certain cases of hyperinsulinism. The dosage has varied from 5–20 mg/kg/d. Side effects include hypertrichosis, advancement of epiphyseal maturation, hyperuricemia, fluid retention, neutropenia, and depression of immunoglobulin G. Failure of adequate response to therapy with diazoxide should prompt consideration of subtotal pancreatectomy.

5. Recent experience suggests that somatostatin analogs may be useful and safe in children with hyperinsulinism. Somatostatin inhibits insulin secretion.

6. Sedatives and anticonvulsant therapy may be helpful to reduce convulsions and neuromuscular irritability. (Phenytoin has the added effect of reducing insulin stimulation.)

C. Diet: In patients with functional fasting "ketotic" hypoglycemia, provide a liberal carbohydrate diet and place a moderate restriction on ketogenic foods.

1. In hyperinsulinemic states, avoid simple sugars and foods high in leucine and arginine. Employ long chain slowly metabolized carbohydrates.

2. Give small frequent feedings (6 or more meals a day). It may be necessary to feed the patient at regular intervals throughout the 24 hours and give small carbohydrate feedings 30–45 minutes after regular meals.

D. Surgical Measures: Surgical removal of a portion of the pancreas (or of a tumor, if present) should be undertaken for any individual with hyperinsulinemia whose condition cannot be controlled by the above measures.

Prognosis

With prompt corrective treatment and normalization of glucose concentrations, the prognosis is good.

GALACTOSEMIA

Galactosemia is an autosomal recessive disease with an incidence of 1:40,000 live births; the condition is due to congenital absence of the activity of the enzyme galactose-1-phosphate uridyl transferase, which is necessary to convert galactose-1-phosphate. There is decreased activity of the enzyme in heterozygous individuals. Galactosemia is characterized by vomiting, feeding difficulties, hepatomegaly, cataracts, mental retardation (not universal), and jaundice during the neonatal period. Untreated *E coli* sepsis and death is frequent. Other findings include renal Fanconi syndrome, ovarian failure, and increased levels of galactose in the blood and galactose-1-phosphate in erythrocytes. A screening test is available to diagnose the condition during the newborn period; this is a part of neonatal screening programs.

A second form of galactosemia is due to galactokinase deficiency and does not affect the liver, kidneys, or central nervous system; cataracts may develop in patients during the first few months of life.

Treatment consists of excluding galactose (especially milk and its derivatives) from the diet. This prevents development of the signs and symptoms of the disease or may result in improvement after they have developed. A more normal diet may be tolerated later in childhood. Ovarian failure is treated at the time of puberty.

The mother of a known galactosemic child should be on a restricted galactose diet during subsequent pregnancies.

GLYCOGEN STORAGE DISEASE

Numerous disorders affecting the biosynthesis and degradation of glycogen have been described, including:

Type I, Von Gierke's Disease: Type I, the most common glycogen storage disease, is an autosomal recessive disorder that involves the liver and kidneys. It starts at birth or in early infancy and is characterized by anorexia, weight loss, vomiting, convulsions, and coma. Organomegaly of the liver and kidneys, growth retardation, obesity with a "doll-like" appearance, and bleeding tendencies may be noted.

Laboratory findings include a deficiency in glucose 6-phosphatase, flat epinephrine and glucagon tolerance curves, elevated blood lipid, lactic and pyruvic acid levels, and abnormal glycogen deposition in the liver. Treatment includes frequent high-carbohydrate feedings, sometimes including nighttime intragastric tube feedings.

Type II, Pompe's Disease (Maltase Deficiency): Findings include muscle weakness, cardiomegaly, macroglossia, hepatomegaly, normal mental development, and deficiency of the lysosomal enzyme α1,4-glucosidase.

Type III, Cori's Disease: Type III involves the liver, striated muscle, and red blood cells. The clinical features are similar to those of type I but less severe. A defect in debranching enzymes (amylo-1,6-glucosidase or oligo-1,4-glucantransferase) and hepatomegaly are typical findings.

Type IV, Andersen's Disease (Amylopectinosis): Findings include abnormal levels of glycogen in the liver and reticuloendothelial system, diminished response to glucagon and epinephrine, a defect in the branching enzyme (amylo-1,4 $\rightarrow$ 1,6-transglucosidase), hepatosplenomegaly, severe cirrhosis, ascites, and typically death in infancy.

Type V, McArdle's Syndrome: Type V (muscle phosphorylase deficiency) involves the skeletal muscle with clinical muscle weakness, stiffness, and easy fatigability. There is a defect in muscle phosphorylase.

Type VI, Hers' Disease: Type VI is clinically similar to type I but is less severe. There is a deficiency in liver phosphorylase.

Type VII: Other types involve reduced activity of phosphoglucomutase, phosphofructokinase, or phosphohexoisomerase. Findings include weak muscles, partial defect of other glycolytic enzymes, and elevated levels of AST (SGOT), serum aldolase, and phosphocreatine kinase.

PHENYLKETONURIA
(Phenylpyruvic Oligophrenia)

Phenylketonuria is an autosomal recessive condition that affects 1:10,000 live Caucasian births. The classic form is due to a deficiency of phenyalanine hydroxylase.

Clinical Findings

Affected children (most often blond and blue-eyed) appear normal at birth but soon develop vomiting, irritability, a "mouse-like" odor, patchy eczematous lesions of the skin, convulsions, schizoid personality, and abnormal findings on EEG. If untreated, mentality is retarded. (An occasional patient may have normal intelligence without treatment.) Affected children are hyperactive and display erratic behavior. Perspiration is excessive. Serum and urinary phenylalanine levels are markedly high. Phenistix Reagent Strips, or Guthrie bacterial inhibition assay (of particular value in young infants). Some normal infants, particularly those with physiologic jaundice of the newborn, may have transiently elevated (> 6 mg/dL) blood levels of phenylalanine. Orthohydroxyphenylacetic acid is usually present in the urine.

Treatment

A diet low in phenylalanine (58 + 18 mg/kg) should be instituted to keep plasma phenylalanine levels between 5 and 10 mg/dL; when started in patients during the first weeks of life, this diet prevents severe retardation. It has also been shown that it is possible to breastfeed an affected infant in combination with a milk substitute that is deficient in phenylalanine. The diet should be titrated against the nutritional status of the child and the serum phenylalanine levels to ensure that the diet is restricted enough to prevent manifestations of the disease but liberal enough to prevent hypophenylalaninemia with resultant malnutrition, retarded growth and development, and cerebral damage. It is now generally recommended that weekly serum phenylalanine assays be done during the first year of life. In established cases, proper diet may arrest the condition and produce improvement in personality and in symptoms other than the mental deficiency. It may be discontinued after several years.

The blood phenylalanine levels of phenylketonuric females should be maintained in the normal range during the childbearing years to decrease the risk of abnormalities (eg, growth and mental retardation, microcephaly) in their offspring who may be nonphenylketonuric.

Hyperphenylalaninemia may be a transient phenomenon in some newborns who have normal urinary metabolites and do not require treatment.

Genetics & Inborn Errors | 24

Eva Sujansky, MD

The identification of genetic disorders often has important implications for the prognosis and management of affected children. A correct diagnosis is also important for the establishment of an accurate recurrence risk and allows parents to make informed reproductive decisions. Traditionally, genetic disorders included chromosomal abnormalities, single gene defects, and multifactorial conditions. The recent progress in molecular genetics allowed the identification of additional causes of genetic disorders collectively called nontraditional modes of inheritance. These include gonadal mosaicism, uniparental disomy, imprinting, contiguous gene syndromes, and mitochondrial inheritance.

CHROMOSOME ABNORMALITIES

Normal humans have 46 chromosomes (23 of maternal and 23 of paternal origin) in every cell except gonads, which have 23 chromosomes. Errors during cell division will result in chromosome abnormalities. Uneven division of chromosomes into two daughter cells (non-disjunction) is responsible for numerical abnormalities; breaks in chromosomes, which rejoin randomly and form new combinations, are responsible for structural aberrations. While only a handful of numerical abnormalities are compatible with livebirth, the number of possible structural abnormalities is infinite. Collectively, chromosome abnormalities can be found in approximately .5% of all newborns.

The numerical chromosome abnormalities (any deviation from the normal 46 chromosomes per cell) are most frequently trisomy or monosomy. Abnormalities of chromosome structure include deletion (a chromosome segment missing), duplication (presence of an additional chromosome segment), and translocation (a segment of one chromosome is attached to another chromosome). Translocation is balanced if the total amount of chromosome material per cell is normal, or unbalanced if translocation resulted in a partial monosomy or duplication of chromosome material. Less common structural abnormalities include inversion (the middle portion of a chromosome is inverted) and ring chromosome (both ends of a chromosome are lost, deleted, and the new ends are reconnected to form a ring).

Mosaicism denotes the presence of 2 different chromosome constitutions in different cells of an individual. For example, a child with Down syndrome mosaicism has some cells with the normal number of chromosomes, others show trisomy 21.

Chromosome Nomenclature

The results of chromosome analysis are routinely reported in a cytogenetic "shorthand," using standard symbols. See examples below:

46,XX: normal female.

46,XY: normal male.

47,XY, + 21: male with trisomy 21 (note: trisomy is depicted by "+" symbol before the chromosome number).

46,XX,4p–: deletion of a short arm (p) of chromosome 4 (note: the symbol "–", indicating deletion, is after the chromosome).

46,XX,5q+: duplication of a long arm (q) of chromosome 5.

45,XX,–14,–21,+ t(14;21): 45 chromosomes with one copy of the normal chromosomes 14 and 21 missing and having one translocation chromosome consisting of 14 and 21.

46,XY,t(1;8)(q32:p22): translocation between the long arm of chromosome 1, at the band 32 and the short arm of chromosome 8, at the band 22.

CLINICAL SIGNIFICANCE

Chromosome abnormality should be suspected in children with any of the following: dysmorphic features, congenital malformations, developmental delay, mental retardation, prenatal and/or postnatal growth retardation, and/or abnormal sexual characteristics. The identification of other potentially etiologic factors in such children, such as fetal exposure to alcohol, parental consanguinity, or perinatal hypoxia, does not rule out the presence of a chromosome abnormality. Fragile X syndrome, XXY, and XYY often are associated with excessive growth. In general, abnormalities of the autosomes (chromosomes number 1 through 22) have more severe consequences for morbidity and mortality than abnormalities of the sex chromosomes (X and Y), some of which may cause only learning and behavioral problems; trisomy or monosomy of a whole chromosome is more deleterious than duplication or deletion of a small segment and deletion is more damaging than duplication. Table 24–1 describes examples of characteristic physical findings associated with some chromosome abnormalities.

DIAGNOSIS

Tissues Used for Chromosome Analysis

1. **Peripheral blood lymphocytes,** obtained from a few milliliters of sterile heparinized blood (green top tube) are the most accessible and most frequently used.
2. **Skin** or other tissue (gonads, thymus) is obtained post mortem or to test for mosaicism. A sterile piece of tissue is placed into tissue culture media or sterile saline (*never* into formalin) and immediately sent to the cytogenetic laboratory.
3. **Bone marrow** is the only tissue with sufficient number of mitoses present to allow an immediate chromosome analysis. Therefore, it is used if immediate results (within 6–12 hours) are needed for appropriate management (eg, a newborn with complex congenital heart disease requiring immediate intervention is suspicious for having trisomy 13).
4. **Amniocytes** or **chorionic villi** are used for prenatal diagnosis.

Techniques of Chromosome Analysis

1. **Routine**, conventional chromosome analysis results in production of a karyotype (a layout of paired chromosomes, arranged from number 1 through 22 and sex chromosomes) in which all chromosomes demonstrate a light and dark stained banding pattern, characteristic for each chromosome pair. This technique is appropriate to detect numerical abnormalities and those structural abnormalities which involve a large chromosome segment.
2. **High resolution** chromosome analysis is a technique by which the chromosomes are more elongated, and therefore, smaller structural abnormalities can be detected.
3. **Fragile X study** is a special technique aimed at the detection of a fragile site at the distal end of the long arm of the X chromosome (Xq27.3) associated with a specific type of X-linked mental retardation, called Fragile X syndrome. The study involves utilization of culture media deficient in folate or thymidine, which enhances fragile sites. The fragile site can be detected in 80% of males and 60% of females with the gene. Recently, molecular analysis be-

Table 24–1. Phenotypic features of selected chromosomal syndromes.

Syndromes	Signs
Trisomy 21 Down syndrome	Mongoloid slant of eyes, brushfield spots of iris, protruding tongue, 3rd fontanelle, low set auricles, excess nuchal skin, Simian lines, single flexion crease and incurving (clinodactyly) of 5th fingers, increased distance between 1st and 2nd toes, mottling of skin, hypotonia, CHD (endocardial cushion defect, VSD, other).
Trisomy 13	IUGR in all 3 parameters, coloboma of iris (pupil of keyhole shape), capillary hemangioma, skin defect of skull, hyperconvex nails, polydactyly, rocker bottom feet, arrhinencephaly, cleft lip and palate, CHD, urinary tract abnormalities.
Trisomy 18	IUGR, anti-mongoloid slant of eyes, short palpebral fissure, small mouth, micrognathia, low set, abnormal auricles, prominent occiput, short sternum, abnormal position of fingers (2nd overlapping 3rd and 5th overlapping 4th), hypoplastic finger nails, rocker bottom feet, CHD, spasticity, feeding problems.
Turner syndrome 45,X	Triangular face, antimongoloid slant of eyes, abnormal shape of ears, webbed or wide neck, broad “shield” chest, wide set nipples, edema of hands and feet, shortened 4th and 5th metacarpals and metatarsals, cubitus valgus; short stature, primary amenorrhea, CHD especially coarctation of aorta. Mostly normal I.Q., infertility.
Klinefelter syndrome 47,XXY	Tall stature, postpubertally small testicles, gynecomastia, eunuchoid build. Increased risk for mild MR, learning and behavior problems, infertility.
47,XYY	No characteristic physical findings, except tall stature. Increased risk for behavior problem, mild MR.
Wolf-Hirschhorn 4p-	IUGR, prominent nasal bridge (“roman warrior profile”) V-shaped glabella with abnormally arched eyebrows, beaked nose, carp shaped mouth, feeding problems.
13q-	IUGR, radial ray defects, if involving q 14 segment; retinoblastoma.
Recombinant 8 syndrome Dup 8q 22→qter Del 8p 23→ pter	Hispanic ancestry, AGA, postnatal FTT; broad forehead, upturned nares, long philtrum, thin upper lip, thick lower lip, low set ears, brachycephaly, deep plantar furrow. CHD, especially conotruncal abnormalities.
18q-	Deep set eyes, atretic ear canals, abnormal auricles.

came available. It has been established that normal individuals have less than 200 base pairs of cytosine phosphate guanosine dinucleotides repeats, carriers of the gene have up to 500 base pairs (premutatin), and individuals affected with Fragile X syndrome have over 600 base pairs repeats (full mutation). The molecular analysis has a much lower frequency of false negative test results than the cytogenetic analysis and is less labor intensive.

4. **Detection of excessive chromosome fragility.** Excessive chromosome breaks and rearrangements can help to diagnose some well defined single gene syndromes such as Bloom syndrome, Fanconi anemia, ataxia-telangiectasia, etc. If the laboratory is informed ahead of time of the clinical suspicion of one of these disorders, techniques known to enhance the abnormality may be used.
5. **Fluorescent in-situ hybridization** (FISH) is a technique for the detection of structural chromosome abnormalities, based on molecular methods. It utilizes fluorescent DNA probes for specific chromosome segments which allow the detection of cryptic rearrangements, invisible by high resolution chromosome analysis. FISH can be used if there is a strong clinical suspicion for a particular chromosome abnormality (example: 4p- or trisomy 21), but the karyotype is normal. In addition, it can identify the origin of abnormal additional chromosome material, either attached to other chromosomes or standing separately as a marker chromosome.
6. **Chromosome painting** is another molecular technique. It is similar in principle to FISH, but identifies a whole chromosome utilizing different color DNA probes for individual chromosomes; ie, the whole chromosome is "painted." This technique is not yet available routinely in every cytogenetic laboratory.

Useful Principle

The cytogenetic laboratory needs to be informed about the indication for chromosome analysis. The more information (description of dysmorphic features, malformations, etc) the laboratory has, the better they can choose the most appropriate technique(s).

RECURRENCE RISKS

1. Numerical abnormalities are most frequently sporadic; however, some families have shown hereditary predisposition to a nondisjunction; therefore, the empirical recurrence risk after the first affected child is 1–2%.

2. Structural chromosome abnormalities: De novo abnormalities (both parents have normal chromosomes) have a very low recurrence risk because of possible gonadal mosaicism. If one parent has a balanced chromosome rearrangement, the recurrence risk is significantly increased. The specific risk varies according to the chromosome involved and the type of rearrangements.

PREVENTION

1. Identification of families with an increased recurrence risk, which includes: previous child with chromosome abnormality, parent with balanced translocation, or a history of multiple fetal losses.
2. Prenatal diagnosis. Amniocentesis at 14–16 weeks of pregnancy or chorionic villi sampling at 9–10 weeks of gestation.

SINGLE GENE DEFECTS

Disorders caused by a mutation of a single gene are responsible for a large number of genetic disorders. Some of these diseases are very rare, but collectively single gene disorders affect approximately 1% of the general population. A complete listing of all known single gene disorders can be found in Victor A. McKusick's text *Mendelian Inheritance in Man.*

All genes are paired (allele) except those on X and Y chromosomes in males. Allele are located in corresponding places (loci) of chromosome pairs; thus, one allele of each pair is of maternal, and the other is of paternal origin. On the basis of gene location and modes of inheritance, we can recognize dominant genes (one copy of abnormal gene, ie, heterozygous state causes morbidity) and recessive genes (both alleles have to be abnormal, ie, homozygous state causes a disease); autosomal genes are located on autosomal chromosomes 1 through 22, and sex-linked genes are located on X chromosome (majority) and Y chromosome (very few). Thus, single-gene disorders include those caused by autosomal dominant, autosomal recessive, X-linked dominant, and X-linked recessive genes.

AUTOSOMAL DOMINANT INHERITANCE

Principles of Inheritance

1. Vertical transmission: multiple generations can be affected.
2. Both sexes equally affected; male to male transmission possible: either parent, if affected, can pass the disorder to male or female offspring.
3. Each offspring of affected has 50% recurrence risk: the affected parent passes the normal or the abnormal allele to each child.
4. Variable clinical expressivity of the disorder: the inter- and intrafamilial severity of the disorder varies.
5. Nonpenetrance-skipped generation: some individuals with the abnormal gene do not show any clinical symptoms of the disorder.

Reasons for Negative Family History

1. New germinal mutation.
2. Non-penetrance.
3. Non-paternity.
4. Phenocopy: clinically similar disorder of different etiology.

Clinical Significance

Autosomal dominant disorders may demonstrate clinical signs and symptoms at birth or later in life, sometimes in the 3rd or 4th decade. Thus, in some disorders, an asymptomatic child of an affected parent might have inherited the abnormal gene. Presymptomatic DNA testing, if available, may be used for clarification of the child's genotype.

Examples of autosomal dominant disorders include: neurofibromatosis, Marfan syndrome, osteogenesis imperfecta, Huntington disease, and adult-type polycystic kidney disease.

AUTOSOMAL RECESSIVE INHERITANCE

Principles of Inheritance

1. Both parents are heterozygous carriers, ie, they have one normal and one abnormal allele of the gene. Carriers are usually clinically normal, but they might show abnormal laboratory findings, which is the basis for carrier testing (sickle cell, Tay-Sachs, etc).
2. Increased frequency of consanguinity: consanguinity between the parents increases the chance for both to be carriers of the same gene.

3. Each offspring of two carrier parents has a 25% risk to inherit both abnormal alleles and to be affected, a 50% chance to inherit the abnormal allele from one parent and the normal from the other and to be carrier, and a 25% chance to inherit both normal alleles.
4. Horizontal transmission: affected siblings, clinically normal parents.
5. All offspring of an affected parent are carriers: a parent with 2 abnormal alleles must pass 1 copy to each offspring.

Clinical Significance

Autosomal recessive disorders are usually more severe than autosomal dominant disorders. If a correct diagnosis of the first affected child is not made, multiple affected siblings may be born before the genetic nature of the disorder is appreciated. Examples of autosomal recessive disorders are infantile polycystic kidney disease, hemoglobinopathies, cystic fibrosis, oculo-cutaneous albinism, Meckel syndrome and other dysmorphic syndromes, and most inborn errors of metabolism.

X-LINKED RECESSIVE INHERITANCE

Principles of Inheritance

1. Mostly males affected: A mutated recessive gene on the only X chromosome of a male will be expressed, as there is not the same allele on his Y chromosome to compensate for the effect of the abnormal gene.
2. Affected males are related to each other through usually unaffected females who have two X chromosomes, one of which is randomly inactivated in each cell. Consequently, in females, the mutated gene is active in approximately 50% of cells, and the normal gene, active in 50% of cells, is sufficient for a normal function.
3. Less severe symptoms in occasionally affected females: females show symptoms if the X inactivation is not random and the abnormal gene is active more frequently.
4. No male to male transmission: a son inherits a Y and not an X chromosome from his father.
5. Affected male passes the gene to *all* daughters who inherit his X chromosome and are then carriers.
6. Carrier female has 50% chance of passing the gene to each offspring: the daughters who inherit the gene are carriers, the sons with the gene are affected.

Clinical Significance

Although X-linked disorders are much more common in males, they must be considered in females with a compatible clinical presentation.

Affected females usually have milder symptoms, caused by the presence of active abnormal and inactive normal X in more than expected 50% of cells. In rare instances, females may be as severely affected as males. In those cases, chromosome analysis, aimed at ruling out monosomy or a structural abnormality of X, is indicated.

Examples of X-linked recessive disorders include hemophilia, Duchenne muscular dystrophy, ocular albinism, and numerous X-linked mental retardation syndromes including fragile X syndrome. However, although the gene is X-linked, the inheritance of the fragile X syndrome does not strictly follow the general principles of X-linked inheritance: Both males and females with the premutation (see chromosome techniques) are asymptomatic carriers and individuals of both sexes with a full mutation are affected. In addition, genomic imprinting plays a role in the clinical expression of the gene: The premutation must be passed through a female to change into a full mutation.

X-LINKED DOMINANT INHERITANCE

1. Principles are similar to the X-linked recessive inheritance with the exception that heterozygous females are also affected.
2. Clinical Significance. This is a rare form of inheritance. Examples include incontinentia pigmenti and vitamin D resistant rickets.

DIAGNOSIS OF SINGLE GENE DISORDERS

1. **Physical examination** leading to the detection of characteristic physical findings. For example, the presence of multiple café-au-lait spots, neurofibromas, and lisch nodules of irises is diagnostic for neurofibromatosis 1.
2. **Family history.** For example, the discovery of members of multiple generations of both sexes affected with a neurodegenerative disorder is compatible with autosomal dominant inheritance even in the absence of a specific diagnosis.
3. **Diagnostic tests**, specific for the given disorder, ie, detection of enzyme defects in inborn errors of metabolism, abnormal sweat

test in cystic fibrosis, abnormal amount of dystrophin in muscle biopsy in Duchenne muscular dystrophy, etc.

Molecular Testing

1. **Direct detection** of the mutation.

   Prerequisites: The specific mutation is known and the mutation is responsible for either adding or abolishing a restriction enzyme recognition site, thus the size of the fragment and its movement on the gel is different from a normal gene. Advantage of this technique is 100% reliability and the ability to make the diagnosis in patients with a negative family history. Examples of disorders with a detectable mutation include Duchenne muscular dystrophy, retinoblastoma, neurofibromatosis, 21-hydroxylase deficiency, hemophilia, myotonic dystrophy, and fragile X syndrome.

2. **Indirect detection** through utilizing linkage analysis is to be considered, if the specific mutation is unknown, but the chromosome location of the gene is known.

   Prerequisites: Multiple family members affected with the disease and the availability of polymorphic DNA markers so closely linked to the disease gene that they are unlikely to segregate independently from the disease gene. The closer the linkage between the markers and the gene in question and the more DNA markers are utilized, the higher the probability that the linkage study is accurate. The disadvantages of linkage study include the necessity of multiple affected and unaffected family members to participate in the study and the possibility of crossing over between the markers and the gene, which results in inaccurate diagnosis. Disorders with available linkage analysis include neurofibromatosis, tuberous sclerosis, retinoblastoma, Duchenne muscular dystrophy without detectable deletion, spinal muscular atrophy, etc.

   DNA testing was greatly advanced by the development of the polymerase chain reaction (PCR) technique which significantly decreased the sample size and the time required for the test, making it less expensive and more accessible. Molecular testing can be helpful for presymptomatic and prenatal diagnosis and for confirmation of a diagnosis in mildly affected patients.

PREVENTION OF SINGLE GENE DISORDERS

The following options are available for couples concerned about having an affected offspring:

1. **Artificial insemination by donor** if the father is affected with X-linked or autosomal dominant disease, or if both parents are carriers of an autosomal recessive gene.
2. **Donor egg** and in vitro fertilization if the mother does not wish to pass her abnormal autosomal dominant or X-linked gene.
3. **Prenatal diagnosis** of disorders with available molecular testing (direct or linkage analysis).
4. **Pre-implantation** testing of a polar body or an early zygote is being developed.

MULTIFACTORIAL INHERITANCE

The inheritance of many frequently familial disorders does not fit the single gene model. Traditionally, the additive effect of multiple common genes with a threshold effect, in combination with further unidentified environmental factors, has been implicated as the cause of these disorders. However, it has been recently suggested, on the basis of statistical evidence, that single major loci are important in at least two traditionally multifactorial defects: cleft lip and palate and congenital heart defects. This information is still tentative, and at the present, the principles of empirical recurrence risk of multifactorial models are still valid.

CLINICAL SIGNIFICANCE

Disorders with multifactorial inheritance include the majority of isolated congenital malformations such as congenital heart disease, cleft lip and/or palate, congenital dislocation of hip, pyloric stenosis, celiac disease, Hirschsprung disease, neural tube defects and club foot; the majority of mental retardation; common, later onset diseases such as hyperlipidemia, hypertension and allergies; and normal traits such as height, pigmentation, and intelligence. Sporadic cases, or multiple family members, scattered throughout the kindred, can be affected with multifactorial disorder. The recurrence risk of relatives of affected person is increased and empirical recurrence risk tables are available for different disorders.

The recurrence risk is not constant, as in single gene defects (ie, each offspring of a parent with autosomal dominant disorder has 50%

recurrence risk, regardless of how many siblings have been already affected), but it is directly related to the number of affected family members, how closely they are related to the person at risk, whether they are of the less commonly affected sex, and how severely they are affected. In general, after one first degree affected relative (parent, child, or sibling) the recurrence risk for most multifactorial disorders is 3–5%; after two affected first degree relatives, the risk is approximately 10%.

PREVENTION

1. Parents of affected children need to be informed about the increased recurrence risk.
2. Prenatal diagnosis (ultrasound, alpha fetoprotein) can be utilized for the detection of congenital malformations.
3. Children at increased risk for a multifactorial disorder must be closely monitored for a recurrence as early intervention may prevent complications.

NON-TRADITIONAL INHERITANCE

GONADAL MOSAICISM

A new gene mutation affecting not one, but a cluster of gametes, will result in gonadal mosaicism. Thus, two clinically normal parents may have two or more affected offspring, mimicking autosomal recessive inheritance. An example is osteogenesis imperfecta, type 2 (lethal), which was previously thought to be caused by an autosomal recessive disorder, but molecular analyses confirmed gonadal mosaicism. The recurrence risk in cases of gonadal mosaicism is unknown, but is estimated to be 5–10%.

UNIPARENTAL DISOMY

Under normal circumstances, one chromosome of each chromosome pair is of maternal, the other of paternal origin. In uniparental disomy, both alleles originated from the same parent and none from the other. Uniparental disomy cannot be detected by chromosome analysis, which is normal. Only molecular analysis, using specific polymorphic markers, can identify the parental origin of the chromosomes. Uniparental disomy has been documented for human chromosomes 7, 11, 15, and X. Uniparental disomy is responsible for Beckwith–Wiedemann, Prader–Willi, and Angelmann syndromes in some patients. It has been found to be responsible for passing homozygosity for cystic fibrosis from a mother to her child, and it has been documented that both X and Y chromosomes have been passed from a father with hemophilia to his affected son. In addition, uniparental disomy has been implicated in some cases of prenatal and postnatal growth retardation (Russell–Silver syndrome) and in fetal demise.

IMPRINTING

Imprinting is a process by which the expression of a gene depends on its parental origin. For example, a uniparental disomy of chromosomes 15 of maternal origin will result in Prader–Willi syndrome, whereas a paternal uniparental disomy of the same chromosome pair will cause Angelmann syndrome.

CONTIGUOUS GENE SYNDROMES

Some well-defined dysmorphic syndromes, previously of unknown etiology, have been found to be caused by a sub-microscopic or visible chromosome deletion. Thus, they are believed to be caused by a number of genes located in linear arrangement on the chromosome, (ie, contiguous genes). Currently recognized contiguous gene syndromes include DiGeorge syndrome (deletion 22q11), Miller-Dieker syndrome (del 17p13), WAGR syndrome (Wilms' tumor, aniridia, genitourinary abnormalities, and retardation) on chromosome 11p13, and retinoblastoma—mental retardation (13q14).

MITOCHONDRIAL INHERITANCE

In addition to mutation of genes found in nuclei of cells, human disorders may be caused by mutation of mitochondrial genes, located in the cytoplasm of cells. The normal function of mitochondrial genes is very important for normal energy metabolism, through oxidative phosphorylation and formation of ATP. This generates energy especially important for a normal function of the central nervous system and cardiac and peripheral muscles. Thus, the mutations of mitochondrial genes have adverse effects predominantly on these organs. Since cytoplasmic mitochondria are inherited through the egg (the sperm contains a minimal amount of cytoplasm), mitochondrial diseases are inherited through the maternal lineage, and affected males usually do not pass the mutation to their offspring. Mitochondrial inheritance is implicated in Leber optic atrophy and a variety of neuromuscular degenerative disorders.

PRINCIPLES OF PEDIGREE ANALYSIS

1. Negative family history does not exclude the presence of single gene disorder. Explanations include a new mutation, or decreased penetrance of a dominant gene, autosomal recessive or multifactorial inheritance.
2. Multiple generations affected are compatible with autosomal or X-linked dominant disorders.
3. Mostly males are affected and they are related to one other through unaffected or mildly affected females: X-linked recessive (can be passed through affected males) or mitochondrial (not passed through affected males) inheritance.
4. Only siblings are affected: Compatible with autosomal recessive inheritance, gonadal mosaicism, or multifactorial.
5. Affected individuals are scattered in irregular fashion through the kindred: multifactorial.

INBORN ERRORS OF METABOLISM

Inborn errors of metabolism (IEM) are disorders caused by blocks in metabolic pathways. The clinical symptoms of these disorders are caused either by the accumulation of a substrate behind the block or by the deficiency of the product of a normal metabolic reaction. The recognition of an IEM, most of which are inherited as autosomal recessive disorders, is extremely important. Inborn errors of metabolism frequently present as a medical emergency, and because many of them can be successfully treated, early diagnosis is paramount to the prevention of significant morbidity and mortality. Although infants with IEM are best managed in centers with expertise in treatment of metabolic diseases, the primary care physicians must suspect the diagnosis of IEM and initiate an appropriate laboratory workup.

WHEN SHOULD IEM BE CONSIDERED?

1. Acutely ill newborn with symptoms of neonatal sepsis: vomiting, poor feeding, jaundice, lethargy, seizures, or jitteriness, especially if the alteration of the mental status is out of the proportion to systemic findings or if there is a peculiar body odor, or history of unexplained neonatal death in a sib or maternal uncle.
2. Typical Reye or Reye-like syndrome: encephalopathy, vomiting, hepatomegaly.
3. Vomiting, especially cyclic, or associated with acidosis.
4. Acutely altered neurologic/mental status, ataxia, seizures, hypertonia in neonate, or hypotonia in a child.
5. Mental retardation, especially if there is slowing or regression of development.
6. Unexplained metabolic imbalance: acidosis, hyperammonemia, or hyperglycemia.
7. Unusual body odor: smell of sweaty feet or mouse-like smell.
8. Coarse facial features and other physical findings compatible with storage disorders (see below).
9. Sudden, unexplained death after rapid deterioration of a previously healthy infant.

The suspicion of inborn errors is heightened by a history of consanguinity, unexplained infant deaths in siblings or maternal male relatives, aversion to certain food, and appearance of symptoms with changes in diet.

Suspicious physical findings include abnormal hair, retinal changes (cherry red spot or retinitis pigmentosa), corneal clouding, coarse facial features, hepatomegaly, skeletal changes, microcephaly or macrocephaly, abnormal muscle tone, and failure to thrive. The presence of another specific cause which can explain the symptoms, such as intercurrent infection, does not exclude IEM as some disorders become symptomatic during infection. Others, like galactosemia, increase the risk of gram-negative septicemia. The presence of facial dysmorphism and/or congenital malformations does not rule out IEM (Table 24–2).

CLASSIFICATION OF IEM'S

Disorders of carbohydrate metabolism (eg, galactosemia, glycogen storage diseases, fructose intolerance, primary lactic acidemias).
Defects of amino acid metabolism (eg, phenylketonuria, tyrosinemia, maple syrup urine disease, homocystinuria, nonketotic hyperglycinemia, urea cycle disorders such as transcarbamoylase deficiency).
Organic acidurias (eg, glutaric acidemia, type I and II, methylmalonic acidemia, primary lactic acidemia, isovaleric acidemia).
Defects of fatty acid oxidation (eg, deficiencies of long chain and medium chain acyl-CoA dehydrogenase: LCAD, MCAD).
Disorders of purine metabolism (eg, Lesch–Nyhan syndrome).
Lysosomal storage disorders (eg, mucopolysaccharidoses such as Hurler syndrome, mucolipidoses such as Mannosidoses or I-cell disease, lipidoses such as Niemann–Pick diseases).
Peroxisomal disorders (eg, Zellweger syndrome).

The clinical and laboratory features of these categories are listed in Table 24–2.

DIAGNOSTIC EVALUATION

1. Acutely ill infant or child: *Blood:* CBC, ammonia, glucose, acid-base status, amino acids, carnitine total, and free. *Urine:* pH, reducing substances, ketones, organic acids, amino acids. Other studies such as CSF glycine, plasma lactate, and pyruvate depending upon age and specific presentations.
2. Stable child with mental retardation/developmental delay: *Blood*: CBC, acid-base status, amino acids. *Urine:* amino acids, organic

acids, mucopolysaccharides, ketones, pH, reducing substances. Consider on the basis of above tests results and clinical findings: urine oligosaccharides, blood lactate and pyruvate, or other studies. Instructions on handling the samples for metabolic evaluations are in Table 24–3.

MANAGEMENT OF ACUTELY ILL INFANT OR CHILD WITH IEM

1. Treatment must be prompt and vigorous. Treatment must be started as soon as hyperammonemia or acid-base imbalance are diagnosed, while waiting for the results of other tests.
2. Stop oral intake (stop intake of all protein and all sugars, except glucose).
3. Give glucose IV in amounts sufficient to stop catabolic process.
4. Treat hyperammonemia with dialysis or pharmacologically.
5. Treat acidosis with bicarbonate.
6. More specific treatment may be instituted after establishment of diagnosis.

SPECIFIC TREATMENT FOR IEM

The goal of the treatment is to compensate the metabolic imbalance caused by the block in the pathway. This can be accomplished by supplementing a deficient metabolite (eg, arginine in disorders of urea cycle), eliminating a harmful substrate from the diet (eg, phenylalanine in phenylketonuria), providing co-enzyme (eg, vitamin B_{12} therapy in some types of methylmalonic acidemia), pharmacologically removing accumulated substrate (isovaleric acidemia), or replacing the missing enzyme (by infusion or transplant). Ideally, a permanent solution would be gene replacement and research trials are underway.

THE EVALUATION OF A DYSMORPHIC CHILD

Disruption of normal morphogenesis during intrauterine life is responsible for the presence of major malformations and dysmorphic features such as single flexion creases of the palms (Simian lines), hy-

Table 24–2. Clinical and laboratory features of inborn errors.[1–4]

	Defects of Carbohydrate Metabolism	Defects of Amino Acid Metabolism[2]	Organic Acid Disorders[3]	Defects of Fatty Acid Oxidation	Defects of Purine Metabolism	Lysosomal Storage Diseases	Disorders of Peroxisomes
Neurodevelopmental							
Mental/developmental retardation	+++	+++	+++	–	++	+++	+++
Developmental regression	–	–	+	–	–	+++	+++
Acute encephalopathy	+++	+++	+++	+++	–	–	–
Seizures	++	+++	+++	+	–	+++	++
Ataxia/movement disorder	–	+	++	–	+++	–	–
Hypotonia	++	++	++	+++	–	+	+++
Hypertonia	–	++	+++	–	++	+	–
Abnormal behavior	–	++	++	–	++	+++	–
Growth							
Failure to thrive	+++	+++	+++	–	–	+	–
Short stature	++	–	+	–	–	++	–
Macrocephaly	–	–	+	–	–	+++	++
Microcephaly	+	++	+++	–	–	+	–
General							
Vomiting/anorexia	++	+++	+++	+++	–	–	++
Food aversion or craving	++	+++	+++	+++	–	–	–
Odor	–	++	++	–	–	–	–
Dysmorphic features	–	+	+	–	–	++	++
Congenital malformations	–	++	++	–	–	–	++
Organ specific							
Hepatomegaly	+++	–	++	+++	–	+++	+++

Liver disease/cirrhosis	+ +	+	–	–	–	–	+
Splenomegaly	–	–	–	–	–	+ +	+
Skeletal dysplasia	–	–	–	–	–	+ +	+ +
Cardiomyopathy	+ +	–	+	+ + +	–	+ +	–
Tachypnea/hyperpnea	+ +	+ +	+ +	+ +	–	–	–
Rash	–	+ +	+ +	–	–	–	–
Alopecia or abnormal hair	–	+	+ +	–	–	–	+
Cataracts or corneal opacity	+ +	–	–	–	–	+ +	–
Retinal abnormality	–	+	+	–	–	+ +	+ +
Frequent infections	+ +	–	+ +	–	+ +	–	–
Deafness	–	–	+	–	–	+ +	–
Laboratory-general							
Hypoglycemia	+ + +	+	+ +	+ +	–	–	–
Hyperammonemia	–	+ +	+ +	+ +	–	–	–
Metabolic acidosis	+ +	+ +	+ + +	+ + +	–	–	–
Respiratory alkalosis	–	+ +	–	–	–	–	–
Elevated lactate/pyruvate	+ +	–	+ + +	+ +	–	–	–
Elevated liver enzymes	+ +	+ +	+ +	+ + +	–	+	+
Neutropenia or thrombocytopenia	+	–	+	–	+ +	+	–
Ketosis	+ + +	+ +	+ + +	–	–	–	–
Hypoketosis	–	–	+	+ + +	–	–	–

[1] + + +, most conditions in group; + +, some; +, one or few; –, not found.
[2] Includes disorders of urea cycle but not maple syrup urine disease.
[3] Includes maple syrup urine disease and disorders of pyruvate oxidation.
[4] From Goodman SI, Greene CL: Inborn errors of metabolism. In: Hathaway WE et al (editors) *Current Pediatric Diagnosis & Treatment,* 11th ed. Appleton & Lange, 1993.

Table 24–3. Obtaining and handling samples to diagnose inborn errors.[1]

Test	Comments
Acid-base status	Accurate estimation of anion gap must be possible. Samples for blood gases should be kept on ice and analyzed immediately.
Blood ammonia	Sample should be collected without a tourniquet, kept on ice, and analyzed immediately.
Blood lactic acid and pyruvic acid	Sample should be collected without a tourniquet, kept on ice, and analyzed immediately. Reduction of pyruvic acid to lactic acid must be prevented. Normal literature values are for the fasting, rested state.
Amino acids	Blood and urine should be examined. CSF glycine should be measured if nonketotic hyperglycinemia is to be ruled out. Normal literature values are for the fasting state. Growth of bacteria in urine should be prevented. At autopsy: liver, kidney, or vitreous may be analyzed if urine is not available.
Organic acids	Urine preferred for analysis. At autopsy: liver, kidney, or vitreous may be analyzed if urine is not available.
Urine mucopolysaccharides	Variations in urine concentration may cause errors in screening tests. Diagnosis requires knowing which mucopolysaccharides are increased. Some patients with Morquio's disease do not have abnormal mucopolysacchariduria.
Enzyme assays	Specific assays must be requested. Exposure to heat may cause loss of enzyme activity. Enzyme activity in whole blood may become normal after transfusion or vitamin therapy. Leukocyte or fibroblast pellets should be kept frozen prior to assays. Fibroblasts may be grown from skin biopsies taken up to 72 hours after death. Tissues such as liver and kidney should be taken as soon as possible after death, frozen immediately, and kept at –70 °C until assayed.

[1] From Goodman SI, Greene CL: Inborn errors of metabolism. In: Hathaway WE et al (editors): *Current Pediatric Diagnosis & Treatment,* 11th ed. Appleton & Lange, 1993.

poplastic finger nails, upslant or downslant of the eyes, epicanthic folds, abnormal shape of auricles, etc.

ETIOLOGY

Dysmorphogenesis can be caused by chromosome abnormalities, single gene defects, adverse environmental factors such as teratogens, or by a combination of multiple factors. In approximately 50% of dysmorphic children, specific etiology cannot be identified.

PATHOGENESIS

On the basis of pathogenesis, dysmorphic features can be classified as malformations, ie, true primarily abnormal development caused by intrinsic factors such as a chromosome abnormality; deformations, caused by external mechanical forces acting upon a normally developing fetus, such as uterine constraint; and disruptions, the result of extrinsic interruption of normal development, such as amniotic bands interfering with normal closure of body cavities or of separation of fingers.

THE VALUE OF RECOGNITION OF DYSMORPHIC FEATURES

1. Recognition of dysmorphic features allows a diagnosis of specific syndromes, thus establishing correct prognosis and recurrence risk (eg, Down syndrome). This is especially valuable in newborns as the correct diagnosis might influence the management (eg, Trisomy 13 or 18).
2. In children with developmental delay or mental retardation, the presence of dysmorphic features helps to establish timing of the harmful insult to prenatal versus perinatal or postnatal periods and aids in the identification of the etiology.
3. Multiple dysmorphic features alert the professionals to look for major malformations. For example, abnormally formed auricles are associated with higher frequency of hearing loss, etc.
4. The presence of dysmorphic features helps to differentiate a child with an isolated multifactorial defect such as CHD from a child with a more complex syndrome, eg, Noonan syndrome with CHD.

PRINCIPLES OF SYNDROME IDENTIFICATION

1. Dysmorphic features must be differentiated from familial features found in normal relatives and normal variations frequent in the general population, such as mongolian spots.
2. Familiarity with a large number of syndromes and their clinical variability is necessary, because the clinician with limited knowledge of syndromes is in danger of misdiagnosing the patient. Excellent extensive reviews of specific syndromes can be found in *Smith's Recognizable Pattern of Human Malformations*, edited by Dr. Ken Jones, and Dr. Gorlin's book entitled *Syndromes of the Head and Neck.*
3. Establishment of a differential diagnosis beginning with that patient's abnormality which has the lowest incidence in the general population is indicated, ie, use radial ray defect rather than more common VSD if both are present. Comparison with known syndromes with radial ray defect helps to find the syndrome most compatible with the patient's diagnosis.
4. Do not over-diagnose. If a specific syndrome cannot be confidently identified, diagnosis must be deferred. The child needs to be periodically re-evaluated (the younger the child, the more frequently). A diagnosis may become apparent later either because the child developed new signs, which aid the diagnosis, or the diagnostic techniques improve.

THE ROLE OF TERATOGENS IN DYSMORPHOGENESIS

The exposure of a genetically susceptible fetus to a potential teratogen increases the chance of malformations. Although many environmental agents are potentially teratogenic, very few are proven teratogens. These include the following:

- Infectious agents (rubella virus, cytomegalic virus, toxoplasma, herpes virus, varicella virus).
- Drugs and medications (including alcohol, cocaine, anticonvulsants, vitamin A derivatives).
- Maternal diseases (such as diabetes mellitus and phenylketonuria).
- Uterine conditions (malformed uterus, twinning).

Prerequisites for Teratogenic Action

1. **Teratogenicity of agents:** Documentation of teratogenicity in humans is important. Information can be obtained from the Teratogen Information Service available in many states or from clinical genetics centers.
2. **Genetic predisposition of the fetus:** All fetuses exposed to known teratogens are not adversely affected; the genetic makeup may influence the absorption, metabolism, excretion, etc, of a teratogen.
3. **Exposure during vulnerable stages of fetal development:** Exposures during the organogenesis may be responsible for major congenital malformations; later exposures may contribute to a neurodevelopmental dysfunction.
4. ***Caution:*** The history of teratogenic exposure does not rule out the contribution of other etiologies to the patient's dysmorphogenesis; a chromosome abnormality or single gene syndrome may need to be considered, if clinically warranted.

MENTAL RETARDATION

The American Association of Mental Deficiency defines mental retardation (MR) as a concurrent presence of intellectual functioning more than 2 standard deviations below the mean (ie, IQ < 70) and a deficit in adaptive behavior. The purpose of this altered definition is to prevent overlabeling with mental retardation children who have learning disability or undetected sensory deficit. While over-diagnosis of MR in a child with normal intellectual potential may be detrimental for the future, lack of detection of MR is also harmful. There are a number of mandated services for MR children which are unavailable without the diagnosis. In everyday practice, the diagnosis of MR is still mostly based on IQ < 70. The incidence of MR is approximately 2–4%.

ETIOLOGY OF MENTAL RETARDATION

Multifactorial mental retardation (physiological, familial MR) comprises 90% of all MR. This group of MR represents the lowest tail of normal Gaussian distribution of IQ of general population. The MR is mild (IQ 70–50), is not associated with minor or major malformations, is more common in lower socio-economic classes, and frequently there is positive family history for mildly MR family members. One parent with multifactorial MR has an approximately 20% chance for affected offspring, and both parents with MR have a 40% chance for affected offspring. Normal parents with one affected child have an approximately 5% recurrence risk.

The remaining categories of MR collectively represent 10% of all MR children and 0.3% of the general population. Most of the children in these categories have severe MR (IQ 50–30), although some are only mildly retarded. The etiologies include chromosome abnormality: Down syndrome is most common and Fragile X syndrome is the second most common genetic syndrome with MR. Other chromosome anomalies are present in 1–4% of severely MR children surviving past 1 year. Examples of single gene defects causing MR include inborn errors of metabolism (3–7% of severe MR), neurocutaneous and other disorders, and syndromes such as Smith–Lemli–Opitz and Rett syndrome. MR caused by teratogenic exposures include fetal alcohol syndrome and fetal hydantoin syndrome, congenital rubella, and CMV. Infections cause 2.8–8.5% of severe MR. Environmental factors such as Rh incompatibility, lead-poisoning, and accidental or non-accidental trauma account for approximately 1% of MR. Syndromes of unknown etiology such as Cornelia de Lange are associated with MR.

MR associated with other CNS dysfunction of heterogeneous etiology includes MR associated with cerebral palsy (over 50% has documented prenatal etiology); MR with multiple congenital malformations (chromosomal, single gene defect, or teratogenic); and MR with CNS malformations such as hydrocephalus, neural tube defects, midline brain defects, etc.

Recurrence risk in these categories corresponds with the genetic mechanisms involved, as discussed under those headings.

Diagnostic evaluation of MR children includes detailed family, pregnancy, medical, and developmental histories and physical examination aimed at detection of dysmorphic features that aid in diagnosing a specific syndrome and detection of signs of single gene disorders (eg, depigmented ash-leaf spots of tuberous sclerosis). Laboratory testing is based on the clinical suspicion of an etiology and may include chromosome analysis, studies for inborn errors of metabolism, brain imaging, etc.

GENETIC EVALUATION AND COUNSELING

Purpose of Referrals to Genetics Clinic

The genetics clinic can assist the primary care provider with any of the following:

1. Establishment of correct diagnosis.
2. Explanation of natural history of the disorder.
3. Management issues.
4. Establishment of recurrence risk.
5. Identification of available reproductive options.
6. Helping families to adjust to having an affected child.

Correct diagnosis is of utmost importance, before the other information about the disorder can be provided. Detailed history (prenatal, developmental, medical, family), and review of the results of previous tests in combination with physical examination and select laboratory studies aid the dysmorphologist/geneticist in establishment of diagnoses.

While the diagnostic features of most genetic diseases and various syndromes are well known, the specific information about the natural history and the impact of various management approaches on the course of many disorders is often inadequate.

The recurrence risk for individual family members is established according to the principles of inheritance of different disorders. In cases with unknown etiology, where a specific diagnosis cannot be established, the genetic evaluation may be reassuring because the absence of a known genetic disorder indicates probable low recurrence risk.

Available reproductive options may include any of the following: (a) taking chances; (b) no reproduction; (c) artificial insemination by donor (paternal chromosomal, autosomal dominant, or X-linked disease, both parents are carriers of autosomal recessive disorder); (d) donor egg and in vitro fertilization (to avoid passing an abnormal maternal gene or chromosome); (e) prenatal diagnosis (ultrasound, amniocentesis, chorionic villi sampling, maternal serum alpha fetoprotein); and (f) pre-implantation genetic evaluation is in a developmental stage.

Genetic counseling should be nondirective. It should provide all available information about all aspects of the disorder. The counselors should support the family in any decision they deem appropriate for their family's goals and moral values.

Indications for Referral to a Genetic Clinic

1. Child with birth defects and/or developmental delay/mental retardation.
2. Dysmorphic child.
3. Parent or child affected with known or suspected genetic disorder (chromosomal or single gene or multifactorial).
4. Positive family history of birth defects or retardation in aunts, uncles, grandparents, or other relatives, especially if multiple members are affected.
5. Possible teratogenic exposure or other abnormalities of pregnancy.
6. Advanced maternal age (over 35 years) or other indications for prenatal diagnosis.

The advantages of a genetic evaluation include (1) the establishment of a diagnosis which in turn may clarify the child's prognosis and indicate the appropriateness of supportive therapies (OT, PT, etc); (2) the clarification of the etiology in helping to identify recurrence risk and the appropriate reproductive options; and (3) provision of extensive information in helping to alleviate parental guilt for producing an abnormal child and helping the parents to accept the situation.

Neoplastic Diseases | 25

Linda C. Stork, MD

Cancer in children differs biologically from cancer in adults (Figure 25–1). Neoplastic disease is the second leading cause of death in the pediatric age group in the United States. Solid tumors represent 70% of cases and acute leukemia represents the remaining 30%.

For solid tumors in general, the less the tumor burden and the more localized the tumor at diagnosis, the better the chance of cure. For the leukemias, various clinical and laboratory features present at diagnosis correlate with ultimate prognosis. Present day treatment of pediatric cancers is complex, multimodal, and multidisciplinary and should be carried out under the direction of centers specializing in the care of children with neoplastic diseases.

BRAIN TUMORS

Brain tumors represent the second most common type of childhood cancer, with leukemia being the most common. About 50% of these arise in the posterior fossa. Cerebellar tumors include medulloblastomas or primitive neuroectodermal tumors (PNET), astrocytomas, and ependymomas. Supratentorial tumors include astrocytomas (high and low grade), optic gliomas, craniopharyngiomas, choroid plexus tumors, ependymomas, PNET, teratomas, and germinomas. Gliomas and astrocytomas occur in the brainstem.

The entire symptom complex of an intracranial space-occupying lesion, which includes vomiting, increased intracranial pressure, and papilledema, can be caused by lesions that are not neoplastic. The principal ones are abscess, hemorrhage, CNS infections, and venous sinus thrombosis. CT scan and MRI can help differentiate between these lesions. Some brain tumors grow slowly over years before diagnosis and others develop quickly over months.

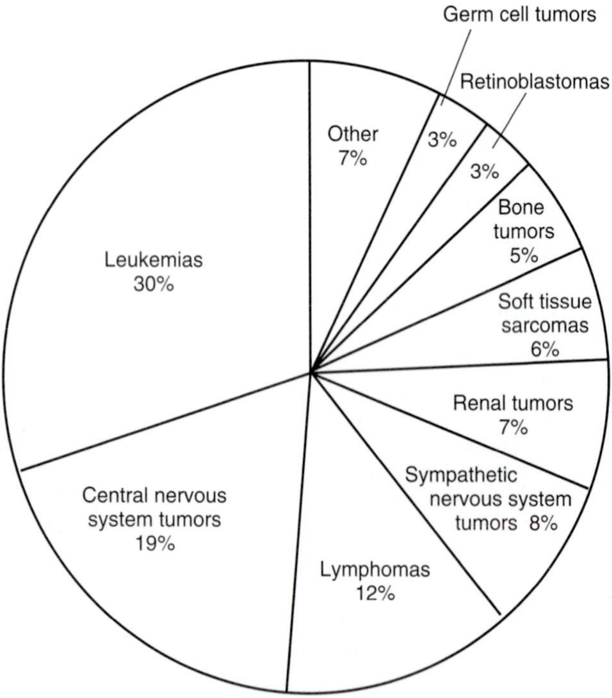

Figure 25–1. Approximate incidence of the principal cancers in children less than 15 years old (SEER program, 1973–1982).

Clinical Findings

A. Symptoms & Signs: Evidence of increased intracranial pressure includes headache, vomiting (often without nausea and before breakfast), diplopia, blurred vision, and papilledema. Personality changes including irritability, apathy, and disturbances in sleep and eating patterns are frequent. Sudden enlargement of the head, if head circumferences have been plotted, is detectable when sutures are still open, or after sutures have split. Alterations of consciousness and stiff neck with tonsillar herniation may be seen.

1. Cerebellar & 4th Ventricle Tumors–Evidence of increased intracranial pressure is often present along with cerebellar signs, including ataxia, dysmetria, and nystagmus. Pressure on adjacent structures may cause head tilt, cranial nerve signs, pyramidal tract signs, and stiff neck.

2. Supratentorial Tumors–Evidence of increased intracranial pressure is usually present, along with seizures (generalized, psychomotor, focal), in about 40% of cases. Hemiparesis, visual field defects, and personality changes often develop. Tumors of the diencephalon (like optic gliomas) are often associated with emaciation despite good oral intake (diencephalic syndrome). Tumors of the suprasellar region are often associated with visual disorders, diabetes insipidus, and pituitary insufficiency.

3. Brainstem Tumors–Cranial nerve palsies are especially common in these tumors, along with hemiparesis and ataxia. Signs of increased intracranial pressure are uncommon.

B. Imaging: CT scan with contrast usually identifies the mass, hydrocephalus, midline shift, and edema. MRI is currently considered the imaging modality that best delineates brain tumors in all locations. The presence of calcification and cysts correlate with specific tumor types. Spinal MRIs are necessary to diagnose "drop mets" in patients with medulloblastoma, ependymomas, and germinomas.

Treatment

In general, complete surgical resection should be attempted whenever the tumor location permits. Ventriculoperitoneal shunts may be necessary to correct hydrocephalus. Many tumors are not resectable, including those of the brainstem and diencephalon. Until the 1980s, radiation therapy was the primary treatment for brain tumors. Unfortunately, severe learning disabilities and endocrine dysfunction often developed in survivors. Chemotherapy along with radiation therapy has been shown to increase survival in incompletely resected medulloblastomas. In addition to radiation therapy to the posterior fossa, radiation therapy to the entire craniospinal axis is necessary to prevent recurrence and "drop mets" in medulloblastomas (PNET). Cooperative clinical trials are currently evaluating the role of intensive chemotherapy in the treatment of many types of brain tumors. Trials are also evaluating whether radiation can be delayed, reduced, or omitted in young children.

Prognosis

The prognosis depends on tumor location, histology, grade (low versus high), and extent of surgical resection. At least 50% of patients with medulloblastoma (PNET) survive 5 years, fewer than 25% of patients with brainstem gliomas survive 5 years, and over 75% of patients with completely resected low-grade astrocytomas survive 5 years.

HODGKIN'S DISEASE

Hodgkin's disease occurs twice as frequently in males than females, with its peak incidence in the third decade. It has been reported in children as young as 3 years of age. The cause is not known. The clinical and surgical staging system is shown in Table 25–1.

Clinical Findings

A. Symptoms & Signs: Painless cervical lymph node enlargement is the most common presentation of Hodgkin's disease in children. Anorexia, weight loss, fatigue, weakness, fever, malaise, pruritus, and night sweats may be associated (Table 25–1). Hodgkin's disease can arise in any lymph node. Involved nodes are usually firm and nontender. Hepatosplenomegaly and extranodal disease, particularly in lung and bone marrow, may be present. Infections and inflammatory causes

Table 25–1. Staging classification for Hodgkin's disease.[1] (Ann Arbor classification.)

Stage[2]	Distinctive Features
I	Involvement of a single lymph node region (I) or a single extralymphatic organ or site (I_E).
II	Invlovement of 2 or more lymph node regions on the same side of the diaphragm (II) or localized involvement of an extralymphatic organ or site and of one or more lymph node regions on the same side of the diaphragm (II_E).
III	Involvement of lymph node regions on both sides of the diaphragm (III), which may be accompanied by localized involvement of an extralymphatic organ or site (III_E) or of spleen (III_S) or both (III_{SE}).
IV	Diffuse or disseminated involvement of one or more extralymphatic organs with or without associated lymph node involvement. The organs involved should be identified by a symbol.

[1] Modified and reproduced, with permission, from Kempe CH, Silver HK, O'Brien D (editors): *Current Pediatric Diagnosis & Treatment*, 8th ed. Lange, 1984.

[2] Stages are also classified as IA, IB, IIA, IIB, etc, on the basis of symptoms and signs: A = asymptomatic; B = fever, night sweats, or weight loss > 10% of body weight in the 6 months prior to diagnosis.

of lymphadenopathy are in the differential diagnosis, including infectious mononucleosis and atypical mycobacterial infections.

B. Laboratory Findings: Hematologic findings may be normal or may show anemia, leukocytosis, leukopenia, thrombocytosis, thrombocytopenia, eosinophilia, or elevated sedimentation rate. Acute phase reactant proteins, including fibrinogen, ceruloplasmin, C-reactive protein, and ferritin, may be elevated in serum and can serve as sensitive markers of response to therapy and early recurrent disease. Cell-mediated immunity is often impaired in patients with Hodgkin's disease. Hemolytic anemia and abnormal levels of immunoglobulins may also occur. The diagnosis of Hodgkin's disease is made by biopsy of the involved node. Clinical staging should include bilateral bone marrow aspirates and biopsies. General anesthesia may be contraindicated if a large mediastinal mass is causing airway compromise.

C. Imaging: Clinical staging includes a number of radiographic modalities. Chest x-rays or chest CT scan may show parenchymal or mediastinal nodal disease. Lymphangiography, rarely performed in children, may reveal a "foamy" enlarged node, which implies tumor filling the node. Abdominal CT scan may show enlarged periaortic nodes or spleen and liver abnormalities. Gallium scan may help identify areas of occult disease.

D. Staging: Surgical staging by laparotomy, with splenectomy, liver biopsy, and lymph node sampling is still reasonable in fully grown patients with low stage disease who may be successfully treated with radiation therapy alone. However, pediatric oncologists prefer to treat growing children with chemotherapy and limited radiation. Such patients do not need surgical staging.

Treatment

Fully grown patients with surgical stages I and II disease can be successfully treated with extended field irradiation alone. Therapy for growing children with low-stage disease remains controversial, but chemotherapy with or without low-dose radiation to involved areas is becoming widely used. Chemotherapy is the primary treatment modality for stages III and IV disease. Chemotherapeutic agents commonly employed in combination are vincristine, mechlorethamine or cyclophosphamide, procarbazine, prednisone, vinblastine, bleomycin, doxorubicin, and dacarbazine (Table 25–2).

Prognosis

In adequately treated patients, 5-year survival rates have improved greatly. In stages I and II disease, rates range from 85 to 90%.

Table 25–2. Antineoplastic agents.[1]

Agent	Indications	Toxicity
Asparaginase (Elspar)	Acute lymphoblastic leukemia.	Nausea, vomiting, fever, hypersensitivity, pancreatitis, hyperglycemia thromboses.
Bleomycin (Blenoxane)	Hodgkin's disease, non-Hodgkin's lymphoma, testicular tumors.	Nausea, vomiting, stomatitis, fever, chills, pulmonary fibrosis, hyperpigmentation, alopecia.
Carmustine (BCNU)	Malignant gliomas, medulloblastoma, advanced Hodgkin's disease and other sarcomas, neuroblastoma, malignant melanoma.	Nausea, vomiting, hepatotoxicity, chemical derrmatitis. Bone marrow depression (3- to 4-wk delay).
Cisplatin (Platinol, CDDP)	Germ cell tumors, osteogenic sarcoma, brain tumors, neuroblastoma.	Nausea, vomiting, anorexia, alopecia, bone marrow depression, renal failure, magnesium and calcium wasting hearing impairment.
Cyclophosphamide (Cytoxan)	Leukemia, Hodgkin's disease, neuroblastoma, sarcomas, retinoblastoma, hepatoma, rhabdomyosarcoma, Ewing's sarcoma.	Nausea, vomiting, anorexia, alopecia, bone marrow depression, hemorrhagic cystitis.
Cytarabine (cytosine arabinoside; Cytosar-U)	Acute myeloblastic and acute lymphocytic leukemia.	Nausea, vomiting, anorexia, bone marrow depression, hepatotoxicity.
Dacarbazine (DTIC)	Hodgkin's disease, neuroblastoma, sarcomas.	Bone marrow depression, flulike syndrome, rash, liver failure, pain at IV infusion site.

(*continued*)

Table 25–2. Antineoplastic agents (*continued*).[1]

Agent	Indications	Toxicity
Dactinomycin (Cosmegan)	Wilms' tumor, sarcomas, rhabdomyosarcoma.	Nausea, vomiting, anorexia, bone marrow depression, alopecia. Chemical dermatitis if leakage at intravenous site. Tanning of skin if used with radiation therapy.
Daunorubicin (daunomycin)	Acute myelogenous, monomyelogenous, and monoblastic leukemias.	Same as for doxorubicin (below).
Doxorubicin (Adriamycin)	Acute lymphoblastic and myelocytic leukemia, lymphoma, Hodgkin's disease, Wilms' tumor neuroblastoma, ovarian or thyroid carcinoma, Ewing's sarcoma, osteogenic sarcoma, rhabdomyosarcoma, other soft tissue sarcomas.	Alopecia, stomatitis, esophagitis, nausea, vomiting. Severe chemical cellulitis and necrosis if extravasated. Bone marrow depression, irreversible myocardial damage (rare if cumulative dose less 350 mg/m^2).
Etoposide (VP-16)	Leukemias, germ cell tumors, neuroblastoma, brain tumors, sarcomas.	Allergic reactions, bone marrow depression, nausea and vomiting, neurotoxicity.
Fluorouracil (Adrucil)	Hepatoma, gastrointestinal carcinoma.	Nausea, vomiting, oral ulceration, bone marrow depression, gastroenteritis, alopecia, anorexia.
Ifosfamide	Sarcomas, recurrent solid tumors.	Bone marrow depression, hemorrhagic cystitis, nausea and vomiting, renal failure, alopecia, neurotoxicity.

(*continued*)

Table 25–2. Antineoplastic agents (*continued*).[1]

Agent	Indications	Toxicity
Lomustine (CCNU; CeeNu)	Brain turmors, Hodgkin's disease.	Nausea, vomiting, alopecia, stomatitis, hepatotoxicity. Bone marrow depression (4- to 6-wk delay).
Mechlorethamine (nitrogen mustard)	Hodgkin's disease, non-Hodgkin's lymphoma.	Nausea, vomiting, bone marrow depression, strong vesicating effect on skin and veins.
Mercaptopurine (Purinethol)	Acute myeloblastic and acute lymphocytic leukemia.	Nausea, vomiting, rare oral ulcerations, bone marrow depression.
Methotrexate	Acute lymphocytic leukemia, central nervous system leukemia, lymphoma, choriocarcinoma, brain tumors, Hodgkin's disease.	Oral ulcers, gastrointestinal irritation, bone marrow depression, hepatotoxicity. Do not use in presence of impaired renal function.
Prednisone	Acute myeloblastic and lymphocytic leukemia, lymphoma, Hodgkin's disease, bone pain from metastatic disease, central nervous system tumors.	Increased appetite, sodium retention, hypertension, osteoporosis, provocation of latent diabetes or tuberculosis.
Procarbazine (Matulane)	Hodgkin's disease, lymphoma.	Nauasea, vomiting, anorexia. Bone marrow depression (3-wk delay). Do not give with narcotics or sedatives; has "disulfiram effect." Monitor liver and renal function.
Vinblastine	Histiocytosis, Hodgkin's disease, germ cell tumors.	Bone marrow depression, alopecia, mucositis, neurotoxicity, chemical dermatitis.

(*continued*)

Table 25–2. Antineoplastic agents (*continued*).[1]

Agent	Indications	Toxicity
Vincristine (Oncovin)	Acute lymphocytic and myeloblastic leukemia, lymphoma, Hodgkin's disease, rhabdomyosarcoma, Wilms' tumor, neuroblastoma, Ewing's sarcoma, retinoblastoma, hepatoma, sarcomas, osteogenic sarcoma, brain tumors.	Alopecia, constipation, abdominal cramps, jaw pain, paresthesia, myalgia, muscle weakness, neurotoxicity, decrease in deep tendon reflexes, chemical dermatitis. Do not use in presence of severe liver impairment.

[1] Since the dosage of these agents varies widely depending on number of drugs used simultaneously, type of tumor being treated, bone marrow reserve, and previous toxicities and therapies (eg, irradiation), the dosages are not given in this handbook.

In stages III and IV disease, rates range from about 50 to 80%. Late side effects of treatment with radiation and chemotherapy include infertility, impaired bony growth, hypothyroidism, and second cancers.

NON-HODGKIN'S LYMPHOMA

Non-Hodgkin's lymphomas encompass a more diverse group of lymphomas in adults than in children. Histologic classification into two main groups, lymphoblastic and nonlymphoblastic, is important for determining appropriate therapy and prognosis in childhood lymphomas.

Burkitt's tumor (African lymphoma) is a nonlymphoblastic lymphoma found principally in Africa and is responsible for half of all cancer deaths in children in Uganda and Central Africa. A viral cause has been assumed, and the Epstein-Barr virus seems to play an important role in this disease. The tumor is characterized by (1) predilection for the facial bones and mandible *or* (2) primary involvement of abdominal nodes and viscera and (3) massive proliferation of primitive lymphoid cells. When Burkitt's lymphoma is seen in patients outside Africa, it presents most often as an abdominal tumor, and occasionally in the nasopharynx.

Clinical Findings

A. Symptoms & Signs: Non-Hodgkin's lymphoma of childhood tends to grow rapidly. The gastrointestinal tract in the region of the terminal ileum, cecum, appendix, ascending colon, and mesenteric nodes is the most common site of nonlymphoblastic lymphoma (aside from African Burkitt's). Acute abdominal pain, intussusception, gastrointestinal tract perforation, and hemorrhage may occur. Lymphoblastic lymphoma presents most commonly with a mediastinal mass, with or without pleural effusion. Chronic cough, dyspnea, and orthopnea are often associated. Involvement of the tonsillar region, cervical nodes, and nasopharynx may be diagnosed by the presence of a mass or compression symptoms. Other less common sites of primary disease include bone, ovaries, skin, and central nervous system (CNS).

B. Laboratory Findings: Spread to the bone marrow and CNS often occurs with lymphoblastic or disseminated non-lymphoblastic lymphoma. Thus, bone marrow aspirates and biopsies and spinal fluid cytology need to be obtained to determine the extent of the disease. The CBC is usually normal in non-Hodgkin's lymphoma unless widespread disease and marrow infiltration is present. Serum uric acid and LDH are often very elevated in patients with Burkitt's lymphoma and moderately elevated in patients with lymphoblastic lymphoma.

C. Imaging: These patients should be evaluated radiographically as is done for Hodgkin's lymphoma, with the exception of lymphangiogram and the addition of bone scan.

Treatment

Staging laparotomy is not performed in non-Hodgkin's lymphoma. Complete surgical resection of isolated nodal, extranodal, or gastrointestinal disease, when possible, is advocated. However, debulking of widespread abdominal disease or mediastinal mass should not be performed. General anesthesia is usually contraindicated in patients with large mediastinal masses. Multiple-drug chemotherapy should be started as soon as possible after diagnosis. Severe tumor lysis syndrome may develop following the initiation of treatment. Hyperuricemia, hyperphosphatemia, hypocalcemia with tetany, and renal failure may develop (see below, Leukemia, Supportive Measures). Duration of therapy depends on location, type of lymphoma, and extent of disease, and currently ranges from 4–18 months. The drugs most commonly employed are vincristine, cyclophosphamide, doxorubicin, prednisone, methotrexate, cytarabine, and etoposide (Table

25–2). In patients at high risk for CNS involvement, presymptomatic intrathecal therapy should be given. Radiation therapy is rarely used in the treatment of lymphomas in children.

Prognosis

The prognosis in children with non-Hodgkin's lymphoma depends primarily on histology and extent of disease. Overall, at least 75% of children with non-Hodgkin's lymphoma can be cured.

NEUROBLASTOMA

Neuroblastoma arises from cells in the sympathetic ganglia and adrenal medulla. It is the third most frequent pediatric neoplasm seen in children less than 5 years old. This tumor may be seen in the newborn period; the highest incidence is at 2 years of age. The tumors may regress spontaneously in infants less than 1 year old. Presentation in the abdominal area is commonly associated with distant metastases and carries a poor prognosis.

Clinical Findings

A. Symptoms & Signs: General symptoms include failure to thrive, anorexia, fatigue, periorbital ecchymoses, chronic diarrhea, hypertension, pallor, irritability, bone pain, limp, and bluish skin nodules. Opsoclonus and myoclonus ("dancing eyes" and "dancing feet") have been associated with neuroblastoma.

1. Cervical Tumors–Involvement of the cervicothoracic ganglion may be associated with Horner's syndrome.

2. Posterior Thoracic Tumors–Tumors may present with respiratory symptoms such as cough, croup, dysphagia, and fatigue, or with symptoms of spinal cord compression.

3. Abdominal Tumors–Tumors may cause abdominal swelling from adrenal or paraspinal tumor. They may be very large and cross the midline or may be deep and difficult to palpate. Other findings include abdominal pain, change in bowel habits, delay in walking, paraplegia, or shock if a large tumor has ruptured.

B. Laboratory Findings: Anemia is common at diagnosis and results from chronic disease, hemorrhage into tumor, or marrow invasion. Thrombocytosis is common. Bone marrow is a common site of metastases and may reveal classic rosettes or sheets of anaplastic neuroblasts. Urine levels of catecholamines (vanillylmandelic acid

[VMA] and homovanillic acid [HVA]) are elevated in nearly 90% of patients. Amplification of the n-*myc* oncogene in the tumor itself indicates a poor prognosis.

C. Imaging: Multiple destructive lesions of bone with a "moth-eaten" appearance may be seen in all bones. Pathologic fracture may also occur. Both skeletal survey and bone scan are necessary to determine extent of bony metastases.

1. Thoracic Tumors–Chest x-ray often shows soft tissue with clear borders and scattered calcifications close to the spine and in the upper chest. There may be erosion and separation of posterior ribs. CT scan or spinal MRI should be obtained to define the tumor mass and its involvement with adjacent vital structures and spinal canal.

2. Abdominal Tumors–Abdominal x-ray may reveal a soft tissue mass in the region of the adrenal gland or along the spine. Many tumors show calcification. CT scan should be obtained to delineate the tumor and to look for hepatic metastases. Spinal MRI may be necessary to evaluate for intercanalicular disease.

Treatment

Current therapeutic recommendations include surgery alone with close follow-up for patients with stage I disease. (See Table 25–3 for staging). Patients with stage II disease and small or microscopic residua after surgery can also be safely treated with surgery alone and close follow-up. Improved treatments for advanced disease continue to be evaluated. Agents shown to be effective in neuroblastoma include vincristine, cylophosphasmide, dacarbazine, etoposide, doxorubicin, cisplatin, and melphalan (Table 25–2). Neuroblastoma is very radiosensitive. Very-high-dose chemotherapy with total body irradiation, followed by autologous bone marrow transplant, is currently being evaluated in treatment of advanced disease. Retinoic acid may help differentiate neuroblastoma cells into ganglion cells, and this drug has recently been studied in clinical trials.

Prognosis

The most important variables for predicting prognosis are age and stage. Children diagnosed at less than 1 year of age have about an 80% survival rate. Patients with stage 1 disease have a survival rate of about 80%. Survival of children diagnosed at older than 2 years (of whom two-thirds present with metastatic disease) is about 25%. Patients whose tumors have n-*myc* amplification have a poor prognosis, regardless of stage.

Table 25–3. International staging system for neuroblastoma.

Stage I:	Localized tumor confined to the area of origin; complete gross excision, with or without microscopic residual disease; identifiable lymph nodes negative microscopically.
Stage IIA:	Unilateral tumor with incomplete gross excision; identifiable lymph nodes negative microscopically.
Stage IIB:	Unilateral tumor with complete or incomplete gross excision; with positive ipsilateral regional lymph nodes; identifiable contralateral lymph nodes negative microscopically.
Stage III:	Tumor infiltrating across the midline with or without regional lymph node involvement; or unilateral tumor with contralateral regional lymph node involvement; or midline tumor with bilateral regional lymph node involvement.
Stage IV:	Dissemination of tumor to distant lymph nodes, bone, bone marrow, liver and/or other organs (except as defined in stage IV).
Stage IVS:	Localized primary tumor as defined for stage 1 or 2 with dissemination limited to liver, skin, and/or bone marrow.

WILMS' TUMOR (Nephroblastoma)

The most common abdominal masses encountered in early childhood are hydronephrosis, neuroblastoma, and Wilms' tumor. Wilms' tumor is believed to be embryonal in origin. It develops within renal parenchyma and enlarges with distortion and invasion of adjacent renal tissue. It occurs most commonly in children between 2 and 5 years old. Bilateral Wilms' tumors occur in up to 5% of patients. This tumor may be associated with congenital anomalies such as hemihypertrophy, aniridia, ambiguous genitalia, hypospadias, undescended testes, duplications of ureters or kidneys, horseshoe kidney, multiple nevi, and Beckwith's syndrome.

Clinical Findings

A. Symptoms & Signs: Ninety percent of patients present with an abdominal mass, but only about 30% complain of abdominal discomfort. Anemia is observed at diagnosis in about 25% of patients, hypertension in 20%, and hematuria in 15%.

B. Laboratory Findings: Urinalyses are usually normal, but hematuria or pyuria may be found. Serum creatinine is usually normal. A normochromic, normocytic anemia may be present.

C. Imaging: A soft tissue mass may be seen on a plain film of the abdomen and calcification may occur in a marginal concentric fashion. Hepatomegaly may be present if the liver has extensive metastases. Abdominal ultrasound and CT scan can define the mass, which usually appears well encapsulated. Ultrasound may demonstrate tumor thrombus in the renal vein or inferior vena cava. CT scan of chest or 4-view chest x-ray may reveal metastases.

Treatment

Surgical excision of the entire mass, without prior biopsy, is the standard surgical procedure in the United States. A transabdominal approach is essential to allow adequate mobilization, prevent excess manipulation of the tumor, and allow examination of abdominal viscera, nodes, and the opposite kidney. Conservative surgery is appropriate when bilateral disease is present at diagnosis.

Treatment of Wilms' tumor depends on surgical staging and histology (Table 25–4). Improvement in survival has resulted from cooperative clinical trials in the United States and Europe. Chemotherapy agents used to treat Wilms' tumor include dactinomycin and vincristine for the lower stages, with the addition of doxorubicin and occasionally cytoxan for the higher stages or unfavorable histology. Radiotherapy to the tumor bed is no longer recommended in stages I and II disease, but appears to be of benefit in stages III and IV disease.

Table 25–4. Wilms' tumor stages.

Stage	Findings
I	Tumor *limited* to kidney; intact capsule; completely resected
II	Tumor extension *beyond capsule* into perirenal soft tissues or renal vessels but *no* residua beyond margin of resection; surgical rupture: *flank* only
III	*Residual* tumor in abdomen: 1) + lymph nodes 2) massive rupture 3) peritoneal implants 4) not fully resected secondary to local infiltration into vital structures
IV	Hematogenous metastases
V	Bilateral; each side staged as above

Prognosis

The survival rate is best in children with localized disease and favorable histology. Survival rates have significantly improved over the past 30 years, and the overall 5-year survival rate is now about 80%.

TUMORS OF SOFT TISSUE

The most common malignant soft tissue tumor seen in children is rhabdomyosarcoma. Rhabdomyosarcoma is one of the tumors associated with neurofibromatosis. The most common primary site of occurrence is the head and neck, followed in decreasing frequency by genitourinary, extremity, trunk, and retroperitoneal sites. Pathologic evaluation of a biopsy specimen or of the completely removed tumor (depending on size and location) is necessary to distinguish rhabdomyosarcoma from other soft tissue sarcomas, lymphomas, and neuroblastoma.

Clinical Findings

A. Symptoms & Signs: The child usually presents with a firm mass in the region of the tumor. Orbital rhabdomyosarcoma often presents with proptosis. Middle ear and parameningeal tumors may present with chronic otitis media, cranial nerve palsies, and headaches.

B. Laboratory Findings: CBC and serum chemistries are usually normal, although LDH may be elevated. Bone marrow aspirates and biopsies need to be performed to evaluate for metastatic disease.

C. Imaging: CT scan or MRI of the primary mass is necessary to determine extent of disease and resectability. Evaluation for metastatic disease should include skeletal survey and bone scan, and CT of the abdomen and lungs.

Treatment & Prognosis

Treatment depends on location of the tumor, histologic type, and extent of disease. Treatment modalities include surgery, chemotherapy, and radiation therapy. Effective chemotherapy includes vincristine, dactinomycin, cytoxan, ifosfamide, etoposide, and doxorubicin (Table 25–2).

The overall disease-free survival is about 70%. Orbital tumors have the best prognosis.

Fibrosarcomas and liposarcomas are rare lesions and should be surgically excised when possible. In certain circumstances, electron beam therapy (4000–6000 rads) may be of benefit. The role of adjuvant chemotherapy is unclear.

Benign tumors are generally slow-growing and nontender. Most commonly seen are the fibromas and lipomas. These may be excised if they are symptomatic.

TUMORS OF BONE

Malignant bone tumors are more common in children over 10 than in younger age groups. Osteogenic sarcoma and Ewing's sarcoma are the most common types of bone tumors; rare tumors include chondrosarcoma, fibrosarcoma, and synovial sarcoma. Osteogenic sarcoma typically arises in the metaphyses of long bones. The distal femur is the most common site, followed by the proximal tibia and proximal humerus. Ewing's sarcoma arises in long and flat bones, including the pelvis.

Clinical Findings

A. Symptoms & Signs: Bone tumors may present with bone pain, with or without associated mass, limitation of motion, and x-ray changes in the involved bones.

B. Laboratory Findings: CBC may show anemia of chronic disease if widespread metastatic disease is present. LDH and sedimentation rate are often elevated in Ewing's sarcoma and alkaline phosphatase and sedimentation rate may be elevated in osteogenic sarcoma.

Imaging

Plain x-rays of osteogenic sarcoma typically display a "sunburst" appearance with lytic and blastic elements within the lesion. X-rays of Ewing's sarcoma typically show a moth-eaten and lytic appearance with elevation of the periosteum ("onion-skinning"). MRI scan of the lesion allows assessment of the extent of disease and involvement of the neurovascular bundle. Metastatic disease to lungs and other bones is not uncommon at diagnosis and should be sought with chest CT scan and bone scan prior to planning therapy.

Treatment & Prognosis

Survival rate for patients with osteosarcoma was less than 20% with surgical amputation alone, but significant improvement has resulted from the combination of aggressive surgery (amputation or complex limb-preservation surgery) and multiple drug chemotherapy. A few courses of chemotherapy is usually given prior to definitive surgery. Effective chemotherapeutic agents for osteogenic sarcoma include high-dose methotrexate with leucovorin rescue, doxorubicin, cisplatin, and ifosfamide (Table 25–2). Radiation therapy is not effective in osteogenic sarcoma. Local high-dose radiation therapy (5000–6000 rads) has traditionally been used along with chemotherapy for Ewing's sarcoma. However, many centers now advocate full surgical resection, when possible, as for osteogenic sarcoma. Effective chemotherapy for Ewing's sarcoma includes cyclophosphamide, doxorubicin, adriamycin, vincristine, ifosfamide, and etoposide (Table 25–2). The 5-year disease-free survival for osteogenic sarcoma and for Ewing's sarcoma is about 60%. Newer chemotherapy regimens may improve these survival rates. Patients who present with metastatic disease have a very poor prognosis. Ewing's sarcoma can recur many years after completion of treatment.

There are a number of fibrous, cartilaginous, and osseous benign tumors. Some have classic x-ray findings. In general, they should be biopsied or excised to rule out the possibility of a malignant tumor.

RETINOBLASTOMA

Retinoblastoma is a malignant ocular tumor that occurs before the age of 5 in over 90% of cases. The tumor may arise sporadically or be inherited. Patients with inherited retinoblastoma often have bilateral disease, while those with the sporadic form have unilateral disease.

Clinical Findings

A. Symptoms & Signs: The most common presenting complaint is leukocoria (white "cat's eye reflex") noted by parents. Strabismus, signs of orbital inflammation, and retinal detachment may be associated. The diagnosis is usually made by inspection of the globe under anesthesia by an ophthalmologist experienced with these tumors. The differential diagnosis includes lesions of ***Toxocara canis***, toxoplasmosis, and retrolental fibroplasia. The tumor is typically confined to the globe but is extraocular in about 15% of cases.

B. Laboratory Findings: Metastatic evaluation should include cerebrospinal fluid cytology and bone marrow aspirate and biopsy. It is very rare, however, for retinoblastoma to spread to the spinal fluid or bone marrow without extra-ocular spread.

C. Imaging: Metastatic evaluation should include orbital CT scan to define extraocular extension and ocular nerve involvement. Head CT or MRI should be obtained in bilateral cases to look for retinoblastoma involving the pineal gland (trilateral retinoblastoma).

Treatment

Eradication of the tumor by enucleation depends on the potential for useful vision. Since the majority of unilateral tumors involve over one-half the retina by the time of diagnosis, enucleation is most commonly advised. For smaller lesions where vision may be saved, cryotherapy, photocoagulation, or radiotherapy have been successful treatments. Combination chemotherapy should be given to patients with regional or distant extraocular spread. Ophthalmologic evaluation of the uninvolved eye should be performed at regular intervals for several years in order to detect early bilateral disease.

Prognosis

Survival of retinoblastoma is greater than 90%. Patients with the inherited form have a high risk of second cancers throughout their lives, the most common being osteogenic sarcoma. Genetic counseling is important for families of patients with retinoblastoma. The risk of a subsequent sibling developing retinoblastoma varies from 1 to 50%, depending on the presence of other affected family members. Siblings should be carefully examined and followed by an ophthalmologist.

GERM CELL TUMORS

Germ cell tumors are derived from primordial germ cells and can be benign or malignant, gonadal (ovarian or testicular), or extragonadal. Extragonadal midline sites are involved in about two-thirds of cases, including the sacrococcygeal area, mediastinum, retroperitoneum, and CNS. Patients with gonadal dysgenesis (as in Turner's syndrome) and those with undescended testes are at increased risk of developing germ cell tumors, particularly gonadoblastomas and germinomas. Teratomas can be benign or malignant, depending on the degree of maturity of the tissue elements involved. Since therapy is different for benign and malignant teratomas, very careful pathologic evaluation of the tumor is necessary. Malignant germ cell tumors characteristically secrete alpha-fetoprotein (AFP) or beta-subunit human chorionic gonadotropin (β-hCG), which are valuable serum markers of disease activity.

Sacrococcygeal teratomas are found more often in neonates than in older infants and children. The majority of these tumors have an external component, allowing for rapid diagnosis. Most of these tumors are benign at the time of diagnosis. However, since benign teratomas have the capacity to become malignant, full surgical excision is necessary. The coccyx should be removed as well since the chance of recurrence in that area is high. Serum AFP should be monitored.

Tumors of the ovary are characterized by an enlarging palpable mass in the lower abdomen or pelvis. Severe abdominal pain may occur due to a twisted pedicle. Treatment of ovarian tumors is by complete surgical removal for localized disease. Postoperative chemotherapy is used to treat malignant germ cell tumors, whether completely or incompletely excised. The best treatment results so far have been obtained with cisplatin, etoposide, and bleomycin. Prognosis is generally very good.

Testicular tumors vary from highly malignant (embryonal carcinoma, germinoma, or malignant teratoma) to relatively benign (Leydig cell tumor or benign teratoma). They are rare in boys under 15 years of age. Paratesticular rhabdomyosarcoma may also present as a scrotal mass in the male child. Tumors are characterized by painless, solid swelling of the testicle, which does not transilluminate and appears to have a purplish discoloration. Hydrocele may be associated.

Orchiectomy with high ligation of the cord is indicated in all testicular tumors. Radiographic staging with abdominal and chest CT scan, bone scan, and skeletal survey is necessary prior to treatment of malignant tumors. Metastases may occur in lungs, mediastinum, bones, and regional and abdominal lymph nodes. For boys without radiographic evidence of lymphatic or hematologic spread, orchiectomy without chemotherapy but with close serial follow-up of serum AFP levels appears to be adequate initial treatment. The most successful chemotherapy for malignant testicular germ cell tumors is as described for ovarian primaries. The prognosis is very good.

LANGERHANS CELL HISTIOCYTOSIS (Histiocytosis X)

The diseases discussed under this heading comprise a heterogeneous group of proliferative disorders of unknown cause, but immune system dysfunction may be involved in their pathogenesis. They differ in behavior from true neoplasms. Eosinophilic granuloma of bone, Hand-Schüller-Christian disease, and Letterer-Siwe disease are names previously given to the differing presentations of histiocytosis X. Langerhans histiocytes—phagocytes normally found in skin—are the proliferating cells in these disorders. Whether these cells are immature, normal, or malignant is unclear. Various immunologic abnormalities have been observed in patients with these diseases.

Clinical Findings

Certain patients present primarily with signs and symptoms of lytic lesions limited to the bones—especially the skull, ribs, clavicles, and vertebrae. These lesions are well demarcated on x-ray and occasionally are painful with overlying soft tissue swelling. Biopsy reveals eosinophilic granuloma, which may be the only lesion the patient will develop, although further bone and even visceral lesions may occur.

Another group of patients present with otitis media, seborrheic skin rash, and evidence of bone lesions, usually in the mastoid or skull area. They also frequently have visceral involvement, lymphadenopathy, and hepatosplenomegaly. The classic triad of Hand-Schüller-Christian disease (bony involvement, exophthalmos, and diabetes insipidus) is rarely seen; however, diabetes insipidus may develop over time.

A third group of patients present early in life primarily with visceral involvement. They often have a petechial or macular skin rash, generalized lymphadenopathy, enlarged liver and spleen, pulmonary involvement, and hematologic abnormalities such as anemia and thrombocytopenia. Bone lesions can occur. This acute visceral form, Letterer-Siwe disease, is often fatal.

The principal diseases to be differentiated from histiocytosis X are infections with histiocyte proliferation (eg, toxoplasmosis, tularemia), bone tumors (primary or metastatic), lymphomas or leukemias, immune deficiency states, and storage diseases. The diagnosis is established by biopsy of abnormal areas of bone, skin, bone marrow, lymph node, or liver. Complete immunologic evaluation is essential to distinguish Letterer-Siwe disease from severe combined immune deficiency.

Treatment

Isolated bony lesions, if progressive or symptomatic (or both), are best treated by curettage and local radiotherapy. Multiple bony involvement and visceral involvement often respond well to prednisone, vinblastine, cyclophosphamide, methotrexate, and etoposide (Table 25–2). Combination chemotherapy does not appear to offer significant advantage over single- or double-agent chemotherapy. If diabetes insipidus occurs, treatment with vasopressin gives good control.

Prognosis

In patients with Langerhans histiocytosis, the prognosis is often unpredictable. Many patients with considerable bony and visceral involvement have shown apparent complete recovery. The disease can also smolder for years, causing significant morbidity without mortality. In general, the younger the patient and the more extensive the visceral involvement, the worse the prognosis.

LEUKEMIAS IN CHILDHOOD

Most leukemias (97.5%) in childhood are acute. The most common type is acute lymphoblastic leukemia (ALL), which accounts for about 80% of cases (Table 25–5). The highest incidence of leukemia occurs in patients between 2 and 5 years of age. There is an increased risk of leukemia in patients with chromosomal abnormalities or immune deficiency states.

Clinical Findings

A. Symptoms & Signs: Initial signs and symptoms, in order of decreasing frequency, include fever, pallor, petechiae and purpura, lymphadenopathy, hepatosplenomegaly, anorexia, fatigue, bone and joint pain, abdominal pain, and weight loss. Nonmalignant conditions in the differential diagnosis include juvenile rheumatoid arthritis, immune thrombocytopenic purpura, Epstein-Barr viral disease, and aplastic anemia. CNS infiltration may cause manifestations simulating meningitis, with increased intracranial pressure and cranial nerve palsies. Septicemia may occur during the course of the disease due to neutropenia.

B. Laboratory Findings:

1. Blood–Red blood cell counts and hemoglobin levels are usually low. The white blood cell count may be elevated, normal, or reduced, but neutropenia is often present. In some cases, large numbers of abnormal cells (blasts) are seen on smear; in others, no peripheral blasts are noted. Thrombocytopenia is very frequent.

2. Bone Marrow–By definition, leukemia is present when more than 25% of cells in a bone marrow aspirate are malignant blasts. In almost all cases, 50–98% of nucleated cells are blast forms with

Table 25–5. Acute leukemias of childhood.

Type	Approximate Frequency	Morphology	Immunophenotype (Histochemical Staining)
Lymphoblastic (ALL)	80%		
B-Cell Precursor ALL	84%[1]	Typically small blasts (≤2 RBC diameters), scant cytoplasm, indistinct nucleoli.[2]	Majority are CALLA (+)
T-Cell ALL	15%		E-rosette or T-cell surface antigen (+)
B-Cell ALL	1%	Blasts with deeply basophilic cytoplasm and vacuolization.	Surface immunoglobulin (+)
Nonlymphoblastic (ANLL)	20%		
Myeloblastic	45%[3]	Blasts with few or many cytoplasmic granules; may have Auer rods.	Myeloperoxidase (MP) (+)
Promyelocytic	4%	Promyelocytes with numerous cytoplasmic granules.	MP (+)
Myelomonocytic	26%	Myeloblasts with cytoplasmic granules and monoblasts.	MP (+) and nonspecific esterase (NSE) (+)
Monocytic	21%	Monoblasts with smooth or irregular, folded nuclear contour.	NSE (+)
Erythroid	2%	Erythroblasts amid dyserythropoiesis.	
Megakaryocytic	2%	Blasts look like lymphoblasts or undifferentiated myeloblasts.	Platelet peroxidase (+) endoplasmic reticulum on electron microscopy

[1] % of ALL.

[2] Some lymphoblasts are larger, with more cytoplasm and more prominent nucleoli, similar morphologically to undifferentiated myeloblasts.

[3] % of ANLL.

[4] Frequency may be underestimated since megakaryocytic leukemia has only recently been recognized.

marked reduction in the normal erythroid, myeloid, and platelet precursors. Blasts from the majority of cases of childhood ALL have an antigen present on the cell surface called the common ALL-antigen (CALLA). These blasts are derived from B-cell precursors early in their development. Less commonly, lymphoblasts are of T-cell origin or of mature B-cell origin.

3. Chromosomes–A variety of chromosome abnormalities have been reported in the blasts of all forms of acute leukemia. Certain abnormalities, including reciprocal translocations [eg, t(4;11) and t(9;22)] or monosomy 7 are associated with a very poor prognosis.

4. Serum–Levels of uric acid and lactate dehydrogenase are often elevated.

5. Cerebrospinal Fluid–Pleocytosis (consisting of blast forms), elevated levels of protein, and decreased levels of glucose may be seen.

Treatment of Leukemias

A. Acute Lymphoblastic Leukemia:

1. Remission Induction–Most patients (95%) achieve complete remission following 4 weeks of treatment with vincristine, prednisone, asparaginase, and intrathecal methotrexate (Table 25–2).

2. Central Nervous System Leukemia–Because of the risk of CNS leukemia, patients should receive presymptomatic CNS treatment with intrathecal chemotherapy. Treatment of frank CNS leukemia requires whole brain and spinal irradiation along with intrathecal drugs.

3. Maintenance–Maintenance therapy lasts 2–3 years, with daily oral mercaptopurine and weekly methotrexate as mainstays of treatment, often with monthly vincristine and prednisone as well.

4. Relapse–If the disease recurs, another remission may be induced with selected combinations of the above drugs or other antineoplastic agents. Ultimate prognosis for patients who relapse depends on when relapse occurs in relation to completion of initial therapy. Allogeneic bone marrow transplant offers the best chance of cure for patients who relapse while receiving chemotherapy.

B. Acute Nonlymphocytic Leukemia (ANLL): ANLL of childhood is more difficult to cure than ALL. Remission induction has been successful with a number of agents; the most commonly used are cytarabine and daunorubicin (Table 25–2). Presymptomatic treatment of CNS with intrathecal cytarabine is necessary. The advantage of bone marrow transplantation over aggressive chemotherapy for long-term cure in patients who achieve remission remains to be determined and may depend on ANLL subtypes and associated chromosomal abnormalities.

C. Supportive Measures: Transfusions of packed red blood cells and platelets should be given as needed. Fevers in the face of neutropenia should be treated with broad-spectrum antibiotics. Allopurinol taken orally is effective in reducing the hyperuricemia of tumor lysis syndrome. Intravenous hydration and alkalinization (to decrease uric acid precipitation in kidneys) is also of value. Hyperkalemia, severe hyperphosphatemia, tetany, or oliguria may develop with tumor lysis syndrome and may require temporary hemodialysis.

Prognosis

Aggressive combination chemotherapy and supportive therapy with blood products and antibiotics have contributed to improved survival. Long-term "cure" rates are now at least 70% for all patients with ALL. In general, children diagnosed with ALL between the ages of 1 and 9 years with a white blood cell count of less than 50,000/μL at diagnosis have the best chance of cure. Children with ANLL have a poorer prognosis, with long-term cure rates between 40% and 60%.

INFECTIONS IN THE ONCOLOGY PATIENT

Immunodeficiency may be congenital in cancer patients but more often is due to suppression of the immune system by the cancer or drugs. Deficiencies of neutrophils, T lymphocytes, or B lymphocytes tend to predispose the host to infection with different agents. Neutropenia caused by chemotherapy predisposes to infection with gram-negative or gram-positive bacteria and fungi. B lymphocyte deficiency can develop from repeated exposure to steroids, cyclophosphamide, and methotrexate, and predisposes to infection with extracellular bacteria such as pneumococci and staphylococci. T lymphocyte deficiency caused especially by exposure to steroids and radiation predisposes to infection with intracellular bacteria (mycobacteria, *Listeria*, etc), fungi (*Candida, Aspergillus*, etc), protozoa (*Pneumocystis*, etc), and viruses (herpes simplex, etc). Patients receiving intensive chemotherapy or steroids require prophylaxis against pneumocystis. Patients non-immune to varicella are at risk for very serious, even fatal, infection if exposed to varicella. Such patients should receive Varicella-Zoster immune globulin (VZIG) within 72 hours after exposure and treatment with IV acyclovir for active infection.

Many opportunistic organisms do not produce disease except in the immunodeficient host. Such hosts are often infected with a number of pathogens simultaneously. Infections caused by common organisms may present uncommon clinical manifestations. Determination of the specific infecting agents is essential for effective treatment.

Approach to Treatment of Febrile Neutropenia

For patients with absolute neutropenia [WBC × (% bands + segs) < 500/μL] and temperature > 38.3° C (oral), broad-spectrum antibiotics should be initiated immediately after cultures are obtained even if the patient appears clinically well. This practice is necessary because signs of infection (ie, exudate, fluctuance, swelling, erythema, and pain) are decreased or absent when neutrophil counts are very low. Thorough physical examination should include close inspection of skin for septic emboli and perirectal area for signs of cellulitis. Most episodes of febrile neutropenia are culture negative. The antibiotics probably control small foci of infection (in the gut or lung) until the WBC recovers enough to eradicate the bacterial overgrowth. No digital rectal exams or rectal temperatures should be performed in neutropenic patients.

Central venous catheters may have to be removed if bacteremia persists despite antibiotics. If disseminated varicella or herpes zoster is suspected, IV acyclovir should be started immediately, prior to culture confirmation. Fungal infection should be suspected in a patient who remains febrile after a number of days on broad-spectrum antibiotics. Once an infectious agent is identified, antimicrobial drug therapy should be specific and lethal for it. Combinations of antibiotics may be necessary, since multiple infectious agents may be involved in some cases.

The hemotopoietic growth factor G-CSF, or Neupogen, stimulates proliferation and maturation of neutrophil precursors in bone marrow and accelerates neutrophil recovery follow chemotherapy. G-CSF given daily, starting about 24 hours after a course of chemotherapy has decreased the incidence of febrile neutropenia following chemotherapy by as much as 40% in both adults and children.

26 | Allergic Diseases

David S. Pearlman, MD

Allergic reactivity, or the specific ability to reject foreign substances, is normal. Some forms of allergy, however, occur only in certain individuals in whom a presumably hereditary predisposition is important. These disorders—**allergic rhinitis**, **asthma**, and **atopic dermatitis**—are called **"atopic disorders."** In most instances, allergic reactivity based on IgE antibody to innocuous inhaled or ingested materials is an important cause of the disorder. The most important of these materials are animal allergens, house dust mite and insect allergens, spores from indoor and outdoor molds, and tree, grass, and weed pollen. Inhalants generally induce symptoms in the upper and/or lower respiratory tract. Sensitivity to foods, drugs, and stinging insects, and other ingested materials contribute to perennial, seasonal, or episodic problems, some of which can be life-threatening.

PRINCIPLES OF DIAGNOSIS

Diagnosis is based first on the history and physical findings. Identification of the allergic antibody that may be involved is helpful and sometimes essential for determining the nature of the reaction and the environmental culprit. **These tests are not diagnostic in themselves, and their interpretation requires knowing the child**, including his or her environmental exposures. Atopic disorders tend to occur in families, and multiple disorders often occur in the same child. A history of time and place (eg, at school or at home) where a reaction occurs is helpful in determining environmental culprits. Some reactions occur within minutes ("early reaction"), but others can develop hours after allergen exposure.

Laboratory Tests

The principal allergic antibody identified belongs to the IgE class, also called **skin sensitizing antibody**. There are two basic kinds of tests for IgE antibody: **skin tests** and **serologic tests**.

A. Skin Tests: These are very sensitive "biologic" tests which measure allergic antibody as a manifestation of the local release of mediators from sensitized cells on which the allergic reaction takes place. Sensitized mediator cells are found throughout the body, including the skin, which provides an extremely convenient site for testing. Prick tests are generally done first. Since these tests are relatively painless, a large number of allergens can be applied conveniently, and they are safer than intradermal tests in highly sensitive children. Intradermal tests are more sensitive than prick tests but are reserved for allergens that do not elicit a positive prick test though are still considered to be likely culprits of the disorder. The end point of these tests is a wheal and erythema reaction (hive), which occurs rapidly and peaks within 15–20 minutes. Skin testing is potentially dangerous in highly sensitive individuals. Most test materials are impure and in high concentration can produce an irritant reaction ("false-positive test"). Positive tests may or may not be of significant clinical relevance, hence it is important to interpret test results strictly within the context of the clinical circumstances of the patient.

B. Serologic Tests: These tests measure serum IgE antibody per se. The best known is the radioallergosorbent test (RAST), a radioimmunoassay, but various enzymatic immunoassay variations are commonly available (ELISAs). Serologic tests correlate best with skin tests when high levels of antibody are present, but are less sensitive than skin tests. Theoretically, these tests should be especially useful for testing severe drug and stinging insect hypersensitivity. However, particularly with drug sensitivity, the important drug metabolites responsible for drug sensitivity rarely are available for serologic or skin testing and the lesser sensitivity of serologic tests make these tests less valuable for determining potentially life-threatening sensitivity.

C. Immunoglobulin Levels: IgE levels are measured by radioimmunosorbent or ELISA tests. Elevated IgE levels do occur in some allergic disorders, but the frequency of this occurrence and correlation with the presence or absence of allergy is so imperfect that this is not generally a useful screening procedure. Greatly elevated IgE levels in infancy are highly predictive of an atopic diathesis but a normal or low IgE level does not rule out either an atopic disorder or specific allergic sensitization.

D. Provocative Testing: Challenging the patient with a suspected allergen and observing the response also is useful, particularly with possible food sensitivity. It should not be used, however, when life-threatening sensitivity is suspected. A positive response can establish a cause-and-effect relationship but not necessarily the mechanism involved (eg, a positive challenge to milk may be due to allergy or lactase deficiency).

Eosinophils are a component of allergic inflammation, and the presence of a large number in secretions or blood is often seen in atopic disorders. Large numbers are suggestive but not diagnostic of an allergic reaction, and their absence does not rule out allergy. Nasal eosinophilia is especially helpful in diagnosing allergic rhinitis, but nasal eosinophilia in infants up to 3 months of age can be normal.

Controversial Techniques for Diagnosis and Treatment

Intracutaneous end-point titration (sometimes called the "Rinkel test"), sublingual and serial intracutaneous provocation titration tests, cytotoxic tests, tests for IgG antibodies for food allergy, and sublingual desensitization—all used for diagnosing or treating "allergy"—are not scientifically validated.

GENERAL PRINCIPLES OF TREATMENT

Controlling the Environment

Avoiding the offending allergen is the most effective treatment of all allergic disorders. Although complete avoidance may be impossible, it is often feasible to reduce the degree of exposure to the point that reactions are trivial. The avoidance of nonallergic add-on irritants such as smoke is also important. The single most important area of exposure is a child's bedroom. Here the greatest effort should be made to control house dust (the most allergenic ingredients of which are house dust mites or insects and animal saliva or dander). Overnight exposure to pollens and molds can be diminished by keeping the bedroom window closed overnight or employing an air conditioner as a partial filter in the bedroom or centrally. Animals should not be allowed in the bedroom if there is any question of animal sensitivity and should be kept out of the house or eliminated from the environment altogether depending upon the degree of the child's sensitivity. A HEPA filter in the child's bedroom may help. The remainder of the house is the second most important environmental area, but exposures at preschools or schools, or at babysitters' or friends' houses can be problematic and may require alternative arrangements.

Hyposensitization (Immunotherapy)

Specific hyposensitization is attempted if the allergen is not sufficiently avoidable and is considered a significant problem. Its value is documented both for upper respiratory tract inhalant allergy and for allergic asthma, and it is effective for Hymenoptera insect sting allergy. Evidence for effectiveness is greatest for pollens, house dust mites, and Hymenoptera venom. It also may be efficacious for mold sensitivity. Injection therapy to foods is experimental and may be dangerous. The use of bacterial extracts is of little value.

The procedure involves injecting extremely small amounts of allergen subcutaneously in gradually increasing dosage at frequent intervals (generally once or twice a week) until a top or maintenance dose is reached. This is usually the highest tolerated dose, or the amount that induces a state of clinical hyporeactivity to the allergen as demonstrated after natural contact. The top dose is used as the maintenance dose with carefully regulated lengthening of intervals, eventually to perhaps every 4 weeks, if tolerated. Injection therapy is given for a minimum of 2 years, often 3–5 years, and occasionally for longer periods.

Drug Therapy

The following are principal groups of therapeutic agents used for the treatment of allergic disorders:

A. Adrenergic Agents: Epinephrine is the single most important agent for treating acute severe allergic reactions. It is used to decrease bronchospasm in acute severe asthma, although more selective beta-2 adrenergic agents such as terbutaline by injection are available. Moreover, selective beta-2 adrenergic drugs used by inhalation are generally as effective as injectable adrenergic agents in relieving asthma and are associated with fewer side effects. Orally active beta-2 agents also can be effective. The vasoconstrictive properties of certain adrenergic agents such as phenylephrine and pseudoephedrine also are useful in decongestion of allergic and nonallergic rhinitis. They can be used topically in the nose for short (5 days or less) periods, or orally, alone or in conjunction with antihistamines.

B. Antihistamines: Antihistamines are specific antagonists of histamine and are therefore useful when histamine is an important mediator of the reaction. Since histamine is only one of the numerous mediators involved, however, antihistamines rarely are completely therapeutic. There are at least two major classes of antihistamines: H1-receptor inhibitors, which are the classic antihistamines used for many years in allergic disorders, and H2-receptor inhibitors, marketed for inhibiting gastric acid secretion but which also have vascular properties. H1 antihistamines are particularly useful for allergic rhinitis and urticaria and as a part of the treatment of anaphylaxis. The addition of H2 antihistamines (eg, cimetidine and ranitidine) to an H1 antihistamine can help control urticaria not controlled by H1 antihistamines alone, and both classes are sometimes recommended for the treatment of anaphylaxis. Antihistamines are *not* the drugs of first choice in allergic emergencies—epinephrine is—but they may be administered after epinephrine has been given. Since antihistamines are competitive antagonists, they are best used in advance of histamine liberation and of anticipated symptoms. Most antihistamines are potentially soporific and they should be used cautiously during school hours. Antihistamines are most effective in reducing symptoms of rhinorrhea, nasal itching and sneezing, eye tearing, itching, and hives. In contrast to general warnings in the *PDR*, antihistamines can be used when asthma is present (and may even have some beneficial effects in asthma!).

C. Theophylline and Aminophylline: Theophylline and its ethylene diamine derivative **aminophylline** are effective but potentially toxic bronchodilators, the improper use of which has been associated with severe reactions and, in some instances, even death. Periodic monitoring of blood theophylline levels is important in patients on long-term theophylline therapy. Theophylline can be therapeutic over a wide range of blood concentrations, but levels between 10 and 20 μg/mL have been considered "optimal" for severe asthma since *major* toxicity rarely occurs with peak blood levels below 20 μg/mL. Since levels can vary significantly owing to viral infections, diet, the use of erythromycin and other drugs, peak levels higher than 15 μg/mL on a long-term basis are discouraged. In early to mid-infancy, metabolism is markedly diminished and these drugs rarely should be employed at these ages.

D. Expectorants: Glyceryl guaiacolate (guaifenesin) is used primarily to thin mucus in asthma and upper respiratory tract disorders but its effectiveness is not clear. Iodides appear to be more effective, but problems such as goiter, salivary gland inflammation, gastric irritation, and acne can occur with prolonged use.

E. Corticosteroids: These are extremely potent antiallergic drugs, but side effects associated with prolonged therapy limit their use mainly to those conditions that are refractory to other measures or are life-threatening. Topically active corticosteroids which are inactivated rapidly upon absorption have been developed, giving them a high local therapeutic potency with low systemic effects. Intranasal topical steroids, and inhalant topical steroids for chronic asthma are relatively safe and effective in these conditions, as are topical steroids for eczema. Significant absorption of active drug occurs with extensive use over inflamed skin or with occlusive dressings, especially with the halogenated preparations. Systemic corticosteroids should be considered for short-term use for acute severe asthma not immediately responsive to nonsteroid therapy, for severe contact dermatitis, and for medical emergencies due to allergic reactions as a second- or third-line medication after adrenergic agents and antihistamines have been given. Long-term use of systemic steroids should be considered when nonsteroid agents or topical steroids cannot control symptoms sufficiently. When long-term use is necessary, alternate-day therapy with a short-acting preparation such as prednisone in the early morning should be attempted, using the least amount necessary to control symptoms.

F. Sedatives: Sedatives have little place in the treatment of allergic disorders and are contraindicated in asthma since they can depress the respiratory center. Anxiety associated with extreme asthma is more a reflection of the severity of asthma than its cause.

G. Oxygen: Oxygen is extremely important in the treatment of severe asthma since hypoxemia virtually always is present with severe obstruction.

H. Antibiotics: There are no special indications for antibiotics in allergic disorders. In most instances, viral infections precipitate respiratory problems such as asthma.

I. Cromolyn Sodium (Intal, Nasalcrom, and Crolom): Cromolyn sodium is a topically active agent useful in treatment of asthma, allergic rhinitis, and conjunctivitis. In asthma it is particularly effective as a preventive when used 15–20 minutes prior to contact with an asthmogenic agent such as an allergen or exercise. It can be used alone or in conjunction with adrenergic or other agents. If used routinely on a long-term basis, it is best given 3–4 times a day, although twice a day usage may be effective. It is a relatively safe and nonirritating drug.

PROPYHLAXIS OF ATOPIC ALLERGIC DISORDERS

There is evidence that avoidance of certain foods in the first few months of life, specifically cow products, eggs, wheat, and chicken, with or without concomitant dust and animal control, can lessen development of food sensitivity, allergic rhinitis, asthma, or eczema in the first year or so of life. Although some studies show no benefit from these procedures, it seems prudent to institute dietary and environmental restrictions in the first few months of life in children with a strong family history of atopy.

MEDICAL EMERGENCIES DUE TO ALLERGIC REACTIONS

Anaphylactic shock, **angioedema** (particularly of the airway), and **bronchial obstruction** are life-threatening manifestations of severe allergic reactions. Sweating, flushing, palpitations, lightheadedness, paresthesias, and urticaria may precede or accompany severe reactions. Shock can occur alone.

Treatment

A. Immediate:

1. Epinephrine, aqueous, 1/1000, 0.2–0.4 mL should be injected intramuscularly without delay, and may be repeated at intervals of 15–20 minutes as necessary. If the reaction is due to the injection of a drug, serum, or sting on an extremity, a tourniquet should be applied proximal to the site to delay absorption and 0.1 mL of adrenaline should be injected into the site to delay absorption.
2. Antihistamines should be given intramuscularly, or **slowly** intravenously. An H1 antihistamine such as diphenhydramine should be used initially; the addition of an H2 antihistamine (eg, cimetidine) is recommended.
3. An asthmatic component should be treated with aminophylline and inhaled adrenergics, and other treatment for asthma as indicated.
4. Tracheostomy can be life-saving in cases of profound laryngeal edema.
5. Hypovolemia secondary to massive transudation of intravascular fluid can be a part of the reaction; maintenance of proper fluid volume by IV replacement may be necessary.

B. Subsequent Measures: Adrenocorticosteroids should be given after epinephrine and antihistamines have been administered. The patient should be watched for 24 hours since there can be a recurrence ("delayed anaphylaxis") many hours after the initial reaction.

Insect Sting Sensitivity

Life-threatening insect allergy is due mostly to the venom of stinging insects of the class Hymenoptera (bees, wasps, hornets, and fire ants). Venom immunotherapy in children is reserved mainly for those instances in which a life-threatening reaction involving the cardiovascular or respiratory tract has occurred. A large local reaction or urticaria without respiratory or cardiovascular compromise probably is not an indication for immunotherapy. Venom antigens for diagnosis and treatment are efficacious although whole body extracts may be useful for fire ant allergy. Treatment kits for anaphylactic reactions (ANA-KIT) or spring-loaded epinephrine injectables (Epi-Pen or Epi-Pen, Jr.) should be made available for immediate use for children with extreme insect sensitivity and should be kept in the home or taken along by a responsible person in times of travel. The single most important item in such a kit is epinephrine.

ALLERGIC RHINITIS

Major symptoms of **allergic rhinitis** include chronic or recurrent nasal congestion generally with nasal itching and sneezing, with serous to mucoid discharge. Itching of the eyes with or without tearing also occurs, particularly in the seasonal or episodic variety. The appearance of the nasal mucosa can vary from somewhat hyperemic to very edematous with purplish pallor. Rhinitis may be perennial, owing to exposure to perennially present allergens; seasonal, owing to pollens or seasonal molds; episodic, owing to occasional encounter with allergens such as animals; or any combination of these. The disease can occur even in infancy, but becomes more frequent and intense with age due to increased exposure to environmental allergens. "Allergic facies" can include allergic shiners, suborbital edema that takes on a bluish discoloration secondary to nasal congestion, flattened malar eminences, and a transverse crease across the nose from pushing the nose upward in an attempt to relieve nasal itching ("allergic salute"). Differential diagnosis includes chronic sinusitis and non-allergic ("vasomotor") rhinitis. Other conditions to be considered in chronic nasal "congestion" include adenoid hypertrophy, foreign bodies (usually unilateral), choanal stenosis or atresia, nasopharyngeal neoplasms, and palatal malformations. Helpful laboratory findings include nasal eosinophilia, but this is not a universal finding, nor does its presence establish an allergic etiology. Allergy tests reveal IgE antibody to offending allergens.

Associated Conditions

Allergic rhinitis is a risk factor for chronic or recurrent **otitis media** with effusion. Nasal polyps are unusual in children and though they often contain eosinophils, generally they are not caused by allergy. They can be associated with cystic fibrosis. Sinusitis may accompany allergic rhinitis.

Table 26–1. Drugs useful in treating rhinitis.

	Decongestant	Antihistamine	Nasal Cromolyn	Anticholinergic	Nasal Steroid
Sneezing	(×)	×	(×)		×
Itching	(×)	×	(×)		×
Rhinorrhea	(×)	(×)	(×)	×	×
Congestion	×	±			×

Treatment

Known or suspected allergens must be avoided. When symptoms are severe or other symptomatic measures have failed, or when associated with complications, immunotherapy should be considered.

A. Drug Therapy: Table 26–1 lists various drugs useful in treating rhinitis and the symptoms and signs most relieved by each. Chronic rhinitis is more of a congestive problem, whereas acute or seasonal rhinitis tends to involve more itching, sneezing, and rhinorrhea. Antihistamines, with or without decongestants, and nasal and ocular cromolyn are first-line drugs, whereas topical corticosteroids are reserved for more resistant cases.

BRONCHIAL ASTHMA

Asthma is an obstructive disorder of the tracheal bronchial tree, in which the obstruction is variable and largely reversible. The major symptoms of asthma are cough and wheezing, a high-pitched squeaky sound from the partially obstructed large airways, shortness of breath, and chest tightness. **Wheezing is not an invariable symptom or sign;** asthma may present with chronic cough ("cough variant asthma"). Obstruction is due to mucosal edema, bronchospasm, increased and unusually viscid secretions, and chronic inflammation of mucosal walls often with sloughing of epithelium. **Asthma is a chronic disorder, the symptoms of which may be only episodic.** It can be mild, severe, infrequent, or constant. Because of great pulmonary reserve, obstruction can be profound without causing death, but deaths from asthma do occur. The adolescent age group is at special risk. It is a very common disorder, grossly underdiagnosed; its severity often is underestimated and generally undertreated, and it may be diagnosed as recurrent bronchitis or pneumonia. A large proportion of childhood asthma begins before age 3, but wheezing is common in this age group and frequently disappears as a problem. Risk factors for persistence (asthma) include parental atopic disease, atopic disposition of the patient, indoor exposure to allergens, and to maternal smoke. Approximately twice as many males are affected as females before adolescence, after which there is no major difference between the sexes.

Most children with asthma eventually demonstrate evidence of allergy, which can play a minor to major role in asthma. Especially early in life viral respiratory infection is a frequent precipitating event; precipitants most often are multifactorial and can include irritants, exercise, some medications (aspirin infrequently), and occasionally emotional factors (mainly indirectly, through maladaptive behaviors with asthma). Asthma can occur alone or with allergic rhinitis and/or atopic dermatitis. Inhalants are most important in causing symptoms, but occasionally foods, especially early in life, may be causative. The prognosis of asthma is variable; the likelihood that asthma will be "outgrown" increases with the milder form of the disorder, **but probably no more than half of even milder asthmatics outgrow the disorder.** Moderate or severe asthma generally is not outgrown. If symptoms *are* lost, the most common time is around puberty.

An important feature of at least chronic symptomatic asthma is an extraordinary generalized hyperreactivity of the tracheobronchial tree. Because of this feature, asthma sometimes is called "reactive airways disorder." Reactions to allergens and irritants may occur within minutes of exposure, but with sufficient sensitization and strong allergen exposure a second kind of reaction occurs 4–12 hours after allergen exposure and can be prolonged. There is a large inflammatory component to chronic asthma, and regular use of antiinflammatory drugs ("controller drugs") is important in moderate and severe asthma. Beta2 agonists are not antiinflammatory and are used to relieve symptoms as needed ("reliever drugs"); their need is a useful indicator of disease activity. Signs and symptoms of asthma are only a crude reflection of the obstructive process, and in many patients, neither the child's, parents' nor the physician's assessment of the asthma are very accurate. *The most accurate indicator of the degree of obstruction is measurement of airflow with a pulmonary function device.* A reliable simple peak flow meter, such as a Wright Peak Flow Meter, *used properly* (by patient and medical personnel), is important to the diagnosis and treatment of children with asthma.

In infancy, predominant symptoms may be dyspnea, excessive secretions, noisy and rattly breathing, cough, and intercostal or suprasternal retractions rather than the typical pronounced expiratory wheezes that occur in older children. Physical findings depend upon the degree of obstruction. Between episodes, findings can be normal. With progressive obstruction, air exchange diminishes, expiration becomes prolonged, and wheezing generally occurs and increases in intensity. With greater obstruction, wheezing will decrease due to poor air exchange, hyperinflation may be apparent, and in later stages retractions and use of accessory respiratory muscles increases. Pulsus paradoxicus may be present. There may be pallor; **cyanosis is a very late sign.** Tachycardia may occur and ultimately there can be respiratory failure. The hallmark of asthma is responsiveness to bronchodilators, both a therapeutic and diagnostic point. In the later stages of an asthmatic paroxysm or simply with severe asthma, response to bronchodilators is poor, a condition sometimes called "status asthmaticus."

Eosinophil accumulations in bronchial secretions and blood are common. The hematocrit can be elevated with dehydration or in severe chronic obstructive disease. In severe asthma, the first blood gas abnormality is hypoxemia without CO_2 retention. Since hyperpnea is usual in an attack. $PaCO_2$ tends to be low with the hypoxemia so that "normal" PCO_2 in an attack should be taken as CO_2 retention. Particularly in young children, some metabolic acidosis is not unusual. Early in asthmatic paroxysms, the pH tends to be alkaline from hyperventilation. If obstruction is severe, there can be CO_2 retention with a respiratory acidosis, often with a metabolic component. X-ray may show bilateral hyperinflation, bronchial thickening, peribronchial infiltration, and areas of density that may represent patchy atelectasis (common) or associated bronchopneumonia. The former is often confused with the latter. In uncomplicated asthma, a chest x-ray is not always necessary. Lung functions reveal a decrease in flow rates, particularly FEV_1. There is hyperinflation of the chest with increased residual volume and functional residual capacity. During asymptomatic intervals, all of the above may be normal, but there frequently is residual hyperinflation on a chronic basis even in asthmatic children asymptomatic for prolonged periods. Allergy tests may reveal IgE antibodies to potentially causative allergens.

Bronchial asthma may be confused with acute bronchiolitis, laryngotracheobronchitis, bronchopneumonia, or pertussis, especially in the very young. Some children with immunodeficiency disease, particularly in the first 3 years of life, have associated cough and wheezing due to chronic lower respiratory tract infection. Nasal wheezes can be transmitted to the chest especially in infants, and other forms of upper airway obstruction such as adenoidal hypertrophy and foreign body may cause wheezing sounds. The predominant wheeze from lower airway obstruction is expiratory, although inspiratory wheezing along with expiratory wheezing can occur. Wheezing that is predominantly inspiratory more often than not is laryngeal or higher in origin. In tracheal or bronchial foreign body obstruction, dyspnea and wheezing is usually of sudden onset and often unilateral, although it may be bilateral. Characteristic x-ray findings are not always present. The differentiation between bronchial asthma and cystic fibrosis is made on the basis of high sweat chloride in the latter, and a history often present in cystic fibrosis of serious pulmonary infections since birth, along with a personal and family history of associated intestinal disturbances with profuse, bulky stools and pancreatic enzyme deficiency. In asthma, chronic inflammatory changes generally are not seen on chest x-ray, in contrast to those seen in cystic fibrosis and other chronic infectious lower pulmonary disorders. Cystic fibrosis and asthma frequently coexist. Tracheal or bronchial compression by extramural forces may be due to the presence of a foreign body in the esophagus, anomalous vessels, or neoplastic or inflammatory lymphadenopathy.

Treatment

A. General: Identify and avoid known or suspected allergens and irritants!

Immunotherapy should be considered for allergens that cannot be avoided and that play a substantial role in the disorder. Educate the parents and the child, if old enough, to understand asthma, the importance of avoidance or other therapy, and the proper use of medications. The major pharmacotherapeutic agents are **bronchodilators** of the **adrenergic** and **methylxanthine** (theophylline or aminophylline) classes, which relieve symptoms ("relievers") and **antiinflammatory drugs** (corticosteroids, cromolyn, and nedocromil) which control disease activity ("controllers").

Adrenergic aerosols are extremely useful but must not be abused. Overreliance on these drugs can lead to delays in obtaining other needed therapy and may possibly make asthma worse. Adrenergic inhalants can be as effective as injected drugs in reversing acute severe asthma and are attended with fewer side effects. These agents should be used on an as needed basis for all degrees of asthma, mild to severe, to relieve symptoms. The frequency at which they are used is an index of disease activity and indicates a need to institute or increase dosage of maintenance controller drugs. As with all children, encourage exercise in those with asthma. Children with frequent overt asthma attacks (eg, 1 or 2 per week other than from exercise alone) and evidence of more or less constant pulmonary obstruction should be on constant pharmacologic therapy.

Cromolyn or nedocromil can be considered firstline drugs for chronic symptomatic asthma. Inhalant corticosteroids can also be considered firstline drugs for long-term therapy and are used for more severe asthma or asthma not controlled by cromolyn or nedocromil, and in addition or in place of theophylline and as a substitute for long-term alternate-day systemic steroid therapy. Systemic corticosteroids are used acutely (days) for the treatment of acute severe asthma not responsive to bronchodilators; they also are employed chronically (weeks to months) and occasionally even longer, mainly on an alternate-day early morning dosing regimen when all other measures are not sufficient to keep the asthma under control. Aminophylline (theophylline) may have some antiinflammatory activity but is used mostly as an adjunct to therapy with other antiinflammatory drugs, to increase control or reduce steroid need.

TREATMENT OF ACUTE SEVERE ASTHMA (Status Asthmaticus)

This is a medical emergency and requires prompt and aggressive treatment. Aerosolized adrenergic drugs given by a compressed air device, or preferably by oxygen, are the drugs of first choice (Table 26–2). If the child is not cooperative or is in extremus, an injectable adrenergic may be used initially. Sensitivity to adrenergic drugs may improve after initiation of other therapy, particularly corticosteroids, and responsiveness may occur even as early as 1–2 hours after their administration.

Hospital or Emergency Room Care

(1) Give moisturized oxygen by face mask or nasal prong, at a flow rate of approximately 4 L/min.

(2) Give 5% dextrose solution with 0.2% saline IV with poor responsiveness to initial therapy, poor fluid intake, vomiting, or dehydration. *Do not overhydrate.* Particularly if corticosteroids are used, add potassium (approximately 10–20 mEq/L of intravenous fluids) after urination is established.

(3) The effectiveness of aminophylline when inhalant beta-adrenergic agents are maximized is debated. If aminophylline is used, give 3–5 mg/kg in intravenous tubing over a 10–20 minute period if not used in the previous 12 hours, and either repeat in 4–6 hours or

Table 26–2. Adrenergic drugs.

Drug	Route[1]	Dose	Frequency
Terbutaline mg/mL (1:1000)	SC	0.01 mg/kg up to 0.30 mL	q 20 min × 2
Epinephrine aqueous 1:200 (Sus-Phrine)	SC	0.01 mg/kg up to 0.30 mL	q 20 min × 3
Epinephrine suspension 1:200 (Sus-Phrine)	SC	0.005 mL/kg up to 0.15 mL	single dose
Albuterol 0.05%[2]	NA	0.25–0.5 mL in 2 mL saline	q 20 min × 3

[1] SC = subcutaneous; NA = nebulized aerosol.
[2] This and other β_2 agents are also available as a metered dose inhaler and can be used two inhalations per dose. For mild to moderate asthma, use every 4 hours as needed only.

give as a constant infusion using a rate of 0.5–0.8 mg/kg/h. The rate should be determined by measurement of theophylline blood levels, aiming for a level of 10 + 3 μg/mL on a constant basis.

(4) Take an arterial blood sample for pH, PCO_2, and PO_2, or use oximetry for PO_2 determination (this does *not*, however, tell you the $PaCO_2$). Repeated monitoring of gases and pH may be necessary.

(5) Correct acidosis of pH of ≤ 7.1 with sodium bicarbonate. The appropriate bicarbonate dose can be calculated with the following formula:

$$\textbf{mEq bicarbonate needed} = \textbf{negative base excess} \times \textbf{0.3} \times \textbf{body weight in kg}$$

(6) Give albuterol 0.5% by inhalation every 30 minutes to 1 hour until there is a response. Interval can be extended to every 4 hours as tolerated.

(7) If the patient is already receiving corticosteroids, increase the dose temporarily. Patients who require hospitalization or who have severe asthma not responsive to other therapy within the first 2 hours should receive corticosteroids promptly. Give the equivalent of 2 mg/kg of prednisone every 4–6 hours until a therapeutic response is obtained, following which taper the dosage as rapidly as possible over a 3–7 day period.

(8) Give antibiotics if specifically indicated.

Table 26–3. Average total daily dose + SD.

Age	Average Total Daily Dose + SD
1–8 yr	25 ± 5 mg/kg
8–16 yr	20 ± 5 mg/kg
> yr	12 ± 3 mg/kg

(9) Mechanical ventilation using a volume respirator capable of producing high expiratory pressures by personnel expert in such use may be necessary with respiratory failure. Failure to respond adequately to the previously defined measures can be considered as CO_2 retention above 45 mm Hg (arbitrary) or increasing arterial $PACO_2$.

(10) Obtain a chest x-ray if there is a question of pneumo-thorax, massive atelectasis, or other *significant* intrathoracic complication.

Do Nots

(1) Do not use narcotics or barbiturates (they depress the respiratory center).

(2) Do not use epinephrine excessively; inhaled beta-2 adrenergic agents are preferred.

(3) **Do not treat acute severe paroxysm as purely an acute problem**. Follow-up therapy including eventually adequate fluid intake with shifting from IV to oral medications and the continued use of pharmacotherapy out of hospital is important until pulmonary functions reverse to essential normality. Treatment in hospital generally is not required for more than 2 or 3 days for acute severe asthmatic paroxysms, but aggressive therapy on an outpatient basis must be continued for many days thereafter. *Make certain adequate follow-up is established before discharge.*

ATOPIC DERMATITIS
(Infantile Eczema)

This ordinarily begins in early infancy after age 2 months. It is a condition of itchy skin in which the threshold for itching is abnormally low, and it is usually associated with skin dryness and sometimes with ichthyosis. The majority of children exhibit evidence of

IgE antibody to a variety of allergens, but the role of IgE antibody in the disease process often is unclear. Food allergens by ingestion, and inhalant allergens (mites, pollens, molds, animal allergens), particularly by direct contact, can play an important role in some children. Foods most often implicated are milk, egg white, peanuts, and, to a lesser extent, peas, wheat, pork, beef, and corn.

Lesions generally begin as erythematous papules, sometimes secondary to scratching, which can result in variable degrees of scaling, vesicular oozing lesions, and, in the more chronic forms, lichenification. In infants, there is predilection for the cheeks and extensor areas; in older children and adolescents, the flexural creases are most commonly affected along with the feet and hands. Pruritus is characteristic and frequently intense. Scratching plays a major role in the pathogenesis and predisposes to secondary infection. Skin dryness, sweating, and contact with rough materials and detergents all can aggravate itching. Psychologic factors also can intensify itching.

Differential Diagnosis

Seborrheic dermatitis, **contact dermatitis**, and **scabies** with a secondary eczematoid reaction may be confused with atopic dermatitis. Disorders in which skin eruptions can resemble atopic dermatitis include **Wiscott-Aldrich syndrome**, **x-linked agammaglobulinemia**, **ataxia-telangiectasia**, **phenylketonuria**, **severe combined immunodeficiency**, **Hurler's and Hartnup syndromes**, and **ahistidinemia**. Although this disorder may be lost by age 3, it persists into later childhood and adulthood more often than is generally appreciated. Various immune abnormalities have been identified, but there are no laboratory findings that are pathognomonic. IgE antibody is found in approximately 80% of patients, and IgE immunoglobulin levels are elevated in many cases as well. Secondary bacterial infections, especially with staphylococci and streptococci, occur frequently. Viral infections, mainly with herpes virus, may produce extensive viral lesions (Kaposi's varicelliform eruption).

Treatment

Good skin care, vigorous specific skin treatment, and identification and elimination of any allergens or irritants that may aggravate the disease are the mainstays of treatment. Hyposensitization is of uncertain value.

Adequate hydration is important, particularly in dry climates. In drier climates, daily baths without soap or with the occasional use of mild soaps (eg, Dove, Basis, Neutrogena) are used to hydrate the skin, and the skin is then patted partly dry and covered with a bland cream or one that contains corticosteroid if there is active inflammation. Topical corticosteroids are the mainstay of control of inflammation by both methods. A strong (eg, fluorinated) corticosteroid is used twice a day initially to control intense inflammation, but with more chronic use, the weakest corticosteroid needed is used. This generally is 1% hydrocortisone in a variety of available bases.

For acute severe dermatitis with weeping, Burow's solution (aluminum subacetate) soaks made up to 1/20 solution is used for 20 minutes at a time, with gauze or cloth thoroughly moistened with solution applied 4 times a day or more for up to 3 days. Systemic antibiotics are used for secondary infections. Antihistamines can be used as antipruritic agents, but are of secondary effectiveness in controlling pruritus compared with topical corticosteroids. The use of potent topical corticosteroids frequently and extensively over inflamed skin can lead to significant systemic absorption. There is a high likelihood that a child with atopic dermatitis will develop allergic rhinitis, asthma, or both.

ADVERSE REACTIONS TO FOODS

Serious allergic reactions to foods include anaphylaxis, hives, angioedema of the upper airway, and severe asthma; however, a wide variety of signs and symptoms can be encountered. The more severe the reaction, the faster it is likely to occur; the majority of severe reactions occur within minutes to a couple of hours after ingestion of the food. Many (and probably most) reactions to foods, however, are caused by nonallergic mechanisms and include pharmacologic or metabolic, toxic, or idiosyncratic reactions. Reactions occur most frequently in infancy. Evidence of IgE antibody to a food allergen can be obtained by skin prick testing (intradermal tests are too nonspecific), serologic tests, or both. The apparent presence of IgE antibody does not in itself establish the diagnosis, nor does the apparent absence rule it out. A reaction may depend upon the amount of food ingested, rate of absorption, and other concurrent factors such as the presence of an enteric infection, which alters the intestinal permeability.

Good evidence for a reaction to a suspected food is improvement of symptoms on avoidance of the food (elimination diet), and aggravation of symptoms on adding back the food (challenge). Food challenges should not be done, however, in cases of life-threatening sensitivity.

Syndromes sometimes associated with food sensitivity include angioedema and urticaria; anaphylaxis; gastrointestinal intolerance;

and allergic rhinitis, asthma, and eczema (see previous sections). In addition, "tension-fatigue syndrome"—a syndrome of symptoms ranging from irritability, disturbed behavior, sleeplessness, fatigue, lassitude, and disinterest, associated with allergic shiners, sometimes with headache and vague abdominal complaints—has been blamed on food allergy. When it occurs, however, it is not clear that allergic mechanisms are involved. There are numerous claims that various foodstuffs including sugar, food dyes, various specific foods, and natural salicylates in foods, can produce hyperactivity or other behavioral changes in children with attention deficit disorder. If these substances do contribute, it would appear to occur in an extremely small subpopulation of children. Various foods contain vasoactive material that can intensify vascular (migraine) headaches on a nonallergic basis; the most common foods implicated are chocolate, cheeses, liver, and some wines and beers. Allergic reactions to foods also may intensify vascular headaches. Eosinophilic enterocolitis, pulmonary hemosiderosis related to milk sensitivity, and villous atrophy with malabsorption also can be caused by foods. The diagnosis is based upon a suspicion that a particular food may be causing a problem, elimination of the food, and then challenge to determine whether symptoms abate and then reappear. Children tend to have sensitivity to only one food at a time, occasionally two; multiple food allergies are rarely documented. A high level of IgE antibody to a food is more likely to be of clinical significance than a low level. The most common allergens implicated in young children are milk, peanut, egg, soy, and wheat. In older children, shellfish, fish, and nuts also are involved with some frequency.

Other disorders from which "food allergy" should be differentiated include those producing gastrointestinal intolerance—carbohydrate enzyme deficiency (eg, lactase), irritable bowel syndrome, gastrointestinal malformations, acute or chronic intestinal infections, celiac disease, pyloric stenosis, and cystic fibrosis.

Treatment

Treatment is based primarily on avoiding the food, although in less sensitive children, small amounts can be tolerated. *It is important to ensure nutritional adequacy when eliminating foods from the diet.* Food allergies can be outgrown—most likely to milk and soy—but when severe allergy exists, especially to peanuts, other nuts, fish, and shellfish, it is not likely. Loss of sensitivity to eggs is highly variable. In children with potential life-threatening sensitivity, an emergency medical kit with epinephrine should be available for use by the older child or a responsible adult.

DRUG SENSITIVITY

Reactions to drugs can be due to toxicity; an idiosyncratic or peculiar response to the usual action of the drug; anaphylactoid (pseudoallergic), in which the mediators associated with allergic reactants occur by nonallergic mechanisms (eg, some reactions to radiocontrast dyes); or allergic, in which IgE and perhaps other immune reactions play an important role. Manifestations of drug allergy are extremely varied. Most commonly, skin eruptions occur. A prolonged syndrome of serum sickness, previously due mostly to foreign serum, can occur particularly with penicillins and sulfonamides. Some drugs given in repository forms or by mouth may linger in the body for weeks and continue to induce symptoms during this period of time. Any drug is a potential sensitizer, but the penicillins and sulfonamides are at the top of the list. Sulfonamides and tetracyclines can be photosensitizing.

It is often difficult to know whether a rash that develops when a drug is administered is, in fact, due to the agent. In many instances, the eruption is unrelated, and there is no drug sensitivity. Unfortunately, diagnostic tests for drugs are highly imperfect, and, particularly with antibiotics, it is usually wisest to make a tentative presumption of drug sensitivity and substitute a structurally different drug. In most instances, drug reactions are due to sensitivity to by-products of the drug, and in only a few instances have these been identified. Penicillin is the best-studied reagents available for testing are useful, but tests are not foolproof.

Treatment

Treatment consists of discontinuing the drug and supportive therapy depending upon the symptoms involved (see other sections). Pretreatment with antihistamines and corticosteroids in cases in which contrast dyes that previously induced reactions must be used has been successful but *is not foolproof*. Reactions to such dyes generally are "pseudoallergic" and tests of the dye, including use of small test doses, are not accurate or advised.

URTICARIA

Urticaria, or "hives," are multiple, although occasionally single, pruritic erythematous wheals of varying sizes, consisting of localized edema and surrounding erythema. Hives can be allergic or nonallergic. Emotional tension may aggravate hives but rarely is the only cause. Angioedema, essentially urticaria of the deeper skin, results in more diffuse edema, and resolves more slowly than hives. It is a problem mainly if it affects the respiratory tract. The most common classes of allergens inducing urticaria are foods and medications. **"Physical" urticarias** include a cold-induced form in which exposure to cold air, cold water, or other cold objects induces localized urticaria or angioedema. In severe forms, death from sudden massive mediator release can occur—for example, from swimming in cold water. **"Cholinergic" urticaria** is a form relating to overheating, characterized by intense itching and small wheals with much erythema. Exercise or fever are precipitants of this form. There is a form of **exercise-anaphylaxis** phenomena in which urticaria and angioedema can occur with exercise, to an extent that it may be part of a more generalized anaphylactic syndrome, but generally without pulmonary involvement; it can be life-threatening. **Papular urticaria** is a term given to multiple papules induced by insect bites, and is found especially on the extremities. Papules secondary to infection from scratching and scabies also occurs. **Dermographism** is a familial or acquired form of "skin sensitivity" in which the threshold of the vascular response to stroking of the skin is lowered. Stroking the skin may produce erythema with or without a wheal; it is not necessarily related to allergy. **Hereditary angioedema** is a rare, nonallergic genetic disorder, characterized by periodic bouts of angioedema that are nonpruritic and can be life-threatening.

Diagnosis depends mainly upon a thorough historical review with implication of possible causative agents, and, if necessary, elimination and challenge. Allergy tests to causative agents can be useful sometimes. Inhalant or contact allergens can occasionally induce hives, the former particularly on a seasonal basis. Treatment consists of avoiding the causative factors and use of H_1 antihistamines such as diphenhydramine or hydroxyzine. With more chronic forms, the addition of an H_2 antihistamine such as cimetidine can be helpful. With severe acute urticaria and angioedema, epinephrine may be necessary. Occasionally, short courses of corticosteroids are necessary.

27 | Collagen Diseases

Elaine Van Gundy, MD

"Collagen diseases" are not limited to pathological alterations of collagen but also involve changes in connective tissue, and therefore are often called "connective tissue diseases." Although many diseases involve connective tissue, seven disorders with similar characteristics can accurately be called collagen diseases: rheumatic fever, rheumatoid arthritis, Lyme disease, polyarteritis (periarteritis) nodosa, systemic lupus erythematosus (SLE), scleroderma, and dermatomyositis.

Arthritis is a common feature seen in the collagen diseases. Therefore, a brief discussion regarding evaluation of childhood arthritis will precede the discussion of the specific collagen diseases.

EVALUATION OF THE CHILD PRESENTING WITH ARTHRITIS

The differential diagnosis for arthritis may be categorized as: (1) orthopedic; (2) rheumatic; (3) infectious; (4) neoplastic; and (5) systemic. Please refer to Table 27–1 for a partial list of conditions that may present with arthritis.

The evaluation of the child presenting with arthritis requires an accurate history and physical which emphasize the character of the presenting symptoms. Historical clues supporting an organic condition include signs of systemic illness (weight loss, fever, night sweats, rash, diarrhea). Initial laboratory evaluation may include a complete blood count (CBC), erythrocyte sedimentation rate (ESR) and antinuclear antibody (ANA) titer. Table 27–2 summarizes laboratory and clinical clues seen with conditions presenting with arthritis.

In summary, the differential diagnosis for evaluating a child with arthritis is broad. The history and physical examination will help to guide in further evaluation. Laboratory screening tests are often abnormal with organic conditions, although they may be normal (early juvenile rheumatoid arthritis (JRA), early leukemia, toxic synovitis). In orthopedic conditions laboratory screening tests will be normal.

Table 27–1. Conditions that may present with arthritis.

Orthopedic	**Infectious disease**
Musculoskeletal trauma	Osteomyelitis
Chondromalacia patella	Septic arthritis
Hypermobility	Viral arthritis
Rheumatic	Lyme disease
JRA	**Neoplastic**
SLE	Leukemia
Juvenile dermatomyositis	Neuroblastoma
Henoch-Schönlein purpura	**Systemic conditions**
Rheumatic fever	Inflammatory bowel disease
Spondyloarthropathy	Sickle cell anemia
	Hemophilia

JRA = juvenile rheumatoid arthritis; SLE = systemic lupus erythematosus.

Chronic arthritis of undetermined etiology requires repeated physical examination together with stepwise laboratory and possible radiographic evaluation.

RHEUMATIC FEVER

Rheumatic fever is the most common cause of symptomatic acquired heart disease in childhood. It is clear that group A β-hemolytic streptococci are implicated in the etiology of rheumatic fever, but the pathogenetic mechanism remains obscure.

The initial attack and subsequent relapses of rheumatic fever are invariably preceded by a β-hemolytic streptococcal infection 1–3 weeks earlier, although not all of these infections are clinically manifest. Since rheumatic heart disease represents a hypersensitivity reaction, one can assume that several infections with group A β-hemolytic streptococci are required to trigger the first episode of rheumatic fever.

Predisposing Factors

Lower socioeconomic status (overcrowding), familial predisposition, and reinfection with β-hemolytic streptococci place a person at increased risk.

Clinical Findings

The diagnosis is usually certain if the child has either: (a) two major manifestations; or (b) one major and two minor manifestations

Table 27–2. Childhood arthritis and associated laboratory and clinical characteristics.

Condition	CBC	ESR	ANA	Other Characteristics
Orthopedic conditions	Normal	Normal	Normal	History of precipitating events
Rheumatic disease	WBC = nl, ↑ or ↓ H/H = nl or ↓	nl or ↑	nl or positive	Arthritis persistent
Leukemia	WBC = nl, ↑ or ↓ H/H = nl or ↓ Abnormal smear	no or ↑	nl or mildly positive	Systemically ill
Inflammatory bowel disease	Anemia	nl or ↑	negative	Diarrhea, wt. loss, monoarthritis
Sickle cell disease	Anemia	nl or ↑	negative	Abnormal hemoglobin electrophoresis
Septic arthritis	↑ WBC	↑ ESR	negative	Child appears toxic, joints warm, ↑ WBC, synovial fluid; purulent with > 50,000 WBC
Viral arthritis	Usually normal	Normal or sl ↑	negative	Usually hip involved (sometimes knee), child appears well
Lyme disease	Normal	Normal or sl ↑	negative	Tick exposure; rash; positive serology

CBC = complete blood count; ESR = erythrocyte sedimentation rate; ANA = antinuclear antibody; WBC = white blood count; H/H = hemoglobin/hematocrit.

(modified after Jones), along with supportive evidence of recent streptococcal infection.

A. Major Manifestations:

1. Signs of active carditis

2. Polyarthritis. Inflammation of the large joints (ankles, knees, hips, wrists, elbows, and shoulders) usually occurs in a migratory fashion.

3. Subcutaneous nodules

4. Erythema marginatum

5. Chorea

B. Minor Manifestations:

1. Fever

2. Arthralgia

3. Previous rheumatic fever

4. Electrocardiographic changes, particularly prolonged PR intervals.

5. Abnormal blood test results: increased ESR, C-reactive protein (CRP), white blood cell (WBC) count, anemia.

C. Supportive Evidence:

1. Recent scarlet fever

2. Throat culture positive for Group A streptococci.

3. Increased antistreptolysin O (ASO) or other streptococcal antibodies.

Diagnosis

There is no specific laboratory test for rheumatic fever. Combined use of clinical and laboratory findings may aid in diagnosis and subsequent evaluation of the degree of rheumatic activity. Echocardiography is helpful in diagnosis by demonstrating subclinical carditis in suspected rheumatic fever.

Treatment

A. Specific Measures:

1. Corticosteroids–Corticosteroids should be administered for management of acute-onset congestive heart failure (CHF) associated with carditis. However, long-term controlled studies show no benefit from corticosteroid therapy in preventing chronic rheumatic heart disease. These drugs are therefore not recommended for patients with carditis who are not in CHF.

2. Salicylates–Salicylates markedly reduce fever, alleviate joint pain, and reduce swelling. Rheumatic fever usually responds with dramatic rapidity to salicylates. This provides useful diagnostic differentiation from rheumatoid arthritis, which responds much more slowly. Salicylates should be continued as long as necessary for the relief of symptoms. The average dose of aspirin is 80–120 mg/kg/d every 4–6 hours. The highest dosage is recommended for the first 48 hours.

3. Penicillin–Penicillin in full dosage should be used in all cases for 10 days, then followed by daily prophylaxis to prevent recurrences (below).

B. General Measures:

Resumption of full activity should be gradual and related to the severity of the attack, particularly if a significant degree of carditis is present.

Prophylaxis

The main principle of prophylaxis is the prevention of recurrent infection with β-hemolytic streptococci.

A. Penicillin: The unequivocal treatment of choice is benzathine penicillin G, given intramuscularly every 28 days; 1.2 million U is sufficient for school-age children. In day care settings or other situations of extreme exposure, the interval should be every 21 days. Oral penicillin G, 200,000 U, may be used twice daily but is less desirable because of possible poor compliance. Therapeutic doses of penicillin are recommended when valvular involvement is present before tooth extraction or other surgery.

B. Erythromycin: Erythromycin, 125–250 mg/d given orally, is useful in children who cannot tolerate penicillin.

Course & Prognosis

The course of rheumatic fever varies markedly. It may be fulminating, leading to death early in the course of an acute episode; or it may be entirely asymptomatic, being diagnosed in retrospect on the basis of pathologic findings. Adequate penicillin prophylaxis virtually eliminates recurrences. Lifetime prognosis depends primarily on the severity of the initial cardiac insult and the prevention of recurrences.

RHEUMATOID ARTHRITIS

Rheumatoid arthritis in childhood, commonly known as **juvenile rheumatoid arthritis (JRA)**, is an inflammatory disease of unknown etiology. Although familial clustering occurs, no definite genetic pattern exists. It is the most common collagen vascular disease found in children.

Table 27–3. Types and clinical presentation of JRA.

Type	Peak Age at Onset (yr)	Sex	Clinical Manifestations
Systemic	no peak	F = M	Fever, rash, hepatosplenomegaly, arthritis, pericarditis, no uveitis
Polyarticular	1–3 & 9	F > M	≥ joints, symmetrical, infrequent systemic features, chronic uveitis in 5%
Pauciarticular	1–3	F > M	< 5 joints, asymmetrical, no systemic features, chronic uveitis in 20%

JRA = juvenile rheumatoid arthritis.

There are three subgroups of JRA, distinguished by their clinical manifestations, course and prognosis, and serologic findings. The three types—systemic, polyarticular, and pauciarticular—are summarized in Table 27–3.

Rheumatoid arthritis should be distinguished from **ankylosing spondylitis**. Ankylosing spondylitis is 10 times more frequent in males. It is sometimes familial and affects the spine (particularly the sacroiliac joints). Transient and nondeforming peripheral arthritis, usually confined to a few large joints—especially in the lower extremities—occurs in 50% of patients; it may occur before back complaints appear. Acute iritis and aortitis are characteristic extra-articular manifestations. Autoantibodies are not present, but 90% of affected individuals will carry the HLA-B27 histocompatibility antigen.

Clinical Findings

All three types of JRA share the common feature of arthritis (which by criteria must be present ≥ 6 weeks), but have very different clinical presentations.

A. Symptoms & Signs:

1. Systemic–This category accounts for 10% of JRA cases. Systemic onset is characterized by high spiking fever (usually to 39 °C or higher) once or twice a day, rapidly returning to baseline or even subnormal temperature. The fever may be associated with a characteristic evanescent morbilliform rash most commonly found on the trunk and proximal extremities. Arthritis may occur at any time during the course of the disease. Other features include hepatosplenomegaly, pleuritis, pericarditis, and abdominal pain. Children with systemic JRA characteristically look very sick while febrile but appear surprisingly healthy the rest of the time.

2. Polyarticular–Polyarticular onset accounts for 50% of cases of JRA. This subgroup is characterized by arthritis in five or more joints. Polyarticular JRA usually is symmetrical, and typically involves the fingers, toes, knees, ankles, wrists, hips, and mandibles. Cervical spondylitis may be present. Joints are slightly swollen and tender, with limited motion. Finger joints become characteristically spindle-shaped with shiny smooth skin. Rheumatoid nodules are infrequent but occur most commonly in older females who are RF (rheumatoid factor) positive. Systemic features are uncommon. Uveitis occurs in a small percentage of patients (5%), although the patients that are ANA positive are at increased risk for eye disease.

3. Pauciarticular–This subgroup accounts for 40% of JRA cases. Its onset is characterized by involvement of four or fewer joints. The knees and ankles are most commonly affected, usually asymmetrically. Children with this form of JRA do not have any systemic symptoms and appear well. Chronic uveitis is most common in this group (20%), with the majority of patients with uveitis (90%) being ANA positive.

B. Laboratory Findings: Findings include polymorphonuclear leukocytosis and accelerated sedimentation rates, especially in active disease. Moderate anemia is present. HLA-B27 antigen is frequently present in ankylosing spondylitis but is not common in JRA. The RF is rarely positive in JRA, although the ANA is commonly positive in the polyarticular and pauciarticular forms of the disease. Synovial fluid may show an inflammatory reaction. Synovial biopsy demonstrates chronic inflammation, although it is not specific for rheumatoid arthritis.

C. Imaging: Findings in the early phase of JRA usually include swelling of periarticular soft structures, synovial effusion, and slight widening of the joint spaces. Accelerated epiphyseal maturation, expansion of ossification centers, and disproportionate longitudinal bone growth may occur. Later findings include obliteration of joint spaces, bone erosion, and generalized osteoporosis of bones in the involved areas.

D. Other Findings: Electrocardiographic findings are usually normal unless cardiac involvement is present. Echocardiography may indicate pericarditis.

Treatment

A. Specific Measures:

1. Nonsteroidal Anti-Inflammatory Drugs (NSAIDs)–Aspirin is the most satisfactory anti-inflammatory agent. Its recommended dose is 80–120 mg/kg/d in divided doses. Levels of 20–30 mg/dL are therapeutic. The response of rheumatoid arthritis to salicylates occurs within 3–4 days but is usually not as dramatic as in rheumatic fever. In patients who cannot tolerate aspirin, other NSAIDs such as tolmetin (Tolectin) 20–30 mg/kg/d, or naproxen (Naprosyn) 10–15 mg/kg/d should be tried.

2. Gold Salts & Penicillamine–These agents are used in patients who do not respond to salicylates or NSAIDs.

3. Methotrexate–Studies indicate that low doses (10.0 mg/m^2/week) of methotrexate in children are beneficial in JRA. It is not yet known whether this drug can induce long-term remission of the disease. Its use in children should be restricted to those who have failed conventional therapy.

4. Corticosteroids–Corticosteroids do not alter the natural remission rate or the length of JRA. They are, however, useful (eg, prednisone 1–2 mg/kg/d) in cases of myocarditis and others in which the disease is life-threatening. Corticosteroids are used topically to treat uveitis, and may be used systemically in low doses (5–10 mg/d) if the uveitis is unresponsive to topical therapy. Low-dose therapy is also helpful in patients with debilitating morning stiffness as well as those beginning on slow-acting anti-inflammatory drugs. Intra-articular corticosteroids have a place in the management of JRA in cases of monarticular involvement or rehabilitation retarded by slow progress in one or two joints.

B. General Measures:

1. Physical Therapy–Overall goals include prevention of deformities and maintenance of muscle strength and function. Acutely inflamed joints should not be subjected to weight-bearing maneuvers, but range-of-motion exercises should be prescribed. Later, stretching and strengthening exercises should be added. Heat and hydrotherapy may be useful adjuncts to a well-planned exercise program.

2. Orthopedic Care–Overnight wearing of splints will ensure proper alignment of joints. Avoid the use of cylinder casts.

3. Ophthalmic Care–Periodic slit-lamp examination is the only means for early diagnosis of iridocyclitis, which may otherwise continue undiagnosed until vision fails.

4. Rest–As fatigue is a frequent symptom, periods of rest should be alternated with periods of activity. Complete bed rest should be discouraged, however, since it can lead to osteoporosis, renal calculi, muscle atrophy, or joint deformities.

Course & Prognosis

Rheumatoid arthritis is a chronic disease with waxing and waning of inflammatory activity. Its systemic features (eg, fever, rash, pericarditis) remit more often than the joint manifestations.

With good medical management, the majority of patients will have complete functional recovery; fewer than 10% will be severely disabled. Deaths are rare in the pediatric population.

LYME DISEASE
(Lyme Arthritis)

Lyme disease is a form of arthritis that may become chronic. The first case was reported in Connecticut in 1975, and is caused by a spirochete transmitted by the deer tick (*Ixodes dammini*).

Onset usually occurs in summer; early symptoms commonly include fever, flu-like malaise, headache, and stiff neck. A target-shaped skin rash (erythema chronicum migrans) develops, usually within 30 days of exposure to the tick, and may be confused with ringworm (Chapter 12). Disseminated disease often involves the heart (myocarditis, AV block), the nervous system (aseptic meningitis, neuropathies), and the joints (arthritis). Later manifestations usually occur within 3 months of exposure. Both early and later symptoms may be recurrent.

Diagnosis of Lyme disease is based on supporting clinical evidence and laboratory findings. An enzyme-linked immunosorbent assay (ELISA) should be performed. If the result is positive, a Western blot (WB) analysis, which is more specific and more sensitive, should be done as confirmation. The combination of a positive ELISA and WB, together with a typical symptom history, supports the diagnosis of Lyme disease.

Treatment involves administration of either amoxicillin, doxycycline (in patients >9 years of age) or erythromycin (in penicillin-allergic children <9). Intravenous antibiotics (eg, ceftriaxone, cefotaxime) are indicated for CNS involvement or arthritis unresponsive to oral treatment. Prompt administration may avoid later complications.

POLYARTERITIS NODOSA

Polyarteritis (periarteritis) nodosa is a rare systemic disease characterized by inflammatory damage to blood vessels, with resulting injury to involved organs. Pathologic findings include segmental inflammation of small- and medium-sized arteries, with fibrinoid changes and (more rarely) necrosis in vessel walls. **Mucocutaneous lymph node syndrome** (Kawasaki disease [Chapter 11]), and infantile polyarteritis nodosa bear many pathologic similarities to polyarteritis nodosa.

Clinical Findings

Clinical manifestations vary, depending on the location of the involved arterioles.

A. Symptoms: The symptoms of polyarteritis nodosa are those of a rapidly progressive wasting disease, eg, fever, lassitude, weight loss, and generalized pains in the extremities, abdomen, or both.

B. Signs: Skin eruptions of the urticarial, purpuric, or macular type develop. Subcutaneous nodules are frequently present along the course of the blood vessels. Involvement of the kidneys, gastrointestinal tract, heart, and nervous system often manifests with features such as hypertension, myocardial infarction, seizures, and peripheral neuropathy.

C. Laboratory Findings: Abnormal test results reflect the organ involved. Findings may include anemia, with moderate leukocytosis and eosinophilia; accelerated sedimentation rate; proteinuria; intermittent microscopic hematuria and showers of casts; elevated levels of nonprotein nitrogen; sterile blood cultures; and cardiomegaly on x-ray. Muscle, skin, or testicular biopsies may show vasculitis and aid in diagnosis.

Treatment

Treatment with corticosteroids usually produces symptomatic improvement; immunosuppressive doses may prolong life, but the response is unpredictable and quite variable.

Prognosis

The prognosis is poor for patients with renal, cardiac, or CNS involvement, although spontaneous and corticosteroid-induced remissions have been reported.

SYSTEMIC LUPUS ERYTHEMATOSUS

Systemic lupus erythematosus (SLE) is a multisystem progressive disease whose protean symptomatology and relentless course present a diagnostic and therapeutic challenge. Pathologically, immune complex vasculitis, extensive fibrinoid degeneration, and necrosis are found. SLE is nine times more common in females than in males. Onset peaks in the pediatric population during the adolescent years. The cause of SLE is unknown. It is thought that multiple factors (viral, immunologic, and genetic) are involved. A lupuslike syndrome (including positive findings in lupus erythematosus (LE) cell preparations and ANA tests) may occur during procainamide or anticonvulsant therapy.

Clinical Findings

A. Symptoms and Signs: Children or adolescents with SLE often present with fever, rash, arthralgia, and arthritis. Myalgia, fatigue, weakness, and weight loss frequently occur. Table 27–4 summarizes typical clinical presentations.

B. Laboratory Findings: Antinuclear antibodies are present in 100% of active cases of SLE. Table 27–5 summarizes common laboratory findings.

Diagnosis & Treatment

Diagnosis of SLE is based on clinical findings and presentation, although specific laboratory abnormalities aid in the diagnosis. Con-

Table 27–4. Clinical manifestations of SLE.

System	Presentation
Cutaneous	Butterfly rash, mucocutaneous ulcers, alopecia, photosensitivity, digital ulcerations, Raynaud's phenomenon
Cardiac	Pericarditis (most common), endocarditis and myocarditis (less common)
Pulmonary	Pleuritis, basilar pneumonitis
Gastrointestinal	Abdominal pain, diarrhea, esophageal dysmotility
Renal	Nephritis, hypertension, uremia, nephrotic syndrome
Musculoskeletal	Arthralgia, arthritis, myalgia
Nervous system	Seizures, organic brain syndrome
Lymphoreticular	Splenomegaly, hepatomegaly, lymphadenopathy

SLE = systemic lupus erythematosus.

Table 27–5. Laboratory findings in SLE.

Autoantibodies
Anemia
Thrombocytopenia
Hypocomplementemia
Leukopenia
Hematuria, proteinuria
Elevated ESR
Positive Coombs' test
False (+) VDRL

ESR = erythrocyte sedimentation rate; VDRL = Venereal Disease Research Laboratory.

sistent features include the episodic nature of the disease, multisystem involvement, and positive ANA.

NSAIDs should be given for joint symptoms. Prednisone, given in doses of at least 60 mg/m^2/d, not only suppresses the acute inflammatory manifestations but also mitigates progressive glomerular involvement in many cases. Antibiotics should be given at the first sign of an infection. Hydroxychloroquine may be useful for skin and joint symptoms.

Azathioprine (Imuran) and cyclophosphamide (Cytoxan) are effective in controlling renal and systemic manifestations of SLE in some children who are resistant to corticosteroids alone. Recent evidence suggests that long-term survival in cases of lupus nephritis has improved when cyclophosphamide and prednisone are used together.

Intravenous pulse therapy with methylprednisolone sodium succinate (Solu-Medrol) may be tried in critically ill patients.

Because of their well-known photosensitivity, SLE patients should use sunscreens when exposed to the sun.

Course & Prognosis

Renal complications and CNS involvement are the most frequent causes of death. With good medical management, the overall survival rate has increased.

SCLERODERMA

Scleroderma is a collagen disease which chiefly affects the skin but may involve any organ. In local benign scleroderma (**morphea**), a linear distribution of lesions appears that first shows erythema and edema with subsequent scarring and shrinking. In the progressive generalized form, there is more extensive thickening and induration of the skin, followed by contractures. Interstitial and perivascular fibrosis may occur in the viscera.

Trophic ulcers, calcific deposits, and **Raynaud's phenomenon** (intermittent attacks of pallor followed by cyanosis in the fingers, usually precipitated by cold or emotional distress) are common. Raynaud's phenomenon is often the initial presenting symptom and may precede other manifestations by years. Disturbances in esophageal motility lead to dysphagia, and small bowel involvement leads to malabsorption. Antinuclear antibodies are frequently observed.

There is no specific therapy for scleroderma. Physiotherapy given early may minimize contractures. Corticosteroids are of little value. Bethanechol, cimetidine, and antacids have been used for dysphagia. Colchicine and D-penicillamine therapy have produced inconsistent results.

The prognosis is excellent for patients with local scleroderma but only fair for those with the severe generalized form, in which death may occur within a year. Some deformity may occur with the former and is the rule with the latter. Renal or cardiac involvement suggests a poor prognosis.

DERMATOMYOSITIS

Juvenile dermatomyositis is a multisystem inflammatory disease of unknown cause, involving primarily the muscles, skin, and subcutaneous tissues; it may be an autoimmune disorder. Since juvenile dermatomyositis appears to be a vascular process leading to arteritis and phlebitis, it may involve any organ. Muscles show segmental or focal necrosis, inflammation, fibrinoid changes in blood vessel capillaries, and finally, atrophy.

Clinical Findings

The diagnostic features of juvenile dermatomyositis are listed in Table 27–6.

A. Symptoms: Symptoms include symmetrical proximal muscle weakness, fever, muscle tenderness and pain, malaise and weight loss, arthralgia and arthritis, dyspnea, and dysphagia.

B. Signs: The pathognomonic rash of this disease is a violaceous (heliotrope) discoloration of the eyelids.

Table 27–6. Diagnostic features of dermatomyositis.

Proximal muscle weakness
Muscle enzyme elevation
Characteristic skin rash
Electromyogram findings
Muscle biopsy histology

C. Laboratory Findings: Elevation of muscle enzymes (serum glutamic-oxaloacetic transaminase [SGOT], creatine phosphokinase [CPK], and aldolase) is a useful laboratory tool. Anemia, increased sedimentation rate, and increased levels of serum globulin may be present. Myopathy on electromyogram and inflammation on muscle biopsy will aid in the diagnosis.

Treatment

Corticosteroid therapy is indicated in all patients with acute or active disease. Prednisone (1–2 mg/kg/d in divided doses) during the first month after diagnosis is usually required. Treatment should be vigorous and modulated to produce normal muscle enzymes. The immunosuppressive drugs methotrexate and azathioprine may be of value in life-threatening disease and in children whose disease is not adequately controlled with corticosteroid therapy alone.

Physiotherapy is a very important part of the treatment; the principles outlined in the section on rheumatoid arthritis should be followed.

Course & Prognosis

The clinical course of juvenile dermatomyositis varies considerably. The prognosis is favorable in most cases with early treatment. A small percentage of children will experience a relapsing course. The majority of patients can be returned to functional normality. Calcinosis, contractures, and atrophy produce long-term residua. Intractable muscle weakness, sepsis, and gastrointestinal vasculitis may issue in death in a small number of patients.

28 | Pediatric Emergencies

F. Keith Battan, MD

The primary mission of a Pediatric Emergency Department (PED) is *resuscitation* and *stabilization* of the life-threatened child. A large amount of definitive care for less serious illnesses and injuries is provided as well. The complete spectrum of illnesses and injuries is seen, from minor acute illnesses to life- or limb-threatening injuries or illnesses. Care provided by the PED to critically ill or injured patients overlaps with that provided in pediatric intensive care units; therefore many of the topics discussed in this chapter relate only to initial stabilization and treatment; more comprehensive treatments are described elsewhere in this book.

Care of the severely injured child is an essential part of the PED mission. Trauma causes more deaths after the first year of life than any other diagnosis.

APPROACH TO THE VERY ILL OR INJURED CHILD

Children, unlike adults, rarely exhibit sudden death from cardiac etiologies. Rather, pediatric cardiopulmonary arrests are usually due to respiratory causes, and are the result of a prolonged period of deterioration, during which significant insults to brain, heart, liver, kidneys, and other vital organs occur. By the time cardiopulmonary arrest occurs, the attendant hypoxia and acidosis that have occurred lead to a very dismal outcome. Very few children suffering total arrest survive or are left without significant neurologic impairments. Therefore the key to good outcomes is early recognition and intervention before an arrest occurs. *Recognition of the child who is at risk for cardiopulmonary arrest, and early intervention, is essential.*

When the arrival of a very sick child occurs abruptly, adequate nursing and physician staff must be assembled. Subspecialists are included as indicated, eg, neurosurgeons or general surgeons. Team roles are assigned, ensuring that the team leader is clearly designated.

Radiology, the blood bank, OR, and the lab are notified, as appropriate.

History

A brief problem-oriented history should be obtained from the parents soon after immediate resuscitation begins and without interrupting the resuscitation. A physician not involved with the resuscitation can obtain a history and counsel the parents on the current status of their child. Essential elements of the history are included in the mnemonic **"AMPLE"**:

A: Allergies and immunizations. Injuries breaking the skin will require determining the status of tetanus immunization.

M: Medications, including over-the-counter and prescription drugs. Many of these agents can produce toxic effects such as altered mental status and cardiorespiratory symptoms.

P: Past illnesses. Determine chronic illnesses, especially bleeding disorders or immunodeficiencies; previous surgeries or hospitalizations; and developmental disabilities.

L: Last meal. Children can be presumed to have a full stomach unless quantity and timing of the last oral intake can be determined. This information has implications for airway management given the risk for vomiting and aspiration.

E: Events preceding the injury or illness. Include timing, duration of symptoms, fever, and treatment. For injured children, determine supervision, witnesses to the event, mechanism of injury, secondary impacts, and pre-hospital course and care.

EXAMINATION: THE ABCS
(Rapid Assessment and Intervention)

Systematic use of the **"Airway, Breathing, Circulation"** method of examination (ABCs) allows rapid assessment of the degree of the child's physiologic derangement and indicates the immediate interventions necessary to prevent further deterioration. In this system, highest priority is to assess the patency of the airway, and if there is obstruction, measures to correct the obstruction are initiated immediately. Once airway patency is assured, the presence and adequacy of breathing is assessed. Again, if respiratory efforts are inadequate, interventions such as bag-valve-mask ventilation are begun to normalize oxygenation and ventilation. Once airway and breathing have been determined to be adequate or have been stabilized, then assessment of and intervention in circulation are done. The ABCs are detailed below. Basic life support measures will not be reviewed here.

Airway

A. Assessment: Assess airway patency by **look, listen, and feel: Look** for adequacy of chest wall movement, signs of upper airway obstruction such as increased work of inspiration, and level of consciousness. **Listen** for abnormal breath sounds such as stridor or gurgling. **Feel** for air movement at the mouth and nose by lowering your face to the child's mouth and nose.

B. Intervention: If airway obstruction is present, begin airway maneuvers in order of increasing invasiveness. If neck injury is possible, immobilize the cervical spine and maintain normal alignment.

(1) Perform head tilt (in non-trauma cases) with chin lift or jaw thrust: Gently extend the head on the neck, and lift the chin with fingers on the mandible or by exerting upward traction on the angle of the jaw. If airway obstruction persists, reposition the head before proceeding.
(2) Suction the mouth of secretions or foreign materials.
(3) Attempt to visualize foreign bodies, with a laryngoscope if necessary, and remove with fingers or Magill forceps. Blind finger sweeps for foreign bodies should not be done.
(4) Insert an oropharyngeal airway. This eliminates obstruction due to posterior prolapse of the tongue into the posterior pharynx, which is the most common cause of upper airway obstruction in the unconscious child. In a conscious child, a nasopharyngeal airway may be used to avoid provoking vomiting and possible aspiration.
(5) Consider performing foreign body maneuvers at this point if the airway remains obstructed.
(6) Place an endotracheal tube (see Table 28–1 for sizes) if obstruction persists, or if the child needs assisted ventilation for other reasons.
(7) Needle cricothyroidotomy may be necessary in the rare patient when endotracheal intubation is not possible.

Table 28–1. Estimation formulas.

Estimated body weight (kg) = (age in yrs × 2) + 8
Median blood pressure (systolic) = (age in yrs × 2) + 90
5th percentile systolic BP (hypotension) = (age in yrs × 2) + 70
Endotracheal tube size = (age + 16)/4

Breathing

A. Assessment: Look for apnea, inadequate chest wall movement, or signs of respiratory distress. Signs include:

(1) Abnormal respiratory rate for age. Tachypnea is common and frequently non-specific, but its cause must be sought. In a sick or injured child, *an abnormally low heart or respiratory rate with or without respiratory distress is a pre-arrest sign and requires aggressive immediate intervention.*
(2) Increased work of breathing, manifested by retractions, flaring of the alae nasae, or grunting. Retractions can be intercostal, supraclavicular, or substernal. An increased reliance on the diaphragm for breathing in children leads to abdominal or "see-saw" respirations, as the stomach protrudes during inspiration and vice-versa.
(3) Adequate and symmetric chest rise and fall (tidal volume).
(4) Altered mental status. Hypercarbia results in lethargy, while early hypoxia is manifested by agitation or restlessness.
(5) Skin color change. Cyanosis is a late finding due to the relative anemia of children and signifies profound hypoxia, whereas less severe alterations in PaO_2 may result in mottled, gray, or pale skin.

Listen for adventitious breath sounds such as wheezing. Auscultate for rales, wheezing, and symmetry of breath sounds. The smaller the chest, the more transmitted breath sounds may impair your ability to localize auscultatory findings.

Feel for subcutaneous crepitus or tracheal deviation, eg, from pneumothorax. The majority of the respiratory assessment comes from inspection; as Yogi Berra said, "You can see a lot by just looking!"

Intervention

(1) Oxygen should be immediately given to any patient exhibiting respiratory distress, or signs of poor perfusion.
(2) For spontaneously breathing patients with minimal distress, a nasal cannula can be used. Non-rebreather masks deliver a higher F_IO_2 and are appropriate for more seriously ill patients.
(3) If there is inadequate or absent breathing, begin positive-pressure ventilation with an appropriate size bag-valve-mask device (Table 28–2). Ensure that there is adequate chest rise and fall, and auscultate for air entry bilaterally. If there is resistance to bagging, repeat the interventions in "Airway" above.

Table 28–2. Equipment sizes and estimated weight by age.

Age (yr)	Weight (kg)	ETT[1] Size	Laryngoscope Blade	Chest Tube (fr.)	Foley (fr.)
Premature newborn	1–2.5	2.5 uncuffed	0	8	5
Term newborn	3.0	3.0	0–1	10	8
1	10	3.5–4.0	1	18	8
2	12	4.5	1	18	10
3	14	4.5	1	20	10
4	16	5.0	2	22	10
5	18	5.0–5.5	2	24	10
6	20	5.5	2	26	12
7	22	5.5–6.0	2	26	12
8	24	6.0 cuffed	2	28	14
10	32	6.0–6.5	2–3	30	14
Adolescent	50	7.0	3	36	14
Adult	70	8.0	3	40	14

[1] ETT = endotracheal tube; NB, cuffed ETTs used about age 8.

(4) Consider needle thoracostomy to alleviate pneumothorax for patients in severe distress or arrest who have asymmetric breath sounds, jugular venous distension, or subcutaneous crepitus.

(5) Endotracheal intubation should be performed for children in severe distress, those unresponsive to bag-mask ventilation, those in coma or who otherwise require airway protection, and in children who will require prolonged mechanical ventilation.

(6) Intravenous access is second in priority to the above interventions but should be established in children with severe distress or respiratory failure (see below). Advanced airway techniques are described in standard texts of pediatric emergency or critical care medicine. Further discussion follows under "respiratory failure," below.

Circulation

Assessment: Unlike respiratory assessment, the assessment of circulatory status is largely by hands-on examination. The diagnosis of shock can and should be made by the following clinical signs without a blood pressure determination. Assess for:

(1) Tachycardia or bradycardia. As mentioned above, bradycardia is ominous and requires aggressive intervention.
(2) Capillary fill time: This is a very useful index of circulatory integrity. CFT > 2 seconds is abnormal.
(3) Warmth of the extremities: Palpate hands or feet. If they are cool, determine the point at which the extremities become warm; the more proximal coolness begins, the more profound the shock.
(4) Pulses: Pulses should be assessed as normal, bounding (as in early phases of warm shock), thready, or absent. If peripheral pulses are absent, more proximal pulses should be sought.
(5) Skin color: Mottling, cyanosis, or grayness reflect hypoxia/ischemia.
(6) Altered mental status: Ischemia or hypoxemia will be reflected in altered levels of consciousness.
(7) Blood pressure: Because of the ability of children to respond to hypovolemia with marked increases in systemic vascular resistance, blood pressure does not fall until very late in the course of shock, making BP an insensitive indicator of shock. It is not necessary to know BP to determine perfusion status: If the patient has an abnormal heart rate and one of the other signs described above, he or she is in shock and should be treated accordingly. Poor perfusion as determined by CFT and the other clinical signs above with a normal BP is compensated shock, when the blood pressure also falls it is decompensated shock. When time permits, BP should be determined with the appropriate-sized cuff. Age-appropriate BP can be determined by charts or the following estimation formula: Systolic BP should be greater than (2 × age in years) + 70 for children over one year of age, newborns to one-month-olds should have a SBP > 60. See discussion of treatment under "Shock," below. *Hypotension is a late finding in shock. The diagnosis of shock can be made by physical examination.*

Interventions

Hypoperfusion or circulatory failure necessitates IV access, volume replacement, and, at times, pressors. Lack of pulses or frank arrest require CPR (external cardiac massage).

To summarize, rapidly assess the ABCs, taking care to sequentially assess each system and intervene appropriately before moving to the next step.

RESPIRATORY FAILURE

Respiratory failure is characterized by the inability of the body to maintain normal partial pressures of oxygen and/or CO_2 in the blood. It can be caused by conditions intrinsic (eg, asthma, pneumonia) or extrinsic (head injury, trauma) to the lungs. Respiratory failure can result from either upper or, more commonly, lower airway obstruction. Early recognition and timely intervention are again key.

Respiratory distress is characterized by increased work of breathing. Minute ventilation is equal to tidal volume times respiratory rate, therefore respiratory failure can occur with a high respiratory rate but inadequate tidal volume, and vice versa. Signs of respiratory distress are listed above in the assessment of breathing. As early respiratory distress progresses into late respiratory distress or respiratory failure, the increased work of breathing will eventually decrease, accompanied by a decrease in mentation. With increasing hypercarbia, there will be lethargy; with hypoxia, initial agitation will give way to increasing obtundation. As the patient tires, or as in the case of insufficient central respiratory drive, there will be decreasing or no respiratory distress. Thus, a child with a history of breathing difficulties may exhibit no respiratory distress and yet be in respiratory failure. *Respiratory failure is characterized by a depressed level of consciousness with or without signs of respiratory distress.*

The vast majority of cardiopulmonary arrests in children are caused by respiratory etiologies, and severe illness or injury of any type almost invariably have associated respiratory failure; therefore, ensuring the patency of the airway and normalizing respiration are essential in any resuscitation. Failure to manage the airway successfully is the leading cause of preventable mortality. *Stabilization of airway and breathing are the keys to successful pediatric resuscitations.*

Assessment

(1) History: Obtain duration of symptoms, history of choking or gagging episode, cough, the presence or absence of fever, past respiratory symptoms or diagnoses, or prematurity.
(2) Physical examination as above is generally sufficient to make the diagnosis of respiratory failure. Frequent reassessment is critical for the child in respiratory distress to ensure that no progression to respiratory failure is occurring.
(3) Labs: Pulse oximetry is mandatory in any child with respiratory distress. Arterial blood gases, if necessary, will confirm hypoxia and determine acid-base status and PCO_2. Radiographs of the

Table 28–3. Common causes of upper and lower airway obstruction.

Upper Airway	
Common	**Uncommon**
Croup Foreign body	Epiglottitis Bacterial tracheitis Retropharyngeal abscess/cellulitis Peritonsillar abscess Congenital defects
Lower Airway	
Common	**Uncommon**
Reactive airway disease Pneumonia Foreign body	Pulmonary edema Acidosis, any cause Pulmonary contusion Congestive heart failure Severe anemia

neck in cases of upper airway obstruction and of the chest in lower airway obstruction may be helpful. Radiographs to rule out foreign-body aspiration should include the entire airway and stomach, and include an assisted expiration view to assess air trapping.

Upper vs. lower airway obstruction causes of respiratory distress. Table 28–3 lists common causes. The upper airway extends from nasopharynx to carina, the lower airway from carina to the most distal gas exchange unit. Upper airway obstruction is characterized by increased work of breathing during inspiration and signs of upper airway narrowing such as stridor. This inspiratory work leads to an increase in the ratio of inspiration to expiration, which is normally roughly 1:1. Conversely, lower airway obstruction will lead to expiratory work and an I:E ratio of 1:2 or more. Wheezing, rales, or other adventitious breath sounds may be heard in lower airway obstruction.

SHOCK

Shock is defined as inadequate tissue perfusion. It is a clinical diagnosis, and does not rely on BP determination or lab values. The diagnosis of shock can and should be made by examination.

Table 28–4. Differentiation of shock states and initial therapy.

	Hypovolemic	Distributive	Cardiogenic
Etiologies	Vomiting/ diarrhea, blood loss	Anaphylaxis, sepsis, neurogenic	Dysrhythmias, congenital heart disease, myocarditis
Pathophysiology	Inadequate intravascular volume	Vasogenic maldistribution of vascular volume	Pump failure, inadequate cardiac output or increase afterload
Diagnosis	History, normal cardiac exam	History (allergic or infectious etc), toxic appearance with septic shock, normal cardiac exam	Exam: poor perfusion, rales, hepatomegaly, abnormal heart sounds
Initial treatment	Crystalloid infusion	Crystalloid infusion, pressors if refractory	Fluid restriction, pressors, diuretics, ± afterload reducers

Assessment

Assessment is described above under "Circulation." See Table 28–4 for differentiation and initial therapy for shock states.

Treatment

(1) Institute ALS care as described above. Maintain a patent airway and support breathing if necessary. Hypotensive or severely acidotic patients should be intubated and ventilated.
(2) Administer 100% oxygen.
(3) Place patient in Trendelenburg position unless respiratory distress is present.
(4) Establish IV access. Two large-bore IV catheters are required for hypotensive patients. Consider intraosseous access if peripheral access cannot be obtained. Follow access guidelines described below.
(5) Rapidly infuse only isotonic crystalloid (LR or NS). Use 20 mL/kg boluses, with reassessment of perfusion between boluses. Colloid infusion, (eg, albumin) can be considered after 3 boluses or if signs of increased capillary permeability are present.
(6) Consider vasopressor support (Table 28–5) if there is inadequate response to volume infusion.

Table 28–5. Emergency pediatric drugs and pressors.[1]

Atropine

Indications:
1) Bradycardia, due to cardiac etiologies
2) Vagal tone excess, eg, during laryngoscopy and intubation
3) Anticholinesterase poisoning
4) Asystole, after epinephrine use.
5) Epinephrine first-line for hypoxic/ischemic induced bradycardia

Dose: 0.01–0.02 mg/kg
maximum 1–2 mg

Route: IV, IO, ET

Note: Atropine may be useful in hemodyanically significant primary cardiac-based bradycardias. Because of paradoxical bradycardia somtimes seen in infants, a minimum 0.1 mg dose is recommended by the American Heart Asociation.

Sodium Bicarbonate

Indications:
1) Documented metabolic acidosis
2) Empiric treatment for presumed acidosis
3) Hyperkalemia

Dose: 1–2 meq/kg empirically, or by ABG

Route: IV, IO

Note: Sodium bicarbonate will be effective only if the patient is adequately oxygenated, ventilated, and perfused. Has some adverse side effects.

Calcium Chloride

Indications:
1) Documented hypocalcemia
2) Calcium-channel blocker overdose
3) Hyperkalemia, hypermagnesemia

Dose: 10–30 mg/kg slowly

Route: IV, preferably centrally; IO

Note: Calcium is no longer indicated for asystole or EMD. Potent tissue necrosis if infiltration occurs. Use with caution.

Epinephrine

Indications:
1) Bradycardia, especially hypoxic-ischemic
2) Hypotension (by infusion)
3) Asystole
4) Fine ventricular fibrillation refractory to initial defibrillation
5) Electromechanical dissociation
6) Anaphylaxis

Dose/route: IV/IO: 0.01 mg/kg of 1:10,000 solution. Repeat at no more than five-minute intervals. If initial dose unsuccessful, use at least twice the initial dose for subsequent doses.
ET: .02–.03 mg/kg
IO: as IV
SC: (anaphylactic shock): 0.01 mg/kg 1:1000 solution = .01 mL/kg max dose 0.3–0.5 mL.
Infusion: 0.1–1.0 µg/kg/min

(*continued*)

Table 28–5. Emergency pediatric drugs and pressors (*continued*).[1]

Note: Epinphrine is the single most important drug in pediatric resuscitation. Evidence from animal studies and small series of human subjects indicates that the present recommended dose may be insufficient and that doses of 0.2–0.3 mg/kg may be a more optimal dose. A randomized controlled trial has not been done.

Glucose

Indications: 1) Hypoglycemia
2) Altered mental status, empirically
3) With insulin, for hyperkalemia

Dose: 0.5–1.0 g/kg

Route: IV, IO

Note: Neonates—2 mL/kg D_{10}
Older child—2–4 mL/kg D_{25}
6–10 mL/kg D_{10}

Naloxone (Narcan)

Indications: 1) Opiate overdose
2) Altered mental status—empiric

Dose: 0.1 mg/kg <10 kg
.01 mg/kg >10 kg

Route: IV, IO, ET

Note: Side effects are few. A dose of 2.0 mg may be given in young children, 4.0 mg in adolescents. Repeat as necessary, or as constant infusion in narcotic overdoses.

Dopamine: Usually first line inotrope. Stimulates beta and dopaminergic receptors. At higher doses alpha effects predominate. Dose: 5–20 μg/kg/minute. Renal and splanchnic vasodilation at low doses. Central access recommended for all pressors.

Dobutamine: Increases stroke volume without increasing myocardial oxygen consumption. Safer than epinephrine or isoproterenol infusions. Beta-adrenergic. Dose: 1–10 μg/kg/minute.

Amrinone: Phosphodiesterase inhibitor. Provides inotropy and afterload reduction. May cause dysrhythmias. Dose: initial bolus 0.75 mg/kg over 3 minutes, then infusion 5–10 μg/kg/minute.

Epinephrine: Very potent inotrope and chronotrope. Increases SVR markedly. Alpha-adrenergic. Significant potential toxicities, eg, dysrhythmias, ischemia. Dose: 0.05–1.0 μg/kg/minute.

Isoproterenol: Pure beta agonist. Useful for resistant heart block. May drop SVR and cause peripheral vasodilation, therefore ensure normal volume status when initiating. Increases myocardial oxygen consumption and may cause tachydysrhythmias. Dose: 0.05–1.0 μg/kg/minute.

[1] ET = endotracheal; IO = intraosseous; IV = intravenous; SC = subcutaneous.

(7) CVP determination will guide therapy in refractory shock states.
(8) Place foley catheter and maintain urine output of > 1 mL/kg/hr.
(9) Send blood for indicated lab determinations.

MONITORING

All very sick or injured children should have a minimum level of monitoring, lines, and tubes: (1) 100% oxygen; (2) continuous cardiorespiratory monitoring; (3) pulse oximetry and end-tidal CO_2 monitoring if intubated; (4) intravenous access of at least one and preferably two short, large-bore peripheral IVs. If peripheral IV access is not established within ninety seconds, initiate attempts at more central access, including intraosseous lines, percutaneous catheterization of the femoral, internal or external jugular, or subclavian veins, or cutdown of the antecubital, saphenous, or femoral veins, depending on the expertise of the providers available. Central access is preferred for infusion of vasopressors or CVP monitoring. Consider arterial access for beat-to-beat BP monitoring or for frequent lab draws. (5) blood pressure determinations every five to ten minutes; (6) nasogastric tube placement for any patients receiving positive-pressure ventilation or with ileus or surgical abdomens; (7) foley catheter placement for children in shock or receiving prolonged ventilation, if no contraindications exist (see Trauma); (8) cervical spine immobilization and placement on a backboard if spinal injury is a consideration.

Empiric Treatment

Patients with altered mental status should receive 100% oxygen, naloxone 1 mg IV in a younger child, 2 mg IV in an older child, and dextrose 0.5–1.0 g/kg (2–4 mL/kg D25). Patients presenting with cardiorespiratory failure without a clear etiology, particularly if there is a history suggestive of infection or if the patient is immunosuppressed, (eg, oncology, transplant, sickle-cell anemia patients), should receive empiric broad-spectrum IV antibiotics such as cefotaxime or ceftriaxone, and ampicillin in infants < 3 mos. Cultures can be obtained after stabilization occurs.

Additional Physical Examination

Following assessment and stabilization of the ABC's, perform a more detailed examination. Keep in mind the possibility of ingestions or exposures for patients without clear etiologies for their deterioration.

Labs & Radiographs

(1) Obtain a bedside glucose determination. Particularly in infants and small children, serious illness is often accompanied by hypoglycemia.
(2) For children presenting with cardiorespiratory collapse, obtain complete blood count, electrolytes, serum glucose, creatinine, BUN, arterial blood gas, and blood culture.
(3) Consider liver function tests and serum ammonia, particularly if there is altered mental status or hypoglycemia.
(4) Do urinalysis and toxicology screen.
(5) Consider calcium, magnesium, and phosphorus determinations if the patient may be postictal or is actively seizing.

Diagnostic imaging is directed by history or exam findings. Consider cranial CT for children with altered mental status if there is a possibility of trauma, if there are lateralizing neurologic findings, or signs of intracranial hypertension.

Summary

Care of the critically ill or injured child is a team effort. An organized approach with strict attention to the stabilization of Airway, Breathing, and Circulation will ensure an optimal outcome. *Frequent reassessment* is mandatory to detect deterioration.

EMERGENCY DRUGS

Maintenance of breathing and circulation remain the mainstays of pediatric resuscitations. Oxygen and epinephrine are the principal drugs of use in pediatrics, although the full complement of ALS medications are used. Principles of use include:

(1) Use the appropriate pediatric dose based on weight in kilograms.
(2) Be aware of different delivery modalities, eg, any drug that can be given intravenously can be given IO, and some drugs can be given via endotracheal tube (naloxone, epinephrine, atropine, and lidocaine).
(3) Administer medications close to the IV catheter and flush in with saline.
(4) Use code cards or sheets with preprinted drug dosages and equipment sizes whenever possible to minimize dosing errors. A resuscitation tape (Broselow tape) is available that uses the child's

height to estimate weight, determined by placing the patient directly on the tape, which enables proper selection of drug doses and equipment sizes.

Table 28–5 contains a list of the most commonly used drugs and vasopressors.

TRAUMA

Background

Death due to injuries is the leading cause of death for children. Previously, trauma care was solely the domain of surgeons. It is now clear that optimal outcomes for this very important subset of the pediatric population come from a multidisciplinary approach utilizing emergency pediatricians, pediatric surgeons, pediatric intensivists, and other essential support services such as neurosurgery and orthopedics. This impressive array of resources can be found at pediatric trauma centers. However, the majority of injured children are not taken care of in these centers; therefore, pediatric care providers must be able to participate in initial assessment and stabilization before transport to a referral facility. Pediatricians must be aware of trauma's sobering statistics and become actively involved in the entire spectrum of care of the traumatized child, from injury prevention to prehospital, hohildren grants are helping to upgrade the pediatric capability of existing EMS services nationwide.

Epidemiology

Common mechanisms of injury include motor vehicle crashes, either as occupants or pedestrians, falls, sporting injuries, and drownings. Blunt injuries predominate over penetrating injuries from gunshot wounds or stabbings by 9:1. Toddlers and teenagers are most at risk, and males are more frequently injured than females. Head injury is common in major injuries and is usually the cause of death. Abdominal injuries are common and frequently difficult to diagnose. Injury prevention efforts at every level of the health-care system are essential.

Approach

(1) Organize a trauma receiving team with appropriate composition and a designated team leader.
(2) Assign roles for the resuscitation, including airway management, establishment of IV access, lab drawing, etc.

(3) Assemble subspecialists, eg, neurosurgeons, as indicated by prehospital communications, and technologists, eg, radiology technicians.
(4) Notify the OR if operative intervention may be needed.
(5) Document interventions with times.
(6) Keep a calm atmosphere in the trauma receiving unit, which will enhance thoughtful care.
(7) Compile a problem list to assist in determining priorities for care.
(8) Never neglect a child's pain and fear. Strongly consider analgesia and sedation in appropriate patients. Constant reassurance is helpful. Enlist the aid of social workers or Child Life workers whenever possible.

Primary Survey

Assessment of the trauma patient is divided into the primary and secondary surveys. This system is useful in the approach to the child with multi-system, life-threatening injuries, as well as to apparently less severely injured children. The primary survey is the rapid initial assessment which identifies and immediately treats life-threatening problems. It ascertains physiologic derangements, eg, respiratory failure or shock, and does not include anatomic diagnoses such as fractured pelvis. The primary survey is the **resuscitation phase**, while the secondary survey represents diagnosis and definitive care for each injury. The primary survey is comprised of:

A: Airway, with cervical spine control.
B: Breathing.
C: Circulation, with hemorrhage control.
D: Disability, a rapid neurologic assessment.
E: Expose and examine.

The approach to the trauma ABCDEs is exactly like the ABCs above, ie, each system is assessed sequentially, and the integrity of that system assured before moving to the next system. Small children are notorious for having significant internal injuries with an initially normal appearance and no cutaneous signs of significant injury. Assessment and initial interventions in the primary survey are described below.

A. Airway With Cervical Spine Control: Considerations are similar to airway assessment and management as discussed above, with the addition of in-line cervical immobilization. (1) Initially, maintain in-line immobilization of the head in neutral position with gentle axial manual traction. (2) Next, provide a rigid collar and tape across the forehead and chin. These precautions should be left in place until appropriate radiologic and clinical exams have been conducted. (3) Pad the head with towel rolls across the top and sides of the head. (4) Strap the entire child tightly to a backboard. If the child vomits, the backboard can then be log-rolled while maintaining the entire spine in-line. (5) Suction the mouth and nose of blood and secretions. (6) Remove foreign bodies in the mouth and loose teeth. (7) Give 100% oxygen to every patient while the assessment proceeds. (8) Intubate the trachea of severely injured patients who have airway obstruction or who are unconscious. Consider rapid-sequence neuroinduction for nonflaccid patients. Oral intubation is generally possible even while maintaining cervical spine precautions and is the route of choice. Nasotracheal intubation is an alternative in teens with spontaneous respirations, if cribriform plate fracture is unlikely. (9) Consider needle cricothyroidotomy if severe midface trauma is present or if endotracheal intubation cannot be achieved.

B. Breathing Assessment: Assessment proceeds just as detailed in the first section. (1) Determine respiratory effort, rate, adequacy and symmetry of chest rise and fall, increased work of breathing, and focal decreases in breath sounds. (2) In the trauma setting, always consider hemo- and/or pneumothorax. Signs include tracheal shift, decreased breath sounds on the side of the pneumothorax, and subcutaneous crepitus. Cyanosis, bradycardia, jugular venous distension, and hypotension may be present. Suspicion of pneumothorax or hemothorax calls for immediate tube thoracostomy placement of sufficient diameter to drain blood. Placement is in the fifth intercostal space in the midaxillary line. (3) Quickly examine the chest for wounds sufficient to cause open pneumothorax (sucking chest wound). Occlude these on three sides with vaseline-impregnated gauze and ensure positive-pressure ventilation.

C. Circulation Assessment With Hemorrhage Control: Circulation is again assessed in an identical fashion to that described above. (1) Bleeding wounds are controlled quickly by direct pressure with a gauze bandage. (2) Remember to detect early signs of shock, eg, tachycardia and delayed CFT. (3) Insert two large-bore, short peripheral IV catheters. Alternatives for access are discussed above in Circulation. If it is necessary to place IO lines, obtain additional personnel to then place a more secure central line. (4) When placing lines, obtain blood for lab work as below. (5) *Shock management of trauma patients:* Begin rapid intravascular replacement with boluses of isotonic crystle. Patients in extremis may receive O-negative blood. Use a fluid warmer for all administered fluids. (6) Muffled heart

Table 28–6. AVPU system for evaluation of level of consciousness.

A—Alert
V—responsive to Voice
P—responsive to Pain
U—Unresponsive

sounds, poor pulses, narrowed pulse pressure, and hypotension suggest cardiac tamponade and mandate immediate pericardiocentesis.

D. Disability: Perform a brief neurologic examination to exclude conditions requiring immediate treatment. (1) Characterize the LOC by the AVPU system (Table 28–6). (2) Determine pupil size and reactivity. If one or both pupils are dilated and unreactive or sluggishly reactive to light, begin treating for presumed intracranial hypertension. (3) Briefly check for spinal cord integrity by looking for spontaneous movement of the extremities or localization of painful stimulus in the legs. (4) Suspected **ICP elevation** treatment is discussed below. Obtain immediate neurosurgical consultation.

E. Expose & Examine: The child should be completely undressed and examined, and logrolling should be used to examine the back. During this time, it is important to maintain temperature with warming lights and/or warmed blankets applied to previously inspected areas.

Secondary Survey

After the resuscitative or primary phase has been completed, a detailed head-to-toe examination is done. Ensure that all appropriate tubes have been placed. Space permits only a brief description below.

A. Skin: Look for abrasions, lacerations, and contusions. Cutaneous findings may signify underlying pathology, eg, a contusion on the thorax may overlie a pulmonary contusion. Careful cleaning and selective debridement is important. Ensure tetanus immunization within the last five years.

B. Head & Neck: Perform a detailed exam. Palpate for bony defects. Look for signs of CSF leak (clear or serosanguinous drainage from ears or nose) or basilar skull fracture (hemotympanum, raccoon eyes, or Battle's sign). Rule out broken or misaligned teeth, nasal septal displacement or hematomas, limitation of extraocular movements, and cranial nerve palsies.

C. Chest: Tamponade and hemopneumothoraces will have been decompressed in the primary survey. Chest x-ray or chest CT may reveal pulmonary contusions. Myocardial contusions are rare but should be considered with blunt direct anterior thorax injury, as should dissecting aortic injuries. Paradoxic chest wall movements suggest flail chest segments.

D. Abdomen: Penetrating injuries violating the peritoneum require operative exploration. Blunt injuries to liver, spleen, kidneys, and hollow viscera represent a diagnostic challenge. Diagnosis depends on: (1) serial examinations for bowel sounds, tenderness, and organ size; (2) plain films to rule out free intra-abdominal air and CT with double contrast; (3) liver functions tests, which have fair sensitivity but good specificity for liver injuries, and amylase testing for traumatic pancreatitis; (4) in selected unstable patients, diagnostic peritoneal lavage (DPL) to look for blood or intestinal contamination.

E. Pelvis & Genitourinary: Palpate for pelvic instability, pain with direct pressure, or crepitus. Blood at the urinary meatus or in the scrotum, an abnormal prostate, or pelvic fracture suggest the possibility of urethral disruption. Urethrogram should be done before foley catheter placement when these signs are present. Examine the vagina for injuries. Rectal examination is always done to assess tone and to hemetest.

F. Musculoskeletal: Inspect for swelling, pain, tenderness, and neurovascular status. Examine the back by logrolling. Assess pulses, perfusion, and neurologic function distal to fractures. Delayed diagnoses of long-bone fractures are not uncommon in unconscious children.

G. Neurologic: Perform a detailed examination of mental status, speech, cranial nerves, tone, strength, sensation, cerebellar signs, and reflexes. Perform serial AVPU assessments or employ pediatric Glasgow coma scales (Table 28–7). Consider high-dose methylprednisolone therapy for acute spinal cord injuries.

Discussion of closed head injury follows.

Labs & Radiographs

(1) Laboratory determinations: Routine tests include complete blood count, amylase, type and crossmatch for one unit of PRBC's for each 10 kg of body weight, and urinalysis for hematuria. Consider coagulation studies, electrolytes, creatinine, and toxicology screens.

(2) Radiographs: Routine films include lateral, anterior-posterior, and odontoid view of the cervical spine. Abdominal (chest and pelvis) and long bone films are performed as indicated.

Table 28–7. Glasgow Coma Scale.

Eye opening response	
Spontaneous	4
To speech	3
To pain	2
None	1
Verbal response	
Oriented	5
Confused conversation	4
Inappropriate words	3
Incomprehensible sounds	2
None	1
Best upper limb motor response	
Obeys	6
Localizes	5
Withdraws	4
Abnormal flexion	3
Extensor response	2
None	1

CT of the head and abdomen has become very common. Special studies such as urethrograms and aortograms are obtained in consultation with members of the trauma team.

CLOSED HEAD INJURY (CHI)

CHI is one of the most common injuries seen in a pediatric ED. Complications include subdural, epidural, and parenchymal hemorrhage, diffuse axonal injury, cerebral edema, and CSF leak and subsequent infection. A clinical classification system (Table 28–8) allows determination of which patients deserve observation, cranial CT, neurosurgical consultation, admission, or emergent neuroresuscitation.

Assessment

Apply the ABCDEs of trauma resuscitation. Historical points to be determined:

(1) Mechanism of injury: How significant was the decelerative force? Shear stresses result from the shaken baby syndrome.
(2) Mental status immediately following the injury: Was there loss of consciousness or subsequent confusion or amnesia?
(3) Behavior since the injury: Has there been vomiting, headache, altered vision, or abnormal mental status?

Table 28–8. Clinical classification of head-injured patients.[1]

Mild:	No LOC[2] or amnesia; alert, oriented; asymptomatic or slight headache with dizziness only
Moderate:	Possible findings: History of LOC,[2] amnesia; posttraumatic seizure; vomiting; more than slight headache; listlessness, lethargy
Severe:	Possible findings: Disoriented, unable to follow commands; decreasing level of consciousness; focal neurologic signs; penetrating skull injury or depressed skull fracture

[1] From Rosenthal BW, Bergman I: Intracranial injury after moderate head trauma in children. *J Pediatr* 1989;115:346–350. By permission.
[2] LOC = loss of consciousness.

Examination should center on:

(1) General level of consciousness and trend: Is the child becoming more obtunded, remaining stable, or gradually lightening?
(2) Rule out associated injuries, eg, mandibular fractures, scalp or skull injuries, CSF leak, signs of basilar skull fracture, or cervical spine injuries.
(3) Complete neurologic examination, including serial mental status assessments and evidence of antero- or retrograde amnesia.
(4) Complete vital signs, paying attention to signs of Cushing's triad (bradycardia, hypertension, irregular respirations).
(5) Consider non-accidental trauma if the injuries observed are inconsistent with the history given.

Diagnostic Imaging

Plain films of the skull are of little therapeutic significance unless there is concern for depressed skull fracture or penetrating injury. Fractures across the distribution of the middle meningeal artery are no longer thought to deserve CT for the perception of increased risk for intracranial bleeding. The morbidity from CHI stems from intracranial processes, not skull fractures per se. Obtain CT of the head for patients with persistent vomiting, an abnormal neurologic exam, or deteriorating level of consciousness.

Concussion

A brief loss or alteration of consciousness followed by a return to the normal state is defined as a concussion. Patients may present with amnesia, pallor, or several episodes of vomiting. The examination is normal and there is no anatomic damage to brain tissue, although subtle neuropsychiatric sequelae may ensue.

Contusion

A bruise of the brain tissue constitutes a cerebral contusion. Level of consciousness is depressed, and focal neurologic findings correspond to the contused area of the brain.

Acute Intracranial Pressure Elevation

Acute ICP elevation occurs not only in the setting of CHI, but also with CNS infections, metabolic derangements (eg, DKA or Reye's syndrome), hydrocephalus, ventriculoperitoneal shunt obstruction, cerebrovascular accident, and tumor. Herniation syndromes may or may not be associated. Early recognition and immediate treatment are essential to avoid disastrous outcomes.

Diagnosis

Symptoms include: (1) increasing headache; (2) decreasing level of consciousness, usually listlessness progressing to lethargy and obtundation; (3) visual changes, eg, diplopia or loss of visual acuity; and (4) vomiting.

Examination findings may include: (1) decreased level of consciousness; (2) stiff neck; (3) cranial nerve palsies; and the late findings of (4) sluggish or frankly unreactive, dilated pupils; (5) Cushing's triad; (6) papilledema.

Management

Measures to control ICP must be immediately instituted. Strict attention to the ABCs is paramount.

(1) Intubate the trachea and hyperventilate to a PCO_2 of 28–30. Use a neuroinductive rapid sequence technique to avoid the elevation in ICP that occurs with laryngoscopy and intubation.
(2) Elevate the head of the bed to 30°.
(3) Keep the head in the midline to avoid impedance of venous flow from the head.
(4) Administer mannitol 0.5–1.0 g/kg IV.
(5) Infuse isotonic fluids at no more than two-thirds of maintenance rates while maintaining normal perfusion with intermittent boluses as needed.
(6) Avoid painful stimuli, if possible.
(7) Treat fever.

(8) Obtain neurosurgical consultation.
(9) Admit to a PICU or operating room.

A common problem is a child who is hypotensive but who appears to have increased ICP. In this case, restoration of circulating volume takes precedence over restriction of fluids in consideration of ICP. Remember that cerebral perfusion pressure is the ICP minus the mean arterial pressure, therefore MAP needs to be maintained to have adequate CPP. Once normal intravascular volume has been restored, fluids can be reduced to two-thirds of the maintenance rates. Invasive monitoring will guide further therapy. Never perform lumbar puncture acutely if there is concern for elevated ICP.

Disposition

(1) Mild injuries: Children with no history of loss of consciousness and no vomiting who have a normal general and neurologic exam on presentation have a very low risk of serious intracranial injuries and can be discharged after a brief period of observation with detailed discharge instructions.
(2) Moderate injuries: Patients with the above risk factors of vomiting or LOC and who may not have a normal mental status on admission to the ED require serial neurologic examinations. If the child's mental status is becoming more normal with time and there are no lateralizing signs, the patient may be observed for a period of hours until normal, then discharged with instructions. Advise the parents that intracranial hemorrhages can slowly accumulate, such that they may not present for several days after the injury. If the child is not responsive to voice commands, has lateralizing signs, or has progressive decrease in level of consciousness, obtain a cranial CT. If CT is normal, the child can be observed further and discharged when completely normal. Abnormal CT's mandate consultation by a neurosurgeon.
(3) Severe injuries: As detailed above, these children deserve cerebral resuscitation, neurosurgical consultation, and admission to PICU.

BURNS

Thermal injury has a horrible morbidity and mortality to children. The nature, extent, and thickness of the burn, as well as associated injuries, should be ascertained in the initial evaluation.

Classification

The depth of thermal injury through epidermis and dermis determines classification. **Superficial** burns (formerly first-degree), as typified by sunburn, are dry, warm, painful, and hypersensitive. They heal without specific treatment. **Partial-thickness** (formerly second-degree) burns affect epidermis and variable but not complete elements of the dermis. Partial thickness burns can be superficial, resulting in burns that are red, painful, and potentially blistered; or deep, resulting in dry, white, and hyposensitive burns. Treatment depends on depth of damage. **Full-thickness** (formerly third-degree) burns affect all epidermal and dermal elements, and are anesthetic, white, avascular, dry, and leathery-appearing. Skin grafting helps ameliorate the uneven and hard fibrotic scar formation as healing proceeds.

Management

A. Superficial Burns: cool compresses and analgesia.

B. Partial-Thickness Burns: These should be aseptically debrided, washed with 1% dilute povidone-iodine solution, copiously irrigated with normal saline, and dressed with topical antibiotic, commonly silver sulfadiazine, although Polysporin or Neosporin can be used in smaller areas. Blisters should be debrided. The wounds should be covered with a bulky dressing and serially examined, starting within 24 hours. Burns of the hands, feet, face, perineum, or other sensitive areas with the potential for contractions or disfiguration should be referred to a burn surgeon. Always provide appropriate analgesia.

C. Full-Thickness Burns & Extensive or Deep Partial-Thickness Burns: These injuries place particular importance on the ABC's of trauma management, as the pediatric airway may become obstructed by thermal injury, there may be hypoxic or smoke inhalation injury to the lungs, and there are substantial fluid management problems associated with major burns. Be aware of the possibility of toxic byproducts of combustion such as cyanide and carbon monoxide. A burn surgeon should be promptly consulted. See the Burn Resuscitation Protocol.

MAJOR BURN RESUSCITATION PROTOCOL

- Secure the airway.
- Administer 100% oxygen.
- Assist ventilation if needed.

- Obtain IV access.
- Normalize perfusion.
- Remove all clothing.
- Stop the burning process (irrigate).
- Perform complete examination.

Fluid Management for Major Burns

Substantial fluid loss occurs through burned skin, and there is increased capillary permeability. It is essential to maintain normal intravascular volume. Figure 28–1 shows percentage of BSA by body part for infants and children. The Parkland formula for fluid replacement is 4 mL/kg/percent BSA burned for the first 24 hours, with half in the first 8 hours, in addition to maintenance rates.

Disposition

Minor superficial burns and superficial partial-thickness burns can be treated as outpatients if appropriate follow-up and analgesia can be provided. Admission will be necessary for major burns, defined as > 10% BSA for superficial partial-thickness burns, or > 2% if full thickness, or burns involving eyes, ears, face, perineum, hands or feet, or associated with fractures.

ELECTRICAL INJURIES

Complications of electrical injuries include:

(1) Burns: even brief contact with a high voltage source will cause thermal damage. Search for exit wounds. Care is the same as that for other burns.
(2) Dysrhythmia: Current traversing the heart can cause non-perfusing ventricular dysrhythmias.
(3) Neurologic injuries: Early signs include disorientation and peripheral nerve injury; late injuries are neuropsychiatric in nature, eg, concentration or memory defects.
(4) Internal injuries: Passage of current through the body can cause an arc of thermal injury with extensive damage to deep tissues.

Electric cord injuries deserve special mention. Commonly a young child will bite an electric cord, sustaining burns to the oral commissure. Initially, the burns appear gray and necrotic. Delayed coagulation around the mouth may occur. Sloughing of the eschar as the wound heals days later may lead to brisk bleeding.

Name________________________Age__________Ward___________

First-degree erythema not to be included.

Shade in second-degree burn areas below.

Shade in third-degree burn areas below.

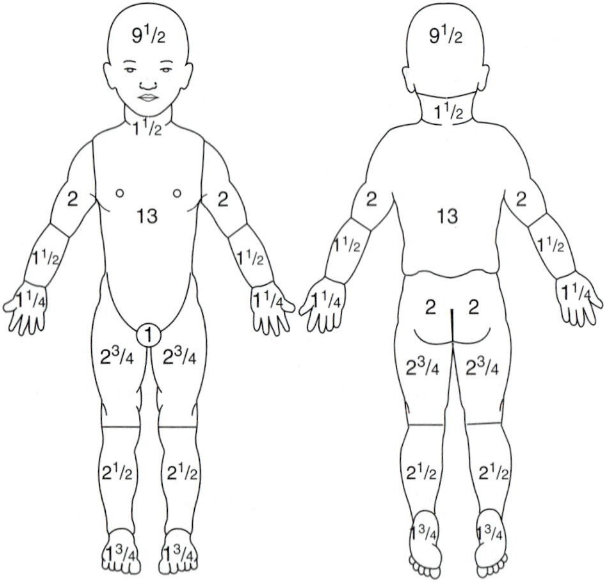

(Above: infant < 1 yr of age)

Area[1]	Age (yr) 0	1	5	10	15	Adult
Head area	19%	17%	13%	11%	9%	7%
Trunk area	26%	26%	26%	26%	26%	26%
Arm area	7%	7%	7%	7%	7%	7%
Thigh area	$5^1/2$%	$6^1/2$%	$8^1/2$%	$8^1/2$%	$9^1/2$%	$9^1/2$%
Leg area	5%	5%	5%	6%	6%	7%

Total third-degree burns________%

Total second-degree burns______%   TOTAL BURNS_______%

[1]The neck, hands, buttocks, genitalia, and feet are not included in this chart.

Disposition

All but the most superficial injuries will require cardiac monitoring and hospital admission. Surgical revision of burns may be necessary.

BITES AND STINGS

Bites

Many ED visits are due to bites, generally from domestic animals. Most fatalities are from dog bites, infectious complications are more common from cat and human bites.

General Care

All wounds require that tetanus immunization be current, administer tetanus immune globulin if unimmunized. The occurrence of rabies is unusual, except in feral animals. Follow local reporting rules. Suture bite wounds, especially cat and human bites, only if necessary for cosmetic reasons. If a bite involves a joint capsule, periosteum, or neurovascular bundle, consult an orthopedic surgeon. All wounds should receive high-pressure, high-volume irrigation with judicious debridement of ragged or devitalized edges, and removal of foreign material.

Dog Bites

Wounds are generally laceration/puncture. Infecting organisms include *Pasteurella multocida*, streptococci, staphylococci, and anaerobes. Prophylactic antibiotics have not been shown to improve outcome in uncomplicated dog bites not involving hands or feet. Dog bites that have become infected can be treated with penicillin for coverage against *P. multocida*, and broader spectrum coverage can be provided by cefalexin or amoxicillin and clavulanic acid. Parenteral therapy is necessary if there is toxicity, bony involvement, or extensive cellulitis. Complications of dog bites include CNS infections, osteomyelitis, septic arthritis, sepsis, and endocarditis.

Cat Bites

Because a cat bite creates a puncture-wound inoculum, there should be even greater reluctance to suture, and prophylactic antibi-

Figure 28–1. Lund and Browder modification of Berkow's scale for estimating extent of burns.

otics are recommended. *P. multocida* is the most common infecting organism, and antibiotic coverage is as recommended for dog bites. Complications include cat scratch disease, cellulitis, tenosynovitis, osteomyelitis, and septic arthritis.

Human Bites

Most human bites stem from assaults, particularly the "fight bite," where the clenched fist strikes teeth, exposing the metacarpophalangeal joint to infection. These wounds should receive operative debridement by a hand surgeon and intravenous antibiotics. Infected human bites commonly grow from culture streptococci, anaerobes, staphylococci, and *Eikenella corrodens*. Coverage against these organisms is recommended.

Insect Stings & Arthropod Bites

Stings are common and generally not serious. Biting arthropods such as spiders, millipedes, scorpions, ticks, and mites abound, but rarely cause serious injury or mortality. Anaphylaxis is the most important sequela.

A. Insect Stings: Bee and wasp stings cause immediate pain, swelling, pruritus, and redness. Myriad home remedies such as meat tenderizer have been advocated but never proven to be effective. Presentation and treatment of anaphylaxis is described below.

B. Spider Bites: Only a few species, such as black widows, tarantulas, and brown recluse spiders commonly cause serious envenomations. Black widow bites may initially pass unnoticed by the child. Local erythema and edema may progress to significant symptoms such as excruciating pain within one hour. Classically, severe abdominal pain and/or thorax and back pain are present. Ulceration at the bite site may appear later.

Treatment

A. General Treatment: (1) Apply cool compresses and elevate the sting or bite site. (2) Cleanse the wound site. (3) Ensure tetanus immunization status is current. (4) Administer oral antihistamines, eg, diphenhydramine or hydroxyzine, for pruritus. (5) Admit children with moderate or severe symptoms to the hospital.

Black widow antivenom is available but has significant side effects. Calcium and benzodiazepines have been used for severe black widow bite symptoms.

B. Anaphylaxis: Anaphylaxis accounts for many deaths per year and requires aggressive therapy. Symptoms include chest or neck tightness, faintness, dizziness, syncope, or disorientation. Signs may include face and neck swelling, upper airway obstruction, wheezing, urticaria, and hypotension. Immediate treatment consists of: (1) 100% oxygen; (2) subcutaneous epinephrine 0.01 mL/kg of 1:1000 solution, up to 0.5 mL maximum dose, or 0.01 mg/kg of 1:10,000 solution IV ephinephrine; (3) endotracheal intubation if upper airway obstruction is evolving; (4) IV access; (5) volume support, and vasopressors if unresponsive to crystalloid infusion; and (6) albuterol or other inhaled beta-adrenergic agents to treat bronchospasm. Children experiencing systemic symptoms should be referred to an allergist for consideration of desensitization and provision of an epinephrine auto-injection pen.

HYPOTHERMIA

Hypothermia is defined as a core temperature less than 35° C. Most often in pediatrics it is associated with cold-water submersion accidents. Other associations include sepsis, static encephalopathy, ingestions, and metabolic disorders. Hypothermia represents a failure of the normally closely-regulated physiologic mechanisms that maintain normal body temperature. As core temperature falls, peripheral vasoconstriction gives way to hypothalamic-mediated increases in muscle tone, metabolism, and shivering.

Clinical Findings

Signs depend on depth of temperature depression. Severe cases (< 28° C.) mimic death: pupils are fixed and dilated, there is no discernable pulse or respirations, and muscles are rigid. If these changes are a *primary* result of hypothermia and are not simply post-mortem changes, then death cannot be declared until the patient has been rewarmed and resuscitative efforts are unsuccessful. Hence the ED saying: "They're not dead until they're warm and dead." Children have survived core temperatures as low as 19° C neurologically intact.

Treatment

(1) Handle the patient gently, as the hypothermic myocardium is prone to ventricular fibrillation. (2) Document rewarming with an indwelling low-reading rectal thermometer. (3) Treat ventricular fibrillation and asystole per PALS protocols including chest compressions. Spontaneous reversion to sinus rhythm may occur at 28–30° C as rewarming proceeds. (4) If peripheral pulses are present in the severely hypothermic patient, even as low as 6 per minute, withhold chest

compressions, as even that low rate may be sufficient to satisfy the metabolic demands of the hypothermic child. (5) Correct hypoxemia and hypercapnia, clotting disturbances, acidemia, and glucose or electrolyte disturbances.

Rewarming

Rewarming interventions are passive or active, and the latter external or core.

Passive rewarming, such as by blankets, is appropriate only for mild cases (> 33° C).

Active external rewarming: use warming lights, hot water bottles, heating pads, and warmed bags of IV fluid. Immersion in warm baths can be used only if monitoring is not necessary. Be aware of the potential for the "core temperature afterdrop" phenomenon as cool acidemic blood is shunted to the core as rewarming proceeds.

Active core rewarming: this is the most effective method, and should be employed in any case of serious hypothermia. Techniques include: warmed humidified oxygen, IV fluids warmed (to 40° C) for gastric, bladder, and mediastinal lavage. Controlled core rewarming and volume and electrolyte disturbances can be managed most effectively with hemodialysis and extracorporeal blood rewarming, and should be used whenever available.

HEAT ILLNESS

Heat injury and illness can be life-threatening, as in heat stroke, or mildly disabling, as in heat cramps. Most mild to moderate forms of heat illness can be avoided by acclimization and liberal salt and water intake during exercise.

Heat Stroke

Heat stroke is a true emergency, and represents a failure of thermoregulation. Diagnosis is based on an exposure history, a rectal temperature greater than 40° C, and associated neurologic findings. Lack of sweating is *not* a necessary criterion. CNS dysfunction is prominent, along with the symptoms of heat exhaustion, described below. Combativeness and disorientation are common, and in more severe cases, coma, nuchal rigidity, seizures, and posturing are present. Cardiac output can be low, normal, or high. Complications are protean, and include rhabdomyolysis, DIC, myocardial and renal tublar necrosis, hepatic degeneration, ARDS, renal failure, electrolyte derangements, and hepatic degeneration. *After* rapid cooling is begun, consider other differential diagnoses: malignant hyperthermia, infection, or neuroleptic malignant syndrome.

A. Management:

(1) Remove the patient from the heat source.
(2) Stabilize the ABCs.
(3) Immediately begin cooling the patient with ice, cooling fans, cool water mist, or other cooling devices.
(4) Administer crystalloid: LR or NS for poor perfusion, 20 mL/kg initially, and D_5NS for maintenance fluid. Consider CVP determination.
(5) Initiate monitoring and tubes as detailed above (Monitoring).
(6) Perform laboratory tests: Electrolytes, liver function tests, glucose, BUN and creatinine, blood culture, PT/PTT, creatine kinase, serum magnesium, phosphate, calcium, arterial blood gases, and urinalysis.
(7) Admit to a PICU.

Heat Cramps

Heat cramps are brief and self-limited, albeit quite painful. Core temperature is normal or only slightly elevated. Cramping occurs in skeletal or abdominal muscles, but there is no muscle rigidity. Treat mild cases with oral salt-containing fluids; severe cases may require isotonic IV fluid.

Heat Exhaustion

Core temperature is normal or slightly elevated. Constitutional symptoms of weakness, disorientation, nausea and vomiting, poor perfusion, headache, and thirst, with or without muscle cramps, occur after exposure to heat and humidity. Patients continue to sweat, but there should be no major CNS dysfunction. Treat with IV isotonic fluids, modified when electrolyte levels have been determined.

ALTERED MENTAL STATUS/COMA

Many important disease entities present with altered mental status (AMS) as the only clue to their etiology. Optimal outcome is dependent on stabilizing the ABCs and empirically treating for entities that are treatable. For example, if one has already empirically treated the AMS with IV dextrose, no excess morbidity will ensue even when it is not possible to diagnose emergently the myriad etiologies that present with hypoglycemia.

Differential Diagnosis

A useful mnemonic is **"AEIOU TIPS"**:

A: Alcohol

E: Electrolyte disorders (principally sodium)

Encephalopathies (eg, Reye's, infectious, progressive)

Endocrine (eg, DKA, thyrotoxicosis, adrenal crisis)

I: Inborn errors

Intussusception (lethargy may precede any gastrointestinal symptoms)

O: Overdose (sedative/hypnotics, barbiturates, cyclic antidepressants, narcotics, OTC medications, cyanide, many others)

U: Uremia

T: Trauma (head injury, hemorrhagic shock, non-accidental)

I: Insulin (hypo/hyperglycemia)

P: Psychogenic (malingering)

S: Sepsis, stroke, shock, seizures

Management

Even with known ingestions, care is largely supportive. (1) Strict attention to the ABCs is vital. (2) Give 100% oxygen, naloxone 1–2 mg IV, dextrose 0.5–1.0 g/kg (2–4 mL/kg D_{25}), the "AMS cocktail." (3) Obtain a bedside glucose determination as soon as possible. (4) Obtain the *history*: duration of symptoms, fever, trauma, possibility of ingestion and drugs in the home, history suggestive of seizures, headaches, chronic illnesses and symptoms thereof. (5) Conduct a *physical examination*: complete vital signs, which often give clues to ingestions; respiratory pattern, eg, hyperventilation, Cheyne-Stokes, etc; posturing; pupillary size and reactivity; eye movements, including brainstem testing; meningismus; other clues to etiologyranial CT if signs of mass lesion, cerebral edema, or meningitis are present. If CT is normal, proceed with a lumbar puncture. (7) Consider empiric broad-spectrum antibiotics. (8) Frequently reassess and maintain vital functions. (9) Consider consultation with neurologists and toxicologists as indicated.

Pediatric Procedures | 29

Mark G. Roback, MD

Procedures in pediatric patients differ from those in adults in two important respects. First, the patients are smaller, making procedures more difficult technically. Second, pediatric patients are not always able to cooperate by holding still, which can make already difficult procedures even more challenging. This second consideration frequently requires the use of restraints.

Restraining pediatric patients may be effectively accomplished physically or pharmacologically depending on individual circumstances. All restrained patients require cardiorespiratory monitoring. Adequate physical restraint requires able assistants and the use of a papoose board with sheets for bundling. There are a number of medications available for conscious sedation; detailed description is beyond the scope of this chapter.

The goal of any procedure is successful completion while subjecting the patient to the least amount of discomfort possible. Pediatric patients will often display distress secondary to fear even in the face of adequate analgesia. Patient anxiety must be considered and addressed with parents whenever a child receives a procedure.

All procedures require fastidious attention to sterile technique. When povidone-iodine (Betadine) solution is used in the neonate, it must be wiped completely from the skin after the procedure to prevent skin irritation or burns. Universal precautions, including gloves and eye protection, are used at all times.

DIAGNOSTIC SPECIMEN COLLECTION

BLOOD SAMPLING

Venipuncture

A. Indications: Blood sampling for chemistry and hematologic laboratory values, blood culture collection, and venous blood gas determination.

B. Sites: Sites commonly used for pediatric venipuncture include small vessels of the hands and feet which are frequently visualized directly, whereas the antecubital and distal saphenous veins may not be visualized and require location by palpation. The saphenous vein predictably runs along the anterior aspect of the medial malleolus and may be accessed blindly. In infants, scalp veins are usually prominent in the pre- and posterior auricular as well as frontal areas. Venipuncture of femoral and external jugular veins is reserved for emergency situations.

C. Equipment: Butterfly needles (25-, 23-, or 21-gauge) are typically used. The flexible tubing facilitates blood collection when access is difficult. A connector piece adapter may be added to allow the use of a Vacutainer system when large volumes of blood are required. Straight needles connected directly to a syringe, with or without a Vacutainer system, may also be used but are technically more difficult.

D. Procedure: Restrain the child in appropriate fashion and prepare the skin with alcohol. Place a tourniquet or rubber band proximally and insert the needle into the vein directed longitudinally toward the heart. If a syringe is connected to the end of the butterfly tubing, apply minimal negative pressure to avoid collapsing small blood vessels.

1. External Jugular Vein–Place the restrained child in the Trendelenburg position, supine with the head turned to one side and extended slightly over the edge of the table (Figure 29–1). When the patient cries, the vein will be visible, extending from the angle of the jaw toward the midpoint of the clavicle. Prepare the area with alcohol and insert a 23- or 21-gauge butterfly or straight needle connected to a syringe into the vein. Apply constant negative pressure with the syringe to avoid air embolus. Distal skin traction may facilitate entry through the skin of the neck into the vein. After you have removed the needle, have the child sit up, and apply direct pressure to the area for approximately 3–5 minutes.

2. Femoral Vein–In emergency situations the femoral vein may be accessed for blood sampling. The child's leg is held slightly flexed at the hip and rotated externally. Palpate the femoral artery inferiolateral to the inguinal ligament in its position lateral to the femoral vein. Prepare the area with Betadine and alcohol. Using sterile technique, palpate the femoral artery again and enter the femoral vein just medial to the artery (Figure 29–2). Apply pressure for several minutes after completion of blood sampling.

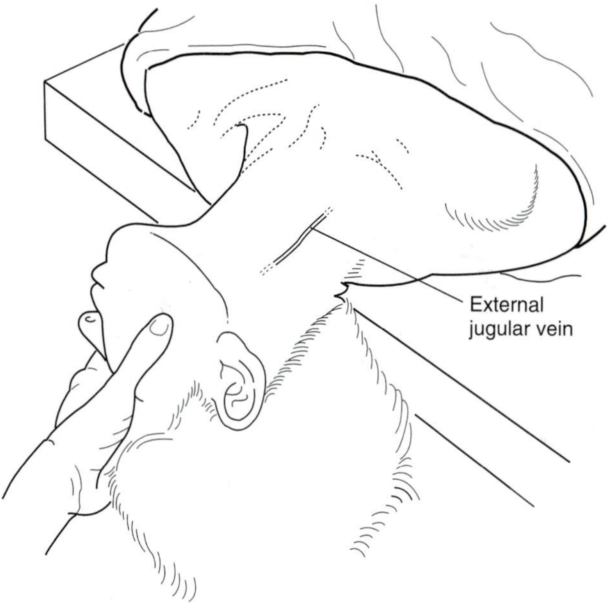

Figure 29–1. External jugular vein procedure.

E. Complications: Complications of venipuncture include infection, hematoma, and local skin irritation. Sampling blood from the external jugular, femoral, and valveless scalp veins increases the possibility of air embolus and requires constant negative pressure while accessing these vessels.

Capillaries

A. Indications: Selected laboratory values may be obtained via capillary vessels in pediatric patients when venous access proves difficult. Electrolytes, glucose, complete blood count, and capillary blood gases may be obtained with certain limitations. Falsely elevated potassium secondary to hemolysis and unreliable pO_2 readings (usually lower than actual) may be expected. Blood cultures should *not* be obtained by this method because of inadequate blood volumes and the risk of contamination.

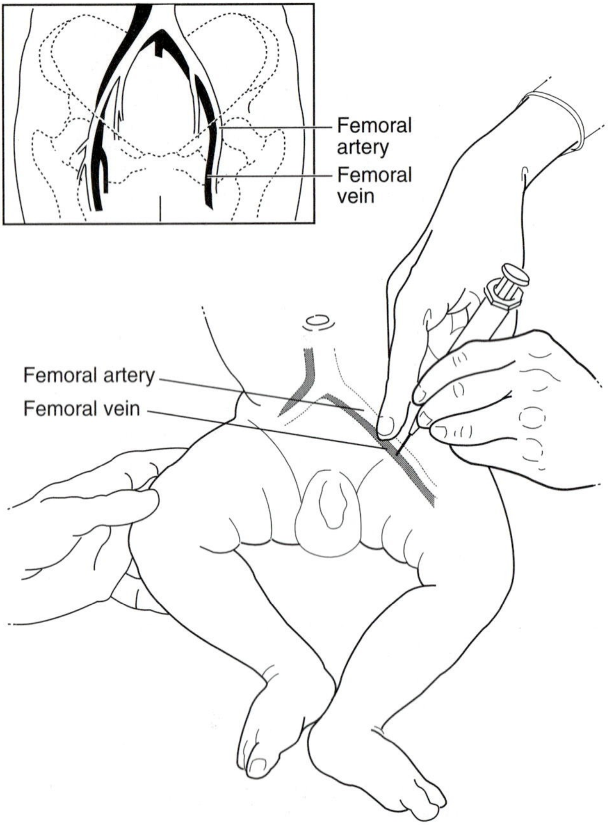

Figure 29–2. Femoral vein procedure.

B. Contraindications: Patients with hypotension or significant vasoconstriction are not candidates for this method. Markedly bruised sites should not be penetrated.

C. Sites: The finger, toe, heel, or ear lobe may be used.

D. Equipment: Puncture the skin with a 3-mm lancet (never use a scalpel blade). Collect the blood with heparinized capillary tubes.

E. Procedure: Before the procedure, the site may be wrapped in warm towels to enhance blood flow through vasodilatation. Clean the site with alcohol wipes and puncture the skin with the 3-mm lancet. Discard the first drop of blood before collecting the specimen in the capillary tube. Do not squeeze the extremity; the pressure will impede blood flow by interfering with capillary refilling, and may dilute the specimen by introducing tissue fluid.

F. Complications: Repeated capillary blood sampling increases the risk of infection, scarring, and calcified nodule formation.

Arterial Blood Sampling

A. Indications: Obtaining blood for arterial blood gas (ABG) determination; inadequacy or difficulty of obtaining capillary specimens.

B. Contraindications: Infection at the site, compromised collateral circulation, bleeding disorder, or previous cutdown at the site.

C. Sites: Sites commonly used include the **radial, dorsalis pedis, temporal,** and **posterior tibial arteries**. The **brachial artery** may be used for blood sampling but is ordinarily avoided because of its anatomic arterial pre-bifurcation position as well as its close proximity to nerves and veins. The **femoral artery** is used *only* during cardiopulmonary resuscitation efforts.

D. Equipment: A 23- or 25-gauge heparinized butterfly needle or standard ABG kit.

E. Procedure: Restrain the patient properly and palpate the artery. After alcohol prep, introduce the needle through the skin and into the artery. Blood will flow briskly from the needle hub. To avoid arterial laceration, do not manipulate the needle laterally while it is in the subcutaneous tissues. Apply direct pressure for a minimum of 5 minutes after completing the procedure.

F. Complications: Possible complications include compromised circulation and injury to associated structures (nerves, veins, and tendons), as well as hematoma, infection, and the formation of arteriovenous fistulae.

URINE SPECIMENS

Bag Specimens

A. Indications: Collection of urine for urinalysis, particularly specific gravity.

B. Procedure: After the skin surrounding the urethra has been cleansed with Betadine or soap and water, a plastic bag with a circular opening and an adhesive covering is positioned around the urethral opening. This technique is of questionable utility for determining the presence of a urinary tract infection (UTI) and is not useful for culture.

C. Complications: Leakage of urine around the adhesion site and local skin irritation.

Clean Catch

A. Indications: Collection of urine for urinalysis and culture in children of an appropriate age, usually over 4 years.

B. Procedure: Retract the foreskin or labia, and clean the area around the distal urethra with Betadine wipes or soap and water. Collect the specimen from a midstream void.

C. Complications: Cooperation is difficult for young children. In addition, contaminated urine specimens are common.

Transurethral Bladder Catheterization

A. Indications: Collection of urine for analysis and culture.

B. Contraindications: In trauma patients, evidence of urethral injury such as blood at the meatus or perineal hematoma; in males, blood in the scrotum or disruption of the prostate detected by rectal examination.

C. Equipment: If a standardized urine catheter kit is not available, a 5- or 8-French sterile feeding tube, for neonates and infants respectively, is used with a sterile drape.

D. Procedure: Unlike the bag and clean catch techniques, transurethral bladder catheterization is a true sterile procedure requiring the use of sterile gloves and equipment. Female patients are held with legs flexed at the hips while males should be in full extension. Separate the labia or hold the penis in a cephalad position, and clean the area around the urethral meatus with betadine and sterile water or saline. (In uncircumcised males, the foreskin must be retracted for prep and replaced on completion). An appropriately sized sterile prelubricated feeding tube is placed through the urethral opening and advanced with slow, steady pressure until urine flow begins. The initial stream of urine is discarded and the remaining sample may be collected for analysis and culture.

If the catheter does not advance readily, it may be pulled back slightly, repositioned, and advanced slowly. *Never* use force to advance the catheter. In males, repositioning the penis may help.

If an indwelling catheter is required, the technique is the same, except that a Foley catheter is used. After urine is obtained, the balloon is inflated using sterile saline in amounts specified on the side of the catheter, and then is pulled back gently to verify placement in the bladder. The catheter is then taped to the thigh and connected to a sterile collecting system.

E. Complications: Injury to the urethra, bleeding, and introduction of infection.

Suprapubic Percutaneous Bladder Aspiration

A. Indications: Collection of urine for analysis and culture, in patients younger than two years but typically infants. Bladder aspiration is the method least likely to yield contaminants; on the other hand, partially-filled bladders are difficult to aspirate.

B. Contraindications: Patients with distended abdomens, previous abdominal surgeries, or bleeding disorders.

C. Site: In the midline, approximately 1 cm superior to the symphysis pubis.

D. Equipment: A 1½-inch, 23-gauge needle attached to a 3-mL syringe.

E. Procedure: The patient is held in the frog-leg position and the suprapubic region is prepared with Betadine. Position the needle and direct it slightly cephalad from perpendicular to the abdominal wall through the midline. Advance the needle firmly while aspirating. If the needle is in the proper location, partial fullness of the bladder is the most common reason for negative aspirations. Repeated attempts are usually unsuccessful.

F. Complications: Bowel penetration and bleeding. Introduction of infection has not been demonstrated using this technique.

CEREBROSPINAL FLUID (CSF)

Lumbar Puncture (LP)

A. Indications: Obtaining CSF for opening and closing pressures, cell count, glucose and protein, cultures, various stains, and special neurologic analyses.

B. Contraindications: Patients with suspected increased intracranial pressure, shock, or infection of the skin at the puncture site.

C. Site: The L4 spinous process located at the midpoint of a line drawn between the posterior superior iliac crests is a good landmark. In older children the spinal cord extends approximately to the level of L2, leaving the interspaces below L2 to the L5-S1 interspace available for puncture. The cord extends to about L3 in infants, thus making interspaces L4-L5 or L5-S1 appropriate for puncture.

D. Equipment: Standardized LP kits contain sterile drapes, collection tubes, and a spinal needle. A 1½-inch, 22-gauge needle is used for infants. For toddlers and younger children, the 22-gauge needle is available in 2½-inch and 3½-inch sizes. A 3½-inch, 20-gauge spinal needle is appropriate for older children and adults. A manometer with a 3-way stopcock is included to obtain opening and closing pressures.

E. Procedure: Careful positioning and adequate patient restraint is essential in successful lumbar punctures. Place the patient on a firm, flat surface in the lateral recumbent position (Figure 29–3). Infants may be held in the sitting position. Hold the patient with the lower back arched. This maneuver widens the lumbar vertebral interspaces and facilitates needle entry into the subarachnoid space. Avoid flexing the patient's neck; this position does not help to open the lumbar interspaces and may impede the patient's airway. Patients receiving this procedure require cardiorespiratory monitoring. Supplemental oxygen must be readily available at all times during this procedure.

Position the patient and identify the puncture site. Prepare the lower back with Betadine; place the sterile drapes using sterile gloves. In patients other than infants, the skin and subcutaneous membranes are usually anesthetized with 1% lidocaine. Position the spinal needle in the midline, bevel up and perpendicular to the back, and direct it slowly through the skin toward the umbilicus until you feel a "pop." This sensation indicates that the needle has penetrated the ligamentum flavum and entered the subarachnoid space. Remove the stylet; clear CSF will flow from the needle hub. If no CSF is elicited, replace the stylet and advance a short distance; or remove the needle and try again.

Complications: The most common complications include bleeding, the "traumatic tap" (perivertebral venous bleeding), and headache in older children. Introduction of infection and epidermoid tumors from using needles without stylets have also been reported.

BONE MARROW

Iliac Crest Aspiration

A. Indications: Diagnostic test in cases of pancytopenia, neutropenia, and idiopathic thrombocytopenia (ITP); and in suspected leukemia, lymphoma, neuroblastoma, or storage disease.

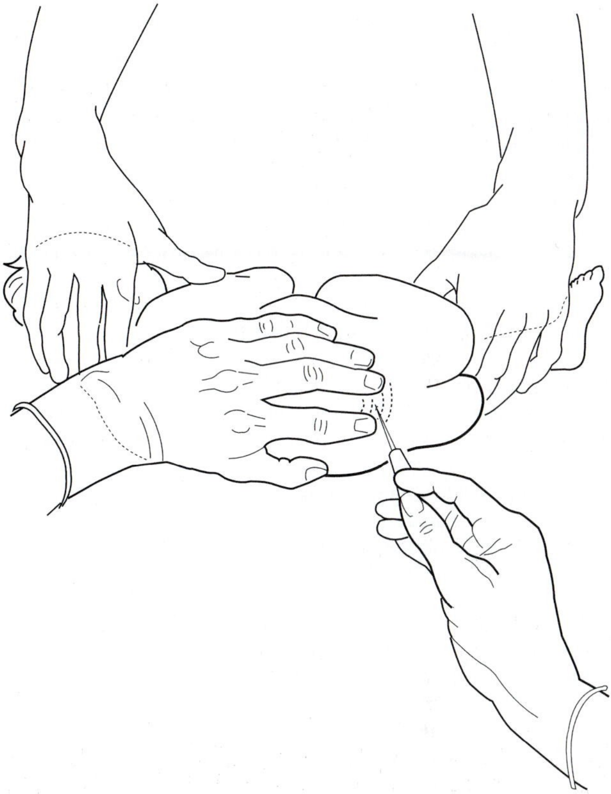

Figure 29–3. Lumbar puncture with assistance of nurse.

B. Contraindications: Infection over the site; or in hemodynamically compromised patients.

C. Sites: The posterior iliac crest is used most frequently for diagnostic purposes.

D. Equipment: Bone marrow needles of various sizes are available, but spinal needles may be used and are sometimes preferred in small infants.

E. Procedure: Anesthetize the skin and tissues down to the periosteum with 1% lidocaine. EMLA (eutectic mixture of lidocaine and prilocaine) cream may be applied 30–45 minutes prior to the procedure to anesthetize the skin. Insert the needle down to the periosteum using a perpendicular approach through the skin and soft tissues. Once the periosteum is reached, apply a twisting downward pressure to penetrate the cortex. At this time remove the stylet. Extract the marrow using a syringe and strong, sustained suction. Smear the marrow sample on a dry glass slide for staining. Remove the needle and apply pressure to the puncture site until bleeding has stopped. Apply a dressing.

F. Complications: Infection and bleeding are most common.

PLEURAL FLUID

Thoracentesis

A. Indications: Sampling of pleural fluid for analysis and culture. Emergent thoracentesis for pneumothorax or hemothorax is discussed under Therapeutic Interventions.

B. Contraindications: Pre-existing skin or chest wall infections should not be punctured.

C. Sites: For pleural fluid aspiration, the posterior axillary line at the seventh intercostal space is located approximately at the tip of the scapula when the arm is raised.

D. Equipment: Attach an 18- or 20- gauge peripheral intravenous catheter (PIV catheter) or 19- to 21-gauge butterfly needle to a 20–60 mL syringe with a 3-way stopcock to facilitate fluid removal.

E. Procedure: The extent of the pleural effusion should be determined using upright chest radiography and ultrasonography when available. Hold the patient in the sitting position or with the pleural effusion side dependent. Prepare the area as for surgery, and anesthetize the skin and subcutaneous tissues down to the pleura with 1% lidocaine. Introduce the needle or PIV catheter into the pleural space by directing the needle over the rib to avoid the inferior vessels and nerves. A hemostat may be clamped to the end of the needle to limit depth of penetration and to avoid parenchymal lung injury. The syringe and 3-way stopcock can be rapidly attached to the needle or PIV catheter to avoid introduction of air and pneumothorax. Large amounts of fluid should be removed at intervals to avoid significant intrapleural fluid and pressure changes. A "dry" tap is one that yields no fluid; in most cases it results from poor positioning, insufficient amounts, or loculated pleural fluid.

F. Complications: Complications include the creation of a pneumothorax or hemothorax secondary to injuring the underlying lung; patients receiving positive pressure ventilation are at increased risk. Introduction of infection and pulmonary edema from rapid removal of large volumes of fluid and excessive pressure changes have been reported.

VASCULAR ACCESS

VENOUS ACCESS

Peripheral Intravenous Catheter (PIV Catheter)

A. Indications: When peripheral intravenous access is required for fluids or medications.

B. Contraindications: Infection at skin puncture site or phlebitis of the vein.

C. Sites: Antecubital and hand veins are usually attempted first, followed by foot and saphenous veins in small children. Scalp veins may be used in infants, while the external jugular (EJ) vein is reserved for emergent access.

D. Equipment: Plastic PIV catheters sized 24- to 20-gauge and 25-gauge butterfly needles for scalp veins are used. Use a 3-mL syringe with a T connector to draw blood through the PIV catheter.

E. Procedure: Immobilize the extremity by taping it to a board prior to entry attempts. PIV catheters consist of a needle inside a plastic catheter. The vein is entered after preparation with alcohol. Blood should accumulate in the catheter hub. While holding the needle steady, advance the catheter and cannulate the vein. Withdraw the needle and attach a 3-mL syringe with T connector for drawing blood or flushing with saline.

1. Scalp Veins–You may use 24-gauge PIV catheters, but you may occasionally need to use a 25-gauge butterfly needle. Place a small rubber band for use as a tourniquet around the patient's head. Cannulate the scalp vein as with a PIV catheter. Advance the needle when blood is visible in the butterfly tubing. Cut the tourniquet. Position the butterfly needle to facilitate infusion; you may need to place a small cotton ball under the butterfly. Tape the apparatus securely to the scalp, using tincture of benzoin to aid adherence.

2. External Jugular (EJ) Vein–Position the patient as described for EJ venipuncture (Figure 29–1). In most cases, a 22- or 20-

gauge PIV catheter is used. Enter and cannulate the vein in the same manner described for other peripheral veins. Tape the apparatus securely. You can expect variations in the infusion flow with changes in the patient's head position.

F. Complications: Extravasation and phlebitis, especially after catheters have been in place a few days; or when large volumes or solute loads (dextrose concentrations > 12.5 gm%) are infused. Tissue necrosis may result.

Percutaneous Central Venous Lines (CVLs)

A. Indications: CVLs are indicated in infants and children receiving long-term parenteral medications or nutrition; for resuscitation; and in patients with limited peripheral venous access.

B. Contraindications: Insertion site infection or burns; known vascular anomalies.

C. Sites: Femoral, subclavian, internal jugular, and **antecubital** veins have been used to enter the central venous circulation in children. This discussion is limited to femoral and antecubital (long-arm) CVLs.

D. Equipment: PIV catheters and CVL catheter kits range in size from 24- to 16-gauge (3–7 French).

E. Procedure:

1. Femoral–Hold the child's leg slightly flexed at the hip and externally rotated. Palpate the femoral artery inferiolateral to the inguinal ligament in its position lateral to the femoral vein. Prepare and drape the area for a surgical procedure. Using strict sterile technique, again palpate the femoral artery. Enter the femoral vein just medial to the artery (Figure 29–2) with a needle, bevel up, connected to a syringe.

If you use the Seldinger technique, insert a wire through the "finder" needle into the vein. Remove the needle. Prepare the site for the catheter with an introducer or vein dilator by inserting the wire through the skin and into the vein. Blood should be readily withdrawn from the catheter hub. Flush the vein with saline and secure the catheter to the leg using 3-0 or 4-0 silk sutures. Obtain a radiograph to confirm catheter position. Another method is to insert a PIV catheter connected to a syringe directly into the vein without using the wire.

2. Antecubital–Long-arm CVL kits contain 18-gauge "breakaway" needles that allow the vein to be entered and cannulated without using a wire. Measure the distance from the insertion site to the patient's right nipple. After sterile prep, draping, and local anesthesia with 1% lidocaine, insert the needle into the vein. Blood flow from the catheter hub confirms position in the vein. Thread the catheter through the needle into the vein to the distance measured. At that point, withdraw the needle from the insertion point and break it away from the catheter. Flush the catheter with saline and secure it in place with tape. Obtain a radiograph to confirm position. The Seldinger wire technique may also be used in a manner similar to that described above for the femoral CVL.

F. Complications: Reported complications of CVLs include infection, ranging from cellulitis and phlebitis to line sepsis, as well as hematomas and edema or thromboses, which may lead to vascular compromise of extremities and air emboli.

Venous Cutdown

A. Indications: When percutaneous vascular access attempts are unsuccessful and rapid venous access is required (eg, resuscitation).

B. Sites: First attempts at venous cutdown usually use the distal saphenous vein as it runs over the anterior aspect of the medial malleolus. The saphenous vein may also be entered in the groin.

C. Equipment: A "cutdown tray" or equivalent with sterile scalpel and blade, fine mosquito hemostat, 3-0 silk ties, and appropriately sized PIV catheters.

D. Procedure: Immobilize leg as shown in Figure 29–4. Prepare and drape the site as for a surgical procedure. Place a tourniquet. Anesthetize the overlying skin using 1% lidocaine. Make a 1-cm transverse incision just through the skin. Using the curved hemostat, isolate 1–2 cm of the vein, using gentle longitudinal (parallel to the vein) blunt dissection. Look for blood flow within the vessel to differentiate the vein from nerves or tendons. Isolate the vein with the hemostat (Figure 29–5) and pull the two silk ties through. Place the ties proximal and distal to the site of catheter insertion. Position the PIV catheter bevel up. Gentle traction on the proximal silk tie will facilitate insertion of the catheter into the vein. Relieve tension on the proximal tie and advance the catheter over the needle. Blood flow from the catheter hub confirms position. If no flow is apparent, release the tourniquet and infuse a small amount of sterile saline. Extravasation of fluid indicates that the catheter is not in the vessel.

Use the proximal tie to secure the catheter in the vein. Tie off the distal vein only if you note excessive bleeding. Close the incision and secure the catheter using 3-0 or 4-0 silk sutures.

E. Complications: Infections of the incision site and phlebitis.

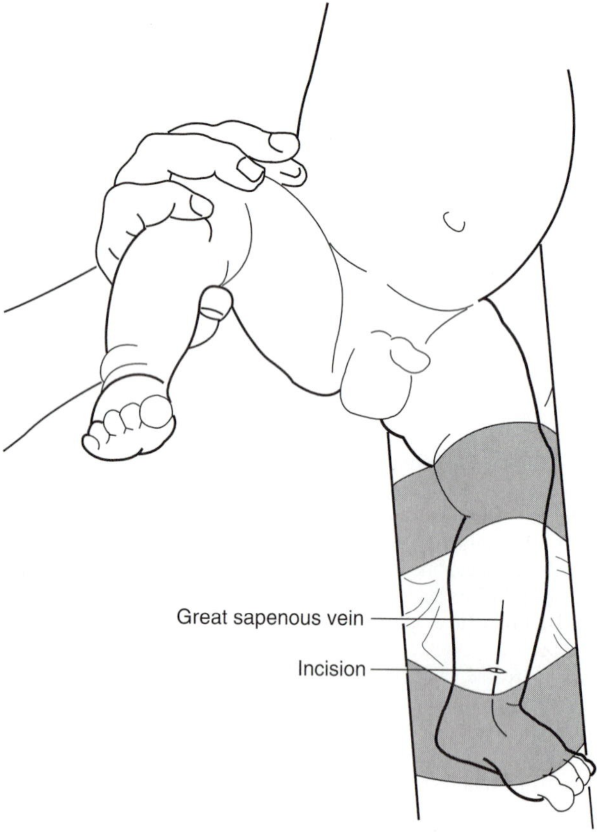

Figure 29–4. Position and taping of leg for venous cutdown.

ARTERIAL ACCESS

Peripheral Arterial Catheter

A. Indications: Continuous blood pressure monitoring and frequent arterial blood sampling.

B. Contraindications: Decreased circulation to the extremity to be catheterized, presence of localized infection, or bleeding disorder.

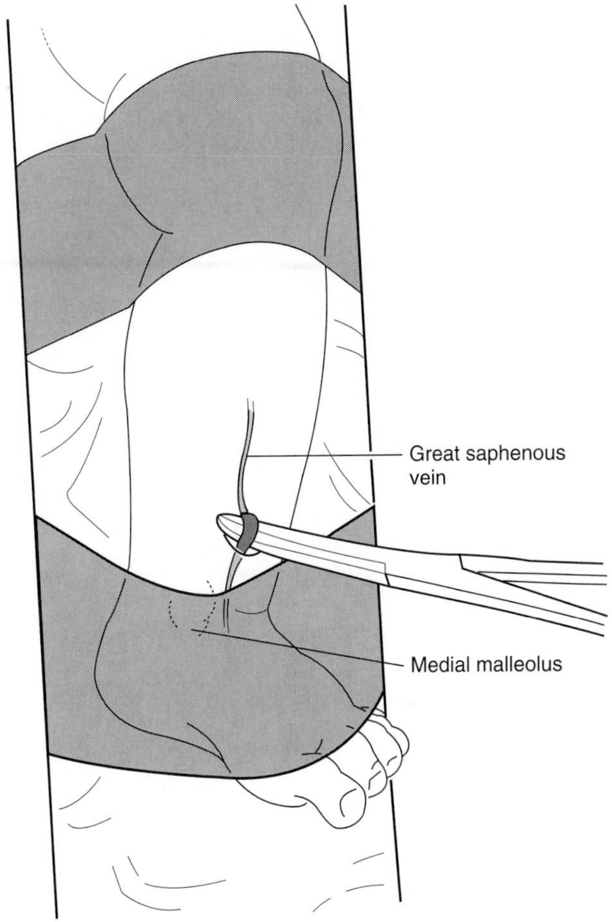

Figure 29–5. Isolation of vein for venous cutdown.

Administration of medications or significant fluid volumes is contraindicated.

C. Sites: The good collateral circulation of the radial and posterior tibial arteries posterior to the medial malleolus makes these vessels the preferred sites for first attempts. You may also use the dorsalis pedis or temporal arteries, but be careful to avoid perfusion compromise. Fiberoptic transilluminators may be used to localize the artery.

D. Equipment: Specific arterial catheter kits are available; however, a 24- or 22-gauge PIV catheter may be used. A T connector and transducer are used for continuous blood pressure monitoring.

E. Procedure: Immobilize the extremity. Prepare the area with Betadine and place a sterile drape. With sterile gloves, palpate the artery and inject a small amount of lidocaine *without* epinephrine just under the skin adjacent to the artery. Position the PIV catheter bevel up at a 45-degree angle to the skin. Insert the catheter into the skin and advance it until blood flows from the hub. If no blood flow is observed, withdraw the catheter slowly in that both sides of the artery may have been pierced. Lower the catheter toward the skin and advance the catheter over the needle. Flush with normal saline, attach the T connector, and secure the catheter with tape or 4-0 silk sutures.

F. Complications: Complications include hemorrhage from the puncture site; thrombus; or spasm leading to occlusion of blood flow to an extremity, infection, air embolus, and nerve damage.

INTRAOSSEOUS (IO) ACCESS

Intraosseous Catheter

A. Indications: IO access is used during cardiopulmonary resuscitation when peripheral venous access has been unsuccessful. IO placement should begin after *no more than two minutes* of attempting PIV access. IO infusion of resuscitation fluids and medications reaches the central circulation rapidly. Crystalloid solutions, blood products, and all drugs may be infused via the IO route.

B. Contraindications: Do not puncture infected skin or attempt to enter bones with preexisting fractures or previous IO punctures.

C. Sites: The preferred site for patients up to 6 years is the proximal tibia, on the flat area just medial and slightly inferior to the tibial tuberosity. Sites appropriate for older children and adults are the medial aspect of the distal femur (Figure 29–6) and the medial aspect of the distal tibia, just proximal to the medial malleolus.

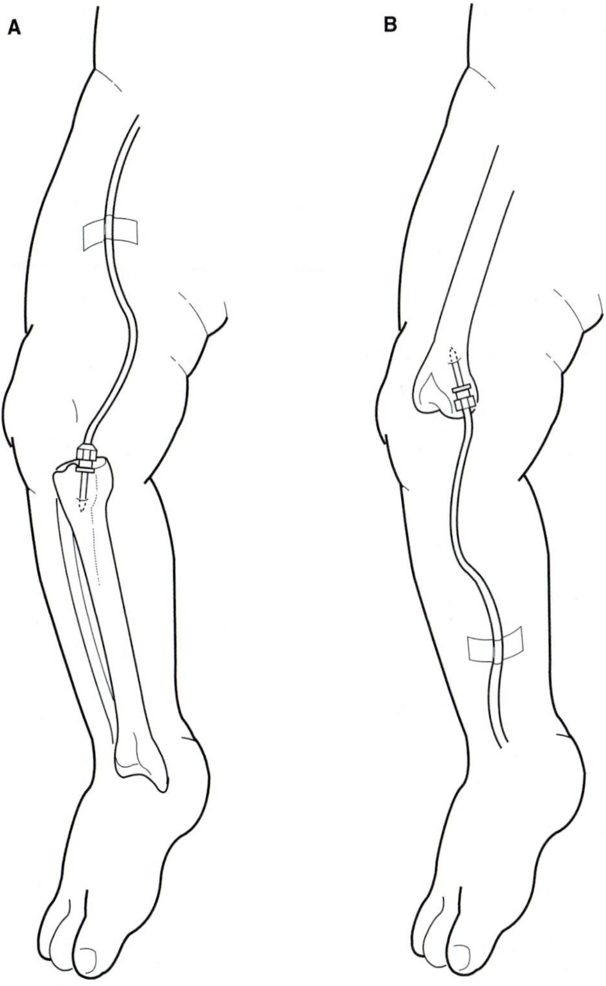

Figure 29–6. Sites for bone marrow infusion. A. Insertion site for an intraosseous tibial line. B. Insertion site for an intraosseous femoral line.

D. Equipment: Age-appropriate IO needles with stylets are preferred, but any large-bore needle may be used. Needle sizes used for infants and small children are 20- or 18-gauge; older children require 16- or 14-gauge needles. Avoid long needles that are easily dislodged.

E. Procedure: Restrain conscious patients securely; use local anesthetic. Prepare the area with Betadine and wipe clean with alcohol. Hold the needle firmly and direct it almost perpendicular to the bone, with a slight deviation away from the growth plate. Apply steady pressure using a slight twisting motion until you penetrate the bone cortex; you will then feel a giving or yielding sensation. Further downward pressure may lead to penetration of the opposite bony cortex and result in infusion of soft tissues.

F. Complications: Extravasation of fluid from the puncture site is a frequent complication and may lead to skin sloughing if sclerosing agents are infused. Cellulitis, osteomyelitis, and bony fracture occur rarely. Improper needle positioning may lead to growth plate injury and impaired bone development. Fat embolism has been reported only in adults.

UMBILICAL VESSEL CATHETERIZATION

Umbilical Vein Catheter

A. Indications: Used for intravenous access in the resuscitation of newborns; may also be used for exchange transfusions.

B. Contraindications: This procedure is contraindicated in patients over one week of age, or who have been discharged from the hospital after birth.

C. Sites: Thin-walled larger single vein of the umbilical stump.

D. Equipment: Umbilical catheters range from 3.5 to 8.0 French. You will also need sterile umbilical tape, a curved hemostat, and curved iris forceps without teeth.

E. Procedure: Keep the infant under a radiant warmer. Restrain the infant and prepare the area as for a surgical procedure. Place umbilical tape or a pursestring suture around the base of the umbilical cord. Cut the cord 3–5 mm from the base. Determine desired position of catheter. Low placement is used for resuscitation and exchange transfusion; the catheter is positioned in the vein just deeply enough for blood return. High placement refers to the position of the catheter tip in the vena cava above the diaphragm to avoid the ductus venosus, portal vein, and hepatic veins. Measure the distance in centimeters from the shoulder to the level of the umbilicus and add the length of

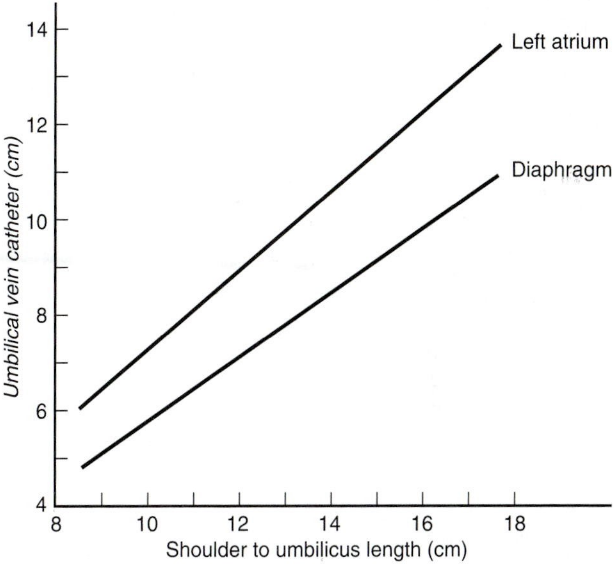

Figure 29–7. Relationship between length of umbilical venous catheter placed and shoulder-umbilicus length in an infant. (Adapted from Dunn P: Arch Dis Child 1966;41:71.)

the umbilical stump. Use Figure 29–7 to determine the length of catheter required. Flush the catheter with heparinized saline.

Identify the vein and remove any clots with the iris forceps. Use the hemostat to hold the umbilicus in position to facilitate vein cannulization. Advance the catheter to desired position; you should be able to withdraw blood easily. Obtain an x-ray to confirm catheter position. Secure the catheter to the umbilical stump with 3-0 silk sutures.

F. Complications: Vessel perforation, hemorrhage, infection, air embolus, vasospasm and hepatic injury secondary to infusion of sclerosing solutions or portal vein thrombosis.

Umbilical Artery Catheter

A. Indications: Frequent blood sampling in newborns.

B. Contraindications: Same as umbilical vein.

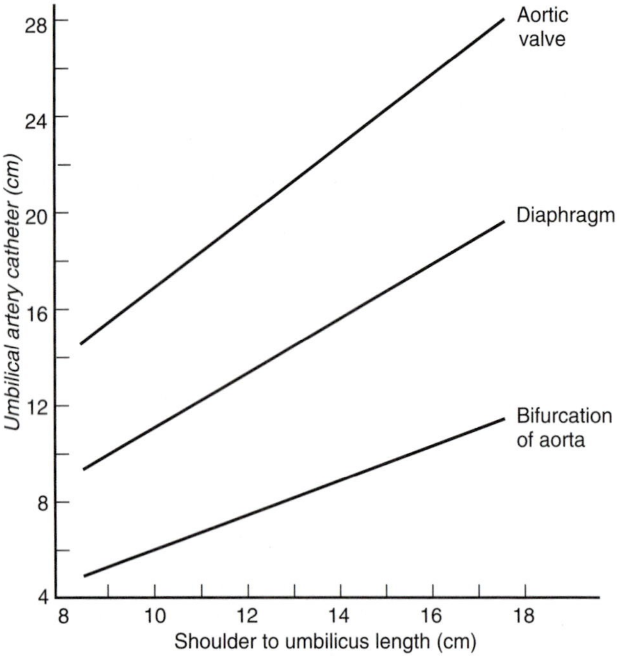

Figure 29–8. Relationship between length of umbilical artery catheter placed and shoulder-umbilicus length in an infant. (Adapted from Dunn P: Arch Dis Child 1966;41:73.)

C. Sites: Thick-walled, usually paired arteries of the umbilical stump.

D. Equipment: Same as for umbilical vein access, except that umbilical artery catheters are 3.5 and 5 French.

E. Procedure: Similar to that for the umbilical vein. Determine the desired position of the catheter. Low placement positions the catheter tip just below the aortic bifurcation (L3–L4). High placement refers to catheter tip position in the thoracic aorta (T6–T9). measure the distance in centimeters from the shoulder to the level of the umbilicus and add the length of the umbilical stump. Use Figure 29–8 to calculate the length of the catheter required.

Dilate the artery gently, using the toothless iris forceps prior to cannulation. Use the hemostat to apply cephalad traction to the cord and advance the catheter toward the feet. When the desired position is obtained, confirm catheter placement with an x-ray. Secure the catheter with 3-0 silk sutures.

F. Complications: Vessel perforation, hemorrhage, infection, air embolus, vasospasm, hypertension, and thromboembolic events to kidneys, gastrointestinal tract, and lower extremities.

THERAPEUTIC INTERVENTIONS

Thoracentesis

A. Indications: Emergent removal of air or blood in pneumothorax or tension pneumothorax and hemothorax. Quantities of pleural fluid large enough to result in respiratory compromise may also require emergent therapeutic thoracentesis.

B. Contraindications: Avoid infected areas of the skin and chest wall.

C. Site: The site for emergent air removal in the supine patient is the second or third intercostal space in the midclavicular line. The anterior axillary or mid-axillary line in the fourth or fifth interspace may also be used. Removal of pleural fluid or blood is best accomplished with the patient sitting; however, in hemodynamically unstable patients, the fourth or fifth intercostal space in the midaxillary line may be punctured with the patient supine.

D. Equipment: You will need a 19- or 21-gauge butterfly needle attached to a 20–60-mL syringe with a 3-way stopcock, to facilitate air or fluid removal.

E. Procedure: The basic procedure for thoracentesis is discussed under Diagnostic Specimen Collection. Enter the pleural cavity by inserting a needle over the appropriate rib until you detect a rush of air or fluid. *Always* direct the needle over the superior aspect of the rib to avoid damage to the neurovascular bundle. Be careful to avoid laceration of the lung parenchyma. When tension pneumothorax or hemothorax is suspected, preparations should be made for immediate chest tube placement after thoracentesis has been performed.

F. Complications: See the discussion of thoracentesis under Diagnostic Specimen Collection.

Table 29–1. Instrument sizes for pediatric procedures.

Age	Butterfly Needle gauge	PIV Catheter gauge	Spinal Needle gauge	Spinal Needle length (inches)	I0 Needle gauge	Foley Catheter French	Chest Tube French
Preterm	25	24	22	1½	20	5	10
Newborn	25 or 23	24 or 22	22	1½	20	5	10–12
1–6 mo	23	22	22	1½	20	8	10–12
6–12 mo	23	22	22	1½	20 or 18	8	12–20
1–2 yr	23	22	22	1½ or 2½	18	8–10	16–20
2–4 yr	23	22	22	2½	18	10	20–24
4–6 yr	23	22	22	2½	18 or 16	10	24–28
6–8 yr	23	22	22	2½	16	10	28
8–10 yr	23	22	22	2½ or 3½	16	10–12	28–32
10–12 yr	23 or 21	22 or 20	22 or 20	3½	16 or 14		32
12–14 yr	21	20	20	3½	14	12	32–36
14–adult	21	20 or 18	20	3½	14	12	36–42

Chest Tube Placement

A. Indications: Definitive treatment for pneumothorax or tension pneumothorax and hemothorax. Used to remove recurrent pleural effusions and empyemas.

B. Contraindications: Bleeding disorders or situations which require surgical intervention.

C. Sites: The sites most commonly used are the second intercostal space in the midclavicular line and the fourth or fifth intercostal space in the midaxillary line.

D. Equipment: You will need a chest tube tray containing a scalpel with No. 10 blade, large and small curved clamps, straight and curved scissors, and a needle holder. Sterile drapes, syringes, needles for anesthetic infiltration, a properly sized chest tube (Table 29–1), tubing, and a drainage system are also required.

E. Procedure: Wear a surgical gown, gloves, and goggles. Restrain the patient adequately, prepare and drape the site as for a surgical procedure. Anesthetize the tissues in layers; include the skin, subcutaneous tissues, muscle, periosteum, and parietal pleura. It is important to provide adequate anesthesia; however, do not use more than 5 mg/kg of lidocaine.

Make a 2–3 cm transverse incision, one rib below the desired site of entry. With a curved clamp, tunnel upwards over the rib superior to the insertion site by firmly spreading the subcutaneous layers. This "tissue tunnel" will help to prevent air leak.

When you reach the muscle overlying the appropriate intercostal space, firmly push the clamp over the rib and into the pleural space. Remove the clamp and place a gloved finger through the opening into the pleural space. Use a sweeping motion to feel for and break down loculations or adhesions.

Clamp the proper sized chest tube (Table 29–1) distal to the last air hole. Using another curved clamp, grasp the proximal end of the tube longitudinally between the jaws of the clamp and follow the gloved finger into the pleural space. Remove the clamp and direct the tube toward the apex of the lung. Advance the tube until all holes are within the pleural space.

Hold the tube in place securely and attach the tubing immediately to a drainage system. Release the clamp attached to the tube. Secure the tube with 1-0 silk pursestring sutures. Confirm tube position by chest x-ray. Cover with an occlusive dressing.

F. Complications: Infection and hematoma at the incision site, empyema, pneumonia, and atelectasis may occur. The incidence of complications is related to the length of time of chest tube placement.

30 | Poisons & Toxins

Richard C. Dart, MD, PhD,
& Barry H. Rumack, MD

Over 1.9 million cases of poisoning were reported to the American Association of Poison Control Centers in 1994, and approximately 60% of those were children under 6 years of age. The most frequent causes of poisoning (each accounting for about 8–9% of the total) were cleaning substances, plants, and analgesics.

Accidents involving household poisons, especially in children under the age of 5, can be attributed to 4 main factors: improper storage, failure to return a poison to its proper place, failure to read the label properly, and failure to recognize the substance as poisonous. It is clearly the responsibility of a parent to create a safe environment for the child.

Although many common exposures do not result in serious symptoms, the child who survives the ingestion of a highly toxic poison may be permanently disabled. Disabilities may include esoph-ageal stricture after ingestion of lye, permanent liver or kidney damage after ingestion of poisons such as chlorinated hydrocarbons, or sequelae of hypoxic brain injury from poison-induced respiratory insufficiency. Table 30–1 lists the symptoms and signs of acute poisoning for various toxins.

GENERAL MANAGEMENT OF POISONINGS

Prophylaxis

Instructions in poison prevention and poison-proofing of homes should be given to the parents prior to or during the child's 6-month checkup. Before the child begins climbing or walking, the danger of storing pharmaceuticals in the medicine cabinet should be discussed, and other areas of storage should also be investigated. Parents should be asked about the contents of such areas as under the sink (drain cleaners), kitchen pantries (cleaning supplies), bathroom cabinets (medicines, antiseptics), basements and utility rooms (paints, thinners, salt), garage (antifreeze, automotive supplies), storage sheds (pesticides, herbicides), and laundry rooms (detergents, ammonia, fabric softeners).

Table 30–1. Symptoms and signs of acute poisoning by various substances.[1]

Symptoms and Signs	Substance or Other Cause
Alopecia	Thallium, arsenic, selenium, radiation sickness.
Blood changes	
Anemia	Lead, naphthalene, chlorates, favism, solanine and other plant poisons, snake venom.
Cherry-red blood	Cyanide. (The lips in carbon monoxide poisoning are usually dusky and not cherry-red.)
Hematuria or hemoglobinuria	Heavy metals, naphthalene, nitrates, chlorates, favism, solanine, and other plant poisons.
Hemorrhage	Warfarin, thallium, snake venom.
Methemoglobinemia	Nitrates, nitrites, aniline dyes, methylene blue, chlorates, pyridium.
Breath odors	
Bitter almond	Cyanide (Odor only detected by 40% of people.)
Garlic	Arsenic, phosphorus, organic phosphate, selenium.
Burns of skin and mucous membranes	Lye, hypochlorite, phenol, sodium bisulfate, etc.
Cyanosis	Barbiturates, opiates, nitrites, aniline dyes, chlorates.
Eye manifestations	
Lacrimation	Organic phosphates, nicotine, mushrooms, riot agents.
Ptosis	Botulism, thallium.
Pupillary constriction	Opiates, parathion and other organic phosphates, mushrooms and some other plant poisons.
Pupillary dilatation	Atropine, nicotine, antihistamines, phenylephrine, mushrooms, thallium, oleander.
Strabismus	Botulism, thallium.
Visual disturbances	Atropine, parathion and other organic phosphates, botulism.

(*continued*)

Table 30–1. Symptoms and signs of acute poisoning by various substances (*continued*).[1]

Symptoms and Signs	Substance or Other Cause
Fever	Atropine, salicylates, food poisoning, antihistamines, tranquilizers, camphor.
Flushing	Atropine, antihistamines, tranquilizers.
Gastrointestinal tract symptoms	
Abdominal cramps	Corrosive substances, food poisoning, lead, arsenic, black widow spider bite, boric acid, carbon tetrachloride, organic phosphates, phosphorus, nicotine, castor beans, fluorides, thallium.
Diarrhea	Food poisoning, iron, organic phosphates, arsenic, napththalene, castor beans, mercury, boric acid, thallium, nicotine, nitrates, solanine and other plant poisons, mushrooms.
Dry mouth	Atropine, antihistamines, ephedrine, furosemide.
Hematemesis	Corrosive substances, warfarin, aminophyline, fluorides.
Stomatis	Corrosive substances, heavy metals.
Vomiting	Aminophyline, food poisoning, organic phosphates, nicotine, digitalis, arsenic, boric acid, lead, mercury, iron, phosphorus, thallium, DDT, dieldrin, nitrates, castor beans, mushrooms, oleander, naphthalene.
Headache	Carbon monoxide, organic phosphates, atropine, lead, dieldrin, carbon tetrachloride.
Heart abnormalities	
Bradycardia	Digitalis, mushrooms, organic phosphates, beta blocker, calcium channel blocker.
Tachycardia	Atropine, tricyclic antidepressants, stimulants.
Other irregularities of rhythm	Nitrates, oleander.
Jaundice	Phosphorus, chlordane, favism, mushrooms, acetaminophen.

(*continued*)

Table 30–1. Symptoms and signs of acute poisoning by various substances (*continued*).[1]

Symptoms and Signs	Substance or Other Cause
Muscle involvement	
Cramps	Lead, black widow spider bite.
Spasm or dystonia	Phenothiazines, scorpion sting, strychnine.
Nervous system involvement	
Ataxia	Lead, organic phosphates, antihistamines, thallium, sedative-hypnotics.
Coma	Barbiturates, carbon monoxide, cyanide, opiates, ethyl alcohol, salicylates, hydrocarbons, parathion and other organic phosphates, lead, mercury, boric acid, antihistamines, digitalis, mushrooms.
Convulsions	Aminophyline, amphetamine and other stimulants, atropine, camphor, boric acid, lead, mercury, parathion and other organic phosphates, nicotine, phenothiazines, antihistamines, arsenic, DDT, dieldrin, kerosene, fluorides, nitrates, barbiturates, digitalis, salicylates, solanine and other plant poisons, thallium.
Delirium	Aminophyline, antihistamines, atropine, salicylates, lead, barbiturates, boric acid.
Depression	Barbiturates, kerosene, tranquilizers, arsenic, lead, boric acid, DDT, naphthalene.
Mental confusion	Alcohol, barbiturates, atropine, nicotine, antihistamines, carbon tetrachloride, mercury, digitalis, mushrooms.
Paresthesias	DDT, heavy metals.
Weakness	Organic phosphates, arsenic, lead, nicotine, thallium, nitrates, fluorides, botulism.
Pallor	Lead, naphthalene, chlorates, favism, solanine and other plant poisons, fluorides.

(*continued*)

Table 30–1. Symptoms and signs of acute poisoning by various substances (*continued*).[1]

Symptoms and Signs	Substance or Other Cause
Proteinuria	Arsenic, mercury, phosphorus.
Respiratory tract symptoms	
Aspiration pneumonia	Kerosene.
Cough	Hydrocarbons, mercury vapor, chlorine.
Respiratory difficulty	Barbiturates, opiates, salicylates, ethyl alcohol, organic phosphates, dieldrin.
Respiratory failure	Cyanide, carbon monoxide, antihistamines, thallium, fluorides.
Respiratory stimulation	Salicylates, amphetamine and other stimulants, atropine, mushrooms.
Salivation and sweating	Parathion and other organic phosphates, muscarine and other mushroom poisoning, nicotine.
Skin erythema	Boric acid.

[1] Adapted from Arana JM: The clinical diagnosis of poison. *Pediatr Clin North Am* 1970;17:477.

Other poison-proofing questions include: Has there been ample provision for locked storage? How should medicines and products be disposed of safely? How should containers be labeled, especially if the product is taken from its original container? What are the best methods of dealing with a child's normal investigation of the environment that may lead to tasting or handling toxic substances?

Treatment issues should also be discussed. Do the parents know of the use of activated charcoal and syrup of ipecac? They should be given the phone number of the local poison center, and urged to obtain poison prevention literature. The physician should provide (or prescribe) a 1-oz bottle of syrup of ipecac for the parent.

Poison prevention is important. The peak age of accidental poisoning is 2 years. If a child ingests a poison, there is a 56% chance of a repeat poisoning in the family within 1 year. When repeated exposures to toxic substances occur, child battering or neglect should be considered.

Diagnosis

Most childhood exposures are not intentional ingestions. Rather, the child "textures" and "tastes" the poison using his or her mouth. Ninety-five percent of all childhood exposures do not result in serious symptoms, most probably because the amount ingested is quite small. In the absence of a definite history of ingestion or of contact with a toxic substance, the diagnosis of poisoning versus another childhood illness presents many difficulties. Most of the symptoms of poisoning are not diagnostic, but certain clues to the presence of an unsuspected poisoning are included below.

A. History: The child is frequently found near the source of the poison. Product containers should be brought to the office or hospital, since the ingredients are often listed on the labels. The physician should call the nearest poison center or manufacturer in cases of exposure, since product formulation and treatment may have changed since the time the label was printed. Poison centers can also be of help if the label does not have specific ingredients. Unfortunately, the initial history correlates with the actual agent ingested less than half the time. It is best to compare the clinical condition of the patient with the probable signs and symptoms of poisoning using a recognized reference, such as the POISINDEX Information System.

B. Symptoms & Signs: The signs and symptoms may vary greatly depending upon what toxic substances are involved in the exposure. Table 30–1 gives examples of common symptoms seen with various toxic agents.

C. Laboratory Findings: Evidence may be obtained from the appearance, smell, or chemical analysis of blood, urine, vomitus, gastric washings, or fat obtained by biopsy. Occasionally, characteristic odors of poisons may be detected on the patient's breath. Blood in vomitus or stool may suggest the ingestion of a strong irritant or corrosive. Other specialized tests are available for specific agents.

D. X-ray Findings: Various x-rays may be helpful. Just a few examples would include location of swallowed coins or other radiopaque pharmaceuticals and foreign objects, x-rays of bones to evaluate chronic lead and bismuth poisoning, and evaluation of pulmonary edema from aspiration of hydrocarbons.

EMERGENCY TREATMENT
(See Table 30–2.)

Emergency care should be supervised by a physician in a hospital, where complete facilities and antidotes are available. Consultation with a certified regional poison center is highly recommended for confusing or difficult cases.

Table 30–2. Emergency treatment for poisoning.

Ingested Poisons

1. Syrup of ipecac may be useful in all cases except corrosives, (ongoing or impending) coma, or seizures.
2. Lavage only if semiconscious or in coma. Endotracheal tube is inserted in larger children.
3. Activated charcoal.
4. Dilute ingested chemicals with water. *Do not* give fluids to dilute ingested medications.

Inhaled Irritants

1. Oxygen therapy.
2. Mouth-to-mouth resuscitation.
3. Humidity.
4. Observe for pneumonitis and pulmonary edema.

Local Irritants

1. Copious water irrigation.
2. Careful eye examination.
3. No chemical "antidotes."

Available Consultants

1. Poison control centers.
2. State health departments.
3. Medical center consultants.
4. Pharmaceutical houses.
5. US agricultural office.
6. Medical examiner (coroner's office, toxicologist).

Specific "Antidote" Treatment Available

1. Amphetamines (see p 956).
2. Arsenic (see p 957).
3. Belladona derivatives (see p 959).
4. Carbon monoxide (see p 961).
5. Cyanide (see p 962).
6. Ferrous sulfate (see p 963).
7. Mercury (see p 967).
8. Narcotics (see p 971).
9. Nitrites and nitrates (see p 971).
10. Phosphates, organic (see p 974).
11. Snake bites (see p 977).
12. Spider bites (see p 978).
13. Tricyclic antidepressants (see p 979).

Ingested Poisons

Speed is essential for effective therapy. The choice of which method to use is not always clear. Induced vomiting is much more effective than lavage with a small-bore nasogastric tube; however, a large-bore nasogastric tube is more effective than emesis.

A. Emesis in the Home: Contraindications to emesis include absent gag reflex, coma, convulsions, and ingestion of strong acids, strong bases, or sharp objects. Emesis should not be induced in patients who may develop altered mental status. Since the induction of emesis may be delayed 30 minutes or more, it is important to instruct the parents on the use of ipecac as early as possible. Syrup of ipecac can be used to induce emesis at a dose of 30 mL for a child 40–45 kg or greater, 15 mL for a child 1–12 years old, and 5–10 mL in a child 6–12 months old (consider administering this dose in a health care facility only). After the dose has been given, the child should be encouraged to drink 4–6 oz of clear fluid, and then should be ambulated. This dose may be repeated once if emesis does not occur within 30 minutes. *Do not* administer more than 30 mL of syrup of ipecac to a young child. *Do not* use mustard water, salt water, or gag a child with a spoon. Consult your local poison center to determine whether or not it is necessary to send the child to a health care facility after emesis. In many cases it will be important to send the child to the hospital whether or not vomiting has occurred. If vomiting has occurred, have the parents recover the regurgitated vomitus in a pan for later analysis.

B. Emesis in the Hospital: Administer syrup of ipecac as outlined above. The use of syrup of ipecac produces an average recovery of 30% of the ingested agent.

C. Lavage: The use of gastric lavage is recommended if performed soon after ingestion, or in comatose or convulsing patients. The patient's airway should be protected by placement in the Trendelenburg and left lateral decubitus position with suction available. In unconscious patients, cuffed, endotracheal intubation is recommended. In children over age 5, lavage should be done with 150–200 mL of lukewarm tap water or saline per wash. In younger children, 50–100 mL of normal saline per wash should be used. Lavage should continue until the return is clear. The amount of fluid returned in the lavage should approximate the amount of fluid given to avoid fluid-electrolyte imbalance.

D. Activated Charcoal: This material has a large surface area on which to adsorb various toxins. Additives such as cherry syrup, ice cream, milk, and cocoa powder or chocolate milk should only be used when there is no other way of getting the child to take the charcoal. In patients with a nasogastric tube in place, use the tube to place the charcoal in the child's stomach. Sorbitol and bentonite do not appear to alter the adsorptive capacity of charcoal.

The most common use of activated charcoal is as a single dose. The dose in children is 15–30 g, with some authors suggesting 1–2 g/kg as a rough guideline, especially in infants. The FDA suggests a minimal dilution of 240 mL of water per 20–30 g of activated charcoal given as an aqueous slurry. A maximum dose has not been recommended. For some poisons, a repeated oral dose of charcoal may enhance total body clearance. A saline cathartic or sorbitol can be given with the first dose, but multiple cathartic doses with charcoal may cause life-threatening complications. When large doses are required and the patient is unable to hold the charcoal down, continuous nasogastric infusion of 0.25–0.5 g/kg/hr. may be successful in ameliorating the vomiting associated with charcoal administration.

Activated charcoal is not absorbed orally, but adverse reactions have occurred, including black stools, vomiting (12–16%), constipation, gastrointestinal obstruction, aspiration pneumonitis, and emphysema.

There are certain classes of poisons in which activated charcoal may not be useful. Small molecular weight agents such as ions (iron, lithium) are not adsorbed effectively. When given with a corrosive, it may cause vomiting, which could cause further damage to esophageal mucous membranes. When given with hydrocarbons, charcoal may cause vomiting, which could lead to aspiration.

E. Catharsis: The dose of the saline cathartics magnesium of sodium sulfate is 250 mg/kg, and the dose of magnesium citrate is 4 mL/kg up to 300 mL per dose. Usually only one dose of a saline cathartic is administered. Sorbitol is also used as a cathartic, both alone and combined with activated charcoal. In a child over 1 year of age, 1 0–1.5 g/kg per dose as a 35% solution may be administered up to a maximum of 50 g per dose. It is best to administer sorbitol in a health care facility so fluids and electrolyte status can be monitored.

Surface Poisons

Remove poisons by washing the area with large volumes of water or soap and water. In cases involving water-insoluble substances, the solubility of that compound in various solvents should be checked before recommending large areas of the skin be washed with alcohol or various hydrocarbons. These substances may defat the skin, and may present more hazard than the toxin itself. *Caution: Do not* use chemical antidotes. Neutralization with liberated heat during the reaction may actually increase the extent of injury.

Inhaled Poisons

Patients exposed to toxic inhalants should be removed from exposure, monitored for respiratory distress, and given emergency airway support, 100% humidified supplemental oxygen with assisted ventilation, or both, as required.

MANAGEMENT OF SPECIFIC COMMON TYPES OF POISONING IN CHILDREN

ACETAMINOPHEN

In large overdose, this commonly used analgesic-antipyretic may produce hepatotoxicity. Because of differences in metabolism, children under age 12 are unlikely to suffer hepatotoxicity even if plasma levels of the drug are in the toxic range. Children over age 12 may develop hepatotoxicity if untreated and if plasma levels are in the toxic range (Figure 30–1).

Symptoms during the first 24 hours may include nausea, vomiting, diaphoresis, and malaise. Coma and metabolic acidosis have been seen. If the patient is not treated, hepatotoxicity may be observed via laboratory tests at approximately 36 hours, with peak AST (SGOT), ALT (SGPT), bilirubin levels, and prothrombin time occurring by 3 days. This hepatotoxic event is transient, and even in children with AST levels as high as 20,000 IU/L, discharge from the hospital with no sequelae usually occurs by the seventh day.

The plasma drug level should be determined 4 or more hours after ingestion, when it will have reached its peak. This assumes there is no further absorption. If the level is in the toxic range, treatment with the antidote must be initiated.

Treatment

Emesis or lavage should be performed upon arrival at the emergency care facility. In general, activated charcoal should be administered in the first 4 hours to ensure the amount of acetaminophen absorbed is small. N-acetylcysteine (Mucomyst), which is antidotal for acetaminophen, does bind to charcoal; the degree of absorption is not clinically significant.

ACIDS, CORROSIVES

The strong mineral acids exert primarily a local corrosive effect on the skin and mucous membranes. Classically, acids cause oral and gastric burns, but seldom produce esophageal damage. The majority of these burns resolve. However, pyloric constriction with obstruction and vomiting may occur at 3 weeks. This response is

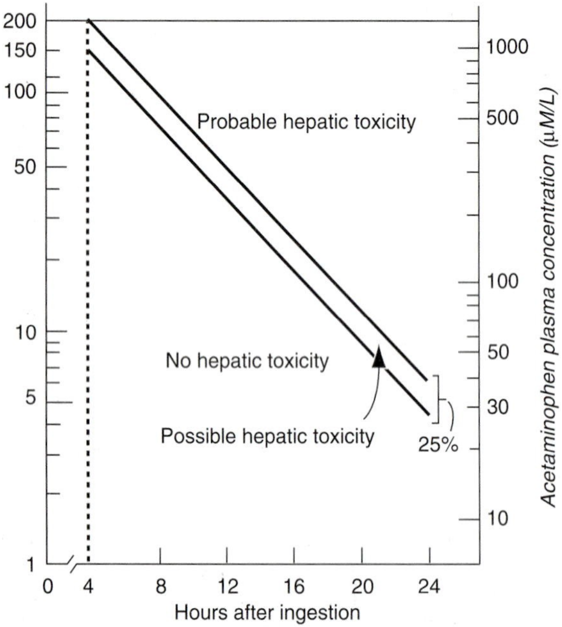

Figure 30–1. Semilogarithmic plot of plasma acetaminophen levels vs. time (Rumack-Matthew nomogram for acetaminophen poisoning). *Cautions for use of this chart:* (1) The time coordinates refer to time of ingestion. (2) Serum levels drawn before 4 hours may not represent peak levels. (3) The graph should be used only in relation to a single acute ingestion. (4) The lower solid line 25% below the standard nomogram is included to allow for possible errors in acetaminophen plasma assays and estimated time from ingestion of an overdose. (Adapted with permission from Rumack BH, Matthew H: Acetaminophen poisoning and toxicity. *Pediatrics* 1975;**55:**871. Copyright Midromedex Inc, 1974–1989.)

thought to be due to pylorospasm occurring immediately after ingestion, which traps the acid in this area and produces a more significant burn.

Symptoms include severe pain in the throat and upper gastrointestinal tract; marked thirst; bloody vomitus; difficulty in swallowing, breathing, and speaking; discoloration and destruction of skin and mucous membranes in and around the mouth; collapse; and shock. Milder burns may result in fewer symptoms but serious sequelae are still possible.

Eye contact may produce severe pain, swelling, corneal erosions, and in some severe cases, blindness. Normally, brief exposures to acidic solutions with a pH of greater than 2 produce no injury to the corneal epithelium. Inhalation of acidic agents may produce dyspnea, chest pain, and pulmonary edema. Bronchospasm and hypoxemia may result.

Treatment

Do not give emetics or lavage. Dilute the acid immediately with 4–8 oz (not over 15 mL/kg) of water or milk. Avoid carbonates or bicarbonates internally, since they may form gas and cause distension of a weakened stomach wall. Do not administer other alkaline or neutralizing agents. Diagnostic endoscopy may be performed as indicated within the first 12–24 hours. This procedure may help grade the extent of damage and predict the necessity of further treatment. The use of steroids is debatable.

ALCOHOL, ETHYL

Incoordination, slow reaction time, blurred vision, staggering gait, slurred speech, hypoglycemia, convulsions, and coma are the potential manifestations of overdosage. The diagnosis of alcoholic intoxication is commonly overlooked in children.

Treatment

Supportive treatment and aggressive management of any degree of hypoglycemia are usually the only treatments required.

AMPHETAMINES

Acute ingestion results in initial hypertension, hyperpyrexia, and hyperactivity. Extreme, unmanageable hyperactivity and anxiety, as well as flushing, various cardiac arrhythmias, cardiac pain, convulsions, and eventual circulatory collapse may occur. Gastrointestinal complaints include nausea, vomiting, diarrhea, and abdominal pain.

Treatment

Standard gastric decontamination should be performed. Hyperactivity is generally managed with diazepam (0.25–0.4 mg/kg, up to a maximum of 5 mg in children 30 days to 5 years old and a maximum of 10 mg in children over 5 years; given intravenously over 2–3 minutes) unless severe hallucinations and agitation are present. In these cases, intravenous haloperidol or droperidol may be more effective. Clorpromazine is generally not recommended. Acid diuresis is not recommended.

ANTIHISTAMINES

The effects of poisoning with these agents are variable, but anticholinergic or sympathomimetic effects are apparent in most cases. Atropine-like toxic effects such as dry mouth, fever, and dilated pupils may predominate. Signs of CNS toxicity include ataxia, hallucinations, and convulsions followed by coma and respiratory depression. Especially in older children, depression may be prominent.

Prolonged toxic manifestations may be caused by sustained-action tablets. Most antihistamines are combined in products that also contain stimulants (phenylpropanolamine, ephedrine) and analgesics (aspirin, acetaminophen). These agents should be considered when treating antihistamines.

Treatment

Treatment consists of emesis or lavage, charcoal, and catharsis; the latter are important when sustained-action tablets have been ingested. Convulsions should be controlled with diazepam. Stimulants are contraindicated. Decrease fever with fluids and sponge baths as required. Avoid salicylates and acetaminophen, especially if found in a combination product. Physostigmine, 0.5–2 mg intravenously, slowly, will reverse coma, hallucinations, dysrhythmias, convulsions, and hypertension, but should only be used to reverse life-threatening manifestations. It may also be useful as a diagnostic test when the cause of symptoms is unclear. Repeat doses should be given only to reverse severe toxic manifestations.

ARSENIC

Acute arsenic ingestion quickly produces gastrointestinal symptoms and may be accompanied by a metallic taste, hoarseness, dysphagia, renal damage, shock, and fever. Increased capillary permeability, dehydration, protein depletion, garlicy odor on the breath, and hypotension may be noted. Chronic toxicity is characterized by peripheral neuritis, weight loss, and, sometimes, involvement of the skin, kidneys, and gastrointestinal tract. Laboratory determination of arsenic levels in vomitus, urine, and tissues is confirmatory. Blood levels below 1 PIgmg/100 mL are within the normal range. Blood levels are generally only useful after acute exposures.

Treatment

Treatment consists of antishock therapy and specific therapy with dimercaptosuccinic acid (DMSA, Chemet) 10 mg/kg/dose, tid for 5 days, followed by the same dose bid for 14 more days. Use of dimercaprol (BAL), 2.5 mg/kg intramuscularly immediately and then 2 mg/kg intramuscularly every 4 hours, may be indicated. After 4–8 injections, give BAL twice daily for 5–10 days or until recovery. BAL produces a reaction similar to serum sickness in over 80% of patients.

BARBITURATES

There are two categories of barbiturate poisoning: (1) intoxication with short-acting drugs (eg, pentobarbitol, secobarbitol), which are detoxified in the liver; and (2) intoxication with long-acting drugs (eg, phenobarbitol), which are cleared via the kidneys. The general symptoms are similar in both types and consist of drowsiness, ataxia, difficulty in thinking clearly, depression of spinal reflexes, respiratory depression, hypotension, and coma. Coma should be classified by the Reed classification (Table 30–3).

Treatment

Any amount in excess of 10–15 mg/kg for long-acting agents or 5–8 mg/kg for short-acting agents may produce more than therapeutic depression. Following suspected ingestion, close observation should be continued for a minimum of 4–6 hours.

A. Short-Acting Drugs:

1. Emesis, lavage, charcoal, and cathartics should be administered as under Emergency Treatment (see p 000). Emesis may be contraindicated because of the short time to CNS depression.
2. Analeptic agents (eg, doxapram, nikethamide, caffeine) are contraindicated in all cases.

Table 30–3. Clinical classification of coma.[1]

Symptoms	Class
Asleep; can be aroused and can answer questions.	0
Comatose; does not withdraw from painful stimuli; reflexes intact.	1
Comatose; does not withdraw from painful stimuli; no respiratory or circulatory depression; most reflexes intact.	2
Comatose; no respiratory or circulatory depression; most or all reflexes absent.	3
Comatose; respiratory depression, with cyanosis; circulatory failure or shock (or both); reflexes absent.	4

[1] After Reed.

3. Respiratory assistance should be provided.
4. Hypotension is common and should be treated with isotonic volume expansion. Vasopressors may be utilized if fluids are inadequate.
5. Shock lung with pulmonary edema may occur.
6. Forced diuresis is ineffective, since less than 3% of the drug is excreted via the kidneys. Fluids should be held to three-fourths of maintenance, since cerebral edema may be a complication, especially following anoxia. Hemodialysis and hemoperfusion may be helpful but should be reserved for severe cases.
7. Vital signs should be monitored continuously until the patient has been free of symptoms for 24 hours and charcoal stools have been passed.
8. Coma lasts approximately 10 hours for each milligram of barbiturate above the therapeutic level of 0.5–2 mg/dL.

B. Long-Acting Drugs:

1–5. As above.

6. Forced alkaline diuresis improves clearance by 3 times. Urine output should be 3–6 mL/kg/hr., preferably 6 mL/kg/hr. If the urine pH is less than 7.5, alkalinization may be performed with sodium bicarbonate.
7. Hemodialysis or charcoal perfusion may be useful if the patient is not responsive to the above measures. These procedures are rarely needed. Their use should be based on deteriorating clinical condition.
8. Therapeutic levels of long-acting barbiturates are 2–4 mg/dL, but patients with tolerance may have considerably higher levels without toxicity. Correlate levels with clinical status.

BELLADONNA DERIVATIVES (Atropine, Scopolamine, Jimson Weed)

Symptoms are dryness of mouth, thirst, difficulty in swallowing, and blurring of vision. Physical signs include dilated pupils, flushed skin, tachycardia, fever, delirium, delusions, weakness, and stupor. Symptoms are rapid in onset but may last for long periods.

Treatment

Induce emesis. Physostigmine, 0.5–2 mg intravenously slowly, dramatically reverses the central and peripheral effects of belladonna alkaloids. Physostigmine should be reserved as a diagnostic agent or for cases of severe toxicity. Owing to a short half-life, its effects usually end within an hour and the patient's symptoms recur. Seizures should respond to diazepam; if not, physostigmine may be used. Forced diuresis and peritoneal and hemodialysis are ineffective. Exchange transfusions may be helpful if very high doses have been taken.

BIRTH-CONTROL PILLS

The only toxic effects noted are nausea, vomiting, and vaginal bleeding. These effects are rare. Treatment is symptomatic.

BORIC ACID

Toxicity can result from ingestion or absorption through inflamed skin. Manifestations include severe gastroenteritis; CNS signs such as irritability, restlessness, and seizures; and a fiery red rash, called toxic epidermal necrolysis. Shock, coma, and death may be seen in more serious ingestions.

Treatment

Gastric lavage or induced emesis (or both) is the immediate therapy. Activated charcoal should be administered. Good supportive care includes maintenance of fluid and electrolyte balance and treatment of hypotension with isotonic fluids and vasopressors as needed. Seizures may be treated with intravenous diazepam. Excretion of ingested or absorbed boric acid can be facilitated with exchange transfusion, hemodialysis, or peritoneal dialysis. Hemodialysis is probably indicated in severely symptomatic patients with impaired renal function, and in patients with severe fluid-electrolyte abnormalities, not amenable to conventional therapy.

CARBON MONOXIDE

Carbon monoxide combines with hemoglobin to form carboxyhemoglobin, which cannot carry oxygen and may result in tissue hypoxia. The cellular cytochrome systems may also be affected. In acute exposures, the patient is generally asymptomatic with levels of 10–20%; levels of 20–30% produce mild symptoms, 30-40% moderate symptoms, and 40–50% severe symptoms. Symptoms are more severe in patients who have exercised or taken alcohol or who reside at high altitudes. Symptoms range from mild flu-like symptoms of headache, nausea, vomiting, to lethargy, depressed sensorium, and occasionally seizures. The heart is particularly sensitive to carbon monoxide and clinical effects include tachycardia, hypotension, peripheral vasodilatation, cyanosis, shock, and cardiac arrest. Early cardiac arrhythmias are thought to be rare. Severe carbon monoxide intoxication may result in pulmonary edema. Residual or delayed neurologic effects may occur after acute carbon monoxide poisoning.

Treatment

Therapy consists of removal from the source and administration of oxygen. The half-life of carboxyhemoglobin is 40–90 minutes in 100% oxygen and 180–360 minutes in room air. The half-life is somewhat dependent on respiratory rate, age, pulmonary health, and physical activity. Hyperbaric oxygen is now considered to be the treatment of choice for symptomatic patients. Hyperbaric oxygen increases the concentration of the oxygen dissolved in the plasma and displaces carbon monoxide from the hemoglobin. Severely symptomatic patients should be referred to a facility with a hyperbaric chamber. Severe symptoms include coma, dizziness, seizures, focal neurologic deficits, severe metabolic acidosis (pH less than 7.25), pulmonary edema, and other cardiovascular signs.

CYANIDE

Cyanide specifically inhibits the cytochrome oxidase system, causing cellular anoxia. The onset of symptoms after inhalation is rapid but may be delayed by minutes to hours after ingestion. Symptoms include giddiness, hyperpnea, headache, palpitation, and unconsciousness. The breath may smell of bitter almonds. Death usually occurs in 15 minutes unless treatment is immediate.

Treatment

Immediately begin 100% oxygen. Obtain the Lilly Cyanide Antidote Kit and prepare it for use. Note that most of the doses are for adults and need to be modified for children. A dosage chart for children is available on the POISINDEX Information System. Intravenous sodium nitrite 3% is given first, followed by intravenous sodium thiosulfate (25%). The amount of sodium nitrite should not exceed that listed in the chart. Fatal methemoglobinemia may result. As an approximation only, the average child with 12 g of hemoglobin would be given 0.33 mL/kg of the 3% sodium nitrite at a rate of 2–5 mL/min. This should produce approximately 30% methemoglobinemia. The initial dose of sodium thiosulfate 25% is 1.65 mL/kg. If clinical response is inadequate, additional sodium nitrite, at half the amount of the initial dose, may be administered 30 minutes following the first dose. These antidotes should only be used in significantly symptomatic patients such as those with seizures, unconsciousness, acidosis, or unstable vital signs. Supportive care is effective in less severe poisonings.

DETERGENTS

Fatalities due to poisoning with anionic and nonanionic detergents have not been reported. The primary symptoms associated with these agents alone include nausea, vomiting, and diarrhea. Occasionally, these detergents may contain alkaline irritants that have the potential for causing alkaline burns.

Cationic detergents may also be found in the home, in products such as antiseptics and antistatic agents. Acute poisoning from these agents may cause gastroenteritis, convulsions, burns, and strictures. Insufficient data are available to determine the nontoxic amount of a cationic detergent or noncorrosive concentration (approximately 7.5%). Burns may occur with benzalkonium chloride in concentrations of 10% or greater.

Treatment

Anionic and nonanionic detergents generally cause minimal effects and require only monitoring for excessive fluid loss if vomiting and diarrhea are extensive.

In cases involving cationic detergents, dilution with water or milk may be initiated first; there is some risk in inducing emesis or performing gastric lavage since many of these compounds are corrosive and if systemic effects occur, seizures and coma may be seen fairly rapidly. These agents are well adsorbed to charcoal and rapid administration of activated charcoal is recommended for large amounts of dilute solutions. With more concentrated solutions, esophagoscopy should be considered and performed within the first 24–48 hours. Definitive burn care may be required if burns are identified on esophagoscopy. Supportive care may be required for seizures, hypotension, and pulmonary edema.

FERROUS SULFATE

Ingestion of ferrous sulfate (elemental iron) in amounts as low as 60 mg/kg may cause serious intoxication. Five phases of intoxication are described: (1) Hemorrhagic gastroenteritis occurs shortly after ingestion (30–120 minutes); shock due to blood loss may be present. (2) A recovery phase occurs and lasts from 2–12 hours after ingestion. (3) Delayed shock may occur 12–24 hours after ingestion and may be due to a vasodepressant action of ferritin or unbound ionic iron. (4) Liver damage occurs at 3–5 days. (5) Delayed gastric obstruction due to scarring of local corrosive injury may occur, usually at 3 weeks after ingestion.

The history is the most important diagnostic clue. X-rays of the abdomen may show the radiopaque tablets in the gastrointestinal tract. Patients with a serum iron level of over 500 µg/dL require chelation therapy.

Treatment

Remove ferrous sulfate by induced vomiting and lavage with a large-bore tube. Supportive measures (blood, plasma, saline, and vasopressors as indicated) are imperative. Exchange transfusion may be useful if the patient does not respond to standard measures. Deferoxamine (Desferal) is useful in cases of severe intoxication. The dose is 15 mg/kg/hr. as a drip—not a push—during the first 12–24 hours. Intramuscular deferoxamine should only be used if intravenous access cannot be established.

FLUORIDES

Fluorides are found in high concentrations in agricultural poisons and insecticides. Lower concentrations are found in such things as toothpaste and fluoride tablets. Clinical reactions produced by fluorides include nausea, vomiting, colicky abdominal pain, diarrhea, cyanosis, excitement, and convulsions. In most instances, gastrointestinal signs and symptoms predominate, but in fatal poisonings, death is usually a result of cardiac failure or respiratory paralysis. In serious poisonings, degeneration of the kidney may occur, as may hypocalcemia, hyperkalemia, and a variable skin rash. In general, ingestion of fluoride tablets used for dental care does not result in severe symptoms owing to their low concentration (1 mg per tablet).

Treatment

Calcium salts (chloride, carbonate, lactate) have been used orally as lavage solutions in concentrations of 5 mL/L of water or a 0.15% calcium hydroxide (lime water) solution. Most household exposures are treated with milk in large quantities (10–15 mL/kg orally). Vomiting may be induced or gastric lavage performed with a large-bore tube. Activated charcoal is not generally of use with fluoride ingestion. For a cathartic, sodium sulfate, sodium citrate, or sorbitol may be used. Monitor serum calcium and observe for clinical signs of hypocalcemia. If necessary, administer calcium gluconate (10%) slowly intravenously, and repeat as necessary. After the initial correction of hypocalcemia, a calcium gluconate infusion at a rate of 15 g/m^2 for 24 hours may be required to compensate for the slow release of fluoride ion from the bone.

GLUE

Toluene was once the most common solvent used in glue, but it has largely been replaced in products by less toxic substances. The most frequent symptoms following glue "sniffing" include weakness, fatigue, confusion, lacrimation, euphoria, headache, dizziness, muscular weakness, nausea, and dilated pupils. Chronic inhalers may develop muscular weakness syndromes, gastrointestinal syndromes, or neuropsychiatric syndromes. Death may occur from respiratory failure.

Treatment

Eliminate exposure to the solvent. Conservative management is indicated, but fluid-electrolyte status should be monitored, as should hepatic, renal, and hematologic parameters. Chronic abusers should receive substance abuse counseling.

HALLUCINOGENS

Marijuana has stimulant, depressant, and hallucinogenic properties, but usually the depressant properties predominate. Euphoria, mood swings, and distortion of time and space commonly occur. Panic states or psychotic reactions are uncommon.

LSD (lysergic acid diethylamide) causes euphoria, mood swings, loss of inhibitions, and depersonalization. Flashbacks (recurrence of initial effects), panic states, and hallucinations occur in some individuals.

Mescaline typically produces mydriasis, salivation, tachypnea, headache, nausea and vomiting, flushing, and diaphoresis. Auditory, gustatory, olfactory, tactile, and visual hallucinations have all been seen with mescaline. These psychologic effects are generally mild in adults, but may be more pronounced in children; they rarely last longer than 6–12 hours.

PCP (phencyclidine) is a veterinary anesthetic that causes agitation, paranoid behavior, nystagmus, hypertension, muscle rigidity, respiratory depression, renal failure, "staring" coma, and occasionally self-destructive behavior. It is often mistakenly taken as or with LSD, mescaline, psilocybin, or marijuana.

Treatment

Treatment of hallucinogenic agents is primarily symptomatic and supportive. Patients should be placed in a low-stimulus environment and given reassurance. Anxiety can be reduced with diazepam (0.04–0.2 mg/kg per dose every 2–4 hours to a maximum of 0.6 mg over 8 hours). Seizures may also be treated with diazepam (0.2–0.5 mg/kg per dose, maximum 5 mg in children under 5 and 10 mg in children over 5). Management of PCP ingestion may include treatments for dystonias, renal failure due to rhabdomyolysis or myoglobinuria, hypoglycemia, and hypertension.

IBUPROFEN

One study states that children who ingest up to 2.4 grams remain asymptomatic. In cases where symptoms occur, abdominal pain, vomiting, drowsiness, and lethargy are seen most frequently. A few case reports, especially in young children, have reported apnea, seizures, metabolic acidosis, and CNS depression leading to coma.

Treatment

For children who have ingested less than 100 mg/kg, only dilution with milk or water is required. Dilution should be with less than 4 oz of fluid in children. If more than 400 mg/kg have been ingested, there is a potential for seizures or CNS depression. In such cases, gastric lavage may be preferred to emesis. A cathartic combined with activated charcoal may also be of some use in adsorbing the material. Patients should be monitored for hypotension, seizures, acidosis, and gastrointestinal bleeding. Hemodialysis and alkalinization of the urine have not been shown effective in treatment of ibuprofen poisoning.

LYE & BLEACHES

Ingestion of lye and bleaches may result in ulceration and perforation of the gastrointestinal tract. Long-term complications are primarily strictures of the upper gastrointestinal tract. Gastric emptying is not recommended because of the potential for vomiting, and thereby further injury to the esophagus. Dilution with a small amount of water is recommended, but excessive amounts may cause vomiting. Perform esophagoscopy after 12 hours but before 24 hours. Use of corticosteroids is controversial. Antibiotics are not indicated unless an infection is demonstrated. Give supportive therapy with sedation and analgesia as necessary. Intravenous nutrition and fluids may be necessary in the early stages of treatment. Early tracheostomy may be indicated in cases of severe ingestion.

MEPROBAMATE
(Equanil, Miltown)

Respiratory depression, coma, arrhythmias, lethargy, headache, hyperactive deep-tendon reflexes, increased heart rate, hypotension, and pulmonary edema may be noted. Death may occur from cardiac or respiratory failure.

Treatment

Emesis or gastric lavage with a large-bore tube may be performed, although supportive treatment may be sufficient in mild intoxications. Hemodialysis, hemoperfusion, or charcoal hemoperfusion may be indicated in severe cases.

MERCURY

Acute symptoms of severe inorganic mercury poisoning include sudden, profound circulatory collapse, increased heart rate, peripheral vasoconstriction, vomiting, decreased blood pressure, and possibly bloody diarrhea. Kidney failure has been seen within 24 hours. Severe acidosis may occur. Some symptoms may be delayed until after 12 hours, including a mercury gum line, lower nephron nephrosis, ulcerative colitis, hepatic damage, and shock. Chronic symptoms generally reported are those of gastrointestinal irritability, a blue-black gum line, salivation, stomatitis, nephrosis, and irritability. Acrodynia occurs in children following chronic exposure to small amounts of mercury, including topically applied mercury.

Treatment

Inorganic mercury salts may produce gastric erosion, and the possibility of perforation should be considered before using emesis or lavage in patients presenting some time after an ingestion. Abdominal x-rays may be helpful in determining whether lavage or emesis is required. Good supportive care should be given for symptoms such as seizures and hypotension. A timed, 24-hour baseline urinary mercury level is a good index of total body burden. For acute poisoning, extrapolating a collection of 2–12 hours is a good initial index. This should be followed by a 24-hour collection. Chelation can be performed with several agents. The first choice is DMSA, 10 mg/kg tid for 5 days followed by the same dose bid for 14 days. Penicillamine, 100 mg/kg/d orally in children, may be given, up to a maximum of 1 g/d in divided doses for 3–10 days. The urine should be monitored daily for urinary excretion of mercury. If the urine mercury decreases rapidly, the body burden is probably small. After 10 days, a repeat baseline collection should be performed to determine whether rebound has occurred and rechelation is necessary. For those individuals cannot take oral medications, BAL may be used in doses of 3–5 mg/kg per dose every 4 hours given deep IM for the first 2 days, 2.5–3 mg/kg per dose IM every 6 hours for the next 2 days, then 2.5–3 mg/kg per dose every 12 hours for a week after that. Again, urine mercury levels should be monitored to assess the effects of therapy.

MUSHROOMS

The most common intoxicating American species of mushrooms are delineated below. Almost 90% of cases of childhood accidental ingestions involve nontoxic puffballs or nontoxic "little brown mushrooms." The services of a mycologist must be obtained through a botanical garden or poison center to identify the species.

Clinical Findings & Treatment

Clinical findings and treatment vary according to the type of mushroom ingested (Table 30–4).

A. Cyclopeptide-containing: Vomiting and severe diarrhea occur after a latent period of 6–20 hours, followed by liver and kidney damage.

B. Muscarinic-containing: These fungi may contain muscarine that may cause parasympathomimetic manifestations. Some may cause an anticholinergic syndrome (see Belladonna Derivatives, above). Hallucinations may occur with ingestion of either type of mushroom. If patients have severe atropinic signs, physostigmine may be tried (see above).

C. Hydrazine-containing: These mushrooms may cause nausea and vomiting, muscle cramps, abdominal pain, severe diarrhea, fever, liver failure, seizures, and coma. Hemolysis may be seen, as may methemoglobinemia. The toxin may be removed or decreased by cooking or drying. Pyridoxine may be antidotal for neurologic symptoms, but there is limited experience with its use. The dose recommended in the literature is 25 mg/kg given as an infusion over 15–30 minutes. Repeat doses up to a maximum daily dose of 15–20 g may be administered for recurring neurologic signs such as seizures and coma. Pyridoxine doses of 0.2–5 g/d for 2–40 months have caused peripheral neuropathy. Methemoglobinemia can be treated with methylene blue in a dose of 1–2 mg/kg per dose (0.1–0.2 mL/kg per dose) given intravenously over a few minutes as needed every 4 hours. Additional doses may be required. Doses of greater than 15 mg/kg may cause hemolysis.

D. Psilocybin-containing: Psilocybin causes nausea, vomiting, headache, and hallucinations. Onset of symptoms is generally within 30–60 minutes, but may be as long as 3 hours. Most cases recover fully within 12 hours. Tonic-clonic seizures, usually intermittent, have occurred in children after ingestion of large quantities.

NARCOTICS
(Opiates)

Narcotic intoxication (eg, morphine, codeine, and diphenoxylate [in Lomotil]) produces respiratory depression, hypotension, pinpoint pupils, skeletal muscle relaxation, decreased urinary output, and, occasionally, shock. Propoxyphene (Darvon) has been associated with

Table 30–4. Mushroom poisoning.

Class	Representatives	Clinical Effects	Treatment
Cyclopepides	*Amanita verna* *Amanita phalloides* *Galerina* species	Vomiting, diarrhea, delayed liver and kidney damage	Supportive care, penicillin, silibinin
Muscarinic	*Boletus satanas* *Clitocybe dealbata* *Inocybe* species	Salivation, bradycardia, miosis, increased peristalsis, hypotension, wheezing	If muscarinic, atropine, 50 μg/kg SC
Hydrazine	*Gyromitra* species	Vomiting, diarrhea, muscle cramps, fever, liver failure, seizures, coma	For CNS effects, pyridoxine
Psilocybin	*Psilocybe* species	Hallucinations	Treatment usually not necessary
Coprine	*Coprinus atramentarius*	Flushing, vomiting, tachycardia, vertigo	Usually symptomatic; for severe cases methylpyrazole (experimental)
Muscimol	*Amanita muscarid* *Amanita patherina*	Drowsiness, delirium, muscle spasms, seizures, coma	Supportive
Orellanine	*Cortinarius* species (some)	Delayed kidney damage	Supportive, hemoperfusion

convulsions in overdoses. Diphenoxylate is especially known for its delayed-onset CNS and respiratory depression.

Treatment

Acute overdosage is treated similarly to barbiturate intoxication. Respiratory assistance and maintenance of adequate blood pressure are mandatory. Naloxone (Narcan) is an effective narcotic antagonist that does not cause respiratory depression and has no known toxicity, even in large doses. The dose of naloxone should be no less than 2.0 mg regardless of the patient's age. If there is no immediate response, the dose may be repeated several times. Patients who have had opiate reversal with naloxone should be observed carefully for recurrence of CNS and respiratory depression.

NITRITES & NITRATES

Sodium nitrite, food preservatives, phenacetin, home remedies such as spirits of nitrite, a high concentration of nitrites in water, as well as various inhalants (amyl, butyl, and isobutyl nitrate) may produce methemoglobinemia. The onset may be gradual and symptoms may be deceiving. Ingestion of as little as 10 mL of isobutyl or amyl nitrate has produced severe methemoglobinemia and death in both adults and children. Clinical signs include hypertension, tachycardia, respiratory depression, methemoglobinemia, headache, nausea, vomiting, diarrhea, and in severe cases, seizures. Symptoms generally do not occur until approximately 30% of the hemoglobin has been converted to methemoglobin. A drop of the patient's blood dried on filter paper may appear brown if levels are 15% or greater.

Treatment

A 1% solution of methylene blue (0.1 mL/kg) is administered intravenously and may be repeated 30 minutes later to reverse symptoms. Persistence of methemoglobinemia at high levels in a symptomatic patient is an indication for exchange transfusion.

PETROLEUM DISTILLATES
(Charcoal Starter, Kerosene, Paint Thinner, Turpentine, & Related Products)

The following products are common causes of poisoning: kerosene, lamp oils, turpentine, other pine products, gasoline, lighter fluid, insecticides with petroleum distillate bases, benzene, naphtha, and mineral spirits.

Ingestion of petroleum distillates causes local irritation with a burning sensation in the mouth, esophagus, and stomach. Vomiting and occasionally diarrhea with blood-tinged stools may occur. Kerosene and similar products are likely to cause spontaneous emesis in 1 hour in about 90% of patients. Just a few drops aspirated into the pulmonary tree can cause a severe pneumonia, a complication to which infants and children are prone. Pulmonary complications are reported with greater frequency among children who ingest kerosene or mineral seal oil than in those who ingest other petroleum distillate products with higher viscosity. Pulmonary involvement is usually indicated by cyanosis, rapid breathing, tachycardia, and fever. Basilar rales may progress rapidly to massive pulmonary edema or hemorrhage, infiltration, and secondary infection.

In general, ingestion of more than 30 mL (1 oz) of a petroleum distillate is associated with a higher incidence of CNS complications such as lethargy, coma, seizures, confusion, disorientation, and peripheral neuropathy. CNS involvement is reported most frequently among patients who ingest lamp oils and kerosene. In severe poisonings, there may be cardiac dilatation, hepatosplenomegaly, proteinuria, formed elements in the urine, and cardiac dysfunction associated with congestive heart failure. In fatal poisonings, death usually occurs in 2–24 hours.

Treatment

Although controversial, induced emesis is useful in cases where systemic toxicity is predicted. The American Academy of Pediatrics recommends emesis if more than 1 mL/kg has been ingested. Estimation of the amount ingested may be difficult in children. Gastric lavage should be performed only if a cuffed endotracheal tube is inserted, because there is no such thing as a "careful gastric lavage" in children. If the amount ingested is small, a saline cathartic is all that is necessary. For CNS depression, supportive care is indicated.

"Prophylactic" antibiotic therapy is of questionable value. Oxygen and mists are helpful. Corticosteroids have not been shown to be of benefit in treating hydrocarbon pneumonitis. Hospitalization is indicated only if the child has taken a large amount or is symptomatic. Fever and other symptoms may continue for as long as 10 days without infection, and pneumatoceles may develop 3–5 weeks after pneumonitis.

Withhold digestible fats, oils, and alcohol, which may promote absorption from the bowel or cause aspiration pneumonitis on their own.

The rapidity of recovery depends upon the degree of pulmonary involvement. Resolution may take as long as 4 weeks.

PHENOTHIAZINES

Phenothiazine compounds produce significant anticholinergic, alpha-adrenergic blocking, and extrapyramidal properties. The symptoms seen will depend on the class of the agent ingested, but may include extrapyramidal motor symptoms (opisthotonos, oculogyric crisis, torticollis, trismus, rigidity) and convulsions.

Treatment

Decontamination should be done either with emesis or gastric lavage depending on the potential for CNS depression and seizures. Activated charcoal and a cathartic will also be useful. Phenytoin (2 mg/kg every 8 hours) may be useful in reversing the depressed intraventricular conductivity of the myocardium. Dystonic disorders may be treated with diphenhydramine at a dose of 1–2 mg/kg to a maximum of 50 mg intravenously. The malignant neuroleptic syndrome may be treated with oral dantrolene at a dose of 2.5 mg/kg intravenously followed by 2.5 mg/kg every six hours.

PHOSPHATES, ORGANIC
(Diazinon, Disyston, Malathion, Parathion, etc)

Many insecticides contain organic phosphates. All inhibit cholinesterases, resulting in parasympathetic and CNS stimulation. Symptoms include headache, dizziness, blurred vision, diarrhea, abdominal pain, dyspnea, chest pain, bronchial constriction, pulmonary edema, respiratory failure, convulsions, cyanosis, coma, loss of reflexes and sphincter control, sweating, salivation, miosis, tearing, muscle fasciculations, and even generalized collapse.

Lowered red cell cholinesterase activity helps to confirm the diagnosis.

Treatment

The patient who has been exposed dermally must be decontaminated with soap and water as soon as possible to prevent further absorption. For children who have ingested an organophosphate, lavage is probably safer than emesis because of the rapid onset of symptoms.

Many organophosphates are dissolved in a hydrocarbon solvent, which could lead to aspiration. Atropine is useful for treatment of the muscarinic effects, but will not reverse nicotinic effects. Early, prompt, and adequate atropinization is of paramount importance in symptomatic patients. Begin with 50 μg/kg intravenously in a small child and 1–2 mg intravenously in an older child. Repeat every 15–30 minutes until dry mouth, mydriasis, and tachycardia appear. Severely poisoned patients may require exceedingly large doses of atropine to achieve adequate atropinization. If anticholinergic findings occur following a diagnostic dose of atropine, the patient is probably not seriously poisoned. In addition, pralidoxime (2-PAM), 500 mg intravenously over 15 minutes, should be given if symptoms are severe.

Supportive measures include oxygen, artificial respiration, postural drainage of secretions, and measures to combat shock and seizures.

RIOT-CONTROL CHEMICALS

Riot-control chemicals consist of an agent in hydrocarbon solvent such as kerosene, and in some cases a propellant such as freon gas. There are a number of chloroacetophenone derivatives as well as chloropicrin agents, dibenzoxazepine compounds, orthochlorobenzylidene malononitrile agents, and capsicum. The chemical agent typically causes lacrimation, photophobia, and in some instances nausea and vomiting. In lower concentration, these materials cause lacrimation and pain but no tissue damage. Skin sensitization and corneal scarring can occur, particularly when the chemical is released close enough to the victim's face or skin to create a high local concentration.

Treatment

The most effective treatment is prompt removal from the sprayed area and careful decontamination of the patient. After removing all clothes, the patient should shower carefully, using copious amounts of soap and water. An ophthalmologist should examine the eyes for possible corneal damage. Medical personnel involved in decontamination should wear protective clothing.

SALICYLATES

Salicylates are still common in pediatric exposures. Acute salicylate poisoning involves vomiting, tinnitus, hyperpnea, acid-base disturbances such as respiratory alkalosis and metabolic acidosis, electrolyte imbalances such as hypokalemia, fever, dehydration, lowered cerebrospinal fluid glucose levels, and pulmonary edema. Severe cases may involve hallucinations, seizures, coma, cerebral edema, and hepatotoxicity.

Salicylates stimulate the respiratory center, causing respiratory alkalosis. Salicylates also interfere with intermediary metabolism and allow the accumulation of organic acids. The two processes together produce a metabolic acidosis that is difficult to treat. In chronic cases or infants, the initial alkalosis may not be evident.

Treatment

The method of gastric decontaimination used depends on the patient's condition (coma, seizures), dosage form (liquid vs tablet), and time since ingestion. Activated charcoal and cathartics are also useful.

Adequate hydration is important, usually with a hypotonic glucose solution such as 0.2–0.45 normal saline. In acidotic patients, administration of sodium bicarbonate (3–6 mL/kg/hr. of a solution containing 88 mEq/L) should be given.

Potassium supplementation may be required because sodium or potassium is excreted with the bicarbonate during the respiratory alkalosis stage. Depletion may be present even with normal serum potassium. Potassium supplements may be at levels of 10–20 mEq/L of fluid, depending on the patient's condition.

Treatment of tetany may require intravenous calcium. The dose depends on serum calcium levels. The pulmonary edema is *not* responsive to digoxin, diuretics, or tourniquets.

Alkalinizing the urine to a pH of 7–8 will enhance salicylate excretion but without proper potassium supplementation may be difficult to maintain. Carbonic anhydrase inhibitors such as Diamox should *not* be used to alkalinize the urine because of negative acid-base reactions.

SCORPION STINGS

The toxin of the bark scorpion (*Centruroides exilicouda*) causes generalized muscular pain, nausea, vomiting, opisthotonos, and a distincitve movement disorder with variable CNS involvement.

Treatment

Keep the patient recumbent and quiet. If the patient is symptomatic, consider administering 0.1 mg/kg of diazepam. Provide adequate sedation and institute supportive measures. Symptomatic measures should be used for control of seizures, hypertension, and supraventricular tachycardia. Antivenin is of some value in cases involving *Centruroides* species, but is only available in Arizona.

SNAKE BITES

In the United States, nearly all snakebites are inflicted by members of the *Crotalidae* family (rattlesnakes, moccasins, copperhead). Bites by the *Elapidae* (coral snakes) are much less common and are not covered here.

Manifestations of crotalid envenomation include local pain, swelling and erythema, nausea and vomiting, abdominal cramps, and a metallic taste. Local wound manifestations usually develop promptly, but may be delayed for several hours. Systemic signs such as hypotension may develop early or late. Hypotension is caused by volume depletion secondary to diffuse capillary injury.

Treatment

Keep the patient recumbent and quiet. Immobilize bitten part below heart level and remove rings and other constrictive items. Transport to medical facility immediately. After arrival at medical facility, the injured part should be immobilized at or above heart level. Do not use ice. Treat shock and respiratory failure with standard resuscitation from shock. Incision and suction are not useful. A high vacuum suction device is available that effectively removes venom through the puncture wound in an animal model. If a constrictive band of any type has been placed, it should not be removed until intravenous access is secured.

The primary methods of treatment are volume resuscitation and Antivenin (*Crotalidae*) polyvalent. Resuscitation should be performed with an isotonic fluid. Antivenin should be given when progressive tissue injury, hemotological injury, or hypotension develop. Antivenin is most effective when given early. After 6–8 hours it is less helpful, but may still be indicated if injury is worsening. The package insert provides directions on its use. The dose ranges from 5–30 vials or more depending on the severity of the envenomation, the species of snake, and the patient's age. If the patient develops an allergic reaction, the antivenin should be discontinued immediately. If indicated, it may be cautiously restarted after treatment with epinephrine and antihistamines. Blood component therapy is rarely needed, but may be indicated for severe anemia, thrombocytopenia or coagulopathy. Steroids are not useful during the acute phase of poisoning. Tetanus prophylaxis and standard local wound care should be provided. Consultation with a physician experienced in the treatment of snakebite and antivenin use is highly recommended for all envenomations.

SPIDER BITES

Black Widow Spider

The bite of a female black widow spider (*Latrodectus mactans*) causes pain at the site of injection. Clinical manifestations include generalized muscle pains with severe abdominal cramps, irritability, nausea and vomiting, variable CNS symptoms, profuse perspiration, labored breathing, and collapse. Examination reveals small maculopapular erythema at the area of bite, abdominal tenderness, restlessness, and hyperactive deep tendon reflexes.

Keep the patient recumbent and quiet with adequate sedation. No first aid measures have proven to be of value. Calcium gluconate in a dose of 50 mg/kg intravenously (up to 250 mg/kg per 24 hours) may be of some value in reducing the muscle spasms. Methocarbamol in a dose of 15 mg/kg every 6 hours has also been of some value. Antivenin (*Latrodectus mactans*) effectively reduces muscle cramping, CNS effects, and hypertension. This antivenin should be reserved for patients who display persistent symptoms that are not relieved by other methods. Instructions for use are included in the package. Tetanus immunization status should be updated. Other methods to reduce muscle spasm and pain include diazepam and narcotics.

Brown Spider

The North American brown recluse spider (violin spider, *Loxosceless reclusa*) is most commonly seen in the central and Midwestern areas of the United States. Its bite characteristically produces a localized reaction with progressively more severe pain over 8 hours. The initial bleb on an erythematous ischemic base may occur before ulceration. Other symptoms may include cyanosis, a morbilliform rash, fever, shock, chills, malaise, weakness, nausea and vomiting, joint pains with hemoglobinuria, jaundice, and delirium.

Medical care is supportive, no specific antivenin is available. Many bites require little treatment other than local care and an antitetanus agent. If there is severe itching, diphenhydramine, 5 mg/kg/d orally (maximum dosage 25–50 mg four times a day) may be used.

The use of steroids is questionable. A polymorphonucular leukocyte inhibitor such as dapsone or colchicine may be helpful. Dapsone may cause hemolysis, which is also a complication of *Loxosceles* envenomation. Surgical intervention should be delayed until 6 or more weeks after the bite. In rare cases, platelets may be needed when thrombocytopenia is present.

TRICYCLIC ANTIDEPRESSANTS
(Amitriptyline, Doxepin, Imipramine, Nortriptyline, etc)

Amitriptyline (Elavil), doxepin (Sinequan), imipramine (Tofranil), nortriptyline (Aventyl), and other tricyclic antidepressants characteristically cause cardiac dysrhythmias, CNS abnormalities (agitation, hallucinations, seizures, and coma), and other signs of atropinism such as dilated pupils, malar flushing, dry mouth, hyperpyrexia, and urinary retention. Some of the newer cyclic antidepressants such as amoxapine have less cardiovascular toxicity but still cause CNS toxicity, with subsequent convulsions.

Treatment

Emesis is not indicated after overdose since rapid neurologic deterioration may occur. Gastric lavage and activated charcoal and a cathartic may be of use. Multiple-dose activated charcoal may be effective with these agents. Sodium bicarbonate is the most useful agent in correcting cardiac dysrhythmias. Lidocaine may be useful for persistent dysrhythmia. The blood pH should be kept at 7.5–7.6. Good supportive care is required for control of seizures, hypertension, hypotension, respiratory depression, and pulmonary edema. Cardiac monitoring should continue until 24 hours after signs of toxicity have resolved.

Drug Therapy (Formulary) | 31

Holly U. Biffl, MD, Alan K. Kamada, PharmD, & Stanley J. Szefler, MD[1]

GENERAL PRINCIPLES OF DRUG ADMINISTRATION IN CHILDREN

The complexity of drug therapy in children has increased over the years. Not only must physicians select the most appropriate medication, they must also individualize the dose and frequency of dosing to ensure the child's safety and obtain optimum efficacy. Thus, all prescribers should have a basic knowledge of each drug. In addition, they must allow for other factors that influence the selection of dose and dosing interval, including patient differences in absorption, distribution, metabolism, and excretion of drugs. Concomitant disease states and physiologic conditions that may vary with age can also influence drug disposition. Because of this, physicians should not simply scale down adult doses when administering medications to children. A brief overview of the major factors involved in selecting medication doses in children is provided, followed by a formulary of medications commonly used in pediatric practice.

DETERMINATION OF DOSE & DOSING INTERVAL

Factors Influencing Dose & Dosing Interval

In pediatric patients, a number of physiologic factors will influence the absorption, distribution, metabolism, or excretion of medica-

[1] The authors would like to acknowledge the assistance of Dr. Wendy Frieling for prior work on this chapter, and Drs. Steve Abman, Paul Bouressa, Ron Gotlin, Taru Hays, Roger Hollister, Gary Lum, Mark Roback, Adam Rosenberg, Michael Schaffer, James Shira, and Judy Sondheimer for their review of drug dosages in the formulary section.

tions. These factors may alter the doses and frequency of dosing required; they are provided in Table 31–1.

Calculation of Dose

Standard doses for most medications are readily available for the treatment of adult patients. Because of the individualization required, however, choosing the appropriate dose for a child is more complex. In the past, pediatric drug doses were based on age; however, it is preferable to determine doses based either on the child's body weight (ie, mg/kg) or body surface area (ie, mg/m^2). The formulary in this chapter bases pediatric doses on body weight. For some medications, however, it is better to dose by body surface area (BSA), according to the following formula:

$$\textbf{pediatric dose} = \textbf{adult dose} \times \frac{\textbf{BSA}}{\textbf{1.73 m}^2}\textbf{BSA}$$

BSA is determined from Figure 31–1 using the patient's height and weight.

For intravenous (IV) medications, **loading doses** are often employed to allow the medication to distribute to the various tissue "compartments" (ie, different types of body tissue; in some cases, organs or groups of organs). Loading doses may also be appropriate for oral medications with long elimination half-lives. To calculate loading doses, you will need to know the **volume of distribution (Vd)**, a theoretical parameter that indicates the space to which the drug distributes. The calculation of a loading dose is as follows:

$$\textbf{loading dose (mg/kg)} = \textbf{desired plasma concentration (mg/L)} \times \textbf{Vd (L/kg)}$$

Volumes of distribution may also be calculated for medications administered by oral or other routes provided bioavailability is relatively complete. For calculation of maintenance doses, the **clearance,** or rate of elimination of the drug must be known. To calculate maintenance infusions, the following equation is used:

$$\textbf{maintenance dose (mg/kg/hour)} = \textbf{desired plasma concentration (mg/L)} \times \textbf{clearance (L/kg/hour)}$$

In general practice, population averages are used for the initial calculation of loading and maintenance doses. Guidelines for loading

Table 31–1. Physiologic factors influencing drug disposition.[1]

Disposition Parameter	Physiologic Variable	Affected Age Group(s)	Pharmacokinetic Result	Example(s)
Absorption	Increased gastric pH	Neonates, infants, young children	Increased bioavailability of basic drugs Decreased bioavailability of acidic drugs	Phenobarbital
	Decreased gastric and intestinal motility	Neonates, infants		
	Increased gastric and intestinal motility	Older infants, children	Unpredictable bioavailability	Digoxin
	Decreased bile acids	Neonates	Decreased bioavilability	Vitamin E
Distribution	Increased total body water and extra-cellular water	Neonates, infants	Increased volume of distribution	Theophylline, aminoglycosides
	Decreased albumin and protein binding	Neonates, infants	Increased volume and increased free drug concentration	Phenytoin
Metabolism	Decreased enzyme capacity	Neonates, infants	Increased elimination half-life and decreased clearance	Phenobarbital
	Increased enzyme capacity	Young children	Decreased elimination half-life and increased clearance	Theophylline
Excretion	Decreased glomerular function	Neonates, infants	Increased elimination half-life	Aminoglycosides
	Decreased tubular function	Neonates, infants	Increased elimination half-life	Penicillins, sulfonamides

[1] Reprinted with permission from *Applied Pharmacokinetics: Principles of Therapeutic Drug Monitoring*, 3rd ed. Evans WF, Schentag JJ, Jusko WJ (editors). Applied Therapeutics, Inc., 1992.

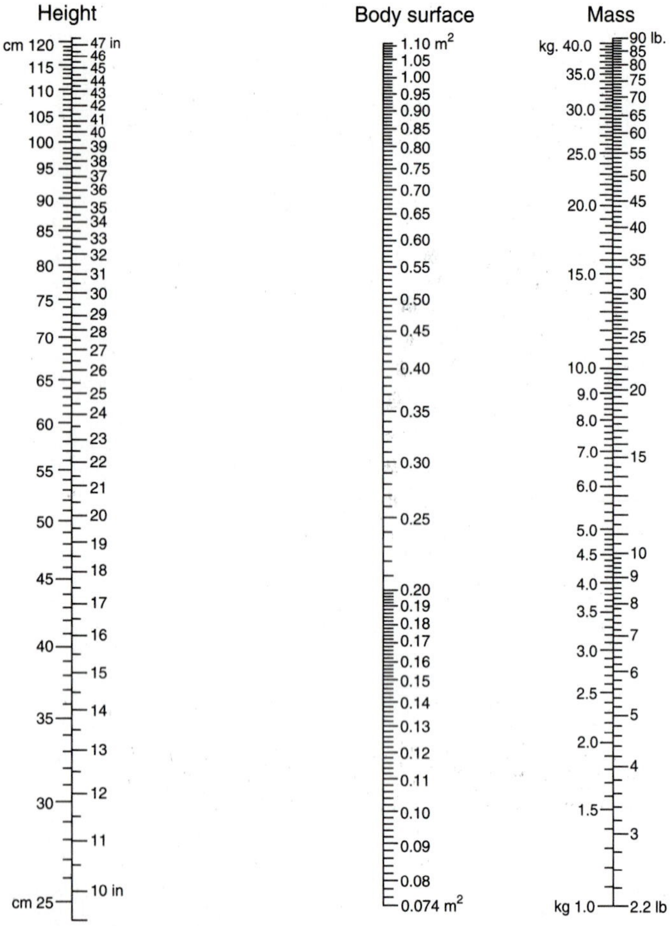

Figure 31–1. Body surface area: Children. To determine the body surface area in a child, use a straight edge to connect the height and mass. The point of intersection on the body surface line gives the area in m^2. (Reproduced with permission from *Geigy Scientific Tables*, 8th ed, vol. 1. Lentner C ed: CIBA-Geigy;1981.)

doses and maintenance doses are included in the formulary within this chapter. Further dosage individualization is then based on measured plasma drug concentrations. A special consideration that may cause some confusion when dosing drugs in pediatric patients is the removal of drugs by dialysis. Drugs that are significantly removed by dialysis are listed in Table 31–2.

When you calculate pediatric doses, *do not exceed the maximum adult doses*, unless clinical situations known to alter drug disposition are present or unless indicated by drug monitoring. Clinical situations that may alter the disposition of some medications (and may require dosage adjustments) include liver and kidney disease, altered fluid status, obesity, and significant drug interactions.

Monitoring Drug Therapy

For some medications, plasma concentrations have been well correlated to their therapeutic activity. Therapeutic ranges, determined from data for both efficacy and safety, have been developed for a number of medications; these are listed in Table 31–3.

For these particular medications, therapeutic drug monitoring is useful in titrating doses to obtain optimum efficacy while ensuring safety from toxicity. Keep in mind that a number of factors, including timing of the last dose and blood samples, bioavailability, distribution, and rate of elimination, can all affect the measured plasma drug concentrations. These factors should be considered when unexpected or seemingly erroneous plasma concentrations are reported. In addition, specific laboratories and institutions usually have their own set of "normal" reference ranges.

Monitoring Medications in Breast-Feeding Mothers

In addition to medications that are directly administered, neonates and infants may also be exposed to drugs through breast feeding, although generally in very low concentrations. Nevertheless, you should consider a number of questions when using medications in mothers who are breast feeding. These include:

1. Does the mother actually require medication(s)?
2. If so, what is the least toxic drug that can be used?
3. Can the dosing schedule be altered to minimize the infant's drug exposure?
4. Are there known adverse effects, and would they be easily identified in the infant?

Table 31–2. Percentage of drugs removed by dialysis.[1]

Drug	Hemodialysis (%)	Peritoneal Dialysis (%)	Drug	Hemodialysis (%)	Peritoneal Dialysis (%)
Acetaminophen	20–50	0–5	Ethosuximide	20–100	
Acetazolamide	20–50		Flecainide	0–5	
Acetohexamide		0–5	Flucytosine	50–100	20–50
Acyclovir	50–100		Flurazepam	0–5	
Amantadine	5–20	5–20	Gentamicin	50–100	20–50
Amikacin	50–100	20–50	Glutethimide	0–20	
Amoxicillin	20–50		Heparin	0–5	0–5
Amphotericin B	0–5		Imipenem/cilastatin	20–50	
Ampicillin	20–50	0–5	Isoniazid	50–100	
Aspirin	50–100	50–100	Kanamycin	50–100	20–50
Atenolol	20–50		Ketoconazole	0–5	0–5
Azathioprine	5–50		Lidocaine	0–5	
Azlocillin	20–50		Lithium	50–100	50–100
Aztreonam	20–50	5–20	Lorazepam	0–20	
Bretylium	20–50		Mebendazole	0–5	
Captopril	20–50		Meprobamate	20–50	5–20
Carbenicillin	20–50		Methicillin	0–5	
Cefaclor	20–50		Methyldopa	5–20	5–20
Cefamandole	20–50		Methylprednisolone	5–20	
Cefazolin	20–50	5–20	Metoclopramide	0–5	
Cefonicid	5–20		Metronidazole	0–5	5–20
Cefoperazone	5–20	0–5	Mexiletine		0–5
Ceforanide	20–50		Mezlocillin		20–50
Cefotaxime	20–50	5–20	Minocycline	0–5	0–5
Cefotetan	5–20		Moxalactam	50–100	5–20
Cefoxitin	20–50	5–20	Nadolol	5–50	

Ceftazidime	50–100	5–20	Nafcillin	0–5	
Ceftizoxime	20–50	5–20	Neomycin	50–100	
Ceftriaxone	0–5		Netilmicin	50–100	
Cefuroxime	20–50	5–20	Oxacillin	0–5	
Cefalexin	20–50	5–20	Oxazepam	0–5	
Cephalothin	20–50		Penicillin G	5–50	
Chloral hydrate	50–100		Pentobarbital	5–20	0–20
Chloramphenicol	5–20	0–5	Phenobarbital	20–100	5–50
Chlordiazepoxide	0–20		Phenothiazines	0–5	
Chlorpropamide		0–5	Phenytoin	0–5	0–5
Cimetidine	5–20	5–20	Piperacillin	20–50	
Ciprofloxacin	5–20		Primidone	20–50	
Clavulanic acid	50–100		Procainamide/N-acetyl-procainamide	5–50	
Clindamycin	0–5	0–5			
Clonidine	0–5		Propoxyphene	0–5	0–5
Cloxacillin	0–5		Propranolol	0–5	
Colchicine	0–5		Quinidine	5–20	5–20
Cyclophosphamide	20–50		Ranitidine	5–20	
Diazepam	0–5		Secobarbital	5–20	0–20
Dicloxacillin	0–5		Sulfamethoxazole		5–20
Digitoxin	0–5		Tetracycline	5–20	
Digoxin	0–5	0–5	Ticarcillin	20–50	
Disopyramide	0–5		Tobramycin	50–100	20–50
Doxycycline	0–5		Tocainide	20–50	
Enalapril	20–50		Tolbutamide	0–5	
Erythromycin	5–20		Trimethoprim	5–50	
Ethambutol	0–5		Valproic acid	0–5	0–5
Ethanol	50–100		Vancomycin	0–5	5–20
Ethchlorvynol	0–20	0–5	Verapamil	0–5	

[1] Adapted with permission from Gambertoglio JG, Rodondi LC. Dialysis of drugs. In: Knoben JE, Anderson PO (editors): *Handbook of Clinical Data*. Drug Intelligence Publications, 1988.

Table 31–3. Suggested therapeutic plasma drug concentrations.[1]

Drug	Concentration
Amikacin[2]	Peak: 20–25 μg/mL Trough: 1–4 μg/mL
Caffeine	5–15 μg/mL
Carbamazepine	5–10 μ/mL
Chloramphenicol	10–20 μg/mL
Digoxin	0.5–2.0 μg/L
Gentamicin[2]	Peak: 6–8 μg/mL Trough: 0.5–1.0 μg/mL
Phenobarbital	10–30 μg/mL
Phenytoin	10–20 μg/mL
Primidone	5–15 μg/mL
Procainamide	4–6 μg/mL
Quinidine	3–5 μg/mL
Theophylline	Asthma: 5–15 μg/mL Apnea: 5–10 μg/mL
Tobramycin[2]	Peak: 6–8 μg/mL Trough: 0.5–1.0 μg/mL
Valproic acid	50–100 μg/mL
Vancomycin	Peak: 25–35 μg/mL Trough: 5–10 μg/mL

[1] References: Yaffe SJ, Aranda JV: *Pediatric Pharmacology: Therapeutic Principles in Practice.* Saunders, 1992; Evans WE, Schentag JJ, Jusko WJ: *Applied Pharmacokinetics; Principles of Therapeutic Drug Monitoring.* Applied Therapeutics, 1992.

[2] Range for serious infections; slightly higher concentrations desired for life-threatening infections.

5. Is the infant likely to have idiosyncratic or allergic reactions to the medication?
6. Are there any physiologic factors present that would result in accumulation of the drug in the infant?
7. Will the amount of drug delivered via breast milk approximate a therapeutic dose to the infant?

Although drug overdose via breast milk exposure is rare, you should be aware that idiosyncratic or allergic reactions are usually *not dose-related*. Of special concern are radiolabeled compounds and chemotherapeutic agents; in most cases these should *not* be given to a mother if she continues to breast-feed. Drugs that are contraindicated in breast-feeding mothers are listed in Table 31–4.

Table 31–4. Drugs contraindicated during breastfeeding.[1]

Contraindicated	Relative Contraindication
Amantadine	Alcohol
Amiodarone	Anti-thyroid drugs
Bromocriptine	Clonidine
Clemastine	Dipasone
Cocaine	Diazepam
Cimetidine	Ethosuximide
Chloramphenicol	Iodides
Cyclophosphamide	Isoniazid
Cyclosporin	Methadone
Doxorubicin	Nicotine
Ergotamine	Nitrofurantoin
Gold salts	Phenobarbital
Isotretinoin	Procainamide
Lithium	Sulfonamides
Methotrexate	
Metronidazole	
Phencyclidine (PCP)	
Phenindione	
Radioactive compounds	
Thiouracil	

[1] References: Anderson PO: Drugs and breastfeeding. In: Knoben JE, Anderson PO (editors): *Handbook of Clinical Drug Data*. Drug Intelligence Publications, 1988; Neibyl JR: Teratology and drugs in pregnancy and lactation. In: Scott JR, DiSaia PJ, Hammond CB et al: *Danforth's Obstetrics and Gynecology*. Lippincott, 1990.

RECOMMENDED RESOURCES

For a more comprehensive discussion of relevant topics related to individualization of pediatric treatment regimens, the following resources are recommended:

Briggs GG, Freeman RK, Yaffe SJ: *Drugs in Pregnancy and Lactation*. Williams & Wilkins, 1990.

Evans WE, Schentag JJ, Jusko WJ: *Applied Pharmacokinetics: Principles of Therapeutic Drug Monitoring*. Applied Therapeutics, 1992.

Knoben JE, Anderson PO: *Handbook of Clinical Drug Data*. Drug Intelligence Publications, 1988.

Roberts RJ: *Drug Therapy in Infants: Pharmacologic Principles and Clinical Experience*. Saunders, 1984.

Yaffe SJ, Aranda JV: Pediatric Pharmacology: Therapeutic Principles in Practice. Saunders, 1992.

FORMULARY[1]

There are a number of variables that alter the disposition of drugs in pediatric patients. Awareness of these factors when prescribing medications to children will minimize toxicities while maximizing the drug's efficacy. This formulary includes suggested doses for children, and in some cases adult doses. Neonatal doses are not always included; other sources should be consulted for specific drug dosing in newborns. *Note that not all cautions and contraindications are listed for each medication.*

(This section of the formulary excludes anti-infectives and antibiotics, which can be found in the section beginning on page xxxx.)[2]

Acetaminophen (many trade names): How supplied: tabs: 80 (chewable), 160, 325, 500 mg; caplets: 160 mg; liquid: 50 mg/15 mL; syrup; 160 mg/5 mL; drops: 80 mg/0.8 mL; suppositories: 120, 125, 130, 300, 325, 500, 600, 650 mg. Dose: Based on weight: 10–15 mg/kg/dose PO, PR q4–6h; Based on age: Neonates, 10 mg/kg/dose; 1–2 yrs, 120 mg/dose; 2–3 yrs, 160 mg/dose; 4–5 yrs, 240 mg/dose; 6–8 yrs, 320 mg/dose; 9–10 yrs, 400 mg/dose; 11–12 yrs, 480 mg/dose; adult, 325–1000 mg/dose.

Acetazolamide (Diamox): How supplied: tabs: 125, 250 mg; caps (sustained release): 500 mg; injection: 500 mg/5 mL. Dose: (1) glaucoma: PO: 8–30 mg/kg/d divided q6–8 h; IM, IV: 5–10 mg/kg/dose q6 h. (2) edema: PO, IV, IM: 5 mg/kg or 150 mg/m^2/d or qod. (3) epilepsy: PO: 8–30 mg/kg/d in 1–4 divided doses. (4) urine alkalinization: 5 mg/kg/dose repeated 2–3 times per 24 h. 5–30 mg/kg/d PO or IV q6–8h; adults: 250–1000 mg/d PO or IV q6h–qod. (5) to reduce cerebrospinal fluid production in post-hemorrhagic ventriculomegaly: begin at 25 mg/kg/d IV or PO q6h, then increase daily

[1] The following sources were used to compile information for this section: *Physicians' Desk Reference,*. Medical Economics Data, 1992; *Formulary of Accepted Drugs and Drug Dosing Handbook,* The Children's Hospital, 1992.

[2] IV: digitalizing doses are 80% of the oral digitalizing doses. Maintenance doses are based on the same percentages of the loading doses as above and divided bid.

to 50, 75, 100 mg/kg/d. *Note*: Safety and efficacy in children have not been established.

Acetylcysteine (Mucomyst): How supplied: vials: 10% and 20% in 4, 10, and 30 mL vials. Dose: nebulization: Infants: 2 mL of 5% solution nebulized tid–qid; children: 3–5 mL of 5–10% solution tid–qid; adolescents: 5–10 mL of 5–10% solution tid–qid. Acetaminophen overdose: 140 mg/kg loading dose PO or NG, then 70 mg/kg/dose PO or NG q4h for a total of 17 doses (dilute 1:4 in water or soft drink).

Acrivastine (Semprex-D): How supplied: caps 8 mg (with 60 mg pseudoephedrine). Dose: 1 cap q8h. *Note:* Safety in children < 12 yr has not been established.

ACTH (Acthar, Cortrophin-Zinc, Cortrosyn, HP-Acthar): How supplied: gel: 40, 80 USP/mL in 1, 5 mL vials; aqueous: 25, 40 USP/vial. Dose: infantile spasms: IM: 20–40 U/d or 80 U (gel) qod.

Adenosine (Adenocard): How supplied: vials 6 mg/2 mL. Dose: Children, 75–225 μg/kg/dose; adults, 6–12 mg (must be administered by rapid IV bolus).

Albumin: How supplied: injection: 5% in 50, 250, 500, 1000 mL vials; 25% in 20, 50, 100 mL vials. Dose: as volume expander 10 mL/kg; hypoproteinuria: 1 gm/kg/d can be given as infusion over 4h or in daily total parenteral nutrition (TPN).

Albuterol (Proventil, Ventolin): How supplied: tabs: 2, 4 mg; extended-release tabs 4, 8 mg; syrup: 2 mg/5 mL; solution for nebulization: 5 mg/mL; inhaler: 90 μg/puff, ~ 200 puffs/inhaler. Dose: PO: Children, 0.1 mg/kg/dose q8h; adults, 2–4 mg q8h; inhalation: 1–2 puffs q4–6h; nebulization: 0.1 mg/kg/dose; max 5 mg/dose, diluted in 2–3 mL of NS, usually bid–qid but may be repeated prn.

Allopurinol (Lopurin, Zyloprim): How supplied: tabs: 100, 300 mg. Dose: hyperuricemia: < 6 yr: 150 mg/d PO q8h; 6–10 yr: 300 mg/d PO q8h; adults: 200–600 mg/d PO q8h (max dose 800 mg/d).

Aluminum Hydroxide (Amphojel, ALternaGEL, others): How supplied: tabs: 320, 640 mg; suspension: 320, 600 mg/5 mL. Dose: hyperacidity: 1–2 tsp PO 4–6 times/d. hyperphosphatemia: 50–150 mg/kg/d divided q4–6h. Caution should be used in patients with renal failure.

Amiodarone (Cordarone): How supplied: tab 200 mg. Dose: 10 mg/kg/d × 7 days, maintenance 5 mg/kg/d.

Aminocaproic Acid (Amicar): How supplied: tabs: 500 mg; syrup: 250 mg/mL; injections: 250 mg/mL. Dose: 100–200 mg/kg/d divided qid. *Note:* Safety and efficacy in children have not been established.

Aminophylline: How supplied: (see also Theophylline) tabs: 100, 200 mg (79% theo); syrup: 105 mg/5 mL (86% theo, 90 mg theo/5 mL; injection: 25 mg/mL (79% theo, 20 mg theo/1 mL). Dose: PO: see Theophylline; IV: loading: 2–6 mg/kg IV; maintenance (IV drip): Neonates, 0.2 mg/kg/h; 1 mo–1 yr, 0.2–0.9 mg/kg/h; 1–9 yr, 1.0–1.2 mg/kg/h; 9–16 yr, 0.8–1.0 mg/kg/h; young adult smokers, 0.8–1.0 mg/kg/h; nonsmoking adults, 0.5–0.7 mg/kg/h. *Note:* Blood levels require monitoring. For apnea of prematurity: 4–6 mg/kg IV over 30 min or PO, then maintenance 1.5–3 mg/kg/dose q8–12h IV or PO. *Note:* Start maintenance 8–12h after loading dose.

Amitriptyline (Elavil, Endep, others): How supplied: tabs: 10, 25, 50, 75, 100, 150 mg; injection: 10 mg/mL. Dose: Adolescents: 10 mg PO tid plus 20 mg PO hs; adults: 75–150 mg PO qd in divided doses. *Note:* Not recommended for children < 12 yr.

Ammonium Chloride: How supplied: tabs: 300, 500, 1000 mg; caps: 300, 500 mg; syrup: 500 mg/5 mL; injection: 0.4, 4.0, 5.0 mEq/mL. Dose: urine acidification: 60–75 mg/kg/d PO or IV q6h (max dose 4–6 g/d).

Aspirin: How supplied: tabs: 81, 165, 325 mg; caps: 356.4 mg with 30 mg caffeine; suppositories: 120, 325, 650 mg. Dose: antipyretic, analgesic: 10–15 mg/kg/dose PO or PR q6–8h; adults, 325–650 mg/dose q4h (max 4–6 doses/d); antirheumatic: 65–100 mg/kg/d PO q6–8h; Kawasaki disease: 100 mg/kg/d PO divided q6h.

Astemizole (Hismanal): How supplied: 10 mg tab. Dose: 1 tab qd. *Note:* Safety in children < 12 yr has not been established. Do not prescribe with macrolide antibiotics or ketoconazole/itraconazole.

Atropine Sulfate: How supplied: tabs: 0.3, 0.4, 0.6 mg; injection; 0.1, 0.3, 0.4, 0.5, 1, 1.2 mg/mL; solution for inhalation 0.2% (2 mg/mL), 0.5% (5 mg/mL); ophthalmic ointment 0.5%, ophthalmic solution 0.5%, 1%, 3%. Dose: bradycardia: Children; 0.01–0.03 mg/kg/dose IV, IM, SC (max 2.0 mg); adults: 0.5–1.0 mg/dose IV, IM, SC (max 2 mg); nebulization: 0.05 mg/kg/dose in 2 mL of NS (max dose 1.0–2.5 mg) given tid–bid; cardiac arrest: 0.01–0.03 mg/kg/dose ET or IV q2–5 min (min dose 0.1 mg); adults, 0.5–2.0 mg/dose.

Azathioprine (Imuran): How supplied: tabs: 50 mg; injection: 100 mg/20 mL. Dose: renal transplant: 1–5 mg/kg/d PO or IV. Dose: rheumatoid arthritis or systemic lupus erythematosus: 1 mg/kg/d PO, increase gradually to 2.5 mg/kg/d PO. Inflammatory bowel disease: 1–2 mg/kg/PO.

Baclofen (Lioresal): How supplied: tabs: 10, 20 mg. Dose: reversible spasticity: 5 mg/dose PO tid and gradually increase as needed to max dose of 20 mg/dose qid.

Beclomethasone (Beclovent, Beconase, Vanceril): How supplied: oral inhaler: 42 µg/puff, ~ 200 puffs/inhaler; nasal inhaler: 42 µg/puff; nasal spray: 42 µg/spray. Dose: 6–12 yr, 1–2 inhalations q6–12h (max 10 inhalations/d); > 12 yr, 2 inhalations q6–12h (max 20 inhalations/d).

Beractant (Survanta): How supplied: vials 200 mg phospholipids/8 mL. Dose: 4 mL/kg endotracheally (infant given ¼ dose in each of 4 body positions); prophylaxis up to 3 additional doses q6–12h; rescue 1 up to 4 additional doses q6–12h. *Note:* Continuous pulse oximeter monitoring recommended.

Bisacodyl (Dulcolax): How supplied: tabs: 5 mg; suppositories: 10 mg. Dose: PO: 0.3 mg/kg/dose; adults, 1–15 mg/dose; PR:< 2 yr, 5 mg/dose; > 2 yr, 10 mg/dose (max one dose qd).

Bretylium (Bretylol): How supplied: injection 50 mg/mL. Dose: 5 mg/kg/dose IV bolus, may repeat q10–20 min up to total of 30 mg/kg; > 12 years, 15–30 µg/kg/min constant infusion.

Budesonide (Rhinocort): How supplied: nasal inhaler: 32 µg/puff, ~ 200 puffs/inhaler. Dose: 1–2 puffs/nasal passage qd–bid.

Caffeine: How supplied: (as citrate) solution: 10 mg/mL; injection: 10 mg/mL. Dose: For apnea of prematurity, loading dose 20 mg/kg/dose PO or IV, then maintenance 5 mg/kg/d. *Note:* Give maintenance dose 24h after loading dose.

Calcium Carbonate: How supplied: tab 300, 500 mg. Dose: 300–500 mg/kg/d PO q6–8h.

Calcium Chloride: How supplied: 10% or 100 mg/mL solution (1.4 mEq Ca^{2+}/mL). Dose: Symptomatic hypocalcemia, elemental Ca 10–20 mg/kg/dose IV; maintenance, elemental Ca 20–80 mg/kg/d as 24h infusion (preferred) or divided qid bolus. Children: 20–50 mg/kg/dose IV or IO q10min.

Calcium Gluconate (9% Ca): Dose: hypocalcemia: Children: 200–1000 mg/kg/d IV in 4 divided doses or as a continuous infusion.

Calcium Lactate (13% Ca): How supplied: tabs: 650 mg. Dose: Children, 400–500 mg/kg/d PO q6–8h; adults, 1.5–3 g/kg/d PO tid.

Captopril (Capoten): How supplied: 12.5, 25, 50, 100 mg. Dose: Infants (< 2 mos): 0.1–0.25 mg/kg/dose q8–24h, titrate up to 0.5 mg/kg/dose q6–24h; Infants (> 2 mos) and children: Initial starting dose of 0.01–0.05 mg/kg/dose PO q8–12h, titrate dose with response; adults: 25 mg/dose PO q8–12h initially and increase as tolerated up to max of 450 mg/d. *Note:* Safety and efficacy in children have not been established.

Carbamazepine (Tegretol): How supplied: tabs: 200 mg; chewable tabs: 100 mg; suspension: 100 mg/5 mL. Dose: 6–12 yr, initial:

100 mg/dose PO bid; increment: weekly increases of 100 mg/d PO tid–qid; maintenance: 400–800 mg/d PO tid–qid (max dose 1000 mg/d); > 12 yr, initial: 200 mg/dose PO bid; increment: weekly increases of 200 mg/d PO tid–qid; maintenance: 800–1200 mg/d PO tid–qid (max dose 1200 mg/d). *Note:* Safety and efficacy in children < 6 years old have not been established.

Charcoal, activated: How supplied: 25, 50 g bottles. Dose: Infants < 1 yr, 1 g/kg q4–6h; children 1–12 yr, 25–50 g q4–6h; adults, 25–50 g q4–6h. Minimum dose 25 g. *Note:* Patient must have intact gag reflex or airway controlled.

Chloral Hydrate: How supplied: tabs: 250, 500 mg; syrup: 500 mg/10 mL, 1000 mg/10 mL; suppository: 325, 500, 650 mg. Dose: Neonates: 25–50 mg/kg/dose PO or PR; children: 25–100 mg/kg/dose PO, NG, PR; adults: 250–2000 mg/dose PO, NG, PR. *Note:* Liver toxicity reported with excessive use.

Chlordiazepoxide (Librium): How supplied: tabs: 5, 10, 25 mg; caps: 5, 10, 25 mg; injection: 100 mg/5 mL. Dose: PO: > 6 yr, 5 mg/dose PO bid–qid; adults, 5–25 mg/dose PO bid–qid; injection: > 12 yr, 25–100 mg/dose IM or IV q2–4h prn.

Chlorothiazide (Diuril): How supplied: tabs: 250, 500 mg; suspension: 250 mg/5 mL; injection: 500 mg/20 mL. Dose: PO: Children, 20 mg/kg/d PO q12h; adults, 500–2000 mg/d PO q12–24h; IV: adults, 500–2000 mg/d IV Q12–24h.

Chlorpheniramine (many trade names): How supplied: tabs: 4 mg; caps, timed release: 8, 12 mg; syrup: 2 mg/5 mL; injection: 10 mg/mL. Dose: 0.35 mg/kg/d PO or SC qid; adults, 2–4 mg/dose tid–qid; 8–12 mg/dose bid (timed-release).

Chlorpromazine (Thorazine): How supplied: tabs: 10, 25, 50, 100, 200 mg; caps: 30, 75, 150, 200, 300 mg; syrup: 10 mg/5 mL; suppositories: 25, 100 mg; injection: 25 mg/mL. Dose: 0.5 mg/kg/dose PO q4–6h; adults, 10–50 mg/dose; 1–2 mg/kg/dose PR q6–8h; adults, 10–50 mg/dose; injection: 0.5 mg/kg/dose IM or IV q6–8h; adults, 25–100 mg/dose (maximum doses: < 5 yr, 40 mg/d; 5–12 yr, 75 mg/d; adults, 1–2 g/d).

Cholestyramine (Questran): How supplied: powder: 4 g/packet, 163 g/tin. Dose: > 6 yr, 240 mg/kg/d PO tid; adults, 4 g/dose PO tid–qid.

Cimetidine (Tagamet): How supplied: tabs: 200, 300, 400, 800 mg; syrup: 300 mg/5 mL; injection: 150 mg/mL. Dose: Premature infants: 2–10 mg/kg/d q8h; infants and children: 20–40 mg/kg/d PO or IV q6h; adults, 300 mg/dose PO or IV q6h. *Note:* Alters theophylline metabolism.

Cisapride (Propulsid): How supplied: tabs: 10 mg. Dose: Infants and children, 0.1–0.2 mg/kg/dose qid; adults 10–20 mg/dose qid a.c.

Citrate (Polycitra, Polycitra K, Bicitra): How supplied: Polycitra: 1 mEq Na, 1 mEq K, 2 mEq bicarbonate/mL; Polycitra K: 0 mEq Na, 2 mEq K, 2 mEq bicarbonate/mL; Bicitra: 1 mEq Na, 0 mEq K, 1 mEq bicarbonate/mL. Dose: 5–15 mL/dose PO q6–8h; adults, 10–30 mL/dose PO q6–8h.

Clemastine (Tavist): How supplied: tabs: 1.34, 2.68 mg; syrup: 0.5 mg/5 mL. Dose: 6–12 yr: 0.5–1.0 mg/dose PO bid (max dose 3 mg/d); > 12 yr: 1–2 mg/dose PO bid (max dose 6 mg/d).

Clonazepam (Klonopin): How supplied: tabs: 0.5, 1.0, 2.0 mg. Dose: < 10 yr: initial dose 0.01–0.03 mg/kg/d PO q8–12h; increments of 0.25–0.50 mg every 3rd day to max maintenance dose of 0.1–0.2 mg/kg/d q8–12h; adults: initial 1.5 mg/day PO tid; increments of 0.5–1.0 mg every 3rd day to max maintenance dose of 20 mg/d PO tid.

Codeine: How supplied: tabs: 15, 30, 60 mg (sulfate); injection: 20, 60 mg/mL (phosphate). Dose: analgesic: Children, 0.5–1.0 mg/kg/dose PO or IV q4–6h; adults, 30–60 mg/dose PO or IV q4–6h; antitussive: Children, 0.2–0.5 mg/kg/dose PO q4–6h max 30 mg/24h; adults, 15–30 mg/dose PO q4–6h.

Colfosceril Palmitate, Cetyl Alcohol, Tyloxapol (Exosurf): How supplied: vial, 8 mL when reconstituted. Dose: 5 mL/kg ET: prophylaxis: birth and up, to 2 additional doses q12h; rescue, 2 doses 12h apart. Give by slow infusion midline/supine; after ½ dose rotate 45 degrees for 30 sec; after second half-dose, rotate 45 degrees to another side for 30 sec. Continuous pulse-oximetry recommended; and slow dosing if $S_aO_2 < 90\%$.

Cromolyn Sodium (Intal, Nasalcrom, Crolom): How supplied: inhaler: 800 µg/puff, 8.1 gm canister (110 puffs), 14.2 canister (200 puffs); liquid for nebulization: 20 mg/2 mL; nasal spray: 5.2 mg/spray, 100 sprays/13 mL container; 200 sprays/26 mL container; eye drops: 40 mg/mL (4%), 10 mL container. Dose: inhalation: 2 puffs tid–qid; nebulization: 20 mg/dose tid–qid; nasal: 1 spray each nostril tid–qid; eyes: 1–2 drops instilled in each eye 4–6 times/d.

Cyclosporine A (Sandimmune): How supplied: caps 25, 50, 100 mg; oral solution 100 mg/mL. Dose: 1 mg/kg/dose q8h IV; 5 mg/kg/dose q12h PO. *Note:* Therapeutic levels vary depending upon indication for use; trough blood levels must be monitored.

Cyproheptadine (Periactin): How supplied: tabs: 4 mg; syrup: 2 mg/5 mL. Dose: 0.25 mg/kg/d PO q8–12h (max dose 0.5 mg/kg/d).

Dantrolene (Dantrium): How supplied: caps: 25, 50, 100 mg; injection: 20 mg/70 mL. Dose: malignant hyperthermia: prophylaxis, 4–8 mg/kg/d PO q6–8h starting 1–2 days before anesthesia; treatment, 1 mg/kg IV repeated prn up to max of 10 mg/kg. Dose: spasticity: PO: Initial 0.5 mg/kg/dose bid; increase frequency to tid–qid at 4–7d intervals; then increase dose by 0.5 mg/kg to max of 3 mg/kg/dose bid–qid up to 400 mg/d. *Note:* Long-term safety of PO administration not established in children < 5 yr.

Deferoxamine Mesylate (Desferal): How supplied: 500 mg/vial. Dose: diagnostic challenge: 1 g IM once; therapeutic: acute iron intoxication: 15 mg/kg/h IV by continuous infusion; 50 mg/kg/dose IM q6h (max 500 mg/dose; except 1000 mg/dose for first dose only).

Desmopressin Acetate (DDAVP): How supplied: nasal solution: 0.1 mg/mL; injection: 4 μg/mL. Dose: diabetes insipidus: Children, 5–30 μg/d q12–24h intranasally; adult, 10–40 μg/d q8–24h intranasally; *or* 2–4 μg/d IV or SC q12–24h; coagulopathy: 0.3 μg/kg/dose IV.

Dexamethasone (Decadron, others): How supplied: tabs: 0.25, 0.5, 0.75, 1.5, 4, 6 mg; elixir: 0.5 mg/5 mL, 1 mg/mL; injection: 4, 10, 24 mg/mL. Dose: for extubation: 0.5–1.0 mg/kg/dose for 3 doses IV or PO.

Dextroamphetamine (Dexedrine, others): How supplied: tabs: 5, 10 mg; caps: 5, 10, 15 mg; elixir: 5 mg/5 mL. Dose: attention deficit disorder: 3–5 yr: 2.5 mg/d PO initially; then increments of 2.5 mg at weekly intervals; daily dose bid–tid; > 5 yr: 5.0 mg/d PO initially; then increments of 5.0 mg at weekly intervals; daily dose bid–tid, max dose 40 mg/d.

Dextromethorphan (many trade names): How supplied: available in many preparations. Dose: 0.5–1 mg/kg/d PO q4–24h.

Diazepam (Valium): How supplied: tabs: 2, 5, 10 mg; injection: 5 mg/mL. Dose: sedation: Children: 0.1–0.8 mg/kg/d PO q6–8h; injection: 0.04–0.2 mg/kg/dose IV q2–4h; adults: 2–10 mg/dose PO q6–8h; injection: 2–10 mg/dose IV q3–4h; seizures: children: < 5 yr, 0.2–0.5 mg/kg/dose IV q15–30 min; total max 5 mg; > 5 yr, 1 mg/dose IV q15–50 min; total max 10 mg, repeat q2–4h prn.

Diazoxide (Hyperstat, Proglycem): How supplied: caps: 50 mg; liquid: 50 mg/mL; injection: 15 mg/mL. Dose: hypertension: Children and adults, 1–3 mg/kg/dose IV rapid bolus; repeat q5–15 min, then q4–24h; hypoglycemia: Infants, 8–20 mg/kg/d PO tid–qid or IV q8–12h; children and adults, 3–8 mg/kg/d PO or IV q8–12h.

Digoxin (Lanoxin): How supplied: tabs: 125, 250, 500 μg (bioavailability 60–80%); caps: 50, 100, 200 μg (bioavailability 90–

100%); elixir: 50 μg/mL (bioavailability 70–85%); injection: 100, 250 mg/mL (IV bioavailability 100%). Dose: tabs or elixir: Premature infants, 20–30 μg/kg PO digitalizing dose; maintenance dose is 20–30% of oral digitalizing dose, bid; full-term infants, 25–35 μg/kg PO digitalizing dose*; 1–24 mo, 35–60 μg/kg PO digitalizing dose*; 2–5 yr, 30–40 μg/kg PO digitalizing dose*; 5–10 yr, 20–35 μg/kg PO digitalizing dose*; > 10 yr, 10–15 μg/kg PO digitalizing dose.* Maintenance dose is 25–35% of oral digitalizing dose, divided bid*; in < 10 yr digitalizing doses are given as ½ the total digitalizing dose initially; then ¼ the total digitalizing dose q8–18h × 2.

Dimenhydrinate (Dramamine, others): How supplied: tabs: 50 mg; syrup: 15 mg/5 mL; injection: 50 mg/mL. Dose: < 12 yr: 5 mg/kg/d PO or IM q6h (max 150 mg/d); > 12 yr: 50–100 mg/dose PO or IM q4h (max 400 mg/d).

Dimercaprol (BAL): How supplied: oil for injection 100 mg/mL. Dose: lead poisoning: 3–4 mg/kg/dose IM q4h for 2–7 days; arsenic poisoning: 2.5 mg/kg/dose IM q4–6h for 2 days, then decrease dose over next few days.

Diphenhydramine (Benadryl, others): How supplied: tabs: 50; caps: 25, 50 mg; elixir: 12.5 mg/5 mL; injection: 10, 50 mg/mL. Dose: Children, 5 mg/kg/d PO, IV, or IM q6–8h (max dose 300 mg/d); adults, 10–50 mg/kg/dose PO, IV, or IM q6–8h (max dose 400 mg/d).

Dobutamine (Dobutrex): How supplied: injection: 12.5 mg/mL. Dose: IV infusion: 2.5–15 μg/kg/min (max dose 40 μg/kg/min).

Docusate Sodium (Colace, others): How supplied: caps: 50, 100, 150 mg; liquid: 10 mg/mL; syrup: 20 mg/5 mL, 50 mg/15 mL. Dose: < 3 yr, 10–40 mg/d PO qd–qid; 3–6 yr, 20–60 mg/d PO qd–qid; 6–12 yr, 40–120 mg/d PO qd–qid; > 12 yr, 50–200 mg/d PO qd–qid.

Dopamine (Intropin): How supplied: injection: 40, 80, 160 mg/mL. Dose: IV infusion: 2–20 μg/kg/min (max dose 20–50 μg/kg/min).

Edrophonium (Tensilon): How supplied: injection: 10 mg/mL. Dose: in diagnosis of myasthenia gravis; Infants: initial 0.1 mg, followed by 0.4 mg if no response; 0.5 mg total dose. Children: initial 0.04 mg/kg followed by 0.16 mg/kg if no response, to max of 10 mg; total dose 0.2 mg/kg.

Enalapril Maleate (Vasotec): How supplied: tabs: 2.5, 5, 10, 20 mg; injection 1.25 mg/mL. Dose: Children: 0.1–0.3 mg/kg/d qd–bid, max 40 mg/24h; IV 0.05–0.1 mg/kg/dose q6h, max 5 mg/dose; adults, 2.5–5 mg/dose PO qd initially; then increase up to 40 mg/d PO qd–bid.

Epinephrine: How supplied: 1/1000 aqueous solution (1 mg/mL) for IM/SC injection, 1/10,000 aqueous solution (0.01 mg/mL) for IV injection, 1/200 glycerine solution (5 mg/mL) for SC injection, 2.25% solution for inhalation. Dose: bronchospasm and acute allergic reactions (hives, angioedema); 1/1000 aqueous solution, 0.01 mg/kg q 15 min SC (max 0.5 mg); 1/200 glycerine solution, 0.005 mg/kg q 6–12h; hypotension/cardiac arrest: 1/10,000 aqueous solution 0.1 mL/kg/dose (5 mL maximum) IV, IO, or ET; infusion 0.1 μg/kg/min.

Epinephrine, Racemic: Dose: > 2 yr: 0.5 mL diluted with 3 mL NS as nebulization; may repeat q2h. < 2 yr: 0.25 mL (as above).

Epoetin alfa (Epogen, Procrit): How supplied: 2000, 3000, 4000 and 10,000 U/mL vials. Dose: Prevention of anemia of prematurity for infants < = 1200 gm at birth; begin when on 2/3 full enteral feeds, 150 U/kg/ SC 3 × wk. Give with therapeutic iron and 25 IU/d PO vitamin E.

Ethacrynic Acid (Edecrin): Dose: difficult-to-control edema, congestive heart failure, hepatic or renal disease: Older children, 25 mg/dose PO initially, then slowly increase in 25 mg/dose increments q2–3 d (max 3 mg/kg/d divided q12h). Contraindicated in infants.

Ethosuximide (Zarontin): Dose: (optimal dose usually 20 mg/kg/d) 3–6 yr, 250 mg/d PO initially, then increase slowly by 250 mg/d increments q4–7 d, daily dose divided q12–24h; > 6 yr, 500 mg/d PO initially, then increase slowly by 250 mg/d increments q4–7d, daily dose divided q12–24h (max dose 1.5 g/d).

Fentanyl (Sublimaze): How supplied: injection: 50 μg/mL. Dose: 1–3 μg/kg/dose IV or IM.

Flecainide (Tambocor): How supplied: tabs 100 mg. Dose: Children 2–6 mg/kg/d or 115–230 $mg/m^2/d$ bid–tid; adults 100 mg bid, increased by 50 mg increments to maximum of 400 mg/d.

Flumazenil (Romazicon): How supplied: 0.1 mg/mL, 5 mL, 10 mL vials. Dose: Infants < 6 mo 0.01–0.02 mg/kg (max 0.2 mg) IV over 15 sec, may repeat q45 sec to max of 1 mg in the first hour; pediatric > 6 mo and adults, 0.2 mg IV over 15 sec, may repeat q45 sec to max of 1 mg in the first hour. *Note:* Contraindicated in patients known or suspected of tricyclic antidepressant overdose, patients treated chronically with benzodiazapines for seizure disorders, and patients whose seizures stopped acutely with benzodiazepines.

Flunisolide (Nasalide, Aerobid): How supplied: nasal spray (0.025%): 25 μg/spray, 200 sprays/bottle. Dose: seasonal or perennial rhinitis: nasal inhalant: Children 6–14 yr, 1 spray each nostril tid or 2 sprays each nostril bid (max dose 4 sprays/nostril/d); adults, 2 sprays each nostril bid–tid (max dose 8 sprays/nostril/d). Asthma: oral inhalation: Children > 6 yr: oral inhalation bid (max 4 inhal/24h); adults: 2 inhalations bid (max 8 inhal/24h).

Fluoride: How supplied: tabs: 0.25, 0.5, 1.0 mg; liquid; 0.5, 2, 4 mg/mL. Dose: Children: 2 wk–2 yr, 0.25 mg/d; 2–3 yr, 0.25–0.5 mg/d; 3–16 yr, 0.5–1.0 mg/d.

9-alpha Fluorocortisol (Florinef): How supplied: tabs: 0.1 mg. Dose: 0.05–0.15 mg/d PO qd–bid.

Flurazepam (Dalmane): How supplied: caps: 15, 30 mg. Dose: > 15 yr, 15–30 mg/dose PO qhs.

Fluticasone (Flonase): How supplied: nasal spray 0.05%, 50 µg/puff; ~ 120 puffs/container. Dose: 1–2 sprays/nasal passage qd. *Note:* Safety in children < 12 yr not established.

Folic Acid: How supplied: tabs: 1 mg. Dose: Children 0.2–1.0 mg/d PO; adults, 1 mg/d PO.

Furosemide (Lasix, others): How supplied: tabs: 20, 40, 80 mg; syrup: 10 mg/mL; injection: 10 mg/mL. Dose: Children, 1–2 mg/kg/dose PO, IV, or IM q6–12h; adults, 20–80 mg/dose PO, IV, or IM q12–24h (max 600 mg/d).

Gamma Benzene Hexachloride (Kwell, Scabene): How supplied: 1% cream, lotion, and shampoo. Dose: skin: a thin layer applied from the neck down, left on the skin 6h for children, 8–12h for adults, then washed off. Usually only one treatment is necessary; an adult usually uses 60 mL; hair: 30–60 mL per application, worked thoroughly into dry hair; allow to stand 4 min, lather with water, rinse thoroughly, remove nits with comb provided. Repeat treatment in 7 days if lice or nits are still present.

Glucagon: How supplied: injection: 1 mg/mL. Dose: 25–300 µg/kg/dose SC, IM, or IV q10–25 min (max 1 mg/dose).

Haloperidol (Haldol): How supplied: tabs: 0.5, 1, 2, 5, 10, 20 mg; syrup: 2 mg/mL; injection: 5 mg/mL. Dose: psychotic disorders: 0.05–0.15 mg/kg/d to be divided PO bid–tid; non-psychotic behavior disorders and Tourette's syndrome: 0.05–0.075 mg/kg/d.

Heparin Sodium: How supplied: injection: 10, 100, 1000, 2500, 5000, 7500, 10,000, 15,000, 20,000, 40,000 U/mL. Dose: For line patency, 1–2 U/mL; for clotting complications: Children, 50 U/kg IV bolus once, then 10–25 U/kg/hr as continuous infusion; adults 10,000 U/dose IV bolus once, then 5000–10,000 U/dose IV q4–6h.

Hydralazine (Apresoline): How supplied: tabs: 10, 25, 50, 100 mg; injection: 20 mg/mL. Dose: Chronic hypertension: Children, 0.75–3.0 mg/kg/d PO q6–12h; adults, 10–50 mg/dose PO qid; hypertensive crisis: Children, 0.1–0.2 mg/kg/dose IM or IV q4–6h; adults, 20–40 mg/dose IM or IV q4–6h.

Hydrochlorothiazide (Esidrix, HydroDiuril, others): How supplied: tabs: 25, 50, 100 mg. Dose: Children, 2–3 mg/kg/d PO bid; adults, 25–100 mg/dose PO qd–bid (max 200 mg/d).

Hydrocortisone [Cortisol] (Solu-Cortef): Dose: Physiologic replacement: ~ 12.5 mg/m^2/d IM or IV qd; asthma: children, initial dose 4–8 mg/kg/dose IV once, then 8 mg/kg/d IV q6h; adults, 100–500 mg/dose IV q2–6h; hypotension/presumed adrenal insufficiency, 10–15 mg/m^2/d IV q8h.

Hydroxyzine (Atarax, Vistaril): How supplied: caps 25, 50, 100 mg; tabs 10, 25, 50, 100 mg; suspension 25 mg/sec; solution 10 mg/sec, injection 25 mg/mL, 50 mg/mL. Dose: Children, 1–2 mg/kg/d PO tid–qid; adults, 25–100 mg/dose PO qid; children, 1 mg/kg/dose, IM; adults, 25–100 mg/dose IM.

Ibuprofen (Advil, Pediaprofen, Motrin): How supplied: tabs 200, 300, 400, 600 mg, liquid 100 mg/5 mL. Dose: antipyretic and anti-inflammatory, 10 mg/kg/dose tid–qid.

Imipramine (Tofranil): How supplied: tabs: 10, 25, 50 mg; caps: 75, 100, 125, 150 mg; injection: 12.5 mg/mL. Dose: depression: Adolescents, initially 30–40 mg/d PO bid–tid, then gradually increase to maintenance of max 100 mg/d PO qd–bid; adults, initially 75–100 mg/d PO bid, then gradually increase to maintenance of 50–300 mg/d PO qd–bid; enuresis: > 6 yr; 25 mg/dose 1h before bedtime may increase to 50 mg/dose for 6–12 yr; 75 mg/dose for > 12 yr (max dose 2.5 mg/kg/d).

Indomethacin (Indocin): How supplied: caps: 25, 50 mg; sustained-release caps 75 mg; suspension: 25 mg/5 mL; injection: 1 mg/vial. Dose: Patent ductus closure, see Table 31–5. Anti-inflammatory: > 14 yr, 1–3 mg/kg/d PO tid–qid; adults, 25–50 mg/kg/d, maximum 200 mg/day PO bid–qid.

Table 31–5. Indomethacin dosing for closure of patent ductus arteriosus.[1]

	Dose No.		
Age at First Dose	**1**	**2**	**3**
< 48 h	0.2	0.1	0.1
2–7 d	0.2	0.2	0.2
>7 d	0.2	0.25	0.25

[1] Dose in mg/kg at intervals of 12–24 h.

[2] Doses given 12–24 h apart, for a total of three doses.

Insulin: How supplied: Many formulations are available including human, pork, and beef products; some are rapid-onset (regular, Semilente), intermediate-onset (Lente, NPH) and delayed-onset (Ultralente). There are many considerations in deciding which type of insulin is optimal. Dose: Diabetic ketoacidosis: usual dose 0.05–0.1 U/kg/hr IV of regular insulin given as continuous IV infusion; maintenance: usual dose range is 0.5–1.0 U/kg/d given in divided doses SC. For glucose intolerance in premature infants, 0.01–0.1 U/kg/h of regular insulin.

Ipecac Syrup: How supplied: 7% syrup in 15 and 30 mL bottles. Dose: Infants 6–12 mo: 10 mL PO once, followed by clear liquids; children 1–12 yr: 15–30 mL PO once, followed by clear liquids; > 12 yr: 30–60 mL PO once, followed by clear liquids; may repeat dose once if no emesis occurs within 20 min.

Ipratropium Bromide (Atrovent): How supplied: oral inhaler 18 μg/puff, 200 puffs/inhaler; aerosol solution 0.02%, 2–5 mL vials. Dose: 2 puffs qid, 1 vial for aerosol treatment qid. *Note:* Safety in children < 12 yr has not been established.

Iron Dextran: How supplied: injection: 50 mg of elemental iron/mL. Dose: iron deficiency anemia: calculated using the following formulae]:

dose in mL:

$$\text{wt (kg)} \times 0.0476 \times (\text{normal Hgb} - \text{patient Hgb});$$

dose in mg of iron:

$$\text{wt (kg)} \times 2.4 \times (\text{normal Hgb} - \text{patient Hgb})$$

Add 1 mL/5 kg (50 mg iron/5 kg) of body weight to the dose calculated above to replenish iron stores, up to max 14 mL total; max IV dose is 2 mL/d; max IM daily dose is based on weight (Table 31–6).

Note: Prior to receiving iron dextran therapy, all patients should receive a test dose, 0.5 mL either IV or IM.

Table 31–6. Maximum intramuscular daily dose of iron dextran.

Weight	Dose (mL)
Children < 5 kg	0.5
Children 5–10 kg	1.0
Children > 10 kg	2.0
Adults	5.0

Table 31–7. Iron supplements.

Ferrous sulfate (Fer-In-Sol):	**Ferrous Sulfate**	**Elemental Iron**
Caps:	190 mg	60 mg
Drops:	75 mg/0.6 mL	15 mg/0.6 mL
Syrup:	90 mg/5 mL	18 mg/5 mL
Ferrous gluconate (Fergon):	**Ferrous Gluconate**	**Elemental Iron**
Tabs:	320 mg	35 mg
Caps:	435 mg	50 mg
Elixir:	300 mg/5 mL	34 mg/5 mL

Iron Supplements: How supplied: Table 31–7.

Dose: dietary supplement (in mg of elemental iron): Premature infants, 2–6 mg/kg/d PO qd–tid: term infants, 1 mg/kg/d PO qd–tid: (US RDA for > 4 yr = 18 mg/d); iron deficiency (in mg of elemental iron): 6 mg/kg/d PO tid; for use with Epoetin alfa, 4–8 mg/kg/d PO.

Isotretinoin (Accutane): How supplied: caps: 10, 20, 40 mg. Dose: severe cystic acne: 0.5–1.0 mg/kg/d PO bid (max dose 2 mg/kg/d). *Note:* Contraindicated in pregnancy.

Ketamine: How supplied: 10, 50, 100 mg/mL for injection. Dose: 0.5–1 mg/kg IV, 2–4 mg/kg/IM. Use in conjunction with anticholinergics: atropine (0.01 mg/kg, minimum 0.2 mg, maximum 0.5 mg) or glycopyrrolate (5 μg/kg, max 250 μg).

Ketorolac Tromethamine (Acular): How supplied: 0.5% ophthalmic solution, 5 mL. Dose: 1 drop in each eye qid for 7 days. *Note:* Safety in children not established.

Lactulose (Cephulac, others): How supplied: syrup: 10 g/15 mL (60 gm%). Dose: Infants: 2.5–10 mL/d PO tid–qid; older children and adolescents: 40–90 mL/d PO tid–qid; adults: 30–45 mL/dose PO tid–qid.

Levocabastine (Livostin): How supplied: 0.05% ophthalmic solution; 2.5, 5, 10 mL. Dose: 1 drop in each eye qid, up to 2 wk. **Note:** Safety in children has not been established.

Levothyroxine (Synthroid): How supplied: tabs: 25, 37.5, 50, 75, 100, 112, 125, 150, 175, 200, 300 μg; injection: 20, 50 μg/mL. Dose: Children, 75–100 $\mu g/m^2/d$; adult, initial dose 25–50 μg/d PO, then increase by increments of 25 μg q2–3 wk to maintenance of 100–200 μg/d. (IV dose is ~ 50% of PO dose.)

Lidocaine (Xylocaine): How supplied: (1% = 10 mg/mL); injection: 0.5%, 1.0%, 1.5%, 2.0%; also 50 mg/5 mL, 100 mg/5 mL prefilled syringes; ointment: 2.5%, 5.0%; oral spray: 10%; topical jelly 2%. Dose: local anesthesia: 3–4.5 mg/kg max total dose; IV for cardiac arrhythmias: 1 mg/kg IV bolus q5 min × 3, may be given as continuous IV infusion of 20–50 μg/kg/min. Maximum with epinephrine, 7 μg/kg/dose.

Lindane: see Gamma Benzene Hexachloride.

Lodoxamide Tromethamine (Alomide): How supplied: 0.1% ophthalmic solution, 10 mL. Dose: 1–2 drops in each eye qid up to three months. *Note:* Safety in children < 2 yr has not been established.

Loperamide (Imodium, Imodium A-D): How supplied: caps: 2 mg: syrup: 1 mg/5 mL. Dose: Children < 20 kg, 0.05 mg/kg/dose up to tid; > 20 kg, 2 mg/dose tid.

Loratidine (Claritin, Claritin-D): How supplied: tabs 10 mg and 5 mg with 120 mg pseudoephedrine (extended-release). Dose: 10 mg qd, extended-release, 1 tab q12h.

Lorazepam (Ativan): How supplied: tabs: 0.5, 1, 2 mg; injection: 2 mg/mL, 4 mg/mL. Dose: 0.05–0.1 mg/kg/dose IV q6h (adults 2–4 mg/dose max); *or* adults 2–6 mg/d PO q8–12h (max 10 mg/d).

Magnesium Citrate: How supplied: solution: 300 mL bottles. Dose: 4 mL/kg/dose PO, max 200 mL dose.

Magnesium Hydroxide (Milk of Magnesia): How supplied: tabs; 311 mg; suspension: 405 mg/5 mL regular strength; 800 mg/5 mL extra strength. Dose: Children < 2 yr: 0.5–1.0 mL/kg/dose PO prn; children 2–5 yr: 5–15 mL/d as a single or divided dose; children 6–11 yr: 15–30 mL/d; adult: 15–60 mL/dose PO prn (1 mL = ~ 80 mg).

Magnesium Sulfate: How supplied: solution: 50% (500 mg/mL). Dose: cathartic: Children, 250 mg/kg/dose PO; adults, 10–30 g/d PO. For hypomagnesemia with refractory hypocalcemia, 0.2–0.4 mEq IV or IM q6h for 3–4 doses.

Mannitol: How supplied: injection: 50, 100, 150, 200, 250 mg/mL. Dose: cerebral edema: 0.5–1.0 g/kg/dose IV prn.

Meclizine (Antivert, Bonine): How supplied: tabs: 12.5, 25, 50 mg. Dose: vertigo: 25–100 mg/d PO q6–12h; motion sickness: 25–50 mg/d PO 1h prior to travel. *Note:* Not recommended in children < 12 yr.

Meperidine (Demerol): How supplied: tabs: 50, 100 mg; syrup: 50 mg/5 mL; injection: 25, 50, 75, 100 mg/mL. Dose: Children: 1–1.5 mg/kg/dose PO, SC, or IM q3–4h prn; adults: 50–150 mg/dose PO, SC, or IM q3–4h prn.

Mesalamine (Asacol): How supplied: delayed-release tabs, 400 mg. Dose: Adults 800 mg qid.

Metaproterenol (Alupent, Metaprel): How supplied: tabs: 10, 20 mg; syrup: 10 mg/5 mL; inhaler: 0.65 mg/puff, 200 puffs/inhaler; solution for nebulization: 5% (50 mg/mL). Dose: Children < 6 yr, 1.3–2.6 mg/kg/d PO tid–qid; 6–9 yr, 10 mg/dose PO tid–qid; > 9 yr, 20 mg/dose PO tid–qid; inhalation (not recommended for children < 12 yr): 2–3 puffs q3–4h, max 12 puffs/d; nebulization: 0.2–0.5 mL/dose in 2.5 mL NS q1–6h prn.

Methadone: How supplied: tabs: 5, 10 mg; liquid: 5, 10 mg/5 mL; injection: 10 mg/mL. Dose: analgesic: Adults, 2.5–10 mg/dose PO, SC, or IM q3–4h. *Note:* Not recommended for use in children.

Methimazole (Tapazole): How supplied: tabs: 5, 10 mg. Dose: hyperthyroidism: Children, initial dose 0.4 mg/kg/d PO q8h, then 50% of initial dose as maintenance; adults, initial dose 15–60 mg/d PO q8h, then 5–30 mg/d PO qd.

Methsuximide (Celontin): How supplied: caps: 150, 300 mg. Dose: Adults: 300 mg/d PO for 1 wk, then increase by 300 mg/d qwk for 3 wk, to max 1200 mg/d; usual maintenance dose is 10–20 mg/kg/d PO; children; 10–20 mg/kg/d divided bid/qid.

Methyldopa (Aldomet): How supplied: tabs: 125, 250, 500 mg; suspension: 250 mg/5 mL; injection: 50 mg/mL. Dose: Children: 10 mg/kg/d PO q6–12h, increase at 2-d intervals to max 65 mg/kg/d or 3 g/d, whichever is less: IV (for hypertensive crisis): 20–40 mg/kg/d IV q6h (max 65 mg/kg/d or 3 g/d, whichever is less); adults, 250 mg/dose PO bid–tid, increase at 2-d intervals to max 3 g/d, usual maintenance dose is 500–2000 mg/d PO bid–qid; IV (for hypertensive crisis): 250–500 mg/dose IV q6h, max 1 gm q6h.

Methylene Blue: How supplied: solution: 1% (10 mg/mL); tabs 65 mg. Dose: antidote for cyanide poisoning and drug-induced methemoglobinemia: 1–2 mg/kg/dose slowly IV. For NADH-methemoglobin reductase deficiency 1.5–5 mg/kg/24h.

Methylphenidate (Ritalin): How supplied: tabs: 5, 10, 20 mg; slow-release caps: 20 mg. Dose (children > 6 yr): 5 mg/dose PO bid (before breakfast and lunch), increase gradually 5–10 mg/wk to max 60 mg/d.

Methylprednisolone (Depo-Medrol, Medrol, Solu-Medrol): How supplied: tabs: 2, 4, 8, 16, 24, 32 mg; injection (Solu-Medrol, as succinate for IV, IM): 40, 125, 500, 1000, 2000 mg/vials; injection (Depo-Medrol, as acetate for IM repository): 20, 40, 80 mg/mL. Dose: asthma: initial dose 1–2 mg/kg/dose IV once, then 0.5–1.0 mg/kg/dose IV q6h; anti-inflammatory: 0.16–1.0 mg/kg/d PO or IV q6–12h.

Metoclopramide (Reglan): How supplied: tabs: 5, 10 mg; syrup: 5 mg/5 mL; injection: 5, 10 mg/mL. Dose: gastroesophageal reflux: 1–6 yr, 0.1 mg/kg/dose PO or IV qid; 6–12 yr, 2.5–5 mg/dose PO or IV qid; adults, 10–15 mg/dose PO or IV qid; antiemetic: 1–2 mg/kg/dose IV q2–3h prn.

Midazolam (Versed): How supplied: injection: 1 mg/mL, 5 mg/mL. Dose: conscious sedation: 0.01–0.06 mg/kg/dose IV, usual adult dose 5 mg/dose; 0.1–0.2 mg/kg/dose IV, usual adult dose 1–5 mg/dose; 0.3 mg/kg/dose intranasal.

Mineral Oil: How supplied: plain and flavored preparations, 4.2 g mineral oil/15 mL. Dose: Children > 6 yr: 5–30 mL PO qd given as single or divided dose. Not recommended for children < 6 yr. Adults 16–30 mL/dose, titrate dose based on stools.

Morphine Sulfate: How supplied: tabs: 10, 15, 30 mg; elixir: 2, 4, 20 mg/mL; suppositories: 5, 10, 20 mg; injection: 8, 10, 15 mg/mL. Dose: Children, 0.1–0.2 mg/kg/dose SC, IM, or IV q2–4h prn; adults, 10–30 mg/dose PO q4h prn, or 2–10 mg/dose IV q2–4h prn.

Naloxone (Narcan): How supplied: injection: 0.02, 0.4, 1.0 mg/mL. Dose: Children, 0.01–0.1 mg/kg/dose IV once, may repeat dose of 0.1 mg/kg if needed, ETT, SC and IM routes acceptable; adults, 0.4–2 mg/dose IV once, may repeat q2–3 min; max dose 4 mg.

Naphazoline (Naphcon-A): How supplied: 0.025% ophthalmic solution with 0.3% pheniramine maleate, 15 mL. Dose: 1–2 drops each eye qid.

Naproxen (Aleve, Naprosyn): How supplied: tabs 200, 250, 375, 500 mg; liquid 125 mg/5 mL. Dose: anti-inflammatory 15 mg/kg/d bid–tid; max 1250 mg/d.

Nedocromil (Tilade): How supplied: oral inhaler 1.75 mg/puff, ~ 112 puffs/inhaler. Dose: 2 puffs qid, may reduce to 2 puffs bid–tid. *Note:* Safety in children < 12 yr has not been established.

Neomycin Sulfate: How supplied: tabs: 500 mg; suspension: 500 mg/5 mL. Dose: hepatic encephalopathy: initial dose 2.5–7 $g/m^2/d$ PO q6h for 5–7 days, then 2.5 $g/m^2/d$ PO q6h.

Neostigmine (Prostigmin): How supplied: tabs: 15 mg; injection: 0.25, 0.5, 1 mg/mL. Dose: myasthenia gravis: test dose: Children, 0.04 mg/kg/dose IM, 0.02 mg/kg/dose IV; adults, 0.02 mg/kg/dose IM; treatment: children: 0.01–0.04 mg/kg/dose SC, IM, or IV q2–3h prn; adults: 0.5 mg/dose SC, IM, or IV q3–4h prn (max 10 mg/d); 15–375 mg/d PO prn. *Note:* Safety and efficacy in children have not been established.

Nifedipine (Adalat, Procardia): How supplied: caps: 10, 20 mg. Dose: hypertension: Children (not FDA approved): 0.25–0.5 mg/kg/dose PO or sublingual q6–8h *for emergent use*, not to exceed adult doses; adults: 10–20 mg/dose PO tid, max 30 mg/dose and 180 mg/d.

Nitroglycerin: How supplied: injection: 5 mg/mL. Dose: 0.25–10 μg/kg/min as continuous IV infusion.

Nitroprusside (Nipride): How supplied: injection: 50 mg/5 mL. Dose: hypertensive crisis: 0.5–10 μg/kg/min as continuous IV infusion.

Norepinephrine (Levophed): How supplied: injection: 1 mg/mL. Dose: shock: 0.05–0.1 μg/kg/min as continuous IV infusion.

Olsalazine (Dipentum): How supplied: caps 250 mg. Dose: Adults 500 mg PO bid.

Omeprazole (Prilosec): How supplied: tabs, 20 mg. Dose: Adults: 20 mg/d.

Pancreatic Enzymes (Cotazym, Creon, Pancrease, Viokase, others): How supplied: powder: Cotazym (in caps), Viokase; enteric-coated spheres: Cotazym-S, Creon, Pancrease; non-enteric coated tabs: Viokase. Dose: 500–2000 U/lipase/kg/meal.

Pancuronium (Pavulon): How supplied: injection: 1 mg/mL, 2 mg/mL. Dose: 0.03–0.1 mg/kg/dose IV q30 min–2h prn, titrate dose based on patient response.

Paraldehyde: How supplied: solution: 1 g/mL; injection 1 g/mL. Dose: seizures: 0.3 mL/kg/dose in oil PO or PR q4–6h (adults 16–32 mL). For rectal dosage, mix paraldehyde 2:1 with oil (peanut, cottonseed, or olive); for oral dosage, dilute in milk or fruit juice.

Paregoric: How supplied: solution: 0.4 mg morphine/mL. Dose: opiate withdrawal in newborns: 0.2–0.5 mL/dose PO q3–4h prn, max 0.7 mL/kg/dose; analgesia: 0.25–0.5 mL/kg/dose PO qd–qid, max 10 mL/dose.

Pemoline (Cylert): How supplied: tabs: 18.75, 37.5, 75 mg; chewable tabs: 37.5 mg. Dose: treatment of ADHD: Children ≥ 6 yrs: initial dose 37.5 mg/d PO qAM, increase by 18.75 mg/d at weekly intervals prn (max dose 112.5 mg/d).

Penicillamine (Cuprimine): Dose: (1) Wilson's disease: Children: 20 mg/kg/d PO divided qid; adults: 0.75–1.5 g/d PO divided qid, adjust dose to result in an initial 24-hour cupriuresis of > 2 mg for 3 months; (2) cystinuria: children: 30 mg/kg/d PO divided qid; adults: 1–4 g/d PO divided qid, adjust dose to limit cystine excretion to 100–200 mg/d if no history of stones and < 100 mg/d with history of stones; (3) rheumatoid arthritis: children: efficacy has not been established; adults, 125–250 mg/d, may increase at 1–3 month intervals by 125–250 mg (max = 1500 mg/d); (4) arsenic poisoning: 100 mg/kg/d PO divided qid (max = 1 g/d); (5) lead poisoning: children: 25–40 mg/kg/d PO divided bid–tid; adults: 1–1.5 g/d for 1–2 months, continue until blood lead level is < 60 μg/dL.

Pentobarbital (Nembutal): How supplied: caps: 50, 100; elixir 20 mg/5 mL; suppositories: 30, 60, 120, 200 mg; injection: 50 mg/mL. Dose: sedation: 2–6 mg/kg/dose PO, max 100 mg/dose; 3–6 mg/kg/dose PR in children < 4 yr, 1.5–3 mg/kg/dose PR > 4 yr.

Phenazopyridine (Pyridium): How supplied: tabs: 100, 200 mg. Dose: symptomatic relief of urinary tract infection: Children > 6 yr: 100 mg/dose PO tid after meals; adults, 200 mg/dose PO tid after meals.

Phenobarbital: How supplied: tabs: 15, 30, 60, 100 mg; elixir: 20 mg/5 mL; injection: 65, 130 mg/mL. Dose: sedation: 2–3 mg/kg/dose PO or IM q6–8h prn; seizures; 10–20 mg/kg/dose IM or IV initially; can give further 5–10 mg/kg increments to serum level of 40 μg/mL, then 3–5 mg/kg/d PO q24h (adults 150–250 mg/d).

Phenytoin (Dilantin): How supplied: tabs: 50 mg; caps: 30, 100 mg; suspension: 30, 125 mg/5 mL; injection: 50 mg/mL. Dose: seizures: 10–20 mg/kg/dose slow IV initially, not to exceed 1 mg/kg/min, then 4–8 mg/kg/d PO or IV qd–tid; adult, 300–600 mg/d PO or IV qd–tid.

Physostigmine Salicylate (Antilirium): How supplied: injection: 1 mg/mL. Dose: reversal of central nervous system effects caused by anticholinergics: 0.01-0.03 mg/kg/dose IM or IV, no more than 0.5 mg/min, repeat q5–10 min up to max total dose of 2 mg. *Note:* Life-threatening situations only.

Potassium Iodide: How supplied: syrup: 325 mg/5 mL; solution: 1 g/mL. Dose: expectorant: Children, 100–300 mg/d PO bid–tid; adults, 300–900 mg/d PO tid.

Potassium Supplement: How supplied: potassium chloride: effervescent tabs: 25, 50 mEq; caps: 4, 8, 10 mEq: liquid: 5%, 10%, 20% (5% = 10 mEq/15 mL); powder: 15, 20 mEq/packet, 25 mEq/scoop; injection: 2 mEq/mL. Dose: maintenance: ~ 1–2 mEq/kg/d PO qd–qid (40–80 mEq/d for adults); hypokalemia: 0.5–1.0 mEq/kg/dose slow IV.

Pralidoxime (Protopam): How supplied: tabs: 500 mg; injection: 1 g/20 mL. Dose: reversal of paralysis due to organophosphates: 20–40 mg/kg/dose slow IV, as 5% solution, repeat q1h prn; adults 1–2 g/dose slow IV, dose may be given SC, IM, or PO if necessary.

Prazosin (Minipress): How supplied: tabs: 1, 2, 5 mg. Dose: hypertension: *Not approved for use in children;* Adults: initial 1 mg/dose PO bid–tid, slowly increase to a total daily dose of 20 mg; usual dose 6–15 mg/d.

Prednisolone: How supplied: tabs 5 mg; syrup 5 mg/mL and 15 mg/mL. Dose: Same as prednisone.

Prednisone: How supplied: tabs: 1, 2.5, 5, 10, 20, 25, 50 mg; syrup: 5 mg/5 mL. Dose: physiologic replacement: 3–4 mg/m^2/d PO bid; asthma: 1–2 mg/kg/d PO qd–bid, max 20–40 mg/d for 3–5 days; anti-inflammatory: 0.5–2 mg/kg/d PO bid–qid.

Primidone (Mysoline): How supplied: tabs: 50, 250 mg; suspension: 250 mg/5 mL. Dose: seizures: < 8 yr, days 1–3; 50 mg/dose PO qhs: days 4–6: 50 mg/dose PO bid; days 7–9: 100 mg/dose PO bid; day 10 on: 125–250 mg/dose PO tid; usual maintenance dose 10–25 mg/kg/d PO tid; > 8 yr, days 1–3: 100–125 mg/dose PO qhs: days 4–6: 100–125 mg/dose PO bid; days 7–9: 100–125 mg/dose PO tid; day 10 on: 250 mg/dose PO tid, slowly increased to max 750–1500 mg/d tid–qid.

Probenecid (Benemid): How supplied: tabs: 500 mg. Dose: hyperuricemia: > 2 yr: 25 mg/kg/dose PO once, then 40 mg/kg/d PO qid; > 14 yr: 1–2 g/dose PO once, then 2 g/d PO qid.

Procainamide (Pronestyl): How supplied: tabs: 250, 375, 500 mg; sustained-release tabs: 500 mg; caps: 250, 375, 500 mg; injection: 100, 500 mg/mL. Dose: cardiac arrhythmias: Children: 15–50 mg/kg/d PO q3–6h, max 4 g/d; IV: 10–15 mg/kg/dose IV over 30 min, then 20–80 μg/kg/min continuous IV infusion; adult: ~ 50 mg/kg/d PO q3–6h, usually 250–500 mg/dose q3–6h, max 4 g/d; IV: 100–200 mg IV over 30 min, max 1 g, then 2–6 mg/min continuous IV infusion.

Prochlorperazine (Compazine): How supplied: tabs: 5, 10, 25 mg; sustained-release caps: 10, 15, 30 mg; syrup: 5 mg/5 mL; suppositories: 2.5, 25 mg; injection: 5 mg/mL. Contraindicated in children < 2 yrs. Dose: antiemetic: Children 9–13 kg: 2.5 mg/dose PO or PR qd–bid; 14–18 kg: 2.5 mg/dose PO or PR bid–tid; 19–40 kg: 2.5–5 mg/dose PO or PR bid–tid; adults: 5–10 mg/dose PO tid–qid or 25 mg PR bid: IM: children: 0.13 mg/kg/dose; adults: 5–10 mg/dose tid–qid (max 40 mg/d).

Promethazine (Phenergan): How supplied: tabs: 12.5, 25, 50 mg; syrup: 6.25, 25 mg/5 mL; suppositories: 12.5, 25, 50 mg; injection: 25, 50 mg/mL. Dose: antihistamine: Children, 0.1 mg/kg/dose PO tid and 0.5 mg/kg/dose PO qhs; adults, 12.5–25 mg/dose PO tid and qhs; nausea: children, 0.25–0.5 mg/kg/dose PO, PR, or IM q4–6h prn; adults, 12.5–25 mg/dose PO, PR, or IM q4–6h prn; sedation: children, 0.5–1 mg/kg/dose PO, PR, or IM q6h prn; adults, 25–50 mg/dose PO, PR, or IM q6h prn; motion sickness: children, 0.5 mg/kg/dose PO, or PR bid prn; adults, 25 mg PO or PR bid prn.

Propranolol (Inderal): How supplied: tabs: 10, 20, 40, 60, 80, 90 mg; extended-release caps: 80, 120, 160 mg; injection: 1 mg/mL. Dose: hypertension and tachyarrhythmias: 0.25 mg/kg/dose PO q6h, can increase to max of 3.5 mg/kg/dose q6h; 0.01 mg/kg IV q6h, max 0.15 mg/kg/dose; Adults: initial 40 mg/dose PO bid, then increase slowly to maintenance dose of 120–240 mg/d PO q8–12h (max dose 640 mg/d); arrhythmias: children: 0.01–0.1 mg/kg/dose slow IV (max 1 mg/dose), then 0.5–4 mg/kg/d; adults: 1–3 mg/dose slow IV, then 10–30 mg/d PO tid–qid; tetralogy spells: 0.15–0.25 mg/kg/dose slow IV, may repeat once, max 10 mg/dose, then 1–2 mg/kg/dose PO q6h; migraine prophylaxis: < 35 kg: 10–20 mg/dose PO tid; > 35 kg: 20–40 mg/dose PO tid; adults: sustained-release 60–160 mg/dose qd.

Propylthiouracil (PTU): How supplied: tabs: 50 mg. Dose: hyperthyroidism: initial dose 6–7 mg/kg/d PO q8h, then maintenance usually ⅓–½ of initial dose; initial adult dose usually 300 mg/d PO q8h.

Prostaglandin E_1 (Prostin): How supplied: injection: 500 µg/mL. Dose: to maintain patency of ductus arteriosus: 0.05–0.1 µg/kg/min as continuous IV infusion.

Protamine sulfate: How supplied: injection: 5, 10 mg/mL. Dose: 1 mg will neutralize ~ 100 U of heparin (max dose is 50 mg per 10-min period).

Pseudoephedrine (Sudafed, Novafed, others): How supplied: tabs: 30, 60 mg; extended-release, 120 mg (dose q12h); syrup: 30 mg/5 mL. Dose: 4 mg/kg/d PO qid; adults, 30–60 mg/dose PO q6–8h.

Pyridostigmine (Mestinon): How supplied: tabs: 60 mg; extended-release tabs: 180 mg; syrup: 60 mg/5 mL; injection: 5 mg/mL. Dose: symptomatic treatment of myasthenia gravis: Children, 7 mg/kg/d PO q4–6, adjust prn; adult: usual dose 600 mg/d PO prn.

Quinidine: How supplied: gluconate (62% quinidine base): tabs: 324 mg (202 mg base); extended-release tabs: 324 mg (202 mg base); sulfate (83% quinidine base): tabs: 100, 200, 300 mg (88, 176, 264 mg base). Dose: (as base) Children, test dose: 2 mg/kg/dose PO once; maintenance dose: 15–60 mg/kg/d PO q6h; adults, test dose: 1 tab PO; maintenance: 100–600 mg/dose PO q6–8h.

Ranitidine (Zantac): How supplied: tabs: 150, 300 mg; oral syrup 15 mg/mL; injection: 25 mg/mL. Dose: Children: 5 mg/kg/d PO bid; parenteral: 1–2 mg/kg/d IM or IV q6–8h; adults: 300–600 mg/d PO qd–bid; parenteral: 50 mg/dose IM or IV q6–8h.

Rocuronium: How supplied: injectable 10 mg/mL. Dose: 0.6–0.9 mg/kg IV.

Salmeterol (Serevent): How supplied: oral inhaler 25 µg/puff, 120 puffs/inhaler. Dose: 2 puffs bid. *Note:* Safety in children < 12 yr has not been established.

Scopolamine Hydrobromide (Transderm-Scōp, others): How supplied: tabs: 400, 600 mg; transderm patch: releases 1.5 mg over 3 days; injection: 0.4 mg/mL; ophthalmic solution 0.25%. Dose: motion sickness: transderm patch 1 per 3 days (apply 4 hours prior to travel); *or* 6 μg/kg PO, IM, SC.

Secobarbital (Seconal): How supplied: tabs: 50, 100 mg; caps: 50, 100 mg; elixir: 22 mg/5 mL; suppositories: 30, 60, 120, 200 mg; injection: 50 mg/mL. Dose: sedation: Children: 6 mg/kg/d PO or PR q8h; adults 20–40 mg/dose PO or PR bid–tid.

Sodium Polystyrene Sulfonate (Kayexalate): How supplied: powder: 3.6 g/tsp (exchanges ~ 1 mEq K/g); suspension 15 g/60 mL. Dose: treatment of hyperkalemia: Children: 1 g/kg/dose PO q6h *or*1 g/kg/dose PR q2–6h; adults: 15–60 g/dose PO qd–qid; *or* 30–50 g/dose PR q6h.

Sotalol (Betapace): How supplied: caplets 80, 160, 240 mg. Dose: 2–8 mg/kg/d bid, max adult dose 960 mg/d.

Spironolactone (Aldactone): How supplied: tabs: 25, 50, 100 mg. Dose: edema associated with mineralocorticoid (aldosterone) excess: 1–3.3 mg/kg/d PO qd–bid; adults 25–200 mg/d PO qd–bid.

Succinylcholine (Anectine): How supplied: injection: 20 mg/mL, 50 mg/mL, 100 mg/mL. Dose: Infants, small children: 1–2 mg/kg/dose IV; adolescents and older children: 0.6–1 mg/kg/dose IV; adults: 0.3–1.1 mg/kg/dose IV; may be given IM if necessary, 3–4 mg/kg/dose IM (max 150 mg/dose).

Sucralfate (Carafate): How supplied: tabs: 1 g; suspension 1 g/10 mL. Dose: short-term treatment of duodenal ulcers: Infants and children 25 mg/kg/dose tid–qid; > 12 yr: 1 g/dose PO qid. *Note:* Drug should be given on an empty stomach.

Sulfasalazine (Azulfidine): How supplied: tabs: 500 mg; enteric-coated tabs: 500 mg. Dose: management of ulcerative colitis: > 2 yr: initial 40–100 mg/kg/d PO q4–8h, then 30 mg/kg/d PO qid; adults: initial dose 3–4 g/d PO q4–8h, then 2 g/d PO qid, max 6 g/d.

Sulfinpyrazone (Anturane): How supplied: tabs 100 mg, caps 200 mg. Dose: 5 mg/kg/d bid.

Terbutaline (Brethine): How supplied: tabs: 2.5, 5 mg; inhaler: 200 μg/puff, ~ 300 puffs/inhaler; injection: 1 mg/mL (may be used for nebulization). Dose: Children: < 12 yr: 0.05–0.1 mg/kg/dose PO tid; > 12 yr: 2.5–5 mg/dose PO tid; inhalation: children > 12 yrs: 2 puffs q4–6h prn; nebulization: *(not FDA-approved for this use)* 0.1 mg/kg/dose q1h prn, max 2.5 mg/dose; 0.005–0.1 mg/kg/dose SC q15–30 min × 2 (max 0.25 mg/dose).

Terfenadine (Seldane): How supplied: tabs: 60 mg. Dose: perennial and seasonal allergic rhinitis and other allergic symptoms. > 12 yr, 60 mg/dose PO bid. *Note:* Safety and efficacy in children

< 12 yrs have not been established. Do *not* prescribe with macrolide antibiotics or ketoconazole/itraconazole.

Theophylline (many trade names): How supplied: (see also Aminophylline) tabs: 100, 200, 300 mg; syrup: 80 mg/15 mL; sustained-release tabs: 100, 200, 300, 450 mg; sustained-release caps: Slo-Bid gyrocaps: 50, 100, 200, 300 mg; Slo-Phyllin gyrocaps: 60, 125, 250 mg; Theo-Dur sprinkles: 50, 75, 125, 200 mg. Dose: neonatal apnea: loading dose 5 mg/kg/dose PO once; maintenance: < 36 wk: 1–2 mg/kg/d PO q8–12h; > 36 wk: 2–4 mg/kg/day PO q8–12h; asthma: loading dose of 1 mg/kg will raise serum level ~ 2 μg/mL; children < 1 yr: dose in mg/kg/d = (0.2) (age in wks) + 5; children > 1 yr: 12–14 mg/kg/d up to 300 mg/d × 3 days, then if tolerated, 400 mg/d (adults, ≥ 45 kg) or 16 mg/kg/d up to 400 mg/day (< 45 kg) × 3 days, then if tolerated, 600 mg/day (adults ≥ 45 kg) or 20 mg/kg/d up to 600 mg/day (< 45 kg). Further dosage adjustments based on symptoms, adverse effects and serum concentrations.

Thioridazine (Mellaril): How supplied: tabs: 10, 15, 25, 50, 100, 150, 200 mg; liquid: 30, 100 mg/1 mL; suspension: 25, 100 mg/5 mL. Dose: psychotic disorders and severe behavioral problems: 2–12 yr: 0.5–3 mg/kg/d PO bid–qid; adults: initial dose 50–100 mg/dose PO tid, then gradually increase to 200–800 mg/d PO bid–qid.

Tolmetin Sodium (Tolectin): How supplied: tabs: 200 mg; caps: 400 mg. Dose: relief of signs and symptoms of rheumatoid arthritis and osteoarthritis: Children: 15–30 mg/kg/d PO tid–qid; adults: 600–1800 mg/d PO tid–qid.

Triamcinolone Acetonide (Azmacort, Nasacort): How supplied: oral inhaler 200 μg/puff, 240 puffs/inhaler; nasal inhaler 55 μg/puff, 100 puffs/inhaler. Dose: oral inhaler 2 puffs tid–qid (not to exceed 12 puffs/day); nasal inhaler 1 puff/nasal passage qd–bid.

Trimethobenzamide (Tigan): How supplied: caps: 100, 250 mg; suppositories: 100, 200 mg; injection: 100 mg/mL. Dose: antiemetic: < 15 kg: 100 mg/dose PR tid–qid; 15–40 kg: 100–200 mg/dose PO or PR tid–qid; adults: 200–250 mg/dose PO or PR tid–qid; 200 mg/dose IM tid–qid.

Valproic Acid (Depakene, Depakote): How supplied: tabs: 250 mg; enteric-coated tabs: 125, 250, 500 mg; syrup: 250 mg/5 mL. Dose: simple and complex absence seizures: initial dose 15 mg/kg/d PO bid, then increments every week of 5–10 mg/kg/d, max 60 mg/kg/d.

Vecuronium (Norcuron): How supplied: 10 mg injection. Dose: to facilitate endotracheal intubation and to provide skeletal muscle relaxation during surgery or mechanical ventilation. 0.08–0.1 mg/kg/dose IV repeated q30–60 min prn.

Verapamil (Calan, Isoptin): How supplied: tabs: 40, 80, 120 mg; sustained-release caplets: 240 mg; injection: 2.5 mg/mL. Dose: supraventricular tachyarrythmias IV: Children > 1 yr: 0.1–0.15 mg/kg/dose slow IV (max 5 mg/dose), may repeat once q30 min; adults: 5–10 mg/dose slow IV, may repeat once q30 min. Dose: hypertension: children: safety and efficacy in children < 18 yrs have not been established; adults: 240–480 mg/d divided tid.

Vitamin K [phytonadione] (AquaMEPHYTON, Konakion): How supplied: tabs: 5 mg; injection: 2, 10 mg/mL. Dose: neonatal prophylaxis: 0.5–1 mg/dose IM, once within 1h of birth; anticoagulant overdose: 2.5–10 mg/dose PO, SC, IM, or IV, may repeat once, up to 25 mg/dose; hypoprothrombinemia: 2.5–25 mg/dose PO, SC, IM, or IV, up to 50 mg/dose. For hemorrhagic disease: 1–10 mg slow IV push.

FORMULARY OF ANTI-INFECTIVES AND ANTIBIOTICS

Note: Where specific doses for premature infants and neonates are not listed, consult other sources.

Acyclovir (Zovirax): How supplied: ointment: 5%; caps: 200 mg; injection: 500 mg. Dose: topical: q3h; 200 mg PO 5 times/d; 30 mg/kg/d IV q8h. Coverage: herpes simplex; varicella-zoster. Comments: Ointment is efficacious only in initial herpes genitalis. Capsules are efficacious in suppression and treatment of initial and recurrent herpes genitalis. Decrease dose in renal failure.

Amantadine (Symmetrel): How supplied: syrup: 50 mg/5 mL; caps: 100 mg. Dose: Children 1–9 yrs: 4.4–8.8 mg/kg/d PO divided q12h (max 150 mg/d); children > 9 and adults: 200 mg/d PO divided bid. Coverage: influenza A. Comments: Must be started within 24–48 h of onset of symptoms.

Amikacin (Amikin): How supplied: injection: 100 mg/2 mL; 500 mg/2 mL; 1 mg/4 mL. Dose: Adults, children and older infants: 15 mg/kg/d IV or IM q8h; max 1.5 g/d. Newborns: loading dose of 10 mg/kg followed by 7.5 mg/kg IV q12h. Coverage: gram-negatives. Toxicity: renal, VIII nerve. Comments: Peak 15–30 μg/mL, trough < 5 μg/mL. Adjust dose in renal failure.

Amoxicillin (Amoxil, Polymox, Trimon, Wymox): How supplied: caps: 250, 500 mg; suspension: 125, 250 mg/5 mL; chewable tabs:

125, 250 mg. Dose: 40 mg/kg/d PO q8h. Coverage: non-penicillinase producing gram-positive cocci *Listeria, E coli, Salmonella, Shigella.*

Amoxicillin and Potassium Clavulanate (Augmentin): How supplied: suspension: 125 mg amox + 31.25 mg clav/5 mL, 250 mg amox + 62.5 mg clav/5 mL; chewable tabs: 125 mg amox + 31.25 mg clav, 250 mg amox + 62.5 mg clav/5 mL; tabs: 250 mg amox + 125 mg clav, 500 mg amox + 125 mg clav. Dose: same as Amoxicillin. Coverage: β-lactamase-producing gram-negatives and gram-positives.

Amphotericin B (Fungizone): How supplied: injection: 50 mg. Dose: 0.25–1 mg/kg/d IV over 2–6 h q24h. Coverage: *Aspergillus; Candida; Cryptococcus; Blastomyces; Sporotrichum; Coccidioides; Histoplasma; mucormycoses.* Toxicity: renal. Use for severe fungal infections only. *Note:* Safety and efficacy in pediatric patients are not well established.

Ampicillin (Omnipen, Polycillin, Principen): How supplied: suspension: 125, 250, 500 mg/5 mL; chewable tabs: 125 mg; drops: 100 mg/mL; caps: 240, 500 mg; injection: 0.125, 0.25, 0.5, 1, 2, 43 g. Dose: 50 mg/kg/d PO q6h; 100–400 mg/kg/d IV or IM q4–6h. Coverage: same as Amoxicillin.

Aztreonam (Azactam): How supplied: injection: 0.5, 1, 2 g. Dose: 90–120 mg/kg/d IV or IM q6–8h. Coverage: gram-negatives including *Pseudomonas aeruginosa.*

Carbenicillin (Geocillin, Geopen): How supplied: tabs: 382 mg; injection: 2, 5 g. Dose: 30–50 mg/kg/d PO q6h. Coverage: gram-negatives except *Klebsiella.* Toxicity: platelet dysfunction. Comments: Some *Serratia* and *Pseudomonas* are resistant.

Cefaclor (Ceclor): How supplied: suspension: 125, 250 mg/5 mL; caps 250, 500 mg. Dose: 40 mg/kg/d PO q8–12h. Coverage: streptococci; some *H influenzae*; some *S aureus.*

Cefamandole (Mandol): How supplied: injection: 0.5, 1, 2 g. Dose: 50–100 mg/kg/d IV or IM q4–8h. Coverage: same as Cefaclor; some *Klebsiella* and *Proteus*; anaerobes.

Cefazolin (Ancef, Kefzol): How supplied: injection: 0.25, 0.5, 1 g. Dose: 50–100 mg/kg/d IM or IV q8h. Coverage: gram-positive cocci; some gram negatives.

Cefixime (Suprax): How supplied: suspension: 100 mg/5 mL; tabs: 400 mg. Dose: 8 mg/kg/d PO q24h. Coverage: gram-negatives including *H influenzae*; gram-positives except staphylococci and enterococci. Comments: Cefixime is the only oral third-generation cephalosporin.

Cefoperazone (Cefobid): How supplied: injection: 1, 2 g. Dose: *Not approved for use in children*; Adults: 2–4 g/d divided q12h IV or IM. Coverage: same as Cefixime.

Cefotaxime (Claforan): How supplied: injection: 1, 2 g. Dose: 100–200 mg/kg/d IM or IV q6–8h; meningitis, 200 mg/kg/d IM or IV q6h. Coverage: same as Cefixime; does not cover *Listeria*.

Cefoxitin (Mefoxin): How supplied: injection: 1, 2 g. Dose: Children > 3 mos: 80–160 mg/kg/d IM or IV q4–6h; adults: 1–2 g q6–8h IV or IM (max 12 g/d). Coverage: same as Cefazolin plus anaerobes.

Ceftazidime (Fortaz, Tazicef, Tazidime): How supplied: injection: 0.5, 1, 2 g. Dose: Children: 30–50 mg/kg IV q8h (max 6 g/d); adults: 1 g q8–12h IV or IM. Coverage: same as Cefotaxime: most *Pseudomonas*.

Ceftriaxone (Rocephin): How supplied: injection: 1.25, 0.5, 1, 2 g. Dose: Children: 50–100 mg/kg/d IM or IV q12–24h; meningitis, 100 mg/kg/d IM or IV q12h; adults: 1–2 g q12–24h IV (max 4 g/24h) Coverage: same as Cefotaxime.

Cefuroxime (Ceftin, Kefurox, Zinacef): How supplied: injection: 0.75, 1.5 g. Dose: Children < 2 yrs: 125 mg/dose bid PO; children > 2 yrs: 250 mg/dose bid PO; adults: 250–500 mg/dose bid PO. Coverage: streptococci; some staphylococci, some gram-negatives. Comments: May result in delayed cerebrospinal fluid sterilization.

Cephalexin (Keflet, Keflex, Keftab): How supplied: drops: 100 mg/mL; suspension: 125, 250 mg/5 mL; tabs/caps: 0.25, 0.5, 1 g. Dose: 25–50 mg/kg/d PO q6h. Coverage: gram-positive cocci.

Cephapirin (Cefadyl): How supplied: injection: 0.5, 1, 2, 4 g. Dose: 40–80 mg/kg/d IM or IV q6h; Adults: 0.5–1 g/dose q4–6h (max 12g/24h). Coverage: gram-positive cocci.

Cephradine (Anspor, Velosef): How supplied: suspension: 125, 250 mg/5 mL; caps: 250, 500 mg; Dose: 25–50 mg/kg/d PO q6h. Coverage: same as Cephalexin.

Chloramphenicol (Chloromycetin): How supplied: suspension: 150 mg/5 mL; caps: 250 mg; injection: 1 g. Dose: 50–75 mg/kg/d PO or IV q6h; meningitis, 75–100 mg/kg/d IV divided q6h. Coverage: gram-positives and gram-negatives; *Rickettsiae; Chlamydiae*. Comments: Peak 10–25 μg/mL, trough 5–10 μg/mL.

Chloroquine (Aralen PO_4, Plaquenil, Aralen HCL): How supplied: tabs: 500 mg (300 mg base); tabs: 200 mg (155 mg base); injection: 250 mg (200 mg base). Dose: malaria: suppression: 5 mg/kg base qwk (max 310 mg base qwk) acute treatment: 10 mg/kg base; 6 h later, 5 mg/kg base; 18 h later, 5 mg/kg base; 24 h later, 5 mg/kg base. Coverage: *Plasmodium* sp (some *P falciparum* resistant); *Entamoeba histolytica* (extraintestinal). Toxicity: retinal. Comments: Suppressive therapy should begin 2 weeks prior to potential exposure.

Ciprofloxacin (Cipro): How supplied: tabs: 250, 500, 750 mg. Dose: *Not approved for use in children*; Adults: 250–500 mg PO q12h. Coverage: gram-negatives including *Pseudomonas*.

Clindamycin (Cleocin): How supplied: solution: 75 mg/5 mL; caps: 75, 100 mg; injection: 150, 300, 600 mg. Dose: Children: 20–30 mg/kg/d PO q6h; 25–40 mg/kg/d IM or IV q6–8h; adults: 150–450 mg/dose q6–8h PO (max 1.8 g/d); 1.2–1.8 g/24h divided bid–tid, IV or IM (max 4.8 g/24h). Coverage: anaerobes and some gram-positive cocci.

Colistin (Coly-Mycin): How supplied: suspension: 125 mg/5 mL. Dose: 5–15 mg/kg/d PO q8h. Coverage: enteropathogenic *E coli; Shigella*.

Dicloxacillin (Dycill, Dynapen, Pathocil): How supplied: suspension: 62.5 mg/5 mL; caps: 125, 250, 500 mg. Dose: 12–25 mg/kg/d PO q6h; Adults: 125–500 mg PO q6h. Coverage: penicillin-resistant staphylococci.

Doxycycline (Doryx, Vibramycin, Vibra-Tabs): How supplied: suspension: 25 mg/mL; syrup: 50 mg/mL; caps: 50, 100 mg; injection: 100, 200 mg. Dose: Children > 8 yr: 4 mg/kg/d PO q12h for 24 h then 2 mg/kg/d PO q24h; 2–4 mg/kg/d IV over 2 hr q24h. Adults: 200 mg/dose q12h on day 1, followed by 100 mg/dose q12h maintenance. Coverage: gram-positives; *Rickettsiae; Chlamydiae; Mycoplasma; Brucella; Bacteroides*. Toxicity: permanent tooth discoloration when given during tooth development.

Erythromycin (E.E.S., E-mycin, EryPed, Ery-Tab, Ethril, others): How supplied: drops: 100 mg/mL, 100 mg/2.5 mL; suspension: 125, 200, 250, 400 mg/5 mL; chewable tabs: 125, 200, 250 mg; tabs: 250, 330, 400, 500 mg; caps: 125, 250 mg; topical solution: 2% ophthalmic solution: 0.5%; ampoules: 0.25, 0.5, 1 g; injection: 1.5, 1g. Dose: 20–40 mg/kg/d PO q6–8h; 20–50 mg/kg/d IV q6h; acne: topical; eye: topical. Coverage: same as Doxycycline: *Legionella; Bordetella pertussis; Corynebacterium diphtheriae; Clostridia*.

Erythromycin and sulfisoxazole (Pediazole): How supplied: suspension: 200 mg ery + 600 mg sulf/5 mL. Dose: 40 mg/kg of ery PO q6–8h. Coverage: same as erythromycin: *H influenzae*.

Ethambutol (Myambutol): How supplied: tabs: 100, 400 mg. Dose: 15 mg/kg/d PO q24h. Coverage: *M tuberculosis*. Toxicity: optic neuritis.

Flucytosine (Ancobon): How supplied: caps: 250, 500 mg. Dose: Adult: 50–150 mg/kg/d PO q6h. Coverage: *Candida; Cryptococcus*. Toxicity: Bone marrow suppression. Comments: Check sensitivities; many *Candida* species are resistant. *Note:* Safety and efficacy in children have not been established.

Furazolidone (Furoxone): How supplied: suspension: 50 mg/15 mL; tabs: 100 mg. Dose: Children > 1 mo: 5–8 mg/kg/d PO q6h; Adults: 100 mg/dose qid PO. Coverage: *Vibrio cholerae; Giardia.* Comments: Turns urine brownish color. *Notes:* Do not combine with alcohol. Do not give to children < 1 mo old.

Gentamicin (Garamycin): How supplied: injection: 20, 60, 80 mg; ophthalmic solution; ophthalmic ointment. Dose: Children: 6.7–7.5 mg/kg/d IM or IV divided q8h; eye: topical solution, q4h; ointment, q6h; adults: 3–5 mg/kg/d IM or IV divided q8h. Coverage: same as Amikacin. Toxicity: same as Amikacin. Comments: Peak 8–10 μg/mL, trough < 2 μg/mL.

Griseofulvin (Fulvicin P/G, Fulvicin U/F, Grifulvin, others): How supplied: suspension: 125 mg/5 mL; tabs: 125, 165, 250, 330, 500 mg; caps: 125, 250, 500 mg. Dose: Children: 10–15 mg/kg/d PO q24h; adults: 500 mg PO qd. Coverage: *Trichophyton* sp; *Microsporum* sp; *Epidermophyton floccosum.* Comments: Contraindicated in patients with porphyria or hepatocellular failure.

Imipenem-Cilastatin (Primaxin): How supplied: injection: 250, 500 mg. Dose: *Not approved for use in children*; Adults: 500–750 mg q12h IM, or 250–500 mg q6–8h IV. Dose is based on imipenem. Coverage: gram-negatives and gram-positives including *Pseudomonas; Serratia; Enterobacter; Proteus.*

Iodoquinol (Yodoxin): How supplied: tabs: 210, 650 mg. Dose: children < 6 yr: (210-mg tabs) one tablet per 15 pounds body weight; Children 6–12 yrs: (210-mg tabs) 2 tablets tid; adults: (210-mg tabs) 3 tablets tid. Coverage: *Entamoeba histolytica* (intestinal).

Isoniazid (INH, Laniazid): How supplied: syrup: 50 mg/5 mL; tabs: 50, 100, 300 mg. Dose: Children: 10–20 mg/kg/d PO q24h; adults: 5 mg/kg/d PO (usual dose 300 mg PO qd). Coverage: *M tuberculosis.* Toxicity: hepatic; neuro due to pyridoxine deficiency. Comments: Supplement with pyridoxine; use < 10 mg/kg/d when given with rifampin.

Kanamycin (Kantrex): How supplied: injection: 75, 500 mg, 1 g; caps: 500 mg. Dose: 15 mg/kg/d IM or IV q8–12h; 50–100 mg/kg/d PO q6h. Coverage: same as Amikacin; *Vibrio, Salmonella, Shigella.* Toxicity: same as Amikacin. Comments: Oral dosing not absorbed; used for bowel sterilization. Peak 15–30 μg/mL, trough < 10 μg/mL.

Ketoconazole (Nizoral): How supplied: cream: 2% in 15, 30, 60 g tubes; tabs: 200 mg. Dose: topical: to affected area q24h; Children > 2 yrs: 3.6–6.6 mg/kg/d PO q24h; adults: 200 mg/24 h (max 400 mg/24h). Coverage: some dermatophytes; *Candida; Blastomyces,*

Coccidioides, Histoplasma. Toxicity: hepatic. *Note:* Should not be used in children < 2 yr and not in children of any age unless potential benefit outweighs risk.

Mebendazole (Vermox): How supplied: chewable tabs: 100 mg. Dose: pinworms: 100 mg PO; one dose; other nematodes: 100 mg q12h for 3 days. Coverage: *Trichuris; Enterobius; Ascaris; Ancylostoma; Necator.*

Metronidazole (Flagyl, Metric-21, Protostat): How supplied: tabs: 250, 500 mg; injection: 500 mg. Dose: anaerobic infections: Adults: 1.5 mg/kg one time, then 7.5 mg/kg q6h IV. Amebiasis: Children: 30–50 mg/kg/d divided tid; adults: 750 mg PO tid. Trichomoniasis: 2 g PO as a single dose *or* 250 mg tid for 7 days. Coverage: anaerobes; *Giardia; Entamoeba histolytica;* trichomoniases. *Note:* Safety and efficacy for IV use in children have not been established.

Mezlocillin (Mezlin): How supplied: injection: 1, 2, 3, 4 g. Dose: Children 1 mo–12 yr: 200–300 mg/kg/d IV q4–6h; adults: 1.5–4 g/dose q4–6h IV (max 24 g/24h). Coverage: gram-negatives.

Miconazole (Monistat): How supplied: cream, lotion: 2%; vaginal cream: 2%; vaginal suppositories: 100, 200 mg; injection: 200 mg. Dose: Children: topical: to affected area q12h; vaginal: 1 applicator qhs; vaginal: 100–200 mg qhs or for systemic fungal infection; 20–40 mg/kg/d IV q8h (max 60 mg/kg/infusion); adults: 200–3600 mg/d divided tid IV. Coverage: some dermatophytes; *Candida; Cryptococcus; Coccidioides.* Comments: May also be administered intrathecally.

Mupirocin (Bactroban): How supplied: ointment: 2% in 15 g tube. Dose: topical q8h. Coverage: Impetigo due to *S aureus*, B-hemolytic strep, *S pyogenes.*

Nafcillin (Nafcil, Unipen): How supplied: solution: 250 mg/5 mL; caps: 250 mg; tabs: 500 mg; injection: 0.5, 1, 2 g. Dose: Children: 50–200 mg/kg/d IM or IV q6h; adults: 500 mg IV or IM q6h. Coverage: penicillinase-producing staphylococci.

Niclosamide (Niclocide): How supplied: tabs: 500 mg. Dose: *Taenia saginata* and *Diphyllobothrium latum*: 11–34 kg; 1 g PO single dose; 34–59 kg: 1.5 g PO single dose; > 59 kg: 2 g PO single dose; for *H nana*, as above, then: 11–34 kg; 0.5 g PO q24h; 34–59 kg: 1 g PO q24h; > 59 kg: 2 g PO q24h. Coverage: *Taenia saginata; Diphyllobothrium latum; Hymenolepis nana. Note:* Safety and efficacy have not been established in children < 2 yrs.

Nitrofurantoin (Furadantin, Macrodantin): How supplied: suspension: 25 mg/5 mL; caps: 25, 50, 100 mg; tabs: 50, 100 mg. Dose: Children: 5–7 mg/kg/d PO q6h; adults: 50–100 mg/dose q6h.

Coverage: gram-negatives. Toxicity: primaquine-sensitive hemolytic anemia. Comments: Used only for UTI.

Nystatin (Mycostatin, Nilstat, Nystex): How supplied: cream, ointment, powder: 100,000 U/g; suspension: 100,000 U/mL; tabs: 500,000 U. Dose: topical: to affected area q12h; for oral thrush: Infants: 2 mL/dose q6h; children: 4–6 mL/dose or 1 tab/dose q6h applied directly to areas of thrush; for treatment of thrush or fungal prophylaxis with central venous catheter in place, 0,5 mL PO Q6h. Coverage: *Candida.* Comments: Also comes in vaginal preparations.

Oxacillin (Bactocill, Prostaphlin): How supplied: suspension: 250 mg/5 mL; caps: 250, 500 mg; injection: 0.25, 0.5, 1, 2, 4 g. Dose: Children: 150–200 mg/kg/d IM or IV q6h; adults: 250–2000 mg/dose q4–6h IV or IM. Coverage: penicillinase-resistant staphylococci.

Oxytetracycline (Terramycin): How supplied: caps: 250 mg; injection: 50, 100, 250 mg. Dose: Children > 8 yr: 20–50 mg/kg/d PO q6h; 15–25 mg/kg/d IM q12h; adults: 1–2 g divided qid PO or 250 mg IM q24h or 300 mg IM divided q8–12h. Coverage: same as Doxycycline. Toxicity: same as Doxycycline.

Penicillin G (Pentids, Pfizerpen G): How supplied: suspension: 125, 250, 500 mg/5 mL; tabs: 125, 150, 250, 500 mg; injection: 1, 2, 5, 10, 20 million U. Dose: 25–50 mg/kg/d PO q6–8h; 0.1–0.25 million U/kg/d divided q4–6h IM or IV. Coverage: some gram-positive cocci; some gram-negative cocci; oral anaerobes. Treatment of meningitis and bacteremia: Meningitis: 75–100,000 IU/kg per dose slow IV push; Bacteremia: 25–50,000 IU/kg per dose. Dosage intervals: see Table 31–8.

Penicillin G, Benzathine (Bicillin): How supplied: injection: 0.6, 0.9, 1.2, 3 million U. Dose: 25,000–50,000 U/kg IM single dose. Coverage: Streptococci groups A, C, G, H, L, M.

Table 31–8. Dosage intervals for administration of Penicillin G.

PCA (wk)	Postnatal Age (d)	Interval (h)
≤ 29	0–28	12
	> 28	8
30–36	0–14	12
	> 14	8
≥ 37	0–7	12
	> 7	8

PCA = post-conceptional age.

Penicillin G, Procaine (Wycillin): How supplied: injection: 0.3, 0.6, 1.2, 2.4 million U. Dose: 25,000–50,000 U/kg/d IM. Coverage: same as penicillin G; spirochetes.

Penicillin V (Betapen-VK, Ledercillin VK, Pen-Vee K, Veetids): How supplied: solution: 125, 250 mg/5 mL; tabs: 125, 250, 500 mg. Dose: 25–50 mg/kg/d PO divided q6–8h. Coverage: streptococci groups A, C, G, H, L, M; oral anaerobes.

Pentamidine (Pentam 300): How supplied: injection: 300 mg. Dose: 4 mg/kg/d IM or IV. Coverage: *Pneumocystis carinii.* Toxicity: hypotension.

Piperacillin (Pipracil): How supplied: injection: 2, 3, 4 g. Dose: *Not approved for use in children*; 200–300 mg/kg/d IV divided q4–6h; Adults: 2–4 g/dose q4–8 (max 24 g/24h). Coverage: gram-negatives; anaerobes.

Praziquantel (Biltricide): How supplied: tabs: 600 mg. Dose: schistosomiasis: 60 mg/kg/d PO q8h for 3 doses; clonorchiasis and opisthorchiasis: 75 mg/kg/d PO q8h for 3 doses. Coverage: *Schistosoma* sp. *Note:* Safety in children < 4 yr has not been established.

Pyrantel (Antiminth): How supplied: suspension: 250 mg/5 mL. Dose: Children and adults: 11 mg/kg PO as single dose; repeat in 2 wks (max 1 g/dose). Coverage: *Enterobius; Ascaris.*

Pyrimethamine (Daraprim): How supplied: tabs: 25 mg. Dose: For prophylaxis of malaria: Children < 4 yr: 1/4 tab PO qwk; 4–10 yr: ½ tab PO qwk; > 10 yr: 1 tab PO qwk. For *T gondii*: 1 mg/kg/d PO q12h with a sulfa; adults: 50–75 mg PO qd. Coverage: *Plasmodium* sp; *Toxoplasma gondii.*

Quinacrine (Atabrine): How supplied: tabs: 100 mg. Dose: 6 mg/kg/d PO q8h. Coverage: *Giardia.* Toxicity: hepatic; hemolysis in G6PD deficiency. Comments: Turns skin yellow.

Ribavirin (Virazole): How supplied: vial: 6 g. Dose: 6 g aerosolized over 12–18 hr q24h. Coverage: Respiratory syncytial virus (RSV). Comments: Must be started within the first 3 days of RSV lower respiratory tract infection.

Rifampin (Rifadin, Rimactane): How supplied: caps: 150, 300 mg. Dose: 10–20 mg/kg/d PO q12–24h, max 600 mg/dose. For *H influenzae* prophylaxis: 20 mg/kg/d q12h for 4 doses. For *N meningitidis* prophylaxis: 20 mg/kg/d q24h for 4 doses. Coverage: *Mycobacterium; Neisseria; H influenzae.* Toxicity: hepatic. Comments: All body secretions may be colored red-orange.

Spectinomycin (Trobicin): How supplied: injection: 2, 4 g. Dose: Adults: 2 g in single dose; max 2 g IM. Coverage: *N gonorrhoeae. Note:* Safety and efficacy in children have not been shown.

Streptomycin: How supplied: injection: 1, 5 g. Dose: tuberculosis: Children: 20–30 mg/kg/d IM q12h (max 2 g/d); adults: 15 mg/kg/d divided q12h IM. Coverage: *M tuberculosis:* some gram-negatives. Toxicity: vestibular.

Sulfadoxine and Pyrimethamine (Fansidar): How supplied: tabs: 500 mg SDX/25 mg PMA. Dose: For prophylaxis:< 4 yr: 1/2 tab PO q2wk; 4–8 yr: 1 tab PO q2wk; 9–14 yr: 1 1/2 tab PO q2wk; > 14 yr: 2 tab PO q2wk; *or* half the above doses qwk. Same quantity may be used as a single dose for an acute attack. Coverage: *Plasmodium* sp including chloroquine-resistant *P falciparum*. Toxicity: hemolysis in G6PD deficiency; Stevens-Johnson syndrome. Comments: Fansidar-resistant *P falciparum* now exist. *Note:* Do not use in infants < 2 mo.

Sulfamethizole (Thiosulfil): How supplied: tabs: 500 mg. Dose: *Contraindicated in infants* < 2 mo; 30–45 mg/kg/d PO q6h; Adults: 500–1000 mg/dose tid–qid. Coverage: *E coli; Klebsiella; Enterobacter; S aureus; Proteus; H influenzae*. Comments: Used only for UTI.

Sulfamethoxazole (Gantanol): How supplied: suspension: 500 mg/5 mL; tabs: 500 mg. Dose: *Contraindicated in infants* < 2 mo; 50–60 mg/kg/d PO q12h; Adults: 2 g PO divided q12h. Coverage: same as sulfamethizole; malaria. Comments: Primarily used for UTI.

Sulfisoxazole (Gantrisin): How supplied: suspension: 500 mg/5 mL; tabs: 500 mg. Dose: *Contraindicated in infants* < 2 MO; 150 mg/kg/d PO Q6H; max 6 g/d; Adults: 4–8 g/24h divided Q6H PO. Coverage: same as sulfamethizole. Comments: Use half daily dose for prophylaxis of otitis media.

Tetracycline (Achromycin, Sumycin): How supplied: syrup: 125 mg/5 mL; suspension: 125 mg/5 mL; caps: 250, 500 mg; tabs: 250, 500 mg; injection: 100, 250, 500 mg. Dose: Children > 8 yr: 25–50 mg/kg/d PO q6h; adults: 250–500 mg/dose PO q6h. Coverage same as Doxycycline. Toxicity: same as Doxycycline.

Thiabendazole (Mintezol): How supplied: suspension: 500 mg/5 mL; chewable tabs: 500 mg. Dose: 50 mg/kg/d PO q12h; max 3 g/d. Coverage: strongyloidiasis; cutaneous larva migrans; visceral larva migrans; trichinosis. *Note:* Safety and efficacy in children < 30 lbs have not been established.

Ticarcillin (Ticar): How supplied: injection: 1, 3, 6 g. Dose: 200–300 mg/kg/d IV q4–6h. Coverage: same as Carbenicillin. Toxicity: Platelet dysfunction.

Ticarcillin and Clavulanate (Timentin): How supplied: injection: 3/0.1, 3/0.2 g. Dose: *Not approved for use in children;* same as Ticarcillin. Coverage: same as Ticarcillin; *Klebsiella, S aureus, H influenzae.*

Tobramycin (Nebcin): How supplied: injection: 20, 80 mg, 1.2 g. Dose: 6–7.5 mg/kg/d IM or IV q6–8h. Coverage: gram-negatives including *Pseudomonas*. Toxicity: same as Amikacin. Comments: May need higher doses in patients with cystic fibrosis; peak 6–8 μg/mL, trough 0.5–1.0 μg/mL.

Trifluridine (Viroptic): How supplied: ophthalmic solutions: 1%. Dose: 1 drop q2h to affected eye. Coverage: herpes simplex.

Trimethoprim (Proloprim, Trimpex): How supplied: tabs: 100, 200 mg. Dose: Adults: 100 mg/dose PO q12h. Coverage: *E coli, Proteus mirabilis, Klebsiella pneumoniae, Enterobacter*, coagulase-negative staphylococci. *Note:* Effectiveness in children < 12 yrs has not been established.

Trimethoprim-sulfamethoxazole (Bactrim, Septra): How supplied: suspension: 40 mg TMP/200 mg SMX/5 mL; tabs: 80 mg TMP/400 mg SMX, 160 mg TMP/800 mg SMX; injection: 400 mg TMP/2000 mg SMX. Dose: *Contraindicated in infants* < 2 mo; Children: 6–12 mg TMP/kg/d PO q12h: 10–20 mg TMP/kg/d IV q6h; adults: 160 mg TMP q12h. Coverage: gram-positives and gram-negatives; *Salmonella; Shigella, P carinii.*

Vancomycin (Vancocin, Vancoled, Vancor): How supplied: pulvules: 125, 250 mg; bottle: 1, 10 g; injection: 0.5, 1 g. Dose: pseudomembranous colitis: 20–40 mg/kg/d PO q6h; max 2 g/d. Staphylococcal infection: 40 mg/kg/d IV q8h. Coverage: *Clostridium difficile*; gram-positive cocci including methicillin-resistant. Toxicity: rash, hypotension, renal, 8th cranial nerve.

Vidarabine (Vira-A): How supplied: ophthalmic ointment: 3%; injection: 1 g. Dose: topical: ½ in. to affected eye 5 times/d; 10–15 mg/kg/d IV over 12–24 hr q24h. Coverage: herpes simplex.

Zidovudine (AZT) (Retrovir): How supplied: solution: 150 mg/5 mL; caps: 100 mg. Dose: 720 mg/m^2/d q6h (max 200 mg q6h). Coverage: HIV. Toxicity: granulocytopenia; anemia.

Appendix: Common Laboratory Values & Useful Formulas

Thomas J. McIntee, MD, Sandra J. Meech, MD,
& Marsha S. Anderson, MD

Tables:

COMMON NORMAL BLOOD CHEMISTRY VALUES & OTHER HEMATOLOGIC VALUES[1]

(Values may vary with the procedure employed.)

The following is a compilation of normal values for some commonly used laboratory tests. Where values differ with age, tables

[1] Adapted from S Meites (editor): *Pediatric Clinical Chemistry*, 3rd ed. American Association for Clinical Chemistry, 1989; and The Children's Hospital of Denver Clinical Laboratory.

have been provided. Some laboratory values that are often ordered together are arranged in tables. It is important to note that the methodology used for various laboratory tests and the units in which they are reported may vary significantly between different laboratories. If any doubt exists, consult your laboratory for normal ranges.

Clinical judgment should be used in interpretation of laboratory results and patient management.

Determinations for:

(S) = Serum
(B) = Whole blood (P) = Plasma
(RBC) = Red blood cells

Acid-Base Measurements at Sea Level (B)

pH: 7.30–7.46: 1 d
7.32–7.46: 2 d–1 mo
7.34–7.43: > 1 mo
PaO_2: 65–76 mm Hg (8.66–10.13 kPa)
$PaCO_2$: 36–38 mm Hg (4.8–5.07 kPa)
Base excess: −2 to +2 meq/L, except in newborns (range, −4 to −0)

Alanine Aminotransferase (ALT, SGPT) (S)

(at 37 °C)
Newborns (1–3 d): 1–25 IU/L
Children 1–3 yr: 5–45 IU/L
4–6 yr: 10–25 IU/L
7–9 yr: 10–35 IU/L
Adult males: 7–46 IU/L
Adult females: 4–35 IU/L

Albumin

Birth–3 mo: 3.2–4.8 g/dL
Over 1 yr: 3.7–5.7 g/dL

Alkaline Phosphate: see Table A–1.

Ammonia (P)

Newborns: 90–150 µg/dL (53–88 µmol/L: higher in premature and jaundiced infants
Thereafter: 0–60 µg/dL (0–35 µmol/L)

Table A–1. Alkaline phosphatase in serum.

Values at 37 °C using *p*-nitrophenyl phosphate buffered with AMP (kinetic).		
Group	**Males (IU/L)**	**Females (IU/L)**
Newborns (1–3 d)	95–368	95–368
2–24 mo	115–460	115–460
2–5 yr	115–391	115–391
6–7 yr	115–460	115–460
8–9 yr	115–345	115–345
10–11 yr	115–336	115–437
12–13 yr	127–403	92–336
14–15 yr	79–446	78–212
16–18 yr	58–331	35–124
Adults	41–137	39–118

Amylase (S)

Neonates: Undetectable
2–12 mo: Levels increase slowly to adult levels
Adults: 28–108 IU/L at 37 °C

α_1-Antitrypsin (S)

1–3 mo: 127–404 mg/dL
3–12 mo: 145–362 mg/dL
1–2 yr: 160–382 mg/dL
2–15 yr: 148–394 mg/dL

Aspartate Aminotransferase (AST, SGOT) (S)

(at 37 °C)
Newborns (1–3 d): 16–74 IU/L
Children 1–3 yr: 20–60 IU/L
4–6 yr: 15–50 IU/L
7–9 yr: 15–40 IU/L
Adult males: 8–46 IU/L
Adult females: 7–34 IU/L

Bicarbonate, Actual (P)

Calculated from pH and $PaCO_2$
Newborns: 18–27 mmol/L

2 mo–2 yr: 19–24 mmol/L
Children: 18–25 mmol/L
Adult males: 20.1–28.9 mmol/L
Adult females: 18.4–28.8 mmol/L

Bilirubin (S)
Levels after 1 mo are as follows:
Conjugated: 0–0.3 mg/dL (0–5 μmol/L)
Unconjugated: 0.1–0.7 mg/dL (2–12 μmol/L)

Calcium (S)
Premature infants (1st wk): 3.5–4.5 meq/L (1.7–2.3 mmol/L)
Full-term infants (1st wk): 4–5 meq/L (2–2.5 mmol/L)
Thereafter: 4.4–5.3 meq/L (2.2–2.7 mmol/L)

Calcium (Ionized)
At pH 7.4: 3.9–4.5 mg/dL (0.9–1.12 mmol/L)

Cation-Anion Gap (S, P)
5–15 mmol/L

Chloride (S, P)
Premature infants: 95–110 mmol/L)
Full-term infants: 96–116 mmol/L
Children: 98–105 mmol/L
Adults: 98–108 mmol/L

Coagulation Factors: see Table A–2.

Complement (S)
C3: 0–6 mo: 53–166 mg/dL
6 mo–adult: 75–195 mg/dL
C4: 0–6 mo: 7–42 mg/dL
6 mo–adult: 9.5–45 mg/dL

Creatine (S, P): see Table A–3.
0.2–0.8 mg/dL (15.2–61 μmol/L)

Table A–2. Coagulation factors.

Values in units/mL. Shown are mean values and −2 SD or lower range (in parentheses).

Factor	Preterm (25–32 wk)	Term Infant	Infant (6 mo)	Adult
II	0.32 (0.18)	0.52 (0.25)	0.88 (0.60)	1.0 (0.7)
V	0.80 (0.43)	1.00 (0.54)	0.91 (0.55)	1.0 (0.6)
VII	0.37 (0.24)	0.57 (0.35)	0.87 (0.50)	1.0 (0.6)
VIII	0.74 (0.40)	1.50 (0.55)	0.90 (0.50)	1.0 (0.6)
vWf	1.50 (0.90)	1.60 (0.84)	1.07 (0.60)	1.0 (0.6)
IX	0.22 (0.17)	0.35 (0.15)	0.86 (0.36)	1.0 (0.5)
X	0.38 (0.20)	0.45 (0.30)	0.78 (0.38)	1.0 (0.6)
XI	0.20 (0.12)	0.42 (0.20)	0.86 (0.38)	1.0 (0.6)
XII	0.22 (0.09)	0.44 (0.16)	0.77 (0.39)	1.0 (0.6)
XIII	. . .	0.61 (0.36)	1.04 (0.50)	1.0 (0.6)
PreK	0.26 (0.14)	0.35 (0.16)	0.86 (0.56)	1.1 (0.6)

vWf = von Willebrand factor; PreK = prekallikrein.

Creatine Kinase (Creatine Phosphokinase) (S, P)

(at 37 °C)
Newborns (1–3 d): 40–474 IU/L
Adult males: 30–210 IU/L
Adult females: 20–128 IU/L

Creatinine Clearance

Values show great variability and depend on specificity of analytical methods used (Table A–3).
Newborns (1 d): 5–50 mL/min/1.73 m^2 (mean, 18 mL/min/1.73 m^2)
Newborns (6 d): 15–90 mL/min/1.73 m^2 (mean, 36 mL/min/1.73 m^2)
Adult males: 85–125 mL/min/1.73 m^2

C-Reactive Protein (CRP)

< 1 mg/dL

Ferritin (S)

Newborns: 20–200 ng/mL (mean, 117 ng/mL)
1 mo: 60–550 ng/mL (mean, 350 ng/mL)
1–15 years: 7–140 ng/mL (mean, 31 ng/mL)

Table A–3. Creatinine in serum and plasma.

Group	Males mg/dL (μmol/L)	Females mg/dL (μmol/L)
Newborns (1–3 d)[1]	0.2–1.0 (17.7–88.4)	0.2–1.0 (17.7–88.4)
1 yr	0.2–0.6 (17.7–53.0)	0.2–0.5 (17.7–44.2)
2–3 yr	0.2–0.7 (17.7–61.9)	0.3–0.6 (26.5–53.0)
4–7 yr	0.2–0.8 (17.7–70.7)	0.2–0.7 (17.7–61.9)
8–10 yr	0.3–0.9 (26.5–79.6)	0.3–0.8 (26.5–70.7)
11–12 yr	0.3–1.0 (26.5–88.4)	0.3–0.9 (26.5–79.6)
13–17 yr	0.3–1.2 (26.5–106.1)	0.3–1.1 (26.5–97.2)
18–20 yr	0.5–1.3 (44.2–115.0)	0.3–1.1 (26.5–97.2)

[1] Values may be higher in premature newborns.

Adult males: 50–225 ng/mL (mean, 140 ng/mL)
Adult females: 10–150 ng/mL (mean, 40 ng/mL)

Glucose (S, P)

Premature infants: 20–80 mg/dL (1.11–4.44 mmol/L)
Full-term infants: 30–100 mg/dL (1.67–5.56 mmol/L)
Children and adults (fasting): 60–105 mg/dL (3.33–5.88 mmol/L)

γ-Glutamyl Transpeptidase (S)

(at 37 °C [kinetic])
0–1 mo: 12–271 IU/L
1–2 mo: 9–159 IU/L
2–4 mo: 7–98 IU/L
4–7 mo: 5–45 IU/L
7–12 mo: 4–27 IU/L
1–15 yr: 3–30 IU/L
Adult males: 9–69 IU/L
Adult females: 3–33 IU/L

Glycohemoglobin (Hemoglobin A_{1c}) (B)

Normal: Less than 6.4% of total hemoglobin. Diabetic patients in good control of their condition ordinarily have levels < 7–8%. *This measurement is very method-dependent.*

Hematologic Values: see Table A–4.

Immunoglobins (S): see Table A–5.

Table A–4. Hematologic values.

Age	Hct (%)	MCV (fL)	HgB (g/dL)
Birth	44–64	85–125	14–24
2 wk–3 mo	30–49	80–102	10–17
6 mo–1 yr	30–40	78	11–15
4 yr–10 yr	31–43	80–82	12.5–15

Iron (S, P)

Newborns: 20–157 μg/dL (3.6–28.1 μmol/L)
6 wk–3 yr: 20–115 μg/dL (3.6–20.6 μmol/L)
3–9 yr: 20–141 μg/dL (3.6–25.2 μmol/L)
9–14 yr: 21–151 μg/dL (3.8–27 μmol/L)
14–16 yr: 20–181 μg/dL (3.6–32.4 μmol/L)
Adults: 44–196 μg/dL (7.9–35.3 μmol/L)

Iron-Binding Capacity (S, P)

Newborns: 59–175 μg/dL (10.6–31.3 μmol/L)
Children and adults: 275–458 μg/dL (45–72 μmol/L)

Lactate (B)

Venous blood: 5–18 mg/dL (0.5–2 mmol/L)
Arterial blood: 3–7 mg/dL (0.3–0.8 mmol/L)

Lactate Dehydrogenase (LDH) (S, P)

Values using lactate substrate (kinetic), at 37 °C:

Table A–5. Immunoglobulins in serum.

Group	IgG (mg/dL)	IgA (mg/dL)	IgM (mg/dL)
Cord blood	766–1693	0.04–9	4–26
2 wk–3 mo	299–852	3–66	15–149
3–6 mo	142–988	4–90	18–118
6–12 mo	418–1142	14–95	43–223
1–2 yr	356–1204	13–118	37–239
2–3 yr	492–1269	23–137	49–204
3–6 yr	564–1381	35–209	51–214
6–9 yr	658–1535	29–384	50–228
9–12 yr	625–1598	60–294	64–278
12–16 yr	660–1548	81–252	45–256

Newborns (1–3 d): 40–348 IU/L
1 mo–5 yr: 150–360 IU/L
5–8 yr: 150–300 IU/L
8–12 yr: 130–300 IU/L
12–14 yr: 130–280 IU/L
14–16 yr: 130–230 IU/L
Adult males: 70–178 IU/L
Adult females: 42–166 IU/L

Lead (B)

< 10 μg/dL (0.48 μmol/L). Levels of 10 μg/dL or greater have been associated with impairment of cognitive functioning.

Lipase (S, P)

20–136 IU/L based on 4-hour incubation.

Lipid profiles: see Table A–6.

Magnesium (S, P)

Newborns: 1.5–2.3 meq/L (0.75–1.15 mmol/L)
Adults: 1.4–2 meq/L (0.7–1 mmol/L)

Methemoglobin (B)

0–0.3 g/dL (0–186 μmol/L)

Osmolality (S, P)

285–295 mosm/kg.

Oxygen Capacity (B)

1.34 mL/g of hemoglobin.

Peripheral Blood Values: see Table A–7.

Phosphorus, Inorganic (S, P)

Premature infants:
At birth: 5.6–8 mg/dL (1.18–2.58 mmol/L)
6–10 d: 6.1–11.7 mg/dL (1.97–3.78 mmol/L)
20–25 d: 6.6–9.4 mg/dL (2.13–3.04 mmol/L)
Full-term infants:
At birth: 5–7.8 mg/dL (1.61–2.52 mmol/L)
3 d: 5.8–9 mg/dL (1.87–2.91 mmol/L)
6–12 d: 4.9–8.9 mg/dL (1.58–2.87 mmol/L)

Table A–6. Lipid profiles for selected ages.

Age Group	Cholesterol (mg/dL)		High-density Lipoprotein (mg/dL)		Low-density Lipoprotein (mg/dL)		Triglyceride Fasting > 12 hr (mg/dL)	
	Male	*Female*	*Male*	*Female*	*Male*	*Female*	*Male*	*Female*
6–7 yr	115–197	126–199	35–77	24–76	56–134	52–149	32–79	24–128
8–9 yr	112–199	124–208	31–80	34–77	52–129	57–143	28–105	34–115
10–11 yr	108–220	115–208	34–81	30–74	45–149	56–140	30–115	39–131
12–13 yr	117–202	114–207	30–82	33–73	55–135	58–138	33–112	36–125
14–15 yr	103–207	102–208	26–72	29–73	48–143	47–140	35–136	36–122
16–17 yr	107–198	106–213	25–66	27–78	53–134	44–147	38–167	34–136

Children:
1 yr: 3.8–6.2 mg/dL (1.23–2 mmol/L)
10 yr: 3.6–5.6 mg/dL (1.16–1.81 mmol/L)
Adults: 3.1–5.1 mg/dL (1–1.65 mmol/L)

Potassium (S, P)
Premature infants: 4.5–7.2 mmol/L
Full-term infants: 3.7–5.2 mmol/L
Children: 3.5–5.5 mmol/L
Adults: 3.5–5.3 mmol/L

Proteins in Serum: see Table A–8.

Pyruvate (B)
Resting adult males (arterial blood): 50.5–60.1 µmol/L
Adults (venous blood): 34–102 µmol/L

Sedimentation Rate (B) [Modified Westergren]
0–20 mm/hr

Sodium (S, P)
Children and adults: 135–148 mmol/L

Thyroid Values: see Table A–9.

Urea Nitrogen (S, P)
1–2 yr: 5–15 mg/dL (1.8–5.4 mmol/L)
Thereafter: 10–20 mg/dL (3.5–7.1 mmol/L)

Uric Acid (S, P)
Males: 0–14 yr: 2–7 mg/dL (119–416 µmol/L)
$>$ 14 yr: 3–8 mg/dL (178–476 µmol/L)
Females: 0–14 yr: 2–7 mg/dL (119–416 µmol/L)
$>$ 14 yr: 2–7 mg/dL (119–416 µmol/L)

Zinc (S)
Males: 83–88 µg/dL (12.7–13.5 µmol/L)
Females: 85–91 µg/dL (13–13.9 µmol/L)
Females taking oral contraceptives: 86–93 µg/dL (13.2–14.2 µmol/L)
At 16 weeks of gestation: 66–70 µg/dL (10.1–10.7 µmol/L)
At 38 weeks of gestation: 54–58 µg/dL (8.3–8.9 µmol/L)

Table A–7. Normal peripheral blood values at various age levels.

Value	1st d	2nd d	6th d	2 wk	1 mo	2 mo
Red blood cells[1] (million/μL)	5.9 (4.1–7.5)	6 (4.0–7.3)	5.4 (3.9–6.8)	5 (4.5–5.5)	4.7 (4.2–5.2)	4.1 (3.6–4.6)
Hemoglobin (g/dL)	19 (14–24)	19 (15–23)	18 (13–23)	16.5 (15–20)	14 (11–17)	12 (11–14)
White blood cells[1] (per μL)	17,000 (8–38)		13,500 (6–17)	12,000	11,500	11,000
PMNs (%)	57	55	50	34	34	33
Eosinophils[1] (total) (per μL)	20–1,000				150–1,150	
Lymphocytes (%)	20	20	37	55	56	56
Monocytes (%)	10	15	9	8	7	7
Immature white blood cells (%)	10	5	0–1	0	0	0

Platelets (per µL)	350,000		325,000	300,000		
Nucleated red blood cells/100 white blood cells[1]	0–10		0.0–0.3	0	0	0
Reticulocytes (%)	3 (2–8)	3 (2–10)	1 (0.5–5.0)	0.4 (0.0–2.0)	0.2 (0.00–0.5)	0.5 (0.2–2.0)
Mean diameter of red blood cells (µm)	8.6				8.1	
MCV (fl)	85–125		89–101	94–102	90	
MCHC (%)	36		35	34		
MCH (pg)	35–40		36	31	30	
Hematocrit (%)	54 ± 10		51	50	35–50	

MCH = mean corpuscular hemoglobin; MCHC = mean corpuscular hemoglobin concentration; MCV = mean corpuscular volume; PMN = polymorphonuclear leukocyte.

[1] Total nucleated red blood cells: first day, <1000/µL.

Table A–7. Normal peripheral blood values at various age levels (*continued*).

Value	3 mo	6 mo	1 yr	2 yr	5 yr	8–12 yr	Adults	
							Males	**Females**
Red blood cells[1] (million/μL)	4 (3.5–4.5)	4.5 (4–5)	4.6 (4.1–5.1)	4.7 (4.2–5.2)	4.7 (4.2–5.2)	5 (4.5–5.4)	5.4 (4.6–6.2)	4.8 (4.2–5.4)
Hemoglobin (g/dL)	11 (10–13)	11.5 (10.5–14.5)	12 (11–15)	13 (12–15)	13.5 (12.5–15.0)	14 (13.0–15.5)	16 (13–18)	14 (11–16)
White blood cells[1] (per μL)	10,500	10,500	10,000	9,500	8,000	8,000	7,000 (5–10)	
PMNs (%)	33	36	39	42	55	60	57–58	
Eosinophils[1] (total) (per μL)	70–550	70–550					100–400	
Lymphocytes (%)	57	55	53	49	36	31	25–33	
Monocytes (%)	7	6	6	7	7	7	3–7	
Immature white blood cells (%)	0	0	0	0	0	0	0	

Platelets (per μL)	260,000			260,000		260,000	260,000
Nucleated red blood cels/100 white blood cells[1]	0	0	0	0	0	0	0
Reticulocytes (%)	2 (0.5–4.0)	8.0 (0.2–1.5)	1 (0.4–1.8)	1 (0.4–1.8)	1 (0.4–1.8)	1 (0.4–1.8)	1 (0.5–2.0)
Mean diameter of red blood cells (μm)	7.7		7.4		7.4		7.5
MCV (fl)	80	78	78	80	80	82	82–92
MCHC (%)		33		32	34	34	34
MCH (pg)	27	26	25	26	27	28	27–31
Hematocrit (%)	35	30–40	36	37	31–43	40	40–54 37–47

MCH = mean corpuscular hemoglobin; MCHC = mean corpuscular hemoglobin concentration; MCV = mean corpuscular volume; PMN = polymorphonuclear leukocyte.

[1] Total nucleated red blood cells: first day, <1000/μL.

Table A–8. Proteins in serum.

Values are for cellulose acetate electrophoresis and are in g/dL. SI conversion factor: g/dL × 10 = g/L.

Group	Total Protein	Albumin
At birth	4.6–7.0	3.2–4.8
3 mo	4.5–6.5	3.2–4.8
1 yr	5.4–7.5	3.7–5.7
>4 yr	5.9–8.0	3.8–5.4

NORMAL VALUES: URINE, SWEAT, & CEREBROSPINAL FLUID[1]

URINE

Calcium

5–15 μg/24 h (2.5–7.5 mmol/24 h)

Chloride

Infants: 1.7–8.5 mmol/24 h
Children: 17–34 mmol/24 h
Adults: 140–240 mmol/24 h

Osmolality

Infants: 50–600 mosm/kg
Older children: 50–1400 mosm/kg

Potassium

26–123 mmol/L

Sodium

Infants: 0.3–3.5 nmol/24h (6–10 mmol/m^2)
Children and adults: 5.6–17 mmol/24h

[1] Adapted from S Meites (editor): *Pediatric Clinical Chemistry*, 3rd ed. American Association for Clinical Chemistry, 1989; and The Children's Hospital of Denver Clinical Laboratory.

Table A–9. Normal thyroid function values in infancy and childhood.[1]

Age	Total T_4 (μg/dL)	Total T_3 (ng/dL)	T_3 Resin Uptake (%)	TBG (mg/dL)	TSH (μU/mL)
Birth (cord blood)	10.2(7.4–13.0)	45(15–75)	0.90(0.75–1.05)	5.6	9.0(<2.5–17.4)
1–3 d	17.2((11.8–22.6)	124(32–216)	1.15(0.90–1.40)	5.0	8.0(<2.5–13.3)
1–2 wk	13.2(9.8–16.6)	250	1.00(0.85–1.15)		
2–4 wk	11.0(7.0–15.0)	160(160–240)	0.95(0.80–1.15)		4.0(0.6–10.0)
1–4 mo	10.3(7.2–14.4)	163(117–209)	0.90(0.75–1.05)		<2.5(<2.5)
4–12 mo	11.0(7.8–16.5)	176(110–280)	0.98(0.88–1.12)	4.4(3.1–5.6)	2.1(0.6–6.3)
1–5 y	10.5(7.3–15.0)	168(105–269)	0.99(0.88–1.12)	4.2(2.9–5.4)	2.0(0.6–6.3)
5–10 y	9.3(6.4–13.3)	150(94–241)	1.00(0.88–1.12)	3.8(2.5–5.0)	2.0(0.6–6.3)
10–15 y	8.1(5.6–11.7)	113(83–213)	1.01(0.88–1.12)	3.3(2.1–4.6)	1.9(0.6–6.3)
Adult	8.4(4.3–12.5)	125(70–204)	1.01(0.85–1.14	3.5(2.1–5.5)	1.8(0.2–7.6)

T_4 = thyroxine; T_3 = triiodothyronine; TBG = thyroid-binding globulin; TSH = thyroid-stimulating hormone. T_4, T_3, TSH, and TBG are measured by radioimmunoassay; T_4 measured by competitive protein binding are 15% lower. Data are means (ranges, which equal ± 2 SD from mean value).

[1] Data from LaFranchi (*Clinical Pediatric and Adolescent Endocrinology.* Philadelphia, PA: WB Saunders Co; 1982;82).

Vanillylmandelic Acid (VMA)

Because of the difficulty in obtaining an accurately timed 24-hour collection, values based on microgram per milligram of creatinine are the most reliable indications of VMA excretion in young children.

1–12 mo: 1–35 μg/mg of creatinine (31–135 μg/kg/24 h)
1–2 yr: 1–30 μg/mg of creatinine
2–5 yr: 1–15 μg/mg of creatinine
5–10 yr: 1–14 μg/mg of creatinine
10–15 yr: 1–10 μg/mg of creatinine
Adults: 1–7 μg/mg of creatinine (1–7 mg/24h: 5–35 μmol/24h)

SWEAT

Electrolytes

Values for chloride; elevated values in the presence of a family history or clinical findings of cystic fibrosis are diagnostic of cystic fibrosis.

Normal: < 40 mmol/L
Borderline: 40–60 mmol/L
Elevated: > 60 mmol/L

CEREBROSPINAL FLUID VALUES

Appearance

clear, colorless

Cells

White blood cells
Birth: 0–30
> 3 mo: 0–5

Red blood cells

Birth: 2–50
> 3 mo: 0

Glucose (mg/dL)

50–80 (two-thirds of blood glucose)

Protein (mg/dL)

Birth: 40–150
1–6 mo: 20–65
> 6 mo: 15–35

BEDSIDE LABORATORY TESTS & USEFUL FORMULAS

1. Clinitest: Used to detect reducing substances in stool; reflects carbohydrate malabsorption. Mix 1 part stool with 2 parts water (use 1N HCl if testing for sucrose). Add 15 drops of this mixture to one Clinitest tablet. Compare color of suspension with chart for percentage of reducing substances. Abnormal if ≥ ½%.

2. Cold Agglutinins: Present in *Mycoplasma* disease. Collect 4–5 drops of blood in small purple-top tube (0.2 mL EDTA). Place tube in ice water for 30–60 seconds. Rotate tube and look for clumping. Agglutination that occurs with cold and resolves with warming is interpreted as a cold agglutinin titer > 1:64.

3. Creatinine Clearance (Ccr)—Spot Urine:

(Schwartz Method)

Estimated Ccr = kL/Pcr
k = proportionality constant
L = height (cm)
Pcr = plasma creatinine (mg/dL)

k values

Low birth weight (LBW) during first year of life	0.33
Term AGA during first year of life	0.45
Children/adolescent girls	0.55
Adolescent boys	0.70

4. Fecal Leukocytes: Present in inflammatory enterocolitis. Place stool mucus on microscope slide. Add 2 drops 0.5% methylene blue. Wait 2–3 minutes. Examine under microscope.

5. Laboratory Hyponatremia With Hyperglycemia: Serum sodium is lowered 1.6 meq/L for each 100 mg% of glucose above baseline due to osmotic dilution of extracellular solute.

6. Mentzer Index:

MCV/RBC > 13.5 suggests iron deficiency anemia
MCV/RBC < 11.5 suggests thalassemia minor

7. Serum Osmolality:

mOsm/L = 2(Na + K) = glucose/18 = BUN/2.8

REFERENCES

Hammond K: Normal biochemical & hematologic values. In: Hay et al (editors): *Current Pediatric Diagnosis &* Treatment. 12th ed. Appleton & Lange, 1995.

LaFranchi S: Hypothyroidism, congenital and acquired. In: Kaplan SA (editor): *Clinical Pediatric and Adolescent Endocrinology*. Saunders, 1982.

Lockitch G et al: Age- and sex-specific pediatric reference intervals for biochemistry analytes as measured with the Ektachem-700 analyzer. Clin Chem 1988;34:1622.

Meites S: *Pediatric Clinical Chemistry*. 3rd ed. American Association for Clinical Chemistry, Inc., 1989.

Schwartz G, Brion L, Spitzer A: The use of plasma creatinine concentration for estimating glomerular filtration rate in infants, children, and adolescents. Pediatr Clin North Am 1987;34:571.

Index

(more on reverse)

HOW TO USE

the Pearson Nurse's Drug Guide 2011

Classifications and Prototype Drugs

> mio-Aqueous,
> cerone
> on: ANTIARRHYTHMIC,
> tic: ANTIARRHYTHMIC,
> , ANTIANGINAL
> **Pregnancy Category:** D

The classifications used in this book are based on the system used by the American Hospital Formulary Servic (AHFS). This book further classif drugs by therapeutic uses, enal the nurse to identify drugs same class that have similar tions for use. Thus, the boo vides a framework for understandi how drugs in a given class are used in clinical practice. The pharmacologic classification appears immediately after the **Classifications** heading, followed by the **Therapeutic** classification. In general, all drugs in a class will have similar actions, uses, adverse effects, and nursing implications. Therefore, we have selected certain drugs that are representative of a classification or its subclassification—**prototype drugs**—to aid the nurse in understanding the classification of drugs. Prototype drug monographs are identified with a small icon. The user can refer to the prototype drug to develop a better understanding of drugs that belong within the same classification or subclassification. When a drug belongs to a classification that has a designated prototype drug, that prototype is identified directly below the therapeutic classification. The table on pages xi–xviii identifies the drug prototype considered to be representative of each class. All prototype drugs are highlighted in **bold** type in the index for quick identification. Some drugs have a unique mechanism of action or therapeutic effect. In these cases, there is no prototype drug to be identified.

Pregnancy Category

Drugs may be described as category A, B, C, D, or X according to the risk to the fetus, with A being the lowest and X the highest risk. If the FDA pregnancy category is known, it is indicated after the Therapeutic classifications. Refer to Appendix C, *FDA Pregnancy Categories*, for a more complete description of each category.

Controlled Substances

In the United States, controlled substances are classified as belonging to one of five Schedules (I to V) according to abuse potential. If a drug is a controlled substance, then its Schedule number is listed below the

Pregnancy Category. Schedule I has the highest and Schedule V has the lowest potential for abuse. Refer to Appendix B, *U.S. Schedules of Controlled Substances*, for a more complete description of each schedule.

Availability

Because drugs come in a variety of dosages and forms, the authors include a section devoted to Availability in each monograph. This section identifies the available forms (e.g., tablets, capsules) and the available dosage strengths for every drug.

> **AVAILABILITY** 100 mg, 200 mg, 400 mg tablets; 50 mg/mL injection

> **ACTION & *THERAPEUTIC EFFECT*** Class III antiarrhythmic; also has antianginal and antiadrenergic properties. Acts directly on all cardiac tissues by prolonging duration of action potential and refractory period without significantly affecting resting membrane potential. Slows conduction time through the AV node and can interrupt the reentry pathways through the AV node. *By direct action on smooth muscle, decreases peripheral resistance and increases coronary blood flow. Blocks effects of sympathetic stimulation.*

Action and *Therapeutic Effect*

Each monograph describes the mechanism by which the specific drug produces physiologic and biochemical changes at the cellular, tissue, and organ levels. This information helps the user understand how the drug works in the body and makes it easier to learn its adverse reactions, and cautious uses. The *therapeutic effects*, which are set in italics for clarity and ease of use, are the reasons why a drug is prescribed. Therapeutic effectiveness of the drug can be determined by monitoring improvement in the condition for which the drug is prescribed.

Uses and Unlabeled Uses

The therapeutic applications of each drug are described in terms of approved (i.e., FDA-labeled) uses and unlabeled uses. An unlabeled use is one that does not appear on the drug label or in the manufacturer's literature. Although currently supported by medical literature, unlabeled uses are not currently approved by the FDA.

> **USES** Prophylaxis and treatment of life-threatening ventricular arrhythmias and supraventricular arrhythmias, particularly with atrial fibrillation.
>
> **UNLABELED USES** Treatment of nonexertional angina, conversion of atrial fibrillation to normal sinus rhythm, paroxysmal supraventricular tachycardia, ventricular rate control due to accessory pathway conduction in pre-excited atrial arrhythmia, after defibrillation and epinephrine in cardiac arrest, AV nodal reentry tachycardia.

Contraindications and Cautious Use

Many drugs have contraindications and therefore should not be used in specific conditions, such as during pregnancy or pathologic disorders. In other cases, the drug should be used with great caution because of a greater than average risk of untoward effects.

CONTRAINDICATIONS Hypersensitivity to amiodarone, or benzyl alcohol; cardiogenic shock, severe sinus bradycardia, advanced AV block unless a pacemaker is available, severe sinus-node dysfunction or sick sinus syndrome, bradycardia, congenital or acquired QR prolongation syndromes, or history of torsades de pointes; severe liver disease, pregnancy (category D), lactation.
CAUTIOUS USE Hepatic disease, cirrhosis; Hashimoto's thyroiditis, goiter, thyrotoxicosis, or history of other thyroid dysfunction; mild to moderate hepatic toxicity; CHF, left ventricular dysfunction; hypersensitivity to iodine; older adults; Fabry disease, especially with visual disturbances; electrolyte imbalance, hypokalemia, hypomagnesemia, hypovolemia; preexisting lung disease, COPD; open heart surgery.

ROUTE & DOSAGE

Arrhythmias

Adult: **PO Loading Dose** 800–1600 mg/day in 1–2 doses for 1–3 wk **PO Maintenance Dose** 400–600 mg/day in 1–2 doses **IV Loading Dose** 150 mg over 10 min followed by 360 mg over next 6 h **IV Maintenance Dose** 540 mg over 18 h (0.5 mg/min), may continue at 0.5 mg/min **Convert IV to PO** Duration of infusion less than 1 wk use 800–1600 mg PO, 1–3 wk use 600–800 mg PO, greater than 3 wk use 400 mg PO
Child: **IV** 5 mg/kg then repeat to max of 300 mg total

Hepatic Impairment Dosage Adjustment

Adjustment only suggested in severe hepatic impairment

Route and Dosage

The routes and dosages are highlighted in a gray box for easy access. Route of administration is specified as subcutaneous, IM, IV, PO, PR, nasal, ophthalmic, vaginal, topical, aural, intradermal, or intrathecal. Dosages are listed according to indication or FDA-approved labeled use(s). One of the hallmarks of this drug guide is the comprehensive dosage information it provides. The guide includes adult, geriatric, and pediatric dosages, as well as dosages for neonates and infants whenever applicable. This section also indicates dosage adjustments for renal impairment (based on creatinine clearance), hepatic impairment, patients undergoing hemodialysis, and obese patients (based on ideal body weight). Information about the need for dosage adjustments based on pharmacogenetic variables [e.g., cytochrome (CYP) system of enzymes] is also provided as available.

ADMINISTRATION

- Note: Correct hypokalemia and hypomagnesemia prior to initiation of therapy.

Oral

- Give consistently with respect to meals.
- Note: Only a physician experienced with the drug and treatment of life-threatening arrhythmias should give loading doses.
- Note: GI symptoms commonly occur during high-dose therapy, especially with loading doses. Symptoms usually respond to dose reduction or divided dose given with food, including milk.

Administration

Drug administration is an important primary role for the nurse. Organized by different routes, this section lists comprehensive instructions for administering, handling, and storing medications.

Intravenous Drug Administration

Within the **Administration** section of appropriate monographs, the authors highlight intravenous drugs, indicated by a vertical red bar. This section provides users with comprehensive instructions on how to **Prepare** and **Administer** direct, intermittent, and continuous intravenous medications. When different from adults, intravenous administration and preparation for pediatric patients is provided. It also includes **Solution/Additive** and **Y-Site** incompatibility for every monograph, where appropriate, to indicate which drugs and solutions should not be mixed with the intravenous drug. This is crucial information for drug administration. A chart for Y-Site compatibility for common intravenous drugs is located inside the back cover of this drug guide. These enhancements eliminate the need for additional resources for intravenous administration.

Intravenous

PREPARE: **IV Infusion: First rapid loading dose infusion:** Add 150 mg (3 mL) amiodarone to 100 mL D5W to yield 1.5 mg/mL. **Second infusion during first 24 h (slow loading dose and maintenance infusion):** Add 900 mg (18 mL) amiodarone to 500 mL D5W to yield 1.8 mg/mL. **Maintenance infusions after the first 24 h:** Prepare concentrations of 1–6 mg/mL amiodarone. Note: Use central line to give concentrations greater than 2 mg/mL.

ADMINISTER: **IV Infusion:** Rapidly infuse initial 150 mg dose over the first 10 min at a rate of 15 mg/min. ▪ Over next 6 h, infuse 360 mg at a rate of 1 mg/min. ▪ Over the remaining 18 h, infuse 540 mg at a rate of 0.5 mg/min. ▪ After the first 24 h, infuse maintenance doses of 720 mg/24 h at a rate of 0.5 mg/min.

INCOMPATIBILITIES **Solution/additive:** **Aminophylline, amoxicillin/clavulanic acid, cefazolin, floxacillin, furosemide, quinidine.** **Y-site:** **Aminophylline, ampicillin/sulbactam, argatroban, atenolol, bivalirudin, cefamandole, cefazolin.**

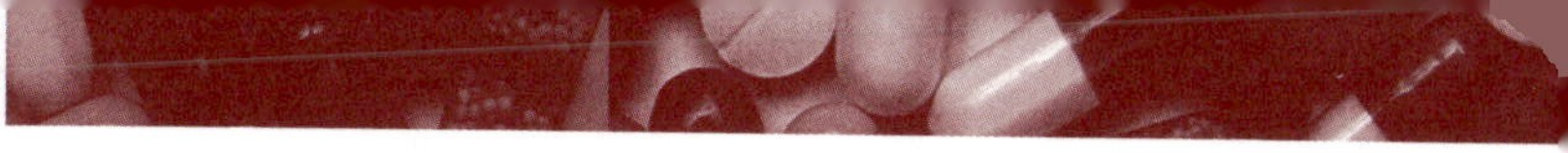

Adverse Effects

Virtually all drugs have adverse side effects that may be bothersome to some individuals but not to others. Adverse effects with an incidence of ≥1% are listed by body system or organs. The most common adverse effects appear in *italic* type, whereas those that are life-threatening are underlined. Users of the drug guide will find a key at the bottom of every page as a quick reminder.

Diagnostic Test Interference

This section describes the effect of the drug on various diagnostic tests and alerts the nurse to possible misinterpretations of test results when applicable. The name of the specific test altered is highlighted in ***bold italic*** type.

INTERACTIONS Drug: Significantly increases **digoxin** levels; enhances pharmacologic effects and toxicities of **disopyramide, procainamide, quinidine, flecainide, lidocaine, lovastatin, simvastatin;** anticoagulant effects of ORAL ANTICOAGULANTS enhanced; **verapamil, diltiazem,** BETA-ADRENERGIC BLOCKING AGENTS may potentiate sinus bradycardia, sinus arrest, or AV block; may increase **phenytoin** levels 2- to 3-fold; **cholestyramine** may decrease amiodarone levels; **fentanyl** may cause bradycardia, hypotension, or decreased output; may increase **cyclosporine** levels and toxicity; **cimetidine** may increase amiodarone levels; **ritonavir** may increase risk of amiodarone toxicity, including cardiotoxicity; **simvastatin** doses over 20 mg increase risk of rhabdomyolysis; **loratadine** use may increase risk of QT prolongation.

ADVERSE EFFECTS (≥1%) **CNS:** Peripheral neuropathy (*muscle weakness,* wasting numbness, tingling), *fatigue,* abnormal gait, dyskinesias, *dizziness,* paresthesia, headache. **CV:** Bradycardia, *hypotension* (IV), sinus arrest, cardiogenic shock, CHF, arrhythmias; AV block. **Special Senses:** *Corneal microdeposits,* blurred vision, optic neuritis, optic neuropathy, permanent blindness, corneal degeneration, macular degeneration, photosensitivity. **GI:** *Anorexia, nausea, vomiting, constipation,* hepatotoxicity. **Metabolic:** Hyperthyroidism or hypothyroidism; may cause neonatal hypo- or hyperthyroidism if taken during pregnancy. **Respiratory:** (Pulmonary toxicity) Alveolitis, pneumonitis (fever, dry cough, dyspnea), interstitial pulmonary fibrosis, *fatal gasping syndrome* with IV in children. **Skin:** Slate-blue pigmentation, *photosensitivity,* rash. **Other:** With chronic use, angioedema.

Interactions

When applicable, this section lists individual drugs, drug classes, foods, and herbs that interact with the drug discussed in the monograph. Drugs may interact to inhibit or enhance one another. Thus, drug interactions may improve the therapeutic response, lead to therapeutic failure, or produce specific adverse reactions. Only drugs that have been shown to cause clinically significant and documented interactions with the drug discussed in the monograph are identified. Note that generic drugs appear in **bold** type, and drug classes appear in SMALL CAPS.

Pharmacokinetics

This section identifies how the drug moves throughout the body. It lists the mechanisms of absorption, distribution, metabolism, elimination, and half-life when known. It also provides information about onset, peak, and duration of the drug action. Where appropriate, information appears for protein-binding and CYP450 metabolism.

> **PHARMACOKINETICS Absorption:** 22–86% absorbed. **Onset (PO):** 2–3 days to 1–3 wk. **Peak:** 3–7 h. **Distribution:** Concentrates in adipose tissue, lungs, kidneys, spleen; crosses placenta; 96% protein bound. **Metabolism:** Extensively in liver; undergoes some enterohepatic cycling; via CYP2C8 and 3A4. **Elimination:** Excreted chiefly in bile and feces; also in breast milk. **Half-Life:** Biphasic, initial 2.5–10 days, terminal 40–55 days.

Nursing Implications

Under the headings **Assessment & Drug Effects** and **Patient & Family Education**, the nurse can quickly and easily identify needed information and incorporate it into the appropriate steps of the nursing process. Before administering a drug, the nurse should read both sections to determine the assessments that should be made before and after administration of the drug, the indicators of drug effectiveness, laboratory tests recommended for individual drugs, and the essential patient and/or family education related to the drug.

Therapeutic Effectiveness

Therapeutic effectiveness of a drug can be determined by monitoring improvement in the condition for which the drug is prescribed, and by using the **Assessment & Drug Effects** section. Drugs have multiple uses or indications. Therefore, it is important to know why a drug is being prescribed for a specific patient (**Uses** and **Unlabeled Uses**). In the italicized sentences at the end of the **Action & *Therapeutic Effect*** section in all monographs, specific indicators of the effectiveness of the drug are provided. Additionally, in the **Route & Dosage** table for each drug, the dosages are listed according to the indications for FDA-labeled use(s) of the drug. Furthermore, the **Therapeutic** classifications listed within the red box at the beginning of the monograph provides the nurse with further assistance in determining and evaluating the therapeutic effectiveness of the drug.

> **NURSING IMPLICATIONS**
>
> **Assessment & Drug Effects**
>
> - Monitor BP carefully during infusion and slow the infusion if significant hypotension occurs; bradycardia should be treated by slowing the infusion or discontinuing if necessary. Monitor heart rate and rhythm and BP until drug response has stabilized; report promptly symptomatic bradycardia. Sustained monitoring is essential because drug has an unusually long half-life.
>
> **Patient & Family Education**
>
> - Check pulse daily once stabilized, or as prescribed. Report a pulse less than 60.
> - Take oral drug consistently with respect to meals.
> - Become familiar with potential adverse reactions and report those that are bothersome to the physician.

PEARSON

NURSE'S DRUG GUIDE 2011

Billie Ann Wilson, BSN, MSN, PhD

Professor Emerita
School of Nursing
Loyola University New Orleans
New Orleans, Louisiana

Margaret T. Shannon, BSN, MSN, PhD

Professor Emeritus of Nursing
Our Lady of Holy Cross College
New Orleans, Louisiana

Kelly M. Shields, PharmD

Associate Professor of Pharmacy Practice
Director of Drug Information Center
Raabe College of Pharmacy
Ohio Northern University
Ada, Ohio

Pearson
New York Boston San Francisco
London Toronto Sydney Tokyo Singapore Madrid
Mexico City Munich Paris Cape Town Hong Kong Montreal

Notice: The authors and the publisher of this volume have taken care to make certain that the doses of drugs and schedules of treatment are correct and compatible with the standards generally accepted at the time of publication. Nevertheless, as new information becomes available, changes in treatment and in the use of drugs become necessary. The reader is advised to carefully consult the instruction and information material included in the package insert of each drug or therapeutic agent before administration. This advice is especially important when using, administering, or recommending new and infrequently used drugs. The authors and publisher disclaim all responsibility for any liability, loss, injury, or damage incurred as a consequence, directly or indirectly, of the use and application of any of the contents of this volume.

www.pearsonhighered.com/drugguides

10 11 / 10 9 8 7 6 5 4 3 2 1

ISBN 0-13-214926-5/978-0-13-214926-6
[retail] ISBN 0-13-214970-2/978-0-13-214970-9

PRINTED IN THE UNITED STATES OF AMERICA

CONTENTS

To

Alvin, Theresa, Ellen, and

Michael, Rick, Kris, and Leah

without whom this work would not have been possible

ABOUT THE AUTHORS

Billie Ann Wilson is Professor Emerita in the School of Nursing at Loyola University in New Orleans, Louisiana. Prior to entering nursing, she taught natural and physical sciences at the secondary and collegiate levels. She holds a BS in Biology from Boston College, an MS in Biology from Purdue University, a BS in Nursing from Northwestern State University of Louisiana, an MSN from Louisiana State University Health Sciences Center, and a PhD in Curriculum and Instruction from the University of New Orleans.

Margaret T. Shannon is Professor Emeritus of Nursing at Our Lady of Holy Cross College, New Orleans, Louisiana. She holds a BS and an MS in Chemistry, both from Saint Louis University; an MA in Teaching Biology from Saint Mary's College, a BS in Nursing from Northwestern State University of Louisiana, an MSN from Louisiana State University Health Sciences Center, and a PhD in Curriculum and Instruction from the University of New Orleans. Prior to entering nursing, she taught physical science, natural science, and mathematics at the secondary and collegiate levels.

Kelly M. Shields is currently Associate Professor of Pharmacy Practice at Ohio Northern University's Raabe College of Pharmacy. She holds a Doctor of Pharmacy from Butler University and completed a fellowship in Natural Product Information and Research at University of Missouri-Kansas City. She has practiced pharmacy in retail, community, and academic settings and has worked as a freelance medical writer.

EDITORIAL REVIEW PANEL

We wish to thank the following individuals for conducting thorough reviews of the drug information in this book for its accuracy, currency, relevance, presentation, accessibility, and use. Their feedback guided us in developing a better book for nurses.

Kim Astroth, PhD, RN
Assistant Professor of Nursing
Illinois State University
Normal, Illinois

Cynthia Bechtel, MS, RN
Professor
MassBay Community College
Framingham, Massachusetts

Melissa Devlin, RPh, PharmD
Clinical Pharmacist
Hospice Pharmacia
Philadelphia, Pennsylvania

Jack Fincham, BS, PhD
Albert W. Jowdy Professor of Pharmacy
The University of Georgia
Athens, Georgia

David Goede, RN, MS, APRN-BC
Instructor
Monroe Community College
Rochester, New York

Tommy Johnson, PharmD, CDE, CDM
Clinical Associate Professor
The University of Georgia
Athens, Georgia

W. Klugh Kennedy, PharmD, BCPP
Clinical Associate Professor
The University of Georgia
Savannah, Georgia

Paul Lockman, PhD
Assistant Professor of Pharmacy
Texas Tech University
Amarillo, Texas

Marge Norquist, RN, MA, MPA
Professor
Community College of Rhode Island
Warwick, Rhode Island

Diane Saleska, MSN, RN
Assistant Clinical Professor
University of Missouri-St. Louis
St. Louis, Missouri

Judy Scott, RN, MSN
Professor
The Community College of Southern Nevada
Las Vegas, Nevada

Greene Shepherd, PharmD
Clinical Associate Professor
The University of Georgia
Athens, Georgia

Valerie Warner, MS, BSN, RN
Professor
College of Southern Idaho
Twin Falls, Idaho

PHARMACY CONSULTANT

A special acknowledgment to **Marc Harrold, PhD, RPh,** Professor of Medicinal Chemistry, School of Pharmacy at Duquesne University in Pittsburgh, Pennsylvania, who is a tremendous addition to the author team as a contributor for all of the monographs for the new drugs in this edition. We are grateful for his expertise and for his valued input.

PREFACE

Pearson Nurse's Drug Guide 2011 is a current and reliable reference designed to provide comprehensive information needed to make appropriate decisions regarding drug administration. This new edition includes 19 monographs for new drugs recently approved by the Food and Drug Administration (FDA) and over 310 updates to drug indications, available forms, adverse effects, dosages, and more. Revised IV administration information has been added and/or updated regarding children. These revisions include subheadings for IV preparation and administration of IV medications for children, which add to the ease of locating appropriate information by age.

On pages xi–xviii, the user will find a current listing of drug classifications and their associated drug prototypes. Prototype drugs are representative of all drugs in a particular classification or subclassification. The classification list serves as a valuable tool, especially for students learning pharmacology and familiarizing themselves with drug families and prototype drugs for classes of drugs.

Each drug monograph provides the necessary information for safe and effective drug administration. The user should read all the information provided. Occasionally, the user will be referred to Appendix F, *Glossary of Key Terms, Clinical Conditions, and Associated Signs and Symptoms*. This unique glossary provides valuable information regarding common assessment findings related to therapeutic effectiveness or ineffectiveness of specific drugs.

The authors recognize that the decision-making process related to drug administration is a cyclical one. For example, assessments are made both prior to and after drug administration. Thus, nursing diagnoses and interventions may change as a result of an *achieved therapeutic effect, therapeutic failure, manifestation of an adverse effect,* or *demonstration of a learning need.* The authors believe that the users of this drug reference will find that the clear and logical design of the drug monographs facilitates decision making and supports the nursing process.

Although some advanced practice nurses and other health professionals now have prescriptive privileges, the term *physician* is used throughout this book to designate the prescriber of medications.

ORGANIZATION

The ***Pearson Nurse's Drug Guide 2011*** is user friendly. Nurses in clinical practice, nursing professors, pharmacists, and nursing students from across the country reviewed the content of this handbook and provided helpful suggestions on how it could be made more useful. Based on these comments, the authors updated and added new information to the monographs in this book. To help readers better understand how to use the drug guide, the authors illustrate and describe all the components of a drug monograph in the **Guide to Using the Pearson Nurse's Guide 2011**, at the beginning of the book.

In this drug guide, all drugs are listed alphabetically according to their generic names. Pharmacologic classifications are paired with therapeutic classifications for every drug monograph for ease of use by nurse clinicians and students alike. Each drug is indexed by both its generic and trade names in the back of the guide to make it easier for the user to locate individual drug monographs. Trade names followed by a maple leaf indicate that brand of the drug is available only in Canada.

If a drug is not listed in the alphabetical section, it may be a combination drug, which is a drug made up of more than one generic component. These combination drugs are listed under their trade names in the index and in Appendix E, *Prescription Combination Drugs*. The appendix identifies the generic components and the amount of each generic drug contained in the combination. Users of this drug guide will find the page numbers for monographs of the component drugs in this appendix to make access to this information easier and faster.

Appendixes

This edition of the drug guide includes several helpful tables and charts in the appendixes, including Appendix A, *Ocular Medications, Low Molecular Weight Heparins, Inhaled Corticosteroids, and Topical Corticosteroids*; Appendix B, *U.S. Schedules of Controlled Substances*; Appendix C, *FDA Pregnancy Categories*; Appendix D, *Oral Dosage Forms That Should Not Be Crushed*; Appendix E, *Prescription Combination Drugs*; Appendix F, *Glossary of Key Terms, Clinical Conditions, and Associated Signs and Symptoms*; Appendix G, *Abbreviations*; and Appendix H, *Herbal and Dietary Supplement Table*. Appendix H identifies name, use, and safety issues associated with herbal products, such as potential drug interactions and side effects. New to this edition is Appendix I, *Look-Alike, Sound-Alike Medications*, which highlights medications that are commonly involved in medication errors.

Index

The index in the ***Pearson Nurse's Drug Guide 2011*** is perhaps the most often-used section in the entire book. All generic, trade, and combination drugs are listed in this index. Whenever a trade name is listed, the generic drug monograph is listed in parentheses. Additionally, classifications are listed and identified in SMALL CAPS, whereas all prototype drugs are highlighted in **bold** type. Drugs belonging to various classifications and subclassifications, including therapeutic classes, are also cross-referenced in this index. As a special feature, the index includes entries for combination drugs (e.g. Tylenol with Codeine) with index references to component drugs as well as the combination drug reference to Appendix E.

ONLINE COMPANION VERSION

The ***Pearson Nurse's Drug Guide 2011*** also comes with an online companion version designed to assist nurses in providing drug information and nursing implications for patients in hospitals, clinics, and all community settings. The online version provides access to many more resources:

- all monographs from the book, including prototypes and newly approved drugs,
- printing capability for use in patient teaching or for quick reference,
- calculators to help nurses do conversions or calculate dosages and IV drip rates,
- audio pronunciation of prototype drug names,
- a link to download trial versions of this drug guide and other references for mobile devices,
- access to drug updates,
- links to drug-related sites,
- drug-related tools,
- medication administration techniques,
- drug classifications,
- principles of pharmacology,
- common herbal remedies, and
- list of look-alike, sound-alike drugs.

You can also send the authors your feedback about the drug guide through this website. **To access this online resource, use the code printed inside the front of this book.**

ACKNOWLEDGMENTS

You can also send the authors your feedback about the drug guide through this website. We wish to express our appreciation to our past and present students who have provided the inspiration for this work. It is for these individuals and all who strive for excellence in patient care that this work was undertaken.

Billie Ann Wilson, BSN, MSN, PhD
Margaret T. Shannon, BSN, MSN, PhD
Kelly M. Shields, PharmD

Classifications	Prototype
ANTIGOUT AGENT	Probenecid
ANTIHISTAMINES	
ANTIHISTAMINES (H_1-RECEPTOR ANTAGONIST)	Diphenhydramine HCl
NON-SEDATING	Loratadine
ANTIPRURITIC	Hydroxyzine HCl
ANTIVERTIGO AGENT	Meclizine HCl
ANTIINFECTIVES	
ANTIBIOTICS	
AMEBICIDE	Paromomycin Sulfate
ANTHELMINTIC	Mebendazole
AMINOGLYCOSIDES	Gentamicin Sulfate
ANTIFUNGALS	Amphotericin B
AZOLE ANTIFUNGAL	Fluconazole
ALLYLAMINE ANTIFUNGAL	Terbinafine
ECHINOCARDIN ANTIFUNGAL	Caspofungin
BETA-LACTAM	Imipenem-Cilastatin
CEPHALOSPORIN	
FIRST GENERATION	Cefazolin Sodium
SECOND GENERATION	Cefaclor
THIRD GENERATION	Cefotaxime Sodium
CLINDAMYCIN	Clindamycin HCl
MACROLIDES	Erythromycin
PENICILLIN	
AMINOPENICILLIN	Ampicillin
ANTIPSEUDOMONAL PENICILLIN	Piperacillin
NATURAL PENICILLIN	Penicillin G Potassium
QUINOLONES	Ciprofloxacin HCl
SULFONAMIDES	Sulfisoxazole
TETRACYCLINE	Tetracycline HCl
URINARY TRACT ANTI-INFECTIVE	Trimethoprim
ANTILEPROSY (SULFONE) AGENT	Dapsone
ANTIMALARIAL	Chloroquine HCl
ANTIPROTOZOAL	Metronidazole
ANTITUBERCULOSIS AGENTS	Isoniazid
ANTITUBERCULOSIS AGENT, ANTIMYCOBACTERIAL	Rifampin
ANTIVIRAL AGENTS	Acyclovir
ADAMANTANES	Amantadine

*Based on the American Hospital Formulary Service Pharmacologic–Therapeutic Classification.
†Prototype drugs are highlighted in tinted boxes in this book.
Complete list of drugs for each classification found in classification index starting on p. 1685.

Classifications	Prototype
ANTIRETROVIRAL AGENTS	
NUCLEOSIDE REVERSE TRANSCRIPTASE INHIBITOR	Lamivudine
NONNUCLEOSIDE REVERSE TRANSCRIPTASE INHIBITOR	Efavirenz
PROTEASE INHIBITOR	Saquinavir
URINARY TRACT ANTI-INFECTIVE	Trimethoprim
VACCINE	Hepatitis B
ANTINEOPLASTICS	
ALKYLATING AGENT	Cyclophosphamide
ANTIANDROGEN	Flutamide
ANTIBIOTIC	Doxorubicin HCl
ANTIMETABOLITES	
ANTIMETABOLITE (ANTIFOLATE)	Methotrexate
ANTIMETABOLITE (PURINE ANTAGONIST)	6-Mercaptopurine
ANTIMETABOLITE (PYRIMIDINE)	5-Fluorouracil
AROMATASE INHIBITOR	Anastrozole
DNA TOPOISOMERASE INHIBITOR (CAMPTOTHECIN)	Topotecan HCl
EPIDERMAL GROWTH FACTOR RECEPTOR-TYROSINE KINASE INHIBITOR (EGFR-TKI)	Gefitinib
HORMONE, SELECTIVE ESTROGEN RECEPTOR MODIFIERS (SERMS)	Tamoxifen Citrate
MITOTIC INHIBITOR	Vincristine Sulfate
TAXANE (TAXOID)	Paclitaxel
ANTITUSSIVES, EXPECTORANTS, & MUCOLYTICS	
ANTITUSSIVE	Benzonatate
EXPECTORANT	Guaifenesin
MUCOLYTIC	Acetylcysteine
AUTONOMIC NERVOUS SYSTEM AGENTS	
ADRENERGIC AGONISTS (SYMPATHOMIMETICS)	
ALPHA-ADRENERGIC AGONIST	Methoxamine HCl
ALPHA- & BETA-ADRENERGIC AGONIST	Epinephrine
BETA-ADRENERGIC AGONIST	Isoproterenol HCl
ADRENERGIC ANTAGONISTS (SYMPATHOLYTICS)	
ALPHA-1 ADRENERGIC ANTAGONIST (GENITOURINARY SMOOTH MUSCLE RELAXANT)	Tamsulosin
ALPHA ANTAGONISTS (BLOCKING AGENT)	Prazosin HCl
BETA ANTAGONISTS	Propranolol HCl

Classifications	Prototype
ERGOT ALKALOID	Ergotamine Tartrate
$5\text{-}HT_1$ SEROTONIN AGONISTS	Sumatriptan
ANTICHOLINERGICS (PARASYMPATHOLYTICS)	
ANTIMUSCARINIC	Atropine Sulfate
ANTISPASMODIC [GENITOURINARY (GU)]	Oxybutynin
CHOLINERGICS (PARASYMPATHOMIMETICS)	
CHOLINESTERASE INHIBITOR	Neostigmine
CENTRAL-ACTING	Donepezil
DIRECT-ACTING CHOLINERGIC	Bethanechol Chloride
AUTONOMIC DRUGS, MISC	Nicotine
BENZODIAZEPINE ANTAGONIST	Flumazenil
BIOLOGICAL RESPONSE MODIFIERS	
FUSION PROTEIN	Alefacept
IMMUNOSUPPRESSANT	Cyclosporine
IMMUNOGLOBULIN	Immune Globulin
IMMUNOMODULATORS	Immune Globulin
INTERFERON	Peginterferon Alfa-2a
TUMOR NECROSIS FACTOR MODIFIER	Etanercept
MONOCLONAL ANTIBODY	Basiliximab
BISPHOSPHONATE (REGULATOR, BONE METABOLISM)	Etidronate Disodium
BLOOD DERIVATIVE, PLASMA VOLUME EXPANDER	Normal Serum Albumin
BLOOD FORMERS, COAGULATORS, & ANTICOAGULANTS	
ANTICOAGULANT	Heparin Sodium
DIRECT THROMBIN INHIBITOR	Lepirudin
LOW MOLECULAR WEIGHT HEPARIN	Enoxaparin
ANTIPLATELET AGENTS	Clopidogrel
GLYCOPROTEIN IIb/IIIa INHIBITOR	Abciximab
COLONY STIMULATING FACTOR	Filgrastim
HEMATOPOIETIC GROWTH FACTOR	Epoetin Alpha
HEMOSTATIC (COAGULATOR)	Aminocaproic Acid
IRON PREPARATION	Ferrous Sulfate
THROMBOLYTIC ENZYME	Alteplase

Classifications	Prototype
BRONCHODILATORS (RESPIRATORY SMOOTH MUSCLE RELAXANT)	
BETA-ADRENERGIC AGONIST	Albuterol
LEUKOTRIENE INHIBITOR	Zafirlukast
XANTHINE	Theophylline
CARDIOVASCULAR AGENTS	
ANGIOTENSIN II RECEPTOR ANTAGONISTS	Losartan Potassium
ANGIOTENSIN-CONVERTING ENZYME INHIBITORS	Enalapril
ANTIARRHYTHMIC AGENTS	
CLASS IA	Procainamide HCl
CLASS IB	Lidocaine HCl
CLASS IC	Flecainide
CLASS II	Propranolol HCl
CLASS III	Amiodarone HCl
ANTILIPEMICS	
BILE ACID SEQUESTRANT	Cholestyramine
FIBRATES	Fenofibrate
HMG-CoA REDUCTASE INHIBITOR (STATIN)	Lovastatin
CALCIUM CHANNEL BLOCKERS	
1,4 DIHYDROPYRIDINE	Nifedipine
MISCELLANEOUS	Verapamil
CARDIAC GLYCOSIDE	Digoxin
CENTRAL-ACTING ANTIHYPERTENSIVE	Methyldopa
INOTROPIC AGENT	Inamrinone
NITRATE VASODILATOR	Nitroglycerin
NONNITRATE VASODILATOR	Hydralazine HCl
RAUWOLFIA ALKALOID	Reserpine
PROSTAGLANDIN (PULMONARY ANTIHYPERTENSIVE)	Epoprostenol sodium
CENTRAL NERVOUS SYSTEM AGENTS	
ANALGESICS, ANTIPYRETICS	
NARCOTIC (OPIATE) AGONISTS	Morphine
NARCOTIC (OPIATE) AGONIST-ANTAGONIST	Pentazocine HCl
NARCOTIC (OPIATE) ANTAGONIST	Naloxone HCl
NONNARCOTIC ANALGESICS	Acetaminophen
NONSTEROIDAL ANTI-INFLAMMATORY DRUGS (NSAIDS)	
COX-1	Ibuprofen
COX-2	Celecoxib
SALICYLATE	Aspirin

Classifications	Prototype
ANESTHETIC	
GENERAL	Thiopental Sodium
LOCAL (ESTER TYPE)	Procaine HCl
LOCAL (AMIDE TYPE)	Lidocaine HCl
ANTIPARKINSON AGENTS	
CENTRALLY ACTING CHOLINERGIC RECEPTOR ANTAGONISTS	Benztropine
CATECHOLAMINE O-METHYL TRANSFERASE (COMT) INHIBITORS	Tolcapone
DOPAMINE RECEPTOR AGONISTS	Levodopa
ANTICONVULSANTS	
BARBITURATE	Phenobarbital
BENZODIAZEPINE	Diazepam
GABA INHIBITOR	Valproic Acid Sodium
GABA ANALOG	Gabapentin
HYDANTOIN	Phenytoin
SUCCINIMIDE	Ethosuximide
SULFONAMIDE	Zonisamide
TRICYCLIC	Carbamazepine
ANXIOLYTICS, SEDATIVE-HYPNOTICS	
BARBITURATE	Secobarbital
BENZODIAZEPINE	Lorazepam
CARBAMATE	Meprobamate
NONBENZODIAZEPINE	Zolpidem
PSYCHOTHERAPEUTIC	
ANTIDEPRESSANTS	
MONOAMINE OXIDASE (MAO) INHIBITORS	Phenelzine Sulfate
SELECTIVE SEROTONIN REUPTAKE INHIBITORS (SSRIS)	Fluoxetine HCl
SEROTONIN NOREPINEPHRINE REUPTAKE INHIBITORS	Venlafaxine
TETRACYCLIC ANTIDEPRESSANTS	Mirtazapine
TRICYCLIC ANTIDEPRESSANTS	Imipramine HCl
ANTIPSYCHOTIC AGENT	
ATYPICAL	Clozapine
BUTYROPHENONE	Haloperidol
MOOD STABILIZER	Lithium Carbonate
PHENOTHIAZINE	Chlorpromazine
CEREBRAL STIMULANT	
AMPHETAMINE	Amphetamine Sulfate
XANTHINE	Caffeine

Classifications	Prototype
ELECTROLYTIC & WATER BALANCE AGENTS	
DIURETIC	
LOOP	Furosemide
OSMOTIC	Mannitol
POTASSIUM-SPARING	Spironolactone
THIAZIDE	Hydrochlorothiazide
VASOPRESSIN ANTAGONIST	Conivaptan
PHOSPHATE BINDER	Sevelamer HCl
REPLACEMENT SOLUTION	Calcium Gluconate
ENZYMES	
ENZYME REPLACEMENT	Pancrelipase
ENZYME INHIBITOR	$Alpha_1$-Proteinase Inhibitor
EYE, EAR, NOSE, & THROAT (EENT) PREPARATIONS	
ANTIHISTAMINE, OCULAR	Emedastine
CARBONIC ANHYDRASE INHIBITOR	Acetazolamide
CYCLOPLEGIC	Cyclopentolate HCl
MIOTIC (ANTIGLAUCOMA AGENT)	Pilocarpine HCl
MYDRIATIC	Homatropine HBr
PROSTAGLANDIN	Latanoprost
VASOCONSTRICTOR, DECONGESTANT	Naphazoline HCl
GASTROINTESTINAL AGENTS	
ANORECTANT	Diethylpropion HCl
ANTACID, ADSORBENT	Aluminum Hydroxide
ANTIDIARRHEAL	Loperamide
ANTIDIARRHEAL, ADSORBENT	Bismuth Subsalicylate
ANTIEMETIC	Prochlorperazine
ANTIEMETIC (5-HT_3 ANTAGONIST)	Ondansetron HCl
ANTISECRETORY (H_2-RECEPTOR ANTAGONIST)	Cimetidine
BULK LAXATIVE	Psyllium Hydrophilic Mucilloid
MUCOUS MEMBRANE ANTIINFLAMMATORY	Mesalamine
PROKINETIC AGENT (GI STIMULANT)	Metoclopramide HCl
PROTON PUMP INHIBITORS	Omeprazole
SALINE CATHARTIC	Magnesium Hydroxide
STIMULANT LAXATIVE	Bisacodyl
STOOL SOFTENER	Docusate Calcium
GOLD COMPOUND	Auranofin

Classifications	Prototype
HORMONES & SYNTHETIC SUBSTITUTES	
ADRENAL CORTICOSTEROID	
GLUCOCORTICOSTEROID	Prednisone
MINERALOCORTICOID	Fludrocortisone Acetate
ANDROGEN/ANABOLIC STEROIDS	Testosterone
ANTIANDROGENS	
5-ALPHA REDUCTASE INHIBITORS	Finasteride
ANTIDIABETIC AGENTS	
ALPHA-GLUCOSIDASE INHIBITOR	Acarbose
BIGUANIDES	Metformin
INCRETIN MODIFIER (DPP-4 INHIBITOR)	Sitagliptan
INSULIN	Insulin Injection
MEGLITINIDES	Repaglinide
SULFONYLUREAS	Glyburide
THIAZOLIDINEDIONES	Rosiglitazone
ESTROGENS	Estradiol
GONADOTROPIN-RELEASING HORMONE ANALOGS	Leuprolide Acetate
GONADOTROPIN-RELEASING HORMONE ANTAGONIST	Ganirelix Acetate
GROWTH HORMONE	Somatropin
OXYTOCIC	Oxytocin Injection
PITUITARY (ANTIDIURETIC)	Vasopressin Injection
PROGESTINS (INJECTABLE PRODUCTS)	Progesterone
PROGESTINS (ORAL PRODUCTS)	Norethindrone
PROSTAGLANDIN (OXYTOCIC)	Carboprost
SOMASTATIN ANALOG	Octreotide
THYROID AGENTS	
ANTITHYROID AGENT	Propylthiouracil
THYROID	Levothyroxine Sodium
VITAMIN D ANALOG	Calcitriol
IMPOTENCE AGENT	
PHOSPHDIESTERASE (PDE-5) INHIBITOR	Sildenafil
RESPIRATORY AGENTS	
LUNG SURFACTANT	Beractant
MAST CELL STABILIZER	Cromolyn Sodium
SKIN & MUCOUS MEMBRANE AGENTS	
ANTIACNE (RETINOID)	Isotretinoin
ANTI-INFLAMMATORY STEROID	Hydrocortisone

Classifications	Prototype
PEDICULICIDE	Permethrin
PSORALEN	Methoxsalen
SCABICIDE	Lindane

SOMATIC NERVOUS SYSTEM AGENTS

SKELETAL MUSCLE RELAXANTS

Classifications	Prototype
CENTRAL-ACTING	Cyclobenzaprine HCl
DEPOLARIZING	Succinylcholine Chloride
NONDEPOLARIZING	Atracurium

ABACAVIR SULFATE

(a-ba'ca-vir)

Ziagen

Classifications: ANTIRETROVIRAL; NUCLEOSIDE REVERSE TRANSCRIPTASE INHIBITOR (NRTI)

Therapeutic: ANTIRETROVIRAL (NRTI)

Prototype: Lamivudine

Pregnancy Category: C

AVAILABILITY 300 mg tablets; 20 mg/mL oral solution

ACTION & *THERAPEUTIC EFFECT* Abacavir is a synthetic nucleoside analogue with inhibitory activity against HIV. It inhibits the activity of viral reverse transcriptase (RT) both by competing with the natural DNA nucleoside and by incorporation into viral DNA. *Abacavir prevents the formation of viral DNA replication. Viral load decreases as measured by an increased CD_4 lymphocyte cell count and suppression of HIV RNA, indicated by decreased HIV RNA copies, in HIV-positive individuals with little or no exposure to zidovudine (AZT).*

USES Treatment of HIV infection in combination with other antiretroviral agents.

CONTRAINDICATIONS Hypersensitivity to abacavir (fatal rechallenge reactions reported); lactic acidosis; creatinine clearance of less than 50 mL/min; severe hepatomegaly; moderate to severe hepatic impairment; lactation; patients with HLA-B*5701 allele (high risk for hypersensitivity reaction).

CAUTIOUS USE Prior resistance to another nucleoside reverse transcriptase inhibitor (NRTI); history of cardiac disease; older adults; pregnancy (category C).

ROUTE & DOSAGE

HIV Infection

Adult: **PO** 300 mg b.i.d.
Child (3 mo–16 y): **PO** 8 mg/kg b.i.d. (max: 300 mg b.i.d.)
Patients weighing 14–21 kg, give 150 mg PO twice daily; *21–30 kg,* give 150 mg PO in the morning and 300 mg in the evening; *over 30 kg,* give 300 mg PO twice daily

Hepatic Impairment Dosage Adjustment

Mild (Child-Pugh score 5–6): 200 mg b.i.d.

ADMINISTRATION

Oral

- Tablets and oral solution are interchangeable on a mg-for-mg basis.
- Store tablets and liquid at 20°–25° C (68°–77° F). Liquid may be refrigerated.

ADVERSE EFFECTS (≥1%) **Body as a Whole:** Hypersensitivity reactions (including fever, skin rash, fatigue, nausea, vomiting, diarrhea, abdominal pain); malaise; lethargy; myalgia; arthralgia; paresthesia; edema; shortness of breath. **CNS:** Insomnia, *headache, fever.* **CV:** Hypotension (associated with hypersensitivity reaction), <u>heart attack</u>. **GI:** <u>Hepatomegaly</u> with steatosis, *nausea, vomiting, diarrhea, anorexia,* pancreatitis, increased GGT, increased liver function tests. **Skin:** *Rash.* **Other:** Lactic acidosis, renal insufficiency.

INTERACTIONS Drug: Alcohol may increase abacavir blood levels.

PHARMACOKINETICS Absorption: Rapidly absorbed, 83% bioavailable. **Distribution:** Distributes into extravascular space and erythrocytes; 50% protein bound. **Metabolism:** Metabolized by alcohol dehydrogenase and glucuronyl transferase to inactive metabolites. **Elimination:** 84% in urine, primarily as inactive metabolites; 16% in feces. **Half-Life:** 1.5 h.

NURSING IMPLICATIONS

Assessment & Drug Effects

- Monitor for S&S of hypersensitivity: fever, skin rash, fatigue, GI distress (nausea, vomiting, diarrhea, abdominal pain). Withhold drug immediately and notify physician if hypersensitivity develops.
- Lab tests: Periodically monitor liver function, BUN and creatinine, CBC with differential, triglyceride levels, and blood glucose, especially in diabetics.
- Withhold drug and notify physician for S&S of acidosis, hepatotoxicity, or renal insufficiency.

Patient & Family Education

- Take drug exactly as prescribed at indicated times. Missed dose: Take immediately, then resume dosing schedule. Do not double a dose.
- Withhold drug immediately and notify physician at first sign of hypersensitivity reaction (see Assessment & Drug Effects).
- Carry Warning Card provided with drug at all times.

ABATACEPT

(a-ba-ta′sept)

Orencia

Classifications: BIOLOGICAL RESPONSE MODIFIER; DISEASE-MODIFYING ANTIRHEUMATIC DRUG (DMARD)

Therapeutic: ANTIRHEUMATIC (DMARD); ANTI-INFLAMMATORY

Pregnancy Category: C

AVAILABILITY 250 mg lyophilized powder for injection

ACTION & *THERAPEUTIC EFFECT* Abatacept inhibits T-cell (T lymphocyte) proliferation and inhibits production of tumor necrosis factor (TNF)-alpha, interferon-gamma, and interleukin-1 (IL-2, IL-6, and IL-15). It suppresses inflammation, decreases anticollagen antibody production, and reduces antigen-specific production of interferon-gamma. *Abatacept is used to reduce the number of activated T lymphocytes found in synovial fluid of rheumatoid arthritis patients. It relieves symptoms and slows progression of structural damage. It improves physical function in adults with active rheumatoid arthritis who have had an inadequate response to other drugs.*

USES Treatment of moderate to severe rheumatoid arthritis in patients with an inadequate response to one or more disease-modifying antirheumatic drugs (DMARDs). It may be used as monotherapy or in combination with other DMARDs, with the exception of TNF antagonists.

CONTRAINDICATIONS Known hypersensitivity to abatacept, live vaccines; active infections; coadministration with anakinra; TNF antagonists; children younger than 6 y; lactation.

CAUTIOUS USE COPD, RA; malignancies; pregnancy (category C).

ROUTE & DOSAGE

Rheumatoid Arthritis

Adult: **IV** Initial dose: *Weight less than 60 kg,* 500 mg; *60–100 kg,* 750 mg; *weight greater than 100 kg,* 1000 mg. Give dose at weeks 2 and 4, then monthly.

Juvenile Idiopathic Arthritis

Child (at least 6 y): **IV** *Weight less than 75 kg,* 10 mg/kg, repeat at weeks 2 and 4, then monthly (max: 1000 mg); *weight 75–100 kg,* 750 mg at weeks 2 and 4, then monthly; *weight at least 100 kg,* 1000 mg at weeks 2 and 4, then monthly

ADMINISTRATION

Intravenous

PREPARE: **IV Infusion:** Use the supplied silicone-free disposable syringe with an 18–21 gauge needle to reconstitute the vial. ▪ Add 10 mL sterile water to each 250 mL to yield 25 mg/mL. ▪ To avoid foaming, gently swirl until completely dissolved. Do not shake or vigorously agitate. ▪ After dissolving, vent the vial with a needle to dissipate any foam. ▪ The reconstituted solution **must be** further diluted to a total of 100 mL as follows: From a 100 mL NS IV bag remove a volume equal to the total volume of abatacept in the reconstituted vials (e.g., for 2 vials, remove 20 mL). Using the supplied silicone-free syringe, slowly add the reconstituted abatacept to the IV bag and gently mix. ▪ The final concentration of the IV solution will be approximately 5, 7.5, or 10 mg/mL, depending on whether 2, 3, or 4 vials are used. ▪ Discard any unused abatacept.

ADMINISTER: **IV Infusion:** Use a 0.2–1.2 micron low-protein-binding filter. Infuse over 30 min.

INCOMPATIBILITIES **Solution/additive:** Should not be infused in the same intravenous line with other agents. **Y-site:** Should not be infused in the same intravenous line with other agents.

▪ Store at 2°–8° C (36°–46° F).

ADVERSE EFFECTS (≥1%) **Body as a Whole:** Infusion-related reactions, <u>malignancies</u>, cough, hypersensitivity reactions. **CNS:** *Headache,* dizziness. **CV:** Hypertension. **GI:** *Nausea,* dyspepsia. **Musculoskeletal:** Back pain, pain in extremity. **Respiratory:** *Upper respiratory tract infection, nasopharyngitis,* sinusitis, influenza, bronchitis. **Skin:** Rash. **Urogenital:** Urinary tract infection.

INTERACTIONS Drug: TNF ANTAGONISTS increase the risk of serious infections.

PHARMACOKINETICS Half-Life: 13.1 days.

NURSING IMPLICATIONS

Assessment & Drug Effects

- Prior to initiating treatment with abatacept, screen for latent TB infection with a TB skin test.
- Monitor for S&S of hypersensitivity (e.g., hypotension, urticaria, and dyspnea); discontinue infusion and notify physician if any of these occur.
- Monitor for S&S of infection. Withhold drug and notify physician if patient develops a serious infection.
- Monitor for deterioration of respiratory status in patients with COPD.

Patient & Family Education

- Report any of the following to a health care provider: Any type of infection, a positive TB skin test, a recent vaccination, a persistent cough, unexplained weight loss, fever, sore throat, or night sweats.
- Report S&S of an allergic reaction that may develop within 24 h of receiving abatacept (e.g., hives swollen face, eyelids, lips, tongue, throat, or trouble breathing).

- Do not accept immunizations with live vaccines while taking or within 3 mo of discontinuing abatacept.

ABCIXIMAB Pr

(ab-cix′i-mab)

ReoPro

Classifications: PLATELET AGGREGATION INHIBITOR; GLYCOPROTEIN IIB/IIIA INHIBITOR

Therapeutic: ANTIPLATELET

Pregnancy Category: C

AVAILABILITY 2 mg/mL in 5 mL vials

ACTION & *THERAPEUTIC EFFECT* Abciximab is a human-murine monoclonal antibody Fab (fragment antigen binding) fragment that binds to the glycoprotein IIb/IIIa (GPIIb/IIIa) receptor sites of platelets. *Abciximab inhibits platelet aggregation by preventing fibrinogen, von Willebrand's factor, and other molecules from adhering to GPIIb/IIIa receptor sites of the platelets.*

USES Adjunct to aspirin and heparin for the prevention of acute cardiac ischemic complications in patients undergoing percutaneous transluminal coronary angioplasty (PTCA).

CONTRAINDICATIONS Hypersensitivity to abciximab or to murine proteins; active internal bleeding; GI or GU bleeding within 6 wk; history of CVA within 2 y or a CVA with severe neurologic deficit; administration of oral anticoagulants unless PT less than 1.2 times control; thrombocytopenia (less than 100,000 cells/mL); recent major surgery or trauma; intracranial neoplasm, aneurysm, severe hypertension; history of vasculitis; use of dextran before or during PTCA; lactation.

CAUTIOUS USE Patients weighing less than 75 kg; older adults; history of previous GI disease; recent thrombolytic therapy; PTCA within 12 h of MI; unsuccessful PTCA; PTCA procedure lasting longer than 70 min; pregnancy (category C).

ROUTE & DOSAGE

PTCA

Adult: **IV** 10–60 min prior to angioplasty, 0.25 mg/kg bolus over 5 min followed by continuous infusion of 0.125 mcg/kg/min (up to 10 mcg/min) for next 12 h

ADMINISTRATION

Intravenous

Do not shake vial. Discard if visible opaque particles are noted.

- Use a nonpyrogenic low protein-binding 0.2- or 0.22-micron filter when withdrawing drug into a syringe from the 2 mg/mL vial and when infusing as continuous IV.

PREPARE: **Direct:** No dilution required. **Continuous:** Inject 5 mL of abciximab (10 mg) into 250 mL of NS or D5W.

ADMINISTER: **Direct:** Give undiluted bolus dose over 5 min. **Continuous:** Infuse at no more than 15 mL/h (10 mcg/min) via an infusion pump over 12 h.

INCOMPATIBILITIES **Solution/additive:** Infuse through separate IV line. **Y-site:** Infuse through separate IV line.

- Discard any unused drug at the end of the 12 h infusion as well as any unused portion left in vial. ▪ Store vials at 2°–8° C (36°–46° F).

ADVERSE EFFECTS (≥1%) **Hematologic:** *Bleeding*, including intracranial, retroperitoneal, and hematemesis; thrombocytopenia.

INTERACTIONS Drug: ORAL ANTICOAGULANTS, NSAIDS, **dipyridamole, ticlopidine, dextran** may increase risk of bleeding.

PHARMACOKINETICS Onset: Greater than 90% inhibition of platelet aggregation within 2 h. **Duration:** Approximately 48 h. **Half-Life:** 30 min.

NURSING IMPLICATIONS

Assessment & Drug Effects

- Monitor for S&S of: Bleeding at all potential sites (e.g., catheter insertion, needle puncture, or cutdown sites; GI, GU, or retroperitoneal sites); hypersensitivity that may occur any time during administration.
- Lab tests: Monitor Hgb, Hct, platelet count, PT, APTT, INR, and activated clotting time, every 2–4 h during first 24 h.
- Avoid or minimize unnecessary invasive procedures and devices to reduce risk of bleeding.
- Elevate head of bed 30° or less and keep limb straight when femoral artery access is used; following sheath removal, apply pressure for 30 min.
- Stop infusion immediately and notify physician if bleeding or S&S of hypersensitivity occurs.

Patient & Family Education

- Report any S&S of bleeding immediately.

ACAMPROSATE CALCIUM

(a-cam-pro′sate)

Campral

Classification: SUBSTANCE ABUSE DETERRENT

Therapeutic: SUBSTANCE ABUSE INHIBITOR

Pregnancy Category: C

AVAILABILITY 333 mg delayed release tablets

ACTION & *THERAPEUTIC EFFECT* May interact with CNS glutamate and GABA neurotransmitter systems and help restore normal balance between neuronal excitation and inhibition. Acamprosate is a neurotransmitter analog. *Reduces craving for alcohol intake due to chronic use, but does not cause alcohol aversion or a disulfiram-like reaction as a result of ethanol ingestion.*

USES Maintenance of abstinence from alcohol in patients with alcoholism.

CONTRAINDICATIONS Hypersensitivity to acamprosate calcium or any of its components; suicidal ideation; severe renal impairment (CrCl less than 30 mL/min).
CAUTIOUS USE Moderate renal impairment; depression; pregnancy (category C); lactation. Safety and efficacy of acamprosate have not been established in adolescents or children younger than 18 y.

ROUTE & DOSAGE

Maintenance of Alcohol Abstinence

Adult: **PO** 666 mg t.i.d.

Renal Impairment Dosage Adjustment

CrCl 30–50 mL/min: 333 mg t.i.d.; less than 30 mL/min: Do not use

ADMINISTRATION

Oral

- Ensure that the drug is not chewed or crushed. It **must be** swallowed whole.
- Store at 15°–30° C (59°–86° F).

ADVERSE EFFECTS (≥1%) **Body as a Whole:** Flu syndrome, chills. **CNS:** Depression, anxiety, insomnia, asthenia, dizziness, paresthesia, headache, somnolence, decreased libido, amnesia, abnormal thinking, tremor. **CV:** Palpitation, syncope. **GI:** *Diarrhea,* nausea, vomiting, anorexia, flatulence, dry mouth, abdominal pain, dyspepsia, constipation, increased appetite. **Metabolic:** Peripheral edema, weight gain. **Musculoskeletal:** Musculoskeletal pain. **Respiratory:** Rhinitis, cough, dyspnea, pharyngitis, bronchitis. **Skin:** Pruritus, diaphoresis, rash. **Special Senses:** Abnormal vision, taste perversion. **Urogenital:** Impotence.

INTERACTIONS Drug: None reported.

PHARMACOKINETICS Absorption: 11% bioavailability. **Metabolism:** Not metabolized. **Elimination:** Renal. **Half-Life:** 20–33 h.

NURSING IMPLICATIONS

Assessment & Drug Effects

- Monitor for S&S depression or suicidal thinking.
- Monitor for dizziness or impaired judgment, thinking, and motor skills; take appropriate protective measures.

Patient & Family Education

- Report any alcohol consumption while taking acamprosate.
- Report promptly any of the following: Unusual anxiousness or nervousness; depression or suicidal thoughts; burning or tingling sensations in arms, legs, hands, or feet; chest pains or palpitations; difficulty urinating.
- Do not drive or engage in other hazardous activities until reaction to the drug is known.

ACARBOSE (Pr)

(a-car′bose)

Precose

Classifications: ANTIDIABETIC; ALPHA-GLUCOSIDASE INHIBITOR

Therapeutic: ANTIDIABETIC

Pregnancy Category: B

AVAILABILITY 25 mg, 50 mg, 100 mg tablets

ACTION & *THERAPEUTIC EFFECT* Acarbose is an oral alpha-glucosidase inhibitor that delays the absorption of sugars from the intestinal tract. The inhibitory effect of acarbose varies according to which enzymes are involved; from most to least inhibited are glucoamylase, sucrase, maltase, and isomaltase. *Acarbose reduces blood sugar by interfering with carbohydrate absorption from the GI tract.*

USES In conjunction with diet and exercise for type 2 diabetes.

UNLABELED USES In combination with other treatments in patients with type 1 or 2 diabetes mellitus.

CONTRAINDICATIONS Inflammatory bowel disease, colon ulcers, partial bowel obstruction, predisposition for obstruction; patients younger than 18 y; lactation.

CAUTIOUS USE GI distress or liver disorders, pregnancy (category B).

ROUTE & DOSAGE

Type 2 Diabetes Mellitus

Adult: **PO** Start with 25 mg daily to t.i.d. with meals, titrate to individual response (max: 150 mg/day for 60 kg or less, 300 mg/day for greater than 60 kg)

ADMINISTRATION

Oral

- Remove drug from foil wrapper immediately before administration.
- Give drug with first bite at each of the three main meals.
- Do not store above 25° C (77° F). Keep tightly closed and protect from moisture.

ADVERSE EFFECTS (≥1%) **CNS:** Sleepiness, weakness, dizziness, headache, vertigo (may be due to poor diabetic control). **Endocrine:** Hypoglycemia (especially in combination with sulfonylureas and insulin). **GI:** *Diarrhea, flatulence, abdominal distention,* borborygmi, increased liver function tests. **Hematologic:** Anemia (especially iron deficiency). **Skin:** Erythema, exanthema, urticaria.

INTERACTIONS Drug: SULFONYLUREAS may increase hypoglycemic effects. Drugs that induce hyperglycemia (e.g., THIAZIDES, CORTICOSTEROIDS, PHENOTHIAZINES, ESTROGENS, **phenytoin, isoniazid**) may decrease effectiveness of acarbose. **Herbal: Ginseng** may increase hypoglycemic effects.

PHARMACOKINETICS Absorption: 0.5–2% is absorbed intact from GI tract. After degradation by intestinal bacteria, up to 35% of dose may be absorbed. **Peak:** Peak blood glucose reduction approximately 70 min after dose. **Metabolism:** In GI tract by intestinal bacteria and digestive enzymes. **Elimination:** 35% in urine, 51% in feces, 5% in air as CO_2. **Half-Life:** 2 h.

NURSING IMPLICATIONS

Assessment & Drug Effects

- Lab tests: Periodically monitor blood glucose, HbA1C liver enzymes, Hct and Hgb.
- Treat hypoglycemia with dextrose; not with sucrose (table sugar).

Patient & Family Education

- Note: Acarbose prevents the breakdown of table sugar. Have a source of dextrose, such as dextrose paste, available to treat low blood sugar.
- Monitor closely blood glucose, especially following dosage changes.
- Report abdominal distress; dietary adjustment or dosage reduction may be warranted.
- Monitor weight and report significant changes.

ACEBUTOLOL HYDROCHLORIDE

(a-se-byoo-toe'lole)

Monitan ♣, Sectral

Classifications: BETA-ADRENERGIC ANTAGONIST; ANTIHYPERTENSIVE; ANTIARRHYTHMIC, CLASS II

Therapeutic: ANTIHYPERTENSIVE; CLASS II ANTIARRYTHMIC

Prototype: Propranolol

Pregnancy Category: B

AVAILABILITY 200 mg, 400 mg capsules

ACTION & *THERAPEUTIC EFFECT*

Beta$_1$-selective adrenergic blocking agent with mild sympathomimetic activity (partial beta-agonist activity). Produces negative chronotropic and inotropic activity (i.e., decreases exercise-induced heart rate, inhibits reflex orthostatic tachycardia, and decreases cardiac output at rest and during exercise). *Decreases both systolic and diastolic BP at rest and during exercise. Exhibits antiarrhythmic activity (class II antiarrhythmic agent).*

USES Treatment of mild to moderate hypertension. Management of recurrent stable ventricular arrhythmias.
UNLABELED USES Supraventricular arrhythmias, chronic stable angina pectoris.

CONTRAINDICATIONS Overt CHF, second- or third-degree AV block, severe bradycardia, cardiogenic shock; acute bronchospasm, pulmonary edema; lactation; children younger than 12 y.
CAUTIOUS USE Impaired cardiac function, well-compensated CHF, mesenteric or peripheral vascular disease; cerebrovascular disease; patients undergoing major surgery involving general anesthesia; renal or hepatic impairment; labile diabetes mellitus; hyperthyroidism; bronchospastic disease (asthma, emphysema); avoid abrupt withdrawal; pregnancy (category B).

ROUTE & DOSAGE

Hypertension
Adult: **PO** 400–800 mg/day in 1–2 divided doses (max: 1200 mg/day)
Geriatric: **PO** 200–400 mg/day (max: 800 mg/day)

Ventricular Arrhythmias
Adult: **PO** 200 mg b.i.d. increased to 600–1200 mg/day

Angina Pectoris
Adult: **PO** 300–400 mg t.i.d.

Renal Impairment Dosage Adjustment
CrCl less than 50 mL/min: Reduce dose by 50%; less than 25 mL/min: Reduce dose by 75%

ADMINISTRATION

Oral
- Check apical pulse before administration. If less than 60 bpm or other ordered parameter, consult physician.
- Discontinue gradually over a period of 2 wk.
- Store at 15°–30° C (59°–86° F).

ADVERSE EFFECTS (≥1%) **Body as a Whole:** *Fatigue.* **CNS:** Dizziness, insomnia, drowsiness, confusion, fainting. **CV:** *Bradycardia,* hypotension, CHF. **GI:** Nausea, *diarrhea, constipation,* flatulence. **Hematologic:** Agranulocytosis, *antinuclear antibodies (ANA).* **Metabolic:** Hypoglycemia (may mask symptoms of a hypoglycemic reaction). **Respiratory:** Bronchospasm, pulmonary edema, dyspnea. **Urogenital:** Decreased libido; impotence.

DIAGNOSTIC TEST INTERFERENCE False-negative test results possible (see **propranolol**).

INTERACTIONS Drug: Other HYPOTENSIVE AGENTS, DIURETICS increase hypotensive effect; with **albuterol, metaproterenol, terbutaline,** or **pirbuterol,** there is mutual antagonism with acebutolol; NSAIDS blunt hypotensive effect; decreases hypoglycemic effect of **glyburide;** increases bradycardia and sinus arrest with **amiodarone.**

PHARMACOKINETICS Absorption: Well absorbed after PO administration; undergoes extensive first-pass metabolism in liver with an average bioavailability of 40%. (In geriatric patients, bioavailability increases twofold.) **Peak:** 3 h. **Distribution:** Minimally into CSF; crosses placenta; is excreted in breast milk. **Metabolism:** In liver to diacetolol with activity equipotent to parent compound. **Elimination:** Metabolite 8–13 h; 50–60% via bile into feces, 30–40% in urine. **Half-Life:** 3–4 h.

NURSING IMPLICATIONS

Assessment & Drug Effects

- Monitor BP and cardiac status throughout therapy. Observe for and report marked bradycardia or hypotension, especially when patient is also receiving a catecholamine-depleting drug (e.g., reserpine).
- Monitor I&O ratio and pattern and report changes to physician (e.g., dysuria, nocturia, oliguria, weight change).
- Monitor for S&S of CHF, especially peripheral edema, dyspnea, activity intolerance.
- Lab tests: Monitor for drug-induced positive ANA titer during long-term therapy, especially in women and older adults; periodic CBC with long-term therapy.

Patient & Family Education

- Know parameters for withholding drug (e.g., pulse less than 60).
- Note: Common adverse effects include insomnia, drowsiness, and confusion.
- Do not drive or engage in potentially hazardous activities until response to drug is known.
- Do not increase, decrease, omit, or discontinue drug regimen without advice from the physician. Abrupt withdrawal may worsen angina or precipitate MI in patient with heart disease.
- Contact physician promptly at the first signs or symptoms of CHF (see Appendix F).
- Report muscle and joint pain to physician. Discontinuation of drug therapy usually reverses these adverse effects.
- Monitor for loss of glycemic control if diabetic.
- Note: Drug may mask symptoms of hypoglycemia (see Appendix F) and potentiate insulin-induced hypoglycemia in diabetics.
- Avoid use of OTC oral cold preparations and topical nasal decongestants unless approved by the physician.

ACETAMINOPHEN, PARACETAMOL (Pr)

(a-seat-a-mee'noe-fen)

Abenol ♣, A'Cenol, Acephen, Anacin-3, Anuphen, APAP, Atasol ♣, Campain ♣, Dolanex, Exdol ♣, Halenol, Liquiprin, Panadol, Pedric, Robigesic ♣, Rounox ♣, Tapar, Tempra, Tylenol, Tylenol Arthritis, Valadol

Classification: NONNARCOTIC ANALGESIC, ANTIPYRETIC

Therapeutic: NONNARCOTIC ANALGESIC; ANTIPYRETIC

Pregnancy Category: B

AVAILABILITY 80 mg, 120 mg, 125 mg, 300 mg, 325 mg, 650 mg suppositories; 80 mg, 160 mg, 325 mg, 500 mg tablets/caplets; 650 mg extended release tablets/capsules; 80 mg/0.8 mL, 80 mg/2.5 mL, 80 mg/5 mL, 120 mg/5 mL, 160 mg/5 mL, 500 mg/5 mL liquid

ACTION & *THERAPEUTIC EFFECT* Produces analgesia by unknown mechanism, but it is centrally acting in the CNS by increasing the pain threshold by inhibiting cyclooxygenase. Reduces fever by direct action on hypothalamus heat-regulating center with consequent peripheral vasodilation, sweating, and dissipation of heat. Unlike aspirin, has little effect on platelet aggregation, does not affect bleeding time, and produces no gastric bleeding. *It provides temporary analgesia for mild to moderate pain. In addition, acetaminophen lowers body temperature in individuals with a fever.*

USES Fever reduction. Temporary relief of mild to moderate pain. Generally as substitute for aspirin when the latter is not tolerated or is contraindicated.

CONTRAINDICATIONS Hypersensitivity to acetaminophen or phenacetin; use with alcohol.

CAUTIOUS USE Repeated administration to patients with anemia, G6PD deficiency, renal or hepatic disease; arthritic or rheumatoid conditions affecting children younger than 12 y; alcoholism; malnutrition; thrombocytopenia; bone marrow depression, immunosuppression; pregnancy (category B).

ROUTE & DOSAGE

Mild to Moderate Pain, Fever

Adult: **PO** 325–650 mg q4–6h (max: 4 g/day) **PR** 650 mg q4–6h (max: 4 g/day)
Child: **PO** 10–15 mg/kg q4–6h **PR** *2–5 y,* 120 mg q4–6h (max: 720 mg/day); *6–12 y,* 325 mg q4–6h (max: 2.6 g/day)
Neonate: **PO** 10–15 mg/kg q6–8h

ADMINISTRATION

Oral

- Administer tablets or caplets whole or crushed and give with fluid of patient's choice.
- Chewable tablets should be thoroughly chewed and wetted before they are swallowed.
- Do not coadminister with a high carbohydrate meal; absorption rate may be significantly retarded.
- Store in light-resistant containers at room temperature, preferably between 15°–30° C (59°–86° F).

Rectal

- Insert suppositories beyond the rectal sphincter.

ADVERSE EFFECTS (≥1%) **Body as a Whole:** Negligible with recommended dosage; rash. **Acute poisoning:** Anorexia, nausea, vomiting, dizziness, lethargy, diaphoresis, chills, epigastric or abdominal pain, diarrhea; onset of hepatotoxicity: elevation of serum transaminases (ALT, AST) and bilirubin; hypoglycemia, hepatic coma, acute renal failure (rare). **Chronic ingestion:** Neutropenia, pancytopenia, leukopenia, thrombocytopenic purpura, *hepatotoxicity in alcoholics,* renal damage.

DIAGNOSTIC TEST INTERFERENCE False increases in ***urinary 5-HIAA*** (5-hydroxyindoleacetic acid) byproduct of serotonin; false decreases in ***blood glucose*** (by ***glucose oxidase–peroxidase procedure***); false increases in ***urinary glucose*** (with certain instruments in glucose analyses); and false increases in ***serum uric acid*** (with ***phosphotungstate method***). High doses or long-term therapy: hepatic, renal, and hematopoietic function (periodically).

INTERACTIONS Drug: Cholestyramine may decrease acetaminophen absorption. With chronic coadministration, BARBITURATES, **carbamazepine, phenytoin,** and **rifampin** may increase potential for chronic hepatotoxicity. Chronic, excessive ingestion of **alcohol** will increase risk of hepatotoxicity.

PHARMACOKINETICS Absorption: Rapid and almost complete absorption from GI tract; less complete absorption from rectal suppository. **Peak:** 0.5–2 h. **Duration:** 3–4 h. **Distribution:** In all body fluids; crosses placenta. **Metabolism:** Extensively in liver. **Elimination:** 90–100% of drug excreted as metabolites in urine; excreted in breast milk. **Half-Life:** 1–3 h.

NURSING IMPLICATIONS

Assessment & Drug Effects

- Monitor for S&S of: Hepatotoxicity, even with moderate acetaminophen doses, especially in individuals with poor nutrition or who have ingested alcohol over prolonged periods; poisoning, usually from accidental ingestion or suicide attempts; potential abuse from psychological dependence (withdrawal has been associated with restless and excited responses).

Patient & Family Education

- Do not take other medications (e.g., cold preparations) containing acetaminophen without medical advice; overdosing and chronic use can cause liver damage and other toxic effects.
- Do not self-medicate adults for pain more than 10 days (5 days in children) without consulting a physician.
- Do not use this medication without medical direction for: Fever persisting longer than 3 days, fever over 39.5° C (103° F), or recurrent fever.
- Do not give children more than 5 doses in 24 h unless prescribed by physician.

ACETAZOLAMIDE Pr

(a-set-a-zole′a-mide)

Acetazolam ♣, Apo-Acetazolamide ♣, Diamox Sequels

ACETAZOLAMIDE SODIUM

(a-set-a-zole′a-mide)

Diamox Parenteral

Classification: CARBONIC ANHYDRASE INHIBITOR

Therapeutic: DIURETIC; ANTICONVULSANT; ANTIGLAUCOMA

Pregnancy Category: C

AVAILABILITY 125 mg, 250 mg tablets; 500 mg sustained release capsules; 500 mg powder for injection

ACTION & *THERAPEUTIC EFFECT* The mechanism of anticonvulsant action is unknown but thought to involve inhibition of CNS carbonic anhydrase, which retards abnormal transmission from CNS neurons. Diuretic effect is due to inhibition of carbonic anhydrase activity in proximal renal tubule, preventing formation of carbonic acid, and therefore the formation of H^+ and HCO_3^-. Inhibition of carbonic anhydrase in eye reduces rate of aqueous humor formation with consequent lowering of intraocular pressure. *Reduces seizure activity and intraocular pressure. Additionally, it has a diuretic effect.*

USES Treatment of seizures: Absence or petit mal, generalized tonic-clonic (grand mal), and focal; reduction of intraocular pressure in open-angle glaucoma and secondary glaucoma; preoperative treatment of acute closed-angle glaucoma; drug-induced edema and as adjunct in treatment of edema due to congestive heart failure; acute high-altitude sickness.

UNLABELED USES Prevent uric acid or cystine renal calculi; to treat acute pancreatitis, premenstrual syndrome (PMS), metabolic alkalosis, and hypokalemic and hyperkalemic forms of familial periodic paralysis; to increase secretion of phenobarbital or lithium; hydrocephalus.

CONTRAINDICATIONS Hypersensitivity to carbonic anhydrase inhibitors, marked renal and hepatic disease; Addison's disease or other types of adrenocortical insufficiency; hyponatremia, hypokalemia, hyperchloremic acidosis; prolonged administration to patients with hyphema; chronic noncongestive angle-closure glaucoma.

CAUTIOUS USE Hypersensitivity to sulfonamides and derivatives (e.g., thiazides), history of hypercalciuria; diabetes mellitus, elderly, gout, patients receiving digitalis, obstructive pulmonary disease, respiratory acidosis; pregnancy (category C).

ROUTE & DOSAGE

Glaucoma

Adult: **PO** 250 mg 1–4 times/day, 500 mg sustained release b.i.d., up to 1 g/day **IM/IV** 500 mg, may repeat in 2–4 h
Child: **PO** 8–30 mg/kg/day in 3 doses **IV** 5–10 mg/kg q6h

Epilepsy

Adult/Child: **PO** 8–30 mg/kg/day in 1–4 doses

Edema

Adult: **PO/IV** 250–375 mg every a.m. (5 mg/kg); may be given every other day if condition improves
Child: **PO/IV** 5 mg/kg or 150 mg/m^2 every a.m.

High Altitude Sickness

Adult: **PO** 250 mg q8–12h or 500 mg sustained release q12–24h, starting 24–48 h before climb and continuing for 48 h at high altitude

Treatment Hydrocephalus

Neonate/Infant: **PO/IV** 20 mg/kg/day in divided doses q8–12h (max: 100 mg/kg/day)

Renal Impairment Dosage Adjustment

CrCl 10–50 mL/min: Extend interval to q12h; less than 10 mL/min: Use not recommended
Hemodialysis Dosage Adjusment: Administer post-dialysis

ADMINISTRATION

Oral

- Administer diuretic dose in morning to avoid interrupted sleep.
- Give with food or meals to minimize GI upset.
- Note: If tablet(s) cannot be swallowed, soften tablet(s) (not sustained release form) in 2 tsp of hot water and add to 2 tsp of honey/syrup to disguise bitter taste; avoid syrups containing alcohol or glycerin, or crush tablet(s) and suspend in syrup (250–500 mg/5 mL syrup). Prepare just before administration. Drug does not dissolve in fruit juices.
- Store oral preparations at 15°–30° C (59°–86° F) unless otherwise directed.

Intramuscular

- Reconstitute as for IV administration. See PREPARE Direct.
- Give IM for rapid lowering of intraocular pressure or in patients unable to take oral dosage.
- Note: The intramuscular dosage is not the route of choice because

the alkalinity of the solution makes the injection painful.

Intravenous

IV administration to neonates, infants, and children: Verify correct IV concentration and rate of infusion/injection with physician.

PREPARE: **Direct:** Reconstitute each 500 mg vial with at least 5 mL of sterile water for injection to yield approximately 100 mg/mL. May be used as prepared or further diluted. **IV Infusion:** Dilute reconstituted solution with D5W or NS. Use within 24 h of reconstitution.

ADMINISTER: **Direct:** Give at a rate of 500 mg or fraction thereof over 1 min. **IV Infusion:** Give as a continuous infusion over 4–8 h.

INCOMPATIBILITIES **Solution/additive: Amino acid. Y-site: Diltiazem, TPN.**

ADVERSE EFFECTS (≥1%) **CNS:** Paresthesias, sedation, malaise, disorientation, depression, fatigue, muscle weakness, flaccid paralysis. **GI:** Anorexia, nausea, vomiting, weight loss, dry mouth, thirst, diarrhea. **Hematologic:** Bone marrow depression with agranulocytosis, hemolytic anemia, aplastic anemia, leukopenia, pancytopenia. **Metabolic:** Increased excretion of calcium, potassium, magnesium, and sodium, metabolic acidosis, hyperglycemia, hyperuricemia. **Ocular:** Transient myopia. **Urogenital:** Glycosuria, urinary frequency, polyuria, dysuria, hematuria, crystalluria. **Other:** Exacerbation of gout, hepatic dysfunction, Stevens-Johnson syndrome.

DIAGNOSTIC TEST INTERFERENCE Monitor for false-positive ***urinary protein*** determinations; falsely high values for ***urine urobilinogen;*** depressed ***iodine uptake*** values (exception: hypothyroidism).

INTERACTIONS Drug: Renal excretion of AMPHETAMINES, **ephedrine, flecainide, quinidine, procainamide,** TRICYCLIC ANTIDEPRESSANTS may be decreased, thereby enhancing or prolonging their effects. Renal excretion of **lithium** is increased. Excretion of **phenobarbital** may be increased. **Amphotericin B** and CORTICOSTEROIDS may accelerate **potassium** loss. DIGITALIS GLYCOSIDES may predispose persons with hypokalemia to **digitalis** toxicity; puts patients on high doses of SALICYLATES at high risk for SALICYLATE toxicity.

PHARMACOKINETICS Absorption: Well absorbed from GI tract. **Onset:** 1 h regular release; 2 h sustained release; 2 min IV. **Peak:** 2–4 h reg; 8–18 h sustained; 15 min IV. **Duration:** 8–12 h reg; 18–24 h sustained; 4–5 h IV. **Distribution:** Distributed throughout body, concentrating in RBCs, plasma, and kidneys; crosses placenta. **Elimination:** Primarily in urine. **Half-Life:** 2.4–5.8 h.

NURSING IMPLICATIONS

Assessment & Drug Effects

- Establish baseline weight before initial therapy and weigh daily thereafter when used to treat edema.
- Monitor for S&S of: Mild to severe metabolic acidosis; potassium loss which is greatest early in therapy (see hypokalemia in Appendix F).
- Monitor I&O especially when used with other diuretics.
- Lab tests: Blood pH, blood gases, urinalysis, CBC, and serum electrolytes (initially and periodically during prolonged therapy or concomitant therapy with other diuretics or digitalis).

Patient & Family Education

- Maintain adequate fluid intake (1.5–2.5 L/24 h; 1 liter is approximately equal to 1 quart) to reduce risk of kidney stones.
- Report any of the following: Numbness, tingling, burning, drowsiness, and visual problems, sore throat or mouth, unusual bleeding, fever, skin or renal problems.
- Eat potassium-rich diet and take potassium supplement when taking this drug in high doses or for prolonged periods.

ACETYLCYSTEINE Pr

(a-se-til-sis'tay-een)

Airbron ✦, Mucomyst, Mucosol, N-Acetylcysteine, Acetadote, Acys-5

Classifications: MUCOLYTIC; ANTIDOTE

Therapeutic: MUCOLYTIC; ANTIDOTE

Pregnancy Category: B

AVAILABILITY 10%, 20% solution for inhalation; 20% solution for injection

ACTION & *THERAPEUTIC EFFECT* Acetylcysteine probably acts by disrupting disulfide linkages of mucoproteins in purulent and nonpurulent bronchial secretions. In acetaminophen overdose, it helps to prevent hepatotoxicity by serving as a substrate for the toxic metabolites of acetaminophen. *Lowers viscosity and facilitates the removal of secretions.*

USES Adjuvant therapy in patients with abnormal, viscid, or inspissated mucous secretions in acute and chronic bronchopulmonary diseases, and in pulmonary complications of cystic fibrosis and surgery, tracheostomy, and atelectasis. Also used in diagnostic bronchial studies and as an antidote for acute acetaminophen poisoning.

UNLABELED USES As an ophthalmic solution for treatment of dry eye (keratoconjunctivitis sicca); as an enema to treat bowel obstruction due to meconium ileus; prevention of radiocontrast-induced renal dysfunction.

CONTRAINDICATIONS Hypersensitivity to acetylcysteine; patients at risk of gastric hemorrhage.

CAUTIOUS USE Patients with asthma, older adults, severe hepatic disease, esophageal varices, peptic ulcer disease; debilitated patients with severe respiratory insufficiency; pregnancy (category B), lactation.

ROUTE & DOSAGE

Mucolytic

Adult: **Inhalation** 1–10 mL of 20% solution q4–6h or 2–20 mL of 10% solution q4–6h **Direct Instillation** 1–2 mL of 10–20% solution q1–4h

Child: **Inhalation** 3–5 mL of 20% solution or 6–10 mL of 10% solution 3–4 times/day

Infant: **Inhalation** 1–2 mL 20% solution or 2–4 mL of 10% solution 3–4 times/day

Acetaminophen Toxicity

Adult/Child: **PO** 140 mg/kg followed by 70 mg/kg q4h for 17 doses (use a 5% solution)

Adult/Adolescent/Child: **IV** 150 mg/kg infused over 60 min, followed by 50 mg/kg over 4 h, then 100 mg/kg over 16 h; total dose 300 mg/kg over 21 h

ADMINISTRATION

Inhalation and Instillation

- Prepare dilution within 1 h of use; drug does not contain an antimicrobial agent. A light purple discoloration does not significantly impair drug's effectiveness.

- Dilute the 20% solution with NS or water for injection. The 10% solution may be used undiluted.
- Give by direct instillation into tracheostomy (1–2 mL of 10–20% solution).
- Instruct patient to clear airway, if possible, coughing productively prior to aerosol administration to ensure maximum effect.
- Store opened vial in refrigerator to retard oxidation; use within 96 h.
- Store unopened vial at 15°–30° C (59°–86° F), unless otherwise directed.

Oral

- Dilute the 20% solution 1:3 with cola, orange juice, or other soft drink to make a 5% solution. If administered via a gastric tube, water may be used as the diluent.
- Freshly prepare all diluted solutions and use within 1 h of preparation.

Intravenous

PREPARE: **IV Infusion:** Acetylcysteine reacts with certain metals and rubber; use IV equipment made of plastic or glass. ▪ Dilute all required doses in D5W as follows: For loading dose, add a dose equal to 150 mg/kg to 200 mL; for first maintenance dose, add a dose equal to 50 mg/kg to 500 mL; for second maintenance dose, add a dose equal to 100 mg/kg to 1000 mL. ▪ Note: The total IV volume should be reduced for patients less than 40 kg and for those with fluid restriction. In small children, individualize the total IV volume to avoid water intoxication and hyponatremia.

ADMINISTER: **IV Infusion:** Give loading dose over 60 min, maintenance dose 1 over 4 h, maintenance dose 2 over 16 h. Complete all infusions over 24 h.

INCOMPATIBILITIES **Y-site:** **Cefepime, ceftazidime.**

- Store reconstituted solution for up to 24 h at 15°–30° C (59°–86° F).

ADVERSE EFFECTS (≥1%) **CNS:** Dizziness, drowsiness. **GI:** Nausea, *vomiting,* stomatitis, hepatotoxicity (urticaria). **Respiratory:** Bronchospasm, rhinorrhea, burning sensation in upper respiratory passages, epistaxis.

PHARMACOKINETICS Onset: 1 min after inhalation or instillation. **Peak:** 5–10 min. **Metabolism:** Deacetylated in liver to cysteine.

NURSING IMPLICATIONS

Assessment & Drug Effects

- During IV infusion, carefully monitor for fluid overload and signs of hyponatremia (i.e., changes in mental status).
- Monitor for S&S of aspiration of excess secretions, and for bronchospasm (unpredictable); withhold drug and notify physician immediately if either occurs.
- Lab tests: Monitor ABGs, pulmonary functions and pulse oximetry as indicated; baseline serum acetaminophen level (for toxicity), LFTs, bilirubin, serum electrolytes, BUN, and plasma glucose.
- Have suction apparatus immediately available. Increased volume of respiratory tract fluid may be liberated; suction or endotracheal aspiration may be necessary to establish and maintain an open airway. Older adults and debilitated patients are particularly at risk.
- Nausea and vomiting may occur, particularly when face mask is used, due to unpleasant odor of

drug and excess volume of liquefied bronchial secretions.

Patient & Family Education

- Report difficulty with clearing the airway or any other respiratory distress.
- Report nausea, as an antiemetic may be indicated.
- Note: Unpleasant odor of inhaled drug becomes less noticeable with continued use.

ACITRETIN

(a-ci-tree'tin)
Soriatane
Classification: RETINOID
Therapeutic: ANTIPSORIATIC
Prototype: Isotretinoin
Pregnancy Category: X

AVAILABILITY 10 mg, 25 mg capsules

ACTION & *THERAPEUTIC EFFECT* Acitretin binds to the retinoic acid receptors in the skin, thus modifying gene expression, epithelial cell growth, and cell differentiation. *Acitretin is a highly toxic metabolite of retinol (vitamin A).*

USES Treatment of severe, recalcitrant psoriasis in adults.

CONTRAINDICATIONS Sensitivity to parabens, papilledema, severe renal impairment or renal failure, development of psychiatric symptoms (depression, etc); pregnancy (category X) for at least 3 y after use, lactation.

CAUTIOUS USE Patients with impaired hepatic function, hepatitis, diabetes mellitus, obesity, alcoholism, history of pancreatitis, hypertriglyceridemia, hypercholesterolemia, coronary artery disease, retinal disease, degenerative joint disease.

ROUTE & DOSAGE

Psoriasis
Adult: **PO** 25–50 mg daily with main meal

ADMINISTRATION

Oral

- Administer as single dose with main meal because food enhances absorption.
- Store at 15°–25° C (59°–77° F) and protect from light. After opening, avoid exposure to high temperatures and humidity.

ADVERSE EFFECTS (≥1%) **Body as a Whole:** *Hyperesthesia, paresthesias, arthralgia, progression of existing spinal hyperostosis, rigors,* back pain, hypertonia, myalgia, fatigue, hot flashes, increased appetite. **CNS:** Headache, depression, aggressive feelings and thoughts of self-harm, insomnia, somnolence. **CV:** Flushing, edema. **GI:** *Dry mouth, increased liver function tests, increased triglycerides and cholesterol,* hepatitis, gingival bleeding, gingivitis, increased saliva, stomatitis, thirst, ulcerative stomatitis, abdominal pain, diarrhea, nausea, tongue disorder. **Special Senses:** Blurred vision, blepharitis, conjunctivitis, decreased night vision/night blindness, eye pain, photophobia; earache, tinnitus; taste perversion. **Respiratory:** Sinusitis. **Skin:** *Alopecia, skin peeling, dry skin, nail disorders, pruritus, rash, cheilitis, skin atrophy, paronychia,* abnormal skin odor and hair texture, cold/clammy skin, increased sweating, purpura, seborrhea, skin ulceration, sunburn. **Other:** *Rhinitis, epistaxis, xerophthalmia.*

INTERACTIONS Drug: Combination with **ethanol** can create **etretinate,** which has a significantly longer half-life than acitretin; interferes with the contraceptive efficacy of **progestin**-only ORAL CONTRACEPTIVES. Use with **methotrexate** increases the risk of hepatitis. **Food:** Excess vitamin A, **ethanol.**

PHARMACOKINETICS Absorption: Rapidly from GI tract, optimal absorption when taken with food. **Peak:** 2–5 h. **Distribution:** Crosses placenta, distributed into breast milk. **Metabolism:** Active metabolite, *cis*-acitretin. **Elimination:** In both urine and feces. **Half-Life:** 49 h acitretin, 63 h *cis*-acitretin.

NURSING IMPLICATIONS

Assessment & Drug Effects

- Monitor for S&S of pancreatitis or loss of glycemic control in diabetics. Report either condition immediately to physician.
- Lab tests: Before initiating therapy and at 1- to 2-wk intervals until response to drug is known, do lipid profile and liver function tests. Monitor blood glucose and HbA1C periodically.

Patient & Family Education

- Note: Transient worsening of psoriasis may occur during early therapy.
- Review common adverse effects of drug; lag time of 2–3 mo may be necessary before drug effect is evident.
- Discontinue drug and report immediately to physician if visual problems develop.
- Note: Dry eyes with decreased tolerance for contact lenses may occur.
- Do not drink alcohol while taking this drug; it increases risk of hepatotoxicity and hypertriglyceridemia; females should avoid alcohol during and for 2 mo following therapy.
- Avoid excessive amounts of vitamin A (consult prescriber).
- Do not donate blood for 3 y following therapy.
- Avoid excessive exposure to sunlight or UV light.
- Use two forms of effective contraception for 1 mo before and at least 3 y following therapy because of the serious risk of fetal deformities that could result from exposure to this medication.

ACRIVASTINE/ PSEUDOEPHEDRINE

(a-cri-vas'teen)

Semprex-D (combination with pseudoephedrine)

Classifications: H_1-RECEPTOR ANTAGONIST; DECONGESTANT

Therapeutic: ANTIHISTAMINE; DECONGESTANT

Prototype: Diphenhydramine

Pregnancy Category: B

AVAILABILITY Acrivastine 8 mg/ pseudoephedrine 60 mg capsules

ACTION & *THERAPEUTIC EFFECT* Acrivastine is an H_1-receptor histamine antagonist that controls histamine-mediated symptoms and acts on sympathetic nerve endings. Pseudoephedrine shrinks swollen nasal mucous membranes and reduces nasal congestion of the mucosa. *It is effective in allergic rhinitis by reducing nasal congestion and decreasing respiratory mucosa swelling.*

USES Seasonal and perennial allergic rhinitis with nasal congestion.

CONTRAINDICATIONS Hypersensitivity to acrivastine, triprolidine, pseudoephedrine, or ephedrine; severe hypertension or severe coronary artery disease; patients on MAO inhibitor drugs; uncontrolled hypertension; tachycardia, acute cardiac arrhythmias; closed-angle glaucoma. **CAUTIOUS USE** Renal insufficiency, hypertension, DM, ischemic heart disease, increased intraocular pressure, hyperthyroidism, BPH, GI disorders, older adults, pregnancy (category B), lactation. Safety and effectiveness in children younger than 12 y have not been established.

ROUTE & DOSAGE

Allergic Rhinitis

Adult: **PO** 1 cap (8 mg acrivastine/60 mg pseudoephedrine) t.i.d.

ADMINISTRATION

Oral

- Do not give to patients with a creatinine clearance of 48 mL/min or less.
- Store at 15°–25° C (59°–77° F); protect from light and moisture.

ADVERSE EFFECTS (≥1%) **CNS:** Headache, vertigo, dizziness, insomnia, jitteriness, *drowsiness*. **GI:** Nausea, diarrhea, dry mouth, dyspepsia.

INTERACTIONS Drug: Alcohol may increase psychomotor impairment.

PHARMACOKINETICS Absorption: Rapidly from GI tract. **Onset:** 1 h. **Duration:** Approximately 12 h. **Metabolism:** In liver. **Elimination:** Approximately 65% excreted unchanged in urine. **Half-Life:** 1.5 h.

NURSING IMPLICATIONS

Assessment & Drug Effects

- Monitor for dizziness, sedation, urinary obstruction, and hypotension, especially in older adults.
- Assess for significant drowsiness, which may necessitate drug discontinuation.

Patient & Family Education

- Do not use this drug in combination with other OTC antihistamines or decongestants.
- Do not drive or engage in potentially hazardous activities until response to drug is known.
- Do not take alcohol or other CNS depressants while taking this drug.

ACYCLOVIR, ACYCLOVIR SODIUM (Pr)

(ay-sye'kloe-ver)

Zovirax

Classification: ANTIVIRAL

Therapeutic: ANTIVIRAL; ANTIHERPES VIRAL

Pregnancy Category: B

AVAILABILITY 200 mg capsules; 400 mg, 800 mg tablets; 200 mg/5 mL suspension; 50 mg/mL injection; 5% ointment, cream

ACTION & *THERAPEUTIC EFFECT* Acyclovir is a synthetic nucleoside analog of guanine. Acyclovir preferentially interferes with DNA synthesis of herpes simplex virus types 1 and 2 (HSV-1 and HSV-2) and varicella-zoster virus, thereby inhibiting viral replication. *Acyclovir reduces viral shedding and formation of new lesions and speeds healing time. It demonstrates antiviral activity against herpes virus simiae (B virus), Epstein-Barr (infectious mononucleosis), varicella-zoster and cytomegalovirus, but does not eradicate the latent herpes virus.*

USES Parenterally for treatment of initial and recurrent mucosal and cutaneous herpes simplex virus (HSV-1 and HSV-2) infections in immunocompromised adults and children and for severe initial episodes of herpes genitalis in immunocompetent (normal immune system) patients. Treatment of herpes encephalitis or neonatal herpes infection. Used orally for treatment of initial episodes of genital herpes, for management of selected patients with severe recurrent episodes, and for prophylaxis to reduce frequency and severity of recurrent infections. Used topically for herpes labialis (cold sores), initial episodes of herpes genitalis and in non-life-threatening mucocutaneous herpes simplex virus infections in immunocompromised patients.

UNLABELED USES Treatment of eczema herpeticum caused by HSV localized and disseminated herpes zoster. Prevention of CMV in transplant patients. Prevention of HSV in immunosuppressed HSV-seropositive patients.

CONTRAINDICATIONS Hypersensitivity to acyclovir and valacyclovir.

CAUTIOUS USE Renal insufficiency, dehydration, seizure disorders, or neurologic disease; pregnancy (category B).

ROUTE & DOSAGE

Cold Sores

Adult/Adolescents (12 y or older): **Topical** Apply 5 times/day for 4 days

Genital Herpes Simplex

Adult: **PO** 400 mg t.i.d. for 7–10 day cycle **IV** 5 mg/kg q8h × 7 days **Topical** Apply q3h 6 times/day × 7 days

Child (younger than 12 y): **IV** 250 mg/m² q8h, 80 mg/kg/day in 2–5 doses

Herpes Simplex Immunocompromised Patient

Adult: **IV** 5 mg/kg q8h × 7 days

Child: **IV** 10 mg/kg q8h × 7 days

Prophylaxis for Genital Herpes Simplex

Adult: **PO** 200 mg 2–5 times/day, 400 mg t.i.d., 800 mg b.i.d.

Child: **PO** 80 mg/kg/day in 2–5 divided doses

Severe Genital Herpes

Adult/Adolescent: **IV** 5 mg/kg q8h × 5 days

Herpes Zoster

Adult: **PO** 800 mg q4h 5 times/day

Child: **PO** 80 mg/kg/day in 5 divided doses

Herpes Simplex Encephalitis

Adult: **IV** 10 mg/kg q8h × 10 days

Child (3 mo–12 y): **IV** 20 mg/kg q8h × 10 days

Neonate (younger than 3 mo): **IV** 10 mg/kg q8h × 10 days

Varicella Zoster

Child/Adolescent: **PO** 20 mg/kg (max: 800 mg) q.i.d. for 5 day cycle initiated within 24 h of onset of rash

Adult: **IV** 10 mg/kg q8h × 7 days

Child: **IV** 20 mg/kg q8h × 7 days

Obesity Dosage Adjustment

Patient dose should be calculated using IBW.

Renal Impairment Dosage Adjustment

CrCl 25–50 mL/min: Standard dose q12h; 10–25 mL/min: Standard dose q24h; less than 10 mL/min: Give half normal dose q24h

Hemodialysis Dosage Adjustment: Administer dose after dialysis

ADMINISTRATION

Oral

- Shake suspension well prior to use.
- Store capsules in tight, light-resistant containers at 15°–30° C (59°–86° F) unless otherwise directed.

Topical

- Wash hands thoroughly before and after treatment of lesions and after handling and disposition of secretions.
- Apply approximately 1/2 inch of cream or ointment ribbon for each 4 square inches of surface area. Use sufficient ointment or cream to completely cover lesions.
- Apply topical preparation with finger cot or surgical glove.
- Store at 15°–25° C (59°–78° F) unless otherwise directed.

Intravenous

PREPARE: **Intermittent:** Reconstitute by adding 10 mL sterile water for injection to 500-mg vial to yield 50 mg/mL. Note: Do not use bacteriostatic water for injection containing benzyl alcohol. Shake well. ▪ Further dilute to 7 mg/mL or less to reduce risk of renal injury and phlebitis. Example: Add 1 mL of reconstituted solution to 9 mL of diluent to yield 5 mg/mL. ▪ Use standard electrolyte and glucose solutions (e.g., NS, LR, D5W) for dilution.

ADMINISTER: **Intermittent:** Administer over at least 1 h to prevent renal tubular damage. Rapid or bolus IV administration **must be** avoided. ▪ Monitor IV flow rate carefully; infusion pump or microdrip infusion set preferred.

INCOMPATIBILITIES **Solution/additive:** Bacteriostatic water for injection, **dobutamine, dopamine, pantoprazole**. **Y-site:** **Amifostine, amsacrine, aztreonam, cefepime, dobutamine, dopamine, fludarabine, foscarnet, gemcitabine, idarubicin, levofloxacin, ondansetron, piperacillin/tazobactam, sargramostim, TPN, vinorelbine.**

▪ Refrigerated reconstituted solution may precipitate; however, crystals will redissolve at room temperature. ▪ Store acyclovir powder and reconstituted solutions at controlled room temperature, preferably at 15°–30° C (59°–86° F) unless otherwise directed by manufacturer. ▪ Use reconstituted solution within 12 h. Use diluted solution within 24 h.

ADVERSE EFFECTS (≥1%) **Body as a Whole:** Generally minimal and infrequent. **CNS:** *Headache,* lightheadedness, lethargy, fatigue, tremors, confusion, seizures, dizziness. **GI:** *Nausea, vomiting, diarrhea.* **Urogenital:** Glomerulonephritis, renal pain, renal tubular damage, acute renal failure. **Skin:** Rash, urticaria, pruritus, burning, stinging sensation, irritation, sensitization. **Other:** Inflammation or phlebitis at IV injection site, sloughing (with extravasation), thrombocytopenic purpura/hemolytic uremic syndrome.

INTERACTIONS Drug: Probenecid decreases acyclovir elimination; **zidovudine** may cause increased drowsiness and lethargy.

PHARMACOKINETICS Absorption: Oral dose is 15–30% absorbed. **Peak:** 1.5–2 h after oral dose. **Distribution:** Into most tissues with lower levels in the CNS; crosses placenta. **Metabolism:** Drug is primarily excreted unchanged. **Elimination:** Renally eliminated; also excreted in breast milk. **Half-Life:** 2.5–5 h.

NURSING IMPLICATIONS

Assessment & Drug Effects

- Observe infusion site during infusion and for a few days following infusion for signs of tissue damage.

- Monitor I&O and hydration status. Keep patient adequately hydrated during first 2 h after infusion to maintain sufficient urinary flow and thus prevent precipitation of drug in renal tubules. Consult physician about amount and length of time oral fluids need to be pushed after IV drug treatment.
- Monitor for S&S of: Reinfection in pregnant patients; acyclovir-induced neurologic symptoms in patients with history of neurologic problems; drug resistance in immunocompromised patients receiving prolonged or repeated therapy; acute renal failure with concomitant use with other nephrotoxic drugs or preexisting renal disease.
- Lab tests: Monitor baseline and periodic renal function studies, particularly with IV administration. Elevations of BUN and serum creatinine and decreases in creatinine clearance indicate need for dosage adjustment, discontinuation of drug, or correction of fluid and electrolyte balance.
- Monitor for adverse effects and viral resistance with long-term prophylactic use of the oral drug.

Patient & Family Education

- Start therapy as soon as possible after onset of S&S for best results.
- Do not exceed recommended dosage, frequency of drug administration, or specified duration of therapy. Contact physician if relief is not obtained or adverse effects appear.
- Cleanse affected areas with soap and water 3–4 times daily prior to topical application; dry well before application. With application to genitals, wear loose-fitting clothes over affected areas.
- Note: Even after HSV infection is controlled, latent virus can be activated by stress, trauma, fever, exposure to sunlight, sexual intercourse, menstruation, or treatment with immunosuppressive drugs.
- Refrain from sexual intercourse if either partner has S&S of herpes infection; neither topical nor systemic drug prevents transmission to other individuals.
- Avoid topical drug contact in or around eyes. Report unexplained eye symptoms to physician immediately (e.g., redness, pain); untreated infection can lead to corneal keratitis and blindness.

ADALIMUMAB (D2E7)

(a-da-lim′u-mab)

Humira

Classifications: BIOLOGICAL RESPONSE MODIFIER; TUMOR NECROSIS FACTOR MODIFIER; DISEASE-MODIFYING ANTIRHEUMATIC DRUG (DMARD)

Therapeutic: ANTIRHEUMATIC AGENT; DMARD; ANTI-INFLAMMATORY

Prototype: Etanercept

Pregnancy Category: B

AVAILABILITY 40 mg/0.8 mL injection

ACTION & *THERAPEUTIC EFFECT*

Adalimumab is a human recombinant IgG1 monoclonal antibody. It neutralizes the effects of tumor necrosis factor (TNF)-alpha, a cytokine, by blocking its interaction with cell surface TNF receptors. This mechanism blocks the normal inflammatory and immune responses controlled by TNF-alpha. In the presence of complement, adalimumab may also lyse TNF-expressing cells. *Reduces the levels of acute phase inflammatory reac-*

tants (C-reactive protein, ESR, interleukin-6) thus decreasing overall joint inflammation; also reduces levels of enzymes that produce tissue remodeling responsible for cartilage destruction. In RA, adalimumab reduces the numerous inflammatory events of polyarthritis. It reduces the overproduction of TNF-alpha principally by macrophages in rheumatoid joints.

USES Treatment of moderate to severe rheumatoid arthritis or psoriatic arthritis and to reduce progression of the disease in patients with or without a disease-modifying antirheumatic drug (DMARD), treatment of Crohn's disease.

CONTRAINDICATIONS Hypersensitivity to adalimumab or mannitol; active infection, either chronic or acute; neoplastic disease; sepsis; lactation. Safe use in children has not been established.

CAUTIOUS USE History of recurrent infection or conditions predisposing to infection; recurrent history of sensitivity to monoclonal antibodies; cardiovascular disease; neurologic disease; patients residing in areas with endemic TB or histoplasmosis; active or latent TB infection prior to therapy; demyelinating disorders; concurrent administration of immunosuppressants; surgery; pregnancy (category B).

ROUTE & DOSAGE

Rheumatoid Arthritis

Adult: **Subcutaneous** 40 mg every other wk (may use 40 mg every wk if not on concomitant methotrexate)

Crohn's Disease

Adult: **Subcutaneous** Initial dose of 160 mg (dose can be administered as 4 injections in 1 day or as 2 injections/day for 2 consecutive days), then 80 mg at wk 2, followed by 40 mg every other wk beginning at wk 4

ADMINISTRATION

Subcutaneous

- Do not administer to persons with active infections. Evaluate for latent TB with TB skin test prior to initiation of therapy.
- Inspect prefilled syringe for particulate matter and discoloration prior to subcutaneous injection.
- Rotate injection sites and do not inject into skin that is red, bruised, tender, or hard. After injecting the drug, do not rub the site.
- Discard any remaining solution in prefilled syringe, as it contains no preservatives.
- Store in original carton at 2°–4° C (38°–48° F). Protect from light. Do not use beyond the expiration date.

ADVERSE EFFECTS (≥1%) **Body as a Whole:** Infections (especially reactivation of latent tuberculosis), sepsis, may see increase in malignancies (lymphoma), back pain, fever, allergic reactions (including <u>anaphylactic shock</u>), *flu-like symptoms, fatigue.* **CNS:** *Headache.* **CV:** Hypertension. **GI:** *Nausea, vomiting,* abdominal pain. **Hematologic:** Development of ANA antibodies. **Respiratory:** *Upper respiratory infection, sinusitis.* **Skin:** *Injection site reactions (erythema, itching, hemorrhage, pain, swelling), rash,* urticaria, fixed drug reaction. **Urogenital:** Urinary tract infection.

INTERACTIONS Drug: Do not give LIVE VIRUS VACCINES to patient on adalimumab; not recommended for use with other TNF BLOCKERS (**etanercept, infliximab, anakinra**).

PHARMACOKINETICS Absorption: 64% absorbed from subcutaneous injection site. **Peak:** 131 h. **Distribution:** Minimal beyond vascular/synovial space. **Elimination:** Higher clearance in presence of anti-adalimumab antibodies, lower clearance with increasing age. **Half-Life:** 11.8 days (10–20 days).

NURSING IMPLICATIONS

Assessment & Drug Effects

- Monitor for and report lupus-like syndrome (e.g., joint pain, rash on cheeks or arms that is sensitive to sun).
- Monitor for and report promptly S&S of infection.
- Monitor neurologic status closely. Report any change in status such as blurred vision or paresthesia.

Patient & Family Education

- Live vaccines should not be accepted by persons taking this drug.
- Report promptly any of the following to the physician: Unexplained joint pain, rash on cheeks or arms, fever, sore throat or other signs of infection, changes in vision, numbness or tingling in extremities.

ADAPALENE

(a-da'pa-leen)

Differin

Classifications: ANTIACNE; RETINOID

Therapeutic: ANTIACNE

Prototype: Isotretinoin

Pregnancy Category: C

AVAILABILITY 0.1%, 0.3% gel; 0.1% cream

ACTION & *THERAPEUTIC EFFECT* Adapalene is a topical retinoid-like compound that modulates cellular differentiation, keratinization, and inflammatory processes related to the pathology of acne vulgaris. Topical adapalene may normalize the differentiation of epithelial follicular cells. *Adapalene decreases the inflammatory process and acne formation.*

USES Topical treatment of acne vulgaris.

CONTRAINDICATIONS Hypersensitivity to adapalene or any of the components of the gel, irritating topical products, and sunburn; skin abrasion, eczema, seborrheic dermatitis.

CAUTIOUS USE Pregnancy (category C), lactation. Safety and effectiveness in children younger than 12 y are not established.

ROUTE & DOSAGE

Acne

Adult: Apply once daily to affected areas in evening

ADMINISTRATION

Topical

- Apply a thin film to clean skin, avoiding eyes, lips, mucous membranes, cuts, abrasions, eczematous or sunburned skin.
- Do not apply to skin recently treated with preparations containing sulfur, resorcinol, or salicylic acid.
- Store at 20°–25° C (68°–77° F).

ADVERSE EFFECTS (≥1%) **Skin:** *Erythema, scaling, dryness, pruritus, burning,* skin irritation, stinging, sunburn, acne flares.

PHARMACOKINETICS Absorption: Minimal through intact skin. **Elimination:** Primarily in bile.

NURSING IMPLICATIONS

Assessment & Drug Effects

- Monitor therapeutic effectiveness, which is indicated by improvement after 8–12 wk of treatment; early therapy may be marked by apparent worsening of acne.
- Note: Cutaneous reactions (e.g., erythema, scaling, pruritus) are common and normally diminish after first month of therapy.

Patient & Family Education

- Apply only as directed; excessive application will not result in faster healing but will cause marked redness, peeling, and discomfort.
- Minimize exposure to sunlight and sunlamps, and use sunscreen and protective clothing as needed.

ADEFOVIR DIPIVOXIL

(a-de'fo-vir)

Hepsera

Classifications: ANTIVIRAL; NUCLEOTIDE ANALOG

Therapeutic: ANTIVIRAL

Pregnancy Category: C

AVAILABILITY 10 mg tablets

ACTION & *THERAPEUTIC EFFECT* Inhibits human hepatitis virus (HBV) DNA polymerase (reverse transcriptase) by competing with its DNA and by causing DNA chain termination after its incorporation into viral DNA. This results in inhibition of HBV DNA replication. *A nucleotide analog with activity against human hepatitis B virus (HBV).*

USES Treatment of chronic hepatitis B.

CONTRAINDICATIONS Hypersensitivity to adefovir; untreated or unknown human immunodeficiency virus (HIV); exacerbations of hepatitis B, especially in patients who have discontinued anti-hepatitis B therapy; lactation. Safety and efficacy in children are not established.

CAUTIOUS USE Decreased cardiac function due to concomitant disease or other drug therapy; elderly; concomitant use of highly nephrotoxic drugs; renal dysfunction; co-administration with drugs that reduce renal function or compete for active tubular secretion; pregnancy (category C). Appropriate infant immunizations should be used to prevent neonatal acquisition of the hepatitis B virus.

ROUTE & DOSAGE

Hepatitis B

Adult: **PO** 10 mg daily

Renal Impairment Dosage Adjustment

CrCl 20–49 mL/min: 10 mg q48h; 10–19 mL/min: 10 mg q72h

Hemodialysis Dosage Adjustment: 10 mg q7days following dialysis

ADMINISTRATION

Oral

- Note that the dosing interval of adefovir should be adjusted in patients with baseline creatinine clearance less than 50 mL/min.
- Store in original container at 15°–30° C (59°–86° F).

ADVERSE EFFECTS (≥1%) **CNS:** *Asthenia,* headache. **GI:** Abdominal pain, nausea, flatulence, diarrhea, dyspepsia, exacerbation of hepatitis after discontinuation of therapy, hepatomegaly. **Metabolic:** *Increased ALT, AST,* increased creatine kinase, amylase, lactic acidosis. **Urogenital:** *Hematuria,* glycosuria, increased serum creatinine, nephrotoxicity. **Other:** HIV resistance in patient with unrecognized HIV, hematuria.

INTERACTIONS Drug: Risk of lactic acidosis when used with NUCLEOSIDE ANALOGS. **Ibuprofen** increases bioavailability of adefovir.

PHARMACOKINETICS Absorption: Adefovir dipivoxil is a prodrug. 59% of dose is absorbed as active drug. **Peak:** 1–4 h. **Distribution:** Minimal protein binding. **Metabolism:** Adefovir dipivoxil is rapidly converted to active adefovir. **Elimination:** Primarily in urine. **Half-Life:** 7.5 h.

NURSING IMPLICATIONS

Assessment & Drug Effects

- Lab tests: Monitor baseline and periodic renal function tests (monitor more often with preexisting impairment or other risk factors for renal impairment); monitor periodic liver function tests, creatinine kinase, serum amylase, and routine blood chemistries including serum electrolytes.
- Withhold drug and notify physician if lactic acidosis is suspected [e.g., hyperventilation, lethargy, plasma pH less than 7.35 and lactate greater than 5–6 mol/L (mEq/L)].

Patient & Family Education

- Report any of the following to physician: Blood in urine, unexplained weakness, or exacerbation of S&S of hepatitis.
- Patients who discontinue adefovir should be monitored at repeated intervals over a period of time for hepatic function.

ADENOSINE

(a-den′o-sin)

Adenocard, Adenoscan
Classification: ANTIARRHYTHMIC
Therapeutic: ANTIARRHYTHMIC
Pregnancy Category: C

AVAILABILITY 3 mg/mL

ACTION & *THERAPEUTIC EFFECT* Slows conduction through the atrioventricular (AV) and sinoatrial (SA) nodes. Can interrupt the reentry pathways through the AV node. *Restores normal sinus rhythm in patients with paroxysmal supraventricular tachycardia.*

USES Conversion to sinus rhythm of paroxysmal supraventricular tachycardia (PSVT) including PSVT associated with accessory bypass tracts (Wolff-Parkinson-White syndrome). "Chemical" thallium stress test.

UNLABELED USES Afterload-reducing agent in low-output states; to prevent graft occlusion following aortocoronary bypass surgery; to produce controlled hypotension during cerebral aneurysm surgery.

CONTRAINDICATIONS AV block, preexisting second- and third-degree heart block or sick sinus rhythm without pacemaker, since a heart block may result. Ineffective for atrial flutter, atrial fibrillation, and ventricular tachycardia.

CAUTIOUS USE Asthmatics, unstable angina, stenotic valvular disease, hypovolemia; hepatic and renal failure; pregnancy (category C).

ROUTE & DOSAGE

Supraventricular Tachycardia

Adult/Adolescent (Weight 50 kg or more): **IV** 6 mg bolus initially; after 1–2 min may give two additional 12 mg bolus doses for a total of 3 doses.

Do not exceed 12 mg in any one dose.
Neonate/Infant/Child: **IV** 0.05–1 mg/kg bolus; additional doses may be increased by 0.05–1 mg/kg q2min (max: 12 mg/dose)

Stress Thallium Test

Adult: **IV** 140 mcg/kg/min × 6 min (max: 0.84 mg/kg total dose)

ADMINISTRATION

Intravenous

Make sure solution is clear at time of use.

- Discard unused portion (contains no preservatives).

PREPARE: **Direct:** No dilution is required.

ADMINISTER: **Direct:** *Supraventricular Tachycardia:* Give rapid bolus over 1–2 sec. *Thallium Stress Test:* Give bolus over 6 min. ▪ If given by IV line, administer as proximally as possible, and follow with a rapid saline flush.

- Store at room temperature 15°–30° C (59°–86° F). Do not refrigerate, as crystallization may occur. If crystals do form, dissolve by warming to room temperature.

ADVERSE EFFECTS (≥1%) **CNS:** Headache, lightheadedness, dizziness, tingling in arms (from IV infusion), apprehension, blurred vision, burning sensation (from IV infusion). **CV:** *Transient facial flushing,* sweating, palpitations, chest pain, atrial fibrillation or flutter. **Respiratory:** Shortness of breath, transient *dyspnea,* chest pressure. **GI:** Nausea, metallic taste, tightness in throat. **Other:** Irritability in children.

INTERACTIONS Drug: Dipyridamole can potentiate the effects of adenosine; **theophylline** will block the electrophysiologic effects of adenosine; **carbamazepine** may increase risk of heart block.

PHARMACOKINETICS Absorption: Rapid uptake by erythrocytes and vascular endothelial cells after IV administration. **Onset:** 20–30 sec. **Metabolism:** Rapid uptake into cells; degraded by deamination to inosine, hypoxanthine, and adenosine monophosphate. **Elimination:** Route unknown. **Half-Life:** 10 sec.

NURSING IMPLICATIONS

Assessment & Drug Effects

- Monitor for S&S of bronchospasm in asthma patients. Notify physician immediately.
- Use a hemodynamic monitoring system during administration; monitor BP and heart rate and rhythm continuously for several minutes after administration.
- Note: Adverse effects are generally self-limiting due to short half-life (10 sec).
- Note: At the time of conversion to normal sinus rhythm, PVCs, PACs, sinus bradycardia, and sinus tachycardia, as well as various degrees of AV block, are seen on the ECG. These usually last only a few seconds and resolve without intervention.

Patient & Family Education

- Note: Flushing may occur along with a feeling of warmth as drug is injected.

AGALSIDASE BETA

(a-gal′si-dase)

Fabrazyme

Classification: ENZYME REPLACEMENT
Therapeutic: ENZYME REPLACEMENT
Prototype: Pancrelipase
Pregnancy Category: B

AVAILABILITY 35 mg/vial injection

ACTION & *THERAPEUTIC EFFECT* Fabry disease is caused by a deficiency of alpha-galactosidase A resulting in accumulation of glycosphingolipids in body tissues causing cardiomyopathy, renal failure, and CVA. Agalsidase beta provides an exogenous source of K-galactosidase A that catalyzes the breakdown of glycosphingolipids including GL-3. *Reduces globotriaosylceramide (GL-3) deposition in capillary endothelium of the kidney and certain other cell types.*

USES Treatment of Fabry disease.

CONTRAINDICATIONS Safety and efficacy in children younger than 16 y have not been established. Lactation.

CAUTIOUS USE Hypersensitivity reaction to agalsidase beta or mannitol; compromised cardiac function, mild to severe hypertension; renal impairment; pregnancy (category B).

ROUTE & DOSAGE

Fabry Disease
Adult: **IV** 1 mg/kg q2wk

ADMINISTRATION

Intravenous

Give antipyretics prior to infusion.

PREPARE: **Infusion:** Bring agalsidase vials and supplied sterile water for injection to room temperature prior to reconstitution. ▪ Reconstitute each 35 mg vial slowly injecting 7.2 mL of sterile water for injection down inside wall of vial. Roll and tilt vial gently to mix but do not shake. ▪ Reconstituted vial contains 5.0 mg/mL of clear, colorless solution. Do not use if there is particulate matter or if discolored. ▪ **Must be** further diluted in NS to a final total volume of 500 mL; prior to adding the volume of reconstituted agalisidase required for the dose, remove an equal volume of NS from the 500 mL infusion bag.

ADMINISTER: **Infusion:** Initial rate should not exceed 0.25 mg/min (15 mg/h; give more slowly if infusion-associated reactions occur). ▪ After tolerance to infusion is established, may increase rate in increments of 0.05–0.08 mg/min (increments of 3 to 5 mg/h) for each subsequent infusion.

INCOMPATIBILITIES **Solution/additive:** Do not infuse with other products.

▪ Store refrigerated until needed. Vials are for single use. Discard any unused portion. Do NOT use after expiration date.

ADVERSE EFFECTS (≥1%) **Body as a Whole:** *Fever, skeletal pain, pallor, rigors, temperature change sensation,* ataxia, stroke. **CNS:** *Dizziness, headache, paresthesia, anxiety, depression,* vertigo. **CV:** *Chest pain, cardiomegaly, hypertension, hypotension, dependent edema,* bradycardia, heart failure, exacerbation of preexisting arrhythmias. **GI:** *Dyspepsia, nausea, abdominal pain.* **Metabolic:** *Antibody development.* **Musculoskeletal:** *Arthrosis, skeletal pain.* **Respiratory:** *Bronchitis,* bronchospasm, laryngitis, *pharyngitis, rhinitis,* sinusitis, dyspnea. **Skin:** Pruritus, urticaria. **Special Senses:** Hearing loss. **Urogenital:** Testicular pain, nephrotic syndrome.

INTERACTIONS Drug: Coadministration with **amiodarone, chloroquine, hydroxychloroquine, gentamicin** is not recommended due to potential of decreased response to agalsidase beta therapy.

PHARMACOKINETICS Metabolism: Degraded through peptide hydrolysis. **Elimination:** Renal elimination expected to be a minor pathway. **Half-Life:** 45–102 min.

NURSING IMPLICATIONS

Assessment & Drug Effects

- During infusion, monitor for infusion-related reactions such as hypertension or hypotension, chest pain or chest tightness, dyspnea, fever and chills, headache, abdominal pain, pruritus and urticaria.
- Slow infusion and notify physician immediately if infusion reaction occurs. Note that additional antipyretic and/or an antihistamine and oral steroid may reduce the symptoms.
- Monitor cardiac status closely, especially with preexisting heart disease.

Patient & Family Education

- Notify physician if you have experienced an unusual reaction to agalsidase beta, agalsidase alfa, mannitol, other drugs, foods, or preservatives.
- Report any of the following to physician immediately: Chest pain or chest tightness, rapid heartbeat, shortness of breath or difficulty breathing; depression; dizziness; skin rash, hives or itching; throat tightness; swelling of the face, lips, neck, ears, or extremities.
- Do not drive or engage in other hazardous activities until reaction to drug is known.

ALBENDAZOLE

(al-ben'da-zole)

Albenza

Classification: ANTHELMINTIC
Therapeutic: ANTHELMINTIC
Prototype: Mebendazole
Pregnancy Category: C

AVAILABILITY 200 mg tablets

ACTION & *THERAPEUTIC EFFECT* A broad-spectrum oral anthelmintic agent. It is the only anthelmintic drug active against all stages of the helminth life cycle (ova, larvae, and adult worms). Its mechanism of action appears to cause selective degeneration of cytoplasmic microtubules in the intestinal cells of the helminths and larvae. *Albendazole ultimately causes decreased ATP production in the helminths, resulting in energy depletion, which kills the worms.*

USES Treatment of neurocysticercosis caused by the larval form of pork tapeworm (*Taenia solium*), hydatid disease caused by the larval form of dog tapeworm (*Echinococcus granulosus*).

CONTRAINDICATIONS Hypersensitivity to the benzimidazole class of compounds or any components of albendazole; children younger than 6 y.

CAUTIOUS USE Retinal lesions, pregnancy (category C), lactation.

ROUTE & DOSAGE

Neurocysticercosis

Adult/Child: **PO** *Older than 6 y, weight less than 60 kg,* 15 mg/kg/day divided b.i.d. for 8–30 day cycle (max: 800 mg/day); *weight 60 kg or more,* 400 mg b.i.d. for 8–30 day cycle

Hydatid Disease

Adult/Child: **PO** *Older than 6 y, weight less than 60 kg,* 15 mg/kg/day divided b.i.d. (max: 800 mg/day); *weight 60 kg or more,* 400 mg b.i.d. for 28-day cycle (then 14 days without drug and repeat regimen for 3 cycles)

ADMINISTRATION

Oral

- Give with meals. Absorption is significantly increased with a fatty meal.
- Do not exceed maximum total daily dose of 800 mg.
- Store at 20°–25° C (68°–77° F).

ADVERSE EFFECTS (≥1%) **Body as a Whole:** Hypersensitivity reactions. **CNS:** *Headache,* dizziness, vertigo, increased intracranial pressure, meningeal signs, alopecia (reversible), fever. **GI:** *Abnormal liver function tests,* abdominal pain, nausea, vomiting. **Hematologic:** (Rare) Reversible leukopenia, granulocytopenia, pancytopenia, agranulocytosis. **Skin:** Rash, urticaria.

INTERACTIONS Drug: Cimetidine, dexamethasone, praziquantel increase albendazole levels.

PHARMACOKINETICS Absorption: Poorly absorbed from GI tract, absorption enhanced with a fatty meal. **Peak:** 2–5 h. **Distribution:** 70% protein bound; widely distributed, including cyst fluid and CSF; secreted into animal breast milk. **Metabolism:** In liver to active metabolite, albendazole sulfoxide. **Elimination:** In bile. **Half-Life:** 8–12 h.

NURSING IMPLICATIONS

Assessment & Drug Effects

- Lab tests: Monitor WBC count, absolute neutrophil count, and liver function tests at start of each 28-day cycle and q2wk during cycle.
- Withhold drug and notify physician if WBC count falls below normal or liver enzymes are elevated.
- Note: Patients should be concurrently treated with appropriate steroid and anticonvulsant therapy.

Patient & Family Education

- Take with meals (see ADMINISTRATION).
- Do not become pregnant during or for at least 1 mo after therapy.

ALBUTEROL (Pr)

(al-byoo′ter-ole)

Accuneb, Novosalmol ♣, ProAir HFA, Proventil, Proventil HFA, ReliOn Ventolin HFA, Ventolin, Ventolin HFA, VoSpire ER

Classifications: BRONCHODILATOR (RESPIRATORY SMOOTH MUSCLE RELAXANT); BETA-ADRENERGIC AGONIST

Theurapeutic: BRONCHODILATOR

Pregnancy Category: C

AVAILABILITY 2 mg, 4 mg tablets; 4 mg, 8 mg extended release tablets; 2 mg/5 mL syrup; 200 mcg capsules for inhalation; 0.083%, 0.5% solution for inhalation; 90 mcg/actuation

ACTION & *THERAPEUTIC EFFECT* Moderately selective $beta_2$-adrenergic agonist with comparatively long action. Acts prominently on $beta_2$ receptors (particularly smooth muscles of trachea, bronchi, uterus, and vascular supply to skeletal muscles). Inhibits histamine release by mast cells. Produces bronchodilation by relaxing smooth muscles of bronchial tree. *Bronchodilation decreases airway resistance, facilitates mucous drainage, and increases vital capacity.*

USES To relieve bronchospasm associated with acute or chronic asthma, bronchitis, or other reversible obstructive airway diseases. Also used to prevent exercise-induced bronchospasm.

CONTRAINDICATIONS Albuterol or levalbuterol hypersensitivity; congenital long QT syndrome. Use of oral syrup in children younger than 2 y.
CAUTIOUS USE Cardiovascular disease, renal impairment, hypertension, hyperthyroidism, diabetes mellitus, elderly, history of seizures; hypersensitivity to sympathomimetic amines or to fluorocarbon propellant used in inhalation aerosols; pregnancy (category C).

ROUTE & DOSAGE

Bronchospasm

Adult: **PO** 2–4 mg 3–4 times/day, 4–8 mg sustained release 2 times/day **Inhaled** 1–2 inhalations q4–6h
Child: **PO** *2–6 y,* 0.1–0.2 mg/kg t.i.d. (max: 4 mg/dose); *6–12 y,* 2 mg 3–4 times/day **Inhaled** *4–12 y,* 1–2 inhalations q4–6h

Prevention of Exercise Induced Brochospasm

Adult: **Inhaled** 2 inhalations 30 min prior to exercise
Child (older than 4 y): **Inhaled** 2 inhalations 30 min prior to exercise

ADMINISTRATION

Oral
- Do not crush extended release tablets. Scored tablets may be broken in half.
- Note: An initial dose of 2 mg t.i.d. or q.i.d. is recommended for older adult patients.
- Store tablets and syrup between 2°–25° C (36°–77° F) in tight, light-resistant container.

Inhalation
- If ordered with beclomethasone, give 20–30 min before beclomethasone unless otherwise directed by physician.
- Administer albuterol inhalation aerosol canister only with the actuator provided.
- Store canisters between 15°–30° C (59°–86° F) away from heat and direct sunlight.

ADVERSE EFFECTS (≥1%) **Body as a Whole:** Hypersensitivity reaction. **CNS:** *Tremor,* anxiety, nervousness, restlessness, convulsions, weakness, headache, hallucinations. **CV:** Palpitation, hypertension, hypotension, bradycardia, reflex tachycardia. **Special Senses:** Blurred vision, dilated pupils. **GI:** Nausea, vomiting. **Other:** Muscle cramps, hoarseness.

DIAGNOSTIC TEST INTERFERENCE Transient small increases in ***plasma glucose*** may occur.

INTERACTIONS Drug: With **epinephrine,** other SYMPATHOMIMETIC BRONCHODILATORS, possible additive effects; MAO INHIBITORS, TRICYCLIC ANTIDEPRESSANTS potentiate action on vascular system; BETA-ADRENERGIC BLOCKERS antagonize the effects of both drugs.

PHARMACOKINETICS Onset: Inhaled: 5–15 min; PO: 30 min. **Peak:** Inhaled: 0.5–2 h; PO: 2.5 h. **Duration:** Inhaled: 3–6 h; PO: 4–6 h (8–12 h with sustained release). **Metabolism:** In liver by CYP3A4; may cross the placenta. **Elimination:** 76% of dose eliminated in urine in 3 days. **Half-Life:** 2.75 h.

NURSING IMPLICATIONS

Assessment & Drug Effects
- Monitor therapeutic effectiveness which is indicated by significant subjective improvement in pulmonary function within 60–90 min after drug administration.
- Monitor for: S&S of fine tremor in fingers, which may interfere with precision handwork; CNS stimula-

tion, particularly in children 2–6 y, (hyperactivity, excitement, nervousness, insomnia), tachycardia, GI symptoms. Report promptly to physician.

- Lab tests: Periodic ABGs, pulmonary functions, and pulse oximetry.
- Consult physician about giving last albuterol dose several hours before bedtime, if drug-induced insomnia is a problem.

Patient & Family Education

- Review directions for correct use of medication and inhaler (see ADMINISTRATION).
- Avoid contact of inhalation drug with eyes.
- Do not increase number or frequency of inhalations without advice of physician.
- Notify physician if albuterol fails to provide relief because this can signify worsening of pulmonary function and a reevaluation of condition/therapy may be indicated.
- Note: Albuterol can cause dizziness or vertigo; take necessary precautions.
- Do not use OTC drugs without physician approval. Many medications (e.g., cold remedies) contain drugs that may intensify albuterol action.

ALCLOMETASONE DIPROPIONATE

(al-clo-met'a-sone)

Aclovate

Pregnancy Category: C

See Appendix A-4.

ALEFACEPT Pr

(a-le'fa-cept)

Amevive

Classifications: BIOLOGICAL RESPONSE MODIFIER; IMMUNOLOGIC

Therapeutic: IMMUNOSUPPRESSANT

Pregnancy Category: B

AVAILABILITY 15 mg vials

ACTION & *THERAPEUTIC EFFECT* Activation of T cells plays a role in chronic plaque psoriasis. Alefacept is thought to bind to CD2 receptors found on all peripheral T cells and to immunoglobulin receptors on cytotoxic cells, such as natural killer cells. Alefacept blocks further activation of T cells and reduces cellular-mediated apoptosis of T cells. *Alefacept modulates the immune response by decreasing activation of T cells that are believed to be the key mediators of psoriasis.*

USES Treatment of moderate to severe chronic plaque psoriasis.

UNLABELED USES Treatment of psoriatic arthritis.

CONTRAINDICATIONS Hypersensitivity to alefacept; CD4+ T lymphocyte count below normal; patients with HIV, history of systemic malignancies; patients with a clinically important infection; serious infections; live or attenuated vaccines; lactation.

CAUTIOUS USE Patients at high risk for malignancies; pregnancy (category B); elderly.

ROUTE & DOSAGE

Chronic Plaque Psoriasis

Adult: **IM** 15 mg once/wk × 12 wk, may repeat course after 12 wk off therapy if CD4 count is above 250 cells/mcL **IV** 7.5 mg once/wk × 12 wk, may repeat course after 12 wk off therapy if CD4 count is above 250 cells/mcL

ADMINISTRATION

- Administer only if CD4+ T lymphocyte count is 250 cells/mcL or more.
- Reconstituted alefacept should be clear and colorless to slightly yellow.

Intramuscular

- Reconstitute the 15 mg vial IM administration with 0.6 mL of the supplied diluent to yield 15 mg/0.5 mL. Gently swirl vial for about 2 min to mix, but do not shake.
- Rotate the injection sites and space at least 1 inch from an old site.
- Never inject into areas where the skin is tender, bruised, red, or hard.

Intravenous

PREPARE: **Direct:** Use supplied needles for preparation and administration. ▪ Reconstitute the 7.5 mg vial for IV administration with 0.6 mL of the supplied diluent to yield 7.5 mg/0.5 mL. ▪ Keeping the needle pointed at the sidewall of the vial, slowly inject the diluent then gently swirl vial for about 2 min to mix, but do not shake.

ADMINISTER: **Direct:** Prime supplied infusion set with 3.0 mL of supplied diluent and insert into vein. ▪ Give reconstituted solution over 5 sec or less and do not use a filter. ▪ Follow with flush using 3 mL of supplied diluent.

INCOMPATIBILITIES **Solution/additive:** Do not add other medications to IV solution.

- Store vials of powder away from light at 15°–30° C (59°–86° F).
- Store reconstituted solution for up to 4 h between 2°–8° C (36°–46° F); discard solution not used within 4 h of reconstitution.

ADVERSE EFFECTS (≥1%) **Body as a Whole:** Secondary malignancies, serious infections, chills, *injection site pain,* injection site inflammation. **CNS:** Dizziness, headache. **GI:** Nausea, vomiting. **Hematologic:** *Lymphopenia,* alefacept antibody formation. **Musculoskeletal:** Myalgia. **Respiratory:** Pharyngitis, increased cough. **Skin:** Pruritus.

INTERACTIONS **Drug:** Additive immunosuppression with other immunosuppressant drugs (e.g., CORTICOSTEROIDS); LIVE VACCINES increase risk of secondary transmission of infection.

PHARMACOKINETICS **Absorption:** 63% from IM injection. **Metabolism:** Presumed to be broken down in plasma. **Half-Life:** 270 h after IV.

NURSING IMPLICATIONS

Assessment & Drug Effects

- Discontinue drug immediately and institute supportive measures if a serious hypersensitivity reaction occurs.
- Note: Drug should be discontinued if CD4+ T lymphocyte counts remain below 250 cells/mcL for 1 mo.
- Lab tests: Weekly WBC with differential during 12-wk dosing period; periodic liver enzymes.
- Monitor for and promptly report S&S of infection.

Patient & Family Education

- Report any of the following promptly: Chest pain or tightness, rapid or irregular heart beat; difficulty breathing or swallowing; swelling of face, tongue, hands, feet or ankles; rapid weight gain; signs of infection (e.g., fever, chills, cough, sore throat, pain or difficulty passing urine); skin rash or itchy skin; severe stomach pain.
- Do not accept live or live-attenuated vaccines while taking this drug.

- Notify physician if you become pregnant while taking this drug or within 8 wk of discontinuing drug.

ALEMTUZUMAB

(a-lem'tu-zu-mab)

Campath

Classifications: BIOLOGICAL RESPONSE MODIFIER; MONOCOLONAL ANTIBODY; ANTINEOPLASTIC

Therapeutic: ANTINEOPLASTIC

Pregnancy Category: C

AVAILABILITY 30 mg/mL injection

ACTION & *THERAPEUTIC EFFECT* Monoclonal antibody that attaches to CD52 cell surface antigens expressed on a variety of leukocytes, including normal and malignant B and T lymphocytes, monocytes, and some granulocytes. Proposed mechanism of action is antibody-dependent lysis of leukemic cells following binding to cell surface antigens. *Initiates antibody-dependent cell lysis, thus inhibiting cell proliferation in chronic lymphocytic leukemia.*

USES Treatment of B-cell chronic lymphocytic leukemia in patients who have failed fludarabine therapy.

UNLABELED USES Treatment of mycosis fungoides, non-Hodgkin's lymphoma.

CONTRAINDICATIONS Type I hypersensitivity to alemtuzumab or its components, hamster protein hypersensitivity; serious infection or exposure to viral infections (i.e., herpes or chickenpox), HIV infection, dental work; infection; lactation.

CAUTIOUS USE History of hypersensitivity to other monoclonal antibodies; ischemic cardiac disease, angina, coronary artery disease; dental disease; history of varicella disease; females of childbearing age; pregnancy (category C). Safety and efficacy in children are not established.

ROUTE & DOSAGE

B-Cell Chronic Lymphocytic Leukemia

Adult: **IV** Start with 3 mg/day, when that is tolerated, increase dose over next 3–7 days to 10 mg/day; when 10 mg/day is tolerated, increase to maintenance dose of 30 mg/day (give 30 mg/day 3 times/wk). Single dose should not exceed 30 mg; cumulative dose should not exceed 90 mg/wk

Toxicity Dosage Adjustment

First time ANC falls below 250/mcL or platelet count falls below 25,000/mcL

- Stop therapy until ANC is at least 500 mcL and platelet count is at least 50,000 mcL, resume at previous dose
- If therapy is stopped for 7 or more days, restart at 3 mg and taper up

Second time ANC below 250/mcL or platelet count falls below 25,000 mcL

- Stop therapy until ANC is at least 500 mcL and platelet count is at least 50,000 mcL, resume at 10 mg dose
- If therapy is stopped for 7 or more days, restart at 3 mg and taper up, do not exceed 10 mg

Third time ANC below 250/mcL or platelet count falls below 25,000 mcL

- Stop therapy permanently

*Patients starting therapy with baseline ANC less than 500 mcL or baseline platelet count less than 25,000 mcL who experience a 50% decrease from baseline should stop therapy until values return to baseline then resume at previous dose. If therapy is stopped for 7 or more days, restart at 3 mg and taper up.

ADMINISTRATION

- Note: Premedication with antihistamines, acetaminophen, antiemetics, and corticosteroids prior to infusion may reduce the severity of adverse side effects.

Intravenous

PREPARE: **IV Infusion:** Do NOT shake ampule prior to use. ▪ Withdraw required dose into a syringe with a sterile, low-protein binding, non-fiber releasing 5 micron filter. Inject into 100 mL NS or D5W. ▪ Gently invert bag to mix. Infuse within 8 h of mixing. ▪ Protect from light. Discard any unused solution. Use within 8 h of mixing.

ADMINISTER: **IV Infusion:** Infuse each dose over 2 h. ▪ Do NOT give single doses greater than 30 mg or cumulative weekly doses greater than 90 mg.

INCOMPATIBILITIES **Solution/additive:** Do not infuse or mix with other drugs.

- Store at 2°–8° C (36°–46° F). Discard if ampule has been frozen. Protect from direct light.

ADVERSE EFFECTS (≥1%) **Body as a Whole:** *Infusion reactions (rigors, fever, nausea, vomiting, hypotension, rash, shortness of breath, bronchospasm, chills), fatigue, pain, sepsis, asthenia, edema, herpes simplex, myalgias,* malaise, moniliasis, temperature change sensation, coma, seizures. **CNS:** *Headache, dysesthesias, dizziness, insomnia,* depression, tremor, somnolence, cerebrovascular accident, subarachnoid hemorrhage. **CV:** *Hypotension, tachycardia, hypertension,* cardiac failure, arrhythmias, MI. **GI:** *Diarrhea, nausea, vomiting, stomatitis, abdominal pain, dyspepsia, anorexia,* constipation. **Hematologic:** *Neutropenia, anemia, thrombocytopenia,* purpura, epistaxis, pancytopenia. **Respiratory:** *Dyspnea, cough, bronchitis, pneumonia, pharyngitis,* bronchospasm, rhinitis. **Skin:** *Rash, urticaria, pruritus, increased sweating.* **Other:** Risk of opportunistic infections.

INTERACTIONS Drug: Additive risk of bleeding with ANTICOAGULANTS, NSAIDS, PLATELET INHIBITORS, SALICYLATES increased risk of opportunistic infections with **fludarabine. Herbal: Feverfew, garlic, ginger, ginkgo** may increase risk of bleeding.

PHARMACOKINETICS Peak: Steady-state levels in approximately 6 wk. **Half-Life:** 12 days.

NURSING IMPLICATIONS

Assessment & Drug Effects

- Monitor for acute infusion-related events, including hypotension, rigors, fever, shortness of breath, bronchospasm, chills, and/or rash. If such a reaction occurs, the infusion should be discontinued and the physician notified.
- Withhold drug and notify physician if absolute neutrophil count less than 250/mcL or platelet count of 25,000/mcL or less.
- Monitor BP closely during infusion period. Careful monitoring of BP and hypotensive symptoms is especially important in patients

Common adverse effects in *italic*, life-threatening effects underlined; generic names in **bold**; classifications in SMALL CAPS; ♣ Canadian drug name; ⓟ Prototype drug

with ischemic heart disease and those on antihypertensives.

- Discontinue infusion and notify physician immediately if any of the following occurs: Hypotension, fever, chills, shortness of breath, bronchospasm, or rash.
- Withhold drug during any serious infection. Therapy may be reinstituted following resolution of the infection.
- Lab tests: CBS with differential and platelet counts weekly or more frequently in the presence of anemia, thrombocytopenia, or neutropenia; periodic blood glucose, serum electrolytes, and alkaline phosphatase.
- Monitor diabetics closely for loss of glycemic control.
- Monitor for S&S of dehydration especially with severe vomiting.

Patient & Family Education

- Do not accept immunizations with live viral vaccines during therapy or if therapy has been recently terminated.
- Use effective methods of contraception to prevent pregnancy during therapy and for at least 6 mo following therapy.
- Report any of the following to physician immediately: Unexplained bleeding, fever, sore throat, flu-like symptoms, S&S of an infection, difficulty breathing, significant GI distress, abdominal pain, fluid retention, or changes in mental status.
- Diabetics should monitor blood glucose levels carefully since loss of glycemic control is a possible adverse reaction.

ALENDRONATE SODIUM

(a-len′dro-nate)

Fosamax, Fosamax D (with 2800 International Units Vitamin D3)

Classifications: BISPHOSPHONATE; BONE METABOLISM REGULATOR
Therapeutic: BONE METABOLISM REGULATOR
Prototype: Etidronate
Pregnancy Category: C

AVAILABILITY 5 mg, 10 mg, 35 mg, 40 mg, 70 mg tablets; 70 mg/75 mL oral solution

ACTION & *THERAPEUTIC EFFECT* A bisphosphonate that inhibits osteoclast-mediated bone resorption. Antiresorption mechanism is thought to be localized to resorption sites of active bone turnover and to have minimal to no interference with bone mineralization. *Alendronate decreases bone resorption, thus minimizing loss of bone density.*

USES Prevention and treatment of osteoporosis in postmenopausal women or in men, Paget's disease. Treatment of glucocorticoid-induced osteoporosis.

CONTRAINDICATIONS Hypersensitivity to alendronate or other bisphosphonates; achalasia, esophageal stricture, severe renal impairment (CrCl less than 35 mL/min); hypocalcemia; abnormalities; lactation.
CAUTIOUS USE Renal impairment, CHF, hyperphosphatemia, liver disease, fever or infection, active upper GI problems; pregnancy (category C).

ROUTE & DOSAGE

Treatment of Osteoporosis

Adult: **PO** 10 mg once/day (max: 40 mg/day) or 70 mg qwk

Prevention of Osteoporosis

Adult: **PO** 5 mg daily or 35 mg qwk

Treatment of Steroid-Induced Osteoporosis

Adult: **PO** 5 mg daily or 35 mg qwk

Treatment of Paget's Disease

Adult: **PO** 40 mg once/day for 6 mo

Renal Impairment Dosage Adjustment

CrCl less than 35 mL/min: Use not recommended

ADMINISTRATION

Oral

- Correct hypocalcemia before administering alendronate.
- Administer in the morning at least 30 min before the first food, beverage, or medication. Do not administer within 2 h of calcium-containing foods, beverages, or medications. At least 30 min should elapse after alendronate dose before taking any other drugs.
- *Oral Solution:* Use oral syringe for accurate dosage. Give with at least 60 mL (2 oz) of plain water.
- *Tablet:* Give with 8 oz of plain water.
- Keep patient sitting up or ambulating for 30 min after taking drug.
- Store according to manufacturer's directions.

ADVERSE EFFECTS (≥1%) **Endocrine:** Hypocalcemia, hypophosphatemia. **GI:** Esophageal irritation and *ulceration, nausea, vomiting, abdominal pain, dyspepsia,* diarrhea, constipation, flatulence. **Other:** Arthralgias, myalgias, headache, rash, alopecia.

INTERACTIONS Drug: Ranitidine increases alendronate availability. **Food: Calcium** and food (especially dairy products) reduce alendronate absorption.

PHARMACOKINETICS Absorption: 0.5–1% from GI tract (absorption significantly decreased by calcium and food). **Onset:** 3–6 wk. **Duration:** 12 wk after discontinuation. **Distribution:** Rapid skeletal uptake. **Metabolism:** Not metabolized. **Elimination:** Up to 50% excreted unchanged in urine. **Half-Life:** Up to 10 h.

NURSING IMPLICATIONS

Assessment & Drug Effects

- Lab tests: Monitor albumin-adjusted serum calcium, serum phosphate, serum alkaline phosphatase, fasting and 24 h urinary calcium, and serum electrolytes. Periodically monitor renal and liver functions.
- Diagnostic test: Bone density scan every 12–18 mo.
- Discontinue drug if the CrCl less than 35 mL/min.

Patient & Family Education

- Review directions for taking drug correctly (see ADMINISTRATION).
- Report fever, especially when accompanied by arthralgia and myalgia.

ALFENTANIL HYDROCHLORIDE

(al-fen′ta-nill)

Alfenta

Classifications: NARCOTIC (OPIATE AGONIST) ANALGESIC; GENERAL ANESTHETIC

Therapeutic: NARCOTIC ANALGESIC; GENERAL ANESTHETIC

Prototype: Morphine

Pregnancy Category: C

Controlled Substance: Schedule II

AVAILABILITY 500 mcg/mL injection

ACTION & *THERAPEUTIC EFFECT* Alfentanil is a narcotic agonist analgesic with rapid onset and short duration of action. CNS effects appear to be related to interaction of drug with opiate receptors. *Analgesia is mediated through changes in the perception of pain at the spinal cord and at higher levels in the CNS. Brief duration of action is advantageous for short surgical procedures, but necessitates incremental injections or continuous infusion for long operations.*

USES Major component of balanced anesthesia; analgesic, analgesic supplement, and primary anesthetic for induction of anesthesia when endotracheal and mechanical ventilation are required.

CONTRAINDICATIONS Coagulation disorders, bacteremia, infection at injection site; lactation. Safety in children younger than 12 y is not established.

CAUTIOUS USE Older adults, history of pulmonary disease; pregnancy (category C).

ROUTE & DOSAGE

Induction of MAC

Adult: **IV** 3–8 mcg/kg; maintenance of MAC: 3–5 mcg/kg q5–20min or 0.25–1 mcg/kg/min; total dose: 3–40 mcg/kg

Obesity Dosage Adjustment

Dose based on IBW

Hepatic Impairment Dosage Adjustment

Maintenance dosage adjustment recommended

ADMINISTRATION

Intravenous

PREPARE: **Direct or Continuous:** Alfentanil is available in a concentration of 500 mcg/mL. Small volumes may be given direct IV undiluted or diluted in 5 mL of NS. ▪ For IV infusion, add 20 mL of alfentanil to 230 mL of compatible IV solution to yield 40 mcg/mL. Compatible IV solutions include NS, D5/NS, D5W, and LR. ▪ Note: Alfentanil may be diluted to concentrations of 25–80 mcg/mL.

ADMINISTER: **Direct:** Administer over at least 3 min. Do not administer more rapidly. **Continuous:** Administer at a rate of 0.25–1 mcg/kg/min. Note: Dose may be individualized.

INCOMPATIBILITIES **Y-site: Amphotericin B, lansoprazole, thiopental.**

▪ Store at 15°–30° C (59°–86° F). Avoid freezing.

ADVERSE EFFECTS (≥1%) **Body as a Whole:** Thoracic muscle rigidity, flushing, diaphoresis; extremities feel heavy and warm. **CNS:** Dizziness, euphoria, drowsiness. **CV:** Hypotension, hypertension, tachycardia, bradycardia. **GI:** *Nausea,* vomiting, anorexia, constipation, cramps. **Respiratory:** Apnea, respiratory depression, dyspnea.

INTERACTIONS Drug: BETA-ADRENERGIC BLOCKERS increase incidence of bradycardia; CNS DEPRESSANTS such as BARBITURATES, TRANQUILIZERS, NEUROMUSCULAR BLOCKING AGENTS, OPIATES, and INHALATION GENERAL ANESTHETICS may enhance the cardiovascular and CNS effects of alfentanil in both magnitude and duration; enhancement or prolongation of postoperative respiratory depression also may result from concomitant administration of any of these agents with alfentanil.

PHARMACOKINETICS Onset: 2 min. **Duration:** Injection 30 min; continuous infusion 45 min. **Distribution:** Crosses placenta. **Metabolism:** In liver by CYP3A4. **Elimination:** Excreted in breast milk. **Half-Life:** 46–111 min.

NURSING IMPLICATIONS

Assessment & Drug Effects

- Monitor for S&S of increased sympathetic stimulation (arrhythmias) and evidence of depressed postoperative analgesia (tachycardia, pain, pupillary dilation, spontaneous muscle movement) if a narcotic antagonist has been administered to overcome residual effects of alfentanil.
- Evaluate adequacy of spontaneous ventilation carefully during postoperative period.
- Monitor vital signs carefully during postoperative period; check for bradycardia, especially if patient is also taking a beta-blocker.
- Note: Narcotic effects wear off quickly with negligible residual effects.
- Note: Dizziness, sedation, nausea, and vomiting are common when drug is used as a postoperative analgesic.

Patient & Family Education

- Report unpleasant adverse effects when drug is used for patient-controlled analgesia.

ALFUZOSIN

(al-fuz'o-sin)

UroXatral, Xatral ♣

Classification: ALPHA-ADRENERGIC ANTAGONIST

Therapeutic: GENITOURINARY SMOOTH MUSCLE RELAXER

Prototype: Tamsulosin

Pregnancy Category: B

AVAILABILITY 10 mg extended release tablet

ACTION & *THERAPEUTIC EFFECT* Alfuzosin is a short-acting, selective antagonist at alpha-1 receptors with a low incidence of hypotension and sexual dysfunction at therapeutic doses. Alpha-1 receptors cause contraction of smooth muscle in the prostate, prostatic capsule, prostatic urethra, bladder base, and bladder neck. Both alpha-1a (70%) and alpha-1b receptors exist in the prostate. *Blockade of alpha-1 receptors by alfuzosin causes smooth muscles in the bladder neck and prostate to relax, thereby reducing pressure on the urethra and improving urine flow rate. This results in a reduction in BPH symptoms.*

USES Treatment of symptomatic benign prostatic hypertrophy (BPH).

CONTRAINDICATIONS Hypersensitivity to alfuzosin; severe hepatic insufficiency; concurrent treatment with potent CYP3A4 inhibitors (e.g., ketoconazole, itraconazole, and ritonavir); angina; QT prolongation.
CAUTIOUS USE Coronary artery disease, cardiac arrhythmias; hepatic disease; dizziness, light-headedness, orthostatic hypotension; pregnancy (category B).

ROUTE & DOSAGE

Benign Prostatic Hypertrophy
Adult: **PO** 10 mg daily

ADMINISTRATION

Oral

- Give immediately after same meal each day.
- Ensure that extended release tablet is not crushed or chewed. It **must be** swallowed whole.

- Store at 15°–30° C (59°–86° F). Protect from light and moisture.

ADVERSE EFFECTS (≥1%) **Body as a Whole:** Fatigue, pain. **CNS:** Dizziness, headache. **GI:** Abdominal pain, dyspepsia, constipation, nausea. **Respiratory:** Upper respiratory infection, bronchitis, sinusitis, pharyngitis. **Urogenital:** Impotence, priapism.

INTERACTIONS Drug: Increased risk of hypotension with other ANTIHYPERTENSIVE AGENTS or **sildenafil, vardenafil,** and **tadalafil; ketoconazole, itraconazole,** PROTEASE INHIBITORS may increase alfuzosin levels and toxicity.

PHARMACOKINETICS Absorption: 49% when taken with food. **Peak:** 8 h. **Metabolism:** In liver by CYP3A4. **Elimination:** 69% in feces, 24% in urine. **Half-Life:** 10 h.

NURSING IMPLICATIONS

Assessment & Drug Effects

- Monitor CV status and BP, especially if on concurrent treatment with antihypertensive drugs or inhibitors of CYP3A4. See INTERACTIONS.
- Check postural vital signs to evaluate for orthostatic hypotension within a few hours following administration.
- Withhold drug and report new or worsening angina to physician.
- Lab tests: Baseline and periodic LFTs.

Patient & Family Education

- Inform physician about all other prescription, nonprescription, or herbal drugs being taken.
- Make position changes slowly to minimize dizziness.
- Do not drive or engage in other hazardous activities until reaction to drug is known.
- Moderate or eliminate grapefruit juice consumption while on this drug.

ALISKIREN

(a-lis′ki-ren)

Tekturna

Classifications: RENIN ANGIOTENSIN SYSTEM ANTAGONIST; ANTIHYPERTENSIVE

Therapeutic: DIRECT RENIN INHIBITOR; ANTIHYPERTENSIVE

Pregnancy Category: C first trimester; D second and third trimester

AVAILABILITY 150 mg, 300 mg tablets

ACTION & *THERAPEUTIC EFFECT* A direct renin inhibitor that reduces plasma renin activity and inhibits the conversion of angiotensinogen to angiotensin I (Ang I) and subsequent production of angiotensin II (Ang II). *Lowers blood pressure by decreasing vasoconstriction and aldosterone production, thus reducing sodium reabsorption and fluid retention.*

USES Treatment of hypertension, either as monotherapy or in combination with other antihypertensive agents.

CONTRAINDICATIONS Hypersensitivity to aliskiren; hyperkalemia; hypercalcemia; dehydration; pregnancy (category D second and third trimester); lactation; children younger than 18 y.

CAUTIOUS USE Cautious use in patients with CrCl less than 30 mL/min; older adults; history of angioedema; respiratory disorders; history of airway surgery; diabetes mellitus; pregnancy (category C first trimester).

ROUTE & DOSAGE

Hypertension
Adult: **PO** 150–300 mg once daily

ADMINISTRATION

Oral
- Give consistently with regard to meals.
- Store at 15°–30° C (59°–86° F) and protect from light.

ADVERSE EFFECTS (≥1%) **CNS:** *Headache, dizziness.* **GI:** *Diarrhea.* **Metabolic:** Hyperkalemia. **Skin:** Angioedema, rash.

INTERACTIONS Drug: Enhances effects of other ANTIHYPERTENSIVE AGENTS. **Atorvastatin** and **ketoconazole** increase the plasma level of aliskiren, while **irbesartan** decreases its plasma level. Aliskiren decreases the plasma level of **furosemide.**

PHARMACOKINETICS Absorption: 2.5%. **Peak:** 1–3 h. **Metabolism:** Less than 10% via liver. **Elimination:** Primarily in stool. **Half-Life:** 24 h.

NURSING IMPLICATIONS

Assessment & Drug Effects
- Monitor for hypotension after the initiation of therapy and following dosage increase.
- Monitor for angioedema, which may occur any time during treatment. Withhold drug and immediately report to physician.
- Lab tests: Periodic serum potassium.

Patient & Family Education
- Full therapeutic effect is usually obtained by 2 wk of therapy.
- Report immediately any of the following: Swelling about the face, lips, tongue; difficulty breathing or swallowing; swelling of hands or feet.
- High fat meals interfere with the absorption of this drug. Do not take drug following a high fat meal.

ALITRETINOIN (9-*cis*-RETINOIC ACID)

(a-li-tre′ti-noyne)
Panretin
Classification: ANTIACNE (RETINOID)
Therapeutic: ANTIACNE
Prototype: Isotretinoin
Pregnancy Category: D

AVAILABILITY 0.1% gel

ACTION & *THERAPEUTIC EFFECT* Naturally occurring retinoid that binds to and activates all known retinoid receptors in cells, which regulate cellular differentiation and proliferation in both healthy and neoplastic cells. *Inhibits the growth of Kaposi's sarcoma (KS) in HIV patients. It does not prevent the development of new KS lesions.*

USES Treatment of cutaneous lesions of AIDS-related Kaposi's sarcoma.
UNLABELED USES Cutaneous T-cell lymphomas.

CONTRAINDICATIONS Hypersensitivity to alitretinoin or other retinoids including vitamin A; when systemic anti-KS therapy is required; pregnancy (category D), lactation.
CAUTIOUS USE Cutaneous T-cell lymphoma. Safety and efficacy in children younger than 18 y, or older adults 65 y or older, are unknown.

ROUTE & DOSAGE

Cutaneous Kaposi's Sarcoma
Adult: **Topical** Apply sufficient gel to cover lesions b.i.d., may increase application to 3–4 times daily if tolerated

ADMINISTRATION

Topical

- Apply gel liberally over lesions; avoid unaffected skin and mucus membranes.
- Dry 3–5 min before covering with clothes. Do not cover with occlusive dressing.
- Store at 15°–30° C (59°–86° F).

ADVERSE EFFECTS (≥1%) **Skin:** Erythema, edema, vesiculation, *rash, burning pain,* pruritus, exfoliative dermatitis, excoriation, paresthesia.

INTERACTIONS Drug: Increased toxicity with insect repellents containing DEET.

PHARMACOKINETICS Absorption: Minimal.

NURSING IMPLICATIONS

Assessment & Drug Effects

- Monitor for S&S of dermal toxicity (e.g., erythema, edema, vesiculation).

Patient & Family Education

- Allow up to 14 wk for therapeutic response.
- Avoid exposure of medicated skin to sunlight or sun lamps.
- Contact physician if inflammation, swelling, or blisters appear on medicated areas.

ALLOPURINOL

(al-oh-pure′i-nole)

Alloprin A ♣, Alloprin, Apo-allopurinol-A ♣, Lopurin, Novo-purinol A, Zyloprim

Classification: ANTIGOUT

Therapeutic: ANTIGOUT

Pregnancy Category: C

AVAILABILITY 100 mg, 300 mg tablets; 500 mg vial

ACTION & *THERAPEUTIC EFFECT* Allopurinol reduces endogenous uric acid by selectively inhibiting action of xanthine oxidase, the enzyme responsible for converting hypoxanthine to xanthine and xanthine to uric acid (end product of purine catabolism). Has no analgesic, anti-inflammatory, or uricosuric actions. *Thus, urate pool is decreased by the lowering of both serum and urinary uric acid levels, and hyperuricemia is prevented.*

USES To control primary hyperuricemia that accompanies severe gout and to prevent possibility of flare-up of acute gouty attack; to prevent recurrent calcium oxalate stones; prophylactically to reduce severity of hyperuricemia associated with antineoplastic and radiation therapies, both of which greatly increase plasma uric acid levels by promoting nucleic acid degradation.

UNLABELED USES To reduce hyperuricemia secondary to Lesch–Nyhan syndrome, polycythemia vera, G6PD deficiency, sarcoidosis, and therapy with thiazides or ethambutol.

CONTRAINDICATIONS Hypersensitivity to allopurinol; as initial treatment for acute gouty attacks; idiopathic hemochromatosis (or those with family history); HLA-B*5801 genotype (strongly associated with allopurinol induced severe cutaneous reactions).

CAUTIOUS USE Impaired hepatic or renal function, history of peptic ulcer, lower GI tract disease, bone marrow depression; pregnancy (category C).

ROUTE & DOSAGE

Treatment of Hyperuricemia
Adult: **PO** 100 mg/day, may increase by 100 mg/wk (max: 800 mg/day), divide doses greater than 300 mg/day **IV** 200–400 mg/m²/day (max: 600 mg/day) in 1–4 divided doses
Child: **PO** *10 y or younger,* 10 mg/kg/day in 2–3 divided doses (max: 800 mg/day) **IV** 200 mg/m²/day in 1–4 divided doses

Treatment of Secondary Hyperuricemia
Adult: **PO** 200–800 mg/day for 2–3 day or longer, divide doses greater than 300 mg/day
Child: **PO** *6–10 y,* 100 mg t.i.d.; *younger than 6 y,* 50 mg t.i.d.

Treatment of Recurrent Renal Calculi
Adult: **PO** 200–300 daily (may divide dose)

Renal Impairment Dosage Adjustment
CrCl 10–20 mL/min: 200 mg/day; 3–9 mL/min: 100 mg daily; less than 3 mL/min: 100 mg with extended interval between doses (24 h or more)
Dialysis Dosage Adjustment: Administer dose after dialysis or use 50% supplemental dose.

ADMINISTRATION

Oral

- Give after meals for best toleration; tablet may be crushed and taken with fluid or mixed with food.
- Store at 15°–30° C (59°–86° F) in a tightly closed container.

Intravenous

PREPARE: **Intermittent:** Reconstitute a single dose vial (500 mg) with 25 mL of sterile water for injection to yield 20 mg/mL. ▪ **Must be** further diluted with NS or D5W to a concentration of 6 mg/mL or less. ▪ Note: Adding 2.3 mL of diluent yields 6 mg/mL.

ADMINISTER: **Intermittent:** Usually administered over 30–60 min.

INCOMPATIBILITIES **Solution/additive: Amikacin, amphotericin B, carmustine, cefotaxime, chlorpromazine, cimetidine, clindamycin, cytarabine, dacarbazine, daunorubicin, diphenhydramine, doxorubicin, doxycycline, droperidol, floxuridine, gentamicin, haloperidol, hydroxyzine, idarubicin, imipenem-cilastatin, mechlorethamine, meperidine, methylprednisolone, metoclopramide, minocycline, nalbuphine, netilmicin, ondansetron, prochlorperazine, promethazine, sodium bicarbonate, streptozocin, tobramycin, vinorelbine.**

ADVERSE EFFECTS (≥1%) **CNS:** Drowsiness, headache, vertigo. **GI:** Nausea, vomiting, diarrhea, abdominal discomfort, indigestion, malaise. **Hematologic:** (Rare) Agranulocytosis, aplastic anemia, bone marrow depression, thrombocytopenia. **Skin:** Urticaria or pruritus, pruritic maculopapular rash, toxic epidermal necrolysis. **Other:** Hepatotoxicity, renal insufficiency.

DIAGNOSTIC TEST INTERFERENCE Possibility of elevated blood levels of ***alkaline phosphatase*** and ***serum transaminases (AST, ALT),*** and decreased blood ***Hct, Hgb, leukocytes.***

INTERACTIONS Drug: Alcohol may inhibit renal excretion of uric acid;

Common adverse effects in *italic*, life-threatening effects underlined; generic names in **bold**; classifications in SMALL CAPS; ♣ Canadian drug name; Ⓟ Prototype drug

ampicillin, amoxicillin increase risk of skin rash; enhances anticoagulant effect of **warfarin;** toxicity from **azathioprine, mercaptopurine, cyclophosphamide, cyclosporin** increased; increases hypoglycemic effects of **chlorpropamide**; THIAZIDES increase risk of allopurinol toxicity and hypersensitivity (especially with impaired renal function); ACE INHIBITORS increase risk of hypersensitivity; high dose vitamin C increases risk of kidney stone formation.

PHARMACOKINETICS Absorption: 80–90% from GI tract. **Onset:** 24–48 h. **Peak:** 2–6 h. **Metabolism:** 75–80% to the active metabolite oxypurinol. **Elimination:** Slowly excreted in urine; excreted in breast milk. **Half-Life:** 1–3 h; oxypurinol, 18–30 h.

NURSING IMPLICATIONS

Assessment & Drug Effects

- Monitor for therapeutic effectiveness which is indicated by normal serum and urinary uric acid levels usually by 1–3 wk (aim of therapy is to lower serum uric acid level gradually to about 6 mg/dL), gradual decrease in size of tophi, absence of new tophaceous deposits (after approximately 6 mo), with consequent relief of joint pain and increased joint mobility.
- Monitor for S&S of an acute gouty attack which is most likely to occur during first 6 wk of therapy.
- Lab tests: Monitor serum uric acid levels q1–2wk to check adequacy of dosage. Perform baseline CBC, liver and kidney function tests before therapy is initiated and then monthly, particularly during first few months. Check urinary pH at regular intervals.
- Monitor patients with renal disorders more often; they tend to have a higher incidence of renal stones and drug toxicity problems.
- Report onset of rash or fever immediately to physician; withdraw drug. Life-threatening toxicity syndrome can occur 2–4 wk after initiation of therapy (more common with impaired renal function) and is generally accompanied by malaise, fever, and aching, a diffuse erythematous, desquamating rash, hepatic dysfunction, eosinophilia, and worsening of renal function.

Patient & Family Education

- Drink enough fluid to produce urinary output of at least 2000 mL/day (fluid intake of at least 3000 mL/day). (Note that 1000 mL is approximately equal to 1 quart.) Report diminishing urinary output, cloudy urine, unusual color or odor to urine, pain or discomfort on urination.
- Report promptly the onset of itching or rash. Stop drug if a skin rash appears, even after 5 or more wk (and reportedly as long as 2 y) of therapy.
- Minimize exposure of eyes to ultraviolet or sunlight, which may stimulate the development of cataracts.
- Do not drive or engage in potentially hazardous activities until response to drug is known.
- Remain under medical supervision while taking allopurinol (generally continued indefinitely); drug can cause severe adverse reactions.

ALMOTRIPTAN

(al-mo-trip′tan)

Axert

Classification: SEROTONIN 5-HT_1 RECEPTOR AGONIST

Therapeutic: ANTIMIGRAINE

Prototype: Sumatriptan

Pregnancy Category: C

AVAILABILITY 6.25 mg, 12.5 mg tablets

ACTION & *THERAPEUTIC EFFECT* Selective agonist that binds with high affinity to serotonin receptors found on extracerebral and intracranial blood vessels. Due primarily to its effects on 5-HT_{1D} and 5-HT_{1B} serotonin receptors on cranial blood vessels, it causes vasoconstriction and decreases inflammation and neurotransmission. *Deactivation of the serotonin receptors results in constriction of cranial vessels that become dilated during a migraine attack and reduces signal transmission in the pain pathways.*

USES Treatment of migraine headache with or without aura.

CONTRAINDICATIONS Hypersensitivity to almotriptan malate. Significant cardiovascular disease such as ischemic heart disease, coronary artery vasospasms, MI, angina, arteriosclerosis, cardiac arrhythmias, diabetes mellitus, colitis, history of cerebrovascular events, or uncontrolled hypertension; stroke, smoking, Wolff-Parkinson-White syndrome, within 24 h of receiving another 5-HT_1 agonist or an ergotamine-containing or ergot-type drug; basilar or hemiplegic migraine.

CAUTIOUS USE Significant risk factors for coronary artery disease unless a cardiac evaluation has been done; hypertension; risk factors for cerebrovascular accident; peripheral vascular disease, impaired liver or kidney function, Raynaud's disease, children, elderly, pregnancy (category C), lactation.

ROUTE & DOSAGE

Migraine Headache

Adult: **PO** 6.25–12.5 mg; if headache returns, may repeat after at least 2 h (max: 2 tabs/24 h)

Renal Impairment Dosage Adjustment

CrCl less than 10 mL/min: 6.25 mg (max: 12.5 mg/day)

Hepatic Impairment Dosage Adjustment

6.25 mg (max: 12.5 mg/day)

ADMINISTRATION

Oral

- Do not give within 24 h of an ergot-containing drug.
- Administer any time after symptoms of migraine appear.
- Do not administer a second dose without consulting the physician for any attack during which the FIRST dose did NOT work.
- Give a second dose if headache was relieved by first dose but symptoms return; however, wait at least 2 h after the first dose before giving a second dose.
- Do not give more than two doses in 24 h.
- Store at 15°–30° C (59°–86° F).

ADVERSE EFFECTS (≥1%) **Body as a Whole:** Flushing. **CNS:** Drowsiness, headache, paresthesia. **CV:** Palpitations, tachycardia, serious cardiac events (including MI) have been reported within a few hours after administration. **GI:** Nausea, vomiting, dry mouth.

INTERACTIONS Drug: Dihydroergotamine, methysergide, other 5-HT_1 AGONISTS may cause prolonged vasospastic reactions; SSRIS, **sibutramine** have rarely caused weakness, hyperreflexia, and incoordination; MAOIS should not be used with 5-HT_1 AGONISTS.

PHARMACOKINETICS Absorption: Well absorbed, 70% reaches systemic circulation. **Peak:** 1–3 h. **Dis-**

tribution: 35% protein bound. **Metabolism:** 27% metabolized by monoamine oxidase. **Elimination:** 75% renally, 13% in feces. **Half-Life:** 3–4 h.

NURSING IMPLICATIONS

Assessment & Drug Effects

- Monitor cardiovascular status carefully following first dose in patients at relatively high risk for coronary artery disease (e.g., postmenopausal women, men over 40 years old, persons with known CAD risk factors) or who have coronary artery vasospasms.
- Report to physician immediately chest pain or tightness in chest or throat that is severe or does not quickly resolve following a dose of almotriptan.
- Pain relief usually begins within 10 min of ingestion, with complete relief in approximately 65% of all patients within 2 h.
- Monitor BP, especially in those being treated for hypertension.

Patient & Family Education

- Review patient information leaflet provided by the manufacturer carefully.
- Notify physician immediately if symptoms of severe angina (e.g., severe or persistent pain or tightness in chest, back, neck, or throat) or hypersensitivity (e.g., wheezing, facial swelling, skin rash, or hives) occur.
- Do not take any other serotonin receptor agonist (e.g., Imitrex, Maxalt, Zomig, Amerge) within 24 h of taking almotriptan.
- Advise physician of any drugs taken within 1 wk of beginning almotriptan.
- Check with physician regarding drug interactions before taking any new OTC or prescription drugs.
- Report any other adverse effects (e.g., tingling, flushing, dizziness) at next physician visit.

ALOSETRON

(a-lo′se-tron)

Lotronex

Classification: SEROTONIN 5-HT_3 RECEPTOR ANTAGONIST

Therapeutic: GI ANTIMOTILITY

Pregnancy Category: B

AVAILABILITY 0.5 mg, 1 mg tablets

ACTION & *THERAPEUTIC EFFECT* Potent and selective serotonin (5-HT_3) receptor antagonist. Serotonin 5-HT_3 receptors are extensively located on enteric neurons of the GI tract. Activation of these receptors affects amount of visceral pain experienced, transit time in the colon, and GI secretions. *Blockage of the serotonin 5-HT_3 receptors by alosetron results in significant control of GI pain, and severe diarrhea related to irritable bowel syndrome.*

USES Treatment of severe chronic irritable bowel syndrome (IBS) in women whose predominant symptom is diarrhea and whose symptoms have lasted longer than 6 mo and have failed to respond to conventional therapy.

CONTRAINDICATIONS Constipation, ischemic colitis, development of ischemic bowel symptoms such as sudden onset of rectal bleeding, bloody diarrhea, new or sudden worsening of abdominal pain; history of chronic or severe constipation, intestinal obstruction, toxic megacolon, GI adhesions, GI perforation, active diverticulitis, history of, or current Crohn's disease or ulcerative colitis; hypersensitivity to

alosetron; thrombophlebitis, hypercoagulable state, inability to comply with Patient–Physician Agreement, severe hepatic impairment.
CAUTIOUS USE Hepatic insufficiency, renal impairment; elderly; pregnancy (category B), lactation. Safety and efficacy in children are not established.

ROUTE & DOSAGE

Irritable Bowel Syndrome

Adult: **PO** Start with 0.5 mg b.i.d. for 4 wk, may increase to 1 mg b.i.d. if tolerated

ADMINISTRATION

Oral

- Ensure that the patient has signed the Patient–Physician Agreement prior to administering alosetron.
- Do not give this drug if the patient has constipation.
- Review the contraindications for this drug and ensure that the patient has none of the conditions for which the drug is contraindicated.
- Store at 25° C (77° F).

ADVERSE EFFECTS (≥1%) **Body as a Whole:** Malaise, fatigue, cramps, pain. **CNS:** Anxiety. **CV:** Tachyarrhythmias. **GI:** *Constipation*, abdominal pain, nausea, distention, reflux, hemorrhoids, hyposalivation, dyspepsia, ischemic colitis. **Skin:** Sweating, urticaria. **Urogenital:** Urinary frequency.

INTERACTIONS Drug: Fluvoxamine increases alosetron serum level.

PHARMACOKINETICS Absorption: Rapidly absorbed, average bioavailability of 50–60%. **Peak:** 1 h. **Distribution:** 82% protein bound. **Metabolism:** Extensively in liver by CYP2C9. **Elimination:** 73% in urine, 24% in feces. **Half-Life:** 1.5 h.

NURSING IMPLICATIONS

Assessment & Drug Effects

- Monitor for and report immediately signs of ischemic colitis such as new or worsening abdominal pain, bloody diarrhea, or blood in the stool.
- Withhold drug and notify physician if patient has not had adequate control of IBS symptoms after 4 wk of treatment with 1 mg twice a day.
- Monitor carefully patients who have decreased GI motility (e.g., older adults, persons receiving other drugs which may decrease GI motility) as they may be at greater risk of serious complications of constipation.
- Monitor carefully patients with any degree of hepatic insufficiency as they may be more susceptible to adverse drug effects.
- Monitor periodically for cardiac arrhythmias, especially with preexisting cardiovascular disease.

Patient & Family Education

- Read the Medication Guide before starting alosetron and each time you refill your prescription.
- Do not start taking alosetron if you are constipated.
- Discontinue alosetron immediately and contact your physician if you experience any of the following: Constipation, new or worsening abdominal pain, bloody diarrhea, or blood in the stool.
- Contact your physician immediately if constipation does not resolve after discontinuation of alosetron. Resume alosetron again only if constipation has resolved and your physician directs you to begin taking the medication again.
- Stop taking alosetron and contact your physician if IBS symptoms are not adequately controlled after 4 wk of taking 1 tablet twice a day.

ALPHA$_1$-PROTEINASE INHIBITOR (HUMAN)

(pro′ten-ase)

Prolastin, Aralast, Zemaira

Classification: RESPIRATORY ENZYME INHIBITOR

Therapeutic: RESPIRATORY ENZYME REPLACEMENT

Pregnancy Category: C

AVAILABILITY **Prolastin:** 25 mg/mL; **Aralast:** 16 mg/mL; **Zemaira:** 50 mg/mL

ACTION & *THERAPEUTIC EFFECT* Alpha$_1$-proteinase inhibitor (alpha$_1$-PI; alpha$_1$-antitrypsin) is extracted from plasma and used in patients with panacinar emphysema who have alpha$_1$-antitrypsin deficiency. Alpha$_1$-antitrypsin deficiency is a chronic, hereditary, and usually fatal autosomal recessive disorder that results in a slowly progressive, panacinar emphysema. *Prevents the progressive breakdown of elastin tissues in the alveoli, thus slowing panacinar emphysema progression.*

USES Indicated for chronic replacement therapy in patients with alpha$_1$-antitrypsin deficiency and demonstrable panacinar emphysema.

CONTRAINDICATIONS Individuals with selective IgA deficiencies; lactation.

CAUTIOUS USE Patients with significant heart disease or other conditions that may be aggravated with slight increases in plasma volume; pregnancy (category C). Safety and efficacy in children are not established.

ROUTE & DOSAGE

Panacinar Emphysema

Adult: **IV** 60 mg/kg once/wk

ADMINISTRATION

Intravenous

Give hepatitis B vaccine prior to utilizing this drug.

PREPARE: **IV Infusion:** Warm unopened diluent and concentrate to room temperature. ▪ Use the supplied, double needle transfer device to reconstitute with sterile water for injection (supplied by manufacturer) to yield a concentration of 20 mg/mL.

ADMINISTER: **IV Infusion:** Give within 3 h after reconstitution. ▪ Give alone, without mixing with other agents. ▪ Administer at rate of 0.08 mL/kg/min or more slowly as determined by response and comfort of the patient. ▪ Note: The recommended dosage takes about 30 min to administer to a 70 kg person.

▪ Store unreconstituted drug at 2°–8° C (35°–46° F). Do not refrigerate after reconstitution. Discard unused solution.

ADVERSE EFFECTS (≥1%) **Hematologic:** Leukocytosis. **CNS:** Dizziness, fever (may be delayed). **Respiratory:** Upper and lower respiratory tract infections. **Other:** Hepatitis B if not immunized.

PHARMACOKINETICS **Distribution:** Crosses placenta; distributed into breast milk. **Metabolism:** Undergoes catabolism in the intravascular space; approximately 33% is catabolized per day. **Half-Life:** 4.5–5.2 days.

NURSING IMPLICATIONS

Assessment & Drug Effects

- Administer with caution in patients at risk for circulatory overload. Monitor cardiac status.
- Monitor respiratory status (rate, dyspnea, lung sounds) throughout therapy.

- Lab tests: Monitor serum alpha$_1$-PI level (minimum serum concentration level should be 80 mg/mL); periodic pulmonary functions and ABGs.

Patient & Family Education

- Avoid smoking and notify physician of any changes in respiratory pattern.

ALPRAZOLAM

(al-pray′zoe-lam)

Niravam, Xanax, Xanax XR

Classifications: ANXIOLYTIC; SEDATIVE-HYPNOTIC; BENZODIAZEPINE

Therapeutic: ANTIANXIETY; SEDATIVE-HYPNOTIC

Prototype: Lorazepam

Pregnancy Category: D

Controlled Substance: Schedule IV

AVAILABILITY 0.25 mg, 0.5 mg, 1 mg, 2 mg tablets; 0.5 mg, 1 mg, 2 mg, 3 mg sustained release tabs; 1 mg/mL oral solution; 0.25 mg, 0.5 mg, 1 mg, 2 mg orally disintegrating tabs

ACTION & *THERAPEUTIC EFFECT* A CNS depressant that appears to act at the limbic, thalamic, and hypothalamic levels of the CNS. *Has antianxiety and sedative effects with addictive potential.*

USES Management of anxiety disorders or for short-term relief of anxiety symptoms. Also used as adjunct in management of anxiety associated with depression and agitation, and for panic disorders, such as agoraphobia.

UNLABELED USES Alcohol withdrawal.

CONTRAINDICATIONS Sensitivity to benzodiazepines; acute narrow angle glaucoma; pulmonary disease; use alone in primary depression or psychotic disorders, bipolar disorders, organic brain disorders; myasthenia gravis; pregnancy (category D), lactation; children younger than 18 y.

CAUTIOUS USE Impaired hepatic function; history of alcoholism; renal impairment, hepatic disease; geriatric and debilitated patients. Effectiveness for long-term treatment (greater than 4 mo) not established.

ROUTE & DOSAGE

Anxiety Disorders

Adult: **PO** 0.25–0.5 mg t.i.d. (max: 4 mg/day)
Geriatric: **PO** 0.125–0.25 mg b.i.d.

Panic Attacks

Adult: **PO** 1–2 mg t.i.d. (max: 8 mg/day); sustained release: Initiate with 0.5–1 mg once/day. Depending on the response, the dose may be increased at intervals of 3 to 4 days in increments of no more than 1 mg/day. Target range 3–6 mg/day (max: 10 mg/day).

Hepatic Impairment Dosage Adjustment

Reduce dose by 50% in hepatic impairment.
Do not discontinue abruptly.

ADMINISTRATION

Oral

- Reduce drug gradually when discontinuing drug.
- Store in light-resistant containers at 15°–30° C (59°–86° F), unless otherwise directed.

ADVERSE EFFECTS (≥1%) **CNS:** *Drowsiness, sedation,* light-headedness, dizziness, syncope, depression,

Common adverse effects in *italic*, life-threatening effects underlined; generic names in **bold**; classifications in SMALL CAPS; ♣ Canadian drug name; ⓟ Prototype drug

headache, confusion, insomnia, nervousness, fatigue, clumsiness, unsteadiness, rigidity, tremor, restlessness, paradoxical excitement, hallucinations. **CV:** Tachycardia, hypotension, ECG changes. **Special Senses:** Blurred vision. **Respiratory:** Dyspnea.

INTERACTIONS Drug: Alcohol and other CNS DEPRESSANTS, ANTICONVULSANTS, ANTIHISTAMINES, BARBITURATES, NARCOTIC ANALGESICS, BENZODIAZEPINES compound CNS depressant effects; **cimetidine, disulfiram, fluoxetine,** TRICYCLIC ANTIDEPRESSANTS increase alprazolam levels (decreased metabolism); ORAL CONTRACEPTIVES may increase or decrease alprazolam effects. **Herbal: Kava, valerian** may potentiate sedation; **St. John's wort** decreases serum level of alprazolam. Cigarette smoking may decrease serum level of alprazolam by 50%.

PHARMACOKINETICS Absorption: Rapidly absorbed. **Peak:** 1–2 h. **Distribution:** Crosses placenta. **Metabolism:** Oxidized in liver to inactive metabolites by CYP3A4. **Elimination:** Renal elimination. **Half-Life:** 12–15 h.

NURSING IMPLICATIONS

Assessment & Drug Effects

- Monitor for S&S of drowsiness and sedation, especially in older adults or the debilitated; they may require supervised ambulation and/or side rails.
- Lab tests: Monitor periodic blood counts, urinalyses, and blood chemistry studies, particularly during continuing therapy.

Patient & Family Education

- Note: Adverse reactions may occur during early high-dose therapy. These usually disappear with continuing therapy, but dosage adjustments may be indicated.
- Make position changes slowly and in stages to prevent dizziness.
- Do not use alcohol, other CNS depressants, or OTC medications containing antihistamines (e.g., sleep aids, cold, hay fever, or allergy remedies) without consulting physician.
- Do not drive or engage in potentially hazardous activities until response to drug is known.
- Taper dosage following continuous use; abrupt discontinuation of drug may cause withdrawal symptoms: Nausea, vomiting, abdominal and muscle cramps, sweating, confusion, tremors, convulsions.

ALPROSTADIL (PGE_1)

(al-pross'ta-dil)

Prostin VR Pediatric, Caverject, Muse, Edex

Classification: PROSTAGLANDIN
Therapeutic: PROSTAGLANDIN
Prototype: Epoprostenol
Pregnancy Category: C

AVAILABILITY 500 mcg/mL injection; 5 mcg/mL, 10 mcg/mL, 20 mcg/mL, 40 mcg/mL powder for injection; 125 mcg, 250 mcg, 500 mcg, 1000 mcg pellets

ACTION & *THERAPEUTIC EFFECT* Preserves ductal patency by relaxing smooth muscle of ductus arteriosus. Alprostadil induces penile erection by relaxing the smooth muscles of the corpus cavernosum and dilating the cavernosal arteries and their penile arterioles. Sufficient rigidity of the penis also requires increased venous outflow resistance. *Preserves ductal patency by relaxing smooth muscle of ductus arteriosus. It induces penile rigidity and erection by penile blood engorgement.*

USES Temporary measure to maintain patency of ductus arteriosus in infants with ductal-dependent congenital heart defects until corrective surgery can be performed. Also used in erectile dysfunction.

CONTRAINDICATIONS Ductus arteriosus respiratory distress syndrome (hyaline membrane disease); neonates with respiratory distress syndrome; hypersensitivity to alprostadil; patients with penile implants. *Muse, Edex:* Women, children, and newborns; lactation. *Muse:* Patients with urethral stricture, inflammation/infection of glans of penis, severe hypospadias, acute or chronic urethritis; sickle cell anemia or trait, thrombocytopenia, thrombocytosis; polycythemia, multiple myeloma.

CAUTIOUS USE Ductus arteriosus; bleeding tendencies; cardiovascular disease; erectile dysfunction; hypersensitivity to alprostadil; leukemia; penile anatomic deformations; patients on anticoagulants, vasoactive or antihypertensive drugs.

ROUTE & DOSAGE

To Maintain Patency of Ductus Arteriosus

Neonate: **IV/Intra-arterial/Intra-aortic** 0.05–0.1 mcg/kg/min, may increase gradually (max: 0.4 mcg/kg/min if necessary)

Erectile Dysfunction of Vasculogenic, Psychogenic, or Mixed Etiology

Adult: **Intracavernosal** Initiate with 2.5 mcg; if inadequate response, increase dose by 2.5 mcg. May then increase dose in 5- to 10-mcg increments until a suitable erection occurs, not exceeding 1 h in duration. Doses greater than 60 mcg not recommended.

Erectile Dysfunction of Pure Neurogenic Etiology

Adult: **Intracavernosal** Initiate with 1.25 mcg; if inadequate response, increase dose by 1.25 mcg, then increase by 2.5 mcg, may then increase dose in 5 mcg increments until a suitable erection occurs, not exceeding 1 h in duration. Doses greater than 60 mcg not recommended.

ADMINISTRATION

Intracavernosal Injection

- Administer only after proper training in the penile injection technique. Refer to information on administration provided to the patient by the manufacturer.
- Use reconstituted solutions immediately.
- Store dry powder at or below 25° C (77° F) for up to 3 mo. Do not freeze.

Transurethral Insertion

- Refer to information on insertion into the urethra provided to the patient by the manufacturer.

Intravenous

PREPARE: **Continuous:** Dilute 500 mcg alprostadil with NS or D5W to volume appropriate for pump delivery system. ▪ Prepare fresh solution q24h. Discard unused portions. ▪ A 500 mcg ampule diluted in 250 mL yields a concentration of 2 mcg/mL.

ADMINISTER: **Continuous:** Infuse at rate of 0.05–0.1 mcg/kg/min up to a maximum of 0.4 mcg/kg/min. ▪ Reduce infusion rate immediately if arterial pressure drops significantly or if fever occurs. ▪ Discontinue promptly, if apnea or bradycardia occurs.

- Store at 2°–8° C (36°–46° F) unless otherwise directed by manufacturer. Protect from freezing.

ADVERSE EFFECTS (≥1%) **CNS:** *Fever,* seizures, lethargy. **CV:** *Flushing,* bradycardia, hypotension, syncope, tachycardia; CHF, ventricular fibrillation, shock. **GI:** Diarrhea, gastric regurgitation. **Hematologic:** Disseminated intravascular coagulation (DIC), thrombocytopenia. **Respiratory:** Apnea. **Urogenital:** Oliguria, anuria. *Penile pain,* prolonged erection, priapism, penile fibrosis, injection site hematoma/ecchymosis, penile rash and edema, prostatitis, perineal pain. **Skin:** Rash on face and arms, alopecia. **Other:** Leg pain.

INTERACTIONS Drug: May increase anticoagulant properties of **warfarin;** ANTIHYPERTENSIVE AGENTS increase risk of hypotension.

PHARMACOKINETICS Onset: 15 min to 3 h. **Metabolism:** Rapidly in lungs. **Elimination:** Through kidneys. **Half-Life:** 5–10 min.

NURSING IMPLICATIONS

Assessment & Drug Effects

Ductus Arteriosus

- Monitor therapeutic effectiveness which is indicated by increase in blood oxygenation (Po_2), usually evident within 30 min, in infants with cyanotic heart disease (restricted pulmonary blood flow). Normal Po_2 for neonates is 60–70 mm Hg. Indicated by increased pH in those with acidosis, increased systemic BP and urinary output, return of palpable pulses, and decreased ratio of pulmonary artery to aortic pressure in infants with restricted systemic blood flow.
- Monitor for arterial pressure, ECG, heart rate, BP, respiratory rate, and rectal temperature, intermittently throughout the infusion.
- Lab tests: Monitor arterial blood gases and arterial blood pH intermittently throughout the infusion.
- Monitor: Systemic BP, pulmonary artery and descending aorta pressures, femoral pulse, and urinary output.

Patient & Family Education

Erectile Dysfunction

- Follow carefully directions for penile injection provided by the manufacturer.
- Do not change dose without consulting the physician.
- Do not use intracavernosal injection more often than 3 times/wk; allow at least 24 h between uses.
- Do not use more than 2 urethral suppository systems in a 24 h period.
- Report nodules or hard tissue in penis; penile pain, redness, swelling, tenderness; or curvature of the erect penis to the physician as soon as possible.
- Seek immediate medical attention if an erection persists longer than 6 h.

ALTEPLASE RECOMBINANT (Pr)

(al′te-plase)

Actilyse, Activase, Cathflo Activase

Classification: THROMBOLYTIC, TISSUE PLASMINOGEN ACTIVATOR
Therapeutic: THROMBOLYTIC ENZYME
Pregnancy Category: C

AVAILABILITY 50 mg, 100 mg vials

ACTION & *THERAPEUTIC EFFECT* This recombinant DNA-derived form of human tissue-type plasminogen activator (t-PA) is a thrombolytic agent. The agent t-PA promotes thrombolysis by forming the active proteolytic enzyme, plasmin. *Plasmin is capable of degrading fibrin, fibrinogen, and factors V, VIII, and XII.*

USES Indicated in selective cases of acute MI, preferably within 6 h of attack for recanalization of the coronary artery; lysis of acute pulmonary emboli; acute ischemic stroke or thrombotic stroke (within 3 h of onset); treatment of acute coronary artery thrombosis in the setting of percutaneous coronary intervention (PCI); reestablishing patency of occluded IV catheter.

UNLABELED USES Lysis of arterial occlusions in peripheral and bypass vessels; DVT.

CONTRAINDICATIONS Active internal bleeding, history of cerebrovascular accident, aneurysm, recent (within 2 mo) intracranial or interspinal surgery or trauma, intracranial neoplasm, increased intracranial pressure; arteriovenous malformation, bleeding disorders, severe uncontrolled hypertension, likelihood of left heart thrombus, acute pericarditis, bacterial endocarditis, severe liver or renal dysfunction, septic thrombophlebitis, current use of oral anticoagulants.

CAUTIOUS USE Recent major surgery (within 10 days), cerebral vascular disease, recent GI or GU bleeding, recent trauma, renal impairment, hypertension, hemorrhagic ophthalmic conditions; age greater than 75 y; pregnancy (category C), lactation.

ROUTE & DOSAGE

Acute MI

Adult: **IV** *Weight 65 kg or more,* 60 mg over first hour, 20 mg/h over second hour, and 20 mg over third hour (for a total of 100 mg over 3 h; *weight less than 65 kg,* 1.25 mg/kg over 3 h (60% of dose over first hour, 20% of dose over second hour, and 20% of dose over third hour). *Accelerated schedule (with heparin and aspirin): Weight greater than 67 kg,* 15 mg bolus, then 50 mg over next 30 min, then 35 mg over next 60 min. *Accelerated schedule (with heparin and aspirin): Weight 67 kg or less,* 15 mg bolus, then 0.75 mg/kg (not to exceed 50 mg) over next 30 min, then 0.5 mg/kg (not to exceed 35 mg) over next 60 min

Acute Ischemic Stroke/ Thrombotic Stroke

Adult: **IV** 0.9 mg/kg over 60 min with 10% of dose as an initial bolus over 1 min (max: 90 mg)

Pulmonary Embolism

Adult: **IV** 100 mg infused over 2 h

Reopen Occluded IV Catheter

Adult/Child (greater than 30 kg): **IV** Instill 2 mg/2 mL into dysfunctional catheter for 2 h. May repeat once if needed.
Child: **IV** *2 y or older, weight 10–29 kg,* Instill 110% of internal lumen volume with 1 mg/mL concentration (max: 2 mg). May repeat if function not restored within 2 h. **IV** *Younger than 2 y, weight less than 10 kg,* 0.5 mg diluted in a volume to fill the lumen of the catheter

ADMINISTRATION

Intravenous

PREPARE: **IV Infusion:** Reconstitute the 50 mg vial as follows:

Do not use if vacuum in vial has been broken. Use a large-bore needle (e.g., 18 gauge) and do not prime needle with air. ▪ Dilute contents of vial with sterile water for injection supplied by manufacturer. ▪ Direct stream of sterile water into the lyophilized cake. Slight foaming is usual. Allow to stand until bubbles dissipate. Resulting concentration is 1 mg/mL. ▪ Reconstitute the 100-mg vial using supplied transfer device for reconstitution. Follow manufacturer's directions.

ADMINISTER: **IV Infusion:** Start IV infusion as soon as possible after the thrombolytic event, preferably within 6 h. ▪ Administer drug as reconstituted (1 mg/mL) or further diluted with an equal volume of NS or D5W to yield 0.5 mg/mL. **Acute MI:** Administer 60% of total dose in the first hour for acute MI, with 6–10% given as a bolus dose over 1–2 min and remainder of first dose infused over hour 1. Follow with second dose (20% of total) over hour 2, and third dose (20% of total) over hour 3. ▪ For patients weighing less than 65 kg calculate dose using 1.25 mg/kg over 3 h. See accelerated schedule under Route & Dosage. **Pulmonary embolism:** Administer entire dose over a 2 h period. **Acute ischemic stroke:** Give 5 mg as an initial bolus over 1 min, then give the remainder of the 0.75 mg/kg dose over 60 min. ▪ Do not exceed a total dose of 100 mg. Higher doses have been associated with intracranial bleeding. ▪ Follow infusion of drug by flushing IV tubing with 30–50 mL of NS or D5W. ▪ Reconstituted drug is stable for 8 h in above solutions at room temperature (2°–30° C; 36°–86° F). Since there are no preservatives, discard any unused solution after that time.

INCOMPATIBILITIES **Solution/additive:** **Dobutamine, dopamine, heparin.** **Y-site:** **Bivalirudin, dobutamine, dopamine, heparin, nitroglycerin.**

▪ Store above reconstituted solutions at room temperature 2°–30° C (36°–86° F) for no longer than 8 h. Discard any unused solution after that time.

ADVERSE EFFECTS (≥1%) **Hematologic:** Internal and superficial bleeding (cerebral, retroperitoneal, GU, GI).

PHARMACOKINETICS **Peak:** 5–10 min after infusion completed. **Duration:** Baseline values restored in 3 h. **Metabolism:** In liver. **Elimination:** In urine. **Half-Life:** 26.5 min.

NURSING IMPLICATIONS

Assessment & Drug Effects

- Monitor for S&S of excess bleeding q15min for the first hour of therapy, q30min for second to eighth hour, then q8h.
- Monitor neurologic checks throughout drug infusion q30min and qh for the first 8 h after infusion.
- Protect patient from invasive procedures because spontaneous bleeding occurs twice as often with alteplase as with heparin. IM injections are contraindicated. Also prevent physical manipulation of patient during thrombolytic therapy to prevent bruising.
- Lab tests: Coagulation tests including APTT, bleeding time, PT, TT, INR, **must be** done before administration of drug. Also check *baseline* Hct, Hgb, and platelet counts, in case of bleeding. Draw Hct following drug administration to detect possible blood loss.

- Keep patient in bed while receiving this medication.
- Check vital signs frequently. Be alert to changes in cardiac rhythm.
- Stop therapy immediately if dysrhythmias occur.
- Report signs of bleeding: Gum bleeding, epistaxis, hematoma, spontaneous ecchymoses, oozing at catheter site, increased pain from internal bleeding. Stop the infusion, then resume when bleeding stops.
- Use the radial artery to draw ABGs. Pressure to puncture sites, if necessary, should be maintained for up to 30 min.
- Continue monitoring vital signs until laboratory reports confirm anticoagulant control; patient is at risk for postthrombolytic bleeding for 2–4 days after intracoronary alteplase treatment.

Patient & Family Education

- Report immediately a sudden severe headache.
- Report blood in urine and bloody or tarry stools.
- Report any signs of bleeding or oozing from cuts or places of injection.
- Remain quiet and on bedrest while receiving this medicine.

ALTRETAMINE, HEXAMETHYLMELAMINE

(al-tre′ta-meen)

Hexalen

Classifications: ANTINEOPLASTIC; ALKYLATING

Therapeutic: ANTINEOPLASTIC

Prototype: Cyclophosphamide

Pregnancy Category: D

AVAILABILITY 50 mg capsules

ACTION & *THERAPEUTIC EFFECT* Altretamine is a synthetic cytotoxic antineoplastic drug. It is metabolized to metabolites with cytotoxic properties. *Altretamine has demonstrated neoplastic activity in patients resistant to alkylating agents.*

USES Ovarian cancer.

UNLABELED USES Breast, cervical, colon, endometrial, head, and neck cancer; small-cell lung cancers and lymphomas.

CONTRAINDICATIONS Hypersensitivity to altretamine, severe bone marrow depression, neurologic toxicity, neurologic disease; intramuscular injections, pregnancy (category D), lactation.

CAUTIOUS USE History of viral infections (i.e., herpes simplex); radiation therapy. Safety and efficacy in children are not established.

ROUTE & DOSAGE

Ovarian Cancer

Adult: **PO** 260 mg/m²/day for 14 or 21 consecutive days in a 28-day cycle

ADMINISTRATION

Oral

- Give only under supervision of a qualified physician experienced in the use of antineoplastics.
- Give in 4 divided doses after meals and at bedtime.
- Discontinue altretamine for 14 days or longer and restart at 200 mg/m²/day if any of the following occur: Severe GI intolerance; WBC count less than 2000/mm³, granulocyte count less than 1000/mm³; or progressive neurotoxicity.
- Store at room temperature, 15°–30° C (59°–86° F).

ADVERSE EFFECTS (≥1%) **CNS:** *Paresthesias, hyporeflexia, muscle weakness, peripheral numbness,* *ataxia, Parkinson-like tremors.* **GI:** *Nausea, vomiting.* **Hematologic:** *Leukopenia, thrombocytopenia.* **Urogenital:** Slight increase in serum creatinine. **Skin:** Alopecia and eczema.

INTERACTIONS Drug: Concomitant administration of altretamine and TRICYCLIC ANTIDEPRESSANTS (**imipramine, amitriptyline**), MONOAMINE OXIDASE INHIBITORS, or **selegiline** have been reported to result in incapacitating dizziness and syncopal episodes during the first week of altretamine treatment. Patients became asymptomatic 24–96 h after discontinuing ANTIDEPRESSANTS.

PHARMACOKINETICS Absorption: Rapidly from GI tract. Approximately 25% reaches systemic circulation due to extensive hepatic first-pass metabolism. **Metabolism:** Rapidly demethylated in the liver. **Elimination:** 62% of the dose is excreted in the urine in 24 h. A small amount is excreted through the lungs. **Half-Life:** 13 h.

NURSING IMPLICATIONS

Assessment & Drug Effects

- Lab tests: Monitor blood counts at least monthly and prior to each course of therapy.
- Perform a neurologic examination regularly; question patient about the presence of paresthesias, hypoesthesias, muscle weakness, peripheral numbness, ataxia, decreased sensations, and alterations in mood or consciousness.
- Withhold medication if neurologic symptoms fail to resolve with dose reduction. Notify physician.
- Monitor for nausea and vomiting, which are related to the cumulative dose of altretamine. After several weeks some patients develop tolerance to the GI effects. Antiemetics may be required to control GI distress.

Patient & Family Education

- Taking altretamine after meals or with food or milk may decrease nausea.
- Report symptoms indicative of neurotoxicity to physician (paresthesias, hypoesthesias, muscle weakness, peripheral numbness, ataxia, decreased sensations, and alterations in mood or consciousness).
- Note: GI, hematologic, and neurologic adverse effects may be severe.

ALUMINUM HYDROXIDE Pr

(a-lu'mi-num)

ALternaGEL, Alu-Cap, Alugel, Alu-Tab, Amphojel, Dialume

ALUMINUM CARBONATE, BASIC

Basaljel

ALUMINUM PHOSPHATE

Phosphaljel

Classifications: ANTACID; ADSORBENT

Therapeutic: ANTACID

Pregnancy Category: C

AVAILABILITY Aluminum Hydroxide: 300 mg, 400 mg, 500 mg, 600 mg tablets; 300 mg, 400 mg, 500 mg, 600 mg capsules; 320 mg/5 mL, 450 mg/5 mL, 600 mg/5 mL, 675 mg/5 mL suspension; **Aluminum Carbonate, Basic:** 608 mg tablets; 608 mg capsules; 400 mg/5 mL suspension; **Aluminum Phosphate:** 608 mg tablets; 608 mg capsules; 400 mg/5 mL suspension

ACTION & *THERAPEUTIC EFFECT* Nonsystemic antacid with moderate neutralizing action. Reduces acid concentration and pepsin activity by raising pH of gastric and intraesophageal secretions. *Reduces gastric acidity by neutralizing the stomach acid content. Aluminum carbonate lowers serum phosphate by binding dietary phosphate to form insoluble aluminum phosphate, which is excreted in feces.*

USES Symptomatic relief of gastric hyperacidity associated with gastritis, esophageal reflux, and hiatal hernia; adjunct in treatment of gastric and duodenal ulcer. More commonly used in combination with other antacids. Aluminum carbonate is used primarily in conjunction with a low phosphate diet to reduce hyperphosphatemia in patients with renal insufficiency and for prophylaxis and treatment of phosphatic renal calculi.

CONTRAINDICATIONS Prolonged use of high doses in presence of low serum phosphate.

CAUTIOUS USE Renal impairment; gastric outlet obstruction; older adults; decreased bowel activity (e.g., patients receiving anticholinergic, antidiarrheal, or antispasmodic agents); patients who are dehydrated or on fluid restriction; pregnancy (category C).

ROUTE & DOSAGE

Antacid (Hydroxide and Phosphate)

Adult: **PO** 600 mg t.i.d. or q.i.d.

Antacid (Carbonate)

Adult: **PO** 10–30 mL of regular suspension or 5–15 mL of extra strength suspension or 2 capsules or tablets q2h

Phosphate Lowering (Carbonate)

Adult: **PO** 10–30 mL of regular suspension or 5–15 mL of extra strength suspension or 2–6 capsules or tablets 1 h p.c. and at bedtime

ADMINISTRATION

Oral

- Tablet **must be** chewed until it is thoroughly wetted before swallowing.
- Note for antacid use: Follow well-chewed tablet with one-half glass of water or milk; follow liquid preparation (suspension) with water to ensure passage into stomach. For phosphate lowering: Follow tablet, capsule, or suspension with full glass of water or fruit juice.
- Store between 15°–30° C (59°–86° F) in tightly closed container.

ADVERSE EFFECTS (≥1%) **GI:** *Constipation*, fecal impaction, intestinal obstruction. **CNS:** Dialysis dementia (thought to be due to aluminum intoxication). **Metabolic:** Hypophosphatemia, hypomagnesemia.

INTERACTIONS Drug: Aluminum will decrease absorption of **chloroquine, cimetidine, ciprofloxacin, digoxin, isoniazid,** IRON SALTS, NSAIDS, **norfloxacin, ofloxacin, phenytoin, phenothiazines, quinidine, tetracycline, thyroxine. Sodium polystyrene sulfonate** may cause systemic alkalosis.

PHARMACOKINETICS Absorption: Minimal absorption. **Peak:** Slow onset. **Duration:** 2 h when taken with food; 3 h when taken 1 h after food. **Elimination:** In feces as insoluble phosphates.

NURSING IMPLICATIONS

Assessment & Drug Effects

- Note number and consistency of stools. Constipation is common and dose related. Intestinal obstruction from fecal concretions has been reported.
- Lab tests: Monitor periodic serum calcium and phosphorus levels

with prolonged high-dose therapy or impaired renal function.

Patient & Family Education

- Increase phosphorus in diet when taking large doses of these antacids for prolonged periods; hypophosphatemia can develop within 2 wk of continuous use of these antacids. The older adult in a poor nutritional state is at high risk.
- Note: Antacid may cause stools to appear speckled or whitish.
- Report epigastric or abdominal pain; it is a clinical guide for adjusting dosage. Keep physician informed. Pain that persists beyond 72 h may signify serious complications.
- Seek medical help if indigestion is accompanied by shortness of breath, sweating, or chest pain, if stools are dark or tarry, or if symptoms are recurrent when taking this medication.
- Seek medical advice and supervision if self-prescribed antacid use exceeds 2 wk.

ALVIMOPAN

(al-vi-mo′pan)

Entereg

Classifications: PERIPHERAL OPIOID RECEPTOR ANTAGONIST; GI MOTILITY STIMULANT

Therapeutic: GI MOTILITY STIMULANT

Pregnancy Category: B

AVAILABILITY 12 mg capsules

ACTION & *THERAPEUTIC EFFECT* Morphine and other post-op analgesics are mu-opioid receptor agonists known to inhibit GI motility and prolong the duration of postoperative ileus. Alvimopan is a selective antagonist of mu-opioid receptors. *It competitively antagonizes the effect of morphine on contractility, shortening the duration of post-op ileus.*

USES To accelerate the time to upper and lower gastrointestinal recovery after partial large or small bowel resection surgery with primary anastomosis.

UNLABELED USES Constipation, opioid-induced constipation.

CONTRAINDICATIONS Therapeutic doses of opioids for greater than 7 consecutive days immediately preop; end-stage renal disease; severe hepatic impairment (Child-Pugh class C).

CAUTIOUS USE Recent exposure to opioids; surgery for complete bowel obstruction; history of CAD or MI; pregnancy (category B); lactation. Safety and efficacy in children not established.

ROUTE & DOSAGE

Acceleration of Postoperative GI Recovery

Adult: **PO** 12 mg 0.5–5 h preoperative; then 12 mg b.i.d. up to 7 days

ADMINISTRATION

Oral

- Give pre-op dose 30 min–5 h before surgery.
- Do not exceed 15 doses (maximum allowed).
- Store at 15°–30° C (59°–86° F).
- Note: Hospitals **must be** registered in and have met all of the requirements for the **Entereg** Access Support and Education (E.A.S.E.) program in order to use alvimopan.

ADVERSE EFFECTS (≥3%) **GI:** Constipation, dyspepsia, flatulence. **Hematologic:** Anemia. **Metabolic:** Hypokalemia. **Musculoskeletal:** Back pain. **Urogenital:** Urinary retention.

INTERACTIONS Food: Decreased extent and rate of absorption if taken with a high fat meal.

PHARMACOKINETICS Absorption: Bioavailability 6%. **Peak:** 2 h. **Distribution:** 90–94% plasma protein bound. **Metabolism:** By intestinal flora. **Elimination:** Fecal (primary) and renal (35%). **Half-Life:** 10–18 h.

NURSING IMPLICATIONS

Assessment & Drug Effects

- Monitor frequently for return of bowel sounds and ability to pass flatus.
- Monitor closely patients with impaired renal function for adverse effects.
- Report to physician increasing abdominal pain, diarrhea, nausea and vomiting.
- Lab tests: Serum potassium in patients predisposed to hypokalemia.

Patient & Family Education

- Report promptly increasing abdominal pain and nausea.

AMANTADINE HYDROCHLORIDE (Pr)

(a-man'ta-deen)

Symmetrel

Classifications: ANTIVIRAL; CENTRAL-ACTING CHOLINERGIC RECEPTOR ANTAGONIST; ANTIPARKINSON

Therapeutic: ANTIVIRAL; ANTIPARKINSON

Pregnancy Category: C

AVAILABILITY 100 mg capsules; 50 mg/5 mL syrup

ACTION & *THERAPEUTIC EFFECT* Because it does not suppress antibody formation, it can be administered for interim protection in combination with influenza A virus vaccine until antibody titer is adequate or to augment prophylaxis in a previously vaccinated individual. Mechanism of action in parkinsonism may be related to release of dopamine and other catecholamines from neuronal storage sites. *Active against several strains of influenza A virus; not effective against influenza B infections. Effective in management of symptoms of parkinsonism when used in conjunction with other antiparkinson agents.*

USES In initial therapy or as adjunct with anticholinergic drugs or levodopa in treatment of all forms of parkinsonism (arteriosclerotic, idiopathic, postencephalitic) and for relief of drug-induced extrapyramidal reactions and symptomatic parkinsonism caused by carbon monoxide poisoning. Also used for prophylaxis and symptomatic treatment of influenza A infections.

UNLABELED USES Primary enuresis, pseudosclerosis, neuroleptic malignant syndrome (NMS), management of cocaine dependency and withdrawal.

CONTRAINDICATIONS Hypersensitivity to amantadine or rimantadine, closed angle glaucoma; suicidal ideation; lactation. Safety in children younger than 1 y for Influenza A is not established.

CAUTIOUS USE History of epilepsy or other types of seizures; CHF, peripheral edema, orthostatic hypotension; recurrent eczematoid dermatitis; psychoses, severe psychoneuroses; hepatic disease; renal impairment; older adults with cerebral arteriosclerosis; pregnancy (category C).

ROUTE & DOSAGE

Influenza A Treatment

Adult (younger than 65 y)/Child (older than 9 y): **PO** 200 mg once/day or 100 mg q12h

Adult (65 y or older): **PO** 100 mg once/day
Child (1–9 y): **PO** 5 mg/kg in 2–3 equal doses (max: 150 mg/day)

Influenza A Prevention

Adult (younger than 65 y): **PO** 200 mg/day or 100 mg q12h; begin as soon as possible after initial exposure and continue for at least 10 days after exposure
Adult (older than 65 y): **PO** 100 mg once daily
HIV-Infected Adult/Adolescent/Child (at least 10 y): **PO** 100 mg twice daily
Child (1–9 y): **PO** 5 mg/kg/day (up to 150 mg/day) given in 2 divided doses (not more than 150 mg/day)

Parkinsonism

Adult: **PO** 100 mg 1–2 times/day, start with 100 mg/day if patient is on other antiparkinsonism medications

Drug-Induced Extrapyramidal Symptoms

Adult: **PO** 100 mg b.i.d. (max: 400 mg/day if needed)

Renal Impairment Dosage Adjustment

CrCl 30–50 mL/min: 200 mg PO for 1st day, then 100 mg PO daily; 15–29 mL/min: 100 mg PO for 1st day, then 100 mg PO on alternate days; less than 15 mL/min: 200 mg q7days

ADMINISTRATION

Oral

- Give with water, milk, or food.
- Use supplied calibrated device for measuring syrup formulation.
- Influenza prophylaxis: Drug should be initiated when exposure is anticipated and continued for at least 10 days.
- Note: Used in conjunction with influenza A vaccine (generally in high-risk patients who have not been vaccinated previously) until protective antibodies develop (10–21 days) after vaccine administration.
- Schedule medication in the morning or, with q12h dosing, schedule 2nd dose several hours before bedtime. If insomnia is a problem, suggest patient limit number of daytime naps.
- Store in tightly closed container preferably at 15°–30° C (59°–86° F) unless otherwise directed by manufacturer. Avoid freezing.

ADVERSE EFFECTS (≥1%) **CNS:** *Dizziness, light-headedness,* headache, ataxia, irritability, anxiety, *nervousness, difficulty in concentrating,* mood or other mental changes, confusion, visual and auditory hallucinations, *insomnia,* nightmares, convulsions. **CV:** Orthostatic hypotension, peripheral edema, dyspnea. **Special Senses:** Blurring or loss of vision. **GI:** Anorexia, *nausea,* vomiting, dry mouth. **Hematologic:** Leukopenia, agranulocytosis.

INTERACTIONS Drug: Alcohol enhances CNS effects; may potentiate effects of ANTICHOLINERGICS.

PHARMACOKINETICS Absorption: Almost completely absorbed from GI tract. **Onset:** Within 48 h. **Peak:** 1–4 h. **Distribution:** Through body fluids. **Metabolism:** Not metabolized. **Elimination:** 90% unchanged in urine. **Half-Life:** 9–37 h (prolonged in renal insufficiency).

NURSING IMPLICATIONS

Assessment & Drug Effects

- Monitor effectiveness. Note that with parkinsonism, maximum response occurs within 2 wk–3 mo. Effectiveness may wane after 6–8 wk of treatment; report change to physician.

- Monitor and report: Mental status changes; nervousness, difficulty concentrating, or insomnia; loss of seizure control; S&S of toxicity, especially with doses above 200 mg/day.
- Establish a baseline profile of the patient's disabilities to accurately differentiate disease symptoms and drug-induced neuropsychiatric adverse reactions.
- Monitor vital signs for at least 3 or 4 days after increases in dosage; also monitor urinary output.
- Lab tests: pH and serum electrolytes.
- Monitor for and report reduced salivation, increased akinesia or rigidity, and psychological disturbances that may develop within 4–48 h after initiation of therapy and after dosage increases with parkinsonism.

Patient & Family Education

- Note: For influenza take within 24 h but no later than 48 h after onset of symptoms for effective response and continue for 24–48 h after symptoms disappear; contact physician if no improvement within this time.
- Make all position changes slowly, particularly from recumbent to upright position, in order to minimize dizziness.
- Report any of the following to physician: Shortness of breath, peripheral edema, significant weight gain, dizziness or lightheadedness, inability to concentrate, and other changes in mental status, difficulty urinating, and visual impairment.
- Do not drive and exercise caution with potentially hazardous activities until response to the drug is known.
- Note: People with Parkinson's disease should not discontinue therapy abruptly; doing so may precipitate a parkinsonian crisis with severe akinesia, rigidity, tremor, and psychic disturbances. Adhere to established dosage regimen.

AMBENONIUM CHLORIDE

(am-be-noe′nee-um)

Mytelase

Classification: CHOLINESTERASE INHIBITOR

Therapeutic: CHOLINESTERASE INHIBITOR

Prototype: Neostigmine

Pregnancy Category: C

AVAILABILITY 10 mg tablets

ACTION & *THERAPEUTIC EFFECT* Inhibits destruction of acetylcholine (ACh) by cholinesterase, thereby prolonging effects of ACh (neurotransmitter) at postsynaptic receptor sites. Has direct stimulant effect on striated muscles. *Improves muscular strength in myasthenia gravis.*

USES Symptomatic treatment of myasthenia gravis for patients who cannot tolerate neostigmine bromide or pyridostigmine bromide because of bromide sensitivity. Has been used in conjunction with corticosteroids, ephedrine sulfate, and potassium chloride to increase muscle strength.

CONTRAINDICATIONS Intestinal or urinary tract obstruction; patients receiving mecamylamine; lactation.

CAUTIOUS USE Epilepsy, bradycardia, cardiac arrhythmias, recent coronary occlusion; bronchial asthma;

hyperthyroidism; older adults; vagotonia; peptic ulcer, megacolon; pregnancy (category C).

ROUTE & DOSAGE

Myasthenia Gravis

Adult: **PO** 2.5–5 mg t.i.d. or q.i.d., may increase q1–2days to 50–75 mg t.i.d. or q.i.d. if necessary
Child: **PO** 0.3 mg/kg/day in 3–4 divided doses, may need up to 1.5 mg/kg/day in 3–4 divided doses

ADMINISTRATION

Oral

- Give with food or milk to minimize adverse effects.
- Schedule larger doses when patient experiences the most fatigue or muscle weakness; to improve ability to eat, give drug 30–45 min before meals.
- Store at 15°–30° C (59°–86° F) unless otherwise directed.

ADVERSE EFFECTS (≥1%) **CNS:** Exaggerated cholinergic (muscarinic) effects; muscle cramps, headache, confusion, dizziness, incoordination, fasciculations, agitation, restlessness, muscle weakness, paralysis, slurred speech, convulsions, respiratory depression. **CV:** Bradycardia. **GI:** Nausea, vomiting, diarrhea, abdominal cramps, excessive salivation. **Special Senses:** Blurred vision, lacrimation. **Respiratory:** Bronchospasm, increased bronchial secretions, dyspnea. **Other:** Diaphoresis.

INTERACTIONS Drug: Demecarium and other CHOLINESTERASE INHIBITORS possibly compound toxicity; **mecamylamine, succinylcholine, procainamide, quinidine,** AMINOGLYCOSIDES increase neuromuscular blocking effects with possibility of respiratory depression; atropine antagonizes effects of ambenonium.

PHARMACOKINETICS Absorption: Poorly absorbed from GI tract. **Onset:** 20–30 min. **Duration:** 3–8 h.

NURSING IMPLICATIONS

Assessment & Drug Effects

- Therapeutic effect may not be apparent for several days after initiation of therapy.
- Keep atropine sulfate immediately available to treat severe cholinergic reactions.
- Monitor for S&S of overdosage (muscle weakness within 1 h; headache, weakness of muscles of neck, chewing, and swallowing, increased salivation) and inadequate ventilation (unusual apprehension, restlessness, rapid pulse and respirations, rising BP).
- Monitor vital signs during dosage adjustment periods.
- Note: Muscle weakness beginning 3 h or more after drug administration is probably due to underdosage or drug resistance.

Patient & Family Education

- Follow directions for taking this drug (see ADMINISTRATION).
- Learn to recognize adverse effects, how to modify the doses accordingly, and when to take atropine.
- Note: During long-term therapy the drug may become ineffective; responsiveness usually returns when dosage is reduced or drug is withdrawn for several days.
- Carry medical identification indicating medical diagnosis and medication(s) being taken.

AMCINONIDE

(am-sin′oh-nide)

Pregnancy Category: C

See Appendix A-4.

AMIFOSTINE

(am-i-fos′teen)

Ethyol

Classification: CYTOPROTECTIVE

Therapeutic: CYTOPROTECTIVE

Pregnancy Category: C

AVAILABILITY 500 mg vial

ACTION & *THERAPEUTIC EFFECT* Amifostine reduces cytotoxic damage induced by radiation or antineoplastic agents in well-oxygenated cells. Protective effects appear to be mediated by the formation of a metabolite of amifostine that removes free radicals from normal cells exposed to cisplatin. *Amifostine is cytoprotective in the kidney, bone marrow, and GI mucosa, but not in the brain or spinal cord. The cytoprotection results in decreased myelosuppression and peripheral neuropathy.*

USES Reduction of the cumulative renal toxicity associated with cisplatin, xerostomia.

UNLABELED USES Reduction of paclitaxel toxicity.

CONTRAINDICATIONS Sensitivity to aminothiol compounds or mannitol, patients with potentially curable malignancies, hypotensive patients or those who are dehydrated, lactation; exfoliated dermatitis.

CAUTIOUS USE Patients at risk for hypocalcemia, cardiovascular disease (i.e., arrhythmias, CHF, TIA, CVA); radiation therapy; renal disease; pregnancy (category C).

ROUTE & DOSAGE

Renal Protection

Adult: **IV** 910 mg/m² once daily prior to chemotherapy

Reduction of Xerostomia

Adult: **IV** 200 mg/m² prior to radiation therapy

ADMINISTRATION

Intravenous

Give antiemetics, adequately hydrate, and defer antihypertensives for 24 h prior to administration.

PREPARE: **IV Infusion:** Reconstitute by adding 9.7 mL of NS injection to a single-dose vial to yield 50 mg/mL. ▪ May be further diluted with NS to a concentration as low as 5 mg/mL.

ADMINISTER: **IV Infusion:** Infuse over no more than 15 min, beginning 30 min before chemotherapy; place patient in supine position prior to and during infusion. ▪ For xerostomia, infuse over 3 min; begin 15–30 min before radiation.

INCOMPATIBILITIES **Solution/additive:** Do not mix with any solutions other than NS. **Y-site:** **Acyclovir, amphotericin B, chlorpromazine, cisplatin, ganciclovir, hydroxyzine, prochlorperazine.**

▪ Store reconstituted solution at 15°–30° C (59°–86° F) for 5 h or refrigerate up to 24 h.

ADVERSE EFFECTS (≥1%) **CV:** *Transient reduction in blood pressure.* **GI:** *Nausea, vomiting.* **Other:** Infusion reactions (flushing, feeling of warmth or coldness, chills, dizziness, somnolence, hiccups, sneezing), hypocalcemia, hypersensitivity reactions.

INTERACTIONS Drug: ANTIHYPERTENSIVES could cause or potentiate hypotension.

PHARMACOKINETICS Onset: 5–8 min. **Metabolism:** In liver to active

Common adverse effects in *italic*, life-threatening effects underlined; generic names in **bold**; classifications in SMALL CAPS; ✤ Canadian drug name; ⊕ Prototype drug

free thiol metabolite. **Elimination:** Renally excreted. **Half-Life:** 8 min.

NURSING IMPLICATIONS

Assessment & Drug Effects

- Monitor for S&S of hypocalcemia and fluid balance if vomiting is significant.
- Monitor BP every 5 min during infusion. Stop infusion if systolic BP drops significantly from baseline (e.g., baseline[drop]: less than 100[20], 100–119[25], 120–139[30], 140–179[40], greater than 180[50]) and place patient flat with legs raised. Restart infusion if BP returns to normal in 5 min.

Patient & Family Education

- Know and understand adverse effects.

AMIKACIN SULFATE

(am-i-kay′sin)

Amikin

Classification: AMINOGLYCOSIDE ANTIBIOTIC

Therapeutic: ANTIBIOTIC

Prototype: Gentamicin

Pregnancy Category: C

AVAILABILITY 250 mg/mL, 50 mg/mL injection

ACTION & *THERAPEUTIC EFFECT* Appears to inhibit protein synthesis in bacterial cells and is usually bactericidal. *Effective against a wide range of gram-negative bacteria, including many strains resistant to other aminoglycosides. Also effective against penicillinase- and non-penicillinase-producing* Staphylococcus.

USES Primarily for short-term treatment of serious infections of respiratory tract, bones, joints, skin, and soft tissue, CNS (including meningitis), peritonitis burns, recurrent urinary tract infections (UTIs).

UNLABELED USES Intrathecal or intraventricular administration, in conjunction with IM or IV dosage.

CONTRAINDICATIONS History of hypersensitivity or toxic reaction with an aminoglycoside antibiotic; lactation.

CAUTIOUS USE Impaired renal function; eighth cranial (auditory) nerve impairment; preexisting vertigo or dizziness, tinnitus, or dehydration; fever; older adults, premature infants, neonates and infants; myasthenia gravis; parkinsonism; hypocalcemia; pregnancy (category C).

ROUTE & DOSAGE

Moderate to Severe Infections

Adult: **IV/IM** 5–7.5 mg/kg loading dose, then 7.5 mg/kg q12h (max: 15 mg/kg/day) for 7–10 days

Child: **IV/IM** 5–7.5 mg/kg loading dose, then 5 mg/kg q8h or 7.5 mg/kg q12h for 7–10 days (max: 1.5 g/day)

Neonate: **IV/IM** 10 mg/kg loading dose, then 7.5 mg/kg q12h for 7–10 days

Uncomplicated UTI

Adult: **IV/IM** 250 mg q12h

Obesity Dosage Adjustment

Calculate dose based on IBW

Renal Impairment Dosage Adjustment

CrCl greater than 60 mL/min: Normal dose q8h; 40–60 mL/min: Normal dose q12h; 20–39 mL/min: Half dose q24h; less than 20 mL/min: Administer loading dose then monitor closely

Dialysis Dosage Adjustment: Administer dose post-dialysis or give 2/3 dose as supplemental dose

ADMINISTRATION

Intramuscular

- Use the 250 mg/mL vials for IM injection. Calculate the required dose and withdraw the equivalent number of mLs from the vial.
- Give deep IM into a large muscle.

Intravenous

Verify correct IV concentration and rate of infusion with physician for neonates, infants, and children.

PREPARE: **Intermittent:** Add contents of 500 mg vial to 100 or 200 mL D5W, NS injection, or other diluent recommended by manufacturer. ▪ For pediatric patients, volume of diluent depends on patient's fluid tolerance. ▪ Note: Color of solution may vary from colorless to light straw color or very pale yellow. Discard solutions that appear discolored or that contain particulate matter.

ADMINISTER: **Intermittent:** Give a single adult dose (including loading dose) over at least 30–60 min by IV infusion. ▪ Increase infusion time to 1–2 h for infants. ▪ Monitor infusion rate carefully. A rapid rise in serum amikacin level can cause respiratory depression (neuromuscular blockade) and other signs of toxicity.

INCOMPATIBILITIES **Solution/additive:** **Aminophylline, amphotericin B, ampicillin,** CEPHALOSPORINS, **chlorothiazide, heparin,** PENICILLINS, **phenytoin, thiopental, vitamin B complex with C.** **Y-site:** **Allopurinol, amphotericin B, azithromycin, hetastarch, propofol, thiopental.**

- Store at 15°–30° C (59°–86° F) unless otherwise directed.

ADVERSE EFFECTS (≥1%) **CNS:** Neurotoxicity: Drowsiness, unsteady gait, weakness, clumsiness, paresthesias, tremors, convulsions, peripheral neuritis. **Special Senses:** *Auditory–ototoxicity,* high-frequency hearing loss, complete hearing loss (occasionally permanent); tinnitus; ringing or buzzing in ears; *Vestibular:* Dizziness, ataxia. **GI:** Nausea, vomiting, <u>hepatotoxicity</u>. **Metabolic:** Hypokalemia, hypomagnesemia. **Skin:** Skin rash, urticaria, pruritus, redness. **Urogenital:** Oliguria, urinary frequency, hematuria, <u>tubular necrosis</u>, azotemia. **Other:** Superinfections.

INTERACTIONS **Drug:** ANESTHETICS, SKELETAL MUSCLE RELAXANTS have additive neuromuscular blocking effects; **acyclovir, amphotericin B, bacitracin, capreomycin, cephalosporins, colistin, cisplatin, carboplatin, methoxyflurane, polymyxin B, vancomycin, furosemide, ethacrynic acid** increase risk of ototoxicity and nephrotoxicity.

PHARMACOKINETICS **Peak:** 30 min IV; 45 min to 2 h IM. **Distribution:** Does not cross blood–brain barrier; crosses placenta; accumulates in renal cortex. **Elimination:** 94–98% renally in 24 h, remainder in 10–30 days. **Half-Life:** 2–3 h in adults, 4–8 h in neonates.

NURSING IMPLICATIONS

Assessment & Drug Effects

- Baseline tests: Before initial dose, C&S; renal function and vestibulocochlear nerve function (and at regular intervals during therapy; closely monitor in the older adult, patients with documented ear problems, renal impairment, or during high dose or prolonged therapy).

- Monitor peak and trough amikacin blood levels: Draw blood 1 h after IM or immediately after completion of IV infusion; draw trough levels immediately before the next IM or IV dose.
- Lab tests: Periodic serum creatinine and BUN, complete urinalysis. With treatment over 10 days, daily tests of renal function, weekly audiograms, and vestibular tests are strongly advised.
- Monitor serum creatinine or creatinine clearance (generally preferred) more often, in the presence of impaired renal function, in neonates, and in the older adult; note that prolonged high trough (greater than 8 mcg/mL) or peak (greater than 30–35 mcg/mL) levels are associated with toxicity.
- Monitor S&S of ototoxicity [primarily involves the cochlear (auditory) branch; high-frequency deafness usually appears first and can be detected only by audiometer]; indicators of declining renal function; respiratory tract infections and other symptoms indicative of superinfections and notify physician should they occur.
- Monitor for and report auditory symptoms (tinnitus, roaring noises, sensation of fullness in ears, hearing loss) and vestibular disturbances (dizziness or vertigo, nystagmus, ataxia).
- Monitor and report any changes in I&O, oliguria, hematuria, or cloudy urine. Keeping patient well hydrated reduces risk of nephrotoxicity; consult physician regarding optimum fluid intake.

Patient & Family Education

- Report immediately any changes in hearing or unexplained ringing/roaring noises or dizziness, and problems with balance or coordination.

AMILORIDE HYDROCHLORIDE

(a-mill'oh-ride)

Midamor

Classification: DIURETIC, POTASSIUM-SPARING

Therapeutic: DIURETIC, POTASSIUM-SPARING; ANTIHYPERTENSIVE

Prototype: Spironolactone

Pregnancy Category: B

AVAILABILITY 5 mg tablets

ACTION & *THERAPEUTIC EFFECT* Potassium-sparing diuretic with mild diuretic and antihypertensive action. Diuretic action is independent of aldosterone and carbonic anhydrase. Induces urinary excretion of sodium and reduces excretion of potassium and hydrogen ions by direct action on distal renal tubules. *Lowers blood pressure by excretion of sodium ion and water from the kidney while sparing potassium excretion.*

USES Potassium-sparing effect in prevention or treatment of diuretic-induced hypokalemia in patients with CHF, hepatic cirrhosis, or hypertension. Also used in management of primary hyperaldosteronism. Usually combined with a potassium-wasting (kaliuretic) diuretic such as a thiazide or loop diuretic.

UNLABELED USES With hydrochlorothiazide for recurrent calcium nephrolithiasis, lithium-induced polyuria.

CONTRAINDICATIONS Elevated serum potassium (greater than 5.5 mEq/L), concomitant use of other potassium-sparing diuretics; anuria, acute or chronic renal insufficiency;

evidence of diabetic nephropathy; type 1 diabetes mellitus; metabolic or respiratory acidosis; lactation. Safety in children is not established.
CAUTIOUS USE Debilitated patients; diet-controlled or uncontrolled diabetes mellitus; cardiopulmonary disease; hepatic disease; older adult; pregnancy (category B).

ROUTE & DOSAGE

Diuretic

Adult: **PO** 5 mg/day, may increase up to 20 mg/day in 1–2 divided doses

ADMINISTRATION

Oral

- Give once/day dose in the morning and schedule the second b.i.d. dose early to avoid interrupting sleep.
- Give with food to reduce possibility of gastric distress.
- Store at 15°–30° C (59°–86° F) in a tightly closed container unless otherwise directed.

ADVERSE EFFECTS (≥1%) **Body as a Whole:** Generally well tolerated. **CNS:** *Headache,* dizziness, nervousness, confusion, paresthesias, drowsiness. **CV:** Cardiac arrhythmias. **Metabolic:** Hyperkalemia, hyponatremia, positive Coombs' test. **Hematologic:** <u>Aplastic anemia</u>. **Special Senses:** Tinnitus; nasal congestion. Visual disturbances, increased intraocular pressure. **GI:** *Diarrhea* or constipation, anorexia, *nausea,* vomiting, abdominal cramps, dry mouth, thirst. **Urogenital:** Polyuria, dysuria, bladder spasms, urinary frequency, impotence, decreased libido. **Respiratory:** Dyspnea, shortness of breath. **Skin:** Rash, pruritus, photosensitivity reactions. **Other:** Weakness, fatigue, muscle cramps.

DIAGNOSTIC TEST INTERFERENCE Manufacturer advises discontinuing amiloride in patients with diabetes mellitus at least 3 days before ***glucose tolerance*** test.

INTERACTIONS Drug: Blood from blood banks, ACE INHIBITORS (e.g., **captopril**), **spironolactone, triamterene,** POTASSIUM SUPPLEMENTS may cause hyperkalemia with cardiac arrhythmias; possibility of increased **lithium** toxicity (decreased renal elimination); possibility of altered **digoxin** response; NSAIDS may attenuate antihypertensive effects. **Food:** POTASSIUM-CONTAINING SALT SUBSTITUTES or foods high in potassium increase risk of hyperkalemia.

PHARMACOKINETICS Absorption: 50% from GI tract. **Onset:** 2 h. **Peak:** 6–10 h. **Duration:** 24 h. **Elimination:** 20–50% unchanged in urine, 40% in feces. **Half-Life:** 6–9 h.

NURSING IMPLICATIONS

Assessment & Drug Effects

- Monitor for S&S of hyperkalemia and hyponatremia (see Appendix F). Hyperkalemia occurs in about 10% of patients receiving amiloride and serum potassium can rise suddenly and without warning. It is more common in older adults and patients with diabetes or renal disease.
- Lab tests: Serum potassium levels, particularly when therapy is initiated, whenever dosage adjustments are made, and during any illness that may affect kidney function. Intermittent evaluations of BUN, creatinine, and ECG for patients with renal or hepatic dysfunction, diabetes mellitus, older adults, or the debilitated.

Patient & Family Education

- Learn S&S of hyperkalemia and hyponatremia (see Appendix F) and report to physician immediately.

- Do not take potassium supplements, salt substitutes, high intake of dietary potassium unless prescribed by physician.
- Do not drive or engage in potentially hazardous activities until response to drug is known.

AMINOCAPROIC ACID (Pr)

(a-mee-noe-ka-proe′ik)

Amicar

Classifications: COAGULATOR; HEMOSTATIC, SYSTEMIC

Therapeutic: ANTIHEMORRHAGIC; ANTIFIBRINOLYTIC

Pregnancy Category: C

AVAILABILITY 250 mg/mL injection; 500 mg, 1000 mg tablets; 250 mg/mL syrup

ACTION & *THERAPEUTIC EFFECT* Synthetic hemostatic with specific antifibrinolysis action. Inhibits plasminogen activator substance, and to a lesser degree plasmin (fibrinolysin), which is concerned with destruction of clots. *Acts as an inhibitor of fibrinolytic bleeding.*

USES To control excessive bleeding resulting from systemic hyperfibrinolysis; also used in urinary fibrinolysis associated with severe trauma, anoxia, shock, urologic surgery, and neoplastic diseases of GU tract.

UNLABELED USES To prevent hemorrhage in hemophiliacs undergoing dental extraction; as a specific antidote for streptokinase or urokinase toxicity; to prevent recurrence of subarachnoid hemorrhage, especially when surgery is delayed; for management of amegakaryocytic thrombocytopenia; and to prevent or abort hereditary angioedema episodes.

CONTRAINDICATIONS Severe renal impairment; active disseminated intravascular clotting (DIC); upper urinary tract bleeding (hematuria); hemophilia; benzyl alcohol hypersensitivity, especially in neonates; paraben hypersensitivity; lactation.

CAUTIOUS USE Cardiac, renal, or hepatic disease; renal impairment; history of pulmonary embolus or other thrombotic diseases; hypovolemia; pregnancy (category C).

ROUTE & DOSAGE

Hemostatic

Adult: **PO/IV** 4–5 g during first hour, then 1–1.25 g qh for 8 h or until bleeding is controlled (max: 30 g/24h)

Child: **PO/IV** 100 mg/kg or 3 g/m² during first hour, then 33.3 mg²/kg qh (max: 18 g/m²/24 h)

Renal Impairment Dosage Adjustment

Reduce dose to 15–25% of normal dose

ADMINISTRATION

Oral

- Note: May need to give patient as many as 10 tablets or 4 tsp for a 5 g dose during the first hour of treatment (each tablet contains 500 mg, syrup contains 250 mg/mL).

Intravenous

PREPARE: **IV Infusion:** Dilute parenteral aminocaproic acid before use. ▪ Each 4 mL (1 g) is diluted with 50 mL of NS, D5W, or LR.

ADMINISTER: **IV Infusion:** Physician orders specific IV flow rate. ▪ Usual rate is 5 g or a fraction thereof over first hour (5 g/250 mL). ▪ Give each additional gram over 1 h. Avoid rapid infusion to prevent hypotension, faintness, and bradycardia or other arrhythmias.

INCOMPATIBILITIES **Solution/additive: Fructose solution.**

- Store in tightly closed containers at 15°–30° C (59°–86° F) unless otherwise directed. Avoid freezing.

ADVERSE EFFECTS (≥1%) **CNS:** Dizziness, malaise, headache, seizures. **CV:** Faintness, orthostatic hypotension; dysrhythmias; thrombophlebitis, thromboses. **Special Senses:** Tinnitus, nasal congestion. Conjunctival erythema. **GI:** Nausea, vomiting, cramps, diarrhea, anorexia. **Urogenital:** Diuresis, dysuria, urinary frequency, oliguria, reddish-brown urine (myoglobinuria), acute renal failure. Prolonged menstruation with cramping. **Skin:** Rash.

DIAGNOSTIC TEST INTERFERENCE ***Serum potassium*** may be elevated (especially in patients with impaired renal function).

INTERACTIONS Drug: ESTROGENS, ORAL CONTRACEPTIVES may cause hypercoagulation.

PHARMACOKINETICS Absorption: Rapidly from GI tract. **Peak:** 2 h. **Distribution:** Readily penetrates RBCs and other body cells. **Elimination:** 80% as unmetabolized drug in 12 h.

NURSING IMPLICATIONS

Assessment & Drug Effects

- Check IV site at frequent intervals for extravasation.
- Observe for signs of thrombophlebitis. Change site immediately if extravasation or thrombophlebitis occurs (see Appendix F).
- Monitor and report S&S of myopathy: Muscle weakness, myalgia, diaphoresis, fever, reddish-brown urine (myoglobinuria), oliguria, as well as thrombotic complications: Arm or leg pain, tenderness or swelling, Homans' sign, prominence of superficial veins, chest pain, breathlessness, dyspnea. Drug should be discontinued promptly.
- Monitor vital signs and urine output.
- Lab tests: With prolonged therapy, monitor creatine phosphokinase activity and urinalyses for early detection of myopathy.

Patient & Family Education

- Report difficulty urinating or reddish-brown urine.
- Report arm or leg pain, chest pain, or difficulty breathing.

AMINOPHYLLINE (THEOPHYLLINE ETHYLENEDIAMIDE)

(am-in-off'i-lin)

Corophyllin ♣, Paladron ♣, Truphylline

Classifications: BRONCHODILATOR; (RESPIRATORY SMOOTH MUSCLE RELAXANT); XANTHINE

Therapeutic: BRONCHODILATOR

Prototype: Theophylline

Pregnancy Category: C

AVAILABILITY 100 mg, 200 mg tablets; 105 mg/5 mL oral liquid; 25 mg/mL injection; 250 mg, 500 mg suppositories

ACTION & *THERAPEUTIC EFFECT* A xanthine derivative that relaxes smooth muscle in the airways of the lungs and suppresses the response of the airways to stimuli that constrict them. *It is a respiratory smooth muscle relaxant that results in bronchodilation.*

USES To prevent and relieve symptoms of acute bronchial asthma and treatment of bronchospasm associ-

Common adverse effects in *italic*, life-threatening effects underlined; generic names in **bold**; classifications in SMALL CAPS; ♣ Canadian drug name; ⊕ Prototype drug

ated with chronic bronchitis and emphysema.

UNLABELED USES As a respiratory stimulant in Cheyne-Stokes respiration; for treatment of apnea and bradycardia in premature infants; as cardiac stimulant and diuretic in treatment of CHF.

CONTRAINDICATIONS Hypersensitivity to xanthine derivatives or to ethylenediamine component; cardiac arrhythmias; lactation.

CAUTIOUS USE Severe hypertension, cardiac disease, arrhythmias; impaired hepatic function; diabetes mellitus; hyperthyroidism; glaucoma; prostatic hypertrophy; fibrocystic breast disease; history of peptic ulcer; neonates and young children, patients over 55 y; COPD, acute influenza or patients receiving influenza immunization; pregnancy (category C).

ROUTE & DOSAGE

Bronchospasm

Adult: **IV Loading Dose** 6 mg/kg over 30 min **IV Maintenance Dose** *Nonsmoker,* 0.5 mg/kg/h; *smoker,* 0.8 mg/kg/h; *CHF or cirrhosis,* 0.1–0.2 mg/kg/h **PO** *Nonsmoker,* 0.5 mg/kg/h times 24 h in 4 divided doses; *smoker,* 0.75 mg/kg/h times 24 h in 4 divided doses; *CHF or cirrhosis,* 0.25 mg/kg/h times 24 h in 4 divided doses

Child: **IV Loading Dose** 6 mg/kg IV over 30 min **IV Maintenance Dose** *1–9 y,* 1 mg/kg/h; *older than 9 y,* 0.8 mg/kg/h **PO** *1–9 y,* 1 mg/kg/h times 24 h in 4 divided doses; *older than 9 y,* 0.75 mg/kg/h times 24 h in 4 divided doses

Infant: **PO/IV** *6–11 mo,* 0.7 g/kg/h; *2–6 mo,* 0.5 mg/kg/h

Neonatal Apnea

Neonate: **PO/IV Loading Dose** 5 mg/kg **PO/IV Maintenance Dose** 5 mg/kg/day divided q12h

Geriatric Patients: **PO** 6.25 mg/kg loading dose, then 2.5 mg/kg q8h

Obesity Dosage Adjustment

Calculate dose based on IBW

ADMINISTRATION

Oral

- Give with a full glass of water on an empty stomach (30 min–1 h before or 2 h after meals) for faster absorption, which is delayed but is not reduced with food.
- Minimize GI symptoms by taking immediately after a meal or with food.
- Do not chew or crush extended (controlled) release preparations before swallowing; however, if tablet is scored, it can be broken in half, then swallowed.
- Do mix contents of extended release capsules with soft, moist food to promote swallowing.

Suppository

- Note: Rectal preparations may be ordered when patient must fast or cannot tolerate the drug orally; absorption is enhanced if rectum is empty.

Intravenous

Verify correct IV concentration and rate of infusion with physician for neonates, infants, and children.

PREPARE: **IV Infusion:** Dilute loading dose in 100–200 mL NS, D5W, D5/NS, or LR. For continuous or intermittent infusion dilute in 500–1000 mL. ▪ Do not use aminophylline solutions if discolored or if crystals are present.

ADMINISTER: **IV Infusion:** Infuse at a rate not to exceed 25 mg/min.

INCOMPATIBILITIES **Solution/additive:** **Amikacin, bleomycin,** CEPHALOSPORINS, **chlorpromazine, ciprofloxacin, clindamycin, dimenhydrinate, dobutamine, doxorubicin, epinephrine, hydralazine, hydroxyzine, insulin, isoproterenol, meperidine, methylprednisolone, morphine, nafcillin, norepinephrine, papaverine, penicillin G, pentazocine, procaine, prochlorperazine, promazine, promethazine, verapamil, vitamin B complex with C, zinc.** **Y-site:** **Amiodarone, ciprofloxacin, clarithromycin, dobutamine, fenoldopam, hydralazine, lansoprazole, ondansetron, TPN, vinorelbine, warfarin.**

- Store at 15°–30° C (59°–86° F) in tightly closed containers unless otherwise directed. - Follow manufacturer's directions regarding storage of suppositories; some can be stored at room temperature; others **must be** refrigerated.

ADVERSE EFFECTS (≥1%) **CNS:** *Nervousness*, restlessness, depression, insomnia, irritability, headache, dizziness, muscle hyperactivity, convulsions. **CV:** Cardiac arrhythmias, tachycardia (with rapid IV), hyperventilation, chest pain, <u>severe hypotension, cardiac arrest</u>. **GI:** *Nausea, vomiting, anorexia*, hematemesis, diarrhea, epigastric pain.

INTERACTIONS **Drug:** Increases **lithium** excretion, lowering **lithium** levels; **cimetidine,** high-dose **allopurinol** (600 mg/day), **ciprofloxacin, erythromycin, troleandomycin** can significantly increase **theophylline** levels. **Herbal: St. John's wort** may decrease effect.

PHARMACOKINETICS **Absorption:** Most products are 100% absorbed from GI tract. **Peak:** IV 30 min; uncoated tablet 1 h; sustained release 4–6 h. **Duration:** 4–8 h; varies with age, smoking, and liver function. **Distribution:** Crosses placenta. **Metabolism:** Extensively in liver; by CYP1A2. **Elimination:** Parent drug and metabolites excreted by kidneys; excreted in breast milk. **Half-Life:** 3.7 h (child); 7.7 h (adult).

NURSING IMPLICATIONS

Assessment & Drug Effects

- Monitor for S&S of toxicity (generally related to theophylline serum levels over 20 mcg/mL). Observe patients receiving parenteral drug closely for signs of hypotension, arrhythmias, and convulsions until serum theophylline stabilizes within the therapeutic range.
- Note: High incidence of toxicity is associated with rectal suppository use due to erratic rate of absorption.
- Monitor and record vital signs and I&O. A sudden, sharp, unexplained rise in heart rate may indicate toxicity.
- Lab tests: Monitor serum theophylline levels.
- Note: Older adults, acutely ill, and patients with severe respiratory problems, liver dysfunction, or pulmonary edema are at greater risk of toxicity due to reduced drug clearance.
- Note: Children appear more susceptible to CNS stimulating effects of xanthines (nervousness, restlessness, insomnia, hyperactive reflexes, twitching, convulsions). Dosage reduction may be indicated.

Patient & Family Education

- Note: Use of tobacco tends to increase elimination of this drug (shortens half-life), necessitating higher dosage or shorter intervals than in nonsmokers.
- Report excessive nervousness or insomnia. Dosage reduction may be indicated.
- Note: Dizziness is a relatively common side effect, particularly in older adults; take necessary safety precautions.
- Do not take OTC remedies for treatment of asthma or cough unless approved by physician.

AMINOSALICYLIC ACID (*PARA*-AMINOSALICYLIC ACID)

(a-mee-noe-sal-i-sil′ik)

Paser

Classification: ANTITUBERCULOSIS

Therapeutic: ANTITUBERCULOSIS

Prototype: Isoniazid

Pregnancy Category: C

AVAILABILITY 4 g packets

ACTION & *THERAPEUTIC EFFECT* Aminosalicylic acid and salts are highly specific bacteriostatic agents that suppress growth and multiplication of *Mycobacterium tuberculosis* by preventing folic acid synthesis. Their mechanism of action resembles that of sulfonamides. Aminosalicylates also reportedly have potent hypolipemic action. *Aminosalicylates are an effective antiinfective alone or in combined therapy and reduce serum cholesterol and triglycerides by lowering LDL and VLDL.*

USES With streptomycin or isoniazid or both in treatment of pulmonary and extrapulmonary tuberculosis to delay drug resistance.

UNLABELED USES Documented for lipid-lowering effect.

CONTRAINDICATIONS Hypersensitivity to aminosalicylates, salicylates, or to compounds containing *para*-aminophenyl groups (e.g., sulfonamides, certain hair dyes); G6PD deficiency, use of the sodium salt in patients on sodium restriction or CHF; lactation.

CAUTIOUS USE Impaired renal and hepatic function; blood dyscrasias; goiter; gastric ulcer; pregnancy (category C).

ROUTE & DOSAGE

Tuberculosis

Adult: **PO** 10–12 g/day in 2–3 divided doses

Child: **PO** 150–300 mg/kg/day in 3–4 divided doses

ADMINISTRATION

Oral

- Give with or immediately following meals to reduce irritative gastric effects. Physician may order an antacid to be given concomitantly. Generally, GI adverse effects disappear after a few days of therapy.
- Store in tight, light-resistant containers in a cool, dry place, preferably at 15°–30° C (59°–86° F), unless otherwise directed.

ADVERSE EFFECTS (≥1%) **Body as a Whole:** Fever, chills, generalized malaise, joint pain, rash, fixed-drug eruptions, pruritus; vasculitis; Loeffler's syndrome. **CNS:** Psychotic reactions. **GI:** *Anorexia, nausea, vomiting, abdominal distress, diarrhea,* peptic ulceration, acute hepatitis, malabsorption. **Hematologic:** Leukopenia, agranulocytosis, eosinophilia, lymphocytosis, thrombocytopenia, hemolytic anemia; (G6PD deficiency), prothrombinemia. **Urogenital:** Renal (irritation), crystalluria. **Other:** With long-term administration, goiter.

DIAGNOSTIC TEST INTERFERENCE Aminosalicylates may interfere with urine ***urobilinogen*** determinations (using ***Ehrlich's reagent***), and may cause false-positive ***urinary protein*** and ***VMA*** determinations (with ***diazoreagent***); false-positive ***urine glucose*** may result with ***cupric sulfate tests*** (e.g., ***Benedict's solution***), but reportedly not with ***glucose oxidase reagents*** (e.g., ***TesTape, Clinistix***). Reduces ***serum cholesterol,*** and possibly ***serum potassium, serum PBI,*** and 24-hour ***I-131 thyroidal uptake*** (effect may last almost 14 days).

INTERACTIONS Drug: Increases hypoprothrombinemic effects of ORAL ANTICOAGULANTS; increased risk of crystalluria with **ammonium chloride, ascorbic acid;** decreased intestinal absorption of **cyanocobalamin, folic acid, digoxin;** ANTIHISTAMINES may inhibit PAS absorption; may increase or decrease **phenytoin** levels; **probenecid, sulfinpyrazone** decrease PAS elimination.

PHARMACOKINETICS Absorption: Almost completely from GI tract; sodium form more rapidly absorbed than the acid. **Peak:** 1.5–2 h. **Duration:** 4 h. **Distribution:** Well distributed to tissue and body fluids except CSF unless meninges are inflamed. **Metabolism:** In liver. **Elimination:** greater than 80% in urine in 7–10 h. **Half-Life:** 1 h.

NURSING IMPLICATIONS

Assessment & Drug Effects

- Monitor for abrupt onset of fever, particularly during the early weeks of therapy, and clinical picture resembling that of infectious mononucleosis (malaise, fatigue, generalized lymphadenopathy, splenomegaly, sore throat), as well as minor complaints of pruritus, joint pains, and headache, which strongly suggest hypersensitivity; report these symptoms promptly.
- Monitor I&O and encourage fluids. High concentrations of drug are excreted in urine, and this can cause crystalluria and hematuria.
- Note: To minimize crystalluria, keep urine neutral or alkaline with adjunctive drugs, such as antacids or with diet.

Patient & Family Education

- Rinse mouth with clear water or chew sugar-free gum or candy to relieve the mildly sour or bitter aftertaste of aminosalicylic acid.
- Note: Hypersensitivity reactions may occur after a few days, but most commonly in the fourth or fifth week; report promptly.
- Notify physician if sore throat or mouth, malaise, unusual fatigue, bleeding or bruising occurs (symptoms of blood dyscrasia).
- Note: Therapy generally lasts about 2 y. Adhere to the established drug regimen, and remain under close medical supervision to detect possible adverse drug effects during the treatment period. Resistant TB strains develop more rapidly when drug regimen is interrupted or is sporadic.
- Note: Urine may turn red on contact with bleach used in commercial toilet bowl cleaners.
- Do not take aspirin or other OTC drugs without physician's approval.
- Discard drug if it discolors (brownish or purplish); this signifies decomposition.

AMIODARONE HYDROCHLORIDE Pr

(a-mee'oh-da-rone)

Cordarone, Amio-Aqueous, Nexterone, Pacerone

Classification: ANTIARRHYTHMIC, CLASS III

Therapeutic: ANTIARRHYTHMIC, CLASS III; ANTIANGINAL

Pregnancy Category: D

AVAILABILITY 100 mg, 200 mg, 400 mg tablets; 50 mg/mL injection

ACTION & *THERAPEUTIC EFFECT* Class III antiarrhythmic; also has antianginal and antiadrenergic properties. Acts directly on all cardiac tissues by prolonging duration of action potential and refractory period without significantly affecting resting membrane potential. Slows conduction time through the AV node and can interrupt the reentry pathways through the AV node. *By direct action on smooth muscle, decreases peripheral resistance and increases coronary blood flow. Blocks effects of sympathetic stimulation.*

USES Prophylaxis and treatment of life-threatening ventricular arrhythmias and supraventricular arrhythmias, particularly with atrial fibrillation.

UNLABELED USES Treatment of nonexertional angina, conversion of atrial fibrillation to normal sinus rhythm, paroxysmal supraventricular tachycardia, ventricular rate control due to accessory pathway conduction in pre-excited atrial arrhythmia, after defibrillation and epinephrine in cardiac arrest, AV nodal reentry tachycardia.

CONTRAINDICATIONS Hypersensitivity to amiodarone, or benzyl alcohol; cardiogenic shock, severe sinus bradycardia, advanced AV block unless a pacemaker is available, severe sinus-node dysfunction or sick sinus syndrome, bradycardia, congenital or acquired QR prolongation syndromes, or history of torsades de pointes; severe liver disease, pregnancy (category D), lactation.

CAUTIOUS USE Hepatic disease, cirrhosis; Hashimoto's thyroiditis, goiter, thyrotoxicosis, or history of other thyroid dysfunction; mild to moderate hepatic toxicity; CHF, left ventricular dysfunction; hypersensitivity to iodine; older adults; Fabry disease, especially with visual disturbances; electrolyte imbalance, hypokalemia, hypomagnesemia, hypovolemia; preexisting lung disease, COPD; open heart surgery.

ROUTE & DOSAGE

Arrhythmias

Adult: **PO Loading Dose** 800–1600 mg/day in 1–2 doses for 1–3 wk **PO Maintenance Dose** 400–600 mg/day in 1–2 doses **IV Loading Dose** 150 mg over 10 min followed by 360 mg over next 6 h **IV Maintenance Dose** 540 mg over 18 h (0.5 mg/min), may continue at 0.5 mg/min **Convert IV to PO** Duration of infusion less than 1 wk use 800–1600 mg PO, 1–3 wk use 600–800 mg PO, greater than 3 wk use 400 mg PO

Child: **IV** 5 mg/kg then repeat to max of 300 mg total

Hepatic Impairment Dosage Adjustment

Adjustment only suggested in severe hepatic impairment

ADMINISTRATION

- Note: Correct hypokalemia and hypomagnesemia prior to initiation of therapy.

Oral

- Give consistently with respect to meals.
- Note: Only a physician experienced with the drug and treatment of life-threatening arrhythmias should give loading doses.
- Note: GI symptoms commonly occur during high-dose therapy, especially with loading doses. Symptoms usually respond to dose reduction or divided dose given with food, including milk.

Intravenous

PREPARE: **IV Infusion: First rapid loading dose infusion:** Add 150 mg (3 mL) amiodarone to 100 mL D5W to yield 1.5 mg/mL. **Second infusion during first 24 h (slow loading dose and maintenance infusion):** Add 900 mg (18 mL) amiodarone to 500 mL D5W to yield 1.8 mg/mL. **Maintenance infusions after the first 24 h:** Prepare concentrations of 1–6 mg/mL amiodarone. Note: Use central line to give concentrations greater than 2 mg/mL.

ADMINISTER: **IV Infusion:** Rapidly infuse initial 150 mg dose over the first 10 min at a rate of 15 mg/min. ▪ Over next 6 h, infuse 360 mg at a rate of 1 mg/min. ▪ Over the remaining 18 h, infuse 540 mg at a rate of 0.5 mg/min. ▪ After the first 24 h, infuse maintenance doses of 720 mg/24 h at a rate of 0.5 mg/min.

INCOMPATIBILITIES **Solution/additive:** **Aminophylline, amoxicillin/clavulanic acid, cefazolin, floxacillin, furosemide, quinidine.** **Y-site:** **Aminophylline, ampicillin/sulbactam, argatroban, atenolol, bivalirudin, cefamandole, cefazolin, ceftazidime, ceftopribole, digoxin, drotrecogin, ertapenem, heparin, imipenem/cilastatin, levofloxacin, magnesium sulfate, methotrexate, piperacillin, piperacillin/tazobactam, potassium phosphate, sodium bicarbonate, sodium nitroprusside, sodium phosphate, tigecycline.**

- Store at 15°–30° C (59°–86° F) protected from light, unless otherwise directed.

ADVERSE EFFECTS (≥1%) **CNS:** Peripheral neuropathy (*muscle weakness,* wasting numbness, tingling), *fatigue,* abnormal gait, dyskinesias, *dizziness,* paresthesia, headache. **CV:** Bradycardia, *hypotension* (IV), <u>sinus arrest, cardiogenic shock</u>, CHF, arrhythmias; AV block. **Special Senses:** *Corneal microdeposits,* blurred vision, optic neuritis, optic neuropathy, permanent blindness, corneal degeneration, macular degeneration, photosensitivity. **GI:** *Anorexia, nausea, vomiting, constipation,* <u>hepatotoxicity</u>. **Metabolic:** Hyperthyroidism or hypothyroidism; may cause neonatal hypo- or hyperthyroidism if taken during pregnancy. **Respiratory:** (Pulmonary toxicity) Alveolitis, pneumonitis (fever, dry cough, dyspnea), interstitial pulmonary fibrosis, <u>*fatal gasping syndrome*</u> with IV in children. **Skin:** Slate-blue pigmentation, *photosensitivity,* rash. **Other:** With chronic use, angioedema.

INTERACTIONS Drug: Significantly increases **digoxin** levels; enhances pharmacologic effects and toxicities of **disopyramide, procainamide, quinidine, flecainide, lidocaine, lovastatin, simvastatin;** anticoagulant effects of ORAL ANTICOAGULANTS enhanced; **verapamil, diltiazem,** BETA-ADRENERGIC BLOCKING AGENTS may potentiate sinus bradycardia, sinus arrest, or AV block; may increase **phenytoin** levels 2- to 3-fold; **cholestyramine** may decrease amiodarone levels; **fentanyl** may cause bradycardia, hypotension, or decreased output; may increase **cyclosporine** levels and toxicity; **cimetidine** may increase amiodarone levels; **ritonavir** may increase risk of amiodarone toxicity, including cardiotoxicity; **simvastatin** doses over 20 mg increase risk of rhabdomyolysis; **loratadine** use may increase risk of QT prolongation. **Food: Grapefruit juice** may increase amidarone concentrations. **Herbal: Echinacea** may increase hepatotoxicity, **St. John's wort** may decrease efficacy. **Lab Test:** Affects thyroid function tests, causing an increase in serum T_4 and serum reverse T_3 levels, and a decline in serum T_3 levels.

PHARMACOKINETICS Absorption: 22–86% absorbed. **Onset (PO):** 2–3 days to 1–3 wk. **Peak:** 3–7 h. **Distribution:** Concentrates in adipose tissue, lungs, kidneys, spleen; crosses placenta; 96% protein bound. **Metabolism:** Extensively in liver; undergoes some enterohepatic cycling; via CYP2C8 and 3A4. **Elimination:** Excreted chiefly in bile and feces; also in breast milk. **Half-Life:** Biphasic, initial 2.5–10 days, terminal 40–55 days.

NURSING IMPLICATIONS

Assessment & Drug Effects

- Monitor BP carefully during infusion and slow the infusion if significant hypotension occurs; bradycardia should be treated by slowing the infusion or discontinuing if necessary. Monitor heart rate and rhythm and BP until drug response has stabilized; report promptly symptomatic bradycardia. Sustained monitoring is essential because drug has an unusually long half-life.
- Monitor for S&S of: Adverse effects, particularly conduction disturbances and exacerbation of arrhythmias, in patients receiving concomitant antiarrhythmic therapy (reduce dosage of previous agent by 30–50% several days after amiodarone therapy is started); drug-induced hypothyroidism or hyperthyroidism (see Appendix F), especially during early treatment period; pulmonary toxicity (progressive dyspnea, fatigue, cough, pleuritic pain, fever) throughout therapy.
- Lab tests: Baseline and periodic assessments should be made of liver, lung, thyroid, neurologic, and GI function. Drug may cause thyroid function test abnormalities in the absence of thyroid function impairment.
- Monitor for elevations of AST and ALT. If elevations persist or if they are 2–3 times above normal baseline readings, reduce dosage or withdraw drug promptly to prevent hepatotoxicity and liver damage.
- Auscultate chest periodically or when patient complains of respiratory symptoms. Check for diminished breath sounds, rales, pleuritic friction rub; observe breathing pattern. Drug-induced pulmonary function problems **must be** distinguished from CHF or pneumonia. Keep physician informed.
- Anticipate possible CNS symptoms within a week after amiodarone therapy begins. Proximal muscle weakness, a common side effect, intensified by tremors presents a great hazard to the ambulating patient. Assess severity of symptoms. Supervision of ambulation may be indicated.

Patient & Family Education

- Check pulse daily once stabilized, or as prescribed. Report a pulse less than 60.
- Take oral drug consistently with respect to meals.
- Become familiar with potential adverse reactions and report those that are bothersome to the physician.
- Use dark glasses to ease photophobia; some patients may not be able to go outdoors in the daytime even with such protection.
- Follow recommendation for regular ophthalmic exams, including funduscopy and slit-lamp exam.
- Wear protective clothing and a barrier-type sunscreen that physically blocks penetration of skin by ultraviolet light (e.g., titanium oxide or zinc formulations) to prevent a photosensitivity reaction (erythema, pruritus); avoid exposure to sun and sunlamps.

AMITRIPTYLINE HYDROCHLORIDE

(a-mee-trip'ti-leen)

Amitril, Apo-Amitriptyline ✦, Emitrip, Endep, Enovil, Levate ✦, Meravil, Novotriptyn ✦, SK-Amitriptyline

Classification: TRICYCLIC ANTIDEPRESSANT

Therapeutic: ANTIDEPRESSANT

Prototype: Imipramine

Pregnancy Category: C

AVAILABILITY 10 mg, 25 mg, 50 mg, 75 mg, 100 mg, 150 mg tablets; 10 mg/mL injection

ACTION & *THERAPEUTIC EFFECT* A tricyclic antidepressant (TCA) that inhibits the reuptake of serotonin (5-HT) and norepinephrine from the synaptic gap; also inhibits norepinephrine reuptake to a moderate degree. Restoration of the levels of these neurotransmitters is a proposed mechanism of its antidepressant action. *Interference with the reuptake of serotonin and norepinephrine results in the antidepressant activity of amitriptyline.*

USES Endogenous depression.

UNLABELED USES Prophylaxis for cluster, migraine, and chronic tension headaches; intractable pain, peptic ulcer disease, to increase muscle strength in myotonic dystrophy, to treat pathologic weeping and laughing secondary to forebrain disease, for eating disorders associated with depression (anorexia or bulimia), and as sedative for nondepressed patients.

CONTRAINDICATIONS TCA hypersensitivity; acute recovery period after MI, cardiac arrhythmias, AV block, long-QT prolongation; suicidal ideation; history of seizure disorders; lactation, children younger than 12 y.

CAUTIOUS USE Prostatic hypertrophy, history of urinary retention or obstruction; angle-closure glaucoma; diabetes mellitus; history of hematologic disorders; history of alcoholism; GERD, BPH; hyperthyroidism; patient with cardiovascular, hepatic, or renal dysfunction; patient with suicidal tendency, electroshock therapy; elective surgery; schizophrenia; respiratory disorders; Parkinson's disease; seizure disorders; older adults, adolescents; pregnancy (category C).

ROUTE & DOSAGE

Antidepressant

Adult: **PO** 25–75 mg/day, may gradually increase to 150–300 mg/day **IM** 20–30 mg q.i.d. until patient can take PO

Common adverse effects in *italic*, life-threatening effects underlined; generic names in **bold**; classifications in SMALL CAPS; ✦ Canadian drug name; ⊕ Prototype drug

Adolescent/Geriatric: **PO** 10 mg t.i.d. with 20 mg at bedtime (max: 150–200 mg/day)

Pharmacogenetic Dosage Adjustment

CYP2D6 poor metabolizers: Dose at 60–75% of normal dose

ADMINISTRATION

Oral

- Give with or immediately after food to reduce possibility of GI irritation. Tablet may be crushed if patient is unable to take it whole; administer with food or fluid.
- Give increased doses preferably in late afternoon or at bedtime due to sedative action that precedes antidepressant effect.
- Give as single dose at bedtime to promote sleep or for patients with dizziness or when daytime sedation interferes with work productivity.
- Note that dose is usually tapered over 2 wk at discontinuation to prevent withdrawal symptoms (headache, nausea, malaise, musculoskeletal pain, panic attack, weakness).

ADVERSE EFFECTS (≥1%) **CNS:** *Drowsiness, sedation, dizziness,* nervousness, restlessness, fatigue, headache, insomnia, abnormal movements (extrapyramidal symptoms), seizures. **CV:** *Orthostatic hypotension,* tachycardia, palpitation, ECG changes. **Special Senses:** Blurred vision, mydriasis. **GI:** *Dry mouth,* increased appetite especially for sweets, *constipation,* weight gain, sour or metallic taste, nausea, vomiting. **Urogenital:** *Urinary retention.* **Other:** (Rare) Bone marrow depression.

INTERACTIONS Drug: ANTIHYPERTENSIVES may decrease some antihypertensive response; CNS DEPRESSANTS, **alcohol,** HYPNOTICS, BARBITURATES, SEDATIVES potentiate CNS depression; ANTICOAGULANTS, ORAL, may increase hypoprothrombinemic effect; **ethchlorvynol,** transient delirium; **levodopa,** SYMPATHOMIMETICS (e.g., **epinephrine, norepinephrine**), possibility of sympathetic hyperactivity with hypertension and hyperpyrexia; MAO INHIBITORS, possibility of severe reactions, toxic psychosis, cardiovascular instability; **methylphenidate** increases plasma TCA levels; THYROID DRUGS may increase possibility of arrhythmias; **cimetidine** may increase plasma TCA levels. **Herbal: Ginkgo** may decrease seizure threshold, **St. John's wort** may cause serotonin syndrome and increase adverse effects.

PHARMACOKINETICS Absorption: Rapidly from GI tract. **Peak:** 2–12 h. **Distribution:** Crosses placenta. **Metabolism:** In liver (CYP2D6). **Elimination:** Primarily in urine; enters breast milk. **Half-Life:** 10–50 h.

NURSING IMPLICATIONS

Assessment & Drug Effects

- Monitor therapeutic effectiveness. It may take 1–6 wk to reduce attacks when used for migraine prophylaxis.
- Monitor for S&S of drowsiness and dizziness (initial stages of therapy); institute measures to prevent falling. Also monitor for overdose or suicide ideation in patients who use excessive amounts of alcohol.
- Lab tests: Baseline and periodic leukocyte and differential counts; renal and hepatic function tests; eye examinations (including glaucoma testing); recommended particularly for older adults, adolescents, and patients receiving high doses/prolonged therapy.

- Monitor BP and pulse rate in patients with preexisting cardiovascular disease. Assess for orthostatic hypotension especially in older adults. Withhold drug if there is a rise or fall in systolic BP (by 10–20 mm Hg), or a sudden increase or a significant change in pulse rate or rhythm. Notify physician.
- Monitor I&O, including bowel elimination pattern.

Patient & Family Education

- Monitor weight; drug may increase appetite or a craving for sweets.
- Understand that tolerance/adaptation to anticholinergic actions (see Appendix F) usually develops with maintenance regimen. Keep physician informed.
- Relieve dry mouth by taking frequent sips of water and increasing total fluid intake.
- Make position change slowly and in stages to prevent dizziness.
- Do not drive or engage in potentially hazardous activities until response to drug is known.
- Do not use OTC drugs without consulting physician while on TCA therapy; many preparations contain sympathomimetic amines.
- Note: Amitriptyline may turn urine blue-green.

AMLEXANOX

(am-lex'a-nox)

Aphthasol, OraDisc A

Classification: ANTI-INFLAMMATORY

Therapeutic: ANTI-INFLAMMATORY

Pregnancy Category: B

AVAILABILITY 5% paste; 2 mg mucoadhesive disc

ACTION & *THERAPEUTIC EFFECT* Amlexanox is a potent inhibitor of inflammatory mediators (e.g., leukotrienes, IgE, IgG). Its mechanism of healing is unknown. *Amlexanox reduces healing time and pain related to aphthous ulcers or canker sores.*

USES Treatment of aphthous ulcers in patients with normal immune systems.

CONTRAINDICATIONS Sensitivity to amlexanox or benzyl alcohol.

CAUTIOUS USE Immunosuppressed patients; pregnancy (category B), lactation. Safety and efficacy in children are not established.

ROUTE & DOSAGE

Aphthous Ulcers

Adult: **Topical** Apply 1/4 in. (0.5 cm) to finger and dab onto each mouth ulcer q.i.d. (after oral hygiene p.c. and at bedtime) for 10-day cycle; apply disc to each mouth ulcer and allow to dissolve

ADMINISTRATION

Topical

- Apply after oral hygiene following each meal and before bedtime.
- Avoid prolonged contact with skin and wash off skin if contact occurs.
- Store at 15°–30° C (59°–86° F) away from heat and moisture. Do not freeze.

ADVERSE EFFECTS (≥1%) **Body as a Whole:** Transient pain, stinging, or burning at application site.

PHARMACOKINETICS Absorption: Minimally absorbed through ulcer. **Onset:** Approximately 3 days. **Elimination:** 17% in urine. **Half-Life:** 3.5 h.

NURSING IMPLICATIONS

Assessment & Drug Effects

- Discontinue use if rash or inflamed membranes develop.

Patient & Family Education

- Use at first sign of canker sore. Wash hands before and immediately after application.
- Flush eyes immediately with large amount of cold water if paste accidentally comes in contact with eyes or eye area.
- Contact physician if healing does not result after 10 days of therapy.

AMLODIPINE

(am-lo′di-peen)

Norvasc

Classifications: CALCIUM CHANNEL BLOCKER; ANTIHYPERTENSIVE

Therapeutic: ANTIHYPERTENSIVE; ANTIANGINAL

Prototype: Nifedipine

Pregnancy Category: C

AVAILABILITY 2.5 mg, 5 mg, 10 mg tablets

ACTION & *THERAPEUTIC EFFECT* Amlodipine is a calcium channel blocking agent that selectively blocks calcium influx across cell membranes of cardiac and vascular smooth muscle without changing serum calcium concentrations. It reduces coronary vascular resistance and increases coronary blood flow. Additionally, amlodipine decreases peripheral vascular resistance, increases oxygen delivery to myocardial tissue, and increases cardiac output. *Amlodipine reduces systolic, diastolic, and mean arterial blood pressure. It also decreases pain due to angina.*

USES Treatment of mild to moderate hypertension and stable angina.

CONTRAINDICATIONS Hypersensitivity to amlodipine; hypotension; severe obstructive coronary artery disease; severe aortic stenosis.

CAUTIOUS USE Liver disease; concomitant use with hypotension; CHF, ventricular dysfunction; lactation; older adults; children younger than 6 y, GERD; hepatic disease; pregnancy (category C).

ROUTE & DOSAGE

Hypertension

Adult: **PO** 5–10 mg once daily

Geriatric: Start with 2.5 mg, adjust dose at intervals of not less than 2 wk

Adolescent/Child (at least 6 y old): **PO** 2.5–5 mg daily (max: 10 mg)

Stable/Vasospastic Angina

Adult: **PO** 5–10 mg daily (usually 10 mg)

Hepatic Impairment Dosage Adjustment

Start with 2.5 mg, adjust dose at intervals of not less than 2 wk

ADMINISTRATION

Oral

- Give drug without regard to meals.
- Prescribed initial dosages of 2.5 mg daily are common if added to a regimen including other antihypertensive drugs.
- Note: Doses are usually titrated over a period of 14 days or more rapidly if warranted.
- Store at 15°–30° C (59°–86° F).

ADVERSE EFFECTS (≥1%) **CV:** Palpitations, flushing tachycardia, *peripheral or facial edema*, bradycardia, chest pain, syncope, postural hypotension. **CNS:** Light-headedness, fatigue, *headache*. **GI:** Abdominal pain, nausea, anorexia, constipation, dyspepsia, dysphagia, diarrhea, flatulence, vomiting. **Urogenital:** Sexual dysfunction, frequency, nocturia. **Respiratory:** Dyspnea. **Skin:** Flushing, rash. **Other:** Arthralgia, cramps, myalgia.

INTERACTIONS Drug: Adenosine may increase the risk of bradycardia; **bosentan** may decrease efficacy of amlodipine; additive hypotensive effects with other ANTIHYPERTENSIVE AGENTS; AZOLE ANTIFUNGALS (e.g., **fluconazole, itraconazole**) may inhibit metabolism of amlodipine; **itraconazole** may increase edema. **Food: Grapefruit juice** may increase amlodipine levels. **Herbal: Ephedra, ma huang, melatonin** may antagonize antihypertensive effects.

PHARMACOKINETICS Absorption: Greater than 90% absorbed from GI tract. **Peak:** 6–9 h. **Duration:** 24 h. **Distribution:** Greater than 95% protein bound. **Metabolism:** In liver (CYP3A4) to inactive metabolites. **Elimination:** In urine (less than 5–10% excreted unchanged), 20–25% in feces. **Half-Life:** Less than 45 y: 28–69 h; greater than 60 y: 40–120 h.

NURSING IMPLICATIONS

Assessment & Drug Effects

- Monitor BP for therapeutic effectiveness. BP reduction is greatest after peak levels of amlodipine are achieved 6–9 h following oral doses.
- Monitor for S&S of dose-related peripheral or facial edema that may not be accompanied by weight gain; rarely, severe edema may cause discontinuation of drug.
- Monitor BP with postural changes. Report postural hypotension. Monitor more frequently when additional antihypertensives or diuretics are added.
- Monitor heart rate; dose-related palpitations (more common in women) may occur.

Patient & Family Education

- Report significant swelling of face or extremities.
- Take care to have support when standing and walking due to possible dose-related light-headedness/dizziness.
- Report shortness of breath, palpitations, irregular heartbeat, nausea, or constipation to physician.

AMMONIUM CHLORIDE

(ah-mo′ni-um)

Classification: ELECTROLYTIC BALANCE AGENT
Therapeutic: ACIDFIER; ELECTROLYTE REPLACEMENT
Pregnancy Category: B

AVAILABILITY 26.75% or 5 mEq/mL solution; 500 mg tablets; 486 mg enteric-coated tablets

ACTION & *THERAPEUTIC EFFECT* Acidifying property is due to conversion of ammonium ion (NH_4^+) to urea in liver with liberation of H^+ and Cl^-. Potassium excretion also increases acid, but to a lesser extent. *Effective as a systemic acidifier in metabolic alkalosis by releasing H^+ ions which lower pH.*

USES Treatment of hypochloremic states and metabolic alkalosis. Diuretic or urinary acidifying agent.

CONTRAINDICATIONS Severe renal or hepatic insufficiency; primary respiratory acidosis.
CAUTIOUS USE Cardiac edema, cardiac insufficiency, pulmonary insufficiency; pregnancy (category B), lactation.

ROUTE & DOSAGE

Urine Acidifier, Diuretic
Adult: **PO** 4–12 g/day divided q4–6h
Child: **PO** 75 mg/kg/day in 4 divided doses

Metabolic Alkalosis and Hypochloremic States
Adult/Child: **IV** Dose calculated on basis of CO_2 combining power or serum Cl deficit, 50% of calculated deficit is administered slowly

ADMINISTRATION

Oral

- Give after meals for best tolerance or use enteric-coated tablets. Tablets should be swallowed whole.
- Store in airtight container.

Intravenous

Check with physician for slower rate for infants.

PREPARE: **Intermittent:** Dilute each 20 mL vial in 500–1000 mL NS. Do not exceed a concentration of 1–2%.

ADMINISTER: **Intermittent:** Give slowly to avoid serious adverse effects (ammonia toxicity) and local irritation and pain. ▪ Give at a rate not to exceed 5 mL/min.

INCOMPATIBILITIES **Solution/additive:** **Codeine phosphate, dimenhydrinate.** **Y-site:** **Warfarin.**

▪ Avoid freezing. ▪ Concentrated solutions crystallize at low temperatures. ▪ Crystals can be dissolved by placing intact container in a warm water bath and warming to room temperature.

ADVERSE EFFECTS (≥1%) **Body as a Whole:** Most secondary to ammonia toxicity. **CNS:** Headache, depression, drowsiness, twitching, excitability; EEG abnormalities. **CV:** Bradycardia and other arrhythmias. **GI:** Gastric irritation, nausea, vomiting, anorexia. **Metabolic:** Metabolic acidosis, hyperammonia. **Respiratory:** Hyperventilation. **Skin:** Rash. **Urogenital:** Glycosuria. **Other:** Pain and irritation at IV site.

DIAGNOSTIC TEST INTERFERENCE Ammonium chloride may increase ***blood ammonia*** and ***AST,*** decrease ***serum magnesium*** (by increasing urinary magnesium excretion), and decrease ***urine urobilinogen.***

INTERACTIONS Drug: Aminosalicylic acid may cause crystalluria; increases urinary excretion of AMPHETAMINES, **flecainide, mexiletine, methadone, ephedrine, pseudoephedrine;** decreased urinary excretion of SULFONYLUREAS, SALICYLATES.

PHARMACOKINETICS Absorption: Completely absorbed in 3–6 h. **Metabolism:** In liver to HCl and urea. **Elimination:** Primarily in urine.

NURSING IMPLICATIONS

Assessment & Drug Effects

- Assess IV infusion site frequently for signs of irritation. Change site as warranted.
- Monitor for S&S of: Metabolic acidosis (mental status changes including confusion, disorientation, coma, respiratory changes including increased respiratory rate and depth, exertional dyspnea); ammonium toxicity (cardiac arrhythmias including bradycardia, irregular respirations, twitching, seizures).
- Monitor I&O ratio and pattern. The diuretic effect of ammonium chloride is compensatory and lasts only 1–2 days.
- Lab tests: Baseline and periodic determinations of CO_2 combining power, serum electrolytes, and

urinary and arterial pH during therapy to avoid serious acidosis.

Patient & Family Education

- Report pain at IV injection site.

AMOXAPINE

(a-mox'a-peen)

Classification: TRICYCLIC ANTIDEPRESSANT
Therapeutic: ANTIDEPRESSANT
Prototype: Imipramine
Pregnancy Category: C

AVAILABILITY 25 mg, 50 mg, 100 mg, 150 mg tablets

ACTION & *THERAPEUTIC EFFECT* Tricyclic antidepressant (TCA) with mixed antidepressant and tranquilizing properties. Antidepressant activity is thought to be due to reduced reuptake of norepinephrine and serotonin at the cell membrane of the neuron, thus increasing the level of both neurotransmitters. *Enhancement of neurotransmitters results in its antidepressant activity.*

USES Neurotic and endogenous depression accompanied by anxiety or agitation.

CONTRAINDICATIONS Hypersensitivity to other tricyclic compounds; acute recovery period after MI; AV block; MAOI therapy, QT prolongation; suicidal ideation; lactation, children younger than 16 y of age.
CAUTIOUS USE History of convulsive disorders, schizophrenia, manic depression, electroshock therapy; alcohol abuse; history of urinary retention, benign prostatic hypertrophy; angle-closure glaucoma or increased intraocular pressure; cardiovascular disorders; impaired renal or hepatic function; elective surgery; pregnancy (category C).

ROUTE & DOSAGE

Antidepressant

Adult: **PO** Start at 50 mg b.i.d. or t.i.d., may increase on third day to 100 mg t.i.d. Maintenance doses less than 300 mg/day as single dose at bedtime.
Geriatric: **PO** 25 mg at bedtime, may increase q3–7days to 50–150 mg/day in divided doses (max: 300 mg/day)

ADMINISTRATION

Oral

- Give with or after food to reduce GI irritation; tablet may be crushed and taken with fluid or mixed with food.
- Give maintenance dose as a single dose at bedtime to minimize daytime sedation and other annoying drug adverse effects.
- Do not abruptly discontinue drug. Doses should be tapered over 2 wk.
- Store at 15°–30° C (59°–86° F) in tightly closed container unless otherwise directed.

ADVERSE EFFECTS (≥1%) **CNS:** *Drowsiness,* dizziness, headache, fatigue, *sedation,* lethargy; extrapyramidal effects (acute dystonic reactions, panic attacks, parkinsonism, tardive dyskinesia), seizures (overdosage). **CV:** Orthostatic hypotension; arrhythmias. **GI:** Constipation, diarrhea, flatulence, *dry mouth,* peculiar taste, nausea, heartburn. **Special Senses:** Blurred vision, dry eyes. **Urogenital:** Nephrotoxicity (overdosage).

INTERACTIONS Drug: May decrease response to ANTIHYPERTENSIVES; CNS DEPRESSANTS, **alcohol,** HYPNOTICS, BARBITURATES, SEDATIVES potentiate CNS depression; may increase hypoprothrombinemic effect of ORAL ANTICOAGULANTS; **ethchlorvynol,** transient delirium; with **levodopa,** SYMPATHOMIMETICS (e.g., **epinephrine, norepinephrine**), possibility of sympathetic hyperactivity with hypertension and hyperpyrexia; with MAO INHIBITORS, possibility of severe reactions: toxic psychosis, cardiovascular instability; **methylphenidate** increases plasma TCA levels; thyroid drugs may increase possibility of arrhythmias; **cimetidine** may increase plasma TCA levels. **Herbal: Ginkgo** may decrease seizure threshold, **St. John's wort** may cause serotonin syndrome.

PHARMACOKINETICS Absorption: Rapidly absorbed. **Peak:** 1–2 h. **Distribution:** Probably crosses placenta; distributed into breast milk. **Metabolism:** Via CYP2D6; active metabolite. **Elimination:** 60% in urine in 6 days; 7–18% in feces. **Half-Life:** 8 h parent drug, 30 h metabolite.

NURSING IMPLICATIONS

Assessment & Drug Effects

- Monitor therapeutic effectiveness. Initial antidepressant effect (mild euphoria, increased energy) may occur within 4–7 days; however, in most patients clinical response does not occur until after 2–3 wk of drug therapy.
- Supervise patient closely during therapy for suicidal ideation and potential serious adverse effects.
- Report immediately signs of neuroleptic malignant syndrome: Fever, sweating, rigidity (catatonia), unstable BP, rapid, irregular pulse; changes in level of consciousness, coma. Although rare, it can be life-threatening if drug is not stopped immediately. Death can result from acute respiratory, renal, or cardiovascular failure.
- Report immediately the onset of signs of tardive dyskinesia (see Appendix F); careful observation/reporting may prevent irreversibility.
- Monitor I&O ratio and bowel elimination pattern. Report continuing constipation.

Patient & Family Education

- Follow directions for taking this drug (see ADMINISTRATION).
- Do not abruptly discontinue drug. Dosage should be tapered over 2 wk. Maintain established dosage regimen. Do not skip, reduce, or double doses or change dose intervals.
- Minimize alcohol intake as it may potentiate drug effects, thus increasing the dangers of overdosage or suicidal ideation.
- Drink at least 2000 mL (approximately 2 qts) fluid daily and eat foods with high fiber content (if allowed) to provide needed roughage.
- Monitor weight at least weekly and report significant weight gain.
- Do not drive or engage in potentially hazardous tasks until response to drug is known.
- Rinse mouth frequently with clear water, especially after eating, to relieve mouth dryness.
- Do not take any prescription or OTC drugs without consulting physician.

AMOXICILLIN

(a-mox-i-sill'in)

Amoxil, Apo-Amoxi ♣, Moxatag, Trimox

Classifications: ANTIBIOTIC; AMINOPENICILLIN
Therapeutic: ANTIBIOTIC
Prototype: Ampicillin
Pregnancy Category: B

AVAILABILITY 125 mg, 200 mg, 250 mg, 400 mg, 500 mg tablets; 250 mg, 500 mg capsules; 50 mg/mL, 125 mg/5 mL, 200 mg/5 mL, 250 mg/5 mL, 400 mg/5 mL powder for suspension; 775 mg extended release tabs

ACTION & *THERAPEUTIC EFFECT* Broad-spectrum semisynthetic aminopenicillin and analog of ampicillin. Like other penicillins, amoxicillin inhibits the final stage of bacterial cell wall synthesis by binding to specific penicillin-binding proteins (PBPs) located inside the cell wall of rapidly multiplying bacteria. It results in bacterial cell lysis and death. *Active against both aerobic gram-positive and aerobic gram-negative bacteria.*

USES Infections of ear, nose, throat, GU tract, skin, and soft tissue caused by susceptible bacteria. Also used in uncomplicated gonorrhea.

CONTRAINDICATIONS Hypersensitivity to penicillins; infectious mononucleosis.

CAUTIOUS USE History of or suspected atopy or allergy (hives, eczema, hay fever, asthma); history of cephalosporin or carbapenem hypersensitivity; colitis, dialysis, diarrhea, GI disease; viral infection, syphilis, severe hepatic impairment; renal impairment or failure, diabetes mellitus, leukemia, pregnancy (category B); lactation.

ROUTE & DOSAGE

Mild to Moderate Infections

Adult: **PO** 250–500 mg q8h
Child/Infant (at least 3 mo): **PO** 25–50 mg/kg/day (max: 60–80 mg/kg/day) divided q8h or 200–400 mg q12h
Neonate/Infant (up to 3 mo): **PO** 20–30 mg/kg/day divided q12h

Gonorrhea

Adult: **PO** 3 g as single dose with 1 g probenecid
Child (2 y or older): **PO** 50 mg/kg as single dose with probenecid 25 mg/kg

Tonsillitis/Pharyngitis (extended release tabs)

Adult/Adolescent: **PO** 775 mg daily with food

Renal Impairment Dosage Adjustment

CrCl 10–30 mL/min: 250–500 mg q12h; less than 10 mL/min: 250–500 mg q24h
Hemodialysis Dosage Adjustment: Admininister extra dose after dialysis

ADMINISTRATION

Oral

- Ensure that chewable tablets are chewed or crushed before being swallowed with a liquid.
- Do not crush or chew extended release tablets.
- Place reconstituted pediatric drops directly on child's tongue or add to formula, milk, fruit juice, water, ginger ale, or other soft drink. Have child drink all the prepared dose promptly.
- Store in tightly covered containers at 15°–30° C (59°–86° F) unless otherwise directed. Reconstituted oral suspensions are stable for 7 days at room temperature.

ADVERSE EFFECTS (≥1%) **Body as a Whole:** As with other penicillins. Hypersensitivity (rash, <u>anaphylaxis</u>), superinfections. **GI:** Diarrhea, nausea, vomiting, <u>pseudomembranous colitis</u> (rare). **Hematologic:** Hemolytic anemia, eosinophilia, <u>agranulocytosis</u> (rare). **Skin:** Pruritus, urticaria, or other skin eruptions. **Special Senses:** Conjunctival ecchymosis.

INTERACTIONS TETRACYCLINES may inhibit activity of amoxicillin; **probenecid** prolongs the activity of amoxicillin.

PHARMACOKINETICS Absorption: Nearly complete absorption. **Peak:** 1–2 h. **Distribution:** Diffuses into most tissues and body fluids, except synovial fluid and CSF (unless meninges are inflamed); crosses placenta; distributed into breast milk in small amounts. **Metabolism:** In liver. **Elimination:** 60% in urine. **Half-Life:** 1–1.3 h.

NURSING IMPLICATIONS

Assessment & Drug Effects

- Determine previous hypersensitivity reactions to penicillins, cephalosporins, and other allergens prior to therapy.
- Lab tests: Baseline C&S tests prior to initiation of therapy, start drug pending results; periodic assessments of renal, hepatic, and hematologic functions should be made during prolonged therapy.
- Monitor for S&S of an urticarial rash (usually occurring within a few days after start of drug) suggestive of a hypersensitivity reaction. If it occurs, look for other signs of hypersensitivity (fever, wheezing, generalized itching, dyspnea), and report to physician immediately.
- Report onset of generalized, erythematous, maculopapular rash (ampicillin rash) to physician. Ampicillin rash is not due to hypersensitivity; however, hypersensitivity should be ruled out.
- Monitor for and report diarrhea which may indicate pseudomembranous colitis.

Patient & Family Education

- Take drug around the clock, do not miss a dose, and continue therapy until all medication is taken, unless otherwise directed by physician.
- Report onset of diarrhea and other possible symptoms of superinfection to physician (see Appendix F).

AMOXICILLIN AND CLAVULANATE POTASSIUM

(a-mox-i-sill′in)

Amoclan, Augmentin, Augmentin-ES600, Augmentin XR, Clavulin ♣

Classifications: BETA-LACTAM ANTIBIOTIC; AMINOPENICILLIN

Therapeutic: ANTIBIOTIC

Prototype: Ampicillin

Pregnancy Category: B

AVAILABILITY 250 mg, 500 mg, 875 mg tablets; 125 mg, 200 mg, 400 mg chewable tablets; 125 mg/5 mL, 200 mg/5 mL, 250 mg/5 mL, 400 mg/5 mL, 600 mg/5 mL oral suspension; 1000 mg amoxicillin/62.5 mg clavulanate sustained release tablets

ACTION & *THERAPEUTIC EFFECT* As a beta-lactam antibiotic, amoxicillin is bactericidal. It inhibits the final stage of bacterial cell wall synthesis by binding with specific penicillin-binding proteins (PBPs) that are located inside the bacterial cell wall that leads to bacterial cell lysis and death. *Effectivenes of ampicillin is synergistic in combination with clavulanic acid. Clavulanic acid in combination with ampicillin inhibits enzyme (beta-lactamase) degradation of amoxicillin and by synergism extends both spectrum of activity and bactericidal effect of* *amoxicillin against many strains of beta-lactamase-producing bacteria resistant to amoxicillin alone.*

USES Infections caused by susceptible beta-lactamase-producing organisms: Lower respiratory tract infections, acute bacterial sinusitis, community acquired pneumonia, otitis media, sinusitis, skin and skin structure infections, and UTI.

CONTRAINDICATIONS Hypersensitivity to penicillins; infectious mononucleosis; patient with previous history of drug-induced cholestasis, jaundice, or other hepatic dysfunction; severe renal impairment.
CAUTIOUS USE Allergic disorders; cephalosporin hypersensitivity; GI disorders; colitis; hepatic or renal disease; elderly; pregnancy (category B), lactation.

ROUTE & DOSAGE

Mild to Moderate Infections

Adult: **PO** 250 or 500 mg tablet (each with 125 mg clavulanic acid) q8–12h; Sustained release tabs: 2 tablets (2000 mg amoxicillin/125 mg clavulanate) q12h × 7–10 days
Child: **PO** *Less than 40 kg,* 20–40 mg/kg/day (based on amoxicillin component) divided q8–12h; *older than 3 mo,* 90 mg/kg/day of 600 ES divided q12h × 10 days
Neonate/Infant (younger than 3 mo): **PO** 30 mg/kg/day (amoxicillin) divided q12h

ADMINISTRATION

Oral

- Give at the start of a meal to minimize GI upset and enhance absorption.
- Note that both 250 and 500 mg tablets contain the exact amount of clavulanic acid (125 mg and potassium salt); therefore, two 250 mg tablets are not equivalent to one 500 mg tablet.
- Reconstitute oral suspension by adding amount of water specified on container to provide a 5 mL suspension. Tap bottle before adding water to loosen powder, then add water in 2 portions, agitating suspension well before each addition.
- Agitate suspension well just before administration of each dose.
- Give dialysis patient an additional 2 doses on the day of dialysis; one dose before and another dose after dialysis.
- Store tablets in tight containers at less than 24° C (71° F). Reconstituted oral suspension should be refrigerated at 2°–8° C (36°–46° F), then discarded after 10 days.

ADVERSE EFFECTS (≥1%) **GI:** *Diarrhea,* nausea, vomiting. **Skin:** Rash, urticaria. **Other:** Candidal vaginitis; moderate increases in serum ALT, AST; hypersensitivity reactions, glomerulonephritis; agranulocytosis (rare).

DIAGNOSTIC TEST INTERFERENCE May interfere with ***urinary glucose*** determinations using ***cupric sulfate, Benedict's solution, Clinitest;*** does not affect ***glucose oxidase methods*** (e.g., Clinistix, TesTape). Positive direct ***antiglobulin*** (***Coombs'***) test results may be reported, a reaction that could interfere with ***hematologic studies*** or with ***transfusion cross-matching*** procedures.

INTERACTIONS Drug: TETRACYCLINES may inhibit activity of amoxicillin; **probenecid** prolongs the activity of amoxicillin.

PHARMACOKINETICS Absorption: Nearly complete absorption. **Peak:** 1–2 h. **Distribution:** Diffuses into most tissues and body fluids, except synovial fluid and CSF (unless meninges are inflamed); crosses placenta; distributed into breast milk in very small amounts. **Metabolism:** In liver. **Elimination:** 50–73% of the amoxicillin and 25–45% of the clavulanate dose excreted in urine in 2 h. **Half-Life:** Amoxicillin 1–1.3 h, clavulanate 0.78–1.2 h.

NURSING IMPLICATIONS

Assessment & Drug Effects

- Determine previous hypersensitivity reactions to penicillins, cephalosporins, and other allergens prior to therapy.
- Lab tests: Baseline C&S tests prior to initiation of therapy; start drug pending results.
- Monitor for S&S of an urticarial rash (usually occurring within a few days after start of drug) suggestive of a hypersensitivity reaction. If it occurs, look for other signs of hypersensitivity (fever, wheezing, generalized itching, dyspnea), and report to physician immediately.
- Monitor for and report diarrhea which may indicate pseudomembranous colitis.

Patient & Family Education

- Female patients should report onset of symptoms of *Candidal vaginitis* (e.g., moderate amount of white, cheesy, nonodorous vaginal discharge; vaginal inflammation and itching; vulvar excoriation, inflammation, burning, itching). Therapy may have to be discontinued.
- Report onset of diarrhea and other possible symptoms of superinfection to physician (see Appendix F).

AMPHETAMINE SULFATE (Pr)

(am-fet'a-meen)

Adderall, Adderall XR

Classifications: CEREBRAL STIMULANT; ANOREXIANT

Therapeutic: CEREBRAL STIMULANT

Pregnancy Category: C

Controlled Substance: Schedule II

AVAILABILITY 5 mg, 10 mg tablets; **Adderall:** 5 mg, 10 mg, 20 mg, 30 mg tablets; 5 mg, 15 mg, 20 mg, 25 mg, 30 mg sustained release capsules

ACTION & *THERAPEUTIC EFFECT* Marked stimulant effect on CNS thought to be due to action on cerebral cortex and possibly the reticular activating system. Acts indirectly on adrenergic receptors by increasing synaptic release of norepinephrine in the brain and by blocking reuptake of norepinephrine at presynaptic membranes. *CNS stimulation results in increased motor activity, diminished sense of fatigue, alertness, wakefulness, and mood elevation. Anorexigenic effect thought to result from direct inhibition of hypothalamic appetite center, as well as mood elevation.*

USES Narcolepsy, attention deficit disorder in children and adults (hyperkinetic behavioral syndrome, minimal brain dysfunction). Use as short-term adjunct to control exogenous obesity not generally recommended because of its potential for abuse.

CONTRAINDICATIONS Hypersensitivity to sympathomimetic amines; history of drug abuse; severe agitation; hyperthyroidism; diabetes mellitus; moderate to severe hypertension, advanced arteriosclerosis, angina pectoris or other cardiovascular disorders; Gilles de la Tourette disorder; glaucoma; during or within 14 days after treatment with MAOIs; lactation.

CAUTIOUS USE Mild hypertension; pregnancy (category C).

ROUTE & DOSAGE

Narcolepsy
Adult: **PO** 5–60 mg/day divided q4–6h in 2–3 doses
Child: **PO** *Older than 12 y,* 10 mg/day, may increase by 10 mg at weekly intervals; *6–12 y,* 5 mg/day, may increase by 5 mg at weekly intervals

Attention Deficit Disorder
Adult/Adolescent: **PO** 10 mg extended release once daily in a.m.; may increase by 5–10 mg at weekly intervals if needed to max of 30 mg/day.
Child: **PO** *6 y,* 5 mg 1–2 times/day, may increase by 5 mg at weekly intervals (max: 40 mg/day); *3–5 y,* 2.5 mg 1–2 times/day, may increase by 2.5 mg at weekly intervals; 10 mg extended release once daily in a.m.; may increase by 5–10 mg at weekly intervals if needed to max of 30 mg/day.

Obesity Dosage Adjustment
Adult: **PO** 5–10 mg 1 h before meals

ADMINISTRATION

Oral

- Give first dose on awakening or early in a.m. when prescribed for narcolepsy.
- Give last dose no later than 6 h before patient retires to avoid insomnia.
- Ensure that sustained release capsules are not crushed or chewed.
- Give drug on an empty stomach 30–60 min before meal to suppress appetite when prescribed for obesity.
- Store at 15°–30° C (59°–86° F) unless otherwise directed.

ADVERSE EFFECTS (≥1%) **Body as a Whole:** Allergy, urticaria, <u>sudden death</u> (reported in children with structural cardiac abnormalities). **CNS:** *Irritability,* psychosis, *restlessness,* nervousness, headache, *insomnia,* weakness, *euphoria,* dysphoria, drowsiness, trembling, hyperactive reflexes. **CV:** *Palpitation,* elevated BP; tachycardia, vasculitis. **Urogenital:** Impotence and change in libido with high doses. **GI:** Dry mouth, anorexia, unusual weight loss, nausea, vomiting, diarrhea, or constipation.

DIAGNOSTIC TEST INTERFERENCE Elevations in ***serum thyroxine (T_4)*** levels with high amphetamine doses.

INTERACTIONS Drug: Acetazolamide, sodium bicarbonate decrease amphetamine elimination; **ammonium chloride, ascorbic acid** increase amphetamine elimination; effects of both amphetamine and BARBITURATES may be antagonized if given together; **furazolidone** may increase BP effects of amphetamines, and interaction may persist for several weeks after furazolidone is discontinued; **guanethidine** antagonizes antihypertensive effects; because MAO INHIBITORS, **selegiline** can precipitate hypertensive crisis (fatalities reported), do not administer amphetamines during or within 14 days of these drugs; PHENOTHIAZINES may inhibit mood elevating effects of amphetamines; TRICYCLIC ANTIDEPRESSANTS enhance amphetamine effects through increased **norepinephrine** release; BETA AGONISTS increase cardiovascular adverse effects.

PHARMACOKINETICS Absorption: Rapid. **Peak effect:** 1–5 h. **Dura-**

tion: Up to 10 h. **Distribution:** All tissues, especially CNS. **Metabolism:** In liver. **Elimination:** Renal; excreted into breast milk. **Half-Life:** 10–30 h.

NURSING IMPLICATIONS

Assessment & Drug Effects

- Monitor for S&S of toxicity in children. Response to this drug is more variable in children than adults; acute toxicity has occurred over a wide range of dosage.
- Monitor for S&S of insomnia or anorexia. Report complaints to physician. Dosage reduction may be required.
- Monitor diabetics closely for loss of glycemic control.
- Monitor growth in children; drug may be discontinued periodically to allow for normal growth.
- Note: Drug's excitatory and euphoric effects are associated with a high abuse potential.

Patient & Family Education

- Keep physician informed of clinical response and persistent or bothersome adverse effects. This drug exerts a stimulating effect that masks fatigue; after exhilaration disappears, fatigue and depression are usually greater than before, and a longer period of rest is needed.
- Report insomnia or undesired weight loss.
- Do not drive or engage in potentially hazardous tasks until response to drug is known.
- Rinse mouth frequently with clear water, especially after eating, to relieve mouth dryness; increase fluid intake, if allowed; chew sugarless gum or sourballs.
- Note: Meticulous oral hygiene is required because decreased saliva encourages demineralization of tooth surfaces and mucosal erosion.
- Avoid caffeine-containing beverages because caffeine increases amphetamine effects.
- Note that drug is usually tapered gradually following prolonged administration of high doses. Abrupt withdrawal may result in lethargy, profound depression, or other psychotic manifestations that may persist for several weeks.

AMPHOTERICIN B Pr

(am-foe-ter′i-sin)

Amphocin, Fungizone

Classification: ANTIFUNGAL

Therapeutic: ANTIFUNGAL

Pregnancy Category: B; C (oral suspension)

AVAILABILITY 50 mg powder for injection; 100 mg/mL suspension; 3% cream, lotion, ointment

ACTION & *THERAPEUTIC EFFECT* Fungistatic antibiotic produced by *Streptomyces nodosus*. Exerts antifungal action on both resting and growing cells at least in part by selectively binding to sterols in fungus cell membrane resulting in cell death. *Fungicidal at higher concentrations, depending on sensitivity of fungus.*

USES Used intravenously for a wide spectrum of potentially fatal systemic fungal (mycotic) infections. Has been used to potentiate antifungal effects of flucytosine (*Ancobon*) and to provide anticandidal prophylaxis in certain susceptible patients receiving immunosuppressive therapy. Used topically for cutaneous and mucocutaneous infections caused by *Candida* (monilia).

UNLABELED USES Treatment of candiduria, fungal endocarditis, meningitis, septicemia; fungal infections of urinary bladder and urinary tract; amebic meningoencephalitis, and paracoccidioidomycosis.

CONTRAINDICATIONS Hypersensitivity to amphotericin; lactation.
CAUTIOUS USE Severe bone marrow depression; renal function impairment; anemia; pregnancy (category B), oral supsension (category C).

ROUTE & DOSAGE

Systemic Infections [Amphocin, Fungizone]

Adult: **IV Test Dose** 1 mg dissolved in 20 mL of D5W by slow infusion (over 10–30 min) **IV Maintenance Dose** 0.25–0.3 mg/kg/day infused over 4–6 h, may gradually increase by 0.125–0.25 mg/kg/day up to 1–1.5 mg/kg/day (max dose: 1.5 mg/mg)
Child: **IV Test Dose** 0.1 mg/kg up to 1 mg dissolved in 20 mL of D5W by slow infusion (over 10–30 min) **IV Maintenance Dose** 0.4 mg/kg/day infused over 4–6 h, may increase by 0.25 mg/kg/day to target dose of 0.25–1 mg/kg/day infused over 2–6 h (max: 1.5 mg/kg)

Candiduria [Amphocin, Fungizone]

Adult: **Irrigation** 5–50 mg/1000 mL sterile water instilled continuously into the bladder via a 3-way closed drainage catheter system at a rate of 1000 mL/24 h

Oral Candidiasis [Fungizone]

Adult/Child: **PO** 100 mg swish and swallow q.i.d.

Cutaneous Candidiasis [Fungizone]

Adult/Child/Infant: **Topical** Apply to lesions 2–4 times/day for 1–4 wk

Renal Impairment Dosage Adjustment

The dose can be reduced or interval extended

ADMINISTRATION

Oral

- Instruct patient not to swallow drug immediately, but swish carefully to coat lesions.
- Store according to manufacturer's recommendations.

Topical Application

- Do not cover with plastic wrap, plastic cloth, rubber, or other occlusive dressings. Ask physician to specify when and how lesions are to be washed.
- Discontinue topical treatment promptly if signs of hypersensitivity, irritation, or worsening of lesions occurs.
- Store topical forms in well-closed containers at room temperature, 15°–30° C (59°–86° F), unless otherwise directed.

Intravenous

PREPARE: Typically prepared by pharmacy service due to complex technique required for IV solution preparation. Each brand of amphotericin is prepared differently according to manufacturer's directions. ▪ Refer to specific manufacturer's guidelines for preparation of IV solutions.
ADMINISTER: **Intermittent:** Use a 1-micron filter. ▪ Infuse total daily dose over 2–6 h. Use longer infusion time for better tolerance. ▪ Alert: Rapid infusion of any amphotericin can cause cardiovascular collapse. If hypotension or arrhythmias develop interrupt infusion and notify physician. ▪ Protect IV solution from light during administration. ▪ Note in-

compatibilities. When given through an existing IV line, flush before and after with D5W. ▪ Initiate therapy using the most distal vein possible and alternate sites with each dose if possible to reduce the risk of thrombophlebitis. ▪ Check IV site frequently for patency.

INCOMPATIBILITIES **Solution/additive:** Any **saline**-containing solution (precipitate will form), PARENTERAL NUTRITION SOLUTIONS, **amikacin, calcium chloride, calcium gluconate, chlorpromazine, cimetidine, ciprofloxacin, diphenhydramine, dopamine, edetate calcium disodium, gentamicin, kanamycin, magnesium sulfate, meropenem, metaraminol, methyldopate, penicillin G, polymyxin, potassium chloride, prochlorperazine, ranitidine, streptomycin, verapamil.** **Y-site:** AMINOGLYCOSIDES, PENICILLINS, PHENOTHIAZINES, **allopurinol, amifostine, amsacrine, aztreonam, bivalirudin, cefepime, cefpirome, cisatracurium, dexmedetomidine, docetaxel, doxorubicin liposome, enalaprilat, etoposide, fenoldopam, filgrastim, fluconazole, fludarabine, foscarnet, gemcitabine, granisetron, heparin** (flush lines with D5W, not NS), **hetastarch, lansoprazole, linezolid, melphalan, meropenem, ondansetron, paclitaxel, pemetrexed, piperacillin/tazobactam, propofol, TPNs, vinorelbine.**

▪ Store according to manufacturer's recommendations for reconstituted and unopened vials.

ADVERSE EFFECTS (≥1%) **Body as a Whole:** Hypersensitivity (pruritus, urticaria, skin rashes, fever, dyspnea, anaphylaxis); *fever, chills.* **CNS:** Headache, sedation, muscle pain, arthralgia, weakness. **CV:** Hypotension, cardiac arrest. **Special Senses:** Ototoxicity with tinnitus, vertigo, loss of hearing. **GI:** Nausea, vomiting, diarrhea, epigastric cramps, anorexia, weight loss. **Hematologic:** Anemia, thrombocytopenia. **Metabolic:** *Hypokalemia, hypomagnesemia.* **Urogenital:** Nephrotoxicity, urine with low specific gravity. **Skin:** Dry, erythema, pruritus, burning sensation; allergic contact dermatitis, exacerbation of lesions. **Other:** Pain; arthralgias, thrombophlebitis (IV site), superinfections.

INTERACTIONS Drug: AMINOGLYCOSIDES, **capreomycin, cisplatin, carboplatin, colistin, cyclosporine, mechlorethamine, furosemide, vancomycin** increase the possibility of nephrotoxicity; CORTICOSTEROIDS potentiate hypokalemia; with DIGITALIS GLYCOSIDES, hypokalemia increases the risk of **digitalis** toxicity.

PHARMACOKINETICS Peak: 1–2 h after IV infusion. **Duration:** 20 h. **Distribution:** Minimal amounts enter CNS, eye, bile, pleural, pericardial, synovial, or amniotic fluids; similar plasma and urine concentrations. **Elimination:** Excreted renally; can be detected in blood up to 4 wk and in urine for 4–8 wk after discontinuing therapy. **Half-Life:** 24–48 h.

NURSING IMPLICATIONS

Assessment & Drug Effects

- Lab tests: Baseline C&S tests prior to initiation of therapy; start drug pending results. Baseline and periodic BUN, serum creatinine, creatinine clearance; during therapy periodic CBC, serum electrolytes (especially K^+, Mg^{++}, Na^+, Ca^{++}), and liver function tests.

- Monitor for S&S of local inflammatory reaction or thrombosis at injection site, particularly if extravasation occurs.
- Monitor cardiovascular and respiratory status and observe patient closely for adverse effects during initial IV therapy. If a test dose (1 mg over 20–30 min) is given, monitor vital signs every 30 min for at least 4 h. Febrile reactions (fever, chills, headache, nausea) occur in 20–90% of patients, usually 1–2 h after beginning infusion, and subside within 4 h after drug is discontinued. The severity of this reaction usually decreases with continued therapy. Keep physician informed.
- Monitor I&O and weight. Report immediately: Oliguria, any change in I&O ratio and pattern, or appearance of urine [e.g., sediment, pink or cloudy urine (hematuria)], abnormal renal function tests, unusual weight gain or loss. Generally, renal damage is reversible if drug is discontinued when first signs of renal dysfunction appear.
- Report to physician and withhold drug, if BUN exceeds 40 mg/dL or serum creatinine rises above 3 mg/dL. Dosage should be reduced or drug discontinued until renal function improves.
- Consult physician about the appearance of mild erythema surrounding topical application to skin lesions. This may be an indication to reduce frequency of topical application.
- Consult physician for guidelines on adequate hydration and adjustment of daily dose as a possible means of avoiding or minimizing nephrotoxicity.
- Report promptly any evidence of hearing loss or complaints of tinnitus, vertigo, or unsteady gait. Tinnitus may not be a complaint in older adults or the very young. Other signs of ototoxicity (i.e., vertigo or hearing loss) are more reliable indicators of ototoxicity in these age groups.

Patient & Family Education

- Notify physician if improvement does not occur within 1–2 wk or if lesions appear to worsen. Nail infections usually require several months or longer to improve.
- Wash towels and clothing that were in contact with affected areas after each treatment.
- Note: Topical cream slightly discolors the skin. Generally, lotion and ointment do not stain skin when rubbed in, but nail lesions may be stained.

AMPHOTERICIN B LIPID-BASED

Abelcet, Amphotec, AmBisome

Classification: ANTIFUNGAL
Therapeutic: ANTIFUNGAL
Prototype: AMPHOTERICIN B
Pregnancy Category: B; C (oral suspension)

AVAILABILITY **Abelcet:** 100 mg/20 mL suspension for injection; **Amphotec:** 50 mg, 100 mg powder for injection; **AmBisome:** 50 mg powder for injection

ACTION & *THERAPEUTIC EFFECT* Fungistatic antibiotic produced by *Streptomyces nodosus*. Exerts antifungal action on both resting and growing cells at least in part by selectively binding to sterols in fungus cell membrane. This results in fungal cell death. *Fungicidal at higher concentrations, depending on sensitivity of fungus.*

USES Used intravenously for a wide spectrum of potentially fatal systemic fungal (mycotic) infections.

UNLABELED USES Treatment of candiduria, fungal endocarditis, meningitis, septicemia; fungal infections of urinary bladder and urinary tract; amebic meningoencephalitis, and paracoccidioidomycosis.

CONTRAINDICATIONS Hypersensitivity to amphotericin; lactation.
CAUTIOUS USE Severe bone marrow depression; renal function impairment; anemia; pregnancy (category B).

ROUTE & DOSAGE

Systemic Infections [Abelcet]
Adult/Child: **IV** 5 mg/kg/day

[Amphotec]
Adult/Child: **IV Test Dose** 10 mL (1.6–8.3 mg) of initial dose infused over 10–30 min **IV Maintenance Dose** 3–4 mg/kg/day (max: 7.5 mg/kg/day) infused at 1 mg/kg/h

[AmBisome]
Adult/Child: **IV** 3–5 mg/kg/day infused over 1–2 h

Cryptococcal Meningitis in HIV [AmBisome]
Adult: **IV** 6 mg/kg/day infused over 2 h

Leishmaniasis [AmBisome]
Adult: **IV** *Immunocompetent patient:* 3 mg/kg/day on days 1–5, 14, and 21; may repeat if necessary *Immunocompromised:* 4 mg/kg/day on days 1–5, 10, 17, 24, 31, and 38

ADMINISTRATION

Oral
- Instruct patient not to swallow drug immediately, but swish carefully to coat lesions.
- Store according to manufacturer's recommendations.

Topical Application
- Do not cover with plastic wrap, plastic cloth, rubber, or other occlusive dressings. Ask physician to specify when and how lesions are to be washed.
- Discontinue topical treatment promptly if signs of hypersensitivity, irritation, or worsening of lesions occurs.
- Store topical forms in well-closed containers at room temperature, 15°–30° C (59°–86° F), unless otherwise directed.

Intravenous

PREPARE: Each brand of amphotericin is prepared differently according to manufacturer's directions. ▪ Refer to specific manufacturer's guidelines for preparation of IV solutions.

ADMINISTER: **Abelcet Intermittent:** Flush existing IV line with D5W before infusion. ▪ Use 5 micron in-line filter. Infuse total daily dose at 2.5 mg/kg/h. ▪ Shake IV bag at least q2h to evenly mix solution.
Amphotec Intermittent: Do not use an in-line filter. ▪ Infuse total daily dose at 1 mg/kg/h. Infusion time may be shortened but should never be less than 2 h. ▪ Infusion time may also be extended for better tolerance.
AmBisome Intermittent: Do not use an in-line filter. ▪ Infuse total daily dose over 2 h. Infusion time may be shortened but should never be less than 1 h. ▪ Alert: Rapid infusion of any amphotericin can cause cardiovascular collapse. If hypotension or arrhythmias develop interrupt infusion and notify physician. ▪ Protect IV solution

from light during administration. ▪ Note incompatibilities. When given through an existing IV line, flush before and after with D5W. ▪ Initiate therapy using the most distal vein possible and alternate sites with each dose if possible to reduce the risk of thrombophlebitis. ▪ Check IV site frequently for patency.

INCOMPATIBILITIES **Solution/additive:** Any **saline**-containing solution (precipitate will form), PARENTERAL NUTRITION SOLUTIONS. **Y-site:** AMINOGLYCOSIDES, PENICILLINS, PHENOTHIAZINES, **alfentanil, amikacin, ampicillin, ampicillin/sulbactam, atenolol, aztreonam, bretylium, buprenorphine, butorphanol, calcium salts, carboplatin, cefazolin, cefepime, ceftazidime, ceftriaxone, chlorpromazine, cimetidine, cisatracurium, cyclophosphamide, cyclosporine, cytarabine, diazepam, digoxin, diphenhydramine, dobutamine, dopamine, doxorubicin, doxorubicin liposome, droperidol, enalaprilat, esmolol, etoposide, famotidine, fluconazole, fluorouracil, haloperidol, heparin** (flush lines with D5W, not NS), **hetastartch, hydromorphone, hydroxyzine, imipenem/cilastatin, labetalol, leucovorin, lidocaine, magnesium sulfate, meperidine, mesna, metoclopramide, midazolam, mitoxantrone, morphone, nalbuphine, naloxone, netilmicin, ofloxacin, ondansetron, paclitaxel, phenytoin, piperacillin, piperacillin/tazobactam, potassium chloride, prochlorperazine, promethazine, propranolol, ranitidine, remifentanil, sodium bicarbonate, ticarcillin/clavulanate, vecuronium, verapamil, vinorelbine.** ▪ Do not mix Abelcet or Amphotec with any other drugs.

▪ Store according to manufacturer's recommendations for reconstituted and unopened vials.

ADVERSE EFFECTS (≥1%) **Body as a Whole:** Hypersensitivity (pruritus, urticaria, skin rashes, fever, dyspnea, anaphylaxis); *fever, chills*. **CNS:** Headache, sedation, muscle pain, arthralgia, weakness. **CV:** Hypotension, cardiac arrest. **Special Senses:** Ototoxicity with tinnitus, vertigo, loss of hearing. **GI:** Nausea, vomiting, diarrhea, epigastric cramps, anorexia, weight loss. **Hematologic:** Anemia, thrombocytopenia. **Metabolic:** *Hypokalemia, hypomagnesemia*. **Urogenital:** Nephrotoxicity, urine with low specific gravity. **Skin:** Dry, erythema, pruritus, burning sensation; allergic contact dermatitis, exacerbation of lesions. **Other:** Pain; arthralgias, thrombophlebitis (IV site), superinfections.

INTERACTIONS Drug: AMINOGLYCOSIDES, **capreomycin, cisplatin, carboplatin, colistin, cyclosporine, mechlorethamine, furosemide, vancomycin** increase the possibility of nephrotoxicity; CORTICOSTEROIDS potentiate hypokalemia; with DIGITALIS GLYCOSIDES, hypokalemia increases the risk of **digitalis** toxicity.

PHARMACOKINETICS Peak: 1–2 h after IV infusion. **Duration:** 20 h. **Distribution:** Minimal amounts enter CNS, eye, bile, pleural, pericardial, synovial, or amniotic fluids; similar plasma and urine concentrations. **Elimination:** Excreted renally; can be detected in blood up to 4 wk and in urine for 4–8 wk after discontinuing therapy. **Half-Life:** 24–48 h.

NURSING IMPLICATIONS

Assessment & Drug Effects

- Lab tests: Baseline C&S tests prior to initiation of therapy; start drug pending results. Baseline and periodic BUN, serum creatinine, creatinine clearance; during therapy periodic CBC, serum electrolytes (especially K^+, Mg^{++}, Na^+, Ca^{++}), and liver function tests.
- Monitor for S&S of local inflammatory reaction or thrombosis at injection site, particularly if extravasation occurs.
- Monitor cardiovascular and respiratory status and observe patient closely for adverse effects during initial IV therapy. If a test dose (1 mg over 20–30 min) is given, monitor vital signs every 30 min for at least 4 h. Febrile reactions (fever, chills, headache, nausea) occur in 20–90% of patients, usually 1–2 h after beginning infusion, and subside within 4 h after drug is discontinued. The severity of this reaction usually decreases with continued therapy. Keep physician informed.
- Monitor I&O and weight. Report immediately oliguria, any change in I&O ratio and pattern, or appearance of urine [e.g., sediment, pink or cloudy urine (hematuria)], abnormal renal function tests, unusual weight gain or loss. Generally, renal damage is reversible if drug is discontinued when first signs of renal dysfunction appear.
- Report to physician and withhold drug, if BUN exceeds 40 mg/dL or serum creatinine rises above 3 mg/dL. Dosage should be reduced or drug discontinued until renal function improves.
- Consult physician about the appearance of mild erythema surrounding topical application to skin lesions. This may be an indication to reduce frequency of topical application.
- Consult physician for guidelines on adequate hydration and adjustment of daily dose as a possible means of avoiding or minimizing nephrotoxicity.
- Report promptly any evidence of hearing loss or complaints of tinnitus, vertigo, or unsteady gait. Tinnitus may not be a complaint in older adults or the very young. Other signs of ototoxicity (i.e., vertigo or hearing loss) are more reliable indicators of ototoxicity in these age groups.

Patient & Family Education

- Notify physician if improvement does not occur within 1–2 wk or if lesions appear to worsen. Nail infections usually require several months or longer to improve.
- Wash towels and clothing that were in contact with affected areas after each treatment.

AMPICILLIN Pr

(am-pi-sill'in)

Novo-Ampicillin ♣, Principen

AMPICILLIN SODIUM

Ampicin ♣, Penbritin ♣

Classifications: ANTIBIOTIC; AMINOPENICILLIN

Therapeutic: ANTIBIOTIC

Pregnancy Category: B

AVAILABILITY 250 mg, 500 mg capsules; 125 mg/5 mL, 250 mg/5 mL oral suspension; 125 mg, 250 mg, 500 mg, 1 gm, 2 gm vials

ACTION & *THERAPEUTIC EFFECT* A broad-spectrum, semisynthetic aminopenicillin that is bactericidal but is inactivated by penicillinase (beta-lactamase). Like other penicillins, ampicillin inhibits the final stage of bacterial cell wall synthesis by binding to specific penicillin-binding proteins (PBPs) located inside the bacterial cell wall resulting in lysis and death of bacteria. *Effective against gram-positive bacteria as well as some gram negative.*

USES Infections of GU, respiratory, and GI tracts and skin and soft tissues; also gonococcal infections, bacterial meningitis, otitis media, sinusitis, and septicemia and for prophylaxis of bacterial endocarditis. Used parenterally only for moderately severe to severe infections.

CONTRAINDICATIONS Hypersensitivity to penicillin derivatives; infectious mononucleosis.

CAUTIOUS USE History of hypersensitivity to cephalosporins; GI disorders; renal disease or impairment; pregnancy (category B), lactation.

ROUTE & DOSAGE

Systemic Infections

Adult: **PO/IV/IM** 250–500 mg q6h

Child (under 40 kg): **PO/IV** 25–50 mg/kg/day divided q6–8h

Neonate: **IV/IM** *Up to 7 days, weight up to 2000 g,* 50 mg/kg/day divided q12h; *up to 7 days, weight greater than 2000 g,* 75 mg/kg/day divided q8h; *older than 7 days, weight less than 1200 g,* 50 mg/kg/day divided q12h; *older than 7 days, weight 1200–2000 g,* 75 mg/kg/day divided q8h; *older than 7 days, weight greater than 2000 g,* 100 mg/kg/day divided q6h

Meningitis

Adult/Child: **IV** 150–200 mg/kg/day divided q3–4h

Neonate: **IV/IM** *Up to 7 days, weight up to 2000 g,* 100 mg/kg/day divided q12h; *up to 7 days, weight greater than 2000 g,* 150 mg/kg/day divided q8h; *older than 7 days, weight less than 1200 g,* 100 mg/kg/day divided 2h; *older than 7 days, weight 1200–2000 g,* 150 mg/kg/day divided q8h; *older than 7 days, weight greater than 2000 g,* 200 mg/kg/day divided q6h

Gonorrhea

Adult: **PO** 3.5 g with 1 g probenecid × 1 **IV/IM** 500 mg q8–12h

Bacterial Endocarditis Prophylaxis

Adult: **IV** 2 g 30 min before procedure

Child: **IV** 50 mg/kg 30 min before procedure (max: 2 g)

Group B Strep Prophylaxis

Adult: **IV** 2 g, then 1 g q4h until delivery

Renal Impairment Dosage Adjustment

CrCl 10–30 mL/min: Give q6–12h; less than 10 mL/min: Give q12h

Dialysis Dosage Adjustment: Dose should be given after dialysis

ADMINISTRATION

Oral

- Give with a full glass of water on an empty stomach (at least 1 h before or 2 h after meals) for maximum absorption. Food hampers rate and extent of oral absorption.

Intramuscular

- Reconstitute each vial by adding the indicated amount of sterile water for injection or bacteriostatic water for injection (1.2 mL to 125 mg; 1 mL to 250 mg; 1.8 mL to 500 mg; 3.5 mL to 1 g; 6.8 mL to 2 g). All reconstituted vials yield 250 mg/mL except the 125 mg vial which yields 125 mg/mL. Administer within 1 h of preparation.

- Withdraw the ordered dose and inject deep IM into a large muscle.

Intravenous

Verify correct IV concentration and rate of infusion with physician for administration to neonates, infants, and children.

PREPARE: **Direct/Intermittent:** Reconstitute as follows with sterile water for injection: Add 5 mL to 500 mg or fraction thereof; add 7.4 mL to 1 g; add 14.8 mL to 2 g. Final concentration **must be** 30 mg/mL or less; may be given direct IV as prepared or further diluted in 50 mL or more of NS, D5W, D5/NS, D5W/0.45NaCl, or LR. ▪ Stability of solution varies with diluent and concentration of solution. Solutions in NS are stable for up to 8 h at room temperature; other solutions should be infused within 2–4 h of preparation. Give direct IV within 1 h of preparation. ▪ Wear disposable gloves when handling drug repeatedly; contact dermatitis occurs frequently in sensitized individuals.

ADMINISTER: **Direct/Intermittent:** Infuse 500 mg or less slowly over 3–5 min. Give 1–2 g over at least 15 min. ▪ With solutions of 100 mL or more, set rate according to amount of solution, but no faster than direct IV rate. ▪ Convulsions may be induced by too rapid administration.

INCOMPATIBILITIES **Solution/additive:** Do not add to a **dextrose**-containing solution unless entire dose is given within 1 h of preparation. **Aztreonam, cefepime, hydrocortisone, prochlorperazine. Y-site: Amphotericin B, epinephrine, fenoldopam, fluconazole, hydralazine, lansoprazole, midazolam, nicardipine, ondansetron, sargramostim, TPN, verapamil, vinorelbine.**

- Store capsules and unopened vials at 15°–30° C (59°–86° F) unless otherwise directed. Keep oral preparations tightly covered.

ADVERSE EFFECTS (≥1%) **Body as a Whole:** Similar to those for penicillin G. Hypersensitivity (pruritus, urticaria, eosinophilia, hemolytic anemia, interstitial nephritis, <u>anaphylactoid reaction</u>); superinfections. **CNS:** Convulsive seizures with high doses. **GI:** *Diarrhea,* nausea, vomiting, <u>pseudomembranous colitis</u>. **Other:** Severe pain (following IM); phlebitis (following IV). **Skin:** *Rash.*

DIAGNOSTIC TEST INTERFERENCE Elevated ***CPK*** levels may result from local skeletal muscle injury following IM injection. ***Urine glucose:*** High urine drug concentrations can result in false-positive test results with ***Clinitest*** or ***Benedict's*** [enzymatic ***glucose oxidase methods*** (e.g., ***Clinistix, Diastix, TesTape***) are not affected]. ***AST*** may be elevated (significance not known).

INTERACTIONS Drug: Allopurinol increases incidence of rash. Effectiveness of the AMINOGLYCOSIDES may be impaired in patients with severe end-stage renal disease. **Chloramphenicol, erythromycin,** and **tetracycline** may reduce bactericidal effects of ampicillin; this interaction is primarily significant when low doses of ampicillin are used. Ampicillin may interfere with the contraceptive action of oral contraceptives (**estrogens**). Female patients should be advised to consider nonhormonal contraception while on antibiotics. **Food:** Food may decrease absorption of ampicillin, so it should be taken 1 h before or 2 h after meals.

PHARMACOKINETICS Absorption: Oral dose is 50% absorbed. Peak effect: 5 min IV, 1 h IM, 2 h PO. **Duration:** 6–8 h. **Distribution:** Most body tissues; high CNS concentrations only with inflamed meninges; crosses the placenta. **Metabolism:** Minimal hepatic metabolism. **Elimination:** 90% in urine; excreted into breast milk. **Half-Life:** 1–1.8 h.

NURSING IMPLICATIONS

Assessment & Drug Effects

- Determine previous hypersensitivity reactions to penicillins, cephalosporins, and other allergens prior to therapy. Monitor closely for signs of hypersensitivity during first 30 min after administration.
- Lab tests: Baseline C&S tests prior to initiation of therapy; start drug pending results. Baseline and periodic assessments of renal, hepatic, and hematologic functions, particularly during prolonged or high-dose therapy.
- Note: Sodium content of IV drug should be considered in patients on sodium restriction.
- Inspect skin daily and instruct patient to do the same. The appearance of a rash should be carefully evaluated to differentiate a nonallergenic ampicillin rash from a hypersensitivity reaction. Report rash promptly to physician.
- Monitor for and report diarrhea which may indicate pseudomembranous colitis.

Patient & Family Education

- Report diarrhea to physician; do not self-medicate. Give a detailed report to the physician regarding onset, duration, character of stools, associated symptoms, temperature and weight loss to help rule out the possibility of drug-induced, potentially fatal pseudomembranous colitis (see Appendix F).
- Report S&S of superinfection (onset of black, hairy tongue; oral lesions or soreness; rectal or vaginal itching; vaginal discharge; loose, foul-smelling stools; or unusual odor to urine).
- Notify physician if no improvement is noted within a few days after therapy is started.
- Take medication around the clock; continue taking medication until it is all gone (usually 10 days) unless otherwise directed by physician or pharmacist.

AMPICILLIN SODIUM AND SULBACTAM SODIUM

(am-pi-sill′in/sul-bak′tam)

Unasyn

Classifications: ANTIBIOTIC; AMINOPENICILLIN

Therapeutic: ANTIBIOTIC

Prototype: Ampicillin

Pregnancy Category: B

AVAILABILITY 1.5 g, 3 g vials

ACTION & *THERAPEUTIC EFFECT*
Ampicillin inhibits the final stage of bacterial cell wall synthesis by binding to specific penicillin-binding proteins (PBPs) located inside the bacterial cell wall, thus destroying the cell wall. Sulbactam inhibits beta-lactamases, most frequently responsible for transferred drug resistance. Thus the spectrum of drugs affected by the combination of the two is increased. *Effective against both gram-positive and gram-negative bacteria including*

Common adverse effects in *italic*, life-threatening effects underlined; generic names in **bold**; classifications in SMALL CAPS; ♣ Canadian drug name; ⓟ Prototype drug

those that produce beta-lactamase and nonbeta-lactamase producers. Ampicillin without sulbactam is not effective against beta-lactamase producing strains.

USES Treatment of infections due to susceptible organisms in skin and skin structures, intra-abdominal infections, and gynecologic infections.

CONTRAINDICATIONS Hypersensitivity to penicillins; mononucleosis. **CAUTIOUS USE** Hypersensitivity to cephalosporins; GI disorders; renal disease or impairment; pregnancy (category B) or lactation.

ROUTE & DOSAGE

Systemic Infections

Adult/Child (weight greater than 40 kg): **IV/IM** 1.5–3 g q6h (max: 4 g sulbactam/day)
Child (1 y or older): **IV** 300 mg/kg/day (200 mg/kg ampicillin and 100 mg/kg sulbactam) divided q6h

Renal Impairment Dosage Adjustment

CrCl greater than 30 mL/min: Give q6–8h; 15–29 mL/min: Give q12h; 5–14 mL/min: Give q24h
Dialysis: Give dose after dialysis

ADMINISTRATION

Intramuscular

- Reconstitute solution with sterile water for injection by adding 6.4 mL diluent to a 3 g vial. Each mL contains 250 mg ampicillin and 125 mg sulbactam.
- Give deep IM into a large muscle. Rotate injection sites.

Intravenous

PREPARE: **Direct/Intermittent:** Reconstitute each 1.5 g vial with 3.2 mL of sterile water for injection to yield 375 mg/mL (250 mg ampicillin/125 mg sulbactam); must further dilute with NS, D5W, D5/NS, D5W/0.45NS, or LR to a final concentration within the range of 3–45 mg/mL.
ADMINISTER: **Direct:** Give slowly over at least 10–15 min. **Intermittent:** Infuse solutions of less than 50 mL over 10–15 min and solutions of 50–100 mL over 15–30 min. With solutions of 100 mL or more, set rate according to amount of solution but no faster than direct IV rate (e.g., 100 mL over 30 min). ▪ Convulsions may be induced by too rapid administration. ▪ Use only freshly prepared solution; administer within 1 h after preparation.
INCOMPATIBILITIES **Solution/additive:** Do not add to a **dextrose**-containing solution unless entire dose is given within 1 h of preparation. **Ciprofloxacin. Y-site: Amiodarone, amphotericin B, ciprofloxacin, idarubicin, lansoprazole, nicardipine, ondansetron, sargramostim.**

- Store powder for injection at 15°–30° C (59°–86° F) before reconstitution. Storage times and temperatures vary for different concentrations of reconstituted solutions; consult manufacturer's directions.

ADVERSE EFFECTS (≥1%) **Body as a Whole:** Hypersensitivity (rash, itching, <u>anaphylactoid reaction</u>), fatigue, malaise, headache, chills, edema. **GI:** *Diarrhea, nausea,* vomiting, abdominal distention, candidiasis. **Hematologic:** Neutropenia, thrombocytopenia. **Urogenital:** Dysuria. **CNS:** Seizures. **Other:** Local pain at injection site; thrombophlebitis.

INTERACTIONS Drug: Allopurinol increases incidence of rash; effectiveness of the AMINOGLYCOSIDES may be impaired in patients with severe end stage renal disease; **chloramphenicol, erythromycin, tetracycline** may reduce bactericidal effects of ampicillin—this interaction is primarily significant when low doses are used; ampicillin may interfere with the contraceptive action of ORAL CONTRACEPTIVES—female patients should be advised to consider nonhormonal contraception while on antibiotics.

PHARMACOKINETICS Peak: Immediate after IV. **Duration:** 6–8 h. **Distribution:** Most body tissues; high CNS concentrations only with inflamed meninges; crosses placenta; appears in breast milk. **Metabolism:** Minimal hepatic metabolism. **Elimination:** In urine. **Half-Life:** 1 h.

NURSING IMPLICATIONS

Assessment & Drug Effects

- Determine previous hypersensitivity reactions to penicillins, cephalosporins, and other allergens prior to therapy.
- Lab tests: Baseline C&S tests prior to initiation of therapy; start drug pending results.
- Report promptly unexplained bleeding (e.g., epistaxis, purpura, ecchymoses).
- Monitor patient carefully during the first 30 min after initiation of IV therapy for signs of hypersensitivity and anaphylactoid reaction (see Appendix F). Serious anaphylactoid reactions require immediate use of emergency drugs and airway management.
- Monitor for and report diarrhea which may indicate pseudomembranous colitis. Observe for and report other S&S of superinfection.
- Monitor I&O ratio and pattern. Report dysuria, urine retention, and hematuria.

Patient & Family Education

- Report chills, wheezing, pruritus (itching), respiratory distress, or palpitations to physician immediately.
- Report diarrhea to physician; do not self-medicate.

AMYL NITRITE

(am′il)

Amyl Nitrite

Classifications: NITRATE VASODILATOR; ANTIDOTE

Therapeutic: ANTIDOTE; NITRATE VASODILATOR

Prototype: Nitroglycerin

Pregnancy Category: X

AVAILABILITY 0.3 mL ampules

ACTION & *THERAPEUTIC EFFECT* Short-acting vasodilator and smooth muscle relaxant. It is converted to nitric oxide, which causes the vasodilation. Action in treatment of cyanide poisoning is based on ability of amyl nitrite to convert hemoglobin to methemoglobin, which forms a nontoxic complex with cyanide ion. *Effective for immediate treatment of cyanide poisoning.*

USES As an adjunct antidote in the immediate treatment of cyanide poisoning. (Because of adverse effects, unpleasant odor, and expense, infrequently used to treat angina pectoris.)

UNLABELED USES Change intensity of heart murmurs.

CONTRAINDICATIONS Hypersensitivity to nitrites or nitrates; severe anemia; uncontrolled hyperthyroidism; acute alcoholism; pregnancy (category X).

CAUTIOUS USE Elderly; recent increase in intracranial pressure; cerebral hemorrhage, head trauma; hypotension; glaucoma; recent MI; lactation, children.

ROUTE & DOSAGE

Acute Angina
Adult: **Inhalation** 0.18–0.3 mL prn

Cyanide Poisoning
Adult/Child: **Inhalation** 0.3 mL perle crushed every minute and inhaled for 15–30 sec until sodium nitrite infusion is ready

ADMINISTRATION

Inhalation

- Crush ampule between fingers to prepare (amyl nitrite is available in 0.18 mL and 0.3 mL perles, which are thin, friable glass ampules enveloped with woven fabric cover).
- Instruct patient to sit a while immediately after drug is administered.
- Note: Amyl nitrite is volatile and highly flammable; when mixed with air or oxygen, it forms a mixture that can explode if ignited.
- Store at 8°–15° C (46°–59° F), unless otherwise directed. Protect from light.

ADVERSE EFFECTS (≥1%) **Body as a Whole:** Transient flushing, weakness. **CV:** Orthostatic hypotension, palpitation, cardiovascular collapse, tachycardia. **GI:** Nausea, vomiting. **Hematologic:** Methemoglobinemia (large doses). **CNS:** *Headache*, dizziness, syncope. **Respiratory:** Respiratory depression.

PHARMACOKINETICS Absorption: Rapidly from mucous membranes. **Onset:** 10–30 sec. **Duration:** 3–5 min.

NURSING IMPLICATIONS

Assessment & Drug Effects

- Monitor for S&S of syncope, due to a sudden drop in systolic BP, which sometimes follows drug inhalation, particularly in older adults.
- Monitor vital signs until stable. Rapid pulse, which usually lasts for a brief period, is an expected response to the fall in BP produced by the drug.
- Chart length of time required for pain to subside after administration of drug.
- Note: Tolerance may develop with repeated use over prolonged periods.

Patient & Family Education

- Note: Drug has a strongly fruity odor.
- Go to the emergency room immediately or consult physician if no relief from angina is experienced after 3 doses 5 min apart.

ANAGRELIDE HYDROCHLORIDE

(a-na′gre-lyde)

Agrylin

Classifications: ANTICOAGULANT; ANTIPLATELET

Therapeutic: ANTIPLATELET; REDUCER OF PLATELET COUNT

Pregnancy Category: C

AVAILABILITY 0.5 mg, 1 mg capsules

ACTION & *THERAPEUTIC EFFECT* Anagrelide action appears to be related to a selective inhibition of platelet production. It inhibits platelet aggregation by affecting several aggregating agents (e.g., thrombin and arachidonic acid, ADP, and collagen). *Anagrelide is associated with significant decreases in plate-*

let counts and is thought to prevent early changes in shape of platelets.

USES Essential thrombocythemia.
UNLABELED USES Polycythemia vera.

CONTRAINDICATIONS Hypotension, severe hepatic impairment, females of childbearing age; lactation.
CAUTIOUS USE Cardiovascular disease, renal and hepatic function impairment, jaundice; pregnancy (category C). Safety and efficacy in patients younger than 16 y are not established.

ROUTE & DOSAGE

Essential Thrombocythemia
Adult (16 y or older): **PO** Start with 0.5 mg q.i.d. or 1 mg b.i.d. × 1 wk, may increase by 0.5 mg/day qwk until platelet count is less than 600,000/mcL (max: 10 mg/day)

Hepatic Impairment Dosage Adjustment
0.5 mg daily for 1 wk

ADMINISTRATION

Oral
- Make sure dosage increments do not exceed 0.5 mg/day in any 1 wk.
- Store at 15°–25° C (59°–77° F) in a light-resistant container.

ADVERSE EFFECTS (≥1%) **Body as a Whole:** *Asthenia, pain, edema (general),* paresthesia, back pain, malaise, fever, chills, photosensitivity. **CNS:** Headache, *dizziness,* CVA, syncope, seizures. **CV:** *Palpitations,* chest pain, tachycardia, peripheral edema, CHF, MI, cardiomyopathy, heart block, atrial fibrillation, pericarditis, arrhythmia, hemorrhage. **GI:** *Diarrhea, abdominal pain, nausea,* flatulence, vomiting, dyspepsia, anorexia, pancreatitis, constipation, GI hemorrhage, and ulceration. **Hematologic:** Anemia, thrombocytopenia, ecchymoses, lymphedema. **Respiratory:** *Dyspnea,* pulmonary infiltrates, pulmonary fibrosis, pulmonary hypertension. **Skin:** Rash, urticaria. **Other:** Dysuria.

PHARMACOKINETICS Absorption: 70% from GI tract. Food reduces bioavailability. **Onset:** 7–14 days. **Duration:** Increased platelet counts were observed 4 days after discontinuing drug. **Metabolism:** Extensively metabolized. **Elimination:** Primarily in urine as metabolites. **Half-Life:** 1.3–1.8 h.

NURSING IMPLICATIONS

Assessment & Drug Effects
- Monitor for therapeutic effectiveness which is indicated by reduction of platelets for at least 4 wk to 600,000/mcL or less or 50% from baseline.
- Monitor for S&S of CHF or myocardial ischemia.
- Monitor for S&S of renal toxicity in patients with renal insufficiency (creatinine 2 mg/dL or more).
- Monitor for S&S of hepatic toxicity in patients with liver functions greater than 1.5 times upper limit of normal.
- Lab tests: Monitor platelet count q2days for first wk, weekly thereafter until maintenance dose reached; closely monitor Hgb, WBC count, liver function tests, and BUN and creatinine while platelet count is being lowered.

Patient & Family Education
- Contact physician if palpitations, fluid retention, breathing difficulty, or any other distressful symptoms develop.
- Avoid excessive exposure to sunlight or UV light.

ANAKINRA

(an-a-kin′ra)

Kineret

Classifications: IMMUNOMODULATOR; INTERLEUKIN-1 RECEPTOR ANTAGONIST; DISEASE-MODIFYING ANTIRHEUMATIC DRUG (DMARD)

Therapeutic: ANTIRHEUMATIC AGENT; DMARD

Pregnancy Category: B

AVAILABILITY 100 mg prefilled syringes

ACTION & *THERAPEUTIC EFFECT* Anakinra is a recombinant human interleukin-1 (IL-1) receptor antagonist (IL-1R1). It blocks the biological activity of IL-1 by inhibiting it from binding to interleukin receptors that are present in both bone and cartilage as well as other kinds of tissues. Interleukin-1 is produced in response to inflammation. IL-1 mediates various responses of tissues, including inflammatory and immunologic responses. *Anakinra competes with interleukin-1 (IL-1) by inhibiting it from binding to its receptor sites in tissues.*

USES Treatment of rheumatoid arthritis in patients failing other disease-modifying antirheumatic drugs (DMARDs). Usually given in combination with another DMARD.

CONTRAINDICATIONS Hypersensitivity to anakinra, *E. coli*–derived products, latex; active infections; live vaccines.

CAUTIOUS USE Neutropenia, immunosuppressed patients, or patients with frequent, serious infections; asthmatics; elderly; renal impairment; concomitant use of tumor necrosis factor (TNF) blocking agents, etanercept, or infliximab; pregnancy (category B), lactation, children.

ROUTE & DOSAGE

Rheumatoid Arthritis
Adult: **Subcutaneous** 100 mg daily

ADMINISTRATION

Subcutaneous

- Do not give anakinra if the patient has an active infection.
- Note that anakinra should not ordinarily be given with tumor necrosis factor (TNF) blocking agents.
- Discard any unused portions as the drug contains no preservative.
- Check expiration date and do not use if expired.
- Store in the refrigerator at 2°–8° C (36°–46° F). DO NOT FREEZE OR SHAKE. Protect from light.

ADVERSE EFFECTS (≥1%) **Body as a Whole:** *Bacterial infections (URI,* sinusitis, flu, *other).* **CNS:** Headache. **GI:** Nausea, diarrhea, abdominal pain. **Hematologic:** Decreased neutrophil count, antibody formation. **Other:** *Injection site reactions (erythema, ecchymosis, edema, inflammation, pain).*

INTERACTIONS Drug: Increased risk of infection with live virus vaccine, **etanercept, infliximab.** Increased risk of neutropenia as well as infection with **etanercept** and **infliximab.**

PHARMACOKINETICS Absorption: 95% absorbed subcutaneous site. **Peak:** 3–7 h. **Elimination:** In urine. **Half-Life:** 4–6 h.

NURSING IMPLICATIONS

Assessment & Drug Effects

- Monitor for S&S of infection (e.g., pneumonia or other URI, cellulitis). Withhold drug and notify physician if these appear.
- Lab tests: Monitor absolute neutrophil count (ANC) prior to initiating

anakinra, monthly for 3 mo, and q3mo thereafter for 1 y; monitor periodically WBC and platelet counts.

- Monitor closely patients with impaired renal function for S&S of adverse drug reactions.
- Assess for injection site reactions manifested by erythema, ecchymosis, inflammation, and pain.

Patient & Family Education

- Review carefully the "Information for Patients and Caregivers" leaflet for detailed instructions on handling and injecting anakinra.
- Give the injection at approximately the same time every day.
- Administer only 1 dose (the entire contents of 1 prefilled glass syringe) per day. Discard any unused portions as the drug contains no preservative. Do not save unused drug.
- Do not permit vaccination with live vaccines while taking anakinra.
- Withhold drug and notify physician for S&S of upper respiratory, skin, or other infection(s).

ANASTROZOLE Pr

(a-nas'tro-zole)

Arimidex

Classifications: ANTINEOPLASTIC; NONSTEROIDAL AROMATASE INHIBITOR

Therapeutic: ANTINEOPLASTIC

Pregnancy Category: D

AVAILABILITY 1 mg tablets

ACTION & *THERAPEUTIC EFFECT* Anastrozole is a potent and selective nonsteroidal aromatase inhibitor that converts estrone to estradiol. It lowers serum estrogen levels in postmenopausal women without interfering with adrenal steroid synthesis. *Inhibiting the biosynthesis of estrogens is one way to deprive tumors of estrogens, and thus restrict tumor growth.*

USES Early and advanced breast cancer with hormone receptor positive or hormone status unknown in postmenopausal women.

CONTRAINDICATIONS Pregnancy (category D), lactation, premenopausal women, postmenopausal hormone replacement therapy; severe hepatic disease, children.

CAUTIOUS USE Mild to moderate hepatic disease; elderly.

ROUTE & DOSAGE

Breast Cancer

Adult: **PO** 1 mg once daily

ADMINISTRATION

Oral

- Give on an empty stomach, 1 h before or 2 h after meals, because food affects extent of absorption.
- Store at 20°–25° C (68°–77° F).

ADVERSE EFFECTS (≥1%) **CNS:** Asthenia, headache, hot flushes, pain, dizziness, depression, paresthesia, malaise, insomnia, confusion, anxiety, nervousness. **CV:** Chest pain, hypertension, thrombophlebitis, <u>ischemic cardiac events</u>, edema. **GI:** *Diarrhea,* nausea, vomiting, constipation, abdominal pain, anorexia, dry mouth, increased liver function tests (ALT, AST, GGT). **Respiratory:** Dyspnea, cough, pharyngitis, bronchitis, rhinitis, sinusitis. **Other:** Rash, peripheral edema, pelvic pain, flu-like syndrome.

PHARMACOKINETICS Absorption: Rapidly absorbed from GI tract. **Distribution:** 40% protein bound. **Metabolism:** 85% metabolized in liver to inactive metabolites. **Elimi-**

nation: 10% excreted unchanged; 60% as metabolites in urine. **Half-Life:** 50 h.

NURSING IMPLICATIONS

Assessment & Drug Effects

- Lab Tests: Monitor periodically liver enzymes, CBC with differential, alkaline phosphatases, total cholesterol, and lipid profile.
- Assess for hypertension, complications of edema, thrombotic events, and signs of liver toxicity.

Patient & Family Education

- Recognize common adverse effects and seek information on measures to control discomfort.
- Seek medical attention if you experience chest pain, calf pain, or shortness of breath; unexplained loss of appetite or nausea; jaundice.

ANIDULAFUNGIN

(a-ni-dul'a-fun-gin)

Eraxis

Classifications: ECHINOCANDIN ANTIFUNGAL

Therapeutic: ANTIFUNGAL ANTIBIOTIC

Prototype: Caspofungin

Pregnancy Category: C

AVAILABILITY 50 mg powder for injection

ACTION & *THERAPEUTIC EFFECT* Anidulafungin is a semisynthetic echinocandin with antifungal activity. It inhibits glucan synthase, an enzyme present in fungal cells. Glucan is an essential component of the fungal cell wall; therefore, anidulafungin causes fungal cell death. *Anidulafungin interferes with reproduction and growth of susceptible fungi.*

USES Treatment of candidemia and other *Candida* infections caused by *C. albicans, C. glabrata, C. parapsilosis*, and *C. tropicalis*. Treatment of esophageal candidiasis.

UNLABELED USES Fungal prophylaxis in immunocompromised children who are hospitalized with neutropenia.

CONTRAINDICATIONS Hypersensitivity to anidulafungin or another echinocandin antifungal agent; lactation.

CAUTIOUS USE Hepatic impairment; pregnancy (category C). Safety and efficacy in children have not been established.

ROUTE & DOSAGE

Candidemia and Other *Candida* Infections

Adult: **IV** 200 mg loading dose on day 1, then 100 mg IV daily for at least 14 days after last positive culture

For the Treatment of Esophageal Candidiasis

Adult: **IV** 100 mg loading dose on day 1, then 50 mg IV daily for at least 14 days (and for at least 7 days after resolution of symptoms)

ADMINISTRATION

Intravenous

PREPARE: **IV Infusion:** Reconstitute each vial with the supplied single-use 15 mL vial of diluent [20% (w/w) dehydrated alcohol in water] to yield 3.33 mg/mL. ▪ Each 50 mg reconstituted vial **must be** further diluted with NS for D5W to a total infusion volume of 100 mL with a concentration of 0.5 mg/mL. ▪ For a 50 mg dose, dilute 15 mL reconstituted solution in 100 mL of IV fluid to yield 0.43 mg/mL. ▪ For a 100 mg dose, dilute 30 mL reconstituted solution in 250 mL of IV fluid to yield 0.36 mg/mL. ▪ For a 200 mg dose, dilute 60 mL reconstituted solution in 500 mL of IV fluid to yield 0.36 mg/mL.

ADMINISTER: **IV Infusion:** Give at a rate **no greater** than 1.1 mg/min. DO NOT give a bolus dose.

INCOMPATIBILITIES **Y-site: Amphotericin B, ertapenem, sodium bicarbonate.**

▪ Store unreconstituted vials, reconstituted vials, and companion diluent vials at 15°–30° C (59°–86° F). Reconstituted vials **must be** further diluted and administered within 24 h.

ADVERSE EFFECTS (≥1%) **Body as a Whole:** Hypersensitivity. **CNS:** Headache. **GI:** Diarrhea, nausea. **Hematologic:** Neutropenia. **Metabolic:** Increased alkaline phosphatase, increased ALT, increased gamma-glutamyl transferase, hypokalemia. **Skin:** Rash.

INTERACTIONS Drug: Cyclosporin increases overall systemic exposure (i.e., area under the curve, or AUC).

PHARMACOKINETICS Distribution: 84% protein bound. **Metabolism:** Nonhepatic degradation to inactive metabolites. **Elimination:** Fecal. **Half-Life:** 40–50 h.

NURSING IMPLICATIONS

Assessment & Drug Effects

- Prior to initiating therapy with anidulafungin, obtain specimen for fungal culture.
- Monitor for and report S&S of hypersensitivity (e.g., dyspnea, flushing, hypotension, swelling about the face, pruritus, rash, and urticaria) or liver dysfunction (e.g., jaundice, clay-colored stools).
- Discontinue infusion if signs of hypersensitivity appear.
- Monitor cardiac status especially with a preexisting history of dysrhythmias.
- Lab tests: Baseline and periodic liver function tests; periodic CBC with differential and platelet count; periodic serum electrolytes, amylase, and lipase.
- Monitor for S&S hypokalemia and hepatic toxicity (see Appendix F).
- Monitor diabetics for loss of glycemic control.

Patient & Family Education

- Report any of the following immediately if experienced during or shortly after infusion: Difficulty breathing, swelling about the face, itching, rash.
- Report S&S of jaundice to the physician: Clay-colored stool, dark urine, yellow skin or sclera, unexplained abdominal pain, or fatigue.

APOMORPHINE HYDROCHLORIDE

(a-po-mor'feen)

Apokyn

Classifications: ANTIPARKINSON; DOPAMINE RECEPTOR AGONIST

Therapeutic: ANTIPARKINSON

Prototype: Levodopa

Pregnancy Category: C

AVAILABILITY 10 mg/mL injection

ACTION & *THERAPEUTIC EFFECT* Apomorphine has central dopamine receptor agonist properties. Its mechanism of action in treatment of Parkinson's is thought to be related to its stimulation of centrally located postsynaptic dopamine D_2-type receptors. *Diminishes hypomobility associated with "off" episodes ("end-of-dose wear-*

ing off" and unpredictable "on/off" episodes) in persons with advanced Parkinson's disease.

USES Rescue of "off" episodes associated with advanced Parkinson's disease.

CONTRAINDICATIONS Concomitant use of drugs of the 5-HT_3 antagonist class (e.g., ondansetron, granisetron, dolasetron, palonosetron, and alosetron); hypersensitivity to the drug or its ingredients (i.e., sodium metabisulfite), benzyl alcohol hypersensitivity; renal failure; QT prolongation; heart failure, or shock; depression, suicidal ideation; decreased alertness, seizures, seizure disorder, unconscious state or coma, decreased alertness; lactation.

CAUTIOUS USE Hypersensitivity to sulfites; cardiovascular, cerebrovascular, respiratory, renal, or hepatic disease; CNS depression, history of (chronic) depression or suicidal ideation; hypotension; vomiting; bradycardia; hypokalemia and hypomagnesemia; older adult; pregnancy (category C).

ROUTE & DOSAGE

"Off" Episodes of Parkinson's Disease

Adult: **Subcutaneous** Start with a test dose where BP can be closely monitored. Escalate test dose no sooner than 2 h after last dose until dose is not tolerated or patient has response. If test dose of 0.2 mL (2 mg) is tolerated and has positive response, continue with 0.2 mL (2 mg); if no response, use test dose of 0.4 mL (4 mg); if tolerated and has a positive response, continue with 0.3 mL (3 mg); if 0.4 mL test dose is not tolerated, try 0.3 mL (3 mg) test dose; if 0.3 mL is tolerated, continue with 0.2 mL (2 mg). May increase by 1 mg every few days, generally should not exceed 0.4 mL (4 mg) as an outpatient. Max dose: 0.6 mL as single injection and max 5 injections/day. If therapy is interrupted for 1 wk, restart with 2 mg dose.

ADMINISTRATION

Subcutaneous

- The dosing pen is marked in mL, not mg, increments; a 1 mg dose is equal to 0.1 mL.
- Aspirate to avoid intravascular injection and ensure the injection is subcutaneous and not intradermal.
- Rotate subcutaneous sites to reduce skin reactions.
- If the patient has not received apomorphine in more than 1 wk, reinstitute it by starting with the initial test dose and titrating to the desired dose.
- Subcutaneous apomorphine causes nausea and vomiting; thus the recommendation is to give 300 mg of trimethobenzamide PO t.i.d., starting 3 days before the first injection and continued for at least the first 2 mo of treatment.
- Store at 15°–30° C (59°–86° F).

ADVERSE EFFECTS (≥1%) **Body as a Whole:** Weakness, yawning, tiredness. **CNS:** CNS depression, dizziness, drowsiness, headache, lightheadedness, euphoria, restlessness, tremor, depression, *dyskinesias, hallucinations*. **CV:** Acute circulatory failure, bradycardia, hypertension, orthostatic hypotension, QT prolongation, vasovagal response, syncope. **GI:** *Nausea, vomiting,* hypersalivation, taste perversions. **Metabolic:** Peripheral edema. **Respiratory:** Respiratory depression, tachypnea, cough, pharyngitis, rhinitis. **Skin:** Contact dermatitis, *bruising,* granuloma, pruritus, sweating. **Urogenital:** *Frequent penile erections,* painful erections.

INTERACTIONS Drug: Alosetron, dolasetron, granisetron, ondansetron, palonosetron may cause severe hypotension and unconsciousness; **alfuzosin, amoxapine, bepridil, chloroquine, clozapine, cyclobenzaprine, droperidol, flecainide, halofantrine, halothane, levomethadyl,** LOCAL ANESTHETICS, MACROLIDES **(clarithromycin, erythromycin, troleandomycin), maprotiline, mefloquine, methadone, pentamidine,** PHENOTHIAZINES, **probucol, gatifloxacin, gemifloxacin, grepafloxacin, levofloxacin, moxifloxacin, sparfloxacin, tacrolimus,** TRICYCLIC ANTIDEPRESSANTS, **amiodarone, clozapine, disopyramide, dofetilide, dolasetron, haloperidol, ibutilide, mesoridazine, palonosetron, pimozide, procainamide, quinidine, thioridazine, sotalol, ziprasidone** may exacerbate QT_c prolongation; may increase CNS depression with other CNS depressants, including TRICYCLIC ANTIDEPRESSANTS, ANXIOLYTICS, SEDATIVES, HYPNOTICS, **dronabinol,** GENERAL ANESTHETICS, **mirtazapine, nefazodone,** OPIATE AGONISTS, **pramipexole, ropinirole,** SKELETAL MUSCLE RELAXANTS, **tramadol, trazodone. Herbal: Kava** may increase the symptoms of Parkinson's disease.

PHARMACOKINETICS Absorption: Subcutaneous absorption dependent on site utilized—abdominal injection absorbed faster than thigh; lowering the temperature of the injection site slows absorption. **Onset:** 7–14 min. **Peak:** 40–60 min. **Duration:** Up to 2 h. **Distribution:** 85–90% protein bound. **Metabolism:** Metabolized by glucuronidation, sulfation, and N-demethylation. **Elimination:** Excreted by kidneys. **Half-Life:** 30–60 min.

NURSING IMPLICATIONS

Assessment & Drug Effects

- Periodic ECG, especially in those with known CV disease.
- Withhold drug and notify physician for S&S of torsades de pointes (i.e., palpitations and syncope), especially in those with bradycardia or suspected hypokalemia or hypomagnesemia.
- Lab tests: Periodic serum electrolytes.
- Monitor closely for orthostatic hypotension, especially when doses are increased, and in patients taking antihypertensive medications and vasodilators (especially nitrates).

Patient & Family Education

- The dosing pen is marked in mL (not mg) increments; a 1 mg dose is equal to 0.1 mL.
- Avoid the use of alcohol while taking this drug.
- Report promptly any of the following: Irregular or fast, pounding heartbeat, or palpitations; dizziness, lightheadedness, or fainting; unexplained weakness, tiredness, or sleepiness; confusion, hallucinations, or depression; unusual body movements; vomiting; or prolonged painful erections.
- Do not engage in potentially hazardous activities until reaction to drug is known.

APRACLONIDINE

(a-pra-clo′ni-deen)

Iopidine

Pregnancy Category: C

See Appendix A-1.

Common adverse effects in *italic,* life-threatening effects underlined; generic names in **bold**; classifications in SMALL CAPS; ♣ Canadian drug name; ⓟ Prototype drug

APREPITANT

(a-pre'pi-tant)

FOSAPREPITANT

(fos-a-pre'pi-tant)

Emend

Classifications: CENTRAL ACTING ANTIEMETIC; SUBSTANCE P/NEUROKININ 1 (NK_1) RECEPTOR ANTAGONIST
Therapeutic: ANTIEMETIC
Pregnancy Category: B

AVAILABILITY 80 mg, 125 mg capsules; 115 mg powder for injection

ACTION & *THERAPEUTIC EFFECT* Aprepitant is a selective substance P/neurokinin 1 (NK_1) receptor antagonist. Substance P and the NK-1 receptors are present in areas in the brain that control the emetic reflex. Aprepitant crosses the blood–brain barrier and occupies brain NK_1 receptors. Peripheral blockade by NK_1 receptor antagonists at receptors located in the GI is an additional hypothesized mechanism of action. *Aprepitant augments the antiemetic activity of the 5-HT_3-receptor antagonist, ondansetron, and inhibits both the acute and delayed phases of emesis induced by chemotherapy agents.*

USES Prevention of acute and delayed nausea and vomiting associated with emetogenic chemotherapy.

CONTRAINDICATIONS Hypersensitivity to aprepitant; concurrent use of pimozide; children younger than 18 y; lactation.
CAUTIOUS USE Chemotherapeutic agents metabolized through CYP3A4; severe hepatic impairment; severe renal impairment without dialysis; pregnancy (category B).

ROUTE & DOSAGE

Chemotherapy-Induced Nausea & Vomiting
Adult: **PO** 125 mg 1 h prior to chemotherapy, then 80 mg qa.m. for the next 2 days in conjunction with other antiemetics **IV** 115 mg substituted for oral dose on day 1

ADMINISTRATION

Oral

- Ensure that capsule is swallowed whole with a full glass of water. Do not crush or sprinkle the contents of the capsule.
- Give 1 h before start of chemotherapy.
- Store at 20°–25° C (68°–77° F). Keep the desiccant in the original bottle.

Intravenous (Fosaprepitant)

PREPARE: **Infusion:** Inject 5 mL NS onto the inside of the vial to prevent foaming. Swirl gently to dissolve. Add to 110 mL of NS to yield 1 mg/mL. Gently invert bag several times to distribute.
ADMINISTER: **Infusion:** Infuse over 15 min or longer if patient complains of burning sensation.

- Reconstituted drug is stable for 24 h at room temperature.

ADVERSE EFFECTS (≥1%) **Body as a Whole:** *Fatigue,* asthenia, malaise, dehydration, fever. **CNS:** Dizziness, insomnia, headache, peripheral neuropathy, sensory neuropathy, anxiety, confusion, depression. **GI:** *Constipation, diarrhea, anorexia, nausea, hiccups,* abdominal pain, gastritis, gastroesophageal reflux, abnormal or impaired taste (dysgeusia), dyspepsia, dysphagia, flatulence, hypersalivation, increased taste disturbance, increased AST and

ALT. **Hematologic:** Neutropenia, anemia. **Musculoskeletal:** Pain, myalgia. **Respiratory:** Cough, dyspnea, upper or lower respiratory infection, pneumonitis, respiratory insufficiency. **Special Senses:** Tinnitus.

INTERACTIONS Drug: Increased risk of cardiovascular toxicity with **dofetilide, pimozide;** may decrease **warfarin** concentrations and INR; may decrease levels and effectiveness of ORAL CONTRACEPTIVES; **carbamazepine, griseofulvin, modafinil, rifabutin, rifapentine, phenobarbital, primidone** may decrease antiemetic efficacy; may increase levels of **dexamethasone.** Because aprepitant is a substrate of CYP3A4, many additional drug interactions are theoretically possible. **Food: Grapefruit juice** may decrease effectiveness of aprepitant. **Herbal: St. John's wort** may decrease effectiveness of aprepitant.

PHARMACOKINETICS Absorption: 60–65% of oral dose reaches systemic circulation. **Peak:** 4 h. **Duration:** 95% protein bound; readily crosses the blood–brain barrier. **Metabolism:** In liver by CYP3A4. **Elimination:** Not renally excreted. **Half-Life:** 9–12 h.

NURSING IMPLICATIONS

Assessment & Drug Effects

- Monitor cardiac status especially with preexisting CV disease or concurrent use of any CYP3A4 substrate drug (e.g., ketoconazole, itraconazole, nefazodone, troleandomycin, clarithromycin).
- Lab tests: Monitor PT/INR 7–10 days after 3-day regimen with concurrent warfarin use; monitor phenytoin level with concurrent use; monitor serum electrolytes, UA, and CBC.

Patient & Family Education

- Report immediately to physician any of the following: Skin rash; difficulty breathing or shortness of breath; rapid, slow, or irregular heartbeat; changes in BP; dizziness or confusion; unexplained sharp or severe pain in leg or stomach; rectal bleeding. Inform physician of all other drugs or herbal products you are using. Do not take new drugs (prescription, OTC, herbal) without first consulting physician.
- Use barrier contraception in addition to oral contraceptives while taking drug.

ARGATROBAN

(ar-ga'tro-ban)

Acova, Novastan

Classifications: ANTICOAGULANT; DIRECT THROMBIN INHIBITOR

Therapeutic: THROMBIN INHIBITOR

Prototype: Lepirudin

Pregnancy Category: C

AVAILABILITY 250 mg/2.5 mL vials

ACTION & *THERAPEUTIC EFFECT* Synthetic derivative of arginine that is a direct thrombin inhibitor. Capable of inhibiting the action of both free and clot-bound thrombin. *Reversibly binds to the thrombin active site, thereby blocking clot-forming activity of thrombin.*

USES Prophylaxis or treatment of thrombosis in patients with heparin-induced thrombocytopenia (HIT); prophylaxis or treatment of coronary artery thrombosis during percutaneous coronary interventions (PCI) in patients at risk for HIT.

UNLABELED USES Treatment of disseminated intravascular coagulation (DIC).

CONTRAINDICATIONS Hypersensitivity to argatroban; lactation. Any bleeding including intracranial bleeding, GI bleeding, retroperitoneal bleeding; severe hepatic impairment. **CAUTIOUS USE** Diseased states with increased risk of hemorrhaging; severe hypertension; GI ulcerations, hepatic impairment; spinal anesthesia, stroke, surgery, trauma; pregnancy (category C). Safety and effectiveness in children younger than 18 y are not established.

ROUTE & DOSAGE

Prevention & Treatment of Thrombosis

Adult: **IV** 2 mcg/kg/min, may be adjusted to maintain an aPTT of 1.5–3 times baseline (max: 10 mcg/kg/min)

Hepatic Impairment Dosage Adjustment

0.5 mcg/kg/min, may be adjusted to maintain an aPTT of 1.5–3 times baseline (max: 10 mcg/kg/min)

Prophylaxis or Treatment of Coronary Thrombosis during PCI

Adult: **IV** Initiate at 25 mcg/kg/min, then bolus of 350 mcg/kg administered via a large bore IV line over 3–5 min, then 25 mcg/kg/min by continuous infusion; maintain activated clotting time (ACT) 300–450 sec; if ACT below 300 sec, increase infusion to 30 mcg/kg/min; if ACT over 450 sec, decrease infusion to 15 mcg/kg/min

ADMINISTRATION

Intravenous

Note: Argatroban is supplied in 100 mg/mL vials which **must be** diluted 100-fold prior to infusion.

PREPARE: **Continuous:** Dilute each 2.5 mL vial by mixing with 250 mL of D5W, NS, or LR to yield 1 mg/mL. ▪ Mix by repeated inversion of the diluent bag for 1 min.

ADMINISTER: **Continuous for Heparin-Induced Thrombocytopenia (HIT/HITTS):** Before administration, discontinue heparin and obtain a baseline aPTT. ▪ Give at a rate of 2 mcg/kg/min, or as ordered. Lower initial doses are required with hepatic impairment. ▪ Check aPTT 2 h after initiation of therapy. After the initial dose, adjust dose (not to exceed 10 mcg/kg/min) until the steady-state aPTT is 1.5 to 3 times baseline (not to exceed 100 sec). Adjust dose to maintain aPTT at 1.5–3 times baseline, but not greater than 100 sec. ▪ Check aPTT 2 h after initiation of therapy to confirm desired therapeutic range. **Continuous for Percutaneous Coronary Intervention:** Start an infusion at 25 mcg/kg/min and give a bolus of 350 mcg/kg, via a large bore IV line, over 3–5 min. ▪ Check ACT 5–10 min after the bolus dose. If the ACT is greater than 450 sec, decrease infusion rate to 15 mcg/kg/min. If ACT is less than 300 sec, give an additional bolus of 150 mcg/kg and increase infusion to 30 mcg/kg/min. ▪ Check ACT q5–10min to maintain an ACT level 300–450 sec.

▪ Diluted solutions are stable for 24 h at 25° C (77° F) in ambient indoor light. ▪ Protect from direct sunlight. Store solutions refrigerated at 2°–8° C (36°–46° F) in the dark.

ADVERSE EFFECTS (≥1%) **Body as a Whole:** Fever, sepsis, pain, allergic reactions (rare). **CV:** Hypotension, <u>cardiac arrest</u>, ventricular tachycardia. **GI:** Diarrhea, nausea, vomiting, coughing, abdominal pain. **Hematologic:** <u>Major GI bleed</u>, *minor GI*

bleeding, hematuria, decrease Hgb/Hct, groin bleed, hemoptysis, brachial bleed. **Respiratory:** Dyspnea. **Urogenital:** UTI.

INTERACTIONS Drug: Heparin results in increased bleeding; may prolong PT with **warfarin;** may increase risk of bleeding with THROMBOLYTICS. **Herbal: Feverfew, garlic, ginger, ginkgo** may increase potential for bleeding.

PHARMACOKINETICS Peak: 1–3 h. **Distribution:** In extracellular fluid; 54% protein bound. **Metabolism:** In liver by CYP3A4/5. **Elimination:** Primarily in bile (78%). **Half-Life:** 39–51 min.

NURSING IMPLICATIONS

Assessment & Drug Effects

- **Heparin-Induced Thrombocytopenia:** Monitor aPTT. Dose adjustment may be needed to reach the target aPTT. Check aPTT 2 h after initiation of therapy. After the initial dose, adjust dose (not to exceed 10 mcg/kg/min), until the steady-state aPTT is 1.5 to 3 times baseline (not to exceed 100 sec).
- Monitor cardiovascular status carefully during therapy.
- Monitor for and report S&S of bleeding: Ecchymosis, epistaxis, GI bleeding, hematuria, hemoptysis.
- Note: Patients with history of GI ulceration, hypertension, recent trauma, or surgery are at increased risk for bleeding.
- Monitor neurologic status and report immediately focal or generalized deficits.
- Lab tests: Baseline and periodic ACT (activated clotting time), thrombin time (TT), platelet count, Hgb and Hct; daily INR when argatroban and warfarin are co-administered; periodic stool test for occult blood; urinalysis.

Patient & Family Education

- Report immediately any of the following to physician: Unexplained back or stomach pain; black, tarry stools; blood in urine, coughing up blood; difficulty breathing; dizziness or fainting spells; heavy menstrual bleeding; nosebleeds; unusual bruising or bleeding at any site.

ARIPIPRAZOLE

(a-rip′-i-pra-zole)

Abilify, Abilify Discmelt

Classifications: ANTIPSYCHOTIC, ATYPICAL; DOPAMINE SYSTEM STABILIZER

Therapeutic: ANTIPSYCHOTIC

Prototype: Clozapine

Pregnancy Category: C

AVAILABILITY 2 mg, 5 mg, 10 mg, 15 mg, 20 mg, 30 mg tablets; 10 mg, 15 mg disintegrating tablets; 1 mg/mL oral solution; 9.75 mg/13 mL injection

ACTION & *THERAPEUTIC EFFECT* Efficacy of aripiprazole may be mediated through a combination of partial agonist activity at D_2 and 5-HT_{1A} receptors and antagonist activity at 5-HT_{2A} receptors. *Partial dopaminergic agonist property of aripiprazole accounts for antipsychotic treatment of schizophrenic and bipolar individuals.*

USES Treatment of schizophrenia, bipolar mania, maintenance in bipolar 1 disorder, adjunct treatment in major depressive disorder.

UNLABELED USES Restless leg syndrome.

CONTRAINDICATIONS Hypersensitivity to aripiprazole; dementia in elderly; QT prolongation; lactation.

CAUTIOUS USE History of seizures or conditions that lower seizure threshold (e.g., Alzheimer's dementia); suicidal ideation; brain tumor; dementia; diabetes mellitus; patients with known cardiovascular disease (history of MI or ischemic heart disease, heart failure, or conduction abnormalities), cerebrovascular disease, or conditions that predispose to hypotension (dehydration, hypovolemia, and treatment with antihypertensive medications); dysphagia; ethanol intoxication; hyperglycemia, hypothermia; obesity, elderly; pregnancy (category C); children younger than 10 y.

ROUTE & DOSAGE

Schizophrenia
Adult: **PO** 10–15 mg once daily, may increase at 2-wk intervals to max of 30 mg/day if needed
Adolescent/Child (at least 10 y old): **PO** 2 mg daily, increase to 5 mg after 2 days, increase to 10 mg after 2 more days. Can increase up to 30 mg.

Bipolar Mania
Adult: **PO** 15–30 mg once daily
Adolescent/Child (at least 10 y old): **PO** 2 mg daily, increase to 5 mg after 2 days, increase to 10 mg after 2 more days. Can increase up to 30 mg.

Agitation Associated with Schizophrenia/Bipolar
Adult: **IM** 9.75 mg (range: 5.25–15 mg)

Adjunct in Major Depression
Adult: **PO** 2–5 mg daily

Pharmacogentic Dosage Adjustment
Reduced CYP2D6 expression (i.e., poor metabolizers): Give 70% of normal starting dose

ADMINISTRATION

Oral

- Note that dose should be reduced by 50% with concurrent treatment with ketoconazole, quinidine, fluoxetine, or paroxetine.
- Store at 15°–30° C (59°–86° F).

ADVERSE EFFECTS (≥1%) **Body as a Whole:** *Headache,* asthenia, fever, flu-like symptoms, peripheral edema, chest pain, neck pain, neck rigidity. **CNS:** *Anxiety, insomnia, lightheadedness, somnolence, akathisia,* tremor, extrapyramidal symptoms, depression, nervousness, increased salivation, hostility, suicidal thought, manic reaction, abnormal gait, confusion, cogwheel rigidity. **CV:** Hypertension, tachycardia, hypotension, bradycardia. Risk of stroke in elderly with dementia-related psychosis. **GI:** *Nausea, vomiting, constipation,* anorexia. **Hematologic:** Ecchymosis, anemia. **Metabolic:** Weight gain, weight loss, hyperglycemia, diabetes mellitus, increased creatine kinase. **Musculoskeletal:** Muscle cramp. **Respiratory:** Rhinitis, cough. **Skin:** Rash. **Special Senses:** Blurred vision.

INTERACTIONS Drug: CYP3A4 inducers (**carbamazepine, phenytoin,** etc.) will decrease aripiprazole levels (may need to double aripiprazole dose); use with CYP2D6 or CYP3A4 inhibitors (**ketoconazole, quinidine, fluoxetine, paroxetine,** etc.) may increase aripiprazole levels (reduce dose by 1/2); may cause additive sedation with other SEDATIVES (alcohol, tramadol, BARBITURATES, etc.); may enhance effects of ANTIHYPERTENSIVE AGENTS. **Herbal: St. John's wort** may decrease aripiprazole levels. **Food:** High fat meals may delay time to peak plasma levels.

PHARMACOKINETICS Absorption: 87% bioavailable. **Peak:** 3–5 h. **Metabolism:** In liver by CYP3A4 and 2D6. Major metabolite, has some activity. **Elimination:** 55% in feces, 25% in urine. **Half-Life:** 75 h (94 h for metabolite); 146 h (poor metabolizers).

NURSING IMPLICATIONS

Assessment & Drug Effects

- Monitor diabetics for loss of glycemic control.
- Monitor cardiovascular status. Assess for and report orthostatic hypotension. Take BP supine then in sitting position. Report systolic drop of greater than 15–20 mm Hg. Patients at increased risk are those who are dehydrated, hypovolemic, or receiving concurrent antihypertensive therapy.
- Monitor body temperature in situations likely to elevate core temperature (e.g., exercising strenuously, exposure to extreme heat, receiving drugs with anticholinergic activity, or being subject to dehydration).
- Monitor for and report signs of tardive dyskinesia.
- Monitor for and immediately report S&S of neuroleptic malignant syndrome (NMS) that include: Hyperpyrexia, muscle rigidity, altered mental status, irregular pulse or blood pressure, tachycardia, diaphoresis, and cardiac dysrhythmia. Withhold drug if NMS is suspected.
- Lab tests: Monitor periodically Hct and Hgb. Monitor periodically blood glucose. Monitor for elevated CPK and myoglobinuria if NMS is suspected.

Patient & Family Education

- Carefully monitor blood glucose levels if diabetic.
- Do not drive or engage in other potentially hazardous activities until reaction to drug is known.
- Avoid situations where you are likely to become overheated or dehydrated.
- Notify physician if you become pregnant or intend to become pregnant while taking this drug.

ASCORBIC ACID (VITAMIN C)

Apo-C ♣, Ascorbicap, Cecon, Cetane, Cevalin, CeVi-Sol ♣, Flavorcee, Redoxon ♣, Schiff Effervescent Vitamin C, Vita-C

ASCORBATE, SODIUM

(a-skor'bate)

Cenolate

Classification: VITAMIN
Therapeutic: VITAMIN SUPPLEMENT; URINARY ACIDIFIER
Pregnancy Category: C

AVAILABILITY 25 mg, 50 mg, 100 mg, 250 mg, 500 mg, 1000 mg tablets; 500 mg/mL injection

ACTION & *THERAPEUTIC EFFECT* Water-soluble vitamin essential for synthesis and maintenance of collagen and intercellular ground substance of body tissue cells, blood vessels, cartilage, bones, teeth, skin, and tendons. Humans are unable to synthesize ascorbic acid in the body therefore, it **must be** consumed daily. *Increases protective mechanism of the immune system, thus supporting wound healing, and resistance to infection.*

USES Prophylaxis and treatment of scurvy and as a dietary supplement.

UNLABELED USES To acidify urine; to prevent and treat cancer; to treat idiopathic methemoglobinemia; as adjuvant during deferoxamine therapy for iron toxicity; in megadoses will possibly reduce severity and duration of common cold. Widely used as an antioxidant in formulations of parenteral tetracycline and other drugs.

Common adverse effects in *italic*, life-threatening effects underlined; generic names in **bold**; classifications in SMALL CAPS; ♣ Canadian drug name; ℗ Prototype drug

CONTRAINDICATIONS Use of sodium ascorbate in patients on sodium restriction; use of calcium ascorbate in patients receiving digitalis.

CAUTIOUS USE Excessive doses in patients with G6PD deficiency; hemochromatosis, thalassemia, sideroblastic anemia, sickle cell anemia; pregnancy (category C); patients prone to gout or renal calculi.

ROUTE & DOSAGE

Therapeutic

Adult: **PO/IV/IM/Subcutaneous** 150–500 mg/day in 1–2 doses

Child: **PO/IV/IM/Subcutaneous** 100–300 mg/day in divided doses

Prophylactic

Adult: **PO/IV/IM/Subcutaneous** 45–60 mg/day

Child: **PO/IV/IM/Subcutaneous** 30–60 mg/day

Urinary Acidifier

Adult: **PO/IV/IM/Subcutaneous** 4–12 g/day in divided doses

Child: **PO/IV/IM/Subcutaneous** 500 mg q6–8h

ADMINISTRATION

Oral

- Give oral solutions mixed with food.
- Dissolve effervescent tablet in a glass of water immediately before ingestion.

Intramuscular, Subcutaneous

- Open ampules with caution. After prolonged storage, decomposition may occur with release of carbon dioxide and resulting increase in pressure within ampule.
- Be aware that ascorbic acid injection may gradually darken on exposure to light; slight coloration reportedly does not affect its therapeutic action.

Intravenous

Verify correct IV concentration and rate of infusion for children with physician.

PREPARE: **Direct/Continuous/Intermittent:** Give undiluted or diluted (preferred) in solutions such as NS, D5W, D5/NS, LR. ▪ Be aware that parenteral vitamin C is incompatible with many drugs. ▪ Consult pharmacist for compatibility information.

ADMINISTER: **Direct:** Give undiluted at a rate of 100 mg or a fraction thereof over 1 min. **Continuous/Intermittent (preferred):** Give at ordered rate determined by volume of solution to be infused.

INCOMPATIBILITIES **Solution/additive: Aminophylline, bleomycin, erythromycin, nafcillin, sodium bicarbonate, theophylline. Y-site: Etomidate, thiopental.**

- Store in airtight, light-resistant, nonmetallic containers, away from heat and sunlight, preferably at 15°–30° C (59°–86° F), unless otherwise specified by manufacturer.

ADVERSE EFFECTS (≥1%) **GI:** Nausea, vomiting, heartburn, diarrhea, or abdominal cramps (high doses). **Hematologic:** Acute hemolytic anemia (patients with deficiency of G6PD); sickle cell crisis. **CNS:** Headache or insomnia (high doses). **Urogenital:** Urethritis, dysuria, crystalluria, hyperoxaluria, or hyperuricemia (high doses). **Other:** Mild soreness at injection site; dizziness and temporary faintness with rapid IV administration.

DIAGNOSTIC TEST INTERFERENCE High doses of ascorbic acid can produce false-negative results for ***urine glucose*** with ***glucose oxidase*** methods (e.g., ***Clinitest, TesTape, Diastix***); false-positive results with

copper reduction methods (e.g., Benedict's solution, Clinitest); and false increases in ***serum uric acid*** determinations (by ***enzymatic methods***). Interferes with ***urinary steroid*** (17-OHCS) determinations (by ***modified Reddy, Jenkins, Thorn procedure***), decreases in ***serum bilirubin,*** and may cause increases in ***serum cholesterol, creatinine,*** and ***uric acid*** (methodologic inferences). May produce false-negative tests for ***occult blood*** in stools if taken within 48–72 h of test.

INTERACTIONS Drug: Large doses may attenuate hypoprothrombinemic effects of ORAL ANTICOAGULANTS; SALICYLATES may inhibit ascorbic acid uptake by leukocytes and tissues, and ascorbic acid may decrease elimination of SALICYLATES; chronic high doses of ascorbic acid may diminish the effects of **disulfiram.**

PHARMACOKINETICS Absorption: Readily absorbed PO; however, absorption may be limited with large doses. **Distribution:** Widely distributed to body tissues; crosses placenta; distributed into breast milk. **Metabolism:** In liver. **Elimination:** Rapidly in urine when plasma level exceeds renal threshold of 1.4 mg/dL.

NURSING IMPLICATIONS

Assessment & Drug Effects

- Lab tests: Periodic Hct and Hgb, serum electrolytes.
- Monitor for S&S of acute hemolytic anemia, sickle cell crisis.

Patient & Family Education

- High doses of vitamin C are not recommended during pregnancy.
- Take large doses of vitamin C in divided amounts because the body uses only what is needed at a particular time and excretes the rest in urine.
- Megadoses can interfere with absorption of vitamin B_{12}.
- Note: Vitamin C increases the absorption of iron when taken at the same time as iron-rich foods.

ASENAPINE

(a-sin′a-peen)

Saphris

Classifications: ANTIPSYCHOTIC, ATYPICAL; SEROTONIN ANTAGONIST; ANTIMANIC; ANTIDEPRESSANT

Therapeutic: ANTIPSYCHOTIC; ANTIMANIC; ANTIDEPRESSANT

Prototype: Clozapine

Pregnancy Category: C

AVAILABILITY 5 mg, 10 mg sublingual tablets

ACTION & *THERAPEUTIC EFFECT* Mechanism of action thought to be related to antagonism to certain CNS dopamine and serotonin receptors. Also causes CNS alpha-1 antagonism resulting in orthostatic hypotension, tachycardia, syncope, and dizziness. *Effect on serotonin may account for activity against the negative symptoms of schizophrenia.*

USES Acute treatment of schizophrenia; acute treatment of manic or mixed episodes associated with bipolar disorder (bipolar I disorder) with or without psychotic features.

CONTRAINDICATIONS Dementia-related psychosis; ketoacidosis; severe neutropenia (ANC less than 1000/mm^3); patients with history of torsades de pointes related to drugs; suicidal ideation; severe hepatic impairment (Child-Pugh class C).

CAUTIOUS USE Tardive dyskinesia, cardiovascular disease (history of MI, ischemic heart disease, HF, conduction abnormalities, bradycardia),

Common adverse effects in *italic*, life-threatening effects underlined; generic names in **bold**; classifications in SMALL CAPS; ♣ Canadian drug name; ⓟ Prototype drug

cerebrovascular disease, dehydration, hypovolemia, diabetes mellitus; concurrent use of drugs that prolong the QT_c interval, including Class IA antiarrhythmics (e.g., quinidine, procainamide) or Class III antiarrhythmics (e.g., amiodarone), antipsychotic medications (e.g., chlorpromazine); history of seizures; Alzheimer's dementia; elderly; history of suicidal tendencies; pregnancy (category C); lactation. Safety and effectiveness in pediatric patients have not been established.

ROUTE & DOSAGE

Schizophrenia

Adult: **SL** 5 mg b.i.d.

Bipolar Disorder

Adult: **SL** Start at 10 mg b.i.d., may decrease to 5 mg b.i.d. if higher dose not tolerated.

ADMINISTRATION

Oral

- Tablet must be placed under tongue and allowed to dissolve completely.
- Ensure that tablet is not chewed or swallowed.
- Eating and drinking should be avoided for 10 min after administration.
- Store at 15°–30° C (59°–86° F).

ADVERSE EFFECTS (≥1%) **Body as a Whole:** Fatigue, irritability, pain in extremities. **CNS:** Agitation, akathisia, anxiety, *dizziness*, dysgeusia, *extrapyramidal symptoms, headache, insomnia, somnolence*. **CV:** Hypertension. **GI:** Constipation, dyspepsia, nausea, vomiting. **Metabolic:** Increased appetite, increased weight. **Musculoskeletal:** Arthralgia. **Respiratory:** Dry mouth, oral hypoesthesia, salivary hypersecretion.

INTERACTIONS Drug: Fluvoxamine and **imipramine** can increase asenapine levels.

PHARMACOKINETICS Absorption: Bioavailability 35%. **Peak:** 0.5–1.5 h. **Distribution:** 95% plasma protein bound. **Metabolism:** In liver via CYP1A2. **Elimination:** 50% renal; 40% fecal. **Half-Life:** 24 h.

NURSING IMPLICATIONS

Assessment & Drug Effects

- Monitor BP, HR, and weight. Monitor orthostatic vital signs with concurrent antihypertensive therapy or any condition that predisposes to hypotension (e.g., advanced age, dehydration).
- Monitor for orthostatic hypotension and syncope, especially early in therapy.
- Monitor diabetics or those at risk for diabetes for loss of glycemic control.
- Withhold drug and report promptly S&S of neuroleptic malignant syndrome (see Appendix F).
- Lab tests: Baseline and periodic CBC.

Patient & Family Education

- Be alert for and report worsening of condition, including ideas of suicide.
- Make position changes slowly, especially from lying or sitting to a standing position.
- If diabetic, monitor blood sugar closely for loss of control.
- Stop taking the drug and report immediately any of the following: High fever, muscle rigidity, altered mental status, or palpitations.
- Avoid engaging in hazardous activities until response to drug is known.
- Avoid alcohol while taking this drug.

ASPARAGINASE

(a-spar'a-gi-nase)

Colaspase, Elspar, Kidrolase A, L-asparaginase

Classifications: ANTINEOPLASTIC; ENZYME; ANTIMETABOLITE

Therapeutic: ANTINEOPLASTIC

Pregnancy Category: C

AVAILABILITY 10,000 international unit vial

ACTION & *THERAPEUTIC EFFECT* A highly toxic drug with a low therapeutic index. Catalyzes asparagine to aspartic acid and ammonia, thus depleting extracellular supply of an amino acid essential to synthesis of DNA and other nucleoproteins. *Reduced availability of asparagine causes death of tumor cells, since unlike normal cells, tumor cells are unable to synthesize their own supply. Resistance to cytotoxic action develops rapidly, and it is not an effective treatment for solid tumors.*

USES Primarily in combination regimens with other antineoplastic agents to treat acute lymphocytic leukemia (ALL).

UNLABELED USES Other leukemias, lymphosarcoma, and (intraarterially) treatment of hypoglycemia due to pancreatic islet cell tumor.

CONTRAINDICATIONS Hypersensitivity to *Escherichia coli* protein; history of or existing pancreatitis; chickenpox (existing or recent illness or exposure), herpetic infection; lactation.

CAUTIOUS USE Liver impairment; diabetes mellitus; anticoagulation therapy, coagulopathy; infections; history of urate calculi or gout; antineoplastic or radiation therapy; pregnancy (category C).

ROUTE & DOSAGE

Induction Agent

Adult: **IV** (sole agent) 200 international units/kg/day for 28 days, inject over at least 30 min into running IV OR 1000 international units/kg/day for days 22–32 (along with prednisone and vincristine)

Child: **IV** 1000 units/kg/day × 10 days starting day 22 (along with prednisone and vincristine)

Desensitization Protocol

Adult/Child: **IV** Schedule begins with 1 international unit, then double the dose q10min until the accumulated total matches the planned dose. See package insert for detailed dosing.

ADMINISTRATION

Intravenous

An intradermal skin test is usually performed prior to initial dose and when drug is readministered after an interval of a week or more; allergic reactions are unpredictable.

- Observe test site for at least 1 h for evidence of positive reaction (wheal, erythema). A negative skin test, however, does not preclude possibility of an allergic reaction.
- Administer test dose and IV infusion under constant supervision by clinician experienced in cancer chemotherapy.
- Use only clear solutions.

***PREPARE:* IV Infusion:** Reconstitute with sterile water or with 0.9% NaCl. ▪Each 10,000 international unit vial is diluted with 5 mL of diluent to yield 2000 international units/mL. ▪ Shake vial well to promote dissolution of powder. Avoid vigorous shaking. Ordinary shaking does not inactivate the enzyme or cause foaming of content.

ADMINISTER: **IV Infusion:** Further dilute reconstituted solution with NS or D5W by administration into tubing of an already free flowing infusion of one of these solutions. ▪ Give over a period of not less than 30 min. ▪ Use a 5-micron filter to remove gelatinous fiber-like particles that can develop in solutions on standing.

▪ Store sealed vial of lyophilized powder below 8° C (46° F) unless otherwise directed by manufacturer. Store reconstituted solutions and solutions diluted for IV infusion at 2°–8° C (36°–46° F) for up to 8 h; then discard.

ADVERSE EFFECTS (≥1%) **Body as a Whole:** Hypersensitivity (*Skin rashes, urticaria*, respiratory distress, anaphylaxis), chills, fever, fatal hyperthermia, perspiration, weight loss. **CNS:** Depression, fatigue, lethargy, drowsiness, confusion, agitation, hallucinations, dizziness, Parkinson-like syndrome with tremor and progressive increase in muscle tone. **GI:** *Severe vomiting, nausea,* anorexia, abdominal cramps, diarrhea, acute pancreatitis, liver function abnormalities. **Urogenital:** Uric acid nephropathy, azotemia, proteinuria, renal failure. **Hematologic:** *Reduced clotting factors* (especially V, VII, VIII, IX), *decreased circulating platelets and fibrinogen,* leukopenia. **Metabolic:** Hyperglycemia, glycosuria, polyuria, hypoalbuminemia, hypocalcemia, hyperuricemia. **Other:** Flank pain, infections.

DIAGNOSTIC TEST INTERFERENCE Asparaginase may interfere with ***thyroid function*** tests: Decreased total ***serum thyroxine*** and increased ***thyroxine-binding globulin index;*** pretreatment values return within 4 wk after drug is discontinued.

INTERACTIONS Drug: Decreased hypoglycemic effects of SULFONYLUREAS, **insulin;** increased potential for toxicity if asparaginase is given concurrently or immediately before CORTICOSTEROIDS, **vincristine;** blocks antitumor effect of **methotrexate** if given concurrently or immediately before it.

PHARMACOKINETICS Distribution: Into intravascular space (80%) and lymph; low levels in CSF, pleural and peritoneal fluids. **Elimination:** Small amounts found in urine. **Half-Life:** 8–30 h.

NURSING IMPLICATIONS

Assessment & Drug Effects

- Have immediately available: Personnel, drugs, and equipment for treating allergic reaction (which may range from urticaria to anaphylactic shock) whenever drug is administered, including skin testing.
- Monitor for S&S and be alert to evidence of hypersensitivity or anaphylactoid reaction (see Appendix F) during drug administration. Anaphylaxis usually occurs within 30–60 min after dose has been given and is more likely with intermittent administrations, particularly at intervals of 7 days or more.
- Monitor I&O and maintain adequate fluid intake.
- Evaluate CNS function (general behavior, emotional status, level of consciousness, thought content, motor function) before and during therapy.
- Note: Toxicity potential is increased when giving drug immediately before a course of prednisone and vincristine; toxicity appears less when given after these drugs.

- Lab tests: Periodic serum amylase, serum calcium blood glucose, coagulation factors, ammonia and uric acid levels, hepatic and renal function tests, peripheral blood counts, and bone marrow function; liver function tests at least twice weekly during therapy.
- Monitor diabetics for loss of glycemic control.
- Monitor for and report S&S of hyperammonemia: Anorexia, vomiting, lethargy, weak pulse, depressed temperature, irritability, asterixis, seizures, coma.
- Anticipate possible prolonged or exaggerated effects of concurrently given drugs or their toxicity because of potential serious hepatic dysfunction that reduces enzymatic detoxification of other drugs. Report incidence promptly.
- Watch for neurotoxic reaction (25% of patients) which usually appears within the first few days of therapy. It is manifested by tiredness and changing levels of consciousness (ranging from confusion to coma).
- Note: Protect from infection during first several days of treatment when circulating lymphoblasts decrease markedly and leukocyte counts may fall below normal. Report promptly S&S of infection: Chill, fever, aches, sore throat.
- Report sudden severe abdominal pain with nausea and vomiting, particularly if these symptoms occur after medication is discontinued (may indicate pancreatitis).

Patient & Family Education

- Note: Therapeutic response will most likely be accompanied by some toxicity in all patients; toxicity is reportedly greater in adults than in children.
- Notify physician of continued loss of weight or onset of foot and ankle swelling.
- Notify physician without delay if nausea or vomiting makes it difficult to take all prescribed medication.
- Report onset of unusual bleeding, bruising, petechiae, melena, skin rash or itching, yellowed skin and sclera, joint pain, puffy face, or dyspnea.
- Do not drive or operate equipment that requires alertness and skill. Exercise caution with potentially hazardous activities. These effects can continue several weeks after last dose of the drug.

ASPIRIN (ACETYLSALICYLIC ACID) Pr

(as′pe-ren)

Alka-Seltzer, A.S.A., Aspergum, Astrin ♣, Bayer, Bayer Children's, Cosprin, Easprin, Ecotrin, Empirin, Entrophen ♣, Halfprin, Measurin, Novasen ♣, St. Joseph Children's, Supasa ♣, Triaphen-10 ♣, ZORprin

Classifications: NONNARCOTIC ANALGESIC, SALICYLATE; ANTIPYRETIC; ANTIPLATELET

Therapeutic: ANALGESIC, ANTIPYRETIC; ANTIPLATELET

Pregnancy Category: D

AVAILABILITY 81 mg chewable tablets; 325 mg, 500 mg tablets; 81 mg, 165 mg, 325 mg, 500 mg, 650 mg, 975 mg enteric-coated tablets; 650 mg, 800 mg sustained release tablets; 120 mg, 200 mg, 300 mg, 600 mg suppositories

ACTION & *THERAPEUTIC EFFECT*

Major action is primarily due to inhibiting the formation of prostaglandins involved in the production of inflammation, pain, and fever. **Anti-inflammatory action:** Inhibits prostaglandin synthesis. As an anti-inflammatory agent, aspirin appears to be involved in enhancing antigen removal and in reducing the spread of inflammatory substances. **Analgesic action:** Principally peripheral with limited action in the CNS in the hypothalamus; results in relief of mild to moderate pain. **Antipyretic action:** Suppress the synthesis of prostaglandin in or near the hypothalamus. Aspirin also lowers body temperature in fever by indirectly causing centrally mediated peripheral vasodilation and sweating. **Antiplatelet action:** Aspirin (but not other salicylates) powerfully inhibits platelet aggregation. High serum salicylate concentrations can impair hepatic synthesis of blood coagulation factors VII, IX, and X. *Reduces inflammation, pain, and fever. Also inhibits platelet aggregation, reducing ability of blood to clot.*

USES To relieve pain of low to moderate intensity. Also for various inflammatory conditions, such as acute rheumatic fever, systemic lupus, rheumatoid arthritis, osteoarthritis, bursitis, and calcific tendonitis, and to reduce fever in selected febrile conditions. Used to reduce recurrence of TIA due to fibrin platelet emboli and risk of stroke in men; to prevent recurrence of MI; as prophylaxis against MI in men with unstable angina.

UNLABELED USES As prophylactic against thromboembolism; to prevent cataract and progression of diabetic retinopathy; and to control symptoms related to gluten sensitivity.

CONTRAINDICATIONS History of hypersensitivity to salicylates including methyl salicylate (oil of wintergreen); sensitivity to other NSAIDs; patients with "aspirin triad" (aspirin sensitivity, nasal polyps, asthma); chronic rhinitis; acute bronchospasm; agranulocytosis; head trauma; increased intracranial pressure; intracranial bleeding; chronic urticaria; history of GI ulceration, bleeding, or other problems; hypoprothrombinemia, vitamin K deficiency, hemophilia, or other bleeding disorders; CHF; pregnancy (category D), especially in third trimester; lactation; in prematures, neonates, or children younger than 2 y, except under advice and supervision of physician; children or teenagers with chickenpox or influenza-like illnesses because of possible association with Reye's syndrome.

CAUTIOUS USE Otic diseases; gout; children with fever accompanied by dehydration; hyperthyroidism; immunosuppressed individuals; asthma; GI disease; history of gout; cardiac disease; renal or hepatic impairment; G6PD deficiency; vitamin K deficiency; anemia; preoperatively; Hodgkin's disease.

ROUTE & DOSAGE

Mild to Moderate Pain, Fever

Adult: **PO/PR** 350–650 mg q4h (max: 4 g/day)
Child: **PO/PR** 10–15 mg/kg in 4–6 h (max: 3.6 g/day)

Arthritic Conditions

Adult: **PO** 3.6–5.4 g/day in 4–6 divided doses
Child: **PO** 80–100 mg/kg/day in 4–6 divided doses (max: 130 mg/kg/day)

Thromboembolic Disorders

Adult: **PO** 81–325 mg daily

TIA Prophylaxis

Adult: **PO** 650 mg b.i.d.

MI Prophylaxis

Adult: **PO** 80–325 mg/day

ADMINISTRATION

Oral

- Give with a full glass of water (240 mL), milk, food, or antacid to minimize gastric irritation.
- Enteric-coated tablets dissolve too quickly if administered with milk and should not be crushed or chewed.
- Store at 15°–30° C (59°–86° F) in airtight container and dry environment unless otherwise directed by manufacturer. Store suppositories in a cool place or refrigerate but do not freeze.

ADVERSE EFFECTS (≥1%) **Body as a Whole:** Hypersensitivity (urticaria, bronchospasm, anaphylactic shock (laryngeal edema). **CNS:** Dizziness, confusion, drowsiness. **Special Senses:** Tinnitus, hearing loss. **GI:** *Nausea*, vomiting, diarrhea, anorexia, *heartburn, stomach pains,* ulceration, occult bleeding, GI bleeding. **Hematologic:** Thrombocytopenia, hemolytic anemia, prolonged bleeding time. **Skin:** Petechiae, easy bruising, rash. **Urogenital:** Impaired renal function. **Other:** Prolonged pregnancy and labor with increased bleeding.

DIAGNOSTIC TEST INTERFERENCE Bleeding time is prolonged 3–8 days (life of exposed platelets) following a single 325-mg (5 grains) dose of aspirin. Large doses of salicylates equivalent to 5 g or more of aspirin per day may cause prolonged ***prothrombin time*** by decreasing prothrombin production; interference with ***pregnancy tests*** (using mouse or rabbit); decreases in ***serum cholesterol, potassium, PBI,*** T_3 and T_4 ***concentrations,*** and an increase in T_3 ***resin uptake. Serum uric acid*** may increase when plasma salicylate levels are below 10 and decrease when above 15 mg/dL using colorimetric methods. ***Urine 5-HIAA:*** Aspirin may interfere with tests using fluorescent methods. ***Urine ketones:*** Salicylates interfere with Gerhardt test (reaction with ferric chloride produces a reddish color that persists after boiling). ***Urine glucose:*** Moderate to large doses of salicylates equivalent to an aspirin dosage 2.4 g/day or more may produce false-negative results with glucose oxidase methods (e.g., ***Clinistix, TesTape***) and false-positive results with copper reduction methods ***(Benedict's solution, Clinitest)***. ***Urinary PSP excretion*** may be reduced by salicylates. Salicylates may cause ***urine VMA*** to be falsely elevated (by most tests), or reduced (by Pisano method). Salicylates may interfere with or cause false decreases in plasma theophylline levels using Schack and Waxler method. High plasma salicylate levels may cause abnormalities in ***liver function tests.***

INTERACTIONS Drug: Aminosalicylic acid increases risk of SALICYLATE toxicity. **Ammonium chloride** and other ACIDIFYING AGENTS decrease renal elimination and increase risk of SALICYLATE toxicity. ANTICOAGULANTS increase risk of bleeding. ORAL HYPOGLYCEMIC AGENTS increase hypoglycemic activity with aspirin doses greater than 2 g/day. CARBONIC ANHYDRASE INHIBITORS enhance SALICYLATE toxicity. CORTICOSTEROIDS add to ulcerogenic effects. **Methotrexate** toxicity is increased. Low doses of SALICYLATES may antagonize uricosuric effects of **probenecid** and **sulfinpyrazone. Herbal: Feverfew, garlic, ginger, ginkgo, evening primrose oil** may increase bleeding potential.

PHARMACOKINETICS Absorption: 80–100% absorbed (depending on formulation), primarily in stomach and upper small intestine. **Peak levels:** 15 min to 2 h. **Distribution:** Widely distributed in most body tissues; crosses placenta. **Metabolism:** Aspirin is hydrolyzed to salicylate in GI mucosa, plasma, and erythrocytes; salicylate is metabolized in liver. **Elimination:** 50% of dose is eliminated in the urine in 2–4 h (low doses) or 15–30 h (high doses). Excreted into breast milk. **Half-Life:** Aspirin 15–20 min; salicylate 2–18 h (dose dependent).

NURSING IMPLICATIONS

Assessment & Drug Effects

- Monitor for loss of tolerance to aspirin. Symptoms usually occur 15 min to 3 h after ingestion: Profuse rhinorrhea, erythema, nausea, vomiting, intestinal cramps, diarrhea.
- Monitor the diabetic child carefully for need to adjust insulin dose. Children on high doses of aspirin are particularly prone to hypoglycemia (see Appendix F).
- Monitor for salicylate toxicity. In adults, a sensation of fullness in the ears, tinnitus, and decreased or muffled hearing are the most frequent symptoms.
- Monitor children for S&S of salicylate toxicity manifested by: hyperventilation, agitation, mental confusion, or other behavioral changes, drowsiness, lethargy, sweating, and constipation.

Patient & Family Education

- Use enteric-coated tablets, extended release tablets, buffered aspirin, or aspirin administered with an antacid to reduce GI disturbances.
- Discontinue aspirin therapy about 1 wk before surgery to reduce risk of bleeding. Do not use aspirin-containing gum or gargles or chew aspirin products for at least 1 wk following oral surgery.
- Discontinue aspirin use with onset of ringing or buzzing in the ears, impaired hearing, dizziness, GI discomfort or bleeding, and report to physician.
- Do not use aspirin for self-medication of pain (adults) beyond 5 days without consulting a physician. Do not use aspirin longer than 3 days for fever (adults and children), never for fever over 38.9° C (102° F) in older adults or 39.5° C (103° F) in children and adults under 60 y or for recurrent fever without medical direction.
- Consult physician before using aspirin for any fever accompanied by rash, severe headache, stiff neck, marked irritability, or confusion (all possible symptoms of meningitis).
- Avoid alcohol when taking large doses of aspirin.
- Observe and report signs of bleeding (e.g., petechiae, ecchymoses, bleeding gums, bloody or black stools, cloudy or bloody urine).
- Maintain adequate fluid intake when taking repeated doses of aspirin.

ATAZANAVIR

(a-ta-zan′a-vir)

Reyataz

Classifications: ANTIRETROVIRAL; PROTEASE INHIBITOR

Therapeutic: PROTEASE INHIBITOR

Prototype: Saquinavir

Pregnancy Category: B

AVAILABILITY 100 mg, 150 mg, 200 mg, 300 mg capsules

ACTION & *THERAPEUTIC EFFECT*

Atazanavir is an HIV-1 protease inhibitor that selectively inhibits the replication of HIV. Protease plays a major role in the virus-specific processing of gene products used in the replication enzymes of HIV-1 infected cells. Thus, protease is necessary for the production of mature viruses. Atazanavir reduces the viral load and increases CD4+ cell count. *Protease inhibition renders the virus noninfectious. Because HIV protease inhibitors inhibit the HIV replication cycle midway in the process, they are active in acutely and chronically infected cells.*

USES Treatment of HIV infection in combination with other antiretroviral agents.

CONTRAINDICATIONS Hypersensitivity to atazanavir; severe hepatic insufficiency; infants younger than 3 mo; lactation; lactase deficiency; severe rash.

CAUTIOUS USE Mild to moderate hepatic impairment, hepatitis B or C; pregnancy (category B); infants older than 3 mo, children younger than 6 y; elderly, females, diabetes mellitus, diabetic ketoacidosis; hemophilia, hepatic disease; hepatitis; jaundice, hypercholesterolemia, hypertriglyceridemia; preexisting conduction system disease (e.g. marked first-degree AV block or second- or third-degree AV block; lactic acidosis, obesity; coadministration with drugs that are highly dependent on CYP3A or UGT1A1 for clearance, and for which elevated plasma concentrations are associated with serious and/or life-threatening events: Cisapride, dihydroergotamine, ergonovine, ergotamine, indinavir, irinotecan, lovastatin, methylergonovine, midazolam (oral use), pimozide, rifampin, St. John's wort, simvastatin, and triazolam.

ROUTE & DOSAGE

HIV Infection

Adult/Adolescent/Child (older than 6 y and weight greater than 39 kg): **PO** 400 mg once/day with a light meal OR 300 mg once/day with 100 mg of ritonavir

Adolescent/Child (at least 6 y and weight 32–39 kg): **PO** 250 mg plus ritonavir (100 mg) once daily

Adolescent/Child (at least 6 y and weight 25–32 kg): **PO** 200 mg plus ritonavir (100 mg) once daily with food (i.e., 7 mg/kg plus ritonavir 4 mg/kg)

Adolescent/Child (6 y or older and weight 20 to less than 25 kg): **PO** 150 mg plus ritonavir (80 mg)

Adolescent/Child (6 y or older and weight 15–20 kg): **PO** 150 mg plus ritonavir (80 mg) once daily with food

Hepatic Impairment Dosage Adjustment

Reduce dose to 300 mg once/day in moderate hepatic insufficiency; not recommended for use in severe hepatic insufficiency

ADMINISTRATION

Oral

- Give with a light meal, not on an empty stomach.
- When co-administered with didanosine buffered formulations, give atazanavir (with food) 2 h before or 1 h after didanosine.
- Give 2 h before/1 h after antacids or buffered drugs.
- Store at 15°–30° C (59°–86° F).

ADVERSE EFFECTS (≥1%) **Body as a Whole:** *Peripheral neuropathy,* fever, pain, fatigue, allergic reaction, angioedema, asthenia, burning sensation, chest pain, edema, facial atrophy, generalized edema, heat sensitivity, infection, malaise, pallor, peripheral edema, photosensitivity, substernal chest pain, sweating. **CNS:** *Headache,* depression, insomnia, dizziness, abnormal dream, abnormal gait, agitation, amnesia, anxiety, confusion, convulsion, decreased libido, emotional lability, hallucination, hostility, hyperkinesia, hypesthesia, increased reflexes, nervousness, psychosis, sleep disorder, somnolence, suicide attempt, twitch. **CV:** Cardiac arrest, heart block (PR prolongation), hypertension, myocarditis, palpitation, syncope, vasodilatation. **GI:** Hyperbilirubinemia, jaundice, *nausea, vomiting, diarrhea,* abdominal pain, anorexia, aphthous stomatitis, colitis, constipation, dental pain, dyspepsia, enlarged abdomen, esophageal ulcer, esophagitis, flatulence, gastritis, gastroenteritis, gastrointestinal disorder, hepatitis, hepatomegaly, hepatosplenomegaly, increased appetite, liver damage, liver fatty deposit, mouth ulcer, pancreatitis, peptic ulcer. **Endocrine:** Decreased male fertility. **Hematologic:** Ecchymosis, purpura. **Metabolic:** Lipodystrophy syndrome, hypercholesterolemia, hypertriglyceridemia. **Musculoskeletal:** Myalgia, arthralgia. **Respiratory:** Cough, dyspnea, hiccup. **Skin:** *Rash,* alopecia, cellulitis, dermatophytosis, dry skin, eczema, nail disorder, pruritus, seborrhea, urticaria, vesiculobullous rash. **Special Senses:** Otitis, taste perversion, tinnitus. **Urogenital:** Abnormal urine, amenorrhea, crystalluria, gynecomastia, hematuria, impotence, kidney calculus, kidney failure, kidney pain, menstrual disorder, oliguria, pelvic pain, polyuria, proteinuria, urinary frequency, urinary tract infection.

INTERACTIONS Drug: There are extensive drug interactions reported; check the package insert for complete listing. May increase levels and toxicity of **cyclosporine,** systemic **lidocaine, sirolimus, tacrolimus, amiodarone, alfuzosin, dronedarone, eplerenone;** increase risk of myopathy and rhabdomyolysis with **atorvastatin, lovastatin, simvastatin;** may increase risk of heart block with **diltiazem;** ANTACIDS, H_2-RECEPTOR ANTAGONISTS, PROTON PUMP INHIBITORS may decrease absorption of atazanavir; **ritonavir** may increase atazanavir levels; may increase toxicity of **irinotecan;** increased risk of prolonged sedations with BENZODIAZEPINES; **indinavir** may increase risk of hyperbilirubinemia; **didanosine, efavirenz, rifampin** may decrease atazanavir levels; **ergotamine, ergonovine dihydroergotamine, bepridil, pimozide** may cause serious adverse reactions; may increase risk of hypotension, visual changes, and priapism with **sildenafil, tadalafil, vardenafil. Herbal: St. John's wort, red yeast rice** may decrease atazanavir levels.

PHARMACOKINETICS Absorption: 68% into systemic circulation; taking with food enhances bioavailability. **Peak:** 2–2.5 h. **Metabolism:** In liver by CYP3A4. **Elimination:** 70% in feces, 13% in urine. **Half-Life:** 7 h.

NURSING IMPLICATIONS

Assessment & Drug Effects

- Monitor CV status and ECG closely, especially with concurrent treatment with other drugs known to prolong the PR interval.
- Lab tests: Baseline and periodic LFTs; total bilirubin if jaundiced; periodic PT/INR with concurrent warfarin therapy; monitor blood glucose closely, especially if diabetic.

Patient & Family Education

- Do not alter the dose or discontinue therapy without consulting physician.
- Inform physician of all prescription, nonprescription, or herbal meds being used.
- Report promptly any of the following: Dizziness or lightheadedness; muscle pain (especially with concurrent statin therapy); severe nausea, vomiting (especially if red or "coffee-ground" in appearance), stomach pain, black tarry stools; yellowing of skin or whites of eyes; skin rash or itchy skin; sore throat, fever, or other S&S of infection; unexplained tiredness or weakness.
- If taking both sildenafil and atazanavir, promptly report any of the following sildenafil-associated adverse effects: Hypotension, visual changes, or prolonged penile erection.

ATENOLOL

(a-ten'oh-lole)

Apo-Atenolol ✤, Tenormin

Classifications: BETA-ADRENERGIC ANTAGONIST; ANTIHYPERTENSIVE AGENT

Therapeutic: ANTIHYPERTENSIVE

Prototype: Propranolol

Pregnancy Category: D

AVAILABILITY 25 mg, 50 mg, 100 mg tablets

ACTION & *THERAPEUTIC EFFECT* Atenolol selectively blocks $beta_1$-adrenergic receptors located chiefly in cardiac muscle. Mechanisms for antihypertensive action include central effect leading to decreased sympathetic outflow to periphery, reduction in renin activity with consequent suppression of the renin-angiotensin-aldosterone system, and competitive inhibition of catecholamine binding at beta-adrenergic receptor sites. *Reduces rate and force of cardiac contractions (negative inotropic action); cardiac output is reduced, as well as systolic and diastolic BP. Atenolol decreases peripheral vascular resistance both at rest and with exercise.*

USES Management of hypertension as a single agent or concomitantly with other antihypertensive agents, especially a diuretic, and in treatment of stable angina pectoris, MI.

UNLABELED USES Antiarrhythmic, mitral valve prolapse, adjunct in treatment of pheochromocytoma and of thyrotoxicosis; and for vascular headache prophylaxis.

CONTRAINDICATIONS Sinus bradycardia, greater than first-degree AV heart block, uncompensated heart failure, cardiogenic shock, peripheral vascular disease, Raynaud's disease, hypotension; abrupt discontinuation, pulmonary edema, acute bronchospasm; pregnancy (category D), lactation.

CAUTIOUS USE Hypertensive patients with CHF controlled by digitalis and diuretics, vasospastic angina (Prinzmetal's angina); asthma, bronchitis, emphysema, and COPD; major depression; diabetes mellitus; impaired renal function, dialysis; myasthenia gravis; pheochromocytoma, hyperthyroidism, thyrotoxicosis; older adults.

ROUTE & DOSAGE

Hypertension, Angina

Adult: **PO** 25–50 mg/day, may increase to 100 mg/day

Child: **PO** 0.8–1.5 mg/kg/day (max: 2 mg/kg/day)

MI

Adult: **PO** Start 50 mg/day

Renal Impairment Dosage Adjustment

CrCl 15–35 mL/min: Max dose of 50 mg/day; less than 15 mL/min: Max dose of 25 mg/day

ADMINISTRATION

Oral

- Crush tablets, if necessary, before administration and give with fluid of patient's choice.
- Store in tightly closed, light-resistant container at 15°–30° C (59°–86° F) unless otherwise directed.

ADVERSE EFFECTS (≥1%) **CNS:** Dizziness, vertigo, light-headedness, syncope, fatigue or weakness, lethargy, drowsiness, insomnia, mental changes, depression. **CV:** *Bradycardia, hypotension, CHF,* cold extremities, leg pains, dysrhythmias. **GI:** Nausea, vomiting, diarrhea. **Respiratory:** Pulmonary edema, dyspnea, <u>bronchospasm</u>. **Other:** May mask symptoms of hypoglycemia; decreased sexual ability.

INTERACTIONS Drug: Atropine and other ANTICHOLINERGICS may increase atenolol absorption from GI tract; NSAIDS may decrease hypotensive effects; may mask symptoms of a hypoglycemic reaction induced by **insulin,** SULFONYLUREAS; may increase **lidocaine** levels and toxicity; pharmacologic and toxic effects of both atenolol and **verapamil** are increased. **Prazosin, terazosin** may increase severe hypotensive response to first dose of atenolol.

PHARMACOKINETICS Absorption: 50% of dose absorbed. **Peak:** 2–4 h. **Duration:** 24 h. **Distribution:** Does not readily cross blood–brain barrier. **Metabolism:** No hepatic metabolism. **Elimination:** 40–50% in urine; 50–60% in feces. **Half-Life:** 6–7 h.

NURSING IMPLICATIONS

Assessment & Drug Effects

- Measure trough BP (just prior to scheduled dose) to determine efficacy.
- Check apical pulse before administration in patients receiving digitalis (both drugs slow AV conduction). If below 60 bpm (or other ordered parameter), withhold dose and consult physician.
- Monitor BP throughout dosage adjustment period. Consult physician for acceptable parameters.

Patient & Family Education

- Adhere rigidly to dose regimen. Sudden discontinuation of drug can exacerbate angina and precipitate tachycardia or MI in patients with coronary artery disease, and thyroid storm in patients with hyperthyroidism.
- Make position changes slowly and in stages, particularly from recumbent to upright posture.

ATOMOXETINE

(a-to-mox′e-teen)

Strattera

Classification: PSYCHOTHERAPEUTIC, MISCELLANEOUS

Therapeutic: ADHD AGENT

Pregnancy Category: C

AVAILABILITY 10 mg, 18 mg, 25 mg, 40 mg, 60 mg, 80 mg, 100 mg capsules

ACTION & *THERAPEUTIC EFFECT* Exact mechanism of action is unknown, but is thought to be related to selective inhibition of the pre-synaptic norepinephrine transporter, resulting in norepinephrine reuptake inhibition. *Improved attentiveness, ability to follow through on tasks*

with less distraction and forgetfulness, and diminished hyperactivity.

USES Acute and maintenance treatment of attention deficit/hyperactivity disorder (ADHD) in adults and children.

CONTRAINDICATIONS Hypersensitive to atomoxetine or any of its constituents; concomitant use or use within 2 wk of MAOIs; narrow angle glaucoma; structural cardiac abnormalities or other serious heart problems; jaundice or elevated liver enzymes; signs or symptoms of liver function impairment (see Appendix F); major depressive disorders; suicidal ideation; major depressive disorder (MDD). Safety and efficacy in children younger than 6 y and the older adult have not been established.

CAUTIOUS USE Severe liver injury may progress to liver failure or death in a small percentage of patients. Hypertension, tachycardia, cardiovascular or cerebrovascular disease; any condition that predisposes to hypotension; urinary retention or urinary hesitancy; concomitant use of CYP2D6 inhibitors (e.g., paroxetine, fluoxetine, quinidine), albuterol or other beta-2 agonists, vasopressor drugs; history of bipolar disorder; history of suicidal tendencies; pregnancy (category C), lactation.

ROUTE & DOSAGE

ADHD

Adult/Adolescent/Child (older than 6 y and weight greater than 70 kg): **PO** Start with 40 mg in morning. May increase after 3 days to target dose of 80 mg/day given either once in the morning or divided morning and late afternoon/early evening. May increase to max of 100 mg/day if needed.

Child/Adolescent (weight less than 70 kg): **PO** Start with 0.5 mg/kg/day. May increase after 3 days to target dose of 1.2 mg/kg/day. Administer once daily in morning or divide dose and give morning and late afternoon/early evening. Max dose is 1.4 mg/kg or 100 mg, whichever is less.

Hepatic Impairment Dosage Adjustment

Child-Pugh Class B: Initial and target doses should be reduced to 50% of the normal dose

Child-Pugh Class C: Initial dose and target doses should be reduced to 25% of normal dose

Pharmacogenetic Dosage Adjustment/Patients Receiving Concurrent CYP2D6 Inhibitors

CYP2D6 poor metabolizers: In children/adolescents (weight up to 70 kg) start at 0.5 mg/kg, adjust upward only after 4 wk if well tolerated; adults/adolescents (weight greater than 70 kg) start at 40 mg/day, adjust upward only after 4 wk if well tolerated; do not exceed 80 mg

ADMINISTRATION

Oral

- Note that total daily dose in children and adolescents is based on weight. Determine that ordered dose is appropriate for weight prior to administration of drug.
- Note manufacturer recommends dosage adjustments with concomitant administration of strong CYP2D6 inhibitors (e.g., paroxetine, fluoxetine, quinidine). Consult physician.
- Store at 15°–30° C (59°–86° F).

ADVERSE EFFECTS (≥1%) **Body as a Whole:** Flu-like syndrome, flushing, fatigue, fever, rigors. **CNS:** Dizziness, *headache,* somnolence, crying, tearfulness, irritability, mood swings, *insomnia,* depression, tremor, early morning awakenings, paresthesias, abnormal dreams, decreased libido, sleep disorder, suicidal ideation. **CV:** Increased blood pressure, sinus tachycardia, palpitations. **GI:** *Upper abdominal pain,* constipation, dyspepsia, *vomiting, decreased appetite,* anorexia, dry mouth, diarrhea, flatulence, severe liver injury (rare). **Endocrine:** Hot flushes, sexual dysfunction. **Metabolic:** Weight loss. **Hepatic:** Hepatotoxicity. **Musculoskeletal:** Arthralgia, myalgia. **Respiratory:** *Cough,* rhinorrhea, nasal congestion, sinusitis. **Skin:** Dermatitis, pruritus, increased sweating. **Special Senses:** Mydriasis. **Urogenital:** Urinary hesitation/retention, dysmenorrhea, ejaculation dysfunction, impotence, delayed onset of menses, irregular menstruation, prostatitis; priapism, male pelvic pain.

INTERACTIONS Drug: Albuterol may potentiate cardiovascular effects of atomoxetine; CYP2D6 inhibitors (**fluoxetine, paroxetine, quinidine**) may increase atomoxetine levels and toxicity; MAOIS may precipitate a hypertensive crisis; may attenuate effects of ANTIHYPERTENSIVE AGENTS.

PHARMACOKINETICS Absorption: Well absorbed from GI tract. **Distribution:** 98% protein bound. **Peak:** 1–2 h. **Metabolism:** In liver by CYP2D6. **Elimination:** Primarily in urine. **Half-Life:** 5.2 h.

NURSING IMPLICATIONS

Assessment & Drug Effects

- Evaluate for continuing therapeutic effectiveness especially with long-term use.
- Monitor children and adolescents for behavior changes that may indicate suicidal ideation, including aggression and anxiety that may be precursors of it.
- Monitor cardiovascular status especially with preexisting hypertension.
- Monitor HR and BP at baseline, following a dose increase, and periodically while on therapy.
- Lab tests: Periodic LFTs.
- Report increased aggression and irritability as these may indicate a need to discontinue the drug.

Patient & Family Education

- Instruct patients on S&S of liver toxicity.
- Report any of the following to the physician: Indicators of suicidal ideation in children and adolescents; chest pains or palpitations, urinary retention or difficulty initiating voiding urine, appetite loss and weight loss, or insomnia.
- Make position changes slowly if you experience dizziness with arising from a lying or sitting position.
- Do not drive or engage in potentially hazardous activities until reaction to the drug is known.

ATORVASTATIN CALCIUM

(a-tor-va′sta-tin)

Lipitor

Classifications: ANTILIPEMIC; HMG-COA; REDUCTASE INHIBITOR (STATIN)

Therapeutic: ANTILIPEMIC; STATIN

Prototype: Lovastatin

Pregnancy Category: X

AVAILABILITY 10 mg, 20 mg, 40 mg tablets

ACTION & *THERAPEUTIC EFFECT* Atorvastatin is an inhibitor of reductase 3-hydroxy-3-methyl-glutaryl coenzyme A (HMG-CoA), which is essential to hepatic production of cholesterol. Atorvastatin increases the number of hepatic low-density-lipid (LDL) receptors, thus increasing LDL uptake and catabolism of LDL. HDL cholesterol blood level increases with use of atorvastatin. *Atorvastatin reduces LDL and total triglyceride (TG) production as well as increases the plasma level of high-density lipids (HDL).*

USES Adjunct to diet for the reduction of LDL cholesterol and triglycerides in patients with primary hypercholesterolemia and mixed dyslipidemia, prevention of cardiovascular disease in patients with multiple risk factors.

CONTRAINDICATIONS Hypersensitivity to atorvastatin, myopathy, active liver disease, unexplained persistent transaminase elevations, renal failure, renal impairment, hepatic encephalopathy, hepatitis, hepatic disease; jaundice, rhabdomyolysis; uncontrolled seizure disorders; pregnancy (category X), lactation.

CAUTIOUS USE Hypersensitivity to other HMG-CoA reductase inhibitors, history of liver disease, patients who consume substantial quantities of alcohol. Safety and efficacy in children younger than 10 y have not been established.

ROUTE & DOSAGE

Hypercholesterolemia/ Prevention of Cardiovascular Disease

Adult: **PO** Start with 10–40 mg daily, may increase up to 80 mg/day

Child/Adolescent (10–17 y): **PO** Start with 10 mg daily, may increase up to 20 mg/day

ADMINISTRATION

Oral

- May be given at any time of day.
- Store at 20°–25° C (68°–77° F).

ADVERSE EFFECTS (≥1%) **Body as a Whole:** Back pain, asthenia, hypersensitivity reaction, myalgia, rhabdomyolysis. **CNS:** Headache. **GI:** Abdominal pain, constipation, diarrhea, dyspepsia, flatulence, increased liver function tests. **Respiratory:** Sinusitis, pharyngitis. **Skin:** Rash.

INTERACTIONS Drug: May increase **digoxin** levels 20%, increases levels of **norethindrone** and **ethinyl estradiol** oral contraceptives; **erythromycin** may increase atorvastatin levels 40%; MACROLIDE ANTIBIOTICS, **cyclosporine, delavirdine, gemfibrozil, niacin, clofibrate,** AZOLE ANTIFUNGALS (**ketoconazole, itraconazole**) may increase risk of rhabdomyolysis; **nelfinavir** may increase atorvastatin levels. **Food: Grapefruit juice** (greater than 1 qt/day) may increase risk of myopathy and rhabdomyolysis.

PHARMACOKINETICS Absorption: Rapidly from GI tract. 30% reaches the systemic circulation. **Onset:** Cholesterol reduction—2 wk. **Peak:** Plasma concentration, 1–2 h; effect 2–4 wk. **Distribution:** 98% or greater protein bound. Crosses placenta, distributed into breast milk of animals. **Metabolism:** In the liver by CYP3A4 to active metabolites. **Elimination:** Primarily in bile; less than 2% in urine. **Half-Life:** 14 h; 20–30 h for active metabolites.

NURSING IMPLICATIONS

Assessment & Drug Effects

- Monitor for therapeutic effectiveness which is indicated by reduction in the level of LDL-C.

- Lab tests: Monitor lipid levels within 2–4 wk after initiation of therapy or upon change in dosage; monitor liver functions at 6 and 12 wk after initiation or elevation of dose, and periodically thereafter.
- Assess for muscle pain, tenderness, or weakness; and, if present, monitor CPK level (discontinue drug with marked elevations of CPK or if myopathy is suspected).
- Monitor carefully for digoxin toxicity with concurrent digoxin use.

Patient & Family Education

- Report promptly any of the following: Unexplained muscle pain, tenderness, or weakness, especially with fever or malaise; yellowing of skin or eyes; stomach pain with nausea, vomiting, or loss of appetite; skin rash or hives.
- Do not take drug during pregnancy because it may cause birth defects. Immediately inform physician of a suspected or known pregnancy.
- Inform physician regarding concurrent use of any of the following drugs: Erythromycin, niacin, antifungals, or birth control pills.
- Minimize alcohol intake while taking this drug.

ATOVAQUONE

(a-to'va-quone)
Mepron
Classification: ANTIPROTOZOAL
Therapeutic: ANTIPROTOZOAL
Prototype: Metronidazole
Pregnancy Category: C

AVAILABILITY 750 mg/5 mL suspension

ACTION & *THERAPEUTIC EFFECT* Atovaquone is an antiprotozoal with antipneumocystic activity, including *Pneumocystis carinii* (PCP) and the *Plasmodium* species. The site of action in PCP is linked to inhibition of the electron transport system in the mitochondria. This results in the inhibition of nucleic acid and ATP synthesis. *Effective against* P. carinii *and the* Plasmodium *species, as well as other protozoans.*

USES Second-line oral therapy of mild to moderate *P. carinii* pneumonia (PCP) in immunocompromised patients intolerant of co-trimoxazole.

UNLABELED USES May be effective in the treatment of cerebral toxoplasmosis.

CONTRAINDICATIONS History of potential life-threatening allergies to atovaquone.

CAUTIOUS USE Severe PCP, concurrent pulmonary diseases, older adults, pregnancy (category C), or lactation; impaired hepatic function; neonates and infants.

ROUTE & DOSAGE

Mild to Moderate *Pneumocystis carinii* Pneumonia (PCP)

Adult: **PO** 750 mg (5 mL) suspension b.i.d. for 21 days

ADMINISTRATION

Oral

- Give with meals because food significantly enhances absorption.
- Store at room temperature 15°–30° C (59°–86° F) unless otherwise directed by the manufacturer.

ADVERSE EFFECTS (≥1%) **Body as a Whole:** *Fever.* **CV:** Hypotension. **CNS:** *Headache, insomnia, dizziness, strange or vivid dreams, anxiety, depression.* **Hematologic:** Anemia, neutropenia. **Metabolic:** Hyponatremia, hypoglycemia. **GI:** *Nausea, diarrhea, vomiting,* abdominal pain, anorexia, dyspepsia, oral candidiasis, oral ulcers. **Skin:** *Rash,* pruritus, erythema multiforme. **Respiratory:** Cough, sinusitis.

DIAGNOSTIC TEST INTERFERENCE May cause increase in **amylase** and other **liver function tests.**

INTERACTIONS Drug: Zidovudine may increase risk of bone marrow toxicity. **Food:** Oral absorption is increased 3- to 4-fold when administered with food, especially with fatty foods.

PHARMACOKINETICS Absorption: Poor, absorption improved when taken with a fatty meal. **Duration:** 6–23 wk after a 3-wk course of therapy. **Distribution:** Penetrates poorly into cerebrospinal fluid; greater than 99.9% protein bound. **Metabolism:** Not metabolized. **Elimination:** Greater than 94% in feces over 21 days (enterohepatically cycled). **Half-Life:** 2–3 days.

NURSING IMPLICATIONS

Assessment & Drug Effects

- Assess for therapeutic failure in patients with GI disorders that may limit absorption of drug.
- Lab tests: Monitor CBC with differential, blood glucose, serum sodium, creatinine, BUN, and serum amylase periodically. Report abnormal elevations in these values; drug may need to be discontinued.

Patient & Family Education

- Note: It is necessary to take this drug exactly as prescribed because it is slowly eliminated from the body.

ATOVAQUONE/PROGUANIL HYDROCHLORIDE

(a-to′va-quone/pro′gua-nil)

Malarone, Malarone Pediatric

Classification: ANTIMALARIAL
Therapeutic: ANTIMALARIAL
Prototype: Chloroquine HCl and Metronidazole
Pregnancy Category: C

AVAILABILITY Atovaquone 250 mg/proguanil HCl 100 mg (adult dose), atovaquone 62.5 mg/proguanil HCl 25 mg (pediatric dose) tablets

ACTION & *THERAPEUTIC EFFECT* Combination of two antimalarial drugs. Atovaquone inhibits electron transport system in mitochondria of the malaria parasite, thus interfering with nucleic acid and ATP synthesis of the parasite. Proguanil interferes with DNA synthesis of the malaria parasite. *This drug combination has synergistic activity toward malarial treatment because each component has a different mode of action.*

USES Prevention and treatment of malaria due to *P. falciparum,* even in chloroquine-resistant areas.

CONTRAINDICATIONS Known hypersensitivity to atovaquone or proguanil; severe malaria.
CAUTIOUS USE Cerebral malaria, complicated malaria, pulmonary edema; renal failure, renal impairment; hepatic disease; lactation; older adults; African Americans, Chinese, Japanese; diarrhea, emesis, GI disease; hepatic disease, infection, sunlight (UV) exposure; pregnancy (category C). Use in children weighing less than 9 kg is not established.

ROUTE & DOSAGE

Prevention of Malaria

Adult: **PO** 1 tablet daily with food starting 1–2 days before travel to malarial area and continuing for 7 days after return

Child: **PO** *Weight 11–20 kg,* 1 pediatric tablet daily; *weight 21–30 kg,* 2 pediatric tablets daily; *weight 31–40 kg,* 3 pediatric tablets daily; *weight greater than 40 kg,* 1 adult tablet daily with food starting 1–2 days before travel to malarial area and continuing for 7 days after return

Treatment of Malaria

Adult: **PO** 4 tablets as a single daily dose for 3 days

Child: **PO** *Weight 5–8 kg,* 2 pediatric tablets; *weight 9–10 kg,* 3 pediatric tablets; *weight 11–20 kg,* 1 adult tablet; *weight 21–30 kg,* 2 adult tablets; *weight 31–40 kg,* 3 adult tablets; *weight greater than 40 kg,* 4 adult tablets as a single daily dose for 3 days

ADMINISTRATION

Oral

- Give at the same time each day with food or a drink containing milk.
- Give a repeat dose if vomiting occurs within 1 h after dosing.

ADVERSE EFFECTS (≥1%) **Body as a Whole:** Fever, *myalgia*, back pain, asthenia, anorexia. **Digestive:** *Nausea, abdominal pain, diarrhea,* dyspepsia. **CNS:** *Headache*. **Respiratory:** Cough. **Skin:** Pruritus. **Other:** Anaphylactic reaction.

INTERACTIONS Drug: Rifampin, rifabutin, tetracycline may decrease serum levels; **metoclopramide** may decrease absorption.

PHARMACOKINETICS Absorption: Atovaquone (A), Poor, absorption improved when taken with a fatty meal; **Proguanil (P),** Extensively absorbed. **Duration: A,** 6–23 wk after a 3-wk course of therapy. **Distribution: A,** Penetrates poorly into cerebrospinal fluid; greater than 99.9% protein bound; **P,** 75% protein bound. **Metabolism: A,** Not metabolized; **P,** Metabolized by CYP2C19 to cycloguanil. **Elimination: A,** Greater than 94% in feces over 21 days (enterohepatically cycled); **P,** Primarily in urine. **Half-Life: A,** 2–3 days; **P,** 12–21 h.

NURSING IMPLICATIONS

Assessment & Drug Effects

- Lab tests: Monitor AST and ALT periodically, especially with long-term therapy.
- Monitor for S&S of parasitemia in patients receiving tetracycline and in those experiencing diarrhea or vomiting.
- Note: Only use metoclopramide to control vomiting if other antiemetics are not available.

Patient & Family Education

- Take this drug at the same time each day for maximum effectiveness.
- Note: Absorption of this drug may be reduced with diarrhea and vomiting. Consult physician if either of these occurs.

ATRACURIUM BESYLATE (Pr)

(a-tra-kyoor′ee-um)

Tracrium

Classifications: SKELETAL MUSCLE RELAXANT, NONDEPOLARIZING; NEUROMUSCULAR BLOCKER

Therapeutic: SKELETAL MUSCLE RELAXANT

Pregnancy Category: C

AVAILABILITY 10 mg/mL injection

ACTION & *THERAPEUTIC EFFECT* Inhibits neuromuscular transmission by binding competitively with acetylcholine to muscle end plate receptors. Has no apparent effect on pain threshold, consciousness, or cerebration. Given in general anesthesia only after unconsciousness has been induced by other drugs. *Synthetic skeletal muscle relaxant that produces short duration of neuromuscular blockade, exhibits minimal direct effects on cardiovascular system, and has less histamine-releasing action.*

USES Adjunct for general anesthesia to produce skeletal muscle relaxation during surgery; to facilitate endotracheal intubation. Especially useful for patients with severe renal or hepatic disease, limited cardiac reserve, and in patients with low or atypical pseudocholinesterase levels.

CONTRAINDICATIONS Myasthenia gravis. Safety during lactation is not established.

CAUTIOUS USE When appreciable histamine release would be hazardous (as in asthma or anaphylactoid reactions, significant cardiovascular disease), neuromuscular disease (e.g., Eaton-Lambert syndrome), carcinomatosis, electrolyte or acid–base imbalances, dehydration, impaired pulmonary function; pregnancy (category C).

ROUTE & DOSAGE

Skeletal Muscle Relaxation

Adult/Child (2 y or older): **IV** 0.4–0.5 mg/kg initial dose, then 0.08–0.1 mg/kg bolus 20–45 min after the first dose and q15–25min thereafter; reduce doses if used with general anesthetics

Child (1 mo–2 y): **IV** 0.3–0.4 mg/kg

Mechanical Ventilation

Adult: **IV** 5–9 mcg/kg/min by continuous infusion

ADMINISTRATION

- Verify correct concentration and rate of infusion for infants and children with physician.

Intravenous

PREPARE: **Direct:** Give initial bolus dose undiluted. **Continuous:** Maintenance dose **must be** diluted with NS, D5W or D5/NS. Maximum concentration should be 0.5 mg/mL. Do not mix in same syringe or administer through same needle as used for alkaline solutions [incompatible with alkaline solutions (e.g., barbiturates)].

ADMINISTER: **Direct:** Give as bolus dose over 30–60 sec. **Continuous:** Give infusion at rate required to maintain desired effect.

INCOMPATIBILITIES **Solution/additive:** **Lactated Ringer's, aminophylline, cefazolin, heparin, quinidine, ranitidine, sodium nitroprusside.** **Y-site:** **Diazepam, propofol, thiopental.**

- Store at 2°–8° C (36°–46° F) to preserve potency unless otherwise directed. Avoid freezing.

ADVERSE EFFECTS (≥1%) **CV:** Bradycardia, tachycardia. **Respiratory:** Respiratory depression. **Other:** Increased salivation, anaphylaxis.

INTERACTIONS Drug: GENERAL ANESTHETICS increase magnitude and duration of neuromuscular blocking action; AMINOGLYCOSIDES, **bacitracin, polymyxin B, clindamycin, lidocaine, parenteral magnesium, quinidine, quinine, tri-**

methaphan, verapamil increase neuromuscular blockade; DIURETICS may increase or decrease neuromuscular blockade; **lithium** prolongs duration of neuromuscular blockade; NARCOTIC ANALGESICS present possibility of additive respiratory depression; **succinylcholine** increases onset and depth of neuromuscular blockade; **phenytoin** may cause resistance to or reversal of neuromuscular blockade.

PHARMACOKINETICS Onset: 2 min. **Peak:** 3–5 min. **Duration:** 60–70 min. **Distribution:** Well distributed to tissues and extracellular fluids; crosses placenta; distribution into breast milk unknown. **Metabolism:** Rapid nonenzymatic degradation in bloodstream. **Elimination:** 70–90% in urine in 5–7 h. **Half-Life:** 20 min.

NURSING IMPLICATIONS

Assessment & Drug Effects

- Lab tests: Baseline serum electrolytes, acid–base balance, and renal function as part of preanesthetic assessment.
- Note: Personnel and equipment required for endotracheal intubation, administration of oxygen under positive pressure, artificial respiration, and assisted or controlled ventilation **must be** immediately available.
- Evaluate degree of neuromuscular blockade and muscle paralysis to avoid risk of overdosage by qualified individual using peripheral nerve stimulator.
- Monitor BP, pulse, and respirations and evaluate patient's recovery from neuromuscular blocking (curare-like) effect as evidenced by ability to breathe naturally or to take deep breaths and cough, keep eyes open, lift head keeping mouth closed, adequacy of hand-grip strength. Notify physician if recovery is delayed.
- Note: Recovery from neuromuscular blockade usually begins 35–45 min after drug administration and is almost complete in about 1 h. Recovery time may be delayed in patients with cardiovascular disease, edematous states, and in older adults.

ATROPINE SULFATE Pr

(a'troe-peen)

Atropair ♣

Classifications: ANTICHOLINERGIC; ANTIMUSCARINIC; ANTIARRHYTHMIC

Therapeutic: ANTISECRETORY; ANTIARRHYTHMIC; BRONCHODILATOR

Pregnancy Category: C

AVAILABILITY 0.4 mg tablets; 0.05 mg/mL, 0.1 mg/mL, 0.3 mg/mL, 0.4 mg/mL, 0.5 mg/mL, 0.8 mg/mL, 1 mg/mL injection

ACTION & *THERAPEUTIC EFFECT*

Acts by selectively blocking all muscarinic responses to acetylcholine (ACh), whether excitatory or inhibitory. Antisecretory action (vagolytic effect) suppresses sweating, lacrimation, salivation, and secretions from nose, mouth, pharynx, and bronchi. Blocks vagal impuse to heart with resulting decrease in AV conduction time, increase in heart rate, and cardiac output, and shortened PR interval. *Potent bronchodilator when bronchoconstriction has been induced by parasympathomimetics, and decreases bronchial secretions. Decreases GI spasm. Produces mydriasis and cycloplegia by blocking responses of iris sphincter muscle and ciliary muscle of lens to cholinergic stimulation. Increases heart rate and cardiac output.*

USES Adjunct in symptomatic treatment of GI disorders (e.g., peptic ulcer, pylorospasm, GI hypermotility, irritable bowel syndrome) and spastic disorders of biliary tract. Relaxes upper GI tract and colon during hypotonic radiography. *Ophthalmic Use:* To produce mydriasis and cycloplegia before refraction and for treatment of anterior uveitis and iritis. *Preoperative Use:* To suppress salivation, perspiration, and respiratory tract secretions; to reduce incidence of laryngospasm, reflex bradycardia arrhythmia, and hypotension during general anesthesia. *Cardiac Uses:* For sinus bradycardia or asystole during CPR or that is induced by drugs or toxic substances (e.g., pilocarpine, beta-adrenergic blockers, organophosphate pesticides, and *Amanita* mushroom poisoning); for management of selected patients with symptomatic sinus bradycardia and associated hypotension and ventricular irritability; for diagnosis of sinus node dysfunction and in evaluation of coronary artery disease during atrial pacing; for management of chronic symptomatic sinus node dysfunction. *Other Uses:* Oral inhalation for short-term treatment and prevention of bronchospasms associated with asthma, bronchitis, and COPD and as drying agent in upper respiratory infection. Adjunctive therapy for hypermotility of GI tract.

CONTRAINDICATIONS Hypersensitivity to belladonna alkaloids; synechiae; angle-closure glaucoma; parotitis; obstructive uropathy (e.g., bladder neck obstruction caused by prostatic hypertrophy); intestinal atony, paralytic ileus, achalasia, pyloric stenosis, obstructive diseases of GI tract, severe ulcerative colitis, toxic megacolon; tachycardia secondary to cardiac insufficiency or thyrotoxicosis; acute hemorrhage; acute MI; myasthenia gravis.

CAUTIOUS USE Myocardial infarction, hypertension, hypotension; coronary artery disease, CHF, tachyarrhythmias; gastric ulcer, GI infections, hiatal hernia with reflux esophagitis; hyperthyroidism; COPD; autonomic neuropathy; hepatic or renal disease; older adults; debilitated patients; children younger than 6 y of age; Down syndrome; autonomic neuropathy, spastic paralysis, brain damage in children; patients exposed to high environmental temperatures; patients with fever; pregnancy (category C).

ROUTE & DOSAGE

Preanesthesia

Adult: **IV/IM/Subcutaneous** 0.4–0.6 mg 30–60 min before surgery
Child: **IV/IM/Subcutaneous** *Weight less than 5 kg,* 0.04 mg/kg; *weight greater than 5 kg,* 0.03 mg/kg 30–60 min before surgery (max: 0.4 mg)

Bradyarrhythmias

Adult: **IV/IM** 1 mg q2–3min (max: 3 mg)
Child: **IV/IM** 0.01–0.03 mg/kg for 1–2 doses

Organophosphate Antidote

Adult: **IV/IM** 1–2 mg q5–60min until muscarinic signs and symptoms subside (may need up to 50 mg)
Child: **IV/IM** 0.05 mg/kg q10–30min until muscarinic signs and symptoms subside

COPD

Adult: **Inhalation** 0.025 mg/kg diluted with 3–5 mL saline, via nebulizer 3–4 times daily (max: 2.5 mg/day)

Child: **Inhalation** 0.03–0.05 mg/kg diluted with 3–5 mL saline, via nebulizer 3–4 times daily

Uveitis

Adult/Child: **Ophthalmic** 1–2 drops of solution or small amount of ointment in eye up to t.i.d.

Cycloplegia

Adult: **Ophthalmic** 1 drop of solution or small amount of ointment in eye 1 h before the procedure
Child: **Ophthalmic** 1–2 drops in eye b.i.d. for 1–3 days prior to procedure or a small amount of ointment in conjunctival sac t.i.d. for 1–3 days prior to procedure with last dose applied several hours before the procedure

ADMINISTRATION

Intravenous

PREPARE: **Direct:** Give undiluted or diluted in up to 10 mL of sterile water.

ADMINISTER: **Direct:** Give 1 mg or fraction thereof over 1 min directly into a Y-site.

INCOMPATIBILITIES **Solution/additive: Pantoprazole.**

- Store at room temperature 15°–30° C (59°–86° F) in protected airtight, light-resistant containers unless otherwise directed by manufacturer.

ADVERSE EFFECTS (≥1%) **CNS:** Headache, ataxia, dizziness, excitement, irritability, convulsions, drowsiness, fatigue, weakness; mental depression, confusion, disorientation, hallucinations. **CV:** Hypertension or hypotension, ventricular tachycardia, palpitation, paradoxical bradycardia, AV dissociation, atrial or <u>ventricular fibrillation</u>. **GI:** Dry mouth with thirst, dysphagia, loss of taste; nausea, vomiting, constipation, delayed gastric emptying, antral stasis, paralytic ileus. **Urogenital:** Urinary hesitancy and retention, dysuria, impotence. **Skin:** Flushed, dry skin; anhidrosis, rash, urticaria, contact dermatitis, allergic conjunctivitis, fixed-drug eruption. **Special Senses:** Mydriasis, blurred vision, photophobia, increased intraocular pressure, cycloplegia, eye dryness, local redness.

DIAGNOSTIC TEST INTERFERENCE ***Upper GI series:*** Findings may require qualification because of anticholinergic effects of atropine (reduced gastric motility and delayed gastric emptying). ***PSP excretion test:*** Atropine may decrease urinary excretion of PSP (phenolsulfonphthalein).

INTERACTIONS Drug: Amantadine, ANTIHISTAMINES, TRICYCLIC ANTIDEPRESSANTS, **quinidine, disopyramide, procainamide** add to anticholinergic effects. **Levodopa** effects decreased. **Methotrimeprazine** may precipitate extrapyramidal effects. Antipsychotic effects of PHENOTHIAZINES are decreased due to decreased absorption.

PHARMACOKINETICS Absorption: Well absorbed from all administration sites. Peak effect: 30 min IM, 2–4 min IV, 1–2 h subcutaneous, 1.5–4 h inhalation, 30–40 min topical. **Duration:** Inhibition of salivation 4 h; mydriasis 7–14 days. **Distribution:** In most body tissues; crosses blood–brain barrier and placenta. **Metabolism:** In liver. **Elimination:** 77–94% in urine in 24 h. **Half-Life:** 2–3 h.

NURSING IMPLICATIONS

Assessment & Drug Effects

- Monitor vital signs. HR is a sensitive indicator of patient's response to atropine. Be alert to changes in quality, rate, and rhythm of HR and respiration and to changes in BP and temperature.

- Initial paradoxical bradycardia following IV atropine usually lasts only 1–2 min; it most likely occurs when IV is administered slowly (more than 1 min) or when small doses (less than 0.5 mg) are used. Postural hypotension occurs when patient ambulates too soon after parenteral administration.
- Note: Frequent and continued use of eye preparations, as well as overdosage, can have systemic effects. Some atropine deaths have resulted from systemic absorption following ocular administration in infants and children.
- Monitor I&O, especially in older adults and patients who have had surgery (drug may contribute to urinary retention). Palpate lower abdomen for distention. Have patient void before giving atropine.
- Monitor CNS status. Older adults and debilitated patients sometimes manifest drowsiness or CNS stimulation (excitement, agitation, confusion) with usual doses of drug or other belladonna alkaloids. In addition to dosage adjustment, side rails and supervision of ambulation may be indicated.
- Monitor infants, small children, and older adults for "atropine fever" (hyperpyrexia due to suppression of perspiration and heat loss), which increases the risk of heatstroke.
- Note: Intraocular tension and depth of anterior chamber should be determined before and during therapy with ophthalmic preparations to avoid glaucoma attacks (ophthalmic solutions and ointments are available in various strengths).
- Patients receiving atropine via inhalation sometimes manifest mild CNS stimulation with doses in excess of 5 mg and mental depression and other mental disturbances with larger doses.

Patient & Family Education

- Follow measures to relieve dry mouth: Adequate hydration; small, frequent mouth rinses with tepid water; meticulous mouth and dental hygiene; gum chewing or sucking sugarless sourballs.
- Note: Drug causes drowsiness, sensitivity to light, blurring of near vision, and temporarily impairs ability to judge distance. Avoid driving and other activities requiring visual acuity and mental alertness.
- Discontinue ophthalmic preparations and notify physician if eye pain, conjunctivitis, palpitation, rapid pulse, or dizziness occurs.

AURANOFIN (Pr)

(au-rane′eh-fin)

Ridaura

Classifications: GOLD COMPOUND; ANTI-INFLAMMATORY; ANTIRHEUMATIC

Therapeutic: ANTI-INFLAMMATORY; ANTIRHEUMATIC

Pregnancy Category: C

AVAILABILITY 3 mg capsules

ACTION & *THERAPEUTIC EFFECT*

Strongly lipophilic and almost neutral in solution, properties that may facilitate transport of agent across cell membranes. Action appears to be immunomodulatory: Serum immunoglobulin concentrations and rheumatoid factor titers are decreased; and anti-inflammatory: Gold is taken up by macrophages with resulting inhibition of phagocytosis and lysosomal enzyme release. *Auranofin is immunomodulatory and anti-inflammatory.*

USES Management of active stage of classic or definite rheumatoid arthritis in adults who do not respond to or tolerate other antiarthritis agents (e.g., NSAIDs, other gold compounds).

UNLABELED USES Juvenile rheumatoid arthritis, active SLE, psoriatic arthritis.

CONTRAINDICATIONS History of gold-induced necrotizing enterocolitis, renal disease, exfoliative dermatitis or bone marrow aplasia; patient who has recently received radiation therapy, history of severe toxicity from previous exposure to gold or other heavy metals; uncontrolled CHF; marked hypertension; SLE; lactation.

CAUTIOUS USE Inflammatory bowel disease, rash, liver disease, renal disease; history of bone marrow depression; older adults; diabetes mellitus, CHF; pregnancy (category C).

ROUTE & DOSAGE

Rheumatoid Arthritis

Adult: **PO** 6 mg/day in 1–2 divided doses, may increase to 6–9 mg/day in 3 divided doses after 6 mo (max: 9 mg/day)
Child: **PO** Initially 0.1 mg/kg/day, may increase to 0.15 mg/kg/day in 1–2 divided doses (max: 0.2 mg/kg/day)

ADMINISTRATION

Oral

- Give capsule with food or fluid of patient's choice.
- Store at 15°–30° C (59°–86° F); protect from light and moisture.
- Note: Expiration date is 4 y after date of manufacture.

ADVERSE EFFECTS (≥1%) **GI:** *Diarrhea, abdominal cramping* and pain; *nausea,* vomiting, anorexia, dysphagia; *stomatitis,* glossitis, metallic taste; flatulence, constipation, GI bleeding, melena. **Hematologic:** <u>Thrombocytopenia, leukopenia</u>, eosinophilia, <u>agranulocytosis, aplastic anemia</u>. **Urogenital:** Proteinuria, hematuria, <u>renal failure</u>. **Skin:** *Rash, pruritus,* dermatitis, urticaria.

DIAGNOSTIC TEST INTERFERENCE Auranofin may enhance response to a ***tuberculin skin test.***

PHARMACOKINETICS Absorption: 20% from small intestine. **Peak:** 2 h. **Distribution:** Highest concentrations in kidneys, spleen, lungs, adrenals, and liver; unknown if crosses placenta; small amounts distributed into breast milk. **Elimination:** 60% of absorbed gold eliminated in urine, remainder in feces. **Half-Life:** 11–23 days.

NURSING IMPLICATIONS

Assessment & Drug Effects

- Monitor for therapeutic effectiveness which develops slowly and is not usually apparent for 3–4 mo.
- Report any of the following S&S promptly: Unexplained bleeding or bruising, metallic taste, sore mouth; pruritus, rash; diarrhea and melena; yellow skin and sclera; unexplained cough or dyspnea.
- Lab tests: Test for signs of possible impending gold toxicity including decreased Hgb; leukocytes less than 4000/mm³; granulocytes less than 1500/mm³; platelets less than 150,000/mm³; proteinuria less than 500 mg/day. Also urinary protein and hepatic function.
- Note: Drug-induced thrombocytopenia is usually spontaneously re-

versible several weeks after drug is withdrawn.

- Continue medical surveillance and supportive therapy after drug is discontinued because adverse effects (such as difficulty in breathing, diarrhea and abdominal pain, fatigue, weakness, unexplained bleeding and bruising, metallic taste) may persist for many months.

Patient & Family Education

- Report adverse effects of therapy, especially abdominal cramping and pain; discontinuance of therapy may be necessary.
- Report metallic taste and pruritus with or without rash. These are among earliest symptoms of impending gold toxicity.
- Do not change dosage (dose or dose interval) by omission, increase, or decrease without first consulting physician.
- Use antidiarrheal OTC drug and high-fiber diet for drug-induced diarrhea.
- Avoid exposure to sunlight (especially between 10 a.m. and 4 p.m.) or to artificial ultraviolet light to prevent photosensitivity reaction.
- Rinse mouth with water frequently for symptomatic treatment of mild stomatitis. Avoid commercial mouth rinses; clean teeth with soft tooth brush and gentle brushing to avoid gingival trauma. Floss at least once daily.

AZACITIDINE

(a-za-ci′ti-deen)

Vidaza

Classifications: ANTINEOPLASTIC AGENT; ANTIMETABOLITE (PYRIMIDINE)

Therapeutic: ANTINEOPLASTIC

Prototype: Fluorouracil

Pregnancy Category: D

AVAILABILITY 100 mg powder for injection

ACTION & *THERAPEUTIC EFFECT* Causes changes in DNA in abnormal blood-forming cells in the bone marrow, resulting in restoration of normal function to tumor-suppressor genes that are responsible for regulating cell differentiation and growth. *Cytotoxic effects of azacitidine cause the death of rapidly dividing cancer cells that are no longer responsive to normal growth control mechanisms.*

USES Treatment of myelodysplastic syndrome, specifically refractory anemia.

UNLABELED USES Refractory acute lymphocytic and myelogenous leukemia.

CONTRAINDICATIONS Hypersensitivity to azacitidine or mannitol; advanced malignant hepatic tumors, myelodysplastic syndrome with hepatic impairment; vaccination; active infection; dental work; intramuscular injections, if platelets less than 50,000 mm^3; pregnancy (category D), lactation. Safety and efficacy in children have not been established.

CAUTIOUS USE Hypoalbuminemia (less than 3 g/dL), hepatic disease; elderly; bone marrow depression; dental disease; history of varicella zoster or other herpes infections; renal impairment, renal failure; older adults.

ROUTE & DOSAGE

Myelodysplastic Syndrome

Adult: **Subcutaneous** 75 mg/m^2 once daily for 7 days every 4 wk; may increase to 100 mg/m^2 if no beneficial response is seen after 2 treatment cycles and no toxicity other than nausea and vomiting has occurred

Renal Impairment Dosage Adjustment

If unexplained elevations of BUN or creatinine occur, the next cycle should be delayed until the values return to normal or baseline, and the dose should be reduced by 50% in the next course

ADMINISTRATION

Subcutaneous

- Reconstitute by slowly injecting 4 mL of sterile water for injection into 100 mg vial to yield 25 mg/mL. Invert 2–3 times and gently rotate until a uniform suspension is achieved. The suspension will be cloudy. If not used immediately, see directions for storage.
- Doses greater than 4 mL should be divided equally into 2 syringes and injected into 2 separate sites. Rotate sites for each injection (thigh, abdomen, or upper arm). Give subsequent injections at least 1 in from an old site and never into areas where the site is tender, bruised, red, or hard.
- Storage: Reconstituted suspension may be kept in the vial or syringe. May refrigerate for up to 8 h. Before use, suspension may be kept at room temperature for up to 30 min. Resuspend by inverting the syringe 2–3 times and gently roll between the palms for 30 sec immediately before administration.

ADVERSE EFFECTS (≥1%) **Body as a Whole:** *Fever, fatigue, malaise, weakness, asthenia, limb pain, back pain,* lymphadenopathy, hematoma, night sweats, cellulitis, lethargy. **CNS:** *Dizziness, headache, depression,* syncope. **CV:** *Chest pain,* cardiac murmur, tachycardia, hypotension. **GI:** *Nausea, vomiting, diarrhea, constipation, anorexia, weight loss, abdominal pain,* stomatitis, dyspepsia. **Hematologic:** *Anemia, thrombocytopenia, leukopenia, neutropenia, ecchymosis, febrile neutropenia.* **Metabolic:** *Peripheral edema.* **Musculoskeletal:** *Myalgia, arthralgia,* muscle cramps. **Respiratory:** *Cough, dyspnea, pharyngitis, nasopharyngitis, pneumonia,* wheezing, pleural effusion, rhonchi. **Skin:** *Injection site erythema, injection site reactions, rash, pruritus, sweating,* urticaria. **Urogenital:** Dysuria, urinary tract infection.

INTERACTIONS Drug: ANTICOAGULANTS, NSAIDS, ANTIPLATELET AGENTS may increase risk of bleeding; **filgrastim, sargramostim** may interfere with the efficacy of azacitidine if given within 24 h of azacitidine dose.

PHARMACOKINETICS Peak: 30 min. **Metabolism:** In liver. **Elimination:** By kidneys. **Half-Life:** 4 h.

NURSING IMPLICATIONS

Assessment & Drug Effects

- Monitor for S&S of drug toxicity in those with renal insufficiency.
- Lab tests: Obtain LFTs and serum creatinine before initiation of therapy; monitor CBC with differential before each treatment cycle and prn.
- Withhold drug and notify physician for S&S of hepatic or renal insufficiency; lab values that indicate leukopenia, neutropenia, thrombocytopenia, or hepatic or renal insufficiency; or serum bicarbonate levels less than 20 mEq/L.

Patient & Family Education

- Promptly report S&S of infection or indication of unusual bleeding tendencies (e.g., dark, tarry stools and easy bruising).
- Women should avoid becoming pregnant and men should not father a child while taking this drug.

AZATHIOPRINE

(ay-za-thye'oh-preen)
Azasan, Imuran
Classifications: IMMUNOSUPPRESSANT; DISEASE-MODIFIYING RHEUMATIC DRUG (DMARD)
Therapeutic: IMMUNOSUPPRESSANT; ANTI-INFLAMMATORY; ANTIRHEUMATIC; DMARD
Prototype: Cyclosporine
Pregnancy Category: D

AVAILABILITY 25 mg, 50 mg, 75 mg, 100 mg tablets; 100 mg vial

ACTION & *THERAPEUTIC EFFECT* Antagonizes purine metabolism and appears to inhibit DNA, RNA, and normal protein synthesis in rapidly growing cells. *Suppresses T cell effects before transplant rejection. Has immunosuppressant and anti-inflammatory properties.*

USES Adjunctive agent to prevent rejection of kidney allografts, usually with other immunosuppressants. Also used in selective adult patients with severe, active rheumatoid arthritis; unresponsive to conventional therapy.

UNLABELED USES SLE, lupus nephritis, psoriatic arthritis; ulcerative colitis, pemphigus, nephrotic syndrome, and other inflammatory and immunologic diseases.

CONTRAINDICATIONS Hypersensitivity to azathioprine or mercaptopurine; clinically active infection, immunization of patient or close family members with live virus vaccines; anuria; pancreatitis; patients receiving alkylating agents (increased risk of neoplasms), concurrent radiation therapy; pregnancy (category D), lactation.

CAUTIOUS USE Impaired kidney and liver function; patients receiving cadaver kidney; myasthenia gravis.

ROUTE & DOSAGE

Renal Transplantation

Adult: **PO** 3–5 mg/kg/day initially, may be able to reduce to 1–3 mg/kg/day **IV** 3–5 mg/kg/day initially, may be able to reduce to 1–3 mg/kg/day; transfer to PO

Rheumatoid Arthritis

Adult: **PO** 1 mg/kg/day initially, may be increased by 0.5 mg/kg/day at 4–6 wk intervals if needed up to 2.5 mg/kg/day

Obesity Dosage Adjustment

Doses calculated on IBW

Renal Impairment Dosage Adjustment

CrCl 10–50 mL/min: 75% of usual dose; less than 10 mL/min: 50% of usual dose
Hemodialysis Dosage Adjustment: Administer after dialysis

ADMINISTRATION

Oral

- Give oral drug in divided doses (as prescribed) with food or immediately after meals to minimize gastric disturbances.

Intravenous

PREPARE: **Direct/Intermittent:** Reconstitute by adding 10 mL sterile water for injection into vial; swirl until dissolved. May be given as prepared or further diluted with 50 mL NS, D5W, or D5/NS. ▪ Reconstituted solution may be stored at room temperature but **must be** used within 24 h after reconstitution (contains no preservatives).

ADMINISTER: **Direct/Intermittent:** May infuse over 30 min to 8 h. Typical infusion time is 30–60 min or longer. ▪ If longer infusion time is ordered, the final volume of the IV solution is increased appropriately. Check with physician.

▪ Store at 15°–30° C (59°–86° F) in tightly closed, light-resistant containers unless otherwise directed.

ADVERSE EFFECTS (≥1%) **Body as a Whole:** Hypersensitivity (skin eruptions, rash, arthralgia). **GI:** Nausea, vomiting, anorexia, esophagitis, diarrhea, steatorrhea, hepatitis with elevations in bilirubin, alkaline phosphatase, AST, ALT, biliary stasis, toxic hepatitis. **Hematologic:** Bone marrow depression, thrombocytopenia, leukopenia, anemia, agranulocytosis, pancytopenia. **Other:** *Secondary infection (immunosuppression);* dysarthria, alopecia; carcinogenic and teratogenic potential reported.

DIAGNOSTIC TEST INTERFERENCE Azathioprine may decrease plasma and urinary ***uric acid*** in patients with gout.

INTERACTIONS Drug: Allopurinol increases effects and toxicity of azathioprine by reducing metabolism of the active metabolite; **allopurinol** doses should be decreased by one third or one fourth; **tubocurarine** and other NONDEPOLARIZING SKELETAL MUSCLE RELAXANTS may reverse or inhibit neuromuscular blocking effects.

PHARMACOKINETICS Absorption: Readily from GI tract. **Distribution:** Crosses placenta. **Metabolism:** Extensively in liver to active metabolite mercaptopurine. **Elimination:** In urine. **Half-Life:** 3 h.

NURSING IMPLICATIONS

Assessment & Drug Effects

- Monitor therapeutic effectiveness which usually requires 6–8 wk of therapy for patients with rheumatoid arthritis (improvement in morning stiffness and grip strength). If no improvement has occurred after 12-wk trial period, drug is generally discontinued.
- Lab tests: Perform CBC, including Hgb and platelet counts, prior to and at least weekly during first month of therapy, twice monthly during second and third months, and monthly, or more frequently thereafter, if indicated (e.g., by dosage or therapy changes).
- Monitor for toxicity. Drug has a high toxic potential. Because it may have delayed action, dosage should be reduced or drug withdrawn at the first indication of an abnormally large or persistent decrease in leukocyte or platelet count to avoid irreversible bone marrow depression.
- Monitor vital signs. Report signs of infection.
- Monitor kidney function (urine protein, urine electrolytes, creatinine clearance, serum creatinine, BUN) periodically.
- Monitor I&O ratio; note color, character, and specific gravity of urine. Report an abrupt decrease in urinary output or any change in I&O ratio.
- Monitor liver function (alkaline phosphatase, AST, ALT, serum bilirubin) and repeat at least every 3 mo or more frequently if indicated. If hepatic toxicity (see Appendix F) develops, therapy may have to be withdrawn.
- Monitor for signs of abnormal bleeding [easy bruising, bleeding gums, petechiae, purpura, melena, epistaxis, dark urine (hematuria), hemoptysis, hematemesis]. If thrombocytopenia occurs, invasive procedures should be withheld, if possible.

- Use protective isolation for the hospitalized patient to reduce risk of infections.

Patient & Family Education

- Avoid contact with anyone who has a cold or other infection and report signs of impending infection. Exercise scrupulous personal hygiene because infection is a constant hazard of immunosuppressive therapy.
- Practice birth control during therapy and for 4 mo after drug is discontinued. This drug is associated with potential hazards in pregnancy.
- Do not receive/take vaccinations or other immunity-conferring agents during therapy because they may precipitate unusually severe reactions due to the immunosuppressive effects of the drug.

AZELAIC ACID

(a'ze-laic)
Azelex, Finacea
Classification: ANTIACNE
Therapeutic: ANTIACNE
Prototype: Isotretinoin
Pregnancy Category: B

AVAILABILITY 20% cream; 15% gel

ACTION & *THERAPEUTIC EFFECT* Azelaic acid is a naturally occurring dicarboxylic acid. Antimicrobial action is attributable to inhibition of the microbial cellular protein synthesis. A normalization of keratinization of the follicle occurs and it reduces the number of acne lesions. *Reduces the number of inflammatory pustules and papules.*

USES Mild to moderate inflammatory acne vulgaris, mild to moderate rosacea.

CONTRAINDICATIONS Hypersensitivity to any component in the drug.
CAUTIOUS USE Dark complexion, pregnancy (category B), lactation. Safety and efficacy in children younger than 12 y are not established.

ROUTE & DOSAGE

Acne Vulgaris, Rosacea
Adult/Child (older than 12 y): **Topical** Apply thin film to clean and dry area b.i.d.

ADMINISTRATION

Topical

- Wash and dry skin thoroughly prior to application of drug.
- Apply by thoroughly massaging a thin film of the cream or gel into the affected area. Avoid occlusive dressing.
- Wash hands before and after application of cream or gel.
- Store at 15°–30° C (59°–86° F).

ADVERSE EFFECTS (≥1%) **Skin:** Pruritus, burning, stinging, tingling, erythema, dryness, rash, peeling, irritation, contact dermatitis, vitiligo depigmentation, hypertrichosis. **Other:** Worsening of asthma.

PHARMACOKINETICS Absorption: Approximately 4% absorbed through the skin. **Onset:** 4–8 wk. **Distribution:** Into all tissues. **Metabolism:** Partially by beta oxidation in liver. **Elimination:** Primarily in urine. **Half-Life:** 12 h.

NURSING IMPLICATIONS

Assessment & Drug Effects

- Assess for signs of hypopigmentation and report immediately.
- Monitor for sensitivity or severe irritation, which may warrant drug dosage reduction or discontinuation.

Patient & Family Education

- Learn proper application of cream or gel and avoid contact with eyes or mucous membranes.
- Wash eyes with copious amounts of water if contact with medication occurs.
- Note: Transient pruritus, burning, and stinging are common; however, severe skin irritation or hypopigmentation should be reported.

AZELASTINE HYDROCHLORIDE

(a-ze-las′teen)

Astelin, Astepro, Optivar

Classifications: ANTIHISTAMINE; H_1-RECEPTOR ANTAGONIST; NASAL AND OCULAR ANTIHISTAMINE

Therapeutic: ANTIHISTAMINE

Prototype: Diphenhydramine

Pregnancy Category: C

AVAILABILITY 137 mcg/spray nasal spray; 0.05% ophth solution; 0.15%, 1% nasal spray

ACTION & *THERAPEUTIC EFFECT* Potent histamine H_1-receptor antagonist and inhibitor of mast cell release of histamine. *Effective in the symptomatic treatment of seasonal allergic rhinitis and as a nasal decongestant.*

USES Seasonal allergic rhinitis, itching associated with allergic conjunctivitis, perennial allergic rhinitis.

CONTRAINDICATIONS Hypersensitivity to azelastine; concurrent use of CNS depressants or alcohol; pregnancy (category C). Safety and efficacy in children younger than 5 y for ophthalmic solution and nasal spray use are not established. **Astepro** nasal spray in children younger than 12 y.

CAUTIOUS USE Hepatic or renal disease; elderly; asthmatics; lactation.

ROUTE & DOSAGE

Allergic Rhinitis

Adult: **Intranasal** 1–2 sprays/nostril b.i.d.

Child (5–11 y): **Intranasal** 1 spray/nostril b.i.d.

Perennial Allergic Rhinitis (Astepro only)

Adult/Adolescent: **Intranasal** 2 sprays/nostril b.i.d.

Allergic Conjunctivitis

See Appendix A-1.

ADMINISTRATION

Intranasal

- Prime delivery unit before first use (see manufacturer's instructions).
- Instruct patient to clear nasal passages prior to drug installation; then tilt head forward slightly and sniff gently when drug is sprayed into each nostril.
- Store the bottle upright at room temperature, 15°–30° C (59°–86° F).

ADVERSE EFFECTS (≥1%) **Body as a Whole:** Fatigue, dizziness. **GI:** Dry mouth, nausea. **Metabolic:** Weight gain. **CNS:** *Headache, somnolence.* **Respiratory:** Pharyngitis, *rhinitis,* paroxysmal sneezing, *cough,* asthma. **Special Senses:** *Bitter taste,* nasal burning, epistaxis, conjunctivitis.

INTERACTIONS Drug: Alcohol and CNS DEPRESSANTS, sedating ANTIHISTAMINES may cause reduced alertness.

PHARMACOKINETICS Absorption: 40% from nasal inhalation. **Peak:** 2–3 h. **Metabolism:** Active metabolites. **Elimination:** Primarily in feces. **Half-Life:** 22 h.

NURSING IMPLICATIONS

Assessment & Drug Effects

- Monitor level of alertness especially in older adults and with concurrent use of other CNS depressants.

Patient & Family Education

- Follow manufacturer's directions for priming the metered dose spray unit before first use and after storage of greater than 3 days.
- Tilt head forward while instilling spray. Avoid getting spray in eyes.
- Do not drive or engage in potentially hazardous activities until response to drug is known.
- Avoid concurrent use of CNS depressants, such as alcohol, while taking this drug.
- Discard spray unit and dispensing package bottle after 3 mo.

AZITHROMYCIN

(a-zi-thro-mye'sin)

AzaSite, Zithromax, Zmax

Classification: MACROLIDE ANTIBIOTIC

Therapeutic: ANTIBIOTIC

Prototype: Erythromycin

Pregnancy Category: B

AVAILABILITY 500 mg, 600 mg tablets; 100 mg/5 mL, 200 mg/5 mL, 1 g/packet oral suspension; 500 mg injection; 1% ophthalmic; **Zmax:** Extended release: 176 mg/5 mL oral suspension

ACTION & *THERAPEUTIC EFFECT* A macrolide antibiotic that reversibly binds to the 50S ribosomal subunit of susceptible organisms and consequently inhibits protein synthesis. *Effective for treatment of mild to moderate infections caused by pyogenic organisms.*

USES Pneumonia, lower respiratory tract infections, pharyngitis/tonsillitis, gonorrhea, nongonococcal urethritis, skin and skin structure infections due to susceptible organisms, otitis media, *Mycobacterium avium–intracellulare* complex infections, acute bacterial sinusitis. **Zmax:** Acute bacterial sinusitis and community acquired pneumonia. **AzaSite:** Bacterial conjunctivitis.

UNLABELED USES Bronchitis, *Helicobacter pylori* gastritis.

CONTRAINDICATIONS Hypersensitivity to azithromycin, erythromycin, or any of the macrolide antibiotics; viral infection; children younger than 6 mo.

CAUTIOUS USE Older adults or debilitated persons, hepatic or renal impairment; GI disease; ventricular arrhythmias, QT prolongation; UV exposure; pregnancy (category B), lactation.

ROUTE & DOSAGE

Bacterial Infections

Adult: **PO** 500 mg on day 1, then 250 mg q24h for 4 more days
IV 500 mg daily for at least 2 days, administer 1 mg/mL over 3 h or 2 mg/mL over 1 h
Child (6 mo or older): **PO** 10 mg/kg on day 1, then 5 mg/kg for 4 more days (max: 250 mg/day)

Acute Bacterial Sinusitis

Adult: **PO** 500 mg once daily × 3 days. Zmax: Single one-time dose of 2 g.
Child (6 mo or older): **PO** 10 mg/kg once daily × 3 days

Otitis Media

Child (older than 6 mo): **PO** 30 mg/kg as a single dose or 10 mg/kg once daily (not to exceed 500 mg/day) for 3 days or 10 mg/kg as a single dose on day 1 followed by 5 mg/kg/day on days 2–5

Gonorrhea

Adult: **PO** 2 g as a single dose

Chancroid

Adult: **PO** 1 g as a single dose
Child: **PO** 20 mg/kg as single dose (max: 1 g)

Bacterial Conjunctivitis

Adult: **Ophthalmic** 1 drop b.i.d × 2 days then daily × 5 days

Renal Impairment Dosage Adjustment

CrCl less than 10 mL/min: Use with caution

ADMINISTRATION

Oral

- Give capsule at least 1 h before or 2 h after a meal. Tablets may be taken without regard to food.
- Do not give within 2 h of an aluminum or magnesium-containing antacid.

Intravenous

PREPARE: **Intermittent:** Reconstitute 500-mg vial with 4.8 mL of sterile water for injection and shake until dissolved. ▪ Final concentration is 100 mg/mL. ▪ Solution **must be** further diluted to 1.0 or 2.0 mg/mL by adding 5 mL of the 100-mg/mL solution to 500 mL or 250 mL, respectively, of D5W, D5/NS, 0.45NaCl, or other compatible solution.

ADMINISTER: **Intermittent:** Administer 1 mg/mL over 3 h. Infuse 2 mg/mL over 1 h. ▪ Note: Do not give a bolus dose.

INCOMPATIBILITIES **Y-site: Amikacin, aztreonam, cefotaxime, ceftazidime, ceftriaxone, cefuroxime, ciprofloxacin, clindamycin, famotidine, fentanyl, furosemide, gentamicin, imipenem/cilastatin, ketorolac, levofloxacin, morphine, ondansetron, piperacillin/tazobactam, potassium, ticarcillin/clavulanate, tobramycin.**

- Store drug when diluted as directed for 24 h at or below 30° C (86° F) or for 7 days under 5° C (41° F).

ADVERSE EFFECTS (≥1%) **CNS:** Headache, dizziness. **GI:** Nausea, vomiting, diarrhea, abdominal pain; <u>hepatotoxicity</u>, mild elevations in liver function tests.

DIAGNOSTIC TEST INTERFERENCE Liver function tests: Reversible, asymptomatic elevations in ***liver enzymes (AST, ALT, gamma glutamyl transferase, alkaline phosphatase)*** have been reported in some patients treated with azithromycin.

INTERACTIONS Drug: ANTACIDS may decrease peak level of azithromycin; may increase toxicity of **digoxin, cyclosporine, phenytoin, dihydroergotamine, ergotamine. Nelfinavir** may increase side effects of azithromycin. Effects of **warfarin** may be potentiated. **Food:** Food will decrease the amount of azithromycin absorbed by 50%.

PHARMACOKINETICS Absorption: 37% of dose reaches the systemic circulation. **Onset:** 48 h. **Peak:** 2.5–4 h. **Distribution:** Extensively into tissues including sputum, blister, and vaginal secretions; tissue concentrations are often higher than serum concentrations. **Metabolism:** In liver. **Elimination:** 5–12% of dose in urine. **Half-Life:** 60–70 h.

NURSING IMPLICATIONS

Assessment & Drug Effects

- Monitor for and report loose stools or diarrhea, since pseudomembranous colitis (see Appendix F) **must be** ruled out.

- Monitor PT and INR closely with concurrent warfarin use.

Patient & Family Education

- Direct sunlight (UV) exposure should be minimized during therapy with drug.
- Take aluminum or magnesium antacids 2 h before or after drug.
- Report onset of loose stools or diarrhea.

AZTREONAM

(az-tree′oh-nam)

Azactam

Classifications: ANTIBIOTIC; BETA-LACTAM ANTIBIOTIC

Therapeutic: ANTIBIOTIC

Prototype: Imipenem-cilastatin

Pregnancy Category: B

AVAILABILITY 1 g, 2 g vials

ACTION & *THERAPEUTIC EFFECT*

Differs structurally from other beta-lactam antibiotics (penicillins and cephalosporins) in having a monocyclic rather than a bicyclic nucleus. Acts by inhibiting synthesis of bacterial cell wall by preferentially binding to specific penicillin-binding proteins (PBP) in the bacterial cell wall. *Highly resistant to beta-lactamases and does not readily induce their formation. Spectrum of activity limited to aerobic, gram-negative bacteria.*

USES Gram-negative infections of urinary tract, lower respiratory tract, skin and skin structures; and for intra-abdominal and gynecologic infections, septicemia, and as adjunctive therapy for surgical infections. Often used in combination with other antibiotics active against gram-positive and anaerobic bacteria in mixed infections.

CONTRAINDICATIONS Lactation, viral infections.

CAUTIOUS USE History of hypersensitivity reaction to penicillin, cephalosporins, or to other drugs; impaired renal or hepatic function, elderly; pregnancy (category B).

ROUTE & DOSAGE

Urinary Tract Infection

Adult: **IV/IM** 0.5–1 g q8–12h

Moderate to Severe Infections

Adult: **IV/IM** 1–2 g q8–12h (max: 8 g/24 h)

Child: **IV** 30 mg/kg/day q6–8h

Renal Impairment Dosage Adjustment

CrCl 10–30 mL/min: Reduce dose 50%; less than 10 mL/min: Reduce dose by 75%

Hemodialysis Dosage Adjustment: Reduce dose to 12.5% and give after hemodialysis

ADMINISTRATION

Intramuscular

- Reconstitute with at least 3 mL of diluent per gram of drug for IM injection. Immediately and vigorously shake vial to dissolve. Suitable diluents include sterile water for injection; bacteriostatic water for injection (with benzyl alcohol and propyl parabens); NS 0.9% for injection.
- Give IM injections deeply into large muscle mass such as the upper outer quadrant of the gluteus maximus or lateral thigh. Rotate injection sites.

Intravenous

Verify correct IV concentration and rate of infusion/injection with physician before giving to neonates, infants, and children.

PREPARE: **Direct:** Reconstitute a single dose with 6–10 mL of sterile water for injection. ▪ Immediately shake vial until solution is dissolved. May be given direct IV as prepared or further diluted for IV infusion. ▪ Reconstituted solutions are colorless to light straw yellow and turn slightly pink on standing. **Intermittent:** Each gram of reconstituted aztreonam **must be** further diluted in at least 50 mL of D5W, NS, or other solution approved by manufacturer to yield a concentration not to exceed 20 mg/mL.

ADMINISTER: **Direct:** Give over 3–5 min. **Intermittent:** Give over 20–60 min through Y-site.

INCOMPATIBILITIES **Solution/additive:** **Ampicillin, metronidazole, nafcillin.** **Y-site:** **Acyclovir, amphotericin B, amphotericin B cholesteryl complex, amsacrine, azithromycin, chlorpromazine, daunorubicin, ganciclovir, lansoprazole, lorazepam, metronidazole, mitomycin, mitoxantrone, streptozocin.**

ADVERSE EFFECTS (≥1%) **Body as a Whole:** Hypersensitivity (urticaria, eosinophilia, anaphylaxis). **CNS:** Headache, dizziness, confusion, paresthesias, insomnia, seizures. **GI:** Nausea, *diarrhea,* vomiting, elevated liver function tests. **Hematologic:** Eosinophilia. **Special Senses:** Tinnitus, nasal congestion, sneezing, diplopia. **Skin:** Rash, purpura, erythema multiforme, exfoliative dermatitis, diaphoresis; petechiae, pruritus. **Other:** Local reactions (phlebitis, thrombophlebitis (following IV), pain at injection sites), superinfections (gram-positive cocci), vaginal candidiasis.

DIAGNOSTIC TEST INTERFERENCE Aztreonam may cause transient elevations of ***liver function tests,*** increases in ***PT*** and ***PTT,*** minor changes in ***Hgb,*** and positive ***Coombs' test.***

INTERACTIONS Drug: **Imipenem-cilastatin, cefoxitin** may be antagonistic, **probenecid** slows renal elimination of aztreonam.

PHARMACOKINETICS Peak: 1 h IM. **Distribution:** Widely distributed including synovial and blister fluid, bile, bronchial secretions, prostate, bone, and CSF; crosses placenta; distributed into breast milk in small amounts. **Metabolism:** Not extensively metabolized. **Elimination:** 60–70% in urine within 24 h. **Half-Life:** 1.6–2.1 h.

NURSING IMPLICATIONS

Assessment & Drug Effects

- Lab tests: Obtain baseline C&S test prior to initiation of therapy. Start drug pending results.
- Baseline and periodic renal function tests, particularly in older adults and in those with history of renal impairment.
- Inspect IV injection sites daily for signs of inflammation. Pain and phlebitis occur in a significant number of patients.

Patient & Family Education

- Determine previous hypersensitivity reactions to penicillins, cephalosporins, and other allergens prior to therapy.
- Monitor for S&S of opportunistic infections (diarrhea, rectal or vaginal itching or discharge, fever, cough) and promptly report onset to physician. Overgrowth of nonsusceptible organisms, particu-

larly *staphylococci, streptococci,* and fungi, is a threat, especially in patients receiving prolonged or repeated therapy.

- Note: IV therapy may cause a change in taste sensation. Report interference with eating.

BACITRACIN

(bass-i-tray'sin)

Baci-IM

Classification: ANTIBIOTIC

Therapeutic: ANTIBIOTIC

Pregnancy Category: C

AVAILABILITY 50,000 unit vial; 500 units/g ophthalmic ointment

ACTION & *THERAPEUTIC EFFECT* Polypeptide antibiotic derived from cultures of *Bacillus subtilis*. Interferes with the bacterial cell membrane by inhibiting cell wall synthesis. *Spectrum of antibacterial activity similar to that of penicillin. Active against many gram-positive organisms. Ineffective against most other gram-negative organisms.*

USES Parenteral therapy restricted to infants with staphylococcal pneumonia and empyema where adequate laboratory facilities and constant supervision are available. Used topically in treatment of superficial infections of skin.

UNLABELED USES Orally for treatment of antibiotic-associated colitis.

CONTRAINDICATIONS Toxic reaction or renal dysfunction associated with bacitracin; pulmonary disease; atopic individuals.

CAUTIOUS USE Hypersensitivity to neomycin; myasthenia gravis or other neuromuscular disease; renal impairment; pregnancy (category C), lactation.

ROUTE & DOSAGE

Systemic Infections

Infant: **IM** *Weight less than 2.5 kg,* up to 900 units/kg/24 h divided q8–12h; *weight greater than 2.5 kg,* up to 1000 units/kg/24h divided q8–12h

Skin Infections

Adult: **Topical** Apply thin layer of ointment b.i.d., t.i.d., as solution of 250–1000 units/mL in wet dressing

ADMINISTRATION

Intramuscular

- Reconstitute with NS containing 2% procaine hydrochloride (prescribed). Do not reconstitute with diluents containing parabens because solution may precipitate or become cloudy.
- Alternate injection sites since injections are painful.
- Dry bacitracin vials should be stored in refrigerator at 2°–8° C (36°–46° F). Store solution for a maximum of 1 wk if refrigerated. Inactivation occurs at room temperature.

Topical

- Clean affected area prior to application. May be covered with a sterile bandage.
- Store ointments in tightly closed containers at 15°–30° C (59°–86° F) unless otherwise directed.

ADVERSE EFFECTS (≥1%) **GI:** Anorexia, nausea, vomiting, diarrhea, rectal itching and burning. **Hematologic:** Systemic use: Bone marrow depression, blood dyscrasias; eosinophilia. **Body as a Whole:** Hypersensitivity (erythema, <u>anaphylaxis</u>). **Urogenital:** <u>Nephrotoxicity</u>; dose related: Increased BUN, uremia, <u>renal</u>

tubular and glomerular necrosis (IM route). **Special Senses:** Tinnitus. **Other:** Pain and inflammation at injection site, fever, superinfection, neuromuscular blockade with respiratory depression.

INTERACTIONS Drug: With AMINOGLYCOSIDES, possibility of additive nephrotoxic and neuromuscular blocking effects; with **tubocurarine** and other NONDEPOLARIZING SKELETAL MUSCLE RELAXANTS, possibility of additive neuromuscular blocking effects.

PHARMACOKINETICS Absorption: Poorly absorbed from intact or denuded skin or mucous membranes. **Peak:** 1–2 h IM. **Duration:** 6–8 h. **Distribution:** Widely distributed including peritoneal and ascitic fluids. **Elimination:** Slow renal excretion (10–40% in 24 h).

NURSING IMPLICATIONS

Assessment & Drug Effects

- Lab tests: Baseline C&S tests prior to initiation of therapy, baseline and periodic kidney function tests.
- Watch for signs of local allergic reaction (itching, burning, redness) with topical skin applications. Local reactions have preceded life-threatening anaphylactic episodes.
- Monitor I&O during parenteral therapy. Adequate urinary output is important to reduce possibility of renal toxicity.
- Inspect urine for turbidity and hematuria, and watch for other S&S of urinary tract dysfunction. Report any changes in urination pattern (e.g., oliguria, urinary frequency, nocturia).
- Note: Prolonged use may result in overgrowth of nonsusceptible organisms, especially *Candida albicans.*

Patient & Family Education

- Report local allergic reactions with topical applications (e.g., itching, burning, redness).

BACLOFEN

(bak'loe-fen)

Kemstro, Lioresal

Classifications: CENTRAL-ACTING SKELETAL MUSCLE RELAXANT; GABA AGONIST

Therapeutic: SKELETAL MUSCLE RELAXANT

Prototype: Cyclobenzaprine

Pregnancy Category: C

AVAILABILITY 10 mg, 20 mg tablets; 10 mg, 20 mg orally disintegrating tablets; 50 mcg/mL, 250 mcg/mL ampules

ACTION & *THERAPEUTIC EFFECT* Centrally acting skeletal muscle relaxant. Depresses monosynaptic and polysynaptic afferent reflex activity at spinal cord level. Baclofen stimulates the GABA receptors, which results in decreased excitatory input into alpha-motor neurons. *Reduces skeletal muscle spasm caused by upper motor neuron lesions.*

USES Symptomatic relief of painful spasms in multiple sclerosis and in the management of detrusor sphincter dyssynergia in spinal cord injury or disease.

UNLABELED USES Treatment of trigeminal neuralgia and of tardive dystonia associated with antipsychotic medications, chronic pain.

CONTRAINDICATIONS Coagulopathy, bacteremia, intramuscular or

B

intrathecal administration, subcutaneous administration.

CAUTIOUS USE Impaired renal and hepatic function; bipolar disorder, psychosis, schizophrenia, seizure disorders, seizures, stroke, cerebral palsy, depression, diabetes mellitus, dialysis, head trauma, PKU, epilepsy; thrombocytopenia; psychiatric or brain disorders; older adults, pregnancy (category C); children younger than 2 y.

ROUTE & DOSAGE

Muscle Spasm

Adult: **PO** 5 mg t.i.d., may increase by 5 mg/dose q3days prn (max: 80 mg/day)
Child: **PO** *2–7 y,* 10–15 mg/day divided q8h, may increase by 5–15 mg/day q3days (max: 40 mg/day); *8 y or older,* 10–15 mg/day divided q8h, may increase by 5–15 mg/day q3days (max: 60 mg/day)
Adult: **Intrathecal** Prior to infusion pump implantation, initiate trial dose of 50 mcg/mL bolus administered in intrathecal space by barbotage over 1 min or less. Observe patient over next 4–8 h for significant decrease in muscle spasm. If response is less than desired, administer second bolus of 75 mcg/1.5 mL and observe 4–8 h. May repeat in 24 h with a 100 mcg/2-mL bolus if necessary. *Post-implant titration:* Use screening dose if response lasted longer than 12 h or double screening dose if response lasted less than 12 h and administer over 24 h. After first 24 h, decrease dose by 10–30% q24h until desired response achieved. Maintenance doses range from 12–1500 mcg/day, with most patients maintained on 300–800 mcg/day.

ADMINISTRATION

Oral

- Give with food or milk to avoid GI distress.

Intrathecal

- Give by direct intrathecal injection (via lumbar puncture or catheter) over at least 1 min or longer.
- Dilute *only* with sterile, preservative free NS injection. Baclofen **must be** diluted to a concentration of 50 mcg/mL when preparing test doses.
- Intrathecal infusion pump: Do not abruptly discontinue as serious adverse effects may develop.
- Store at 15°–30° C (59°–86° F) in tightly closed container unless otherwise directed.

ADVERSE EFFECTS (≥1%) **CNS:** *Transient drowsiness,* vertigo, dizziness, weakness, fatigue, headache, confusion, insomnia; ataxia, loss of seizure control in epileptic patients; abrupt discontinuation of intrathecal administration may result in high fever, altered mental status, exaggerated rebound spasticity, and muscle rigidity, that in rare cases has advanced to rhabdomyolysis, multiple organ-system failure, and death. **CV:** Hypotension. **Special Senses:** Tinnitus, nasal congestion; blurred vision, mydriasis, nystagmus, diplopia, strabismus, miosis. **GI:** Nausea, constipation, vomiting; mild increases in AST, and alkaline phosphatase, jaundice. **Urogenital:** Urinary frequency.

DIAGNOSTIC TEST INTERFERENCE Possibility of increases in ***blood glucose,*** serum ***alkaline phosphatase,*** and ***AST*** levels.

INTERACTIONS Drug: Alcohol, CNS DEPRESSANTS, MAO INHIBITORS, ANTIHISTAMINES compound CNS depression; baclofen may increase blood **glucose** levels, making it necessary to increase dosage of SULFONYLUREAS, **insulin.**

PHARMACOKINETICS Absorption: Readily from GI tract. **Peak:** 2–3 h. **Duration:** 8 h. **Distribution:** Minimal amounts cross blood–brain barrier; crosses placenta; distribution into breast milk unknown. **Metabolism:** 15% in liver. **Elimination:** 70–85% in urine within 72 h; some elimination in feces. **Half-Life:** 3–4 h.

NURSING IMPLICATIONS

Assessment & Drug Effects

- Supervise ambulation. Initially, the loss of spasticity induced by baclofen may affect patient's ability to stand or walk.
- Lab tests: Baseline and periodic BP, weight, blood sugar, hepatic function tests, and urine.
- Monitor for adverse neuropsychiatric or genitourinary symptoms that resemble those of the underlying disease. Assess them carefully and report to the physician.
- Observe carefully for side effects: Mental confusion, depression, hallucinations. Older adults are especially sensitive to this drug.
- Monitor patients with epilepsy closely for possible loss of seizure control.

Patient & Family Education

- Note: CNS depressant effects will be additive to other CNS depressants, including alcohol.
- Monitor blood glucose for loss of glycemic control if diabetic.
- Do not drive or engage in other potentially hazardous activities until the response to drug is known.
- Report adverse reactions to physician. Most can be reduced by decreasing dosage. Incidence of CNS symptoms (drowsiness, dizziness, ataxia) are reportedly high in patients older than 40 y.
- Do not self-dose with OTC drugs without physician's approval.
- Do not stop this drug unless directed to do so by physician. Drug withdrawal needs to be accomplished gradually over a period of 2 wk or more. Abrupt withdrawal following prolonged administration may cause anxiety, agitated behavior, auditory and visual hallucinations, severe tachycardia, acute exacerbation of spasticity, and seizures.

BALSALAZIDE

(bal-sal′a-zide)

Colazal

Classifications: MUCOUS MEMBRANE AGENT; ANTI-INFLAMMATORY

Therapeutic: ANTI-INFLAMMATORY

Prototype: Mesalamine (5-ASA)

Pregnancy Category: B

AVAILABILITY 750 mg capsules

ACTION & *THERAPEUTIC EFFECT* A prodrug of mesalamine that remains intact until it reaches the lumen of the colon. Thought to decrease inflammation of the mucous lining of the colon by blocking cyclooxygenase and inhibiting prostaglandin synthesis in the lining of the colon. *An anti-inflammatory agent and a prodrug of 5-ASA.*

USES Treatment of mild to moderate active ulcerative colitis.

B

CONTRAINDICATIONS Prior hypersensitivity to salicylates, balsalazide; children younger than 5 y.
CAUTIOUS USE Hypersensitivity to mesalamine, sulfasalazine, olsalazine, salicylate. Allergic response to any medications; hepatic or renal impairment; pregnancy (category B), lactation; pyloric stenosis.

ROUTE & DOSAGE

Ulcerative Colitis

Adult: **PO** 2250 mg (three 750 mg caps) t.i.d. for 8–12 wk
Adolescent/Child (older than 5 y): 750–2250 mg (1–3 caps) t.i.d. for up to 8 wk

ADMINISTRATION

Oral
- Give in a consistent manner with respect to food intake (i.e., either always with or always without food).
- Store at room temperature, preferably between 15°–30° C (59°–86° F).

ADVERSE EFFECTS (≥1%) **Body as a Whole:** Arthralgia, fatigue, fever, pain, back pain. **CNS:** Headache, insomnia. **GI:** Abdominal pain, nausea, diarrhea, vomiting, rectal bleeding, flatulence, dyspepsia, coughing, anorexia. **Respiratory:** Rhinitis, pharyngitis.

INTERACTIONS Avoid for 6 wk after VARICELLA VACCINE.

PHARMACOKINETICS Absorption: Low and variable absorption from the colon. **Distribution:** 99% protein bound. **Metabolism:** Metabolized in colon by bacterial azoreduction to release 5-aminosalicylic acid. **Elimination:** Feces (55%), urine (25%).

NURSING IMPLICATIONS

Assessment & Drug Effects
- Monitor for S&S of myelosuppression in patients also receiving azathioprine.
- Lab tests: Closely monitor CBC with concomitant azathioprine therapy; monitor renal and liver functions when used with other aminosalicylates.

Patient & Family Education
- Report worsening of S&S of colitis to physician (e.g., diarrhea, abdominal pain, fever, rectal bleeding).

BASILIXIMAB (Pr)

(bas-i-lix'i-mab)
Simulect
Classifications: IMMUNOSUPPRESSANT; MONOCLONAL ANTIBODY; INTERLEUKIN-2 RECEPTOR ANTAGONIST
Therapeutic: IMMUNOSUPPRESSANT
Pregnancy Category: B

AVAILABILITY 20 mg vials

ACTION & *THERAPEUTIC EFFECT* Immunosuppressant agent that is an interleukin-2 receptor monoclonal antibody produced by recombinant DNA technology. Binds to and blocks interleukin-2R-alpha chain (CD-25 antibodies) on surface of activated T lymphocytes. *Binding to CD-25 antibodies inhibits a critical pathway in the immune response of the lymphocytes involved in allograft rejection.*

USES Prophylaxis of acute renal transplant rejection.

CONTRAINDICATIONS Hypersensitivity to mannitol or murine protein; serious infection or exposure to viral infections (e.g., chickenpox, herpes zoster); lactation.

CAUTIOUS USE History of untoward reactions to dacliximab or other monoclonal antibodies; pregnancy (category B).

ROUTE & DOSAGE

Transplant Rejection Prophylaxis

Adult/Child (weight greater than 35 kg): **IV** 20 mg times 2 doses (1st dose 2 h before surgery, 2nd dose 4 days after transplant)

Child (weight less than 35 kg, 2–15 y): **IV** 12 mg/m² (max: 20 mg/dose) times 2 doses (1st dose 2 h before surgery, 2nd dose 4 days after transplant)

ADMINISTRATION

Intravenous

PREPARE: **Direct/IV infusion:** Add 2.5 mL or 5 mL sterile water for injection to the 10 mg or 20 mg vial, respectively. Rock vial gently to dissolve. ▪ May be given as prepared direct IV as a bolus dose or further diluted in an infusion bag to a volume of 50 mL in NS or D5W. The resulting solution has a concentration of 2.5 mg/mL. ▪ Invert IV bag to dissolve but do not shake. ▪ Discard if diluted solution is colored or has particulate matter. ▪ Use IV solution immediately.

ADMINISTER: **Direct:** Give bolus over 20–30 sec. **IV Infusion:** Infuse the ordered dose of diluted drug over 20–30 min.

▪ If necessary, the diluted solution may be stored at room temperature for 4 h or at 2°–8° C (36°–46° F) for 24 h. Discard after 24 h. ▪ Store undiluted drug at 2°–8° C (36°–46° F).

ADVERSE EFFECTS (≥1%) **Body as a Whole:** Pain, peripheral edema, edema, fever, viral infection, asthenia, arthralgia, acute hypersensitivity reactions with any dose. **CNS:** Headache, tremor, dizziness, insomnia, paresthesias, agitation, depression. **CV:** Hypertension, chest pain, hypotension, arrhythmias. **GI:** Constipation, nausea, diarrhea, abdominal pain, vomiting, dyspepsia, moniliasis, flatulence, GI hemorrhage, melena, esophagitis, erosive stomatitis. **Hematologic:** Anemia, thrombocytopenia, thrombosis, polycythemia. **Respiratory:** Dyspnea, URI, cough, rhinitis, pharyngitis, bronchospasm. **Skin:** Poor wound healing, acne. **Urogenital:** Dysuria, UTI, albuminuria, hematuria, oliguria, frequency, renal tubular necrosis, urinary retention. **Other:** Cataract, conjunctivitis. **Metabolic:** Hyperkalemia, hypokalemia, hyperglycemia, hyperuricemia, hypophosphatemia, hypocalcemia, increased weight, hypercholesterolemia, acidosis.

PHARMACOKINETICS Duration: 36 days. **Distribution:** Binds to interleukin-2R-alpha sites on lymphocytes. **Half-Life:** 7.2 ± 3.2 days in adults, 11.5 ± 6.3 days in children.

NURSING IMPLICATIONS

Assessment & Drug Effects

- Monitor carefully for and immediately report S&S of opportunistic infection or anaphylactoid reaction (see Appendix F).

Patient & Family Education

- Report any distressing adverse effects.
- Avoid vaccination for 2 wk following last dose of drug.

BCG (BACILLUS CALMETTE-GUÉRIN) VACCINE

(ba-cil′lus cal′met-te guer′in)

B

Tice, TheraCys
Classifications: VACCINE; IMMUNOMODULATOR; BIOLOGICAL RESPONSE MODIFIER
Therapeutic: ANTINEOPLASTIC; IMMUNOMODULATOR
Pregnancy Category: C

AVAILABILITY 50 mg, 81 mg, 120 mg powder for suspension

ACTION & *THERAPEUTIC EFFECT* BCG vaccine is an immunization agent for tuberculosis (TB). This vaccine is also active immunotherapy. BCG vaccine stimulates the reticuloendothelial system (RES) to produce macrophages that do not allow mycobacteria to multiply. BCG live is thought to cause a local, chronic inflammatory response involving macrophage and leukocyte infiltration of the bladder. This leads to destruction of superficial tumor cells. *BCG vaccine is an immunization agent for tuberculosis (TB). BCG is active immunotherapy that stimulates the immune mechanism to reject the tumor. It enhances the cytotoxicity of macrophages. BCG live is used intravesically as a biological response modifier for bladder cancer in situ.*

USES To protect tuberculin skin test-negative infants and children, and groups with an excessive rate of new TB infections; carcinoma in situ of the bladder.

UNLABELED USES Malignant melanoma.

CONTRAINDICATIONS Impaired immune responses, immunosuppressive corticosteroid therapy, active TB, concurrent infections; recent TURP, severe hematuria; asymptomatic carriers with positive HIV serology; fever; UTI; lactation.

CAUTIOUS USE Hypersensitivity to BCG; high risk for HIV; aneurysm or prosthesis; pregnancy (category C).

ROUTE & DOSAGE

Prevention of Tuberculosis (Tice only)

Adult: **Intradermal** 0.1 mL
Adult/Child (older than 1 mo): **Percutaneous** After reconstitution, 0.2–0.3 mL of vaccine is dropped onto the cleansed surface of the skin and administered using a multiple-puncture disk applied through the vaccine
Child: **Intradermal** *Younger than 3 mo,* 0.05 mL; *older than 3 mo,* 0.1 mL
Child (younger than 1 mo): **Percutaneous** Reduce adult dose by 1/2 (reconstitute with 2 mL), may need to revaccinate with full dose at 1 y; same as adult

Carcinoma of the Bladder

Adult: **Intravesical** 3 vials of **TheraCys** at 27 mg each (81 mg total) of BCG reconstituted with accompanying diluent 7–14 days after biopsies/transurethral resections once/wk for 6 wk plus one treatment at 3, 6, 12, 18, and 24 mo; 1 vial of **Tice** per intravesical instillation once/wk for 6 wk plus one treatment/mo for 6–12 mo

ADMINISTRATION

WARNING: DO NOT INJECT INTRAVENOUSLY, SUBCUTANEOUSLY, OR INTRADERMALLY.

Percutaneous

- Prepare solution: Add 1 mL sterile water for injection to 1 ampule of vaccine. Draw into syringe and expel back into ampule 3 times to mix.

- Administer drug by dropping 0.2–0.3 mL onto clean surface of skin; then use a sterile multiple-puncture disk to create percutaneous skin punctures.
- Instruct to keep vaccination site dry for 24 h; no dressing is needed.
- Important: Avoid contact with BCG vaccine during preparation and administration.
- Store dry BCG powder, reconstituted vaccine, and diluent refrigerated at 2°–8° C (35°–46° F). Use reconstituted solution within 2 h.

Intravesical Instillation

- **TheraCys:** Dilute 3 vials of **TheraCys** in 50 mL of sterile preservative free NS and instill into bladder slowly by gravity flow via urethral catheter. Patient retains suspension for 2 h and then voids.
- **Tice:** Instill 1 vial of **Tice** intravesically once/wk for 6 wk plus one per mo for 6–12 mo.
- Important: Exercise care when handling BCG vaccine to avoid contact with the product.

ADVERSE EFFECTS (≥1%) **CNS:** Intravesical administration: *Malaise*, dizziness, headache, weakness. **Endocrine:** Hyperpyrexia. **GI:** Abdominal pain, anorexia, constipation, nausea, vomiting, diarrhea; hepatic dysfunction following intratumor injection, granulomatous hepatitis. **Urogenital:** Intravesical administration: Bladder spasms, clot retention, decreased bladder capacity, decreased urine flow, *dysuria, hematuria,* incontinence, nocturia, UTI, cystitis, hemorrhagic cystitis, penile pain, prostatism. **Hematologic:** Thrombocytopenia, eosinophilia, *anemia,* leukopenia, disseminated intravascular coagulation. **Respiratory:** Cough (rare), pulmonary granulomas, pulmonary infection. **Skin:** Abscess with recurrent discharge, red papule that scales or ulcerates in about 5–6 wk, dermatomyositis, granulomas at injection site 4–6 wk after inoculation, keloid formation, lupus vulgaris. **Body as a Whole:** Systemic BCG infection, *chills, flu-like syndrome,* anaphylaxis (rare), allergic reactions, lymphadenitis.

DIAGNOSTIC TEST INTERFERENCE Prior BCG vaccination may result in false-positive ***tuberculin skin test (PPD).*** Following BCG vaccination, tuberculin sensitivity may persist for months to years.

INTERACTIONS Drug: Concurrent antimycobacterial therapy (**aminosalicylic acid, capreomycin, cycloserine, ethambutol, ethionamide, isoniazid, pyrazinamide, rifabutin, rifampin, streptomycin**) that inhibits multiplication of BCG bacilli has the potential to antagonize or altogether negate the BCG vaccine-mediated immune response. **Cyclosporine** may reduce the immunologic response to BCG vaccine. ***Cytomegalovirus* immune globulin** and other live vaccines (measles/mumps/rubella, oral polio) may interfere with immune response to BCG. Previous vaccination with or other exposure to BCG may induce variable sensitivity to tuberculin. A greater booster effect following repeat tuberculin testing has been reported in individuals with prior BCG vaccination when compared with individuals without prior vaccination.

NURSING IMPLICATIONS

Assessment & Drug Effects

- Monitor for S&S of systemic BCG infection: Fever, chills, severe malaise, or cough.

B

- Culture blood and urine, if systemic infection is suspected.
- Assess for regional lymph node enlargement and report fistula formation.

Patient & Family Education

- Review potential adverse effects.
- Keep vaccination site clean until local reaction has subsided.

BECAPLERMIN

(be-cap'ler-min)

Regranex

Classification: PLATELET-DERIVED GROWTH FACTOR (PDGF)

Therapeutic: GROWTH FACTOR

Pregnancy Category: C

AVAILABILITY 0.01% gel

ACTION & *THERAPEUTIC EFFECT* Recombinant human platelet-derived growth factor B in a topical gel. It induces fibroblast proliferation in new granulation tissue. *It is effective against diabetic neuropathic ulcers that involve subcutaneous or deeper tissue, and also have an adequate blood supply. Hence it promotes wound healing of diabetic ulcers.*

USES Lower-extremity diabetic neuropathic ulcers, wound management.

CONTRAINDICATIONS Hypersensitivity to drug or any component in formulation; cresol or paraben hypersensitivity; neoplasms at site of application; wounds that close by primary intention; increased risk of death in patients with diabetes mellitus; children younger than 16 y.

CAUTIOUS USE Concurrent use of corticosteroids, cancer chemotherapy, or other immunosuppressive agents; systemic infection; peripheral vascular disease; ulcer wounds related to arterial or venous insufficiency; thermal, electrical, or radiation burns at wound site; malignancy; elderly; children older than 16 y; pregnancy (category C), lactation.

ROUTE & DOSAGE

Diabetic Neuropathic Ulcers

Adult/Adolescent (older than 16 y): **Topical** Calculate the length of gel based on ulcer size and apply once/day until healed; reassess if ulcer not completely healed in 20 wk

ADMINISTRATION

Topical

- Squeeze calculated length of gel onto clean, firm, nonabsorbable surface.
- Apply even layer to ulcer area with clean tongue depressor or cotton swab and cover with saline-moistened dressing. After 12 h, remove dressing, clean ulcer by rinsing with water or saline to remove residual gel, and apply new saline-moistened dressing without becaplermin for next 12 h. Repeat cycle.
- Apply only to ulcers with good blood supply.
- Dosage calculation: Measure greatest length (*L*) and greatest width (*W*) of ulcer in inches or centimeters; using 15- or 7.5-g tube multiply $(L \times W) \times 0.6$ for dose in inches or $(L \times W)/4$ for dose in cm; using 2-g tube multiply $(L \times W) \times 1.3$ for dose in inches or $(L \times W)/2$ for dose in cm.
- Recalculate weekly/biweekly the amount of drug needed.
- Store at 2°–8° C (36°–46° F). Do not freeze and do not use beyond expiration date.

ADVERSE EFFECTS (≥1%) **Skin:** Erythematous rash.

PHARMACOKINETICS Absorption: Less than 3% absorbed into systemic circulation.

NURSING IMPLICATIONS

Assessment & Drug Effects

- Therapeutic effectiveness: 30% decrease in ulcer size after 10 wk or complete healing after 20 wk.
- Monitor for and report appearance of erythematous rash.

Patient & Family Education

- Consult wound care provider who typically recalculates dosage weekly/biweekly.
- Follow directions for application carefully. Gel may be measured out on waxed paper.
- Wash hands prior to application and do not allow tip of tube to contact ulcer or any surface.
- Report worsening ulceration or development of skin rash.

BECLOMETHASONE DIPROPIONATE

(be-kloe-meth′a-sone)

Beconase AQ, QVAR, Vancenase AQ

Pregnancy Category: C

See Appendix A-3.

BELLADONNA TINCTURE

(bell-a-don′na)

Classifications: ANTICHOLINERGIC; ANTIMUSCARINIC, ANTISPASMODIC

Therapeutic: ANTISPASMODIC

Prototype: Atropine

Pregnancy Category: C

AVAILABILITY 27–33 mg/100 mL tincture

ACTION & *THERAPEUTIC EFFECT* Reversibly blocks action of acetylcholine at parasympathetic neuroeffector sites. *Belladonna inhibits smooth muscle contractions and suppresses secretions of secretory glands.*

USES Adjunct in treatment of peptic ulcer disease, irritable bowel syndrome, and neurogenic bowel disturbances. Also for dysmenorrhea, nocturnal enuresis, spasms of urinary tract, nausea and vomiting of pregnancy, vertigo, and for symptomatic relief of parkinsonism.

CONTRAINDICATIONS Hypersensitivity to anticholinergic drugs; obstructive uropathy, atony of urinary bladder; esophageal reflux, obstructive disease of GI tract, intestinal atony, paralytic ileus, severe ulcerative colitis, toxic megacolon; myasthenia gravis; narrow-angle glaucoma; unstable cardiovascular status in acute hemorrhages; lactation.

CAUTIOUS USE Autonomic neuropathy; heart disease, hypertension; patients older than 40 y (higher incidence of glaucoma); pregnancy (category C).

ROUTE & DOSAGE

Antispasmodic

Adult: **PO** 0.6–1 mL t.i.d. or q.i.d.
Child: **PO** 0.1 mL/kg/day in 3–4 divided doses (max: 3.5 mL/day)

ADMINISTRATION

Oral

- Administer 30–60 min before meals and at bedtime.
- Space administration of antacid and belladonna preparations at least 2 h apart.

B

- Store at 15°–30° C (59°–86° F) in tightly covered, light-resistant containers, unless otherwise directed.

ADVERSE EFFECTS (≥1%) **All:** Dose related. **CNS:** Excitement (young children and older adults), confusion, delirium. **CV:** Rapid heartbeat, tachycardia, palpitation. **Special Senses:** Blurred vision, mydriasis, photophobia. **GI:** *Dry mouth, constipation*. **Urogenital:** Urinary retention, urgency.

INTERACTIONS Drug: Amantadine, ANTIHISTAMINES, TRICYCLIC ANTIDEPRESSANTS, **quinidine, disopyramide, procainamide** have additive anticholinergic effects; **levodopa** effects decreased; **methotrimeprazine** may precipitate extrapyramidal effects; antipsychotic effects of PHENOTHIAZINES decreased (decreased absorption).

PHARMACOKINETICS Absorption: Readily from GI tract. **Onset:** 1–2 h. **Distribution:** Well distributed in body; crosses blood–brain barrier. **Elimination:** Unchanged in urine.

NURSING IMPLICATIONS

Assessment & Drug Effects

- Monitor ambulation of older adults or debilitated patients carefully, since drug may cause drowsiness and confusion.
- Monitor I&O and assess for urinary retention.

Patient & Family Education

- Note: Increase in fluid intake and bulk in diet may prevent or relieve constipation. Notify physician if constipation persists.
- Do not drive or engage in potentially hazardous activities until response to drug is known.
- Practice meticulous oral hygiene. Sugarless gum, lemon drops, and frequent sips of water may help dry mouth.

BENAZEPRIL HYDROCHLORIDE

(ben-a′ze-pril)

Lotensin

Classifications: ANTIHYPERTENSIVE; RENIN ANGIOTENSIN SYSTEM ANTAGONIST

Therapeutic: ANTIHYPERTENSIVE

Prototype: Enalapril

Pregnancy Category: D

AVAILABILITY 5 mg, 10 mg, 20 mg, 40 mg tablets

ACTION & *THERAPEUTIC EFFECT* Lowers blood pressure by specific inhibition of the angiotensin-converting enzyme (ACE) and thus by decreasing angiotensin II (a potent vasoconstrictor) and aldosterone secretion. *Achieves an antihypertensive effect by suppression of the renin-angiotensin-aldosterone system.*

USES Treatment of mild to moderate hypertension.

UNLABELED USES CHF, reno-protective agent.

CONTRAINDICATIONS Hypersensitivity to benazepril or another ACE inhibitor; pregnancy (category D), lactation, or in children younger than 6 y or with a GFR less than 30 mL/h.

CAUTIOUS USE Renal impairment, renal-artery stenosis; patients with hypovolemia, receiving diuretics, undergoing dialysis; patients in whom excessive hypotension would present a hazard (e.g., cerebrovascular insufficiency); CHF; hepatic impairment; diabetes mellitus.

B

ROUTE & DOSAGE

Hypertension

Adult/Adolescent: **PO** 10–40 mg/day in 1–2 divided doses (max: 80 mg/day)

Child (older than 6 y): **PO** 0.1–0.6 mg/kg daily (max: 40 mg/day)

Renal Impairment Dosage Adjustment

CrCl less than 30 mL/min: Use 5 mg starting dose. Do not use in children with CrCl less than 30 mL/min.

ADMINISTRATION

Oral

- Consult physician about initial dose if patient is also receiving diuretics. Typically an initial dose of 5 mg is used to minimize the risk of hypotension.
- Store at room temperature, but not above 30° C (86° F).

ADVERSE EFFECTS (≥1%) **CV:** Hypotension. **CNS:** *Headache,* dizziness, fatigue, weakness. **Endocrine:** Hyperkalemia (at higher doses). **GI:** Nausea, diarrhea or constipation, gastritis. **Urogenital:** Azotemia, oliguria, renal failure in patients with CHF. **Respiratory:** Cough, rhinitis, bronchitis. **Other:** Back pain.

DIAGNOSTIC TEST INTERFERENCE Elevations in ***serum bilirubin*** have been observed after benazepril administration. Benazepril inhibits ***aldosterone*** secretion, which causes an increase in ***serum potassium.***

INTERACTIONS Drug: POTASSIUM-SPARING DIURETICS may increase the risk of hyperkalemia. Benazepril may increase **lithium** toxicity. Use with **azathioprine** increases risk of myelosuppression.

PHARMACOKINETICS Absorption: Readily from GI tract; 37% reaches the systemic circulation. **Peak:** 2–6 h. **Duration:** 20–24 h. **Distribution:** Small amounts cross the blood–brain barrier; crosses placenta; small amount excreted in breast milk. **Metabolism:** In liver to active metabolite, benazeprilat. **Elimination:** Benazeprilat is primarily excreted in urine. **Half-Life:** Benazepril 0.6 h; benazeprilat 22 h.

NURSING IMPLICATIONS

Assessment & Drug Effects

- Assess for hypotension, especially in patients who may be volume depleted (e.g., prolonged diuretic therapy, recent vomiting or diarrhea, salt restriction) or who have CHF.
- Lab tests: Monitor serum potassium levels for hyperkalemia (see Appendix F).

Patient & Family Education

- Do not use salt substitutes unless recommended by physician.
- Report swelling of face, eyes, lips, or tongue or difficulty breathing immediately to physician.

BENDAMUSTINE

(ben-da-mus′teen)

Treanda

Classifications: ANTINEOPLASTIC; ALKYLATING AGENT

Therapeutic: ANTINEOPLASTIC

Prototype: Cyclophosphamide

Pregnancy Category: D

AVAILABILITY 100 mg powder for injection

ACTION & *THERAPEUTIC EFFECT* Alkylating agent that causes the formation of intrastrand and interstrand crosslinks between DNA

B

molecules, thus resulting in inhibition of DNA replication, repair and transcription. *Active against both dividing and resting neoplastic lymphocytes.*

USES Treatment of chronic lymphocytic leukemia, indolent B cell non-Hodgkin's lymphoma.

UNLABELED USES Treatment of relapsed, rituximab-refractory, indolent non-Hodgkin's lymphoma; first-line treatment for follicular lymphoma, indolent lymphoma, and mantle cell lymphoma (MCL) in combination with rituximab.

CONTRAINDICATIONS Grade 2 or greater nonhematologic toxicity; moderate-to-severe hepatic impairment (ALT or AST 2.5–10 × ULN + total bilirubin 1.5–3 × ULN, or bilirubin greater than 3 × ULN); CrCl of less than 40 mL/min; severe or progressive skin reactions; infusion reaction; pregnancy (category D).

CAUTIOUS USE Myelosuppression; mild hepatic or mild-to-moderate renal impairment; grade 3 or 4 infusion reaction; infection; poorly managed hypertension; and lactation. Safety and efficacy in children not established.

ROUTE & DOSAGE

Chronic Lymphocytic Leukemia

Adult: **IV** 100 mg/m^2 on days 1 and 2 of a 28-day cycle, up to 6 cycles

Hematologic Toxicity Dosage Adjustment

Grade 3 or higher: Reduce dose to 50 mg/m^2 on days 1 and 2 of each cycle; if grade 3 or higher toxicity recurs, reduce the dose to 25 mg/m^2 on days 1 and 2 of each cycle.

Indolent B Cell Non-Hodgkin's Lymphoma

Adult: **IV** 120 mg/m^2 on days 1 and 2 q21days

Nonhematologic Toxicity Dosage Adjustment

Clinically significant grade 3 or higher: Reduce dose to 50 mg/m^2 on days 1 and 2 of each cycle.

Toxicity Dosage Adjustment

- For grade 3 or greater nonhematologic toxicity or grade 4 hematologic toxicity: Reduce dose to 90 mg/m^2
- For recurrent grade 3 or greater non-hematologic toxicity or recurrent grade 4 hematologic toxicity: Reduce dose to 60 mg/m^2

ADMINISTRATION

Intravenous

Exercise caution in handling and disposal. Avoid contact with skin. Wash immediately with soap and water if contact occurs.

- Withhold dose for grade 4 hematologic toxicity or clinically significant grade 2 or higher nonhematologic toxicity until nonhematologic toxicity has recovered to grade 1 or less and/or the blood cell counts have improved (ANC count 1000 or more and platelets 75,000 or more).

PREPARE: **IV Infusion:** Reconstitute by adding 20 mL of sterile water for injection to the 100 mg vial to yield 5 mg/mL; should dissolve completely in 5 min. ▪ Withdraw required dose within 30 min of reconstitution and immediately add to 500 mL of NS.

ADMINISTER: **IV Infusion:** Infuse over 30 min.

ADVERSE EFFECTS (≥5%) **Body as a Whole:** Herpes simplex infection, hypersensitivity, infection, *pyrexia.* **CNS:** Asthenia, chills, fatigue. **GI:** Diarrhea, *nausea, vomiting.* **Hematologic:** *Anemia, leukopenia,* lymphopenia, *neutropenia, thrombocytopenia.* **Metabolic:** Hyperuricemia, weight loss. **Respiratory:** Cough, nasopharyngitis. **Skin:** Pruritus, rash.

INTERACTIONS Drug: Compounds that inhibit CYP1A2 (**atazanavir, cimetidine, ciprofloxacin, fluvoxamine, omeprazole, tacrine, zileuton**) will increase levels of bendamustine but decrease levels of its active metabolite. **Clozapine** can cause additive bone marrow suppression.

PHARMACOKINETICS Distribution: 95% protein bound. **Metabolism:** Hepatic oxidation by CYP1A2. **Elimination:** Primarily fecal (90%). **Half-Life:** 40 min.

NURSING IMPLICATIONS

Assessment & Drug Effects

- Monitor closely for infusion reactions (i.e., chills, fever, pruritus, rash) and signs of anaphylaxis. Reactions are more likely with the second and subsequent cycles. Discontinue infusion immediately and notify physician for severe reactions.
- Maintain adequate hydration status to minimize risk of tumor lysis syndrome.
- Monitor for and report S&S of infection.
- Lab tests: Baseline and weekly Hgb, WBC with differential, platelet count during each cycle; frequent serum potassium and uric acid; frequent renal function tests with preexisting renal impairment.

Patient & Family Education

- Men and women should use reliable contraception to avoid pregnancy during and for 3 mo after bendamustine therapy is completed.
- Do not drive or engage in other dangerous activities until reaction to drug is known.
- Report promptly any of the following: Signs of infection, nausea, vomiting, diarrhea, worsening rash or itching.

BENZALKONIUM CHLORIDE

(benz-al-koe′nee-um)

Benza, Benzalchlor-50, Germicin, Pharmatex ✤, Sabol, Zephiran

Classification: TOPICAL ANTIBIOTIC

Therapeutic: ANTIBIOTIC

Pregnancy Category: C

AVAILABILITY 17% concentrate, 1:750 solution, 1:750 tincture/tincture spray

ACTION & *THERAPEUTIC EFFECT* Bactericidal or bacteriostatic action (depending on concentration), probably due to inactivation of bacterial enzyme. *Effective against bacteria, some fungi (including yeasts) and certain protozoa. Generally not effective against spore-forming organisms.*

USES Antisepsis of intact skin, mucous membranes, superficial injuries, and infected wounds; also for irrigations of the eye and body cavities and for vaginal douching.

B

A component of several contact lens wetting and cushioning solutions, and a preservative for ophthalmic solutions.

CONTRAINDICATIONS Casts, occlusive dressings, anal or vaginal packs, lactation.
CAUTIOUS USE Irrigation of body cavities; pregnancy (category C).

ROUTE & DOSAGE

Minor Wounds or Preoperative Disinfection

Adult: **Topical** 1:750 tincture or spray

Preoperative Disinfection of Denuded Skin and Mucous Membranes

Adult: **Topical** 1:10,000–1:2000 solution

Wet Dressings

Adult: **Topical** 1:5000 solution

Urinary Bladder Irrigation

Adult: **Topical** 1:20,000–1:5000 solution

Urinary Bladder Instillation

Adult: **Topical** 1:40,000–1:20,000 solution

Irrigation of Deep Infected Wounds

Adult: **Topical** 1:20,000–1:3000 solution

Vaginal Irrigation

Adult: **Topical** 1:5000–1:2000 solution

Sterile Storage of Instruments, Thermometers, Ampules

Adult: **Topical** 1:750 solution

ADMINISTRATION

Topical

- Use sterile water for injection as diluent for aqueous solutions to be instilled in wounds or body cavities. For other uses, fresh sterile distilled water is used.
- Irrigate eyes immediately and repeatedly with water if medication solution stronger than 1:5000 enters eyes; see a physician promptly.
- Rinse first with water, then with 70% alcohol, before applying benzalkonium for preoperative skin preparation.
- Consult physician about proper dilution of solutions used on denuded skin or inflamed or irritated tissues.
- Store at room temperature, preferably between 15°–30° C (59°–86° F) in airtight container, protected from light.

ADVERSE EFFECTS (≥1%) **Body as a Whole:** Few or no toxic effects in recommended dilutions. **Skin:** Erythema, local burning, hypersensitivity reactions.

NURSING IMPLICATIONS

Assessment & Drug Effects

- Monitor wounds carefully. Report increasing signs of infection or lack of healing.

BENZOCAINE

(ben′zoe-caine)

Americaine, Americaine Anesthetic Lubricant, Americaine-Otic, Anbesol Cold Sore Therapy, Chigger-Tox, Dermoplast, Foille, Hurricaine, Orabase with Benzocaine, Orajel, Solarcaine, T-Caine

Classifications: LOCAL ANESTHETIC (ESTER TYPE); ANTIPRURITIC
Therapeutic: LOCAL ANESTHETIC; ANTIPRURITIC
Prototype: Procaine
Pregnancy Category: C

AVAILABILITY 5% spray, cream, ointment; 6% cream; 8% lotion, 20% spray, ointment, gel, liquid; 20% otic solution

ACTION & *THERAPEUTIC EFFECT* Produces surface anesthesia by inhibiting conduction of nerve impulses from sensory nerve endings. Almost identical to procaine in chemical structure, but has prolonged duration of anesthetic action. *Temporary relief of pain and discomfort.*

USES Temporary relief of pain and discomfort in pruritic skin problems, minor burns and sunburn, minor wounds, and insect bites. Otic preparations are used to relieve pain and itching in acute congestive and serous otitis media, swimmer's ear, and otitis externa. Preparations are also available for toothache, minor sore throat pain, canker sores, hemorrhoids, rectal fissures, pruritus ani or vulvae, as male genital desensitizer to slow onset of ejaculation, and for use as anesthetic-lubricant for passage of catheters and endoscopic tubes.

CONTRAINDICATIONS Hypersensitivity to benzocaine or other PABA derivatives (e.g., sunscreen preparations), or to any of the components in the formulation; use of ear preparation in patients with perforated eardrum or ear discharge; applications to large areas; use in children younger than 2 y.

CAUTIOUS USE History of drug sensitivity; denuded skin or severely traumatized mucosa; pregnancy (category C); children younger than 6 y.

ROUTE & DOSAGE

Anesthetic

Adult: **Topical** Lowest effective dose
Child: **Topical** Lower strengths

ADMINISTRATION

Topical

- Avoid contact of all preparations with eyes and be careful not to inhale mist when spray form is used.
- Do not use spray near open flame or cautery and do not expose to high temperatures. Hold can at least 12 inches (30 cm) away from affected area when spraying.
- Wash and neutralize chemical burns before benzocaine is applied.
- Clean and dry rectal area before administration of hemorrhoidal preparation. Usually administered morning and evening and after each bowel movement.
- Store at 15°–30° C (59°–86° F) in tight, light-resistant containers unless otherwise specified.

ADVERSE EFFECTS (≥1%) **Body as a Whole:** Low toxicity; sensitization in susceptible individuals; allergic reactions, anaphylaxis. **Hematologic:** Methemoglobinemia reported in infants.

INTERACTIONS Drug: Benzocaine may antagonize antibacterial activity of SULFONAMIDES.

PHARMACOKINETICS Absorption: Poorly absorbed through intact skin; readily absorbed from mucous

B

membranes. **Peak:** 1 min. **Duration:** 15–30 min. **Metabolism:** By plasma cholinesterases and to a lesser extent by hepatic cholinesterases. **Elimination:** In urine.

NURSING IMPLICATIONS

Assessment & Drug Effects

- Assess swallowing when used on oral mucosa, as benzocaine may interfere with second (pharyngeal) stage of swallowing; hold food and liquids accordingly.
- Assess for sensitivity. Local anesthetics are potentially sensitizing to susceptible individuals when applied repeatedly or over extensive areas.

Patient & Family Education

- Use specific benzocaine preparation ONLY as prescribed or recommended by manufacturer.
- Discontinue medication if the condition persists, worsens, or if signs of sensitivity, irritation, or infection occur.

BENZONATATE (Pr)

(ben-zoe′na-tate)

Tessalon

Classification: ANTITUSSIVE

Therapeutic: COUGH SUPPRESSANT

Pregnancy Category: C

AVAILABILITY 100 mg capsules

ACTION & *THERAPEUTIC EFFECT* Nonnarcotic antitussive activity reported to be somewhat less effective than that of codeine. Does not inhibit respiratory center at recommended doses. *Decreases frequency and intensity of nonproductive cough.*

USES Decreases frequency and intensity of nonproductive cough in acute and chronic respiratory conditions. Also used in bronchoscopy, thoracentesis, and other procedures when coughing **must be** avoided.

CONTRAINDICATIONS Children younger than 10 y.

CAUTIOUS USE Pregnancy (category C), lactation.

ROUTE & DOSAGE

Antitussive

Adult/Child (older than 10 y): **PO** 100 mg t.i.d. prn up to 600 mg/day

ADMINISTRATION

Oral

- Ensure that soft capsules called perles are swallowed whole.
- Store in airtight containers protected from light.

ADVERSE EFFECTS (≥1%) **Body as a Whole:** Low incidence. **CNS:** Drowsiness, sedation headache, mild dizziness. **GI:** Constipation, nausea. **Skin:** Rash, pruritus.

PHARMACOKINETICS Onset: 15–20 min. **Duration:** 3–8 h.

NURSING IMPLICATIONS

Assessment & Drug Effects

- Auscultate lungs anteriorly and posteriorly at scheduled intervals.
- Observe character and frequency of coughing and volume and quality of sputum. Keep physician informed.

Patient & Family Education

- Do not chew or allow perle to dissolve in mouth; swallow whole. If perle dissolves in mouth, the mouth, tongue, and pharynx will be anesthetized. Also, it is unpleasant to taste.

BENZPHETAMINE HYDROCHLORIDE

(benz-fet'a-meen)

Didrex

Classifications: CEREBRAL STIMULANT; ANOREXIANT

Therapeutic: ANOREXIANT

Prototype: Amphetamine

Pregnancy Category: X

Controlled Substance: Schedule III

AVAILABILITY 50 mg tablets

ACTION & *THERAPEUTIC EFFECT* Indirect acting sympathomimetic amine with amphetamine-like actions but with fewer side effects than amphetamine. Anorexiant effect thought to be secondary to stimulation of hypothalamus to release stored catecholamines in the CNS. *Effective as an appetite suppressant.*

USES Short-term adjunct in management of exogenous obesity.

CONTRAINDICATIONS Known hypersensitivity to sympathomimetic amines; angle-closure glaucoma; advanced arteriosclerosis, angina pectoris, severe cardiovascular disease, moderate to severe hypertension; hyperthyroidism, agitated states; history of drug abuse; children younger than 12 y; lactation; pregnancy (category X).

CAUTIOUS USE Diabetes mellitus; older adults; psychosis.

ROUTE & DOSAGE

Obesity

Adult: **PO** 25–50 mg 1–3 times/day

ADMINISTRATION

Oral

- Give as a single daily dose, preferably midmorning or midafternoon, according to patient's eating habits.
- Schedule daily dose no later than 6 h before patient retires to avoid insomnia.
- Store in tight, light-resistant containers at 15°–30° C (59°–86° F) unless otherwise directed.

ADVERSE EFFECTS (≥1%) **CNS:** Euphoria, irritability, hyperactivity, nervousness, *restlessness, insomnia,* tremor, headache, light-headedness, dizziness, depression following stimulant effects. **CV:** *Palpitation,* tachycardia, elevated BP, irregular heartbeat. **GI:** Xerostomia, nausea, vomiting, diarrhea or constipation, abdominal cramps. **Chronic Intoxication:** Marked insomnia, irritability, hyperactivity, personality changes, psychosis, severe dermatoses.

INTERACTIONS Drug: Acetazolamide, sodium bicarbonate decrease AMPHETAMINE elimination; **ammonium chloride, ascorbic acid** increase AMPHETAMINE elimination; BARBITURATES may antagonize the effects of both drugs; **furazolidone** may increase BP effects of AMPHETAMINES, and interaction may persist for several weeks after discontinuation of **furazolidone; guanethidine** antagonizes antihypertensive effects; because MAO INHIBITORS, **selegiline** can cause hypertensive crisis (fatalities reported); do not administer AMPHETAMINES during or within 14 days of these drugs; PHENOTHIAZINES may inhibit mood-elevating effects of AMPHETAMINES; TRICYCLIC ANTIDEPRESSANTS enhance AMPHETAMINE effects because they increase **norepinephrine** release; BETA AGONISTS increase AMPHETAMINE'S adverse cardiovascular effects.

PHARMACOKINETICS Absorption: Readily absorbed from GI tract.

B

Duration: 4 h. **Metabolism:** Via CYP3A4. **Elimination:** Renal elimination.

NURSING IMPLICATIONS

Assessment & Drug Effects

- Assess for signs of excessive CNS stimulation: Insomnia, restlessness, tremor, palpitations. These may indicate need for dosage adjustment.
- Monitor vital signs; report elevated BP, tachycardia, and irregular heart rhythm.
- Monitor diabetics for loss of glycemic control.

Patient & Family Education

- Note: Anorexiant effects are temporary and tolerance may occur; long-term use is not indicated.
- Do not drive or engage in potentially hazardous activities until response to drug is known.
- Do not terminate high dosage therapy abruptly; GI distress, stomach cramps, trembling, unusual tiredness, weakness, and mental depression may result.

BENZTROPINE MESYLATE

(benz'troe-peen)

Apo-Benztropine ♣, Cogentin, PMS Benztropine ♣

Classifications: CENTRALLY ACTING CHOLINERGIC RECEPTOR ANTAGONIST; ANTIPARKINSON

Therapeutic: ANTIPARKINSON

Prototype: Benztropine

Pregnancy Category: C

AVAILABILITY 0.5 mg, 1 mg, 2 mg tablets; 1 mg/mL ampules

ACTION & *THERAPEUTIC EFFECT* Synthetic centrally acting anticholinergic agent. Acts by diminishing excess cholinergic effect associated with dopamine deficiency. *Suppresses tremor and rigidity; does not alleviate tardive dyskinesia.*

USES Symptomatic treatment of all forms of parkinsonism (arteriosclerotic, idiopathic, postencephalitic) and to relieve extrapyramidal symptoms associated with neuroleptic drugs [e.g., haloperidol (Haldol)], phenothiazines, thiothixene (Navane), acute dystonia. Commonly used as supplement with trihexyphenidyl, carbidopa, or levodopa therapy.

CONTRAINDICATIONS Narrow-angle glaucoma; myasthenia gravis; obstructive diseases of GU and GI tracts; tendency to tachycardia; tardive dyskinesia, children younger than 3 y.

CAUTIOUS USE Older children, older adults or debilitated patients, patients with poor mental outlook, mental disorders; tachycardia; autonomic neuropathy; enlarged prostate; hypertension; history of renal or hepatic disease; pregnancy (category C), lactation.

ROUTE & DOSAGE

Parkinsonism

Adult: **PO** 0.5–1 mg/day, may gradually increase as needed up to 6 mg/day **IM/IV** 1–2 mg/day

Extrapyramidal Reactions

Adult: **PO** 1–2 mg b.i.d. **IM/IV** 1–4 mg 1–2 times daily as needed
Child (older than 3 y): **PO/IM/IV** 1–2 mg/day

Acute Dystonia

Adult: **IV** 1–2 mg daily

ADMINISTRATION

Oral

- Give immediately after meals or with food to prevent gastric irrita-

tion. Tablet can be crushed and sprinkled on or mixed with food.
- Initiate and withdraw drug therapy gradually; effects are cumulative.
- Store in tightly covered, light-resistant container at 15°–30° C (59°–86° F) unless otherwise directed.

Intravenous

IV administration to infants and children: Verify correct IV concentration with physician.

PREPARE: **Direct:** Give undiluted.
ADMINISTER: **Direct:** Give 1 mg or a fraction thereof over 1 min.

ADVERSE EFFECTS (≥1%) **CNS:** *Sedation*, drowsiness, dizziness, paresthesias; agitation, irritability, restlessness, nervousness, insomnia, hallucinations, delirium, mental confusion, toxic psychosis, muscular weakness, ataxia, inability to move certain muscle groups. **CV:** Palpitation, tachycardia, flushing. **Special Senses:** Blurred vision, mydriasis, photophobia. **GI:** Nausea, vomiting, *constipation, dry mouth*, distention, <u>paralytic ileus</u>. **Urogenital:** Dysuria.

INTERACTIONS Drug: Alcohol, CNS DEPRESSANTS have additive sedation and depressant effects; **amantadine,** TRICYCLIC ANTIDEPRESSANTS, MAO INHIBITORS, PHENOTHIAZINES, **procainamide, quinidine** have additive anticholinergic effects and cause confusion, hallucinations, paralytic ileus.

PHARMACOKINETICS Onset: 15 min IM/IV; 1 h PO. **Duration:** 6–10 h.

NURSING IMPLICATIONS

Assessment & Drug Effects
- Monitor I&O ratio and pattern. Advise patient to report difficulty in urination or infrequent voiding. Dosage reduction may be indicated.
- Closely monitor for appearance of S&S of onset of paralytic ileus including intermittent constipation, abdominal pain, diminution of bowel sounds on auscultation, and distention.
- Monitor for and report muscle weakness or inability to move certain muscle groups. Dosage reduction may be needed.
- Supervise ambulation and use protective measures as necessary.
- Report immediately S&S of CNS depression or stimulation. These usually require interruption of drug therapy.

Patient & Family Education
- Do not drive or engage in potentially hazardous activities until response to drug is known. Seek help walking as necessary.
- Avoid alcohol and other CNS depressants because they may cause additive drowsiness. Do not take OTC cold, cough, or hay fever remedies unless approved by physician.
- Sugarless gum, hard candy, and rinsing mouth with tepid water will help dry mouth.
- Avoid strenuous exercise in hot weather; diminished sweating may require dose adjustments because of possibility of heat stroke.

BERACTANT (Pr)

(ber-ac'tant)
Survanta
Classification: LUNG SURFACTANT
Therapeutic: LUNG SURFACTANT
Pregnancy Category: Not applicable

AVAILABILITY 25 mg/mL suspension

B

ACTION & *THERAPEUTIC EFFECT* Beractant is a sterile pulmonary surfactant. Endogenous pulmonary surfactant lowers surface tension on alveolar surfaces during respiration and stabilizes the alveoli against collapse at resting pressures. Deficiency of surfactant causes respiratory distress syndrome (RDS) in premature infants. *Beractant lowers minimum surface tension and restores pulmonary compliance and oxygenation in premature infants.*

USES Prevention and treatment of RDS in premature infants, especially those weighing less than 1250 g.

UNLABELED USES Infants weighing less than 600 g or greater than 1750 g; treatment of RDS in adults.

CONTRAINDICATIONS Nosocomial infections; bovine protein hypersensitivity.

CAUTIOUS USE Lactation.

ROUTE & DOSAGE

Neonate: **Intratracheal** Instill 100 mg/kg (4 mL/kg) birth weight through endotracheal tube, may repeat no more frequently than q6h (max: 4 doses in the first 48 h of life)

ADMINISTRATION

Intratracheal

- Place refrigerated drug at room temperature for at least 20 min or warm in the hand for at least 8 min. Do not use artificial warming methods.
- Suction infant before administration of beractant.
- Follow specific dosing procedure recommended by the manufacturer. Carefully read and follow exactly accompanying drug administration literature.
- Do not suction for 1 h after drug is administered unless signs of significant airway obstruction occur.
- Unopened vials warmed to room temperature will not lose potency if refrigerated within 8 h of warming. Drug should not be warmed and returned to refrigerator more than once.
- Store unopened vials inside carton to protect from light and refrigerated at 2°–8° C (36°–46° F) until ready to use.

ADVERSE EFFECTS (≥1%) **CV:** *Transient bradycardia.* **Respiratory:** *Oxygen desaturation.* **Other:** Increased probability of post-treatment nosocomial sepsis in surfactant-treated infants was observed in the controlled clinical trials but was not associated with increased mortality.

PHARMACOKINETICS **Absorption:** Absorbed from the alveolus into lung tissue, where it can be extensively catabolized and reutilized for further phospholipid synthesis and secretion. **Onset:** 0.5–4 h. **Peak:** 2 h. **Duration:** 48–72 h; may need multiple doses to sustain improvement. **Distribution:** Not distributed to the systemic circulation. **Metabolism:** Surfactant is recycled and metabolized exclusively in the lungs. **Elimination:** Recycling may be a dominant metabolic pathway by which surfactant is taken up by type II pneumocytes and reused. **Half-Life:** 20–30 h.

NURSING IMPLICATIONS

Assessment & Drug Effects

- Monitor heart rate, color, chest expansion, facial expressions, oximeter, and endotracheal tube patency and position, during administration. Most adverse effects occur during dosing.

- Monitor frequently with arterial or transcutaneous measurement of systemic oxygen and CO_2.
- Note: Rales and moist breath sounds may occur transiently following drug administration. These do not necessarily indicate a need for suctioning.

BETAMETHASONE

(bay-ta-meth'a-sone)

Betnelan ♣, Celestone

BETAMETHASONE ACETATE AND BETAMETHASONE SODIUM PHOSPHATE

Celestone Soluspan

BETAMETHASONE BENZOATE

Beben ♣

BETAMETHASONE DIPROPIONATE

Alphatrex, Diprolene

BETAMETHASONE SODIUM PHOSPHATE (PH 8.5)

Betameth, Betnesol ♣, Celestone S

BETAMETHASONE VALERATE

Betaderm ♣, Beta-Val, Betnovate ♣, Celestoderm ♣, Ectosone Lotion ♣, Luxiq, Metaderm ♣, Novobetamet ♣, Valnac

Classifications: ANTI-INFLAMMATORY; ADRENAL CORTICOSTEROID; GLUCOCORTICOID

Therapeutic: ANTI-INFLAMMATORY; ADRENAL CORTICOSTEROID

Prototype: Hydrocortisone

Pregnancy Category: C

AVAILABILITY **Betamethasone:** 0.6 mg tablets; 0.6 mg/5 mL syrup; **Betamethasone Acetate and Betamethasone Sodium:** 3 mg acetate, 3 mg sodium phosphate/mL suspension; **Betamethasone Benzoate and Betamethasone Dipropionate:** 4 mg/mL injection; **Betamethasone Valerate:** 0.1% ointment; 0.01%, 0.05%, 0.1% cream; 0.1% lotion; 1.2 mg/g foam; **Betamethasone Sodium Phosphate:** 0.6 mg/5 mL syrup

ACTION & *THERAPEUTIC EFFECT* Synthetic, long-acting glucocorticoid with minor mineralocorticoid properties but strong immunosuppressive, anti-inflammatory, and metabolic actions. *Relieves anti-inflammatory manifestations and is an immunosuppressive agent.*

USES Reduces serum calcium in hypercalcemia, suppresses undesirable inflammatory or immune responses, produces temporary remission in nonadrenal disease, and blocks ACTH production in diagnostic tests. Topical use provides relief of inflammatory manifestations of corticosteroid-responsive dermatoses.

UNLABELED USES Prevention of neonatal respiratory distress syndrome (hyaline membrane disease).

CONTRAINDICATIONS In patients with systemic fungal infections; acne vulgaris; acne rosacea; Cushing's syndrome; periorbital dermatitis; vaccines; lactation.

CAUTIOUS USE Ocular herpes simplex; concomitant use of aspirin; osteoporosis; diverticulitis, nonspecific ulcerative colitis, abscess or

B

other pyrogenic infection, peptic ulcer disease; asthmatics; diabetes mellitus; hypertension; renal insufficiency; myasthenia gravis; pregnancy (category C).

ROUTE & DOSAGE

Anti-inflammatory Agent

Adult: **PO** 0.6–7.2 mg/day **IM/IV** Up to 9 mg/day as sodium phosphate

Topical (See Appendix A-4)

Child: **PO** 0.0175–0.25 mg/kg/day or 0.5–0.75 mg/m²/day divided q6–8h **IM** 0.0175–0.125 mg/kg/day or 0.5–0.75 mg/m²/day divided q6–8h

Respiratory Distress Syndrome

Adult: **IM** 2 mL of sodium phosphate to mother once daily 2–3 days before delivery

ADMINISTRATION

Oral

- Give with food or milk to lessen stomach irritation.

Intra-articular/Intramuscular/Intralesional

- Use Celestone Soluspan for intra-articular, IM, and intralesional injection. The preparation is not intended for IV use. Do not mix with diluents containing preservatives (e.g., parabens, phenol).
- Use 1% or 2% lidocaine hydrochloride if prescribed. Withdraw betamethasone mixture first, then lidocaine; shake syringe briefly.

Intravenous

PREPARE: **Direct/IV Infusion:** Give by direct IV undiluted or further diluted for infusion in D5W or NS.

ADMINISTER: **Direct:** Give at a rate of 1 dose/min. **IV Infusion:** Give at a rate determined by the total amount of IV fluid.

INCOMPATIBILITIES **Solution/additive and Y-site:** Do not infuse with other drugs.

ADVERSE EFFECTS (≥1%) **Body as a Whole:** Hypersensitivity or anaphylactoid reactions; aggravation or masking of infections; malaise, weight gain, obesity. Most adverse effects are dose and treatment duration dependent. **CNS:** Vertigo, headache, nystagmus, ataxia (rare), increased intracranial pressure with papilledema (usually after discontinuation of medication), mental disturbances, aggravation of preexisting psychiatric conditions, insomnia. **CV:** Hypertension; syncopal episodes, thrombophlebitis, thromboembolism or fat embolism, palpitation, tachycardia, necrotizing angiitis; CHF. **Endocrine:** Suppressed linear growth in children, decreased glucose tolerance; hyperglycemia, manifestations of latent diabetes mellitus; hypocorticism; amenorrhea and other menstrual difficulties. **Special Senses:** Posterior subcapsular cataracts (especially in children), glaucoma, exophthalmos, increased intraocular pressure with optic nerve damage, perforation of the globe, fungal infection of the cornea, decreased or blurred vision. **Metabolic:** Hypocalcemia; *sodium and fluid retention;* hypokalemia and hypokalemic alkalosis; negative nitrogen balance. **GI:** *Nausea,* increased appetite, ulcerative esophagitis, pancreatitis, abdominal distention, peptic ulcer with perforation and hemorrhage, melena; decreased serum concentration of vitamins A and C. **Hematologic:** Thrombocytopenia. **Musculoskeletal:** Osteoporosis, compression fractures, muscle wasting and weakness, tendon rupture, aseptic necrosis of femoral and humeral heads (all resulting from long-term use). **Skin:** Skin thinning and atrophy, *acne, impaired wound healing;* petechiae, ecchymosis, easy bruising; suppression of skin test reaction; hypopigmentation or hyperpigmentation, hirsutism, acneiform eruptions, subcutaneous fat atrophy; allergic dermatitis, urticaria, angioneurotic edema, increased sweating. **Urogenital:** Increased or decreased motility and number of sperm; urinary frequency and urgency, enuresis. **With parenteral therapy, IV site:** Pain, irritation, necrosis, atrophy, sterile abscess; Charcot-like arthropathy following intra-articular use; burning and tingling in perineal area (after IV injection).

DIAGNOSTIC TEST INTERFERENCE May increase ***serum cholesterol, blood glucose, serum sodium, uric acid*** (in acute leukemia) and ***calcium*** (in bone metastasis). It may decrease ***serum calcium, potassium, PBI, thyroxin*** (T_4), ***tri-iodothyronine*** (T_3) ***and reduce thyroid I 131*** uptake. It increases ***urine glucose*** level and ***calcium*** excretion; decreases ***urine 17-OHCS*** and ***17-KS*** levels. May produce false-negative results with ***nitroblue tetrazolium test*** for systemic bacterial infection and may suppress reactions to skin tests.

INTERACTIONS Drug: BARBITURATES, **phenytoin, rifampin** may reduce pharmacologic effect of betamethasone by increasing its metabolism.

PHARMACOKINETICS Peak: 1–2 h **Half-Life:** 35–54 h

NURSING IMPLICATIONS

Assessment & Drug Effects

- Assess therapeutic effectiveness. Response following intra-articular, intralesional, or intrasynovial administration occurs within a few hours and persists for 1–4 wk. Following IM administration response occurs in 2–3 h and persists for 3–7 days.

Patient & Family Education

- Monitor weight at least weekly.
- Discontinue slowly after systemic use of 1 wk or longer. Abrupt withdrawal, especially following high doses or prolonged use, can cause dizziness, nausea, vomiting, fever, muscle and joint pain, weakness.

BETAXOLOL HYDROCHLORIDE

(be-tax'oh-lol)

Betoptic, Betoptic-S, Kerlone

Classifications: EYE PREPARATION; MIOTIC (ANTIGLAUCOMA); BETA-ADRENERGIC ANTAGONIST; ANTIHYPERTENSIVE

Therapeutic: ANTIGLAUCOMA (MIOTIC); ANTIHYPERTENSIVE

Prototype: Propranolol

Pregnancy Category: C

AVAILABILITY 10 mg, 20 mg tablets; 0.25%, 0.5% ophthalmic solution

ACTION & *THERAPEUTIC EFFECT* Acts as a $beta_1$-selective adrenergic receptor blocking agent, especially in the cardioselective $beta_1$ receptors. Its antihypertensive effect is thought to be due to: (1) decreasing cardiac output, (2) reducing sympathetic nervous system outflow to the periphery resulting in vasodilatation, and (3) suppression of renin activity in the kidney. It reduces intraocular pressure within the eye by decreasing the production of aqueous humor. *All three mechanisms result in its antihypertensive effect.*

USES Hypertension. Ocular use for intraocular hypertension, chronic open angle glaucoma (see Appendix A-1).

CONTRAINDICATIONS Hypersensitivity to beta-blockers; sinus bradycardia, AV block greater than first degree, cardiogenic shock, overt cardiac failure; CHF unless secondary to tachyarrhythmia treatable with beta-blockers; glaucoma, angle closure (unless with a miotic); children younger than 18 y; lactation.

CAUTIOUS USE Concomitant use of systemic beta-adrenergic blocking agents; history of heart failure; renal impairment, hepatic impairment; elderly; hyperthyroidism or thyrotoxicosis; diabetes mellitus; with evidence of airflow obstruction or reactive airway disease; depression; pregnancy (category C).

ROUTE & DOSAGE

Hypertension

Adult: **PO** 10–20 mg daily (max: 40 mg/day in 1–2 divided doses)
Elderly: **PO** Start with 5 mg/day and taper up

Renal Impairment Dosage Adjustment

CrCl less than 60 mL/min: Administer 50% of dose (max: 20 mg/day)

Chronic Open-Angle Glaucoma/Ocular Hypertension

See Appendix A-1.

ADMINISTRATION

Oral

- Check pulse before administering betaxolol, oral or ophthalmic. If there are extremes (rate or rhythm), withhold medication and call the physician.

ADVERSE EFFECTS (≥1%) **CV:** Bradycardia, hypotension. **CNS:** Depression. **Respiratory:** Increased airway resistance. **Special Senses:** With ophthalmic solution, *mild ocular stinging* and discomfort, tearing.

INTERACTIONS Drug: Reserpine and other CATECHOLAMINE-DEPLETING AGENTS may cause additive hypotensive effects or bradycardia. **Verapamil** may cause additive heart block.

PHARMACOKINETICS Absorption: 90% of PO dose reaches systemic circulation. **Onset:** 0.5–1 h. **Peak:** 2 h. **Duration:** Greater than 12 h. **Metabolism:** In liver. **Elimination:** 30–40% in urine, 50–60% in bile and feces. **Half-Life:** 12–22 h.

NURSING IMPLICATIONS

Assessment & Drug Effects

- Monitor pulse rate and BP at regular intervals in patients with severe heart disease.
- Report promptly onset of bradycardia or signs of CHF.
- Monitor therapeutic effectiveness. Some patients develop tolerance during long-term therapy.

Patient & Family Education

- Report unusual pulse rate or significant changes to physician according to parameters provided.
- Adhere to regimen EXACTLY as prescribed. Do not stop drug abruptly; angina may be exacer-

bated; dosage is reduced over a period of 1–2 wk.

- Report difficulty in breathing promptly to physician. Drug withdrawal may be indicated.

BETHANECHOL CHLORIDE Pr

(be-than′e-kole)

Duvoid, Urecholine

Classification: DIRECT-ACTING CHOLINERGIC

Therapeutic: CHOLINERGIC

Pregnancy Category: C

AVAILABILITY 5 mg, 10 mg, 25 mg, 50 mg tablets

ACTION & *THERAPEUTIC EFFECT* Synthetic choline ester with effects similar to those of acetylcholine (ACh). Acts directly on postsynaptic receptors, and since it is not hydrolyzed by cholinesterase, its actions are more prolonged than those of ACh. Produces muscarinic effects primarily on GI tract and urinary bladder. Increases tone and peristaltic activity of esophagus, stomach, and intestine; contracts detrusor muscle of urinary bladder, usually enough to initiate micturition. *Bethanechol is a synthetic parasympathomimetic indicated for the treatment of urinary retention associated with neurogenic bladder.*

USES Acute postoperative and postpartum nonobstructive (functional) urinary retention, and for neurogenic atony of urinary bladder with retention.

UNLABELED USES In selected cases of adynamic ileus, gastric atony and retention, reflux esophagitis, congenital megacolon, familial dysautonomia; for prevention and treatment of bladder and salivary gland inhibition induced by tricyclic antidepressants, and for prophylaxis and treatment of phenothiazine-induced bladder dysfunction.

CONTRAINDICATIONS COPD; history of or active bronchial asthma; hyperthyroidism; recent urinary bladder surgery, cystitis, bacteriuria, urinary bladder neck or intestinal obstruction, peptic ulcer, recent GI surgery, peritonitis; marked vagotonia, pronounced vasomotor instability, AV conduction defects, severe bradycardia, hypotension or hypertension, coronary artery disease, recent MI; epilepsy, parkinsonism; lactation, children younger than 8 y.

CAUTIOUS USE Urinary retention; bacteriemia; patients at risk for syncopy; pregnancy (category C).

ROUTE & DOSAGE

Urinary Retention

Adult: **PO** 10–50 mg b.i.d. to q.i.d. (max: 120 mg/day)

Child: **PO** 0.2 mg/kg or 0.6 mg/m^2 t.i.d.

ADMINISTRATION

Oral

- Give on an empty stomach (1 h before or 2 h after meals) to lessen possibility of nausea and vomiting, unless otherwise advised by physician.

ADVERSE EFFECTS (≥1%) **Body as a Whole:** (Dose-related) Increased sweating, malaise, headache, substernal pain or pressure, hypothermia. **CV:** Hypotension with dizziness, faintness, flushing, orthostatic hypotension (large doses); mild reflex tachycardia, atrial fibrillation (hyperthyroid patients), transient complete heart block. **Special Senses:** Blurred vision, miosis, lacrimation. **GI:** Nausea, vomiting, abdominal cramps, diarrhea, borborygmi, belching, salivation, fecal incontinence (large doses), urge to defecate (or urinate). **Respiratory:** Acute asthmatic attack, dyspnea (large doses).

DIAGNOSTIC TEST INTERFERENCE Bethanechol may cause increases in ***serum amylase*** and ***serum lipase,*** by stimulating pancreatic secretions, and may increase ***AST, serum bilirubin,*** and ***BSP retention*** by causing spasms in sphincter of Oddi.

INTERACTIONS Drug: Ambenonium, neostigmine, other CHOLINESTERASE INHIBITORS compound cholinergic effects and toxicity; **mecamylamine** may cause abdominal symptoms and hypotension; **procainamide, quinidine, atropine, epinephrine** antagonize effects of bethanechol.

PHARMACOKINETICS Absorption: Well absorbed. **Onset:** 30 min. **Peak:** 60–90 min. **Duration:** 1–6 h. **Distribution:** Does not cross blood–brain barrier. **Metabolism:** Unknown. **Elimination:** Unknown.

NURSING IMPLICATIONS

Assessment & Drug Effects

- Monitor BP and pulse. Report early signs of overdosage: Salivation, sweating, flushing, abdominal cramps, nausea.
- Monitor I&O. Observe and record patient's response to bethanechol.
- Monitor respiratory status. Promptly report dyspnea or any other indication of respiratory distress.
- Supervise ambulation as indicated by patient response to drug.

Patient & Family Education

- Make position changes slowly and in stages, particularly from lying down to standing.
- Do not stand still for prolonged periods; sit or lie down at first indication of faintness.
- Do not drive or engage in potentially hazardous activities until response to drug is known.
- Note: Drug may cause blurred vision; take appropriate precautions.

BEVACIZUMAB

(be-va-ci-zu′mab)

Avastin

Classifications: ANTINEOPLASTIC; BIOLOGICAL RESPONSE MODIFIER; MONOCLONAL ANTIBODY

Therapeutic: ANTINEOPLASTIC

Pregnancy Category: C

AVAILABILITY 25 mg/mL injection

ACTION & *THERAPEUTIC EFFECT* Binds to vascular endothelial growth factor (VEGF) and prevents the interaction of VEGF to its receptors on the surface of endothelial cells. This blocks endothelial cell proliferation and new blood vessel formation in tumor cells. *Believed to cause reduction of microvascularization in the tumor inhibiting the progression of metastatic disease.*

USES Metastatic colorectal cancer, non–small-cell lung cancer, HER2 negative breast cancer, malignant glioblastoma.

UNLABELED USES Metastatic renal cell cancer, age-related macular degeneration.

CONTRAINDICATIONS Nephrotic syndrome; active bleeding, GI perforation; nephritic syndrome; leucopenia; surgery within 28 days; dental work within 20 days; neonates; lactation. Safety and effectiveness in children and infants are not established.

CAUTIOUS USE Hypersensitivity to bevacizumab; renal disease; hypertension, history of arterial thromboembolic, cardiovascular, or cerebrovascular disease; CHF; history of GI bleeding; pregnancy (category C).

ROUTE & DOSAGE

Metastatic Colorectal Cancer

Adult: **IV** 5–10 mg/kg q14days until disease progression; in conjunction with other chemotherapy

Non–Small-Cell Lung Cancer

Adult: **IV** 15 mg/kg q3wk

Metastatic HER2 Negative Breast Cancer

Adult: **IV** 10 mg/kg q14days

Glioblastoma

Adult: **IV** 10 mg/kg q14days in 28-day cycle

ADMINISTRATION

Intravenous

PREPARE: **IV Infusion:** Withdraw the desired dose of 5 mg/kg and dilute in 100 mL of NS injection. ▪ Do not shake and do NOT mix or administer with dextrose solutions. Discard any unused portion.

ADMINISTER: **IV Infusion:** DO NOT administer IV push or bolus. ▪ Infuse first dose over 90 min; if well tolerated, infuse second dose over 60 min; if well tolerated, infuse all subsequent doses over 30 min.

INCOMPATIBILITIES **Solution/additive:** **Dextrose**-containing solutions. **Y-site:** **Dextrose**-containing solutions.

▪ Store diluted solution at 2°–8° C (36°–46° F) for up to 8 h. Store vials at 2°–8° C (36°–46° F) and protect from light.

ADVERSE EFFECTS (≥1%) **Body as a Whole:** *Asthenia,* pain, wound dehiscence, tracheoesophageal (TE) fistula formation. **CNS:** Syncope, headache, dizziness, confusion, abnormal gait, <u>leukoencephalopathy</u>. **CV:** DVT, *hypertension,* heart failure, intra-abdominal thrombosis, <u>cerebrovascular events.</u> **GI:** Abdominal pain, *diarrhea,* constipation, nausea, vomiting, anorexia, stomatitis, dyspepsia, weight loss, flatulence, dry mouth, colitis, <u>gastrointestinal perforation</u>. **Hematologic:** *Leukopenia, neutropenia,* thrombocytopenia, hemorrhage, *thromboembolism*. **Metabolic:** Hypokalemia, hyperbilirubinemia. **Musculoskeletal:** Myalgia. **Respiratory:** Upper respiratory infection, epistaxis, dyspnea, <u>hemoptysis</u>. **Skin:** Exfoliative dermatitis, alopecia. **Special Senses:** Taste disorder, increased tearing. **Urogenital:** *Proteinuria,* urinary frequency/urgency.

PHARMACOKINETICS Half-Life: 20 days (11–50 days).

NURSING IMPLICATIONS

Assessment & Drug Effects

▪ Monitor for S&S of an infusion reaction (hypersensitivity); infusion should be interrupted in all pa-

B

tients with severe infusion reactions and appropriate therapy instituted.

- Monitor BP at least every 2–3 wk; if hypertension develops, monitor more frequently, even after discontinuation of bevacizumab.
- Withhold drug and promptly notify physician for S&S of CHF, hemorrhage (e.g., epistaxis, hemoptysis, or GI bleeding), or unexplained abdominal pain.
- Lab tests: Urinalysis for proteinuria and 24 h urine if protein 2+ or greater.
- Monitor for dizziness, lightheadedness, or loss of balance. Take appropriate safety measures.

Patient & Family Education

- Report any of the following to the physician: Bloody or black, tarry stool; changes in patterns of urination; swelling of legs or ankles; increased shortness of breath; severe abdominal pain; change in mental awareness, inability to talk or move one side of the body.

BEXAROTENE

(bex-a-ro'teen)

Targretin

Classifications: ANTINEOPLASTIC
Therapeutic: ANTINEOPLASTIC
Prototype: Isotretinoin
Pregnancy Category: X

AVAILABILITY 75 mg capsules; 1% gel

ACTION & *THERAPEUTIC EFFECT* Selectively binds to retinoid X receptors (RXR). Activation of the RXR pathway leads to cell death by interfering with cellular differentiation and proliferation of cells. *Inhibits the growth of tumor cells of squamous (skin) cell origin inducing tumor regression.*

USES Treatment of cutaneous manifestations of cutaneous T-cell lymphoma.

CONTRAINDICATIONS Hypersensitivity to bexarotene; pregnancy (category X), lactation. Safety and efficacy in children are not established.

CAUTIOUS USE Hypersensitivity to retinoid agents; coronary artery disease; diabetes mellitus; alcoholism, history of pancreatitis, hepatitis; elevated triglycerides, hepatic impairment.

ROUTE & DOSAGE

T-Cell Lymphoma
Adult: **PO** 300 mg/m²/day as a single dose with a meal, if no response after 8 wk, may increase to 400 mg/m²/day. Adjust dose downward in 100 mg/m²/day increments if toxicity occurs. **Topical** Apply once every other day × 1 week, increase frequency at weekly intervals to once/day, b.i.d., t.i.d., and q.i.d.

ADMINISTRATION

Oral
- Give drug with or immediately following a meal.
- Do not initiate therapy in a woman of childbearing age until the possibility of pregnancy has been completely ruled out.

Topical
- Apply a generous coating only to skin lesions; avoid normal skin.
- Do not cover with clothing until gel dries.

- Store capsules and gel at 20°–25° C (36°–77° F). Protect from light and avoid high temperatures and humidity after bottle or tube is opened.

ADVERSE EFFECTS (≥1%) **Body as a Whole:** *Headache, asthenia, infection,* chills, fever, flu-like syndrome, back pain, bacterial infection. **CNS:** Insomnia. **CV:** *Peripheral edema.* **GI:** *Abdominal pain, nausea,* diarrhea, vomiting, anorexia. **Endocrine:** *Hyperthyroidism.* **Hematologic:** *Leukopenia,* anemia, hypochromic anemia. **Metabolic:** *Hyperlipidemia, hypercholesterolemia,* increased LDH. **Skin:** *Rash, dry skin,* exfoliative dermatitis, alopecia, photosensitivity.

INTERACTIONS No clinically significant interactions established.

PHARMACOKINETICS Absorption: Best with a fat-containing meal. **Peak:** 2 h. **Distribution:** Greater than 99% protein bound. **Metabolism:** Metabolized by CYP3A4. **Elimination:** Primarily in bile. **Half-Life:** 7 h.

NURSING IMPLICATIONS

Assessment & Drug Effects

- Monitor (with oral dose) for S&S of: Hypothyroidism, hypertriglyceridemia, hypercholesterolemia, and pancreatitis.
- Lab tests (with oral dose): Baseline blood lipids, then weekly for 2–4 wk, and every 8 wk thereafter; baseline liver function tests, then repeat at 1, 2, 4 wk, and every 8 wk thereafter; baseline WBC and thyroid function tests, then repeat periodically thereafter; periodic serum calcium; for females, pregnancy test monthly throughout therapy.
- Withhold oral drug and notify physician if triglycerides greater than 400 mg/dL or AST, ALT, or bilirubin greater than 3 times upper limit of normal.

Patient & Family Education

- Use effective methods of contraception (both men and women) while taking/using this drug and for at least 1 mo after the last dose of the drug.
- Do not take this drug if you are or could be pregnant.
- Report immediately any of the following: Swelling in the face, lips, or wheezing; persistent bloating, constipation, diarrhea, vomiting, or stomach pain; persistent headache, severe drowsiness or weakness.
- Report changes in vision to the physician. An ophthalmologic evaluation may be needed.
- Limit exposure to sunlight or sun lamps and wear sunscreen.
- Report significant skin irritation.

BICALUTAMIDE

(bi-ca-lu'ta-mide)

Casodex

Classification: ANTINEOPLASTIC HORMONE

Therapeutic: ANTINEOPLASTIC; NONSTEROIDAL ANTIANDROGEN

Prototype: Flutamide

Pregnancy Category: X

AVAILABILITY 50 mg tablets

ACTION & *THERAPEUTIC EFFECT* Bicalutamide is a nonsteroidal antiandrogen. It inhibits the pharmacologic effects of androgen by binding to the androgen receptors in the target tissue. *Prostatic carcinoma is androgen sensitive; it re-*

B

sponds to removal of the source of androgen or treatment that counteracts the effects of androgen.

USES In combination with a luteinizing hormone-releasing hormone (LHRH) analog for advanced prostate cancer.

CONTRAINDICATIONS Hypersensitivity to bicalutamide, pregnancy (category X), hepatic failure; lactation.

CAUTIOUS USE Moderate to severe hepatic impairment; glucose intolerance; diabetes mellitus. Safety and efficacy in children are not established.

ROUTE & DOSAGE

Advanced Prostate Cancer

Adult: **PO** 50 mg once/day

ADMINISTRATION

Oral

- Give drug at the same time each day.
- Start treatment with bicalutamide at the same time as treatment with a luteinizing hormone-releasing hormone (LHRH) analog.
- Store at 15°–30° C (59°–86° F).

ADVERSE EFFECTS (≥1%) **CNS:** Dizziness, paresthesia, insomnia, anxiety, decreased libido, confusion, neuropathy, somnolence, nervousness, headache. **CV:** *Hot flashes,* hypertension, chest pain, CHF. **GI:** *Constipation, nausea, diarrhea,* vomiting, increased liver function tests, abdominal pain, anorexia, dyspepsia, dry mouth, melena. **Urogenital:** Nocturia, hematuria, UTI, impotence, gynecomastia, incontinence, frequency, dysuria, urinary retention, urgency. **Metabolic:** Peripheral edema, hyperglycemia, weight loss, weight gain, gout. **Musculoskeletal:** Myasthenia, arthritis, myalgia, leg cramps, pathologic fractures. **Skin:** Rash, sweating, dry skin, pruritus, alopecia. **Body as a Whole:** Flu syndrome, bone pain, infection, anemia.

INTERACTIONS Drug: May increase effects of ORAL ANTICOAGULANTS. Bicalutamide concentrations may be increased by PROTEASE INHIBITORS, **fluoxetine, fluvoxamine, erythromycin** and other CYP3A4 inhibitors. Efficacy of bicalutamide may be decreased by **bosentan, carbamazapine,** BARBITUATES and other CYP3A4 inducers.

PHARMACOKINETICS Absorption: Readily from GI tract. **Metabolism:** In liver. **Elimination:** In urine and feces. **Half-Life:** 5.8 days.

NURSING IMPLICATIONS

Assessment & Drug Effects

- Monitor for S&S of disease progression.
- Lab tests: Periodic PSA levels, CBC, liver functions, renal functions; with concurrent Coumadin therapy, closely monitor PT and INR.

Patient & Family Education

- Report jaundice or any other troubling adverse effects immediately.

BIMATOPROST

(bi-mat′o-prost)

Lumigan

Pregnancy Category: C

See Appendix A-1.

Common adverse effects in *italic*, life-threatening effects underlined; generic names in **bold**; classifications in SMALL CAPS; ♣ Canadian drug name; ℞ Prototype drug

B

BIPERIDEN HYDROCHLORIDE

(bye-per′i-den)
Akineton

BIPERIDEN LACTATE

Akineton
Classifications: ANTICHOLINERGIC; ANTIPARKINSON
Therapeutic: ANTIPARKINSON
Prototype: Levodopa
Pregnancy Category: C

AVAILABILITY 2 mg tablets

ACTION & *THERAPEUTIC EFFECT* Synthetic tertiary amine, antimuscarinic. In common with other antiparkinsonism drugs has atropine-like (anticholinergic) action. Antiparkinsonism activity is thought to be caused by reducing central excitatory action of acetylcholine on cholinergic receptors in the extrapyramidal system. *This action helps to establish some balance between cholinergic (excitatory) and dopaminergic (inhibitory) activity in the basal ganglia with the result of controlling the effect of extrapyramidal symptoms.*

USES Adjunct in all forms of parkinsonism, particularly postencephalitic and idiopathic parkinsonism (appears to be less effective in arteriosclerotic type). Also used to control drug-induced parkinsonism (extrapyramidal symptoms) associated with reserpine and phenothiazine therapy.

CONTRAINDICATIONS Narrow-angle glaucoma; GI or GU obstruction, megacolon; tardive dyskinesia; lactation.
CAUTIOUS USE Older adults or debilitated patients; prostatic hypertrophy; glaucoma; cardiac arrhythmias; epilepsy; pregnancy (category C).

ROUTE & DOSAGE

Parkinsonism
Adult: **PO** 2 mg 1–4 times/day
Geriatric: **PO** 2 mg 1–2 times/day

ADMINISTRATION

Oral
- Give with or after meals to relieve GI disturbances.
- Store in tightly closed, light-resistant containers at 15°–30° C (59°–86° F) unless otherwise directed.

ADVERSE EFFECTS (≥1%) **CNS:** Drowsiness, dizziness, muscle weakness, lack of coordination, disorientation, euphoria, agitation, confusion. **CV:** Mild, transient postural hypotension, tachycardia. **Special Senses:** *Blurred vision,* photophobia. **GI:** *Dry mouth,* nausea, vomiting, constipation.

INTERACTIONS Drug: Alcohol and other CNS DEPRESSANTS INCREASE SEDATION; **haloperidol,** PHENOTHIAZINES, OPIATES, TRICYCLIC ANTIDEPRESSANTS, **quinidine** increase risk of anticholinergic side effects.

NURSING IMPLICATIONS

Assessment & Drug Effects
- Advise patient to make position changes slowly and in stages, particularly from recumbent to upright position.
- Monitor for and report immediately: Mental confusion, drowsiness, dizziness, agitation, hematuria, and decrease in urinary flow.
- Assess for and report blurred vision.
- Monitor I&O ratio and pattern.

B

- Note: Biperiden usually reduces muscle rigidity. In patients with severe parkinsonism, tremors may increase as spasticity is relieved.

Patient & Family Education

- Do not drive or engage in potentially hazardous activities until response to drug is known.
- Note: Patients on prolonged therapy can develop tolerance; an increase in dosage may be required.

BISACODYL

(bis-a-koe'dill)

Apo-Bisacodyl ✤, Bisacolax, Bisco-Lax ✤, Dacodyl, Deficol, Doxidan, Dulcolax, Fleet Bisacodyl, Laxit ✤, Theralax

Classification: STIMULANT LAXATIVE

Therapeutic: LAXATIVE

Pregnancy Category: C

AVAILABILITY 5 mg tablets, enteric coated; 5 mg tablets, delayed release; 10 mg suppository; 10 mg/30 mL enema

ACTION & *THERAPEUTIC EFFECT* Expands intestinal fluid volume by increasing epithelial permeability. *Induces peristaltic contractions by direct stimulation of sensory nerve endings in the colonic wall.*

USES Temporary relief of acute constipation and for evacuation of colon before surgery, proctoscopic, sigmoidoscopic, and radiologic examinations. Also used to cleanse colon before delivery and to relieve constipation in patients with spinal cord damage.

CONTRAINDICATIONS Acute surgical abdomen, nausea, vomiting, abdominal cramps, intestinal obstruction, fecal impaction; use of rectal suppository in presence of anal or rectal fissures, ulcerated hemorrhoids, proctitis, bowel obstruction or perforation, ileus; children younger than 1 y.

CAUTIOUS USE Pregnancy (category C), lactation.

ROUTE & DOSAGE

Laxative

Adult: **PO** 5–15 mg prn (max: 30 mg for special procedures) **PR** 10 mg prn
Child: **PO** *6 y or older,* 5–10 mg prn **PR** *2 y or older,* 10 mg; *younger than 2 y,* 5 mg

ADMINISTRATION

Oral

- Give in the evening or before breakfast because of action time required.
- Give enteric-coated tablets whole to avoid gastric irritation; do not cut or crush. Patient should not chew tablets. Preferably give with a full glass (240 mL) of water or other liquid.
- Do not give within 1 h of antacids or milk. These substances may cause premature dissolution of enteric coating; early release of drug in stomach may result in gastric irritation and loss of cathartic action.
- Store tablets in tightly closed containers at temperatures not exceeding 30° C (86° F).

Rectal

- Suppository may be inserted at time bowel movement is desired.
- Storage is same as tablets.

ADVERSE EFFECTS (≥1%) Systemic effects not reported. Mild cramping, nausea, diarrhea, fluid and electrolyte disturbances (especially potassium and calcium).

INTERACTIONS Drug: ANTACIDS will cause early dissolution of enteric-coated tablets, resulting in abdominal cramping.

PHARMACOKINETICS Absorption: 5–15% from GI tract. **Onset:** 6–8 h PO; 15–60 min PR. **Metabolism:** In liver. **Elimination:** In urine, bile, and breast milk.

NURSING IMPLICATIONS

Assessment & Drug Effects

- Evaluate periodically patient's need for continued use of drug; bisacodyl usually produces 1 or 2 soft formed stools daily.
- Monitor patients receiving concomitant anticoagulants. Indiscriminate use of laxatives results in decreased absorption of vitamin K.

Patient & Family Education

- Add high-fiber foods slowly to regular diet to avoid gas and diarrhea. Adequate fluid intake includes at least 6–8 glasses/day.

BISMUTH SUBSALICYLATE (Pr)

(bis′muth)

Pepto-Bismol

Classifications: ANTIDIARRHEAL; SALICYLATE

Therapeutic: ANTIDIARRHEAL

Pregnancy Category: C

AVAILABILITY 262 mg tablets/caplets; 130 mg/15 mL, 262 mg/15 mL, 524 mg/15 mL liquid

ACTION & *THERAPEUTIC EFFECT* Hydrolyzed in GI tract to salicylate, which is believed to inhibit synthesis of prostaglandins responsible for GI hypermotility and inflammation. It is also a direct mucosal protective agent. *Effectiveness as an antidiarrheal also appears to be due to direct antimicrobial action and to an antisecretory effect on intestinal secretions exposed to toxins.*

USES Prophylaxis and treatment of traveler's diarrhea (turista) and for temporary relief of indigestion.

UNLABELED USES *Helicobacter pylori* associated with peptic ulcer disease.

CONTRAINDICATIONS Hypersensitivity to aspirin or other salicylates; concurrent use with aspirin; coagulopathy, severe hepatic impairment; use for more than 2 days in presence of high fever or in children younger than 3 y unless prescribed by physician; chickenpox or flu; dysentery.

CAUTIOUS USE Diabetes and gout; concurrent use with salicylates and anticoagulants; alcoholism; renal impairment; elderly; smoking; pregnancy (category C), lactation.

ROUTE & DOSAGE

Diarrhea

Adult: **PO** 30 mL or 2 tab q30–60min prn (max: 8 doses/day)

Child: **PO** *3–6 y,* 5 mL or 1/2 tab q30–60min prn (max: 8 doses/day); *6–9 y,* 2/3 tab or 10 mL q30–60min prn (max: 8 doses/day); *9–12 y,* 15 mL or 1 tab q30–60min prn (max: 8 doses/day)

Traveler's Diarrhea

Adult: **PO** 2–4 tab or 15–30 mL q.i.d. for 3 wk

Peptic Ulcer Disease

Adult: **PO** 2 tablets q.i.d. with 2 additional antibiotics for 10–14 days

Child (younger than 10 y): **PO** 15 mL q.i.d. × 6 wk

B

ADMINISTRATION

Oral

- Ensure chewable tablets are chewed or crushed before being swallowed and followed with at least 8 oz water or other liquid.
- Store at 15°–30° C (59°–86° F) unless otherwise directed.

ADVERSE EFFECTS (≥1%) **GI:** Temporary *darkening of stool* and tongue, metallic taste, bluish gum line; bleeding tendencies. With high doses: Fecal impaction. **CNS:** Encephalopathy (disorientation, muscle twitching). **Hematologic:** Bleeding tendency. **Special Senses:** Tinnitus, hearing loss.

DIAGNOSTIC TEST INTERFERENCE Because bismuth subsalicylate is radiopaque, it may interfere with ***radiographic studies*** of GI tract.

INTERACTIONS Drug: Bismuth may decrease the absorption of TETRACYCLINES, QUINOLONES (**ciprofloxacin, norfloxacin, ofloxacin**). May increase level of **aspirin.**

PHARMACOKINETICS Absorption: Undergoes chemical dissociation in GI tract to bismuth subcarbonate and sodium salicylate; bismuth is minimally absorbed, but the salicylate is readily absorbed.

NURSING IMPLICATIONS

Assessment & Drug Effects

- Monitor bowel function; note that stools may darken and tongue may appear black. These are temporary effects and will disappear without treatment.
- Lab tests: *H. pylori* breath test when used for peptic ulcers.

Patient & Family Education

- Note: Bismuth contains salicylate. Use caution when taking aspirin and other salicylates. Many OTC medications for colds, fever, and pain contain salicylates.
- Consult physician if diarrhea is accompanied by fever or continues for more than 2 days.
- Note: Temporary grayish black discoloration of tongue and stool may occur.

BISOPROLOL FUMARATE

(bis-o-pro′lol fum′a-rate)

Zebeta

Classifications: BETA-ADRENERGIC ANTAGONIST; ANTIHYPERTENSIVE

Therapeutic: ANTIHYPERTENSIVE

Prototype: Propranolol

Pregnancy Category: C

AVAILABILITY 5 mg, 10 mg tablets

ACTION & *THERAPEUTIC EFFECT* Long-acting cardioselective ($beta_1$) adrenoreceptor blocking agent. To maintain $beta_1$ cardioselectivity, the lowest effective dose is necessary. Bisoprolol decreases heart rate, blood pressure, contractile force, and cardiac workload, which reduces myocardial oxygen consumption and increases blood flow to myocardium. *Bisoprolol has antianginal properties, especially improving exercise tolerance. It reduces both systolic and diastolic blood pressure at rest and with exercise.*

USES Hypertension.

UNLABELED USES Angina.

CONTRAINDICATIONS History of hypersensitivity to bisoprolol, severe sinus bradycardia, second- and third-degree AV block, overt cardiac failure, cardiogenic shock; pulmonary edema.

CAUTIOUS USE Asthma or COPD, peripheral vascular disease, diabetes mellitus, Prinzmetal's angina;

hyperthyroidism, renal or hepatic insufficiency, cerebrovascular disease, stroke; pregnancy (category C), lactation.

ROUTE & DOSAGE

Hypertension, Angina

Adult: **PO** 2.5–5 mg once daily, may increase to 20 mg/day if necessary

ADMINISTRATION

Oral

- Note: The half-life of the drug is increased in those with significant liver dysfunction; usual initial dose is 2.5 mg and may be carefully titrated upward if necessary.
- Discontinue drug gradually over a period of 1–2 wk to avoid rebound, withdrawal angina, or hypertension.
- Store at room temperature, 15°–30° C (59°–86° F).

ADVERSE EFFECTS (≥1%) **CNS:** Dizziness, fatigue, tiredness, vertigo, anxiety, headache, sleep disturbances. **CV:** Bradycardia, orthostatic hypotension, rebound/withdrawal angina or hypertension following abrupt discontinuation, may exacerbate intermittent claudication. **Endocrine:** Increases serum levels of VLDL-C and decreases levels of HDL-C lipoproteins, may cause slight rise in serum potassium. **GI:** Abdominal pain, dyspepsia, nausea, vomiting, constipation, diarrhea. **Respiratory:** Asthma, bronchospasm, cough, dyspnea, pharyngitis, sinusitis. **Skin:** Rash, acne, pruritus, eczema. **Other:** Arthralgia.

INTERACTIONS Drug: Amiodarone may cause significant bradycardia; BETA-BLOCKERS may reduce **glucose** tolerance, inhibit **insulin** secretion, alter rate of recovery from hypoglycemia, reduce peripheral circulation, and suppress hypoglycemic symptoms; **rifampin** decreases bisoprolol blood levels.

PHARMACOKINETICS Absorption: Readily from GI tract; 82–94% reaches systemic circulation. **Peak:** Therapeutic effect 2–4 wk. **Duration:** 24 h. **Distribution:** Some CNS penetration. **Metabolism:** 50% in liver by CYP3A4. **Elimination:** 50–60% unchanged in urine. **Half-Life:** 10–12.4 h.

NURSING IMPLICATIONS

Assessment & Drug Effects

- Monitor BP frequently during periods of dose adjustment or drug withdrawal.
- Monitor for activity-induced angina both during therapy and following discontinuation of drug.
- Monitor for and report severe hypotension and bradycardia. Dosage adjustment may be required.
- Monitor for bronchospasms in patients with a history of asthma or COPD.
- Monitor diabetics for loss of glycemic control.
- Lab tests: Periodic CBC, electrolytes, renal function, liver function, lipid profile.

Patient & Family Education

- Report orthostatic hypotension and dizziness to physician.
- Do not discontinue drug abruptly unless specifically instructed to do so.
- Note: Drug-induced nightmares and unpleasant dreams are possible when taking this drug.
- Monitor blood glucose for loss of glycemic control.

B

BIVALIRUDIN

(bi-val'i-ru-den)

Angiomax

Classifications: ANTICOAGULANT; DIRECT THROMBIN INHIBITOR

Therapeutic: ANTITHROMBOTIC

Prototype: Lepirudin

Pregnancy Category: B

AVAILABILITY 250 mg vial

ACTION & *THERAPEUTIC EFFECT*

Direct inhibitor of thrombin similar to lepirudin. Capable of inhibiting the action of both free and clot-bound thrombin. *Reversibly binds to the thrombin active site, thereby blocking the thrombogenic activity of thrombin.*

USES Used with aspirin as an anticoagulant in patients undergoing PTCA or PCR, patients at risk for HIT undergoing PCI.

UNLABELED USES DVT prevention.

CONTRAINDICATIONS Hypersensitivity to bivalirudin; cerebral aneurysm, intracranial hemorrhage; patients with increased risk of bleeding (e.g., recent surgery, trauma, CVA, hepatic disease); coagulopathy; lactation. Safety and efficacy in children are not established.

CAUTIOUS USE Asthma or allergies; blood dyscrasia or thrombocytopenia; GI ulceration, serious hepatic disease; hypertension, renal impairment, pregnancy (category B).

ROUTE & DOSAGE

Anticoagulation

Adult: **IV** 0.75 mg/kg bolus (5 min after the bolus, ACT should be performed and 0.3 mg/kg given if needed) followed by 1.75 mg/kg/h for the duration of the procedure, may continue at 0.2 mg/kg/h up to 20 h if needed; intended for use with aspirin 300–325 mg

Renal Impairment Dosage Adjustment

If CrCl less than 30 mL/min, give maintenance dose of 1 mg/kg/h

Hemodialysis Dosage Adjustment: Give 0.25 mg/kg/h maintenance dose

ADMINISTRATION

Intravenous

PREPARE: **Direct/Continuous:** Direct IV bolus dose and initial 4-h continuous infusion: Reconstitute each 250 mg vial with 5 mL of sterile water for injection; gently swirl until dissolved. ▪ Must further dilute each reconstituted vial in 50 mL of D5W or NS to yield 5 mg/mL. **Continuous:** Subsequent low-dose, continuous infusions: Reconstitute each 250 mg vial as above. ▪ Further dilute each reconstituted vial in 500 mL of D5W or NS to yield 0.50 mg/mL.

ADMINISTER: **Direct:** Give bolus dose over 3–5 sec. **Continuous:** Give 1.75 mg/kg/h for the duration of the PTCA procedure. ▪ Subsequent doses, give 0.2 mg/kg/h for up to 20 h as ordered.

INCOMPATIBILITIES **Y-site: Alteplase, amiodarone, amphotericin B, chlorpromazine, diazepam, prochlorperazine, reteplase, streptokinase, vancomycin.**

▪ Store reconstituted vials refrigerated at 2°–8° C (35.6°–46.4° F) for up to 24 h. Store diluted concentrations between 0.5 mg/mL and 5 mg/mL at room temperature, 15°–30° C (59°–86° F), for up to 24 h.

ADVERSE EFFECTS (≥1%) **Body as a Whole:** *Back pain,* pain, fever. **CV:** *Hypotension,* hypertension, bradycardia. **GI:** *Nausea,* vomiting, dyspepsia, abdominal pain. **Hematologic:** Bleeding. **CNS:** *Headache,* anxiety, nervousness. **Urogenital:** Urinary retention, pelvic pain. **Other:** Injection site pain.

INTERACTIONS No clinically significant interactions established.

PHARMACOKINETICS Duration: 1 h. **Distribution:** No protein binding. **Metabolism:** Proteolytic cleavage and renal metabolism. **Elimination:** Renal. **Half-Life:** 25 min.

NURSING IMPLICATIONS

Assessment & Drug Effects

- Monitor cardiovascular status carefully during therapy.
- Monitor for and report S&S of bleeding: Ecchymosis, epistaxis, GI bleeding, hematuria, hemoptysis.
- Patients with history of GI ulceration, hypertension, recent trauma or surgery are at increased risk for bleeding.
- Monitor neurologic status and report immediately: Focal or generalized deficits.
- Lab tests: Baseline and periodic ACT (activated clotting time), APTT, PT, INR, thrombin time (TT), plasma fibrinopeptide A (especially in unstable angina), platelet count, Hgb and Hct; periodic serum creatinine, stool for occult blood, urinalysis.

Patient & Family Education

- Report any of the following immediately: Unexplained back or stomach pain; black, tarry stools; blood in urine, coughing up blood; difficulty breathing; dizziness or fainting spells; heavy menstrual bleeding; nosebleeds; unusual bruising or bleeding at any site.

BLEOMYCIN SULFATE

(blee-oh-mye'sin)

Blenoxane

Classifications: ANTINEOPLASTIC; ANTIBIOTIC

Therapeutic: ANTINEOPLASTIC

Prototype: Doxorubicin

Pregnancy Category: D

AVAILABILITY 15 units, 30 units powder for injection

ACTION & *THERAPEUTIC EFFECT* A toxic drug with low therapeutic index; intensely cytotoxic. By unclear mechanism, blocks DNA, RNA, and protein synthesis. A cell cycle-phase nonspecific agent. Widely used in combination with other chemotherapeutic agents because it lacks significant myelosuppressive activity. *This mixture of cytotoxic antibiotics from a strain of* Streptomyces verticillus *has strong affinity for skin and lung tumor cells, in contrast to its low affinity for cells in hematopoietic tissue.*

USES As single agent or in combination with other chemotherapeutic agents, as adjunct to surgery and radiation therapy. Squamous cell carcinomas of head, neck, penis, cervix, and vulva; lymphomas (including reticular cell sarcoma, lymphosarcoma, Hodgkin's); testicular carcinoma; malignant pleural effusions.

UNLABELED USES *Mycosis fungoides* and *Verruca vulgaris* (common warts), AIDS-related Kaposi's sarcoma.

B

CONTRAINDICATIONS History of hypersensitivity or idiosyncrasy to bleomycin; pulmonary infection; concurrent radiation therapy; women of childbearing age, pregnancy (category D), lactation.
CAUTIOUS USE Compromised hepatic, renal, or pulmonary function; peripheral vascular disease; history of tobacco use; previous cytotoxic drug or radiation therapy.

ROUTE & DOSAGE

Squamous Cell Carcinoma, Testicular Carcinoma

Adult/Child: **Subcutaneous/IM/IV** 10–20 units/m² or 0.25–0.5 units/kg 1–2 times/wk (max: 300–400 units)

Lymphomas

Adult/Child: **Subcutaneous/IM/IV** 10–20 units/m² 1–2 times/wk after a 1–2 units test dose times 2 doses

Hodgkin's Disease, Maintenance

Adult/Child: **Subcutaneous/IM/IV** 1 unit IM or IV/day or 5 units/wk

Renal Impairment Dosage Adjustment

CrCl 10–50 mL/min: Use 75% of dose; less than 10 mL/min: Use 50% of dose

ADMINISTRATION

Note: Due to risk of anaphylactoid reaction, give lymphoma patients 2 units or less for first two doses. If no reaction, follow regular dosage schedule.

Subcutaneous/Intramuscular

- Reconstitute with sterile water, NS, or bacteriostatic water by adding 1–5 mL to the 15 units vial or 2–10 mL to the 30 units vial. Amount of diluent is determined by the total volume of solution that will be injected.
- Inject IM deeply into upper outer quadrant of buttock; change sites with each injection.

Intravenous

IV administration to infants and children: Verify correct IV concentration and rate of infusion with physician.

PREPARE: **Intermittent:** Dilute each 15 units with at least 5 mL of sterile water or NS. ▪ May be further diluted in 50–100 mL of the chosen diluent. ▪ Do not dilute with any solution containing D5W.

ADMINISTER: **Intermittent:** Give each 15 units or fraction thereof over 10 min through Y-tube of free-flowing IV.

INCOMPATIBILITIES **Solution/additive:** **Aminophylline, ascorbic acid, carbenicillin, cephalosporins, diazepam, hydrocortisone, methotrexate, mitomycin, nafcillin, penicillin G, terbutaline.**

- Store unopened ampules at 15°–30° C (59°–86° F) unless otherwise specified by manufacturer.

ADVERSE EFFECTS (≥1%) **Body as a Whole:** Hypersensitivity (anaphylactoid reaction); *mild febrile reaction.* **CNS:** Headache, mental confusion. **GI:** Stomatitis, ulcerations of tongue and lips, anorexia, nausea, vomiting, diarrhea, weight loss. **Hematologic:** Thrombocytopenia, leukopenia, (rare). **Respiratory:** Pulmonary toxicity (dose and age-related); interstitial pneumonitis, pneumonia, or fibrosis. **Skin:** Diffuse alopecia (reversible), *hyperpig-*

mentation, pruritic erythema, vesiculation, acne, thickening of skin and nail beds, *patchy hyperkeratosis,* striae, peeling, bleeding. **Other:** Pain at tumor site; phlebitis; necrosis at injection site, shivering.

INTERACTIONS Drug: Other ANTINEOPLASTIC AGENTS increase bone marrow toxicity; decreases effects of **digoxin, phenytoin,** avoid use with LIVE VACCINES.

PHARMACOKINETICS Distribution: Concentrates mainly in skin, lungs, kidneys, lymphocytes, and peritoneum. **Metabolism:** Unknown. **Elimination:** 60–70% recovered in urine as parent compound. **Half-Life:** 2 h.

NURSING IMPLICATIONS

Assessment & Drug Effects

- Monitor closely for an acute reaction (hypotension, hyperpyrexia, chills, confusion, wheezing, cardiopulmonary collapse). Anaphylactoid reaction can be fatal (see Appendix F). It may occur immediately or several hours after first or second dose, especially in lymphoma patients.
- Monitor temperature. Febrile reaction (mild chills and fever) is relatively common in patients receiving bleomycin therapy. It usually occurs within the first few hours after administration of a large single dose and lasts about 4–12 h. Reaction tends to become less frequent with continued drug administration, but can recur at any time.
- Monitor for and report any of the following: Unexplained bleeding or bruising; evidence of deterioration of renal function (changed I&O ratio and pattern, decreasing creatinine clearance, weight gain or edema); evidence of pulmonary toxicity (nonproductive cough, chest pain, dyspnea).
- Check weight at regular intervals under standard conditions. Weight loss and anorexia may persist a long time after therapy has been discontinued.
- Report symptoms of skin toxicity (hypoesthesia, urticaria, tender swollen hands) promptly. May develop in second or third week of treatment and after 150–200 units of bleomycin have been administered. Therapy may be discontinued.

Patient & Family Education

- Avoid OTC drugs during antineoplastic treatment period unless approved by physician.
- Report skin irritation which may not develop for several weeks after therapy begins.
- Hyperpigmentation may occur in areas subject to friction and pressure, skin folds, nail cuticles, scars, and intramuscular sites.

BORTEZOMIB

(bor-te-zo′mib)

Velcade

Classifications: ANTINEOPLASTIC; BIOLOGICAL RESPONSE MODIFIER; PROTEOSOME INHIBITOR

Therapeutic: ANTINEOPLASTIC; SIGNAL TRANSDUCTION INHIBITOR (STI)

Pregnancy Category: D

AVAILABILITY 3.5 mg powder for injection

ACTION & *THERAPEUTIC EFFECT* Bortezomib is an inhibitor of proteasome, which is responsible for regulation of protein expression and degradation of damaged or obsolete

B

proteins within the cell; its activity is critical to activation or suppression of cellular functions including the cell cycle, oncogene expression, and apoptosis. *Proteasome inhibition may reverse some of the changes that allow proliferation of malignant cells and suppress apoptosis (programmed cell death) in malignant cells.*

USES Treatment of relapsed or refractory multiple myeloma or mantle cell lymphoma.
UNLABELED USES Myelomatous pleural effusion.

CONTRAINDICATIONS Hypersensitivity to bortezomib, boron, or mannitol; acute diffuse infiltrative pulmonary and pericardial disease; pregnancy (category D); lactation. Safety and effectiveness in children are not established.
CAUTIOUS USE Peripheral neuropathy; history of syncope, dehydration, hypotension; concurrent antihypertensive drugs; history of allergies, asthma; preexisting electrolyte or acid-base disturbances, especially hypokalemia or hyponatremia; diabetic mellitus; liver disease; myelosuppression, renal impairment; risk factors for cardiac disease; history of peripheral neuropathy or other neurologic disorders; risk factors for pulmonary disorders; GI toxicities.

ROUTE & DOSAGE

Multiple Myeloma/Mantle Cell Lymphoma (failed previous therapy)

Adult: **IV** 1.3 mg/m² days 1, 4, 8, and 11 followed by a 10-day rest period; at least 72 h should elapse between consecutive doses; 3 wk period is a treatment cycle

Previously Untreated Multiple Myeloma

Adult: **IV** 1.3 mg/m²/dose on days 1, 4, 8, and 11 followed by a 10-day rest period (days 12–21) then on days 22, 25, 29, and 32 followed by a 10-day rest period; 6 wk is one course

Toxicity Dosage Adjustment

Withhold dose with grade 3 or 4 hematologic toxicity, when symptoms resolve dose may be reduced 25% and restarted.
Hemodialysis Dosage Adjustment: Administer after hemodialysis

ADMINISTRATION

Intravenous

Wear protective gloves and prevent contact with skin.

PREPARE: **Direct:** Reconstitute 3.5 mg vial with 3.5 mL of NS for injection to yield 1 mg/mL. ▪ Discard if not clear and colorless. Give within 8 h of reconstitution.
ADMINISTER: **Direct:** Give as a bolus dose over 3–5 sec. Flush before/after with NS.
INCOMPATIBILITIES **Solution/additive:** Do not recommend mixing or injecting with any other drugs.

▪Store unopened vials at 15°–30° C (59°–86° F). Protect from light. ▪Store reconstituted vials at 15°–30° C (59°–86° F). ▪ Give within 8 h of reconstitution. May store up to 3 h in a syringe; however, total storage time must not exceed 8 h when exposed to normal indoor lighting.

ADVERSE EFFECTS (≥1%) **Body as a Whole:** *Asthenia, weakness, fa-*

tigue, malaise, fever, dehydration, peripheral neuropathy, rigors, herpes zoster. **CNS:** *Insomnia, headache, paresthesia, dizziness, anxiety.* **CV:** *Edema, hypotension, orthostatic hypotension.* **GI:** *Nausea, vomiting, diarrhea, anorexia, abdominal pain, constipation, dyspepsia, dysphagia.* **Hematologic:** *Thrombocytopenia, neutropenia, anemia.* **Musculoskeletal:** *Arthralgia, musculoskeletal pain, bone pain, myalgia, back pain, muscle cramps.* **Respiratory:** *Dyspnea, cough, upper respiratory infection.* **Skin:** *Rash, pruritus.* **Special Senses:** *Blurred vision, diplopia.*

INTERACTIONS **Drug:** Hypoglycemia and hyperglycemia have been reported with ANTIDIABETIC AGENTS; ANTIHYPERTENSIVE AGENTS may exacerbate hypotension; ANTICOAGULANTS, **antithymocyte globulin,** NSAIDS, PLATELET INHIBITORS, **aspirin,** THROMBOLYTIC AGENTS may increase risk of bleeding. **Food: Grapefruit juice** may increase drug levels.

PHARMACOKINETICS **Distribution:** 85% protein bound. **Metabolism:** In the liver (CYP3A4, CYP2C19, CYP1A2). **Half-Life:** 9–15 h.

NURSING IMPLICATIONS

Assessment & Drug Effects

- Monitor for and report S&S of neuropathy (e.g., hyperesthesia, hypoesthesia, paresthesia, discomfort or neuropathic pain).
- Monitor diabetics for loss of glycemic control.
- Monitor postural vital signs for orthostatic hypotension.
- Monitor for S&S of developing a pulmonary disorder.
- Monitor I&O and assess for S&S of dehydration or electrolyte imbalance if vomiting and/or diarrhea develop.
- Monitor for exacerbation of CHF, or acute onset of CHF.
- Lab tests: Frequent CBC with platelet count; baseline and periodic LFTs; frequent blood glucose in diabetics.

Patient & Family Education

- Report promptly any of the following: Dizziness, light-headedness or fainting spells; numbness, tingling, or other unusual sensations; signs of infection (e.g., fever, chills, cough, sore throat); bruising, pinpoint red spots on the skin; black, tarry stools, nosebleeds, or any other sign of bleeding.
- Monitor closely blood glucose level if diabetic.
- Report increased S&S of CHF, or acute onset of these S&S.
- Do not drive or engage in other hazardous activities until reaction to drug is known.
- Report any S&S of respiratory difficulty.
- Females should use reliable methods of contraception to avoid pregnancy while on this drug.

BOTULINUM TOXIN TYPE A

(bo′tul-i-num)

Botox, BOTOX Cosmetic

Classifications: SKELETAL MUSCLE RELAXANT; ANTISPASMODIC

Therapeutic: MUSCLE RELAXANT; ANTISPASMODIC

Pregnancy Category: C

AVAILABILITY 100 units powder for injection

B

ACTION & *THERAPEUTIC EFFECT*

Botulinum toxin type A blocks neuromuscular transmission by binding to receptor sites on motor nerve terminals, entering the nerve terminals, and inhibiting the release of acetylcholine. This inhibition occurs as the neurotoxin splits a protein molecule integral to the successful docking and releasing of acetylcholine from storage areas located within nerve endings. *When injected intramuscularly at therapeutic doses, botulinum toxin type A produces partial chemical denervation of the muscle resulting in a localized reduction in muscle activity.*

USES Treatment of blepharospasm, cervical dystonia, strabismus, glabellar frown wrinkles, severe axillary hyperhidrosis.

UNLABELED USES Treatment of other types of wrinkles, migraine headache, achalasia, focal spasticity associated with cerebral palsy with concurrent equinus gait, spasticity associated with stroke.

CONTRAINDICATIONS Presence of infection at the proposed injection site(s); hypersensitivity to Botox. Patients with dysphagia or respiratory compromise.

CAUTIOUS USE Hypersensitivity to albumin; individuals with peripheral motor neuropathic diseases (e.g., amyotrophic lateral sclerosis, or motor neuropathy), or neuromuscular junctional disorders (e.g., myasthenia gravis or Lambert-Eaton syndrome); neuromuscular disorders; ocular disease; cardiovascular disease; elderly; inflammation at the proposed injection site; weakness in the target muscle(s); pregnancy (category C), lactation.

ROUTE & DOSAGE

Blepharospasm

Adult/Child (older than 12 y): **Intradermal** 1.25–2.5 units injected at each site, may repeat in 3 mo if needed; cumulative dose should not exceed 200 units in a 30-day period

Cervical Dystonia

Adult/Adolescent (older than 16 y): **IM** 198–300 units divided among affected muscles

Frown Wrinkles

Adult: **IM** 25 units divided among affected muscles in 5 step doses, may repeat in 3–4 mo if needed

Other Wrinkles

Adult: **Subcutaneous** 1–2 units per site

Spasticity

Adult: **IM** 20–50 units per affected site
Child (2–18 y): **IM** 4 units/kg (max: 200 units per treatment) q3mo

Axillary Hyperhidrosis

Adult: **IM** 50 units per site, may repeat in 4 mo

ADMINISTRATION

Intramuscular, Intradermal, Subcutaneous

- Slowly inject required amount of nonpreserved NS (see dilution calculation) into vial. Discard vial if a vacuum does not pull diluent into vial. Gently rotate to mix. Discard if not clear, colorless, and free of particulate matter. Dilution calculation: Add 1, 2, 4, or 6 mL of NS to yield, respectively, 10 units/0.1 mL, 5 units/0.1 mL, 2.5 units/0.1 mL, 1.25 units/0.1 mL.

- Note: Injection intervals of BOTOX® Cosmetic should be at least 3 mo apart.
- Store at 2°–8° C (36°–46° F) (refrigerated). Administer within 4 h of reconstitution.

INCOMPATIBILITIES Do not mix with other solutions/additives.

ADVERSE EFFECTS (≥1%) **Body as a Whole:** Injection site reactions (localized pain, tenderness, bruising), neck pain, flu-like symptoms, hypertonia, asthenia, fever. **CNS:** *Headache,* drowsiness. **GI:** *Dysphagia,* dry mouth, fever, nausea, vomiting. **Hematologic:** Ecchymosis. **Musculoskeletal:** Local muscle weakness, dysarthria. **Respiratory:** Cough, rhinitis, upper respiratory infection. **Special Senses:** *Ptosis,* superficial punctate keratitis, dry eyes, ocular irritation, lacrimation, photophobia, keratitis, diplopia.

INTERACTIONS Drug: AMINOGLYCOSIDES, NEUROMUSCULAR BLOCKING AGENTS may potentiate neuromuscular blockade; **chloroquine** may antagonize blocking effects.

NURSING IMPLICATIONS

Assessment & Drug Effects

- Evaluate for therapeutic effectiveness, maximal at about 1–2 wk (lasting 3–4 mo).

Patient & Family Education

- Inform physician about all prescription, nonprescription, and herbal drugs being taken.
- Report immediately any of the following: Difficulty breathing or swallowing, problem with speech; unusual bleeding, bruising, or swelling around injection site.
- Note: Effects of the injection generally last 3–4 mo and then repeat treatments may be given.

BRETYLIUM TOSYLATE

(bre-til′ee-um)

Classification: ANTIARRHYTHMIC, CLASS III

Therapeutic: ANTIARRHYTHMIC, CLASS III

Prototype: Amiodarone

Pregnancy Category: C

AVAILABILITY 2 mg/mL, 4 mg/mL, 50 mg/mL injection

ACTION & *THERAPEUTIC EFFECT* Suppresses ventricular fibrillation by direct action on the myocardium and ventricular tachycardia by adrenergic blockade. Shortly after administration, norepinephrine is released from adrenergic postganglionic nerve terminals, resulting in a moderate increase in BP, heart rate, and ventricular irritability. Subsequently (1–2 h), drug-induced release and reuptake of norepinephrine are blocked, leading to a state resembling surgical sympathectomy. *Suppresses arrhythmias with a reentry mechanism and decreases dispersion of ectopic foci. PR, QT, and QRS intervals are unchanged. Because onset of desired action is delayed, bretylium is not a first-line antiarrhythmic agent.*

USES Short-term prophylaxis and treatment of ventricular fibrillation; life-threatening arrhythmias such as ventricular fibrillation not responsive to conventional therapy [e.g., lidocaine, procainamide, direct current (cardioversion)].

CONTRAINDICATIONS No contraindications for use in life-threatening

B

refractory ventricular arrhythmias; digitalis toxicity.

CAUTIOUS USE Digitalis-induced arrhythmias, patients with fixed cardiac output (e.g., severe aortic stenosis or severe pulmonary hypertension because profound hypotension may result), sinus bradycardia, patients on digitalis maintenance, angina pectoris, impaired renal function, renal disease; pregnancy (category C), lactation.

ROUTE & DOSAGE

Ventricular Fibrillation

Adult: **IV** 5 mg/kg rapid IV injection, may increase to 10 mg/kg and repeat q15–30min (max: 30 mg/kg/day); may also give by continuous infusion at 1–2 mg/min **IM** 5–10 mg/kg, may repeat in 1–2 h if arrhythmia persists, then 5–10 mg/kg q6–8h for maintenance
Child: **IV** 5 mg/kg, may repeat q15–30min (max: 30 mg/kg) **IM** 2–5 mg/kg as single dose

ADMINISTRATION

Intramuscular

- Administer no more than 5 mL in any one IM site.
- Keep a record of injection sites. Injection into same site can cause muscle atrophy, necrosis, and fibrosis.

Intravenous

IV administration to infants and children: Verify correct IV concentration and rate of infusion/injection with physician.

PREPARE: **Direct:** Give undiluted. **Continuous:** Give diluted in 50 mL or more of NS or D5W.

ADMINISTER: **Direct:** Give undiluted at a rate of 1 dose/15 seconds. **Continuous:** Give diluted at a rate of 1–2 mg/min.

INCOMPATIBILITIES **Solution/additive: Dobutamine, pantoprazole, phenytoin, procainamide. Y-site: Amphotericin B, cholestryl, propofol, warfarin.**

- Store at 15°–30° C (59°–86° F) unless otherwise directed.

ADVERSE EFFECTS (≥1%) **CV:** Both supine and postural *hypotension* with dizziness, vertigo, lightheadedness, faintness, syncope, transitory hypertension, bradycardia, increased frequency of PVCs, exacerbation of digitalis-induced arrhythmias. **GI:** *Nausea, vomiting* (particularly with rapid IV). **Respiratory:** Respiratory depression.

DIAGNOSTIC TEST INTERFERENCE ***Urinary VMA, epinephrine,*** and ***norepinephrine*** levels may be decreased during bretylium therapy.

INTERACTIONS Drug: Lidocaine, procainamide, quinidine, propranolol may antagonize antiarrhythmic effects and compound hypotension; ANTIHYPERTENSIVE AGENTS will add to hypotensive effects; DIGITALIS GLYCOSIDES may worsen arrhythmias through **digitalis** toxicity. MACROLIDES, QUINOLONES increase the risk of arrhythmias.

PHARMACOKINETICS Onset: Minutes after IV; up to 6 h IM. **Peak:** 6–9 h. **Duration:** 6–24 h. **Distribution:** Does not cross blood–brain barrier; not known if crosses placenta or distributed into breast milk. **Metabolism:** Not metabolized. **Elimination:** 70–80% in urine in 24 h. **Half-Life:** 4–17 h.

NURSING IMPLICATIONS

Assessment & Drug Effects

- Anticipate vomiting. IV administration is associated with a high incidence of nausea and vomiting. These side effects can be minimized by slow administration of drug (10 min or longer).
- Establish baseline readings and monitor BP and ECG when drug is administered. Observe for initial transient rise in BP, increased heart rate, PVCs and other arrhythmias, or worsening of existing arrhythmias, which may occur within a few minutes to 1 h after drug administration. Initial effect of hypertension is usually followed within 1 h by a fall in supine BP and by orthostatic hypotension.
- Use supine position until patient develops tolerance to hypotensive effect of bretylium (generally in several days). Hypotension can occur in the supine position, particularly in patients with severely compromised cardiac function. It may not readily respond to therapy (e.g., vasopressors, fluids); early reporting is essential.
- Raise or lower head of bed slowly; advise patient to make position changes slowly in order to prevent orthostatic hypotension.
- Monitor I&O, particularly in patients with impaired renal function.

Patient & Family Education

- Make position changes slowly. If allowed to be out of bed, dangle legs for a few minutes before standing, but do not stand still for prolonged periods. Men should sit on toilet to urinate.

BRIMONIDINE TARTRATE

(bry-mon′i-deen)

Alphagan P

Pregnancy Category: B

See Appendix A-1.

BRINZOLAMIDE

(brin-zol′a-mide)

Azopt

Pregnancy Category: C

See Appendix A-1.

BROMFENAC

(brom′fen-ac)

Xibrom

Pregnancy Category: C

See Appendix A-1.

BROMOCRIPTINE MESYLATE

(broe-moe-krip′teen)

Cycloset, Parlodel

Classifications: ERGOT ALKALOID; DOPAMINE RECEPTOR AGONIST; ANTIPARKINSON

Therapeutic: ERGOT REPLACEMENT; ANTIDYSKINETIC; ANTIPARKINSON; GLYCEMIC CONTROL AGENT

Prototype: Ergotamine

Pregnancy Category: C

AVAILABILITY 0.8 mg, 2.5 mg tablets; 5 mg capsules

ACTION & *THERAPEUTIC EFFECT*

Semisynthetic ergot alkaloid that is a synthetic dopamine (D_2) receptor agonist. Reduces elevated serum prolactin levels in men and women by activating postsynaptic dopaminergic receptors in hypothalamus to stimulate release of prolactin-inhibiting factor. Activates dopaminergic

B

receptors (D_2 receptors) in neostriatum of CNS, which may explain action in parkinsonism. *Restores ovulation and ovarian function in amenorrheic women, thus correcting female infertility secondary to elevated prolactin levels. Activates dopaminergic receptors in CNS resulting in antiparkinsonism effect. Improves glycemic control in type 2 diabetics.*

USES Short-term management of amenorrhea/galactorrhea or female infertility associated with hyperprolactinemia (when there is no indication of pituitary tumor). Also used as adjunctive to levodopa or levodopa/carbidopa therapy to relieve symptoms of Parkinson's disease and to lower plasma growth hormone in patients with acromegaly. As adjunct to diet and exercise in Type II diabetes.

UNLABELED USES To prevent postpartum lactation, to relieve premenstrual symptoms, to treat hypogonadism and galactorrhea in hyperprolactinemic men; for management of hepatic encephalopathy, Cushing's syndrome, drug-induced neuroleptic malignant syndrome, and cocaine withdrawal.

CONTRAINDICATIONS Hypersensitivity to ergot alkaloids; uncontrolled hypertension; severe ischemic heart disease or peripheral vascular disease; pituitary tumor; **Cycloset:** type 1 diabetes mellitus or diabetic ketoacidosis. Normal prolactin levels, lactation; preeclampsia, eclampsia. Safe use in children younger than 15 y is not established.

CAUTIOUS USE Hepatic and renal dysfunction; history of psychiatric disorder; history of GI bleeding or peptic ulcer; history of MI with residual arrhythmia; pregnancy (category C).

ROUTE & DOSAGE

Amenorrhea or Galactorrhea, Female Infertility

Adult: **PO** 1.25–2.5 mg/day (max: 2.5 mg 2–3 times/day)

Parkinson's Disease

Adult: **PO** 1.25–2.5 mg/day (max: 100 mg/day in divided doses)

Acromegaly

Adult: **PO** 1.25–2.5 mg/day for 3 days, then increase by 1.25–2.5 mg q3–7days until desired effect is achieved, usually 30–60 mg/day in divided doses

Adjunct in Type II Diabetes

Adult: **PO** 0.8 mg daily in the a.m., titrate up (max dose: 1.6–4.8 mg)

ADMINISTRATION

Oral

- Do not administer during the postpartum period until vital signs are stabilized.
- Give with meals, milk, or other food to reduce incidence of GI side effects.
- Have patient in supine position before receiving first dose because dizziness and fainting may occur. For this reason, initial dose is usually prescribed for evening administration.
- Store in tightly closed, light-resistant containers, preferably at 15°–30° C (59°–86° F) unless otherwise directed.

ADVERSE EFFECTS (≥1%) **Body as a Whole:** Mostly dose related. **CNS:** Headache, dizziness, vertigo, lightheadedness, fainting, sedation, nightmares, insomnia, dyskinesia, ataxia; mania, nervousness, anxiety, depression. **CV:** *Orthostatic hypotension*, shock, postpartum hypertension, palpitation, extrasystoles, Raynaud's phenomenon, red, tender, hot, edematous extremities (erythromelalgia), exacerbation of angina, arrhythmias, acute MI. **Special Senses:** Blurred vision, burning sensation in eyes, blepharospasm, diplopia. **GI:** *Nausea*, vomiting, abdominal cramps, epigastric pain, constipation (long-term use) or diarrhea; metallic taste, dry mouth, dysphagia, anorexia, peptic ulcers. **Skin:** Urticaria, rash, mottling, livedo reticularis. **Other:** Fatigue, nasal congestion, asthenia.

INTERACTIONS Drug: Possibility of decreased tolerance to **alcohol;** ANTIHYPERTENSIVE AGENTS add to hypotensive effects; ORAL CONTRACEPTIVES, **estrogen, progestins** may interfere with effect of bromocriptine by causing amenorrhea and galactorrhea; PHENOTHIAZINES, TRICYCLIC ANTIDEPRESSANTS, **methyldopa, reserpine** can cause an increase in **prolactin,** which may interfere with bromocriptine activity.

PHARMACOKINETICS Absorption: 28% from GI tract. **Peak:** 1–2 h. **Duration:** 4–8 h. **Metabolism:** In liver by CYP3A4. **Elimination:** 85% in feces in 5 days; 3–6% in urine. **Half-Life:** 50 h.

NURSING IMPLICATIONS

Assessment & Drug Effects

- Monitor vital signs closely during the first few days and periodically throughout therapy.
- Lab tests: Periodic CBC, liver functions and renal functions with prolonged therapy.
- Monitor for and report psychotic symptoms and other adverse reactions in Parkinson's patients.
- Improvement in Parkinson's disease may be noted in 30–90 min following administration of bromocriptine, with maximum effect in 2 h.

Patient & Family Education

- Make position changes slowly and in stages, especially from lying down to standing, and to dangle legs over bed for a few minutes before walking. Lie down immediately if light-headedness or dizziness occurs.
- Do not drive or engage in other potentially hazardous activities until response to drug is known.
- Avoid exposure to cold and report the onset of pallor of fingers or toes.
- Note: Use barrier-type contraceptive measures until normal ovulating cycle is restored. Oral contraceptives are contraindicated.

BROMPHENIRAMINE MALEATE

(brome-fen-ir′a-meen)

Veltane

Classifications: ANTIHISTAMINE; H_1-RECEPTOR ANTAGONIST

Therapeutic: ANTIHISTAMINE

Prototype: Diphenhydramine

Pregnancy Category: C

AVAILABILITY 10 mg/mL injection; 2 mg/5 mL elixir; 4 mg tablet; ingredient in many oral combination products containing a decongestant, expectorant, and/or analgesic

ACTION & *THERAPEUTIC EFFECT* Antihistamine that has less sedative effect than diphenhydramine. Competes with histamine for H_1-receptor sites on effector cells in the

B

bronchi and bronchioles, thus blocking histamine-mediated responses. *Effective against upper respiratory symptoms and allergic manifestations.*

USES Symptomatic treatment of allergic manifestations. Also used in various cough mixtures and antihistamine-decongestant cold formulations.

CONTRAINDICATIONS Hypersensitivity to antihistamines; acute asthma; newborns.

CAUTIOUS USE Older adults; prostatic hypertrophy; GI obstruction; asthma; narrow-angle glaucoma; COPD, cardiovascular or renal disease; seizure disorders; hyperthyroidism; pregnancy (category C), lactation.

ROUTE & DOSAGE

Allergy

Adult: **PO** 4–8 mg t.i.d. or q.i.d. or 8–12 mg of sustained release b.i.d. or t.i.d. **Subcutaneous/IM/IV** 5–20 mg q6–12h (max: 40 mg/24 h)

Geriatric: **PO** 4 mg 1–2 times/day

Child: **PO** *Older than 6 y,* 2–4 mg t.i.d. or q.i.d. or 8–12 mg of sustained release b.i.d. (max: 12 mg/24 h); *younger than 6 y,* 0.5 mg/kg in 3–4 divided doses

ADMINISTRATION

Oral

- Give with meals or a snack to prevent gastric irritation.

Subcutaneous/Intramuscular

- Give without further dilution or diluted to a 1:10 ratio with NS.

Intravenous

PREPARE: **Direct:** Give undiluted or diluted with 10 mL D5W or NS.
ADMINISTER: **Direct:** Give IV push slowly over 1 min to a recumbent patient.
INCOMPATIBILITIES **Solution/additive:** **Radio-contrast media (diatrizoate, iothalamate), insulin, pentobarbital.**

- Store in tightly covered container at 15°–30° C (59°–86° F) unless otherwise directed. Elixir and parenteral form should be protected from light. Avoid freezing.

ADVERSE EFFECTS (≥1%) **Body as a Whole:** Hypersensitivity reaction (urticaria, increased sweating, agranulocytosis). **CNS:** *Sedation,* drowsiness, dizziness, headache, disturbed coordination. **GI:** Dry mouth, throat, and nose, stomach upset, constipation. **Special Senses:** Ringing or buzzing in ears. **Skin:** Rash, photosensitivity.

DIAGNOSTIC TEST INTERFERENCE May cause false-negative **allergy skin tests.**

INTERACTIONS Drug: Alcohol and other CNS DEPRESSANTS add to sedation.

PHARMACOKINETICS Peak: 3–9 h. **Duration:** Up to 48 h. **Distribution:** Crosses placenta. **Elimination:** 40% in urine within 72 h; 2% in feces. **Half-Life:** 12–34 h.

NURSING IMPLICATIONS

Assessment & Drug Effects

- Drowsiness, sweating, transient hypotension, and syncope may follow IV administration; reaction to drug should be evaluated. Keep physician informed.

B

- Note: Older adults tend to be particularly susceptible to drug's sedative effect, dizziness, and hypotension. Most symptoms respond to reduction in dosage.
- Lab tests: Periodic CBC in patients receiving long-term therapy.

Patient & Family Education

- Acute hypersensitivity reaction can occur within minutes to hours after drug ingestion. Reaction is manifested by high fever, chills, and possible development of ulcerations of mouth and throat, pneumonia, and prostration. Patient should seek medical attention immediately.
- Follow diligent mouth care. Sugarless gum, lemon drops, or frequent rinses with warm water may relieve dry mouth.
- Do not drive a car or perform other potentially hazardous activities until response to drug is known.
- Do not take alcoholic beverages or other CNS depressants (e.g., tranquilizers, sedatives, pain or sleeping medicines) without consulting physician.

BUDESONIDE

(bu-des′o-nide)

Entocort EC, Pulmicort Flexhaler, Rhinocort, Rhinocort Aqua, Rhinocort Turbuhaler

Classifications: ANTI-INFLAMMATORY; ADRENAL CORTICOSTEROID; GLUCOCORTICOID

Therapeutic: ANTI-INFLAMMATORY; ADRENAL CORTICOSTEROID

Prototype: Hydrocortisone

Pregnancy Category: B (inhaled); C (oral)

AVAILABILITY 32 mcg/inhalation; 3 mg capsule

ACTION & *THERAPEUTIC EFFECT*

Has potent glucocorticoid activity. Its anti-inflammatory action on nasal mucosa is thought to be a result of decreased IgE synthesis and decreased arachidonic acid metabolism. *Glucocorticoids have a wide range of inhibitory activities against multiple cell types (e.g., neutrophils, macrophages) and mediators (e.g., histamine, cytokines) involved in allergic and nonallergic/irritant-mediated inflammation.*

USES Treatment of allergic and perennial rhinitis, maintain remission in mild to moderate Crohn's disease; prophylaxis for asthma.

CONTRAINDICATIONS Hypersensitivity to budesonide, status asthmaticus, acute bronchospasms; peptic ulcer disease; lactation.

CAUTIOUS USE Concomitant administration of systemic oral steroids; active or quiescent tuberculosis; infections of respiratory tract; in sun-treated fungal, bacterial, or systemic viral infections or ocular herpes simplex; recent nasal septal ulcers; recurrent epistaxis; nasal surgery or trauma; psychosis; myasthenia gravis; diabetes mellitus; seizure disorders; **oral:** pregnancy (category C); **nasal:** pregnancy (category B).

ROUTE & DOSAGE

Crohn's Disease

Adult: **PO** 9 mg once/day in a.m. for up to 8 wk, may taper to 6 mg daily for 2 wk prior to discontinuing. May repeat 8-wk course for recurring episodes of active Crohn's disease.

B

Asthma Prophylaxis, Rhinitis
See Appendix A-3.

ADMINISTRATION

Oral

- Ensure that capsules are swallowed whole and not chewed.
- Give only in the morning.
- Patients with moderate to severe liver disease should be monitored for increased signs and/or symptoms of hypercorticism. Reducing the dose of Entocort EC capsules should be considered in these patients.
- Store at 25° C (77° F); excursions permitted to 15°–30° C (59°–86° F).

ADVERSE EFFECTS (≥1%) **Body as a Whole:** Arthralgia, fatigue, fever, hyperkinesis, myalgia, asthenia, paresthesia, tremor. **CNS:** Dizziness, emotional lability, facial edema, nervousness, *headache,* agitation, confusion, insomnia, drowsiness. **CV:** Chest pain, hypertension, palpitations, sinus tachycardia. **GI:** Abdominal pain, dyspepsia, gastroenteritis, oral candidiasis, xerostomia, diarrhea, nausea, vomiting, cramps. **Hematologic:** Epistaxis. **Metabolic:** Hypokalemia, weight gain. **Respiratory:** Bronchospasms, *infections,* cough, rhinitis, sinusitis, dyspnea, hoarseness, wheezing. **Skin:** Eczema, pruritus, purpura, rash, alopecia. **Special Senses:** Contact dermatitis, reduced sense of smell, nasal pain. **Urogenital:** Intermenstrual bleeding, dysuria.

INTERACTIONS Drug: Ketoconazole may increase oral budesonide concentrations and toxicity; toxicity may also occur with **anastrozole** (high doses only), **clarithromycin, cyclosporine, danazol, delavirdine, diltiazem, erythromycin, fluconazole, fluoxetine, fluvoxamine, indinavir, isoniazid, INH, itraconazole, mibefradil, nefazodone, nelfinavir, nicardipine, norfloxacin, oxiconazole, quinidine, quinine, ritonavir, saquinavir, troleandomycin, verapamil, and zafirlukast. Food: Grapefruit juice** will significantly increase bioavailability of oral budesonide.

PHARMACOKINETICS Absorption: 20% (nasal) dose, 6–13% of (orally inhaled) dose, 9% PO dose reaches systemic circulation; PO form is absorbed from duodenum at pH greater than 5.5; oral bioavailability increases 2.5 times in hepatic cirrhosis. **Onset:** 8–12 h inhaled, 2 wk oral. **Peak:** 2 wk inhaled, 8 wk oral delayed by high-fat meal. **Distribution:** 90% protein bound. **Metabolism:** 85% of absorbed dose undergoes first pass metabolism by CYP3A4. **Elimination:** 60% in urine, 40% in feces. **Half-Life:** 2–3.6 h.

NURSING IMPLICATIONS

Assessment & Drug Effects

- Monitor closely for S&S of hypercorticism if concomitant doses of ketoconazole or other CYP3A4 inhibitors (see Drug Interactions) are being given.
- Monitor patients with moderate to severe liver disease for increased S&S of hypercorticism.
- Lab tests: Periodic serum potassium.

Patient & Family Education

- Notify the physician immediately for any of the following: Itching, skin rash, fever, swelling of face and neck, difficulty breathing, or if you develop S&S of infection.

- Do not drink grapefruit juice or eat grapefruit regularly.
- Avoid people with infections, especially those with chickenpox or measles if you have never had these conditions.

BUMETANIDE

(byoo-met'a-nide)

Bumex

Classifications: FLUID AND WATER BALANCE AGENT; LOOP DIURETIC

Therapeutic: DIURETIC; ANTIHYPERTENSIVE

Prototype: Furosemide

Pregnancy Category: C

AVAILABILITY 0.5 mg, 1 mg, 2 mg tablets; 0.25 mg/mL injection

ACTION & *THERAPEUTIC EFFECT* Sulfonamide derivative structurally related to furosemide that causes both potassium and magnesium wastage. Inhibits sodium and chloride reabsorption by direct action on proximal ascending limb of the loop of Henle. Also appears to inhibit phosphate and bicarbonate reabsorption. *Produces only mild hypotensive effects at usual diuretic doses. Controls formation of edema.*

USES Edema associated with CHF; hepatic or renal disease, including nephrotic syndrome. Has been used in management of postoperative and premenstrual edema, edema accompanying disseminated carcinoma, and mild hypertension. May be used concomitantly with a potassium-sparing diuretic.

CONTRAINDICATIONS Hypersensitivity to bumetanide or to other sulfonamides; anuria, markedly elevated BUN; hepatic coma; acute MI, ventricular arrhythmias; severe electrolyte deficiency; severe renal disease; diabetes mellitus; lactation.

CAUTIOUS USE Hepatic cirrhosis, as history of gout; history of hypersensitivity to furosemide; elderly; pregnancy (category C).

ROUTE & DOSAGE

Edema

Adult: **PO** 0.5–2 mg once/day, may repeat at 4–5 h intervals if needed (max: 10 mg/day) **IV/IM** 0.5–1 mg over 1–2 min, repeated q2–3h prn (max: 10 mg/day)

ADMINISTRATION

Oral

- Give with food or milk to reduce risk of gastrointestinal irritation.
- Administered in the morning as a single dose, either daily or by intermittent schedule.

Intramuscular

- Use undiluted solution for injection.

Intravenous

PREPARE: **Direct/Continuous:** Give direct IV undiluted (typical) or diluted for infusion with D5W, NS, LR.

ADMINISTER: **Direct:** Give IV push at a rate of a single dose over 1–2 min. **Continuous:** Give diluted solution over 5 min or at prescribed rate.

INCOMPATIBILITIES **Solution/additive: Dobutamine. Y-site: Fenoldopam, midazolam.**

- Diluted infusion should be used within 24 h after preparation.

B

- Store in tight, light-resistant container at 15°–30° C (59°–86° F) unless otherwise directed.

ADVERSE EFFECTS (≥1%) **Body as a Whole:** Sweating, hyperventilation, glycosuria. **CNS:** Dizziness, headache, weakness, fatigue. **CV:** Hypotension, ECG changes, chest pain, *hypovolemia*. **GI:** Nausea, vomiting, abdominal or stomach pain, GI distress, diarrhea, dry mouth. **Metabolic:** *Hypokalemia*, hyponatremia, hyperuricemia, hyperglycemia; *hypomagnesemia;* decreased calcium, chloride. **Musculoskeletal:** Muscle cramps, muscle pain, stiffness or tenderness; arthritic pain. **Special Senses:** Ear discomfort, ringing or buzzing in ears, impaired hearing.

INTERACTIONS Drug: AMINOGLYCOSIDES, **cisplatin** increase risk of ototoxicity; bumetanide increases risk of hypokalemia-induced **digoxin** toxicity; NONSTEROIDAL ANTI-INFLAMMATORY DRUGS (NSAIDS) may attenuate diuretic and hypotensive response; **probenecid** may antagonize diuretic activity; bumetanide may decrease renal elimination of **lithium; sotalol** may increase risk of cardiotoxicity.

PHARMACOKINETICS Absorption: Readily from GI tract. **Onset:** 30–60 min PO; 40 min IV. **Peak:** 0.5–2 h. **Duration:** 4–6 h. **Distribution:** Distributed into breast milk. **Metabolism:** In liver. **Elimination:** 80% in urine in 48 h, 10–20% in feces. **Half-Life:** 60–90 min.

NURSING IMPLICATIONS

Assessment & Drug Effects

- Monitor I&O and report onset of oliguria or other changes in I&O ratio and pattern promptly.
- Monitor weight, BP, and pulse rate. Assess for hypovolemia by taking BP and pulse rate while patient is lying, sitting, and standing. Older adults are particularly at risk for hypovolemia with resulting thrombi and emboli.
- Lab tests: Serum electrolytes, blood studies, liver and kidney function tests, uric acid (particularly patients with history of gout), and blood glucose. Determine values initially and at regular intervals.
- Monitor for S&S of hypomagnesemia and hypokalemia (see Appendix F) especially in those receiving digitalis or who have CHF, hepatic cirrhosis, ascites, diarrhea, or potassium-depleting nephropathy.
- Question patient about hearing difficulty or ear discomfort. Patients at risk of ototoxic effects include those receiving the drug IV, especially at high doses, those with severely impaired renal function, and those receiving other potentially ototoxic or nephrotoxic drugs (see Appendix F).
- Monitor diabetics for loss of glycemic control.

Patient & Family Education

- Report symptoms of electrolyte imbalance to physician promptly (e.g., weakness, dizziness, fatigue, faintness, confusion, muscle cramps, headache, paresthesias).
- Eat potassium-rich foods such as fruit juices, potatoes, cereals, skim milk, and bananas while taking bumetanide.
- Report S&S of ototoxicity promptly to physician (see Appendix F).
- Monitor blood glucose for loss of glycemic control if diabetic.

BUPIVACAINE HYDROCHLORIDE

(byoo-piv'a-kane)

Marcaine, Sensorcaine

Classification: LOCAL ANESTHETIC (AMIDE-TYPE)

Therapeutic: ANESTHETIC, LOCAL

Prototype: Procaine

Pregnancy Category: C

AVAILABILITY 0.25%, 0.5%, 0.75% injection

ACTION & *THERAPEUTIC EFFECT* Anesthetic of the amide type that decreases sodium flux into nerve cell, inhibiting initial depolarization, and prevents propagation and conduction of the nerve impulse. Progression of anesthesia, related to diameter, myelination, and conduction velocity of affected fibers is manifested clinically as sequential loss of nerve function. *Primary depressant effect is in medulla and higher centers affecting patient's reaction to pain, temperature, and touch, as well as proprioception and skeletal muscle tone.*

USES Infiltration anesthesia; peripheral, sympathetic nerve, and epidural (including caudal) block anesthesia; 0.75% bupivacaine solution in dextrose is used for spinal anesthesia.

CONTRAINDICATIONS Known sensitivity to bupivacaine, local anesthetics, other amide-type anesthetics; parabens, or metabisulfites; acidosis; heart block; severe hemorrhage, uncontrolled coagulopathy; hypotension and shock; hypertension, cerebrospinal diseases; use of 0.75% dose in obstetric anesthesia; spinal anesthesia in septicemia; topical or IV regional anesthesia; concurrent or intercurrent use of any other local anesthesia; history of malignant hyperthermia.

CAUTIOUS USE Older adults or debilitated patients, dehydration; hepatic or renal disease, neurologic diseases; known drug allergies and sensitivities; pregnancy (category C); dysrhythmias; lactation, children older than 12 y; obstetrical delivery.

ROUTE & DOSAGE

Infiltration Anesthesia

Adult: **IM Local infiltration, sympathetic block** 0.25% solution; **Lumbar epidural** 0.25%, 0.5%, 0.75% solutions; **Caudal block, peripheral nerve block** 0.25%, 0.5% solutions; **Retrobulbar block** 0.75% solution

Child: **IM** 1–3.7 mg/kg

ADMINISTRATION

Intramuscular

- Inject slowly with frequent aspirations to avoid intravascular injection.

Intrathecal

- Do not use preparations containing preservatives for epidural or spinal anesthesia.
- Do not use multiple-dose vial for lumbar or caudal epidural block.
- Store ampules at 15°–30° C (59°–86° F); protect from freezing. Solutions with epinephrine should be protected from light.

INCOMPATIBILITIES **Solution/additive: Sodium bicarbonate.**

ADVERSE EFFECTS (≥1%) **Body as a Whole:** Hypersensitivity [cutaneous lesions, urticaria, sneezing, diaphoresis, syncope, hyperthermia,

B

angioneurotic edema (including laryngeal edema), anaphylaxis, anaphylactoid reaction]. **CNS:** Nervousness, unusual anxiety, excitement, dizziness, drowsiness, tremors, convulsions, unconsciousness, respiratory arrest. **Special Senses:** Pupillary constriction; blurred or double vision; tinnitus. **GI:** Nausea, vomiting. **Other:** Inflammation or sepsis at injection site, chills, pupillary constriction. **Associated with Epidural Anesthesia, Body as a Whole:** Total spinal block, persistent analgesia, paresthesia. **Urogenital:** Urinary retention, fecal incontinence, loss of perineal sensation and sexual function. **Other:** Slowing of labor, increased incidence of forceps delivery, cranial nerve palsies (with inadvertent intrathecal injection).

INTERACTIONS Drug: CNS DEPRESSANTS augment CNS depression; with **isoproterenol, ergonovine** there is persistent hypertension and a risk of CVA if bupivacaine used with **epinephrine.** MAO INHIBITORS, TRICYCLIC ANTIDEPRESSANTS, PHENOTHIAZINES cause severe or prolonged hypotension or hypertension if bupivacaine used with **epinephrine.**

PHARMACOKINETICS Onset: 4–17 min (epidural, caudal, peripheral, or sympathetic block); within 1 min (spinal block). **Duration:** 3–5 h (epidural, caudal, peripheral, or sympathetic block); 1.25–2.5 h (spinal block). **Distribution:** Crosses placenta. **Metabolism:** In liver. **Elimination:** 6% unchanged in urine. **Half-Life:** 1.5–5.5 h in adults, 8.1 h in neonates.

NURSING IMPLICATIONS

Assessment & Drug Effects

- Monitor for signs of inadvertent intravascular injection, which can produce a transient "epinephrine response" (increased heart rate or systolic BP or both, circumoral pallor, palpitations, nervousness) within 45 seconds in the unsedated patient and an increase by 20 bpm or more in heart rate for at least 15 seconds in sedated patient.
- Monitor for toxicity: CNS stimulation (unusual anxiety, excitement, restlessness) usually occurs first, followed by CNS depression (drowsiness, unconsciousness, respiratory arrest). However, because stimulation is apt to be transient or absent, drowsiness may be the first sign in some patients (especially children and older adults).
- Monitor BP and fetal heart rate continuously during labor because maternal hypotension may accompany regional anesthesia. Place mother on left side with legs elevated.
- Monitor cardiac and respiratory status continuously in patients receiving retrobulbar and dental blocks.

Patient & Family Education

- After spinal anesthesia, sensation to lower extremities may not return for 2.5–3.5 h.

BUPRENORPHINE HYDROCHLORIDE

(byoo-pre-nor′feen)

Buprenex, Suboxone, Subutex

Classifications: ANALGESIC; NARCOTIC (OPIATE AGONIST-ANTAGONIST)

Therapeutic: NARCOTIC ANALGESIC;

Prototype: Pentazocine

Pregnancy Category: C

Controlled Substance: Schedule III

AVAILABILITY 0.3 mg (base)/mL injection; 2 mg, 8 mg sublingual tablets

ACTION & *THERAPEUTIC EFFECT* Opiate agonist–antagonist with agonist activity approximately 30 times that of morphine and antagonist activity equal to or up to 3 times that of naloxone. Respiratory depression occurs infrequently, probably due to drug's opiate antagonist activity. Has a low level of physical dependence. *Dose-related analgesia results from a high affinity of buprenorphine for mu-opioid receptors and as an antagonist at the kappa-opiate receptors in the CNS. Naloxone is an antagonist at the mu-opioid receptor.*

USES *Injectable* used for moderate to severe pain. *Sublingual tablets* used for treatment of opioid dependence.

UNLABELED USES *Injectable* to reverse fentanyl-induced anesthesia. *Sublingual tablets* may be used to ease cocaine withdrawal.

CONTRAINDICATIONS Hypersensitivity to buprenorphine or hypersensitivity to naloxone; lactation, children younger than 2 y.

CAUTIOUS USE Patient with history of opiate use; compromised respiratory function [e.g., chronic obstructive pulmonary disease (COPD), cor pulmonale, decreased respiratory reserve, hypoxia, hypercapnia, or preexisting respiratory depression]; concomitant use of other respiratory depressants; hypothyroidism, myxedema, Addison's disease; severe renal or hepatic impairment; geriatric or debilitated patients; acute alcoholism, delirium tremens; prostatic hypertrophy, urethral stricture; comatose patient; patients with CNS depression, head injury, or intracranial lesion; biliary tract dysfunction; pregnancy (category C).

ROUTE & DOSAGE

Postoperative Pain

Adult/Adolescent (older than 12 y): **IV/IM** 0.3 mg q6h up to 0.6 mg q4h or 25–50 mcg/h by IV infusion
Geriatric: **IV/IM** 0.15 mg q6h
Child (2–12 y): **IV/IM** 2–6 mcg/kg q4–6h prn

Opioid Dependence/Cocaine Withdrawal

Adult: **SL** Initiate with 8 mg daily on day 1 at least 4 h after last opioid dose, 16 mg daily on day 2, then switch to maintenance therapy at the same buprenorphine dose as day 2 (e.g., 16 mg daily). Adjust dose daily until opiate withdrawal effects are suppressed. Maintenance dose range 4–24 mg/day buprenorphine.

ADMINISTRATION

Sublingual

- Place **Suboxone** and **Subutex** tablets under tongue until dissolved. For doses requiring more than two tablets, place all tablets at once under tongue, or if patient cannot accommodate all tablets, place two tablets at a time under tongue.
- Instruct to hold the tablets under tongue until dissolved; advise not to swallow.

Intramuscular

- Give undiluted, deep IM into a large muscle.

B

Intravenous

PREPARE: **Direct/IV Infusion:** May be given undiluted direct IV or further dilute each 1 mL (0.3 mg) ampule in 50 mL of D5W, NS, D5NS, or LR to yield 6 mcg/ mL for infusion. ▪ Do not use if discolored or contains particulate matter.

ADMINISTER: **Direct:** Give slowly at a rate of 0.3 mg over 2 min to a patient in a recumbent position. **IV Infusion:** Give by slow infusion over 3 min or longer depending on volume of IV solution.

INCOMPATIBILITIES **Solution/additive: Diltiazem, floxacillin, furosemide, lorazepam. Y-site: Amphotericin B cholesteryl sulfate complex, doxorubicin liposome, lansoprazole.**

▪ Store at 15°–30° C (59°–86° F); avoid freezing.

ADVERSE EFFECTS (≥1%) **CNS:** *Sedation, drowsiness,* dizziness, vertigo, *headache,* amnesia, euphoria, asthenia, *insomnia, pain* (when used for withdrawal), *withdrawal symptoms.* **CV:** Hypotension, vasodilation. **Special Senses:** Miosis. **GI:** *Nausea,* vomiting, diarrhea, *constipation.* **Respiratory:** Respiratory depression, hyperventilation. **Skin:** Pruritus, injection site reactions, *sweating.*

INTERACTIONS Drug: Alcohol, OPIATES, other CNS DEPRESSANTS, BENZODIAZEPINES augment CNS depression; **diazepam** may cause respiratory or cardiovascular collapse; AZOLE ANTIFUNGALS (e.g., **fluconazole**), MACROLIDE ANTIBIOTICS (e.g., **erythromycin**), and PROTEASE INHIBITORS (e.g., **saquinavir**) may increase buprenorphine levels.

PHARMACOKINETICS Absorption: Widely variable sublingual absorption. **Onset:** 10–30 min IM/IV. **Peak:** 1 h IM/IV; 2–6 h SL. **Duration:** 6–10 h. **Metabolism:** Extensively in liver by CYP3A4 to active metabolite norbuprenorphine. **Elimination:** 70% in feces, 30% in urine in 7 days. **Half-Life:** 2.2 h IM/IV; 37 h SL.

NURSING IMPLICATIONS

Assessment & Drug Effects

- Monitor respiratory status during therapy. Buprenorphine-induced respiratory depression is about equal to that produced by 10 mg morphine, but onset is slower, and if it occurs, it lasts longer.
- Note: Respiratory depression in the healthy adult plateaus or may even decrease in severity with doses more than 1.2 mg because of antagonist activity of the drug.
- Monitor I&O ratio and pattern during buprenorphine therapy; urinary retention is a potential adverse effect.
- Lab tests: Baseline liver function, renal function, alkaline phosphatase, and PSA.
- Supervise ambulation; drowsiness occurs in 66% of patients taking this drug.

Patient & Family Education

- Do not drive or engage in other potentially hazardous activities until response to drug is known.
- Do not use alcohol or other CNS depressing drugs without consulting physician. An additive effect exists between buprenorphine hydrochloride and other CNS depressants including alcohol.

BUPROPION HYDROCHLORIDE

(byoo-pro′pi-on)

B

Wellbutrin, Wellbutrin SR, Wellbutrin XL, Zyban

BUPROPION HYDROBROMIDE

Aplenzin

Classification: ANTIDEPRESSANT

Therapeutic: ANTIDEPRESSANT

Pregnancy Category: B

AVAILABILITY 75 mg, 100 mg tablets; 100 mg, 150 mg, 200 mg sustained release tablets; 150 mg, 300 mg extended release tablets; Hydrobromide form: 174 mg, 348 mg, 522 mg extended release tablet

ACTION & *THERAPEUTIC EFFECT* The neurochemical mechanism of bupropion is not fully understood. It selectively inhibits the neuronal reuptake of dopamine. *Its antidepressive effect is related to CNS stimulant effects.*

USES Indicated for mental depression; since it has been associated with increased risk of seizures, it is not the agent of first choice; adjunct for smoking cessation; seasonal affective disorder.

UNLABELED USES Schizoaffective disorders.

CONTRAINDICATIONS Hypersensitivity to bupropion; history of seizure disorder; current or prior diagnosis of bulimia or anorexia nervosa; suicidal ideation; concurrent administration of an MAO inhibitor; head trauma; seizure disorder; CNS tumor; recent MI; abrupt discontinuation, anorexia nervosa, bulimia nervosa, children younger than 18 y; lactation.

CAUTIOUS USE Renal or hepatic function impairment; drug abuse or dependence; cardiac disease, MI, hepatic disease, biliary cirrhosis; hypertension, bipolar disorder, mania, psychosis, diabetes mellitus, older adults, ethanol intoxication, tics, Tourette's syndrome; pregnancy (category B).

ROUTE & DOSAGE

Depression/Seasonal Affective Disorder

Adult: **PO** 75–100 mg t.i.d., start with 75 mg t.i.d., or 100 mg SR b.i.d., or 150 mg XL daily, and increase dose q3days to 300 mg/day; doses greater than 450 mg/day are associated with an increased risk of adverse reactions including seizures; Aplenzin: 174 mg daily can increase to 348 mg daily

Geriatric: **PO** 50–100 mg/day, may increase by 50–100 mg q3–4days (max: 150 mg/dose)

Smoking Cessation

Adult: **PO** Start with 150 mg once daily × 3 days, then increase to 150 mg b.i.d. (max: 300 mg/day) for 7–12 wk

Hepatic Impairment Dosage Adjustment

Aplenzin max dose: 174 mg in severe cirrhosis patients

ADMINISTRATION

Oral

- Give with meals to decrease incidence of nausea and vomiting.
- Ensure that extended release and sustained release tablets are not chewed or crushed. They **must be** swallowed whole.
- Store away from heat, direct light, and moisture.

B

ADVERSE EFFECTS (≥1%) **Body as a Whole:** Weight loss, weight gain. **CNS:** Seizures. The risk of seizure appears to be strongly associated with dose (especially greater than 450 mg/day) and may be increased by predisposing factors (e.g., head trauma, CNS tumor) or a history of prior seizure; *agitation, insomnia, dry mouth, blurred vision, headache, dizziness, tremor.* **GI:** *Nausea, vomiting, constipation.* **CV:** Tachycardia. **Skin:** Rash.

INTERACTIONS Drug: May increase metabolism of **carbamazepine, cimetidine, phenytoin, phenobarbital,** decreasing their effect; may increase incidence of adverse effects of **levodopa,** MAO INHIBITORS.

PHARMACOKINETICS Absorption: Readily from GI tract. **Onset:** 3–4 wk. **Peak:** 1–3 h. **Metabolism:** In liver (including first pass metabolism) to active metabolites by CYP2B6. **Elimination:** 80% in urine as inactive metabolites **Half-Life:** 8–24 h.

NURSING IMPLICATIONS

Assessment & Drug Effects

- Monitor for therapeutic effectiveness. The full antidepressant effect of drug may not be realized for 4 or more weeks.
- Monitor for and report promptly worsening of depression or suicidal ideation.
- Use extreme caution when administering drug to patient with history of seizures, cranial trauma, or other factors predisposing to seizures; during sudden and large increments in dose, seizure potential is increased.
- Report significant restlessness, agitation, anxiety, and insomnia. Symptoms may require treatment or discontinuation of drug.
- Monitor for and report delusions, hallucinations, psychotic episodes, confusion, and paranoia.
- Lab tests: Monitor hepatic and renal function tests while patient is taking this drug.

Patient & Family Education

- Monitor your weight at least weekly. Report significant changes in weight (±5 lb) to physician.
- Minimize or avoid alcohol because it increases the risk of seizures.
- Do not drive or engage in potentially hazardous activities until response to drug is known because judgment or motor and cognitive skills may be impaired.
- Do not abruptly discontinue drug. Gradual dosage reduction may be necessary to prevent adverse effects.
- Do not take any OTC drugs without consulting physician.

BUSPIRONE HYDROCHLORIDE

(byoo-spye'rone)
BuSpar
Classification: ANXIOLYTIC
Therapeutic: ANTIANXIETY
Prototype: Lorazepam
Pregnancy Category: B

AVAILABILITY 5 mg, 10 mg, 15 mg tablets

ACTION & *THERAPEUTIC EFFECT* An anxiolytic that focuses mainly on the brain D_2-dopamine receptors. It has agonist effects on presynaptic dopamine receptors and also a high affinity for serotonin (5-HT_{1A}) receptors. *Antianxiety effect* *is due to serotonin reuptake inhibition and agonist effects on dopamine receptors of the brain.*

USES Management of anxiety disorders and for short-term treatment of generalized anxiety.
UNLABELED USES Adjuvant for nicotine withdrawal, premenstrual syndrome.

CONTRAINDICATIONS Concomitant use of alcohol and buspirone; concomitant use of MAOI therapy. Safety during labor and delivery, lactation, or in children younger than 18 y is not established.
CAUTIOUS USE Moderate to severe renal or hepatic impairment, pregnancy (category B).

ROUTE & DOSAGE

Anxiety
Adult: **PO** 7.5–15 mg/day in divided doses, may increase by 5 mg/day q2–3days as needed (max: 60 mg/day)
Geriatric: **PO** 5 mg b.i.d., may increase to max of 60 mg/day

ADMINISTRATION

Oral
- Give with food to decrease nausea.
- Store at 15°–30° C (59°–86° F) in tightly closed container unless otherwise directed.

ADVERSE EFFECTS (≥1%) **CNS:** Numbness, paresthesia, tremors, *dizziness, headache,* nervousness, *drowsiness,* lightheadedness, dream disturbances, decreased concentration, excitement, mood changes. **CV:** Tachycardia, palpitation. **Special Senses:** Blurred vision. **GI:** *Nausea,* vomiting, dry mouth, abdominal/gastric distress, diarrhea, constipation. **Urogenital:** Urinary frequency, hesitancy. **Musculoskeletal:** Arthralgias. **Respiratory:** Hyperventilation, shortness of breath. **Skin:** Rash, edema, pruritus, flushing, easy bruising, hair loss, dry skin. **Other:** Fatigue, weakness.

DIAGNOSTIC TEST INTERFERENCE Buspirone may increase serum concentrations of ***hepatic aminotransferases (ALT, AST).***

INTERACTIONS **Drug:** May cause hypertension with MAO INHIBITORS, **trazodone,** possible increase in liver transaminases; increased **haloperidol** serum levels. **Food: Grapefruit juice** may increase drug levels. **Herbal: St. John's wort** may increase drug levels.

PHARMACOKINETICS **Absorption:** Readily from GI tract, undergoes first pass metabolism. **Onset:** 5–7 days. **Peak:** 1 h. **Metabolism:** In liver. **Elimination:** 30–63% in urine as metabolites within 24 h. **Half-Life:** 2–4 h.

NURSING IMPLICATIONS

Assessment & Drug Effects
- Monitor for therapeutic effectiveness. Desired response may begin within 7–10 days; however, optimal results take 3–4 wk. Reinforce the importance of continuing treatment to patient.
- Monitor for and report dystonia, motor restlessness, and involuntary repetitious movement of facial or cervical muscle.
- Observe for and report swollen ankles, decreased urinary output, changes in voiding pattern, jaundice, itching, nausea, or vomiting.

Patient & Family Education
- Report any of the following immediately: Involuntary, repetitive

B

movements of face or neck; weakness, nervousness, nightmares, headache, or blurred vision; depression or thoughts of suicide.
- Do not use OTC drugs without advice of the physician while taking buspirone.
- Do not drive or engage in other potentially hazardous activities until response to drug is known.
- Discuss limits of alcohol intake with physician; cautious use is generally advised.

BUSULFAN

(byoo-sul'fan)

Busulfex, Myleran

Classifications: ANTINEOPLASTIC; ALKYLATING AGENT

Therapeutic: ANTINEOPLASTIC

Prototype: Cyclophosphamide

Pregnancy Category: D

AVAILABILITY 2 mg tablets; 6 mg/mL injection

ACTION & *THERAPEUTIC EFFECT* Potent cytotoxic alkylating agent that may be mutagenic or carcinogenic, and cell cycle nonspecific. Reduces total granulocyte mass but has little effect on lymphocytes and platelets except in large doses. May cause widespread epithelial cellular dysplasia severe enough to make it difficult to interpret exfoliative cytologic examinations. *Causes cell death by acting predominantly on slowly proliferating stem cells by inducing cross linkage in DNA, thus blocking replication.*

USES Palliative treatment of chronic myelogenous (myeloid, granulocytic, myelocytic) leukemia for patients no longer responsive to radiation therapy or to previously tried antineoplastics. Does not appreciably extend survival time. Stem cell transplant conditioning.

UNLABELED USES Polycythemia vera, severe thrombocytosis, as adjunct in treatment of myelofibrosis, allogeneic bone transplantation in patients with acute nonlymphocytic leukemia.

CONTRAINDICATIONS Therapy-resistant chronic lymphocytic leukemia; lymphoblastic crisis of chronic myelogenous leukemia; bone marrow depression, immunizations (patient and household members), chickenpox (including recent exposure), herpetic infections; pregnancy (category D), lactation.

CAUTIOUS USE Men and women in childbearing years; hepatic disease; history of gout or urate renal stones; prior irradiation or chemotherapy.

ROUTE & DOSAGE

Chronic Myelogenous Leukemia

Adult: **PO** 4–8 mg/day until maximal clinical and hematologic improvement, may use 1–4 mg/day if remission is shorter than 3 mo

Child: **PO** 0.06–0.12 mg/kg/day or 1.8–4.6 mg/m²

Stem Cell Transplant Conditioning

Adult: **IV** (used with cyclophosphamide) 0.8 mg/kg IBW or ABW (whichever is lower) q6h × 4 days

Obesity Dosage Adjustment

In severely obese patients, use adjusted ideal body weight = IBW + 0.25 × (actual weight − IBW)

B

ADMINISTRATION

Oral

- Give at same time each day.
- Give on an empty stomach to minimize nausea and vomiting.
- Store in tightly capped, light-resistant container at 15°–30° C (59°–86° F), unless otherwise specified.

Intravenous

PREPARE: **Intermittent:** Prepare a volume of NS or D5W IV solution that is 10 times the volume of busulfan needed. ▪ Using a 5 micron nylon filter (supplied), withdraw the needed dose of busulfan. Remove needle and filter and use a new, nonfiltered needle to add busulfan to the IV fluid. (Always add busulfan to IV fluid rather than IV fluid to busulfan.) ▪ Mix by inverting the IV bag several times.

ADMINISTER: **Intermittent:** Infuse via a central venous catheter over 2 h. ▪ Flush line before/after infusion with at least 5 mL D5W or NS.

ADVERSE EFFECTS (≥1%) **Hematologic:** Major toxic effects are related to <u>bone marrow failure; agranulocytosis</u> (rare), pancytopenia, thrombocytopenia, leukopenia, *anemia*. **Urogenital:** Flank pain, renal calculi, uric acid nephropathy, <u>acute renal failure</u>, gynecomastia, testicular atrophy, azoospermia, impotence, sterility in males, ovarian suppression, menstrual changes, amenorrhea (potentially irreversible), menopausal symptoms. **Respiratory:** Irreversible <u>pulmonary fibrosis</u> ("busulfan lung"). **Skin:** Alopecia, hyperpigmentation. **Other:** Endocardial fibrosis, dizziness, cholestatic jaundice, infections.

DIAGNOSTIC TEST INTERFERENCE Busulfan may decrease ***urinary 17-OHCS*** excretion, and may increase ***blood and urine uric acid*** levels. Drug-induced cellular dysplasia may interfere with interpretation of ***cytologic studies.***

INTERACTIONS Drug: Probenecid, sulfinpyrazone may increase uric acid levels.

PHARMACOKINETICS Absorption: Readily from GI tract. **Peak:** 4 h. **Duration:** 4 h. **Metabolism:** In liver by CYP3A4. **Elimination:** 10–50% in urine within 48 h.

NURSING IMPLICATIONS

Assessment & Drug Effects

- Monitor the following: Vital signs, weight, I&O ratio and pattern. Urge patient to increase fluid intake to 10–12 (8 oz) glasses daily (if allowed) to assure adequate urinary output.
- Monitor for and report symptoms suggestive of superinfection (see Appendix F), particularly when patient develops leukopenia.
- Lab test: Baseline Hgb, Hct, WBC with differential, platelet count, liver function, kidney function, serum uric acid; repeat at least weekly.
- Avoid invasive procedures during periods of platelet count depression.

Patient & Family Education

- Report to physician any of the following: Easy bruising or bleeding, cloudy or pink urine, dark or black stools; sore mouth or throat, unusual fatigue, blurred vision, flank or joint pain, swelling of lower legs and feet; yellowing white of eye, dark urine, light-colored stools,

B

abdominal discomfort, or itching (hepatotoxicity).

- Use contraceptive measures during busulfan therapy and for at least 3 mo after drug is withdrawn.

BUTABARBITAL SODIUM

(byoo-ta-bar′bi-tal)

Butisol Sodium

Classifications: BARBITURATE; ANXIOLYTIC; SEDATIVE-HYPNOTIC

Therapeutic: ANTIANXIETY; SEDATIVE-HYPNOTIC

Prototype: Phenobarbital

Pregnancy Category: C

Controlled Substance: Schedule III

AVAILABILITY 30 mg, 50 mg tablets; 30 mg/5 mL elixir

ACTION & *THERAPEUTIC EFFECT* Intermediate-acting barbiturate that appears to act at thalamus level, where it interferes with transmission of impulses to the cerebral cortex. *Preoperative sedative agent that also is an effective antianxiety agent.*

USES Hypnotic in short-term treatment of simple insomnia, as sedative for relief of anxiety, and to provide sedation preoperatively.

CONTRAINDICATIONS Porphyria; uncontrolled pain; severe respiratory disease; history of addiction; lactation.

CAUTIOUS USE Severe renal or hepatic impairment; acute abdominal conditions; head trauma, history of seizures; history of herpes infection; older adults or debilitated patients; pregnancy (category C).

ROUTE & DOSAGE

Daytime Sedation

Adult: **PO** 15–30 mg t.i.d. or q.i.d.

Preoperative Sedation

Adult: **PO** 50–100 mg 60–90 min before surgery

Child: **PO** 2–6 mg/kg/dose (max: 100 mg)

Hypnotic

Adult: **PO** 50–100 mg at bedtime

ADMINISTRATION

Oral

- Schedule slow withdrawal following long-term use to avoid precipitating withdrawal symptoms.
- Store in tightly covered containers, preferably at 15°–30° C (59°–86° F), unless otherwise directed.

ADVERSE EFFECTS (≥1%) **CNS:** Drowsiness, ***residual sedation*** ("hangover"), headache. **GI:** Nausea, vomiting, constipation, diarrhea. **Skin:** Urticaria, skin rash. **Musculoskeletal:** Muscle or joint pain.

INTERACTIONS Drug: Alcohol and other CNS DEPRESSANTS add to CNS and respiratory depression; butabarbital increases the metabolism of ORAL ANTICOAGULANTS, BETA-BLOCKERS, CORTICOSTEROIDS, **doxycycline, griseofulvin, quinidine,** THEOPHYLLINES, ORAL CONTRACEPTIVES, decreasing their effectiveness. **Herbal: Kava, valerian** may potentiate sedation.

PHARMACOKINETICS Absorption: Readily from GI tract. **Onset:** 40–60 min. **Peak:** 3–4 h. **Duration:** 6–8 h. **Distribution:** Crosses placenta; distributed into breast milk. **Metabo-**

lism: In liver. **Elimination:** In urine primarily as metabolites. **Half-Life:** Average 100 h.

NURSING IMPLICATIONS

Assessment & Drug Effects

- Assess for adverse effects. Older adults and debilitated patients sometimes manifest excitement, confusion, or depression. Children also may react with paradoxical excitement. Side rails may be advisable. Report these reactions to physician.

Patient & Family Education

- Do not drive or engage in other potentially hazardous activities until response to drug is known.
- Do not drink alcoholic beverages while taking this drug. Other CNS depressants may produce additive drowsiness; do not take without approval of physician.
- Note: Prolonged use is not recommended because tolerance to drug occurs in about 14 days.

BUTENAFINE HYDROCHLORIDE

(bu-ten'a-feen)

Lotrimin Ultra, Mentax

Classification: ANTIFUNGAL ANTIBIOTIC

Therapeutic: ANTIFUNGAL

Prototype: Terbinafine

Pregnancy Category: B

AVAILABILITY 1% cream

ACTION & *THERAPEUTIC EFFECT*

Exerts antifungal action by inhibiting fungal sterol synthesis that is needed in formation of the fungal cell membrane. *Antifungal effectiveness against interdigital tinea pedis (athlete's foot), tinea corporis (ringworm), and tinea cruris (jock itch).*

USES Treatment of tinea pedis, tinea corporis, and tinea cruris due to *Epidermophyton floccosum, Trichophyton mentagrophytes, Trichophyton rubrum.*

CONTRAINDICATIONS Hypersensitivity to butenafine; ophthalmic or vaginal administration.

CAUTIOUS USE Hypersensitivity to naftifine or tolnaftate; pregnancy (category B); lactation. Safety and efficacy in children younger than 12 y are not established.

ROUTE & DOSAGE

Tinea Pedis

Adult/Child (older than 12 y): **Topical** Apply to affected area and surrounding skin b.i.d. × 7 days or daily × 4 wk

Tinea Corporis, Tinea Cruris

Adult/Child (younger than 12 y): **Topical** Apply to affected area and surrounding skin once daily

ADMINISTRATION

Topical

- Apply sufficient cream to cover affected skin and surrounding areas.
- Do not use occlusive dressing unless specifically directed to do so.
- Store at 5°–30° C (41°–86° F).

ADVERSE EFFECTS (≥1%) **Skin:** Burning/stinging at application site, contact dermatitis, erythema, irritation, itching.

NURSING IMPLICATIONS

Assessment & Drug Effects

- Note: 2–4 wk of therapy are usually required for effective treatment.

Patient & Family Education

- Discontinue medication and notify physician if irritation or sensitivity develops.
- Avoid contact with mucous membranes.
- Wash hands thoroughly before and after application of cream.

BUTOCONAZOLE NITRATE

(byoo-toe-koe′na-zole)

Femstat 3, Gynazole 1

Classification: AZOLE ANTIFUNGAL ANTIBIOTIC

Therapeutic: ANTIFUNGAL

Prototype: Fluconazole

Pregnancy Category: C

AVAILABILITY 2% cream

ACTION & *THERAPEUTIC EFFECT* Imidazole derivative with antifungal activity. Alters fungal cell membrane permeability, permitting loss of phosphorous compounds, potassium, and other essential intracellular constituents with consequent loss of ability to replicate. Action takes place primarily on medicated infected surface tissues. *Has fungicidal effect as well as effectiveness against some gram-positive bacteria.*

USES Local treatment of vulvovaginal candidiasis.

CONTRAINDICATIONS Safety in children younger than 12 y is not established.

CAUTIOUS USE Hypersensitivity to azole antifungals; HIV patients; diabetes mellitus; pregnancy (category C), lactation.

ROUTE & DOSAGE

Vulvovaginal Candidiasis

Adult: **Topical** 1 applicator full intravaginally at bedtime for 3 days, may be extended another 3 days if needed

Pregnant women: **Topical** 1 applicator full intravaginally at bedtime for 6 days

ADMINISTRATION

Topical Intravaginal

- Continue treatment even during menstruation.
- Store medication at 15°–30° C (59°–86° F); avoid extreme temperature and freezing.

ADVERSE EFFECTS (≥1%) **Urogenital:** Vulvar or vaginal burning, vulvar itching, discharge, soreness, swelling; urinary frequency and burning. **Skin:** Itching of fingers. **CNS:** Headache.

PHARMACOKINETICS Absorption: Small amount absorbed systemically from intravaginal administration. **Distribution:** Crosses placenta in animals. **Metabolism:** In liver. **Elimination:** In both urine and feces within 4–7 days. **Half-Life:** 21–24 h.

NURSING IMPLICATIONS

Assessment & Drug Effects

- Monitor for therapeutic effectiveness. Candidiasis in nonpregnant women is usually controlled in 3 days.

Patient & Family Education

- Take medication exactly as prescribed; do not increase or decrease dosage or discontinue or extend treatment period. Contact physician if symptoms (vaginal burning, discharge, or itching) persist; drug may be discontinued if acute irritation occurs.
- Patient's sexual partner should wear a condom during intercourse.

BUTORPHANOL TARTRATE

(byoo-tor'fa-nole)

Stadol, Stadol NS

Classifications: ANALGESIC; NARCOTIC (OPIATE AGONIST-ANTAGONIST)

Therapeutic: NARCOTIC ANALGESIC

Prototype: Pentazocine

Pregnancy Category: C

Controlled Substance: Schedule IV

AVAILABILITY 1 mg/mL, 2 mg/mL injection; 10 mg/mL spray

ACTION & *THERAPEUTIC EFFECT* Synthetic, centrally acting analgesic with mixed narcotic agonist and antagonist actions. Acts as agonist on one type of opioid receptor and as a competitive antagonist at others. Site of analgesic action believed to be subcortical, possibly in the limbic system. Respiratory depression does not increase appreciably with higher doses, as it does with morphine, but duration of action increases. *Narcotic analgesic that relieves moderate to severe pain with apparently low potential for physical dependence.*

USES Relief of moderate to severe pain, preoperative or preanesthetic sedation and analgesia, obstetric analgesia during labor, cancer pain, renal colic, burns.

UNLABELED USES Musculoskeletal and post-episiotomy pain.

CONTRAINDICATIONS Narcotic-dependent patients; opiate agonist hypersensitivity. Safety in children younger than 18 y is not established.

CAUTIOUS USE History of drug abuse or dependence; emotionally unstable individuals; head injury, increased intracranial pressure; acute MI, ventricular dysfunction, coronary insufficiency, hypertension; patients undergoing biliary tract surgery; respiratory depression, bronchial asthma, obstructive respiratory disease; and renal or hepatic dysfunction; prior to labor, pregnancy (category C).

ROUTE & DOSAGE

Pain Relief

Adult: **IM** 1–4 mg q3–4h as needed (max: 4 mg/dose) **IV** 0.5–2 mg q3–4h as needed
Geriatric: **IM/IV** 0.25–1 mg q6–8h **Intranasal** 1 mg (1 spray) in one nostril, may repeat in 90 sec, then may repeat these 2 doses q3–4h prn

Adjunct to Balanced Anesthesia

Adult: **IV** 2 mg before induction or 0.5–1 mg in increments during anesthesia

B

Labor

Adult: **IV/IM** 1–2 mg may repeat in 4 h

Renal Impairment Dosage Adjustment

For GFR less than 10 mL/min, use 50% of dose

Hepatic Impairment Dosage Adjustment

Use half normal dose and at least 6 h interval

ADMINISTRATION

Intranasal

- Give 1 spray into one nostril only. One spray provides a 1 mg dose.

Intramuscular

- Give preoperative IM injection 60–90 min before surgery.

Intravenous

PREPARE: **Direct:** Give undiluted.
ADMINISTER: **Direct:** Give at a rate of 2 mg over 3–5 min.
INCOMPATIBILITIES **Y-site: Amphotericin B cholesteryl, lansoprazole, midazolam.**

- Store at 15°–30° C (59°–86° F) unless otherwise directed. Protect from light.

ADVERSE EFFECTS (≥1%) **CNS:** Drowsiness, *sedation,* headache, vertigo, dizziness, floating feeling, weakness, lethargy, confusion, lightheadedness, insomnia, nervousness, <u>respiratory depression</u>. **CV:** Palpitation, bradycardia. **GI:** Nausea. **Skin:** Clammy skin, tingling sensation, flushing and warmth, cyanosis of extremities, diaphoresis, sensitivity to cold, urticaria, pruritus. **Genitourinary:** Difficulty in urinating, biliary spasm.

INTERACTIONS Drug: Alcohol and other CNS DEPRESSANTS augment CNS and respiratory depression.

PHARMACOKINETICS Onset: 10–30 min IM; 1 min IV. **Peak:** 0.5–1 h IM; 4–5 min IV. **Duration:** 3–4 h IM; 2–4 h IV. **Distribution:** Crosses placenta; distributed into breast milk. **Metabolism:** In liver in inactive metabolites. **Elimination:** Primarily in urine. **Half-Life:** 3–4 h.

NURSING IMPLICATIONS

Assessment & Drug Effects

- Monitor for respiratory depression. Do not administer drug if respiratory rate is less than 12 breaths/min.
- Monitor vital signs. Report marked changes in BP or bradycardia.
- Note: If used during labor or delivery, observe neonate for signs of respiratory depression.
- Note: Drug can induce acute withdrawal symptoms in opiate-dependent patients.
- Drug is usually withdrawn gradually following chronic administration. Abrupt withdrawal may produce vomiting, loss of appetite, restlessness, abdominal cramps, increase in BP and temperature, mydriasis, faintness. Withdrawal symptoms peak 48 h after discontinuation of drug.

Patient & Family Education

- Lie down to control drug-induced nausea.
- Do not take alcohol or other CNS depressants with this drug without consulting physician because of possible additive effects.
- Do not drive or engage in other potentially hazardous activities until response to drug is known.

CABERGOLINE

(ka-ber′go-leen)

Dostinex

Classifications: ERGOT ALKALOID; DOPAMINE RECEPTOR AGONIST

Therapeutic: ERGOT ALKALOID; ANTIPARKINSON

Prototype: Ergotamine

Pregnancy Category: B

AVAILABILITY 0.5 mg tablets

ACTION & *THERAPEUTIC EFFECT* Cabergoline is a synthetic ergot derivative, long-acting dopamine receptor agonist with a high affinity for D_2 receptors in the anterior pituitary. It also suppresses prolactin secretion. *Cabergoline inhibits both puerperal lactation and pathologic hyperprolactinemia. Exhibits antiparkinsonism effects due to increased levels of dopamine.*

USES Treatment of hyperprolactinemia (idiopathic or secondary to pituitary adenomas).

UNLABELED USES Treatment of Parkinson's disease.

CONTRAINDICATIONS Uncontrolled hypertension and hypersensitivity to ergot derivatives; pregnancy-induced hypertension, preeclampsia, eclampsia, lactation.

CAUTIOUS USE Hepatic function impairment; elderly, psychosis; pregnancy (category B). Safety and efficacy in pediatric patients are unknown.

ROUTE & DOSAGE

Hyperprolactinemia

Adult: **PO** Start with 0.25 mg 2 times/wk, may increase by 0.25 mg 2 times/wk to a max of 1 mg 2 times/wk

Parkinson's Disease

Adult: **PO** Start with 0.5 mg daily, may increase up to 2.5 mg daily (max: 5 mg/day)

ADMINISTRATION

Oral

- Give on same days each week.

ADVERSE EFFECTS (≥1%) **Body as a Whole:** Asthenia, fatigue, hot flashes. **CV:** Postural hypotension. **GI:** *Nausea, constipation,* abdominal pain, dyspepsia, vomiting, dry mouth, diarrhea, flatulence. **Endocrine:** Breast pain, dysmenorrhea. **CNS:** *Headache, dizziness,* paresthesia, somnolence, depression, nervousness.

INTERACTIONS **Drug:** Concurrent use with PHENOTHIAZINES, BUTYROPHENONES, THIOXANTHINES, and **metoclopramide** decreases therapeutic effects of both drugs.

PHARMACOKINETICS **Absorption:** Rapidly absorbed in GI tract, undergoes first-pass metabolism. **Peak:** 2–3 h. **Distribution:** 40–42% protein bound. Crosses placenta. **Metabolism:** Extensively metabolized. **Elimination:** Approximately 22% in urine, 60% in feces. **Half-Life:** 63–69 h.

NURSING IMPLICATIONS

Assessment & Drug Effects

- Lab tests: Monitor serum prolactin levels to assess response to each dosing level.
- Monitor for hypotension, especially when given with other drugs known to lower BP.

Patient & Family Education

- Discontinue this drug once physician advises that serum prolactin level has been maintained for 6 mo.

C

CAFFEINE

(kaf-een′)

Caffedrine, Dexitac, NoDoz, Quick Pep, S-250, Tirend, Vivarin

CAFFEINE AND SODIUM BENZOATE

CITRATED CAFFEINE

Cafcit

Classifications: RESPIRATORY AND CEREBRAL STIMULANT; XANTHINE

Therapeutic: RESPIRATORY AND CEREBRAL STIMULANT

Pregnancy Category: C

AVAILABILITY 100 mg, 150 mg, 200 mg tablets; 200 mg capsules; 10 mg/mL caffeine citrate oral solution; 10 mg/mL caffeine citrate injection

ACTION & *THERAPEUTIC EFFECT* Chief action is thought to be related to inhibition of the enzyme phosphodiesterase, which results in higher concentrations of cyclic AMP. Releases epinephrine and norepinephrine from adrenal medulla, producing CNS stimulation. Small doses improve psychic and sensory awareness and reduce drowsiness and fatigue by stimulating cerebral cortex. Higher doses stimulate medullary, respiratory, vasomotor, and vagal centers. Produces smooth muscle relaxation by direct action on vascular musculature. Mild diuretic action may result from increase in renal blood flow and glomerular filtration rate and decrease in renal tubular reabsorption of sodium and water. *Effective in managing neonatal apnea, and as an adjuvant for pain control in headaches and following dural puncture. Relief of headache is perhaps due to mild cerebral vasoconstriction action and increased vascular tone. It acts as a bronchodilator in asthma.*

USES Orally as a mild CNS stimulant to aid in staying awake and restoring mental alertness, and as an adjunct in narcotic and nonnarcotic analgesia. Used parenterally as an emergency stimulant in acute circulatory failure, as a diuretic, and for neonatal apnea.

UNLABELED USES Topical treatment of atopic dermatitis; to releave spinal puncture headache.

CONTRAINDICATIONS Acute MI, symptomatic cardiac arrhythmias, palpitations; peptic ulcer; pulmonary disease; insomnia, panic attacks. Safe use (**OTC**) in children under 12 y not established.

CAUTIOUS USE Diabetes mellitus; hiatal hernia; psychotic disorders; dementia; depressive disorders; hepatic disease; hypertension with heart disease; pregnancy (category C), lactation.

ROUTE & DOSAGE

Mental Stimulant

Adult: **PO** 100–200 mg q3–4h prn

Circulatory Stimulant

Adult: **IM** 200–500 mg prn

Apnea of Prematurity (Caffeine Citrate Only)

Neonate (28–33 wk gestation): **PO/IV** 20 mg/kg (loading dose); then, after 24 h, 5 mg/kg/day

ADMINISTRATION

Oral

- Powdered form may be dissolved in the patient's liquid of choice.

C

Intramuscular
- Give deep IM into a large muscle.

Intravenous
Note: IV route reserved for emergency situations only.

PREPARE: **IV Infusion:** May be diluted for infusion in D5W.

ADMINISTER: **IV Infusion:** A syringe infusion pump is recommended. ▪ Give loading dose over 30 min and maintenance dose over at least 10 min.

INCOMPATIBILITIES **Y-site: Acyclovir, furosemide, lorazepam, nitroglycerin, oxacillin, pantoprazole.**

ADVERSE EFFECTS (≥1%) **CV:** Tingling of face, flushing, palpitation, tachycardia, arrhythmia, angina, ventricular ectopic beats. **GI:** Nausea, vomiting; epigastric discomfort, gastric irritation (oral form), diarrhea, hematemesis, kernicterus (neonates). **CNS:** *Nervousness, insomnia,* restlessness, irritability, confusion, agitation, fasciculations, delirium, twitching, tremors, clonic convulsions. **Respiratory:** Tachypnea. **Special Senses:** Scintillating scotomas, tinnitus. **Urogenital:** Increased urination, diuresis.

DIAGNOSTIC TEST INTERFERENCE Caffeine reportedly may interfere with diagnosis of pheochromocytoma or neuroblastoma by increasing urinary excretion of ***catecholamines, VMA,*** and ***5-HIAA*** and may cause false positive increases in ***serum urate*** (by ***Bittner method***).

INTERACTIONS Drug: Increases effects of **cimetidine;** increases cardiovascular stimulating effects of BETA-ADRENERGIC AGONISTS; possibly increases **theophylline** toxicity.

PHARMACOKINETICS Absorption: Rapid. **Peak:** 15–45 min. **Distribution:** Widely throughout body; crosses blood–brain barrier and placenta. **Metabolism:** In liver. **Elimination:** In urine as metabolites; excreted in breast milk in small amounts. **Half-Life:** 3–5 h in adults, 36–144 h in neonates.

NURSING IMPLICATIONS

Assessment & Drug Effects
- Monitor vital signs closely as large doses may cause intensification rather than reversal of severe drug-induced depressions.
- Observe children closely following administration as they are more susceptible than adults to the CNS effects of caffeine.
- Lab tests: Monitor blood glucose and HbA1c levels in diabetics.

Patient & Family Education
- Caffeine in large amounts may impair glucose tolerance in diabetics.
- Do not consume large amounts of caffeine as headache, dizziness, anxiety, irritability, nervousness, and muscle tension may result from excessive use, as well as from abrupt withdrawal of coffee (or oral caffeine). Withdrawal symptoms usually occur 12–18 h following last coffee intake.

CALCIPOTRIENE
(cal-ci′po-tri-een)

Dovonex

Classification: VITAMIN D ANALOG

Therapeutic: VITAMIN D ANALOG

Prototype: Calcitriol

Pregnancy Category: C

AVAILABILITY 0.005% ointment and cream

ACTION & *THERAPEUTIC EFFECT* Calcipotriene is a synthetic vitamin D_3 analog for the treatment of

C

moderate plaque psoriasis. *Calcipotriene controls psoriasis by inhibiting proliferation of psoiatic skin, reducing the number of polymorphonuclear leukocytes (PMNs) in the skin cells, and decreasing the number of epithelial cells.*

USES Treatment of moderate plaque psoriasis.

CONTRAINDICATIONS Hypersensitivity to calcipotriene, hypercalcemia or vitamin D toxicity, lactation.

CAUTIOUS USE History of nephrolithiasis; dermatoses other than psoriasis; patients older than 65 y; pregnancy (category C). Safety and efficacy in children not established.

ROUTE & DOSAGE

Adult: **Topical** Apply a thin layer to affected area once or twice daily

ADMINISTRATION

Topical

- A thin layer should be applied to the affected skin and rubbed in gently and completely.
- Calcipotriene should not be applied to the face.
- Wash hands before and after application of medication.

ADVERSE EFFECTS (≥1%) **Skin:** Facial dermatitis, burning, stinging, erythema, folliculitis, mild transient itching.

INTERACTIONS No clinically significant interactions established.

PHARMACOKINETICS Absorption: 6% absorbed systemically. **Onset:** 1 wk. **Peak:** 8 wk. **Duration:** 4 wk. **Metabolism:** Recycled via liver. **Elimination:** In bile.

NURSING IMPLICATIONS

Assessment & Drug Effects

- Observe reductions in scaling, erythema, and lesion thickness indicating a positive therapeutic response.
- Significant reduction in psoriatic lesions usually occurs following 1 wk of treatment. Marked improvement is generally noted by the 8th wk of treatment.
- Lab tests: Monitor periodically serum calcium, phosphate, and calcitriol levels during long-term therapy.

Patient & Family Education

- Treatment with calcipotriene may be indefinite, as reappearance of psoriatic lesions is common following discontinuation of the drug.
- Adverse effects may include burning and stinging with drug application; these are usually transient.
- Do not mix calcipotriene with any other topical medicine.
- Report appearance of facial dermatitis (redness and scaling around mouth and nose).

CALCITONIN (SALMON)

Fortical, Miacalcin

Classification: BONE METABOLISM REGULATOR

Therapeutic: BONE METABOLISM REGULATOR

Pregnancy Category: C

AVAILABILITY 200 international units/mL injection; 200 international units/spray

ACTION & *THERAPEUTIC EFFECT* Calcitonin opposes the effects of parathyroid hormone on bone and kidneys, reduces serum calcium by binding to a specific receptor site on osteoclast cell membrane, and alters transmembrane passage of calcium and phosphorus. Promotes renal excretion of calcium and phosphorus. *Effective in osteoporosis due to inhibition of bone resorption. Effective in symptomatic hypercalcemia by rapidly lowering serum calcium.*

USES Symptomatic Paget's disease of bone (osteitis deformans), postmenopausal osteoporosis. Orphan drug approval (calcitonin human): Short-term adjunctive treatment of severe hypercalcemic emergencies.

UNLABELED USES Diagnosis and management of medullary carcinoma of thyroid; treatment of osteogenesis imperfecta.

CONTRAINDICATIONS Hypersensitivity to fish proteins or to calcitonin; hypocalcemia. Safe use in children under 12 y not established.

CAUTIOUS USE Renal impairment; osteoporosis; pernicious anemia; Zollinger-Ellison syndrome; pregnancy (category C), lactation.

ROUTE & DOSAGE

Paget's Disease

Adult: **Subcutaneous/IM** 100 international units/day, may decrease to 50–100 international units/day or every other day

Hypercalcemia

Adult: **Subcutaneous/IM** 4 international units/kg q12h, may increase to 8 international units/kg q6h if needed

Postmenopausal Osteoporosis

Adult: **Subcutaneous/IM** 100 international units/day **Intranasal** 1 spray (200 international units) daily, alternate nostrils

ADMINISTRATION

Allergy Test Dose

- An allergy skin test is usually done prior to initiation of therapy. The appearance of more than mild erythema or wheal 15 min after intracutaneous injection indicates that the drug should not be given.

Intranasal

- Activate the pump prior to first use; hold bottle upright and depress white side arms 6 times.
- The nasal spray is administered in one nostril daily; alternate nostrils.

Subcutaneous

- Calcitonin human is administered only by subcutaneous injection; calcitonin salmon may be administered by subcutaneous or IM injection.

Intramuscular

- Use IM route when the volume to be injected is greater than 2 mL.
- Rotate injection sites.
- Store calcitonin (human) at or below 25° C (77° F), protected from light, unless otherwise specified by manufacturer.
- Store calcitonin (salmon) in refrigerator, preferably at 2°–8° C (36°–46° F) unless otherwise directed.

ADVERSE EFFECTS (≥1%) **Body as a Whole:** Headache, eye pain, feverish sensation, hypersensitivity reactions, <u>anaphylaxis</u>. Reported for calcitonin human only: Urinary frequency, chills, chest pressure, weakness, paresthesias, tender palms and soles, dizziness, nasal congestion, shortness of breath. **GI:** *Transient nausea,* vomiting, anorexia, unusual taste sensation, abdominal pain, diarrhea. **Skin:** Inflammatory reactions at injection site, flushing of face or hands, pruritus of earlobes, edema of feet, skin rashes. **Urogenital:** Nocturia, diuresis, abnormal urine sediment.

C

INTERACTIONS Drug: May decrease serum **lithium** levels.

PHARMACOKINETICS Onset: 15 min. **Peak:** 4 h. **Duration:** 8–24 h. **Distribution:** Does not cross placenta; distribution into breast milk unknown. **Metabolism:** In kidneys. **Elimination:** In urine. **Half-Life:** 1.25 h.

NURSING IMPLICATIONS

Assessment & Drug Effects

- Have readily available parenteral calcium, particularly during early therapy. Hypocalcemic tetany is a theoretical possibility.
- Examine urine specimens periodically for sediment with long-term therapy.
- Lab tests: Monitor for hypocalcemia (see Signs & Symptoms, Appendix F). Theoretically, calcitonin can lead to hypocalcemic tetany. Latent tetany may be demonstrated by Chvostek's or Trousseau's signs and by serum calcium values: 7–8 mg/dL (latent tetany); below 7 mg/dL (manifest tetany).
- Examine nasal passages prior to treatment with the nasal spray and anytime nasal irritation occurs.
- Nasal ulceration or heavy bleeding are indications for drug discontinuation.

Patient & Family Education

- Watch for redness, warmth, or swelling at injection site and report to physician, as these may indicate an inflammatory reaction. The transient flushing that commonly occurs following injection of calcitonin, particularly during early therapy, may be minimized by administering the drug at bedtime. Consult physician.
- Maintain your drug regimen to prevent early relapses even though symptoms have improved.
- Ensure that you feel comfortable using the nasal pump properly. Notify physician if significant nasal irritation occurs.
- Consult physician before using OTC preparations. Some supervitamins, hematinics, and antacids contain calcium and vitamin D (vitamin may antagonize calcitonin effects).

CALCITRIOL (Pr)

(kal-si-trye′ole)

Calcijex, Rocaltrol

Classification: VITAMIN D ANALOG

Therapeutic: VITAMIN D ANALOG

Pregnancy Category: C

AVAILABILITY 0.25 mcg, 0.5 mcg tablets; 1 mcg/mL oral solution; 1 mcg/mL, 2 mcg/mL injection

ACTION & *THERAPEUTIC EFFECT*
Synthetic form of an active metabolite of ergocalciferol (vitamin D_2). In the liver, cholecalciferol (vitamin D_3) and ergocalciferol (vitamin D_2) are enzymatically metabolized to calcifediol, an activated form of vitamin D_3 in the kidney. Patients with nonfunctioning kidneys are unable to synthesize sufficient calcitriol. *By promoting intestinal absorption and renal retention of calcium, calcitriol elevates serum calcium levels, decreases elevated blood levels of phosphate and parathyroid hormone. Thus it decreases subperiosteal bone resorption and mineralization defects.*

USES Management of hypocalcemia in patients undergoing chronic renal dialysis and in patients with hypoparathyroidism or pseudohypoparathyroidism. Patients with hyperparathyroidism in moderate to severe chronic renal failure not on dialysis.

UNLABELED USES Selected patients with vitamin D–dependent rickets, familial hypophosphatemia (vitamin D–resistant rickets); management of hypocalcemia in premature infants.

CONTRAINDICATIONS Hypercalcemia or vitamin D toxicity.

CAUTIOUS USE Hyperphosphatemia, renal failure; elderly; sarcoidosis; patients receiving digitalis glycosides; pregnancy (category C).

ROUTE & DOSAGE

Hypocalcemia

Adult: **PO** 0.25 mcg/day, may be increased by 0.25 mcg/day q4–8wk for dialysis patients or q2–4wk for hypoparathyroid patients if necessary **IV** 0.5 mcg 3 times/wk at the end of dialysis, may need up to 3 mcg 3 times/wk
Child: **PO** *On hemodialysis:* 0.25–2 mcg/day **IV** 0.01–0.05 mcg/kg 3 times/wk **PO** *Renal failure without dialysis:* 0.014–0.041 mcg/kg/day

ADMINISTRATION

Oral

- Oral dose can be taken either with food or milk or on an empty stomach. Discuss with physician.
- When given for hypoparathyroidism, the dose is given in the morning.
- Capsules should be protected from heat, light, and moisture. Store in tightly closed container.

Intravenous

PREPARE: **Direct:** Give undiluted.
ADMINISTER: **Direct:** Give IV push over 30–60 sec.

ADVERSE EFFECTS (≥1%) **Body as a Whole:** Muscle or bone pain. **CV:** Palpitation. **GI:** Anorexia, nausea, vomiting, dry mouth, thirst, constipation, abdominal cramps, metallic taste. **Metabolic:** Vitamin D intoxication, hypercalcemia, hypercalciuria, hyperphosphatemia. **CNS:** Headache, weakness. **Special Senses:** Blurred vision, photophobia. **Urogenital:** Increased urination.

INTERACTIONS Drug: THIAZIDE DIURETICS may cause hypercalcemia; calcifediol-induced hypercalcemia may precipitate digitalis arrhythmias in patients receiving DIGITALIS GLYCOSIDES.

PHARMACOKINETICS Absorption: Readily absorbed from GI tract. **Onset:** 2–6 h. **Peak:** 10–12 h. **Duration:** 3–5 days. **Metabolism:** In liver. **Elimination:** Mainly in feces. **Half-Life:** 3–6 h.

NURSING IMPLICATIONS

Assessment & Drug Effects

- Lab tests: Determine baseline and periodic levels of serum calcium, phosphorus, magnesium, alkaline phosphatase, creatinine; measure urinary calcium and phosphorus levels q24h.
- Effectiveness of therapy depends on an adequate daily intake of calcium and phosphate. The physician may prescribe a calcium supplement on an as-needed basis.
- Monitor for hypercalcemia (see Signs & Symptoms, Appendix F). During dosage adjustment period, monitor serum calcium levels particularly twice weekly to avoid hypercalcemia.

C

- If hypercalcemia develops, withhold calcitriol and calcium supplements and notify physician. Drugs may be reinitiated when serum calcium returns to normal.

Patient & Family Education

- Discontinue the drug if experiencing any symptoms of hypercalcemia (see Appendix F) and contact physician.
- Do not use any other source of vitamin D during therapy, since calcitriol is the most potent form of vitamin D_3. This will avoid the possibility of hypercalcemia.
- Consult physician before taking an OTC medication. (Many products contain calcium, vitamin D, phosphates, or magnesium, which can increase adverse effects of calcitriol.)
- Maintain an adequate daily fluid intake unless you have kidney problems, in which case consult your physician about fluids.

CALCIUM CARBONATE

Apo-Cal ♣, BioCal, Calcite-500, Calsan ♣, Cal-Sup, Caltrate ♣, Chooz, Dicarbosil, Equilet, Mallamint, Mega-Cal, Nu-Cal, Os-Cal, Oystercal, Titralac, Tums

CALCIUM ACETATE

PhosLo

CALCIUM CITRATE

Citracal

CALCIUM PHOSPHATE TRIBASIC (TRICALCIUM PHOSPHATE)

Posture

CALCIUM LACTATE

Cal-Lac

Classifications: FLUID AND ELECTROLYTIC REPLACEMENT SOLUTION; ANTACID
Therapeutic: NUTRITIONAL SUPPLEMENT; ANTACID
Prototype: Calcium gluconate
Pregnancy Category: B for calcium acetate; other salts not rated

AVAILABILITY Calcium carbonate: 125 mg, 250 mg, 650 mg, 750 mg, 1.25 g, 1.5 g tablets; **Calcium acetate:** 667 mg tablets; **Calcium citrate:** 950 mg, 2376 mg tablets; **Calcium phosphate tribasic:** 1565.2 mg tablets

ACTION & *THERAPEUTIC EFFECT* Calcium carbonate is a rapid-acting antacid with high neutralizing capacity and relatively prolonged duration of action. Decreases gastric acidity, thereby inhibiting proteolytic action of pepsin on gastric mucosa. All forms of calcium salts are used for calcium replacement therapy. *Effectively relieves symptoms of acid indigestion and useful as a calcium supplement.*

USES Relief of transient symptoms of hyperacidity as in acid indigestion, heartburn, peptic esophagitis, and hiatal hernia. Also used as calcium supplement when calcium intake may be inadequate and in treatment of mild calcium deficiency states. Control of hyperphosphatemia in chronic renal failure (calcium acetate).
UNLABELED USES For treatment of hyperphosphatemia in patients with chronic renal failure and to lower BP in selected patients with hypertension.

CONTRAINDICATIONS Hypercalcemia and hypercalciuria (e.g., hyperparathyroidism, vitamin D overdosage, decalcifying tumors, bone metastases), calcium loss due to immobilization, severe renal failure, renal calculi, GI hemorrhage or obstruction, dehydration, digitalis toxicity; hypochloremic alkalosis, ventricular fibrillation, cardiac disease.

CAUTIOUS USE Decreased bowel motility (e.g., with anticholinergics, antidiarrheals, antispasmodics), the older adult; **Calcium acetate:** pregnancy (category B).

ROUTE & DOSAGE

All doses are in terms of *elemental calcium:* 1 g calcium carbonate = 400 mg (20 mEq, 40%) elemental calcium; 1 g calcium acetate = 250 mg (12.6 mEq, 25%) elemental calcium; 1 g calcium citrate = 210 mg (12 mEq, 21%) elemental calcium; 1 g tricalcium phosphate = 390 mg (19.3 mEq, 39%) elemental calcium; calcium lactate = 130 mg (6.5 mEq, 13%) elemental calcium

Supplement for Osteoporosis

Adult: **PO** 1–2 g b.i.d. or t.i.d.

Antacid

Adult: **PO** 0.5–2 g 4–6 times/day

Hyperphosphatemia

Adult: **PO** Calcium acetate 2–4 tablets with each meal

Supplement for Mild Hypercalcemia

Child: **PO** 500 mg/kg/day in divided doses (lactate)

ADMINISTRATION

Oral

- When used as antacid, give 1 h after meals and at bedtime. When used as calcium supplement, give 1–1½ h after meals, unless otherwise directed by physician.
- Chewable tablet should be chewed well before swallowing or allowed to dissolve completely in mouth, followed with water. Powder form may be mixed with water.
- Ensure that sustained release form of drug is not chewed or crushed. It **must be** swallowed whole.

ADVERSE EFFECTS (≥1%) **GI:** *Constipation* or laxative effect, acid rebound, nausea, eructation, *flatulence,* vomiting, fecal concretions. **Metabolic:** Hypercalcemia with alkalosis, metastatic calcinosis, hypercalciuria, hypomagnesemia, hypophosphatemia (when phosphate intake is low). **CNS:** Mood and mental changes. **Urogenital:** Polyuria, renal calculi.

INTERACTIONS Drug: May enhance inotropic and toxic effects of **digoxin; magnesium** may compete for GI absorption; decreases absorption of TETRACYCLINES, QUINOLONES (**ciprofloxacin**).

PHARMACOKINETICS Absorption: Approximately 1/3 of dose absorbed from small intestine. **Distribution:** Crosses placenta. **Elimination:** Primarily in feces; small amounts in urine, pancreatic juice, saliva, breast milk.

NURSING IMPLICATIONS

Assessment & Drug Effects

- Note number and consistency of stools. If constipation is a problem, physician may prescribe alternate or combination therapy with a magnesium antacid or advise patient to take a laxative or stool softener as necessary.
- Lab tests: Determine serum and urine calcium weekly in patients receiving prolonged therapy and in patients with renal dysfunction.

C

- Record amelioration of symptoms of hypocalcemia (see Signs & Symptoms, Appendix F).
- Observe for S&S of hypercalcemia in patients receiving frequent or high doses, or who have impaired renal function (see Appendix F).

Patient & Family Education

- Do not continue this medication beyond 1–2 wk, since it may cause acid rebound, which generally occurs after repeated use for 1 or 2 wk and leads to chronic use. It is potentially dangerous to self-medicate. Do not take antacids longer than 2 wk without medical supervision.
- Avoid taking calcium carbonate with cereals or other foods high in oxalates. Oxalates combine with calcium carbonate to form insoluble, nonabsorbable compounds.
- Do not use calcium carbonate repeatedly with foods high in vitamin D (such as milk) or sodium bicarbonate, as it may cause milk-alkali syndrome: hypercalcemia, distaste for food, headache, confusion, nausea, vomiting, abdominal pain, metabolic alkalosis, hypercalciuria, polyuria, soft tissue calcification (calcinosis), hyperphosphatemia and renal insufficiency. Predisposing factors include renal dysfunction, dehydration, electrolyte imbalance, and hypertension.

CALCIUM CHLORIDE

Classification: FLUID AND ELECTROLYTIC REPLACEMENT SOLUTION
Therapeutic: FLUID AND ELECTROLYTE REPLACEMENT
Prototype: Calcium gluconate
Pregnancy Category: A; C in high doses

AVAILABILITY 10% injection

ACTION & *THERAPEUTIC EFFECT*
Ionizes readily and provides excess chloride ions that promote acidosis and temporary (1–2 days) diuresis secondary to excretion of sodium. *Rapidly and effectively restores serum calcium levels in acute hypocalcemia of various origins and an effective cardiac stabilizer under conditions of hyperkalemia or resuscitation.*

USES Treatment of cardiac resuscitation when epinephrine fails to improve myocardial contractions; for treatment of acute hypocalcemia (as in tetany due to parathyroid deficiency, vitamin D deficiency, alkalosis, insect bites or stings, and during exchange transfusions), for treatment of hypermagnesemia, and for cardiac disturbances of hyperkalemia.

CONTRAINDICATIONS Ventricular fibrillation, hypercalcemia, digitalis toxicity, injection into myocardium or other tissue.
CAUTIOUS USE Digitalized patients; sarcoidosis, renal insufficiency, history of renal stone formation; cardiac arrhythmias; dehydration; diarrhea; cor pulmonale, respiratory acidosis, respiratory failure; pregnancy (category A; category C in high doses).

ROUTE & DOSAGE

All doses are in terms of *elemental calcium:* 1 g calcium chloride = 272 mg (13.6 mEq) elemental calcium

Hypocalcemia

Adult: **IV** 0.5–1 g (7–14 mEq) at 1–3 day intervals as determined by patient response and serum calcium levels
Child: **IV** 2.7–5 mg/kg administered slowly
Neonate: **IV** Less than 1 mEq/day

C

Hypocalcemic Tetany
Adult: **IV** 4.5–16 mEq prn
Child: **IV** 0.5–0.7 mEq/kg t.i.d. or q.i.d.
Neonate: **IV** 2.4 mEq/kg/day in divided doses

CPR
Adult: **IV** 2–4 mg/kg, may repeat in 10 min
Child: **IV** 20 mg/kg, may repeat in 10 min

ADMINISTRATION

Intravenous

IV administration to neonates, infants, and children: Verify correct IV concentration and rate of infusion with physician.

PREPARE: **Direct:** May be given undiluted or diluted (preferred) with an equal volume of NS for injection. ▪ Solution should be warmed to body temperature before administration.

ADMINISTER: **Direct:** Give at 0.5–1 mL/min or more slowly if irritation develops. Avoid rapid administration. ▪ Use a small-bore needle and inject into a large vein to minimize venous irritation and undesirable reactions.

INCOMPATIBILITIES **Solution/additive: Amphotericin B, chlopheniramine, dobutamine,** concentration-dependent incompatibility with other ELECTROLYTES. **Y-site: Amphotericin B cholesteryl complex, propofol, sodium bicarbonate.**

ADVERSE EFFECTS (≥1%) **Body as a Whole:** Tingling sensation. With rapid IV, sensations of heat waves (peripheral vasodilation), fainting. **CV:** (With rapid infusion) hypotension, bradycardia, cardiac arrhythmias, cardiac arrest. **Skin:** Pain and burning at IV site, severe venous thrombosis, necrosis and sloughing (with extravasation).

INTERACTIONS Drug: May enhance inotropic and toxic effects of **digoxin;** antagonizes the effects of **verapamil** and possibly other CALCIUM CHANNEL BLOCKERS.

PHARMACOKINETICS Distribution: Crosses placenta. **Elimination:** Primarily in feces; small amounts in urine, pancreatic juice, saliva, and breast milk.

NURSING IMPLICATIONS

Assessment & Drug Effects

- Monitor ECG and BP and observe patient closely during administration. IV injection may be accompanied by cutaneous burning sensation and peripheral vasodilation, with moderate fall in BP.
- Advise ambulatory patient to remain in bed for 15–30 min or more depending on response following injection.
- Observe digitalized patients closely since an increase in serum calcium increases risk of digitalis toxicity.
- Lab tests: Determine serum pH, calcium, and other electrolytes frequently as guides to dosage adjustments.

Patient & Family Education

- Remain in bed for 15–30 min or more following injection and depending on response.
- Symptoms of mild hypercalcemia, such as loss of appetite, nausea, vomiting, or constipation may occur. If hypercalcemia becomes severe, call health care provider if feeling confused or extremely excited.
- Do not use other calcium supplements or eat foods high in calcium, like milk, cheese, yogurt,

C

eggs, meats, and some cereals, during therapy.

CALCIUM GLUCONATE Pr

(gloo'koe-nate)

Classification: ELECTROLYTE AND WATER BALANCE

Therapeutic: ELECTROLYTE REPLACEMENT SOLUTION

Pregnancy Category: A; C in high doses

AVAILABILITY 500 mg, 650 mg, 975 mg, 1 g tablets; 10% injection

ACTION & *THERAPEUTIC EFFECT* Calcium gluconate acts like digitalis on the heart, increasing cardiac muscle tone and force of systolic contractions (positive inotropic effect). *Rapidly and effectively restores serum calcium levels in acute hypocalcemia of various origins and effective as a cardiac stabilizer under conditions of hyperkalemia or resuscitation.*

USES Negative calcium balance (as in neonatal tetany, hypoparathyroidism, vitamin D deficiency, alkalosis). Also to overcome cardiac toxicity of hyperkalemia, for cardiopulmonary resuscitation, to prevent hypocalcemia during transfusion of citrated blood. Also as antidote for magnesium sulfate, for acute symptoms of lead colic, to decrease capillary permeability in sensitivity reactions, and to relieve muscle cramps from insect bites or stings. Oral calcium may be used to maintain normal calcium balance during pregnancy, lactation, and childhood growth and to prevent primary osteoporosis. Also in osteoporosis, osteomalacia, chronic hypoparathyroidism, rickets, and as adjunct in treatment of myasthenia gravis and Eaton-Lambert syndrome.

UNLABELED USES To antagonize aminoglycoside-induced neuromuscular blockage, and as "calcium challenge" to diagnose Zollinger-Ellison syndrome and medullary thyroid carcinoma.

CONTRAINDICATIONS Ventricular fibrillation, metastatic bone disease, injection into myocardium; administration by subcutaneous or IM routes; renal calculi, hypercalcemia, predisposition to hypercalcemia (hyperparathyroidism, certain malignancies); digitalis toxicity.

CAUTIOUS USE Digitalized patients, renal or cardiac insufficiency, arrhythmias; dehydration; diarrhea; hyperphosphatemia; sarcoidosis, history of lithiasis, immobilized patients; pregnancy (category A; category C in high doses).

ROUTE & DOSAGE

All doses are in terms of *elemental calcium:* 1 g calcium gluconate = 90 mg (4.5 mEq, 9.3%) elemental calcium

Supplement for Osteoporosis

Adult: **PO** 1–2 g b.i.d. to q.i.d. **IV** 7 mEq q1–3days

Child: **PO** 45–65 mg/kg/day in divided doses **IV** 1–7 mEq q1–3days

Neonate: **PO** 50–130 mg/kg/day (max: 1 g)

Hypocalcemia

Adult: **IV** 2–15 g/day continuous or divided dose

Child: **IV** 200–500 mg/kg/day (max: 2–3 g/dose)

Neonate: **IV** Not more than 0.93 mEq

Hypocalcemic Tetany

Adult: **IV** 1–3 g prn

Child: **IV** 100–200 mg/kg/dose, may repeat q6–8h

C

Neonate: **IV** 200 mg followed by 500 mg/kg/day infusion

CPR

Adult: **IV** 2.3–3.7 mEq x 1

Hyperkalemia with Cardiac Toxicity

Adult: **IV** 500–800 mg (max dose: 3 g)

Exchange Transfusions with Citrated Blood

Adult: **IV** 500–1000 mg for each 500 mL of blood

Neonate: **IV** 98 mg for each 100 mL of blood

ADMINISTRATION

Oral

- Ensure that chewable tablets are chewed or crushed before being swallowed with a liquid.
- Give with meals to enhance absorption.

Intravenous

PREPARE: **Direct:** May be given undiluted. **Intermittent/Continuous:** May be diluted in 1000 mL of NS.

ADMINISTER: **Direct:** Give direct IV at a rate of 0.5 mL or a fraction thereof over 1 min. ▪ Do not exceed 2 mL/min. **Intermittent/Continuous:** Give slowly, not to exceed 200 mg/min for adults or 100 mg/min for children. Use a small-bore needle into a large vein to avoid possibility of extravasation and resultant necrosis. ▪ With children, scalp veins should be avoided. Avoid rapid infusion. ▪ High concentrations of calcium suddenly reaching the heart can cause fatal cardiac arrest.

INCOMPATIBILITIES **Solution/additive: Amphotericin B, cefamandole, dobutamine, methylprednisolone, metoclopramide,** concentration-dependent incompatibility with other ELECTROLYTES. **Y-site: Amphotericin B cholesteryl complex, fluconazole, indomethacin, lansoprazole, meropenem.**

- Injection should be stopped if patient complains of any discomfort.
- Patient should be advised to remain in bed for 15–30 min or more following injection, depending on response.

ADVERSE EFFECTS (≥1%) **Body as a Whole:** Tingling sensation. With rapid IV, sensations of heat waves (peripheral vasodilation), fainting. **GI:** PO preparation: Constipation, increased gastric acid secretion. **CV:** (With rapid infusion) hypotension, bradycardia, cardiac arrhythmias, <u>cardiac arrest</u>. **Skin:** Pain and burning at IV site, severe venous thrombosis, necrosis and sloughing (with extravasation).

DIAGNOSTIC TEST INTERFERENCE IV calcium may cause false decreases in ***serum and urine magnesium*** (by ***Titan yellow method***) and transient elevations of ***plasma 11-OHCS*** levels by ***Glenn-Nelson technique.*** Values usually return to control levels after 60 min; ***urinary steroid values (17-OHCS)*** may be decreased.

INTERACTIONS Drug: May enhance inotropic and toxic effects of **digoxin; magnesium** may compete for GI absorption; decreases absorption of TETRACYCLINES, QUINOLONES (**ciprofloxacin**); antagonizes the effects of **verapamil** and possibly other CALCIUM CHANNEL BLOCKERS (IV administration).

PHARMACOKINETICS Absorption: 30% from small intestine. **Onset:** Immediately after IV. **Distribution:** Crosses placenta. **Elimination:** Primarily in feces; small amounts in urine, pancreatic juice, saliva, and breast milk.

NURSING IMPLICATIONS

Assessment & Drug Effects

- Assess for cutaneous burning sensations and peripheral vasodilation, with moderate fall in BP, during direct IV injection.
- Monitor ECG during IV administration to detect evidence of hypercalcemia: Decreased QT interval associated with inverted T wave.
- Observe IV site closely. Extravasation may result in tissue irritation and necrosis.
- Monitor for hypocalcemia and hypercalcemia (see Signs & Symptoms, Appendix F).
- Lab tests: Determine levels of calcium and phosphorus (tend to vary inversely) and magnesium frequently, during sustained therapy. Deficiencies in other ions, particularly magnesium, frequently coexist with calcium ion depletion.

Patient & Family Education

- Report S&S of hypercalcemia (see Appendix F) promptly to your care provider.
- Milk and milk products are the best sources of calcium (and phosphorus). Other good sources include dark green vegetables, soy beans, tofu, and canned fish with bones.
- Calcium absorption can be inhibited by zinc-rich foods: Nuts, seeds, sprouts, legumes, soy products (tofu).
- Check with physician before self-medicating with a calcium supplement.

CALCIUM POLYCARBOPHIL

(pol-ee-kar'boe-fil)

FiberCon

Classifications: BULK LAXATIVE; ANTIDIARRHEAL

Therapeutic: BULK LAXATIVE; ANTIDIARRHEAL

Prototype: Psyllium hydrophilic mucilloid

Pregnancy Category: A; C in high doses

AVAILABILITY 500 mg, 625 mg tablets

ACTION & *THERAPEUTIC EFFECT* Hydrophilic, bulk-producing laxative that restores normal moisture level and bulk content of intestinal tract. In constipation, retains free water in intestinal lumen, thereby indirectly opposing dehydrating forces of the bowel; in diarrhea, when intestinal mucosa is incapable of absorbing fluid, drug absorbs fecal fluid to form a gel. *Relieves constipation or diarrhea associated with bowel disorders and acute nonspecific diarrhea.*

USES Constipation or diarrhea associated with diverticulitis or irritable bowel syndrome; acute nonspecific diarrhea.

CONTRAINDICATIONS GI obstruction; children younger than 6 y.

CAUTIOUS USE Pregnancy (category A; category C in high doses), lactation.

ROUTE & DOSAGE

Constipation or Diarrhea

Adult: **PO** 1 g q.i.d. as needed (max: 6 g/24 h)

Child: **PO** *6–12 y,* 500 mg 1–3 times/day (max: 3 g/24 h); *younger than 6 y,* 500 mg 1–2 times/day (max: 1.5 g/24 h)

C

ADMINISTRATION

Oral

- Administer with at least 180–240 mL (6–8 oz) water or other fluid of patient's choice when used as a laxative and with at least 60–90 mL (2–3 oz) of fluid when used as an antidiarrheal. Chewed tablets should not be swallowed dry.
- If diarrhea is severe, dose can be repeated every half hour up to maximum daily dose.

ADVERSE EFFECTS (≥1%) **GI:** *Flatulence,* abdominal fullness, intestinal obstruction; laxative dependence (long-term use).

PHARMACOKINETICS Absorption: Not absorbed from the intestine. Bowel movement usually occurs within 12–72 h. **Elimination:** In feces.

NURSING IMPLICATIONS

Assessment & Drug Effects

- Evaluate effectiveness of medication. If it is ineffective as an antidiarrheal, report to physician.
- Report rectal bleeding, very dark stools, or abdominal pain promptly.

Patient & Family Education

- You will likely have a bowel movement within 12–72 h.
- This is an OTC product. Take this drug exactly as ordered. Do not increase the dose if response is inadequate. Consult physician. Do not use other laxatives while you are taking calcium polycarbophil.

CALFACTANT

(cal-fac′tant)

Infasurf

Classification: LUNG SURFACTANT

Therapeutic: LUNG SURFACTANT

Prototype: Beractant

Pregnancy Category: Not applicable

AVAILABILITY 35 mg/mL suspension

ACTION & *THERAPEUTIC EFFECT* Pulmonary surfactant. Lowers the surface tension on alveolar surfaces during respiration and stabilizes the alveoli against collapse at resting pressure. Deficiency of surfactant causes respiratory disease syndrome (RDS) in premature infants. *Effectively relieves and prevents RDS in neonates.*

USES Prevention and treatment of RDS in infants at high risk for RDS.

CONTRAINDICATIONS Bovine protein hypersensitivity; nosocomial infections.

CAUTIOUS USE Lactation.

ROUTE & DOSAGE

Prevention & Treatment of RDS

Infant: **Intratracheal** 3 mL/kg of birth weight administered through an endotracheal tube q12h × 3 doses

ADMINISTRATION

Intratracheal

- Swirl vial to disperse suspension; do not dilute and DO NOT SHAKE. Withdraw with 20-gauge or larger needle. Avoid excess foaming. Instill into the endotracheal tube, preferably within 30 min of birth.
- Stop administration of calfactant if reflux into endotracheal tube occurs as indicated by cyanosis, bradycardia, or other signs of airway obstruction.

ADVERSE EFFECTS (≥1%) **CV:** *Bradycardia.* **Respiratory:** *Cyanosis, airway obstruction, reflux of surfactant* into endotracheal tube.

INTERACTIONS Drug: No clinically significant interactions established.

PHARMACOKINETICS Absorption: Absorbs rapidly to air; liquid interface of lung surface.

NURSING IMPLICATIONS

Assessment & Drug Effects

- Monitor closely during and after administration; adjustments in oxygen therapy and ventilator pressures are usually needed.

Patient & Family Education

- This drug will help baby to breathe properly and support normal respiratory function.

CANDESARTAN CILEXETIL

(can-de-sar′tan ci-lex′e-til)

Atacand

Classification: ANGIOTENSIN II RECEPTOR ANTAGONIST, ANTIHYPERTENSIVE

Therapeutic: ANTIHYPERTENSIVE

Prototype: Losartan

Pregnancy Category: C first trimester; D second and third trimester

AVAILABILITY 4 mg, 8 mg, 16 mg, 32 mg tablets

ACTION & *THERAPEUTIC EFFECT* Angiotensin II receptor (type AT_1) antagonist. Angiotensin II is a potent vasoconstrictor and primary vasoactive hormone of the renin–angiotensin–aldosterone system. Candesartan selectively blocks binding of angiotensin II to the AT_1 receptors found in many tissues (e.g., vascular smooth muscle, adrenal glands). *Results in blocking the vasoconstricting and aldosterone-secreting effects of angiotensin II, resulting in an antihypertensive effect. Effectively lowers BP from hypertensive to normotensive range.*

USES Hypertension, heart failure in conjunction with ACE inhibitor.

CONTRAINDICATIONS Known sensitivity to candesartan or any other angiotensin II (AT_1) receptor antagonist (e.g., losartan, valsartan); primary hyperaldosteronism; bilateral renal artery stenosis; pregnancy (category D second and third trimesters); lactation; children younger than 1 y for hypertension, or children with GFR less than 30 mL/min/1.73 m^2.

CAUTIOUS USE Concurrent administration with high-dose diuretics, potassium-sparing diuretics, or potassium salt substitutes; unilateral renal artery stenosis; aortic or mitral valve stenosis; hypertrophic cardiomyopathy; CHF; diabetes; lactation; moderate heptic or renal impairment, significant renal failure; pregnancy (category C first trimester).

ROUTE & DOSAGE

Hypertension

Adult: **PO** Start at 16 mg daily (range 8–32 mg divided once or twice daily)

Adolescent/Child: **PO** *At least 6 y, weighing more than 50 kg,* 8–16 mg given in single or divided doses; adjust based on response; *at least 6 y, weighing less than 50 kg,* 4–8 mg given in single or divided doses; adjust based on response

Child (1–6 y): **PO** 0.2 mg/kg/day; adjust based on response

Heart Failure

Adult: **PO** Start at 4 mcg once daily, double the dose at 2 wk intervals as tolerated by the patient until a dose of 32 mg is reached

Hepatic Impairment Dosage Adjustment

For patients with moderate hepatic impairment, initiate therapy at lower dose

C

ADMINISTRATION

Oral

- Volume depletion should be corrected prior to initiation of therapy to prevent hypotension.
- Dose is individualized and may be given once or twice daily. The daily dose may be titrated up to 32 mg; larger doses are not likely to provide additional benefit.

ADVERSE EFFECTS (≥1%) **Body as a Whole:** Fatigue, peripheral edema, back pain, arthralgia. **CV:** Chest pain. **GI:** Nausea, abdominal pain, diarrhea, vomiting. **CNS:** Headache, dizziness. **Respiratory:** Cough, sinusitis, upper respiratory infection, pharyngitis, rhinitis. **Urogenital:** Albuminuria.

INTERACTIONS Drug: Use with **lithium** may increase risk of **lithium** toxicity.

PHARMACOKINETICS Absorption: Rapidly from GI tract; activated by ester hydrolysis; 15% reaches systemic circulation. **Peak:** Serum concentration, 3–4 h; therapeutic effect, 2–4 wk. **Duration:** 24 h. **Distribution:** Greater than 99% protein bound; crosses placenta; distributed into breast milk. **Metabolism:** Minimally in liver. **Elimination:** Primarily unchanged in bile (67%) and urine (33%). **Half-Life:** 9 h.

NURSING IMPLICATIONS

Assessment & Drug Effects

- Monitor BP as therapeutic effectiveness is indicated by decreases in systolic and diastolic BP within 2 wk with maximal effect at 4–6 wk.
- Monitor for transient hypotension in volume/salt-depleted patients; if hypotension occurs, place in supine position and notify physician.
- Monitor BP periodically; trough readings, just prior to the next scheduled dose, should be made when possible.
- Lab tests: Periodically monitor BUN and creatinine, serum potassium, liver enzymes, and CBC with differential.

Patient & Family Education

- Inform your physician immediately if you become pregnant.
- You may not notice maximum pressure-lowering effect for 6 wk.
- Report episodes of dizziness especially when making position changes.

CAPECITABINE

(cap-e-si′ta-been)

Xeloda

Classifications: ANTINEOPLASTIC; ANTIMETABOLITE, PYRIMIDINE

Therapeutic: ANTINEOPLASTIC

Prototype: 5-Fluorouracil (5-FU)

Pregnancy Category: D

AVAILABILITY 150 mg, 500 mg tablets

ACTION & *THERAPEUTIC EFFECT* Pyrimidine antagonist and cell cycle-specific antimetabolite. Prodrug of 5-FU. Blocks actions of enzymes essential to normal DNA and RNA synthesis. May become incorporated into RNA molecules of tumor cells, thereby interfering with RNA and protein synthesis. *Reduces or stabilizes tumor size in metastatic breast cancer.*

USES Metastatic breast cancer refractory to other treatments, colorectal cancer, single-agent adjuvant therapy for colon cancer after surgery.

CONTRAINDICATIONS Hypersensitivity to capecitabine, doxifluridine, 5-FU; myelosuppression; dihydropyrimidine dehydrogenase (DPD) deficiency; females of childbearing age;

C

active infection; jaundice; severe renal failure; pregnancy (category D); lactation, children younger than 18 y. **CAUTIOUS USE** Mild to moderate renal or hepatic dysfunction; bacterial or viral infection; coronary artery disease, angina, cardiac arrhythmias; history of varicella zoster or other herpes infections; older adults.

ROUTE & DOSAGE

Breast Cancer, Colorectal Cancer

Adult: **PO** 2500 mg/m²/day in 2 divided doses × 2 wk, then 1 wk off. Repeat.

Renal Impairment Dosage Adjustment

CrCl 30–50 mL/min: Reduce dose by 25%; less than 30 mL/min: Do not use

ADMINISTRATION

Oral

- Morning and evening doses (about 12 h apart) should be given within 30 min of the end of a meal. Water is the preferred liquid for taking this drug.

ADVERSE EFFECTS (≥1%) **Body as a Whole:** *Fatigue,* pyrexia, pain, myalgia. **CV:** Edema. **GI:** *Severe diarrhea, nausea, vomiting, stomatitis,* abdominal pain, constipation, dyspepsia, *anorexia.* **Hematologic:** Neutropenia, thrombocytopenia, anemia, lymphopenia. **Metabolic:** Dehydration, hyperbilirubinemia. **CNS:** Paresthesias, headache, dizziness, insomnia. **Skin:** Hand-and-foot syndrome, *dermatitis,* nail disorder. **Special Senses:** Eye irritation.

INTERACTIONS Drug: Leucovorin increases concentration and toxicity of **5-FU,** altered coagulation and/or bleeding reported with **warfarin. Food:** Food decreases extent of absorption.

PHARMACOKINETICS Absorption: Absorption significantly reduced by food. **Peak:** 1.5–2 h. **Distribution:** Approx 35% protein bound. **Metabolism:** Extensively metabolized to 5-FU. **Elimination:** In urine. **Half-Life:** 45 min.

NURSING IMPLICATIONS

Assessment & Drug Effects

- Lab tests: Monitor periodically CBC with differential and liver functions including bilirubin, transaminases, alkaline phosphatase.
- Monitor carefully for S&S of grade 2 or greater toxicity: Diarrhea greater than 4 BMs/day or at night; vomiting greater than 1 time/24 h; significant loss of appetite or anorexia; stomatitis; hand-and-foot syndrome (pain, swelling, erythema, desquamation, blistering); temperature = 100.5° F; and S&S of infection.
- Withhold drug and immediately report S&S of grade 2 or greater toxicity.
- Monitor for dehydration and replace fluids as needed.
- Monitor carefully patients with coronary artery disease for S&S of cardiotoxicity (e.g., increasing angina).

Patient & Family Education

- Report immediately significant nausea, loss of appetite, diarrhea, soreness of tongue, fever of 100.5° F or more, or signs of infection. Review patient drug package insert carefully for more detail.
- Inform physician immediately if you become pregnant.

CAPREOMYCIN

(kap-ree-oh-mye′sin)

Capastat

Classifications: ANTIBIOTIC; ANTITUBERCULOSIS

C

Therapeutic: ANTITUBERCULOSIS
Prototype: Isoniazid
Pregnancy Category: C

AVAILABILITY 1 g powder for injection

ACTION & *THERAPEUTIC EFFECT* Polypeptide antibiotic that is bacteriostatic; action is unclear. Should not be used alone. *Bacteriostatic against human strains of* Mycobacterium tuberculosis *and other species of* Mycobacterium. *Effective second-line antimycobacterial in conjunction with other antitubercular drugs.*

USES Treatment of active tuberculosis when primary agents cannot be tolerated or when causative organism has become resistant.

CONTRAINDICATIONS Lactation. Safe use in infants and children younger than 2 y is not established.
CAUTIOUS USE Hypersensitivity to antibiotics, including capreomycin, or to other drugs; renal insufficiency (extreme caution); acoustic nerve impairment; history of allergies (especially to drugs); preexisting liver disease; myasthenia gravis; parkinsonism; pregnancy (category C).

ROUTE & DOSAGE

Tuberculosis
Adult: **IM/IV** 1 g/day (not to exceed 20 mg/kg/day) for 60–120 days, then 1 g 2–3 times/wk × 18–24 mo. See prescribing information for dose adjustments for renal insufficiency.

Renal Impairment Dosage Adjustment
CrCl 25–50 mL/min: Reduce dose by 50%; 10–24 mL/min: Reduce dose by 50% and give q48h; less than 10 mL/min: Reduce dose by 50% and give twice weekly

ADMINISTRATION

Intramuscular
- Reconstitute by adding 2 mL of NS injection or sterile water for injection to each 1 g vial. Allow 2–3 min for drug to dissolve completely.
- Make IM injections deep into large muscle mass. Superficial injections are more painful and are associated with sterile abscess. Rotate injection sites.
- Solution may become pale straw color and darken with time, but this does not indicate loss of potency.
- After reconstitution, solution may be stored 48 h at room temperature and up to 14 days under refrigeration unless otherwise directed.

Intravenous

PREPARE: **IV Infusion:** Reconstitute by adding 2 mL of NS or sterile water to each 1 g to yield 370 mg/mL. ▪ Allow 2–3 min to dissolve, then add required dose to 100 mL of NS.

ADMINISTER: **IV Infusion:** Give over 60 min. Avoid rapid infusion.

ADVERSE EFFECTS (≥1%) **Skin:** Urticaria, maculopapular rash, photosensitivity. **Hematologic:** Leukocytosis, leukopenia, *eosinophilia*. **CNS:** Neuromuscular blockage (large doses: Skeletal muscle weakness, respiratory depression or arrest). **Urogenital:** Nephrotoxicity (long-term therapy), tubular necrosis. **Special Senses:** *Ototoxicity,* eighth nerve (auditory and vestibular) damage. **Metabolic:** Hypokalemia, and other electrolyte imbalances. **Other:** Impaired hepatic function (decreased BSP excretion); IM site reactions: Pain, induration, excessive bleeding, sterile abscesses.

C

DIAGNOSTIC TEST INTERFERENCE ***BSP*** and ***PSP*** excretion tests may be decreased.

INTERACTIONS Drug: Increased risk of nephrotoxicity and ototoxicity with AMINOGLYCOSIDES, **amphotericin B, colistin, polymyxin B, cisplatin, vancomycin.**

PHARMACOKINETICS Peak: 1–2 h. **Distribution:** Does not cross blood–brain barrier; crosses placenta. **Elimination:** 52% in urine unchanged in 12 h; small amount in bile. **Half-Life:** 4–6 h.

NURSING IMPLICATIONS

Assessment & Drug Effects

- Observe injection sites for signs of excessive bleeding and inflammation.
- Lab tests: Perform the following as guidelines for therapy before drug is started and at regular intervals during therapy: Appropriate bacterial sensitivity tests; CBC; weekly renal function studies (BUN, NPN, creatinine clearance, sediment); liver function tests (periodically); serum potassium levels (monthly).
- Dosage of capreomycin is typically reduced in patients with impaired renal function, as it is cumulative. Follow renal function tests closely.
- Monitor I&O rates and pattern: Report immediately any change in output or I&O ratio, any unusual appearance of urine, or elevation of BUN above 30 mg/dL.
- Evaluate hearing and balance by audiometric measurements (twice weekly or weekly) and tests of vestibular function (periodically).

Patient & Family Education

- Report any change in hearing or disturbance of balance. These effects are sometimes reversible if drug is withdrawn promptly when first symptoms appear.
- Ensure that you know about adverse reactions and what to do about them. Report immediately the appearance of any unusual symptom, regardless of how vague it may seem.

CAPSAICIN

(cap-say'i-sin)

Axsain, Capsaicin, Capsin, Capsacin-P, Dolorac, Zostrix, Zostrix-HP

Classification: TOPICAL ANALGESIC

Therapeutic: TOPICAL ANALGESIC

AVAILABILITY 0.025%, 0.075% lotion; 0.025%, 0.075%, 0.25% cream; 0.025%, 0.05% gel

ACTION & *THERAPEUTIC EFFECT* Capsaicin depletes and prevents reaccumulation of Substance P, the primary chemical mediator of pain impulses from the periphery to the CNS. *Renders skin and joints insensitive to pain; therefore, it serves as an effective peripheral analgesic.*

USES Temporary relief of pain from arthritis, neuralgias, diabetic neuropathy, and herpes zoster.

UNLABELED USES Phantom limb pain, psoriasis, intractable pruritus.

CONTRAINDICATIONS Hypersensitivity to capsaicin or any ingredient in the cream.

CAUTIOUS USE Patients on ACE inhibitors. Safety and efficacy in children younger than 2 y have not been established.

ROUTE & DOSAGE

Analgesia

Adult/Child (older than 2 y): **Topical** Apply to affected area not more than 3–4 times/day

ADMINISTRATION

Topical

- Apply to affected areas only and avoid contact with eyes or broken or irritated skin.
- If applied with bare hand, wash immediately following application. An applicator or gloved hand may be used to apply cream.
- Avoid tight bandages over areas of application of the cream.

ADVERSE EFFECTS (≥1%) **CNS:** Concentration greater than 1%: Neurotoxicity, hyperalgesia. **Skin:** *Burning, stinging, redness,* itching. **Other:** Cough.

INTERACTIONS Drug: May increase incidence of cough with ACE INHIBITORS.

PHARMACOKINETICS Onset: Postherpetic neuralgia: 2–6 wk.

NURSING IMPLICATIONS

Assessment & Drug Effects

- Monitor for significant pain relief, which may require 4–6 wk of application three or four times daily.
- Monitor for and report signs of skin breakdown as these generally indicate need for drug discontinuation.

Patient & Family Education

- Report local discomfort at site of application if discomfort is distressing or persists beyond the first 3–4 days of use.
- Use caution in handling contact lenses following application of cream. Wash hands thoroughly before touching lenses.
- Notify physician if symptoms do not improve or condition worsens within 14–28 days.
- Apply frequently three or four times daily to maximize therapeutic effectiveness.

CAPTOPRIL

(kap′toe-pril)

Capoten

Classifications: RENIN ANGIOTENSIN SYSTEM ANTAGONIST; ANTIHYPERTENSIVE AGENT

Therapeutic: ANTIHYPERTENSIVE; ACE INHIBITOR

Prototype: Enalapril

Pregnancy Category: D

AVAILABILITY 12.5 mg, 25 mg, 50 mg, 100 mg tablets

ACTION & *THERAPEUTIC EFFECT*

Lowers blood pressure by specific inhibition of the angiotensin-converting enzyme (ACE) utilized by renin in the formation of angiotensin II, a potent vasoconstrictor. ACE inhibition alters hemodynamics without compensatory changes in cardiac output (except in patients with CHF). Inhibition of ACE also leads to decreased circulating aldosterone. In heart failure, captopril administration is followed by a fall in CVP and pulmonary wedge pressure; hypotensive action appears to be unrelated to plasma renin levels. *Effective in management of hypertension, and in congestive heart failure with resulting decreases in dyspnea and improved exercise tolerance.*

C

USES Hypertension; CHF (with digitalis and diuretics), diabetic nephropathy, left ventricular dysfunction post MI.

UNLABELED USES Idiopathic edema.

CONTRAINDICATIONS Angioedema, hypersensitivity to captopril or ACE inhibitors; hypotension; jaundice, or marked elevations of hepatic enzymes; pregnancy (category D), lactation.

CAUTIOUS USE Impaired renal function, patient with solitary kidney; collagen-vascular diseases (scleroderma, SLE); patients receiving immunosuppressants or other drugs that cause leukopenia or agranulocytosis; autoimmune disease, bone marrow suppression, coronary or cerebrovascular disease; cardiomyopathy, aortic stenosis; severe salt/volume depletion; heart failure, renal artery stenosis, renal disease, renal failure, renal impairment; hyperkalemia, elderly.

ROUTE & DOSAGE

Hypertension

Adult: **PO** 6.25–25 mg t.i.d., may increase to 50 mg t.i.d. (max: 450 mg/day)
Child: **PO** 0.3–12.5 mg/kg q12–24h, may titrate up to max of 6 mg/kg/day in 2–4 divided doses
Infant: **PO** 0.15–0.3 mg/kg, may titrate up to 6 mg/kg/day in 1–4 divided doses
Neonate: **PO** 0.05–0.1 mg/kg q8–24h, may titrate up to 0.5 mg/kg q6–24h
Premature Infant: **PO** 0.01 mg/kg q8–12h

Congestive Heart Failure

Adult: **PO** 6.25–12.5 mg t.i.d., may increase to 100 mg t.i.d. (max: 450 mg/day)

Renal Insufficiency Dosage Adjustment

CrCl 10–50 mL/min: 75% of dose; less than 10 mL/min: 50% of dose

ADMINISTRATION

Oral

- Give captopril 1 h before meals. Food reduces absorption by 30–40%.
- Store in light-resistant containers at no more than 30° C (86° F) unless otherwise directed.

ADVERSE EFFECTS (≥1%) **Body as a Whole:** Hypersensitivity reactions, serum sickness-like reaction, arthralgia, skin eruptions. **CV:** Slight increase in heart rate, first dose hypotension, dizziness, fainting. **GI:** Altered taste sensation (loss of taste perception, persistent salt or metallic taste); weight loss, intestinal angioedema. **Hematologic:** Hyperkalemia, neutropenia, <u>agranulocytosis</u> (rare). **Respiratory:** *Cough*. **Skin:** *Maculopapular rash,* urticaria, pruritus, <u>angioedema</u>, photosensitivity. **Urogenital:** Azotemia, impaired renal function, nephrotic syndrome, membranous glomerulonephritis. **Other:** Positive antinuclear antibody (ANA) titers.

DIAGNOSTIC TEST INTERFERENCE Elevated ***urine protein levels*** may persist even after captopril has been discontinued. Possibility of transient elevations of ***BUN*** and ***serum creatinine,*** slight increase in ***serum potassium,*** and ***serum prolactin,*** increases in ***liver enzymes,*** and false-positive ***urine acetone*** (using ***sodium nitroprusside re-***

agent). Captopril may decrease ***fasting blood sugar*** in the nondiabetic and cause hypoglycemia in the diabetic patient controlled with antidiabetic drug therapy.

INTERACTIONS Drug: NITRATES, DIURETICS, and ANTIHYPERTENSIVES enhance hypotensive effects. **Aspirin** and other NSAIDS may antagonize hypotensive effects. POTASSIUM-SPARING DIURETICS (**spironolactone, amiloride**) increase **potassium** levels. **Probenecid** decreases elimination and increases effects. May increase risk of angioedema when used with **pregabalin. Food:** Food decreases absorption; take 30–60 min before meals.

PHARMACOKINETICS Absorption: 60–75% absorbed; food may decrease absorption 25–40%. **Onset:** 15 min. **Peak:** 1–2 h. **Duration:** 6–12 h. **Distribution:** To all tissues except CNS; crosses placenta. **Metabolism:** Some liver metabolism. **Elimination:** Primarily in urine; excreted in breast milk.

NURSING IMPLICATIONS

Assessment & Drug Effects

- Monitor BP closely following the first dose. A sudden exaggerated hypotensive response may occur within 1–3 h of first dose, especially in those with high BP or on a diuretic and restricted salt intake.
- Advise bed rest and BP monitoring for the first 3 h after the initial dose.
- Monitor therapeutic effectiveness. At least 2 wk of therapy may be required before full therapeutic effects are achieved.
- Lab tests: Establish baseline urinary protein levels before initiation of therapy and check at monthly intervals for the first 8 mo of treatment and then periodically thereafter. Perform WBC and differential counts before therapy is begun and at approximately 2-wk intervals for the first 3 mo of therapy and then periodically thereafter.

Patient & Family Education

- Report to physician without delay the onset of unexplained fever, unusual fatigue, sore mouth or throat, easy bruising or bleeding (pathognomonic of agranulocytosis).
- Mild skin eruptions are most likely to appear during the first 4 wk of therapy and may be accompanied by fever and eosinophilia.
- Consult physician promptly if vomiting or diarrhea occur.
- Report darkening or crumbling of nailbeds (reversible with dosage reduction).
- Taste impairment occurs in 5–10% of patients and generally reverses in 2–3 mo even with continued therapy.
- Use OTC medications only with approval of the physician. Inform surgeon or dentist that captopril is being taken. Alert diabetic patient that captopril may produce hypoglycemia. Monitor blood glucose and HbA1C closely during first few weeks of therapy.

CARBACHOL INTRAOCULAR

(kar′ba-kole)
Miostat
Pregnancy Category: C
See Appendix A-1.

CARBAMAZEPINE (Pr)

(kar-ba-maz′e-peen)
Apo-Carbamazepine ♣, Carbatrol, Epitol, Equetro, Mazepine ♣, PMS-Carbamazepine ♣, Tegretol, Tegretol XR

C

Classification: ANTICONVULSANT TRICYCLIC
Therapeutic: ANTICONVULSANT; ANTIMANIA
Pregnancy Category: D

AVAILABILITY 100 mg chewable tablets; 200 mg tablets; 100 mg, 200 mg, 400 mg sustained release tablets; 100 mg, 200 mg, 300 mg sustained release capsules; 100 mg/ 5 mL suspension

ACTION & *THERAPEUTIC EFFECT* Anticonvulsant action appears to inhibit sustained repetitive impulses and reduces post-tetanic synaptic transmission in the spinal cord. It limits the spread of seizure activity. Provides relief in trigeminal neuralgia by reducing synaptic transmission within trigeminal nucleus. Unknown mechanism in regard to bipolar disorder. *Effective anticonvulsant for a range of seizure disorders and as an adjuvant reduces depressive signs and symptoms and stabilizes mood. It is effective for pain and other symptoms associated with neurologic disorders.*

USES Alone or with other anticonvulsants in treatment of grand mal and psychomotor or temporal lobe epilepsy and mixed seizures. Also used for symptomatic treatment of trigeminal neuralgia and for pain and paroxysmal symptoms associated with multiple sclerosis and other neurologic disorders, bipolar I disorder.

UNLABELED USES Certain psychiatric disorders including prophylaxis and treatment of manic-depressive illness, treatment of schizoaffective illness, resistant schizophrenia, dyscontrol syndrome; for management of alcohol withdrawal, rage outbursts, and for antidiuretic effect in diabetes insipidus.

CONTRAINDICATIONS Hypersensitivity to carbamazepine and to TCAs or MAOI therapy; history of myelosuppression or hematologic reaction to other drugs; leukopenia; bone marrow depression; increased IOP; SLE; cardiac, hepatic, or renal disease; coronary artery disease; hypertension; pregnancy (category D); children younger than 6 y.

CAUTIOUS USE The older adult; history of cardiac disease, alcoholism; hepatic disease; cardiac arrhythmias; presence of HLA-B*1502 gene increases risk of Stevens-Johnson syndrome or toxic epidermal necrolysis.

ROUTE & DOSAGE

Epilepsy

Adult: **PO** 200 mg b.i.d., gradually increased to 800–1200 mg/ day in 3–4 divided doses. Tegretol XR dosed b.i.d.
Child: **PO** *Younger than 6 y:* 10–20 mg/kg/day, may gradually increase weekly (recommended max: 35 mg/kg/day in 3–4 divided doses); *6–12 y:* 100 mg b.i.d., gradually increased to 400–800 mg/day in 3–4 divided doses (max: 1 g/day); *younger than 6 y:* 20–30 mg/kg/day in 3–4 divided doses

Trigeminal Neuralgia

Adult: **PO** 100 mg b.i.d., gradually increased by 100 mg increments q12h until relief; usual dose 200–800 mg/day in 3–4 divided doses (max: 1.2 g/day). Tegretol XR dosed b.i.d.

C

Bipolar Disorder (Equetro)
Adult: **PO** 200 mg b.i.d.

ADMINISTRATION

Oral

- Do not administer within 14 days of patient receiving a MAO inhibitor.
- Give with a meal to increase absorption.
- Ensure that chewable tablets are chewed or crushed before being swallowed with a liquid.
- Ensure that sustained release form of drug is not chewed or crushed. It **must be** swallowed whole.
- Do not administer carbamazepine suspension simultaneously with other liquid medications: A precipitate may form in the stomach.

ADVERSE EFFECTS (≥1%) **Body as a Whole:** Myalgia, arthralgia, leg cramps, carbamazepine-induced SLE. **CV:** Edema, syncope, arrhythmias, heart block. **GI:** Nausea, vomiting, anorexia, abdominal pain, diarrhea, constipation, dry mouth and pharynx, abnormal liver function tests, hepatitis, cholestatic and hepatocellular jaundice, pancreatitis. **Endocrine:** Hypothyroidism, SIADH. **Hematologic:** Aplastic anemia, *leukopenia* (transient), leukocytosis, agranulocytosis, eosinophilia, thrombocytopenia. **CNS:** Dizziness, vertigo, drowsiness, disturbances of coordination, ataxia, confusion, headache, fatigue, listlessness, speech difficulty, development of minor motor seizures, hyperreflexia, akathisia, involuntary movements, tremors, visual hallucinations, activation of latent psychosis, aggression; agitation, respiratory depression. **Skin:** Skin rashes, urticaria, petechiae, erythema multiforme, Stevens-Johnson syndrome, photosensitivity reactions, altered skin pigmentation, exfoliative dermatitis, alopecia. **Special Senses:** Abnormal hearing acuity, scotomas, conjunctivitis, blurred vision, transient diplopia, oculomotor disturbances, oscillopsia, nystagmus. **Urogenital:** Urinary frequency or retention, oliguria, impotence.

DIAGNOSTIC TEST INTERFERENCE False-negative ***pregnancy test*** results with tests involving ***human chorionic gonadotropin.***

INTERACTIONS Drug: Serum concentrations of other ANTICONVULSANTS may decrease because of increased metabolism; **verapamil, erythromycin, ketoconazole, nefazodone** may increase carbamazepine levels; decreases hypoprothrombinemic effects of ORAL ANTICOAGULANTS; increases metabolism of ESTROGENS, thus decreasing effectiveness of ORAL CONTRACEPTIVES. **Food: Grapefruit juice** may increase drug levels. **Herbal: Ginkgo** may decrease anticonvulsant effectiveness.

PHARMACOKINETICS Absorption: Slowly from GI tract. **Peak:** 2–8 h. **Distribution:** Widely distributed; high concentrations in CSF; crosses placenta; distributed into breast milk. **Metabolism:** In liver by CYP3A4; can induce liver microsomal enzymes. **Elimination:** In urine and feces. **Half-Life:** Variable due to autoinduction: 25–65 h then 14–16 h (with repeated use).

NURSING IMPLICATIONS

Assessment & Drug Effects

- Lab tests: Baseline and periodic CBCs including platelets, reticulocytes, serum electrolytes and serum iron, liver function tests, BUN, and complete urinalysis.
- At least 3 mo into therapy, it is recommended that physician attempt dosage reduction or termination of drug therapy, if possible, in pa-

C

tients with trigeminal neuralgia. Some patients develop tolerance to the effects of carbamazepine.

- Monitor for the following reactions, which commonly occur during early therapy: Drowsiness, dizziness, light-headedness, ataxia, gastric upset. If these symptoms do not subside within a few days, dosage adjustments may be indicated.
- Withhold drug and notify physician if any of the following signs of myelosuppression occur: RBC less than 4 million/mm^3, Hct less than 32%, Hgb less than 11 g/dL, WBC less than 4000/mm^3, platelet count less than 100,000/mm^3, reticulocyte count less than 20,000/mm^3, serum iron greater than 150 mg/dL.
- Monitor for toxicity, which can develop when serum concentrations are even slightly above the therapeutic range.
- Monitor I&O ratio and vital signs during period of dosage adjustment. Report oliguria, signs of fluid retention, changes in I&O ratio, and changes in BP or pulse patterns.
- Cardiac syncope may resemble epileptic seizures. Therefore, it is recommended that patients who experience an apparent increase in frequency of seizures or a change in their character should be checked by continuous ECG monitoring for 24 h.
- Doses higher than 600 mg/day may precipitate arrhythmias in patients with heart disease.
- Confusion and agitation may be aggravated in the older adult; therefore, side rails and supervision of ambulation may be indicated.

Patient & Family Education

- Discontinue drug and notify physician immediately if early signs of toxicity or a possible hematologic problem appear, (e.g., anorexia, fever, sore throat or mouth, malaise, unusual fatigue, tendency to bruise or bleed, petechiae, ecchymoses, bleeding gums, nose bleeds).
- Avoid hazardous tasks requiring mental alertness and physical coordination until reaction to drug is known, since dizziness, drowsiness, and ataxia are common adverse effects.
- Remain under close medical supervision throughout therapy.
- Avoid excessive sunlight, as photosensitivity reactions have been reported. Apply a sunscreen (if allowed) with SPF of 12 or above.
- Carbamazepine may cause breakthrough bleeding and may also affect the reliability of oral contraceptives.
- Be aware that abrupt withdrawal of any anticonvulsant drug may precipitate seizures or even status epilepticus.

CARBIDOPA-LEVODOPA

(kar-bi-doe′pa)

Sinemet, Sinemet-CR, Parcopa

CARBIDOPA

Lodosyn

Classifications: DOPAMINE RECEPTOR AGONIST; ANTIPARKINSON

Therapeutic: ANTIPARKINSON

Pregnancy Category: C

AVAILABILITY **Carbidopa:** 25 mg tablet; **Carbidopa/Levodopa:** 10 mg/100 mg, 25 mg/100 mg, 25 mg/250 mg tablets; 25 mg/100 mg, 50 mg/200 mg sustained release tablets and orally disintegrating tablets

ACTION & *THERAPEUTIC EFFECT* When levodopa is given alone, large doses **must be** administered. Carbidopa prevents peripheral metabolism (decarboxylation) of levodopa and thereby makes more levodopa available for transport to the brain. Carbidopa does not cross blood–brain barrier and therefore does not affect metabolism of levodopa within the brain. *Effective in management of symptoms of Parkinson's disease and parkinsonism of secondary origin while improving life expectancy and quality of life.*

USES Symptomatic treatment of idiopathic Parkinson's disease (paralysis agitans), postencephalitic parkinsonism, and parkinsonism following carbon dioxide and manganese intoxication. Carbidopa is available alone from manufacturer, on request by physician, for use with levodopa when separate titration of each agent is indicated, and for investigational purposes.

CONTRAINDICATIONS Hypersensitivity to carbidopa or levodopa; narrow-angle glaucoma; history of or suspected melanoma; lactation. Safe use in women of childbearing potential and in children younger than 18 y not established.

CAUTIOUS USE Cardiovascular, hepatic, pulmonary, or renal disorders; history of MI; urinary retention; history of peptic ulcer; psychiatric states; endocrine disease; chronic wide-angle glaucoma; seizure disorders; pregnancy (category C).

ROUTE & DOSAGE

Parkinson's Disease in Patients Not Currently Receiving Levodopa

Adult: **PO** 1 tablet containing 10 mg carbidopa/100 mg levodopa or 25 mg carbidopa/100 mg levodopa t.i.d., increased by 1 tablet daily or every other day up to 6 tablets/day

Patients Receiving Levodopa

Adult: **PO** 1 tablet of the 25/250 mixture t.i.d. or q.i.d., adjusted by 1/2–1 tablet as needed up to 8 tablets/day (start at 20–25% of initial dose of levodopa)

ADMINISTRATION

Oral

- Ensure that sustained release form of drug (Sinemet CR) is not chewed or crushed. It may be broken in half but otherwise swallowed whole.
- Give consistently with respect to food. High protein meals may interfere with absorption of levodopa.
- When patient has been taking levodopa alone, carbidopa-levodopa is usually initiated with a morning dose after patient has been without levodopa for at least 8 h.
- Store in tight, light-resistant containers.

ADVERSE EFFECTS (≥1%) **Body as a Whole:** Hoarseness, unusual breathing patterns, <u>neuroleptic malignant syndrome</u>. **CV:** Orthostatic hypotension, irregular heartbeat, palpitation, arrhythmias, phlebitis, edema. **GI:** Nausea, anorexia, dry mouth, bruxism, vomiting, excess salivation. **Hematologic:** Hemolytic and nonhemolytic anemia, thrombocytopenia, <u>agranulocytosis</u>. **Metabolic:** Abnormal liver function tests, abnormal BUN. **CNS:** *Involuntary movements (dyskinetic, dystonic, choreiform),* ataxia, muscle twitching, increase in hand tremor, numbness, headache, dizziness, euphoria, fatigue, confusion, insomnia, nightmares, mental disturbances, anxiety, <u>depression with suicidal tenden-</u>

cies, delirium, seizures. **Skin:** Body odor, skin rash, dark sweat, loss of hair. **Special Senses:** Blepharospasm, mydriasis, miosis, blurred vision, diplopia, oculogyric crisis. **Urogenital:** Dark urine, priapism, urinary frequency, retention, incontinence.

DIAGNOSTIC TEST INTERFERENCE
Urine glucose: False-negative tests may result with use of ***glucose oxidase methods*** (e.g., ***Clinistix, TesTape***) and false-positive results with ***copper reduction methods*** (e.g., ***Benedict's, Clinitest***), especially in patients receiving large doses. It is reported that ***Clinistix*** and ***TesTape*** may be used if reading is taken at margin of wet and dry tape. There is also the possibility of false-positive tests for ***urinary ketones*** by ***dipstick tests*** [e.g., ***Acetest*** (equivocal), ***Ketostix, Labstix***] false elevation of ***serum*** and ***urinary uric acid*** levels by ***colorimetric methods*** (***not*** with ***uricase***); and interference with ***urine PKU test*** results.

INTERACTIONS Drug: MAO INHIBITORS may precipitate hypertensive crisis; TRICYCLIC ANTIDEPRESSANTS potentiate postural hypotension; ANTICHOLINERGIC AGENTS may enhance levodopa effects but can exacerbate involuntary movements; **methyldopa, guanethidine** increase hypotensive and CNS effects; PHENOTHIAZINES, haloperidol, **phenytoin, papaverine** may interfere with levodopa effects.

PHARMACOKINETICS Absorption: 40–70% of carbidopa absorbed after PO dose; carbidopa may enhance absorption of levodopa. **Distribution:** Widely distributed in most body tissues except CNS; crosses placenta; excreted in breast milk. **Elimination:** In urine. **Half-Life:** 2 h.

NURSING IMPLICATIONS

Assessment & Drug Effects

- Make accurate observations and report promptly adverse reactions and therapeutic effects. Rate of dosage increase is determined primarily by patient's tolerance and response to levodopa.
- Monitor vital signs, particularly during period of dosage adjustment. Report alterations in BP, pulse, and respiratory rate and rhythm.
- Monitor all patients closely for behavior changes. Patients in depression should be closely observed for suicidal tendencies.
- Monitor for changes in intraocular pressure in patients with chronic wide-angle glaucoma.
- Monitor patients with diabetes carefully for alterations in diabetes control. Frequent monitoring of blood sugar is advised.
- Lab tests: Periodic blood glucose, hepatic and renal function tests, CBC with differential, Hgb and Hct.
- Report promptly abnormal involuntary movement such as facial grimacing, exaggerated chewing, protrusion of tongue, rhythmic opening and closing of mouth, bobbing of head, jerky arm and leg movements, and exaggerated respiration.
- Assess for "on-off" phenomenon: Sudden, unpredictable loss of drug effectiveness ("off" effect), which lasts 1 min–1 h. This is followed by an equally abrupt return of function ("on" effect). Sometimes symptoms can be controlled by increasing number of doses per day.
- Monitor therapeutic effects. Some patients manifest increase in bradykinesia ("leg freezing" or slow body movement). The patient is unable to start walking and fre-

quently falls. Reduction of dosage may be indicated in these patients.

- Patients who require more frequent drug administration are most likely to manifest gradual return of parkinsonian symptoms toward the end of a dose period.

Patient & Family Education

- Follow physician's directions regarding continuation or discontinuation of levodopa. Both adverse reactions and therapeutic effects occur more rapidly with carbidopa-levodopa combination than with levodopa alone.
- Make positional changes slowly and in stages, particularly from recumbent to upright position, dangle your legs a few minutes before standing, and walk in place before ambulating, as some patients experience weakness, dizziness, and faintness. Tolerance to this effect usually develops within a few months of therapy. Support stockings may help. Consult physician.
- Report muscle twitching and spasmodic winking promptly, as these may be early signs of overdosage.
- You may notice elevation of mood and sense of well-being before any objective improvement. Resume activities gradually and observe safety precautions to avoid injury.
- Maintain your prescribed drug regimen. Abrupt withdrawal can lead to parkinsonian crisis with return of marked muscle rigidity, akinesia, tremor, hyperpyrexia, mental changes.
- Avoid driving or other hazardous activities until reaction to drug is determined.
- Levodopa may cause urine to darken on standing and may also cause sweat to be dark-colored. This effect is not clinically significant.
- Wear medical identification. Inform all health care providers that you are taking carbidopa-levodopa.

CARBOPLATIN

(car-bo-pla′tin)

Paraplatin

Classifications: ANTINEOPLASTIC; ALKYLATING AGENT

Therapeutic: ANTINEOPLASTIC

Prototype: Cyclophosphamide

Pregnancy Category: D

AVAILABILITY 50 mg, 150 mg, 450 mg vials

ACTION & *THERAPEUTIC EFFECT* Carboplatin is a platinum compound that is a chemotherapeutic agent. It produces interstrand DNA cross-linkages, thus interfering with DNA, RNA, and protein synthesis. Carboplatin is cell-cycle nonspecific and induces programmed cell death. *Full or partial activity against a variety of cancers resulting in reduction or stabilization of tumor size and useful in patients with impaired renal function, patients unable to accommodate high-volume hydration, or patients at high risk for neurotoxicity and/or ototoxicity.*

USES Monotherapy or combination therapy for ovarian cancer.

UNLABELED USES Combination therapy for breast, cervical, colon, endometrial, head and neck, and lung cancer; leukemia, lymphoma, and melanoma.

CONTRAINDICATIONS History of severe reactions to carboplatin or other platinum compounds, severe bone marrow depression; significant bleeding; impaired renal function; pregnancy (category D), and lactation.

CAUTIOUS USE Use with other nephrotoxic drugs; coagulopathy; previous radiation therapy; renal impairment.

ROUTE & DOSAGE

Ovarian Cancer

Adult: **IV** 360 mg/m² once q4wk. May be repeated when neutrophil count is at least 2000 mm³ and platelet count is at least 100,000 mm³. If neutrophil and platelet counts are lower, dose of carboplatin should be reduced by 50–75% of initial dose. Alternatively, 400 mg/m² as a 24-h infusion for 2 consecutive days can be used.

Renal Impairment Dosage Adjustment

CrCl 41–59 mL/min: Dose 250 mg/m²; 16–40 mL/min: Dose 200 mg/m²

Hemodialysis Dosage Adjustment: Initial dose not to exceed 150 mg/m²

ADMINISTRATION

Intravenous

PREPARE: **IV Infusion:** Do not use needles or IV sets containing aluminum. ▪ Immediately before use, reconstitute with either sterile water for injection or D5W or NS as follows: 50-mg vial plus 5 mL diluent; 150-mg vial plus 15 mL diluent; 450-mg vial plus 45 mL diluent. All dilutions yield 10 mg/mL. ▪ **Must be** further diluted for infusion with D5W or NS to concentrations as low as 0.5 mg/mL.

ADMINISTER: **IV Infusion:** Give IV solution over 15 min or longer, depending on total amount of solution and patient tolerance. ▪ Lengthening duration of administration may decrease nausea and vomiting. ▪ Premedication with a parenteral antiemetic 30 min before and on a scheduled basis thereafter is normally used. ▪ Do not repeat doses until the neutrophil count is at least 2000/mm³ and platelet count at least 100,000/mm³.

INCOMPATIBILITIES **Solution/additive: Sodium bicarbonate, fluorouracil, mesna. Y-site: Amphotericin B cholesteryl complex, lansoprazole.**

▪ Protect from light. Reconstituted solutions are stable for 8 h at room temperature; discard solutions 8 h after dilution.

ADVERSE EFFECTS (≥1%) **Body as a Whole:** Hypersensitivity reactions. **GI:** *Mild to moderate nausea and vomiting,* anorexia, hypogeusia, dysgeusia, mucositis, diarrhea, constipation, elevated liver enzymes. **Hematologic:** *Thrombocytopenia, leukopenia, neutropenia, anemia.* **Metabolic:** *Mild hyponatremia, hypomagnesemia, hypocalcemia, and hypokalemia.* **CNS:** Peripheral neuropathy. **Skin:** Rash, alopecia. **Special Senses:** Tinnitus. **Urogenital:** Nephrotoxicity.

DIAGNOSTIC TEST INTERFERENCE Decreased ***calcium levels;*** mild increases in ***liver function tests;*** decreased levels of ***magnesium, potassium,*** and ***sodium.***

INTERACTIONS Drug: AMINOGLYCOSIDES may increase the risk of ototoxicity and nephrotoxicity. May decrease **phenytoin** levels.

PHARMACOKINETICS Onset: 8 wk (2 cycles). **Duration:** 2–16 mo. **Distribution:** Highest concentration in the liver, lung, kidney, skin, and tumors. Not bound to plasma proteins. **Metabolism:** Hydrolyzed in the serum. **Elimination:** Primarily by the kidneys; 60–80% excreted in urine within 24 h. **Half-Life:** 3 h.

NURSING IMPLICATIONS

Assessment & Drug Effects

- Monitor closely during first 15 min of infusion, since allergic reactions have occurred within minutes of carboplatin administration.
- Lab tests: Baseline and periodic CBC with differential, platelet count, Hgb and Hct. Monitor kidney function periodically with creatinine clearance tests and serum electrolytes.
- Monitor results of peripheral blood counts. Median nadir occurs at day 21. Leukopenia, neutropenia, and thrombocytopenia are dose related and may produce dose-limiting toxicity.
- Monitor for peripheral neuropathy (e.g., paresthesias), ototoxicity, and visual disturbances.
- Monitor serum electrolyte studies, because carboplatin has been associated with decreases in sodium, potassium, calcium, and magnesium. Special precautions may be warranted for patients on diuretic therapy.

Patient & Family Education

- Learn about the range of potential adverse effects. Strategies for nausea prevention should receive special attention.
- During therapy you are at risk for infection and hemorrhagic complications related to bone marrow suppression. Avoid unnecessary exposure to crowds or infected persons during the nadir period.
- Report paresthesias (numbness, tingling), visual disturbances, or symptoms of ototoxicity (hearing loss and/or tinnitus).

CARBOPROST TROMETHAMINE (Pr)

(kar'boe-prost)

Hemabate

Classifications: PROSTAGLANDIN; OXYTOCIC

Therapeutic: OXYTOCIC

Pregnancy Category: D

AVAILABILITY 250 mcg/mL injection

ACTION & *THERAPEUTIC EFFECT* Synthetic analog of naturally occurring prostaglandin F_2 alpha with longer duration of biological activity. Stimulates myometrial contractions of gravid uterus at term labor. Mean time to abortion 16 h; mean dose required 2.6 mL. *Effectively stimulates uterine contraction and is used to induce abortion. Useful in treatment of postpartum hemorrhage due to uterine atony unresponsive to usual measures.*

USES To induce abortion between 13th and 20th week of pregnancy, as calculated from first day of last menstrual period. Also for refractory postpartum bleeding.

UNLABELED USES To reduce blood loss secondary to uterine atony; to induce labor in intrauterine fetal death and hydatidiform mole.

CONTRAINDICATIONS Acute pelvic inflammatory disease; active cardiac, pulmonary, renal, or hepatic disease; pregnancy (category D); lactation.

CAUTIOUS USE History of asthma; adrenal disease; anemia; hypotension; hypertension; diabetes mellitus; epilepsy; history of uterine surgery; cervical stenosis; fibroids.

ROUTE & DOSAGE

Abortion, Postpartum Bleeding
Adult: **IM** Initial: 250 mcg (1 mL) repeated at 1.5–3.5-h intervals if indicated by uterine response. Dosage may be increased to 500 mcg (2 mL) if uterine contractility is inadequate after several doses of 250 mcg (1 mL), not to exceed total dose of 12 mg or continuous administration for more than 2 days.

ADMINISTRATION

- Give deep IM into a large muscle. Aspirate carefully before injecting drug to avoid inadvertent entry into blood vessel which can result in bronchospasm, tetanic contractions, and shock. Do not use same site for subsequent doses.
- Store drug in refrigerator at 2°–4° C (36°–39° F) unless otherwise specified.

ADVERSE EFFECTS (≥1%) **Body as a Whole:** Fever, flushing, chills, cough, headache, pain (muscles, joints, lower abdomen, eyes), hiccups, breast tenderness. **GI:** *Nausea,* diarrhea, vomiting.

PHARMACOKINETICS Peak: 30–90 min. **Elimination:** Renal within 24 h.

NURSING IMPLICATIONS

Assessment & Drug Effects

- Monitor uterine contractions and observe and report excessive vaginal bleeding and cramping pain. Save all clots and tissue for physician inspection and laboratory analysis.
- Check vital signs at regular intervals. Carboprost-induced febrile reaction occurs in more than 10% of patients and **must be** differentiated from endometritis, which occurs around third day after abortion.

Patient & Family Education

- Report promptly onset of bleeding, foul-smelling discharge, abdominal pain, or fever.
- Since ovulation may reoccur as early as 2 wk post-abortion, consider appropriate contraception.

CARISOPRODOL

(kar-eye-soe-proe′dole)
Soma
Classification: SKELETAL MUSCLE RELAXANT, CENTRAL-ACTING
Therapeutic: SKELETAL MUSCLE RELAXANT
Prototype: Cyclobenzaprine
Pregnancy Category: C

AVAILABILITY 350 mg tablets

ACTION & *THERAPEUTIC EFFECT* Centrally acting skeletal muscle relaxant that appears to cause slight reduction in muscle tone leading to relief of pain and discomfort of muscle spasm. *Effective spasmolytic and reduces pain associated with acute musculoskeletal disorders.*

USES Skeletal muscle spasm, stiffness, and pain in a variety of musculoskeletal disorders and to relieve spasticity and rigidity in cerebral palsy.

CONTRAINDICATIONS Hypersensitivity to carisoprodol and related compounds (e.g., meprobamate, tybamate); acute intermittent porphyria; children younger than 5 y.

CAUTIOUS USE Impaired liver or kidney function, addiction-prone individuals; seizure disorder; pregnancy (category C), lactation.

ROUTE & DOSAGE

Muscle Spasm
Adult: **PO** 350 mg t.i.d.
Child (older than 5 y): **PO** 25 mg/kg/day in 4 divided doses

ADMINISTRATION

Oral
- Give with food, as needed, to reduce GI symptoms. Last dose should be taken at bedtime.
- Store in tightly closed container.

ADVERSE EFFECTS (≥1%) **Body as a Whole:** Eosinophilia, asthma, fever, anaphylactic shock. **CV:** Tachycardia, postural hypotension, facial flushing. **GI:** Nausea, vomiting, hiccups. **CNS:** *Drowsiness, dizziness,* vertigo, ataxia, tremor, headache, irritability, depressive reactions, syncope, insomnia. **Skin:** Skin rash, erythema multiforme, pruritus.

INTERACTIONS Drug: Alcohol, CNS DEPRESSANTS potentiate CNS effects.

PHARMACOKINETICS Onset: 30 min. **Duration:** 4–6 h. **Distribution:** Crosses placenta. **Metabolism:** In liver by CYP2C19. **Elimination:** By kidneys; excreted in breast milk (2–4 times the plasma concentrations). **Half-Life:** 8 h.

NURSING IMPLICATIONS

Assessment & Drug Effects
- Monitor for allergic or idiosyncratic reactions that generally occur from the first to the fourth dose in patients taking the drug for the first time. Symptoms usually subside after several hours; they are treated by supportive and symptomatic measures.

Patient & Family Education
- Avoid driving and other potentially hazardous activities until response to the drug has been evaluated. Drowsiness is a common side effect and may require reduction in dosage.
- Report to physician if symptoms of dizziness and faintness persist. Symptoms may be controlled by making position changes slowly and in stages.
- Do not take alcohol or other CNS depressants (effects may be additive) unless otherwise directed by physician.
- Discontinue drug and notify physician if skin rash, diplopia, dizziness, or other unusual signs or symptoms appear.

CARMUSTINE
(kar-mus'teen)
BiCNU, Gliadel
Classifications: ANTINEOPLASTIC; ALKYLATING
Therapeutic: ANTINEOPLASTIC
Prototype: Cyclophosphamide
Pregnancy Category: D

AVAILABILITY 100 mg injection; 7.7 mg wafer

ACTION & *THERAPEUTIC EFFECT* Highly lipid-soluble compound with cell-cycle-nonspecific activity against rapidly proliferating cells. Produces cross-linkage of DNA strands, thereby blocking DNA, RNA, and protein synthesis in tumor cells. *Drug metabolites thought to be responsible for antineoplastic activities. Full or partial activity against a variety of cancers resulting in reduction or stabiliza-*

C

tion of tumor size and increased survival rates.

USES As single agent or with other antineoplastics in treatment of Hodgkin's disease and other lymphomas, melanoma, primary and metastatic tumors of brain, and GI tract malignancies.

UNLABELED USES Treatment of carcinomas of breast and lungs, Ewing's sarcoma, Burkitt's tumor, malignant melanoma, and topically for mycosis fungoides.

CONTRAINDICATIONS History of pulmonary function impairment; recent illness with or exposure to chickenpox or herpes zoster; infection; severe bone marrow depression, decreased circulating platelets, leukocytes, or erythrocytes; pregnancy (category D), lactation.

CAUTIOUS USE Hepatic and renal insufficiency; patient with previous cytotoxic medication, or radiation therapy; history of herpes infections.

ROUTE & DOSAGE

Previously Untreated Patients—Carcinoma

Adult: **IV** 150–200 mg/m² q6wk in one dose *or* given over 2 days; adjust for hematologic toxicity

Mycosis Fungoides

Adult: **Topical** 0.05–0.4% solution in 30% alcohol to paint entire body (60 mL) or ointment 1–2 times/day for 6–8 wk (10 mg/day) (**must be** specially compounded)

ADMINISTRATION

Note: When administering IV to infants and children, verify correct IV concentration and rate of infusion with physician.

Intravenous

PREPARE: **IV Infusion:** Wear disposable gloves; contact of drug with skin can cause burning, dermatitis, and hyperpigmentation. ▪ Add supplied diluent to the 100 mg vial. Further dilute with 27 mL of sterile water for injection to yield a concentration of 3.3 mg/mL. ▪ Each dose is then added to 100–500 mL of D5W or NS. ▪ If possible avoid using PVC IV tubing and bags.

ADMINISTER: **IV Infusion:** Infuse a single dose over at least 1 h. Slow infusion over 1–2 h and adequate dilution will reduce pain of administration. ▪ Avoid starting infusion into dorsum of hand, wrist, or the antecubital veins; extravasation in these areas can damage underlying tendons and nerves leading to loss of mobility of entire limb.

INCOMPATIBILITIES Solution/additive: **Dextrose 5%, sodium bicarbonate.** Y-site: **Allopurinol.**

▪ Reconstituted solutions of carmustine are clear and colorless and may be stored at 2°–8° C (36°–46° F) for 8 h protected from light. ▪ Store unopened vials at 2°–8° C (36°–46° F), protected from light, unless otherwise directed by manufacturer. ▪ Signs of decomposition of carmustine in unopened vial: Liquefaction and appearance of oil film at bottom of vial. Discard drug in this condition.

ADVERSE EFFECTS (≥1%) **Hematologic:** Delayed myelosuppression (dose-related); thrombocytopenia. **CNS:** Dizziness, ataxia. **Respiratory:** Pulmonary infiltration or fibrosis. **Skin:** Skin flushing and burning pain at injection site, hyperpigmentation of skin (from contact). **Special Senses:** (With high doses) Eye infarctions, retinal hemorrhage, suffusion of conjunctiva. **GI:** Stomatitis, *nausea, vomiting*.

INTERACTIONS Drug: Cimetidine may potentiate neutropenia and thrombocytopenia.

PHARMACOKINETICS Distribution: Readily crosses blood–brain barrier; CSF concentrations 15–70% of plasma concentrations. **Metabolism:** Rapidly metabolized. **Elimination:** 60–70% in urine in 96 h; 6% via lungs, 1% in feces; excreted in breast milk.

NURSING IMPLICATIONS

Assessment & Drug Effects

- Frequently check rate of flow and blood return; monitor injection site for extravasation. If there is any question about patency, line should be restarted.
- Monitor for nausea and vomiting (dose related), which may occur within 2 h after drug administration and persist for up to 6 h.
- Lab tests: Baseline CBC with differential and platelet count, repeat blood studies following infusion at weekly intervals for at least 6 wk. Baseline and periodic tests of hepatic and renal function.
- Platelet nadir usually occurs within 4–5 wk, and leukocyte nadir within 5–6 wk after therapy is terminated.
- Check temperature daily. Avoid use of rectal thermometer to prevent injury to mucosa. An elevation of 0.6° F or more above normal temperature warrants reporting.
- Report symptoms of lung toxicity (cough, shortness of breath, fever) to the physician immediately.
- Be alert to signs of hepatic toxicity (jaundice, dark urine, pruritus, light-colored stools) and renal insufficiency (dysuria, oliguria, hematuria, swelling of lower legs and feet).

Patient & Family Education

- Report burning sensation immediately, as carmustine can cause burning discomfort even in the absence of extravasation. Infusion will be discontinued and restarted in another site. Ice application over the area may decrease the discomfort.
- Intense flushing of skin may occur during IV infusion. This usually disappears in 2–4 h.
- You will be highly susceptible to infection and to hemorrhagic disorders. Be alert to hazardous periods that occur 4–6 wk after a dose of carmustine. If possible, avoid invasive procedures (e.g., IM injections, enemas, rectal temperatures) during this period.
- Report promptly the onset of sore throat, weakness, fever, chills, infection of any kind, or abnormal bleeding (ecchymosis, petechiae, epistaxis, bleeding gums, hematemesis, melena).

CARTEOLOL HYDROCHLORIDE

(car'tee-oh-lole)

Cartrol, Ocupress

Classifications: BETA-ADRENERGIC ANTAGONIST; ANTIHYPERTENSIVE

Therapeutic: ANTIHYPERTENSIVE; BETA-ADRENERGIC BLOCKER

Prototype: Propranolol

Pregnancy Category: C

AVAILABILITY 2.5 mg, 5 mg tablets; 1% solution

ACTION & *THERAPEUTIC EFFECT* Carteolol is a beta-adrenergic blocking agent (antagonist) that competes for available beta receptor sites. It inhibits both $beta_1$ receptors (chiefly in cardiac muscle) and $beta_2$ receptors (chiefly in the bronchial and vascular musculature). It decreases standing and supine hypertension. *Effective antihypertensive agent by reducing BP to normotensive range and useful in managing angina by decreasing myocardial oxygen demand and lowering cardiac work load.*

USES For hypertension, either alone or in combination with other drugs, particularly a thiazide diuretic (not indicated for hypertensive crisis); chronic open-angle glaucoma.

UNLABELED USES To reduce the frequency of anginal attacks.

CONTRAINDICATIONS Sinus bradycardia, severe CHF; greater than first-degree heart block, cardiogenic shock, CHF secondary to tachycardia treatable with beta-blockers, overt cardiac failure, hypersensitivity to beta-blocking agents, persistent severe bradycardia, bronchial asthma or bronchospasm, and severe COPD; pulmonary edema.

CAUTIOUS USE CHF patients treated with digitalis and diuretics, peripheral vascular disease; diabetes, hypoglycemia, thyrotoxicosis; renal disease; CVA; pregnancy (category C), lactation.

ROUTE & DOSAGE

Hypertension

Adult: **PO** 2.5 mg once/day, may increase to 5–10 mg if needed (max: 10 mg/day)

Open-Angle Glaucoma

Adult: **Ophthalmic** 1 drop in affected eye b.i.d.

ADMINISTRATION

Oral

- Administer capsule or tablet whole. Do not crush or break and instruct patient not to chew before swallowing.
- Store away from heat, light, or moisture.

ADVERSE EFFECTS (≥1%) **Body as a Whole:** Rash, muscle cramps, bronchospasm. **CV:** Increased angina, hypotension, CHF, bradycardia. **GI:** Abdominal pain, diarrhea, nausea. **Endocrine:** Hyperglycemia. **CNS:** *Headache, dizziness,* drowsiness, insomnia, anxiety, tremor, paresthesia, weakness.

INTERACTIONS Drug: DIURETICS and other HYPOTENSIVE AGENTS increase hypotensive effect; carteolol and **albuterol, metoproterenol, terbutaline, pirbuterol** are mutually antagonistic; NSAIDS may blunt hypotensive effect; decreases hypoglycemic effect of **glyburide;** may increase bradycardia and sinus arrest with **amiodarone.**

PHARMACOKINETICS Absorption: Readily from GI tract; 85% reaches systemic circulation. **Peak:** 1–3 h. **Duration:** 24–48 h. **Distribution:** Crosses placenta; distributed into breast milk. **Metabolism:** In liver to active metabolite. **Elimination:** Primarily in urine. **Half-Life:** 4–6 h.

NURSING IMPLICATIONS

Assessment & Drug Effects

- Assess heart rate prior to administration. If pulse is less than 50 bpm, withhold drug and notify physician.
- Monitor BP and pulse frequently during period of adjustment and periodically throughout therapy.
- If hypotension (systolic BP less than 90 mm Hg) occurs, withhold

the drug and notify physician, and carefully assess the hemodynamic status of the patient.
- Monitor daily weight and assess for evidence of fluid overload since drug may precipitate CHF (see Signs & Symptoms, Appendix F).
- Monitor diabetic for loss of diabetic control. Drug may prevent the appearance of early S&S of acute hypoglycemia (see Appendix F).
- Drug may reduce tolerance to cold temperatures in older adults or in those who have circulatory problems.

Patient & Family Education
- Report the first sign or symptom of impending CHF (see Signs & Symptoms, Appendix F) or unexplained respiratory symptoms.
- Do not discontinue medication abruptly, since sudden withdrawal may precipitate or exacerbate angina.
- Report slow pulse rate, confusion or depression, dizziness or lightheadedness, skin rash, fever, sore throat, or unusual bleeding or bruising.
- Be cautious while driving or performing other hazardous activities until response to drug is known.
- Take your pulse before and after taking the medication. If it is much slower than normal rate (or less than 50 bpm), check with your physician.

CARVEDILOL

(car-ve-di′lol)

Coreg, Coreg CR, Kredex ♣

Classifications: ALPHA- AND BETA-ADRENERGIC ANTAGONIST; ANTIHYPERTENSIVE

Therapeutic: ANTIHYPERTENSIVE; ADRENERGIC BLOCKER

Prototype: Propanolol HCl

Pregnancy Category: C

AVAILABILITY 3.125 mg, 6.25 mg, 12.5 mg, 25 mg tablets; 10 mg, 20 mg, 40 mg, 80 mg extended release capsule

ACTION & *THERAPEUTIC EFFECT* Adrenergic receptor blocking agent that contributes to blood pressure reduction. Peripheral vasodilatation and, therefore, decreased peripheral resistance results from alpha$_1$-blocking activity of Coreg. It is 3–5 times more potent than labetalol in lowering blood pressure. *An effective antihypertensive agent reducing BP to normotensive range and useful in managing some angina, dysrhythmias, and CHF by decreasing myocardial oxygen demand and lowering cardiac work load.*

USES Management of essential hypertension, CHF, in conjunction with other heart failure medications, left ventricular dysfunction post MI.

CONTRAINDICATIONS Patients with class IV decompensated cardiac failure, bronchial asthma, or related bronchospastic conditions (e.g., chronic bronchitis and emphysema), pulmonary edema; second- and third-degree AV block, sick sinus syndome, cardiogenic shock or severe bradycardia; lactation.

CAUTIOUS USE Patients on MAOI agents, diabetes, hypoglycemia; patients at high risk for anaphylactic reaction, peripheral vascular disease, cerebrovascular insufficiencies, major depression, hepatic or renal impairment; elderly; pregnancy (category C); children younger than 18 y.

C

ROUTE & DOSAGE

CHF

Adult: **PO** Start with 3.125 mg b.i.d. × 2 wk, may double dose q2wk as tolerated up to 25 mg b.i.d. if weight less than 85 kg *or* 50 mg b.i.d. if weight greater than 85 kg

Left Ventricular Dysfunction Post-MI

Adult: **PO** 6.25 mg bid, can double every 3–10 days as tolerated

Hypertension

Adult: **PO** Start with 6.25 mg b.i.d., may increase by 6.25 mg b.i.d. to max of 50 mg/day

ADMINISTRATION

Oral

- Give with food to slow absorption and minimize risk of orthostatic hypotension.
- Dose increments should be made at 7- to 14-day intervals.

ADVERSE EFFECTS (≥1%) **Body as a Whole:** Increased sweating, fatigue, chest pain, pain, arthralgia. **CV:** Bradycardia, hypotension, syncope, hypertension, AV block, angina. **GI:** Diarrhea, nausea, abdominal pain, vomiting. **Respiratory:** Sinusitis, bronchitis. **Hematologic:** Thrombocytopenia. **Metabolic:** Hyperglycemia, weight increase, gout. **CNS:** *Dizziness,* headache, paresthesias.

INTERACTIONS Drug: Rifampin significantly decreases **carvedilol** levels; **cimetidine** may increase **carvedilol** levels; **clonidine, reserpine,** MAO INHIBITORS may cause hypotension or bradycardia; **carvedilol** may increase **digoxin** levels and may enhance hypoglycemic effects of **insulin** and oral HYPOGLYCEMIC AGENTS, may enhance the effects of ANTIHYPERTENSIVES. **Amiodarone** and **fluconazole** increase side effects.

PHARMACOKINETICS Absorption: Rapidly from GI tract, 25–35% reaches the systemic circulation. **Peak:** Antihypertensive effect 7–14 days. **Distribution:** Greater than 98% protein bound. **Metabolism:** In the liver by CYP2D6 and CYP2C9. **Elimination:** Primarily through feces. **Half-Life:** 7–10 h.

NURSING IMPLICATIONS

Assessment & Drug Effects

- Monitor for therapeutic effectiveness which is indicated by lessening of S&S of CHF and improved BP control.
- Lab tests: Monitor liver function tests periodically; at first sign of hepatic toxicity (see Appendix F) stop drug and notify physician.
- Monitor for worsening of symptoms in patients with PVD.
- Monitor digoxin levels with concurrent use; plasma digoxin concentration may increase.

Patient & Family Education

- Do not abruptly discontinue taking this drug.
- Make position changes slowly due to the risk of orthostatic hypotension.
- Do not engage in hazardous activities while experiencing dizziness.
- If you have diabetes, the drug may increase effects of hypoglycemic drugs and mask S&S of hypoglycemia.

C

CASCARA SAGRADA

(kas-kar'a)
Classification: GI STIMULANT, LAXATIVE
Therapeutic: LAXATIVE
Prototype: Bisacodyl
Pregnancy Category: C

AVAILABILITY 325 mg tablets; liquid

ACTION & *THERAPEUTIC EFFECT* Acts principally in large intestine by stimulating propulsive movements of colon through direct chemical irritation. Casanthrol is a derivative of cascara sagrada. *Effective laxative with results in 6–12 h. Useful in conditions where straining at stool is to be avoided.*

USES Temporary relief of constipation and to prevent straining at stool in various disease conditions. Sometimes used with milk of magnesia.

CONTRAINDICATIONS Abdominal pain, fecal impaction; GI bleeding, ulcerations; appendicitis, gastroenteritis, intestinal obstruction, CHF.
CAUTIOUS USE Lactation; renal impairment; diabetic patients; rectal bleeding; concomitant laxative use; pregnancy (category C).

ROUTE & DOSAGE

Laxative

Adult: **PO** Tablet: 325–1000 mg/day; fluid extract: 0.5–1.5 mL/day; aromatic fluid extract: 2–6 mL/day
Child: **PO** 2–12 y, 1/2 of adult dose; *younger than 2 y,* 1/4 of adult dose
Infant: **PO** Aromatic fluid extract: 1.25 mL/day as single dose

ADMINISTRATION

Oral

- Administer with a full glass of water on an empty stomach for best results. Results may be delayed somewhat by food.
- Store in tightly covered, light-resistant containers, unless otherwise directed by manufacturer.

ADVERSE EFFECTS (≥1%) **GI:** Anorexia, nausea, gripping, abnormally loose stools, constipation rebound, melanosis of colon. **Metabolic:** Hypokalemia, impaired glucose tolerance, calcium deficiency. **Urogenital:** Discoloration of urine.

DIAGNOSTIC TEST INTERFERENCE Possibility of interference with ***PSP excretion test*** because of urine discoloration.

INTERACTIONS Drug: Decreased effect of ORAL ANTICOAGULANTS.

PHARMACOKINETICS Absorption: Minimal from GI tract. **Onset:** 6–12 h. **Metabolism:** In liver. **Elimination:** In feces and urine; excreted in breast milk.

NURSING IMPLICATIONS

Assessment & Drug Effects

- Monitor electrolyte balance if significant diarrhea occurs, especially with frail older adults.
- Monitor restoration of normal bowel function.

Patient & Family Education

- A single dose taken before retiring usually results in evacuation of soft stool 6–12 h later.
- Frequent or prolonged use of irritant cathartics disrupts normal reflex activity of colon and rectum and can lead to drug dependence for evacuation.
- See bisacodyl for additional information.

C

CASPOFUNGIN (Pr)

(cas-po-fun′gin)

Cancidas

Classifications: ANTIBIOTIC; ECHINOCANDIN ANTIFUNGAL

Therapeutic: ANTIFUNGAL ANTIBIOTIC

Pregnancy Category: C

AVAILABILITY 50 mg and 70 mg powder for injection

ACTION & *THERAPEUTIC EFFECT* Caspofungin is an antifungal agent that inhibits the synthesis of an integral component of the fungal cell wall of susceptible species. *Interferes with reproduction and growth of susceptible fungi.*

USES Treatment of invasive aspergillosis in those refractory to or intolerant of other antifungal therapies; empirical therapy for presumed fungal infection with febrile neutropenia; treatment of candidemia and intra-abdominal abscesses, peritonitis, and pleural space infections due to *Candida.*

UNLABELED USES Treatment of esophageal candidiasis with or without oropharyngeal candidiasis (thrush).

CONTRAINDICATIONS Hypersensitivity to any component of this product; mannitol; not studied in patients with ESRF, or children younger than 18 y.

CAUTIOUS USE Patients with moderate hepatic insufficiency; cholestasis; concomitant use of cyclosporine; pregnancy (category C); lactation.

ROUTE & DOSAGE

Invasive *Aspergillosis,* Empirical Therapy, *Candida*

Adult: **IV** 70 mg on day 1, then 50 mg daily thereafter

ADMINISTRATION

Intravenous

Allow vial to come to room temperature.

PREPARE: **IV Infusion:** Reconstitute a 50 mg or 70 mg vial with 10.5 mL of NS, sterile water for injection, or bacteriostatic water for injection to yield 5 mg/mL and 7 mg/mL, respectively. Mix gently until clear. ▪ Withdraw the required dose of reconstituted solution and add to 250 mL of NS, 1/2NS, or 1/4NaCl, or LR. **DO NOT** use diluents or IV solutions containing dextrose.

ADMINISTER: **IV Infusion:** Give slowly over at least 1 h. Do not co-infuse with any other medication.

INCOMPATIBILITIES **Solution/additive:** Any **dextrose**-containing solution. Do not mix or co-infuse with any other medications.

▪ Reconstituted solution should be stored at or below 25° C (77° F) for 1 h prior to preparing the IV solution for infusion.
▪ Store IV solution for up to 24 h at or below 25° C (77° F) or 48 h at 2°–8° C (36°–46° F).

ADVERSE EFFECTS (≥1%) **Body as a Whole:** Anaphylaxis, chills, *injection site reaction,* sensation of warmth. **CNS:** Headache. **CV:** Sinus tachycardia. **GI:** *Nausea, vomiting,* diarrhea, abdominal pain. **Hematologic/Lymphatic:** *Phlebitis, thrombophlebitis,* vasculitis, anemia. **Hepatic:** Elevated liver enzymes. **Metabolic:** Anorexia, *hypokalemia.* **Musculoskeletal:** Pain, myalgia. **Respiratory:** <u>Acute respiratory distress syndrome,</u> dyspnea. **Skin:** Rash, facial swelling, pruritus.

INTERACTIONS Drug: Cyclosporine increases overall systematic exposure to caspofungin; inducers of drug clearance or mixed inducer/inhibitors (e.g., **carbamazepine, dexamethasone, efavirenz, nelfinavir, nevirapine, phenytoin, rifampin**) can decrease caspofungin levels; caspofungin decreases the overall systematic exposure to **tacrolimus.**

PHARMACOKINETICS Distribution: 97% protein bound. **Metabolism:** Liver and plasma to inactive metabolites. **Elimination:** Both in urine and feces. **Half-Life:** 9–11 h.

NURSING IMPLICATIONS

Assessment & Drug Effects

- Monitor for S&S of hypersensitivity during IV infusion; frequently monitor IV site for thrombophlebitis.
- Monitor for and report S&S of fluid retention (e.g., weight gain, swelling, peripheral edema), especially with known cardiovascular disease.
- Lab tests: Baseline and periodic LFTs; periodic kidney function tests, serum electrolytes, and CBC with differential, platelet count.
- Monitor blood levels of tacrolimus with concurrent therapy.

Patient & Family Education

- Report immediately any of the following: Facial swelling, wheezing, difficulty breathing or swallowing, tightness in chest, rash, hives, itching, or sensation of warmth.

CEFACLOR (Pr)

(sef'a-klor)

Ceclor, Ceclor CD

Classifications: ANTIBIOTIC; SECOND-GENERATION CEPHALOSPORIN

Therapeutic: ANTIBIOTIC

Pregnancy Category: B

AVAILABILITY 250 mg, 500 mg tablets; 375 mg, 500 mg sustained release tablets; 125 mg/5 mL, 187 mg/5 mL, 250 mg/5 mL, 375 mg/5 mL suspension

ACTION & *THERAPEUTIC EFFECT* Semisynthetic, second-generation oral cephalosporin antibiotic. Possibly more active than other oral cephalosporins against gram-negative bacilli, especially beta-lactamase-producing *Haemophilus influenzae,* including ampicillin-resistant strains and certain gram-positive strains. Preferentially binds to one or more of the penicillin-binding proteins (PBPs) located on cell walls of susceptible organisms. This inhibits third and final stage of bacterial cell wall synthesis, thus killing the bacterium. *Effective in treating acute otitis media and acute sinusitis where the causative agent is resistant to other antibiotics. Useful in treating respiratory and urinary tract infections.*

USES Treatment of otitis media and infections of upper and lower respiratory tract, urinary tract, and skin and skin structures caused by ampicillin-resistant *H. influenzae;* acute uncomplicated UTI.

CONTRAINDICATIONS Hypersensitivity to cephalosporins and related antibiotics. Safe use in infants younger than 1 mo not established. **CAUTIOUS USE** History of sensitivity to penicillins or other drug allergies; GI disease, colitis; markedly impaired renal function; older adults; coagulopathy; pregnancy (category B), lactation.

ROUTE & DOSAGE

Mild to Moderate Infections

Adult: **PO** 250–500 mg q8h, or Ceclor CD 250–500 mg/q12h

C

Child (older than 1 mo): **PO** 20–40 mg/kg/day divided q8h (max: 2 g/day)

ADMINISTRATION

Oral

- Give sustained release tablets with food to enhance absorption. Food does not affect absorption of capsules.
- Ensure that sustained release tablets are not chewed or crushed. They **must be** swallowed whole.
- After stock oral suspension is prepared, it should be kept refrigerated. Expiration date should appear on label. Discard unused portion after 14 days. Shake well before pouring.
- Store pulvules in tightly closed container unless otherwise directed.

ADVERSE EFFECTS (≥1%) **Body as a Whole:** Serum sickness-like reaction, eosinophilia, joint pain or swelling, fever, superinfections. **GI:** *Diarrhea,* nausea, vomiting, anorexia, <u>pseudomembranous colitis</u> (rare). **Skin:** Urticaria, pruritus, morbilliform eruptions.

DIAGNOSTIC TEST INTERFERENCE Cefaclor may produce positive ***direct Coombs' test,*** which can complicate ***cross-matching procedures*** and ***hematologic studies.*** False-positive ***urine glucose*** determinations may result with use of ***copper sulfate reduction methods*** (e.g., ***Clinitest*** or ***Benedict's reagent***) but not with ***glucose oxidase*** (enzymatic) ***tests*** such as ***Clinistix, Diastix, TesTape.***

INTERACTIONS Drug: Probenecid decreases renal excretion of cefaclor.

PHARMACOKINETICS Absorption: Well absorbed; acid stable. **Peak:** 30–60 min. **Elimination:** 60% of dose eliminated renally in 8 h; crosses placenta; excreted in breast milk. **Half-Life:** 0.5–1 h.

NURSING IMPLICATIONS

Assessment & Drug Effects

- Determine previous hypersensitivity to cephalosporins, penicillins, and other drug allergies before therapy is initiated.
- Lab tests: Perform culture and sensitivity tests prior to and periodically during therapy.
- Report persistent diarrhea, as interruption of therapy may be necessary.
- Monitor for manifestations of drug hypersensitivity (see Appendix F). Discontinue drug and promptly report them if they appear.
- Monitor for manifestations of superinfection (see Appendix F). Promptly report their appearance.

Patient & Family Education

- Report promptly any signs or symptoms of superinfection (see Appendix F).
- Yogurt or buttermilk (if allowed) may serve as a prophylactic against intestinal superinfections by helping to maintain normal intestinal flora.

CEFADROXIL

(sef-a-drox′ill)

Duricef

Classifications: ANTIBIOTIC; FIRST-GENERATION CEPHALOSPORIN
Therapeutic: ANTIBIOTIC
Prototype: Cefazolin
Pregnancy Category: B

AVAILABILITY 500 mg capsules; 1 g tablets; 125 mg/5 mL, 250 mg/5 mL, 500 mg/5 mL suspension

ACTION & *THERAPEUTIC EFFECT* Semisynthetic, first-generation cephalosporin antibiotic. Bactericidal action (similar to that of penicillins): Drug penetrates bacterial cell wall, resists beta-lactamases, and inactivates enzymes essential to cell wall synthesis. *Active against organisms that liberate cephalosporinase and penicillinase (beta-lactamases). Effective in reducing signs and symptoms of urinary tract infections, bone and joint infections, skin and soft tissue infections, and pharyngitis.*

USES Primarily in treatment of urinary tract infections caused by *Escherichia coli, Proteus mirabilis,* and *Klebsiella* sp.; infections of skin and skin structures caused by *Staphylococci* and *Streptococci;* and for treatment of group A beta-hemolytic streptococcal pharyngitis and tonsillitis.

CONTRAINDICATIONS Hypersensitivity to cephalosporins and penicillin.

CAUTIOUS USE Sensitivity to penicillins or other drug allergies; impaired renal function, elderly; GI disease, history of colitis, coagulopathy; pregnancy (category B).

ROUTE & DOSAGE

Uncomplicated Urinary Tract Infection

Adult: **PO** 1–2 g/day in 1–2 divided doses
Child: **PO** 30 mg/kg/day in 2 divided doses

Skin and Skin Structure Infections, Streptococcal Pharyngitis, or Tonsillitis

Adult: **PO** 1 g/day in 1–2 divided doses
Child: **PO** 30 mg/kg/day in 2 divided doses

Renal Impairment Dosage Adjustment

CrCl less than 25 mL/min:
Adult: **PO** 1 g q24h
Child: **PO** 15 mg/kg q24h

ADMINISTRATION

Oral

- Give with food or milk to reduce nausea. If nausea persists, termination of therapy may be necessary.
- Follow directions for mixing oral suspension found on drug label. Reconstituted suspension contains 125 mg or 250 mg cefadroxil per 5 mL.
- Shake suspension well before use; discard after 14 days.
- Store in tight container unless otherwise directed. Oral suspensions are stable for 14 days under refrigeration at 2°–8° C (36°–46° F). Avoid freezing. Note expiration date on label.

ADVERSE EFFECTS (≥1%) **Body as a Whole:** Hypersensitivity [rash, swollen eyelids (angioedema), pruritus, chills], superinfections. **GI:** Nausea, *diarrhea,* vomiting, heartburn, gastritis, bloating, abdominal cramps.

DIAGNOSTIC TEST INTERFERENCE False-positive ***urine glucose*** determinations using ***copper sulfate reduction reagents,*** such as ***Clinitest*** or ***Benedict's reagent,*** but not with ***glucose oxidase tests*** (e.g., ***Clinistix, Diastix, TesTape***). ***Cefadroxil-induced positive direct Coombs' test*** may interfere with ***cross-matching procedures*** and ***hematologic studies.***

INTERACTIONS Drug: Probenecid decreases renal excretion of cefadroxil.

PHARMACOKINETICS Absorption: Acid stable; rapidly absorbed from

C

GI tract. **Peak:** 1 h. **Elimination:** 90% unchanged in urine within 8 h; bacterial inhibitory levels persist 20–22 h; crosses placenta; excreted in breast milk. **Half-Life:** 1–12 h.

NURSING IMPLICATIONS

Assessment & Drug Effects

- Determine previous hypersensitivity to cephalosporins, penicillins, and other drug allergies, before therapy is initiated.
- Lab tests: Perform culture and sensitivity testing prior to and periodically during therapy.
- Lab tests: Perform baseline and periodic renal function studies in patients with renal function impairment, and monitor I&O ratio and pattern.
- Monitor for manifestations of drug hypersensitivity (see Signs & Symptoms, Appendix F). Discontinue drug and promptly report them if they appear.
- Monitor for manifestations of superinfection (see Signs & Symptoms, Appendix F). Promptly report their appearance.

Patient & Family Education

- Report promptly the onset of rash, urticaria, pruritus, or fever, as the possibility of an allergic reaction is high, if you are allergic to penicillin.
- Take medication for the full course of therapy as directed by your physician.
- Report promptly S&S of superinfections (see Appendix F).

CEFAZOLIN SODIUM (Pr)

(sef-a'zoe-lin)

Ancef

Classifications: ANTIBIOTIC; FIRST-GENERATION CEPHALOSPORIN

Therapeutic: ANTIBIOTIC

Pregnancy Category: B

AVAILABILITY 250 mg, 500 mg, 1 g injection

ACTION & *THERAPEUTIC EFFECT* Semisynthetic, first-generation cephalosporin C with limited activity against gram-negative organisms. Bactericidal action: Preferentially binds to one or more of the penicillin-binding proteins (PBP) located on cell walls of susceptible organisms. This inhibits third and final stage of bacterial cell wall synthesis, thus killing the bacterium. *Effective treatment for bone and joint infections, biliary tract infections, endocarditis prophylaxis and treatment, respiratory tract and genital tract infections, septicemia and skin infections, and surgical prophylaxis.*

USES Severe infections of urinary and biliary tracts, skin, soft tissue, and bone, and for bacteremia and endocarditis caused by susceptible organisms; also perioperative prophylaxis in patients undergoing procedures associated with high risk of infection (e.g., open heart surgery).

CONTRAINDICATIONS Hypersensitivity to any cephalosporin and related antibiotics.

CAUTIOUS USE History of penicillin sensitivity, impaired renal function, patients on sodium restriction; coagulopathy; GI disease, colitis; pregnancy (category B).

ROUTE & DOSAGE

Moderate to Severe Infections

Adult: **IV/IM** 250 mg–2 g q8h, up to 2 g q4h (max: 12 g/day)

C

Child: **IV/IM** 25–100 mg/kg/day in 3–4 divided doses, up to 100 mg/kg/day (not to exceed adult doses)
Neonate: **IV** *Younger than 7 days,* 40 mg/kg/day divided q12h; *7 days or older,* 40–60 mg/kg/day divided q8–12h

Surgical Prophylaxis

Adult: **IV/IM** 1–2 g 30–60 min before surgery, then 0.5–1 g q8h
Child: **IV/IM** 25–50 mg/kg 30–60 min before surgery, then q8h for 24 h

Renal Impairment Dosage Adjustment

CrCl less than 35 mL/min: Dose q12h; 10 mL/min: Dose q24h

ADMINISTRATION

Intramuscular

- Preparation of IM solution: Reconstitute with sterile water for injection, bacteriostatic water for injection, or 0.9% sodium chloride injection. ▪ Reconstituted solutions are stable for 24 hr at room temperature and for 96 hr refrigerated.
- IM injections should be made deep into large muscle mass. Pain on injection is usually minimal. Rotate injection sites.

Intravenous

IV administration to neonates, infants, and children: Verify correct IV concentration and rate of infusion with physician.

PREPARE: **Direct:** Add 2 mL sterile water for injection to the 500 mg vial to yield 225 mg/mL, or add 2.5 mL to the 1 g vial to yield 330 mg/mL. Shake well to dissolve. ▪ Further dilute with 5 mL sterile water for injection. **Intermittent:** After initial vial reconstitution, add required dose to 50–100 mL of NS or D5W.

ADMINISTER: **Direct/Intermittent:** Infuse 1 g over 5 min or longer as determined by the amount of solution. ▪ The risk of IV site reactions may be reduced by proper dilution of IV solution, use of small bore IV needle in a large vein, and by rotating injection sites.

INCOMPATIBILITIES **Solution/additive:** AMINOGLYCOSIDES, **atracurium, bleomycin, cimetidine, clindamycin, lidocaine, ranitidine. Y-site: Amiodarone,** AMINOGLYCOSIDES, **amphotericin B cholesteryl complex, cisatracurium, hydromorphone, idarubicin, pentamidine, high dose vancomycin, vinorelbine.**

ADVERSE EFFECTS (≥1%) **Body as a Whole:** <u>Anaphylaxis</u>, fever, eosinophilia, superinfections, seizure (high doses in patients with renal insufficiency). **GI:** *Diarrhea,* anorexia, abdominal cramps. **Skin:** Maculopapular rash, urticaria.

DIAGNOSTIC TEST INTERFERENCE Because of cefazolin effect on the ***direct Coombs' test,*** transfusion ***cross-matching procedures*** and ***hematologic studies*** may be complicated. False-positive ***urine glucose*** determinations are possible with use of ***copper sulfate tests*** (e.g., ***Clinitest*** or ***Benedict's reagent***) but not with ***glucose oxidase tests*** such as ***TesTape, Diastix,*** or ***Clinistix.***

INTERACTIONS Drug: Probenecid decreases renal elimination of cefazolin.

PHARMACOKINETICS Peak: 1–2 h after IM; 5 min after IV. **Distribution:** Poor CNS penetration even

C

with inflamed meninges; high concentrations in bile and in diseased bone; crosses placenta. **Elimination:** 70% unchanged in urine in 6 h; small amount excreted in breast milk. **Half-Life:** 90–130 min.

NURSING IMPLICATIONS

Assessment & Drug Effects

- Determine history of hypersensitivity to cephalosporins, penicillins, and other drugs, before therapy is initiated.
- Lab tests: Perform culture and sensitivity testing prior to and during therapy. Therapy may be initiated pending results.
- Monitor I&O rates and pattern: Be alert to changes in BUN, serum creatinine.
- Prompt attention should be given to onset of signs of hypersensitivity (see Appendix F).
- Promptly report the onset of diarrhea. Pseudomembranous colitis, a potentially life-threatening condition, starts with diarrhea.

Patient & Family Education

- Report promptly any signs or symptoms of superinfection (see Appendix F).
- Report signs of coagulation problems such as easy bruising and nosebleeds.

CEFDINIR

(cef′di-nir)

Omnicef

Classifications: ANTIBIOTIC; THIRD-GENERATION CEPHALOSPORIN

Therapeutic: ANTIBIOTIC

Prototype: Cefotaxime sodium

Pregnancy Category: B

AVAILABILITY 300 mg capsules; 125 mg/5 mL, 250 mg/5 mL suspension

ACTION & *THERAPEUTIC EFFECT* Broad-spectrum semisynthetic third-generation beta-lactamase cephalosporin antibiotic. *Effective against a wide variety of gram-positive and gram-negative bacteria.*

USES Community-acquired pneumonia, acute exacerbations of chronic bronchitis, acute maxillary sinusitis, pharyngitis, tonsillitis, uncomplicated skin infections, bacterial otitis media.

CONTRAINDICATIONS Hypersensitivity to cefdinir and other cephalosporins.

CAUTIOUS USE Hypersensitivity to penicillins, penicillin derivatives; renal impairment; ulcerative colitis or antibiotic-induced colitis; bleeding disorders; GI disorders; liver or kidney disease; pregnancy (category B), lactation. Safety and efficacy in neonates and infants younger than 6 mo old not established.

ROUTE & DOSAGE

Community-Acquired Pneumonia, Skin Infections

Adult: **PO** 300 mg q12h × 10 days

Child/Infant (6 mo–12 y): **PO** 7 mg/kg q12h × 10 days

Chronic Bronchitis, Maxillary Sinusitis, Pharyngitis, Tonsillitis

Adult/Adolescent: **PO** 600 mg q24h or 300 mg q12h × 10 days

Child/Infant (6 mo–12 y): **PO** 14 mg/kg q24h or 7 mg/kg q12h × 10 days

Renal Impairment Dosage Adjustment

CrCl less than 10 mL/min: 300 mg daily

C

Hemodialysis Dosage Adjustment: 300 mg or 7 mg/kg dose PO every other day; dose given at the end of each session

ADMINISTRATION

Oral

- Do not give within 2 h of aluminum- or magnesium-containing antacids or iron supplements.
- Reconstitute oral suspension to 125 mg/mL by adding water (38 mL to 60 mL bottle or 63 mL to 100 mL bottle). Shake well before each use.
- Store in tightly closed container. Discard after 10 days.

ADVERSE EFFECTS (≥1%) **GI:** *Diarrhea,* nausea, abdominal pain. **Metabolic:** Increased GGT, increased urine protein, hematuria. **CNS:** Headache. **Skin:** Rash, cutaneous moniliasis. **Urogenital:** Vaginal moniliasis, vaginitis.

DIAGNOSTIC TEST INTERFERENCE False positive for ***ketones*** or ***glucose*** in urine using ***nitroprusside*** or ***Clinitest.***

INTERACTIONS Drug: ANTACIDS should be taken at least 2 h before or after cefdinir; **probenecid** prolongs cefdinir elimination; **iron** decreases absorption.

PHARMACOKINETICS Absorption: 16–25% bioavailability. **Peak:** 2–4 h. **Distribution:** 60–70% protein bound; penetrates sinus tissue, blister fluid, lung tissue, middle ear fluid. **Metabolism:** Hepatic. **Elimination:** In urine. **Half-Life:** 1.6 h.

NURSING IMPLICATIONS

Assessment & Drug Effects

- Determine previous hypersensitivity to cephalosporins, penicillins, and other drug allergies before therapy is initiated.
- Carefully monitor for and immediately report S&S of: Hypersensitivity, superinfection, or pseudomembranous colitis (see Appendix F).
- Discontinue drug and notify physician if seizures associated with drug therapy occur.

Patient & Family Education

- Allow a minimum of 2 h between cefdinir and antacids containing aluminum or magnesium, or drugs containing iron.
- Immediately contact physician if a rash, diarrhea, or new infection (e.g., yeast infection) develops.

CEFDITOREN PIVOXIL

(cef-ditor′en)

Spectracef

Classifications: ANTIBIOTIC; THIRD-GENERATION CEPHALOSPORIN

Therapeutic: ANTIBIOTIC

Prototype: Cefotaxime sodium

Pregnancy Category: B

AVAILABILITY 200 mg, 400 mg tablets

ACTION & *THERAPEUTIC EFFECT* Semisynthetic cephalosporin. Bactericidal activity results from the inhibition of cell wall synthesis through an affinity for penicillin-binding proteins (PBPs). Stable in the presence of a variety of bacterial beta-lactamase enzymes, including penicillinases and some cephalosporinases. *Antibacterial activity is effective against both aerobic gram-positive and aerobic gram-negative bacteria.*

USES Acute exacerbation of bacterial chronic bronchitis, pharyngitis, tonsillitis, uncomplicated skin and skin-structure infections.

CONTRAINDICATIONS Known allergy to cephalosporins or any of the components of cefditoren; carnitine deficiency; milk protein hypersensitivity.
CAUTIOUS USE History of hypersensitivity to penicillin or other drugs; renal or hepatic impairment; poor nutritional status; coagulopathy; diabetes mellitus; colitis, GI disease; older adults; concurrent anticoagulant therapy; pregnancy (category B), lactation. Safety and efficacy in children younger than 12 y are not established.

ROUTE & DOSAGE

Chronic Bronchitis
Adult/Adolescent: **PO** 400 mg b.i.d. × 10 days

Pharyngitis, Tonsillitis, Skin Infections
Adult: **PO** 200 mg b.i.d. × 10 days

Uncomplicated Skin/Soft Tissue Infections
Adult/Adolescent: **PO** 200–400 mg b.i.d. × 10 days

Renal Impairment Dosage Adjustment
CrCl 30–49 mL/min: 200 mg b.i.d.; less than 30 mL/min: 200 mg daily

ADMINISTRATION

Oral
- Give with food to enhance absorption.
- Do not give within 2 h of an antacid or H_2-receptor antagonist (such as cimetidine).
- Store at 15°–30° C (58°–86° F). Protect from light and moisture.

ADVERSE EFFECTS (≥1%) **GI:** *Diarrhea,* nausea, abdominal pain, dyspepsia, vomiting. **Hematologic:** Anemia, leukocytosis. **CNS:** Headache. **Urogenital:** Vaginal moniliasis, hematuria.

INTERACTIONS Drug: ANTACIDS, H_2-RECEPTOR ANTAGONISTS may decrease absorption; **probenecid** will decrease elimination.

PHARMACOKINETICS Absorption: 14% reaches systemic circulation. **Distribution:** 88% protein bound, distributes into blister fluid, tonsils. **Metabolism:** Hydrolyzed. **Elimination:** Primarily in urine. **Half-Life:** 1.6 h.

NURSING IMPLICATIONS

Assessment & Drug Effects
- Obtain history of hypersensitivity to cephalosporins, penicillins, and other drug allergies.
- Lab tests: Baseline C&S tests recommended prior to and periodically during therapy. Baseline and periodic studies of kidney function; frequent PT determinations in patients at risk for increased prothrombin time; as indicated, Hct and Hgb, CBC with differential, urinalysis, serum electrolytes, and liver enzymes.
- Monitor for manifestations of drug hypersensitivity (see Appendix F). Withhold drug and report promptly to physician if they appear.
- Monitor for and report promptly manifestations of superinfection (see Appendix F), especially diarrhea. Diarrhea may indicate a change in intestinal flora and development of enterocolitis.
- Monitor for and report immediately signs of seizure activity or loss of seizure control.

Patient & Family Education

- Do not take within 2 h of antacids or other drugs used to reduce stomach acids.
- Discontinue drug and report to physician signs of an allergic reaction (e.g., rash, urticaria, pruritus, fever).
- Report promptly S&S of superinfection (see Appendix F), especially unexplained diarrhea. Antibiotic-associated colitis is a superinfection that may occur in 4–9 days or as long as 6 wk after drug is discontinued.
- Use daily yogurt or buttermilk (if allowed) as a prophylactic against intestinal superinfections.

CEFEPIME HYDROCHLORIDE

(cef′e-peem)

Maxipime

Classifications: ANTIBIOTIC; FOURTH-GENERATION CEPHALOSPORIN

Therapeutic: ANTIBIOTIC; CEPHALOSPORIN

Prototype: Cefotaxime sodium

Pregnancy Category: B

AVAILABILITY 500 mg, 1 g, 2 g vials

ACTION & *THERAPEUTIC EFFECT* Cefepime, considered to be a fourth-generation cephalosporin antibiotic that preferentially binds to one or more of the penicillin-binding proteins (PBPs) located on cell walls of susceptible organisms. This inhibits the third and final stage of bacterial cell wall synthesis, thus killing the bacteria (bactericidal). *Cefepime is similar to third-generation cephalosporins with respect to broad gram-negative coverage; however, cefepime has broader gram-positive coverage than third-generation cephalosporins. It is highly resistant to hydrolysis by most beta-lactamase bacteria.*

USES Uncomplicated and complicated UTI, skin and soft tissue infections, pneumonia caused by susceptible organisms. Empiric monotherapy for febrile neutropenic patients.

CONTRAINDICATIONS Hypersensitivity to cefepime, other cephalosporins, severe reaction to penicillins, or other beta-lactam antibiotics.

CAUTIOUS USE Patients with history of GI disease, particularly colitis; renal insufficiency; pregnancy (category B), lactation. Safety and efficacy of cefepime in children younger than 12 y not known.

ROUTE & DOSAGE

Mild to Moderate Infections

Adult: **IV/IM** 0.5–1g q12h for 7–10 days

Moderate to Severe Infections

Adult: **IV** 1–2g q12h for 10 days

Febrile Neutropenia

Adult: **IV** 2 g q8h for 7 days or until resolution of neutropenia

Child: **IV** 50 mg/kg q8h until resolution of neutropenia

UTI/Pneumonia

Child: **IV** 50 mg/kg q12h for 7–10 days

Renal Impairment Dosage Adjustment

CrCl 30–60 mL/min: Dose q24h; 11–29 mL/min: Give 50% of normal dose q24h; less than 10 mL/min: 250–500 mg q24h

Hemodialysis Dosage Adjustment: Administer dose after dialysis

C

ADMINISTRATION

Intramuscular

- Reconstitute 500-mg vial and 1-g vial, respectively, with 1.3 or 2.4 mL of one of the following: Sterile water for injection, 0.9% NaCl injection, bacteriostatic water for injection with parabens or benzyl alcohol, or other compatible solution.

Intravenous

PREPARE: **Intermittent:** Dilute with 50–100 mL of one of the following: NS, D5W, D5/NS or other compatible solution.
ADMINISTER: **Intermittent:** Infuse over 30 min; with Y-type administration set, discontinue other compatible solutions while infusing cefepime.
INCOMPATIBILITIES **Solution/additive:** AMINOGLYCOSIDES, **ampicillin, aminophylline, metronidazole.** **Y-site:** **Acyclovir, amphotericin B, amphotericin B cholesteryl complex, chlordiazepoxide, chlorpromazine, cimetidine, ciprofloxacin, cisplatin, dacarbazine, daunorubicin, diazepam, diphenhydramine, dobutamine, dopamine, doxorubicin, droperidol, enalaprilat, etoposide, famotidine, filgrastim, floxuridine, ganciclovir, haloperidol, hydroxyzine, idarubicin, ifosfamide, magnesium sulfate, mannitol, mechlorethamine, meperidine, metoclopramide, mitomycin, mitoxantrone, morphine, nalbuphine, ofloxacin, ondansetron, plicamycin, prochlorperazine, promethazine, streptozocin, vancomycin, vinblastine, vincristine.**

- Store reconstituted solution at 20°–25° C (68°–77° F) for 24 h or in refrigerator at 2°–8° C (36°–46° F) for 7 days. Protect from light.

ADVERSE EFFECTS (≥1%) **Body as a Whole:** Eosinophilia. **GI:** Antibiotic-associated colitis, diarrhea, nausea, oral moniliasis, vomiting, elevated liver function tests (ALT, AST). **CNS:** Headache, fever. **Skin:** Phlebitis, pain, inflammation, rash, pruritus, urticaria. **Urogenital:** Vaginitis.

DIAGNOSTIC TEST INTERFERENCE Positive ***Coombs' test*** without hemolysis. May cause false-positive ***urine glucose test*** with ***Clinitest.***

INTERACTIONS Drug: AMINOGLYCOSIDES may increase risk of nephrotoxicity and have additive/synergistic effects. May decrease efficacy of ORAL CONTRACEPTIVES. **Probenecid** may increase levels.

PHARMACOKINETICS Absorption: Well absorbed after IM administration; serum levels significantly lower than after equivalent IV dose. **Distribution:** Widely distributed, may cross inflamed meninges; crosses placenta, secreted into breast milk. **Metabolism:** In liver. **Elimination:** In urine. **Half-Life:** 2 h.

NURSING IMPLICATIONS

Assessment & Drug Effects

- Determine history of hypersensitivity reactions to cephalosporins, penicillins, or other drugs before therapy is initiated.
- Lab tests: Perform culture and sensitivity tests before initiation of therapy.
- Monitor for S&S of hypersensitivity (see Appendix F). Report their appearance promptly and discontinue drug.
- Monitor for S&S of superinfection or pseudomembranous colitis (see Appendix F); immediately report either to physician.

- With concurrent high-dose aminoglycoside therapy, closely monitor for nephrotoxicity and ototoxicity.

Patient & Family Education

- Promptly report S&S of hypersensitivity (e.g., rash) or superinfection, especially unexplained diarrhea (see Appendix F).

CEFIXIME

(ce-fix′ime)

Suprax

Classifications: ANTIBIOTIC, BETA-LACTAM; THIRD-GENERATION CEPHALOSPORIN
Therapeutic: ANTIBIOTIC
Prototype: Cefotaxime sodium
Pregnancy Category: B

AVAILABILITY 100 mg/5 mL, 200 mg/5 mL suspension; 400 mg tablet

ACTION & *THERAPEUTIC EFFECT* Cefixime is a third-generation cephalosporin. As a beta-lactam antibiotic like the penicillins, it is mainly bactericidal. It inhibits the third and final stage of bacterial cell wall synthesis by preferentially binding to specific penicillin-binding proteins (PBPs) located inside the bacterial cell wall. *Cefixime is highly stable in the presence of beta-lactamases (penicillinases and cephalosporinases) and therefore has excellent activity against a wide range of gram-negative bacteria. It is bactericidal against susceptible bacteria.*

USES Uncomplicated UTI, otitis media, pharyngitis, tonsillitis, and bronchitis.

CONTRAINDICATIONS Patients with known allergy to the cephalosporin group of antibiotics, severe reaction to penicillin.

CAUTIOUS USE Allergy to penicillin, history of colitis, renal insufficiency, GI disease, coagulopathy, pregnancy (category B), lactation. Safety and effectiveness in infants younger than 6 mo have not been established.

ROUTE & DOSAGE

Infection

Adult: **PO** 400 mg/day in 1–2 divided doses
Child: **PO** 8 mg/kg/day in 1–2 divided doses

Renal Impairment Dosage Adjustment

CrCl 21–60 mL/min: Give 75% of dose; less than 20 mL/min: Give 50% of dose

ADMINISTRATION

Oral

- Do not substitute tablets for liquid in treatment of otitis media because of lack of bioequivalence.
- After reconstitution, suspension may be kept for 14 days at room temperature or refrigerated. Store away from heat and light. Keep tightly closed and shake well before using.

ADVERSE EFFECTS (≥1%) **GI:** *Diarrhea,* loose stools, nausea, vomiting, dyspepsia, flatulence. **CNS:** Drug fever, headache, dizziness. **Skin:** Rash, pruritus. **Urogenital:** Vaginitis, genital pruritus.

INTERACTIONS Drug: AMINOGLYCOSIDES may increase risk of nephrotoxicity and have additive/synergistic effects. May decrease efficacy of ORAL CONTRACEPTIVES. **Probenecid** may increase levels.

C

PHARMACOKINETICS Absorption: 40–50% from GI tract. **Peak:** 2–6 h. **Distribution:** Into breast milk. **Elimination:** 50% in urine, 50% in bile. **Half-Life:** 3–4 h.

NURSING IMPLICATIONS

Assessment & Drug Effects

- Determine previous hypersensitivity reactions to cephalosporins, penicillins, and history of other allergies, particularly to drugs prior to initiation of therapy.
- Lab tests: Perform culture and sensitivity tests prior to initiation of therapy.
- Monitor for superinfections (see Appendix F) caused by overgrowth of nonsusceptible organisms, particularly during prolonged use.
- Monitor I&O rates and pattern: Nephrotoxicity occurs more frequently in patients older than 50 y, with impaired renal function, in the debilitated, and in patients receiving high doses or other nephrotoxic drugs.
- Carefully monitor anyone with a history of allergies. Report manifestations of hypersensitivity (see Appendix F).
- Promptly report loose stools or diarrhea, which may indicate pseudomembranous colitis (see Appendix F). Discontinuation of drug may be necessary.

Patient & Family Education

- Report loose stools or diarrhea during drug therapy and for several weeks after. Older adult patients are especially susceptible to pseudomembranous colitis.

CEFOPERAZONE SODIUM

(sef-oh-per′a-zone)
Cefobid

Classifications: ANTIBIOTIC; THIRD-GENERATION CEPHALOSPORIN
Therapeutic: ANTIBIOTIC
Prototype: Cefotaxime sodium
Pregnancy Category: B

AVAILABILITY 1 g, 2 g injection

ACTION & *THERAPEUTIC EFFECT* Semisynthetic third-generation cephalosporin antibiotic. Preferentially binds to one or more of the penicillin-binding proteins (PBP) located on cell walls of susceptible organisms. This inhibits third and final stage of bacterial cell wall synthesis, thus killing the bacterium. Spectrum of activity is similar to that of cefotaxime. *Generally active against a wide variety of gram-negative bacteria, including some strains of* Pseudomonas aeruginosa. *Also active against some organisms resistant to first- and second-generation cephalosporins, some aminoglycoside antibiotics and penicillins.*

USES Infections of skin and skin structures, urinary tract, respiratory tract; peritonitis and other intra-abdominal infections, pelvic inflammatory disease, endometritis and other infections of the female genital tract; bacterial septicemia.
UNLABELED USES Children younger than 12 y.

CONTRAINDICATIONS Hypersensitivity to cephalosporins and related beta-lactam antibiotics.
CAUTIOUS USE History of hypersensitivity to penicillins, history of allergy, particularly to drugs; hepatic disease, history of colitis or other GI disease, history of bleeding disorders; pregnancy (category B), lactation.

ROUTE & DOSAGE

Moderate to Severe Infections

Adult: **IV/IM** 1–2 g q12h; up to 16 g/day in 2–4 divided doses

Simultaneous Hepatic and Renal Impairment Dosage Adjustment

Reduce total dose to 1–2 g/day

Hemodialysis Dosage Adjustment: Administer dose after dialysis

ADMINISTRATION

Intramuscular

- To prepare IM injections, appropriate diluents include sterile water for injection, bacteriostatic water for injection, and 0.5% lidocaine. See package insert for reconstitution procedure.
- Reconstitute for IM: Dilute each 1 g with 5 mL sterile water. Shake vigorously to dissolve. If concentrations of 250 mg/mL or more are needed for IM injection, 2% lidocaine should be added. See manufacturer's directions.

Intravenous

IV administration to neonates, infants, and children: Verify correct IV concentration and rate of infusion with physician.

- Rapid, direct (bolus) IV injections are not recommended.

PREPARE: **Intermittent:** Dilute each 1 g with 5 mL sterile water. Shake vigorously to dissolve, then dilute in 50–100 mL of D5W or NS. **Continuous:** Prepare as for intermittent infusion then **further** dilute in 500–1000 mL of the selected IV solution.

ADMINISTER: **Intermittent:** Give over 15–30 min. **Continuous:** Give 500–1000 mL over 6–24 h.

INCOMPATIBILITIES **Solution/additive:** AMINOGLYCOSIDES, **doxapram. Y-site:** AMINOGLYCOSIDES, **amifostine, amphotericin B cholesteryl complex, cisatracurium, diltiazem, doxorubicin liposome, filgrastim, gemcitabine, hetastarch, labetalol, meperidine, ondansetron, pentamidine, perphenazine, promethazine, sargramostim, vinorelbine.**

- Protect sterile powder and piggyback units from light and store at or below 25° C (77° F). Reconstituted solutions may be stored in original containers for 24 h at 15°–25° C (59°–77° F); for 5 days under refrigeration at or below 5° C (41° F), or for at least 3 wk in freezer.

ADVERSE EFFECTS (≥1%) **Body as a Whole:** Fever, eosinophilia, phlebitis (IV site), transient pain (IM site), superinfections. **GI:** Abdominal cramps, bloating, loose stools or *diarrhea,* pseudomembranous colitis, elevated liver function tests (AST, ALT, alkaline phosphatase). **Hematologic:** Abnormal PT/INR and PTT; hypoprothrombinemia. **Skin:** Skin rash, urticaria, pruritus. **Urogenital:** Transient increases in serum creatinine and BUN, oliguria.

DIAGNOSTIC TEST INTERFERENCE Cefoperazone can cause positive ***direct Coombs' test,*** which may result in interferences with ***hematologic studies*** and ***cross-matching*** procedures. False-positive results for ***urine glucose*** using ***copper sulfate tests (Benedict's, Clinitest),*** but not with ***glucose enzymatic tests*** (e.g., ***Clinistix, TesTape, Diastix***). Also causes ***prolonged prothrombin*** twice during therapy.

INTERACTIONS Drug: Alcohol produces disulfiram reaction.

PHARMACOKINETICS Peak: 1–2 h after IM; 15–20 min after IV. **Distri-**

C

bution: Low CNS penetration except with inflamed meninges; highest concentrations in bile; crosses placenta. **Elimination:** 70–75% excreted unchanged in bile in 6–12 h, small amount excreted in breast milk. **Half-Life:** 2 h.

NURSING IMPLICATIONS

Assessment & Drug Effects

- Determine hypersensitivity to cephalosporins, penicillins, and other drug allergies before therapy begins.
- Lab tests: Perform culture and sensitivity studies before initiation of therapy. Monitor PTT, or PT/INR as appropriate.
- Observe for and question patient about signs of hemostatic defects: Wound bleeding (e.g., surgical patient), nose bleeds, bleeding gums, bloody sputum, hematuria. Hypoprothrombinemia and vitamin K deficiency are possible complications of therapy and can result in significant blood loss in some patients.
- Report the onset of loose stools or diarrhea. Discontinuation of drug may be required for some patients.

Patient & Family Education

- Do not ingest alcohol within 72 h after drug administration as this will cause a disulfiram-like reaction (see Signs & Symptoms, Appendix F). Effects generally appear within 15–30 min after alcohol is taken and disappear spontaneously 1–2 h later.
- Report promptly any signs or symptoms of superinfection (see Appendix F).

CEFOTAXIME SODIUM Pr

(sef-oh-taks′eem)
Claforan

Classifications: BETA-LACTAM ANTIBIOTIC; THIRD-GENERATION CEPHALOSPORIN
Therapeutic: ANTIBIOTIC
Pregnancy Category: B

AVAILABILITY 500 mg, 1 g, 2 g injection

ACTION & *THERAPEUTIC EFFECT*
Broad-spectrum semi-synthetic third-generation cephalosporin antibiotic. Preferentially binds to one or more of the penicillin-binding proteins (PBP) located on cell walls of susceptible organisms. This inhibits third and final stage of bacterial cell wall synthesis, thus killing the bacteria. *Generally active against a wide variety of gram-negative bacteria including most of the Enterobacteriaceae. Also active against some organisms resistant to first- and second-generation cephalosporins, and currently available aminoglycoside antibiotics and penicillins.*

USES Serious infections of lower respiratory tract, skin and skin structures, bones and joints, CNS (including meningitis and ventriculitis), gynecologic and GU tract infections, including uncomplicated gonococcal infections caused by penicillinase-producing *Neisseria gonorrhoeae* (PPNG). Also used to treat bacteremia or septicemia, intra-abdominal infections, and for perioperative prophylaxis.

UNLABELED USES Treatment of disseminated gonococcal infections (gonococcal arthritis-dermatitis syndrome) and as drug of choice for gonococcal ophthalmia caused by PPNG in adults, children, and neonates.

CONTRAINDICATIONS Hypersensitivity to cefotaxime, cephalosporins and other beta-lactam antibiotics.

CAUTIOUS USE History of type I hypersensitivity reactions to penicillin; history of allergy to other beta-lactam; antibiotics; coagulopathy; renal impairment; history of colitis or other GI disease; pregnancy (category B).

ROUTE & DOSAGE

Moderate to Severe Infections

Adult: **IV/IM** 1–2 g q8–12h, up to 2 g q4h (max: 12 g/day)
Child: **IV/IM** *1 wk or younger,* 50 mg/kg q12h; *1–4 wk,* 50 g/kg/q8h; *1 mo–12 y,* 50–200 mg/kg/day divided q4–8h (max: 12 g/24 h)

Disseminated Gonorrhea

Adult: **IV** 1 g q8h

Surgical Prophylaxis

Adult: **IV/IM** 1 g 30–90 min before surgery

Renal Impairment Dosage Adjustment

CrCl less than 20 mL/min: Give 1/2 normal dose
Hemodialysis Dosage Adjustment: Supplemental dose may be needed

ADMINISTRATION

Intramuscular

- Add 3 mL sterile water for injection or bacteriostatic water for injection to vial containing 1 g drug, providing a solution of approximately 300 mg cefotaxime/mL.
- Administer IM injection deeply into large muscle mass (e.g., upper outer quadrant of gluteus maximus). Aspirate to avoid inadvertent injection into blood vessel. If IM dose is 2 g, divide dose and administer into 2 different sites.

Intravenous

IV administration to neonates, infants, and children: Verify correct IV concentration and rate of infusion with physician.

- Do not admix cefotaxime with sodium bicarbonate or any fluid with a pH greater than 7.5.
- Risk of phlebitis may be reduced by use of a small needle in a large vein.

PREPARE: **Direct:** Add 10 mL diluent to vial with 1 or 2 g drug providing a solution containing 95 or 180 mg/mL, respectively. **Intermittent:** To 1 or 2 g drug add 50 or 100 mL D5W, NS, D5/NS, D5/.45% NaCl, LR, or other compatible diluent. **Continuous:** Dilute in 500–1000 mL compatible IV solution.

ADMINISTER: **Direct:** Give over 3–5 min. **Intermittent:** Give over 20–30 min, preferably via butterfly or scalp vein-type needles. **Continuous:** Infuse over 6–24 h.

INCOMPATIBILITIES **Solution/additive:** AMINOGLYCOSIDES, **aminophylline. Y-site: Allopurinol, azithromycin, cisatracurium, filgrastim, fluconazole, gemcitabine, hetastarch, pentamidine, vancomycin.**

- Protect from excessive light. Reconstituted solutions may be stored in original containers for 24 h at room temperature; for 10 days under refrigeration at or below 5° C (41° F); or for at least 13 wk in frozen state.

ADVERSE EFFECTS (≥1%) **Body as a Whole:** Fever, nocturnal perspiration, inflammatory reaction at IV site, phlebitis, thrombophlebitis; pain, induration, and tenderness at IM site, superinfections. **GI:** Nausea, vomiting, *diarrhea,* abdominal pain, colitis, <u>pseudomembranous colitis</u>, anorexia. **Metabolic:** Transient increases in serum AST, ALT, LDH, bilirubin, alkaline phosphatase concentrations. **Skin:** Rash, pruritus.

DIAGNOSTIC TEST INTERFERENCE May cause falsely elevated ***serum*** or ***urine creatinine*** values ***(Jaffe reaction).*** False-positive reactions for ***urine glucose*** have not been reported using ***copper sulfate reduction methods*** (e.g., ***Benedict's, Clinitest***); however, since it has occurred with other cephalosporins, it may be advisable to use ***glucose oxidase tests (Clinistix, TesTape, Diastix).*** Positive ***direct antiglobulin (Coombs') test*** results may interfere with ***hematologic studies*** and ***cross-matching*** procedures.

INTERACTIONS Drug: Probenecid decreases renal elimination; **alcohol** produces disulfiram reaction.

PHARMACOKINETICS Peak: 30 min after IM; 5 min after IV. **Distribution:** CNS penetration except with inflamed meninges; also penetrates aqueous humor, ascitic and prostatic fluids; crosses placenta. **Metabolism:** In liver to active metabolites. **Elimination:** 50–60% unchanged in urine in 24 h; small amount excreted in breast milk. **Half-Life:** 1 h.

NURSING IMPLICATIONS

Assessment & Drug Effects

- Determine previous hypersensitivity reactions to cephalosporins and penicillins, and history of other allergies, particularly to drugs, before therapy is initiated.
- Lab tests: Perform culture and sensitivity tests before initiation of therapy. Serum creatinine, creatinine clearance, BUN should be evaluated at regular intervals during therapy and for several months after drug has been discontinued. Perform periodic hematologic studies (including PT and/or PTT) and evaluation of hepatic functions with high doses or prolonged therapy.
- Monitor I&O rates and patterns, especially with higher doses or concurrent aminoglycoside therapy. Report significant changes in I&O.
- Superinfection due to overgrowth of nonsusceptible organisms may occur, particularly with prolonged therapy.
- Report onset of diarrhea promptly. Check for fever. If diarrhea is mild, discontinuation of cefotaxime may be sufficient.
- If diarrhea is severe, suspect antibiotic-associated pseudomembranous colitis, a life-threatening superinfection (may occur in 4–9 days or as long as 6 wk after cephalosporin therapy is discontinued).

Patient & Family Education

- Report any early signs or symptoms of superinfection promptly. Superinfections caused by overgrowth of nonsusceptible organisms may occur, particularly during prolonged use.
- Yogurt or buttermilk, 120 mL (4 oz) of either (if allowed), may serve as a prophylactic against intestinal superinfection by helping to maintain normal intestinal flora.
- Report loose stools or diarrhea.

CEFOTETAN DISODIUM

(sef′oh-tee-tan)

Cefotan

Classifications: ANTIBIOTIC; SECOND-GENERATION CEPHALOSPORIN

Therapeutic: ANTIBIOTIC

Prototype: Cefotaxime sodium

Pregnancy Category: B

AVAILABILITY 1 g, 2 g, 10 g injection

ACTION & *THERAPEUTIC EFFECT* Semisynthetic beta-lactam antibiotic, classified as a second-generation cephalosporin. Preferentially binds to one or more of the penicillin-binding proteins (PBP) located on cell walls of susceptible organisms. This inhibits third and final stage of bacterial cell wall synthesis, thus killing the bacterium. *Generally less active against susceptible Staphylococci than first-generation cephalosporins, but has broad spectrum of activity against gram-negative bacteria when compared to first- and second-generation cephalosporins. It also shows moderate activity against gram-positive organisms. Although it is generally inactive against* Pseudomonas, *it is active against the Enterobacteriaceae and anaerobes.*

USES Infections caused by susceptible organisms in urinary tract, lower respiratory tract, skin and skin structures, bones and joints, gynecologic tract; also intra-abdominal infections, bacteremia, and perioperative prophylaxis.

CONTRAINDICATIONS Hypersensitivity to cephalosporins and related beta-lactam antibiotics.

CAUTIOUS USE Preexisting coagulopathy; colitis, GI disease; renal impairment; pregnancy (category B); lactation.

ROUTE & DOSAGE

Moderate to Severe Infections
Adult: **IV/IM** 1–2 g q12h

UTI
Adult: **IV** 500 mg q12h or 1–4 g/day

Surgical Prophylaxis
Adult/Adolescent: **IV/IM** 1–2 g 30–60 min before surgery

Renal Impairment Dosage Adjustment
CrCl greater than 30 mL/min: Regular dose q12h; 10–30 mL/min: Regular dose q24h; less than 10 mL/min: Regular dose q48h
Hemodialysis Dosage Adjustment: Give 1/4 dose q24h on days between sessions, 1/2 dose on day of dialysis

ADMINISTRATION

Intramuscular
- For IM reconstitution (follow manufacturer's directions for selection of diluent), add 2 mL diluent to 1 g vial; yields approximately 2.4 mL (375 mg/mL).
- For IM administration, inject well into body of large muscle such as upper outer quadrant of buttock (gluteus maximus).

Intravenous

IV administration to infants and children: Verify correct IV concentration and rate of infusion with physician.

PREPARE: **Direct:** Dilute each 1 g with 10 mL of sterile water for injection. **Intermittent:** Dilute each 1 g with 50–100 mL of D5W or NS.

ADMINISTER: **Direct:** Give over 3–5 min. **Intermittent:** Give a single dose over 30 min. ▪ For IV infusion, solution may be given for longer period of time through tubing system through which other IV solutions are being given.

INCOMPATIBILITIES **Solution/additive:** AMINOGLYCOSIDES, **heparin, promethazine,** TETRACYCLINES. **Y-site:** AMINOGLYCOSIDES, **cistracurium, lansoprazole, pemetrexed, promethazine, vancomycin, vinorelbine.**

C

▪ Protect sterile powder from light; store at or below 22° C (71.6° F); remains stable 24 mo after date of manufacture. May darken with age, but potency is unaffected. ▪ Reconstituted solutions: Stable for 24 h at 25° C (77° F); 96 h when refrigerated at 5° C (41° F); or at least 1 wk when frozen at –20° C (–4° F).

ADVERSE EFFECTS (≥1%) **Body as a Whole:** Fever, chills, injection site pain, inflammation, disulfiram-like reaction. **GI:** Nausea, vomiting, *diarrhea,* abdominal pain, antibiotic-associated colitis. **Hematologic:** Thrombocytopenia, prolongation of bleeding time or prothrombin time. **Skin:** Rash, pruritus.

DIAGNOSTIC TEST INTERFERENCE May cause falsely elevated ***serum*** or ***urine creatinine*** values ***(Jaffe reaction).*** False-positive reactions for ***urine glucose*** have not been reported using ***copper sulfate reduction methods*** (e.g., ***Benedict's, Clinitest***); however, since it has occurred with other cephalosporins, it may be advisable to use ***glucose oxidase tests (Clinistix, TesTape, Diastix).*** Positive ***direct antiglobulin (Coombs') test*** results may interfere with ***hematologic studies*** and ***cross-matching*** procedures.

INTERACTIONS Drug: Probenecid decreases renal elimination of cefotetan; **alcohol** produces disulfiram reaction; **chloramphenicol** may effect therapeutic activity.

PHARMACOKINETICS Peak: 1.5–3 h after IM. **Distribution:** Poor CNS penetration; widely distributed to body tissues and fluids, including bile, sputum, prostatic and peritoneal fluids; crosses placenta. **Elimination:** 51–81% unchanged in urine; 20% in bile; small amount in breast milk. **Half-Life:** 180–270 min.

NURSING IMPLICATIONS

Assessment & Drug Effects

- Determine history of hypersensitivity to cephalosporins and penicillins, and other drug allergies, before therapy begins.
- Lab tests: Perform culture and sensitivity studies before initiation of therapy. Perform periodic hematologic studies (including PT/INR and PTT) and evaluation of renal function, especially if cefotetan dose is high or if therapy is prolonged in order to recognize symptoms of nephrotoxicity and ototoxicity (see Appendix F).
- Report onset of loose stools or diarrhea. If diarrhea is severe, suspect pseudomembranous colitis (see Appendix F) caused by *Clostridium difficile*. Check temperature. Report fever and severe diarrhea to physician; drug should be discontinued.

Patient & Family Education

- Report promptly S&S of superinfection (see Appendix F).
- Report loose stools or diarrhea.

CEFOXITIN SODIUM

(se-fox'i-tin)

Mefoxin

Classifications: ANTIBIOTIC; SECOND-GENERATION CEPHALOSPORIN
Therapeutic: ANTIBIOTIC
Prototype: Cefaclor
Pregnancy Category: B

AVAILABILITY 1 g, 2 g injection

ACTION & *THERAPEUTIC EFFECT* Semisynthetic, broad-spectrum beta-lactam antibiotic classified as second-generation cephalosporin; structurally and pharmacologically related to cephalosporins and penicillins. Preferentially binds to one or more of the penicillin-binding proteins (PBP) located on cell walls of susceptible organisms, thus making it bactericidal. *It shows enhanced activity against a wide variety of gram-negative organisms and is effective for mixed aerobic-anaerobic infections.*

USES Infections caused by susceptible organisms in the lower respiratory tract, urinary tract, skin and skin structures, bones and joints; also intra-abdominal endocarditis, gynecologic infections, septicemia, uncomplicated gonorrhea, and perioperative prophylaxis in prosthetic arthroplasty or cardiovascular surgery. May be cephalosporin of choice for mixed aerobic-anaerobic infections (e.g., *Bacteroides fragilis*).

CONTRAINDICATIONS Hypersensitivity to cephalosporins and related antibiotics.

CAUTIOUS USE History of sensitivity to penicillin or other allergies, particularly to drugs; impaired renal function; coagulopathy; GI disease, colitis; pregnancy (category B).

ROUTE & DOSAGE

Moderate to Severe Infections

Adult: **IV/IM** 1–2 g q6–8h, up to 12 g/day

Child (older than 3 mo): **IV/IM** 80–160 mg/kg/day in 4–6 divided doses (max: 12 g/day)

Surgical Prophylaxis

Adult: **IV/IM** 2 g 30–60 min before surgery, then 2 g q6h for 24 h

Child: **IV/IM** 30–40 mg/kg 30–60 min before surgery, then 30–40 mg q6h for 24 h

Cesarean Surgery

Adult: **IV/IM** 2 g after clamping umbilical cord

Renal Impairment Dosage Adjustment

CrCl 30–50 mL/min: 1–2 g q8–12h; 10–29 mL/min: 1–2 g q12–24h; 5–9 mL/min: 0.5–1 g q12–24h; greater than 5 mL/min: 0.5–1 g q24–48h

Hemodialysis Dosage Adjustment: Dose of 1–2 g post dialysis

ADMINISTRATION

Intramuscular

- Reconstitute each 1 g with 2 mL sterile water for injection or 0.5 or 1% lidocaine hydrochloride (without epinephrine), used to reduce discomfort of IM injection. After reconstitution for IM use, shake vial and allow solution to stand until it becomes clear.
- Administer IM injections deep into large muscle mass such as upper outer quadrant of gluteus maximus. Aspirate before injecting drug. Rotate injection sites.

Intravenous

IV administration to neonates, infants and children: Verify correct IV concentration and rate of infusion/injection with physician.

PREPARE: **Direct:** Rconstitue each 1 g with 10 mL sterile water, D5W, or NS. **Intermittent:** Following reconstitution, dilute 1–2 g in 50–100 mL of D5W or NS. **Continuous:** Dilute large doses in 1000 mL of D5W or NS.

ADMINISTER: **Direct:** Give over 3–5 min. **Intermittent:** Give over 15 min. **Continuous:** Give at a rate determined by the volume of solution.

C

▪ Reconstituted solution may become discolored (usually light yellow to amber) if exposed to high temperatures; however, potency is not affected. ▪ Solution may be cloudy immediately after reconstitution; let stand and it will clear.

INCOMPATIBILITIES **Solution/additive:** AMINOGLYCOSIDES, **ranitidine. Y-site:** AMINOGLYCOSIDES, **cisatracurium, fenoldopam, filgrastim, hetastarch, lansoprazole, pentamidine, vancomycin.**

▪ After reconstitution, solution is stable for 24 h at 25° C (77° F); 7 days when refrigerated at 4° C (39° F), or 30 wk when frozen at –20° C (–4° F).

ADVERSE EFFECTS (≥1%) **Body as a Whole:** Drug fever, eosinophilia, superinfections, local reactions: pain, tenderness, and induration (IM site), thrombophlebitis (IV site). **GI:** *Diarrhea*, pseudomembranous colitis. **Skin:** Rash, exfoliative dermatitis, pruritus, urticaria. **Urogenital:** Nephrotoxicity, interstitial nephritis.

DIAGNOSTIC TEST INTERFERENCE Cefoxitin causes false-positive (black-brown or green-brown color) ***urine glucose*** reaction with ***copper reduction reagents*** such as ***Benedict's*** or ***Clinitest***, but not with ***enzymatic glucose oxidase reagents (Clinistix, TesTape).*** With high doses, falsely elevated ***serum and urine creatinine*** (with ***Jaffe reaction***) reported. False-positive ***direct Coombs' test*** (may interfere with ***cross-matching procedures*** and ***hematologic studies***) has also been reported.

INTERACTIONS Drug: Probenecid decreases renal elimination of cefoxitin.

PHARMACOKINETICS Peak: 20–30 min after IM; 5 min after IV. **Distribution:** Poor CNS penetration even with inflamed meninges; widely distributed in body tissues including pleural, synovial, and ascitic fluid and bile; crosses placenta. **Elimination:** 85% unchanged in urine in 6 h, small amount in breast milk. **Half-Life:** 45–60 min.

NURSING IMPLICATIONS

Assessment & Drug Effects

- Determine previous hypersensitivity to cephalosporins, penicillins, and other drug allergies before therapy is initiated.
- Lab tests: Perform culture and sensitivity testing prior to therapy; periodic renal function tests.
- Inspect injection sites regularly. Report evidence of inflammation and patient's complaint of pain.
- Monitor I&O rates and pattern: Nephrotoxicity occurs most frequently in patients older than 50 y, in patients with impaired renal function, the debilitated, and in patients receiving high doses or other nephrotoxic drugs.
- Be alert to S&S of superinfections (see Appendix F). This condition is most apt to occur in older adult patients, especially when drug has been used for prolonged period.
- Report onset of diarrhea (may be dose related). If severe, pseudomembranous colitis (see Signs & Symptoms, Appendix F) **must be** ruled out. Older adult patients are especially susceptible.

Patient & Family Education

- Report promptly S&S of superinfection (see Appendix F).
- Report watery or bloody loose stools or severe diarrhea.
- Report severe vomiting or stomach pain.
- Report infusion site swelling, pain, or redness.

C

CEFPODOXIME

(cef-po-dox'eem)

Vantin

Classifications: ANTIBIOTIC; THIRD-GENERATION CEPHALOSPORIN

Therapeutic: ANTIBIOTIC

Prototype: Cefotaxime sodium

Pregnancy Category: B

AVAILABILITY 100 mg, 200 mg tablets; 10 mg/mL, 20 mg/mL suspension

ACTION & *THERAPEUTIC EFFECT* Semisynthetic beta-lactam cephalosporin antibiotic that inhibits the final stage of bacterial cell wall synthesis by preferentially binding to specific penicillin-binding proteins (PBPs) within the bacterial cell wall. *Has antibacterial activity resembling that of other third-generation cephalosporins. Highly active against gram-negative bacteria.*

USES Gonorrhea, otitis media, lower and upper respiratory tract infections, urinary tract infections.

UNLABELED USES Skin and soft tissue infections.

CONTRAINDICATIONS Hypersensitivity to cephalosporins and other beta-lactam antibiotics.

CAUTIOUS USE Renal impairment, history of type I hypersensitivity reactions to penicillins; coagulopathy; history of colitis or other GI disease; lactation, pregnancy (category B).

ROUTE & DOSAGE

Respiratory Tract, Skin, and Soft Tissue Infections

Adult: **PO** 200 mg q12h for 10 days

Child: **PO** 10 mg/kg/day divided q12h

Urinary Tract Infections

Adult: **PO** 100 mg q12h

Gonorrhea

Adult: **PO** 200 mg as single dose

Otitis Media

Child (5 mo–12 y): **PO** 10 mg/kg/day divided q12–24h

ADMINISTRATION

Oral

- Give with food to enhance absorption.
- Give 1 h before or 2 h after an antacid.
- Consult physician regarding patients with renal impairment (i.e., creatinine clearance less than 30 mL/min); dosage intervals should be every 12 h.
- Preparation of suspension: To either the 50 mg/5 mL strength or the 100 mg/5 mL strength, add 25 mL of distilled water, then shake vigorously for 15 seconds. Next, to the 50 mg/5 mL strength add 33 mL, or to the 100 mg/5 mL strength add 32 mL, of distilled water, and shake for at least 3 minutes.
- Store suspension for up to 14 days in a refrigerator [2°–8° C (36°–46° F)]. Shake well before using.

ADVERSE EFFECTS (≥1%) **Body as a Whole:** Eye itching, cough, epistaxis, fever, decreased appetite, malaise. **GI:** Diarrhea, nausea, vomiting, abdominal pain, soft stools, flatulance, <u>pseudomembranous colitis</u> (rare). **CNS:** Rare: Headache, asthenia, dizziness, fatigue, anxiety, insomnia, flushing, nightmares, weakness. **Urogenital:** Vaginal candidiasis. **Skin:** Urticaria, rash, scaling, peeling.

C

INTERACTIONS Drug: ANTACIDS, **ranitidine** may decrease absorption. **Food:** Food may increase the absorption.

PHARMACOKINETICS Absorption: 40–50% absorbed from GI tract. **Onset:** Therapeutic effect in 3 days. **Distribution:** Distributes well into inflammatory, pulmonary, and pleural fluid, and tonsils. Some distribution into prostate. 40% bound to plasma proteins. Distributed into breast milk. **Elimination:** 80% in urine. **Half-Life:** 2–3 h.

NURSING IMPLICATIONS

Assessment & Drug Effects

- Determine history of hypersensitivity reactions to cephalosporins and penicillins, and history of allergies, particularly to drugs, before therapy is initiated.
- Lab tests: Perform culture and sensitivity tests before initiation of therapy. Therapy may be instituted pending test results.
- Report onset of loose stools or diarrhea. Although pseudomembranous enterocolitis (see Appendix F) rarely occurs, this potentially life-threatening complication should be ruled out.
- Monitor for manifestations of hypersensitivity (see Appendix F). Discontinue drug and report S&S of hypersensitivity promptly.
- Monitor I&O (especially with high doses). Report significant changes.

Patient & Family Education

- Report any signs or symptoms of hypersensitivity immediately.
- Report loose stools or diarrhea.

CEFPROZIL

(cef'pro-zil)

Cefzil

Classifications: ANTIBIOTIC; SECOND-GENERATION CEPHALOSPORIN
Therapeutic: ANTIBIOTIC
Prototype: Cefaclor
Pregnancy Category: B

AVAILABILITY 250 mg, 500 mg tablets; 125 mg/5 mL, 250 mg/5 mL suspension

ACTION & *THERAPEUTIC EFFECT* Semisynthetic, second-generation cephalosporin antibiotic with drug structure characterized by a beta-lactam ring; generally resistant to hydrolysis by beta-lactamases. Preferentially binds to proteins in cell walls of susceptible organisms, thus killing the bacteria. *Third-generation cephalosporins are more active and have a broader spectrum against gram-negative bacteria than first- or second-generation of cephalosporins.*

USES Upper and lower respiratory tract infections, otitis media, skin infections.

CONTRAINDICATIONS Hypersensitivity to cephalosporin and related antibiotics; severely impaired renal or hepatic function; phenylketonuria (PKU); infants younger than 6 mo.

CAUTIOUS USE Patients with delayed reaction to penicillin or other drugs; coagulopathy; renal impairment, renal disease; GI disease, especially colitis; pregnancy (category B).

ROUTE & DOSAGE

Mild to Moderate Infections

Adult: **PO** 250–500 mg q12–24h for 10–14 days
Child (older than 6 mo): **PO** 15 mg/kg q12h

Common adverse effects in *italic*, life-threatening effects underlined; generic names in **bold**; classifications in SMALL CAPS; ♣ Canadian drug name; ⓟ Prototype drug

Renal Impairment Dosage Adjustment

CrCl less than 29 mL/min: Reduce dose 50%

ADMINISTRATION

Oral

- Drug may be given without regard to meals.
- Consult physician for patients with impaired renal function. Dose is reduced by 50% when creatinine clearance is 0–29 mL/min.
- Administer after hemodialysis since drug is partially removed by dialysis.
- After reconstitution, oral suspension is refrigerated. Discard unused portion after 14 days.

ADVERSE EFFECTS (≥1%) **Body as a Whole:** Hypersensitivity reactions, superinfections. **GI:** Nausea, vomiting, diarrhea, abdominal pain. **Hematologic:** Eosinophilia. **CNS:** Headache. **Skin:** Rash, diaper rash. **Urogenital:** Genital pruritus, vaginal candidiasis.

DIAGNOSTIC TEST INTERFERENCE May cause a positive ***direct Coombs' test;*** false-negative results in the ferricyanide assay for ***blood glucose;*** false-positive reactions for ***urine glucose*** with ***copper reduction tests*** such as ***Benedict's*** or ***Fehling's solution*** or ***Clinitest tablets;*** increased ***partial thromboplastin time,*** indicating thrombocytosis, eosinophilia; minor elevations in ***serum alanine aminotransferase (ALT), aspartate aminotransferase (AST),*** and ***bilirubin.***

INTERACTIONS Drug: Probenecid prolongs the elimination of cefprozil.

PHARMACOKINETICS Absorption: Readily from GI tract. **Peak:** 1–2 h. **Distribution:** Distributes into blister fluid at 50% of the serum level. **Elimination:** Primarily by kidneys. **Half-Life:** 1–2 h.

NURSING IMPLICATIONS

Assessment & Drug Effects

- Determine previous hypersensitivity to cephalosporins or penicillins before treatment.
- Withhold drug and notify physician if hypersensitivity occurs (e.g., rash, urticaria).
- Lab tests: Perform culture and sensitivity tests before therapy. Therapy may be initiated while results are pending.
- Monitor for and report diarrhea, as pseudomembranous colitis is a potential adverse effect.
- Monitor for and report signs of superinfection (see Appendix F).
- When given concurrently with other cephalosporins or aminoglycosides, monitor for signs of nephrotoxicity.

Patient & Family Education

- Report rash or other signs of hypersensitivity immediately.
- Report signs of superinfection (see Appendix F).
- Report loose stools and diarrhea even after completion of drug therapy.

CEFTAZIDIME

(sef'tay-zi-deem)

Fortaz, Tazicef

Classifications: ANTIBIOTIC; THIRD-GENERATION CEPHALOSPORIN

Therapeutic: ANTIBIOTIC

Prototype: Cefotaxime sodium

Pregnancy Category: B

AVAILABILITY 500 mg, 1 g, 2 g injection

C

ACTION & *THERAPEUTIC EFFECT* Semisynthetic, third-generation broad-spectrum cephalosporin antibiotic. Preferentially binds to one or more of the penicillin-binding proteins (PBP) located on cell walls of susceptible microbes; this inhibits the final stage of bacterial cell wall synthesis, leading to cell death of the bacterium. *More active and have a broader spectrum against aerobic gram-negative bacteria than do either first- or second-generation agents.*

USES To treat infections of lower respiratory tract, skin and skin structures, urinary tract, bones, and joints; also used to treat bacteremia, gynecologic, intra-abdominal, and CNS infections (including meningitis).

UNLABELED USES Surgical prophylaxis.

CONTRAINDICATIONS Hypersensitivity to cephalosporins and related beta-lactam antibiotics; viral disease.

CAUTIOUS USE Pregnancy (category B); elderly; coagulopathy, renal disease, renal impairment; GI disease; colitis.

ROUTE & DOSAGE

Moderate to Severe Infections
Adult: **IV/IM** 1–2 g q8–12h, up to 2 g q6h
Geriatric: **IV/IM** 1–2 g q12h
Child: **IV/IM** 30–50 mg/kg/day q8h (max: 6 g/day)
Neonate (4 wk or younger): **IV** 30 mg/kg q12h

Very Severe Infection
Adult: **IV** 2 g q8h

Renal Impairment Dosage Adjustment
CrCl 30–50 mL/min: Dose q12h; 10–30 mL/min: Dose q24h; less than 10 mL/min: Dose q48–72h

Hemodialysis Dosage Adjustment: Removed by dialysis

ADMINISTRATION

Intramuscular

- Reconstitute by adding 3 mL sterile water or bacteriostatic water for injection or 0.5% or 1% lidocaine HCl injection to 1 g vial to yield 280 mg/mL.
- Inject into large muscle mass (e.g., upper outer quadrant of gluteus maximus or lateral part of thigh).

Intravenous

PREPARE: **Direct:** Add 10 mL of sterile water for injection to 1 g to yield 280 mg/mL. **Intermittent:** Prepare as for direct injection then further dilute with 50–100 mL of D5W, NS, or LR.

ADMINISTER: **Direct:** Give over 3–5 min. **Intermittent:** Give over 30–60 min. ▪ If given through a Y-type set, discontinue other solutions during infusion of ceftazidime.

INCOMPATIBILITIES **Solution/additive:** AMINOGLYCOSIDES, **aminophylline, ciprofloxacin, ranitidine, sodium bicarbonate. Y-site: Alatrofloxacin, amiodarone,** AMINOGLYCOSIDES, **amphotericin B cholesteryl complex, amsacrine, azithromycin, clarithromycin, doxorubicin liposome, fluconazole, idarubicin, midazolam, pentamidine, sargramostim, vancomycin, warfarin.**

- Protect sterile powder from light. Reconstituted solution is stable 7 days when refrigerated at 4°–5° C (39°–41° F); for 18–24 h when stored at 15°–30° C (59°–86° F).

ADVERSE EFFECTS (≥1%) **Body as a Whole:** Fever, phlebitis, pain or inflammation at injection site, superinfections. **GI:** Nausea, vomiting, *di-*

arrhea, abdominal pain, metallic taste, drug-associated pseudomembranous colitis. **Skin:** Pruritus, rash, urticaria. **Urogenital:** Vaginitis, candidiasis.

DIAGNOSTIC TEST INTERFERENCE False-positive reactions for ***urine glucose*** have been reported using ***copper sulfate*** (e.g., ***Benedict's solution, Clinitest***). ***Glucose oxidase tests (Clinistix, TesTape)*** are unaffected. May cause positive ***direct antiglobulin (Coombs') test*** results, which can interfere with ***hematologic studies*** and ***transfusion cross-matching procedures.***

INTERACTIONS Drug: Probenecid decreases renal elimination of ceftazidine.

PHARMACOKINETICS Peak: 1 h. **Distribution:** CNS penetration with inflamed meninges; also penetrates bone, gallbladder, bile, endometrium, heart, skin, and ascitic and pleural fluids; crosses placenta. **Metabolism:** Not metabolized. **Elimination:** 80–90% unchanged in urine in 24 h; small amount in breast milk. **Half-Life:** 25–60 min.

NURSING IMPLICATIONS

Assessment & Drug Effects

- Determine history of hypersensitivity to cephalosporins and penicillins, and other drug allergies, before therapy begins.
- Lab tests: Perform culture and sensitivity studies before initiation of therapy. Therapy may begin pending test results.
- If administered concomitantly with another antibiotic, monitor renal function and report if symptoms of dysfunction appear (e.g., changes in I&O ratio and pattern, dysuria).
- Be alert to onset of rash, itching, and dyspnea. Check patient's temperature. If it is elevated, suspect onset of hypersensitivity reaction (see Appendix F).
- Monitor for superinfection. (See Appendix F.)
- If diarrhea occurs and is severe, suspect pseudomembranous colitis (caused by *Clostridium difficile*). Report severe diarrhea to physician.

Patient & Family Education

- Report loose stools or diarrhea promptly.
- Report any signs or symptoms of superinfection promptly (see Appendix F).

CEFTIBUTEN

(sef-ti-bu′ten)

Cedax

Classifications: BETA-LACTAM ANTIBIOTIC; THIRD-GENERATION CEPHALOSPORIN

Therapeutic: ANTIBIOTIC

Prototype: Cefotaxime sodium

Pregnancy Category: B

AVAILABILITY 400 mg capsules; 90 mg/5 mL suspension

ACTION & *THERAPEUTIC EFFECT* Ceftibuten is a broad-spectrum, third-generation beta-lactam antibiotic. Preferentially binds to one or more of the penicillin-binding proteins located in the cell wall of susceptible organisms. This inhibits the final stage of bacterial cell wall synthesis, killing the bacterium. *It has antibacterial activity against both gram-negative and gram-positive bacteria.*

USES Acute bacterial exacerbations of chronic bronchitis caused by *H. influenzae, Moraxella catarrhalis,* or *S. pneumoniae;* acute bacterial

C

otitis media caused by *H. influenzae, M. catarrhalis,* or *S. pyogenes;* pharyngitis or tonsillitis caused by *S. pyogenes.*

CONTRAINDICATIONS Hypersensitivity to ceftibuten or cephalosporins. **CAUTIOUS USE** Renal dysfunction, penicillin hypersensitivity, history of colitis or diabetes; renal impairment; GI disease; coagulopathy; elderly; pregnancy (category B), lactation. Safety and efficacy in infants younger than 6 mo not established.

ROUTE & DOSAGE

Mild to Moderate Infections

Adult: **PO** 400 mg once daily for 10 days

Renal Impairment Dosage Adjustment

CrCl 30–49 mL/min: 200 mg q24h; less than 30 mL/min: 100 mg q24h

Child (6 mo–12 y): **PO** 9 mg/kg once daily (max: 400 mg) for 10 days

Renal Impairment Dosage Adjustment

CrCl 30–49 mL/min: 4.5 mg/kg q24h; less than 30 mL/min: 2.25 mg/kg q24h

ADMINISTRATION

Oral

- Give oral suspension 1 h before or 2 h after a meal.
- Children weighing more than 45 kg may receive maximum daily dose.
- Hemodialysis patients should receive drug at the end of dialysis.
- Store capsules at 2°–25° C (36°–77° F); keep container tightly closed. Reconstituted oral suspension is stable for 14 days under refrigeration at 2°–8° C (36°–46° F).

ADVERSE EFFECTS (≥1%) **Body as a Whole:** Dyspnea, dysuria, fatigue, vaginitis, moniliasis, urticaria, pruritus, rash, paresthesia, taste perversion. **GI:** Nausea, vomiting, diarrhea, dyspepsia, abdominal pain, anorexia, constipation, dry mouth, eructation, flatulence. **CNS:** Headache, dizziness, nasal congestion, somnolence.

INTERACTIONS Drug: AMINOGLYCOSIDES may increase risk of nephrotoxicity and have additive/synergistic effects. May decrease efficacy of ORAL CONTRACEPTIVES. **Probenecid** may increase levels.

PHARMACOKINETICS Absorption: Rapidly from GI tract. **Peak:** Approx. 2–3 h. **Distribution:** Bronchial mucosa levels are approx 37% of plasma levels, middle ear levels approx 50% of plasma levels. **Elimination:** Primarily in urine. **Half-Life:** 1.5–2.5 h.

NURSING IMPLICATIONS

Assessment & Drug Effects

- Determine history of hypersensitivity reactions to cephalosporins, penicillins, or other drugs, before therapy is initiated. Monitor for S&S of hypersensitivity (see Appendix F); report their appearance promptly and discontinue drug.
- Lab tests: Perform culture and sensitivity tests before initiation of therapy. Dosage may be started pending test results.
- Monitor for S&S of superinfection or pseudomembranous colitis (see Appendix F); immediately report either to physician.
- Closely monitor patients with renal impairment; if seizures develop, discontinue drug and notify physician.

Patient & Family Education

- If on dialysis treatment, take this drug after dialysis.
- Report any S&S of hypersensitivity, superinfection, and pseudomembranous colitis promptly.

CEFTIZOXIME SODIUM

(sef-ti-zox′eem)

Cefizox

Classifications: ANTIBIOTIC; THIRD-GENERATION CEPHALOSPORIN

Therapeutic: ANTIBIOTIC

Prototype: Cefotaxime sodium

Pregnancy Category: B

AVAILABILITY 1 g, 2 g injection

ACTION & *THERAPEUTIC EFFECT* Semisynthetic third-generation cephalosporin antibiotic. Preferentially binds to one or more of the penicillin-binding proteins (PBP) located on cell walls of susceptible organisms. This inhibits third and final stage of bacterial cell wall synthesis, thus killing the bacterium. *Its spectrum includes some gram-positive organisms but has predominantly gram-negative coverage.*

USES Infections caused by susceptible organisms in lower respiratory tract, skin and skin structures, urinary tract, bones and joints; also used to treat intra-abdominal infections, pelvic inflammatory disease, uncomplicated gonorrhea, meningitis *(Haemophilus influenzae, Streptococcus pneumoniae),* and for surgical prophylaxis.

UNLABELED USES Meningitis caused by *Neisseria meningitidis* and *E. coli.*

CONTRAINDICATIONS Hypersensitivity to cephalosporins and other beta-lactam antibiotics; viral disease. Safe use in infants younger than 6 mo not established.

CAUTIOUS USE Penicillin hypersensitivity; coagulopathy; GI disease, colitis; elderly; renal disease, renal impairment; lactation; pregnancy (category B).

ROUTE & DOSAGE

Moderate to Severe Infections

Adult: **IV/IM** 1–2 g q8–12h, up to 2 g q4h

Child (6 mo or older): **IV/IM** 50 mg/kg q6–8h, up to 200 mg/kg/day

Life Threatening Infections

Adult: **IV** 3–4 g q8h

Renal Impairment Dosage Adjustment

Use lower dose.

Hemodialysis Dosage Adjustment: Administer dose after dialysis

ADMINISTRATION

Intramuscular

- Reconstitute as follows with sterile water for injection: Add 1.5 mL to 500 mg to yield 280 mg/mL; add 3 mL to 1 g or 6 mL to 2 g to yield 270 mg/mL.
- Give deep IM into a large muscle. Give no more than 1 g into a single injection site.

Intravenous

PREPARE: **Direct:** Reconstitute each 1 g with 10 mL sterile water. Shake well. **Intermittent:** Further dilute reconstituted solution in 50–100 mL D5W, NS, D5/NS, D5/.45% NaCl, LR, or other compatible IV solution.

C

ADMINISTER: **Direct:** Give over 3–5 min. **Intermittent:** Give over 30 min.
INCOMPATIBILITIES **Solution/additive: Promethazine. Y-site: Filgrastim, lansoprazole, vancomycin.**

- Protect from light. Consult manufacturer's directions concerning storage of reconstituted solutions.

ADVERSE EFFECTS (≥1%) **Body as a Whole:** Fever, phlebitis, vaginitis, pain and induration at injection site, paresthesia. **GI:** Nausea, vomiting, diarrhea, <u>pseudomembranous colitis</u>. **Skin:** Rash, pruritus.

DIAGNOSTIC TEST INTERFERENCE Ceftizoxime causes false-positive ***direct Coombs' test*** (may interfere with ***cross-matching procedures*** and ***hematologic studies***).

INTERACTIONS Drug: Probenecid decreases renal elimination of ceftizoxime.

PHARMACOKINETICS Peak: 1 h. **Distribution:** Crosses placenta. **Metabolism:** Not metabolized. **Elimination:** 80–90% unchanged in urine in 24 h; small amount in breast milk. **Half-Life:** 25–60 min.

NURSING IMPLICATIONS

Assessment & Drug Effects

- Determine history of hypersensitivity reactions to cephalosporins, penicillin, or other drugs before therapy is instituted. Report to physician history of allergy, particularly to drugs.
- Lab tests: Perform culture and sensitivity tests before initiation of therapy. Therapy may be instituted pending test results.
- Be alert to symptoms of hypersensitivity reaction (see Appendix F). Serious reactions may require emergency measures.

Patient & Family Education

- Report loose stools or diarrhea promptly.
- Report any signs or symptoms of hypersensitivity (see Appendix F) promptly.

CEFTRIAXONE SODIUM

(sef-try-ax'one)
Rocephin
Classifications: ANTIBIOTIC; THIRD-GENERATION CEPHALOSPORIN
Therapeutic: ANTIBIOTIC
Prototype: Cefotaxime sodium
Pregnancy Category: B

AVAILABILITY 250 mg, 500 mg, 1 g, 2 g injection

ACTION & *THERAPEUTIC EFFECT* Semisynthetic third-generation cephalosporin antibiotic. Preferentially binds to one or more of the penicillin-binding proteins (PBP) located on cell walls of susceptible organisms. This inhibits third and final stage of bacterial cell wall synthesis, thus killing the bacterium. *Similar to other third-generation cephalosporins, ceftriaxone is effective against serious gram-negative organisms and also penetrates the CSF in concentrations useful in treatment of meningitis.*

USES Infections caused by susceptible organisms in lower respiratory tract, skin and skin structures, urinary tract, bones and joints; also intra-abdominal infections, pelvic inflammatory disease, uncomplicated gonorrhea, meningitis, and surgical prophylaxis.

CONTRAINDICATIONS Hypersensitivity to cephalosporins; viral infections; neonates with hyperbilirubinemia, especially premature neonates; neonates with calcium-containing infusions such as parenteral nutrition; signs and symptoms of gallbladder disease.

CAUTIOUS USE Coagulopathy, hypersensitivity to penicillin or other drugs; impaired vitamin K synthesis; chronic hepatic disease; history of GI disease, colitis; renal disease, renal impairment; pregnancy (category B).

ROUTE & DOSAGE

Moderate to Severe Infections
Adult: **IV/IM** 1–2 g q12–24h × 4–14 days (max: 4 g/day)
Child: **IV/IM** 50–75 mg/kg/day in 2 divided doses × 4–14 days (max: 2 g/day)

Bacterial Otitis Media
Child: **IM** 50 mg/kg (max: 1 g)

Meningitis
Adult: **IV/IM** 2 g q12h
Child: **IV/IM** 100 mg/kg/day in 2 divided doses (max: 4 g/day)

Surgical Prophylaxis
Adult: **IV/IM** 1 g 30–120 min before surgery

Uncomplicated Gonorrhea
Adult: **IM** 250 mg as single dose
Child: **IM** 125 mg as single dose

ADMINISTRATION

Intramuscular

- Reconstitute the 1 g or 2 g vial by adding 2.1 mL or 4.2 mL, respectively, of sterile water for injection. Yields 350 mg/mL. See manufacturer's directions for other dilutions.
- Give deep IM into a large muscle.

Intravenous

IV administration to infants and children: Verify correct IV concentration and rate of infusion with physician.

PREPARE: **Intermittent:** Reconstitute each 250 mg with 2.4 mL of sterile water, D5W, NS, or D5/NS to yield 100 mg/mL. ▪ Further dilute with 50–100 mL of the selected IV solution.

ADMINISTER: **Intermittent:** Give over 30 min.

INCOMPATIBILITIES **Solution/additive:** AMINOGLYCOSIDES, **aminophylline, clindamycin, lidocaine, linezolid, metronidazole, theophylline, calcium**-containing products such as parenteral nutrition. **Y-site:** AMINOGLYCOSIDES, **amphotericin B cholesteryl complex, amsacrine, azithromycin, calcium**-containing products, **filgrastim, fluconazole, labetalol, pentamidine, vancomycin, vinorelbine.**

- Protect sterile powder from light. Store at 15°–25° C (59°–77° F).
- Reconstituted solutions: Diluent, concentration of solutions are determinants of stability. See manufacturer's instructions for storage.

ADVERSE EFFECTS (≥1%) **Body as a Whole:** Pruritus, fever, chills, pain, induration at IM injection site; phlebitis (IV site). **GI:** *Diarrhea,* abdominal cramps, <u>pseudomembranous colitis</u>, biliary sludge. **Urogenital:** Genital pruritus; moniliasis.

DIAGNOSTIC TEST INTERFERENCE Causes prolonged ***PT/INR*** during therapy.

INTERACTIONS Drug: Probenecid decreases renal elimination of ceftriaxone; **alcohol** produces disulfiram reaction; effect of **warfarin** may be increased.

PHARMACOKINETICS Peak: 1.5–4 h after IM; immediately after IV. **Distribution:** Widely in body tissues and fluids; good CNS penetration; crosses placenta. **Metabolism:** Not metabolized. **Elimination:** 33–65% unchanged in urine; also in bile and breast milk. **Half-Life:** 5–10 h.

NURSING IMPLICATIONS

Assessment & Drug Effects

- Determine history of hypersensitivity reactions to cephalosporins and penicillins and history of other allergies, particularly to drugs, before therapy is initiated.
- Lab tests: Perform culture and sensitivity tests before initiation of therapy. Dosage may be started pending test results. Periodic coagulation studies (PT and INR) should be done when on concurrent warfarin.
- Inspect injection sites for induration and inflammation. Rotate sites. Note IV injection sites for signs of phlebitis (redness, swelling, pain).
- Monitor for manifestations of hypersensitivity (see Appendix F). Report promptly.
- Watch for and report: Petechiae, ecchymotic areas, epistaxis, or any unexplained bleeding. Ceftriaxone appears to alter vitamin K–producing gut bacteria; therefore, hypoprothrombinemic bleeding may occur.
- Report promptly development of diarrhea. The incidence of antibiotic-produced pseudomembranous colitis (see Appendix F) is higher than with most cephalosporins.

Patient & Family Education

- Report any signs of bleeding.
- Report loose stools or diarrhea promptly.

CEFUROXIME SODIUM

(se-fyoor-ox′eem)

Zinacef

CEFUROXIME AXETIL

Ceftin

Classifications: ANTIBIOTIC; SECOND-GENERATION CEPHALOSPORIN
Therapeutic: ANTIBIOTIC
Prototype: Cefaclor
Pregnancy Category: B

AVAILABILITY 125 mg, 250 mg, 500 mg tablets; 125 mg/5 mL, 250 mg/5 mL suspension; 750 mg, 1.5 g injection

ACTION & *THERAPEUTIC EFFECT* Semisynthetic second-generation cephalosporin beta-lactam antibiotic. Preferentially binds to one or more of the penicillin-binding proteins (PBP) located on cell walls of susceptible organisms. This inhibits third and final stage of bacterial cell wall synthesis, thus killing the bacterium. *Similar to other second-generation cephalosporins, cefuroxime is more active against gram-negative bacteria than are the first-generation cephalosporins but not as active as the third-generation cephalosporins.*

USES Infections caused by susceptible organisms in the lower respiratory tract, urinary tract, skin, and skin structures; also used for treatment of meningitis, gonorrhea, and otitis media and for perioperative prophylaxis (e.g., open-heart surgery), early Lyme disease.

CONTRAINDICATIONS Hypersensitivity to cephalosporins and related antibiotics; viral infections.
CAUTIOUS USE History of allergy, particularly to drugs; penicillin sen-

sitivity; renal insufficiency; history of colitis or other GI disease; potent diuretics; pregnancy (category B), lactation.

ROUTE & DOSAGE

Moderate to Severe Infections

Adult: **PO** 250–500 mg q12h **IV/IM** 750 mg–1.5 g q6–8h
Child (3 mo–12 y): **PO** 10–15 mg/kg (125–250 mg) q12h **IV/IM** 50–100 mg/kg/day divided q8h (max: 6 g/day)

Bacterial Meningitis

Adult: **IV/IM** 1.5–3 g q8h
Child/Infant (older than 3 mo): **IV/IM** 200–240 mg/kg/day divided q6–8h; reduced to 100 mg/kg/day upon improvement

Surgical Prophylaxis

Adult/Adolescent: **IV/IM** 1.5 g 30–60 min before surgery, then 750 mg q8h for 24 h

Renal Impairment Dosage Adjustment

CrCl 10–20 mL/min: Give q12h; less than 10 mL/min: Give q24h
Hemodialysis Dosage Adjustment: Give supplemental dose

ADMINISTRATION

Oral

- Cefuroxime tablets and oral suspension are not substitutable on a mg-for-mg basis.
- The oral suspension is for infants and children 3 mo to 12 y. Each teaspoon (5 mL) contains the equivalent of 125 mg cefuroxime. Shake oral suspension well before each use.

Intramuscular

- Shake IM suspension gently before administration. IM injections should be made deeply into large muscle mass. Rotate injection sites.

Intravenous

IV administration to neonates, infants and children: Verify correct IV concentration and rate of infusion/injection with physician.

PREPARE: **Direct:** Dilute each 750 mg with 8 mL sterile water, D5W, or NS. **Intermittent:** Further dilute in 50–100 mL of compatible solution. **Continuous:** May be added to 1000 mL of IV compatible solution.

ADMINISTER: **Direct:** Give slowly over 3–5 min. **Intermittent:** Give over 30 min. **Continuous:** Give over 6–24 h.

INCOMPATIBILITIES **Solution/additive:** AMINOGLYCOSIDES, **ciprofloxacin, ranitidine. Y-site:** AMINOGLYCOSIDES, **azithromycin, cisatracurium, clarithromycin, filgrastim, fluconazole, midazolam, vancomycin, vinorelbine.**

- Store powder protected from light unless otherwise directed. After reconstitution, store suspension at 2°–30° C (36°–86° F). Discard after 10 days.

ADVERSE EFFECTS (≥1%) **Body as a Whole:** Thrombophlebitis (IV site); pain, burning, cellulitis (IM site); superinfections, positive Coombs' test. **GI:** *Diarrhea,* nausea, antibiotic-associated colitis. **Skin:** Rash, pruritus, urticaria. **Urogenital:** Increased serum creatinine and BUN, decreased creatinine clearance.

DIAGNOSTIC TEST INTERFERENCE Cefuroxime causes false-positive (black-brown or green-brown color) ***urine glucose*** reaction with

copper reduction reagents (e.g., ***Benedict's*** or ***Clinitest***). but not with ***enzymatic glucose oxidase reagents*** (e.g., ***Clinistix, TesTape***). False-positive ***direct Coombs' test*** (may interfere with ***cross-matching procedures*** and ***hematologic studies***) has been reported.

INTERACTIONS Drug: Probenecid decreases renal elimination of cefuroxime, thus prolonging its action.

PHARMACOKINETICS Absorption: Well absorbed from GI tract; hydrolyzed to active drug in GI mucosa. **Peak:** PO 2 h; IM 30 min. **Distribution:** Widely distributed in body tissues and fluids; adequate CNS penetration with inflamed meninges; crosses placenta. **Elimination:** 66–100% in 24 h; in breast milk. **Half-Life:** 1–2 h.

NURSING IMPLICATIONS

Assessment & Drug Effects

- Determine history of hypersensitivity reactions to cephalosporins, penicillins, and history of allergies, particularly to drugs, before therapy is initiated.
- Lab tests: Perform culture and sensitivity tests before initiation of therapy. Therapy may be instituted pending test results. Monitor periodically BUN and creatinine clearance.
- Report onset of loose stools or diarrhea. Pseudomembranous colitis (see Signs & Symptoms, Appendix F) should be ruled out as the cause of diarrhea during and after antibiotic therapy.
- Monitor for manifestations of hypersensitivity (see Appendix F). Discontinue drug and report their appearance promptly.

Patient & Family Education

- Report loose stools or diarrhea promptly.
- Report any signs or symptoms of hypersensitivity (see Appendix F).

CELECOXIB (Pr)

(cel-e-cox′ib)

Celebrex

Classifications: ANALGESIC, NONSTEROIDAL ANTI-INFLAMMMATORY DRUG (NSAID); CYCLOOXYGENASE-2 (COX-2) INHIBITOR; ANTI-INFLAMMATORY

Therapeutic: ANALGESIC, NSAID; COX-2 INHIBITOR; ANTI-INFLAMMATORY; ANTIRHEUMATIC

Pregnancy Category: C first and second trimester; D third trimester

AVAILABILITY 50 mg, 100 mg, 200 mg, 400 mg capsules

ACTION & *THERAPEUTIC EFFECT* Although an NSAID, unlike ibuprofen celecoxib inhibits prostaglandin synthesis by inhibiting cyclooxygenase-2 (COX-2), but does not inhibit cyclooxygenase-1 (COX-1). *Exhibits anti-inflammatory, analgesic, and antipyretic activities. Reduces or eliminates the pain of rheumatoid and osteoarthritis.*

USES Relief of S&S of osteoarthritis and rheumatoid arthritis. Treatment of acute pain and primary dysmenorrhea. Reduction of polyp formation in familial adenomatous polyposis (FAP), ankylosing spondylitis, juvenile rheumatoid arthritis.

CONTRAINDICATIONS Severe hepatic impairment; hypersensitivity to celecoxib, salicylate, or sulfonamide; asthmatic patients with aspirin triad; GI bleeding; advanced renal disease; severe hepatic impairment; anemia; pain from CABG surgery; pregnancy (category D third trimester); lactation; children younger than 18 y; lactation.

CAUTIOUS USE Patients who are P450 2C9 poor metabolizers; patients who weigh less than 50 kg; mild or moderate hepatic impairment; renal insufficiency; aspirin use; prior history of GI bleeding or peptic ulcer disease; alcoholics; asthmatics; bone marrow suppression; CVA; PVD; elevated liver function tests; fluid retention and/or heart failure; known risks for cardiovascular disease; kidney disease; hypertension; fluid retention; pregnancy (category C first and second trimester); children with systemic-onset juvenile rheumatoid arthritis.

ROUTE & DOSAGE

Osteoarthritis/Arthritis/ Ankylosing Spondylitis

Adult: **PO** 100 mg b.i.d. or 200 mg daily

Rheumatoid Arthritis

Adult: **PO** 100–200 mg b.i.d.

Acute Pain, Dysmenorrhea

Adult: **PO** 400 mg 1st dose, then 200 mg same day if needed, then 200 mg b.i.d. prn

FAP

Adult: **PO** 400 mg b.i.d.

Juvenile Rheumatoid Arthritis

Adolescent/Child (older than 2 y, weight greater than 25 kg): **PO** 100 mg b.i.d.

Child (older than 2 y, weight 10–25 kg): **PO** 50 mg b.i.d.

Hepatic Dosage Adjustment

Child-Pugh Class B: Reduce dose by 50%

Pharmacogenetic Dosage Adjustment

Poor CYP2C9 metabolizers: Start with 1/2 normal dose

ADMINISTRATION

Oral

- Give 2 h before/after magnesium or aluminum-containing antacids.
- Store in tightly closed container and protect from light.

ADVERSE EFFECTS (≥1%) **Body as a Whole:** Back pain, peripheral edema. Increased risk of cardiovascular events. **GI:** Abdominal pain, diarrhea, dyspepsia, flatulence, nausea. **CNS:** Dizziness, headache, insomnia. **Respiratory:** Pharyngitis, rhinitis, sinusitis, URI. **Skin:** Rash.

INTERACTIONS Drug: May diminish effectiveness of ACE INHIBITORS; **fluconazole** increases celecoxib concentrations; may increase **lithium** concentrations; may increase INR in older patients on **warfarin.**

PHARMACOKINETICS Peak: 3 h. **Distribution:** 97% protein bound; crosses placenta. **Metabolism:** In liver by CYP2C9. **Elimination:** Primarily in feces (57%), 27% in urine. **Half-Life:** 11.2 h.

NURSING IMPLICATIONS

Assessment & Drug Effects

- Lab tests: Periodically monitor Hct and Hgb, liver functions, BUN and creatinine, and serum electrolytes.
- Monitor closely lithium levels when the two drugs are given concurrently.
- Monitor closely PT/INR when used concurrently with warfarin.
- Monitor for fluid retention and edema especially in those with a history of hypertension or CHF.

Patient & Family Education

- Promptly report any of the following: Unexplained weight gain, edema, skin rash.
- Stop taking celecoxib and promptly report to physician if any of

C

the following occurs: S&S of liver dysfunction including nausea, fatigue, lethargy, itching, jaundice, abdominal pain, and flulike symptoms; S&S of GI ulceration including black, tarry stools and upper GI distress.

- Avoid using celecoxib during the third trimester of pregnancy.

CEPHALEXIN

(sef-a-lex′in)

Ceporex A, Keflex, Novolexin A

Classifications: BETA-LACTAM ANTIBIOTIC; FIRST-GENERATION CEPHALOSPORIN

Therapeutic: ANTIBIOTIC

Prototype: Cefazolin

Pregnancy Category: B

AVAILABILITY 250 mg, 500 mg capsules; 250 mg, 500 mg, 1 g tablets; 125 mg/5 mL, 250 mg/5 mL suspension

ACTION & *THERAPEUTIC EFFECT* Semisynthetic beta-lactam cephalosporin. Preferentially binds to one or more of the penicillin-binding proteins (PBP) located on cell walls of susceptible organisms. This inhibits third and final stage of bacterial cell wall synthesis, thus killing the bacterium. *Broad-spectrum, first-generation cephalosporin antibiotic active against many gram-positive aerobic cocci and much less active against gram-negative bacteria or anaerobic organisms.*

USES To treat infections caused by susceptible pathogens in respiratory and urinary tracts, middle ear, skin, soft tissue, and bone.

CONTRAINDICATIONS Hypersensitivity to cephalosporins and related antibiotics; viral infections. Safe use in infants younger than 1 mo not established.

CAUTIOUS USE History of hypersensitivity to penicillin or other drug allergy; severely impaired renal function; GI disease, colitis; hepatic disease; coagulopathy; pregnancy (category B), lactation.

ROUTE & DOSAGE

Mild to Moderate Infection

Adult: **PO** 250–500 mg q6h

Child: **PO** 25–100 mg/kg/day in 4 divided doses

Skin and Skin Structure Infections

Adult: **PO** 500 mg q12h

Otitis Media

Child: **PO** 75–100 mg/kg/day in 4 divided doses

ADMINISTRATION

Oral

- Cephalexin oral suspension should be refrigerated; discard unused portions 14 days after preparation. Label should indicate expiration date. Keep tightly covered. Shake suspension well before pouring.

ADVERSE EFFECTS (≥1%) **Body as a Whole:** Angioedema, <u>anaphylaxis</u>, superinfections. **GI:** *Diarrhea* (generally mild), nausea, vomiting, anorexia, abdominal pain. **CNS:** Dizziness, headache, fatigue. **Skin:** Rash, urticaria.

DIAGNOSTIC TEST INTERFERENCE False-positive ***urine glucose*** determinations using ***copper sulfate reagents*** (e.g., ***Clinitest, Benedict's reagent***), but not with ***glucose oxidase (enzymatic) tests*** (e.g., ***TesTape, Diastix, Clinistix***). Positive ***direct Coombs' test*** may complicate transfusion ***cross-matching procedures*** and ***hematologic studies.***

INTERACTIONS Drug: Probenecid decreases renal elimination of cephalexin.

PHARMACOKINETICS Absorption: Rapidly from GI tract; stable in stomach acid. **Peak:** 1 h. **Distribution:** Widely distributed in body fluids with highest concentration in kidney; crosses placenta. **Elimination:** 80–100% unchanged in urine in 8 h; excreted in breast milk. **Half-Life:** 38–70 min.

NURSING IMPLICATIONS

Assessment & Drug Effects

- Determine history of hypersensitivity reactions to cephalosporins and penicillin and history of other drug allergies before therapy is initiated.
- Lab tests: Evaluate renal and hepatic function periodically in patients receiving prolonged therapy.
- Monitor for manifestations of hypersensitivity (see Signs & Symptoms, Appendix F). Discontinue drug and report their appearance promptly.

Patient & Family Education

- Keep physician informed if adverse reactions appear.
- Be alert to S&S of superinfections (see Appendix F). These symptoms should be reported promptly and appropriate therapy instituted.

CEPHRADINE

(sef'ra-deen)

Anspor, Velosef

Classifications: ANTIBIOTIC; FIRST-GENERATION CEPHALOSPORIN

Therapeutic: ANTIBIOTIC

Prototype: Cefazolin

Pregnancy Category: B

AVAILABILITY 250 mg, 500 mg capsules; 125 mg/5 mL, 250 mg/5 mL suspension

ACTION & *THERAPEUTIC EFFECT* Semisynthetic acid-stable, first-generation cephalosporin. Preferentially binds to one or more of the penicillin-binding proteins (PBP) located on cell walls of susceptible organisms. This inhibits third and final stage of bacterial cell wall synthesis, thus killing the bacterium. *Broad-spectrum antibiotic that is active against many gram-positive aerobic cocci and much less active against gram-negative bacteria.*

USES Serious infections of respiratory and urinary tracts, skin and soft tissues, and for otitis media caused by susceptible pathogens; for perioperative prophylaxis, in cesarean section (intraoperative and postoperative); in septicemia (due to *Streptococcus pneumoniae, Staphylococcus aureus, Proteus mirabilis,* and *Escherichia coli*). Also used to treat urinary tract infections due to *Klebsiella* sp. and enterococci *(Streptococcus faecalis)*.

CONTRAINDICATIONS Hypersensitivity to cephalosporins and related antibiotics; viral infections. Safe use in children younger than 9 mo not established.

CAUTIOUS USE History of penicillin or other allergies, particularly to drugs; impaired renal function, sodium restriction (parenteral cephradine); coagulopathy, GI disease, colitis, pregnancy (category B), lactation.

ROUTE & DOSAGE

Mild to Moderate Infection

Adult: **PO** 250–500 mg q6h or 500 mg–1 g q12h up to 4 g/day

Child: **PO** 25–50 mg/kg/day in 2–4 divided doses up to 4 g/day

C

Perioperative Prophylaxis
Adult: **PO** 1 g 30–60 min before surgery; 1 g during surgery; then 1 g q4–6h for 24 h

ADMINISTRATION

Oral

- Oral cephradine may be given without regard to meals (acid stable); however, the presence of food may delay absorption.

ADVERSE EFFECTS (≥1%) **Body as a Whole:** Joint pains, eosinophilia, tightness in chest, pain, induration and tissue sloughing (IM injection site); thrombophlebitis (IV site); paresthesias, superinfections. **GI:** *Diarrhea* or loose stools, abdominal pain, heartburn. **CNS:** Dizziness. **Skin:** Urticaria, rash, pruritus.

DIAGNOSTIC TEST INTERFERENCE Cephradine causes false-positive (black-brown or green-brown color) ***urine glucose*** reaction with ***copper reduction reagents*** (e.g., as ***Benedict's*** or ***Clinitest***), but not with ***enzymatic glucose oxidase reagents*** (e.g., ***Clinistix, Tes-Tape***). False-positive ***direct Coombs' test*** (may interfere with ***cross-matching procedures*** and ***hematologic studies***) has also been reported.

INTERACTIONS Drug: Probenecid decreases renal elimination of cephradine.

PHARMACOKINETICS Absorption: Well absorbed from GI tract. **Peak:** 1 h. **Distribution:** Widely distributed in body fluids, with highest concentration in kidney; crosses placenta. **Elimination:** 80–90% eliminated unchanged in urine in 6 h; excreted in breast milk. **Half-Life:** 1–2 h.

NURSING IMPLICATIONS

Assessment & Drug Effects

- Determine history of previous hypersensitivity to cephalosporins, penicillins, and other drug allergies before therapy is initiated.
- Lab tests: Perform culture and sensitivity tests and renal function studies before drug therapy. Baseline and periodic creatinine clearance with impaired renal function.
- Pseudomembranous enterocolitis, a potentially life-threatening superinfection caused by *Clostridium difficile,* may occur during or after cephalosporin therapy. Report diarrhea and fever promptly.
- Monitor for signs of superinfection (see Appendix F). Report their appearance promptly.

Patient & Family Education

- Superinfections caused by overgrowth of nonsusceptible organisms may occur. Report early S&S (see Appendix F) promptly.
- Report loose stools or diarrhea promptly.

CERTOLIZUMAB

(cer-to′li-zu-mab)
Cimzia
Classifications: BIOLOGICAL RESPONSE MODIFIER; IMMUNOMODULATOR; TUMOR NECROSIS FACTOR (TNF) MODIFIER
Therapeutic: TNF MODIFIER; IMMUNOLOGIC; ANTIRHEUMATIC
Prototype: Etanercept
Pregnancy Category: B

AVAILABILITY 400 mg lyophilized powder for injection; 200 mg/mL prefilled syringe

ACTION & *THERAPEUTIC EFFECT* A fragment of an antibody Fab fragment with specificity for tumor necrosis factor (TNF)-alpha. This causes a reduction in the production of proinflammatory cytokines. Increased levels of TNF-alpha are found in the bowel wall areas that are affected by Crohn's disease and RA. *Reduces the inflammatory cytokine production in Crohn's disease. It decreases the serum level of C-reactive protein, a direct measure of the inflammatory process related to Crohn's disease. Effective for treatment of adults with moderately to severely active rheumatoid arthritis.*

USES Reduction of signs and symptoms, as well as maintenance of clinical response, in patients with moderately to severely active Crohn's disease who have experienced an inadequate response to conventional therapy. For treatment of moderate to severely active rheumatoid arthritis.

UNLABELED USES Psoriasis.

CONTRAINDICATIONS Active chronic or localized infections (e.g., TB, histoplasmosis, other fungal infections); HBV reactivation; lupus-like syndrome.

CAUTIOUS USE History of recurrent infection; concurrent immunosuppressive therapy; past/current residence in region where TB and histoplasmosis are endemic; CNS demyelinating disease; neurologic disorders, including seizure disorder, optic neuritis, peripheral neuropathy; recurrent/previous hematologic disorders; heart failure; hypersensitivity response to other TNF blocker(s); pregnancy (category B); lactation; older adult. Safety and efficacy in children not established.

ROUTE & DOSAGE

Crohn's Disease

Adult: **Subcutaneous** 400 mg (two 200 mg injections) at weeks 0, 2, and 4, then q4wk if clinical response occurs

Rheumatoid Arthritis

Adult: **Subcutaneous** Two 200 mg injections, at weeks 0, 2, and 4, then 200 mg every other week

ADMINISTRATION

Subcutaneous

- Reconstitute two 200 mg vials by adding 1 mL sterile water to each using a 20-gauge needle. Swirl gently then allow to sit to dissolve (may require up to 30 min); yields 200 mg/mL. Use within 2 h of reconstitution.
- Use two separate syringes with 20-gauge needles; withdraw 1 mL from each vial. Change to 23-gauge needles and inject into two separate sites on the abdomen or thigh.
- Store reconstituted solution. May be kept at room temperature for no longer than 2 h and refrigerated for up to 24 h.

ADVERSE EFFECTS (≥1%) **Body as a Whole:** Erythema nodosum, injection-site pain, pain in extremity, peripheral edema, pneumonia, *upper respiratory infection, urinary tract infection,* viral infections. **GI:** Abdominal pain. **Musculoskeletal:** *Arthralgia.* **Urogenital:** Pyelonephritis.

DIAGNOSTIC TEST INTERFERENCE Certolizumab may cause erroneously elevated ***activated partial thromboplastin time (aPTT)*** assay results.

INTERACTIONS Drug: Coadministration of **anakinra** may cause increased risks of serious infections and neutropenia.

PHARMACOKINETICS Absorption: 80% bioavailable. **Peak:** 54–171 h. **Half-Life:** 14 days.

C

NURSING IMPLICATIONS

Assessment & Drug Effects

- Prior to initiating therapy, patient should be evaluated for TB risk factors and latent TB. Monitor for S&S of TB throughout therapy.
- Report promptly any S&S of infection or hypersensitivity reaction. (See Appendix F for S&S.)
- Monitor closely carriers of HBV for signs of active infection. If suspected, withhold injection and notify physician.
- Monitor closely patients with heart failure for worsening cardiac status.
- Monitor for and report promptly any abnormal neurologic finding or unexplained bruising or bleeding.
- Lab tests: Baseline TB test; periodic CBC with platelet count.

Patient & Family Education

- Report promptly any of the following: S&S of infections, such as persistent fever; signs of an allergic reaction (e.g., hives, itching, swelling); unexplained bleeding or bruising.
- Do not accept vaccination with live (or attenuated) vaccines while on certolizumab.

CETIRIZINE

(ce-tir′i-zeen)

Reactine ✦, Zyrtec

LEVOCETIRIZINE

(lev-o-ce-tir′i-zeen)

Xyzal

Classifications: ANTIHISTAMINE; H_1-RECEPTOR ANTAGONIST; NON-SEDATING

Therapeutic: ANTIHISTAMINE, NON-SEDATING

Prototype: Loratadine

Pregnancy Category: B

AVAILABILITY 5 mg, 10 mg tablets; 5 mg, 10 mg chewable tablets; 5 mg/5 mL, 2.5 mg/5 mL syrup; **Levocetirizine:** 2.5 mg/mL syrup; 5 mg tablet

ACTION & *THERAPEUTIC EFFECT* Cetirizine is a potent H_1-receptor antagonist and thus an antihistamine without significant anticholinergic or CNS activity. Low lipophilicity combined with its H_1-receptor selectivity probably accounts for its relative lack of anticholinergic and sedative properties. *Effectively treats allergic rhinitis and chronic urticaria by eliminating or reducing the local and systemic effects of histamine release.*

USES Seasonal and perennial allergic rhinitis and chronic idiopathic urticaria.

CONTRAINDICATIONS Hypersensitivity to H_1-receptor antihistamines or hydroxyzine; concurrent use of alcohol; lactation, infants younger than 6 mo.

CAUTIOUS USE Moderate to severe renal impairment, hepatic impairment, pregnancy (category B), children.

ROUTE & DOSAGE

Allergic Rhinitis

Adult: **PO** 5–10 mg once/day
Child: **PO** *2–5 y,* 2.5 mg daily (max: 5 mg/day); *6 y or older,* 5–10 mg daily

Allergic Rhinitis (Levocetirizine)

Adult/Adolescent/Child (older than 6 y): **PO** 2.5–5 mg once/day
Child (2–5 y): **PO** 1.25 mg each evening

Chronic Urticaria

Adult: **PO** 10 mg daily or b.i.d.

Chronic Urticaria (Levocetirizine)

Adult/Adolescent/Child (older than 6 y): **PO** 2.5–5 mg each evening

Child (6 mo–5 y): **PO** 1.25 mg each evening

Renal Impairment Dosage Adjustment (Levocetirizine)

CrCl 51–80 mL/min: 2.5 mg daily; 30–50 mL/min: 2.5 mg every other day; 10–29 mL/min: 2.5 mg twice a week; less than 10 mL/min: Do not use

ADMINISTRATION

Oral

- Consult physician about dosage if significant adverse effects appear. As elimination half-life is prolonged in the older adult, dosage adjustments may be warranted.

ADVERSE EFFECTS (≥1%) **GI:** Constipation, diarrhea, dry mouth. **CNS:** *Drowsiness, sedation, headache,* depression.

INTERACTIONS Drug: Theophylline may decrease cetirizine clearance leading to toxicity. Use with **scopolamine** or **atropine** may cause anticholinergic effects.

PHARMACOKINETICS Absorption: Readily from GI tract. **Peak:** 1 h. **Distribution:** 93% protein bound; minimal CNS concentrations. **Metabolism:** Minimal (by CYP3A4). **Elimination:** 60% unchanged in urine within 24 h, 5% in feces. **Half-Life:** 7.4 h (cetirazine), 8–9 h (levocetirizine).

NURSING IMPLICATIONS

Assessment & Drug Effects

- Monitor for drug interactions. As the drug is highly protein bound, the potential for interactions with other protein-bound drugs exists.
- Monitor for sedation, especially the older adult.

Patient & Family Education

- Do not use in combination with OTC antihistamines.
- Do not engage in driving or other hazardous activities, before experiencing your responses to the drug.

CETRORELIX

(ce-tro-re'lix)

Cetrotide

Classification: GONADOTROPIN-RELEASING HORMONE ANTAGONIST

Therapeutic: LUTEINIZING HORMONE-RELEASING HORMONE RECEPTOR (LRHR) ANTAGONIST

Pregnancy Category: X

AVAILABILITY 0.25 mg, 3 mg injection

ACTION & *THERAPEUTIC EFFECT* Cetrotide is a luteinizing hormone-releasing hormone (LHRH) antagonist. *Prevents premature LH surges in patients undergoing controlled ovarian hyperstimulation for assisted reproduction.*

USES Treatment of infertility as part of an assisted reproduction program.

CONTRAINDICATIONS Hypersensitivity to cetrorelix, extrinsic peptide hormones, mannitol, gonadotropin-releasing hormone analogs; primary ovarian failure; renal failure; pregnancy (category X); known or suspected pregnancy; lactation.

CAUTIOUS USE Hepatic insufficiency; polycystic ovary syndrome.

ROUTE & DOSAGE

Infertility

Adult: **Subcutaneous** 0.25 mg/days during early to mid follicular phase of the cycle (stimulation

C

day 5 or 6) following the initiation of FSH or 3 mg as a single dose is administered when the serum estradiol level is indicative of an appropriate stimulation response, usually on FSH stimulation day 7 (range day 5–9). If HCG has not been administered within 4 days after the injection of 3 mg, then 0.25 mg should be administered once daily until HCG administration.

ADMINISTRATION

Subcutaneous

- Reconstitute the 0.25 or 3 mL vial with 1 or 3 mL, respectively, of sterile water for injection.
- Inject into lower abdominal wall following reconstitution. Rotate injection sites.
- Store the 3 mg dose at room temperature, 15°–30° C (59°–86° F). Store the 0.25 mg dose in the refrigerator.

ADVERSE EFFECTS (≥1%) **CNS:** Headache. **GI:** Nausea, vomiting, abdominal pain. **Endocrine:** Hot flashes. **Skin:** Pruritus at injection site. **Urogenital:** Ovarian enlargement, ovarian hyperstimulation syndrome, pelvic pain.

INTERACTIONS Drug: Cimetidine, methyldopa, metoclopramide, reserpine, PHENOTHIAZINES may interfere with fertility efforts. **Herbal: Black cohosh, DHEA** may antagonize fertility efforts.

PHARMACOKINETICS Absorption: 85% absorbed from subcutaneous injection site. **Peak:** 1–2 h. **Metabolism:** Metabolized by peptidases. **Elimination:** 2–4% in urine, 5–10% in bile. **Half-Life:** 62 h after single dose, 20 h after multiple doses.

NURSING IMPLICATIONS

Assessment & Drug Effects

- Lab test: Monitor routine blood chemistries.
- Monitor weight and report development of edema and/or shortness of breath.

Patient & Family Education

- Contact physician immediately for any of the following: Abdominal or stomach pain, persistent or severe nausea, vomiting or diarrhea; decreased urination; pelvic pain; moderate to severe bloating, rapid weight gain; shortness of breath; swelling of lower legs.

CETUXIMAB

(ce-tux'i-mab)

Erbitux

Classifications: ANTINEOPLASTIC; MONOCLONAL ANTIBODY; EPIDERMAL GROWTH FACTOR RECEPTOR (EGFR) INHIBITOR

Therapeutic: ANTINEOPLASTIC

Prototype: Gefitinib

Pregnancy Category: C

AVAILABILITY 100 mg/50 mL injection

ACTION & *THERAPEUTIC EFFECT* Cetuximab is a recombinant, monoclonal antibody that binds specifically to the epidermal growth factor receptor (EGFR, HER1, c-ErbB-1) on both normal and tumor cells. Binding to the EGFR results in inhibition of cell growth, induction of apoptosis, and decreased vascular endothelial growth factor production. *Overexpression of EGFR is detected in many human cancers, including those of the colon and rectum. Cetuximab inhibits the growth and survival of tu-*

mor cells that overexpress the EGFR.

USES Treatment of EGFR-expressing metastatic colorectal cancer in combination with irinotecan in patients who are refractory to irinotecan-based chemotherapy or as monotherapy in patients who are intolerant to irinotecan-based chemotherapy. Used in combination with radiation for squamous cell cancer of head and neck.

CONTRAINDICATIONS Lactation within 60 days of using cetuximab; worsening of preexisting pulmonary edema or interstitial lung disease. Safety and efficacy in children have not been established.

CAUTIOUS USE Infusion reaction, especially with first-time users; history of hypersensitivity to murine proteins or cetuximab; cardiac disease, coronary artery disease, CHF, arrhythmias; pulmonary disease, pulmonary fibrosis; UV exposure, radiation therapy; pregnancy (category C).

ROUTE & DOSAGE

Colorectal Cancer/Head and Neck Cancer

Adult: **IV** Start with 400 mg/m² over 2 h; continue with 250 mg/m² over 1 h weekly

ADMINISTRATION

Intravenous

Administer with full resuscitation equipment available and under the supervision of a physician experienced with chemotherapy.

- Premedication with an H_1-receptor antagonist (e.g., diphenhydramine 50 mg IV) is recommended.
- Monitor for an infusion reaction for at least 1 h following completion of infusion.

PREPARE: **IV Infusion:** Do not shake or further dilute vial. Do not mix with other medication. ▪ Inject cetuximab solution into a sterile, evacuated container or bag (i.e., glass, polyolefin, ethylene vinyl acetate, DEHP plasticized PVC, or PVC); repeat until needed dose has been added to container, using a new needle for each vial. ▪ Attach to infusion set with a low-protein-binding 0.22-micron filter and prime line with cetuximab. May also administer by syringe and syringe pump; use a new needle and filter for each vial.

ADMINISTER: **IV Infusion:** Do NOT administer a bolus dose. ▪ Give IV infusion via an infusion pump or syringe pump at 5 mL/min or less; piggyback into the patient's IV line. ▪ Flush line with NS after infusion. ▪ Note: Slow infusion rate by 50% if a prior, mild infusion reaction occurred.

INCOMPATIBILITIES **Solution/additive:** Do not mix with other additives.

- Store unopened vials at 2°–8° C (36°–46° F). Note: Vials may contain a small amount of easily visible, white particles. ▪ Cetuximab in IV bag is stable for up to 12 h refrigerated and up to 8 h at 20°–25° C (68°–77° F).

ADVERSE EFFECTS (≥1%) **Body as a Whole:** Infusion reactions (allergic reaction, anaphylactoid reaction, fever, chills, dyspnea, bronchospasm stridor, hoarseness, urticaria, hypotension), *fever,* sepsis, *asthenia, malaise,* pain, infection. **CNS:** *Headache,* insomnia, depression. **CV:** Cardiopulmonary arrest. **GI:** *Nausea, vomiting, diarrhea, abdominal pain, constipation,* stomatitis, dyspepsia. **Hematologic:** Leukopenia, anemia. **Metabolic:** Weight loss, peripheral edema, dehydration, hypomag-

C

nesemia, hypokalemia. **Respiratory:** Pulmonary embolism, pulmonary fibrosis (rare), *dyspnea,* cough. **Skin:** *Rash,* alopecia, pruritus. **Urogenital:** Kidney failure.

PHARMACOKINETICS Half-Life: 114 h (75–188 h).

NURSING IMPLICATIONS

Assessment & Drug Effects

- Discontinue infusion and notify physician for S&S of a severe infusion reaction: Chills, fever, bronchospasm, stridor, hoarseness, urticaria, and/or hypotension. Carefully monitor until complete resolution of all S&S.
- Monitor pulmonary status and report onset of acute or worsening pulmonary symptoms.
- Lab tests: Periodic CBC with differential, electrolytes, Hct and Hgb. Closely Monitor serum electrolytes, including serum magnesium, potassium, and calcium, during and for 1 h after administration of this drug. Additionally, electrolytes need to be monitored for 8 wk after completion of therapy.

Patient & Family Education

- Report immediately: Difficulty breathing, wheezing, shortness of breath, hives, faintness and/or dizziness anytime during IV infusion.
- Report promptly any of the following: Eye inflammation, mouth sores, skin rash, redness, or severe dry skin.
- Wear sunscreen and a hat and limit sun exposure while being treated with this drug.

CEVIMELINE HYDROCHLORIDE

(cev-i-may′leen)

Evoxac

Classifications: CHOLINERGIC AGONIST; CHOLINERGIC ENHANCER
Therapeutic: CHOLINERGIC RECEPTOR ENHANCER
Pregnancy Category: C

AVAILABILITY 30 mg capsules

ACTION & *THERAPEUTIC EFFECT* Cholinergic agent that binds to muscarinic receptors. *Increases secretion of exocrine glands, such as salivary and sweat glands. It relieves severe dry mouth.*

USES Treatment of dry mouth in patients with Sjögren's syndrome.

CONTRAINDICATIONS Hypersensitivity to cevimeline; uncontrolled asthma; acute iritis; narrow-angle glaucoma; lactation.
CAUTIOUS USE Controlled asthma; chronic bronchitis, COPD; cardiac disease, cardiac arrhythmias, myocardial infarction; history of nephrolithiasis or cholelithiasis; elderly; pregnancy (category C); older adults. Safety and effectiveness in children are not established.

ROUTE & DOSAGE

Dry Mouth
Adult: **PO** 30 mg t.i.d.

ADMINISTRATION

Oral
- Give without regard to food.
- Store refrigerated at 2°–8° C (35.6°–46.4° F) with occasional fluctuations between 15°–30° C (59°–86° F).

ADVERSE EFFECTS (≥1%) **Body as a Whole:** *Excessive sweating, headache,* back pain, dizziness, fatigue, pain, hot flushes, rigors, tremor, hypertonia, myalgia, fever, eye pain, earache, flu-like symptoms.

CNS: Insomnia, anxiety, vertigo, depression, hyporeflexia.: **CV:** Peripheral edema, chest pain.: **GI:** *Nausea, diarrhea,* excessive salivation, dyspepsia, abdominal pain, coughing, vomiting, constipation, anorexia, dry mouth, hiccup.: **Respiratory:** *Rhinitis, sinusitis, upper respiratory tract infection,* pharyngitis, bronchitis. **Skin:** Rash, conjunctivitis, pruritus. **Special Senses:** Abnormal vision. **Urogenital:** Urinary tract infection.

INTERACTIONS Drug: BETA-ADRENERGIC AGONISTS may cause conduction disturbances; PARASYMPATHOMIMETIC DRUGS may have additive effects.

PHARMACOKINETICS Absorption: Rapidly absorbed. **Peak:** 1.5–2 h. **Distribution:** Less than 20% protein bound. **Metabolism:** In liver by CYP2D6 and 3A3/4. **Elimination:** Primarily in urine. **Half-Life:** 5 h.

NURSING IMPLICATIONS

Assessment & Drug Effects

- Monitor for S&S of increased airway resistance, especially in patient with asthma, bronchitis, emphysema, or COPD.
- Lab tests: Routine blood chemistry during long-term therapy.
- Report S&S of excess cholinergic activity (e.g., diaphoresis, frequent urge to urinate, nausea and/or diarrhea).

Patient & Family Education

- Do not drive or engage in potentially hazardous activities until response to drug is known.
- Consult physician if confusion, dizziness, or faintness occur.
- Report diminished night vision or depth perception.
- Drink fluids liberally (2000–3000 mL/day) in the event of excessive sweating.

CHARCOAL, ACTIVATED (LIQUID ANTIDOTE)

Actidose, CharcoAid, Charcocaps, Charcodote, Insta-Char
Classifications: ANTIDOTE; ADSORBENT
Therapeutic: ANTIDOTE
Pregnancy Category: C

AVAILABILITY 208 mg/mL, 15 g, 30 g, 50 mg liquid/suspension

ACTION & *THERAPEUTIC EFFECT* Activated charcoal (carbon) is a chemically inert, odorless, tasteless, fine black powder with wide spectrum of adsorptive activity. Acts by binding (adsorbing) toxic substances, thereby inhibiting their GI absorption, enterohepatic circulation, and thus bioavailability. *Action appears to result from drug diffusion from plasma into GI tract where it is adsorbed by activated charcoal. Effectively adsorbs toxins in the gut preventing their systemic absorption and impact.*

USES General purpose emergency antidote in the treatment of poisonings by most drugs and chemicals. Gastric dialysis (repetitive doses) in uremia to adsorb various waste products from GI tract; severe acute poisoning. Has been used to adsorb intestinal gases in treatment of dyspepsia, flatulence, and distention (value in these conditions not established). Sometimes used topically as a deodorant for foul-smelling wounds and ulcers.

CONTRAINDICATIONS Reportedly not effective for poisonings by cyanide, mineral acids, caustic alkalis, organic solvents, iron, ethanol, methanol; gag reflex depression, coma; GI obstruction; quinidine or quinine hypersensitivity.

C

CAUTIOUS USE Pregnancy (category C); lactation.

ROUTE & DOSAGE

Acute Poisonings
Adult: **PO** 30–100 g in at least 180–240 mL (6–8 oz) of water or 1 g/kg
Child (1–12 y): **PO** 1–2 g/kg or 15–30 g in at least 6–8 oz of water
Infant (younger than 1 y): **PO** 1 g/kg
Gastric Dialysis
Adult: **PO** 20–40 g q6h for 1 or 2 days
GI Disturbances
Adult: **PO** 520–975 mg p.c. up to 5 g/day

ADMINISTRATION

Oral

- In an emergency, dose may be approximated by stirring sufficient activated charcoal into tap water to make a slurry the consistency of soup (about 20–30 g in at least 240 mL of water).
- Activated charcoal can be swallowed or given through a nasogastric tube. If administered too rapidly, patient may vomit.
- Store in tightly covered container.

ADVERSE EFFECTS (≥1%) **GI:** Vomiting (rapid ingestion of high doses), constipation, diarrhea (from sorbitol).

INTERACTIONS Drug: May decrease absorption of all other oral medications—administer at least 2 h apart.

PHARMACOKINETICS Absorption: Not absorbed. **Elimination:** In feces.

NURSING IMPLICATIONS

Assessment & Drug Effects

- Record appearance, color, consistency, frequency, and relative amount of stools. Inform patient that activated charcoal will color feces black.

CHLORAL HYDRATE

(klor′al hye′drate)
Aquachloral Supprettes, Noctec, Novochlorhydrate ♣
Classification: ANXIOLYTIC, SEDATIVE-HYPNOTIC
Therapeutic: ANTIANXIETY; SEDATIVE-HYPNOTIC
Prototype: Secobarbital
Pregnancy Category: C
Controlled Substance: Schedule IV

AVAILABILITY 500 mg capsules; 250 mg/5 mL, 500 mg/5 mL syrup; 324 mg, 500 mg, 648 mg suppositories

ACTION & *THERAPEUTIC EFFECT* Produces "physiologic sleep" by mild cerebral depression with little effect on respirations or BP and little or no hangover. *Chloral hydrate in low doses is a sedative-hypnotic that does not affect sleep physiology (e.g., REM sleep).*

USES Short-term management of insomnia, general sedation (especially in the young and the older adult), sedation before and after surgery, to reduce anxiety associated with drug withdrawal, and alone or with paraldehyde to prevent or suppress alcohol withdrawal symptoms.

CONTRAINDICATIONS Known hypersensitivity to chloral hydrate or chloral derivatives; severe hepatic, renal, or cardiac disease; rectal dosage form in patients with proctitis; oral use in patients with esophagitis, gastritis, gastric or duodenal ulcers.

CAUTIOUS USE History of intermittent porphyria, asthma, history of or proneness to drug dependence, depression, suicidal tendencies; pregnancy (category C).

ROUTE & DOSAGE

Sedative

Adult: **PO/PR** 250 mg t.i.d. p.c.
Child: **PO/PR** 25–50 mg/kg/day divided q6–8h (max: 500 mg/dose)

Hypnotic

Adult: **PO/PR** 500 mg–1 g 15–30 min before bedtime or 30 min before surgery
Geriatric: **PO/PR** 250 mg at bedtime
Child: **PO/PR** 50 mg/kg 15–30 min before bedtime or 30 min before surgery (max: 1 g)

EEG Premedication

Child: **PO/PR** 20–25 mg/kg 30–60 min prior to procedure

ADMINISTRATION

Oral

- Dilute liquid preparations in chilled fluids to minimize unpleasant taste.
- Watch to see that drug is not cheeked and hoarded.

Rectal

- Moisten suppository with a water-based lubricant, such as K-Y jelly, prior to insertion.

ADVERSE EFFECTS (≥1%) **Body as a Whole:** Angioedema, eosinophilia, breath odor, leukopenia, ketonuria, renal and hepatic damage, sudden death. **CV:** Arrhythmias, cardiac arrest. **GI:** *Nausea, vomiting, diarrhea,* severe gastritis. **CNS:** Dizziness, motor incoordination, headache. **Skin:** Purpura, urticaria, erythematous rash, eczema, erythema multiforme, fixed drug eruptions. **Special Senses:** Conjunctivitis.

DIAGNOSTIC TEST INTERFERENCE False-positive results for ***urine glucose*** with ***Benedict's solutions,*** and possibly with ***Clinitest*** but not with ***glucose oxidase methods*** (e.g., ***Clinistix, Diastix, Tes-Tape***). Possible interference with fluorometric test for ***urine catecholamines*** (if chloral hydrate is administered within 48 h of test) and ***urinary 17-OHCS*** determinations (by modification of ***Reddy, Jenkins, Thorn procedure***).

INTERACTIONS Drug: Alcohol, BARBITURATES, **paraldehyde,** other CNS DEPRESSANTS potentiate CNS depression; tachycardia may also occur with **alcohol;** increases anticoagulant effect of ORAL ANTICOAGULANTS; **furosemide** IV can produce flushing, diaphoresis, BP changes.

PHARMACOKINETICS Absorption: Readily from oral or rectal administration. **Onset:** 30–60 min. **Peak:** 1–3 h. **Duration:** 4–8 h. **Distribution:** Well distributed to all tissues; 70–80% protein bound; crosses placenta. **Metabolism:** In liver to the active metabolite trichloroethanol. **Elimination:** Primarily by kidneys; small amount excreted in feces via bile. **Half-Life:** 8–11 h.

NURSING IMPLICATIONS

Assessment & Drug Effects

- Do not discontinue abruptly following prolonged use. Sudden withdrawal from dependent patients may produce delirium, mania, or convulsions.
- Monitor for S&S of allergic skin reactions, which may occur within several hours or as long as 10 days after drug administration.

Patient & Family Education

- Do not ambulate without assistance until response to drug is known.

C

- Avoid concomitant use of alcoholic beverages.
- Avoid driving and other potentially hazardous activities while under the influence of chloral hydrate.

CHLORAMBUCIL

(klor-am′byoo-sil)
Leukeran
Classifications: ANTINEOPLASTIC; ALKYLATING AGENT
Therapeutic: ANTINEOPLASTIC; NITROGEN MUSTARD
Prototype: Cyclophosphamide
Pregnancy Category: D

AVAILABILITY 2 mg tablets

ACTION & *THERAPEUTIC EFFECT* Potent aromatic derivative of the alkylating agent nitrogen mustard which is slowest acting and least toxic of the nitrogen mustards. A cell-cycle nonspecific drug (kills both resting and dividing cells), it causes cytotoxic cross linkage in DNA, thus preventing synthesis of DNA, RNA, and proteins. Myelosuppression in therapeutic doses is moderate and rapidly reversible. *Lymphocytic effect is marked; thus it is effective in treatment of various lymphomas.*

USES As single agent or with other antineoplastics in treatment of chronic lymphocytic leukemia, malignant lymphomas including lymphosarcoma, Hodgkin's disease, and giant follicular lymphoma, and in treatment of carcinoma of the ovary, breast, and testes.

UNLABELED USES Nonneoplastic conditions: Vasculitis complicating rheumatoid arthritis, autoimmune hemolytic anemias associated with cold agglutinins, lupus glomerulonephritis, idiopathic nephrotic syndrome, polycythemia vera, macroglobulinemia.

CONTRAINDICATIONS Hypersensitivity to chlorambucil or to other alkylating agents; administration within 4 wk of a full course of radiation or chemotherapy; full dosage if bone marrow is infiltrated with lymphomatous tissue or is hypoplastic; smallpox and other vaccines; pregnancy (category D), lactation.

CAUTIOUS USE Excessive or prolonged dosage, pneumococcus vaccination, history of seizures or head trauma.

ROUTE & DOSAGE

Malignant Diseases (Lymphomas, Hodgkin's Disease, etc.)
Adult: **PO** 0.1–0.2 mg/kg/day (usual dose 4–10 mg/day)
Child: **PO** 0.1–0.2 mg/kg/day in single or divided doses

ADMINISTRATION

Oral

- Control nausea and vomiting by giving entire daily dose at one time, 1 h before breakfast or 2 h after evening meal, or at bedtime. Consult physician.
- Store in tightly closed, light-resistant container.

ADVERSE EFFECTS (≥1%) **Body as a Whole:** Drug fever, skin rashes, papilledema, alopecia, peripheral neuropathy, sterile cystitis, pulmonary complications, seizures (high doses). **GI:** Low incidence of gastric discomfort, <u>hepatotoxicity.</u> **Hematologic:** <u>Bone marrow depression</u>: *Leukopenia,* thrombocytopenia, anemia. **Metabolic:** Sterility, hyperuricemia.

INTERACTIONS Drug: May have to adjust dose of **allopurinol, col-**

chicine because of chlorambucil-associated hyperuricemia.

PHARMACOKINETICS Absorption: Rapidly and completely from GI tract. **Peak:** 1 h. **Distribution:** Extensively bound to plasma and tissue proteins; crosses placenta. **Metabolism:** In liver. **Elimination:** 60% in urine as metabolites within 24 h. **Half-Life:** 1.5–2.5 h.

NURSING IMPLICATIONS

Assessment & Drug Effects

- Lab tests: CBC, Hgb, total and differential leukocyte counts, and serum uric acid initially and at least once weekly during treatment.
- Leukopenia usually develops after the third week of treatment; it may continue for up to 10 days after last dose, then rapidly return to normal.
- Avoid or reduce to minimum injections and other invasive procedures (e.g., rectal temperatures, enemas) when platelet count is low.

Patient & Family Education

- Notify physician if the following symptoms occur: Unusual bleeding or bruising, sores on lips or in mouth; flank, stomach, or joint pain; fever, chills, or other signs of infection, sore throat, cough, dyspnea.
- Report immediately the onset of a skin reaction.
- Drink at least 10–12 glasses [240 mL (8 oz) each] of fluid per day, if not contraindicated.

CHLORAMPHENICOL

(klor-am-fen′i-kole)

Chloromycetin, Novo-chlorocap ✦

CHLORAMPHENICOL SODIUM SUCCINATE

Chloromycetin Sodium Succinate

Classification: ANTIBIOTIC

Therapeutic: ANTIBIOTIC, BROAD-SPECTRUM

Pregnancy Category: C

AVAILABILITY 250 mg capsules; 100 mg/mL injection; 5 mg/mL ophth solution; 10 mg/g ointment

ACTION & *THERAPEUTIC EFFECT* Synthetic broad-spectrum antibiotic believed to act by binding to the 50S ribosome of bacteria and thus interfering with protein synthesis. *Effective against a wide variety of gram-negative and gram-positive bacteria and most anaerobic microorganisms.*

USES Severe infections when other antibiotics are ineffective or are contraindicated. Particularly effective against *Salmonella typhi* and other *Salmonella* sp., *Streptococcus pneumoniae, Neisseria,* meningeal infections caused by *H. influenzae,* and infections involving *Bacteroides fragilis* and other anaerobic organisms, *Rickettsia rickettsii* (cause of Rocky Mountain spotted fever) and other rickettsiae, the lymphogranuloma-psittacosis group *(Chlamydia),* and *Mycoplasma*. Also used in cystic fibrosis anti-infective regimens and topically for infections of skin, eyes, and external auditory canal.

CONTRAINDICATIONS History of hypersensitivity or toxic reaction to chloramphenicol; treatment of minor infections, prophylactic use; typhoid carrier state, history or family history of drug-induced bone marrow depression, concomitant therapy with drugs that produce bone marrow depression; lactation.

CAUTIOUS USE Impaired hepatic or renal function, premature and full-term infants, children; intermittent porphyria; patients with G6PD deficiency; patient or family history of drug-induced bone marrow depression; pregnancy (category C).

ROUTE & DOSAGE

Serious Infections

Adult: **PO/IV** 50 mg/kg/day in 4 divided doses
Infant/Child: **PO/IV** 50–75 mg/kg/day divided q6h (max: 4 g/day)
Neonate: **IV** 25–50 mg/kg/day divided q12–24h

Meningitis

Adult/Child: **IV** 75–100 mg/kg/day divided q6h

ADMINISTRATION

Oral

- Give preferably with a full glass of water on an empty stomach, at least 1 h before or 2 h after a meal, to achieve optimum blood levels.

Ophthalmic

- Apply light pressure to lacrimal duct after instillation for 1–2 min to prevent drainage into nasopharynx and systemic absorption. This is an extremely important step to decrease absorption. Several cases of aplastic anemia have been associated with use of ophthalmic preparations.

Intravenous

IV administration to neonates, infants, children: Verify correct IV concentration and rate of infusion with physician.

PREPARE: **Direct:** Dilute each 1 g with 10 mL of sterile water or D5W. **Intermittent:** Further dilute in 50–100 mL of D5W.

ADMINISTER: **Direct:** Give slowly over a period of at least 1 min. **Intermittent:** Give over 30–60 min.

INCOMPATIBILITIES **Solutions/additives:** **Chlorpromazine, glycopyrrolate, metoclopramide, polymyxin B, prochlorperazine, promethazine,** TETRACYCLINES, **vancomycin.** **Y-site:** **Fluconazole.**

- Solution for infusion may form crystals or a second layer when stored at low temperatures. Solution can be clarified by shaking vial.
- Do not use cloudy solutions.

- Store topical ophthalmic, otic, and skin preparations, PO forms, and unopened ampuls at room temperature and protected from light unless otherwise directed by manufacturer.

ADVERSE EFFECTS (≥1%) **Body as a Whole:** Hypersensitivity, angioedema, dyspnea, fever, anaphylaxis, superinfections, Gray syndrome. **GI:** Nausea, vomiting, diarrhea, perianal irritation, enterocolitis, glossitis, stomatitis, unpleasant taste, xerostomia. **Hematologic:** Bone marrow depression (dose-related and reversible): Reticulocytosis, leukopenia, granulocytopenia, thrombocytopenia, increased plasma iron, reduced Hgb, hypoplastic anemia, hypoprothrombinemia. Non-dose-related and irreversible pancytopenia, agranulocytosis, aplastic anemia, paroxysmal nocturnal hemoglobinuria, leukemia. **CNS:** Neurotoxicity: Headache, mental depression, confusion, delirium, digital paresthesias, peripheral neuritis. **Skin:** Urticaria, contact dermatitis, maculopapular and vesicular rashes, fixed-drug eruptions. **Special Senses:** Visual disturbances, optic neuritis, optic nerve atrophy, contact conjunctivitis.

DIAGNOSTIC TEST INTERFERENCE Possibility of false-positive results for ***urine glucose*** by ***copper reduction methods*** (e.g., ***Benedict's solution, Clinitest***). Chloramphenicol may interfere with ***17-OHCS*** (urinary steroid) determinations (modification of ***Reddy, Jenkins, Thorn procedure*** not affected), with ***urobilinogen excretion,*** and with responses to ***tetanus toxoid*** and possibly other active immunizing agents.

INTERACTIONS Drug: The metabolism of **chlorpropamide, dicumarol, phenytoin, tolbutamide** may be decreased, prolonging their activity. **Phenobarbital** decreases chloramphenicol levels. The response to **iron** preparations, **folic acid,** and **vitamin** B_{12} may be delayed.

PHARMACOKINETICS Absorption: Rapidly from GI tract. **Peak:** PO: 1–3 h; IV: 1 h. **Distribution:** Widely distributed to most body tissues including saliva and ascitic, pleural and synovial fluid; concentrates in liver and kidneys; penetrates CNS; crosses placenta. **Metabolism:** Primarily inactivated in liver. **Elimination:** Much longer in neonates; metabolite and free drug excreted in urine; excreted in breast milk. **Half-Life:** 1.5–4.1 h.

NURSING IMPLICATIONS

Assessment & Drug Effects

- Lab tests: Perform bacterial culture and susceptibility tests prior to first dose. Baseline CBC, platelets, serum iron, and reticulocyte cell counts before initiation of therapy, at 48 h intervals during therapy, and periodically. Monitor chloramphenicol blood levels weekly or more frequently with hepatic dysfunction and in patients receiving therapy for longer than 2 wk. Desired concentrations: Peak 10–20 mcg/mL; through 5–10 mcg/mL.
- Check temperature at least q4h. Usually chloramphenicol is discontinued if temperature remains normal for 48 h.
- Monitor I&O ratio or pattern: Report any appreciable change.
- Monitor for S&S of gray syndrome, which has occurred 2–9 days after initiation of high dose chloramphenicol therapy in premature infants and neonates and in children 2 y or younger. Report early signs: Abdominal distention, failure to feed, pallor, changes in vital signs.

Patient & Family Education

- A bitter taste may occur 15–20 sec after IV injection; it usually lasts only 2–3 min.
- Report immediately sore throat, fever, fatigue, petechiae, nose bleeds, bleeding gums, or other unusual bleeding or bruising, or any other suspicious sign of symptom.
- Watch for S&S of superinfection (see Appendix F).
- Notify physician immediately if signs of hypersensitivity reaction (see Appendix F), irritation, superinfection, or other adverse reactions appear.

CHLORDIAZEPOXIDE HYDROCHLORIDE

(klor-dye-az-e-pox′ide)

Librium, Solium ♣

Classifications: ANXIOLYTIC; SEDATIVE-HYPNOTIC; BENZODIAZEPINE
Therapeutic: ANTIANXIETY; SEDATIVE-HYPNOTIC
Prototype: Lorazepam
Pregnancy Category: D
Controlled Substance: Schedule IV

AVAILABILITY 5 mg, 10 mg, 25 mg capsules

ACTION & *THERAPEUTIC EFFECT* Benzodiazepine derivative that acts on the limbic, thalamic, and hypothalamic areas of the CNS. Has long-acting hypnotic properties. Causes mild suppression of REM sleep and of deeper phases, particularly stage 4, while increasing total sleep time. *Produces mild anxiolytic (reduces anxiety), sedative, anticonvulsant, and skeletal muscle relaxant effects.*

USES Relief of various anxiety and tension states, preoperative apprehension and anxiety, and for management of alcohol withdrawal.

UNLABELED USES Essential, familial, and senile action tremors.

CONTRAINDICATIONS Hypersensitivity to chlordiazepoxide and other benzodiazepines; narrow-angle glaucoma, prostatic hypertrophy, shock, comatose states, primary depressive disorder or psychoses, pregnancy (category D), lactation, oral use in children younger than 6 y, parenteral use in children younger than 12 y, acute alcohol intoxication.

CAUTIOUS USE Anxiety states associated with impending depression, history of impaired hepatic or renal function; addiction-prone individuals, blood dyscrasias; in the older adult, debilitated patients, children; aggressive or hyperactive children; hyperkinesis, COPD.

ROUTE & DOSAGE

Mild Anxiety, Preoperative Anxiety

Adult: **PO** 5–10 mg t.i.d. or q.i.d.
Geriatric: **PO** 5 mg b.i.d. to q.i.d.
Child: **PO** 5 mg b.i.d. to q.i.d.; may be increased to 10 mg t.i.d.

Severe Anxiety and Tension

Adult: **PO** 20–25 mg t.i.d. or q.i.d.

Alcohol Withdrawal Syndrome

Adult: **PO** 50–100 mg prn up to 300 mg/day

ADMINISTRATION

Oral

- Give with or immediately after meals or with milk to reduce GI distress. If an antacid is prescribed, it should be taken at least 1 h before or after chlordiazepoxide to prevent delay in drug absorption.
- Store in tight, light-resistant containers at room temperature unless otherwise specified by manufacturer.

ADVERSE EFFECTS (≥1%) **Body as a Whole:** Edema, pain in injection site, jaundice, hiccups, <u>respiratory depression</u>. **CV:** Orthostatic hypotension, tachycardia, changes in ECG patterns seen with rapid IV administration. **GI:** Nausea, dry mouth, vomiting, constipation, increased appetite. **CNS:** *Drowsiness,* dizziness, *lethargy,* changes in EEG pattern; vivid dreams, nightmares, headache, vertigo, syncope, tinnitus, confusion, hallucinations, parodoxic rage, depression, delirium, ataxia. **Skin:** Photosensitivity, skin rash. **Urogenital:** Urinary frequency.

DIAGNOSTIC TEST INTERFERENCE Chlordiazepoxide increases ***serum bilirubin, AST*** and ***ALT;*** decreases ***radioactive iodine uptake;*** and may falsely increase readings for ***urinary 17-OHCS*** (modified ***Glenn-Nelson*** technique).

INTERACTIONS Drug: Alcohol, CNS DEPRESSANTS, ANTICONVULSANTS potentiate CNS depression; **cimetidine** increases **chlordiazepoxide** plasma levels, thus increasing toxicity; may decrease antiparkinson effects of **levodopa;** may increase **phenytoin** levels; smoking decreases sedative and antianxiety effects. **Herbal: Kava, valerian** may potentiate sedation.

PHARMACOKINETICS Absorption: Well absorbed from GI tract. **Peak:** 1–4 h. **Distribution:** Widely distributed throughout body; crosses placenta. **Metabolism:** In liver via CYP3A4 to long-acting active metabolite. **Elimination:** Slowly excreted in urine (may last several days); excreted in breast milk. **Half-Life:** 5–30 h.

NURSING IMPLICATIONS

Assessment & Drug Effects

- Monitor for S&S of orthostatic hypotension and tachycardia, observe closely and monitor vital signs.
- Check BP and pulse before giving benzodiazepine in early part of therapy. If blood pressure falls 20 mm Hg or more or if pulse rate is above 120 bpm, notify physician.
- Lab tests: Periodic blood cell counts and liver function tests are recommended during prolonged therapy.
- Monitor I&O until drug dosage is stabilized. Report changes in I&O ratio and dysuria to physician.
- Monitor for S&S of paradoxic reactions—excitement, stimulation, disturbed sleep patterns, acute rage—which may occur during first few weeks of therapy in psychiatric patients and in hyperactive and aggressive children receiving chlordiazepoxide. Withhold drug and report to physician.
- Assess patient's sleep pattern. If dreams or nightmares interfere with rest, notify physician.
- Supervise ambulation, especially with older adults & debilitated patients.

Patient & Family Education

- Abrupt discontinuation of drug in patients receiving high doses for long periods (4 mo or longer) has precipitated withdrawal symptoms, but not for at least 5–7 days because of slow elimination.
- Long-term use of this drug may cause mouth soreness. Good oral hygiene can alleviate the discomfort.
- Avoid activities requiring mental alertness until reaction to the drug has been evaluated.
- Avoid drinking alcoholic beverages. When combined with chlordiazepoxide, effects of both are potentiated.
- Avoid excessive sunlight. Use sunscreen lotion (SPF 12 or above) if allowed.

CHLOROPROCAINE HYDROCHLORIDE

(klor-oh-proe′kane)

Nesacaine, Nesacaine-CE ♣

Classification: LOCAL ANESTHETIC (ESTER-TYPE)

Therapeutic: LOCAL ANESTHETIC

Prototype: Procaine

Pregnancy Category: C

AVAILABILITY 1%, 2%, 3% injection

C

ACTION & *THERAPEUTIC EFFECT* Short-acting ester-type local anesthetic that decreases sodium influx into nerve cells, thus preventing initial depolarization, propagation, and conduction of the nerve impulse. *Produces anesthetic effect, but not used for spinal, topical, or IV regional anesthesia.*

USES Infiltration anesthesia and for peripheral, sympathetic, and epidural (including caudal) block anesthesia.

CONTRAINDICATIONS Known sensitivity to ester-type anesthetics, bisulfites, parabens (preservative) or PABA; intercurrent use of bupivacaine; coagulopathy; anticoagulant therapy. Safe use in children younger than 12 y not established.

CAUTIOUS USE Cardiac function impairment; history of drug hypersensitivity; debilitated, older adult, or acutely ill patients; neurologic disease, myasthenia gravis; dysrhythmias; sepsis; pregnancy (category C); lactation.

ROUTE & DOSAGE

Infiltration and Nerve Block

Adult: 1–2% solution: Max of 800 mg without epinephrine, 1 g with epinephrine

Caudal and Epidural Block (Without Preservatives)

Adult: 2–3% solution: Max of 800 mg without epinephrine, 1 g with epinephrine

ADMINISTRATION

Caudal/Epidural

- A test dose (3 mL of 3% solution or 5 mL of 2% solution) may be given before epidural use to check for intravascular or subarachnoid injection. Signs of intravascular injection: "Epinephrine response" (tachycardia, circumoral pallor, palpitations, nervousness). Signs of subarachnoid injection: Motor paralysis and extensive sensory anesthesia.
- Nesacaine formulation incorporates parabens (preservative) and sodium bisulfite; Nesacaine-CE is preservative-free but incorporates sodium bisulfite. Determine patient's sensitivity to parabens before administration of drug.
- Do not administer solution that is colored. Discard partially used solutions that are preservative-free.
- Store vials at 15°–30° C (59°–86° F); protect from freezing and from direct light.

ADVERSE EFFECTS (≥1%) **Body as a Whole: Sneezing**, <u>anaphylactoid reactions</u>. **CV:** Myocardial depression, hypotension, arrhythmias, bradycardia, <u>cardiac arrest</u>. **GI:** Nausea, vomiting. **CNS:** Anxiety, nervousness, tremors, sedation, circumoral paresthesia, convulsions followed by drowsiness, <u>respiratory arrest</u>. **Skin:** Cutaneous lesions of delayed onset; urticaria. **Special Senses:** Blurred or double vision, tinnitus. **Other:** With caudal or epidural anesthesia: Urinary retention, fecal or urinary incontinence, slowing of labor and increased incidence of forceps delivery, headache, backache, edema, status asthmaticus.

INTERACTIONS Drug: May antagonize effects of SULFONAMIDES; increased risk of hypotension with MAO INHIBITORS, ANTIHYPERTENSIVE AGENTS.

PHARMACOKINETICS Onset: 6–12 min. **Duration:** 30–60 min without epinephrine; 60–90 min with epinephrine. **Metabolism:** Hydrolyzed by plasma pseudocholinesterases. **Elimination:** Excreted by kidneys.

NURSING IMPLICATIONS

Assessment & Drug Effects

- Monitor vital signs throughout period of drug use.
- Have immediately available resuscitation equipment, oxygen, resuscitative drugs, and vasopressors when chloroprocaine is in use.

Patient & Family Education

- Report urinary retention or urinary or fecal incontinence.

CHLOROQUINE PHOSPHATE (Pr)

(klor'oh-kwin)

Aralen

Classification: ANTIMALARIAL

Therapeutic: ANTIMALARIAL; AMEBICIDE

Pregnancy Category: C

AVAILABILITY 250 mg (150 mg base), 500 mg (300 mg base) tablets

ACTION & *THERAPEUTIC EFFECT* Antimalarial activity is believed to be based on its ability to form complexes with DNA of parasite, thereby inhibiting replication and transcription to RNA and nucleic acid synthesis. *Acts as a suppressive agent in patient with* P. vivax *or* P. malariae *malaria; terminates acute attacks and increases intervals between treatment and relapse of malaria. Abolishes the acute attack of* P. falciparum *malaria but does not prevent the infection. Chloroquine-resistant strains have been reported.*

USES Suppression and treatment of malaria caused by *P. malariae, P. ovale, P. vivax,* and susceptible forms of *P. falciparum,* and in the treatment of extraintestinal amebiasis. Concomitant therapy with primaquine is necessary for radical cure of *P. vivax* and *P. malariae* malarias.

UNLABELED USES Discoid and systemic lupus erythematosus, porphyria cutanea tarda, solar urticaria, polymorphous light eruptions, and in rheumatoid arthritis (as second-line therapy).

CONTRAINDICATIONS Hypersensitivity to 4-aminoquinolines, psoriasis; porphyria, renal disease, 4-aminoquinoline-induced retinal or visual field changes; long-term therapy in children. Safe use in women of childbearing potential not established.

CAUTIOUS USE Impaired hepatic function, alcoholism, eczema, patients with G6PD deficiency, infants and children, hematologic, GI, and neurologic disorders; pregnancy (category C).

ROUTE & DOSAGE

Doses are expressed in terms of chloroquine base.

Acute Malaria

Adult: **PO** 600 mg base followed by 300 mg base at 6, 24, and 48 h

Child: **PO** 10 mg base/kg, then 5 mg base/kg at 6, 24, and 48 h

Malaria Suppression

Adult: **PO** 300 mg base the same day each week starting 2 wk before exposure and continuing for 4–6 wk after leaving the area of exposure (max: 300 mg base/wk)

Child: **PO** 5 mg base/kg the same day each week starting 2 wk before exposure and continuing for 4–6 wk after leaving the area of exposure (max: 300 mg base/wk)

C

Extraintestinal Amebiasis

Adult: **PO** 600 mg base/day for 2 days, then 300 mg base/day for 2–3 wk
Child: **PO** 10 mg base/kg/day for 2–3 wk

Rheumatoid Arthritis, SLE

Adult: **PO** 150 mg base/day with evening meal

ADMINISTRATION

Oral

- Give immediately before or after meals to minimize GI distress.
- Monitor child's dose closely. Children are extremely susceptible to overdosage.

ADVERSE EFFECTS (≥1%) **Body as a Whole:** Slight weight loss, myalgia, lymphedema of upper limbs. **CV:** Hypotension; ECG changes. **GI:** *Diarrhea,* abdominal cramps, *nausea,* vomiting, anorexia. **Hematologic:** Hemolytic anemia in patients with G6PD deficiency. **CNS:** Mild transient headache, fatigue, irritability, confusion, nightmares, skeletal muscle weakness, paresthesias, reduced reflexes, vertigo. **Skin:** Bleaching of scalp, eyebrows, body hair, and freckles, pruritus, patchy alopecia (reversible). **Special Senses:** (Usually reversible): Blurred vision, disturbances of accommodation, night blindness, scotomas, visual field defects, photophobia, corneal edema, opacity or deposits, ototoxicity (rare).

INTERACTIONS Drug: Aluminum- and **magnesium**-containing ANTACIDS and LAXATIVES decrease chloroquine absorption, so separate administration by at least 4 h; chloroquine may interfere with response to **rabies vaccine. Food:** Taking **lemon juice** decreases therapeutic effect.

PHARMACOKINETICS Absorption: Rapidly and almost completely absorbed. **Peak:** 1–2 h. **Distribution:** Widely distributed; concentrates in lungs, liver, erythrocytes, eyes, skin, and kidneys; crosses placenta. **Metabolism:** Partially in liver to active metabolites. **Elimination:** In urine; excreted in breast milk. **Half-Life:** 70–120 h.

NURSING IMPLICATIONS

Assessment & Drug Effects

- Lab tests: CBC and ECG are advised before initiation of therapy and periodically thereafter in patients on long-term therapy.
- Monitor for changes in vision. Retinopathy (generally irreversible) can be progressive even after termination of therapy. Patient may be asymptomatic or complain of night blindness, scotomas, visual field changes, blurred vision, or difficulty in focusing. Withhold drug and report immediately to physician.

Patient & Family Education

- Report promptly visual or hearing disturbances, muscle weakness, or loss of balance, symptoms of blood dyscrasia (fever, sore mouth or throat, unexplained fatigue, easy bruising or bleeding).
- Use of dark glasses in sunlight or bright light may provide comfort (because of photophobia) and reduce risk of ocular damage.
- Avoid driving or other potentially hazardous activities until reaction to drug is known.
- May cause rusty yellow or brown discoloration of urine.
- Do not drink lemon juice along with chloroquine. It decreases the drug's effectiveness.

CHLOROTHIAZIDE
(klor-oh-thye'a-zide)

CHLOROTHIAZIDE SODIUM
Diuril

Classifications: ELECTROLYTE & WATER BALANCE AGENT; THIAZIDE DIURETIC; ANTIHYPERTENSIVE

Therapeutic: THIAZIDE DIURETIC; ANTIHYPERTENSIVE

Prototype: Hydrochlorothiazide

Pregnancy Category: C

AVAILABILITY 250 mg, 500 mg tablets; 500 mg injection

ACTION & *THERAPEUTIC EFFECT* Thiazide diuretic whose primary action is production of diuresis by direct action on the distal convoluted tubules. Inhibits reabsorption of sodium, potassium, and chloride ions. *Promotes renal excretion of sodium (and water), bicarbonate, and potassium. Antihypertensive mechanism is due to decreased peripheral resistance and reduced blood pressure.*

USES Adjunctively to manage edema associated with CHF, hepatic cirrhosis, renal dysfunction, corticosteroid, or estrogen therapy. Used alone as step 1 agent in stepped-care approach, or in combination with other agents for treatment of hypertension.

UNLABELED USES To reduce polyuria of central and nephrogenic diabetes insipidus, to prevent calcium-containing renal stones, and to treat renal tubular acidosis.

CONTRAINDICATIONS Hypersensitivity to thiazide or sulfonamides; anuria; hypokalemia; renal failure; jaundiced neonates; SLE.

CAUTIOUS USE History of sulfa allergy; impaired renal or hepatic function or gout; hypercalcemia, diabetes mellitus, older adult or debilitated patients, pancreatitis, sympathectomy; pregnancy (category C).

ROUTE & DOSAGE

Hypertension, Edema

Adult: **PO** 250 mg–1 g/day in 1–2 divided doses **IV** 500 mg–1 g/day in 1–2 divided doses

Geriatric: **PO** 500 mg daily or 1 g 3 times/wk

Edema

Child: **PO** *Younger than 6 mo,* 20–40 mg/kg/day in 1–2 divided doses; *older than 6 mo,* 20 mg/kg/day in 2 divided doses

ADMINISTRATION

Oral

- Give with or after food to prevent gastric irritation. Extent of absorption appears to be increased by taking it with food.
- Schedule daily doses to avoid nocturia and interrupted sleep.

Intravenous

- Reserve for emergency or when patient unable to take oral medication. - IV administration to infants and children: Verify correct IV concentration and rate of infusion with physician.

PREPARE: **Intermittent:** Reconstitute the 500-mg vial with at least 18 mL sterile water for injection. - May be further diluted with D5W or NS.

ADMINISTER: **Intermittent:** Give at a rate of 500 mg over 5 min. - Thiazide preparations are extremely irritating to the tissues, and great care **must be** taken to avoid extravasation. - If infiltration occurs, stop medication, remove needle, and apply ice if area is small.

C

INCOMPATIBILITIES **Solution/additive: Amikacin, chlorpromazine, codeine, fluorouracil, hydralazine, insulin, levorphanol, methadone, morphine, norepinephrine, pentobarbital, polymyxin B, procaine, prochlorperazine, promazine, promethazine, streptomycin, triflupromazine, vancomycin, vitamin B complex with C, warfarin.**

▪ Store tablets, PO solutions, and parenteral dosage forms at 15°–30° C (59°–86° F) unless otherwise directed by manufacturer. ▪ Unused reconstituted IV solutions may be stored at room temperature up to 24 h. Use only clear solutions.

ADVERSE EFFECTS (≥1%) **Body as a Whole:** Fever, respiratory distress, <u>anaphylactic reaction</u>. **CV:** Irregular heart beat, weak pulse, orthostatic hypotension. **GI:** Vomiting, acute pancreatitis, diarrhea. **Hematologic:** <u>Agranulocytosis</u> (rare), <u>aplastic anemia</u> (rare), asymptomatic hyperuricemia, hyperglycemia, glycosuria, SIADH secretion. **Metabolic:** *Hypokalemia,* hypercalcemia, hyponatremia, hypochloremic alkalosis, elevated cholesterol and triglyceride levels. **CNS:** Unusual fatigue, dizziness, mental changes, vertigo, headache. **Skin:** Urticaria, photosensitivity, skin rash.

DIAGNOSTIC TEST INTERFERENCE Chlorothiazide (thiazides) may cause: marked increases in ***serum amylase*** values, decrease in ***PBI*** determinations; increase in excretion of ***PSP;*** increase in ***BSP retention;*** false-negative ***phentolamine*** and ***tyramine*** tests; interference with ***urine steroid*** determinations, and possibly the ***histamine test*** for pheochromocytoma. Thiazides should be discontinued at least 3 days before ***bentiromide test*** (thiazides can invalidate test) and before ***parathyroid function tests*** because they tend to decrease calcium excretion.

INTERACTIONS Drug: Amphotericin B, CORTICOSTEROIDS increase hypokalemic effects of chlorothiazide; the hypoglycemic effects of SULFONYLUREAS and **insulin** may be antagonized; **cholestyramine, colestipol** decrease thiazide absorption; intensifies hypoglycemic and hypotensive effects of **diazoxide;** increased potassium and magnesium loss may cause **digoxin** toxicity; decreases **lithium** excretion, increasing its toxicity; increases risk of NSAID-induced renal failure and may attenuate diuresis.

PHARMACOKINETICS Absorption: Incompletely absorbed PO. **Onset:** 2 h PO; 15 min IV. **Peak:** 3–6 h PO; 30 min IV. **Duration:** 6–12 h PO; 2 h IV. **Distribution:** Throughout extracellular tissue; concentrates in kidney; crosses placenta. **Metabolism:** Does not appear to be metabolized. **Elimination:** In urine and breast milk. **Half-Life:** 45–120 min.

NURSING IMPLICATIONS

Assessment & Drug Effects

- Monitor for therapeutic effect. Antihypertensive action of a thiazide diuretic requires several days before effects are observed; usually optimum therapeutic effect is not established for 3–4 wk.
- Lab tests: Baseline and periodic blood count, serum electrolytes, CO_2, BUN, creatinine, uric acid, and blood glucose.
- Monitor for hyperglycemia. Thiazide therapy can cause hyperglycemia (see Appendix F) and glycosuria in diabetic and diabetic-prone individuals.

- Monitor patients with gout. Asymptomatic hyperuricemia can be produced because of interference with uric acid excretion.
- Establish baseline weight before initiation of therapy. Weigh patient at the same time each a.m. under standard conditions. A gain of more than 1 kg (2.2) within 2 or 3 days and a gradual weight gain over the week's period is reportable.
- Monitor BP closely during early drug therapy.
- Inspect skin and mucous membranes daily for evidence of petechiae in patients receiving large doses and those on prolonged therapy.
- Monitor I&O rates and patterns: Excessive diuresis may cause electrolyte imbalance and necessitate prompt dosage adjustment.
- Monitor patients on digitalis therapy for S&S of hypokalemia (see Appendix G), which can precipitate digitalis intoxication.

Patient & Family Education

- Urination will occur in greater amounts and with more frequency than usual, and there will be an unusual sense of tiredness. With continued therapy, diuretic action decreases; BP lowering effects usually are maintained, and sense of tiredness diminishes.
- Make position changes slowly to minimize risks associated with orthostatic hypotension.
- Report to physician any illness accompanied by prolonged vomiting or diarrhea.
- Avoid drinking large quantities of coffee or other caffeine drinks. Caffeine has a diuretic effect.
- Report S&S of hypokalemia, hypercalcemia, or hyperglycemia (see Appendix F).
- Hypokalemia may be prevented if the daily diet contains potassium-rich foods. Eat a banana and drink at least 6 oz orange juice every day.
- Report photosensitivity reaction to physician. Photosensitivity may occur 1½–2 wk after initial sun exposure.

CHLORPHENIRAMINE MALEATE

(klor-fen-eer′a-meen)

Aller-Chlor, Chlo-Amine, Chlor-Trimeton, Chlor-Tripolon ♣, Novopheniram ♣, Phenetron, Telachlor, Teldrin, Trymegan

Classification: ANTIHISTAMINE (H_1-RECEPTOR ANTAGONIST)

Therapeutic: ANTIHISTAMINE

Prototype: Diphenhydramine

Pregnancy Category: C

AVAILABILITY 2 mg, 4 mg tablets; 8 mg, 12 mg sustained release tablets; 2 mg/5 mL syrup

ACTION & *THERAPEUTIC EFFECT* Antihistamine that competes with histamine for H_1-receptor sites on effector cells; thus it promotes capillary permeability and edema formation and constrictive action on respiratory, gastrointestinal, and vascular smooth muscles. *Has effective antihistamine reaction resulting in decreasing allergic symptomatology.*

USES Symptomatic relief of various uncomplicated allergic conditions; to prevent transfusion and drug reactions in susceptible patients, and as adjunct to epinephrine and other standard measures in anaphylactic reactions.

CONTRAINDICATIONS Hypersensitivity to antihistamines of similar

C

structure; lower respiratory tract symptoms, narrow-angle glaucoma, obstructive prostatic hypertrophy or other bladder neck obstruction, GI obstruction or stenosis; premature and newborn infants; during or within 14 days of MAO INHIBITOR therapy.

CAUTIOUS USE Convulsive disorders, increased intraocular pressure, hyperthyroidism, cardiovascular disease, hepatic disease; BPH; GI obstruction; hypertension, diabetes mellitus, history of bronchial asthma, COPD, older adult patients, patients with G6PD deficiency, pregnancy (category C), lactation.

ROUTE & DOSAGE

Symptomatic Allergy Relief

Adult: **PO** 2–4 mg t.i.d. or q.i.d. *or* 8–12 mg b.i.d. or t.i.d. (max: 24 mg/day)
Geriatric: **PO** 4 mg daily or b.i.d. *or* 8 mg sustained release at bedtime
Child: **PO** *6–12 y,* 2 mg q4–6h (max: 12 mg/day); *2–6 y,* 1 mg q4–6h

ADMINISTRATION

Oral

- Give on an empty stomach for fastest response.
- Sustained release tablets should be swallowed whole and not crushed or chewed.
- Ensure that chewable tablets are chewed or crushed before being swallowed with a liquid.

ADVERSE EFFECTS (≥1%) **Body as a Whole:** Sensation of chest tightness. **CV:** Palpitation, tachycardia, mild hypotension or hypertension. **GI:** Epigastric distress, anorexia, nausea, vomiting, constipation, or diarrhea. **CNS:** *Drowsiness,* sedation, headache, dizziness, vertigo, fatigue, disturbed coordination, tremors, euphoria, nervousness, restlessness, insomnia. **Special Senses:** *Dryness of mouth,* nose, and throat, tinnitus, vertigo, acute labyrinthitis, thickened bronchial secretions, blurred vision, diplopia. **Urogenital:** Urinary frequency or retention, dysuria.

DIAGNOSTIC TEST INTERFERENCE Antihistamines should be discontinued 4 days before ***skin testing*** procedures for allergy because they may obscure otherwise positive reactions.

INTERACTIONS Drug: Alcohol (ethanol) and other CNS DEPRESSANTS produce additive sedation and CNS depression.

PHARMACOKINETICS Absorption: Well absorbed from GI tract; about 45% of dose reaches systemic circulation intact. **Onset:** Within 6 h. **Peak:** 2–6 h. **Distribution:** Highest concentrations in lung, heart, kidney, brain, small intestine, and spleen. **Metabolism:** By CYP3A4. **Half-Life:** 12–43 h.

NURSING IMPLICATIONS

Assessment & Drug Effects

- Monitor for CNS depression and sedation, especially when chlorpheniramine is given in combination with other CNS depressants.
- Monitor BP in hypertensive patients since chlorpheniramine may elevate BP.

Patient & Family Education

- Avoid driving a car and other potentially hazardous activities until drug response has been determined.
- Avoid or minimize alcohol intake. Antihistamines have additive effects with alcohol.

- Report any of the following: Tinnitus or palpitations.
- Consult physician before taking additional OTC drugs for allergy relief.

CHLORPROMAZINE (Pr)

(klor-proe′ma-zeen)

CHLORPROMAZINE HYDROCHLORIDE

Sonazine, Thorazine

Classifications: ANTIPSYCHOTIC; PHENOTHIAZINE; ANTIEMETIC

Therapeutic: ANTIPSYCHOTIC; ANTIEMETIC

Pregnancy Category: C

AVAILABILITY 10 mg, 25 mg, 50 mg, 100 mg, 200 mg tablets; 30 mg, 75 mg, 150 mg, 200 mg, 300 mg sustained release capsules; 10 mg/5 mL syrup; 30 mg/mL, 100 mg/mL oral concentrate; 25 mg/mL injection

ACTION & *THERAPEUTIC EFFECT* Phenothiazine derivative with actions at all levels of CNS with a mechanism that produces strong antipsychotic effects. Antiemetic effect due to suppression of the chemoreceptor trigger zone (CTZ). Antipsychotic drugs are sometimes called neuroleptics because they tend to reduce initiative and interest in the environment, decrease displays of emotions or affect, suppress spontaneous movements and complex behavior, as well as decrease psychotic symptoms. *Mechanism thought to be related to blockade of postsynaptic dopamine receptors in the brain. Also has antiemetic effects due to its action on the CTZ.*

USES To control manic phase of manic-depressive illness, for symptomatic management of psychotic disorders, including schizophrenia, in management of severe nausea and vomiting, to control excessive anxiety and agitation before surgery, and for treatment of severe behavior problems in children (e.g., attention deficit disorder). Also used for treatment of acute intermittent porphyria, intractable hiccups, and as adjunct in treatment of tetanus.

CONTRAINDICATIONS Hypersensitivity to phenothiazine derivatives, sulfite, or benzyl alcohol; withdrawal states from alcohol; CNS depression; comatose states, brain damage, bone marrow depression, Reye's syndrome; children younger than 6 mo; lactation.

CAUTIOUS USE Agitated states accompanied by depression, seizure disorders, respiratory impairment due to infection or COPD; glaucoma, diabetes, hypertensive disease, peptic ulcer, prostatic hypertrophy; thyroid, cardiovascular, and hepatic disorders; patients exposed to extreme heat or organophosphate insecticides; previously detected breast cancer; pregnancy (category C).

ROUTE & DOSAGE

Psychotic Disorders, Agitation

Adult: **PO** 25–100 mg t.i.d. or q.i.d., may need up to 1000 mg/day **IM/IV** 25–50 mg up to 600 mg q4–6h

Child: **PO** *Older than 6 mo,* 0.55 mg/kg q4–6h prn up to 500 mg/day **IM/IV** *Older than 6 mo,* 0.5–1 mg/kg q6–8h

Nausea and Vomiting

Adult: **PO** 10–25 mg q4–6h prn **IM/IV** 25–50 mg q4–6h prn

C

Child: **PO** *Older than 6 mo,* 0.55 mg/kg q4–6h prn up to 500 mg/day **IM/IV** *Older than 6 mo,* 0.55 mg/kg q6–8h

Dementia

Geriatric: **PO** Initial 10–25 mg 1–2 times/day, may increase q4–7days by 10–25 mg/day (max: 800 mg/day)

Intractable Hiccups

Adult: **PO/IM** 25–50 mg t.i.d. or q.i.d.

Tetanus

Adult: **IM/IV** 25–50 mg q6–8h
Child: **IM/IV** 0.5 mg/kg q6–8h

Nausea and Vomiting during Surgery

Adult/Adolescent: **IV** 2 mg q2min prn (max total: 25 mg)
Child/Infant (older than 6 mo): **IV** 1 mg q2min prn (max total: 0.25 mg/kg)

Intractable Hiccups

Adult/Adolescent: **IV** 25–50 mg in 500–1000 mL NS, not to exceed 1 mg/min

ADMINISTRATION

Oral

- Give with food or a full glass of fluid to minimize GI distress.
- Mix chlorpromazine concentrate just before administration in at least 1/2 glass juice, milk, water, coffee, tea, carbonated beverage, or with semisolid food.
- Ensure that sustained release form of drug is not chewed or crushed. It **must be** swallowed whole.

Intramuscular/Intravenous

- Avoid parenteral drug contact with skin, eyes, and clothing because of its potential for causing contact dermatitis.
- Keep patient recumbent for at least 30 min after parenteral administration. Observe closely. Report hypotensive reactions.

Intramuscular

- Inject IM preparations slowly and deep into upper outer quadrant of buttock. If irritation is a problem, consult physician about diluting medication with normal saline or 2% procaine. Rotate injection sites.

Intravenous

PREPARE: **Direct:** Dilute 25 mg with 24 mL of NS to yield 1 mg/mL. **Continuous:** May be further diluted in up to 1000 mL of NS.

ADMINISTER: **Direct:** Administer 1 mg or fraction thereof over 1 min for adults and over 2 min for children. **Continuous:** Give slowly at a rate not to exceed 1 mg/min.

- Lemon yellow color of parenteral preparation does not alter potency; if otherwise colored or markedly discolored, solution should be discarded.

INCOMPATIBILITIES **Solution/additive:** **Aminophylline, amphotericin B, ampicillin, chloramphenicol, chlorothiazide, methohexital, penicillin G, pentobarbital, phenobarbital.** **Y-site:** **Allopurinol, amifostine, amphotericin B cholesteryl complex, aztreonam, bivalirudin, cefepime, etoposide, fludarabine, furosemide, lansoprazole, linezolid, melphalan, methotrexate, paclitaxel, piperacillin/tazobactam, remifentanil, sargramostim.**

- All forms are stored preferably between 15°–30° C (59°–86° F) protected from light, unless otherwise specified by the manufacturer. Avoid freezing.

ADVERSE EFFECTS (≥1%) **Body as a Whole:** Idiopathic edema, muscle necrosis (following IM), SLE-like syndrome, sudden unexplained death. **CV:** Orthostatic hypotension, palpitation, tachycardia, ECG changes (usually reversible): Prolonged QT and PR intervals, blunting of T waves, ST depression. **GI:** Dry mouth; constipation, adynamic ileus, cholestatic jaundice, aggravation of peptic ulcer, dyspepsia, increased appetite. **Hematologic:** Agranulocytosis, thrombocytopenic purpura, pancytopenia (rare). **Metabolic:** Weight gain, hypoglycemia, hyperglycemia, glycosuria (high doses), enlargement of parotid glands. **CNS:** *Sedation, drowsiness,* dizziness, restlessness, neuroleptic malignant syndrome, tardive dyskinesias, tumor, syncope, headache, weakness, insomnia, reduced REM sleep, bizarre dreams, cerebral edema, convulsive seizures, hypothermia, inability to sweat, depressed cough reflex, *extrapyramidal symptoms,* EEG changes. **Respiratory:** Laryngospasm. **Skin:** Fixed-drug eruption, urticaria, reduced perspiration, contact dermatitis, exfoliative dermatitis, photosensitivity, eczema, anaphylactoid reactions, hypersensitivity vasculitis; hirsutism (long-term therapy). **Special Senses:** Blurred vision, lenticular opacities, mydriasis, photophobia. **Urogenital:** Anovulation, infertility, pseudopregnancy, menstrual irregularity, gynecomastia, galactorrhea, priapism, inhibition of ejaculation, reduced libido, urinary retention and frequency.

DIAGNOSTIC TEST INTERFERENCE Chlorpromazine (phenothiazines) may increase ***cephalin flocculation,*** and possibly other ***liver function tests;*** also may increase ***PBI.*** False-positive result may occur for ***amylase, 5-hydroxyindole acetic acid, phenylketonuria, porphobilinogens, urobilinogen (Ehrlich's reagent),*** and ***urine bilirubin (Bili-Labstix).*** False-positive or false-negative ***pregnancy test*** results possibly caused by a metabolite of phenothiazines, which discolors urine depending on test used.

INTERACTIONS Drug: Alcohol, CNS DEPRESSANTS increase CNS depression; ANTACIDS, ANTIDIARRHEALS decrease absorption—space administration 2 h before or after administration of chlorpromazine; **phenobarbital** increases metabolism of phenothiazine; GENERAL ANESTHETICS increase excitation and hypotension; antagonizes antihypertensive action of **guanethidine; phenylpropanolamine** poses possibility of sudden death; TRICYCLIC ANTIDEPRESSANTS intensify hypotensive and anticholinergic effects; ANTICONVULSANTS decrease seizure threshold—may need to increase anticonvulsant dose. **Herbal: Kava** increases risk and severity of dystonic reaction.

PHARMACOKINETICS Absorption: Rapid absorption with considerable first pass metabolism in liver; rapid absorption after IM. **Onset:** 30–60 min. **Peak:** 2–4 h PO; 15–20 min IM. **Duration:** 4–6 h. **Distribution:** Widely distributed; accumulates in brain; crosses placenta. **Metabolism:** In liver by CYP2D6. **Elimination:** In urine as metabolites; excreted in breast milk. **Half-Life:** Biphasic 2 and 30 h.

NURSING IMPLICATIONS

Assessment & Drug Effects

- Establish baseline BP (in standing and recumbent positions), and pulse, before initiating treatment.

- Monitor BP frequently. Hypotensive reactions, dizziness, and sedation are common during early therapy, particularly in patients on high doses and in the older adult receiving parenteral doses.
- Lab tests: Periodic CBC with differential, liver function tests, and blood glucose.
- Monitor cardiac status with baseline ECG in patients with preexisting cardiovascular disease.
- Be alert for signs of neuroleptic malignant syndrome (see Appendix G). Report immediately.
- Report extrapyramidal symptoms that occur most often in patients on high dosage, the pediatric patient with severe dehydration and acute infection, the older adult, and women. Reduce smoking, if possible.
- Monitor I&O ratio and pattern: Urinary retention due to mental depression and compromised renal function may occur.
- Be alert to complaints of diminished visual acuity, reduced night vision, photophobia, and a perceived brownish discoloration of objects. Patient may be more comfortable with dark glasses.
- Monitor diabetics or prediabetics on long-term, high-dose therapy for reduced glucose tolerance and loss of diabetes control.
- Ocular examinations, and EEG (in patients older than 50 y) are recommended before and periodically during prolonged therapy.

Patient & Family Education

- Take medication as prescribed and keep appointments for follow-up evaluation of dosage regimen. Improvement may not be experienced until 7 or 8 wk into therapy.
- May cause pink to red-brown discoloration of urine.
- Wear protective clothing and sunscreen lotion with SPF above 12 when outdoors, even on dark days. Photosensitivity causes exposed skin areas to have appearance of an exaggerated sunburn. If reaction occurs, report to physician.
- Practice meticulous oral hygiene. Oral candidiasis occurs frequently in patients receiving phenothiazines.
- Avoid driving a car or undertaking activities requiring precision and mental alertness until drug response is known.
- Do not abruptly stop this drug. Abrupt withdrawal of drug or deliberate dose skipping, especially after prolonged therapy with large doses, can cause onset of extrapyramidal symptoms (see Appendix F) and severe GI disturbances. When drug is to be discontinued, dosage **must be** tapered off gradually over a period of several weeks.

CHLORPROPAMIDE

(klor-proe′pa-mide)

Apo-Chlorpropamide ♣, Diabinese, Novopropamide ♣

Classification: ANTIDIABETIC SULFONYLUREA

Therapeutic: ANTIDIABETIC

Prototype: Glyburide

Pregnancy Category: C

AVAILABILITY 100 mg, 250 mg tablets

ACTION & *THERAPEUTIC EFFECT*

Longest-acting first-generation sulfonylurea compound. Lowers blood glucose by stimulating beta cells in pancreas to synthesize and release endogenous insulin. *Antidiabetic effect is due to the ability of the drug to stimulate the beta cells of the pancreas to manufacture and release insulin. Therapeutic effectiveness is indicated by HbA1C levels greater than 7%.*

USES Stable non-insulin-dependent diabetes mellitus (type 2) in patients who cannot be controlled by diet alone and who do not have complications of diabetes.

UNLABELED USES Neurogenic diabetes insipidus.

CONTRAINDICATIONS Known hypersensitivity to sulfonylureas and to sulfonamides; diabetes complicated by severe infection; acidosis; severe renal, hepatic, or thyroid insufficiency; lactation. Safe use in children not established.

CAUTIOUS USE Older adult patients, Addison's disease, CHF, and hepatic porphyria; pregnancy (category C).

ROUTE & DOSAGE

Antidiabetic

Adult: **PO** Initial: 100–250 mg/day with breakfast, adjust by 50–125 mg/day q3–5days until glycemic control is achieved, up to 750 mg/day

ADMINISTRATION

Oral

- Give as a single morning dose with breakfast or 3 doses and taken with meals.
- Store at 15°–30° C (59°–86° F) in a tightly closed container, unless otherwise directed.

ADVERSE EFFECTS (≥1%) **Body as a Whole:** Flushing, photosensitivity, alcohol intolerance. **GI:** GI distress, anorexia, nausea, diarrhea, constipation, cholestatic jaundice. **Hematologic:** Leukopenia, thrombocytopenia, agranulocytosis. **Metabolic:** Hypoglycemia, antidiuretic effect (SIADH), dilutional hyponatremia, water intoxication. **CNS:** Drowsiness, muscle cramps, weakness, paresthesias. **Skin:** Rash, pruritus.

INTERACTIONS Drug: Adverse effects of ORAL ANTICOAGULANTS, **phenytoin,** SALICYLATES, NSAIDS may be increased along with those of chlorpropamide; THIAZIDE DIURETICS may increase blood sugar; **alcohol** produces disulfiram reaction; **probenecid,** MAO INHIBITORS may increase hypoglycemic effects. **Herbal: Garlic, ginseng** may increase hypoglycemic effects.

PHARMACOKINETICS Absorption: Readily from GI tract. **Onset:** 1 h. **Peak:** 3–6 h. **Distribution:** Highly protein bound; distributed into breast milk. **Metabolism:** In liver. **Elimination:** 80–90% in urine in 96 h. **Half-Life:** 36 h.

NURSING IMPLICATIONS

Assessment & Drug Effects

- Lab tests: Periodic fasting and postprandial blood glucose; HbA1C every 3 mo; baseline and periodic hematologic and hepatic studies are advisable, particularly in patients receiving high doses. A CBC should be performed if symptoms of anemia appear.
- Report dizziness, shortness of breath, malaise, fatigue.
- Monitor for S&S of hypoglycemia (see Appendix F).
- Monitor I&O ratio and pattern: Infrequently, chlorpropamide produces an antidiuretic effect, with resulting severe hyponatremia, edema, and water intoxication. If fluid intake far exceeds output

and edema develops (weight gain), report to the physician.

C

Patient & Family Education

- Report hypoglycemic episodes to physician. Because chlorpropamide has a long half-life, hypoglycemia can be severe.
- Report any of the following immediately to physician: Skin eruptions, malaise, fever, or photosensitivity. Immediately report these symptoms to physician. A change to another hypoglycemic agent may be indicated.

CHLORTHALIDONE

(klor-thal′i-done)

Thalitone

Classifications: ELECTROLYTE & WATER BALANCE AGENT; DIURETIC; ANTIHYPERTENSIVE

Therapeutic: DIURETIC; ANTIHYPERTENSIVE

Prototype: Hydrochlorothiazide

Pregnancy Category: B

AVAILABILITY 15 mg, 25 mg, 50 mg, 100 mg tablets

ACTION & *THERAPEUTIC EFFECT* Sulfonamide derivative that increases excretion of sodium and chloride by inhibiting their reabsorption in the cortical diluting segment of the ascending loop of Henle. *Antihypertensive effect is correlated to the decrease in extracellular and intracellular volumes. Decreased volume results in reduced cardiac output with subsequent decrease in peripheral resistance.*

USES Edema associated with CHF, renal decompensation, hepatic cirrhosis, corticosteroid and estrogen therapy; as sole agent or with other antihypertensives to treat hypertension.

CONTRAINDICATIONS Hypersensitivity to sulfonamide or thiazide derivatives; anuria, hypokalemia; toxemia; hyperparathroidism; lactation; neonates with jaundice.

CAUTIOUS USE History of renal and hepatic disease, hyponatremia, hypochloremia; gout, SLE, diabetes mellitus; history of allergy or bronchial asthma; pregnancy (category B).

ROUTE & DOSAGE

Hypertension

Adult: **PO** 12.5–25 mg/day, may be increased to 100 mg/day if needed

Child: **PO** 2 mg/kg 3 times/wk

Edema

Adult: **PO** 50–100 mg/day, may be increased to 200 mg/day if needed

ADMINISTRATION

Oral

- Administer as single dose in a.m. to reduce potential for interrupted sleep because of diuresis.
- Consult physician when chlorthalidone is used as a diuretic; an intermittent dose schedule may reduce incidence of adverse reactions.
- Store tablets in tightly closed container at 15°–30° C (59°–86° F) unless otherwise advised.

ADVERSE EFFECTS (≥1%) **CV:** Orthostatic hypotension. **GI:** Anorexia, nausea, vomiting, diarrhea, constipation, cramping, jaundice. **Hematologic:** Agranulocytosis, thrombocytopenia, aplastic anemia. **CNS:** Dizziness, vertigo, paresthesias, headache. **Metabolic:** *Hypokalemia,* hyponatremia, hypochloremia, hypercalcemia, glycosuria, hyperglycemia, exacerbation of gout. **Skin:** Rash, urticaria, photosensitivity, vasculitis. **Urogenital:** Impotence.

INTERACTIONS Drug: Increased risk of **digoxin** toxicity because of hypokalemia; CORTICOSTEROIDS, **amphotericin B** increases hypokalemia; decreases **lithium** elimination; may antagonize the hypoglycemic effects of SULFONYLUREAS; NSAIDS may attenuate diuretic effects; **cholestyramine** decreases thiazide absorption.

PHARMACOKINETICS Absorption: Readily from GI tract. **Onset:** 2 h. **Peak:** 3–6 h. **Duration:** 24–72 h. **Distribution:** Crosses placenta; appears in breast milk. **Elimination:** 30–60% in urine in 24 h. **Half-Life:** 54 h.

NURSING IMPLICATIONS

Assessment & Drug Effects

- Establish baseline BP measurements and check at regular intervals during period of dosage adjustment when chlorthalidone is used for hypertension.
- Be alert to signs of hypokalemia (see Appendix F). Older adult patients are more sensitive to adverse effects of drug-induced diuresis because of age-related changes in the cardiovascular and renal systems.
- Lab tests: Baseline and periodic: Serum electrolytes (particularly K^+, Mg^{2+}, Ca^{2+}, Na^+), serum uric acid, creatinine, BUN, and uric acid and blood glucose (especially in patients with diabetes).
- Monitor lithium and digoxin levels closely when either of these drugs is used concurrently.

Patient & Family Education

- Maintain adequate potassium intake, monitor weight, and make a daily estimate of I&O ratio.

C

CHLORZOXAZONE

(klor-zox'a-zone)

Classification: CENTRALLY ACTING SKELETAL MUSCLE RELAXANT

Therapeutic: SKELETAL MUSCLE RELAXER; ANTISPASMODIC

Prototype: Cyclobenzaprine

Pregnancy Category: C

AVAILABILITY 250 mg, 500 mg tablets

ACTION & *THERAPEUTIC EFFECT* Centrally acting skeletal muscle relaxant that acts indirectly by depressing nerve transmission through polysynaptic pathways in spinal cord, subcortical centers, and brainstem; also possibly has a sedative effect. *Effectively controls muscle spasms and pain associated with musculoskeletal conditions.*

USES Symptomatic treatment of muscle spasm and pain associated with various musculoskeletal conditions.

CONTRAINDICATIONS Impaired liver function; alcoholism; hepatic disease, jaundice; lactation.
CAUTIOUS USE Patients with known allergies or history of drug allergies; renal impairment or failure; CNS depression; older adult patients; pregnancy (category C).

ROUTE & DOSAGE

Skeletal Muscle Relaxant

Adult: **PO** 250–500 mg t.i.d. or q.i.d. (max: 3 g/day)

Child: **PO** 20 mg/kg/day in 3–4 divided doses

ADMINISTRATION

Oral

- Give with food or meals to prevent gastric distress. If necessary, tablet may be crushed and mixed with food or liquid (e.g., milk, fruit juice).
- Store in tight container at 15°–30° C (59°–86° F) unless otherwise directed.

ADVERSE EFFECTS (≥1%) **GI:** Anorexia, heartburn, nausea, vomiting, constipation, diarrhea, abdominal pain, hepatotoxicity: Jaundice, liver damage. **CNS:** *Drowsiness, dizziness,* light-headedness, headache, malaise, overstimulation. **Skin:** Erythema, rash, pruritus, urticaria, petechiae, ecchymoses.

INTERACTIONS Drug: Alcohol, CNS DEPRESSANTS add to CNS depression.

PHARMACOKINETICS Absorption: Readily absorbed from GI tract. **Onset:** 1 h. **Peak:** 1–4 h. **Duration:** 3–4 h. **Distribution:** Not known if crosses placenta or distributed into breast milk. **Metabolism:** In liver. **Elimination:** In urine. **Half-Life:** 66 min.

NURSING IMPLICATIONS

Assessment & Drug Effects

- Monitor ambulation during early drug therapy; some patients may require supervision.
- Lab tests: Periodic liver function tests are advised in patients receiving long-term therapy even if sporadic.
- Note: Since chlorzoxazone metabolite may discolor urine, dark urine cannot be a reliable sign of a hepatotoxic reaction.

Patient & Family Education

- Avoid activities requiring mental alertness, judgment, and physical coordination until reaction to drug is known, since sedation, drowsiness, and dizziness may occur.
- Drug may discolor urine orange to purplish red, but this is of no clinical significance.
- Discontinue drug and notify physician if signs of hypersensitivity (see Appendix F) or of liver dysfunction appear (abdominal discomfort, yellow sclerae or skin, pruritus, malaise, nausea, vomiting).
- Check with physician before taking an OTC depressant (e.g., antihistamine, sedative, alcohol) since effects may be additive.

CHOLESTYRAMINE RESIN (Pr)

(koe-less-tear′a-meen)

LoCHOLEST, Questran, Questran Light, Prevalite

Classifications: ANTILIPEMIC; BILE ACID SEQUESTRANT

Therapeutic: CHOLESTEROL-LOWERING

Pregnancy Category: C

AVAILABILITY 4 g powder for suspension; 1 g tablet

ACTION & *THERAPEUTIC EFFECT* Anion-exchange resin used for its cholesterol-lowering effect. Adsorbs and combines with intestinal bile acids in exchange for chloride ions to form an insoluble, nonabsorbable complex that is excreted in the feces. As a result, bile salts are continually (but not entirely) prevented from reentry into the enterohepatic circulation, thus increasing fecal loss of bile acids. This leads to lowered serum total cholesterol by decreasing low-density lipoprotein (LDL) cholesterol.

The resin anion-exchange agent increases fecal loss of bile acids, which leads to lowered serum total cholesterol by decreasing (LDL) cholesterol, and reducing bile acid deposit in dermal tissues (decreasing pruritus). Serum triglyceride levels may increase or remain unchanged.

USES As adjunct to diet therapy in management of patients with primary hypercholesterolemia (type IIa hyperlipidemia) with a significant risk of atherosclerotic heart disease and MI; for relief of pruritus secondary to partial biliary stasis.

UNLABELED USES To control diarrhea caused by excess bile acids in colon; for hyperoxaluria.

CONTRAINDICATIONS Complete biliary obstruction or biliary cirrhosis, cholelithiasis; GI obstruction; hypersensitivity to bile acid sequestrants; coagulopathy; lactation. Safe use in children 6 y or younger not established.

CAUTIOUS USE Bleeding disorders; hemorrhoids; impaired GI function, decreased GI motility; peptic ulcer, malabsorption states (e.g., steatorrhea); phenylketonuria (Questran Light only); renal disease; pregnancy (category C).

ROUTE & DOSAGE

Hypercholesterolemia

Adult: **PO** 4 g b.i.d. to q.i.d. a.c. and at bedtime, may need up to 24 g/day

Child: **PO** 240 mg/kg/day in 3 divided doses

Hyperlipoproteinemia

Adult: **PO** 4–8 g b.i.d. to q.i.d. a.c. and at bedtime (32 g/day or less)

Pruritus

Adult: **PO** 4 g b.i.d. to q.i.d. a.c. and at bedtime (16 g/day or less)

ADMINISTRATION

Oral

- Place contents of one packet or one level scoopful on surface of at least 120 to 180 mL (4–6 oz) of water or other preferred liquid. Permit drug to hydrate by standing without stirring 1–2 min, twirling glass occasionally, then stir until suspension is uniform. Rinse glass with small amount of liquid and have patient drink remainder to ensure entire dose is taken. Administer before meals.
- Store in tightly closed container at 15°–30° C (59°–86° F) unless otherwise specified.

ADVERSE EFFECTS (≥1%) **GI:** *Constipation,* fecal impaction, hemorrhoids, abdominal pain and distension, flatulence, bloating sensation, belching, nausea, vomiting, heartburn, anorexia, diarrhea, steatorrhea. **Endocrine:** Increased libido. **Metabolic:** Weight loss or gain, iron, calcium, vitamin A, D, and K deficiencies (from poor absorption); hypoprothrombinemia, hyperchloremic acidosis, decreased erythrocyte folate levels. **Skin:** Rash, irritations of skin, tongue, and perianal areas. **Special Senses:** Arcus juvenilis, uveitis.

DIAGNOSTIC TEST INTERFERENCE Cholestyramine therapy may be accompanied by increased ***serum AST, phosphorus, chloride,*** and ***alkaline phosphatase*** levels; decreased ***serum calcium, sodium,*** and ***potassium*** levels.

INTERACTIONS Drug: Decreases the absorption of ORAL ANTICOAGULANTS, **digoxin,** TETRACYCLINES, **penicillins, phenobarbital,** THYROID HORMONES, THIAZIDE DIURETICS, IRON SALTS, FAT-SOLUBLE VITAMINS (A, D, E, K) from the GI tract—administer cholestyramine 4 h before or 2 h after these drugs. Can bind to and affect absorption of any drug.

PHARMACOKINETICS Absorption: Not absorbed from GI tract. **Elimination:** Excreted in feces as insoluble complex.

NURSING IMPLICATIONS

Assessment & Drug Effects

- Be alert to early symptoms of hypoprothrombinemia (petechiae, ecchymoses, abnormal bleeding from mucous membranes, tarry stools) and report their occurrence promptly. Long-term use of cholestyramine resin can increase bleeding tendency.
- Monitor bowel function. Preexisting constipation may be worsened in the older adult and women.
- Consult physician regarding supplemental vitamins A and D and folic acid that may be required by patient on long-term therapy.
- Lab tests: Periodic CBC, platelet count, serum electrolytes, and lipid profile.

Patient & Family Education

- Report constipation to physician. High-bulk diet with adequate fluid intake is an essential adjunct to cholestyramine treatment and generally resolves the problems of constipation and bloating sensation.
- Do not omit doses. Sudden withdrawal can promote uninhibited absorption of other drugs taken concomitantly, leading to toxicity or overdosage.
- GI adverse effects usually subside after the first month of drug therapy.
- The following symptoms may be drug-induced and should be reported promptly: Severe gastric distress with nausea and vomiting, unusual weight loss, black stools, severe hemorrhoids (GI bleeding), sudden back pain.

CHOLINE MAGNESIUM TRISALICYLATE

(cho'leen mag-ne'si-um tri-sal'i-ci-late)

Trilisate

Classifications: ANALGESIC (SALICYLATE), NONSTEROIDAL ANTI-INFLAMMATORY DRUG (NSAID); ANTIPYRETIC

Therapeutic: ANALGESIC, NSAID

Prototype: Aspirin

Pregnancy Category: C first and second trimester; D third trimester

AVAILABILITY 500 mg, 750 mg, 1000 mg tablets; 500 mg/5 mL liquid

ACTION & *THERAPEUTIC EFFECT* Choline magnesium trisalicylate, a nonsteroidal, anti-inflammatory preparation, acts by inhibiting prostaglandin synthesis by reversibly inhibiting cyclooxygenase (both COX-1 and COX-2), resulting in its anti-inflammatory properties as well as its analgesic property. *Has anti-inflammatory, analgesic, and antipyretic action.*

USES Osteoarthritis, rheumatoid arthritis, and other arthrides. Preferable to aspirin for patients with GI bleeding.

CONTRAINDICATIONS Hypersensitivity to nonacetylated salicylates; children younger than 6 y; children and teenagers with chickenpox, influenza, or flu symptoms because of the potential for Reye's syndrome; coagulopathy, anticoagulant therapy, G6PD deficiency; pregnancy (category D third trimester); contraindicated in late pregnancy, near term, or in labor and delivery.

CAUTIOUS USE Chronic renal and hepatic failure, history of GI disease, peptic ulcer; patients on coumadin or heparin, anemia; hypovolemic states; older adults; pregnancy (category C first and second trimester); lactation.

ROUTE & DOSAGE

Arthritis

Adult: **PO** 1.5–2.5 g/day in 1–3 divided doses (max: 4.5 g/day)

Mild to Moderate Pain, Fever

Adult: **PO** 2–3 g/day in 2 divided doses

Child: **PO** 30–60 mg/kg/day in 3–4 divided doses

ADMINISTRATION

Oral

- Give with food to reduce gastric upset. Do not give with antacids.
- Store at 59°–86° F (15°–30° C).

ADVERSE EFFECTS (≥1%) **GI:** Vomiting, diarrhea. **CNS:** Headache, vertigo, confusion, drowsiness. **Special Senses:** Tinnitus.

INTERACTIONS Drug: Aminosalicylic acid increases risk of salicylate toxicity; **ammonium chloride** and other **acidifying agents** decrease its renal elimination, increasing risk of salicylate toxicity; ANTICOAGULANTS increase risk of bleeding; CARBONIC ANHYDRASE INHIBITORS enhance salicylate toxicity; CORTICOSTEROIDS compound ulcerogenic effects; increases **methotrexate** toxicity; low doses of salicylates may antagonize uricosuric effects of **probenecid, sulfinpyrazone.**

PHARMACOKINETICS Absorption: Readily absorbed from small intestine. **Onset:** 30 min. **Peak:** 1–3 h. **Metabolism:** In liver. **Elimination:** In urine. **Half-Life:** 2–3 h.

NURSING IMPLICATIONS

Assessment & Drug Effects

- As with other NSAIDS, the antipyretic and anti-inflammatory effects may mask usual S&S of infection or other diseases.
- Assess for GI discomfort; nausea, gastric irritation, indigestion, diarrhea, and constipation are frequent complaints.
- Monitor for S&S of bleeding. Closely monitor PT if used concurrently with warfarin.

Patient & Family Education

- Avoid taking aspirin, NSAIDS, or acetaminophen concurrently with drug.
- Avoid dangerous activities until reaction to drug is determined, due to possible CNS effects (e.g., vertigo, drowsiness).
- Report tinnitus or persistent gastric irritation and epigastric pain.
- Report any unexplained bruising or bleeding to physician.
- Hypoglycemic effects may be enhanced for those with type 2 diabetes taking an oral hypoglycemic agent (OHA).
- Do not give to children or teenagers with chickenpox, influenza, or flu symptoms because of association with Reye's syndrome.

CHORIONIC GONADOTROPIN

(go-nad'oh-troe-pin)

Pregnyl

Classification: HUMAN CHORIONIC GONADOTROPIN (HCG) HORMONE

Therapeutic: HCG HORMONE

Pregnancy Category: X

AVAILABILITY 10,000 unit vial

ACTION & *THERAPEUTIC EFFECT* Human chorionic gonadotropin (HCG) is a polypeptide hormone produced by the placenta and extracted from urine during first trimester of pregnancy. Actions nearly identical to those of pituitary luteinizing hormone (LH). Promotes production of gonadal steroid hormones by stimulating interstitial cells of the testes to produce androgen, and the corpus luteum of the ovary to produce progesterone. *Administration of HCG to women of childbearing age with normal functioning ovaries causes maturation of the ovarian follicle and triggers ovulation.*

USES Prepubertal cryptorchidism not due to anatomic obstruction and male hypogonadism secondary to pituitary deficiency. Also used in conjunction with menotropins to induce ovulation and pregnancy in infertile women in whom the cause of anovulation is secondary; ovulation usually occurs within 18 h. To stimulate spermatogenesis in males with hypogonadism.

UNLABELED USES Corpus luteum dysfunction.

CONTRAINDICATIONS Known hypersensitivity to HCG, hypogonadism of testicular origin, hamster protein hypersensitivity; hypertrophy or tumor of pituitary, prostatic carcinoma or other androgen-dependent neoplasms, precocious puberty; ovarian failure; dysfunctional uterine bleeding; adrenal insufficiency; uncontrolled thyroid disease; children younger than 4 y; neonates; pregnancy (category X).

CAUTIOUS USE Epilepsy, migraine, asthma, cardiac or renal disease; endometriosis; thrombophlebitis; lactation.

ROUTE & DOSAGE

Prepubertal Cryptorchidism

Child: **IM** 4000 units 3 times/wk for 3 wk, *or* 5000 units every other day for 4 doses, *or* 500–1000 units 3 times/wk for 4–6 wk

Hypogonadotropic Hypogonadism

Adult: **IM** 500–1000 units 3 times/wk for 3 wk, then 2 times/wk for 3 wk *or* 4000 units 3 times/wk for 6–9 mo followed by 2000 units 3 times/wk for 3 mo

Stimulation of Spermatogenesis

Adult: **IM** 5000 units 3 times/wk until normal testosterone levels are achieved (4–6 mo), then 2000 units 2 times/wk with menotropins for 4 mo

Induction of Ovulation

Adult: **IM** 500–1000 units 1 day following last dose of menotropins

ADMINISTRATION

- Reconstitute only with diluent supplied by manufacturer.
- Following reconstitution solution is stable for 30–90 day, depending on manufacturer, when refrigerated; thereafter potency decreases.
- Store powder for injection at 15°–30° C (59°–86° F) unless otherwise directed.

ADVERSE EFFECTS (≥1%) **Body as a Whole:** Edema, pain at injection site, <u>arterial thromboembolism</u>. **Endocrine:** Gynecomastia, precocious puberty, increased urinary steroid excretion, ectopic pregnancy (incidence low). When used with menotropins (human menopausal gonadotropin): Ovarian hyperstimulation (ascites with or without pain, pleural effusion, ruptured ovarian cysts with resultant hemoperitoneum, multiple births). **CNS:** Headache, irritability, restlessness, depression, fatigue.

DIAGNOSTIC TEST INTERFERENCE ***Pregnancy tests:*** Possibility of false results.

INTERACTIONS Drug: No clinically significant drug interactions established. **Herbal: Black cohosh** may antagonize fertility effects.

PHARMACOKINETICS Onset: 2 h. **Peak:** 6 h. **Distribution:** Testes in males, ovaries in females. **Elimination:** 10–12% in urine within 24 h. **Half-Life:** 23 h.

NURSING IMPLICATIONS

Assessment & Drug Effects

- Assess prepubescent males for development of secondary sex characteristics.
- Assess females for and report excessive menstrual bleeding, irregular menstrual cycles, and abdominal/pelvic distention or pain.

Patient & Family Education

- Report promptly onset of abdominal pain and distension (ovarian hyperstimulation syndrome).
- Report to physician if the following appear: Axillary, facial, pubic hair; penile growth; acne; deepening of voice. Induction of androgen secretion by HCG may induce precocious puberty in patient treated for cryptorchidism.
- Observe for signs of fluid retention. A weight chart should be maintained for a biweekly record. Report to physician if weight gain is associated with edema.

CICLESONIDE

(ci-cle-so'nide)

Alvesco, Omnaris

Pregnancy Category: C

See Appendix A-3.

CICLOPIROX OLAMINE

(sye-kloe-peer'ox)

Loprox, Penlac Nail Lacquer

Classification: ANTIFUNGAL ANTIBIOTIC

Therapeutic: ANTIFUNGAL ANTIBIOTIC

Pregnancy Category: B

AVAILABILITY 1% cream, ointment; 8% nail lacquer; 1% shampoo

ACTION & *THERAPEUTIC EFFECT* Synthetic broad-spectrum antifungal agent with activity against pathogenic fungi. Inhibits transport of amino acids within fungal cell, thereby interfering with synthesis of fungal protein, RNA, and DNA. *Effective against the following organisms: Dermatophytes, yeasts, some species of* Mycoplasma *and* Trichomonas vaginalis, *and certain strains of gram-positive and gram-negative bacteria.*

USES Topically for treatment of tinea cruris and tinea corporis (ringworm) due to *Trichophyton rubrum, Trichophyton mentagrophytes, Epidermophyton floccosum,* and *Microsporum canis,* and for tinea (pityriasis) versicolor due to *M. furfur;* also cutaneous candidiasis (moniliasis) caused by *Candida albicans.* Nail lacquer indicated for onychomycosis of fingernails and toenails due to *T. rubrum;* seborrheic dermatitis of the scalp.

C

CONTRAINDICATIONS Hypersensitivity to ciclopirox olamine or to any component in the formulation; concurrent administration of corticosteroid therapy. Safe use in children younger than 10 y not established.
CAUTIOUS USE Type 1 diabetic patient; history of seizure disorder; immunosuppression; pregnancy (category B); lactation.

ROUTE & DOSAGE

Tinea

Adult: **Topical** Massage cream into affected area and surrounding skin twice daily, morning and evening

Onychomycosis

Adult: **Topical** Paint affected nail(s) under the surface of the nail and on the nail bed once daily at bedtime (at least 8 h before washing). After 7 days, remove lacquer with alcohol and remove or trim away unattached nail. Continue up to 48 wk.

Seborrheic Dermatitis

Adult: **Topical** Wet hair and apply approximately 1 tsp (5 mL) to the scalp (may use up to 10 mL for long hair), leave on scalp for 3 min, then rinse. Repeat treatment twice/wk × 4 wk, with a minimum of 3 days between applications.

ADMINISTRATION
- Wash hands thoroughly before and after treatments.
- Consult with physician about specific procedure for cleansing the skin before medication is applied. Regardless of method used, dry skin thoroughly before drug application.
- Avoid occlusive dressing, wrapping, or clothing over site where cream is applied.
- Store at 15°–30° C (59°–86° F) unless otherwise directed.

ADVERSE EFFECTS (≥1%) **Skin:** Irritation, pruritus, burning, worsening of clinical condition.

PHARMACOKINETICS Absorption: 1.3% absorbed through intact skin. **Distribution:** Distributed to epidermis, corium (dermis), including hair and hair follicles and sebaceous glands; not known if crosses placenta or is distributed into breast milk. **Elimination:** Excreted primarily by kidneys. **Half-Life:** 1.7 h.

NURSING IMPLICATIONS

Assessment & Drug Effects
- Monitor for therapeutic effectiveness. Tinea versicolor generally responds to drug treatment in about 2 wk. Tinea pedis ("athlete's foot"), tinea corporis (ringworm), tinea cruris ("jock itch"), and candidiasis (moniliasis) require about 4 wk of therapy.

Patient & Family Education
- Use medication for the prescribed time even though symptoms improve.
- Report skin irritation or other possible signs of sensitization. A reaction suggestive of sensitization warrants drug discontinuation.
- Do not use occlusive dressings or wrappings.
- Avoid contact of drug in or near the eyes.
- Wear light clothing and footwear that will allow ventilation. Loose-fitting cotton underwear or socks are preferred.

CIDOFOVIR

(cye-do′fo-ver)
Vistide
Classification: ANTIVIRAL
Therapeutic: ANTIVIRAL
Prototype: Acyclovir
Pregnancy Category: C

AVAILABILITY 75 mg/mL injection

ACTION & *THERAPEUTIC EFFECT* Cidofovir, a nucleotide analog, suppresses cytomegalovirus (CMV) replication by inhibiting CMV DNA polymerase. *Cidofovir reduces the rate of viral DNA synthesis of CMV. It is limited for use in treating CMV retinitis in patients with AIDS. Also effective against herpes viruses and other viruses.*

USES Treatment of CMV retinitis in patients with AIDS.

CONTRAINDICATIONS Hypersensitivity to cidofovir, history of severe hypersensitivity to probenecid or other sulfa-containing medications; childbearing women and men without barrier contraception; lactation; severe renal dysfunction. Safety and effectiveness in children not established.

CAUTIOUS USE Renal function impairment, history of diabetes, myelosuppression, previous hypersensitivity to other nucleoside analogs; older adults; pregnancy (category C).

ROUTE & DOSAGE

CMV Retinitis: Induction & Maintenance

Adult: **IV** 5 mg/kg once weekly for 2 wk. Also give 2 g probenecid 3 h prior to infusion and 1 g 8 h after infusion (4 g total). Continue every 2 wk.

Renal Impairment Dosage Adjusment

If serum Cr increases by 0.3–0.4, lower dose to 3 mg/kg

ADMINISTRATION

- Pretreatment: Prehydrate with IV of 1 L NS infused over 1–2 h immediately before cidofovir infusion. If able to tolerate fluid load, infuse second liter over 1–3 h starting at beginning (or end) of cidofovir infusion.

Intravenous

PREPARE: **IV Infusion:** Dilute the calculated dose in 100 mL of NS.
ADMINISTER: **IV Infusion:** Give over 1 h at constant rate. ▪ Do not coadminister with other agents with significant nephrotoxic potential.

- Store vials at 20°–25° C (68°–77° F); may store diluted IV solution at 2°–8° C (36°–46° F) for up to 24 h.

ADVERSE EFFECTS (≥1%) **Body as a Whole:** Infection, allergic reactions. **GI:** Nausea, vomiting, diarrhea. **Metabolic:** Metabolic acidosis. **Hematologic:** Neutropenia. **CNS:** *Fever, headache,* asthenia. **Respiratory:** Dyspnea, pneumonia. **Special Senses:** Ocular hypotony. **Urogenital:** *Nephrotoxicity, proteinuria.*

INTERACTIONS Drug: AMINOGLYCOSIDES, **amphotericin B, foscarnet, pentamidine** can increase risk of nephrotoxicity.

PHARMACOKINETICS Duration: Probenecid increases serum levels and area under concentration–time curve. **Elimination:** 80–100% in urine; probenecid delays urinary excretion.

NURSING IMPLICATIONS

Assessment & Drug Effects

- Lab tests: Baseline and periodic serum creatinine, urine protein;

periodic and WBC count with differential prior to each dose. Dose adjustments or discontinuation may be required.

- Periodic visual acuity tests and measurement of intraocular pressure are recommended.
- Monitor for S&S of hypersensitivity (see Appendix F). Report their appearance promptly.

Patient & Family Education

- Initiate or continue regular ophthalmologic exams.
- Be alert to potential adverse reactions caused by probenecid (e.g., headache, nausea, vomiting, hypersensitivity reactions) and cidofovir.

CILOSTAZOL

(sil-os′tah-zol)

Pletal

Classifications: ANTIPLATELET; PHOSPHODIESTERASE INHIBITOR

Therapeutic: PERIPHERAL VASODILATOR; PLATELET AGGREGATION INHIBITOR

Pregnancy Category: C

AVAILABILITY 50 mg, 100 mg tablets

ACTION & *THERAPEUTIC EFFECT* Inhibition of an isoenzyme which results in vasodilatation and inhibition of platelet aggregation induced by collagen or arachidonic acid. *Increases the skin temperature of the extremities and improves claudication. Effectiveness is indicated by increased ability to walk further without claudication.*

USES Intermittent claudication.

CONTRAINDICATIONS Congestive heart failure of any severity; hypersensitivity to cilostazol; acute MI; hemostatic disorders or pathologic bleeding; lactation.

CAUTIOUS USE Cardiac arrhythmias, MI within 6 mo; valvular heart disease; peptic ulcer disease; renal failure; pregnancy (category C). Safety and efficacy in children younger than 18 y are not established.

ROUTE & DOSAGE

Intermittent Claudication

Adult: **PO** 100 mg b.i.d., may need to reduce to 50 mg b.i.d. with concomitant CYP3A4 or CYP2C19 inhibitors

ADMINISTRATION

Oral

- Give at least 30 min before or 2 h after a meal. Do not give with grapefruit juice.
- Store at 20°–25° C (68°–77° F).

ADVERSE EFFECTS (≥1%) **Body as a Whole:** Back pain, *headache,* infection, myalgia. **CNS:** Dizziness, vertigo. **CV:** Palpitations, tachycardia. **GI:** Abdominal pain, *abnormal stools, diarrhea,* dyspepsia, flatulence, nausea. **Respiratory:** Cough, pharyngitis, rhinitis.

INTERACTIONS Drug: Diltiazem, erythromycin, fluconazole, fluvoxamine, fluoxetine, ketoconazole, itraconazole, MACROLIDE ANTIBIOTICS, **nefazodone, omeprazole, sertraline,** PROTEASE INHIBITORS may increase cilostazol levels and adverse effects. **Herbal: Evening primrose oil** may increase bleeding risk. **Food:** High fat meals may increase peak concentrations. **Grapefruit juice** may increase concentration.

PHARMACOKINETICS Absorption: Well absorbed from GI tract. **Onset:** 2–4 wk. **Distribution:** 95–98% protein bound. Smoking may decrease serum levels. May be excreted in breast milk. **Metabolism:** Metabolized by CYP3A4 to active metabolites. **Elimination:** Metabolites primarily excreted in urine and feces. **Half-Life:** 11–13 h.

NURSING IMPLICATIONS

Assessment & Drug Effects

- Monitor therapeutic effectiveness indicated by ability to walk farther without leg pain.
- Monitor for S&S of CHF. Do not give cilostazol to patients with preexisting CHF.

Patient & Family Education

- Avoid grapefruit or grapefruit juice while taking cilostazol.
- Allow 2–12 wk for therapeutic response.

CIMETIDINE Pr

(sye-met′i-deen)

Tagamet, Tagamet HB

Classification: ANTISECRETORY (H_2-RECEPTOR ANTAGONIST)

Therapeutic: ANTISECRETORY

Pregnancy Category: B

AVAILABILITY 100 mg, 200 mg, 400 mg, 800 mg tablets; 300 mg/5 mL liquid; 150 mg/mL injection

ACTION & *THERAPEUTIC EFFECT* Has high selectivity for inhibition of histamine H_2-receptors on parietal cells of the stomach, thus suppressing all phases of daytime and nocturnal basal gastric acid secretion in the stomach. Indirectly reduces pepsin secretion. *Blocks the H_2-receptors on the parietal cells of the stomach, thus decreasing gastric acid secretion; raises the pH of the stomach and thereby reduces pepsin secretion.*

USES Short-term treatment of active duodenal ulcer and prevention of ulcer recurrence (at reduced dosage) after it is healed. Also used for short-term treatment of active benign gastric ulcer, pathologic hypersecretory conditions such as Zollinger-Ellison syndrome, and heartburn.

UNLABELED USES Prophylaxis of stress-induced ulcers, upper GI bleeding, and aspiration pneumonitis; gastroesophageal reflux; chronic urticaria; acetaminophen toxicity.

CONTRAINDICATIONS Known hypersensitivity to cimetidine or other H_2-receptor antagonists.

CAUTIOUS USE Older adults or critically ill patients; impaired renal or hepatic function; organic brain syndrome; gastric ulcers; immunocompromised patients, pregnancy (category B).

ROUTE & DOSAGE

Duodenal Ulcer

Adult: **PO** 300 mg q.i.d. *or* 400 mg b.i.d. *or* 800 mg at bedtime **IM/IV** 300 mg q6–8h

Child: **PO/IM/IV** 20–40 mg/kg/day in 4 divided doses

Neonate: **PO/IM/IV** 5–10 mg/kg/day divided q8–12h

Infant: **PO/IM/IV** 10–20 mg/kg/day divided q6–12h

Duodenal Ulcer, Maintenance Therapy

Adult: **PO** 400 mg at bedtime

Gastric Ulcer

Adult: **PO** 300 mg q.i.d. with meals and at bedtime **IM/IV** 300 mg q6–8h

Upper GI Bleed

Adult: **IV** 37.5 mg/h

Heartburn

Adult: **PO** 200 mg 2–4 times/day

C

Pathologic Hypersecretory Disease

Adult: **PO** 300 mg q.i.d. with meals and at bedtime, may increase up to 2400 mg/day **IM/IV** 300 mg q6–8h, may increase up to 2400 mg/day

Renal Impairment Dosage Adjustment

CrCl less than 20 mL/min: Dose q12h

Hemodialysis Dosage Adjustment: Give scheduled dose after dialysis

ADMINISTRATION

Oral

- Give 1 h before or 2 h after an antacid.

Intramuscular

- Give IM injection undiluted into a large muscle.

Intravenous

IV administration to neonates, infants and children: Verify correct IV concentration and rate of infusion/injection with physician.

PREPARE: **Direct:** Dilute 300 mg in 18 mL D5W or NS to yield 300 mg/20 mL. **Intermittent:** Dilute 300 mg in 50 mL D5W or NS. **Continuous:** Further dilute in up to 1000 mL of selected IV solution.

ADMINISTER: **Direct:** Give 300 mg or fraction thereof over at least 5 min. **Intermittent:** Give over 15–20 min. **Continuous:** Give a loading dose of 150 mg at the intermittent infusion rate; then give continuous infusion equally spaced over 24 h.

INCOMPATIBILITIES **Solution/additive:** **Amphotericin B, cefazolin, chlorpromazine, pentobarbital, phenobarbital, secobarbital.** **Y-site:** **Allopurinol, amphotericin B cholesteryl complex, amsacrine, cefepime, indomethacin, lansoprazole, phenytoin, warfarin.**

- Parenteral solutions are stable for 48 h at room temperature when added to commonly used IV solutions for dilution. Follow manufacturer's directions. ▪ Store all forms of cimetidine at 15°–30° C (59°–86° F) protected from light unless otherwise directed by manufacturer.

ADVERSE EFFECTS (≥1%) **Body as a Whole:** Fever. **CV (rare):** Cardiac arrhythmias and cardiac arrest after rapid IV bolus dose. **GI:** Mild transient diarrhea; severe diarrhea, constipation, abdominal discomfort. **Hematologic:** Increased prothrombin time; neutropenia (rare), thrombocytopenia (rare), aplastic anemia. **Metabolic:** Slight increase in serum uric acid, BUN, creatinine; transient pain at IM site; hypospermia. **Musculoskeletal:** Exacerbation of joint symptoms in patients with preexisting arthritis. **CNS:** Drowsiness, dizziness, light-headedness, depression, headache, reversible confusional states, paranoid psychosis. **Skin:** Rash, Stevens-Johnson syndrome, reversible alopecia. **Urogenital:** Gynecomastia and breast soreness, galactorrhea, reversible impotence.

DIAGNOSTIC TEST INTERFERENCE Cimetidine may cause false-positive ***Hemoccult test for gastric bleeding*** if test is performed within 15 min of oral cimetidine administration.

INTERACTIONS **Drug:** Cimetidine decreases the hepatic metabolism of **warfarin, phenobarbital, phenytoin, diazepam, propranolol, lidocaine, theophylline,** thus increasing their activity and toxicity; ANTACIDS may decrease absorption of cimetidine.

PHARMACOKINETICS Absorption: 70% of PO dose absorbed from GI tract. **Peak:** 1–1.5 h. **Distribution:** Widely distributed; crosses blood–brain barrier and placenta. **Metabolism:** In liver by CYP1A2 and 3A4. **Elimination:** Most of drug excreted in urine in 24 h; excreted in breast milk. **Half-Life:** 2 h.

NURSING IMPLICATIONS

Assessment & Drug Effects

- Monitor pulse of patient during first few days of drug regimen. Bradycardia should be reported. Pulse usually returns to normal within 24 h after drug discontinuation.
- Monitor I&O ratio and pattern: Particularly in the older adult, severely ill, and in patients with impaired renal function.
- Lab tests: Periodic evaluations of blood count and renal and hepatic function are advised during therapy.
- Be alert to onset of confusional states, particularly in the older adult or severely ill patient. Symptoms occur within 2–3 days after first dose; report immediately. Symptoms usually resolve within 3–4 days after therapy is discontinued.
- Check BP and report an elevation to the physician, if patient complains of severe headache.

Patient & Family Education

- Seek advice about self-medication with any OTC drug.
- Report breast tenderness or enlargement. Mild bilateral gynecomastia and breast soreness may occur after 1 mo or more of therapy. It may disappear spontaneously or remain throughout therapy.
- Report recurrence of gastric pain or bleeding (black, tarry stools or "coffee ground" vomitus) immediately, and notify physician if diarrhea continues more than 1 day.
- Avoid driving and other potentially hazardous activities until reaction to drug is known.
- Duodenal or gastric ulcer is a chronic, recurrent condition that requires long-term maintenance drug therapy.

CINACALCET HYDROCHLORIDE

(sin-a-kal′set)

Sensipar

Classifications: PARATHYROID HORMONE; CALCIUM RECEPTOR AGONIST

Therapeutic: PARATHYROID HORMONE

Pregnancy Category: C

AVAILABILITY 30 mg, 60 mg, 90 mg tablets

ACTION & *THERAPEUTIC EFFECT* Directly lowers parathyroid hormone (PTH) levels by increasing the sensitivity of calcium-sensing receptors on the parathyroid gland to extracellular calcium. This causes decreased calcium and phosphate adsorption from bone, and thus decreased serum calcium and phosphate levels. *Lowers PTH production; this also decreases rate of bone turnover and bone fibrosis in chronic renal failure disease (CRFD).*

USES Treatment of secondary hyperparathyroidism in patients with chronic kidney disease on dialysis; hypercalcemia in patients with parathyroid cancer.

CONTRAINDICATIONS Hypersensitivity to cinacalcet; lactation, children younger than 18 y.

C

CAUTIOUS USE Moderate and severe hepatic impairment, hypocalcemia, history of seizures; hypotension; heart failure; history of arrhythmias; pregnancy (category C).

ROUTE & DOSAGE

Secondary Hyperparathyroidism
Adult: **PO** Start with 30 mg once daily; may increase q2–4wk until target iPTH of 150–300 pg/mL (max: 300 mg/day)

Parathyroid Cancer
Adult: **PO** 30 mg twice daily; titrate q2–4wk as 60 mg b.i.d., 90 mg b.i.d., then 90 mg 3–4 times daily as needed to normalize calcium concentrations

ADMINISTRATION

Oral

- Give with food or shortly after a meal.
- Tablets should be swallowed whole and not divided, crushed, or chewed.
- Store at 15°–30° C (59°–86° F).

ADVERSE EFFECTS (≥1%) **Body as a Whole:** Dizziness, asthenia, noncardiac chest pain, dialysis access infection. **CV:** Hypertension. **GI:** *Nausea, vomiting, diarrhea,* anorexia. **Metabolic:** Hypocalcemia. **Musculoskeletal:** *Myalgia,* adynamic bone disease (renal osteodystrophy).

INTERACTIONS Drug: May increase **amoxapine, atomoxetine, carvedilol, clozapine, codeine, cyclobenzaprine, dexfenfluramine, dextromethorphan, donepezil, encainide, fenfluramine, flecainide, fluoxetine, haloperidol, hydrocodone, maprotiline, meperidine, methadone, methamphetamine, metoprolol, mexiletine, morphine, oxycodone, paroxetine, perphenazine, propafenone, propranolol, risperidone, thioridazine** (use may be contraindicated with cinacalcet), **timolol, tramadol, trazodone,** TRICYCLIC ANTIDEPRESSANTS, **venlafaxine, zolpidem** levels; cinacalcet levels may be increased by strong CYP3A4 inhibitors such as **amiodarone, aprepitant, clarithromycin, dalfopristin; diltiazem, erythromycin, fluconazole, fluvoxamine, itraconazole, ketoconazole, miconazole, nefazodone, quinupristin, troleandomycin, verapamil, voriconazole, zafirlukast, zileuton. Food: Grapefruit juice** may increase cinacalcet levels.

PHARMACOKINETICS Peak: 2–6 h. **Distribution:** 93–97% protein bound. **Metabolism:** In liver by CYP3A4. **Elimination:** 80% by kidneys, 15% in feces. **Half-Life:** 30–40 h.

NURSING IMPLICATIONS

Assessment & Drug Effects

- Monitor for S&S of hypocalcemia (e.g., paresthesias, myalgias, cramping, tetany, convulsions).
- Withhold drug and notify physician for serum calcium less than 7.5 mg/dL or symptoms of hypocalcemia. Drug should not be resumed until serum calcium levels reach 8 mg/dL, and/or symptoms of hypocalcemia resolve.
- Lab tests: Serum calcium and phosphorus within 1 wk after and iPTH 1–4 wk after initiation of drug or dose adjustment; thereafter, monthly serum calcium and phosphorus (more often with a history of a seizure disorder), and iPTH every 1–3 mo.
- Closely monitor iPTH and serum calcium with concurrent administration of a strong CYP3A4 (e.g.,

ketoconazole, erythromycin, itraconazole).

Patient & Family Education

- Report promptly any of the following: Seizure or convulsion; muscle spasms or cramping of the abdomen, back, legs, face; burning, numbness, pricking, tickling, or tingling of the face, lips, tongue, hands, or feet; changes in mental status.

CIPROFLOXACIN HYDROCHLORIDE (Pr)

(ci-pro-flox′a-cin)

Cipro, Cipro IV, Cipro XR, Proquin XR

CIPROFLOXACIN OPHTHALMIC

Ciloxan

Classification: QUINOLONE ANTIBIOTIC

Therapeutic: ANTIBIOTIC

Pregnancy Category: C

AVAILABILITY 100 mg, 250 mg, 500 mg, 750 mg tablets; 500 mg extended release tablets; 50 mg/mL, 100 mg/mL suspension; 200 mg, 400 mg injection; 3.5 mg/mL ophth solution

ACTION & *THERAPEUTIC EFFECT* Synthetic quinolone that is a broad-spectrum bactericidal agent. Inhibits DNA-gyrase, an enzyme necessary for bacterial DNA replication and some aspects of transcription, repair, recombination, and transposition. *Effective against many gram-positive and aerobic gram-negative organisms. Not active against anaerobes.*

USES UTIs, lower respiratory tract infections, skin and skin structure infections, bone and joint infections, GI infection or infectious diarrhea, chronic bacterial prostatitis, nosocomial pneumonia, acute sinusitis. Post-exposure prophylaxis for anthrax. **Ophthalmic:** Corneal ulcers, bacterial conjunctivitis caused by *Staphylococci, Streptococci,* and *Pseudomonas aeruginosa.*

CONTRAINDICATIONS Known hypersensitivity to ciprofloxacin or other quinolones, syphilis, viral infection; tendon inflammation or tendon pain; lactation.

CAUTIOUS USE Known or suspected CNS disorders (i.e., severe cerebral arteriosclerosis or seizure disorders); myasthenia gravis; myocardial ischemia, atrial fibrillation, QT prolongation, CHF; GI disease, colitis; CVA; uncorrected hypokalemia; patients receiving theophylline derivatives or caffeine, severe renal impairment and crystalluria during ciprofloxacin therapy, and patients on coumarin therapy; pregnancy (category C); children.

ROUTE & DOSAGE

Uncomplicated UTI

Adult: **PO** 250 mg q12h or 500 mg XR daily × 3 days **IV** 200 mg q12h × 7–14 days

Complicated UTI

Adult: **PO** 1000 mg XR daily × 7–14 days **IV** 400 mg q12h × 7–14 days

Acute Sinusitis

Adult: **PO** 500 mg b.i.d. × 10 days

Moderate to Severe Systemic Infection

Adult: **PO** 500–750 mg q12h **IV** 200–400 mg q8–12h

C

Renal Impairment Dosage Adjustment

CrCl 30–50 mL/min: **PO** 250–500 mg q12h, **IV** No change in dose; less than 30 mL/min: **PO** 250–500 mg q18h, **IV** 200–400 mg q18–24h

Bacterial Conjunctivitis

Adult: **Ophthalmic** 1–2 drops in conjunctival sac q2h while awake for 2 days, then 1–2 drops q4h while awake for the next 5 days **Ointment** 1/2-inch ribbon into conjunctival sac t.i.d. × 2 days, then b.i.d. × 5 days

Corneal Ulcers

Adult: **Ophthalmic** 2 drops q15min for 6 h, 2 drops q30min for the next 18 h, then 2 drops q1h for 24 h, then 2 drops q4h for 14 days

ADMINISTRATION

- For patients with renal impairment, oral and IV doses are lowered according to creatinine clearance.

Oral

- Do not give an antacid within 4 h of the oral ciprofloxacin dose.

Intravenous

PREPARE: **Intermittent:** Dilute in NS or D5W to a final concentration of 0.5–2 mg/mL. ▪ Typical dilutions are 200 mg in 100–250 mL and 400 mg in 250–500 mL.
ADMINISTER: **Intermittent:** Give slowly over 60 min. Avoid rapid infusion and use of a small vein.
INCOMPATIBILITIES **Solution/additive: Aminophylline, amoxicillin, amoxicillin/clavulanate potassium, amphotericin B, ampicillin/sulbactam, ceftazidime, cefuroxime, clindamycin, heparin, metronidazole, piperacillin, sodium bicarbonate, ticarcillin. Y-site: Aminophylline, ampicillin, ampicillin/sulbactam, azithromycin, cefepime, dexamethasone, drotrecogin alfa, furosemide, heparin, hydrocortisone, lansoprazole, phenytoin, propofol, sodium bicarbonate, theophylline, TPN, warfarin.**

- Discontinue other IV infusion while infusing ciprofloxacin or infuse through another site. ▪ Reconstituted IV solution is stable for 14 days refrigerated.

ADVERSE EFFECTS (≥1%) **GI:** Nausea, vomiting, diarrhea, cramps, gas, pseudomembranous colitis. **Metabolic:** Transient increases in liver transaminases, alkaline phosphatase, lactic dehydrogenase, and eosinophilia count. **Musculoskeletal:** Tendon rupture, cartilage erosion. **CNS:** Headache, vertigo, malaise, peripheral neuropathy, seizures (especially with rapid IV infusion). **Skin:** Rash, phlebitis, pain, burning, pruritus, and erythema at infusion site; photosensitivity. **Special Senses:** *Local burning and discomfort, crystalline precipitate on superficial portion of cornea,* lid margin crusting, scales, foreign body sensation, itching, and conjunctival hyperemia.

DIAGNOSTIC TEST INTERFERENCE Ciprofloxacin does not interfere with ***urinary glucose*** determinations using ***cupric sulfate solution*** or with ***glucose oxidase tests;*** may cause false positive on ***opiate screening tests.***

INTERACTIONS Drug: May increase **theophylline** levels 15–30%; ANTACIDS, **sulcralfate, iron** decrease absorption of ciprofloxacin; may increase PT for patients on **warfarin.** **Food:** Calcium decreases the levels of ciprofloxacin.

PHARMACOKINETICS Absorption: 60–80% from GI tract. **Ophthalmic:** Minimal absorption through cornea or conjunctiva. **Onset:** Topical 0.5–2 h. **Duration:** Topical 12 h. **Peak:** Immediate release: 0.5–2 h; Cipro XR: 1–2.5 h; Proquin XR: 3.5–8.7 h. **Distribution:** Widely distributed including prostate, lung, and bone; crosses placenta; distributed into breast milk. **Elimination:** Primarily in urine with some biliary excretion. **Half-Life:** 3.5–4 h.

NURSING IMPLICATIONS

Assessment & Drug Effects

- Report tendon inflammation or pain. Drug should be discontinued.
- Lab tests: Culture and sensitivity tests should be done prior to initial dose. Treatment may be implemented pending results.
- Monitor urine pH; it should be less than 6.8, especially in the older adult and patients receiving high dosages of ciprofloxacin, to reduce the risk of crystalluria.
- Monitor I&O ratio and patterns: Patients should be well hydrated; assess for S&S of crystalluria.
- Monitor plasma theophylline concentrations, since drug may interfere with half-life.
- Administration with theophylline derivatives or caffeine can cause CNS stimulation.
- Assess for S&S of GI irritation (e.g., nausea, diarrhea, vomiting, abdominal discomfort) in clients receiving high dosages and in older adults.
- Monitor PT and INR in patients receiving coumarin therapy.
- Assess for S&S of superinfections (see Appendix F).

Patient & Family Education

- Immediately report tendon inflammation or pain. Drug should be discontinued.
- Fluid intake of 2–3 L/day is advised, if not contraindicated.
- Report sudden, unexplained joint pain.
- Restrict caffeine due to the following effects: Nervousness, insomnia, anxiety, tachycardia.
- Use sunscreen and avoid overexposure to sunlight.
- Report nausea, diarrhea, vomiting, and abdominal pain or discomfort.
- Use caution with hazardous activities until reaction to drug is known. Drug may cause lightheadedness.

CISATRACURIUM BESYLATE

(cis-a-tra-kyoo-ri′um)

Nimbex

Classifications: SKELETAL MUSCLE RELAXANT, NONDEPOLARIZING; NEUROMUSCULAR BLOCKER

Therapeutic: SKELETAL MUSCLE RELAXANT

Prototype: Atracurium

Pregnancy Category: B

AVAILABILITY 2 mg/mL, 10 mg/mL injection

ACTION & *THERAPEUTIC EFFECT* Cisatracurium is a neuromuscular blocking agent with intermediate onset and duration of action compared with similar agents. It binds competitively to cholinergic receptors on the motor endplate of neurons, antagonizing the action of acetylcholine. *Antagonism of acetylcholine blocks neuromuscular transmission of nerve impulses.*

USES Adjunct to general anesthesia to facilitate tracheal intubation and provide skeletal muscle relaxation during surgery or mechanical ventilation.

CONTRAINDICATIONS Hypersensitivity to cisatracurium or other related agents; rapid-sequence endotracheal intubation. Not studied in infants younger than 1 mo.

CAUTIOUS USE History of hemiparesis, electrolyte imbalances, burn patients, pulmonary disease, COPD; neuromuscular diseases (e.g., myasthenia gravis), older adults, renal function impairment, pregnancy (category B), lactation.

ROUTE & DOSAGE

Intubation

Adult: **IV** 0.15 or 0.20 mg/kg
Child (2–12 y): **IV** 0.1–0.15 mg/kg
Infant (older than 1 mo): **IV** 0.15 mg/kg

Maintenance

Adult: **IV** 0.03 mg/kg q20min prn *or* 1–2 mcg/kg/min
Child (2 y or older): **IV** 1–2 mcg/kg/min

Mechanical Ventilation in ICU

Adult: **IV** 3 mcg/kg/min (can range from 0.5 to 10.2 mcg/kg/min)

ADMINISTRATION

- Administer carefully adjusted, individualized doses using a peripheral nerve stimulator to evaluate neuromuscular function.
- Given only by or under supervision of expert clinician familiar with the drug's actions and potential complications.
- Have immediately available personnel and facilities for resuscitation and life support and an antagonist of cisatracurium.
- Note that 10-mL multiple-dose vials contain benzyl alcohol and should not be used with neonates.

Intravenous

PREPARE: **Direct:** Give undiluted. **IV Infusion:** Dilute 10 mg in 95 mL or 40 mg in 80 mL of compatible IV fluid to prepare 0.1 mg/mL or 0.4 mg/mL, respectively, IV solution. ▪ Compatible IV fluids include D5W, NS, D5/NS, D5/LR. **ICU IV Infusion (Mechanical Ventilation):** Dilute the contents of the 200 mg vial (i.e., 10 mg/mL) in 1000 mL or 500 mL of compatible IV fluid to prepare 0.2 mg/mL or 0.4 g/mL, respectively, IV solutions.

ADMINISTER: **Direct:** Give a single dose over 5–10 sec. **IV Infusion:** Adjust the rate based on patient's weight.

INCOMPATIBILITIES Solution/additive: **Ketorolac, propofol (dose dependent).** Y-site: **Amphotericin B, amphotericin B cholesteryl complex, ampicillin, cefazolin, cefotaxime, cefotetan, cefuroxime, diazepam, furosemide, ganciclovir, heparin, methylprednisolone, sodium bicarbonate, thiopental, trimethoprim/sulfamethoxazole.**

- Refrigerate vials at 2°–8° C (36°–46° F). Protect from light. Diluted solutions may be stored refrigerated or at room temperature for 24 h.

ADVERSE EFFECTS (≥1%) **CV:** Bradycardia, hypotension, flushing. **Respiratory:** Bronchospasm. **Skin:** Rash.

PHARMACOKINETICS Onset: Varies from 1.5 to 3.3 min (higher dose has faster onset). **Peak:** Varies from 1.5 to 3.3 min (higher dose has faster peak). **Duration:** Varies with dose from 46 to 121 min (higher dose, longer recovery time). **Metabolism:** Undergoes Hoffman elimination (pH- and temperature-dependent degradation) and hydrolysis by plasma esterases. **Elimination:** In urine. **Half-Life:** 22 min.

NURSING IMPLICATIONS

Assessment & Drug Effects

- Time-to-maximum neuromuscular block is ≈1 min slower in the older adult.
- Monitor for bradycardia, hypotension, and bronchospasms; monitor ICU patients for spontaneous seizures.

CISPLATIN (cis-DDP, cis-PLATINUM II)

(sis′pla-tin)

Abiplatin ♣, Platinol

Classifications: ANTINEOPLASTIC; ALKYLATING AGENT

Therapeutic: ANTINEOPLASTIC

Prototype: Cyclophosphamide

Pregnancy Category: D

AVAILABILITY 1 mg/mL injection

ACTION & *THERAPEUTIC EFFECT* A heavy metal complex with platinum as central atom surrounded by 2 chloride atoms and 2 ammonia molecules in the cis chemical position. Produces interstrand and intrastrand cross linkage in DNA of rapidly dividing cells, thus preventing DNA, RNA, and protein synthesis. *Cell cycle-nonspecific (i.e., effective throughout the entire cell life cycle).*

USES Established combination therapy (cisplatin, vinblastine, bleomycin) in patient with metastatic testicular tumors and with doxorubicin for metastatic ovarian tumors following appropriate surgical or radiation therapy.

UNLABELED USES Carcinoma of endometrium, bladder, head, and neck.

CONTRAINDICATIONS History of hypersensitivity to cisplatin or other platinum-containing compounds; impaired renal function; severe myelosuppression; impaired hearing; active infection; history of gout and urate renal stones, renal failure; hypomagnesia; concurrent administration with loop diuretics; Raynaud syndrome; pregnancy (category D). Safe use in children not established, although experimental regimens have been used.

CAUTIOUS USE Previous cytotoxic drug or radiation therapy with other ototoxic and nephrotoxic drugs; peripheral neuropathy; hyperuricemia; electrolyte imbalances, moderate renal impairment; hepatic impairment; history of circulatory disorders.

ROUTE & DOSAGE

Testicular Neoplasms

Adult: **IV** 20 mg/m²/day for 5 days q3–4wk for 3 courses

Ovarian Neoplasms

Adult: **IV** *With cyclophosphamide:* 75–100 mg/m² once q4wk; *single agent:* 100 mg/m² once q4wk

Advanced Bladder Cancer

Adult: **IV** 50–75 mg/m² q3–4 wk

ADMINISTRATION

- Usually a parenteral antiemetic agent is administered 30 min before cisplatin therapy is instituted and given on a scheduled basis throughout day and night as long as necessary.
- Before the initial dose is given, hydration is started with 1–2 L IV

infusion fluid to reduce risk of nephrotoxicity and ototoxicity.

C

Intravenous

PREPARE: **IV Infusion:** Use disposable gloves when preparing cisplatin solutions. If drug accidentally contacts skin or mucosa, wash immediately and thoroughly with soap and water. ▪ Do not use any equipment containing aluminum. ▪ Withdraw required dose and dilute in 2 L D5W 5% dextrose in 1/2 or 1/3 normal saline containing 37.5 g mannitol.

ADMINISTER: **IV Infusion:** Give 2 L over 6–8 h.

INCOMPATIBILITIES **Solution/additive: 5% dextrose, fluorouracil, mesna, metoclopramide, sodium bicarbonate, thiotepa. Y-site: Amifostine, amphotericin B, cholesteryl, cefepime, lansoprazole, piperacillin/tazobactam, thiotepa, TPN.**

▪ Hydration and forced diuresis are continued for at least 24 h after drug administration to ensure adequate urinary output.

▪ Store at 15°–30° C (59°–86° F). Do not refrigerate. Protect from light. Once vial is opened, solution is stable for 28 days protected from light or 7 days in fluorescent light.

ADVERSE EFFECTS (≥1%) **Body as a Whole:** Anaphylactic-like reactions. **CV:** Cardiac abnormalities. **GI:** *Marked nausea, vomiting,* anorexia, stomatitis, xerostomia, diarrhea, constipation. **Hematologic:** Myelosuppression (25–30% patients): Leukopenia, thrombocytopenia; hemolytic anemia, hemolysis. **Metabolic:** Hypocalcemia, *hypomagnesemia,* hyperuricemia, elevated AST, SIADH. **CNS:** Seizures, headache; peripheral neuropathies (may be irreversible): Paresthesia, unsteady gait, clumsiness of hands and feet, exacerbation of neuropathy with exercise, loss of taste. **Special Senses:** Ototoxicity (may be irreversible): Tinnitus, hearing loss, deafness, vertigo, blurred vision, changes in ability to see colors (optic neuritis, papilledema). **Urogenital:** Nephrotoxicity.

INTERACTIONS Drug: AMINOGLYCOSIDES, **amphotericin B, vancomycin,** other **nephrotoxic drugs** increase nephrotoxicity and acute renal failure—try to separate by at least 1–2 wk; AMINOGLYCOSIDES, **furosemide** increase risk of ototoxicity.

PHARMACOKINETICS Peak: Immediately after infusion. **Distribution:** Widely distributed in body fluids and tissues; concentrated in kidneys, liver, and prostate; accumulated in tissues. **Metabolism:** Not known. **Elimination:** 15–50% in urine within 24–48 h. **Half-Life:** 73–290 h.

NURSING IMPLICATIONS

Assessment & Drug Effects

- Obtain baseline ECG and cardiac monitoring during induction therapy because of possible myocarditis or focal irritability.
- Lab tests: The following tests should be done *before* initiating every course of therapy and repeated each week during treatment period: Serum uric acid, serum creatinine, BUN, urinary creatinine clearance. CBC and platelet counts are done weekly for 2 wk after each course of treatment. Monitor periodically serum electrolytes and liver function tests.
- A repeat course of therapy should not be given until (1) serum creatinine is below 1.5 mg/dL; (2) BUN is below 25 mg/dL; (3) platelets 100,000/mm^3 or more; (4) WBC

4000/mm^3 or more; (5) audiometric test is within normal limits.

- Monitor urine output and specific gravity for 4 consecutive hours before treatment and for 24 h after therapy. A urine output of less than 75 mL/h necessitates medical intervention to avert a renal emergency.
- Audiometric testing should be performed before the first dose and before each subsequent dose. Ototoxicity (reported in 31% of patients) may occur after a single dose of 50 mg/m^2. Children who receive repeated doses are especially susceptible.
- Monitor for anaphylactoid reactions (particularly in patient previously exposed to cisplatin), which may occur within minutes of drug administration.
- Monitor closely for dose-related adverse reactions. Drug action is cumulative; therefore severity of most adverse effects increases with repeated doses.
- Suspect ototoxicity if patient manifests tinnitus or difficulty hearing in the high frequency range.
- Monitor results of blood studies. The nadirs in platelet and leukocyte counts occur between day 18 and 23 (range: 7.5–45) with most patients recovering in 13–62 days.
- Monitor and report abnormal bowel elimination; diarrhea is a possible response to GI irritation.
- Inspect oral membranes for xerostomia (white patches and ulcerations) and tongue for signs of fungal overgrowth (black, furry appearance).
- Weigh the patient under standard conditions every day. A gradual ascending weight profile occurring over a period of several days should be reported.

Patient & Family Education

- Continue maintenance of adequate hydration (at least 3000 mL/24 h oral fluid if physician agrees) and report promptly: Reduced urinary output, flank pain, anorexia, nausea, vomiting, dry mucosae, itching skin, urine odor on breath, fluid retention, and weight gain.
- Avoid rapid changes in position to minimize risk of dizziness or falling.
- Tingling, numbness, and tremors of extremities, loss of position sense and taste, and constipation are early signs of neurotoxicity. Report their occurrence promptly to prevent irreversibility.
- Report tinnitus or any hearing impairment.
- Report promptly evidence of unexplained bleeding and easy bruising.
- Report unusual fatigue, fever, sore mouth and throat, abnormal body discharges.

CITALOPRAM HYDROBROMIDE

(cit-a-lo′pram)

Celexa

Classification: SELECTIVE SEROTONIN-REUPTAKE INHIBITOR (SSRI)

Therapeutic: ANTIDEPRESSANT

Prototype: Fluoxetine

Pregnancy Category: C

AVAILABILITY 20 mg, 40 mg tablets; 10 mg/5 mL oral solution

ACTION & *THERAPEUTIC EFFECT*
Selective serotonin reuptake inhibitor (SSRI) in the CNS. Antidepressant effect is presumed to be linked to its inhibition of CNS presynaptic neuronal uptake of serotonin which results in antidepressant activity. *Selective serotonin reuptake inhibition mechanism results in the*

C

antidepressant activity of citalopram.

USES Depression.
UNLABELED USES Anxiety, hot flashes, obsessive-compulsive disorder, post-traumatic stress disorder, panic disorder.

CONTRAINDICATIONS Hypersensitivity to citalopram; unstable heart disease, recent MI; concurrent use of MAOIs or use within 14 days of discontinuing MAOIs; mania; volume depleted, hyponatremia; suicidal ideation; bipolar depression; children younger than 18 y.
CAUTIOUS USE Hypersensitivity to other SSRIs; renal or hepatic insufficiency; history of potential suicide; older adults; concurrent use of diuretics, NSAIDs; dehydration; severe renal impairment or renal failure; cardiovascular disease (e.g., dysrhythmias, conduction defects, myocardial ischemia); history of drug abuse; history of seizure disorders or suicidal tendencies; bipolar disorder, history of mania; ECT treatments; pregnancy (category C), lactation.

ROUTE & DOSAGE

Depression
Adult: **PO** Start at 20 mg daily, may increase to 40 mg daily if needed
Geriatric: **PO** 20 mg daily

ADMINISTRATION

Oral
- Do not begin this drug within 14 days of stopping an MAOI.
- Reduced doses are advised for the older adult and those with hepatic or renal impairment.
- Dose increments should be separated by at least 1 wk.
- Store at 15°–30° C (59°–86° F) in tightly closed container and protect from light.

ADVERSE EFFECTS (≥1%) **Body as a Whole:** Asthenia, fatigue, fever, arthralgia, myalgia. **CV:** Tachycardia, postural hypotension, hypotension. **GI:** *Nausea,* vomiting, diarrhea, dyspepsia, abdominal pain, *dry mouth,* anorexia, flatulence. **CNS:** Dizziness, *insomnia, somnolence,* agitation, tremor, anxiety, paresthesia, migraine, neuromalignant syndrome. **Respiratory:** URI, rhinitis, sinusitis. **Skin:** Increased sweating. **Urogenital:** Dysmenorrhea, decreased libido, ejaculation disorder, impotence.

INTERACTIONS **Drug:** Combination with MAOIS could result in hypertensive crisis, hyperthermia, rigidity, myoclonus, autonomic instability; **cimetidine** may increase citalopram levels; **linezolid** may cause serotonin syndrome. **Herbal:** **St. John's wort** may cause serotonin syndrome.

PHARMACOKINETICS **Absorption:** Rapidly absorbed from GI tract; approximately 80% reaches systemic circulation. **Peak:** Steady-state serum concentrations in 1 wk; peak blood levels at 4 h. **Distribution:** 80% protein bound; crosses placenta; distributed into breast milk. **Metabolism:** In liver by CYP3A4 and CYP2C9 enzymes. **Elimination:** 20% in urine, 80% in bile. **Half-Life:** 35 h.

NURSING IMPLICATIONS

Assessment & Drug Effects
- Watch closely for worsening of depression or emergence of suicidal ideations.
- Monitor for therapeutic effectiveness: Indicated by elevation of

mood; 1–4 wk may be needed before improvement is noted.

- Lab tests: Monitor periodically hepatic functions, CBC, serum sodium, and lithium levels when the two drugs are given concurrently.
- Monitor periodically HR and BP, and carefully monitor complete cardiac status in person with known or suspected cardiac disease.
- Monitor closely older adult patients for adverse effects especially with doses greater than 20 mg/day.

Patient & Family Education

- Do not engage in hazardous activities until reaction to this drug is known.
- Avoid using alcohol while taking citalopram.
- Report immediately worsening of clinical condition, including suicidal ideation or other unusual changes in behavior.
- Report distressing adverse effects including any changes in sexual functioning or response.
- Periodic ophthalmology exams are advised with long-term treatment.

CLADRIBINE

(cla′dri-been)

Leustatin

Classifications: ANTINEOPLASTIC; ANTIMETABOLITE, PURINE ANTAGONIST

Therapeutic: ANTINEOPLASTIC; ANTIMETABOLITE

Prototype: 6-Mercaptopurine

Pregnancy Category: D

AVAILABILITY 1 mg/mL injection

ACTION & *THERAPEUTIC EFFECT* Cladribine is a synthetic antineoplastic agent with selective toxicity toward certain normal and malignant lymphocytes and monocytes. It accumulates intracellularly, preventing repair of single-stranded DNA breaks and ultimately interfering with cellular metabolism and DNA synthesis. *Cladribine is cytotoxic to both actively dividing and quiescent lymphocytes and monocytes, inhibiting both DNA synthesis and repair.*

USES Treatment of hairy cell leukemia, chronic lymphocytic leukemia, non-Hodgkin's lymphomas.

UNLABELED USES Advanced cutaneous T-cell lymphomas, acute myeloid leukemia, autoimmune hemolytic anemia, mycosis fungoides.

CONTRAINDICATIONS Hypersensitivity to cladribine; severe bone marrow suppression; pregnancy (category D).

CAUTIOUS USE Hepatic or renal impairment; previous radiation therapy or chemotherapy. Safety and efficacy in children not established.

ROUTE & DOSAGE

Hairy Cell Leukemia

Adult: **IV** 0.09 mg/kg/day by 7 days continuous infusion

Chronic Lymphocytic Leukemia/ Non-Hodgkin's Lymphoma

Adult: **IV** 0.1 mg/kg/day by 7 days continuous infusion repeated monthly

ADMINISTRATION

- Use disposable gloves and protective clothing when handling the drug.
- Wash immediately if skin contact occurs.

Intravenous

PREPARE: **IV Infusion (single daily dose):** Add the required dose to 500 mL of NS. IV infusion (7-day dose): The calculated dose of cladribine is injected into an infusion reservoir using a 0.22 micron filter. An amount of bacteriostatic NS is added through a 0.22 micron filter to bring the total to 100 mL. (Note: Reservoir usually prepared by the pharmacist.)

ADMINISTER: **IV Infusion (single daily dose):** Distribute evenly over ordered time (i.e., 2 h or 24 h). **IV infusion (7-day dose):** Give through a central line and control by a pump device (e.g., Deltec pump) to deliver 100 mL evenly over 7 days.

INCOMPATIBILITIES **Solution/additive:** Do not mix with any other diluents or drugs.

- Diluted solutions of cladribine may be stored refrigerated for up to 8 h prior to administration. - Store unopened vials in refrigerator [2°–8° C (36°–46° F)], and protect from light.

ADVERSE EFFECTS (≥1%) **CNS:** Headache, dizziness. **GI:** Nausea, diarrhea. **Hematologic:** *Myelosuppression (neutropenia)*, *anemia*, thrombocytopenia. **Metabolic:** *Fever*. **CNS:** Headache, dizziness. **Urogenital:** Elevated serum creatinine.

INTERACTIONS Drug: Additive risk of bleeding with ANTICOAGULANTS, NSAIDS, PLATELET INHIBITORS, SALICYLATES.

PHARMACOKINETICS Onset: Therapeutic effect 10 days to 4 mo. **Duration:** 7–25+ mo. **Distribution:** Crosses placenta; distributed into breast milk. **Metabolism:** In malignant leukocytes, cladribine is phosphorylated to active forms, which are subsequently incorporated into cellular DNA. **Half-Life:** Initial 35 min, terminal 6.7 h.

NURSING IMPLICATIONS

Assessment & Drug Effects

- Monitor vital signs during and after drug infusion. Fever (above 100° F) is common during the 5th to 7th day in patients with hairy cell leukemia, and severe fever (above 104° F) may develop within the first month of therapy.
- Lab tests: Frequent hematologic studies; periodic serum creatinine and liver function tests.
- Closely monitor hematologic status; myelosuppression is common during the first month after starting therapy.
- Monitor for and report S&S of infection. Note that within the first month, fever may occur in the absence of infection.
- With high doses of cladribine, monitor for neurologic toxicity and acute nephrotoxicity.

Patient & Family Education

- Be fully informed regarding adverse responses to the drug.
- Understand the need for close follow-up during and after treatment with the drug.

CLARITHROMYCIN

(clar′i-thro-my-sin)

Biaxin, Biaxin XL

Classification: MACROLIDE ANTIBIOTIC

Therapeutic: ANTIBIOTIC

Prototype: Erythromycin

Pregnancy Category: C

AVAILABILITY 250 mg, 500 mg tablets; 500 mg, 1000 mg sustained release tablets; 125 mg/5 mL, 250 mg/5 mL suspension

ACTION & *THERAPEUTIC EFFECT* A semisynthetic macrolide antibiotic that binds to the 50S ribosomal subunit of susceptible bacterial organisms and, thereby, blocks RNA-mediated bacterial protein synthesis of the bacteria. *It is active against both aerobic and anaerobic gram-positive and gram-negative organisms.*

USES Treatment of upper respiratory, lower respiratory infections; acute maxillary sinusitis; otitis media; and skin and soft tissue infections. Prevention and treatment of *Mycobacterium avium* complex (MAC) infections in patients with HIV. Used in combination for *Helicobacter pylori*.

CONTRAINDICATIONS Hypersensitivity to clarithromycin, erythromycin, or any other macrolide antibiotics; patients receiving pimozide; suspected or potential bacteremias; acute porphyria; severe hepatic or biliary disease; congenital QT prolongation, torsades de pointes; viral infections. Safety and efficacy in infants younger than 20 mo not established.

CAUTIOUS USE Renal impairment, older adults, GI disease, colitis; pregnancy (category C), lactation.

ROUTE & DOSAGE

Mild to Moderate Infections

Adult: **PO** 250–500 mg b.i.d. × 7–14 days or 1000 mg XL daily for 7–14 days
Child: **PO** 7.5 mg/kg q12h

MAC Infections

Adult: **PO** 500 mg q12h
Child: **PO** 7.5 mg/kg q12h

***H. pylori* Infections (with other medications)**

Adult: **PO** 500 mg b.i.d. to t.i.d.

Renal Impairment Dosage Adjustment

CrCl less than 30 mL/min: Decrease dose by 1/2 or double the dosing interval

ADMINISTRATION

Oral

- Ensure that sustained release form of drug is not chewed or crushed. It **must be** swallowed whole.
- Shake suspension well before use.
- Store at 15°–30° C (59°–86° F).

ADVERSE EFFECTS (≥1%) **GI:** Diarrhea, abdominal discomfort, nausea, abnormal taste, dyspepsia. **Hematologic:** Eosinophilia. **CNS:** Headache. **Skin:** Rash, urticaria.

DIAGNOSTIC TEST INTERFERENCE May increase ***serum AST*** and ***ALT levels***.

INTERACTIONS Drug: May increase **theophylline** levels; drugs known to interact with **erythromycin** (i.e., **digoxin, carbamazepine, triazolam, warfarin, ergotamine, dihydroergotamine**) should be monitored carefully for increased levels and toxicity; **pimozide** may increase risk of arrhythmias. **Food: Grapefruit juice** increases risk of adverse effects.

PHARMACOKINETICS Absorption: Readily from GI tract; 50% reaches the systemic circulation. **Peak:** 2–4 h. **Distribution:** Into most body tissue (excluding CNS); high pulmonary tissue concentrations. **Metabolism:** Partially in the liver; active 14-OH metabolite acts synergistically with the parent compound against *H. influenzae*. **Elimination:** 20% unchanged in urine; 10–15% of 14-OH metabolite excreted in urine. **Half-Life:** 3–5 h.

C

NURSING IMPLICATIONS

Assessment & Drug Effects

- Inquire about previous hypersensitivity to other macrolides (e.g., erythromycin) before treatment.
- Withhold drug and notify physician, if hypersensitivity occurs (e.g., rash, urticaria).
- Monitor for and report loose stools or diarrhea, since pseudomembranous colitis **must be** ruled out.
- When clarithromycin is given concurrently with anticoagulants, digoxin, or theophylline, blood levels of these drugs may be elevated. Monitor appropriate serum levels and assess for S&S of drug toxicity.

Patient & Family Education

- Complete prescribed course of therapy.
- Report rash or other signs of hypersensitivity immediately.
- Report loose stools or diarrhea even after completion of drug therapy.

CLEMASTINE FUMARATE

(klem′as-teen)

Tavist-1

Classification: ANTIHISTAMINE (H_1-RECEPTOR ANTAGONIST)

Therapeutic: ANTIHISTAMINE

Prototype: Diphenhydramine

Pregnancy Category: B

AVAILABILITY 1.34 mg, 2.68 mg tablets; 0.67 mg/5 mL syrup

ACTION & *THERAPEUTIC EFFECT* An antihistamine (H_1-receptor antagonist) that competes for H_1-receptor sites on cells, thus blocking histamine effectiveness. Has greater selectivity for peripheral H_1-receptors and, consequently, it produces little sedation. Has prominent antipruritic activity and low incidence of unpleasant adverse effects. *Effective in controlling various allergic reactions (e.g., nasal congestion, sneezing, itching).*

USES Symptomatic relief of allergic rhinitis (sneezing, rhinorrhea, pruritus) and mild uncomplicated allergic skin manifestations such as urticaria and angioedema.

CONTRAINDICATIONS Hypersensitivity to clemastine or to other antihistamines of similar chemical structure; lower respiratory tract symptoms, including acute asthma; concomitant MAOI therapy; closed-angle glaucoma; children younger than 6 y; lactation.

CAUTIOUS USE History of bronchial asthma, COPD; increased intraocular pressure; GI or GU obstruction; hyperthyroidism; hepatic disease; cardiovascular disease, hypertension, older adults; children, pregnancy (category B).

ROUTE & DOSAGE

Allergic Rhinitis

Adult: **PO** 1.34 mg b.i.d., may increase up to 8.04 mg/day
Child: **PO** *Older than 6 y,* 0.67 mg b.i.d., may increase up to 4.02 mg/day; *younger than 6 y,* 0.335–0.67 mg/kg/day in 2 divided doses (max: 1.34 mg/day)

Allergic Urticaria

Adult: **PO** 2.68 mg b.i.d. or t.i.d., may increase up to 8.04 mg/day
Child: **PO** 1.34 mg b.i.d., may increase up to 4.02 mg/day

ADMINISTRATION

Oral

- Drug may be administered with food, water, or milk to reduce possibility of gastric irritation.

- Older adult patients usually require less than average adult dose.
- Store at 15°–30° C (59°–86° F) unless otherwise directed.

ADVERSE EFFECTS (≥1%) **Body as a Whole:** Anaphylaxis, excess perspiration, chills. **CV:** Hypotension, palpitation, tachycardia, extrasystoles. **GI:** *Dry mouth,* epigastric distress, anorexia, nausea, vomiting, diarrhea, constipation. **Hematologic:** Hemolytic anemia, thrombocytopenia, agranulocytosis. **CNS:** Sedation, *transient drowsiness,* dry nose and throat, headache, dizziness, weakness, fatigue, disturbed coordination; confusion, restlessness, nervousness, hysteria, convulsions, tremors, irritability, euphoria, insomnia, paresthesias, neuritis. **Respiratory:** Dry nose and throat, thickening of bronchial secretions, tightness of chest, wheezing, nasal stuffiness. **Skin:** Urticaria, rash, photosensitivity. **Special Senses:** Vertigo, tinnitus, acute labyrinthitis, blurred vision, diplopia. **Urogenital:** Difficult urination, urinary retention, early menses.

INTERACTIONS Drug: Alcohol and other CNS DEPRESSANTS increase sedation; MAO INHIBITORS may prolong and intensify anticholinergic effects.

PHARMACOKINETICS Absorption: Readily from GI tract. **Peak:** 5–7 h. **Duration:** 10–12 h. **Distribution:** Into breast milk. **Metabolism:** In liver. **Elimination:** In urine.

NURSING IMPLICATIONS

Assessment & Drug Effects

- Monitor for drowsiness, poor coordination, or dizziness, especially in the older adult or debilitated. Supervision of ambulation may be warranted.
- Assess for symptomatic relief with use of the medication.
- Lab tests: Periodic hematologic studies with long-term use.

Patient & Family Education

- Check with physician before taking alcohol or other CNS depressants, since effects may be additive.
- Clemastine may cause lethargy and drowsiness; therefore, necessary safety precautions should be taken.
- Older adults should make position changes slowly and in stages, particularly from recumbent to upright posture, as dizziness and hypotension occur more frequently than in younger patients.
- Avoid driving and other potentially hazardous activities until response to the drug has been established.

CLEVIDIPINE BUTYRATE

(cle-vi-di′peen bu-ti′rate)

Cleviprex

Classifications: CALCIUM CHANNEL BLOCKER; ANTIHYPERTENSIVE

Therapeutic: ANTIHYPERTENSIVE

Prototype: Nifedipine

Pregnancy Category: C

AVAILABILITY 0.5 mg/mL emulsion for injection

ACTION & *THERAPEUTIC EFFECT* An L-type calcium channel blocker that interferes with the influx of calcium during depolarization of arterial smooth muscle. Decreases systemic vascular resistance, thus lowering mean arterial pressure. *Decreases blood pressure.*

USES Treatment of hypertension when oral administration is neither feasible nor desired.

CONTRAINDICATIONS Hypersensitivity to soybeans, soy products, eggs/egg products; defective lipid metabolism (e.g., pathologic hyperlipidemia, lipid nephrosis, acute pancreatitis); severe aortic stenosis.

CAUTIOUS USE Reflex tachycardia, hypotension, heart failure; lipid intake restriction; rebound hypertension following drug discontinuation; elderly; pregnancy (category C); lactation. Safety and efficacy in children not established.

ROUTE & DOSAGE

Hypertension
Adult: **IV** Initial dose of 1–2 mg/h. Titrate dose to desired BP: May initially double dose every 90 sec; as BP approaches goal, decrease dose increments to less than double the previous dose and lengthen time intervals between doses to q5–10min.

ADMINISTRATION

Intravenous

PREPARE: **IV Infusion:** Supplied premixed, ready to use. Invert vial gently to produce a uniform emulsion.

ADMINISTER: **IV Infusion:** Use infusion device that permits calibrated rates. ▪ May infuse through a central or peripheral line using NS, D5W, D5W/NS, D5W/LR, LR, or 10% amino acid solution. ▪ Complete infusion within 4 h of entering vial.

INCOMPATIBILITIES **Solution/additive:** Do not dilute in any IV solution. **Y-site:** Unknown; do not mix.

▪ Store refrigerated at 2°–8° C (36°–46° F). Do not return unopened vials to refrigeration once they have reached room temperature.

ADVERSE EFFECTS (≥1%) **CNS:** Headache. **CV:** Hypotension, reflex tachycardia. **GI:** Nausea, vomiting.

PHARMACOKINETICS Distribution: 99.5% plasma protein bound. **Metabolism:** In the plasma. **Elimination:** Renal (63–74%) and fecal (7–22%). **Half-Life:** 15 min.

NURSING IMPLICATIONS

Assessment & Drug Effects

- Monitor HR and BP continuously during infusion. Increases in HR is a normal response to vasodilation and rebound hypertension may occur for at least 8 h after infusion is stopped.
- Monitor cardiac status continuously during infusion, especially with preexisting HF. Clevidipine may have a negative inotropic effect and exacerbate HF.

Patient & Family Education

- Report promptly any of the following: Signs of heart failure; visual changes, weakness, or other signs of neurologic impairment.

CLINDAMYCIN HYDROCHLORIDE (Pr)

(klin-da-mye'sin)

Cleocin, Dalacin C ♣

CLINDAMYCIN PALMITATE HYDROCHLORIDE

Cleocin Pediatric

CLINDAMYCIN PHOSPHATE

Cleocin Phosphate, Cleocin T, Dalacin C, Evoclin, Cleocin Vaginal Ovules or Cream

Classification: LINCOSAMIDE ANTIBIOTIC
Therapeutic: ANTIBIOTIC
Pregnancy Category: B

AVAILABILITY 75 mg, 150 mg, 300 mg capsules; 75 mg/5 mL oral suspension; 150 mg/mL injection; 2% vaginal cream; 100 mg suppositories; 10 mg gel, lotion; 1% foam

ACTION & *THERAPEUTIC EFFECT* Semisynthetic derivative of lincomycin that suppresses protein synthesis by binding to 50 S subunits of bacterial ribosomes, and, therefore, inhibits other antibiotics (e.g., erythromycin) that act at this site. *Particularly effective against susceptible strains of anaerobic streptococci as well as aerobic gram-positive cocci.*

USES Serious infections when less toxic alternatives are inappropriate. Topical applications are used in treatment of acne vulgaris. Vaginal applications are used in treatment of bacterial vaginosis in nonpregnant women.

UNLABELED USES In combination with pyrimethamine for toxoplasmosis in patients with AIDS.

CONTRAINDICATIONS History of hypersensitivity to clindamycin or lincomycin; history of regional enteritis, ulcerative colitis, or antibiotic-associated colitis; viral infection.

CAUTIOUS USE History of GI disease, renal or hepatic disease; atopic individuals (history of eczema, asthma, hay fever); older patients over 60 y; pregnancy (category B); lactation.

ROUTE & DOSAGE

Moderate to Severe Infections

Adult: **PO** 150–450 mg q6h **IM/IV** 600–1200 mg/day in divided doses (max: 2700 mg/day)
Child: **PO** 10–30 mg/kg/day q6–8h **IM/IV** 20–40 mg/kg/day in divided doses
Neonate: **IM/IV** *7 days or younger, weight 2000 g or less,* 10 mg/kg/day q12h; *7 days or younger, weight greater than 2000 g,* 15 mg/kg/day q8h; *older than 7 days, weight less than 1200 g,* 10 mg/kg/day q12h; *older than 7 days, weight 1200 g–2000 g,* 15 mg/kg/day q8h; *older than 7 days, weight greater than 2000 g,* 20 mg/kg/day q6–8h

Acne Vulgaris

Adult: **Topical** Apply to affected areas b.i.d.; 1% foam daily application

Bacterial Vaginosis

Adult: **Topical** Insert 1 suppository intravaginally at bedtime × 3 days, or insert 1 applicator full of cream intravaginally at bedtime × 7 days

ADMINISTRATION

Oral

- Administer clindamycin capsules with a full [240 mL (8 oz)] glass of water to prevent esophagitis.
- Note expiration date of oral solution; retains potency for 14 days at room temperature. Do not refrigerate, as chilling causes thickening and thus makes pouring it difficult.

Intramuscular

- Deep IM injection is recommended. Rotate injection sites and observe daily for evidence of inflammatory reaction. Single IM doses should not exceed 600 mg.

Intravenous

IV administration to neonates, infants, and children: Verify correct IV concentration and rate of infusion with physician.

PREPARE: **Intermittent:** Each 18 mg **must be** diluted with at least 1 mL of D5W, NS, D5/.45% NaCl, or other compatible solution. ▪ Final concentration should never exceed 18 mg/mL.

ADMINISTER: **Intermittent:** Never give a bolus dose. ▪ Do not give more than 1200 mg in a single 1-h infusion. ▪ Infusion rate should not exceed 30 mg/min.

INCOMPATIBILITIES **Solution/additive: Aminophylline,** BARBITURATES, **calcium gluconate, ceftriaxone, ciprofloxacin, gentamicin, magnesium sulfate, ranitidine. Y-site: Allopurinol, azithromycin, doxapram, filgrastim, fluconazole, idarubicin, lansoprazole.**

▪ Store in tight containers at 15°–30° C (59°–86° F) unless otherwise directed.

ADVERSE EFFECTS (≥1%) **Body as a Whole:** Fever, serum sickness, sensitization, swelling of face (following topical use), generalized myalgia, superinfections, proctitis, vaginitis, pain, induration, sterile abscess (following IM injections); thrombophlebitis (IV infusion). **CV:** Hypotension (following IM), cardiac arrest (rapid IV). **GI:** *Diarrhea,* abdominal pain, flatulence, bloating, *nausea, vomiting,* pseudomembranous colitis; esophageal irritation, loss of taste, medicinal taste (high IV doses), jaundice, abnormal liver function tests. **Hematologic:** Leukopenia, eosinophilia, agranulocytosis, thrombocytopenia. **Skin:** *Skin rashes,* urticaria, pruritus, dryness, contact dermatitis, gram-negative folliculitis, irritation, oily skin.

DIAGNOSTIC TEST INTERFERENCE Clindamycin may cause increases in ***serum alkaline phosphatase, bilirubin, creatine phosphokinase (CPK)*** from muscle irritation following IM injection; ***AST, ALT.***

INTERACTIONS Drug: Chloramphenicol, erythromycin possibly are mutually antagonistic to clindamycin; neuromuscular blocking action enhanced by NEUROMUSCULAR BLOCKING AGENTS **(atracurium, tubocurarine, pancuronium).**

PHARMACOKINETICS Absorption: Approximately 90% absorbed from GI tract; 10% of topical application is absorbed through skin. **Peak:** 45–60 min PO; 3 h IM. **Duration:** 6 h PO; 8–12 h IM. **Distribution:** Widely distributed except for CNS; crosses placenta; distributed into breast milk. **Metabolism:** In liver. **Elimination:** In urine and feces. **Half-Life:** 2–3 h.

NURSING IMPLICATIONS

Assessment & Drug Effects

- Lab tests: Culture and susceptibility testing should be performed initially. Periodic CBC with differential, liver, and kidney function tests.
- Monitor BP and pulse in patients receiving drug parenterally. Hypotension has occurred following IM injection. Advise patient to remain recumbent following drug administration until BP has stabilized.
- Severe diarrhea and colitis, including pseudomembranous colitis, have been associated with oral (highest incidence), parenteral, and topical clindamycin. Report immediately the onset of watery diarrhea, with or without fever. Symptoms may appear within a few days to 2 wk after therapy is begun or up to several weeks following cessation of therapy.
- Be alert to signs of superinfection (see Appendix F).

- Be alert for signs of anaphylactoid reactions (see Appendix F), that require immediate attention.

Patient & Family Education

- Report loose stools or diarrhea promptly.
- Stop drug therapy if significant diarrhea develops (more than 5 loose stools daily) and notify physician.
- Do not self-medicate with antidiarrheal preparations. Antiperistaltic agents may prolong and worsen diarrhea by delaying removal of toxins from colon.

CLOBETASOL PROPIONATE

(cloe-bay′ta-sol)

Clobex, Temovate, Embeline gel; Olux Foam

Pregnancy Category: C

See Appendix A-4.

CLOCORTOLONE PIVALATE

(kloe-kor′toe-lone)

Cloderm

Pregnancy Category: C

See Appendix A-4.

CLOFARABINE

(clo-fa-ra′been)

Clolar

Classifications: ANTINEOPLASTIC; PURINE ANTIMETABOLITE

Therapeutic: ANTINEOPLASTIC; ANTIMETABOLITE

Prototype: 6-Mercaptopurine

Pregnancy Category: D

AVAILABILITY 1 mg/mL injection

ACTION & *THERAPEUTIC EFFECT* Clofarabine inhibits DNA repair within cancer cells, thus interfering with mitosis; it also disrupts the mitochondrial membrane, leading to cancer cell death. *Cytotoxic to rapidly proliferating and quiescent cancer cells.*

USES Treatment of persons 1–21 y of age with relapsed or refractory acute lymphocytic leukemia (ALL) after at least 2 prior regimens.

CONTRAINDICATIONS Severe bone marrow suppression; active infection; pregnancy (category D); lactation.

CAUTIOUS USE Renal or hepatic function impairment; thrombocytopenia; neutropenia; previous chemotherapy or radiation therapy; females of childbearing age; history of viral infections such as herpes; history of cardiac disease or hypotension.

ROUTE & DOSAGE

Acute Lymphocytic Leukemia

Adult/Adolescent/Child: **IV** 52 mg/m^2/day for 5 days

ADMINISTRATION

- Do not give drugs with known renal toxicity during the 5 days of clofarabine administration.

Intravenous

PREPARE: **IV Infusion:** Withdraw required dose from vial using a 0.2 micron filter syringe. ▪ Further dilute in 100 mL or more of D5W or NS prior to infusion.

ADMINISTER: **IV Infusion:** Give over 2 h. ▪ Note: It is recommended that IV fluids be given continuously throughout the 5 days of clofarabine administration.

- Store diluted solution at room temperature. Use within 24 h of mixing.

C

ADVERSE EFFECTS (≥1%) **CNS:** Anxiety, depression, dizziness, headache, irritability, somnolence. **CV:** *Tachycardia,* pericardial infusion, left ventricular systolic dysfunction (LSVT). **GI:** *Vomiting, nausea,* and *diarrhea,* abdominal pain, constipation. **Hematologic/Lymphatic:** *Anemia, leukopenia, thrombocytopenia, neutropenia, febrile neutropenia.* **Hepatic:** Jaundice, hepatomegaly. **Metabolic:** Anorexia, decreased appetite, edema, decreased weight. **Musculoskeletal:** Arthralgia, back pain, myalgia. **Respiratory:** Cough, dyspnea, epistaxis, pleural effusion, respiratory distress. **Skin:** Dermatitis, contusion, dry skin, erythema, palmar-plantar erythrodysesthesia syndrome, pruritus. **Body as a Whole:** Increased risk of infection.

PHARMACOKINETICS Distribution: 47% protein bound. **Metabolism:** Negligible. **Elimination:** Primarily unchanged in the urine. **Half-Life:** 5.2 h.

NURSING IMPLICATIONS

Assessment & Drug Effects

- Monitor vital signs frequently during infusion of clofarabine.
- Monitor closely for S&S of capillary leak syndrome or systemic inflammatory response syndrome (e.g., tachypnea, tachycardia, hypotension, pulmonary edema). If either is suspected, immediately DC IV, institute supportive measures and notify physician.
- Monitor I&O rates and pattern and watch for S&S of dehydration, including dizziness, lightheadedness, fainting spells, or decreased urine output.
- Withhold drug and notify physician if hypotension develops for any reason during 5-day period of drug administration.
- Lab tests: Baseline and periodic CBC and platelet counts (more frequent with cytopenias); frequent LFTs and kidney function test during the 5 days of clofarabine therapy.

Patient & Family Education

- Report any distressing adverse effect of therapy to physician.
- Use effective measures to avoid pregnancy while taking this drug.

CLOFIBRATE

(kloe-fy'brate)

Atromid-S, Claripex ♣, Novofibrate ♣

Classifications: ANTILIPEMIC; FIBRATE

Therapeutic: CHOLESTEROL-LOWERING; ANTIHYPERLIPIDEMIC

Prototype: Fenofibrate

Pregnancy Category: C

AVAILABILITY 500 mg capsules

ACTION & *THERAPEUTIC EFFECT* Mechanism of action appears to inhibit cholesterol biosynthesis prior to transfer of triglycerides from liver to serum. Interferes with binding of free fatty acids to albumin and increases fecal excretion of neutral sterols. It affects the mobilization of cholesterol from tissue. *Clofibrate reduces very low density lipoproteins (VLDL) to a greater extent than it reduces low density lipoproteins (LDL). It also lowers serum triglycerides more dramatically than cholesterol.*

USES Adjunct for treatment of severe primary (type III) hyperlipidemia.

UNLABELED USES Management of diabetes insipidus.

CONTRAINDICATIONS Severely impaired renal function or significant hepatic dysfunction, primary biliary cirrhosis; hypothyroidism; peptic ulcer disease; lactation. Safe use in children younger than 14 y not established.

CAUTIOUS USE History of jaundice or mild to moderate hepatic disease; gallstones; peptic ulcer; hypothyroidism; cardiovascular disease; pregnancy (category C).

ROUTE & DOSAGE

Hyperlipidemia

Adult: **PO** 2 g/day in 2–4 divided doses

Diabetes Insipidus

Adult: **PO** 1.5–2 g/day in 2–4 divided doses

ADMINISTRATION

Oral

- If gastric distress is a problem, administer drug with meals.
- Preserve in closed, light-resistant containers at 15°–30° C (59°–86° F) unless otherwise directed.

ADVERSE EFFECTS (≥1%) **CV:** Increase or decrease in angina, CHF, arrhythmias. **GI:** *Nausea,* vomiting, loose stools, diarrhea, flatulence, abdominal distress, gastritis, stomatitis, cholelithiasis. **Hematologic:** Neutropenia, leukopenia, anemia, eosinophilia, agranulocytosis, potentiation of anticoagulant effect. **Metabolic:** Elevated AST and ALT. **Musculoskeletal:** Flu-like symptoms. **CNS:** Drowsiness, dizziness, headache. **Skin:** Swelling and phlebitis at xanthoma sites, skin rash, allergy, urticaria, pruritus. **Urogenital:** Renal insufficiency, impotence, decreased libido.

DIAGNOSTIC TEST INTERFERENCE Clofibrate therapy may lead to increased ***BSP*** retention, ***thymol*** turbidity; increased ***serum creatine phosphokinase (CPK); proteinuria,*** parodoxical increase in ***LDL*** or ***cholesterol*** levels (if there is a large decrease in VLDL level). Lower fasting ***blood glucose*** and ***serum insulin*** levels in patients with diabetes mellitus.

INTERACTIONS Drug: ORAL ANTICOAGULANTS increase hypoprothrombinemia and increase risk of bleeding; **probenecid** increases effects of clofibrate; SULFONYLUREAS increase hypoglycemic effects.

PHARMACOKINETICS Absorption: Readily absorbed from GI tract. **Peak:** 4–6 h. **Distribution:** Distributed to extracellular space; crosses placenta; distribution into breast milk unknown. **Metabolism:** Hydrolyzed in plasma to clofibric acid, which is further metabolized in liver. **Elimination:** In urine. **Half-Life:** 12–35 h.

NURSING IMPLICATIONS

Assessment & Drug Effects

- Lab tests: Baseline and periodic lipid profile; periodic liver function tests, CBC, renal function tests, and determinations of plasma and urine steroid levels, serum electrolyte levels, and blood glucose.

Patient & Family Education

- Report flu-like symptoms (malaise, muscle soreness, aching, weakness) promptly to physician. Other reportable conditions include leukopenia, pulmonary edema, and renal insufficiency (see Appendix F) and gastric pain, nausea, and vomiting.

CLOMIPHENE CITRATE

(kloe′mi-feen)

Clomid, Milophene, Serophene

Classifications: OVULATION STIMULANT; NONSTEROID SELECTIVE ESTROGEN RECEPTOR MODULATOR (SERM)
Therapeutic: OVULATION STIMULANT; ANTIESTROGENIC
Pregnancy Category: X

AVAILABILITY 50 mg tablets

ACTION & *THERAPEUTIC EFFECT* Oral nonsteroidal selective estrogen receptor modulator (SERM). Induces ovulation in selected infrequently ovulating or anovulatory women. Clomiphene blocks the normal negative feedback of circulating estradiol on the hypothalamus, preventing estrogen from lowering the output of gonadotropin releasing hormone (GnRH). It acts by binding to hypothalamic estrogen receptors, decreasing their numbers, and thereby inhibiting receptor replenishment. *Inhibition of receptor replenishment results in a false hypoestrogenic state which stimulates pituitary release of luteinizing hormone (LH), follicle-stimulating hormone (FSH), and gonadotropins, leading to ovarian stimulation.*

USES Infertility in appropriately selected women desiring pregnancy whose partners are fertile and potent.

UNLABELED USES Male infertility, menstrual abnormalities, gynecomastia, fibrocystic breast disease, regulation of cycles in patients using rhythm method of contraception, endometrial hyperplasia, persistent lactation.

CONTRAINDICATIONS Neoplastic lesions, ovarian cyst; hepatic disease or dysfunction; abnormal uterine bleeding; endometriosis; primary ovarian failure; men with testicular failure; untreated thyroid disease; visual abnormalities; major depression or psychosis; thrombophlebitis; pregnancy (category X); lactation.

CAUTIOUS USE Polycystic ovarian enlargement, pelvic discomfort, sensitivity to pituitary gonadotropins.

ROUTE & DOSAGE

Infertility

Adult: **PO First course:** 50 mg/day for 5 days; start on 5th day of cycle following start of spontaneous or induced bleeding (with progestin) or at any time in the patient who has had no recent uterine bleeding **Second course if ovulation:** Repeat first course until conception or for 3 cycles **Second course if no ovulation:** 100 mg/day for 5 days as above (max: 100 mg/day)

ADMINISTRATION

Oral

- Each course of therapy should start on or about the 5th cycle day once ovulation has been established.
- Store at 15°–30° C (59°–86° F) in tightly capped, light-resistant container.

ADVERSE EFFECTS (≥1%) **Body as a Whole:** *Vasomotor flushes,* breast discomfort, abdominal pain, heavy menses, exacerbation of endometriosis; mental depression, headache, fatigue, insomnia, dizziness, vertigo. **GI:** Nausea, vomiting, increased appetite with weight gain, constipation, bloating. **Endocrine:** Spontaneous abortion, multiple ovulations, ovarian failure, *ovarian hyperstimulation syndrome, enlarged ovaries with multiple follicular cysts.* **Special Senses:** Transient blurring, diplopia, scotomas, photophobia, floaters, prolonged after-images. **Urogenital:** Urinary frequency, polyuria.

DIAGNOSTIC TEST INTERFERENCE Clomiphene may increase BSP retention; ***plasma transcortin, thyroxine*** and ***sex hormone binding globulin*** levels. Also increases ***follicle-stimulating*** and ***luteinizing hormone*** secretion in most patients.

INTERACTIONS Drug: No clinically significant drug interactions established. **Herbal: Black cohosh** may antagonize infertility treatments.

PHARMACOKINETICS Absorption: Readily absorbed from GI tract. **Metabolism:** In liver. **Elimination:** Primarily in feces in 5 days; the remainder is excreted slowly from enterohepatic pool or is stored in body fat for later release. **Half-Life:** 5 days.

NURSING IMPLICATIONS

Assessment & Drug Effects

- Monitor for abnormal bleeding. Report it immediately.
- Monitor for visual disturbances. Their occurrence indicates the need for a complete ophthalmologic evaluation. Drug will be stopped until symptoms subside.
- Pelvic pain indicates the need for immediate pelvic examination for diagnostic purposes.

Patient & Family Education

- Take the medicine at same time every day to maintain drug levels and prevent forgetting a dose.
- Missed dose: Take drug as soon as possible. If not remembered until time for next dose, double the dose, then resume regular dosing schedule. If more than one dose is missed, check with physician.
- Report these symptoms: Hot flushes resembling those associated with menopause; nausea, vomiting, headache.
- Report promptly yellowing of eyes, light-colored stools, yellow, itchy skin, and fever symptomatic of jaundice.
- Stop taking clomiphene if pregnancy is suspected.
- Because of the possibility of lightheadedness, dizziness, and visual disturbances, do not perform hazardous tasks requiring skill and coordination in an environment with variable lighting.
- Report promptly excessive weight gain, signs of edema, bloating, decreased urinary output.
- If clomiphene is continued more than 1 y, patient should have an ophthalmologic examination at regular intervals.

CLOMIPRAMINE HYDROCHLORIDE

(clo-mi′pra-meen)

Anafranil

Classification: TRICYCLIC ANTIDEPRESSANT

Therapeutic: ANTIPSYCHOTIC; TRICYCLIC ANTIDEPRESSANT

Prototype: Imipramine

Pregnancy Category: C

AVAILABILITY 25 mg, 50 mg, 75 mg capsules

ACTION & *THERAPEUTIC EFFECT* Inhibits the reuptake of norepinephrine and serotonin at the presynaptic neuron. Of the tricyclic antidepressants (TCAs), it is the most selective and potent inhibitor of serotonin (5-HT) reuptake. *The basis of its antidepressant effects is thought to be due to the elevated serum levels of norepinephrine and serotonin.*

USES Obsessive-compulsive disorder (OCD).

UNLABELED USES Panic disorder, autism, agoraphobia.

C

CONTRAINDICATIONS Hypersensitivity to other tricyclic compounds; acute recovery period after MI, QT elongation, cardiac arrhythmias (AV block, bundle-branch block); suicidal ideation; children younger than 10 y.

CAUTIOUS USE History of convulsive disorders, prostatic hypertrophy, urinary retention, cardiovascular, hepatic, GI, or blood disorders; history of seizure disorder; respiratory depression; older adults; diabetes mellitus; GERD; Parkinson's disease; closed-angle glaucoma; asthma; bipolar disorder; history of suicidal ideation; pregnancy (category C), lactation.

ROUTE & DOSAGE

Obsessive-Compulsive Disorder

Adult: **PO** 25 mg daily, gradually increase to 100 mg daily as tolerated over 2 wk, then up to 250 mg daily

Adolescent/Child (older than 10 y): **PO** 25 mg daily, gradually increase to 100 mg daily or 3 mg/kg (whichever is less) as tolerated over 2 wk, then up to 200 mg or 3 mg/kg daily (whichever is less)

Depression

Adult: **PO** 50–150 mg/day in single or divided doses

Pharmacogenetic Dosage Adjustment

Poor CYP2D6 metabolizers should receive 60% of normal dose

ADMINISTRATION

Oral

- Give with meals to reduce GI adverse effects.
- Following titration to the full dose, drug may be given as a single dose at bedtime to reduce daytime sedation.
- Store at 15°–30° C (59°–86° F).

ADVERSE EFFECTS (≥1%) **Body as a Whole:** Diaphoresis. **CV:** Hypotension, tachycardia. **GI:** Constipation, *dry mouth*. **Endocrine:** Galactorrhea, hyperprolactinemia, amenorrhea, *weight gain*. **Hematologic:** Leukopenia, <u>agranulocytosis</u>, thrombocytopenia, anemia. **CNS:** Mania, *tremor*, dizziness, hyperthermia, <u>neuroleptic malignant syndrome</u>, seizures (especially with abrupt withdrawal). **Urogenital:** Delayed ejaculation, anorgasmia.

DIAGNOSTIC TEST INTERFERENCE Clomipramine appears to elevate serum ***prolactin*** levels. ***Serum AST*** and ***ALT*** are elevated. Serum levels of ***triiodothyronine (T_3)*** and ***free triiodothyronine (FT_3)*** have been significantly reduced from baseline. ***Thyroxine-binding globulin (TBG)*** levels were increased from baseline, whereas ***thyroxine (T_4)***, ***free thyroxine (FT_4)***, and reverse ***T_3*** were unchanged.

INTERACTIONS Drug: MAO INHIBITORS may precipitate hyperpyrexic crisis, tachycardia, or seizures; ANTIHYPERTENSIVE AGENTS potentiate orthostatic hypotension; CNS DEPRESSANTS, **alcohol** add to CNS depression; **norepinephrine** and other SYMPATHOMIMETICS may increase cardiac toxicity; **cimetidine** decreases hepatic metabolism, thus increasing imipramine levels; **methylphenidate** inhibits metabolism of **imipramine** and thus may increase its toxicity. **Herbal: Ginkgo** may decrease seizure threshold; **St. John's wort** may cause serotonin syndrome.

PHARMACOKINETICS Absorption: Rapidly from GI tract; 20–78%

Common adverse effects in *italic*, life-threatening effects <u>underlined</u>; generic names in **bold**; classifications in SMALL CAPS; ♣ Canadian drug name; ● Prototype drug

reaches systemic circulation. **Onset:** Approx 4–10 wk. **Peak:** 2–6 h. **Distribution:** Widely distributed including the CSF; crosses placenta. **Metabolism:** Extensive first-pass metabolism in the liver; active metabolite is desmethylclomipramine. **Elimination:** 50–60% in urine, 24–32% in feces. **Half-Life:** 20–30 h.

NURSING IMPLICATIONS

Assessment & Drug Effects

- Monitor for seizures, especially in those with predisposing factors or concurrent therapy with other drugs that lower seizure threshold.
- Lab tests: Periodic CBC with differential, platelet count, and Hct and Hgb. Monitor liver functions, especially with long-term therapy.
- Monitor for and report signs of neuroleptic malignant syndrome (see Appendix F).
- Monitor for sedation and vertigo, especially at the beginning of therapy and following dosage increases. Supervision of ambulation may be indicated.
- Notify physician of fever and complaints of sore throat since these may indicate need to rule out adverse hematologic changes.

Patient & Family Education

- Do not take nonprescribed drugs or discontinue therapy without consent of physician. Abrupt discontinuation may cause nausea, headache, malaise, or seizures.
- Men should understand that the drug may cause impotence or ejaculation failure.
- Report promptly a sore throat accompanied by fever.
- Use caution with ambulation until response to drug is known.
- Moderate alcohol intake since it may potentiate adverse drug effects.

CLONAZEPAM

(kloe-na′zi-pam)

Klonopin, Klonopin Wafers, Rivotril ♣

Classifications: ANTICONVULSANT; BENZODIAZEPINE

Therapeutic: ANTICONVULSANT

Prototype: Diazepam

Pregnancy Category: D

Controlled Substance: Schedule IV

AVAILABILITY 0.5 mg, 1 mg, 2 mg tablets; 0.125 mg, 0.25 mg, 0.5 mg, 1 mg, and 2 mg orally disintegrating wafers

ACTION & *THERAPEUTIC EFFECT* Benzodiazepine derivative with strong anticonvulsant activity that prevents seizures by potentiation of the effects of GABA, an inhibitory neurotransmitter. Suppresses the spread of seizure activity in the cortex, thalamus, and limbic regions of the brain. *Suppresses spike and wave discharge in absence seizures (petit mal) and decreases amplitude, frequency, duration, and spread of discharge in minor motor seizures.*

USES Alone or with other drugs in absence, myoclonic, and akinetic seizures, Lennox-Gastaut syndrome, absence seizures refractory to succinimides or valproic acid, and for infantile spasms and restless legs.

UNLABELED USES Panic disorder, complex partial seizure pattern, and generalized tonic-clonic convulsions.

CONTRAINDICATIONS Hypersensitivity to benzodiazepines; liver disease; acute narrow-angle glaucoma; pulumonary disease, COPD; coma or CNS depression; pregnancy (category D), lactation; children younger than 10 y.

C

CAUTIOUS USE Renal or hepatic disease; COPD; drug-controlled open-angle glaucoma; bipolar disorder, preexisting depression; addiction-prone individuals; neuromuscular disease; mixed seizure disorders; children.

ROUTE & DOSAGE

Seizures

Adult: **PO** 1.5 mg/day in 3 divided doses, increased by 0.5–1 mg q3days until seizures are controlled or until intolerable adverse effects (max recommended dose: 20 mg/day)
Child (younger than 10 y): **PO** 0.01–0.03 mg/kg/day (not to exceed 0.05 mg/kg/day) in 3 divided doses; may increase by 0.25–0.5 mg q3days until seizures are controlled or until intolerable adverse effects (max recommended dose: 0.2 mg/kg/day)

Panic Disorders

Adult: **PO** 1–2 mg/day in divided doses (max: 4 mg/day)

ADMINISTRATION

Oral

- Give largest dose at bedtime if daily dose cannot be equally divided.
- Place wafer form on tongue to dissolve.
- Store in tightly closed container protected from light at 15°–30° C (59°–86° F) unless otherwise specified.

ADVERSE EFFECTS (≥1%) **CV:** Palpitations. **GI:** Dry mouth, sore gums, anorexia, coated tongue, increased salivation, increased appetite, nausea, constipation, diarrhea. **Hematologic:** Anemia, leukopenia, thrombocytopenia, eosinophilia. **CNS:** *Drowsiness, sedation, ataxia,* insomnia, aphonia, choreiform movements, coma, dysarthria, "glassy-eyed" appearance, headache, hemiparesis, hypotonia, slurred speech, tremor, vertigo, confusion, depression, hallucinations, aggressive behavior problems, hysteria, suicide attempt. **Respiratory:** Chest congestion, respiratory depression, rhinorrhea, dyspnea, hypersecretion in upper respiratory passages. **Skin:** Hirsutism, hair loss, skin rash, ankle and facial edema. **Special Senses:** Diplopia, nystagmus, abnormal eye movements. **Urogenital:** Increased libido, dysuria, enuresis, nocturia, urinary retention.

DIAGNOSTIC TEST INTERFERENCE Clonazepam causes transient elevations of ***serum transaminase*** and ***alkaline phosphatase.***

INTERACTIONS Drug: Alcohol and other CNS DEPRESSANTS increase sedation and CNS depression; may increase **phenytoin** levels. **Herbal: Kava, valerian** may potentiate sedation.

PHARMACOKINETICS Absorption: Readily absorbed from GI tract. **Onset:** 60 min. **Peak:** 1–2 h. **Duration:** Up to 12 h in adults; 6–8 h in children. **Distribution:** Crosses placenta; distributed into breast milk. **Metabolism:** In liver. **Elimination:** In urine primarily as metabolites. **Half-Life:** 18–40 h.

NURSING IMPLICATIONS

Assessment & Drug Effects

- Monitor for signs of suicidal ideation in depressive individuals.
- Lab tests: Periodic liver function tests, platelet counts, blood counts, and renal function tests.

- Both psychological and physical dependence may occur in the patient on long-term, high-dose therapy.
- Monitor for S&S of overdose, including somnolence, confusion, irritability, sweating, muscle and abdominal cramps, diminished reflexes, coma.

Patient & Family Education

- Report loss of seizure control promptly. Anticonvulsant activity is often lost after 3 mo of therapy; dosage adjustment may reestablish efficacy.
- Do not abruptly discontinue this drug. Abrupt withdrawal can precipitate seizures. Other withdrawal symptoms include convulsion, tremor, abdominal and muscle cramps, vomiting, sweating.
- Do not drive a car or engage in other activities requiring mental alertness and physical coordination until reaction to the drug is known. Drowsiness occurs in approximately 50% of patients.

CLONIDINE HYDROCHLORIDE

(kloe′ni-deen)

Catapres, Catapres-TTS, Dixaril ✦, Duraclon

Classifications: CENTRAL-ACTING ANTIHYPERTENSIVE; ANALGESIC

Therapeutic: ANTIHYPERTENSIVE, CENTRAL-ACTING; ANALGESIC

Prototype: Methyldopa

Pregnancy Category: C

AVAILABILITY 0.1 mg, 0.2 mg, 0.3 mg tablets; 0.1 mg/24 h, 0.2 mg/24 h, 0.3 mg/24 h transdermal patch; 100 mcg/mL, 500 mcg/mL injection

ACTION & *THERAPEUTIC EFFECT* Centrally acting receptor agonist that stimulates alpha$_2$-adrenergic receptors in CNS to inhibit sympathetic cardioaccelerator and vasomotor centers. Central actions reduce plasma concentrations of norepinephrine. It decreases systolic and diastolic BP and heart rate. *Decreases systolic and diastolic BP and heart rate. Reportedly minimizes or eliminates many of the common clinical S&S associated with withdrawal of heroin, methadone, or other opiates.*

USES Step 2 drug in stepped-care approach to treatment of hypertension, either alone or with diuretic or other antihypertensive agents. Epidural administration as adjunct therapy for severe pain.

UNLABELED USES Prophylaxis for migraine; treatment of dysmenorrhea, menopausal flushing, diarrhea, paroxysmal localized hyperhidroses; alcohol, smoking, opiate, and benzodiazepine withdrawal; in the clonidine suppression test for diagnosis of pheochromocytoma; Tourette's syndrome; attention deficit disorder with hyperactivity (ADDH) in children.

CONTRAINDICATIONS Anticoagulant therapy, coagulopathy; lactation; **Patch:** Polyarteritis nodosa, scleroderma, SLE on affected areas; **Epidural:** Severe cardiovascular disease, or those who are hemodynamically unstable; infection at injection site; obstetric, postpartum, perioperative pain management; use above the C_4 dermatome. May be a rare case when use outweighs possible serious risk.

CAUTIOUS USE Severe coronary insufficiency, recent MI, sinus node dysfunction, cerebrovascular disease; diabetes mellitus; older adult; chronic renal failure; hepatic function impairment; Raynaud's disease, thromboangiitis obliterans; history of depression; pregnancy (category C); children.

ROUTE & DOSAGE

Hypertension

Adult: **PO** 0.1 mg b.i.d. or t.i.d., may increase by 0.1–0.2 mg/day until desired response is achieved (max: 2.4 mg/day) **Transdermal** 0.1 mg patch once q7days, may increase by 0.1 mg q1–2wk
Geriatric: **PO** Start with 0.1 mg once daily
Child: **PO** 5–10 mcg/kg/day divided q8–12h, may increase to 5–25 mcg/kg/day divided q6h (max: 0.9 mg/day)

Severe Pain

Adult: **Epidural** Start infusion at 30 mcg/h and titrate to response. Use rates greater than 40 mcg/h with caution.
Child: **Epidural** Start infusion at 0.5 mcg/kg/h and titrate to response

ADDH

Child: **PO** 5 mcg/kg/day in 4 divided doses (average dose, 0.15–0.2 mg/day) **Transdermal** 0.2–0.3 mg/day q5–7days

ADMINISTRATION

- Give last PO dose immediately before patient retires to ensure overnight BP control and to minimize daytime drowsiness.
- Oral dosage is increased gradually over a period of weeks so as not to lower BP abruptly (especially important in the older adult).
- Apply transdermal patch to dry skin, free of hair and rash. Avoid irritated, abraded, or scarred skin. Recommended areas for applying transdermal patch are upper outer arm and anterior chest. Rotate application sites and keep a record.
- During change from PO clonidine to transdermal system, PO clonidine should be maintained for at least 24 h after patch is applied. Consult physician.
- Do not abruptly discontinue drug. It should be withdrawn over a period of 2–4 days. Abrupt withdrawal may result in a hypertensive crisis within 8–18 h.
- Store in tightly closed container at 15°–30° C (59°–86° F) unless otherwise directed.

ADVERSE EFFECTS (≥1%) **CV:** *Hypotension (epidural),* postural hypotension (mild), peripheral edema, ECG changes, tachycardia, bradycardia, flushing, rapid increase in BP with abrupt withdrawal. **GI:** *Dry mouth, constipation,* abdominal pain, pseudo-obstruction of large bowel, altered taste, nausea, vomiting, hepatitis, hyperbilirubinemia, weight gain (sodium retention). **CNS:** *Drowsiness, sedation,* dizziness, headache, fatigue, weakness, sluggishness, dyspnea, vivid dreams, nightmares, insomnia, behavior changes, agitation, hallucination, nervousness, restlessness, anxiety, mental depression. **Skin:** Rash, pruritus, thinning of hair, exacerbation of psoriasis; with transdermal patch: Hyperpigmentation, recurrent herpes simplex, skin irritation, contact dermatitis, mild erythema. **Special Senses:** Dry eyes. **Urogenital:** Impotence, loss of libido.

DIAGNOSTIC TEST INTERFERENCE

Avoid use of transdermal patch during MRI. Possibility of decreased urinary excretion of ***aldosterone, catecholamines,*** and ***VMA*** (however, sudden withdrawal of clonidine may cause increases in these values); transient increases in ***blood glucose;*** weakly positive ***direct antiglobulin (Coombs') tests.***

INTERACTIONS Drug: Alcohol and other CNS DEPRESSANTS add to CNS depression; TRICYCLIC ANTIDEPRESSANTS may reduce antihypertensive effects. OPIATE ANALGESICS increase hypotension with epidural clonidine. Increased risk of bradycardia or AV block when epidural clonidine is used with **digoxin,** CALCIUM CHANNEL BLOCKERS, or BETA BLOCKERS.

PHARMACOKINETICS Absorption: Readily absorbed from GI tract. **Onset:** 30–60 min PO; 1–3 days transdermal. **Peak:** 2–4 h PO; 2–3 days transdermal. **Duration:** 8 h PO; 7 days transdermal. **Distribution:** Widely distributed; crosses blood–brain barrier; not known if crosses placenta or distributed into breast milk. **Metabolism:** In liver. **Elimination:** 80% in urine, 20% in feces. **Half-Life:** 6–20 h.

NURSING IMPLICATIONS

Assessment & Drug Effects

- Monitor BR closely. Determine positional changes (supine, sitting, standing).
- With epidural administration, frequently monitor BP and HR. Hypotension is a common side effect that may require intervention.
- Monitor BP closely whenever a drug is added to or withdrawn from therapeutic regimen.
- Monitor I&O during period of dosage adjustment. Report change in I&O ratio or change in voiding pattern.
- Determine weight daily. Patients not receiving a concomitant diuretic agent may gain weight, particularly during first 3 or 4 days of therapy, because of marked sodium and water retention.
- Supervise closely patients with history of mental depression, as they may be subject to further depressive episodes.

Patient & Family Education

- Although postural hypotension occurs infrequently, make position changes slowly, and in stages, particularly from recumbent to upright position, and dangle and move legs a few minutes before standing. Lie down immediately if faintness or dizziness occurs.
- Avoid potentially hazardous activities until reaction to drug has been determined due to possible sedative effects.
- Do not omit doses or stop the drug without consulting the physician.
- Do not take OTC medications, alcohol, or other CNS depressants without prior discussion with physician.
- Examine site when transdermal patch is removed and report to physician if erythema, rash, irritation, or hyperpigmentation occurs.
- If transdermal patch loosens, tape it in place with adhesive. The patch should never be cut or trimmed.

CLOPIDOGREL BISULFATE (Pr)

(clo-pi′do-grel)

Plavix

Classification: ANTIPLATELET

Therapeutic: PLATELET AGGREGATION INHIBITOR; ANTITHROMBOTIC

Pregnancy Category: B

AVAILABILITY 75 mg, 300 mg tablets

ACTION & *THERAPEUTIC EFFECT* Inhibits platelet aggregation by se-

C

lectively preventing the binding of adenosine diphosphate to its platelet receptor. The drug's effect on the adenosine diphosphate receptor of a platelet is irreversible. *Clopidogrel prolongs bleeding time, thereby reducing atherosclerotic events in high-risk patients.*

USES Acute coronary syndrome (ST or non-ST elevations). Secondary prevention of MI, stroke, and vascular death in patients with recent MI, stroke, unstable angina or established peripheral arterial disease.

UNLABELED USES Reduction of restenosis after stent placement.

CONTRAINDICATIONS Hypersensitivity to clopidogrel; intracranial hemorrhage, peptic ulcer, or any other active pathologic bleeding. Discontinue clopidogrel 7 days before surgery and during lactation. Safety and efficacy not established in children.

CAUTIOUS USE Concurrent use with drugs that might induce gastrointestinal bleeding; GI bleeding, peptic ulcer disease; hepatic impairment (moderate to severe); severe renal impairment; patients at risk for increased bleeding; pregnancy (category B).

ROUTE & DOSAGE

Secondary Prevention

Adult: **PO** 75 mg daily

Acute Coronary Syndrome (Non-ST Elevation)

Adult: **PO** 300 mg loading dose then 75 mg daily (use with aspirin)

ADMINISTRATION

Oral

- Do not administer to persons with active pathologic bleeding.
- Discontinue drug 7 days prior to surgery.
- Store at 15°–30° C (59°–86° F) in tightly closed container and protect from light.

ADVERSE EFFECTS (≥1%) **Body as a Whole:** Flu-like syndrome, fatigue, pain, arthralgia, back pain. **CV:** Chest pain, edema, hypertension, thrombocytopenic purpura. **GI:** Abdominal pain, dyspepsia, diarrhea, nausea, hypercholesterolemia. **Hematologic:** Thrombotic thrombocytopenic purpura, epistaxis. **CNS:** Headache, dizziness, depression. **Respiratory:** URI, dyspnea, rhinitis, bronchitis, cough. **Skin:** Rash, pruritus.

INTERACTIONS Drug: NSAIDS may increase risk of bleeding events. **Herbal: Garlic, ginger, ginkgo, evening primrose oil** may increase risk of bleeding.

PHARMACOKINETICS Absorption: Rapidly from GI tract. **Onset:** 2 h; reaches steady state in 3–7 days. **Distribution:** 94–98% protein bound. **Metabolism:** Rapidly hydrolyzed in plasma to active metabolite. **Elimination:** 50% in urine and 50% in feces. **Half-Life:** 8 h.

NURSING IMPLICATIONS

Assessment & Drug Effects

- Carefully monitor for and immediately report S&S of GI bleeding, especially when coadministered with NSAIDS, aspirin, heparin, or warfarin.
- Lab tests: Periodic platelet count and lipid profile.
- Evaluate patients with unexplained fever or infection for myelotoxicity.

Patient & Family Education

- Report promptly any unusual bleeding (e.g., black, tarry stools).

- Avoid chronic aspirin or NSAID use unless approved by physician.

CLORAZEPATE DIPOTASSIUM

(klor-az′e-pate)

Novoclopate ✦, Tranxene, Tranxene-SD

Classifications: ANXIOLYTIC; SEDATIVE-HYPNOTIC; ANTICONVULSANT; BENZODIAZEPINE

Therapeutic: ANTIANXIETY; SEDATIVE-HYPNOTIC; ANTICONVULSANT

Prototype: Lorazepam

Pregnancy Category: D

Controlled Substance: Schedule IV

AVAILABILITY 3.75 mg, 7.5 mg, 15 mg capsules and tablets; 11.25 mg, 22.5 mg long acting tablets

ACTION & *THERAPEUTIC EFFECT* Anxiolytic benzodiazepine exerts its effects through enhancement of GABA-benzodiazepine receptor complex, an inhibitory neurotransmitter. Clorazepate has depressant effects on the CNS, thus controlling anxiety associated with stress and also resulting in sedative effects. *Effective in controlling anxiety and withdrawal symptoms of alcohol.*

USES Management of anxiety disorders, short-term relief of anxiety symptoms, as adjunct in management of partial seizures, and symptomatic relief of acute alcohol withdrawal.

CONTRAINDICATIONS Hypersensitivity to clorazepate and other benzodiazepines; acute narrow-angle glaucoma; depressive neuroses; pulmonary disease, COPD; psychotic reactions, drug abusers. Safe use during pregnancy (category D), lactation, and in children younger than 9 y not established.

CAUTIOUS USE Older adults; debilitated patients; hepatic disease; kidney disease; Parkinson's disease; neuromuscular disease; seizure disorders; bipolar disorder, mania, history of suicidal ideation.

ROUTE & DOSAGE

Anxiety

Adult: **PO** 15 mg/day at bedtime, may increase to 15–60 mg/day in divided doses (max: 60 mg/day)

Acute Alcohol Withdrawal

Adult: **PO** 30 mg followed by 30–60 mg in divided doses (max: 90 mg/day), taper by 15 mg/day over 4 days to 7.5–15 mg/day until patient is stable

Partial Seizures

Adult: **PO** 7.5 mg t.i.d.
Child (9–12 y): **PO** 3.75–7.5 mg b.i.d., may increase by no more than 3.75 mg/wk (max: 60 mg/day)

ADMINISTRATION

Oral

- Give with food to minimize gastric distress.
- Ensure that sustained-release form of drug is not chewed or crushed. It **must be** swallowed whole.
- Taper drug dose gradually over several days when drug is to be discontinued.
- Store in light-resistant container at 15°–30° C (59°–86° F) unless otherwise specified.

ADVERSE EFFECTS (≥1%) **Body as a Whole:** Allergic reactions. **CV:** Hypotension. **GI:** GI disturbances, abnormal liver function tests, xerostomia. **Hematologic:** Decreased Hct, blood dyscrasias. **CNS:** *Drowsiness,* ataxia, dizziness, headache, paradoxical excitement, mental confusion, insomnia. **Special Senses:** Diplopia, blurred vision.

INTERACTIONS Drug: Alcohol and other CNS DEPRESSANTS compound CNS depression; clorazepate increases effects of **cimetidine, disulfiram,** causing excessive sedation. **Herbal: Ginkgo** may decrease anticonvulsant effectiveness.

PHARMACOKINETICS Absorption: Decarboxylated in stomach; absorbed as active metabolite, desmethyldiazepam. **Peak:** 1 h. **Duration:** 24 h. **Distribution:** Crosses placenta; distributed into breast milk. **Metabolism:** In liver to oxazepam. **Elimination:** Primarily in urine. **Half-Life:** 30–200 h.

NURSING IMPLICATIONS

Assessment & Drug Effects

- Drowsiness, a common side effect, is more likely to occur at initiation of therapy and with dose increments on successive days.
- Lab tests: Periodic blood counts and tests of liver function should be performed throughout therapy.
- Monitor patient with history of cardiovascular disease in early therapy for drug-induced responses. If systolic BP drops more than 20 mm Hg or if there is a sudden increase in pulse rate, withhold drug and notify physician.

Patient & Family Education

- Take drug as prescribed and do not change dose or abruptly stop taking the drug without physician's approval.
- Do not self-dose with OTC drugs (cold remedies, sleep medications, antacids) without consulting physician.
- Avoid driving and other potentially hazardous activities until reaction to drug is known.
- Do not use alcohol and other CNS depressants while on clorazepate therapy.
- If a woman becomes pregnant during therapy or intends to become pregnant, communicate with physician about the desirability of discontinuing the drug.

CLOTRIMAZOLE

(kloe-trim′a-zole)

Canesten ♣, Gyne-Lotrimin, Gyne-Lotrimin-3, Lotrimin, Mycelex, Mycelex-G

Classifications: ANTIBIOTIC; AZOLE ANTIFUNGAL

Therapeutic: AZOLE ANTIFUNGAL

Prototype: Fluconazole

Pregnancy Category: B (topical); C (oral)

AVAILABILITY 1% cream, solution, lotion; 10 mg troches; 100 mg, 200 mg, 500 mg vaginal tablets; 1% vaginal cream

ACTION & *THERAPEUTIC EFFECT* Acts by altering fungal cell membrane permeability, permitting loss of phosphorous compounds, potassium, and other essential intracellular constituents with consequent loss of ability to replicate. *Has broad-spectrum fungicidal activity. Active against a wide variety of fungi, yeast, dermatophytes and certain gram-positive bacteria.*

USES Dermal infections including tinea pedis, tinea cruris, tinea corporis, tinea versicolor; also vulvovaginal and oropharyngeal candidiasis.

UNLABELED USES Trichomoniasis.

CONTRAINDICATIONS Ophthalmic uses; systemic mycoses. Safe use in children younger than 3 y not established.

CAUTIOUS USE Hyersensitivity to other azole antifungals; hepatic impairment, diabetes mellitus; HIV; pregnancy (category C for oral troches; category B for topical use); lactation.

ROUTE & DOSAGE

Dermal Infections

Adult: **Topical** Apply small amount onto affected areas b.i.d. a.m. and p.m.

Vulvovaginal Infections

Adult: **Intravaginal** Insert 1 applicator full or one 100 mg vaginal tablet into vagina at bedtime for 7 days, or one 500 mg vaginal tablet at bedtime for 1 dose

Oropharyngeal Candidiasis

Adult/Child: **PO** 1 troche (lozenge) 5 times/day q3h for 14 days

ADMINISTRATION

- Instruct patient taking the oral lozenge to allow it to dissolve slowly in mouth over 15–30 min for maximum effectiveness.
- Apply skin cream and solution preparations sparingly. Protect hands with latex gloves when applying medication.
- Avoid contact of clotrimazole preparations with the eyes.
- Do not use occlusive dressings unless directed by physician to do so.
- Consult physician about skin cleansing procedure before applying medication. Regardless of procedure used, dry skin thoroughly.
- Store cream and solution formulations at 15°–30° C (59°–86° F); do not store troches or vaginal tablets above 35° C (95° F) unless otherwise directed.

ADVERSE EFFECTS (≥1%) **GI:** Abnormal liver function tests; occasional nausea and vomiting (with oral troche). **Skin:** Stinging, erythema, edema, vesication, desquamation, pruritus, urticaria, skin fissures. **Urogenital:** Mild burning sensation, lower abdominal cramps, bloating, cystitis, urethritis, mild urinary frequency, vulval erythema and itching, pain and vaginal soreness during intercourse.

INTERACTIONS Drug: Intravaginal preparations may inactivate SPERMICIDES.

PHARMACOKINETICS Absorption: Minimal systemic absorption; minimally absorbed topically. **Peak:** High saliva concentrations less than 3 h; high vaginal concentrations in 8–24 h. **Metabolism:** In liver. **Elimination:** Eliminated as metabolite in bile.

NURSING IMPLICATIONS

Assessment & Drug Effects

- Evaluate effectiveness of treatment. Report any signs of skin irritation with dermal preparations.
- Anticipate signs of clinical improvement within the first week of drug use.

Patient & Family Education

- Use clotrimazole as directed and for the length of time prescribed by physician.
- Generally, clinical improvement is apparent during first week of therapy. Report to physician if condition worsens or if signs of irritation or sensitivity develop, or if no improvement is noted after 4 wk of therapy.

C

- If receiving the drug vaginally, your sexual partner may experience burning and irritation of penis or urethritis; refrain from sexual intercourse during therapy or have sexual partner wear a condom.

CLOXACILLIN, SODIUM

(klox-a-sill'in)

Apo-Cloxi ♣, Cloxapen, Novo-cloxin ♣

Classifications: ANTIBIOTIC, PENICILLIN; BETA-LACTAM

Therapeutic: ANTIBIOTIC

Prototype: Penicillin G

Pregnancy Category: B

AVAILABILITY 250 mg, 500 mg capsules; 125 mg/5 mL oral suspension

ACTION & *THERAPEUTIC EFFECT* Cloxacillin inhibits final stage of bacterial cell wall synthesis by preferentially binding to specific penicillin-binding proteins (PBPs) that are located within the bacterial cell wall, which results in cell lysis and therefore cell death. *Effective against most gram-positive bacteria. Highly active against most penicillinase-producing staphylococci, and generally ineffective against gram-negative bacteria and methicillin-resistant staphylococci (MRSA).*

USES Primarily in infections caused by penicillinase-producing staphylococci and penicillin-resistant staphylococci. May be used to initiate therapy in suspected staphylococcal infections pending culture and susceptibility test results.

CONTRAINDICATIONS Sensitivity to penicillins; lactation. Safe use in neonates not established.

CAUTIOUS USE History of or suspected atopy or allergy (asthma, eczema, hives, hay fever), renal or hepatic function impairment, history of allergy to cephalosporins, pregnancy (category B).

ROUTE & DOSAGE

Mild to Moderate Infections

Adult: **PO** 250–500 mg q6h

Child (weight less than 20 kg): **PO** 12.5–25 mg/kg q6h (max: 4 g/day)

ADMINISTRATION

Oral

- Give on an empty stomach (at least 1 h before or 2 h after meals) unless otherwise advised by physician. Food reduces rate and extent of drug absorption.
- After reconstitution PO solution retains potency for 14 days if refrigerated (shake well before pouring).
- Unless otherwise advised, store capsules at 15°–30° C (59°–86° F).

ADVERSE EFFECTS (≥1%) **Body as a Whole:** Wheezing, sneezing, chills, drug fever, <u>anaphylaxis</u>, superinfections. **GI:** *Nausea,* vomiting, flatulence, *diarrhea*. **Hematologic:** Eosinophilia, leukopenia, <u>agranulocytosis</u>. **Metabolic:** Elevated AST, ALT; jaundice (possibly of allergic etiology). **Skin:** Pruritus, urticaria, rash.

INTERACTIONS Drug: Probenecid decreases cloxacillin elimination.

PHARMACOKINETICS Absorption: 37–60% from GI tract. **Peak:** 0.5–2 h. **Duration:** 4–6 h. **Distribution:** Distributed throughout body with highest concentrations in liver, kidney, spleen, bone, bile, and pleural fluid; low CSF penetration; crosses placenta; distributed into breast milk. **Metabolism:** In liver. **Elimination:** Primarily in urine; some elimination via bile. **Half-Life:** 30–60 min.

NURSING IMPLICATIONS

Assessment & Drug Effects

- Determine previous exposure and sensitivity to penicillins and cephalosporins and other allergic reactions of any kind before treatment is initiated.
- Monitor for S&S of anaphylactoid reaction (see Appendix F) or other signs or symptoms of hypersensitivity reaction (see Appendix F) as with other penicillins.
- Lab tests: Periodic assessments of renal, hepatic, and hematopoietic function are advised in patients on long-term therapy.

Patient & Family Education

- Take medication around the clock, do not miss a dose, and continue taking the medication until it is finished.
- Report to physician the onset of hypersensitivity reaction (see Appendix F) and superinfections.
- Check with physician if GI adverse effects (nausea, vomiting, diarrhea) appear.

CLOZAPINE Pr

(clo′za-pin)

Clozaril, Fazaclo

Classification: ANTIPSYCHOTIC, ATYPICAL

Therapeutic: ATYPICAL ANTIPSYCHOTIC

Pregnancy Category: B

AVAILABILITY 25 mg, 50 mg, 100 mg tablets and 12.5 mg, 25 mg, 50 mg, 100 mg orally disintegrating tablets

ACTION & *THERAPEUTIC EFFECT* Interferes with binding of dopamine to D_1 and D_2 receptors in the limbic region of brain. It binds primarily to nondopaminergic sites (e.g., alpha-adrenergic, serotonergic, and cholinergic receptors). *Limited to treatment of schizophrenia uncontrolled by other agents.*

USES Management of severely ill schizophrenic patients who have failed to respond to other neuroleptic agents.

UNLABELED USES Schizo-affective disorder, severe obsessive-compulsive disorder, bipolar disorder, dementia-related behavioral disorders.

CONTRAINDICATIONS Severe CNS depression, blood dyscrasia, history of bone marrow depression; patients with myeloproliferative disorders, uncontrolled epilepsy; clozapine-induced agranulocytosis, severe granulocytosis, chemotherapy, coma, leukemia, leukopenia, neutropenia, myocarditis, concurrent administration of benzodiazepines or other psychotropic drugs; renal failure, dialysis, hepatitis, jaundice; infants, lactation.

CAUTIOUS USE Arrhythmias, GI disorders, narrow-angle glaucoma, hepatic and renal impairment, prostatic hypertrophy, history of seizures; patients with cardiovascular and/or pulmonary disease; cerebrovascular disease, cardiac arrhythmias, tachycardia, dehydration, neurologic disease, tardive dyskinesia, previous history of agranulocytosis; surgery, glaucoma, infection, pregnancy (category B); older adults. Safety and efficacy in children younger than 9 y have not been established.

ROUTE & DOSAGE

Schizophrenia

Adult (older than 16 y): **PO** Initiate at 12.5 mg daily or b.i.d.

C

then increase by 25–50 mg/day and titrate to a target dose of 350–450 mg/day in 3 divided doses, further increases (not more than twice weekly) can be made if necessary (max: 900 mg/day)

ADMINISTRATION

Oral

- Drug is usually withdrawn gradually over 1–2 wk if therapy must be discontinued.
- Store the drug away from heat or light.

ADVERSE EFFECTS (≥1%) **CV:** Orthostatic hypotension, *tachycardia,* ECG changes, increased risk of myocarditis especially during first month of therapy, pericarditis, pericardial effusion, cardiomyopathy, heart failure, MI, mitral insufficiency. **GI:** Nausea, dry mouth, constipation, hypersalivation. **Hematologic:** Agranulocytosis. **CNS:** Seizures, *transient fever,* sedation, neuroleptic malignant syndrome (rare), dystonic reactions (rare). **Metabolic:** Hyperglycemia, diabetes mellitus. **Urogenital:** Urinary retention. **Other:** Increased mortality from severe hematologic, cardiovascular, and respiratory adverse effects.

INTERACTIONS Drug: Alcohol and other CNS DEPRESSANTS compound depressant effects; ANTICHOLINERGIC AGENTS potentiate anticholinergic effects; ANTIHYPERTENSIVE AGENTS may potentiate hypotension. **Herbal: St. John's wort** and **kava** may increase sedation.

PHARMACOKINETICS Absorption: Readily absorbed from GI tract. **Onset:** 2–4 wk. **Peak:** 2.5 h. **Distribution:** Possibly distributed into breast milk. **Metabolism:** In liver. **Elimination:** 50% in urine, 30% in feces. **Half-Life:** 8–12 h.

NURSING IMPLICATIONS

Assessment & Drug Effects

- Lab tests: Baseline WBC and absolute neutrophil count **must be** made before initial treatment, every week for first 6 mo, then every 2 wk for next 6 mo, then every 4 wk, and weekly for 4 wk after the drug is discontinued. Periodically monitor blood glucose.
- Monitor diabetics for loss of glycemic control.
- Monitor for seizure activity; seizure potential increases at the higher dose level.
- Closely monitor for recurrence of psychotic symptoms if the drug is being discontinued.
- Monitor cardiovascular and respiratory status, especially during the first month of therapy. Report promptly S&S of potential cardiac problems.
- Monitor for development of tachycardia or hypotension, which may pose a serious risk for patients with compromised cardiovascular function.

Patient & Family Education

- Carefully monitor blood glucose levels if diabetic.
- Do not engage in any hazardous activity until response to the drug is known. Drowsiness and sedation are common adverse effects.
- Due to the risk of agranulocytosis (see Appendix F) it is important to comply with blood test regimen. Report flulike symptoms, fever, sore throat, lethargy, malaise, or other signs of infection.
- Rise slowly to avoid orthostatic hypotension.
- Report immediately any of the following: Unexplained fatigue, especially with activity; shortness of breath, sudden weight gain or edema of the lower extremities.
- Take drug exactly as ordered.

- Do not use OTC drugs or alcohol without permission of physician.

COCAINE

(koe-kane′)

COCAINE HYDROCHLORIDE

Classification: ANESTHETIC, LOCAL
Therapeutic: TOPICAL ANESTHETIC
Prototype: Procaine
Pregnancy Category: C
Controlled Substance: Schedule II

AVAILABILITY 4%, 10% topical solution

ACTION & *THERAPEUTIC EFFECT* Alkaloid obtained from leaves of *Erythroxylon coca*. Topical application blocks nerve conduction and produces surface anesthesia accompanied by local vasoconstriction. Exerts adrenergic effect by potentiating action of endogenous (and injected) epinephrine and norepinephrine, possibly by inhibiting reuptake of catecholamines into sympathetic nerve terminals. Topical form of cocaine is a local anesthetic. *Systemic absorption produces descending CNS stimulation, with intense, short-lived euphoria accompanied by indifference to pain or hunger and with illusions of great strength, endurance, and mental capacity, all the basis for drug abuse.*

USES Surface anesthesia of ear, nose, throat, rectum, and vagina. Ophthalmic use largely abandoned because of its tendency to cause corneal sloughing. Sometimes used as ingredient in Brompton's cocktail.

CONTRAINDICATIONS Hypersensitivity to local anesthetics; sepsis in region of proposed application; acute MI, history of cardiac arrhythmias, cardiac disease; seizures or seizure disorders; thyrotoxicosis cerebrovascular disease; Tourette's syndrome; MAOI therapy; lactation.

CAUTIOUS USE History of drug sensitivities, history of drug abuse; pregnancy (category C).

ROUTE & DOSAGE

Surface Anesthesia

Adult: **Topical** 1–10% solution (use greater than 4% solution with caution), max single dose of 1 mg/kg

ADMINISTRATION

Topical

- Exercise caution to ensure that drug is taken as prescribed.
- Preserve in tightly closed, light-resistant containers.

ADVERSE EFFECTS (≥1%) **Body as a Whole:** Formication ("cocaine bugs"), hypersensitivity reactions. **CV:** Tachycardia, <u>ventricular fibrillation, MI</u>, angina pectoris. **GI:** Nausea, vomiting, anorexia, abdominal pain. **CNS:** *CNS stimulation* and <u>CNS depression (respiratory and circulatory failure)</u>. **Respiratory:** Pneumonia, lung damage (chronic cocaine smoking). **Special Senses:** Runny nose, perforated nasal septum; clouding, pitting, and ulceration of cornea.

INTERACTIONS **Drug: Epinephrine** entails risk of severe hypertension and arrhythmias; MAO INHIBITORS potentiate pharmacologic effects of cocaine.

PHARMACOKINETICS **Absorption:** Readily absorbed from mucous membranes; absorption limited by vasoconstriction. **Onset:** 1 min. **Peak:** 15–120 min. **Duration:** 30 min–2 h. **Distribution:** Crosses placenta; distributed into breast milk. **Metabolism:** Hydrolyzed in serum. **Elimination:** In urine; detectable for up to 30 h. **Half-Life:** 1–2.5 h.

NURSING IMPLICATIONS

Assessment & Drug Effects

- When used for anesthesia of throat, cocaine causes temporary paralysis of cilia of respiratory tract cells, reducing protection against aspiration. It also may interfere with pharyngeal stage of swallowing. Give nothing by mouth until sensation returns.
- Monitor cardiovascular status, especially in patients with known cardiac disease. Report promptly cardiac arrhythmias.

Patient & Family Education

- Promptly report angina or chest pain or respiratory distress.

CODEINE

(koe′deen)

CODEINE PHOSPHATE

Paveral ♣

CODEINE SULFATE

Classifications: NARCOTIC (OPIATE AGONIST) ANALGESIC; ANTITUSSIVE
Therapeutic: NARCOTIC ANALGESIC; ANTITUSSIVE
Prototype: Morphine
Pregnancy Category: C
Controlled Substance: Schedule II

AVAILABILITY 15 mg, 30 mg, 60 mg tablets; 15 mg/5 mL oral solution; 30 mg, 60 mg injection

ACTION & *THERAPEUTIC EFFECT*
Opium agonist in the CNS. Analgesia is mediated through changes in the perception of pain at the spinal cord and higher levels in the CNS. The antitussive effects are mediated through direct action on receptors in the cough center of the medulla. *Analgesic potency is about one-sixth that of morphine; antitussive activity is also a little less than that of morphine.*

USES Symptomatic relief of mild to moderately severe pain when control cannot be obtained by nonnarcotic analgesics and to suppress hyperactive or nonproductive cough.

CONTRAINDICATIONS Hypersensitivity to codeine or other morphine derivatives; acute asthma, COPD; increased intracranial pressure, head injury, acute alcoholism, hepatic or renal dysfunction, hypothyroidism. Safe use in neonates not established.
CAUTIOUS USE Prostatic hypertrophy, G6PD deficiency; GI disease; hepatic disease; hepatitis; immunosuppression; debilitated patients, very young and very old patients; history of drug abuse; pregnancy (category C), lactation.

ROUTE & DOSAGE

Analgesic

Adult: **PO/IM/Subcutaneous** 15–60 mg q.i.d.
Child: **PO/IM/Subcutaneous** 0.5–1 mg/kg q4–6h prn (max: 60 mg/dose)

Antitussive

Adult: **PO** 10–20 mg q4–6h prn (max: 120 mg/24 h)

Child: **PO** *6–12 y,* 5–10 mg q4–6h (max: 60 mg/24 h); *2–6 y,* 2.5–5 mg q4–6h (max: 30 mg/24 h)

ADMINISTRATION

Oral

- Administer PO codeine with milk or other food to reduce possibility of GI distress.

Subcutaneous/Intramuscular

- Give parenterally to achieve greatest effectiveness. An oral dose is about 60% as effective as an equal parenteral dose.
- Preserve in tight, light-resistant containers at 15°–30° C (59°–86° F) unless otherwise directed.

ADVERSE EFFECTS (≥1%) **Body as a Whole:** Shortness of breath, anaphylactoid reaction. **CV:** Palpitation, hypotension, orthostatic hypotension, bradycardia, tachycardia, circulatory collapse. **GI:** *Nausea,* vomiting, *constipation.* **CNS:** *Dizziness,* light-headedness, *drowsiness,* sedation, lethargy, euphoria, agitation; restlessness, exhilaration, convulsions, narcosis, respiratory depression. **Skin:** Diffuse erythema, rash, urticaria, *pruritus,* excessive perspiration, facial flushing, fixed-drug eruption. **Special Senses:** Miosis. **Urogenital:** Urinary retention.

INTERACTIONS Drug: Alcohol and other CNS DEPRESSANTS augment CNS depressant effects. **Herbal: St. John's wort** may cause increased sedation.

PHARMACOKINETICS Absorption: Readily from GI tract. **Onset:** 15–30 min. **Peak:** 1–1.5 h. **Duration:** 4–6 h. **Distribution:** Crosses placenta; distributed into breast milk. **Metabolism:** In liver. **Elimination:** In urine. **Half-Life:** 2.5–4 h.

NURSING IMPLICATIONS

Assessment & Drug Effects

- Record relief of pain and duration of analgesia.
- Evaluate effectiveness as cough suppressant. Treatment of cough is directed toward decreasing frequency and intensity of cough without abolishing cough reflex, need to remove bronchial secretions.
- Supervise ambulation and use other safety precautions as warranted since drug may cause dizziness and light-headedness.
- Monitor for nausea, a common side effect. Report nausea accompanied by vomiting. Change to another analgesic may be warranted.

Patient & Family Education

- Make position changes slowly and in stages, particularly from recumbent to upright posture. Lie down immediately if light-headedness or dizziness occurs.
- Lie down when feeling nauseated and to notify physician if this symptom persists. Nausea appears to be aggravated by ambulation.
- Avoid driving and other potentially hazardous activities until reaction to drug is known. Codeine may impair ability to perform tasks requiring mental alertness.
- Do not take alcohol or other CNS depressants unless approved by physician.

COLCHICINE

(kol′chi-seen)

Novocolchine ♣

Classification: ANTIGOUT

Therapeutic: ANTIGOUT

Pregnancy Category: C

AVAILABILITY 0.5 mg, 0.6 mg tablets

C

ACTION & *THERAPEUTIC EFFECT*

Has antimitotic and indirect anti-inflammatory properties. Colchicine inhibits the migration of neutrophils into the area of inflammation. It does appear to prevent the release of an inflammatory glycoprotein from phagocytes in the inflammatory process. *Inhibition of inflammation and reduction of pain and swelling, which occurs in gouty arthritis. Colchicine is nonanalgesic and nonuricosuric.*

USES Prophylactically for recurrent gouty arthritis and for acute gout, either as single agent or in combination with a uricosuric such as probenecid, allopurinol, or sulfinpyrazone.

UNLABELED USES Sarcoid arthritis, chondrocalcinosis (pseudogout), arthritis associated with erythema nodosum, leukemia, adenocarcinoma, acute calcific tendonitis, familial Mediterranean fever, multiple sclerosis, primary biliary cirrhosis, mycosis fungoides, and in experimental studies of normal and abnormal cell division.

CONTRAINDICATIONS Blood dyscrasias; severe GI, renal, hepatic, or cardiac disease. Safe use in children not established.

CAUTIOUS USE Older adult and debilitated patients, early manifestations of GI, renal, hepatic, or cardiac disease; pregnancy (category C).

ROUTE & DOSAGE

Acute Gouty Attack

Adult: **PO** 0.5–1.2 mg followed by 0.5–0.6 mg q1–2h until pain relief or intolerable GI symptoms (max: 4 mg/attack)

Prophylaxis

Adult: **PO** 0.5 or 0.6 mg every night or every other night as needed (up to 1.8 mg/day may be needed for severe cases)

Surgical Patients

Adult: **PO** 0.5 or 0.6 mg t.i.d. starting 3 days before surgery and continuing for 3 days after surgery

Renal Impairment Dosage Adjustment

CrCl 10–50 mL/min: Prolonged use is not recommended; less than 10 mL/min: Reduce recommended dose by 50%

ADMINISTRATION

Oral

- Administer oral drug with milk or food to reduce possibility of GI upset.
- Preserve in tight, light-resistant containers preferably between 15°–30° C (59°–86° F), unless otherwise directed by manufacturer.

ADVERSE EFFECTS (≥1%) **GI:** *Nausea, vomiting, diarrhea, abdominal pain,* anorexia, hemorrhagic gastroenteritis, steatorrhea, hepatotoxicity, pancreatitis. **Hematologic:** Neutropenia, <u>bone marrow depression</u>, thrombocytopenia, <u>agranulocytosis, aplastic anemia</u>. **CNS:** Mental confusion, peripheral neuritis, syndrome of muscle weakness (accompanied by elevated serum creatine kinase). **Skin:** Severe irritation and tissue damage if IV administration leaks around injection site. **Urogenital:** Azotemia, proteinuria, hematuria, oliguria.

DIAGNOSTIC TEST INTERFERENCE Possible interference with ***urinary steroid (17-OHCS)*** determinations when done by modifications of ***Reddy, Jenkins, Thorn procedure.*** False-positive ***urine tests for RBCs and Hgb*** reported.

INTERACTIONS Drug: May decrease intestinal absorption of vitamin B_{12}.

PHARMACOKINETICS Absorption: Rapidly from GI tract. **Peak:** 0.5–2 h; may have multiple peaks because of enterohepatic cycling. **Distribution:** Widely distributed; concentrates in leukocytes, kidney, liver, spleen, and intestinal tract. **Metabolism:** Partially metabolized in liver. **Elimination:** Primarily in feces; 10–20% in urine in 24 h.

NURSING IMPLICATIONS

Assessment & Drug Effects

- Lab tests: Baseline and periodic determinations of serum uric acid and creatinine are advised, as well as CBC, including Hgb, platelet count, serum electrolytes, and urinalysis.
- Monitor for dose-related adverse effects; they are most likely to occur during the initial course of treatment.
- Monitor for early signs of colchicine toxicity including weakness, abdominal discomfort, anorexia, nausea, vomiting, and diarrhea. Report to physician. To avoid more serious toxicity, drug should be discontinued promptly until symptoms subside.
- Monitor I&O ratio and pattern (during acute gouty attack): High fluid intake promotes excretion and reduces danger of crystal formation in kidneys and ureters.

Patient & Family Education

- Withhold drug and report to the physician the onset of GI symptoms or signs of bone marrow depression (nausea, sore throat, bleeding gums, sore mouth, fever, fatigue, malaise, unusual bleeding or bruising).
- Avoid fermented beverages such as beer, ale, and wine as they may precipitate gouty attack.

COLESEVELAM HYDROCHLORIDE

(co-less′e-ve-lam)

Welchol

Classifications: ANTIHYPERLIPIDEMIC; BILE ACID SEQUESTRANT
Therapeutic: CHOLESTEROL-LOWERING; BILE ACID SEQUESTRANT
Prototype: Cholestyramine resin
Pregnancy Category: B

AVAILABILITY 625 mg tablets; 3.75 mg powder for suspension

ACTION & *THERAPEUTIC EFFECT* Anion exchange resin used for its cholesterol-lowering effect. Binds with bile salts in the intestinal tract to form an insoluble complex that is excreted in the feces, thus reducing circulating cholesterol and increasing serum LDL removal rate. Serum triglyceride levels may increase slightly. *Decreases serum LDL and total cholesterol level. Removes bile salts from the intestine.*

USES Adjunctive therapy to diet and exercise for reduction of elevated LDL cholesterol alone or in combination; adjunct to diet and exercise for control of type 2 diabetes

CONTRAINDICATIONS Hypersensitivity to colesevelam; complete biliary obstruction; history of hypertriglyceridemia-induced pancreatitis; serum triglyceride concentrations greater than 500 mg/dL; bowel obstruction; children younger than 2 y of age.

C

CAUTIOUS USE Preexisting GI disorders or bowel disease, primary biliary cirrhosis, partial biliary obstruction, biliary atresia; diabetes mellitus; hypertriglyceridemia; older adults, pregnancy (category B); malabsorption states; bleeding disorders.

ROUTE & DOSAGE

Hypercholesterolemia, Monotherapy or Combination Therapy

Adult: **PO** 3 tablets b.i.d. with meals or 6 tablets daily with a meal, may be increased to 7 tablets/day

Type 2 Diabetes

Adult: **PO** 3 tablets b.i.d. or 6 tablets daily

ADMINISTRATION

Oral

- Give with meals (mandatory) and adequate liquid (e.g., 8 oz).
- Store at 15°–30° C (59°–86° F) with occasional fluctuations to 40° C (90° F); protect from moisture.

ADVERSE EFFECTS (≥1%) **Body as a Whole:** Infection, pain, flu-like syndrome, asthenia, myalgia. **CNS:** Headache. **GI:** Abdominal pain, *flatulence, constipation,* diarrhea, nausea, dyspepsia. **Respiratory:** Sinusitis, rhinitis, cough, pharyngitis.

INTERACTIONS Drug: May decrease absorption of **verapamil.** Can bind and affect absorption of any drug.

PHARMACOKINETICS Absorption: Not absorbed. **Metabolism:** Not metabolized. **Elimination:** 0.05% in urine.

NURSING IMPLICATIONS

Assessment & Drug Effects

- Lab tests: Monitor total cholesterol, LDL-C, HDL-C, and triglycerides periodically; periodic blood glucose monitoring and HbA1C.
- Withhold drug and notify physician for triglycerides greater than 300 mg/dL.

Patient & Family Education

- Report S&S of GI distress (see Appendix F), especially constipation.

COLESTIPOL HYDROCHLORIDE

(koe-les′ti-pole)

Cholestabyl ♣, Colestid, Lestid ♣

Classifications: ANTIHYPERLIPIDEMIC; BILE ACID SEQUESTRANT

Therapeutic: CHOLESTEROL-LOWERING AGENT; BILE ACID SEQUESTRANT

Prototype: Cholestyramine

Pregnancy Category: C

AVAILABILITY 1 g tablets; 5 g powder for suspension

ACTION & *THERAPEUTIC EFFECT* Insoluble chloride salt of a basic anion exchange resin with high molecular weight, which adsorbs and combines with intestinal bile acids in exchange for chloride ions to form an insoluble, nonabsorbable complex that is excreted in the feces. *Reduces circulating cholesterol and increases serum LDL removal rate. Serum triglycerides are not affected or are minimally increased.*

USES Pruritus associated with partial biliary obstruction; biliary cirrhosis; also as adjunct to diet therapy of patient with primary hypercholesterolemia (type IIa hyperlipoproteinemia) or with coronary artery disease unresponsive to diet or other measures alone.

UNLABELED USES Digitoxin overdose and hyperoxaluria and to control postoperative diarrhea caused by excess bile acids in colon.

CONTRAINDICATIONS Complete biliary obstruction, biliary cirrhosis; hypersensitivity to bile acid sequestrants; renal disease. Safe use in children not established.

CAUTIOUS USE Hemorrhoids; bleeding disorders; malabsorption states; GI motility disorders, dysphagia; older adult; pregnancy (category C).

ROUTE & DOSAGE

Hypercholesterolemia

Adult: **PO** 15–30 g/day in 2–4 doses a.c. and at bedtime, or 1–2 tabs 1–2 times/day

Digitalis Toxicity

Adult: **PO** 10 g followed by 5 g q6–8h as needed

ADMINISTRATION

Oral

- Give 30 min before a meal when ordered a.c.
- Ensure that tablets are not chewed or crushed. They **must be** swallowed whole.
- Always mix granule form with liquids, juices, soups, cereals, or pulpy fruits. Add powder to at least 90 mL fluid. When carbonated drink is used, slowly stir in a large glass because excess foaming may occur. Rinse glass with small amount extra fluid to be sure all the drug is taken.
- Drugs given concomitantly should be scheduled at least 1 h before or 4 h after ingestion of colestipol to reduce interference with their absorption (see drug interactions).
- Store at 15°–30° C (59°–86° F) in tightly closed container unless otherwise instructed.

ADVERSE EFFECTS (≥1%) **Body as a Whole:** Joint and muscle pain, arthritis, shortness of breath. **GI:** *Constipation,* abdominal pain or distention, belching, flatulence, nausea, vomiting, diarrhea. **Metabolic:** Transient increases in liver enzyme tests, serum phosphorus and chloride; decreases in serum sodium and potassium. **Skin:** Dermatitis, urticaria.

INTERACTIONS Drug: Because it decreases the absorption from the GI tract of ORAL ANTICOAGULANTS, **digoxin,** TETRACYCLINES, PENICILLINS, **phenobarbital,** THYROID HORMONES, THIAZIDE DIURETICS, IRON SALTS, FAT-SOLUBLE VITAMINS (A, D, E, K), administer cholestyramine 4 h before or 2 h after these drugs. Can bind and affect absorption of any drug.

PHARMACOKINETICS Absorption: Not absorbed from GI tract. **Elimination:** In feces as insoluble complex.

NURSING IMPLICATIONS

Assessment & Drug Effects

- Watch for changes in bowel elimination pattern. Constipation should not be allowed to persist without medical attention.
- Lab tests: Periodic total cholesterol, LDL-C, HDL-C, and triglycerides; periodic serum electrolytes. Report S&S of hyponatremia and hypokalemia (see Appendix F).

Patient & Family Education

- To prevent drug interactions, it is important to keep to established schedule for taking colestipol and other drugs. See Drug Interactions.
- If receiving prolonged therapy, report unusual bleeding (vitamin K deficiency). Colestipol prevents absorption of fat-soluble vitamins (A, D, E, K).

C

COLFOSCERIL PALMITATE

(col-fos'ce-ril)
Exosurf Neonatal
Classification: LUNG SURFACTANT
Therapeutic: LUNG SURFACTANT
Prototype: Beractant
Pregnancy Category: Not applicable

AVAILABILITY 108 mg powder for injection

ACTION & *THERAPEUTIC EFFECT* Synthetic lung surfactant. Endogenous pulmonary surfactant lowers surface tension on alveolar surfaces during respiration and stabilizes the alveoli against collapse at resting pressures. Colfosceril lowers minimum surface tension on alveolar surfaces and restores pulmonary compliance and oxygenation in premature infants. *Helps to reverse the effects of the deficiency of surfactant that causes respiratory distress syndrome (RDS) in premature infants.*

USES Prophylactic treatment of infants with birth weights less than 1350 g who are at risk of developing RDS. Prophylactic therapy of infants with birth weights greater than 1350 g who show evidence of pulmonary immaturity.

UNLABELED USES Rescue treatment of infants with established RDS; RDS in adults.

CONTRAINDICATIONS Infants who have major congenital abnormalities or who are suspected of having congenital infections.

ROUTE & DOSAGE

Prophylaxis

Infant: **Intratracheal** 3 doses of 5 mL/kg are recommended, with the first dose being given as soon as possible after birth and repeat doses 12 and 24 h later to infants who remain on mechanical ventilation

Rescue Therapy

Infant: **Intratracheal** 2 doses of 5 mL/kg are recommended, the first dose being initiated as soon as the diagnosis of RDS is confirmed and the second 12 h later in infants remaining on mechanical ventilation

ADMINISTRATION

Intratracheal

- Reconstitute immediately before use if possible. Use only supplied diluent for reconstitution.
- Reconstitute as follows: (1) Withdraw diluent with 18–19-gauge needle attached to 10–12-mL syringe; (2) inject into vial by allowing vacuum to draw diluent in; (3) do not withdraw needle and aspirate as much of solution as possible back into syringe; (4) maintain vacuum and quickly release plunger. Repeat steps 3 and 4 three or four times to ensure adequate mixing.
- Reconstituted drug is a milky white suspension. Gently shake if needed to resuspend it.
- Withdraw entire ordered dose into syringe while maintaining vacuum in vial.
- Before administration of drug, ensure that endotracheal tube tip is in the trachea.
- Before administration of drug, the infant should be suctioned. If possible, avoid suctioning for 2 h after drug administration.
- Drug is administered without interrupting mechanical ventilation. Use side port on the endotracheal tube adaptor.

- Administer dose in halves, each half over 1–2 min. Give first half dose with head in midline position; then turn head and torso to the right. Wait 30 sec; then return to midline position for second half dose. Give each dose in short bursts timed with inspiration. After second half dose, turn head and torso to left for 30 sec; then return to midline.
- Slow or stop drug administration and adjust ventilator rate or FIO_2 if any of the following occur: Heart rate decreases, infant becomes dusky or agitated, or O_2 saturation drops.
- Store at 15°–30° C (59°–86° F) in a dry place. Reconstituted solution is stable for 12 h.

INCOMPATIBILITIES **Solution/additive:** Do not mix any antibiotics with surfactant; this may inactivate surfactant.

ADVERSE EFFECTS (≥1%) **CV:** Bradycardia, tachycardia. **Respiratory:** Decreased oxygen saturation, mucous plugging, apnea, pulmonary hemorrhage.

INTERACTIONS Drug: No clinically significant interactions established.

PHARMACOKINETICS Absorption: Absorbed from the alveolus into lung tissue. **Duration:** At least 7 days. **Distribution:** Distributes uniformly to all lobes of the lung, distal airways, and alveolar spaces. **Metabolism:** Recycled and metabolized exclusively in the lungs. **Half-Life:** 20–36 h.

NURSING IMPLICATIONS

Assessment & Drug Effects

- During administration of drug, continuous ECG and transcutaneous monitoring are required. Also monitor chest expansion and facial expression.
- Monitor pulmonary function during administration. Rapid changes may require immediate adjustment of peak inspiratory pressure, ventilator rate, or FIO_2.
- Monitor continuously for 30 min following administration. Frequent arterial blood gas sampling is required to prevent hyperoxia and hypocarbia.

COLISTIMETHATE SODIUM

(koe-lis-ti-meth′ate)

Coly-Mycin M

Classifications: URINARY TRACT ANTIINFECTIVE; ANTIBIOTIC

Therapeutic: URINARY TRACT ANTI-INFECTIVE

Prototype: Trimethoprim

Pregnancy Category: B

AVAILABILITY 150 mg injection

ACTION & *THERAPEUTIC EFFECT* Believed to act by affecting phospholipid component in bacterial cytoplasmic membranes with resulting damage and leakage of essential intracellular components. *Bactericidal against most gram-negative organisms, but not effective against* Proteus *or* Neisseria *species.*

USES Particularly for severe, acute and chronic UTIs caused by susceptible strains of gram-negative organisms resistant to other antibiotics. Has been used with carbenicillin for *Pseudomonas* sepsis in children with acute leukopenia.

CONTRAINDICATIONS Hypersensitivity to polypeptide antibiotics; concomitant use of drugs that potentiate neuromuscular blocking effect (aminoglycoside antibiotics, other polymyxins, anticholinesterases, curariform muscle relaxants, ether, sodium citrate); nephrotoxic and ototoxic drugs; pregnancy (category B).

CAUTIOUS USE Impaired renal function; myasthenia gravis; older adult patients, infants; lactation.

ROUTE & DOSAGE

Urinary Tract Infections

Adult/Child: **IM/IV** 2.5–5 mg/kg/day divided in 2–4 doses (max: 5 mg/kg/day)

Renal Impairment Dosage Adjustment

Serum Cr 1.3–1.5 mg/dL: 2.5–3.8 mg/kg/day in 2 divided doses; 1.6–2.5 mg/dL: 2.5 mg/kg/day in a single dose or 2 divided doses; 2.6–4 mg/dL: 1.5 mg/kg q36h

ADMINISTRATION

Intramuscular

- Reconstitute each 150-mg vial with 2 mL of sterile water for injection to yield a concentration of 75 mg/mL. Swirl vial gently during reconstitution to avoid bubble formation. IM injection should be made deep into upper outer quadrant of buttock. ▪ Patients commonly experience pain at injection site. Rotate sites.

Intravenous

PREPARE: **Direct/Intermittent:** Prepare first half of total daily dose as directed for IM then further dilute with 20 mL sterile water for injection. ▪ Prepare second half of total daily dose by diluting further in 50 mL or more of D5W, NS, D5/NS, LR or other compatible solution. ▪ IV infusion solution should be freshly prepared and used within 24 h.

ADMINISTER: **Direct/Intermittent:** First half of total daily dose: Give slowly over 3–5 min. ▪ Second half of total daily dose: Starting 1–2 h after the first half dose has been given, infuse the second half dose over the next 22–23 h.

INCOMPATIBILITIES **Solution/additive: Cefazolin, cephapirin, erythromycin, hydrocortisone, hydroxyzine, kanamycin.**

- Reconstituted solution may be stored in refrigerator at 2°–8° C (36°–46° F) or at controlled room temperature of 15°–30° C (59°–86° F). Use within 7 days. ▪ Store unopened vials at controlled room temperature.

ADVERSE EFFECTS (≥1%) **Body as a Whole:** Drug fever, pain at IM site. **GI:** GI disturbances. **CNS:** Circumoral, lingual, and peripheral paresthesias; visual and speech disturbances, <u>neuromuscular blockade</u> (generalized muscle weakness, dyspnea, <u>respiratory depression or paralysis</u>), seizures, psychosis. **Respiratory:** <u>Respiratory arrest</u> after IM injection. **Skin:** Pruritus, urticaria, dermatoses. **Special Senses:** Ototoxicity. **Urogenital:** <u>Nephrotoxicity</u>.

INTERACTIONS Drug: Tubocurarine, pancuronium, atracurium, AMINOGLYCOSIDES may compound and prolong respiratory depression; AMINOGLYCOSIDES, **amphotericin B, vancomycin** augment nephrotoxicity.

PHARMACOKINETICS Peak: 1–2 h IM. **Duration:** 8–12 h. **Distribution:** Widely distributed in most tissues except CNS; crosses placenta; distributed into breast milk in low concentrations. **Metabolism:** In liver.

Elimination: 66–75% in urine within 24 h. **Half-Life:** 2–3 h.

NURSING IMPLICATIONS

Assessment & Drug Effects

- Lab tests: Culture and susceptibility tests should be performed initially. Baseline renal function tests should be performed prior to therapy; frequent monitoring of renal function and urine drug levels is advisable during therapy.
- Report restlessness or dyspnea promptly. Respiratory arrest has been reported after IM administration.
- Monitor I&O ratio and patterns: Decrease in urine output or change in I&O ratio and rising BUN, serum creatinine, and serum drug levels (without dosage increase) are indications of renal toxicity. If they occur, withhold drug and report to physician.
- Be alert to neurologic symptoms: Changes in speech and hearing, visual changes, drowsiness, dizziness, ataxia, and transient paresthesias, and keep physician informed.
- Monitor closely postoperative patients who have received curariform muscle relaxants, ether, or sodium citrate for signs of neuromuscular blockade (delayed recovery, muscle weakness, depressed respiration).

Patient & Family Education

- Avoid operating a vehicle or other potentially hazardous activities while on drug therapy because of the possibility of transient neurologic disturbances.

CONIVAPTAN HYDROCHLORIDE (Pr)

(con-i-vap'tin)
Vaprisol

Classifications: ELECTROLYTIC & WATER BALANCE AGENT; DIURETIC; VASOPRESSIN ANTAGONIST
Therapeutic: VASOPRESSIN ANTAGONIST; DIURETIC
Pregnancy Category: C

AVAILABILITY 5 mg/mL solution for injection

ACTION & *THERAPEUTIC EFFECT* Conivaptan is a vasopressin receptor (V2) antagonist that reduces the effect of vasopressin in the kidney, thus increasing the excretion of free water into the renal collecting ducts. *Conivaptan increases urine output and decreases urine osmolality in patients with euvolemic hyponatremia, thus restoring serum sodium balance.*

USES Treatment of euvolemic hyponatremia (e.g., syndrome of inappropriate secretion of antidiuretic hormone, or SIADH) in hospitalized patients.

CONTRAINDICATIONS Hypersensitivity to conivaptan; CHF; hyponatremia associated with hypovolemia; hypotension, syncope; intravenous use only; concurrent administration of potent CYP3A4 inhibitors such as ketoconazole, itraconazole, ritonavir, etc; lactation. Safety and efficacy in children not established.

CAUTIOUS USE Renal or hepatic function impairment; pregnancy (category C).

ROUTE & DOSAGE

Euvolemic Hyponatremia
Adult: **IV** 20 mg loading dose followed by 20 mg IV over 24 h. May repeat 20 mg/day dose for 1–3 days, or may titrate up to 40 mg/day based on response. Total duration of infusion should not exceed 4 days.

C

ADMINISTRATION

Intravenous

PREPARE: **IV Infusion:** Use a filter needle when withdrawing a drug from an ampule. *Loading dose infusion:* Withdraw 4 mL (20 mg) from one ampule and add to 100 mL of D5W. Gently invert the bag several times to mix. *Initial maintenance infusion:* Withdraw 4 mL (20 mg) from one ampule and add to 250 mL of D5W. Gently invert the bag several times to mix. *Maximum maintenance dose infusion:* Withdraw 8 mL (40 mg) from two ampules and add to 250 mL of D5W. Gently invert the bag several times to mix.

ADMINISTER: **IV Infusion:** Give via a large vein and change infusion site every 24 h. *Loading dose:* Give over 30 min. *Maintenance dose:* Give over 24 h. ▪ Frequently monitor the serum sodium level. A reduction in dose or discontinuation of infusion may be required if the serum sodium rises too rapidly. Discontinue infusion immediately and notify physician of a rise in serum sodium greater than 12 mEq/L/24 h. DO NOT resume infusion if serum sodium continues to rise. ▪ Infusion may be resumed ONLY if hyponatremia persists or reoccurs and patient demonstrates no indication of neurologic impairment. If the serum sodium rises too slowly, the dose may be titrated up to 40 mg over 24 h.

INCOMPATIBILITIES **Solution/additive: Lactated Ringer's solution, sodium chloride 0.9%.**

▪ Store vials at 25° C (77° F). Ampules should be stored in the original container and protected from light until ready for use. ▪ After diluting with D5W, the solution should be used immediately, with infusion completed within 24 h of mixing.

ADVERSE EFFECTS (≥2%) **Body as a Whole:** Cannula-site reaction, *infusion-site reaction,* pain, peripheral edema, pyrexia, *thirst.* **CNS:** Confusional state, *headache,* insomnia. **CV:** Atrial fibrillation, hypertension, hypotension, orthostatic hypotension, phlebitis. **GI:** Constipation, diarrhea, dry mouth, nausea, vomiting. **Hematologic:** Anemia. **Metabolic:** Dehydration, hyperglycemia, hypoglycemia, *hypokalemia,* hypomagnesemia, hyponatremia. **Respiratory:** Pneumonia. **Skin:** Erythema. **Special Senses:** Oral candidiasis.

INTERACTIONS Drug: Compounds that inhibit CYP3A4 (e.g., **ketoconazole, itraconazole, clarithromycin, ritonavir, indinavir**) can increase conivaptan levels. Conivaptan can increase the levels of **digoxin** and drugs that require CYP3A4 for metabolism (e.g., **midazolam,** HMG COA REDUCTASE INHIBITORS, **amlodipine**). **Food: Grapefruit juice** may increase the level of conivaptan. **Herbal: St. John's wort** may decrease the level of conivaptan.

PHARMACOKINETICS Distribution: 99% protein bound. **Metabolism:** Extensive hepatic metabolism. **Elimination:** Primarily fecal elimination (83%) with minor renal elimination. **Half-Life:** 5 h.

NURSING IMPLICATIONS

Assessment & Drug Effects

- Monitor infusion site for erythema, phlebitis, or other site reaction.
- Monitor vital signs and neurologic status frequently; report immediately S&S of hypernatremia (see Appendix F).

- Lab tests: Baseline and frequent serum sodium, serum potassium, and urine osmolality.
- Monitor digoxin blood levels with concurrent therapy and assess for S&S of digoxin toxicity.
- Monitor I&O closely. Effective treatment is accompanied by increased urine output, whereas decreasing urine output and oliguria may indicate developing hypernatremia.

Patient & Family Education

- Report any of the following to a health care provider: Pain at the infusion site, dizziness, confusion, palpitations, swelling of hands or feet.

CORTISONE ACETATE

(kor′ti-sone)

Cortistan, Cortone

Classifications: ADRENOCORTICAL STEROID; ANTI-INFLAMMATORY

Therapeutic: ANTI-INFLAMMATORY; GLUCOCORTICOID REPLACEMENT; IMMUNOSUPPRESSANT

Prototype: Prednisone

Pregnancy Category: D

AVAILABILITY 5 mg, 10 mg, 25 mg tablets; 50 mg/mL injection

ACTION & *THERAPEUTIC EFFECT*
Short-acting synthetic steroid with prominent glucocorticoid activity and minimal mineralocorticoid effects. Cortisone is converted in the body to cortisol, resulting in metabolic effects including promotion of protein, carbohydrate, and fat metabolism and interference with linear growth in children. *Has anti-inflammatory and immunosuppressive actions. Suppresses inflammation caused by radiant, mechanical, chemical, and infectious stimuli. Also suppress immune responses in diseases, such as in asthma, urticaria, or renal allograft.*

USES Replacement therapy for primary or secondary adrenocortical insufficiency and inflammatory and allergic disorders.

CONTRAINDICATIONS Hypersensitivity to glucocorticoids; psychoses; viral, fungal, or bacterial diseases of skin; Cushing's syndrome, immunologic procedures; pregnancy (category D), lactation.

CAUTIOUS USE Diabetes mellitus; hypertension, CHF; older adults; active or arrested tuberculosis; coagulopathy; hepatic disease; psychosis, emotional instability; renal disease, seizure disorders; active or latent peptic ulcer.

ROUTE & DOSAGE

Replacement or Inflammatory Disorders

Adult: **PO/IM** 20–300 mg/day in 1 or more divided doses, try to reduce periodically by 10–25 mg/day to lowest effective dose

Child: **PO** 2.5–10 mg/kg/day divided q6–8h **IM** 1–5 mg/kg/day divided q12–24h

ADMINISTRATION

Oral

- Administer cortisone (usually in a.m.) with food or fluid of patient's choice to reduce gastric irritation.
- Sodium chloride and a mineralocorticoid are usually given with cortisone as part of replacement therapy.

Intramuscular

- Shake bottle well before withdrawing dose.

C

- Give deep IM into a large muscle.
- Drug **must be** gradually tapered rather than withdrawn abruptly.
- Store at 15°–30° C (59°–86° F) in tightly closed container unless otherwise directed by manufacturer. Protect from heat and freezing.

ADVERSE EFFECTS (≥1%) **CV:** CHF, hypertension, *edema*. **GI:** *Nausea*, peptic ulcer, pancreatitis. **Endocrine:** Hyperglycemia. **Hematologic:** Thrombocytopenia. **Musculoskeletal:** *Compression fracture*, osteoporosis, muscle weakness. **CNS:** Euphoria, insomnia, vertigo, nystagmus. **Skin:** Impaired wound healing, petechiae, ecchymosis, acne. **Special Senses:** *Cataracts*, glaucoma, blurred vision.

INTERACTIONS Drug: BARBITURATES, **phenytoin, rifampin** decrease effects of cortisone.

PHARMACOKINETICS Absorption: Readily absorbed from GI tract. **Onset:** Rapid PO; 24–48 h IM. **Peak:** 2 h PO; 24–48 h IM. **Duration:** 1.25–1.5 days. **Distribution:** Concentrated in many tissues; crosses placenta; distributed into breast milk. **Metabolism:** In liver. **Elimination:** In urine. **Half-Life:** 0.5 h; HPA suppression: 8–12 h.

NURSING IMPLICATIONS

Assessment & Drug Effects

- Monitor for S&S of Cushing's syndrome (see Appendix F), especially in patients on long-term therapy.
- Lab tests: Periodic blood glucose and CBC with platelet count.
- Cortisone may mask some signs of infection, and new infections may appear.
- Be alert to clinical indications of infection: Malaise, anorexia, depression, and evidence of delayed healing. (Classic signs of inflammation are suppressed by cortisone.)
- Report ecchymotic areas, unexplained bleeding, and easy bruising.

Patient & Family Education

- Take drug exactly as prescribed. Do not alter dose intervals or stop therapy abruptly.
- Monitor weight and report a steady gain especially if it is accompanied by signs of fluid retention (e.g., edema of ankles or hands).
- Report changes in visual acuity, including blurring, promptly.
- Inform physician or dentist that cortisone is being taken.

CROMOLYN SODIUM Pr

(kroe'moe-lin)

Crolom, Fivent ♣, Gastrocom, Intal, Opticrom, Rynacrom ♣, Vistacrom ♣

Classifications: RESPIRATORY AGENT; MAST CELL STABILIZER; ANTI-INFLAMMATORY; ANTIASTHMATIC

Therapeutic: ANTIASTHMATIC; ANTI-INFLAMMATORY

Pregnancy Category: B

AVAILABILITY 20 mg/2 mL solution for nebulization; 800 mcg spray; 40 mg/mL nasal solution; 4% ophth solution; 100 mg/5 mL oral concentrate.

ACTION & *THERAPEUTIC EFFECT* Synthetic asthma prophylactic agent with unique action. Inhibits release of bronchoconstrictors—histamine and SRS-A (slow-reacting substance of anaphylaxis) from sensitized pulmonary mast cells, thereby suppressing an allergic response. Additionally, cromolyn may also reduce the release of inflammatory leukotrienes.

Particularly effective for IgE-mediated or "extrinsic asthma" precipitated by exposure to specific allergen (e.g., pollens, dust, animal dander), by inhibiting the release of bronchoconstrictors.

USES Primarily for prophylaxis of mild to moderate seasonal and perennial bronchial asthma and allergic rhinitis. Also used for prevention of exercise-related bronchospasm, prevention of acute bronchospasm induced by known pollutants or antigens, and for prevention and treatment of allergic rhinitis. Orally for systemic mastocytosis. **Ophthalmic use:** Allergic ocular disorders, conjunctivitis, vernal keratoconjunctivitis.

UNLABELED USES Orally for prophylaxis of GI and systemic reactions to food allergy.

CONTRAINDICATIONS Use of aerosol (because of fluorocarbon propellants) in patients with coronary artery disease or history of arrhythmias; dyspnea, acute asthma, status asthmaticus, or acute bronchospasm; patients unable to coordinate actions or follow instructions. Safe use in children younger than 2 y not determined.

CAUTIOUS USE Renal or hepatic dysfunction; pregnancy (category B), lactation.

ROUTE & DOSAGE

Allergies

Adult: **Inhalation** Metered dose inhaler or capsule: 1 spray or 1 capsule inhaled q.i.d.; nasal solution: 1 spray in each nostril 3–6 times/day at regular intervals

Child: **Inhalation** *Older than 6 y,* Metered dose inhaler or capsule: Same as for adult; *older than 6 y,* nasal solution: Same as for adult

Conjunctivitis

Adult: **PO** 2 ampules q.i.d. 30 min a.c. and at bedtime

Child (2–12 y): **PO** 1 ampule q.i.d. 30 min a.c. and at bedtime

Mastocytosis

See Appendix A-1

ADMINISTRATION

Oral

- Give at least 30 min before meals.

Inhalation

- Patients should receive detailed instructions for each inhalation device. See manufacturer's instructions. Therapeutic effect is dependent on proper inhalation technique.
- Advise patient to clear as much mucus as possible before inhalation treatments.
- Instruct patient to exhale as completely as possible before placing inhaler mouthpiece between lips, tilt head backward and inhale rapidly and deeply with steady, even breaths. Remove inhaler from mouth, hold breath for a few seconds, then exhale into the air. Repeat until entire dose is taken.
- Protect cromolyn from moisture and heat. Store in tightly closed, light-resistant container at 15°–30° C (59°–86° F) unless otherwise directed.

ADVERSE EFFECTS (≥1%) **Body as a Whole:** Peripheral eosinophilia, angioedema, bronchospasm, anaphylaxis (rare). **GI:** Swelling of parotid glands, dry mouth, slightly bitter aftertaste, *nausea,* vomiting, esophagitis. **CNS:** Headache, dizziness, peripheral neuritis. **Skin:** Erythema, urticaria, rash, contact dermatitis. **Special Senses:** *Sneezing, nasal stinging and burning,* dryness and *irritation of throat and trachea;*

cough; nasal congestion, itchy, puffy eyes, lacrimation, *transient ocular burning, stinging.*

INTERACTIONS Drug: No clinically significant interactions established.

PHARMACOKINETICS Absorption: Approximately 8% of dose absorbed from lungs. **Onset:** 1 wk with regular use. **Peak:** 15 min. **Duration:** 4–6 h; may last as long as 2–3 wk. **Elimination:** In bile and urine in equal amounts. **Half-Life:** 80 min.

NURSING IMPLICATIONS

Assessment & Drug Effects

- Withhold drug and notify physician if any of the following occur; angioedema or bronchospasm.
- Monitor for exacerbation of asthmatic symptoms including breathlessness and cough that may occur in patients receiving cromolyn during corticosteroid withdrawal.
- For patients with asthma, therapeutic effects may be noted within a few days but generally not until after 1–2 wk of therapy.

Patient & Family Education

- Throat irritation, cough, and hoarseness can be minimized by gargling with water, drinking a few swallows of water, or by sucking on a lozenge after each treatment.
- Talk to your physician about what to do in the event of an acute asthmatic attack. Cromolyn is of no value in acute asthma.
- Cromolyn does not eliminate the continued need for therapy with bronchodilators, expectorants, antibiotics, or corticosteroids, but the amount and frequency of use of these medications may be appreciably reduced.
- Report any unusual signs or symptoms. Hypersensitivity reactions (see Signs & Symptoms, Appendix F) can be severe and life-threatening. Drug should be discontinued if an allergic reaction occurs.

CROTAMITON

(kroe-tam′i-ton)

Eurax

Classifications: SCABICIDE; ANTIPRURITIC

Therapeutic: SCABICIDE; ANTIPRURITIC

Prototype: Lindane

Pregnancy Category: C

AVAILABILITY 10% cream, lotion

ACTION & *THERAPEUTIC EFFECT* By unknown mechanisms, drug eradicates *Sarcoptes scabiei* and effectively relieves itching. *Scabicidal and antipruritic agent.*

USES Treatment of scabies and for symptomatic treatment of pruritus.

CONTRAINDICATIONS Application to acutely inflamed skin, raw or weeping surfaces, eyes, or mouth; history of previous sensitivity to crotamiton.

CAUTIOUS USE Pregnancy (category C); children.

ROUTE & DOSAGE

Scabies

Adult/Child: **Topical** Apply a thin layer of cream from neck to toes; apply a second layer 24 h later. Bathe 48 h after last application to remove drug.

ADMINISTRATION

Topical

- Shake container well before use of solution.

- The skin **must be** thoroughly dry before applying medication.
- If drug accidentally contacts eyes, thoroughly flush out medication with water.
- Pruritus treatment: Massage medication gently into affected areas until it is completely absorbed. Repeat as needed (usually effective for 6–10 h).
- Store in tightly closed containers at 15°–30° C (59°–86° F). Do not freeze.

ADVERSE EFFECTS (≥1%) **Skin:** Skin irritation (particularly with prolonged use), rash, erythema, sensation of warmth, allergic sensitization.

INTERACTIONS Drug: No clinically significant interactions established.

NURSING IMPLICATIONS

Assessment & Drug Effects

- Monitor for and report significant skin irritation or allergic sensitization.

Patient & Family Education

- Review package insert before treatment begins.
- Discontinue medication and report to physician if irritation or sensitization develops.

CYANOCOBALAMIN

(sye-an-oh-koe-bal′a-min)

Anacobin ✤, Bedoz ✤, Nascobal, Rubion ✤

Classification: VITAMIN B_{12}

Therapeutic: VITAMIN B_{12}

Pregnancy Category: A (PO or nasal spray); C (parenteral)

AVAILABILITY 25 mcg, 50 mcg, 100 mcg, 250 mcg tablets; 400 mcg/unit, 500 mcg/0.1 mL nasal gel; 500 mcg/0.1 mL nasal spray

ACTION & *THERAPEUTIC EFFECT* Vitamin B_{12} is a cobalt-containing B complex vitamin essential for normal growth, cell reproduction, maturation of RBCs, nucleoprotein synthesis, maintenance of nervous system (myelin synthesis), and believed to be involved in protein and carbohydrate metabolism. Vitamin B_{12} deficiency results in megaloblastic anemia, dysfunction of spinal cord with paralysis, GI lesions. *Therapeutically effective for treatment of vitamin B_{12} deficiency and pernicious anemia.*

USES Vitamin B_{12} deficiency due to malabsorption syndrome as in pernicious (Addison's) anemia, sprue; GI pathology, dysfunction, or surgery; fish tapeworm infestation, and gluten enteropathy. Also used in B_{12} deficiency caused by increased physiologic requirements or inadequate dietary intake, and in vitamin B_{12} absorption (Schilling) test.

UNLABELED USES To prevent and treat toxicity associated with sodium nitroprusside.

CONTRAINDICATIONS History of sensitivity to vitamin B_{12}, other cobalamins, or cobalt; early Leber's disease (hereditary optic nerve atrophy), indiscriminate use in folic acid deficiency.

CAUTIOUS USE Heart disease, anemia, pulmonary disease; pregnancy (category A for PO and oral routes; category C for parenteral).

ROUTE & DOSAGE

Vitamin B_{12} Deficiency

Adult: **IM/Deep Subcutaneous** 30 mcg/day for 5–10 days, then 100–200 mcg/mo

C

Child: **IM/Deep Subcutaneous** 100 mcg doses to a total of 1–5 mg over 2 wk, then 60 mcg/mo

Pernicious Anemia

Adult: **IM/Deep Subcutaneous** 100–1000 mcg/day for 2–3 wk, then 100–1000 mcg q2–4wk
Intranasal one pump in one nostril once weekly
Child: **IM** 30–50 mcg/day × 2 wk to total of 1000 mcg, then 100 mcg/mo
Infant: **IM** 1000 mcg/day × at least 2 wk, then 50 mcg/mo

Diagnosis of Megaloblastic Anemia

Adult: **IM/Deep Subcutaneous** 1 mcg/day for 10 days while maintaining a low folate and vitamin B_{12} diet

Schilling Test

Adult: **IM/Deep Subcutaneous** 1000 mcg × 1 dose

Nutritional Supplement

Adult: **PO** 1–25 mcg/day
Child: **PO** *Younger than 1 y,* 0.3 mcg/day; *1 y or older,* 1 mcg/day

ADMINISTRATION

Oral

- PO preparations may be mixed with fruit juices. However, administer promptly since ascorbic acid affects the stability of vitamin B_{12}.
- Administration of oral vitamin B_{12} with meals increases its absorption.

Subcutaneous/Intramuscular

- Give deep subcutaneous by slightly tenting the skin at the injection site.
- IM may be given into any normal IM injection site.
- Preserved in light-resistant containers at room temperature preferably at 15°–30° C (59°–86° F) unless otherwise directed by manufacturer.

ADVERSE EFFECTS (≥1%) **Body as a Whole:** Feeling of swelling of body, <u>anaphylactic shock, sudden death</u>. **CV:** Peripheral vascular thrombosis, pulmonary edema, CHF. **GI:** Mild transient diarrhea. **Hematologic:** Unmasking of polycythemia vera (with correction of vitamin B_{12} deficiency). **Metabolic:** Hypokalemia. **Skin:** Itching, rash, flushing. **Special Senses:** Severe optic nerve atrophy (patients with Leber's disease).

DIAGNOSTIC TEST INTERFERENCE Most antibiotics, methotrexate, and pyrimethamine may produce invalid diagnostic ***blood assays for vitamin B_{12}***. Possibility of false-positive test for ***intrinsic factor antibodies.***

INTERACTIONS Drug: Alcohol, aminosalicylic acid, neomycin, colchicine may decrease absorption of oral cyanocobalamin; **chloramphenicol** may interfere with therapeutic response to cyanocobalamin.

PHARMACOKINETICS Absorption: Intestinal absorption requires presence of intrinsic factor in terminal ileum. **Distribution:** Widely distributed; principally stored in liver, kidneys, and adrenals; crosses placenta, excreted in breast milk. **Metabolism:** Converted in tissues to active co-enzymes; enterohepatically cycled. **Elimination:** 50–95% of doses 100 mcg or more are excreted in urine in 48 h. **Half-Life:** 6 days (400 days in liver).

C

NURSING IMPLICATIONS

Assessment & Drug Effects

- Lab tests: Before initiation of therapy, reticulocyte and erythrocyte counts, Hgb, Hct, vitamin B_{12}, and serum folate levels should be determined; then repeated between 5 and 7 days after start of therapy and at regular intervals during therapy. Monitor potassium levels during the first 48 h. Conversion to normal erythropoiesis increases erythrocyte potassium requirement and can result in severe hypokalemia and sudden death.
- Obtain a careful history of sensitivities. Sensitization to cyanocobalamin can take as long as 8 y to develop.
- Monitor vital signs in patients with cardiac disease and in those receiving parenteral cyanocobalamin, and be alert to symptoms of pulmonary edema, which generally occur early in therapy.
- Characteristically, reticulocyte concentration rises in 3–4 days, peaks in 5–8 days, and then gradually declines as erythrocyte count and Hgb rise to normal levels (in 4–6 wk).
- Obtain a complete diet and drug history and inquire into alcohol drinking patterns for all patients receiving cyanocobalamin to identify and correct poor habits.

Patient & Family Education

- Notify physician of any intercurrent disease or infection. Increased dosage may be required.
- To prevent irreversible neurologic damage resulting from pernicious anemia, drug therapy **must be** continued throughout life.
- Rich food sources of B_{12} are nutrient-added breakfast cereals, vitamin B_{12}-fortified soy milk, organ meats, clams, oysters, egg yolk, crab, salmon, sardines, muscle meat, milk, and dairy products.

CYCLIZINE HYDROCHLORIDE

(sye′kli-zeen)

Marezine, Marzine ✤

CYCLIZINE LACTATE

Marezine Lactate, Marzine

Classifications: ANTIHISTAMINE (H_1-RECEPTOR ANTAGONIST); ANTIVERTIGO AGENT; ANTIEMETIC

Therapeutic: ANTIVERTIGO; ANTIEMETIC; ANTIHISTAMINE

Prototype: Meclizine

Pregnancy Category: B

AVAILABILITY 50 mg tablets; 50 mg/mL injection

ACTION & *THERAPEUTIC EFFECT*

Piperazine antihistamine (H_1-receptor antagonist) that exhibits CNS depression and anticholinergic, antispasmodic, local anesthetic, and antihistaminic activity. Has prominent depressant action on labyrinthine excitability and on conduction in vestibular-cerebellar pathways. *Produces marked antimotion and antiemetic effects.*

USES Chiefly for prevention and treatment of motion sickness and postoperative nausea and vomiting.

CONTRAINDICATIONS Increased intraocular pressure; asthma, closed-angle glaucoma; children younger than 6 y.

CAUTIOUS USE Narrow-angle glaucoma; prostatic hypertrophy; elderly; obstructive disease of GU or GI tracts; postoperative patients; pregnancy (category B), lactation.

ROUTE & DOSAGE

Motion Sickness

Adult: **PO** 50 mg 30 min before travel, then q4–6h prn (max: 200 mg/day) **IM** 50 mg q4–6h prn
Child: **PO** *6–12 y,* 25 mg q4–6h prn (max: 75 mg/day) **IM** *6–12 y,* 1 mg/kg t.i.d. prn (max: 75 mg/day)

Postoperative Vomiting

Adult: **IM** 50 mg 15–30 min before end of operation, may repeat q4–6h (t.i.d.) prn during first few days after surgery

ADMINISTRATION

Oral

- Give dose 30 min prior to any activity likely to cause motion sickness.

Intramuscular

- Aspirate needle carefully before injecting IM. Anaphylactic reactions following inadvertent IV injection have been reported.
- For prophylaxis of postoperative nausea and vomiting, drug usually prescribed with preoperative medication or is administered 20–30 min before expected termination of surgery.
- Store tablets in tight, light-resistant container at 15°–30° C (59°–86° F) unless otherwise directed. Store parenteral form in a cold place at 5°–10° C (41°–50° F). When parenteral solution is stored at room temperature for prolonged periods, it may become slightly yellow, but this does not indicate loss of potency.

ADVERSE EFFECTS (≥1%) **CV:** Hypotension, palpitation, tachycardia. **GI:** Anorexia, nausea, vomiting, diarrhea, or constipation, cholestatic jaundice. **CNS:** *Drowsiness,* excitement, euphoria, auditory and visual hallucinations, hyperexcitability alternating with drowsiness, convulsions, respiratory paralysis (rare). **Skin:** Urticaria, rash. **Special Senses:** *Dry mouth,* nose, and throat; blurred vision, diplopia; tinnitus. **Other:** Pain at IM injection site.

DIAGNOSTIC TEST INTERFERENCE Because cyclizine is an antihistamine, inform patient that ***skin testing*** procedures should not be scheduled for about 4 days after drug is discontinued or false-negative reactions may result.

INTERACTIONS Drug: Alcohol, BARBITURATES, CNS DEPRESSANTS (e.g., HYPNOTICS, SEDATIVES, and ANXIOLYTICS) may compound effects of cyclizine.

PHARMACOKINETICS Onset: Rapid. **Duration:** 4–6 h. **Metabolism:** Unknown.

NURSING IMPLICATIONS

Assessment & Drug Effects

- Monitor postoperative patient's vital signs closely, as cyclizine can cause hypotension.
- Monitor for and report signs of CNS stimulation (e.g., hyperexcitability, euphoria). Dose reduction or discontinuation of drug may be indicated.

Patient & Family Education

- Take cyclizine with food or a glass of milk or water to minimize GI irritation.
- Do not drive a car or engage in other potentially hazardous activities until reaction to the drug is known. Adverse effects include drowsiness and dizziness.
- Alcohol, barbiturates, narcotic analgesic, and other CNS depressants may compound sedative action.

C

CYCLOBENZAPRINE HYDROCHLORIDE Pr

(sye-kloe-ben′za-preen)

Amrix, Flexeril

Classification: SKELETAL MUSCLE RELAXANT, CENTRAL ACTING

Therapeutic: SKELETAL MUSCLE RELAXANT; ANTISPASMODIC

Pregnancy Category: B

AVAILABILITY 5 mg, 10 mg tablets; 15 mg, 30 mg extended release capsules

ACTION & *THERAPEUTIC EFFECT* Relieves skeletal muscle spasm of local origin without interfering with muscle function. Believed to act primarily within CNS at brain stem. Depresses tonic somatic motor activity, although both gamma and alpha motor neurons are affected. *Cyclobenzaprine is a skeletal muscle relaxant approved for the relief of muscle spasm associated with acute, painful musculoskeletal conditions.*

USES Short-term adjunct to rest and physical therapy for relief of muscle spasm associated with acute musculoskeletal conditions. Not effective in treatment of spasticity associated with cerebral palsy or cerebral or cord disease.

UNLABELED USES Fibromyalgia.

CONTRAINDICATIONS Acute recovery phase of MI, patients with cardiac arrhythmias, heart block or conduction disturbances, QT prolongation; CHF, hyperthyroidism; closed-angle glaucoma, increased intraocular pressure; moderate or severe hepatic impairment; MAOI therapy; cerebral palsy. Safe use in children younger than 15 y not established.

CAUTIOUS USE Prostatic hypertrophy, history of urinary retention, seizures; cardiovascular disease; mild hepatic impairment; older adults, debilitated patients; history of psychiatric illness; pregnancy (category B), lactation.

ROUTE & DOSAGE

Muscle Spasm

Adult/Adolescent (at least 15 y old): **PO** 5–10 mg t.i.d. (max: 30 mg/day) or 15–30 mg daily extended release

Geriatric: Start with 5 mg, adjust dose slowly

Mild Hepatic Impairment Dosage Adjustment

Start with 5 mg

Moderate to Severe Hepatic Impairment Dosage Adjustment

Not recommended

ADMINISTRATION

Oral

- Do not administer drug if patient is receiving an MAO inhibitor (e.g., furazolidone, isocarboxazid, pargyline, tranylcypromine).
- Do not open extended release capsules. They **must be** swallowed whole.
- Cyclobenzaprine is intended for short-term (2 or 3 wk) use.
- Store in tightly closed container, preferably at 15°–30° C (59°–86° F) unless otherwise directed by manufacturer.

ADVERSE EFFECTS (≥1%) **Body as a Whole:** Edema of tongue and face, sweating, myalgia, hepatitis, alopecia. Shares toxic potential of tricyclic antidepressants. **CV:** Tachycardia, syncope, palpitation, vasodilation, chest pain, orthostatic hypotension, dyspnea; with high doses, possibility of severe arrhythmias. **GI:** *Dry mouth*, indigestion, unpleasant taste, coated tongue, tongue discoloration, vomiting, anorexia, abdominal pain, flatulence, diarrhea, paralytic ileus. **CNS:** *Drowsiness, dizziness,* weakness, fatigue, asthenia, paresthesias, tremors, muscle twitching, insomnia, euphoria, disorientation, mania, ataxia. **Skin:** Pruritus, urticaria, skin rash. **Urogenital:** Increased or decreased libido, impotence.

INTERACTIONS Drug: Alcohol, BARBITURATES, other CNS DEPRESSANTS enhance CNS depression; potentiates anticholinergic effects of **phenothiazine** and other ANTICHOLINERGICS; MAO INHIBITORS may precipitate hypertensive crisis—use with extreme caution.

PHARMACOKINETICS Absorption: Well absorbed from GI tract with some first-pass elimination in liver. **Onset:** 1 h. **Peak:** 3–8 h. **Duration:** 12–24 h. **Distribution:** 93% protein bound. **Metabolism:** In liver to inactive metabolites. **Elimination:** Slowly in urine with some elimination in feces; may be excreted in breast milk. **Half-Life:** 1–3 days.

NURSING IMPLICATIONS

Assessment & Drug Effects

- Supervision of ambulation may be indicated, especially in the older adult because of risk of drowsiness and dizziness.
- Withhold drug and notify physician if signs of hypersensitivity (e.g., pruritus, urticaria, rash) appear.

Patient & Family Education

- Avoid driving and other potentially hazardous activities until reaction to drug is known. Adverse effects include drowsiness and dizziness.
- Avoid alcohol and other CNS depressants (unless otherwise directed by physician) because cyclobenzaprine enhances their effects.
- Dry mouth may be relieved by increasing total fluid intake (if not contraindicated).
- Keep physician informed of therapeutic effectiveness. Spasmolytic effect usually begins within 1 or 2 days and may be manifested by lessening of pain and tenderness, increase in range of motion, and ability to perform ADL.

CYCLOPENTOLATE HYDROCHLORIDE (Pr)

(sye-kloe-pen′toe-late)

Ak-Pentolate, Cyclogyl, Pentalair

Classifications: EYE PREPARATION; CYCLOPLEGIC

Therapeutic: CYCLOPLEGIC

Pregnancy Category: C

AVAILABILITY 0.5%, 1%, 2% ophth solution

ACTION & *THERAPEUTIC EFFECT* Tertiary amine antimuscarinic compound with systemic side effects and CNS toxicity. Acts by blocking response of iris sphincter muscle, and muscle of accommodation in the ciliary body to cholinergic stimulation. *Results in dilation and paralysis of accommodation of the eyes.*

USES Induction of cycloplegia or mydriasis for ophthalmic diagnostic procedures.

C

CONTRAINDICATIONS Narrow-angle glaucoma, excessively increased intraocular pressure; lactation; children with a history of epilepsy.
CAUTIOUS USE Elderly patients, brain damage (in children), Down's syndrome, spastic paralysis in children, blue-eyed individuals; infants; seizure disorders; pregnancy (category C).

ROUTE & DOSAGE

Cycloplegia or Mydriasis
Adult: **Topical** 1 drop of 1% solution in eye 40–50 min before procedure, followed by 1 drop in 5 min; may need 2% solution in patients with darkly pigmented eyes
Child: **Topical** 1 drop of 0.5–1% solution in eye 40–50 min before procedure, followed by 1 drop in 5 min; may need 2% solution in patients with darkly pigmented eyes

ADMINISTRATION

Topical
- Clarify with physician which strength (1% or 2%) should be used.
- Ask patient to remove soft contact lenses prior to installation of drops.

ADVERSE EFFECTS (≥1%) **Body as a Whole:** Flushing, fever. **CNS:** Drowsiness dysarthria, disorientation, ataxia, hallucinations, hyperkinesis, psychosis, seizures. **CV:** Sinus tachycardia, hypotension. **GI:** Dry mouth, abdominal distention in infants. **Skin:** Rash, contact urticaria. **Special Senses:** Burning, stinging, transient increases in intraocular pressure, irritation, punctate keratitis, blurred vision, hyperemia, synechiae, conjunctivitis, photophobia. **Urogenital:** Urinary retention.

INTERACTIONS Drug: May interfere with the ocular antihypertensive effects of **carbachol, pilocarpine, physostigmine.**

PHARMACOKINETICS Peak: 15–60 min. **Duration:** 24 h.

NURSING IMPLICATIONS

Assessment & Drug Effects
- Monitor cardiac status especially with preexisting heart disease.

Patient & Family Education
- Do not touch the dropper to any surface, including your skin or eyes.
- Exercise caution when driving or engaging in other potentially hazardous activities as cyclopentolate ophthalmic may cause blurred vision. If you experience blurred vision, avoid these activities.
- Protect your eyes when in bright light. Cyclopentolate ophthalmic may cause increased light sensitivity.
- Do not wear soft contact lenses when the eyedrops are being inserted.
- Report immediately any of the following: Difficulty breathing, swelling of your lips, tongue, face or hives; palpitations; and unusual behavior.

CYCLOPHOSPHAMIDE Pr

(sye-kloe-foss'fa-mide)
Cytoxan, Neosar, Procytox ♣
Classifications: ANTINEOPLASTIC; ALKYLATING AGENT
Therapeutic: ANTINEOPLASTIC
Pregnancy Category: D

AVAILABILITY 25 mg, 50 mg tablets; 100 mg, 200 mg, 500 mg, 1 g, 2 g vials

C

ACTION & *THERAPEUTIC EFFECT*
Cell-cycle–nonspecific alkylating agent chemically related to the nitrogen mustards that causes cross-linkage of DNA strands, thereby blocking synthesis of DNA, RNA, and protein. *Has pronounced immunosuppressive activity and antineoplastic effects.*

USES As single agent or in combination with other chemotherapeutic agents in treatment of malignant lymphoma, multiple myeloma, leukemias, mycosis fungoides (advanced disease), neuroblastoma, adenocarcinoma of ovary, carcinoma of breast, or malignant neoplasms of lung.

UNLABELED USES To prevent rejection in homotransplantation; to treat severe rheumatoid arthritis, multiple sclerosis, systemic lupus erythematosus, Wegener's granulomatosis, nephrotic syndrome.

CONTRAINDICATIONS Men and women in childbearing years; serious infections (including chickenpox, herpes zoster); live virus vaccines; myelosuppression; dehydration; lactation.

CAUTIOUS USE History of radiation or cytotoxic drug therapy; hepatic and renal impairment, elderly; recent history of steroid therapy; bone marrow infiltration with tumor cells; history of urate calculi and gout; patients with leukopenia, thrombocytopenia; pregnancy (category D).

ROUTE & DOSAGE

Neoplasm

Adult: **PO Initial** 1–5 mg/kg/day; **Maintenance** 1–5 mg/kg q7–10days **IV Initial** 40–50 mg/kg in divided doses over 2–5 days up to 100 mg/kg; **Maintenance** 10–15 mg/kg q7–10days *or* 3–5 mg twice weekly

Child: **PO Initial** 2–8 mg/kg or 60–250 mg/m²; **Maintenance** 2–5 mg/kg *or* 50–150 mg/m² twice weekly **IV Initial** 2–8 mg/kg *or* 60–250 mg/m²

Renal Impairment Dosage Adjustment

CrCl less than 10 mL/min: Give 50% of dose; administer post-dialysis, give supplemental dose of 35%

ADMINISTRATION

Oral

- Administer PO drug on empty stomach. If nausea and vomiting are severe, however, it may be taken with food. An antiemetic medication may be prescribed to be given before the drug.
- Store cyclophosphamide PO solution in refrigerator at 2°–8° C (36°–46° F) and use within 14 days.

Intravenous

PREPARE: **Direct:** Add 5 mL bacteriostatic water for injection (paraben-preserved only) to each 100 mg and shake gently to dissolve. **Intermittent:** May be further diluted with 100–250 mL D5W, NS, D5/NS, LR, or other compatible solution.

ADMINISTER: **Direct/Intermittent:** Give each 100 mg or fraction thereof over 10–15 min.

INCOMPATIBILITIES **Y-site: Amphotericin B cholesteryl complex, lansoprazole.**

- Store at temperature between 2° and 30° C (36° and 86° F) unless otherwise recommended by the manufacturer.

ADVERSE EFFECTS (≥1%) **Body as a Whole:** Transient dizziness, fatigue, facial flushing, diaphoresis, drug fever, anaphylaxis, secondary neoplasia. **GI:** *Nausea, vomiting,* mucositis, *anorexia,* hepatotoxicity, diarrhea. **Hematologic:** Leukopenia, *neutropenia,* acute myeloid leukemia, anemia, thrombophlebitis, interference with normal healing. **Metabolic:** Severe hyperkalemia, SIADH, hyponatremia, weight gain (but without edema) or weight loss, hyperuricemia. **Respiratory:** Pulmonary emboli and edema, pneumonitis, interstitial pulmonary fibrosis. **Skin:** *Alopecia* (reversible), transverse ridging of nails, pigmentation of nail beds and skin (reversible), nonspecific dermatitis, toxic epidermal necrolysis, Stevens-Johnson syndrome. **Urogenital:** Sterile hemorrhagic and nonhemorrhagic cystitis, bladder fibrosis, nephrotoxicity.

DIAGNOSTIC TEST INTERFERENCE Cyclophosphamide suppresses positive reactions to **Candida,** ***mumps, trichophytons,*** and ***tuberculin PPD skin tests. Papanicolaou (PAP)*** smear may be falsely positive.

INTERACTIONS Drug: Succinylcholine, prolonged neuromuscular blocking activity; **doxorubicin** may increase cardiac toxicity.

PHARMACOKINETICS Absorption: Readily from GI tract. **Peak:** 1 h PO. **Distribution:** Widely distributed, including brain, breast milk; crosses placenta. **Metabolism:** In liver by CYP3A4. **Elimination:** In urine as active metabolites and unchanged drug. **Half-Life:** 4–6 h.

NURSING IMPLICATIONS

Assessment & Drug Effects

- Lab tests: Total and differential leukocyte count, platelet count, and Hct are determined initially and at least 2 times per week during maintenance period. Baseline and periodic determinations of liver and kidney function and serum electrolytes also should be made. Microscopic urine examinations are recommended after large IV doses.
- Thrombocytopenia is rare, but if it occurs (count of 100,000/mm³ or lower), assess for signs of unexplained bleeding or easy bruising. If platelet count indicates thrombocytopenia (100,000/mm³ or less), drug will be discontinued.
- Marked leukopenia is the most serious side effect. It can be fatal. Nadir may occur in 2–8 days after first dose but may be as late as 1 mo after a series of several daily doses. Leukopenia usually reverses 7–10 days after therapy is discontinued.
- During severe leukopenic period, protect patient from infection and trauma and from visitors and medical personnel who have colds or other infections.
- Report onset of unexplained chills, sore throat, tachycardia. Monitor temperature carefully and report an elevation immediately. The development of fever in a neutropenic patient (granulocyte count less than 1000) is a medical emergency because sepsis can develop quickly in these patients.
- Observe and report character of wound drainage. During period of neutropenia, purulent drainage may become serosanguineous because there are not enough WBC to create pus. Because of suppressed immune mechanisms, wound healing may be prolonged or incomplete.
- Monitor I&O ratio and patterns: Since the drug is a chemical irritant, PO and IV fluid intake is generally increased to help prevent renal irritation and hemorrhagic cystitis. Have patient void fre-

C

quently, especially after each dose and just before retiring to bed.
- Watch for symptoms of water intoxication or dilutional hyponatremia; patients are usually well hydrated as part of the therapy.
- Promptly report hematuria or dysuria. Drug schedule is usually interrupted and fluids are forced.
- Record body weight at least twice weekly (basis for dose determination). Alert physician to sudden change or slow, steady weight gain or loss over a period of time that appears inconsistent with caloric intake.
- Diarrhea may signal onset of hyperkalemia, particularly if accompanied by colicky pain, nausea, bradycardia, and skeletal muscle weakness. These symptoms warrant prompt reporting to physician.
- Monitor for hyperuricemia, which occurs commonly during early treatment period in patients with leukemias or lymphoma. Report edema of lower legs and feet; joint, flank, or stomach pain.
- Protect patient from potential sources of infection. Cyclophosphamide makes the patient particularly susceptible to varicella-zoster infections (chickenpox, herpes zoster).
- Report any sign of overgrowth with opportunistic organisms, especially in patient receiving corticosteroids or who has recently been on steroid therapy.
- Report fever, dyspnea, and nonproductive cough. Pulmonary toxicity is not common, but the already debilitated patient is particularly susceptible.

Patient & Family Education
- Adhere to dosage regimen and do not omit, increase, decrease, or delay doses. If for any reason drug cannot be taken, notify physician.
- Alopecia occurs in about 33% of patients on cyclophosphamide therapy. Hair loss may be noted 3 wk after therapy begins; regrowth (often differs in texture and color) usually starts 5–6 wk after drug is withdrawn and may occur while on maintenance doses.
- Use adequate means of contraception during and for at least 4 mo after termination of drug treatment. Breast-feeding should be discontinued before cyclophosphamide therapy is initiated.
- Amenorrhea may last up to 1 y after cessation of therapy in 10–30% of women.

CYCLOSERINE
(sye-kloe-ser'een)
Seromycin
Classification: ANTITUBERCULOSIS AGENT
Therapeutic: ANTITUBERCULOSIS
Pregnancy Category: C

AVAILABILITY 250 mg capsules

ACTION & *THERAPEUTIC EFFECT* Broad-spectrum anti-infective that inhibits cell wall synthesis in susceptible strains. It competitively interferes with the incorporation of D-alanine into the bacterial cell wall, resulting in cell death. *Effective against gram-positive and gram-negative bacteria and* Mycobacterium tuberculosis.

USES In conjunction with other tuberculostatic drugs in treatment of active pulmonary and extrapulmonary tuberculosis when primary agents have failed. Also used in treatment of acute UTI unresponsive to conventional treatment.

UNLABELED USES Treatment of tuberculosis meningitis and nocardiosis.

CONTRAINDICATIONS Epilepsy; depression, severe anxiety, history of psychoses; severe renal insufficiency; chronic alcoholism. Safe use in children not established.

CAUTIOUS USE Renal impairment, lactation; anemia; pregnancy (category C).

ROUTE & DOSAGE

Tuberculosis

Adult: **PO** 250 mg q12h for 2 wk, may increase to 500 mg q12h (max: 1 g/day)

Urinary Tract Infection

Adult: **PO** 250 mg q12h for 2 wk

ADMINISTRATION

Oral

- Pyridoxine 200–300 mg/day may be ordered concurrently to prevent neurotoxic effects of cycloserine.
- Store in tightly closed container at 15°–30° C (59°–86° F) unless otherwise directed.

ADVERSE EFFECTS (≥1%) **CV:** Arrhythmias, CHF. **Hematologic:** Vitamin B_{12} and folic acid deficiency, megaloblastic or sideroblastic anemia. **CNS:** *Drowsiness,* anxiety, *headache,* tremors, myoclonic jerking, convulsions, vertigo, visual disturbances, speech difficulties (dysarthria), lethargy, depression, disorientation with loss of memory, confusion, nervousness, psychoses, tic episodes, character changes, hyperirritability, aggression, hyperreflexia, peripheral neuropathy, paresthesias, paresis, dyskinesias. **Skin:** Dermatitis, photosensitivity. **Special Senses:** Eye pain (optic neuritis), photophobia.

INTERACTIONS Drug: Alcohol increases risk of seizures; **ethionamide, isoniazid** potentiate neurotoxic effects; may inhibit **phenytoin** metabolism, increasing its toxicity.

PHARMACOKINETICS Absorption: 70–90% from GI tract. **Peak:** 3–4 h. **Distribution:** Distributed to lung, ascitic, pleural and synovial fluids, and CSF; crosses placenta; distributed into breast milk. **Metabolism:** Not metabolized. **Elimination:** 60–70% in urine within 72 h; small amount in feces. **Half-Life:** 10 h.

NURSING IMPLICATIONS

Assessment & Drug Effects

- Lab tests: Culture and susceptibility tests should be performed before initiation of therapy and periodically thereafter to detect possible bacterial resistance. Monitor plasma drug levels weekly and hematologic, renal, and hepatic function at regular intervals.
- Maintenance of blood-drug level below 30 mg/mL considerably reduces incidence of neurotoxicity. Possibility of neurotoxicity increases when dose is 500 mg or more or when renal clearance is inadequate.
- Observe patient carefully for signs of hypersensitivity and neurologic effects. Neurotoxicity generally appears within first 2 wk of therapy and disappears after drug is discontinued.
- Drug should be withheld and physician notified or dosage reduced if symptoms of CNS toxicity or hypersensitivity reaction (see Appendix F) develop.

C

Patient & Family Education

- Take cycloserine after meals to prevent GI irritation.
- Notify physician immediately of the onset of skin rash and early signs of CNS toxicity (see Appendix F).
- Avoid potentially hazardous tasks such as driving until reaction to cycloserine has been determined.
- Take drug precisely as prescribed and to keep follow-up appointments. Continuous therapy may extend into months or years.

CYCLOSPORINE (Pr)

(sye'kloe-spor-een)

Gengraf, Neoral, Sandimmune, Restasis

Classifications: BIOLOGICAL RESPONSE MODIFIER; IMMUNOSUPPRESSANT

Therapeutic: IMMUNOSUPPRESSANT; ANTIRHEUMATIC; ANTIPSORIATIC

Pregnancy Category: C

AVAILABILITY Sandimmune: 25 mg, 50 mg, 100 mg capsules; 100 mg/mL oral solution; **Gengraf, Neoral:** (Microemulsion) 25 mg, 100 mg capsules; 100 mg/mL oral solution; 50 mg/mL injection; **Restasis:** 0.05% ophth emulsion

ACTION & *THERAPEUTIC EFFECT* Has immunosuppressant action by reducing transplant rejection due to selective and reversible inhibition of the first phase of T-cell activation with T-lymphocytes (which normally stimulate antibody production). *It is used to prevent allograft rejection in transplant patients. Additionally, it is a disease-modifying antirheumatic drug (DMARD).*

USES In conjunction with adrenal corticosteroids to prevent organ rejection after kidney, liver, and heart transplants (allografts). Has had limited use in pancreas, bone marrow, and heart/lung transplantations. Also used for treatment of chronic transplant rejection in patients previously treated with other immunosuppressants; rheumatoid arthritis, severe psoriasis. Ophthalmic emulsion for the treatment of keratoconjunctivitis sicca.

UNLABELED USES Sjögren's syndrome, to prevent rejection of heart-lung and pancreatic transplants, ulcerative colitis.

CONTRAINDICATIONS Hypersensitivity to cyclosporine; recent contact with or bout of chickenpox, herpes zoster; administration of live virus vaccines to patient or family members; **Gengraf** and **Neoral** in psoriasis or RA patients with abnormal renal function, uncontrolled hypertension, or malignancies; ocular infection, **PO form:** Lactation.

CAUTIOUS USE Renal, hepatic, pancreatic, or bowel dysfunction; biliary tract disease, jaundice, hyperkalemia; electrolyte imbalance, hyperuricemia, hypertension; infection; radiation therapy, older adults, encephalopathy, females of childbearing age, fungal or viral infection, gout, herpes infection, lymphoma; neoplastic disease, malabsorption problems (e.g., liver transplant patients); pregnancy (category C).

ROUTE & DOSAGE

Prevention of Organ Rejection

Adult/Child: **PO** 14–18 mg/kg beginning 4–12 h before transplantation and continued for 1–2 wk after surgery, then gradual reduction by 5%/wk, max dose of microemulsion: 10 mg/kg/day; **Maintenance** 5–10 mg/kg/day **IV** 5–6 mg/kg beginning 4–12 h before transplantation and continued after surgery until patient can take orally

Rheumatoid Arthritis (Neoral)
Adult: **PO** 2.5 mg/kg/day divided into 2 doses. May increase by 0.5–0.75 mg/kg/day q4wk to a max of 4 mg/kg/day.

Severe Psoriasis (Neoral)
Adult: **PO** 1.25 mg/kg b.i.d. If significant improvement has not occurred after 4 wk, may increase dose by 0.5 mg/kg/day every 2 wk to max of 4 mg/kg/day.

Keratoconjunctivitis Sicca
Adult: **Ophthalmic** 1 drop in affected eye(s) twice daily approximately 12 h apart

ADMINISTRATION

Oral

- Do not dilute oral solution with grapefruit juice. Dilute with orange or apple juice, stir well, then administer immediately.
- The various product brands may not be bioequivalent on a mg for mg basis. Do not interchange without physician supervision.

Intravenous

PREPARE: **IV Infusion:** Dilute each 1 mL immediately before administration in 20–100 mL of D5W or NS.
ADMINISTER: **IV Infusion:** Give by slow infusion over approximately 2–6 h. ▪ Rapid IV can result in nephrotoxicity.

INCOMPATIBILITIES **Solution/additive: Magnesium sulfate. Y-site: Amphotericin B cholesteryl complex, TPN.**

▪ Store preferably at 15°–30° C (59°–86° F) in well-closed containers. Do not refrigerate. ▪ Protect ampules from light.

ADVERSE EFFECTS (≥1%) **Body as a Whole:** Lymphoma, gynecomastia, chest pain, leg cramps, edema, fever, chills, weight loss, increased risk of skin malignancies in psoriasis patients previously treated with methotrexate, psoralens, or UV light therapy. **CV:** *Hypertension,* MI (rare). **GI:** Gingival hyperplasia, diarrhea, nausea, *vomiting,* abdominal discomfort, anorexia, gastritis, constipation. **Hematologic:** Leukopenia, anemia, thrombocytopenia, *hypermagnesemia, hyperkalemia,* hyperuricemia, *decreased serum bicarbonate,* hyperglycemia. **CNS:** *Tremor,* convulsions, headache, paresthesias, hyperesthesia, flushing, night sweats, insomnia, visual hallucinations, confusion, anxiety, flat affect, depression, lethargy, weakness, paraparesis, ataxia, amnesia. **Skin:** *Hirsutism,* acne, oily skin, flushing. **Special Senses:** Sinusitis, tinnitus, hearing loss, sore throat. **Urogenital:** Urinary retention, frequency, *nephrotoxicity (oliguria).*

DIAGNOSTIC TEST INTERFERENCE ***Hyperlipidemia*** and abnormalities in ***electrophoresis*** reported; believed to be due to polyoxyl 35 castor oil (Cremophor) in IV cyclosporine.

INTERACTIONS Drug: AMINOGLYCOSIDES, **danazol, diltiazem, doxycycline, erythromycin, ketoconazole, methylprednisolone, metoclopramide, nicardipine,**

NSAIDS, **prednisolone, verapamil** may increase cyclosporine levels; **carbamazepine, isoniazid, octreotide, phenobarbital, phenytoin, rifampin** may decrease cyclosporine levels; **acyclovir,** AMINOGLYCOSIDES, **amphotericin B, cimetidine, erythromycin, ketoconazole, melphalan, ranitidine, cotrimoxazole, trimethoprim** may increase risk of nephrotoxicity; POTASSIUM-SPARING DIURETICS, ACE INHIBITORS **(captopril, enalapril)** may potentiate hyperkalemia. **Food: Grapefruit juice** may increase concentration. **Herbal: St. John's wort** may decrease cyclosporine levels; **berberine** may increase toxicities.

PHARMACOKINETICS Absorption: Variably and incompletely absorbed (30%). Microemulsion formulation (Neoral) has less variability and may produce significantly higher serum levels compared with the standard formulation. **Peak:** 3–4 h. **Distribution:** Widely distributed; 33–47% distributed to plasma; 41–50% to RBCs; crosses placenta; distributed into breast milk. **Metabolism:** In liver by CYP3A4, including significant first pass metabolism; considerable enterohepatic circulation. **Elimination:** Primarily in bile and feces; 6% in urine. **Half-Life:** 19–27 h.

NURSING IMPLICATIONS

Assessment & Drug Effects

- Observe patients receiving the drug parenterally for at least 30 min continuously after start of IV infusion, and at frequent intervals thereafter to detect allergic or other adverse reactions.
- Monitor I&O ratio and pattern: Nephrotoxicity has been reported in about one third of transplant patients. It has occurred in mild forms as late as 2–3 mo after transplantation. In severe form, it can be irreversible, and therefore early recognition is critical.
- Monitor vital signs. Be alert to indicators of local or systemic infection that can be fungal, viral, or bacterial. Also report significant rise in BP.
- Lab tests: Baseline and periodic tests are advised for (1) renal function (BUN, serum creatinine), (2) liver function (AST, ALT, serum amylase, bilirubin, and alkaline phosphatase), and (3) serum potassium.
- Lab tests: In psoriasis patients, CBC, BUN, uric acid, potassium, lipids, and magnesium should be monitored biweekly during first 3 mo.
- Periodic tests should be made of neurologic function. Neurotoxic effects generally occur over 13–195 days after initiation of cyclosporine therapy. Signs and symptoms are reportedly fully reversible with dosage reduction or discontinuation of drug.
- Monitor blood or plasma drug concentrations at regular intervals, particularly in patients receiving the drug orally for prolonged periods, as drug absorption is erratic.

Patient & Family Education

- Take medication with meals to reduce nausea or GI irritation.
- Enhance palatability of oral solution by mixing it with milk, chocolate milk, or orange juice, preferably at room temperature. Mix in a glass rather than a plastic container. Stir well, drink immediately, and rinse glass with small quantity of diluent to assure getting entire dose.
- Take medication at same time each day to maintain therapeutic blood levels.

- Practice good oral hygiene. Inspect mouth daily for white patches, sores, swollen gums.
- Hirsutism is reversible with discontinuation of drug.

CYPROHEPTADINE HYDROCHLORIDE

(si-proe-hep'ta-deen)

Periactin, Vimicon ✤

Classifications: ANTIHISTAMINE (H_1-RECEPTOR ANTAGONIST); ANTIPRURITIC

Therapeutic: ANTIHISTAMINE

Prototype: Diphenhydramine

Pregnancy Category: B

AVAILABILITY 4 mg tablets

ACTION & *THERAPEUTIC EFFECT* Potent piperidine antihistamine with pharmacologic actions that acts by competing with histamine for H_1-receptor sites, thus preventing histamine-mediated responses. *Has significant antipruritic, local anesthetic, and antiserotonin activity.*

USES Symptomatic relief of various allergic conditions, including hay fever, vasomotor rhinitis, allergic conjunctivitis, urticaria caused by cold sensitivity, and pruritus of allergic dermatoses. Effective in treatment of anaphylactoid reactions as adjunct to epinephrine and other standard measures after acute symptoms have been controlled.

UNLABELED USES Cushing's disease, carcinoid syndrome, vascular headaches, appetite stimulant.

CONTRAINDICATIONS Hypersensitivity to cyproheptadine or other H_1-receptor antagonist antihistamines; acute asthma attack; newborns, premature infants, lactation. Safe use in children younger than 2 y not established.

CAUTIOUS USE Older adult and debilitated patients; patients predisposed to urinary retention; glaucoma; asthma; COPD; hyperthyroidism; cardiovascular or hepatic disease, hypertension; GI or GU tract obstruction, children with a family history of SIDS; pregnancy (category B), children.

ROUTE & DOSAGE

Allergies

Adult: **PO** 4 mg t.i.d. or q.i.d. (4–20 mg/day), max: 0.5 mg/kg/day

Geriatric: **PO** Start with 4 mg b.i.d.

Child: **PO** 0.25 mg/kg/day in 3–4 divided doses (max: 12 mg/day for 2–6 y, 16 mg/day for 6–12 y)

ADMINISTRATION

Oral

- GI adverse effects may be minimized by administering drug with food or milk.
- Store in tightly covered container at 15°–30° C (59°–86° F) unless otherwise directed.

ADVERSE EFFECTS (≥1%) **GI:** *Dry mouth,* nausea, vomiting, epigastric distress, appetite stimulation, weight gain, transient decrease in fasting blood sugar level, increased serum amylase level, cholestatic jaundice. **CNS:** *Drowsiness,* dizziness, faintness, headache, tremulousness, fatigue, disturbed coordination. **Respiratory:** Thickened bronchial secretions.

Skin: Skin rash. **Special Senses:** Dry nose and throat. **Urogenital:** Urinary frequency, retention, and difficult urination.

DIAGNOSTIC TEST INTERFERENCE As a general rule, antihistamines are discontinued about 4 days before ***skin testing procedures*** are to be performed because they may produce false-negative results.

INTERACTIONS Drug: Alcohol and CNS DEPRESSANTS add to CNS depression; TRICYCLIC ANTIDEPRESSANTS and other ANTICHOLINERGICS have additive anticholinergic effects; may inhibit pressor effects of **epinephrine.**

PHARMACOKINETICS Absorption: Readily absorbed from GI tract. **Duration:** 6–9 h. **Distribution:** Distribution into breast milk not known. **Metabolism:** In liver. **Elimination:** In urine.

NURSING IMPLICATIONS

Assessment & Drug Effects

- Monitor level of alertness. In some patients, the sedative effect disappears spontaneously after 3–4 days of drug administration.
- Since drug may cause dizziness, supervision of ambulation and other safety precautions may be warranted.

Patient & Family Education

- Avoid activities requiring mental alertness and physical coordination, such as driving a car, until reaction to the drug is known.
- Drug causes sedation, dizziness, and hypotension in older adults. Report these symptoms. Children are more apt to manifest CNS stimulation (e.g., confusion, agitation, tremors, hallucinations). Reduction in dosage may be indicated.
- Cyproheptadine may increase and prolong the effects of alcohol, barbiturates, narcotic analgesics, and other CNS depressants.
- Maintain sufficient fluid intake to help to relieve dry mouth and also reduce risk of cholestatic jaundice.

CYTARABINE

(sye-tare′a-been)

Cytosar-U, DepoCyt

Classifications: ANTINEOPLASTIC; ANTIMETABOLITE, PURINE ANTAGONIST

Therapeutic: ANTINEOPLASTIC

Prototype: 6-Mercaptopurine

Pregnancy Category: D

AVAILABILITY 10 mg/mL liposomal, 20 mg/mL, 100 mg, 500 mg, 1 g, 2 g injection

ACTION & *THERAPEUTIC EFFECT* Pyrimidine analog with cell phase specificity affecting rapidly dividing cells in S phase (DNA synthesis). In certain conditions prevents development of cell from G_1 to S phase. Interferes with DNA and RNA synthesis in rapidly growing cells. *Antineoplastic agent which has strong myelosuppressant activity. Immunosuppressant properties are exhibited by obliterated cell-mediated immune responses, such as delayed hypersensitivity skin reactions.*

USES To induce and maintain remission in acute myelocytic leukemia, acute lymphocytic leukemia, and meningeal leukemia and for treatment of lymphomas. Used in combination with other antineoplastics in established chemotherapeutic protocols.

CONTRAINDICATIONS History of drug-induced myelosuppression; immunization procedures; active meningeal infection (**liposomal cy-**

tarabine); pregnancy (category D) particularly during first trimester, lactation. Safe use in infants not established.

CAUTIOUS USE Impaired renal or hepatic function, elderly; neurologic disease; gout, drug-induced myelosuppression.

ROUTE & DOSAGE

Leukemias

Adult/Child: **IV** 100–200 mg/m² by continuous infusion over 24 h **Subcutaneous** 1 mg/kg 1–2 times/wk **Intrathecal** 5–75 mg once q4days or once/day for 4 days

Renal Impairment Dosage Adjustment

Serum Cr of 1.5–1.9 mg/dL (or from baseline of 0.5–1.2 mg/dL): Reduce to 1 g/m²/dose.
Serum Cr of 2 or more (or greater than 1.2 mg/dL change): Do not exceed 100 mg/m²/day.

ADMINISTRATION

Intrathecal

- For intrathecal injection, reconstitute with an isotonic, buffered diluent without preservatives. Follow manufacturer's recommendations.

Intravenous

PREPARE: **Direct:** Reconstitute with bacteriostatic water for injection (without benzyl alcohol for neonates) as follows: Add 5 mL to the 100-mg vial to yield 20 mg/mL; add 10 mL to the 500 mg vial to yield 50 mg/mL. **IV Infusion:** May be further diluted with 100 mL or more of D5W or NS.

ADMINISTER: **Direct:** Give at a rate of 100 mg or a fraction thereof over 3 min. **IV Infusion:** Give over 30 min or longer depending on the total volume of IV solution to be infused.

INCOMPATIBILITIES **Solution/additive: Fluorouracil, gentamicin, heparin, hydrocortisone, insulin, nafcillin, oxacillin, penicillin G. Y-site: Allopurinol, amphotericin B cholesteryl sulfate complex, gallium, ganciclovir, lansoprazole, TPN.**

- Store cytarabine in refrigerator until reconstituted. - Reconstituted solutions may be stored at 15°–30° C (59°–86° F) for 48 h. Discard solutions with a slight haze.

ADVERSE EFFECTS (≥1%) **Body as a Whole:** Weight loss, sore throat, fever, thrombophlebitis and pain at injection site; pericarditis, bleeding (any site), pneumonia. Potentially carcinogenic and mutagenic. **GI:** *Nausea, vomiting,* diarrhea, stomatitis, oral or anal inflammation or ulceration, esophagitis, anorexia, <u>hemorrhage</u>, hepatotoxicity, jaundice. **Hematologic:** *Leukopenia, thrombocytopenia,* anemia, megaloblastosis, myelosuppression (reversible); transient hyperuricemia. **CNS:** Headache, <u>neurotoxicity</u>; peripheral neuropathy, brachial plexus neuropathy, personality change, neuritis, vertigo, lethargy, somnolence, confusion. **Skin:** Rash, erythema, freckling, cellulitis, skin ulcerations, pruritus, urticaria, bulla formation, desquamation. **Special Senses:** Conjunctivitis, keratitis, photophobia. **Urogenital:** Renal dysfunction, urinary retention.

INTERACTIONS Drug: GI toxicity may decrease **digoxin** absorption; decreases AMINOGLYCOSIDES activity against *Klebsiella pneumoniae.*

PHARMACOKINETICS Peak: 20–60 min subcutaneous. **Distribution:** Crosses blood–brain barrier and placenta. **Metabolism:** In liver. **Elimination:** 80% in urine in 24 h. **Half-Life:** 1–3 h.

NURSING IMPLICATIONS

Assessment & Drug Effects

- Inspect patient's mouth before the administration of each dose. Toxicity necessitating dosage alterations almost always occurs. Report adverse reactions immediately.
- Lab tests: Hct and platelet counts and total and differential leukocyte counts should be evaluated daily during initial therapy. Serum uric acid and hepatic function tests should be performed at regular intervals throughout treatment period.
- Hyperuricemia due to rapid destruction of neoplastic cells may accompany cytarabine therapy. A regimen that includes a uricosuric agent such as allopurinol, urine alkalinization, and adequate hydration may be started. To reduce potential for urate stone formation, fluids are forced in excess of 2 L, if tolerated. Consult physician.
- Monitor I&O ratio and pattern.
- Monitor body temperature. Be alert to the most subtle signs of infection, especially low-grade fever, and report promptly.
- When platelet count falls below 50,000/mm^3 and polymorphonuclear leukocytes to below 1000/mm^3, therapy may be suspended. WBC nadir is usually reached in 5–7 days after therapy has been stopped. Therapy is restarted with appearance of bone marrow recovery and when preceding cell counts are reached.
- Provide good oral hygiene to diminish adverse effects and chance of superinfection. Stomatitis and cheilosis usually appear 5–10 days into the therapy.

Patient & Family Education

- Report promptly protracted vomiting or signs of nephrotoxicity (see Appendix F).
- Flu-like syndrome occurs usually within 6–12 wk after drug administration and may recur with successive therapy. Report chills, fever, achy joints and muscles.
- Practice good oral hygiene to minimize discomfort from stomatitis.
- Report any S&S of superinfection (see Appendix F).

CYTOMEGALOVIRUS IMMUNE GLOBULIN (CMVIG, CMV-IVIG)

(cy-to-meg'a-lo-vi-rus)

CytoGam

Classifications: BIOLOGICAL RESPONSE MODIFIER; IMMUNOGLOBULIN

Therapeutic: IMMUNOGLOBULIN

Prototype: Peginterferon alfa-2a

Pregnancy Category: C

AVAILABILITY 50 mg/mL injection

ACTION & *THERAPEUTIC EFFECT* Cytomegalovirus immune globulin (CMVIG) is a preparation of immunoglobulin G (IgG) antibodies with high concentrations of antibodies directed against cytomegalovirus (CMV). *The CMV antibodies attenuate or reduce the incidence of serious CMV disease, such as CMV-associated pneumonia, CMV-associated hepatitis, and concomitant fungi and parasitic superinfections.*

USES Attenuation of primary cytomegalovirus (CMV) disease associated with kidney transplantation.

UNLABELED USES Prevention of CMV disease in other organ transplants (especially heart) when the recipient is seronegative for CMV and the donor is seropositive.

CONTRAINDICATIONS History of previous severe reactions associated with CMVIG or other human immunoglobulin preparations, selective immunoglobulin A (IgA) deficiency.

CAUTIOUS USE Myelosuppression, maltose or sucrose hypersensitivity; renal insufficiency, diabetes mellitus, age older than 65, volume depletion, sepsis, paraproteinemia; cardiac disease; pregnancy (category C), lactation.

ROUTE & DOSAGE

Prevention of CMV Disease

Adult: **IV** 150 mg/kg within 72 h of transplantation, then 100 mg/kg 2, 4, 6, and 8 wk post-transplant, then 50 mg/kg 12 and 16 wk post-transplant

ADMINISTRATION

Intravenous

CMVIG should be administered through a separate IV line using an infusion pump. See manufacturer's directions if this is not possible.

PREPARE: **IV Infusion:** Use a double-ended transfer needle or large syringe to reconstitute with 50 mL sterile water. ▪ Gently rotate vial to dissolve; do not shake. Allow 30 min to dissolve powder. Reconstituted solution contains 50 mg/mL. ▪ **Must be** completely infused within 12 h since solution contains no preservative.

ADMINISTER: **IV Infusion:** Use a constant infusion pump and give at rate of 15, 30, 60 mg/kg/h over first 30 min, second 30 min, third 30 min, respectively. Monitor closely during and after each rate change. ▪ If flushing, nausea, back pain, fever, or chills develops, slow or temporarily discontinue infusion. ▪ If BP begins to decrease, stop infusion and institute emergency measures. **Infusion of Subsequent IV Doses:** The intervals for increasing the dose from 15 to 30 to 60 mg may be shortened from 30 to 15 min.
▪ Never infuse more than 75 mL/h of CMVIG.
▪ Reconstituted solution should be started within 6 h and completed within 12 h of preparation. Discard solution if cloudy.

ADVERSE EFFECTS (≥1%) **Body as a Whole:** Muscle aches, back pain, anaphylaxis (rare), fever and chills during infusion. **CV:** Hypotension, palpitations. **GI:** Nausea, vomiting, metallic taste. **CNS:** Headache, anxiety. **Respiratory:** Shortness of breath, wheezing. **Skin:** Flushing.

INTERACTIONS Drug: May interfere with the immune response to LIVE VIRUS VACCINES **(BCG, measles/mumps/rubella, live polio),** defer vaccination with live viral vaccines for approximately 3 mo after administration of CMVIG; revaccination may be necessary if these vaccines were given shortly after CMVIG.

NURSING IMPLICATIONS

Assessment & Drug Effects

- Monitor vital signs preinfusion, before increases in infusion rate, periodically during infusion, and postinfusion.
- Notify physician immediately if any of the following occur: Flushing, nausea, back pain, fall in BP, other signs of anaphylaxis.
- Emergency drugs should be available for treatment of acute anaphylactic reactions.

- Monitor for CMV-associated syndromes (e.g., leukopenia, thrombocytopenia, hepatitis, pneumonia) and for superinfections.

Patient & Family Education

- Familiarize yourself with potential adverse effects and know which to report to physician.
- Defer vaccination with live viral vaccines for 3 mo after administration of CMVIG.

DACARBAZINE

(da-kar'ba-zeen)

DTIC-Dome

Classifications: ANTINEOPLASTIC; ALKYLATING AGENT

Therapeutic: ANTINEOPLASTIC

Prototype: Cyclophosphamide

Pregnancy Category: C

AVAILABILITY 10 mg/mL injection

ACTION & *THERAPEUTIC EFFECT* Cytotoxic agent that may have alkylating properties and is cell-cycle nonspecific. Another possible mechanism may be as an antimetabolite (purine) analog. Either mechanism would interfere with DNA replication, RNA transcription, and protein synthesis in rapidly proliferating cells. *Has carcinogenic, mutagenic, and teratogenic effects.*

USES As single agent or in combination with other antineoplastics in treatment of metastatic malignant melanoma, refractory Hodgkin's disease.

UNLABELED USES Various sarcomas and malignant glucagonoma.

CONTRAINDICATIONS Hypersensitivity to dacarbazine; severe bone marrow suppression; active infection; live vaccine; lactation.

CAUTIOUS USE Hepatic or renal impairment; previous radiation or chemotherapy; pregnancy (category C).

ROUTE & DOSAGE

Neoplasms

Adult: **IV** 2–4.5 mg/kg/day for 10 days repeated at 4-wk intervals or 250 mg/m²/day for 5 days repeated at 3-wk intervals

Hodgkin's Disease

Adult: **IV** 150 mg/m²/day × 5 days; repeat at 4-wk intervals

ADMINISTRATION

Intravenous

IV administration to infants and children: Verify correct IV concentration and rate of infusion with physician.

- Wear gloves when handling this drug. If solution gets into the eyes, wash them with soap and water immediately, then irrigate with water or isotonic saline.

PREPARE: **Direct:** Reconstitute drug with sterile water for injection to make a solution containing 10 mg/mL dacarbazine (pH 3.0–4.0) by adding 9.9 mL to 100 mg or 19.7 mL to 200 mg. **IV Infusion:** Dilute further reconstituted solution in 50–250 mL of D5W or NS.

ADMINISTER: **Direct:** Give by direct IV over at least 15 min. **IV Infusion (*preferred*):** Infuse IV over 30–60 min. ▪ If possible, avoid using antecubital vein or veins on dorsum of hand or wrist where extravasation could lead to loss of mobility of entire limb. ▪ Avoid veins in extremity with compromised venous or lymphatic drainage and veins near joint spaces.

INCOMPATIBILITIES **Solution/additive:** **Allopurinol, heparin, hydrocortisone.** **Y-site:** **Allopurinol, cefepime, heparin, piperacillin/tazobactam.**

▪ Administer dacarbazine only to patients under close supervision because close observation and frequent laboratory studies are required during and after therapy. ▪ ***IV extravasation:*** Monitor injection site frequently (instruct patient to do so, if able). Give prompt attention to patient's complaint of swelling, stinging, and burning sensation around injection site. ▪ Extravasation can occur painlessly and without visual signs. Danger areas for extravasation are dorsum of hand or ankle (especially if peripheral arteriosclerosis is present), joint spaces, and previously irradiated areas. ▪ If extravasation is suspected, infusion should be stopped immediately and restarted in another vein. Report to the physician. Prompt institution of local treatment is IMPERATIVE.

▪ Store reconstituted solution up to 72 h at 4° C (39° F) or at room temperature 15°–30° C (59°–86° F) for up to 8 h. ▪ Store diluted reconstituted solution for 24 h at 4° C (39° F) or at room temperature for up to 8 h. Protect from light.

ADVERSE EFFECTS (≥1%) **Body as a Whole:** Hypersensitivity (erythematosus, urticarial rashes, hepatotoxicity, photosensitivity); facial paresthesia and flushing, flu-like syndrome, myalgia, malaise, anaphylaxis. **CNS:** Confusion, headache, seizures, blurred vision. **GI:** *Anorexia, nausea, vomiting*. **Hematologic:** <u>Severe leukopenia and thrombocytopenia</u>, mild anemia. **Skin:** Alopecia. **Other:** *Pain along injected vein*.

PHARMACOKINETICS **Distribution:** Localizes primarily in liver. **Metabolism:** In liver by CYP1A2. **Elimination:** 35–50% in urine in 6 h. **Half-Life:** 5 h.

NURSING IMPLICATIONS

Assessment & Drug Effects

- Monitor IV site carefully for extravasation; if suspected, discontinue IV immediately and notify physician.
- Note: Skin damage by dacarbazine can lead to deep necrosis requiring surgical debridement, skin grafting, and even amputation. Older adults, the very young, comatose, and debilitated patients are especially at risk. Other risk factors include establishing an IV line in a vein previously punctured several times and the use of nonplastic catheters.
- Lab tests: Monitor for hematopoietic toxicity that usually appears about 4 wk after first dose. Generally, a leukocyte count of less than 3000/mm^3 and a platelet count of less than 100,000/mm^3 require suspension or cessation of therapy.
- Avoid, if possible, all tests and treatments during platelet nadir requiring needle punctures (e.g., IM). Observe carefully and report evidence of unexplained bleeding.
- Monitor for severe nausea and vomiting (greater than 90% of patients) that begin within 1 h after drug administration and may last for as long as 12 h.
- Check patient's mouth for ulcerative stomatitis prior to the administration of each dose.

D

- Monitor I&O ratio and pattern and daily temperature. Renal impairment extends the half-life and increases danger of toxicity. Report symptoms of renal dysfunction and even a slight elevation of temperature.

Patient & Family Education

- Learn about all potential adverse drug effects.
- Report flu-like syndrome that may occur during or even a week after treatment is terminated and last 7–21 days. Symptoms frequently recur with successive treatments.
- Avoid prolonged exposure to sunlight or to ultraviolet light during treatment period and for at least 2 wk after last dose. Protect exposed skin with sunscreen lotion (SPF 15) and avoid exposure in midday.
- Report promptly the onset of blurred vision or paresthesia.

DACLIZUMAB

(dac'li-zu-mab)

Zenapax

Classifications: BIOLOGICAL RESPONSE MODIFIER; MONOCLONAL ANTIBODY; IMMUNOSUPPRESSANT; INTERLEUKIN-2 (IL-2) RECEPTOR ANTAGONIST

Therapeutic: IMMUNOSUPPRESSANT; IL-2 RECEPTOR ANTAGONIST

Pregnancy Category: C

AVAILABILITY 5 mg/mL injection

ACTION & *THERAPEUTIC EFFECT* Immunosuppressant IgG-1 monoclonal antibody produced by recombinant DNA technology. Binds to interleukin-2 (IL-2) receptor complex of lymphocytes. *Daclizumab inhibits IL-2–mediated activation of lymphocytes which is the major pathway for cellular immune rejection of allografts.*

USES Prophylaxis of acute organ rejection in renal transplant.

CONTRAINDICATIONS Hypersensitivity to daclizumab; murine protein hypersensitivity; lactation.

CAUTIOUS USE Moderate to severe renal impairment; allergies, asthma, or history of allergic responses to medications; previously administered daclizumab to the same patient; fungal or herpes infection, lymphoma, neoplastic disease; elderly; vaccination, varicella, viral infection; pregnancy (category C).

ROUTE & DOSAGE

Renal Transplant

Adult/Child (older than 11 mo): **IV** 1 mg/kg. Start first dose no more than 24 h prior to transplant; repeat q14days for 4 more doses.

ADMINISTRATION

Intravenous

PREPARE: **IV Infusion:** Add calculated amount of drug (based on patient's body weight) to 50 mL of NS. ▪ Invert infusion bag to dissolve, but do not shake. Discard if diluted solution is colored or has particulate matter.

ADMINISTER: **IV Infusion:** Infuse diluted drug over 15 min.

- Use diluted solution immediately or store at room temperature for 4 h or at 2°–8° C (36°–46° F) for 24 h. Discard after 24 h. ▪ Store unopened vials at 2°–8° C (36°–46° F) and protect from light.

ADVERSE EFFECTS (≥1%) **Body as a Whole:** Edema (general and in extremities), pain, fever, fatigue, shivering, generalized weakness, arthralgia, myalgia, hypersensitivity reactions. **CNS:** Tremor, headache, dizziness, insomnia, anxiety, depression. **CV:** Chest pain, hypertension, hypotension, tachycardia, thrombosis, bleeding. **GI:** Constipation, nausea, diarrhea, vomiting, abdominal pain, dyspepsia, abdominal distention, epigastric pain, flatulence, gastritis, hemorrhoids. **Urogenital:** Oliguria, dysuria, renal tubular necrosis, hydronephrosis, urinary tract bleeding, renal insufficiency. **Respiratory:** Dyspnea, pulmonary edema, cough, atelectasis, congestion, pharyngitis, rhinitis, hypoxia, rales, abnormal breath sounds, pleural effusion. **Skin:** Impaired wound healing, acne, pruritus, hirsutism, rash, night sweats. **Other:** Diabetes mellitus, dehydration, blurred vision.

INTERACTIONS Drug: Mycophenolate, cyclosporine may increase mortality.

PHARMACOKINETICS Duration: 120 days. **Half-Life:** 20 days (11–38 days).

NURSING IMPLICATIONS

Assessment & Drug Effects

- Monitor carefully for and immediately report S&S of opportunistic infection or anaphylactoid reaction (see Appendix F).

Patient & Family Education

- Use effective contraception before beginning daclizumab therapy, during therapy, and for 4 mo after completion of therapy.
- Avoid vaccinations during daclizumab therapy.

DACTINOMYCIN

(dak-ti-noe-mye'sin)
Cosmegen

Classifications: ANTINEOPLASTIC; ANTIBIOTIC
Therapeutic: ANTINEOPLASTIC
Prototype: Doxorubicin
Pregnancy Category: D

AVAILABILITY 0.5 mg injection

ACTION & *THERAPEUTIC EFFECT* Potent cytotoxic cell cycle nonspecific antibiotic. Complexes with DNA, thereby inhibiting DNA, RNA, and protein synthesis in actively proliferating cells. Potentiates effects of x-ray therapy and the converse also appears likely. *Has antineoplastic properties that result from inhibiting DNA and RNA synthesis.*

USES As single agent or in combination with other antineoplastics or radiation to treat Wilms' tumor, rhabdomyosarcoma, carcinoma of testes and uterus, Ewing's sarcoma, solid malignancies, gestational trophoblastic neoplasia, and sarcoma botryoides.

UNLABELED USES Malignant melanoma, Kaposi's sarcoma, osteogenic sarcoma, among others.

CONTRAINDICATIONS Acute infection; pregnancy (category D), lactation, infants younger than 6 mo.

CAUTIOUS USE Previous therapy with antineoplastics or radiation within 3–6 wk, bone marrow depression; infections; history of gout; impairment of kidney or liver function; obesity; chickenpox, herpes zoster, and other viral infections.

ROUTE & DOSAGE

Neoplasms

Adult/Adolescent/Child/Infant (older than 6 mo): **IV** 500 mcg/day for 5 days max, may repeat at 2–4 wk intervals if tolerated (if patient is obese or edematous, give 400–600 mcg/m²/day to relate dosage to lean body mass); monitor for symptoms of toxicity from overdosage

Wilms' Tumor, Childhood Rhabdomyosarcoma, Ewing's Sarcoma, Nephroblastoma

Adult/Child: **IV** 15 mcg/kg/day × 5 days with other agents

Gestational Trophoblastic Neoplasia

Adult: **IV** 12 mcg/kg/day × 5 days or 500 mcg × 2 days with other agents

Solid Tumor

Adult/Adolescent/Child/Infant (older than 6 mo): **IV** 50 mcg/kg (lower extremity) or 35 mcg/kg (upper extremity)

ADMINISTRATION

Intravenous

Use gloves and eye shield when preparing solution. If skin is contaminated, rinse with running water for 10 min; then rinse with buffered phosphate solution. ▪ If solution gets into the eyes, wash with water immediately; then irrigate with water or isotonic saline for 10 min.

PREPARE: **Direct:** Reconstitute 0.5 mg vial by adding 1.1 mL sterile water (without preservative) for injection; the resulting solution will contain approximately 0.5 mg/mL. **IV Infusion:** Further dilute reconstituted solution in 50 mL of D5W or NS for infusion.

ADMINISTER: **Direct:** Use two-needle technique for direct IV: Withdraw calculated dose from vial with one needle, change to new needle to give directly into vein without using an infusion. Give over 2–3 min. ▪ Or give directly into an infusing solution of D5W or NS, or into tubing or side arm of a running IV infusion. **IV Infusion:** Give diluted solution as a single dose over 15–30 min.

INCOMPATIBILITIES **Y-site: Filgrastim.**

▪ Store drug at 15°–30° C (59°–86° F) unless otherwise directed. Protect from heat and light.

ADVERSE EFFECTS (≥1%) **GI:** *Nausea, vomiting*, anorexia, abdominal pain, diarrhea, proctitis, GI ulceration, *stomatitis*, cheilitis, glossitis, dysphagia, hepatitis. **Hematologic:** Anemia (including aplastic anemia), agranulocytosis, *leukopenia, thrombocytopenia*, pancytopenia, reticulopenia. **Skin:** Acne, desquamation, hyperpigmentation and reactivation of erythema especially over previously irradiated areas, *alopecia* (reversible). **Other:** Malaise, fatigue, lethargy, fever, myalgia, anaphylaxis, gonadal suppression, hypocalcemia, hyperuricemia, thrombophlebitis; *necrosis, sloughing, and contractures at site of extravasation;* hepatitis, hepatomegaly.

INTERACTIONS Drug: Elevated **uric acid** level produced by dactinomycin may necessitate dose adjustment of ANTIGOUT AGENTS; effects of both dactinomycin and other MYELOSUPPRESSANTS are potentiated; effects of both **radiation** and dactinomycin are potentiated, and dactinomycin may reactivate erythema from previous radiation therapy; **vitamin K** effects (antihemorrhagic) decreased, leading to prolonged clotting time and potential hemorrhage.

PHARMACOKINETICS Distribution: Concentrated in liver, spleen, kidneys, and bone marrow; does not cross blood–brain barrier; crosses placenta. **Elimination:** 50% unchanged in bile and 10% in urine; only 30% in urine over 9 days. **Half-Life:** 36 h.

NURSING IMPLICATIONS

Assessment & Drug Effects

- Observe injection site frequently; if extravasation occurs, stop infusion immediately. Restart infusion in another vein. Report to physician. Institute prompt local treatment to prevent thrombophlebitis and necrosis.
- Monitor for severe toxic effects that occur with high frequency. Effects usually appear 2–4 days after a course of therapy is stopped and may reach maximal severity 1–2 wk following discontinuation of therapy.
- Use antiemetic drugs to control nausea and vomiting, which often occur a few hours after drug administration. Vomiting may be severe enough to require intermittent therapy. Observe patient daily for signs of drug toxicity.
- Lab tests: Frequent renal, hepatic, and bone marrow function tests are advised. Perform WBC counts daily, and platelet counts every 3 days to detect hematopoietic depression.
- Monitor temperature and inspect oral membranes daily for stomatitis.
- Monitor for stomatitis, diarrhea, and severe hematopoietic depression. These may require prompt interruption of therapy until drug toxicity subsides.
- Report onset of unexplained bleeding, jaundice, and wheezing. Also, be alert to signs of agranulocytosis (see Appendix F). Report to physician. Antibiotic therapy, protective isolation, and discontinuation of the antineoplastic are indicated.
- Observe and report symptoms of hyperuricemia (see Appendix F). Urge patient to increase fluid intake up to 3000 mL/day if allowed.

Patient & Family Education

- Note: Infertility is a possible, irreversible adverse effect of this drug.
- Learn preventative measures to minimize nausea and vomiting.
- Note: Alopecia (hair loss) is an anticipated reversible adverse effect of this drug. Seek appropriate supportive guidance.

DALTEPARIN SODIUM

(dal-tep-a′rin)

Fragmin

Pregnancy Category: B

See Appendix A-2.

DANAZOL

(da′na-zole)

Cyclomen ♣

Classification: ANDROGEN/ANABOLIC STEROID

Therapeutic: ANABOLIC STEROID

Prototype: Testosterone

Pregnancy Category: X

AVAILABILITY 50 mg, 100 mg, 200 mg capsules

ACTION & *THERAPEUTIC EFFECT*

Synthetic androgen steroid; derivative of testosterone with dose-related mild androgenic effects. Suppresses pituitary output of FSH and LH, resulting in anovulation and associated amenorrhea. *Interrupts progress and pain of endometriosis by causing atrophy and involution of both normal and ectopic endometrial tissue.*

USES Palliative treatment of endometriosis when alternative hormonal therapy is ineffective, contraindicated, or intolerable. Also used to treat fibrocystic breast disease and hereditary angioedema.

UNLABELED USES To treat precocious puberty, gynecomastia, menorrhagia, premenstrual syndrome (PMS), chronic immune thrombocytopenic purpura (ITP), autoimmune hemolytic anemia, hemophilia A and B.

CONTRAINDICATIONS Pregnancy (category X), lactation; children; undiagnosed abnormal genital bleeding; impaired renal, cardiac, or hepatic function; porphyria; vaginal bleeding.

CAUTIOUS USE Migraine headache, epilepsy; seizure disorders; history of strokes; elderly.

ROUTE & DOSAGE

Endometriosis

Adult: **PO** 400 mg b.i.d. for 3–6 mo, start during menstruation or if pregnancy test is negative, may extend to 9 mo if necessary. Do not repeat regimen

Fibrocystic Breast Disease

Adult: **PO** 100–400 mg in 2 divided doses, start during menstruation or if pregnancy test is negative

Hereditary Angioedema

Adult: **PO** 200 mg b.i.d. or t.i.d., may decrease by 50% at intervals of 1–3 mo or longer, start during menstruation or if pregnancy test is negative

ADMINISTRATION

Oral

- Start therapy during menstruation, or after a negative pregnancy test.
- Store capsules at 15°–30° C (59°–86° F) in tightly closed container.

ADVERSE EFFECTS (≥1%) **Body as a Whole:** Hypersensitivity (skin rashes, nasal congestion). **Endocrine:** Androgenic effects (acne, mild hirsutism, deepening of voice, oily skin and hair, hair loss, edema, weight gain, pitch breaks, voice weakness, decrease in breast size); hypoestrogenic effects (*hot flashes;* sweating; emotional lability; nervousness; vaginitis with itching, drying, burning, or bleeding; *amenorrhea, irregular menstrual patterns*); impairment in glucose tolerance. **CNS:** Dizziness, sleep disorders, fatigue, tremor, irritability. **Special Senses:** Conjunctival edema. **CV:** Elevated BP. **GI:** Gastroenteritis, <u>hepatic damage</u> (rare), increased LDL, decreased HDL. **Urogenital:** Decreased libido. **Musculoskeletal:** Joint lock-up, joint swelling.

INTERACTIONS Herbal: Echinacea possibility of increased hepatotoxicity.

PHARMACOKINETICS Elimination: Other pharmacokinetic information is not known. **Half-Life:** 4.5 h.

NURSING IMPLICATIONS

Assessment & Drug Effects

- Routine breast examinations should be carried out during therapy. Carcinoma of the breast should be ruled out prior to start of therapy for fibrocystic breast disease. Advise patient to report to physician if any nodule enlarges or becomes tender or hard during therapy.

- Because danazol may cause fluid retention, patients with cardiac or renal dysfunction, epilepsy, or migraine should be observed closely during therapy, as these problems could worsen. Monitor weight.
- Drug-induced edema may compress the median nerve, producing symptoms of carpal tunnel syndrome. If patient complains of wrist pain that worsens at night, paresthesias in radial palmar aspect of the hand and fingers, consult physician.
- Lab tests: Baseline and periodic liver function tests should be performed in all patients. Patients with diabetes (or history of) should have blood glucose tests.

Patient & Family Education

- Note: Pain and discomfort are usually relieved in 2 or 3 mo; the nodularity in 4–6 mo. Menses may be regular or irregular in pattern during therapy.
- Note: Drug-induced amenorrhea is reversible. Ovulation and cyclic bleeding usually return within 60–90 days after therapeutic regimen is discontinued as well as the potential for conception.
- Use a nonhormonal contraceptive during treatment because ovulation may not be suppressed until 6–8 wk after therapy is begun. If pregnancy occurs while taking this drug, contact physician immediately.
- Report voice changes promptly. Virilizing adverse effects may persist even after drug therapy is terminated.

DANTROLENE SODIUM

(dan'troe-leen)

Dantrium

Classification: DIRECT-ACTING SKELETAL MUSCLE RELAXANT
Therapeutic: SKELETAL MUSCLE RELAXANT; ANTISPASMODIC
Pregnancy Category: C

AVAILABILITY 25 mg, 50 mg, 100 mg capsules; 20 mg vial

ACTION & *THERAPEUTIC EFFECT* Hydantoin derivative with peripheral skeletal muscle relaxant action. Directly relaxes the spastic muscle by interfering with calcium ion release from sarcoplasmic reticulum within skeletal muscle. *Relief of muscle spasticity, however, may be accompanied by muscle weakness sufficient to affect overall functional capacity of the patient.*

USES Orally for the symptomatic treatment of skeletal muscle spasms secondary to spinal cord injury, stroke, cerebral palsy, multiple sclerosis. Used intravenously for the management of malignant hyperthermia. Oral dantrolene can be used prophylactically for patients with a history of malignant hyperthermia or with a family history of the disorder.

UNLABELED USES Neuroleptic malignant syndrome, exercise-induced muscle pain, and flexor spasms.

CONTRAINDICATIONS Active hepatic disease; when spasticity is necessary to sustain upright posture and balance in locomotion or to maintain increased body function; spasticity due to rheumatic disorders; lactation. Safe use in children younger than 5 y is not established.

CAUTIOUS USE Impaired cardiac or pulmonary function, muscular sclerosis; neuromuscular disease; myopathy; patients older than 35 y, especially women; pregnancy (category C).

ROUTE & DOSAGE

Relief of Spasticity

Adult: **PO** 25 mg once/day, increase to 25 mg b.i.d. to q.i.d., may increase q4–7days up to 100 mg b.i.d. to q.i.d.

Child: **PO** 0.5 mg/kg b.i.d., increase to 0.5 mg/kg t.i.d. or q.i.d., may increase by 0.5 mg/kg up to 3 mg/kg b.i.d. to q.i.d. (max: 100 mg q.i.d.)

Malignant Hyperthermia Treatment

Adult/Child: **IV** 1 mg/kg rapid direct IV push repeated prn up to a total of 10 mg/kg **PO** May be necessary to continue orally with 1–2 mg/kg q.i.d. for 1–3 days to prevent recurrence

Malignant Hyperthermia Prophylaxis

Adult: **IV** 1.5 mg/kg infusion over 1 h may be repeated

Hepatic Impairment Dosage Adjustment

Do not use in active liver disease

ADMINISTRATION

Oral

- Prepare oral suspension for a single dose, when necessary, by emptying contents of capsule(s) into fruit juice or other liquid. Shake suspension well before pouring. ▪ Avoid contamination, keep refrigerated, and use within several days, since it does not contain a preservative.

Intravenous

PREPARE: **Direct:** Dilute each 20 mg with 60 mL sterile water without preservatives. Shake until clear. **Infusion:** Large volume used for prophylaxis may be transferred to plastic (not glass) infusion bags.

ADMINISTER: **Direct:** Give by rapid direct IV push. Avoid extravasation; solution has a high pH and therefore is extremely irritating to tissue. ▪ Ensure IV patency prior to giving drug direct IV. **Infusion:** Give over 1 h.

- Store capsules in tightly closed, light-resistant container. Contents of vial (for IV use) **must be** protected from direct light and used within 6 h after reconstitution, since it does not contain a preservative. ▪ Store both PO and parenteral forms at 15°–30° C (59°–86° F) unless otherwise directed.

ADVERSE EFFECTS (≥1%) **Body as a Whole:** Hypersensitivity (pruritus, urticaria, eczematoid skin eruption, photosensitivity, eosinophilic pleural effusion). **CNS:** Drowsiness, *muscle weakness,* dizziness, lightheadedness, unusual fatigue, speech disturbances, headache, confusion, nervousness, mental depression, insomnia, euphoria, seizures. **CV:** Tachycardia, erratic BP. **Special Senses:** Blurred vision, diplopia, photophobia. **GI:** *Diarrhea,* constipation, nausea, vomiting, anorexia, swallowing difficulty, alterations of taste, gastric irritation, abdominal cramps, GI bleeding; hepatitis, jaundice, hepatomegaly, <u>hepatic necrosis</u> (all related to prolonged use of high doses). **Urogenital:** Crystalluria with pain or burning with urination, urinary frequency, urinary retention, nocturia, enuresis, difficult erection.

INTERACTIONS Drug: Alcohol and other CNS DEPRESSANTS compound CNS depression; **estrogens** increase risk of hepatotoxicity in women older than 35 y; **verapamil** and other CALCIUM CHANNEL BLOCKERS increase risk of ventricular fibrillation and cardiovascular collapse with IV dantrolene.

PHARMACOKINETICS Absorption: Incompletely absorbed from GI tract. **Peak:** 5 h. **Distribution:** Crosses placenta. **Metabolism:** In liver. **Elimination:** In urine chiefly as metabolites. **Half-Life:** 8.7 h.

NURSING IMPLICATIONS

Assessment & Drug Effects

- Monitor for therapeutic effectiveness. Improvement may not be apparent until 1 wk or more of drug therapy.
- Monitor vital signs during IV infusion. Also monitor ECG, CVP, and serum potassium.
- Supervise ambulation until patient's reaction to drug is known. Relief of spasticity may be accompanied by some loss of strength.
- Note: Most common adverse effects are generally transient, lasting up to 14 days after initiation of therapy. Keep physician informed.
- Monitor patients with impaired cardiac or pulmonary function closely for cardiovascular or respiratory symptoms such as tachycardia, BP changes, feeling of suffocation.
- Monitor for and report symptoms of allergy and allergic pleural effusion: Shortness of breath, pleuritic pain, dry cough.
- Alert physician if improvement is not evident within 45 days. Drug may be discontinued because of the possibility of hepatotoxicity (see Appendix F).
- Lab tests: Perform baseline and regularly scheduled hepatic function tests (alkaline phosphatase, AST, ALT, total bilirubin), blood cell counts, and renal function tests.
- Monitor bowel function. Persistent diarrhea may necessitate drug withdrawal. Severe constipation with abdominal distention and signs of intestinal obstruction have been reported.

Patient & Family Education

- Report promptly the onset of jaundice: Yellow skin or sclerae; dark urine, clay-colored stools, itching, abdominal discomfort. Hepatotoxicity frequently occurs between 3rd and 12th mo of therapy.
- Do not drive or engage in other potentially hazardous activities until response to drug is known.
- Do not use OTC medications, alcoholic beverages, or other CNS depressants unless otherwise advised by physician. Liver toxicity occurs more commonly when other drugs are taken concurrently.

DAPSONE (Pr)

(dap′sone)

Aczone, Avlosulfon ✦, DDS

Classification: ANTILEPROSY (SULFONE)

Therapeutic: ANTILEPROSY

Pregnancy Category: C

AVAILABILITY 25 mg, 100 mg tablets; 5% gel

ACTION & *THERAPEUTIC EFFECT* Sulfone derivative chemically related to sulfonamides, with bacteriostatic and bactericidal activity similar to that group. Interferes with bacterial cell growth by competitive inhibition of folic acid synthesis by susceptible organisms. It also interferes with alternative pathways of complement system. *Drug is effective against dapsone-sensitive multibacillary (borderline, borderline lepromatous, or* *lepromatous) leprosy, and dapsone-sensitive paucibacillary (indeterminate, tuberculoid, or borderline tuberculoid) leprosy.* ***Gel form*** *is effective against acne vulgaris.*

USES Drug of choice for treatment of all forms of leprosy (unless organism is dapsone resistant). Used in dapsone-sensitive multibacillary leprosy (with clofazimine and rifampin) and in dapsone-sensitive paucibacillary leprosy (with rifampin, clofazimine, or ethionamide). Also used prophylactically in contacts of patients with all forms of leprosy except tuberculoid and indeterminate leprosy. Used for treatment of dermatitis herpetiformis. Gel used for acne vulgaris.

UNLABELED USES Chemoprophylaxis of malaria (with pyrimethamine), systemic and discoid lupus erythematosus, pemphigus vulgaris, dermatosis (especially those associated with bullous eruptions, mucocutaneous lesions, inflammation or pustules); rheumatoid arthritis, allergic vasculitis; treatment of initial episodes of *P. carinii* pneumonia (with trimethoprim) in limited number of adults with AIDS.

CONTRAINDICATIONS Hypersensitivity to sulfones or its derivatives; advanced renal amyloidosis, anemia, methemoglobin reductase deficiency.

CAUTIOUS USE Sulfonamide hypersensitivity; chronic renal, hepatic, pulmonary, or cardiovascular disease, refractory anemias, albuminuria, G6PD deficiency; pregnancy (category C), lactation.

ROUTE & DOSAGE

Tuberculoid and Indeterminate-Type Leprosy
Adult: **PO** 100 mg/day (with 6 mo of rifampin 600 mg/day) for a minimum of 3 y

Lepromatous and Borderline Lepromatous Leprosy
Adult: **PO** 100 mg/day for 10 y or more
Child: **PO** 1–2 mg/kg/day once daily in combination therapy (max: 100 mg/day)

Dermatitis Herpetiformis
Adult: **PO** 50 mg/day, may be increased to 300 mg/day if necessary (max: 500 mg/day)

Prophylaxis for Close Contacts of Patient with Multibacillary Leprosy
Adult: **PO** 50 mg/day
Child: **PO** *Younger than 6 mo,* 6 mg 3 times/wk; *6–23 mo,* 12 mg 3 times/wk; *2–5 y,* 25 mg 3 times/wk; *6–12 y,* 25 mg/day

***P. carinii* Pneumonia Prophylaxis**
Adult: **PO** 50 mg b.i.d. or 100 mg daily
Child: **PO** 2 mg/kg once daily (max: 100 mg/day)

Acne
Apply pea-sized amount of gel to affected area b.i.d.

ADMINISTRATION

Oral

- Give with food to reduce possibility of GI distress.
- Store in tightly covered, light-resistant containers at 15°–30° C (59°–86° F). Drug discoloration apparently does not indicate a chemical change.

Topical

- Clean skin with soap and water before application.

ADVERSE EFFECTS (≥1%) **Body as a Whole:** Hypersensitivity (cutaneous reactions); erythema multiforme, exfoliative dermatitis, toxic epidermal necrolysis (rare), allergic rhinitis, urticaria, fever, infectious mononucleosis-like syndrome. **CNS:** Headache, nervousness, insomnia, vertigo; paresthesia, *muscle weakness.* **CV:** Tachycardia. **GI:** Anorexia, nausea, vomiting, abdominal pain; toxic hepatitis, cholestatic jaundice (reversible with discontinuation of drug therapy); increased ALT, AST, LDH; hyperbilirubinemia. **Hematologic:** In patient with or without G6PD deficiency; *dose-related hemolysis,* Heinz body formation, *methemoglobinemia with cyanosis,* hemolytic anemia; aplastic anemia (rare), agranulocytosis. **Skin:** Drug-induced lupus erythematosus, phototoxicity. **Special Senses:** Blurred vision, tinnitus. **Other:** Male infertility; sulfone syndrome (fever, malaise, exfoliative dermatitis, hepatic necrosis with jaundice, lymphadenopathy, methemoglobinemia, anemia).

INTERACTIONS Drug: Activated charcoal decreases dapsone absorption and enterohepatic circulation; **pyrimethamine, trimethoprim** increase risk of adverse hematologic reactions; **rifampin** decreases dapsone levels 7–10 fold.

PHARMACOKINETICS Absorption: Rapidly and nearly completely absorbed from GI tract. **Peak:** 2–8 h. **Distribution:** Distributed to all body tissues; high concentrations in kidney, liver, muscle, and skin; crosses placenta; distributed into breast milk. **Metabolism:** In liver by CYP3A4. **Elimination:** 70–85% in urine; remainder in feces; traces of drug may be found in body for 3 wk after repeated doses. **Half-Life:** 20–30 h.

NURSING IMPLICATIONS

Assessment & Drug Effects

- Monitor for therapeutic effectiveness that may not appear for leprosy until after 3–6 mo of therapy.
- Lab tests: Perform baseline then weekly CBC during the first month of therapy, at monthly intervals for at least 6 mo, and semiannually thereafter.
- Determine periodic dapsone blood levels.
- Perform liver function tests in patients who complain of malaise, fever, chills, anorexia, nausea, vomiting, and have jaundice.
- Monitor severity of anemia. Nearly all patients demonstrate hemolysis.
- Monitor temperature during first few weeks of therapy. If fever is frequent or severe, leprosy reactional state should be ruled out.

Patient & Family Education

- Report symptoms of leprosy that do not improve within 3 mo or get worse to physician.
- Report the appearance of a rash with bullous lesions around elbows and other joints promptly. Drug-induced or worsening skin lesions require withdrawal of dapsone.
- Report symptoms of peripheral neuropathy with motor loss (muscle weakness) promptly.

DAPTOMYCIN

(dap-to-my′sin)

Cubicin

Classifications: ANTIBIOTIC; LIPOPEPTIDE

Therapeutic: ANTIBIOTIC

Pregnancy Category: B

AVAILABILITY 500 mg vial

ACTION & *THERAPEUTIC EFFECT*

Daptomycin is cyclic lipopeptide antibiotic. It binds to bacterial membranes of gram-positive bacteria causing rapid depolarization of the membrane potential leading to inhibition of protein, DNA, and RNA synthesis and bacterial cell death. *Daptomycin is effective against a broad spectrum of gram-positive organisms, including both susceptible and resistant strains of* S. aureus.

USES Complicated skin and skin structure infections, bacteremia.
UNLABELED USES Vancomycin-resistant enterococci.

CONTRAINDICATIONS Pseudomembranous colitis; myopathy. Safe use in infants or children younger than 18 y is not known.
CAUTIOUS USE Severe renal or hepatic impairment, end-stage renal failure; peripheral neuropathy; GI disease; history of rhabdomyolysis, myopathy; elderly; pregnancy (category B), lactation.

ROUTE & DOSAGE

Skin Infections
Adult: **IV** 4 mg/kg q24h × 7–14 days
Bacteremia (*S. aureus*)
Adult: **IV** 6 mg/kg × 2–6 wk
Renal Impairment Dosage Adjustment
Skin infection: CrCl less than 30 mL/min: 4 mg/kg q48h; *bacteremia:* CrCl less than 30 mL/min: 6 mg/kg q48h
Hemodialyis Dosage Adjustment: Dose by CrCl, administer after dialysis

ADMINISTRATION

Intravenous

PREPARE: **IV Infusion:** Reconstitute the 250 mg vial or the 500 mg vial with 5 mL or 10 mL, respectively, of NS to yield 50 mg/mL. ▪ Further dilute the 50 mg/mL solution in 50–100 mL of NS.

ADMINISTER: **IV Infusion:** Infuse over 30 min; if same IV line is used for infusion of other drugs, flush line before/after with NS.
INCOMPATIBILITIES **Solution/additive:** **Dextrose**-containing solutions.

▪ Store unopened vials in 2°–8° C (36°–46° F). Avoid excessive heat. ▪ May store reconstituted, single-use vials or IV solution for 12 h at room temperature or 48 h if refrigerated.

ADVERSE EFFECTS (≥1%) **Body as a Whole:** Injection site reactions, fever, fungal infections. **CNS:** Headache, insomnia, dizziness. **CV:** Hypotension, hypertension. **GI:** Constipation, nausea, vomiting, diarrhea, abnormal liver function tests. **Hematologic:** Anemia. **Metabolic:** Elevated CPK. **Musculoskeletal:** Limb pain, arthralgia. **Respiratory:** Dyspnea. **Skin:** Rash, pruritus. **Urogenital:** UTIs, renal failure.

INTERACTIONS Drug: Significant reactions not identified.

PHARMACOKINETICS Elimination: Primarily renal. **Half-Life:** 8 h.

NURSING IMPLICATIONS

Assessment & Drug Effects

- Monitor for and report: Muscle pain or weakness, especially with concurrent therapy with HMG-CoA reductase inhibitors (statin drugs); S&S of peripheral neuropathy, superinfection such as candidiasis.
- Lab tests: Perform C&S before treatment is begun; baseline renal function tests; weekly CPK levels; PT/INR during first few days of daptomycin therapy with concurrent warfarin use; daily blood glucose monitoring in diabetics;

serum electrolytes if S&S of hypokalemia or hypomagnesemia (see Appendix F) appear.

- Withhold drug and notify physician if S&S of myopathy develop with CPK elevation greater than 1000 units/L (~5 × ULN), or if CPK level is 10 × ULN or greater.

Patient & Family Education

- Report any of the following to the physician: Muscle pain, weakness or unusual tiredness; numbness or tingling; difficulty breathing or shortness of breath; severe diarrhea or vomiting; skin rash or itching.

DARBEPOETIN ALFA

(dar-be-po-e'tin)

ARANESP

Classifications: BLOOD FORMER; HEMATOPOIETIC GROWTH FACTOR

Therapeutic: ANTIANEMIC

Prototype: Epoetin alfa

Pregnancy Category: C

AVAILABILITY 25 mcg/mL, 40 mcg/mL, 60 mcg/mL, 100 mcg/mL, 150 mcg/mL, 200 mcg/mL, 300 mcg/mL, 500 mcg/mL vials; 40 mcg/0.4 mL, 60 mcg/0.3 mL, 100 mcg/0.5 mL, 150 mcg/0.3 mL, 200 mcg/0.4 mL, 300 mcg/0.6 mL, 500 mcg/mL syringe

ACTION & *THERAPEUTIC EFFECT* An erythropoiesis-stimulating protein that stimulates red blood cell production in the bone marrow in response to hypoxia. Production of endogenous erythropoietin is impaired in patients with chronic renal failure (CRF) resulting in anemia. *Darbepoetin stimulates release of reticulocytes from the bone marrow into the blood stream where they mature into RBCs.*

USES Treatment of anemia in patients with chronic renal failure or chemotherapy-associated anemia, treatment of chemotherapy-induced anemia in nonmyeloid malignancies.

CONTRAINDICATIONS Patients with uncontrolled hypertension; hypersensitivity to darbepoetin or human albumin; antibody-mediated anemia due to anti-erythropoietin antibodies.

CAUTIOUS USE Controlled hypertension, elevated hemoglobin, folic acid or vitamin B_{12} deficiencies, hematologic diseases; infections, inflammatory or malignant processes, osteofibrosis, occult blood loss, hemolysis, severe aluminum toxicity, bone marrow fibrosis, chronic renal failure patients not on dialysis; pregnancy (category C), lactation.

ROUTE & DOSAGE

Anemia

Adult: **IV/Subcutaneous** Initially, 0.45 mcg/kg once/wk. Reduce dose by 25% if there is a rapid increase (i.e., more than 1 g/dL in any 2-wk period) in Hgb or if the Hgb is approaching 12 g/dL. If the Hgb does not increase by 1 g/dL after 4 wk of therapy and iron stores are adequate, increase the dose by 25%. Maintenance dose is 0.26–0.65 mcg/kg once/wk.

Converting Epoetin Alfa to Darbepoetin

Adults: **IV/Subcutaneous** Estimate the starting dose of darbepoetin alfa based on the total weekly dose of epoetin alfa at the time of conversion. If the patient was receiving epoetin alfa 2–3

times/wk, administer darbepoetin alfa once/week; if the patient was receiving epoetin alfa once/week, administer darbepoetin alfa once every 2 wk. The route of administration (i.e., subcutaneous or IV) should be maintained. Note: The following darbepoetin alfa dosage recommendations are estimates based on total amount of epoetin alfa administered per week. Because of individual variability, titrate doses to maintain the target Hgb.

Estimated Starting Dose (titrate to maintain target Hgb)

Previous weekly dose of epoetin alfa: 1500–2499 units/wk:
- Darbepoetin dose: 6.25 mcg/wk

Previous weekly dose of epoetin alfa: 2500–4999 units/wk:
- Darbepoetin dose: 10–12.5 mcg/wk

Previous weekly dose of epoetin alfa: 5000–10,999 units/wk:
- Darbepoetin dose: 20–25 mcg/wk

Previous weekly dose of epoetin alfa: 11,000–17,999 units/wk:
- Darbepoetin dose: 40 mcg/wk

Previous weekly dose of epoetin alfa: 18,000–33,999 units/wk:
- Darbepoetin dose: 60 mcg/wk

Previous weekly dose of epoetin alfa: 34,000–89,999 units/wk:
- Darbepoetin dose: 100 mcg/wk

Previous weekly dose of epoetin alfa: Greater than 90,000 units/wk:
- Darbepoetin dose: 200 mcg/wk

ADMINISTRATION

All Routes
- Correct deficiencies of folic acid or vitamin B_{12} prior to initiation of therapy.

Subcutaneous
- Do not shake solution. Shaking may denature the darbepoetin, rendering it biologically inactive.
- Inspect solution for particulate matter prior to use. Do not use if solution is discolored or if it contains particulate matter.
- Use only one dose per vial, and do not reenter vial.
- Do not give with any other drug solution.

Intravenous

PREPARE: **Direct:** Without shaking vial, withdraw the desired dose and give undiluted. ▪ Discard the unused portion.

ADMINISTER: **Direct:** Give direct IV as a bolus dose over 1 min. ▪ Discard any unused portion of the vial. It contains no preservatives.

- Store at 2°–8° C (36°–46° F). Do not freeze or shake. Protect from light.

ADVERSE EFFECTS (≥1%) **Body as a Whole:** Injection site pain, *peripheral edema,* fatigue, fever, death, chest pain, fluid overload, access infection, access hemorrhage, flu-like symptoms, asthenia, *infection.* **CNS:** *Headache,* dizziness. **CV:** *Hypertension, hypotension, arrhythmias,* cardiac arrest, angina, chest pain, vascular access thrombosis, CHF, red cell aplasia. **GI:** *Nausea, vomiting, diarrhea,* constipation. **Musculoskeletal:** *Myalgia, arthralgia,* limb pain, back pain. **Respiratory:** *Upper respiratory infection, dyspnea, cough,* bronchitis. **Skin:** Pruritus. **Other:** Increased risk of thrombotic events and mortality in cancer patients.

INTERACTIONS Drug: No clinically significant reactions reported.

PHARMACOKINETICS Absorption: 37% absorbed from **subcutaneous**

site. **Peak:** 24–72 h **Subcutaneous**. **Distribution:** Distribution confined primarily to intravascular space. **Elimination:** 10% in urine. **Half-Life:** 21 h **IV**, 49 h **Subcutaneous**.

NURSING IMPLICATIONS

Assessment & Drug Effects

- Control BP adequately prior to initiation of therapy and closely monitor and control during therapy. Report immediately S&S of CHF, cardiac arrhythmias, or sepsis. Note that hypertension is an adverse effect that **must be** controlled.
- Notify physician of a rapid rise in Hgb as dosage will need to be reduced because of risk of serious hypertension. Note that BP may rise during early therapy as Hgb increases.
- Monitor for premonitory neurologic symptoms (i.e., aura, and report their appearance promptly). The potential for seizures exists during periods of rapid Hgb increase (e.g., greater than 1.0 g/dL in any 2-wk period).
- Monitor closely and report immediately S&S of thrombotic events (e.g., MI, CVA, TIA), especially for patients with CRF.
- Lab tests: At baseline and periodically thereafter, evaluate iron stores, including transferrin and serum ferritin; Hgb twice weekly until stabilized and maintenance dose is established, then weekly for at least 4 wk, and at regular intervals thereafter; CBC with differential and platelet count at regular interval; periodic BUN, creatinine, serum phosphorus, and serum potassium.

Patient & Family Education

- Adhere closely to antihypertensive drug regimen and dietary restrictions.
- Monitor BP as directed by physician.
- Do not drive or engage in other potentially hazardous activity during the first 90 days of therapy because of possible seizure activity.
- Report any of the following to the physician: Chest pain, difficulty breathing, shortness of breath, severe or persistent headache, fever, muscle aches and pains, or nausea.

DARIFENACIN HYDROBROMIDE

(dar-i-fen'a-sin)

Enablex

Classifications: ANTICHOLINERGIC; MUSCARINIC RECEPTOR ANTAGONIST; BLADDER ANTISPASMODIC

Therapeutic: BLADDER ANTISPASMODIC

Prototype: Oxybutin

Pregnancy Category: C

AVAILABILITY 7.5 mg and 15 mg extended release tablets

ACTION & *THERAPEUTIC EFFECT* Darifenacin is a selective M3 muscarinic receptor antagonist. Muscarinic M3 receptors play an important role in contraction of the urinary bladder smooth muscle and stimulation of salivary secretion. *Control of urinary incontinence due to urgency and frequency.*

USES Treatment of overactive bladder with symptoms of urge urinary incontinence, urgency, and frequency.

CONTRAINDICATIONS Hypersensitivity to the drug; severe hepatic impairment (Child-Pugh C class); urinary retention; gastric obstruction; pyloric stenosis, ileus; urinary retention; uncontrolled narrow-angle glaucoma.

CAUTIOUS USE Risk of urinary retention, clinically significant bladder outflow obstruction, renal disease; decreased GI motility, GERD, severe constipation, ulcerative colitis; myasthenia gravis; controlled narrow-angle glaucoma; pregnancy (category C), lactation.

ROUTE & DOSAGE

Overactive Bladder
Adult: **PO** 7.5–15 mg daily

Moderate Hepatic Impairment (Child-Pugh B Class) Dosage Adjustment
Max dose: 7.5 mg or less daily

ADMINISTRATION

Oral

- Ensure that the drug is not chewed or crushed. It **must be** swallowed whole.
- Note: Dosage should not exceed 7.5 mg daily with moderate hepatic impairment (i.e., Child-Pugh B class) or concurrent therapy with potent inhibitors of CYP3A4 (e.g., itraconazole, clarithromycin, nefazodone, nelfinavir, ritonavir).
- Store 15°–30° C (59°–86° F). Protect from light.

ADVERSE EFFECTS (≥1%) **Body as a Whole:** Flu-like symptoms, urinary tract infection. **CNS:** *Headache,* asthenia, dizziness. **GI:** *Constipation, dry mouth, dyspepsia, nausea,* abdominal pain, diarrhea.

INTERACTIONS Drug: Potent inhibitors of CYP3A4 (e.g., **clarithromycin, erythromycin, itraconazole, ketoconazole, nefazodone, nelfinavir,** and **ritonavir**) increase darifenacin levels. Darifenacin will cause additive anticholinergic effects with other ANTICHOLINERGIC drugs. Darifenacin can increase **digoxin** concentrations. **Food: Grapefruit juice** may increase darifenacin levels.

PHARMACOKINETICS Absorption: 15–19% bioavailability. **Peak:** 7 h. **Distribution:** 98% protein bound. **Metabolism:** Extensive hepatic metabolism. **Elimination:** Renal and fecal. **Half-Life:** 13–19 h.

NURSING IMPLICATIONS

Assessment & Drug Effects

- Monitor for adverse effects of concurrently used drugs that have a narrow therapeutic window and are metabolized by CYP26D (e.g., flecainide, thioridazine, or TRICYCLIC ANTIDEPRESSANTS).
- Lab tests: Monitor blood levels of digoxin with concurrent therapy and assess for S&S of digoxin toxicity.

Patient & Family Education

- Follow directions for taking the drug (see ADMINISTRATION).
- Do not drive or engage in potentially hazardous activities until response to drug is known.
- Use caution in hot environments to minimize the risk of heat prostration.
- Report any of the following to a health care provider: Difficulty passing urine, unexplained nausea, or persistent constipation.

DARUNAVIR

(da-run'a-ver)

Prezista

Classifications: ANTIRETROVIRAL; HIV PROTEASE INHIBITOR
Therapeutic: ANTIRETROVIRAL; PROTEASE INHIBITOR
Prototype: Saquinavir
Pregnancy Category: C

AVAILABILITY 75 mg, 150 mg, 300 mg, 600 mg tablets

D

ACTION & *THERAPEUTIC EFFECT* Darunavir is an inhibitor of HIV-1 protease that selectively inhibits the cleavage of HIV polyproteins in infected cells, thereby preventing the maturation of virus particles. *Darunavir reduces the viral load (decreases the number of RNA copies) and increases the number of T helper CD4 cells.*

USES Treatment of HIV infection with ritonavir and other antiretroviral agents.

CONTRAINDICATIONS Hypersensitivity to darunavir or protease inhibitors, ritonavir; pancreatitis; lactation. Safety and efficacy in children have not been established.

CAUTIOUS USE Hepatic function impairment, hepatitis; severe renal impairment, chronic renal failure; hemophilia A or B; diabetes mellitus; diabetes ketoacidosis; hyperglycemia; elderly; pregnancy (category C).

ROUTE & DOSAGE

HIV Infection, Treatment Naive
Adult: **PO** 800 mg daily with 100 mg ritonavir PO

HIV Infection, Treatment Experienced
Adult: **PO** 600 mg b.i.d. with 100 mg ritonavir PO
Adolescent/Child (weight greater than 40 kg): **PO** 600 mg b.i.d. with 100 mg ritonavir PO
Adolescent/Child (weight 30–40 kg): **PO** 450 mg b.i.d. with 60 mg ritonavir PO
Child (older than 6 y, weight 20–30 kg): **PO** 375 mg b.i.d. with 50 mg ritonavir PO

ADMINISTRATION

Oral
- Give with food and coadminister with 100 mg ritonavir.
- Tablets **must be** swallowed whole.
- Store at 15°–30° C (59°–86° F). Protect from light and moisture.

ADVERSE EFFECTS (≥2%) **CNS:** *Headache.* **GI:** Abdominal pain, constipation, *diarrhea, vomiting.* **Skin:** Stevens-Johnson syndrome. **Hepatic:** Acute hepatitis.

INTERACTIONS Drug: AZOLE ANTIFUNGALS and **indinavir** increase the levels of darunavir. Coadministration of other inhibitors of CYP3A4 may also increase darunavir. ANTICONVULSANTS (e.g., **carbamazepine, phenobarbital, phenytoin**), CORTICOSTEROIDS (e.g., **dexamethasone**), **efavirenz,** RIFAMYCINS (e.g., **rifampin, rifabutin**), and **saquinavir** may decrease darunavir levels. Darunavir may increase the levels of AZOLE ANTIFUNGALS, CORTICOSTEROIDS, **efavirenz, indinavir,** RIFAMYCINS, **amiodarone, bepridil, lidocaine, quinidine,** CALCIUM CHANNEL BLOCKERS (e.g., **nifedipine, nicardipine, felodipine**), **clarithromycin,** IMMUNOSUPPRESSANTS (e.g., **cyclosporine, sirolimus, tacrolimus**), PHOSPHODIESTERASE TYPE 5 INHIBITORS (e.g., **sildenafil, tadalafil, vardenafil**), and trazodone, due in part to its ability to inhibit CYP3A4. Darunavir decreases the levels of the **lopinavir/ritonavir** combination, ORAL CONTRACEPTIVES (e.g., **ethinyl estradiol, norethindrone**), **methadone,** SELECTIVE SEROTONIN REUPTAKE INHIBITORS [SSRIS (e.g., **paroxetine, sertraline**)], and **warfarin.** Use of BENZODIAZEPINES (e.g., **midazolam, triazolam**) increases the risk of prolonged or increased sedation or respiratory depression. Use of ERGOT ALKALOIDS may increase ergot toxicity. Coadministration with HMG COA REDUCTASE INHIBITORS increases the risk of myopathy. Combination use with **pimozide** increases the risk of cardiac arrhythmias. **Food:** Food enhances the bioavailability of darunavir. **Herbal: St. John's wort** decreases the level of darunavir.

PHARMACOKINETICS Absorption: 82% absorbed (in combination with ritonavir). **Peak:** 2.5–4 h. **Distribution:** 95% protein bound. **Metabolism:** In the liver. **Elimination:** Primarily fecal (80%) with minor elimination in urine. **Half-Life:** 15 h.

NURSING IMPLICATIONS

Assessment & Drug Effects

- Monitor for and report S&S of pancreatitis, as this may be an indication for discontinuation of darunavir.
- Monitor for S&S of skin rash. Notify physician immediately if a severe rash appears.
- Monitor diabetics for loss of glycemic control.
- Lab tests: Periodic CD4+ cell count, plasma HIV-RNA, lipid profile, LFTs; and plasma glucose.
- Increase monitoring of INR with concurrent warfarin therapy.
- Monitor for adverse effects or loss of efficacy of concurrent medications, as many drug interactions occur with darunavir.

Patient & Family Education

- Follow directions for taking the drug (see Administration). If a dose is missed by more than 6 h, wait until the next regularly scheduled dose. If a dose is missed by less than 6 h, take a dose and continue with the next regularly scheduled dose.
- Ensure that you know which medicines should NOT be taken with darunavir, as serious consequences could occur.
- Report any of the following to a health care provider: Blistering, redness, or peeling skin or mucus membranes; severe skin rash.
- Use or add a barrier contraceptive if using an estrogen-containing oral contraceptive if you wish to prevent pregnancy.

DASATINIB

(das-a'ti-nib)

Sprycel

Classifications: ANTINEOPLASTIC AGENT; BIOLOGICAL RESPONSE MODIFIER; TYROSINE KINASE INHIBITOR (TKI)

Therapeutic: ANTINEOPLASTIC; TKI

Prototype: Gefitinib

Pregnancy Category: D

AVAILABILITY 20 mg, 50 mg, 70 mg, 100 mg tablets

ACTION & *THERAPEUTIC EFFECT* Dasatinib is a BCR-ABL tyrosine kinase inhibitor. BCR-ABL tyrosine kinase is an enzyme produced by a chromosomal translocation associated with chronic myeloid leukemia (CML) and certain types of acute lymphocytic leukemias (Ph^+ ALL). *Dasatinib inhibits the growth of CML and ALL cell lines overexpressing BCR-ABL kinase.*

USES Treatment of chronic, accelerated, or myeloid or lymphoid blast phase chronic myelogenous leukemia (CML) in adults resistant or intolerant to prior therapy. Treatment of Philadelphia chromosome–positive (Ph^+) acute lymphocytic leukemia (ALL) in adults resistant or intolerant to prior therapy.

CONTRAINDICATIONS Hypersensitivity to dasatinib; pregnancy (category D); lactation; active bleeding. Concurrent use of anticoagulants or antiplatelet drugs; hypokalemia; hypomagnesemia. Safety and efficacy in children younger than 18 y have not been established.

CAUTIOUS USE Hepatic impairment; bacterial or viral infection; history of GI bleeding; interstitial pneumonia; pleural effusion; QT prolongation; concurrent use of antiarrhythmic drugs.

ROUTE & DOSAGE

CML and Philadelphia Chromosome-Positive ALL

Adult: **PO** Starting dose 70 mg b.i.d. May increase/decrease dose by 20 mg based on response.

Chronic Phase CML

Adult: **PO** 100 mg daily

Dosage Adjustments for Neutropenia and Thrombocytopenia

Chronic phase CML where absolute neutrophil count (ANC) less than 500/m³ and/or platelets less than 50,000/mm³

Step 1: DC dasatinib until the ANC 1000/mm³ or more and platelets 50,000/mm³ or more

Step 2: If cell recovery occurs in 7 days or less, restart at original dose

Step 3: If platelets less than 25,000 mm³ and/or recurrence of ANC less than 500/mm³, resume at dose of 80 mg daily

Accelerated phase CML, blast phase CML, and Ph⁺ ALL where ANC less than 500/mm³ and/or platelets less than 10,000/mm³

Step 1: Assure that cytopenia is unrelated to the underlying leukemia. If so, DC until ANC 1000/mm³ or more and platelets 20,000/mm³ or more.

Step 2: Resume at starting dose

Step 3: If cytopenia recurs, repeat step 1 and resume at 50 mg b.i.d. (second episode) or 40 mg b.i.d. (third episode)

Step 4: If cytopenia is related to the underlying leukemia, may increase to 180 mg daily

ADMINISTRATION

Oral

- Do not crush or break tablets. They should be swallowed whole.
- Ensure that hypokalemia and hypomagnesemia are corrected prior to administering dasatinib.
- Store at 15°–30° C (59°–86° F).

ADVERSE EFFECTS (≥1%) **Body as a Whole:** Chills, contusion, febrile neutropenia, *hemorrhage, infection,* malaise, *pain, pyrexia,* tumor lysis syndrome, weight gain or weight loss. **CNS:** *Asthenia,* anxiety, confusional state, CNS bleeding, depression, dizziness, dysgeusia, *fatigue, headache,* insomnia, neuropathy, somnolence, syncope, tremor, vertigo. **CV:** Arrhythmia, chest pain, angina, <u>congestive heart failure</u>, pericardial effusion, cardiomegaly, hypertension, hypotension, <u>myocardial infarction</u>, palpitations. **GI:** *Abdominal distention and pain,* anal fissure, *anorexia,* ascites, colitis, constipation, *diarrhea,* dysphagia, gastritis, *GI bleeding, nausea,* oral soft tissue disorder, *vomiting, mucosal inflammation.* **Hematologic:** *Anemia, neutropenia,* pancytopenia, *thrombocytopenia,* elevated ALT and AST, hypocalcemia, hypophosphatemia. **Metabolic:** Appetite disturbances, *fluid retention, edema,* hyperuricemia. **Musculoskeletal:** *Arthralgia, musculoskeletal pain,* muscle inflammation, myalgia, musculoskele-

D

tal stiffness. **Respiratory:** Asthma, *cough, dyspnea,* lung infiltration, *plural effusion,* pneumonia, pulmonary edema, pulmonary hypertension, *upper respiratory tract infection.* **Skin:** Acne, alopecia, dermatitis, dry skin, hyperhidrosis, nail disorder, photosensitivity reaction, pigmentation disorder, pruritus, *skin rash.* **Special Senses:** Conjunctivitis, dry eye, tinnitus. **Urogenital:** Gynecomastia, renal failure, urinary frequency.

INTERACTIONS Drug: Aluminum- and **magnesium**-based ANTACIDS decrease dasatinib absorption. AZOLE ANTIFUNGAL AGENTS (e.g., **ketoconazole, itraconazole**), MACROLIDE ANTIBIOTICS (e.g., **clarithromycin, erythromycin, telithromycin**), HIV PROTEASE INHIBITORS (e.g., **indinavir, nelfinavir, ritonavir, saquinavir**), **nefazodone,** and other inhibitors of CYP3A4 may increase dasatinib levels. Compounds that induce CYP3A4 (e.g., **carbamazepine, dexamethasone, phenobarbital, phenytoin, rifampin**) may decrease dasatinib levels. PROTON PUMP INHIBITORS and H_2 ANTAGONISTS may reduce the absorption of dasatinib due to long-term suppression of gastric acid secretion. Dasatinib may alter the plasma concentrations of other drugs that require CYP3A4 and have a narrow therapeutic window (e.g., **cyclosporine,** ERGOT ALKALOIDS). Dasatinib increases the levels of **simvastatin**. **Food:** Food enhances the bioavailability of dasatinib. **Herbal: St. John's wort** may decrease the level of dasatinib.

PHARMACOKINETICS Peak: 0.5–6 h. **Distribution:** 93–96% protein bound. **Metabolism:** Extensive hepatic metabolism. **Elimination:** Fecal. **Half-Life:** 3–5 h.

NURSING IMPLICATIONS

Assessment & Drug Effects

- Monitor for and report S&S of fluid retention (e.g., pleural or pericardial effusion, peripheral or pulmonary edema, ascites).
- Monitor for S&S of cardiac dysfunction (e.g., heart failure, arrhythmias). ECG monitoring may be needed to evaluate potential QT interval prolongation.
- Monitor for numerous adverse side effects of dasatinib. Immediately report suspected bleeding or infection.
- Lab tests: Baseline and periodic serum potassium and magnesium; baseline CBC with differential (including ANC and platelet count), weekly for first 2 mo, then monthly; periodic LFTs.

Patient & Family Education

- Take antacids (if needed for GI distress) 2 h before or after dasatinib.
- Do not use OTC medications for heartburn (other than antacids) without consulting physician.
- Inform your physician if you are pregnant or planning to become pregnant, as dasatinib may harm the fetus.
- Report immediately to your health care provider any of the following: Bleeding (including wine- or coke-colored urine, or black tarry stools) or easy bruising, fever or other signs of an infection, severe lethargy or weakness.

DAUNORUBICIN HYDROCHLORIDE

(daw-noe-roo′bi-sin)

Cerubidine

D

DAUNORUBICIN CITRATED LIPOSOMAL

DaunoXome
Classifications: ANTINEOPLASTIC; ANTIBIOTIC; ANTHRACYCLINE
Therapeutic: ANTINEOPLASTIC
Prototype: Doxorubicin HCl
Pregnancy Category: D

AVAILABILITY Daunorubicin HCl: 10 mg, 20 mg, 50 mg, 100 mg lyophilized vials; **Daunorubicin Citrated Liposomal:** 2 mg/mL (equivalent to 50 mg daunorubicin base) injection

ACTION & *THERAPEUTIC EFFECT* Cytotoxic and antimitotic anthracycline antibiotic that is cell-cycle specific for S-phase of cell division. Has rapid interaction with the DNA molecule changing its shape, thus resulting in inhibition of DNA, RNA, and protein synthesis. *Antineoplastic effects against acute leukemias with decreased incidence of cardiotoxicity than doxorubicin.*

USES To induce remission in acute nonlymphocytic/lymphocytic leukemia, advanced HIV-associated Kaposi's sarcoma.
UNLABELED USES Non-Hodgkin's lymphoma.

CONTRAINDICATIONS Severe myelosuppression; immunizations (patient, family), and preexisting cardiac disease unless risk-benefit is evaluated; uncontrolled systemic infection; pregnancy (category D), lactation.
CAUTIOUS USE History of gout, urate calculi, hepatic or renal function impairment; older adult patients with inadequate bone reserve due to age or previous cytotoxic drug therapy, tumor cell infiltration of bone marrow, patient who has received potentially cardiotoxic drugs or related antineoplastics.

ROUTE & DOSAGE

Neoplasms
Adult: **IV** *Younger than 60 y,* 45 mg/m²/day on days 1, 2, and 3 of first course then days 1 and 2 of subsequent courses (max total cumulative dose: 500–600 mg/m²); *60 y or older,* 30 mg/m²/day on days 1, 2, and 3 of first course then days 1 and 2 of subsequent courses
Child: **IV** As combination therapy, *2 y or older,* 25 mg/m² weekly; *younger than 2 y,* 1 mg/kg

Kaposi's Sarcoma (DaunoXome)
Adult: **IV** 40 mg/m² over 1 h, repeat q2wk (withhold therapy if granulocyte count less than 750 cells/mm³)

Renal Impairment Dosage Adjustment
If serum Cr greater than 3 mg/dL, give 50% of dose

Hepatic Impairment Dosage Adjustment
For total bilirubin 1.2–3 mg/dL, give 50% of dose; greater than 3–5 mg/dL, give 25% of dose; greater than 5 mg/dL, omit dose

ADMINISTRATION

Intravenous
Use gloves during preparation for infusion to prevent skin contact with this drug. If contact occurs, decontaminate skin with copious amounts of water with soap.

Daunorubicin HCl

***PREPARE:* Direct:** Reconstitute 20 mg vial with 4 mL sterile water for injection. The concentration of the solution will be 5 mg/mL. ▪ Withdraw dose into syringe containing 10–15 mL normal saline. **IV Infusion:** Dilute further in 100 mL NS as required.

ADMINISTER: **Direct:** Inject over approximately 3 min into the tubing or side arm of a rapidly flowing IV infusion of D5W or NS. **Infusion:** Give a single dose over 30–45 min.

Specific to DaunoXome

PREPARE: **IV Infusion:** Each vial of DaunoXome contains the equivalent of 50 mg daunorubicin base. Dilute with enough D5W to produce a concentration of 1 mg/1 mL.

ADMINISTER: **IV Infusion:** Give DaunoXome over 60 min. Do not use a filter with DaunoXome.

INCOMPATIBILITIES **Solution/additive:** **Dexamethasone, heparin.** **Y-site:** **Allopurinol, aztreonam, cefepime, fludarabine, lansoprazole, piperacillin/tazobactam.**

▪ Avoid extravasation because it can cause severe tissue necrosis.

▪ Store reconstituted solution at room temperature (15°–30° C; 59°–86° F) for 24 h and under refrigeration at 2°–8° C (36°–46° F) for 48 h. Protect from light.

ADVERSE EFFECTS (≥1%) **Body as a Whole:** Fever. **CNS:** Amnesia, anxiety, ataxia, confusion, hallucinations, emotional lability, tremors. **CV:** Pericarditis, myocarditis, arrhythmias, peripheral edema, CHF, hypertension, tachycardia. **GI:** *Acute nausea and vomiting* (mild), anorexia, *stomatitis,* mucositis, diarrhea (occasionally) hemorrhage. **Urogenital:** Dysuria, nocturia, polyuria, dry skin. **Hematologic:** *Bone marrow depression thrombocytopenia, leukopenia*, anemia, **Skin:** Generalized *alopecia* (reversible), transverse pigmentation of nails, severe cellulitis or tissue necrosis at site of drug extravasation. **Endocrine:** Hyperuricemia, gonadal suppression.

PHARMACOKINETICS **Distribution:** Highest concentrations in spleen, kidneys, liver, lungs, and heart; does not cross blood–brain barrier; crosses placenta. **Metabolism:** In liver to active metabolite. **Elimination:** 25% in urine, 40% in bile. **Half-Life:** 18.5–26.7 h.

NURSING IMPLICATIONS

Assessment & Drug Effects

- Monitor for therapeutic effectiveness. A profound suppression of bone marrow is required to induce a complete remission. Nadirs for thrombocytes and leukocytes are usually reached in 10–14 days.
- Monitor serum bilirubin; drug dose needs to be reduced when bilirubin is greater than 1.2 mg/dL.
- Lab tests: Perform Hct, platelet count, total and differential leukocyte count, serum uric acid, chest x-ray, and cardiac, hepatic, and renal function tests prior to and periodically during therapy.
- Monitor BP, temperature, pulse, and respiratory function during treatment.
- Monitor for S&S of acute CHF. It can occur suddenly, especially when total dosage exceeds 550 mg/m^2, or in patients with compromised heart function because of previous radiation therapy to heart area.
- Report immediately: Breathlessness, orthopnea, change in pulse and BP parameters. Early clinical diagnosis of drug-induced CHF is essential for successful treatment.
- Report promptly S&S of superinfections including elevation of

temperature, chills, upper respiratory tract infection, tachycardia, overgrowth with opportunistic organisms because myelosuppression imposes risk of superimposed infection (see Appendix F).

- Protect patient from contact with persons with infections. The most hazardous period is during nadirs of thrombocytes and leukocytes.
- Control nausea and vomiting (usually mild) by antiemetic therapy.
- Inspect oral membranes daily. Mucositis may occur 3–7 days after drug is administered.

Patient & Family Education

- Note: Loss of hair is probable; recovery is usual in 6–10 wk.
- Use barrier contraceptives during treatment because this drug is teratogenic. Tell your physician immediately if you become pregnant during therapy.
- Note: A transient effect of the drug is to turn urine red on the day of infusion.

DECITABINE

(de-sit′a-bine)

Dacogen

Classifications: ANTINEOPLASTIC; ANTIMETABOLITE; PYRIMIDINE

Therapeutic: ANTINEOPLASTIC

Prototype: 5-Fluorouracil

Pregnancy Category: D

AVAILABILITY 50 mg lyophilized powder for injection

ACTION & *THERAPEUTIC EFFECT* Decitabine is an antimetabolite that exerts antineoplastic effects after its direct incorporation into DNA and inhibition of DNA transferase, causing loss of cell differentiation and cell death. Nonproliferating cells are resistant to the effects of decitabine. *Decitabine-induced changes in neoplastic cells may restore normal function to genes that are critical for control of cellular differentiation and proliferation.*

USES Treatment of patients with myelodysplastic syndrome (MDS). This includes previously treated and untreated patients with de novo and secondary MDS of all French-American-British (FAB) subtypes (i.e., refractory anemia, refractory anemia with ringed sideroblasts, refractory anemia with excess blasts, refractory anemia with excess blasts in transformation, and chronic myelomonocytic leukemia) and intermediate-1, intermediate-2, and high-risk International Prognostic Scoring System (IPSS) groups.

UNLABELED USES Treatment of chronic myelogenous leukemia (CML).

CONTRAINDICATIONS Hypersensitivity to decitabine; conception within 2 mo of drug use; renal failure patients with CrCl less than 2 mg/mL; liver dysfunction with transaminase greater than 2 × upper limit of normal (ULN), or serum bilirubin greater than 1.5 mg/dL; active infection; pregnancy (category D), lactation. Safety and efficacy in children not established.

CAUTIOUS USE Moderate to severe renal failure; hepatic impairment.

ROUTE & DOSAGE

Myelodysplastic Syndrome

Adult: **IV** 15 mg/m^2 q8h × 3 days. Patient should receive a minimum of 4 cycles of therapy repeated q6wk.

ADMINISTRATION

Intravenous

PREPARE: **IV Infusion:** Caution should be exercised when han-

D

dling and preparing decitabine. Procedures for proper handling and disposal of antineoplastic drugs should be applied. ▪ Reconstitute each vial with 10 mL sterile water for injection to yield approximately 5 mg/mL at pH 6.7–7.3. Immediately after reconstitution, further dilute with NS, D5W, or LR to a final drug concentration of 0.1–1 mg/mL. ▪ Use within 15 min of reconstitution (see Storage).

ADMINISTER: **IV infusion:** Premedicate with standard antiemetic therapy. Give decitabine over 3 h. ▪ **NOTE:** Withhold dose and notify physician of any of the following: Absolute neutrophil count (ANC) less than 1000/mcL; platelet count less than 50,000/mcL; serum creatinine at 2 mg/dL or higher; ALT, total bilirubin 2 × ULN or more; or an active or uncontrolled infection.

▪ Store vials at 15°–30° C (59°– 86° F). Unless used within 15 min of reconstitution, the diluted solution **must be** prepared using cold (2°–8° C) infusion fluids and stored at 2°–8° C (36°–46° F) for up to a maximum of 7 h until administration.

ADVERSE EFFECTS (≥5%) **Body as a Whole:** *Fatigue, pyrexia, Mycobacterium avium* complex infection, peripheral edema, bacteremia, candidal infection, cellulitis, injection site reactions, rigors, tenderness, transfusion reaction, sinusitis, staphylococcal infection. **CNS:** Intracranial hemorrhage, anxiety, confusional state, dizziness, headache, hypesthesia, insomnia, pyrexia. **CV:** Cardiorespiratory arrest, cardiac murmur, hypotension. **GI:** *Nausea, vomiting, constipation, diarrhea,* abdominal distention and discomfort, anorexia, dyspepsia, gastroesophageal reflux disease, glossodynia, gingival bleeding, hemorrhoids, lip ulceration, stomatitis, tongue ulceration. **Hematologic:** *Anemia, neutropenia, thrombocytopenia,* hematoma, leukopenia, lymphadenopathy, thrombocythemia. **Metabolic:** *Hyperglycemia,* increased AST, decreased blood albumin, increased blood alkaline phosphatase, altered blood bicarbonate, decreased blood bilirubin, decreased blood chloride, increased blood lactate dehydrogenase, increased blood urea, decreased total protein, dehydration, hyperbilirubinemia, altered potassium levels, hypoalbuminemia, hypomagnesemia, hyponatremia. **Musculoskeletal:** Arthralgia, back pain, chest wall pain, musculoskeletal discomfort, myalgia, pain in limb. **Respiratory:** *Cough,* lung crackles, hypoxia, pharyngitis, pneumonia, pulmonary edema, rales. **Skin:** Alopecia, ecchymosis, erythema, pallor, *petechiae,* pruritus, rash, skin lesion, swelling face, urticaria. **Special Senses:** Blurred vision. **Urogenital:** Dysuria, urinary frequency, urinary tract infection.

PHARMACOKINETICS Distribution: Negligible plasma protein binding. **Half-Life:** 0.2–0.8 h.

NURSING IMPLICATIONS

Assessment & Drug Effects

- Monitor for and report S&S of pulmonary or peripheral edema, cardiac arrhythmias, new-onset depression, or infection.
- Lab tests: CBC with differentials and platelet count prior to each chemotherapy cycle; baseline and periodic LFTs and serum creatinine.
- Avoid IM injections with platelet counts less than 50,000/mcL.

- Monitor diabetics for loss of glycemic control.

Patient & Family Education

- Do not accept vaccinations during treatment with decitabine.
- Avoid contact with anyone who recently received the oral poliovirus vaccine.
- Women of childbearing age should avoid becoming pregnant while receiving decitabine.
- Men should not father a child while receiving decitabine and for 2 mo after the end of therapy.
- Report any of the following to a health care provider: Signs of infection such as fever, chills, sore throat; signs of bleeding such as easy bruising, black, tarry stools, blood in the urine; irregular heart rate; significant tiredness or weakness.

DEFEROXAMINE MESYLATE

(de-fer-ox'a-meen)

Desferal

Classifications: CHELATING AGENT; ANTIDOTE

Therapeutic: ANTIDOTE

Pregnancy Category: C

AVAILABILITY 500 mg, 2 g powder for injection

ACTION & *THERAPEUTIC EFFECT* Chelating agent isolated from *Streptomyces pilosus* with specific affinity for ferric ion and low affinity for calcium. Binds ferric ions to form a stable water soluble chelate readily excreted by kidneys. *Main effect is removal of iron from ferritin, hemosiderin, and transferrin of patient in iron toxicity.*

USES Adjunct in treatment of acute iron intoxication or iron overload.

UNLABELED USES To promote aluminum excretion.

CONTRAINDICATIONS Severe renal disease, anuria, pyelonephritis; primary hemochromatosis; acute infection.

CAUTIOUS USE History of pyelonephritis; infants and children younger than 3 y; elderly, cardiac dysfunction; pregnancy (category C), lactation.

ROUTE & DOSAGE

Acute Iron Intoxication

Adult: **IM/IV** 1 g followed by 500 mg at 4 h intervals for 2 doses, subsequent doses of 500 mg q4–12h may be given if necessary (max: 6 g/24 h), infuse at 15 mg/kg/h or less

Child (older than 3 y): **IV** 15 mg/kg/h (max: 6 g/24 h) **IM** 40–90 mg/kg (up to 1 g) q4–8h

Chronic Iron Overload

Adult: **IM** 500 mg–1 g/day **Subcutaneous** 1–2 g/day (20–40 mg/kg/day) infused over 8–24 h

Child (older than 3 y): **IM** 500 mg–1 g/day **Subcutaneous** 20–40 mg/kg/day over 8–12 h

ADMINISTRATION

Subcutaneous

- Reconstitute by adding 5 mL sterile water for injection to each 500 mg vial or 20 mL to each 2 gram vial to yield 100 mg/mL. Dissolve completely.
- Give subcutaneously over 8–24 h using a portable minipump device.

Intramuscular

- Reconstitute by adding 2 mL sterile water for injection to 500 mg vial

D

or 8 mL to the 2 g vial to yield 250 mg/mL. Dissolve completely.

- Use IM route for all patients not in shock; preferred route for acute intoxication.

Intravenous

For infants and children: Verify correct IV concentration and rate with physician.

PREPARE: **IV Infusion:** Reconstitute by adding 5 mL sterile water for injection to 500 mg vial to yield 100 mg/mL. ▪ After drug is completely dissolved, withdraw prescribed amount from vial and add to NS, D5W, or LR solution.

ADMINISTER: **IV Infusion:** *Adult:* Give initial dose at a rate not to exceed 15 mg/kg/h; give two subsequent 500 mg dose at 125 mg/h; give any additional doses over 4–12 h. *Child:* Give at 15 mg/kg/h. ▪ Do not infuse IV rapidly; such infusion is associated with the occurrence of more adverse effects.

INCOMPATIBILITIES **Solution/admixture: Iron dextran.**

- Store at room temperature 15°–30° C (59°–86° F) for not longer than 1 wk. Protect from light.

ADVERSE EFFECTS (≥1%) **Body as a Whole:** Hypersensitivity (generalized itching, cutaneous wheal formation, rash, fever, <u>anaphylactoid reaction</u>). **CV:** Hypotension, tachycardia. **Special Senses:** Decreased hearing; blurred vision, decreased visual acuity and visual fields, color vision abnormalities, night blindness, retinal pigmentary degeneration. **GI:** Abdominal discomfort, diarrhea. **Urogenital:** Dysuria, exacerbation of pyelonephritis, orange-rose discoloration of urine. **Other:** *Pain and induration at injection site.*

INTERACTIONS Drug: Use with **ascorbic acid** increases cardiac risk, **prochlorperazine** may cause loss of consciousness.

PHARMACOKINETICS Distribution: Widely distributed in body tissues. **Metabolism:** Forms nontoxic complex with iron. **Elimination:** Primarily in urine; some in feces.

NURSING IMPLICATIONS

Assessment & Drug Effects

- Lab tests: Perform baseline kidney function tests prior to drug administration.
- Monitor injection site. If pain and induration occur, move infusion to another site.
- Monitor I&O ratio and pattern. Report any change. Observe stools for blood (iron intoxication frequently causes necrosis of GI tract).
- Note: Periodic ophthalmoscopic (slit lamp) examinations and audiometry are advised for patients on prolonged or high-dose therapy for chronic iron overload.

Patient & Family Education

- Deferoxamine chelate makes urine turn a reddish color.
- Report blurred vision or any other visual abnormality.

DEGARELIX ACETATE

(de-ga′re-lix)

Firmagon

Classification: GONADOTROPIN-RELEASING HORMONE (GNRH) ANTAGONIST

Therapeutic: GNRH ANTAGONIST

Prototype: Ganirelix acetate

Pregnancy Category: X

AVAILABILITY 80 mg, 240 mg powder for injection

ACTION & *THERAPEUTIC EFFECT* A gonadotropin-releasing hormone (GnRH) receptor antagonist. It binds reversibly to pituitary GnRH receptors, reducing the release of gonadotropins and, consequently, testosterone. *Testosterone suppression slows the growth of androgen-sensitive prostate cancer cells as indicated by PSA values.*

USES Treatment of advanced prostate cancer.

CONTRAINDICATIONS Hypersensitivity to degarelix; women who are or may become pregnant (category X); lactation.

CAUTIOUS USE Congenital long QT syndrome; electrolyte abnormalities; CHF; elderly. Safety and effectiveness in pediatric patients have not been established.

ROUTE & DOSAGE

Prostate Cancer

Adult: **Subcutaneous** Initial dose of 240 mg in two 120 mg injections, followed by 80 mg q28days

ADMINISTRATION

Subcutaneous

- Glove should be worn for reconstitution. Follow carefully manufacturer's guidelines for reconstitution of the powder vial.
- Administer into the abdominal area within 1 h of reconstitution.
- Initial dose: Give as 2 subcutaneous injections of 120 mg each (at a concentration of 40 mg/mL).
- Maintenance dose: Give 1 subcutaneous injection of 80 mg (at a concentration of 20 mg/mL).
- Store at 25° C (77° F), excursions permitted between 15°–30° C (59°–86° F).

ADVERSE EFFECTS (≥1%) **Body as a Whole:** *Injection-site reactions*, night sweats. **CNS:** Asthenia, chills, dizziness, fatigue, fever, headache, insomnia. **CV:** *Hot flashes*, hypertension. **GI:** Constipation, nausea, diarrhea. **Metabolic:** Increases in ALT, AST, and GGT, *weight gain*. **Musculoskeletal:** Arthralgia, back pain. **Urogenital:** Erectile dysfunction, gynecomastia, testicular atrophy, urinary tract infections.

INTERACTIONS Drug: Degarelix may cause an additive effect with other drugs that prolong the QT interval prolongation (e.g., ANTIARRHYTHMIC AGENTS, **chlorpromazine, dolasetron, droperidol, mefloquine, mesoridazine, moxifloxacin, pentamidine, pimozide, tacrolimus, thioridazine, ziprasidone**).

PHARMACOKINETICS Peak: 2 days. **Distribution:** 90% Plasma protein bound. **Metabolism:** Hepatobiliary. **Elimination:** Biliary excretion 70–80%; urinary excretion 20–30%. **Half-Life:** 53 days.

NURSING IMPLICATIONS

Assessment & Drug Effects

- Monitor ECG and QT interval, especially with electrolyte imbalances, a history of CHF, and concurrent Class IA (e.g., quinidine) or III (e.g., amiodarone) antiarrhythmics.
- Lab tests: Baseline and periodic PSA and serum testosterone, periodic LFTs.

Patient & Family Education

- Hot flashes are a common side effect that usually subside spontaneously.
- Degarelix can decrease bone density leading to osteoporosis. With

long-term therapy, bone density tests are advisable.

D

DELAVIRDINE MESYLATE

(del-a-vir′deen)

Rescriptor

Classifications: ANTIVIRAL; NONNUCLEOSIDE REVERSE TRANSCRIPTASE INHIBITOR (NNRTI)

Therapeutic: ANTIVIRAL; NNRTI

Prototype: Efavirenz

Pregnancy Category: C

AVAILABILITY 100 mg tablets

ACTION & *THERAPEUTIC EFFECT* Nonnucleoside reverse transcriptase inhibitor (NNRTI) of HIV-1 binds directly to reverse transcriptase (RT) and disrupts RNA- and DNA-dependent DNA polymerase activities. *It prevents replication of the HIV-1 virus. Resistant strains appear rapidly.*

USES Treatment of HIV infection in combination with other antiretroviral agents.

CONTRAINDICATIONS Hypersensitivity to delavirdine; concurrent administration with drugs that are highly dependent on CYP3A for clearance, and for which elevated plasma concentrations are associated with serious or life-threatening events; lactation.

CAUTIOUS USE Impaired liver function; elderly; achlorhydria; pregnancy (category C).

ROUTE & DOSAGE

HIV Infection

Adult/Adolescent: **PO** 400 mg t.i.d.

ADMINISTRATION

Oral

- Disperse in water by adding a single dose to at least 3 oz of water, let stand for a few minutes, then stir to create a uniform suspension just prior to administration.
- Give drug to patients with achlorhydria with an acid beverage such as orange or cranberry juice.
- Store at 20°–25° C (68°–77° F) and protect from high humidity in a tightly closed container.

ADVERSE EFFECTS (≥1%) **Body as a Whole:** Headache, fatigue, allergic reaction, chills, edema, arthralgia. **CNS:** Abnormal coordination, agitation, amnesia, anxiety, confusion, dizziness. **CV:** Chest pain, bradycardia, palpitations, postural hypotension, tachycardia. **GI:** Nausea, vomiting, diarrhea, increased LFTs, abdominal cramps, anorexia, aphthous stomatitis. **Hematologic:** Neutropenia. **Respiratory:** Bronchitis, cough, dyspnea. **Skin:** *Rash,* pruritus.

INTERACTIONS Drug: ANTACIDS, H_2-RECEPTOR ANTAGONISTS decrease absorption; **didanosine** and **delavirdine** should be taken 1 h apart to avoid decreased delavirdine levels; **clarithromycin, fluoxetine, ketoconazole** may increase delavirdine levels; **carbamazepine, phenobarbital, phenytoin, rifabutin, rifampin** may decrease delavirdine levels; delavirdine may increase levels of **clarithromycin, indinavir, saquinavir, dapsone, rifabutin, alprazolam, midazolam, triazolam,** DIHYDROPYRIDINE, CALCIUM CHANNEL BLOCKERS (e.g., **nifedipine, nicardipine,** etc.), **quinidine, warfarin.** Use with HMG-COA REDUCTASE INHIBITORS may increase the risk of rhabdomyolysis. Use with **pimozide** may cause cardiac arrhythmias. Use with **trazodone** may increase **tra-**

zodone levels. Use with inhaled **fluticasone** may increase **fluticasone** levels. Use with HYPNOTICS, **alprazolam, midazolam, triazolam** can cause respiratory depression. **Herbal: St. John's wort** may decrease antiretroviral activity.

PHARMACOKINETICS Absorption: Rapidly from GI tract, 80% reaches systemic circulation. **Peak:** 1 h. **Distribution:** 98% protein bound. **Metabolism:** In the liver by CYP3A4. **Elimination:** Half in urine, 44% in feces. **Half-Life:** 2–11 h.

NURSING IMPLICATIONS

Assessment & Drug Effects

- Therapeutic effectiveness: Indicated by decreased viral load.
- Monitor for and immediately report appearance of a rash, generally within 1–3 wk of starting therapy; rash is usually diffuse, maculopapular, erythematous, and pruritic.

Patient & Family Education

- Take this drug exactly as prescribed. Missed doses increase risk of drug resistance.
- Do not take antacids and delavirdine at the same time; separate by at least 1 h.
- Report all prescription and nonprescription drugs used to physician because of multiple drug interactions.
- Discontinue medication and notify physician if rash is accompanied by any of the following: Fever, blistering, oral lesions, conjunctivitis, swelling, muscle or joint pain.

DEMECLOCYCLINE HYDROCHLORIDE

(dem-e-kloe-sye'kleen)

Declomycin

Classifications: ANTIBIOTIC; TETRACYCLINE

Therapeutic: TETRACYCLINE ANTIBIOTIC

Prototype: Tetracycline

Pregnancy Category: D

AVAILABILITY 150 mg capsules; 150 mg, 300 mg tablets

ACTION & *THERAPEUTIC EFFECT* Demeclocycline is a broad-spectrum, tetracycline antibiotic. It is pumped through the inner cytoplasmic membrane of bacteria. Demeclocycline blocks the binding of transfer RNA (tRNA) to the messenger RNA (mRNA) of the bacteria. Therefore, bacterial protein synthesis is inhibited and bacterial cells are destroyed. *Effective against both gram-positive and gram-negative bacteria.*

USES Similar to those of tetracycline.

UNLABELED USES Treatment of chronic SIADH (syndrome of inappropriate antidiuretic hormone) secretion.

CONTRAINDICATIONS Hypersensitivity to any of the tetracyclines; severe renal or hepatic disease; cirrhosis, common bile duct obstruction; period of tooth development in fetus; pregnancy (category D), lactation, children younger than 8 y (causes permanent yellow discoloration of teeth, enamel hypoplasia, and retarded bone growth).

CAUTIOUS USE Mild or moderate impaired renal or hepatic function; nephrogenic diabetes insipidus; use of capsule or tablet formulations in patients with esophageal compression or obstruction.

ROUTE & DOSAGE

Anti-infective

Adult: **PO** 150 mg q6h or 300 mg q12h (max: 2.4 g/day)

Child (older than 8 y): **PO** 8–12 mg/kg/day divided q8–12h

Gonorrhea

Adult: **PO** 600 mg followed by 300 mg q12h for 4 days

SIADH

Adult: **PO** 600–1200 mg/day in 3–4 divided doses

ADMINISTRATION

Oral

- Give not less than 1 h before or 2 h after meals. Foods rich in iron (e.g., red meat or dark green vegetables) or calcium (e.g., milk products) impair absorption.
- Concomitant therapy: Do not give antacids with tetracyclines.
- Check expiration date before giving drug. Renal damage and death have resulted from use of outdated tetracyclines.
- Store in tight, light-resistant containers, preferably at 15°–30° C (59°–86° F) unless otherwise directed. Tetracyclines form toxic products when outdated or exposed to light, heat, or humidity.

ADVERSE EFFECTS (≥1%) **Body as a Whole:** Hypersensitivity [*photosensitivity,* pericarditis, anaphylaxis (rare)]. **GI:** *Nausea,* vomiting, *diarrhea,* esophageal irritation or ulceration, enterocolitis, abdominal cramps, anorexia. **Urogenital:** Diabetes insipidus, azotemia, hyperphosphatemia. **Skin:** Pruritus, erythematous eruptions, exfoliative dermatitis.

DIAGNOSTIC TEST INTERFERENCE Like other tetracyclines, demeclocycline may cause false increases in ***urine catecholamines*** (***fluorometric*** methods); false decreases in ***urine urobilinogen;*** and false-negative ***urine glucose*** with ***glucose oxidase*** methods (e.g., ***Clinistix, TesTape***).

INTERACTIONS Drug: ANTACIDS, IRON PREPARATION, **calcium, magnesium, zinc, kaolin-pectin, sodium bicarbonate** can significantly decrease demeclocycline absorption; effects of **desmopressin** and demeclocycline antagonized; increases **digoxin** absorption, increasing risk of **digoxin** toxicity; **methoxyflurane** increases risk of renal failure. **Food:** Dairy products significantly decrease demeclocycline absorption; food may decrease drug absorption also.

PHARMACOKINETICS Absorption: 60–80% absorbed from GI tract. **Peak:** 3–4 h. **Distribution:** Concentrated in liver; crosses placenta; distributed into breast milk. **Metabolism:** In liver; enterohepatic circulation. **Elimination:** 40–50% excreted in urine and 31% in feces in 48 h. **Half-Life:** 10–17 h.

NURSING IMPLICATIONS

Assessment & Drug Effects

- Lab tests: C&S prior to initial therapy and periodically during prolonged therapy. With prolonged therapy, add periodic evaluations of serum drug levels, electrolytes, and renal, hepatic, and hematopoietic systems.
- Monitor I&O ratio and pattern and record weights in patients with impaired kidney or liver function, or on prolonged or high dose therapy.

Patient & Family Education

- Do not use antacids while taking this drug.
- Take drug on an empty stomach to enhance absorption. Because esophageal irritation and ulceration have been reported, take each dose with a full glass (240 mL) of water; remain upright for at

least 90 sec after taking medication; and avoid taking drug within 1 h of lying down or bedtime.

- Notify physician if gastric distress is a problem; a snack or light meal free of dairy products may be added to the regimen.
- Report symptoms of superinfections (see Appendix F).
- Demeclocycline-induced phototoxic reaction can be unusually severe. Avoid sunlight as much as possible and use sunscreen.

DENILEUKIN DIFTITOX

(den-i-leu′kin dif′ti-tox)

Ontak

Classifications: ANTINEOPLASTIC; INTERLEUKIN-2 (IL-2) RECEPTOR INHIBITOR

Therapeutic: ANTINEOPLASTIC; IMMUNOMODULATOR; IL-2 RECEPTOR INHIBITOR

Pregnancy Category: C

AVAILABILITY 150 mcg/mL vial

ACTION & *THERAPEUTIC EFFECT* A recombinant DNA cytotoxic protein that is an interleukin-2 (IL-2) receptor-specific protein that acts as an antineoplastic agent. It acts against malignant cells that express particular high-affinity IL-2 receptors on the cell surface, thus inhibiting cellular protein synthesis and causing cell death in malignant cells. *Effectiveness is indicated by reduced tumor burden. Interacts with high affinity to IL-2 receptors on the cell surface in particular leukemias and lymphomas.*

USES Persistent or recurrent T-cell lymphoma.

CONTRAINDICATIONS Hypersensitivity to denileukin, diphtheria toxin, or interleukin-2; serum albumin levels below 3 g/dL; lactation.

CAUTIOUS USE Cardiovascular disease; peripheral vascular disease, coronary artery disease; hepatic and renal impairment, elderly; preexisting lowering of serum albumin levels; pregnancy (category C). Safety and efficacy in children younger than 18 y are unknown.

ROUTE & DOSAGE

T-Cell Lymphoma

Adult: **IV** 9 or 18 mcg/kg/day for 5 days every 21 days

ADMINISTRATION

Intravenous

PREPARE: **IV Infusion:** Bring vials to room temperature (solution will be clear when room temperature is reached). Swirl to mix, but do not shake. ▪ Use only plastic syringe and plastic IV bag. Withdraw the calculated dose and inject it into an <u>empty</u> IV bag. Add NO MORE THAN 9 mL sterile saline without preservative to IV bag for each 1 mL of drug. ▪ Use within 6 h of preparation.

ADMINISTER: **IV Infusion:** Infuse over <u>at least</u> 15 min without an in-line filter. ▪ Stop infusion and notify physician if S&S of hypersensitivity occur.

INCOMPATIBILITIES **Solution/additive:** Do not physically mix with any other drug.

ADVERSE EFFECTS (≥1%) **Body as a Whole:** *Chills, fever, asthenia, infection, pain, headache, chest pain,* flu-like syndrome; injection site reaction; *acute hypersensitivity reaction (hypotension, back pain, dyspnea, vasodilation, rash, chest pain or tightness, tachycardia, dysphagia, syncope, <u>anaphylaxis</u>),* myalgia, ar-

D

thralgia. **CNS:** *Dizziness, paresthesia, nervousness,* confusion, insomnia. **CV:** *Vascular leak syndrome (hypotension, edema, hypoalbuminemia); hypotension, vasodilation, tachycardia,* thrombotic events, hypertension, arrhythmia. **GI:** *Nausea, vomiting, anorexia, diarrhea,* constipation, dyspepsia, dysphagia. **Hematologic:** *Anemia,* thrombocytopenia, leukopenia. **Metabolic:** *Hypoalbuminemia; transaminase increase; edema; hypocalcemia; weight loss;* dehydration; hypokalemia. **Respiratory:** *Dyspnea, cough, pharyngitis, rhinitis,* lung disorder. **Skin:** *Rash, pruritus, sweating.* **Urogenital:** *Hematuria, albuminuria, pyuria, increased creatinine.* **Special Senses:** Loss of visual acuity.

INTERACTIONS No clinically significant interactions established.

PHARMACOKINETICS Distribution: Primarily distributed to liver and kidneys. **Metabolism:** By proteolytic degradation. **Half-Life:** 70–80 min.

NURSING IMPLICATIONS

Assessment & Drug Effects

- Monitor and notify physician immediately for S&S of hypersensitivity or anaphylaxis that occur during/within 24 h of infusion.
- Monitor and notify physician immediately for S&S of flu-like syndrome that occur within several hours to days following infusion.
- Monitor outpatients for weight gain, developing edema, or declining blood pressure. Notify physician immediately for S&S of vascular leak syndrome (e.g., edema PLUS hypotension or hypoalbuminemia) that may occur within 2 wk of infusion.
- Lab tests: Baseline and weekly CBC with differential, platelet count, blood chemistry panel (including serum electrolytes, serum albumin, renal and liver functions).

Patient & Family Education

- Report S&S of infection promptly to physician.
- Check weight daily and report rapid weight gain or swelling of extremities promptly.
- Report bothersome adverse effects or S&S of infection or flu-like symptoms (e.g., fever, nausea, vomiting, diarrhea, rash).

DESIPRAMINE HYDROCHLORIDE

(dess-ip′ra-meen)

Norpramin

Classification: TRICYCLIC ANTIDEPRESSANT

Therapeutic: TRICYCLIC ANTIDEPRESSANT

Prototype: Imipramine

Pregnancy Category: C

AVAILABILITY 10 mg, 25 mg, 50 mg, 75 mg, 100 mg, 150 mg tablets

ACTION & *THERAPEUTIC EFFECT* Desipramine is a tricyclic antidepressant (TCA) and the active metabolite of imipramine. Antidepressant activity appears to be related to blocking reuptake of norepinephrine and serotonin in the CNS, thus increasing their levels. *In common with other TCAs, it has antidepressant activity.*

USES Endogenous depression and various depression syndromes.

UNLABELED USES Attention deficit disorder in children older than 6 y and adolescents; to prevent depression in cocaine withdrawal.

CONTRAINDICATIONS Hypersensitivity to tricyclic compounds; recent MI, QT prolongation, cardiac arrhythmias, AV block, bundle branch block; concurrent use of MAOI therapy; suicidal ideation; lactation. Safe use in children younger than 6 y is not established.

CAUTIOUS USE Urinary retention, prostatic hypertrophy; narrow-angle glaucoma; epilepsy; alcoholism; adolescents, older adults; bipolar disease; thyroid; cardiovascular, renal, and hepatic disease; suicidal tendency; ECT; elective surgery; pregnancy (category C).

ROUTE & DOSAGE

Antidepressant

Adult: **PO** 75–100 mg/day at bedtime or in divided doses, may gradually increase to 150–300 mg/day (use lower doses in older adult patients)
Adolescent: **PO** 25–50 mg/day in divided doses (max: 100 mg/day)
Child (6–12 y): **PO** 1–3 mg/kg/day in divided doses (max: 5 mg/kg/day)

Pharmacogenetic Dosage Adjustment

CYP2D6 poor metabolizers: Start with 40% of normal dose

ADMINISTRATION

Oral

- Give drug with or immediately after food to reduce possibility of gastric irritation.
- Give maintenance dose at bedtime to minimize daytime sedation.
- Store drug in tightly closed container at 15°–30° C (59°–86° F) unless otherwise specified.

ADVERSE EFFECTS (≥1%) **Body as a Whole:** Hypersensitivity (rash, urticaria, photosensitivity). **CNS:** *Drowsiness,* dizziness, weakness, fatigue, headache, insomnia, confusional states, depressive reaction, paresthesias, ataxia. **CV:** *Postural hypotension,* hypotension, palpitation, tachycardia, ECG changes, flushing, heart block. **Special Senses:** Tinnitus, parotid swelling; blurred vision, disturbances in accommodation, mydriasis, increased IOP. **GI:** *Dry mouth, constipation,* bad taste, diarrhea, nausea. **Urogenital:** *Urinary retention,* frequency, delayed micturition, nocturia; impaired sexual function, galactorrhea. **Hematologic:** Bone marrow depression and agranulocytosis (rare). **Other:** Sweating, craving for sweets, weight gain or loss, SIADH secretion, hyperpyrexia, eosinophilic pneumonia.

INTERACTIONS Drug: May somewhat decrease response to ANTIHYPERTENSIVES; CNS DEPRESSANTS, **alcohol,** HYPNOTICS, BARBITURATES, SEDATIVES potentiate CNS depression; may increase hypoprothrombinemic effect of ORAL ANTICOAGULANTS; **ethchlorvynol** may cause transient delirium; **levodopa,** SYMPATHOMIMETICS (e.g., **epinephrine, norepinephrine**) pose possibility of sympathetic hyperactivity with hypertension and hyperpyrexia; MAO INHIBITORS pose possibility of severe reactions, toxic psychosis, cardiovascular instability; **methylphenidate** increases plasma TCA levels; THYROID AGENTS may increase possibility of arrhythmias; **cimetidine** may increase plasma TCA levels. **Herbal: Ginkgo** may decrease seizure threshold; **St. John's wort** may cause **serotonin** syndrome.

PHARMACOKINETICS Absorption: Rapidly from GI tract and injection sites. **Peak:** 4–6 h. **Distribution:** Crosses placenta. **Metabolism:** In liver. **Elimination:** Primarily in urine. **Half-Life:** 7–60 h.

D

NURSING IMPLICATIONS

Assessment & Drug Effects

- Monitor children and adolescents for signs of suicidal ideation.
- Monitor for therapeutic effectiveness: Usually not realized until after at least 2 wk of therapy.
- Monitor BP and pulse rate during early phase of therapy, particularly in older adult, debilitated, or cardiovascular patients. If BP rises or falls more than 20 mm Hg or if there is a sudden increase in pulse rate or change in rhythm, withhold drug and inform physician.
- Note: Drowsiness, dizziness, and orthostatic hypotension are signs of impending toxicity in patient on long-term, high dosage therapy. Prolonged QT or QRS intervals indicate possible toxicity. Report to physician.
- Observe patient with history of glaucoma. Report symptoms that may signal acute attack: Severe headache, eye pain, dilated pupils, halos of light, nausea, vomiting.
- Monitor bowel elimination pattern and I&O ratio. Severe constipation and urinary retention are potential problems of TCA therapy.
- Note: Norpramin tablets may contain tartrazine, which can cause allergic-type reactions including bronchial asthma in susceptible individuals. Such individuals are frequently also sensitive to aspirin.

Patient & Family Education

- Make all position changes slowly and in stages, particularly from recumbent to standing position.
- Do not drive or engage in other potentially hazardous activities until reaction to drug is known.
- Take medication exactly as prescribed; do not change dose or dose intervals.
- Note: Patients who receive high doses for prolonged periods may experience withdrawal symptoms including headache, nausea, musculoskeletal pain, and weakness if drug is discontinued abruptly.
- Do not take OTC drugs unless physician has approved their use.
- Stop, or at least limit, smoking because it may increase the metabolism of desipramine, thereby diminishing its therapeutic action.

DESLORATADINE

(des-lor-a-ta′deen)

Clarinex, Clarinex Reditabs

Classifications: ANTIHISTAMINE, NONSEDATING; H_1-RECEPTOR ANTAGONIST

Therapeutic: ANTIHISTAMINE; ANTIALLERGIC

Prototype: Loratadine

Pregnancy Category: C

AVAILABILITY 5 mg tablets; 2.5 mg, 5 mg orally dissolving tablets; 0.5 mg/mL syrup

ACTION & *THERAPEUTIC EFFECT*

A long-acting, nonsedating antihistamine with selective H_1-receptor antagonist properties. The drug reduces human mast cell release of the inflammatory cytokines. Therefore, it also exhibits antiallergic effects. *Desloratadine is effective in controlling allergic rhinitis and inhibiting histamine-induced wheals and flare (hives).*

USES Treatment of seasonal or perennial allergic rhinitis and idiopathic urticaria.

CONTRAINDICATIONS Hypersensitivity to desloratadine or loratadine; neonates; infants; lactation.
CAUTIOUS USE Renal and hepatic insufficiencies; bladder neck obstruction or urinary retention; prostatic hypertrophy; asthma; glaucoma; pregnancy (category C). Safety and efficacy in children younger than 12 y not known.

ROUTE & DOSAGE

Allergic Rhinitis, Idiopathic Urticaria

Adult: **PO** 5 mg daily

Renal Impairment Dosage Adjustment

CrCl less than 50 mL/min: 5 mg every other day

Hepatic Impairment Dosage Adjustment

5 mg every other day

ADMINISTRATION

Oral
- Note that drug should be given every other day to patients with significant renal or hepatic impairment.
- Store between 2°–25° C (36°–77° F).

ADVERSE EFFECTS (≥1%) **Body as a Whole:** Pharyngitis, fatigue, flu-like symptoms, myalgia. **CNS:** Somnolence, dizziness. **GI:** Dry mouth, nausea, dry throat. **Urogenital:** Dysmenorrhea.

INTERACTIONS Drug: No clinically significant interactions established.

PHARMACOKINETICS Absorption: Well absorbed. **Peak:** 3 h. **Distribution:** 85–89% protein bound. **Metabolism:** Extensively metabolized in liver to 3-hydroxydesloratadine, an active metabolite. **Elimination:** Equally in urine and feces. **Half-Life:** 27 h.

NURSING IMPLICATIONS

Assessment & Drug Effects
- Monitor cardiovascular status and report significant changes in BP and palpitations or tachycardia.
- Lab tests: Monitor periodically renal and liver function tests.
- Concurrent drugs: Monitor ECG when used in combination with any other drug that can produce an additive effect causing QT interval prolongation.

Patient & Family Education
- Drug may cause significant drowsiness in older adult patients and those with liver or kidney impairment.
- Note: Concurrent use of alcohol and other CNS depressants may have an additive effect.
- Do not take this drug more often than every other day if you have renal impairment.

DESMOPRESSIN ACETATE

(des-moe-pres′sin)
DDAVP, Stimate
Classification: POSTERIOR PITUITARY HORMONE
Therapeutic: ANTIDIURETIC HORMONE (ADH)

Prototype: Vasopressin
Pregnancy Category: B

AVAILABILITY 0.1 mg, 0.2 mg tablets; 0.1% nasal solution; 0.15 mg/spray nasal spray; 4 mcg/mL, 15 mcg/mL injection

D

ACTION & *THERAPEUTIC EFFECT*

Synthetic analog of the natural human posterior pituitary (antidiuretic) hormone, arginine vasopressin. Reduces urine volume and osmolality of serum in patients with central diabetes insipidus by increasing reabsorption of water by kidney collecting tubules. Produces a dose-related increase in factor VIII (antihemophilic factor) and von Willebrand's factor. *Desmopressin is an effective replacement for antidiuretic hormone. It also can shorten or normalize bleeding time, and correct platelet adhesion abnormalities in certain patients with bleeding disorders.*

USES To control and prevent symptoms and complications of central (neurohypophyseal) diabetes insipidus, and to relieve temporary polyuria and polydipsia associated with trauma or surgery in the pituitary region.

UNLABELED USES To increase factor VIII activity in selected patients with mild to moderate hemophilia A and in type I von Willebrand's disease or uremia, and to control enuresis in children.

CONTRAINDICATIONS Nephrogenic diabetes insipidus, type II B von Willebrand's disease; renal failure, renal impairment; **PO form:** Patients with fluid and electrolyte imbalance; **intranasal form:** Children with primary nocturnal enuresis (PNE).

CAUTIOUS USE Coronary artery insufficiency, hypertensive cardiovascular disease; history of hyponatremia; water intoxication with hyponatremia; severe CHF; older adults; history of thromboembolic disease; pregnancy (category B).

ROUTE & DOSAGE

Diabetes Insipidus

Adult: **Intranasal** 0.1–0.4 mL (10–40 mcg) in 1–3 divided doses **IV/Subcutaneous** 2–4 mcg in 2 divided doses **PO** 0.2–0.4 mg/day
Child: **Intranasal** *3 mo–12 y,* 0.05–0.3 mL in 1–2 divided doses **IV/Subcutaneous** 0.3 mcg/kg infused over 15–30 min **PO** 0.05 mg titrated to response

Enuresis

Adult: **Intranasal** 5–40 mcg at bedtime
Child (6 y or older): **PO** 0.2 mg at bedtime, may titrate up to 0.6 mg at bedtime

Von Willebrand's Disease

Adult/Child (older than 3 mo): **IV/Subcutaneous** 0.3 mcg/kg 30 min preop, may repeat in 48 h if needed

Renal Impairment Dosage Adjustment

Do not use if CrCl is less than 50 mL/min

ADMINISTRATION

Oral

- Note that 0.2 mg PO is equivalent to 10 mcg (0.1 mL) intranasal.

Intranasal

- Follow manufacturer's instructions for proper technique with nasal spray.
- Give initial dose in the evening, and observe antidiuretic effect. Dose is increased each evening until uninterrupted sleep is obtained. If daily urine volume is more than 2 L after nocturia is controlled, morning dose is started

and adjusted daily until urine volume does not exceed 1.5–2 L/24 h.

Subcutaneous

- Give undiluted.

Intravenous

PREPARE: **Direct:** Give undiluted for diabetes insipidus. **IV Infusion:** Dilute 0.3 mcg/kg in 10 mL of NS (children weighing 10 kg or less) or 50 mL of NS (children greater than 10 kg and adults) for von Willebrand's disease (type I).

ADMINISTER: **Direct:** Give direct IV over 30 s for diabetes insipidus. **IV Infusion:** Give over 15–30 min for von Willebrand's disease (type I).

- Store parenteral and nasal solution in refrigerator preferably at 4° C (39.2° F) unless otherwise directed. Avoid freezing. ▪ Nasal spray can be stored at room temperature. ▪ Discard solutions that are discolored or contain particulate matter.

ADVERSE EFFECTS (≥1%) **All:** Dose related. **CNS:** Transient headache, drowsiness, listlessness. **Special Senses:** Nasal congestion, rhinitis, nasal irritation. **GI:** Nausea, heartburn, mild abdominal cramps. **Other:** Vulval pain, shortness of breath, slight rise in BP, facial flushing, pain and swelling at injection site, hyponatremia.

INTERACTIONS Drug: Demeclocycline, lithium, other VASOPRESSORS may decrease antidiuretic response; **carbamazepine, chlorpropamide, clofibrate** may prolong antidiuretic response.

PHARMACOKINETICS Absorption: 10–20% through nasal mucosa. **Onset:** 15–60 min. **Peak:** 1–5 h. **Duration:** 5–21 h. **Distribution:** Small amount crosses blood–brain barrier; distributed into breast milk. **Half-Life:** 76 min.

NURSING IMPLICATIONS

Assessment & Drug Effects

- Monitor I&O ratio and pattern (intervals). Fluid intake **must be** carefully controlled, particularly in older adults and the very young to avoid water retention and sodium depletion.
- Weigh patient daily and observe for edema. Severe water retention may require reduction in dosage and use of a diuretic.
- Monitor BP during dosage-regulating period and whenever drug is administered parenterally.
- Lab tests: Monitor urine and plasma osmolality. An increase in urine osmolality and a decrease in plasma osmolality indicate effectiveness of treatment in diabetes insipidus.

Patient & Family Education

- Report upper respiratory tract infection or nasal congestion.
- Follow manufacturer's instructions for insertion to ensure delivery of drug high into nasal cavity and not down throat. A flexible calibrated plastic tube is provided.

DESONIDE

(dess′oh-nide)

DesOwen, Tridesilon

Pregnancy Category: C

See Appendix A-4.

DESOXIMETASONE

(des-ox-i-met′a-sone)

Topicort, Topicort-LP

Pregnancy Category: C
See Appendix A-4.

D

DEXAMETHASONE

(dex-a-meth'a-sone)

Decadron, Dexamethasone Intensol, Maxidex, Mymethasone

DEXAMETHASONE SODIUM PHOSPHATE

Decadron Phosphate, Maxidex Ophthalmic

Classifications: ADRENAL CORTICOSTEROID; GLUCOCORTICOID
Therapeutic: ADRENAL CORTICOSTEROID
Prototype: Prednisone
Pregnancy Category: C

AVAILABILITY **Dexamethasone:** 0.25 mg, 0.5 mg, 0.75 mg, 1 mg, 1.5 mg, 2 mg, 4 mg, 6 mg tablets; 0.5 mg/5 mL, 0.5 mg/0.5 mg oral solution; 0.01%, 0.04% topical aerosol; **Dexamethasone sodium phosphate:** 4 mg/mL, 10 mg/mL, 20 mg/mL, 24 mg/mL injection; 0.1% cream; 0.1% ophth solution, suspension; 0.05% ophth ointment

ACTION & *THERAPEUTIC EFFECT* Long-acting synthetic adrenocorticoid with intense anti-inflammatory (glucocorticoid) activity and minimal mineralocorticoid activity. ***Anti-inflammatory action:*** Prevents accumulation of inflammatory cells at sites of infection; inhibits phagocytosis, lysosomal enzyme release, and synthesis of potent mediators of inflammation, prostaglandins, and leukotrienes; reduces capillary dilation and permeability. ***Immunosuppression:*** May be due to prevention or suppression of delayed hypersensitivity immune reaction. *Has anti-inflammatory and immunosuppression properties.*

USES Adrenal insufficiency concomitantly with a mineralocorticoid; inflammatory conditions, allergic states, collagen diseases, hematologic disorders, cerebral edema, and addisonian shock. Also palliative treatment of neoplastic disease, as adjunctive short-term therapy in acute rheumatic disorders and GI diseases, and as a diagnostic test for Cushing's syndrome and for differential diagnosis of adrenal hyperplasia and adrenal adenoma.
UNLABELED USES As an antiemetic in cancer chemotherapy; as a diagnostic test for endogenous depression; and to prevent hyaline membrane disease in premature infants.

CONTRAINDICATIONS Systemic fungal infection, acute infections, active or resting tuberculosis, vaccinia, varicella, administration of live virus vaccines (to patient, family members), latent or active amebiasis; Cushing's syndrome; neonates or infants weighing less than 1300 g; lactation. ***Topical use:*** Rosacea, perioral dermatitis; venous statis ulcers. ***Ophthalmic use:*** Primary open-angle glaucoma, eye infections, superficial ocular herpes simplex, keratitis, and tuberculosis of eye.
CAUTIOUS USE Stromal herpes simplex, keratitis, GI ulceration, renal disease, diabetes mellitus, hypothyroidism, myasthenia gravis, CHF, cirrhosis, psychic disorders, seizures; children; coagulopathy; pregnancy (category C).

D

ROUTE & DOSAGE

Allergies, Inflammation, Neoplasias

Adult: **PO** 0.25–4 mg b.i.d. to q.i.d. **IM** 8–16 mg q1–3wk or 0.8–1.6 mg intralesional q1–3wk **IV** 0.75–0.9 mg/kg/day divided q6–12h
Child: **PO/IV/IM** 0.08–0.3 mg/kg/day divided q6–12h

Cerebral Edema

Adult: **IV** 10 mg followed by 4 mg q6h, reduce dose after 2–4 days then taper over 5–7 days
Child: **PO/IV/IM** 1–2 mg/kg loading dose, then 1–1.5 mg/kg/day divided q4–6h × 5 days (max: 16 mg/day)

Shock

Adult: **IV** 1–6 mg/kg as a single dose or 40 mg repeated q2–6h if needed or 20 mg bolus then 3 mg/kg/day

Dexamethasone Suppression Test

Adult: **PO** 0.5 mg q6h for 48 h

Inflammation

Adult/Child: **Ophthalmic/Topical/Inhalation/Intranasal** See Appendix A

ADMINISTRATION

Oral

- Give the once-daily dose in the a.m. with food or liquid of patient's choice.
- Taper dosage over a period of time before discontinuing because adrenal suppression can occur with prolonged use.
- Do not store or expose aerosol to temperature above 48.9° C (120° F); do not puncture or discard into a fire or an incinerator.

Intramuscular

- Give IM injection deep into a large muscle mass (e.g., gluteus maximus). Avoid subcutaneous injection: Atrophy and sterile abscesses may occur.
- Use repository form, dexamethasone acetate, for IM or local injection only. The white suspension settles on standing; mild shaking will resuspend drug.

Intravenous

PREPARE: **Direct:** Give undiluted. **Intermittent:** Dilute in D5W or NS for infusion.

ADMINISTER: **Direct:** Give direct IV push over 30 sec or less. **Intermittent:** Set rate as prescribed or according to amount of solution to infuse.

INCOMPATIBILITIES **Solution/additive:** **Daunorubicin, diphenhydramine, doxorubicin, doxapram, glycopyrrolate, metaraminol, phenobarbital, vancomycin.** **Y-site:** **Ciprofloxacin, fenoldopam, idarubicin, midazolam, topotecan.**

- Store at 15°–30° C (59°–86° F) unless otherwise directed.

ADVERSE EFFECTS (≥1%) **Aerosol Therapy:** *Nasal irritation,* dryness, epistaxis, rebound congestion, bronchial asthma, anosmia, perforation of nasal septum. ***Systemic Absorption*—CNS:** Euphoria, insomnia, convulsions, increased ICP, vertigo, headache, psychic disturbances. **CV:** CHF, hypertension, *edema.* **Endocrine:** Menstrual irregularities, *hyperglycemia;* cushingoid state; growth suppression in children; hirsutism. **Special Senses:** *Posterior subcapsular cataract,* increased IOP, glaucoma, exophthalmos. **GI:** Peptic ulcer with possible perforation, abdominal distension, nausea, increased appetite, heartburn, dyspepsia, pancreatitis, bowel perforation, *oral candidiasis.* **Musculoskeletal:** Muscle weakness, loss of muscle mass, vertebral compression fracture, pathologic fracture of long bones, tendon rupture. **Skin:** Acne, *impaired wound healing,* petechiae, ecchymoses, diaphoresis, allergic dermatitis, hypo- or hyperpigmentation, subcutaneous and cutaneous atrophy, burning and tingling in perineal area (following IV injection).

DIAGNOSTIC TEST INTERFERENCE ***Dexamethasone suppression test for endogenous depression:*** False-positive results may be caused by **alcohol, glutethimide, meprobamate;** false-negative results may be caused by high doses of benzodiazepines (e.g., **chlordiazepoxide** and **cyproheptadine**), long-term glucocorticoid treatment, **indomethacin, ephedrine,** estrogens or hepatic enzyme-inducing agents **(phenytoin)** may also cause false-positive results in ***test for Cushing's syndrome.***

INTERACTIONS Drug: BARBITURATES, **phenytoin, rifampin** increase steroid metabolism—dosage of dexamethasone may need to be increased; **amphotericin B,** DIURETICS compound potassium loss; **ambenonium, neostigmine, pyridostigmine** may cause severe muscle weakness in patients with myasthenia gravis; may inhibit antibody response to VACCINES, TOXOIDS.

PHARMACOKINETICS Absorption: Readily from GI tract. **Onset:** Rapid. **Peak:** 1–2 h PO; 8 h IM. **Duration:** 2.75 days PO; 6 days IM; 1–3 wk intralesional, intra-articular. **Distribution:** Crosses placenta; distributed into breast milk. **Elimination:** Hypothalamus-pituitary axis suppression: 36–54 h. **Half-Life:** 3–4.5 h.

NURSING IMPLICATIONS

Assessment & Drug Effects

- Monitor and report S&S of Cushing's syndrome (see Appendix F) or other systemic adverse effects.
- Monitor neonates born to a mother who has been receiving a corticosteroid during pregnancy for symptoms of hypoadrenocorticism.
- Monitor for S&S of a hypersensitivity reaction (see Appendix F). The acetate and sodium phosphate formulations may contain bisulfites, parabens, or both; these inactive ingredients are allergenic to some individuals.

Patient & Family Education

- Take drug exactly as prescribed.
- Report lack of response to medication or malaise, orthostatic hypotension, muscular weakness and pain, nausea, vomiting, anorexia, hypoglycemic reactions (see Appendix F), or mental depression to physician.
- Report changes in appearance and easy bruising to physician.
- Add potassium-rich foods to diet; report signs of hypokalemia (see Appendix F). Concomitant potassium-depleting diuretic can enhance dexamethasone-induced potassium loss.
- Note: Dexamethasone dose regimen may need to be altered during stress (e.g., surgery, infections, emotional stress, illness, acute bronchial attacks, trauma). Consult physician if change in living or working environment is anticipated.
- Discontinue drug gradually under the guidance of the physician.
- Note: It is important to prevent exposure to infection, trauma, and sudden changes in environmental factors, as much as possible, because drug is an immunosuppressor.

DEXCHLORPHENIRAMINE MALEATE

(dex-klor-fen-eer'a-meen)

Classifications: ANTIHISTAMINE; H_1-RECEPTOR ANTAGONIST
Therapeutic: ANTIHISTAMINE
Prototype: Diphenhydramine
Pregnancy Category: B

AVAILABILITY 4 mg sustained release tablets; 2 mg/5 mL syrup

ACTION & *THERAPEUTIC EFFECT* H_1-receptor antagonist that competes for H_1-receptor sites on cells, thus blocking histamine release. *Has high antihistamine effects and moderate anticholinergic effects.*

USES Perennial and seasonal allergic rhinitis, other manifestations of allergy, and vasomotor rhinitis. Also as adjunct to epinephrine in treatment of anaphylactic reactions.

CONTRAINDICATIONS Hypersensitivity to antihistamines of similar class; closed-angle glaucoma; acute asthmatic attack, lower respiratory tract symptoms, newborns, premature infants, children younger than 2 y (**syrup** and **tablets**), **extended release tablets:** children younger than 6 y for 4 mg and 12 y for 6 mg.
CAUTIOUS USE Increased intraocular pressure; prostatic hypertrophy; hyperthyroidism; asthma, COPD; renal, hepatic, and cardiovascular disease; serious GI disorders; older adults; pregnancy (category B), lactation.

ROUTE & DOSAGE

Allergic Rhinitis

Adult: **PO** 4–6 mg at bedtime or q8–10h during the day

Child: **PO** *2–5 y,* 0.5 mg q4–6h (max: 3 mg/24 h); *6–11 y,* 1 mg q4–6h (max: 6 mg/24 h) or 4 mg at bedtime

ADMINISTRATION

Oral
- Ensure that sustained release form of drug is not chewed or crushed. It **must be** swallowed whole.
- Give medication with food, water, or milk to lessen GI distress.
- Store at 15°–30° C (59°–86° F) unless otherwise directed.

ADVERSE EFFECTS (≥1%) **CNS:** *Drowsiness,* dizziness, weakness, headache, excitation, neuritis, disturbed coordination, insomnia, euphoria, paresthesias. **Special Senses:** Vertigo, tinnitus, acute labyrinthitis; blurred vision. **CV:** Palpitations, tachycardia, hypotension, extrasystoles. **GI:** Nausea, vomiting, anorexia, *dry mouth,* constipation, diarrhea. **Urogenital:** Difficulty in urinating, *urinary retention,* urinary frequency, early menses. **Hematologic:** <u>Agranulocytosis</u> (rare), hemolytic or hypoplastic anemia. **Skin:** Skin eruptions, photosensitivity.

DIAGNOSTIC TEST INTERFERENCE In common with other antihistamines, dexchlorpheniramine may interfere with ***skin tests for allergy;*** discontinue dexchlorpheniramine at least 72 h before tests.

INTERACTIONS Drug: Alcohol and other CNS DEPRESSANTS, MAO INHIBITORS compound CNS depression.

PHARMACOKINETICS Absorption: Readily from GI tract. **Onset:** 15–30 min. **Peak:** 3 h. **Distribution:** Small amounts into breast milk. **Metabolism:** In liver. **Elimination:** In urine within 24 h.

NURSING IMPLICATIONS

Assessment & Drug Effects

- Supervise ambulation and take safety precautions, especially with older adult patients.
- Monitor I&O and assess for difficulty voiding (e.g., frequency or retention).

Patient & Family Education

- Swallow timed or sustained release tablet whole. Do not break, crush, or chew.
- Do not drive or engage in other potentially hazardous activities until reaction to drug is known.
- Ask physician about the use of alcohol, tranquilizers, sedatives, or other CNS depressants because the effects of dexchlorpheniramine will be additive.

DEXMEDETOMIDINE HYDROCHLORIDE

(dex-med-e-to′mi-deen)

Precedex

Classifications: ALPHA$_2$-ADRENERGIC AGONIST; SEDATIVE-HYPNOTIC
Therapeutic: SEDATIVE-HYPNOTIC
Prototype: Methoxamine HCl
Pregnancy Category: C

AVAILABILITY 100 mcg/mL injection

ACTION & *THERAPEUTIC EFFECT* Dexmedetomidine stimulates alpha$_2$-adrenergic receptors in the CNS (primarily in the medulla oblongata) causing inhibition of the sympathetic vasomotor center of the brain. Hemodynamic responses of the heart affected by alpha$_2$ receptors are better controlled with dexmedetomidine than with other related drugs (e.g., midazolam). *Sedative properties utilized in intubating patients and for initially maintaining them on a mechanical ventilator.*

USES Sedation of initially intubated or mechanically ventilated patients.

CONTRAINDICATIONS Hypersensitivity to dexmedetomidine; labor and delivery, including cesarean section.

CAUTIOUS USE Patients with arrhythmias or cardiovascular disease, uncontrolled hypertension; hypotension; cerebrovascular disease; renal or hepatic insufficiency; signs of light anesthesia; pregnancy (category C), lactation; older adults over 65 y. Safety and efficacy in children younger than 18 y are unknown.

ROUTE & DOSAGE

Sedation

Adult: **IV** 1 mcg/kg loading dose infused over 10 min, then continue with infusion of 0.2–0.7 mcg/kg/h for up to 24 h adjusted to maintain sedation

Hepatic Impairment Dosage Adjustment

Reduce initial dosage

Renal Impairment Dosage Adjustment

CrCl less than 30 mL/min: Reduce initial dose

ADMINISTRATION

Intravenous

***PREPARE:* Continuous:** Withdraw 2 mL of dexmedetomidine and add to 48 mL of NS to yield 4 mcg/mL. Shake gently to mix.

***ADMINISTER:* Continuous:** Administer using a controlled infusion device. ▪ A loading dose of 1 mcg/kg is infused over 10 min followed by the ordered maintenance dose. Do **NOT** use administration set containing natural rubber. Do **NOT** infuse longer than 24 h.

INCOMPATIBILITIES **Y-site: Amphotericin B, diazepam.**

- Store at 15°–30° C (59°–86° F).

ADVERSE EFFECTS (≥1%) **Body as a Whole:** Pain, infection. **CV:** *Hypotension,* bradycardia, atrial fibrillation. **GI:** *Nausea,* thirst. **Respiratory:** Hypoxia, pleural effusion, pulmonary edema. **Hematologic:** Anemia, leukocytosis. **Urogenital:** Oliguria.

INTERACTIONS Drug: BARBITURATES, BENZODIAZEPINES, GENERAL ANESTHETICS, OPIATE AGONISTS, ANXIOLYTICS, SEDATIVES/HYPNOTICS, **ethanol,** TRICYCLIC ANTIDEPRESSANTS, **tramadol,** PHENOTHIAZINES, SKELETAL MUSCLE RELAXANTS, **azatadine, brompheniramine, carbinoxamine, chlorpheniramine, clemastine, cyproheptadine, dexchlorpheniramine, dimenhydrinate, diphenhydramine, doxylamine, hydroxyzine, methdilazine, phenindamine, promethazine, tripelennamine** enhance CNS depression possibly prolong recovery from anesthesia.

PHARMACOKINETICS Metabolism: Extensively in liver (CYP2A6). **Elimination:** Primarily in urine. **Half-Life:** 2 h.

NURSING IMPLICATIONS

Assessment & Drug Effects

- Monitor for hypertension during loading dose; reduction of loading dose may be required.
- Monitor cardiovascular status continuously; notify physician immediately if hypotension or bradycardia occur.

DEXMETHYLPHENIDATE

(dex-meth-ill-fen′i-date)

Focalin, Focalin XR

Classification: CEREBRAL STIMULANT
Therapeutic: CEREBRAL STIMULANT
Prototype: Amphetamine
Pregnancy Category: C
Controlled Substance: Schedule II

AVAILABILITY 2.5 mg, 5 mg, 10 mg tablets; 5 mg, 10 mg, 20 mg extended release capsules

ACTION & *THERAPEUTIC EFFECT* Thought to block the reuptake of norepinephrine and dopamine into the presynaptic neurons and, thereby, increases release of these substances into the synapse. The mode of action in controlling the symptoms of attention deficit hyperactivity disorder (ADHD) is not fully understood. *Is effective in controlling ADHD syndrome in conjunction with other measures (psychological, educational, and social).*

USES Attention deficit hyperactivity disorder (ADHD).

CONTRAINDICATIONS Hypersensitivity to dexmethylphenidate or methylphenidate; known structural cardiac abnormalities in children or adults, cardiomyopathy, congenital heart disease; coronary heart disease; severe agitation, anxiety, or tension; psychotic symptomatology; substance abuse; glaucoma; motor tics other than Tourette's syndrome; concurrent MAOI therapy; children younger than 6 y; seizures; lactation.

CAUTIOUS USE Moderate to severe hepatic insufficiency; Tourette's syndrome; depression; emotional instability; alcoholism or drug dependence; history of seizure disorders; hypertension, CHF, cardiac arrhythmias; hyperthyroidism; pregnancy (category C).

D

ROUTE & DOSAGE

Attention Deficit Hyperactivity Disorder

Adult: **PO** 2.5 mg b.i.d., may increase by 2.5–5 mg/day at weekly intervals to max of 20 mg/day. If converting from methylphenidate, start with 1/2 of methylphenidate dose. Extended release: 10 mg daily, may increase by 5 mg at weekly intervals to max of 20 mg/day.

Child (older than 6 y): **PO** 2.5 mg b.i.d., may increase by 2.5–5 mg/day at weekly intervals to max of 20 mg/day. If converting from methylphenidate, start with 1/2 of methylphenidate dose. Extended release: 5 mg daily, may increase by 5 mg at weekly intervals to max of 20 mg/day.

ADMINISTRATION

Oral

- Do not administer with or within 14 days following discontinuation of an MAO inhibitor.
- Give sustained release capsules whole. They should not be crushed or chewed.
- Give b.i.d. doses at least 4 h apart.
- Store at 15°–30° C (59°–86° F).

ADVERSE EFFECTS (≥1%) **Body as a Whole:** Fever, allergic reactions. **CNS:** Dizziness, insomnia, nervousness, tics, abnormal thinking, hallucinations, emotional lability, CNS overstimulation or sympathomimetic effects [angina, anxiety, agitation, biting, blurred vision, delirium, diaphoresis, flushing or pallor, hallucinations, hyperthermia, labile blood pressure and heart rate (hypotension or hypertension), mydriasis, palpitations, paranoia, purposeless movements, psychosis, sinus tachycardia, tachypnea, or tremor]. **CV:** Hypertension, tachycardia. **GI:** *Abdominal pain,* decreased appetite, nausea, vomiting.

INTERACTIONS Drug: Additive stimulant effects with other STIMULANTS (including **amphetamine, caffeine**); increased vasopressor effects with **dopamine, epinephrine, norepinephrine, phenylpropanolamine, pseudoephedrine;** MAO INHIBITORS may cause hypertensive crisis; antagonizes hypotensive effects of **guanethidine, bretylium;** may inhibit metabolism and increase serum levels of **fosphenytoin, phenytoin, phenobarbital,** and **primidone, warfarin,** TRICYCLIC ANTIDEPRESSANTS.

PHARMACOKINETICS Absorption: Well absorbed. **Peak:** 1–1.5 h. **Metabolism:** De-esterified in liver. No interaction with CYP450 system. **Elimination:** Primarily in urine. **Half-Life:** 2.2 h.

NURSING IMPLICATIONS

Assessment & Drug Effects

- Withhold drug and notify physician if patient has a seizure. Monitor closely for loss of seizure control with a prior history of seizures.
- Monitor BP in all patients receiving this drug. Monitor cardiac status and report palpitations or other signs of arrhythmias.
- Monitor for potential abuse and dependence on this drug. Careful supervision is needed during drug withdrawal since severe depression may occur.
- Monitor for signs of aggression or psychotic behavior in adolescents and children.
- Lab tests: Periodic CBC, differential, platelet counts, and LFTs during prolonged therapy.

- Concurrent drugs: Monitor patients on BP-lowering drugs for loss of BP control. Monitor plasma levels of oral anticoagulants and anticonvulsants; doses of these drugs may need to be decreased.

Patient & Family Education

- Withhold drug and report immediately any of the following signs of overdose: Vomiting, agitation, tremors, muscle twitching, convulsions, confusion, hallucinations, delirium, sweating, flushing, headache, or high temperature.
- Note that drug is usually discontinued if improvement is not observed after appropriate dosage adjustment over 1 mo.

DEXRAZOXANE

(dex-ra-zox′ane)

Zinecard

Classifications: CHELATING AGENT; CHEMOPROTECTIVE AGENT; CARDIOPROTECTIVE

Therapeutic: CARDIOPROTECTIVE FOR DOXORUBICIN

Pregnancy Category: C

AVAILABILITY 250 mg, 500 mg vials for injection

ACTION & *THERAPEUTIC EFFECT* A derivative of EDTA that readily penetrates cell membranes. Dexrazoxane is converted intracellularly to a chelating agent that interferes with iron-mediated free radical generation thought to be partially responsible for one form of cardiomyopathy. *Cardioprotective effect is related to its chelating activity.*

USES Reduction of cardiomyopathy associated with a cumulative doxorubicin dose of 300 mg/m^2.

CONTRAINDICATIONS Chemotherapy regimens that do not contain anthracycline; lactation.

CAUTIOUS USE Myelosuppression, elderly; prior radiation or chemotherapy; renal failure or impairment; pregnancy (category C). Safety and efficacy in children have not been established.

ROUTE & DOSAGE

Cardiomyopathy

Adult: **IV** 10 parts dexrazoxane to 1 part doxorubicin or 500 mg/m^2 for every 50 mg/m^2 of doxorubicin

Renal Impairment Dosage Adjustment

CrCl less than 40 mL/min: Use a 5:1 ratio of dexrazoxane to doxorubicin

ADMINISTRATION

Intravenous

Wear gloves when handling dexrazoxane. Immediately wash with soap and water if drug contacts skin or mucosa.

- Doxorubicin dose **must be** started within 30 min of beginning dexrazoxane.

PREPARE: **Direct:** Reconstitute by adding 25 or 50 mL of 0.167 M sodium lactate injection (provided by manufacturer) to the 250- or 500-mg vial, respectively, to produce a 10-mg/mL solution. **IV Infusion:** Further dilute reconstituted solution with NS or D5W to a concentration of 1.3–5 mg/mL for infusion.

ADMINISTER: **Direct:** Give bolus dose slowly. **IV Infusion:** Give over 10–15 min.

- Store reconstituted solutions for 6 h at 15°–30° C (59°–86° F).

ADVERSE EFFECTS (≥1%) **All:** Adverse effects of dexrazoxane are difficult to distinguish from those of the chemotherapeutic agents. Pain at injection site, leukopenia, granulocytopenia, and thrombocytopenia appear to occur more frequently with the addition of dexrazoxane than with placebo.

PHARMACOKINETICS Distribution: Not protein bound. **Metabolism:** In liver. **Elimination:** 42% in urine. **Half-Life:** 2–2.5 h.

NURSING IMPLICATIONS

Assessment & Drug Effects

- Monitor cardiac function. Drug does not eliminate risk of doxorubicin cardiotoxicity.
- Lab tests: Monitor hepatic, renal, and hematopoietic status throughout course of therapy.
- Note: Adverse effects are likely due to concurrent cytotoxic drugs rather than dexrazoxane.

Patient & Family Education

- Report any of the following to physician: Worsening shortness of breath, swelling extremities, or chest pains.

DEXTRAN 40

(dex'tran)

Gentran 40, 10% LMD, Rheomacrodex

Classification: PLASMA VOLUME EXPANDER

Therapeutic: PLASMA VOLUME EXPANDER

Prototype: Albumin

Pregnancy Category: C

AVAILABILITY 10% solution in D5W or NS

ACTION & *THERAPEUTIC EFFECT* Low-molecular-weight polysaccharide. As a hypertonic colloidal solution, produces immediate and short-lived expansion of plasma volume by increasing colloidal osmotic pressure and drawing fluid from interstitial to intravascular space. *Cardiovascular response to volume expansion includes increased BP, pulse pressure, CVP, cardiac output, venous return to heart, and urinary output.*

USES Adjunctively to expand plasma volume and provide fluid replacement in treatment of shock or impending shock. Also used in prophylaxis and therapy of venous thrombosis and pulmonary embolism. Used as priming fluid or as additive to other primers during extracorporeal circulation.

CONTRAINDICATIONS Hypersensitivity to dextrans, severe renal failure, hypervolemic conditions, severe CHF, significant anemia, hypofibrinogenemia or other marked hemostatic defects including those caused by drugs, (e.g., heparin, warfarin); lactation.

CAUTIOUS USE Active hemorrhage; severe dehydration; chronic liver disease; impaired renal function; thrombocytopenia; patients susceptible to pulmonary edema or CHF; pregnancy (category C).

ROUTE & DOSAGE

Shock

Adult/Adolescent/Child: **IV** Up to 20 mL/kg in the first 24 h (doses up to 10 mL/kg/day may be given for a maximum of 4 additional days if needed)

Prophylaxis for Thromboembolic Complications

Adult: **IV** 500–1000 mL (10 mL/kg) on the day of operation

Common adverse effects in *italic*, life-threatening effects underlined; generic names in bold; classifications in SMALL CAPS; ♣ Canadian drug name; Ⓟ Prototype drug

followed by 500 mL/day for 2–3 days, may continue with 500 mL q2–3days for up to 2 wk if necessary

Priming for Extracorporeal Circulation

Adult: **IV** 10–20 mL/kg added to perfusion circuit

ADMINISTRATION

Intravenous

If blood is to be administered, draw a cross-match specimen before dextran infusion.

PREPARE: **IV Infusion:** Use only if seal is intact, vacuum is detectable, and solution is absolutely clear. ▪ No dilution required.

ADMINISTER: **IV Infusion:** Specific flow rate should be prescribed by physician. ▪ For emergency treatment of shock in adults give first 500 mL rapidly (e.g., 20–40 mL/min); give remaining portion of the daily dose over 8–24 h or at the rate prescribed.

INCOMPATIBILITIES **Solution/additive:** **Amoxicillin, ampicillin, oxacillin, penicillin.**

▪ Store at a constant temperature, preferably 25° C (77° F). Once opened, discard unused portion because dextran contains no preservative.

ADVERSE EFFECTS (≥1%) **Body as a Whole:** Hypersensitivity (mild to generalized urticaria, pruritus, <u>anaphylactic shock</u> (rare), <u>angioedema</u>, dyspnea). **Other:** Renal tubular vacuolization (osmotic nephrosis), stasis, and blocking; oliguria, <u>renal failure</u>; increased AST and ALT, interference with platelet function, prolonged bleeding and coagulation times.

DIAGNOSTIC TEST INTERFERENCE When blood samples are drawn for study, notify laboratory that patient has received dextran. ***Blood glucose:*** False increases (utilizing ***ortho-toluidine methods*** or ***sulfuric*** or ***acetic acid*** hydrolysis). ***Urinary protein:*** False increases (utilizing ***Lowry method***). ***Bilirubin assays:*** False increases when alcohol is used. ***Total protein assays:*** False increases using ***biuret reagent. Rh testing, blood typing*** and ***cross-matching*** procedures: Dextran may interfere with results (by inducing rouleaux formation) when ***proteolytic enzyme techniques*** are used (***saline agglutination*** and ***indirect antiglobulin methods*** reportedly not affected).

INTERACTIONS Drug: May potentiate **abciximab** anticoagulant effects.

PHARMACOKINETICS Onset: Volume expansion within minutes of infusion. **Duration:** 12 h. **Metabolism:** Degraded to glucose and metabolized to CO_2 and water over a period of a few weeks. **Elimination:** 75% excreted in urine within 24 h; small amount excreted in feces.

NURSING IMPLICATIONS

Assessment & Drug Effects

- Evaluate patient's state of hydration before dextran therapy begins. Administration to severely dehydrated patients can result in renal failure.
- Lab tests: Baseline Hct prior to and after initiation of dextran (dextran usually lowers Hct). Notify physician if Hct is depressed below 30% by volume.
- Monitor vital signs and observe patient closely for at least the first 30 min of infusion. Hypersensitivity reaction is most likely to occur during the first few minutes of administration. Terminate therapy at

the first sign of a hypersensitivity reaction (see Appendix F).

- Monitor CVP as an estimate of blood volume status and a guide for determining dosage. Normal CVP: 5–10 cm H_2O.
- Observe for S&S of circulatory overload (see Appendix F).
- Note: When sodium restriction is indicated, know that 500 mL of dextran 40 in 0.9% normal saline contains 77 mEq of both sodium and chloride.
- Monitor I&O ratio and check urine specific gravity at regular intervals. Low urine specific gravity may signify failure of renal dextran clearance and is an indication to discontinue therapy.
- Report oliguria, anuria, or lack of improvement in urinary output (dextran usually causes an increase in urinary output). Discontinue dextran at first sign of renal dysfunction.
- High doses are associated with transient prolongation of bleeding time and interference with normal blood coagulation.

Patient & Family Education

- Report immediately S&S of bleeding: Easy bruising, blood in urine or dark tarry stool.

DEXTROAMPHETAMINE SULFATE

(dex-troe-am-fet′a-meen)

Dexampex, Dexedrine, Oxydess II ✤, Spancap No. 1

Classifications: RESPIRATORY AND CEREBRAL STIMULANT; AMPHETAMINE; ANOREXIANT

Therapeutic: AMPHETAMINE; ANOREXIANT

Prototype: Amphetamine

Pregnancy Category: C

Controlled Substance: Schedule II

AVAILABILITY 5 mg, 10 mg tablets; 5 mg, 10 mg, 15 mg sustained release capsules

ACTION & *THERAPEUTIC EFFECT* Has anorexigenic action; this is thought to result from CNS stimulation and possibly from loss of acuity of smell and taste. *Is a more potent appetite suppressant than amphetamine. CNS stimulating effect approximately twice that of racemic amphetamine. In hyperkinetic children, amphetamines reduce motor restlessness by an unknown mechanism.*

USES Adjunct in short-term treatment of exogenous obesity, narcolepsy, and attention deficit disorder with hyperactivity in children (also called minimal brain dysfunction or hyperkinetic syndrome).

UNLABELED USES Adjunct in epilepsy to control ataxia and drowsiness induced by barbiturates; to combat sedative effects of trimethadione in absence seizures.

CONTRAINDICATIONS Hypersensitivity to sympathomimetic amines, closed-angle glaucoma, agitated states, psychoses (especially in children), structural cardiac abnormalities, valvular heart disease; congenital heart disease, coronary heart disease, advanced arteriosclerosis, symptomatic heart disease, moderate to severe hypertension, hyperthyroidism, history of drug abuse, during or within 14 days of MAOI therapy, as anorexiant in children younger than 12 y, for attention deficit disorder in children younger than 3 y; lactation.

CAUTIOUS USE Bipolar disease; salicylate hypersensitivity; seizure disorders; suicidal ideation, depression; salicylate hypersensitivity; pregnancy (category C). Safety and efficacy in children younger than 3 y have not been established.

ROUTE & DOSAGE

Narcolepsy

Adult: **PO** 5–20 mg 1–3 times/day at 4–6 h intervals
Child: **PO** *6–12 y,* 5 mg/day, may increase by 5 mg at weekly intervals; *older than 12 y,* 10 mg/day, may increase by 10 mg at weekly intervals

Attention Deficit Disorder

Child: **PO** *3–5 y,* 2.5 mg 1–2 times/day, may increase by 2.5 mg at weekly intervals; *6 y or older,* 5 mg 1–2 times/day, may increase by 5 mg at weekly intervals (max: 40 mg/day)

Obesity

Adult: **PO** 5–10 mg 1–3 times/day or 10–15 mg of sustained release once/day 30–60 min a.c.

ADMINISTRATION

Oral

- Ensure that sustained release capsule is not chewed or crushed. It **must be** swallowed whole.
- Give 30–60 min before meals for treatment of obesity. Give long-acting form in the morning.
- Give last dose no later than 6 h before patient retires (10–14 h before bedtime for sustained release form) to avoid insomnia.
- Store in tightly closed containers at 15°–30° C (59°–86° F) unless otherwise directed.

ADVERSE EFFECTS (≥1%) **CNS:** Nervousness, *restlessness,* hyperactivity, *insomnia,* euphoria, dizziness, headache; ***with prolonged use:*** Severe depression, psychotic reactions. **CV:** Palpitations, tachycardia, elevated BP. **GI:** Dry mouth, unpleasant taste, anorexia, weight loss, diarrhea, constipation, abdominal pain. **Other:** Impotence, changes in libido, unusual fatigue, increased intraocular pressure, marked dystonia of head, neck, and extremities; sweating.

DIAGNOSTIC TEST INTERFERENCE Dextroamphetamine may cause significant elevations in ***plasma corticosteroids*** (evening levels are highest) and increases in ***urinary epinephrine*** excretion (during first 3 h after drug administration).

INTERACTIONS Drug: Acetazolamide, sodium bicarbonate decrease dextroamphetamine elimination; **ammonium chloride, ascorbic acid** increase dextroamphetamine elimination; effects of both BARBITURATES and dextroamphetamine may be antagonized; **furazolidone** may increase BP effects of AMPHETAMINES—interaction may persist for several weeks after discontinuing **furazolidone;** antagonizes antihypertensive effects of **guanethidine;** MAO INHIBITORS, **selegiline** can cause—hypertensive crisis (fatalities reported)—do not administer AMPHETAMINES during or within 14 days of these drugs; PHENOTHIAZINES may inhibit mood elevating effects of AMPHETAMINES; TRICYCLIC ANTIDEPRESSANTS enhance dextroamphetamine effects because of increased **norepinephrine** release; BETA-ADRENERGIC AGONISTS increase cardiovascular adverse effects.

PHARMACOKINETICS Absorption: Rapid. **Peak:** 1–5 h. **Duration:** Up to 10 h. **Distribution:** All tissues, especially the CNS. **Metabolism:** In liver. **Elimination:** Renal elimination; excreted in breast milk. **Half-Life:** 10–30 h.

D

NURSING IMPLICATIONS

Assessment & Drug Effects

- Monitor children, adolescents, and adults for signs and symptoms of adverse cardiac reactions (e.g., arrhythmias).
- Monitor growth rate closely in children.
- Monitor children and adolescents for development of aggressive or abnormal behaviors.
- Note: Tolerance to anorexiant effects may develop after a few weeks; however, tolerance does not appear to develop when dextroamphetamine is used to treat narcolepsy.

Patient & Family Education

- Swallow sustained release capsule whole with a liquid; do not chew or crush.
- Do not drive or engage in other potentially hazardous activities until response to drug is known.
- Drug is usually tapered off gradually following long-term use to avoid extreme fatigue, mental depression, and prolonged sleep pattern.

DEXTROMETHORPHAN HYDROBROMIDE

(dex-troe-meth-or′fan)

Balminil DM ♣, Benylin DM, Cremacoat 1, Delsym, DM Cough, Hold, Koffex ♣, Mediquell, Neo-DM ♣, Ornex DM ♣, Pedia Care, Pertussin 8 Hour Cough Formula, Robidex ♣, Robitussin DM, Romilar CF, Romilar Children's Cough, Sedatuss ♣, Sucrets Cough Control

Classification: ANTITUSSIVE
Therapeutic: ANTITUSSIVE
Prototype: Benzonatate
Pregnancy Category: C

AVAILABILITY 30 mg capsules; 2.5 mg, 5 mg, 7.5 mg, 15 mg lozenges; 10 mg/15 mL, 3.5 mg/5 mL, 7.5 mg/5 mL, 15 mg/5 mL liquid; 15 mg/15 mL, 10 mg/5 mL syrup

ACTION & *THERAPEUTIC EFFECT* Nonnarcotic derivative of levorphanol. Chemically related to morphine but without central hypnotic or analgesic effect. Controls cough spasms by depressing the cough center in medulla. Antitussive activity comparable to that of codeine but is less likely than codeine to cause constipation, drowsiness, or GI disturbances. *Temporarily relieves coughing spasm.*

USES Temporary relief of cough spasms in nonproductive coughs due to colds, pertussis, and influenza.

CONTRAINDICATIONS Children younger than 2 y, infants and neonates; asthma, COPD, productive cough, persistent or chronic cough; severe hepatic function impairment; concurrent MAOI therapy.

CAUTIOUS USE Chronic pulmonary disease; enlarged prostate; patients on MAOI; mild or moderate hepatic impairment; pregnancy (category C); lactation.

ROUTE & DOSAGE

Cough

Adult: **PO** 10–20 mg q4h or 30 mg q6–8h (max: 120 mg/day) or 60 mg of sustained action liquid b.i.d.
Child: **PO** *2–6 y,* 2.5–5 mg q4h or 7.5 mg q6–8h (max: 30 mg/day) or 15 mg sustained action liquid b.i.d.; *6–12 y,* 5–10 mg q4h or 15 mg q6–8h (max: 60 mg/day) or 30 mg sustained action liquid b.i.d.

ADMINISTRATION

Oral

- Do not give lozenges to children younger than 6 y.
- Ensure that extended release form of drug is not chewed or crushed. It **must be** swallowed whole.
- Note: Although soothing local effect of the syrup may be enhanced if given undiluted, depression of cough center depends only on systemic absorption of drug.

ADVERSE EFFECTS (≥1%) **CNS:** Dizziness, drowsiness, CNS depression with very large doses; excitability, especially in children. **GI:** GI upset, constipation, abdominal discomfort.

INTERACTIONS Drug: High risk of excitation, hypotension, and hyperpyrexia with MAO INHIBITORS.

PHARMACOKINETICS Absorption: Readily from GI tract. **Onset:** 15–30 min. **Duration:** 3–6 h. **Metabolism:** In liver. **Elimination:** In urine.

NURSING IMPLICATIONS

Assessment & Drug Effects

- Monitor for dizziness and drowsiness, especially when concurrent therapy with CNS depressant is used.

Patient & Family Education

- Note: Treatment aims to decrease the frequency and intensity of cough without completely eliminating protective cough reflex.
- While dextromethorphan is available OTC, any cough persisting longer than 1 wk–10 days needs to be medically diagnosed.

DIAZEPAM Pr

(dye-az′e-pam)

Diastat, Diazemuls ♣, Valium

Classifications: BENZODIAZEPINE ANTICONVULSANT; ANXIOLYTIC

Therapeutic: ANTICONVULSANT; ANTIANXIETY

Pregnancy Category: D

Controlled Substance: Schedule IV

AVAILABILITY 2 mg, 5 mg, 10 mg tablets; 1 mg/mL, 5 mg/mL, 5 mg/ 5 mL oral solution; 5 mg/mL injection; 2.5 mg, 5 mg, 10 mg, 15 mg, 20 mg rectal gel

ACTION & *THERAPEUTIC EFFECT* Long-acting benzodiazepine psychotherapeutic agent. Benzodiazepines act at the limbic, thalamic, and hypothalamic regions of the CNS and produce CNS depression resulting in sedation, hypnosis, skeletal muscle relaxation, and anticonvulsant activity dependent on the dosage. *Has antianxiety, anticonvulsant, and skeletal muscle relaxation properties.*

USES Drug of choice for status epilepticus. Management of anxiety disorders, for short-term relief of anxiety symptoms, to allay anxiety and tension prior to surgery, cardioversion and endoscopic procedures, as an amnesic, and treatment for restless legs. Also used to alleviate acute withdrawal symptoms of alcoholism, voiding problems in older adults, and adjunctively for relief of skeletal muscle spasm associated with cerebral palsy, paraplegia, athetosis, stiffman syndrome, tetanus.

CONTRAINDICATIONS Acute narrow-angle glaucoma, untreated open-angle glaucoma; during or within 14 days of MAOI therapy; pregnancy (category D), lactation. **Injectable form:** Shock, coma, acute alcohol intoxication, depressed vital signs, obstetric patients, infants younger than 30 days of age. **Tablet form:** Infants younger than 6 mo of age.

CAUTIOUS USE Epilepsy, psychoses, mental depression; myasthenia gravis; impaired hepatic or renal function; neuromuscular disease; bipolar disorder, dementia, Parkinson's disease; organic brain syndrome, psychosis, suicidal ideation; drug abuse, addiction-prone individuals. Use injectable diazepam with extreme caution in older adults, the very ill, and patients with COPD, or asthma.

ROUTE & DOSAGE

Status Epilepticus

Adult: **IV/IM** 5–10 mg, repeat if needed at 10–15 min intervals up to 30 mg, then repeat if needed q2–4h
Child (5 y or older): **IV** 1 mg/kg q2–5min (max: 10 mg), may repeat in 2–4 h
Child/Infant (1 mo–5 y): **IV** 0.2–0.5 mg slowly q2–5min up to 5 mg
Neonate: **IV** 0.1–0.3 mg/kg q15–30min (max total dose: 2 mg)

Muscle Spasm

Adult/Adolescent/Child (5 y or older): **IV** 5–10 mg q3–4h prn (larger dose for tetanus)
Child/Infant (1 mo–5 y): **IV** 1–2 mg q3–4h prn

Anxiety

Adult/Adolescent: **IV** 2–10 mg, repeat if needed in 3–4 h
Child/Infant (6 mo or older): **IV** 0.04–0.3 mg q2–4h (max: 0.6 mg/kg/8 h)

Alcohol Withdrawal

Adult: **IV** 10 mg then 5–10 mg in 3–4 h

Preoperative

Adult: **IV** 5–15 mg 5–10 min before procedure

ADMINISTRATION

Oral

- Ensure that sustained release form is not chewed or crushed. It **must be** swallowed whole. Give other tablets crushed with fluid or mixed with food if necessary.
- Supervise oral ingestion to ensure drug is swallowed.
- Avoid abrupt discontinuation of diazepam. Taper doses to termination.

Intramuscular

- Give deep into large muscle mass. Inject slowly. Rotate injection sites.

Intravenous

PREPARE: **Direct:** Do not dilute or mix with any other drug.
ADMINISTER: **Direct:** Give direct IV by injecting drug slowly, taking at least 1 min for each 5 mg (1 mL) given to adults and taking at least 3 min to inject 0.25 mg/kg body weight of children. ▪ If injection cannot be made directly into vein, inject slowly through infusion tubing as close as possible to vein insertion. ▪ The emulsion form is incompatible with PVC infusion sets. ▪ Avoid small veins and take extreme care to avoid intra-arterial administration or extravasation.
INCOMPATIBILITIES **Solution/additive: Bleomycin, dobutamine, doxorubicin, epinephrine, fluorouracil, furosemide, glycopyrrolate, nalbuphine, sodium bicarbonate.** Emulsion also incompatible with **morphine. Y-site: Amphotericin B cholesteryl complex, atracu-**

rium, bivalirudin, cefepime, dexmedetomidine, diltiazem, fenoldopam, fluconazole, foscarnet, furosemide, heparin, hetastarch, lansoprazole, linezolid, meropenem, oxaliplatin, pancuronium, potassium chloride, propofol, remifentanil, tirofiban, vecuronium, vitamin B complex with C. Do not mix emulsion with any other drugs. Do not administer through **polyvinyl chloride (PVC)** infusion sets.

- Store in tight, light-resistant containers at 15°–30° C (59°–86° F), unless otherwise specified by manufacturer.

ADVERSE EFFECTS (≥1%) **Body as a Whole:** Throat and chest pain. **CNS:** *Drowsiness,* fatigue, ataxia, confusion, paradoxic rage, dizziness, vertigo, amnesia, vivid dreams, headache, slurred speech, tremor; EEG changes, tardive dyskinesia. **CV:** Hypotension, tachycardia, edema, <u>cardiovascular collapse</u>. **Special Senses:** Blurred vision, diplopia, nystagmus. **GI:** Xerostomia, nausea, constipation, hepatic dysfunction. **Urogenital:** Incontinence, urinary retention, gynecomastia (prolonged use), menstrual irregularities, ovulation failure. **Respiratory:** Hiccups, coughing, <u>laryngospasm</u>. **Other:** Pain, venous thrombosis, phlebitis at injection site.

INTERACTIONS Drug: Alcohol, CNS DEPRESSANTS, ANTICONVULSANTS potentiate CNS depression; **cimetidine** increases diazepam plasma levels, increases toxicity; may decrease antiparkinson effects of **levodopa;** may increase **phenytoin** levels; smoking decreases sedative and antianxiety effects. **Herbal: Kava, valerian** may potentiate sedation.

PHARMACOKINETICS Absorption: Readily from GI tract; erratic IM absorption. **Onset:** 30–60 min PO; 15–30 min IM; 1–5 min IV. **Peak:** 1–2 h PO. **Duration:** 15 min–1 h IV; up to 3 h PO. **Distribution:** Crosses blood–brain barrier and placenta; distributed into breast milk. **Metabolism:** In liver to active metabolites. **Elimination:** Primarily in urine. **Half-Life:** 20–50 h.

NURSING IMPLICATIONS

Assessment & Drug Effects

- Monitor for adverse reactions. Most are dose related.
- Monitor for therapeutic effectiveness. Maximum effect may require 1–2 wk; patient tolerance to therapeutic effects may develop after 4 wk of treatment.
- Observe necessary preventive precautions for suicidal tendencies that may be present in anxiety states accompanied by depression.
- Observe patient closely and monitor vital signs when diazepam is given parenterally; hypotension, muscular weakness, tachycardia, and respiratory depression may occur.
- Lab tests: Periodic CBC and liver function tests during prolonged therapy.
- Supervise ambulation. Adverse reactions such as drowsiness and ataxia are more likely to occur in older adults and debilitated or those receiving larger doses. Dosage adjustment may be necessary.
- Monitor I&O ratio, including urinary and bowel elimination.
- Note: Psychic and physical dependence may occur in patients on long-term high dosage therapy, in those with histories of alcohol or drug addiction, or in those who self-medicate.

D

Patient & Family Education

- Avoid alcohol and other CNS depressants during therapy unless otherwise advised by physician. Concomitant use of these agents can cause severe drowsiness, respiratory depression, and apnea.
- Do not drive or engage in other potentially hazardous activities or those requiring mental precision until reaction to drug is known.
- Tell physician if you become or intend to become pregnant during therapy; drug may need to be discontinued.
- Take drug as prescribed; do not change dose or dose intervals.

DIAZOXIDE

(dye-az-ox'ide)

Hyperstat I.V., Proglycem

Classifications: VASODILATOR; ANTIHYPERTENSIVE; SULFONYLUREA; ANTIDIABETIC

Therapeutic: ANTIHYPERTENSIVE; HYPOGLYCEMIC AGENT

Prototype: Hydralazine

Pregnancy Category: C

AVAILABILITY 50 mg capsules; 50 mg/mL suspension; 15 mg/mL injection

ACTION & *THERAPEUTIC EFFECT* Rapid-acting thiazide nondiuretic hypotensive and hyperglycemic agent. In contrast to thiazide diuretics, causes sodium and water retention, thus decreasing urinary output. This is probably due to its increase of proximal tubular reabsorption of sodium and decrease of glomerular filtration rate. Hypotensive effect may be accompanied by marked reflex increase in heart rate, cardiac output, and stroke volume; thus cerebral and coronary blood flows are usually maintained. *Reduces peripheral vascular resistance and BP by direct vasodilatory effect on peripheral arteriolar smooth muscles, perhaps by direct competition for calcium receptor sites.*

USES Intravenously for emergency lowering of BP in hospitalized patients with malignant hypertension, particularly when associated with renal impairment. Not effective in pheochromocytoma. Commonly used with a diuretic such as furosemide (Lasix) to counteract diazoxide-induced sodium and water retention. Orally in treatment of various diagnosed hypoglycemic states due to hyperinsulinism when other medical treatment or surgical management has been unsuccessful or is not feasible.

CONTRAINDICATIONS Hypersensitivity to diazoxide; cerebral bleeding, eclampsia; aortic coarctation; AV shunt, significant coronary artery disease; pheochromocytoma; lactation. Use of oral diazoxide for functional hypoglycemia or in presence of increased bilirubin in newborns.

CAUTIOUS USE Diabetes mellitus; impaired cerebral or cardiac circulation; impaired renal function; patients taking corticosteroids or estrogen–progestogen combinations; hyperuricemia, history of gout, uremia; thiazide diuretic hypersensitivity; pregnancy (category C).

ROUTE & DOSAGE

Severe Hypertension

Adult/Child: **IV** 1–3 mg/kg up to 150 mg, repeat at 5–15 min intervals if necessary

Hypoglycemia

Adult/Child: **PO** 3–8 mg/kg/day divided q8–12h

Neonate/Infant: **PO** 8–15 mg/kg/day divided q8–12h

ADMINISTRATION

Intravenous

Note: Give any prescribed diuretic 30–60 min prior to IV diazoxide. ▪ Keep patient recumbent 8–10 h because of possible additive hypotensive effect.

PREPARE: **Direct:** Give undiluted.
ADMINISTER: **Direct:** Give IV by rapid direct injection over 10–30 sec. ▪ Keep patient recumbent while receiving IV and for at least 30 min following administration. ▪ Check IV injection site frequently. Solution is strongly alkaline. Extravasation of medication into tissues can cause severe inflammatory reaction. ▪ Administer drug by peripheral vein ONLY.
INCOMPATIBILITIES **Y-site: Hydralazine, lidocaine, propranolol.**

▪ Do not give darkened solutions. Store capsules, oral suspension, and injectables at 2°–30° C (36°–86° F) unless otherwise directed. Protect from light, heat, and freezing.

ADVERSE EFFECTS (≥1%) **CNS:** Headache, weakness, malaise, *dizziness,* polyneuritis, sleepiness, insomnia, euphoria, anxiety, extrapyramidal signs. **CV:** Palpitations, atrial and ventricular arrhythmias, flushing, shock; *orthostatic hypotension,* CHF, transient hypertension. **Special Senses:** Tinnitus, momentary hearing loss; blurred vision, transient cataracts, subconjunctival hemorrhage, ring scotoma, diplopia, lacrimation, papilledema. **GI:** *Nausea, vomiting,* abdominal discomfort, diarrhea, constipation, ileus, anorexia, transient loss of taste, impaired hepatic function. **Hematologic:** Transient neutropenia, eosinophilia, decreased Hgb/Hct, decreased IgG. **Body as a Whole:** Hypersensitivity (rash, fever, leukopenia); chest and back pain, muscle cramps. **Urogenital:** Decreased urinary output, nephrotic syndrome (reversible), hematuria, increased nocturia, proteinuria, azotemia; inhibition of labor. **Skin:** Pruritus, flushing, monilial dermatitis, herpes, hirsutism; loss of scalp hair, sweating, sensation of warmth, burning, or itching. **Endocrine:** Advance in bone age (children), *hyperglycemia, sodium and water retention, edema,* hyperuricemia, glycosuria, enlargement of breast lump, galactorrhea; decreased immunoglobulinemia, hirsutism.

DIAGNOSTIC TEST INTERFERENCE Diazoxide can cause false-negative response to ***glucagon.***

INTERACTIONS Drug: SULFONYLUREAS antagonize effects; THIAZIDE DIURETICS may intensify hyperglycemia and antihypertensive effects; **phenytoin** increases risk of hyperglycemia, and diazoxide may increase **phenytoin** metabolism, causing loss of seizure control.

PHARMACOKINETICS Onset: 30–60 s IV; 1 h PO. **Peak:** 5 min IV. **Duration:** 2–12 or more h IV; 8 h PO. **Distribution:** Crosses blood–brain barrier and placenta. **Metabolism:** Partially metabolized in the liver. **Elimination:** In urine. **Half-Life:** 21–45 h.

NURSING IMPLICATIONS

Assessment & Drug Effects

- Lab tests: Initial blood glucose, serum electrolytes, and CBC and at regular intervals in patients receiving multiple doses.
- Following IV injection, monitor BP q5min for the first 15–30 min

or until stabilized, then hourly for balance of drug effect.

- Notify physician immediately if BP continues to fall 30 min or more after IV drug administration. Cause other than drug effect is probable.
- Monitor pulse: Tachycardia has occurred immediately following IV; palpitation and bradycardia have also been reported.
- Report promptly any change in I&O ratio.
- Oral administration usually does not produce marked effects on BP. However, do make periodic measurements of BP and vital signs.
- Observe patient closely for S&S of CHF (see Appendix F).
- Monitor diabetics carefully for loss of glycemic control.
- Evaluate serum electrolyte levels at regular intervals, particularly in patients with impaired renal function; hypokalemia potentiates hyperglycemic effect of diazoxide.

Patient & Family Education

- Note: Drug may cause hyperglycemia and glycosuria in diabetic and diabetic-prone individuals. Closely monitor blood and urine glucose; report any abnormalities to physician.
- Report palpitations, chest pain, dizziness, fainting, or severe headache.

DIBUCAINE

(dye'byoo-kane)

Nupercainal

Classification: ANESTHETIC, LOCAL (AMIDE-TYPE)

Therapeutic: LOCAL ANESTHETIC

Prototype: Procaine

Pregnancy Category: C

AVAILABILITY 1% ointment

ACTION & *THERAPEUTIC EFFECT* Long-acting anesthetic of the amide type that appears to inhibit initiation and conduction of nerve impulses by reducing permeability of nerve cell membrane to sodium ions. *Relief of pain and itching due to inhibiting conduction of nerve impulses.*

USES Fast, temporary relief of pain and itching due to hemorrhoids and other anorectal disorders, nonpoisonous insect bites, sunburn, minor burns, cuts, and scratches.

CONTRAINDICATIONS Hypersensitivity to amide-type anesthetics, children younger than 1 y.

CAUTIOUS USE Pregnancy (category C), lactation, children younger than 12 y.

ROUTE & DOSAGE

Itching Due to Insect Bites or Hemorrhoids

Adult: **Topical** Apply skin cream or ointment to affected area as needed [max: 1 oz (28 g)/24 h]; insert rectal ointment morning and evening and after each bowel movement

Child: **Topical** Apply skin cream or ointment to affected area as needed [max: 1/4 oz (7 g)/24 h]

ADMINISTRATION

Topical

- Apply cream preparation after bathing or swimming (water soluble).
- Store at 15°–30° C (59°–86° F) in tight, light-resistant containers.

ADVERSE EFFECTS (≥1%) **Skin:** Irritation, contact dermatitis; rectal bleeding (suppository).

PHARMACOKINETICS Absorption: Poorly absorbed from intact skin; readily absorbed from mucous membranes or abraded skin. **Onset:** 15 min. **Duration:** 2–4 h.

NURSING IMPLICATIONS

Patient & Family Education

- Discontinue if irritation or rectal bleeding (following use of rectal preparations) develops and consult physician.
- Physician may prescribe sitz baths 3–4 times/day to reduce the swelling and pain of hemorrhoids.
- Note: Medication is intended for temporary relief of mild to moderate itching or pain. Seek medical advice for continuing discomfort, pain, bleeding, or sensation of rectal pressure.

DICLOFENAC SODIUM

(di-klo′fen-ak)

Solaraze, Voltaren, Voltaren-XR

DICLOFENAC POTASSIUM

Cataflam

DICLOFENAC EPOLAMINE

Flector

Classifications: ANALGESIC, NONSTEROIDAL ANTI-INFLAMMATORY DRUG (NSAID); ANTIPYRETIC

Therapeutic: ANALGESIC, NSAID; ANTIPYRETIC

Prototype: Ibuprofen

Pregnancy Category: B

AVAILABILITY Diclofenac Sodium: 25 mg, 50 mg, 75 mg delayed release tablets 100 mg sustained release tablets 0.1% ophth solution 1%, 3% gel; **Diclofenac Potassium:** 50 mg tablets; **Diclofenac Epolamine:** 1.3% transdermal patch

ACTION & *THERAPEUTIC EFFECT* Diclofenac competitively inhibits both cyclooxygenase (COX) isoenzymes, COX-1 and COX-2, by blocking arachidonic acid conversion to other chemicals, thus leading to its analgesic, antipyretic, and anti-inflammatory effects. It appears to be a potent inhibitor of cyclooxygenase, thereby decreasing the synthesis of prostaglandins. *Nonsteroidal anti-inflammatory drug (NSAID) with analgesic and antipyretic activity.*

USES Analgesic and antipyretic effects in symptomatic treatment of rheumatoid arthritis, osteoarthritis, and ankylosing spondylitis. Also acute gout; juvenile rheumatoid arthritis; various rheumatic conditions. **Ophthalmic:** Cataract surgery; photophobia associated with refractive surgery. **Topical:** Treatment of actinic keratosis. **Transdermal:** Acute pain.

CONTRAINDICATIONS Hypersensitivity to diclofenac, NSAIDS, or salicylate; patients in whom asthma, urticaria, angioedema, bronchospasm, severe rhinitis, history of GI bleeding; hepatic porphyria; shock, or other sensitivity reaction is precipitated by aspirin or other NSAIDS; postoperative CABG pain.

CAUTIOUS USE Geriatric patients and children; patients receiving anticoagulant therapy; diabetes mellitus; history of GI disease; hepatic disease; GU tract problems such as dysuria, cystitis, hematuria, nephritis, nephrotic syndrome, patients who must restrict their sodium intake; impaired hepatic function; SLE; heart failure, cardiac disease; hypertension; pregnancy (category B), lactation.

D

ROUTE & DOSAGE

Rheumatoid Arthritis

Adult: **PO** 150–200 mg/day in 3–4 divided doses or 75 mg delayed release daily or 100 mg sustained release daily
Child: **PO** 25 mg b.i.d. or t.i.d.

Osteoarthritis

Adult: **PO** 100–150 mg/day in 3–4 divided doses; 75 mg delayed release daily; 100 mg sustained release daily **Topical** 4 g for each knee, ankle or foot q.i.d.

Ankylosing Spondylitis

Adult: **PO** 25 mg q.i.d. and 25 mg at bedtime

Cataract Surgery

Adult: **Ophthalmic** 1 drop of 0.1% solution in affected eye q.i.d. beginning 24 h after surgery and continuing for 2 wk

Actinic Keratosis

Adult: **Topical** Apply to affected area b.i.d. for 60–90 days

Acute Pain (Flector)

Adult: **Transdermal** Apply one patch to most painful area b.i.d.

ADMINISTRATION

Oral

- Ensure that sustained release forms of drug are not chewed or crushed. **Must be** swallowed whole.
- Give on an empty stomach, 1 h before or after a meal; absorption is delayed markedly by food. Minimize gastric irritation by administering it with a full glass of milk or water.
- Schedule administration 30 min before physical therapy or planned exercise to keep discomfort at a minimum.
- Discontinue therapy about 1 wk before surgery to reduce risk of bleeding.
- Store at 15°–30° C (59°–86° F) away from heat and direct light.

ADVERSE EFFECTS (≥1%) **CNS:** Dizziness, headache, drowsiness. **Special Senses:** Tinnitus. **Skin:** Rash, pruritus. **GI:** *Dyspepsia,* nausea, vomiting, abdominal pain, cramps, constipation, diarrhea, indigestion, abdominal distension, flatulence, peptic ulcer; liver enzymes, transaminases increased, liver test abnormalities. **CV:** Fluid retention, hypertension, CHF. **Respiratory:** Asthma. **Body as a Whole:** Back, leg, or joint pain. **Endocrine:** Hyperglycemia. **Hematologic:** Prolonged bleeding time; inhibits platelet aggregation.

DIAGNOSTIC TEST INTERFERENCE ***Liver function test*** values may be increased. ***Liver function test*** abnormalities may return to normal despite continued use; however, if significant abnormalities occur, clinical signs and symptoms consistent with liver disease develop, or systemic manifestations such as eosinophilia or rash occur, the medication should be discontinued. ***Serum uric acid*** concentrations may be decreased because of increased ***renal clearance***.

INTERACTIONS Drug: Increases **cyclosporine**-induced nephrotoxicity; increases **methotrexate** levels (increases toxicity); may decrease BP-lowering effects of DIURETICS; may increase levels and toxicity of **lithium;** may increase **digoxin** levels. **Herbal: Feverfew, garlic, ginger, ginkgo** may increase risk of bleeding.

PHARMACOKINETICS Absorption: Readily absorbed from GI tract; 50–60% reaches systemic circulation. **Peak:** 2–3 h. **Distribution:** Widely distributed including synovial fluid and into breast milk; 99% protein bound. **Metabolism:** Extensively metabolized in liver. **Elimination:** 50–70% in urine, 30–35% in feces. **Half-Life:** 1.2–2 h (PO); 12 h (transdermal).

NURSING IMPLICATIONS

Assessment & Drug Effects

- Lab tests: Periodic LFTs, serum uric acid concentrations, Hct, PT/INR, and blood glucose.
- Observe and report signs of bleeding (e.g., petechiae, ecchymoses, bleeding gums, bloody or black stools, cloudy or bloody urine).
- Monitor BP for hypertension and blood sugar for hyperglycemia.
- Monitor diabetics closely for loss of diabetic control.
- Monitor for increased serum sodium and potassium in patients receiving potassium-sparing diuretics.
- Monitor for S&S of CHF, including weight gains greater than 1 kg (2 lb)/24 h.
- Monitor for signs and symptoms of GI irritation and ulceration.

Patient & Family Education

Oral Form

- Do not lie down for 15–30 min after taking medicine to decrease esophageal irritation.
- Discontinue use with onset of ringing or buzzing in the ears, impaired hearing, dizziness, GI discomfort, or bleeding and notify physician.
- Do not take aspirin or other OTC analgesics without permission of the physician.
- Avoid alcohol or other CNS depressants.
- Do not drive or engage in other potentially hazardous activities until reaction to drug is known.
- Note: Diabetics need to monitor blood glucose carefully for loss of glycemic control.

D

DICLOXACILLIN SODIUM

(dye-klox-a-sill′in)

Dycill, Dynapen, Pathocil

Classification: ANTIBIOTIC, PENICILLIN

Therapeutic: PENICILLIN ANTIBIOTIC

Prototype: Penicillin G potassium

Pregnancy Category: B

AVAILABILITY 125 mg, 250 mg, 500 mg capsules; 62.5 mg/5 mL suspension

ACTION & *THERAPEUTIC EFFECT* Semisynthetic, acid-stable, penicillinase-resistant penicillin. It inhibits the final stage of bacterial cell wall synthesis by preferentially binding to specific penicillin-binding proteins (PBPs) that are located inside the bacterial cell wall; this leads to cell death. *Effective against penicillinase-producing staphylococci.*

USES Primarily in systemic infections caused by penicillinase-producing staphylococci and penicillin-resistant staphylococci.

CONTRAINDICATIONS Hypersensitivity to penicillins.

CAUTIOUS USE History of or suspected atopy or allergy (asthma, eczema, hives, hay fever); history of hypersensitivity to cephalosporins or carbapenem; GI disease, colitis; lactation; renal or hepatic impairment; pregnancy (category B).

ROUTE & DOSAGE

Mild to Moderate Infections

Adult: **PO** 125–500 mg q6h
Child (weight less than 40 kg): **PO** 12.5–25 mg/kg q6h (max: 4 g/day)

ADMINISTRATION

Oral

- Give on an empty stomach at least 1 h before or 2 h after meals. Food reduces drug absorption.
- Reconstitute powder for oral suspension by shaking container to loosen powder. Add water according to label starting with half of the amount, then shake vigorously. Add remaining half and shake again vigorously. Shake well before each use.
- Store reconstituted oral suspensions for 7 days at room temperature (15°–30° C; 59°–86° F) or 14 days under refrigeration at 2°–8° C (36°–46° F). Date and label container. Store capsules at room temperature in tight containers unless otherwise directed.

ADVERSE EFFECTS (≥1%) **Body as a Whole:** Hypersensitivity (pruritus, urticaria, rash, wheezing, sneezing, anaphylaxis; eosinophilia). **GI:** Nausea, vomiting, flatulence, *diarrhea*, abdominal pain. **Other:** Transient elevations of ALT, superinfections.

INTERACTIONS Drug: Probenecid decreases dicloxacillin elimination.

PHARMACOKINETICS Absorption: 35–76% absorbed from GI tract. **Peak:** 0.5–2 h. **Duration:** 4–6 h. **Distribution:** Distributed throughout body with highest concentrations in liver and kidney; low CSF penetration; crosses placenta; distributed into breast milk. **Metabolism:** In liver. **Elimination:** Primarily in urine with some elimination through bile. **Half-Life:** 30–60 min.

NURSING IMPLICATIONS

Assessment & Drug Effects

- Note: Take care to establish previous exposure and sensitivity to penicillins and cephalosporins as well as other allergic reactions of any kind before initiating therapy.
- Obtain C&S prior to initiation of therapy to determine susceptibility of causative organism. Therapy may begin pending test results.
- Lab tests: Baseline blood cultures, WBC, and differential counts and at least weekly for patients on prolonged therapy. Periodic ALT and AST determinations, urinalysis, BUN, and creatinine are also advised for these patients.

Patient & Family Education

- Take medication around the clock. Do not miss a dose and continue taking medication until it is all gone, unless otherwise directed by physician.
- Check with physician if GI side effects appear.
- Watch for and report the signs of hypersensitivity reactions and superinfections (see Appendix F).

DICYCLOMINE HYDROCHLORIDE

(dye-sye'kloe-meen)

Bentyl, Bentylol ✦, Byclomine, Dibent, Dilomine, Formulex ✦, Lomine ✦, Nospaz, Protylol ✦, Spasmoject

Classifications: ANTICHOLINERGIC; ANTISPASMODIC
Therapeutic: GI ANTISPASMODIC
Prototype: Atropine
Pregnancy Category: B

AVAILABILITY 10 mg, 20 mg capsules; 20 mg tablets; 10 mg/5 mL syrup; 10 mg/mL injection

ACTION & *THERAPEUTIC EFFECT* Synthetic tertiary amine with antispasmodic properties. Relieves smooth muscle spasm in GI and biliary tracts, uterus, and ureters by nonspecific direct relaxant action. *Exerts antispasmodic effect of the GI as well as the urinary tract.*

USES Adjunctively in treatment of functional bowel disorders/irritable bowel syndrome.

UNLABELED USES Acute enterocolitis, peptic ulcer, and infant colic, urinary incontinence.

CONTRAINDICATIONS Hypersensitivity to anticholinergic drugs; obstructive diseases of GU and GI tracts, paralytic ileus, intestinal atony, biliary tract disease; closed-angle glaucoma; unstable cardiovascular status; severe ulcerative colitis, toxic megacolon, esophagitis; myasthenia gravis; peripheral neuropathy; infants younger than 6 mo; lactation.

CAUTIOUS USE Prostatic hypertrophy; autonomic neuropathy; hyperthyroidism; coronary heart disease, CHF, arrhythmias, hypertension; hepatic or renal disease; GERD, hiatal hernia associated with esophageal reflux; pregnancy (category B).

ROUTE & DOSAGE

Irritable Bowel Disorders
Adult: **PO** 20–40 mg q.i.d. **IM** 20 mg q.i.d.
Child: **PO** 10 mg t.i.d. or q.i.d. (max: 40 mg/day)
Infant (older than 6 mo): **PO** 5 mg t.i.d. or q.i.d.

ADMINISTRATION

Oral
- Give 30 min before meals and at bedtime.

Intramuscular
- Give deep IM into a large muscle. Do NOT give IV.
- Store below 30° C (86° F) unless otherwise directed.

ADVERSE EFFECTS (≥1%) **All:** Dose related. **Body as a Whole:** Allergic reactions; curare-like effect (cyanosis, apnea, respiratory arrest); decreased sweating; suppression of lactation; urticaria. **CNS:** Lightheadedness, drowsiness, headache, insomnia, brief euphoria, fever, restlessness, irritability, coma, seizures. **CV:** Fluctuations in heart rate, palpitation, tachycardia. **GI:** *Dry mouth,* nausea, *constipation,* paralytic ileus, vomiting, diminished sense of taste, bloated feeling. **Urogenital:** Urinary hesitancy, *urinary retention,* impotence. **Special Senses:** Blurred vision.

PHARMACOKINETICS Absorption: Readily from GI tract. **Onset:** 1–2 h. **Duration:** 4 h. **Metabolism:** In liver. **Elimination:** 80% in urine, 10% in feces. **Half-Life:** 9–10 h.

NURSING IMPLICATIONS

Assessment & Drug Effects
- Monitor for adverse effects especially in infants. Treatment of infant colic with dicyclomine includes some risk, especially in infants younger than 2 mo of age. Infants younger than 6 wk have developed respiratory symptoms

as well as seizures, fluctuations in heart rate, weakness, and coma within minutes after taking syrup formulation. Symptoms generally last 20–30 min and are believed to be due to local irritation.

- Monitor I&O to assess for urinary retention.
- If drug produces drowsiness and light-headedness, supervision of ambulation and other safety precautions are warranted.

Patient & Family Education

- Exercise caution in hot weather. Dicyclomine may increase risk of heatstroke by decreasing sweating, especially in older adults.
- Do not drive or engage in other potentially hazardous activities until reaction to drug is known.
- Report changes in urine volume, voiding pattern.

DIDANOSINE (DDI)

(di-dan′o-sine)

Videx, Videx EC

Classifications: ANTIRETROVIRAL; NUCLEOSIDE REVERSE TRANSCRIPTASE INHIBITOR (NRTI)

Therapeutic: ANTIRETROVIRAL (NRTI)

Prototype: Lamivudine

Pregnancy Category: B

AVAILABILITY 125 mg, 200 mg, 250 mg, 400 mg delayed release capsules; 10 mg/mL powder for oral solution

ACTION & *THERAPEUTIC EFFECT* DDI interferes with the HIV RNA-dependent DNA polymerase (reverse transcriptase), thus preventing replication of the virus. *Synthetic purine nucleotide that inhibits replication of HIV.*

USES Advanced HIV infection in patients who are intolerant to zidovudine (AZT) or who demonstrate significant clinical or immunologic deterioration during zidovudine therapy.

CONTRAINDICATIONS Hypersensitivity to any of the components in the formulation; pancreatitis; PKU; lactation.

CAUTIOUS USE Individuals with peripheral vascular disease, history of neuropathy, chronic pancreatitis, renal impairment, or any liver impairment; patients on sodium restriction; renal failure, renal impairment; alcoholism; elderly; gout; concurrent use with stavudine in pregnancy; pregnancy (category B).

ROUTE & DOSAGE

HIV Infection

Adult/Adolescent/Child: **PO** *Weight 60 kg or more,* tablets, 400 mg daily or 200 mg b.i.d.; *weight 60 kg or more,* powder, 250 mg b.i.d.; *weight 25–60 kg,* tablets, 250 mg daily or 125 mg b.i.d.; *weight 20–25 kg,* 200 mg daily

Child/Infant (older than 8 mo): **PO (solution)** 120 mg/m² b.i.d.

Neonate/Infant (2 wk–8 mo): **PO** 100 mg/m² q8h

Renal Impairment Dosage Adjustment

Varies based on patient weight and dosage form used; see package insert

ADMINISTRATION

Oral

- Give drug on an empty stomach. Food should not be consumed

within 15–30 min of drug administration.
- Give with water. Do NOT give with fruit juice or any other acid-containing liquid.
- Ensure that delayed release forms are swallowed whole. They must not be crushed or chewed.
- Mix powder for oral solution (buffered) with at least 120 mL (4 oz) of water, stir until dissolved (requires 2–3 min), and immediately swallowed.
- Dosage reduction may be indicated in those with renal impairment.
- Store reconstituted liquid in a tightly closed container in refrigerator for up to 30 days.

ADVERSE EFFECTS (≥1%) **CV:** Palpitations, thrombophlebitis, arrhythmias, *vasodilation*. **CNS:** *Headache, dizziness, nervousness, insomnia, peripheral neuropathy,* lethargy, poor coordination, seizures. **Special Senses:** Retinal depigmentation, photophobia, blurred vision, optic neuritis, diplopia, blindness. **GI:** *Abdominal pain, nausea, vomiting, diarrhea,* constipation, stomatitis, dry mouth, <u>pancreatitis</u>, increased liver enzymes. **Hematologic:** Increased WBC, neutrophil, lymphocyte, and platelet counts; increased Hgb, thrombocytopenia, ecchymosis, hemorrhage, petechiae. **Metabolic:** Hypocalcemia, hypokalemia, hypomagnesemia, hyperuricemia (asymptomatic), *hypertriglyceridemia*. **Musculoskeletal:** Muscle atrophy, myalgia, arthritis, decreased strength. **Respiratory:** *Asthma, cough, dyspnea, epistaxis, rhinitis, rhinorrhea,* hypoventilation, pharyngitis, rhonchi or rales, sinusitis, congestion. **Skin:** Rash, impetigo, eczema, *pruritus, sweating,* erythema.

INTERACTIONS Drug: ALUMINUM- and MAGNESIUM-CONTAINING ANTACIDS may increase the aluminum- and magnesium-associated adverse effects of tablets. The effectiveness of **dapsone** in prophylaxis of *Pneumocystis carinii* pneumonia may be reduced by concomitant didanosine. May cause additive neuropathy with **zalcitabine** (ddC). **Food:** Absorption is significantly decreased by food. Take on an empty stomach.

PHARMACOKINETICS Absorption: Rapidly absorbed from GI tract when administered to fasting patient with antacids; 23–40% reaches systemic circulation. **Peak:** 0.6–1 h. **Distribution:** Distributed primarily to body water; 21% reaches CSF; crosses placenta. **Elimination:** 36% in urine. **Half-Life:** 0.8–1.5 h.

NURSING IMPLICATIONS

Assessment & Drug Effects

- Monitor for S&S of pancreatitis (e.g., abdominal pain, nausea, vomiting, elevated serum amylase). Report immediately to physician and withhold drug until ruled out.
- Monitor for S&S of peripheral neuropathy (e.g., numbness, tingling, burning, pain in hands or feet). Report to physician; dose reduction may be indicated.
- Monitor patients with renal impairment for drug toxicity and hypermagnesemia manifested by muscle weakness and confusion.
- Lab tests: Periodic CBC with differential, serum electrolytes including magnesium, uric acid, and lipid profile.

Patient & Family Education

- Report immediately to physician any of the following: Abdominal pain, nausea, or vomiting.

DIETHYLPROPION HYDROCHLORIDE

(dye-eth-il-proe′pee-on)

Nobesine ✦, Propion, Ten-Tab, Tenuate, Tenuate Dospan, Tepanil

Classification: ANOREXIANT

Therapeutic: ANOREXIANT

Pregnancy Category: B

Controlled Substance: Schedule IV

AVAILABILITY 25 mg tablets; 75 mg sustained release tablets

ACTION & *THERAPEUTIC EFFECT* Sympathomimetic amine chemically related to amphetamine. Anorexigenic action probably secondary to direct (CNS) stimulation of appetite control center in hypothalamus and limbic regions. *Suppresses appetite as a result of drug action on CNS appetite control center.*

USES Used solely in management of exogenous obesity as short-term (a few weeks) adjunct in a regimen of weight reduction based on caloric restriction.

CONTRAINDICATIONS Known hypersensitivity or idiosyncrasy to sympathomimetic amines; severe hypertension, advanced arteriosclerosis, valvular heart disease; hyperthyroidism; glaucoma; history of drug abuse; anorexia nervosa; symptomatic cardiovascular disease, arrhythmias; MAOI therapy; pulmonary hypertension; children younger than 6 y.

CAUTIOUS USE Hypertension, psychosis, mania, agitated states, epilepsy; diabetes mellitus; elderly, renal failure or impairment; seizure disorder; pregnancy (category B), lactation.

ROUTE & DOSAGE

Obesity

Adult: **PO** 25 mg t.i.d. 30–60 min a.c. or 75 mg sustained release daily midmorning

ADMINISTRATION

Oral

- Give on an empty stomach, 30 min–1 h before meals.
- Note: Additional dose sometimes prescribed in midevening to control nighttime hunger. Rarely causes insomnia except in high doses.
- Store between 15°–30° C (59°–86° F) in well-closed container unless otherwise specified.

ADVERSE EFFECTS (≥1%) **Body as a Whole:** Hypersensitivity (urticaria, rash, erythema); muscle pain, dyspnea, hair loss, blurred vision, severe dermatoses (chronic intoxication), increased sweating. **CNS:** Mild euphoria, restlessness, *nervousness,* dizziness, headache, irritability, hyperactivity, insomnia, drowsiness, mood changes, lethargy, increase in convulsive episodes in patients with epilepsy. **CV:** Palpitation, tachycardia, precordial pain, rise in BP. **GI:** Nausea, vomiting, diarrhea, constipation, dry mouth, unpleasant taste. **Urogenital:** Impotence, changes in libido, gynecomastia, menstrual irregularities; polyuria, dysuria.

INTERACTIONS Drug: Acetazolamide, sodium bicarbonate decreases diethylpropion elimination; **ammonium chloride, ascorbic acid** increases diethylpropion elimination; a BARBITURATE and diethylpropion taken together may antagonize the effects of both drugs; **furazolidone** may increase blood pressure effects of AMPHETAMINES, and interaction may persist for several weeks after discontinuation of **furazolidone; guanethidine** antagonizes antihypertensive effects; MAO INHIBITORS, **selegiline** can cause hypertensive crisis (fatalities reported)—AMPHETAMINES should not be administered at the same time as or within 14 days of these drugs; PHENOTHIAZINES may inhibit mood elevating effects of AMPHETAMINES; TRICYCLIC ANTIDEPRESSANTS enhance AMPHETAMINES' effects by increasing **norepinephrine** release; BETA AGONISTS increase cardiovascular adverse effects.

PHARMACOKINETICS Absorption: Readily from GI tract. **Duration:** 4 h, regular tablets; 10–14 h, sustained release. **Elimination:** In urine. **Half-Life:** 4–6 h.

NURSING IMPLICATIONS

Assessment & Drug Effects

- Observe patients with epilepsy closely for reduction in seizure control.
- Monitor diabetics for loss of glycemic control.
- Note: Varying degrees of psychologic and rarely physical dependence can occur.

Patient & Family Education

- Swallow sustained release tablets whole; do NOT chew.
- Do not drive or engage in other potentially hazardous activities until reaction to drug is known.
- If diabetic, closely monitor blood glucose values.

DIFLORASONE DIACETATE

(dye-flor'a-sone)

Florone, Florone E, Maxiflor, Psorcon

Pregnancy Category: C

See Appendix A-4.

DIFLUNISAL

(dye-floo'ni-sal)

Dolobid

Classifications: ANALGESIC, NONSTEROIDAL ANTI-INFLAMMATORY DRUG (NSAID); ANTIPYRETIC

Therapeutic: ANALGESIC, NSAID; ANTIPYRETIC

Prototype: Ibuprofen

Pregnancy Category: C; D third trimester

AVAILABILITY 250 mg, 500 mg tablets

ACTION & *THERAPEUTIC EFFECT* A long-acting nonsteroidal anti-inflammatory drug (NSAID); unlike aspirin, inhibition of platelet function and effect on bleeding time are dose related and reversible, lasting only about 24 h after drug is discontinued. Is a nonnarcotic analgesic agent. Exerts mild antipyretic effect; therefore it is not used clinically for this purpose. This NSAID has peripheral analgesic properties due to interfering with prostaglandin synthesis by inhibiting cyclooxygenase (COX) isoenzymes, COX-1 and COX-2. *Has analgesic and anti-inflammatory properties.*

USES Acute and long-term relief of mild to moderate pain and symptomatic treatment of osteoarthritis and rheumatoid arthritis.

CONTRAINDICATIONS Patients in whom aspirin or other NSAIDs precipitate an acute asthmatic attack (bronchospasm), urticaria, angioedema, severe rhinitis, or shock; active peptic ulcer, GI bleeding; severe salicylate hypersensitivity; treatment of perioperative pain in CABG perioperative care; pregnancy (category D third trimester). Safe use in children younger than 12 y is not established.

CAUTIOUS USE History of upper GI disease; preexisting renal disease; impaired renal or hepatic function; alcoholics; compromised cardiac function, and other conditions associated with fluid retention; patients receiving diuretics; bone marrow suppression; geriatric patients; hypertension; patients who may be adversely affected by prolonged bleeding time; elderly; pregnancy (category C first and second trimester), lactation.

ROUTE & DOSAGE

Pain Relief
Adult: **PO** 1000 mg followed by 500 mg q8–12h

Arthritis
Adult: **PO** 500–1000 mg/day in 2 divided doses (max: 1500 mg/day)

ADMINISTRATION

Oral

- Give with water, milk, or food to reduce GI irritation. Food causes slight reduction in absorption rate, but does not affect total amount absorbed.
- Store at 15°–30° C (59°–86° F) in tightly closed containers unless otherwise directed.

ADVERSE EFFECTS (≥1%) **Body as a Whole:** Hypersensitivity syndrome (fever, chills, rash, eosinophilia, changes in renal and hepatic function, <u>anaphylactic reactions with bronchospasm</u>). **CNS:** Headache, drowsiness, insomnia, dizziness, vertigo, light-headedness, fatigue, weakness, nervousness, confusion, disorientation. **CV:** Palpitation, tachycardia, *peripheral edema*. **Special Senses:** Tinnitus, hearing loss; blurred vision, reduced visual acuity, changes in color vision, scotomas, corneal deposits, retinal disturbances. **GI:** *Nausea,* GI pain, flatulence, GI bleeding, peptic ulcer, anorexia, eructation, cholestatic jaundice. **Urogenital:** Hematuria, proteinuria, interstitial nephritis, <u>renal failure</u>. **Hematologic:** Prolonged PT, anemia, decreased serum uric acid, transient elevations of liver function tests. **Skin:** Rash, toxic epidermal necrolysis, exfoliative dermatitis, urticaria. **Other:** Weight gain, hyperventilation, dyspnea, photosensitivity.

DIAGNOSTIC TEST INTERFERENCE Diflunisal can lower ***serum uric acid*** concentrations by as much as 1.4 mg/dL and increased renal clearance of uric acid.

INTERACTIONS Drug: ANTACIDS decrease diflunisal absorption; **aspirin** and other NSAIDS increase risk of GI bleeding; increases risk of **warfarin**-induced hypoprothrombinemia; increases **methotrexate** levels and toxicity.

PHARMACOKINETICS Absorption: Readily from GI tract. **Onset:** 1 h. **Peak:** 2–3 h. **Duration:** 12 h. **Distribution:** Probably crosses placenta; distributed into breast milk. **Metabolism:** In liver. **Elimination:** In urine. **Half-Life:** 8–12 h.

NURSING IMPLICATIONS

Assessment & Drug Effects

- Monitor for therapeutic effectiveness: Full anti-inflammatory effect for arthritis may not occur until 8 days to several weeks into therapy.
- Lab test: With prolonged use, periodic Hgb and Hct, PT/INR, and renal function tests.
- Note: Although the antipyretic effect is mild, chronic or high doses may mask fever in some patients.

Patient & Family Education

- Swallow tablet whole; do not crush or chew.
- Report onset of visual or auditory problems immediately to physician.
- Be aware of I&O ratio and pattern and check for and report peripheral edema and unusual weight gain.
- Report promptly to physician the onset of melena (i.e., dark, tarry stools) or hematemesis (i.e., bloody or dark brown vomitus) or severe stomach pain.
- Do not drive or engage in other potentially hazardous activities until reaction to drug is known.

DIGOXIN Pr

(di-jox'in)

Lanoxicaps, Lanoxin

Classifications: CARDIAC GLYCOSIDE; INOTROPIC

Therapeutic: CARDIAC GLYCOSIDE; ANTIARRYTHMIC

Pregnancy Category: C

AVAILABILITY 0.05 mg, 0.1 mg, 0.2 mg capsules; 0.125 mg, 0.25 mg, 0.5 mg tablets; 0.05 mg/mL elixir; 0.25 mg/mL, 0.1 mg/mL injection

ACTION & *THERAPEUTIC EFFECT* Widely used cardiac glycoside that acts by increasing the force and velocity of myocardial systolic contraction (positive inotropic effect). It also decreases conduction velocity through the atrioventricular node. *Increases the contractility of the heart muscle (positive inotropic effect). Has antiarrhythmic properties that result from its effects on the AV node.*

USES Rapid digitalization and for maintenance therapy in CHF, atrial fibrillation, atrial flutter, paroxysmal atrial tachycardia.

CONTRAINDICATIONS Digitalis hypersensitivity, sick sinus syndrome, Wolff-Parkinson-White syndrome; ventricular fibrillation, ventricular tachycardia unless due to CHF. Full digitalizing dose not given if patient has received digoxin during previous week or if slowly excreted cardiotonic glycoside has been given during previous 2 wk.

CAUTIOUS USE Renal insufficiency, hypokalemia, advanced heart disease, cardiomyopathy, acute MI, incomplete AV block, cor pulmonale; hypothyroidism; lung disease; premature and immature infants, children, older adults, or debilitated patients; pregnancy (category C).

ROUTE & DOSAGE

Digitalizing Dose (Give 1/2 dose initially followed by 1/4 at 8–12 h intervals)

Adult: **PO** 0.75–1.5 mg **IV** 0.5–1 mg
Child: **IV** *2–10 y,* 20–35 mcg/kg; *older than 10 y,* 8–12 mcg/kg
PO *2–10 y,* 30–40 mcg/kg; *older than 10 y,* 10–15 mcg/kg

Infant: **IV** 30–50 mcg/kg **PO** 35–60 mcg/kg
Neonate: **IV** *Preterm,* 15–25 mcg/kg; *full-term,* 20–30 mcg/kg

Maintenance Dose

Adult: **PO/IV** 0.1–0.375 mg/day
Child: **PO/IV** *Younger than 2 y,* 7.5–9 mcg/kg/day; *2–10 y,* 6–7.5 mcg/kg/day; *older than 10 y,* 0.125–0.25 mg/day
Neonate: **IV** 4–8 mcg/kg/day

ADMINISTRATION

Oral

- Give without regard to food. Administration after food may slightly delay rate of absorption, but total amount absorbed is not affected.
- Crush and mix with fluid or food if patient cannot swallow it whole.

Intravenous

PREPARE: **Direct:** Give undiluted or diluted in 4 mL of sterile water, D5W, or NS (less diluent may cause precipitation).

ADMINISTER: **Direct:** Give each dose over at least 5 min. ▪ Monitor IV site frequently. Infiltration of parenteral drug into subcutaneous tissue can cause local irritation and sloughing.

INCOMPATIBILITIES **Solution/additive: Dobutamine. Y-site: Amiodarone, amphotericin B cholesteryl complex, fluconazole, foscarnet, propofol.**

- Store tablets, elixir, and injection solution at 25° C (77° F) or at 15°–30° C (59°–86° F).

ADVERSE EFFECTS (≥1%) **CNS:** Fatigue, muscle weakness, headache, facial neuralgia, mental depression, paresthesias, hallucinations, confusion, drowsiness, agitation, dizziness. **CV:** Arrhythmias, hypotension, AV block. **Special Senses:** Visual disturbances. **GI:** Anorexia, *nausea,* vomiting, diarrhea. **Other:** Diaphoresis, recurrent malaise, dysphagia.

INTERACTIONS Drug: ANTACIDS, **cholestyramine, colestipol** decrease digoxin absorption; DIURETICS, CORTICOSTEROIDS, **amphotericin B,** LAXATIVES, **sodium polystyrene sulfonate** may cause hypokalemia, increasing the risk of digoxin toxicity; **calcium IV** may increase risk of arrhythmias if administered together with digoxin; **quinidine, verapamil, amiodarone, flecainide** significantly increase digoxin levels, and digoxin dose should be decreased by 50%; **erythromycin** may increase digoxin levels; **succinylcholine** may potentiate arrhythmogenic effects; **nefazodone** may increase digoxin levels. **Food:** High fiber intake may decrease absorption. **Herbal: Ginseng** increase digoxin toxicity; **ma huang, ephedra** may induce arrhythmias; **St. John's wort** decreases plasma concentration. **Lab Test: Panax ginseng** can falsely elevate concentrations with fluorescence polarization immunoassay (FPIA) or falsely lower concentrations when microparticle enzyme immunoassay (MEIA).

PHARMACOKINETICS Absorption: 70% PO tablets; 90% PO liquid and capsules. **Onset:** 1–2 h PO; 5–30 min IV. **Peak:** 6–8 h PO; 1–5 h IV. **Duration:** 3–4 days in fully digitalized patient. **Distribution:** Widely distributed; tissue levels significantly higher than plasma levels; crosses placenta. **Metabolism:** 14% in liver. **Elimination:** 80–90% by kidneys; may appear in breast milk. **Half-Life:** 34–44 h.

NURSING IMPLICATIONS

Assessment & Drug Effects

- Take apical pulse for 1 full min, noting rate, rhythm, and quality before administering drug.

- Withhold medication and notify physician if apical pulse falls below ordered parameters (e.g., less than 50 or 60/min in adults and less than 60 or 70/min in children).
- Be familiar with patient's baseline data (e.g., quality of peripheral pulses, blood pressure, clinical symptoms, serum electrolytes, creatinine clearance) as a foundation for making assessments.
- Lab tests: Baseline and periodic serum digoxin, potassium, magnesium, and calcium. Draw blood samples for determining plasma digoxin levels at least 6 h after daily dose and preferably just before next scheduled daily dose.
- Monitor for S&S of drug toxicity: In children, cardiac arrhythmias are usually reliable signs of early toxicity. Early indicators in adults (anorexia, nausea, vomiting, diarrhea, visual disturbances) are rarely initial signs in children.
- Monitor I&O ratio during digitalization, particularly in patients with impaired renal function. Also monitor for edema daily and auscultate chest for rales.
- Monitor serum digoxin levels closely during concurrent antibiotic–digoxin therapy, which can precipitate toxicity because of altered intestinal flora.
- Observe patients closely when being transferred from one preparation (tablet, elixir, or parenteral) to another; when tablet is replaced by elixir potential for toxicity increases since 30% or more of drug is absorbed.

Patient & Family Education

- Report to physician if pulse falls below 60 or rises above 110 or if you detect skipped beats or other changes in rhythm, when digoxin is prescribed for atrial fibrillation.
- Suspect toxicity and report to physician if any of the following occur: Anorexia, nausea, vomiting, diarrhea, or visual disturbances.
- Weigh each day under standard conditions. Report weight gain greater than 1 kg (2 lb)/day.
- Take digoxin PRECISELY as prescribed. Do not skip or double a dose or change dose intervals, and take it at same time each day.
- Do not to take OTC medications, especially those for coughs, colds, allergy, GI upset, or obesity, without prior approval of physician.
- Continue with brand originally prescribed unless otherwise directed by physician.

DIGOXIN IMMUNE FAB (OVINE)

(di-jox'in)

Digibind, DigiFab

Classification: ANTIDOTE

Therapeutic: ANTIDOTE

Pregnancy Category: C

AVAILABILITY 38 mg, 40 mg vial

ACTION & *THERAPEUTIC EFFECT*

Fragments of antidigoxin antibodies (Fab) used instead of whole antibody molecules permits more extensive and faster distribution to serum and toxic cellular sites. Fab acts by selectively complexing with circulating digoxin or digitoxin, thereby preventing drug from binding at receptor sites; the complex is then eliminated in urine. *Used as an antidote for digitalis toxicity.*

USES Treatment of potentially life-threatening digoxin or digitoxin intoxication in carefully selected patients.

CONTRAINDICATIONS Hypersensitivity to sheep products; renal or cardiac failure.
CAUTIOUS USE Prior treatment with sheep antibodies or ovine Fab fragments; mannitol hypersensitivity; history of allergies; impaired renal function or renal failure; elderly; pregnancy (category C), lactation.

ROUTE & DOSAGE

Serious Digoxin Toxicity Secondary to Overdose
Adult/Child: **IV** Dosages vary according to amount of digoxin to be neutralized; dosages are based on total body load or steady state serum digoxin concentrations (see package insert); some patients may require a second dose after several hours

ADMINISTRATION

Intravenous
PREPARE: **Direct:** Dilute each vial with 4 mL of sterile water for injection to yield 9.5 mg/mL for Digibind and 10 mg/mL for DigiFab; mix gently. **IV Infusion:** Dilute further with any volume of NS compatible with cardiac status. ▪ For those receiving less than 3 mg, further dilute to a concentration of 1 mg/mL by adding an additional 34 mL of NS to Digibind or 36 mL of NS to DigiFab. ▪ For very small doses for infants, reconstitute to a concentration of 10 mg/mL.
ADMINISTER: **Direct:** Give undiluted bolus only if cardiac arrest is imminent. **IV Infusion:** Give IV infusion over 30 min, preferably through a 0.22-micron membrane filter. ▪ For administration to infants: Reconstitute as for direct IV and administer with a tuberculin syringe. ▪ For small doses (e.g., 2 mg or less), dilute the reconstituted 40 mg vial with 36 mL of NS to yield 1 mg/mL. ▪ Closely monitor for fluid overload.

▪ Use reconstituted solutions promptly or refrigerated at 2°–8° C (36°–46° F) for up to 4 h.

ADVERSE EFFECTS (≥1%) Adverse reactions associated with use of digoxin immune Fab are related primarily to the effects of **digitalis** withdrawal on the heart (see Nursing Implications). Allergic reactions have been reported rarely. Hypokalemia.

DIAGNOSTIC TEST INTERFERENCE Digoxin immune Fab may interfere with ***serum digoxin*** determinations by immunoassay tests.

PHARMACOKINETICS Onset: Less than 1 min after IV administration. **Elimination:** In urine over 5–7 days. **Half-Life:** 14–20 h.

NURSING IMPLICATIONS

Assessment & Drug Effects
- Perform skin testing for allergy prior to administration of immune Fab, particularly in patients with history of allergy or who have had previous therapy with immune Fab.
- Keep emergency equipment and drugs immediately available before skin testing is done or first dose is given and until patient is out of danger.
- Monitor for therapeutic effectiveness: Reflected in improvement in cardiac rhythm abnormalities,

mental orientation and other neurologic symptoms, and GI and visual disturbances. S&S of reversal of digitalis toxicity occurs in 15–60 min in adults and usually within minutes in children.
- Baseline and frequent vital signs and EGG during administration.
- Lab tests: Baseline and periodic serum potassium and serum digoxin; serum digoxin or digitoxin concentration (this measurement will not be accurate for at least 5–7 days after therapy begins because of test interference by immune Fab).
- Note: Serum potassium is particularly critical during first several hours following administration of immune Fab. Monitor closely.
- Monitor closely: Cardiac status may deteriorate as inotropic action of digitalis is withdrawn by action of immune Fab. CHF, arrhythmias, increase in heart rate, and hypokalemia can occur.
- Make sure serum digoxin levels and ECG readings are obtained for at least 2–3 wk.

Patient & Family Education
- Tell your prescriber or health care professional about all other medications you are taking, including non-prescription medications, nutritional supplements, or herbal products.
- Check with your prescriber before stopping or starting any of your medicines.

DIHYDROERGOTAMINE MESYLATE

(dye-hye-droe-er-got'a-meen)

D.H.E. 45, Migranal

Classifications: ALPHA-ADRENERGIC ANTAGONIST; ERGOT ALKALOID
Therapeutic: ANTIMIGRAINE

Prototype: Ergotamine
Pregnancy Category: X

AVAILABILITY 4 mg/mL nasal spray; 1 mg/mL injection

ACTION & *THERAPEUTIC EFFECT* Alpha-adrenergic blocking agent and ergot alkaloid with direct constricting effect on smooth muscle of peripheral and cranial blood vessels. Additionally, its ergot properties act as selective serotonin agonists at the 5-HT_1 receptors located on intracranial blood vessels, which may also cause vasoconstriction of large intracranial conductance arteries; this correlates with relief of migraine headaches. *Reduces rate of serotonin-induced platelet aggregation. Has somewhat weaker vasoconstrictor action than ergotamine but greater adrenergic blocking activity, resulting in relief from migraine headaches.*

USES To prevent or abort vascular headache (e.g., migraine or histaminic cephalalgia) when rapid control is desired or other routes are not feasible. With low-dose heparin therapy to prevent postoperative deep-vein thrombosis and pulmonary embolism.

UNLABELED USES To treat postural hypotension.

CONTRAINDICATIONS History of hypersensitivity to ergot preparations; peripheral vascular disease, coronary heart disease, MI, hypertension; peptic ulcer; severely impaired hepatic or renal function; sepsis; within 48 h of surgery; pregnancy (category X), lactation. Safe use in children younger than 6 y is not established.

CAUTIOUS USE Moderate or mild renal or hepatic impairment; obesity; diabetes mellitus; postmenopausal women; males older than 40 y; pulmonary heart disease; valvular heart disease; smokers.

ROUTE & DOSAGE

Migraine Headache

Adult: **IV/IM/Subcutaneous** 1 mg, may be repeated at 1 h intervals to a total of 3 mg IM or 2 mg IV/subcutaneous (max: 6 mg/wk) **Intranasal** 1 spray (0.5 mg) in each nostril, may repeat with additional spray in 15 min if no relief (max: 4 sprays/attack); wait 6–8 h before treating another attack (max: 8 sprays/24 h, 24 sprays/wk)

ADMINISTRATION

Intranasal

- Give at first warning of migraine headache.

Intramuscular/Subcutaneous

- Give at first warning of migraine headache.
- Withdraw IM or subcutaneous dose directly from ampule. Do not dilute.
- Note: Onset of action is about 20 min; when rapid relief is required, the IV route is prescribed.

Intravenous

PREPARE: **Direct:** Give undiluted.
ADMINISTER: **Direct:** Give at a rate of 1 mg/60 sec.

- Store at 15°–30° C (59°–86° F) unless otherwise directed. - Protect ampules from heat and light; do not freeze. - Discard ampule if solution appears discolored.

ADVERSE EFFECTS (≥1%) **CV** Vasospasm: Coldness, numbness and tingling in fingers and toes, muscle pains and weakness of legs, precordial distress and pain, transient tachycardia or bradycardia, hypertension (large doses). **GI:** *Nausea, vomiting.* **Body as a Whole:** Dizziness, dysphoria, *localized edema and itching;* ergotism (excessive doses).

INTERACTIONS Drug: BETA-BLOCKERS, **erythromycin** increase peripheral vasoconstriction with risk of ischemia; increased **ergotamine** toxicity with drugs that inhibit CYP3A4 (e.g., PROTEASE INHIBITORS, **amprenavir, ritonavir, nelfinavir, indinavir, saquinavir**), MACROLIDE ANTIBIOTICS **(erythromycin, azithromycin, clarithromycin),** AZOLE ANTIFUNGALS **(ketoconazole, itraconazole, fluconazole, clotrimazole), nefazodone, fluoxetine, fluvoxamine. Food: Grapefruit juice** may increase toxicity.

PHARMACOKINETICS Onset: 15–30 min IM; less than 5 min IV. **Duration:** 3–4 h. **Distribution:** Probably distributed into breast milk. **Metabolism:** In liver by CYP3A4. **Elimination:** Primarily in urine; some in feces. **Half-Life:** 21–32 h.

NURSING IMPLICATIONS

Assessment & Drug Effects

- Monitor cardiac status, especially when large doses are given.
- Monitor for and report numbness and tingling of fingers and toes, extremity weakness, muscle pain, or intermittent claudication.

Patient & Family Education

- Take at first warning of migraine headache.
- Lie down in a quiet, darkened room for several hours after drug administration for best results.
- Report immediately if any of the following S&S develop: Chest pain, nausea, vomiting, change in heartbeat, numbness, tingling, pain or

weakness of extremities, edema, or itching.

- Women should use effective means of contraception while using this drug. Notify physician if you become pregnant.

DILTIAZEM

(dil-tye'a-zem)

Cardizem, Cardizem CD, Cardizem LA, Cartia XT, Dilacor XR, Tiazac, Taztia XT

DILTIAZEM IV

Cardizem IV

Classifications: CALCIUM CHANNEL BLOCKING AGENT; ANTIANGINAL; ANTIHYPERTENSIVE

Therapeutic: ANTIHYPERTENSIVE; ANTIANGINAL; ANTIARRHYTHMIC

Prototype: Verapamil

Pregnancy Category: C

AVAILABILITY 30 mg, 60 mg, 90 mg, 120 mg tablets; 120 mg, 180 mg, 240 mg sustained release tablets; 60 mg, 90 mg, 120 mg, 180 mg, 240 mg, 300 mg, 360 mg sustained release capsules; 120 mg, 180 mg, 240 mg, 300 mg, 360 mg, 420 mg extended release tablets; 25 mg, 50 mg vials

ACTION & *THERAPEUTIC EFFECT* Inhibits calcium ion influx through slow channels into cell of myocardial and arterial smooth muscle. Improves myocardial perfusion, and reduces left ventricular workload. *Slows SA and AV node conduction (antiarrhythmic effect). Dilates coronary arteries and arterioles and inhibits coronary artery spasm; thus myocardial oxygen delivery is increased (antianginal effect). By vasodilation of peripheral arterioles, drug decreases total peripheral vascular resistance and reduces arterial BP at rest (antihypertensive effect).*

USES Vasospastic angina (Prinzmetal's variant or at rest angina), chronic stable (classic effort-associated) angina, essential hypertension. **IV form:** Atrial fibrillation, atrial flutter, supraventricular tachycardia.

UNLABELED USES Prevention of reinfarction in non-Q-wave MI.

CONTRAINDICATIONS Known hypersensitivity to drug; sick sinus syndrome (unless pacemaker is in place and functioning); acute MI; CHF; left ventricular dysfunction; second- or third-degree AV block, Wolff-Parkinson-White syndrome, Lown-Ganong-Levine syndrome; severe hypotension (systolic less than 90 mm Hg or diastolic less than 60 mm Hg); patients undergoing intracranial surgery; bleeding aneurysms. Safe use in children is not established.

CAUTIOUS USE Sinoatrial nodal dysfunction, sick sinus syndrome; right ventricular dysfunction, severe bradycardia; conduction abnormalities; renal or hepatic impairment; older adults; pregnancy (category C).

ROUTE & DOSAGE

Angina

Adult: **PO** 30 mg q.i.d., may increase q1–2days as required (usual range: 180–360 mg/day in divided doses)

Hypertension

Adult: **PO** 60–120 mg sustained release b.i.d. (usual range: 240–360 mg/day) or 120–540 mg of CD or LA once daily

Atrial Fibrillation

Adult: **IV** 0.25 mg/kg IV bolus over 2 min, if inadequate response, may repeat in 15 min with 0.35 mg/kg, followed by a continuous infusion of 5–10 mg/h (max: 15 mg/h for 24 h)

ADMINISTRATION

Oral

- Do not crush sustained release capsules or tablets. They **must be** swallowed whole.
- Withhold if systolic BP is less than 90 mm Hg or diastolic is less than 60 mm Hg.
- Give before meals and at bedtime.
- Store at 15°–30° C (59°–86° F).

Intravenous

PREPARE: **Direct:** Give undiluted. **Continuous:** For IV infusion, add to a volume of D5W, NS, or D5/0.45% NaCl that can be administered in 24 h or less.

ADMINISTER: **Direct:** Give as a bolus dose over 2 min. A second bolus may be given after 15 min. **Continuous:** Give at a rate 5–15 mg/h. Infusion duration longer than 24 h and infusion rate greater than 15 mg/h are not recommended.

INCOMPATIBILITIES **Solution/additive: Furosemide. Y-site: Acetazolamide, acyclovir, aminophylline, ampicillin, ampicillin/sulbactam, cefoperazone, diazepam, furosemide, hydrocortisone, insulin, methylprednisolone, mezlocillin, nafcillin, phenytoin, rifampin, sodium bicarbonate, thiopental.**

ADVERSE EFFECTS (≥1%) **CNS:** *Headache,* fatigue, dizziness, asthenia, drowsiness, nervousness, insomnia, confusion, tremor, gait abnormality. **CV:** Edema, arrhythmias, angina, second- or third-degree AV block, bradycardia, CHF, flushing, hypotension, syncope, palpitations. **GI:** Nausea, constipation, anorexia, vomiting, diarrhea, impaired taste, weight increase. **Skin:** Rash.

INTERACTIONS Drug: BETA-BLOCKERS, **digoxin** may have additive effects on av node conduction prolongation; may increase **digoxin** or **quinidine** levels; **cimetidine** may increase diltiazem levels, thus increasing effects; may increase **cyclosporine** levels.

PHARMACOKINETICS Absorption: Approximately 80% absorbed from GI tract, with 40% reaching systemic circulation. **Peak:** 2–3 h; 6–11 h sustained release; 11–18 h Cardizem LA. **Distribution:** Into breast milk. **Metabolism:** In liver (CYP3A4). **Elimination:** Primarily in urine with some elimination in feces. **Half-Life:** Oral 3.5–9 h, IV 2 h.

NURSING IMPLICATIONS

Assessment & Drug Effects

- Check BP and ECG before initiation of therapy and monitor particularly during dosage adjustment period.
- Lab tests: With concurrent therapy, monitor digoxin levels when initiating, adjusting, and discontinuing diltiazem.
- Monitor for and report S&S of CHF.
- Monitor for headache. An analgesic may be required.
- Supervise ambulation as indicated.

Patient & Family Education

- Make position changes slowly and in stages; light-headedness and dizziness (hypotension) are possible.
- Do not drive or engage in other potentially hazardous activities until reaction to drug is known.

D

DIMENHYDRINATE

(dye-men-hye′dri-nate)

Calm-X, Dimenhydrinate Injection, Dramamine

Classifications: ANTIHISTAMINE (H_1-RECEPTOR ANTAGONIST); ANTIVERTIGO

Therapeutic: ANTIVERTIGO; ANTIEMETIC

Prototype: Diphenhydramine

Pregnancy Category: B

AVAILABILITY 50 mg tablets; 50 mg chewable; 50 mg/mL injection; 15.62 mg/5 mL, 12.5 mg/4 mL, 12.5 mg/5 mL liquid

ACTION & *THERAPEUTIC EFFECT* H_1-receptor antagonist. Precise mode of antiemetic action is thought to involve ability to inhibit cholinergic stimulation in vestibular and associated neural pathways. It has been reported to inhibit labyrinthine stimulation for up to 3 h. *Has antihistamine, antiemetic, and antivertigo activity.*

USES Chiefly in prevention and treatment of motion sickness. Also has been used in management of vertigo, nausea, and vomiting associated with radiation sickness, labyrinthitis, Ménière's syndrome, stapedectomy, anesthesia, and various medications.

CONTRAINDICATIONS Narrow-angle glaucoma, BPH; GI obstruction; urinary tract obstruction; CNS depression; lactation, neonates. Safe use in children younger than 2 y is not established.

CAUTIOUS USE Convulsive disorders; asthma, COPD; severe hepatic disease; PKU; history of porphyria; closed-angle glaucoma; elderly; pregnancy (category B).

ROUTE & DOSAGE

Motion Sickness

Adult: **PO** 50–100 mg q4–6h (max: 400 mg/24 h) **IV/IM** 50 mg as needed

Child: **PO** *2–6 y,* up to 25 mg q6–8h (max: 75 mg/24 h); *6–12 y,* 25–50 mg q6–8h (max: 150 mg/24 h) **IM** 1.25 mg/kg q.i.d. up to 300 mg/day

ADMINISTRATION

- First dose should be given 30–60 min before starting activity.

Oral

- Ensure that chewable tablets are chewed and not swallowed whole.

Intramuscular

- Give undiluted and inject deep IM into a large muscle.

Intravenous

PREPARE: **Direct:** Dilute each 50 mg in 10 mL of NS.

ADMINISTER: **Direct:** Give each 50 mg or fraction thereof over 2 min.

INCOMPATIBILITIES **Solution/additive:** **Aminophylline, amobarbital, chlorpromazine, glycopyrrolate, hydrocortisone, hydroxyzine, pentobarbital, phenobarbital, phenytoin, prochlorperazine, promazine, promethazine, thiopental.**

- Store preferably at 15°–30° C (59°–86° F), unless otherwise directed by manufacturer. ▪ Examine parenteral preparation for particulate matter and discoloration. Do not use unless absolutely clear.

ADVERSE EFFECTS (≥1%) **CNS:** *Drowsiness,* headache, incoordination, dizziness, blurred vision, nervousness, restlessness, *insomnia (especially children).* **CV:** Hypotension, palpitation. **GI:** Dry mouth, nose, throat; anorexia, constipation or diarrhea. **Urogenital:** Urinary frequency, dysuria.

DIAGNOSTIC TEST INTERFERENCE ***Skin testing*** procedures should not be performed within 72 h after use of an antihistamine.

INTERACTIONS Drug: Alcohol and other CNS DEPRESSANTS enhance CNS depression, drowsiness; TRICYCLIC ANTIDEPRESSANTS compound anticholinergic effects.

PHARMACOKINETICS Absorption: Readily absorbed from GI tract. **Onset:** 15–30 min PO; immediate IV; 20–30 min IM. **Duration:** 3–6 h. **Distribution:** Distributed into breast milk. **Elimination:** In urine.

NURSING IMPLICATIONS

Assessment & Drug Effects

- Use falls precautions and supervise ambulation; drug produces high incidence of drowsiness.
- Note: Tolerance to CNS depressant effects usually occurs after a few days of drug therapy; some decrease in antiemetic action may result with prolonged use.
- Monitor for dizziness, nausea, and vomiting; these may indicate drug toxicity.

Patient & Family Education

- Do not drive or engage in other potentially hazardous activities until response to drug is known.
- Take 30–60 min before departure to prevent motion sickness; repeat before meals and upon retiring.

DIMERCAPROL

(dye-mer-kap′role)

BAL in Oil, British Anti-Lewisite

Classifications: CHELATING AGENT; ANTIDOTE
Therapeutic: ANTIDOTE
Pregnancy Category: C

AVAILABILITY 100 mg/mL injection

ACTION & *THERAPEUTIC EFFECT* Dithiol compound that combines with ions of various heavy metals to form relatively stable, nontoxic, soluble complexes called chelates, which can be excreted; inhibition of enzymes by toxic metals is thus prevented. *Neutralizes the effects of various heavy metals.*

USES Acute poisoning by arsenic, gold, and mercury; as adjunct to edetate calcium disodium (EDTA) in treatment of lead encephalopathy.

UNLABELED USES Chromium dermatitis; ocular and dermatologic manifestations of arsenic poisoning, as adjunct to penicillamine to increase rate of copper excretion in Wilson's disease, and for poisoning with antimony, bismuth, chromium, copper, nickel, tungsten, zinc.

CONTRAINDICATIONS Hepatic insufficiency (with exception of postarsenical jaundice); history of peanut oil hypersensitivity; severe renal insufficiency; poisoning due to cadmium, iron, selenium, or uranium; lactation.

CAUTIOUS USE Hypertension; oliguria; patients with G6PD deficiency; preexisting renal disease; rheumatoid arthritis; pregnancy (category C).

ROUTE & DOSAGE

Arsenic or Gold Poisoning

Adult/Child: **IM** 2.5–3 mg/kg q4h for first 2 days, then q.i.d. on third day, then b.i.d. for 10 days

Common adverse effects in *italic*, life-threatening effects underlined; generic names in **bold**; classifications in SMALL CAPS; ♣ Canadian drug name; ⓟ Prototype drug

Mercury Poisoning
Adult/Child: **IM** 5 mg/kg initially, followed by 2.5 mg/kg 1–2 times/day for 10 days

Acute Lead Encephalopathy
Adult/Child: **IM** 4 mg/kg initially, then 3–4 mg/kg q4h with EDTA for 2–7 days depending on response

ADMINISTRATION

Intramuscular

- Initiate therapy ASAP (within 1–2 h) after ingestion of the poison because irreversible tissue damage occurs quickly, particularly in mercury poisoning.
- Give by deep IM injection only. Local pain, gluteal abscess, and skin sensitization possible. Rotate injection sites and observe daily.
- Determine if a local anesthetic may be given with the injection to decrease injection site pain.
- Handle with caution; contact of drug with skin may produce erythema, edema, dermatitis.

ADVERSE EFFECTS (≥1%) **CNS:** Headache, anxiety, muscle pain or weakness, restlessness, paresthesias, tremors, *convulsions,* shock. **CV:** *Elevated BP,* tachycardia. **Special Senses:** Rhinorrhea; burning sensation, feeling of pain and constriction in throat. **GI:** Nausea, *vomiting;* burning sensation in lips and mouth, halitosis, salivation; abdominal pain, metabolic acidosis. **Urogenital:** Burning sensation in penis, <u>renal damage</u>. **Other:** Pains in chest or hands, pain and sterile abscess at injection site, sweating, reduction in polymorphonuclear leukocytes, dental pain.

DIAGNOSTIC TEST INTERFERENCE ***I^{131} thyroid uptake*** values may be decreased if test is done during or immediately following dimercaprol therapy.

INTERACTIONS Drug: Iron, cadmium, selenium, uranium form toxic complexes with dimercaprol.

PHARMACOKINETICS Peak: 30–60 min. **Distribution:** Distributed mainly in intracellular spaces, including brain; highest concentrations in liver and kidneys. **Elimination:** Completely excreted in urine and bile within 4 h. **Half-Life:** Short.

NURSING IMPLICATIONS

Assessment & Drug Effects

- Monitor vital signs. Elevations of systolic and diastolic BPs accompanied by tachycardia frequently occur within a few minutes following injection and may remain elevated up to 2 h.
- Note: Fever occurs in approximately 30% of children receiving treatment and may persist throughout therapy.
- Monitor I&O. Drug is potentially nephrotoxic. Report oliguria or change in I&O ratio to physician.
- Check urine daily for albumin, blood, casts, and pH. Blood and urinary levels of the metal serve as guides for dosage adjustments.
- Minor adverse reactions generally reach maximum 15–20 min after drug administration and subside in 30–90 min.

Patient & Family Education

- Drink as much fluid as the physician will permit.

DIMETHYL SULFOXIDE

(dye-meth′il sul-fox′ide)

DMSO, Rimso-50

Classifications: GENITOURINARY; LOCAL ANTI-INFLAMMATORY
Therapeutic: INTERSTITIAL CYSTITIS AGENT
Pregnancy Category: C

AVAILABILITY 50% solution

ACTION & *THERAPEUTIC EFFECT* Reported effects include anti-inflammatory effects, membrane penetration, collagen dissolution, vasodilation, muscle relaxation, diuresis, initiation of histamine release at administration site, cholinesterase inhibition. *Has symptomatic relief of interstitial cystitis with local anti-inflammatory properties.*

USES Symptomatic treatment of interstitial cystitis.

UNLABELED USES Topical treatment of a variety of musculoskeletal disorders, arthritis, scleroderma, tendinitis, breast and prostate malignancies, retinitis pigmentosa, herpesvirus infections, head and spinal cord injuries, shock, and as a carrier to enhance penetration and absorption of other drugs. Also used to protect living cells and tissues during cold storage (cryo-protection). Widely used as an industrial solvent and in veterinary medicine for treatment of musculoskeletal injuries.

CONTRAINDICATIONS Urinary tract malignancy; lactation. Safe use in children is not established.

CAUTIOUS USE Hepatic or renal dysfunction; pregnancy (category C).

ROUTE & DOSAGE

Interstitial Cystitis

Adult: **Instillation** 50 mL of 50% solution instilled slowly into urinary bladder and retained for 15 min; may repeat q2wk until maximum relief obtained, then increase intervals between treatments

ADMINISTRATION

Instillation

- Apply analgesic lubricant such as lidocaine jelly to urethra to facilitate insertion of catheter.
- Instruct patient to retain instillation for 15 min and then expel it by spontaneous voiding.
- Note: Discomfort associated with instillation usually lessens with repeated administration. Physician may prescribe an oral analgesic or suppository containing belladonna and an opiate prior to instillation to reduce bladder spasm.
- Store at 15°–30° C (59°–86° F) unless otherwise directed. Protect from strong light. Avoid contact with plastics.

ADVERSE EFFECTS (≥1%) **Special Senses:** Transient disturbances in color vision, photophobia. **GI:** Nausea, diarrhea. Hypersensitivity: Local or generalized rash, erythema, pruritus, urticaria, swelling of face, dyspnea (anaphylactoid reaction). **Other:** Nasal congestion, headache, sedation, drowsiness. **Following instillation:** *Garlic-like odor on breath and skin; garlic-like taste;* discomfort during administration; transient cystitis. **Following topical application:** Vesicle formation.

INTERACTIONS **Drug:** Decreases effectiveness of **sulindac,** possibly causing severe peripheral neuropathy.

PHARMACOKINETICS **Absorption:** Readily absorbed systemically. **Peak:** 4–8 h. **Distribution:** Widely distributed in tissues and body fluids; penetrates blood–brain barrier; distributed into breast milk. **Metabolism:** Metabolized to dimethyl sulfide (garlic breath) and dimethyl sulfone. **Elimination:** Dimethyl sulfide excreted through lungs and skin; dimethyl sulfone may remain in serum longer than 2 wk and is excreted in urine and feces.

NURSING IMPLICATIONS

Assessment & Drug Effects

- Monitor and report level of bladder discomfort. In cases of severe discomfort physician may elect to do instillation under anesthesia.
- Monitor for visual disturbances. Complete eye evaluation, including slit-lamp examination, is recommended prior to and at regular intervals during therapy.

Patient & Family Education

- Note: Garlic-like taste may be experienced within minutes after drug instillation and may last for several hours. Garlic-like odor on breath and skin may last as long as 72 h.

DINOPROSTONE (PGE_2, PROSTAGLANDIN E_2)

(dye-noe-prost′one)

Cervidil, Prostin E_2, Prepidil

Classification: OXYTOCIC

Therapeutic: PROSTAGLANDIN; OXYTOCIC

Prototype: Oxytocin

Pregnancy Category: C

AVAILABILITY 20 mg suppository; **Prepidil:** 0.5 mg gel; **Cervidil:** 10 mg vaginal insert

ACTION & *THERAPEUTIC EFFECT* Synthetic prostaglandin E_2 that appears to act directly on myometrium and vascular smooth muscle. Stimulation of gravid uterus in early weeks of gestation is more potent than that of oxytocin. *Contractions are qualitatively similar to those that occur during term labor. Has high success rate when used as abortifacient before twentieth week and for stimulation of labor in cases of intrauterine fetal death.*

USES To terminate pregnancy from twelfth week through second trimester as calculated from first day of last regular menstrual period; to evacuate uterine contents in management of missed abortion or intrauterine fetal death up to 28 wk gestational age; to manage benign hydatidiform mole; cervical ripening prior to labor induction.

CONTRAINDICATIONS Acute pelvic inflammatory disease; abnormal fetal position; history of pelvic surgery, uterine fibroids, cervical stenosis, active cardiac, pulmonary, renal, or hepatic disease.

CAUTIOUS USE History of hypertension, hypotension, asthma, epilepsy, anemia, diabetes mellitus; jaundice, history of hepatic, renal, or cardiovascular disease; cervicitis, acute vaginitis, infected endocervical lesion; previous history of caesarean section; pregnancy (category C).

ROUTE & DOSAGE

Induction of Labor

Adult: **Endocervical** Place *Prepidil* 0.5 mg endocervically, may repeat q6h (max: 1.5 mg); place *Cervidil* insert 10 mg transversely in the posterior fornix of the vagina, remove on onset of active labor or 12 h after insertion

Evacuation of Uterus

Adult: **Intravaginal** Insert suppository high in vagina, repeat q2–5h until abortion occurs or membranes rupture (max total dose: 240 mg)

ADMINISTRATION

Endocervical & Intravaginal

- Antiemetic and antidiarrheal medication may be prescribed to be given before dinoprostone to minimize GI side effects.

- Place vaginal insert in the vagina immediately after removal from the foil package. DO NOT use without retrieval system.
- Keep patient in supine position for 10 min after administration of suppository to prevent expulsion and enhance absorption.
- Store suppositories in freezer at temperature not exceeding –20° C (–4° F) unless otherwise specified.

ADVERSE EFFECTS (≥1%) **CNS:** Headache, tremor, tension. **CV:** Transient hypotension, flushing, cardiac arrhythmias. **GI:** *Nausea, vomiting, diarrhea.* **Urogenital:** Vaginal pain, endometritis, uterine rupture. **Respiratory:** Dyspnea, cough, hiccups. **Body as a Whole:** Chills, *fever,* dehydration, diaphoresis, rash.

INTERACTIONS Drug: OXYTOCICS used with extreme caution.

PHARMACOKINETICS Absorption: Slowly absorbed from vagina; Cervidil insert releases approximately 0.3 mg/h. **Onset:** 10 min. **Duration:** 2–3 h. **Distribution:** Widely distributed in body. **Metabolism:** Rapidly metabolized in lungs, kidneys, spleen, and other tissues. **Elimination:** Mainly in urine; some in feces.

NURSING IMPLICATIONS

Assessment & Drug Effects

- Observe patient carefully, after insertion of the drug. Rupture of the membranes is not a contraindication to drug, but be aware that profuse bleeding may result in expulsion of the suppository. Report wheezing, chest pain, dyspnea, and significant changes in BP and pulse to the physician.
- Monitor uterine contractions and observe for and report excessive vaginal bleeding and cramping pain.
- Monitor vital signs. Fever is a physiologic response of the hypothalamus to use of dinoprostone and occurs within 15–45 min after insertion of suppository. Temperature returns to normal within 2–6 h after discontinuation of medication.

Patient & Family Education

- Continue taking your temperature (late afternoon) for a few days after discharge. Contact physician with onset of fever, bleeding, abdominal cramps, abnormal or foul-smelling vaginal discharge.
- Avoid douches, tampons, intercourse, and tub baths for at least 2 wk. Clarify with physician.

DIPHENHYDRAMINE HYDROCHLORIDE (Pr)

(dye-fen-hye′dra-meen)

Allerdryl ✦, Benadryl, Benadryl Dye-Free, Sleep-Eze 3, Sominex Formula 2, Tusstat, Twilite, Valdrene

Classifications: CENTRALLY ACTING CHOLINERGIC ANTAGONIST; ANTIHISTAMINE; H$_1$-RECEPTOR ANTAGONIST

Therapeutic: ANTIHISTAMINE; SEDATIVE-HYPNOTIC; ANTIPARKINSON; ANTIDYSKINETIC; NONNARCOTIC ANTITUSSIVE

Pregnancy Category: C

AVAILABILITY 25 mg, 50 mg capsules, tablets; 6.25 mg/5 mL, 12.5 mg/5 mL syrup; 50 mg/mL injection

ACTION & *THERAPEUTIC EFFECT* Diphenhydramine competes for H$_1$-receptor sites on effector cells, thus blocking histamine release. Effects in parkinsonism and drug-induced extrapyramidal symptoms are apparently related to its ability to suppress central cholinergic activity and to prolong action of dopamine by inhibiting its reuptake and storage. *Has antihistamine, antivertigo, antiemetic, antianaphylactic, antitussive, antidyskinetic, and sedative-hypnotic effects.*

USES Temporary symptomatic relief of various allergic conditions and to treat or prevent motion sickness, vertigo, and reactions to blood or plasma in susceptible patients. Also used in anaphylaxis as adjunct to epinephrine and other standard measures after acute symptoms have been controlled; in treatment of parkinsonism and drug-induced extrapyramidal reactions; as a nonnarcotic cough suppressant; as a sedative-hypnotic; and for treatment of intractable insomnia.

CONTRAINDICATIONS Hypersensitivity to antihistamines of similar structure; lower respiratory tract symptoms (including acute asthma); narrow-angle glaucoma; prostatic hypertrophy, bladder neck obstruction; GI obstruction or stenosis; lactation, premature neonates, and neonates; use as nighttime sleep aid in children younger than 2 y.

CAUTIOUS USE History of asthma; COPD; convulsive disorders; increased IOP; hyperthyroidism; hypertension, cardiovascular disease; hepatic disease; diabetes mellitus; older adults, infants, and young children; pregnancy (category C).

ROUTE & DOSAGE

Allergy Symptoms, Antiparkinsonism, Motion Sickness, Nighttime Sedation

Adult: **PO** 25–50 mg t.i.d. or q.i.d. (max: 300 mg/day) **IV/IM** 10–50 mg q4–6h (max: 400 mg/day)

Child: **PO** *2–6 y*, 6.25 mg q4–6h (max: 300 mg/24 h); *6–12 y*, 12.5–25 mg q4–6h (max: 300 mg/24 h) **IV/IM** 5 mg/kg/day divided into 4 doses (max: 300 mg/day)

Nonproductive Cough

Adult: **PO** 25 mg q4–6h (max: 100 mg/day)

Child: **PO** *2–6 y*, 6.25 mg q4–6h (max: 25 mg/24 h); *6–12 y*, 12.5 mg q4–6h (max: 50 mg/24 h)

ADMINISTRATION

Oral

- Give with food or milk to lessen GI adverse effects.
- For motion sickness: Give the first dose 30 min before exposure to motion; give remaining doses before meals and at bedtime.

Intramuscular

- Give IM injection deep into large muscle mass; alternate injection sites. Avoid perivascular or subcutaneous injections because of its irritating effects.
- Note: Hypersensitivity reactions (including anaphylactic shock) are more likely to occur with parenteral than PO administration.

Intravenous

PREPARE: **Direct:** Give undiluted.
ADMINISTER: **Direct:** Give at a rate of 25 mg or a fraction thereof over 1 min.
INCOMPATIBILITIES **Solution/additive:** **Amphotericin B, dexamethasone, iodipamide, methylprednisolone, pentobarbital, phenobarbital, phenytoin, thiopental.** **Y-site:** **Allopurinol, amphotericin B cholesteryl complex, cefmetazole, foscarnet, furosemide.**

D

- Store in tightly covered containers at 15°–30° C (59°–86° F) unless otherwise directed by manufacturer. Keep injection and elixir formulations in light-resistant containers.

ADVERSE EFFECTS (≥1%) **CNS:** *Drowsiness,* dizziness, headache, fatigue, disturbed coordination, tingling, heaviness and weakness of hands, tremors, euphoria, nervousness, restlessness, insomnia; confusion; (especially in children): Excitement, fever. **CV:** Palpitation, *tachycardia,* mild hypotension or hypertension, cardiovascular collapse. **Special Senses:** Tinnitus, vertigo, dry nose, throat, nasal stuffiness; blurred vision, diplopia, photosensitivity, dry eyes. **GI:** *Dry mouth,* nausea, epigastric distress, anorexia, vomiting, constipation, or diarrhea. **Urogenital:** Urinary frequency or retention, dysuria. **Body as a Whole:** Hypersensitivity (skin rash, urticaria, photosensitivity, anaphylactic shock). **Respiratory:** Thickened bronchial secretions, wheezing, sensation of chest tightness.

DIAGNOSTIC TEST INTERFERENCE Diphenhydramine should be discontinued 4 days prior to ***skin testing*** procedures for allergy because it may obscure otherwise positive reactions.

INTERACTIONS Drug: Alcohol and other CNS DEPRESSANTS, MAO INHIBITORS compound CNS depression.

PHARMACOKINETICS Absorption: Readily absorbed from GI tract but only 40–60% reaches systemic circulation. **Onset:** 15–30 min. **Peak:** 1–4 h. **Duration:** 4–7 h. **Distribution:** Crosses placenta; distributed into breast milk. **Metabolism:** In liver; some degradation in lung and kidney. **Elimination:** Mostly in urine within 24 h.

NURSING IMPLICATIONS

Assessment & Drug Effects

- Monitor cardiovascular status especially with preexisting cardiovascular disease.
- Monitor for adverse effects especially in children and the older adult.
- Supervise ambulation and institute falls precautions as necessary. Drowsiness is most prominent during the first few days of therapy and often disappears with continued therapy. Older adults are especially likely to manifest dizziness, sedation, and hypotension.

Patient & Family Education

- Do not use alcohol and other CNS depressants because of the possible additive CNS depressant effects with concurrent use.
- Do not drive or engage in other potentially hazardous activities until the response to drug is known.
- Increase fluid intake, if not contraindicated; drug has an atropine-like drying effect (thickens bronchial secretions) that may make expectoration difficult.

DIPHENOXYLATE HYDROCHLORIDE WITH ATROPINE SULFATE

(dye-fen-ox'i-late)

Diphenatol, Lofene, Lomanate, Lomotil, Lonox, Lo-Trol, Low-Quel, Nor-Mil

Classification: ANTIDIARRHEAL
Therapeutic: ANTIDIARRHEAL
Pregnancy Category: C
Controlled Substance: Schedule V

AVAILABILITY 2.5 mg tablets; 2.5 mg/5 mL liquid

ACTION & *THERAPEUTIC EFFECT* Diphenoxylate is a synthetic narcotic opiate agonist. Commercially available only with atropine sulfate to discourage deliberate overdosage. Inhibits mucosal receptors responsible for peristaltic reflex, thereby reducing GI motility. *Reduces GI motility.*

USES Adjunct in symptomatic management of diarrhea.

CONTRAINDICATIONS Hypersensitivity to diphenoxylate or atropine; severe dehydration or electrolyte imbalance, advanced liver disease, obstructive jaundice, diarrhea caused by pseudomembranous enterocolitis; diarrhea induced by poisons; glaucoma; children younger than 2 y of age; lactation.

CAUTIOUS USE Advanced hepatic disease, abnormal liver function tests; renal function impairment, MAOI therapy; addiction-prone individuals, or those whose history suggests drug abuse; ulcerative colitis; young children; pregnancy (category C).

ROUTE & DOSAGE

Diarrhea

Adult: **PO** 1–2 tablets or 1–2 teaspoons full (5 mL) 3–4 times/day (each tablet or 5 mL contains 2.5 mg diphenoxylate HCl and 0.025 mg atropine sulfate)
Child (2–12 y): **PO** 0.3–0.4 mg/kg/day of liquid in divided doses

ADMINISTRATION

Oral

- Crush tablet if necessary and give with fluid of patient's choice.
- Reduce dosage as soon as initial control of symptoms occurs.
- Withhold drug in presence of severe dehydration or electrolyte imbalance until appropriate corrective therapy has been initiated.
- Note: Treatment is generally continued for 24–36 h before it is considered ineffective.
- Store in tightly covered, light-resistant container, preferably 15°–30° C (59°–86° F), unless otherwise directed by manufacturer.

ADVERSE EFFECTS (≥1%) **Body as a Whole:** Hypersensitivity (pruritus, angioneurotic edema, giant urticaria, rash). **CNS:** Headache, sedation, drowsiness, dizziness, lethargy, numbness of extremities; restlessness, euphoria, mental depression, weakness, general malaise. **CV:** Flushing, palpitation, tachycardia. **Special Senses:** Nystagmus, mydriasis, blurred vision, miosis (toxicity). **GI:** Nausea, vomiting, anorexia, dry mouth, abdominal discomfort or distension, paralytic ileus, toxic megacolon. **Other:** Urinary retention, swelling of gums.

INTERACTIONS Drug: MAO INHIBITORS may precipitate hypertensive crisis; **alcohol** and other CNS DEPRESSANTS may enhance CNS effects; also see **atropine.**

PHARMACOKINETICS Absorption: Readily absorbed from GI tract. **Onset:** 45–60 min. **Peak:** 2 h. **Duration:** 3–4 h. **Distribution:** Distributed into breast milk. **Metabolism:** Rapidly metabolized to active and inactive metabolites in liver. **Elimination:** Slowly through bile into feces; small amount in urine. **Half-Life:** 4.4 h.

NURSING IMPLICATIONS

Assessment & Drug Effects

- Assess GI function; report abdominal distention and signs of decreased peristalsis.
- Monitor for S&S of dehydration (see Appendix F). It is essential to monitor young children closely; dehydration occurs more rapidly in this age group and may influence variability of response to diphenoxylate and predispose patient to delayed toxic effects.
- Monitor frequency and consistency of stools.

Patient & Family Education

- Take medication only as directed by physician.
- Notify physician if diarrhea persists or if fever, bloody stools, palpitation, or other adverse reactions occur.
- Do not drive or engage in other potentially hazardous activities until response to drug is known.

DIPIVEFRIN HYDROCHLORIDE

(dye-pi've-frin)

Propine

Pregnancy Category: B

See Appendix A-1.

DIPYRIDAMOLE

(dye-peer-id'a-mole)

Apo-Dipyridamole ♣, Persantine

Classifications: ANTIPLATELET; PLATELET AGGREGATE INHIBITOR

Therapeutic: PLATELET AGGREGATE INHIBITOR

Pregnancy Category: B

AVAILABILITY 25 mg, 50 mg, 75 mg tablets; 10 mg injection

ACTION & *THERAPEUTIC EFFECT* Nonnitrate coronary vasodilator that increases coronary blood flow by selectively dilating coronary arteries, thereby increasing myocardial oxygen supply. Additionally, it exhibits mild inotropic action as well as antiplatelet aggregation activity. *Has antiplatelet, and coronary vasodilator effects.*

USES To prevent postoperative thromboembolic complications associated with prosthetic heart valves and as adjunct for thallium stress testing.

UNLABELED USES To reduce rate of reinfarction following MI; to prevent TIAs (transient ischemic attacks) and coronary bypass graft occlusion.

CONTRAINDICATIONS Safety and efficacy in children younger than 12 y are not established.

CAUTIOUS USE Hypotension, anticoagulant therapy; aspirin sensitivity; elderly; severe hepatic dysfunction; syncope; pregnancy (category B), lactation.

ROUTE & DOSAGE

Prevention of Thromboembolism in Cardiac Valve Replacement

Adult: **PO** 75–100 mg q.i.d.
Child: **PO** 1–2 mg t.i.d.

Thromboembolic Disorders

Adult: **PO** 150–400 mg/day in divided doses

Thallium Stress Test

Adult: **IV** 0.142 mg/kg/min for 4 min

ADMINISTRATION

Oral

- Give on an empty stomach at least 1 h before or 2 h after meals, with a full glass of water. Physician may prescribe with food if gastric distress persists.

Intravenous

PREPARE: **Direct:** Dilute to at least a 1:2 ratio with 0.45% NaCl, NS, or D5W to yield a final volume of 20–50 mL.

ADMINISTER: **Direct:** Give a single dose over 4 min (0.142 mg/kg/min).

- Store in tightly closed container at 15°–30° C (59°–86° F) unless otherwise directed. Protect injection from direct light.

ADVERSE EFFECTS (≥1%) Usually dose related, minimal, and transient. **CNS:** Headache, dizziness, faintness, syncope, weakness. **CV:** Peripheral vasodilation, flushing. **GI:** Nausea, vomiting, diarrhea, abdominal distress. **Skin:** Skin rash, pruritus.

INTERACTIONS Drug: Other ANTICOAGULANTS can increase bleeding risk. **Herbal: Evening primrose oil, ginseng** can increase bleeding risk.

PHARMACOKINETICS Absorption: Readily absorbed from GI tract. **Peak:** 45–150 min. **Distribution:** Small amount crosses placenta. **Metabolism:** In liver. **Elimination:** Mainly in feces. **Half-Life:** 10–12 h.

NURSING IMPLICATIONS

Assessment & Drug Effects

- Monitor therapeutic effectiveness. Clinical response may not be evident before second or third month of continuous therapy. Effects include reduced frequency or elimination of anginal episodes, improved exercise tolerance, reduced requirement for nitrates.

Patient & Family Education

- Notify physician of any adverse effects.
- Make all position changes slowly and in stages, especially from recumbent to upright posture, if postural hypotension or dizziness is a problem.

DISOPYRAMIDE PHOSPHATE

(dye-soe-peer'a-mide)

Napamide, Norpace, Norpace CR, Rythmodan ♣, Rythmodan-LA ♣

Classification: ANTIARRHYTHMIC, CLASS IA

Therapeutic: ANTIARRHYTHMIC, CLASS IA

Prototype: Procainamide

Pregnancy Category: C

AVAILABILITY 100 mg, 150 mg regular and sustained release capsules

ACTION & *THERAPEUTIC EFFECT* Class IA antiarrhythmic agent that decreases myocardial conduction velocity and excitability in the atria, ventricles, and accessory pathways. It prolongs the QRS and QT intervals in normal sinus rhythm and atrial arrhythmias. *Acts as myocardial depressant by reducing rate of spontaneous diastolic depolarization in pacemaker cells, thereby suppressing ectopic focal activity.*

USES To suppress and prevent recurrence of premature ventricular contractions (unifocal, multifocal, paired) and ventricular tachycardia not severe enough to require cardioversion.

UNLABELED USES In combination with other antiarrhythmic drugs to treat or prevent serious refractory arrhythmias. To convert atrial fibrillation, atrial flutter, and paroxysmal atrial tachycardia to normal sinus rhythm.

CONTRAINDICATIONS Cardiogenic shock, preexisting 2nd or 3rd degree AV block (if no pacemaker is present); sick sinus syndrome (bradycardia-tachycardia); Wolff-Parkinson-White (WPW) syndrome or bundle branch block, history of torsades de pointes; cardiogenic shock; QT prolongation; uncompensated or inadequately compensated CHF, hypotension (unless secondary to cardiac arrhythmia), hypokalemia.
CAUTIOUS USE Myocarditis or other cardiomyopathy, underlying cardiac conduction abnormalities; hepatic or renal impairment; urinary tract disease (especially prostatic hypertrophy); diabetes mellitus; myasthenia gravis; elderly; narrow-angle glaucoma; family history of glaucoma; pregnancy (category C), lactation.

ROUTE & DOSAGE

Arrhythmias
Adult: **PO** *Weight greater than 50 kg,* 100–200 mg q6h or 300 mg loading dose*; weight less than 50 kg,* 100 mg q6h
Adolescent: **PO** 6–15 mg/kg/day in divided doses q6h
Child: **PO** *Younger than 1 y,* 10–30 mg/kg/day in divided doses q6h; *1–4 y,* 10–20 mg/kg/day in divided doses q6h; *4–12 y,* 10–15 mg/kg/day in divided doses q6h

ADMINISTRATION

Oral
- Start drug 6–12 h after last quinidine dose and 3–6 h after last procainamide dose for patients who have been receiving either quinidine or procainamide.
- Give sustained release capsules whole.
- Do not use sustained release capsules in loading doses when rapid control is required or in patients with creatinine clearance of 40 mL/min or less.
- Start sustained release capsules 6 h after last dose of conventional capsule if change in drug form is made.
- Store at 15°–30° C (59°–86° F) unless otherwise directed.

ADVERSE EFFECTS (≥1%) **Body as a Whole:** Hypersensitivity (pruritus, urticaria, rash, photosensitivity, <u>laryngospasm</u>). **CNS:** Dizziness, headache, fatigue, muscle weakness, convulsions, paresthesias, nervousness, acute psychosis, peripheral neuropathy. **CV:** *Hypotension,* chest pain, edema, dyspnea, syncope, bradycardia, tachycardia; worsening of CHF or cardiac arrhythmia; <u>cardiogenic shock, heart block</u>; edema with weight gain. **Special Senses:** *Blurred vision,* dry eyes, increased IOP, precipitation of acute angle-closure glaucoma. **GI:** *Dry mouth, constipation,* epigastric or abdominal pain, cholestatic jaundice. **Urogenital:** *Hesitancy* and *retention,* urinary frequency, urgency, renal insufficiency. **Other:** Dry nose and throat, drying of bronchial secretions, initiation of uterine contractions (pregnant patient); muscle aches, precipitation of myasthenia gravis, <u>agranulocytosis</u> (rare), thrombocytopenia.

INTERACTIONS Drug: ANTICHOLINERGIC DRUGS (e.g., TRICYCLIC ANTIDEPRESSANTS, ANTIHISTAMINES) compound anticholinergic effects; other ANTIARRHYTHMICS compound toxicities; **phenytoin, rifampin** may increase disopyramide metabolism and decrease levels; may increase **warfarin**-induced hypoprothrombinemia.

PHARMACOKINETICS Absorption: Readily from GI tract; 60–83% reaches systemic circulation. **Onset:** 30 min–3.5 h. **Peak:** 1–2 h. **Duration:** 1.5–8.5 h. **Distribution:** Distributed in extracellular fluid; crosses placenta; distributed into breast milk. **Metabolism:** In liver. **Elimination:** 80% in urine, 10% in feces. **Half-Life:** 4–10 h.

NURSING IMPLICATIONS

Assessment & Drug Effects

- Check apical pulse before administering drug. Withhold drug and notify physician if pulse rate is slower than 60 bpm, faster than 120 bpm, or if there is any unusual change in rate, rhythm, or quality.
- Monitor ECG closely. The following signs are indications for drug withdrawal: Prolongation of QT interval and worsening of arrhythmia interval, QRS widening (greater than 25%).
- Monitor for rapid weight gain or other signs of fluid retention.
- Lab tests: Baseline and periodic blood glucose, and serum potassium. Correct hypokalemia or other imbalances before initiation of therapy.
- Monitor BP closely in all patients during periods of dosage adjustment and in those receiving high dosages.
- Monitor I&O, particularly in older adults and patients with impaired renal function or prostatic hypertrophy. Persistent urinary hesitancy or retention may necessitate lower dosage or discontinuation of drug.
- Report S&S of hyperkalemia (see Appendix F); it enhances drug's toxic effects.
- Monitor for S&S of CHF.

Patient & Family Education

- Take drug precisely as prescribed to maintain regularity of heartbeat.
- Weigh daily under standard conditions and check ankles for edema. Report to physician a weekly weight gain of 1–2 kg (2–4 lb) or more.
- Make position changes slowly, particularly when getting up from lying down because of the possibility of hypotension; dangle legs for a few minutes before walking, and do not stand still for prolonged periods.
- Do not drive or engage in other potentially hazardous activities until response to drug is known.

D

DISULFIRAM

(dye-sul'fi-ram)

Antabuse, Cronetal, Ro-sulfiram

Classifications: ENZYME INHIBITOR; ANTIALCOHOL AGENT

Therapeutic: ALCOHOL ABUSE DETERRANT

Pregnancy Category: B

AVAILABILITY 250 mg, 500 mg tablets

ACTION & *THERAPEUTIC EFFECT* Acts as a deterrent to alcohol ingestion by inhibiting the enzyme acetaldehyde dehydrogenase, which normally metabolizes alcohol in the body. *When a small amount of alcohol is ingested, a complex of highly unpleasant symptoms known as the disulfiram reaction occurs, which serves as a deterrent to further drinking.*

D

USES Adjunct in treatment of the patient with chronic alcoholism who sincerely wants to maintain sobriety.

CONTRAINDICATIONS Severe myocardial disease; cardiac disease; psychosis; patients who have recently ingested alcohol, metronidazole, paraldehyde; multiple drug dependence.

CAUTIOUS USE Diabetes mellitus; epilepsy; seizure disorders; hypothyroidism; coronary artery disease, cerebral damage; chronic and acute nephritis; renal disease; hepatic cirrhosis or insufficiency; abnormal EEG; pregnancy (category B), lactation.

ROUTE & DOSAGE

Alcoholism

Adult: **PO** 500 mg/day for 1–2 wk, then 125–500 mg/day (max: 500 mg/day)

ADMINISTRATION

Oral

- Daily does may be given at bedtime to minimize sedative effect of the drug. Decrease in dose may also reduce sedative effect.
- Make sure patient has abstained from alcohol and alcohol-containing preparations for at least 12 h and preferably 48 h before initiating therapy.
- Store at 15°–30° C (59°–86° F) unless otherwise directed. Protect tablets from light.

ADVERSE EFFECTS (≥1%) **Reaction with alcohol ingestion:** Flushing of face, chest, arms, pulsating headache, nausea, violent vomiting, thirst, sweating, marked uneasiness, confusion, weakness, vertigo, blurred vision, pruritic skin rash, hyperventilation, abnormal gait, slurred speech, disorientation, confusion, personality changes, bizarre behavior, psychoses, tachycardia, palpitation, chest pain, <u>hypotension to shock level arrhythmias, acute congestive failure</u>. **Severe reactions:** <u>Marked respiratory depression, unconsciousness, convulsions, sudden death</u>. **Body as a Whole:** Hypersensitivity (allergic or acneiform dermatitis; urticaria, fixed-drug eruption). **CNS:** Drowsiness, fatigue, restlessness, headache, tremor, psychoses (usually with high doses), polyneuritis, peripheral neuropathy, optic neuritis. **GI:** Mild GI disturbances, garlic-like or metallic taste, <u>hepatotoxicity</u>, hypersensitivity hepatitis.

DIAGNOSTIC TEST INTERFERENCE Disulfiram can reduce ***uptake of*** I^{131}***;*** or decreases ***PBI*** test results (rare).

INTERACTIONS Drug: Alcohol (including in liquid OTC drugs, **IV nitroglycerin, IV cotrimoxazole**), **metronidazole, paraldehyde** will produce disulfiram reaction; **isoniazid** can produce neurologic symptoms; may increase blood levels and toxicity of **warfarin, paraldehyde,** BARBITURATES, **phenytoin.**

PHARMACOKINETICS Absorption: Readily absorbed from GI tract. **Onset:** Up to 12 h. **Duration:** Up to 2 wk. **Distribution:** Initially deposited in fat. **Metabolism:** Metabolized slowly in liver. **Elimination:** 5–20% excreted in feces; 20% remains in body for 1–2 wk; some may be excreted in breath as carbon disulfide.

NURSING IMPLICATIONS

Assessment & Drug Effects

- Lab tests: Baseline and follow-up transaminase studies every 10–14 days to detect hepatic dysfunction.

Common adverse effects in *italic*, life-threatening effects <u>underlined</u>; generic names in **bold**; classifications in SMALL CAPS; ♣ Canadian drug name; ℗ Prototype drug

- Note: Disulfiram reaction occurs within 5–10 min following ingestion of alcohol and may last 30 min to several hours. Intensity of reaction varies with each individual, but is generally proportional to the amount of alcohol ingested.
- Treat patient with severe disulfiram reaction as though in shock. Monitor potassium levels, especially if patient has diabetes mellitus.

Patient & Family Education

- Understand fully the possible dangers if alcohol is ingested during disulfiram treatment before consenting to therapy.
- Report promptly to physician the onset of nausea with right upper quadrant pain or discomfort, itching, jaundiced sclerae or skin, dark urine, clay-colored stools. Withhold drug pending liver function tests.
- Note: Ingestion of even small amounts of alcohol or use of external applications that contain alcohol may be sufficient to produce a reaction. Read all labels and avoid use of anything containing alcohol.
- Alcohol sensitivity may last as long as 2 wk after disulfiram has been discontinued.
- Note: Adverse effects of drug are often experienced during first 2 wk of therapy; symptoms usually disappear with continued therapy or with dose reduction.
- Do not drive or engage in other potentially hazardous activities until response to drug is known.

DOBUTAMINE HYDROCHLORIDE

(doe-byoo'ta-meen)

Dobutrex

Classifications: ADRENERGIC AGONIST; VASOPRESSOR
Therapeutic: CARDIAC STIMULANT; IONOTROPIC
Prototype: Isoproterenol
Pregnancy Category: C

AVAILABILITY 12.5 mg/mL injection

ACTION & *THERAPEUTIC EFFECT* Produces inotropic effect by acting on beta receptors and primarily on myocardial alpha-adrenergic receptors. Increases cardiac output and decreases pulmonary wedge pressure and total systemic vascular resistance. Also increases conduction through AV node, and has lower potential for precipitating arrhythmias than dopamine. *In CHF or cardiogenic shock it increases cardiac output, enhances renal perfusion, increases renal output, and renal sodium excretion.*

USES Inotropic support in short-term treatment of adults with cardiac decompensation due to depressed myocardial contractility (cardiogenic shock) resulting from either organic heart disease or from cardiac surgery.

UNLABELED USES To augment cardiovascular function in children undergoing cardiac catheterization, stress thallium testing.

CONTRAINDICATIONS History of hypersensitivity to other sympathomimetic amines or sulfites, ventricular tachycardia, idiopathic hypertrophic subaortic stenosis; hypovolemia; children younger than 2 y.

CAUTIOUS USE Preexisting hypertension, hypotension; atrial fibrillation; acute MI; unstable angina, severe coronary artery disease; pregnancy (category C).

D

ROUTE & DOSAGE

Cardiac Decompensation
Adult: **IV** 0.5–1 mcg/kg/min then titrate up to 2.5–15 mcg/kg/min (max: 40 mcg/kg/min)
Adolescent/Child: **IV** 2–20 mcg/kg/min

ADMINISTRATION

Intravenous

PREPARE: **Continuous:** Reconstitute by adding 10 mL sterile water for injection or D5W to 250-mg vial; if not completely dissolved, add an additional 10 mL of diluent. ▪ Further dilution is typical (e.g., 250 mg in 1000 mL yields 250 mcg/mL; 250 mg in 500 mL yields 500 mcg/mL; 250 mg in 250 mL yields 1000 mcg/mL). ▪ Use IV solutions within 24 h.

ADMINISTER: **Continuous:** Rate of infusion is determined by body weight and controlled by an infusion pump (preferred) or a microdrip IV infusion set. ▪ IV infusion rate and duration of therapy are determined by heart rate, blood pressure, ectopic activity, urine output, and whenever possible, by measurements of cardiac output and central venous or pulmonary wedge pressures.

INCOMPATIBILITIES **Solution/additive:** **Acyclovir, alteplase, aminophylline, bretylium, bumetanide, calcium chloride, calcium gluconate, diazepam, digoxin, furosemide, heparin, insulin, magnesium sulfate, phenytoin, potassium chloride, potassium phosphate, sodium bicarbonate.** **Y-site:** **Acyclovir, alteplase, aminophylline, amphotericin B cholesteryl sulfate, cefepime, foscarnet, furosemide, heparin, indomethacin, lansoprazole, pantoprazole, pemetrexed, phytonadione, piperacillin/tazobactam, thiopental, warfarin.**

▪ Refrigerate reconstituted solution at 2°–15° C (36°–59° F) for 48 h or store for 6 h at room temperature.

ADVERSE EFFECTS (≥1%) **All:** Generally dose related. **CNS:** Headache, tremors, paresthesias, mild leg cramps, nervousness, fatigue (with overdosage). **CV:** *Increased heart rate and BP,* premature ventricular beats, palpitation, *anginal pain.* **GI:** Nausea, vomiting. **Other:** Nonspecific chest pain, shortness of breath.

INTERACTIONS Drug: GENERAL ANESTHETICS (especially **cyclopropane** and **halothane**) may sensitize myocardium to effects of CATECHOLAMINES such as dobutamine and lead to serious arrhythmias—use with extreme caution; BETA-ADRENERGIC BLOCKING AGENTS (e.g., **metoprolol, propranolol**) may make dobutamine ineffective in increasing cardiac output, but total peripheral resistance may increase—concomitant use generally avoided; MAO INHIBITORS, TRICYCLIC ANTIDEPRESSANTS potentiate pressor effects—use with extreme caution.

PHARMACOKINETICS Onset: 2–10 min. **Peak:** 10–20 min. **Metabolism:** Metabolized in liver and other tissues by COMT. **Elimination:** In urine. **Half-Life:** 2 min.

NURSING IMPLICATIONS

Assessment & Drug Effects

▪ Correct hypovolemia by administration of appropriate volume expanders prior to initiation of therapy.

- Monitor therapeutic effectiveness. At any given dosage level, drug takes 10–20 min to produce peak effects.
- Monitor ECG and BP continuously during administration.
- Note: Marked increases in blood pressure (systolic pressure is the most likely to be affected) and heart rate, or the appearance of arrhythmias or other adverse cardiac effects are usually reversed promptly by reduction in dosage.
- Observe patients with preexisting hypertension closely for exaggerated pressor response.
- Monitor I&O ratio and pattern. Urine output and sodium excretion generally increase because of improved cardiac output and renal perfusion.

Patient & Family Education

- Report anginal pain to physician promptly.

DOCETAXEL

(doc-e-tax′el)

Taxotere

Classifications: ANTINEOPLASTIC; TAXANE

Therapeutic: ANTINEOPLASTIC

Prototype: Paclitaxel

Pregnancy Category: D

AVAILABILITY 20 mg, 80 mg injection

ACTION & *THERAPEUTIC EFFECT* Docetaxel is a semisynthetic analog of paclitaxel. Docetaxel, like paclitaxel, binds to the microtubule network essential for interphase and mitosis of the cell cycle. *Docetaxel stabilizes the microtubules involved in cell division and prevents their normal functioning; this results in inhibiting mitosis in cancer cells.*

USES Metastatic breast cancer, metastatic prostate cancer, non-small cell lung cancer.

CONTRAINDICATIONS Hypersensitivity to docetaxel or other drugs formulated with polysorbate 80, paclitaxel; neutrophil count less than 1500 cells/mm^3, biliary tract disease, hepatic disease, jaundice, intramuscular injections, thrombocytopenia, acute infection, pregnancy (category D), lactation.

CAUTIOUS USE Bone marrow suppression, bone marrow transplant patients; CHF, ascites, peripheral edema, pleural effusion; radiation therapy; pulmonary disorders, acute bronchospasm; cardiac tamponade; dental disease, dental work, herpes infection; hypotension, elderly; infection. Safety and effectiveness in children younger than 16 y are not established.

ROUTE & DOSAGE

Breast Cancer

Adult: **IV** 60–100 mg/m^2 q3wk (premedicate patients with dexamethasone 8 mg b.i.d. × 5 days, starting 1 day prior to docetaxel)

Prostate Cancer

Adult: **IV** 75 mg/m^2 q21days plus prednisone (5 mg PO twice daily) for 10 cycles (premedicate patients with dexamethasone 8 mg 12h, 3h, and 1h prior to starting docetaxel infusion)

Non–Small-Cell Lung Cancer

Adult: **IV** 75 mg/m^2 q3wk

ADMINISTRATION

- Note: If drug contacts skin during preparation, wash immediately with soap and water.

Intravenous

PREPARE: **IV Infusion:** Bring vials to room temperature for 5 min; add provided diluent to yield 10 mg/mL, gently rotate for 45 sec; let stand until surface foam dissipates. ▪ Inject required amount of diluted solution into a 250-mL, or larger, bag of NS or D5W; the final concentration should be between 0.3–0.74 mg/mL. Mix completely by manual rotation. ▪ Use glass or polypropylene bottles or polypropylene or polyolefin plastic bags and administer through polyethylene-lined administration sets. Do not use PVC administration sets or containers. ▪ Mix completely by manual rotation. ▪ Use within 4 h (including the 1 h infusion time).

ADMINISTER: **IV Infusion:** Give at a constant rate over 1 h. ▪ Administer ONLY after premedication with corticosteroids to prevent hypersensitivity. ▪ Reduce dose by 25% following severe neutropenia (less than 500 cells/mm³) for 7 days or longer for febrile neutropenia, severe cutaneous reactions, or severe peripheral neuropathy.

INCOMPATIBILITIES **Y-site: Amphotericin B, doxorubicin, methylprednisolone, nalbuphone.**

- Refrigerate vials at 2°–8° C (36°–46° F). Protect from light. Do not store in PVC bags. ▪ Store diluted solutions in refrigerator or at room temperature for 8 h.

ADVERSE EFFECTS (≥1%) **CNS:** Paresthesia, pain, burning sensation, weakness, confusion. **CV:** Hypotension, *fluid retention (peripheral edema, weight gain),* pleural effusion. **GI:** *Nausea, vomiting, diarrhea, stomatitis,* abdominal pain; increased liver function tests (AST or ALT). **Hematologic:** *Neutropenia, leukopenia, thrombocytopenia, anemia*, febrile neutropenia. **Skin:** Rash, localized eruptions, desquamation, *alopecia*, nail changes (hyper/hypopigmentation, onycholysis). **Body as a Whole:** *Hypersensitivity reactions,* infusion site reactions (hyperpigmentation, inflammation, redness, dryness, phlebitis, extravasation).

INTERACTIONS Drug: Possibility of interacting with other drugs metabolized by CYP3A4.

PHARMACOKINETICS Distribution: 97% protein bound. **Metabolism:** In liver by CYP3A4. **Elimination:** 80% in feces, 20% renally. **Half-Life:** 11.1 h.

NURSING IMPLICATIONS

Assessment & Drug Effects

- Lab tests: Monitor bilirubin, AST or ALT, and alkaline phosphatase prior to each drug cycle. Monitor frequently CBCs with differential. Withhold drug and notify physician if platelets less than 100,000 or neutrophils less than 1500 cells/mm³.
- Monitor for S&S of hypersensitivity (see Appendix F), which may develop within a few minutes of initiation of infusion. It is usually not necessary to discontinue infusion for minor reactions (i.e., flushing or local skin reaction).
- Assess throughout therapy and report cardiovascular dysfunction, respiratory distress; fluid retention; development of neurosensory symptoms; severe, cutaneous eruptions on feet, hands, arms, face, or thorax; and S&S of infection.

Patient & Family Education

- Learn common adverse effects and measures to control or minimize them when possible. Report immediately any distressing adverse effects.
- Note: It is extremely important to comply with corticosteroid therapy and monitoring of lab values.
- Avoid pregnancy during therapy.

DOCOSANOL

(doc′os-a-nol)

Abreva

Classification: ANTIVIRAL-LIKE

Therapeutic: ANTIVIRAL-LIKE

Pregnancy Category: C

AVAILABILITY 10% cream

ACTION & *THERAPEUTIC EFFECT* Docosanol inhibits viral replication by interfering with the early intracellular events surrounding viral entry into target cells. It exhibits preferential activity against lipid-enveloped viruses that use fusion mechanisms for entry into target cells. *Believed to exert its antiviral effect by inhibiting fusion of the HSV (herpesvirus) envelope with the human cell plasma membrane, therefore making it difficult for the virus to enter the cell and replicate.*

USES Treatment of herpes simplex infections of the face and lips (i.e., cold sores).

CONTRAINDICATIONS Hypersensitivity to docosanol or any of the inactive ingredients in the ointment; immunosuppressant patients; lactation.

CAUTIOUS USE Pregnancy (category C). Safety and efficacy in children are not established.

ROUTE & DOSAGE

Herpes Simplex Infections

Adult: **Topical** Apply to lesions 5 times/day for up to 10 days, starting at onset of symptoms

ADMINISTRATION

Topical

- Apply cream only to the affected areas using a gloved finger. Rub in gently but completely.
- Do not apply near or in the eyes.
- Avoid application to the mucous membranes inside of the mouth.
- Store at 20°–25° C (68°–77° F).

ADVERSE EFFECTS (≥1%) **CNS:** Headache. **Skin:** Skin irritation, burning.

INTERACTIONS Drug: No clinically significant interactions established.

NURSING IMPLICATIONS

Assessment & Drug Effects

- Monitor severity and extent of infection.
- Notify physician if improvement is not seen within 10 days of initiating treatment

Patient & Family Education

- Wash hands before and after applying cream.
- Do not share this cream with any other individual as this may spread the herpes virus.
- Report to physician if your condition worsens or does not improve within 10 days of beginning treatment.

DOCUSATE CALCIUM (DIOCTYL CALCIUM SULFOSUCCINATE) Pr

(dok′yoo-sate)

DCS, PMS-Docusate Calcium, Pro-Cal-Sof, Surfak

DOCUSATE POTASSIUM

Dialose, Diocto-K, Kasof

DOCUSATE SODIUM

Colace, Colace Enema, Dio-Sul, Disonate, DGSS, D-S-S, Duosol, Lax-gel, Laxinate 100, Modane Soft, Pro-Sof, Regulax ♣, Regutol, Therevac-Plus, Therevac-SB

Classification: STOOL SOFTENER
Therapeutic: STOOL SOFTENER
Pregnancy Category: C

AVAILABILITY Docusate Calcium: 50 mg, 240 mg capsules; **Docusate Potassium:** 100 mg tablets; 240 mg capsules; **Docusate Sodium:** 100 mg tablets; 50 mg, 100 mg, 240 mg, 250 mg capsules; 50 mg/15 mL 60 mg/15 mL, 150 mg/15 mL syrup

ACTION & *THERAPEUTIC EFFECT* Anionic surface-active agent with emulsifying and wetting properties. *Detergent action lowers surface tension, permitting water and fats to penetrate and soften stools for easier passage.*

USES Prophylactically in patients who should avoid straining during defecation and for treatment of constipation associated with hard, dry stools (e.g., following anorectal surgery, MI).

CONTRAINDICATIONS Atonic constipation, nausea, vomiting, abdominal pain, fecal impaction, structural anomalies of colon and rectum, intestinal obstruction or perforation; use of docusate sodium in patients on sodium restriction; use of docusate potassium in patients with renal dysfunction; concomitant use of mineral oil.

CAUTIOUS USE History of CHF, edema, diabetes mellitus; pregnancy (category C).

ROUTE & DOSAGE

Stool Softener
Adult: **PO** 50–500 mg/day **PR** 50–100 mg added to enema fluid
Child: **PO** *Younger than 3 y,* 10–40 mg/day; *3–6 y,* 20–60 mg/day; *6–12 y,* 40–120 mg/day

ADMINISTRATION

Oral
- Give with a full glass of water if allowed.
- Store syrup formulations in tight, light-resistant containers at 15°–30° C (59°–86° F) unless directed otherwise.

Rectal
- Microenema: Insert full length of nozzle (half length for children) into the rectum. Squeeze entire contents of tube and remove completely before releasing grip on tube.
- Store in tightly covered containers.

ADVERSE EFFECTS (≥1%) **GI:** Occasional mild abdominal cramps, *diarrhea,* nausea, bitter taste. **Other:** Throat irritation (liquid preparation), rash.

INTERACTIONS Drug: Docusate will increase systemic absorption of **mineral oil.**

PHARMACOKINETICS Not studied.

NURSING IMPLICATIONS

Assessment & Drug Effects
- Withhold drug if diarrhea develops and notify physician.
- Therapeutic effectiveness: Usually apparent 1–3 days after first dose.

Patient & Family Education

- Take sufficient liquid with each dose and increase fluid intake during the day, if allowed. Oral liquid (NOT syrup) may be administered in milk, fruit juice, or infant formula to mask bitter taste.
- Do not take concomitantly with mineral oil.
- Do not take for prolonged periods in lieu of proper dietary management or treatment of underlying causes of constipation.

DOFETILIDE

(do-fe-ti′lyde)

Tikosyn

Classifications: ANTIARRHYTHMIC, CLASS III; POTASSIUM CHANNEL BLOCKER

Therapeutic: ANTIARRHYTHMIC, CLASS III

Prototype: Amiodarone HCl

Pregnancy Category: C

AVAILABILITY 125 mcg, 250 mcg, 500 mcg capsules

ACTION & *THERAPEUTIC EFFECT* Class III antiarrhythmic agent that prolongs the cardiac action potential by blocking the potassium channels and thus one or more of the potassium currents. Action results in suppression of arrhythmias dependent upon reentry of potassium ions. *Effectiveness indicated by correction of atrial arrhythmias.*

USES Symptomatic atrial fibrillation and flutter.

CONTRAINDICATIONS QT prolongation; ventricular arrhythmias; history of torsades de pointes; hypersensitivity to dofetilide; electrolyte imbalances (e.g., hypokalemia, hypomagnesemia, etc.); renal failure; lactation.

CAUTIOUS USE Atrioventricular block, bradycardia, CHF, concurrent administration of potassium depleting diuretics, hepatic or renal impairment; history of moderate QT_c interval prolongation; moderate to severe hypertension; recent MI or unstable angina; vascular heart disease; older adults; pregnancy (category C). Safety and efficacy in children younger than 18 y are unknown.

ROUTE & DOSAGE

Atrial Fibrillation/Flutter

Adult: **PO** Based on creatinine clearance (CrCl) and QT_c interval, if QT_c increases by more than 15% from baseline or is greater than 500 milliseconds 2–3 h after initial dose. Decrease subsequent doses by 50%.

Renal Impairment Dosage Adjustment

CrCl greater than 60 mL/min: 500 mcg b.i.d.; 40–60 mL/min: 250 mcg b.i.d.; 20–39 mL/min: 125 mcg b.i.d.

ADMINISTRATION

Oral

- Do not give dofetilide if QT/QT_c interval greater than 420 milliseconds (or greater than 500 milliseconds with ventricular conduction abnormalities).
- Administer only with continuous ECG monitoring.
- Do not initiate therapy until 3 mo after withdrawal of previous antiarrhythmic therapy.
- Do not initiate therapy until 3 mo after amiodarone has been with-

drawn or plasma level is less than 0.3 mcg/mL.

- Store at 15°–30° C (59°–86° F); protect from moisture and humidity.

ADVERSE EFFECTS (≥1%) **Body as a Whole:** Flu-like syndrome, back pain. **CNS:** *Headache,* dizziness, insomnia. **CV:** Torsades de pointes arrhythmia, *ventricular arrhythmias,* AV block, *chest pain*. **GI:** Nausea, diarrhea, abdominal pain. **Respiratory:** Respiratory infection, dyspnea. **Skin:** Rash.

INTERACTIONS Drug: Dofetilide levels increased by **verapamil, cimetidine, trimethoprim, ketoconazole, prochlorperazine, megestrol;** do not give with drugs known to increase the QT_c interval such as **bepridil,** PHENOTHIAZINES, TRICYCLIC ANTIDEPRESSANTS, ORAL MACROLIDES, other ANTIARRHYTHMICS.

PHARMACOKINETICS Absorption: Greater than 90% bioavailable. **Peak:** 2–3 h. **Distribution:** 60–70% protein bound. **Metabolism:** In liver. **Elimination:** Primarily excreted unchanged in urine. **Half-Life:** 10 h.

NURSING IMPLICATIONS

Assessment & Drug Effects

- Monitor ECG continuously during first 3 mo of therapy; then periodically.
- Do not discharge patient until 12 h after conversion to normal sinus rhythm.
- Lab tests: Baseline and periodic serum electrolytes (including magnesium), periodic CBC, and routine blood chemistry. Serum potassium **must be** within normal limits prior to and throughout therapy with dofetilide.
- Notify physician immediately of electrolyte imbalances, especially hypokalemia and hypomagnesemia.

Patient & Family Education

- Report immediately conditions that cause potassium loss (e.g., prolonged vomiting, diarrhea, excessive sweating).
- Do **NOT** take concurrently cimetidine, verapamil, ketoconazole, trimethoprim.

DOLASETRON MESYLATE

(dol-a-se′tron)

Anzemet

Classifications: SELECTIVE SEROTONIN ($5-HT_3$) RECEPTOR ANTAGONIST; ANTIEMETIC

Therapeutic: ANTIEMETIC

Prototype: Ondansetron

Pregnancy Category: B

AVAILABILITY 50 mg, 100 mg tablets; 20 mg/mL injection

ACTION & *THERAPEUTIC EFFECT* Dolasetron is a selective serotonin ($5-HT_3$) receptor antagonist used for control of nausea and vomiting associated with cancer chemotherapy. Serotonin receptors affected are located in the chemoreceptor trigger zone (CTZ) of the brain and peripherally on the vagal nerve terminal. Serotonin, released from the cells of the small intestine, activate $5-HT_3$ receptors located on vagal efferent neurons, thus initiating the vomiting reflex. *Has antiemetic properties that help patients on chemotherapy.*

USES Prevention of nausea and vomiting from emetogenic chemotherapy, prevention and treatment of postoperative nausea and vomiting.

CONTRAINDICATIONS Hypersensitivity to dolasetron. Safety and efficacy in children younger than 2 y are not established.

D

CAUTIOUS USE Patients who have or may develop prolongation of cardiac conduction intervals, particularly QT_c (i.e., patients with hypokalemia, hypomagnesemia, diuretics, congenital QT syndrome; patients taking antiarrhythmic drugs and high-dose anthracycline therapy, etc.), pregnancy (category B), and lactation.

ROUTE & DOSAGE

Prevention of Chemotherapy-Induced Nausea and Vomiting

Adult/Child (older than 2 y): **IV** 1.8 mg/kg or 100 mg administered 30 min prior to chemotherapy (not more than 100 mg/dose) **PO** 100 mg 1 h prior to chemotherapy

Pre-/Postoperative Nausea and Vomiting

Adult: **IV** 12.5 mg 15 min before cessation of anesthesia or when postoperative nausea and vomiting occurs **PO** 100 mg within 2 h prior to surgery

Child (older than 2 y): **IV** 0.35 mg/kg up to 12.5 mg 15 min before cessation of anesthesia or when postoperative nausea and vomiting occurs **PO** 1.2 mg/kg up to 100 mg starting 2 h prior to surgery (may also mix IV formulation in apple or apple-grape juice and administer orally)

ADMINISTRATION

Oral

- Give within 2 h before surgery, when used for postoperative nausea.

Intravenous

PREPARE: **Direct:** Give undiluted. **IV Infusion:** Dilute in 50 mL of any of the following: NS, D5W, D5/0.45% NaCl, LR.

ADMINISTER: **Direct:** Inject undiluted drug over 30 sec. **IV Infusion:** Infuse diluted drug over 15 min.

INCOMPATIBILITIES **Solution/additive:** **Potassium chloride.**

- Store at 20°–25° C (66°–77° F) and protect from light. - Diluted IV solution may be stored refrigerated up to 48 h.

ADVERSE EFFECTS (≥1%) **Body as a Whole:** Fever, fatigue, pain, chills or shivering. **CNS:** *Headache,* dizziness, drowsiness. **CV:** Hypertension. **GI:** *Diarrhea,* increased LFTs, abdominal pain. **Genitourinary:** Urinary retention.

INTERACTIONS Drugs: Avoid use with **apomorphine** due to hypotension; **ziprasidone** may prolong QT interval.

PHARMACOKINETICS Absorption: Rapidly absorbed from GI tract. **Peak:** 0.6 h IV, 1 h PO. **Distribution:** Crosses placenta, distributed into breast milk. **Metabolism:** Metabolized to hydrodolasetron by carbonyl reductase. Hydrodolasetron is metabolized in the liver by CYP2D6. **Elimination:** Primarily in urine as hydrodolasetron. **Half-Life:** 10 min dolasetron, 7.3 h hydrodolasetron.

NURSING IMPLICATIONS

Assessment & Drug Effects

- Lab tests: Determine serum electrolytes before initiating drug. Hypokalemia and hypomagnesemia should be correct before initiating therapy. With prolonged therapy, periodically monitor LFTs, PTT, CBC with platelet count, and alkaline phosphatase.
- Monitor closely cardiac status especially with vomiting, excess diuresis, or other conditions that

may result in electrolyte imbalances.
- Monitor ECG, especially in those taking concurrent antiarrhythmic or other drugs that may cause QT prolongation.
- Monitor for and report signs of bleeding (e.g., hematuria, epistaxis, purpura, hematoma).

Patient & Family Education
- Headache requiring analgesic for relief is a common adverse effect.

DONEPEZIL HYDROCHLORIDE (Pr)

(don-e'pe-zil)

Aricept, Aricept ODT

Classifications: CENTRAL ACTING CHOLINERGIC; CHOLINESTERASE INHIBITOR

Therapeutic: ANTIDEMENTIA; ALZHEIMER'S AGENT

Pregnancy Category: C

AVAILABILITY 5 mg, 10 mg tablets and orally disintegrating tablets

ACTION & *THERAPEUTIC EFFECT* In early stages of Alzheimer's disease, pathologic changes in neurons result in deficiency of acetylcholine. Aricept, a cholinesterase inhibitor, presumably elevates acetylcholine concentration in the cerebral cortex by slowing degrading acetylcholine released by remaining intact neurons. *Improves global function, cognition, and behavior of patients with mild to moderate Alzheimer's.*

USES Mild, moderate, or severe dementia of Alzheimer's type.

UNLABELED USES Vascular dementia, poststroke aphasia, memory improvement in multiple sclerosis patients.

CONTRAINDICATIONS Hypersensitivity to donepezil or tacrine; lactation; children; GI bleeding, jaundice.

CAUTIOUS USE Anesthesia, sick sinus rhythm, AV block, bradycardia, cardiac arrhythmias, cardiac disease, hypotension; hyperthyroidism, history of ulcers, abnormal liver function; patients with asthma or obstructive pulmonary disease, history of seizures, seizures, urinary tract obstruction, intestinal obstruction; diarrhea, emesis, GI disease, renal failure, renal impairment, surgery; pregnancy (category C).

ROUTE & DOSAGE

Alzheimer's Disease Related Dementia (Mild to Moderate)

Adult: **PO** 5–10 mg at bedtime

Alzheimer's Disease Related Dementia (Severe)

Adult: **PO** 10 mg daily

ADMINISTRATION

Oral
- Give at bedtime just prior to going to bed.
- Dosage increase from 5 to 10 mg is usually made only after 4–6 wk of therapy.
- Store at 15°–30° C (59°–86° F).

ADVERSE EFFECTS (≥1%) **Body as a Whole:** *Headache,* fatigue. **CNS:** *Insomnia,* dizziness, depression, tremor, irritability, vertigo, ataxia. **CV:** Syncope, hypertension, atrial fibrillation, hot flashes, hypotension. **GI:** *Nausea, diarrhea, vomiting, muscle cramps, anorexia,* GI bleeding, bloating, fecal incontinence, epigastric pain. **Respiratory:** Dyspnea. **Skin:** Pruritus, sweating, urticaria. **Other:** Ecchymoses, muscle cramps, dehydration, blurred vision, urinary incontinence, nocturia.

INTERACTIONS Drug: Ketoconazole, quinidine may inhibit donepezil metabolism; **carbamazepine, dexamethasone, phenobarbital, phenytoin, rifampin** may increase donepezil elimination; donepezil may interfere with the action of ANTICHOLINERGIC AGENTS.

PHARMACOKINETICS Absorption: Rapidly absorbed from GI tract. **Peak:** 3–4 h. **Distribution:** 96% protein bound. **Metabolism:** Metabolized in the liver by CYP2D6 and CYP3A4 to at least 2 active metabolites. **Elimination:** Primarily in urine. **Half-Life:** 70 h.

NURSING IMPLICATIONS

Assessment & Drug Effects

- Monitor closely for S&S of GI ulceration and bleeding, especially with concurrent use of NSAIDs.
- Monitor carefully patients with a history of asthma or obstructive pulmonary disease.
- Monitor cardiovascular status; drug may have vagotonic effect on the heart, causing bradycardia, especially in presence of conduction abnormalities.

Patient & Family Education

- Exercise caution. Fainting episodes related to slowing the heart rate may occur.
- Report immediately to physician any S&S of GI ulceration or bleeding (e.g., "coffee-grounds" emesis, tarry stools, epigastric pain).

DOPAMINE HYDROCHLORIDE

(doe′pa-meen)

Classifications: ALPHA- AND BETA-ADRENERGIC AGONIST; INOTROPIC
Therapeutic: CARDIAC STIMULANT; VASOPRESSOR

Prototype: Epinephrine
Pregnancy Category: C

AVAILABILITY 40 mg/mL, 80 mg/mL, 160 mg/mL injection

ACTION & *THERAPEUTIC EFFECT* Major cardiovascular effects produced by direct action on alpha- and beta-adrenergic receptors and on specific dopaminergic receptors in mesenteric and renal vascular beds. Positive inotropic effect on myocardium increases cardiac output with increase in systolic and pulse pressure and little or no effect on diastolic pressure. Improves circulation to renal vascular bed by decreasing renal vascular resistance with resulting increase in glomerular filtration rate and urinary output. *Due to its potential for inotropic, chronotropic, and vasopressor effects, dopamine has several clinical uses, including decreased cardiac output as well as correction of hypotension associated with cardiogenic and septic shock.*

USES To correct hemodynamic imbalance in shock syndrome due to MI (cardiogenic shock), trauma, endotoxic septicemia (septic shock), open heart surgery, and CHF.

UNLABELED USES Acute renal failure; cirrhosis; hepatorenal syndrome; barbiturate intoxication.

CONTRAINDICATIONS Pheochromocytoma; tachyarrhythmias or ventricular fibrillation; children younger than 2 y.

CAUTIOUS USE Patients with history of occlusive vascular disease (e.g., Buerger's or Raynaud's disease); CAD; cold injury; acute MI; diabetic endarteritis, arterial embolism; neonates; pregnancy (category C), lactation.

ROUTE & DOSAGE

Shock/Surgery

Adult: **IV** 2–5 mcg/kg/min increased gradually up to 20–50 mcg/kg/min if necessary
Adolescent/Child: **IV** 1–5 mcg/kg/min increased gradually up to 20 mcg/kg/min

CHF

Adult: **IV** 3–10 mcg/kg/min

ADMINISTRATION

Intravenous

PREPARE: **Continuous:** Dilute just prior to administration. ▪ Dilute each ampule in one of the following: D5W, D5/NS, D5/LR, D5/0.45% NaCl, NS. ▪ Dilute 200 mg ampule in 250 mL, 500 mL, or 1000 mL IV solution to yield 800 mcg/mL, 400 mcg/mL, or 200 mcg/mL, respectively. Dilute 400 mg ampule in 250 mL, 500 mL, or 1000 mL IV solution to yield 1600 mcg/mL, 800 mcg/mL or 400 mcg/mL, respectively. ▪ Dilute 400 mg ampule in 250 mL, 500 mL, or 1000 mL IV solution to yield 1600 mcg/mL, 800 mcg/mL, or 400 mcg/mL, respectively. ▪ Dilute 800 mg ampule in 250 mL, 500 mL, or 1000 mL IV solution to yield 3200 mcg/mL, 1600 mcg/mL or 800 mcg/mL, respectively. ▪ Consult package information for other dilutions.

ADMINISTER: **Continuous:** Infusion rate is based on body weight. ▪ Infusion rate and guidelines for adjusting rate relative changes in blood pressure are prescribed by physician. ▪ Microdrip and other reliable metering device should be used for accuracy of flow rate.

INCOMPATIBILITIES **Solution/additive: Acyclovir, alteplase, amphotericin B, ampicillin, metronidazole, penicillin G, sodium bicarbonate. Y-site: Acyclovir, alteplase, amphotericin B cholesteryl complex, cefepime, doxycycline, furosemide, indomethacin, insulin, lansoprazole, sodium bicarbonate, thiopental.**

▪ Correct hypovolemia, if possible, with either whole blood or plasma before initiation of dopamine therapy. ▪ Monitor infusion continuously for free flow, and take care to avoid extravasation, which can result in tissue sloughing and gangrene. Use a large vein of the antecubital fossa. ▪ Antidote for extravasation: Stop infusion promptly and remove needle. Immediately infiltrate the ischemic area with 5–10 mg phentolamine mesylate in 10–15 mL of NS, using syringe and fine needle. Pediatric dosage of phentolamine should be 0.1–0.2 mg/kg (max: 10 mg per dose). ▪ Protect dopamine from light. Discolored solutions should not be used.

▪ Store reconstituted solution for 24 h at 2°–15° C (36°–59° F) or 6 h at room temperature 15°–30° C.

ADVERSE EFFECTS (≥1%) **CV:** *Hypotension,* ectopic beats, *tachycardia,* anginal pain, palpitation, vasoconstriction (indicated by disproportionate rise in diastolic pressure), cold extremities; less frequent: <u>Aberrant conduction</u>, bradycardia, widening of QRS complex, elevated blood pressure. **GI:** Nausea, vomiting. **CNS:** Headache. **Skin:** Necrosis, tissue sloughing with extravasation, <u>gangrene</u>, piloerection. **Other:** Azotemia, dyspnea, dilated pupils (high doses).

DIAGNOSTIC TEST INTERFERENCE Dopamine may modify test response when histamine is used as a control for ***intradermal skin tests.***

INTERACTIONS Drug: MAO INHIBITORS, ERGOT ALKALOIDS, increase alpha-adrenergic effects (headache, hyperpyrexia, hypertension); **guanethidine, phenytoin** may decrease dopamine action; BETA-BLOCKERS antagonize cardiac effects; ALPHA BLOCKERS antagonize peripheral vasoconstriction; **halothane, cyclopropane** increase risk of hypertension and ventricular arrhythmias.

PHARMACOKINETICS Onset: Less than 5 min. **Duration:** Less than 10 min. **Distribution:** Widely distributed; does not cross blood–brain barrier. **Metabolism:** Inactive in the liver, kidney, and plasma by monoamine oxidase and COMT. **Elimination:** In urine. **Half-Life:** 2 min.

NURSING IMPLICATIONS

Assessment & Drug Effects

- Monitor blood pressure, pulse, peripheral pulses, and urinary output at intervals prescribed by physician. Precise measurements are essential for accurate titration of dosage.
- Report the following indicators promptly to physician for use in decreasing or temporarily suspending dose: Reduced urine flow rate in absence of hypotension; ascending tachycardia; dysrhythmias; disproportionate rise in diastolic pressure (marked decrease in pulse pressure); signs of peripheral ischemia (pallor, cyanosis, mottling, coldness, complaints of tenderness, pain, numbness, or burning sensation).
- Monitor therapeutic effectiveness. In addition to improvement in vital signs and urine flow, other indices of adequate dosage and perfusion of vital organs include loss of pallor, increase in toe temperature, adequacy of nail bed capillary filling, and reversal of confusion or comatose state.

D

DORIPENEM

(dor-i-pen′em)

Doribax

Classifications: BETA-LACTAM ANTIBIOTIC; CARBAPENEM ANTIBIOTIC

Therapeutic: ANTIBIOTIC

Prototype: Imipenem-cilastatin

Pregnancy Category: B

AVAILABILITY 500 mg single-use vials

ACTION & *THERAPEUTIC EFFECT* Inhibits essential penicillin-binding proteins resulting in inhibition of bacterial cell wall synthesis, resulting in bacterial cell death. *Bactericidal against aerobic and anaerobic gram-negative and gram-positive bacteria, and effectively resolves infection.*

USES Single-agent treatment of complicated intra-abdominal infections and urinary tract infections, including pyelonephritis caused by susceptible organisms.

UNLABELED USES Hospital acquired pneumonia.

CONTRAINDICATIONS Hypersensitivity to doripenem, or beta-lactam antibiotics; multiple allergies; inhalation route.

CAUTIOUS USE Hypersensitivity to cephalosporins, penicillins; moderate to severe renal impairment; GI disease, colitis, IBD; older adults; history of a seizure disorder; bacterial meningitis; pregnancy (category B); lactation. Safe use in children and adolescents is not established.

ROUTE & DOSAGE

Complicated Intra-Abdominal Infection

Adult: **IV** 500 mg q8h × 5–14 days

Complicated UTI, Including Pyelonephritis

Adult: **IV** 500 mg q8h × 10 days

Renal Impairment Dosage Adjustment

CrCl 30–50 mL/min: 250 mg q8h; greater than 10 mL/min but less than 30 mL/min: 250 mg q12h

ADMINISTRATION

Intravenous

PREPARE: **Intermittent:** Add 10 mL of sterile water for injection or NS to the vial, gently shake to form suspension; yields 50 mg/mL. ▪ *Preparation of 500 mg dose:* Withdraw contents of vial with a 21-gauge needle and add to infusion bag of 100 mL of NS or D5W, gently shake until clear. Final concentration is 4.5 mg/mL. ▪ *Preparation of 250 mg dose:* Prepare as for the 500 mg dose then remove 55 mL of solution from IV bag and discard. ▪ Infuse the remaining solution, which contains 250 mg (4.5 mg/mL).

ADMINISTER: **Intermittent:** Infuse over 15–30 min.

INCOMPATIBILITIES **Solution/additive:** Do not combine with any other drug. **Y-site:** Do not add to Y-site.

ADVERSE EFFECTS (≥1%) **Body as a Whole:** Anaphylaxis, hypersensitivity reactions. **CNS:** *Headache*. **CV:** Phlebitis. **GI:** Diarrhea, nausea, oral candidiasis. **Hematologic:** Anemia. **Metabolic:** Elevated hepatic enzymes. **Skin:** Rash. **Urogenital:** Vulvomycotic infection

INTERACTIONS Drug: Doripenem decreases plasma levels of **valproic acid. Probenecid** increases doripenem plasma levels.

PHARMACOKINETICS Distribution: Minimal protein binding. **Metabolism:** In liver (18%) to inactive metabolite. **Elimination:** Urine (primarily unchanged). **Half-Life:** 1 h.

NURSING IMPLICATIONS

Assessment & Drug Effects

- Lab tests: Perform C&S tests prior to therapy. Monitor periodically LFTs, Hct and Hgb.
- Determine history of hypersensitivity reactions to other beta-lactams, cephalosporins, penicillins, or other drugs.
- Discontinue drug and immediately report S&S of hypersensitivity (see Appendix F).
- Report S&S of superinfection or pseudomembranous colitis (see Appendix F).

Patient & Family Education

- Learn S&S of hypersensitivity, superinfection, and pseudomembranous colitis; report any of these to physician promptly.

DORNASE ALFA

(dor'naze)

Pulmozyme

Classifications: RESPIRATORY ENZYME; MUCOLYTIC

Therapeutic: MUCOLYTIC

Pregnancy Category: B

AVAILABILITY 1 mg/mL solution for inhalation

ACTION & *THERAPEUTIC EFFECT* Dornase is a solution of recombinant human deoxyribonuclease (DNAse), an enzyme that selectively cleaves DNA. In cystic fibrosis (CF) patients, viscous, purulent secretions in the airway reduce pulmonary function and lead to exacerbations of infection. Purulent pulmonary secretions contain very high concentrations of DNA released by degenerating leukocytes that are present in response to infection. *Dornase hydrolyzes the DNA in sputum of CF patients and reduces sputum viscosity, thus reducing incidence of VRI.*

USES In combination with standard therapies to reduce the frequency of respiratory infections in patients with CF and to improve pulmonary function.
UNLABELED USES Chronic bronchitis.

CONTRAINDICATIONS Hypersensitivity to dornase or hamster protein; infants younger than 3 mo.
CAUTIOUS USE Pregnancy (category B), lactation.

ROUTE & DOSAGE

Cystic Fibrosis
Adult/Child (older than 3 mo): **Inhalation** 2.5 mg (1 ampule) inhaled once daily using a recommended nebulizer, may increase to twice daily (do not mix with other agents in nebulizer)

ADMINISTRATION

Inhalation
- Do not dilute or mix with any other drugs or solutions in the nebulizer.
- Use only with nebulizer systems recommended by the drug manufacturer.
- Do not shake ampules; do not use ampules that have been at room temperature longer than 24 h or have become cloudy or discolored.
- Store refrigerated at 2°–8° C (36°–46° F) in protective foil pouch.

ADVERSE EFFECTS (≥1%) **Respiratory:** Hoarseness, sore throat, voice alterations, pharyngitis, laryngitis, cough, rhinitis. **Other:** Conjunctivitis, chest pain, rash.

PHARMACOKINETICS Absorption: Minimal systemic absorption. **Onset:** 3–8 days. **Duration:** Benefit lasts up to 4 days after discontinuing treatment.

NURSING IMPLICATIONS

Assessment & Drug Effects
- Monitor for improvement in dyspnea and sputum clearance.
- Monitor for S&S of hypersensitivity (see Appendix F). Patients with a history of hypersensitivity to bovine pancreatic dornase are at high risk.
- Monitor for adverse effects; rarely, dosage adjustments may be required.

Patient & Family Education
- Report rash, hives, itching, or other S&S of hypersensitivity to physician immediately.
- Know potential adverse effects and report those that are bothersome or do not disappear.
- Take a missed dose as soon as possible; if it is almost time for the next dose, skip the missed dose.

DORZOLAMIDE HYDROCHLORIDE
(dor-zol'a-mide)

Trusopt
Classifications: EYE PREPARATION; CARBONIC ANHYDRASE INHIBITOR
Therapeutic: CARBONIC ANHYDRASE INHIBITOR
Prototype: Acetazolamide
Pregnancy Category: C

AVAILABILITY 2% ophth solution

ACTION & *THERAPEUTIC EFFECT* Dorzolamide is a sulfonamide and inhibits carbonic anhydrase in the eye, thus reducing the rate of aqueous humor formation with subsequent lowering of IOP. Elevated IOP is a major risk factor in the pathogenesis of optic nerve damage and visual field loss due to glaucoma. *Lowers IOP in glaucoma or ocular hypertension.*

USES Elevated intraocular pressure in patients with ocular hypertension or open-angle glaucoma.

CONTRAINDICATIONS Previous hypersensitivity to dorzolamide.
CAUTIOUS USE History of hypersensitivity to other carbonic anhydrase inhibitors, sulfonamides, or thiazide diuretics; ocular infection or inflammation; recent ocular surgery; moderate to severe renal or hepatic insufficiency; angle-closure glaucoma; concomitant use of oral carbonic anhydrase inhibitors; older adults, corneal abrasion; pregnancy (category C).

ROUTE & DOSAGE

Glaucoma, Ocular Hypertension
Adult/Child: **Ophthalmic** 1 drop in affected eye t.i.d.

ADMINISTRATION

Instillation
- Apply gentle pressure to lacrimal sac during and immediately following drug instillation for about 1 min to lessen degree of systemic absorption.
- Administer at least 10 min apart, if another ophthalmic drug is being used concurrently.
- Store at 15°–30° C (59°–86° F).

ADVERSE EFFECTS (≥1%) **CNS:** Headache. **GI:** Bitter taste, nausea. **Special Senses:** *Transient burning or stinging, transient blurred vision,* superficial punctate keratitis, tearing, dryness, photophobia, ocular allergic reaction. **Skin:** Rash.

PHARMACOKINETICS Absorption: Some systemic absorption from topical instillation. **Onset:** 2 h. **Duration:** 8–12 h. **Distribution:** Distributes into red blood cells. **Elimination:** In urine. **Half-Life:** RBC elimination about 4 mo.

NURSING IMPLICATIONS

Assessment & Drug Effects
- Inquire about previous hypersensitivity to sulfonamides prior to therapy.
- Withhold drug and notify physician if S&S of local or systemic hypersensitivity occur (see Appendix F).
- Withhold the drug and notify the physician if ocular irritation occurs.

Patient & Family Education
- Learn proper technique for applying eyedrops.
- Do not allow tip of drug dispenser to come in contact with the eye.
- Discontinue drug and report to physician: Ocular irritation, infection, or S&S of systemic hypersensitivity occur (see Appendix F).

DOXAPRAM HYDROCHLORIDE
(dox′a-pram)

Dopram
Classifications: CEREBRAL STIMULANT; RESPIRATORY STIMULANT
Therapeutic: CEREBRAL STIMULANT; RESPIRATORY STIMULANT
Prototype: Caffeine
Pregnancy Category: B

AVAILABILITY 20 mg/mL injection

ACTION & *THERAPEUTIC EFFECT*
Short-acting analeptic capable of stimulating all levels of the cerebrospinal axis. Respiratory stimulation by direct medullary action or possibly by indirect activation of peripheral chemoreceptors increases tidal volume and slightly increases respiratory rate. *Decreases Pco_2 and increases Po_2 by increasing alveolar ventilation; may elevate BP and pulse rate by stimulation of brainstem vasomotor area. It is used to stimulate respiration postanesthesia, for drug-induced CNS depression, and for chronic pulmonary disease associated with acute hypercapnia.*

USES Short-term adjunctive therapy to alleviate postanesthesia and drug-induced respiratory depression. Also as a temporary measure (approximately 2 h) in hospitalized patients with COPD associated with acute respiratory insufficiency as an aid to prevent elevation of $Paco_2$ during administration of oxygen. (Not used with mechanical ventilation.)

UNLABELED USES Neonatal apnea refractory to xanthine therapy.

CONTRAINDICATIONS Epilepsy and other convulsive disorders; of ventilatory mechanism due to muscle paresis, pulmonary fibrosis, flail chest, pneumothorax, airway obstruction, extreme dyspnea, or acute bronchial asthma; severe hypertension, coronary artery disease, uncompensated heart failure, CVA; MAOI; lactation; children younger than 12 y.

CAUTIOUS USE History of bronchial asthma, COPD; cardiac disease, severe tachycardia, arrhythmias, hypertension; hyperthyroidism; pheochromocytoma; head injury, cerebral edema, increased intracranial pressure; peptic ulcer, patients undergoing gastric surgery; acute agitation; pregnancy (category B).

ROUTE & DOSAGE

Postanesthesia

Adult: **IV** 0.5–1 mg/kg single injection (not more than 1.5 mg/kg), may repeat q5min up to 2 mg/kg total dose; infusion of 0.5–1 mg/kg (max total dose: 4 mg/kg)

Drug-Induced CNS Depression

Adult: **IV** 1–2 mg/kg repeat in 5 min, then q1–2h until patient awakens [if relapse occurs, resume q1–2h injections (max total dose: 3 g), if no response after priming dose, may give 1–3 mg/min for up to 2 h until patient awakens]

Chronic Obstructive Pulmonary Disease

Adult: **IV** 0.5–2 mg/kg OR 1–2 mg/min for a max of 2 h (max rate: 3 mg/min)

ADMINISTRATION

- IV administration to neonates: Verify correct IV concentration and rate of infusion with physician. Generally do not use in newborns because doxapram contains benzyl alcohol.
- Ensure adequacy of airway and oxygenation before initiation of doxapram therapy.

Intravenous

PREPARE: **Direct:** Give undiluted. **IV Infusion for CNS Depression:** Dilute 250 mg (12.5 mL) in 250 mL of D5W or NS. **IV Infusion for COPD:** Add 400 mg doxapram to 180 mL of D5W, D10W, or NS to yield 2 mg/mL.

ADMINISTER: **Direct for CNS Depression:** Give undiluted over 5 min. **IV Infusion for CNS Depression:** Give at a rate of 1–3 mg/min, depending on patient response. Never exceed 3 mg/min. ▪ Infusion should not be administered for longer than 2 h. **IV Infusion for COPD:** Infuse at 0.5–1.5 mL/min.

INCOMPATIBILITIES **Solution/additive:** **Aminophylline, ascorbic acid,** CEPHALOSPORINS, **carbenicillin, dexamethasone, diazepam, digoxin, dobutamine, folic acid, furosemide, hydrocortisone, ketamine, methylprednisolone, minocycline, thiopental, ticarcillin.** **Y-site:** **Clindamycin.**

▪ Store at 15°–30° C (59°–86° F) unless otherwise directed.

ADVERSE EFFECTS (≥1%) **CNS:** Dizziness, sneezing, apprehension, confusion, *involuntary movements,* hyperactivity, paresthesias; feeling of warmth and burning, especially of genitalia and perineum; flushing, sweating, hyperpyrexia, headache, pilomotor erection, pruritus, muscle tremor, rigidity, convulsions, *increased deep-tendon reflexes,* bilateral Babinski sign, *carpopedal spasm,* pupillary dilation, mild delayed narcosis. **CV:** *Mild to moderate increase in BP, sinus tachycardia,* bradycardia, extrasystoles, lowered T waves, PVCs, chest pains, tightness in chest. **GI:** Nausea, vomiting, diarrhea, salivation, sour taste. **Urogenital:** Urinary retention, frequency, incontinence. **Respiratory:** Dyspnea, tachypnea, cough, laryngospasm, bronchospasm, hiccups, rebound hypoventilation, hypocapnia with tetany. **Other:** Local skin irritation, thrombophlebitis with extravasation; decreased Hgb, Hct, and RBC count; elevated BUN; albuminuria.

INTERACTIONS Drug: MAO INHIBITORS, SYMPATHOMIMETIC AGENTS add to pressor effects.

PHARMACOKINETICS Onset: 20–40 s. **Peak:** 1–2 min. **Duration:** 5–12 min. **Metabolism:** Rapidly metabolized. **Elimination:** In urine as metabolites.

NURSING IMPLICATIONS

Assessment & Drug Effects

- Monitor IV site frequently. Extravasation or use of same IV site for prolonged periods can cause thrombophlebitis (see Appendix F) or tissue irritation.
- Monitor carefully and observe accurately: BP, pulse, deep tendon reflexes, airway, and arterial blood gases. All are essential guides for determining minimum effective dosage and preventing overdosage. Make baseline determinations for comparison.
- Lab tests: Draw arterial Po_2 and Pco_2 and O_2 saturation prior to both initiation of doxapram infusion and oxygen administration in patients with COPD, and then at least every 30 min during infusion.
- Discontinue doxapram if arterial blood gases show evidence of deterioration and when mechanical ventilation is initiated.
- Observe patient continuously during therapy and maintain vigilance until patient is fully alert (usually about 1 h) and protective pharyn-

geal and laryngeal reflexes are completely restored.

- Notify physician immediately of any adverse effects. Be alert for early signs of toxicity: Tachycardia, muscle tremor, spasticity, hyperactive reflexes.
- Note: A mild to moderate increase in BP commonly occurs.
- Discontinue if sudden hypotension or dyspnea develops.

DOXAZOSIN MESYLATE

(dox-a′zo-sin)

Cardura

Classification: ALPHA-ADRENERGIC ANTAGONIST

Therapeutic: ANTIHYPERTENSIVE

Prototype: Prazosin

Pregnancy Category: B

AVAILABILITY 1 mg, 2 mg, 4 mg, 8 mg tablets

ACTION & *THERAPEUTIC EFFECT* By selective competitive inhibition of alpha$_1$-adrenoreceptors, it produces vasodilation in both arterioles and veinous vessels resulting in both peripheral vascular resistance and reduced blood pressure. *Long-acting effect of lowering blood pressure in supine or standing individuals with most pronounced effect on diastolic pressure.*

USES Mild to moderate hypertension, benign prostatic hypertrophy.

UNLABELED USES CHF.

CONTRAINDICATIONS Hypersensitivity to doxazosin, prazosin, and terazosin; hypotension, syncope. Safe use in children is not established.

CAUTIOUS USE Hepatic impairment or disease; renal disease, impairment, or failure; pregnancy (category B); lactation.

ROUTE & DOSAGE

Hypertension

Adult: **PO** Start with 1 mg at bedtime and titrate up to maximum of 16 mg/day in 1–2 divided doses

Geriatric: **PO** Start with 0.5 mg at bedtime

ADMINISTRATION

Oral

- Give initial dose at bedtime to minimize problems with postural hypotension and syncope.
- Individualize maintenance dose according to the standing BP response.
- Store at 15°–30° C (59°–86° F).

ADVERSE EFFECTS (≥1%) **CV:** *Orthostatic hypotension,* edema. **CNS:** Vertigo, *headache,* dizziness, somnolence, fatigue, nervousness, anxiety. **GI:** Nausea, abdominal pain. **Hematologic:** Leukopenia. **Skin:** Pruritus, eczema.

INTERACTIONS Drug: Sildenafil, vardenafil, and **tadalafil** may enhance hypotensive effects.

PHARMACOKINETICS Absorption: Readily absorbed from GI tract; 62–69% of dose reaches systemic circulation. **Peak:** 2–6 h. **Duration:** Up to 24 h. **Distribution:** Highly protein bound (98–99%). **Metabolism:** Approximately 35% of dose is metabolized in liver. **Elimination:** 9% in urine, 63% in feces. **Half-Life:** 9–12 h.

NURSING IMPLICATIONS

Assessment & Drug Effects

- Monitor BP with patient lying down and standing; doses above 4 mg increase the risk of postural hypotension.
- Monitor BP 2–6 h after initial dose or any dose increase. This is when

postural hypotension is most likely to occur.

Patient & Family Education

- Do not drive or engage in other potentially hazardous activities for 12–24 h after the first dose or an increase in dosage or when medication is restarted after an interruption in dosage.
- Use caution when rising from a sitting or supine position in order to avoid orthostatic hypotension and syncope; make position and directional changes slowly and in stages.
- Report to the physician episodes of dizziness or palpitations. These will require a dosage adjustment.

DOXEPIN HYDROCHLORIDE

(dox′e-pin)

Prudoxin, Sinequan, Triadapin ♣, Zonalon

Classifications: TRICYCLIC ANTIDEPRESSANT; ANXIOLYTIC

Therapeutic: ANTIDEPRESSANT; ANTIANXIETY

Prototype: Imipramine

Pregnancy Category: C

AVAILABILITY 10 mg, 25 mg, 50 mg, 75 mg, 100 mg, 150 mg capsules; 10 mg/mL oral concentrate; 5% topical cream

ACTION & *THERAPEUTIC EFFECT* Dibenzoxepin is a tricyclic antidepressant (TCA) that inhibits serotonin reuptake from the synaptic gap; also inhibits norepinephrine reuptake to a moderate degree. Recent evidence suggests that the upset of monoamine oxidase output seen in depressed patients may be regulated by long-term treatment with antidepressants due to their action on beta-adrenergic receptors. This action on beta-receptors may be a better explanation than the reuptake theory for TCAs' antidepressant effects. *Effective for treatment of both depression and anxiety.*

USES Psychoneurotic anxiety or depressive reactions; mixed symptoms of anxiety and depression; anxiety or depression associated with alcoholism; organic disease; psychotic depressive disorders; topical for treatment of pruritus.

UNLABELED USES Peptic ulcer disease, neuralgia.

CONTRAINDICATIONS Prior sensitivity to any TCA; during acute recovery phase following MI; bundle-branch block, cardiac arrhythmias, QT prolongation; ileus; glaucoma; increased intraocular pressure; prostatic hypertrophy; tendency for urinary retention; lactation. Safe use in children younger than 12 y is not established.

CAUTIOUS USE Patients receiving electroconvulsive therapy, patients with suicidal tendency, bipolar disorder, schizophrenia, psychosis; diabetes mellitus; GI disease; GERD; Parkinson's disease; seizure disorders; renal, cardiovascular, or hepatic dysfunction; pregnancy (category C).

ROUTE & DOSAGE

Antidepressant

Adult: **PO** 30–150 mg/day at bedtime or in divided doses, may gradually increase to 300 mg/day (use lower doses in older adult patients)

Geriatric: **PO** 10–25 mg at bedtime, may gradually increase to 75 mg/day

Child: **PO** 1–3 mg/kg/day in single or divided doses

Pruritus

Adult: **Topical** Apply a thin film q.i.d. with at least 3–4 h between applications, may use up to 8 days

Pharmacogenetic Dosage Adjustment

CYP2D6 Poor metabolizers: Give 40% of normal starting oral dose

ADMINISTRATION

Oral

- Give oral concentrate diluted with approximately 120 mL water, milk, or fruit juice.
- Empty capsule and swallow contents with fluid or mix with food as necessary if it cannot be swallowed whole.
- Inform physician if daytime sedation is pronounced. Entire daily dose (up to 150 mg) may be prescribed for bedtime administration.

Topical

- Apply a thin film to affected areas; allow 3–4 h between applications.
- Store all forms at 15°–30° C (59°–86° F) in tightly closed, light-resistant container.

ADVERSE EFFECTS (≥1%) **All:** Anticholinergic. **CNS:** *Drowsiness,* dizziness, weakness, fatigue, headache, hypomania, confusion, tremors, paresthesias. **CV:** *Orthostatic hypotension,* palpitation, hypertension, tachycardia, ECG changes. **Special Senses:** Mydriasis, blurred vision, photophobia. **GI:** *Dry mouth,* sour or metallic taste, epigastric distress, constipation. **Urogenital:** Urinary retention, delayed micturition, urinary frequency. **Other:** Increased perspiration, tinnitus, weight gain, photosensitivity reaction, skin rash, agranulocytosis, *burning or stinging at application site,* edema.

INTERACTIONS Drug: May decrease some antihypertensive response to ANTIHYPERTENSIVES; CNS DEPRESSANTS, **alcohol,** HYPNOTICS, BARBITURATES, SEDATIVES potentiate CNS depression; may increase hypoprothrombinemic effect of ORAL ANTICOAGULANTS; **ethchlorvynol** may cause transient delirium; **levodopa,** SYMPATHOMIMETICS (e.g., **epinephrine, norepinephrine**) introduce possibility of sympathetic hyperactivity with hypertension and hyperpyrexia; MAO INHIBITORS introduce possibility of severe reactions, toxic psychosis, cardiovascular instability; **methylphenidate** increases plasma TCA levels; THYROID AGENTS may increase possibility of arrhythmias; **cimetidine** may increase plasma TCA levels. **Herbal: Ginkgo** may decrease seizure threshold; **St. John's wort** may cause **serotonin** syndrome.

PHARMACOKINETICS Absorption: Rapidly from GI sites and through intact skin. **Peak:** 2 h. **Distribution:** Crosses placenta; distributed into breast milk. **Metabolism:** In liver. **Elimination:** Primarily in urine. **Half-Life:** 6–8 h.

NURSING IMPLICATIONS

Assessment & Drug Effects

- Monitor use of other CNS depressants, including alcohol. Danger of overdosage or suicide attempt is increased when patient uses excessive amounts of alcohol.
- Be alert to changes in voiding and evaluate patient for constipation and abdominal distention; drug has moderate to strong anticholinergic effects.

Patient & Family Education

- Maintain established dosage regimen and avoid change of intervals, doubling, reducing, or skipping doses.

- Consult physician about safe amount of alcohol, if any, that can be taken. The actions of both alcohol and doxepin are potentiated when used together and for up to 2 wk after doxepin is discontinued.
- Do not drive or engage in other potentially hazardous activities until response to drug is known.

DOXERCALCIFEROL

(dox-er-kal'si-fe-rol)

Hectorol

Classification: VITAMIN D ANALOG

Therapeutic: ANTIHYPERPARATHYROID; VITAMIN D ANALOG

Prototype: Calcitriol

Pregnancy Category: B

AVAILABILITY 0.5 mcg, 2.5 mcg capsule; 2 mcg/mL injection

ACTION & *THERAPEUTIC EFFECT* Vitamin D_2 analog that is activated by the liver. Activated vitamin D is needed for absorption of dietary calcium in the intestine, and the parathyroid hormone (PTH), which mobilizes calcium from the bone tissue. *Regulates the blood calcium level.*

USES Reduction of elevated iPTH in secondary hyperparathyroidism in patients undergoing chronic renal dialysis; secondary hyperparathyroidism in chronic kidney disease not on dialysis.

CONTRAINDICATIONS Hypersensitivity to doxercalciferol or other vitamin D analogs; recent hypercalcemia, recent hyperphosphatemia, hypervitaminosis D.

CAUTIOUS USE Renal or hepatic insufficiency; renal osteodystrophy with hyperphosphatemia, prolonged hypercalcemia; pregnancy (category B), lactation. Safety and efficacy in children are not established.

ROUTE & DOSAGE

Secondary Hyperparathyroidism

Adult: **PO** 10 mcg 3 times/wk at dialysis, adjust dose as needed to lower iPTH into the range of 150–300 pg/mL by increasing the dose in 2.5 mcg increments every 8 wk (max: 60 mcg/wk) **IV** 4 mcg 3 times/wk at end of dialysis (max: 18 mcg/wk)

ADMINISTRATION

Oral

- Give at time of dialysis.
- Withhold drug and notify physician if any of the following occurs: iPTH less than 100 pg/mL, hypercalcemia, hyperphosphatemia, or product of serum calcium times serum phosphorus greater than 70.
- Store at 20°–25° C (66°–77° F); excursions to 15°–30° C (59°–86° F) are permitted.

Intravenous

PREPARE: **Direct:** No dilution is needed. ▪ Withdraw appropriate dose from ampule using a filter needle. ▪ Change needles before injecting as an IV bolus. Discard any unused portion.

ADMINISTER: **Direct:** Give a bolus injection at the end of dialysis sessions.

- Store at 15°–20° C (59°–77° F).

ADVERSE EFFECTS (≥1%) **Body as a Whole:** Abscess, *headache, malaise,* arthralgia. **CNS:** *Dizziness,* sleep disorder. **CV:** Bradycardia, *edema.* **GI:** Anorexia, constipation, dyspepsia, *nausea, vomiting.* **Respi-**

ratory: *Dyspnea.* **Skin:** Pruritus. **Other:** Weight gain.

INTERACTIONS Drug: Cholestyramine, mineral oil may decrease absorption; MAGNESIUM-CONTAINING ANTACIDS may cause hypermagnesemia; other VITAMIN D ANALOGS may increase toxicity and hypercalcemia.

PHARMACOKINETICS Absorption: Absorbed from GI tract and is activated in the liver. **Peak:** 11–12 h. **Metabolism:** Activated by CYP 27 to form 1alpha, 25-$(OH)_2D_2$ (major metabolite) and 1alpha, 24-dihydroxy vitamin D_2 (minor metabolite). **Half-Life:** 32–37 h.

NURSING IMPLICATIONS

Assessment & Drug Effects

- Lab tests: Baseline and periodic iPTH, serum calcium, serum phosphorus. Monitor levels weekly during dose titration.
- Monitor for S&S of hypercalcemia (see Appendix F).

Patient & Family Education

- Do not take antacids without consulting the physician.
- Notify the physician if you become pregnant while taking this drug.
- Do not use mineral oil on the days doxercalciferol is taken. Mineral oil may decrease absorption of drug.
- Do not take nonprescription drugs containing magnesium while taking doxercalciferol.
- Report S&S of hypercalcemia immediately: Bone or muscle pain, dry mouth with metallic taste, rhinorrhea, itching, photophobia, conjunctivitis, frequent urination, anorexia and weight loss.

DOXORUBICIN HYDROCHLORIDE (Pr)

(dox-oh-roo'bi-sin)

Adriamycin, Rubex

DOXORUBICIN LIPOSOME

Doxil

Classifications: ANTINEOPLASTIC; ANTIBIOTIC

Therapeutic: ANTINEOPLASTIC

Pregnancy Category: D

AVAILABILITY 10 mg, 20 mg, 50 mg, 100 mg, 150 mg powder for injection; 2 mg/mL injection; 20 mg liposomal injection

ACTION & *THERAPEUTIC EFFECT* Cytotoxic antibiotic with wide spectrum of antitumor activity. Intercalates with preformed DNA residues, blocking effective DNA and RNA transcription. A potent radiosensitizer capable of enhancing radiation reactions. *Highly destructive to rapidly proliferating cells and slowly developing carcinomas; selectively toxic to cardiac tissue.*

USES Doxorubicin: To produce regression in neoplastic conditions, including acute lymphoblastic and myeloblastic leukemias, transitional cell bladder cancer, breast cancer, Hodgkin's disease, ovarian cancer, small-cell lung cancer, non-Hodgkin's lymphoma, thyroid cancer, Wilms' tumor, soft tissue and bone sarcomas. Generally used in combined modalities with surgery, radiation, and immunotherapy. Effective pretreatment to sensitize superficial tumors to local radiation therapy. **Doxorubicin Liposome:** Kaposi's sarcoma, progressive/refractory ovarian cancer, relapsed/refractory multiple myeloma.

CONTRAINDICATIONS Myelosuppression, thrombocytopenia; impaired cardiac function, obstructive jaundice, previous treatment with complete cumulative doses of doxorubicin or daunorubicin; pregnancy (category D), lactation.

CAUTIOUS USE Impaired hepatic or renal function; patients who have received cyclophosphamide or pelvic irradiation or radiotherapy to areas surrounding heart; history of atopic dermatitis.

ROUTE & DOSAGE

CONVENTIONAL DOXORUBICIN

Acute Lymphatic Leukemia

Adult/Child: **IV** 30 mg/m^2 weekly × 4 wk

Acute Myelogenous Leukemia

Adult/Child: **IV** 30 mg/m^2 × 3 days (with cytarabine)

Transitional Bladder Cell Cancer

Adult: **IV** 30 mg/m^2/dose once monthly

Hodgkin's Disease

Adult/Child: **IV** 25 mg/m^2 days 1 and 15, repeat q28days

Thyroid Cancer

Adult/Child: **IV** 60–75 mg/m^2 q3wk

Other Neoplasms

Adult: **IV** 40–50 mg/m^2 usually in combination with other agents (max total cumulative lifetime dose: 500–550 mg/m^2)
Child: **IV** 35–75 mg/m^2 as single dose, repeat at 21-day interval, or 20–30 mg/m^2 once weekly (max total cumulative lifetime dose: 500–550 mg/m^2)

Hepatic Impairment Dosage Adjustment

Bilirubin 1.2–3 mg/dL: Reduce dose by 50%; bilirubin 3–5 mg/dL: Reduce dose by 75%; bilirubin greater than 5 mg/dL: Stop therapy

DOXORUBICIN LIPOSOME

Kaposi's Sarcoma

Adult: **IV** 20 mg/m^2 q3wk. Infuse over 30 min (do not use in-line filters).

Progressive/Refractory Ovarian Cancer

Adult: **IV** 50 mg/m^2 q4wk, minimum of 4 courses

Relapsed/Refractory Multiple Myeloma

Adult: **IV** 45 mg/m^2 q4wk, up to 6 cycles

Hepatic Impairment Dosage Adjustment

Bilirubin 1.2–3 mg/dL: Reduce dose 50%; bilirubin 3–5 mg/dL: Reduce dose by 75%

ADMINISTRATION

Intravenous

▪ IV administration to children: Verify correct IV concentration and rate of infusion with physician. ▪ Wear gloves and use caution when preparing drug solution. If powder or solution contacts skin or mucosa, wash copiously with soap and water.

Conventional Doxorubicin

PREPARE: **Direct:** *Vial reconsitution:* Dilute with 1 mL of nonbacteriostatic NS for each 2 mg of doxorubicin to yield a final concentraion of 2 mg/mL. ▪ For each mL of NS added, withdraw an equal volume of air from vial to minimize pressure buildup. Shake to dissolve. ▪ *Doxorubicin solutions:* Solutions of 2 mg/mL are available that can be further diluted in 50 mL or more of NS or D5W.

D

ADMINISTER: **Direct:** Give bolus dose slowly into Y-site of freely running IV infusion of NS or D5W. ▪ If possible, use IV tubing attached to a needle inserted into a larger vein with a butterfly needle. ▪ Usually infused over 3–5 min. ▪ Monitor for red streaking along vein or facial flushing which indicates need to slow infusion rate.

Lyophilized Doxorubicin

PREPARE: **IV Infusion:** Dilute doses up to 90 mg in 250 mL of D5W and doses greater than 90 mg in 500 mL D5W. Solution will be translucent but not clear, and will be red in color. ▪ DO NOT use filters during preparation or administration.

ADMINISTER: **IV Infusion:** DO NOT give bolus injection or undiluted solution. ▪ Infuse at 1 mg/min initially; may increase rate to complete infusion in 1 h if no adverse reactions occur. Slow infusion rate as warranted if an adverse reaction occurs. ▪ Do not use a filter.

INCOMPATIBILITIES **Solution/additive:** *Conventional doxorubicin:* **Aminophylline, diazepam, fluorouracil.** **Y-site:** *Conventional doxorubicin:* **Allopurinol, amphotericin B cholesteryl sulfate, cefepime, gallium, ganciclovir, lansoprazole, pemetrexed, prochlorperazine, propofol, TPN.** *Doxorubicin liposome:* **Amphotericin B, amphotericin B cholesteryl complex, hydroxyzine, mannitol, meperidine, metoclopramide, mitoxantrone, morphine, paclitaxel, piperacillin/tazobactam, promethazine, sodium bicarbonate.**

▪ Facial flushing and local red streaking along the vein may occur if drug is administered too rapidly. ▪ Avoid using antecubital vein or veins on dorsum of hand or wrist, if possible, where extravasation could damage underlying tendons and nerves. ▪ Also avoid veins in extremity with compromised venous or lymphatic drainage.

▪ Store reconstituted solution for 24 h at room temperature; refrigerated at 4°–10° C (39°–50° F) for 48 h. Protect from sunlight; discard unused solution.

ADVERSE EFFECTS (≥1%) **Body as a Whole:** Hypersensitivity (red flare around injection site, erythema, skin rash, pruritus, angioedema, urticaria, eosinophilia, fever, chills, <u>anaphylactoid reaction</u>). **CV:** <u>Serious, irreversible myocardial toxicity with delayed CHF, ventricular arrhythmias, acute left ventricular failure</u>, hypertension, hypotension, cardiomyopathy. **GI:** *Stomatitis,* esophagitis with ulcerations; nausea, vomiting, anorexia, inanition, diarrhea. **Hematologic:** *Severe myelosuppression* (60–85% of patients); *<u>leukopenia (principally granulocytes)</u>,* thrombocytopenia, anemia. **Skin:** Hyperpigmentation of nail beds, tongue, and buccal mucosa (especially in blacks); *complete alopecia* (reversible), hyperpigmentation of dermal creases (especially in children), rash, *recall phenomenon (skin reaction due to prior radiotherapy).* **Other:** Lacrimation, drowsiness, fever, facial flush with too rapid IV infusion rate, microscopic hematuria, hyperuricemia, *hand-foot syndrome. With extravasation: severe cellulitis, vesication, tissue necrosis,* lymphangitis, phlebosclerosis.

INTERACTIONS Drug: BARBITURATES may decrease effects by increasing its hepatic metabolism; **streptozo-**

cin may prolong doxorubicin half-life; agents affecting QT interval (e.g., **Bepridil, droperidol, erythromycin, haloperidol, methadone,** PHENOTHIAZINES, etc.) may increase risk of cardiac side effects. Conventional formulation: Avoid use with **zidovudine.**

PHARMACOKINETICS Distribution: Widely distributed; does not cross blood–brain barrier; 75% protein binding; does not cross placenta; passes into breast milk. **Metabolism:** In liver to active metabolite. **Elimination:** Primarily in bile. **Half-Life:** 30–50 h. *Doxorubicin Liposome:* **Distribution:** Vascular fluid. **Metabolism:** In plasma and liver. **Elimination:** In urine. **Half-Life:** 44–55 h.

NURSING IMPLICATIONS

Assessment & Drug Effects

- Care should be taken to avoid extravasation. Stop infusion, remove IV needle, and notify physician promptly if patient complains of stinging or burning sensation at the injection site.
- Monitor any area of extravasation closely for 3–4 wk. If ulceration begins (usually 1–4 wk after extravasation), a plastic surgeon should be consulted.
- Establish baseline data. Include temperature, pulse, respiration, BP, body weight, laboratory values, and I&O ratio and pattern.
- Lab tests: Baseline and periodic hepatic function, renal function, CBC with differential throughout therapy.
- Note: The nadir of leukopenia (an expected 1000/mm^3) typically occurs 10–14 days after single dose, with recovery occurring within 21 days.
- Cardiac function must be evaluated prior to initiation of therapy, at regular intervals, and at end of therapy.
- Be alert to and report early signs of cardiotoxicity (see Appendix F). Acute life-threatening arrhythmias may occur within a few hours of drug administration.
- Report promptly objective signs of hepatic dysfunction (jaundice, dark urine, pruritus) or kidney dysfunction (altered I&O ratio and pattern, local discomfort with voiding).
- Report signs of superinfection (see Appendix F) promptly; these may result from antibiotic therapy during leukopenic period.
- Avoid rectal medications and use of rectal thermometer; rectal trauma is associated with bloody diarrhea resulting from an antiblastic effect on rapidly growing intestinal mucosal cells.

Patient & Family Education

- Note: Complete loss of hair (reversible) is an expected adverse effect. It may also involve eyelashes and eyebrows, beard and mustache, pubic and axillary hair. Regrowth of hair usually begins 2–3 mo after drug is discontinued.
- Drug turns urine red for 1–2 days after administration.
- Keep hands away from eyes to prevent conjunctivitis. Increased tearing for 5–10 days after a single dose is possible.
- Maintain fastidious oral hygiene, especially before and after meals. Stomatitis, generally maximal in second week of therapy, frequently begins with a burning sensation accompanied by erythema of oral mucosa that may progress to ulceration and dysphagia in 2 or 3 days.
- Exposure to doxorubicin during the first trimester of pregnancy can result in fetal abnormalities or fetal loss.

DOXYCYCLINE HYCLATE

(dox-i-sye'kleen)

Apo-Doxy ♣, Doryx, Doxy, Doxycin ♣, Monodox, Novodoxylin ♣, Vibramycin, Vibra-Tabs

Classifications: ANTIBIOTIC; TETRACYCLINE

Therapeutic: ANTIBIOTIC

Prototype: Tetracycline

Pregnancy Category: D

AVAILABILITY 50 mg, 75 mg, 100 mg capsules, tablets; 200 mg injection

ACTION & *THERAPEUTIC EFFECT* Semisynthetic broad-spectrum long-acting tetracycline antibiotic that is more lipophilic than the other tetracyclines, which allows it to pass easily through the lipid layer of bacteria where reversible binding to the 30 S ribosomal subunits of bacteria occurs. This blocks the binding of transfer RNA (tRNA) to the messenger RNA (mRNA) of the bacteria, resulting in inhibition of bacterial protein synthesis. *Primarily bacteriostatic against both gram-positive and gram-negative bacteria. Similar in use to tetracycline.*

USES Similar to those of tetracycline (e.g., chlamydial and mycoplasmal infections); gonorrhea, syphilis in penicillin-allergic patients; rickettsial diseases; acute exacerbations of chronic bronchitis.

UNLABELED USES Treatment of acute PID, leptospirosis, prophylaxis for rape victims, suppression and chemoprophylaxis of chloroquine-resistant *Plasmodium falciparum* malaria, short-term prophylaxis and treatment of travelers' diarrhea caused by enterotoxigenic strains of *Escherichia coli.* Intrapleural administration for malignant pleural effusions, post-exposure anthrax treatment and prophylaxis.

CONTRAINDICATIONS Sensitivity to any of the tetracyclines; use during period of tooth development including last half of pregnancy; pregnancy (category D), lactation, infants, and children younger than 8 y (causes permanent yellow discoloration of teeth, enamel hypoplasia, and retardation of bone growth).

CAUTIOUS USE Alcoholism; hepatic disease; GI disease; sulfite hypersensitivity; sunlight (UV) exposure.

ROUTE & DOSAGE

Anti-infective

Adult: **PO/IV** 100 mg q12h on day 1, then 100 mg/day as single dose (max: 100 mg q12h)

Child (older than 8 y): **PO/IV** 4.4 mg/kg in 1–2 doses on day 1, then 2.2–4.4 mg/kg/day in 1–2 divided doses

Gonorrhea

Adult: **PO** 200 mg immediately, followed by 100 mg at bedtime, then 100 mg b.i.d. for 3 days

Primary and Secondary Syphilis

Adult: **PO** 300 mg/day in divided doses for at least 10 days

Travelers' Diarrhea

Adult: **PO** 100 mg/day during risk period (up to 2 wk) beginning day 1 of travel

Acute Pelvic Inflammatory Disease

Adult: **IV** 100 mg q12h until improved, then 100 mg PO b.i.d. to complete 14 days

Acne

Adult: **PO** 100 mg q12h on day 1, then 100 mg daily

Child: **PO** *Older than 8 y, weight greater than 45 kg,* 100 mg q12h on day 1, then 100 mg daily; *older than 8 y, weight less than 45 kg,* 2.2 mg/kg q12h on day 1, then 2.2 mg/kg/daily

Anthrax Post-Exposure

Adult/Adolescent/Child (older than 8 y, weight greater than 45 kg): **IV** 100 mg q12h, then switch to PO for a total of 60

Child (weight 45 kg or less or 8 y): **IV** 2.2 mg/kg q12h, then switch to PO for a total of 60

ADMINISTRATION

Oral

- Check expiration date. Degradation products of tetracycline are toxic to the kidneys.
- Give with food or a full glass of milk to minimize nausea without significantly affecting bioavailability of drug (UNLIKE MOST TETRACYCLINES).
- Consult physician about ordering the oral suspension for patients who are bedridden or have difficulty swallowing.

Intravenous

PREPARE: **Intermittent:** Reconstitute by adding 10 mL sterile water for injection, or D5W, NS, LR, D5/LR, or other diluent recommended by manufacturer, to each 100 mg of drug. ▪ Further dilute with 100–1000 mL (per 100 mg of drug) of compatible infusion solution to produce concentrations ranging from 0.1 to 1 mg/mL.

ADMINISTER: **Intermittent:** IV infusion rate will usually be prescribed by physician. Duration of infusion varies with dose but is usually 1–4 h. ▪ Recommended minimum infusion time for 100 mg of 0.5 mg/mL solution is 1 h. Infusion should be completed within 12 h of dilution. ▪ When diluted with LR or D5/LR, infusion **must be** completed within 6 h to ensure adequate stability. ▪ Protect all solutions from direct sunlight during infusion.

INCOMPATIBILITIES **Solution/additive: Potassium phosphate. Y-site: Allopurinol, heparin, meropenem, piperacillin/tazobactam, TPN.**

▪ Store oral and parenteral forms (prior to reconstitution) in tightly covered, light-resistant containers at 15°–30° C (59°–86° F) unless otherwise directed. ▪ Refrigerate reconstituted solutions for up to 72 h. After this time, infusion **must be** completed within 12 h.

ADVERSE EFFECTS (≥1%) **Special Senses:** Interference with color vision. **GI:** Anorexia, *nausea,* vomiting, diarrhea, enterocolitis; esophageal irritation (oral capsule and tablet). **Skin:** Rashes, photosensitivity reaction. **Other:** Thrombophlebitis (IV use), superinfections.

DIAGNOSTIC TEST INTERFERENCE Like other ***tetracyclines,*** doxycycline may cause false increases in ***urinary catecholamines*** (fluorometric methods); false decreases in ***urinary urobilinogen;*** false-negative ***urine glucose*** with ***glucose oxidase methods*** (e.g., ***Clinistix, TesTape***); parenteral doxycycline (containing ascorbic acid) may cause false-positive determinations using ***Benedict's reagent*** or ***Clinitest.***

INTERACTIONS Drug: ANTACIDS, **iron** preparation, **calcium, magnesium, zinc, kaolin-pectin, sodium bicarbonate** can significantly decrease absorption; effects of both doxycycline and **desmopressin** antagonized; increases **digoxin** absorption, thus increasing risk of **digoxin** toxicity; **methoxyflurane** increases risk of renal failure.

PHARMACOKINETICS Absorption: Completely absorbed from GI tract. **Peak:** 1.5–4 h. **Distribution:** Penetrates eye, prostate, and CSF; crosses placenta; distributed into breast milk. **Metabolism:** In GI tract. **Elimination:** 20–30% in urine and 20–40% in feces in 48 h. **Half-Life:** 14–24 h.

NURSING IMPLICATIONS

Assessment & Drug Effects

- Report sudden onset of painful or difficult swallowing promptly to physician. Doxycycline (capsule and tablet forms) is associated with a comparatively high incidence of esophagitis, especially in patients older than 40 y.
- Report evidence of superinfections (see Appendix F).

Patient & Family Education

- Take capsule or tablet forms with a full glass (240 mL) of water to ensure passage into stomach and prevent esophageal ulceration. Avoid taking capsule or tablet within 1 h of lying down or retiring.
- Avoid exposure to direct sunlight and ultraviolet light during and for 4 or 5 days after therapy is terminated to reduce risk of phototoxic reaction. Phototoxic reaction appears like an exaggerated sunburn. Sunscreens provide little protection.

DRONABINOL

(droe-nab′i-nol)

Marinol, THC

Classifications: CANNABINOID; ANTIEMETIC
Therapeutic: ANTIEMETIC; APPETITE STIMULANT

Pregnancy Category: C
Controlled Substance: Schedule III

AVAILABILITY 2.5 mg, 5 mg, 10 mg capsules

ACTION & *THERAPEUTIC EFFECT* Synthetic derivative of tetrahydrocannabinol (THC), the principal psychoactive constituent of marijuana *(Cannabis sativa)*. Inhibits vomiting through the control mechanism in the medulla oblongata, producing potent antiemetic effect. Has complex CNS effect that necessitates close supervision of the patient during drug use. Decreases REM sleep; effect on BP is unpredictable; oral temperature may be decreased, and heart rate may be increased. Risk of drug abuse is high. *Produces potent antiemetic effect and is used to treat chemotherapy-induced nausea and vomiting.*

USES To treat chemotherapy-induced nausea and vomiting in cancer patients who fail to respond to conventional antiemetic therapy. Appetite stimulant for AIDS patients.
UNLABELED USES Glaucoma.

CONTRAINDICATIONS Nausea and vomiting caused by other than chemotherapeutic agents; hypersensitivity to dronabinol or sesame oil; lactation.
CAUTIOUS USE First exposure, especially in the older adult or cardiac patient; hypertension, cardiovascular disorders; epilepsy; psychiatric illness, patient receiving other psychoactive drugs; severe hepatic dysfunction; pregnancy (category C).

ROUTE & DOSAGE

Chemotherapy-Induced Nausea
Adult/Child: **PO** 5 mg/m^2 1–3 h before administration of chemo

therapy, then q2–4h after chemotherapy for a total of 4–6 doses, dose may be increased by 2.5 mg/m² (max: 15 mg/m² if necessary)

Appetite Stimulant

Adult: **PO** 2.5 mg b.i.d., before lunch and dinner

ADMINISTRATION

Oral

- Do not repeat dose following a CNS adverse reaction until patient's mental state has returned to normal and the circumstances have been evaluated.
- Store at 8°–15° C (46°–59° F).

ADVERSE EFFECTS (≥1%) **CNS:** *Drowsiness,* psychologic high, dizziness, anxiety, confusion, euphoria, sensory or perceptual difficulties, impaired coordination, depression, irritability, headache, ataxia, memory lapse, paresthesias, paranoia, depersonalization, disorientation, tinnitus, nightmares, speech difficulty, facial flush, diaphoresis. **CV:** Tachycardia, orthostatic hypotension, hypertension, syncope. **GI:** Dry mouth, diarrhea, fecal incontinence. **Other:** Muscular pains.

INTERACTIONS Drug: Alcohol and other CNS DEPRESSANTS may exaggerate psychoactive effects of dronabinol; TRICYCLIC ANTIDEPRESSANTS, **atropine** may cause tachycardia.

PHARMACOKINETICS Absorption: Rapidly absorbed from GI tract, with bioavailability of 10–20%. **Peak:** 2–3 h. **Distribution:** Fat soluble; distributed to many organs; distributed into breast milk. **Metabolism:** In liver; extensive first-pass metabolism. **Elimination:** Principally in bile; 50% in feces within 72 h; 10–15% in urine. **Half-Life:** 25–36 h.

NURSING IMPLICATIONS

Assessment & Drug Effects

- Monitor patients with hypertension or heart disease for BP and cardiac status.
- Response to dronabinol is varied, and previous uneventful use does not guarantee that adverse reactions will not occur. Effects of drug may persist an unpredictably long time (days). Extended use at therapeutic dosage may cause accumulation of toxic amounts of dronabinol and its metabolites.
- Watch for disturbing psychiatric symptoms if dose is increased: Altered mental state, loss of coordination, evidence of a psychologic high (easy laughing, elation and heightened awareness), or depression.
- Note: Abrupt withdrawal is associated with symptoms (within 12 h) of irritability, insomnia, restlessness. Peak intensity occurs at about 24 h: Hot flashes, diaphoresis, rhinorrhea, watery diarrhea, hiccups, anorexia. Usually, syndrome is over in 96 h.

Patient & Family Education

- Do not drive or engage in other potentially hazardous activities that require alertness and judgment because of high incidence of dizziness and drowsiness.
- Understand potential (reversible) for drug-induced mood or behavior changes that may occur during dronabinol use.
- Do not ingest alcohol during period of systemic dronabinol effect. Effect on blood ethanol levels is complex and unpredictable.

DRONEDARONE

(dro-ne′da-rone)

Multaq
Classification: ANTIARRHYTHMIC, CLASS III
Therapeutic: ANTIARRHYTHMIC, CLASS III
Prototype: Amiodarone
Pregnancy Category: X

AVAILABILITY 400 mg tablets

ACTION & *THERAPEUTIC EFFECT* Has antiarrhythmic properties of all four classes of antiarrhythmic drugs. Known to inhibit potassium currents, sodium channels, and slow-L type calcium channels. Also has antiadrenergic properties. *Reduces risk of hospitalization in patients with recent paroxysmal or persistent atrial fibrillation (AF) or atrial flutter (AFL).*

USES Recent episode of paroxysmal or persistent atrial fibrillation or atrial flutter in patients with associated CV risk factors and who are in sinus rhythm or who will be cardioverted.

CONTRAINDICATIONS NYHA class IV HF or NYHA class II-III HF with a recent decompensation requiring hospitalization or referral to a specialized HF clinic; second and third degree AV block or sick sinus syndrome (except with used in conjunction with a functioning pacemaker); bradycardia less than 40 bpm; QT_c interval elongation; severe hepatic impairment; pregnancy (category X), lactation.

CAUTIOUS USE HF; prolonged QT interval; hypokalemia, hypomagnesium; potassium-depleting diuretics; women of child-bearing age. Safety and efficacy of children younger than 18 y have not been established.

ROUTE & DOSAGE

Atrial Fibrillation or Atrial Flutter

Adult: **PO** 400 mg b.i.d. with meals

ADMINISTRATION

Oral

- Give with morning and evening meal. Do NOT give with grapefruit juice.
- Store at 15°–3° C (56°–89° F).

ADVERSE EFFECTS (≥1%) **Body as a Whole:** Asthenia. **CV:** Bradycardia, *QT_c prolongation.* **GI:** Abdominal pain, diarrhea, dyspepsia, nausea, vomitting. **Metabolic:** *Increased serum creatinine.* **Skin:** Dermatitis, eczema, erythematous, maculapapular rash, pruritus.

INTERACTIONS Drug: Concomitant use of CYP3A4 inducers (e.g., **rifampin, phenobarbital, carbamazepine, phenytoin**) can increase the levels of dronedarone. **Ketoconazole, itraconazole, clarithromycin**, and other inhibitors of CYP3A4 can increase the levels of dronedarone. Dronedarone can increase the levels of **digoxin** and other compounds requiring P-glycoprotein (P-gp) transport. BETA-BLOCKERS may provoke excessive bradycardia. **Verapamil** and **diltiazem** can potentiate dronedarone's effects on conduction. **Food: Grapefruit juice** can increase the levels of dronedarone. **Herbal: St. John's wort** can decrease the levels of dronedarone.

PHARMACOKINETICS Peak: 3–6 h. **Distribution:** 98% Plasma protein bound. **Metabolism:** Extensive hepatic metabolism to active and inactive compounds. **Elimination:** 84% in the feces; 6% in the urine. **Half-Life:** 13–19 h.

NURSING IMPLICATIONS

Assessment & Drug Effects

- Monitor vital signs and ECG. Report promptly prolongation of the QT_c interval.
- Report promptly S&S of worsening HF (e.g., rapid weight gain, dependent edema, increasing shortness of breath).
- Lab tests: Baseline and periodic potassium and magnesium levels; periodic serum creatinine; periodic digoxin levels with concurrent therapy.
- Withhold drug and notify physician if hypokalemia or hypomagnesemia develops.

Patient & Family Education

- Report immediately any of the following: Shortness of breath, wheezing, chest tightness, coughing up frothy sputum, rapid weight gain, requiring more pillows to sleep at night.
- Women of childbearing age should use effective contraception while on this drug.
- Avoid grapefruit and grapefruit juice while taking this drug.

DROPERIDOL

(droe-per'i-dole)

Inapsine

Classifications: BUTYROPHENONE; ANTIEMETIC; ANXIOLYTIC

Therapeutic: ANTIEMETIC; ANTIANXIETY

Prototype: Haloperidol

Pregnancy Category: C

AVAILABILITY 2.5 mg/mL injection

ACTION & *THERAPEUTIC EFFECT* Antagonizes emetic effects of morphine-like analgesics and other drugs that act on chemoreceptor trigger zone. *Sedative property reduces anxiety and motor activity without necessarily inducing sleep; patient remains responsive. Has antiemetic properties.*

USES To produce tranquilizing effect and to reduce nausea and vomiting during surgical and diagnostic procedures. Also for premedication, during induction, and as adjunct in maintenance of general or regional anesthesia. Principally used in fixed combination with the potent narcotic analgesic fentanyl (Innovar) to produce neuroleptanalgesia (quiescence, reduced motor activity, and indifference to pain and environmental stimuli) to permit carrying out a variety of diagnostic and minor surgical procedures.

UNLABELED USES IV antiemetic in cancer chemotherapy.

CONTRAINDICATIONS Known or suspected QT elongation; history of torsades de pointes; known intolerance to droperidol; hypokalemia, hypomagnesia, lactation. Safe use in children younger than 2 y is not established.

CAUTIOUS USE Older adult, debilitated, alcoholism, and other poor-risk patients; MAOI therapy; Parkinson's disease; cardiac disease; cardiac bradyarrhythmias, cardiac arrhythmias, CHF, hypotension; liver and kidney impairment or disease; pregnancy (category C).

ROUTE & DOSAGE

Postoperative Nausea and Vomiting Prevention Using Continual ECG Monitoring

Adult: **IV/IM** 2.5 mg; additional doses of 1.25 mg may be given
Child: **IV/IM** 0.1 mg/kg (max: 2.5 mg)

Renal Impairment Dosage Adjustment

Due to increased risk of QT prolongation and torsades de points continuous monitoring is required

ADMINISTRATION

Intramuscular

- Give undiluted.
- Give deep IM into a large muscle.

Intravenous

IV administration to infants and children: Verify correct rate of IV injection with physician.

PREPARE: **Direct:** Give undiluted. ***ADMINISTER:*** **Direct:** *Adult:* Give at a rate of 2.5 mg or fraction thereof over 1–2 min. *Child:* Give a single dose over at least 2 min. ***INCOMPATIBILITIES*** **Solution/additive:** BARBITURATES. **Y-site:** **Allopurinol, amphotericin B cholesteryl complex, cefepime, cefotetan, fluorouracil, foscarnet, furosemide, heparin, leucovorin, methotrexate, nafcillin, piperacillin/tazobactam.**

- Store at 15°–30° C (59°–86° F), unless otherwise directed by manufacturer. Protect from light.

ADVERSE EFFECTS (≥1%) **CNS:** *Postoperative drowsiness, extrapyramidal symptoms:* dystonia, akathisia, oculogyric crisis; dizziness, restlessness, anxiety, hallucinations, mental depression. **CV:** *Hypotension, tachycardia,* irregular heartbeats *(prolonged QTc interval even at low doses).* **Other:** Chills, shivering, laryngospasm, bronchospasm.

INTERACTIONS Drugs: Additive effect with CNS depressants, **metoclopramide** may increase extrapyramidal symptoms, closely monitor other drugs affecting QT interval.

PHARMACOKINETICS Onset: 3–10 min. **Peak:** 30 min. **Duration:** 2–4 h; may persist up to 12 h. **Distribution:** Crosses placenta. **Metabolism:** In liver. **Elimination:** In urine and feces.

NURSING IMPLICATIONS

Assessment & Drug Effects

- Monitor ECG throughout therapy. Report immediately prolongation of QT_c interval.
- Monitor vital signs closely. Hypotension and tachycardia are common adverse effects.
- Exercise care in moving medicated patients because of possibility of severe orthostatic hypotension. Avoid abrupt changes in position.
- Observe patients for signs of impending respiratory depression carefully when receiving a concurrent narcotic analgesic.
- Note: EEG patterns are slow to return to normal during the postoperative period.
- Observe carefully and report promptly to physician early signs of acute dystonia: Facial grimacing, restlessness, tremors, torticollis, oculogyric crisis. Extrapyramidal symptoms may occur within 24–48 h postoperatively.
- Note: Droperidol may aggravate symptoms of acute depression.

DROTRECOGIN ALFA (ACTIVATED)

(dro-tree′co-gin)

Xigris
Classifications: BIOLOGICAL RESPONSE MODIFIER; THROMBOLYTIC; RECOMBINANT HUMAN ACTIVATED PROTEIN C
Therapeutic: ANTI-INFLAMMATORY; ANTITHROMBOLYTIC
Pregnancy Category: C

AVAILABILITY 5 mg, 20 mg vials

ACTION & *THERAPEUTIC EFFECT* Drotrecogin alfa is a recombinant form of human activated protein C (APC). Protein C deficiencies are found in most septic patients and result in a higher mortality rate. Activated protein C exerts antithrombotic and anticoagulant effects by inhibiting clotting factor Va and VIIIa. Activated protein C may exert an anti-inflammatory effect by inhibiting human tumor necrosis factor (TNF) produced by monocytes, and by limiting the thrombin-induced inflammatory responses of the endothelial lining of the vasculature. *Drotrecogin alfa possesses profibrinolytic and anti-inflammatory properties.*

USES Reduction in mortality in patients with severe sepsis and evidence of organ dysfunction.

CONTRAINDICATIONS Prior hypersensitivity to drotrecogin alfa; chronic severe hepatic disease; active internal bleeding or trauma; recent hemorrhagic stroke (within 3 months); invasive surgery or invasive procedures; recent intracranial or intraspinal surgery, or severe head trauma (within 2 mo); intracranial neoplasm, lesion, aneurysm, or herniation; presence of an epidural catheter; lactation.

CAUTIOUS USE Immunosuppression; increased risk of bleeding, hypercoagulability; concurrent use of anticoagulants, or aspirin; thrombocytopenia; children younger than 18 y; recent ischemic stroke, or intracranial aneurysm; pregnancy (category C).

ROUTE & DOSAGE

Sepsis
Adult: **IV** 24 mcg/kg/h continuous infusion for 96 h

ADMINISTRATION

Intravenous

PREPARE: **Continuous:** Prepare immediately prior to use. ▪Reconstitute 5 mg or 20 mg vials with 2.5 mL or 10 mL, respectively, of sterile water for injection to yield approximate concentration of 2 mg/mL. ▪Slowly add sterile water to vial, avoid inverting or shaking vial, gently swirl until powder is completely dissolved. Slowly withdraw calculated dose from vial, add to infusion bag of NS by directing stream to side of bag to minimize agitation, then gently invert to mix. ▪ Final concentration should be 100–200 mcg/mL. ▪Do not transport infusion bag between locations attached to mechanical pump. ▪Note: When using a syringe pump, solution is typically diluted to a final concentration of 100–1000 mcg/mL.

ADMINISTER: **Continuous:** Give over 96 h. ▪ Dose adjustment based on clinical or laboratory parameters is not recommended. ▪IV **must be** completed within 12 h after solution is prepared.

INCOMPATIBILITIES **Solution/additive:** Do not mix with any other drugs. **Y-site:** **Amiodarone, ampicillin/sulbactam sodium, ceftazidime, ciprofloxacin, clindamycin, cyclosporine, dobutamine, dopamine, epinephrine, fosphenytoin, furosemide, gentamicin, heparin**

sodium, human serum albumin, imipenem/cilastatin, insulin human (regular), levofloxacin, magnesium sulfate, metronidazole, midazolam, nitroprusside sodium, norepinephrine bitartrate, piperacillin/tazobactam sodium, potassium phosphate, ranitidine, ticarcillin/clavulanate, tobramycin sulfate, vancomycin.

- Storage: Reconstituted vial may be held at 15°–30° C (59°–86° F), but **must be** used within 3 h of preparation.

ADVERSE EFFECTS (≥1%) **Hematologic:** *Bleeding* (including intracranial).

DIAGNOSTIC TEST INTERFERENCE May affect the ***APTT assay.*** This interference may result in an apparent factor concentration that is lower than the true concentration.

INTERACTIONS Drug: ANTICOAGULANTS, NSAIDS, ANTIPLATELET AGENTS may increase risk of bleeding.

PHARMACOKINETICS Absorption: Steady state reached in 2 h. **Duration:** Serum levels undetectable 2 h after end of infusion. **Half-Life:** 1.6 h.

NURSING IMPLICATIONS

Assessment & Drug Effects

- Monitor closely for S&S of hemorrhage. Stop infusion immediately should clinically important bleeding occur. There is no antidote for drotrecogin alfa.
- Discontinue drotrecogin alfa 2 h prior to invasive procedures with an inherent risk of bleeding. Reinitiation may be reconsidered 12 h after major invasive procedure or immediately after uncomplicated less invasive procedures.
- Lab tests: Monitor closely PT; APTT is not a reliable indication of coagulation.

DULOXETINE HYDROCHLORIDE

(du-lox′e-teen)

Cymbalta

Classifications: ANTIDEPRESSANT; SEROTONIN NOREPINEPHRINE REUPTAKE INHIBITOR (SNRI)

Therapeutic: ANTIDEPRESSANT; SNRI; ANTIANXIETY; NEUROPATHIC PAIN RELIEVER

Prototype: Venlafaxine

Pregnancy Category: C

AVAILABILITY 20 mg, 30 mg, 60 mg capsules

ACTION & *THERAPEUTIC EFFECT* As a selective serotonin and norepinephrine reuptake inhibitor (SSNRI), duloxetine causes potentiation of serotonergic and noradrenergic activity in the CNS. Antidepressant and antianxiety effects are presumed to be due to its dual inhibition of CNS presynaptic neuronal uptake of serotonin and norepinephrine, thus increasing the serum levels of both substances. *Effective as an antidepressant, antianxiety, and neuropathic pain reliever.*

USES Treatment of major depression, generalized anxiety, fibromyalgia, diabetic peripheral neuropathy.

UNLABELED USES Stress urinary incontience.

CONTRAINDICATIONS Concurrent administration of MAOI therapy; uncontrolled narrow-angle glaucoma; alcoholism; end-stage renal disease; hepatitis; jaundice; abrupt discontinuation; third trimester of pregnancy, lactation. Safety and efficacy in children younger than 18 y not established.

CAUTIOUS USE Anorexia nervosa, bipolar disease; history of mania, history of suicidal ideation; cardiac disease; renal impairment or renal failure; hypertension; pregnancy (category C).

ROUTE & DOSAGE

Depression

Adult: **PO** 40–60 mg/day in one or two divided doses

Generalized Anxiety/Diabetic Neuropathy

Adult: **PO** 60 mg once daily

Fibromyalgia

Adult: **PO** 30 mg/day × 1 wk then 60 mg/day

ADMINISTRATION

Oral

- Do not initiate therapy within 14 days of the last dose of an MAOI.
- **Must be** swallowed whole. Do not cut, chew, or crush. Do not sprinkle on food or mix with liquids.
- Store at 15°–30° C (59°–86° F).

ADVERSE EFFECTS (≥1%) **Body as a Whole:** Fatigue, hot flashes. **CNS:** Dizziness, somnolence, tremor, *insomnia*. **GI:** *Nausea, dry mouth, constipation,* diarrhea, vomiting. **Metabolic:** Decreased appetite, weight loss. **Skin:** Increased sweating. **Special Senses:** Blurred vision. **Urogenital:** Decreased libido, abnormal orgasm, erectile dysfunction, ejaculatory dysfunction. Cholestatic jaundice and hepatitis.

INTERACTIONS Drug: Alcohol may result in increased liver function tests; MAOIS may result in hyperthermia, rigidity, mental status changes, myoclonus, autonomic instability, features resembling neuroleptic malignant syndrome; **cimetidine, fluoxetine, fluvoxamine, paroxetine, quinidine,** QUINOLONES may increase levels and half-life of duloxetine; may increase levels and toxicity of **thioridazine,** TRICYCLIC ANTIDEPRESSANTS. **Amphetamine, dextroamphetamine, buspirone, cocaine, dexfenfluramine, fenfluramine, lithium, phentermine, sibutramine, nefazodone,** SSRIS, TRIPTANS, **tramadol, trazodone** may cause serotonin syndrome. **Herbal: St. John's wort, tryptophan** may cause serotonin syndrome.

PHARMACOKINETICS Peak: 6 h. **Metabolism:** In the liver by CYP2D6 and CYP1A2. **Elimination:** 70% in urine, 20% in feces. **Half-Life:** 12 h (8–17 h).

NURSING IMPLICATIONS

Assessment & Drug Effects

- Ensure that a complete list of all concurrent medications is obtained.
- Monitor for S&S of numerous drug-drug interactions (see Interaction section).
- Lab test: LFTs for unexplained abdominal pain or enlarged liver.
- Monitor closely for and report suicide ideation, especially when drug is initiated or dosage changed.
- Report emergence of any of the following: Anxiety, agitation, panic attacks, insomnia, irritability, hostility, psychomotor restlessness, hypomania, and mania.
- Monitor BP, especially in those being treated for hypertension.

Patient & Family Education

- The beneficial effects of this drug may not be felt for approximately 4 wk.
- Report any of the following: Suicidal ideation (especially early in treatment or when dosage is changed), palpitations, anxiety, hyperactivity, agitation, panic attacks, insomnia, irritability, hostility, restlessness.

- Do not abruptly discontinue taking this drug. Notify physician if side effects are bothersome.
- Avoid or minimize use of alcohol while taking this drug.
- Do not self-treat for coughs, colds, or allergies. Consult physician.

DUTASTERIDE

(du-tas′ter-ide)

Avodart

Classifications: ANTIANDROGEN; 5-ALPHA REDUCTASE INHIBITOR

Therapeutic: BENIGN PROSTATIC HYPERPLASIA (BPH) AGENT

Prototype: Finasteride

Pregnancy Category: X

AVAILABILITY 0.5 mg capsules

ACTION & *THERAPEUTIC EFFECT* Specific inhibitor of the steroid 5-alpha-reductase, an enzyme necessary to convert testosterone into the potent androgen 5-alpha-dihydrotestosterone (DHT) in the prostate gland. *Decreases the production of testosterone in the prostate gland.*

USES Treatment of benign prostatic hypertrophy (BPH) with or without tamsulosin.

UNLABELED USES Treatment of male pattern baldness.

CONTRAINDICATIONS Hypersensitivity to dutasteride or finasteride; pregnancy (category X), lactation, and children younger than 18 y.

CAUTIOUS USE Hepatic impairment, obstructive uropathy.

ROUTE & DOSAGE

BPH

Adult: **PO** 0.5 mg once daily

ADMINISTRATION

Oral

- Do not handle capsules if you are or may become pregnant because of the potential for absorption of dutasteride and the subsequent risk to a developing male fetus.
- Do not open or crush capsules. They **must be** swallowed whole.
- Store at 15°–30° C (59°–86° F).

ADVERSE EFFECTS (≥1%) **Endocrine:** Gynecomastia. **Urogenital:** Ejaculation dysfunction, impotence, decreased libido.

INTERACTIONS Drug: Diltiazem, verapamil may decrease clearance of dutasteride. **Herbal:** May see exaggerated effects with **saw palmetto.**

PHARMACOKINETICS Absorption: Rapidly; 60% bioavailability. **Peak:** 2–3 h. **Distribution:** 99% protein bound. **Metabolism:** In liver by CYP3A4 to 1 active and 2 inactive metabolites. **Elimination:** Primarily in feces. **Half-Life:** 5 wk.

NURSING IMPLICATIONS

Assessment & Drug Effects

- Monitor voiding patterns, assessing for ease of starting a stream, frequency, and urgency.
- Lab tests: Monitor baseline PSA and again at 3–6 mo to establish new baseline to use to assess potentially cancer-related changes in PSA. After 6 mo of treatment, obtained PSA values should be doubled for comparison with normal values in untreated men.

Patient & Family Education

- Do not donate blood until at least 6 mo following last dose to prevent administration of dutasteride to a pregnant female transfusion recipient.
- Ejaculate volume might be decreased during treatment but this

does not seem to interfere with normal sexual function.

- Note that the incidence of most drug-related sexual adverse events (impotence, decreased libido, and ejaculation disorder) typically decrease with duration of treatment.

D

DYPHYLLINE

(dye′fi-lin)

Lufyllin, Protophylline ♣

Classifications: RESPIRATORY SMOOTH MUSCLE RELAXANT, XANTHINE; BRONCHODILATOR

Therapeutic: BRONCHODILATOR; ANTIASTHMA

Prototype: Theophylline

Pregnancy Category: C

AVAILABILITY 200 mg, 400 mg tablets

ACTION & *THERAPEUTIC EFFECT* Xanthine and derivative of theophylline that results in bronchodilation, myocardial stimulation, and smooth muscle relaxation. *Effective bronchodilator and antiasthmatic agent.*

USES Acute bronchial asthma and reversible bronchospasm associated with chronic bronchitis and emphysema.

CONTRAINDICATIONS Hypersensitivity to xanthine compounds; apnea in newborns; children 6 y or younger.

CAUTIOUS USE Severe cardiac disease, hypertension, acute myocardial injury; renal or hepatic dysfunction; glaucoma; seizure disorders; hyperthyroidism; peptic ulcer; in the older adults or children; concomitant administration of other xanthine formulations or other CNS-stimulating drugs; pregnancy (category C), lactation.

ROUTE & DOSAGE

Asthma

Adult: **PO** 200–800 mg q6h up to 15 mg/kg q.i.d.

Child (6 y or older): **PO** 4.4–6.6 mg/kg/day in divided doses

ADMINISTRATION

Oral

- Give oral preparation with a full glass of water on an empty stomach (e.g., 1 h before or 2 h after meals) to enhance absorption. However, administration after meals may help to relieve gastric discomfort.
- Exercise care in the amount of elixir given to children because it has a high alcohol content (18–20%).

ADVERSE EFFECTS (≥1%) **CNS:** Headache, irritability, restlessness, dizziness, insomnia, light-headedness, muscle twitching, convulsions. **CV:** Palpitation, *tachycardia,* extrasystoles, flushing, hypotension. **GI:** *Nausea,* vomiting, diarrhea, anorexia, epigastric distress. **Respiratory:** Tachypnea. **Other:** Albuminuria, fever, dehydration.

INTERACTIONS Drug: BETA-BLOCKERS may antagonize bronchodilating effects of dyphylline; **halothane** increases risk of cardiac arrhythmias; **probenecid** may decrease dyphylline elimination.

PHARMACOKINETICS Absorption: Readily from GI tract. **Peak:** 1 h. **Metabolism:** In liver (but not to theophylline). **Elimination:** In urine. **Half-Life:** 2 h.

NURSING IMPLICATIONS

Assessment & Drug Effects

- Lab tests: Baseline and periodic pulmonary function tests to assess therapeutic effectiveness.
- Monitor therapeutic effectiveness; usually occurs at a blood level of at least 12 mcg/mL.
- Note: Toxic dyphylline plasma levels, although rare with normal dosage, are a risk in patients with a diminished capacity for dyphylline clearance (e.g., those with CHF or hepatic impairment or who are older than 55 y or younger than 1 y).

Patient & Family Education

- Take medication consistently with or without food at the same time each day.
- Notify physician of adverse effects: Nausea, vomiting, insomnia, jitteriness, headache, rash, severe GI pain, restlessness, convulsions, or irregular heartbeat.
- Avoid alcohol and also large amounts of coffee and other xanthine-containing beverages (e.g., tea, cocoa, cola) during therapy.
- Consult physician before taking OTC preparations. Many OTC drugs for coughs, colds, and allergies contain nervous system stimulants.

ECHOTHIOPHATE IODIDE

(ek-oh-thye′oh-fate)

Phospholine Iodide

Pregnancy Category: C

See Appendix A-1.

ECONAZOLE NITRATE

(e-kone′a-zole)

Ecostatin ♣, Spectazole

Classifications: ANTIBIOTIC; AZOLE ANTIFUNGAL

Therapeutic: AZOLE ANTIFUNGAL

Prototype: Fluconazole

Pregnancy Category: C

AVAILABILITY 1% cream

ACTION & *THERAPEUTIC EFFECT* Azole antifungal antibiotic with broad spectrum of activity similar to that of miconazole. It disrupts normal fungal cell membrane permeability. *Active against dermatophytes, yeasts, and many other fungi.*

USES Topically for treatment of tinea pedis (athlete's foot or ringworm of foot), tinea cruris ("jock itch" or ringworm of groin), tinea corporis (ringworm of body), tinea versicolor, and cutaneous candidiasis (moniliasis).

UNLABELED USES Has been used for topical treatment of erythrasma and with corticosteroids for fungal or bacterial dermatoses associated with inflammation.

CONTRAINDICATIONS Infants younger than 3 mo.

CAUTIOUS USE Pregnancy (category C), lactation.

ROUTE & DOSAGE

Tinea Cruris, Tinea Corporis, Tinea Pedis, Cutaneous Candidiasis

Adult/Child: **Topical** Apply sufficient amount to affected areas twice daily, morning and evening

Tinea Versicolor

Adult: **Topical** Apply sufficient amount to affected areas once daily

ADMINISTRATION

Topical

- Cleanse skin with soap and water and dry thoroughly before applying medication (unless otherwise directed by physician). Wash hands thoroughly before and after treatments.
- Do not use occlusive dressings unless prescribed by physician.
- Store at less than 30° C (86° F) unless otherwise directed.

ADVERSE EFFECTS (≥1%) **Skin:** Burning, stinging sensation, pruritus, erythema.

INTERACTIONS Drug: No clinically significant interactions established.

PHARMACOKINETICS Absorption: Minimal percutaneous absorption through intact skin; increased absorption from denuded skin. **Peak:** 0.5–5 h. **Elimination:** Less than 1% of applied dose is eliminated in urine and feces.

NURSING IMPLICATIONS

Patient & Family Education

- Use medication for the prescribed time even if symptoms improve and report to physician skin reactions suggestive of irritation or sensitization.
- Notify physician if full course of therapy does not result in improvement. Diagnosis should be reevaluated.
- Do not to apply the topical cream in or near the eyes or intravaginally.

ECULIZUMAB

(e-cul-i-zu′mab)

Soliris

Classifications: BIOLOGICAL RESPONSE MODIFIER; MONOCLONAL ANTIBODY; IMMUNOGLOBULIN

Therapeutic: IMMUNOGLOBULIN
Prototype: Immune globulin
Pregnancy Category: C

AVAILABILITY 30 mL vials containing 10 mg/mL solution for IV injection

ACTION & *THERAPEUTIC EFFECT* A monoclonal antibody (IgG) immunoglobulin molecule that binds with high affinity to complement C5 inhibiting formation of the terminal complement complex, C5b-9. *Inhibition of C5b-9 complement complex prevents complement-mediated hemolysis in those with RBC deficiency in patients with paroxysmal nocturnal hemoglobinuria (PNH), resulting from genetic mutation.*

USES Reduction of hemolysis in patients with paroxysmal nocturnal hemoglobinuria.

CONTRAINDICATIONS Serious meningococcal infections; children younger than 18 y.

CAUTIOUS USE History of hypersensitivity to protein components; older adults; systemic infection; pregnancy (category C), lactation.

ROUTE & DOSAGE

Paroxysmal Nocturnal Hemoglobinuria

Adult: **IV** 600 mg IV infusion every 7 days × 4 wk (a total of 4 doses); then 900 mg IV on day 7 after the 4th dose, and then 900 mg IV every 14 days thereafter

ADMINISTRATION

Intravenous

Note: Patients **must be** vaccinated against *Neisseria meningitidis* **at least 2 wk prior to** the first dose of eculizumab. Prior to initiating treatment, patients and prescribers **must be** enrolled in the Soliris™ Safety Registry.

PREPARE: **IV Infusion:** Dilute to a final concentration of 5 mg/mL in NS, D5/0.45% NaCl, or LR by adding the required volume of eculizumab to an EQUAL volume of IV fluid. Invert bag to mix. ▪ Final infusion volumes will be 600 mg in 120 mL or 900 mg in 180 mL. ▪ Allow to come to room temperature prior to infusion

ADMINISTER: **IV Infusion:** Do NOT give direct IV. ▪ Give over 35 min via infusion pump or syringe pump. If infusion is slowed for an infusion reaction, the total infusion time should not exceed 2 h.

INCOMPATIBILITIES **Solution/additive/Y-site:** Do not mix with any other drugs or solutions.

▪ Store infusion bags for 24 h at 2°–8° C (36°–46° F).

ADVERSE EFFECTS (≥1%) **Body as a Whole:** Herpes simplex infections, influenza-like illness, pain in extremity. **CNS:** *Fatigue, headache.* **GI:** Constipation, *nausea.* **Musculoskeletal:** *Back pain,* myalgia. **Respiratory:** *Cough, nasopharyngitis,* respiratory tract infection, sinusitis.

PHARMACOKINETICS Half-Life: 272 ± 82 h.

NURSING IMPLICATIONS

Assessment & Drug Effects

- Monitor for a hypersensitivity reaction throughout infusion and for at least 1 h after completion of the infusion.
- Monitor for early signs of meningococcal infection. Report immediately if an infection is suspected.
- Lab tests: Baseline and periodic serum LDH and RBC blood studies.

Patient & Family Education

- Although patient must be vaccinated against *N. meningitidis* prior to therapy with eculizumab, vaccination may not prevent meningitis. Report immediately any of the following: Moderate to severe headache with nausea or vomiting, stiff neck or stiff back, fever, rash, confusion, severe muscle aches with flu-like symptoms, and sensitivity to light.

EDETATE CALCIUM DISODIUM

(ed′e-tate)

Calcium Disodium Versenate

Classification: CHELATING AGENT

Therapeutic: CHELATING AGENT; ANTIPOISON AGENT

Pregnancy Category: B

AVAILABILITY 200 mg/mL injection

ACTION & *THERAPEUTIC EFFECT* Chelating agent that combines with divalent and trivalent metals to form stable, nonionizing soluble complexes that can be readily excreted by kidneys. Action is dependent on ability of heavy metal to displace the less strongly bound calcium in the drug molecules. *Chelating agent that binds with heavy metals such as lead to form a soluble complex that can be excreted through the kidney, thereby ridding the body of the poisonous substance.*

USES As adjunct in treatment of acute and chronic lead poisoning (plumbism). Generally used in combination with dimercaprol (BAL) in treatment of lead encephalopathy or when blood lead level exceeds 100 mcg/dL. Also used to diagnose suspected lead poisoning.

UNLABELED USES Treatment of poisoning from other heavy metals such as chromium, manganese, nickel, zinc, and possibly vanadium; removal of radioactive and nuclear fission products such as plutonium, yttrium, uranium. Not effective in poisoning from arsenic, gold, or mercury.

CONTRAINDICATIONS Severe kidney disease, active renal disease, anuria, oliguria; hepatitis; IV use in patients with lead encephalopathy not generally recommended (because of possible increase in intracranial pressure).

CAUTIOUS USE Kidney dysfunction; active tubercular lesions; history of gout; cardiac arrhythmias; pregnancy (category B), lactation.

ROUTE & DOSAGE

Diagnosis of Lead Poisoning

Adult: **IV/IM** 500 mg/m² (max: 1 g) over 1 h, then collect urine for 24 h (if mcg lead:mg EDTA ratio in urine is greater than 1, the test is positive)

Child: **IM** 50 mg/kg (max: 1 g), then collect urine for 6–8 h, (if mcg lead:mg EDTA ratio in urine is greater than 0.5, the test is positive)

Treatment of Lead Poisoning

Adult/Child: **IV** 1–1.5 g/m²/day infused over 8–24 h for up to 5 days **IM** 1–1.5 g/m²/day divided q8–12h

Asymptomatic Lead Poisoning

Adult/Child: **IV** 1 g/m²/day infused over 8–24 h for up to 5 days

Lead Nephropathy/Renal Impairment Dosage Adjustment

Adult: **IV** *Based on serum creatinine less than 2 mg/dL:* 1 g/m²/day × 5 days; *2–3 mg/dL,* 500 mg/m²/day × 5 days; *3.1–4 × 3 doses mg/dL,* 500 mg/m² q48h; *greater than 4 mg/dL,* 500 mg/m² once/wk. Infuse over 8–24 h, may repeat monthly.

ADMINISTRATION

- Note: Calcium disodium edetate can produce potentially fatal effects when higher than recommended doses are used or when it is continued after toxic effects appear.

Intramuscular

- IM route preferred for symptomatic children and recommended for patients with incipient or overt lead-induced encephalopathy.
- Add Procaine HCl to minimize pain at injection site (usually 1 mL of procaine 1% to each 1 mL of concentrated drug). Consult physician.

Intravenous

PREPARE: **IV Infusion:** Dilute the 5 mL ampule with 250–500 mL of NS or D5W.

ADMINISTER: **IV Infusion:** Warning: Rapid IV infusion may be LETHAL by suddenly increasing intracranial pressure in patients who already have cerebral edema. Manufacturer recommends total daily dose over 8–12 h. Consult physician for specific rate.

INCOMPATIBILITIES **Solution/additive:** **Amphotericin B, D10W hydralazine, lactated Ringer's.**

ADVERSE EFFECTS (≥1%) **CV:** Hypotension, thrombophlebitis. **GI:** Anorexia, nausea, vomiting, diarrhea, abdominal cramps, cheilosis. **Hematologic:** Transient bone marrow depression, depletion of blood metals. **Urogenital:** Nephrotoxicity (renal tubular necrosis), proteinuria, hematuria. **Body as a Whole:** *Febrile reaction* (excessive thirst, fever, chills, severe myalgia, arthralgia, GI distress), *histamine-like reactions* (flushing, throbbing headache, sweating, sneezing, nasal congestion, lacrimation, postural hypotension, tachycardia).

DIAGNOSTIC TEST INTERFERENCE Edetate calcium disodium may decrease ***serum cholesterol, plasma lipid*** levels (if elevated), and ***serum potassium*** values. ***Glycosuria*** may occur with toxic doses.

INTERACTIONS Drug: May affect **insulin** requirements.

PHARMACOKINETICS Absorption: Well absorbed IM. **Onset:** 1 h. **Peak:** Peak chelation 24–48 h. **Distribution:** Distributed to extracellular fluid; does not enter CSF. **Metabolism:** Not metabolized. **Elimination:** Chelated lead excreted in urine; 50% excreted in 1 h. **Half-Life:** 20–60 min IV, 90 min IM.

NURSING IMPLICATIONS

Assessment & Drug Effects

- Determine adequacy of urinary output prior to therapy. This may be done by administering IV fluids before giving first dose.
- Increase fluid intake to enhance urinary excretion of chelates. Avoid excess fluid intake, however, in patients with lead encephalopathy because of the danger of further increasing intracranial pressure. Consult physician regarding allowable intake.
- Monitor I&O. Since drug is excreted almost exclusively via kidneys, toxicity may develop if output is inadequate. Stop therapy if urine flow is markedly diminished or absent. Report any change in output or I&O ratio to physician.
- Lab tests: Obtain serum creatinine, calcium, and phosphorus before and during each course of therapy. Monitor baseline and frequent BUN levels and ECG during therapy. With prolonged therapy determine periodic determinations of blood trace element metals (e.g., copper, zinc, magnesium).
- Be alert for occurrence of febrile reaction that may appear 4–8 h after drug infusion (see ADVERSE EFFECTS).

EDROPHONIUM CHLORIDE

(ed-roe-foe′nee-um)

Enlon, Reversol

Classifications: CHOLINERGIC MUSCLE STIMULANT; CHOLINESTERASE INHIBITOR

Therapeutic: ANTICHOLINESTERASE MUSCLE STIMULANT

Prototype: Neostigmine

Pregnancy Category: C

AVAILABILITY 10 mg/mL injection

ACTION & *THERAPEUTIC EFFECT* Facilitates transmission of impulses across the myoneural junction by inhibiting the destruction of acetylcholine by cholinesteratse. *Acts as antidote to curariform drugs by displacing them from muscle cell receptor sites, thus permitting resumption of normal transmission of neuromuscular impulses.*

USES Differential diagnosis and as adjunct in evaluation of treatment requirements of myasthenia gravis; curare antagonist.

CONTRAINDICATIONS Hypersensitivity to anticholinesterase agents; cholinesterase inhibitor toxicity; intestinal and urinary obstruction; lactation.

CAUTIOUS USE Sulfite hypersensitivity; bronchial asthma; cardiac arrhythmias; bradycardia; peptic ulcer disease; hypotension; patients receiving digitalis; pregnancy (category C).

ROUTE & DOSAGE

Myasthenia Gravis Diagnosis

Adult: **IV** Prepare 10 mg in a syringe; inject 2 mg over 15–30 sec, if no reaction after 45 sec, inject the remaining 8 mg, may repeat test after 30 min **IM** Inject 10 mg, if cholinergic reaction occurs, retest after 30 min with 2 mg to rule out false-negative reaction

Child: **IV** *Weight 34 kg or less,* 1 mg, if no response after 45 sec, dose may be titrated up to 5 mg **IM** 2 mg **IV** *Weight greater than 34 kg,* 2 mg, if no response after 45 sec, dose may be titrated up to 10 mg **IM** 5 mg

Evaluation of Myasthenia Treatment

Adult: **IV** 1–2 mg administered 1 h after last PO dose of anticholinesterase medication

Curare Antagonist

Adult: **IV** 1 mL (10 mg) over 30–45 sec, repeat as necessary. Max dose: 4 mL (40 mg).

ADMINISTRATION

- Note: Have antidote (atropine sulfate) immediately available and facilities for endotracheal intubation, tracheostomy, suction, assisted respiration, and cardiac monitoring for treatment of cholinergic reaction.

Intramuscular

- Give undiluted. IM route used if IV route not accessible.

Intravenous

PREPARE: **Direct/Infusion:** May be given undiluted or diluted in D5W or NS for infusion.

ADMINISTER: **Direct:** Inject 2 mg (adult and child weighing more than 34 kg) or 1 mg (child weighing 34 kg or less) over 15–30 sec; if no reaction after 45 sec, inject additional 8 mg (adult) or titrate up to a total of 8 mg additional (child weighing more than 34 kg) or titrate in 1 mg increments up to a total of 4 mg additional (child weighing 34 kg or less), may repeat test after 30 min. ▪ If cholinergic reaction (increased muscle weakness) is obtained after initial 1 or 2 mg, discontinue test and give atropine IV (as ordered).

IV Infusion: Infuse over 1 h.

ADVERSE EFFECTS (≥1%) **Body as a Whole:** Severe adverse effects uncommon with usual doses. **CNS:** Weakness, muscle cramps, dysphoria, fasciculations, incoordination, dysarthria, dysphagia, convulsions, <u>respiratory paralysis</u>. **CV:** Bradycardia, irregular pulse, hypotension, pulmonary edema. **Special Senses:** Miosis, blurred vision, diplopia, lacrimation. **GI:** Diarrhea, abdominal cramps, nausea, vomiting, excessive salivation. **Respiratory:** Increased bronchial secretions, <u>bronchospasm, laryngospasm</u>, pulmonary edema. **Other:** Excessive sweating, urinary frequency, incontinence.

INTERACTIONS Drug: Procainamide, quinidine may antagonize the effects of edrophonium; DIGITALIS GLYCOSIDES increase the sensitivity of the heart to edrophonium; **succinylcholine, decamethonium** may prolong neuromuscular blockade.

PHARMACOKINETICS Onset: 30–60 sec IV; 2–10 min IM. **Duration:** 5–10 min IV; 5–30 min IM.

NURSING IMPLICATIONS

Assessment & Drug Effects

- Monitor vital signs. Observe for signs of respiratory distress. Patients older than 50 y are particularly likely to develop bradycardia, hypotension, and cardiac arrest.
- Edrophonium test for myasthenia gravis: All cholinesterase inhibitors (anticholinesterases) should be discontinued for at least 8 h before test. Positive response to edrophonium test consists of brief improvement in muscle strength unaccompanied by lingual or skeletal muscle fasciculations.
- Evaluation of myasthenic treatment: *Myasthenic response* (immediate subjective improvement with increased muscle strength, absence of fasciculations; generally indicates that patient requires larger dose of anticholinesterase agent or longer-acting drug); *Cholinergic response* [muscarinic adverse effects (lacrimation, diaphoresis, salivation, abdominal cramps, diarrhea, nausea, vomiting; accompanied by decrease in muscle strength; usually indicates over-treatment with cholinesterase inhibitor)]; *Adequate response* [no change in muscle strength; fasciculations may be present or absent; minimal cholinergic adverse effects (observed in patients at or near optimal dosage level)].

EFAVIRENZ (Pr)

(e-fa′vi-renz)

Sustiva

Classifications: ANTIRETROVIRAL; NONNUCLEOSIDE REVERSE TRANSCRIPTASE INHIBITOR (NNRTI)
Therapeutic: ANTIRETROVIRAL; NNRTI

Pregnancy Category: D (including first trimester)

AVAILABILITY 50 mg, 200 mg capsules; 600 mg tablets

ACTION & *THERAPEUTIC EFFECT* Nonnucleoside reverse transcriptase inhibitor (NNRTI) of HIV-1. Binds directly to reverse transcriptase and blocks RNA polymerase activities of the HIV-1 virus, thus preventing replication of the virus. *Prevents replication of the HIV-1 virus. Resistant strains appear rapidly. Effectiveness is indicated by reduction in viral load (plasma level HIV RNA).*

USES HIV-1 infection in combination with other antiretroviral agents.

CONTRAINDICATIONS Hypersensitivity to efavirenz; coadministration with bepridil, midazolam, pimozide, triazolam, or ergot derivative; coadministration with standard doses of variconazole; pregnancy (category D, including fetal harm in first trimester), lactation.

CAUTIOUS USE Liver disease, alcoholism, hepatitis B or C, hypertriglyceridemia, hypercholesterolemia, substance abuse, antimicrobial resistance, bipolar disorder, depression, suicidal ideation, exfoliative dermatitis; females of childbearing age, CNS disorders; history of seizures; older adults. Safety and efficacy in children younger than 3 y or who weigh less than 13 kg (29 lb) are not known.

ROUTE & DOSAGE

HIV Infection
Adult/Adolescent: **PO** 600 mg daily

Child: **PO** *3 y or older, weight 10–15 kg,* 200 mg daily; *weight 15–20 kg,* 250 mg daily; *weight 20–25 kg,* 300 mg daily; *weight 25–32.5 kg,* 350 mg daily; *weight 32.5–40 kg,* 400 mg daily; *weight greater than 40 kg,* 600 mg daily

ADMINISTRATION

Oral

- Use bedtime dosing to increase tolerability of CNS adverse effects.
- Give exactly as ordered. Do not skip a dose or discontinue therapy without consulting the physician.
- Do not give efavirenz following a high fat meal.
- Store at 15°–30° C (59°–86° F) in a tightly closed container and protect from light.

ADVERSE EFFECTS (≥1%) **Body as a Whole:** Fatigue, fever. **CNS:** Dizziness, headache, hypoesthesia, impaired concentration, insomnia, abnormal dreams, somnolence, depression, nervousness, adverse psychiatric experiences. **CV:** Hypercholesterolemia. **GI:** *Nausea,* vomiting, *diarrhea,* dyspepsia, abdominal pain, flatulence, anorexia, increased liver function tests (ALT, AST). **Respiratory:** Cough. **Skin:** *Rash* (erythematous rash, pruritus, *maculopapular rash,* <u>erythema multiforme, Stevens-Johnson syndrome, toxic epidermal necrolysis</u>), increased sweating. **Urogenital:** Renal calculus, hematuria.

DIAGNOSTIC TEST INTERFERENCE False-positive urine tests for **marijuana.**

INTERACTIONS Drug: Decreased concentrations of **clarithromycin, indinavir, nelfinavir, saquinavir, voriconazole;** increased concentrations of **ritonavir, azithromycin, ethinyl estradiol.** Efavirenz levels are increased by **ritonavir, fluconazole** and decreased by **saquinavir, rifampin.** Additional drugs not recommended for administration with efavirenz include **midazolam, triazolam,** ERGOT DERIVATIVES, **warfarin. Herbal: St. John's wort** may decrease antiretroviral activity.

PHARMACOKINETICS Peak: 5 h; steady-state 6–10 days. **Distribution:** 99% protein bound. **Metabolism:** In liver by cytochrome P450 3A4 and 2B6; can induce (increase) its own metabolism. **Elimination:** 14–34% in urine, 16–61% in feces. **Half-Life:** 52–76 h after single dose, 40–55 h after multiple doses.

NURSING IMPLICATIONS

Assessment & Drug Effects

- Monitor for suicidal ideation in patients who are depressed, or who have a history of depression.
- Monitor GI status and evaluate ability to maintain a normal diet.
- Lab tests: Periodic liver functions and lipid profile.

Patient & Family Education

- Contact physician promptly if any of the following occurs: Skin rash, delusions, inappropriate behavior, suicidal ideation.
- Avoid pregnancy because of fetal harm in first trimester of pregnancy.
- Use or add barrier contraception if using hormonal contraceptive.
- Notify physician immediately if you become pregnant.
- Do not drive or engage in potentially hazardous activities until response to the drug is known. Dizziness, impaired concentration, and drowsiness usually improve with continued therapy.

EFLORNITHINE HYDROCHLORIDE

(e-flor'ni-theen)

Vaniqa

Classification: DERMATOLOGIC

Therapeutic: FACIAL HIRSUTISM AGENT

Pregnancy Category: C

AVAILABILITY 13.9% cream

ACTION & *THERAPEUTIC EFFECT* Inhibits enzyme activity in the skin that is required for hair growth. *Results in retarding the rate of hair growth.*

USES Reduction of unwanted facial hair in women.

CONTRAINDICATIONS Hypersensitivity to eflornithine or its components; children younger than 12 y.
CAUTIOUS USE Bone marrow suppression; HIV; pregnancy (category C), lactation.

ROUTE & DOSAGE

Hair Removal

Adult: **Topical** Apply thin layer to affected areas of the face and adjacent involved areas under the chin and rub in thoroughly b.i.d. at least 8 h apart

ADMINISTRATION

Topical

- Apply thin layer to affected skin areas on face and under chin and rub in thoroughly.
- Do not wash treated areas for at least 4 h after application.
- Store at 15°–30° C (59°–86° F).

ADVERSE EFFECTS (≥1%) **Body as a Whole** Facial edema. **CNS** Dizziness. **GI:** Dyspepsia, anorexia. **Skin:** *Acne, pseudofolliculitis barbae,* stinging, burning, pruritus, erythema, tingling, irritation, rash, alopecia, folliculitis, ingrown hair.

INTERACTIONS No clinically significant interactions established.

PHARMACOKINETICS Absorption: Less than 1% absorbed through intact skin. **Metabolism:** Not metabolized. **Elimination:** Primarily in urine. **Half-Life:** 8 h.

NURSING IMPLICATIONS

Assessment & Drug Effects

- Monitor for and report skin irritation.
- Note: Drug slows growth of facial hair, but is not a depilatory.

Patient & Family Education

- Note: Effect of drug is usually not apparent for 4–8 wk.
- Reduce frequency of drug application to once daily if skin irritation occurs. If irritation continues, contact physician.

ELETRIPTAN HYDROBROMIDE

(e-le-trip'tan)

Relpax

Classification: SEROTONIN 5-HT_1 RECEPTOR AGONIST

Therapeutic: ANTIMIGRAINE

Prototype: Sumatriptan

Pregnancy Category: C

AVAILABILITY 20 mg, 40 mg tablets

ACTION & *THERAPEUTIC EFFECT* Eletriptan is a potent agonist at central serotonin 5-HT_{1B}, 5-HT_{1D}, and 5-HT_{1F} receptors. Eletriptan stimulates presynaptic 5-HT_{1D} receptors inhibiting dural vasodilation and agonizes vascular 5-HT_{1B} receptors causing vasoconstriction of intracranial extracerebral vessels. *Inhibits dural vasodilation and inflammation, and causes vasoconstriction of painfully dilated intracranial extracerebral vessels, thus relieving the migraine headache. Also relieves photophobia, phonophobia, and nausea and vomiting associated with migraine attacks.*

USES Treatment of acute migraine attacks with or without aura.

CONTRAINDICATIONS Hypersensitivity to eletriptan; history of coronary artery disease; ischemic or vasospastic coronary artery disease, arteriosclerosis, history of MI; ischemic colititis, Raynaud's disease uncontrolled hypertension; CVA or TIA; within 24 h of administering of another ergotamine; lactation within 24 h after dose; children younger than 18 y; severe hepatic insufficiency; hemiplegic or basilar migraine; peripheral vascular disease; concurrent MAOI therapy.

CAUTIOUS USE Hypotension in the elderly; older adults over 65 y; mild to moderate hepatic impairment; diabetes, obesity, smoking, high cholesterol; men older than 40 y; postmenopausal women. Use within 72 h of potent CYP3A4 metabolizing drugs; pregnancy (category C), lactation.

ROUTE & DOSAGE

Acute Migraine

Adult: **PO** 20 mg or 40 mg at onset of migraine (max: 40 mg/dose and 80 mg/day), may repeat dose in 2 h if partial response
Geriatric: Use not recommended

Hepatic Impairment Dosage Adjustment

Use not recommended in severe hepatic impairment

ADMINISTRATION

Oral

- Give one tablet as soon as the migraine begins.
- May give 2nd tablet if headache improves but returns after 2 h.
- If 1st tablet is ineffective, do not give a 2nd without consulting physician.
- Do not give within 72 h of potent CYP3A4 inhibitors (see INTERACTIONS).
- Store at 15°–30° C (59°–86° F). Protect from light and moisture.

ADVERSE EFFECTS (≥1%) **Body as a Whole:** *Asthenia,* paresthesia, flushing, back pain, chills. **CNS:** Dizziness, drowsiness, headache, somnolence, hypertonia, hypesthesia. **CV:** Chest tightness/pressure, palpitation, hypertension. The following are rare, usually seen in patients with cardiovascular disease risk factors: Coronary vasospasm, transient myocardial ischemia, MI, ventricular tachycardia, atrial fibrillation, ventricular fibrillation. **GI:** Abdominal pain, dyspepsia, dysphagia, nausea, vomiting, dry mouth. **Respiratory:** Pharyngitis. **Skin:** Sweating.

INTERACTIONS Drug: Drugs that inhibit CYP3A4 may increase eletriptan levels and toxicity, do not administer eletriptan within 72 h of AZOLE ANTIFUNGALS (especially **itraconazole, ketoconazole, voriconazole**), **amiodarone, cimetidine, dalfopristin, quinupristin, diltiazem, metronidazole, nicardipine, norfloxacin, quinine, verapamil, zafirlukast, zileuton,** MACROLIDE ANTIBIOTICS, NONNUCLEOTIDE REVERSE TRANSCRIPTASE INHIBITORS, PROTEASE INHIBITORS, SELECTIVE SEROTONIN REUPTAKE INHIBITORS, **sibutramine;** ERGOT ALKALOIDS may prolong vasospastic adverse reactions (do not use within 24 h of ergot-containing drugs); do not administer within 24 h of other 5-HT_1 AGONISTS (may cause increased adverse effects). **Food: Grapefruit juice** may increase eletriptan levels and toxicity. **Herbal: Gingko, ginseng, echinacea, St. John's wort** may increase triptan toxicity.

PHARMACOKINETICS Absorption: Rapidly absorbed, 50% reaches systemic circulation. **Onset:** 1–2 h. **Peak:** 1.5 h. **Distribution:** 85% protein bound. **Metabolism:** In liver by CYP3A4. **Elimination:** 90% cleared by nonrenal routes, 9% eliminated in urine. **Half-Life:** 4–5 h.

NURSING IMPLICATIONS

Assessment & Drug Effects

- Monitor CV status carefully following first dose in patients at risk for coronary artery disease (e.g., history of hypertension, postmenopausal women, men older than 40 y, persons with known CAD risk factors) or who have coronary artery vasospasms.
- Report immediately chest pain, tightness in chest or throat that is severe or does not quickly resolve following a dose of eletriptan.
- Monitor therapeutic effectiveness. Pain relief is usually achieved within 1 h.

Patient & Family Education

- Note: If first dose is ineffective, do not take a second dose as it will not work for the same attack.
- Inform physician of all prescription, nonprescription, and herbal drugs you are taking. Do not add additional drugs without informing physician as many drugs interact with eletriptan.
- Report promptly any of the following: Headache more severe than usual, migraine; dizziness, faintness, blurred vision; chest, neck, or throat pain; irregular heart beat, palpitations; shortness of breath, wheezing, difficulty breathing; tingling, pain, or numbness in the face, hands, or feet; seizures; severe stomach pain, cramping, or bloody diarrhea.
- Do not drive or engage in any potentially hazardous task until reaction to drug is known.

EMEDASTINE DIFUMARATE (Pr)

(em-e-das′teen di-foom′a-rate)

Emadine

Classifications: EYE PREPARATION; ANTIHISTAMINE, OCULAR; H_1-RECEPTOR ANTAGONIST

Therapeutic: OCULAR ANTIHISTAMINE

Pregnancy Category: B

AVAILABILITY 0.05% ophth solution

ACTION & *THERAPEUTIC EFFECT* Emedastine is a selective antagonist at H_1-receptors. It blocks H_1-receptors and inhibits histamine-stimulated vascular permeability in the conjunctiva. *Relieves ocular pruritus related to allergic response to histamine.*

USES Temporary relief of seasonal allergic conjunctivitis.

CONTRAINDICATIONS Hypersensitivity to emedastine.

CAUTIOUS USE Hypersensitivity to other antihistamines, soft contact lenses; pregnancy (category B), lactation. Safety and efficacy in children younger than 3 y are not established.

ROUTE & DOSAGE

Allergic Conjunctivitis

Adult: **Ophthalmic** 1 drop in affected eye q.i.d.

E

ADMINISTRATION

Instillation

- Wash hands before and after use. ▪ Shake well before using. Apply drops in the center of the lower conjunctional sac. Do not touch eyelids with dropper.
- Gently close eyes for 1–2 min after installation of drops.
- Wait 10 min after installation of drug before inserting soft lenses into eyes
- Store in a tightly closed bottle. Protect the solution from light.
- Do not use if discolored.

ADVERSE EFFECTS (≥1%) **CNS:** Headache. **Special Senses:** *Ocular irritation, mild transient stinging and burning,* conjunctival congestion, eyelid edema, eye pain, photophobia, abnormal lacrimation.

INTERACTIONS Drug: No clinically significant interactions established.

PHARMACOKINETICS Absorption: Minimal. **Half-Life:** 3–4 h.

NURSING IMPLICATIONS

Assessment & Drug Effects

- Monitor for S&S of hypersensitivity to the drug (see Appendix F).
- Evaluate safety of engaging in hazardous activities since drowsiness is a potential adverse effect.

Patient & Family Education

- Learn potential adverse responses to emedastine.
- Eye drops contain benzalkonium chloride, which may damage soft contact lenses. After instillation of drops, wait 10 min before inserting these contact lenses into the eye.
- Contact your physician if symptoms do not start to improve in 2 or 3 days.

EMLA (EUTECTIC MIXTURE OF LIDOCAINE AND PRILOCAINE)

EMLA Cream

Classification: LOCAL ANESTHETIC
Therapeutic: LOCAL ANESTHETIC
Prototype: Procaine
Pregnancy Category: B

AVAILABILITY 2.5% lidocaine/2.5% prilocaine cream

ACTION & *THERAPEUTIC EFFECT* EMLA cream is a mixture of lidocaine and prilocaine. The mixture forms a liquid at room temperature. *EMLA is a topical analgesic.*

USES Topical anesthetic on normal intact skin for local anesthesia.
UNLABELED USES Topical anesthetic prior to leg ulcer debridement; treatment of postherpetic neuralgia.

CONTRAINDICATIONS Patients with known sensitivity to local anesthetics; patients with congenital or idiopathic methemoglobinemia; tympanic membrane perforation; children younger than 1 mo of age.
CAUTIOUS USE Acutely ill, debilitated, or older adult patients; severe liver disease; pregnancy (category B), lactation.

ROUTE & DOSAGE

Topical Anesthetic

Adult/Child (older than 1 mo): **Topical** Apply 2.5 g of cream (1/2 of 5-g tube) over 20–25 cm² of skin, cover with occlusive dressing and wait at least 1 h, then remove dressing and wipe off cream, cleanse area with an antiseptic solution and prepare patient for the procedure

ADMINISTRATION

Topical

- Apply a thick layer to skin (approximately 1/2 of 5-g tube per 20–25 cm^2 or 2 × 2 in) at site of procedure. Apply an occlusive dressing. Do not spread out cream. Seal edges of dressing well to avoid leakage.
- Apply EMLA cream 1 h before routine procedure and 2 h before painful procedure.
- Remove EMLA cream prior to skin puncture and clean area with an aseptic solution.
- Store at room temperature 15°–30° C (59°–86° F).

ADVERSE EFFECTS (≥1%) **Hematologic:** Methemoglobinemia, especially in infants, small children, and patients with G6PD deficiency. **Skin:** *Blanching and redness,* itching, heat sensation. **Body as a Whole:** Edema, soreness, aching, numbness, heaviness. **Other:** The adverse effects of lidocaine could occur with large doses or if there is significant systemic absorption.

INTERACTIONS Drug: May cause additive toxicity with CLASS I ANTIARRHYTHMICS; may increase risk of developing methemoglobin when used with **acetaminophen, chloroquine, dapsone, fosphenytoin,** NITRATES and NITRITES, **nitric oxide, nitrofurantoin, nitroprusside, pamaquine, phenobarbital, phenytoin, primaquine, quinine,** or SULFONAMIDES.

PHARMACOKINETICS Absorption: Penetrates intact skin. **Onset:** 15–60 min. **Peak:** 2–3 h. **Duration:** 1–2 h after removal of cream. **Distribution:** Crosses blood–brain barrier and placenta, distributed into breast milk. **Metabolism:** In liver. **Elimination:** 98% of absorbed dose is excreted in urine. **Half-Life:** 60–150 min.

NURSING IMPLICATIONS

Assessment & Drug Effects

- Monitor for local skin reactions including erythema, edema, itching, abnormal temperature sensations, and rash. These reactions are very common and usually disappear in 1–2 h.
- Note: Patients taking Class I antiarrhythmic drugs may experience toxic effects on the cardiovascular system. EMLA should be used with caution in these patients.
- Wash immediately with water or saline if contact with the eye occurs; protect the eye until sensation returns.

Patient & Family Education

- Skin analgesia lasts for 1 h following removal of the occlusive dressing. Analgesia may be accompanied by temporary loss of all sensation in the treated skin. Advise caution until sensation returns.

EMTRICITABINE

(em-tri′ci-ta-been)

Emtriva

Classifications: ANTIRETROVIRAL; NUCLEOSIDE REVERSE TRANSCRIPTASE INHIBITOR (NRTI)

Therapeutic: ANTIRETROVIRAL, NRTI

Prototype: Zidovudine

Pregnancy Category: D

AVAILABILITY 200 mg capsules; 10 mg/mL oral solution

ACTION & *THERAPEUTIC EFFECT* Emtricitabine is a synthetic nucleoside reverse transcriptase analogue with inhibitory activity against HIV-1. It inhibits HIV-1 reverse transcriptase (RT), both by competing with the natural DNA nucleoside and by incorporation into viral DNA, which terminates the formation of the viral DNA chain. *The viral load is decreased as measured by an increase in CD4 leukocyte count and suppression of viral RNA.*

USES Treatment of HIV in combination with other antiretroviral agents.

UNLABELED USES Treatment of chronic hepatitis B in HIV-positive patients.

CONTRAINDICATIONS Children younger than 3 mo; suicidal ideation; HBV infection; pregnancy (category D); lactation.

CAUTIOUS USE Renal impairment, and with end-stage renal disease; hepatic impairment; history of mental illness including bipolar disorder, psychosis; alcoholism; substance abuse; seizure disorders; hypercholesterolemia, hypertriglyceridemia.

ROUTE & DOSAGE

HIV

Adult: **PO** 200 mg once/day
Child (3 mo–17 y): **PO** 6 mg/kg days (max: 240 mg/day) OR if *weight greater than 33 kg,* 200 mg daily

Renal Impairment Dosage Adjustment

CrCl 30–49 mL/min: 200 mg q48h; 15–29 mL/min: 200 mg q72h; less than 15 mL/min: 200 mg q96h

ADMINISTRATION

Oral

- Give at the same time daily.
- Store between 15°–30° C (59°–86° F) in a tightly closed container.

ADVERSE EFFECTS (≥1%) **Body as a Whole:** Asthenia, neuropathy, peripheral neuritis. **CNS:** *Headache,* depression, dizziness, insomnia. **GI:** *Diarrhea, nausea,* dyspepsia, abdominal pain, hepatomegaly. **Metabolic:** Lactic acidosis. **Musculoskeletal:** Arthralgia, myalgia, paresthesias. **Respiratory:** Cough, rhinitis. **Skin:** *Rash,* hyperpigmentation of palms and soles of feet.

INTERACTIONS None yet reported.

PHARMACOKINETICS Absorption: 93% reaches systemic circulation. **Peak:** 1–2 h. **Distribution:** 4% protein bound. **Metabolism:** In liver. **Elimination:** Urine. **Half-Life:** 10 h (active metabolite has intracellular half-life of 39 h).

NURSING IMPLICATIONS

Assessment & Drug Effects

- Monitor individuals with a history of depression for S&S of suicidal ideation.
- Monitor closely for S&S of lactic acidosis, especially in persons with known risk factors such as female gender, obesity, alcoholism, or hepatic disease.
- Withhold drug and notify physician if S&S suggestive of lactic acidosis or hepatotoxicity occur.
- Lab tests: Baseline renal function tests; frequent LFTs and serum electrolytes during the last trimester of pregnancy; complete blood chemistry if lactic acidosis is suspected; and periodic lipid profile; serum cholesterol and triglycerides; bone density monitoring for history of osteoporosis.
- Monitor closely for severe exacerbation of hepatitis B in coinfected patients if this drug is discontinued.

Patient & Family Education

- May cause serious CNS effects. Avoid driving or operating machinery until individual reaction to the drug is known.
- Report any of the following to the physician: Difficulty breath-

ing, shortness of breath, fast or irregular heartbeat; weight gain with fullness around waist and/or face; vomiting or diarrhea; unexplained muscle aches, pains, weakness, or fatigue; yellow eyes or skin.
- Avoid alcoholic drinks while taking this drug.
- Do not self-treat nausea, vomiting, or stomach pain. Contact physician for guidance.

ENALAPRIL MALEATE Pr

(e-nal′a-pril)
Vasotec

ENALAPRILAT

Vasotec I.V.
Classifications: ANGIOTENSIN-CONVERTING ENZYME (ACE) INHIBITOR; ANTIHYPERTENSIVE
Therapeutic: ANTIHYPERTENSIVE
Pregnancy Category: C first trimester; D second and third trimester

AVAILABILITY 2.5 mg, 5 mg, 10 mg, 20 mg tablets; 1.25 mg/mL injection

ACTION & *THERAPEUTIC EFFECT* Angiotensin-converting enzyme (ACE) inhibitor that catalyzes the conversion of angiotensin I to angiotensin II, a vasoconstrictor substance. Therefore, inhibition of ACE decreases angiotensin II levels, thus decreasing vasopressor activity and aldosterone secretion. Both actions achieve an antihypertensive effect by suppression of the renin–angiotensin–aldosterone system. ACE inhibitors also reduce peripheral arterial resistance (afterload), pulmonary capillary wedge pressure (PCWP), a measure of preload, pulmonary vascular resistance, and improve cardiac output as well as exercise tolerance. *Antihypertensive effect lowers blood pressure. Improvement in cardiac output results in increased exercise tolerance.*

USES Management of mild to moderate hypertension. Malignant, refractory, accelerated, and renovascular hypertension (except in bilateral renal artery stenosis or renal artery stenosis in a solitary kidney), CHF.
UNLABELED USES Hypertension or renal crisis in scleroderma.

CONTRAINDICATIONS Hypersensitivity to enalapril or captopril; hypotension. There has been evidence of fetotoxicity and kidney damage in newborns exposed to ACE inhibitors during pregnancy (category D second and third trimester); infants and children with CrCl less than 30 mL/min/1.73 m^2; lactation.
CAUTIOUS USE Renal impairment, renal artery stenosis; patients with hypovolemia, receiving diuretics; undergoing dialysis; hepatic disease; bone marrow suppression; patients in whom excessive hypotension would present a hazard (e.g., cerebrovascular insufficiency); CHF; aortic stenosis, cardiomyopathy hepatic impairment; diabetes mellitus; pregnancy (category C first trimester).

ROUTE & DOSAGE

Hypertension
Adult: **PO** 2.5–5 mg/day, may increase to 10–40 mg/day in 1–2 divided doses **IV** 0.625–1.25 mg q6h, may give up to 5 mg q6h in hypertensive emergencies
Neonate: **PO** 0.1 mg/kg q24h

E

Child: **PO** 0.08 mg/kg/day in 1–2 divided doses, may increase (max: 5 mg/kg/day) **IV** 5–10 mcg/kg/dose q8–24h

Congestive Heart Failure

Adult: **PO** 2.5 mg b.i.d., may increase up to 5–20 mg/day in 1–2 divided doses (max: 40 mg/day)

Renal Impairment Dosage Adjustment

Enalapril: CrCl less than 30 mL/min, start with 2.5 mg dose then titrate

Enalaprilat: CrCl less than 30 mL/min, start with dose of 0.625 mg q6h then titrate

Hemodialysis Dosage Adjustment: Administer post-dialysis or give 20–25% supplemental dose

ADMINISTRATION

Oral

- Discontinue diuretics, if possible, for 2–3 days prior to initial oral dose to reduce incidence of hypotension. If the diuretic cannot be discontinued, give an initial dose of 2.5 mg. Keep patient under medical supervision for at least 2 h and until BP has stabilized for at least an additional hour.
- Give with food or drink of patient's choice.
- Protect from heat and light. Expiration date: 30 mo following date of manufacture if stored at less than 30° C.
- Store tablets at 30° C (86° F); protect from heat and light.

Intravenous

Note: Verify correct IV concentration and rate of infusion/injection with physician for neonates, infants, children.

PREPARE: **Direct:** Give undiluted. **Intermittent:** Dilute in 50 mL of D5W, NS, D5/NS, D5/LR.

ADMINISTER: **Direct/Intermittent:** Give direct IV slowly over at least 5 min through a port of a free flowing infusion of D5W or NS or as an infusion over 5 min. ▪ Longer infusion time decreases risk of severe hypotension.

INCOMPATIBILITIES **Y-site: Amphotericin B, amphotericin B cholesteryl, caspofungin, cefepime, dantrolene, diazepam, lansoprazole, phenytoin.**

ADVERSE EFFECTS (≥1%) **CNS:** *Headache, dizziness,* fatigue, nervousness, paresthesias, asthenia, insomnia, somnolence. **CV:** *Hypotension including postural hypotension;* syncope, palpitations, chest pain. **GI:** Diarrhea, nausea, abdominal pain, loss of taste, dyspepsia. **Hematologic:** Decreased Hgb and Hct. **Urogenital:** Acute kidney failure, deterioration in kidney function. **Skin:** Pruritus with and without *rash,* angioedema, erythema. **Metabolic:** Hyperkalemia. **Respiratory:** Cough. **Whole Body:** Angioedema.

INTERACTIONS Drug: Indomethacin and other NSAIDS may decrease antihypertensive activity; POTASSIUM SUPPLEMENTS, POTASSIUM-SPARING DIURETICS may cause hyperkalemia; may increase **lithium** levels and toxicity.

PHARMACOKINETICS Absorption: 70% from GI tract. **Onset:** 1 h PO; 15 min IV. **Peak:** 4–8 h PO; 4 h IV. **Duration:** 12–24 h PO; 6 h IV. **Distribution:** Limited amount crosses blood–brain barrier; crosses placenta. **Metabolism:** PO dose undergoes first-pass metabolism in liver to active form, enalaprilat. **Elimina-**

tion: 60% in urine, 33% in feces within 24 h. **Half-Life:** 2 h.

NURSING IMPLICATIONS

Assessment & Drug Effects

- Monitor for therapeutic effectiveness. Peak effects after the first IV dose may not occur for up to 4 h; peak effects of subsequent doses may exceed those of the first.
- Maintain bedrest and monitor BP for the first 3 h after the initial IV dose. First-dose phenomenon (i.e., a sudden exaggerated hypotensive response) may occur within 1–3 h of first IV dose, especially in the patient with very high blood pressure or one on a diuretic and controlled salt intake regimen. An IV infusion of normal saline for volume expansion may be ordered to counteract the hypotensive response. This initial response is not an indicator to stop therapy.
- Monitor BP for first several days of therapy. If antihypertensive effect is diminished before 24 h, the total dose may be given as 2 divided doses.
- Report transient hypotension with lightheadedness. Older adults are particularly sensitive to drug-induced hypotension. Supervise ambulation until BP has stabilized.
- Lab tests: Monitor serum potassium and be alert to symptoms of hyperkalemia (K^+ greater than 5.7 mEq/L). Patients who have diabetes, impaired kidney function, or CHF are at risk of developing hyperkalemia during enalapril treatment. Monitor kidney function closely during first few weeks of therapy.

Patient & Family Education

- Full antihypertensive effect may not be experienced until several weeks after enalapril therapy starts.
- When drug is discontinued due to severe hypotension, the hypotensive effect may persist a week or longer after termination because of long duration of drug action.
- Do not follow a low-sodium diet (e.g., low-sodium foods or low-sodium milk) without approval from physician.
- Avoid use of salt substitute (principal ingredient: potassium salt) and potassium supplements because of the potential for hyperkalemia.
- Notify physician of a persistent nonproductive cough, especially at night, accompanied by nasal congestion.
- Report to physician promptly if swelling of face, eyelids, tongue, lips, or extremities occurs. Angioedema is a rare adverse effect and, if accompanied by laryngeal edema, may be fatal.
- Do not drive or engage in other potentially hazardous activities until response to drug is known.

E

ENFUVIRTIDE

(en-fu-vir′tide)

Fuzeon

Classifications: ANTIRETROVIRAL; FUSION INHIBITOR

Therapeutic: ANTIRETROVIRAL; FUSION INHIBITOR

Pregnancy Category: C

AVAILABILITY 90 mg/mL injection

ACTION & *THERAPEUTIC EFFECT*

Enfuvirtide interferes with entry of HIV-1 into host cells by inhibiting fusion of the virus with the host cell membranes. In order for HIV-1 to enter and infect a human cell, the viral surface glycoprotein (gp41) must bind to the host CD4+ cells. Then, the viral glycoprotein undergoes a change in shape facilitating the fusion of viral membranes with the host cell membrane. Prevents entry of the HIV-1 virus into host cells. *Effectiveness is measured in reduction of viral load as measured by an increase in CD4 leucocyte count and suppression of viral RNA.*

USES Treatment of advanced HIV disease with evidence of resistance to other therapies.

CONTRAINDICATIONS Hypersensitivity to enfuvirtide or any of its components; HIV/HBV co-infected patients; severe hepatomegaly; lactation.

CAUTIOUS USE Renal and hepatic impairment; renal clearance of less than 35 mL/min; bacterial pneumonia, low initial CD4 count, past history of lung disease, high initial viral load, IV drug use; mannitol hypersensitivity; history of pulmonary disease; pregnancy (category C).

ROUTE & DOSAGE

Advanced HIV Disease

Adult/Adolescent (16 y or older or weight 42.6 kg or more): Subcutaneous 90 mg b.i.d.

Child/Adolescent (6–16 y or weight less than 42.6 kg): Subcutaneous 2 mg/kg (up to 90 mg) b.i.d.

ADMINISTRATION

Subcutaneous

- Reconstitute by adding 1.1 mL sterile water for injection into vial. Mix by gently tapping vial for 10 sec, then gently rolling in palms of hands. Ensure that no drug is remaining on vial wall. Allow vial to stand until powder completely dissolves (up to 45 min). Solution should be clear, colorless, and without bubbles or particulate matter.
- Bring refrigerated reconstituted solution to room temperature before injection. Ensure that powder is fully dissolved and solution is clear, colorless, and without bubbles or particulate matter.
- Inject into upper arm, abdomen, or anterior thigh.
- Rotate injection sites and inject in an area with no current injection site reaction.
- Store unreconstituted vials at 15°–30° C (59°–86° F) or refrigerated at 2°–6° C (3°–46° F); do not freeze.

ADVERSE EFFECTS (≥1%) **Body as a Whole**: Injection site reactions (pain, induration, erythema, nodules, cysts, pruritus, ecchymoses), infection at injection site, fatigue, systemic hypersensitivity reactions, Guillain-Barré syndrome, asthenia, herpes simplex infections, influenza, lymphadenopathy, myalgia, peripheral neuropathy. **CNS**: Anxiety, depression, insomnia. **GI**: Diarrhea, nausea, abdominal pain, anorexia, constipation, dysgeusia, pancreatitis, weight loss. **Hematologic**: Eosinophilia, anemia. **Metabolic**: Increased amylase, increased lipase, increased ALT and AST, hypertriglyceridemia. **Respiratory**: Bacterial pneumonia, acute respiratory distress syndrome, cough, sinusitis. **Skin**: Pruritus, skin papilloma. **Special Senses**: Conjunctivitis. **Urogenital**: Glomerulonephritis.

INTERACTIONS Increases levels of **tripranavir** (dose adjustment not needed).

PHARMACOKINETICS Absorption: 84.3% absorbed from subcutaneous site. **Peak**: Average 4–8 h. **Distribution**: 92% protein bound. **Metabolism**: Catabolized into constituent amino acids. **Half-Life**: 4 h.

NURSING IMPLICATIONS

Assessment & Drug Effects

- Inspect subcutaneous sites for S&S of site reactions (e.g., itching, swelling, redness, pain, tenderness, or hardened skin) that usually last for less than 7 days postinjection.
- Monitor closely for S&S of pneumonia, especially with low initial CD4 count, high initial viral load, IV drug use, smoking, or prior history of lung disease.
- Lab tests: Periodic LFTs, serum lipase and amylase, lipid profile, and CBC with differential.

Patient & Family Education

- Report promptly S&S of infection at subcutaneous injection sites: Increased heat, redness, pain, or oozing.
- Report promptly S&S of pneumonia: Cough with fever, rapid breathing, shortness of breath.

ENOXAPARIN Pr

(e-nox′a-pa-rin)

Lovenox

Classifications: ANTICOAGULANT; LOW MOLECULAR WEIGHT HEPARIN

Therapeutic: ANTICOAGULANT; ANTITHROMBOTIC

Pregnancy Category: B

AVAILABILITY 30 mg/0.3 mL, 40 mg/0.4 mL, 60 mg/0.6 mL, 80 mg/0.8 mL, 100 mg/1 mL injection

ACTION & *THERAPEUTIC EFFECT* Low molecular weight heparin with antithrombotic properties. Does affect thrombin time (TT) and activated thromboplastin time (aPTT) up to 1.8 times the control value. Antithrombotic properties are due to its antifactor Xa and antithrombin (antifactor IIa) in the coagulation activities. *An effective anticoagulation agent, it is used for prophylactic treatment as an antithrombotic agent following certain types of surgery.*

USES Prevention of deep vein thrombosis (DVT) after hip, knee, or abdominal surgery, treatment of DVT and pulmonary embolism, management of acute ST elevation myocardial infarction (STEMI), non-Q wave MI.

CONTRAINDICATIONS Patients with active major bleeding, GI bleeding, hemophilia, heparin hypersensitivity, heparin-induced thrombocytopenia (HIT), thrombocytopenia associated with an antiplatelet antibody in the presence of enoxaparin, bleeding disorders, idiopathic thrombocytopenic purpura (ITP), hypersensitivity to enoxaparin; porcine protein hypersensitivity, neonates, infants and children.

CAUTIOUS USE Uncontrolled arterial hypertension, recent history of GI disease, conditions or surgery with increased risk of bleeding, hepatic disease, hypertension, coagulopathy, thrombocytopenia, dental disease, diabetic retinopathy, dialysis, diverticulitis, inflammatory bowel disease, peptic ulcer disease, older adults, endocarditis, renal disease, renal impairment, stroke, surgery, pregnancy (category B), lactation.

ROUTE & DOSAGE

Prevention of DVT after Hip or Knee Surgery

Adult: **Subcutaneous** 30 mg b.i.d. for 10–14 days starting 12–24 h post-surgery

Prevention of DVT after Abdominal Surgery

Adult: **Subcutaneous** 40 mg daily starting 2 h before surgery and continuing for 7–10 days (max: 12 days)

Treatment of DVT and Pulmonary Embolus

Adult: **Subcutaneous** 1 mg/kg q12h or 1.5 mg/kg/day; monitor anti-Xa activity to determine appropriate dose

Non-Q Wave MI

Adult: **Subcutaneous** 1 mg/kg q12h for 2–8 days, give concurrently with aspirin 100–325 mg/day

Acute STEMI

Adult: **IV** 30 mg bolus plus 1 mg/kg subcutaneously, then 1 mg/kg q12h subcutaneously

Renal Impairment Dosage Adjustment

CrCl less than 30 mL/min: 30 mg or 1 mg/kg q24h

E

ADMINISTRATION

Subcutaneous

- Use a TB syringe or prefilled syringe to ensure accurate dosage.
- Do not expel the air bubble from the 30 or 40 mg prefilled syringe before injection.
- Place patient in a supine position for injection of the drug.
- Alternate injections between left and right anterolateral and posterolateral abdominal wall.
- Hold the skin fold between the thumb and forefinger and insert the whole length of the needle into the skin fold. Hold skin fold throughout the injection. Do not rub site post-injection.
- Store at 15°–30° C (59°–86° F).

Intravenous

PREPARE: **Direct:** Give undiluted.

ADMINISTER: **Direct:** Give bolus dose direct IV through an IV line. Flush before and after with NS or D5W to ensure that the IV line has been cleared. Do not mix with any other drugs or solutions.

ADVERSE EFFECTS (≥1%) **Body as a Whole:** Allergic reactions (rash, urticaria), fever, angioedema, arthralgia, pain and inflammation at injection site, peripheral edema, fever. **Digestive:** Abnormal liver function tests. **Hematologic:** *Hemorrhage,* thrombocytopenia, ecchymoses, anemia. **Respiratory:** Dyspnea. **Skin:** Rash, pruritus.

INTERACTIONS Drug: Aspirin, NSAIDS, **warfarin** can increase risk of hemorrhage. **Herbal: Garlic, ginger, ginkgo, feverfew, horse chestnut** may increase risk of bleeding.

PHARMACOKINETICS Absorption: 91% absorbed from subcutaneous injection site. **Peak:** 3 h. **Duration:** 4.6 h. **Distribution:** Appears to accumulate in liver, kidneys, and spleen. Does not cross placenta. **Elimination:** Primarily in urine. **Half-Life:** 4.6 h.

NURSING IMPLICATIONS

Assessment & Drug Effects

- Lab tests: Baseline coagulation studies; periodic CBC, platelet count, urine and stool for occult blood.
- Monitor platelet count closely. Withhold drug and notify physician if platelet count less than 100,000/mm^3.
- Monitor closely patients with renal insufficiency and older adults who are at higher risk for thrombocytopenia.
- Monitor for and report immediately any sign or symptom of unexplained bleeding.

Patient & Family Education

- Report to physician promptly signs of unexplained bleeding such as: Pink, red, or dark brown urine; red or dark brown vomitus; bleeding gums or bloody sputum; dark, tarry stools.
- Do not take any OTC drugs without first consulting physician.

ENTACAPONE

(en-ta′ca-pone)

Comtan

Classifications: CATECHOLAMINE O-METHYLTRANSFERASE (COMT) INHIBITOR; ANTIPARKINSON

Therapeutic: ANTIPARKINSON

Prototype: Tolcapone

Pregnancy Category: C

AVAILABILITY 200 mg tablets

ACTION & *THERAPEUTIC EFFECT* Selective inhibitor of catecholamine O-methyltransferase (COMT). COMT is responsible for metabolizing levodopa to an intermediate compound 3-O-methyldopa, a chemical which interferes with the availability of levodopa to the brain. Therefore, it increases availability of levodopa in CNS. *Taken with levodopa, it decreases the formation of 3-O-methyldopa, thus increasing the duration of the motor response of the brain to levodopa in Parkinson's disease, diminishing Parkinson's manifestations.*

USES Adjunct to levodopa/carbidopa to treat Parkinson's disease.

CONTRAINDICATIONS Hypersensitivity to entacapone; concurrent MAO inhibitors; children.

CAUTIOUS USE Hepatic impairment; biliary obstruction; concomitant administration with CNS depressants; drugs metabolized by COMT (e.g., isoproterenol, epinephrine, etc.); history of hypotension or syncope; pregnancy (category C), lactation.

ROUTE & DOSAGE

Parkinson's Disease

Adult: **PO** 200 mg administered with each dose of levodopa/carbidopa up to 8 times/day

ADMINISTRATION

Oral

- Give simultaneously with each levodopa/carbidopa dose.
- **Must be** tapered if discontinued. Never discontinue abruptly.
- Do not administer to patients receiving nonselective MAO inhibitors.
- Store at 15°–30° C (59°–86° F).

ADVERSE EFFECTS (≥1%) **Body as a Whole:** Back pain, fatigue, asthenia. **CNS:** *Dyskinesia, hyperkinesia,* hypokinesia, dizziness, anxiety, somnolence, agitation. **GI:** Taste perversion, *nausea, diarrhea,* abdominal pain, constipation, vomiting, dry mouth, dyspepsia, flatulence, gastritis. **Respiratory:** Dyspnea. **Skin:** Increased sweating. **Other:** *Urine discoloration,* purpura.

INTERACTIONS Drug: Extreme caution **must be** used if administered with a nonselective MAOI; **bitolterol, dobutamine, dopamine, epinephrine, isoetharine, isoproterenol, methyldopa, norepinephrine** may increase heart rates, possibly cause arrhythmias, excessive changes in BP.

PHARMACOKINETICS Absorption: Rapidly absorbed, 35% bioavailable. **Peak:** 1 h. **Distribution:** Highly protein bound. **Metabolism:** Extensively metabolized in plasma and erythrocytes. **Elimination:** Primarily in feces. **Half-Life:** 2.4 h (terminal).

NURSING IMPLICATIONS

Assessment & Drug Effects

- Monitor carefully for hyperpyrexia, confusion, or emergence of Parkinson's S&S during drug withdrawal.
- Monitor for orthostatic hypotension and worsening of dyskinesia or hyperkinesia.
- Lab tests: Hgb and serum ferritin levels with prolonged therapy.

Patient & Family Education

- Take with levodopa/carbidopa; not effective alone.
- Do not discontinue abruptly; gradually reduce dosage.
- Exercise caution when rising from a sitting or lying position because faintness/dizziness can occur.
- Exercise caution with hazardous activities until reaction to the drug is known.
- Harmless brownish-orange discoloration of urine is possible.
- Report unusual adverse effects (e.g., hallucinations/unexplained diarrhea).

ENTECAVIR

(en-te'ca-vir)

Baraclude

Classifications: ANTIRETROVIRAL; NUCLEOSIDE REVERSE TRANSCRIPTASE INHIBITOR (NRTI)

Therapeutic: ANTIRETROVIRAL; NRTI

Prototype: Lamivudine

Pregnancy Category: C

AVAILABILITY 0.5 and 1 mg tablets; 0.05 mg/mL oral solution

ACTION & *THERAPEUTIC EFFECT* Inhibits hepatitis B viral (HBV) DNA polymerase by inhibiting viral reverse transcriptase of messenger RNA that ultimately results in inhibiting the synthesis of HBV DNA. *The antiviral activity of entecavir inhibits HBV DNA synthesis.*

USES Treatment of chronic hepatitis B infection in patients who have shown resistance to lamivudine or in nucleoside-treatment-naïve patients.

CONTRAINDICATIONS Hypersensitivity to entecavir; lactic acidosis; severe hepatomegaly; HIV/HVB co-infected patients, if HIV is not being treated; lactation. Safety and effectiveness in children younger than 16 y have not been established.

CAUTIOUS USE Liver transplant patients; HIV patients; concurrent use of cyclosporine; renal impairment, ESRF, dialysis; labor and delivery; pregnancy (category C).

ROUTE & DOSAGE

Chronic Hepatitis B (nucleoside-treatment–naïve patients)

Adult/Adolescent (16 y or older): **PO** 0.5 mg daily

Chronic Hepatitis B (lamivudine-resistant patients)

Adult/Adolescent (16 y or older): **PO** 1 mg daily

Renal Impairment Dosage Adjustment

CrCl 30–49 mL/min: Decrease dose by 50%; 10–29 mL/min: Decrease dose by 70%; less than 10 mL/min: Decrease dose by 90%

ADMINISTRATION

Oral

- Give on an empty stomach (at least 2 h before/after a meal).

- Administer after hemodialysis.
- Store in a tightly closed container at 15°–30° C (59°–86° F)

ADVERSE EFFECTS (≥1%) **CNS:** Dizziness, fatigue, headache, insomnia, somnolence. **GI:** Diarrhea, dyspepsia, nausea, vomiting. **Metabolic:** Elevated liver enzymes (ALT, AST), hyperamylasemia, elevated lipase concentration, hyperbilirubinemia, fasting hyperglycemia, glycosuria, hematuria, lactic acidosis.

INTERACTIONS Drug: Use of entecavir with drugs that reduce renal function or compete for active tubular secretion may increase serum concentrations of either drug. **Food:** High-fat meal reduces oral absorption.

PHARMACOKINETICS Peak: 0.5–1 h. **Distribution:** 13% protein bound. **Metabolism:** Minimal. **Elimination:** Primarily in the urine. **Half-Life:** 128–149 h.

NURSING IMPLICATIONS

Assessment & Drug Effects

- Monitor closely for adverse reactions when drugs that are known to affect renal function are taken concurrently.
- Lab tests: Periodic LFTs during treatment and for several months after drug is discontinued; periodic fasting plasma glucose.
- Monitor for S&S of lactic acidosis, including respiratory distress, tachycardia, and irregular HR.

Patient & Family Education

- Follow directions for taking the drug (see ADMINISTRATION).
- Do not discontinue medication without consent of physician.
- Do not drive or engage in potentially hazardous activities until response to drug is known.
- Inform physician if you are or plan to become pregnant.
- Report any of the following to a health care provider: Unexplained tiredness or weakness, unusual muscle pain, difficulty breathing, cold extremities, dizziness or lightheadedness, irregular heartbeat, loss of appetite, stomach pain, nausea, vomiting, clay-colored stool, dark urine, or jaundice.

E

EPHEDRINE HYDROCHLORIDE

(e-fed′rin)
Efedron

EPHEDRINE SULFATE

Ectasule, Ephedsol, Vatronol
Classifications: ALPHA- AND BETA-ADRENERGIC AGONIST; BRONCHODILATOR
Therapeutic: BRONCHODILATOR
Prototype: Epinephrine HCl
Pregnancy Category: C

AVAILABILITY 25 mg capsules; 50 mg/mL injection; 0.25% nasal spray; 1% nasal gel

ACTION & *THERAPEUTIC EFFECT* Both indirect- and direct-acting sympathomimetic amine. Thought to act indirectly by releasing tissue stores of norepinephrine and directly by stimulation of alpha-, $beta_1$-, and $beta_2$-adrenergic receptors. Like epinephrine, contracts dilated arterioles of nasal mucosa, thus reducing engorgement and edema and facilitating ventilation and drainage. *Ephedrine relaxes bronchial smooth muscle, relieving mild bronchospasm, improving air exchange and increasing vital capacity.*

USES Temporary relief of congestion of hay fever, allergic rhinitis, and sinusitis; and in treatment and prophylaxis of mild cases of acute asthma and in patients with chronic asthma requiring continuing treatment. Also has been used for its CNS stimulant actions in treatment of narcolepsy, to improve respiration in narcotic and barbiturate poisoning, to combat hypotensive states, especially those associated with spinal anesthesia; in management of enuresis or impaired bladder control; as adjunct in treatment of myasthenia gravis; as mydriatic; to relieve dysmenorrhea; and for temporary support of ventricular rate in Adams-Stokes syndrome; for peripheral edema secondary to type I diabetic neuropathy.

CONTRAINDICATIONS History of hypersensitivity to ephedrine or other sympathomimetics; narrow-angle glaucoma; angina pectoris, coronary insufficiency, chronic heart disease, uncontrolled hypertension, cardiac arrhythmias, cardiomyopathy; hypovolemia; concurrent MAOI therapy; lactation.

CAUTIOUS USE Hypertension, arteriosclerosis, closed-angle glaucoma; diabetes mellitus; hyperthyroidism; prostatic hypertrophy; pregnancy (category C).

ROUTE & DOSAGE

Bronchodilator, Nasal Decongestant

Adult: **PO** 25–50 mg q3–4h prn (max: 150 mg/24 h)
IM/IV/Subcutaneous 12.5–25 mg

Child: **PO** *Older than 2 y,* 2–3 mg/kg/day in 4–6 divided doses; *6–12 y,* 6.25–12.5 mg q4h (max: 75 mg/24 h)

Hypotension

Adult: **PO** 25 mg 1–4 times/day (max: 150 mg/24 h)
IM/Subcutaneous/IV 10–50 mg IM/Subcutaneous or 10–25 mg slow IV, may repeat in 5–10 min if necessary (max: 150 mg/24 h)

Child: **PO/IM/Subcutaneous/IV** 3 mg/kg/day in 4–6 divided doses (max: 75 mg/24 h)

Myasthenia Gravis

Adult: **PO** 25 mg t.i.d. or q.i.d.

Enuresis

Adult: **PO** 25 mg at bedtime

Urinary Incontinence

Geriatric: **PO** 25–50 mg q6h

Nasal Decongestant

Adult: **Intranasal** 2–4 drops or a small amount of jelly in each nostril no more than q.i.d. for 3–4 consecutive days

ADMINISTRATION

Oral

- Administer last dose a few hours before bedtime, if possible, to minimize insomnia.
- Store at 15°–30° C (59°–86° F) in tightly closed, light-resistant containers unless otherwise directed by the manufacturer.

Intranasal

- Have patient clear nose before instilling nasal preparation.

Subcutaneous/Intramuscular

- Give undiluted.

Intravenous

PREPARE: **Direct:** Give undiluted.
ADMINISTER: **Direct:** Direct IV at a rate of 10 mg or fraction thereof over 30–60 sec.
INCOMPATIBILITIES **Solution/additive:** **Hydrocortisone, pentobarbital, phenobarbital, secobarbital, thiopental.** **Y-site:** **Thiopental.**

- Store in tightly closed, light-resistant containers. Do not use liquid formulation unless it is absolutely clear.

ADVERSE EFFECTS (≥1%) **CNS:** Headache, insomnia, *nervousness,* anxiety, tremulousness, giddiness. **CV:** Palpitation, tachycardia, precordial pain, cardiac arrhythmias. **GU:** Difficult or painful urination, acute urinary retention (especially older men with prostatism). **GI:** Nausea, vomiting, anorexia. **Body as a Whole:** Sweating, thirst, overdosage: Euphoria, confusion, delirium, convulsions, pyrexia, hypertension, rebound hypotension, respiratory difficulty. **Skin:** Fixed-drug eruption. **Topical Use:** *Burning, stinging,* dryness of nasal mucosa, sneezing, rebound congestion.

DIAGNOSTIC TEST INTERFERENCE Ephedrine is generally withdrawn at least 12 h before ***sensitivity tests*** are made to prevent false-positive reactions.

INTERACTIONS Drug: MAO INHIBITORS, TRICYCLIC ANTIDEPRESSANTS, **furazolidone, guanethidine** may increase alpha-adrenergic effects (headache, hyperpyrexia, hypertension); **sodium bicarbonate** decreases renal elimination of ephedrine, increasing its CNS effects; **epinephrine, norepinephrine** compound sympathomimetic effects; effects of ALPHA and BETA-BLOCKERS and ephedrine antagonized.

PHARMACOKINETICS Absorption: Readily absorbed from GI tract. **Peak:** 15 min–1 h. **Duration:** Bronchodilation 2–4 h; cardiac and pressor effects up to 4 h PO and 1 h IV. **Distribution:** Widely distributed; crosses blood–brain barrier and placenta; distributed into breast milk. **Metabolism:** Small amounts metabolized in liver. **Elimination:** In urine. **Half-Life:** 3–6 h.

NURSING IMPLICATIONS

Assessment & Drug Effects

- Supervise continuously patients receiving ephedrine IV. Take baseline BP and other vital signs. Check BP repeatedly during first 5 min, then q3–5min until stabilized.
- Monitor I&O ratio and pattern, especially in older male patients. Encourage patient to void before taking medication (see ADVERSE EFFECTS).
- Monitor for systemic effects of nose drops that can occur because of excessive dosage from rapid absorption of drug solution through nasal mucosa. This is most likely to occur in older adults.

Patient & Family Education

- Note: Ephedrine is a commonly abused drug. Learn adverse effects and dangers; take medication ONLY as prescribed.
- Do not take OTC medications for coughs, colds, allergies, or asthma unless approved by physician. Ephedrine is a common ingredient in these preparations.

EPINASTINE HYDROCHLORIDE

(e-pi-nas'teen)

Elestat

Pregnancy Category: C

See Appendix A-1.

EPINEPHRINE Pr

(ep-i-ne'frin)

Epinephrine Pediatric, EpiPen Auto-Injector, Primatene Mist Suspension

E

EPINEPHRINE BITARTRATE

AsthmaHaler, Bronkaid Mist Suspension, Bronitin Mist Suspension, Epitrate

EPINEPHRINE HYDROCHLORIDE

Adrenalin Chloride, Bronkaid Mistometer, Dysne-Inhal, Epifrin, SusPhrine ♣

EPINEPHRINE, RACEMIC

Vaponefrin ♣

Classifications: ALPHA- AND BETA-ADRENERGIC AGONIST; CARDIAC STIMULANT; VASOPRESSOR

Therapeutic: ANTI-ANAPHYLACTIC; VASOPRESSOR

Pregnancy Category: C

AVAILABILITY 1:100, 1:1000, 2.25% solution for inhalation; 0.35 mg, 0.2 mg spray; 1:1000, 1:2000, 1:10,000, 1:100,000 injection; 1:200 suspension; 0.1%, 0.5%, 1%, 2% ophth solution; 0.1% nasal solution

ACTION & *THERAPEUTIC EFFECT* A catecholamine that acts directly on both alpha and beta receptors; the most potent activator of alpha receptors. Strengthens myocardial contraction; increases systolic but may decrease diastolic blood pressure; increases cardiac rate and cardiac output. Constricts bronchial arterioles and inhibits histamine release, thus reducing congestion and edema and increasing tidal volume and vital capacity. Relaxes uterine smooth musculature and inhibits uterine contractions. *Reverses analphylatic reactions and provides temporary relief from acute asthmatic attack. Restores normal cardiac rhythm.*

USES Temporary relief of bronchospasm, acute asthmatic attack, mucosal congestion, hypersensitivity and anaphylactic reactions, syncope due to heart block or carotid sinus hypersensitivity, and to restore cardiac rhythm in cardiac arrest. Relaxes myometrium and inhibits uterine contractions; prolongs action and delays systemic absorption of local and intraspinal anesthetics. Used topically to control superficial bleeding. Ophthalmic preparation is used in management of simple (open-angle) glaucoma, generally as an adjunct to topical miotics and oral carbonic anhydrase inhibitors; also used as ophthalmic decongestant.

CONTRAINDICATIONS Hypersensitivity to sympathomimetic amines; narrow-angle glaucoma; hemorrhagic, traumatic, or cardiogenic shock; cardiac dilatation, cerebral arteriosclerosis, coronary insufficiency, arrhythmias, organic heart or brain disease; during second stage of labor; for local anesthesia of fingers, toes, ears, nose, genitalia.

CAUTIOUS USE Older adults or debilitated patients; prostatic hypertrophy; hypertension; diabetes mellitus; hyperthyroidism; Parkinson's disease; tuberculosis; psychoneurosis; in patients with long-standing bronchial asthma and emphysema with degenerative heart disease; pregnancy (category C), lactation.

ROUTE & DOSAGE

Anaphylaxis

Adult: **Subcutaneous** 0.1–0.5 mg q10–15min prn **IV** 0.1–0.25 mg q5–15min

Child: **Subcutaneous** 0.01 mL/kg of, 1:1000 q10–15min prn **IV** 0.01 mL/kg of 1:1000 q10–15min

Neonate: **IV Intratracheal** 0.01–0.05 mg/kg q3–5min prn

Cardiac Arrest

Adult: **IV** 1 mg q3–5min as needed **Intracardiac** 0.1–1 mg
Child: **IV** 0.01 mg/kg q3–5min as needed (max: 1 mg) **Intracardiac** 0.05–0.1 mg/kg

Asthma

Adult: **Subcutaneous** 0.1–0.5 mg q20min–4h **Inhalation** 1 inhalation q4h prn
Child: **Subcutaneous** 0.01 mL/kg of 1:1000 q20min–4h **Inhalation** 1 inhalation q4h prn

Glaucoma

Adult/Child: **Instillation** 1–2 drops 0.25–2% solution 1/day or b.i.d.

Ocular Mydriasis

See Appendix A-1

Nasal Hemostasis

Adult/Child: **Instillation** 1–2 drops 0.1% ophthalmic or 0.1% nasal solution

Topical Hemostatic

Adult/Child: **Topical** 1:50,000–1:1000 applied topically or 1:500,000–1:50,000 mixed with a local anesthetic

ADMINISTRATION

Inhalation

- Have patient in an upright position when aerosol preparation is used. The reclining position can result in overdosage by producing large droplets instead of fine spray.
- Instruct patient to rinse mouth and throat with water immediately after inhalation to avoid swallowing residual drug (may cause epigastric pain and systemic effects from the propellant in the aerosol preparation) and to prevent dryness of oropharyngeal membranes.

Instillation

- Instill nose drops with head in lateral, head-low position to prevent entry of drug into throat.
- Instruct patient to rinse nose dropper or spray tip with hot water after each use to prevent contamination of solution with nasal secretions.

Ophthalmic

- Remove soft contact lenses before instilling eye drops.
- Instruct patient to apply gentle finger pressure against nasolacrimal duct immediately after drug is instilled for at least 1 or 2 min following instillation to prevent excessive systemic absorption.

Subcutaneous

- Use tuberculin syringe to ensure greater accuracy in measurement of parenteral doses.
- Protect epinephrine injection from exposure to light at all times. Do not remove ampule or vial from carton until ready to use.
- Shake vial or ampule thoroughly to disperse particles before withdrawing epinephrine suspension into syringe; then inject promptly.
- Aspirate carefully before injecting epinephrine. Inadvertent IV injection of usual subcutaneous doses can result in sudden hypertension and possibly cerebral hemorrhage.
- Rotate injection sites and observe for signs of blanching. Vascular constriction from repeated injections may cause tissue necrosis.

Intravenous

Note: Verify correct rate of IV injection to neonates, infants, children with physician.

- Note: 1:1000 solution contains 1 mg/1 mL. 1:10,000 solution contains 0.1 mg/1 mL.

PREPARE: **Direct:** Dilute each 1 mg of 1:1000 solution with 10 mL of NS to yield 1:10,000 solution. ▪ The 1:10,000 solution may be given undiluted. **IV Infusion:** Dilute required dose in 250–500 mL of D5W.

ADMINISTER: **Direct:** Give each 1 mg over 1 min or longer; may give more rapidly in cardiac arrest. **IV Infusion:** 1–10 mcg/min titrated according to patient's condition.

INCOMPATIBILITIES **Solution/additive: Aminophylline, cephapirin, hyaluronidase, mephentermine, sodium bicarbonate, warfarin. Y-site: Ampicillin, thiopental, sodium bicarbonate.**

ADVERSE EFFECTS (≥1%) **Special Senses:** *Nasal burning or stinging,* dryness of nasal mucosa, sneezing, rebound congestion. *Transient stinging or burning of eyes,* lacrimation, brow ache, headache, rebound conjunctival hyperemia, allergy, iritis; with prolonged use: Melanin-like deposits on lids, conjunctiva, and cornea; corneal edema; loss of lashes (reversible); maculopathy with central scotoma in aphakic patients (reversible). **Body as a Whole:** *Nervousness,* restlessness, sleeplessness, fear, anxiety, *tremors,* severe headache, cerebrovascular accident, weakness, dizziness, syncope, pallor, sweating, dyspnea. **GI:** Nausea, vomiting. **CV:** Precordial pain, *palpitations,* hypertension, MI, tachyarrhythmias including ventricular fibrillation. **Respiratory:** Bronchial and pulmonary edema. **Urogenital:** Urinary retention. **Skin:** Tissue necrosis with repeated injections. **Metabolic:** Metabolic acidoses, elevated serum lactic acid, transient elevations of blood glucose. **CNS:** Altered state of perception and thought, psychosis.

INTERACTIONS Drug: May increase hypotension in circulatory collapse or hypotension caused by PHENOTHIAZINES, **oxytocin, entacapone.** Additive toxicities with other SYMPATHOMIMETICS **(albuterol, dobutamine, dopamine, isoproterenol, metaproterenol, norepinephrine, phenylephrine, phenylpropanolamine, pseudoephedrine, ritodrine, salmeterol, terbutaline),** MAO INHIBITORS, TRICYCLIC ANTIDEPRESSANTS. ALPHA- AND BETA-ADRENERGIC BLOCKING AGENTS (e.g., **ergotamine, propranolol**) antagonize effects of epinephrine. GENERAL ANESTHETICS increase cardiac irritability.

PHARMACOKINETICS Absorption: Inactivated in GI tract. **Onset:** 3–5 min, 1 h on conjunctiva. **Peak:** 20 min, 4–8 h on conjunctiva. **Duration:** 12–24 h topically. **Distribution:** Widely distributed; does not cross blood–brain barrier; crosses placenta. **Metabolism:** In tissue and liver by monoamine oxidase (MAO) and catecholamine-methyltransferase (COMT). **Elimination:** Small amount unchanged in urine; excreted in breast milk.

NURSING IMPLICATIONS

Assessment & Drug Effects

- Check BP repeatedly when epinephrine is administered IV during first 5 min, then q3–5min until stabilized.
- Monitor BP, pulse, respirations, and urinary output and observe patient closely following IV administration. Continuous cardiac monitoring is recommended during IV infusion. If disturbances in cardiac rhythm occur, withhold

epinephrine and notify physician immediately.
- Keep physician informed of any changes in intake-output ratio.
- Advise patient to report bronchial irritation, nervousness, or sleeplessness. Dosage should be reduced.
- Monitor blood glucose and HbA1C for loss of glycemic control if diabetic.

Patient & Family Education
- Report to physician if symptoms of asthma are not relieved in 20 min or if they become worse following inhalation.
- Be aware intranasal application may sting slightly.
- Administer ophthalmic drug at bedtime or following prescribed miotic to minimize mydriasis, with blurred vision and sensitivity to light (possible in some patients being treated for glaucoma).
- Transitory stinging may follow initial ophthalmic administration and that headache and browache occur frequently at first but usually subside with continued use. Notify physician if symptoms persist.
- Discontinue epinephrine eye drops and consult a physician if signs of hypersensitivity develop (edema of lids, itching, discharge, crusting eyelids).
- Learn how to administer epinephrine subcutaneously. Keep medication and equipment available for home emergency. Confer with physician.
- Advise patient to report bronchial irritation, nervousness, or sleeplessness. Dosage should be reduced.
- Report tolerance to physician; may occur with repeated or prolonged use. Continued use of epinephrine in the presence of tolerance can be dangerous.
- Take medication only as prescribed and immediately notify physician of onset of systemic effects of epinephrine.
- Discard discolored or precipitated solutions.

EPIRUBICIN HYDROCHLORIDE

(e-pi-roo′bi-sin)

Ellence

Classifications: ANTINEOPLASTIC; ANTIBIOTIC

Therapeutic: ANTINEOPLASTIC

Prototype: Doxorubicin HCl

Pregnancy Category: D

AVAILABILITY 2 mg/mL

ACTION & *THERAPEUTIC EFFECT* Cytotoxic antibiotic with wide spectrum of antitumor activity and strong immunosuppressive properties. Complexes with DNA causing the DNA helix to change shape, thus blocking effective DNA and RNA transcription. *Highly destructive to rapidly proliferating cells. Effectiveness indicated by tumor regression.*

USES Adjunctive therapy for axillary node-positive breast cancer.

CONTRAINDICATIONS Hypersensitivity to epirubicin and other related drugs; marked myelosuppression, severely impaired cardiac function, severe cardiac arrhythmias, recent MI; severe hepatic disease, jaundice; previous treatment with maximum doses of epirubicin, doxorubicin, or daunorubicin; pregnancy (category D), lactation.
CAUTIOUS USE Arrhythmias; mild or moderate liver dysfunction; severe renal insufficiency or renal failure.

ROUTE & DOSAGE

Breast Cancer

Adult: **IV** 100–120 mg/m² infused on day 1 of a 3–4 wk cycle or 50–60 mg/m² on day 1 and 8 of a 3–4 wk cycle (max cumulative dose: 900 mg/m²)

Hepatic Impairment Dosage Adjustment

Bilirubin 1.2–3 mg/dL: Give 50% of dose; bilirubin over 3 mg/dL: Give 25% of dose; bilirubin greater than 5 mg/dL: Skip dose

Toxicity Dosage Adjustment

Reduce dose by 25% if platelets less than 50,000/mm³, ANC less than 250/mm³, neutropenic fever, or grade 3 or 4 hematologic toxicity

ADMINISTRATION

Intravenous

Note: Pregnant women should **NOT** prepare or administer this drug. Wear protective goggles, gowns and disposable gloves and masks when handling this drug. Discard **ALL** equipment used in preparation of this drug in high-risk, waste-disposal bags for incineration. Treat accidental contact with skin or eyes by rinsing with copious amounts of water followed by prompt medical attention.

- Note: Reduce dosages when serum creatinine greater than 5 mg/dL or AST 2–4 times the upper limit of normal.

PREPARE: **IV Infusion:** Epirubicin is manufactured as a preservative-free ready-to-use solution. The contents of a vial **must be** used within 24 h of first penetrating the rubber stopper. Discard unused solution.

ADMINISTER: **IV Infusion:** Measure ordered dose and inject into a port of a freely flowing IV solution of D5W or NS over 3–20 min. ▪ **DO NOT** give by direct IV push into a vein. ▪ Avoid IV sites that enter small veins or repeated injections into the same vein. ▪ Monitor IV site closely for S&S of extravasation and if suspected, notify physician immediately.

INCOMPATIBILITIES **Solution/additive:** ALKALINE SOLUTIONS (including **sodium bicarbonate**), **fluorouracil, heparin.**

- Store between 2°–8° C (36°–46° F). Protect from light.

ADVERSE EFFECTS (≥1%) **Body as a Whole:** *Lethargy,* fever. **CV:** Asymptomatic decrease in LVEF, CHF. **GI:** *Nausea, vomiting, mucositis, diarrhea,* anorexia. **Hematologic:** <u>Leukopenia, neutropenia, anemia, thrombocytopenia, AML</u>. **Skin:** *Alopecia, injection site reaction,* rash, itching, skin changes. **Other:** *Amenorrhea, hot flashes, infection, conjunctivitis/keratitis,* <u>secondary acute myelogenous leukemia</u> (related to cumulative dose).

INTERACTIONS Drug: Cimetidine increases epirubicin levels; concomitant use with cardioactive drugs (e.g., CALCIUM CHANNEL BLOCKERS) may affect cardiac function.

PHARMACOKINETICS Distribution: Widely distributed, 77% protein bound, concentrated in red blood cells. **Metabolism:** Extensively in liver, blood and other organs. Clearance is reduced in patients with hepatic impairment. **Elimination:** Primarily in bile, some urinary excretion; clearance decreases in older adult female patients. **Half-Life:** 33 h.

NURSING IMPLICATIONS

Assessment & Drug Effects

- Withhold drug and notify physician of any of the following: Neutrophil count less than 1500 cells/mm^3, recent MI, suspicion of severe myocardial insufficiency.
- Obtain baseline and periodic (before each cycle of therapy) cardiac evaluation: Left ventricular ejection fraction, ECG and ECHO (tests are recommended especially in the presence of risk factors of cardiac toxicity).
- Monitor cardiac status closely throughout therapy as the risk of developing severe CHF increases rapidly when cumulative doses approach 900 mg/m^2. Report significant ECG changes immediately. Report immediately S&S of the following: Tachycardia, gallop rhythm, pleural effusion, pulmonary edema, dependent edema, ascites, or hepatomegaly.
- Lab tests: Baseline and periodic (before each cycle of therapy) CBC with differential, platelet count, serum total bilirubin, AST, serum creatinine.

Patient & Family Education

- Review all literature regarding the adverse effects of epirubicin therapy carefully.
- Report any of the following to physician immediately: Pain at the site of IV infusion, chest pain, palpitations, shortness of breath or difficulty breathing, sudden weight gain, swelling of hands, feet or legs, or any unexplained bleeding.
- Be aware that your urine may turn red for 1–2 days after receiving this drug. This change is expected and harmless.
- Do not take OTC cimetidine or any other OTC drug without consulting physician.
- Use effective means of contraception (both men and women) while on epirubicin therapy.

E

EPLERENONE

(e-ple′re-none)

Inspra

Classifications: ELECTROLYE & WATER BALANCE AGENT; SELECTIVE ALDOSTERONE RECEPTOR ANTAGONIST (SARA); ANTIHYPERTENSIVE

Therapeutic: ANTIHYPERTENSIVE; DIURETIC; SARA

Prototype: Spironolactone

Pregnancy Category: B

AVAILABILITY 25 mg, 50 mg, 100 mg tablets

ACTION & *THERAPEUTIC EFFECT*
Binds to mineralocorticoid receptors and blocks the binding of aldosterone, a component of the renin-angiotensin-aldosterone system (RAAS). Thus eplerenone blocks the primary effect of aldosterone which is sodium reabsorption. *Lowers blood pressure by inhibiting sodium and water retention, thus reducing total plasma volume.*

USES Treatment of hypertension, alone or with other antihypertensive agents. Adjunctive therapy for post MI heart failure.

CONTRAINDICATIONS Serum potassium greater than 5.5 mEq/L; type 2 diabetes with microalbuminuria; serum creatinine greater than 2 mg/dL in males or greater than 1.8 mg/dL in females; creatinine clearance less than 50 mL/min; lactation.

CAUTIOUS USE Hepatic impairment; concomitant use of another mineralocorticoid receptor blocker and ACE inhibitors or angiotensin II antagonists; severe hepatic disease; pregnancy (category B); safety and efficacy in children, infants, or neonates are not established.

ROUTE & DOSAGE

Hypertension

Adult: **PO** 50 mg once daily, may be increased to 50 mg b.i.d. or 100 mg daily, if inadequate response after 4 wk

Renal Impairment Dosage Adjustment

Do not administer if CrCl less than 50 mL/min due to risk of hyperkalemia

ADMINISTRATION

Oral

- Do not administer in combination with potassium supplements or potassium-sparing diuretics.
- Manufacturer recommends dosage reduction to 25 mg once daily with concurrent administration of erythromycin, saquinavir, verapamil, or fluconazole.
- Store at 15°–30° C (59°–86° F).

ADVERSE EFFECTS (≥1%) **Body as a Whole:** Fatigue, flu-like syndrome. **CNS:** Headache, dizziness. **CV:** Angina, <u>MI</u>. **GI:** Diarrhea, abdominal pain. **Endocrine:** Gynecomastia. **Metabolic:** *Hyperkalemia*, increased GGT, hypercholesterolemia, hypertriglyceridemia, decreased sodium levels. **Respiratory:** Cough. **Urogenital:** Albuminuria, abnormal vaginal bleeding.

INTERACTIONS Drug: ACE INHIBITORS, ANGIOTENSIN II RECEPTOR BLOCKERS, AZOLE ANTIFUNGALS (e.g., **fluconazole, itraconazole, ketoconazole**), **erythromycin, saquinavir, verapamil** may increase risk of hyperkalemia. **Food: Potassium**-containing SALT SUBSTITUTES may increase risk of hyperkalemia.

PHARMACOKINETICS Absorption: Rapidly absorbed. **Peak:** 1.5 h. **Distribution:** 50% protein bound, primarily to $alpha_1$-acid glycoproteins. **Metabolism:** In liver by CYP3A4. **Elimination:** 32% in feces, 67% in urine. **Half-Life:** 4–6 h.

NURSING IMPLICATIONS

Assessment & Drug Effects

- Monitor cardiovascular status with frequent BP determinations. Note that BP lowering usually occurs within 2 wk with maximal antihypertensive effects achieved within 4 wk.
- Lab tests: Monitor baseline and periodic serum potassium, serum sodium, renal function tests, lipid profile, and LFTs. Monitor type 2 diabetics for microalbuminuria.
- Concurrent drugs: Monitor serum potassium levels more frequently when patient also receiving an ACE inhibitor or an angiontensin II receptor antagonist. Monitor frequently for lithium toxicity with concurrent use.
- Withhold drug and notify physician for any of the following: Serum potassium greater than 5.5 mEq/L, serum creatinine greater than 2 mg/dL in males or greater than 1.8 mg/dL in females, creatinine clearance less than 50 mL/min, microalbuminuria in type 2 diabetics.

Patient & Family Education

- Do not use potassium supplements, salt substitutes containing potassium, or contraindicated drugs (e.g., ketoconazole, itraconazole) without consulting physician.
- Do not use OTC nonsteroidal anti-inflammatory drugs without consulting physician.
- Do not drive or operate machinery until reaction to drug is known. It may cause dizziness.

EPOETIN ALFA (HUMAN RECOMBINANT ERYTHROPOIETIN) Pr

(e-po-e-tin)

Epogen, Eprex ✦, Procrit

Classification: HEMATOPOIETIC GROWTH FACTOR

Therapeutic: ANTIANEMIC; HUMAN ERYTHROPOIETIN

Pregnancy Category: C

AVAILABILITY 2000 units/mL, 3000 units/mL, 4000 units/mL, 10,000 units/mL, 20,000 units/mL

ACTION & *THERAPEUTIC EFFECT* Human erythropoietin is produced in the kidney and stimulates bone marrow production of RBCs (erythropoiesis). Hypoxia and anemia generally increase the production of erythropoietin. Epoetin alpha stimulates RBC production. *Stimulates the production of RBCs in the bone marrow of severely anemic patients.*

USES Elevates the hematocrit of patients with anemia secondary to chronic renal failure (CRF); patients may or may not be on dialysis; other anemias related to malignancies and AIDS. Autologous blood donations for anticipated transfusions. Reduces need for blood in anemic surgical patients; anemia secondary to chronic renal failure (CRF); malignancy, other diseases, with or without current dialysis.

CONTRAINDICATIONS Uncontrolled hypertension and known hypersensitivity to mammalian cell–derived products and albumin (human); hamster protein hypersensitivity; iron-deficiency anemia; lactation; neonates.

CAUTIOUS USE Leukemia, sickle cell disease; coagulopathy; seizure disorders; pregnancy (category C).

ROUTE & DOSAGE

Anemia

Adult: **Subcutaneous/IV** Start with 50–100 units/kg/dose until target Hct range of 30–33% (max: 36%) is reached. [Hct should not increase by more than 4 points in any 2-wk period, rapid increase in Hct increases the risk of serious adverse reactions (hypertension, seizures).] May increase dose if Hct has not increased 5–6 points after 8 wk of therapy, reduce dose after target range is reached or the Hct increases by more than 4 points in any 2-wk period, dose usually increased or decreased by 25 units/kg increments.

Child: **Subcutaneous/IV** 50 units/kg/dose 3 times/wk initially, when Hct increased to 35%, decrease dose by 25 units/kg/dose until Hct reaches 40%

Anemia of CRF

Adult: **Subcutaneous/IV** Start with 50–100 units/kg/dose until target Hct range of 30–33% (max: 36%) is reached; if Hgb increases more than 1 g/dL and approaches 12 g/dL, reduce dose by 25%. If after 4 wk there is less than 1 g/dL, increase dose by 25%.

ADMINISTRATION

Subcutaneous

- Do not shake solution. Shaking may denature the glycoprotein, rendering it biologically inactive.
- Inspect solution for particulate matter prior to use. Do not use if solution is discolored or if it contains particulate matter.
- Use only one dose per vial, and do not reenter vial.
- Do not give with any other drug solution.

Intravenous

PREPARE: **Direct:** Give undiluted.
ADMINISTER: **Direct:** Give direct IV as a bolus dose over 1 min.
INCOMPATIBILITIES **Solution/additive:** D10W, normal saline.

- Discard any unused portion of the vial. It contains no preservatives.

- Store at 2°–8° C (36°–46° F). Do not freeze or shake.

ADVERSE EFFECTS (≥1%) **CNS:** Seizures, *headache*. **CV:** *Hypertension*. **GI:** Nausea, diarrhea. **Hematologic:** *Iron deficiency*, thrombocytosis, pure red cell aplasia, *clotting of AV fistula*. **Other:** Sweating, bone pain, arthralgias.

INTERACTIONS Drug: Do not give concurrently with **darbepoetin alfa.**

PHARMACOKINETICS Onset: 7–14 days. **Metabolism:** In serum. **Elimination:** Minimal recovery in urine. **Half-Life:** 4–13 h.

NURSING IMPLICATIONS

Assessment & Drug Effects

- Control BP adequately prior to initiation of therapy and closely monitor and control during therapy. Hypertension is an adverse effect that **must be** controlled.
- Be aware that BP may rise during early therapy as the Hct increases. Notify physician of a rapid rise in Hct (more than 4 points in 2 wk). Dosage will need to be reduced because of risk of serious hypertension.
- Monitor for hypertensive encephalopathy in patients with CRF during period of increasing Hct.
- Monitor for premonitory neurologic symptoms (i.e., aura, and report their appearance promptly). The potential for seizures exists during periods of rapid Hct increase (more than 4 points in 2 wk).
- Monitor closely for thrombotic events (e.g., MI, CVA, TIA), especially for patients with CRF.
- Lab tests: Baseline transferrin and serum ferritin. Determine Hct twice weekly until it is stabilized in the target range (30–33%) and the maintenance dose of epoetin alfa has been determined; then monitor at regular intervals. Perform CBC with differential and platelet count regularly. Monitor BUN, creatinine, and serum electrolytes regularly.

Patient & Family Education

- Important to comply with antihypertensive medication and dietary restrictions.
- Do not drive or engage in other potentially hazardous activity during the first 90 days of therapy because of possible seizure activity.
- Note: As Hct increases, there is an improved sense of well-being and quality of life. It is important to continue compliance with dietary and dialysis prescriptions.
- Understand that headache is a common adverse effect. Report if

severe or persistent, may indicate developing hypertension.

- Keep all follow-up appointments.

EPOPROSTENOL SODIUM (Pr)

(e-po-pros'te-nol)

Flolan

Classifications: PROSTAGLANDIN; PULMONARY ANTIHYPERTENSIVE

Therapeutic: PULMONARY ANTIHYPERTENSIVE

Pregnancy Category: B

AVAILABILITY 0.5 mg, 1.5 mg powder for injection

ACTION & *THERAPEUTIC EFFECT* Naturally occurring prostaglandin that reduces right and left ventricular afterload, increases cardiac output, and increases stroke volume through its vasodilation effect. Potent pulmonary vasodilator that reduces pulmonary hypertension. *Potent vasodilator of pulmonary and systemic arterial vascular beds and an inhibitor of platelet aggregation.*

USES Long-term treatment of primary pulmonary hypertension in NYHA Class III and IV patients.

CONTRAINDICATIONS Chronic use with left ventricular systolic dysfunction in CHF patients, hypersensitivity to epoprostenol or related compounds.

CAUTIOUS USE Older adults, pregnancy (category B), concurrent use of hypotensive drugs. Safety and efficacy in children are not established.

ROUTE & DOSAGE

Primary Pulmonary Hypertension

Adult: **IV** *Acute dose,* Initiate with 2 ng/kg/min, increase by 2 ng/kg/min q15min until dose-limiting effects occur (e.g., nausea, vomiting, headache, hypotension, flushing); *Chronic administration,* Start infusion at 4 ng/kg/min less than the maximum tolerated infusion; if maximum tolerated infusion is 5 ng/kg/min or less, start *maintenance infusion* at 50% of maximum tolerated dose

ADMINISTRATION

- Note: Anticoagulation therapy is generally initiated along with epoprostenol to reduce the risk of developing thromboembolic disease.

Intravenous

PREPARE: **Continuous:** Note: **Must be** reconstituted using sterile diluent for epoprostenol; must not be mixed with any other medications or solution prior to or during administration. ▪ To make 100 mL of 3000 ng/mL, add 5 mL of the supplied diluent to one 0.5 mg vial; withdraw 3 mL and add to enough diluent to make a total of 100 mL. ▪ To make 100 mL of 5000 ng/mL, add 5 mL of diluent to one 0.5 mg vial; withdraw contents of vial and add to enough diluent to make a total of 100 mL. ▪ To make 100 mL of 10,000 ng/mL, add 5 mL of diluent to each of two 0.5 mg vials; withdraw contents of each vial and add to enough diluent to make a total of 100 mL. ▪ To make 100 mL of 15,000 ng/mL, add 5 mL of diluent to a 1.5 mg vial; withdraw contents of vial and add to enough diluent to make a total of 100 mL.

ADMINISTER: **Continuous:** Give at ordered rate using an infusion control device. Avoid abrupt infusion interruption or large dosage reduction.

INCOMPATIBILITIES **Solution/additive:** Do not mix or infuse with any other parenteral drugs or solutions prior to or during administration.

▪ Store unopened vials at 15°–25° C (59°–77° F). Protect from light. ▪ See manufacturer's directions for stability or storage of reconstituted solutions.

ADVERSE EFFECTS (≥1%) **CNS:** *Chills, fever, flu-like syndrome, dizziness,* syncope, *headache, anxiety/nervousness,* hyperesthesia, paresthesia, dizziness. **CV:** *Tachycardia, hypotension, flushing, chest pain,* bradycardia. **GI:** *Diarrhea, nausea, vomiting,* abdominal pain. **Musculoskeletal:** *Jaw pain, myalgia, nonspecific musculoskeletal pain.* **Respiratory:** Dyspnea. **Other:** Dose-limiting effects.

INTERACTIONS Drug: Hypotension if administered with other VASODILATORS or ANTIHYPERTENSIVES.

PHARMACOKINETICS Peak: Approximately 15 min. **Metabolism:** Rapidly hydrolyzed at neutral pH in blood; also subject to enzyme degradation. **Elimination:** 82% in urine. **Half-Life:** Approximately 6 min.

NURSING IMPLICATIONS

Assessment & Drug Effects

- Assess carefully for development of pulmonary edema during dose ranging.
- Monitor respiratory and cardiovascular status frequently during entire period of chronic use of epoprostenol.
- Monitor for and report recurrence or worsening of symptoms associated with primary pulmonary hypertension (e.g., dyspnea, dizziness, exercise intolerance) or adverse effects of drug; dosage adjustments may be needed.

Patient & Family Education

- Learn correct techniques for storage, reconstitution, and administration of drug, and maintenance of catheter site (see ADMINISTRATION).
- Notify physician immediately of S&S of worsening primary pulmonary hypertension, adverse drug reactions, and S&S of infection at catheter site or sepsis.

EPROSARTAN MESYLATE

(e-pro-sar′tan)

Teveten

Classifications: RENIN ANGIOTENSIN SYSTEM ANTAGONIST; ANGIOTENSIN II RECEPTOR ANTAGONIST, ANTIHYPERTENSIVE

Therapeutic: ANTIHYPERTENSIVE

Prototype: Losartan potassium

Pregnancy Category: C first trimester; D second and third trimester

AVAILABILITY 400 mg, 600 mg tablets

ACTION & *THERAPEUTIC EFFECT* Selectively blocks the binding of angiotensin II to the AT_1 receptors found in many tissues. This blocks the vasoconstricting and aldosterone-secreting effects of angiotensin II, thus resulting in an antihypertensive effect. *It decreases both the systolic and diastolic BP.*

USES Treatment of hypertension.

CONTRAINDICATIONS Hypersensitivity to eprosartan, losartan, or other angiotensin II receptor antagonists; pregnancy (category D second and third trimester), lactation; children younger than 18 y.

CAUTIOUS USE Angioedema, aortic or mitral value stenosis, coronary artery disease, cardiomyopathy, hypotension, CHF; biliary obstruction; older adults; severe hepatic dysfunction, renal artery stenosis, renal disease, renal impairment; pregnancy (category C first trimester).

ROUTE & DOSAGE

Hypertension
Adult: **PO** 600 mg daily or 400 mg daily to b.i.d. (max: 800 mg/day)

ADMINISTRATION

Oral
- Correct volume depletion prior to therapy to prevent hypotension.
- Store at 15°–30° C (59°–86° F); protect from moisture and direct light.

ADVERSE EFFECTS (≥1%) **Body as a Whole:** Viral infection, fatigue, arthralgia. **CNS:** Depression. **GI:** Abdominal pain, hypertriglyceridemia. **Respiratory:** Upper respiratory infection, rhinitis, pharyngitis, cough.

PHARMACOKINETICS Absorption: Only 13% of oral dose reaches systemic circulation. **Peak:** 1–2 h. **Metabolism:** Minimal metabolism. **Elimination:** 61% in feces and 37% in urine. **Half-Life:** 5–9 h.

NURSING IMPLICATIONS

Assessment & Drug Effects
- Monitor BP periodically; do trough readings just before scheduled dose when possible.
- Monitor for S&S of angioedema (may occur within 30 min or as long as 30 days after initial dose).
- Lab tests: Monitor liver function, BUN and creatinine, serum potassium, CBC with differential periodically.

Patient & Family Education
- Inform physician immediately of pregnancy.
- Report episodes of dizziness especially associated with position changes.
- Report swelling of lips, tongue, face, or feeling of obstruction in neck immediately.

EPTIFIBATIDE

(ep-ti-fib′a-tide)
Integrilin
Classifications: ANTIPLATELET; PLATELET GLYCOPROTEIN (GP IIB/IIIA) INHIBITOR
Therapeutic: ANTIPLATELET
Prototype: Abciximab
Pregnancy Category: B

AVAILABILITY 0.75 mg/mL, 2 mg/mL injection

ACTION & *THERAPEUTIC EFFECT* Binds to the glycoprotein IIb/IIIa (GPIIb/IIIa) receptor sites of platelets. *Inhibits platelet aggregation by preventing fibrinogen, von Willebrand's factor, and other molecules from adhering to GPIIb/IIIa receptor sites on platelets.*

USES Treatment of acute coronary syndromes (unstable angina, non-Q-wave MI) and patients undergoing percutaneous coronary interventions (PCIs).

CONTRAINDICATIONS Hypersensitivity to eptifibatide; active bleeding; GI or GU bleeding within 6 wk; thrombocytopenia; renal failure requiring dialysis; coagulopathy; recent major surgery or trauma; intracranial neoplasm, intracranial bleeding within 6 mo; concurrent administration of another GPIIb/IIIa receptor inhibitor (e.g., abciximab); severe hypertension (systolic blood pressure greater than 200 mm Hg or diastolic blood pressure greater than 110 mm Hg), aneurysm.
CAUTIOUS USE Hypersensitivity to related compounds (e.g., abcix-

imab, tirofiban, lamifiban); concurrent administration of other anticoagulants; pregnancy (category B), lactation. Safety and effectiveness in children are not established.

ROUTE & DOSAGE

Acute Coronary Syndromes (ACS)

Adult: **IV** 180 mcg/kg initial bolus (max: 22.6 mg) followed by 2 mcg/kg/min until hospital discharge or up to 72 h

Percutaneous Coronary Interventions (PCI)

Adult: **IV** 180 mcg/kg initial bolus followed by 2 mcg/kg/min; after 10 min, a second 180 mcg/kg bolus should be given; the infusion should continue up to 24 h after the end of the procedure

Renal Impairment Dosage Adjustment

If CrCl 10–49 mL/min, then give 1 mcg/kg/min continuous infusion

ADMINISTRATION

- Note: Review contraindications to administration prior to giving this drug.

Intravenous

PREPARE: **Direct:** Give undiluted.
ADMINISTER: **Direct:** Give bolus doses IV push over 1–2 min. **Continuous:** Start continuous infusion immediately following bolus dose. ▪ Give undiluted directly from the 100-mL vial (at a rate based on patient's weight) using a vented infusion set. ▪ May be given in the same IV line with NS or D5/NS (either solution may contain up to 60 mEq KCl).

- Store unopened vials at 2°–8° C (36°–46° F) and protect from light. Discard any unused portion in opened vial.

ADVERSE EFFECTS (≥1%) **CNS:** Intracranial bleed (rare). **GI:** GI bleeding. **Hematologic:** *Bleeding* (major bleeding 4.4–11%), anemia, thrombocytopenia.

INTERACTIONS Drug: ORAL ANTICOAGULANTS, NSAIDS, **dipyridamole, ticlopidine, dextran** may increase risk of bleeding.

PHARMACOKINETICS Duration: 6–8 h after stopping infusion. **Metabolism:** Minimally metabolized. **Elimination:** 50% in urine. **Half-Life:** 2.5 h.

NURSING IMPLICATIONS

Assessment & Drug Effects

- Lab tests: Prior to infusion determine PT/aPTT and INR, activated clotting time (ACT) for those undergoing percutaneous coronary intervention (PCI); Hct or Hgb; platelet count; and serum creatinine.
- Lab tests: Monitor aPTT and INR (target aPPT, 50–70 sec); during PCI (target ACT, 300–350 sec).
- Minimize all vascular and other trauma during treatment. When obtaining IV access, avoid using a noncompressible site such as the subclavian vein.
- Monitor carefully for and immediately report S&S of bleeding (e.g., femoral artery access site bleeding, intracerebral hemorrhage, GI bleeding).
- Immediately stop infusion of eptifibatide and heparin if bleeding at the arterial access site cannot be controlled by pressure.
- Achieve hemostasis at the arterial access site by standard compression for a minimum of 4 h prior to hospital discharge following discontinuation of eptifibatide and heparin.

ERGOCALCIFEROL

(er-goe-kal-si'fe-role)

Activated Ergosterol, Drisdol, D-ViSol, Ostoforte ♣, Radiostol ♣, Radiostol Forte ♣, Vitamin D_2

Classification: VITAMIN D ANALOG

Therapeutic: VITAMIN D ANALOG

Prototype: Calcitriol

Pregnancy Category: C

AVAILABILITY 8000 international units/mL oral liquid; 50,000 units capsules, tablets; 500,000 international units/mL injection

ACTION & *THERAPEUTIC EFFECT* The name vitamin D encompasses two related fat-soluble substances. Vitamin D acts like a hormone in that it is distributed through the circulation and plays a major regulatory role. Responsible for regulation of serum calcium level. *Maintains normal blood calcium and phosphate ion levels by enhancing their intestinal absorption and by promoting mobilization of calcium from bone and renal tubular resorption of phosphate.*

USES Familial hypophosphatemia (vitamin D–resistant rickets), osteomalacia (adult rickets), anticonvulsant-induced rickets and osteomalacia, osteoporosis, renal osteodystrophy, hypocalcemia associated with hypoparathyroidism; prophylaxis and treatment of nutritional rickets. Also hypophosphatemia in Fanconi's syndrome.

UNLABELED USES With varying clinical results in lupus vulgaris, psoriasis, and rheumatoid arthritis.

CONTRAINDICATIONS Hypersensitivity to vitamin D, hypervitaminosis D, hypercalcemia, hyperphosphatemia, renal osteodystrophy with hyperphosphatemia, malabsorption syndrome, decreased kidney function. Safe use of amounts in excess of 400 international units (10 mcg) daily during pregnancy (category C) is not established.

CAUTIOUS USE Coronary disease; arteriosclerosis (especially in older adults); history of kidney stones; biliary tract disease; lactation.

ROUTE & DOSAGE

Nutritional Rickets, Osteomalacia

Adult: **PO** 25–125 mcg/day for 6–12 wk, may need up to 7.5 mg/day in patients with malabsorption

Child: **PO** 50–125 mcg/day, may need up to 250–625 mcg/day in patients with malabsorption

Vitamin D–Dependent Rickets

Adult: **PO** 250 mcg–1.5 mg/day, may need up to 12.5 mg/day (prolonged therapy with greater than 2.5 mg/day increases risk of toxicity)

Child: **PO** 75–125 mcg/day, may need up to 1.5 mg/day

Hypoparathyroidism, Pseudohypoparathyroidism

Adult: **PO** 625 mcg–5 mg/day, may need up to 10 mg/day (prolonged therapy with greater than 2.5 mg/day increases risk of toxicity)

Child: **PO** 1.25–5 mg/day, (prolonged therapy with greater than 2.5 mg/day increases risk of toxicity)

ADMINISTRATION

Oral

- Preserve in tightly covered, light-resistant containers. Drug decomposes when exposed to light and air.

ADVERSE EFFECTS (≥1%) **Body as a Whole:** Fatigue, weakness, vertigo, tinnitus, ataxia, muscle and joint pain, hypotonia (infants), exanthema, rhinorrhea; pruritus; mild acidosis. **CNS:** Headache, drowsiness, convulsions. **GI:** Metallic taste, dry mouth, anorexia, nausea, vomiting, diarrhea, constipation, abdominal cramps. **Hematologic:** Anemia. **Musculoskeletal:** Calcification of soft tissues (kidneys, blood vessels, myocardium, lungs, skin). **Urogenital:** Nephrotoxicity (polyuria, hyposthenuria, polydipsia, nocturia, casts, albuminuria, hematuria), kidney failure. **CV:** Hypertension, cardiac arrhythmias. **Special Senses:** Conjunctivitis (calcific); photophobia. **Metabolic:** Osteoporosis (adults); weight loss, chronic hypervitaminosis D in children (mental and physical retardation, suppression of linear growth).

DIAGNOSTIC TEST INTERFERENCE Vitamin D may cause false increase in ***serum cholesterol*** measurements ***(Zlatkis-Zak reaction).***

INTERACTIONS Drug: Cholestyramine, colestipol, mineral oil may decrease absorption of vitamin D.

PHARMACOKINETICS Absorption: Readily from GI tract. **Peak:** After 4 wk. **Duration:** 2 mo or more. **Distribution:** Most of drug first appears in lymph, stored chiefly in liver and in skin, brain, spleen, and bones. **Metabolism:** In liver and kidney to active metabolites. **Elimination:** About 50% of PO dose in bile; may be stored in tissues for months. **Half-Life:** 12–24 h.

NURSING IMPLICATIONS

Assessment & Drug Effects

- Monitor closely patients receiving therapeutic doses of vitamin D; must remain under close medical supervision.
- Lab tests: When high therapeutic doses are used, progress is followed by frequent determinations (q2wk or more often) of serum calcium, phosphorus, magnesium, alkaline phosphatase, BUN, and determinations of urine calcium, casts, albumin, and RBC. Blood calcium concentration is generally kept between 9 and 10 mg/dL.
- Monitor for hypercalcemia; in patients with osteomalacia a decrease in serum alkaline phosphatase may signal the onset of hypercalcemia.

Patient & Family Education

- Avoid magnesium-containing antacids and laxatives with chronic kidney failure when receiving vitamin D preparations since vitamin D increases the risk of magnesium intoxication than other patients.
- Do not use OTC medications unless approved by physician.

ERGOLOID MESYLATE

(er'goe-loid mess'i-late)

Gerimal

Classifications: ALPHA-ADRENERGIC ANTAGONIST; ERGOT ALKALOID
Therapeutic: ANTIDEMENTIA; ALZHEIMER'S AGENT
Prototype: Ergotamine tartrate
Pregnancy Category: X

AVAILABILITY 1 mg tablets

ACTION & *THERAPEUTIC EFFECT* Produces peripheral vasodilation primarily by central action and may cause slight reduction in BP and heart rate. Relieves symptoms of cerebral arteriosclerosis. *Some improvements in Alzheimer's dementia symptoms, possibly by increasing cerebral metabolism with consequent increase in blood flow. Improvement may not be apparent until after 3–4 wk of therapy.*

USES Senile dementia of Alzheimer type.

CONTRAINDICATIONS Acute or chronic psychosis; hypersensitivity to ergoloid; pregnancy (category X), lactation.
CAUTIOUS USE Acute intermittent porphyria; elderly; hepatic disease; hypotension; bradycardia.

ROUTE & DOSAGE

Senile Dementia of Alzheimer Type
Adult: **PO** 1 mg t.i.d.; doses up to 4.5–12 mg/day have been used

ADMINISTRATION

Oral
- Store in tightly closed container.

ADVERSE EFFECTS (≥1%) **Body as a Whole:** Mostly dose related. **CV:** Orthostatic hypotension, dizziness or light-headedness, flushing, sinus bradycardia. **Special Senses:** Blurred vision, nasal stuffiness. **GI:** Anorexia, stomach cramps, transient nausea and vomiting, heartburn. **Skin:** Skin rash.

INTERACTIONS Drug: Use with other ERGOT ALKALOIDS may increase toxicities.

PHARMACOKINETICS Absorption: Incompletely from GI tract; 50% reaches systemic circulation. **Peak:** 1.5–3 h. **Metabolism:** Undergoes rapid first-pass metabolism in liver. **Elimination:** Primarily in feces. **Half-Life:** 2–12 h.

NURSING IMPLICATIONS

Assessment & Drug Effects
- Establish baseline values of BP and pulse; check at regular intervals throughout therapy.
- Report to physician sinus bradycardia (40 bpm); has been reported in patients receiving 1.5 mg doses. Pulse rate usually returns to normal within 2 days after drug is discontinued.
- Withdraw drug permanently if marked bradycardia or hypotension occurs.

Patient & Family Education
- Make position changes slowly, particularly from recumbent to upright posture, and move ankles and feet for a few minutes before walking.

ERGOTAMINE TARTRATE (Pr)

(er-got'a-meen)
Ergomar
Classifications: ALPHA-ADRENERGIC ANTAGONIST; ERGOT ALKALOID
Therapeutic: ANTIMIGRAINE
Pregnancy Category: X

AVAILABILITY 2 mg sublingual tablets

ACTION & *THERAPEUTIC EFFECT* Natural amino acid alkaloid of ergot. Alpha-adrenergic blocking agent with direct stimulating action on cranial and peripheral vascular smooth muscles and depressant effect on central vasomotor centers. *In vascular headache, exerts vasoconstrictive action on previously dilated cerebral vessels, reduces amplitude of arterial pulsations, and antagonizes effects of serotonin.*

USES As single agent or in combination with caffeine to prevent or abort migraine, cluster headache (histamine cephalalgia), and other vascular headaches.

CONTRAINDICATIONS Hypersensitivity to ergotamine; sepsis, obliterative vascular disease, thromboembolic disease, prolonged use of excessive dosage, liver and kidney disease, severe pruritus, diabetes mellitus; marked arteriosclerosis, history of MI, peripheral vascular disease; coronary artery disease, angina; basilar/hemiplegic migraine; hepatic disease; biliary tract disease; cholestasis; hypertension; infectious states, anemia, malnutrition; pregnancy (category X), use in children.
CAUTIOUS USE Lactation, older adult patients.

ROUTE & DOSAGE

Vascular Headaches
Adult: **SL** 1–2 mg followed by 1–2 mg q30min until headache abates or until max of 6 mg/24 h or 10 mg/wk

ADMINISTRATION

Sublingual

- Instruct patient to allow sublingual (SL) tablet to dissolve under tongue and not to drink, eat, or smoke while tablet is in place. Do not crush SL tablets.

ADVERSE EFFECTS (≥1%) **Body as a Whole:** Paresthesias; pain (spasms) of facial muscles, tongue, limbs, and lumbar region with difficulty in walking; muscle pains, *weakness,* numbness, coldness and cyanosis of digits (Raynaud's phenomenon). **CNS:** Delirium; convulsive seizures; confusion; depression; drowsiness. **GI:** *Nausea; vomiting;* diarrhea; abdominal pain; unquenchable thirst; partial necrosis of tongue, disagreeable aftertaste. **CV:** Rapid, weak, or irregular pulse; intermittent claudication, complete absence of medium- and large-vessel pulsations in extremities; precordial distress and pain; angina pectoris, transient bradycardia or tachycardia; elevated or lowered BP. **Skin:** Itching and cold skin; gangrene of nose, digits, ears. **Urogenital:** Kidney failure. **Other:** Symptoms of ergotism.

INTERACTIONS Drug: With high doses of BETA-ADRENERGIC BLOCKERS, SYMPATHOMIMETICS, possibility of additive vasoconstrictor effects; **erythromycin, troleandomycin** may cause severe peripheral vasospasm. **Eletriptan, naratriptan, rizatriptan, sumatriptan, or zolmitriptan** may increase risk of coronary ischemia, separate drugs by 24 h; AZOLE ANTIFUNGALS **(ketoconazole, itraconazole, fluconazole, clotrimazole), nefazodone, fluoxetine, fluvoxamine, amprenavir, delavirdine, efavirenz, indinavir, nelfinavir, ritonavir, and saquinavir,** may inhibit ergot metabolism and increase toxicity; **sibutramine, dexfenfluramine, nefazodone, fluvoxamine** may increase risk of serotonin syndrome. **Food: Grapefruit juice** may increase toxicity.

PHARMACOKINETICS Absorption: Variable. **Peak:** 0.5–3 h. **Distribution:** Crosses blood–brain barrier. **Metabolism:** Extensive first-pass metabolism in liver. **Elimination:** 96% in feces; excreted in breast milk. **Half-Life:** 2.7 h initial phase, 21 h terminal phase.

NURSING IMPLICATIONS

Assessment & Drug Effects

- Monitor adverse GI effects. Nausea and vomiting are adverse reactions that occur in about 10% of patients after they take ergotamine. Patient may need an antiemetic. Consult with physician.

- Monitor patients with PVD carefully for development of peripheral ischemia.
- Monitor long-term effectiveness. Patients receiving high ergotamine doses for prolonged periods may experience increased frequency of headaches, fatigue, and depression. Discontinuation of the drug in these patients results in severe withdrawal headache that may last a few days.
- Overdose symptoms: Nausea, vomiting, weakness, and pain in legs, numbness and tingling in fingers and toes, tachycardia or bradycardia, hypertension or hypotension, and localized edema.

Patient & Family Education

- Begin drug therapy as soon after onset of migraine attack as possible, preferably during migraine prodrome (scintillating scotomas, visual field defects, nausea, paresthesias usually on side opposite to that of the migraine).
- Notify physician if migraine attacks occur more frequently or are not relieved.
- Lie down in a quiet, dark room for 2–3 h after drug administration.
- Report muscle pain or weakness of extremities, cold or numb digits, irregular heartbeat, nausea, or vomiting. Carefully protect extremities from exposure to cold temperatures; provide warmth, but not heat, to ischemic areas.
- Do NOT increase dosage without consulting physician; overdosage is the chief cause of adverse effects from the drug.

ERLOTINIB

(er-lo′ti-nib)

Tarceva

Classifications: ANTINEOPLASTIC; TYROSINE KINASE INHIBITOR-EPIDERMAL GROWTH FACTOR RECEPTOR (TKI-EGFR) INHIBITOR

Therapeutic: ANTINEOPLASTIC

Prototype: Gefitinib

Pregnancy Category: D

AVAILABILITY 25 mg, 100 mg, 150 mg tablets

ACTION & *THERAPEUTIC EFFECT*

Erlotinib is a human epidermal growth factor receptor type 1 (HER1/EGFR) inhibitor. Antitumor action is believed to be due to inhibition of phosphorylation of tyrosine kinase associate with the EGFR present on the cell surface of both normal and cancer cells. *Inhibition of EGFR in cancer cells diminishes their capacity for cell proliferation, cell survival, and decreases metastases.*

USES Treatment of patients with locally advanced or metastatic non–small cell lung cancer (NSCLC) after failure of at least one prior chemotherapy regimen, pancreatic cancer.

CONTRAINDICATIONS Hypersensitivity to erlotinib; severe hepatic impairment; pregnancy (category D); lactation.

CAUTIOUS USE Mild or moderate hepatic impairment; interstitial pulmonary disease (interstitial pneumonia, pneumonitis, alveolitis); myelosuppression; ocular toxicities (corneal ulcer, eye pain).

ROUTE & DOSAGE

Metastatic Non–Small-Cell Lung Cancer

Adult: **PO** 150 mg once daily

Pancreatic Cancer (with Gemcitabine)

Adult: **PO** 100 mg daily

Hepatic Impairment Dosage Adjustment

Discontinue use in patient with severe change in liver function

ADMINISTRATION

Oral

- Give at least 1 h before or 2 h after eating.
- Store at 15°–30° C (59°–86° F). Keep container tightly closed. Protect from light.

ADVERSE EFFECTS (≥1%) **Body as a Whole:** Infection. **GI:** *Diarrhea, anorexia, fatigue,* nausea, vomiting, stomatitis, abdominal pain. **Metabolic:** Increased LFTs. **Respiratory:** *Dyspnea,* cough, interstitial lung disease (sometimes fatal). **Skin:** *Acneiform rash,* pruritus, dry skin. **Special Senses:** Conjunctivitis, dry eyes.

INTERACTIONS Drug: Atazanavir, clarithromycin, indinavir, itraconazole, ketoconazole, nefazodone, nelfinavir, ritonavir, saquinavir, telithromycin, troleandomycin, voriconazole may increase erlotinib levels and toxicity; **rifampin, rifabutin, rifapentine, phenytoin, carbamazepine, phenobarbital** may decrease erlotinib levels, increased bleeding with **warfarin. Herbal: St. John's wort** may decrease erlotinib levels.

PHARMACOKINETICS Absorption: 60% absorbed orally; food can increase to 100%. **Peak:** 4 h. **Metabolism:** In liver by CYP3A4. **Elimination:** Primarily in feces (83%). **Half-Life:** 36.2 h.

NURSING IMPLICATIONS

Assessment & Drug Effects

- Monitor closely changes in pulmonary function.
- Withhold drug and notify physician for acute onset of new or progressive pulmonary symptoms (e.g., dyspnea, cough, or fever) or significant changes in liver functions as indicated by elevated transaminases, bilirubin, and alkaline phosphatase.
- Lab tests: Periodic LFTs. Discontinue drug in patients with severe liver impairment.

Patient & Family Education

- Report promptly any of the following: Severe or persistent diarrhea, nausea, anorexia, or vomiting; onset or worsening of unexplained shortness of breath or cough; eye irritation.
- Monitor closely PT/INR values with concurrent warfarin therapy.
- Women should use effective means to avoid pregnancy while taking this drug.

ERTAPENEM SODIUM

(er-ta-pen′em)

Invanz

Classification: BETA-LACTAM ANTIBIOTIC

Therapeutic: ANTIBIOTIC

Prototype: Imipenem-cilastatin

Pregnancy Category: B

AVAILABILITY 1 g vial

ACTION & *THERAPEUTIC EFFECT* Broad-spectrum carbapenem antibiotic that inhibits the cell wall synthesis of gram-positive and gram-negative bacteria by its strong affinity for penicillin-binding proteins (PBPs) of the bacterial cell wall. *Effective against both gram-positive* *and gram-negative bacteria. Highly resistant to most bacterial beta-lactamases.*

USES Complicated intra-abdominal infections, complicated skin and skin structure infections, community-acquired pneumonia, complicated UTI (including pyelonephritis), and acute pelvic infections due to susceptible bacteria.

CONTRAINDICATIONS Hypersensitivity to ertapenem, penicillins, or carbapenem antibiotics; hypersensitivity to amide-type local anesthetics such as lidocaine; hypersensitivity to meropenem or imipenem; children younger than 3 mo.

CAUTIOUS USE Renal impairment; history of CNS disorders; history of seizures; hypersensitivity to other beta-lactam antibiotics (penicillins, cephalosporins); hypersensitivity to other allergens; meningitis; pregnancy (category B); lactation (bottle feed during and for 5 days after therapy ends).

ROUTE & DOSAGE

Community-Acquired Pneumonia; Complicated UTI

Adult/Adolescent: **IV/IM** 1 g daily × 10–14 days; may switch to appropriate PO antibiotic after 3 days if responding

Child/Infant (older than 3 mo): **IV/IM** 15 mg/kg q12h × 10–14 days

Intra-Abdominal Infection

Adult/Adolescent: **IV/IM** 1 g daily × 5–14 days

Child/Infant (older than 3 mo): **IV/IM** 15 mg/kg b.i.d. × 5–14 days; max: 1 g/day

Skin and Skin Structure Infections

Adult/Adolescent: **IV/IM** 1 g daily × 7–14 days

Child/Infant (older than 3 mo): **IV/IM** 15 mg/kg b.i.d. × 7–14 days (max: 1 g/day)

Acute Pelvic Infections

Adult: **IV/IM** 1 g daily × 3–10 days

Renal Impairment Dosage Adjustment

CrCl less than 30 mL/min: Reduce dose to 500 mg daily

ADMINISTRATION

Intramuscular

- Reconstitute 1 g vial with 3.2 mL of 1% lidocaine HCl injection (without epinephrine). Shake vial thoroughly to form solution. Use immediately.
- Inject deep IM into a large muscle mass (such as the gluteal muscles or lateral part of the thigh).
- The reconstituted IM solution should be used within 1 h after preparation. Note: DO NOT use this solution for IV administration.

Intravenous

PREPARE: **Intermittent for Adult/Child:** Reconstitute 1 g vial with 10 mL of sterile water for injection, NS, or bacteriostatic water for injection. Shake well to dissolve. **Intermittent for Adult/Child (13 y or older):** Immediately after reconstition, transfer contents to 50 mL of NS injection solution. **Intermittent for Child (3 mo–12 y):** Immediately after reconstition, transfer required dose to enough NS injection solution to yield a final concentration of 20 mg/mL or less.

ADMINISTER: **Intermittent:** Infuse over 30 min. Note: Infusion should be completed within 6 h of reconstitution.

INCOMPATIBILITIES **Solution/additive: Dextrose, mannitol, lactated Ringer's injection. Y-site:** Do not mix or infuse with any other drugs.

- Store lyophilized powder above 25° C (77° F). ▪Must use reconstituted solution stored at room temperature (not above 25° C/77° F) within 6 h. ▪May store for 24 h under refrigeration. Use within 4 h of removal from refrigeration. ▪ Do not freeze.

ADVERSE EFFECTS (≥1%) **Body as a Whole:** Phlebitis or thrombosis at injection site, asthenia, fatigue, death, fever, leg pain. **CNS:** Anxiety, altered mental status, dizziness, headache, insomnia. **CV:** Chest pain, hypertension, hypotension, tachycardia, edema. **GI:** Abdominal pain, *diarrhea*, acid regurgitation, constipation, dyspepsia, nausea, vomiting, increased AST and ALT. **Respiratory:** Cough, dyspnea, pharyngitis, rales/rhonchi, and respiratory distress. **Skin:** Erythema, pruritus, rash. **Urogenital:** Vaginitis.

INTERACTIONS Drug: Probenecid decreases renal excretion.

PHARMACOKINETICS Absorption: 90% from IM site. **Peak:** 2.3 h. **Distribution:** 95% protein bound, distributes into breast milk, may cross placenta. **Metabolism:** Hydrolysis of beta-lactam ring. **Elimination:** 80% in urine, 10% in feces. **Half-Life:** 4.5 h.

NURSING IMPLICATIONS

Assessment & Drug Effects

- Lab tests: Perform C&S tests prior to therapy. Monitor periodically liver and kidney function.
- Determine history of hypersensitivity reactions to other beta-lactams, cephalosporins, penicillins, or other drugs.
- Discontinue drug and immediately report S&S of hypersensitivity (see Appendix F).
- Report S&S of superinfection or pseudomembranous colitis (see Appendix F).
- Monitor for seizures especially in older adults and those with renal insufficiency.
- Lab tests: Monitor AST, ALT, alkaline phosphatase, CBC, platelet count, and routine blood chemistry during prolonged therapy.

Patient & Family Education

- Learn S&S of hypersensitivity, superinfection, and pseudomembranous colitis (see Appendix F); report any of these to physician promptly.

ERYTHROMYCIN Pr

(er-ith-roe-mye'sin)

Apo-Erythro Base ♣, A/T/S, E-Mycin, Eryc, EryDerm, EryTab, Erythrocin, Erythromid ♣, Erythromycin Base, Novo-Rythro ♣, PCE, Ro-Mycin ♣

ERYTHROMYCIN ESTOLATE

Novo-Rythro Estolate ♣

ERYTHROMYCIN STEARATE

Apo-Erythro-S ♣, Erythrocin Stearate, SK-Erythromycin

Classification: MACROLIDE ANTIBIOTIC

Therapeutic: ANTIBIOTIC

Pregnancy Category: B

AVAILABILITY Erythromycin: 250 mg, 333 mg, 500 mg tablets, capsules 2% topical solution 2% gel; 2% ointment 2% pledgets; 5% ophth ointment; **Erythromycin Estolate:** 125 mg, 250 mg capsules 125 mg/mL, 250 mg/mL suspension; **Erythromycin Stearate:** 250 mg, 500 mg tablets

ACTION & *THERAPEUTIC EFFECT* Macrolide antibiotic that binds to the 50S ribosomal subunit, thus inhibiting bacterial protein synthesis. *More active against gram-positive organisms than against gram-negative organisms due to its superior penetration into gram-positive organisms.*

USES Pneumococcal pneumonia, *Mycoplasma pneumoniae* (primary atypical pneumonia), acute pelvic inflammatory disease caused by *Neisseria gonorrhoeae* in females sensitive to penicillin, infections caused by susceptible strains of staphylococci, streptococci, and certain strains of *Haemophilus influenzae.* Also used in intestinal amebiasis, Legionnaires' disease, uncomplicated urethral, endocervical, and rectal infections caused by *Chlamydia trachomatis,* for prophylaxis of ophthalmia neonatorum caused by *N. gonorrhoeae, C. trachomatis,* and for chlamydial conjunctivitis in neonates. Considered an acceptable alternative to penicillin for treatment of streptococcal pharyngitis, for prophylaxis of rheumatic fever and bacterial endocarditis, for treatment of diphtheria as adjunct to antitoxin and for carrier state, and as alternate choice in treatment of primary syphilis in patients allergic to penicillins. **Topical applications:** Pyodermas, acne vulgaris, and external ocular infections, including neonatal chlamydial conjunctivitis and gonococcal ophthalmia.

CONTRAINDICATIONS Hypersensitivity to erythromycins or other macrolide antibiotics; congenital QT prolongation; electrolyte imbalances. **Estolate:** History of hepatotoxicity in patients with hepatic disease.

CAUTIOUS USE Impaired liver function; seizure disorders; history of GI disorders; pregnancy (category B).

ROUTE & DOSAGE

Moderate to Severe Infections

Adult: **PO** 250–500 mg q6h; 333 mg q8h

Child: **PO** 30–50 mg/kg/day divided q6h **Topical** Apply ointment to infected eye 1 or more times/day

Neonate: **PO** *7 days or younger,* 10 mg/kg q12h; *older than 7 days,* 10 mg/kg q8–12h **Topical** 0.5–1 cm in conjunctival sac once

***Chlamydia trachomatis* Infections**

Adult: **PO** 500 mg q.i.d. or 666 mg q8h

Child: **Topical** Apply 0.5–1 cm ribbon in lower conjunctival sacs shortly after birth

ADMINISTRATION

Oral

- Erythromycin base or stearate should be given on an empty stomach 1 h before or 3 h after meals. Do not give with, or immediately before or after, fruit juices.
- Erythromycin estolate and enteric-coated tablets may be given without regard to meals.
- Ensure that capsules and tablets are not chewed or crushed. They **must be** swallowed whole.

Topical

- Prophylaxis for neonatal eye infection: Ribbon of ointment approximately 0.5–1 cm long is placed into lower conjunctival sac of neonate shortly after birth. Use a new tube of erythromycin for each neonate.

- Store all forms at 15°–30° C (59°–86° F) in tightly capped containers unless otherwise directed by manufacturer.

ADVERSE EFFECTS (≥1%) **GI:** *Nausea, vomiting, abdominal cramping,* diarrhea, heartburn, anorexia. **Body as a Whole:** Fever, eosinophilia, urticaria, skin eruptions, fixed drug eruption, anaphylaxis. Superinfections by nonsusceptible bacteria, yeasts, or fungi. **Special Senses:** Ototoxicity: Reversible bilateral hearing loss, tinnitus, vertigo. **Digestive:** (Estolate) Cholestatic hepatitis syndrome. **Skin:** (Topical use) Erythema, desquamation, burning, tenderness, dryness or oiliness, pruritus.

DIAGNOSTIC TEST INTERFERENCE False elevations of ***urinary catecholamines, urinary steroids,*** and ***AST, ALT*** (by ***colorimetric methods***).

INTERACTIONS Drug: Serum levels and toxicities of **alfentanil, bexarotene, carbamazepine, cevimeline, cilostazol, clozapine, cyclosporine, disopyramide, estazolam, fentanyl, midazolam, methadone, modafinil, quinidine, sirolimus, digoxin, theophylline, triazolam, warfarin** are increased. **Ergotamine, dihydroergotamine** may increase peripheral vasospasm. **Food: Grapefruit juice** may increase side effects.

PHARMACOKINETICS Absorption: Most erythromycins are absorbed in small intestine. **Peak:** 1–4 h PO. **Distribution:** Widely distributed to most body tissues; low concentrations in CSF; concentrates in liver and bile; crosses placenta. **Metabolism:** Partially in liver. **Elimination:** Primarily in bile; excreted in breast milk. **Half-Life:** 1.5–2 h.

NURSING IMPLICATIONS

Assessment & Drug Effects

- Report onset of GI symptoms after PO administration. These are dose related; if symptoms persist after dosage reduction, physician may prescribe drug to be given with meals in spite of impaired absorption.
- Monitor for adverse GI effects. Pseudomembranous enterocolitis (see Appendix F), a potentially life-threatening condition, may occur during or after antibiotic therapy.
- Observe for S&S of superinfection by overgrowth of nonsusceptible bacteria or fungi. Emergence of resistant staphylococcal strains is highly predictable during prolonged therapy.
- Lab tests: Periodic liver function tests during prolonged therapy.
- Monitor for S&S of hepatotoxicity. Premonitory S&S include: Abdominal pain, nausea, vomiting, fever, leukocytosis, and eosinophilia; jaundice may or may not be present. Symptoms may appear a few days after initiation of drug but usually occur after 1–2 wk of continuous therapy. Symptoms are reversible with prompt discontinuation of erythromycin.
- Monitor for ototoxicity that appears to develop most frequently in patients receiving 4 g/day or more, older adults, female patients, and patients with kidney or liver dysfunction. It is reversible with prompt discontinuation of drug.

Patient & Family Education

- Notify physician for S&S of superinfection (see Appendix F).
- Notify physician immediately for S&S of pseudomembranous enterocolitis (see Appendix F), which may occur even after the drug is discontinued.

- Report any ototoxic effects including dizziness, vertigo, nausea, tinnitus, roaring noises, hearing impairment (see Appendix F).

ERYTHROMYCIN ETHYLSUCCINATE

(er-ith-roe-mye'sin)

Apo-Erythro-ES ✦, E.E.S., E.E.S.-200, E.E.S.-400, EryPed, Pediamycin

Classification: MACROLIDE ANTIBIOTIC

Therapeutic: ANTIBIOTIC

Prototype: Erythromycin

Pregnancy Category: B

AVAILABILITY 200 mg chewable tablet, 400 mg tablets; 100 mg/2.5 mL, 200 mg/5 mL, 400 mg/5 mL suspension

ACTION & *THERAPEUTIC EFFECT* Macrolide antibiotic that binds to the 50S ribosomal subunit of bacteria, thus inhibiting bacterial protein synthesis. *More active against gram-positive than gram-negative bacteria.*

USES See ERYTHROMYCIN.

CONTRAINDICATIONS Hypersensitivity to erythromycins or any macrolide antibiotic; history of erythromycin-associated hepatitis; preexisting liver disease; congenital QT prolongation; electrolyte imbalances. **CAUTIOUS USE** Myasthenia gravis; history of GI disease; seizure disorders; pregnancy (category B), lactation.

ROUTE & DOSAGE

Infection

Adult: **PO** 400 mg q6h up to 4 g/day according to severity of infection

Child: **PO** 30–50 mg/kg/day in 4 divided doses (max: 100 mg/kg/day) for severe infections

ADMINISTRATION

- Note: 400 mg erythromycin ethylsuccinate is approximately equal to 250 mg erythromycin base.

Oral

- Chewable tablets should be chewed and not swallowed whole.
- Suspensions are stable for 14 days at room temperature unless otherwise stated by manufacturer. Note expiration date.
- Store tablets in tight containers unless otherwise directed.

ADVERSE EFFECTS (≥1%) **GI:** Diarrhea, *nausea,* vomiting, stomatitis, *abdominal cramps,* anorexia, hepatotoxicity. **Skin:** Skin eruptions. **Special Senses:** Ototoxicity. **Body as a Whole:** Potential for superinfections.

INTERACTIONS Drug: Serum levels and toxicities of **alfentanil, bexarotene, carbamazepine, cevimeline, cilostazol, clozapine, cyclosporine, disopyramide, estazolam, fentanyl, midazolam, methadone, modafinil, quinidine, sirolimus, digoxin, theophylline, triazolam, warfarin** are increased. **Ergotamine** may increase peripheral vasospasm and may increase risk of arrhythmias.

PHARMACOKINETICS Absorption: Readily absorbed from GI tract. **Peak:** 2 h. **Distribution:** Concentrates in liver; crosses placenta; distributed into breast milk. **Metabolism:** In liver. **Elimination:** Primarily in bile and feces. **Half-Life:** 2–5 h.

NURSING IMPLICATIONS

Assessment & Drug Effects

- Lab tests: Determine C&S prior to treatment. Periodic liver function

tests and blood cell counts if therapy is prolonged 10 days.
- Cholestatic hepatitis syndrome is most likely to occur in adults who have received erythromycin estolate for more than 10 days or who have had repeated courses of therapy. The condition generally clears within 3–5 days after cessation of therapy.

E

Patient & Family Education
- Advise patient to report immediately the onset of adverse reactions and to be on the alert for signs and symptoms associated with jaundice (see Appendix F).
- Ototoxicity is most likely to occur in patients receiving high dosage or who have impaired kidney function. Report immediately the onset of tinnitus, vertigo, or hearing impairment.

ERYTHROMYCIN GLUCEPTATE
(er-ith-roe-mye'sin)
Ilotycin Gluceptate

ERYTHROMYCIN LACTOBIONATE
Erythrocin Lactobionate-I.V.
Classification: MACROLIDE ANTIBIOTIC
Therapeutic: ANTIBIOTIC
Prototype: Erythromycin
Pregnancy Category: B

AVAILABILITY 500 mg, 1 g injection

ACTION & *THERAPEUTIC EFFECT* Soluble salt of erythromycin. It binds to the 50S ribosome subunits of susceptible bacteria, resulting in the suppression of protein synthesis of bacteria. *More active against gram-positive than gram-negative bacteria.*

USES When oral administration is not possible or the severity of infection requires immediate high serum levels. See erythromycin.

CONTRAINDICATIONS Hypersensitivity to erythromycin or macrolide antibiotics; congenital QT prolongation; electrolyte imbalances.
CAUTIOUS USE Impaired liver function; seizure disorders; pregnancy (category B), lactation.

ROUTE & DOSAGE

Infections
Adult/Child: **IV** 15–20 mg/kg/day in 4 divided doses

Legionnaires' Disease
Adult: **IV** 0.5–1 g q6h × 21 days

Pelvic Inflammatory Disease
Adult: **IV** 500 mg q6h × 3d, then convert to PO

ADMINISTRATION

Intravenous

PREPARE: **Intermittent/Continuous:** Initial solution is prepared by adding 10 mL sterile water for injection without preservatives to each 500 mg or fraction thereof. ▪ Shake vial until drug is completely dissolved. **Intermittent:** Further dilute each 1 g dose in 100–250 mL of LR or NS. **Continuous (*preferred*):** Further dilute each 1 g in 1000 mL LR or NS. ▪Give within 4 h.

ADMINISTER: **Intermittent:** Give 1 g or fraction thereof over 20–60 min. ▪Slow rate if pain develops along course of vein. **Continuous (*preferred*):** Continuous infusion is administered slowly, usually over 6–24 h.

INCOMPATIBILITIES **Solution/additive:** **Dextrose**-containing solutions, **ascorbic acid, carbenicil-**

lin, colistimethate, clindamycin, furosemide, heparin, linezolid, metaraminol, metoclopramide, tetracycline, vitamin B complex with C. Y-site: Cefepime, ceftazidime, fluconazole.

- Store: **Gluceptate,** reconstituted solution is stable up to 7 days if refrigerated at 2°–8° C (36°–46° F); use solution diluted for infusion within 4 h. **Lactobionate,** reconstituted solution is stable up to 14 days if refrigerated at 2°–8° C (36°–46° F); use solution diluted for infusion within 8 h.

ADVERSE EFFECTS (≥1%) **Body as a Whole:** *Pain and venous irritation after IV injection;* allergic reactions, anaphylaxis (rare); superinfections. **GI:** *Nausea,* vomiting, diarrhea, *abdominal cramps,* variations in liver function tests following prolonged or repeated therapy. (See also ERYTHROMYCIN.)

INTERACTIONS Drug: Serum levels and toxicities of **alfentanil, bexarotene, carbamazepine, cevimeline, cilostazol, clozapine, cyclosporine, disopyramide, estazolam, fentanyl, midazolam, methadone, modafinil, quinidine, sirolimus, digoxin, theophylline, triazolam, warfarin** are increased. **Ergotamine** may increase peripheral vasospasm, and may increase risk of arrhythmias.

PHARMACOKINETICS Peak: 1 h. **Distribution:** Concentrates in liver; crosses placenta; distributed into breast milk. **Metabolism:** In liver. **Elimination:** Primarily in bile and feces; 12–15% in urine. **Half-Life:** 3–5 h.

NURSING IMPLICATIONS

Assessment & Drug Effects

- Lab tests: Determine C&S prior to initiation of therapy. Periodic liver function tests with daily high doses or prolonged or repeated therapy.
- Monitor hearing impairment may occur with large doses of this drug. It may occur as early as the second day and as late as the third week of therapy.
- Monitor for S&S of thrombophlebitis (see Appendix F). IV infusion of large doses is reported to increase risk.

Patient & Family Education

- Notify physician immediately of tinnitus, dizziness, or hearing impairment.

ESCITALOPRAM OXALATE

(es-ci-tal′o-pram)

Lexapro

Classifications: ANTIDEPRESSANT; SELECTIVE SEROTONIN REUPTAKE INHIBITOR (SSRI)

Therapeutic: ANTIDEPRESSANT; SSRI

Prototype: Fluoxetine

Pregnancy Category: C

AVAILABILITY 5 mg, 10 mg, 20 mg tablets; 5 mg/5 mL liquid

ACTION & *THERAPEUTIC EFFECT* Selective serotonin reuptake inhibitor (SSRI) in the CNS. Antidepressant effect is presumed to be linked to its inhibition of CNS presynaptic neuronal uptake of serotonin. *Selective serotonin reuptake inhibition mechanism results in the antidepressant activity with or without anxiety symptoms.*

USES Depression, generalized anxiety disorder.

UNLABELED USES Treatment of panic disorders, social anxiety disorders.

CONTRAINDICATIONS Hypersensitivity to citalopram; concurrent use of MAOIS or use within 14 days of discontinuing MAOIS; abrupt discontinuation; suicidal ideations; mania; bipolar depression; volume depleted; suicidal ideation.

CAUTIOUS USE Hypersensitivity to other SSRIs; suicidal tendencies; bipolar disorder; obsessive-compulsive disorder, major depressive disorder, all major psychiatric disorders especially pediatric patients; depression, history of mania, hypomania; hyponatremia, ethanol intoxication, ECT, dehydration, severe renal impairment, hepatic disease; older adults; history of seizure disorders; elderly; pregnancy (category C), lactation (not within 4 h of drug ingestion). Safety and efficacy in children younger than 12 y are unknown.

ROUTE & DOSAGE

Depression, Generalized Anxiety

Adult/Adolescent: **PO** 10 daily, may increase to 20 mg daily if needed after 1 wk
Geriatric: **PO** 10 mg daily

Panic Disorder

Adult: **PO** 5 daily, may increase to 20 mg daily if needed after 1 wk

Hepatic Impairment Dosage Adjustment

Adult: **PO** 10 daily

ADMINISTRATION

Oral

- Do not begin this drug within 14 days of stopping an MAOI.
- Dose increments should be separated by at least 1 wk.
- Store at 15°–30° C (59°–86° F) in tightly closed container and protect from light.

ADVERSE EFFECTS (≥1%) **Body as a Whole:** Fatigue, fever, arthralgia, myalgia. **CV:** Palpitation, hypertension. **GI:** *Nausea,* diarrhea, dyspepsia, abdominal pain, dry mouth, vomiting, flatulence, reflux. **CNS:** Dizziness, *insomnia, somnolence,* paresthesia, migraine, tremor, vertigo. **Metabolic:** Increased or decreased weight, hyponatremia. **Respiratory:** URI, rhinitis, sinusitis. **Skin:** Increased sweating. **Urogenital:** Dysmenorrhea, decreased libido, ejaculation disorder, impotence, menstrual cramps.

INTERACTIONS Drug: Combination with MAOI could result in hypertensive crisis, hyperthermia, rigidity, myoclonus, autonomic instability; **cimetidine** may increase escitalopram levels; **linezolid** may cause serotonin syndrome. Use with drugs affecting hemostasis (**aspirin**, **warfarin**) increases bleeding risk. **Herbal: St. John's wort** may cause serotonin syndrome.

PHARMACOKINETICS Absorption: Rapidly absorbed from GI tract. **Onset:** Approximately 1 wk. **Peak:** 3 h. **Distribution:** 80% protein bound; crosses placenta; distributed into breast milk. **Metabolism:** In liver by CYP3A4, 2C19, and 2D6 enzymes. **Elimination:** 20% in urine, 80% in bile. **Half-Life:** 25 h.

NURSING IMPLICATIONS

Assessment & Drug Effects

- Closely observe for worsening of depression or emergence of suicidality especially in adolescents or children.
- Lab tests: Monitor periodically hepatic functions, CBC, serum sodium, and lithium levels when the two drugs are given concurrently.
- Monitor periodically HR and BP, and carefully monitor complete

cardiac status in person with known or suspected cardiac disease.

- Monitor closely older adult patients for adverse effects, especially with doses greater than 20 mg/day.

Patient & Family Education

- Report promptly changes in behavior such as anxiety, agitation, depression, panic attacks, aggressiveness, and suicidal ideation.
- Do not engage in hazardous activities until reaction to this drug is known.
- Avoid using alcohol while taking escitalopram.
- Inform physician of commonly used OTC drugs as there is potential for drug interactions. The use of aspirin and NSAIDs can affect coagulation and cause increased risk of bleeding.
- Report distressing adverse effects including any changes in sexual functioning or response.
- Periodic ophthalmology exams are advised with long-term treatment.

ESMOLOL HYDROCHLORIDE

(ess′moe-lol)

Brevibloc

Classifications: BETA-ADRENERGIC ANTAGONIST; ANTIARRHYTHMIC

Therapeutic: ANTIARRHYTHMIC

Prototype: Propranolol

Pregnancy Category: C

AVAILABILITY 10 mg/mL, 250 mg/mL injection

ACTION & *THERAPEUTIC EFFECT* Ultrashort-acting beta$_1$-adrenergic blocking agent with cardioselective properties. Inhibits the agonist effect of catecholamines by competitive binding at beta-adrenergic receptors. Antiarrhythmic properties occur at the AV node. *Effective as an antiarrhythmic agent on the AV-nodal conduction system. Blocks sympathetically mediated increases in cardiac rate and BP since it binds predominantly to beta$_1$-receptors in cardiac tissue.*

USES Supraventricular tachyarrhythmias (SVT) in perioperative and postoperative periods or in other critical situations. Also short-term treatment of noncompensating sinus tachycardia and in the control of heart rate for patients with MI.

UNLABELED USES Moderate postoperative hypertension; treatment of intense transient adrenergic response to surgical stress in cardiac as well as noncardiac surgery.

CONTRAINDICATIONS Hypersensitivity to esmolol; heart block greater than first degree, sinus bradycardia, cardiogenic shock; decompensated CHF; acute bronchospasm; pregnancy (category C). Safety in children is not established.

CAUTIOUS USE History of allergy; CHF; pulmonary disease such as bronchial asthma, COPD, or pulmonary edema; diabetes mellitus; kidney function impairment; lactation.

ROUTE & DOSAGE

Supraventricular Tachyarrhythmias

Adult: **IV** 500 mcg/kg loading dose followed by 50 mcg/kg/min, may increase dose q5–10min prn if response inadequate, may repeat loading dose followed by 100 mcg/kg/min × 4 min; may continue repeating loading dose and increasing

4-min dose by 50 mcg/kg/min prn (max: 200 mcg/kg/min)

Intraoperative/Postoperative Tachycardia

Adult: **IV** 80 mg bolus followed by 150 mcg/kg/min; increase if needed (max: 300 mcg/kg/min)

ADMINISTRATION

Intravenous

Note: Do not use the 2500 mg ampule for direct IV injection.

PREPARE: **Direct:** Use the 10 mg/mL vial undiluted for the loading dose. **IV Infusion:** Use the concentrate (250 mg/mL) for infusion. ▪Prepare maintenance infusion by adding 2.5 g to 250 mL or 5 g to 500 mL of IV solution to yield 10 mg/mL. Compatible diluents include D5W, D5/LR, D5/NS, D5/.45NS, LR.

ADMINISTER: **Direct:** Give loading dose over 1 min. **IV Infusion:** Give maintenance infusion over 4 min. ▪If adequate response is noted, continue maintenance infusion with periodic adjustments as needed. ▪If an adequate response has not occurred, repeat loading dose and follow with an increased maintenance infusion of 100 mcg/kg/min. ▪May continue titration cycle with same loading dose while increasing maintenance infusion by 50 mcg/kg/min until desired end point is near. ▪Then omit loading dose and titrate maintenance dose up or down by 25 to 50 mcg/kg/min until desired heart rate is reached.

INCOMPATIBILITIES **Solution/additive:** **Diazepam, procainamide, thiopental.** **Y-site:** **Amphotericin B cholesteryl, furosemide, warfarin.**

▪ Diluted infusion solution is stable for at least 24 h at room temperature.

ADVERSE EFFECTS (≥1%) **CNS:** Headache, *dizziness,* somnolence, confusion, agitation. **CV:** *Hypotension* (dose related), cold hands and feet, bradyarrhythmias, flushing, myocardial depression. **GI:** Nausea, vomiting. **Respiratory:** Dyspnea, chest pain, rhonchi, <u>bronchospasm</u>. **Skin:** *Infusion site inflammation* (redness, swelling, induration).

INTERACTIONS Drug: May increase **digoxin** IV levels 10–20%; **morphine** IV may increase esmolol levels by 45%; **succinylcholine** may prolong neuromuscular blockade.

PHARMACOKINETICS Onset: Less than 5 min. **Peak:** 10–20 min. **Duration:** 10–30 min. **Metabolism:** Hydrolyzed by RBC esterases. **Elimination:** In urine. **Half-Life:** 9 min.

NURSING IMPLICATIONS

Assessment & Drug Effects

- Monitor BP, pulse, ECG, during esmolol infusion. Hypotension may have its onset during the initial titration phase; thereafter the risk increases with increasing doses. Usually the hypotension experienced during esmolol infusion is resolved within 30 min after infusion is reduced or discontinued.
- Change injection site if local reaction occurs. IV site reactions (burning, erythema) or diaphoresis may develop during infusion. Both reactions are temporary. Blood chemistry abnormalities have not been reported.
- Overdose symptoms: Discontinue administration if the following symptoms occur: Bradycardia, severe dizziness or drowsiness, dyspnea, bluish-colored fingernails or palms of hands, seizures.

E

ESOMEPRAZOLE MAGNESIUM

(e-so-me′pra-zole)

Nexium

Classification: PROTON PUMP INHIBITOR

Therapeutic: ANTIULCER

Prototype: Omeprazole

Pregnancy Category: B

AVAILABILITY 20 mg, 40 mg capsules; 20 mg, 40 mg powder for injection; 10 mg, 20 mg, 40 mg oral suspensions

ACTION & *THERAPEUTIC EFFECT*

Isomer of omeprazole. A weak base that is converted to the active form in the highly acidic environment of the gastric parietal cells. Inhibits the enzyme H^+K^+-ATPase (the acid pump), thus suppressing gastric acid secretion. *Due to inhibition of the H^+K^+-ATPase, esomeprazole substantially decreases both basal and stimulated acid secretion through inhibition of the acid pump in parietal cells.*

USES Erosive esophagitis, gastrointestinal reflux disease (GERD), hypersecretory diseases, duodenal ulcer associated with *H. pylori* in combination with antibiotics.

CONTRAINDICATIONS Hypersensitivity to esomeprazole magnesium, omeprazole, or other proton pump inhibitors; gastric malignancy; lactation; children younger than 1 y.

CAUTIOUS USE Severe renal insufficiency; severe hepatic impairment; treatment for more than a year; gastric ulcers; elderly; IBD, GI disease; pregnancy (category B).

ROUTE & DOSAGE

Healing of Erosive Esophagitis

Adult/Adolescent: **PO/IV** 20–40 mg daily at least 1 h before meals times 4–8 wk

GERD, Erosive Esophagitis Maintenance

Adult/Adolescent: **PO/IV** 20–40 mg daily at least 1 h before meals times 4–8 wk

Child/Infant (older than 1 y): **PO** *20 kg or more:* 10–20 mg daily at least 1 h before meals up to 8 wk; *weight less than 20 kg:* 10 mg daily at least 1 h before meals up to 8 wk

Duodenal Ulcer

Adult: **PO** 40 mg daily times 10 days

Hypersecretory Disease (Zollinger-Ellison)

Adult: **PO** 40 mg b.i.d.

NSAID Ulcer Prophylaxis

Adult: **PO** 20–40 mg daily

Hepatic Impairment Dosage Adjustment

Child-Pugh class C: Do not exceed 20 mg/day

ADMINISTRATION

Oral

- Give at least 1 h before eating.
- Do not crush or chew capsule. **Must be** swallowed whole.
- Open capsule and mix pellets with applesauce (cold or room temperature) if patient cannot swallow capsules. Do NOT crush pellets. Applesauce should be swallowed immediately after mixing without chewing.
- May take with antacids.
- Store in the original blister package 15°–30° C (59°–86° F).

Intravenous

PREPARE: **Direct:** Reconstitute powder with 5 mL of NS. **IV Infusion:** Further dilute reconstituted solution in 50 mL of NS, LR, or D5W.

ADMINISTER: **Direct:** Withdraw required dose from reconstituted solution and give over no less than 3 min. **IV Infusion:** Give IV solution over 10–30 min.

INCOMPATIBILITIES Do not give simultaneously with any other medication through the same IV site or line.

- Flush IV line with NS, LR, or D5W before/after infusion.
- Store reconstituted solution at room temperature up to 30° C (86° F); give within 12 h of reconstitution with NS or LR and within 6 h of reconstitution with D5W.

ADVERSE EFFECTS (≥1%) **CNS:** Headache. **GI:** Nausea, vomiting, diarrhea, constipation, abdominal pain, flatulence, dry mouth.

INTERACTIONS Drug: May increase **diazepam, phenytoin, warfarin** levels. May decrease levels of **atazanavir** and **nelfinavir**. **Food:** Food decreases absorption by up to 35%.

PHARMACOKINETICS Absorption: Destroyed in acidic environment, therefore capsules are designed for delayed absorption in the small intestine. 70% reaches systemic circulation. **Metabolism:** In liver by CYP2C19. **Elimination:** Inactive metabolites excreted in both urine and feces. **Half-Life:** 1.5 h.

NURSING IMPLICATIONS

Assessment & Drug Effects

- Monitor for S&S of adverse CNS effects (vertigo, agitation, depression) especially in severely ill patients.
- Monitor phenytoin levels with concurrent use.
- Monitor INR/PT with concurrent warfarin use.
- Lab tests: Periodic liver function tests, CBC, Hct and Hbg, urinalysis for hematuria and proteinuria.

Patient & Family Education

- Report any changes in urinary elimination such as pain or discomfort associated with urination to physician.
- Report severe diarrhea. Drug may need to be discontinued.

ESTAZOLAM

(es-ta-zo′lam)

Classifications: ANXIOLYTIC; SEDATIVE-HYPNOTIC; BENZODIAZEPINE
Therapeutic: ANTIANXIETY; SEDATIVE-HYPNOTIC
Prototype: Lorazepam
Pregnancy Category: X
Controlled Substance: Schedule IV

AVAILABILITY 1 mg, 2 mg tablets

ACTION & *THERAPEUTIC EFFECT* Benzodiazepine whose effects (anxiolytic, sedative, hypnotic, skeletal muscle relaxant) are mediated by the inhibitory neurotransmitter gamma-aminobutyric acid (GABA). GABA acts at the thalamic, hypothalamic, and limbic levels of CNS. *Benzodiazepines generally decrease the number of awakenings from sleep. Stage 2 sleep is increased with all benzodiazepines. Estazolam shortens stages 3 and 4 (slow-wave sleep), and REM sleep is shortened. The total sleep time, however, is increased.*

USES Short-term management of insomnia.

CONTRAINDICATIONS Known sensitivity to benzodiazepines; acute closed-angle glaucoma, primary depressive disorders or psychosis; abrupt discontinuation; coma, shock, acute alcohol intoxication; children younger than 18 y; pregnancy (category X), lactation.

CAUTIOUS USE Renal and hepatic impairment, renal failure; organic brain syndrome, alcoholism, benzodiazepine dependence, suicidal ideations, CNS depression, seizure disorder, status epilepticus; substance abuse; shock, coma; dementia, mania, psychosis; myasthenia gravis, Parkinson's disease; sleep apnea; open-angle glaucoma, GI disorders, older adult and debilitated patients; limited pulmonary reserve, pulmonary disease, COPD.

ROUTE & DOSAGE

Insomnia

Adult: **PO** 1 mg at bedtime, may increase up to 2 mg if necessary (some debilitated older adult patients should start with 0.5 mg at bedtime)

ADMINISTRATION

Oral

- For older adult patients in good health, a 1 mg dose is indicated; reduce initial dose to 0.5 mg for debilitated or small older adult patients.
- Dosage reduction also may be needed in the presence of hepatic impairment.

ADVERSE EFFECTS (≥1%) **CNS:** Headache, dizziness, impaired coordination, hypokinesia, *somnolence,* hangover, weakness. **CV:** Palpitations, arrhythmias, syncope (all rare). **Hematologic:** Leukopenia, <u>agranulocytosis</u>. **GI:** Constipation, xerostomia, anorexia, flatulence, vomiting. **Musculoskeletal:** Arthritis, arthralgia, myalgia, muscle spasm.

INTERACTIONS Drug: Cimetidine may decrease metabolism of estazolam and increase its effects; **alcohol** and other CNS DEPRESSANTS may increase drowsiness; CYP3A4 inhibitors **(ketoconazole, itraconazole, nefazodone, diltiazem, fluvoxamine, cimetidine, isoniazid, erythromycin)** can increase concentrations and toxicity of estazolam; **carbamazepine, phenytoin, rifampin,** BARBITURATES may decrease estazolam concentrations. **Food: Grapefruit juice** greater than 1 quart may increase toxicity. **Herbal: Kava, valerian** may potentiate sedation.

PHARMACOKINETICS Absorption: Rapidly absorbed from GI tract. **Onset:** 20–30 min. **Peak:** 2 h. **Distribution:** Crosses rapidly into brain; crosses placenta; distributed into breast milk. **Metabolism:** Extensively in liver. **Elimination:** In urine. **Half-Life:** 10–24 h.

NURSING IMPLICATIONS

Assessment & Drug Effects

- Monitor for improvement in S&S of insomnia.
- Assess for excess CNS depression or daytime sedation.
- Assess for safety, especially with older adult or debilitated patients, as dizziness and impaired coordination are known adverse effects.

Patient & Family Education

- Learn adverse effects and report those experienced to the physician.
- Avoid using this drug in combination with other CNS depressant drugs or alcohol.
- Do not drive or engage in other potentially hazardous activities until response to drug is known.

ESTRADIOL (Pr)

(ess-tra-dye′ole)

Alora, Climara, Divigel, Estrace, Estraderm, Estring, EstroGel, Evamist, Menostar, Vivelle, Vivelle DOT, Vagifem

ESTRADIOL ACETATE
Femring, Femtrace

ESTRADIOL CYPIONATE
Depo-Estradiol Cypionate, Estro-Cyp

ESTRADIOL VALERATE
Delestrogen, Femogex ♦

ESTRADIOL HEMIHYDRATE
Estrasorb

Classification: ESTROGEN
Therapeutic: ESTROGEN REPLACEMENT
Pregnancy Category: X

AVAILABILITY Estradiol: 0.025 mg, 0.0375 mg, 0.05 mg, 0.06 mg, 0.075 mg, 0.1 mg patch; 14 mcg/24 h transdermal patch; 0.5 mg, 1 mg, 2 mg tablets; 25 mcg vaginal tablets, 2 mg vaginal ring, 0.1 mg vaginal cream; 2.5 mg/g topical emulsion; 0.06%, 0.1% topical gel; 1.53 mg/actuation transdermal spray; **Cypionate:** 5 mg/mL injection; **Valerate:** 10 mg/mL, 20 mg/mL, 40 mg/mL injection; **Acetate:** 0.45 mg, 0.9 mg, 1.8 mg tablets; 0.05 mg/day, 0.1 mg/day vaginal insert; **Hemihydrate:** 0.25% topical emulsion

ACTION & *THERAPEUTIC EFFECT* Natural or synthetic steroid hormone secreted principally by the ovarian follicles, and also by the adrenals, corpus luteum, placenta, and testes. Estrogen binds to a specific intracellular receptor, forming a complex that stimulates synthesis of proteins responsible for estrogenic effects. Promotes endometrial lining development, but long-time use leads to abnormal endometrial hyperplasia, and abnormal bleeding. Conversely, estrogen-stimulated endometrium suddenly deprived of estrogen may bleed within 48–72 h. *Estradiol (estrogens) effects simulate those produced by the endogenous hormone. May mask onset of climacteric.*

USES Natural or surgical menopausal symptoms, kraurosis vulvae, atrophic vaginitis, primary ovarian failure, female hypogonadism, castration. Used adjunctively with diet, calcium, and physical therapy to prevent and treat postmenopausal osteoporosis; also for palliation in advanced prostatic carcinoma and inoperable metastatic breast cancer in women at least 5 y after menopause. Combined with progestins in many oral contraceptive formulations.

CONTRAINDICATIONS Known or suspected pregnancy (category X); estrogenic-dependent neoplasms, breast cancer (except in selected patients being treated for metastatic disease). History of thromboembolic disorders; active arterial thrombosis or thrombophlebitis; undiagnosed abnormal genital bleeding; uterine fibroids; endometriosis; history of cholestatic disease; hepatic disease; thyroid dysfunction; blood dyscrasias; hypercalcemia; lupus (SLE).
CAUTIOUS USE Adolescents with incomplete bone growth; endometriosis; hypertension, cardiac insufficiency; diseases of calcium and phosphate metabolism (metabolic bone disease); cerebrovascular disease; mental depression; benign breast disease, family history of breast or genital tract neoplasm; diabetes mellitus; gallbladder disease; preexisting leiomyoma, abnormal mammogram, history of idiopathic jaundice of pregnancy; varicosities; asthma; epilepsy; migraine headaches; liver or kidney dysfunction; jaundice, acute intermittent porphyria, pyridoxine deficiency.

ROUTE & DOSAGE

Menopause, Atrophic Vaginitis, Kraurosis Vulvae, Female Hypogonadism, Female Castration, Primary Ovarian Failure

Adult: **PO** 0.45–2 mg/day in a cyclic regimen **Topical** 2–4 g vaginal cream intravaginally once/day for 1–2 wk, then 1–2 g/day for 1–2 wk, then 1 g 1–3 times/wk; Transdermal patch **Estraderm** twice weekly; **Climara, FemPatch, Menostar** qwk in a cyclic regimen; **Estrasorb** Apply 1 packet to the left thigh and calf and 1 packet to the right thigh and calf once daily in the morning; **EstroGel** Apply 1.25 g (one-half applicatorful) to one arm every day (usually in the morning). **IM Cypionate** 1–5 mg once q3–4wk; **Valerate** 10–25 mg once q4wk; **Acetate** Insert 1 vaginal ring into the upper third of the vaginal vault. Keep in place continuously for 3 mo, then remove. **Divigel** Apply one packet to upper thigh daily (alternate legs). **Evamist** Apply one spray to inner forearm daily, dose may be increased to 2–3 sprays daily

Metastatic Breast Cancer

Adult: **PO** 10 mg t.i.d.

Prostatic Cancer

Adult: **PO** 1–2 mg t.i.d. **IM Valerate** 30 mg once q1–2wk

Postpartum Breast Engorgement

Adult: **IM Valerate** 10–25 mg at end of first stage of labor

ADMINISTRATION

Oral

- Give with or immediately after solid food to reduce nausea.
- Protect tablets from light and moisture in well-closed container. Protect from freezing, unless otherwise directed by manufacturer.

Intravaginal

- Insert calibrated dosage applicator approximately 5 cm (2 in.) into vagina, directing it slightly back toward sacrum. Instill medication by pushing plunger. Patient should remain in recumbent position about 30 min to prevent losing the medication. Observe perineal area before each administration: If mucosa is red, swollen, or excoriated or if there is a change in vaginal discharge, report to physician.

Topical

- Cleanse and dry selected skin area. Apply as directed under Route & Dosage.

Transdermal

- Cleanse and dry selected skin area on trunk of body, preferably the abdomen. Avoid application to the breasts, to an irritated, abraded, oily area, or to the waistline. If system falls off, it may be reapplied, or if necessary, a new one can be applied. Return to original treatment schedule. Rotate application site with an interval of at least 1 wk between applications to a particular site.

Intramuscular

- Give deep into a large muscle.
- Store at 15°–30° C (59°–86° F); protect from light and freezing.

ADVERSE EFFECTS (≥1%) **CNS:** Headache, migraine, dizziness, mental depression, chorea, convulsions, increased risk of dementia. **CV:** <u>Thromboembolic disorders</u>, stroke, CAD, hypertension. **Special Senses:** Intolerance to contact lenses, worsening of myopia or astigmatism, scotomas. **GI:** *Nausea,* vomiting, anorexia, increased appetite, diarrhea, abdominal cramps or pain, constipation, bloating, colitis, acute pancreatitis, cholestatic jaundice, benign hepatoadenoma. **Urogenital:** Mastodynia, breast secretion, spotting, changes in menstrual flow, dysmenorrhea, amenorrhea, cervical erosion, altered cervical secretions, premenstrual-like syndrome, vaginal candidiasis, endometrial cystic hyperplasia, reactivation of endometriosis, increased size of preexisting fibromyomas, cystitis-like syndrome, hemolytic uremic syndrome, change in libido; in men: Gynecomastia, testicular atrophy, feminization, impotence (reversible). **Metabolic:** Reduced carbohydrate tolerance, hyperglycemia, hypercalcemia, folic acid deficiency, fluid retention. **Skin:** Dermatitis, pruritus, seborrhea, oily skin, acne; photosensitivity, chloasma, loss of scalp hair, hirsutism. **Body as a Whole:** Pain and postinjection flare at injection site; sterile abscess; leg cramps, weight changes. **Hematologic:** Acute intermittent porphyria.

DIAGNOSTIC TEST INTERFERENCE Estradiol reduces response of ***metyrapone*** test and excretion of ***pregnanediol. Increases: BSP*** retention, norepinephrine-induced ***platelet aggregability, hydrocortisone, PBI, T_4, sodium, thyroxine-binding globulin (TBG), prothrombin and factors VII, VIII, IX,*** and ***X; serum triglyceride,*** and ***phospholipid*** concentrations, ***renin*** substrate. ***Decreases: Antithrombin III, pyridoxine*** and ***serum folate*** concentrations, serum ***cholesterol,*** values for the ***T_3 resin uptake*** test, ***glucose tolerance.*** May cause false-positive test for ***LE cells*** or ***antinuclear antibodies (ANA).***

INTERACTIONS Drug: BARBITURATES, **phenytoin, rifampin** decrease estrogen effect by increasing its metabolism; ORAL ANTICOAGULANTS may decrease hypoprothrombinemic effects; interfere with effects of **bromocriptine;** may increase levels and toxicity of **cyclosporine,** TRICYCLIC ANTIDEPRESSANTS, **theophylline;** decrease effectiveness of **clofibrate.**

PHARMACOKINETICS Absorption: Rapid from GI tract; readily through skin and mucous membranes; slow from IM injections. **Distribution:** Throughout body tissues, especially in adipose tissue; crosses placenta. **Metabolism:** Primarily in liver. **Elimination:** In urine; in breast milk.

NURSING IMPLICATIONS

Assessment & Drug Effects

- Monitor adverse GI effects. Nausea, frequently at breakfast time, usually disappears after 1 or 2 wk of drug use.
- Check BP on a regular basis in patients with cardiac or kidney dysfunction or hypertension; monitored carefully.
- Note: Severe hypercalcemia (greater than 15 mg/dL) may be caused by estradiol therapy in patients with breast cancer and bone metastasis.

Patient & Family Education

- Comply with established dosage schedule. Do not alter unless physician prescribes a change.
- Notify physician of intermittent breakthrough bleeding, spotting, bleeding, or unexplained and sudden pain.
- Determine weight under standard conditions 1 or 2 times/wk; report sudden weight gain or other signs of fluid retention.
- Notify physician of calf pain upon flexing foot and the following

symptoms of thromboembolic disorders: Tenderness, swelling, and redness in extremity; sudden, severe headache or chest pain; slurring of speech; change in vision; tenderness, pain, sudden shortness of breath.

- Monitor blood glucose for loss of glycemic control if diabetic.
- Decrease caffeine intake, since estrogen depresses caffeine metabolism.
- Learn self-examination of breasts and follow a monthly schedule.
- Estrogen-induced feminization and impotence in male patients are reversible with termination of therapy.

ESTRAMUSTINE PHOSPHATE SODIUM

(ess-tra-muss'teen)

Emcyt

Classifications: ANTINEOPLASTIC; ALKYLATING AGENT; NITROGEN MUSTARD

Therapeutic: ANTINEOPLASTIC

Prototype: Cyclophosphamide

Pregnancy Category: D

AVAILABILITY 140 mg capsules

ACTION & *THERAPEUTIC EFFECT*

Conjugate of estradiol and the carbamate of nitrogen mustard. Incorporation of estramustine in tumor tissues is probably due to the presence of estramustine-binding protein (EMBP), which is found in prostate carcinoma, glioma, melanoma, and breast carcinoma. Binds to proteins and microtubulin resulting in microtubule changes in the cell division cycle, thus arresting cell division in the G2/M phase of the cell cycle. *Major effectiveness reported to be in patients who have been refractory to estrogen therapy alone.*

USES Palliative treatment of metabolic or progressive carcinoma of prostate.

CONTRAINDICATIONS Hypersensitivity to either estradiol or nitrogen mustard; active thrombophlebitis or thromboembolic disorders; pregnancy (category D), lactation.

CAUTIOUS USE History of thrombophlebitis, thromboses, or thromboembolic disorders; cerebrovascular or coronary artery disease; gallstones or peptic ulcer; impaired liver function; metabolic bone diseases associated with hypercalcemia; diabetes mellitus; hypertension, conditions that might be aggravated by fluid retention (e.g., epilepsy, migraine, kidney dysfunction); older adult patients.

ROUTE & DOSAGE

Neoplasm

Adult: **PO** 14 mg/kg/day in 3–4 divided doses

ADMINISTRATION

Oral

- Give with meals to reduce incidence of GI adverse effects. Some patients require drug withdrawal because of intolerable GI effects.
- Store at 2°–8° C (38°–46° F) in tight, light-resistant containers, unless otherwise directed by manufacturer.

ADVERSE EFFECTS (≥1%) **CNS:** Lethargy, emotional lability, insomnia, headache, anxiety. **CV:** CVA, MI, *thrombophlebitis,* CHF, *peripheral edema.* **GI:** *Nausea,* diarrhea, anorexia, flatulence, vomiting, thirst, GI bleeding. **Hematologic:** Leukopenia, thrombocytopenia, *abnormalities in liver function tests,* hypercalcemia, bone marrow depression (rare). **Respiratory:** Hoarseness, burning sensation in throat, dyspnea, upper respiratory discharge, pulmonary emboli. **Skin:** Rash, pruritus, urticaria, dry skin, easy bruising, flushing, peeling skin and fingertips, thinning hair. **Special Senses:** Tearing of eyes. **Urogenital:** Gynecomastia, breast tenderness, impotence. **Endocrine:** Decrease in glucose tolerance. **Musculoskeletal:** Leg cramps.

INTERACTIONS Food: Milk, dairy products, calcium supplements may decrease estramustine absorption.

PHARMACOKINETICS Absorption: Readily absorbed from GI tract. **Peak:** 2–3 h. **Metabolism:** Dephosphorylated in intestines to estramustine, estradiol, estrone, and nitrogen mustard; further metabolized in liver. **Elimination:** In feces via bile. **Half-Life:** 20 h.

NURSING IMPLICATIONS

Assessment & Drug Effects

- Monitor weight and examine for peripheral edema. Be mindful that drug can cause CHF.
- Monitor I&O ratio and pattern to prevent dehydration and electrolyte imbalance, especially with vomiting or diarrhea.
- Observe diabetics closely because of possibility of estramustine-induced reduction in glucose tolerance. Monitor baseline and periodic glucose tolerance tests.
- Lab tests: Perform baseline and periodic liver enzymes and bilirubin tests; repeat after drug has been discontinued for 2 mo.

Patient & Family Education

- Eat small meals at frequent intervals to reduce drug-induced nausea, eat slowly, and try cold food if food odors are offensive.
- Drink liquids 1 h before or 1 h after rather than with meals; clear liquids may be more palatable.

ESTROGEN-PROGESTIN COMBINATIONS (CONTRACEPTIVES)

Oral

Monophasic: Apri, Alesse, Aviane, Balziva, Brevicon, Cryselle, Demulen, Desogen, Gencept, Junel, Lessina, Levlite, Levora, Loestrin, Lo/Ovral, Low-Ogestrel, Microgestin, Modicon, Nordette, Norethin, Norinyl, Nortrel, Ogestrel, Ortho-Cept, Ortho-Cyclen, Ortho-Novum, Ovcon, Portia, Previfem, Seasonale, Sprintec, Yasmin, Yaz, Zovia
Biphasic: LoSeasonique, Kariva, Mircette, Ortho-Novum 10/11
Triphasic: Aranelle, Cyclessa, Enpresse, Estrostep, Estrostep Fe, Lybrel, Ortho-Novum 7/7/7, Ortho Tri-Cyclen, Ortho Tri-Cyclen Lo, Tri-Norinyl, Tri-Previfem, Tri-Sprintec, Triphasil, Trivora, Velivet
Postcoital Contraceptives: Plan B, Preven

Transdermal

Ortho Evra

Intravaginal

NuvaRing

Classification: ESTROGEN-PROGESTIN COMBINATIONS
Therapeutic: CONTRACEPTIVE
Prototype: Estradiol, Norethindrone
Pregnancy Category: X

AVAILABILITY Combination oral contraceptives contain one of the following estrogens and one of the following progestins. **Estrogen:** Ethinyl estradiol 10 mcg, 20 mcg, 25 mcg, 30 mcg, 35 mcg, 40 mcg, 50 mcg; mestranol 50 mcg; **Progestin:** Desogestrel 0.15 mg; drospirenone 3 mg; ethynodiol diacetate 1 mg; levonorgestrel 0.05 mg, 0.075 mg, 0.1 mg, 0.125 mg, 0.15 mg, 0.25 mg, 0.75 mg; norethindrone 0.4 mg, 0.5 mg, 0.75 mg, 1 mg; norethindrone acetate 1 mg, 1.5 mg; norgestimate 0.18 mg, 0.215 mg, 0.25 mg; norgestrel 0.3 mg, 0.5 mg; **Transdermal:** Norelgestromin 6 mg/0.75 mg ethinyl estradiol patch; **Vaginal:** Etonogestrel 11.7 mg/2.7 mg ethinyl estradiol vaginal insert

ACTION & *THERAPEUTIC EFFECT* Three types of estrogen-progestin combinations are available: (1) monophasic, fixed dosage of estrogen-progestin throughout the cycle; (2) biphasic, amount of estrogen remains the same throughout cycle, less progestin in first half of cycle and increased progestin in second half; (3) triphasic, estrogen amount is the same or varies throughout cycle, progestin amount varies. *Fixed combination of estrogen and progestin produces contraception by preventing ovulation and rendering reproductive tract structures hostile to sperm penetration and zygote implantation.*

USES To prevent conception and to treat hypermenorrhea and endometriosis; postcoital contraceptive or "morning after pill"; moderate acne in females 15 y or older (Tri-Cyclen).

CONTRAINDICATIONS Familial or personal history of or existence of breast or other estrogen-dependent neoplasm, recurrent chronic cystic mastitis, history of or existence of thrombophlebitis or thromboembolic disorders, cerebral vascular or coronary artery disease, MI, serious hepatic dysfunction, hepatic neoplasm, family history of hepatic porphyria, undiagnosed abnormal vaginal bleeding, women age 40 and over, adolescents with incomplete epiphyseal closure; pregnancy (category X), lactation, missed abortion. **CAUTIOUS USE** History of depression, preexisting hypertension, or cardiac or renal disease; impaired liver function, history of migraine, convulsive disorders, or asthma; multiparous women with grossly irregular menses, diabetes, or familial history of diabetes; gallbladder disease, lupus erythematosus, rheumatic disease, varicosities, smokers.

ROUTE & DOSAGE

Contraception

Adult: **PO** 1 active tablet daily for 21 days, then placebo tablet or no tablets for 7 days, repeat cycle **Continuous regimen** (Seasonale) 1 tablet daily × 84 consecutive days. Wait 7 days for withdrawal bleeding before starting next cycle **Topical** Apply one patch once weekly for 3 wk, then have 1 wk patch-free before repeating the cycle **Intravaginal** Insert 1 ring on or before day 5 of the cycle. Remove ring after 3 wk, followed by a 1 wk rest. Then insert new ring.

Postcoital Contraception (Plan B, Preven, Ovral)

Adult: **PO** Ovral, 2 tablets within 72 h of intercourse, then 2 tablets 12 h later; 1 (Plan B) or 2 (Preven) tablets within 72 h of unprotected intercourse, take second dose of 1 (Plan B) or 2 (Preven) tablets 12 h later

ADMINISTRATION

- Give without regard to meals.
- Do not exceed 24-h intervals between the daily doses; taking with a meal or at bedtime is a helpful reminder.

ADVERSE EFFECTS (≥1%) **Body as a Whole:** Paresthesias. **CV:** Malignant hypertension, thrombotic and thromboembolic disorders, *mild to moderate increase in BP,* increase in size of varicosities, edema. **Endocrine:** Estrogen excess (*nausea,* bloating, menstrual tension, cervical mucorrhea, polyposis, *chloasma, hypertension,* migraine headache, breast fullness or tenderness, edema); estrogen deficiency (hypomenorrhea, *early or mid-cycle breakthrough bleeding,* increased spotting); progestin excess (hypomenorrhea, breast regression, *vaginal candidiasis,* depression, fatigue, weight gain, increased appetite, acne, oily scalp, hair loss); progestin deficiency (late-cycle breakthrough bleeding, amenorrhea). **GI:** *Nausea,* cholelithiasis, gallbladder disease, cholestatic jaundice, benign hepatic adenomas; diarrhea, constipation, abdominal cramps. **Metabolic:** *Decreased glucose tolerance,* pyridoxine deficiency (see also diagnostic test interferences), acute intermittent porphyria. **Skin:** Rash (allergic), photosensitivity (photoallergy or phototoxicity), irritation from patch. **Special Senses:** Unexplained loss of vision, optic neuritis, proptosis, diplopia, change in corneal curvature (steepening), intolerance to contact lenses, retinal thrombosis, papilledema. **Urogenital:** Ureteral dilation, increased incidence of urinary tract infection, hemolytic uremia syndrome, renal failure, increased risk of congenital anomalies, decreased quality and quantity of breast milk, dysmenorrhea, increased size of preexisting uterine fibroids, *menstrual disorders.* Foreign body sensation, coital problems, device expulsion, vaginal discomfort, vaginitis, leukorrhea from ring.

DIAGNOSTIC TEST INTERFERENCE ORAL CONTRACEPTIVES (OCS) increase ***BSP*** retention, ***prothrombin*** and ***coagulation factors II, VII, VIII, IX, X; platelet agregability, thyroid-binding globulin, PBI, T_4: transcortin; corticosteroid, triglyceride*** and ***phospholipid*** levels; ***ceruloplasmin, aldosterone, amylase, transferrin; renin*** activity, ***vitamin A.*** OCS decrease ***antithrombin III, T_3*** resin uptake, ***serum folate, glucose tolerance, albumin, vitamin B_{12}*** and reduce the ***metyrapone*** test response.

INTERACTIONS Drug: Aminocaproic acid may increase clotting factors, leading to hypercoagulable state; BARBITURATES, ANTICONVULSANTS, ANTIBIOTICS, **rifampin,** ANTIFUNGALS reduce efficacy of OCS and increase incidence of breakthrough bleeding and risk of pregnancy. May decrease efficacy of **lamotrigine. Herbal: St. John's wort** may decrease efficacy of OCS.

PHARMACOKINETICS Absorption: Oral: Readily from GI tract; or from transdermal patch placed on abdomen, buttock, upper outer arm and upper torso (excluding breast). Vaginal insert: Norgestrel 100% absorbed, ethinyl estradiol 56% absorbed. **Peak:** Patch: 48 h. **Duration:** Patch: 1 wk. **Distribution:** Widely distributed; crosses placenta; small amount distributed into breast milk. **Metabolism:** In liver. **Elimination:** In urine and feces. **Half-Life:** 6–45 h oral. Following removal of the patch: Norelgestromin 28 h, ethinyl estradiol 17 h; vaginal ring: Norgestrel 29 h; ethinyl estradiol 45 h.

NURSING IMPLICATIONS

Assessment & Drug Effects

- Check BP periodically. In some women, changes in BP occur

within each cycle; in others, slow increase of pressure, particularly diastolic, over several months is significant. Drug-induced BP elevation is usually reversible with cessation of OCs.

- Nausea with or without vomiting occurs in approximately 10% of patients during the first cycle and is reportedly one of the major reasons for voluntary discontinuation of therapy. Most adverse effects tend to disappear in third or fourth cycle of use. Instruct patient to report symptoms that persist after fourth cycle. Dose adjustment or a different product may be indicated.
- Hirsutism and loss of hair are reversible with discontinuation of OCs or by change of selected combination.
- Acne may improve, worsen, or develop for first time. In women on OCs for at least 1 y, postcontraceptive acne sometimes occurs 3–4 mo after stopping drug and may continue for 6–12 mo.
- Anovulation or amenorrhea following termination of OC regimen may persist more than 6 mo. The user with pretreatment oligomenorrhea or secondary amenorrhea is most apt to have oversuppression syndrome.

Patient & Family Education

- Use an additional method of birth control during the first week of the initial cycle.
- Consult patient information supplied with drug for management of missed doses.
- Ovulation is unlikely with omission of 1 daily dose; however, the possibility of escaped ovulation, spotting, or breakthrough bleeding increases with each missed dose.
- Discontinue medication if intracycle bleeding resembling menstruation occurs. Begin taking tablets from a new compact on day 5. If bleeding persists, see physician.
- Transdermal patches: Apply only one patch at a time and never cut or otherwise alter a patch prior to application.
- See physician to rule out pregnancy if 2 consecutive periods are missed, before continuing on OCs.
- Learn breast self-examination and do every month.
- Record frequent weight checks to permit early recognition of fluid retention.
- Understand the increased risk of thromboembolic and cardiovascular problems and increased incidence of gallbladder disease with OC use. Be alert to manifestations of thrombotic or thromboembolic disorders: Severe headache (especially if persistent and recurrent), dizziness, blurred vision, leg or chest pain, respiratory distress, unexplained cough. Discontinue drug if any of these symptoms appear and report them promptly to physician.
- Report sudden abdominal pain immediately to physician in order to rule out ectopic pregnancy.
- Stop drug and contact physician if unexplained partial or complete, sudden or gradual loss of vision, protrusion of eyeballs, or blurred vision occurs.
- If OC use is accompanied by vaginal itching and irritation, report to physician promptly to rule out candidiasis.
- Monitor blood glucose closely if diabetic. Adjustment of antidiabetic medication may be necessary.
- Use alternate method of birth control when breast feeding until infant is weaned.

E

ESTROGENS, CONJUGATED

(ess'tro-jenz)

C.E.S. ♣, Cenestin, Enjuvia, Premarin, Progens, SCE-A Vaginal Cream

Classification: ESTROGENS

Therapeutic: FEMALE HORMONE REPLACEMENT THERAPY (HRT)

Prototype: Estradiol

Pregnancy Category: X

AVAILABILITY 0.3 mg, 0.45 mg, 0.625 mg, 0.9 mg, 1.25 mg, 2.5 mg tablets; 25 mg injection; 0.625 mg/g vaginal cream

ACTION & *THERAPEUTIC EFFECT* Circulating estrogens modulate the pituitary secretion of the gonadotropins luteinizing hormone (LH) and follicle stimulating hormone (FSH) through a negative feedback mechanism. Estrogens act to reduce the elevated levels of these gonadotropins seen in postmenopausal women. *Binds to intracellular receptors that stimulate DNA and RNA to synthesize proteins responsible for effects of estrogen.*

USES Atrophic vaginitis, kraurosis vulvae, and abnormal bleeding (hormonal imbalance); also female hypogonadism, primary ovarian failure, vasomotor symptoms associated with menopause; to retard progression of osteoporosis and as palliative therapy of breast and prostatic carcinomas.

UNLABELED USES Infertility, hyperparathyroidism.

CONTRAINDICATIONS Breast cancer, except for palliative therapy; vaginal and cervical cancers; endometrial cancer; endometrial hyperplasia; abnormal vaginal bleeding; hepatic disease or cancer; hypercalcemia; ovarian cancer; history of thromboembolic disease; known or suspected pregnancy (category X).

CAUTIOUS USE Hypertension; gallbladder disease; diabetes mellitus; heart failure; kidney dysfunction.

ROUTE & DOSAGE

Menopause, Osteoporosis, Atrophic Vaginitis, Kraurosis Vulvae

Adult: **PO** 0.3–1.25 mg/day for 21 days each month, adjust to lowest level that gives symptom control (0.625 mg/day or less) **IV/IM** 25 mg, repeated in 6–12 h if needed **Topical** 2–4 g of cream/day

Female Hypogonadism

Adult: **PO** 2.5–7.5 mg/day in 1–3 divided doses for 20 days, followed by a 10-day rest period

Breast Cancer

Adult: **PO** 10 mg t.i.d. for at least 3 mo

Prostatic Cancer Palliation

Adult: **PO** 1.25–2.5 mg t.i.d.

ADMINISTRATION

Oral

- Give at the same time each day.

Topical

- Use calibrated dosage applicator dispensed with the cream.

Intramuscular

- Reconstitute by first removing approximately 5 mL of air from the dry-powder vial, then slowly inject the supplied diluent to the vial by aiming it at the side of the vial. Gently agitate to dissolve but DO NOT SHAKE.
- Use within a few hours of reconstitution.

Intravenous

PREPARE: **Direct:** Reconstitute as for IM injection.

ADMINISTER: **Direct:** Give slowly at a rate of 5 mg/min. ▪ Estrogen solution is compatible with D5W and NS and may be added to IV tubing just distal to the needle if necessary.

INCOMPATIBILITIES **Solution/additive: Ascorbic acid. Y-site: Pantoprazole.**

▪ Store ampule and reconstituted solution at 2°–8° C (38°–46° F) and protected from light; stable for 60 days. ▪ Discard precipitated or discolored solution.

ADVERSE EFFECTS (≥1%) **CNS:** Headache, dizziness, depression, *libido changes*. **CV:** Thromboembolic disorders, hypertension. **GI:** *Nausea,* vomiting, diarrhea, bloating, cholestatic jaundice. **Urogenital:** Mastodynia, spotting, changes in menstrual flow, dysmenorrhea, amenorrhea. **Metabolic:** Reduced carbohydrate tolerance, fluid retention. **Other:** Leg cramps, intolerance to contact lenses.

INTERACTIONS Drug: BARBITURATES, **carbamazepine, phenytoin, rifampin** decrease estrogen effect by increasing its metabolism; ORAL ANTICOAGULANTS may decrease hypoprothrombinemic effects; interfere with effects of **bromocriptine;** may increase levels and toxicity of **cyclosporine,** TRICYCLIC ANTIDEPRESSANTS, **theophylline;** decrease effectiveness of **clofibrate.**

PHARMACOKINETICS Absorption: Rapid absorption from GI tract; readily absorbed through skin and mucous membranes (including vaginal mucosa); slow absorption from IM injections. **Distribution:** Distributed throughout body tissues, especially in adipose tissue; crosses placenta, excreted in breast milk. Conjugated estrogens are bound primarily to albumin. **Metabolism:** Metabolized primarily in liver to glucuronide and sulfate conjugates of estradiol, estrone, and estriol. **Elimination:** In urine. **Half-Life:** 4–18 h.

NURSING IMPLICATIONS

Assessment & Drug Effects

- See additional implications under estradiol.
- Monitor for and report breakthrough vaginal bleeding.
- Assess for relief of menopausal symptoms.
- Lab tests: Monitor serum phosphatase levels with prostate cancer.
- Monitor bone density annually when used for osteoporosis prophylaxis.

Patient & Family Education

- Be aware of importance of taking drug exactly as prescribed: Specifically, do not omit, increase, or decrease doses without advice of physician.
- Intravaginal administration: For self-administration, wash hands well before and after application, and avoid contact of denuded areas with the cream. Do not use tampons while on vaginal cream therapy.
- Notify physician promptly of adverse symptoms.
- Know signs of thrombophlebitis (see Appendix F) and report promptly if suspected.
- Review package insert to ensure understanding of estrogen therapy.

ESTROGENS, ESTERIFIED

(ess′tro-jenz)

Estratab, Menest, Menrium, Neo-Estrone ♣

Classification: ESTROGEN
Therapeutic: ESTROGEN; FEMALE HORMONE REPLACEMENT THERAPY (HRT)
Prototype: Estradiol
Pregnancy Category: X

AVAILABILITY 0.3 mg, 0.625 mg, 1.25 mg, 2.5 mg tablets

ACTION & *THERAPEUTIC EFFECT* At the cellular level, estrogens increase cervical secretions, result in proliferation of the endometrium, and increase uterine tone. Estrogens also can affect bone calcium deposition and accelerate epiphyseal closure. Estrogens appear to prevent osteoporosis associated with the onset of menopause; they generally do not reverse bone density loss that has already developed. *Binds to intracellular receptors that stimulate DNA and RNA to synthesize proteins responsible for effects of estrogen.*

USES Atrophic vaginitis, kraurosis vulvae and abnormal bleeding (hormonal imbalance), female hypogonadism, castration, primary ovarian failure, vasomotor symptoms associated with menopause, palliative therapy of breast and prostatic carcinomas; prevention of osteoporosis.

CONTRAINDICATIONS Breast cancer; cervical cancer; endometrial cancer; endometrial hyperplasia; prostate cancer; hepatic disease or cancer; hypercalcemia; lupus (SLE); history of thromboembolic disease; known or suspected pregnancy (category X); lactation.
CAUTIOUS USE Hypertension; gallbladder disease; diabetes mellitus; heart failure; kidney dysfunction; migraine headaches; seizure disorders.

ROUTE & DOSAGE

Menopause
Adult: **PO** 0.3–1.25 mg/day for 21 days each month, adjust to lowest level that gives symptom control (0.625 mg/day or less)

Female Hypogonadism, Primary Ovarian Failure, Female Castration
Adult: **PO** 2.5–7.5 mg/day in 1–3 divided doses for 20 days followed by a 10-day rest period, during last 5 days of estrogen, give a PO progestin

Breast Cancer
Adult: **PO** 10 mg t.i.d. for 2–3 mo

Prostatic Cancer (palliation)
Adult: **PO** 1.25–2.5 mg t.i.d. for several weeks

Prevention of Osteoporosis
Adult: **PO** 0.3 mg daily

ADMINISTRATION

Oral
- Give with food or fluid of patient's choice.
- Store tablets at 15°–30° C (59°–86° F) in a tightly closed container.

ADVERSE EFFECTS (≥1%) **CNS:** Headache, dizziness, depression, *libido changes*. **CV:** Thromboembolic disorders, hypertension. **GI:** *Nausea*, vomiting, diarrhea, bloating, cholestatic jaundice. **Urogenital:** Mastodynia, spotting, changes in menstrual flow, dysmenorrhea, amenorrhea. **Metabolic:** Reduced carbohydrate tolerance, fluid retention. **Other:** Leg cramps, intolerance to contact lenses.

INTERACTIONS Drug: BARBITURATES, **phenytoin, rifampin** decrease estrogen effect by increasing its metabolism; ORAL ANTICOAGULANTS may decrease hypoprothrombinemic effects; interfere with effects of **bromocriptine;** may increase levels and toxicity of **cyclosporine,** TCAS, **theophylline;** decrease effectiveness of **clofibrate.**

PHARMACOKINETICS Absorption: Well absorbed with first pass metabolism. **Metabolism:** Metabolized in GI mucosa and liver to estrone, further metabolized to inactive metabolites. **Elimination:** In urine and bile. **Half-Life:** 4–18.5 h.

NURSING IMPLICATIONS

Assessment & Drug Effects

- See nursing implications under estradiol.
- Monitor for and report breakthrough vaginal bleeding.
- Assess for relief of menopausal symptoms.
- Lab tests: Monitor serum phosphatase levels with prostate cancer.
- Monitor bone density annually when used for osteoporosis prophylaxis.

Patient & Family Education

- Be aware of importance of taking drug exactly as prescribed: Specifically, do not omit, increase, or decrease doses without advice of physician. Know what to do when a dose is missed.
- Review package insert to ensure understanding of estrogen therapy.

ESTRONE

(ess'trone)

Classification: ESTROGEN
Therapeutic: ESTROGEN; FEMALE HORMONE REPLACEMENT THERAPY (HRT)
Prototype: Estradiol
Pregnancy Category: X

AVAILABILITY 5 mg/mL injection

ACTION & *THERAPEUTIC EFFECT* Due to increased risk of serious complications from extended use, estrogen HRT or estrogen-progestin HRT should be prescribed for the shortest duration possible consistent with the treatment goals of post menopausal symptoms. *Replaces estrogen in postmenopausal women, relieving symptoms of menopause.*

USES Atrophic vaginitis, kraurosis vulvae, and abnormal bleeding (hormonal imbalance); also female hypogonadism, primary ovarian failure, vasomotor symptoms associated with menopause, and as palliative therapy of prostatic carcinoma.

CONTRAINDICATIONS Breast cancer; liver dysfunction; history of thromboembolic disease; known or suspected pregnancy (category X), lactation.

CAUTIOUS USE Hypertension; gallbladder disease; diabetes mellitus; heart failure; kidney dysfunction; seizure disorders.

ROUTE & DOSAGE

Menopause

Adult: **IM** 0.1–0.5 mg 2–3 times/wk

Female Hypogonadism, Primary Ovarian Failure

Adult: **IM** 0.1–1 mg/wk in single or divided doses

Inoperable Prostatic Cancer Palliation

Adult: **IM** 2–4 mg/day 2–3 times/wk

ADMINISTRATION

Intramuscular

- Shake vial and syringe well to suspend medication before withdrawing and injecting medication.
- Give deep into a large muscle.

- Store at 15°–30° C (59°–86° F); protect from light and do not freeze.

ADVERSE EFFECTS (≥1%) **CNS:** Headache, dizziness, depression, *libido changes*. **CV:** Thromboembolic disorders, hypertension. **GI:** *Nausea,* vomiting, diarrhea, bloating, cholestatic jaundice. **Urogenital:** Mastodynia, spotting, changes in menstrual flow, dysmenorrhea, amenorrhea. **Metabolic:** Reduced carbohydrate tolerance, fluid retention. **Other:** Leg cramps, intolerance to contact lenses.

INTERACTIONS Drug: Carbamazepine, phenytoin, rifampin decrease estrogen levels because they increase metabolism; may enhance steroid effects of CORTICOSTEROIDS; may decrease anticoagulant effects of ORAL ANTICOAGULANTS.

PHARMACOKINETICS Absorption: Occurs over several days. **Metabolism:** Converts to estradiol in GI mucosa. **Half-Life:** 4–18.5 h.

NURSING IMPLICATIONS

Assessment & Drug Effects

- See nursing implications under estradiol.
- Monitor for and report breakthrough vaginal bleeding.
- Assess for relief of menopausal symptoms.
- Lab tests: Monitor serum phosphatase levels with prostate cancer.
- Monitor patients with conditions that may be influenced by fluid retention carefully (e.g., migraine, cardiac or kidney dysfunction, asthma, epilepsy, hypertension). Check BP on a regular basis.

Patient & Family Education

- Review package insert to assure understanding of estrogen therapy.
- Determine weight under standard conditions 1 or 2 times/wk and report sudden weight gain or other signs of fluid retention.
- Notify physician of the following symptoms of thromboembolic disorders immediately: Tenderness, swelling, and redness in extremity; calf pain upon flexing foot; sudden, severe headache or chest pain; slurring of speech; change in vision; sudden shortness of breath.
- Report symptoms of vaginal candidiasis (thick, white, curd-like secretions and inflamed, congested introitus) to permit appropriate treatment.

ESTROPIPATE

(es-troe-pi'pate)

Ogen, Ortho-Est

Classification: ESTROGEN

Therapeutic: ESTROGEN; FEMALE HORMONE REPLACEMENT THERAPY (HRT)

Prototype: Estradiol

Pregnancy Category: X

AVAILABILITY 0.625 mg, 1.25 mg, 2.5 mg, 5 mg tablets; 1.5 mg/g cream

ACTION & *THERAPEUTIC EFFECT* Water-soluble preparation of pure crystalline estrone. Due to increased risk of serious complications from extended use, estrogen HRT or estrogen-progestin HRT should be prescribed for the shortest duration possible consistent with the treatment goals of postmenopausal symptoms. *Replaces estrogen in postmenopausal women relieving symptoms of menopause.*

USES Atrophic vaginitis, kraurosis vulvae, and abnormal bleeding (hormonal imbalance); also female hypogonadism, primary ovarian failure, vasomotor symptoms associated with menopause, and as palliative therapy of prostatic carcinoma.

CONTRAINDICATIONS Estrogen hypersensitivity; breast cancer; vaginal cancer; endometrial hyperplasia; history of thromboembolic disease; known or suspected pregnancy (category X); lactation.

CAUTIOUS USE Hypertension; gallbladder disease; diabetes mellitus; heart failure; kidney dysfunction; seizure disorders.

ROUTE & DOSAGE

Menopause, Atrophic Vaginitis, Kraurosis Vulvae

Adult: **PO** 0.75–6 mg/day for 21 days each month; adjust to lowest level that gives symptom control **Intravaginal** 2–4 g of cream once/day in a cyclic regimen

Female Hypogonadism, Primary Ovarian Failure, Female Castration

Adult: **PO** 1.5–9 mg/day in 1–3 divided doses for 21 days, followed by an 8–10-day drug-free period

ADMINISTRATION

Oral

- Give with food or fluid of patient's choice.

Intravaginal

- Apply vaginal cream using calibrated dosage applicator dispensed with drug. Squeeze tube of cream to force sufficient amount into applicator so that number on plunger indicating prescribed dose is level with top of barrel.
- Store at 15°–30° C (59°–86° F) in tightly closed containers unless otherwise directed.

ADVERSE EFFECTS (≥1%) **CNS:** Headache, dizziness, depression, *libido changes*. **CV:** <u>Thromboembolic disorders</u>, edema, hypertension. **GI:** *Nausea*, vomiting, diarrhea, bloating, cholestatic jaundice. **Urogenital:** Mastodynia, spotting, changes in menstrual flow, dysmenorrhea, amenorrhea. **Metabolic:** Reduced carbohydrate tolerance, fluid retention. **Other:** Leg cramps, intolerance to contact lenses.

INTERACTIONS Drug: Carbamazepine, phenytoin, rifampin decrease estrogen levels because they increase its metabolism; may enhance steroid effects of CORTICOSTEROIDS; may decrease anticoagulant effects of ORAL ANTICOAGULANTS. **Herbal: St. John's wort** may decrease blood levels. **Dong quai, red clover, black cohosh,** and **saw palmetto** may have additive hormonal effects.

PHARMACOKINETICS Absorption: Absorbed with some metabolism occuring in GI tract. Some systemic absorption from vaginal administration. **Metabolism:** In GI tract and liver. **Half-Life:** 4–18.5 h.

NURSING IMPLICATIONS

Assessment & Drug Effects

- See nursing implications under estradiol.
- Monitor for and report breakthrough vaginal bleeding.
- Assess for relief of menopausal symptoms.
- Lab tests: Monitor serum phosphatase levels with prostate cancer.

Patient & Family Education

- Do not use tampons while on vaginal cream therapy.
- Intravaginal administration: For self-administration, wash hands well before and after application.

- Pull plunger out of barrel and wash applicator in warm soapy water after use.
- Note: Sudden discontinuation of vaginal cream after high dosage or prolonged use may evoke withdrawal bleeding.

ESZOPICLONE

(es-zo′pi-clone)
Lunesta
Classifications: SEDATIVE-HYPNOTIC
Therapeutic: SEDATIVE-HYPNOTIC
Pregnancy Category: C
Controlled Substance: Schedule IV

AVAILABILITY 1 mg, 2 mg, 3 mg tablets

ACTION & *THERAPEUTIC EFFECT* Eszopiclone is a nonbenzodiazepine sedative-hypnotic agent. Mechanism of action believed to result from its interaction with GABA-receptor complexes at binding sites close to or coupled to benzodiazepine receptors in the brain. *Improves sleep maintenance in transient insomnia.*

USES Treatment of insomnia.

CONTRAINDICATIONS Hypersensitivity to eszopiclone; concurrent administration with CYP3A4 inhibitor drugs; alcohol intoxication; alcoholism; eszopiclone induced angioedema; children younger than 18 y; suicidal tendencies or ideation.

CAUTIOUS USE Hepatic impairment; elderly or debilitated patients; concurrent administration of CNS depressants; signs and symptoms of depression; COPD; pregnancy (category C), lactation.

ROUTE & DOSAGE

Insomnia
Adult: **PO** 2–3 mg at bedtime
Geriatric: **PO** 1–2 mg at bedtime

Severe Hepatic Impairment Dosage Adjustment
Start with 2 mg or less

ADMINISTRATION

Oral
- Give immediately prior to bedtime.
- Store at 15°–30° C (59°– 86° F).

ADVERSE EFFECTS (≥1%) **CNS:** Anxiety, confusion, depression, dizziness, hallucinations, *headache,* irritability, decreased libido, nervousness, *somnolence.* **CV:** *Tachycardia,* pericardial infusion, left ventricular systolic dysfunction (LVSD). **GI:** Dry mouth, dyspepsia, nausea, vomiting. **GU:** Dysmenorrhea, gynecomastia. **Respiratory:** Infection. **Skin:** Rash, pruritus. **Special Senses:** *Unpleasant taste.*

INTERACTIONS Drug: Inhibitors of CYP3A4, including (but not limited to) **amiodarone,** ANTIRETROVIRAL PROTEASE INHIBITORS, **aprepitant, clarithromycin, dalfopristin/quinupristin, delavirdine, diltiazem, efavirenz** (inducer or inhibitor), **erythromycin, fluconazole, fluoxetine, fluvoxamine, itraconazole, ketoconazole, mifepristone, nefazodone, norfloxacin,** other systemic AZOLE ANTIFUNGALS (**miconazole** and **voriconazole**), **troleandomycin,** and **zafirlukast** increase eszopiclone levels. **Ethanol** and other CNS DEPRESSANT agents can produce additive effects in combination with eszopiclone. **Herbal: St. John's wort** can increase eszopiclone levels.

PHARMACOKINETICS Absorption: Rapidly absorbed from GI tract. **Distribution:** 52–59% protein bound. **Peak:** 1 h. **Metabolism:** Extensive hepatic metabolism. **Elimination:** Primarily in the urine. **Half-Life:** 5–6 h.

NURSING IMPLICATIONS

Assessment & Drug Effects

- Monitor for and report worsening insomnia and cognitive or behavioral changes.
- Monitor for suicidal ideation in depressive patients.
- Monitor for S&S of CNS depression when other CNS depressants are used concurrently.
- Supervise ambulation if patient is out of bed after taking eszopiclone.

Patient & Family Education

- Follow directions for taking the drug (see Administration).
- Do not take this drug unless you can get at least 8 h of sleep.
- Do not consume alcohol while taking this drug.
- Do not drive or engage in potentially hazardous activities until response to drug is known.
- Report any of the following to a health care provider: Worsening insomnia, cognitive or behavioral changes, problem with reproductive function.

ETANERCEPT (Pr)

(e-tan′er-cept)

Enbrel

Classifications: BIOLOGICAL RESPONSE MODIFIER; IMMUNOMODULATOR; TUMOR NECROSIS FACTOR (TNF) MODIFIER

Therapeutic: DISEASE-MODIFYING ANTIRHEUMATIC DRUG (DMARD); ANTIPSORIATIC

Pregnancy Category: B

AVAILABILITY 25 mg, 50 mg injection; 50 mg/mL prefilled syringe

ACTION & *THERAPEUTIC EFFECT* Fusion protein produced by recombinant DNA technology. Binds specifically to tumor necrosis factor (TNF) and blocks it from attaching to cell surface TNF receptors. This naturally occurring cytokine (e.g., TNF) is part of the normal immune and inflammatory response. TNF mediates inflammation and modulates cellular immune responses. Elevated levels of TNF are found in the synovial fluids of rheumatoid arthritis (RA) patients. *Effectiveness is indicated by improved RA symptomatology and/or decreased inflammation in other inflammatory disorders.*

USES Reduction of the signs and symptoms of RA and psoriatic RA in adults, and polyarticular juvenile RA (JRA) in children with inadequate response to other disease-modifying antirheumatic drugs. Treatment of ankylosing spondylitis, moderate-severe chronic plaque psoriasis.

CONTRAINDICATIONS Patients with sepsis or other active infection; agranulocytosis; hypersensitivity to etanercept; malignancy; benzyl alcohol hypersensitivity; bleeding, hematologic disease, intramuscular administration, intravenous administration; latex hypersensitivity; sepsis; varicella; lactation.

CAUTIOUS USE Immunosuppression; autoimmune disease, bone marrow suppression; diabetes mellitus; hamster protein hypersensitivity; heart failure; multiple sclerosis, neoplastic disease, neurologic disease, seizure disorder, seizures; vaccination, varicella, vasculitis; pregnancy (category B). Safety and efficacy in children younger than 2 y are not established.

E

ROUTE & DOSAGE

Rheumatoid Arthritis, Psoriatic Arthritis, Ankylosing Spondylitis

Adult: **Subcutaneous** 25 mg twice weekly; or 50 mg once weekly

Juvenile RA

Adolescent/Child (2–17 y): **Subcutaneous** 0.4 mg/kg (max: 25 mg/dose) twice weekly or 0.8 mg/kg weekly

Plaque Psoriasis

Adult: **Subcutaneous** 50 twice weekly (3–4 days apart) for 3 mo, then 50 mg weekly

ADMINISTRATION

Subcutaneous

- Reconstitute by slowly injecting the supplied diluent into the vial. Swirl gently to dissolve and do not shake. Reconstituted solution should be clear and colorless. Use within 6 h.
- Inject into thigh, abdomen, upper arm; rotate injection sites and never inject into an old injection site or where skin is tender, bruised, red, or hard.
- Store reconstituted solution up to 6 h refrigerated at 2°–8° C (36°–46° F). Store unopened dose tray refrigerated at 2°–8° C (36°–46° F).

ADVERSE EFFECTS (≥1%) **Body as a Whole:** Asthenia, serious *infections,* sepsis, monitor for reactivation of tuberculosis, <u>increased malignancy risk</u>. **CNS:** Headache, dizziness, cerebral ischemia, depression, demyelinating disorders (multiple sclerosis, myelitis, optic neuritis). **CV:** Heart failure, <u>MI</u>, myocardial ischemia, hypertension, hypotension. **GI:** Abdominal pain, dyspepsia, cholecystitis, pancreatitis, GI hemorrhage. **Respiratory:** Rhinitis, URI, pharyngitis, cough, respiratory disorder, sinusitis, dyspnea may reactivate latent tuberculosis (TB). **Skin:** Rash; injection site reactions *(erythema, itching, pain, swelling).* **Musculoskeletal:** Bursitis. **Hematologic:** <u>Pancytopenia</u>.

INTERACTIONS Drug: Concurrent or recent use with **azathioprine, cyclophosphamide, leflunomide, methotrexate** has been associated with pancytopenia.

PHARMACOKINETICS Onset: 1–2 wk. **Peak:** 72 h. **Half-Life:** 115 h.

NURSING IMPLICATIONS

Assessment & Drug Effects

- Monitor carefully for and immediately report S&S of infection.

Patient & Family Education

- A PPD test is recommended before starting therapy to check for TB.
- Discard all needles and syringes after use; do not reuse.
- Withhold etanercept and notify physician before resuming drug if you develop an infection or are exposed to varicella virus.
- Avoid vaccinations, in general, and live vaccines, in particular, while on etanercept.
- Note: Injection site reactions (e.g., redness, pain, swelling) are common in the first month of therapy but generally decrease over time.

ETHACRYNIC ACID

(eth-a-krin′ik)

Edecrin

ETHACRYNATE SODIUM

Sodium Edecrin

Classifications: ELECTROLYTIC AND WATER BALANCE AGENT; LOOP DIURETIC

Therapeutic: LOOP DIURETIC
Prototype: Furosemide
Pregnancy Category: B

AVAILABILITY 25 mg, 50 mg tablet; 50 mg injection

ACTION & *THERAPEUTIC EFFECT* Inhibits sodium and chloride reabsorption in proximal tubule and most segments of loop of Henle. Promotes significant fluid excretion by inhibiting reabsorption of a large proportion of filtered sodium. *Rapid and potent diuretic effect resulting in hypotensive effect. Fluid and electrolyte loss may exceed that caused by thiazides.*

USES Severe edema associated with CHF, hepatic cirrhosis, ascites of malignancy, kidney disease, nephrotic syndrome, lymphedema.

UNLABELED USES Treatment of nephrogenic diabetes insipidus, hypercalcemia, mild to moderate hypertension, and as adjunct in therapy of hypertensive crisis complicated by pulmonary edema.

CONTRAINDICATIONS History of hypersensitivity to ethacrynic acid; increasing azotemia, anuria; hepatic coma; severe diarrhea, dehydration, electrolyte imbalance, hypotension; lactation, infants, and neonates; parenteral use in pediatric patients.

CAUTIOUS USE Hepatic cirrhosis, history of hepatic encephalopathy; severe myocardial disease; older adult cardiac patients; diabetes mellitus; history of gout; pulmonary edema associated with acute MI; diabetic mellitus; hyperaldosteronism; nephrotic syndrome; history of pancreatitis; pregnancy (category B).

ROUTE & DOSAGE

Edema

Adult: **PO** 50–100 mg 1–2 times/day, may increase by 25–50 mg prn up to 400 mg/day
IV 0.5–1 mg/kg or 50 mg up to 100 mg, may repeat if necessary
Child: **PO** 1 mg/kg daily, may increase to 3 mg/kg/day

ADMINISTRATION

Oral

- Give after a meal or food to prevent gastric irritation.
- Schedule doses to avoid nocturia and thus sleep interference. Avoid administration within at least 4 h of bedtime, if possible. This recommendation may not apply to the patient who accumulates fluid and develops respiratory symptoms during sleep.

Intravenous

PREPARE: **Direct:** Reconstitute by adding 50 mL of D5W or NS to vial. ▪ Use solution within 24 h. ▪ Vials reconstituted with D5W may turn cloudy; if so, discard the vial.

ADMINISTER: **Direct:** Give at a rate of 10 mg/min. May give through tubing of a freely flowing, compatible infusion. ▪ If a second IV dose is required, a new site should be selected to prevent thrombophlebitis.

INCOMPATIBILITIES **Solution/additive:** **Hydralazine, procainamide, ranitidine, tolazoline, triflupromazine.**

- Store oral and parenteral form at 15°–30° C (59°–86° F) unless otherwise directed.

ADVERSE EFFECTS (≥1%) **CNS:** Headache, fatigue, apprehension, confusion. **CV:** *Postural hypoten-*

sion (dizziness, light-headedness). **Metabolic:** Hyponatremia, *hypokalemia,* hypochloremic alkalosis, hypomagnesemia, hypocalcemia, hypercalciuria, hyperuricemia, hypovolemia, hematuria, glycosuria, hyperglycemia, gynecomastia, elevated BUN, creatinine, and urate levels. **Special Senses:** Vertigo, tinnitus, sense of fullness in ears, temporary or permanent deafness. **GI:** Anorexia, diarrhea, nausea, vomiting, dysphagia, abdominal discomfort or pain, GI bleeding (IV use), abnormal liver function tests. **Hematologic:** Thrombocytopenia, agranulocytosis (rare), severe neutropenia (rare). **Skin:** Skin rash, pruritus. **Body as a Whole:** Fever, chills, acute gout; local irritation and thrombophlebitis with IV injection.

INTERACTIONS Drug: THIAZIDE DIURETICS increase potassium loss; increased risk of **digoxin** toxicity from hypokalemia; CORTICOSTEROIDS, **amphotericin B** increase risk of hypokalemia; decreased **lithium** clearance, so increased risk of lithium toxicity; SULFONYLUREA effect may be blunted, causing hyperglycemia; ANTIHYPERTENSIVE AGENTS increase risk of orthostatic hypotension; AMINOGLYCOSIDES may increase risk of ototoxicity; **warfarin** potentiates hypoprothrombinemia.

PHARMACOKINETICS Absorption: Rapidly absorbed from GI tract. **Onset:** 30 min PO; 5 min IV. **Peak:** 2 h PO; 15–30 min IV. **Duration:** 6–8 h PO; 2 h IV. **Distribution:** Does not cross CSF. **Metabolism:** Metabolized to cysteine conjugate. **Elimination:** 30–65% in urine; 35–40% in bile. **Half-Life:** 30–70 min.

NURSING IMPLICATIONS

Assessment & Drug Effects

- Observe closely following IV infusion. Rapid, copious diuresis following IV administration can produce hypotension.
- Monitor IV site closely. Extravasation of IV drug causes local pain and tissue irritation from dehydration and blood volume depletion.
- Monitor BP during initial therapy. Because orthostatic hypotension can occur, supervise ambulation.
- Monitor BP and pulse throughout therapy in patients with impaired cardiac function. Diuretic-induced hypovolemia may reduce cardiac output, and electrolyte loss promotes cardiotoxicity in those receiving digitalis (cardiac) glycosides.
- Establish baseline weight prior to start of therapy; weigh patient under standard conditions. Keep physician informed of weight loss or gain in excess of 1 kg (2 lb)/day.
- Monitor I&O ratio. Report promptly excessive diuresis, oliguria, hematuria, or sudden profuse diarrhea. Report signs to physician.
- Lab tests: Determine baseline and periodic blood count, serum electrolytes, CO_2, BUN, creatinine, blood glucose, uric acid, and liver function.
- Observe for and report S&S of electrolyte imbalance: Anorexia, nausea, vomiting, thirst, dry mouth, polyuria, oliguria, weakness, fatigue, dizziness, faintness, headache, muscle cramps, paresthesias, drowsiness, mental confusion.
- Report immediately possible signs of thromboembolic complications (see Appendix F).
- Impaired glucose tolerance with hyperglycemia and glycosuria has occurred in patients receiving doses in excess of 200 mg/day.

Patient & Family Education

- Learn S&S of hypokalemia and hyponatremia (see Appendix F), and report any of these promptly to physician.

- Make position changes slowly, particularly from lying to upright posture.
- Notify physician immediately of any evidence of impaired hearing. Hearing loss may be preceded by vertigo, tinnitus, or fullness in ears; it may be transient, lasting 1–24 h, or it may be permanent.

ETHAMBUTOL HYDROCHLORIDE

(e-tham′byoo-tole)

Etibi ✦, Myambutol

Classification: ANTITUBERCULOSIS

Therapeutic: ANTITUBERCULAR

Prototype: Isoniazid

Pregnancy Category: B

AVAILABILITY 100 mg, 400 mg tablets

ACTION & *THERAPEUTIC EFFECT* Mode of action not completely understood, but it appears to inhibit RNA synthesis and thus arrests multiplication of tubercle bacilli. The emergence of resistant strains is delayed by administering ethambutol in combination with other antituberculosis drugs. *Synthetic antituberculosis agent that is also effective against atypical mycobacterial infections.*

USES In conjunction with other antituberculosis agents in treatment of pulmonary tuberculosis.

UNLABELED USES Atypical mycobacterial infections.

CONTRAINDICATIONS Optic neuritis; hypersensitivity to ethambutol; optic neuritis, patients unable to report changes in vision (young children, or unconscious patients); children younger than 6 y.

CAUTIOUS USE Renal impairment, hepatic disease; gout; ocular defects (e.g., cataract, recurrent ocular inflammatory conditions, diabetic retinopathy); pregnancy (category B).

ROUTE & DOSAGE

Tuberculosis

Adult: **PO** 15 mg/kg q24h; for retreatment start with 25 mg/kg/day for 60 days, then decrease to 15 mg/kg/day

Child (6–12 y): **PO** 10–15 mg/kg/day

ADMINISTRATION

Oral

- Give with food if GI irritation occurs.
- Protect ethambutol from light, moisture, and excessive heat. Store at 15°–30° C (59°–86° F) in tightly closed container unless otherwise directed.

ADVERSE EFFECTS (≥1%) **CNS:** Headache, dizziness, confusion, hallucinations, paresthesias, joint pains. **Special Senses:** Ocular toxicity: *Retrobulbar optic neuritis;* possibility of anterior optic neuritis with decrease in visual acuity, temporary loss of vision, constriction of visual fields, red–green color blindness, central and peripheral scotomas, eye pain, photophobia; retinal hemorrhage and edema. **GI:** Anorexia, nausea, vomiting, abdominal pain. **Body as a Whole:** Hypersensitivity (pruritus, dermatitis, <u>anaphylaxis</u>).

INTERACTIONS Drug: Aluminum-containing antacids can decrease absorption.

PHARMACOKINETICS Absorption: 70–80% from GI tract. **Peak:** 2–4 h. **Distribution:** Distributes to most body tissues; highest concentrations in erythrocytes, kidney, lungs, saliva; crosses placenta; distributed into breast milk. **Metabolism:** In liver. **Elimination:** 50% in urine within 24 h; 20–22% in feces. **Half-Life:** 3–4 h.

E

NURSING IMPLICATIONS

Assessment & Drug Effects

- Perform C&S prior to and periodically throughout therapy.
- Ophthalmoscopic examination is recommended prior to and at monthly intervals during therapy.
- Monitor I&O ratio in patients with renal impairment. Report oliguria or any significant changes in ratio or in laboratory reports of kidney function. Systemic accumulation with toxicity can result from delayed drug excretion.
- Lab tests: Perform liver and kidney function tests, CBC, and serum uric acid levels at regular intervals throughout therapy.

Patient & Family Education

- Adhere to drug regimen exactly and keep follow-up appointments.
- Notify physician promptly of the onset of blurred vision, changes in color perception, constriction of visual fields, or any other visual symptoms. Have eyes checked periodically. Ethambutol can cause irreversible blindness due to optic neuritis.

ETHINYL ESTRADIOL

(eth′in-il ess-tra-dye′ole)

Estinyl, Feminone

Classification: ESTROGEN
Therapeutic: ESTROGEN; FEMALE HORMONE REPLACEMENT THERAPY (HRT)
Prototype: Estradiol
Pregnancy Category: X

AVAILABILITY 0.02 mg, 0.05 mg, 0.5 mg tablets

ACTION & *THERAPEUTIC EFFECT* Potent oral estrogen given cyclically for short-term use. Ethinyl estradiol is not commonly used as a single agent, but most commonly found in combination oral contraceptives. *May be used to prevent osteoporosis and relieve symptoms associated with menopause.*

USES Moderate to severe vasomotor symptoms associated with menopause; also postmenopausal osteoporosis, female hypogonadism, and as palliation for inoperable, metastatic cancer of female breast (at least 5 y postmenopause) and of the prostate.

UNLABELED USES Postcoital contraceptive.

CONTRAINDICATIONS Breast, ovarian, cervical, or endometrial cancer; endometrial hyperplasia; uterine or vaginal cancer; abnormal vaginal bleeding; hepatic disease or cancer; jaundice; MI; history of thromboembolic disease; heart failure; coagulopathies; lupus; known or suspected pregnancy (category X), lactation.

CAUTIOUS USE Hypertension; gallbladder disease; diabetes mellitus; kidney dysfunction.

ROUTE & DOSAGE

Menopause, Postmenopausal Osteoporosis

Adult: **PO** 0.02–0.05 mg/day for 21 days each month, adjust to lowest level that gives symptom control

Female Hypogonadism

Adult: **PO** 0.05 mg 1–3 times/day for 2 wk, followed by 2 wk of progestin, continue this regimen for 3–6 mo

Breast Cancer

Adult: **PO** 1 mg t.i.d. for 2–3 mo

Prostatic Cancer Palliation

Adult: **PO** 0.15–2 mg/day

Postcoital Contraceptive

Adult: **PO** 5 mg/day for 5 consecutive days beginning within 72 h of coitus

ADMINISTRATION

Oral

- Morning-after pill: Start drug within 24 h and not later than 72 h after sexual exposure when used as an emergency postcoital contraceptive. Perform a pregnancy test prior to dosing.
- Store at 15°–30° C (59°–86° F) in tight, light-resistant container.

ADVERSE EFFECTS (≥1%) **CNS:** Headache, dizziness, depression, *libido changes.* **CV:** Thromboembolic disorders, hypertension. **GI:** *Nausea,* vomiting, diarrhea, anorexia, weight changes, bloating, cholestatic jaundice. **Urogenital:** Mastodynia, breakthrough bleeding, changes in menstrual flow, dysmenorrhea, amenorrhea; in men: Impotence, gynecomastia, testicular atrophy. **Metabolic:** Reduced carbohydrate tolerance, fluid retention. **Body as a Whole:** Leg cramps, edema, intolerance to contact lenses.

INTERACTIONS Drug: Carbamazepine, phenytoin, rifampin decrease estrogen levels because they increase its metabolism; may enhance steroid effects of CORTICOSTEROIDS; may decrease anticoagulant effects of ORAL ANTICOAGULANTS.

PHARMACOKINETICS Absorption: 83% absorbed. **Metabolism:** Extensively metabolized in liver. **Elimination:** In urine and feces. **Half-Life:** 3–27 h.

NURSING IMPLICATIONS

Assessment & Drug Effects

- Check BP on a regular basis in patients with conditions that may be influenced by fluid retention (migraine, cardiac or kidney dysfunction, asthma, epilepsy, hypertension).

Patient & Family Education

- Be aware that risk of blood clot formation is high. Notify physician immediately of calf pain upon foot flexion and the following symptoms of thromboembolic disorders: Tenderness, pain, swelling, and redness in extremity; sudden, severe headache or chest pain, slurring of speech; change in vision; sudden shortness of breath.
- Determine weight under standard conditions 1 or 2 times/wk and report sudden weight gain or other signs of fluid retention.
- Notify physician of yellow skin and sclera, pruritus, dark urine, and light-colored stools; history of jaundice in pregnancy increases the possibility of estrogen-induced jaundice.
- Report symptoms of vaginal candidiasis (thick, white, curd-like secretions and inflamed congested introitus) to permit appropriate treatment.
- Note: Estrogen-induced feminization and impotence in male patients are reversible with termination of therapy.
- Decrease caffeine intake from sources such as tea, coffee, and cola; estrogenic depression of caffeine metabolism may cause caffeinism.

ETHIONAMIDE

(e-thye-on-am'ide)

E

Trecator
Classifications: ANTITUBERCULOSIS; ANTILEPROSY (SULFONE)
Therapeutic: ANTITUBERCULAR; ANTILEPROSY
Prototype: Isoniazid
Pregnancy Category: C

AVAILABILITY 250 mg tablets

ACTION & *THERAPEUTIC EFFECT* Ethionamide appears to inhibit mycolic acid synthesis, which disrupts the formation of the mycobacterial cell wall. *Effective against human and bovine strains of* Mycobacterium tuberculosis *and* M. kansasii *and some strains of* Mycobacterium avium-intracellulare *complex. Also active against* M. leprae.

USES Any form of active tuberculosis when treatment with primary antituberculosis drugs (e.g., isoniazid, streptomycin, ethambutol, rifampin) has failed. **Must be** given with at least one other effective antituberculosis agent.
UNLABELED USES Atypical mycobacterial infections and tuberculous meningitis.

CONTRAINDICATIONS Hypersensitivity to ethionamide and chemically related drugs [e.g., isoniazid, niacin (nicotinamide)]; severe liver damage; hepatic encephalopathy.
CAUTIOUS USE Diabetes mellitus, liver dysfunction, history of psychiatric illnesses including depression; history of thyroid disease; pregnancy (category C), lactation, children younger than 12 y.

ROUTE & DOSAGE

Tuberculosis
Adult: **PO** 0.5–1 g/day divided q8–12h
Child: **PO** 15–20 mg/kg/day in 2–3 equally divided doses (max: 1 g/day)

ADMINISTRATION

Oral
- Give with or after meals to minimize GI adverse effects. Some patients tolerate ethionamide best when it is taken as a single dose after the evening meal or as a single dose at bedtime.
- About 50% of patients cannot tolerate a single dose larger than 500 mg because of GI adverse effects.
- Store in a cool, dry place at 8°–15° C (46°–59° F) in a tightly closed container unless otherwise directed.

ADVERSE EFFECTS (≥1%) **CNS:** Headache, restlessness, mental depression, drowsiness, dizziness, ataxia, hallucinations, paresthesias, convulsions. **GI:** Dose related and frequent; symptoms may be due to CNS stimulation rather than to GI irritation: Anorexia, *epigastric distress, nausea, vomiting,* metallic taste, *diarrhea,* stomatitis, sialorrhea. **Metabolic:** Elevated ALT, AST; hepatitis (with jaundice), hypothyroidism. **Urogenital:** Menorrhagia, impotence. **Body as a Whole:** Postural hypotension.

INTERACTIONS Drug: Cycloserine, isoniazid may increase neurotoxic effects.

PHARMACOKINETICS Absorption: 80% absorbed from GI tract. **Peak:** 3 h. **Duration:** 9 h. **Distribution:** Widely distributed including CSF; crosses placenta; distribution into breast milk unknown. **Metabolism:** In liver. **Elimination:** In urine. **Half-Life:** 3 h.

NURSING IMPLICATIONS

Assessment & Drug Effects

- Lab tests: Perform C&S prior to start of therapy. Baseline liver function tests (AST and ALT), CBC, and kidney function tests including urinalysis and every 2–4 wk during therapy.
- Report onset of skin rash. Progression to exfoliative dermatitis can occur if drug is not promptly discontinued.
- Monitor blood glucose closely in the diabetic until response to drug is established. Diabetics appear to be especially prone to hepatotoxicity (see Appendix F).

Patient & Family Education

- Avoid alcohol or use in moderation because ethionamide may increase potential for liver dysfunction.
- Notify physician of S&S of hepatotoxicity (see Appendix F); generally reversible if drug is promptly withdrawn.
- Make position changes slowly and in stages, particularly from lying to upright posture if experiencing hypotension.

ETHOSUXIMIDE (Pr)

(eth-oh-sux'i-mide)

Zarontin

Classification: SUCCINIMIDE ANTICONVULSANT

Therapeutic: ANTICONVULSANT

Pregnancy Category: C

AVAILABILITY 250 mg capsules; 250 mg/5 mL syrup

ACTION & *THERAPEUTIC EFFECT* Succinimide anticonvulsant that reduces the current in T-type calcium channel found on primary afferent neurons. Activation of the T channel causes low-threshold calcium spikes in neurons, believed to play a role in the spike-and-wave pattern observed during absence (petit mal) seizures. *Reduces frequency of epileptiform attacks, apparently by depressing motor cortex and elevating CNS threshold to stimuli.*

USES Management of absence (petit mal) seizures, myoclonic seizures, and akinetic epilepsy. May be administered with other anticonvulsants when other forms of epilepsy coexist with petit mal.

CONTRAINDICATIONS Hypersensitivity to succinimides; severe liver or kidney disease; bone marrow suppression; use alone in mixed types of epilepsy (may increase frequency of grand mal seizures); children younger than 3 y.

CAUTIOUS USE Hematologic disease; preexisting hepatic disease; intermittent porphyria; renal disease; pregnancy (category C).

ROUTE & DOSAGE

Absence Seizures

Adult/Child (6–12 y): **PO** 250 mg b.i.d., may increase q4–7days prn (max: 1.5 g/day)

Child (3–6 y): **PO** 250 mg/day, may increase q4–7days prn (max: 1.5 g/day)

ADMINISTRATION

Oral

- Give with food if GI distress occurs.
- Store all forms at 15°–30° C (59°–86° F); capsules in tight containers, and syrup in light-resistant containers; avoid freezing.

E

ADVERSE EFFECTS (≥1%) **CNS:** Drowsiness, hiccups, ataxia, dizziness, headache, euphoria, restlessness, irritability, anxiety, hyperactivity, aggressiveness, inability to concentrate, lethargy, confusion, sleep disturbances, night terrors, hypochondriacal behavior, muscle weakness, fatigue. **Special Senses:** Myopia. **GI:** Nausea, vomiting, *anorexia, epigastric distress,* abdominal pain, *weight loss,* diarrhea, constipation, gingival hyperplasia. **Urogenital:** Vaginal bleeding. **Hematologic:** Eosinophilia, leukopenia, thrombocytopenia, agranulocytosis, pancytopenia, aplastic anemia, positive direct Coombs' test. **Skin:** Hirsutism, pruritic erythematous skin eruptions, urticaria, alopecia, erythema multiforme, exfoliative dermatitis.

INTERACTIONS Drug: Carbamazepine decreases ethosuximide levels; **isoniazid** significantly increases ethosuximide levels; levels of both **phenobarbital** and ethosuximide may be altered with increased seizure frequency. **Herbal: Ginkgo** may decrease anticonvulsant effectiveness.

PHARMACOKINETICS Absorption: Readily from GI tract. **Peak:** 4 h; steady state: 4–7 days. **Metabolism:** In liver. **Elimination:** In urine; small amounts in bile and feces. **Half-Life:** 30 h (child), 60 h (adult).

NURSING IMPLICATIONS

Assessment & Drug Effects

- Lab tests: Perform baseline and periodic hematologic studies, liver and kidney function.
- Monitor adverse drug effects. GI symptoms, drowsiness, ataxia, dizziness, and other neurologic adverse effects occur frequently and indicate the need for dosage adjustment.
- Observe closely during period of dosage adjustment and whenever other medications are added or eliminated from the drug regimen. Therapeutic serum levels: 40–80 mcg/mL.
- Observe patients with prior history of psychiatric disturbances for behavioral changes. Close supervision is indicated. Drug should be withdrawn slowly if these symptoms appear.

Patient & Family Education

- Discontinue drug only under physician supervision; abrupt withdrawal of ethosuximide (whether used alone or in combination therapy) may precipitate seizures or petit mal status.
- Do not drive or engage in other potentially hazardous activities until response to drug is known.
- Monitor weight on a weekly basis. Report anorexia and weight loss to physician; may indicate need to reduce dosage.

ETIDRONATE DISODIUM Pr

(e-ti-droe'nate)

Didronel, EHDP

Classifications: BISPHOSPHONATE; REGULATOR, BONE METABOLISM

Therapeutic: BONE METABOLISM REGULATOR

Pregnancy Category: C

AVAILABILITY 200 mg, 400 mg tablets

ACTION & *THERAPEUTIC EFFECT* Diphosphate preparation with primary action on bone. Reduces elevated cardiac output associated with Paget's disease by decreasing vascularity of bone. Induces reversible hyperphosphatemia without adverse effects. *Slows rate of bone*

resorption and new bone formation in pagetic bone lesions and in normal remodeling process. Response of Paget's disease may be slow (1–3 mo) and may continue for months after treatment is discontinued.

USES Symptomatic Paget's disease and heterotopic ossification due to spinal cord injury or after total hip replacement.

UNLABELED USES Prevention and treatment of corticosteroid-induced osteoporosis.

CONTRAINDICATIONS Enterocolitis; pathologic fractures; renal failure; lactation. Safety and effectiveness in children are not established.

CAUTIOUS USE Renal impairment; asthma; colitis; dysphagia; esophagitis; gastritis; patients on restricted calcium and vitamin D intake; pregnancy (category C).

ROUTE & DOSAGE

Paget's Disease

Adult: **PO** 5–10 mg/kg/day for up to 6 mo or 11–20 mg/kg/day for up to 3 mo, may repeat after 3–6 mo off the drug if necessary

Heterotopic Ossification Due to Spinal Cord Injury

Adult: **PO** 20 mg/kg/day for 2 wk, then 10 mg/kg/day for an additional 10 wk

Heterotopic Ossification Due to Total Hip Arthroplasty

Adult: **PO** 20 mg/kg/day starting 1 mo before the procedure and continuing for 3 mo after

ADMINISTRATION

Oral

- Give as single dose on empty stomach 2 h before meals with full glass of water or juice to reduce gastric irritation.
- Relieve GI adverse effects by dividing total oral daily dose.

ADVERSE EFFECTS (≥1%) **GI:** Nausea, diarrhea, *loose bowel movements,* metallic or altered taste. **Musculoskeletal:** Increased or recurrent bone pain in pagetic sites, onset of bone pain in previously asymptomatic sites, increased risk of fractures in patient with Paget's disease. **Metabolic:** Hypocalcemia, hyperphosphatemia, elevated serum phosphatase, suppressed mineralization of uninvolved skeleton (focal osteomalacia). **Urogenital:** Renal insufficiency (high doses).

INTERACTIONS Drug: CALCIUM SUPPLEMENTS, ANTACIDS, IRON AND OTHER MINERAL SUPPLEMENTS may decrease absorption of etidronate (give etidronate 2 h before other drugs). **Food:** Food, especially milk and dairy products, will decrease absorption of etidronate (give 2 h before meals).

PHARMACOKINETICS Absorption: Variably from GI tract. **Distribution:** 50% distributed to bone. **Metabolism:** Not metabolized. **Elimination:** 50% in urine. **Half-Life:** 6 h.

NURSING IMPLICATIONS

Assessment & Drug Effects

- Report persistent nausea or diarrhea; GI adverse effects may interfere with adequate nutritional status and need to be treated promptly.
- Monitor I&O ratio, serum creatinine, or BUN of patient with impaired kidney function.
- Lab tests: Periodic serum calcium and phosphate.
- Monitor for signs of hypocalcemia. Latent tetany (hypocalcemia) may be detected by Chvostek's

and Trousseau's signs and a serum calcium value of 7–8 mg/dL.

- Note: Serum phosphate levels generally return to normal 2–4 wk after medication is discontinued.

Patient & Family Education

- Avoid eating 2 h before or after taking etidronate. Drug absorption is decreased by food, especially milk, milk products, and other foods high in calcium, mineral supplements, and antacids.
- Notify physician promptly of sudden onset of unexplained pain. Risk of pathological fractures increases when daily dose of 20 mg/kg is taken longer than 3 mo.
- Report promptly if bone pain, restricted mobility, heat over involved bone site occur.

ETODOLAC

(e-to′do-lac)

Classifications: ANALGESIC, NONSTEROIDAL ANTI-INFLAMMATORY AGENT (NSAID); DISEASE-MODIFYING ANTIRHEUMATIC DRUG (DMARD)
Therapeutic: ANALGESIC, NSAID; DMARD; ANTIPYRETIC
Prototype: Ibuprofen
Pregnancy Category: C first and second trimester; D third trimester

AVAILABILITY 400 mg, 500 mg tablets; 200 mg, 300 mg capsules; 400 mg, 500 mg, 600 mg sustained release tablets

ACTION & *THERAPEUTIC EFFECT* Inhibits cyclooxygenase (COX-1 and COX-2) enzyme activity and prostaglandin synthesis. NSAIDs may also suppress production of rheumatoid factor. *Produces analgesic and anti-inflammatory effects of an NSAID.*

USES Osteoarthritis and acute pain, rheumatoid arthritis.
UNLABELED USES Temporal arteritis.

CONTRAINDICATIONS Hypersensitivity to NSAIDS, salicylates; ulceration or inflammation; perioperative CABG pain; asthma, urticaria, or other allergic reactions to aspirin or other NSAIDs; S&S of developing liver disease; pregnancy (category D third trimester). Safety and efficacy in children younger than 6 y are not established.
CAUTIOUS USE Renal impairment, liver function impairment, GI disorders, history of GI ulceration, GI bleeding; cardiac disorders including fluid retention, hypertension, heart failure; dehydration; preexisting hematologic diseases (e.g., coagulopathy and hemophilia) or thrombocytopenia; IM injections; dental work; diabetes mellitus; surgery when hemostasis is required; immunosuppression, neutropenia; patients over 65 y, pregnancy (category C first and second trimester), lactation.

ROUTE & DOSAGE

Acute Pain
Adult: **PO** 200–400 mg q6–8h prn

Osteoarthritis
Adult: **PO** 600–1200 mg/day in 2–4 divided doses, (max: 1200 mg/day or 20 mg/kg for patients weighing 60 kg or less; Lodine XL 400–1000 mg once daily)

Rheumatoid Arthritis
Adult: **PO** 500 mg b.i.d.

ADMINISTRATION

Oral

- Give with food or antacid to reduce risk of GI ulceration.

- Ensure that sustained release form of drug is not chewed or crushed. It **must be** swallowed whole.
- Store at 15°–25° C (59°–77° F); tablets and capsules in bottles; sustained release capsules in unit-dose packages. Protect all forms from moisture.

ADVERSE EFFECTS (≥1%) **CV:** Fluid retention, edema. **CNS:** Dizziness, headache, drowsiness, insomnia. **GI:** *Dyspepsia, nausea, vomiting, diarrhea,* indigestion, heartburn, abdominal pain, constipation, flatulence, gastritis, melena, peptic ulcer, GI bleeding. **Hematologic:** Thrombocytopenia, increased bleeding time. **Skin:** Rash, pruritus. **Urogenital:** Urinary frequency. **Metabolic:** Hepatotoxicity. **Special Senses:** Blurred vision; tinnitus. **Respiratory:** Asthma.

DIAGNOSTIC TEST INTERFERENCE May cause a false-positive ***urinary bilirubin*** test and a false-positive ***ketone*** test done with the dipstick method. May cause a small decrease (1 to 2 mg/dL) in ***serum uric acid*** levels.

INTERACTIONS Drug: May reduce effects of **diuretics** and antihypertensive effects of **beta-blockers** and other ANTIHYPERTENSIVE MEDICATIONS. May increase **digoxin** and **lithium** levels and nephrotoxicity due to **cyclosporine. Herbal: Feverfew, garlic, ginger, ginkgo** may increase bleeding.

PHARMACOKINETICS Absorption: Readily from GI tract. **Onset:** 30 min. **Peak:** 1–2 h. **Duration:** 4–12 h. **Distribution:** Widely distributed; 99% protein bound; not known if crosses placenta or if distributed into breast milk. **Metabolism:** Extensively in liver. **Elimination:** 72% in urine, 16% in feces. **Half-Life:** 6–7 h.

NURSING IMPLICATIONS

Assessment & Drug Effects

- Assess for signs of GI ulceration and bleeding. Risk factors include high doses of etodolac, history of peptic ulcer disease, alcohol use, smoking, and concomitant use of aspirin.
- Assess carefully for fluid retention by monitoring weight and observing for edema in patients with a history of CHF.
- Monitor for decreased BP control in hypertensive patients.
- Lab tests: Periodic CBC and kidney and liver function.
- Monitor for drug toxicity when used concurrently with either digoxin or lithium.
- Monitor for rhinitis, urticaria, or other signs of allergic reactions.
- Monitor carefully increases in etodolac dosage with older adult patients; adverse effects are more pronounced.

Patient & Family Education

- Learn S&S of GI ulceration. Stop medication in presence of bleeding and contact the physician immediately.
- Do not take aspirin, which may potentiate ulcerogenic effects.

ETOPOSIDE

(e-toe-po'side)

Etopophos, VePesid

Classifications: ANTINEOPLASTIC; MITOTIC INHIBITOR

Therapeutic: ANTINEOPLASTIC, CELL-CYCLE SPECIFIC

Prototype: Vincristine

Pregnancy Category: D

AVAILABILITY 50 mg capsules; 20 mg/mL injection; 100 mg lyophilized powder for injection

ACTION & *THERAPEUTIC EFFECT* Produces cytotoxic action by arresting G_2 (resting or premitotic) phase of cell cycle; also acts on S phase of DNA synthesis. High doses cause lysis of cells entering mitotic phase, and lower doses inhibit cells from entering prophase. *Antineoplastic effect is due to its ability to arrest mitosis (cell division).*

USES Treatment of refractory testicular neoplasms, in patients who have already received appropriate surgical, chemotherapeutic, and radiation therapy; for treatment of choriocarcinoma in women and small cell carcinoma of the lung.

UNLABELED USES Hodgkin's and non-Hodgkin's lymphomas, acute myelogenous (nonlymphocytic) leukemia.

CONTRAINDICATIONS Severe bone marrow depression; severe hepatic or renal impairment; existing or recent viral infection, bacterial infection; intraperitoneal, intrapleural, or intrathecal administration; pregnancy (category D), lactation. Safe use in children is not established.

CAUTIOUS USE Impaired kidney or liver function; gout; radiation therapy.

ROUTE & DOSAGE

Testicular Carcinoma
Adult: **IV** 100 mg/m²/day for 5 consecutive days or 100 mg/m² on days 1, 3, and 5 q3–4wk for 3–4 courses **PO** Twice the IV dose rounded to the nearest 50 mg

Small Cell Lung Carcinoma
Adult: **IV** 35 mg/m²/day for 4 consecutive days to 50 mg/m²/day for 5 consecutive days q3–4wk **PO** Twice the IV dose rounded to the nearest 50 mg

Hepatic Impairment Dosage Adjustment
Total bilirubin 1.5–3 mg/dL: Decrease by 50%, 3.1–5 mg/dL: Decrease by 75%, over 5 mg/dL hold dose

Renal Impairment Dosage Adjustment
CrCl 45–60 mL/min: Reduce dose 15%; 30–44 mL/min: Reduce dose 20%; less than 30 mL/min: Reduce dose 25%

ADMINISTRATION

Oral

- Oral dose is usually in the range of 70–100 mg/m² daily, rounded to nearest 50 mg.
- Refrigerate capsules at 2°–8° C (36°–46° F) unless otherwise directed. Do not freeze.

Intravenous

Note: Wear disposable surgical gloves when preparing or disposing of etoposide. Wash immediately with soap and water if skin comes in contact with drug.

PREPARE: **IV Infusion:** *Etoposide concentration for injection:* Each 100 mg **must be** diluted with 250–500 mL of D5W or NS to produce final concentrations of 0.2–0.4 mg/mL. *Etoposide phosphate:* Add 5 or 10 mL of sterile water for injection, D5W, NS, bacteriostatic water for injection, or bacteriostatic NS for injection to yield 20 or 10 mg/mL etoposide, respectively. ▪ May be given as prepared or further diluted to as low as 0.1 mg/mL in either D5W or NS.

ADMINISTER: **IV Infusion:** Give by slow IV infusion over 30–60 min to reduce risk of hypotension and bronchospasm. ▪ Before administration, inspect solution for particulate matter and discoloration. Solution should be clear and yellow. If crystals are present, discard. ***INCOMPATIBILITIES*** **Y-site: Cefepime, filgrastim, gallium, idarubicin.**

▪ Diluted solutions with concentration of 0.2 mg/mL are stable for 96 h, and the 0.4 mg/mL solutions are stable for 24 h under normal room fluorescent light in glass or plastic (PVC) containers. ▪ Phosphate solution is stable for 24 h at room temperature or refrigerated.

ADVERSE EFFECTS ($\geq$1%) **Body as a Whole:** Hypersensitivity (sweating, chills, fever, coryza, tachycardia; throat, back and general body pain; abdominal cramps, flushing, substernal chest pain, dyspnea, <u>bronchospasm</u>, pulmonary edema, <u>anaphylactoid reaction</u>). **CNS:** Peripheral neuropathy, paresthesias, weakness, somnolence, unusual tiredness, transient confusion. **CV:** Transient hypotension; thrombophlebitis with extravasation. **GI:** *Nausea, vomiting,* dyspepsia, anorexia, diarrhea, constipation, stomatitis. **Hematologic:** *Leukopenia (principally granulocytopenia), thrombocytopenia,* <u>severe myelosuppression</u>, *anemia, pancytopenia, neutropenia.* **Respiratory:** Pleural effusion, bronchospasm. **Skin:** *Reversible alopecia* (can progress to total baldness); radiation recall dermatitis; necrosis, *pain at IV site.*

INTERACTIONS Drug: ANTICOAGULANTS, ANTIPLATELET AGENTS, NSAIDS, **aspirin** may increase risk of bleeding. Avoid concurrent use of LIVE VACCINES. **Food: Grapefruit juice** may decrease effect.

PHARMACOKINETICS Absorption: Approximately 50% from GI tract. **Peak:** 1–1.5 h. **Distribution:** Variable penetration into CSF. **Metabolism:** In liver. **Elimination:** 44–60% in urine, 2–16% in feces over 3 days. **Half-Life:** 5–10 h.

NURSING IMPLICATIONS

Assessment & Drug Effects

- Check IV site during and after infusion. Extravasation can cause thrombophlebitis and necrosis.
- Be prepared to treat an anaphylactoid reaction (see Appendix F). Stop infusion immediately if the reaction occurs.
- Monitor vital signs during and after infusion. Stop infusion immediately if hypotension occurs.
- Lab tests: Perform baseline all prior to and at regular intervals during therapy, and before each subsequent treatment course. Tests include: CBC with differential; liver and kidney function tests (AST, ALT, serum bilirubin, LDH, BUN, serum creatinine).
- Withhold therapy when an absolute neutrophil count is below 500/mm^3 or a platelet count below 50,000/mm^3.
- Be alert to evidence of patient complaints that might suggest development of leukopenia (see Appendix F), infection (immunosuppression), and bleeding.
- Protect patient from any trauma that might precipitate bleeding during period of platelet nadir particularly. Withhold invasive procedures if possible.

Patient & Family Education

- Learn possible adverse effects of etoposide, such as blood dyscrasias, alopecia, carcinogenesis, before treatment begins.
- Make position changes slowly, particularly from lying to upright position because transient hypotension after therapy is possible.
- Inspect mouth daily for ulcerations and bleeding. Avoid obvi-

ous irritants such as hot or spicy foods, smoking, alcohol.

E

ETRAVIRINE

(e-tra'vi-reen)

Intelence

Classifications: ANTIRETROVIRAL; NONNUCLEOSIDE REVERSE TRANSCRIPTASE INHIBITOR (NNRTI)

Therapeutic: ANTIRETROVIRAL; NNRTI

Prototype: Efavirenz

Pregnancy Category: B

AVAILABILITY 100 mg tablets

ACTION & *THERAPEUTIC EFFECT* Prevents replication of HIV-1 viruses by binding directly to reverse transcriptase, thus blocking RNA- and DNA-dependent polymerase activities. *Effectiveness is indicated by reduction in viral load (plasma level HIV RNA).*

USES HIV-1 infection in combination with other antiretroviral agents in treatment-experienced adult patients resistant to other antiretroviral agents (including other NNRTIs).

CONTRAINDICATIONS Severe skin reactions; lactation.

CAUTIOUS USE Moderate to severe hepatic impairment (Child-Pugh class C); concurrent hepatitis B or C, dyslipidemia; elderly; pregnancy (category B). Safety and efficacy in children not established.

ROUTE & DOSAGE

HIV Infection

Adult: **PO** 200 mg b.i.d. p.c.

ADMINISTRATION

Oral

- Give after a meal. Ensure that tablets are not chewed.
- May dissolve in water if patient cannot swallow tablets. Once dissolved, should be swallowed immediately. Rinse glass several times and instruct to swallow each time to ensure entire dose has been administered.
- Store at 15°–30° C (59°–86° F). Keep bottles closed tightly to protect from moisture. Do not remove desiccant pouches from bottle.

ADVERSE EFFECTS (≥2%) **Body as a Whole:** Peripheral neuropathy. **CNS:** Fatigue, headache. **CV:** Hypertension. **GI:** Abdominal pain, *diarrhea, nausea,* vomiting. **Metabolic:** Elevated creatinine, elevated LDL, elevated total cholesterol, elevated triglycerides, elevated glucose, elevated ALT. **Skin:** *Rash.*

INTERACTIONS Drug: Compounds that inhibit CYP3A4, CYP2C9, and/or CYP2C19 (e.g., **itraconazole, ketoconazole**) may increase plasma levels of etravirine. Compounds that induce CYP3A4, CYP2C9, and/or CYP2C19 (e.g., **carbamazepine, phenobarbital, phenytoin**) may decrease plasma levels of etravirine. Etravirine may decrease the plasma levels of other compounds that require CYP3A4 for metabolism (e.g., **HIV protease inhibitors**) and may increase the plasma levels of other compounds that require CYP2C9 and/or CYP2C19 for metabolism (e.g., **diazepam, warfarin**). **Herbal: St. John's wort** may decrease etravirine levels.

PHARMACOKINETICS Peak: 2.5 to 4 h. **Distribution:** 99.9% protein bound. **Metabolism:** In liver by CYP2C9, CYP2C19, and CYP3A4.

Elimination: 93.7% in feces, 1.2% in urine. **Half-Life:** 41 h.

NURSING IMPLICATIONS

Assessment & Drug Effects

- Monitor for and report promptly potentially serious adverse reactions, including skin hypersensitivity reactions and S&S of hepatic dysfunction.
- Monitor for and report S&S of opportunistic infections.
- Lab tests: Periodic CD4+ T cell count, plasma HIV RNA, CBC with platelet count, serum amylase, hepatic and renal function tests, and lipid profile.

Patient & Family Education

- Do not take on an empty stomach.
- Do not remove drying-agent pouches from medication bottle.
- Report promptly any of the following: Rash, S&S of infection.
- Report use of all prescription and nonprescription medications, as well as herbs, to physician.

EVEROLIMUS

(e-ver-o-li'mus)

Afinitor

Classifications: BIOLOGICAL RESPONSE MODIFIER; IMMUNOMODULATOR; ANTINEOPLASTIC; IMMUNOSUPPRESSANT

Therapeutic: ANTINEOPLASTIC

Pregnancy Category: D

AVAILABILITY 5 mg, 10 mg tablets

ACTION & *THERAPEUTIC EFFECT* Binds to an intracellular protein of cancer cells of the kidney that inhibits a major dysfunctional kinase pathway in renal cancer development. It also reduces the expression of vascular endothelial growth factor (VEGF) in these cells. *Reduces cell proliferation, angiogenesis, and glucose uptake in renal carcinoma cells.*

USES Treatment of patients with advanced renal cell cancer who have failed treatment with sunitinib or sorafenib.

CONTRAINDICATIONS Hypersensitivity to everolimus, or other rapamycin derivatives; Child-Pugh class C, hepatic impairment; severe non-infection pneumonitis; fungal infection; live vaccine; pregnancy (category D), lactation.

CAUTIOUS USE Child-Pugh class B hepatic impairment; renal impairment.

ROUTE & DOSAGE

Renal Cell Cancer

Adult: **PO** 10 mg once daily. 15–20 mg daily for patients taking a strong CYP3A4 inducer.

Hepatic Impairment Dosage Adjustment

Moderate impairment (Child-Pugh class B): Reduce to 5 mg once daily.
Severe impairment (Child-Pugh class C): Not recommended.

ADMINISTRATION

Oral

- Give at the same time each day with/without food.
- Ensure that the tablet is swallowed whole. It should not be crushed or chewed.
- Store at 15°–30° C (59°–86° F). Protect from light and moisture.

ADVERSE EFFECTS (≥3%) **Body as a Whole** *Asthenia,* chest pain, chills, epistaxis, *fatigue, infection,* peripheral edema, pyrexia. **CNS:** Dizzi-

E

ness, dysgeusia, headache, insomnia, paresthesia. **CV:** Hypertension, tachycardia. **GI:** Abdominal pain, *diarrhea,* dry mouth, dysphagia, hemorrhoids, *mucosal inflammation,* nausea, *stomatitis,* vomiting. **Hematologic:** *Anemia, decreased hemoglobin,* decreased neutrophils, decreased platelets, *lymphopenia,* hemorrhage. **Metabolic:** Decreased weight, elevated AST and ALT, elevated bilirubin, elevated creatinine, *hypercholesterolemia, hypertriglyceridemia, hyperglycemia, hypophosphatemia.* **Musculoskeletal:** Jaw pain, pain in extremity. **Respiratory:** Alveolitis, bronchitis, *cough, dyspnea,* interstitial lung disease, lung infiltration, nasopharyngitis, pneumonia, *pneumonitis,* pulmonary alveolar hemorrhage, pulmonary effusion, pharyngolaryngeal pain, rhinorrhea, sinusitis. **Skin:** Acneiform dermatitis, dry skin, erythema, hand-foot syndrome, nail disorder, onychoclasis, pruritus, *rash,* skin lesion. **Special Senses:** Eyelid edema. **Urogenital:** Renal failure

INTERACTIONS Drug: Strong inhibitors of CYP3A4 and P-glycoprotein (e.g., **ketoconazole, erythromymin, veramapil**) increase everolimus levels. Strong inducers (e.g., **rifampin**) decrease everolimus levels.

PHARMACOKINETICS Peak: 1–2 h. **Distribution:** 74% plasma protein bound. **Metabolism:** In liver to inactive metabolites. **Elimination:** Fecal (80%) and renal (5%). **Half-Life:** 30 h.

NURSING IMPLICATIONS

Assessment & Drug Effects

- Monitor for and promptly report S&S of a hypersensitivity reaction (e.g., anaphylaxis, dyspnea, flushing, chest pain, angioedema).
- Monitor pulmonary status and report promptly unexplained cough, shortness of breath, pain on inspiration, or diminished breath sounds.
- Monitor for and promptly report S&S of infection.
- Lab tests: Baseline and periodic CBC with differential, renal function tests, blood glucose, and lipid profile.

Patient & Family Education

- Report promptly any signs of infections, including sore throat, fever, and flu-like symptoms.
- Avoid live vaccinations and close contact with those who have received live vaccines.
- Practice meticulous oral hygiene. Do not use mouthwashes that contain alcohol or peroxide.
- Women should use adequate means of contraception to avoid pregnancy while on this drug and for 8 wk after ending treatment.

EXEMESTANE

(ex-e-mes'tain)

Aromasin

Classifications: ANTINEOPLASTIC; AROMATASE INHIBITOR

Therapeutic: ANTINEOPLASTIC

Prototype: Anastrozole

Pregnancy Category: D

AVAILABILITY 25 mg tablet

ACTION & *THERAPEUTIC EFFECT*

Steroidal aromatase inhibitor that suppresses plasma estrogens estradiol and estrone. The enzyme, aromatase converts estrone to estradiol. *Tumor regression is possible in postmenopausal women with estrogen dependent breast cancer. Effectiveness is indicated by evidence of reduction in tumor size.*

USES Estrogen-receptor positive early breast cancer following treatment with tamoxifen, treatment of advanced breast cancer in postmenopausal women whose disease has progressed following tamoxifen therapy.

CONTRAINDICATIONS Hypersensitivity to exemestane; coadministration of estrogen-containing drugs; pregnancy (category D). Safety and efficacy in children not established.
CAUTIOUS USE Hepatic or renal insufficiency; GI disorders; cardiovascular disease; hyperlipidemia; lactation.

ROUTE & DOSAGE

Early and Advanced Breast Cancer
Adult: **PO** 25 mg daily after a meal

ADMINISTRATION

Oral
- Give following a meal.
- Store at 15°–30° C (59°–86° F).

ADVERSE EFFECTS (≥1%) **Body as a Whole:** *Fatigue, hot flashes, pain,* flu-like symptoms; edema; fever; paresthesia. **CNS:** *Depression, insomnia, anxiety;* dizziness; headache. **CV:** Hypertension. **GI:** *Nausea,* vomiting, abdominal pain, anorexia, constipation, diarrhea, increased appetite. **Respiratory:** Dyspnea, cough, bronchitis, sinusitis. **Skin:** Increased sweating, rash, itching. **Other:** UTI; lymphedema.

PHARMACOKINETICS Absorption: Rapidly, approximately 42% reaches systemic circulation. **Distribution:** Extensive tissue distribution, 90% protein bound. **Metabolism:** Extensively in liver (CYP3A4). **Elimination:** Equally in urine and feces. **Half-Life:** 24 h.

NURSING IMPLICATIONS

Assessment & Drug Effects
- Lab tests: Baseline liver function, BUN and creatinine; periodic WBC with differential, lipid profile, routine blood chemistry.

Patient & Family Education
- Review manufacturer's patient literature thoroughly to reinforce understanding of likely adverse effects.
- Report bothersome adverse effects to physician.

EXENATIDE

(e-xe′na-tide)
Byetta
Classification: ANTIDIABETIC, INCRETIN MIMETIC
Therapeutic: ANTIDIABETIC
Pregnancy Category: C

AVAILABILITY 250 mcg/mL injection

ACTION & *THERAPEUTIC EFFECT* Improves glycemic control in type 2 diabetes mellitus by mimicking the functions of incretin, a glucagon-like peptide-1 (GLP-1). Exenatide enhances glucose-dependent insulin secretion by pancreatic beta-cells, suppresses inappropriately elevated glucagon secretion, and slows gastric emptying. These actions decrease glucagon stimulation of hepatic glucose output and decrease insulin demand. *Improves glycemic control by reducing fasting and postprandial glucose concentrations in patients with type 2 diabetes.*

USES Adjunct treatment of type 2 diabetes mellitus in those inadequately managed by metformin, a sulfonylurea, or a combination of these agents.

CONTRAINDICATIONS Hypersensitivity to exenatide, or cresol; type I diabetes; severe GI disease, diabetic ketoacidosis; gastroparesis; end-stage renal disease, severe renal impairment (CrCl less than 30 mL/min).

CAUTIOUS USE Elderly; renal impairment; renal disease; thyroid disease; lactation; pregnancy (category C). Safety and efficacy are not established in children.

ROUTE & DOSAGE

Type 2 Diabetes Mellitus
Adult: **Subcutaneous** Initial dose of 5 mcg b.i.d., within 60 min prior to the morning and evening meal. After 1 mo, may increase to 10 mcg b.i.d., within 60 min prior to the morning and evening meal.

ADMINISTRATION

- Give subcutaneously into thigh, abdomen, or upper arm within 60 min before the morning and evening meals. Do not administer after a meal.
- Do not give within 1 h of oral antibiotics, an oral contraceptive, or acetaminophen.
- Store at 36°–46° F (2°–8° C) and protect from light. Discard pen 30 days after first use. Do not use if pen has been frozen. After first use, pen may be kept at or below 77° F (25° C).

ADVERSE EFFECTS (≥1%) **CNS:** Asthenia, dizziness, restlessness, jittery feeling. **GI:** Nausea, vomiting, diarrhea, dyspepsia, anorexia, gastroesophageal reflux. **Metabolic:** Hypoglycemia, excessive sweating (hyperhidrosis or diaphoresis).

INTERACTIONS Drug: Due to its ability to slow gastric emptying, exenatide can decrease the rate and/or serum levels of oral medications that require GI absorption.

PHARMACOKINETICS Peak: 2 h. **Elimination:** Primarily in urine. **Half-Life:** 2.4 h.

NURSING IMPLICATIONS

Assessment & Drug Effects

- Monitor for and report S&S of significant GI distress, including NV&D.
- Monitor for S&S of hypoglycemia and S&S of acute pancreatitis (acute abdominal pain with/without vomiting). If pancreatitis is suspected, withhold drug and notify physician immediately.
- Lab tests: Periodic fasting and postprandial plasma glucose and periodic HbA1C; baseline and periodic renal function tests.

Patient & Family Education

- If a dose is missed, wait for the next scheduled dose.
- Discard any pen that has been in use for greater than 30 days.
- Exenatide may cause decreased appetite and some weight loss.
- Report significant GI distress to physician. Report promptly persistent, severe abdominal pain that my be accompanied by vomiting.

EZETIMIBE

(e-ze-ti'mibe)

Zetia, Ezetrol ♣

Classifications: ANTILIPEMIC; CHOLESTEROL ABSORPTION INHIBITOR

Therapeutic: CHOLESTEROL LOWERING

Pregnancy Category: C

AVAILABILITY 10 mg tablets

ACTION & *THERAPEUTIC EFFECT* Selectively blocks the lining of the small intestine by inhibiting the absorption of cholesterol, but does not inhibit cholesterol synthesis in the liver or increase bile acid excretion. Thus it decreases the amount of intestinal cholesterol available to the liver. *Lowers both total cholesterol and low-density lipid (LDL) cholesterol, apo B, triglycerides, and increases HDL-C; its mechanism of action is complementary to statins.*

USES Treatment of primary hypercholesterolemia alone or with an HMG-CoA reductase inhibitor (statin); treatment of homozygous sitosterolemia as an adjunct to diet.

CONTRAINDICATIONS Hypersensitivity to ezetimibe; concurrent use with HMG-CoA reductase inhibitor in patients with active liver disease or elevated serum transaminases; moderate to severe hepatic disease; lactation; children younger than 10 y.

CAUTIOUS USE Mild hepatic insufficiency; elderly; pregnancy (category C).

ROUTE & DOSAGE

Hypercholesterolemia
Adult: **PO** 10 mg daily

ADMINISTRATION

Oral

- Give no sooner than 2 h before or 4 h after administration of a bile acid sequestrant such as cholestyramine.
- Store at 15°–30° C (59°–86° F). Protect from moisture.

ADVERSE EFFECTS (≥1%) **Body as a Whole** Fatigue, arthralgia, back pain, myalgia, angioedema, myopathy. **CNS** Dizziness, headache. **GI:** Abdominal pain, diarrhea. **Respiratory:** Pharyngitis, sinusitis, cough. **Hematologic:** Thrombocytopenia. **Skin:** Rash. **Other:** Hepatitis, pancreatitis, rhabdomyolysis.

INTERACTIONS Drug: BILE ACID SEQUESTRANTS (e.g., **cholestyramine**) may decrease absorption (give ezetimibe 2 h before or 4 h after these drugs); **cyclosporine** or FIBRIC ACID DERIVATIVES can significantly increase ezetimibe levels.

PHARMACOKINETICS Absorption: Well absorbed from the small intestine. **Peak:** 4–12 h. **Distribution:** Ezetimibe-glucuronide is 99% protein bound. **Metabolism:** Extensively conjugated to an active glucuronide compound (ezetimibe-glucuronide). Metabolized in small intestine and liver. **Elimination:** Primarily in feces. **Half-Life:** 22 h.

NURSING IMPLICATIONS

Assessment & Drug Effects

- Lab tests: Monitor baseline and periodic lipid profile; periodic Hgb and Hct and platelet count. Monitor baseline LFTs and when used with a statin, monitor periodic LFTs in accordance with the monitoring schedule for that statin.
- Assess for and report unexplained muscle pain, especially when used in combination with a statin drug.
- Monitor closely patients who take both ezetimibe and cyclosporine.

Patient & Family Education

- Report unexplained muscle pain, tenderness, or weakness.
- Females should use effective methods of contraception to prevent pregnancy while taking this drug in combination with a statin.

FAMCICLOVIR

(fam-ci'clo-vir)

Famvir

Classification: ANTIVIRAL
Therapeutic: ANTIVIRAL
Prototype: Acyclovir
Pregnancy Category: B

F

AVAILABILITY 125 mg, 250 mg, 500 mg tablets

ACTION & *THERAPEUTIC EFFECT* Prodrug of the antiviral agent penciclovir that prevents viral replication by inhibition of DNA synthesis in herpes virus–infected cells. *Effectiveness is indicated by decreasing pain and crusting of lesions followed by loss of vesicles, ulcers, and crusts. Interferes with DNA synthesis of herpes simplex virus type 1 and 2 (HSV-1 and HSV-2) infections, varicella-zoster virus, and cytomegalovirus.*

USES Management of acute herpes zoster, genital herpes, recurrent episodes of genital herpes in immunocompromised adults. Suppression of recurrent episodes of genital herpes in immunocompetent adults.

CONTRAINDICATIONS Hypersensitivity to famciclovir, lactation.
CAUTIOUS USE Renal or hepatic impairment, carcinoma, older adults, pregnancy (category B). Safety in children younger than 18 y is not established.

ROUTE & DOSAGE

Herpes Zoster, Treatment

Adult: **PO** 500 mg q8h for 7 days, start within 48–72 h of onset of rash

Renal Impairment Dosage Adjustment

CrCl 40–59 mL/min: 500 mg q12h; 20–39 mL/min: 500 mg q24h

Treatment of Recurrent Genital Herpes

Adult: **PO** 125 mg b.i.d. × 5 days

Suppression of Recurrent Genital Herpes

Adult: **PO** 250 mg b.i.d. for up to 1 y

ADMINISTRATION

Oral

- Most effective when given within 72 h of appearance of a rash or within 6 h of onset of a genital lesion.
- Store at room temperature, 15°–30° C (59°–86° F).

ADVERSE EFFECTS (≥1%) **CNS:** *Headache,* somnolence, dizziness, paresthesias, fatigue, fever, rigors. **Hematologic:** Purpura. **GI:** Nausea, diarrhea, vomiting, constipation, anorexia, abdominal pain. **Body as a Whole:** Pharyngitis, sinusitis, pruritus.

INTERACTIONS Drug: Probenecid may decrease elimination; famciclovir may increase **digoxin** levels.

PHARMACOKINETICS Absorption: Readily absorbed from GI tract and rapidly converted to penciclovir in intestinal and liver tissue. **Onset:** Median times to full crusting of lesions, loss of vesicles, loss of ulcers, and loss of crusts were 6, 5, 7, and 19 days, respectively; median time to loss of acute pain was 21 days. **Peak:** 1 h. **Distribution:** Distributes into breast milk of animals. **Metabolism:** Metabolized in liver and intestinal tissue to penciclovir, which is the active antiviral agent. **Elimination:** Approximately 60% recovered in urine as penciclovir. **Half-Life:** Penciclovir 2–3 h.

NURSING IMPLICATIONS

Assessment & Drug Effects

- Lab tests: Baseline CBC and routine blood chemistry studies prior to and after short courses of therapy; periodically during prolonged treatment.
- Monitor digoxin level and assess for S&S of digoxin toxicity when digoxin is used concurrently with famciclovir.

Patient & Family Education

- Learn potential adverse effects and report those that are bothersome to physician.
- Be aware that a full therapeutic response may take several weeks.

FAMOTIDINE

(fa-moe'ti-deen)

Pepcid, Pepcid AC

Classification: ANTISECRETORY (H_2-RECEPTOR ANTAGONIST)

Therapeutic: ANTIULCER

Prototype: Cimetidine

Pregnancy Category: B

AVAILABILITY 10 mg, 20 mg, 40 mg tablets; 40 mg/5 mL suspension; 10 mg/mL, 20 mg/50 mL injection

ACTION & *THERAPEUTIC EFFECT* A potent competitive inhibitor of histamine at its H_2 receptor sites in gastric parietal cells. Inhibits basal, nocturnal, meal-stimulated, and pentagastrin-stimulated gastric secretion as well as pepsin secretion. *Reduces parietal cell output of hydrochloric acid; thus, detrimental effects of acid on gastric mucosa are diminished.*

USES Short-term treatment of active duodenal ulcer. Maintenance therapy for duodenal ulcer patients on reduced dosage after healing of an active ulcer. Treatment of pathologic hypersecretory conditions (e.g., Zollinger-Ellison syndrome), benign gastric ulcer, gastroesophageal reflux disease (GERD), gastritis.

UNLABELED USES Stress ulcer prophylaxis.

CONTRAINDICATIONS Hypersensitivity to famotidine or other H_2-receptor antagonists; sudden GI bleeding; lactation.

CAUTIOUS USE Renal insufficiency; renal failure; PKU; hepatic disease; elderly; pregnancy (category B).

ROUTE & DOSAGE

Duodenal Ulcer

Adult: **PO** 40 mg at bedtime or 20 mg b.i.d. **PO Maintenance Therapy** 20 mg at bedtime **IV** 20 mg q12h

Child: **PO/IV** 0.25–0.5 mg/kg q12h (max: 40 mg/day)

Pathological Hypersecretory Conditions

Adult: **PO** 20–160 mg q6h **IV** 20 mg q6h

GERD, Gastritis

Adult: **PO** 10 mg b.i.d.

Child: **PO** 1 mg/kg/day in 2 divided doses (max: 40 mg b.i.d.)

Renal Impairment Dosage Adjustment

CrCl less than 50 mL/min: 50% of usual dose or usual dose q36–48h

ADMINISTRATION

Oral

- Give with liquid or food of patient's choice; an antacid may also be given if patient is also on antacid therapy.
- Store at 15°–30° C (59°–86° F). Protect from moisture and strong light; do not freeze.

Intravenous

Note: Verify correct IV concentration and rate of infusion/injection with physician before administration to infants or children.

PREPARE: **Direct:** Dilute each 20 mg (2 mL) famotidine IV solution (containing 10 mg/mL) with D5W, NS, or other compatible IV diluent (see manufacturer's directions) to a total volume of 5 or 10 mL. **Intermittent:** Dilute required dose with 100 mL compatible IV solution.

ADMINISTER: **Direct:** Give over not less than 2 min. **Intermittent:** Infuse over 15–30 min.

INCOMPATIBILITIES **Y-site:** **Amphotericin B cholesteryl complex, azithromycin, cefepime, piperacillin/tazobactam.**

- Store IV solution at 2°–8° C (36°–46° F); reconstituted IV solution is stable for 48 h at room temperature 15°–30° C (59°–86° F).

ADVERSE EFFECTS (≥1%) **CNS:** Dizziness, headache, confusion, depression. **GI:** Constipation, diarrhea. **Skin:** Rash, acne, pruritus, dry skin, flushing. **Hematologic:** Thrombocytopenia. **Urogenital:** Increases in BUN and serum creatinine.

INTERACTIONS Drug: May inhibit absorption of **itraconazole** or **ketoconazole.**

PHARMACOKINETICS Absorption: Incompletely from GI tract (40–50% reaches systemic circulation). **Onset:** 1 h. **Peak:** 1–3 h PO; 0.5–3 h IV. **Duration:** 10–12 h. **Metabolism:** In liver. **Elimination:** In urine. **Half-Life:** 2.5–4 h.

NURSING IMPLICATIONS

Assessment & Drug Effects

- Monitor for improvement in GI distress.
- Monitor for signs of GI bleeding.

Patient & Family Education

- Be aware that pain relief may not be experienced for several days after starting therapy.

FAT EMULSION, INTRAVENOUS

(fat e-mul′sion)

Intralipid, Liposyn II, Soyacal

Classifications: CALORIC AGENT; LIPID EMULSION

Therapeutic: NUTRITIONAL SUPPLEMENT; LIPID

Pregnancy Category: C

AVAILABILITY 10%, 20%, 30% emulsion

ACTION & *THERAPEUTIC EFFECT* Soybean oil in water emulsion containing egg yolk phospholipids and glycerin. Liposyn 10% is safflower oil in water emulsion containing egg phosphatides and glycerin. *Used as a nutritional supplement.*

USES Fatty acid deficiency. Also to supply fatty acids and calories in high-density form to patients receiving prolonged TPN therapy who cannot tolerate high dextrose concentrations or when fluid intake **must be** restricted as in renal failure, CHF, ascites.

CONTRAINDICATIONS Hyperlipemia; bone marrow dyscrasias; impaired fat metabolism as in pathological hyperlipemia, lipoid nephrosis, acute pancreatitis accompanied by hyperlipemia.

CAUTIOUS USE Severe hepatic or pulmonary disease; coagulation disorders; anemia; newborns, premature neonates, infants with hyperbilirubinemia; when danger of fat embolism exists; history of gastric ulcers; diabetes mellitus; thrombocytopenia; pregnancy (category C).

ROUTE & DOSAGE

Prevention of Essential Fatty Acid Deficiency

Adult: **IV** 500 mL of 10% or 250 mL of 20% solution twice/wk (max: rate of 100 mL/h)
Child: **IV** 5–10 mL/kg/day twice/wk (max: 3–4 g/kg/day; max: rate of 100 mL/h)

Calorie Source in Fluid-Restricted Patients

Adult: **IV** Up to 2.5 g/kg or 60% of nonprotein calories daily (max: rate of 100 mL/h)
Child: **IV** Up to 4 g/kg or 60% of nonprotein calories daily (max: rate of 100 mL/h)
Premature Neonate: **IV** 0.25–0.5 g/kg/day, increase by 0.25–0.5 g/kg/day (max: 3–4 g/kg/day; max: infusion 0.15 g/kg/h)

ADMINISTRATION

Intravenous

Do not use if oil appears to be separating out of the emulsion.

PREPARE: **IV Infusion:** Allow preparations that have been refrigerated to stand at room temperature for about 30 min before using whenever possible. ▪ Check with a pharmacist before mixing fat emulsions with electrolytes, vitamins, drugs, or other nutrient solutions.

ADMINISTER: **IV Infusion for Adult:** *10% emulsion:* Infuse at 1 mL/min for first 15–30 min; increase to 2 mL/min if no adverse reactions. ▪ *20% emulsion:* Infuse at 0.5 mL/min for first 15–30 min; increase to 2 mL/min if no adverse reactions occur. **IV Infusion for Child:** *10% emulsion:* Infuse at 0.1 mL/min for first 10–15 min; increase to 1 g/kg in 4 h if no adverse reactions occur. ▪ Do not exceed 100 mL/h. ▪ *20% emulsion:* Infuse at 0.05 mL/min for first 10–15 min; increase to 1 g/kg in 4 h if no adverse reactions occur. ▪ Do not exceed 50 mL/h. **IV Infusion for Premature Neonate:** Infuse at rate not to exceed 0.15 g/kg/h. **IV Infusion for All Patients:** Give fat emulsions via a separate peripheral site or by piggyback into same vein receiving amino acid injection and dextrose mixtures or give by piggyback through a Y-connector near infusion site so that the two solutions mix only in a short piece of tubing proximal to needle. ▪ Must hang fat emulsions higher than hyperalimentation solution bottle to prevent backup of fat emulsion into primary line. ▪ Do not use an in-line filter because size of fat particles is larger than pore size. ▪ Control flow rate of each solution by separate infusion pumps. ▪ Use a constant rate over 20–24 h to reduce risk of hyperlipemia in neonates and prematures because they tend to metabolize fat slowly.

INCOMPATIBILITIES **Solution/additive:** **Aminophylline, amphotericin B, ampicillin, calcium**

chloride, calcium gluconate, dextrose 10%, gentamicin, hetastarch, magnesium chloride, penicillin G, phenytoin, ranitidine, vitamin B complex. Y-site: **Acyclovir, albumin, amphotericin B, cyclosporine, doxorubicin, doxycycline, droperidol, ganciclovir, haloperidol, heparin, hetastarch, hydromorphone, levorphanol, lorazepam, midazolam, minocycline, nalbuphine, ondansetron, pentobarbital, phenobarbital, potassium phosphate, sodium phosphate.**

▪ Discard contents of partly used containers. ▪ Store, unless otherwise directed by manufacturer, Intralipid 10% and Liposyn 10% at room temperature [25° C (77° F) or below]; refrigerate Intralipid 20%. Do not freeze.

ADVERSE EFFECTS (≥1%) **Body as a Whole:** Hypersensitivity reactions (to egg protein), irritation at infusion site. **Hematologic:** Hypercoagulability, thrombocytopenia in neonates. **GI:** *Transient increases in liver function tests, hyperlipemia.* **[Long-Term Administration]** Sepsis, jaundice (cholestasis), hepatomegaly, kernicterus (infants with hyperbilirubinemia), <u>shock</u> (rare).

DIAGNOSTIC TEST INTERFERENCE Blood samples drawn during or shortly after fat emulsion infusion may produce abnormally high ***hemoglobin MCH and MCHC*** values. Fat emulsions may cause transient abnormalities in ***liver function tests*** and may interfere with estimations of ***serum bilirubin*** (especially in infants).

INTERACTIONS Drug: No clinically significant interactions established.

NURSING IMPLICATIONS

Assessment & Drug Effects

- Observe patient closely. Acute reactions tend to occur within the first 2½ h of therapy.
- Lab tests: Determine baseline values for hemoglobin, platelet count, blood coagulation, liver function, plasma lipid profile (especially serum triglycerides and cholesterol, free fatty acids in plasma). Repeat 1 or 2 times weekly during therapy in adults; more frequently in children. Report significant deviations promptly.
- Lab tests: Obtain daily platelet counts in neonates during first week of therapy, then every other day during second week, and 3 times a week thereafter because newborns are prone to develop thrombocytopenia.
- Note: Lipemia must clear after each daily infusion. Degree of lipemia is measured by serum triglycerides and cholesterol levels 4–6 h after infusion has ceased.

Patient & Family Education

- Report difficulty breathing, nausea, vomiting, or headache to physician.

FEBUXOSTAT

(fee-bux'o-stat)

Uloric

Classifications: ANTIGOUT; XANTHINE OXIDASE INHIBITOR
Therapeutic: ANTIGOUT
Prototype: Allopurinol
Pregnancy Category: C

AVAILABILITY 40 mg, 80 mg tablets

ACTION & *THERAPEUTIC EFFECT* Febuxostat decreases serum uric acid by inhibiting the enzyme needed to convert xanthine to uric acid (the end product of protein catabolism). *Effectiveness is measured by decreasing serum uric acid level to less than 6 mg/dL.*

USES Management of hyperuricemia in patients with chronic gout.

CONTRAINDICATIONS Asymptomatic hyperuricemia.
CAUTIOUS USE History of MI or stroke; severe renal impairment (CrCl less than 30 mL/min); severe hepatic dysfunction (Child-Pugh class C); pregnancy (category C); lactation. Safety and effectiveness in children younger than 18 y have not been established.

ROUTE & DOSAGE

Gout
Adult: **PO** 40 mg once daily; can be increased to 80 mg once daily

ADMINISTRATION

Oral
- Concurrent therapy with an NSAID or colchicine is recommended to prevent gout flares during the first 6 mo of therapy.
- Store at 15°–30° C (59°–86° F) away from light.

ADVERSE EFFECTS (≥1%) **CV:** <u>Atrial fibrilation, AV block, thromboembolic events</u>. **GI:** Nausea. **Metabolic:** Elevated AST and ALT levels. **Musculoskeletal:** Arthralgia. **Skin:** Rash.

INTERACTIONS Drug: Febuxostat will increase the levels of drugs requiring xanthine oxidase for normal metabolism (e.g., **6-mercaptopurine, theophylline, azathioprine**)

PHARMACOKINETICS Absorption: 49%. **Peak:** 1–1.5 h. **Distribution:** Greater than 99% plasma protein bound. **Metabolism:** Extensive hepatic metabolism via oxidation and glucuronide conjugation. **Elimination:** Renal (49%) and fecal (45%). **Half-Life:** 5–8 h.

NURSING IMPLICATIONS

Assessment & Drug Effects
- Monitor for and report gout flares.
- Monitor CV status throughout therapy.
- Lab tests: Baseline serum uric acid, again at 2 wk, and periodically thereafter. LFTs at 2 and 4 mo from start of therapy and periodically thereafter.

Patient & Family Education
- Notify physician if you experience a gout flare, but do not stop taking this drug.
- NSAIDs are typically used to control gout flares. Consult physician.

FELBAMATE

(fel′ba-mate)
Felbatol
Classification: ANTICONVULSANT
Therapeutic: ANTICONVULSANT
Prototype: Phenytoin
Pregnancy Category: C

AVAILABILITY 400 mg, 600 mg tablets; 600 mg/5 mL suspension

ACTION & *THERAPEUTIC EFFECT* Anticonvulsant that blocks repetitive firing of neurons and increases seizure threshold; prevents seizure spread. *Increases seizure threshold and prevents seizure spread.*

USES Treatment of Lennox–Gastaut syndrome and partial seizures.
UNLABELED USES Monotherapy or in combination with other anticonvulsants for the treatment of generalized tonic/clonic seizures.

CONTRAINDICATIONS Hypersensitivity to felbamate, history of blood dyscrasia or hepatic dysfunction.
CAUTIOUS USE Renal impairment, renal failure; older adults; hypersensitivity to other carbamates; thrombocytopenia; iron-deficiency anemia; pregnancy (category C), lactation. Safety and effectiveness in children other than those with Lennox–Gastaut syndrome are not established.

ROUTE & DOSAGE

Partial Seizures

Adult: **PO** Initiate with 1200 mg/day in 3–4 divided doses, may increase by 600 mg/day q2wk (max: 3600 mg/day); when converting to monotherapy, reduce dose of concomitant anticonvulsants by 1/3 when initiating felbamate, then continue to decrease other anticonvulsants by 1/3 with each increase in felbamate q2wk; when using as adjunctive therapy, decrease other anticonvulsants by 20% when initiating felbamate and note that further reductions in other anticonvulsants may be required to minimize side effects and drug interactions

Lennox–Gastaut Syndrome

Child: **PO** Start at 15 mg/kg/day in 3 or 4 divided doses, reduce concurrent antiepileptic drugs by 20%, further reductions may be required to minimize side effects due to drug interactions, may increase felbamate by 15 mg/kg/day at weekly intervals (max: 45 mg/kg/day)

ADMINISTRATION

Oral

- Titrate dose under close clinical supervision.
- Shake suspension well before giving a dose.
- Store in airtight container at room temperature, 15°–30° C (59°–86° F).

ADVERSE EFFECTS (≥1%) **CNS:** Mild tremors, headache, dizziness, ataxia, diplopia, blurred vision; agitation, aggression, hallucinations, fatigue, psychological disturbances. **Endocrine:** Slight elevation of serum cholesterol, hyponatremia, hypokalemia, weight gain and loss. **GI:** *Nausea and vomiting,* anorexia, constipation, hiccup, taste disturbance, indigestion, esophagitis, increased appetite, <u>acute liver failure</u>. **Hematologic:** <u>*Aplastic anemia*</u>.

INTERACTIONS Drug: Felbamate reduces serum **carbamazepine** levels by a mean of 25%, but increases levels of its active metabolite, increases serum **phenytoin** levels approximately 20%, and increases **valproic acid** levels. **Herbal: Gingko** may decrease anticonvulsant effectiveness.

PHARMACOKINETICS Absorption: 90% from GI tract. Absorption of tablet not affected by food. **Onset:** Therapeutic effect approximately 14 days. **Peak:** Peak plasma levels at 1–6 h. **Distribution:** 20–25% protein bound, readily crosses the blood–brain barrier. **Metabolism:** In the liver via the cytochrome P450 system. **Elimination:** 40–50% excreted unchanged in urine, rest excreted in urine as metabolites. **Half-Life:** 20–23 h.

NURSING IMPLICATIONS

Assessment & Drug Effects

- Lab tests: Obtain baseline values for liver function and complete hematologic studies before initiating therapy, repeat frequently during therapy, and for a lengthy period after discontinuation of fel-

bamate. Monitor serum sodium and potassium levels periodically.
- Report immediately any hematologic abnormalities.
- Note: When used concomitantly with either phenytoin or carbamazepine, carefully monitor serum levels of these drugs when felbamate is added, when adjustments in felbamate dosing are made, or when felbamate is discontinued.
- Monitor weight, because both weight gain and loss have been reported.
- Monitor for S&S of drug toxicity including GI distress and CNS toxicity.

Patient & Family Education
- Report promptly signs of liver dysfunction including jaundice, anorexia, GI discomfort, and fatigue.
- Report promptly signs of bone marrow suppression including infection, bleeding, easy bruising or signs of anemia.

FELODIPINE
(fel-o′di-peen)
Plendil
Classifications: CALCIUM CHANNEL BLOCKER; ANTIHYPERTENSIVE
Therapeutic: ANTIHYPERTENSIVE
Prototype: Nifedipine
Pregnancy Category: C

AVAILABILITY 2.5 mg, 5 mg, 10 mg sustained release tablets

ACTION & *THERAPEUTIC EFFECT* Calcium antagonist with high vascular selectivity that reduces systolic, diastolic, and mean arterial pressure at rest and during exercise. Felodipine inhibits influx of extracellular calcium across myocardial and vascular smooth muscle cell membranes. Resultant decrease in intracellular calcium inhibits contractility of smooth muscle, resulting in dilation of coronary and systemic arteries. *BP reduction is due to reduction in peripheral vascular resistance (afterload) against which the heart works. This reduces oxygen demand by the heart and may account for its effectiveness in chronic stable angina.*

USES Treatment of hypertension.
UNLABELED USES Angina, CHF, pulmonary hypertension.

CONTRAINDICATIONS Hypersensitivity to felodipine; sick sinus rhythm or second- or third-degree heart block except with the use of a pacemaker; abnormal aortic stenosis; hypotension; bradycardia; cardiogenic shock; acute MI; left ventricular dysfunction. Safety and efficacy in children are not established.
CAUTIOUS USE Hypotension, CHF, angina; aortic stenosis, cardiomyopathy; older adults; GERD; hiatal hernia; hepatic impairment; pregnancy (category C), lactation.

ROUTE & DOSAGE

Hypertension
Adult: **PO** 5–10 mg once/day (max: 20 mg/day)

Hepatic Impairment Dosage Adjustment
Start older adults and patients with impaired liver function at 2.5 mg daily

ADMINISTRATION

Oral
- Give tablet whole. Do not crush or chew tablets.
- Store at or below 30° C (86° F) in a tightly closed, light-resistant container.

ADVERSE EFFECTS (≥1%) **Body as a Whole:** Most adverse effects appear to be dose dependent. **CV:** Tachycardia, *palpitations, flushing, peripheral edema*. **CNS:** *Dizziness, fatigue,* headache. **GI:** Nausea, flatulence, diarrhea, dyspepsia. **Hematologic:** Small but significant decreases in Hct, Hgb, and RBC count.

F

DIAGNOSTIC TEST INTERFERENCE Serum ***alkaline phosphatase*** may be slightly but significantly increased. Plasma total and ionized ***calcium*** levels rise significantly. Serum ***gamma-glutamyl transferase*** may increase.

INTERACTIONS Drug: Adenosine may cause prolonged bradycardia if it is used to treat patients with toxic concentrations of CALCIUM CHANNEL BLOCKERS. **Carbamazepine, phenobarbital, phenytoin** may decrease felodipine effect. **Cimetidine** may increase felodipine bioavailability and adverse effect risk. Concomitant felodipine and **digoxin** administration produces only transient increases in plasma **digoxin** concentrations (35–40% increase), which are not sustained with continued administration. **Food: Grapefruit juice** may increase adverse effects.

PHARMACOKINETICS Absorption: Completely from GI tract; it undergoes extensive first-pass metabolism with only about 15% of dose reaching systemic circulation. **Onset:** Less than 1 h. **Peak:** 2–4 h. **Duration:** 20–24 h (sustained release formulation). **Distribution:** Greater than 99% bound to plasma proteins. **Metabolism:** Metabolized via hepatic cytochrome P-450 mixed function oxidase system. **Elimination:** 60–70% of metabolites are excreted in urine within 72 h. **Half-Life:** 10 h.

NURSING IMPLICATIONS

Assessment & Drug Effects

- Monitor BP carefully, especially at initiation of drug therapy, in patients older than 64 y, and in those with impaired liver function.
- Anticipate BP reduction with possible reflex heart rate increase (5–10 bpm) 2–5 h after dosing.
- Report sustained hypotension promptly; more common with concurrent beta-blocker therapy.
- Assess for and report reflex tachycardia; may precipitate angina.
- Monitor patients for possible digoxin toxicity when taking concurrent digoxin.

Patient Education

- Report peripheral edema, headache, or flushing to physician. These may necessitate discontinuation of drug.
- Get up from lying down slowly and in stages; there is potential for dizziness and hypotension.

FENOFIBRATE (Pr)

(fen-o-fi'brate)

Antara, Lofibra, Tricor, Triglide, TriLipix

Classifications: ANTILIPEMIC; FIBRATE

Therapeutic: CHOLESTEROL-LOWERING

Pregnancy Category: C

AVAILABILITY 48 mg, 50 mg, 154 mg, 160 mg tablets; 43 mg, 67 mg, 87 mg, 134 mg, 200 mg capsules or 50 mg, 100 mg, 150 mg, 160 mg capsules; 45 mg, 135 mg delayed release capsules

ACTION & *THERAPEUTIC EFFECT* Fibric acid derivative with lipid-regulating properties. Lowers plasma triglycerides by inhibiting triglyceride synthesis and, as a result, lowers VLDL production as well as stimulates the catabolism of triglyceride-rich lipoprotein (e.g., VLDL). Produces a moderate increase in HDL cholesterol levels in most patients. *Effectiveness indicated by reduction in the level of serum triglycerides and VLDL production.*

USES Adjunctive therapy to diet for patients with high triglycerides.

CONTRAINDICATIONS Hypersensitivity to fenofibrate or other fibric acid derivatives (e.g., clofibrate, benzofibrate); liver or severe kidney dysfunction; unexplained liver function abnormality; preexisting hepatic disease; primary biliary cirrhosis; preexisting gallbladder disease; lactation; thrombocytopenia. Safety and efficacy in children younger than 10 y (**capsules**), younger than 18 y (**Tricor tablets**) are not established.

CAUTIOUS USE Renal impairment, older adults; history of bleeding disorders; myelosuppression; pregnancy (category C).

ROUTE & DOSAGE

Hypertriglyceridemia

Adult: **PO** 43–200 mg/day depending on product

ADMINISTRATION

Oral

- Drug is usually discontinued after 2 mo if adequate lipid reduction is not achieved with the maximum recommended dose.
- Give at least 1 h before or 4–6 h after cholestyramine.
- Store at 15°–30° C (59°–86° F) in a tightly closed container and protect from light.

ADVERSE EFFECTS (≥1%) **Body as a Whole:** Asthenia, fatigue, infections, flu-like syndrome, localized pain, arthralgia. **CNS:** Headache, paresthesia, dizziness, insomnia. **CV:** Arrhythmia. **GI:** Dyspepsia, eructation, flatulence, nausea, vomiting, abdominal pain, constipation, diarrhea, increased appetite. **Respiratory:** Cough, rhinitis, sinusitis. **Skin:** Pruritus, rash. **Special Senses:** Earache, eye floaters, blurred vision, conjunctivitis, eye irritation, **Urogenital:** Decreased libido, polyuria, vaginitis.

INTERACTIONS Drug: May potentiate anticoagulant effects of **warfarin;** combination with an HMG-COA REDUCTASE INHIBITOR (STATIN) may result in rhabdomyolysis; **cholestyramine, colestipol** may decrease absorption (give fenofibrate 1 h before or 4–6 h after BILE ACID SEQUESTRANTS); may increase risk of nephrotoxicity of **cyclosporine.**

PHARMACOKINETICS Absorption: Well absorbed from the GI tract; increased with food. **Peak:** 6–8 h. **Distribution:** 99% protein bound; excreted in breast milk. **Metabolism:** Rapidly hydrolyzed by esterases to active metabolite, fenofibric acid. **Elimination:** 60% in urine, 25% in feces. **Half-Life:** 20 h.

NURSING IMPLICATIONS

Assessment & Drug Effects

- Lab tests: Periodically monitor lipid levels, liver functions, and CBC with differential.
- Assess for muscle pain, tenderness, or weakness and, if present, monitor CPK level. Withdraw drug with marked elevations of CPK or if myopathy is suspected.

- Monitor patients on coumarin-type drugs closely for prolongation of PT/INR.

Patient & Family Education

- Contact physician immediately if any of the following develops: Unexplained muscle pain, tenderness, or weakness, especially with fever or malaise; yellowing of skin or eyes; nausea or loss of appetite; skin rash or hives.
- Inform physician regarding concurrent use of cholestyramine, oral anticoagulants, or cyclosporine.

FENOLDOPAM MESYLATE

(fen-ol′do-pam mes′y-late)

Corlopam

Classifications: NON-NITRATE VASODILATOR; DOPAMINE AGONIST; ANTIHYPERTENSIVE

Therapeutic: ANTIHYPERTENSIVE

Pregnancy Category: B

AVAILABILITY 10 mg/mL injection

ACTION & *THERAPEUTIC EFFECT* Rapid-acting vasodilator that is a dopamine D_1-like receptor agonist. Exerts hypotensive effects by decreasing peripheral vascular resistance while increasing renal blood flow, diuresis, and natriuresis. *Indicated by rapid reduction in BP. Decreases both systolic and diastolic pressures.*

USES Short-term (up to 48 h) management of severe hypertension.

CONTRAINDICATIONS Hypersensitivity to fenoldopam. Avoid concomitant use with beta-blockers.

CAUTIOUS USE Asthmatic patients; hepatic cirrhosis, portal hypertension, or variceal bleeding; arrhythmias, tachycardia, or angina, particularly unstable angina; elevated IOP; angular-closure glaucoma; hypotension; hypokalemia; acute cerebral infarct or hemorrhage; pregnancy (category B), lactation.

ROUTE & DOSAGE

Severe Hypertension

Adult: **IV** 0.1–0.3 mcg/kg/min by continuous infusion for up to 48 h, may increase by 0.05–0.1 mcg/kg/min q15min (dosage range: 0.01–1.6 mcg/kg/min)

Child: **IV** 0.2 mcg/kg/min, may increase to 0.3–0.5 mcg/kg/min

ADMINISTRATION

Intravenous

PREPARE: **Continuous for Adult:** Dilute to a final concentration of 40 mcg/mL by adding 1 mL (10 mg), 2 mL (20 mg), or 3 mL (30 mg) of fenoldopam to 250, 500, or 1000 mL, respectively, of NS or D5W. **Continuous for Child:** Dilute to a final concentration of 60 mcg/mL by adding 0.6 mL (6 mg), 1.5 mL (15 mg) or 3 mL (3 mg) of fenoldopam to 100, 250, or 500 mL, respectively, of NS or D5W.

ADMINISTER: **Continuous for Adult/Child:** Give only by continuous infusion; never give a direct or bolus dose. ▪ Titrate initial dose up or down no more frequently than q15min.

INCOMPATIBILITIES **Y-site:** **Aminophylline, amphotericin B, ampicillin, bumetanide, cefoxitin, dexamethasone, diazepam, fosphenytoin, furosemide, ketorolac, methohexital, methylprednisolone, pentobarbital, phenytoin, pro-**

chlorperazine, sodium bicarbonate, thiopental.

▪ Note: Diluted solution is stable under normal room temperature and light for 24 h. Discard any unused solution after 24 h. ▪ Store at 15°–30° C (59°–86° F) in a tightly closed container and protect from light.

ADVERSE EFFECTS (≥1%) **Body as a Whole:** Injection site reaction, pyrexia, nonspecific chest pain. **CNS:** Headache, nervousness, anxiety, insomnia, dizziness. **CV:** *Hypotension, tachycardia,* T-wave inversion, flushing, postural hypotension, extrasystoles, palpitations, bradycardia, heart failure, ischemic heart disease, MI, angina. **GI:** Nausea, vomiting, abdominal pain or fullness, constipation, diarrhea. **Metabolic:** Increased creatinine, BUN, glucose, transaminases, LDH; hypokalemia. **Respiratory:** Nasal congestion, dyspnea, upper respiratory disorder. **Skin:** Sweating. **Other:** UTI, leukocytosis, bleeding.

INTERACTIONS Use with BETA-BLOCKERS increases risk of hypotension.

PHARMACOKINETICS Onset: 5 min. **Peak:** 15 min. **Duration:** 15–30 min. **Distribution:** Crosses placenta. **Metabolism:** Conjugated in liver. **Elimination:** 90% in urine, 10% in feces. **Half-Life:** 5 min.

NURSING IMPLICATIONS

Assessment & Drug Effects

- Monitor BP and HR carefully at least q15min or more often as warranted; expect dose-related tachycardia.
- Lab tests: Carefully monitor serum electrolytes (especially serum potassium), BUN and creatinine, liver enzymes, and blood glucose and HbA1C.

FENOPROFEN CALCIUM

(fen-oh-proe′fen)

Nalfon

Classifications: ANALGESIC, NONSTEROIDAL ANTI-INFLAMMATORY DRUG (NSAID); ANTIPYRETIC

Therapeutic: ANALGESIC, NSAID; ANTIPYRETIC

Prototype: Ibuprofen

Pregnancy Category: B first and second trimester; D third trimester

AVAILABILITY 200 mg, 300 mg capsules; 600 mg tablets

ACTION & *THERAPEUTIC EFFECT* Exhibits anti-inflammatory, analgesic, and antipyretic properties of an NSAID. Fenoprofen competitively inhibits both cyclooxygenase COX-1 and COX-2 enzymes by blocking arachidonate binding to prostaglandin G_2 resulting in its pharmacologic effects. *Has nonsteroidal, anti-inflammatory, antipyretic, antiarthritic properties that provide relief from mild to severe pain.*

USES Anti-inflammatory and analgesic effects in the symptomatic treatment of acute and chronic rheumatoid arthritis and osteoarthritis; relief of mild to moderate pain.

UNLABELED USES Juvenile rheumatoid arthritis, acute gouty arthritis, ankylosing spondylitis; fever associated with pulmonary tuberculosis, type A influenza, colds; neoplasms.

CONTRAINDICATIONS Hypersensitivity to fenoprofen or other NSAIDs; salicylate; history of nephrotic syndrome associated with aspirin or other NSAIDS; patient in whom urticaria, severe rhinitis, bronchospasm, angioedema, nasal polyps are precipitated by aspirin or other NSAIDS; severe renal or

F

hepatic dysfunction; perioperative pain associated in CABG; pregnancy (category D third trimester). Safety in lactation or children is not established.

CAUTIOUS USE History of upper GI tract disorders; lupus; older adults; renal failure; renal impairment; hemophilia or other bleeding tendencies; compromised cardiac function, hypertension; impaired hearing; pregnancy (category B first and second trimester); lactation.

ROUTE & DOSAGE

Inflammatory Disease

Adult: **PO** 300–600 mg t.i.d. or q.i.d. (max: 3200 mg/day)
Child: **PO** 900 mg/m² in divided doses, may increase over 4 wk to 1.8 g/m²

Mild to Moderate Pain

Adult: **PO** 200 mg q4–6h prn

ADMINISTRATION

Oral

- Give on an empty stomach 30–60 min before or 2 h after meals. Give with meals, milk, or antacid (prescribed) if patient experiences GI disturbances.
- May crush tablets or empty capsule and mix with fluid or mix with food.
- Store capsules and tablets in tightly closed containers at 15°–30° C (59°–86° F); avoid freezing.

ADVERSE EFFECTS (≥1%) **CNS:** *Headache, drowsiness,* dizziness, fatigue, lassitude, tremor, confusion, insomnia, nervousness, depression. **Special Senses:** Tinnitus, decreased hearing, deafness; blurred vision. **GI:** *Indigestion, nausea, vomiting,* anorexia, *constipation,* diarrhea, flatulence, abdominal pain, dry mouth; infrequent: Gastritis, peptic ulcer, GI bleeding. **Urogenital:** Dysuria, cystitis, hematuria, oliguria, azotemia, anuria, allergic nephritis, papillary necrosis, nephrotoxicity (rare). **Hematologic:** (Infrequent) Thrombocytopenia, hemolytic anemia, agranulocytosis, pancytopenia. **Skin:** (May or may not be hypersensitivity reaction) Pruritus, rash, purpura, increased sweating, urticaria. **Body as a Whole:** Dyspnea, malaise, anaphylaxis, edema.

INTERACTIONS Drug: Fenoprofen may prolong bleeding time; should not be given with ORAL ANTICOAGULANTS, **heparin;** action and side effects of **phenytoin,** SULFONYLUREAS, SULFONAMIDES, and fenoprofen may be potentiated. **Herbal: Feverfew, garlic, ginger, gingko** may increase bleeding potential.

PHARMACOKINETICS Absorption: 80% from GI tract. **Onset:** 2 h. **Peak:** 2 h. **Duration:** 4–6 h. **Distribution:** Small amounts distributed into breast milk. **Metabolism:** In liver. **Elimination:** Primarily in urine; some biliary excretion. **Half-Life:** 3 h.

NURSING IMPLICATIONS

Assessment & Drug Effects

- Lab tests: Baseline evaluations of Hct and Hgb, kidney and liver function.
- Baseline and periodic auditory and ophthalmic examinations are recommended in patients receiving prolonged or high-dose therapy.
- Monitor for S&S of GI bleeding.

Patient & Family Education

- Do not drive or engage in potentially hazardous activities until response to drug is known; fenoprofen may cause dizziness and drowsiness.
- Report immediately the onset of unexplained fever, rash, arthralgia, oliguria, edema, weight gain

to physician. Possible symptoms of nephrotic syndrome are rapidly reversible if drug is promptly withdrawn.

- Understand that alcohol and aspirin may increase risk of GI ulceration and bleeding tendencies; avoid both unless otherwise advised by physician.

FENTANYL CITRATE

(fen′ta-nil)

Actiq Oralet, Duragesic, Fentora, Ionsys, Onsolis, Sublimaze

Classifications: ANALGESIC; NARCOTIC (OPIATE AGONIST)

Therapeutic: NARCOTIC ANALGESIC

Prototype: Morphine

Pregnancy Category: C (B for fentanyl injection)

Controlled Substance: Schedule II

AVAILABILITY 0.05 mg/mL injection; 100 mcg, 200 mcg, 300 mcg, 400 mcg lozenges; 200 mcg, 400 mcg, 600 mcg, 800 mcg, 1200 mcg, 1600 mcg lozenges on a stick; 12 mcg/h, 25 mcg/h, 50 mcg/h, 75 mcg/h, 100 mcg/h transdermal patch; 100 mcg, 200 mcg, 300 mcg, 400 mcg, 600 mcg, 800 mcg buccal tablet; 0.2 mg, 0.4 mg. 0.6 mg, 0.8 mg, 1.2 mg buccal film

ACTION & *THERAPEUTIC EFFECT* Synthetic, potent narcotic agonist analgesic that causes analgesia and sedation. Its alterations in respiratory rate and alveolar ventilation may persist beyond the analgesic effect. *Provides analgesia for moderate to severe pain as well as sedation.*

USES Short-acting analgesic during operative and perioperative periods, as a narcotic analgesic supplement in general and regional anesthesia, and with droperidol or with diazepam to produce neuroleptanalgesia. Also given with oxygen and a skeletal muscle relaxant (neuroleptanesthesia) to selected high-risk patients (e.g., those undergoing open heart surgery) when attenuation of the response to surgical stress without use of additional anesthesia agents is important.

CONTRAINDICATIONS Patients who have received MAO inhibitors within 14 days; substance abuse; myasthenia gravis; labor and delivery; pregnancy (category C).

CAUTIOUS USE Head injuries, increased intracranial pressure; older adults, debilitated, poor-risk patients; cardiac diseases, angina, hypotension, or cardiac arrhythmias; COPD, other respiratory problems; liver and kidney dysfunction; bradyarrhythmias; children; pregnancy (category B for fentanyl injection).

ROUTE & DOSAGE

Premedication

Adult: **IV** 50–100 mcg 30–60 min before surgery **PO** Suck on 400 mcg lozenge until sedated

Child: **PO** Suck on lozenge until sedated, *weight 10–25 kg,* 200 mcg lozenge; *weight 25–35 kg,* 300 mcg lozenge; *weight 35–40 kg,* 400 mcg lozenge

Adjunct for Regional Anesthesia

Adult: **IM/IV** 50–100 mcg

General Anesthesia

Adult: **IV** 2–20 mcg/kg, additional doses of 25–100 mcg as required

Child: **IV** 2–3 mcg/kg as needed

Postoperative Pain

Adult: **IM/IV** 50–100 mcg q1–2h prn
Child: **IM** 1.7–3.3 mcg/kg q1–2h prn

Chronic Pain

Adult: **Transdermal** Individualize and regularly reassess doses of transdermal fentanyl; for patient not already receiving an opioid, the initial dose is 25 mcg/h patch q3days; for patients already on opioids, see package insert for conversions **Stick lozenge (Actiq)** Place in mouth between cheek and lower gum and suck on lozenge; should be consumed over 15-min period

ADMINISTRATION

Oral

- *Buccal tablet:* Do not push tablet through blister, as this may cause damage to tablet. *Lozenge:* Place unit between cheek and lower gum, moving it from one side to the other using the handle. Instruct the patient to suck, not chew, the lozenge. Should be consumed over a 15-min period.

Intramuscular

- Inject undiluted into a large muscle.

Transdermal

- Place on nonirritated flat surface (e.g., chest, back, upper arm). The upper back is preferred to minimize unintended patch removal. Clip (not shave) hair at application site prior to system application. If needed, clean site prior to application only with clear water. Press patch in place for 30 sec. If gel from patch leaks out and contacts skin of patient or caregiver, wash thoroughly with water.

Intravascular

PREPARE: **Direct:** Give parenteral doses undiluted or diluted in 5 mL sterile water or NS.
ADMINISTER: **Direct:** Infuse over 3–5 min.
INCOMPATIBILITIES **Solution/additive: Fluorouracil, lidocaine. Y-site: Azithromycin, phenytoin.**

- Store at 15°–30° C (59°–86° F) unless otherwise directed. Protect drug from light.

ADVERSE EFFECTS (≥1%) **CNS:** *Sedation,* euphoria, dizziness, diaphoresis, delirium, convulsions with high doses. **CV:** Hypotension, bradycardia, circulatory depression, cardiac arrest. **Special Senses:** Miosis, blurred vision. **GI:** *Nausea,* vomiting, constipation, ileus. **Respiratory:** Laryngospasm, bronchoconstriction, respiratory depression or arrest. **Body as a Whole:** Muscle rigidity, especially muscles of respiration after rapid IV infusion, urinary retention. **Skin:** Rash, contact dermatitis from patch.

INTERACTIONS Drug: Alcohol and other CNS DEPRESSANTS potentiate effects; MAO INHIBITORS may precipitate hypertensive crisis.

PHARMACOKINETICS Absorption: Absorbed through the skin, leveling off between 12–24 h. **Onset:** Immediate IV; 7–15 min IM; 12–24 h transdermal. **Peak:** 3–5 min IV; 24–72 h transdermal. **Duration:** 30–60 min IV; 1–2 h IM; 72 h transdermal. **Metabolism:** In liver by CYP3A4. **Elimination:** In urine. **Half-Life:** 17 h transdermal.

NURSING IMPLICATIONS

Assessment & Drug Effects

- Monitor vital signs and observe patient for signs of skeletal and thoracic muscle (depressed respirations) rigidity and weakness.

- Watch carefully for respiratory depression and for movements of various groups of skeletal muscle in extremities, external eye, and neck during postoperative period. These movements may present patient management problems; report promptly.
- Note: Duration of respiratory depressant effect may be considerably longer than narcotic analgesic effect. Have immediately available oxygen, resuscitative and intubation equipment, and an opioid antagonist such as naloxone.

Patient & Family Education

- Follow exactly instructions for taking fentanyl and for disposal of unit provided in patient information.
- Exercise caution when engaging in hazardous activities until reaction to drug is known.
- Children exposed to buccal tablets are at high risk for respiratory depression. Keep out of reach of children.

FERROUS SULFATE Pr

(fer′rous sul′fate)

Feosol, Fer-In-Sol, Fer-Iron, Fero-Gradumet, Ferospace, Ferralyn, Ferra-TD, Fesofor, Hematinic, Mol-Iron, Novoferrosulfa ✦, Slow-Fe

FERROUS FUMARATE

(fer′rous foo′ma-rate)

Feco-T, Femiron, Feostat, Fersamal, Fumasorb, Fumerin, Hemocyte, Ircon-FA, Neo-Fer-50 ✦, Novofumar ✦, Palafer ✦, Palmiron

FERROUS GLUCONATE

(fer′rous gloo′koe-nate)

Fergon, Fertinic ✦, Novoferrogluc ✦, Simron

Classification: IRON PREPARATION

Therapeutic: ANTIANEMIC; IRON SUPPLEMENT

Pregnancy Category: A

AVAILABILITY Ferrous Sulfate: 167 mg, 200 mg, 324 mg, 325 mg tablets; 160 mg sustained release tablets, capsules; 90 mg/5 mL syrup; 220 mg/5 mL elixir; 75 mg/0.6 mL drops; **Ferrous Fumarate:** 63 mg, 100 mg, 200 mg, 324 mg, 325 mg, 350 mg tablets; 100 mg/5 mL suspension; 45 mg/0.6 mL drops; **Ferrous Gluconate:** 240 mg, 325 mg tablets

ACTION & *THERAPEUTIC EFFECT* ***Ferrous sulfate:*** Standard iron preparation that corrects erythropoietic abnormalities induced by iron deficiency but does not stimulate erythropoiesis. ***Ferrous gluconate:*** Claimed to cause less gastric irritation and be better tolerated than ferrous sulfate. *Effectiveness is experienced within 48 h as a sense of well-being, increased vigor, improved appetite, and decreased irritability (in children). Reticulocyte response begins in about 4 days; it usually peaks in 7–10 days and returns to normal after 2 or 3 wk.*

USES To correct simple iron deficiency and to treat iron deficiency (microcytic, hypochromic) anemias. Also may be used prophylactically during periods of increased iron needs, as in infancy, childhood, and pregnancy.

CONTRAINDICATIONS Peptic ulcer, regional enteritis, ulcerative colitis; hemolytic anemias (in absence of iron deficiency), hemochromatosis, hemosiderosis, patients receiving repeated transfusions, pyridoxine-responsive anemia; cirrhosis of liver.

CAUTIOUS USE Hepatic disease; GI diseases; sulfite hypersensitivity; pregnancy (category A).

ROUTE & DOSAGE

Iron Deficiency

Adult: **PO Sulfate (30% elemental iron)** 750–1500 mg/day in 1–3 divided doses; **Fumarate (33% elemental iron)** 200 mg t.i.d. or q.i.d.; **Gluconate (12% elemental iron)** 325–600 mg q.i.d., may be gradually increased to 650 mg q.i.d. as needed and tolerated

Child: **PO Sulfate (30% elemental iron)** *Younger than 6 y,* 75–225 mg/day in divided doses; *6–12 y,* 600 mg/day in divided doses; **Fumarate (33% elemental iron)** 3 mg/kg t.i.d.; **Gluconate (12% elemental iron)** *Younger than 6 y,* 100–300 mg/day in divided doses; *6–12 y,* 100–300 mg t.i.d.

Iron Supplement

Adult: **PO Sulfate** *Pregnancy,* 300–600 mg/day in divided doses; **Fumarate** 200 mg once/day; **Gluconate** 325–600 mg once/day

Child: **PO Fumarate** 3 mg/kg once/day; **Gluconate** *Younger than 6 y,* 100–300 mg/day in divided doses; *6–12 y,* 100–300 mg once/day

Infant: **PO Fumarate** *Low birth weight,* 2 mg/kg/day up to 15 mg/day; *3 y or younger,* 1 mg/kg/day (max: 15 mg/day)

ADMINISTRATION

Oral

- Give on an empty stomach if possible because oral iron preparations are best absorbed then (i.e., between meals). Minimize gastric distress if needed by giving with or immediately after meals with adequate liquid.
- Do not crush tablet or empty contents of capsule when administering.
- Do not give tablets or capsules within 1 h of bedtime.
- Consult physician about prescribing a liquid formulation or a less corrosive form, such as ferrous gluconate, if the patient experiences difficulty in swallowing tablet or capsule.
- Dilute liquid preparations well and give through a straw or placed on the back of tongue with a dropper to prevent staining of teeth and to mask taste. Instruct the patient to rinse mouth with clear water immediately after ingestion.
- Mix ferosol elixir with water; not compatible with milk or fruit juice. Fer-In-Sol (drops) may be given in water or in fruit or vegetable juice, according to manufacturer.
- Do not use discolored tablets.
- Store in tightly closed containers and protect from moisture. Store at 15°–30° C (59°–86° F).

ADVERSE EFFECTS (≥1%) **GI:** *Nausea, heartburn,* anorexia, *constipation,* diarrhea, epigastric pain, abdominal distress, *black stools.* **Special Senses:** Yellow-brown discoloration of eyes and teeth (liquid forms). **Large Chronic Doses in Infants** Rickets (due to interference with phosphorus absorption). **Massive Overdosage** Lethargy, drowsiness, nausea, vomiting, abdominal pain, diarrhea, local corrosion of stomach and small intestines, pallor or cyanosis, metabolic acidosis, shock, cardiovascular collapse, convulsions, liver necrosis, coma, renal failure, death.

DIAGNOSTIC TEST INTERFERENCE By coloring feces black, large iron doses may cause false-positive tests for ***occult blood with orthotoluidine (Hematest, Occultist, Labstix); guaiac reagent benzidine test*** is reportedly not affected.

INTERACTIONS Drug: ANTACIDS decrease iron absorption; iron decreases absorption of TETRACYCLINES, **ciprofloxacin, ofloxacin; chloramphenicol** may delay iron's effects; iron may decrease absorption of **penicillamine. Food:** Food decreases absorption of iron; **ascorbic acid (vitamin C)** may increase iron absorption.

PHARMACOKINETICS Absorption: 5–10% absorbed in healthy individuals; 10–30% absorbed in iron-deficiency; food decreases amount absorbed. **Distribution:** Transported by transferrin to bone marrow, where it is incorporated into hemoglobin; crosses placenta. **Elimination:** Most of iron released from hemoglobin is reused in body; small amounts are lost in desquamation of skin, GI mucosa, nails, and hair; 12–30 mg/mo lost through menstruation.

NURSING IMPLICATIONS

Assessment & Drug Effects

- Lab tests: Monitor Hgb and reticulocyte values during therapy. Investigate the absence of satisfactory response after 3 wk of drug treatment.
- Continue iron therapy for 2–3 mo after the hemoglobin level has returned to normal (roughly twice the period required to normalize hemoglobin concentration).
- Monitor bowel movements as constipation is a common adverse effect.

Patient & Family Education

- Note: Ascorbic acid increases absorption of iron. Consuming citrus fruit or tomato juice with iron preparation (except the elixir) may increase its absorption.
- Be aware that milk, eggs, or caffeine beverages when taken with the iron preparation may inhibit absorption.
- Be aware that iron preparations cause dark green or black stools.
- Report constipation or diarrhea to physician; symptoms may be relieved by adjustments in dosage or diet or by change to another iron preparation.

FESOTERODINE

(fes-o-ter-o-deen)

Toviaz

Classifications: ANTICHOLINERGIC; MUSCARINIC RECEPTOR ANTAGONIST; BLADDER ANTISPASMODIC
Therapeutic: BLADDER ANTISPASMODIC
Prototype: Oxybutynin
Pregnancy Category: C

AVAILABILITY 4 mg, 8 mg extended release tablets

ACTION & *THERAPEUTIC EFFECT* A muscarinic receptor antagonist that reduces urinary incontinence, urgency, and frequency. It helps regulate the involuntary contractions of the bladder associated with sudden urges to urinate. *It controls urinary incontinence or overactive bladder (OAB).*

USES Treatment of overactive bladder in patients with urinary urge, incontinence, urgency, and frequency.

CONTRAINDICATIONS Severe hepatic impairment (Child-Pugh class C); gastric obstruction, paralytic ileus, uncontrolled narrow-angle glaucoma; urinary retention; severe BPH; severe renal insufficiency (CrCl less than 30 mL/min) use should be avoided or requires a dosage reduction. Safety and efficacy in children have not been established.

CAUTIOUS USE Mild to moderate hepatic impairment (Child-Pugh class A and B); mild to moderate renal insufficiency; history of constipation; bladder outlet obstruction; history of decreased GI motility; severe constipation; palpitations; narrow-angle glaucoma; myasthenia gravis; concomitant administration of an anticholinergic agent; pregnancy (category C).

ROUTE & DOSAGE

Overactive Bladder

Adult: **PO** 4–8 mg daily. Do not exceed 4 mg daily with concurrent potent CYP3A4 inhibitors.

Hepatic Impairment Dosage Adjustment

Severe hepatic impairment (Child-Pugh class C): Not recommended

Renal Impairment Dosage Adjustment

CrCl less than 30 mL/min: Not recommended

ADMINISTRATION

Oral

- Give with water without regard to food.
- Do not break or crush extended release tablet. Ensure that it is swallowed whole.
- Store at 15°–30° C (59°–86° F).

ADVERSE EFFECTS (≥1%) **Body as a Whole:** Peripheral edema, upper respiratory tract infection, urinary tract infection. **CNS:** Insomnia. **GI:** Constipation, *dry mouth*, dyspepsia, nausea. **Metabolic:** Elevated ALT levels, elevated GGT levels. **Musculoskeletal:** Back pain. **Respiratory:** Cough, dry throat. **Skin:** Rash. **Special Senses:** Dry eyes. **Urogenital:** Dysuria, urinary retention.

INTERACTIONS Drug: Potent CYP3A4 INHIBITORS (e.g., **clarithromycin, itraconazole, ketoconazole, nefazodone, nelfinavir,** and **ritonavir**) increase fesoterodine levels. INDUCERS OF CYP3A4 (e.g., **rifampin**) can decrease fesoterodine levels.

PHARMACOKINETICS Absorption: 52% bioavailable. **Peak:** 5 h. **Distribution:** 50% plasma protein bound. **Metabolism:** Hepatic metabolism to active and inactive metabolites. **Elimination:** Renal (70%) and fecal (7%). **Half-Life:** 7 h.

NURSING IMPLICATIONS

Assessment & Drug Effects

- Monitor bowel and bladder function as urinary retention and constipation are potential adverse effects. Older adults are at greater risk for adverse effects, especially with the 8 mg dose.
- Monitor for and report bothersome anticholinergic effects (see Appendix F).

Patient & Family Education

- Use caution in hot environments to avoid heat prostration as fesoterodine causes decreased sweating and reduces body cooling in excessive heat.
- Exercise caution with hazardous activities until response to drug is known.

- Moderate alcohol consumption as it may enhance drowsiness caused by fesoterodine.

FEXOFENADINE

(fex-o-fen′a-deen)

Allegra

Classifications: ANTIHISTAMINE; H_1-RECEPTOR ANTAGONIST, NONSEDATING

Therapeutic: NONSEDATING ANTIHISTAMINE

Prototype: Loratadine

Pregnancy Category: C

AVAILABILITY 30 mg, 60 mg, 180 mg tablets; 60 mg capsules; 30 mg orally disintegrating tablet; 30 mg/5 mL oral suspension

ACTION & *THERAPEUTIC EFFECT* Competes with histamine for binding at the H_1-receptor. This blocks effects of histamine on H_1-receptors in bronchial smooth muscle. It also results in decreased formation of edema, flare, and pruritus that result from histaminic activity. *Inhibits antigen-induced bronchospasm and histamine release from mast cells. Efficacy is indicated by reduction of the following: Nasal congestion and sneezing; watery or red eyes; itching nose, palate, or eyes.*

USES Relief of symptoms associated with seasonal allergic rhinitis, and chronic urticaria.

CONTRAINDICATIONS Hypersensitivity to fexofenadine or terfenadine; neonates.

CAUTIOUS USE Mild to severe renal and hepatic insufficiency, hypertension, diabetes mellitus, ischemic heart disease, increased ocular pressure, hyperthyroidism, renal impairment, prostatic hypertrophy; elderly, pregnancy (category C), lactation; young children.

ROUTE & DOSAGE

Allergic Rhinitis

Adult/Adolescent: **PO** 60 mg b.i.d. OR 180 mg daily

Child (2–11 y): **PO** 30 mg b.i.d.

Child (6–11 y): **PO (oral disintegrating tablet)** 30 mg b.i.d.

Chronic Urticaria

Adult: **PO** 60 mg b.i.d. OR 180 mg daily

Child (2–11 y): **PO** 30 mg b.i.d.

Child (611 y): **PO (oral disintegrating tablet)** 30 mg b.i.d.

Child (younger than 2 y)/Infant (older than 6 mo): **PO** 15 mg b.i.d.

Renal Impairment Dosage Adjustment

CrCl less than 80 mL/min: Give normal dose only once per day

ADMINISTRATION

Oral

- Reduce starting dose for those with decreased kidney function.
- Do not give within 15 min of an aluminum- or magnesium-containing antacid.
- Store at 20°–25° C (68°–77° F). Protect from excess moisture.

ADVERSE EFFECTS (≥1%) **CNS:** *Headache,* drowsiness, fatigue. **GI:** Nausea, dyspepsia, throat irritation.

INTERACTIONS Drug: ANTACIDS will decrease serum level of fexofenadine. **Herbal: St. John's wort** will decrease serum level of fexofenadine. **Food: Grapefruit juice** or **apple juice** may decrease efficacy.

PHARMACOKINETICS Absorption: Rapidly from GI tract, 33% reaches systemic circulation. **Onset:** 1 h. **Peak:** 2–3 h. **Duration:** At least 12 h. **Distribution:** 60–70% bound to plasma proteins. **Metabolism:** Only 5% of dose metabolized in liver. **Elimination:** 80% in urine, 11% in feces. **Half-Life:** 14.4 h.

F

NURSING IMPLICATIONS

Assessment & Drug Effects

- Monitor therapeutic effectiveness, which is indicated by decreased nasal congestion, sneezing, watery or red eyes, and itching nose, palate, or eyes.

Patient & Family Education

- Note: Drug is well tolerated and causes minimal adverse effects.

FILGRASTIM Pr

(fil-gras'tim)

Neupogen

Classification: HEMATOPOIETIC GROWTH FACTOR

Therapeutic: ANTINEUTROPENIC; GRANULOCYTE COLONY-STIMULATING FACTOR (G-CSF)

Pregnancy Category: C

AVAILABILITY 300 mcg/mL injection

ACTION & *THERAPEUTIC EFFECT* Human granulocyte colony-stimulating factor (G-CSF) produced by recombinant DNA technology. Endogenous G-CSF regulates production of neutrophils within the bone marrow; primarily affects neutrophil proliferation, differentiation, and selected end-cell functional activity (including enhanced phagocytic activity and antibody-dependent killing). *Increases neutrophil proliferation and differentiation within the bone marrow.*

USES To decrease the incidence of infection, as manifested by febrile neutropenia, in patients with nonmyeloid malignancies receiving myelosuppressive anticancer drugs associated with a significant incidence of severe neutropenia with fever; to decrease neutropenia associated with bone marrow transplant; to treat chronic neutropenia; to mobilize peripheral blood stem cells (PBSCs) for autologous transplantation.

CONTRAINDICATIONS Hypersensitivity to *Escherichia coli*–derived proteins, concurrent administration with chemotherapy, radiation; ARDS.

CAUTIOUS USE Sickle cell disease; respiratory insufficiency; pregnancy (category C); lactation.

ROUTE & DOSAGE

Neutropenia

Adult/Child: **IV** 5 mcg/kg/day by 30 min infusion, may increase by 5 mcg/kg/day (max: 30 mcg/kg/day) **Subcutaneous** 5 mcg/kg/day as single dose, may increase by 5 mcg/kg/day (max: 20 mcg/kg/day)

Bone Marrow Transplant

Adult: **IV** 10 mcg/kg/day given 24 h after cytotoxic therapy and 24 h after bone marrow transfusion

ADMINISTRATION

Subcutaneous & Intravenous

- Do not administer filgrastim 24 h before or after cytotoxic chemotherapy. ▪ Use only one dose per vial; do not reenter the vial. ▪ Prior to injection, filgrastim may be allowed to reach room temperature for a maximum of 6 h. ▪ Discard any vial left at room temperature for longer than 6 h.

PREPARE: **Intermittent/Continuous:** May dilute with 10–50 mL D5W to yield 15 mcg/mL or greater. ▪ If more diluent is used to yield concentrations of 5–15 mcg/mL, 2 mL of 5% human albumin **must be** added for each 50 mL D5W (prior to adding filgrastim) to prevent adsorption to plastic IV infusion materials.

ADMINISTER: **Intermittent:** Give a single dose over 15–30 min. ▪ Flush line before/after with D5W. **Continuous:** Give a single dose over 4–24 h. ▪ Flush line before/after with D5W.

INCOMPATIBILITIES **Y-site:** **Amphotericin B, cefepime, cefoperazone, cefotaxime, cefoxitin, ceftizoxime, ceftriaxone, cefuroxime, clindamycin, dactinomycin, etoposide, fluorouracil, furosemide, gentamicin, heparin, imipenem, mannitol, methylprednisolone, metronidazole, mitomycin, piperacillin, prochlorperazine, thiotepa.**

▪ Store refrigerated at 2°–8° C (36°–46° F). Do not freeze. Avoid shaking.

ADVERSE EFFECTS (≥1%) **CV:** Abnormal ST segment depression. **Hematologic:** Anemia. **GI:** Nausea, anorexia. **Body as a Whole:** *Bone pain,* hyperuricemia, *fever.*

DIAGNOSTIC TEST INTERFERENCE Elevations in **leukocyte alkaline phosphatase, serum alkaline phosphatase, lactate dehydrogenase,** and **uric acid** have been reported. These elevations appear to be related to increased bone marrow activity.

INTERACTIONS Drug: Can interfere with activity of CYTOTOXIC AGENTS, do not use 24 h before or after CYTOTOXIC AGENTS.

PHARMACOKINETICS Absorption: Readily from subcutaneous site. **Onset:** 4 h. **Peak:** 1 h. **Elimination:** Probably in urine. **Half-Life:** 1.4–7.2 h.

F

NURSING IMPLICATIONS

Assessment & Drug Effects

- Lab tests: Obtain a baseline CBC with differential and platelet count prior to administering drug. Obtain CBC twice weekly during therapy to monitor neutrophil count and leukocytosis. Monitor Hct and platelet count regularly.
- Discontinue filgrastim if absolute neutrophil count exceeds 10,000/mm^3 after the chemotherapy-induced nadir. Neutrophil counts should then return to normal.
- Assess degree of bone pain if present. Consult physician if nonnarcotic analgesics do not provide relief.

Patient & Family Education

- Report bone pain and, if necessary, to request analgesics to control pain.
- Note: Proper drug administration and disposal are important. A puncture-resistant container for the disposal of used syringes and needles should be available to the patient.

FINASTERIDE (Pr)

(fin-as′te-ride)

Propecia, Proscar

Classifications: ANTIANDROGEN; 5-ALPHA REDUCTASE INHIBITOR

Therapeutic: ANTIANDROGEN

Pregnancy Category: X

AVAILABILITY 1 mg, 5 mg tablets

ACTION & *THERAPEUTIC EFFECT*
Specific inhibitor of the steroid 5-alpha-reductase, an enzyme necessary to convert testosterone into the potent androgen 5-alpha-dihydrotestosterone (DHT) in the prostate gland. *Decreases the production of testosterone in the prostate gland.*

F

USES Benign prostatic hypertrophy, male pattern hair loss (androgenetic alopecia).

CONTRAINDICATIONS Hypersensitivity to finasteride; females, pregnancy (category X), lactation, children.

CAUTIOUS USE Hepatic impairment, obstructive uropathy.

ROUTE & DOSAGE

Benign Prostatic Hypertrophy
Adult: **PO** 5 mg/day

Male Pattern Hair Loss
Adult: **PO** 1 mg daily

ADMINISTRATION

Oral
- Crush tablets if necessary. Pregnant women should not handle the crushed drug; if absorbed through the skin it may be harmful to a male fetus.
- Store at 15°–30° C (59°–86° F) unless otherwise directed.

ADVERSE EFFECTS (≥1%) **Urogenital:** Impotence, decreased libido, decreased volume of ejaculate.

DIAGNOSTIC TEST INTERFERENCE
Depresses levels of **DHT** and **prostate-specific antigen (PSA). Testosterone** levels usually are increased.

INTERACTIONS Drug: No clinically significant interactions established. **Herbal: Saw palmetto** may potentiate effects of finasteride.

PHARMACOKINETICS Absorption: Readily from GI tract. **Onset:** 3–6 mo. **Duration:** 5–7 days. **Elimination:** 39% in urine, 57% in feces. **Half-Life:** 5–7 h.

NURSING IMPLICATIONS

Assessment & Drug Effects
- Evaluate carefully any sustained increase in serum PSA levels while patient is taking finasteride. It may indicate the presence of prostate cancer or noncompliance with the therapy.
- Monitor patients with a large residual urinary volume or decreased urinary flow. These patients may not be candidates for this therapy.

Patient & Family Education
- Use a barrier contraceptive to prevent pregnancy in a sexual partner.
- Be aware that impotence and decreased libido may occur with treatment.

FLAVOXATE HYDROCHLORIDE

(fla-vox'ate)
Urispas
Classification: SMOOTH MUSCLE RELAXANT
Therapeutic: URINARY TRACT ANTISPASMODIC
Prototype: Oxybutynin
Pregnancy Category: B

AVAILABILITY 100 mg tablets

ACTION & *THERAPEUTIC EFFECT*
Exerts spasmolytic action on smooth muscle. Increases urinary bladder capacity in patients with spastic bladder, possibly by direct action on detrusor muscle. Also demonstrates local anesthetic and

analgesic action. *Has antispasmodic action on the urinary bladder.*

USES Symptomatic relief of dysuria, frequency, urgency, nocturia, incontinence, and suprapubic pain associated with various urologic disorders.

CONTRAINDICATIONS Pyloric or duodenal obstruction, obstructive intestinal lesions, ileus, achalasia, GI hemorrhage; obstructive uropathies of lower urinary tract. Safety in children younger than 12 y is not established.

CAUTIOUS USE Elderly; suspected or closed-angle glaucoma; myasthenia gravis; autonomic neuropathy; dehydration; pregnancy (category B).

ROUTE & DOSAGE

Dysuria, Nocturia, Incontinence
Adult: **PO** 100–200 mg t.i.d. or q.i.d.

ADMINISTRATION

Oral
- Give without regard to meals.
- Store at 15°–30° C (59°–86° F) unless otherwise directed.

ADVERSE EFFECTS (≥1%) **CNS:** Headache, vertigo, drowsiness, mental confusion (especially in older adults). **CV:** Palpitation, tachycardia. **Special Senses:** Blurred vision, increased intraocular tension, disturbances of eye accommodation. **GI:** Nausea, vomiting, dry mouth (and throat), constipation (with high doses). **Skin:** Dermatosis, urticaria. **Other:** Dysuria, hyperpyrexia, eosinophilia, leukopenia (rare).

INTERACTIONS Drug: May antagonize the GI motility effects of **metoclopramide,** may add to GI slowing caused by ANTIDIARRHEALS

PHARMACOKINETICS Elimination: 10–30% in urine within 6 h.

NURSING IMPLICATIONS

Assessment & Drug Effects
- Monitor heart rate. Report tachycardia.
- Those with suspected glaucoma should be closely monitored for increased intraocular tension.

Patient & Family Education
- Do not drive or engage in potentially hazardous activities until response to drug is known.
- Report adverse reactions to physician as well as clinical improvement or the lack of a favorable response.

FLECAINIDE (Pr)

(fle-kay'nide)
Tambocor
Classification: ANTIARRHYTHMIC, CLASS IC
Therapeutic: ANTIARRHYTHMIC, CLASS IC
Pregnancy Category: C

AVAILABILITY 50 mg, 100 mg, 150 mg tablets

ACTION & *THERAPEUTIC EFFECT* Local (membrane) anesthetic and antiarrhythmic with electrophysiologic properties similar to other class IC antiarrhythmic drugs. Slows conduction velocity throughout myocardial conduction system, increases ventricular refractoriness. *Is an effective suppressant of PVCs and a variety of atrial and ventricular arrhythmias.*

USES Life-threatening ventricular arrhythmias.

UNLABELED USES Atrial tachycardia and other arrhythmias unresponsive to standard agents (e.g., quinidine), Wolff-Parkinson-White syndrome, and recurrent ventricular tachycardias.

CONTRAINDICATIONS Hypersensitivity to flecainide; preexisting second- or third-degree AV block, right bundle branch block when associated with a left hemiblock unless a pacemaker is present; cardiogenic shock, left ventricular dysfunction; recent acute MI; QT prolongation syndromes; electrolyte imbalances.
CAUTIOUS USE Hypersensitivity to amide local anesthetics; atrial fibrillation; cardiac arrhythmias; cardiac disease; elderly; sick sinus syndrome; severe or moderate hepatic or renal impairment; pregnancy (category C), children and infants.

ROUTE & DOSAGE

Life-Threatening Ventricular Arrhythmias

Adult: **PO** 100 mg q12h, may increase by 50 mg b.i.d. q4days (max: 400 mg/day)
Child: **PO** 1–3 mg/kg/day in 3 divided doses (max: 8 mg/kg/day)

ADMINISTRATION

Oral

- Do not increase dosage more frequently than every 4 days.
- Store in tightly covered, light-resistant containers at 15°–30° C (59°–86° F) unless otherwise directed.

ADVERSE EFFECTS (≥1%) **CNS:** *Dizziness,* headache, light-headedness, unsteadiness, paresthesias, fatigue. **CV:** <u>Arrhythmias</u>, chest pain, worsening of CHF. **Special Senses:** *Blurred vision, difficulty in focusing,* spots before eyes. **GI:** *Nausea,* constipation, change in taste perception. **Body as a Whole:** Dyspnea, fever, edema.

INTERACTIONS Drug: Cimetidine may increase flecainide levels; may increase **digoxin** levels 15–25%; BETA-BLOCKERS may have additive negative inotropic effects.

PHARMACOKINETICS Absorption: Readily from GI tract. **Peak:** 2–3 h. **Distribution:** Crosses placenta; distributed into breast milk. **Metabolism:** In liver. **Elimination:** Mainly in urine. **Half-Life:** 7–22 h.

NURSING IMPLICATIONS

Assessment & Drug Effects

- Correct preexisting hypokalemia or hyperkalemia before treatment is initiated.
- Note: ECG monitoring, including Holter monitor for ambulating patients, is recommended because of the possibility of drug-induced arrhythmias.
- Lab tests: Monitor plasma level, especially in patients with severe CHF or renal failure because drug elimination may be delayed in these patients.
- Note: Effective trough plasma levels are between 0.7–1 mcg/mL. The probability of adverse reactions increases when trough levels exceed 1 mcg/mL.
- Monitor carefully during period of dose adjustment.

Patient & Family Education

- Note: It is VERY important to take this drug at the prescribed times.
- Report visual disturbances to physician.

FLOXURIDINE

(flox-yoor'i-deen)

FUDR

Classifications: ANTINEOPLASTIC; ANTIMETABOLITE, PYRIMIDINE
Therapeutic: ANTINEOPLASTIC

Prototype: Fluorouracil
Pregnancy Category: D

AVAILABILITY 500 mg powder for injection

ACTION & *THERAPEUTIC EFFECT* Pyrimidine antagonist and cell-cycle specific. Catabolized to fluorouracil in the body; highly toxic because it blocks an enzyme essential to normal DNA and RNA synthesis. *Proliferative cells of neoplasms are affected more than healthy tissue cells.*

USES Palliative agent in management of selected patients with GI metastasis to liver.

UNLABELED USES Carcinoma of breast, ovary, cervix, urinary bladder, and prostate not responsive to other antimetabolites.

CONTRAINDICATIONS Existing or recent viral infections; pregnancy (category D); lactation.

CAUTIOUS USE Poor nutritional status, bone marrow depression, serious infections; high-risk patients: Prior high-dose pelvic irradiation, use of alkylating agents; impaired kidney or liver function.

ROUTE & DOSAGE

Carcinoma

Adult: **Intra-arterial** 0.1–0.6 mg/kg/day by continuous intra-arterial infusion

ADMINISTRATION

Intra-arterial Infusion

PREPARE: **Direct:** Reconstitute with 5 mL sterile distilled water for injection; further dilute with D5W or NS injection to a volume appropriate for the infusion apparatus to be used.

ADMINISTER: **Direct:** It is administered by pump to overcome pressure in large arteries and to ensure a uniform rate. ▪ Examine infusion site frequently for signs of extravasation. If this occurs, stop infusion and restart in another vessel.

INCOMPATIBILITIES **Y-site: Allopurinol, cefepime.**

▪ Keep reconstituted solutions, which are stable at 2°–8° C (36°–46° F), for no more than 2 wk. ▪ Store at 15°–30° C (59°–86° F) unless otherwise directed.

ADVERSE EFFECTS (≥1%) **CNS:** Vertigo, convulsions, depression, hemiplegia. **CV:** Myocardial ischemia, angina. **GI:** *Nausea, vomiting, stomatitis,* diarrhea, cramps, anorexia, enteritis, gastritis, esophagopharyngitis. **Hematologic:** <u>Leukopenia</u>, *thrombocytopenia.* **Skin:** Dermatitis, alopecia (usually reversible), *erythema* or increased skin pigmentation (photosensitivity), dry skin, pruritic ulcerations, rash. **Body as a Whole:** Hiccups, fever, epistaxis, decreased resistance to disease. **Urogenital:** Renal insufficiency.

INTERACTIONS Drug: Metronidazole may increase general floxuridine toxicity; may increase or decrease serum levels of **phenytoin, fosphenytoin; hydroxyurea** can decrease conversion to active metabolite.

PHARMACOKINETICS Distribution: Distributed to tumor, intestinal mucosa, bone marrow, liver, and CSF; probably crosses placenta. **Metabolism:** Rapidly metabolized in liver to fluorouracil. **Elimination:** 15% in urine, 60–80% through lungs as carbon dioxide. **Half-Life:** 16 min.

NURSING IMPLICATIONS

Assessment & Drug Effects

- Discontinue therapy promptly with onset of any of the following: Stomatitis, esophagopharyngitis, intractable vomiting, diarrhea, leukopenia (WBC less than 3500/mm^3), or rapidly falling WBC count, thrombocytopenia (platelets 100,000/mm^3), GI bleeding, hemorrhage from any site.

- Lab tests: Obtain baseline and periodic total and differential leukocyte counts, Hct, platelet count, serum uric acid creatinine, and liver function tests.

Patient & Family Education

- Be aware that floxuridine sometimes causes temporary thinning of hair.

FLUCONAZOLE (Pr)

(flu-con′a-zole)

Diflucan

Classification: AZOLE ANTIFUNGAL

Therapeutic: AZOLE ANTIFUNGAL

Pregnancy Category: C

AVAILABILITY 50 mg, 100 mg, 150 mg, 200 mg tablets; 10 mg/mL, 40 mg/mL suspension; 2 mg/mL injection

ACTION & *THERAPEUTIC EFFECT* Interferes with formation of ergosterol, the principal sterol in the fungal cell membrane leading to cell death. *Antifungal properties are related to the drug effect on the functioning of fungal cell membrane.*

USES Cryptococcal meningitis and oropharyngeal and systemic candidiasis, both commonly found in AIDS and other immunocompromised patients; vaginal candidiasis.

CONTRAINDICATIONS Hypersensitivity to fluconazole or other azole antifungals.

CAUTIOUS USE AIDS or malignancy; hepatic impairment; structural cardiac disease; history of torsades de pointes or QT prolongation; renal impairment or failure; pregnancy (category C), lactation.

ROUTE & DOSAGE

Oropharyngeal Candidiasis

Adult: **PO/IV** 200 mg day 1, then 100 mg/day × 14 days
Child: **PO/IV** 3–6 mg/kg/day × 14 days

Esophageal Candidiasis

Adult: **PO/IV** 200 mg day 1, then 100 mg daily × 3 wk
Child/Infant: **PO/IV** 3–6 mg/kg/day × 21 days

Systemic Candidemia

Adult: **PO/IV** 400 mg day 1, then 200 mg daily × 4 wk
Child/Infant/Neonate (older than 14 days): **PO/IV** 6 mg/kg q12h × 28 days
Neonate (0–14 days): **IV** 6 mg/kg q72h

Vaginal Candidiasis

Adult: **PO** 150 mg × 1 dose

Cryptococcal Meningitis

Adult: **PO/IV** 400 mg day 1, then 200 mg daily × 10–12 wk
Child/Infant/Neonate (older than 14 days): **PO/IV** 12 mg/kg day 1, then 6–12 mg/kg/day × 10–12 wk
Neonate (0–14 days): **IV** 6–12 mg/kg day 1, then 6–12 mg/kg q48h
Premature Neonates (0–14 days): **IV** 5–6 mg/kg q72h

Renal Impairment Dosage Adjustment

CrCl 50 mL/min or less (without concurrent dialysis): Give 50% of maintenance dose

Dialysis Dosage Adjustment: Administer full dose post-dialysis

ADMINISTRATION

Oral

- Take this medication for the full course of therapy, which may take weeks or months.
- Take next dose as soon as possible if you miss a dose; however, do not take a dose if it is almost time for next dose. Do not double dose.

Intravenous

PREPARE: **Continuous:** Packaged ready for use as a 2 mg/mL solution. Remove wrapper just prior to use.

ADMINISTER: **Continuous:** Give at a maximum rate of approximately 200 mg/h. Give after hemodialysis is completed.

- Do not use IV admixtures of fluconazole and other medications.

INCOMPATIBILITIES **Solution/additive:** **Trimethoprim-sulfamethoxazole.** **Y-site:** **Amphotericin B, amphotericin B cholesteryl, ampicillin, calcium gluconate, cefotaxime, ceftazidime, ceftriaxone, cefuroxime, chloramphenicol, clindamycin, diazepam, digoxin, erythromycin, furosemide, haloperidol, hydroxyzine, imipenem-cilastatin, pentamidine, piperacillin, ticarcillin, trimethoprim-sulfamethoxazole.**

ADVERSE EFFECTS ($\geq$1%) **CNS:** Headache. **GI:** Nausea, vomiting, abdominal pain, diarrhea, increase in AST in patients with cryptococcal meningitis and AIDS. **Skin:** Rash.

INTERACTIONS Drug: Increased PT in patients on **warfarin;** may increase **alosetron, bexarotene, phenytoin, cevimeline, cilostazol, cyclosporine, dihydroergotamine, ergotamine, dofetilide, haloperidol, levobupivacaine, modafinil, zonisamide** levels and toxicity; hypoglycemic reactions with ORAL SULFONYLUREAS; decreased fluconazole levels with **rifampin, cimetidine;** may prolong the effects of **fentanyl, alfentanil, methadone.**

PHARMACOKINETICS Absorption: 90% from GI tract. **Peak:** 1–2 h. **Distribution:** Widely distributed, including CSF. **Metabolism:** 11% of dose metabolized in liver. **Elimination:** In urine. **Half-Life:** 20–50 h.

NURSING IMPLICATIONS

Assessment & Drug Effects

- Monitor for allergic response. Patients allergic to other azole antifungals may be allergic to fluconazole.
- Lab tests: Monitor BUN, serum creatinine, and liver function.
- Note: Drug may cause elevations of the following laboratory serum values: ALT, AST, alkaline phosphatase, bilirubin.
- Monitor for S&S of hepatotoxicity.

Patient & Family Education

- Monitor carefully for loss of glycemic control if diabetic.
- Inform physician of all medications being taken.

FLUCYTOSINE

(floo-sye′toe-seen)

Ancobon, Ancotil ♣

Classification: ANTIFUNGAL

Therapeutic: ANTIFUNGAL
Prototype: Fluconazole
Pregnancy Category: C

AVAILABILITY 250 mg, 500 mg capsules

ACTION & *THERAPEUTIC EFFECT* Selectively penetrates fungal cell and is converted to fluorouracil, an antimetabolite believed to be responsible for antifungal activity. *Has antifungal activity against* Cryptococcus *and* Candida *as well as chromomycosis.*

USES Alone or in combination with amphotericin B for serious systemic infections caused by susceptible strains of *Cryptococcus* and *Candida* species.

UNLABELED USES *Chromomycosis.*

CONTRAINDICATIONS Lactation.

CAUTIOUS USE Extreme caution in impaired kidney function; hepatic disease; electrolyte imbalance; bone marrow depression, hematologic disorders, patients being treated with or having received radiation or bone marrow depressant drugs; dental disease; pregnancy (category C).

ROUTE & DOSAGE

Fungal Infection
Adult: **PO** 50–150 mg/kg/day divided q6h
Child: **PO** *Weight less than 50 kg,* 1.5–4.5 g/m²/day divided q6h; *weight greater than 50 kg,* 50–150 mg/kg/day divided q6h
Neonate: **PO** 50–100 mg/kg/day in 1–2 divided doses

ADMINISTRATION

Oral

- Lower dosages with longer dosage intervals are recommended in patients with serum creatinine of 1.7 mg/dL or higher. Check with physician.
- Give capsules a few at a time over 15 min to decrease incidence and severity of nausea and vomiting.
- Store in light-resistant containers at 15°–30° C (59°–86° F).

ADVERSE EFFECTS (≥1%) **CNS:** Confusion, hallucinations, headache, sedation, vertigo. **GI:** Nausea, vomiting, diarrhea, abdominal bloating, enterocolitis. **Hematologic:** Hypoplasia of bone marrow: Anemia, leukopenia, thrombocytopenia, agranulocytosis, eosinophilia. **Skin:** Rash. **Metabolic:** Elevated levels of serum alkaline phosphatase, AST, ALT, BUN, serum creatinine. **GI:** Hepatomegaly, hepatitis.

DIAGNOSTIC TEST INTERFERENCE False elevations of ***serum creatinine*** can occur with ***Ektachem analyzer.***

INTERACTIONS Drug: Amphotericin B produces additive or synergistic effects and can increase flucytosine toxicity by inhibiting its renal clearance.

PHARMACOKINETICS Absorption: Readily from GI tract. **Peak:** 2 h. **Distribution:** Widely distributed in body tissues including aqueous humor and CSF; crosses placenta. **Metabolism:** Minimal. **Elimination:** 75–90% in urine unchanged. **Half-Life:** 3–6 h.

NURSING IMPLICATIONS

Assessment & Drug Effects

- C&S tests should be performed before initiation of therapy and at weekly intervals during therapy. Organism resistance has been reported.
- Lab tests: Obtain baseline hematology, kidney and liver function on all patients before and at fre-

quent intervals during therapy. Twice weekly leukocyte and differential counts with WBC with differential and platelet counts are recommended.

- Frequent assays of blood drug level are recommended, especially in patients with impaired kidney function to determine adequacy of drug excretion (therapeutic range: 25–120 mg/mL).
- Monitor I&O. Report change in I&O ratio or pattern. Because most of drug is eliminated unchanged by kidneys, compromised function can lead to drug accumulation.

Patient & Family Education

- Report fever, sore mouth or throat, and unusual bleeding or bruising tendency to physician.
- Be aware that the general duration of therapy is 4–6 wk, but it may continue for several months.

FLUDARABINE

(flu-dar'a-bine)

Fludara, Oforta

Classifications: ANTINEOPLASTIC; ANTIMETABOLITE, PURINE ANALOG
Therapeutic: ANTINEOPLASTIC; IMMUNOSUPPRESSANT
Prototype: Mercaptopurine
Pregnancy Category: D

AVAILABILITY 50 mg powder for injection; 25 mg/mL solution for injection; 10 mg tablet

ACTION & *THERAPEUTIC EFFECT* Inhibits DNA polymerase alpha, ribonucleotide reductase, and DNA primase, thus inhibiting DNA synthesis in tumor-sensitive cells. *Fludarabine has cytotoxic effects on lymphocytic leukemia and lymphoma as well as immunosuppressant properties.*

USES Treatment of B-cell chronic lymphocytic leukemia (CLL) in patients who fail to respond to a regimen containing at least one standard alkylating agent.

UNLABELED USES Non-Hodgkin's lymphoma; in combination therapy for the treatment of primary resistant or relapsing acute myelogenous leukemia (AML), acute lymphoblastic leukemia (ALL), and secondary AML; cutaneous T-cell lymphoma; macroglobulinemia; myelodysplastic syndrome; prolymphocytic leukemia (PLL); stem-cell transplant preparation.

CONTRAINDICATIONS Hypersensitivity to fludarabine; concomitant administration of pentostatin; pregnancy (category D); live vaccines; lactation. Safety and efficacy in children have not been established.

CAUTIOUS USE Renal impairment; patients at risk for tumor lysis syndrome; history of herpes or viral infection.

ROUTE & DOSAGE

Treatment of Unresponsive B-cell Chronic Lymphocytic Leukemia

Adult: **IV** 25 mg/m² daily × 5 days; repeat q28days **PO** 40 mg/m² daily × 5 days; repeat q28days

Renal Impairment Dosage Adjustment

CrCl 30–70 mL/min: 20% dose reduction; less than 30 mL/min: Should not receive IV fludarabine; oral dose given at 50% of dose

ADMINISTRATION

Intravenous

PREPARE: **IV Infusion:** Exercise caution in the preparation and handling of fludarabine. Avoid exposure by inhalation or direct contact with skin or mucous membranes. ▪ Reconstitute each 50 mg vial by adding 2 mL of sterile water for injection to yield 25 mg/mL. The solution should dissolve within 15 sec and have a pH of 7.2-8.2. ▪ Further dilute in 100–125 mL of D5W or NS. ▪ Administer within 8 h of reconstitution.

ADMINISTER: **IV Infusion:** Give over 30 min.

INCOMPATIBILITIES **Y-site: Acyclovir, amiodarone, amphotericin B, chlorpromazine, dantrolene, daunorubicin, diazepam, ganciclovir, hydroxyzine, idarubicin, pantoprazole, phenytoin, prochlorperazine, quinupristin-dalfopristin, trastuzumab.**

▪ Store unreconstituted vials at 2°–8° C (36°–46° F). ▪ Discard any unused reconstituted product.

ADVERSE EFFECTS (≥1%) **Body as a Whole:** *Fever, chills, fatigue, infection, pain,* malaise, diaphoresis, anaphylaxis, hyperglycemia, dehydration. **CNS:** *Weakness,* paresthesia. **CV:** *Edema.* **GI:** *Nausea, vomiting, diarrhea, anorexia, stomatitis,* GI bleeding, esophagitis, mucositis. **Hematologic:** *Neutropenia, thrombocytopenia,* hemolytic anemia. **Musculoskeletal:** Myalgia. **Respiratory:** *Cough, pneumonia, dyspnea,* sinusitis, pharyngitis, upper respiratory tract infection. **Skin:** *Rash,* pruritus. **Special Senses:** Visual disturbance, hearing loss. **Urogenital:** Dysuria, urinary infection, hematuria.

INTERACTIONS Drug: Use with **pentostatin** increases risk of severe pulmonary toxicity. Do not give LIVE VACCINES due to decreased immune response. Use with **natalizumab** increases immunosuppression.

PHARMACOKINETICS Metabolism: Rapid conversion to active metabolite (2-fluoro-ara-A). **Elimination:** Renal. **Half-Life:** 7–12 h.

NURSING IMPLICATIONS

Assessment & Drug Effects

- Monitor for and report S&S of hemolysis, infection, tumor lysis syndrome (e.g., flank pain, hematuria), peripheral neuropathy, or respiratory distress.
- Lab tests: Baseline creatinine clearance and CBC with differential and platelet count, repeat prior to each treatment cycle, and more often as indicated; periodic serum electrolytes, serum uric acid, and renal function tests.

Patient & Family Education

- Report any of the following to a health care provider: Fever, chills, cough, sore throat, or other signs of infection; pain or difficulty passing urine; signs of bleeding such as easy bruising, black, tarry stools, nosebleeds; signs of anemia such as excessive weakness, lightheadedness, or confusion; difficulty breathing or shortness of breath; decreased vision; mouth sores or skin rash.
- Avoid activities that could cause physical injury and predispose to severe bleeding.
- Women of childbearing age should avoid becoming pregnant while receiving fludarabine.

FLUDROCORTISONE ACETATE (Pr)

(floo-droe-kor′ti-sone)

Florinef Acetate

Classifications: ADRENOCORTICAL STEROID; MINERALOCORTICOID

Therapeutic: ANTI-INFLAMMATORY; MINERALOCORTICOID
Pregnancy Category: C

AVAILABILITY 0.1 mg tablets

ACTION & *THERAPEUTIC EFFECT* Long-acting synthetic steroid with potent mineralocorticoid activity. Small doses produce marked sodium retention, increased urinary potassium excretion, and elevated BP. *Synthetic corticosteroid replacement product for adrenocortical insufficiency.*

USES Partial replacement therapy for adrenocortical insufficiency and for treatment of salt-losing forms of congenital adrenogenital syndrome.
UNLABELED USES To increase systolic and diastolic blood pressure in patients with severe hypotension secondary to diabetes mellitus or to levodopa therapy.

CONTRAINDICATIONS Hypersensitivity to glucocorticoids, idiopathic thrombocytopenic purpura, psychoses, acute glomerulonephritis, viral or bacterial diseases of skin, infections not controlled by antibiotics, active or latent amebiasis, hypercorticism, smallpox vaccination or other immunologic procedures.
CAUTIOUS USE Diabetes mellitus; chronic, active hepatitis positive for hepatitis B surface antigen; hyperlipidemia; cirrhosis; stromal herpes simplex; glaucoma, tuberculosis of eye; osteoporosis; convulsive disorders; hypothyroidism; diverticulitis; nonspecific ulcerative colitis; fresh intestinal anastomoses; active or latent peptic ulcer; gastritis; esophagitis; thromboembolic disorders; CHF; metastatic carcinoma; hypertension; renal insufficiency; history of allergies; active or arrested tuberculosis; systemic fungal infection; myasthenia gravis; pregnancy (category C), lactation; children.

ROUTE & DOSAGE

Adrenocortical Insufficiency
Adult: **PO** 0.1 mg/day, may range from 0.1 mg 3 times/wk to 0.2 mg/day
Child: **PO** 0.05–0.1 mg/day

Salt-Losing Adrenogenital Syndrome
Adult: **PO** 0.1–0.2 mg/day
Child: **PO** 0.05–0.1 mg/day

ADMINISTRATION

Oral
- Note: Concomitant oral cortisone or hydrocortisone therapy may be advisable to provide substitute therapy approximating normal adrenal activity.
- Store in airtight containers at 15°–30° C (59°–86° F). Protect from light.

ADVERSE EFFECTS (≥1%) **CNS:** Vertigo, headache, nystagmus, increased intracranial pressure with papilledema (usually after discontinuation of medication), mental disturbances, aggravation of preexisting psychiatric conditions, insomnia, ataxia (rare). **CV:** CHF, hypertension, <u>thromboembolism</u> (rare), tachycardia. **Endocrine:** Suppressed linear growth in children, decreased glucose tolerance; hyperglycemia, manifestations of latent diabetes mellitus; hypocorticism; amenorrhea and other menstrual difficulties. **Special Senses:** Posterior subcapsular cataracts (especially in children), glaucoma, exophthalmos, increased intraocular pressure with optic nerve damage, perforation of the globe. **Metabolic:** Hypocalcemia; *sodium and fluid retention;* hypoka-

F

lemia and hypokalemic alkalosis, negative nitrogen balance, decreased serum concentration of vitamins A and C. **GI:** *Nausea,* increased appetite, ulcerative esophagitis, pancreatitis, abdominal distension, peptic ulcer with perforation and hemorrhage, melena. **Hematologic:** Thrombocytopenia. **Musculoskeletal:** (Long-term use) Osteoporosis, compression fractures, muscle wasting and weakness, tendon rupture, aseptic necrosis of femoral and humeral heads. **Skin:** Skin thinning and atrophy, *acne, impaired wound healing;* petechiae, ecchymosis, easy bruising; suppression of skin test reaction; hypopigmentation or hyperpigmentation, hirsutism, acneiform eruptions, subcutaneous fat atrophy; allergic dermatitis, urticaria, angioneurotic edema, increased sweating. **Body as a Whole:** Anaphylactoid reactions (rare), aggravation or masking of infections; malaise, weight gain, obesity. **Urogenital:** Increased or decreased motility and number of sperm.

INTERACTIONS Drug: The antidiabetic effects of **insulin** and SULFONYLUREAS may be diminished; **amphotericin B,** DIURETICS may increase **potassium** loss; **warfarin** may decrease prothrombin time; **indomethacin, ibuprofen** can potentiate the pressor effect of fludrocortisone; ANABOLIC STEROIDS increase risk of edema and acne; **rifampin** may increase the hepatic metabolism of fludrocortisone.

PHARMACOKINETICS Absorption: Readily from GI tract. **Peak:** 1.7 h. **Metabolism:** In liver. **Half-Life:** 3.5 h.

NURSING IMPLICATIONS

Assessment & Drug Effects

- Monitor weight and I&O ratio to observe onset of fluid accumulation, especially if patient is on unrestricted salt intake and without potassium supplement. Report weight gain of 2 kg (5 lb)/wk.
- Monitor and record BP daily. If hypertension develops as a consequence of therapy, report to physician. Usually, the dose will be reduced to 0.05 mg/day.
- Check BP q4–6h and weight at least every other day during periods of dosage adjustment.
- Lab tests: Periodic serum electrolytes and ABGs during prolonged therapy.
- Monitor for S&S of hypokalemia and hyperkalemic metabolic alkalosis (see Appendix F).

Patient & Family Education

- Report signs of hypokalemia (see Appendix F).
- Be aware of signs of potassium depletion associated with high sodium intake: Muscle weakness, paresthesias, circumoral numbness; fatigue, anorexia, nausea, mental depression, polyuria, delirium, diminished reflexes, arrhythmias, cardiac failure, ileus, ECG changes.
- Eat foods with high potassium content.
- Signs of edema should be reported immediately. Sodium intake may or may not require regulation, depending on individual needs and clinical situation.
- Weigh daily under standard conditions and report steady weight gain.
- Report intercurrent infection, trauma, or unexpected stress of any kind promptly when taking maintenance therapy.
- Carry medical identification at all times.

FLUMAZENIL Pr

(flu-ma′ze-nil)

Mazicon ♣, Romazicon

Common adverse effects in *italic,* life-threatening effects underlined; generic names in **bold**; classifications in SMALL CAPS; ♣ Canadian drug name; Pr Prototype drug

Classification: BENZODIAZEPINE ANTAGONIST
Therapeutic: BENZODIAZEPINE ANTIDOTE
Pregnancy Category: C

AVAILABILITY 0.1 mg/mL injection

ACTION & *THERAPEUTIC EFFECT* Antagonizes the effects of benzodiazepine on the CNS, including sedation, impairment of recall, and psychomotor impairment. Does not reverse the effects of opioids. *Reverses the action of a benzodiazepine.*

USES Reversal of sedation induced by benzodiazepine for anesthesia or diagnostic or therapeutic procedures as well as through overdose.
UNLABELED USES Seizure disorders, alcohol intoxication, hepatic encephalopathy, facilitation of weaning from mechanical ventilation.

CONTRAINDICATIONS Hypersensitivity to flumazenil or to benzodiazepines; patients given a benzodiazepine for control of a life-threatening condition; patients showing signs of cyclic antidepressant overdose; seizure-prone individuals; during labor and delivery.
CAUTIOUS USE Hepatic function impairment, older adults, lactation, intensive care patients, head injury, anxiety or pain disorder; drug- and alcohol-dependent patients, and physical dependence upon benzodiazepines; pregnancy (category C); children.

ROUTE & DOSAGE

Reversal of Sedation
Adult: **IV** 0.2 mg over 15 sec, may repeat 0.2 mg each min for 4 additional doses or a cumulative dose of 1 mg
Child: **IV** 0.01 mg/kg may repeat each min (max: 1 mg)

Benzodiazepine Overdose
Adult: **IV** 0.2 mg over 30 sec, if no response after 30 sec, then 0.3 mg over 30 sec, may repeat with 0.5 mg each min (max cumulative dose: 3 mg)

ADMINISTRATION

Intravenous

PREPARE: **Direct:** May give undiluted or diluted. If diluted use D5W, lactated Ringer's, NS.
ADMINISTER: **Direct for Reversal of Anesthesia:** Ensure patency of IV before administration of flumazenil, since extravasation will cause local irritation. ▪ Do not give as bolus dose. Give through an IV that is freely flowing into a large vein.
Direct for Reversal of Anesthesia or Sedation: Give each dose slowly over 15 sec. ▪ In high-risk patients, slow the rate to provide the smallest effective dose.
Direct for Benzodiazepine Overdose: Give each dose slowly over 30 sec.

▪ Use all diluted solutions within 24 h of dilution.

ADVERSE EFFECTS (≥1%) **CNS:** Emotional lability, headache, *dizziness,* agitation, *resedation,* seizures, blurred vision. **GI:** *Nausea, vomiting,* hiccups. **Other:** Shivering, pain at injection site, hypoventilation.

INTERACTIONS Drug: May antagonize effects of **zaleplon, zolpidem;** may cause convulsions or arrhythmias with TRICYCLIC ANTIDEPRESSANTS.

PHARMACOKINETICS Onset: 1–5 min. **Peak:** 6–10 min. **Duration:** 2–4 h. **Metabolism:** In the liver to inactive metabolites. **Elimination:** 90–

95% in urine, 5–10% in feces within 72 h. **Half-Life:** 54 min.

NURSING IMPLICATIONS

Assessment & Drug Effects

- Monitor respiratory status carefully until risk of resedation is unlikely (up to 120 min). Drug may not fully reverse benzodiazepine-induced ventilatory insufficiency.
- Monitor carefully for seizures and take appropriate precautions.

Patient & Family Education

- Do not drive or engage in potentially hazardous activities until at least 18–24 h after discharge following a procedure.
- Do not ingest alcohol or nonprescription drugs for 18–24 h after flumazenil is administered or if the effects of the benzodiazepine persist.

FLUNISOLIDE

(floo-niss'oh-lide)

AeroBid, Nasalide, Nasarel

Pregnancy Category: C

See Appendix A-3.

FLUOCINOLONE ACETONIDE

(floo-oh-sin'oh-lone)

Fluoderm ♣, Synalar

Prototype: Hydrocortisone

Pregnancy Category: C

See Appendix A-4.

FLUOCINONIDE

(floo-oh-sin'oh-nide)

Lidemol, Lidex, Lidex-E, Lyderm, Topsyn, Vanos

Pregnancy Category: C

See Appendix A-4.

FLUORESCEIN SODIUM

(flure'e-seen)

Fluorescite

Classification: OPHTHALMIC DIAGNOSTIC AGENT

Therapeutic: OPHTHALMIC DIAGNOSTIC AGENT

Pregnancy Category: X

AVAILABILITY 100 mg/mL injection

ACTION & *THERAPEUTIC EFFECT* Mildly antiseptic fluorescent dye that demonstrates defects of the corneal epithelium. *Any break in the epithelial tissue allows the dye to enter the tissue. Epithelial damage will appear as a bright green area.*

USES Used intravenously as a diagnostic aid in retinal angiography. Also used as an antidote for aniline dye.

CONTRAINDICATIONS Intra-arterial administration; intrathecal administration; pregnancy (category X).

CAUTIOUS USE History of hypersensitivity, allergies, bronchial asthma.

ROUTE & DOSAGE

Retinal Angiography

Adult: **IV** 5 mL of 10% solution or 3 mL of 25% solution injected rapidly in antecubital vein

Child: **IV** 7.5 mg/kg injected rapidly in antecubital vein

ADMINISTRATION

Intravenous

ADMINISTER: **IV Direct for Adult:** 5 mL of 10% solution or 3 mL of 25% solution injected rapidly in antecubital vein. **IV Direct for Child:** 7.5 mg/kg injected rapidly in antecubital vein.

ADVERSE EFFECTS (≥1%) **CNS:** Headache, paresthesias, pyrexia, convulsions. **CV:** Hypotension, transient dyspnea, acute pulmonary edema, basilar artery ischemia, syncope, <u>severe shock, cardiac arrest</u>. **GI:** Nausea, vomiting, strong metallic taste following high dosage. **Body as a Whole:** Hypersensitivity (urticaria, pruritus, angioneurotic edema, <u>anaphylactic reaction</u>). **Skin:** Thrombophlebitis at injection site, temporary discoloration of skin and urine.

NURSING IMPLICATIONS

Assessment & Drug Effects

- Have facilities for treatment of anaphylactic reaction immediately available (e.g., epinephrine 1:1000 for IV or IM use, an antihistamine, and oxygen).
- Discontinue fluorescein immediately if S&S of sensitivity develop.

Patient & Family Education

- Note: IV administration may impart a yellowish orange discoloration to skin and to urine. Skin discoloration usually fades in 6–12 h; urine clears in 24–36 h.

FLUOROMETHOLONE

(flure-oh-meth'oh-lone)

Fluor-Op, FML Forte, FML Liquifilm Ophthalmic

Pregnancy Category: C

See Appendix A-1.

FLUOROURACIL [5-FLUOROURACIL (5-FU)] (Pr)

(flure-oh-yoor'a-sil)

Carac, Efudex, Fluoroplex

Classifications: ANTINEOPLASTIC; ANTIMETABOLITE, PYRIMIDINE

Therapeutic: ANTINEOPLASTIC

Pregnancy Category: D

AVAILABILITY 50 mg/mL injection; 1%, 2%, 5% topical solution; 0.5%, 1%, 5% topical cream

ACTION & *THERAPEUTIC EFFECT* Pyrimidine antagonist and cell-cycle specific. Blocks action of enzymes essential to normal DNA and RNA synthesis and may become incorporated in RNA to form a fraudulent molecule; unbalanced growth and death of cell follow. Exhibits higher affinity for tumor tissue than healthy tissue. *Highly toxic, especially to proliferative cells in neoplasms, bone marrow, and intestinal mucosa.*

USES Systemically as single agent or in combination with other antineoplastics for treatment of patients with inoperable neoplasms of breast, colon or rectum, stomach, pancreas, urinary bladder, ovary, cervix, liver. Also topically for solar or actinic keratoses and superficial basal cell carcinoma.

UNLABELED USES To induce repigmentation in vitiligo; actinic cheilitis; malignant effusions; mucosal leukoplakia.

CONTRAINDICATIONS Poor nutritional status; myelosuppression; pregnancy (category D), lactation.

CAUTIOUS USE Major surgery during previous month; history of high-dose pelvic irradiation, metastatic cell infiltration of bone marrow, previous use of alkylating agents; cardiac disease, CAD, angina; men and women in childbearing ages; hepatic or renal impairment.

ROUTE & DOSAGE

Carcinoma

Adult: **IV** 12 mg/kg/day for 4 consecutive days up to 800 mg or until toxicity develops or 12 days therapy, may repeat at 1-mo intervals; if toxicity occurs, 15 mg/kg once weekly can be given until toxicity subsides

Actinic and Solar Keratosis

Adult: **Topical** Apply cream or solution b.i.d. for 2–4 wk; apply Carac once daily

Superficial Basal Cell Carcinoma

Adult: **Topical** Apply 5% cream b.i.d. for 3–6 wk

Obesity Dosage Adjustment

Dose patient based on lean body mass

ADMINISTRATION

Topical

- Use gloved fingers to apply topical drug.
- Do not use occlusive dressings with topical drug. Use a porous gauze dressing for cosmetic purposes.
- Store at 15°–30° C (59°–86° F) unless otherwise directed. Protect from light and freezing.

Intravenous

Note: Parenteral dose is determined by actual weight unless patient is obese, in which case ideal weight is used.

- Safe handling: Double-glove with latex gloves, and change the double set after every 30 min of exposure. If a drug spill occurs, change gloves immediately after it is cleaned up.

PREPARE: **Direct/Infusion:** This drug may be given undiluted or further diluted in D5W or NS for infusion. ▪ If a precipitate forms, redissolve drug by heating to 60° C (140° F) and shake vigorously. Allow to cool to body temperature before administration.

ADMINISTER: **Direct/Infusion:** Give by direct IV injection over 1–2 min. ▪ Infuse over 2–24 h as ordered. **IV Extravasation:** Inspect injection site frequently; avoid extravasation. If it occurs, stop infusion and restart in another vein. ▪ Ice compresses may reduce danger of local tissue damage from infiltrated solution.

INCOMPATIBILITIES **Solution/additive:** **Carboplatin, chlorpromazine, cisplatin, cytarabine, diazepam, doxorubicin, epirubicin, fentanyl, leucovorin calcium, metoclopramide, morphine.** **Y-site:** **Aldesleukin, amphotericin B cholesteryl, droperidol, filgrastim, gallium, lansoprazole, ondansetron, TPN, topotecan, vinorelbine.**

- Fluorouracil solution is normally colorless to faint yellow. Slight discoloration during storage does not appear to affect potency or safety. ▪ Discard dark yellow solution.

ADVERSE EFFECTS (≥1%) **CNS:** Euphoria, acute cerebellar syndrome (dysmetria, nystagmus, ataxia, severe mental deterioration); pustular contact hypersensitivity. **CV:** Cardiotoxicity (rare), angina. **GI:** Anorexia, *nausea, vomiting, stomatitis,* esophagopharyngitis, medicinal taste, *diarrhea,* proctitis. **Hematologic:** Anemia, leukopenia, thrombocytopenia, eosinophilia. **Body as a Whole:** Hypersensitivity: Pustular contact eruption, edema of face, eyes, tongue, legs. **Skin:** SLE-like dermatitis, *alopecia,* photosensitivity, erythema, increased pigmentation, skin dryness and fissuring, pruritic maculopapular rash. **[Topi-**

cal] Local pain, pruritus, hyperpigmentation, burning at site of application, dermatitis, suppuration, swelling, scarring, toxic granulation.

DIAGNOSTIC TEST INTERFERENCE Fluorouracil may increase excretion of ***5-hydroxyindoleacetic acid (5-HIAA)*** and decrease ***plasma albumin*** (because of drug-induced protein malabsorption).

INTERACTIONS Drug: Metronidazole may increase general floxuridine toxicity; may increase or decrease serum levels of **phenytoin, fosphenytoin; hydroxyurea** can decrease conversion to active metabolite.

PHARMACOKINETICS Distribution: Distributed to tumor, intestinal mucosa, bone marrow, liver, and CSF; probably crosses placenta. **Metabolism:** In liver. **Elimination:** 15% in urine, 60–80% through lungs as carbon dioxide. **Half-Life:** 16 min.

NURSING IMPLICATIONS

Assessment & Drug Effects

- Lab tests: Obtain total and differential leukocyte counts before each dose is administered. Discontinue drug if leukopenia occurs (WBC less than 3500/mm³) or if patient develops thrombocytopenia (platelet count less than 100,000/mm³). Baseline and periodic checks of Hct and liver and kidney function are also advised.
- Use protective isolation of patient during leukopenic period (WBC less than 3500/mm³).
- Watch for and report signs of abnormal bleeding from any source during thrombocytopenic period (day 7–17); inspect skin for ecchymotic and petechial areas. Protect patient from trauma.
- Report disorientation or confusion; drug should be withdrawn immediately.
- Indications to discontinue drug: Severe stomatitis, leukopenia (WBC less than 3500/mm³ or rapidly decreasing count), intractable vomiting, diarrhea, thrombocytopenia (platelets less than 100,000/mm³), and hemorrhage from any site.
- Inspect patient's mouth daily. Promptly report cracked lips, xerostomia, white patches, and erythema of buccal membranes.
- Report development of maculopapular rash; it usually responds to symptomatic treatment and is reversible.
- Be aware of expected response of lesion to topical 5-FU: Erythema followed in sequence by vesiculation, erosion, ulceration, necrosis, epithelialization. Applications of drug are continued until ulcerative stage is reached (2–6 wk after initial applications) and then discontinued.

Patient & Family Education

- Understand that it is very important to report the first signs of toxicity: Anorexia, vomiting, nausea, stomatitis, diarrhea, GI bleeding.
- Avoid exposure to sunlight or ultraviolet lamp treatments. Protect exposed skin. Photosensitivity usually subsides 2–3 mo after last dose.
- Report promptly to physician any difficulty in maintaining balance while ambulating.
- Use contraception during 5-FU treatment. If you suspect you are pregnant, tell your physician.

FLUOXETINE HYDROCHLORIDE (Pr)

(flu'ox-e-tine)

Prozac, Prozac Weekly, Sarafem
Classifications: SELECTIVE SEROTONIN REUPTAKE INHIBITOR (SSRI); ANTIDEPRESSANT
Therapeutic: ANTIDEPRESSANT; SSRI
Pregnancy Category: C

AVAILABILITY 10 mg, 15 mg tablets; 10 mg, 20 mg, 40 mg capsules; 20 mg/5 mL solution; 90 mg sustained release capsules (Prozac Weekly)

ACTION & *THERAPEUTIC EFFECT*
A selective serotonin reuptake inhibitor (SSRI). Antidepressant effect is presumed to be linked to its inhibition of CNS neuronal uptake of serotonin, a neurotransmitter. *Effectiveness may take from several days to 5 wk to develop fully. Drug has antidepressant, antiobsessive-compulsive, and antibulimic actions.*

USES Depression, geriatric depression, obsessive-compulsive disorder (OCD), bulimia nervosa, premenstrual dysphoric disorder, panic disorder.

UNLABELED USES Obesity, fibromyalgia, hot flashes.

CONTRAINDICATIONS Hypersensitivity to fluoxetine or other SSRI drugs; concurrent administration with MAOIs, or thioridazine; children younger than 7 y for OCD, children younger than 8 y for depression.

CAUTIOUS USE Hepatic and renal impairment, renal failure, abrupt discontinuation, anorexia nervosa, mania, bleeding; hyponatremia, cardiac disease, dehydration, diabetes mellitus, patients with history of suicidal ideations or current suicidal tendencies; seizure disorders, ECT, hepatic disease. Older adults may require dose adjustments; pregnancy (category C), lactation.

ROUTE & DOSAGE

Depression, Obsessive-Compulsive Disorder

Adult: **PO** 20 mg/day in a.m., may increase by 20 mg/day at weekly intervals (max: 80 mg/day); 20 mg/day in a.m.; when stable may switch to 90 mg sustained release capsule qwk (max: 90 mg/wk)
Child (older than 7 y): **PO** 10–20 mg/day in a.m. (max: 60 mg/day for OCD)
Geriatric: **PO** Start with 10 mg/day

Premenstrual Dysphoric Disorder

Adult: **PO** 10–20 mg daily (max: 60 mg/day)

Bulimia Nervosa

Adult: **PO** 60 mg daily

Panic Disorder

Adult: **PO** 10 mg daily may increase to 20 mg daily

Pharmacogenetic Dosage Adjustment

CYP2D6 poor metabolizers: Start at 80% of normal dose

ADMINISTRATION

Oral

- Give as a single dose in morning. Give in two divided doses; one in a.m. and one at noon to prevent insomnia, when more than 20 mg/day prescribed.
- Provide suicidal or potentially suicidal patient with small quantities of prescription medication.
- Monitor for worsening of depression or expression of suicidal ideations.
- Store at 15°–25° C (59°–77° F).

ADVERSE EFFECTS (≥1%) **CNS:** *Headache, nervousness, anxiety, in-*

somnia, drowsiness, fatigue, tremor, dizziness. **CV:** Palpitations, hot flushes, chest pain. **GI:** *Nausea, diarrhea,* anorexia, dyspepsia, increased appetite, dry mouth. **Skin:** Rash, pruritus, sweating, hypersensitivity reactions. **Special Senses:** Blurred vision. **Body as a Whole:** Myalgias, arthralgias, flu-like syndrome, hyponatremia. **Urogenital:** Sexual dysfunction, menstrual irregularities.

INTERACTIONS Drug: Concurrent use of **tryptophan** may cause agitation, restlessness, and GI distress; MAO INHIBITORS, **selegiline** may increase risk of severe hypertensive reaction and death; increases half-life of **diazepam;** may increase toxicity of TRICYCLIC ANTIDEPRESSANTS; AMPHETAMINES, **cilostazol, nefazodone, pentazocine, propafenone, sibutramine, tramadol, venlafaxine** may increase risk of serotonin syndrome; may inhibit metabolism of **carbamazepine, phenytoin, ritonavir;** increased ergotamine toxicity with **dihydroergotamine, ergotamine.** ANTIPSYCHOTICS like **pimozide** can cause QT prolongation. **Herbal: St. John's wort** may cause serotonin syndrome.

PHARMACOKINETICS Absorption: 60–80% from GI tract. **Onset:** 1–3 wk. **Peak:** 4–8 h. **Distribution:** Widely distributed, including CNS. **Metabolism:** In liver to active metabolite, norfluoxetine. **Elimination:** Greater than 80% in urine; 12% in feces. **Half-Life:** Fluoxetine 2–3 days, norfluoxetine 7–9 days.

NURSING IMPLICATIONS

Assessment & Drug Effects

- Monitor children and adolescents for changes in behavior and suicidal ideation.
- Use with caution in the older adult patient or patient with impaired renal or hepatic function (may need lower dose).
- Supervise patients closely who are high suicide risks; especially during initial therapy.
- Monitor for S&S of anaphylactoid reaction (see Appendix F).
- Lab tests: Periodic serum electrolytes; monitor closely plasma glucose in diabetes.
- Monitor serum sodium level for development of hyponatremia, especially in patients who are taking diuretics or are otherwise hypovolemic.
- Monitor diabetics for loss of glycemic control; hypoglycemia has occurred during initiation of therapy, and hyperglycemia during drug withdrawal.
- Weigh weekly to monitor weight loss, particularly in the older adult or nutritionally compromised patient. Report significant weight loss to physician.
- Observe for and promptly report rash or urticaria and S&S of fever, leukocytosis, arthralgias, carpal tunnel syndrome, edema, respiratory distress, and proteinuria.
- Observe for dizziness and drowsiness and employ safety measures as indicated.
- Monitor for and report increased anxiety, nervousness, or insomnia; may need modification of drug dose.
- Monitor for seizures in patients with a history of seizures. Use appropriate safety precautions.

Patient & Family Education

- Notify physician of any rash; possible sign of a serious group of adverse effects.
- Do not drive or engage in potentially hazardous activities until response to drug is known; especially if dizziness noted.

- Monitor blood glucose for loss of glycemic control if diabetic.
- Note: Drug may increase seizure activity in those with history of seizure.

F

FLUOXYMESTERONE

(floo-ox-ee-mess′te-rone)
Androxy, Ora Testryl ♣
Classification: ANDROGEN/ANABOLIC STEROID
Therapeutic: ANABOLIC STEROID; MALE HORMONE REPLACEMENT
Prototype: Testosterone
Pregnancy Category: X
Controlled Substance: Schedule III

AVAILABILITY 10 mg tablets

ACTION & *THERAPEUTIC EFFECT* Short-acting, orally effective derivative of testosterone with hypercholesterolemic effect. *Replacement therapy for endogenous testosterone. Promotes recalcification of osseous metastases and regression of soft tissue lesions.*

USES In men as replacement therapy in conditions associated with testicular hormone deficiency; in women to antagonize effects of estrogen in androgen-responsive inoperable breast cancer.

CONTRAINDICATIONS Breast cancer in men, prostatic cancer, benign obstructive prostatic hypertrophy; hypercalcemia; diabetes mellitus; severe cardiorenal disease or liver damage; nephrosis or nephrotic phase of nephritis; history of MI; athletes; infants; women with inoperable mammary cancer less than 1 y or greater than 5 y after menopause; pregnancy (category X), lactation.

CAUTIOUS USE Children, older males, history of MI, or coronary disease, hepatic, renal or congestive heart failure, women.

ROUTE & DOSAGE

Male Hypogonadism

Adult: **PO** 5 mg 1–4 times per day

Metastatic Carcinoma of Female Breast

Adult: **PO** 10–40 mg/day in divided doses

ADMINISTRATION

Oral
- Give immediately before or with meals to diminish GI distress.

ADVERSE EFFECTS (≥1%) **Endocrine:** Virilization (women), gynecomastia (men). **Urogenital:** Priapism, impotence. **Metabolic:** Jaundice (reversible), hypoglycemia, hypercalcemia. **GI:** Hepatocellular carcinoma, peliosis hepatitis, nausea, vomiting, diarrhea, symptoms resembling peptic ulcer. **Body as a Whole:** Anaphylactic reactions (rare), *edema, acne.*

INTERACTIONS Drug: ORAL ANTICOAGULANTS increase risk of bleeding. Possibly increases risk of **cyclosporine** toxicity. **Insulin** and ORAL HYPOGLYCEMIC AGENTS may decrease **glucose** level; dose will need to be adjusted. **Herbal: Echinacea** may increase hepatotoxicity.

PHARMACOKINETICS Absorption: Readily from GI tract. **Metabolism:** In liver. **Half-Life:** 9.5 h.

NURSING IMPLICATIONS

Assessment & Drug Effects

- Lab test: Obtain baseline and periodic liver function and serum electrolytes, Hgb, Hct, and serum and urine calcium; also serial serum cholesterol in patients with history of MI or coronary artery disease.
- Monitor I&O ratio and pattern and weight, and check for edema; report significant changes.
- Monitor for S&S of hypercalcemia (see Appendix F); particularly likely in patients with metastatic breast carcinoma.
- Watch for symptoms of hypoglycemia (see Appendix F) and report to physician. Drug may reduce blood glucose in diabetic patients.
- Observe patient on concomitant anticoagulant therapy for ecchymotic areas, petechiae, or abnormal bleeding from any site. Close monitoring of PT and INR is essential.

Patient & Family Education

- Good personal hygiene, including meticulous skin care is very important (females and prepubertal males are especially likely to develop acne).
- Note and report symptoms of jaundice (see Appendix F) to physician. Dose adjustment may reverse the condition.
- Report menstrual irregularities.
- Report priapism (prolonged erection) to physician promptly, it is a symptom of overdosage. A temporary interruption of regimen may be indicated. Also report persistent GI distress, diarrhea, or the onset of jaundice.
- Be aware that virilization usually occurs. Report to physician any voice change (hoarseness or deepening), increased libido (associated with clitoral enlargement), hirsutism immediately. Usually, stopping therapy will end further development of symptoms but will not reverse hirsutism or voice change.

F

FLUPHENAZINE DECANOATE

(floo-fen′a-zeen)

Prolixin Decanoate, Modecate Decanoate ✦

FLUPHENAZINE HYDROCHLORIDE

Moditen HCl ✦, Permitil, Prolixin

Classifications: ANTIPSYCHOTIC; PHENOTHIAZINE

Therapeutic: ANTIPSYCHOTIC

Prototype: Chlorpromazine

Pregnancy Category: C

AVAILABILITY 1 mg, 2.5 mg, 5 mg, 10 mg tablets; 2.5 mg/5 mL elixir; 5 mg/mL oral concentrate; 2.5 mg/mL, 25 mg/mL injection; **Decanoate:** 25 mg/mL injection

ACTION & *THERAPEUTIC EFFECT* Potent phenothiazine, antipsychotic agent that blocks postsynaptic dopamine receptors in the brain. Similar to other phenothiazines with the following exceptions: More potent per weight, higher incidence of extrapyramidal complications, and lower frequency of sedative, hypotensive, and antiemetic effects. *Effective for treatment of antipsychotic symptoms including schizophrenia.*

USES Management of manifestations of psychotic disorders.

UNLABELED USES As antineuralgia adjunct.

CONTRAINDICATIONS Known hypersensitivity to phenothiazines; subcortical brain damage, comatose or severely depressed states, blood dyscrasias, renal or hepatic disease; lactation. **Parenteral form** not recommended for children younger than 12 y.

CAUTIOUS USE With anticholinergic agents, other CNS depressants; older adults, previously diagnosed breast cancer; closed-angle glaucoma; GI disorders; significant pulmonary disease; renal failure; seizure disorders; history of suicidal ideation or high risk for suicide attempt; cardiovascular diseases; pheochromocytoma; history of convulsive disorders; patients exposed to extreme heat or phosphorous insecticides; peptic ulcer; respiratory impairment; pregnancy (category C).

ROUTE & DOSAGE

Psychosis

Adult: **PO** 0.5–10 mg/day in 1–4 divided doses (max: of 20 mg/day) **IM/Subcutaneous HCl** 2.5–10 mg/day divided q6–8h (max: 10 mg/day); **Decanoate** 12.5–25 mg q1–4wk; **Enanthate** 25 mg q2wk

Dementia Behavior

Geriatric: **PO** 1–2.5 mg/day, may increase every 4–7 days by 1–2.5 mg/day (max: 20 mg/day in 2–3 divided doses)

ADMINISTRATION

Oral

- Dilute oral concentrate in fruit juice, water, carbonated beverage, milk, soup. Avoid caffeine-containing beverages (cola, coffee) as a diluent, also tannic acid (tea) or pectinates (apple juice).
- Be careful not to contact skin or clothing with drug when preparing oral concentrate or liquid preparations for injection. Warn patient to avoid spilling drug. If drug contacts skin, rinse/flush skin promptly with warm water.
- Protect all preparations from light and freezing. Solutions may safely vary in color from almost colorless to light amber. Discard dark or otherwise discolored solutions.
- Store in tightly closed container at 15°–30° C (59°–86° F) unless otherwise specified by manufacturer. Protect all forms from light.

Intramuscular/Subcutaneous

- Fluphenazine hydrochloride (HCl) is given IM and fluphenazine decanoate may be given IM or subcutaneously.

ADVERSE EFFECTS (≥1%) **CNS:** *Extrapyramidal symptoms* (resembling Parkinson's disease), tardive dyskinesia, sedation, drowsiness, dizziness, headache, mental depression, catatonic-like state, impaired thermoregulation, grand mal seizures. **CV:** Tachycardia, hypertension, hypotension. **GI:** Dry mouth, nausea, epigastric pain, constipation, fecal impaction, cholecystic jaundice. **Urogenital:** Urinary retention, polyuria, inhibition of ejaculation. **Hematologic:** Transient leukopenia, agranulocytosis. **Skin:** Contact dermatitis. **Body as a Whole:** Peripheral edema. **Special Senses:** Nasal congestion, blurred vision, increased intraocular pressure, *photosensitivity*. **Endocrine:** Hyperprolactinemia.

INTERACTIONS Drug: Alcohol and other CNS DEPRESSANTS may potentiate depressive effects; decreases seizure threshold, may need to adjust dosage of ANTICONVULSANTS. **Herbal: Kava** may increase risk and severity of dystonic reactions.

PHARMACOKINETICS Absorption: HCl is readily absorbed PO and IM; decanoate, enanthate have delayed IM absorption. **Onset:** 1 h HCl; 24–72 h decanoate, enanthate. **Peak:** 0.5 h PO; 1.5–2 h IM HCl. **Duration:** 6–8 h HCl; 1–6 wk decanoate; 2–4 wk enanthate. **Distribution:** Crosses blood–brain barrier and placenta. **Metabolism:** In liver. **Half-Life:** 15 h HCl; 3.6 days enanthate; 7–10 days decanoate.

NURSING IMPLICATIONS

Assessment & Drug Effects

- Report immediately onset of mental depression and extrapyramidal symptoms.
- Be alert for appearance of acute dystonia (see Appendix F). Symptoms can be controlled by reducing dosage or by adding an antiparkinsonism drug such as benztropine.
- Lab tests: Monitor kidney function in patients on long-term treatment. Withhold drug and notify physician if BUN is elevated. Also perform WBC with differential, liver function tests, periodically.
- Monitor BP during early therapy. If systolic drop is more than 20 mm Hg, inform physician.
- Monitor I&O ratio and bowel elimination pattern. Check for abdominal distension and pain. Monitor for xerostomia and constipation.

Patient & Family Education

- Do not drive or engage in potentially hazardous activities until response to drug is known.
- Do not alter dosage regimen or stop taking drug abruptly.
- Be alert for adverse effects, early detection is critical because drug has a long duration of action. Inform physician promptly if following symptoms appear: Light-colored stools, changes in vision, sore throat, fever, cellulitis, rash, any interference with movement.
- Be aware that it may be difficult for you to adjust to extremes in temperature. Extended exposure to high environmental temperature, to sun's rays, or to a high fever places the patient taking this drug at risk for heat stroke.
- Avoid exposure to sun; wear protective clothing and cover exposed skin surfaces with sun screen lotion (SPF above 12).
- Avoid alcohol while on fluphenazine therapy.
- Note: Fluphenazine may discolor urine pink to red or reddish brown.
- Periodic ophthalmologic exams are recommended.

FLURANDRENOLIDE

(flure-an-dren′oh-lide)

Cordran, Cordran SP, Drenison ♣

Pregnancy Category: C

See Appendix A-4.

FLURAZEPAM HYDROCHLORIDE

(flure-az′e-pam)

Apo-Flurazepam ♣, Dalmane, Novoflupam ♣

Classifications: SEDATIVE-HYPNOTIC; ANXIOLYTIC; BENZODIAZEPINE

Therapeutic: SEDATIVE-HYPNOTIC

Prototype: Lorazepam

Pregnancy Category: X

Controlled Substance: Schedule IV

AVAILABILITY 15 mg, 30 mg capsules

F

ACTION & *THERAPEUTIC EFFECT* Benzodiazepine derivative that enhances the GABA-benzodiazepine receptor complex. GABA is an inhibitory neurotransmitter involved in anxiolytic and sedative effects. Flurazepam appears to act at limbic and subcortical levels of CNS to produce sedation. *Reduces sleep induction time; produces marked reduction of stage 4 sleep (deepest sleep stage) while at the same time increasing duration of total sleep time.*

USES Hypnotic in management of all kinds of insomnia (e.g., difficulty in falling asleep, frequent nocturnal awakening or early morning awakening or both). Also for treatment of poor sleeping habits.

CONTRAINDICATIONS Prolonged administration; sleep apnea; benzodiazepine hypersensitivity; ethanol intoxication; COPD, sleep apnea; respiratory depression; shock; coma; major depression or psychosis; intermittent porphyria; children younger than 15 y; pregnancy (category X), lactation.
CAUTIOUS USE Impaired renal or hepatic function; glaucoma; mental depression, psychoses, history of suicidal tendencies, bipolar disorder; intermittent porphyria; addiction-prone individuals; older adult or debilitated patients; COPD.

ROUTE & DOSAGE

Sedative, Hypnotic
Adult (15 y or older): **PO** 15–30 mg at bedtime
Geriatric: **PO** 15 mg at bedtime

ADMINISTRATION

Oral
- Give once patient is in bed and ready to fall asleep.
- Store in light-resistant container with childproof cap at 15°–30° C (59°–86° F) unless otherwise specified.

ADVERSE EFFECTS (≥1%) **CNS:** *Residual sedation, drowsiness,* lightheadedness, dizziness, ataxia, headache, nervousness, apprehension, talkativeness, irritability, depression, hallucinations, nightmares, confusion, paradoxic reactions: Excitement, euphoria, hyperactivity, disorientation, <u>coma</u> (overdosage). **Special Senses:** Blurred vision, burning eyes. **GI:** Heartburn, nausea, vomiting, diarrhea, abdominal pain. **Body as a Whole:** Immediate allergic reaction, hypotension, granulocytopenia (rare), jaundice (rare).

DIAGNOSTIC TEST INTERFERENCE Flurazepam may increase serum levels of ***total and direct bilirubin, alkaline phosphatase, AST,*** and ***ALT.*** False-negative ***urine glucose*** reactions may occur with ***Clinistix*** and ***Diastix;*** no effect with ***TesTape.***

INTERACTIONS Drug: Alcohol, CNS DEPRESSANTS, ANTICONVULSANTS potentiate CNS depression; **cimetidine, disulfiram** may increase flurazepam levels, thus increasing its toxicity. **Herbal: Kava, valerian** may potentiate sedation.

PHARMACOKINETICS Absorption: Readily from GI tract. **Onset:** 15–45 min. **Duration:** 7–8 h. **Distribution:** Crosses blood–brain barrier and placenta; distributed into breast milk. **Metabolism:** In liver to active metabolites. **Elimination:** Primarily in urine. **Half-Life:** 47–100 h.

NURSING IMPLICATIONS

Assessment & Drug Effects
- Monitor effectiveness. Hypnotic effect is apparent on second or third

night of consecutive use and continues 1–2 nights after drug is stopped (drug has a long half-life).
- Supervise ambulation. Residual sedation and drowsiness are relatively common. Excessive drowsiness, ataxia, vertigo, and falling occur more frequently in older adults or debilitated patients.
- Lab tests: Obtain blood counts and liver and kidney function with repeated use.
- Be aware that withdrawal symptoms have occurred 3 days after abrupt discontinuation after prolonged use and include worsening of insomnia, dizziness, blurred vision, anorexia, GI upset, nasal congestion, paresthesias.

Patient & Family Education

- Avoid potentially hazardous activities until response to drug is known.
- Avoid alcohol. Concurrent ingestion with flurazepam intensifies CNS depressant effects; symptoms may occur even when alcohol is ingested as long as 10 h after last flurazepam dose.
- Be aware of the possible additive depressant effects when drug is combined with barbiturates, tranquilizers, or other CNS depressants.

FLURBIPROFEN SODIUM

(flure-bi′proe-fen)

Ansaid, Ocufen

Classifications: ANALGESIC, NONSTEROIDAL ANTI-INFLAMMATORY DRUG (NSAID); COX-1 AND COX-2 INHIBITOR; ANTIPYRETIC

Therapeutic: ANALGESIC, NSAID

Prototype: Ibuprofen

Pregnancy Category: B first or second trimester; D third trimester

AVAILABILITY 50 mg, 100 mg tablets; 0.03% ophth solution

ACTION & *THERAPEUTIC EFFECT* Inhibits prostaglandin synthesis including in the conjunctiva and uvea by inhibiting the COX-1 or COX-2 enzymes. Ocular flurbiprofen reduces miosis, permitting maintenance of drug-induced mydriasis during surgical procedures. *An anti-inflammatory, nonsteroidal analgesic. Also inhibits migration of leukocytes into inflamed tissues, depresses monocyte function, and may inhibit platelet aggregation.*

USES Inhibition of intraoperative miosis; arthritis and other inflammatory diseases; mild to moderate pain.

UNLABELED USES Management of postoperative ocular inflammation, prevention of postcystoid macular edema.

CONTRAINDICATIONS Hypersensitivity to NSAIDs, or salicylates; epithelial herpes simplex; keratitis; perioperative pain from CABG; pregnancy (category D third trimester), lactation. Safety in children is not established.

CAUTIOUS USE Concomitant use with other NSAIDs; patient who may be adversely affected by prolonged bleeding time; patient in whom asthma, rhinitis, or urticaria is precipitated by aspirin or other NSAIDs; pregnancy (category B first and second trimester).

ROUTE & DOSAGE

Inflammatory Disease

Adult: **PO** 200–300 mg/day in 2–4 divided doses (max: 300 mg/day)

F

Mild to Moderate Pain
Adult: **PO** 50–100 mg q6–8h
Inhibition of Intraoperative Miosis
Adult: **Topical** 1 drop in eye approximately q30min beginning 2 h before surgery for a total of 4 drops per affected eye

ADMINISTRATION

Topical

- Instill ophthalmic preparation with great care to avoid contamination of solution. Do not touch eye surface with dropper.

Oral

- Use the 300 mg dose for initiation of therapy or for acute exacerbations of disease.
- Store at 15°–30° C (59°–86° F) in tight, light-resistant container.

ADVERSE EFFECTS (≥1%) **Special Senses:** *Mild ocular stinging,* burning, itching, or foreign body sensation (transient). **Other:** Slowed corneal healing; increased bleeding time. **For adverse effects to oral preparations, see ibuprofen.**

INTERACTIONS Drug: ORAL ANTICOAGULANTS, **heparin** may prolong bleeding time; actions and side effects of both flurbiprofen and **phenytoin,** SULFONYLUREAS, or SULFONAMIDES may be potentiated. **Herbal: Feverfew, garlic, ginger, gingko** may increase bleeding potential.

PHARMACOKINETICS Absorption: 80% absorbed from GI tract. **Onset:** 2 h. **Peak:** 2 h. **Duration:** 6–8 h. **Distribution:** Small amounts distributed into breast milk. **Metabolism:** In liver. **Elimination:** Primarily in urine; some biliary excretion. **Half-Life:** 5 h.

NURSING IMPLICATIONS

Assessment & Drug Effects

- Observe patients with history of cardiac decompensation closely for evidence of fluid retention and edema.
- Lab tests: Baseline and periodic evaluations of Hgb, renal and hepatic function, and auditory and ophthalmologic examinations are recommended in patients receiving prolonged or high-dose therapy.
- Monitor for GI distress and S&S of GI bleeding.

Patient & Family Education

- Report ocular irritation that persists after flurbiprofen use during surgery (tearing, dry eye sensation, dull eye pain, photophobia) to physician.
- Be alert for bleeding tendency and report unexplained bleeding, prolongation of bleeding time, or bruises.
- Notify physician immediately of passage of dark tarry stools, "coffee ground" emesis, frankly bloody emesis, or other GI distress, as well as blood or protein in urine, and onset of skin rash, pruritus, jaundice.
- Do not drive or engage in potentially hazardous activities until response to the drug is known.
- Avoid alcohol. Concurrent use may increase risk of GI ulceration and bleeding tendencies.

FLUTAMIDE (Pr)

(flu'ta-mide)
Eulexin
Classifications: ANTINEOPLASTIC; ANTIANDROGEN
Therapeutic: ANTINEOPLASTIC
Pregnancy Category: D

AVAILABILITY 125 mg capsules

ACTION & *THERAPEUTIC EFFECT* Nonsteroidal, nonhormonal, antiandrogenic drug that inhibits androgen uptake or binding of androgen to target tissues (i.e., prostatic cancer cells). *Interferes with the binding of both testosterone and dihydrotestosterone to target tissue (i.e., prostate cancer cells).*

USES In combination with luteinizing hormone-releasing hormone agonists (i.e., leuprolide) or castration for early stage and metastatic prostate cancer.

CONTRAINDICATIONS Hypersensitivity to flutamide; severe liver impairment if ALT is equal to twice the normal value; females; pregnancy (category D), lactation.
CAUTIOUS USE Lactase deficiency.

ROUTE & DOSAGE

Prostate Cancer
Adult: **PO** 250 mg (2 caps) q8h

ADMINISTRATION

Oral
- Use with caution in patients with severe hepatic impairment.
- Store at 2°–30° C (36°–86° F) in a tightly closed, light-resistant container.

ADVERSE EFFECTS (≥1%) **CNS:** Drowsiness, confusion, depression, anxiety, nervousness. **GI:** Diarrhea, nausea, vomiting, anorexia, hepatitis, cholestatic jaundice, encephalopathy, hepatic necrosis, <u>acute hepatic failure</u>, may increase ALT, AST, bilirubin. **Urogenital:** *Hot flashes, loss of libido, impotence.* **Hematologic:** Anemia, leukopenia, thrombocytopenia. **Skin:** Rash. **Body as a Whole:** Edema. **Endocrine:** Gynecomastia, galactorrhea.

INTERACTIONS Drug: May increase INR in patients on **warfarin.**

PHARMACOKINETICS Absorption: Readily absorbed from GI tract. **Onset:** Antiandrogenic activity 2.2 h; symptomatic relief 2–4 wk. **Duration:** 3 mo–2.5 y, with an average of 10.5 mo. **Metabolism:** Metabolized in liver to at least 10 different metabolites; the major metabolite, 2-hydroxyflutamide (SCH-16423), is an alpha-hydroxylated derivative that is biologically active. **Elimination:** 98% in urine. **Half-Life:** 5–6 h.

NURSING IMPLICATIONS

Assessment & Drug Effects
- Monitor for symptomatic relief of bone pain.
- Assess for development of gynecomastia and galactorrhea; if these become bothersome, dosage reduction may be warranted.
- Lab tests: Monitor liver function and serum bilirubin periodically.
- Monitor for and report development of a lupus-like syndrome.

Patient & Family Education
- Be aware of potential adverse effects of therapy.
- Notify physician immediately of the following: Pain in upper abdomen, yellowing of skin and eyes, dark urine, respiratory problems, rashes on face, difficulty urinating, sore throat, fever, chills.

FLUTICASONE
(flu-ti-ca′sone)
Advair, Flonase, Flovent, Flovent HFA, Cutivate, Veramyst
Pregnancy Category: C
See Appendixes A-3, A-4.

FLUVASTATIN

(flu-vah-stat'in)

Lescol, Lescol XL

Classifications: HMG-COA REDUCTASE INHIBITOR (STATIN); ANTIHYPERLIPEMIC

Therapeutic: CHOLESTEROL-LOWERING (STATIN)

Prototype: Lovastatin

Pregnancy Category: X

AVAILABILITY 20 mg, 40 mg capsules; 80 mg extended release tablet

ACTION & *THERAPEUTIC EFFECT* Inhibits reductase 3-hydroxy-3-methylglutaryl coenzyme A (HMG-CoA) that is essential to hepatic production of cholesterol. Cholesterol-lowering effect triggers induction of LDL receptors, which promotes removal of LDL and VLDL remnants (precursors of LDL) from plasma. *Results in an increase in plasma HDL concentration. HDLs collect excess cholesterol from body cells and transport it to the liver for excretion.*

USES Adjunct to diet for the reduction of elevated total LDL cholesterol in patients with primary hypercholesterolemia (types IIa and IIb).

UNLABELED USES Other types of hyperlipidemias.

CONTRAINDICATIONS Hypersensitivity to fluvastatin, lovastatin, pravastatin, or simvastatin; active liver disease or unexplained persistent elevated liver function tests; pregnancy (category X), lactation; children 10 y or younger.

CAUTIOUS USE Patients who consume substantial quantities of alcohol; history of liver disease; renal impairment.

ROUTE & DOSAGE

Hypercholesterolemia

Adult: **PO** 20 mg at bedtime, may increase up to 80 mg/day in 1–2 doses

ADMINISTRATION

Oral

- Ensure the extended release tablet is not chewed or crushed. It **must be** swallowed whole.
- Separate doses of this drug and bile-acid resin (e.g., cholestyramine) by at least 2 h when given concomitantly.
- Note: Dosage adjustments may be required in patients with significant renal or hepatic impairment.
- Store at room temperature, 15°–30° C (59°–86° F).

ADVERSE EFFECTS (≥1%) **CNS:** Headache, fatigue. **Body as a Whole:** Myalgia. **GI:** Dyspepsia, diarrhea, abdominal pain. **Skin:** Rash.

INTERACTIONS Drug: May increase risk of bleeding with **warfarin; cholestyramine** decreases fluvastatin absorption; **rifampin** increases metabolism of fluvastatin; may increase risk of myopathy and rhabdomyolysis with **gemfibrozil, fenofibrate, clofibrate.**

PHARMACOKINETICS Absorption: Readily from GI tract; about 24% reaches systemic circulation after first-pass metabolism. **Onset:** 3–6 wk. **Peak:** Serum level 0.5–1 h. **Distribution:** 98% protein bound; distributed into breast milk. **Metabolism:** In liver. **Elimination:** 95% in bile; 5% in urine. **Half-Life:** 0.5–1 h.

F

NURSING IMPLICATIONS

Assessment & Drug Effects

- Lab tests: Monitor lipoprotein levels; maximal lipid-lowering effect occurs in 4–6 wk. Monitor serum transaminase and CPK levels every 3–4 mo for the first year and periodically thereafter.
- Monitor PT and INR in patients on concurrent warfarin therapy; PT & INR may be prolonged.

Patient & Family Education

- Take fluvastatin at bedtime.
- Be alert and report signs of bleeding immediately when also taking warfarin.
- Notify physician immediately of the following: Fever; rash; muscle pain, weakness, tenderness, or cramping.
- Reduce or eliminate alcohol consumption while taking fluvastatin.

FLUVOXAMINE

(flu-vox'a-meen)

Luvox, Luvox CR

Classifications: SELECTIVE SEROTONIN REUPTAKE INHIBITOR (SSRI); ANTIDEPRESSANT

Therapeutic: ANTIDEPRESSANT; SSRI

Prototype: Fluoxetine

Pregnancy Category: C

AVAILABILITY 25 mg, 50 mg, 100 mg tablets; 100 mg, 150 mg extended release capsules

ACTION & *THERAPEUTIC EFFECT* Antidepressant with potent, selective, inhibitory activity on neuronal (5-HT) serotonin reuptake (SSRI). *Effective as an antidepressant and for control of obsessive-compulsive disorders.*

USES Treatment of obsessive-compulsive disorders, social anxiety disorder.

UNLABELED USES Post-traumatic stress disorder, depression, panic attacks.

CONTRAINDICATIONS Hypersensitivity to fluvoxamine or fluoxetine; suicidal ideation; concurrent MAOI therapy; bipolar disorder; children 8 y or younger for use with obsessive-compulsive disorder.

CAUTIOUS USE Liver disease, renal impairment, abrupt discontinuation; cardiac disease, dehydration, hyponatremia, older adults, ECT, seizure disorders, history of suicidal ideation, tobacco smoking; pregnancy (category C), lactation.

ROUTE & DOSAGE

Obsessive-Compulsive Disorder

Adult: **PO** Start with 50 mg daily, may increase slowly up to 300 mg/day given every night or divided b.i.d. OR 100 mg extended release every night, may increase up (max: 300 mg/day)

Adolescent: **PO** Start with 25 mg daily, may increase up to 300 mg/day in divided doses

Child (8–11 y): **PO** Start with 25 mg every night, may increase by 25 mg q4–7days (max: 200 mg/day in divided doses)

Social Anxiety Disorder

Adult: **PO** 100 mg extended release caps every night, may increase as needed up to 300 mg/day

Pharmacogenetic Dosage Adjustment

Poor CYP2D6 metabolizers: Start with 70% of dose

ADMINISTRATION

Oral

- Do not open extended release capsules. They **must be** swallowed whole.
- Give starting doses at bedtime to improve tolerance to nausea and vomiting; both are common early in therapy.
- Store at room temperature, 15°–30° C (59°–86° F), away from moisture and light.

F

ADVERSE EFFECTS (≥1%) **CNS:** *Somnolence, headache, agitation, insomnia, dizziness,* seizures. **CV:** Orthostatic hypotension, slight bradycardia. **GI:** *Nausea, vomiting, dry mouth, constipation, anorexia.* **Urogenital:** Sexual dysfunction. **Skin:** Stevens-Johnson syndrome, toxic epidermal necrolysis (rare).

DIAGNOSTIC TEST INTERFERENCE ***Gamma-glutamyl transferase*** increased by more than 3-fold following 3 wk of therapy.

INTERACTIONS Drug: Fluvoxamine has been shown to significantly increase plasma levels of **amitriptyline, clomipramine,** and other TRICYCLIC ANTIDEPRESSANTS to mildly increase levels of their metabolites. May antagonize the blood pressure-lowering effects of **atenolol** and other BETA-BLOCKERS. May increase levels and toxicity of **carbamazepine, mexiletine.** May increase **lithium** levels causing neurotoxicity, **serotonin** syndrome, somnolence, and mania. One report of increased **theophylline** levels with toxicity. Increases prothrombin time in patients on **warfarin;** increased ergotamine toxicity with **dihydroergotamine, ergotamine.** Use with CYP1A2 INHIBITORS **(thioridazine, pimozide, alosetron, tizanidine)** increases **fluvoxamine** levels and toxicity. **Food: Grapefruit juice** may increase risk of side effects. **Herbal: Melatonin** may increase and prolong drowsiness; **St. John's wort** may cause **serotonin** syndrome.

PHARMACOKINETICS Absorption: Almost completely absorbed from GI tract. **Onset:** 4–7 days. **Distribution:** Approximately 77% bound to plasma proteins; excreted in human breast milk but in an amount that poses little risk to the nursing infant. **Metabolism:** In liver. **Elimination:** Completely in urine. **Half-Life:** 16–24 h.

NURSING IMPLICATIONS

Assessment & Drug Effects

- Monitor for significant nausea and vomiting, especially during initial therapy.
- Monitor for worsening of depression or emergence of suicidal ideations especially in adolescents and children.
- Assess safety; drowsiness and dizziness are common adverse effects.
- Monitor PT and INR carefully with concurrent warfarin therapy; adjust warfarin as needed.

Patient & Family Education

- Note: Nausea and vomiting are common in early therapy. Notify physician if these adverse effects last more than a few days.
- Exercise caution with hazardous activity until response to the drug is known.

FOLIC ACID (VITAMIN B_9, PTEROYLGLUTAMIC ACID)

(fol'ic)

Apo-Folic ♣, Folacin, Novofolacid ♣

Common adverse effects in *italic*, life-threatening effects underlined; generic names in **bold**; classifications in SMALL CAPS; ♣ Canadian drug name; ⓟ Prototype drug

FOLATE SODIUM

Folvite Sodium

Classification: VITAMIN B_9

Therapeutic: VITAMIN SUPPLEMENT

Pregnancy Category: A

AVAILABILITY 0.4 mg, 0.8 mg, 1 mg tablets; 5 mg/mL injection

ACTION & *THERAPEUTIC EFFECT* Vitamin B_9 essential for nucleoprotein synthesis and maintenance of normal erythropoiesis. Acts against folic acid deficiency that results in production of defective DNA that leads to megaloblast formation and arrest of bone marrow maturation. *Stimulates production of RBCs, WBCs, and platelets in patients with megaloblastic anemias.*

USES Folate deficiency, macrocytic anemia, and megaloblastic anemias associated with malabsorption syndromes, alcoholism, primary liver disease, inadequate dietary intake, pregnancy, infancy, and childhood.

CONTRAINDICATIONS Folic acid alone for pernicious anemia or other vitamin B_{12} deficiency states; normocytic, refractory, aplastic, or undiagnosed anemia; neonates.

CAUTIOUS USE Pregnancy (category A).

ROUTE & DOSAGE

Therapeutic

Adult: **PO/IM/Subcutaneous/IV** 1 mg/day or less

Child: **PO/IM/Subcutaneous/IV** 1 mg/day or less

Maintenance

Adult: **PO/IM/Subcutaneous/IV** 0.4 mg/day or less

Child: **PO/IM/Subcutaneous/IV** *4 y or younger*, up to 0.3 mg/day; *older than 4 y*, up to 0.1 mg/day

Infant: **PO/IM/Subcutaneous/IV** 0.1 mg/day

ADMINISTRATION

Oral

- Oral route is preferred to other routes.

Intramuscular/Subcutaneous

- Give undiluted. Use caution not to inject intradermally.

Intravenous

PREPARE: **Direct/Continuous:** Given undiluted.

ADMINISTER: **Direct/Continuous:** Give over 30–60 sec. ▪ May also add to a continuous infusion.

INCOMPATIBILITIES **Solution/additive:** **Calcium gluconate, chlorpromazine, dextrose 40% in water, doxapram.**

- Store at 15°–30° C (59°–86° F) in tightly closed containers protected from light, unless otherwise directed.

ADVERSE EFFECTS (≥1%) Reportedly nontoxic. Slight flushing and feeling of warmth following IV administration.

DIAGNOSTIC TEST INTERFERENCE Falsely low serum ***folate levels*** may occur with ***Lactobacillus casei assay*** in patients receiving antibiotics such as TETRACYCLINES.

INTERACTIONS **Drug: Chloramphenicol** may antagonize effects of **folate** therapy; **phenytoin** metabolism may be increased, thus decreasing its levels.

PHARMACOKINETICS **Absorption:** Readily from proximal small intestine. **Peak:** 30–60 min PO. **Distribution:** Distributed to all body tissues;

high concentrations in CSF; crosses placenta; distributed into breast milk. **Metabolism:** In liver to active metabolites. **Elimination:** Small amounts in urine in folate-deficient patients; large amounts excreted in urine with high doses.

NURSING IMPLICATIONS

Assessment & Drug Effects

- Obtain a careful history of dietary intake and drug and alcohol usage prior to start of therapy.
- Keep physician informed of patient's response to therapy.
- Monitor patients on phenytoin for subtherapeutic plasma levels.

Patient & Family Education

- Remain under close medical supervision while taking folic acid therapy. Adjustment of maintenance dose should be made if there is threat of relapse.

FONDAPARINUX SODIUM

(fon-da-par'i-nux)

Arixtra

Classification: ANTICOAGULANT, SELECTIVE FACTOR XA INHIBITOR

Therapeutic: ANTICOAGULANT; ANTITHROMBOTIC

Pregnancy Category: B

AVAILABILITY 2.5 mg/0.5 mL, 5 mg/0.4 mL, 7.5 mg/0.6 mL, 10 mg/0.8 mL syringe

ACTION & *THERAPEUTIC EFFECT* Fondaparinux sodium causes antithrombin III (ATIII)-mediated selective inhibition of Factor Xa. It potentiates the innate neutralization of Factor Xa by ATIII. This interrupts the blood coagulation cascade, inhibiting thrombin formation and, thus, thrombus development. *Effective in the prevention and treatment of deep-vein thrombosis measured by the laboratory value of the amount of anti-Xa assay expressed in mg.*

USES Prophylaxis for DVT or pulmonary embolism (PE) in patients undergoing hip or knee replacement surgery or abdominal surgery; treatment of acute DVT without PE with warfarin, treatment of PE with warfarin.

CONTRAINDICATIONS Hypersensitivity to fondaparinux; active bleeding; GI bleeding; severe renal impairment with a creatinine clearance of less than 30 mL/min; weight less than 50 kg; active major bleeding; bacterial endocarditis; intramuscular administration; thrombocytopenia associated with fondaparinux. Safety and effectiveness in children have not been established.

CAUTIOUS USE Renal impairment or disease; older adult; indwelling epidural catheter; dental disease, dental work; diabetic retinopathy; diverticulitis; endocarditis, epidural anesthesia; hemophilia, heparin-induced thrombocytopenia (HIT), hepatic disease, hypertension, idiopathic thrombocytopenia purpura (ITP); inflammatory bowel disease, lumbar puncture, spinal anesthesia; stroke, surgery; thrombocytopenia, thrombolytic therapy; vaginal bleeding, menstruation; peptic ulcer disease; bleeding disorders including a history of GI ulceration, etc., history of heparin-induced thrombocytopenia; pregnancy (category B), lactation.

ROUTE & DOSAGE

DVT, Pulmonary Embolism Prophylaxis

Adult: **Subcutaneous** *Weight greater than 50 kg,* 2.5 mg daily starting at least 6 h postsurgery × 5–9 days; *for hip fracture patients,* up to 24 days additional use

Treatment of DVT, Pulmonary Embolism

Adult: **Subcutaneous** *Weight less than 50 kg,* 5 mg; *50–100 kg,* 7.5 mg; *weight greater than 100 kg,* 10 mg once daily × 5–9 days

Renal Impairment Dosage Adjustment

CrCl 30–50 mL/min: Use with caution; less than 30 mL/min: Use is contraindicated

ADMINISTRATION

Subcutaneous

- Give no sooner than 6 h after surgery.
- Inspect visually for particulate matter and discoloration prior to administration.
- Do not expel the air bubble from the syringe before the injection.
- Use prefilled syringe to inject into fatty tissue, alternating injection sites (e.g., between L and R abdominal wall).
- Store at 25° C (77° F); excursions permitted to 15°–30° C (59°–86° F).

ADVERSE EFFECTS (≥1%) **Body as a Whole:** Fever, edema. **CNS:** Insomnia, dizziness, confusion, headache. **CV:** Hypotension. **GI:** Nausea, constipation, vomiting, diarrhea, dyspepsia, elevated LFTs. **Endocrine:** Hypokalemia. **Hematologic:** Hemorrhage, *anemia,* hematoma. **Skin:** Irritation at injection site, rash, purpura, bullous eruption. **Urogenital:** UTI, urinary retention.

INTERACTIONS Drug: ANTICOAGULANTS, ANTIPLATELETS, NSAIDS, **aspirin** may increase risk of bleeding. **Herbal: Feverfew, ginkgo, ginger, evening primrose oil** may potentiate bleeding.

PHARMACOKINETICS Absorption: Rapidly and completely absorbed from subcutaneous injection site. **Peak:** 2–3 h. **Distribution:** Primarily in blood. **Metabolism:** Negligible metabolism. **Elimination:** In urine. **Half-Life:** 18 h.

NURSING IMPLICATIONS

Assessment & Drug Effects

- Monitor for S&S of bleeding or hemorrhage. If noted, withhold fondaparinux and notify physician immediately.
- Withhold fondaparinux and notify physician if platelet count falls below 100,000/mm^3.
- Lab tests: Monitor baseline and periodic renal function rests; periodic CBC including platelet count, serum creatinine level, and stool occult blood tests. Lab test for measuring drug effectiveness is amount of anti-Xa assay expressed in mg.

Patient & Family Education

- Report any of the following to a health care provider: Signs of unexplained bleeding such as: Pink, red, or dark brown urine; red or dark brown vomitus; bleeding gums or bloody sputum; dark, tarry stools.
- Learn proper injection technique if you are to self-administer this drug.
- Do not take any OTC drugs without first consulting physician.

F

FORMOTEROL FUMARATE

(for-mo-ter'ol)

Foradil Aerolizer

Classifications: BETA-ADRENERGIC AGONIST; BRONCHODILATOR

Therapeutic: BRONCHODILATOR

Prototype: Albuterol

Pregnancy Category: C

AVAILABILITY 12 mcg inhalation capsules

ACTION & *THERAPEUTIC EFFECT* Long-acting selective $beta_2$-adrenergic receptor agonist that stimulates production of intracellular cyclic AMP, which causes relaxation of bronchial smooth muscle. It also inhibits release of mediators of immediate hypersensitivity (e.g., histamine and leukotrienes) from mast cells in the lung. *Acts locally in lung as a bronchodilator; prevents bronchoconstriction that occurs during an asthma attack.*

USES Treatment of asthma, prevention of exercise induced asthma, prevention of bronchospasm in COPD.

UNLABELED USES Bronchitis.

CONTRAINDICATIONS Hypersensitivity to formoterol; significantly worsening or acutely deteriorating asthma; severe asthmatic attacks; paradoxical bronchospasm; children 5 y or younger.

CAUTIOUS USE Cardiovascular disorders (especially coronary insufficiency, cardiac arrhythmias, and hypertension), QT prolongation; convulsive disorders; thyrotoxicosis; heightened responsiveness to sympathomimetic amines; diabetes mellitus; pregnancy (category C), lactation.

ROUTE & DOSAGE

Treatment of Asthma, COPD

Adult/Child (5 y or older): **Inhaled** Inhale contents of 1 capsule q12h

Prevention of Exercise-Induced Asthma

Adult/Child (12 y or older): **Inhaled** Inhale contents of 1 capsule at least 15 min before exercise, do not repeat for at least 12 h

ADMINISTRATION

Oral Inhalation

- Remove capsule from blister IMMEDIATELY before use.
- Avoid exposing capsules to moisture.
- Give capsules only by the oral inhalation route and only by using the Aerolizer Inhaler™. Review use of the Aerolizer Inhaler in *Patient Instructions for Use* provided by manufacturer. Do not use a spacer with the Aerolizer.
- Instruct patient not to swallow capsule and not to exhale into the Aerolizer.
- Store capsules in the blister at 20°–25° C (86°–77° F).

ADVERSE EFFECTS (≥1%) **Body as a Whole:** *Viral infections,* chest infection, chest pain, fatigue. **CNS:** Headache, tremor, dizziness, insomnia. **GI:** Abdominal pain, dyspepsia, nausea. **Respiratory:** Pharyngitis, bronchitis, dyspnea, tonsillitis, dysphonia, fatal exacerbation of asthma. **Skin:** Rash.

INTERACTIONS Drug: Effects may be antagonized by NONSELECTIVE BETA-BLOCKERS; XANTHINES, STEROIDS; DIURETICS may potentiate hypokalemia.

PHARMACOKINETICS Absorption: Rapidly absorbed into plasma after oral inhalation. **Onset:** 1–3 min. **Peak:** 1–3 h. **Metabolism:** Metabolized by glucuronidation in the liver. **Elimination:** 60% in urine, 33% in feces. **Half-Life:** 10 h.

NURSING IMPLICATIONS

Assessment & Drug Effects

- Monitor cardiovascular status with periodic ECG, BP, and HR determinations.
- Withhold drug and notify physician immediately of S&S of bronchospasm.
- Lab tests: Monitor serum potassium and blood glucose periodically.
- Monitor diabetics closely for loss of glycemic control.

Patient & Family Education

- Do not take this drug more frequently than every 12 h.
- Use a short-acting inhaler if symptoms develop between doses of formoterol.
- Seek medical care immediately if a previously effective dosage regimen fails to provide the usual response, or if swelling about the face and neck and difficulty breathing develop.
- Report any of the following immediately to the physician: Rash, hives, palpitations, chest pain, rapid heart rate, tremor or nervousness.
- Note to diabetics: Monitor blood glucose levels carefully since hyperglycemia is a possible adverse reaction.

FOSAMPRENAVIR CALCIUM

(fos-am-pre′na-vir)

Lexiva

Classifications: ANTIRETROVIRAL; PROTEASE INHIBITOR

Therapeutic: ANTIRETROVIRAL; PROTEASE INHIBITOR

Prototype: Saquinavir

Pregnancy Category: C

AVAILABILITY 700 mg tablet; 50 mg/mL oral suspension

ACTION & *THERAPEUTIC EFFECT* Fosamprenavir is a prodrug rapidly converted to amprenavir. Amprenavir is an HIV-1 protease inhibitor that binds to the active site of HIV-1 protease. Binding prevents processing of viral Gag and Gag-Pol polyprotein precursors, resulting in formation of immature noninfectious viral particles. *Inhibits normal replication of the HIV virus rending the virus noninfectious.*

USES Treatment of HIV infection in combination with other antiretroviral agents.

CONTRAINDICATIONS Hypersensitivity to amprenavir; sulfonamide hypersensitivity; ergot derivatives, pimozide, midazolam, triazolam; coadministration of ritonavir, flecainide, and propafenone; severe hepatic impairment; hypercholesterolemia, hypertriglyceridemia; lactation. Safety and efficacy in children younger than 18 y have not been established.

CAUTIOUS USE Sulfonamide allergy; mild to moderate hepatic impairment; diabetes mellitus; diabetic ketoacidosis; elderly; hemophilia; pregnancy (category C).

ROUTE & DOSAGE

HIV Infection

Adult: **PO** 700 mg b.i.d. in combination with 100 mg ritonavir b.i.d. (preferred if previously on a protease inhibitor); or 1400 mg b.i.d.; or 1400 mg daily in combination with 200 mg ritonavir daily

HIV Prophylaxis (Occupational Exposure to HIV)

Adult: **PO** 700 mg with ritonavir 100 mg b.i.d.; 1400 mg with ritonavir 200 mg daily; or 1400 mg b.i.d. for basic prophylaxis regimen

Mild to Moderate Hepatic Impairment Dosage Adjustment

Reduce dose to 700 mg b.i.d. without ritonavir; not recommended in severe hepatic impairment.

F

ADMINISTRATION

Oral

- Ensure that patient is not receiving drugs contraindicated with fosamprenavir.
- Store at 15°–30° C (59°–86° F) in a tightly closed container.

ADVERSE EFFECTS (≥1%) **Body as a Whole:** Fatigue. **CNS:** *Oral/perioral paresthesia,* peripheral paresthesia, depression, mood disorders. **GI:** *Nausea, vomiting, diarrhea,* abdominal pain, taste disorders, increased triglycerides, and hyperglycemia. **Skin:** *Rash,* pruritus, <u>Stevens-Johnson syndrome</u>.

INTERACTIONS Note: Interaction profile can be significantly affected by coadministration with ritonavir. Metabolite is a strong inhibitor of CYP3A4. **Drug:** Administration with **amiodarone, bepridil, dihydroergotamine, ergotamine, flecainide, itraconazole, ketoconazole, lidocaine, midazolam, pimozide, propafenone, quinidine, triazolam,** and TRICYCLIC ANTIDEPRESSANTS may cause life-threatening reactions; **rifampin, rifabutin,** ORAL CONTRACEPTIVES, **phenobarbital, phenytoin, carbamazepine** decrease **amprenavir** concentrations; **amprenavir** may increase **dihydroergotamine, ergotamine, sildenafil** concentrations and toxicity; **amprenavir** may decrease **methadone** levels; monitor INR with **warfarin;** increased risk of myopathy and rhabdomyolysis with **lovastatin, simvastatin;** may decrease antiviral effectiveness of **delavirdine** or **lopinavir/ritonavir. Herbal: St. John's wort** may decrease antiretroviral activity.

PHARMACOKINETICS Absorption: Prodrug is rapidly hydrolyzed to amprenavir (active component) by gut enzymes during absorption. **Peak:** 2.5 h. **Metabolism:** In liver by CYP3A4. **Elimination:** 14% in urine, 75% in feces. **Half-Life:** 7.7 h.

NURSING IMPLICATIONS

Assessment & Drug Effects

- Ensure that patient has provided a complete list of all prescription, nonprescription, or herbal drugs being used.
- Monitor closely diabetics for loss of glycemic control.
- Monitor males taking PDE5 inhibitors for erectile dysfunction for adverse events including hypotension, visual changes, and priapism. Report promptly.
- Lab test: Baseline and periodic LFTs; periodic lipid profile; periodic blood glucose.

Patient & Family Education

- If you miss a dose by more than 4 h, wait and take the next dose at the regular time.
- Do not take other prescription, nonprescription, or herbal drugs without consulting physician.
- Monitor blood glucose more often than usual if diabetic.

- To prevent pregnancy, use a barrier contraceptive in addition to hormonal contraception.

FOSCARNET

(fos′car-net)

Classification: ANTIVIRAL
Therapeutic: ANTIVIRAL
Pregnancy Category: C

AVAILABILITY 24 mg/mL injection

ACTION & *THERAPEUTIC EFFECT* Selectively inhibits the viral-specific DNA polymerases and reverse transcriptases of susceptible viruses, thus preventing elongation of the viral DNA chain. *Effective against cytomegalovirus (CMV), herpes simplex virus types 1 and 2 (HSV-1, HSV-2), human herpesvirus 6 (HHV-6), Epstein-Barr virus (EBV), and varicella-zoster virus (VZV).*

USES CMV retinitis, mucocutaneous HSV, acyclovir-resistant HSV in immunocompromised patients.

UNLABELED USES Other CMV infections, herpes zoster infections in AIDS patients.

CONTRAINDICATIONS Hypersensitivity to foscarnet; lactation.

CAUTIOUS USE Kidney function impairment, cardiac disease; mineral and electrolyte imbalances, seizures, older adults; pregnancy (category C). Safety and efficacy in children are not established.

ROUTE & DOSAGE

CMV Retinitis

Adult: **IV Induction** 60 mg/kg q8h for 2–3 wk OR 90 mg/kg q12h for 2–3 wk; induction may be repeated if relapse occurs

Recurrent CMV Retinitis

Adult: **IV** 90–120 mg/kg/day

Acyclovir-Resistant HSV in Immunocompromised Patients

Adult: **IV** 40 mg/kg q8–12h for up to 3 wk or until lesions heal

Renal Impairment Dosage Adjustment

See package insert.

ADMINISTRATION

- Note: Dose **must be** adjusted for renal insufficiency. See package insert for specific dosing adjustment.

Intravenous

PREPARE: **Direct:** Given undiluted (24 mg/mL) through a central line. ▪ For peripheral infusion, dilute to 12 mg/mL with D5W or NS. ▪ Do not give other IV solution or drug through the same catheter with foscarnet.

ADMINISTER: **Direct:** Give at a constant rate not to exceed 1 mg/kg/min over the specified period of infusion with an infusion pump. ▪ Do not increase the rate of infusion or shorten the specified interval between doses. ▪ Use prepared IV solutions within 24 h.

INCOMPATIBILITIES **Solution/additive:** **Lactated Ringer's, acyclovir, amphotericin B, diazepam, digoxin, diphenhydramine, dobutamine, droperidol, ganciclovir, haloperidol, leucovorin, lorazepam, midazolam, pentamidine, phenytoin, prochlorperazine, promethazine, sulfamethoxazole/trimethoprim, TPN, trimetrexate, vancomycin.** **Y-site:** **Acyclovir, amphotericin B, diazepam, digoxin, diphenhydramine, dobutamine, droperidol, gan-**

ciclovir, haloperidol, leucovorin, lorazepam, midazolam, pentamidine, phenytoin, prochlorperazine, promethazine, sulfamethoxazole/trimethoprim, trimetrexate, vancomycin.

- Prehydrate and continue daily hydration with 2.5 L of NS to reduce nephrotoxicity.
- Store according to manufacturer's directions.

ADVERSE EFFECTS (≥1%) **CV:** Thrombophlebitis if infused through a peripheral vein. **CNS:** Tremor, muscle twitching, headache, weakness, fatigue, confusion, anxiety. **Endocrine:** *Hyperphosphatemia,* hypophosphatemia, hypocalcemia. **GI:** Nausea, vomiting, diarrhea. **Urogenital:** Penile ulceration. **Hematologic:** *Anemia,* leukopenia, thrombocytopenia. **Renal:** *Nephrotoxicity* (acute renal failure, tubular necrosis). **Skin:** Fixed drug eruption, rash.

DIAGNOSTIC TEST INTERFERENCE May cause increase or decrease in serum ***calcium, phosphorus,*** and ***magnesium.*** Decreases ***Hct*** and ***Hgb.*** Increased serum ***creatinine.***

INTERACTIONS Drug: AMINOGLYCOSIDES, **amphotericin B, vancomycin** may increase risk of nephrotoxicity. **Etidronate, pamidronate, pentamidine (IV)** may exacerbate hypocalcemia.

PHARMACOKINETICS Onset: 3–7 days. **Duration:** Relapse usually occurs 3–4 wk after end of therapy. **Distribution:** 3–28% of dose may be deposited in bone; variable penetration into CSF; crosses placenta; distributed into breast milk. **Metabolism:** Not metabolized. **Elimination:** 73–94% in urine. **Half-Life:** 3–4 h.

NURSING IMPLICATIONS

Assessment & Drug Effects

- Report serum creatinine and creatinine clearance values. Drug dose will be decreased in response to decreased clearance.
- Lab tests: Periodic CBC, serum electrolytes, serum creatinine, and creatinine clearance throughout therapy.
- Monitor for electrolyte imbalances.
- Monitor for seizures and take appropriate precautions.
- Question patients regarding local irritation of the penile or vulvovaginal epithelium. If either occurs, increase hydration and better personal hygiene.

Patient & Family Education

- Report perioral tingling, numbness, and paresthesia to physician immediately.
- Understand that drug is not a cure for CMV retinitis; regular ophthalmologic exams are necessary.
- Note: Good hydration is important to maintain adequate output of urine.

FOSFOMYCIN TROMETHAMINE

(fos-fo-my'sin)

Monurol

Classification: ANTI-INFECTIVE
Therapeutic: URINARY TRACT ANTI-INFECTIVE
Prototype: Nitrofurantoin
Pregnancy Category: B

AVAILABILITY 3 g packets

ACTION & *THERAPEUTIC EFFECT* Synthetic, broad-spectrum, bactericidal agent that blocks the first steps in bacterial cell wall synthesis. *Acts as a bactericidal agent against* Enterococcus faecalis, E.

faecium, *and* Escherichia coli. *In addition, it is effective against* Klebsiella, Proteus, *and* Serratia. *Effectiveness is indicated by improvement in cystitis symptoms within 2–3 days.*

USES Treatment of uncomplicated UTIs in women due to susceptible strains of *E. coli* and *E. faecalis.*

CONTRAINDICATIONS Hypersensitivity to fosfomycin.
CAUTIOUS USE Pregnancy (category B); lactation. Safety and efficiency in children younger than 12 y are not established.

ROUTE & DOSAGE

UTI
Adult: **PO** 3 g sachet dissolved in 3–4 oz of water as a single dose given once

ADMINISTRATION

Oral
- Pour entire contents of a single dose into 3–4 oz water (not hot), stir to dissolve completely, and give immediately. Drug must not be taken in the dry form.
- Store at 15°–30° C (59°–86° F).

ADVERSE EFFECTS (≥1%) **Body as a Whole:** Pain. **CNS:** *Headache,* dizziness. **GI:** *Diarrhea,* nausea, abdominal pain, dyspepsia. **Respiratory:** Rhinitis, pharyngitis. **Urogenital:** Vaginitis, dysmenorrhea.

INTERACTIONS Drug: Metoclopramide may decrease urinary excretion of fosfomycin.

PHARMACOKINETICS Absorption: Rapidly from GI tract, 37% of dose reaches systemic circulation as free acid. **Peak Urine Concentration:** 2–4 h. **Distribution:** Not protein bound, distributed to kidneys, bladder wall, prostate, and seminal vesicles. **Elimination:** Primarily in urine. **Half-Life:** 5.7 h.

NURSING IMPLICATIONS

Assessment & Drug Effects
- Lab tests: Obtain urine C&S before and after therapy.

Patient & Family Education
- Notify physician if symptoms do not improve in 2–3 days.

FOSINOPRIL

(fos-in′o-pril)
Monopril
Classifications: ANGIOTENSIN-CONVERTING ENZYME (ACE) INHIBITOR; ANTIHYPERTENSIVE AGENT
Therapeutic: ANTIHYPERTENSIVE; ACE INHIBITOR
Prototype: Enalapril
Pregnancy Category: D

AVAILABILITY 10 mg, 20 mg, 40 mg tablets

ACTION & *THERAPEUTIC EFFECT* Lowers BP by interrupting conversion sequences initiated by renin that leads to formation of angiotensin II, a potent vasoconstrictor. Inhibition of ACE also leads to decreased circulating aldosterone, a secretory response to angiotensin II stimulation. *Lowers blood pressure and reduces peripheral arterial resistance (afterload) and improves cardiac output as well as activity tolerance.*

USES Mild to moderate hypertension, CHF.

CONTRAINDICATIONS Hypersensitivity to fosinopril or any other ACE inhibitor(s); history of angioedema; renal artery stenosis; pregnancy (category D), lactation.

CAUTIOUS USE Impaired kidney function, autoimmune disease; concomitant immunosuppression; collagen-vascular disease; hepatic disease; hyperkalemia, or surgery and anesthesia; black patients; aortic stenosis or cardiomyopathy; dialysis; elderly. Safety in children is not established.

F

ROUTE & DOSAGE

Hypertension, CHF

Adult: **PO** 5–40 mg once/day (max: 80 mg/day)

ADMINISTRATION

Oral

- An initial 5 mg dose is preferred in HF patients with moderate to severe renal failure or in those who have been recently diuresed.
- Store at 15°–30° C (59°–86° F) and protect from moisture.

ADVERSE EFFECTS (≥1%) **CV:** Hypotension. **CNS:** Headache, fatigue, dizziness. **Endocrine:** Hyperkalemia. **GI:** Nausea, vomiting, diarrhea. **Urogenital:** Proteinuria. **Respiratory:** Cough. **Skin:** Rash.

INTERACTIONS Drug: NSAIDS may decrease antihypertensive effects of fosinopril. POTASSIUM SUPPLEMENTS, POTASSIUM-SPARING DIURETICS increase risk of hyperkalemia. ACE inhibitors may increase **lithium** levels and toxicity.

PHARMACOKINETICS Absorption: Readily absorbed from GI tract; converted to its active form, fosinoprilat, in the liver. **Peak:** 3 h. **Duration:** 24 h. **Distribution:** Approximately 90% protein bound; crosses placenta. **Metabolism:** Hydrolyzed by intestinal and hepatic esterases to its active form, fosinoprilat. **Elimination:** 44% in urine, 46% in feces. **Half-Life:** 3–4 h (fosinoprilat).

NURSING IMPLICATIONS

Assessment & Drug Effects

- Monitor for at least 2 h after initial dose for first-dose hypotension, especially in salt- or volume-depleted patients.
- Monitor BP at the time of peak effectiveness, 2–6 h after dosing and at the end of the dosing interval just before next dose.
- Report diminished antihypertensive effect toward the end of the dosing interval. An inadequate trough response may be an indication for dividing the daily dose.
- Lab tests: Obtain BUN and serum creatinine periodically. Increases may necessitate dose reduction or discontinuation of the drug. Monitor serum potassium.
- Observe for S&S of hyperkalemia (see Appendix F).

Patient & Family Education

- Discontinue fosinopril and report to physician any of the following: S&S of angioedema (e.g., swelling of face or extremities, difficulty breathing or swallowing); syncope; chronic, nonproductive cough.
- Maintain adequate fluid intake and avoid potassium supplements or salt substitutes unless specifically prescribed by the physician.
- Report vomiting or diarrhea to physician immediately.

FOSPHENYTOIN SODIUM

(fos-phen'i-toin)

Cerebyx

Classification: HYDANTOIN ANTICONVULSANT

Therapeutic: ANTICONVULSANT

Prototype: Phenytoin

Pregnancy Category: D

AVAILABILITY 150 mg, 750 mg vials

ACTION & *THERAPEUTIC EFFECT* Prodrug of phenytoin that converts to the anticonvulsant phenytoin that modulates the sodium channels of neurons, calcium flux across neuronal membranes, and enhances the sodium–potassium ATPase activity of neurons and glial cells. *Effective as an anticonvulsant agent by preventing seizure activity.*

USES Control of generalized convulsive status epilepticus and the prevention and treatment of seizures during neurosurgery, or as a parenteral short-term substitute for oral phenytoin.

UNLABELED USES Antiarrhythmic agent especially in treatment of digitalis-induced arrhythmia; treatment of trigeminal neuralgia (tic douloureux).

CONTRAINDICATIONS Hypersensitivity to hydantoin products, rash, seizures due to hypoglycemia, sinus bradycardia, complete or incomplete heart block; Adams-Stokes syndrome; pregnancy (category D).

CAUTIOUS USE Impaired liver or kidney function, alcoholism, hypotension, heart block, bradycardia, severe CAD, diabetes mellitus, hyperglycemia, respiratory depression, acute intermittent porphyria; lactation.

ROUTE & DOSAGE

Status Epilepticus

Adult: **IV Loading Dose** 15–20 mg PE/kg (PE = phenytoin sodium equivalents) administered at 100–150 mg PE/min **IV Maintenance Dose** 4–6 mg PE/kg/day

Substitution for Oral Phenytoin Therapy

Adult: **IV/IM** Substitute fosphenytoin at the same total daily dose in mg PE as the oral dose at a rate of infusion not greater than 150 mg PE/min

ADMINISTRATION

- Note: All dosing is expressed in phenytoin sodium equivalents (PE) to avoid the need to calculate molecular weight adjustments between fosphenytoin and phenytoin sodium doses. **Always** prescribe and fill fosphenytoin in PE units.

Intramuscular

- Follow institutional policy regarding maximum volume to inject into one IM site.

Intravenous

PREPARE: **Direct:** Dilute in D5W or NS to a concentration of 1.5–25 mg PE/mL.

ADMINISTER: **Direct:** Give 100–150 mg PE/min. Do not administer at a rate greater than 150 mg PE/min.

INCOMPATIBILITIES **Y-site: Fenoldopam, midazolam.**

- Store at 2°–8° C (36°–46° F); may store at room temperature not to exceed 48 h.

ADVERSE EFFECTS (≥1%) **CNS:** Usually dose related. Paresthesia, tinnitus, *nystagmus, dizziness, somnolence, drowsiness,* ataxia, mental confusion, tremors, insomnia, headache, seizures, increased reflexes, dysarthria, intracranial hypertension. **CV:** Bradycardia, tachycardia, asystole, hypotension, hypertension, <u>cardiovascular collapse, cardiac arrest</u>, heart block, ventricular fibrillation, phlebitis. **Special Senses:** Photophobia, conjunctivitis, diplopia, blurred vision. **GI:** *Gingival hyperplasia,* nausea, vomiting, constipation, epigastric pain, dysphagia, loss of taste, weight loss, hepatitis, liver necrosis. **Hematologic:** Thrombocytopenia, leukopenia, leukocytosis, agranulocytosis, pancytopenia, eosinophilia; megaloblastic, hemolytic, or aplastic anemias. **Metabolic:** Fever, hyperglycemia, glycosuria, weight gain, edema, transient increase in serum thyrotropic (TSH) level, hyperkalemia, osteomalacia or rickets associated with hypocalcemia and elevated alkaline phosphatase activity. **Skin:** Alopecia, hirsutism (especially in young female); rash: Scarlatiniform, maculopapular, urticarial, morbilliform (may be fatal); bullous, exfoliative, or purpuric dermatitis; Stevens-Johnson syndrome, toxic epidermal necrolysis, keratosis, neonatal hemorrhage, *pruritus.* **Urogenital:** Acute renal failure, Peyronie's disease. **Respiratory:** Acute pneumonitis, pulmonary fibrosis. **Musculoskeletal:** Periarteritis nodosum, acute systemic lupus erythematosus, craniofacial abnormalities (with enlargement of lips). **Other:** Lymphadenopathy, injection site pain, chills.

DIAGNOSTIC TEST INTERFERENCE Fosphenytoin may produce lower than normal values for ***dexamethasone*** or ***metyrapone*** tests; may increase serum levels of ***glucose, BSP,*** and ***alkaline phosphatase*** and may decrease ***PBI*** and ***urinary steroid*** levels.

INTERACTIONS Drug: Alcohol decreases effects; OTHER ANTICONVULSANTS may increase or decrease fosphenytoin levels; fosphenytoin increases metabolism of CORTICOSTEROIDS, ORAL ANTICOAGULANTS, and ORAL CONTRACEPTIVES, decreasing their effectiveness; **amiodarone, chloramphenicol, omeprazole** increase fosphenytoin levels; antituberculosis agents, **voriconazole** decrease fosphenytoin levels. **Food: Folic acid, calcium, vitamin D** absorption may be decreased by fosphenytoin; fosphenytoin absorption may be decreased by enteral nutrition supplements. **Herbal: Ginkgo** may decrease anticonvulsant effectiveness.

PHARMACOKINETICS Absorption: Completely absorbed after IM administration. **Peak:** 30 min IM. **Distribution:** 95–99% bound to plasma proteins, displaces phenytoin from protein binding sites; crosses placenta, small amount in breast milk. **Metabolism:** Converted to phenytoin by phosphatases; phenytoin is oxidized in liver to inactive metabolites. **Elimination:** Half-life 15 min to convert fosphenytoin to phenytoin, 22 h phenytoin; phenytoin metabolites excreted in urine.

NURSING IMPLICATIONS

Note: See **phenytoin** for additional nursing implications.

Assessment & Drug Effects

- Monitor ECG, BP, and respiratory function continuously during and for 10–20 min after infusion.
- Discontinue infusion and notify physician if rash appears. Be prepared to substitute alternative therapy rapidly to prevent withdrawal-precipitated seizures.
- Lab tests: Monitor CBC with differential, platelet count, serum electrolytes, and blood glucose.
- Allow at least 2 h after IV infusion and 4 h after IM injection before monitoring total plasma phenytoin concentration.
- Monitor diabetics for loss of glycemic control.

- Monitor carefully for adverse effects, especially in patients with renal or hepatic disease or hypoalbuminemia.

Patient & Family Education

- Be aware of potential adverse effects. Itching, burning, tingling, or paresthesia are common during and for some time following IV infusion.

FROVATRIPTAN

(fro-va-trip'tan)

Frova

Classification: SEROTONIN 5-HT_1 RECEPTOR AGONIST

Therapeutic: ANTIMIGRAINE

Prototype: Sumatriptan

Pregnancy Category: C

AVAILABILITY 2.5 mg tablets

ACTION & *THERAPEUTIC EFFECT* Selective agonist that binds with high affinity to 5-HT_{1D}, 5-HT_{1B}, 5-HT_{1F} serotonin receptors, which are found on extracerebral and intracranial blood vessels, and on other structures in the CNS. This results in vasoconstriction and agonist effects on nerve terminals in trigeminal system. *Activation of 5-HT_1 receptors results in constriction of cranial vessels that become dilated during a migraine attack, and reduced signal transmission in the pain pathways.*

USES Treatment of migraine headache with or without aura.

CONTRAINDICATIONS Hypersensitivity to frovatriptan; significant cardiovascular disease such as ischemic heart disease, coronary artery vasospasms, peripheral vascular disease, history of cerebrovascular events, or uncontrolled hypertension; within 24 h of receiving another 5-HT_1 agonist or an ergotamine-containing or ergot-type drug; basilar or hemiplegic migraine. Safety and efficacy in children younger than 18 y are not established.

CAUTIOUS USE Significant risk factors for coronary artery disease unless a cardiac evaluation has been done; hypertension; risk factors for cerebrovascular accident; impaired liver or kidney function; pregnancy (category C), lactation.

ROUTE & DOSAGE

Migraine Headache

Adult: **PO** 2.5 mg. If headache returns, may repeat after at least 2 h (max: 7.5 mg/24 h).

ADMINISTRATION

Oral

- Do not give within 24 h of an ergot-containing drug.
- Administer any time after symptoms of migraine appear.
- Do not administer a second dose without consulting the physician for any attack during which the FIRST dose did NOT work.
- Give a second dose if headache was relieved by first dose but symptoms return; however, wait at least 2 h after the first dose before giving a second dose.
- Do not give more than two doses in 24 h.
- Store at 15°–30° C (59°–86° F).

ADVERSE EFFECTS (≥1%) **Body as a Whole:** Fatigue, hot or cold sensation, flushing. **CNS:** Dizziness, headache, paresthesia, somnolence, insomnia, anxiety. **CV:** Chest pain, palpitation. **GI:** Dyspepsia, nausea, vomiting, diarrhea, dry mouth. **Musculoskeletal:** Skeletal pain. **Special Senses:** Abnormal vision. **Skin:** Sweating.

INTERACTIONS Drug: Dihydroergotamine, methysergide, other 5-HT_1 AGONISTS may cause prolonged vasospastic reactions; SSRIS, **sibutramine** have rarely caused weakness, hyperreflexia, and incoordination; MAOIS should not be used with 5-HT_1 AGONISTS. **Herbal: Gingko, ginseng, echinacea, St. John's wort** may increase triptan toxicity.

PHARMACOKINETICS Absorption: 20–30% bioavailability. **Peak:** 2–4 h. **Distribution:** 15% protein bound. **Metabolism:** In liver by CYP1A2. **Elimination:** 30% renally, 60% in feces. **Half-Life:** 26 h.

NURSING IMPLICATIONS

Assessment & Drug Effects

- Monitor cardiovascular status carefully following first dose in patients at relatively high risk for coronary artery disease (e.g., postmenopausal women, men older than 40 y, persons with known CAD risk factors), or who have coronary artery vasospasms.
- Report to physician immediately chest pain or tightness in chest or throat that is severe, or does not quickly resolve following a dose of frovatriptan.
- Pain relief usually begins within 10 min of ingestion, with complete relief in approximately 65% of all patients within 2 h.
- Monitor BP, especially in those being treated for hypertension.

Patient & Family Education

- Review patient information leaflet provided by the manufacturer carefully.
- Notify physician immediately if symptoms of severe angina (e.g., severe or persistent pain or tightness in chest, back, neck, or throat) or hypersensitivity (e.g., wheezing, facial swelling, skin rash, itching, or hives) occur.
- Do not take any other serotonin receptor agonist (e.g., Imitrex, Maxalt, Zomig, Amerge) within 24 h of taking frovatriptan.
- Report any other adverse effects (e.g., tingling, flushing, dizziness) at next physician visit.

FULVESTRANT

(ful-ves′trant)

Faslodex

Classifications: ANTINEOPLASTIC; ANTIESTROGEN

Therapeutic: ANTINEOPLASTIC

Prototype: Tamoxifen citrate

Pregnancy Category: D

AVAILABILITY 50 mg/mL

ACTION & *THERAPEUTIC EFFECT*
Fulvestrant is an estrogen receptor antagonist that selectively binds to the estrogen receptors (ER) of breast cancer cells. Estrogen stimulates the tumor growth of estrogen-sensitive breast tissue cancer cells in postmenopausal women. *In postmenopausal women, many breast cancers have estrogen receptors (ERs), and the growth of these tumors is stimulated by estrogen. Therefore, fulvestrant decreases estrogen-sensitive breast tissue tumor growth.*

USES Treatment of hormone receptor-positive metastatic breast cancer in postmenopausal women with disease progression following antiestrogen therapy.

CONTRAINDICATIONS Hypersensitivity to fulvestrant; pregnancy (category D); lactation.

CAUTIOUS USE Moderate to severe liver impairment; biliary disease; coagulopathy; anticoagulant therapy. Safety and effectiveness in children not established.

ROUTE & DOSAGE

Metastatic Breast Cancer
Adult: **IM** 250 mg once/mo

ADMINISTRATION

Intramuscular
- Break the seal of the white plastic cover on the syringe luer connector to remove the cover with the attached rubber tip cap. Twist to lock the needle to the luer connector. Remove excess gas from the syringe (a small gas bubble may remain).
- Administer slowly in the buttock.
- Immediately activate needle protection device upon withdrawal from patient by pushing lever arm completely forward until needle tip is fully covered.
- Store in a refrigerator, 2°–8° C (36°–46° F) in original container.

ADVERSE EFFECTS (≥1%) **Body as a Whole:** *Asthenia, pain, injection site pain,* flu-like syndrome, fever, peripheral edema. **CNS:** Dizziness, insomnia, paresthesia, depression, anxiety. **CV:** *Vasodilation.* **GI:** *Nausea, vomiting, constipation, diarrhea,* anorexia. **Hematologic:** Anemia. **Musculoskeletal:** *Bone pain,* arthritis. **Respiratory:** *Pharyngitis, dyspnea, cough.* **Skin:** Rash, sweating.

PHARMACOKINETICS Peak: 7 days. **Duration:** 1 mo. **Distribution:** 99% protein bound. **Metabolism:** In liver via CYP3A4. **Elimination:** 90% in feces. **Half-Life:** 40 days.

NURSING IMPLICATIONS

Assessment & Drug Effects
- Monitor for S&S of tumor progression.
- Lab tests: Monitor periodic CBC with differential.

Patient & Family Education
- Use two methods of contraception while taking this drug. Immediately notify physician if you think you are pregnant.
- Report vaginal bleeding to physician. Understand the possibility of drug-induced menstrual irregularities before starting treatment.

FUROSEMIDE Pr

(fur-oh'se-mide)

Fumide ✤, Furomide ✤, Lasix, Luramide ✤

Classifications: ELECTROLYTIC AND WATER BALANCE AGENT; LOOP DIURETIC; ANTIHYPERTENSIVE

Therapeutic: LOOP DIURETIC; ANTIHYPERTENSIVE

Pregnancy Category: C

AVAILABILITY 20 mg, 40 mg, 80 mg tablets; 10 mg/mL, 40 mg/5 mL oral solution; 10 mg/mL injection

ACTION & *THERAPEUTIC EFFECT* Rapid-acting potent sulfonamide "loop" diuretic and antihypertensive. Inhibits reabsorption of sodium and chloride primarily in loop of Henle and also in proximal and distal renal tubules. *An antihypertensive that decreases edema and intravascular volume.*

USES Treatment of edema associated with CHF, cirrhosis of liver, and kidney disease, including nephrotic syndrome. May be used for management of hypertension, alone or in combination with other antihypertensive agents, and for treatment of hypercalcemia. Has been used concomitantly with mannitol for treatment of severe cerebral edema, particularly in meningitis.

CONTRAINDICATIONS History of hypersensitivity to furosemide or sulfonamides; increasing oliguria, anuria, fluid and electrolyte depletion states; hepatic coma; preeclampsia, eclampsia.

CAUTIOUS USE Infants, older adults; hepatic disease; hepatic cirrhosis; renal disease, nephrotic syndrome; cardiogenic shock associated with acute MI; ventricular arrhythmias, CHF, diarrhea; history of SLE, history of gout; diabetes mellitus; pregnancy (category C), lactation.

ROUTE & DOSAGE

Edema

Adult: **PO** 20–80 mg in 1 or more divided doses up to 600 mg/day if needed **IV/IM** 20–40 mg in 1 or more divided doses up to 600 mg/day
Child: **PO** 2 mg/kg, may be increased by 1–2 mg/kg q6–8h (max: 6 mg/kg/dose) **IV/IM** 1–2 mg/kg, may be increased by 1 mg/kg q2h if needed (max: 6 mg/kg/dose)
Neonate: **PO** 1–4 mg/kg q12–24h **IV/IM** 1 mg/kg q12–24h

Hypertension

Adult: **PO** 10–40 mg b.i.d. (max: 480 mg/day)

ADMINISTRATION

Oral

- Give with food or milk to reduce possibility of gastric irritation.
- Schedule doses to avoid sleep disturbance (e.g., a single dose is generally given in the morning; twice-a-day doses at 8 a.m. and 2 p.m.).
- Store tablets at controlled room temperature, preferably at 15°–30° C (59°–86° F) unless otherwise directed. Protect from light.
- Store oral solution in refrigerator, preferably at 2°–8° C (36°–46° F). Protect from light and freezing.

Intramuscular

- Protect syringes from light once they are removed from package.
- Discard yellow or otherwise discolored injection solutions.

Intravenous

Note: Verify correct IV concentration and rate of infusion/injection with physician before administration to infants or children.

PREPARE: **Direct:** Give undiluted.
ADMINISTER: **Direct:** Give undiluted at a rate of 20 mg or a fraction thereof over 1 min. ▪ With high doses a rate of 4 mg/min is recommended to decrease risk of ototoxicity.
INCOMPATIBILITIES **Solution/additive:** **Amiodarone, buprenorphine, chlorpromazine, diazepam, dobutamine, erythromycin, fructose, gentamicin, isoproterenol, meperidine, metoclopramide, milrinone, netilmicin, pancuronium, papaveretum, prochlorperazine, promethazine, quinidine, thiamine.** **Y-site:** **Amrinone, amsacrine, azithromycin, chlorpromazine, ciprofloxacin, clarithromycin, diltiazem, dobutamine, dopamine, doxoru-**

bicin, droperidol, esmolol, fenoldopam, filgrastim, fluconazole, gemcitabine, gentamicin, hydralazine, idarubicin, labetalol, lansoprazole, levofloxacin, meperidine, methocarbamol, metoclopramide, midazolam, milrinone, morphine, netilmicin, nicardipine, ondansetron, quinidine, tetracycline, thiopental, tobramycin, vecuronium, vinblastine, vincristine, vinorelbine, TPN.

- Use infusion solutions within 24 h.
- Store parenteral solution at controlled room temperature, preferably at 15°–30° C (59°–86° F) unless otherwise directed. Protect from light.

ADVERSE EFFECTS (≥1%) **CV:** Postural hypotension, dizziness with excessive diuresis, acute hypotensive episodes, circulatory collapse. **Metabolic:** Hypovolemia, dehydration, hyponatremia, *hypokalemia,* hypochloremia, metabolic alkalosis, hypomagnesemia, hypocalcemia (tetany), hyperglycemia, glycosuria, elevated BUN, hyperuricemia. **GI:** Nausea, vomiting, oral and gastric burning, anorexia, diarrhea, constipation, abdominal cramping, acute pancreatitis, jaundice. **Urogenital:** Allergic interstitial nephritis, irreversible renal failure, urinary frequency. **Hematologic:** Anemia, leukopenia, thrombocytopenic purpura; aplastic anemia, agranulocytosis (rare). **Special Senses:** Tinnitus, vertigo, feeling of fullness in ears, hearing loss (rarely permanent), blurred vision. **Skin:** Pruritus, urticaria, exfoliative dermatitis, purpura, photosensitivity, porphyria cutanea tarda, necrotizing angiitis (vasculitis). **Body as a Whole:** Increased perspiration; paresthesias; activation of SLE, muscle spasms, weakness; thrombophlebitis, pain at IM injection site.

DIAGNOSTIC TEST INTERFERENCE Furosemide may cause elevations in ***BUN, serum amylase, cholesterol, triglycerides, uric acid*** and ***blood glucose*** levels, and may decrease ***serum calcium, magnesium, potassium,*** and ***sodium*** levels.

INTERACTIONS Drug: OTHER DIURETICS enhance diuretic effects; with **digoxin** increased risk of toxicity because of hypokalemia; NONDEPOLARIZING NEUROMUSCULAR BLOCKING AGENTS (e.g., **tubocurarine**) prolong neuromuscular blockage; CORTICOSTEROIDS, **amphotericin B** potentiate hypokalemia; decreased **lithium** elimination and increased toxicity; SULFONYLUREAS, **insulin** blunt hypoglycemic effects; NSAIDS may attenuate diuretic effects.

PHARMACOKINETICS Absorption: 60% PO dose from GI tract. **Peak:** 60–70 min PO; 20–60 min IV. **Onset:** 30–60 min PO; 5 min IV. **Duration:** 2 h. **Distribution:** Crosses placenta. **Metabolism:** Small amount in liver. **Elimination:** Rapidly in urine; 50% of oral dose and 80% of IV dose excreted within 24 h; excreted in breast milk. **Half-Life:** 30 min.

NURSING IMPLICATIONS

Assessment & Drug Effects

- Observe patients receiving parenteral drug carefully; closely monitor BP and vital signs. Sudden death from cardiac arrest has been reported.
- Monitor for S&S of hypokalemia (see Appendix F).
- Monitor BP during periods of diuresis and through period of dosage adjustment.

- Observe older adults closely during period of brisk diuresis. Sudden alteration in fluid and electrolyte balance may precipitate significant adverse reactions. Report symptoms to physician.
- Lab tests: Obtain frequent blood count, serum and urine electrolytes, CO_2, BUN, blood sugar, and uric acid values during first few months of therapy and periodically thereafter.
- Monitor I&O ratio and pattern. Report decrease or unusual increase in output. Excessive diuresis can result in dehydration and hypovolemia, circulatory collapse, and hypotension. Weigh patient daily under standard conditions.
- Monitor urine and blood glucose and HbA1C closely in diabetics and patients with decompensated hepatic cirrhosis. Drug may cause hyperglycemia.

Patient & Family Education

- Consult physician regarding allowable salt and fluid intake.
- Ingest potassium-rich foods daily (e.g., bananas, oranges, peaches, dried dates) to reduce or prevent potassium depletion.
- Learn S&S of hypokalemia (see Appendix F). Report muscle cramps or weakness to physician.
- Make position changes slowly because high doses of antihypertensive drugs taken concurrently may produce episodes of dizziness or imbalance.
- Avoid replacing fluid losses with large amounts of water.
- Avoid prolonged exposure to direct sun.

GABAPENTIN Pr

(gab-a-pen′tin)

Neurontin, Gabarone

Classifications: ANTICONVULSANT; GABA ANALOG
Therapeutic: ANTICONVULSANT
Pregnancy Category: C

AVAILABILITY 100 mg, 300 mg, 400 mg capsules; 100 mg, 300 mg, 400 mg, 600 mg, 800 mg tablets; 250 mg/5 mL solution

ACTION & *THERAPEUTIC EFFECT*
Gabapentin is a GABA neurotransmitter analog; however, it does not inhibit GABA uptake or degradation. Mechanism of action is unknown. It appears to interact with GABA cortical neurons, but its relationship to functional activity as an anticonvulsant is unknown. *Used in conjunction with other anticonvulsants to control certain types of seizures in patients with epilepsy. Effective in controlling painful neuropathies.*

USES Adjunctive therapy for partial seizures with or without secondary generalization in adults, post-herpetic neuralgia.
UNLABELED USES Add-on therapy for generalized seizures, peripheral neuropathy, migraine prophylaxis.

CONTRAINDICATIONS Hypersensitivity to gabapentin; suicidal ideations; lactation. Safety and efficacy in infants and children younger than 3 y are not established.
CAUTIOUS USE Status epilepticus, renal impairment, older adults; suicidal tendencies; psychiatric disorders; children; pregnancy (category C).

ROUTE & DOSAGE

Adjunctive Therapy for Seizure Disorder

Adult/Child (older than 12 y):
PO Start 300 mg on day 1, 300 mg b.i.d. on day 2, 300 mg t.i.d. on day 3, and continue to

increase over a week to an initial total dose of 400 mg t.i.d. (1200 mg/day); may increase to 1800–2400 mg/day depending on response (most patients receive 900–1800 mg/day in 3 divided doses) 400 mg t.i.d. (1200 mg/day)
Child (3–12 y): **PO** Start 10–15 mg/kg/day in 3 divided doses, titrate q3days to target dose of 40 mg/kg/day in pts 3–4 y or 25–35 mg/kg/day in pts 5 y or older in 3 divided doses

Post-Herpetic Neuralgia

Adult: **PO** Start 300 mg day 1, 300 mg b.i.d. day 2, and 300 mg t.i.d. day 3; may increase up to 600 mg t.i.d. if needed

Renal Impairment Dosage Adjustment

CrCl greater than 60 mL/min: 400 mg t.i.d.; 30–60 mL/min: 300 mg b.i.d.; 15–30 mL/min: 300 mg daily; less than 15 mL/min: 300 mg every other day
Hemodialysis Dosage Adjustment: 200–300 mg following dialysis

ADMINISTRATION

Oral

- Separate doses of gabapentin and antacids by 2 h.
- Withdraw drug gradually over 1 wk; abrupt discontinuation may cause status epilepticus.
- Store at 15°–30° C (59°–86° F); protect from heat, moisture, and direct light.

ADVERSE EFFECTS (≥1%) **CNS:** *Drowsiness, fatigue,* dizziness, tremor, slurred speech, impaired concentration, headache, increased frequency of partial seizures. **Endocrine:** Weight gain. **GI:** Nausea, gastric upset, vomiting. **Special Senses:** Blurred vision, nystagmus. **Skin:** Rash, eczema.

INTERACTIONS Drug: Increase in **phenytoin** levels at higher doses (300–600 mg/day gabapentin). Does not affect serum levels of other ANTICONVULSANTS. ANTACIDS reduce absorption of gabapentin. **Herbal: Ginkgo** may decrease effectiveness.

PHARMACOKINETICS Absorption: 50–60% from GI tract. **Peak:** Peak level 1–3 h; peak effect 2–4 wk. **Distribution:** Crosses the blood–brain barrier; readily passes into cerebrospinal fluid; not bound to plasma proteins; highest concentrations found in pancreas and kidneys. **Metabolism:** Does not appear to be metabolized. **Elimination:** 76–81% unchanged in 96 h; 10–23% recovered in feces. **Half-Life:** 5–6 h.

NURSING IMPLICATIONS

Assessment & Drug Effects

- Monitor for therapeutic effectiveness; may not occur until several weeks following initiation of therapy.
- In those treated for seizure disorders, assess frequency of seizures: In rare cases, the drug has increased the frequency of partial seizures.
- Monitor for and report dizziness, somnolence, or other signs of CNS depression. Assess safety: Vision, concentration, and coordination impairment increase the risk for injury.
- Monitor for changes in behavior that may be indicative of suicidal ideation.

Patient & Family Education

- Learn potential adverse effects of drug.

G

- Notify physician immediately if any of the following occur: Increased seizure frequency, visual changes, unusual bruising or bleeding.
- Do not drive or engage in other potentially hazardous activities until response to drug is known.
- Do not abruptly discontinue use of drug; do not take drug within 2 h of an antacid.

GALANTAMINE HYDROBROMIDE

(ga-lan′ta-meen)

Razadyne, Razadyne ER

Classifications: CENTRALLY ACTING CHOLINERGIC; CHOLINESTERASE INHIBITOR; ANTIDEMENTIA

Therapeutic: ANTIALZHEIMER'S; ANTIDEMENTIA

Prototype: Donezepril HCl

Pregnancy Category: B

AVAILABILITY 4 mg, 8 mg, 12 mg tablets; 8 mg, 16 mg, 24 mg extended release capsules; 4 mg/mL oral solution

ACTION & *THERAPEUTIC EFFECT* Competitive and reversible inhibitor of acetylcholinesterase, which is the enzyme responsible for the hydrolysis (breakdown) of the neurotransmitter, acetylcholine. The cholinergic system is used in the processing needed for attention, memory, and modulation of excitatory neurotransmission. *In Alzheimer's disease cholinesterase inhibitors are designed to offset loss of presynaptic cholinergic function, slowing decline of memory and maintaining ability to perform functions of daily living.*

USES Treatment of mild to moderate dementia of Alzheimer's type.

UNLABELED USES Vascular dementia.

CONTRAINDICATIONS Hypersensitivity to galantamine; lactation, or in children.

CAUTIOUS USE Bradycardia, heart block or other cardiac conduction disorders; asthma, COPD; potential bladder outflow obstruction; a history of seizures or GI bleeding; pregnancy (category B).

ROUTE & DOSAGE

Alzheimer's Disease

Adult: **PO** Initiate with 4 mg b.i.d. times at least 4 wks, if tolerated may increase by 4 mg b.i.d. q4wk to target dose of 12 mg b.i.d. (8–16 mg b.i.d.)

Hepatic Impairment Dosage Adjustment

Not recommended with severe hepatic impairment

Renal Impairment Dosage Adjustment

CrCl less than 9 mL/min: Not recommended

ADMINISTRATION

Oral

- Give with meals (breakfast and dinner) to reduce the risk of nausea.
- Extended release capsules should be swallowed whole and not crushed or chewed.
- Make increases in dosage increments at 4-wk intervals.
- If drug is interrupted for several days or more, restart at the lowest dose and gradually increase to the current dose.
- Store at 15°–30° C (59°–86° F).

ADVERSE EFFECTS (≥1%) **Body as a Whole:** Weight loss, fatigue, rhinitis, syncope, malaise, asthenia, fever. **CNS:** Dizziness, headache, depression, insomnia, somnolence, tremor. **CV:** Bradycardia, chest pain. **GI:** *Nausea, vomiting,* diarrhea, anorexia, abdominal pain, dyspepsia, flatulence. **Hematologic:** Anemia. **Urogenital:** UTI, hematuria, incontinence. **Nervous System:** Tinnitus, leg cramps. **Other:** Increased mortality in patients with mild cognitive impairment.

INTERACTIONS Drug: Additive effects with other CHOLINESTERASE INHIBITORS (e.g., **succinylcholine, bethanecol**); **cimetidine, erythromycin, ketoconazole, paroxetine** may increase levels and toxicity.

PHARMACOKINETICS Absorption: Rapidly and completely. **Peak:** 1 h. **Distribution:** Mainly distributes to red blood cells. **Metabolism:** In liver by CYP2D6 and CYP3A4. **Elimination:** 95% in urine. **Half-Life:** 7 h (4.4–10 h).

NURSING IMPLICATIONS

Assessment & Drug Effects

- Monitor cardiovascular status including baseline and periodic EKG and BP readings. Assess for postural hypotension.
- Monitor I&O rates and pattern for urinary incontinence or urinary retention.
- Monitor appetite and food intake. Weigh weekly and report significant weight loss.
- Lab tests: Baseline ALT/AST, BUN and creatinine; periodic blood glucose, alkaline phosphatase, urinalysis, stool for occult blood.

Patient & Family Education

- Report any of the following to a health care provider immediately: Loss of weight, urinary retention, chest pain, palpitations, difficulty breathing, fainting, dark stools, blood in the urine.

GALLIUM NITRATE

(gal'li-um)

Ganite

Classification: BONE RESORPTION INHIBITOR

Therapeutic: BONE RESORPTION INHIBITOR; CALCIUM REGULATOR

Pregnancy Category: C

AVAILABILITY 25 mg/mL injection

ACTION & *THERAPEUTIC EFFECT* Exerts a hypocalcemic effect by inhibition of calcium resorption from bone, possibly by reducing the rate of bone metabolism. *Lowers calcium serum levels by inhibiting calcium resorption from bone.*

USES Hypercalcemia of malignancy.
UNLABELED USES Paget's disease, painful bone metastases, adjuvant therapy for bladder cancer and lymphomas.

CONTRAINDICATIONS Severe renal impairment (serum creatinine greater than 2.5 mg/dL); hypovolemia; hypocalcemia; lactation.
CAUTIOUS USE Renal function impairment; pregnancy (category C). Safety and efficacy in children are not established.

ROUTE & DOSAGE

Hypercalcemia

Adult: **IV** 100–200 mg/m²/day × 5 days

Bone Metastases

Adult: **IV** 200 mg/m²/day × 7 days

ADMINISTRATION

Intravenous

Hydrate patient with oral or IV NS to produce a urine output of 2 L/day; maintain adequate hydration throughout treatment.

PREPARE: **Continuous:** Dilute each daily dose with 1000 mL NS (preferred if not contraindicated) or D5W.

ADMINISTER: **Continuous:** Infuse over 24 h taking care to avoid rapid infusion. ▪ Control rate with infusion pump or microdrip device.

INCOMPATIBILITIES **Y-site: Cisplatin, cytarabine, doxorubicin, haloperidol, hydromorphone.**

▪ Do not administer concurrently with potentially nephrotoxic drugs.

▪ Store IV solutions at 15°–30° C (59°–86° F) for 48 h or refrigerated at 2°–8° C (36°–46° F) for 7 days. Discard unused portions.

ADVERSE EFFECTS (≥1%) **CNS:** *Fatigue,* paresthesia, hyperthermia. **CV:** Hypotension. **GI:** *Nausea, vomiting, diarrhea,* anorexia, stomatitis, dysgeusia, mucositis, metallic taste. **Hematologic:** Anemia, granulocytopenia, thrombocytopenia. **Metabolic:** Hypocalcemia, hypophosphatemia, hypomagnesemia. **Urogenital:** Nephrotoxicity, acute renal failure. **Other:** Optic neuritis, maculopapular rash.

INTERACTIONS Drug: AMINOGLYCOSIDES, **amphotericin B, vancomycin** increase the risk of nephrotoxicity.

PHARMACOKINETICS Onset: 48 h. **Duration:** 4–14 days after discontinuation of therapy. **Distribution:** Concentrates in tumors; distributed to lung, skin, muscle, and heart with high concentrations in liver and kidney; not known if crosses placenta or is distributed into breast milk. **Metabolism:** Not metabolized. **Elimination:** 35–71% via kidneys within first 24 h. **Half-Life:** 25–111 h.

NURSING IMPLICATIONS

Assessment & Drug Effects

- Ensure that patient is well hydrated. A urine output of 2 L/day is desirable throughout treatment.
- Lab tests: Monitor BUN and serum creatinine throughout therapy. Notify physician if serum creatinine exceeds 2.5 mg/dL; discontinue drug if this occurs. Also, check baseline serum calcium and serum phosphorus; follow with assessments daily and twice weekly, respectively.
- Note: If hypocalcemia occurs, withhold gallium nitrate and notify physician.

Patient & Family Education

- Learn S&S of hypocalcemia (see Appendix F). Notify physician immediately if any occur.

GANCICLOVIR

(gan-ci′clo-vir)

Cytovene

Classification: ANTIVIRAL
Therapeutic: ANTIVIRAL
Prototype: Acyclovir
Pregnancy Category: C

AVAILABILITY 250 mg, 500 mg capsules; 500 mg powder for injection

ACTION & *THERAPEUTIC EFFECT*

Ganciclovir is a synthetic purine nucleoside analog that is an antiviral drug active against cytomegalovirus (CMV). It inhibits the replication of CMV DNA. *Sensitive human viruses include CMV, herpes simplex virus-1 and -2 (HSV-1, HSV-2), Epstein-Barr virus, and varicella-zoster virus.*

USES CMV retinitis, prophylaxis and treatment of systemic CMV infections in immunocompromised patients including HIV-positive and transplant patients.

CONTRAINDICATIONS Hypersensitivity to ganciclovir or acyclovir; infection; severe thrombocytopenia.
CAUTIOUS USE Valacyclovir or penciclovir hypersensitivity; renal impairment, older adults, bone marrow suppression; chemotherapy; radiation therapy; dehydration; secondary malignancy; pregnancy (category C), lactation.

ROUTE & DOSAGE

Induction Therapy

Adult/Child (older than 3 mo): **IV** 5 mg/kg q12h for 14–21 days (doses may range from 2.5–5 mg/kg q8–12h for 10–35 days)

Maintenance Therapy

Adult/Child: **IV** 5 mg/kg daily 7 days/wk or 6 mg/kg daily 5 days/wk **PO** 1000 mg t.i.d. or 500 mg 6 times/day q3h while awake

Prevention of CMV Disease in Transplant Recipients

Adult/Child: **IV** 5 mg/kg q12h 7–14 days, then 5 mg/kg daily or 6 mg/kg/day 5 days/wk

Renal Impairment Dosage Adjustment

CrCl 50–70 mL/min: Use 50% of dose; 25–50 mL/min: Use 50% of dose and q24h interval; 10–25 mL/min: Use 25% of dose and q24h interval
Hemodialysis Dosage Adjustment: Give dose post-dialysis

ADMINISTRATION

- Note: Do not administer if neutrophil count falls below 500/mm³ or platelet count falls below 25,000/mm³.
- Avoid direct contact of powder in capsules or solution with skin and mucous membranes. Wash thoroughly with soap and water if contact occurs.

Oral

- Give with food.

Intravenous

IV administration to infants and children: Verify correct IV concentration and rate of infusion with physician.

PREPARE: **Intermittent:** Reconstitute the 500-mg vial using only 10 mL of sterile water (supplied) for injection immediately before use to yield 50 mg/mL. ▪ Shake well to dissolve. ▪ Withdraw the ordered amount and add to 100 mL of NS, D5W, or LR (volume less than 100 mL may be used, but the final concentration should be less than 10 mg/mL).
ADMINISTER: **Intermittent:** Give at a constant rate over 1 h. Avoid rapid infusion or bolus injection.
INCOMPATIBILITIES **Solution/additive:** Amino acid solutions (TPN), bacteriostatic water for injection, **foscarnet.** **Y-site:** **Amifostine, amsacrine, aztreonam, cefepime, cytarabine, doxorubicin, fludarabine, foscarnet, gemcitabine, ondansetron, piperacillin/tazobactam, sargramostim, tacrolimus, TPN, vinorelbine.**

▪ Store reconstituted solutions refrigerated at 4° C; use within 12 h. ▪ Store infusion solution refrigerated up to 24 h of preparation.

ADVERSE EFFECTS (≥1%) **CNS:** *Fever,* headache, disorientation, mental status changes, ataxia, coma, confusion, dizziness, paresthesia, nervousness, somnolence, tremor. **CV:** Edema, phlebitis. **GI:** *Nausea, diarrhea,* anorexia, elevated liver enzymes. **Hematologic:** *Bone marrow suppression, thrombocytopenia, granulocytopenia, eosinophilia, leukopenia,* hyperbilirubinemia. **Metabolic:** Hyperthermia, hypoglycemia. **Urogenital:** Infertility. **Skin:** Rash.

G

INTERACTIONS Drug: ANTINEOPLASTIC AGENTS, **amphotericin B, didanosine, trimethoprim-sulfamethoxazole (TMP-SMZ), dapsone, pentamidine, probenecid, zidovudine** may increase bone marrow suppression and other toxic effects of ganciclovir; may increase risk of nephrotoxicity from **cyclosporine;** may increase risk of seizures due to **imipenem-cilastatin.** Oral product increases **didanosine** levels.

PHARMACOKINETICS Onset: 3–8 days. **Duration:** Clinical relapse can occur 14 days to 3.5 mo after stopping therapy; positive blood and urine cultures recur 12–60 days after therapy. **Distribution:** Distributes throughout body including CSF, eye, lungs, liver, and kidneys; crosses placenta in animals; not known if distributed into breast milk. **Metabolism:** Not metabolized. **Elimination:** Unchanged in urine. **Half-Life:** 2.5–4.2 h.

NURSING IMPLICATIONS

Assessment & Drug Effects

- Lab tests: Neutrophil and platelet counts at least every other day during twice-daily dosing and weekly thereafter; more frequent monitoring may be indicated in certain patients. Monitor serum creatinine or creatinine clearance at least q2wk. Closely monitor renal function in the older adult.
- Inspect IV insertion site throughout infusion for signs and symptoms of phlebitis.

Patient & Family Education

- Note: Drug is not a cure for CMV retinitis; follow regular ophthalmologic examination schedule.
- Drink lots of fluids during therapy.
- Use barrier contraception throughout therapy and for at least 90 days afterwards.
- Maintain frequent hematologic monitoring.

GANIRELIX ACETATE (Pr)

(gan-i-rel′ix)

Antagon

Classification: GONADOTROPIN-RELEASING HORMONE (GnRH) ANTAGONIST

Therapeutic: GnRH ANTAGONIST

Prototype: Ganirelix

Pregnancy Category: X

AVAILABILITY 250 mcg/0.5 mL syringe

ACTION & *THERAPEUTIC EFFECT* Ganirelix is a gonadotropin-releasing hormone (GnRH) antagonist that suppresses pituitary gonadotropins and sex hormones. *It prevents LH surges in reproductive protocols, and causes shrinkage of uterine fibroids.*

USES Infertility treatment.

CONTRAINDICATIONS Prior hypersensitivity to ganirelix, LHRH, or other LHRH analogs, mannitol hypersensitivity; ovarian cyst; primary ovarian failure; pregnancy (category X), lactation.

CAUTIOUS USE History of current allergic disorders (e.g., asthma, hay fever, urticaria, eczema) or a history of allergic reactions to medications; renal/hepatic dysfunction; endocrine disorders; alcohol consumption.

ROUTE & DOSAGE

Infertility
Adult: **Subcutaneous** After initiating follicle-stimulating hormone (FSH) therapy on day 2 or 3 of the cycle, give 250 mcg once daily during the early-to-mid-follicular phase

ADMINISTRATION
- Note: The packaging of the product, Antagon, contains natural rubber latex which may cause allergic reactions.

Subcutaneous
- Inject into subcutaneous tissue in the abdomen around the umbilicus or into the upper thigh.
- Rotate injection sites.
- Store at 5°–30° C (59°–86° F) and protect from light.

ADVERSE EFFECTS (≥1%) **CNS:** Headache. **GI:** Abdominal pain, nausea. **Endocrine:** Ovarian hyperstimulation syndrome. **Skin:** Injection site reaction. **Urogenital:** Vaginal bleeding.

INTERACTIONS Drug: No clinically significant interactions established.

PHARMACOKINETICS Absorption: 91% from subcutaneous site. **Peak:** 1 h. **Distribution:** 81% protein bound. **Elimination:** 75% in feces; 22% in urine. **Half-Life:** 13–16 h.

NURSING IMPLICATIONS

Assessment & Drug Effects
- Exercise caution with patients with hypersensitivity to GnRH or with known allergic disorders (e.g., asthma, hay fever). These patients should be carefully monitored after the first injection for S&S of an anaphylactic reaction.
- Lab tests: Monitor baseline and periodic CBC with differential, and periodic total bilirubin.

Patient & Family Education
- Report menstrual disorders (e.g., spotting, frank vaginal bleeding) to physician.
- Notify physician immediately if you think you are pregnant.

GATIFLOXACIN
(gat-i-flox'a-sin)
Zymer
Classifications: ANTIBIOTIC; QUINOLONE
Therapeutic: ANTIBIOTIC
Prototype: Ciprofloxacin
Pregnancy Category: C

AVAILABILITY 200 mg, 400 mg tablets; 0.3% ophth solution

ACTION & *THERAPEUTIC EFFECT* Synthetic quinolone that is a broad-spectrum bactericidal agent. Inhibits topoisomerase II (DNA-gyrase), an enzyme necessary for bacterial replication, transcription, repair, and recombination. *Effective against gram-positive and gram-negative bacteria.*

USES Acute bacterial exacerbation of chronic bronchitis; acute sinusitis; community-acquired pneumonia; uncomplicated or complicated UTI; pyelonephritis; gonorrhea due to susceptible organisms.

CONTRAINDICATIONS Hypersensitivity to gatifloxacin or other quinolone antibiotics; diabetes mellitus; viral infections; lactation. Safety and efficacy in children younger than 18

y are unknown. **Ophthalmic** use in infants younger than 1 mo.

CAUTIOUS USE Patients with CNS disorders including seizures or epilepsy; myasthenia gravis; GI disorders, renal dysfunction; hypersensitivity to other medications; concurrent administration of aluminum-containing antacids; pregnancy (category C).

G

ROUTE & DOSAGE

Acute Bacterial Exacerbation of Chronic Bronchitis, Complicated

Adult: **PO** 400 mg daily × 5 days

Complicated UTI, Acute Pyelonephritis

Adult: **PO** 400 mg daily × 7–10 days

Acute Sinusitis

Adult: **PO** 400 mg daily × 10 days

Community-Acquired Pneumonia

Adult: **PO** 400 mg daily × 7–14 days

Uncomplicated UTI

Adult: **PO** 400 mg as a single dose or 200 mg daily × 3 days

Uncomplicated Gonorrhea

Adult: **PO** 400 mg as a single dose

Renal Impairment Dosage Adjustment

CrCl less than 40 mL/min or on dialysis: 400 mg × 1 day, then 200 mg daily

ADMINISTRATION

Oral

- Give at least 4 h before or after an aluminum- or magnesium-containing antacid, or iron-containing products.
- Store at 15°–30° C (59°–86° F).

ADVERSE EFFECTS (≥1%) **Body as a Whole:** Headache, allergic reactions, chills, fever; back pain, chest pain. **CNS:** Dizziness, abnormal dreams, insomnia, paresthesia, tremor, vasodilatation, vertigo. **CV:** Palpitation; peripheral edema. **GI:** Nausea, diarrhea, abdominal pain, constipation, dyspepsia, glossitis, oral moniliasis, stomatitis, vomiting. **Respiratory:** Dyspnea, pharyngitis. **Skin:** Rash, sweating. **Urogenital:** Vaginitis, dysuria, hematuria. **Special Senses:** Abnormal vision, taste perversion, tinnitus. **Metabolic:** Hyperglycemia, hypoglycemia. **Other:** Cartilage erosion.

DIAGNOSTIC TEST INTERFERENCE May cause false positive on ***opiate screening tests.***

INTERACTIONS Drug: Probenecid decreases elimination of gatifloxacin; **ferrous sulfate,** ALUMINUM- or MAGNESIUM-CONTAINING ANTACIDS reduce absorption of gatifloxacin; gatifloxacin may cause slight increase in **digoxin** levels.

PHARMACOKINETICS Absorption: 96% from GI tract. **Peak:** 1–2 h PO. **Distribution:** 20% protein bound. **Metabolism:** Minimal metabolism (less than 1%). **Elimination:** Primarily in urine. **Half-Life:** 7–14 h (up to 35–40 h in severe renal failure).

NURSING IMPLICATIONS

Assessment & Drug Effects

- Monitor for S&S of CNS disturbance especially with history of cerebrovascular disease or seizures.
- Lab tests: C&S prior to initiation of therapy; baseline and periodic WBC with differential.
- Monitor diabetics for loss of glycemic control.
- Monitor for changes in digoxin blood levels with coadministered drugs.

Patient & Family Education

- Be aware that increased risk of seizures are associated with drug use in patient with history of seizures.
- Report unexplained dizziness or problems with balance, tendon pain, severe diarrhea, skin rash, mental status changes.

GEFITINIB (Pr)

(ge-fi′ti-nib)

Iressa

Classifications: ANTINEOPLASTIC; EPIDERMAL GROWTH FACTOR RECEPTOR-TYROSINE KINASE INHIBITOR (EGFR-TKI)

Therapeutic: ANTINEOPLASTIC

Pregnancy Category: D

AVAILABILITY 250 mg tablets

ACTION & *THERAPEUTIC EFFECT* Gefitinib is a selective epidermal growth factor receptor-tyrosine kinase inhibitor (EGFR-TKI). EGFR is expressed or overexpressed in many cancers. EGFR expression is associated with poor prognosis for cancer, development of metastasis, and resistance to chemotherapy, hormonal therapy, and radiation therapy. *Inhibits upregulation or overexpression of EGRF in cancer cells, thus diminishing their capacity for cell proliferation, cell survival, and decreasing their invasive capacity and metastases.*

USES Treatment of locally advanced or metastatic non–small-cell lung cancer after failure of both platinum and docetaxel therapy in patients who have previously used gefitinib.

UNLABELED USES Treatment of head and neck and other solid tumors.

CONTRAINDICATIONS Hypersensitivity to gefitinib; pregnancy (category D), lactation; children younger than 18 y.

CAUTIOUS USE Severe renal impairment; hepatic impairment; bacterial/viral infection; dermatologic toxicities; GI disorders; hepatic insufficiency; interstitial lung disease (interstitial pneumonia, pneumonitis, and alveolitis), pulmonary fibrosis, respiratory insufficiency; myelosuppression; females of childbearing age; prior chemotherapy, radiation therapy; ocular toxicities (corneal ulcer, eye pain).

ROUTE & DOSAGE

Non–Small-Cell Lung Cancer

Adult: **PO** 250 mg daily, may increase to 500 mg daily if on enzyme-inducing drugs

Head and Neck Cancers

Adult: **PO** 500 mg/day

ADMINISTRATION

Oral

- Give without regard to meals.
- Store tablets at 15°–30° C (59°–86° F).

ADVERSE EFFECTS (≥1%) **Body as a Whole:** Asthenia, peripheral edema. **GI:** *Diarrhea, nausea, vomiting,* anorexia, weight loss, stomatitis. **Respiratory:** Dyspnea, <u>interstitial lung disease.</u> **Skin:** *Acne/acneiform rash, dry skin,* pruritus, vesicular/bullous rash. **Special Senses:** Amblyopia, conjunctivitis, aberrant eyelash growth.

INTERACTIONS Drug: BARBITURATES, **bosentan, carbamazepine, dexamethasone, nevirapine, oxcarbazepine, phenytoin** or **fosphenytoin, rifampin, rifabutin, rifapentine** may increase metabolism and decrease levels of gefitinib; **amiodarone,** PROTEASE INHIBI-

TORS, **cimetidine, clarithromycin, dalfopristin; quinupristin, delavirdine, efavirenz, erythromycin, fluconazole, fluvoxamine, fluoxetine, imatinib, itraconazole, ketoconazole, mifepristone, nefazodone,** and **voriconazole** may increase levels and toxicity of gefitinib; may increase INR with **warfarin;** H_2-RECEPTOR ANTAGONISTS, PROTON PUMP INHIBITORS may decrease absorption of gefitinib. **Food: Grapefruit juice** may increase levels and toxicity of gefitinib. **Herbal: St. John's wort** may decrease levels of gefitinib.

PHARMACOKINETICS Absorption: Slowly absorbed, 60% reaches systemic circulation. **Peak:** 3–7 h. **Metabolism:** In liver primarily by CYP3A4. **Elimination:** 86% in feces. **Half-Life:** 48 h.

NURSING IMPLICATIONS

Assessment & Drug Effects

- Monitor pulmonary status and report promptly dyspnea, cough, and fever.
- Withhold drug and notify physician for significant elevations of transaminases, bilirubin, or alkaline phosphatase.
- Monitor for adverse effects, especially with concurrent use of drugs that may inhibit CYP3A4 (e.g., amiodarone, cimetidine, erythromycin, fluconazole, grapefruit juice, etc.). See INTERACTIONS.
- Lab tests: Periodic LFTs; frequent PT/INR with concurrent warfarin.

Patient & Family Education

- Report promptly any of the following: Eye pain or irritation; fever; breathing difficulty or shortness of breath; mouth sores.
- Inform physician of all prescription, nonprescription, or herbal drugs you are taking.
- Females should use reliable contraceptives while taking this drug.
- Minimize or avoid intake of grapefruit juice while taking this drug.

GEMCITABINE HYDROCHLORIDE

(gem-ci'ta-been)

Gemzar

Classifications: ANTINEOPLASTIC AGENT; ANTIMETABOLITE, PYRIMIDINE

Therapeutic: ANTINEOPLASTIC

Prototype: Fluorouracil

Pregnancy Category: D

AVAILABILITY 20 mg/mL injection

ACTION & *THERAPEUTIC EFFECT* Pyrimidine analog with cell phase specificity by affecting rapidly dividing cells in S phase (DNA synthesis). It also blocks the progression of cells from G_1 phase to S phase of cell cycle. Gemcitabine interferes with DNA synthesis by inhibiting ribonucleotide. In addition, if gemcitabine is incorporated into the DNA strand, it inhibits further growth of the strand. *Gemcitabine induces DNA fragmentation in dividing cells, resulting in the cell death of tumor cells.*

USES Locally advanced or metastatic adenocarcinoma of the pancreas, non–small-cell lung cancer, breast cancer.

CONTRAINDICATIONS Hypersensitivity to gemcitabine, severe thrombocytopenia, acute infection, pregnancy (category D), lactation.

CAUTIOUS USE Myelosuppression, renal or hepatic dysfunction, older adults; neutropenia; history of bleeding disorders, infection, previous cytotoxic or radiation treatment. Safety and effectiveness in children are not established.

ROUTE & DOSAGE

Pancreatic Cancer
Adult: **IV** 1000 mg/m² once weekly for up to 7 wk, followed by 1 wk rest from treatment; may repeat once weekly for 3 of every 4 wk

Non–Small-Cell Lung Cancer
Adult: **IV** 1000 mg/m² on days 1, 8, 15 of 28-day cycle OR 1250 mg/m² on days 1 and 8 of 21-day cycle. Given with cisplatin.

Breast Cancer
Adult: **IV** 1250 mg/m² on days 1 and 8 of 21-day cycle. Given with paclitaxel.

ADMINISTRATION

Intravenous

PREPARE: **IV Infusion:** Dilute with NS without preservatives by adding 5 mL or 25 mL to the 200 mg or 1 g vial, respectively, to yield 38 mg/mL. ▪ Shake to dissolve. ▪ Dilute further if necessary with NS to concentrations as low as 0.1 mg/mL.

ADMINISTER: **IV Infusion:** Infuse over 30 min. Infusion time greater than 60 min is associated with increased toxicity.

INCOMPATIBILITIES **Y-site: Acyclovir, amphotericin B, cefoperazone, cefotaxime, furosemide, ganciclovir, imipenem/cilastatin, irinotecan, methotrexate, methylprednisolone, mitomycin, piperacillin, piperacillin/tazobactam, prochlorperazine.**

▪ Store reconstituted solutions unrefrigerated at 20°–25° C (68°–77° F). Use within 24 h of reconstitution.

ADVERSE EFFECTS (≥1%) **CNS:** *Fever, flu-like syndrome (anorexia, headache, cough, chills, myalgia),* paresthesias. **GI:** *Nausea, vomiting, diarrhea,* stomatitis, *transient elevations of liver transaminases.* **Hematologic:** *Myelosuppression (anemia, leukopenia, neutropenia, thrombocytopenia).* **Skin:** Bullous skin eruption, desquamation. **Urogenital:** Mild proteinuria and hematuria. **Other:** *Dyspnea, edema, peripheral edema, infection,* elevated liver function tests.

INTERACTIONS Drug: May increase effect of **warfarin** or ORAL ANTICOAGULANTS.

PHARMACOKINETICS Peak: Peak concentrations reached 30 min after infusion; lower clearance in women and older adult results in higher concentrations at any given dose. **Distribution:** Crosses placenta, distributed into breast milk. **Metabolism:** Intracellularly by nucleoside kinases to active diphosphate and triphosphate nucleosides. **Elimination:** 92–98% recovered in urine within 1 wk. **Half-Life:** 32–94 min.

NURSING IMPLICATIONS

Assessment & Drug Effects

- Lab tests: Monitor CBC with differential and platelet count prior to each dose. Monitor baseline and periodic renal and hepatic function.

Patient & Family Education

- Learn about common adverse effects and measures to control or minimize when possible. Notify physician immediately of any distressing adverse effects.
- Note: Fever with flu-like symptoms, rash, and GI distress are very common.
- Females should use reliable contraception while taking this drug.

GEMFIBROZIL

(gem-fi'broe-zil)

Lopid

Classifications: ANTILIPEMIC; FIBRATE

Therapeutic: CHOLESTEROL-LOWERING

Prototype: Fenofibrate

Pregnancy Category: C

G

AVAILABILITY 600 mg tablets

ACTION & *THERAPEUTIC EFFECT* Fibric acid derivative with lipid regulating properties. Blocks lipolysis of stored triglycerides in adipose tissue and inhibits hepatic uptake of fatty acids. *Decreases VLDL and therefore triglyceride synthesis. Produces a moderate increase in HDL cholesterol levels and reduces levels of total and LDL cholesterol and triglycerides.*

USES Patients with very high serum triglyceride levels (above 750 mg/dL) (type IV and V hyperlipidemia) who have not responded to intensive diet restriction and are at risk of pancreatitis and abdominal pain. Also severe familial hypercholesterolemia (type IIa or IIb) that developed in childhood and has failed to respond to dietary control or to other cholesterol-lowering drugs.

CONTRAINDICATIONS Gallbladder disease, biliary cirrhosis, hepatic or severe renal dysfunction. Safety and efficacy in children younger than 18 y are not established.

CAUTIOUS USE Diabetes mellitus, hypothyroidism; renal impairment, cholelithiasis; pregnancy (category C), lactation.

ROUTE & DOSAGE

Hypertriglyceridemia

Adult: **PO** 600 mg b.i.d. 30 min before morning and evening meal, may increase up to 1500 mg/day

ADMINISTRATION

Oral

- Give 30 min before breakfast and evening meal.
- Store at 15°–30° C (59°–86° F) unless otherwise directed.

ADVERSE EFFECTS (≥1%) **CNS:** Headache, dizziness, blurred vision. **GI:** *Abdominal* or *epigastric pain,* diarrhea, nausea, vomiting, flatulence. **Hematologic:** Eosinophilia, mild decreases in Hct, Hgb. **Musculoskeletal:** Painful extremities, back pain, muscle cramps, myalgia, arthralgia, swollen joints. **Skin:** Rash, dermatitis, pruritus, urticaria. **Endocrine:** Hypokalemia, moderate hyperglycemia.

INTERACTIONS Drug: May potentiate hypoprothrombinemic effects of ORAL ANTICOAGULANTS; **lovastatin** increases risk of myopathy and rhabdomyolysis; may increase hypoglycemic effects of ANTIDIABETIC MEDICATIONS.

PHARMACOKINETICS Absorption: Readily from GI tract. **Peak:** 1–2 h. **Metabolism:** Undergoes enterohepatic circulation. **Elimination:** In urine; 6% in feces. **Half-Life:** 1.3–1.5 h.

NURSING IMPLICATIONS

Assessment & Drug Effects

- Lab tests: Monitor baseline and at regular intervals during first year of therapy for serum LDL and VLDL, triglycerides, total cholesterol, CBC, blood glucose, liver function tests.
- Note: Mild decreases in WBC, Hgb, Hct may occur during early stage of treatment but generally stabilize with continued therapy.

- Note: Drug is usually withdrawn if lipid response is inadequate after 3 mo of therapy.
- Notify physician if patient presents S&S suggestive of cholelithiasis or cholecystitis; gallbladder studies may be indicated. Symptoms often occur during the night or early morning; jaundice may or may not be present.

Patient & Family Education

- Do not drive or engage in other potentially hazardous activities until response to drug is known.
- Report promptly if you develop jaundice, pruritis, or unexplained, upper abdominal discomfort.

GEMIFLOXACIN

(gem-i-flox'a-cin)

Factive

Classifications: ANTIBIOTIC; QUINOLONE

Therapeutic: ANTIBIOTIC

Prototype: Ciprofloxacin HCl

Pregnancy Category: C

AVAILABILITY 320 mg tablet

ACTION & *THERAPEUTIC EFFECT* Gemifloxacin inhibits bacterial DNA gyrases (topoisomerase II), enzymes essential in replication, transcription, and repair of bacterial DNA. *Gemifloxacin is active against a wide range of gram-positive and gram-negative bacteria. It has greater activity against gram-positive cocci and against penicillin- and ciprofloxacin-resistant* Streptococcus pneumoniae *than other fluoroquinolones.*

USES Treatment of acute exacerbations of chronic bronchitis, mild to moderate community-acquired pneumonia.

UNLABELED USES Acute sinusitis, UTI, acute pyelonephritis.

CONTRAINDICATIONS Hypersensitivity to gemifloxacin or other fluoroquinolone antibiotics; known QT prolongation; tendon pain; viral disease; lactation. Safety and effectiveness in children younger than 18 y have not been established.

CAUTIOUS USE Hypokalemia, hypomagnesemia, or concurrent use of Class IA or III antiarrhythmic agents; bradycardia, acute myocardial ischemia; renal disease or impairment; hepatic disease; central nervous system disorders such as epilepsy; glucose 6-phosphate dehydrogenase deficiency; tendonitis, elderly, concurrent use of corticosteroids; pregnancy (category C).

ROUTE & DOSAGE

Acute Exacerbation of Chronic Bronchitis

Adult: **PO** 320 mg daily × 5 days

Community-Acquired Pneumonia

Adult: **PO** 320 mg daily × 7 days

Sinusitis

Adult: **PO** 320 mg daily × 10 days

UTI

Adult: **PO** 320 mg daily × 3 days

Renal Impairment Dosage Adjustment

CrCl 40 mL/min or less: 160 mg daily

ADMINISTRATION

Oral

- Give 2 h before/3 h after drugs containing aluminum, magne-

sium, iron, zinc, or buffered tablets of any type.
- Give at least 2 h before sucralfate.
- Store at 15°–30° C (59°–86° F) and protect from light.

ADVERSE EFFECTS (≥1%) **CNS:** Headache. **GI:** Nausea, vomiting, diarrhea, elevated liver enzymes. **Skin:** Rash.

G

INTERACTIONS Drug: ANTACIDS, **didanosine (tablets and powder), iron, sevelamer, sulcralfate** decrease absorption; may prolong the QT interval with **amiodarone, bretylium, disopyramide, dofetilide, ibutilide, quinidine, procainamide, sotalol** leading to arrhythmias; may augment phototoxicity of RETINOIDS.

PHARMACOKINETICS Absorption: 71% absorbed. **Peak:** 0.5–2 h. **Metabolism:** Minimally in liver. **Elimination:** Primarily renal. **Half-Life:** 7 h.

NURSING IMPLICATIONS

Assessment & Drug Effects

- Monitor cardiac status with concurrent use of drugs that may prolong the QT interval. Report immediately bradycardia or S&S of heart failure.
- Withhold drug and report to physician any of the following: Tremors, restlessness, lightheadedness, confusion, hallucinations, paranoia, depression, nightmares, and insomnia.
- Lab tests: C&S prior to initiation of therapy; baseline and periodic serum electrolytes; frequent blood glucose levels in diabetics; CBC with differential and platelet count with prolonged treatment.

Patient & Family Education

- Use sunscreen and protective clothing outdoors. Avoid sun lamps.
- Stop gemifloxacin and notify physician for pain or swelling of a tendon or around a joint.
- Drink fluid liberally (unless contraindicated) while taking this drug.
- Do not drive or engage in other hazardous activities until reaction to drug is known.

GEMTUZUMAB OZOGAMICIN

(gem-tu′zu-mab)
Mylotarg
Classifications: ANTINEOPLASTIC; MONOCLONAL (IgG_4) ANTIBODY
Therapeutic: ANTINEOPLASTIC; IMMUNOSUPPRESSANT
Pregnancy Category: D

AVAILABILITY 5 mg vial

ACTION & *THERAPEUTIC EFFECT* Chemotherapeutic agent composed of recombinant IgG_4 antibodies, which bind specifically to CD33 antigens that are expressed on the surface of leukemic myeloblasts and immature normal cells of myelomonocytic origin. *Cytotoxic to the CD33 positive human leukemia cells in the bone marrow. CD33 antigens are found on the surface of leukemic cells.*

USES Treatment of CD33 positive acute myeloid leukemia (AML) in first relapse in patients 60 y or older.

CONTRAINDICATIONS Hypersensitivity to gemtuzumab or anti-CD33 antibody therapy, murine protein hypersensitivity; systemic infections; pregnancy (category D), lactation.
CAUTIOUS USE Hepatic impairment including jaundice; renal dysfunction; pulmonary disease; moderate or severe thrombocytopenia or

neutropenia; history of asthma or allergies.

ROUTE & DOSAGE

Acute Myeloid Leukemia (AML)
Adult: **IV** 9 mg/m² infused over 2 h, repeat in 14 days

ADMINISTRATION

Intravenous
Protect gemtuzumab from sunlight and unshielded fluorescent light during preparation and administration. ▪ Allow vials to come to room temperature before reconstitution. ▪ Acetaminophen 650 mg orally and diphenhydramine 25–50 mg IV are normally given prior to infusion to control adverse effects.

PREPARE: **Continuous:** Reconstitute each vial with 5 mL of sterile water for injection to yield 1 mg/mL. Gently swirl to dissolve. Dilute the reconstituted drug further just prior to administration by withdrawing the required amount of drug and adding it to 100 mL of NS. Cover the IV bag with a UV protectant cover.
ADMINISTER: **Continuous:** Infuse over 2 h through a separate IV line with a nonpyrogenic low-protein-binding 0.2–1.2 micron filter. Do not give push as a bolus dose.
INCOMPATIBILITIES **Solution/additive & Y-site:** Do not mix with other drugs.

▪ Store unopened vials refrigerated at 2°–8° C (36°–46° F). Store reconstituted drug refrigerated at 2°–8° C (36°–46° F) and protected from light for up to 8 h.

ADVERSE EFFECTS (≥1%) **Body as a Whole:** Severe hypersensitivity *anaphylaxis, chills, fever, asthenia, infection, sepsis.* **CV:** *Hypotension,* hypertension, tachycardia. **GI:** *Nausea, vomiting, mucositis, abdominal pain, anorexia, constipation, diarrhea, stomatitis.* **Hematologic:** *<u>Neutropenia, thrombocytopenia, anemia</u>, bleeding,* epistaxis, cerebral hemorrhage, hematuria, ecchymosis. **Metabolic:** Hyperglycemia, *hyperbilirubinemia,* abnormal AST, ALT, hypokalemia, hypomagnesemia, increased lactic dehydrogenase. **Musculoskeletal:** Arthralgia. **CNS:** *Headache,* depression, dizziness, *insomnia.* **Respiratory:** Hypoxia, *dyspnea, cough,* pharyngitis, rhinitis, pneumonia, *fatal pulmonary events.* **Skin:** *Rash, herpes simplex, local reactions from infusion, peripheral edema, petechiae.*

INTERACTIONS PLATELET INHIBITORS, ANTICOAGULANTS, **aspirin,** and NSAIDS may potentiate bleeding.

PHARMACOKINETICS Metabolism: Hydrolyzed in liver to calicheamicin. **Half-Life:** 45–100 h.

NURSING IMPLICATIONS

Assessment & Drug Effects

- Monitor for S&S of postinfusion syndrome: Fever, chills, and rigors which occur 2–4 h after initiation of infusion; hypotension and dyspnea which may occur during first 24 h after infusion.
- Monitor vital signs during and for at least 2 h after infusion.
- Lab tests: Monitor CBC with differential, platelet count, lymphoblast smears at least weekly. Periodically monitor liver functions and routine blood chemistry.

Patient & Family Education

- Report S&S of infection immediately to physician (e.g., chills, fever, sore throat, lower back or side pain).

- Report unusual bleeding or bruising, black tarry stools, or pinpoint red spots on skin to physician immediately.
- Avoid exposure to infections.
- Avoid immunizations unless approved by physician; avoid contact with anyone who has received oral polio virus vaccine.
- Avoid situations that could result in injury during periods of bone marrow suppression.

G

GENTAMICIN SULFATE (Pr)

(jen-ta-mye′sin)

Garamycin Ophthalmic, Genoptic

Classification: AMINOGLYCOSIDE ANTIBIOTIC

Therapeutic: ANTIBIOTIC

Pregnancy Category: D

AVAILABILITY 10 mg/mL, 40 mg/mL; 0.1% ointment, cream; 3 mg/mL ophth solution; 3 mg/g ophth ointment

ACTION & *THERAPEUTIC EFFECT* Broad-spectrum aminoglycoside antibiotic that binds irreversibly to 30S subunit of bacterial ribosomes, blocking a vital step in protein synthesis, and attachment of RNA molecules to bacterial ribosomes resulting in cell death. *Active against a wide variety of aerobic gram-negative but not anaerobic gram-negative bacteria. Also effective against certain gram-positive organisms, particularly penicillin-sensitive.*

USES Parenteral use restricted to treatment of serious infections of GI, respiratory, and urinary tracts, CNS, bone, skin, and soft tissue (including burns) when other less toxic antimicrobial agents are ineffective or are contraindicated. Has been used in combination with other antibiotics. Also used topically for primary and secondary skin infections and for superficial infections of external eye and its adnexa.

UNLABELED USES Prophylaxis of bacterial endocarditis in patients undergoing operative procedures or instrumentation.

CONTRAINDICATIONS History of hypersensitivity to, or toxic reaction with any aminoglycoside antibiotic; pregnancy (category D), lactation.

CAUTIOUS USE Impaired renal function; history of eighth cranial (acoustic) nerve impairment; preexisting vertigo or dizziness or tinnitus; dehydration, fever; renal impairment, dehydration; Fabry disease; use in older adults, premature infants, neonates, and infants; obesity, neuromuscular disorders: Myasthenia gravis, parkinsonian syndrome; hypocalcemia, heart failure, topical applications to widespread areas.

ROUTE & DOSAGE

Moderate to Severe Infection

Adult: **IV/IM** 1–2 mg/kg loading dose followed by 3–5 mg/kg/day in 3 divided doses **Intrathecal** 4–8 mg preservative free daily **Topical** 1–2 drops of solution in eye q4h up to 2 drops q1h or small amount of ointment b.i.d. or t.i.d.

Child: **IV/IM** 6–7.5 mg/kg/day in 3 divided doses **Intrathecal** *Older than 3 mo,* 1–2 mg preservative free daily

Neonate: **IV/IM** 2.5 mg/kg/day

Prophylaxis of Bacterial Endocarditis

Adult: **IV/IM** 1.5 mg/kg 30 min before procedure, may repeat in 8 h

Child (weight less than 27 kg):
IV/IM 2 mg/kg 30 min before procedure, may repeat in 8 h

Obesity Dosage Adjustment

Dose based on IBW, in morbid obesity use IBW +0.4 (TBW–IBW)

Renal Impairment Dosage Adjustment

Reduce dose or extend dosing interval

ADMINISTRATION

Ophthalmic

- Apply pressure to inner canthus for 1 min immediately after instillation of drops.
- Have patient keep eyes closed for 1–2 min after administration of ophthalmic ointment to assure medication contact. Caution patient that vision will be blurred for a few minutes.

Topical

- Wash affected area with mild soap and water, rinse, and dry thoroughly. Gently apply small amount of medication to lesions; cover with sterile gauze.
- Do not apply topical preparations, particularly cream, to large denuded body surfaces because systemic absorption and toxicity are possible.

Intramuscular

- Give deep into a large muscle.
- Do not use solutions that are discolored or that contain particulate matter; drug for IV or IM is clear and colorless or slightly yellow.

Intrathecal

- Note: Intrathecal formulation is a clear and colorless solution.
- Use promptly after opening; contains no preservatives and any unused portion should be discarded.

Intravenous

PREPARE: **Intermittent:** Dilute a single dose with 50–200 mL of D5W or NS. ▪ For pediatric patients, amount of infusion fluid may be proportionately smaller depending on patient's needs but should be sufficient to be infused over the same time period as for adults.

ADMINISTER: **Intermittent:** Give over 30 min–1 h. May extend infusion time to 2 h for a child.

INCOMPATIBILITIES **Solution/additive:** Fat emulsion, **TPN, amphotericin B, ampicillin, carbenicillin,** CEPHALOSPORINS, **cytarabine, heparin, ticarcillin.** **Y-site:** **Allopurinol, amphotericin B cholesteryl, azithromycin, furosemide, heparin, hetastarch, idarubicin, indomethacin, iodipamide, propofol, warfarin.**

- Store all gentamicin solutions between 2°–30° C (36°–86° F) unless otherwise directed by manufacturer.

ADVERSE EFFECTS (≥1%) **Special Senses:** Ototoxicity (vestibular disturbances, impaired hearing), optic neuritis. **CNS:** Neuromuscular blockade: Skeletal muscle weakness, apnea, respiratory paralysis (high doses); arachnoiditis (intrathecal use). **CV:** Hypotension or hypertension. **GI:** Nausea, vomiting, transient increase in AST, ALT, and serum LDH and bilirubin; hepatomegaly, splenomegaly. **Hematologic:** Increased or decreased reticulocyte counts; granulocytopenia, thrombocytopenia (fever, bleeding tendency), thrombocytopenic purpura, anemia. **Body as a Whole:** Hypersensitivity (rash, pruritus, urticaria, exfoliative dermatitis, eosinophilia, burning sensation of skin, drug fe-

G

ver, joint pains, laryngeal edema, anaphylaxis). **Urogenital:** Nephrotoxicity: Proteinuria, tubular necrosis, cells or casts in urine, hematuria, rising BUN, nonprotein nitrogen, serum creatinine; *decreased creatinine clearance*. **Other:** Local irritation and pain following IM use; thrombophlebitis, abscess, superinfections, syndrome of hypocalcemia (tetany, weakness, hypokalemia, hypomagnesemia). **Topical and Ophthalmic:** Photosensitivity, sensitization, erythema, pruritus; burning, stinging, and lacrimation (ophthalmic formulation).

INTERACTIONS Drug: Amphotericin B, capreomycin, cisplatin, methoxyflurane, polymyxin B, vancomycin, ethacrynic acid, and **furosemide** increase risk of nephrotoxicity. GENERAL ANESTHETICS and NEUROMUSCULAR BLOCKING AGENTS (e.g., **succinylcholine**) potentiate neuromuscular blockade. **Indomethacin** may increase gentamicin levels in neonates.

PHARMACOKINETICS Absorption: Well absorbed from IM site. **Peak:** 30–90 min IM. **Distribution:** Widely distributed in body fluids, including ascitic, peritoneal, pleural, synovial, and abscess fluids; poor CNS penetration; concentrates in kidney and inner ear; crosses placenta. **Metabolism:** Not metabolized. **Elimination:** Excreted unchanged in urine; small amounts accumulate in kidney and are eliminated over 10–20 days; small amount excreted in breast milk. **Half-Life:** 2–4 h.

NURSING IMPLICATIONS

Assessment & Drug Effects

- Lab tests: Perform C&S and renal function prior to first dose and periodically during therapy. Determine creatinine clearance and serum drug concentrations at frequent intervals.
- Note: Dosages are generally adjusted to maintain peak serum gentamicin concentrations of 4–10 mcg/mL, and trough concentrations of 1–2 mcg/mL. Prolonged peak concentrations above 12 mcg/mL and trough concentrations above 2 mcg/mL are associated with toxicity.
- Draw blood specimens for peak serum gentamicin concentration 30 min–1h after IM administration, and 30 min after completion of a 30–60 min IV infusion. Draw blood specimens for trough levels just before the next IM or IV dose.
- Monitor vital signs and I&O. Keep patient well hydrated to prevent chemical irritation of renal tubules. Report oliguria, unusual appearance of urine, change in I&O ratio or pattern, and presence of edema (prolongs elimination time).
- Report promptly S&S of ototoxic effect (e.g., headache, dizziness or vertigo, nausea and vomiting with motion, ataxia, nystagmus, tinnitus, roaring noises, sensation of fullness in ears, hearing impairment).
- Watch for S&S of bacterial overgrowth (opportunistic infections) with resistant or nonsusceptible organisms (diarrhea, anogenital itching, vaginal discharge, stomatitis, glossitis).

Patient & Family Education

- Note: When using topical applications: Avoid excessive exposure to sunlight because of danger of photosensitivity; withhold medication and notify physician if condition fails to improve within 1 wk, worsens, or signs of irritation or sensitivity occur; and apply medication as directed and only for length of time prescribed (overuse can result in superinfections).

GLATIRAMER ACETATE

(gla-tir′a-mer)

Copaxone, Copolymer-1

Classifications: BIOLOGICAL RESPONSE MODIFIER; IMMUNOLOGIC

Therapeutic: IMMUNOSUPPRESSANT

Pregnancy Category: B

AVAILABILITY 20 mg injection

ACTION & *THERAPEUTIC EFFECT* Glatiramer is a random synthetic copolymer of L-alanine, L-glutamic acid, L-lysine, and L-tyrosine. It modifies immune processes that are responsible for the pathogenesis of multiple sclerosis. *Its function is to reduce the relapse rate of multiple sclerosis (MS), a demyelinating disease of the CNS of unknown origin.*

USES Reduction of the frequency of relapses in patients with relapsing–remitting multiple sclerosis.

CONTRAINDICATIONS Hypersensitivity to glatiramer acetate or mannitol. Safety and effectiveness in children younger than 18 y have not been established.

CAUTIOUS USE Immunosuppression, history of asthma or other respiratory disorders; pregnancy (category B), lactation.

ROUTE & DOSAGE

Multiple Sclerosis

Adult: **Subcutaneous** 20 mg daily

ADMINISTRATION

Subcutaneous

- Use recommended subcutaneous injection sites: Arms, abdomen, hips, and thighs.
- Reconstitute with supplied diluent, swirl gently, let stand at room temperature until completely dissolved, then use immediately.
- Do not store reconstituted drug. Before reconstitution, store vials at –20° to –10° C (–4° to –14° F).

ADVERSE EFFECTS (≥1%) **Body as a Whole:** *Asthenia, back pain,* chills, facial edema, fever, *flu-like syndrome, infection, pain, arthralgia.* **CNS:** Migraine, agitation, *anxiety, hypotonia.* **CV:** *Chest pain, palpitations,* syncope, tachycardia, *vasodilation.* **GI:** *Diarrhea, nausea,* anorexia, gastroenteritis, vomiting. **Respiratory:** *Dyspnea, rhinitis,* bronchitis. **Skin:** *Rash, pruritus, sweating.* **Other:** *Postinjection reaction (flushing, chest pain, palpitations, anxiety, dyspnea, constriction of throat, urticaria), injection site reactions (erythema, hemorrhage, pain, pruritus, urticaria, swelling),* ecchymoses, *lymphadenopathy,* ear pain, dysmenorrhea, urinary urgency.

NURSING IMPLICATIONS

Assessment & Drug Effects

- Monitor for therapeutic effectiveness: Indicated by longer remission periods and reduced frequency of attacks.
- Assess for systemic postinjection reactions (see PATIENT & FAMILY EDUCATION). Assure patient that reaction is self-limiting. Assess for local reactions at injection sites including erythema, itching, induration, and soreness.

- Monitor for S&S of compromised immune response (e.g., increasing frequency of infections).

Patient & Family Education

- Note: Systemic postinjection reaction with chest pain, palpitations, flushing, urticaria, anxiety, dyspnea, and laryngeal constriction may occur immediately after injection. These symptoms are transient (lasting from 30 sec–30 min), require no treatment, and resolve spontaneously.
- Report any distressing adverse drug effects.

G

GLIMEPIRIDE

(gli-me′pi-ride)

Amaryl

Classifications: HORMONE; ANTIDIABETIC; SULFONYLUREA

Therapeutic: ANTIDIABETIC

Prototype: Glyburide

Pregnancy Category: C

AVAILABILITY 1 mg, 2 mg, 4 mg tablets

ACTION & *THERAPEUTIC EFFECT* Second-generation sulfonylurea hypoglycemic agent that directly stimulates functioning pancreatic beta cells to secrete insulin, leading to a direct drop in blood glucose. Indirect action leads to increased sensitivity of peripheral insulin receptors, resulting in increased insulin binding in peripheral tissues. *Lowers blood sugar by increasing secretion of insulin from pancreatic beta cells. Glimepiride improves postprandial glycemic control.*

USES Adjunct to diet and exercise in patients with type 2 diabetes, may also be used in combination with insulin in type 2 diabetes.

CONTRAINDICATIONS Hypersensitivity to glimepiride, diabetic ketoacidosis; lactation, nondiabetic patients with renal glycosuria.

CAUTIOUS USE Previous hypersensitivity to other sulfonylureas, sulfonamides, or thiazide diuretics; hypoglycemia or conditions predisposing to hypoglycemia (e.g., prolonged nausea and vomiting, alcohol ingestion, renal or hepatic function impairment, severe infections, surgery); pregnancy (category C). Safe use in children is not established.

ROUTE & DOSAGE

Type 2 Diabetes Mellitus

Adult: **PO** Start with 1–2 mg once daily with breakfast or first main meal, may increase to usual maintenance dose of 1–4 mg once daily (max: 8 mg/day)

ADMINISTRATION

Oral

- Give with breakfast or first main meal.
- Note: Maximum starting dose is 2 mg or less. With renal or hepatic insufficiency, initial recommended dose is 1 mg.
- Store in tightly closed container at 15°–30° C (59°–86° F).

ADVERSE EFFECTS (≥1%) **CNS:** Dizziness, asthenia, headache, blurred vision, changes in accommodation. **GI:** Nausea, vomiting, diarrhea, abdominal pain. **Hematologic:** Leukopenia, <u>agranulocytosis</u> (rare), thrombocytopenia. **Metabolic:** Hypoglycemia. **Skin:** Rash, pruritus, erythema, urticaria, maculopapular eruptions.

INTERACTIONS Drug: Hypoglycemic effects may be potentiated by other highly protein-bound drugs (e.g., ADRENERGIC ANTAGONISTS, **chloramphenicol,** MAO INHIBITORS, NSAIDS, **probenecid,** SALICYLATES, SULFONAMIDES, **warfarin**). CORTICOSTEROIDS, **phenytoin, isoniazid, nicotinic acid,** SYMPATHOMIMETIC AMINES, THIAZIDE DIURETICS may attenuate effects of glimepiride. **Herbal: Ginseng, garlic** may increase hypoglycemic effects.

PHARMACOKINETICS Absorption: Completely absorbed from GI tract. **Onset:** 1 h. **Peak:** 2–3 h. **Distribution:** Greater than 99.5% protein bound; probably secreted into breast milk. **Metabolism:** In liver by CYP2C9. **Elimination:** 60% in urine, 40% in feces. **Half-Life:** 5–9 h.

NURSING IMPLICATIONS

Assessment & Drug Effects

- Lab tests: Monitor fasting and postprandial blood glucose frequently. Monitor HgbA1C every 3–6 mo. Monitor periodically during long-term therapy: Liver function tests, serum osmolarity, serum sodium, and CBC with differential.
- Monitor for hypoglycemia especially with concurrent drugs which enhance hypoglycemic effects.

Patient & Family Education

- Take a missed dose as soon as possible unless it is almost time for next dose; NEVER take two doses at the same time.
- Avoid drinking alcohol or using OTC drugs without informing physician.
- Learn about adverse reactions and drug interactions.

GLIPIZIDE

(glip'i-zide)

Glucotrol, Glucotrol XL

Classifications: ANTIDIABETIC; SULFONYLUREA

Therapeutic: ANTIDIABETIC

Prototype: Glyburide

Pregnancy Category: C

AVAILABILITY 5 mg, 10 mg tablets; 5 mg, 10 mg sustained release tablets

ACTION & *THERAPEUTIC EFFECT* Second-generation sulfonylurea hypoglycemic agent that directly stimulates functioning pancreatic beta cells to secrete insulin, leading to an acute drop in blood glucose. Indirect action leads to altered numbers and sensitivity of peripheral insulin receptors, resulting in increased insulin binding. It also causes inhibition of hepatic glucose production and reduction in serum glucagon levels. *It lowers blood glucose level by stimulating pancreatic beta cells.*

USES Adjunct to diet for control of hyperglycemia in patient with type 2 diabetes mellitus after dietary control alone has failed; also used to treat transient loss of control in patient usually controlled well on diet.

CONTRAINDICATIONS Hypersensitivity to sulfonylureas; diabetic ketoacidosis; lactation. Safe use in children is not established.

CAUTIOUS USE Impaired renal and hepatic function; thyroid disease; older adults; debilitated, malnourished patients; G6PD deficiency; trauma; surgery; patients with adrenal or pituitary insufficiency; pregnancy (category C).

ROUTE & DOSAGE

Control of Hyperglycemia

Adult: **PO** 2.5–5 mg/day 30 min before breakfast, may increase by 2.5–5 mg q1–2wk; greater than 15 mg/day in divided doses 30 min before morning and evening meal (max: 40 mg/day); 5–10 mg sustained release tablets once/day

ADMINISTRATION

Oral

- Give once-daily dosing 30 min before the first meal of the day.
- Ensure that sustained release form of drug is not chewed or crushed. It **must be** swallowed whole.
- Store in tightly closed, light-resistant container at 15°–30° C (59°–86° F).

ADVERSE EFFECTS (≥1%) **GI:** Nausea, diarrhea, constipation, gastralgia, cholestatic jaundice (rare). **Metabolic:** Hepatic porphyria, <u>hypoglycemia</u>. **Skin:** Erythema, morbilliform or maculopapular rash, pruritus, urticaria, eczema (transient). **Body as a Whole:** Hypersensitivity (fatigue, drowsiness, hunger, GI distress with heartburn, abdominal pain, anorexia). **CNS:** Transient drowsiness, headache, anxiety, ataxia, confusion; seizures, <u>coma</u>. **CV:** Tachycardia. **Special Senses:** Visual disturbances.

INTERACTIONS Drug: Alcohol produces **disulfiram**-like reaction in some patients; ORAL ANTICOAGULANTS, **chloramphenicol, clofibrate, phenylbutazone,** MAO INHIBITORS, SALICYLATES, **probenecid,** SULFONAMIDES may potentiate hypoglycemic actions; THIAZIDES may antagonize hypoglycemic effects; **cimetidine** may increase glipizide levels, causing hypoglycemia. **Herbal: Ginseng, garlic** may increase hypoglycemic effects.

PHARMACOKINETICS Absorption: Readily from GI tract. **Onset:** 15–30 min. **Peak:** 1–2 h. **Duration:** Up to 24 h. **Metabolism:** Metabolized extensively in liver. **Elimination:** Mainly in urine with some excretion via bile in feces. **Half-Life:** 3–5 h.

NURSING IMPLICATIONS

Assessment & Drug Effects

- Observe response to the initial dose, especially in older adult or debilitated patients; early signs of hypoglycemia are easily overlooked.
- Lab tests: Monitor fasting and postprandial blood glucose, and HgbA1C. Monitor periodically during long-term therapy: Liver function tests, serum electrolytes, and serum osmolarity.
- Patients transferred from a sulfonylurea with a long half-life (e.g., chlorpropamide, half-life: 30–40 h) **must be** made aware of the potential for hypoglycemic responses (see Appendix F) for 1–2 wk because of potential overlapping of drug effect.
- Note: The first signs of hypoglycemia may be hard to detect in patients receiving concurrent beta-blockers or older adults.

Patient & Family Education

- Treat mild hypoglycemia (reaction without loss of consciousness or neurologic symptoms) with PO glucose and adjustment of dosage and meal pattern; monitor closely for at least 5–7 days to assure reestablishment of safe control. Severe hypoglycemia requires emergency hospitalization to permit treatment to maintain a blood glucose level above 100 mg/dL.

- Test fasting and postprandial blood glucose frequently.
- Keep all follow-up medical appointments and adhere to dietary instructions, regular exercise program, and scheduled and blood testing.
- When a drug that affects the hypoglycemic action of sulfonylureas (see DRUG INTERACTIONS) is withdrawn or added to the glipizide regimen, be alert to the added danger of loss of control. Urine and blood glucose tests and test for ketone bodies should be carefully monitored.
- Report promptly severe skin rash and pruritus as these may indicate a need for discontinuation of drug. Symptoms usually subside rapidly when drug is withdrawn.

GLUCAGON

(gloo′ka-gon)
GlucaGen
Classification: ANTIHYPOGLYCEMIC
Therapeutic: ANTIHYPOGLYCEMIC; DIAGNOSTIC TEST AID
Pregnancy Category: B

AVAILABILITY 1 mg powder for injection

ACTION & *THERAPEUTIC EFFECT* Recombinant glucagon identical to glucagon produced by alpha cells of islets of Langerhans. Stimulates uptake of amino acids and their conversion to glucose precursors. Promotes lipolysis in liver and adipose tissue with release of free fatty acid and glycerol, which further stimulates ketogenesis and hepatic gluconeogenesis. Action in hypoglycemia relies on presence of adequate liver glycogen stores. *Increases blood glucose secondary to gluconeogenesis, the breakdown of glycogen to glucose in the liver.*

USES Emergency treatment of severe hypoglycemic reactions in diabetic patients who are unconscious or unable to swallow food or liquids and in psychiatric patients receiving insulin shock therapy. Also radiologic studies of GI tract to relax smooth muscle and thereby allow finer detail of mucosa; to diagnose insulinoma.

UNLABELED USES GI disturbances associated with spasm, cardiovascular emergencies, and to overcome cardiotoxic effects of beta-blockers, quinidine, tricyclic antidepressants; as an aid in abdominal imaging.

CONTRAINDICATIONS Hypersensitivity to glucagon or protein compounds; depleted glycogen stores in liver; insulinemia; pheochromocytoma.

CAUTIOUS USE Cardiac disease, CAD; adrenal insufficiency; malnutrition; children; pregnancy (category B), lactation.

ROUTE & DOSAGE

Hypoglycemia
Adult: **IM/IV/Subcutaneous** 1 mg, may repeat q5–20min if no response for 1–2 more doses
Child: **IM/IV/Subcutaneous** *Weight greater than 20 kg,* 1 mg; *weight less than 20 kg,* 20–30 mcg/kg (max: 1 mg/dose), may repeat q5–20min if no response for 1–2 more doses

Insulin Shock Therapy
Adult: **IM/IV/Subcutaneous** 1 mg usually 1 h after coma develops, may repeat in 25 min if no response

Diagnostic Aid to Relax Stomach or Upper GI Tract

Adult: **IM/IV** 0.25–2 mg 10 min before procedure

Diagnostic Aid for Colon Exam

Adult: **IM/IV** 2 mg 10 min before procedure

G

ADMINISTRATION

Note: 1 mg = 1 unit

Subcutaneous/Intramuscular

- Dilute 1 unit (1 mg) of glucagon with 1 mL of diluent supplied by manufacturer.
- Use immediately after reconstitution of dry powder. Discard any unused portion.
- Note: Glucagon is incompatible in syringe with any other drug.

Intravenous

PREPARE: **Direct:** Prepare as noted for intramuscular injection. Do not use a concentration greater than 1 unit/mL.

ADMINISTER: **Direct:** Give 1 unit or fraction thereof over 1 min.
- May be given through a Y-site D5W (not NS) infusing.

INCOMPATIBILITIES **Solution/additive: Sodium chloride.**

- Store unreconstituted vials and diluent at 20°–25° C (68°–77° F).

ADVERSE EFFECTS (≥1%) **GI:** Nausea and vomiting. **Body as a Whole:** Hypersensitivity reactions. **Skin:** Stevens-Johnson syndrome (erythema multiforme). **Metabolic:** Hyperglycemia, hypokalemia.

INTERACTIONS Drug: May enhance effect of ORAL ANTICOAGULANTS.

PHARMACOKINETICS Onset: 5–20 min. **Peak:** 30 min. **Duration:** 1–1.5 h. **Metabolism:** In liver, plasma, and kidneys. **Half-Life:** 3–10 min.

NURSING IMPLICATIONS

Assessment & Drug Effects

- Be prepared to give IV glucose if patient fails to respond to glucagon. Notify physician immediately.
- Note: Patient usually awakens from (diabetic) hypoglycemic coma 5–20 min after glucagon injection. Give PO carbohydrate as soon as possible after patient regains consciousness.
- Note: After recovery from hypoglycemic reaction, symptoms such as headache, nausea, and weakness may persist.

Patient & Family Education

- Note: Physician may request that a responsible family member be taught how to administer glucagon subcutaneously or IM for patients with frequent or severe hypoglycemic reactions. Notify physician promptly whenever a hypoglycemic reaction occurs so the reason for the reaction can be determined.
- Review package insert and directions (see ADMINISTRATION).

GLYBURIDE Pr

(glye′byoor-ide)

DiaBeta, Euglucon ✦, Glynase, Micronase

Classifications: ANTIDIABETIC; SULFONYLUREA

Therapeutic: ANTIDIABETIC

Pregnancy Category: C

AVAILABILITY 1.25 mg, 2.5 mg, 5 mg tablets; 1.5 mg, 3 mg, 4.5 mg, 6 mg micronized tablets

ACTION & *THERAPEUTIC EFFECT* One of the most potent of the second-generation sulfonylurea hypoglycemic agents. Appears to lower blood sugar concentration in both diabetic and nondiabetic individuals by sensitizing pancreatic beta cells to release insulin in the presence of elevated serum glucose levels. *Blood glucose-lowering effect persists during long-term glyburide treatment, but there is a gradual decline in meal-stimulated secretion of endogenous insulin toward pretreatment levels.*

USES Adjunct to diet and exercise to lower blood glucose in patients with type 2 diabetes mellitus.

CONTRAINDICATIONS Hypersensitivity to glyburide or sulfonylureas; diabetic ketoacidosis; as sole therapy for type 2 diabetes mellitus; type I diabetes mellitus; major surgery; severe trauma; severe infection; moderate or severe renal impairment (CrCl less than 50 mL/min) or renal failure; withhold 14 days before labor and delivery; lactation. Safe use in children is not established.
CAUTIOUS USE History of sulfonamide hypersensitivity; cardiovascular disease; thyroid disease; mild renal impairment or hepatic disease; older adults, debilitated, or malnourished patients; adrenal or pituitary insufficiency; pregnancy (category C).

ROUTE & DOSAGE

Control of Hyperglycemia
Adult: **PO** 1.25–5 mg/day with breakfast, may increase by 2.5–5 mg q1–2wk; greater than 15 mg/day should be given in divided doses with morning and evening meal (max: 20 mg/day); Micronized 1.5–3 mg/day (max: 12 mg/day)

ADMINISTRATION

Oral
- Give once daily in the morning with breakfast or with first main meal.
- Store in tightly closed, light-resistant container at 15°–30° C (59°–86° F).

ADVERSE EFFECTS (≥1%) **Metabolic:** Hypoglycemia. **GI:** Epigastric fullness, heartburn, nausea, vomiting. **Skin:** Pruritus, erythema, urticarial or cholestatic jaundice (rare) morbilliform eruptions. **Special Senses:** Blurred vision.

INTERACTIONS Drug: Alcohol causes disulfiram-like reaction in some patients; ORAL ANTICOAGULANTS, **chloramphenicol, clofibrate, phenylbutazone,** MAO INHIBITORS, SALICYLATES, **probenecid,** SULFONAMIDES, **clarithromycin** may potentiate hypoglycemic actions; THIAZIDES may antagonize hypoglycemic effects; **cimetidine** may increase glyburide levels, causing hypoglycemia. **Herbal: Ginseng, garlic** may increase hypoglycemic effects.

PHARMACOKINETICS Absorption: Readily absorbed from GI tract. **Onset:** 15–60 min. **Peak:** 1–2 h. **Duration:** Up to 24 h. **Distribution:** Distributed in highest concentrations in liver, kidneys, and intestines; crosses placenta. **Metabolism:** Extensively in liver. **Elimination:** Equally in urine and feces. **Half-Life:** 10 h.

NURSING IMPLICATIONS

Assessment & Drug Effects
- Monitor blood glucose levels carefully during the dangerous early treatment period when dosage is being individualized. Older adults are especially vulnerable to glyburide-induced hypoglycemia (see Appendix F) because the antidiabetic agent is long-acting.

- Note: The first signs of hypoglycemia may be hard to detect when the patient is also receiving a beta-blocker or is an older adult.
- Lab tests: Monitor at regular intervals: Fasting and postprandial blood glucose, HbA1C, and liver function tests.

Patient & Family Education

- Eat or drink some form of sugar (e.g., corn syrup, orange juice with 2 or 3 tsp of table sugar) when symptoms of hypoglycemia occur. Report reaction to physician promptly.
- Remember that loss of control of diabetes may result from stress such as fever, surgery, trauma, or infection. Check blood glucose more frequently during stress periods.
- Keep all follow-up medical appointments and adhere to dietary instructions, regular exercise program, and scheduled blood testing.
- Report blurred vision to physician.

G

GLYCERIN

(gli'ser-in)

Fleet Babylax, Glycerol, Osmoglyn

GLYCERIN ANHYDROUS

Ophthalgan

Classifications: HYPEROSMOTIC LAXATIVE; ANTIGLAUCOMA

Therapeutic: HYPEROSMOTIC LAXATIVE; ANTIGLAUCOMA

Pregnancy Category: C

AVAILABILITY 50% oral solution; suppositories; 4 mL/applicator, ophth solution

ACTION & *THERAPEUTIC EFFECT*
When administered orally, glycerin raises plasma osmotic pressure by withdrawing fluid from extravascular spaces; lowers ocular tension by decreasing volume of intraocular fluid. May also reduce CSF pressure. Topical application to eye reduces edema by hydroscopic effect. Glycerin suppositories apparently work by causing dehydration of exposed tissue, which produces an irritant effect, and by absorbing water from tissues, thus creating more bowel mass. Both actions stimulate peristalsis in the large bowel. *Reduces intraocular pressure by lowering intraocular fluid. Relieves constipation by absorption of water and stimulation of peristalsis.*

USES Orally to reduce elevated intraocular pressure (IOP) before or after surgery in patients with acute narrow-angle glaucoma, retinal detachment, or cataract and to reduce elevated CSF pressure. Sterile glycerin (anhydrous) is used topically to reduce superficial corneal edema resulting from trauma, surgery, or disease and to facilitate ophthalmoscopic examination. Used rectally (suppository or enema) to relieve constipation.

UNLABELED USES To reduce mortality due to strokes in older adults.

CONTRAINDICATIONS Diabetic ketoacidosis; moderate or severe renal impairment (CrCl less than 50 mL/min), renal failure.

CAUTIOUS USE Cardiac disease, mild renal impairment; hepatic disease; diabetes mellitus; thyroid disease; dehydrated or older adults; pregnancy (category C); lactation.

ROUTE & DOSAGE

Decrease IOP

Adult/Child: **PO** 1–1.8 g/kg 1–1.5 h before ocular surgery, may repeat q5h

Constipation
Adult/Child (6 y or older): **PR** Insert 1 suppository or 5–15 mL of enema high into rectum and retain for 15 min
Child (younger than 6 y): **PR** Insert 1 infant suppository or 2–5 mL of enema high into rectum and retain for 15 min
Neonate: **PR** 0.5 mL of rectal solution (enema)

Reduction of Corneal Edema
Adult: **Topical** 1–2 drops instilled into eye q3–4h

ADMINISTRATION

Oral
- Pour oral solution over crushed ice and have patient sip through a straw.
- Prevent or relieve headache (from cerebral dehydration) by having patient lie down during and after administration of drug.

Rectal
- Ensure that suppository is inserted beyond rectal sphincter.

ADVERSE EFFECTS (≥1%) **CNS:** Headache, dizziness, disorientation. **CV:** Irregular heartbeat. **GI:** Nausea, vomiting, thirst, diarrhea, abdominal cramps, rectal discomfort, hyperemia of rectal mucosa. **Metabolic:** Hyperglycemia, glycosuria, dehydration, hyperosmolar nonketotic coma.

PHARMACOKINETICS Absorption: Readily absorbed from GI tract after oral administration; rectal preparations are poorly absorbed. **Onset:** 10 min PO. **Peak:** 30 min–2 h. **Duration:** 4–8 h. **Metabolism:** 80% metabolized in liver; 10–20% metabolized in kidneys to CO_2 and water or utilized in glucose or glycogen synthesis. **Elimination:** 7–14% excreted unchanged in urine. **Half-Life:** 30–40 min.

NURSING IMPLICATIONS

Assessment & Drug Effects
- Consult physician regarding fluid intake in patients receiving drug for elevated IOP. Although hypotonic fluids will relieve thirst and headache caused by the dehydrating action of glycerin, these fluids may nullify its osmotic effect.
- Monitor glycemic control in diabetics. Drug may cause hyperglycemia (see Appendix F).

Patient & Family Education
- Evacuation usually comes 15–30 min after administration of glycerin rectal suppository or enema.
- Note: Slight hyperglycemia and glycosuria may occur with PO use; adjustment in antidiabetic medication dosage may be required.

GLYCOPYRROLATE

(glye-koe-pye'roe-late)
Robinul, Robinul Forte
Classifications: ANTICHOLINERGIC; ANTIMUSCARINIC; ANTISPASMODIC
Therapeutic: GI ANTISPASMODIC
Prototype: Atropine
Pregnancy Category: B

AVAILABILITY 1 mg, 2 mg tablets; 0.2 mg/mL injection

ACTION & *THERAPEUTIC EFFECT* Synthetic anticholinergic (antimuscarinic) that inhibits muscarinic action of acetylcholine on autonomic neuroeffector sites innervated by postganglionic cholinergic nerves. *Inhibits motility of GI and genitourinary tract; it also decreases volume of gastric and pan-*

creatic secretions, saliva, and perspiration.

USES Adjunctive management of peptic ulcer and other GI disorders associated with hyperacidity, hypermotility, and spasm. Also used parenterally as preanesthetic and intraoperative medication and to reverse neuromuscular blockade.

CONTRAINDICATIONS Glaucoma; asthma; prostatic hypertrophy, obstructive uropathy; obstructive lesions or atony of GI tract; achalasia; severe ulcerative colitis; myasthenia gravis; BPH; urinary tract obstruction; during cyclopropane anesthesia; neonates younger than 1 mo.

CAUTIOUS USE Autonomic neuropathy, hepatic or renal disease; cardiac arrhythmias; pregnancy (category B), lactation.

ROUTE & DOSAGE

Peptic Ulcer

Adult: **PO** 1 mg t.i.d or 2 mg b.i.d. or t.i.d. in equally divided intervals (max: 8 mg/day), then decrease to 1 mg b.i.d. **IM/IV** 0.1–0.2 mg 3–4 times/day

Reversal of Neuromuscular Blockade

Adult/Child: **IV** 0.2 mg administered with 1 mg of neostigmine or 5 mg pyridostigmine

Preanesthetic

Child: **PO** 40–100 mcg/kg t.i.d.–q.i.d. **IM** 4–10 mcg/kg q3–4h
Adult: **IM** 4 mcg/kg 30–60 min before procedure

ADMINISTRATION

Oral

- Give without regard to meals.

Intramuscular

- Give undiluted, deep into a large muscle.

Intravenous

PREPARE: **Direct:** Give undiluted.
- Inspect for cloudiness and discoloration. Discard if present.

ADMINISTER: **Direct:** Give 0.2 mg or fraction thereof over 1–2 min.

INCOMPATIBILITIES **Solution/additive: Chloramphenicol, dexamethasone, diazepam, dimenhydrinate, methohexital, methylprednisolone, pentazocine, phenobarbital, secobarbital, sodium bicarbonate, thiopental. Y-site: Propofol.**

- Store at 20°–25° C (68°–77° F).

ADVERSE EFFECTS (≥1%) **Body as a Whole:** *Decreased sweating,* weakness. **CNS:** Dizziness, drowsiness, overdosage (neuromuscular blockade with curare-like action leading to muscle weakness and paralysis is possible). **CV:** Palpitation, tachycardia. **GI:** *Xerostomia,* constipation. **GU:** *Urinary hesitancy or retention.* **Special Senses:** Blurred vision, mydriasis.

INTERACTIONS Drug: Amantadine, ANTIHISTAMINES, TRICYCLIC ANTIDEPRESSANTS, **quinidine, disopyramide, procainamide** compound anticholinergic effects; decreases **levodopa** effects; **methotrimeprazine** may precipitate extrapyramidal effects; decreases antipsychotic effects (decreased absorption) of PHENOTHIAZINES.

PHARMACOKINETICS Absorption: Poorly and incompletely absorbed from GI tract. **Onset:** 1 min IV; 15–30 min IM/Subcutaneous; 1 h PO. **Peak:** 30–45 min IM/Subcutaneous; 1 h PO. **Duration:** 2–7 h IM/Subcutaneous; 8–12 h PO. **Distribution:** Crosses placenta. **Metabolism:** Minimally in liver. **Elimination:** 85% in urine. **Half-Life:** 30–70 min (adult), 20–99 min (child), 20–120 min (infant).

NURSING IMPLICATIONS

Assessment & Drug Effects

- Incidence and severity of adverse effects are generally dose related.
- Monitor I&O ratio and pattern particularly in older adults. Watch for urinary hesitancy and retention.
- Monitor vital signs, especially when drug is given parenterally. Report any changes in heart rate or rhythm.

Patient & Family Education

- Avoid high environmental temperatures (heat prostration can occur because of decreased sweating).
- Do not drive or engage in other potentially hazardous activities requiring mental alertness until response to drug is known.
- Use good oral hygiene, rinse mouth with water frequently and use a saliva substitute to lessen effects of dry mouth.

GOLD SODIUM THIOMALATE

(thye-oh-mah'late)

Myochrysine ♣

Classifications: BIOLOGICAL RESPONSE MODIFIER; IMMUNOMODULATOR; DISEASE-MODIFYING ANTIRHEUMATIC DRUG (DMARD)

Therapeutic: ANTIRHEUMATIC; GOLD COMPOUND

Prototype: Auranofin

Pregnancy Category: C

AVAILABILITY 50 mg/mL injection

ACTION & *THERAPEUTIC EFFECT* Water-soluble gold compound. Drug appears to act by suppression of phagocytosis, altered immune responses, and possibly by inhibition of prostaglandin synthesis. *Has immunomodulatory and anti-inflammatory effects.*

USES Selected patients (adults and juveniles) with acute rheumatoid arthritis.

UNLABELED USES Psoriatic arthritis, Felty's syndrome.

CONTRAINDICATIONS History of severe toxicity from previous exposure to gold or other heavy metals; severe debilitation; SLE, Sjögren's syndrome in rheumatoid arthritis; renal disease; hepatic dysfunction, history of infectious hepatitis or hematologic disorders; uncontrolled diabetes or CHF.

CAUTIOUS USE History of drug allergies or hypersensitivity, marked hypertension; previous kidney or liver disease; compromised cerebral or cardiovascular circulation; pregnancy (category C).

ROUTE & DOSAGE

Rheumatoid Arthritis

Adult: **IM** 10 mg wk 1, 25 mg wk 2, then 25–50 mg/wk to a cumulative dose of 1 g (if improvement occurs, continue at 25–50 mg q2wk for 2–20 wk, then q3–4wk indefinitely or until adverse effects occur)

Child: **IM** 10 mg test dose, then 1 mg/kg/wk or 2.5–5 mg for wk 1 and 2, followed by 1 mg/kg q1–4wk (max single dose: 50 mg)

ADMINISTRATION

Intramuscular

- Agitate vial before withdrawing dose to ensure uniform suspension.
- Give deep into upper outer quadrant of gluteus maximus with patient lying down. Patient should remain recumbent for at least 30 min after injection because of the danger of "nitritoid reaction" (tran-

sient giddiness, vertigo, facial flushing, fainting).

- Observe for allergic reactions.
- Store in tight, light-resistant containers at 15°–30° C (59°–86° F). Do not use if any darker than pale yellow.

ADVERSE EFFECTS (≥1%) **CNS:** Dizziness, syncope, sweating, flushing. **CV:** Bradycardia. **GI:** Hepatitis, metallic taste, *stomatitis,* nausea, vomiting. **Hematologic:** Agranulocytosis, aplastic anemia, eosinophilia (all rare). **Urogenital:** Nephrotic syndrome, glomerulitis with hematuria, *proteinuria.* **Skin:** Transient pruritus, *erythema, dermatitis,* fixed drug eruption, alopecia, shedding of nails, gray to blue pigmentation of skin (chrysiasis). **Special Senses:** Gold deposits in ocular tissues, *photosensitivity.* **Body as a Whole:** Peripheral neuritis, angioneurotic edema, interstitial pneumonitis, anaphylaxis (rare). **Respiratory:** Pulmonary fibrosis.

INTERACTIONS Drug: ANTIMALARIALS, IMMUNOSUPPRESSANTS, **penicillamine, phenylbutazone** increase risk of blood dyscrasias.

PHARMACOKINETICS Absorption: Slowly and irregularly absorbed from IM site. **Peak:** 3–6 h. **Distribution:** Widely distributed, especially to synovial fluid, kidney, liver, and spleen; does not cross blood–brain barrier; crosses placenta. **Metabolism:** Not studied. **Elimination:** 60–90% of dose ultimately excreted in urine; also eliminated in feces; traces may be found in urine for 6 mo. **Half-Life:** 3–168 days.

NURSING IMPLICATIONS

Assessment & Drug Effects

- Lab tests: Prior to each injection, urinalysis for protein, blood, and sediment. Withhold drug and notify physician promptly if proteinuria or hematuria develops. Also do baseline Hgb and RBC, WBC count, differential count, platelet count before initiation of therapy and at regular intervals.
- Note: Rapid reduction in hemoglobin level, WBC count below 4000/mm^3, eosinophil count above 5%, and platelet count below 100,000/mm^3 signify possible toxicity.
- Interview and examine patient before each injection to detect occurrence of transient pruritus or dermatitis (both are common early indications of toxicity), stomatitis (sore tongue, palate, or throat), metallic taste, indigestion, or other signs and symptoms of possible toxicity. Interrupt treatment immediately and notify physician if any of these reactions occurs.
- Observe for allergic reaction, which may occur almost immediately after injection, 10 min after injection, or at any time during therapy. Withhold drug and notify physician if observed. Keep antidote dimercaprol (BAL) on hand during time of injection.

Patient & Family Education

- Therapeutic effects may not appear until after 2 mo of therapy.
- Notify physician of rapid improvement in joint swelling; this is indicative that you are closely approaching drug tolerance level.
- Use protective measures in sunlight. Exposure to sunlight may aggravate gold dermatitis.
- Notify physician at the appearance of unexplained skin bruising; this is always an indication for doing a platelet count.
- Know possible adverse reactions and report any symptom suggestive of toxicity immediately to physician.

GOLIMUMAB

(go-li-mu′mab)
Simponi
Classifications: BIOLOGICAL RESPONSE MODIFIER; MONOCLONAL ANTIBODY; TUMOR NECROSIS FACTOR (TNF) MODIFIER; DISEASE-MODIFYING ANTIRHEUMATIC DRUG (DMARD)
Therapeutic: ANTIRHEUMATIC (DMARD); ANTIPSORIATIC
Prototype: Etanercept
Pregnancy Category: B

AVAILABILITY 50 mg/0.5 mL prefilled syringe solution; 50 mg/0.5 mL SmartJect auto injector solution

ACTION & *THERAPEUTIC EFFECT* A monoclonal antibody that binds to TNF-alpha, thus preventing it from binding to its receptors. TNF (a cytokine) is part of the immune and inflammatory response. However, elevated levels of TNF are found in the synovial fluids of rheumatoid arthritis (RA) patients. *Effectiveness is indicated by improved RA symtomatology and/or decreased inflammation in other inflammatory disorders.*

USES Treatment of moderately to severely active rheumatoid arthritis in combination with methotrexate, active ankylosing spondylitis, and active psoriatic arthritis

CONTRAINDICATIONS Hypersensitivity to golimumab; serious infection or sepsis; fungal infection; live vaccines; agranulocytosis; malignancy; lactation.
CAUTIOUS USE History of hepatitis B; rheumatoid arthritis; CHF; demyelization disorders, multiple sclerosis; cytopenia; pregnancy (category B).

ROUTE & DOSAGE

Rheumatoid Arthritis
Adult: **Subcutaneous** 50 mg qmo

Ankylosing Spondylitis
Adult: **Subcutaneous** 50 mg qmo

Psoriatic Arthritis
Adult: **Subcutaneous** 50 mg qmo

ADMINISTRATION

Subcutaneous
- Allow prefilled syringe/autoinjector to come to room temperature for 30 min prior to injection. Do not warm any other way.
- Do not shake the autoinjector at any time. After injection, do not pull autoinjector away from skin until a second click sound (3–15 sec after the first sound) is heard.
- Rotate injection sites. Do not inject into areas that are tender, bruised, red, or hard.
- Do not initiate treatment in anyone with an active infection.
- Store refrigerated at 2°–8° C (36°–46° F) and protect from light by keeping in carton until use.

ADVERSE EFFECTS (≥1%) **Body as a Whole:** Influenza, injection site erythema. **CNS:** Dizziness, pyrexia. **CV:** Hypertension. **GI:** Oral herpes. **Metabolic:** Elevated ALT and AST levels. **Respiratory:** Bronchitis, *nasopharyngitis,* sinusitis, *upper respiratory tract infection.* **Skin:** Paraesthesia.

INTERACTIONS Drug: Abatacept, anakinra and other TNF-ALPHA BLOCKERS may increase the risk of serious infection.

PHARMACOKINETICS Peak: 2–6 days. **Half-Life:** 2 wk.

G

NURSING IMPLICATIONS

Assessment & Drug Effects

- Monitor closely for S&S of infection.
- Withhold drug and notify physician if symptoms of an infection develop.
- Monitor for and report new-onset and exacerbations of psoriasis.
- Lab tests: Baseline and periodic TB tests, periodic LFTs.

Patient & Family Education

- Contact physician immediately for any of the following: Symptoms of infection; jaundice; extreme fatigue; poor appetite or vomiting; or pain in the upper, right abdomen.
- If a case of pre-existing psoriasis worsens or if a new rash develops, contact physician.

GOSERELIN ACETATE

(gos-er′e-lin)

Zoladex

Classification: GONADOTROPIN-RELEASING HORMONE (GnRH) ANALOG

Therapeutic: GnRH ANALOG

Prototype: Leuprolide

Pregnancy Category: X

AVAILABILITY 3.6 mg, 10.8 mg subcutaneous implant

ACTION & *THERAPEUTIC EFFECT*
A synthetic form of luteinizing hormone-releasing hormone (LHRH or GnRH) that inhibits pituitary gonadotropin secretion. *With chronic administration, serum testosterone levels fall into the range normally seen with surgically castrated men.*

USES Prostate cancer, breast cancer. Endometrial thinning agent prior to endometrial ablation for dysfunctional uterine bleeding.

UNLABELED USES Endometriosis, uterine leiomyomas.

CONTRAINDICATIONS Known hypersensitivity to an LHRH; vaginal bleeding; endometriosis or endometrial thinning; hypercalcemia; pregnancy (category X); lactation.

CAUTIOUS USE Urinary tract obstruction; family history of osteoporosis; osteoporosis; patients at risk for spinal cord compression or urinary tract obstruction. Safety and efficacy in children are not established.

ROUTE & DOSAGE

Prostate Cancer, Breast Cancer, Endometriosis, Uterine Leiomyomas

Adult: **Subcutaneous** 3.6 mg q28days, 10.8 mg depot q12wk

Endometrial Thinning Prior to Endometrial Ablation

Adult: **Subcutaneous** 3.6 mg q28days

ADMINISTRATION

Subcutaneous

- Follow manufacturer's directions exactly for implanting the drug subcutaneously in the upper abdominal wall.
- Store at room temperature not to exceed 25° C (77° F).

ADVERSE EFFECTS (≥1%) **CNS:** Headache, tumor flare. **Endocrine:** Gynecomastia, breast swelling and tenderness, *postmenopausal symptoms* (*hot flashes*, vaginal dryness). **GI:** Nausea. **Urogenital:** Vaginal spotting, breakthrough bleeding, decreased libido, *impotence*. **Musculoskeletal:** Bone pain, bone loss.

DIAGNOSTIC TEST INTERFERENCE Increased levels of ***alkaline phosphatase*** and ***estradiol*** in the first 1–8 days; initial increase then decrease in ***FSH, LH,*** and ***testosterone.***

INTERACTIONS Drug: No clinically significant interactions established.

PHARMACOKINETICS Absorption: Rapidly absorbed following subcutaneous administration. **Duration:** 29 days. **Elimination:** Excreted by kidneys. **Half-Life:** 4.9 h.

NURSING IMPLICATIONS

Assessment & Drug Effects

- Monitor carefully during the first month of therapy for S&S of spinal cord compression or ureteral obstruction in patients with prostate cancer. Report immediately to physician.
- Anticipate a transient worsening of symptoms (e.g., bone pain) during the first weeks of therapy in patients with prostate cancer.

Patient & Family Education

- Note: Sexual dysfunction in men and hot flashes may accompany drug use.
- Notify physician immediately of symptoms of spinal cord compression or urinary obstruction.

GRANISETRON

(gran'i-se-tron)

Granisol, Kytril, Sancuso

Classifications: ANTIEMETIC; $5\text{-}HT_3$ ANTAGONIST

Therapeutic: ANTIEMETIC

Prototype: Ondansetron

Pregnancy Category: B

AVAILABILITY 1 mg tablets; 1 mg/mL injection; 2 mg/10 mL oral solution; 3.1 mg transdermal patch

ACTION & *THERAPEUTIC EFFECT* Granisetron is a selective serotonin ($5\text{-}HT_3$) receptor antagonist. Serotonin receptors of the $5\text{-}HT_3$ type are located centrally in the chemoreceptor trigger zone, and peripherally on the vagal nerve terminals. Serotonin released from the wall of the small intestine stimulates these vagal afferent neurons through the serotonin receptors, and initiates the vomiting reflex. *Effective in preventing nausea and vomiting associated with cancer chemotherapy.*

USES Prevention of nausea and vomiting associated with initial and repeat courses of emetogenic cancer therapy, including high-dose cisplatin, postoperative nausea and vomiting.

CONTRAINDICATIONS Hypersensitivity to granisetron, or benzyl alcohol; GI obstruction; neonates; children younger than 2 y.

CAUTIOUS USE Hypersensitivity to ondansetron or similar drugs; liver disease; pregnancy (category B), lactation.

ROUTE & DOSAGE

Chemotherapy-Related Nausea and Vomiting

Adult/Child: **IV** *Older than 2 y,* 10 mcg/kg, beginning at least 30 min before initiation of chemotherapy (up to 40 mcg/kg per dose has been used) **PO** 1 mg b.i.d., start 1 mg up to 1 h prior to chemotherapy, then second tab 12 h later OR 2 mg daily

Adult: **Transdermal** Apply 1 patch q5days

Postoperative Nausea and Vomiting

Adult: **IV** 1 mg before anesthesia induction or before reversal of anesthesia

G

ADMINISTRATION

Oral

- Give only on the day of chemotherapy.

Transdermal

- Apply patch to upper outer arm 24–48 h before start of chemotherapy.
- Remove patch no sooner than 24 h after completion of chemotherapy.
- Patch may be left in place for up to 7 days.

Intravenous

PREPARE: **Direct:** Give undiluted. **IV Infusion:** Dilute in NS or D5W to a total volume of 20–50 mL. ▪ Prepare infusion at time of administration; do not mix in solution with other drugs.

ADMINISTER: **Direct:** Give a single dose over 30 sec. **IV Infusion:** Infuse diluted drug over 5 min or longer; complete infusion 20–30 min prior to initiation of chemotherapy.

INCOMPATIBILITIES **Y-site: Amphotericin B, doxorubicin.**

- Store at 15°–30° C (59°–86° F) for 24 h after dilution under normal lighting conditions.

ADVERSE EFFECTS (≥1%) **CNS:** *Headache,* dizziness, somnolence, insomnia, labile mood, anxiety, fatigue. **GI:** Constipation, diarrhea, elevated liver function tests.

INTERACTIONS Drug: Ketoconazole may inhibit metabolism.

PHARMACOKINETICS Onset: Several minutes. **Duration:** Approximately 24 h. **Distribution:** Widely distributed in body tissues. **Metabolism:** Appears to be metabolized in liver. **Elimination:** Excreted in urine as metabolites. **Half-Life:** 10–11 h in cancer patients, 4–5 h in healthy volunteers.

NURSING IMPLICATIONS

Assessment & Drug Effects

- Monitor the frequency and severity of nausea and vomiting.
- Lab tests: Monitor liver function; elevated AST and ALT values usually normalize within 2 wk of last dose.
- Assess for headache, which usually responds to nonnarcotic analgesics.

Patient & Family Education

- Note: Headache requiring an analgesic for relief is a common adverse effect.
- Learn ways to manage constipation.

GRISEOFULVIN MICROSIZE

(gri-see-oh-ful'vin)

Fulvicin-U/F, Grifulvin V, Grisactin, Grisovin-FP ♣

GRISEOFULVIN ULTRAMICROSIZE

Fulvicin P/G, Grisactin Ultra, Gris-PEG

Classification: ANTIFUNGAL ANTIBIOTIC

Therapeutic: ANTIFUNGAL

Pregnancy Category: C

AVAILABILITY Griseofulvin Microsize: 250 mg, 500 mg tablets, 250 mg capsules; 125 mg/5 mL suspension; **Griseofulvin Ultramicrosize:** 125 mg, 165 mg, 250 mg, 330 mg tablets.

ACTION & *THERAPEUTIC EFFECT* Arrests metaphase of cell division by disrupting mitotic spindle structure in fungal cells. Deposits in keratin precursor cells and has special affinity for diseased tissue. It is tightly bound to new keratin of skin, hair, and nails that becomes highly resistant to fungal invasion. *Effective against various species of* Epidermophyton, Microsporum, *and* Trichophyton *(has no effect on other fungi, including* Candida, *bacteria, and yeasts).*

USES Mycotic disease of skin, hair, and nails not amenable to conventional topical measures. Concomitant use of appropriate topical agent may be required, particularly for tinea pedis.

UNLABELED USES Raynaud's disease, angina pectoris, and gout.

CONTRAINDICATIONS Hypersensitivity to griseofulvin; porphyria; hepatocellular failure; SLE; lactation, children 2 y or younger, prophylaxis against fungal infections.

CAUTIOUS USE Penicillin-sensitive patients (possibility if cross-sensitivity with penicillin exists; however, reportedly penicillin-sensitive patients have been treated without difficulty); hepatic impairment; pregnancy (category C).

ROUTE & DOSAGE

Tinea Corporis, Tinea Cruris, Tinea Capitis

Adult: **PO** 500 mg microsize or 330–375 mg ultramicrosize daily in single or divided doses
Child: **PO** 10–20 mg/kg/day microsize or 5–10 mg/kg/day ultramicrosize in single or divided doses

Tinea Pedis, Tinea Unguium

Adult: **PO** 0.75–1 g microsize or 660–750 mg ultramicrosize daily in single or divided doses (decrease microsize dose to 500 mg/day after response is noted)
Child: **PO** 10–20 mg/kg/day microsize or 5–10 mg/kg/day ultramicrosize in single or divided doses

ADMINISTRATION

Oral

- Give with or after meals to allay GI disturbances.
- Give the microsize formulations with a high fat content meal (increases drug absorption rate) to enhance serum levels. Consult physician.
- Store at 15°–30° C (59°–86° F) in tightly covered containers unless otherwise directed.

ADVERSE EFFECTS (≥1%) **Body as a Whole:** Hypersensitivity (urticaria, photosensitivity, skin rashes, pruritus, fixed drug eruption, serum sickness syndromes, severe angioedema). **CNS:** *Severe headache,* insomnia, fatigue, mental confusion, impaired performance of routine functions, psychotic symptoms, vertigo. **GI:** Heartburn, nausea, vomiting, diarrhea, flatulence, dry mouth, thirst, decreased taste acuity, anorexia, unpleasant taste, furred tongue, oral thrush. **Hematologic:** Leukopenia, neutropenia, granulocytopenia, punctate basophilia, monocytosis. **Urogenital:** Nephrotoxicity (proteinuria); hepatotoxicity; estrogen-like effects (in children); aggravation of SLE. **Other:** Overgrowth of nonsusceptible organisms; candidal intertrigo.

INTERACTIONS Drug: Alcohol may cause flushing and tachycardia; BARBITURATES may decrease activity of griseofulvin; may decrease hypoprothrombinemic effects of ORAL ANTICOAGULANTS; may increase **estrogen** metabolism, resulting in breakthrough bleeding, and decrease contraceptive efficacy of ORAL CONTRACEPTIVES.

PHARMACOKINETICS Absorption: Absorbed primarily from duodenum; microsize is variably and unpredictably absorbed; ultramicrosize is almost completely absorbed. **Peak:** 4–8 h. **Distribution:** Concentrates in skin, hair, nails, fat, and skeletal muscle; crosses placenta. **Metabolism:** In liver. **Elimination:** Mainly in urine; some excretion in perspiration. **Half-Life:** 9–24 h.

G

NURSING IMPLICATIONS

Assessment & Drug Effects

- Inquire about history of sensitivity to griseofulvin, penicillins, or other allergies prior to initiating treatment.
- Monitor food intake. Drug may alter taste sensations, and this may cause appetite suppression and inadequate nutrient intake.
- Lab tests: WBC with differential at least once weekly during first month of therapy or longer; periodic renal and hepatic function tests are also advised.

Patient & Family Education

- Continuing treatment as prescribed to prevent relapse, even if you experience symptomatic relief after 48–96 h of therapy.
- Note: Duration of treatment depends on time required to replace infected skin, hair, or nails, and thus varies with infection site. Average duration of treatment for tinea capitis (scalp ringworm), 4–6 wk; tinea corporis (body ringworm), 2–4 wk; tinea pedis (athlete's foot), 4–8 wk; tinea unguium (nail fungus), at least 4 mo for fingernails, depending on rate of growth, and 6 mo or more for toenails.
- Avoid exposure to intense natural or artificial sunlight, because photosensitivity-type reactions may occur.
- Note: Headaches often occur during early therapy but frequently disappear with continued drug administration.
- Avoid alcohol while taking this drug. Disulfiram-type reaction (see Appendix F) are possible with ingestion of alcohol during therapy.
- Pharmacologic effects of oral contraceptives may be reduced. Breakthrough bleeding and pregnancy may occur. Alternative forms of birth control should be used during therapy.

GUAIFENESIN (Pr)

(gwye-fen′e-sin)

Anti-Tuss, GG-Cen, Glyceryl Guaiacolate, Glycotuss, Glytuss, Guiatuss, Humibid, Hytuss, Malotuss, Mytussin, Mucinex, Resyl ♣, Robitussin

Classification: EXPECTORANT

Therapeutic: EXPECTORANT

Pregnancy Category: C

AVAILABILITY 100 mg/5 mL syrup; 100 mg/5 mL, 200 mg/5 mL liquid; 200 mg capsules; 300 mg sustained release capsules; 100 mg, 200 mg, 1200 mg tablets; 600 mg sustained release tablets

ACTION & *THERAPEUTIC EFFECT* Enhances reflex outflow of respiratory tract fluids by irritation of gastric mucosa. *Aids in expectoration by reducing adhesiveness and surface tension of secretions.*

USES To combat dry, nonproductive cough associated with colds and bronchitis. A common ingredient in cough mixtures.

CONTRAINDICATIONS Hypersensitivity to guaifenesin; cough due to

CHF, ACE inhibitor therapy, or tobacco smoking; children younger than 6 y.

CAUTIOUS USE Chronic cough; asthma; pregnancy (category C), lactation.

ROUTE & DOSAGE

Cough
Adult: **PO** 200–400 mg q4h up to 2.4 g/day
Child: **PO** *Younger than 2 y,* 12 mg/kg/day in 6 divided doses; *2–5 y,* 50–100 mg q4h up to 600 mg/day; *6–11 y,* 100–200 mg q4h up to 1.2 g/day

ADMINISTRATION

Oral
- Ensure that sustained release form of drug is not chewed or crushed. It **must be** swallowed whole.
- Follow dose with a full glass of water if not contraindicated.
- Carefully observe maximum daily doses for adults and children.

ADVERSE EFFECTS (≥1%) **GI:** Low incidence of nausea. **CNS:** Drowsiness.

DIAGNOSTIC TEST INTERFERENCE Guaifenesin may produce color interference with certain laboratory determinations of ***urinary 5-hydroxyindoleacetic acid (5-HIAA)*** and ***vanillylmandelic acid (VMA).***

INTERACTIONS Drug: By inhibiting platelet function, guaifenesin may increase risk of hemorrhage in patients receiving **heparin** therapy.

NURSING IMPLICATIONS

Assessment & Drug Effects
- Monitor for therapeutic effectiveness. Persistent cough may indicate a serious condition requiring further diagnostic work.
- Notify physician if high fever, rash, or headaches develop.

Patient & Family Education
- Increase fluid intake to help loosen mucus; drink at least 8 glasses of fluid daily.
- Contact physician if cough persists beyond 1 wk.
- Contact physician if high fever, rash, or headache develops.

GUANABENZ ACETATE

(gwan'a-benz)

Wytensin

Classifications: ALPHA-ADRENERGIC AGONIST; CENTRAL-ACTING ANTIHYPERTENSIVE

Therapeutic: ANTIHYPERTENSIVE

Prototype: Methyldopa

Pregnancy Category: C

AVAILABILITY 4 mg, 8 mg tablets

ACTION & *THERAPEUTIC EFFECT* Centrally acting alpha$_2$-adrenergic agonist that lowers BP, primarily by stimulating central alpha-adrenergic receptors that lead to inhibition of sympathetic outflow from brain. *Reduces both supine and standing BP, usually without producing postural hypotension, and slightly lowers pulse rate. Since central adrenergic hyperactivity causes symptoms of narcotic withdrawal, guanabenz appears to help control abstinence symptoms by reducing norepinephrine output.*

USES Used alone in treatment of hypertension or in combination with a thiazide diuretic.

UNLABELED USES Opiate detoxification, analgesic for chronic pain.

CONTRAINDICATIONS Lactation. Safe use in children is not established.

CAUTIOUS USE Severe coronary insufficiency, recent MI, cerebrovascular disease, severe hepatic or renal failure; older adults; concurrent use of MAOI therapy; pregnancy (category C).

ROUTE & DOSAGE

Hypertension

Adult: **PO** 4 mg b.i.d., may increase by 4–8 mg/day q1–2wk up to 32 mg b.i.d.
Geriatric: **PO** 4 mg once daily, may increase q1–2wk

Opiate Withdrawal

Adult: **PO** 4 mg b.i.d. to q.i.d.

ADMINISTRATION

Oral

- One dose is usually given at bedtime to ensure overnight control and reduce possibility of daytime drowsiness or sedation.
- Store at 15°–30° C (59°–86° F) in tightly closed containers unless otherwise directed.

ADVERSE EFFECTS (≥1%) **CNS:** *Drowsiness* or *sedation,* dizziness, weakness, headache, anxiety, ataxia, depression, sleep disturbances, somnolence. **CV:** Chest pain, edema, arrhythmias, palpitation, hypotension, bradycardia, nervousness. **GI:** *Dry mouth,* nausea, epigastric pain, diarrhea, vomiting, constipation, abdominal discomfort, taste disorders. **Urogenital:** Increased urination, urinary frequency, sexual dysfunction. **Special Senses:** Blurred vision, miosis, nasal congestion. **Body as a Whole:** Dyspnea, muscle aches, aches in extremities, lethargy, irritability, unusual fatigue or weakness. **Skin:** Rash, pruritus.

INTERACTIONS Drug: Alcohol and other CNS DEPRESSANTS compound CNS depression; TRICYCLIC ANTIDEPRESSANTS may reduce antihypertensive effects of guanabenz.

PHARMACOKINETICS Absorption: 75% absorbed from GI tract. **Onset:** 60 min. **Peak:** 2–5 h. **Duration:** 6–12 h. **Distribution:** Widely distributed; crosses blood–brain barrier; not known if crosses placenta or distributed into breast milk. **Metabolism:** Extensively metabolized. **Elimination:** 80% in urine; 20% in feces. **Half-Life:** 4–14 h.

NURSING IMPLICATIONS

Assessment & Drug Effects

- Monitor BP and HR. Report palpitations or hypotension to physician.
- Evaluate mental status and alertness.
- Lab tests: Baseline and periodic blood chemistry (serum potassium, CBC, creatinine, uric acid, cholesterol, glucose), urinalysis for protein and sugar.
- Give early attention and specific treatment to dry mouth. It can interfere with patient's food and fluid intake; deprivation of normal salivary flow is a potential dental hazard since it favors demineralization of teeth; and it can be a factor in noncompliance.

Patient & Family Education

- Make all position changes slowly and in stages in the event that you experience orthostatic hypotension. This is important in older adults, who tend to be more sensitive to normal adult doses of antihypertensive drugs.
- Do not omit a dose or stop drug therapy without consulting physician. Do not discontinue therapy abruptly; can cause sympathetic overactivity (anxiety, nervousness, palpitation, chest pain, fast or ir-

regular heartbeat, trembling, flushing, headache, increased sweating and salivation, elevation of BP, usually above basal level).

- Do not drive or engage in potentially hazardous activities until response to drug is known. Also, guanabenz may reduce tolerance to alcohol and other CNS depressants.

GUANFACINE HYDROCHLORIDE

(gwahn′fa-seen)

Intuniv, Tenex

Classifications: ALPHA-ADRENERGIC AGONIST; CENTRAL-ACTING ANTIHYPERTENSIVE

Therapeutic: ANTIHYPERTENSIVE

Prototype: Methyldopa

Pregnancy Category: B

AVAILABILITY 1 mg, 2 mg tablets; 1 mg, 2 mg, 3 mg, 4 mg extended release tablets

ACTION & *THERAPEUTIC EFFECT* In cerebral cortex, stimulation of alpha$_2$-adrenoreceptors triggers inhibitory neurons to reduce central sympathetic outflow (i.e., impulses from vasomotor center to heart and blood vessels). **Extended release form:** Targets ADHD symptoms through central alpha$_2$-receptor activity in the prefrontal cortex. *Results in decreased peripheral vascular resistance, thus lowering blood pressure, and a slightly reduced (5 bpm) heart rate. Minimizes the signs and symptoms of ADHD in children.*

USES Management of mild-to-moderate hypertension; attention deficit hyperactivity disorder (ADHD) (**extended form** only).

UNLABELED USES Adjunct in heroin withdrawal; Tourette's syndrome.

CONTRAINDICATIONS Treatment of acute hypertension associated with toxemia of pregnancy; psychiatric disorders that mimic ADHD; children younger than 6 y (**extended release form**) and younger than 12 y (**tablet**).

CAUTIOUS USE Severe coronary insufficiency, recent MI, cerebrovascular disease; chronic renal or hepatic failure; older adult; pregnancy (category B), lactation.

ROUTE & DOSAGE

Hypertension

Adult: **PO** 1 mg/day at bedtime, may be gradually increased to 3 mg/day if needed

Attention Deficit Hyperactivity Disorder

Adult/Adolescent/Child (older than 6 y): **PO** 1 mg daily, titrate up (normal range: 1–4 mg daily)

ADMINISTRATION

Oral

- Usually given as a single dose at bedtime to reduce effect of somnolence.
- Discontinue treatment gradually with planned tapering of schedule.
- Store tablets at 15°–30° C (59°–86° F) in tightly closed container; protect from light.

ADVERSE EFFECTS (≥1%) **CNS:** Confusion, amnesia, mental depression, drowsiness, *dizziness, sedation,* headache, asthenia, *fatigue,* insomnia. **CV:** Bradycardia, palpitation, substernal pain. **Special Senses:** Rhinitis, tinnitus, taste change; vision disturbances, conjunctivitis, iritis. **GI:** *Dry mouth, constipation,* abdominal pain, diarrhea, dysphagia, nausea. **Urogenital:** *Impotence,* testicular disorder, urinary incontinence. **Musculoskeletal:** Leg cramps, hypokinesia. **Skin:** Dermatitis, pruritus, purpura, sweating. **Other:** Dyspnea.

INTERACTIONS Drug: Alcohol and other CNS DEPRESSANTS compound sedation and CNS depression. May increase **valproic acid** levels. Use cautiously with CYP3A4 INHIBITORS or INDUCERS.

G

PHARMACOKINETICS Absorption: Readily absorbed from GI tract; 70% protein bound. **Onset:** 2 h; 6 hr (extended release). **Peak:** 6 h. **Duration:** Up to 24 h. **Distribution:** Crosses placenta. **Metabolism:** In liver. **Elimination:** 80% in the urine in 24 h. **Half-Life:** 17 h.

NURSING IMPLICATIONS

Assessment & Drug Effects

- Do not discontinue abruptly; may cause plasma and urinary catecholamine increases leading symptoms of tachycardia, insomnia, anxiety, nervousness. Rebound hypertension (i.e., increases in BP to levels significantly greater than those before therapy) may occur 2–7 days after abrupt drug withdrawal, but serious effects rarely develop.
- Monitor BP until it is stabilized. Report a rise in pressure that occurs toward end of dose interval; a divided dose schedule may be ordered.
- Assess mental status and alertness. Adverse effects tend to be dose-dependent, increasing significantly with doses above 3 mg/day.

Patient & Family Education

- Continue drug even after you feel well. This is a maintenance dosage regimen (dose and dose intervals). If 2 or more doses are missed, consult physician about how to re-establish dosage regimen.
- Employ measures to keep mouth moist; saliva substitutes (e.g., Moi-Stir, Xero-Lube) are available OTC. If dry mouth persists longer than 2 wk, patient should check with dentist.
- Do not drive or engage in other potentially hazardous tasks requiring alertness until response to drug is known.
- Avoid alcohol and do not self-medicate with OTC drugs such as sleeping medications, or cough medications without consulting physician.

HAEMOPHILUS b CONJUGATE VACCINE (Hib)

(hee-mof′il-us)

HibTITER, PedvaxHIB, ProHIBiT

Classification: VACCINE

Therapeutic: VACCINE

Prototype: Hepatitis B vaccine

Pregnancy Category: C

AVAILABILITY 7.5 mcg, 10 mcg, 15 mcg, 25 mcg injection

ACTION & *THERAPEUTIC EFFECT* A polysaccharide extracted from *Haemophilus influenzae* type b (Hib). Hib, principal antigen in the vaccine, promotes production of Hib anticapsular antibodies. It mediates complement-dependent bacteriolyses of *H. influenzae* type b organism. *Vaccine produces antibodies effective against* H. influenza *type b.*

USES To provide active immunity to *H. influenzae* type b (Hib) infection in children 2 mo–5 y.

UNLABELED USES Adults at risk of Hib infection who have Hodgkin's disease, before immunosuppressive chemotherapy.

CONTRAINDICATIONS Hypersensitivity to any component of vaccine (e.g., thiomersal); febrile illness (other than upper respiratory tract infection); active infection; immunosuppression; infants younger than 2 mo.

CAUTIOUS USE Latex hypersensitivity; pregnancy (category C).

ROUTE & DOSAGE

Immunoprophylaxis for *H. influenzae* type b Infection
Child: IM *2–6 mo,* **HibTITER** 0.5 mL, 3 doses 2 mo apart with booster at 15 mo; **PedvaxHIB** 0.5 mL, 2 doses 2 mo apart with booster at 12 mo; *7–11 mo,* **HibTITER** 0.5 mL, 2 doses 2 mo apart with booster at 15 mo; **PedvaxHIB** 0.5 mL, 2 doses 2 mo apart with booster at 15 mo; *12–14 mo,* **HibTITER** 0.5 mL, 1 dose with booster at 15 mo; **PedvaxHIB** 0.5 mL, 1 dose with booster at 15 mo; *15 mo–5 y,* all vaccines 0.5 mL as 1 dose

ADMINISTRATION

Intramuscular
- Reconstitute lyophilized powder with supplied diluent.
- Note: Use different sites when giving Hib polysaccharide vaccine and DPT (diphtheria, pertussis, tetanus) at the same time.
- Store at 2°–8° C (36°–46° F); may be frozen without loss of potency. Do not freeze the diluent.

ADVERSE EFFECTS (≥1%) **Skin:** Irritation at injection site (4–9%). **Other:** Acute febrile reactions (13%), irritability, anorexia, anaphylactoid reaction (rare).

DIAGNOSTIC TEST INTERFERENCE Hib polysaccharide vaccine may interfere with interpretation of ***antigen detection tests*** (e.g., latex agglutination) used in diagnosis of systemic Hib disease.

INTERACTIONS Drug: IMMUNOSUPPRESSANT DRUGS, STEROIDS may decrease antibody response.

PHARMACOKINETICS Onset: Antibody levels detected within 2 wk. **Peak:** 3 wk. **Duration:** 1.5–3.5 y. **Distribution:** Crosses placenta; distributed into breast milk.

NURSING IMPLICATIONS

Assessment & Drug Effects
- Be prepared for anaphylactoid reaction (see Appendix F) by having epinephrine 1:1000 available.

Patient & Family Education
- Note: Local reactions to the vaccine at the injection site (erythema, tenderness, induration, swelling, pain) may appear within 6 h after administration; usually symptoms are mild and disappear in 24 h.
- Monitor temperature after injection. An acute febrile reaction with temperature above 38.3° C (101° F) may follow vaccination (less than 1% of recipients). Notify physician.

H

HALCINONIDE

(hal-sin′oh-nide)
Halog
Classifications: ANTI-INFLAMMATORY; FLUORINATED STEROID
Therapeutic: ANTI-INFLAMMATORY
Prototype: Hydrocortisone
Pregnancy Category: C

AVAILABILITY 0.1% ointment, cream, solution

ACTION & *THERAPEUTIC EFFECT* Fluorinated steroid with substituted 17-hydroxyl group. Crosses cell membranes, complexes with nuclear DNA and stimulates synthesis of enzymes thought to be responsible for anti-inflammatory effects. *Exhibits* *anti-inflammatory, antipyretic, and vasocontrictive properties.*

USES Relief of pruritic and inflammatory manifestations of corticosteroid-responsive dermatoses.

CONTRAINDICATIONS Use on large body surface area; long-term use; infection; acne vulgaris, acne rosacea, perioral dermatitis.

CAUTIOUS USE Hypersensitivity to corticosteroids; diabetes mellitus; older adults; skin abrasion; pregnancy (category C), lactation.

H

ROUTE & DOSAGE

Inflammation
Adult: **Topical** Apply thin layer b.i.d. or t.i.d.
Child: **Topical** Apply thin layer once/day

ADMINISTRATION

Topical

- Wash skin gently and dry thoroughly before each application.
- Note: Ointment is preferred for dry scaly lesions. Moist lesions are best treated with solution.
- Do not apply in or around the eyes.
- Do not apply occlusive dressings over areas covered with halcinonide unless specifically prescribed.
- Store at 15°–30° C (59°–86° F).

ADVERSE EFFECTS (≥1%) **Endocrine:** Reversible HPA axis suppression, hyperglycemia, glycosuria. **Skin:** Burning, itching, irritation, erythema, dryness, folliculitis, hypertrichosis, pruritus, acneiform eruptions, hypopigmentation, perioral dermatitis, allergic contact dermatitis, stinging cracking/tightness of skin, secondary infection, skin atrophy, striae, miliaria, telangiectasia.

PHARMACOKINETICS Absorption: Minimum through intact skin; increased from axilla, eyelid, face, scalp, scrotum, or with occlusive dressing.

NURSING IMPLICATIONS

Assessment & Drug Effects

- Discontinue if signs of infection or irritation occur.
- Monitor for systemic corticosteroid effects that may occur with occlusive dressings or topical applications over large areas of skin.

Patient & Family Education

- Do not use an occlusive dressing with this drug unless specifically directed to do so by physician.
- Wash your hands before and after applying this topical medicine.
- Do not get any of the medication in your eyes. If you do, rinse it out with plenty of cool tap water.

HALOPERIDOL (Pr)

(ha-loe-per'i-dole)

Haldol, Peridol ♣

HALOPERIDOL DECANOATE

Haldol LA

Classification: ANTIPSYCHOTIC; BUTYROPHENONE

Therapeutic: ANTIPSYCHOTIC

Pregnancy Category: C

AVAILABILITY 0.5 mg, 1 mg, 2 mg, 5 mg, 10 mg, 20 mg tablets; 2 mg/mL oral solution; 5 mg/mL, 50 mg/mL, 100 mg/mL injection

ACTION & *THERAPEUTIC EFFECT* Blocks postsynaptic dopamine (D_2) receptors in the limbic system of the brain. Decrease in dopamine neurotransmission has been correlated with its antipsychotic effects, and its higher instance of extrapyramidal effects. *Decreases psychotic manifestations and exerts strong antiemetic effect.*

USES Management of manifestations of psychotic disorders and for control of tics and vocal utterances of Gilles de la Tourette's syndrome; for treatment of agitated states in acute and chronic psychoses. Used for short-term treatment of hyperactive children and for severe behavior problems in children of combative, explosive hyperexcitability.

UNLABELED USES Cancer chemotherapy as an antiemetic in doses smaller than those required for antipsychotic effects; treatment of autism; alcohol dependence; chorea.

CONTRAINDICATIONS Parkinson's disease, seizure disorders, coma; severe neutropenia (ANC less than 1000/mm^3); alcoholism; severe mental depression, CNS depression. Safe use in children younger than 3 y is not established.

CAUTIOUS USE Older adult or debilitated patients, urinary retention, pulmonary disease; history of hypocalcemia; glaucoma, severe cardiovascular disorders, long QT syndrome, AV block, bundle-branch block, cardiac arrhythmias, uncompensated heart failure, recent acute MI; hematologic disease; thyrotoxicosis, or hyperthyroidism; pregnancy (category C), lactation.

ROUTE & DOSAGE

Psychosis

Adult: **PO** 0.2–5 mg b.i.d. or t.i.d. **IM** 2–5 mg repeated q4h prn; Decanoate: 50–100 mg q4wk
Child: **PO** 0.5 mg/day in 2–3 divided doses, may be increased by 0.5 mg q5–7days to 0.05–0.15 mg/kg/day

Severe Psychosis

Adult: **PO** 3–5 mg b.i.d. or t.i.d., may need up to 100 mg/day **IM** 2–5 mg, may repeat q.h. prn; Decanoate: 50–100 mg q4wk
Child: **PO** 0.05–0.15 mg/kg/day in 2–3 divided doses

Dementia

Geriatric: **PO** 0.25–0.5 mg 1–2 times daily, may increase every 4–7 days (max: 4 mg/day in 2–3 divided doses)

Tourette's Disorder

Adult: **PO** 0.2–5 mg b.i.d. or t.i.d.
Child: **PO** 0.05–0.075 mg/kg/day in 2–3 divided doses

Pharmacogenetic Dosage Adjustment

CYP3D6 poor metabolizers: Start with 75% of initial dose

ADMINISTRATION

Oral

- Give with a full glass (240 mL) of water or with food or milk.
- Taper dosing regimen when discontinuing therapy. Abrupt termination can initiate extrapyramidal symptoms.

Intramuscular

- Give by deep injection into a large muscle. Do not exceed 3 mL per injection site.
- Have patient recumbent at time of parenteral administration and for about 1 h after injection. Assess for orthostatic hypotension.
- Store in light-resistant container at 15°–30° C (59°–86° F), unless otherwise specified by manufacturer. Discard darkened solutions.

ADVERSE EFFECTS (≥1%) **CNS:** *Extrapyramidal reactions:* Parkinsonian symptoms, dystonia, akathisia, <u>tardive dyskinesia</u> (after long-term use); insomnia, restlessness, anxiety, euphoria, agitation, drowsiness, mental depression, lethargy, fatigue, weakness, tremor, ataxia, headache, confusion, vertigo; <u>neu-</u>

roleptic malignant syndrome, hyperthermia, grand mal seizures, exacerbation of psychotic symptoms. **CV:** Tachycardia, ECG changes, hypotension, hypertension (with overdosage). **Endocrine:** Menstrual irregularities, galactorrhea, lactation, gynecomastia, impotence, increased libido, hyponatremia, hyperglycemia, hypoglycemia. **Special Senses:** Blurred vision. **Hematologic:** Mild transient leukopenia, agranulocytosis (rare). **GI:** Dry mouth, anorexia, nausea, vomiting, constipation, diarrhea, hypersalivation. **Urogenital:** Urinary retention, priapism. **Respiratory:** Laryngospasm, bronchospasm, increased depth of respiration, bronchopneumonia, respiratory depression. **Skin:** Diaphoresis, maculopapular and acneiform rash, photosensitivity. **Other:** Cholestatic jaundice, variations in liver function tests, decreased serum cholesterol.

INTERACTIONS Drug: CNS DEPRESSANTS, OPIATES, **alcohol** increase CNS depression; may antagonize activity of ORAL ANTICOAGULANTS; ANTICHOLINERGICS may increase intraocular pressure; **methyldopa** may precipitate dementia.

PHARMACOKINETICS Absorption: Well absorbed from GI tract; 60% reaches systemic circulation. **Onset:** 30–45 min IM. **Peak:** 2–6 h PO; 10–20 min IM; 6–7 days decanoate. **Distribution:** Distributes mainly to liver with lower concentration in brain, lung, kidney, spleen, heart. **Metabolism:** In liver. **Elimination:** 40% excreted in urine within 5 days; 15% eliminated in feces; excreted in breast milk. **Half-Life:** 13–35 h.

NURSING IMPLICATIONS

Assessment & Drug Effects

- Monitor for therapeutic effectiveness. Because of long half-life, therapeutic effects are slow to develop in early therapy or when established dosing regimen is changed. "Therapeutic window" effect (point at which increased dose or concentration actually decreases therapeutic response) may occur after long period of high doses. Close observation is imperative when doses are changed.
- Target symptoms expected to decrease with successful haloperidol treatment include hallucinations, insomnia, hostility, agitation, and delusions.
- Monitor patient's mental status daily.
- Monitor for neuroleptic malignant syndrome (NMS) (see Appendix F), especially in those with hypertension or taking lithium. Symptoms of NMS can appear suddenly after initiation of therapy or after months or years of taking neuroleptic (antipsychotic) medication. Immediately discontinue drug if NMS suspected.
- Monitor for parkinsonism and tardive dyskinesia (see Appendix F). Risk of tardive dyskinesia appears to be greater in women receiving high doses and in older adults. It can occur after long-term therapy and even after therapy is discontinued.
- Monitor for extrapyramidal (neuromuscular) reactions that occur frequently during first few days of treatment. Symptoms are usually dose related and are controlled by dosage reduction or concomitant administration of antiparkinson drugs.
- Be alert for behavioral changes in patients who are concurrently receiving antiparkinson drugs.
- Monitor for exacerbation of seizure activity.
- Observe patients closely for rapid mood shift to depression when haloperidol is used to control mania

or cyclic disorders. Depression may represent a drug adverse effect or reversion from a manic state.
- Lab tests: Monitor WBC count with differential and liver function in patients on prolonged therapy.

Patient & Family Education
- Avoid use of alcohol during therapy.
- Do not drive or engage in other potentially hazardous activities until response to drug is known.
- Discuss oral hygiene with health care provider; dry mouth may promote dental problems. Drink adequate fluids.
- Avoid overexposure to sun or sunlamp and use a sunscreen; drug can cause a photosensitivity reaction.

HEMIN
(hee′min)
Panhematin
Classifications: HEMATOLOGIC; BLOOD DERIVATIVE; ENZYME INHIBITOR
Therapeutic: ENZYME INHIBITOR
Pregnancy Category: C

AVAILABILITY 7 mg/mL injection

ACTION & *THERAPEUTIC EFFECT* Derived from processed red blood cells. Represses synthesis of porphyrin in liver or bone marrow by blocking production of delta-aminolevulinic acid (ALA) synthetase, an essential enzyme in the porphyrin-heme biosynthetic pathway. *Effective in ameliorating recurrent attacks of acute intermittent porphyria (AIP).*

USES Recurrent attacks of acute intermittent porphyria (AIP) only after an appropriate period of alternate therapy has been tried (i.e., glucose 400 g/day for 1–2 days).

CONTRAINDICATIONS History of hypersensitivity to hemin; anticoagulation therapy; porphyria cutanea tarda.

CAUTIOUS USE Pregnancy (category C), lactation. Safe use in children younger than 16 y is not established.

ROUTE & DOSAGE

Acute Intermittent Porphyria
Adult: **IV** 1–4 mg/kg/day administered over 10–15 min for 3–14 days, do not repeat dose earlier than q12h (max: 6 mg/kg in 24 h)

ADMINISTRATION

Intravenous

PREPARE: **IV Infusion:** Reconstitute immediately before use by aseptically adding 43 mL sterile water for injection to vial to yield 7 mg/mL. Shake well for 2–3 min to dissolve all particles. ▪ Terminal filtration through a sterile 0.45 micron or smaller filter is recommended. ▪ Discard unused portions.

ADMINISTER: **IV Infusion:** Give a single dose over 10–15 min.

- Freeze and store lyophilized powder until time of use.

ADVERSE EFFECTS (≥1%) **Body as a Whole:** *Phlebitis* (when administered into small veins). **Hematologic:** Decreased Hct, anticoagulant effect (prolonged PT, thromboplastin time, thrombocytopenia, hypofibrinogenemia). **Urogenital:** Reversible renal shutdown (with excessive doses).

INTERACTIONS Drug: Potentiates anticoagulant effects of ANTICOAGULANTS; BARBITURATES, ESTROGENS, CORTICOSTEROIDS may antagonize hemin effect.

PHARMACOKINETICS Duration: Can be detected in plasma up to 5 days. **Elimination:** Excess amounts eliminated in bile and urine.

NURSING IMPLICATIONS

Assessment & Drug Effects

- Monitor IV site for signs and symptoms of thrombophlebitis (see Appendix F).
- Monitor throughout therapy (decrease in these values indicates favorable clinical response): ALA, UPG (uroporphyrinogen), PBG (porphobilinogen or coproporphyrin).
- Monitor clinical effect of drug therapy by checking patient's symptoms and complaints associated with acute porphyria, which may include depression, insomnia, anxiety, disorientation, hallucinations, psychoses; dark urine, nausea, vomiting, abdominal pain, low back and leg pain, pareses (neuropathy), seizures.
- Monitor I&O and promptly report the onset of oliguria or anuria.

Patient & Family Education

- Notify physician of bruising, hematuria, tarry black stools, and nosebleeds.

H

HEPARIN SODIUM ⓟ

(hep′a-rin)

Hepalean ♣, Heparin Sodium Lock Flush Solution, Hep-Lock

Classification: ANTICOAGULANT

Therapeutic: ANTICOAGULANT

Pregnancy Category: C

AVAILABILITY 10 units/mL, 100 units/mL, 1000 units/mL, 2000 units/mL, 5000 units/mL, 10,000 units/mL, 20,000 units/mL, 40,000 units/mL injection

ACTION & *THERAPEUTIC EFFECT* Exerts direct effect on the cascade of blood coagulation by enhancing the inhibitory actions of antithrombin III (heparin cofactor) on several factors essential to normal blood clotting. This blocks the conversion of prothrombin to thrombin and fibrinogen to fibrin. *Inhibits formation of new clots. Has rapid anticoagulant effect. Does not lyse already existing thrombi but may prevent their extension and propagation.*

USES Prophylaxis and treatment of venous thrombosis and pulmonary embolism and to prevent thromboembolic complications arising from cardiac and vascular surgery, frostbite, and during acute stage of MI. Also used in treatment of disseminated intravascular coagulation (DIC), atrial fibrillation with embolization, and as anticoagulant in blood transfusions, extracorporeal circulation, and dialysis procedures.

UNLABELED USES Prophylaxis in hip and knee surgery. Heparin Sodium Lock Flush Solution is used to maintain potency of indwelling IV catheters in intermittent IV therapy or blood sampling. It is not intended for anticoagulant therapy.

CONTRAINDICATIONS History of hypersensitivity to heparin (white clot syndrome); active bleeding, bleeding tendencies; jaundice; ascorbic acid deficiency; inaccessible ulcerative lesions; visceral carcinoma; open wounds, extensive denudation of skin, suppurative thrombophlebitis; advanced kidney, liver, or biliary disease; active tuberculosis; bacterial endocarditis; continuous tube drainage of stomach or small intestines; threatened abortion; suspected intracranial hemorrhage, severe hypertension;

recent surgery of eye, brain, or spinal cord; spinal tap; shock.

CAUTIOUS USE Alcoholism; history of allergy; during menstruation; immediate postpartum period; patients with indwelling catheters; older adults; use of acid-citrate-dextrose (ACD)-converted blood (may contain heparin); patients in hazardous occupations; cerebral embolism; pregnancy (category C), especially the third trimester, lactation.

ROUTE & DOSAGE

Treatment of Thromboembolism

Adult: **IV** 5000-unit bolus dose, then 20,000–40,000 units infused over 24 h, dose adjusted to maintain desired APTT or 5000–10,000 units IV piggyback q4–6h **Subcutaneous** 10,000–20,000 units followed by 8000–20,000 units q8–12h
Child: **IV** 50 units/kg bolus, then 20,000 units/m^2/24 h or 50–100 units/kg q4h

Open Heart Surgery

Adult: **IV** 150–400 units/kg

Prophylaxis of Embolism

Adult: **Subcutaneous** 5000 units q8–12h until patient is ambulatory

ADMINISTRATION

- Note: Before administration, check coagulation test values; if results are not within therapeutic range, notify physician for dosage adjustment.
- Do not use solutions of heparin or heparin lock-flush that contain benzyl alcohol preservative in neonates.

Subcutaneous

- Use more concentrated heparin solutions for subcutaneous injection.
- Make injections into the fatty layer of the abdomen or just above the iliac crest. Avoid injecting within 5 cm (2 in.) of umbilicus or in a bruised area. Insert needle into tissue roll perpendicular to skin surface. Do not withdraw plunger to check entry into blood vessel.
- Systematically rotate injection sites and keep record.
- Exercise caution to avoid IM injection.

Intravenous

PREPARE: **Direct:** Give undiluted. **Intermittent/Continuous:** May add to any amount of NS, D5W, or LR for injection. ▪ Invert IV solution container at least 6 times to ensure adequate mixing.

ADMINISTER: **Direct:** Give a single dose over 60 sec. **Intermittent/Continuous (*preferred*):** Use infusion pump and give over 4–24 h.

INCOMPATIBILITIES **Solution/additive:** **Alteplase, amikacin, atracurium, ciprofloxacin, codeine, cytarabine, dobutamine, doxorubicin, erythromycin, gentamicin, haloperidol, hyaluronidase, hydrocortisone, kanamycin, levorphanol, meperidine, methicillin, morphine, netilmicin, polymyxin B, promethazine, streptomycin, tetracycline, tobramycin, vancomycin.** **Y-site:** **Alteplase, amiodarone, amphotericin B cholesteryl, amsacrine, ciprofloxacin, clarithromycin, dacarbazine, diazepam, dobutamine, doxorubicin, doxycycline, droperidol, ergotamine, filgrastim, gatifloxacin, gentamicin, haloperidol, idarubicin, isosorbide, levofloxacin, methotrimeprazine, mexiletine, nitroglycerin, phenytoin, polymyxin B, tobramycin, tra-**

madol, triflupromazine, vancomycin, vinorelbine.

▪ Store at 15°–30° C (59°–86° F). Protect from freezing.

ADVERSE EFFECTS (≥1%) **Hematologic:** Spontaneous bleeding, *transient thrombocytopenia,* hypofibrinogenemia, "white clot syndrome." **Body as a Whole:** Fever, chills, urticaria, pruritus, skin rashes, itching and burning sensations of feet, numbness and tingling of hands and feet, elevated BP, headache, nasal congestion, lacrimation, conjunctivitis, chest pains, arthralgia, bronchospasm, anaphylactoid reactions. **Endocrine:** Osteoporosis, hypoaldosteronism, suppressed renal function, hyperkalemia; rebound hyperlipidemia (following termination of heparin therapy). **GI:** Increased AST, ALT. **Urogenital:** Priapism (rare). **Skin:** Injection site reactions: Pain, itching, ecchymoses, tissue irritation and sloughing; cyanosis and pains in arms or legs (vasospasm), reversible transient alopecia (usually around temporal area).

DIAGNOSTIC TEST INTERFERENCE Notify laboratory that patient is receiving heparin, when a test is to be performed. Possibility of false-positive rise in ***BSP*** test and in ***serum thyroxine;*** and increases in ***resin*** T_3 **uptake;** false-negative ***^{125}I fibrinogen uptake.*** Heparin prolongs ***PT.*** Valid readings may be obtained by drawing blood samples at least 4–6 h after an IV dose (but at any time during heparin infusion) and 12–24 h after a subcutaneous heparin dose.

INTERACTIONS Drug: May prolong PT, which is used to monitor therapy with ORAL ANTICOAGULANTS; **aspirin,** NSAIDS increase risk of bleeding; **nitroglycerin** IV may decrease anticoagulant activity; **protamine** antagonizes effects of heparin. **Herbal: Evening primrose oil, feverfew, ginkgo, ginger** may potentiate bleeding.

PHARMACOKINETICS Onset: 20–60 min subcutaneous. **Peak:** Within minutes. **Duration:** 2–6 h IV; 8–12 h subcutaneous. **Distribution:** Does not cross placenta; not distributed into breast milk. **Metabolism:** In liver and by reticuloendothelial system. **Elimination:** In urine. **Half-Life:** 90 min.

NURSING IMPLICATIONS

Assessment & Drug Effects

- Lab tests: Baseline blood coagulation tests, Hct, Hgb, RBC, and platelet counts prior to initiation of therapy and at regular intervals throughout therapy.
- Monitor APTT levels closely.
- Note: In general, dosage is adjusted to keep APTT between 1.5–2.5 times normal control level.
- Draw blood for coagulation test 30 min before each scheduled subcutaneous or intermittent IV dose and approximately q4h for patients receiving continuous IV heparin during dosage adjustment period. After dosage is established, tests may be done once daily.
- Patients vary widely in their reaction to heparin; risk of hemorrhage appears greatest in women, all patients older than 60 y, and patients with liver disease or renal insufficiency.
- Monitor vital signs. Report fever, drop in BP, rapid pulse, and other S&S of hemorrhage.
- Observe all needle sites daily for hematoma and signs of inflammation (swelling, heat, redness, pain).
- Antidote: Have on hand protamine sulfate (1% solution), specific heparin antagonist.

Patient & Family Education

- Protect from injury and notify physician of pink, red, dark brown, or cloudy urine; red or dark brown vomitus; red or black stools; bleeding gums or oral mucosa; ecchymoses, hematoma, epistaxis, bloody sputum; chest pain; abdominal or lumbar pain or swelling; unusual increase in menstrual flow; pelvic pain; severe or continuous headache, faintness, or dizziness.
- Note: Menstruation may be somewhat increased and prolonged; usually, this is not a contraindication to continued therapy if bleeding is not excessive.
- Learn correct technique for subcutaneous administration if discharged from hospital on heparin.
- Engage in normal activities such as shaving with a safety razor in the absence of a low platelet (thrombocyte) count. Usually, heparin does not affect bleeding time.
- Caution: Smoking and alcohol consumption may alter response to heparin and are not advised.
- Do not take aspirin or any other OTC medication without physician's approval.

HEPATITIS A VACCINE

(hep'a-ti-tis)
Havrix, Vaqta
Classification: VACCINE
Therapeutic: VACCINE
Prototype: Hepatitis B vaccine
Pregnancy Category: C

AVAILABILITY 720 EIU/0.5 mL, 1440 EIU/1 mL (Havrix); 25 units/0.5 mL, 50 units/1 mL (Vaqta)

ACTION & *THERAPEUTIC EFFECT* Anti-hepatitis A virus antibody titers following administration of hepatitis A vaccine (inactivated) are comparable to those observed after natural hepatitis A virus infection. *Antibody levels are 50- to 300-fold higher with inactivated hepatitis A vaccine than with passive immunity with human immune globulin.*

USES Active immunization against hepatitis A.

CONTRAINDICATIONS Hypersensitivity to any component in vaccine, children younger than 12 mo.
CAUTIOUS USE Severe cardiac disease; coagulopathy; vitamin K deficiency; pregnancy (category C), lactation.

ROUTE & DOSAGE

Hepatitis A Immunization
Adult: **IM** 1 mL in deltoid muscle; booster dose (1 mL) at 6–12 mo after primary dose
Child (1–18 y): **IM** 2 doses of 0.5 mL in deltoid muscle given 1 mo apart; booster dose (0.5 mL) at 6–12 mo after primary doses

ADMINISTRATION

Intramuscular

- Give only in deltoid for adults and children older than 2 y. DO NOT give IV, subcutaneously, or intradermally.
- Use vaccine as packaged without dilution.
- Shake vial and syringe well before withdrawal and injection, respectively. Vaccine should be an opaque white suspension; discard if it looks otherwise.
- Store at 2°–8° C (36°–47° F). Discard vaccine if it has been frozen.

ADVERSE EFFECTS (≥1%) **CNS:** *Headache,* fatigue, fever, malaise, somnolence vertigo, insomnia, photophobia, convulsions, neuropathy, paresthesia. **GI:** Anorexia, nausea, abdominal pain, diarrhea, dysgeusia, vomiting. **Skin:** Pruritus, rash, urticaria, erythema multiforme, hyperhidrosis, angioedema (rare). **Other:** *Soreness at injection site, pain, swelling, redness at injection site,* pharyngitis, lymphadenopathy.

INTERACTIONS Drug: No clinically significant interactions established.

PHARMACOKINETICS Onset: 3 wk. **Duration:** 1–3 y with single dose, 5–10 y with booster.

NURSING IMPLICATIONS

Assessment & Drug Effects

- Do not administer during a febrile illness.
- Assess for S&S of anaphylaxis and have epinephrine available.

Patient & Family Education

- Note: Injection site soreness is common; most adverse reactions are mild and usually last less than 24 h.
- Get booster injection within 6–12 mo if risk of exposure is still present.

HEPATITIS B IMMUNE GLOBULIN

(hep'a-ti-tis)

HepaGam B, HyperHep, Nabi-HB

Classification: VACCINE

Therapeutic: VACCINE

Prototype: Hepatitis B vaccine

Pregnancy Category: C

AVAILABILITY 1 mL, 4 mL, 5 mL vials

ACTION & *THERAPEUTIC EFFECT* Sterile solution of immunoglobulins [immunoglobulin G (IgG)] prepared by using pooled human plasma. The possibility of transmission of hepatitis infection or AIDS from H-BIG is remote. *Preparation contains a high antibody titer specific to hepatitis B surface antigen (anti-HBs); plasma does not show serologic evidence of hepatitis B surface antigen (HBsAg).*

USES Prophylactically to provide passive immunity to hepatitis B infection in individuals exposed to HBV or HBsAg-positive materials (blood plasma, serum). Also as postexposure prophylaxis after bite or percutaneous exposure, ingestion, direct mucous membrane contact, sexual or intimate contact, and in neonates born to HBsAg-positive women. Prevention of hepatitis B reccurrence following liver transplant (HepaGam B only).

CAUTIOUS USE History of systemic allergic reactions to immune globulin; thrombocytopenia or bleeding disorders, HBsAg-positive individuals, patients with specific immunoglobulin A (IgA) deficiency; pregnancy (category C), lactation.

ROUTE & DOSAGE

Hepatitis B Prophylaxis

Adult/Child: **IM** 0.06 mL/kg as soon as possible after exposure, preferably within 24 h, but no later than 7 days, repeat 28–30 days after exposure

Newborn Exposure

Child: **IM** 0.5 mL as soon as possible after birth, but no later than 24 h, repeat dose 3 and 6 mo later

Prevention of Recurrence Post-Liver Transplant (HepaGram B)

Adult: **IV** 20,000 units/dose daily (days 1–7), every 2 wk (week 2–12), monthly thereafter

ADMINISTRATION

Intramuscular

- *Adult:* Give into anterolateral upper thigh or deltoid. *Neonates:* Give into anterolateral thigh.

Intravenous

PREPARE: **Infusion:** Give undiluted.

ADMINISTER: **Infusion:** Give via infusion pump at 2 mL/min; decrease to 1 mL/min if infusion-related adverse events occur.

- Store at 2°–8° C (36°–46° F) unless otherwise directed. Avoid freezing.

ADVERSE EFFECTS (≥1%) **Body as a Whole:** Muscle stiffness; pain, tenderness, swelling, erythema of injection site, nausea, faintness, fever, dizziness, malaise, lassitude, body and joint pain, leg cramps. **Skin:** Urticaria, rash, angioedema, pruritus, erythema, sensitization (following large or repeated doses), anaphylaxis (rare).

INTERACTIONS Drug: May interfere with immune response to LIVE-VIRUS VACCINES (measles/mumps/rubella/poliovirus).

PHARMACOKINETICS Absorption: Slowly absorbed from IM site. **Onset:** 1–6 days. **Peak:** 3–11 days. **Duration:** 2–6 mo. **Elimination:** Half-life 21 days.

NURSING IMPLICATIONS

Assessment & Drug Effects

- Have epinephrine 1:1000 readily available; hypersensitivity reactions are most likely to occur in patients receiving large doses or repeated injections.

Patient & Family Education

- Learn potential adverse reactions.

HEPATITIS B VACCINE (RECOMBINANT) Pr

(hep'a-ti-tis)

Engerix-B, Recombivax HB

Classification: VACCINE

Therapeutic: VACCINE

Pregnancy Category: C

AVAILABILITY 10 mcg/mL, 5 mcg/0.5 mL, 40 mcg/mL (Recombivax); 20 mcg/mL, 10 mcg/0.5 mL (Engerix-B)

ACTION & *THERAPEUTIC EFFECT* Suspension of inactivated and purified hepatitis B surface antigen (HBsAg) derived from human plasma of screened asymptomatic HBsAg-positive carriers of hepatitis B virus. Hepatitis B vaccine recombinant is the first vaccine produced by gene splicing. *The recommended 3-dose regimen produces active immunity against hepatitis B infection by inducing protective antibody (anti-HBs) formation.*

USES To promote active immunity in individuals at high risk of potential exposure to hepatitis B virus or HBsAg-positive materials. Has been used simultaneously (into different sites) with hepatitis B immune globulin (H-BIG) for post-exposure prophylaxis in selected patients and in infants born to HBsAg-positive mothers.

CONTRAINDICATIONS History of allergic reaction to hepatitis B vaccine or to any ingredient in the formulation; HBsAg carriers.

CAUTIOUS USE Compromised cardiopulmonary status, serious active infection or fever; renal disease, renal failure; thrombocytopenia or other bleeding disorders; pregnancy (category C), lactation.

ROUTE & DOSAGE

Hepatitis B Prophylaxis

Adult: IM **Recombivax** 1 mL (10 mcg) at 0, 1, and 6 mo; **Engerix-B** 1 mL (20 mcg) at 0, 1, and 6 mo or 0, 1, 2, and 12 mo
Child: IM **Recombivax** 0.5 mL (5 mcg) at 0, 1, and 6 mo; **Engerix-B** 0.5 mL (10 mcg) at 0, 1, and 6 mo or 0, 1, 2, and 12 mo

Dialysis and Immunodeficient Patients

Adult: IM **Recombivax** 2 mL (20 mcg) at 0, 1, and 6 mo; **Engerix-B** 2 mL (40 mcg) at 0, 1, and 6 mo or 0, 1, 2, and 12 mo

ADMINISTRATION

Intramuscular

- Give preferably into the deltoid and in neonates into the anterolateral thigh, avoiding blood vessels and nerves. Carefully aspirate to prevent inadvertent intravascular injection.
- Have epinephrine immediately available to treat anaphylaxis.
- Shake vial well before withdrawing dose to assure uniform suspension.
- Store unopened and opened vials at 2°–8° C (36°–46° F) unless otherwise directed. Avoid freezing (freezing destroys potency).

ADVERSE EFFECTS (≥1%) **Body as a Whole:** *Mild local tenderness at injection site, local inflammatory reaction* (swelling, heat, redness, induration, pain); *fever, malaise, fatigue,* headache, dizziness, faintness, leg cramps, myalgia, arthralgia. **GI:** Nausea, vomiting, diarrhea. **Skin:** Rash, urticaria, pruritus.

INTERACTIONS Drug: No clinically significant interactions established.

PHARMACOKINETICS Absorption: Slowly absorbed from IM site. **Onset:** 2 wk. **Peak:** 6 mo. **Duration:** At least 3 y.

NURSING IMPLICATIONS

Assessment & Drug Effects

- Note: The ACIP recommends serologic confirmation of postvaccination immunity in patients undergoing dialysis and in immunodeficient patients.
- Monitor temperature. Some patients develop a temperature elevation of 38.3° C (101° F) following vaccination that may last 1 or 2 days.

Patient & Family Education

- Learn potential adverse reaction.

HETASTARCH

(het'a-starch)

HES, Hespan, Hydroxyethyl Starch, Hextend

Classification: PLASMA EXPANDER
Therapeutic: PLASMA EXPANDER
Prototype: Albumin
Pregnancy Category: C

AVAILABILITY 6 g/100 mL injection

ACTION & *THERAPEUTIC EFFECT*
Synthetic starch closely resembling human glycogen. Acts much like albumin and dextran but is claimed to be less likely to produce anaphylaxis or to interfere with cross matching or blood typing procedures. *Causes no significant alterations in fibrinogen or clotting time but may prolong the PTT and PT. Not a substitute for blood or plasma. In hypovolemic patients, it increases arterial and venous pressures, heart rate, cardiac output, urine output, as well as colloidal osmotic pressure. Colloidal*

osmotic properties are approximately equal to those of human serum albumin.

USES Early fluid replacement and plasma volume expansion when whole blood is not available or when there is no time for necessary cross matching. Used to expand plasma volume during cardiopulmonary bypass and in adjunctive treatment of shock caused by hemorrhage, burns, surgery, sepsis, or other trauma. Also used as an agent for sediment agent in preparation of granulocytes by leukapheresis.

UNLABELED USES As a priming fluid in pump oxygenators for perfusion during extracorporeal circulation and as a cryoprotective agent for long-term storage of whole blood.

CONTRAINDICATIONS Severe bleeding disorders, CHF, renal failure with oliguria and anuria, treatment of shock not accompanied by hypovolemia, intracranial bleeding. Safe use in children is not established.

CAUTIOUS USE Hepatic or renal insufficiency, pulmonary edema in the very young or older adults, patients on sodium restriction; pregnancy (category C), lactation.

ROUTE & DOSAGE

Plasma Volume Expansion
Adult: **IV** 500–1000 mL or 20 mL/kg/day (max: 1500 mL/day)

Leukapheresis
Adult: **IV** 250–750 mL infused at a constant fixed ratio of 1:8 to venous whole blood

Renal Impairment Dosage Adjustment
CrCl less than 10 mL/min: Use original initial dose, then reduce doses by 25–50%

ADMINISTRATION

Intravenous

PREPARE: **IV Infusion:** Use undiluted as prepared by manufacturer.

ADMINISTER: **IV Infusion:** Specific flow rate is prescribed by physician. Rate may be as high as 20 mL/kg/h in acute hemorrhagic shock. ▪ Rate is usually reduced in patients with burns or septic shock.

INCOMPATIBILITIES **Y-site:** **Amikacin, amphotericin B, cefoperazone, cefotaxime, cefoxitin, diazepam, gentamicin, ranitidine, sodium bicarbonate, theophylline, tobramycin.**

▪ Store at room temperature; avoid extremes of heat or cold. ▪ Discard partially used bags.

ADVERSE EFFECTS (≥1%) **CV:** Peripheral edema, circulatory overload, heart failure. **Hematologic:** With large volumes, prolongation of PT, PTT, clotting time, and bleeding time; decreased Hct, Hgb, platelets, calcium, and fibrinogen; dilution of plasma proteins, hyperbilirubinemia, increased sedimentation rate. **Body as a Whole:** Pruritus, anaphylactoid reactions (periorbital edema, urticaria, wheezing), vomiting, mild fever, chills, influenza-like symptoms, headache, muscle pains, submaxillary and parotid glandular swelling.

INTERACTIONS Drug: No clinically significant interactions established.

PHARMACOKINETICS Duration: 24–36 h. **Distribution:** Remains in intravascular space. **Metabolism:** In reticuloendothelial system. **Elimination:** In urine with some biliary excretion.

NURSING IMPLICATIONS

Assessment & Drug Effects

- Monitor for S&S of hypersensitivity reaction (see Appendix F).
- Measure and record I&O. Report oliguria or significant changes in I&O ratio.
- Monitor BP and vital signs and observe patient for unusual bruising or bleeding.
- Lab tests: Monitor WBC count with differential, platelet count, and PT & PTT during leukapheresis.
- Observe for signs of circulatory overload (see Appendix F).
- Check laboratory reports of Hct values. Notify physician if there is an appreciable drop in Hct or if value approaches 30% by volume. Hct should not be allowed to drop below 30%.

Patient & Family Education

- Notify physician for any of the following: Difficulty breathing, nausea, chills, headache, itching.

H

HOMATROPINE HYDROBROMIDE (Pr)

(hoe-ma'troe-peen)

AK-Homatropine, Homatrine, Homatropine, Isopto Homatropine

Pregnancy Category: C

See Appendix A-1.

HYALURONIDASE, OVINE

(hi-a-lu-ron'i-dase)

Amphadase, Vitrase

Classifications: HYALURONIC ACID DERIVATIVE; ABSORPTION AND DISPERSING ENHANCER

Therapeutic: ABSORPTION AND DISPERSING ENHANCER

Pregnancy Category: C

AVAILABILITY 150 units/mL and 200 units/mL for injection; lyophilized powder, 6200 units

ACTION & *THERAPEUTIC EFFECT* Hyaluronidase is a diffusing substance that modifies the permeability of connective tissue through the hydrolysis of hyaluronic acid found in the intercellular substance of connective tissue. *It increases the absorption and dispersion of solutions in the intercellular spaces.*

USES Adjuvant to increase the absorption and dispersion of other injected drugs; hypodermoclysis; adjunct in subcutaneous urography for improving resorption of radiopaque agents.

UNLABELED USES Adjunct for ophthalmic anesthesia, treatment of vitreous hemorrhage and diabetic retinopathy.

CONTRAINDICATIONS Hypersensitivity to hyaluronidase or any other ingredient in formulation; injection into infected or acutely inflamed area, area of swelling due to bites or stings; corneal injection; injection by IV.

CAUTIOUS USE Pregnancy (category C), lactation.

ROUTE & DOSAGE

Adjuvant to Increase the Absorption and Dispersion of Other Drugs

Adult: 150 units (range: 50–300) added to solution

Child: 150 units (range: 50–300) added to solution

Hypodermoclysis
Adult: 15 units added to each 100 mL of fluid
Child (3 y or older): 15 units added to each 100 mL of fluid

Subcutaneous Urography
Adult: **Subcutaneous** 75 units prior to contrast medium
Child: **Subcutaneous** 75 units prior to contrast medium

ADMINISTRATION

Subcutaneous or Solution Additive

- Reconstitute vial with 6.2 mL NS for injection to yield 1000 units/mL. Apply the 5-micron filter needle to the 1 mL syringe in injection kit and further dilute: To produce 50 units/mL, withdraw 0.05 mL reconstituted solution and add 0.95 mL NS. ▪ To produce 75 units/mL, withdraw 0.075 mL reconstituted solution and add 0.925 mL NS. ▪ To produce 150 units/mL, withdraw 0.15 mL reconstituted solution and add 0.85 mL NS. ▪ To produce 300 units/mL, withdraw 0.3 mL reconstituted solution and add 0.7 mL NS. ▪ Use immediately after preparation.
- Give subcutaneously prior to contrast media. Do not inject near an infected or acutely inflamed area.
- Store unopened vial at 2°–8° C (35°–46° F). After reconstitution, store at 20°–25° C (59°–77° F), and use within 6 h. Protect from light.

ADVERSE EFFECTS (≥1%) **CV:** Edema. **Other:** Injection site reaction (e.g., erythema, irritation); enhanced adverse events associated with coadministered drugs.

INTERACTIONS Drug: SALICYLATES, CORTICOSTEROIDS, ESTROGENS, or H_1-BLOCKERS may confer partial resistance to the action of hyaluronidase in some tissues.

NURSING IMPLICATIONS

Assessment & Drug Effects

- Monitor for S&S of hypersensitivity: Urticaria, erythema, chills, nausea, vomiting, dizziness, tachycardia, and hypotension. Withhold and notify physician if hypersensitivity occurs.
- Note: Those receiving large doses of salicylates, cortisone, ACTH, estrogens, or antihistamines may require larger amounts of hyaluronidase for equivalent dispersing effect.

Patient & Family Education

- Report immediately any of the following: Rash, itching, chills, nausea, vomiting, dizziness, or palpitations.

H

HYDRALAZINE HYDROCHLORIDE (Pr)

(hye-dral′a-zeen)

Classifications: NONNITRATE VASODILATOR; ANTIHYPERTENSIVE
Therapeutic: ANTIHYPERTENSIVE
Pregnancy Category: C

AVAILABILITY 10 mg, 25 mg, 50 mg, 100 mg tablets; 20 mg/mL vial

ACTION & *THERAPEUTIC EFFECT* Reduces BP mainly by direct effect on vascular smooth muscles of arterial-resistance vessels, resulting in vasodilatation. *Reduces BP with diastolic response often being greater than systolic response. Vasodilation reduces peripheral resistance and substantially improves cardiac output, and renal and cerebral blood flow.*

USES Most commonly in stepped-care approach to treat moderate to

severe hypertension. Also in early malignant hypertension and resistant hypertension that persists after sympathectomy.
UNLABELED USES Conjunctively with cardiac glycosides and other vasodilators in short-term treatment of acute CHF; unexplained pulmonary hypertension; eclampsia.

CONTRAINDICATIONS Monotherapy for CHF, mitral valvular rheumatic heart disease, MI, tachycardia.
CAUTIOUS USE Coronary heart disease; cerebrovascular accident, advanced renal impairment, coronary heart disease, renal disease; renal failure; SLE; use with MAO inhibitors; pregnancy (category C), lactation.

ROUTE & DOSAGE

Hypertension
Adult: **PO** 10–50 mg q.i.d. **IM** 10–50 mg q4–6h **IV** 10–20 mg q4–6h, may increase to 40 mg
Geriatric: **PO** Start with 10 mg 2–3 times/day
Child: **PO** 3–7.5 mg/kg/day in 4 divided doses **IV/IM** 0.1–0.2 mg/kg in divided doses (max: 20 mg)

Renal Impairment Dosage Adjustment
CrCl 10–50 mL/min: Dose q8h

ADMINISTRATION

Oral
- Give with food; bioavailability is increased by taking it with food.
- Discontinue gradually to avoid sudden rise in BP and acute heart failure.
- Inform patients of the dangers of abrupt withdrawal.

Intramuscular
- Give deep into a large muscle.

Intravenous

PREPARE: **Direct:** Give undiluted. Use immediately after being drawn into syringe. ▪ Do not add to IV solutions.
ADMINISTER: **Direct:** Give each 10 mg or fraction thereof over 1 min.
INCOMPATIBILITIES **Solution/additive:** **Aminophylline, ampicillin, chlorothiazide, edetate calcium disodium, ethacrynate, hydrocortisone, mephentermine, methohexital, nitroglycerin, phenobarbital, verapamil, D5W.** **Y-site:** **Aminophylline, ampicillin, diazoxide, furosemide.**

- Store at 15°–30° C (59°–86° F) in tight, light-resistant containers unless otherwise directed. Avoid freezing.

ADVERSE EFFECTS (≥1%) **Body as a Whole:** Hypersensitivity (rash, urticaria, pruritus, fever, chills, arthralgia, eosinophilia, cholangitis, hepatitis, obstructive jaundice). **CNS:** *Headache,* dizziness, tremors. **CV:** *Palpitation,* angina, *tachycardia,* flushing, paradoxical pressor response. Overdose: Arrhythmia, <u>shock</u>. **Special Senses:** Lacrimation, conjunctivitis. **GI:** Anorexia, nausea, vomiting, diarrhea, constipation, abdominal pain, paralytic ileus. **Urogenital:** Difficulty in urination, glomerulonephritis. **Hematologic:** Decreased hematocrit and hemoglobin, anemia, <u>agranulocytosis</u> (rare). **Other:** Nasal congestion, muscle cramps, SLE-like syndrome, fixed drug eruption, edema.

DIAGNOSTIC TEST INTERFERENCE Positive ***direct Coombs' tests*** in patients with hydralazine-induced SLE. Hydralazine interferes with urinary ***17-OHCS*** determinations ***(modified Glenn-Nelson technique).***

INTERACTIONS Drug: BETA-BLOCKERS and other ANTIHYPERTENSIVE AGENTS compound hypotensive effects.

PHARMACOKINETICS Absorption: Readily absorbed from GI tract. **Onset:** 20–30 min. **Peak:** 2 h. **Duration:** 2–6 h. **Distribution:** Crosses placenta; distributed into breast milk. **Metabolism:** In liver. **Elimination:** 90% in urine; 10% in feces. **Half-Life:** 2–8 h.

NURSING IMPLICATIONS

Assessment & Drug Effects

- Monitor BP and HR closely. Check every 5 min until it is stabilized at desired level, then every 15 min thereafter throughout hypertensive crisis.
- Lab tests: Baseline and periodic determinations of BUN, creatinine clearance, uric acid, serum potassium, blood glucose, and ECG. Baseline and periodic antinuclear antibody titer recommended with prolonged therapy.
- Monitor for S&S of SLE, especially with prolonged therapy.
- Monitor I&O when drug is given parenterally and in those with renal dysfunction.

Patient & Family Education

- Monitor weight, check for edema, and report weight gain to physician.
- Note: Some patients experience headache and palpitations within 2–4 h after first PO dose; symptoms usually subside spontaneously.
- Make position changes slowly and avoid standing still, hot baths/showers, strenuous exercise, and excessive alcohol intake.
- Do not drive or engage in other potentially hazardous activities until response to drug is known.

HYDROCHLOROTHIAZIDE (HCTZ) Pr

(hye-droe-klor-oh-thye′a-zide)

Apo-Hydro ♣, Esidrix, Oretic, Urozide ♣

Classifications: ELECTROLYTIC AND WATER BALANCE; THIAZIDE DIURETIC

Therapeutic: DIURETIC

Pregnancy Category: B

AVAILABILITY 12.5 mg capsules; 25 mg, 50 mg, 100 mg tablets; 50 mg/5 mL oral solution

ACTION & *THERAPEUTIC EFFECT* Diuretic action is associated with drug interference with absorption of sodium ions across the distal renal tubular segment of the nephron. This enhances excretion of sodium, chloride, potassium, bicarbonates, and water. It also decreases cardiac output and reduces plasma and extracellular fluid volume. *Therapeutic effectiveness is measured by decrease in edema and lowering of blood pressure.*

USES Adjunct in treatment of edema associated with CHF, hepatic cirrhosis, renal failure, and in the management of hypertension.

UNLABELED USES Nephrogenic diabetes insipidus, hypercalciuria, and treatment of electrolyte disturbances associated with renal tubular acidosis.

CONTRAINDICATIONS Hypersensitivity to thiazides or other sulfonamides; anuria; electrolyte imbalance.

CAUTIOUS USE Bronchial asthma, allergy; hepatic cirrhosis; renal dysfunction; acid/base imbalance; CHF; stroke, CVA; history of gout, SLE; diabetes mellitus; older adults;

excessive sunlight UV exposure; neonates with jaundice; pregnancy (category B), lactation.

ROUTE & DOSAGE

Edema

Adult: **PO** 25–200 mg/day in 1–3 divided doses

Hypertension

Adult: **PO** 12.5–100 mg/day in 1–2 divided doses
Child: **PO** 2.2 mg/kg/day in 2 divided doses
Neonate (younger than 6 mo): **PO** 2–4 mg/kg/day in 2 divided doses

ADMINISTRATION

Oral

- Give with food or milk to reduce GI upset.
- Schedule doses to avoid nocturia and interrupted sleep. If given in 2 doses, schedule second dose no later than 3 p.m.
- Store tablets in tightly closed container at 15°–30° C (59°–86° F) unless otherwise directed.

ADVERSE EFFECTS (≥1%) **CNS:** Mood changes, unusual tiredness or weakness, dizziness, light-headedness, paresthesias. **CV:** Irregular heartbeat, weak pulse, orthostatic hypotension. **GI:** Dry mouth, increased thirst, nausea, vomiting, anorexia, diarrhea, pancreatitis, jaundice. **Hematologic:** Agranulocytosis, thrombocytopenia, aplastic anemia, leukopenia. **Metabolic:** *Hyperglycemia,* glycosuria, *hyperuricemia, hypokalemia.* **Other:** Hypersensitivity reactions, photosensitivity, blurred vision, yellow vision (xanthopsia), muscle spasm.

DIAGNOSTIC TEST INTERFERENCE Falsely decreased value in ***total-urinary estrogen*** by ***spectrophotometric assay.*** See ***chlorothiazide.***

INTERACTIONS Drug: Amphotericin B, CORTICOSTEROIDS increase hypokalemic effects; SULFONYLUREAS, **insulin** may antagonize hypoglycemic effects; **cholestyramine, colestipol** decrease THIAZIDE absorption; **diazoxide** intensifies hypoglycemic and hypotensive effects; increased **potassium** and **magnesium** loss may cause **digoxin** toxicity; decreases **lithium** excretion and increases toxicity; increases risk of NSAID-induced renal failure and may attenuate diuresis.

PHARMACOKINETICS Absorption: Incompletely absorbed. **Onset:** 2 h. **Peak:** 4 h. **Duration:** 6–12 h. **Distribution:** Distributed throughout extracellular tissue; concentrates in kidney; crosses placenta; distributed in breast milk. **Metabolism:** Does not appear to be metabolized. **Elimination:** In urine. **Half-Life:** 45–120 min.

NURSING IMPLICATIONS

Assessment & Drug Effects

- Monitor for therapeutic effectiveness. Antihypertensive effects may be noted in 3–4 days; maximal effects may require 3–4 wk.
- Lab tests: Baseline and periodic determinations of serum electrolytes, blood counts, BUN, blood glucose, uric acid, CO_2, are recommended.
- Check BP at regular intervals.
- Monitor closely for hypokalemia; it increases the risk of digoxin toxicity.
- Monitor I&O and check for edema.
- Note: Drug may cause hyperglycemia and loss of glycemic control in diabetics.
- Note: Drug may cause orthostatic hypotension, dizziness.

Common adverse effects in *italic*, life-threatening effects underlined; generic names in **bold**; classifications in SMALL CAPS; ♣ Canadian drug name; ● Prototype drug

Patient & Family Education

- Monitor weight daily.
- Note: Diabetic patients need to monitor blood glucose closely. This drug causes impaired glucose tolerance.
- Report signs of hypokalemia (see Appendix F) to physician.
- Change positions slowly; avoid hot baths or showers, extended exposure to sunlight, and sitting or standing still for long periods.
- Note: Photosensitivity reaction may occur 10–14 days after initial sun exposure.

HYDROCODONE BITARTRATE

(hye-droe-koe′done)

Dihydrocodeinone Bitartrate, Hycodan, Robidone A, Vicodin (with acetaminophen)

Classifications: NARCOTIC (OPIATE AGONIST) ANALGESIC; ANTITUSSIVE

Therapeutic: NARCOTIC ANALGESIC; ANTITUSSIVE

Prototype: Morphine

Pregnancy Category: C

Controlled Substance: Schedule II

AVAILABILITY 5 mg hydrocodone usually with 500 mg or more acetaminophen

ACTION & *THERAPEUTIC EFFECT* CNS depressant with moderate to severe relief of pain. Available in the United States only in combination with other drugs. *Suppresses cough reflex by direct action on cough center in medulla. CNS depressant with moderate to severe relief of pain.*

USES Symptomatic relief of hyperactive or nonproductive cough and for relief of moderate to moderately severe pain. A common ingredient in a variety of proprietary mixtures.

CONTRAINDICATIONS Hypersensitivity to hydrocodone; acute or severe asthmatic bronchitis; COPD; upper airway obstruction; children younger than 2 y.

CAUTIOUS USE Respiratory depression, asthma, emphysema; history of drug abuse or dependence; postoperative patients; hepatic or renal disease; renal impairment or failure; older adults, debilitated patients; children weighing less than 50 kg; G6PD deficiency; GI disease; patients with preexisting increased intracranial pressure; pregnancy (category C), lactation.

ROUTE & DOSAGE

Mild to Moderate Pain, Cough

Adult: **PO** 5–10 mg q4–6h prn (max: 15 mg/dose)

Child (2–12 y): **PO** 1.25–5 mg q4–6h (max: 10 mg/dose)

ADMINISTRATION

Oral

- Give with food or milk to prevent GI irritation.
- Preserve in tight, light-resistant containers.

ADVERSE EFFECTS (≥1%) **GI:** Dry mouth, *constipation, nausea,* vomiting. **CNS:** Light-headedness, sedation, dizziness, *drowsiness,* euphoria, dysphoria. **Respiratory:** <u>*Respiratory depression*</u>. **Skin:** Urticaria, rash, pruritus.

INTERACTIONS Drug: Alcohol and other CNS DEPRESSANTS compound sedation and CNS depression. **Herbal: St. John's wort** increases sedation.

PHARMACOKINETICS Onset: 10–20 min. **Duration:** 3–6 h. **Distribu-**

tion: Crosses placenta; distributed into breast milk. **Metabolism:** In liver. **Elimination:** In urine. **Half-Life:** 3.8 h.

NURSING IMPLICATIONS

Assessment & Drug Effects

- Monitor for effectiveness of drug for pain relief.
- Monitor for nausea and vomiting, especially in ambulatory patients.
- Monitor respiratory status and bowel elimination.

Patient & Family Education

- Avoid hazardous activities until response to drug is determined.
- Do not use alcohol or other CNS depressants; may cause additive CNS depression.
- Drink plenty of liquids for adequate hydration.
- Do not take larger doses than prescribed since abuse potential is high.

HYDROCORTISONE (Pr)

(hye-droe-kor′ti-sone)

Aeroseb-HC, Cetacort, Cortaid, Cortenema, Dermolate, Hytone, Rectocort ♣, Synacort

HYDROCORTISONE ACETATE

Anusol HC, Carmol HC, Cortaid, Cort-Dome, Corticaine, Cortifoam, Cortiment ♣, Epifoam

HYDROCORTISONE CYPIONATE

Cortef

HYDROCORTISONE SODIUM SUCCINATE

A-Hydrocort, Solu-Cortef

HYDROCORTISONE VALERATE

Westcort

HYDROCORTISONE BUTYRATE

Locoid

Classification: ADRENOCORTICAL STEROID

Therapeutic: ANTI-INFLAMMATORY; IMMUNOSUPPRESSANT

Pregnancy Category: D first trimester; C second and third trimester

AVAILABILITY Hydrocortisone: 5 mg, 10 mg, 20 mg tablets; 0.5%, 1%, 2.5% cream, lotion, ointment, spray; **Hydrocortisone Acetate:** 25 mg/mL, 50 mg/mL suspension; 0.5%, 1% cream, ointment; **Hydrocortisone Cypionate:** 5 mg, 20 mg tablet; **Hydrocortisone Sodium Succinate:** 100 mg/2 mL, 250 mg/2 mL, 500 mg/4 mL, 1000 mg/8 mL vials; **Hydrocortisone Valerate:** 0.2% cream, ointment; **Hydrocortisone Butyrate:** 0.1% cream, ointment, topical solution

ACTION & *THERAPEUTIC EFFECT*

Short-acting synthetic steroid with both glucocorticoid and mineralocorticoid properties that affect nearly all systems of the body. **Anti-inflammatory (glucocorticoid) action:** Stabilizes leukocyte lysosomal membranes; inhibits phagocytosis and release of allergic substances; suppresses fibroblast formation and collagen deposition; reduces capillary dilation and permeability; and increases responsiveness of cardiovascular system to circulating catecholamines. **Immunosuppressive action:** Modifies immune response to various stimuli; reduces antibody titers; and suppresses cell-mediated hypersensitivity reactions. **Mineralocorticoid action:** Promotes sodium retention, but under certain circumstances (e.g., sodium loading), enhances sodium excretion; promotes potassium excretion; and increases glomerular filtration rate (GFR).

Metabolic action: Promotes hepatic gluconeogenesis, protein catabolism, redistribution of body fat, and lipolysis. *Has anti-inflammatory, immunosuppressive, and metabolic functions in the body.*

USES Replacement therapy in adrenocortical insufficiency; to reduce serum calcium in hypercalcemia, to suppress undesirable inflammatory or immune responses, to produce temporary remission in nonadrenal disease, and to block ACTH production in diagnostic tests. Use as anti-inflammatory or immunosuppressive agent largely replaced by synthetic glucocorticoids that have minimal mineralocorticoid activity. Topically for atopic dermatitis or inflammatory conditions.

CONTRAINDICATIONS Hypersensitivity to glucocorticoids, idiopathic thrombocytopenic purpura, psychoses, acute glomerulonephritis, viral or bacterial diseases of skin, infections not controlled by antibiotics, active or latent amebiasis, hypercorticism (Cushing's syndrome), smallpox vaccination or other immunologic procedures; acne. Topical steroids contraindicated in presence of varicella, vaccinia, on surfaces with compromised circulation; pregnancy (category D first trimester), lactation (except for topical use).

CAUTIOUS USE Children; diabetes mellitus; chronic, active hepatitis positive for hepatitis B surface antigen; hyperlipidemia; cirrhosis; stromal herpes simplex; glaucoma, tuberculosis of eye; osteoporosis; convulsive disorders; hypothyroidism; diverticulitis; nonspecific ulcerative colitis; fresh intestinal anastomoses; active or latent peptic ulcer; gastritis; esophagitis; thromboembolic disorders; CHF; metastatic carcinoma; hypertension; renal insufficiency; history of allergies; active or arrested tuberculosis; systemic fungal infection; myasthenia gravis; pregnancy (category C second and third trimester).

ROUTE & DOSAGE

Adrenal Insufficiency, Anti-inflammatory

Adult: **PO** 10–320 mg/day in 3–4 divided doses **IV/IM** 15–800 mg/day in 3–4 divided doses (max: 2 g/day) **Subcutaneous** Sodium phosphate only, 15–240 mg/day
Child: **PO** 2.5–10 mg/kg/day in 3–4 divided doses **IV/IM** 1–5 mg/kg/day divided q12–24h

Intra-articular, Intralesional (Acetate Salt)

Adult: **IM** 5–50 mg q3–5days for bursae; 5–50 mg once q1–4wk for joints

Anti-inflammatory Agent

Adult: **Topical** Apply a small amount to the affected area 1–4 times/day **PR** Insert 1% cream, 10% foam, 10–25 mg suppository, or 100 mg enema nightly

Atopic Dermatitis

Adult/Adolescent/Child/Infant (older than 3 mo): **Topical** Apply sparingly b.i.d.

ADMINISTRATION

Note: Hydrocortisone phosphate may be given subcutaneously, IM, or IV. Hydrocortisone succinate may be given IM or IV.

Oral

- Give oral drug with food.

Rectal

- Administer retention enema preferably after a bowel movement;

retain at least 1 h or all night if possible.

Topical

- Apply medication sparingly, rub until it disappears, and then reapply, leaving a thin coat over lesion. Cover area with transparent plastic or other occlusive device or vehicle only when so ordered.
- Avoid covering a weeping or exudative lesion.
- Note: Occlusive dressings usually are not applied to face, scalp, scrotum, axilla, and groin.
- Inspect skin carefully between applications for ecchymotic, petechial, and purpuric signs, maceration, secondary infection, skin atrophy, striae or miliaria; if present, stop medication and notify physician.
- Store medication at 15°–30° C (59°–86° F) unless otherwise directed by manufacturer; protect from light and freezing.

Intramuscular

- Inject deep into gluteal muscle.

Intravenous

IV administration to infants, children: Verify correct IV concentration and rate of infusion/injection with physician.

PREPARE: **Direct (preferred):** Give undiluted. **Intermittent:** Dilute in 50–1000 mL of D5W, NS, or D5/NS.

ADMINISTER: **Direct:** Give each dose at a rate of 500 mg or fraction thereof over 1 min. **Intermittent:** Give over 10 min.

INCOMPATIBILITIES **Solution/additive: Amobarbital, ampicillin, bleomycin, colistimethate, dimenhydrinate, doxapram, doxorubicin, ephedrine, heparin, hydralazine, metaraminol, methicillin, nafcillin, pentobarbital, phenobarbital, prochlorperazine, promethazine, secobarbital, tetracycline. Y-site: Ergotamine, phenytoin.**

- Administer solutions that have been diluted for IV infusion within 24 h.

ADVERSE EFFECTS (≥1%) **Body as a Whole:** Hypersensitivity or anaphylactoid reactions; aggravation or masking of infections; malaise, weight gain, obesity; urogenital urinary frequency and urgency, enuresis increased or decreased motility and number of sperm. **CNS:** Vertigo, headache, nystagmus, ataxia (rare), increased intracranial pressure with papilledema (usually after discontinuation of medication), mental disturbances, aggravation of preexisting psychiatric conditions, insomnia, anxiety, mental confusion, depression. **CV:** Syncopal episodes, thrombophlebitis, thromboembolism or fat embolism, palpitation, tachycardia, necrotizing angiitis, CHF, hypertension edema. **Endocrine:** Suppressed linear growth in children, decreased glucose tolerance; hyperglycemia, manifestations of latent diabetes mellitus; hypocorticism; amenorrhea and other menstrual difficulties; moon facies. **Special Senses:** Posterior subcapsular cataracts (especially in children), glaucoma, exophthalmos, increased intraocular pressure with optic nerve damage, perforation of the globe, fungal infection of the cornea, decreased or blurred vision. **Metabolic:** Hypocalcemia; *sodium* and *fluid retention;* hypokalemia and hypokalemic alkalosis decreased serum concentration of vitamins A and C; hyperglycemia, hypernatremia. **GI:** Cramping, bleeding, *nausea,* increased appetite, ulcerative esophagitis, pancreatitis, abdominal distention, peptic ulcer with perforation and hemorrhage, melena. **Hematologic:** Thrombocytopenia, polycythemia, ecchymoses. **Musculoskeletal:** Osteoporosis, compression fractures, muscle wasting and weakness, tendon rupture, aseptic necrosis of femoral and humeral heads. **Skin:** Skin thinning and atrophy, *acne, impaired wound healing;* petechiae, ecchymosis, easy bruising; suppression of skin test reaction; hypopigmentation or hyperpigmentation, hirsutism, acneiform eruptions, subcutaneous fat atrophy; allergic dermatitis, urticaria, angioneurotic edema, increased sweating. With parenteral therapy at IV site–pain, irritation, necrosis, atrophy, sterile abscess; Charcot-like arthropathy following intra-articular use; burning and tingling in perineal area (after IV injection).

DIAGNOSTIC TEST INTERFERENCE Hydrocortisone (corticosteroids) may increase serum ***cholesterol, blood glucose,*** serum ***sodium, uric acid*** (in acute leukemia) and ***calcium*** (in bone metastasis). It may decrease serum ***calcium, potassium, PBI, thyroxin (T_4), triiodothyronine (T_3) and reduce thyroid I 131*** uptake. It increases ***urine glucose*** level and ***calcium*** excretion; decreases ***urine 17-OHCS*** and ***17-KS*** levels. May produce false-negative results with ***nitroblue tetrazolium test*** for systemic bacterial infection and may suppress reactions to skin tests.

INTERACTIONS Drug: BARBITURATES, **phenytoin, rifampin** may increase hepatic metabolism, thus decreasing cortisone levels; ESTROGENS potentiate the effects of hydrocortisone; NSAIDS compound ulcerogenic effects; **cholestyramine, colestipol** decrease hydrocortisone absorption; DIURETICS, **amphotericin B** exacerbate hypokalemia; ANTICHOLINESTERASE AGENTS (e.g., **neostigmine**) may produce severe weakness; immune response to VACCINES and TOXOIDS may be decreased.

PHARMACOKINETICS Absorption: Readily from GI tract and IM injection site. **Onset:** 1–2 h PO; immediately IV; 3–5 days PR. **Peak:** 1 h PO; 4–8 h IM. **Duration:** 1–1.5 days PO/IM; 0.5–4 wk intra-articular. **Distribution:** Distributed primarily to muscles, liver, skin, intestines, kidneys; crosses placenta. **Metabolism:** In liver. **Elimination:** HPA suppression 8–12 h; metabolites excreted in urine; excreted in breast milk. **Half-Life:** 1.5–2 h.

NURSING IMPLICATIONS

Assessment & Drug Effects

- Establish baseline and continuing data on BP, weight, fluid and electrolyte balance, and blood glucose.
- Lab tests: Periodic serum electrolytes blood glucose, Hct and Hgb, platelet count, and WBC with differential.
- Monitor for adverse effects. Older adults and patients with low serum albumin are especially susceptible to adverse effects.
- Be alert to signs of hypocalcemia (see Appendix F).
- Ophthalmoscopic examinations are recommended every 2–3 mo, especially if patient is receiving ophthalmic steroid therapy.
- Monitor for persistent backache or chest pain; compression and spontaneous fractures of long bones and vertebrae present hazards.
- Monitor for and report changes in mood and behavior, emotional instability, or psychomotor activity, especially with long-term therapy.

- Be alert to possibility of masked infection and delayed healing (anti-inflammatory and immunosuppressive actions).
- Note: Dose adjustment may be required if patient is subjected to severe stress (serious infection, surgery, or injury).
- Note: Single doses of corticosteroids or use for a short period (less than 1 wk) do not produce withdrawal symptoms when discontinued, even with moderately large doses.

Patient & Family Education

- Expect a slight weight gain with improved appetite. After dosage is stabilized, notify physician of a sudden slow but steady weight increase [2 kg (5 lb)/wk].
- Avoid alcohol and caffeine; may contribute to steroid-ulcer development in long-term therapy.
- Do not ignore dyspepsia with hyperacidity. Report symptoms to physician and do NOT self-medicate to find relief.
- Do NOT use aspirin or other OTC drugs unless prescribed specifically by the physician.
- Note: A high protein, calcium, and vitamin D diet is advisable to reduce risk of corticosteroid-induced osteoporosis.
- Notify physician of slow healing, any vague feeling of being sick, or return to pretreatment symptoms.
- Do not abruptly discontinue drug; doses are gradually reduced to prevent withdrawal symptoms.
- Report exacerbation of disease during drug withdrawal.
- Apply topical preparations sparingly in small children. The hazard of systemic toxicity is higher because of the greater ratio of skin surface area to body weight.

HYDROMORPHONE HYDROCHLORIDE

(hye-droe-mor′fone)

Dilaudid, Dilaudid-HP

Classifications: NARCOTIC (OPIATE) AGONIST; ANALGESIC

Therapeutic: NARCOTIC ANALGESIC; ANTITUSSIVE

Prototype: Morphine

Pregnancy Category: C; D in prolonged use or high doses at term

Controlled Substance: Schedule II

AVAILABILITY 2 mg, 4 mg, 8 mg tablets; 5 mg/5 mL oral liquid; 1 mg/mL, 10 mg/mL injection

ACTION & *THERAPEUTIC EFFECT* Has more rapid onset and shorter duration of action than morphine, and is reported to have less hypnotic effect. *An effective narcotic analgesic that controls mild to moderate pain. Also has antitussive properties.*

USES Relief of moderate to severe pain and control of persistent nonproductive cough.

CONTRAINDICATIONS Intolerance to opiate agonists; opiate-naïve patients; acute bronchial asthma, COPD, upper airway obstruction, decreased respiratory reserve, severe respiratory depression; pregnancy (category D if used for prolonged periods or in high does at term); lactation.

CAUTIOUS USE Abrupt discontinuation, alcoholism; angina; biliary tract disease; older adults; epidural administration; GI disease, GI obstruction; head trauma; heart failure; hepatic disease; hypotension, hypovolemia, oliguria, prostatic hypertrophy; pulmonary disease; renal disease, renal impairment; paralytic ileus; increased intracranial pressure; inflammatory bowel disease; labor; latex hypersensitivity; obstetric delivery; bladder obstruction; cardiac arrhythmias, cardiac disease; respiratory depression; seizure disorder, seizures; substance abuse; surgery; ulcerative colitis; urethral stricture, urinary retention; pregnancy (category C).

ROUTE & DOSAGE

Moderate to Severe Pain

Adult: **PO** 2–4 mg q4–6h prn in naïve patients **Subcutaneous/IM/IV** 0.75–2 mg q4–6h depending on patient response
Child: **PO** 0.03–0.08 mg/kg q4–6h (max: 5 mg/dose) **IV** 0.015 mg/kg q4–6h prn

Antitussive

Adult: **PO** 1 mg q3–4h prn
Child (6–12 y): **PO** 0.5 mg q3–4h prn

ADMINISTRATION

Oral

- For chronic pain, around-the-clock dosing is recommended.

Subcutaneous/Intramuscular

- High-potency hydromorphone is highly concentrated, making delivery of exact small doses difficult. Use high-potency hydromorphone only if an accurate dose can be measured and delivered.
- Store at room 15°–30° C (59°–86° F) and protect from light.

Intravenous

IV administration to children: Verify correct IV concentration and rate of infusion with physician.

PREPARE: **Direct:** May be given undiluted or diluted in 5 mL of sterile water or NS. **IV Infusion:** Solution typically diluted to 1 mg/mL (specific concentration is ordered by physician) in D5W, NS, or other compatible solution. ▪ *For Dilaudid-HP:* Reconstitute 250 mg dry powder vial immediately prior to use with 25 mL sterile water for injection to yield 10 mg/mL. ▪ Final dilution of Dilaudid-HP 250 and HP 500 (supplied 500 mg/50 mL) **must be** ordered by physician.

ADMINISTER: **Direct:** Give 2 mg or fraction thereof over 3–5 min. **IV Infusion:** Both final volume and rate of infusion **must be** ordered by physician.

INCOMPATIBILITIES **Solution/additive: Prochlorperazine, sodium bicarbonate, thiopental. Y-site: Amphotericin B cholesteryl, minocycline, phenytoin, sargramostim, tetracycline, thiopental.**

- A slight discoloration in ampules or multidose vials causes no loss of potency. ▪ Store in tight, light-resistant containers at 15°–30° C (59°–86° F).

ADVERSE EFFECTS (≥1%) **GI:** Nausea, vomiting, constipation. **CNS:** Euphoria, dizziness, sedation, *drowsiness.* **CV:** Hypotension, bradycardia or tachycardia. **Respiratory:** Respiratory depression. **Special Senses:** Blurred vision.

INTERACTIONS Drug: Alcohol and other CNS DEPRESSANTS compound sedation and CNS depression. **Herbal: St. John's wort, kava** may increase sedation.

PHARMACOKINETICS Absorption: 60% absorbed from GI tract. **Onset:** 15 min IV, 30 min PO. **Peak:** 30–90 min. **Duration:** 3–4 h. **Distribution:** Crosses placenta; distributed into breast milk. **Metabolism:** In liver. **Elimination:** In urine. **Half-Life:** 2–3 h.

NURSING IMPLICATIONS

Assessment & Drug Effects

- Note baseline respiratory rate, rhythm, and depth and size of pupils before administration. Respirations of 12/min or less and mitosis are signs of toxicity. Withhold drug and promptly notify physician.
- Monitor vital signs at regular intervals. Drug-induced respiratory depression may occur even with small doses and increases progressively with higher doses.
- Assess effectiveness of pain relief 30 min after medication administration.
- Monitor drug effects carefully in older adult or debilitated patients and those with impaired renal and hepatic function.
- Assess effectiveness of cough. Drug depresses cough and sigh reflexes and may induce atelectasis, especially in postoperative patients and those with pulmonary disease.
- Note: Nausea and orthostatic hypotension most often occur in ambulatory patients or when a supine patient assumes the head-up position.
- Monitor I&O ratio and pattern. Assess lower abdomen for bladder distension. Report oliguria or urinary retention.
- Monitor bowel pattern; drug-induced constipation may require treatment.

Patient & Family Education

- Request medication at the onset of pain and do not wait until pain is severe.
- Use caution with activities requiring alertness; drug may cause drowsiness, dizziness, and blurred vision.
- Avoid alcohol and other CNS depressants while taking this drug.

H

HYDROQUINONE

(hye′droe-kwin-one)

Eldopaque, Eldoquin, Esoterica Regular, Melanex, Porcelana, Solaquin

Classifications: PIGMENT AGENT; DEPIGMENTOR

Therapeutic: DEPIGMENTOR

Pregnancy Category: C

AVAILABILITY 1.5%, 2%, 3%, 4% cream, gel, solution

ACTION & *THERAPEUTIC EFFECT* Topical agent that causes reversible bleaching of hyperpigmented skin due to increased melanin. Interferes with formation of new melanin but does not destroy existing pigment. Depresses melanin synthesis and melanocytic growth, possibly by increasing excretion of melanin from melanocytes. *Interferes with formation of new melanin but does not destroy existing pigment.*

USES Gradual bleaching of hyperpigmented skin conditions such as chloasma or melasma, severe freckling, senile lentigines (age spots or liver spots). Also as an antioxidant in topical preparations. Some formulations include a sunscreening agent (e.g., Porcelana with Sunscreen, Mercolized Cocrema, Pabaquinone, and Solaquin).

CONTRAINDICATIONS Hyersensitivity to hydroquinone, PABA, paraben, or sulfite; prickly heat, sunburn, irritated skin, depilatory usage.

CAUTIOUS USE Pregnancy (category C), lactation. Safe use in children younger than 12 y not established.

ROUTE & DOSAGE

Bleaching of Hyperpigmented Skin
Adult: **Topical** Apply thin layer and rub into hyperpigmented skin b.i.d., a.m. and p.m.

ADMINISTRATION

Topical

- Test skin for sensitivity before treatment is initiated. Apply small amount of drug (about 25 mm in diameter) to an unbroken patch of skin and check in 24 h. Do not use drug if vesicle formation, itching, or excessive inflammation occur. Minor redness is not a contraindication.
- Limit applications to an area no larger than that of face and neck.

ADVERSE EFFECTS (≥1%) **Skin:** Dryness and fissuring of paranasal and infraorbital areas, inflammatory reaction, erythema; stinging, tingling, burning sensations; irritation, sensitization, and contact dermatitis.

INTERACTIONS Drug: No clinically significant interactions established.

NURSING IMPLICATIONS

Assessment & Drug Effects

- Monitor for therapeutic effectiveness: In general, complete depigmentation occurs in 1–4 mo and lasts 2–6 mo after hydroquinone is discontinued. Once desired results are obtained, reduce amount and frequency of applications to the least that will maintain depigmentation.
- Discontinue if bleaching or skin lightening does not occur after 2 or 3 mo of therapy.

Patient & Family Education

- Use a sunscreen agent or a hydroquinone formulation containing a sunscreen for daytime applications.
- Wash drug off if rash or irritation develops and consult physician.
- Avoid contact with the eyes and not to use on open lesions, sunburned, irritated, or otherwise damaged skin.
- Continue use of protective clothing and sunscreening agent after treatment is terminated to reduce possibility of repigmentation.

HYDROXOCOBALAMIN (VITAMIN $B_{12 ALPHA}$)

(hye-drox-oh-koe-bal'a-min)

Hydrobexan, Hydroxo-12, LA-12

Classification: VITAMIN SUPPLEMENT

Therapeutic: VITAMIN B_{12} REPLACEMENT

Prototype: Cyanocobalamin

Pregnancy Category: A (C if greater than RDA)

AVAILABILITY 1000 mcg/mL injection

ACTION & *THERAPEUTIC EFFECT* Cobalamin derivative similar to cyanocobalamin (vitamin B_{12}). Essential for normal cell growth, cell reproduction maturation of RBCs, myelin synthesis, and believed to be involved in protein synthesis. *Effective in vitamin B_{12} deficiency that results in megaloblastic anemia.*

USES Treatment of vitamin B_{12} deficiency.

UNLABELED USES Cyanide poisoning and tobacco amblyopia.

CONTRAINDICATIONS History of sensitivity to vitamin B_{12}, other cobalamins, or cobalt; indiscriminate use in folic acid deficiency.

CAUTIOUS USE Pregnancy (category A; category C in greater than RDA), lactation, children.

ROUTE & DOSAGE

Vitamin B_{12} Deficiency
Adult: **IM** 30 mcg/day for 5–10 days and then 100–200 mcg/mo or 1000 mcg every other day until remission and then 1000 mcg/mo
Child: **IM** 100 mcg doses to a total of 1–5 mg over 2 wk and then 30–50 mcg/mo

ADMINISTRATION

Intramuscular
- Give deep into a large muscle.

INTERACTIONS **Drug: Chloramphenicol** may interfere with therapeutic response to hydroxocobalamin.

PHARMACOKINETICS **Distribution:** Widely distributed; principally stored in liver, kidneys, and adrenals; crosses placenta. **Metabolism:** Converted in tissues to active coenzymes; enterohepatically cycled. **Elimination:** 50–95% of doses 100 mcg or greater are excreted in urine in 48 h; excreted in breast milk.

NURSING IMPLICATIONS

Assessment & Drug Effects
- Monitor for therapeutic effectiveness: Response to drug therapy is usually dramatic, occurring within 48 h. Effectiveness is measured by laboratory values and improvement in manifestations of vitamin B_{12} deficiency.
- Lab tests: Prior to therapy determine reticulocyte and erythrocyte counts, Hgb, Hct, vitamin B_{12}, and serum folate levels; repeated 5–7 days after start of therapy and at regular intervals during therapy.
- Obtain a careful history of sensitivities. Sensitization can take as long as 8 y to develop.
- Monitor potassium levels during the first 48 h, particularly in patients with Addisonian pernicious anemia or megaloblastic anemia. Conversion to normal erythropoiesis can result in severe hypokalemia and sudden death.
- Monitor vital signs in patients with cardiac disease and be alert to symptoms of pulmonary edema; generally occur early in therapy.
- Monitor bowel function. Bowel regularity is essential for consistent absorption of oral preparations.

Patient & Family Education
- Notify physician of any intercurrent disease or infection. Increased dosage may be required.
- Note: It is imperative to understand that drug therapy **must be** continued throughout life for pernicious anemia to prevent irreversible neurologic damage.
- Neurologic damage is considered irreversible if there is no improvement after 1–1.5 y of adequate therapy.
- Dietary deficiency of vitamin B_{12} has been observed in strict vegetarians (vegans) and their breastfed infants as well as in the elderly.

HYDROXYCHLOROQUINE

(hye-drox-ee-klor'oh-kwin)

Plaquenil Sulfate

Classifications: BIOLOGICAL RESPONSE MODIFIER; ANTIMALARIAL; DISEASE MODIFYING RHEUMATIC DRUG (DMARD)

Therapeutic: ANTIMALARIAL; ANTIRHEUMATIC

Prototype: Chloroquine
Pregnancy Category: C

AVAILABILITY 200 mg tablets

ACTION & *THERAPEUTIC EFFECT* Antimalarial activity is believed to be based on ability to form complexes with DNA of parasite, thereby inhibiting replication and transcription to RNA and DNA synthesis of the parasite. *Effective against* Plasmodium vivax *and* Plasmodium malariae. *Also is effective as second line of defense for treatment of rheumatoid arthritis and SLE.*

USES Suppressive prophylaxis and treatment of acute malarial attacks due to all forms of susceptible malaria. Used adjunctively with primaquine for eradication of *Plasmodium vivax* and *Plasmodium malariae*. More commonly prescribed than chloroquine for treatment of rheumatoid arthritis and lupus erythematosus (usually in conjunction with salicylate or corticosteroid therapy).
UNLABELED USES Porphyria cutanea tarda.

CONTRAINDICATIONS Known hypersensitivity to retinal or visual field changes associated with quinoline compounds; psoriasis, porphyria, G6PD deficiency; long-term therapy in children.
CAUTIOUS USE Hepatic disease; alcoholism, use with hepatotoxic drugs; impaired renal function, porphoria; metabolic acidosis; patients with tendency to dermatitis; pregnancy (category C).

ROUTE & DOSAGE

Note: Doses are expressed in terms of hydroxychloroquine base: 400 mg tablet = 310 mg base; 800 mg tablet = 620 mg base

Acute Malaria

Adult: **PO** 620 mg base followed by 310 mg base at 6, 18, and 24 h
Child: **PO** 10 mg base/kg, then 5 mg base/kg at 6, 18, and 24 h

Malaria Suppression

Adult: **PO** 310 mg base the same day each week starting 2 wk before exposure and continuing for 4–6 wk after leaving the area of exposure
Child: **PO** 5 mg base/kg the same day each week starting 2 wk before exposure and continuing for 4–8 wk after leaving the area of exposure

Lupus Erythematosus

Adult: **PO** 310 mg base 1–2 times/day
Child: **PO** 3–5 mg/kg/day in 1–2 divided doses (max: 400 mg/day or 7 mg/kg/day)

Rheumatoid Arthritis

Adult: **PO** 400–600 mg/day until response, then decrease to lowest maintenance levels possible
Child: **PO** 3–5 mg/kg/day in 1–2 divided doses (max: 400 mg/day or 7 mg/kg/day)

ADMINISTRATION

Oral

- Give drug with meals or milk to reduce incidence of GI distress.
- Give antacids and laxatives at least 4 h before or after hydroxychloroquine.
- Store at 15°–30° C (59°–86° F) unless otherwise directed.

ADVERSE EFFECTS (≥1%) **CNS:** Fatigue, vertigo, headache, mood or mental changes, anxiety, *retinopathy,* blurred vision, difficulty focusing. **GI:** Anorexia, nausea, vomiting, diarrhea, abdominal cramps, weight loss. **Hematologic:** Hemolysis in patients with G6PD deficiency, <u>agranulocytosis</u> (rare), <u>aplastic anemia</u> (rare), thrombocytopenia. **Skin:** Bleaching or loss of hair, unusual pigmentation (blue-black) of skin or inside mouth, skin rash, itching.

INTERACTIONS Drug: Aluminum- and **magnesium**-containing ANTACIDS and LAXATIVES decrease hydroxychloroquine absorption; separate administrations by at least 4 h; hydroxychloroquine may interfere with response to **rabies vaccine.**

PHARMACOKINETICS Absorption: Rapidly and almost completely absorbed. **Peak:** 1–2 h. **Distribution:** Widely distributed; concentrates in lungs, liver, erythrocytes, eyes, skin, and kidneys; crosses placenta. **Metabolism:** Partially in liver to active metabolite. **Elimination:** In urine; excreted in breast milk. **Half-Life:** 70–120 h.

NURSING IMPLICATIONS

Assessment & Drug Effects

- Monitor for therapeutic effectiveness; may not appear for several weeks, and maximal benefit may not occur for 6 mo.
- Lab tests: Baseline and periodic blood cell counts on all patients on long-term therapy.
- Withhold drug and notify physician if weakness, visual symptoms, hearing loss, unusual bleeding, bruising, or skin eruptions occur.

Patient & Family Education

- Learn about adverse effects and their symptoms when taking prolonged therapy.
- Follow drug regimen exactly as prescribed by the physician.

HYDROXYUREA

(hye-drox′ee-yoo-ree-ah)

Hydrea, Droxia

Classifications: ANTINEOPLASTIC; ANTIMETABOLITE

Therapeutic: ANTINEOPLASTIC

Pregnancy Category: D

AVAILABILITY 500 mg capsules

ACTION & *THERAPEUTIC EFFECT* A cell-cycle-phase antineoplastic agent; hydroxyurea causes an immediate inhibition of DNA synthesis by acting as an RNA reductase inhibitor, necessary for DNA synthesis but without interfering with the synthesis of RNA or protein. *Cytotoxic effect limited to tissues with high rates of cell proliferation.*

USES Palliative treatment of metastatic melanoma, chronic myelocytic leukemia; recurrent metastatic, or inoperable ovarian cancer. Also used as adjunct to x-ray therapy for treatment of advanced primary squamous cell (epidermoid) carcinoma of head (excluding lip), neck, lungs.

UNLABELED USES Psoriasis; combination therapy with radiation of lung carcinoma; sickle cell anemia.

CONTRAINDICATIONS Pregnancy (category D), lactation, severe myelosuppression. Safety and effectiveness in children not established.

CAUTIOUS USE Recent use of other cytotoxic drugs or irradiation; bone marrow depression; renal dysfunction; HIV patients; older adults; history of gout.

ROUTE & DOSAGE

Palliative Therapy

Adult: **PO** 80 mg/kg q3days or 20–30 mg/kg/day

Sickle Cell Anemia

Adult: **PO** 15 mg/kg/day, may increase by 5 mg/kg/day (max: 35 mg/kg/day or until toxicity develops)

Renal Impairment Dosage Adjustment

CrCl 10–50 mL/min: Administer 50% of dose; less than 10 mL/min: Administer 20% of dose

Hemodialysis Dosage Adjustment: Administer dose after hemodialysis; no supplemental dose needed

ADMINISTRATION

Oral

- Open, mix with water, and give immediately when patient has difficulty swallowing capsule.
- Store in tightly covered container at 15°–30° C (59°–86° F) unless otherwise directed.

ADVERSE EFFECTS (≥1%) **CNS:** Rare: Headache, dizziness, hallucinations, convulsions. **GI:** Stomatitis, anorexia, nausea, vomiting, diarrhea, constipation. **Hematologic:** Bone marrow suppression (*leukopenia,* anemia, thrombocytopenia), megaloblastic erythropoiesis. **Skin:** Maculopapular rash, facial erythema, postirradiation erythema. **Urogenital:** Renal tubular dysfunction, elevated BUN, serum, creatinine levels, hyperuricemia. **Body as a Whole:** Fever, chills, malaise.

INTERACTIONS Drug: No clinically significant interactions established.

PHARMACOKINETICS Absorption: Readily absorbed from GI tract. **Peak:** 2 h. **Distribution:** Crosses blood–brain barrier. **Metabolism:** In liver. **Elimination:** As respiratory CO_2 and as urea in urine.

NURSING IMPLICATIONS

Assessment & Drug Effects

- Lab tests: Determine status of kidney, liver, and bone marrow function before and periodically during therapy; monitor hemoglobin, WBC, platelet counts at least once weekly.
- Interrupt therapy if WBC drops to $2500/mm^3$ or platelets to $100,000/mm^3$.
- Monitor I&O. Advise patients with high serum uric acid levels to drink at least 10–12 240 mL (8 oz) glasses of fluid daily to prevent uric acid nephropathy.
- Note: Patients with marked renal dysfunction may rapidly develop visual and auditory hallucinations and hematologic toxicity.

Patient & Family Education

- Notify physician of fever, chills, sore throat, nausea, vomiting, diarrhea, loss of appetite, and unusual bruising or bleeding.
- Use barrier contraceptive during therapy. Drug is teratogenic.

HYDROXYZINE HYDROCHLORIDE (Pr)

(hye-drox′i-zeen)

Atarax Syrup, Hyzine-50, Vistaril Intramuscular, Vistacon, Vistaject-25 & -50

HYDROXYZINE PAMOATE

Vistaril Oral

Classifications: ANTIHISTAMINE; H_1-RECEPTOR ANTAGONIST

Therapeutic: ANTIHISTAMINE; ANTIPRURITIC; ANTIANXIETY; ANTIEMETIC

Pregnancy Category: C

AVAILABILITY Hydroxyzine HCl: 10 mg, 25 mg, 50 mg tablets; 10 mg/5 mL syrup; 25 mg/5 mL oral suspension; 25 mg/mL, 50 mg/mL injection; **Hydroxyzine Pamoate:** 25 mg, 50 mg, 100 mg capsules; 25 mg/5 mL suspension

ACTION & *THERAPEUTIC EFFECT* H_1-receptor antagonist effective in treatment of histamine-mediated pruritus or other allergic reactions. Its tranquilizing effect is produced primarily by depression of hypothalamus and brain-stem reticular formation, rather than cortical areas. *Effective as an antianxiety agent and sedative. Additionally, it is an effective agent for pruritus.*

USES Emotional or psychoneurotic states characterized by anxiety, tension, or psychomotor agitation; to relieve anxiety, control nausea and emesis, and reduce narcotic requirements before or after surgery or delivery. Also used in management of pruritus due to allergic conditions (e.g., chronic urticaria), atopic and contact dermatoses, and in treatment of acute and chronic alcoholism with withdrawal symptoms or delirium tremens.

CONTRAINDICATIONS Known hypersensitivity to hydroxyzine; use as sole treatment in psychoses or depression; lactation.

CAUTIOUS USE History of allergies; GI disorders; cardiac disease; COPD; older adults; pregnancy (category C).

ROUTE & DOSAGE

Anxiety
Adult: **PO** 25–100 mg t.i.d. or q.i.d. **IM** 25–100 mg q4–6h
Child: **PO** *Younger than 6 y,* 50 mg/day in divided doses; *older than 6 y,* 50 mg/day in divided doses **IM** 1.1 mg/kg q4–6h

Pruritus
Adult: **PO** 25 mg t.i.d. or q.i.d. **IM** 25 mg q4–6h
Geriatric: **PO** 10 mg 3–4 times daily
Child: **PO** *Older than 6 y,* 50–100 mg/day in divided doses; *younger than 6 y,* 50 mg/day in divided doses **IM** 1.1 mg/kg q4–6h

Nausea
Adult: **IM** 25–100 mg q4–6h
Child: **IM** 1.1 mg/kg q4–6h

ADMINISTRATION

Oral
- Note: Tablets may be crushed and taken with fluid of patient's choice. Capsule may be emptied and contents swallowed with water or mixed with food. Liquid formulations are available.

Intramuscular
- Give deep into body of a relatively large muscle. The Z-track technique of injection is recommended to prevent subcutaneous infiltration.
- Recommended site: In adult, the gluteus maximus or vastus lateralis; in children, the vastus lateralis.
- Protect all forms from light. Store at 15°–30° C (59°–86° F) unless otherwise specified.

INCOMPATIBILITIES Solution/additive: **Aminophylline, amobarbital, chloramphenicol, dimenhydrinate, penicillin G, pentobarbital, phenobarbital.**

ADVERSE EFFECTS (≥1%) **CNS:** *Drowsiness* (usually transitory), sedation, dizziness, headache. **CV:** Hypotension. **GI:** *Dry mouth.* **Body as a Whole:** Urticaria, dyspnea, chest tightness, wheezing, involuntary motor activity (rare). **Hemato-**

logic: Phlebitis, hemolysis, thrombosis. **Skin:** Erythematous macular eruptions, erythema multiforme, digital gangrene from inadvertent IV or intra-arterial injection, injection site reactions.

DIAGNOSTIC TEST INTERFERENCE Possibility of false-positive ***urinary 17-hydroxycorticosteroid*** determinations (modified ***Glenn-Nelson technique***).

INTERACTIONS Drug: Alcohol and CNS DEPRESSANTS add to CNS depression; TRICYCLIC ANTIDEPRESSANTS and other ANTICHOLINERGICS have additive anticholinergic effects; may inhibit pressor effects of **epinephrine.**

PHARMACOKINETICS Absorption: Readily from GI tract. **Onset:** 15–30 min PO. **Duration:** 4–6 h. **Distribution:** Not known if it crosses placenta or is distributed into breast milk. **Metabolism:** In liver. **Elimination:** In bile.

NURSING IMPLICATIONS

Assessment & Drug Effects

- Evaluate alertness. Drowsiness may occur and usually disappears with continued therapy or following reduction of dosage.
- Monitor condition of oral membranes daily when patient is on high dosage of hydroxyzine.
- Reduce dosage of the depressant up to 50% when CNS depressants are prescribed concomitantly.

Patient & Family Education

- Do not drive or engage in other potentially hazardous activities until response to drug is known.
- Do NOT take alcohol and hydroxyzine at the same time.
- Relieve dry mouth by frequent warm water rinses, increasing fluid intake, and use of a salivary substitute (e.g., Moi-Stir, Xero-Lube).
- Give teeth scrupulous care. Avoid irritation or abrasion of gums and other oral tissues.

HYOSCYAMINE SULFATE

(hye-oh-sye'a-meen)

Anaspaz, Cystospaz, Levsin, Levsinex, NuLev

Classifications: ANTICHOLINERGIC; ANTIMUSCARINIC; ANTISPASMODIC

Therapeutic: ANTISPASMODIC

Prototype: Atropine

Pregnancy Category: C

AVAILABILITY 0.125 mg, 0.150 mg tablets; 0.125 mg sublingual tablets; 0.375 sustained release capsules; 0.125 mg orally disintegrating tablet 0.125 mg/mL oral solution; 0.125 mg/5 mL elixir; 0.5 mg/mL injection

ACTION & *THERAPEUTIC EFFECT* Competitive inhibitor of acethycholine at autonomic postganglionic cholinergic receptors. It decreases motility (smooth muscle tone) in GI, biliary, and urinary tracts. Specific anticholingenric responses are dose-related. *Has both anticholinergic and antispasmodic activity.*

USES GI tract disorders caused by spasm and hypermotility, as conjunct therapy with diet and antacids for peptic ulcer management, and as an aid in the control of gastric hypersecretion and intestinal hypermotility. Also symptomatic relief of biliary and renal colic, as a "drying agent" to relieve symptoms of acute rhinitis, to control preanesthesia salivation and respiratory tract secretions, to treat symptoms of parkinsonism, and to reduce pain and hypersecretion in pancreatitis.

CONTRAINDICATIONS Hypersensitivity to belladonna alkaloids, prostatic hypertrophy, obstructive diseases of GI or GU tract, ulcerative colitis, paralytic ileus or intestinal atony; myasthenia gravis; children younger than 2 y.

CAUTIOUS USE Diabetes mellitus, cardiac disease, cardiac arrhythmias; autonomic neuropathy; closed-angle glaucoma; GERD, hiatal hernia; pulmonary disease; renal or hepatic disease; pregnancy (category C), lactation.

ROUTE & DOSAGE

GI Spasms

Adult: **IV/IM/Subcutaneous** 0.25–0.5 mg q4h **PO/SL** 0.125–0.25 mg t.i.d. or q.i.d. prn

Child (2–12 y): **PO** 0.0625–0.125 mg q4h prn (max: 0.75 mg/day)

ADMINISTRATION

- Note: Dose for older adults may need to be less than the standard adult dose. Observe patient carefully for signs of paradoxic reactions.

Oral

- Give preparations about 1 h before meals and at bedtime (at least 2 h after last meal).
- Ensure that sustained release form of drug is not chewed or crushed. It **must be** swallowed whole.

Intramuscular/Subcutaneous

- May be given undiluted.

Intravenous

PREPARE: **Direct:** Give undiluted.
ADMINISTER: **Direct:** Give a single dose over 60 sec.

- Store 15°–30° C (59°–86° F).

ADVERSE EFFECTS (≥1%) **CNS:** Headache, unusual tiredness or weakness, confusion, *drowsiness,* excitement in older adult patients. **CV:** Palpitations, tachycardia. **Special Senses:** *Blurred vision,* increased intraocular tension, cycloplegia, mydriasis. **GI:** *Dry mouth, constipation,* paralytic ileus. **Other:** *Urinary retention,* anhidrosis, suppression of lactation.

INTERACTIONS Drug: Amantadine, ANTIHISTAMINES, TRICYCLIC ANTIDEPRESSANTS, **quinidine, disopyramide, procainamide** add anticholinergic effects; decreases **levodopa** effects; **methotrimeprazine** may precipitate extrapyramidal effects; decreases antipsychotic effects of PHENOTHIAZINES (decreased absorption).

PHARMACOKINETICS Absorption: Well absorbed from all administration sites. **Onset:** 2–3 min IV; 20–30 min PO. **Peak:** 15–30 min IV; 30–60 min PO. **Duration:** 4–6 h (up to 12 h with sustained release form). **Distribution:** Distributed in most body tissues; crosses blood–brain barrier and placenta; distributed in breast milk. **Metabolism:** In liver. **Elimination:** In urine. **Half-Life:** 3.5–13 h.

NURSING IMPLICATIONS

Assessment & Drug Effects

- Monitor bowel elimination; may cause constipation.
- Monitor urinary output.
- Lessen risk of urinary retention by having patient void prior to each dose.
- Assess for dry mouth and recommend good practices of oral hygiene.

Patient & Family Education

- Avoid excessive exposure to high temperatures; drug-induced heatstroke can develop.
- Do not drive or engage in other potentially hazardous activities until response to drug is known.
- Use dark glasses if experiencing blurred vision, but if this adverse effect persists, notify physician for dose adjustment or possible drug change.

IBANDRONATE SODIUM

Boniva

Classifications: BISPHOSPHONATE; BONE METABOLISM REGULATOR

Therapeutic: BONE METABOLISM REGULATOR

Prototype: Etidronate

Pregnancy Category: C

AVAILABILITY 2.5 mg and 150 mg tablets

ACTION & *THERAPEUTIC EFFECT* Ibandronate is a potent third-generation bisphosphonate. It inhibits activity of osteoclasts and reduces bone resorption and turnover in the matrix of the bone. *In postmenopausal women, it reduces the rate of bone turnover, resulting in a net gain in bone mass.*

USES Prevention and treatment of osteoporosis in postmenopausal women.

UNLABELED USES Treatment of metastatic bone disease in breast cancer.

CONTRAINDICATIONS Hypersensitivity to ibandronate; severe renal impairment; hypocalcemia, vitamin D deficiency; inability to stand or sit up straight for 60 min; achalasia, esophageal stricture, dysphagia; concurrent administration with antacids, supplements, or vitamins; children younger than 18 y.

CAUTIOUS USE Mild or moderate renal impairment; history of GI bleeding or disease, esophagitis, esophageal or gastric ulcers; older adults; pregnancy (category C), lactation.

ROUTE & DOSAGE

Postmenopausal Osteoporosis

Adult: **PO** 2.5 mg daily or 150 mg once monthly on the same day each month

Renal Impairment Dosage Adjustment

CrCl less than 30 mL/min: Use not recommended

ADMINISTRATION

- Correct hypocalcemia before administering ibandronate.
- Give at least 60 min before food, beverage, or other medications (including vitamins).
- Instruct to swallowed whole with a full glass of plain water (180–240 mL; 6–8 oz) while standing or sitting in an upright position.
- Keep patient sitting up or ambulating for 60 min after taking drug.
- Store 15°–30° C (59°–86° F).

ADVERSE EFFECTS (≥1%) **CNS:** Dizziness, headache, nerve root lesion, vertigo. **GI:** Dyspepsia, constipation, diarrhea, esophagitis, gastritis, pharyngitis, nausea, vomiting. **Respiratory:** Upper respiratory infection, pharyngitis. **Skin:** Rash. **Body as a Whole:** Back pain. **Other:** Tooth disorder.

DIAGNOSTIC TEST INTERFERENCE Interferes with the use of bone-imaging agents.

INTERACTIONS Drug: Concurrent administration of **calcium, magnesium,** or **iron** reduces ibandronate adsorption. **Food:** Food reduces ibandronate absorption (ibandronate should be taken in a fasting state).

PHARMACOKINETICS Absorption: Bioavailability poor (0.6%). **Peak:** 0.5–2 h. **Distribution:** 86–99% protein bound. **Metabolism:** None. **Elimination:** Renal. **Half-Life:** 10–60 h.

NURSING IMPLICATIONS

Assessment & Drug Effects

- Lab tests: Monitor albumin-adjusted serum calcium, serum phosphate, serum alkaline phosphatase, fasting and 24 h urinary calcium, and serum electrolytes; baseline and periodic renal function.

- Withhold drug and notify physician if the CrCl less than 30 mL/min.
- Diagnostic test: Bone density scan every 12–18 mo.
- Monitor for S&S of upper GI distress, especially with concurrent use of NSAIDs or aspirin.

Patient & Family Education

- Take the monthly dose (150 mg) on the same day each month. Carefully follow directions for taking the drug (see ADMINISTRATION).
- If a monthly dose is missed, and the next scheduled dose is more than 7 days away, take one 150 mg tablet the next morning then resume the original monthly schedule. Do not take two 150 mg tablets in the same week.
- Report to physician any of the following: Severe bone, joint, or muscle pain; heartburn, pain behind the sternum, difficulty or pain with swallowing.

I

IBUPROFEN Pr

(eye-byoo′proe-fen)

Advil, Amersol ✤, Caldolor, Children's Motrin, Ibuprin, Junior Strength Motrin Caplets, Motrin, Nuprin, Pediaprofen, Pamprin-IB, Rufen, Trendar

Classifications: ANALGESIC, NONSTEROIDAL ANTI-INFLAMMATORY DRUG (NSAID) (COX-1 AND COX-2 INHIBITOR); ANTIPYRETIC

Therapeutic: ANALGESIC, NSAID; ANTI-INFLAMMATORY; ANTIPYRETIC

Pregnancy Category: B

AVAILABILITY 100 mg, 200 mg, 400 mg, 600 mg, 800 mg tablets; 50 mg, 100 mg chewable tablets; 100 mg/5 mL, 100 mg/2.5 mL suspension; 40 mg/mL drops; 100 mg/mL injection

ACTION & *THERAPEUTIC EFFECT*

Prototype of the propionic acid NSAIDs (COX-1 and COX-2) inhibitor with nonsteroidal anti-inflammatory activity that blocks prostaglandin synthesis. Ibuprofen activity also includes modulation of T-cell function, inhibition of inflammatory cell chemotaxis, decreased release of superoxide radicals, or increased scavenging of these compounds at inflammatory sites. *Has nonsteroidal anti-inflammatory, analgesic, and antipyretic effects. Inhibits platelet aggregation and prolongs bleeding time.*

USES Chronic, symptomatic rheumatoid arthritis and osteoarthritis; relief of mild to moderate pain; primary dysmenorrhea; reduction of fever.

UNLABELED USES Gout, juvenile rheumatoid arthritis, psoriatic arthritis, ankylosing spondylitis, vascular headache.

CONTRAINDICATIONS Patient in whom urticaria, severe rhinitis, bronchospasm, angioedema, nasal polyps are precipitated by aspirin or other NSAIDs; active peptic ulcer, bleeding abnormalities; perioperative pain related to CABG. Safe use in children younger than 6 mo is not established.

CAUTIOUS USE Hypertension, history of GI ulceration; diabetes mellitus, impaired hepatic or renal function, history of coronary artery disease, angina, MI cardiac decompensation; chronic renal failure, patients with SLE; pregnancy (category B).

ROUTE & DOSAGE

Inflammatory Disease

Adult: **PO** 400–800 mg t.i.d. or q.i.d. (max: 3200 mg/day)
Child: **PO** *Weight less than 20 kg,* up to 400 mg/day in divided doses; *weight 20–30 kg,* up to 600 mg/day in divided doses; *weight 30–40 kg,* up to 800 mg/day in divided doses

Dysmenorrhea

Adult: **PO** 400 mg q4–6h up to 1200 mg/day

Mild to Moderate Pain

Adult: **PO** 400 mg q4–6h up to 1200 mg/day **IV** 400 mg q4–6h prn or 100–200 mg q4h prn

Fever

Adult: **PO** 200–400 mg t.i.d. or q.i.d. (max: 1200 mg/day)
Child (6 mo–12 y): **PO** 5–10 mg/kg q4–6h up to 40 mg/kg/day

ADMINISTRATION

Oral

- Give on an empty stomach, 1 h before or 2 h after meals. May be taken with meals or milk if GI intolerance occurs.
- Ensure that chewable tablets are chewed or crushed before being swallowed.
- Note: Tablet may be crushed if patient is unable to swallow it whole and mixed with food or liquid before swallowing.
- Store in tightly closed, light-resistant container unless otherwise directed by manufacturer.

Intravenous

Patients should be well hydrated before IV infusion to prevent renal damage.

PREPARE: **Infusion:** Dilute required dose with NS, D5W or LR to a final concentration of 4 mg/mL or less.

ADMINISTER: **Infusion:** Infuse over at least 30 min.

ADVERSE EFFECTS (≥1%) **CNS:** Headache, dizziness, light-headedness, anxiety, emotional lability, fatigue, malaise, drowsiness, anxiety, confusion, depression, aseptic meningitis. **CV:** Hypertension, palpitation, congestive heart failure (patient with marginal cardiac function); thrombotic events (MI, stroke); peripheral edema. **Special Senses:** Amblyopia (blurred vision, decreased visual acuity, scotomas, changes in color vision); nystagmus, visual-field defects; tinnitus, impaired hearing. **GI:** Dry mouth, gingival ulcerations, dyspepsia, *heartburn, nausea,* vomiting, anorexia, diarrhea, constipation, bloating, flatulence, epigastric or abdominal discomfort or pain, GI ulceration, *occult blood loss.* **Hematologic:** Thrombocytopenia, neutropenia, hemolytic or aplastic anemia, leukopenia; decreased Hgb, Hct; transitory rise in AST, ALT, serum alkaline phosphatase; rise in (Ivy) bleeding time. **GU:** Acute renal failure, polyuria, azotemia, cystitis, hematuria, nephrotoxicity, decreased creatinine clearance. **Skin:** Maculopapular and vesicobullous skin eruptions, erythema multiforme, pruritus, rectal itching, acne. **Body as a Whole:** Fluid retention with edema, Stevens-Johnson syndrome, toxic hepatitis, hypersensitivity reactions, anaphylaxis, bronchospasm, serum sickness, SLE, angioedema.

INTERACTIONS Drug: ORAL ANTICOAGULANTS, **heparin** may prolong bleeding time; may increase **lithium** and **methotrexate** toxicity.

Herbal: Feverfew, garlic, ginger, ginkgo may increase bleeding potential.

PHARMACOKINETICS Absorption: 80% from GI tract (oral product). **Onset:** 1 h (antipyretic). **Peak:** 1–2 h. **Duration:** 6–8 h. **Metabolism:** In liver. **Elimination:** Primarily in urine; some biliary excretion. **Half-Life:** 2–4 h.

NURSING IMPLICATIONS

Assessment & Drug Effects

- Monitor for therapeutic effectiveness. Optimum response generally occurs within 2 wk to anti-inflammatory and/or analgesic effect (e.g., relief of pain, stiffness, or swelling; or improved joint flexion and strength).
- Observe patients with history of cardiac decompensation closely for evidence of fluid retention and edema.
- Lab tests: Baseline and periodic evaluations of Hgb, renal and hepatic function, and auditory and ophthalmologic examinations are recommended in patients receiving prolonged or high-dose therapy.
- Monitor for GI distress and S&S of GI bleeding.
- Note: Symptoms of acute toxicity in children include apnea, cyanosis, response only to painful stimuli, dizziness, and nystagmus.

Patient & Family Education

- Notify physician immediately of passage of dark tarry stools, "coffee ground" emesis, frankly bloody emesis, or other GI distress, as well as blood or protein in urine, and onset of skin rash, pruritus, jaundice.
- Do not drive or engage in other potentially hazardous activities until response to the drug is known.
- Do not self-medicate with ibuprofen if taking prescribed drugs or being treated for a serious condition without consulting physician.
- Do not give to children younger than 3 mo or for longer than 2 days without consulting physician.
- Do not take aspirin concurrently with ibuprofen.
- Avoid alcohol and NSAIDs unless otherwise advised by physician. Concurrent use may increase risk of GI ulceration and bleeding tendencies.

IBUTILIDE FUMARATE

(i-bu'ti-lide)

Corvert

Classification: ANTIARRHYTHMIC, CLASS III

Therapeutic: ANTIARRHYTHMIC, CLASS III

Prototype: Amiodarone HCl

Pregnancy Category: C

AVAILABILITY 0.1 mg/mL injection

ACTION & *THERAPEUTIC EFFECT* Ibutilide is a Class III antiarrhythmic agent that prolongs the cardiac action potential and increases both atrial and ventricular refractoriness without affecting conduction. *Effect in treating recently occurring atrial arrhythmias. Like other Class III antiarrhythmic drugs it may produce proarrhythmic effects that can be life threatening.*

USES Rapid conversion of atrial fibrillation or atrial flutter of recent onset.

CONTRAINDICATIONS Hypersensitivity to ibutilide, hypokalemia, hypomagnesemia. Safety and effectiveness in children younger than 18 y are not established.

CAUTIOUS USE History of CHF, cardiac ejection fraction of 35% or less, recent MI, prolonged QT intervals, ventricular arrhythmias; renal or liver disease, cardiovascular disorder other than atrial arrhythmias; pregnancy (category C), lactation.

ROUTE & DOSAGE

Atrial Fibrillation or Flutter

Adult: IV *Weight less than 60 kg,* 0.01 mg/kg, may repeat in 10 min if inadequate response; *weight 60 kg or greater,* 1 mg, may repeat in 10 min if inadequate response

ADMINISTRATION

- Hypokalemia and hypomagnesemia should be corrected prior to treatment with ibutilide.

Intravenous

PREPARE: **Direct:** Give undiluted. **IV Infusion:** Contents of 1 mg vial may be diluted in 50 mL of D5W or NS to yield 0.017 mg/mL.
ADMINISTER: **Direct/IV Infusion:** Give a single dose by direct injection or infusion over 10 min. ▪Stop injection/infusion as soon as presenting arrhythmia is terminated or with appearance of ventricular tachycardia or marked prolongation of QT or QT_c.

- Store diluted solution up to 24 h at 15°–30° C (59°–86° F) or 48 h refrigerated at 2°–8° C (36°–46° F).

ADVERSE EFFECTS (≥1%) **CNS:** Headache. **CV:** Proarrhythmic effects (sustained and nonsustained polymorphic ventricular tachycardia), AV block, bundle branch block, ventricular extrasystoles, hypotension, postural hypotension, bradycardia, tachycardia, palpitations, prolonged QT segment. **GI:** Nausea.

INTERACTIONS Drug: Increased potential for proarrhythmic effects when administered with PHENOTHIAZINES, TRICYCLIC ANTIDEPRESSANTS, **amiodarone, disopyramide, quinidine, procainamide, sotalol** may cause prolonged refractoriness if given within 4 h of ibutilide.

PHARMACOKINETICS Onset: 30 min. **Metabolism:** In liver. **Elimination:** 82% in urine, 19% in feces. **Half-Life:** 6 h (range 2–21 h).

I

NURSING IMPLICATIONS

Assessment & Drug Effects

- Observe with continuous ECG, BP, and HR monitoring during and for at least 4 h after infusion or until QT_c has returned to baseline. Monitor for longer periods with liver dysfunction or if proarrhythmic activity is observed.
- Lab tests: Baseline serum potassium and magnesium are recommended, as hypokalemia and hypomagnesemia should be corrected prior to beginning treatment with ibutilide.
- Monitor for therapeutic effectiveness. Conversion to normal sinus rhythm normally occurs within 30 min of initiation of infusion.

Patient & Family Education

- Consult physician and understand the potential risks of ibutilide therapy.

IDARUBICIN

(i-da-a-roo'bi-cin)

Idamycin PFS

Classifications: ANTINEOPLASTIC; ANTIBIOTIC
Therapeutic: ANTINEOPLASTIC
Prototype: Doxorubicin
Pregnancy Category: D

AVAILABILITY 5 mg, 10 mg, 20 mg vials; 1 mg/mL injection

ACTION & *THERAPEUTIC EFFECT* Cytotoxic anthracycline antibiotic that exhibits inhibitory effects on DNA topoisomerase II, an enzyme responsible for repairing faulty sections of DNA. It results in breaks in the helix of the DNA, and thus it affects RNA and protein synthesis in rapidly dividing cells. *It exhibits inhibitory effects on DNA and RNA polymerase, thus affecting nuceleic acid and protein syntheses in rapidly dividing cells.*

USES In combination with other antineoplastic drugs for treatment of AML.
UNLABELED USES Breast cancer, other solid tumors.

CONTRAINDICATIONS Myelosuppression, hypersensitivity to idarubicin or doxorubicin, children younger than 2 y, pregnancy (category D), lactation.
CAUTIOUS USE Impaired renal or hepatic function; patients who have received irradiation or radiotherapy to areas surrounding heart; cardiac disease.

ROUTE & DOSAGE

Acute Myelogenous Leukemia (AML)

Adult: **IV** 12 mg/m² daily for 3 days injected slowly over 10–15 min

Acute Nonlymphocytic Leukemia, Acute Lymphocytic Leukemia

Child: **IV** 10–12 mg/m²/day for 3 days

Renal Impairment Dosage Adjustment

Creatinine greater than 2 mg/dL: Give 75% of dose

Hepatic Impairment Dosage Adjustment

Bilirubin 1.5–5 mg/dL: Give 50% of dose; if greater than 5 mg/dL: Do not use drug

ADMINISTRATION

Intravenous

IV administration to infants, children: Verify correct IV concentration and rate of infusion with physician.

PREPARE: **IV Infusion:** Reconstitute by adding 1 mL of nonbacteriostatic NS for each 1 mg of idarubicin to yield 1 mg/mL. ▪ Vials are under negative pressure, therefore, carefully insert needle into vial to reconstitute. ▪ Wash skin accidentally exposed with soap and water.

ADMINISTER: **IV Infusion:** Give slowly over 10–15 min into tubing of free flowing IV of NS or D5W. ▪ If extravasation is suspected, immediately stop infusion, elevate the arm, and apply ice pack for 30 min then q.i.d. for 30 min × 3 days.

INCOMPATIBILITIES **Solution/additive:** ALKALINE SOLUTIONS (i.e., **sodium bicarbonate**), **heparin. Y-site: Acyclovir, allopurinol, ampicillin/sulbactam, cefazolin, cefepime, ceftazidime, clindamycin, dexamethasone,**

etoposide, furosemide, gentamicin, heparin, hydrocortisone, imipenem/cilastatin, lorazepam, meperidine, methotrexate, mezlocillin, piperacillin/tazobactam, sargramostim, sodium bicarbonate, teniposide, vancomycin, vincristine.

- Store reconstituted solutions up to 7 days refrigerated at 2°–8° C (36°–46° F) and 72 h at room temperature 15°–30° C (59°–86° F).

ADVERSE EFFECTS (≥1%) **CV:** CHF, atrial fibrillation, chest pain, MI. **GI:** *Nausea, vomiting, diarrhea, abdominal pain,* mucositis. **Hematologic:** *Anemia, leukopenia*, thrombocytopenia. **Other:** Nephrotoxicity, hepatotoxicity, *alopecia,* rash.

INTERACTIONS Drug: IMMUNOSUPPRESSANTS cause additive bone marrow suppression; ANTICOAGULANTS, NSAIDS, SALICYLATES, **aspirin,** THROMBOLYTIC AGENTS increase risk of bleeding; idarubicin may blunt the effects of **filgrastim, sargramostim.**

PHARMACOKINETICS Onset: Median time to remission 28 days. **Peak:** Serum level 4 h. **Duration:** Serum levels 120 h. **Distribution:** Concentrates in nucleated blood and bone marrow cells. **Metabolism:** In liver to idarubicinol, which may be as active as idarubicin. **Elimination:** 16% in urine; 17% in bile. **Half-Life:** Idarubicin 15–45 h, idarubicinol 45 h.

NURSING IMPLICATIONS

Assessment & Drug Effects

- Monitor infusion site closely, as extravasation can cause severe local tissue necrosis. Notify physician if pain, erythema, or edema develops at insertion site.
- Lab tests: Monitor hepatic and renal function, CBC with differential and coagulation studies periodically.
- Monitor cardiac status closely, especially in older adult patients or those with preexisting cardiac disease.
- Monitor hematologic status carefully; during the period of myelosuppression, patients are at high risk for bleeding and infection.
- Monitor for development of hyperuricemia secondary to lysis of leukemic cells.

Patient & Family Education

- Learn all potential adverse reactions to idarubicin.
- Anticipate possible hair loss.
- Discuss interventions to minimize nausea, vomiting, diarrhea, and stomatitis with health care providers.

IFOSFAMIDE

(i-fos'fa-mide)

Classifications: ANTINEOPLASTIC; ALKYLATING AGENT
Therapeutic: ANTINEOPLASTIC
Prototype: Cyclophosphamide
Pregnancy Category: D

AVAILABILITY 1 g, 3 g vials

ACTION & *THERAPEUTIC EFFECT* The alkylated metabolite of ifosfamide interacts with DNA as a cell cycle nonspecific agent. Antineoplastic action is primarily due to cross-linking of strands of DNA and RNA, as well as inhibition of protein synthesis. *It has antineoplastic and cytotoxic action on cancer cells that results in cell death.*

USES In combination with other agents in various regimens for germ cell testicular cancer, soft tissue sarcomas, Ewing's sarcoma, and non-Hodgkin's lymphoma. Also for lung and pancreatic sarcoma.

CONTRAINDICATIONS Patients with severe bone marrow depression or who have demonstrated previous hypersensitivity to ifosfamide; dehydration; pregnancy (category D), lactation.

CAUTIOUS USE Impaired renal function, renal failure; hepatic disease; prior radiation or prior therapy with other cytotoxic agents.

ROUTE & DOSAGE

Antineoplastic

Adult: **IV** 1.2 g/m²/day for 5 consecutive days; administer over at least 30 min, repeat q3wk or after recovery from hematologic toxicity (platelets 100,000/mm³ or greater; WBC 4000/mm³ or greater)

ADMINISTRATION

Intravenous

PREPARE: **IV Infusion:** Dilute each 1 g in 20 mL of sterile water or bacteriostatic water to yield 50 mg/mL. ▪Shake well to dissolve. ▪May be further diluted with D5W, NS, or LR to achieve concentrations of 0.6–20 mg/mL. ▪Use solution prepared with sterile water within 6 h.

ADMINISTER: **IV Infusion:** Give slowly over 30 min. ▪Note: Mesna is always given concurrently with ifosfamide; never give ifosfamide alone.

INCOMPATIBILITIES **Y-site:** **Cefepime, methotrexate.**

- Store reconstituted solution prepared with bacteriostatic solution up to a week at 30° C (86° F) or 6 wk at 5° C (41° F).

ADVERSE EFFECTS (≥1%) **CNS:** *Somnolence, confusion, hallucinations,* coma, dizziness, seizures, cranial nerve dysfunction. **GI:** *Nausea, vomiting,* anorexia, diarrhea, metabolic acidosis, hepatic dysfunction. **Hematologic:** Neutropenia, thrombocytopenia. **Urogenital:** Hemorrhagic cystitis, nephrotoxicity. **Skin:** *Alopecia,* skin necrosis with extravasation.

INTERACTIONS Drug: HEPATIC ENZYME INDUCERS (BARBITURATES, **phenytoin, chloral hydrate**) may increase hepatic conversion of ifosfamide to active metabolite; CORTICOSTEROIDS may inhibit conversion to active metabolites.

PHARMACOKINETICS Distribution: Distributed into breast milk. **Metabolism:** In liver via CYP3A4. **Elimination:** 70–86% in urine. **Half-Life:** 7–15 h.

NURSING IMPLICATIONS

Assessment & Drug Effects

- Lab tests: Monitor CBC with differential prior to each dose and at regular intervals; urinalysis prior to each dose for microscopic hematuria.
- Hold drug and notify physician if WBC count is below 2000/mm³ or platelet count is below 50,000/mm³.
- Reduce risk of hemorrhagic cystitis by hydrating with 3000 mL of fluid daily prior to therapy and for at least 72 h following treatment to ensure ample urine output.
- Monitor for and repost promptly any of the following CNS symptoms: Somnolence, confusion, depressive psychosis, and hallucinations.

Patient & Family Education

- Void frequently to lessen contact of irritating chemical with bladder mucosa by keeping well hydrated.

- Note: Susceptibility to infection may increase. Avoid people with infection. Notify physician of any infection, fever or chills, cough or hoarseness, lower back or side pain, painful or difficult urination.
- Check with physician immediately if there is any unusual bleeding or bruising, black tarry stools, or blood in urine or if pinpoint red spots develop on skin.
- Discuss possible adverse effects (e.g., alopecia, nausea, and vomiting) and measures that can minimize them with health care provider.

ILOPERIDONE

(i-lo-per'i-done)

Fanapt

Classification: ANTIPSYCHOTIC, ATYPICAL

Therapeutic: ATYPICAL ANTIPSYCHOTIC

Prototype: Clozapine

Pregnancy Category: C

AVAILABILITY 1 mg, 2 mg, 4 mg, 6 mg, 8 mg, 10 mg, 12 mg tablets.

ACTION & *THERAPEUTIC EFFECT* Is a both a dopamine (D_2) and serotonin (5-HT_2) antagonist. *Effect in treating acute schizophrenia uncontrolled by other agents.*

USES Acute treatment of schizophrenia in patients who have not responded to other antipsychotic agents.

CONTRAINDICATIONS Dementia-related psychosis; hypersensitivity to iloperidone; suicidal ideation; recent acute MI; ANC less than 100 mm_3; lactation

CAUTIOUS USE Elderly; congenital long QT syndrome; history of cardiac arrhythmias; history of suicidal tendencies; cardiovascular disease; CVA; CHF; cerebrovascular disease; tardive dykinesia; DM; history of seizures; history of leucopenia/neutropenia; hepatic impairment; patients at risk for aspiration pneumonia; pregnancy (category C). Safety and efficacy in children have not been established.

ROUTE & DOSAGE

Schizophrenia

Adult: **PO** Initial 1 mg b.i.d., then titrated to 6–12 mg b.i.d. Recommended titration schedule: Increase each b.i.d. dose by 2 mg a day from day 2 through 7 or until desired dose reached (max: 12 mg b.i.d.). Note: Reduce dose by 50% with concurrent use of a strong CYP2D6 inhibitor (e.g., fluoxetine or paroxetine) or strong CYP3A4 inhibitor (e.g., ketoconazole or clarithromycin).

ADMINISTRATION

Oral

- Note that gradual dose titration is recommended initially and whenever patient has been off drug for more than 3 days.
- Store at 15°–30° C (59°–86° F) and protect from light.

ADVERSE EFFECTS (≥1%) **Body as a Whole:** Fatigue. **CNS:** *Dizziness,* extrapyramidal disorder, lethargy, *somnolence,* tremor. **CV:** Hypotension, orthostatic hypotension, <u>*tachycardia*</u>. **GI:** Abdominal discomfort, diarrhea, *dry mouth, nausea*. **Metabolic:** Increased weight. **Musculoskeletal:** Arthralgia, musculoskeletal stiffness. **Respiratory:** Dyspnea, nasal congestion, nasopharyngitis, upper respiratory infection. **Skin:** Rash. **Special Senses:** Blurred vision. **Urogenital:** Ejaculation failure.

INTERACTIONS Drug: Potential additive QT prolongation if used in combination with drugs with similar effects (e.g., **disopyramide, procainamide, amiodarone, bretylium**). Inhibitors of CYP3A4 (e.g., **ketoconazole, itraconazole, clarithromycin**) or CYP2D6 (e.g., **fluoxetine, paroxetine**) can increase iloperidone levels. **Food: Grapefruit juice** may increase iloperidone levels.

PHARMACOKINETICS Peak: 2–4 h. **Distribution:** 95% plasma protein bound. **Metabolism:** Extensive hepatic metabolism to active and inactive metabolites. **Elimination:** Renal (major) and fecal. **Half-Life:** 18–33 h.

NURSING IMPLICATIONS

Assessment & Drug Effects

- Monitor for suicidal ideation and report promptly if suspected.
- Monitor BP, HR, and weight. Monitor orthostatic vital signs with concurrent antihypertensive therapy or any condition that predisposes to hypotension (e.g., advanced age, dehydration).
- Monitor for orthostatic hypotension and syncope, especially early in therapy.
- Monitor ECG for prolongation of the QT_c interval.
- Monitor diabetics and those at risk for diabetes for loss of glycemic control.
- Lab tests: Baseline and periodic CBC with differential.

Patient & Family Education

- Be alert for and report worsening of condition, including ideas of suicide.
- Make position changes slowly, especially from a lying or sitting position to a standing position.
- If diabetic, monitor blood sugar closely for loss of control.
- Stop taking the drug and report immediately any of the following: Feeling faint or fainting, high fever, muscle rigidity, altered mental status, or palpitations.
- Do not drink alcohol while taking this drug.
- Avoid engaging in hazardous activities until response to drug is known.

ILOPROST

(i'lo-prost)

Classifications: PROSTAGLANDIN; ANTIHYPERTENSIVE, PULMONARY
Therapeutic: PULMONARY ANTIHYPERTENSIVE
Prototype: Epoprostenol
Pregnancy Category: C

AVAILABILITY 2 mcg/2 mL ampule

ACTION & *THERAPEUTIC EFFECT* Iloprost is a synthetic analog of prostaglandin. It dilates systemic and pulmonary arterial vascular beds. *Dilation of the pulmonary arterial vessels reduces pulmonary hypertension.*

USES Treatment of pulmonary arterial hypertension in patients with New York Heart Association (NYHA) Class III or IV symptoms.

UNLABELED USES Treatment of severe Raynaud phenomenon associated with systemic sclerosis.

CONTRAINDICATIONS Systolic blood pressure less than 85 mm Hg; lactation; children.

CAUTIOUS USE Impaired hepatic function, elderly, renal impairment with inhaled iloprost; asthma, acute respiratory infection, COPD; elderly; dialysis; pregnancy (category C).

ROUTE & DOSAGE

Pulmonary Hypertension

Adult: **Inhaled** 2.5–5 mcg 6–9 times daily, but no more than q2h during waking hours

ADMINISTRATION

Inhalation

- Transfer the contents of one ampule to the drug delivery system medication chamber immediately before use. Follow instructions provided by manufacturer for the delivery system. Do not allow contact with skin or eyes.
- Do not administer if systolic BP is less than 85 mg Hg.
- Do not administer any sooner than 2 h after the previous dose.
- Discard any solution remaining in the medication chamber after the inhalation session.
- Store at 20°–25° C (68°–77° F).

ADVERSE EFFECTS (≥1%) **CNS:** *Headache*, insomnia. **CV:** *Hypotension, vasodilation (flushing)*, palpitations, syncope, chest pain, tachycardia, congestive heart failure. **GI:** *Nausea, vomiting*. **Hepatic:** Increased alkaline phosphatase, increased gamma-glutamyltransferase (GGT). **Musculoskeletal:** Back pain, muscle cramps, *trismus*. **Renal:** Kidney failure. **Respiratory:** *Cough*, dyspnea, hemoptysis, pneumonia, peripheral edema. **Body as a Whole:** *Flu-like syndrome*, tongue pain.

INTERACTIONS Drug: Enhanced hypotension when given with other VASODILATORS or ANTIHYPERTENSIVE agents; increased risk of bleeding when given with other ANTICOAGULANTS or ANTITHROMBOTIC agents.

PHARMACOKINETICS Distribution: 60% protein bound. **Metabolism:** Completely metabolized to inactive products. **Elimination:** Urine (major) and feces. **Half-Life:** 20–30 min.

NURSING IMPLICATIONS

Assessment & Drug Effects

- Supervise ambulation, especially with concurrent use of other drugs known to cause dizziness or syncope.
- Monitor vital signs closely during initiation of drug therapy.
- Monitor for and report S&S of heart failure.
- Withhold drug and notify physician if S&S of pulmonary edema appear.
- Lab tests: Monitor blood levels of anticoagulants when used concurrently.

Patient & Family Education

- Follow directions for taking the drug (see Administration). Iloprost inhalation should be used with the Prodose AAD system. Do not use it with other types of nebulizers.
- Make position changes slowly, especially when arising from a chair or bed.
- Do not drive or engage in potentially hazardous activities until response to drug is known.
- Report any of the following to a health care provider: Dizziness or fainting, especially upon exertion, or increased difficulty breathing.

IMATINIB MESYLATE

(i-ma'ti-nib)

Gleevec

Classifications: ANTINEOPLASTIC; MONOCLONAL ANTIBODY; EPIDERMAL GROWTH FACTOR RECEPTOR-TYROSINE KINASE INHIBITOR (EGFR-TKI)
Therapeutic: ANTINEOPLASTIC
Prototype: Gefitinib
Pregnancy Category: D

AVAILABILITY 100 mg, 400 mg tablet

ACTION & *THERAPEUTIC EFFECT*
Epidermal growth factor receptor-tyrosine kinase inhibitor (EGFR-TKI) that interferes with intracellular signaling pathways that are involved in the development of malignancies. Imatinib inhibits abnormal Bcr-Abl tyrosine kinase created by the Philadelphia chromosome abnormality in chronic myeloid leukemia (CLM). Tyrosine kinase is required for activation of a wide variety of intracellular activities vital to cell functioning and intracellular metabolic pathways. *Inhibits WBC cell proliferation and induces cell death in Bcr-Abl tyrosine kinase positive cells as well as in newly formed leukemic cells. Thus, it interferes with progression of chronic myeloid leukemia (CML). Additionally, imatinib inhibits proliferation and induces cell death in gastrointestinal stomal tumor (GIST) that express a mutation of an activated cKit tyrosine kinase.*

USES Treatment of CML in blast crisis, or in chronic phase after failure of interferon-alpha therapy; unresectable and/or metastatic malignant gastrointestinal stromal tumors (GISTs), acute lymphoblastic leukemia.
UNLABELED USES Acute lymphocytic leukemia (ALL), soft tissue sarcoma, recurrence of stomach and intestinal tumors.

CONTRAINDICATIONS Hypersensitivity to imatinib or any of its components; viral infections; intramuscular injections with concurrent thrombocytopenia; pregnancy (category D), lactation; children younger than 3 y.
CAUTIOUS USE History of hypersensitivity to other monoclonal antibodies; hepatic or renal impairment; bleeding, bone marrow suppression; cardiac disease; dental disease, dental work; older adults, females of childbearing age; fungal infections; GI bleeding; heart failure; hepatic disease; infection; jaundice; peripheral edema, renal disease; vaccination, history of viral infection.

ROUTE & DOSAGE

CML Chronic Phase
Adult: **PO** 400–800 mg daily with a meal and large glass of water
Child (older than 3 y): **PO** 260 or 340 mg/m^2/day in 1 or 2 divided dose(s)

CML Accelerated Phase or Blast Crisis
Adult: **PO** 600 mg daily with a meal and large glass of water

Acute Lymphoblastic Leukemia
Adult: **PO** 600 mg/day

GISTs
Adult: **PO** 400 mg daily

Hepatic Impairment Dosage Adjustment
Reduce dose to 300–400 mg daily

ADMINISTRATION

Oral
- Give with meal and large glass of water (at least 8 oz).

- Store at 15°–30° C (59°–86° F).

ADVERSE EFFECTS (≥1%) **Body as a Whole:** *Fluid retention, edema, fatigue,* weight gain, *fever,* night sweats, weakness. **CNS:** CNS hemorrhage, *headache.* **GI:** *Nausea, vomiting, diarrhea,* GI hemorrhage, dyspepsia, *abdominal pain, constipation, anorexia,* increased AST, ALT, and bilirubin. **Hematologic:** Hemorrhage, *neutropenia, thrombocytopenia,* petechiae, epistaxis, pancytopenia (rare), thrombocytopenia (rare). **Metabolic:** Hypokalemia. **Musculoskeletal:** *Muscle cramps, pain, arthralgia,* myalgia. **Respiratory:** *Cough, dyspnea,* pharyngitis, pneumonia. **Skin:** *Rash,* pruritus.

INTERACTIONS Drug: Clarithromycin, erythromycin, ketoconazole, itraconazole may increase imatinib levels and toxicity; **carbamazepine, dexamethasone, phenobarbital, phenytoin, rifampin** may decrease imatinib levels; may increase levels of BENZODIAZEPINES, DIHYDROPYRIDINE, CALCIUM CHANNEL BLOCKERS (e.g., **nifedipine**), **warfarin. Herbal: St. John's wort** may decrease imatinib levels.

PHARMACOKINETICS Absorption: Well absorbed, 98% reaches systemic circulation. **Peak:** 2–4 h. **Metabolism:** Primarily by CYP3A4 in liver. **Elimination:** Primarily in feces. **Half-Life:** 18 h imatinib, 40 h active metabolite.

NURSING IMPLICATIONS

Assessment & Drug Effects

- Monitor for S&S of fluid retention. Weigh daily and report rapid weight gain immediately.
- Lab tests: CBC with platelet count and differential weekly times 1 mo, biweekly for the 2nd mo, periodically thereafter as clinically indicated; baseline and monthly AST, ALT, alkaline phosphatase, bilirubin; periodic serum creatinine and electrolytes.
- Withhold drug and notify physician for any of the following: Bilirubin greater than 3 × ULN, AST/ALT greater than 5 × ULN; treatment may be reinstituted when bilirubin less than 1.5 × ULN and AST/ALT less than 2.5 × ULN.

Patient & Family Education

- Do not take any OTC drugs (e.g., acetaminophen, St. John's wort) without consulting physician.
- Report any S&S of bleeding immediately to physician (e.g., black tarry stool, bright red or cola-colored urine, bleeding from gums).
- Report immediately to physician any unexplained change in mental status.
- Use effective means of contraception while taking this drug. Women of childbearing age should avoid becoming pregnant.

IMIPENEM-CILASTATIN SODIUM (Pr)

(i-mi-pen'em sye-la-stat'in)

Primaxin

Classification: BETA-LACTAM ANTIBIOTIC

Therapeutic: ANTIBIOTIC

Pregnancy Category: C

AVAILABILITY 250 mg, 500 mg vials

ACTION & *THERAPEUTIC EFFECT* Fixed combination of imipenem, a beta-lactam antibiotic, and cilastatin. Action of imipenem: Inhibition of mucopeptide synthesis in bacterial cell walls leading to cell death. Cilastatin increases the serum half-life of imipenem. *Effectively used for severe or resistant infections. Acts synergistically with aminoglycoside antibiotics against some isolates of* Pseudomonas aeruginosa. *Infections resistant to cephalosporins, penicillins, and aminoglycosides have responded to treatment with this combination.*

USES Treatment of serious infections caused by susceptible organisms in the urinary tract, lower respiratory tract, bones and joints, skin and skin structures; also intra-abdominal, gynecologic, and mixed infections; bacterial septicemia and endocarditis.

CONTRAINDICATIONS Hypersensitivity to any component of product, multiple allergens; carbapenem hypersensitivity; penicillin hypersensitivity.

CAUTIOUS USE Patients with CNS disorders (e.g., seizures, brain lesions, history of recent head injury); seizures; renal failure, renal impairment, renal disease; patients with history of cephalosporin allergies; pregnancy (category C), lactation.

ROUTE & DOSAGE

Serious Infections

Adult: **IV:** 250–500 mg infused over 20–30 min q6–8h (max dose: 4 g/day): **IM:** 500 or 750 mg q12h (max dose: 4 g/day)
Child: **IV** *Older than 3 mo,* 25 mg/kg q6h; *1–3 mo,* 100 mg/kg/day in divided doses **IM** 15–25 mg/kg q12h
Neonate: **IV** *Weight greater than 1500 g,* 25 mg/kg q8–12h

Renal Impairment Dosage Adjustment

Make adjustments per package insert (based on CrCl)

ADMINISTRATION

Caution: IM and IV solutions are NOT interchangeable; do NOT give IM solution by IV, and do NOT give IV solution as IM.

Intramuscular

- Reconstitute powder for IM injection as follows: Add 2 mL or 3 mL of 1% lidocaine HCl solution without epinephrine, respectively, to the 500 mg vial or the 750 mg vial. Agitate to form a suspension then withdraw and inject entire contents of the vial IM.
- Give IM suspension by deep injection into the gluteal muscle or lateral thigh.
- Use reconstituted IM injection within 1 h after preparation.

Intravenous

PREPARE: **Intermittent:** Reconstitute each dose with 10 mL of D5W, NS, or other compatible infusion solution. ▪ Agitate the solution until clear. Color should range from colorless to yellow. ▪ Further dilute with 100 mL of same solution used for initial dilution.

ADMINISTER: **Intermittent:** Give each 500 mg or fraction thereof over 20–30 min. Infuse larger doses over 40–60 min. ▪ DO NOT give as a bolus dose. ▪ Nausea appears to be related to infusion rate, and if it presents during infusion, slow the rate (occurs most frequently with 1-g doses).

INCOMPATIBILITIES **Solution/additive: Lactated Ringer's,** some **dextrose**-containing solutions, **sodium bicarbonate, TPN. Y-**

site: **Allopurinol, amiodarone, amphotericin B cholesteryl, azithromycin, etoposide, fluconazole, gemcitabine, lorazepam, meperidine, midazolam, milrinone, sargramostim, sodium bicarbonate.**

▪ Store according to manufacturer's recommendations; stability of IV solutions depends on diluent used for reconstitution. ▪ Most IV solutions retain potency for 4 h at 15°–30° C (59°–86° F) or for 24 h if refrigerated at 4° C (39° F). Avoid freezing.

ADVERSE EFFECTS (≥1%) **Body as a Whole:** Hypersensitivity (rash, fever, chills, dyspnea, pruritus), weakness, oliguria/anuria, polyuria, polyarthralgia; *phlebitis and pain at injection site,* superinfections. **CNS:** Seizures, dizziness, confusion, somnolence, encephalopathy, myoclonus, tremors, paresthesia, headache. **GI:** *Nausea, vomiting,* diarrhea, pseudomembranous colitis, hemorrhagic colitis, gastroenteritis, abdominal pain, glossitis, heartburn. **Respiratory:** Chest discomfort, hyperventilation, dyspnea. **Skin:** Rash, pruritus, urticaria, candidiasis, flushing, increased sweating, skin texture change, facial edema. **Metabolic:** Hyponatremia, hyperkalemia. **Special Senses:** Transient hearing loss; increased WBC, AST, ALT, alkaline phosphatase, BUN, LDH, creatinine; decreased Hgb, Hct, eosinophilia.

INTERACTIONS Drug: Aztreonam, cephalosporins, penicillins may antagonize the antibacterial effects. May affect **cyclosporine** levels.

PHARMACOKINETICS Distribution: Widely distributed; limited concentrations in CSF; crosses placenta; in breast milk. **Elimination:** 70% in urine within 10 h. **Half-Life:** 1 h.

NURSING IMPLICATIONS

Assessment & Drug Effects

- Determine previous hypersensitivity reaction to beta-lactam antibiotics (penicillins and cephalosporins) or to other allergens.
- Monitor for S&S of hypersensitivity (see Appendix F). Discontinue drug and notify physician if S&S occur.
- Monitor closely patients vulnerable to CNS adverse effects.
- Notify physician if focal tremors, myoclonus, or seizures occur; dosage adjustment may be needed.
- Monitor for S&S of superinfection (see Appendix F).
- Notify physician promptly to rule out pseudomembranous enterocolitis if severe diarrhea accompanied by abdominal pain and fever occurs (see Appendix F).
- Note: Sodium content derived from drug is high; consider in patient on restricted sodium intake.
- Monitor renal, hematologic, and liver function periodically.

Patient & Family Education

- Notify physician immediately to report pruritus or symptoms of respiratory distress.
- Report pain or discomfort at IV infusion site.
- Report loose stools or diarrhea promptly.

IMIPRAMINE HYDROCHLORIDE

(im-ip′ra-meen)

Impril ♣, Novopramine ♣, Tofranil

IMIPRAMINE PAMOATE

Tofranil-PM

Classification: TRICYCLIC ANTIDEPRESSANT

Therapeutic: TRICYCLIC ANTIDEPRESSANT
Pregnancy Category: D

AVAILABILITY 10 mg, 25 mg, 50 mg tablets; 25 mg/mL oral product; **Imipramine pamoate:** 75 mg, 100 mg, 125 mg, 150 mg capsules

ACTION & *THERAPEUTIC EFFECT* TCAs potentiate both norepinephrine and serotonin in the CNS by blocking their reuptake by presynaptic neurons. Imipramine decreases number of awakenings from sleep, markedly reduces time in REM sleep, and increases stage 4 sleep. *Effective as an antidepressant. Relief of nocturnal enuresis is due to anticholinergic activity and to nervous system stimulation, resulting in earlier arousal to sensation of full bladder.*

USES Endogenous depression and occasionally for reactive depression. Imipramine is the only TCA used as temporary adjuvant treatment of enuresis in children older than 6 y.

UNLABELED USES Certain syndromes that mimic or overlap diagnostically with depression: Alcoholism, cocaine withdrawal; attention deficit disorder with or without hyperactivity (children older than 6 y and adolescents); with amphetamines or methylphenidate for narcolepsy; phobic anxiety syndromes such as panic disorders and agoraphobia; obsessive-compulsive neurosis; chronic intractable pain.

CONTRAINDICATIONS Hypersensitivity to tricyclic drugs; concomitant use of MAOIs within 14 days; suicidal ideation; acute recovery period after MI, defects in bundle-branch conduction, QT prolongation; severe renal or hepatic impairment; use of imipramine HCl in children younger than 12 y except to treat enuresis; use of pamoate in children of any age; pregnancy (category D), lactation.

CAUTIOUS USE History of hypersensitivity to dibenzazepine compounds; respiratory difficulties; cardiovascular, hepatic, or GI diseases; blood disorders; increased intraocular pressure, narrow-angle glaucoma; schizophrenia, hypomania or manic episodes, patient with suicidal tendency, seizure disorders; prostatic hypertrophy, urinary retention; alcoholism, hyperthyroidism; electroshock therapy; older adults; children, adolescents.

ROUTE & DOSAGE

Depression

Adult: **PO** 75–100 mg/day (max: 300 mg/day) in 1 or more divided doses
Child: **PO** 1.5 mg/kg/day, may increase by 1 mg/kg/day q3–4days (max: 5 mg/kg/day)

Enuresis in Childhood

Child: **PO** 25 mg 1 h before bedtime; *younger than 12 y,* may increase to 50 mg nightly (max: 2.5 mg/kg); *older than 12 y,* may increase to 75 mg nightly (max: 2.5 mg/kg)

Pharmacogenetic Dosage Adjustment

Poor CYP2D6 metabolizers: Start at 30% of normal dose

ADMINISTRATION

Oral

- Give with or immediately after food.

- Note: Single doses can be given at bedtime or q.a.m., respectively, if drowsiness or insomnia results.

ADVERSE EFFECTS (≥1%) **Body as a Whole:** Hypersensitivity (skin rash, erythema, petechiae, urticaria, pruritus, photosensitivity, angioedema of face, tongue, or generalized; drug fever). **CNS:** *Sedation, drowsiness,* dizziness, headache, fatigue, numbness, tingling (paresthesias) of extremities; incoordination, ataxia, tremors, peripheral neuropathy, extrapyramidal symptoms (including parkinsonism effects and tardive dyskinesia); lowered seizure threshold, altered EEG patterns, delirium, disturbed concentration, confusion, hallucinations, anxiety, nervousness, insomnia, vivid dreams, restlessness, agitation, shift to hypomania, mania; exacerbation of psychoses; hyperpyrexia. **CV:** *Orthostatic hypotension,* mild sinus tachycardia; *arrhythmias,* hypertension or hypotension, palpitation, MI, CHF, *heart block,* ECG changes, stroke, flushing, cold cyanotic hands and feet (peripheral vasospasm). **Endocrine:** Testicular swelling, gynecomastia (men), galactorrhea and breast enlargement (women), increased or decreased libido, ejaculatory and erectile disturbances, delayed or absent orgasm (male and female); elevation or depression of blood glucose levels. **Special Senses:** Nasal congestion, tinnitus; *blurred vision,* disturbances of accommodation, *slight mydriasis,* nystagmus. **GI:** *Dry mouth,* constipation, heartburn, excessive appetite, weight gain, nausea, vomiting, diarrhea, slowed gastric emptying time, flatulence, abdominal cramps, esophageal reflux, anorexia, stomatitis, increased salivation, black tongue, peculiar taste, paralytic ileus. **Urogenital:** *Urinary retention,* delayed micturition, nocturia, paradoxic urinary frequency. **Hematologic:** Bone marrow depression; agranulocytosis, eosinophilia, thrombocytopenia. **Other:** Excessive perspiration, cholestatic jaundice, precipitation of acute intermittent porphyria; dyspnea, changes in heat and cold tolerance, hair loss, syndrome of inappropriate antidiuretic hormone secretion (SIADH).

DIAGNOSTIC TEST INTERFERENCE Imipramine elevates ***serum bilirubin, alkaline phosphatase*** and may increase or decrease ***blood glucose.*** It decreases ***urinary 5-HIAA*** and ***VMA*** excretion and may falsely increase excretion of ***urinary catecholamines.***

INTERACTIONS Drug: MAO INHIBITORS may precipitate hyperpyrexic crisis, tachycardia, or seizures; ANTIHYPERTENSIVE AGENTS potentiate orthostatic hypotension; CNS DEPRESSANTS, **alcohol** add to CNS depression; **norepinephrine** and other SYMPATHOMIMETICS may increase cardiac toxicity; **cimetidine** decreases hepatic metabolism, thus increasing imipramine levels; **methylphenidate** inhibits metabolism of imipramine and thus may increase its toxicity. **Herbal: Ginkgo** may decrease seizure threshold; **St. John's wort** may cause **serotonin** syndrome.

PHARMACOKINETICS Absorption: Completely absorbed from GI tract. **Peak:** 1–2 h. **Metabolism:** Metabolized to the active metabolite desipramine in liver. **Elimination:** Primarily in urine, small amount in feces; crosses placenta; may be secreted in breast milk. **Half-Life:** 8–16 h.

NURSING IMPLICATIONS

Assessment & Drug Effects

- Monitor for therapeutic effectiveness: May not occur for 2 wk or more.
- Monitor children and adolescents for increase in suicidality.
- Note: Dose sensitivity and adverse effects are most likely to occur in adolescents and older adults; lower initial doses are recommended for these patients.
- Lab tests: Monitor periodically hepatic and renal function, CBC with differential, and fluid and electrolyte balance.
- Monitor HR and BP frequently. Orthostatic hypotension may be marked in pretreatment hypertensive or cardiac patients.
- Note: During the first 2 wk of therapy, older adults may develop confusion, restlessness, disturbed sleep, forgetfulness. Symptoms last 3–20 days. Report to physician.
- Weigh patient under standard conditions biweekly: Report a gain of 0.5–1 kg (1.5–2 lb) within 2–3 days and frank edema.
- Monitor urinary and bowel elimination, at least until maintenance dosage is stabilized, to detect urinary retention or frequency, constipation, or paralytic ileus.
- Notify physician of extrapyramidal symptoms (tremors, twitching, ataxia, incoordination, hyperreflexia, drooling) in patients receiving large doses and especially in older adults.
- Monitor diabetic patients for loss of glycemic control. Hyperglycemia or hypoglycemia (see Appendix F) occur in some patients.

Patient & Family Education

- Report promptly signs of a worsening condition, suicidal ideation, or unusual changes in behavior, especially in children and adolescents.
- Change position slowly and in stages, especially from lying down to upright posture and dangle legs over bed for a few minutes before walking.
- Note: Effectiveness can decrease with continued drug administration in some patients. Inform physician if this occurs.
- Do NOT use OTC drugs while on a TCA without physician approval.
- Do not drive or engage in other potentially hazardous activities until response to drug is known.
- Avoid exposure to strong sunlight because of potential photosensitivity. Use sunscreen with at least SPF of 12–15 if allowed.

IMIQUIMOD

(i-mi′qui-mod)

Aldara

Classifications: KERATOLYTIC AGENT; IMMUNE RESPONSE MODIFIER

Therapeutic: IMMUNE RESPONSE MODIFIER; KERATOLYTIC

Pregnancy Category: C

AVAILABILITY 5% cream in 250 mg single use packets

ACTION & *THERAPEUTIC EFFECT* An immune response modifier that is thought to induce cytokine production, including interferon-alfa, which may interfere with viral replication. *Does not totally eradicate HPV. Despite destruction of HPV warts, latent or subclinical HPV infection can persist, and recurrence of visible warts is common.*

USES Treatment of external genital and perianal warts *(Condylomata acuminata)*, actinic keratosis on the face and scalp of immunocompetent adults, and superficial basal cell carcinoma.

UNLABELED USES Treatment of common warts.

CONTRAINDICATIONS Occlusive dressing; ocular exposure; excessive sun exposure or sunburn; UV exposure; surgery or drug treatment on affected area; children younger than 12 y.

CAUTIOUS USE Hypersensitivity to benzyl alcohol or paraben; HIV infection; pregnancy (category C), lactation

ROUTE & DOSAGE

Genital and Perianal Warts

Adult/Adolescent (older than 12 y): **Topical** Apply a thin layer to the affected areas once daily 3 times/wk just before bedtime. Wash off cream after 6–10 h (max: 16 wk therapy).

Actinic Keratosis

Adult: **Topical** Apply a thin layer to the affected areas once daily 2 times/wk just before sleep for 16 wk. Wash off cream after 8 h.

Superficial Basal Cell Carcinoma

Adult: **Topical** Apply a thin layer to the affected areas once daily 5 times/wk just before sleep for 6 wk. Wash off cream after 8 h.

ADMINISTRATION

Topical

- Hand washing before and after application is recommended.
- Wash treatment area with soap and water and allow to dry thoroughly (at least 10 min).
- Single-use packets contain sufficient cream to cover an area of up to 20 cm^2 (approx. 8 in. by 8 in.).
- Instruct patient to apply a thin layer of cream (avoid using excessive cream), and work into area until no longer visible. Do not occlude the application site.
- After each treatment period, remove the cream by washing the treated area with soap and water.
- Store below 25° C (77° F).

ADVERSE EFFECTS (≥1%) **Body as a Whole:** Fungal infections, flu-like symptoms, myalgia. **CNS:** Headache. **Skin:** *Application site reactions, pruritus,* burning, bleeding, stinging, redness, tenderness, irritation, *erythema,* edema, weeping/exudates, dry skin, scabbing/crusting, hyperkeratosis.

PHARMACOKINETICS Absorption: Minimal absorption through intact skin.

NURSING IMPLICATIONS

Patient & Family Education

- Uncircumcised males with warts under the foreskin: Pull back the foreskin and clean the area daily to help avoid penile skin reactions.
- Females should not apply cream directly into the vagina. Application to the labia may cause pain or swelling and may cause difficulty in passing urine.
- When being treated for actinic keratosis, avoid or minimize UV light exposure (artificial and sunlight) during treatment of actinic keratosis. Wear protective clothing. If sunburn develops, avoid using imiquimod cream until fully recovered.

IMMUNE GLOBULIN INTRAMUSCULAR [IGIM, GAMMA GLOBULIN, IMMUNE SERUM GLOBULIN (ISG)] Pr

(im'mune glob'u-lin)

BayGam

IMMUNE GLOBULIN INTRAVENOUS (IGIV)

Flebogamma, Gammagard, Gammar-P IV, Gamunex, IGIV, Iveegam, Octagam, Sandoglobulin

Classifications: BIOLOGICAL RESPONSE MODIFIER; IMMUNOGLOBULIN
Therapeutic: IMMUNOGLOBULIN
Pregnancy Category: C

AVAILABILITY IGIM: 2 mL, 10 mL vials **IGIV:** 5%, 10% solution; 50 mg/mL powder for injection

I

ACTION & *THERAPEUTIC EFFECT*
Sterile concentrated solution containing globulin (primarily IgG) prepared from human plasma of either venous or placental origin and processed by a special fractionating technique. *Like hepatitis B immune globulin (H-BIG), contains antibodies specific to hepatitis B surface antigen but in lower concentrations. Therefore, not considered treatment of first choice for postexposure prophylaxis against hepatitis B but usually an acceptable alternative when H-BIG is not available.*

USES IGIM: In susceptible persons to provide passive immunity or to modify severity of certain infectious diseases [e.g., rubeola (measles), rubella (German measles), varicella-zoster (chickenpox), type A (infectious) hepatitis], and as replacement therapy in congenital agammaglobulinemia or IgG deficiency diseases. May be used as an alternative to H-BIG to provide passive immunity in hepatitis B infection. Also for postexposure prophylaxis of hepatitis non-A, non-B, and nonspecific hepatitis. **IGIV:** Principally as maintenance therapy in patients unable to manufacture sufficient quantities of IgG antibodies, in patients requiring an immediate increase in immunoglobulin levels, and when IM injections are contraindicated as in patients with bleeding disorders or who have small muscle mass. Also in chronic autoimmune thrombocytopenia and idiopathic thrombocytopenic purpura (ITP). Treatment of primary immunodeficiency disorders associated with defects in humoral immunity.

UNLABELED USES Kawasaki syndrome, chronic lymphocytic leukemia, AIDS, premature and low-birth-weight neonates, autoimmune neutropenia, or hemolytic anemia.

CONTRAINDICATIONS History of anaphylaxis or severe reaction to human immune serum globulin (IG) or to any ingredient in the formulations; persons with clinical hepatitis A; IGIV for patients with class-specific anti-IgA deficiencies; IGIM in severe thrombocytopenia or other bleeding disorders; intramuscular injection.

CAUTIOUS USE Dehydration, diabetes mellitus, children, older adults, hypovolemia, IgA deficiency, infection; renal disease, renal impairment; sepsis; sucrose hypersensitivity; vaccination, viral infection; pregnancy (category C), lactation.

ROUTE & DOSAGE

Hepatitis A Exposure

Adult/Child: **IM** 0.02 mL/kg as soon as possible after exposure; if period of exposure will be 3 mo or longer, give 0.05–0.06 mL/kg once q4–6mo

Hepatitis B Exposure

Adult/Child: **IM** 0.02–0.06 mL/kg as soon as possible after exposure if H-BIG is unavailable

Rubella Exposure

Adult: **IM** 20 mL as single dose in susceptible pregnant women

Rubeola Exposure

Adult/Child: **IM** 0.25 mL/kg within 6 days of exposure

Varicella-Zoster Exposure

Adult/Child: **IM** 0.6–1.2 mL/kg promptly

Immunoglobulin Deficiency

*Dosages may vary between brands

Adult/Child: **IV** 200–400 mg/kg monthly **IM** 1.2 mL/kg followed by 0.6 mL/kg q2–4wk

Idiopathic Thrombocytopenia Purpura

Adult/Child: **IV** 400 mg/kg/day for 5 consecutive days or 1 g/kg × 1–2 days

Obesity Dosage Adjustment

Dose based on IBW or adjusted IBW

ADMINISTRATION

▪ Note: In hepatitis A (infectious hepatitis), immune globulin is most effective when given before or as soon as possible after exposure but not more than 2 wk after (incubation period for hepatitis A is 15–50 days). ▪ Do not give immune globulin to those presenting clinical manifestations of hepatitis A. ▪ For hepatitis B (serum hepatitis), give immune globulin within 24 h and not more than 7 days after exposure. ▪ Note: IGIM and IGIV formulations are NOT interchangeable.

Intramuscular

▪ Give adults and older children injections into deltoid or anterolateral aspect of thigh; neonates and small children, into anterolateral aspect of thigh.
▪ Avoid gluteal injections; however, when large volumes of immune globulin are prescribed or when large doses **must be** divided into several injections, the upper outer quadrant of the gluteus has been used in adults.

Intravenous

PREPARE: **IV Infusion:** Refer to manufacturer's directions for information on reconstitution and dilution of the specific product.

ADMINISTER: **IV Infusion:** Flow rates vary with product being infused. Refer to manufacturer's directions for the specific product.
▪ Do not mix with other drugs.
▪ Discard partially used vial.

INCOMPATIBILITIES Do not mix other drugs with immunoglobulin.

▪ Store as directed by manufacturer for specific product. Avoid freezing. ▪ Do not use if turbidity has occurred or if product has been frozen.

ADVERSE EFFECTS (≥1%) **Body as a Whole:** *Pain, tenderness, muscle stiffness at IM site;* local inflammatory reaction, erythema, urticaria, angioedema, headache, malaise, fever, arthralgia, nephrotic syndrome, hypersensitivity (fever, chills, anaphylactic shock), infusion reactions (*nausea, flushing, chills,* headache, chest tightness, wheezing, skeletal pain, back pain, abdominal cramps, anaphylaxis), renal dysfunction, renal failure.

INTERACTIONS Drug: May interfere with antibody response to LIVE VIRUS VACCINES (measles/mumps/rubella);

give VACCINES 14 days before or 3 mo after IMMUNE GLOBULINS.

PHARMACOKINETICS **Peak:** 2 days. **Distribution:** Rapidly and evenly distributed to intravascular and extravascular fluid compartments. **Half-Life:** 21–23 days.

NURSING IMPLICATIONS

Assessment & Drug Effects

- Make sure emergency drugs and appropriate emergency facilities are immediately available for treatment of anaphylaxis or sensitization.
- Note: Hypersensitivity reactions (see Appendix F) are most likely in patients receiving large IM doses, repeated injections, or rapid IV infusion.
- Monitor vital signs and infusion rate closely when patient is receiving IGIV.
- Note: IGIV has a mild diuretic effect in some patients due to presence of maltose.

Patient & Family Education

- Report immediately S&S of hypersensitivity (see Appendix F).
- Report immediately infusion symptoms of nausea, chills, headache, and chest tightness; these are indications to slow rate of infusion.
- Note: Passive immunity to measles (rubeola) lasts about 3–4 wk after immune globulin. In general, children 15 mo or younger need active immunization with measles virus vaccine 3 mo after IGIM.

INAMRINONE LACTATE ℗

(in-am′ri-none)

Amrinone

Classifications: CARDIAC INOTROPIC; VASODILATOR

Therapeutic: CARDIAC INOTROPIC

Pregnancy Category: C

AVAILABILITY 5 mg/mL injection

ACTION & *THERAPEUTIC EFFECT* A cardiac inotropic agent with vasodilator activity. Mode of action appears to differ from that of the digitalis glycosides and beta-adrenergic stimulants. In patients with depressed myocardial function, it enhances myocardial contractility, increases cardiac output and stroke volume, and reduces right and left ventricular filling pressure, pulmonary capillary wedge pressure (PCWP), and systemic vascular resistance. *It reduces preload and afterload by its direct relaxant effect on vascular smooth muscle. Inamrinone produces hemodynamic improvements as well as symptomatic relief in patients in CHF due to ischemic heart disease.*

USES Short-term management of CHF in patients not adequately controlled by traditional therapy, such as digitalis, diuretics, and vasodilators, and may be used in conjunction with these agents.

CONTRAINDICATIONS Hypersensitivity to inamrinone or to bisulfites; severe aortic or pulmonic valvular disease in lieu of appropriate surgery, acute MI; uncorrected hypokalemia or dehydration. Safe use in children is not established.

CAUTIOUS USE Compromised renal or hepatic function, arrhythmias, hypertrophic subaortic stenosis; decreased platelets; pregnancy (category C), lactation.

ROUTE & DOSAGE

Congestive Heart Failure

Adult: **IV** 0.75 mg/kg bolus given slowly over 2–3 min, then start infusion at 5–10 mcg/kg/min, may repeat bolus in 30 min (max: 10 mg/kg/day)

Renal Impairment Dosage Adjustment

CrCl less than 10 mL/min: Give 50–75% of dose

ADMINISTRATION

Intravenous

PREPARE: **Direct:** Give loading dose undiluted or diluted by adding 1 mL of NS or 0.45% NS to each 5 mg (1 mL). **IV Infusion:** Dilute 300 mg (60 mL) in 60 mL of NS or 0.45% NS to yield 2.5 mg/mL. ▪Natural color is clear yellow. Discard discolored solutions and those with precipitate.

ADMINISTER: **Direct:** Give loading dose over 2–3 min. May inject into a running D5W infusion through Y-connector or directly. **IV Infusion:** Give diluted solution at a rate of 5–10 mg/kg/min. ▪Use infusion pump to regulate rate.

INCOMPATIBILITIES **Solution/additive:** **Sodium bicarbonate, dextrose**-containing solutions. **Y-site:** **Furosemide, sodium bicarbonate.**

▪ Use all diluted solutions within 24 h. ▪Protect ampules from light.

ADVERSE EFFECTS (≥1%) **Body as a Whole:** Hypersensitivity (pericarditis, pleuritis; myositis with interstitial shadows on chest x-ray and elevated sedimentation rate; vasculitis with nodular pulmonary densities, hypoxemia, ascites, jaundice). **CV:** Hypotension, arrhythmias. **Endocrine:** Nephrogenic diabetes insipidus. **GI:** Nausea, vomiting, anorexia, abdominal cramps, hepatotoxicity. **Hematologic:** Asymptomatic thrombocytopenia.

INTERACTIONS **Drug:** Possibility of excessive hypotension with disopyramide.

PHARMACOKINETICS **Onset:** 2–5 min. **Peak:** 10 min. **Duration:** About 2 h. **Distribution:** Unknown if it crosses placenta or into breast milk. **Metabolism:** In liver. **Elimination:** Primarily in urine. **Half-Life:** 3.6–7.5 h.

NURSING IMPLICATIONS

Assessment & Drug Effects

- Monitor for therapeutic effectiveness: Increased cardiac output, decreased PCWP, relief of symptoms of CHF. Central venous pressure may be used to assess hypotension and blood volume.
- Monitor BP, heart rate, and respirations and keep physician informed. Rate of administration and duration of therapy are prescribed according to clinical response and adverse effects.
- Consult physician for guidelines. In general, rate of infusion should be slowed or stopped with excessive drop in BP or arrhythmias.
- Monitor infusion site to prevent extravasation.
- Monitor I&O ratio and pattern and daily weights. Improvement in cardiac output enhances diuresis with consequent danger of hypokalemia and arrhythmias, particularly in digitalized patients.
- Lab tests: Monitor closely platelet counts, liver enzymes, fluid and electrolyte balances, renal function.
- Correct hypokalemia before and during therapy.
- Note: If platelet count falls below 150,000/mm³, report immediately to physician; may indicate thrombocytopenia.
- Allergy alert: IV preparation contains sodium metabisulfite, a reducing agent to which certain susceptible individuals are allergic.

I

Discontinue immediately if patient shows hypersensitivity reactions.

- Observe patient closely when drug is withdrawn after prolonged therapy; clinical deterioration may occur within hours.

INDAPAMIDE

(in-dap'a-mide)

Lozide ♣, Lozol

Classifications: ELECTROLYTIC AND WATER BALANCE AGENT; DIURETIC

Therapeutic: THIAZIDE-LIKE DIURETIC; ANTIHYPERTENSIVE

Prototype: Hydrochlorothiazide

Pregnancy Category: B

AVAILABILITY 1.25, 2.5 mg tablets

ACTION & *THERAPEUTIC EFFECT* Sulfonamide derivative that has both diuretic and direct vascular effects. Action mechanism is similar to thiazide diuretics. Acts on the proximal portion of the distal renal tubules. Enhances excretion of sodium, potassium, and water by interfering with sodium transfer across renal epithelium of tubules. *Hypotensive activity appears to result from a decrease in plasma and extracellular fluid volume, decreased peripheral vascular resistance, direct arteriolar dilation, and calcium channel blockade.*

USES Alone or with other antihypertensives in the management of hypertension in patients who have failed to respond to diet, exercise, or weight reduction.

UNLABELED USES Edema associated with CHF.

CONTRAINDICATIONS Hypersensitivity to indapamide or other sulfonamide derivatives, anuria, renal failure; lactation.

CAUTIOUS USE Electrolyte imbalance, hypokalemia, severe renal disease; impaired hepatic function or progressive liver disease; prediabetic and type II diabetic patient, hyperparathyroidism, thyroid disorders; SLE; sympathectomized patient; history of gout; pregnancy (category B). Safe use in children is not established.

ROUTE & DOSAGE

Hypertension, Edema

Adult: **PO** 2.5 mg once/day, may increase to 5 mg/day if needed

ADMINISTRATION

Oral

- Give with food or milk to reduce GI irritation.
- Administer in a.m. to prevent nocturia. Urge patient to take at least 240 mL (8 oz) of fluid (if allowed) with the medication.
- Store in tight, light-resistant container unless otherwise directed.

ADVERSE EFFECTS (≥1%) **CNS:** Headache, dizziness, fatigue, weakness, muscle cramps or spasm, paresthesia, tension, anxiety, nervousness, agitation, vertigo, insomnia, mental depression, blurred vision, drowsiness. **CV:** Orthostatic hypotension, PVCs, dysrhythmias, flushing, palpitation. **GI:** Dry mouth, anorexia, nausea, vomiting, diarrhea, constipation, abdominal cramps or pain. **Urogenital:** Urinary frequency, nocturia, polyuria, glycosuria, impotence or reduced libido. **Skin:** Rash, hives, pruritus, vasculitis, photosensitivity. **Metabolic:** Dilutional hyponatremia, *hyperuricemia,* exacerbation of gout; *hypokalemia,* hyperglycemia, hypochloremia, hypercalcemia, increased BUN or creatinine, weight loss, exacerbation of SLE; increased cholesterol.

DIAGNOSTIC TEST INTERFERENCE Since indapamide may cause hypercalcemia (and hypophosphatemia), it is generally withheld before tests for ***parathyroid function*** are performed.

INTERACTIONS Drug: Effects of **diazoxide** and indapamide intensified; increased risk of **digoxin** toxicity with hypokalemia; decreased renal **lithium** clearance may increase risk of **lithium** toxicity.

PHARMACOKINETICS Absorption: Readily from GI tract. **Peak:** 2–2.5 h. **Duration:** Up to 36 h. **Metabolism:** In liver. **Elimination:** 60% in urine; 16–23% in feces. **Half-Life:** 14–18 h.

NURSING IMPLICATIONS

Assessment & Drug Effects

- Monitor BP periodically throughout therapy.
- Lab tests: Obtain baseline and periodic BUN, serum creatinine, uric acid, blood glucose, serum electrolytes, and fluid balance.
- Monitor for digitalis toxicity with concurrent therapy.
- Note: Electrolyte imbalances may be clinically serious with protracted vomiting and diarrhea, excessive sweating, GI drainage, and paracentesis.
- Report promptly signs of hyponatremia or hypokalemia (see Appendix F).
- Monitor diabetics for loss of glycemic control.

Patient & Family Education

- Notify physician of decreased urine output, dizziness, weakness or muscle cramps, nausea, jaundice, or blurred vision.
- Take precautions from sun exposure because of risk of photosensitivity.
- Record weight at least every other day; inspect ankles and legs for edema. Report unexplained, progressive weight gain [e.g., 1–1.5 kg (2–3 lb) in 2–3 days].

INDINAVIR SULFATE

(in-din'a-vir)

Crixivan

Classification: ANTIVIRAL; PROTEASE INHIBITOR

Therapeutic: PROTEASE INHIBITOR

Prototype: Saquinavir

Pregnancy Category: C

AVAILABILITY 100 mg, 200 mg, 333 mg, 400 mg capsules

ACTION & *THERAPEUTIC EFFECT* Indinavir is an HIV protease inhibitor. HIV protease is an enzyme required to produce the polyprotein precursors of the functional proteins in infectious HIV. Indinavir binds to the protease active site and thus inhibits its activity. *Protease inhibitors prevent cleavage of the HIV viral polyproteins, resulting in formation of immature noninfectious virus particles.*

USES Treatment of HIV infection, usually in combination with other antiretroviral agents or protease inhibitors.

CONTRAINDICATIONS Hypersensitivity to indinavir; severe leukocyturia of greater than 100 cells/high power field; lactation.

CAUTIOUS USE Hepatic dysfunction, hepatitis; renal impairment, history of nephrolithiasis, diabetes mellitus; hyperglycemia; concurrent HBV infection; history of adverse responses to other protease inhibitors; pregnancy (category C). Safety and efficacy in children are not established.

ROUTE & DOSAGE

HIV

Adult: **PO** 800 mg (2 × 400 mg) q8h 1 h before or 2 h after meal
With ritonavir: 800 mg b.i.d. plus 100–200 mg ritonavir b.i.d.

ADMINISTRATION

Oral

- Give with water on an empty stomach 1 h before or 2 h after meal; if needed, may be given with a very light meal or beverage.
- Note: When didanosine and indinavir are ordered concurrently, give each on empty stomach at least 1 h apart.
- Do not administer concurrently with midazolam or triazolam.
- Store tightly closed with desiccant in original bottle.

ADVERSE EFFECTS (≥1%) **CNS:** Fatigue, headache, insomnia, dizziness, somnolence, nervousness, agitation, anxiety, paresthesia, peripheral neuropathy, tremor, vertigo. **CV:** Palpitations. **Hematologic:** Anemia, splenomegaly, lymphadenopathy. **GI:** *Nausea,* diarrhea, abdominal discomfort, dyspepsia, stomatitis, anorexia, dry mouth, cholecystitis, cholestasis, constipation, flatulence. **Skin:** Body odor, rash, pruritus, seborrhea, skin ulceration, dry skin, sweating, urticaria. **Other:** Myalgia, allergic reaction, bronchitis, cough, rhinitis, taste alterations, visual disturbances, hyperglycemia, diabetes, kidney stones.

INTERACTIONS Drug: Rifabutin, rifampin significantly decrease indinavir levels. **Ketoconazole** significantly increases indinavir levels. Indinavir could inhibit the metabolism and increase the toxicity of **midazolam, sildenafil, tadalafil, trazodone, triazolam, vardenafil.** Indinavir and **didanosine** should be administered at least 1 h apart on empty stomach to permit full absorption of each; increased **ergotamine** toxicity with indinavir. **Rosuvastatin** should not be used concurrently. **Herbal: St. John's wort,** garlic decreases ANTIRETROVIRAL activity of indinavir.

PHARMACOKINETICS Absorption: Rapidly absorbed from GI tract; a meal high in calories, fat, and protein significantly reduces absorption. **Distribution:** 60% protein bound. **Metabolism:** In liver by CYP3A4. **Elimination:** Primarily in feces (greater than 80%), 20% in urine.

NURSING IMPLICATIONS

Assessment & Drug Effects

- Lab tests: Monitor CBC with differential and platelet count, liver function tests, CPK, urinalysis, and serum amylase periodically.
- Assess for S&S of renal dysfunction, respiratory dysfunction, GI distress, and other common adverse effects.

Patient & Family Education

- Learn drug interactions and potential adverse reactions. Drink plenty of liquids to minimize risk of renal stones.
- Notify physician of flank pain, hematuria, S&S of jaundice, or other distressing adverse effects.

INDOMETHACIN

(in-doe-meth′a-sin)

Indocid ✤, Indocin, Indocin SR

Classification: ANALGESIC, NONSTEROIDAL ANTI-INFLAMMATORY (NSAID)

Therapeutic: ANALGESIC, NSAID; ANTIRHEUMATIC

Prototype: Ibuprofen
Pregnancy Category: B first and second trimester; D third trimester

AVAILABILITY 25 mg, 50 mg capsules; 75 mg sustained release capsules; 25 mg/5 mL oral suspension; 50 mg suppositories; 1 mg injection

ACTION & *THERAPEUTIC EFFECT* Potent nonsteroidal compound that competes with COX-1 and COX-2 enzymes, thus interfering with formation of prostaglandin. Appears to reduce motility of polymorphonuclear leukocytes, development of cellular exudates, and vascular permeability in injured tissue resulting in its anti-inflammatory effects. Inhibition of prostaglandins is thought to promote closure of the patency of the ductus arterious. Antipyretic and anti-inflammatory actions may be related to its ability to inhibit prostaglandin biosynthesis. *It is a potent analgesic, anti-inflammatory, and antipyretic agent. Promotes closure of persistent patent ductus arteriosus.*

USES Palliative treatment in active stages of moderate to severe rheumatoid arthritis, ankylosing rheumatoid spondylitis, acute gouty arthritis, and osteoarthritis of hip in patients intolerant to or unresponsive to adequate trials with salicylates and other therapy. Also used IV to close patent ductus arteriosus in the premature infant.

UNLABELED USES To relieve biliary pain and dysmenorrhea, Paget's disease, athletic injuries, juvenile arthritis, idiopathic pericarditis.

CONTRAINDICATIONS Allergy to indomethacin, aspirin, or other NSAID; nasal polyps associated with angioedema; history of recurrent GI lesions; perioperative pain with CABG; pregnancy (D third trimester), lactation.

CAUTIOUS USE History of psychiatric illness, epilepsy, parkinsonism; impaired renal or hepatic function; hypertension; history of ulcer disease or GI bleeding; infection; coagulation disorders; uncontrolled infections; coagulation defects, CHF; older adults, persons in hazardous occupations; pregnancy (category B first and second trimester).

ROUTE & DOSAGE

Rheumatoid Arthritis

Adult: **PO** 25–50 mg b.i.d or t.i.d. (max: 200 mg/day) or 75 mg sustained release 1–2 times/day

Pediatric Arthritis

Child: **PO** 1–2 mg/kg/day in 2–4 divided doses (max: 4 mg/kg/day) or 150–200 mg/day

Acute Gouty Arthritis

Adult: **PO/PR** 50 mg t.i.d. until pain is tolerable, then rapidly taper

Bursitis

Adult: **PO** 25–50 mg t.i.d. or q.i.d. (max: 200 mg/day) or 75 mg sustained release 1–2 times/day

Close Patent Ductus Arteriosus

Premature neonate: **IV** *Younger than 48 h,* 0.2 mg/kg followed by 2 doses of 0.1 mg/kg q12–24h; *2–7 days,* 0.2 mg/kg followed by 2 doses of 0.2 mg/kg q12–24h; *younger than 7 days,* 0.2 mg/kg followed by 2 doses of 0.25 mg/kg q12–24h

ADMINISTRATION

Oral

- Give immediately after meals, or with food, milk, or antacid (if prescribed) to minimize GI side effects.

Rectal

- Indomethacin rectal suppository use is contraindicated with history of proctitis or recent bleeding.

Intravenous

PREPARE: **Direct:** Dilute 1 mg with 1 mL of NS or sterile water for injection without preservatives. Resulting concentration (1 mg/mL) may be further diluted with an additional 1 mL for each 1 mg to yield 0.5 mg/mL.

ADMINISTER: **Direct:** Give by direct IV with a single dose given over 20–30 min.

INCOMPATIBILITIES **Y-site: Amino acid, calcium gluconate, cimetidine, dobutamine, dopamine, gentamicin, levofloxacin, tobramycin, tolazoline.**

- Avoid extravasation or leakage; drug can be irritating to tissue. - Discard any unused drug, since it contains no preservative.

- Store oral and rectal forms in tight, light-resistant containers unless otherwise directed. Do not freeze.

ADVERSE EFFECTS (≥1%) **Body as a Whole:** Hypersensitivity (rash, purpura, pruritus, urticaria, angioedema, angiitis, rapid fall in blood pressure, dyspnea, asthma syndrome in aspirin-sensitive patients), edema, weight gain, flushing, sweating. **CNS:** Headache, *dizziness,* vertigo, light-headedness, syncope, fatigue, muscle weakness, ataxia, insomnia, nightmares, drowsiness, confusion, coma, convulsions, peripheral neuropathy, psychic disturbances (hallucinations, depersonalization, depression), aggravation of epilepsy, parkinsonism. **CV:** Elevated BP, palpitation, chest pains, tachycardia, bradycardia, CHF. **Special Senses:** Blurred vision, lacrimation, eye pain, visual field changes, corneal deposits, retinal disturbances including macula, *tinnitus,* hearing disturbances, epistaxis. **GI:** *Nausea, vomiting,* diarrhea, anorexia, bloating, abdominal distention, ulcerative stomatitis, proctitis, rectal bleeding, <u>GI ulceration, hemorrhage, perforation, toxic hepatitis</u>. **Hematologic:** Hemolytic anemia, <u>aplastic anemia</u> (sometimes fatal), <u>agranulocytosis</u>, leukopenia, thrombocytopenic purpura, inhibited platelet aggregation. **Urogenital:** Renal function impairment, hematuria, urinary frequency; vaginal bleeding, breast changes. **Skin:** Hair loss, exfoliative dermatitis, erythema nodosum, tissue irritation with extravasation. **Metabolic:** Hyponatremia, hypokalemia, hyperkalemia, hypoglycemia or hyperglycemia, glycosuria (rare).

DIAGNOSTIC TEST INTERFERENCE Increased ***AST, ALT, bilirubin, BUN;*** positive direct ***Coombs' test.***

INTERACTIONS Drug: ORAL ANTICOAGULANTS, **heparin, alcohol** may prolong bleeding time; may increase **lithium** toxicity; effects of ORAL ANTICOAGULANTS, **phenytoin,** SALICYLATES, SULFONAMIDES, SULFONYLUREAS increased because of protein-binding displacement; increased toxicity including GI bleeding with SALICYLATES, NSAIDS; may blunt effects of ANTIHYPERTENSIVES and DIURETICS. **Herbal: Feverfew, garlic, ginger, ginkgo** may increase bleeding potential.

PHARMACOKINETICS Absorption: Completely absorbed from GI tract. **Onset:** 1–2 h. **Peak:** 3 h. **Duration:** 4–6 h. **Metabolism:** In liver. **Elimination:** Primarily in urine. **Half-Life:** 2.5–124 h.

NURSING IMPLICATIONS

Assessment & Drug Effects

- Monitor for therapeutic effectiveness: In acute gouty attack, relief of joint tenderness and pain is usually apparent in 24–36 h; swelling generally disappears in 3–5 days. In rheumatoid arthritis: Reduced fever, increased strength, reduced stiffness, and relief of pain, swelling, and tenderness.

- Question patient carefully regarding aspirin sensitivity before initiation of therapy.
- Observe patients carefully; instruct to report adverse reactions promptly to prevent serious and sometimes irreversible or fatal effects.
- Lab tests: Monitor renal function, hepatic function, CBC with differential, BP and HR, visual and hearing acuity periodically.
- Monitor weight and observe dependent areas for signs of edema in patients with underlying cardiovascular disease.
- Monitor I&O closely and keep physician informed during IV administration for patent ductus arteriosus. Significant impairment of renal function is possible; urine output may decrease by 50% or more. Also monitor BUN, serum creatinine, glomerular filtration rate, creatinine clearance, and serum electrolytes.

Patient & Family Education

- Notify physician of S&S of GI bleeding, visual disturbance, tinnitus, weight gain, or edema.
- Do not take aspirin or other NSAIDs; they increase possibility of ulcers.
- Note: Frontal headache is the most frequent CNS adverse effect; if it persists, dosage reduction or drug withdrawal may be indicated. Take drug at bedtime with milk to reduce the incidence of morning headache.
- Do not drive or engage in other potentially hazardous activities until response to drug is known.

INFLIXIMAB

(in-flix'i-mab)

Remicade

Classifications: BIOLOGICAL RESPONSE MODIFIER; MONOCLONAL ANTIBODY (IgG); TUMOR NECROSIS FACTOR (TNF) MODIFIER

Therapeutic: IMMUNOMODULATOR; ANTI-INFLAMMATORY; DISEASE-MODIFYING ANTIRHEUMATIC DRUG (DMARD)

Pregnancy Category: B

AVAILABILITY 100 mg powder for injection

ACTION & *THERAPEUTIC EFFECT* An IgG_1-K is a monoclonal antibody that binds specifically to tumor necrosis factor-alpha (TNF-alpha), a cytokine. Thus, it prevents TNF-alpha from binding to its receptors. TNF-alpha induces proinflammatory cytokines. Infliximab reduces infiltration of inflammatory cells and TNF-alpha production in inflamed areas of the intestine as seen in Crohn's disease. *Infliximab decreases GI inflammation in Crohn's and related diseases. It is also a disease-modifying antirheumatic drug (DMARD).*

USES Moderately to severely active Crohn's disease, including fistulizing Crohn's disease, rheumatoid arthritis, ankylosing spondylitis, ulcerative colitis.

CONTRAINDICATIONS Hypersensitivity to infliximab; CHF; infection, sepsis; murine protein hypersensitivity; lactation.

CAUTIOUS USE History of allergic phenomena or untoward responses to monoclonal antibody preparation; renal or hepatic impairment; multiple sclerosis (potential exacerbation); fungal infection; heart failure, human antichimeric antibody

(HACA); leukopenia, thrombocytopenia; immunosuppressed patients; neoplastic disease; tuberculosis; vaccination; vasculitis; neurologic disease; neutropenia; seizure disorder, seizures; older adults; pregnancy (category B).

ROUTE & DOSAGE

Crohn's Disease

Adult: **IV** 5 mg/kg infused over at least 2 h, repeat at 2 and 6 wk for fistulizing disease, then q8wk
Child: **IV** 5 mg/kg at weeks 0, 2, and 6, then 5 mg/kg q8wk

Rheumatoid Arthritis

Adult: **IV** 3 mg/kg at weeks 0, 2, and 6, then q8wk

Ulcerative Colitis

Adult: **IV** 5 mg/kg at weeks 0, 2, and 6, then 5 mg/kg q8wk

Ankylosing Spondylitis

Adult: **IV** 5 mg/kg at weeks 0, 2, and 6, then 5 mg/kg q6wk

ADMINISTRATION

▪ Note: Do not administer to a patient who has known or suspected sepsis.

Intravenous

PREPARE: **IV Infusion:** Reconstitute each 100 mg vial with 10 mL of sterile water for injection using a 21-gauge or smaller syringe. Inject sterile water against wall of vial, then gently swirl to dissolve but do not shake. ▪Let stand for 5 min. ▪Solution should be colorless to light yellow with a few translucent particles. Discard if particles are opaque. ▪Further dilute by first removing from a 250-mL IV bag of NS a volume of NS equal to the volume of reconstituted infliximab to be added to the IV bag. Slowly add the total volume of reconstituted infliximab solution to the 250-mL infusion bag and gently mix. ▪ Infusion concentration should be 0.4 to 4 mg/mL. ▪Begin infusion within 3 h of preparation.

ADMINISTER: **IV Infusion:** Give over at least 2 h using a polyethylene-lined infusion set with an in-line, low-protein-binding filter (pore size 1.2 micron or less). ▪Flush infusion set before and after with NS to ensure delivery of total drug dose. ▪ Discard unused infusion solution.

INCOMPATIBILITIES **Y-site:** Do not infuse with any other drugs.

▪ Store unopened vials at 2°–8° C (36°–46° F).

ADVERSE EFFECTS (≥1%) **Body as a Whole:** Fatigue, fever, pain, myalgia, back pain, chills, hot flashes, arthralgia; infusion-related reactions (fever, chills, pruritus, urticaria, chest pain, hypotension, hypertension, dyspnea). Increased risk of lymphoma and opportunistic infections, including tuberculosis. **CNS:** Headache, dizziness, involuntary muscle contractions, paresthesias, vertigo, anxiety, depression, insomnia. **CV:** Chest pain, peripheral edema, hypotension, hypertension, tachycardia, anemia, CHF, pericardial effusion, systemic and cutaneous vasculitis. **GI:** Nausea, diarrhea, abdominal pain, vomiting, constipation, dyspepsia, flatulence, intestinal obstruction, ulcerative stomatitis, increased hepatic enzymes. **Hematologic:** Leukopenia, neutropenia, thrombocytopenia, pancytopenia. **Respiratory:** URI, pharyngitis, bronchitis, rhinitis, coughing, sinusitis, dyspnea. **Skin:** Rash, pruritus, acne, alopecia, fungal dermatitis, eczema, dry skin, increased sweating, urticaria. **Other:** Infections, development of autoantibodies, lupus-like syndrome, conjunctivitis, dysuria, urinary frequency.

INTERACTIONS Drug: May blunt effectiveness of VACCINES given concurrently.

PHARMACOKINETICS Distribution: Distributed primarily to the vascular compartment. **Half-Life:** 9.5 days.

NURSING IMPLICATIONS

Assessment & Drug Effects

- Discontinue IV infusion and notify physician for fever, chills, pruritus, urticaria, chest pain, dyspnea, hypo/hypertension.
- Monitor for up to 2 h post-infusion for an acute infusion reaction (e.g., chest pain, hypotension, hypertension, dyspnea).
- Monitor for and immediately report S&S of generalized infection.

Patient & Family Education

- Seek medical evaluation immediately if you suspect an infection.

INSULIN ASPART

(in′su-lyn)

NovoLog, NovoLog 50/50, NovoLog 70/30

Classifications: ANTIDIABETIC; INSULIN, RAPID-ACTING
Therapeutic: RAPID-ACTING INSULIN
Prototype: Insulin injection
Pregnancy Category: B (**NovoLog**); C (**NovoLog 70/30**)

AVAILABILITY 100 units/mL injection; insulin aspart/insulin aspart protamine injection

ACTION & *THERAPEUTIC EFFECT* A recombinant insulin analog that is more rapidly absorbed than human insulin, with a more rapid onset and shorter duration than regular human insulin. *Provides better blood glucose control than regular human insulin when given before a meal.*

USES Treatment of diabetes mellitus.

CONTRAINDICATIONS Systemic allergic reactions; history of allergic reactions to insulin; hypoglycemia.
CAUTIOUS USE Fever, hyperthyroidism, surgery or trauma; decreased insulin requirements due to diarrhea, nausea, or vomiting, malabsorption; renal or hepatic impairment, hypokalemia; pregnancy [category B (**NovoLog**) and category C (**NovoLog 70/30**)], lactation.

ROUTE & DOSAGE

Diabetes

Adult: **Subcutaneous** 0.25–0.7 units/kg/day injected 5–10 min before each meal **IV** Use only under close medical supervision in a clinical setting

ADMINISTRATION

- Use only if solution is absolutely clear.

Subcutaneous

- **Must be** given **no sooner** than 5–10 min before a meal.
- Draw up insulin aspart first when mixing with NPH insulin. Give injection immediately after it is mixed.
- Store refrigerated at 2°–8° C (36°–46° F); may be stored at room temperature, 15°–30° C (59°–86° F) for up to 28 days. Do not expose to excessive heat or sunlight, and do not freeze.

Intravenous

PREPARE: **Infusion:** Dilute with NS or D5W in a polypropylene infusion bag to a final concentration of 0.05–1 unit/mL.

ADMINISTER: **Infusion:** Give at rate ordered by physician.

ADVERSE EFFECTS (≥1%) **Body as a Whole:** Allergic reactions. **Endocrine:** Hypoglycemia, hypokalemia. **Skin:** Injection site reaction, lipodystrophy, pruritus, rash.

INTERACTIONS Drug: ORAL ANTIDIABETIC AGENTS, ACE INHIBITORS, **disopyramide, fluoxetine,** MAO INHIBITORS, **propoxyphene,** SALICYLATES, SULFONAMIDE ANTIBIOTICS, **octreotide** may enhance hypoglycemia; CORTICOSTEROIDS, **niacin, danazol,** DIURETICS, SYMPATHOMIMETIC AGENTS, PHENOTHIAZINES, THYROID HORMONES, ESTROGENS, PROGESTOGENS, **isoniazid, somatropin** may decrease hypoglycemic effects; BETA-BLOCKERS, **clonidine, lithium, alcohol** may either potentiate or weaken effects of insulin; **pentamidine** may cause hypoglycemia followed by hyperglycemia. **Herbal: Garlic, ginseng** may potentiate hypoglycemic effects.

PHARMACOKINETICS Absorption: Rapidly absorbed from subcutaneous injection site. **Onset:** 15 min. **Peak:** 1–3 h. **Duration:** 3–5 h. **Distribution:** Low protein binding. **Metabolism:** In liver with some metabolism in the kidneys. **Half-Life:** 81 min.

NURSING IMPLICATIONS

Assessment & Drug Effects

- Monitor for S&S of hypoglycemia (see Appendix F). Initial hypoglycemic response begins within 15 min and peaks 45–90 min after injection.
- Lab tests: Periodic postprandial blood glucose and HbA1C.
- Withhold drug and notify physician if patient is hypokalemic.

Patient & Family Education

- Eat immediately after injecting insulin aspart because it has a fast onset and short duration of action.
- Do not inject into areas with redness, swelling, itching, or dimpling.
- Ingest some form of sugar (e.g., orange juice, dissolved table sugar, honey) if symptoms of hypoglycemia develop, and seek medical assistance.
- Check blood sugar as prescribed, especially postprandial values; make note of and notify physician of fasting blood glucose less than 80 and greater than 120 mg/dL.
- Notify the physician of any of the following: Fever, infection, trauma, diarrhea, nausea or vomiting. Dosage adjustment may be needed.
- Do not take any other medication unless approved by the physician.

INSULIN DETEMIR

(in′su-lyn det′e-mir)

Levemir

Classifications: ANTIDIABETIC; INSULIN, LONG-ACTING

Therapeutic: LONG-ACTING INSULIN

Prototype: Insulin injection

Pregnancy Category: C

AVAILABILITY 100 units/mL available in 10 mL multidose vials and 3 mL prefilled syringes

ACTION & *THERAPEUTIC EFFECT* Insulin detemir, a long-acting human insulin, exerts its action by binding to insulin receptors. Receptor-bound insulin lowers blood glucose by facilitating cellular uptake of glucose into skeletal muscle and fat, and inhibiting the output of glucose from the liver. *Insulin detemir is effective as a glucose-lowering agent, with glycemic control equivalent to that of NPH insulin.*

USES Treatment of type 1 and type 2 diabetes mellitus.

CONTRAINDICATIONS Hypersensitivity to insulin detemir, or cresol; use in insulin infusion pumps; diabetic ketoacidosis, coma, hyperosmolar hyperglycemic state, hypoglycemia. Safe and effective use in children with type 2 diabetes has not been established.

CAUTIOUS USE Renal and hepatic impairment; older adults; cardiac disease, CHF, illness, stress; pregnancy (category C), lactation.

ROUTE & DOSAGE

Diabetes

Adult/Child: **Subcutaneous** Insulin-naïve patients: 0.1–0.2 units/kg daily in evening or 10 units daily or b.i.d. in evenly spaced doses. For those taking a basal insulin product (i.e., NPH insulin, insulin glargine), a unit-to-unit dose conversion can be used.

ADMINISTRATION

Subcutaneous

- Once-daily injections should be given with the evening meal or at bedtime. With twice-daily dosing, the evening dose may be given with the evening meal, at bedtime, or 12 h after the morning dose.
- Do not administer IV or IM. With thin patients, inject at a 45-degree angle into a pinched fold of skin to avoid IM injection.
- Do not mix with any other type of insulin. Do not use with an insulin infusion pump.
- Store unopened vials under refrigeration at 2°–8° C (36°–46° F). Once removed from refrigeration, pens, cartridges, and other delivery devices **must be** kept at room temperature (not to exceed 30° C or 85° F) and either used within 42 days or discarded.

INCOMPATIBILITIES **Solution/additive:** Insulin detemir should not be mixed with any other insulin preparations.

ADVERSE EFFECTS (≥1%) **[See** INSULIN (REGULAR)**] Body as a Whole:** Allergic reactions. **Metabolic:** Hypoglycemia, weight gain. **Skin:** Lipodystrophy, pruritus, rash.

DIAGNOSTIC TEST INTERFERENCE See INSULIN INJECTION (REGULAR).

INTERACTIONS Drug: See INSULIN INJECTION (REGULAR). **Herbal: Garlic** and **green tea** may potentiate hypoglycemic effects.

PHARMACOKINETICS Absorption: Slow, prolonged absorption over 24 h. **Peak:** 6–8 h. **Distribution:** 98–99% protein bound. **Half-Life:** 5–7 h.

NURSING IMPLICATIONS

Assessment & Drug Effects

- Monitor for S&S of hypoglycemia (see Appendix F), especially after changes in insulin dose or type.
- Lab tests: Periodic fasting blood glucose and HbA1C; periodic serum potassium with concurrent potassium-lowering drugs.
- Monitor weight periodically.

Patient & Family Education

- Follow directions for taking the drug (see Administration). Rotate injection sites and never inject into an area with redness, swelling, itching, or dimpling.
- Know parameters for withholding drug. Check blood sugar as prescribed; notify physician of fasting blood glucose below 80 or above 120 mg/dL.
- Ingest some form of sugar (e.g., orange juice, dissolved table sugar,

honey) if symptoms of hypoglycemia develop; and seek medical assistance.

- Notify the physician of any of the following: Fever, infection, trauma, diarrhea, nausea, or vomiting.
- Do not take any other medication unless approved by physician.

INSULIN GLARGINE

(in′su-lyn glar′geen)

Lantus, Lantus SoloStar

Classifications: ANTIDIABETIC; INSULIN, LONG-ACTING

Therapeutic: LONG-ACTING INSULIN

Prototype: Insulin injection

Pregnancy Category: C

AVAILABILITY 100 units/mL injection; 3 mL cartridge; prefilled, disposable pen

ACTION & *THERAPEUTIC EFFECT* A recombinant human insulin analog with a long duration of action. Lowers blood glucose levels over an extended period of time by stimulating peripheral glucose uptake especially in muscle and fat tissue. In addition, insulin inhibits hepatic glucose production. *Lowers blood glucose levels over an extended period of time. It also prevents the conversion of glucagon to glucose in the liver.*

USES Bedtime dosing of adults and children with type 1 diabetes, or adults with type 2 diabetes.

CONTRAINDICATIONS Prior hypersensitivity to insulin glargine; hypoglycemia. Safety and efficacy in children with type 2 diabetes are unknown.

CAUTIOUS USE Renal and hepatic impairment; pregnancy (category C), lactation. Safety and efficacy in children younger than 6 y of age in type 1 diabetes.

ROUTE & DOSAGE

Type 1 Diabetes

Adult/Child: **Subcutaneous** If not taking insulin, give 10 units at same time each day (usually at bedtime) once daily; if taking NPH or ultralente insulin once daily, give same dose at same time each day (usually at bedtime); if taking NPH insulin twice daily, give 80% of total daily dose at same time each day (usually at bedtime)

Type 2 Diabetes

Adult: **Subcutaneous** If already taking oral hypoglycemic drugs, start with 10 units at same time each day (usually at bedtime) once daily and adjust according to patient's needs

ADMINISTRATION

Subcutaneous

- Do not give this product IV.
- Give at same time each day (usually at bedtime) and do not mix with any other insulin product.
- Store in refrigerator at 2°–8° C (36°–46° F), may store at room temperature, 15°–30° C (59°–86° F). Discard opened refrigerated vials after 28 days and unrefrigerated vials after 14 days. Do not expose to excessive heat or sunlight, and do not freeze.

ADVERSE EFFECTS (≥1%) **Body as a Whole:** Allergic reactions. **Endocrine:** Hypoglycemia, hypokalemia. **Skin:** Injection site reaction, lipodystrophy, pruritus, rash.

INTERACTIONS Drug: ORAL ANTIDIABETIC AGENTS, ACE INHIBITORS,

disopyramide, fluoxetine, MAO INHIBITORS, **propoxyphene,** SALICYLATES, SULFONAMIDE ANTIBIOTICS, **octreotide** may enhance hypoglycemia; CORTICOSTEROIDS, **niacin, danazol,** DIURETICS, SYMPATHOMIMETIC AGENTS, PHENOTHIAZINES, THYROID HORMONES, ESTROGENS, PROGESTOGENS, **isoniazid, somatropin** may decrease hypoglycemic effects; BETA-BLOCKERS, **clonidine, lithium, alcohol** may either potentiate or weaken effects of insulin; **pentamidine** may cause hypoglycemia followed by hyperglycemia. **Herbal: Garlic, ginseng** may potentiate hypoglycemic effects.

PHARMACOKINETICS Absorption: Slowly absorbed from subcutaneous injection site. **Onset:** 3–4 h. **Duration:** 10.4–24 h. **Metabolism:** In liver to active metabolites.

NURSING IMPLICATIONS

Assessment & Drug Effects

- Monitor for S&S of hypoglycemia (see Appendix F), especially after changes in insulin dose or type.
- Lab tests: Monitor fasting blood glucose and HbA1C periodically.
- Withhold drug and notify physician if patient is hypokalemic.

Patient & Family Education

- Do not inject into areas with redness, swelling, itching, or dimpling.
- Absorption patterns for this drug are not dependent on the injection site.
- Ingest some form of sugar (e.g., orange juice, dissolved table sugar, honey) if symptoms of hypoglycemia develop and seek medical assistance.
- Check blood sugar as prescribed; notify physician of fasting blood glucose less than 80 and greater than 120 mg/dL.
- Notify the physician of any of the following: Fever, infection, trauma, diarrhea, nausea, or vomiting. Dosage adjustment may be needed.
- Do not take any other medication unless approved by physician.

INSULIN GLULISINE

(in'su-lyn glu-li'seen)

Apidra, Apidra SoloSTAR

Classifications: ANTIDIABETIC; INSULIN, RAPID-ACTING

Therapeutic: ANTIDIABETIC; RAPID-ACTING INSULIN

Prototype: Insulin injection (Regular)

Pregnancy Category: C

AVAILABILITY 100 units/mL multidose (10 mL) vials; 3 mL cartridge system

ACTION & *THERAPEUTIC EFFECT* Insulin glulisine, formed by recombinant DNA, is a rapid-acting insulin. Insulin lowers blood glucose by stimulating peripheral glucose uptake by skeletal muscle and fat and by inhibiting hepatic glucose production. Insulin causes lipolysis in the adipocytes, inhibits proteolysis, and enhances protein synthesis. *Insulin glulisine has a more rapid onset of action and a shorter duration of action than regular human insulin; thus, it provides good postprandial blood glucose control.*

USES Treatment of diabetes mellitus; type I diabetes mellitus in children.

CONTRAINDICATIONS Hypoglycemia; systemic allergy to insulin; children younger than 4 y

CAUTIOUS USE Renal impairment, hepatic dysfunction; thyroid disease; fever; older adults; children older than 4 y; pregnancy (category C), lactation.

ROUTE & DOSAGE

Diabetes

Adult/Adolescent/Child (4 y and older): **Subcutaneous** 5–10 units within 15 min before starting a meal or within 20 min after starting a meal. Dose should be individualized.
Adult/Adolescent/Child: **IV** 0.05–1 unit/mL via infusion; use under close supervision

ADMINISTRATION

Subcutaneous

- Give within 15 min before or up to 20 min after a meal.
- Store refrigerated at 36°–46° F (2°–8° C). Discard vial if frozen. Protect from light.

Intravenous

PREPARE: **Infusion:** Dilute with NS in a PVC bag to a final concentration of 0.05–1 unit/mL.
ADMINISTER: **Infusion:** Give at rate ordered by physician.

ADVERSE EFFECTS (≥1%) [See INSULIN (REGULAR)] **Body as a Whole:** Allergic reactions. **Metabolic:** Hypoglycemia. **Skin:** Injection site reactions, lipodystrophy, pruritus, rash.

DIAGNOSTIC TEST INTERFERENCE See INSULIN INJECTION (REGULAR).

PHARMACOKINETICS Absorption: 70% bioavailable from injection sites. **Onset:** 15–30 min. **Peak:** 55 min. **Duration:** 3–4 h. **Metabolism:** In liver with some metabolism in the kidney. **Half-Life:** 42 min subcutaneous.

NURSING IMPLICATIONS

Assessment & Drug Effects

- Monitor for S&S of hypoglycemia (see Appendix F). Initial hypoglycemic response begins within 15 min and peaks, on average, 40–60 min after injection.
- Lab tests: Periodically monitor fasting and postprandial blood glucose and HbA1C.

Patient & Family Education

- Follow exactly directions for timing injection in relation to each meal.
- Do not inject into areas with redness, swelling, itching, or dimpling.
- If mixing with NPH human insulin, draw up insulin glulisine first. Inject immediately after mixing.
- Ingest some form of sugar (e.g., orange juice, dissolved table sugar, honey) if symptoms of hypoglycemia develop, and seek medical assistance.
- Check blood sugar as prescribed, especially postprandial values; notify physician of fasting blood glucose less than 80 and greater than 140 mg/dL.
- Notify the physician of any of the following: Fever, infection, trauma, diarrhea, nausea, or vomiting. Dosage adjustment may be needed.
- Do not take any other medication unless approved by the physician.

INSULIN (REGULAR) Pr

(in'su-lyn)

Humulin R, Novolin R, Regular Insulin, Velosulin BR

Classifications: ANTIDIABETIC; INSULIN, SHORT-ACTING
Therapeutic: SHORT-ACTING INSULIN
Pregnancy Category: B

AVAILABILITY 100 units/mL

ACTION & *THERAPEUTIC EFFECT* Short-acting, clear, colorless solution of exogenous unmodified insulin extracted from beta cells in pork pancreas or synthesized by recombinant DNA technology (human). Enhances transmembrane passage of glucose across cell membranes in muscle and adipose tissue. Promotes conversion of glucose to glycogen in the liver. *It lowers blood glucose levels by increasing peripheral glucose uptake and by inhibiting the liver from changing glycogen to glucose.*

USES Emergency treatment of diabetic ketoacidosis or coma, to initiate therapy in patient with insulin-dependent diabetes mellitus, and in combination with intermediate-acting or long-acting insulin to provide better control of blood glucose concentrations in the diabetic patient. Used IV to stimulate growth hormone secretion (glucose counter-regulatory hormone) to evaluate pituitary growth hormone reserve in patient with known or suspected growth hormone deficiency. Other uses include promotion of intracellular shift of potassium in treatment of hyperkalemia (IV) and induction of hypoglycemic shock as therapy in psychiatry.

CONTRAINDICATIONS Hypersensitivity to insulin.

CAUTIOUS USE Renal impairment, renal failure; hepatic impairment, fever, thyroid disease; older adults; pregnancy (category B), children and infants.

ROUTE & DOSAGE

Diabetes Mellitus

Adult: **Subcutaneous** 5–10 units 30–60 min a.c. and at bedtime (dose adjustments based on blood glucose determinations)
Child: **Subcutaneous** 2–4 units 30–60 min a.c. and at bedtime (dose adjustments based on blood glucose determinations)

Ketoacidosis

Adult: **IV** 2.4–7.2 units loading dose, followed by 2.4–7.2 units/h continuous infusion
Child: **IV** 0.1 units/kg loading dose, followed by 0.1 units/h continuous infusion

ADMINISTRATION

- Note: Insulins should not be mixed unless prescribed by physician. In general, regular insulin is drawn up into syringe first. ▪ Any change in the strength (e.g., U-40, U-100), brand (manufacturer), purity, type (regular, etc.), species (pork, human), or sequence of mixing two kinds of insulin is made by the physician only, since a simultaneous change in dosage may be necessary.

Subcutaneous

- Use an insulin syringe.
- Give regular insulin 30–60 min before a meal.
- Avoid injection of cold insulin; it can lead to lipodystrophy, reduced rate of absorption, and local reactions.
- Common injection sites: Upper arms, thighs, abdomen [avoid area over urinary bladder and 2 in. (5 cm) around navel], buttocks, and upper back (if fat is loose enough to pick up). Rotate sites.

Intravenous

PREPARE: **Direct:** Give undiluted. **Continuous:** Typically diluted in NS or 0.45% NaCl. 100 units added to 1000 mL yields 0.1 units/mL.

ADMINISTER: **Direct:** Give 50 units or a fraction thereof over 1 min. **Continuous:** Rate **must be** ordered by physician.

INCOMPATIBILITIES **Solution/additive:** **Aminophylline, amo-**

barbital, chlorothiazide, cytarabine, dobutamine, pentobarbital, phenobarbital, phenytoin, secobarbital, sodium bicarbonate, thiopental. Y-site: **Dobutamine.**

▪ Regular insulin may be adsorbed into the container or tubing when added to an IV infusion solution. ▪ Amount lost is variable and depends on concentration of insulin, infusion system, contact duration, and flow rate. ▪ Monitor patient response closely.

I

▪ Insulin is stable at room temperature up to 1 mo. Avoid exposure to direct sunlight or to temperature extremes [safe range is wide: 5°–38° C (40°–100° F)]. Refrigerate but do not freeze stock supply. Insulin tolerates temperatures above 38° C with less harm than freezing.

ADVERSE EFFECTS (≥1%) **Body as a Whole:** Most adverse effects are related to hypoglycemia; <u>anaphylaxis</u> (rare), hyperinsulinemia (*profuse sweating,* hunger, headache, *nausea, tremulousness,* tremors, *palpitation,* tachycardia, weakness, fatigue, nystagmus, circumoral pallor); numb mouth, tongue, and other paresthesias; visual disturbances (diplopia, blurred vision, mydriasis), staring expression, confusion, personality changes, ataxia, incoherent speech, apprehension, irritability, inability to concentrate, personality changes, uncontrolled yawning, loss of consciousness, delirium, hypothermia, convulsions, Babinski reflex, <u>coma</u>. (Urine glucose tests will be negatives.) **CNS:** With overdose, psychic disturbances (i.e., aphasia, personality changes, maniacal behavior). **Metabolic:** Posthypoglycemia or rebound hyperglycemia (Somogyi effect), lipoatrophy and lipohypertrophy of injection sites; insulin resistance. **Skin:** Localized allergic reactions at injection site; generalized urticaria or bullae, lymphadenopathy.

DIAGNOSTIC TEST INTERFERENCE Large doses of insulin may increase urinary excretion of ***VMA.*** Insulin can cause alterations in ***thyroid function tests*** and ***liver function test*** and may decrease ***serum potassium*** and ***serum calcium.***

INTERACTIONS Drug: Alcohol, ANABOLIC STEROIDS, MAO INHIBITORS, **guanethidine,** SALICYLATES may potentiate hypoglycemic effects; **dextrothyroxine,** CORTICOSTEROIDS, **epinephrine** may antagonize hypoglycemic effects; **furosemide,** THIAZIDE DIURETICS increase **serum glucose** levels; **propranolol** and other BETA-BLOCKERS may mask symptoms of hypoglycemic reaction. **Herbal: Garlic, ginseng** may potentiate hypoglycemic effects.

PHARMACOKINETICS Absorption: Rapidly absorbed from IM and subcutaneous injections. **Onset:** 0.5–1 h. **Peak:** 2–4 h. **Duration:** 5–7 h. **Distribution:** Throughout extracellular fluids. **Metabolism:** In liver with some metabolism in kidneys. **Elimination:** Less than 2% excreted in urine. **Half-Life:** Biological, up to 13 h.

NURSING IMPLICATIONS

Assessment & Drug Effects

- Note: Frequency of blood glucose monitoring is determined by the insulin regimen and health status of the patient.
- Lab tests: Periodic fasting and postprandial blood glucose and HbA1C. Test urine for ketones in new, unstable, and type 1 diabetes; if patient has lost weight, exercises vigorously, or has an illness; whenever blood glucose is substantially elevated.

- Notify physician promptly for markedly elevated blood sugar or presence of acetone with sugar in the urine; may indicate onset of ketoacidosis.
- Monitor for hypoglycemia (see Appendix F) at time of peak action of insulin. Onset of hypoglycemia (blood sugar: 50–40 mg/dL) may be rapid and sudden.
- Check BP, I&O ratio, and blood glucose and ketones every hour during treatment for ketoacidosis with IV insulin.
- Patients with severe hypoglycemia are usually treated with glucagon, epinephrine, or IV glucose 10–50%. As soon as patient is fully conscious, oral carbohydrate (e.g., orange juice with sugar, Gatorade, or Pedialyte) to prevent secondary hypoglycemia may be used.

Patient & Family Education

- Learn correct injection technique.
- Inject insulin into the abdomen rather than a near muscle that will be heavily taxed, if engaged in active sports.
- Notify physician of local reactions at injection site; may develop 1–3 wk after therapy starts and last several hours to days, usually disappear with continued use.
- Do not change prescription lenses during early period of dosage regulation; vision stabilizes, usually 3–6 wk.
- Check your blood glucose often as directed by the physician. Hypoglycemia can result from excess insulin, insufficient food intake, vomiting, diarrhea, unaccustomed exercise, infection, illness, nervous or emotional tension, or overindulgence in alcohol.
- Respond promptly to beginning symptoms of hypoglycemia. Severe hypoglycemia is an emergency situation. Take 4 oz (120 mL) of any fruit juice or regular carbonated beverage [1.5–3 oz (45–90 mL) for child] followed by a meal of longer-acting carbohydrate or protein food. Failure to show signs of recovery within 30 min indicates need for emergency treatment.
- Carry some form of fast-acting carbohydrate (e.g., lump sugar, Life-Savers, or other candy) at all times to treat hypoglycemia.
- Check blood glucose regularly during menstrual period; loss of diabetes control (hyperglycemia or hypoglycemia) is common; adjust insulin dosage accordingly, as prescribed by physician.
- Notify physician immediately of S&S of diabetic ketoacidosis.
- Continue taking insulin during an illness, go to bed, and drink noncaloric liquids liberally (every hour if possible). Consult physician for insulin regulation if unable to eat prescribed diet.
- Avoid OTC medications unless approved by physician.

INSULIN, ISOPHANE (NPH)

(in′su-lyn)

Humulin N, Novolin N, ReliOn N

Classifications: ANTIDIABETIC; INSULIN, INTERMEDIATE ACTING

Therapeutic: INTERMEDIATE ACTING INSULIN

Prototype: Insulin

Pregnancy Category: B

AVAILABILITY 100 units/mL

ACTION & *THERAPEUTIC EFFECT*

Intermediate-acting, cloudy suspension of zinc insulin crystals modified by protamine in a neutral buffer. NPH Iletin II (pork), and Insulatard NPH are "purified" or "single component" insulins that have been purified and are less likely to cause allergic reactions than nonpurified preparations. Lowers blood glucose levels by increasing peripheral glucose uptake, especially by skeletal muscle and fat tissue, and by inhibiting the liver from changing glycogen to glucose. *Controls postprandial hyperglycemia, usually without supplemental doses of insulin injection.*

USES Used to control hyperglycemia in the diabetic patient. Mixtard and Novolin 70/30 are fixed combinations of purified regular insulin 30% and NPH 70%.

CONTRAINDICATIONS During episodes of hypoglycemia or in patients sensitive to any ingredient in the formulation; intravenous route; diabetic ketoacidosis; hyperosmolar hyperglycemic state.
CAUTIOUS USE In insulin-resistant patients, hyperthyroidism or hypothyroidism; fever; older adults, pregnancy (category B), renal or hepatic impairment; children.

ROUTE & DOSAGE

Diabetes Mellitus
Adult: **Subcutaneous** Individualized doses (see INSULIN, REGULAR)

ADMINISTRATION

Subcutaneous
- Give isophane insulin 30 min before first meal of the day. If necessary, a second smaller dose may be prescribed 30 min before supper or at bedtime.
- Ensure complete dispersion by mixing thoroughly by gently rotating vial between palms and inverting it end to end several times. Do not shake.
- Do NOT mix insulins unless prescribed by physician. In general, when insulin injection (regular insulin) is to be combined, it is drawn first.
- Note: Isophane insulin may be mixed with insulin injection without altering either solution.
- Store unopened vial at 2°–8° C (36°–46° F). Avoid freezing and exposure to extremes in temperature or to direct sunlight.

ADVERSE EFFECTS (≥1%) (see INSULIN, REGULAR).

INTERACTIONS (see INSULIN, REGULAR).

PHARMACOKINETICS Onset: 1–2 h. **Peak:** 4–12 h NPH. **Duration:** 18–24 h NPH. **Metabolism:** In liver and kidney. **Elimination:** Less than 2% excreted unchanged in urine. **Half-Life:** Up to 13 h.

NURSING IMPLICATIONS

(see INSULIN, REGULAR)

Assessment & Drug Effects
- Suspect hypoglycemia if fatigue, weakness, sweating, tremor, or nervousness occur.

Patient & Family Education
- If insulin was given before breakfast, a hypoglycemic episode is most likely to occur between mid-afternoon and dinnertime, when insulin effect is peaking. Advise to eat a snack in mid-afternoon and to carry sugar or candy to treat a reaction. A snack at bedtime will prevent insulin reaction during the night.
- Learn the S&S of hypoglycemia and hyperglycemia (see Appendix F).

INSULIN LISPRO
(in′su-lyn lis′pro)

Humalog
Classifications: ANTIDIABETIC; INSULIN, RAPID-ACTING
Therapeutic: RAPID-ACTING INSULIN
Prototype: Insulin injection
Pregnancy Category: B

AVAILABILITY 100 units/mL

ACTION & *THERAPEUTIC EFFECT* Insulin lispro of recombinant DNA origin is a human insulin that is a rapid-acting, glucose-lowering agent of shorter duration than human regular insulin. It lowers blood glucose levels by increasing peripheral glucose uptake, especially by skeletal muscle and fat tissue, and by inhibiting the liver from changing glycogen to glucose. *It lowers blood glucose levels and inhibits liver from changing glycogen to glucose.*

USES Treatment of diabetes mellitus.

CONTRAINDICATIONS During episodes of hypoglycemia or in patients sensitive to any ingredient in the formulation; intravenous administration.

CAUTIOUS USE In insulin-resistant patients, hyperthyroidism or hypothyroidism; older adults, renal or hepatic impairment; children, pregnancy (category B), lactation.

ROUTE & DOSAGE

Diabetes Mellitus (type 1)
Adult: **Subcutaneous** 5–10 units 0–15 min a.c. (dose adjustments based on blood glucose determinations)

ADMINISTRATION

Subcutaneous
- Give within 15 min before or immediately after a meal.
- Note: May be given in same syringe with longer-acting insulins but absorption may be delayed.

ADVERSE EFFECTS (≥1%) See INSULIN INJECTIONS, REGULAR.

INTERACTIONS See INSULIN INJECTION, REGULAR.

PHARMACOKINETICS Absorption: Rapidly absorbed from IM and subcutaneous injection sites. **Onset:** Less than 15 min. **Peak:** 0.5–1 h. **Duration:** 3–4 h. **Distribution:** Throughout extracellular fluids. **Metabolism:** Metabolized in liver with some metabolism in kidneys. **Elimination:** Less than 2% excreted in urine. **Half-Life:** Biological, up to 13 h.

NURSING IMPLICATIONS

(see INSULIN INJECTION, REGULAR)

Assessment & Drug Effects
- Assess for hypoglycemia from 1 to 3 h after injection.
- Assess highly insulin-dependent patients for need for increases in intermediate/long-acting insulins.

Patient & Family Education
- Note: Risk of hypoglycemia is greatest 1–3 h after injection.

INSULIN ZINC SUSPENSION (LENTE)

(in'su-lyn)
Humulin L, Novolin L
Classifications: ANTIDIABETIC; INSULIN, INTERMEDIATE-ACTING
Therapeutic: INSULIN, INTERMEDIATE-ACTING
Prototype: Insulin injection
Pregnancy Category: B

AVAILABILITY 100 units/mL

ACTION & *THERAPEUTIC EFFECT* Intermediate-acting human insulin created by adding zinc ions to human regular insulin. It lowers blood glucose levels by increasing peripheral glucose uptake, especially by skeletal muscle and fat tissue, and by inhibiting the liver from changing glycogen to glucose. It is not the ideal basal insulin since its absorption is variable. *It lowers glucose level over a longer period of time than regular human insulin.*

USES Hyperglycemia in diabetic patients allergic to other preparations of insulin. Also for patients with evidence of thrombotic phenomena in which protamine may be a factor.

CONTRAINDICATIONS During episodes of hypoglycemia or in patients sensitive to any ingredient in the formulation; insulin pump; intravenous administration; hyperosmolar hyperglycemic state; diabetic ketoacidosis. **CAUTIOUS USE** In insulin resistant patients, hyperthyroidism or hypothyroidism; lactation, older adults, pregnancy (category B), renal or hepatic impairment; children.

ROUTE & DOSAGE

Diabetes Mellitus

Adult: **IM/Subcutaneous** Individualized doses (see INSULIN INJECTION, REGULAR)

ADMINISTRATION

Subcutaneous/Intramuscular

- Give insulin zinc suspensions 30 min before breakfast. Some patients require another injection 30 min before supper time or at bedtime.
- Note: Zinc insulin preparation (Lente) is compatible with regular insulin.
- Ensure complete dispersion by mixing thoroughly by gently rotating the vial between the palms and by inverting it end-to-end several times. Do not shake.
- Note: Time of action of insulin zinc (Lente) approximates that of isophane insulin suspension (NPH) allowing patients usually to be transferred directly to the latter on a unit-for-unit basis.
- Store unopened vial at 2°–8° C (36°–46° F). Avoid freezing and exposure to extremes in temperature or to direct sunlight.

ADVERSE EFFECTS (≥1%) See INSULIN INJECTION, REGULAR.

INTERACTIONS See INSULIN INJECTION.

PHARMACOKINETICS Onset: 1–2 h. **Peak:** 8–12 h. **Duration:** 18–24 h. **Metabolism:** In liver and kidney. **Elimination:** Less than 2% excreted unchanged in urine. **Half-Life:** Up to 13 h.

NURSING IMPLICATIONS

(see INSULIN INJECTION, REGULAR)

Patient & Family Education

- Be alert for S&S of hypoglycemia (see Appendix F); most apt to occur between mid-afternoon and dinner time (an early symptom may be a sense of extreme fatigue). Immediately take soluble carbohydrate (e.g., orange juice, honey). If the time between the midday and evening meal is prolonged, an afternoon snack may be needed.
- Do not overlook possibility of nocturnal hypoglycemia, especially during dose adjustment. Signs include restlessness or profuse sweating during sleep.

INTERFERON ALFA-2b

(in-ter-feer'on)

Intron A

Classifications: BIOLOGICAL RESPONSE MODIFIER; IMMUNOMODULATOR; INTERFERON; ANTINEOPLASTIC

Therapeutic: INTERFERON; ANTINEOPLASTIC; IMMUNOMODULATOR; ANTIVIRAL

Prototype: Peg-interferon alfa-2a

Pregnancy Category: C

AVAILABILITY 5 million international units, 10 million international units, 18 million international units, 25 million international units, 50 million international units vials

ACTION & *THERAPEUTIC EFFECT*
Interferon (IFN) alfa-2b, one of 4 types of alpha interferons, is a highly purified protein and natural product of human leukocytes within 4–6 h after viral stimulation. Produced by recombinant DNA technology (rIFN-A). **Antiviral action:** Reprograms virus-infected cells to inhibit various stages of virus replication. **Antitumor action:** Suppresses cell proliferation. **Immunomodulating action:** Enhances phagocytic activity of macrophages and augments specific cytotoxicity of lymphocytes for target cells. The immune system and the interferon system of defense are complementary. *Has a broad spectrum of antiviral, cytotoxic, and immunomodulating activity (i.e., favorably adjusts immune system to better combat foreign invasion of antigens, cancers, and viruses).*

USES Hairy cell leukemia in splenectomized and non-splenectomized patients 18 y or older, chronic hepatitis B or C, malignant melanoma, condylomata acuminata, AIDS-related Kaposi's sarcoma.

UNLABELED USES Multiple sclerosis, condylomata acuminata.

CONTRAINDICATIONS Hypersensitivity to interferon alfa-2b or to any components of the product; colitis; severe cytopenia; pancreatitis; suicidal ideation; neonates.

CAUTIOUS USE Severe, preexisting cardiac, renal, or hepatic disease; pulmonary disease (e.g., COPD); diabetes mellitus, patients prone to ketoacidosis; coagulation disorders; severe myelosuppression; recent MI; previous dysrhythmias; history of depression or suicidal tendencies; pregnancy (category C), lactation.

ROUTE & DOSAGE

Hairy Cell Leukemia

Adult: **IM/Subcutaneous** 2 million units/m² 3 times/wk

Kaposi's Sarcoma

Adult: **IM/Subcutaneous** 30 million units/m² 3 times/wk

Condylomata Acuminata

Adult: **IM/Subcutaneous** 1 million units/m² 3 times/wk

Chronic Hepatitis B or C

Adult: **Subcutaneous** 3 million units 3 times/wk x 18–24 mo

Malignant Melanoma

Adult: **IV** 20 million international units/m² daily for 5 days/wk x 4 wk; maintenance dose is 10 million international units/m² given subcutaneously weekly x 48 wk

Renal Impairment Dosage Adjustment

Not removed by dialysis

ADMINISTRATION

Subcutaneous/Intramuscular

- Reconstitution: The final concentration with the amount of required diluent is determined by the condition being treated (see manufacturer's directions). Inject diluent (bacteriostatic water for injection) into interferon alfa-2b vial; gently agitate solution before withdrawing dose with a sterile syringe.
- Make sure reconstituted solution is clear and colorless to light yellow and free of particulate material; discard if there are particles or solution is discolored.
- Store vials and reconstituted solutions at 2°–8° C (36°–46° F); remains stable for 1 mo. Discard any remaining drug in reconstituted vials.

Intravenous

***PREPARE:* IV Infusion:** Prepare **immediately** before use. Select the appropriate number of vials (i.e., 10, 18, or 50 million international units) of recombinant powder for injection and add to each the 1 mL of supplied diluent. Swirl gently to dissolve but do not shake. ▪ Further dilute by adding the required dose to 100 mL of NS. The final concentration should be less than 10 million international units/100 mL.

***ADMINISTER:* IV Infusion:** Infuse over 20 min.

***INCOMPATIBILITIES* Solution/additive: Dextrose**-containing solutions.

ADVERSE EFFECTS (≥1%) **Body as a Whole:** *Flu-like syndrome (fever, chills) associated with myalgia and arthralgia,* leg cramps. **CNS:** Depression, nervousness, anxiety, confusion, *dizziness, fatigue,* somnolence, insomnia, altered mental states, ataxia, tremor, paresthesias, *headache.* **CV:** Hypertension, dyspnea, *hot flushes.* **Special Senses:** Epistaxis, pharyngitis, sneezing; abnormal vision. **GI:** Taste alteration, *anorexia,* weight loss, *nausea,* vomiting, stomatitis, *diarrhea,* flatulence. **Hematologic:** Mild thrombocytopenia, transient granulocytopenia, anemia, *neutropenia,* leukemia. **Skin:** Mild pruritus, mild alopecia, rash, dry skin, herpetic eruptions, nonherpetic cold sores, urticaria.

INTERACTIONS Drug: May increase **theophylline** levels; additive myelosuppression with ANTINEOPLASTICS, **zidovudine** may increase hematologic toxicity, increase **doxorubicin** toxicity, increase neurotoxicity with **vinblastine.** Use with **ribavirin** increases risk of hemolytic anemia; do not use in combination with **ribavirin** if CrCl less than 50 mL/min.

PHARMACOKINETICS Peak: 6–8 h. **Metabolism:** In kidneys. **Half-Life:** 6–7 h.

NURSING IMPLICATIONS

(see INTERFERON ALFA-2A)

Assessment & Drug Effects

- Assess hydration status; patient should be well hydrated, especially during initial stage of treatment and if vomiting or diarrhea occurs.
- Lab tests: Closely monitor CBC with differential and platelet counts.
- Monitor for and promptly report any of the following: Chest pain, dyspnea, ecchymoses, petechiae, fever, severe abdominal pain, or psychic disturbances.
- Assess for flu-like symptoms, which may be relieved by acetaminophen (if prescribed).
- Monitor level of GI distress and ability to consume fluids and food.

- Monitor mental status and alertness; implement safety precautions if needed.

Patient & Family Education

- Learn techniques for reconstitution and administration of drug.
- Seek medical attention promptly for any of the following: Chest pain, shortness of breath, easy bruising, persistent fever, decrease or loss of vision, severe abdominal pain, depression or suicidal ideation.
- Note: If flu-like symptoms develop, take acetaminophen as advised by physician and take interferon at bedtime.
- Use caution with hazardous activities until response to drug is known.
- Learn about adverse effects and notify physician about those that cause significant discomfort.

INTERFERON ALFACON-1

(in-ter-fer′on al′fa-con)

Infergen

Classifications: BIOLOGICAL RESPONSE MODIFIER; IMMUNOMODULATOR; ANTIVIRAL; INTERFERON

Therapeutic: ANTIVIRAL; IMMUNOMODULATOR

Prototype: Peg-interferon alfa-2a

Pregnancy Category: C

AVAILABILITY 9 mcg, 15 mcg injection

ACTION & *THERAPEUTIC EFFECT* DNA recombinant Type 1 interferon. Its antiviral, antiproliferative, and natural killer (NK) cell activity is five times greater than interferon alpha-2b. *Effectiveness is measured by normalization of ALT level and serum HCV RNA less than 100 copies/mL. Type 1 interferons bind to the cell surface receptors inducing biological responses including antiviral, antiproliferative, and immunomodulatory activities.*

USES Treatment of chronic hepatitis C.

CONTRAINDICATIONS Hypersensitivity to alpha interferons or *E. coli* products; decompensated liver disease such as jaundice, ascites, etc.; suicidal tendencies or severe psychiatric disorder; lactation, children younger than 18 y.

CAUTIOUS USE History of severe psychiatric disorder, depression, or suicidal ideation; preexisting cardiac disease, elderly, myelosuppression, previous hypersensitivity to interferon therapy; history of endocrine disorders; ophthalmic disorders or autoimmune disorders; pregnancy (category C).

ROUTE & DOSAGE

Chronic Hepatitis C

Adult: **Subcutaneous** 9 mcg 3 times/wk × 24 wk

ADMINISTRATION

Subcutaneous

- Allow at least 24 h to elapse between doses of interferon alfacon-1.
- Give only one dose per vial or per prefilled syringe. Enter each vial only once. Discard unused portion of a vial or prefilled syringe immediately.
- Initiate treatment only if acceptable baseline lab values are obtained: Platelet count 75 × 10^9/L or greater, Hgb 100 g/L or greater, ANC 1500 × 10^6/L or greater, serum creatinine less than 2 mg/dL, serum albumin 25 g/L or greater, bilirubin WNL, TSH, and T_4 WNL.

- Store vials and syringes at 2°–8° C (36°–46° F). Avoid direct sunlight and vigorous shaking.

ADVERSE EFFECTS (≥1%) **Body as a Whole:** *Asthenia, headache, fatigue, fever, chills, injection site reaction (pain, edema, hemorrhage, inflammation), pain, myalgia, arthralgia,* increased sweating. **CNS:** *Insomnia, depression, dizziness, paresthesia, nervousness, depression, anxiety,* agitation. **CV:** Hypertension, palpitation. **GI:** *Nausea, diarrhea, abdominal pain, anorexia, vomiting, dyspepsia,* constipation, flatulence, toothache, hemorrhoids, weight loss, hepatotoxicity. **Hematologic:** *Granulocytopenia, thrombocytopenia, leukopenia,* ecchymosis, lymphadenopathy, lymphocytosis. **Respiratory:** *Cough, bronchitis, dyspnea, pneumonia, rhinitis,* pharyngitis. **Skin:** *Alopecia, rash,* dry skin, *pruritus,* erythema. **Urogenital:** Dysmenorrhea, vaginitis, menstrual disorder.

INTERACTIONS No clinically significant interactions established.

PHARMACOKINETICS Peak: 24–36 h.

NURSING IMPLICATIONS

Assessment & Drug Effects

- Monitor for and report any of the following S&S immediately: Depression, suicidal ideation, suicide attempt, or other indications of psychiatric disturbance.
- Withhold drug and notify physician if symptoms of hepatic decompensation such as jaundice or ascites develop. Withhold drug and notify physician if any other severe adverse reaction occurs.
- Lab tests: Baseline, 2 wk after initiation of therapy, and periodically thereafter: Platelet count, Hgb and Hct, WBC and ANC, serum creatinine, serum albumin, bilirubin, thyroid function, and triglyceride; periodic ALT to determine liver functions.

Patient & Family Education

- Report immediately any signs of psychiatric disturbance including depression, thoughts of suicide, nervousness, anxiety, agitation, apathy, or significant mood swings to physician.

INTERFERON BETA-1a

(in-ter-fer′on)

Avonex, Rebif

Classifications: BIOLOGICAL RESPONSE MODIFIER; IMMUNOMODULATOR; INTERFERON

Therapeutic: IMMUNOMODULATOR

Prototype: Peg-interferon alfa-2a

Pregnancy Category: C

AVAILABILITY Avonex: 33 mcg vial; 30 mcg/5 mL prefilled syringe; **Rebif:** 22 mcg, 44 mcg vial

ACTION & *THERAPEUTIC EFFECT* Interferon beta-1a is produced by recombinant DNA technology. Interferon beta-1a inhibits expression of pro-inflammatory cytokines including INF-G, thought to be a major factor in triggering the autoimmune reaction that leads to multiple sclerosis. It is believed that INF-G stimulates cytotoxic T-cells and causes degradation by macrophages' enzymes on the myelin sheath of neurons in the spinal cord. *Effective in improving time of onset of progression in disability; it was significantly longer in patients treated with interferon beta-1a.*

USES Relapsing-remitting multiple sclerosis.

CONTRAINDICATIONS Previous hypersensitivity to interferon beta or human albumin, albumin hypersensitivity, hamster protein hypersensitivity; lactation (using **Rebif**).
CAUTIOUS USE Suicidal tendencies, depression, preexisting psychiatric disorders; bone marrow depression; cardiac disease; seizure disorders; thyroid disease; hepatic impairment; pregnancy (category C), lactation (using **Avonex**). Safety and efficacy in children younger than 18 y are not established.

ROUTE & DOSAGE

Multiple Sclerosis
Adult: **IM Avonex** 30 mcg qwk
Subcutaneous Rebif 44 mcg 3 times/wk

ADMINISTRATION

Intramuscular

- **Avonex:** Reconstitute single use Avonex vial (33 mcg of lyophilized powder) with 1.1 mL of supplied diluent and swirl gently to dissolve.
- Withdraw 1 mL for administration.
- Discard any residual drug as the product contains no preservatives.
- Use within 6 h of reconstitution.

Subcutaneous

- **Rebif:** Give at the same time each day (preferably in the late afternoon or evening) on the same three days of the week at least 48 h apart each week.
- Dose is usually titrated up from 8.8 mcg to 44 mcg three times a week over a 4-wk period.
- Inject subcutaneously using either a 22 or 44 mcg prefilled syringe. Discard any residual drug as the product contains no preservatives.
- Store unreconstituted vials or prefilled syringes at 2°–8° C (36°–46° F).
- May store for up to 30 days at room temperature up to 25° C (77° F). Do not use beyond expiration date.

ADVERSE EFFECTS (≥1%) **Body as a Whole:** Alopecia, myalgias, *flu-like syndrome,* anaphylaxis. **CNS:** Headache, *fever,* fatigue, lethargy, depression, somnolence, weakness, agitation, malaise, confusion or reduced ability to concentrate, anxiety, dementia, emotional lability, depersonalization, suicide attempts, worsening of psychiatric disorders. **CV:** Tachycardia, CHF (rare). **GI:** Nausea, vomiting, *diarrhea, hepatic injury.* **Hematologic:** *Leukopenia, thrombocytopenia,* anemia, pancytopenia (rare), thrombocytopenia (rare). **Metabolic:** Hypocalcemia, elevated serum creatinine, elevated liver transaminases. **Skin:** Local skin necrosis at injection site, *pain at injection site.*

PHARMACOKINETICS Peak: Avonex 7.8–9.8 h; **Rebif** 16 h. **Metabolism:** Rapidly inactivated in body fluids and tissue. **Half-Life: Avonex** 8.6–10 h; **Rebif** 69 h.

NURSING IMPLICATIONS

Assessment & Drug Effects

- Withhold drug and notify physician if depression or suicidal ideation develops or if there is a worsening of psychiatric symptoms.
- Monitor patients with cardiac disease carefully for worsening cardiac function.
- Lab tests: Monitor periodically liver function tests, renal function tests, routine blood chemistry, and CBC with differential, and platelet count. Monitor thyroid function tests q6mo with preexisting thyroid dysfunction or when clinically indicated.

Patient & Family Education

- Take a missed dose as soon as possible but not within 48 h of next scheduled dose.
- Learn about common adverse effects, especially flu-like syndrome (headache, fatigue, fever, rigors, chest pain, back pain, myalgia).
- Withhold drug and notify physician of depression or suicidal ideation or exacerbation of a preexisting seizure disorder.
- Women who become pregnant should notify physician promptly.

I

INTERFERON BETA-1b

(in-ter-fer'on)

Betaseron, Extavia

Classifications: BIOLOGICAL RESPONSE MODIFIER; IMMUNOMODULATOR; INTERFERON; ANTINEOPLASTIC

Therapeutic: IMMUNOMODULATOR

Prototype: Peg-interferon alfa-2a

Pregnancy Category: C

AVAILABILITY 0.3 mg vial

ACTION & *THERAPEUTIC EFFECT*

Interferon beta-1b is a glycoprotein produced by recombinant DNA techniques using a strain of *E. coli. Both natural and recombinant DNA interferon beta-1b possess antiviral, antiproliferative, antitumor, and immunomodulatory activity. The effectiveness of interferon beta-1b for multiple sclerosis (MS) is based on the assumption that MS is an immunologically mediated illness.*

USES Relapsing and relapsing-remitting multiple sclerosis.

UNLABELED USES AIDS, AIDS-related Kaposi's sarcoma, metastatic renal cell carcinoma, malignant melanoma, cutaneous T-cell lymphoma, acute hepatitis C.

CONTRAINDICATIONS Previous hypersensitivity to interferon beta-1b or human albumin, mannitol hypersensitivity; history of depression of suicidal tendencies; lactation.

CAUTIOUS USE Suicidal/mental disorders especially chronic depression; seizures; cardiac disease; pregnancy (category C) but may cause a spontaneous abortion. Safety and efficacy in children younger than 18 y are not established.

ROUTE & DOSAGE

Multiple Sclerosis

Adult: **Subcutaneous** 0.25 mg (8 million international units) every other day

ADMINISTRATION

Subcutaneous

- Reconstitute by adding 1.2 mL of the supplied diluent (0.54% NaCl) to vial and gently swirl. Do NOT shake. The resultant solution contains 0.25 mg (8 million units)/mL.
- Discard reconstituted solution if it contains particulate matter or is discolored. Also discard unused solution.
- Rotate injection sites; use 27-gauge needle to administer drug.
- Store vials under refrigeration, 2°–8° C (36°–46° F) or at room temperature.

ADVERSE EFFECTS (≥1%) **CNS:** Headache, *fever,* fatigue, dizziness, lethargy, depression, somnolence, weakness, agitation, malaise, confusion or reduced ability to concentrate, anxiety, dementia, emotional lability, depersonalization, suicide attempts. **CV:** Tachycardia, peripheral edema, CHF (rare). **GI:** Nausea, vomiting, *diarrhea.* **Hematologic:** *Leukopenia, thrombocytopenia,* anemia. **Metabolic:** Hypocalcemia, elevated serum creatinine, elevated liver transaminases, autoimmune hepatitis, hepatic failure. **Skin:** Local skin necrosis at injection site, rash, *pain at injection site*. **Body as a Whole:** Alopecia, myalgias, *flu-like syndrome*.

INTERACTIONS Drug: Zidovudine (AZT) levels are increased, resulting in toxicity.

PHARMACOKINETICS Absorption: About 50% absorbed from subcutaneous sites. **Distribution:** Penetrates intact blood–brain barrier poorly; crosses placenta; distributed into breast milk. **Metabolism:** Rapidly inactivated in body fluids and tissue.

NURSING IMPLICATIONS

Assessment & Drug Effects

- Monitor vital signs, neurologic status, and neuropsychiatric status frequently during therapy.
- Lab tests: Monitor liver function at 1, 3, and 6 mo after initiation of therapy and as clinically warranted thereafter; monitor renal function, complete blood counts, and serum electrolytes periodically.
- Assess for and promptly treat flu-like symptom complex (fever, chills, myalgia, etc.).
- Assess injection sites; pain and redness are common reactions. Report tissue ulceration promptly.

Patient & Family Education

- Learn and understand potential adverse drug reactions.
- Learn proper technique for solution preparation and injection.
- Self-medicate with acetaminophen (if not contraindicated) if flu-like symptom complex develops.
- Avoid prolonged exposure to sunlight.
- Use caution when performing hazardous activities until response to drug is known.

INTERFERON GAMMA-1b

(in-ter-feer'on)

Actimmune

Classifications: BIOLOGICAL RESPONSE MODIFIER; IMMUNOMODULATOR; INTERFERON; ANTINEOPLASTIC

Therapeutic: IMMUNOMODULATOR; ANTINEOPLASTIC

Prototype: Peg-interferon alfa-2a

Pregnancy Category: C

AVAILABILITY 100 mcg (2 million IU)/0.5 mL vial

ACTION & *THERAPEUTIC EFFECT* **Immunomodulatory:** Interferon gamma is produced by T-cells and natural killer (NK) cells after activation with immune or inflammatory stimuli. Interferon gamma stimulates macrophages to increase IL-12 and TNF-alpha production, which enhances interferon gamma synthesis. Interleukin-10 downregulates interferon gamma production by NK and T-cells by preventing macrophage secretion of IL-12 and TNF-alpha. **Antineoplastic:** It also exerts antitumor effects by increasing expression of tumor suppressor genes and activating macrophages to lyse tumor cells. **Antiviral:** Has potent phagocyte-activating effects that include stimulating macrophages and generation of toxic oxygen metabolites (i.e., free radicals) capable of destroying virally infected cells. *Is a naturally occurring cytokine with antiviral, immunomodulatory, and antiproliferative activity. It enhances phagocyte function in chronic granulomatous disease and improves killing of viruses; also enhances osteoclast function in malignant osteopetrosis.*

USES Chronic granulomatous disease, severe malignant osteopetrosis.

UNLABELED USES Idiopathic pulmonary fibrosis, refractory mycobacterium infection, ovarian cancer.

CONTRAINDICATIONS Hypersensitivity to interferon gamma or products derived from *E. coli;* suicidal ideation; pre-existing severe psychiatric disorder or the development of one; lactation.

CAUTIOUS USE Preexisting cardiac disease, CHF, cardiac arrhythmias; seizure disorders and compromised CNS function; elderly; myelosuppression; pregnancy (category C). Safety and efficacy in infants younger than 1 y are not established.

I

ROUTE & DOSAGE

Chronic Granulomatous Disease, Osteopetrosis

Adult/Child: **Subcutaneous** BSA 0.5 m^2 or greater, 50 mcg/m^2 3 times weekly

Adult/Child: **Subcutaneous** BSA 0.5 m^2 or less, 1.5 mcg/kg 3 times weekly

Idiopathic Pulmonary Fibrosis

Adult: **Subcutaneous** 180–200 mcg 3 times weekly

ADMINISTRATION

- Note: Pretreatment (4 h before) with acetaminophen is recommended to reduce headache, myalgia, and fever. Treatment should be continued 24 h postinjection.

Subcutaneous

- Do not shake vial. Inject subcutaneously undiluted into right or left deltoid area or anterior thigh area.
- Avoid intradermal or IV injection. Rotate injection sites.
- Store 2°–8° C (36°–46° F); do not freeze. Discard any unused portions or any vial left at room temperature for more than 12 h.

ADVERSE EFFECTS (≥1%) **Body as a Whole:** *Fever, fatigue, chills,* myalgia, arthralgia, night sweats. **CNS:** *Headache,* altered mental status, ataxia, confusion, dizziness, Parkinsonian symptoms, disorientation, seizures, hallucinations. **CV:** Heart block, heart failure, DVT, hypotension, MI, syncope, tachyarrhythmia. **GI:** *Nausea, vomiting, diarrhea.* **Hematologic:** *Leukopenia, thrombocytopenia.* **Respiratory:** Bronchospasm, interstitial pneumonitis, pulmonary embolism, tachypnea. **Skin:** Local skin necrosis at injection site, *pain at injection site, rash.* **Urogenital:** Reversible renal insufficiency.

INTERACTIONS Drug: Use cautiously with **aminophylline, fosphenytoin, phenytoin, theophylline, warfarin.**

PHARMACOKINETICS Absorption: 90% absorbed from subcutaneous site. **Peak:** 7 h. **Half-Life:** 5.9 h.

NURSING IMPLICATIONS

Assessment & Drug Effects

- Monitor CV status frequently. Report promptly severe hypotension and/or syncope.
- Monitor for and report S&S of infection.
- Lab tests: Baseline and at 3 mo CBC with differential and platelet counts; complete blood chemistry (including renal and liver function tests), and urinalysis.

Patient & Family Education

- Report promptly: Skin rash, itching, unusual weakness or tiredness, chest pain or palpitations, or signs of an infection.
- Do not accept vaccination with a live vaccine during or for 3 mo following the end of therapy.

IODOQUINOL

(eye-oh-do-kwin'ole)
Yodoxin
Classification: AMEBICIDE
Therapeutic: AMEBICIDE
Prototype: Emetine
Pregnancy Category: C

AVAILABILITY 210 mg, 650 mg tablets

ACTION & *THERAPEUTIC EFFECT*
Direct-acting (contact) amebicide. *Effective against both trophozoites and cyst forms of* Entamoeba histolytica *in intestinal lumen. Not useful for extraintestinal amebiasis.*

USES Intestinal amebiasis and for asymptomatic passers of cysts. Commonly used either concurrently or in alternating courses with another intestinal amebicide.

UNLABELED USES Balantidiasis and *Acrodermatitis enteropathica;* traveler's diarrhea; shampoo preparation (Sebaquin) used for control of seborrheic dermatitis of scalp.

CONTRAINDICATIONS Hypersensitivity to any 8-hydroxyquinoline or to iodine-containing preparations or foods; hepatic or renal damage; lactation.

CAUTIOUS USE Severe thyroid disease; minor self-limiting problems; prolonged high-dosage therapy; preexisting optic neuropathy; pregnancy (category C).

ROUTE & DOSAGE

Intestinal Amebiasis

Adult: **PO** 650 mg t.i.d. for 20 days (max: 2 g/day); may repeat after a 2–3 wk drug-free interval
Child: **PO** 30–40 mg/kg/day in 2–3 divided doses for 20 days (max: 1.95 g/day); may repeat after a 2–3 wk drug-free interval

ADMINISTRATION

Oral

- Give drug after meals. If patient has difficulty swallowing tablet, crush and mix with applesauce.

ADVERSE EFFECTS (≥1%) **Body as a Whole:** Hypersensitivity (urticaria, pruritus). **CNS:** Headache, agitation, retrograde amnesia, vertigo, ataxia, peripheral neuropathy (especially in children); muscle pain, weakness usually below T12 vertebrae, dysesthesias especially of lower limbs, paresthesias, increased sense of warmth. **Special Senses:** Blurred vision, optic atrophy, optic neuritis, permanent loss of vision. **GI:** Nausea, vomiting, anorexia, abdominal cramps, diarrhea, constipation, rectal irritation and itching. **Skin:** Discoloration of hair and nails, acne, hair loss, urticaria, various forms of skin eruptions. **Hematologic:** Agranulocytosis (rare). **Endocrine:** Thyroid hypertrophy, iodism [generalized furunculosis (iodine toxiderma), skin eruptions, fever, chills, weakness].

DIAGNOSTIC TEST INTERFERENCE
Iodoquinol can cause elevations of ***PBI*** and decrease of ***I-131 uptake*** (effects may last for several weeks to 6 mo even after discontinuation of therapy). ***Ferric chloride test for PKU*** (phenylketonuria) may yield false-positive results if iodoquinol is present in urine.

PHARMACOKINETICS Absorption: Small amount from GI tract. **Elimination:** In feces.

NURSING IMPLICATIONS

Assessment & Drug Effects

- Monitor I&O ratio. Record characteristics of stools: Color, consistency, frequency, presence of blood, mucus, or other material.

- Note: Ophthalmologic examinations are recommended at regular intervals during prolonged therapy.
- Monitor and report immediately the onset of blurred or decreased vision or eye pain. Also report symptoms of peripheral neuropathy: Pain, numbness, tingling, or weakness of extremities.

Patient & Family Education

- Report any of the following: Skin rash, blurred vision, fever or other signs of infection.
- Complete full course of treatment. Stool needs be examined again 1, 3, and 6 mo after termination of treatment.
- Note: Intestinal amebiasis is spread mainly by contaminated water, raw fruits or vegetables, flies, roaches, and hand-to-mouth transfer of infected feces. It is very important to wash hands after defecation and before eating.

IPECAC SYRUP

(ip′e-kak)

Ipecac Syrup

Classifications: ANTIDOTE; EMETIC

Therapeutic: EMETIC

Pregnancy Category: C

AVAILABILITY 15 mL, 30 mL doses

ACTION & *THERAPEUTIC EFFECT* Derived from dried roots of *Cephaelis ipecacuanha.* Contains cephaeline (produces emesis) and emetine, a toxic alkaloid that is excreted slowly from the body. Emetine can cause potentially fatal cumulative toxicity with repeated use. It appears to inhibit protein synthesis and energy production in muscle tissue with resultant skeletal and cardiac muscle toxicity. *Acts locally on gastric mucosa and centrally on chemoreceptor trigger zone (CTZ) in the medulla to induce vomiting.*

USES Emergency emetic to remove unabsorbed ingested poisons.

CONTRAINDICATIONS Comatose, semicomatose, inebriated, deeply sedated patients; patients in shock; patients with depressed gag reflex; seizures, active or impending; treatment of ingested strong alkali, acids, or other corrosives, strychnine, petroleum distillates, volatile oils, or rapid-acting CNS depressants; infants younger than 6 mo

CAUTIOUS USE Impaired cardiac function; elderly; arteriosclerosis; cerebovascular disease; head trauma; pregnancy (category C), lactation.

ROUTE & DOSAGE

Emergency Emesis

Adult: **PO** 30 mL followed by 1–2 240 mL (8 oz) glasses of water, may repeat once in 20 min if necessary

Child: **PO** *Older than 1 y,* 15 mL followed by 1–2 240 mL (8 oz) glasses of water, may repeat once in 20 min if necessary; *younger than 1 y,* 5–10 mL followed by 120–240 mL (4–8 oz) of water, may repeat once in 20 min if necessary

ADMINISTRATION

Oral

- Do not confuse with ipecac fluid extract, which is 14 times stronger and has caused deaths when mistakenly given at the same dosage as ipecac syrup.
- Do not induce vomiting if victim is unconscious, semiconscious, or convulsing.
- Store in tight containers at temperature not exceeding 25° C (77° F).

ADVERSE EFFECTS (≥1%) **Body as a Whole:** Achy, stiff muscles, severe myopathy, convulsions, coma. **CV:** Cardiomyopathy, cardiotoxicity, cardiac arrhythmias, atrial fibrillation, tachycardia, chest pain, dyspnea, hypotension, fatal myocarditis. **GI:** Diarrhea, mild GI upset. If drug is not vomited but absorbed or if ipecac overdosage: *persistent vomiting,* gastroenteritis, bloody diarrhea, sensory disturbances, stomach cramps, tremor.

PHARMACOKINETICS Onset: 15–30 min. **Duration:** 25 min. **Elimination:** Metabolite can be detected in urine up to 60 days after excessive doses.

NURSING IMPLICATIONS

Assessment & Drug Effects

- Note: Emetic effect occurs in 15–30 min and continues for 20–25 min. If vomiting does not occur in 20–30 min, repeat dose once.
- Contact physician immediately if vomiting does not occur within 15–20 min after a second dose. Dosage should be recovered by gastric lavage and activated charcoal if necessary.
- Note: Ipecac syrup can be cardiotoxic if not vomited and allowed to be absorbed.
- Report immediately to physician if vomiting persists longer than 2–3 h after ipecac syrup is given.

Patient & Family Education

- Call an emergency room, poison control center, or physician before using ipecac syrup.

IPRATROPIUM BROMIDE

(i-pra-troe'pee-um)

Atrovent, Atrovent HFA

Classifications: ANTICHOLINERGIC; ANTIMUSCARINIC; BRONCHODILATOR

Therapeutic: BRONCHODILATOR

Prototype: Atropine

Pregnancy Category: B

AVAILABILITY 0.02% solution for inhalation; 18 mcg inhaler; 0.03%, 0.06% nasal spray

ACTION & *THERAPEUTIC EFFECT* Results in bronchodilation by inhibiting acetylcholine at its receptor sites, thereby blocking cholinergic bronchomotor tone (bronchoconstriction); also abolishes vagally mediated reflex bronchospasm triggered by such nonspecific agents as cigarette smoke, inert dusts, cold air, and a range of inflammatory mediators (e.g., histamine). *Produces local, site-specific effects on the larger central airways including bronchodilation and prevention of bronchospasms.*

USES Maintenance therapy in COPD including chronic bronchitis and emphysema; nasal spray for perennial rhinitis and symptomatic relief of rhinorrhea associated with the common cold.

UNLABELED USES Perennial nonallergic rhinitis.

CONTRAINDICATIONS Use as primary treatment for acute episodes; hypersensitivity to atropine, bromides, peanut oils, soy lecithin. Safe use in children 3 y or younger (inhalation) or 5 y or younger (intranasal) is not established.

CAUTIOUS USE Narrow-angle glaucoma; prostatic hypertrophy, bladder neck obstruction; pregnancy (category B).

ROUTE & DOSAGE

COPD

Adult: **Inhalation** 2 inhalations of MDI q.i.d. at no less than 4 h intervals (max: 12 inhalations in 24 h)

Nebulizer 500 mcg (1 unit dose vial) q6–8h
Child (3–12 y): **Inhalation** 1–2 inhalations t.i.d. (max: 6/day)
Nebulizer 125–250 mcg t.i.d.

Rhinitis

Adult (5 y or older): **Intranasal** 2 sprays of 0.03% each nostril b.i.d. or t.i.d.

Common Cold

Adult: **Intranasal** 2 sprays of 0.06% each nostril t.i.d. or q.i.d. up to 4 days

I

ADMINISTRATION

Intranasal/Inhalation/Nebulizer

- Demonstrate aerosol use and check return demonstration.
- Wait 3 min between inhalations if more than one inhalation per dose is ordered.
- Avoid contact with eyes.

ADVERSE EFFECTS (≥1%) **Special Senses:** Blurred vision (especially if sprayed into eye), difficulty in accommodation, acute eye pain, worsening of narrow-angle glaucoma. **GI:** Bitter taste, dry oropharyngeal membranes. With higher doses: Nausea, constipation. **Respiratory:** *Cough,* hoarseness, exacerbation of symptoms, drying of bronchial secretions, mucosal ulcers, epistaxis, nasal dryness. **Skin:** Rash, hives. **Urogenital:** Urinary retention. **CNS:** Headache.

PHARMACOKINETICS Absorption: 10% of inhaled dose reaches lower airway; approximately 0.5% of dose is systemically absorbed. **Peak:** 1.5–2 h. **Duration:** 4–6 h. **Elimination:** 48% of dose excreted in feces; less than 5% excreted in urine. **Half-Life:** 1.5–2 h.

NURSING IMPLICATIONS

Assessment & Drug Effects

- Monitor respiratory status; auscultate lungs before and after inhalation.
- Report treatment failure (exacerbation of respiratory symptoms) to physician.

Patient & Family Education

- Note: This medication is not an emergency agent because of its delayed onset and the time required to reach peak bronchodilation.
- Review patient information sheet on proper use of nasal spray.
- Allow 30–60 sec between puffs for optimum results. Do not let medication contact your eyes.
- Wait 5 min between this and other inhaled medications. Check with physician about sequence of administration.
- Take medication only as directed, noting some leniency in number of puffs within 24 h. Supervise child's administration until certain all of dose is being administered.
- Rinse mouth after medication puffs to reduce bitter taste.
- Discuss changes in normal urinary pattern with the physician (more common in older adults).
- Call physician if you note changes in sputum color or amount, ankle edema, or significant weight gain.

IRBESARTAN

(ir-be-sar'tan)

Avapro

Classifications: ANGIOTENSIN II RECEPTOR ANTAGONIST; ANTIHYPERTENSIVE
Therapeutic: ANTIHYPERTENSIVE
Prototype: Losartan

Pregnancy Category: C first trimester; D second and third trimester

AVAILABILITY 75 mg, 150 mg, 300 mg tablets

ACTION & *THERAPEUTIC EFFECT* Irbesartan is an angiotensin II receptor (type AT_1) antagonist. Irbesartan selectively blocks the binding of angiotensin II to the AT_1 receptors found in many tissues (e.g., vascular smooth muscle, adrenal glands), resulting in vasodilation of vascular smooth muscle. *This results in blocking the vasoconstricting and aldosterone-secreting effects of angiotensin II, thus resulting in an antihypertensive effect.*

USES Hypertension, treatment of diabetic nephropathy in patients with hypertension and type 2 diabetes.

UNLABELED USES CHF.

CONTRAINDICATIONS Hypersensitivity to irbesartan, losartan, or valsartan; hypovolemia; pregnancy (category D second and third trimester), lactation, children.

CAUTIOUS USE Patients on diuretics, arterial stenosis of the renal artery, hepatic disease; severe CHF, African American patients; pregnancy (category C first trimester).

ROUTE & DOSAGE

Hypertension

Adult: **PO** Start with 150 mg once daily, may increase to 300 mg/day

ADMINISTRATION

Oral

- Correct volume depletion prior to initiation of therapy to prevent hypotension. Titrate daily dose up to 300 mg; larger doses, however, are not likely to provide additional benefit.

ADVERSE EFFECTS (≥1%) **Body as a Whole:** Edema, fatigue, pain. **CNS:** Dizziness, headache, anxiety, nervousness. **CV:** Tachycardia, chest pain. **GI:** Diarrhea, dyspepsia, nausea, vomiting, abdominal pain. **Respiratory:** Upper respiratory infection, cough, sinus disorder, pharyngitis, rhinitis. **Skin:** Rash. **Other:** UTI, hepatitis.

PHARMACOKINETICS Absorption: Rapidly absorbed from GI tract, 60–80% bioavailability. **Distribution:** 90% protein bound. **Metabolism:** In the liver primarily by CYP2C9. **Elimination:** Primarily in feces. **Half-Life:** 11–15 h.

NURSING IMPLICATIONS

Assessment & Drug Effects

- Monitor for therapeutic effectiveness: Maximum pressure lowering effect may not be evident for 6–12 wk; indicated by decreases in systolic and diastolic BP.
- Monitor BP periodically; trough readings, just prior to the next scheduled dose, should be made when possible.
- Lab tests: Monitor periodically BUN and creatinine, serum potassium, and CBC with differential.

Patient & Family Education

- Inform physician immediately if you become pregnant.
- Notify physician of episodes of dizziness, especially when making position changes.

IRINOTECAN HYDROCHLORIDE

(eye-ri-no′te-can)

Camptosar

Classifications: ANTINEOPLASTIC; CAMPTOTHECIN ANALOG

Therapeutic: ANTINEOPLASTIC
Prototype: Topotecan
Pregnancy Category: D

AVAILABILITY 20 mg/mL injection

ACTION & *THERAPEUTIC EFFECT* Irinotecan is a camptothecin analog that displays antitumor activity by inhibiting the intranuclear enzyme topoisomerase I (DNA gyrase). By inhibiting topoisomerase I, irinotecan and its active metabolite SN-38 cause double-stranded DNA damage during the synthesis (S) phase of DNA synthesis. *Irinotecan inhibits both DNA and RNA synthesis.*

USES Metastatic carcinoma of colon or rectum.

CONTRAINDICATIONS Previous hypersensitivity to irinotecan, topotecan, or other camptothecin analogs; acute infection, diarrhea, pregnancy (category D), lactation. Safety and effectiveness in children are not established.

CAUTIOUS USE Gastrointestinal disorders, myelosuppression, renal or hepatic function impairment, history of bleeding disorders, previous cytotoxic or radiation therapy.

ROUTE & DOSAGE

Metastatic Carcinoma

Adult: **IV** 125 mg/m² once weekly for 4 wk, then a 2-wk rest period (future courses may be adjusted to range from 50 to 150 mg/m² depending on tolerance; see complete prescribing information for specific dosage adjustment recommendations based on toxic effects)

Pharmacogenetic Dosage Adjustment

Patients with UGT1A1*28 allele have increased risk of side effects, start with decreased dose

ADMINISTRATION

Intravenous

Administer only after premedication (at least 30 min prior) with an antiemetic.

- Wash immediately with soap and water if skin contacts drug during preparation.

PREPARE: **IV Infusion:** Dilute the ordered dose in enough D5W (preferred) or NS to yield a concentration of 0.12–2.8 mg/mL. ▪ Typical amount of diluent used is 250–500 mL.

ADMINISTER: **IV Infusion:** Infuse over 90 min. ▪ Closely monitor IV site; if extravasation occurs, immediately flush with sterile water and apply ice.

INCOMPATIBILITIES **Y-site:** **Gemcitabine.**

- Store undiluted at 15°–30° C (59°–86° F) and protect from light. Use reconstituted solutions within 24 h.

ADVERSE EFFECTS (≥1%) **Body as a Whole:** *Asthenia, fever, pain,* chills, edema, abdominal enlargement, back pain. **CNS:** Headache, *insomnia, dizziness.* **CV:** Vasodilation/flushing. **GI:** *Diarrhea (early and late onset), dehydration, nausea, vomiting, anorexia, weight loss, constipation, abdominal cramping and pain,* flatulence, stomatitis, dyspepsia, increased alkaline phosphatase and AST. **Hematologic:** *<u>Leukopenia, neutropenia</u>, anemia.* **Respiratory:** *Dyspnea,* cough, rhinitis. **Skin:** *Alopecia,* sweating, rash.

INTERACTIONS Drug: ANTICOAGULANTS, ANTIPLATELET AGENTS, NSAIDS may increase risk of bleeding; **carbamazepine, phenytoin, phenobarbital** may decrease irinotecan levels. **Herbal: St. John's wort** may decrease irinotecan levels.

PHARMACOKINETICS Peak: 1 h. **Distribution:** Irinotecan is 30% protein bound; active metabolite SN-38 is 95% protein bound. **Metabolism:** In liver by carboxylesterase enzyme to active metabolite SN-38. **Elimination:** 10 h for SN-38; 20% excreted in urine. **Half-Life:** 10–20 h.

NURSING IMPLICATIONS

Assessment & Drug Effects

- Lab tests: Monitor WBC with differential, Hgb, and platelet count before each dose; monitor closely coagulation parameters especially with concurrent use of other drugs which affect these parameters.
- Lab tests: Monitor fluid and electrolyte balance closely during and after periods of diarrhea. Monitor liver and renal function tests and blood glucose periodically.
- Monitor for acute GI distress, especially early diarrhea (within 24 h of infusion), which may be preceded by diaphoresis and cramping, and late diarrhea (more than 24 h after infusion).

Patient & Family Education

- Learn about common adverse effects and measures to control or minimize when possible.
- Notify physician immediately when you experience diarrhea, vomiting, and S&S of infection. Diarrhea requires prompt treatment to prevent serious fluid and electrolyte imbalances.

IRON DEXTRAN

(i'ern dek'stran)

DexFerrum, INFeD, Proferdex

Classifications: BLOOD FORMER; IRON SUPPLEMENT; ANTIANEMIC

Therapeutic: ANTIANEMIC; IRON SUPPLEMENT

Prototype: Ferrous sulfate

Pregnancy Category: C

AVAILABILITY 50 mg elemental iron/mL

ACTION & *THERAPEUTIC EFFECT* A dark brown, slightly viscous liquid complex of ferric hydroxide with dextran in 0.9% NaCl solution for injection. Reticuloendothelial cells of liver, spleen, and bone marrow dissociate iron from iron dextran complex. The released ferric ion combines with transferrin and is transported to bone marrow, where it is incorporated into hemoglobin. *Effective in replacement of iron needed in iron deficiency anemia, thus replenishing hemoglobin and depleted iron stores.*

USES Only in patients with clearly established iron deficiency anemia when oral administration of iron is unsatisfactory or impossible.

CONTRAINDICATIONS Hypersensitivity to the product; all anemias except iron-deficiency anemia; acute phase of infectious renal disease; infants weighing less than 5 kg, and neonates.

CAUTIOUS USE Rheumatoid arthritis, ankylosing spondylitis; renal disease; SLE; impaired hepatic function; cardiac disease; history of allergies or asthma; pregnancy (category C), lactation.

ROUTE & DOSAGE

Iron Deficiency

Adult: **IM/IV** Dose is individualized and determined based on patient's weight and hemoglobin (see package insert); do not administer more than 100 mg (2 mL) of iron dextran within 24 h
Child: **IM/IV** *Weight less than 5 kg,* no more than 0.5 mL (25 mg)/day; *weight 5–10 kg,* no more than 1 mL (50 mg)/day; *weight greater than 10 kg,* no more than 2 mL (100 mg)/day

ADMINISTRATION

Note: The multiple-dose vial is used ONLY for IM injections. It is not suitable for IV use because it contains a preservative (phenol).

Test Dose

- Give a test dose of 0.5 mL over a 5 min period before the first IM or IV therapeutic dose to observe patient's response to the drug. Have epinephrine (0.5 mL of a 1:1000 solution) immediately available for hypersensitivity emergency.
- Note: Although anaphylactic reactions (see Appendix F) usually occur within a few minutes after injection, it is recommended that 1 h or more elapse before remainder of initial dose is given following test dose.

Intramuscular

- Use the multiple-dose vial ONLY for IM injections. It is not suitable for IV use because it contains a preservative (phenol).
- Give injection only into the muscle mass in upper outer quadrant of buttock (never in the upper arm). In small child, use the lateral thigh. Use a 2- or 3-inch, 19- or 20-gauge needle. The Z-track technique is recommended. Use one needle to withdraw drug from container and another needle for injection.
- Note: If patient is receiving IM in standing position, patient should be bearing weight on the leg opposite the injection site; if in bed, patient should be in the lateral position with injection site uppermost.

Intravenous

Ensure that ONLY the vial for IV use is selected.

PREPARE: **Direct:** Give undiluted. **IV Infusion:** Dilute in 250–1000 mL of NS.

ADMINISTER: **Direct:** *Test Dose:* A test dose is given before the first IV therapeutic dose. ▪ *DexFerrum:* Give test dose of 25 mg (0.5 mL) slowly over 5 min. ▪ *INFeD:* Give test dose over 30 sec. Wait 1–2 h and if no adverse reaction occurs, give the remainder of the first dose by IV infusion.

IV Infusion: Infuse at a rate not to exceed 50 mg (1 mL) or fraction thereof over 60 sec. Avoid rapid infusion.

INCOMPATIBILITIES **Solution/additive: TPN.**

- After infusion is completed, flush vein with 10 mL of NS.
- Have patient remain in bed for at least 30 min after IV administration to prevent orthostatic hypotension. Monitor BP and pulse.

- Store below 30° C (86° F) unless otherwise directed.

ADVERSE EFFECTS (≥1%) **Body as a Whole:** Hypersensitivity (urticaria, skin rash, allergic purpura, pruritus, fever, chills, dyspnea, arthralgia, myalgia; anaphylaxis). **CNS:** Headache, shivering, transient paresthesias, syncope, dizziness, coma, seizures. **CV:** *Peripheral vas-*

cular flushing (rapid IV), hypotension, precordial pain or pressure sensation, tachycardia, fatal cardiac arrhythmias, circulatory collapse. **GI:** Nausea, vomiting, transient loss of taste perception, metallic taste, diarrhea, melena, abdominal pain, hemorrhagic gastritis, intestinal necrosis, hepatic damage. **Skin:** Sterile abscess and brown skin discoloration (IM site), local phlebitis (IV site), lymphadenopathy, *pain at IM injection site.* **Metabolic:** Hemosiderosis, metabolic acidosis, hyperglycemia, reactivation of quiescent rheumatoid arthritis, exogenous hemosiderosis. **Hematologic:** Bleeding disorder with severe toxicity.

DIAGNOSTIC TEST INTERFERENCE Falsely elevated ***serum bilirubin*** and falsely decreased ***serum calcium*** values may occur. Large doses of iron dextran may impart a brown color to serum drawn 4 h after iron administration. ***Bone scans*** involving Tc-99m diphosphonate have shown dense areas of activity along contour of iliac crest 1–6 days after IM injections of iron dextran.

INTERACTIONS May decrease absorption of oral **iron, chloramphenicol** may decrease effectiveness of iron, a toxic complex may form with **dimercaprol.**

PHARMACOKINETICS Absorption: 60% from IM site by 3 days; 90% absorbed by 1–3 wk. **Distribution:** Crosses placenta; distributed into breast milk. **Metabolism:** In reticuloendothelial system. **Half-Life:** 6 h.

NURSING IMPLICATIONS

Assessment & Drug Effects

- Monitor for therapeutic effectiveness: Anticipated response to parenteral iron therapy is an average weekly hemoglobin rise of about 1 g/day. Peak levels are generally reached in about 4–8 wk.
- Note: Systemic reactions may occur over 24 h after parenteral iron has been administered. Large IV doses are associated with increased frequency of adverse effects.
- Lab tests: Periodic determinations of Hgb and Hct, and reticulocyte count should be made.

Patient & Family Education

- Do not take oral iron preparations when receiving iron injections.
- Eat foods high in iron and vitamin C.
- Notify physician of any of the following: Backache or muscle ache, chills, dizziness, fever, headache, nausea or vomiting, paresthesias, pain or redness at injection site, skin rash or hives, or difficulty breathing.

IRON SUCROSE INJECTION

(i′ron su′crose)

Venofer

Classifications: BLOOD FORMER; IRON REPLACEMENT; ANTIANEMIC

Therapeutic: ANTIANEMIC; IRON DEFICIENCY REPLACEMENT

Prototype: Ferrous sulfate

Pregnancy Category: B

AVAILABILITY 20 mg elemental iron/mL

ACTION & *THERAPEUTIC EFFECT* A complex of polynuclear iron (III) hydroxide in sucrose. It is dissociated by the reticuloendothelial system (RES) into iron and sucrose. Normal erythropoiesis depends on the concentration of iron and erythropoietin available in the plasma; both are decreased in renal failure. Exogenous administration of erythropoietin increases red blood cell production and iron utilization, contributing to iron deficiency in hemodialized patients. *Increases serum iron level in chronic renal failure patients, and results in increased hemoglobin level.*

USES Treatment of iron deficiency anemia in patients with chronic renal failure (with or without concurrent administration of erythropoietin).

CONTRAINDICATIONS Patients with iron overload, hypersensitivity to Venofer, or for anemia not caused by iron deficiency; hemochromatosis.

CAUTIOUS USE Patients with a history of hypotension; older adults, decreased renal, hepatic, or cardiac function; pregnancy (category B), lactation. Safety and effectiveness in infants or children are not established.

ROUTE & DOSAGE

Iron Deficiency Anemia

Adult: **IV Hemodialysis dependent (HDD-CKD):** 100 mg given at least 15 min per hemodialysis session (cumulative dose: 1000 mg). **Non-hemodialysis dependent (NDD-CKD):** 200 mg on 5 different occasions within the 14-day period. **Peritoneal dialysis dependent (PDD-CKD):** 300 mg on days 1 and 15, then 400 mg 14 days later

ADMINISTRATION

Intravenous

PREPARE: **Direct/Infusion: HDD-CKD:** Give direct IV undiluted or diluted immediately prior to infusion in a maxiumum of 100 mL NS. ▪ **NDD-CKD:** Give direct IV undiluted. ▪ **PDD-CKD:** Dilute 300–400 mg in a maxiumum of 250 mL of NS for infusion.

ADMINISTER: **Direct:** Give the undiluted solution slowly by direct IV over 2–5 min. **IV Infusion:** Infusion diluted solution for **HDD-CKD patient** over at least 15 min and for **PDD-CKD patient** over 90 min. ▪ Avoid rapid infusion.

INCOMPATIBILITIES **Solution/additive:** Do not mix with other medications or parenteral nutrition solutions.

▪ Store unopened vials preferably at 25° C (77° F), but room temperature permitted. Discard unused portion in opened vial.

ADVERSE EFFECTS (≥1%) **Body as a Whole:** Fever, pain, asthenia, malaise, <u>anaphylactoid reactions</u>. **Cardiovascular:** *Hypotension,* chest pain, hypertension, hypervolemia. **Digestive:** Nausea, vomiting, diarrhea, abdominal pain, elevated liver function tests. **Musculoskeletal:** *Leg cramps,* muscle pain. **CNS:** Headache, dizziness. **Respiratory:** Dyspnea, pneumonia, cough. **Skin:** Pruritus, injection site reaction.

INTERACTIONS Drug: May reduce absorption of ORAL IRON PREPARATIONS.

PHARMACOKINETICS Peak: 4 wk. **Distribution:** Primarily to blood with some distribution to liver, spleen, bone marrow. **Metabolism:** Dissociated to iron and sucrose in reticuloendothelial system. **Elimination:** Sucrose is eliminated in urine, 5% of iron excreted in urine. **Half-Life:** 6 h.

NURSING IMPLICATIONS

Assessment & Drug Effects

- Withhold drug and notify physician when serum ferritin level equals or exceeds established guidelines.
- Stop infusion and notify physician for S&S overdosage or infusing too

rapidly: Hypotension, edema; headache, dizziness, nausea, vomiting, abdominal pain, joint or muscle pain, and paresthesia.

- Lab tests: Periodic serum ferritin, transferrin saturation, Hct, and Hgb.
- Monitor patient carefully during the first 30 min after initiation of IV therapy for signs of hypersensitivity and anaphylactoid reaction (see Appendix F).

Patient & Family Education

- Report any of the following promptly: Itching, rash, chest pain, headache, dizziness, nausea, vomiting, abdominal pain, joint or muscle pain, and numbness and tingling.

ISOCARBOXAZID

(eye-soe-kar-box′a-zid)

Marplan

Classifications: ANTIDEPRESSANT; MONOAMINE OXIDASE INHIBITOR (MAOI)

Therapeutic: ANTIDEPRESSANT

Prototype: Phenelzine

Pregnancy Category: C

AVAILABILITY 10 mg tablets

ACTION & *THERAPEUTIC EFFECT* Inhibits monoamine oxidase, the enzyme involved in the catabolism of catecholamine neurotransmitters and serotonin. *Effectiveness as an antidepressant is due to its inhibition of MAO.*

USES Symptomatic treatment of depressed patients refractory to or intolerant of TCAs or electroconvulsive therapy.

CONTRAINDICATIONS Hypersensitivity to MAO inhibitors; pheochromocytoma; children (younger than 16 y); older adults (over 60 y) or debilitated patients; cardiac arrhythmias, hypertension, CVA; severe renal or hepatic impairment; history of headache; increased intracranial pressure, surgery; stroke, head trauma; suicidal ideation; lactation.

CAUTIOUS USE Hyperthyroidism, parkinsonism, epilepsy, schizophrenia; bipolar disorder; psychosis; suicidal risks; dental work; pregnancy (category C).

ROUTE & DOSAGE

Refractory Depression

Adult: **PO** 10–30 mg/day in 1–3 divided doses (max: 30 mg/day)

ADMINISTRATION

Oral

- Note: Dosage is individualized on the basis of patient response. Lowest effective dosage should be used.
- Store in a tight, light-resistant container.

ADVERSE EFFECTS (≥1%) **CNS:** Dizziness, light-headedness, tiredness, weakness, *drowsiness,* vertigo, headache, *overactivity,* hyperreflexia, muscle twitching, tremors, mania hypomania, *insomnia,* confusion, memory impairment. **CV:** *Orthostatic hypotension,* <u>paradoxical hypertension</u>, palpitation, tachycardia, other arrhythmias. **Special Senses:** *Blurred vision,* nystagmus, glaucoma. **GI:** Increased appetite, weight gain, *nausea,* diarrhea, *constipation, anorexia,* black tongue, *dry mouth,* abdominal pain. **Urogenital:** Dysuria, *urinary retention,* incontinence, sexual disturbances. **Body as a Whole:** Peripheral edema, excessive sweating, chills, skin rash, hepatitis, jaundice.

INTERACTIONS Drug: TRICYCLIC ANTIDEPRESSANTS, **fluoxetine,** AMPHETAMINES, **ephedrine, reserpine,**

guanethidine, buspirone, methyldopa, dopamine, levodopa, tryptophan may precipitate hypertensive crisis, headache, or hyperexcitability; **alcohol** and other CNS DEPRESSANTS compound CNS depressant effects; **meperidine** can cause fatal cardiovascular collapse; ANESTHETICS exaggerate hypotensive and CNS depressant effects; **metrizamide** increases risk of seizures; compounds hypotensive effects of DIURETICS and other ANTIHYPERTENSIVE AGENTS. **Food:** All **tyramine**-containing foods (aged cheeses, processed cheeses, sour cream, wine, champagne, beer, pickled herring, anchovies, caviar, shrimp, liver, dry sausage, figs, raisins, overripe bananas or avocados, chocolate, soy sauce, bean curd, yeast extracts, yogurt, papaya products, meat tenderizers, broad beans) may precipitate hypertensive crisis. **Herbal: Ginseng, ephedra, ma huang, St. John's wort** may precipitate hypertensive crisis.

PHARMACOKINETICS Duration: Up to 2 wk. **Metabolism:** In liver.

NURSING IMPLICATIONS

Assessment & Drug Effects

- Monitor for and report promptly signs of clinical deterioration or suicidal ideation. Children and adolescents are at particular risk.
- Monitor for therapeutic effectiveness: May be apparent within 1 wk or less, but in some patients there may be a time lag of 3–4 wk before improvement occurs.
- Monitor BP. Monitor for orthostatic hypotension by evaluating BP with patient recumbent and standing.
- Check for peripheral edema daily and monitor weight several times weekly.
- Note: Toxic symptoms from overdosage or from ingestion of contraindicated substances (e.g., foods high in tyramine) may occur within hours.
- Monitor I&O and bowel elimination patterns.

Patient & Family Education

- Monitor closely behavior of children and adolescents; report immediately unusual changes in behavior or suicidal ideation.
- Make position changes slowly and in stages; lie down or sit down if faintness occurs.
- Use caution when performing potentially hazardous activities.
- Consult physician before self-medicating with OTC agents (e.g., cough, cold, hay fever, or diet medications).
- Avoid alcohol and excessive caffeine-containing beverages and tryptophan and tyramine-containing foods including cheeses, yeast, meat extracts, smoked or pickled meat, poultry, or fish, fermented sausages, and overripe fruit.

ISOMETHEPTENE/ DICHLORALPHENAZONE/ ACETAMINOPHEN

(i-so-meth′ep-tene/di-chlor-al-phen′a-zone/a-cet′a-min-o-phen)

Isopap, Duradrin, Midrin, Migratine

Classifications: SYMPATHOMIMETIC; ANALGESIC, NON-NARCOTIC
Therapeutic: ANTIMIGRAINE; NON-NARCOTIC ANALGESIC
Pregnancy Category: C
Controlled Substance: Schedule C-IV

AVAILABILITY 65 mg; **isometheptene mucate,** 100 mg; **dichloralphenazone,** 325 mg; **APAP** capsules

ACTION & *THERAPEUTIC EFFECT* Isometheptene is a sympathomimetic amine that acts by constricting cranial and cerebral arterioles. Isometheptene relieves vascular headaches. Dichloralphenazone is a mild sedative that helps reduce headache pain. Acetaminophen is a mild analgesic. *Effective as a mild sedative, reduces headache pain as well as being a mild analgesic.*

USES Relief for tension, vascular, and migraine headaches.

CONTRAINDICATIONS Patients with glaucoma; severe renal disease, organic heart disease; hepatic disease; concurrent MAO inhibitors.

CAUTIOUS USE Hypertension; peripheral vascular disease, and recent cardiovascular attacks; older adults; pulmonary disease; pregnancy (category C), lactation.

ROUTE & DOSAGE

Tension Headache

Adult: **PO** 1–2 capsules q4h up to 8 capsules/24 h

Migraine Headache

Adult: **PO** 2 capsules at onset, then 1 capsule qh until relief (max: 5 capsules/12 h)

ADMINISTRATION

Oral

- Do not give this drug to anyone who is concurrently using an MAOI. Allow 14 days to elapse between discontinuation of the MAOI and administration of this drug.
- Do not give more than 8 capsules in a 24 h period.
- Store at 15°–30° C (59°–86° F) in a dry place.

ADVERSE EFFECTS (≥1%) **CNS:** Transient dizziness. **GI:** Acetaminophen hepatotoxicity. **Skin:** Rash.

INTERACTIONS Drug: MAOIS may cause hypertensive crisis; other **acetaminophen**-containing drugs (including OTC) may increase risk of hepatotoxicity.

PHARMACOKINETICS Absorption: Rapidly absorbed. **Metabolism:** Dichloralphenazone is metabolized to chloral hydrate and antipyrine. See ACETAMINOPHEN and CHLORAL HYDRATE for more detail. **Elimination:** Renal and hepatic. **Half-Life:** 12 h.

NURSING IMPLICATIONS

Assessment & Drug Effects

- Monitor BP closely with preexisting hypertension.
- Monitor lower extremity perfusion with a history of PVD.

Patient & Family Education

- Avoid, or moderate, alcohol use while taking this drug.
- Do not drive or engage in other potentially hazardous activities until response to drug is known.
- Report any decrease in tolerance to walking if you have a history of PVD.

ISONIAZID (ISONICOTINIC ACID HYDRAZIDE) Pr

(eye-soe-nye'a-zid)

INH, Isotamine ♣, Laniazid, Nydrazid, PMS Isoniazid ♣

Classifications: ANTI-INFECTIVE; ANTITUBERCULOSIS

Therapeutic: ANTITUBERCULOSIS

Pregnancy Category: C

AVAILABILITY 50 mg, 100 mg, 300 mg tablets; 50 mg/5 mL syrup; 100 mg/mL injection

ACTION & *THERAPEUTIC EFFECT* Hydrazide of isonicotinic acid with highly specific action against *Myco-*

bacterium tuberculosis. Postulated to act by interfering with biosynthesis of bacterial proteins, nucleic acid, and lipids. *Exerts bacteriostatic action against actively growing tubercle bacilli; may be bactericidal in higher concentrations.*

USES Treatment of all forms of active tuberculosis caused by susceptible organisms and as preventive in high-risk persons (e.g., household members, persons with positive tuberculin skin test reactions). May be used alone or with other tuberculostatic agents.

UNLABELED USES Treatment of atypical mycobacterial infections; tuberculous meningitis; action tremor in multiple sclerosis.

CONTRAINDICATIONS History of isoniazid-associated hypersensitivity reactions, including hepatic injury; acute liver damage of any etiology; lactation.

CAUTIOUS USE Chronic liver disease; HIV infection; hepatitis; severe renal dysfunction; history of convulsive disorders; chronic alcoholism; persons older than 50 y; pregnancy (category C).

ROUTE & DOSAGE

Treatment of Active Tuberculosis

Adult: **PO/IM** 5 mg/kg (max: 300 mg/day)
Child: **PO/IM** 10–20 mg/kg (max: 300–500 mg/day)

Preventive Therapy

Adult: **PO** 300 mg/day
Child: **PO** 10 mg/kg up to 300 mg/day or 15 mg/kg 3 times/wk

ADMINISTRATION

Oral

- Give on an empty stomach at least 1 h before or 2 h after meals. If GI irritation occurs, drug may be taken with meals.

Intramuscular

- Note: Isoniazid solution for IM injection tends to crystallize at low temperatures; if this occurs, solution should be allowed to warm to room temperature to redissolve crystals before use.
- Give deep into a large muscle and rotate injection sites; local transient pain may follow IM injections.
- Store in tightly closed, light-resistant containers.

ADVERSE EFFECTS (≥1%) **Body as a Whole:** Drug-related fever, rheumatic and lupus erythematosus-like syndromes, irritation at injection site; hypersensitivity (fever, chills, skin eruption, vasculitis). **CNS:** *Paresthesias, peripheral neuropathy,* headache, unusual tiredness or weakness, tinnitus, dizziness, hallucinations. **Special Senses:** Blurred vision, visual disturbances, optic neuritis, atrophy. **GI:** Nausea, vomiting, epigastric distress, dry mouth, constipation; hepatotoxicity (*elevated AST, ALT;* bilirubinemia, jaundice, <u>hepatitis</u>). **Hematologic:** <u>Agranulocytosis</u>, hemolytic or <u>aplastic anemia</u>, thrombocytopenia, eosinophilia, methemoglobinemia. **Metabolic:** Decreased vitamin B_{12} absorption, pyridoxine (vitamin B_6) deficiency, pellagra, gynecomastia, hyperglycemia, glycosuria, hyperkalemia, hypophosphatemia, hypocalcemia, acetonuria, metabolic acidosis, proteinuria. **Other:** Dyspnea, urinary retention (males).

DIAGNOSTIC TEST INTERFERENCE Isoniazid may produce false-positive results using ***copper sulfate tests*** (e.g., ***Benedict's solution, Clinitest***) but not with **glucose oxidase methods** (e.g., ***Clinistix, Dextrostix, TesTape***).

INTERACTIONS Drug: Cycloserine, ethionamide enhance CNS toxicity; may increase **phenytoin** levels, resulting in toxicity; ALUMINUM-CONTAINING ANTACIDS decrease GI absorption; **disulfiram** may cause coordination difficulties or psychotic reactions; **alcohol** increases risk of hepatotoxicity. **Food:** Food decreases rate and extent of isoniazid absorption; should be taken 1 h before meals.

PHARMACOKINETICS Absorption: Readily from GI tract; food may reduce rate and extent of absorption. **Peak:** 1–2 h. **Distribution:** Distributed to all body tissues and fluids including the CNS; crosses placenta. **Metabolism:** Inactivated by acetylation in liver. **Elimination:** 75–96% in urine in 24 h; excreted in breast milk. **Half-Life:** 1–4 h.

NURSING IMPLICATIONS

Assessment & Drug Effects

- Monitor for therapeutic effectiveness: Evident within the first 2–3 wk of therapy. Over 90% of patients receiving optimal therapy have negative sputum by the sixth month.
- Withhold drug and notify physician immediately of a hypersensitivity reaction; generally occurs within 3–7 wk after initiation of therapy.
- Perform appropriate susceptibility tests before initiation of therapy and periodically thereafter to detect possible bacterial resistance.
- Lab tests: Monitor hepatic function periodically. Isoniazid hepatitis (sometimes fatal) usually develops during the first 3–6 mo of treatment, but may occur at any time during therapy; much more frequent in patients 35 y or older, especially in those who ingest alcohol daily.
- Monitor for and report promptly signs of hepatic toxicity (see Appendix F).
- Monitor for and report promptly signs of peripheral neuritis (e.g., paresthesias of feet and hands with numbness, tingling, burning).
- Monitor BP during period of dosage adjustment. Some experience orthostatic hypotension; therefore, caution against rapid positional changes.
- Monitor diabetics for loss of glycemic control.
- Check weight at least twice weekly under standard conditions.

Patient & Family Education

- Report promptly any of the following signs of liver toxicity: Unexplained weakness, nausea/vomiting, loss of appetite, dark urine, jaundice, clay-colored stools.
- Avoid or at least reduce alcohol intake while on isoniazid therapy because of increased risk of hepatotoxicity.

ISOPROTERENOL HYDROCHLORIDE (Pr)

(eye-soe-proe-ter′e-nole)

Isuprel

Classifications: BETA-ADRENERGIC AGONIST; BRONCHODILATOR; CARDIAC STIMULATOR

Therapeutic: BRONCHODILATOR; ANTIARRHYTHMIC; CARDIAC STIMULATOR

Pregnancy Category: C

AVAILABILITY 0.2 mg/mL, 0.02 mg/mL injection

ACTION & *THERAPEUTIC EFFECT* Synthetic sympathomimetic amine that acts directly on $beta_1$- and $beta_2$-adrenergic receptors that relaxes bronchospasm, and, by increasing ciliary motion, facilitates expectoration of pulmonary secretions. Induces stimulation of $beta_1$-adrenergic receptors and results in increased cardiac output and cardiac workload by increasing strength of contraction through positive inotropic and chronotropic effects on the heart. It also shortens AV conduction time and its refractory period in patients with heart block. *Reverses bronchospasm and facilitates removal of bronchial secretion. Increases cardiac output and cardiac workload. Also has antiarrhythmic properties by affecting AV node conduction.*

USES Reversible bronchospasm induced by anesthesia. As cardiac stimulant in cardiac arrest, carotid sinus hypersensitivity, cardiogenic and bacteremic shock, Adams-Stokes syndrome, or ventricular arrhythmias. Used in treatment of shock that persists after replacement of blood volume.

UNLABELED USES Treatment of status asthmaticus in children.

CONTRAINDICATIONS Preexisting cardiac arrhythmias associated with tachycardia; tachycardia caused by digitalis intoxication, central hyperexcitability, cardiogenic shock secondary to coronary artery occlusion and MI; ventricular fibrillation.

CAUTIOUS USE Sensitivity to sympathomimetic amines; older adult and debilitated patients, hypertension, coronary insufficiency and other cardiovascular disorders, angina; renal dysfunction, hyperthyroidism, diabetes, prostatic hypertrophy, glaucoma, tuberculosis; pregnancy (category C), lactation.

ROUTE & DOSAGE

Bronchospasm

Adult: **IV** 0.01–0.02 mg prn

Cardiac Arrhythmias/Cardiac Resuscitation

Adult: **IV** 0.02–0.06 mg bolus, followed by 5 mcg/min infusion
Child: **IV** 0.1 mcg/kg/min by continuous infusion

Shock/Hypoperfusion

Adult: **IV** 0.5–5 mcg/min

ADMINISTRATION

Intravenous

Note: Maximum concentration on IV solution for both adults and children: 20 mcg/mL (0.02 mg/mL)

PREPARE: **Direct IV Injection for Adult with AV Block/Arrhythmia/Bradycardia/Cardiac Arrest:** Dilute 1 mL (0.2) of 1:5000 solution with 9 mL NS or D5W to produce a 1:50,000 (0.02 mg/mL) solution or use 1:50,000 solution undiluted. **Continuous Infusion for Adult with AV Block/Arrhythmia/Bradycardia/Cardiac Arrest:** Dilute 10 mL (2 mg) of 1:5000 solution in 500 mL D5W to produce a 1:250,000 (4 mcg/mL) solution. **IV Infusion for Adult with Shock Hypoperfusion:** Dilute 5 mL (1 mg) of 1:5000 solution in 500 mL D5W to produce a 1:500,000 (2 mcg/mL) solution. **Direct IV Injection for Adult with Bronchospasm:** Dilute 1 mL (0.2 mg) of 1:5000 solution with 9 mL NS or D5W to produce a 1:50,000 solution undiluted. **Continuous Infusion for Child with AV Block/Bradycardia:** Dilute to a range of 4–12 mcg/mL in 100 mL of D5W or NS.

ADMINISTER: **Direct IV for Adult/Child:** Give at a rate of 0.2 mg or fraction thereof over 1 min. ▪ Flush with 15–20 mL NS. **Continuous IV Infusion for Adult/Child:** Rate is adjusted according to patient response. Infusion rate is generally decreased or infusion may be temporarily discontinued if heart rate exceeds 110 bpm, because of the danger of precipitating arrhythmias. ▪ Microdrip or constant-infusion pump is recommended to prevent sudden influx of large amounts of drug. ▪ IV administration is regulated by continuous ECG monitoring. ▪ Patient **must be** observed and response to therapy **must be** monitored continuously.

INCOMPATIBILITIES **Solution/additive: Sodium bicarbonate, aminophylline, carbenicillin, diazepam, furosemide.**

▪ Isoproterenol solutions lose potency with standing. ▪ Discard if precipitate or discoloration is present.

ADVERSE EFFECTS (≥1%) **CNS:** Headache, mild tremors, nervousness, anxiety, insomnia, excitement, fatigue. **CV:** Flushing, palpitations, tachycardia, unstable BP, anginal pain, <u>ventricular arrhythmias</u>. **GI:** Swelling of parotids (prolonged use), bad taste, buccal ulcerations (sublingual administration), nausea. **Other:** Severe prolonged asthma attack, sweating, bronchial irritation and edema. **Acute Poisoning:** Overdosage, especially after excessive use of aerosols (*tachycardia,* palpitations, nervousness, nausea, vomiting).

INTERACTIONS Drug: Epinephrine and other SYMPATHOMIMETIC AMINES, TRICYCLIC ANTIDEPRESSANTS increase effects and cause cardiac toxicity. HALOGENATED GENERAL ANESTHETICS exacerbate arrhythmias; while BETA-BLOCKERS antagonize effects.

PHARMACOKINETICS Absorption: Rapidly from parenteral administration. **Onset:** Immediate. **Metabolism:** Metabolized by COMT in liver, lungs, and other tissues. **Elimination:** 40–50% unchanged in urine.

NURSING IMPLICATIONS

Assessment & Drug Effects

- Check pulse before and during IV administration. Rate greater than 110 usually indicates need to slow infusion rate or discontinue infusion. Consult physician for guidelines.
- Incidence of arrhythmias is high, particularly when drug is administered IV to patients with cardiogenic shock or ischemic heart disease, digitalized patients, or to those with electrolyte imbalance.
- Note: Tolerance to bronchodilating effect and cardiac stimulant effect may develop with prolonged use.
- Note: Once tolerance has developed, continued use can result in serious adverse effects including rebound bronchospasm.

ISOSORBIDE DINITRATE

(eye-soe-sor′bide)

Coronex ♣, Dilatrate-SR, Iso-Bid, Isordil, Novosorbide ♣

Classification: NITRATE VASODILATOR

Therapeutic: VASODILATOR; ANTIANGINAL

Prototype: Nitroglycerin

Pregnancy Category: C

AVAILABILITY 2.5 mg, 5 mg, 10 mg sublingual tablets; 5 mg, 10 mg chewable tablets; 5 mg, 10 mg, 20 mg, 30 mg, 40 mg tablets; 40 mg sustained release tablets, capsules

ACTION & *THERAPEUTIC EFFECT* Relaxes vascular smooth muscle with resulting vasodilation. Dilation of peripheral blood vessels tends to cause peripheral pooling of blood, decreased venous return to heart, and decreased left ventricular end-diastolic pressure, with consequent reduction in myocardial oxygen consumption. *Has an antianginal effect as a result of vasodilation of the coronary arteries.*

USES Relief of acute anginal attacks and for management of long-term angina pectoris.

UNLABELED USES Alone or in combination with a cardiac glycoside or with other vasodilators (e.g., hydralazine, prazosin, for refractory CHF; diffuse esophageal spasm without gastroesophageal reflux and heart failure).

CONTRAINDICATIONS Hypersensitivity to nitrates or nitrites; severe anemia; hyperthyroidism; head trauma; increased intracranial pressure; recent MI; GI disease; children.

CAUTIOUS USE Glaucoma, hypotension, hypovolemia; hyperthyroidism; hepatic disease; elderly; pregnancy (category C), lacation. **Extended release form:** GI disease such as hypermotility or malabsorption syndrome.

ROUTE & DOSAGE

Angina Prophylaxis

Adult: **PO** Regular tablets 2.5–30 mg q.i.d. a.c. and at bedtime; Sublingual tablet 2.5–10 mg q4–6h; Chewable tablet 5–30 mg chewed q2–3h; Sustained release tablets 40 mg q6–12h

Acute Anginal Attack

Adult: **PO** Sublingual tablet 2.5–10 mg q2–3h prn; Chewable tablet 5–30 mg chewed prn for relief

ADMINISTRATION

Oral

- Do not confuse with isosorbide, an oral osmotic diuretic.
- Give regular oral forms on an empty stomach (1 h a.c. or 2 h p.c.). If patient complains of vascular headache, however, it may be taken with meals.
- Advise patient not to eat, drink, talk, or smoke while sublingual tablet is under tongue.
- Instruct patient to place sublingual tablet under tongue at first sign of an anginal attack. If pain is not relieved, repeat dose at 5–10 min intervals to a maximum of 3 doses. If pain continues, notify physician or go to nearest hospital emergency room.
- Chewable tablet **must be** thoroughly chewed before swallowing.
- Do not crush sustained release form. It **must be** swallowed whole.
- Have patient sit when taking rapid-acting forms of isosorbide dinitrate (sublingual and chewable tablets) because of the possibility of faintness.
- Store in tightly closed container in a cool, dry place. Do not expose to extremes of temperature.

ADVERSE EFFECTS (≥1%) **Body as a Whole:** Hypersensitivity reaction, paradoxical increase in anginal pain, methemoglobinemia (overdose). **CNS:** Headache, dizziness, weakness, *lightheadedness,* restlessness. **CV:** Palpitation, postural hypotension, tachycardia. **GI:** Nausea, vomiting. **Skin:** *Flushing,* pallor, perspiration, rash, exfoliative dermatitis.

INTERACTIONS Drug: Alcohol may enhance hypotensive effects and lead to cardiovascular collapse; ANTIHYPERTENSIVE AGENTS, PHENOTHIAZINES add to hypotensive effects.

PHARMACOKINETICS Absorption: Significant first pass metabolism with PO absorption, with 10–90% reaching systemic circulation. **Onset:** 2–5 min SL; within 1 h regular tabs; within 3 min chewable tabs; 30 min sustained release tabs. **Duration:** 1–2 h SL; 4–6 h regular tabs; 0.5–2 h chewable tabs; 6–8 h sustained release tabs. **Metabolism:** In liver. **Elimination:** 80–100% in urine within 24 h.

NURSING IMPLICATIONS

Assessment & Drug Effects

- Monitor effectiveness of drug in relieving angina.
- Note: Headaches tend to decrease in intensity and frequency with continued therapy but may require administration of analgesic and reduction in dosage.
- Note: Chronic administration of large doses may produce tolerance and thus decrease effectiveness of nitrate preparations.

Patient & Family Education

- Make position changes slowly, particularly from recumbent to upright posture, and dangle feet and ankles before walking.
- Lie down at the first indication of lightheadedness or faintness.
- Keep a record of anginal attacks and the number of sublingual tablets required to provide relief.
- Do not drink alcohol because it may increase possibility of lightheadedness and faintness.

ISOSORBIDE MONONITRATE

(eye-soe-sor'bide)

Ismo, Imdur, Monoket

Classification: NITRATE VASODILATOR

Therapeutic: ANTIANGINAL

Prototype: Nitroglycerin

Pregnancy Category: C

AVAILABILITY 10 mg, 20 mg tablets; 30 mg, 60 mg, 120 mg sustained release tablets

ACTION & *THERAPEUTIC EFFECT* Isosorbide mononitrate is a long-acting metabolite of the coronary vasodilator isosorbide dinitrate. It decreases preload as measured by pulmonary capillary wedge pressure (PCWP), and left ventricular end volume and diastolic pressure (LVEDV), with a consequent reduction in myocardial oxygen consumption. *It is equally or more effective than isosorbide dinitrate in the treatment of chronic, stable angina. It is a potent vasodilator with antianginal and antiischemic effects.*

USES Prevention of angina. Not indicated for acute attacks.

CONTRAINDICATIONS Hypersensitivity to nitrates; severe anemia; closed-angle glaucoma; recent MI; postural hypotension, head trauma, cerebral hemorrhage (increases intracranial pressure).

CAUTIOUS USE Older adults, hypotension; pregnancy (category C), lactation. **Extend form** should not be used in patients with GI disease (e.g. GI motility, malabsorption syndrome).

ROUTE & DOSAGE

Prevention of Angina

Adult: **PO** Regular release (ISMO, Monoket) 20 mg b.i.d. 7 h apart; Sustained release (Imdur) 30–60 mg every morning, may increase up to 120 mg once daily after several days if needed (max dose: 240 mg)

ADMINISTRATION

Oral

- Give first dose in morning on arising and second dose 7 h later with twice daily dosing regimen. Give in morning on arising with once daily dosing.

- Store sustained release tablets in a tight container.

ADVERSE EFFECTS (≥1%) **CNS:** Headache, agitation, anxiety, confusion, loss of coordination, hypoesthesia, hypokinesia, insomnia or somnolence, nervousness, migraine headache, paresthesia, vertigo, ptosis, tremor. **CV:** Aggravation of angina, abnormal heart sounds, murmurs, MI, transient hypotension, palpitations. **Hematologic:** Hypochromic anemia, purpura, thrombocytopenia, methemoglobinemia (high doses). **GI:** Nausea, vomiting, dry mouth, abdominal pain, constipation, diarrhea, dyspepsia, flatulence, tenesmus, gastric ulcer, hemorrhoids, gastritis, glossitis. **Metabolic:** Hyperuricemia, hypokalemia. **GU:** Renal calculus, UTI, atrophic vaginitis, dysuria, polyuria, urinary frequency, decreased libido, impotence. **Respiratory:** Bronchitis, pneumonia, upper respiratory tract infection, nasal congestion, bronchospasm, coughing, dyspnea, rales, rhinitis. **Skin:** Rash, pruritus, hot flashes, acne, abnormal texture. **Special Senses:** Diplopia, blurred vision, photophobia, conjunctivitis.

INTERACTIONS Drug: Alcohol may cause severe hypotension and cardiovascular collapse. **Aspirin** may increase nitrate serum levels. CALCIUM CHANNEL BLOCKERS may cause orthostatic hypotension.

PHARMACOKINETICS Absorption: Completely and rapidly absorbed from GI tract; 93% reaches systemic circulation. **Onset:** 1 h. **Peak:** Regular release 30–60 min; sustained release 3–4 h. **Duration:** Regular release 5–12 h; sustained release 12 h. **Metabolism:** In liver by denitration and conjugation to inactive metabolites. **Elimination:** Primarily by kidneys. **Half-Life:** 4–5 h.

NURSING IMPLICATIONS

Assessment & Drug Effects

- Monitor cardiac status, frequency and severity of angina, and BP.
- Assess for and report possible S&S of toxicity, including orthostatic hypotension, syncope, dizziness, palpitations, lightheadedness, severe headache, blurred vision, and difficulty breathing.
- Lab tests: Monitor serum electrolytes periodically.

Patient & Family Education

- Do not crush or chew sustained release tablets. May break tablets in two and take with adequate fluid (4–8 oz).
- Do not withdraw drug abruptly; doing so may precipitate acute angina.
- Maintain correct dosing interval with twice daily dosing.
- Note: Geriatric patients are more susceptible to the possibility of developing postural hypotension.
- Avoid alcohol ingestion and aspirin unless specifically permitted by physician.

ISOTRETINOIN (13-*cis*-RETINOIC ACID) Pr

(eye-soe-tret′i-noyn)

Amnesteem, Claravis, Sotret

Classification: ANTIACNE (RETINOID)

Therapeutic: ANTIACNE; ANTINEOPLASTIC

Pregnancy Category: X

AVAILABILITY 10 mg, 20 mg, 40 mg capsules

ACTION & *THERAPEUTIC EFFECT* Highly toxic metabolite of retinol (vitamin A). Principal actions: Regulation of cell (e.g., epithelial) differentiation and proliferation and of altered lipid composition on skin surface. Decreases sebum secretion by reducing sebaceous gland size; inhibits gland cell differentiation; blocks follicular keratinization. *Has antiacne properties and may be used as a chemotherapeutic agent for epithelial carcinomas.*

USES Treatment of severe recalcitrant cystic or conglobate acne in patient unresponsive to conventional treatment, including systemic antibiotics.

UNLABELED USES Lamellar ichthyosis, oral leukoplakia, hyperkeratosis, acne rosacea, scarring gram-negative folliculitis; adjuvant therapy of basal cell carcinoma of lung and cutaneous T-cell lymphoma (mycosis fungoides); psoriasis; chemoprevention for prostate cancer.

CONTRAINDICATIONS Tinnitus; hypersensitivity to parabens (preservatives in the formulation), retinoid hypersensitivity, leukopenia, neutropenia; UV exposure; pregnancy (category X), females of childbearing age, lactation.

CAUTIOUS USE Coronary artery disease; major depression, psychosis, history of suicides, alcoholism; hepatitis, hepatic disease; visual disturbance; rheumatologic disorders, osteoporosis; history of pancreatitis, inflammatory bowel disease; diabetes mellitus; obesity; retinal disease; elevated triglycerides, hyperlipidemia.

ROUTE & DOSAGE

Cystic Acne

Adult: **PO** 0.5–1 mg/kg/day in 2 divided doses (max recommended dose: 2 mg/kg/day) for 15–20 wk

Disorders of Keratinization

Adult: **PO** Up to 4 mg/kg/day in divided doses

ADMINISTRATION

Oral

- Give with or shortly after meals.
- Note: A single course of therapy provides adequate control in many patients. If a second course is necessary, it is delayed at least 8 wk because improvement may continue without the drug.
- Store in tight, light-resistant container. Capsules remain stable for 2 y.

ADVERSE EFFECTS (≥1%) **Body as a Whole:** Most are dose-related (i.e., occurring at doses greater than 1 mg/kg/day), reversible with termination of therapy. **CNS:** Lethargy, headache, fatigue, visual disturbances, pseudotumor cerebri, paresthesias, dizziness, depression, psychosis, <u>suicide</u> (rare). **Special Senses:** Reduced night vision, dry eyes, papilledema, eye irritation, *conjunctivitis,* corneal opacities. **GI:** *Dry mouth,* anorexia, nausea, vomiting, abdominal pain, nonspecific GI symptoms, <u>acute hepatotoxic reactions</u> (rare), inflammation and bleeding of gums, increased AST, ALT, acute pancreatitis. **Hematologic:** Decreased Hct, Hgb, elevated sedimentation rate. **Musculoskeletal:** Arthralgia; bone, joint, and muscle pain and stiffness; chest pain, skeletal hyperostosis (especially in athletic people and with prolonged therapy), mild bruising, decreased bone mineral density. **Skin:** *Cheilitis,* skin fragility, dry skin, pruritus, peeling of face, palms, and soles; photosensitivity (photoallergic and phototoxic), erythema, skin infections, petechiae, rash, urticaria, exaggerated healing response (painful exuberant granulation tissue with crusting), brittle nails, alopecia **Respiratory:** Epistaxis, *dry nose.* **Metabolic:** Hyperuricemia, *increased serum concentrations of triglycerides by 50–70%,* serum cholesterol by 15–20%, VLDL cholesterol by 50–60%, LDL cholesterol by 15–20%.

INTERACTIONS Drug: VITAMIN A SUPPLEMENTS increase toxicity; decreases effectiveness of ESTROGEN hormonal contraceptives in oral form as well as topical/injectable/implantable/insertable ESTROGEN hormonal birth control. Use with systemic CORTICOSTEROIDS or **phenytoin** may increase bone loss.

PHARMACOKINETICS Absorption: Rapid absorption after slow dissolution in GI tract; 25% of administered drug reaches systemic circulation. **Peak:** 3.2 h. **Distribution:** Not fully understood; appears in liver, ureters, adrenals, ovaries, and lacrimal glands. **Metabolism:** In liver; enterohepatically cycled. **Elimination:** In urine and feces in equal amounts. **Half-Life:** 10–20 h.

NURSING IMPLICATIONS

Assessment & Drug Effects

- Lab tests: Determine baseline blood lipids at outset of treatment, then at 2 wk, 1 mo, and every month thereafter throughout course of therapy; liver function tests at 2- or 3-wk intervals for 6 mo and once a month thereafter during treatment.
- Report signs of liver dysfunction (jaundice, pruritus, dark urine) promptly.
- Monitor closely for loss of glycemic control in diabetic and diabetic-prone patients.
- Monitor for development of depression and suicidal ideation.
- Note: Persistence of hypertriglyceridemia (levels above 500–800 mg/dL) despite a reduced dose indicates necessity to stop drug to prevent onset of acute pancreatitis.

Patient & Family Education

- Maintain drug regimen even if during the first few weeks transient exacerbations of acne occur. Recurring symptoms may signify response of deep unseen lesions.
- Discontinue medication at once and notify physician if visual disturbances occur along with nausea, vomiting, and headache.
- Rule out pregnancy within 2 wk of starting treatment. Use a reliable contraceptive 1 mo before, throughout, and 1 mo after therapy is discontinued.
- Do not self-medicate with multivitamins, which usually contain vitamin A. Toxicity of isotretinoin is enhanced by vitamin A supplements.
- Avoid or minimize exposure of the treated skin to sun or sunlamps. Photosensitivity (photoallergic and phototoxic) potential is high.
- Notify physician immediately of abdominal pain, rectal bleeding, or severe diarrhea, which are possible symptoms of drug-induced inflammatory bowel disease.
- Keep lips moist and softened (use thin layer of lubricant such as petroleum jelly); dry mouth and cheilitis (inflamed, chapped lips), frequent adverse effects of isotretinoin.
- Notify physician of joint pain, such as pain in the great toe (symptom of gout and hyperuricemia).

ISOXSUPRINE HYDROCHLORIDE

(eye-sox′syoo-preen)

Tri Soxuprine

Classifications: BETA-ADRENERGIC AGONIST; ALPHA-ADRENERGIC RECEPTOR INHIBITOR; VASODILATOR
Therapeutic: VASODILATOR
Prototype: Isoprotenerol
Pregnancy Category: C

AVAILABILITY 10 mg, 20 mg tablets

ACTION & *THERAPEUTIC EFFECT* Sympathomimetic with beta-adrenergic stimulant activity and with an inhibitory effect on alpha receptors. Vasodilating action on arteries within skeletal muscles is greater than on cutaneous vessels. *Has both cerebral and peripheral vasodilatory properties.*

USES Adjunctive therapy in treatment of cerebral vascular insufficiency and peripheral vascular disease, such as Raynaud's disease.

CONTRAINDICATIONS Immediately postpartum; presence of arterial bleeding; parenteral use in presence of hypotension, fetal distress; intrauterine fetal death; vaginal bleeding; tachycardia.
CAUTIOUS USE Bleeding disorders; severe cerebrovascular disease, severe obliterative coronary artery disease, recent MI; pregnancy (category C), lactation.

ROUTE & DOSAGE

Cerebral Vascular Insufficiency, Peripheral Vascular Disease

Adult: **PO** 10–20 mg t.i.d. or q.i.d.

ADMINISTRATION

Oral

- May give without regard to meals.

ADVERSE EFFECTS (≥1%) **CV:** Flushing, orthostatic hypotension with lightheadedness, faintness; palpitation, tachycardia. **CNS:** Dizziness, nervousness, trembling, weakness. **GI:** Nausea, vomiting, abdominal distress, abdominal distention.

PHARMACOKINETICS Absorption: Readily from GI tract. **Peak:** 1 h. **Duration:** 3 h. **Distribution:** Crosses placenta. **Metabolism:** In blood. **Elimination:** In urine. **Half-Life:** 1.25 h.

NURSING IMPLICATIONS

Assessment & Drug Effects

- Monitor for therapeutic effectiveness: Response to treatment of peripheral vascular disorders may take several weeks. Evaluate clinical manifestations of arterial insufficiency.
- Monitor BP and pulse; may cause hypotension and tachycardia. Supervise ambulation.
- Observe both mother and baby for hypotension and irregular and rapid heartbeat if isoxsuprine is used to delay premature labor. Hypocalcemia, hypoglycemia, and ileus have been observed in babies born of mothers taking isoxsuprine.

Patient & Family Education

- Notify physician of adverse reactions (skin rash, palpitation, flushing) promptly; symptoms are usually effectively controlled by dosage reduction or discontinuation of drug.
- Prevent orthostatic hypotension by making position changes slowly and in stages, particularly from lying down to sitting upright and avoid standing still.
- Note: For treatment of menstrual cramps, isoxsuprine is usually started 1–3 days before onset of menstruation and continued until pain is relieved or menstrual flow stops.

ISRADIPINE

(is-ra′di-peen)

DynaCirc CR

Classifications: CALCIUM CHANNEL BLOCKER; ANTIHYPERTENSIVE

Therapeutic: ANTIHYPERTENSIVE; ANTIANGINAL

Prototype: Nifedipine

Pregnancy Category: C

AVAILABILITY 2.5 mg, 5 mg capsules; 5 mg, 10 mg sustained release tablets

ACTION & *THERAPEUTIC EFFECT* Inhibits calcium ion influx into cardiac muscle and smooth muscle without changing calcium concentrations, thus affecting contractility. Isradipine relaxes coronary vascular smooth muscle. It significantly decreases systemic vascular resistance and reduces BP at rest and during isometric and dynamic exercise. *Reduces BP and has an antianginal effect.*

USES Mild to moderate hypertension.

UNLABELED USES Angina, CHF.

CONTRAINDICATIONS Hypersensitivity to isradipine or other calcium channel drugs.

CAUTIOUS USE CHF, acute MI, severe bradycardia, cardiogenic shock, ventricular dysfunction; older adult; mild renal impairment, hepatic impairment; GERD, hiatal hernia with esophageal reflux; pregnancy (category C), lactation. Safety and effectiveness in adolescents and children are not established.

ROUTE & DOSAGE

Hypertension

Adult: **PO** 1.25–10 mg b.i.d. (max: 20 mg/day); DynaCirc CR dosed daily

Angina

Adult: **PO** 2.5–7.5 mg t.i.d. (max: 15 mg/day)

ADMINISTRATION

Oral

- Do not crush sustained release form. It **must be** swallowed whole.
- Note: After the first 2–4 wk of therapy, dose may be increased for improved BP control in increments of 5 mg/day at 2–4 wk intervals up to a maximum dose of 20 mg/day.
- Store in tight, light-resistant container.

ADVERSE EFFECTS (≥1%) **CNS:** Headache, dizziness, fainting, fatigue, sleep disturbances, vertigo. **CV:** Flushing, ankle edema, palpitations, tachycardia, hypotension, chest pain, CHF. **GI:** Nausea, vomiting, abdominal discomfort, constipation, increased liver enzymes. **Respiratory:** Dyspnea. **Skin:** Rash, decreased skin sensation.

INTERACTIONS Drug: Adenosine may prolong bradycardia. May increase **cyclosporine** levels and toxicity.

PHARMACOKINETICS Absorption: Rapidly and completely absorbed from GI tract, but only 15–24% reaches systemic circulation because of first-pass metabolism. **Onset:** 1 h. **Peak:** 2–3 h. **Duration:** 12 h. **Distribution:** Not known if crosses placenta or is distributed into breast milk. **Metabolism:** Extensive first-pass metabolism in liver. **Elimination:** 70% in urine as inactive metabolites; 30% in feces. **Half-Life:** 5–11 h.

NURSING IMPLICATIONS

Assessment & Drug Effects

- Monitor BP throughout course of therapy.

- Monitor patients with a history of CHF carefully, especially with concurrent beta-blocker use. Promptly report S&S of worsening heart failure.
- Monitor ambulation, especially with older adult patients, until response to drug is known.

Patient & Family Education

- Notify physician promptly of shortness of breath, palpitations, or other signs of adverse cardiovascular effects.
- Do not drive or engage in other potentially hazardous activities until response to drug is known.

ITRACONAZOLE

(i-tra-con'a-zole)

Sporanox

Classifications: ANTIBIOTIC; AZOLE ANTIFUNGAL

Therapeutic: AZOLE ANTIFUNGAL

Prototype: Fluconazole

Pregnancy Category: C

AVAILABILITY 100 mg capsules; 10 mg/mL oral solution

ACTION & *THERAPEUTIC EFFECT*

Interferes with formation of ergosterol, the principal sterol in the fungal cell membrane that, when depleted, interrupts fungal membrane functioning. *Antifungal properties affect the fungal cell membrane functioning.*

USES Treatment of systemic fungal infections caused by blastomycosis, histoplasmosis, aspergillosis, onychomycosis due to dermatophytes of the toenail with or without fingernail involvement; oropharyngeal and esophageal candidiasis; orally to treat superficial mycoses (*Candida,* pityriasis versicolor).

UNLABELED USES Systemic and vaginal candidiasis.

CONTRAINDICATIONS Hypersensitivity to itraconazole; hypotension; CrCl less than 30 mL/min; ventricular dysfunction as in CHF; or history of CHF when treating onychomycosis; neuropathy; systemic candidiasis; lactation.

CAUTIOUS USE Hypersensitivity to other azole antifungals, achlorhydria; GERD; COPD, cystic fibrosis; dialysis; older adults, females of childbearing age; hepatic disease, hepatitis, HIV infection; hypochlorhydria; pulmonary disease; renal disease, renal impairment; valvular heart disease, ventricular dysfunction; angina, cardiac disease; pregnancy (category C), children.

ROUTE & DOSAGE

Blastomycosis, Nonmeningeal Histoplasmosis, Aspergillosis

Adult: **PO** 200 mg once daily (increase to max 200 mg b.i.d. if no apparent improvement). Continue for at least 3 mo; for life-threatening infections, start with 200 mg t.i.d. for 3 days, then 200–400 mg/day.
Child: **PO** 3–5 mg/kg/day for 3–6 mo

Oropharyngeal Candidiasis

Adult: **PO** 200 mg daily for 1–2 wk

Esophageal Candidiasis

Adult: **PO** 100 mg daily for at least 3 wk (max: 200 mg/day)

Vaginal Candidiasis

Adult: **PO** 200 mg daily for 3 days

Life-Threatening Infections
Adult: **PO** 200 mg t.i.d. × 3 days
Onychomycosis
Adult: **PO** 200 mg daily × 3 mo

ADMINISTRATION

Oral

- Give capsules with a full meal.
- Give oral solution without food. Liquid should be vigorously swished for several seconds and swallowed.
- Do not interchange oral solution and capsules.
- Divide dosages greater than 200 mg/day into two doses.
- Store liquid at or below 25° C (77° F).

I

ADVERSE EFFECTS (≥1%) **CV:** Hypertension with higher doses. **CNS:** Headache, dizziness, fatigue, somnolence, hearing loss (euphoria, drowsiness less than 1%). **Endocrine:** Gynecomastia, hypokalemia (especially with higher doses), hypertriglyceridemia. **GI:** *Nausea, vomiting, dyspepsia, abdominal pain, diarrhea, anorexia, flatulence, gastritis;* elevations of serum transaminases, alkaline phosphatase, and bilirubin. **Urogenital:** Decreased libido, impotence. **Skin:** Rash, pruritus. **Acute Poisoning:** Severe toxicity (doses exceeding 400 mg daily have been associated with higher risk of hypokalemia, hypertension, adrenal insufficiency).

INTERACTIONS Drug: Use with oral **midazolam, nisoldipine, pimozide, quinidine, dofetilide, triazolam** is contraindicated. Itraconazole may increase levels and toxicity of **ergotamine, dihydroergotamine,** ORAL HYPOGLYCEMIC AGENTS **warfarin, ritonavir, indinavir, vinca alkaloids, busulfan, ergonovine, methylergonovine, midazolam, triazolam, diazepam, nifedipine, nicardipine, amlodipine, felodipine, lova–statin, simvastatin, cyclosporine, tacrolimus, methylprednisolone, digoxin.** Combination with **dofetilide, levomethadyl, oral midazolam, pimozide, quinidine, triazolam** may cause severe cardiac events including cardiac arrest or sudden death. Itraconazole levels are decreased by **carbamazepine, phenytoin, phenobarbital, isoniazid, rifabutin, rifampin. Herbal: St. John's wort** and **garlic** may decrease itraconazole levels.

PHARMACOKINETICS Absorption: Well absorbed from GI tract when taken with food. **Onset:** 2 wk–3 mo. **Peak:** Peak levels at 1.5–5 h. Steady-state concentrations reached in 10–14 days. **Distribution:** Highly protein bound, minimal concentrations in CSF. Higher concentrations in tissues than in plasma. **Metabolism:** Extensively in liver by CYP3A4, may undergo enterohepatic recirculation. **Elimination:** 35% in urine, 55% in feces. **Half-Life:** 34–42 h.

NURSING IMPLICATIONS

Assessment & Drug Effects

- Lab tests: C&S tests should be done before initiation of therapy. Drug may be started pending results. Monitor hepatic functions especially in those with preexisting hepatic abnormalities.
- Monitor for digoxin toxicity when given concurrently with digoxin.
- Monitor PT and INR carefully when given concurrently with warfarin.
- Monitor for S&S of hypersensitivity (see Appendix F); discontinue drug and notify physician if noted.

Patient & Family Education

- Take capsules, but NOT oral solution, with food.
- Notify physician promptly for S&S of liver dysfunction, including anorexia, nausea, and vomiting; weakness and fatigue; dark urine and clay-colored stool.
- Note: Risk of hypoglycemia may increase in diabetics on oral hypoglycemic agents.

IVERMECTIN

(i-ver-mec'tin)

Stromectol

Classification: ANTHELMINTIC

Therapeutic: ANTHELMINTIC; ANTI-PARASITIC

Prototype: Mebendazole

Pregnancy Category: C

AVAILABILITY 3 mg tablets

ACTION & *THERAPEUTIC EFFECT* A semisynthetic anthelmintic agent which is a broad-spectrum antiparasitic agent that causes an increase in permeability to chloride ions of the parasitic cell membrane, resulting in hyperpolarization of nerve or muscle cells of parasites. This results in their paralysis and cell death. *Causes cell death of parasites.*

USES Treatment of strongyloidiasis of the intestinal tract, onchocerciasis.

CONTRAINDICATIONS Hypersensitivity to ivermectin. Safety and efficacy in children weighing 15 kg or less are not established.

CAUTIOUS USE Asthma; older adults; moderate or severe hepatic disease; hyperreactive onchodermatitis; pregnancy (category C); lactation; children greater than or equal to 15 kg of weight.

ROUTE & DOSAGE

Strongyloides

Adult/Child (weight 15 kg or greater): **PO** 200 mcg/kg × 1 dose

Onchocerciasis

Adult/Child (weight 15 kg or greater): **PO** 150 mcg/kg × 1 dose, may repeat q3–12mo prn

ADMINISTRATION

Oral

- Give tablets with water rather than any other type of liquid.
- Store below 30° C (86° F).

ADVERSE EFFECTS (≥1%) **Body as a Whole:** *Fever,* peripheral edema. **CNS:** Dizziness. **CV:** Tachycardia. **GI:** Diarrhea, nausea. **Skin:** *Pruritus, rash.* **Other:** Arthralgia/synovitis, lymphadenopathy.

INTERACTIONS Drug: May increase effect of **warfarin.**

PHARMACOKINETICS Peak: 4 h. **Distribution:** Distributed into breast milk. **Metabolism:** In the liver. **Elimination:** In feces over 12 days. **Half-Life:** 16 h.

NURSING IMPLICATIONS

Assessment & Drug Effects

- Monitor for therapeutic effectiveness: Indicated by negative stool samples.
- Monitor for cardiovascular effects such as orthostatic hypotension and tachycardia.
- Monitor for and report inflammatory conditions of the eyes.

Patient & Family Education

- Get a follow-up stool examination to determine effectiveness of treatment. Treatment for worms does not kill adult parasites; repeated follow-up and retreatment are usually needed.

- Notify physician if eye discomfort develops.

IXABEPILONE

(ix-a-be-pi'lone)

Ixempra

Classifications: ANTINEOPLASTIC AGENT; EPOTHILONE

Therapeutic: ANTINEOPLASTIC AGENT; ANTIMITOTIC

Pregnancy Category: D

AVAILABILITY 15 mg and 45 mg lyophilized powder, single-use vials

ACTION & *THERAPEUTIC EFFECT* Binds directly to microtubules needed to form the spindles required in mitosis of dividing cells. *Blocks new cell formation during the mitotic phase of their cell division cycle, thus leading to cancer cell death.*

USES Treatment of metastatic or locally advanced breast cancer either alone or in combination with capecitabine in patients who have failed therapy with an anthracycline and a taxane. Monotherapy is indicated only if a patient has also failed with capecitabine therapy.

CONTRAINDICATIONS Hepatic impairment in patients with AST or ALT greater than 10 × ULN, and/or bilirubin greater than 3 × ULN; concomitant use of capecitabine and bilirubin greater than 1 × ULN, or AST or ALT greater than 2.5 × ULN; grade 4 neuropathy or any other grade 4 toxicity; pregnancy (category D); lactation.

CAUTIOUS USE Hypersensitivity to ixabepilone; monotherapy of patients with hepatic impairment baseline values of AST or ALT greater than 5 × ULN.

ROUTE & DOSAGE

Breast Cancer

Adult: **IV** 40 mg/m² over 3 h q3wk

Obesity Dosage Adjustment

BSA greater than 2.2 m²: Dosage should be calculated based on 2.2 m² instead of actual m²

Dosage Adjustments

- **Grade 2 neuropathy 7 days or more, or grade 3 neuropathy less than 7 days, or grade 3 toxicity other than neuropathy:** 32 mg/m²
- **Neutrophil less than 500 cells/mm³ 7 days or more, or febrile neutropenia, or platelets less than 25,000/mm³ or platelets less than 50,000/mm³ with bleeding:** Decrease dose by 20%
- **Grade 3 neuropathy 7 days or more or disabling neuropathy, or any grade 4 toxicity:** Do not administer
- **Regimen with a strong CYP3A4 inhibitor:** 20 mg/m²

Hepatic Impairment Dosage Adjustment in Monotherapy

- **AST and ALT 10 × ULN or less and bilirubin 1.5 × ULN or less:** 32 mg/m²
- **AST and ALT 10 × ULN or less and bilirubin greater than 1.5 × ULN but 3 × ULN or less:** 20–30 mg/m²
- **AST and ALT greater than 10 × ULN or bilirubin greater than 3 × ULN:** Do not administer

ADMINISTRATION

Intravenous

Use gloves when handling vials containing ixabepilone.

PREPARE: **IV Infusion:** Supplied in kit containing a powder vial and diluent vial. Allow kit to come to room temperature for 30 min before reconstitution. ▪ Slowly inject diluent into the powder vial to yield 2 mg/mL. Swirl gently and invert vial to dissolve. ▪ Further dilute in LR solution in DEHP-free bags. Select a volume of LR to produce a final concentration of 0.2–0.6 mg/mL. Mix thoroughly.

ADMINISTER: **IV Infusion:** Use DEHP-free infusion line with a 0.2–1.2 micron in-line filter. ▪ Infuse at a rate appropriate to the total volume of solution. Complete infusion within 6 h of preparation.

INCOMPATIBILITIES **Solution/additive:** Diluents other than **lactated Ringer's injection** should not be combined with ixabepilone. **Y-site:** Do not use a Y-site connection with this drug.

▪ Store drug kit refrigerated at 2°–8° C (36°–46° F) in original packaging. ▪ Reconstituted solution may be stored in the vial for a maximum of only 1 h at room temperature/light. ▪ Once further diluted with lactated Ringer's injection, solution is stable at room temperature/light for 6 h.

ADVERSE EFFECTS (≥1%) **Body as a Whole:** Chest pain, dehydration, edema, *fatigue,* hypersensitivity reactions, pain, *peripheral neuropathy,* pyrexia. **CNS:** Dizziness, *headache,* insomnia. **CV:** Flushing. **GI:** *Abdominal pain, anorexia, constipation, diarrhea,* gastroesophageal reflux disease (GERD), *mucositis, nausea, stomatitis, vomiting,* taste disorder. **Hematologic:** Anemia, *leukopenia, neutropenia,* thrombocytopenia. **Metabolic:** Weight loss. **Musculoskeletal:** *Arthralgia, myalgia, musculoskeletal pain.* **Respiratory:** Cough, dyspnea, upper respiratory tract infection. **Skin:** *Alopecia,* exfoliation, hyperpigmentation, nail disorder, palmar-plantar erythrodysesthesia syndrome, pruritus, rash. **Special Senses:** Lacrimation.

INTERACTIONS Drug: Inhibitors of CYP3A4 (e.g., HIV PROTEASE INHIBITORS, MACROLIDE ANTIBIOTICS, AZOLE ANTIFUNGAL AGENTS) increase the plasma level of ixabepilone. Strong CYP3A4 inducers (e.g., **dexamethasone, phenytoin, carbamazepine, rifampin, rifabutin, phenobarbital**) decrease the plasma level of ixabepilone. **Food: Grapefruit** and **grapefruit juice** increase the plasma level of ixabepilone. **Herbal: St. John's wort** decreases the plasma level of ixabepilone.

PHARMACOKINETICS Distribution: 67–77% protein bound. **Metabolism:** In liver. **Elimination:** Stool (major) and urine (minor). **Half-Life:** 52 h.

NURSING IMPLICATIONS

Actions & Drug Effects

- Monitor for signs of an infusion-related hypersensitivity reaction.
- Monitor for and promptly report signs of neuropathy.
- Lab tests: Baseline and periodic WBC count with differential, platelet count, LFTs; periodic serum electrolytes.

Patient & Family Education

- Report promptly any of the following: Numbness and tingling of the hands or feet, S&S of infection (e.g., fever of 100.5° F or greater, chills, cough, burning or pain on

urination), hives, itching, rash, flushing, swelling, shortness of breath, difficulty breathing, chest tightness or pain, palpitations or unusual weight gain.
- Use effective contraceptive measures to prevent pregnancy.

KANAMYCIN

(kan-a-mye'sin)
Kantrex
Classifications: ANTIBIOTIC; AMINOGLYCOSIDE
Therapeutic: ANTIBIOTIC
Prototype: Gentamicin
Pregnancy Category: D

AVAILABILITY 1 g vials

ACTION & *THERAPEUTIC EFFECT* Broad-spectrum, aminoglycoside antibiotic that binds irreversibly to aminoglycoside-binding sites on 30 S ribosomal subunit of bacteria, subsequently inhibiting bacterial protein synthesis. *Usually bactericidal in action. Active against many aerobic gram-negative microorganisms, as well as some gram-positive bacteria. It is not effective against anaerobic gram-negative bacteria.*

USES Parenterally for short-term treatment of serious infections; intraperitoneally after fecal spill during surgery; as irrigation solution; and as aerosol treatment. In conjunction with other drugs to treat tuberculosis in patients resistant to conventional therapy.

CONTRAINDICATIONS History of hypersensitivity to kanamycin or other aminoglycosides; history of drug-induced ototoxicity, preexisting hearing loss, vertigo, or tinnitus; long-term therapy; intraperitoneally to patients under effects of inhalation anesthetics or skeletal muscle relaxants; pregnancy (category D); infant younger than 1 y.
CAUTIOUS USE Impaired renal function; older adults, neonates, and infants (immature renal systems); myasthenia gravis; parkinsonian syndrome; lactation.

ROUTE & DOSAGE

Serious Infection

Adult/Child: **IV/IM** 15 mg/kg/day in equally divided doses q8–12h
Adult: **Intraperitoneal** 500 mg diluted in 20 mL sterile water instilled through wound catheter **Inhalation** 250 mg diluted in 3 mL NS administered per nebulizer q6–12h **Irrigation** 0.25% solution prn

Renal Impairment Dosage Adjustment

CrCl 50–80 mL/min: Give 60–90% of dose; 10–50 mL/min: Give 30–70% of dose or q12h; less than 10 mL/min: Give 20–30% of dose or q24–48h

ADMINISTRATION

Intramuscular
- Administer IM injection deep into upper outer quadrant of gluteal muscle (often painful).
- Observe sites daily for signs of irritation; rotate injection sites.

Intravenous

PREPARE: **Intermittent for Adult:** Dilute each 500 mg with at least 100 mL NS, D5W, D5/NS, or other compatible solution. **Inter-**

mittent for Child: Dilute each 2.5–5 mg in 1 mL of NS, D5W, D5/SW, or other compatible solution.

ADMINISTER: **Intermittent for Adult/Child:** Over 30–60 min. **Intermittent for Child:** Use a constant-rate volumetric infusion device for administration.

INCOMPATIBILITIES **Solution/additive: Amphotericin B, cefazolin, cefoxitin, ceftazidime, cefuroxime, cephalothin, cephapirin, chlorpheniramine, colistimethate, heparin, hyaluronidase, hydrocortisone, lincomycin, methicillin, methohexital, nitrofurantoin, pentobarbital, phenobarbital, prochlorperazine, sodium bicarbonate, thiopental, warfarin.**

- Store vials at 15°–30° C (59°–86° F) unless otherwise directed. Some vials may darken with time, but this does not affect potency. ▪ Discard partially used vials within 48 h.

ADVERSE EFFECTS (≥1%) **All:** Dose related. **Body as a Whole:** Eosinophilia, maculopapular rash, pruritus, urticaria, drug fever, <u>anaphylaxis</u>. **CNS:** Dizziness, circumoral and other paresthesias, optic neuritis, peripheral neuritis, headache, restlessness, tremors, lethargy, convulsions; <u>neuromuscular paralysis, respiratory depression</u> (rarely). **Special Senses:** Deafness (can be irreversible), *tinnitus, vertigo* or *dizziness,* ataxia, nystagmus. **GI:** Nausea, vomiting, diarrhea, appetite changes, abdominal discomfort, stomatitis, proctitis, malabsorption syndrome (with prolonged oral administration). **Hematologic:** Anemia, increased or decreased reticulocytes, granulocytopenia, <u>agranulocytosis</u>, thrombocytopenia, purpura. **Urogenital:** <u>Nephrotoxicity</u>; hematuria, urine casts and cells, proteinuria; elevated serum creatinine and BUN. **Other:** Superinfections; local pain; nodular formation at injection site.

INTERACTIONS Drug: Amphotericin B, cisplatin, methoxyflurane, vancomycin add to nephrotoxicity; GENERAL ANESTHETICS, SKELETAL MUSCLE RELAXANTS add to neuromuscular blocking effects; **capreomycin** compounds ototoxicity and nephrotoxicity; LOOP AND THIAZIDE DIURETICS, carboplatin may increase risk of ototoxicity.

PHARMACOKINETICS Absorption: Readily absorbed from peritoneal cavity, bronchial tree, and wounds. **Peak:** 1–2 h. **Distribution:** Crosses placenta; distributed into breast milk. **Elimination:** 80–90% in urine within 24 h. **Half-Life:** 2–4 h.

NURSING IMPLICATIONS

Assessment & Drug Effects

- Lab tests: Monitor baseline C&S, urinalysis, and kidney function prior to initiation of therapy and periodically thereafter. Monitor serum sodium, potassium, calcium, and magnesium.
- Notify physician immediately of signs of renal irritation: Albuminuria, casts, red and white cells in urine, increasing BUN, and serum creatinine, decreasing creatinine clearance, oliguria, and edema.
- Monitor peak and trough serum kanamycin concentrations: Assess peak specimen 30–60 min after IM administration; 30 min after completion of a 30–60 min IV infusion. Assess trough levels just before the next IM or IV dose.
- Keep patient well hydrated to prevent chemical irritation of renal tubules.
- Monitor I&O. Report decrease in urine output or change in I&O ratio.

- Determine baseline weight and vital signs and monitor at regular intervals during therapy.
- Report signs of superinfection (see Appendix F).
- Monitor for hearing and balance problems; stop drug if ototoxicity occurs. Tinnitus is not a reliable index of ototoxicity in the very elderly. Risk of ototoxicity is high in patients with impaired renal function, older adults, poorly hydrated patients, and with therapy 5 days or longer.
- Note: Deafness has occurred 2–7 days or more after termination of therapy in patients with impaired renal function.

K

Patient & Family Education

- Report ototoxic symptoms such as dizziness, hearing loss, weakness, or loss of balance; drug may need to be discontinued.

KAOLIN AND PECTIN

(kay'oh-lin and pek'tin)

Kaolin w/Pectin

Classification: ANTIDIARRHEAL
Therapeutic: ANTIDIARRHEAL
Prototype: Loperamide
Pregnancy Category: C

AVAILABILITY 5.2 g kaolin/260 mg pectin/30 mL, 90 g kaolin/2 g pectin/30 mL

ACTION & *THERAPEUTIC EFFECT* Kaolin is hydrated aluminum silicate adsorpant. Kaolin is reported to have adsorbent, protectant, and demulcent properties. Mechanism of action of pectin may help consolidate stool. *Effective as an antidiarrheal agent.*

USES Adjunct in symptomatic treatment of mild to moderately severe acute diarrhea. Commonly used in antidiarrheal combination products.

CONTRAINDICATIONS Suspected obstructive bowel lesion, pseudomembranous colitis, diarrhea associated with bacterial toxins; presence of fever; use for more than 48 h without medical direction; lactation.

CAUTIOUS USE Older adults; infants or children 3 y or younger, pregnancy (category C).

ROUTE & DOSAGE

Diarrhea

Adult: **PO** 60–120 mL of regular suspension or 45–90 mL of concentrated suspension after each loose bowel movement

Child: **PO** *3–5 y,* 15–30 mL regular suspension or 15 mL concentrated suspension after each loose bowel movement; *6–11 y,* 30–60 mL regular suspension or 30 mL concentrated suspension after each loose bowel movement; *12 y or older,* 60 mL regular suspension or 45 mL concentrated suspension after each loose bowel movement

ADMINISTRATION

Oral

- Administer at least 2–4 h before other oral medications.
- Shake suspension well before pouring.
- Store in tightly closed container at 15°–30° C (59°–86° F) unless otherwise directed. Protect from freezing.

ADVERSE EFFECTS (≥1%) **GI:** Constipation usually mild and transient.

INTERACTIONS Drug: Chloroquine, digoxin, penicillamine,

tetracycline, ciprofloxacin, and most other drugs.

PHARMACOKINETICS Absorption: Not absorbed from GI tract.

NURSING IMPLICATIONS

Assessment & Drug Effects

- Assess for abdominal distention and number of stools per day.
- Note: Fecal impaction may result from taking kaolin and pectin, especially in older adults.
- Note: Drug may decrease absorption of any orally administered medication.

Patient & Family Education

- Do not exceed prescribed dosage.
- Notify physician if diarrhea is not controlled within 48 h or if fever develops.

KETOCONAZOLE

(ke-to-con'a-zol)

Extina, Kuric, Nizoral, Nizoral A-D, Xolegel

Classification: ANTIFUNGAL, AZOLE

Therapeutic: AZOLE ANTIFUNGAL

Prototype: Fluconazole

Pregnancy Category: C

AVAILABILITY 200 mg tablets; 2% cream; 2% shampoo; 2% foam; 2% gel

ACTION & *THERAPEUTIC EFFECT* Interferes with formation of ergosterol, the principal sterol in the fungal cell membrane that, when depleted, interrupts membrane function by increasing its permeability. *Antifungal properties are related to the drug effect on the fungal cell membrane functioning.*

USES Oral—Severe systemic fungal infections including candidiasis (e.g., oral thrush, candiduria), chronic mucocutaneous candidiasis, pulmonary and disseminated coccidioidomycosis, histoplasmosis, paracoccidioidomycosis, blastomycosis, and chromomycosis. **Topical**—Tinea corporis and tinea cruris (caused by *Epidermophyton floccosum, Trichophyton mentagrophytes,* and *Trichophyton rubrum*) and in treatment of tinea versicolor (pityriasis) caused by *Malassezia furfur (Pityrosporum obiculare),* seborrheic dermatitis.

UNLABELED USES Oral—Onychomycosis, vaginal candidiasis, Cushing's syndrome associated with adrenal or pituitary adenoma; precocious puberty, dysfunctional hirsutism, and as swish and swallow preparation for prophylaxis against fungal infections in patients with neutropenia induced by cancer chemotherapy and in patients with AIDS.

CONTRAINDICATIONS Hypersensitivity to ketoconazole or any component in the formulation; chronic alcoholism, fungal meningitis; onychomycosis; ocular exposure, ophthalmic administration.

CAUTIOUS USE Azole antifungal hypersensitivity; achlorhydria, hypochlorhydria; asthma; severe hepatic impairment; alcoholism; older adult; HIV infection; hyperactive onchodermatitis; pregnancy (category C), lactation. Safe use in children younger than 2 y is not established.

ROUTE & DOSAGE

Fungal Infections

Adult: **PO:** 200–400 mg once/day: **Topical:** Apply 1–2 times/day to affected area and surrounding skin

K

Child (older than 2 y): **PO** 3.3–6.6 mg/kg/day as single dose

Dandruff

Adult/Child: **Topical** Shampoo twice a week for 4 wk with at least 3 days between shampoos
Topical (Extina) Apply b.i.d. × 4 wk; (Xolegel) Apply daily × 2 wk

ADMINISTRATION

Oral

- Give with water, fruit juice, coffee, or tea; drug requires an acid medium for dissolution and absorption.
- Relieve nausea and vomiting during early therapy by taking drug with food and dividing into 2 daily doses.
- Do not give with antacids.
- Store in tightly covered container at 15°–30° C (59°–86° F) unless otherwise directed.

Topical

- Apply sufficient shampoo to produce lather to wash scalp and hair and gently massage over entire scalp area for 1 min, rinse hair thoroughly and repeat, leaving shampoo on scalp for 3 min. Rinse thoroughly.

ADVERSE EFFECTS (≥1%) **Oral—Body as a Whole:** Skin rash, erythema, urticaria, pruritus, angioedema, anaphylaxis. **GI:** *Nausea, vomiting,* anorexia, epigastric or abdominal pain, constipation, diarrhea, transient elevation in serum liver enzymes, fatal hepatic necrosis (rare). **Hematologic:** With high doses, lowers serum testosterone and ACTH-induced corticosteroid serum levels, transient decreases in serum cholesterol and triglycerides; hyponatremia (rare). **Urogenital:** Gynecomastia (males), breast pain; uterine bleeding, loss of libido, impotence, oligospermia, hair loss. **Other:** Acute hypoadrenalism (reduction of adrenal stress syndrome), renal hypofunction. **Topical—Skin:** Mild transient erythema, severe irritation, pruritus, stinging.

INTERACTIONS Drug: Alcohol may cause sunburnlike reaction; ANTACIDS, ANTICHOLINERGICS, H_2-RECEPTOR ANTAGONISTS decrease ketoconazole absorption; **isoniazid, rifampin** increase ketoconazole metabolism, thus decreasing its activity; levels of **phenytoin** and ketoconazole decreased; may increase levels of **cyclosporine** or **carbamazepine,** increasing the risk of toxicity; **warfarin** may potentiate hypoprothrombinemia; may increase ergotamine toxicity of **dihydroergotamine, ergotamine;** may increase concentration and toxicity of **trazodone. Herbal: Echinacea** may increase risk of hepatotoxicity.

PHARMACOKINETICS Absorption: Erratically from GI tract (needs an acid pH); minimal absorption topically. **Peak:** 1–2 h. **Distribution:** Distributed to saliva, urine, sebum, and cerumen; CSF levels unpredictable; distributed into breast milk. **Metabolism:** In liver (CYP3A4). **Elimination:** Primarily in feces, 13% in urine. **Half-Life:** 8 h.

NURSING IMPLICATIONS

Assessment & Drug Effects

- Lab tests: Monitor baseline liver function tests (AST, ALT, alkaline phosphatase, and bilirubin) and repeat at least monthly throughout therapy.
- Monitor for S&S of hepatotoxicity (see Appendix F). Discontinue drug immediately to prevent irreversible liver damage and report to physician.

Patient & Family Education

- Report S&S of hepatotoxicity promptly to physician (see Appendix F).
- Note: Drowsiness and dizziness are early and time-limited adverse effects.
- Do not drive or engage in potentially hazardous activities until response to drug is known.
- Avoid OTC drugs for gastric distress, such as Rolaids, Tums, Alka-Seltzer and check with physician before taking any other nonprescription medicines.
- Do not alter dose or dose interval and do not stop taking ketoconazole before consulting the physician.
- Notify physician if skin condition fails to respond to topical therapy or worsens or if signs of irritation or sensitivity occur.

KETOPROFEN

(kee-toe-proe′fen)

Oruvail

Classifications: ANALGESIC, NONSTEROIDAL ANTI-INFLAMMATORY DRUG (NSAID); ANTIPYRETIC

Therapeutic: ANALGESIC, NSAID

Prototype: Ibuprofen

Pregnancy Category: B first and second trimester; D in third trimester

AVAILABILITY 25 mg, 50 mg, 75 mg capsules; 100 mg, 150 mg, 200 mg sustained release capsules

ACTION & *THERAPEUTIC EFFECT* Nonsteroidal anti-inflammatory drug (NSAID) that inhibits both COX-1 and COX-2 enzymes; thus it also inhibits prostaglandin synthesis, and therefore interferes with the inflammatory process. It inhibits platelet aggregation and prolongs bleeding time. *Has analgesic, anti-inflammatory, and antiplatelet properties.*

USES Acute or long-term treatment of rheumatoid arthritis and osteoarthritis; primary dysmenorrhea; headache; symptomatic relief of postoperative, dental, and postpartum pain; visceral pain associated with cancer.

UNLABELED USES Reiter's syndrome, juvenile arthritis, acute gouty arthritis, biliary pain, renal colic.

CONTRAINDICATIONS Patient in whom aspirin, salicylate, or another NSAID induces asthma, urticaria, bronchospasm, severe rhinitis, shock; perioperatively for CABG surgery; renal nephritis, nephritic syndrome; pregnancy (category D third trimester); lactation. Safety in children younger than 16 y is not established.

CAUTIOUS USE History of GI disease, GI bleeding, active ulcer; renal or hepatic impairment, patient who may be adversely affected by prolongation of bleeding time; heart failure, fluid retention; hypertension; patient receiving diuretics; geriatric patient; anemia; dental work; myasthenia gravis; pregnancy (category B first and second trimester).

ROUTE & DOSAGE

Inflammatory Disease

Adult: **PO** 75 mg t.i.d. or 50 mg q.i.d. (max: 300 mg/day) or 200 mg sustained release daily
Geriatric: **PO** Start with 25 mg q.i.d., may also start with 50 mg t.i.d.

Mild to Moderate Pain, Dysmenorrhea

Adult: **PO** 12.5–50 mg q6–8h

K

ADMINISTRATION

Oral

- Do not crush.
- Give with food, milk, or prescribed antacid to reduce GI irritation.
- Store drug at 15°–30° C (59°–86° F) in tightly closed, light-resistant container unless otherwise directed.

ADVERSE EFFECTS (≥1%) **CNS:** Trouble in sleeping, nervousness, *headache,* dizziness; depression, drowsiness, confusion, migraine, vertigo. **CV:** Peripheral edema, palpitations, hypertension, tachycardia. **Special Senses:** Visual disturbances, conjunctivitis, eye pain, retinal hemorrhage, pigmentation changes; dry nose or throat, tinnitus, hearing impairment. **GI:** *Dyspepsia,* <u>drug-induced peptic ulcer, GI bleeding</u>, nausea, vomiting, diarrhea, constipation, flatulence, stomach pain, anorexia, dry mouth, gingivitis, rectal burning and hemorrhage, melena, jaundice, elevated ALT, AST. **Hematologic:** Prolonged bleeding time, anemia, purpura, <u>agranulocytosis</u>, thrombocytosis. **Urogenital:** Gynecomastia, changes in libido, urinary tract irritation (dysuria, frequency/urgency), renal impairment. **Respiratory:** <u>Laryngospasm, bronchospasm, laryngeal edema</u>, pharyngitis. **Skin:** Rash, pruritus, urticaria, erythema, photosensitivity. **Endocrine:** Aggravation of diabetes mellitus.

INTERACTIONS Drug: ORAL ANTICOAGULANTS, **heparin** may prolong bleeding time; may increase **lithium** toxicity; may increase **methotrexate** toxicity. **Herbal: Feverfew, garlic, ginger, ginkgo** increases bleeding potential.

PHARMACOKINETICS Absorption: Readily from GI tract. **Onset:** 1–2 h. **Peak:** 1–2 h. **Duration:** 4–6 h. **Metabolism:** In liver. **Elimination:** Primarily in urine, some biliary excretion. **Half-Life:** 1.1–4 h.

NURSING IMPLICATIONS

Assessment & Drug Effects

- Lab tests: Monitor baseline and periodic evaluations of hemoglobin, renal and hepatic function.
- Monitor for and report tinnitus, hearing impairment, and visual disturbance, especially during prolonged or high-dose therapy.
- Monitor for S&S of GI ulceration (e.g., stool for occult blood, persistent indigestion).

Patient & Family Education

- Report promptly signs of jaundice (see Appendix F) as well as the following: Blurred vision, tinnitus, urinary urgency or frequency, unexplained bleeding, weight gain with edema.
- Note: Possible CNS adverse effects (e.g., lightheadedness, dizziness, drowsiness).
- Do not drive or engage in potentially hazardous activities until response to drug is known.
- Note: Alcohol, aspirin, or other NSAIDs may increase risk of GI ulceration and bleeding tendencies and therefore should be avoided.
- Tell dentist or surgeon that you are taking ketoprofen.

KETOROLAC TROMETHAMINE

(ke-tor′o-lac)

Acular, Acular LS, Acuvail, Toradol

Common adverse effects in *italic*, life-threatening effects <u>underlined</u>; generic names in **bold**; classifications in SMALL CAPS; ♣ Canadian drug name; ⓟ Prototype drug

Classifications: ANALGESIC, NONSTEROIDAL ANTI-INFLAMMATORY DRUG (NSAID); ANTIPYRETIC
Therapeutic: NONNARCOTIC ANALGESIC, NSAID
Prototype: Ibuprofen
Pregnancy Category: C first and second trimester; D third trimester

AVAILABILITY 10 mg tablets; 15 mg/mL, 30 mg/mL injection; 0.4%, 0.5% ophth solution

ACTION & *THERAPEUTIC EFFECT* It inhibits synthesis of prostaglandins by inhibiting both COX-1 and COX-2 enzymes. Is a peripherally acting analgesic. It inhibits platelet aggregation and prolongs bleeding time. *Exhibits analgesic, anti-inflammatory, and antipyretic activity. Effective in controlling acute postoperative pain.*

USES *Short-term* management of pain; ocular itching due to seasonal allergic conjunctivitis, reduction of postoperative pain and photophobia after refractive surgery.

CONTRAINDICATIONS Hypersensitivity to ketorolac; hypersensitivity reaction to aspirin, salicylates, or other NSAIDs; during labor and delivery; surgery; patients with severe renal impairment or at risk for renal failure due to volume depletion; perioperative use in CABG surgery for 10–14 days after; patients with risk of bleeding; history of GI bleeding or peptic ulcer; pre- or intraoperatively; intrathecal or epidural administration; in combination with other NSAIDs; pregnancy (category D third trimester); children younger than 2 y.

CAUTIOUS USE Impaired renal or hepatic function; Crohn's disease or IBD; bleeding disorders; corticosteroid therapy; myelosuppressive chemotherapy; older adults; debilitated patients; diabetes mellitus; lactase deficiency; coagulation disorders; SLE; CHF; history of hypertension, MI or stroke; pregnancy (category C first and second trimester); children younger than 3 y with ophthalmic solution.

ROUTE & DOSAGE

Pain

Adult: **IV Loading Dose** 30 mg (15 mg if less than 50 kg) **IM** 30–60 mg loading dose, then 15–30 mg q6h [max: 150 mg/day on first day, then 120 mg subsequent days (30 mg load, then 15 mg q6h if less than 50 kg)] **PO** 10 mg q6h prn (max: 40 mg/day) max duration all routes 5 days
Geriatric: **IV Loading Dose** 15 mg **IM** 30 mg loading dose, then 15 mg q6h **PO** 5–10 mg q6h prn (max: 40 mg/day) max duration all routes 5 days

Pain after Refractive Surgery

Adult: **Ophthalmic** *Acular LS only* 1 drop in operative eye q.i.d. up to 4 days

Allergic Conjunctivitis

Adult: **Ophthalmic** 1 drop 0.5% solution q.i.d.

ADMINISTRATION

WARNING: DO NOT ADMINISTER IV, IM, OR PO KETOROLAC LONGER THAN 5 DAYS.

Oral
- Give with food to reduce GI effects.

Instillation
- Do not touch container to the eye when applying ophthalmic drops.

Intramuscular
- Inject IM drug slowly and deeply into a large muscle.
- Rotate injection sites to avoid injection site pain in patients receiving multiple doses.

Intravenous

PREPARE: **Direct:** Give undiluted.
ADMINISTER: **Direct:** Give IV bolus dose over at least 15 sec. Preferred method is to give through a Y-tube in a free-flowing IV.
INCOMPATIBILITIES **Solution/additive:** **Haloperidol, hydroxyzine, meperidine, morphine, prochlorperazine, promethazine.** **Y-site:** **Azithromycin, fenoldopam.**

- Store all forms at 15°–30° C (59°–86° F).

ADVERSE EFFECTS (≥1%) **CNS:** *Drowsiness,* dizziness, headache. **GI:** *Nausea,* dyspepsia, GI pain, hemorrhage. **Other:** Edema, sweating, pain at injection site.

INTERACTIONS Drug: May increase **methotrexate** levels and toxicity; may increase **lithium** levels and toxicity. **Herbal:** **Feverfew, garlic, ginger, ginkgo** increased bleeding potential.

PHARMACOKINETICS Peak: 45–60 min. **Distribution:** Into breast milk. **Metabolism:** In liver. **Elimination:** In urine. **Half-Life:** 4–6 h.

NURSING IMPLICATIONS

Assessment & Drug Effects
- Correct hypovolemia prior to administration of ketorolac.
- Lab tests: Periodic serum electrolytes and liver functions; urinalysis (for hematuria and proteinuria) with long-term use.
- Monitor urine output in older adults and patients with a history of cardiac decompensation, renal impairment, heart failure, or liver dysfunction as well as those taking diuretics. Discontinuation of drug will return urine output to pretreatment level.
- Monitor for S&S of GI distress or bleeding including nausea, GI pain, diarrhea, melena, or hematemesis. GI ulceration with perforation can occur anytime during treatment. Drug decreases platelet aggregation and thus may prolong bleeding time.
- Monitor for fluid retention and edema in patients with a history of CHF.

Patient & Family Education
- Watch for S&S of GI ulceration and bleeding (e.g., bloody emesis, black tarry stools) during long-term therapy.
- Note: Possible CNS adverse effects (e.g., lightheadedness, dizziness, drowsiness).
- Do not drive or engage in potentially hazardous activities until response to drug is known.
- Do not use other NSAIDs while taking this drug.

KETOTIFEN FUMARATE
(kee-toe-tye′fen)
Zaditor
Pregnancy Category: C
See Appendix A-1.

LABETALOL HYDROCHLORIDE
(la-bet′a-lole)

Trandate
Classifications: ALPHA- & BETA-ADRENERGIC ANTAGONIST; ANTIHYPERTENSIVE
Therapeutic: ANTIHYPERTENSIVE
Prototype: Propranolol
Pregnancy Category: B first and second trimester; D third trimester

AVAILABILITY 100 mg, 200 mg, 300 mg tablet; 5 mg/mL injection

ACTION & *THERAPEUTIC EFFECT* Acts as an adrenergic receptor blocking agent that combines selective alpha activity and nonselective beta-adrenergic blocking actions. The alpha blockade results in vasodilation, decreased peripheral resistance, and orthostatic hypotension. It has beta-blocking effects on the sinus node, AV node, and ventricular muscle, which lead to bradycardia, delay in AV conduction, and depression of cardiac contractility. *Effective in reducing blood pressure by vasodilation as well as depression of cardiac contractility.*

USES Mild, moderate, and severe hypertension. May be used alone or in combination with other antihypertensive agents, especially thiazide diuretics.

CONTRAINDICATIONS NSAID or salicylate hypersensitivity; bronchial asthma; uncontrolled cardiac failure, heart block (greater than first degree), cardiogenic shock, severe bradycardia; systolic blood pressure less than 100 mm Hg; perioperative CABG pain; pregnancy (category D third trimester). Safe use in children is not established.

CAUTIOUS USE Nonallergic bronchospastic disease (e.g., COPD); renal disease, renal failure, hepatic disease; well-compensated patients with history of heart failure; acute MI; coronary artery disease; pheochromocytoma; severe liver dysfunction, jaundice; diabetes mellitus; SLE; myasthenia gravis; older adults; peripheral vascular disease; pregnancy (category B first and second trimester); lactation.

ROUTE & DOSAGE

Hypertension
Adult: **PO** 100 mg b.i.d., may gradually increase to 200–400 mg b.i.d. (max: 1200–2400 mg/day). **IV** 20 mg slowly over 2 min, with 40–80 mg q10min if needed up to 300 mg total or 2 mg/min continuous infusion (max: 300 mg total dose)
Geriatric: **PO** Start with 100 mg daily **IV** 20 mg slowly over 2 min, with 40–80 mg q10min if needed up to 300 mg total or 2 mg/min continuous infusion (max: 300 mg total dose)

ADMINISTRATION

Oral
- Give with or immediately after food consistently. Food increases drug bioavailability.

Intravenous
Note: Amount of IV solution may be changed depending on patient status.

PREPARE: **Direct:** Give undiluted. **Continuous:** Dilute 300 mg in 240 mL of D5W, NS, D5/NS, LR, or other compatible IV solution to yield 1 mg/mL.

ADMINISTER: **Direct:** Give a 20-mg dose slowly over 2 min. ▪ Maximum hypotensive effect occurs 5–15 min after each administration. **Continuous:** Normal rate is 2 mg/min. ▪ Controlled infusion pump device is recommended for maintaining accurate flow rate during IV infusion. ▪ Keep patient supine when receiving labetalol IV. ▪ Take BP immediately before administration. Rate is adjusted according to BP response. ▪ Discontinue drug once the desired BP is attained.

INCOMPATIBILITIES **Solution/additive: Sodium bicarbonate, ceftriaxone, tenecteplase. Y-site: Amphotericin B cholesteryl, cefoperazone, furosemide, heparin, nafcillin, thiopental, warfarin.**

L

▪ Store at 2°–30° C (36°–86° F) unless otherwise advised. Do not freeze. ▪ Protect tablets from moisture.

ADVERSE EFFECTS (≥1%) **CNS:** Dizziness, fatigue/malaise, headache, tremors, transient paresthesias (especially scalp tingling), hypoesthesia (numbness) following IV, mental depression, drowsiness, sleep disturbances, nightmares. **CV:** *Postural hypotension,* angina pectoris, palpitation, bradycardia, syncope, pedal or peripheral edema, pulmonary edema, CHF, flushing, cold extremities, arrhythmias (following IV), paradoxical hypertension (patients with pheochromocytoma). **Special Senses:** Dry eyes, vision disturbances, nasal stuffiness, rhinorrhea. **GI:** Nausea, vomiting, dyspepsia, constipation, diarrhea, taste disturbances, cholestasis with or without jaundice, increases in serum transaminases, dry mouth. **Urogenital:** Acute urinary retention, difficult micturition, impotence, ejaculation failure, loss of libido, Peyronie's disease. **Respiratory:** Dyspnea, <u>bronchospasm</u>. **Skin:** Rashes of various types, increased sweating, pruritus. **Body as a Whole:** Myalgia, muscle cramps, toxic myopathy, antimitochondrial antibodies, positive antinuclear antibodies (ANA), SLE syndrome, pain at IV injection site.

DIAGNOSTIC TEST INTERFERENCE False increases in ***urinary catecholamines*** when measured by ***nonspecific trihydroxyindole (THI) reaction*** (due to labetalol metabolites) but not with specific ***radioenzymatic*** or ***high-performance liquid chromatography assay techniques.***

INTERACTIONS Drug: Cimetidine may increase effects of labetalol; **glutethimide** decreases effects of labetalol; **halothane** adds to hypotensive effects; may mask symptoms of hypoglycemia caused by ORAL SULFONYLUREAS, **insulin;** BETA AGONISTS antagonize effects of labetalol.

PHARMACOKINETICS Absorption: Readily from GI tract, only 25% reaches systemic circulation due to first pass metabolism. **Onset:** 20 min–2 h PO; 2–5 min IV. **Peak:** 1–4 h PO; 5–15 min IV. **Duration:** 8–24 h PO; 2–4 h IV. **Distribution:** Crosses placenta; distributed into breast milk. **Metabolism:** In liver (CYP-2D6). **Elimination:** 60% in urine, 40% in bile. **Half-Life:** 3–8 h.

NURSING IMPLICATIONS

Assessment & Drug Effects

▪ Monitor BP and pulse during dosage adjustment period. Use standing BP as indicator for making dosage adjustments for oral drugs and assessing patient's tolerance of dosage increases. Take after patient stands for 10 min. Clarify with physician.

- Monitor BP at 5 min intervals for 30 min after IV administration; then at 30 min intervals for 2 h; then hourly for about 6 h; and as indicated thereafter.
- Monitor diabetic patients closely; drug may mask usual cardiovascular response to acute hypoglycemia (e.g., tachycardia).
- Maintain patient in supine position for at least 3 h after IV administration. Then determine patient's ability to tolerate elevated and upright positions before allowing ambulation. Manage this slowly.
- Lab tests: Periodic liver function tests.

Patient & Family Education

- Note: Postural hypotension is most likely to occur during peak plasma levels (i.e., 2–4 h after drug administration).
- Make all position changes slowly and in stages, particularly from lying to upright position. Older adult patients are especially sensitive to hypotensive effects.
- Do not drive or engage in other potentially hazardous activities until response to drug is known.
- Diabetics should closely monitor blood sugar for loss of glycemic control.
- Do not abruptly stop taking this drug. It is usually discontinued gradually.

LACOSAMIDE

(lac-os′a-mide)

Vimpat
Classification: ANTICONVULSANT
Therapeutic: ANTICONVULSANT
Pregnancy Category: C
Controlled Substance: Schedule V

AVAILABILITY 50 mg, 100 mg, 150 mg, 200 mg tablets; 200 mg/20 mL single dose vial.

ACTION & *THERAPEUTIC EFFECT* Lacosamide selectively enhances slow inactivation of voltage-gated sodium channels, thus stabilizing hyper-excitable membranes and inhibiting repetitive neuronal firing. *Decreases frequency of partial-onset seizures in those treated with multiple antiepileptic drugs.*

USES Adjunctive therapy in the treatment of partial-onset seizures in patients 18 y or older.

UNLABELED USES Neuropathic pain.

CONTRAINDICATIONS Severe hepatic impairment; suicidal ideation; lactation. Safety and effectiveness in children younger than 17 y is not established.

CAUTIOUS USE History of multiorgan hypersensitivity reactions; CrCl 30 mL/min or less; renal disease; mild to moderate hepatic impairment; history of suicidal tendencies, history of chronic depression; cardiovascular disease, cardiac conduction problems (e.g. second-degree AV block); myocardial ischemia, heart failure; seizure disorders; diabetic neuropathy; older adults; pregnancy (category C).

ROUTE & DOSAGE

Partial-Onset Seizures
Adult: **PO or IV** 50 mg b.i.d.; may increase by 100 mg/day qwk to

L

100–200 mg b.i.d. Note: Patients may be switched from PO to IV (or vice versa) using equivalent doses and administration frequency.

Hepatic Impairment Dosage Adjustment

Mild to moderate impairment: Maximum daily dose of 300 mg
Severe impairment: Not recommended

Renal Impairment Dosage Adjustment

CrCl less than 30 mL/min: Maximum daily dose of 300 mg

L

ADMINISTRATION

Oral

- Do not abruptly stop medication; it should be withdrawn gradually, over a minimum of 1 wk.
- Store tablets at 15°–30° C (59°–86° F).

Intravenous

PREPARE: **IV Infusion:** May give undiluted or diluted in NS, D5W, LR.
ADMINISTER: **IV Infusion:** Give over 30–60 min.
INCOMPATIBILITIES **Solution/additive:** Do not mix with other drugs.

- May be stored diluted for up to 26 h at 15°–30° C (59°–86° F).

ADVERSE EFFECTS (≥1%) **Body as a Whole:** Asthenia, contusion, *fatigue*, gait disturbance, injection site pain and irritation, skin laceration. **CNS:** *Ataxia*, balance disorder, depression, *dizziness, headache*, memory impairment, nystagmus, somnolence, tremor, vertigo. **GI:** Diarrhea, *nausea*, vomiting. **Skin:** Pruritus. **Special Senses:** *Blurred vision, diplopia*.

INTERACTIONS Drug: May prolong QT interval when given with other drugs known to affect QT interval (e.g., ANTIARRYTHMICS, **astemizole, bepridil, droperidol**).

PHARMACOKINETICS Absorption: Approximately 100% oral absorption. **Peak:** 1–4 h. **Distribution:** Less than 15% protein bound. **Metabolism:** Hepatic oxidation to less active metabolite. **Elimination:** Primarily fecal (95%). **Half-Life:** 13 h.

NURSING IMPLICATIONS

Assessment & Drug Effects

- Monitor for and record all seizure activity.
- Monitor for and report promptly suicidal behavior and ideation.
- Monitor closely patients with known cardiac conduction abnormalities. Baseline and periodic ECGs are recommended
- Lab test: Periodic CBC with differential, especially with long-term therapy.
- Monitor older adults for adverse reactions after each upward dose titration. Institute safety precautions as needed to avoid injury from falls.

Patient & Family Education

- Exercise caution with hazardous activities until reaction to drug is known.
- Report promptly feelings of depression, unusual changes in mood or behavior, or thoughts of inflicting harm to self.
- Report bothersome neurologic symptoms such as dizziness, loss of balance, and blurred vision.
- Do not abruptly stop taking this drug. It **must be** tapered off.

LACTULOSE

(lak′tyoo-lose)

Cephulac, Chronulac

Classifications: HYPEROSMOTIC LAXATIVE; NEUROLOGIC

Therapeutic: LAXATIVE; AMMONIUM DETOXICANT

Pregnancy Category: B

AVAILABILITY 10 g/15 mL solution, syrup

ACTION & *THERAPEUTIC EFFECT* Reduces blood ammonia by acidifying colon contents, thus retarding diffusion of nonionic ammonia (NH_3) from colon to blood while promoting its migration from blood to colon. In the acidic colon, NH_3 is converted to nonabsorbable ammonium ions (NH^{4+}) and is then expelled in feces. *Osmotic effect of lactulose moves water from plasma to intestines, softening stools, and stimulates peristalsis by pressure from water content of stool. Decreases blood ammonia in a patient with hepatic encephalopathy. Effectiveness is marked by improved EEG patterns and mental state (clearing of confusion, apathy, and irritation).*

USES Prevention and treatment of portal-systemic encephalopathy (PSE), including stages of hepatic precoma and coma, and by prescription for relief of chronic constipation.

UNLABELED USES To restore regular bowel habit posthemorrhoidectomy; to evacuate bowel in older adult patients with severe constipation after barium studies; and for treatment of chronic constipation in children.

CONTRAINDICATIONS Low galactose diet.

CAUTIOUS USE Diabetes mellitus; concomitant use with electrocautery procedures (proctoscopy, colonoscopy); older adult and debilitated patients; pediatric use; pregnancy (category B), lactation.

ROUTE & DOSAGE

Prevention and Treatment of Portal-Systemic Encephalopathy

Adult: **PO** 30–45 mL t.i.d. or q.i.d. adjusted to produce 2–3 soft stools/day

Adolescent/Child: **PO** 40–90 mL/day in divided doses adjusted to produce 2–3 soft stools/day

Infant: **PO** 2.5–10 mL/day in 3–4 divided doses adjusted to produce 2–3 soft stools/day

Management of Acute Portal-Systemic Encephalopathy

Adult: **PO** 30–45 mL q1–2h until laxation is achieved, then adjusted to produce 2–3 soft stools/day **Rectal** 300 mL diluted with 700 mL water given via rectal balloon catheter, and retained for 30–60 min, may repeat in 4–6 h if necessary or until patient can take PO

Chronic Constipation

Adult: **PO** 30–60 mL/day prn

Child: **PO** 7.5 mL/day after breakfast

ADMINISTRATION

Oral

- Give with fruit juice, water, or milk (if not contraindicated) to increase palatability. Laxative effect is enhanced by taking with ample liquids. Avoid meal times.

Rectal

- Administer as a retention enema via a rectal balloon catheter. If so-

lution is evacuated too soon, instillation may be promptly repeated.
- Do not freeze. Avoid prolonged exposure to temperatures above 30° C (86° F) or to direct light. Normal darkening does not affect action, but discard solution that is very dark or cloudy.

ADVERSE EFFECTS (≥1%) **GI:** Flatulence, borborygmi, belching, abdominal cramps, pain, and distention (initial dose); *diarrhea* (excessive dose); nausea, vomiting, colon accumulation of hydrogen gas; hypernatremia.

INTERACTIONS Drug: LAXATIVES may incorrectly suggest therapeutic action of lactulose.

PHARMACOKINETICS Absorption: Poorly absorbed from GI tract. **Metabolism:** In gut by intestinal bacteria.

NURSING IMPLICATIONS

Assessment & Drug Effects
- In children if the initial dose causes diarrhea, dosage is reduced immediately. Discontinue if diarrhea persists.
- Promote fluid intake (1500–2000 mL/day or greater) during drug therapy for constipation; older adults often self-limit liquids. Lactulose-induced osmotic changes in the bowel support intestinal water loss and potential hypernatremia. Discuss strategy with physician.

Patient & Family Education
- Laxative action is not instituted until drug reaches the colon; therefore, about 24–48 h is needed.
- Do not self-medicate with another laxative due to slow onset of drug action.
- Notify physician if diarrhea (i.e., more than 2 or 3 soft stools/day) persists more than 24–48 h. Diarrhea is a sign of overdosage. Dose adjustment may be indicated.

LAMIVUDINE (Pr)

(lam-i-vu'deen)
Epivir, Epivir-HBV, Heptovir ♣
Classifications: ANTIRETROVIRAL; NUCLEOSIDE REVERSE TRANSCRIPTASE INHIBITOR (NRTI)
Therapeutic: ANTIRETROVIRAL; NRTI
Pregnancy Category: C

AVAILABILITY 100 mg, 150 tablets; 5 mg/mL, 10 mg/mL oral solution

ACTION & *THERAPEUTIC EFFECT* Lamivudine is a synthetic nucleoside analog reverse transcriptase inhibitor. It inhibits the transcription of the HIV viral RNA chain as well as the hepatitis B viral RNA chain. *Antiviral action is effective against HIV viruses and hepatitis B (HBV) viral infections.*

USES HIV infection in combination with zidovudine; treatment of chronic hepatitis B.

CONTRAINDICATIONS Hypersensitivity to lamivudine, lactation.
CAUTIOUS USE Renal impairment, renal failure; diabetes mellitus, diabetes mellitus; obesity; pregnancy (category C).

ROUTE & DOSAGE

HIV Infection
Adult: Epivir **PO** 150 mg b.i.d.
Child (3 mo–16 y): Epivir **PO** 4 mg/kg b.i.d. (max: 150 mg b.i.d.)

Renal Impairment Dosage Adjustment

CrCl 30–49 mL/min: 150 mg daily; 15–29 mL/min: 150 mg first dose, then 100 mg daily; 5–14 mL/min: 150 mg first dose, then 50 mg daily; less than 5 mL/min: 50 mg first dose, then 25 mg daily

Chronic Hepatitis B

Adult: Epivir-HBV **PO** 100 mg daily

Renal Impairment Dosage Adjustment

CrCl 30–49 mL/min: 100 mg first dose, then 50 mg daily; 15–29 mL/min: 100 mg first dose, then 25 mg daily; 5–14 mL/min: 35 mg first dose, then 15 mg daily; less than 5 mL/min: 35 mg first dose, then 10 mg daily

ADMINISTRATION

Oral

- Give Epivir b.i.d. in combination with AZT. The recommended dose for adults who weigh less than 50 kg (110 lb) is 2 mg/kg. Give Epivir-HBV daily; do NOT give in combination with AZT.
- Store solution at 2°–25° C (36°–77° F) tightly closed.

ADVERSE EFFECTS (≥1%) **CNS:** *Neuropathy, insomnia,* sleep disorders, *dizziness,* depression, *headache,* fatigue, *fever, chills.* **GI:** *Nausea, diarrhea,* vomiting, anorexia, abdominal pain, cramps, dyspepsia, increased LFTs (ALT, amylase), hepatomegaly with steatosis. **Hematologic:** Neutropenia, anemia, thrombocytopenia. **Musculoskeletal:** Myalgia, arthralgia, malaise, pain. **Skin:** Rash. **Respiratory:** Nasal symptoms, cough. **Metabolic:** Lactic acidosis.

INTERACTIONS Drug: Increases the C_{max} of **zidovudine. Trimethoprim-sulfamethoxazole** increases serum levels of lamivudine. Increased risk of lactic acidosis in combination with other REVERSE TRANSCRIPTASE INHIBITORS and ANTIRETROVIRAL AGENTS.

PHARMACOKINETICS Absorption: Rapidly absorbed from GI tract (86% reaches systemic circulation). **Distribution:** Low binding to plasma proteins. **Metabolism:** Minimal. **Elimination:** Excreted primarily unchanged in urine. **Half-Life:** 2–4 h.

NURSING IMPLICATIONS

Assessment & Drug Effects

- Monitor children closely for S&S of pancreatitis; if they occur, immediately stop drug and notify physician.
- Lab tests: Monitor CBC with differential, kidney & liver function, and serum amylase throughout therapy.
- Monitor for and report all significant adverse reactions.

Patient & Family Education

- Report any of the following immediately: Nausea, vomiting, anorexia, abdominal pain, jaundice.
- Note: The long-term effects of lamivudine are unknown.

LAMOTRIGINE

(la-mo'tri-geen)

Lamictal, Lamictal CD, Lamictal XR

Classification: ANTICONVULSANT
Therapeutic: ANTICONVULSANT
Pregnancy Category: C

AVAILABILITY 25 mg, 100 mg, 150 mg, 200 mg tablets; 2 mg, 5 mg, 25 mg chewable tablets; 25 mg, 50 mg, 100 mg, 200 mg orally disintegrating tablet; 25 mg, 50 mg, 100 mg, 200 mg extended release tablet

ACTION & *THERAPEUTIC EFFECT* May act by inhibiting the release of glutamate and aspartate, excitatory neurotransmitters at voltage-sensitive sodium channels, resulting in decreased seizure activity in the brain. *This stabilizes neuronal membranes. Effectiveness is measured by decreasing seizure activity.*

USES Adjunctive therapy for partial seizures in adults and children (older than 2 y). Generalized tonic–clonic, grand mal, or myoclonic seizures in adults, treatment of bipolar disorder (immediate release only).
UNLABELED USES Absence seizures, prevention of migraines.

L

CONTRAINDICATIONS Hypersensitivity to lamotrigine, suicidal ideation; development of any skin rash unless it is clearly not related to the drug; lactation. Safety and efficacy for treatment of seizures in children 2 y or younger are not established.
CAUTIOUS USE Renal insufficiency, concomitant administration of other anticonvulsants, bipolar disorder, history of suicidal tendencies; elderly; CHF, cardiac or liver function impairment; pregnancy (category C). Safety and efficacy of lamotrigine in the acute treatment of mood episode have not been established. Safety and efficacy have not been established in children with a mood disorder who are younger than 18 y.

ROUTE & DOSAGE

Partial Seizures, Patients Receiving Anticonvulsants Other Than Valproic Acid

Adult/Adolescent: **PO** Start with 50 mg daily for 2 wk, then 50 mg b.i.d. for 2 wk, may titrate up to 300–500 mg/day in 2 divided doses (max: 700 mg/day)
Child (2–12 y): **PO** 0.3 mg/kg/day in divided doses × 2 wk, then 0.6 mg/kg/day in divided doses × 2 wk (max: 15 mg/kg/day or 400 mg/day)

Partial Seizures, Patients Receiving Valproic Acid

Adult: **PO** Start with 25 mg every other day for 2 wk, then 25 mg daily for 2 wk, may titrate up to 150 mg/day in 2 divided doses (max: 200 mg/day)
Child (2–16 y): **PO** 0.15 mg/kg/day in divided doses × 2 wk, then increase to 0.3 mg/kg/day in divided doses × 2 wk (max: 5 mg/kg/day or 250 mg/day)

Bipolar Disorder, Patients Not Receiving Valproate or Carbamazepine

Adult: **PO** Start with 25 mg daily for 2 wk, then 50 mg daily for 2 wk, then 100 mg/day for 1 wk, then 200 mg daily

Bipolar Disorder, Patients Receiving Valproic Acid

Adult/Adolescent (older than 16 y): **PO** Start with 25 mg every other day for 2 wk, then 25 mg daily for 2 wk, then 50 mg daily for 1 wk, then 100 mg daily

Bipolar Disorder, Patients Receiving Carbamazepine

Adult/Adolescent (older than 16 y): **PO** Start with 50 mg daily for 2 wk, then 50 mg b.i.d. for 2 wk, then 100 b.i.d for 1 wk, then 150 mg b.i.d. for 1 wk, then 200 mg b.i.d.

Hepatic Impairment Dosage Adjustment

Reduce dose by 25% in patients with moderate or severe impairment (without ascites); reduce by 50% in patients with severe impairment and ascites

ADMINISTRATION

Oral

- Ensure that chewable tablets are chewed or crushed before being swallowed with a liquid.
- When discontinued, drug should be tapered off gradually over a 2-wk period, unless patient safety is at risk.

ADVERSE EFFECTS (≥1%) **CNS:** *Dizziness, ataxia, somnolence, headache,* aphasia, vertigo, confusion, slurred speech, irritability, depression, incoordination, hostility. **GI:** *Nausea,* vomiting, anorexia, abdominal pain, diarrhea, dyspepsia, constipation. **Urogenital:** Hematuria, dysmenorrhea, vaginitis. **Special Senses:** *Diplopia, blurred vision.* **Musculoskeletal:** Peripheral neuropathy, chills, tremor, arthralgia. **Skin:** Rash (including Stevens-Johnson syndrome, toxic epidermal necrolysis), urticaria, pruritus, alopecia, acne. **Respiratory:** *Rhinitis,* pharyngitis, cough.

INTERACTIONS Drug: Carbamazepine, phenobarbital, primidone, phenytoin, fosphenytoin, rifampin, ORAL CONTRACEPTIVES may decrease lamotrigine levels. **Valproic acid** may increase lamotrigine levels. Lamotrigine may decrease serum levels of **valproic acid.** May affect efficacy of ORAL CONTRACEPTIVES. Chronic **acetaminophen** use may affect serum concentrations of lamotrigine. **Herbal: Ginkgo** may decrease anticonvulsant effectiveness. **Evening primrose** oil may affect seizure threshold.

PHARMACOKINETICS Absorption: Readily absorbed from GI tract; 98% reaches systemic circulation. **Onset:** 12 wk. **Peak:** 1–4 h. **Distribution:** 55% protein bound; crosses placenta; distributed into breast milk. **Metabolism:** In liver to inactive metabolite. **Elimination:** Can induce own metabolism; excreted in urine. **Half-Life:** 25–30 h.

NURSING IMPLICATIONS

Assessment & Drug Effects

- Withhold drug if rash develops and immediately report to physician.
- Monitor the plasma levels of lamotrigine and other anticonvulsants when given concomitantly.
- Monitor patients with bipolar disorder for worsening of their symptoms and suicidal ideation. Withhold the drug and immediately report to physician.
- Monitor for adverse reactions when lamotrigine is used with other anticonvulsants, especially valproic acid.
- Be aware of drug interactions and closely monitor when interacting drugs are added or discontinued.

Patient & Family Education

- Do not take drug if a skin rash develops. Contact your physician immediately.
- Notify physician for any of the following: Worsening seizure control, skin rash, ataxia, blurred vision or diplopia, fever or flu-like symptoms.
- Do not drive or engage in other potentially hazardous activities until response to the drug is known.
- Use protection from sunlight or ultraviolet light until tolerance is known; drug increases photosensitivity.
- Women using oral contraceptives to avoid pregnancy should add a barrier contraceptive.

- Schedule periodic ophthalmologic exams with long-term use.
- Do not discontinue abruptly.

LANREOTIDE ACETATE

(lan-re'o-tide)

Somatuline Depot

Classifications: SOMATOSTATIN ANALOG; ANTIGROWTH HORMONE

Therapeutic: ACROMEGALY AGENT; SOMATOSTATIN HORMONE REPLACEMENT

Prototype: Octreotide

Pregnancy Category: C

AVAILABILITY 60 mg, 90 mg, 120 mg single-dose prefilled syringe

ACTION & *THERAPEUTIC EFFECT* An analog of natural somatostatin produced by the hypothalamus. Somatostatin inhibits the secretion of growth hormone (GH) that in turn inhibits secretion of insulin-like growth factor-1 (IGF-1). *Inhibition of IGF-1 suppresses proliferation of chondrocytes and stops bone growth.*

USES Long-term treatment of acromegaly in those who have not responded to surgery and/or radiotherapy, or for whom surgery and/or radiotherapy is not an option.

UNLABELED USES Treatment of symptoms, specifically diarrhea and cutaneous flushing, with carcinoid neuroendocrine tumors

CONTRAINDICATIONS Hypersensitivity to lanreotide; lactation. Safety and efficacy in children have not been established.

CAUTIOUS USE Cholelithiasis, gallbladder disease; gastroparesis; hypothyroidism; diabetes mellitus; cardiac disease; moderate to severe renal impairment; moderate to severe hepatic impairment; older adults; pregnancy (category C).

ROUTE & DOSAGE

Acromegaly

Adult: **Subcutaneous** 90 mg q4wk × 3 mo; then 60–120 mg q4wk depending on response

Hepatic/Renal Impairment Dosage Adjustment

Initial dose: 60 mg with moderate and severe impairment

ADMINISTRATION

Subcutaneous

- Remove from refrigeration 30 min before injection to allow to come to room temperature, but keep in sealed pouch.
- Inject deeply into subcutaneous tissue in the upper, outer quadrant of the buttock. Do not fold skin. Insert needle rapidly and to its full length at a right angle to skin. Alternate right and left sides.
- Store refrigerated and protect from light in original package.

ADVERSE EFFECTS (≥1%) **Body as a Whole:** Injection site pain. **CNS:** Headache. **CV:** Bradycardia. **GI:** *Abdominal pain, cholelithiasis,* constipation, *diarrhea,* flatulence, loose stools, *nausea,* vomiting. **Hematologic:** Anemia. **Metabolic:** Decreased weight. **Musculoskeletal:** Arthralgia. **Skin:** Pruritus.

INTERACTIONS Drug: BETA-BLOCKERS have an additive effect on the reduction of heart rate. Lanreotide may increase the bioavailability of **bromocriptine.** Coadministration may decrease the bioavailability of **cyclosporine.** Lanreotide may increase the plasma level of drugs metabolized by CYP 450 enzymes.

PHARMACOKINETICS Absorption: 69–79% depending on dose. **Peak:** Within 24 h. **Metabolism:** Extensive, only 5% excreted unchanged. **Elimination:** Stool (95%) and urine (5%). **Half-Life:** 23–30 days.

NURSING IMPLICATIONS

Assessment & Drug Effects

- Monitor cardiovascular status as bradycardia and hypertension are potential adverse effects.
- Lab tests: Baseline and periodic GH, IGF-1, blood glucose; baseline LFTs and renal function tests; periodic thyroid function tests, HCT and Hgb.
- Periodic gallbladder motility tests are recommended.
- Monitor diabetics for loss of glycemic control.

Patient & Family Education

- Ensure that proper technique for subcutaneous drug administration is utilized.
- Diabetics should monitor blood glucose values often as this drug may elevate or lower blood glucose.
- Report to physician severe pain in the upper right area of the stomach/abdomen, along with nausea and vomiting. These symptoms could indicate the presence of gallstones.

LANSOPRAZOLE

(lan′so-pra-zole)

Prevacid, Prevacid 24 HR, Prevacid IV

DEXLANSOPRAZOLE

Kapidex

Classifications: ANTISECRETORY; PROTON PUMP INHIBITOR
Therapeutic: ANTIULCER; ANTISECRETORY
Prototype: Omeprazole
Pregnancy Category: B

AVAILABILITY 15 mg, 30 mg sustained release capsules; 15 mg, 30 mg orally disintegrating tablets; 15 mg, 30 mg packets for suspension; 30 mg powder for injection; **Dexlansoprazole (delayed release):** 30 mg, 60 mg capsules

ACTION & *THERAPEUTIC EFFECT* Suppresses gastric acid secretion by inhibiting the H^+, K^+-ATPase enzyme [the acid (proton H^+) pump] in the parietal cells. *Suppresses gastric acid formation in the stomach.*

USES Short-term treatment of duodenal ulcer (up to 4 wk) and erosive esophagitis (up to 8 wk), pathologic hypersecretory disorders, gastric ulcers; in combination with antibiotics for *Helicobacter pylori.* Gastroesophageal reflux disease (GERD).

CONTRAINDICATIONS Hypersensitivity to lansoprazole or dexlansoprazole; gastric malignancy; severe hepatic impairment (Child-Pugh class B), proton pump inhibitors (PPIs) hypersensitivity, lactation, infants.

CAUTIOUS USE Mild to moderat hepatic disease (Child-Pugh class A and B), pregnancy (category B).

ROUTE & DOSAGE

Duodenal Ulcer

Adult: **PO** 15 mg once daily × 4 wk (treatment) or longer (maintenance)

Erosive Esophagitis

Adult: **PO** 30 mg once daily × 8 wk, then decrease to 15 mg once daily **IV** 30 mg once daily for up to 7 days

Healing Erosive Esophagitis (Dexlansoprazole)

Adult: **PO** 60 mg daily for up to 8 wk

Maintenance of Healed Erosive Esophagitis (Dexlansoprazole)

Adult: **PO** 30 mg daily

Non-Erosive GERD (Dexlansoprazole)

Adult: **PO** 30 mg daily for 4 wk

GERD

Adult: **PO** 15 mg once daily for up to 8 wk
Child (1–11 y): **PO** 15–30 mg daily for up to 12 wk (max: 30 mg/day)

Hypersecretory Disorder

Adult: **PO** 60 mg once daily (max: 120 mg/day in divided doses), may need to be adjusted for hepatic impairment

NSAID-Associated Gastric Ulcer

Adult: **PO** 30 mg daily for up to 8 wk

H. pylori

Adult: **PO** 30 mg b.i.d. × 2 wk, in combination with antibiotics

Hepatic Impairment Dosage Adjustment

Dose reduction required in severe hepatic disease. Child-Pugh class B: Max dose 30 mg/day (dexlansoprazole).

ADMINISTRATION

Oral

- *All forms:* Administer dosage 30 min a.c. Give once daily dose before breakfast.
- Give at least 30 min prior to any concurrent sucralfate therapy.
- Do not crush or chew capsules. Capsules can be opened and granules sprinkled on food or mixed with 40 mL of apple juice and administered through an NG tube. Do not crush or chew granules.
- Note: Disintegrating tablets contain phenylalanine and should not be used for patients with PKU. Capsule and syrup formulations do not contain phenylalanine.

Intravenous

PREPARE: **IV Infusion:** Reconstitute by adding 5 mL of sterile water for injection to each 30 mg vial to yield 6 mg/mL. Swirl gently to mix. ▪ Further dilute in 50 mL of NS, LR, or D5W. If reconstituted with NS or LR, administer within 24 h. If reconstituted with D5W, administer within 12 h.

ADMINISTER: **IV Infusion:** Infuse over 30 min through the in-line filter provided. ▪ Use a dedicated line or a Y-site; flush Y-site with NS before and after administration. ▪ Do NOT give IV push. Immediately stop infusion if precipitation or discoloration occurs.

INCOMPATIBILITIES **Solution/additive & Y-site:** Do not administer with other drugs or diluents.

- Reconstituted solution can be held for 1 h at 25° C (77° F) before further dilution.

ADVERSE EFFECTS (≥1%) **CNS:** Fatigue, dizziness, headache. **GI:** Nausea, *diarrhea,* constipation, anorexia, increased appetite, thirst, elevated serum transaminases (AST, ALT). **Skin:** Rash.

INTERACTIONS Drug: May decrease **theophylline** levels. **Sucralfate** decreases lansoprazole bioavailability. May interfere with absorption of **ketoconazole, digoxin, ampicillin,** or IRON SALTS. Use with **warfarin** may increase INR. May alter **tacrolimus** concentration. **Food:** Food reduces peak lansoprazole levels by 50%.

PHARMACOKINETICS Absorption: Rapidly from GI tract after leaving stomach; unstable in acidic media. **Onset:** Acid reduction within 2 h; ulcer relief within 1 wk. **Peak:** 1.5–3 h. Dexlansoprazole has 2 peaks, at 1–2 h then at 4–5 h. **Duration:** 24 h. **Distribution:** 97% bound to plasma proteins. **Metabolism:** In liver via CYP2C19 and 3A4. **Elimination:** 14–25% in urine as metabolites; part of dose eliminated in bile and feces. **Half-Life:** 1.5 h.

NURSING IMPLICATIONS

Assessment & Drug Effects

- Lab tests: Monitor CBC, kidney and liver function tests, and serum gastric levels periodically.
- Monitor for therapeutic effectiveness of concurrently used drugs that require an acid medium for absorption (e.g., digoxin, ampicillin, ketoconazole).

Patient & Family Education

- Inform physician of significant diarrhea.

LANTHANUM CARBONATE

(lan-tha′num)

Fosrenol

Classifications: ELECTROLYTE AND WATER BALANCE AGENT; PHOSPHATE BINDER

Therapeutic: PHOSPHATE BINDER

Prototype: Sevelamer hydrochloride

Pregnancy Category: C

AVAILABILITY 250 mg, 500 mg, 750 mg, 1 g chewable tablets

ACTION & *THERAPEUTIC EFFECT* Lanthanum is used for the management of hyperphosphatemia in end-stage renal disease; it is a calcium/aluminum-free phosphate binding agent. It has a higher affinity for binding to phosphate than calcium or aluminum. Low systemic absorption minimizes the risk of aluminum intoxication and hypercalcemia. Lanthanum decreases phosphate absorption from the diet. Dietary phosphate bound to lanthanum carbonate is excreted in the feces. *Lowers serum phosphate.*

USES Reduce serum phosphate levels in patients with end-stage renal disease.

CONTRAINDICATIONS Prior hypersensitivity to lanthanum carbonate; children younger than 18 y.

CAUTIOUS USE Bowel obstruction, Crohn's disease, acute peptic ulcer, ulcerative colitis; lactation; pregnancy (category C).

ROUTE & DOSAGE

Hyperphosphatemia

Adult: **PO** 250–500 mg t.i.d. with or immediately after meals; may titrate up every 2–3 wk in increments of 750 mg/day to achieve acceptable serum phosphate levels (max: 3750 mg/day)

ADMINISTRATION

Oral

- Give with or immediately after a meal.
- Tablets **must be** chewed completely before swallowing. Whole tablets should not be swallowed.
- Store at 15°–30° C (59°–86° F).

ADVERSE EFFECTS (≥1%) **CNS:** Headache. **CV:** Hypotension. **GI:** *Nausea, vomiting, diarrhea,* abdominal pain, constipation. **Respiratory:** Bronchitis, rhinitis. **Other:** Dialysis graft occlusion.

PHARMACOKINETICS Absorption: Minimal from GI tract. **Metabolism:** Not metabolized. **Elimination:** In feces. **Half-Life:** 53 h.

NURSING IMPLICATIONS

Assessment & Drug Effects

- Monitor for dialysis graft occlusion, as lanthanum therapy may increase occlusion risk.
- Lab tests: Serum phosphate levels during dosage titration and regularly throughout treatment; periodic serum calcium, bicarbonate, and chloride.

Patient & Family Education

- Chew chewable tablets completely, then swallow.
- Report promptly any of the following: Headache, drowsiness, dizziness, fainting, confusion, irritability, nausea, vomiting, or loss of appetite.

L

LAPATINIB DITOSYLATE

(la-pa'ti-nib di-toe'si-late)

Tykerb

Classifications: BIOLOGICAL RESPONSE MODIFIER; ANTINEOPLASTIC; EPIDERMAL GROWTH FACTOR RECEPTOR-TYROSINE KINASE INHIBITOR (EGFR-TKI)

Therapeutic: ANTINEOPLASTIC

Prototype: Gefitinib

Pregnancy Category: D

AVAILABILITY 250 mg tablets

ACTION & *THERAPEUTIC EFFECT* An inhibitor of intracellular tyrosine kinase domains of both epidermal growth factor receptors [EGFR (ErbB1) and HER2 (ErbB2)] required for cell proliferation of certain breast cancers. *Inhibits ErbB-driven tumor cell growth in those who are positive for the HER2 receptor.*

USES Treatment of advanced or metastatic breast cancer in patients whose tumor overexpresses the human epidermal receptor type 2 (HER2) protein and who have received prior therapy including an anthracycline, a taxane, and trastuzumab.

CONTRAINDICATIONS Hypersensitivity to lapatinib, capecitabine, doxifluridine, 5-FU; decreased left ventricular ejection fraction (LVEF) of grade 1, that is below lower limits of normal (LLN); myelosuppression; dihydropyrimidine dehydrogenase (DPD) deficiency; active infection; jaundice; severe renal failure or impairment; hypokalemia, hypomagnesemia; females of childbearing age; pregnancy (category D), lactation; children younger than 18 y.

CAUTIOUS USE Moderate to severe hepatic impairment; coronary artery disease; angina, cardiac arrhythmias, congenital QT_c prolongation syndrome.

ROUTE & DOSAGE

Breast Cancer

Adult: **PO** 1250 mg daily on days 1–21 with capecitabine 2000 mg/m^2/day q12h on days 1–14; repeat in 21-day cycle.

Hepatic Impairment Dosage Adjustment

750 mg/day with severe hepatic function impairment (Child-Pugh class C).

ADMINISTRATION

Oral

- Give lapatinib at least 1 h before/after a meal.
- Give capecitabine with food or within 30 min after food.
- Note that concurrent use with strong CYP3A4 inhibitors/inducers should be avoided (see Drug Interactions). If concurrent use is necessary, dosage adjustments are required.
- Store at 15°–30° C (59°–86° F) in a tightly closed container.

ADVERSE EFFECTS (≥1%) **CNS:** Insomnia, *fatigue*. **CV:** QT prolongation. **GI:** *Diarrhea*, dyspepsia, mucosal inflammation, *nausea*, stomatitis, *vomiting*. **Hematologic:** Neutropenia, thrombocytopenia. **Metabolic:** Elevated ALT and AST levels, hyperbilirubinemia. **Musculoskeletal:** Back pain, pain in extremities. **Respiratory:** Dyspnea, pneumonitis. **Skin:** Dry skin, *palmar-plantar erythrodysesthesia, rash*.

INTERACTIONS Drug: INHIBITORS OF CYP3A4 (**ketoconazole, clarithromycin, atazanavir, indinavir, nefazodone, nelfinavir, ritonavir, saquinavir, telithromycin, voriconazole**) will increase lapatinib plasma level. INDUCERS OF CYP3A4 (**dexamethasone, phenytoin, carbamazepine, rifampin, rifabutin, rifapentine, phenobarbital**) will decrease lapatinib plasma level. Lapatinib can increase plasma levels of **theophylline** and **warfarin. Food: Grapefruit juice** may increase the plasma level of lapatinib; co-administration with food increases lapatinib plasma levels. **Herbal: St. John's wort** will decrease plasma levels of lapatinib.

PHARMACOKINETICS Peak: 4 h. **Distribution:** 9% Plasma protein bound. **Metabolism:** Extensive hepatic metabolism. **Elimination:** Fecal (major) and renal (minor). **Half-Life:** 24 h.

NURSING IMPLICATIONS

Assessment & Drug Effects

- Prior to initiating therapy, hypokalemia and hypomagnesemia should be corrected.
- Monitor cardiac status (i.e., LV ejection fraction, ECG with QT measurement) throughout therapy.
- Monitor for and report severe diarrhea as it may cause dehydration and serious electrolyte imbalances.
- Lab tests: Baseline and periodic serum electrolytes; periodic CBC with differential and platelet count, Hgb, Hct, LFTs.
- Monitor for theophylline and warfarin toxicity with concurrent use.

Patient & Family Education

- Adhere to directions regarding medication and food.
- Report promptly any of the following: Palpitations, shortness of breath, severe diarrhea.
- Do not eat grapefruit or drink grapefruit juice while taking lapatinib.
- Do not take St. John's wort or OTC medications for stomach ulcers while taking lapatinib unless approved by the physician.
- Women are advised to use effective means of contraception while taking lapatinib.

LARONIDASE

(la-ron'i-dase)

Aldurazyme

Classification: ENZYME REPLACEMENT THERAPY

Therapeutic: ENZYME REPLACEMENT THERAPY

Prototype: Pancrelipase
Pregnancy Category: B

AVAILABILITY 2.9 mg/5 mL injection

ACTION & *THERAPEUTIC EFFECT* Laronidase is a recombinant form of human alpha-L-iduronidase used for enzyme replacement therapy in individuals with mucopolysaccharidosis I (MPSI). This is an inherited lysosomal storage disease caused by deficiency of the enzyme alpha-L-iduronidase. *Replacement therapy for individuals lacking the enzyme alpha-L-iduronidase in mucopolysaccharidosis.*

USES Treatment of Hurler and Hurler-Scheie forms of mucopolysaccharidosis I (MPS I); treatment of moderate to severe Scheie form of MPS I.

L

CONTRAINDICATIONS Hypersensitivity to laronidase; children younger than 5 y.
CAUTIOUS USE Renal or hepatic dysfunction; acute illness; history of allergies, asthma; COPD or history of compromised respiratory function; hypersensitivity to drugs, especially recombinant forms; pregnancy (category B), lactation.

ROUTE & DOSAGE

Mucopolysaccharidosis
Adult/Child (older than 5 y): **IV** 0.58 mg/kg infused over 3–4 h once/wk

ADMINISTRATION

Intravenous

- Pretreatment with antipyretics and/or antihistamines 60 min prior to infusion is recommended.

PREPARE: **IV Infusion:** Determine volume of infusion based on the patient's body weight (100 mL if weight 20 kg or less or 250 mL if weight greater than 20 kg). ▪ Prepare IV infusion of 0.1% albumin (human) in NS injection as follows: 1) Remove and discard a volume of NS injection equal to the volume of albumin (human) to be added to the IV bag (for 100 mL infusion use 2 mL of 5% albumin or 0.4 mL of 25% albumin, for 250 mL infusion use 5 mL of 5% albumin or 1 mL of 25% albumin); 2) add the appropriate volume of albumin to the IV bag and gently rotate to mix; 3) withdraw and discard a volume of fluid from the IV bag equal to the volume of laronidase concentrate to be added; 4) slowly withdraw the required amount of laronidase from vials (avoid excessive agitation), then slowly add laronidase to the IV solution. ▪ Gently rotate to mix. Use immediately.

ADMINISTER: **IV Infusion:** Infuse initially at 10 mcg/kg/h; may increase q15min during first hour, as tolerated, to a max rate of 200 mcg/kg/h. ▪ Maintain max for remainder of the infusion (2–3 h). ▪ Use a PVC set with an in-line, low-protein-binding 0.2 micron filter.

INCOMPATIBILITIES **Solution/additive:** Do not recommend mixing or infusing with other drugs.

- Store at 2°–8° C (36°–46° F). Do not freeze or shake. Discard any unused drug.

ADVERSE EFFECTS (≥1%) **Body as a Whole:** Infusion reactions (flushing, fever, headache, rash), injection site pain, hypersensitivity reactions. **CNS:** Hyperreflexia, paresthesias. **CV:** Chest pain, hypotension, edema. **Hematologic:** Thrombocytopenia. **Respiratory:** Upper respiratory tract infection. **Skin:** Rash.

PHARMACOKINETICS Half-Life: 1.5–3.6 h.

NURSING IMPLICATIONS

Assessment & Drug Effects

- Monitor for infusion-related reactions. Slow or stop infusion and notify physician for any of the following: Cough, bronchospasm, dyspnea, urticaria, angioedema, pruritus, or other signs of hypersensitivity.
- Lab tests: Periodic platelet count.

Patient & Family Education

- Report promptly difficulty breathing, rash, or itching.

LATANOPROST (Pr)

(la-tan′o-prost)

Xalatan

Classifications: EYE PREPARATION; PROSTAGLANDIN

Therapeutic: PROSTAGLANDIN

Pregnancy Category: B

AVAILABILITY 0.005% solution

ACTION & *THERAPEUTIC EFFECT* Prostaglandin analog that is thought to reduce intraocular pressure (IOP) by increasing the outflow of aqueous humor. *Reduces elevated intraocular pressure in patients with open-angle glaucoma.*

USES Treatment of open-angle glaucoma, ocular hypertension, and elevated intraocular pressure (IOP).

CONTRAINDICATIONS Hypersensitivity to latanoprost or another component in the solution; intraocular infection; conjunctivitis.

CAUTIOUS USE Active intraocular inflammation such as iritis or uveitis; patients at risk for macular edema; hepatic or renal impairment; pregnancy (category B), lactation. Safety and effectiveness in children are not established.

ROUTE & DOSAGE

Glaucoma

Adult: **Ophthalmic** 1 drop in affected eye(s) daily in evening

ADMINISTRATION

Installation

- Ensure that contact lenses are removed prior to installation and not reinserted for 15 min after installation.
- Apply only to affected eye(s). Ensure that only one drop is instilled.
- Do not allow tip of dropper to touch eye.
- Wait at least 5 min before/after instillation of other eyedrops.
- Refrigerate at 2°–8° C (36°–46° F). Protect from light.

ADVERSE EFFECTS (≥1%) **Body as a Whole:** Headaches, asthenia, flu-like symptoms. **GI:** Abnormal liver function tests. **Skin:** Rash. **Special Senses:** *Conjunctival hyperemia, growth of eyelashes, ocular pruritus,* ocular dryness, visual disturbance, ocular burning, foreign body sensation, eye pain, pigmentation of the periocular skin, blepharitis, cataract, superficial punctate keratitis, eyelid erythema, ocular irritation, and eyelash darkening, eye discharge, tearing, photophobia, allergic conjunctivitis, increases in iris pigmentation (brown pigment), conjunctival edema.

INTERACTIONS Drug: Precipitation may occur if mixed with eyedrops containing **thimerosal;** space other EYE PREPARATIONS at least 5 min apart.

PHARMACOKINETICS Absorption: Absorbed through the cornea. **Onset:** 3–4 h. **Peak IOP Reduction:** 8–12 h. **Distribution:** Minimal systemic distribution. **Metabolism:** Hydrolyzed in aqueous humor to active form. **Elimination:** Renally excreted. **Half-Life:** 17 min.

NURSING IMPLICATIONS

Assessment & Drug Effects

- Withhold eyedrops and notify physician if acute intraocular inflammation (iritis or uveitis) or external eye inflammation are noted.
- Note that increased pigmentation of the iris and eyelid, and additional growth of eyelashes on the treated eye are adverse effects that may develop gradually over months to years.

Patient & Family Education

- Contact physician immediately if any ocular reaction occurs, especially conjunctivitis and lid reactions.
- Note: Increased pigmentation of the iris and eyelid, and additional growth of eyelashes on the treated eye, are possible adverse effects of this drug. Persons with light colored eyes receiving treatment to one eye may develop a darker eye.

L

LEFLUNOMIDE

(le-flu′no-mide)

Arava

Classifications: BIOLOGICAL RESPONSE MODIFIER; IMMUNOMODULATOR; ANTI-INFLAMMATORY

Therapeutic: DISEASE-MODIFYING ANTIRHEUMATIC DRUG (DMARD)

Pregnancy Category: X

AVAILABILITY 10 mg, 20 mg, 100 mg tablets

ACTION & *THERAPEUTIC EFFECT* An immunomodulator that demonstrates anti-inflammatory effects. Suppression of pyrimidine synthesis in T and B lymphocytes interferes with RNA and protein synthesis in cells that are involved in the inflammatory process within affected joints. Reduction in activity of these lymphocytes leads to reduced cytokine and antibody-mediated destruction of the synovial joints as well as attenuation of the inflammatory process. *Reduces the S&S of rheumatoid arthritis (RA), retards structural joint damage, and improves physical function.*

USES Active RA.

CONTRAINDICATIONS Hepatic disease; jaundice; lactase deficiency; hypersensitivity to leflunomide; patients with positive hepatitis B or C serology; malignancy, particularly lymphoproliferative disorders; severe immunosuppression; vaccination, infants; uncontrolled infection; pregnancy (category X), lactation.

CAUTIOUS USE Renal insufficiency; renal failure; alcoholism; immunosuppression; lactase deficiency; infection. Use in patients younger than 18 y has not been fully studied.

ROUTE & DOSAGE

Rheumatoid Arthritis

Adult: **PO** Initiate with a loading dose of 100 mg/day × 3 days, then maintenance dose of 20 mg daily, may decrease to 10 mg/day if higher dose is not tolerated

ADMINISTRATION

Oral

- Initiate with a 3-day loading dose followed by a lower maintenance dose.

ADVERSE EFFECTS (≥1%) **Body as a Whole:** Allergic reaction, asthenia, flu-like syndrome, infection, pain, back pain, arthralgia, leg cramps, synovitis, tenosynovitis. **CNS:** Dizziness, headache, paresthesias, peripheral neuropathy. **CV:** Hypertension, chest pain. **GI:** *Diarrhea,* increased LFTs (ALT and AST), abdominal pain, anorexia, dyspepsia, gastroenteritis, nausea, mouth ulcer, vomiting, weight loss, hepatotoxicity. **Metabolic:** Hypokalemia. **Respiratory:** Bronchitis, cough, respiratory infection, pharyngitis, pneumonia, rhinitis, sinusitis. **Skin:** Rash, alopecia, eczema, pruritus, dry skin, Stevens-Johnson syndrome, toxic epidermal necrolysis (rare). **Urogenital:** UTI.

INTERACTIONS Drug: Rifampin may significantly increase leflunomide levels; **cholestyramine, charcoal** decrease absorption; caution should be used with other hepatotoxic drugs.

PHARMACOKINETICS Absorption: Approximately 80% reaches systemic circulation. **Peak:** 6–12 h for active metabolite. **Distribution:** Greater than 99% protein bound. **Metabolism:** Metabolized primarily to M1 (active metabolite). **Elimination:** 43% in urine, 48% in feces. **Half-Life:** 19 days for active metabolite.

NURSING IMPLICATIONS

Assessment & Drug Effects

- Lab tests: Baseline screening to rule out hepatitis B or C; baseline and monthly liver enzymes × 12 mo, then every 6 mo thereafter.
- Monitor carefully for and report immediately S&S of infection; withhold leflunomide if infection is suspected.
- Monitor BP and weight periodically. Doses greater than 25 mg/day are associated with a greater incidence of side effects such as alopecia, weight loss, and elevated liver enzymes.

Patient & Family Education

- Use reliable contraception while taking leflunomide.
- Note: Both women and men need to discontinue leflunomide and undergo a drug elimination procedure prescribed by the physician BEFORE conception.
- Withhold drug if you develop an infection and notify the physician before resuming the drug.
- Notify physician about any of the following: Hair loss, weight loss, GI distress, rash, or itching.

LEPIRUDIN (Pr)

(le-pir′u-din)

Refludan

Classifications: ANTICOAGULANT; DIRECT THROMBIN INHIBITOR

Therapeutic: ANTITHROMBOTIC; THROMBIN INHIBITOR

Pregnancy Category: B

AVAILABILITY 50 mg powder for injection

ACTION & *THERAPEUTIC EFFECT* Highly specific direct inhibitor of thrombin, including thrombin entrapped within established clots. One molecule of lepirudin binds to one molecule of thrombin and thereby blocks the thrombogenic activity of thrombin. Increases PT/INR and aPTT values in relation to the dose given. *Has antithrombotic activity. Its effectiveness is indicated by aPTT value in target range of 1.5 to 2.5.*

USES Anticoagulation in patients with heparin-induced thrombocytopenia (HIT).

L

CONTRAINDICATIONS Hypersensitivity to lepirudin; intracranial bleeding; patients with increased risk of bleeding (e.g., recent surgery, CVA, advanced kidney impairment); lactation. Safety and efficacy in children not established.

CAUTIOUS USE Serious liver injury (e.g., cirrhosis); renal impairment; pregnancy (category B).

ROUTE & DOSAGE

Anticoagulation

Adult: **IV** 0.4 mg/kg initial bolus (max: 44 mg) followed by 0.15 mg/kg/h (max: 16.5 mg/h) for 2–10 days, adjust rate to maintain aPTT of 1.5–2.5

Renal Impairment Dosage Adjustment

CrCl 45–60 mL/min: Initial dose 0.2 mg/kg, then 0.075 mg/kg/h; 30–44 mL/min: Initial dose 0.2 mg/kg then 0.045 mg/kg/h; 15–29 mL/min: Initial dose 0.2 mg/kg, then 0.0225 mg/kg/h; less than 15 mL/min: Do not use

ADMINISTRATION

Intravenous

PREPARE: **Direct:** Reconstitute by adding 1 mL of sterile water for injection or NS to the 50-mg vial. ▪ To prepare bolus dose, withdraw reconstituted solution into a 10-mL syringe and dilute to 10 mL with sterile water for injection, NS or D5W to yield 5 mg/mL. **Continuous:** Transfer the contents of two reconstituted vials into 250 or 500 mL of D5W or NS to yield 0.4 or 0.2 mg/mL, respectively.

ADMINISTER: **Direct:** Give over 15–20 sec. **Continuous:** Give at a rate determined by body weight. If aPTT ratio is above the target range (1.5–2.5), stop infusion for 2 h, then restart at 50% of original rate (no additional IV bolus should be given). The aPTT ratio should be determined again in 4 h. ▪ If aPTT ratio is below the target range (1.5–2.5), the infusion rate should be stepped up in 20% increments. The aPTT ratio should be determined again 4 h later. ▪ Note: An infusion rate greater than 0.21 mg/kg/h is not advised without checking for coagulation abnormalities that might impair an appropriate aPTT response.

▪ Diluted solution is stable for 24 h during infusion. Store unopened vials at 2°–25° C (36°–77° F).

ADVERSE EFFECTS (≥1%) **CNS:** Intracranial bleeding. **CV:** Heart failure, ventricular fibrillation, pericardial effusion, MI. **GI:** Abnormal LFTs. **Hematologic:** Bleeding from injection site, anemia, hematoma, bleeding, hematuria, GI and rectal bleeding, epistaxis, hemothorax, vaginal bleeding. **Respiratory:** Pneumonia, cough, bronchospasm, stridor, dyspnea. **Skin:** Allergic skin reactions. **Body as a Whole:** Sepsis, abnormal kidney function, multiorgan failure.

INTERACTIONS **Drug:** **Warfarin**, NSAIDS, SALICYLATES, ANTIPLATELET AGENTS increases risk of bleeding. **Herbal:** **Feverfew, ginkgo, ginger, valerian** may potentiate bleeding.

PHARMACOKINETICS **Distribution:** Distributed primarily to extracellular compartment. **Metabolism:** By catabolic hydrolysis in serum. **Elimination:** 48% in urine. **Half-Life:** 1.3 h.

NURSING IMPLICATIONS

Assessment & Drug Effects

▪ Lab tests: Baseline aPTT prior to initiation of therapy (withhold

Common adverse effects in *italic*, life-threatening effects underlined; generic names in **bold**; classifications in SMALL CAPS; ♣ Canadian drug name; ⓟ Prototype drug

therapy and notify physician if baseline aPTT ratio 2.5 or greater); aPTT 4 h after start of therapy and at least once daily (more often with renal or hepatic impairment) thereafter.

- Give with extreme caution to those at increased risk for bleeding.
- Monitor carefully for bleeding events (e.g., from puncture wounds, hematoma, hematuria); and report immediately.
- Do not give oral anticoagulants until lepirudin dose has been reduced and aPTT ratio lowered to just above 1.5.

LETROZOLE

(le'tro-zole)

Femara

Classifications: ANTINEOPLASTIC; AROMATASE INHIBITOR

Therapeutic: ANTINEOPLASTIC

Prototype: Anastrozole

Pregnancy Category: D

AVAILABILITY 2.5 mg tablets

ACTION & *THERAPEUTIC EFFECT* Nonsteroid competitive inhibitor of aromatase, the enzyme that converts androgens to estrogens. It does not inhibit adrenal steroid synthesis. *Results in the regression of estrogen-dependent tumors.*

USES Advanced breast cancer in postmenopausal women following antiestrogen therapy, first-line treatment of locally advanced or metastasized breast cancer in postmenopausal women.

CONTRAINDICATIONS Hypersensitivity to letrozole; pregnancy (category D), pregnant women, women of childbearing age, premenopausal females, hormone replacement therapy (HRT).

CAUTIOUS USE Moderate to severe hepatic impairment; elderly; lactation. Safety and efficacy in children are not established.

ROUTE & DOSAGE

Breast Cancer

Adult: **PO** 2.5 mg daily

Hepatic Impairment Dosage Adjustment

Reduce the dose in severe hepatic impairment (Child-Pugh C class) by 50%

ADMINISTRATION

Oral

- Give without regard to food.

ADVERSE EFFECTS (≥1%) **Body as a Whole:** Fatigue, peripheral edema, asthenia, weight increase, *musculoskeletal pain,* arthralgia, angioedema. **CNS:** Headache, somnolence, dizziness. **CV:** Chest pain, hypertension, hypercholesterolemia. **GI:** Nausea, vomiting, constipation, diarrhea, abdominal pain, anorexia, dyspepsia. **Respiratory:** Dyspnea, cough. **Skin:** Hot flushes, rash, pruritus.

INTERACTIONS Drug: ESTROGENS, ORAL CONTRACEPTIVES could interfere with the pharmacologic action of letrozole.

PHARMACOKINETICS Absorption: Rapidly from GI tract. **Metabolism:** In liver (CYP3A4 and 2A6). **Elimination:** 90% in urine. **Half-Life:** 2 days.

NURSING IMPLICATIONS

Assessment & Drug Effects

- Lab tests: Periodically monitor serum calcium and CBC with differential.

- Monitor carefully for S&S of thrombophlebitis or thromboembolism; report immediately.

Patient & Family Education

- Notify physician immediately if S&S of thrombophlebitis develop (see Appendix F).

LEUCOVORIN CALCIUM

(loo-koe-vor′in)

LEVOLEUCOVORIN

(levo-loo-koe-vor′in)

Classifications: BLOOD FORMER; ANTIANEMIC

Therapeutic: ANTIANEMIC; CHEMOTHERAPEUTIC PROTECTANT

Pregnancy Category: C

L

AVAILABILITY 5 mg, 10 mg, 15 mg, 25 mg tablets; 50 mg, 100 mg, 350 mg vials

ACTION & *THERAPEUTIC EFFECT* Both leucovorin and levoleucovorin are reduced forms of folic acid. Unlike folic acid, they do not require enzymatic reduction by dihydrofolate reductase. Thus, they are readily available as an essential cell growth factor. During antineoplastic therapy, both forms of the drug prevent serious toxicity by protecting cells from the action of folic acid antagonists such as methotrexate. *Antidote against folic acid antagonists such as methotrexate.*

USES Folate-deficient megaloblastic anemias due to sprue, pregnancy, and nutritional deficiency when oral therapy is not feasible. Also to prevent or diminish toxicity of antineoplastic folic acid antagonists, particularly methotrexate. Also to treat advanced colorectal cancer when given concurrently with 5-fluorouracil (5-FU).

CONTRAINDICATIONS Hypersensitivity to folic acid or folinic acid; undiagnosed anemia, pernicious anemia, or other megaloblastic anemias secondary to vitamin B_{12} deficiency; intrathecal administration; oral form with stomatitis.

CAUTIOUS USE Renal dysfunction, third space fluid collection (i.e., ascites, pleural effusion), renal function impairment, or inadequate hydration; elderly; seizure disorders; pregnancy (category C), lactation.

ROUTE & DOSAGE

Megaloblastic Anemia

Adult/Child: **IV/IM** Up to 1 mg/day

Leucovorin Rescue for Methotrexate Toxicity

Adult/Child: **PO/IM/IV** 10 mg/m² q6h until serum methotrexate levels are reduced

Levoleucovorin Rescue

Adult/Adolescent/Child (older than 6 y): **IV** 7.5 mg q6h × 10 doses

Inadvertent Overdose of Methotrexate (Levoleucovorin)

Adult/Adolescent/Child (older than 6 y): **IV** 7.5 mg q6h until serum methotrexate levels are below 0.01 micromolar

Leucovorin Rescue for Other Folate Antagonist Toxicity

Adult/Child: **PO/IM/IV** 5–15 mg/day

Advanced Colorectal Cancer

Adult: **IV** 200 mg/m² followed by fluorouracil 370 mg/m²

ADMINISTRATION

Oral

- Note: Oral route is NOT recommended for doses higher than 25 mg or if patient is likely to vomit.

Intramuscular

- Give deep into a large muscle.

Intravenous

PREPARE: **Leucovorin Direct:** Give 1 mL (3 mg) ampules, which contain benzyl alcohol, undiluted. **Leucovorin IV Infusion:** For doses less than 10 mg/m^2, reconstitute each 50 mg in 5 mL (10 mg/1 mL in 10 mL) of bacteriostatic water for injection with benzyl alcohol as a preservative. ▪ For doses greater than 10 mg/m^2 reconstitute, as above, but with sterile water for injection without a preservative. Final concentration is 10 mg/mL. ▪Further dilute in 100–500 mL of IV solutions (e.g., D5W, NS, LR) to yield a concentration of 10–20 mg/mL of IV solution. **Levoleucovorin Direct:** Reconstitute the 50-mg vial with 5.3 mL NS injection to yield 10 mg/mL. ▪ May further dilute, immediately, in NS or D5W to 0.5–5 mg/mL. ▪Do not mix with other solutions or additives.

ADMINISTER: **Leucovorin/Levoleucovorin Direct:** Give 160 mg or fraction thereof over 1 min. **Leucovorin/Levoleucovorin IV Infusion:** Do not exceed direct IV rate. ▪Give more slowly if the volume of IV solution to be infused is large.

INCOMPATIBILITIES **Solution/additive:** **Fluorouracil.** **Y-site:** **Amphotericin B cholesteryl complex, droperidol, foscarnet, sodium bicarbonate.**

▪**Leucovorin:** Use solution reconstituted with bacteriostatic water within 7 days. ▪Use solution reconstituted with sterile water for injection immediately. **Levoleucovorin:** Solutions with NS may be held at 15°–30° C (59°–86° F) for up to 12 h. Solutions with D5W may be held at 15°–30° C (59°–86° F) for up to 4 h. ▪Protect from light.

ADVERSE EFFECTS (≥1%) **Body as a Whole:** Allergic sensitization (urticaria, pruritus, rash, wheezing). **Hematologic:** Thrombocytosis.

INTERACTIONS Drug: May enhance adverse effects of **fluorouracil;** may reverse therapeutic effects of **trimethoprim-sulfamethoxazole.**

PHARMACOKINETICS Onset: Within 30 min. **Peak:** 0.9 h (levoleucovorin). **Duration:** 3–6 h. **Distribution:** Crosses placenta; distributed into breast milk. **Metabolism:** In liver and intestinal mucosa to tetrahydrofolic acid derivatives. **Elimination:** 80–90% in urine, 5–8% in feces. **Half-Life:** 6 h; 0.77 h (levoleucovorin).

NURSING IMPLICATIONS

Assessment & Drug Effects

- Monitor neurologic status. Use of leucovorin alone in treatment of pernicious anemia or other megaloblastic anemias associated with vitamin B_{12} deficiency can result in an apparent hematological remission while allowing already present neurologic damage to progress.
- Lab tests: Baseline and daily serum creatinine and methotrexate levels; frequent urine pH to ensure urinary alkalinization (pH at or above 7).

Patient & Family Education

- Notify physician of S&S of a hypersensitivity reaction immediately (see Appendix F).

L

LEUPROLIDE ACETATE (Pr)

(loo-proe'lide)

Eligard, Lupron, Lupron Depot, Lupron Depot-Ped

Classification: GONADOTROPIN-RELEASING HORMONE (GnRH) ANALOG

Therapeutic: GnRH ANALOG

Pregnancy Category: X

AVAILABILITY 5 mg/mL injection; 3.75 mg, 7.5 mg, 11.25 mg, 15 mg, 22.5 mg, 30 mg microspheres for injection (depot formulations)

ACTION & *THERAPEUTIC EFFECT* Occupies and desensitizes pituitary GnRH receptors, resulting initially in release of gonadotropins LH and FSH and stimulation of ovarian and testicular steroidogenesis. ***Antitumor effect:*** *May inhibit growth of hormone-dependent tumors as indicated by reduction in concentrations of PSA and serum testosterone to levels equal to or less than pretreatment levels.* ***Contraceptive effect:*** *By inhibiting gonadotropin release, ovulation or spermatogenesis is suppressed. Has antitumor effect in males and contraceptive effects in both males and females.*

USES Palliative treatment of advanced prostatic carcinoma as alternative to orchiectomy or estrogen administration; endometriosis; anemia caused by leiomyomata.

UNLABELED USES Breast cancer; male contraceptive; delayed puberty.

CONTRAINDICATIONS Known hypersensitivity to benzyl alcohol, GnRH analog hypersensitivity; following orchiectomy or estrogen therapy; metastatic cerebral lesions; menstruation, abnormal vaginal bleeding, pregnancy (category X), lactation.

CAUTIOUS USE Life-threatening carcinoma in which rapid symptomatic relief is necessary; osteoporosis; elderly.

ROUTE & DOSAGE

Palliative Treatment for Prostate Cancer

Adult: **Subcutaneous** 1 mg/day **IM** 7.5 mg/mo or 22.5 mg q3mo or 30 mg q4mo (depot preparation)

Endometriosis, Anemia

Adult: **IM** 3.75 mg qmo or 11.25 mg q3mo

Precocious Puberty

Child: **IM** Depot-Ped, 0.15–0.3 mg/kg q28days (min: 7.5 mg), titrate by 3.75-mg increments q4wk

ADMINISTRATION

Subcutaneous

- Do not use Depot-Ped form for subcutaneous injection.
- Rotate injection sites.

Intramuscular

- Prepare solution for Depot-Ped injection using a 22-gauge needle (or syringe provided by manufacturer), withdraw 1.5 mL of diluent from the supplied ampule and inject it into the vial. Shake well to form a uniform suspension. Withdraw entire contents and administer immediately.
- Do not administer parenteral drug formulation if particulate matter or discoloration is present.
- Refrigerate unopened vials. Store vial in use at room temperature for several months with minimal loss of potency. Protect from light and freezing.

ADVERSE EFFECTS (≥1%) **Body as a Whole:** *Disease flare (worsening of S&S of carcinoma),* injection site irritation, asthenia, fatigue, fever, facial swelling. **CNS:** Dizziness, pain, headache, paresthesia. **CV:** *Peripheral edema,* cardiac arrhythmias, MI. **Endocrine:** *Hot flushes, impotence, decreased libido,* gynecomastia, breast tenderness, amenorrhea, vaginal bleeding, thyroid enlargement, hypoglycemia. **GI:** Nausea, vomiting, constipation, anorexia, sour taste, GI bleeding, diarrhea. **Musculoskeletal:** Increased bone pain, myalgia. **Renal:** Increased hematuria, dysuria, flank pain. **Respiratory:** Pleural rub, pulmonary fibrosis flare. **Hematologic:** Decreased Hct, Hgb. **Skin:** Pruritus, rash, hair loss.

INTERACTIONS Drug: ANDROGENS, ESTROGENS counteract therapeutic effects.

PHARMACOKINETICS Absorption: Readily absorbed from subcutaneous or IM sites. **Metabolism:** By enzymes in hypothalamus and anterior pituitary. **Half-Life:** 3 h.

NURSING IMPLICATIONS

Assessment & Drug Effects

- Monitor PSA and testosterone levels in males with prostate cancer. A gradual rise in values after their decrease may signify treatment failure.
- Inspect injection site. If local hypersensitivity reactions occur (erythema, induration), suspect sensitivity to benzyl alcohol. Report to physician.
- Monitor I&O ratio and pattern. Report hematuria and decreased output. Carefully monitor voiding problems.

Patient & Family Education

- When used for prostate cancer, bone pain and voiding problems (i.e., symptoms of tumor obstruction) usually increase during first several weeks of continuous treatment but are transient. Hot flushes also may be experienced.
- Notify physician of neurologic S&S (paresthesia and weakness in lower limbs). Exercise caution when walking without assistance.
- When used for endometriosis, continuous treatment may cause amenorrhea and other menstrual irregularities.

LEVALBUTEROL HYDROCHLORIDE

(lev-al-bu′ter-ole)

Xopenex, Xopenex HFA

Classifications: SHORT-ACTING BETA-ADRENERGIC AGONIST; BRONCHODILATOR

Therapeutic: BRONCHODILATOR

Prototype: Albuterol

Pregnancy Category: C

AVAILABILITY 0.63 mg/3 mL, 1.25 mg/3 mL inhalation solution

ACTION & *THERAPEUTIC EFFECT* An isomer of albuterol with $beta_2$-adrenergic agonist properties; drug acts on the $beta_2$ receptors of the smooth muscles of the bronchial tree, thus resulting in bronchodilation. *Effective bronchodilator that decreases airway resistance, facilitates mucous drainage, and increases vital capacity.*

USES Treatment or prevention of bronchospasm in patients with reversible obstructive airway disease.

CONTRAINDICATIONS Hypersensitivity to levalbuterol or albuterol; angioedema; children younger than 6 y; lactation.

CAUTIOUS USE Cardiovascular disorders especially coronary insufficiency, cardiac arrhythmias, hyper-

L

tension, QT elongation, convulsive disorders; diabetes mellitus, diabetic ketoacidosis; older adults; seizures, status asthmaticus, tachycardia; hypersensitivity to sympathetic amines; hyperthyroidism, thyrotoxicosis; pregnancy (category C).

ROUTE & DOSAGE

Bronchospasm

Adult: **Inhalation** 0.63 mg by nebulization t.i.d. q6–8h, may increase to 1.25 mg t.i.d. if needed
Child (6–11 y): **Inhalation** 0.31 mg by nebulization t.i.d. q6–8h (max: 0.63 mg t.i.d.)

ADMINISTRATION

Inhalation

- Use vials within 2 wk of opening pouch. Protect vial from light and use within 1 wk after removal from pouch. Use only if solution in vial is colorless.

INCOMPATIBILITIES **Solution/additive:** Compatibility when mixed with other drugs in a nebulizer has not been established.

- Store at 15°–25° C (59°–77° F) in protective foil pouch.

ADVERSE EFFECTS (≥1%) **Body as a Whole:** Allergic reactions, flu syndrome, pain. **CNS:** Migraine, dizziness, nervousness, tremor, anxiety. **CV:** Tachycardia. **GI:** Dyspepsia. **Respiratory:** Increased cough, viral infection, rhinitis, sinusitis, turbinate edema, <u>paradoxical bronchospasm</u>. **Endocrine:** Increase in serum glucose.

INTERACTIONS Drug: BETA-ADRENERGIC BLOCKERS may antagonize levalbuterol effects; MAOI, TRICYCLIC ANTIDEPRESSANTS may potentiate levalbuterol effects on vascular system; ECG changes or hypokalemia may be exacerbated by LOOP or THIAZIDE DIURETICS.

PHARMACOKINETICS Onset: 5–15 min. **Duration:** 3–6 h. **Half-Life:** 3.3 h.

NURSING IMPLICATIONS

Assessment & Drug Effects

- Monitor for S&S of CNS or cardiovascular stimulation (e.g., BP, HR, respiratory status).
- Lab tests: Periodic serum potassium levels especially with coadministered loop or thiazide diuretics.
- Monitor diabetics for loss of glycemic control.

Patient & Family Education

- Seek medical advice immediately if a previously effective dose becomes ineffective.
- Report immediately to physician: Chest pains or palpitations, swelling of the eyelids, tongue, lips, or face; increased wheezing or difficulty breathing.
- Do not use drug more frequently than prescribed.
- Exercise caution with hazardous activities; dizziness and vertigo are possible side effects.
- Check with physician before taking OTC cold medication.

LEVETIRACETAM

(lev-e-tir′a-ce-tam)

Keppra, Keppra XR

Classification: ANTICONVULSANT
Therapeutic: ANTICONVULSANT
Pregnancy Category: C

AVAILABILITY 250 mg, 500 mg, 750 mg, 1000 mg tablets; 500 mg, 700 mg extended release tablets; 100 mg/mL oral solution; 100 mg/mL injection

ACTION & *THERAPEUTIC EFFECT*

The precise mechanism of antiepileptic effects is unknown. It is a broad spectrum antiepileptic agent that does not involve GABA inhibition. It prevents epileptiform burst firing and propagation of seizure activity. *Inhibits complex partial seizures and prevents epileptic and seizure activity.*

USES Adjunctive therapy for partial onset, myoclonic, tonic clonic seizures.

CONTRAINDICATIONS Hypersensitivity to levetiracetam; labor; pregnancy (category C), lactation; children younger than 4 y; **Extended release tablets:** children younger than 12 y; suicidal ideation.
CAUTIOUS USE Renal impairment; renal disease; renal failure; older adults; history of psychosis or depression, suicidal tendencies.

ROUTE & DOSAGE

Partial Onset Seizures

Adult/Adolescent (older than 16 y): **PO** 500 mg b.i.d., may increase by 500 mg b.i.d. q2wk (max: 3000 mg/day) **IV** 500 mg b.i.d., may increase q2wk (max: 3000 mg/day)
Child (4–15 y): **PO** 10 mg/kg b.i.d.; may increase by 20 mg/kg q2wk up to 60 mg/kg/day

Tonic Clonic Seizures

Adult/Adolescent (older than 16 y): **PO/IV** 500 mg b.i.d., increase by 1000 mg q2wk to dose of 3000 mg/day
Child (older than 6 y): **PO** 10 mg/kg b.i.d., increase by 20 mg/kg q2wk to dose of 60 mg/kg/day in 2 doses

Myoclonic Seizures

Adult/Adolescent/Child (at least 12 y): **PO** 500 mg b.i.d., increase by 1000 mg/day q2wk to recommended dose of 3000 mg/day in divided doses

Renal Impairment Dosage Adjustment

CrCl 50–80 mL/min: 500–1000 mg q12h (IR or IV form), 1000–2000 mg q24 (XR form); 30–49 mL/min: 250–750 mg q12h (IR or IV form), 500–1500 mg q24h (XR form); less than 30 mL/min: 250–500 mg q12h (IR or IV form), 500–1000 mg q24h (XR form)
Hemodialysis Dosage Adjustment: 500–1000 mg q24h; 250–500 mg supplemental following hemodialysis

Hepatic Impairment Dosage Adjustment

Child-Pugh class C: Reduce to 1/2 dose

ADMINISTRATION

Oral

- Dose increment changes should be made no more often than at 2-wk intervals.
- Taper dose if discontinued.
- Give supplemental doses to dialysis patients after dialysis.
- Store at 15°–30° C (59°–86° F).

ADVERSE EFFECTS (≥1%) **Body as a Whole:** *Asthenia, headache, infection,* pain. **CNS:** *Somnolence,* amnesia, anxiety, ataxia, depression, dizziness, emotional lability, hostility, nervousness, vertigo, paradoxical increase in seizures (as add-on therapy). **GI:** Anorexia. **Respiratory:** Cough, pharyngitis, rhinitis, sinusitis. **Special Senses:** Diplopia. **Other:** Increased symptoms of depression; suicidal ideation.

INTERACTIONS Drug: Levetiracetam does not affect **estrogen, warfarin,** or **digoxin** levels or affect levels of other antiepileptic drugs.

Sevelamer, colesevelam may decrease effectiveness.

PHARMACOKINETICS Absorption: Rapidly and almost completely absorbed. **Peak:** 1 h; steady-state 2 days. **Distribution:** Less than 10% protein bound. **Metabolism:** Minimal hepatic metabolism. **Elimination:** Renally eliminated. **Half-Life:** 7.1 h (9.6 h in older adults).

NURSING IMPLICATIONS

Assessment & Drug Effects

- Monitor individuals with a history of psychosis or depression for signs and symptoms of suicidal tendencies, suicidal ideation, and suicidality. Report any of these symptoms to the physician.
- Monitor and notify physician of difficulty with gait or coordination.
- Lab tests: Periodic CBC with differential, Hct and Hgb, LFTs.

Patient & Family Education

- Monitor for signs and symptoms of suicidality, especially in children with a history of depression or psychosis.
- Do not drive or engage in potentially hazardous activities until response to drug is known.
- Do not abruptly discontinue drug. MUST use gradual dose reduction/taper.

LEVOBETAXOLOL HYDROCHLORIDE

(le-vo-be-tax′oh-lol)
Betaxon
Pregnancy Category: C
See Appendix A-1.

LEVOBUNOLOL

(lee-voe-byoo′noe-lole)
Betagan
Pregnancy Category: C
See Appendix A-1.

LEVOCETIRIZINE

(lev-o-ce-tir′i-zeen)
Xyzal
Pregnancy Category: B
See Cetirizine.

LEVODOPA (L-DOPA) (Pr)

(lee-voe-doe′pa)
Classifications: DOPAMINE RECEPTOR AGONIST; ANTIPARKINSON
Therapeutic: ANTIPARKINSON
Pregnancy Category: C

AVAILABILITY 100 mg, 250 mg, 500 mg tablets and capsules

ACTION & *THERAPEUTIC EFFECT* A metabolic precursor of dopamine, a catecholamine neurotransmitter. Levodopa readily crosses the blood–brain barrier; it is believed that the dopamine level is severely reduced in parkinsonism. *Levodopa restores dopamine levels in extrapyramidal centers of the brain.*

USES Idiopathic Parkinson's disease, postencephalitic and arteriosclerotic parkinsonism, and parkinsonism symptoms associated with manganese and carbon monoxide poisoning.

UNLABELED USES To relieve pain of herpes zoster (shingles), liver coma (caused by cirrhosis or fulminating hepatitis), bone pain in metastatic breast carcinoma, adjunctive therapy in CHF.

CONTRAINDICATIONS Known hypersensitivity to levodopa; narrow-angle glaucoma patients with suspicious pigmented lesion or history of melanoma; acute psychoses, within 2 wk of use of MAOIs, suicidal ideation; lactation. Safe use in children is not established.

CAUTIOUS USE Cardiovascular, kidney, liver, or endocrine disease, history of MI with residual arrhythmias; peptic ulcer; convulsions; history of suicidal tendencies; depression; bipolar disorder; psychiatric disorders; chronic wide-angle glaucoma; diabetes; pulmonary diseases, bronchial asthma; pregnancy (category C).

ROUTE & DOSAGE

Parkinson's Disease

Adult: **PO** 500 mg to 1 g daily in 2 or more equally divided doses, may be increased by 100–750 mg q3–7days (max: 8 g/day); used in combination with carbidopa, decrease levodopa dose by 75–80%

ADMINISTRATION

Oral

- Give with food to reduce nausea. Absorption is decreased with high-protein meals.
- Crush tablets or empty capsule content into fruit juice as needed.
- Store in tight, light-resistant containers.

ADVERSE EFFECTS (≥1%) **CNS:** *Choreiform and involuntary movements,* increased hand tremor, bradykinetic episodes (on–off phenomena), trismus, grinding of teeth (bruxism), ataxia, muscle twitching, numbness, weakness, fatigue, headache, opisthotonos, confusion, agitation, anxiety, euphoria, insomnia, nightmares; psychotic episodes with paranoid delusions or hallucinations, severe depression, including suicidal tendencies, hypomania. **CV:** *Orthostatic hypotension;* palpitations, tachycardia, hypertension. **Special Senses:** *Blepharospasm,* diplopia, blurred vision, dilated pupils. **GI:** *Anorexia, nausea, vomiting,* abdominal distress, flatulence, dry mouth, dysphagia, sialorrhea; burning sensation of tongue, bitter taste, diarrhea or constipation; GI bleeding, hepatotoxicity. **Body as a Whole:** Flushing, increased sweating, weight gain or loss, edema, dark sweat or urine. **Urogenital:** Urinary retention or incontinence, increased sexual drive, priapism, postmenopausal bleeding. **Skin:** Skin rashes, loss of hair. **Respiratory:** Rhinorrhea, bizarre breathing patterns.

DIAGNOSTIC TEST INTERFERENCE Elevated ***BUN, AST, ALT, alkaline phosphatase, LDH, bilirubin, protein-bound iodine,*** serum level of ***growth hormone;*** decreased ***glucose tolerance; hypokalemia,*** decreased ***WBC, Hgb, Hct. Urine glucose:*** False-negative tests may result with use of ***glucose oxidase methods*** (e.g., ***Clinistix, TesTape***) and false-positive results with the ***copper reduction method*** (e.g., ***Clinitest***), especially in patients receiving large doses. It is reported that ***Clinistix*** and ***TesTape*** may be used if reading is taken at margin of wet and dry tape. ***Urinary ketones:*** There is possibility of false-positive tests by dipsticks [e.g., ***Acetest*** (equivocal), ***Ketostix, Labstix***]; ***Serum and urinary uric acid:*** False elevations by ***colorimetric methods,*** but not with ***uricase; Urinary protein:*** False increases by ***Lowry method; Urinary VMA:*** False decreases by ***Pisano method; Urinary catecholamine:*** False increases by ***Hingerty method. PKU urine test:*** Interference.

INTERACTIONS Drug: MAO INHIBITORS may precipitate hypertensive crisis; TRICYCLIC ANTIDEPRESSANTS augment postural hypotension; PHENOTHIAZINES, **haloperidol** may antagonize the therapeutic effects of levodopa; **pyridoxine** can reverse effects of levodopa; ANTICHOLINERGICS may exacerbate abnormal involuntary movements; **methyldopa** may increase toxic CNS effects; HALOGENATED GENERAL ANESTHETICS increase risk of arrhythmias. **Food:** Food decreases the rate and extent of levodopa absorption. **Herbal: Kava** may worsen parkinsonian symptoms.

PHARMACOKINETICS Absorption: Rapidly and well absorbed from GI tract; lower absorption if taken with food. **Peak:** 1–3 h. **Distribution:** Widely distributed in body. **Metabolism:** Most of drug is decarboxylated to dopamine in lumen of GI tract, liver, and serum. **Elimination:** 80–85% of dose excreted in urine in 24 h. **Half-Life:** 1 h.

NURSING IMPLICATIONS

Assessment & Drug Effects

- Monitor vital signs, particularly during period of dosage adjustment. Report alterations in BP, pulse, and respiratory rate and rhythm.
- Supervise ambulation as indicated. Orthostatic hypotension is usually asymptomatic, but some patients experience dizziness and syncope. Tolerance to this effect usually develops within a few months of therapy.
- Make accurate observations and report adverse reactions and therapeutic effects promptly. Rate of dosage increase is determined primarily by patient's tolerance and response to drug.
- Monitor all patients closely for behavior changes.
- Lab tests: Monitor blood glucose and HbA1C, CBC, Hgb and Hct, serum potassium, and liver and kidney function periodically.
- Report promptly muscle twitching and spasmodic winking (blepharospasm); these are early signs of overdosage. Patients on full therapeutic doses for longer than 1 y may develop such abnormal involuntary movements as well as jerky arm and leg movements. Symptoms tend to increase if dosage is not reduced.
- Report to physician any S&S of the on–off phenomenon sometimes associated with chronic management: Rapid unpredictable swings in intensity of motor symptoms of parkinsonism evidenced by increase in bradykinesia (attacks of "leg freezing" or slow body movement).
- Monitor mental status for S&S of drug-induced neuropsychiatric adverse reactions.

Patient & Family Education

- Do not take with high-protein foods. Also avoid high consumption of food sources of pyridoxine, including wheat germ, green vegetables, bananas, whole-grain cereals, muscular and glandular meats (especially liver), legumes.
- Do not take OTC preparations or fortified cereals unless approved by physician. Multivitamins, antinauseants, and fortified cereals usually contain vitamin B_6.
- Make positional changes slowly, particularly from lying to upright position, and dangle legs a few minutes before standing.
- Resume activities gradually, observing safety precautions to avoid injury. Elevation of mood and sense of well-being may precede objective improvement. Significant improvement usually occurs during second or third wk of therapy, but may not occur for 6 mo or more in some patients.

- Follow prescribed drug regimen. Sudden withdrawal of medication can lead to parkinsonism crisis (with return of marked rigidity, akinesia, tremor, hyperpyrexia) or neuroleptic malignant syndrome (NMS).
- A metabolite of levodopa may cause urine to darken and sweat to be dark-colored.

LEVOFLOXACIN

(lev-o-flox′a-sin)

Levaquin, Iquix, Quixin

Classifications: ANTIBIOTIC; QUINOLONE

Therapeutic: ANTIBIOTIC

Prototype: Ciprofloxacin

Pregnancy Category: C

AVAILABILITY 250 mg, 500 mg, 750 mg tablets; 25 mg/mL solution; 25 mg/mL injection; 0.5%, 1.5% ophth solution

ACTION & *THERAPEUTIC EFFECT*

A broad-spectrum fluoroquinolone antibiotic that inhibits DNA-gyrase, an enzyme necessary for bacterial replication, transcription, repair, and recombination. *Effective against many aerobic gram-positive and aerobic gram-negative organisms.*

USES Treatment of maxillary sinusitis, acute exacerbations of bacterial bronchitis, community-acquired pneumonia, uncomplicated skin/skin structure infections, UTI, acute pyelonephritis caused by susceptible bacteria; acute bacterial sinusitis; chronic bacterial prostatitis; bacterial conjunctivitis.

CONTRAINDICATIONS Hypersensitivity to levofloxacin and quinolone antibiotics; tendon pain, inflammation or rupture; syphilis; viral infections; phototoxicity; suicidal ideation; psychotic manifestations; manifestations of peripheral neuropathy; hypoglycemic reaction to drug; QT prolongation, hypokalemia; lactation. Safety and efficacy in infants younger than 6 mo are not established.

CAUTIOUS USE History of suicidal ideation; psychosis; anxiety, confusion, depression; known or suspected CNS disorders predisposed to seizure activity; risk factors associated with potential seizures (e.g., some drug therapy, renal insufficiency), dehydration, renal impairment (CrCl less than 50 mL/min); colitis; cardiac arrhythmias; older adults; pregnancy (category C).

ROUTE & DOSAGE

Infections

Adult: **PO** 500 mg q24h × 10 days **IV** 500 mg infused over 60 min q24h × 7–14 days

Community-Acquired Pneumonia

Adult: **PO/IV** 750 mg q24h × 5 days

Uncomplicated UTI

Adult: **PO/IV** 250 mg q24h × 14 days

Complicated UTI, Pyelonephritis

Adult: **PO/IV** 250 mg q24h × 10 days

Acute Bacterial Sinusitis

Adult: **PO/IV** 750 mg daily × 5 days

Chronic Bacterial Prostatitis

Adult: **PO/IV** 500 mg q24h × 28 days

Skin & Skin Structure Infections

Adult: **PO** 750 mg q24h × 14 days

Inhaled Anthrax

Adult/Adolescent/Child (weight at least 50 kg): **IV** 500 mg daily × 60 days

Infant/Child (older than 6 mo and weight less than 50 kg): **IV** 8 mg/kg q12h (no more than 250 mg/dose)

Renal Impairment Dosage Adjustment

For initial dose of 500 mg, adjust as follows: CrCl 20–50 mL/min: 250 mg q24h; less than 20 mL/min: 250 mg q48h
For initial dose of 750 mg, adjust as follows: CrCl 20–50 mL/min: 750 mg q48h; 10–19 mL/min: 500 mg q48h; less than 20 mL/min: 250 mg q48h

Bacterial Conjunctivitis

Adult: **Ophthalmic** Days 1–2, 1–2 drops in affected eye(s) q2h while awake (max: 8 times/day), days 3–7, 1–2 drops in affected eye(s) q4h while awake (max: 4 times/day)

ADMINISTRATION

Oral

- Do not give oral drug within 2 h of drugs containing aluminum or magnesium (antacids), iron, zinc, or sucralfate.

Intravenous

PREPARE: **Intermittent:** Withdraw the desired dose from 500 or 750 mg (25 mg/mL) single-use vial. ▪ Add to enough D5W, NS, D5/NS, D5/LR, or other compatible solutions to produce a concentration of 5 mg/mL [e.g., 500 mg (or 20 mL) added to 80 mL]. ▪ Discard any unused drug remaining in the vial.

ADMINISTER: **Intermittent:** Infuse 500 mg or less over 60 min. ▪ Infuse 750 mg over at least 90 min. ▪ Do NOT give a bolus dose or infuse too rapidly.

INCOMPATIBILITIES **Y-site:** Do not add any drugs to levofloxacin solution or infuse simultaneously through the same line (manufacturer recommendation). **Azithromycin, furosemide, heparin, indomethacin, insulin, nitroglycerin, nitroprusside, propofol.**

- Store tablets in a tightly closed container. IV solution is stable for 72 h at 25° C (77° F).

ADVERSE EFFECTS (≥1%) **CNS:** Headache, insomnia, dizziness. **GI:** Nausea, diarrhea, constipation, vomiting, abdominal pain, dyspepsia. **Skin:** Rash, pruritus. **Special Senses:** Decreased vision, foreign body sensation, transient ocular burning, ocular pain, photophobia. **Urogenital:** Vaginitis. **Body as a Whole:** Injection site pain or inflammation, chest or back pain, fever, pharyngitis. **Other:** Cartilage erosion.

DIAGNOSTIC TEST INTERFERENCE May cause false positive on ***opiate screening tests.***

INTERACTIONS Drug: Magnesium or **aluminum**-containing antacids, **sucralfate, iron, zinc** may decrease levofloxacin absorption; NSAIDS may increase risk of CNS reactions, including seizures; may cause hyper- or hypoglycemia in patients on ORAL HYPOGLYCEMIC AGENTS.

PHARMACOKINETICS Absorption: Rapidly from GI tract. **Peak:** PO 1–2 h. **Distribution:** Penetrates lung tissue, 24–38% protein bound. **Metabolism:** Minimally in the liver. **Elimination:** Primarily unchanged in urine. **Half-Life:** 6–8 h.

NURSING IMPLICATIONS

Assessment & Drug Effects

- Lab tests: Do C&S test prior to beginning therapy.

- Withhold therapy and report to physician immediately any of the following: Skin rash or other signs of a hypersensitivity reaction (see Appendix F); CNS symptoms such as seizures, restlessness, confusion, hallucinations, depression; skin eruption following sun exposure; symptoms of colitis such as persistent diarrhea; joint pain, inflammation, or rupture of a tendon.
- Monitor diabetics on oral hypolgycemic agents for loss of glycemic control.

Patient & Family Education

- Learn important indications for discontinuing drug and immediately notifying physician.
- If tendon pain occurs, discontinue the drug and notify the physician.
- Consume fluids liberally while taking levofloxacin.
- Allow a minimum of 2 h between drug dosage and taking any of the following: Aluminum or magnesium antacids, iron supplements, multivitamins with zinc, or sucralfate.
- Avoid exposure to excess sunlight or artificial UV light.
- Closely monitor blood glucose if taking oral hypoglycemic agents for diabetic control.

LEVOLEUCOVORIN

(levo-loo-koe-vor′in)

Fusilev

Pregnancy Category: C

See Leucovorin.

LEVONORGESTREL-RELEASING INTRAUTERINE SYSTEM

(lee′vo-nor-jes-trel)

Mirena

Classification: PROGESTIN HORMONE

Therapeutic: PROGESTIN

Prototype: Norgestrel

Pregnancy Category: X

AVAILABILITY 52 mg unit

ACTION & *THERAPEUTIC EFFECT* A progestogen that induces morphological changes in the endometrium including glandular atrophy, leukocytic infiltration, and decrease in glandular and stromal mitoses. Contraceptive effect may result by preventing follicular maturation and ovulation, thickening of the cervical mucus of the uterus, thus preventing passage of sperm into the uterus, or decreasing ability of sperm to survive in an environment of altered endometrium. *Effective contraceptive.*

USES Hormonal contraception.

CONTRAINDICATIONS Hypersensitivity to any component of the product; previously inserted IUD which has not been removed; suspicion of pregnancy, within 6 wk of giving birth or prior to complete involution of the uterus; history of ectopic pregnancy or any condition which predisposes to ectopic pregnancy; history of uterine anomalies which distort the uterine cavity; acute PID or history of PID unless there has been a subsequent intrauterine pregnancy; cervicitis or vaginitis or other lower genital tract infection; genital actinomycosis; woman or partner has multiple sex partners; vaginal bleeding of unknown etiology; postpartum endometriosis or septic abortion in past 3 mo; abnormal Pap or suspected/known cervical neoplasm; known or suspected carcinoma of

L

the breast; acute liver disease or liver tumor; immune deficiency states; pregnancy (category X).

CAUTIOUS USE Women at risk for venereal disease; anemia; diabetes mellitus; history of psychic depression; intermittent porphyria; fluid retention; history of migraines; impaired liver function; presence or history of salpingitis; venereal disease; genital bleeding of unknown etiology; coagulopathy; previous pelvic surgery.

ROUTE & DOSAGE

Contraception

Adult: **Intrauterine** Insert device on 7th day of menstrual cycle; may leave in place up to 5 y

ADMINISTRATION

Intrauterine

- Inserted only by physician or other person qualified by special training in the intrauterine system.

ADVERSE EFFECTS (≥1%) **CV:** Hypertension. **GI:** Abdominal pain, nausea. **Endocrine:** Breast tenderness/pain. **Hematologic:** Anemia. **Metabolic:** Weight gain. **CNS:** Depression, emotional lability, headache (including migraine), nervousness. **Skin:** Acne, alopecia, eczema. **Urogenital:** Amenorrhea, dysmenorrhea, leukorrhea, decreased libido, vaginal moniliasis, vulvovaginal disorders, cervicitis, dyspareunia.

INTERACTIONS Drug: No clinically significant interactions established.

PHARMACOKINETICS Peak: Few weeks. **Duration:** 5 y. **Distribution:** 86% protein bound. **Metabolism:** In liver. **Elimination:** In both urine and feces. **Half-Life:** 37 h.

NURSING IMPLICATIONS

Assessment & Drug Effects

- Monitor for decreased pulse, perspiration, or pallor during insertion. Keep patient supine until these signs have disappeared.
- Monitor BP especially with preexisting hypertension.

Patient & Family Education

- Report S&S of PID immediately: (e.g., prolonged or heavy bleeding, unusual vaginal discharge, abdominal or pelvic pain or tenderness, painful sexual intercourse, chills, fever, and flu-like symptoms).
- Report any of the following to physician immediately: Migraine (if not experienced before) or exceptionally severe headache, or jaundice.

LEVORPHANOL TARTRATE

(lee-vor'fa-nole)

Levo-Dromoran

Classifications: ANALGESIC; NARCOTIC (OPIATE AGONIST)

Therapeutic: NARCOTIC ANALGESIC

Prototype: Morphine sulfate

Pregnancy Category: B; D with long-time use or high doses

Controlled Substance: Schedule II

AVAILABILITY 2 mg tablets; 2 mg/mL injection

ACTION & *THERAPEUTIC EFFECT*
A potent synthetic morphine derivative with agonist activity only. Reported to cause less nausea, vomiting, and constipation than equivalent doses of morphine but may produce more sedation, smooth-muscle relaxation, and respiratory depression. *More potent as an analgesic and has somewhat longer duration of action than morphine.*

USES To relieve moderate to severe pain. Also preoperatively to allay apprehension.

CONTRAINDICATIONS Hypersensitivity to levorphanol; labor and delivery, pregnancy (category D with long time use or high doses); lactation.

CAUTIOUS USE Patients with impaired respiratory reserve, or depressed respirations from another cause (e.g., severe infection, obstructive respiratory conditions, chronic bronchial asthma). Patients with head injury or increased intracranial pressure; acute MI, cardiac dysfunction; liver disease, biliary surgery, alcohol or delirium tremens; liver or kidney dysfunction, hypothyroidism, Addison's disease, toxic psychosis, prostatic hypertrophy, or urethral stricture; concurrent use with CNS depressant drugs; older adults, other vulnerable populations; pregnancy (category B short term use of low doses).

ROUTE & DOSAGE

Moderate to Severe Pain
Adult: **PO** 1 mg q3–6h prn **IV** 1 mg q3–6h prn **IM/Subcutaneous** 1–2 mg q6–8h

ADMINISTRATION

Oral/Intramuscular/Subcutaneous

- Give in the smallest effective dose to minimize the possibility of tolerance and physical dependence.
- Rotate injection sites.
- Store tablets at 15°–30° C (59°–86° F) unless otherwise directed. Store in tightly covered, light-resistant containers.

Intravenous

PREPARE: **Direct:** May be given undiluted or diluted in 5 mL of NS or sterile water.

ADMINISTER: **Direct:** Give at a rate of 2 mg or fraction thereof over 5 min. ▪ AVOID rapid injection. ▪ May inject into Y-site of compatible infusion solution.

INCOMPATIBILITIES **Solution/additive:** **Aminophylline, ammonium chloride, amobarbital, chlorothiazide, heparin, methicillin, nitrofurantoin, novobiocin, pentobarbital, perphenazine, phenobarbital, phenytoin, secobarbital, sodium bicarbonate, sodium iodide, sulfadiazine, sulfisoxazole diethanolamine, thiopental.**

ADVERSE EFFECTS (≥1%) **CNS:** Euphoria, *sedation, drowsiness,* nervousness, confusion. **CV:** Hypotension, arrhythmias. **GI:** *Nausea,* vomiting, dry mouth, cramps, *constipation.* **Urogenital:** Urinary frequency, urinary retention, sedation. **Special Senses:** Blurred vision. **Respiratory:** Respiratory depression. **Body as a Whole:** Physical dependence.

INTERACTIONS **Drug:** **Alcohol** and other CNS DEPRESSANTS compound sedation and CNS depression. **Herbal:** **St. John's wort** may increase sedation.

PHARMACOKINETICS **Peak:** 60–90 min (PO); 15–30 min (IM). **Duration:** 6–8 h. **Distribution:** Crosses placenta; distributed into breast milk. **Metabolism:** In liver. **Elimination:** In urine. **Half-Life:** 11–16 h.

NURSING IMPLICATIONS

Assessment & Drug Effects

- Assess degree of pain relief. Drug is most effective when peaks and valleys of pain relief are avoided.
- Monitor bowel function.
- Monitor ambulation, especially in older adult patients.

L

Patient & Family Education

- Do not drive or engage in other potentially hazardous activities.
- Avoid alcohol and other CNS depressants unless approved by physician.
- Note: Ambulation may increase frequency of nausea and vomiting.
- Increase fluid and fiber intake to offset constipating effects of the drug.

LEVOTHYROXINE SODIUM (T_4) Pr

(lee-voe-thye-rox′een)

Eltroxin ✦, Levoxyl, Levolet, Novothyrox, Synthroid, Unithroid

Classification: THYROID HORMONE REPLACEMENT

Therapeutic: THYROID HORMONE REPLACEMENT

Pregnancy Category: A

AVAILABILITY 25 mcg, 50 mcg, 75 mcg, 88 mcg, 100 mcg, 112 mcg, 125 mcg, 137 mcg, 150 mcg, 175 mcg, 200 mcg, 300 mcg tablets; 200 mcg, 500 mcg injection

ACTION & *THERAPEUTIC EFFECT* Synthetically prepared levo-isomer of thyroxine (T_4, principal component of thyroid gland secretions, determines normal thyroid function). Principal effects include diuresis, loss of weight and puffiness, increased sense of well-being and activity tolerance, plus rise of T_3 and T_4 serum levels toward normal. *By replacing decreased or absent thyroid hormone, it restores metabolic rate of a hypothyroid individual.*

USES Specific replacement therapy for diminished or absent thyroid function resulting from primary or secondary atrophy of gland, surgery, excessive radiation or antithyroid drugs, congenital defect. Administered orally for hypothyroid state; administered IV for myxedematous coma or other thyroid dysfunctions demanding rapid replacement, as well as in failure to respond to oral therapy.

CONTRAINDICATIONS Hypersensitivity to levothyroxine; thyrotoxicosis; severe cardiovascular conditions, acute MI; obesity treatment; adrenal insufficiency.

CAUTIOUS USE Cardiac disease, angina pectoris, cardiac arrhythmias, hypertension; diabetes mellitus; older adult, impaired kidney function, pregnancy (category A).

ROUTE & DOSAGE

Thyroid Replacement

Adult: **PO** 25–50 mcg/day, gradually increased by 50–100 mcg q1–4wk to usual dose of 100–400 mcg/day **IV/IM** 1/2 established oral dose (usually 50–100 mcg daily)

Child: **PO** *0–6 mo,* 8–10 mcg/kg/day or 25–50 mcg/day; *6–12 mo,* 6–8 mcg/kg/day or 50–75 mcg/day; *1–5 y,* 5–6 mcg/kg/day or 75–100 mcg/day; *6–12 y,* 4–5 mcg/kg/day or 100–150 mcg/day; *older than 12 y,* 2–3 mcg/kg/day or greater than 150 mcg/day

Myxedematous Coma

Adult: **IV** 200–500 mcg day 1, additional 100–300 mcg on day 2 if needed

ADMINISTRATION

Oral

- Give as a single dose, preferably 1 h before or 2 h after breakfast. Give consistently with respect to meals.

- Maintenance dosage for older adults may be 25% lower than for heavier and younger adults.
- Store in tight, light-resistant container.

Intravenous

PREPARE: **Direct:** Reconstitute vial by adding 5 mL of NS for injection to each 100 mcg. Shake well to dissolve. Use immediately.
ADMINISTER: **Direct:** Give bolus dose over 1 min.
INCOMPATIBILITIES Do not mix with other medications.

- Store dry powder at 15°–30° C (59°–86° F).

ADVERSE EFFECTS (≥1%) **CNS:** Irritability, nervousness, *insomnia,* headache (pseudotumor cerebri in children), tremors, craniosynostosis (excessive doses in children). **CV:** Palpitations, tachycardia, arrhythmias, angina pectoris, hypertension. **GI:** Nausea, diarrhea, change in appetite. **Urogenital:** Menstrual irregularities. **Body as a Whole:** Weight loss, heat intolerance, sweating, fever, leg cramps, temporary hair loss (children).

INTERACTIONS Drug: Cholestyramine, colestipol decrease absorption of levothyroxine; **epinephrine, norepinephrine** increase risk of cardiac insufficiency; ORAL ANTICOAGULANTS may potentiate hypoprothrombinemia.

PHARMACOKINETICS Absorption: Variable and incompletely absorbed from GI tract (50–80%). **Peak:** 3–4 wk. **Duration:** 1–3 wk. **Distribution:** Gradually released into tissue cells. **Half-Life:** 6–7 days.

NURSING IMPLICATIONS

Assessment & Drug Effects

- Monitor HR and BP. Report promptly tachycardia or suspected arrhythmias.
- Monitor for adverse effects during early adjustment. If metabolism increases too rapidly, especially in older adults and heart disease patients, symptoms of angina or cardiac failure may appear.
- Lab tests: Baseline and periodic tests of thyroid function. Closely monitor PT/INR and assess for evidence of bleeding if patient is receiving concurrent anticoagulant therapy. A decrease in anticoagulant dosage may be needed 1–4 wk after concurrent levothyroxine is started.
- Monitor bone age, growth, and psychomotor function in children.
- Some children have partial hair loss after a few months; it returns even with continued therapy.
- Synthroid 100 and 300 mcg tablets contain tartrazine, which may cause an allergic-type reaction in certain patients; particularly those who are hypersensitive to aspirin.

Patient & Family Education

- Thyroid replacement therapy is usually lifelong.
- Notify physician immediately of signs of toxicity (e.g., chest pain, palpitations, nervousness).
- Avoid OTC medications unless approved by physician.

LIDOCAINE HYDROCHLORIDE (Pr)

(lye′doe-kane)

Anestacon, Dilocaine, L-Caine, Lidoderm, Lida-Mantle, Lidoject-1, LidoPen Auto Injector, Nervocaine, Octocaine, Xylocaine, Xylocard ♣

Classifications: ANTIARRHYTHMIC, CLASS IB; LOCAL ANESTHETIC (AMIDE TYPE)

Therapeutic: ANTIARRHYTHMIC, CLASS IB; LOCAL ANESTHETIC; ANTICONVULSANT
Pregnancy Category: B

AVAILABILITY Antidysrhythmic: 300 mg/3 mL auto-injector; 0.2%, 0.4%, 0.8%, 1%, 2%, 4%, 10%, 20% injections; **Local Anesthetic:** 0.5%, 1%, 1.5%, 2%, 4% injection; **Topical:** 2%, 2.5%, 4%, 5% solution; 2.5%, 5% ointment; 0.5%, 4% cream; 0.5%, 2.5% gel; 0.5%, 10% spray; 2% jelly; 0.5% patch; 0.5 mg intradermal patch

ACTION & *THERAPEUTIC EFFECT* Exerts antiarrhythmic action (Class IB) by suppressing automaticity in His-Purkinje system. Combines with fast sodium channels in myocardial cell membranes, thus inhibiting sodium influx into myocardial cells. Thus it decreases ventricular depolarization, automaticity, and excitability during diastole. As a local anesthetic, it decreases pain through a reversible nerve conduction blockade. *Suppresses automaticity in His-Purkinje system of the heart and elevates electrical stimulation threshold of ventricle during diastole. Prompt, intense, and longer-lasting local anesthetic than procaine.*

USES Rapid control of ventricular arrhythmias occurring during acute MI, cardiac surgery, and cardiac catheterization and those caused by digitalis intoxication. Also as surface and infiltration anesthesia and for nerve block, including caudal and spinal block anesthesia and to relieve local discomfort of skin and mucous membranes. **Patch** for relief of pain associated with post-herpetic neuralgia.

UNLABELED USES Refractory status epilepticus.

CONTRAINDICATIONS History of hypersensitivity to amide-type local anesthetics; application or injection of lidocaine anesthetic in presence of severe trauma or sepsis, blood dyscrasias, post-MI; supraventricular arrhythmias, Stokes-Adams syndrome, untreated sinus bradycardia, severe degrees of sinoatrial, atrioventricular, and intraventaricular heart block.

CAUTIOUS USE Liver or kidney disease, CHF, marked hypoxia, respiratory depression, hypovolemia, shock; myasthenia gravis; debilitated patients, older adults; family history of malignant hyperthermia (fulminant hypermetabolism); pregnancy (category B), lactation. **Topical use:** in eyes, over large body areas, over prolonged periods, in severe or extensive trauma or skin disorders.

ROUTE & DOSAGE

Ventricular Arrhythmias

Adult: **IV** 50–100 mg bolus at a rate of 20–50 mg/min, may repeat in 5 min, then start infusion of 1–4 mg/min immediately after first bolus, not more than 300 mg/h **IM** 200–300 mg, may repeat once after 60–90 min
Child: **IV** 1 mg/kg bolus dose, then 20–50 mcg/kg/min infusion

Anesthetic Uses

Adult: **Infiltration** 0.5–1% solution **Nerve Block** 1–2% solution **Epidural** 1–2% solution **Caudal** 1–1.5% solution **Spinal** 5% with glucose **Saddle Block** 1.5% with dextrose **Topical** 2.5–5% jelly, ointment, cream, or solution

Post-Herpetic Neuralgia

Adult: **Topical** Apply up to 3 patches over intact skin in most painful areas once for up to 12 h per 24 h period

ADMINISTRATION

Intramuscular

- Give in deltoid muscle as preferred site.

Topical

- Do not apply topical lidocaine to large areas of skin or to broken or abraded surfaces. Consult physician about covering area with a dressing.
- Avoid topical preparation contact with eyes.

Intravenous

- Note: Do not use lidocaine solutions containing preservatives for spinal or epidural (including caudal) block. Use ONLY lidocaine HCl injection without preservatives or epinephrine that is specifically labeled for IV injection or infusion.

PREPARE: **Direct:** Give undiluted. **IV Infusion:** Use D5W for infusion. For adults, add 1 g to 250 or 500 mL to yield 2 or 4 mg/mL, respectively; for children, add 120 mg to 100 m to yield 1.2 mg/mL. ▪ Do not use solutions with particulate matter or discoloration.

ADMINISTER: **Direct:** Give at a rate of 50 mg or fraction thereof over 1 min. **IV Infusion:** Use microdrip and infusion pump. *Adult:* Rate of flow is usually 4 mg/min or less. *Child:* Infuse at 30 mcg/kg/min.

INCOMPATIBILITIES **Solution/additive:** **Ampicillin, cefazolin, methohexital, phenytoin.** **Y-site:** **Amphotericin B cholesteryl complex, phenytoin, thiopental.**

- Discard partially used solutions of lidocaine without preservatives.

ADVERSE EFFECTS (≥1%) **CNS:** Drowsiness, dizziness, lightheadedness, restlessness, confusion, disorientation, irritability, apprehension, euphoria, wild excitement, numbness of lips or tongue and other paresthesias including sensations of heat and cold, chest heaviness, difficulty in speaking, <u>difficulty in breathing or swallowing</u>, muscular twitching, tremors, psychosis. With high doses: <u>Convulsions, respiratory depression and arrest</u>. **CV:** With high doses: hypotension, bradycardia, conduction disorders including heart block, <u>cardiovascular collapse, cardiac arrest</u>. **Special Senses:** Tinnitus, decreased hearing; blurred or double vision, impaired color perception. **Skin:** Site of topical application may develop erythema, edema. **GI:** Anorexia, nausea, vomiting. **Body as a Whole:** Excessive perspiration, soreness at IM site, local thrombophlebitis (with prolonged IV infusion), hypersensitivity reactions (urticaria, rash, edema, <u>anaphylactoid reactions</u>).

DIAGNOSTIC TEST INTERFERENCE Increases in ***creatine phosphokinase (CPK)*** level may occur for 48 h after IM dose and may interfere with test for presence of MI.

INTERACTIONS Drug: Lidocaine patch may increase toxic effects of **tocainide, mexiletine;** BARBITURATES decrease lidocaine activity; **cimetidine,** BETA-BLOCKERS, **quinidine** increase pharmacologic effects of lidocaine; **phenytoin** increases cardiac depressant effects; **procainamide** compounds neurologic and cardiac effects.

PHARMACOKINETICS Absorption: Topical application is 3% absorbed through intact skin. **Onset:** 45–90 sec IV; 5–15 min IM; 2–5 min topical. **Duration:** 10–20 min IV; 60–90 min IM; 30–60 min topical; greater than 100 min injected for anesthesia. **Distribution:** Crosses blood–brain barrier and placenta; distributed into breast milk. **Metabolism:** In liver via CYP3A4 and 2D6. **Elimination:** In urine. **Half-Life:** 1.5–2 h.

NURSING IMPLICATIONS

Assessment & Drug Effects

- Stop infusion immediately if ECG indicates excessive cardiac depression (e.g., prolongation of PR interval or QRS complex and the appearance or aggravation of arrhythmias).
- Monitor BP and ECG constantly; assess respiratory and neurologic status frequently to avoid potential overdosage and toxicity.
- Auscultate lungs for basilar rales, especially in patients who tend to metabolize the drug slowly (e.g., CHF, cardiogenic shock, hepatic dysfunction).
- Watch for neurotoxic effects (e.g., drowsiness, dizziness, confusion, paresthesias, visual disturbances, excitement, behavioral changes) in patients receiving IV infusions or with high lidocaine blood levels.

Patient & Family Education

- Swish and spit out when using lidocaine solution for relief of mouth discomfort; gargle for use in pharynx, may be swallowed (as prescribed).
- Oral topical anesthetics (e.g., Xylocaine Viscous) may interfere with swallowing reflex. Do NOT ingest food within 60 min after drug application; especially pediatric, geriatric, or debilitated patients.

LINCOMYCIN HYDROCHLORIDE

(lin-koe-mye'sin)
Lincocin

Classification: LINCOSAMIDE ANTIBIOTIC
Therapeutic: ANTIBIOTIC
Prototype: Clindamycin
Pregnancy Category: B

AVAILABILITY 300 mg injection

ACTION & *THERAPEUTIC EFFECT* Derived from *Streptomyces lincolnensis* and binds to the 50S ribosomal subunits of the bacteria inhibiting protein synthesis, eventually resulting in inhibition of bacterial cell growth or bacterial cell death. *Effective against most of the common gram-positive pathogens. Also effective against many anaerobic bacteria.*

USES Reserved for treatment of serious infections caused by susceptible bacteria in penicillin-allergic patients or patients for whom penicillin is inappropriate.

CONTRAINDICATIONS Previous hypersensitivity to lincomycin and clindamycin; impaired liver function, known monilial infections (unless treated concurrently); use in newborns, lactation.

CAUTIOUS USE Impaired kidney function; history of GI disease, particularly colitis; history of liver, endocrine, or metabolic diseases; history of asthma, hay fever, eczema, drug or other allergies; older adult patients, pregnancy (category B).

ROUTE & DOSAGE

Infections

Adult: **IM** 600 mg q12–24 h **IV** 600 mg–1 g q8–12h (max: 8 g/day)
Child: **IM** 10 mg/kg q12–24h **IV** 10–20 mg/kg/day q8–12h

ADMINISTRATION

Intramuscular

- Give injection deep into large muscle mass; inject slowly to minimize pain. Rotate injection sites.

Intravenous

PREPARE: **Intermittent:** Dilute each 1 g of lincomycin in at least 100 mL of D5W, NS, or other compatible solution.

ADMINISTER: **Intermittent:** Give at a rate of 1 g/h or less.

INCOMPATIBILITIES **Solution/additive: Carbenicillin, kanamycin, methicillin, penicillin G, phenytoin.**

- Follow manufacturer's directions for further information on reconstitution, storage time, compatible IV fluids, and IV administration rates.

ADVERSE EFFECTS (≥1%) **Body as a Whole:** Hypersensitivity [pruritus, urticaria, skin rashes, exfoliative and vesiculobullous dermatitis, erythema multiforme (rare), angioedema, photosensitivity, <u>anaphylactoid reaction</u>, serum sickness]; superinfections (proctitis, pruritus ani, vaginitis); vertigo, dizziness, headache, generalized myalgia, thrombophlebitis following IV use; pain at IM injection site. **CV:** Hypotension, syncope, <u>cardiopulmonary arrest</u> (particularly after rapid IV). **GI:** Glossitis, stomatitis, *nausea, vomiting,* anorexia, decreased taste acuity, unpleasant or altered taste, abdominal cramps, *diarrhea,* acute enterocolitis, <u>pseudomembranous colitis (potentially fatal)</u>. **Hematologic:** Neutropenia, leukopenia, <u>agranulocytosis</u>, thrombocytopenic purpura, <u>aplastic anemia</u>. **Special Senses:** Tinnitus.

INTERACTIONS Drug: Kaolin and pectin decrease lincomycin absorption; **tubocurarine, pancuronium** may enhance neuromuscular blockade.

PHARMACOKINETICS Peak: 30 min IM. **Duration:** 12–14 h IM; 14 h IV. **Distribution:** High concentrations in bone, aqueous humor, bile, and peritoneal, pleural, and synovial fluids; crosses placenta; distributed into breast milk. **Metabolism:** Partially in liver. **Elimination:** In urine and feces. **Half-Life:** 5 h.

NURSING IMPLICATIONS

Assessment & Drug Effects

- Lab tests: Perform C&S initially and during therapy to determine continued microbial susceptibility. Periodic liver and kidney function tests and CBC are indicated during prolonged drug therapy.
- Take a careful history of previous sensitivities to drugs or other allergens.
- Monitor BP and pulse. Have patient remain recumbent following drug administration until BP stabilizes.
- Monitor closely and report changes in bowel frequency. Discontinue drug if significant diarrhea occurs.
- Diarrhea, acute colitis, or pseudomembranous colitis (see Appendix F) may occur up to several weeks after cessation of therapy.
- Examine IM/IV injection sites daily for signs of inflammation.
- Monitor serum drug levels closely in patients with severe impairment of kidney function.
- Monitor for S&S of superinfections that are most likely to occur when therapy exceeds 10 days (see Appendix F).

Patient & Family Education

- Notify physician immediately of symptoms of hypersensitivity (see Appendix F). Drug should be discontinued.

- Notify physician promptly of the onset of perianal irritation, diarrhea, or blood and mucus in stools.

LINDANE (Pr)

(lin′dane)

Gamma Benzene, Kwell, Scabene

Classifications: SCABICIDE; PEDICULICIDE

Therapeutic: ANTIPARASITIC; PEDICULICIDE

Pregnancy Category: C

AVAILABILITY 1% lotion, shampoo

ACTION & *THERAPEUTIC EFFECT* Related to its direct absorption by parasites and ova (nits). Drug absorption through the parasite exoskeleton results in death of parasites and their ova. *Has ectoparasitic and ovicidal activity against the two variants of* Pediculus humanus, Pediculus capitis *(head louse) and* Pediculus pubis *(crab louse), and the arthropod* Sarcoptes scabiei *(scabies).*

USES To treat head and crab lice and scabies infestations and to eradicate their ova.

CONTRAINDICATIONS Premature neonates, patient with known seizure disorders; application to eyes, face, mucous membranes, urethral meatus, open cuts or raw, weeping surfaces; prolonged or excessive applications or simultaneous application of creams, ointments, oils; extensive dermatitis; uncontrolled seizures; lactation, infants, neonates, children younger than 10 y, individuals weighing less than 110 lb.

CAUTIOUS USE History of seizures; HIV infection; alcoholism; pregnancy (category C).

ROUTE & DOSAGE

Lice and Scabies Infestation

Adult/Child: **Topical** Apply to all body areas except the face, leave lotion on 8–12 h, then rinse off; leave shampoo on 5 min, then rinse thoroughly; do NOT repeat in less than 1 wk

ADMINISTRATION

Note: Caregiver needs to wear plastic disposable or rubber gloves when applying lindane, especially if pregnant or applying medication to more than one patient, to avoid prolonged skin contact.

Topical

- Remove all skin lotions, creams, and oil-based hair dressings completely and allow skin to dry and cool before applying lindane; this will reduce percutaneous absorption.
- Shake cream or lotion container well. *Scabies:* Apply thin film from neck down over entire body surface including soles of feet. Avoid face and urethral meatus. Pay particular attention to intertriginous areas (finger webs and other body creases and folds), wrists, elbows, and belt line. Rub drug in; allow skin to dry and cool after application. After 8–12 h, remove medication by bath or shower. *Crab lice:* Apply thin film of drug to hair and skin of pubic area and, if infected, to thighs, trunk, axillary areas. Leave in place 8–12 h and follow with bath or shower. Observation of living lice after 7 days indicates the need for reapplication.
- Shampoo *(head lice):* Apply sufficient quantity to wet hair and skin. Work drug thoroughly onto hair shafts and scalp and allow to remain in place 4 min. Add small

amounts of water sufficient to make a thick lather; then rinse well with water. Pay particular attention to areas above and behind ears and occipital region. Use fine-tooth comb or tweezers to remove remaining nit shells. If necessary, treatment may be repeated after 7 days but not more than twice in 1 wk. *Crab lice:* See above. Repeat treatment after 7 days only if live lice can be demonstrated.

- Store in tight container away from direct light and heat. Protect from freezing.

ADVERSE EFFECTS (≥1%) **CNS:** CNS stimulation (usually after accidental ingestion or misuse of product): Restlessness, dizziness, tremors, convulsions; seizures; <u>death</u>. **Body as a Whole:** Inhalation (headache, nausea, vomiting, irritation of ENT). **Skin:** Eczematous eruptions.

INTERACTIONS Drug: No clinically significant interactions established.

PHARMACOKINETICS Absorption: Slowly and incompletely absorbed through intact skin; maximum absorption from face, scalp, axillae. **Distribution:** Stored in body fat. **Metabolism:** In liver. **Elimination:** In urine and feces.

NURSING IMPLICATIONS

Assessment & Drug Effects

- Monitor for seizure activity in individuals with a history of seizures. Withhold drug and report to physician immediately.
- Burrows made by scabies mites (may or may not be visible) appear as grayish black straight or S-shaped lines with a papule containing the mite at one end and surrounded by a mild erythematous area.

Patient & Family Education

- Lindane is highly toxic drug if topical applications are excessive or if swallowed or inhaled. Keep out of reach of children.
- Note: Lindane shampoo is an effective disinfectant for personal items such as combs, brushes.
- Skin penetration with scabies mites causes an intolerable itching that may persist 2–3 wk after they have been killed.
- Discontinue medication and notify physician if skin eruptions appear.
- Do not apply medication to face, mouth, open skin lesions, or to eyelashes; avoid contact with eyes. If accidental eye contact occurs, flush with water.

L

LINEZOLID

(lin-e-zo′lid)

Zyvox, Zyvoxam ♣

Classification: ANTIBIOTIC, OXAZOLIDINONE

Therapeutic: ANTIBIOTIC

Pregnancy Category: C

AVAILABILITY 400 mg, 600 mg tablets; 100 mg/5 mL suspension; 200 mg, 400 mg, 600 mg injection

ACTION & *THERAPEUTIC EFFECT* Synthetic antibiotic that binds to a site on the 23S ribosomal RNA of the bacteria which prevents the bacterial RNA translation process, thus preventing further growth. *Is bactericidal against gram-positive, gram-negative, and anaerobic bacteria. Bacteriostatic against enterococci and staphylococci, and bactericidal against streptococci.*

USES Treatment of vancomycin-resistant *Enterococcus faecium* (VREF), nosocomial pneumonia, complicated and uncomplicated skin and skin structure infections, community-acquired pneumonia due to susceptible gram-positive organisms.

CONTRAINDICATIONS Hypersensitivity to linezolid; concurrent MAOI therapy.

CAUTIOUS USE Lactation, history of thrombocytopenia, thrombocytopenia; patients on serotonin reuptake inhibitors, or adrenergic agents, active alcoholism, anemia, bleeding, bone marrow suppression, cardiac arrhythmias, cardiac disease, cerebrovascular disease, chemotherapy, coagulopathy, colitis, diarrhea, hypertension, hyperthyroidism, leukopenia, MI, radiographic contrast administration, spinal anesthesia, surgery, hypertension; phenylketonuria; carcinoid syndrome; pregnancy (category C), lactation.

L

ROUTE & DOSAGE

Vancomycin-Resistant *Enterococcus faecium*

Adult/Adolescent (older than 12 y): **PO/IV** 600 mg q12h × 14–28 days

Child (2–11 y): **PO/IV** 10 mg/kg q8h × 14–28 days

Nosocomial or Community-Acquired Pneumonia, Complicated Skin Infections

Adult/Adolescent (older than 12 y): **PO/IV** 600 mg q12h × 10–14 days

Child (5–11 y): **PO/IV** 10 mg/kg q8h × 10–14 days

Uncomplicated Skin Infections

Adult: **PO** 400 mg q12h × 10–14 days

Adolescent: **PO** 600 mg q12h × 10–14 days

Child: **PO** *Younger than 5 y,* 10 mg/kg q8h × 10–14 days; *5–11 y,* 10 mg/kg q12h × 10–14 days

ADMINISTRATION

Note: No dosage adjustment is necessary when switching from IV to oral administration.

Oral

- Reconstitute suspension by adding 123 mL distilled water in two portions; after adding first half, shake to wet all of the powder, then add second half of water and shake vigorously to produce a uniform suspension with a concentration of 100 mg/5 mL.
- Before each use, mix suspension by inverting bottle 3–5 times, but DO NOT SHAKE. Discard unused suspension after 21 days.

Intravenous

PREPARE: **Intermittent:** IV solution is supplied in a single-use, ready-to-use infusion bag. Remove from protective wrap immediately prior to use. ▪Check for minute leaks by firmly squeezing bag. Discard if leaks are detected.

ADMINISTER: **Intermittent:** Do not use infusion bag in a series connection. ▪Give over 30–120 min. If IV line is used to infuse other drugs, flush before and after with D5W, NS, or LR.

INCOMPATIBILITIES **Solution/additive:** **Ceftriaxone, erythromycin, trimethoprim-sulfamethoxazole.** **Y-site:** **Amphotericin B, ceftriaxone, chlorpromazine, diazepam, pentamidine, phenytoin.**

- Store at 25° C (77° F) preferred; 15°–30° C (59°–86° F) permitted. Protect from light and keep bottles tightly closed.

ADVERSE EFFECTS (≥1%) **Body as a Whole:** Fever. **GI:** Diarrhea, nausea, vomiting, constipation, taste alteration, abnormal LFTs, tongue discoloration. **Hematologic:** Thrombocytopenia, leukopenia. **CNS:** Headache, insomnia, dizziness. **Skin:** Rash. **Urogenital:** Vaginal moniliasis.

INTERACTIONS Drug: MAO INHIBITORS may cause hypertensive crisis; **pseudoephedrine** may cause elevated BP; may cause **serotonin** syndrome with SELECTIVE SEROTONIN REUPTAKE INHIBITORS. **Food:** Tyramine-containing food may cause elevated BP. **Herbal: Ginseng, ephedra, ma huang** may lead to elevated BP, headache, nervousness.

PHARMACOKINETICS Absorption: Rapidly or extensively absorbed, 100% bioavailable. **Peak:** 1–2 h PO. **Distribution:** 31% protein bound. **Metabolism:** By oxidation. **Elimination:** Primarily in urine. **Half-Life:** 6–7 h.

NURSING IMPLICATIONS

Assessment & Drug Effects

- Monitor for S&S of: Bleeding; hypertension; or pseudomembranous colitis that begins with diarrhea.
- Lab tests: C&S before initiating therapy and during therapy as indicated; drug may be started pending results. Monitor complete blood count, including platelet count and Hgb and Hct, in those at risk for bleeding or with longer than 2 wk of linezolid therapy.

Patient & Family Education

- Report any of the following to physician promptly: Onset of diarrhea; easy bruising or bleeding of any type; or S&S of superinfection (see Appendix F), S&S of seizure activity.
- Avoid foods and beverages high in tyramine (e.g., aged, fermented, pickled, or smoked foods, and beverages). Limit tyramine intake to less than 100 mg per meal (see *Information for Patients* provided by the manufacturer).
- Do not take OTC cold remedies or decongestants without consulting physician.
- Note for phenylketonurics: Each 5 mL oral suspension contains 20 mg phenylalanine.

LIOTHYRONINE SODIUM (T_3)

(lye-oh-thye'roe-neen)

Cytomel, Triostat

Classification: THYROID HORMONE

Therapeutic: THYROID HORMONE REPLACEMENT

Prototype: Levothyroxine sodium

Pregnancy Category: A

AVAILABILITY 5 mcg, 25 mcg, 50 mcg tablets; 10 mcg/mL injection

ACTION & *THERAPEUTIC EFFECT* Synthetic form of natural thyroid hormone (T_3). Shares actions and uses of thyroid but has more rapid action and more rapid disappearance of effect, permitting quick dosage adjustment, if necessary. *Replacement therapy for absent or decreased thyroid hormone. Principal effect is an increase in the metabolic rate of all body tissues.*

USES Replacement or supplemental therapy for cretinism, myxedema, goiter, secondary (pituitary) or tertiary (hypothalamic) hypothyroidism, and T_3 suppression test.

CONTRAINDICATIONS Hypersensitivity to liothyronine; thyrotoxicosis; obesity treatment; severe cardiovascular conditions, acute MI, uncon-

L

trolled hypertension; adrenal insufficiency.

CAUTIOUS USE Angina pectoris, hypertension; diabetes mellitus; impaired kidney function, renal failure; older adult; pregnancy (category A), lactation.

ROUTE & DOSAGE

Thyroid Replacement

Adult: **PO** 25–75 mcg/day
Geriatric: **PO** 5 mcg/day, increase by 5 mcg/day every 1–2 wk
Child: **PO** 5 mcg/day gradually increased by 5 mcg/day q3–4days until desired response

Myxedema

Adult: **PO** 5–100 mcg/day **IV** 25–50 mcg, may repeat between 4 and 12 h after previous dose. Target dose greater than 65 mcg/day (max: 100 mcg/day).
Geriatric: **PO** Start at 5 mcg/day

Goiter

Adult: **PO** 5–75 mcg/day
Geriatric: **PO** Start at 5 mcg/day
Child: **PO** 5 mcg/day, increase by 5 mcg q1–2 wk (usual maintenance dose 15–20 mcg/day)

T_3 Suppression Test

Adult: **PO** 75–100 mcg/day × 7 days

ADMINISTRATION

Oral

- Give daily before breakfast.

Intravenous

PREPARE: **Direct:** Give undiluted.
ADMINISTER: **Direct:** Give each 10 mcg or fraction thereof over 1 min.

- Store tablets in heat-, light-, and moisture-proof container.

ADVERSE EFFECTS (≥1%) **Endocrine:** Result from overdosage evidenced as S&S of hyperthyroidism (see Appendix F). **Musculoskeletal:** Accelerated rate of bone maturation in children.

INTERACTIONS Drug: Cholestyramine, colestipol decrease absorption; **epinephrine, norepinephrine** increase risk of cardiac insufficiency; ORAL ANTICOAGULANTS may potentiate hypoprothrombinemia.

PHARMACOKINETICS Absorption: Completely absorbed from GI tract. **Peak:** 24–72 h. **Duration:** Up to 72 h. **Distribution:** Gradually released into tissue cells. **Half-Life:** 6–7 days.

NURSING IMPLICATIONS

Assessment & Drug Effects

- Watch for possible additive effects during the early period of liothyronine substitution for another preparation, particularly in older adults, children, and patients with cardiovascular disease. Residual actions of other thyroid preparations may persist for weeks.
- Metabolic effects of liothyronine persist a few days after drug withdrawal.
- Withhold drug and notify physician at onset of overdosage symptoms (hyperthyroidism, see Appendix F); usually therapy can be resumed with lower dosage.

Patient & Family Education

- Take medication exactly as ordered.
- Learn S&S of hyperthyroidism (see Appendix F); notify physician promptly if they appear.

LIOTRIX (T_3-T_4)

(lye'oh-trix)

Thyrolar
Classification: THYROID HORMONE
Therapeutic: THYROID HORMONE REPLACEMENT
Prototype: Levothyroxine sodium
Pregnancy Category: A

AVAILABILITY 0.0125 mcg, 3.1 mcg, 6.25 mcg, 12.5 mcg, 25 mcg, 37.5 mcg

ACTION & *THERAPEUTIC EFFECT* Synthetic levothyroxine (T_4) and liothyronine (T_3) that influence growth and maturation of tissues, increase energy expenditure, and affect turnover of essentially all substrates. These hormones play an integral role in metabolic processes, and are important to development of the CNS in newborns. *Increases metabolic rate of all body tissues.*

USES Replacement or supplemental therapy for cretinism, myxedema, goiter, and secondary (pituitary) or tertiary (hypothalamic) hypothyroidism. Also with antithyroid agents in thyrotoxicosis and to prevent goitrogenesis and hypothyroidism.

CONTRAINDICATIONS Untreated thyrotoxicosis, acute MI, morphologic hypogonadism, nephrosis, adrenal deficiency due to hypopituitarism; tartrazine dye hypersensitivity, obesity treatment.
CAUTIOUS USE Myxedema; hypertension, angina, cardiac arrhythmias, cardiac disease, coronary artery disease; older adults; hypertension; arteriosclerosis; kidney dysfunction, pregnancy (category A), lactation; neonates, infants, children.

ROUTE & DOSAGE

Thyroid Replacement
Adult/Child: **PO** 12.5–30 mcg/day, gradually increase to desired response

ADMINISTRATION

Oral
- Give as a single daily dose, preferably before breakfast.
- Make dose increases at 1- to 2-wk intervals.
- Store in heat-, light-, and moisture-proof container. Shelf-life: 2 y.

ADVERSE EFFECTS (≥1%) **CNS:** Nervousness, headache, tremors, insomnia. **CV:** Palpitation, tachycardia, angina pectoris, cardiac arrhythmias, hypertension, CHF. **GI:** Nausea, abdominal cramps, diarrhea. **Body as a Whole:** Weight loss, heat intolerance, fever, sweating, menstrual irregularities. **Musculoskeletal:** Accelerated rate of bone maturation in infants and children.

INTERACTIONS Drug: Cholestyramine, colestipol decrease absorption; **epinephrine, norepinephrine** increase risk of cardiac insufficiency; ORAL ANTICOAGULANTS may potentiate hypoprothrombinemia.

NURSING IMPLICATIONS

Assessment & Drug Effects
- Watch for possible additive effects during the early period of liothyronine substitution for another preparation, particularly in older adults, children, and patients with cardiovascular disease. Residual actions of other thyroid preparations may persist for weeks.

- Note: Metabolic effects of liotrix persist a few days after drug withdrawal.
- Withhold drug and notify physician at onset of overdosage symptoms (hyperthyroidism, see Appendix F); usually therapy can be resumed with lower dosage.
- Monitor diabetics for glycemic control; an increase in insulin or oral hypoglycemic may be required.

Patient & Family Education

- Notify physician of headache (euthyroid patients); may indicate need for dosage adjustment or change to another thyroid preparation.
- Take medication exactly as ordered.
- Learn S&S of hyperthyroidism (see Appendix F); notify physician if they appear.

LISDEXAMFETAMINE DIMESYLATE

(lis-dex-am-fet′a-meen)

Vyvanse

Classifications: CEREBRAL STIMULANT; AMPHETAMINE; ANOREXIGENIC

Therapeutic: STIMULANT; ANOREXIGENIC

Prototype: Amphetamine

Pregnancy Category: C

Controlled Substance: Schedule II

AVAILABILITY 20 mg, 30 mg, 40 mg, 50 mg, 60 mg, and 70 mg capsules

ACTION & *THERAPEUTIC EFFECT* An isomer of amphetamine that has anorexigenic action; this is thought to result from CNS stimulation and possibly from loss of acuity of smell and taste. *In hyperkinetic children, amphetamines reduce motor restlessness by an unknown mechanism.*

USES Treatment of attention-deficit hyperactivity disorder (ADHD).

CONTRAINDICATIONS Hypersensitivity to sympathomimetic amines, dextroamphetamine, or amphetamine; advanced arteriosclerosis; structural cardiac abnormalities, cardiomyopathy, cardiac arrhythmias, or symptomatic cardiovascular disease; moderate to severe hypertension; glaucoma; agitated states; patients with history of drug abuse; during or within 14 days of administering MAOIs; hyperthyroidism; seizure disorders; tics or Tourette syndrome; substance abuse; emergence of new psychotic or manic symptoms caused by amphetamine use; lactation; children younger than 6 y.

CAUTIOUS USE Controlled hypertension, heart failure, recent MI, or recent ventricular arrhythmia; preexisting psychotic disorder; suicidal tendencies; bipolar disorder, depression; history of aggressive or hostile behavior; alcoholism; pregnancy (category C).

ROUTE & DOSAGE

Attention-Deficit Hyperactivity Disorder

Adult/Child (6–12 y): **PO** 30 mg daily in a.m.; may increase to 50–70 mg daily at weekly intervals (max: 70 mg daily)

ADMINISTRATION

Oral

- Give daily dose in the morning.
- Capsule may be taken whole or opened and dissolved in a glass of water.
- Store at 15°–30° C (59°–86° F) and protect from light.

ADVERSE EFFECTS (≥1%) **Body as a Whole:** Pyrexia. **CNS:** Affect lability, dizziness, *headache, insomnia, irritability,* somnolence, tic. **GI:** *Abdominal pain,* dry mouth, nausea, vomiting. **Metabolic:** Decreased appetite, weight loss. **Skin:** Rash.

DIAGNOSTIC TEST INTERFERENCE Can cause a significant elevation in plasma CORTICOSTEROID levels and may interfere with ***urinary steroid determinations.***

INTERACTIONS Drug: Chlorpromazine and **haloperidol** inhibit the CNS stimulant effects of amphetamines. **Furazolidone** and MAO INHIBITORS can increase adverse effects. **Lithium** may inhibit the effects of lisdexamfetamine. **Propoxyphene** can potentiate the CNS stimulation of lisdexamfetamine. Compounds that acidify the urine lower the plasma levels of lisdexamfetamine. Lisdexamfetamine inhibits the actions of **adrenergic blockers.** Co-administration of ANTIHISTAMINES with lisdexamfetamine can counteract desired sedative effects. Lisdexamfetamine may antagonize the hypotensive effects of ANTIHYPERTENSIVE AGENTS. Lisdexamfetamine may delay the absorption of **ethosuximide** and **phenytoin.** Lisdexamfetamine may potentiate the actions of TRICYCLIC ANTIDEPRESSANTS, **meperidine** and **norepinephrine.**

PHARMACOKINETICS Absorption: Rapidly from GI tract. **Peak:** 1 h. **Distribution:** Extensive throughout body. **Metabolism:** Prodrug converted in liver to dextroamphetamine. **Elimination:** Urine (96%). **Half-Life:** 1 h (lisdexamfetamine) 6–8 h (dextroamphetamine).

NURSING IMPLICATIONS

Assessment & Drug Effects

- Monitor children, adolescents, and adults for signs and symptoms of adverse cardiac reactions (e.g., hypertension, arrhythmias). Report promptly exertional chest pain or syncope.
- Monitor closely growth rate in children.
- Typically therapy is interrupted or dosage reduced periodically to assess effectiveness in behavior disorders.
- Monitor children and adolescents for development of aggressive or abnormal behaviors.

Patient & Family Education

- Do not drive or engage in other potentially hazardous activities until response to drug is known.
- Report promptly any of the following: Chest pain with activity, new or worse behavior or thought problems, psychotic symptoms (e.g., hearing voices, believing things that are not true).
- Taper drug gradually following long-term use to avoid extreme fatigue, mental depression, and prolonged abnormal sleep pattern.

LISINOPRIL

(ly-sin′o-pril)

Prinivil, Zestril

Classifications: ANTIHYPERTENSIVE; ANGIOTENSIN-CONVERTING ENZYME (ACE) INHIBITOR

Therapeutic: ANTIHYPERTENSIVE

Prototype: Enalapril

Pregnancy Category: D

AVAILABILITY 2.5 mg, 5 mg, 10 mg, 20 mg, 30 mg, 40 mg tablets

ACTION & *THERAPEUTIC EFFECT* Lowers BP by specific inhibition of the angiotensin-converting enzyme (ACE). This interrupts conversion sequences initiated by renin that form angiotensin II, a potent vasoconstrictor. ACE inhibition alters hemodynamics without compensatory reflex tachycardia or changes in cardiac output (except in patients with CHF). *Improves cardiac output and exercise tolerance. Aldosterone is also reduced, thus permitting a potassium-sparing effect.*

USES Hypertension, alone or concomitantly with other classes of antihypertensive agents; CHF; to improve MI survival.

L

CONTRAINDICATIONS Patients with a history of angioedema related to treatment with an ACE inhibitor, ACE inhibitor hypersensitivity; pregnancy (category D), children younger than 6 y; lactation.

CAUTIOUS USE Impaired kidney function, renal artery stenosis, renal disease, renal failure, hyperkalemia, aortic stenosis, cardiomyopathy; cerebrovascular disease; collagen vascular disease; coronary artery disease, dialysis; older adults; heart failure, hyperkalemia, hypotension, hypovolemia; African Americans; autoimmune diseases, especially systemic lupus erythematosus (SLE).

ROUTE & DOSAGE

Hypertension

Adult: **PO** 10 mg once/day, may increase up to 20–40 mg 1–2 times/day (max: 80 mg/day)
Child (6–16 y): **PO** Start at 0.07 mg/kg (max: 5 mg) once/day (max: 40 mg/day)
Geriatric: **PO** Initial 2.5–5 mg/day, may increase by 2.5–5 mg/day every 1–2 wk (max: 40 mg/day)

Heart Failure

Adult: **PO** 5–40 mg/day

ADMINISTRATION

Oral

- Monitor drug effect for several hours or until the BP is stabilized for at least 1 additional hour. Concurrent administration with a diuretic may compound hypotensive effect.
- Store away from both moisture and heat.

ADVERSE EFFECTS (≥1%) **CNS:** Headache, dizziness, fatigue. **CV:** Hypotension, chest pain. **GI:** Nausea, vomiting, diarrhea, anorexia, constipation, intestinal angioedema. **Hematologic:** Neutropenia. **Respiratory:** Dyspnea, cough. **Skin:** Rash. **Metabolic:** Azotemia, hyperkalemia, increased BUN, and creatinine levels.

INTERACTIONS Drug: Indomethacin and other NSAIDS may decrease antihypertensive activity; POTASSIUM SUPPLEMENTS, POTASSIUM-SPARING DIURETICS may cause hyperkalemia; may increase **lithium** levels and toxicity.

PHARMACOKINETICS Absorption: 25% absorbed from GI tract. **Onset:** 1 h. **Peak:** 6–8 h. **Duration:** 24 h. **Distribution:** Limited amount crosses blood–brain barrier; crosses placenta; small amount distributed in breast milk. **Metabolism:** Is not metabolized. **Elimination:** Primarily in urine. **Half-Life:** 12 h.

NURSING IMPLICATIONS

Assessment & Drug Effects

- Place patient in supine position and notify physician if sudden and severe hypotension occurs within the first 1–5 h after initial drug dose; greatest risk for hypotension is in patients who are sodium- or volume-depleted because of diuretic therapy.
- Measure BP just prior to dosing to determine whether satisfactory control is being maintained for 24 h. If the antihypertensive effect is diminished in less than 24 h, an increase in dosage may be necessary.
- Monitor closely for angioedema of extremities, face, lips, tongue, glottis, and larynx. Discontinue drug promptly and notify physician if such symptoms appear; carefully monitor for airway obstruction until swelling is relieved.
- Monitor serum sodium and serum potassium levels for hyponatremia and hyperkalemia.
- Lab tests: Determine WBC count prior to initiation of treatment, every month for the first 3–6 mo of therapy, and at periodic intervals for 1 y. Withhold therapy and notify physician if neutropenia (neutrophil count less than 1000/mm^3) develops; kidney function tests at periodic intervals, especially in patients with severe volume or sodium replacement or those with severe CHF.

Patient & Family Education

- Discontinue drug and contact physician immediately for severe hypersensitivity reaction (e.g., hoarseness, swelling of the face, mouth, hands, or feet, or sudden trouble breathing).
- Be aware of importance of proper diet, including sodium and potassium restrictions. Do NOT use salt substitute containing potassium.
- Continued compliance with high BP medication is very important. If a dose is missed, take it as soon as possible but not too close to next dose.
- Do not drive or engage in other potentially hazardous activities until response to the drug is known.
- With concomitant therapy, lisinopril increases the risk of lithium toxicity.
- Notify physician promptly of any indication of infection (e.g., sore throat, fever).
- Do not store drug in a moist area. Heat and moisture may cause the medicine to break down.

L

LITHIUM CARBONATE Pr

(li′thee-um)

Eskalith, Eskalith CR, Lithane, Lithobid, Lithonate, Lithotabs

LITHIUM CITRATE

Cibalith-S

Classification: ANTIPSYCHOTIC; MOOD STABILIZER

Therapeutic: ANTIPSYCHOTIC; ANTIMANIC; ANTIDEPRESSANT

Pregnancy Category: D

AVAILABILITY Lithium Carbonate: 150 mg, 300 mg, 600 mg capsules; 300 mg, 450 mg sustained release tablets; **Lithium Citrate:** 300 mg/5 mL syrup

ACTION & *THERAPEUTIC EFFECT*

The lithium ion behaves in the body much like the sodium ion; but its exact mechanism of action is unclear. Competes with various physiologically important cations: Na^+, K^+, Ca^{2+}, Mg^{2+}; therefore, it affects cell membranes, body water, and neurotransmitters. At the synapse, it accelerates catecholamine destruction, inhibits the release of neurotransmitters and decreases sensitivity of postsynaptic receptors. Decreases overactivity of receptors involved in stimulating manic states. *Effective response evidenced by changed facial affect, improved posture, assumption of self-care, improved ability to concentrate, improved sleep pattern.*

USES Control and prophylaxis of acute mania and the acute manic phase of mixed bipolar disorder.

UNLABELED USES Acute and recurrent depression (unipolar affective disorder), schizophrenic disorders, disorders of impulse control, alcohol dependence, antineoplastic drug-induced neutropenia, aplastic anemia, SIADH, cyclic neutropenia.

CONTRAINDICATIONS History of ACE inhibitor induced angioedema; significant cardiovascular or kidney disease, brain damage, severe debilitation, dehydration or sodium depletion; patients on low-salt diet or receiving diuretics; pregnancy (category D), lactation, children younger than 12 y.

CAUTIOUS USE Older adults; thyroid disease; epilepsy; concomitant use with haloperidol and other antipsychotics; cardiac disease, cardiac arrhythmias, dehydration, diarrhea; older adults; fever, hyponatremia, hypothyroidism, concurrent infection; leukemia; mental status changes, organic brain syndrome, parkinsonism; psoriasis; renal disease, renal impairment; seizure disorder, sick sinus syndrome, sodium restriction, risk of suicidal ideation, thyroid disease, urinary retention; diabetes mellitus; severe infections; urinary retention.

ROUTE & DOSAGE

Mania

Adult: **PO Loading Dose** 600 mg t.i.d. or 900 mg sustained release b.i.d. or 30 mL (48 mEq) of solution t.i.d. **PO Maintenance Dose** 300 mg t.i.d. or q.i.d. or 15–20 mL (24–32 mEq) solution in 2–4 divided doses (max: 2.4 g/day)
Child: **PO** 15–60 mg/kg/day in divided doses

ADMINISTRATION

Oral

- Give with meals.
- Ensure that sustained release tablets are not chewed or crushed; **must be** swallowed whole.
- Protect from light and moisture.

ADVERSE EFFECTS (≥1%) **CNS:** Dizziness, *headache, lethargy,* drowsiness, *fatigue,* slurred speech, psychomotor retardation, giddiness, incontinence, restlessness, seizures, confusion, blackout spells, disorientation, recent memory loss, stupor, coma, EEG changes. **CV:** Arrhythmias, hypotension, vasculitis, peripheral circulatory collapse, ECG changes. **Special Senses:** Impaired vision, transient scotomas, tinnitus. **Endocrine:** Diffuse thyroid enlargement, hypothyroidism, *nephrogenic diabetes insipidus,* transient hyperglycemia, glycosuria, hyponatremia. **GI:** *Nausea, vomiting, anorexia, abdominal pain, diarrhea, dry mouth,* metallic taste. **Musculoskeletal:** *Fine hand tremors,* coarse tremors, choreoathetotic movements; fasciculations, clonic movements, incoordination including ataxia, *muscle weakness,* hyperreflexia, encephalopathic syndrome (weakness, lethargy, fever, tremors, confusion, extrapyramidal symptoms). **Skin:** Thought to be toxicity rather than allergy: Pruritus, maculopapular rash, hyperkeratosis, chronic folliculitis, transient acneiform papules (face, neck, intertriginous areas), anesthesia of skin, cutaneous ulcers, drying and thinning of hair, allergic vasculitis. **Hematologic:** *Reversible leukocytosis* (14,000 to 18,000/ mm³). **Urogenital:** Albuminuria, oliguria, urinary incontinence, polyuria, polydipsia, increased uric acid excretion. **Body as a Whole:** Edema, weight gain (common) or loss, exacerbation of psoriasis; flu-like symptoms.

INTERACTIONS Drug: Carbamazepine, haloperidol, PHENOTHIAZINES increase risk of neurotoxicity, extrapyramidal effects, and tardive dyskinesias; DIURETICS, NSAIDS, **methyldopa, probenecid,** TETRACYCLINES decrease renal clearance of lithium, increasing pharmacologic and toxic effects; THEOPHYLLINES, **urea, sodium bicarbonate, sodium or potassium citrate** increase renal clearance of lithium, decreasing its pharmacologic effects.

PHARMACOKINETICS Absorption: Readily absorbed from GI tract. **Peak:** 0.5–3 h carbonate; 15–60 min citrate. **Distribution:** Crosses blood–brain barrier and placenta; distributed into breast milk. **Metabolism:** Not metabolized. **Elimination:** 95% in urine, 1% in feces, 4–5% in sweat. **Half-Life:** 20–27 h.

NURSING IMPLICATIONS

Assessment & Drug Effects

- Monitor response to drug. Usual lag of 1–2 wk precedes response to lithium therapy. Keep physician informed of progress.
- Lab test: Periodic lithium levels (draw blood sample prior to next dose or 8–12 h after last dose); periodic thyroid function tests.
- Monitor for S&S of lithium toxicity (e.g., vomiting, diarrhea, lack of coordination, drowsiness, muscular weakness, slurred speech when level is 1.5–2 mEq/L; ataxia, blurred vision, giddiness, tinnitus, muscle twitching, coarse tremors, polyuria when greater than 2 mEq/ L). Withhold one dose and call physician. Drug should not be stopped abruptly.
- Monitor older adults carefully to prevent toxicity, which may occur at serum levels ordinarily tolerated by other patients.
- Be alert to and report symptoms of hypothyroidism (see Appendix F).
- Weigh patient daily; check ankles, tibiae, and wrists for edema. Report changes in I&O ratio, sudden weight gain, or edema.
- Report early signs of extrapyramidal reactions promptly to physician.

Patient & Family Education

- Be alert to increased output of dilute urine and persistent thirst. Dose reduction may be indicated.
- Contact physician if diarrhea or fever develops. Avoid practices that may encourage dehydration: Hot environment, excessive caffeine beverages (diuresis).
- Drink plenty of liquids (2–3 L/ day) during stabilization period and at least 1–1.5 L/day during ongoing therapy.
- Avoid self-prescribed low-salt regimen, self-dosing with antacids containing sodium, and high-sodium foods (e.g., prepared meats and diet soda).
- Do not drive or engage in other potentially hazardous activities until response to drug is known. Lithium may impair both physical and mental ability.
- Use effective contraceptive measures during lithium therapy. If

therapy is continued during pregnancy, serum lithium levels **must be** closely monitored to prevent toxicity.

LODOXAMIDE

(lo-dox′a-mide)

Alomide

Pregnancy Category: B

See Appendix A-1.

LOMEFLOXACIN

(lo-me-flox′a-cin)

Maxaquin

Classification: FLUOROQUINOLONE ANTIBIOTIC

Therapeutic: ANTIBIOTIC

Prototype: Ciprofloxacin

Pregnancy Category: C

AVAILABILITY 400 mg tablets

ACTION & *THERAPEUTIC EFFECT* A fluoroquinolone broad spectrum bactericidal agent that inhibits DNA gyrase, an enzyme necessary for bacterial DNA replication and some aspects of its transcription, repair, recombination, and transposition. *Inhibits replication of susceptible gram-negative and gram-positive bacteria.*

USES Urinary tract infections, transurethral surgery prophylaxis.

UNLABELED USES Lower respiratory tract infections.

CONTRAINDICATIONS Known hypersensitivity to lomefloxacin or any other quinolone; tendon pain; QT prolongation; renal failure or CrCl less than 10 mL/min; lactation.

CAUTIOUS USE Kidney disease; acute MI, atrial fibrillation, bradycardia; cerebrovascular disease; myasthenia gravis; patients with a history of epilepsy, psychosis, or increased intracranial pressure; pregnancy (categeroy C); children and adolescents.

ROUTE & DOSAGE

Urinary Tract and Lower Respiratory Tract Infections

Adult: **PO** 400 mg daily × 10 days

Transurethral Surgery Prophylaxis

Adult: **PO** 400 mg 2–6 h before surgery

ADMINISTRATION

Oral

- Avoid giving mineral supplements or vitamins with iron or zinc within 2 h of lomefloxacin.
- Do not give antacids with magnesium, aluminum, or sucralfate within 4 h before or 2 h after drug.
- Give hemodialysis patients an initial 400 mg loading dose followed by a 200 mg/day maintenance dose.

ADVERSE EFFECTS (≥1%) **CNS:** *Headache, peripheral neuropathy.* **GI:** Nausea, abdominal discomfort. **Skin:** Photosensitivity. **Musculoskeletal:** Risk of tendon rupture (rare).

DIAGNOSTIC TEST INTERFERENCE May cause false positive on ***opiate screening tests.***

INTERACTIONS Drug: ALUMINUM- and MAGNESIUM-CONTAINING ANTACIDS decrease systemic bioavailability of lomefloxacin. Concurrent CORTICOSTEROID use may increase the risk of tendon rupture.

PHARMACOKINETICS Absorption: Readily from GI tract. **Peak:** 1–2 h. **Distribution:** Crosses placenta; distributed into breast milk. **Elimina-**

tion: 76% in urine within 48 h. **Half-Life:** 6.35–7.77 h.

NURSING IMPLICATIONS

Assessment & Drug Effects

- Lab tests: Draw C&S prior to first dose; drug may be started pending results of C&S.
- Take thorough history of hypersensitivity reactions to quinolones or other drugs prior to therapy.
- Discontinue lomefloxacin and notify physician at the first sign of a skin rash or other allergic reaction.
- Monitor for tendon pain. If it occurs, hold the drug and report to physician.
- Monitor for seizures, especially in patients with known or suspected CNS disorders. Discontinue lomefloxacin and notify physician immediately if a seizure occurs.
- Assess for S&S of superinfection (see Appendix F).

Patient & Family Education

- Notify physician of loose stools or diarrhea promptly.
- Drink fluids liberally, if not contraindicated.
- Take appropriate cautions, dizziness or light-headedness may occur.
- Be aware of the possibility of phototoxicity; avoid excessive sunlight or artificial ultraviolet light.

LOMUSTINE

(loe-mus'teen)

CeeNU, CCNU

Classifications: ANTINEOPLASTIC; ALKYLATING AGENT; NITROSOUREA
Therapeutic: ANTINEOPLASTIC
Prototype: Cyclophosphamide
Pregnancy Category: D

AVAILABILITY 10 mg, 40 mg, 100 mg capsules

ACTION & *THERAPEUTIC EFFECT* Lipid-soluble alkylating nitrosourea with actions like those of carmustine (e.g., cell-cycle-nonspecific activity against rapidly proliferating cell populations). Inhibits synthesis of both DNA and RNA. *Has antineoplastic and myelosuppressive effect.*

USES Palliative therapy in addition to other modalities or with other chemotherapeutic agents in primary and metastatic brain tumors and as secondary therapy in Hodgkin's disease.

UNLABELED USES GI, lung, and renal carcinomas, non-Hodgkin's lymphomas, malignant melanoma, and multiple myeloma.

CONTRAINDICATIONS Immunization with live virus vaccines, viral infections; severe bone marrow suppression; active infection; pregnancy (category D), lactation.

CAUTIOUS USE Patients with decreased circulating platelets, leukocytes, or erythrocytes; kidney or liver function impairment; previous cytotoxic or radiation therapy; pulmonary disease.

ROUTE & DOSAGE

Palliative Therapy

Adult: **PO** 130 mg/m² as single dose, repeated in 6 wk; subsequent doses based on hematologic response (WBC greater than 4000/mm³, platelets greater than 100,000/mm³)
Child: **PO** 75–150 mg/m² q6wk

ADMINISTRATION

Oral

- Give on an empty stomach to reduce possibility of nausea, may also give an antiemetic before drug to prevent nausea.

L

- Store capsules away from excessive heat (over 40° C).

ADVERSE EFFECTS (≥1%) **CNS:** Lethargy, ataxia, disorientation. **GI:** Anorexia, *nausea, vomiting,* stomatitis, transient elevations of LFTs. **Hematologic:** Delayed (cumulative) myelosuppression: (Thrombocytopenia, leukopenia); anemia. **Skin:** Alopecia, skin rash, itching. **Urogenital:** Nephrotoxicity. **Respiratory:** Pulmonary toxicity (rare).

INTERACTIONS Drug: Cimetidine can increase bone marrow toxicity; ANTICOAGULANTS, NSAIDS, SALICYLATES increase risk of bleeding.

PHARMACOKINETICS Absorption: Readily absorbed from GI tract. **Peak:** 1–6 h. **Distribution:** Readily crosses blood–brain barrier; crosses placenta; distributed into breast milk. **Metabolism:** In liver to several active metabolites. **Elimination:** In urine. **Half-Life:** 16–48 h.

NURSING IMPLICATIONS

Assessment & Drug Effects

- Lab tests: Monitor blood counts weekly for at least 6 wk after last dose. Liver and kidney function tests should be performed periodically.
- A repeat course is not given until platelets have returned to above 100,000/mm^3 and leukocytes to above 4000/mm^3.
- Avoid invasive procedures during nadir of platelets.
- Thrombocytopenia occurs about 4 wk and leukopenia about 6 wk after a dose, persisting 1–2 wk.
- Inspect oral cavity daily for S&S of superinfections (see Appendix F) and stomatitis or xerostomia.

Patient & Family Education

- Nausea and vomiting may occur 3–5 h after drug administration, usually lasting less than 24 h.
- Anorexia may persist for 2 or 3 days after a dose.
- Notify physician of signs of sore throat, cough, fever. Also report unexplained bleeding or easy bruising.
- Use reliable contraceptive measures during therapy.
- Be aware of the possibility of hair loss while taking this drug.
- A given dose may include capsules of different colors; the pharmacist prepares prescribed dose by combining various capsule strengths.

LOPERAMIDE (Pr)

(loe-per'a-mide)

Imodium, Imodium AD, Kaopectate III, Maalox Anti-diarrheal, Pepto Diarrhea Control

Classification: ANTIDIARRHEAL

Therapeutic: ANTIDIARRHEAL

Pregnancy Category: C

AVAILABILITY 2 mg tablets, capsules; 1 mg/mL, 1 mg/5 mL liquid

ACTION & *THERAPEUTIC EFFECT* Inhibits GI peristaltic activity by direct action on circular and longitudinal intestinal muscles. Prolongs transit time of intestinal contents, increases consistency of stools, and reduces fluid and electrolyte loss. *Effectiveness as an antidiarrheal agent is due to prolonging transit time in the colon.*

USES Acute nonspecific diarrhea, chronic diarrhea associated with inflammatory bowel disease, and to reduce fecal volume from ileostomies.

CONTRAINDICATIONS Conditions in which constipation should be avoided, ileus, severe colitis, bacterial gastroenteritis; acute diarrhea caused by broad-spectrum antibiotics (pseudomembranous colitis) or associated with microorganisms that penetrate intestinal mucosa (e.g., toxigenic *Escherichia coli, Salmonella,* or *Shigella*); GI bleeding; lactation. Safe use in children younger than 2 y is not established. **CAUTIOUS USE** Dehydration; diarrhea caused by invasive bacteria; ulcerative colitis; impaired liver function; prostatic hypertrophy; history of narcotic dependence; pregnancy (category C).

ROUTE & DOSAGE

Acute Diarrhea

Adult: **PO** 4 mg followed by 2 mg after each unformed stool (max: 16 mg/day)
Child: **PO** *2–6 y,* 1 mg t.i.d.; *6–8 y,* 2 mg b.i.d.; *8–12 y,* 2 mg t.i.d.

Chronic Diarrhea

Adult: **PO** 4 mg followed by 2 mg after each unformed stool until diarrhea is controlled (max: 16 mg/day)
Child: **PO** 0.1 mg/kg after each unformed stool (usually 1 mg)

ADMINISTRATION

Oral

- Do not give prn doses to a child with acute diarrhea.

ADVERSE EFFECTS (≥1%) **Body as a Whole:** Hypersensitivity (skin rash); fever. **CNS:** Drowsiness, fatigue, dizziness, CNS depression (overdosage). **GI:** Abdominal discomfort or pain, abdominal distention, bloating, constipation, nausea, vomiting, anorexia, dry mouth; toxic megacolon (patients with ulcerative colitis).

INTERACTIONS Drug: No clinically significant interactions established.

PHARMACOKINETICS Absorption: Poorly absorbed from GI tract. **Onset:** 30–60 min. **Peak:** 2.5 h solution; 4–5 h capsules. **Duration:** 4–5 h. **Metabolism:** In liver. **Elimination:** Primarily in feces, less than 2% in urine. **Half-Life:** 11 h.

NURSING IMPLICATIONS

Assessment & Drug Effects

- Monitor therapeutic effectiveness. Chronic diarrhea usually responds within 10 days. If improvement does not occur within this time, it is unlikely that symptoms will be controlled by further administration.
- Discontinue if there is no improvement after 48 h of therapy for acute diarrhea.
- Monitor fluid and electrolyte balance.
- Notify physician promptly if the patient with ulcerative colitis develops abdominal distention or other GI symptoms (possible signs of potentially fatal toxic megacolon).

Patient & Family Education

- Notify physician if diarrhea does not stop in a few days or if abdominal pain, distention, or fever develops.
- Record number and consistency of stools.
- Do not drive or engage in other potentially hazardous activities until response to drug is known.
- Do not take alcohol and other CNS depressants concomitantly unless otherwise advised by physician; may enhance drowsiness.
- Learn measures to relieve dry mouth; rinse mouth frequently with water, suck hard candy.

LOPINAVIR/RITONAVIR

(lop-i-na′ver/rit-o-na′ver)

Kaletra
Classifications: ANTIRETROVIRAL; PROTEASE INHIBITOR
Therapeutic: PROTEASE INHIBITOR
Prototype: Saquinavir mesylate
Pregnancy Category: C

AVAILABILITY 200 mg lopinavir/50 mg ritonavir, 100 mg lopinavir/25 mg ritonavir tablets; 400 mg lopinavir/100 mg ritonavir/5 mL suspension

ACTION & *THERAPEUTIC EFFECT* Lopinavir, an HIV protease inhibitor that inhibits the activity of HIV protease and prevents the cleavage of viral polyproteins essential for the maturation of HIV. Ritonavir inhibits the CYP3A metabolism of lopinavir, thereby, increasing the blood level of lopinavir. *Decreases plasma HIV RNA level; reduces viral load as a result of the combined therapy of the two drugs in HIV infected patients.*

L

USES Treatment of HIV infection in combination with other antiretroviral agents.

CONTRAINDICATIONS Hypersensitivity to lopinavir or ritonavir; lactation. Safe use in other cases in infants younger than 14 days are not established.

CAUTIOUS USE Hepatic impairment, patients with hepatitis B or C, older adults; diabetes mellitus; history of pancreatitis; cardiac disease; potential for PR prolongation and QT prolongation; conduction abnormalities, ischemic heart disease, and cardiomyopathy; pregnancy (category C).

ROUTE & DOSAGE

HIV Infection—Treatment Naïve
Adult: **PO** 800/200 mg or 400/100 mg b.i.d. daily

HIV Infection—Treatment Experienced
Adult: **PO** 400/100 mg (3 tablets or 5 mL suspension) b.i.d., increase dose to 533/133 mg (4 tablets or 6.5 mL) b.i.d., with concurrent efavirenz or nevirapine
Child: **PO** with concurrent efavirenz or nevirapine *6 mo–12 y, weight 7–15 kg,* 12/3 mg/kg b.i.d.; *weight 15–40 kg,* 10/2.5 mg/kg; *weight greater than 40 kg,* 400/100 mg b.i.d., increase dose *weight 7–15 kg,* 13/3.25 mg/kg; *weight 15–40 kg,* 11/2.75 mg/kg; *weight greater than 40 kg,* 533/133 mg b.i.d.
Adolescent/Child/Infant (6 mo to 18 y): **PO** Without concurrent efavirenz, nevirapine, fosamprenavir, or nelfinavir 230/57.5 mg/m^2 b.i.d.
Infant (14 days to 6 mo): **PO** 16/4 mg/kg or 300/75 mg/m^2 b.i.d.

ADMINISTRATION

Note: Take with food.

Oral

- Give with a meal or light snack.
- Note: If didanosine is concurrently ordered, give didanosine 1 h before or 2 h after lopinavir/ritonavir.
- Store refrigerated at 2°–8° C (36°–46° F). If stored at room temperature 25° C (77° F) or below, discard after 2 mo.

ADVERSE EFFECTS (≥1%) **Body as a Whole:** Asthenia, pain. **GI:** Abdominal pain, abnormal stools, *diarrhea, nausea,* vomiting. **CNS:** Headache, insomnia, abnormal taste. **Skin:** Rash. **Metabolic:** Hypercholesterolemia, increased triglycerides, ALT increased, weakness. **Hematologic:** Platelets decreased, amenorrhea.

INTERACTIONS Drug: Flecainide, propafenone, pimozide may lead to life-threatening arrhythmias; **rifampin** may decrease antiretroviral response; **dihydroergotamine, ergonovine, ergotamine, methylergonovine** may lead to acute ergot toxicity; HMG-COA REDUCTASE INHIBITORS may increase risk of myopathy and rhabdomyolysis; BENZODIAZEPINES may have prolonged sedation or respiratory depression; **efavirenz, nevirapine,** ANTICONVULSANTS, STEROIDS may decrease lopinavir levels; **delavirdine, ritonavir** may increase lopinavir levels; may increase levels of **amprenavir, indinavir, saquinavir, ketoconazole, itraconazole, midazolam, triazolam, rifabutin, sildenafil, atorvastatin, cerivastatin,** IMMUNOSUPPRESSANTS; may decrease levels of **atovaquone, methadone, ethinyl estradiol;** may increase trazodone toxicity; decrease efficacy of hormonal contraceptives, increases midazolam concentration and toxicity. Also see INTERACTIONS in **ritonavir** monograph. **Herbal: St. John's wort, garlic** may decrease effect.

PHARMACOKINETICS Absorption: Increased absorption when taken with food. **Peak:** 4 h. **Distribution:** 98–99% protein bound. **Metabolism:** Extensively metabolized by CYP3A. **Elimination:** Primarily in feces. **Half-Life:** 5–6 h lopinavir.

NURSING IMPLICATIONS

Assessment & Drug Effects

- Monitor for S&S of: Pancreatitis, especially with marked triglyceride elevations; new onset diabetes or loss of glycemic control; hypothyroidism or Cushing's syndrome.
- Lab test: Periodically monitor fasting blood glucose, AST and ALT, total cholesterol and triglycerides, serum amylase, inorganic phosphorus, CBC with differential, and thyroid functions.

Patient & Family

- Report all prescription and nonprescription drugs being taken. Do not use herbal products, especially St. John's wort, without first consulting the physician.
- Become familiar with the potential adverse effects of this drug; report those that are bothersome to physician.
- Concurrent use of sildenafil (Viagra) increases risk for adverse effects such as hypotension, changes in vision, and sustained erection; promptly report any of these to the physician.
- Use additional or alternative contraceptive measures if estrogen-based hormonal contraceptives are being used.

LORATADINE (Pr)

(lor'a-ta-deen)

Alavert, Claritin, Claritin Reditabs

Classifications: NONSEDATING ANTIHISTAMINE; H_1-RECEPTOR ANTAGONIST
Therapeutic: NONSEDATING ANTIHISTAMINE
Pregnancy Category: B

AVAILABILITY 10 mg tablets; 1 mg/mL syrup

ACTION & *THERAPEUTIC EFFECT* Long-acting nonsedating antihistamine with selective peripheral H_1-receptor sites, thus blocking histamine release. Loratadine is a long-acting H_1-receptor antagonist of histamine that disrupts capillary permeability, edema formation, and constriction of respiratory, GI, and vascular smooth muscle. *Effective in relieving allergic reactions related to histamine release.*

USES Relief of symptoms of seasonal allergic rhinitis; idiopathic chronic urticaria.

CONTRAINDICATIONS Hypersensitivity to loratadine, lactation.
CAUTIOUS USE Hepatic and renal impairment, renal disease, renal failure; asthma; pregnancy (category B).

ROUTE & DOSAGE

Allergic Rhinitis
Adult: **PO** 10 mg once/day on an empty stomach; start patients with liver disease with 10 mg every other day
Child: **PO** *Weight less than 30 kg,* 5 mg daily; *weight greater than 30 kg,* 10 mg daily

ADMINISTRATION

Oral
- Give on an empty stomach, 1 h before or 2 h after a meal.
- Store in a tightly closed container.

ADVERSE EFFECTS (≥1%) **CNS:** Dizziness, dry mouth, fatigue, headache, somnolence, altered salivation and lacrimation, thirst, flushing, anxiety, depression, impaired concentration. **CV:** Hypotension, hypertension, palpitations, syncope, tachycardia. **GI:** Nausea, vomiting, flatulence, abdominal distress, constipation, diarrhea, weight gain, dyspepsia. **Body as a Whole:** Arthralgia, myalgia. **Special Senses:** Blurred vision, earache, eye pain, tinnitus. **Skin:** Rash, pruritus, photosensitivity.

PHARMACOKINETICS Absorption: Readily from GI tract. **Onset:** 1–3 h. **Peak:** 8–12 h; reaches steady state levels in 3–5 days. **Duration:** 24 h. **Distribution:** Distributed into breast milk. **Metabolism:** In liver to active metabolite, descarboethoxyloratidine. **Elimination:** In urine and feces. **Half-Life:** 12–15 h.

NURSING IMPLICATIONS

Assessment & Drug Effects
- Assess carefully for and report distressing or dangerous S&S that occur after initiation of the drug. A variety of adverse effects, although not common, are possible. Some are an indication to discontinue the drug.
- Monitor cardiovascular status and report significant changes in BP and palpitations or tachycardia.

Patient & Family Education
- Drug may cause significant drowsiness in older adult patients and those with liver or kidney impairment.
- Note: Concurrent use of alcohol and other CNS depressants may have an additive effect.

LORAZEPAM (Pr)

(lor-a′ze-pam)
Ativan
Classifications: ANXIOLYTIC; SEDATIVE-HYPNOTIC; BENZODIAZEPINE
Therapeutic: ANTIANXIETY; SEDATIVE-HYPNOTIC
Pregnancy Category: D
Controlled Substance: Schedule IV

AVAILABILITY 0.5 mg, 1 mg, 2 mg tablets; 2 mg/mL oral solution; 2 mg/mL, 4 mg/mL injection

ACTION & *THERAPEUTIC EFFECT*
Most potent of the available benzo-

diazepines. Effects (antianxiety, sedative, hypnotic, and skeletal muscle relaxant) are mediated by the inhibitory neurotransmitter GABA. Action sites are thalamic, hypothalamic, and limbic levels of CNS. *Antianxiety agent that also causes mild suppression of REM sleep, while increasing total sleep time.*

USES Management of anxiety disorders and for short-term relief of symptoms of anxiety. Also used for preanesthetic medication to produce sedation and to reduce anxiety and recall of events related to day of surgery; for management of status epilepticus.

UNLABELED USES Chemotherapy-induced nausea and vomiting.

CONTRAINDICATIONS Known sensitivity to benzodiazepines; acute narrow-angle glaucoma; primary depressive disorders or psychosis; COPD; children younger than 12 y (**PO** preparation); coma, shock, sleep apnea; acute alcohol intoxication; dementia; pregnancy (category D), and lactation.

CAUTIOUS USE Renal or hepatic impairment; renal failure; organic brain syndrome; myasthenia gravis; narrow-angle glaucoma; pulmonary disease; mania; psychosis; suicidal tendency; history of seizure disorders; GI disorders; older adult and debilitated patients; limited pulmonary reserve.

ROUTE & DOSAGE

Antianxiety

Adult: **PO** 2–6 mg/day in divided doses (max: 10 mg/day)
Geriatric: **PO** 0.5–1 mg/day (max: 2 mg/day)
Child: **PO/IV** 0.05 mg/kg q4–8h (max: 2 mg/dose)

Insomnia

Adult: **PO** 2–4 mg at bedtime
Geriatric: **PO** 0.5–1 mg at bedtime

Premedication

Adult: **IM** 2–4 mg (0.05 mg/kg) at least 2 h before surgery **IV** 0.044 mg/kg up to 2 mg 15–20 min before surgery
Child: **PO/IV/IM** 0.05 mg/kg (range: 0.02–0.09 mg/kg)

Status Epilepticus

Adult: **IV** 4 mg injected slowly at 2 mg/min, may repeat dose once if inadequate response after 10 min

ADMINISTRATION

Oral

- Increase the evening dose when higher oral dosage is required, before increasing daytime doses.

Intramuscular

- Injected undiluted, deep into a large muscle mass.

Intravenous

- IV administration to neonates, infants, children: Verify correct IV concentration and rate of infusion with physician. ▪ Patients older than 50 y may have more profound and prolonged sedation with IV lorazepam (usual max initial dose: 2 mg).

PREPARE: **Direct:** Prepare lorazepam immediately before use. Dilute with an equal volume of sterile water, D5W, or NS.

ADMINISTER: **Direct:** Inject directly into vein or into IV infusion tubing at rate not to exceed 2 mg/min and with repeated aspiration to confirm IV entry. ▪ Take extreme precautions to PREVENT intra-arterial injection and perivascular extravasation.

INCOMPATIBILITIES **Solution/additive: Dexamethasone. Y-site: Aldesleukin, aztreonam, fluconazole, foscarnet, gallium, idarubicin, imipenem/cilastatin, omeprazole, ondansetron, sargramostim, sufentanil, thiopental, TPN with albumin.**

▪ Keep parenteral preparation in refrigerator; do not freeze. ▪ Do not use a discolored solution or one with a precipitate.

ADVERSE EFFECTS (≥1%) **Body as a Whole:** Usually disappear with continued medication or with reduced dosage. **CNS:** Anterograde amnesia, *drowsiness, sedation,* dizziness, weakness, unsteadiness, disorientation, depression, sleep disturbance, restlessness, confusion, hallucinations. **CV:** Hypertension or hypotension. **Special Senses:** Blurred vision, diplopia; depressed hearing. **GI:** Nausea, vomiting, abdominal discomfort, anorexia.

INTERACTIONS Drug: Alcohol, CNS DEPRESSANTS, ANTICONVULSANTS potentiate CNS depression; **cimetidine** increases lorazepam plasma levels, increases toxicity; lorazepam may decrease antiparkinsonism effects of **levodopa;** may increase **phenytoin** levels; smoking decreases sedative and antianxiety effects. **Herbal: Kava, valerian** may potentiate sedation.

PHARMACOKINETICS Absorption: Readily absorbed from GI tract. **Onset:** 1–5 min IV; 15–30 min IM. **Peak:** 60–90 min IM; 2 h PO. **Duration:** 12–24 h. **Distribution:** Crosses placenta; distributed into breast milk. **Metabolism:** Not metabolized in liver. **Elimination:** In urine. **Half-Life:** 10–20 h.

NURSING IMPLICATIONS

Assessment & Drug Effects

- IM or IV lorazepam injection of 2–4 mg is usually followed by a depth of drowsiness or sleepiness that permits patient to respond to simple instructions whether patient appears to be asleep or awake.
- Supervise ambulation of older adult patients for at least 8 h after lorazepam injection to prevent falling and injury.
- Lab tests: Assess CBC and liver function tests periodically for patients on long-term therapy.
- Supervise patient who exhibits depression with anxiety closely; the possibility of suicide exists, particularly when there is apparent improvement in mood.

Patient & Family Education

- Do not drive or engage in other hazardous activities for a least 24–48 h after receiving IM injection of lorazepam.
- Do not consume alcoholic beverages for at least 24–48 h after an injection and avoid when taking an oral regimen.
- Notify physician if daytime psychomotor function is impaired; a change in regimen or drug may be needed.
- Terminate regimen gradually over a period of several days. Do not stop long-term therapy abruptly; withdrawal may be induced with feelings of panic, tonic–clonic seizures, tremors, abdominal and muscle cramps, sweating, vomiting.
- Discuss discontinuation of drug with physician if you wish to become pregnant.

LOSARTAN POTASSIUM Pr

(lo-sar'tan)

Cozaar

Classifications: ANGIOTENSIN II RECEPTOR ANTAGONIST; ANTIHYPERTENSIVE

Therapeutic: ANTIHYPERTENSIVE

Pregnancy Category: C first trimester; D second and third trimester

AVAILABILITY 25 mg, 50 mg tablets

ACTION & *THERAPEUTIC EFFECT*
Angiotensin II receptor (type AT_1) antagonist acts as a potent vasoconstrictor and primary vasoactive hormone of the renin–angiotensin–aldosterone system. Selectively blocks the binding of angiotensin II to the AT_1 receptors found in many tissues (e.g., vascular smooth muscle, adrenal glands). *Antihypertensive effect is due to vasodilation and inhibition of aldosterone effects on sodium and water retention.*

USES Hypertension.

CONTRAINDICATIONS Hypersensitivity to losartan, children younger than 6 y or children with CrCl less than 30 mL/min/1.73 m²; pregnancy (category D second and third trimester), lactation.

CAUTIOUS USE Patients on diuretics, heart failure; hyperkalemia; hypovolemia; renal or hepatic impairment pregnancy (category C first trimester).

ROUTE & DOSAGE

Hypertension

Adult: **PO** 25–50 mg in 1–2 divided doses (max: 100 mg/day); start with 25 mg/day if volume depleted (i.e., on diuretics)

ADMINISTRATION

Oral

- Note: Starting dose is reduced 50% in patients with possible volume depletion or a history of liver disease.

ADVERSE EFFECTS (≥1%) **CNS:** Dizziness, insomnia, headache. **GI:** Diarrhea, dyspepsia. **Musculoskeletal:** Muscle cramps, myalgia, back or leg pain. **Respiratory:** Nasal congestion, cough, upper respiratory infection, sinusitis.

INTERACTIONS Drug: Phenobarbital decreases serum levels of losartan and its metabolite.

PHARMACOKINETICS Absorption: Rapidly absorbed from GI tract; approximately 25–33% reaches systemic circulation. **Peak:** 6 h. **Duration:** 24 h. **Distribution:** Highly bound to plasma proteins; does not appear to cross blood–brain barrier. **Metabolism:** Extensively metabolized in liver by cytochrome P450 enzymes to an active metabolite. **Elimination:** 35% in urine, 60% in feces. **Half-Life:** Losartan 1.5–2 h; metabolite 6–9 h.

NURSING IMPLICATIONS

Assessment & Drug Effects

- Monitor BP at drug trough (prior to a scheduled dose).
- Inadequate response may be improved by splitting the daily dose into twice-daily dose.
- Lab tests: Monitor CBC, electrolytes, liver & kidney function with long-term therapy.

Patient & Family Education

- Do not use potassium supplements or salt substitutes without consulting physician.
- Notify physician of symptoms of hypotension (e.g., dizziness, fainting).
- Notify physician immediately of pregnancy.

LOTEPREDNOL ETABONATE

(lo-te′pred-nol e-ta-bo′nate)

Alrex, Lotemax
Pregnancy Category: C
See Appendix A-1.

LOVASTATIN

(loe-vah-stat′in)

Altoprev, Mevacor

Classifications: ANTILIPEMIC; LIPID-LOWERING; HMG-COA REDUCTASE INHIBITOR (STATIN)

Therapeutic: LIPID-LOWERING; STATIN

Pregnancy Category: X

AVAILABILITY 10 mg, 20 mg, 40 mg tablets; 10 mg, 20 mg, 40 mg, 60 mg extended release tablets

ACTION & *THERAPEUTIC EFFECT* Reduces plasma cholesterol levels by interfering with body's ability to produce its own cholesterol. This cholesterol-lowering effect triggers induction of LDL receptors, which promote removal of LDL and VLDL remnants (precursors of LDL) from plasma. Also results in an increase in plasma HDL concentrations (HDL collects excess cholesterol from body cells and transports it to liver for excretion). *Reduces plasma cholesterol levels by interfering with body's ability to produce its own cholesterol, and it also lowers LDL and VLDL cholesterol.*

USES Adjunct to diet for treatment of primary moderate hypercholesterolemia (types IIa and IIb) when diet and other nonpharmacologic measures have failed to reduce elevated total LDL cholesterol levels. Lovastatin is less effective in treatment of homozygous familial hypercholesterolemia than primary hypercholesterolemia, possibly because in these persons LDL receptors are not functional.

CONTRAINDICATIONS Active liver disease, unexplained elevations of serum transaminases; cholestasis, hepatic encephalopathy, hepatic disease, hepatitis, jaundice; rhabdomyolysis; surgery, trauma; hypotension, renal failure; pregnancy (category X), lactation, children younger than 10 y.

CAUTIOUS USE Patient who consumes substantial quantities of alcohol; history of liver disease; electrolyte imbalance, endocrine disease, females of childbearing age, infection, myopathy, renal disease, renal impairment, seizure disorder. Patient with risk factors predisposing to development of kidney failure secondary to rhabdomyolysis.

ROUTE & DOSAGE

Hypercholesterolemia
Adult: **PO** 20–40 mg 1–2 times/day

ADMINISTRATION

Oral

- Give with the evening meal if daily. Give the first of 2 daily doses with breakfast.
- Ensure that extended release tablets are not crushed or chewed. They **must be** swallowed whole.
- Store tablets at 5°–30° C (41°–86° F) in light-resistant, tightly closed container.

ADVERSE EFFECTS (≥1%) **Body as a Whole:** Generally well tolerated. **CNS:** Dizziness, mild transient headache, insomnia, fatigue. **Special Senses:** Blurred vision. **GI:** Dyspepsia, dysgeusia, heartburn, nausea, constipation, diarrhea, flatus, abdominal pain, and cramps. **Metabolic:** Increases in serum transaminases, elevated creatine phosphokinase (CPK). **Skin:** Rash, pruritus.

INTERACTIONS Drug: Clarithromycin, clofibrate, cyclosporine, danazol, erythromycin, fenofibrate, fluconazole, gemfibrozil, itraconazole, ketoconazole, miconazole, niacin, and PROTEASE INHIBITORS increase risk of myopathy and rhabdomyolysis; potentiate hypoprothrombinemia with **warfarin. Food: Grapefruit juice** (greater than 1 qt/day) may increase risk of myopathy and rhabdomyolysis.

PHARMACOKINETICS Absorption: 30% from GI tract; extensive first-pass metabolism. **Onset:** 2 wk. **Peak:** 4–6 wk. **Distribution:** Crosses blood–brain barrier and placenta; distributed into breast milk. **Metabolism:** In liver to active metabolites. **Elimination:** 83% in feces; 10% in urine. **Half-Life:** 1.1–1.7 h.

NURSING IMPLICATIONS

Assessment & Drug Effects

- Lab tests: Perform liver function tests q4–6wk during first 15 mo of therapy. Monitor blood cholesterol levels and lipid profile periodically.
- Drug-induced increases in serum transaminases, usually not associated with jaundice or other clinical S&S, return to normal when drug is discontinued. If these values rise and remain at 3 times upper level of normal, drug will be discontinued and liver biopsy considered.

Patient & Family Education

- Notify physician promptly of muscle tenderness or pain, especially if accompanied by fever or malaise. If CPK is elevated or if myositis is diagnosed, drug will be discontinued.
- Avoid or at least reduce alcohol consumption.
- Understand that lovastatin is not a substitute for, but an addition to, diet therapy.

LOXAPINE HYDROCHLORIDE

(lox'a-peen)

Loxitane C, Loxitane IM

LOXAPINE SUCCINATE

Loxitane, Loxapac ♣

Classification: ANTIPSYCHOTIC
Therapeutic: ANTIPSYCHOTIC
Prototype: Chlorpromazine
Pregnancy Category: C

AVAILABILITY 5 mg, 10 mg, 25 mg, 50 mg capsules; 25 mg/mL oral solution; 50 mg/mL injection

ACTION & *THERAPEUTIC EFFECT* This antipsychotic blocks postsynaptic dopamine receptors in limbic system and increases dopamine turnover by blockade of D_2-receptors in that region. After approximately 12 wk of chronic therapy, depolarization blockade of dopamine occurs, decreasing dopamine neurotransmission, correlating with its antipsychotic effects. *Stabilizes emotional component of schizophrenia by acting on subcortical level of CNS.*

USES Manifestations of psychotic disorders.

UNLABELED USES Anxiety associated with mental depression.

CONTRAINDICATIONS Severe drug-induced CNS depression; Parkinson's disease; comatose states, children younger than 16 y, lactation.

CAUTIOUS USE Glaucoma, prostatic hypertrophy, urinary retention, history of convulsive disorders, cardiovascular disease; alcoholism;

brain tumor; older adults; hematologic disease; hepatic disease; peptic ulcer disease; renal impairment; thyroid disease; pregnancy (category C).

ROUTE & DOSAGE

Psychosis

Adult: **PO** Start with 10 mg b.i.d. and rapidly increase to maintenance levels of 60–100 mg/day in 2–4 divided doses (max: 250 mg/day) **IM** 12.5–50 mg q4–6h

Dementia Behavior

Geriatric: **PO** 5–10 mg 1–2 times/day, may increase q4–7days (max: 125 mg/day)

L

ADMINISTRATION

Oral

- Give with food, milk, or water to reduce possibility of stomach irritation.
- Dilute oral concentrate in about 2–3 oz (60–90 mL) water or orange or grapefruit juice shortly before administration. Measure concentrate with calibrated dropper dispensed with drug. Do not store diluted solution.

Intramuscular

- Use only with acute psychosis or when oral route not feasible.
- Reduce dosage gradually over period of several days when therapy is to be terminated.
- Protect from light and freezing. Intensification of straw color to light amber is acceptable. Discard if solution is noticeably discolored.

ADVERSE EFFECTS (≥1%) **CNS:** *Drowsiness,* sedation, dizziness, syncope, EEG changes, paresthesias, staggering gait, muscle weakness, *extrapyramidal effects,* akathisia, tardive dyskinesia, neuroleptic malignant syndrome. **CV:** *Orthostatic hypotension,* hypertension, tachycardia. **Special Senses:** Nasal congestion, tinnitus; blurred vision, ptosis. **GI:** Constipation, dry mouth. **Skin:** Dermatitis, facial edema, pruritus, photosensitivity. **Urogenital:** Urinary retention, menstrual irregularities. **Body as a Whole:** Polydipsia, weight gain or loss, hyperpyrexia, transient leukopenia.

INTERACTIONS Drug: Alcohol and other CNS DEPRESSANTS potentiate CNS depression; will inhibit vasopressor effects of **epinephrine.**

PHARMACOKINETICS Absorption: Readily absorbed from GI tract. **Onset:** 20–30 min. **Peak:** 1.5–3 h. **Duration:** 12 h. **Distribution:** Widely distributed; crosses placenta; distributed into breast milk. **Metabolism:** In liver. **Elimination:** 50% in urine, 50% in feces. **Half-Life:** 19 h.

NURSING IMPLICATIONS

Assessment & Drug Effects

- Monitor baseline BP pattern prior and during therapy; both hypotension and hypertension have been reported as adverse reactions.
- Observe carefully for extrapyramidal effects such as acute dystonia (see Appendix F) during early therapy. Most symptoms disappear with dose adjustment or with antiparkinsonism drug therapy.
- Discontinue therapy and report promptly to physician the first signs of impending tardive dyskinesia (fine vermicular movements of the tongue) when patient is on long-term treatment.
- Monitor I&O and bowel elimination patterns and check for bladder distention. Depressed patients often fail to report urinary retention or constipation.

- Risk of seizures is increased in those with history of convulsive disorders.

Patient & Family Education

- Do NOT change dosage regimen in any way without physician approval.
- Avoid self-dosing with OTC drugs unless approved by the physician.
- Drowsiness usually decreases with continued therapy. If it persists and interferes with daily activities, consult physician. A change in time of administration or dose may help.
- Avoid potentially hazardous activity until response to drug is known.
- Learn measures to relieve dry mouth; rinse mouth frequently with water, suck hard candy. Avoid commercial products that may contain alcohol and enhance drying and irritation.
- Notify physician of blurred or colored vision.
- Do not take drug dose and notify physician of following: Light-colored stools, bruising, unexplained bleeding, prolonged constipation, tremor, restlessness and excitement, sore throat and fever, rash.
- Stay out of bright sun; cover exposed skin with sunscreen.

LUBIPROSTONE

(lu-bi-pros'tone)

Amitiza

Classifications: LAXATIVE AND STOOL SOFTENER; CHLORIDE CHANNEL ACTIVATOR

Therapeutic: LAXATIVE AND STOOL SOFTENER

Pregnancy Category: C

AVAILABILITY 24 mcg capsule

ACTION & *THERAPEUTIC EFFECT*
Lubiprostone activates chloride channels in the intestine that enhance chloride-rich intestinal fluid secretion without changing serum sodium and potassium concentrations. *The increase in intestinal fluid secretion enhances intestinal motility, thereby increasing the passage of stool and alleviating symptoms associated with chronic idiopathic constipation.*

USES Treatment of chronic idiopathic constipation; constipation predominant irritable bowel syndrome (IBS-C).

CONTRAINDICATIONS Hypersensitivity to lubiprostone; history of mechanical GI obstruction: Crohn's disease, volvulus, diverticulitis, etc.; severe diarrhea; lactation. Safe use in children is unknown.
CAUTIOUS USE GI disease, pregnancy (category C).

ROUTE & DOSAGE

Chronic Idiopathic Constipation
Adult: **PO** 24 mcg b.i.d.

IBS-C
Adult: **PO** 8 mcg daily

ADMINISTRATION

Oral

- Administer with food to minimize nausea.
- Capsule should be swallowed whole.
- Do not administer to a patient with severe diarrhea or suspected bowel obstruction.
- Store at 15°–30° C (59°–86° F).

ADVERSE EFFECTS (≥1%) **Body as a Whole:** Chest pain, peripheral edema, pyrexia. **CNS:** Anxiety, depression, dizziness, fatigue, *headache,* insomnia. **CV:** Hypertension. **GI:** *Abdominal pain and discomfort,* constipation, *diarrhea,* dry mouth, dyspepsia, *flatulence,* viral gastroenteritis, gastroesophageal reflux disease, loose stools, *nausea,* vomiting. **Musculoskeletal:** Arthralgia, back pain, pain in extremities. **Respiratory:** Bronchitis, cough, dyspnea, nasopharyngitis, sinusitis, upper respiratory infection. **Urogenital:** Urinary tract infection.

PHARMACOKINETICS Absorption: Very low. **Peak:** 1.1 h (M3). **Distribution:** 94% protein bound. **Metabolism:** Extensive nonhepatic metabolism. **Elimination:** Urine (major) and feces. **Half-Life:** 0.9–1.4 h.

NURSING IMPLICATIONS

Assessment & Drug Effects

- Monitor for and report S&S of bowel obstruction.
- Lab tests: Baseline LFTs.

Patient & Family Education

- Report to physician if you experience severe or prolonged diarrhea, or new or worsening abdominal pain or dyspnea following dosing.
- Do not drive or engage in potentially hazardous activities until response to drug is known.

LYMPHOCYTE IMMUNE GLOBULIN

(lim′fo-site)

Antithymocyte Globulin, ATG, Atgam

Classifications: BIOLOGICAL RESPONSE MODIFIER; IMMUNOGLOBULIN

Therapeutic: LYMPHOCYTE IMMUNOGLOBULIN; ANTITHYMOCYTE GLOBULIN; IMMUNOSUPPRESSANT

Prototype: Immune globulin

Pregnancy Category: C

AVAILABILITY 50 mg/mL injection

ACTION & *THERAPEUTIC EFFECT* An immunoglobulin (IgG) and lymphocyte-selective immunosuppressant derived from human thymus lymphocytes. During rejection of allografts, human leukocyte antigens (HLAs) bind to peptides and form complexes. Helper T-lymphocytes activate these complexes and produce interleukins, cytotoxic T-cells, and natural killer cells, resulting in destruction of transplanted tissue. *Alters the formation of T-lymphocytes, thus reversing acute allograft rejection.*

USES Primarily to prevent or delay onset or to reverse acute renal allograft rejection.

UNLABELED USES Moderate and severe aplastic anemia in patients unsuitable for bone marrow transplantation, T-cell malignancy, acute and chronic graft-vs-host disease, and to prevent rejection of skin allografts.

CONTRAINDICATIONS Hypersensitivity to lymphocyte immune globulin or other equine gamma globulin preparations; history of previous systemic reaction to ATG, hemorrhagic diatheses; leporine protein hypersensitivity; use in kidney transplant patient not receiving a concomitant immunosuppressant; fungal or viral infections.

CAUTIOUS USE Hypotension, infection, leukopenia, lymphoma, neoplastic disease, thrombocytopenia, vaccination, varicella; pregnancy (category C), lactation; children (experience limited).

ROUTE & DOSAGE

Renal Allotransplantation

Adult: **IV** 10–30 mg/kg/day by slow IV infusion
Child: **IV** 5–25 mg/kg/day by slow IV infusion

Prevention of Allograft Rejection

Adult: **IV** 15 mg/kg/day for 14 days followed by 15 mg/kg every other day for 14 days

Treatment of Allograft Rejection

Adult: **IV** 10–15 mg/kg/day for 14 days followed by 15 mg/kg every other day for 14 days if needed

Aplastic Anemia

Adult/Child: **IV** 10–20 mg/kg/day × 8–14 days followed by 10–20 mg/kg every other day for 7 doses

ADMINISTRATION

Intravenous

Note: Administer lymphocyte immune globulin (ATG) ONLY if experienced with immunosuppressant therapy and management of kidney transplant patients.

▪ Do an intradermal skin test to rule out allergy to the drug before first dose. ▪ Inject 0.1 mL of a 1:1000 dilution (5 mcg equine IgG in normal saline) and a saline control. ▪ If local reaction occurs (wheal or erythema more than 10 mm) or if there is pseudopod formation, itching, or local swelling, use caution during infusion. ▪ Discontinue infusion if systemic reaction develops (generalized rash, tachycardia, dyspnea, hypotension, anaphylaxis).

PREPARE: **IV Infusion:** Withdraw required dose of ATG concentrate and inject into IV solution container of 0.45% NaCl or NS. Invert IV container during injection of ATG to prevent its contact with air inside container. Use enough IV solution to create a concentration 4 mg/mL or less. ▪ Inspect concentrate and diluted solution for particulate matter (may develop during storage) and discoloration; discard if present.

ADMINISTER: **IV Infusion:** Give through an in-line 0.2–1 micron filter into a high-flow vein to decrease potential for phlebitis and thrombosis. Give over 4 h or longer (usually 4–8 h). ▪ Must finish infusion within 12 h of preparation.

▪ Total storage time for diluted solutions: NO MORE than 12 h (including storage time and actual infusion time). ▪ Refrigerate ampules and diluted solutions (if prepared before time of infusion) at 2°–8° C (35°–46° F). Do not freeze.

ADVERSE EFFECTS (≥1%) **CNS:** Headache, paresthesia, seizures. **CV:** Peripheral thrombophlebitis, hypotension, <u>hypertension</u>. **GI:** Nausea, vomiting, diarrhea, stomatitis, hiccups, epigastric pain, abdominal distention. **Hematologic:** *Leukopenia, thrombocytopenia.* **Musculoskeletal:** Arthralgia, myalgias, chest or back pain. **Respiratory:** Dyspnea, <u>laryngospasm, pulmonary edema</u>. **Skin:** *Rash, pruritus,* urticaria, wheal and flare. **Body as a Whole:** *Chills, fever,* night sweats, pain at infusion site, hyperglycemia, systemic infection, wound dehiscence; <u>anaphylaxis</u>, *serum sickness,* herpes simplex virus reactivation.

INTERACTIONS Drug: Azathioprine, CORTICOSTEROIDS, other IMMU-

NOSUPPRESSANTS increase degree of immunosuppression.

PHARMACOKINETICS Distribution: Poorly distributed into lymphoid tissues (spleen, lymph nodes); probably crosses placenta and into breast milk. **Elimination:** About 1% of dose is excreted in urine. **Half-Life:** Approximately 6 days.

NURSING IMPLICATIONS

Assessment & Drug Effects

- Discontinue infusion and initiate appropriate therapy promptly with onset of anaphylactic response (respiratory distress; pain in chest, flank, back; hypotension, anxiety).
- Monitor closely BP, vital signs, and patient's complaints during entire administration period. Prompt treatment is indicated for symptoms of anaphylaxis (incidence: 1%), serum sickness, or allergic response. Always have equipment for assisted respiration, epinephrine, antihistamines, corticosteroid, and vasopressor available at bedside.
- Watch closely for S&S of serum sickness: Fever, malaise, arthralgia, nausea, vomiting, lymphadenopathy and morbilliform eruptions on trunk and extremities. Rash begins as asymptomatic pale pink macules in periumbilical region, axilla, and groin, then rapidly becomes generalized. Serum sickness usually occurs 6–18 days after initiation of therapy; may occur during drug administration or when treatment is stopped.
- Monitor carefully for S&S of thrombocytopenia, concurrent infection, and leukopenia; patient usually receives concomitant corticosteroids and antimetabolites.
- Monitor patient's temperature and attend to complaints of sore throat or rhinorrhea. Report to physician.

Patient & Family Education

- Notify physician immediately of pain in chest, flank, or back; chills; pruritus; night sweats; sore throat.

MAFENIDE ACETATE

(ma′fe-nide)
Sulfamylon
Classification: ANTIBIOTIC, SULFONAMIDE
Therapeutic: ANTIBIOTIC
Prototype: Sulfisoxazole
Pregnancy Category: C

AVAILABILITY 5% solution; cream

ACTION & *THERAPEUTIC EFFECT* Produce marked reduction of bacterial growth in vascular tissue. Active in presence of purulent matter and serum. *Bacteriostatic against many gram-positive and gram-negative organisms, including* Pseudomonas aeruginosa*, and certain strains of anaerobes.*

USES Adjunctive therapy in second- and third-degree burns to prevent sepsis.

CONTRAINDICATIONS History of hypersensitivity to mafenide; respiratory (inhalation) injury, pulmonary infection; lactation, children younger than 3 mo.
CAUTIOUS USE Impaired kidney or pulmonary function, burn patients with acute kidney failure; pregnancy (category C).

ROUTE & DOSAGE

Burns
Adult: **Topical** Apply aseptically to burn areas to a thickness of

approximately 15 mm ($^1/_{16}$ in) once or twice daily

ADMINISTRATION

Topical

- Apply cream or solution aseptically to cleansed, debrided burn areas with sterile gloved hand.
- Cover burn areas with cream at all times. Make reapplications to areas from which cream has been removed as necessary.
- Store in tight, light-resistant containers. Avoid extremes of temperature.

ADVERSE EFFECTS (≥1%) **Hypersensitivity:** Pruritus, rash, urticaria, blisters, facial edema, eosinophilia. **Skin:** *Intense pain, burning, or stinging at application sites,* bleeding of skin, excessive body water loss, delayed eschar separation, excoriation of new skin, superinfections. **Hematologic:** Hemolytic anemia, bone marrow suppression (rare). **Other:** Metabolic acidosis.

INTERACTIONS Drug: No clinically significant interactions established.

PHARMACOKINETICS Absorption: Rapidly from burn surface. **Peak:** 2–4 h. **Metabolism:** Rapidly inactivated in blood to a weak carbonic anhydrase inhibitor. **Elimination:** Via kidneys.

NURSING IMPLICATIONS

Assessment & Drug Effects

- Monitor vital signs. Report immediately changes in BP, pulse, and respiratory rate and volume.
- Monitor I&O. Report oliguria or changes in I&O ratio and pattern.
- Lab tests: Monitor fluid and electrolyte status throughout therapy; acid–base balance should be monitored in patients with extensive burns and in those with pulmonary or kidney dysfunction.
- Be alert to S&S of metabolic acidosis (see Appendix F).
- Be alert to evidence of superinfections (see Appendix F), particularly in and below burn eschar.
- Observe carefully; accuracy is critical. It is frequently difficult to distinguish between adverse reactions to mafenide and the effects of severe burns.
- Note: Allergic reactions have reportedly occurred 10–14 days after initiation of mafenide therapy. Temporary discontinuation of drug may be necessary.
- Report intense local pain to physician; pain caused by drug may require administration of analgesic.

Patient & Family Education

- Apply only a thin dressing over burns unless otherwise directed.
- Therapy is usually continued until healing is progressing well (usually 60 days) or site is ready for grafting (after about 35–40 days). It is not withdrawn while there is a possibility of infection unless adverse reactions intervene.
- Report any of the following to the physician immediately: Foul-smelling drainage from wounds, bleeding at wound site, unexplained fever.

MAGALDRATE

(mag′al-drate)

Riopan

Classification: ANTACID

Therapeutic: ANTACID

Prototype: Aluminum hydroxide

Pregnancy Category: B with occasional use

AVAILABILITY 540 mg/5 mL suspension

ACTION & *THERAPEUTIC EFFECT* By reducing gastric acidity, stomach pH increases and proteolytic activity of pepsin is inhibited. *Nonsystemic antacid with true buffering action and high acid-neutralizing capacity.*

USES Symptomatic relief of hyperacidity associated with peptic ulcer, gastritis, peptic esophagitis, and hiatal hernia, particularly in patients who need to restrict sodium.

CONTRAINDICATIONS Sensitivity to components; hypermagnesia; appendicitis, colostomy, diverticulitis, ileostomy, ulcerative colitis; pregnancy (category B) with occasional use; children younger than 16 y.

CAUTIOUS USE Impaired kidney function, dialysis patients; CHF; biliary cirrhosis, GI obstruction, constipation.

M

ROUTE & DOSAGE

Antacid

Adult: **PO** 480–1080 mg (5–10 mL suspension or 1–2 tablets) q.i.d. (max: 20 tablets or 100 mL/day)

ADMINISTRATION

Oral

- Shake suspension vigorously before pouring. Preferably give between meals and at bedtime.
- Give suspension with sufficient water to ensure passage of drug into stomach.
- Make sure chewable tablets are chewed thoroughly before being swallowed. Give tablet to be swallowed whole with enough water to ensure prompt swallowing without chewing.

ADVERSE EFFECTS (≥1%) **GI:** Infrequent constipation or diarrhea (with prolonged use). **Urogenital:** Hypermagnesemia (in patients with impaired kidney function).

INTERACTIONS Drug: Will decrease absorption of TETRACYCLINES.

PHARMACOKINETICS Absorption: Minimally from GI tract. **Duration:** Buffering action up to 60 min.

NURSING IMPLICATIONS

Assessment & Drug Effects

- Question patient about effectiveness of medication in relieving GI distress.
- Lab tests: Check patients on prolonged therapy periodically for electrolyte imbalance (i.e., hypermagnesemia).

Patient & Family Education

- Be aware that, in common with other antacids, magaldrate may cause premature dissolution and absorption of enteric-coated tablets and interfere with the absorption of oral tetracyclines and other oral medications.
- Do not take other oral drugs, generally, within 1–2 h of an antacid.

MAGNESIUM CITRATE

(mag-nes′i-um)

Citrate of Magnesia, Citroma, Citro-Nesia

Classification: SALINE CATHARTIC

Therapeutic: LAXATIVE

Prototype: Magnesium hydroxide

Pregnancy Category: A

AVAILABILITY 1.75 g/30 mL solution

ACTION & *THERAPEUTIC EFFECT* Hyperosmotic laxative that promotes bowel evacuation by causing osmotic retention of fluid; this distends colon and stimulates peristaltic activity. *Evacuates bowels.*

USES To evacuate bowel prior to certain surgical and diagnostic procedures and to help eliminate parasites and toxic materials after treatment with a vermifuge.

CONTRAINDICATIONS Severe renal impairment, renal failure; nausea, vomiting, diarrhea, abdominal pain, acute surgical abdomen; intestinal impaction, obstruction or perforation; rectal bleeding; use of solutions containing sodium bicarbonate in patients on sodium-restricted diets; children younger than 2 y.

CAUTIOUS USE Mild or moderate renal impairment; cardiac disease; older adults; pregnancy (category A), lactation.

ROUTE & DOSAGE

Bowel Evacuation
Adult: **PO** 240 mL once
Child: **PO** *2–6 y,* 4–12 mL; *6–12 y,* 50–100 mL

ADMINISTRATION

Oral

- Give on an empty stomach with a full (240 mL) glass of water. Time dosing so that it does not interfere with sleep. Drug produces a watery or semifluid evacuation in 2–6 h.
- Chill solution by pouring it over ice or refrigerate it until ready to use to increase palatability.
- Be aware that once container is opened, effervescence will decrease. This does not effect the quality of preparation.
- Store at 2°–30° C (36°–86° F) in tightly covered containers.

ADVERSE EFFECTS (≥1%) **GI:** Abdominal cramps, nausea, fluid and electrolyte imbalance, hypermagnesemia (prolonged use).

INTERACTIONS Drug: May decrease effectiveness of **digoxin,** ORAL ANTICOAGULANTS, PHENOTHIAZINES; will decrease absorption of **ciprofloxacin,** TETRACYCLINES; **sodium polystyrene sulfonate** will bind magnesium, decreasing its effectiveness.

PHARMACOKINETICS Onset: 0.5–2 h.

NURSING IMPLICATIONS

Assessment & Drug Effects

- Monitor for dehydration, hypokalemia, and hyponatremia (see Appendix F) since drug may cause intense bowel evacuation.

Patient & Family Education

- Do not use for routine treatment of constipation (especially in older adult).
- Expect some degree of abdominal cramping.

MAGNESIUM HYDROXIDE Pr

(mag-nes′i-um)

Magnesia, Magnesia Magma, Milk of Magnesia, M.O.M.

Classifications: SALINE CATHARTIC; ANTACID

Therapeutic: LAXATIVE; ANTACID

Pregnancy Category: A

AVAILABILITY 311 mg tablets; 400 mg/5 mL, 800 mg/5 mL suspension

ACTION & *THERAPEUTIC EFFECT* Aqueous suspension of magne-

M

sium hydroxide with rapid and long-acting neutralizing action. Causes osmotic retention of fluid, which distends colon, resulting in mechanical stimulation of peristaltic activity. *Acts as antacid in low doses and as mild saline laxative at higher doses.*

USES Short-term treatment of occasional constipation, for relief of GI symptoms associated with hyperacidity, and as adjunct in treatment of peptic ulcer. Also has been used in treatment of poisoning by mineral acids and arsenic, and as mouthwash to neutralize acidity.

CONTRAINDICATIONS Abdominal pain, nausea, vomiting, chronic diarrhea, severe kidney dysfunction, fecal impaction, intestinal obstruction or perforation, rectal bleeding, colostomy, ileostomy, children younger than 2 y is not established. **CAUTIOUS USE** Older adults, renal impairment, renal disease; pregnancy (category A), lactation.

ROUTE & DOSAGE

Laxative
Adult: **PO** 2.4–4.8 g (30–60 mL)/day in 1 or more divided doses
Child: **PO** *2–5 y,* 0.4–1.2 g (5–15 mL)/day in 1 or more divided doses; *6–11 y,* 1.2–2.4 g (15–30 mL)/day in 1 or more divided doses

ADMINISTRATION

Oral
- Shake bottle well before pouring to assure mixing of suspension.
- Follow drug with at least a full glass of water to enhance drug action for laxative effect. Administer in the morning or at bedtime. Most effective when taken on an empty stomach.
- Store at 15°–30° C (59°–86° F) in tightly covered container. Slowly absorbs carbon dioxide on exposure to air. Avoid freezing.

ADVERSE EFFECTS (≥1%) **GI:** Nausea, vomiting, abdominal cramps, *diarrhea.* **Urogenital:** Alkalinization of urine. **Body as a Whole:** Weakness, lethargy, mental depression, hyporeflexia, dehydration, coma. **Metabolic:** Electrolyte imbalance with prolonged use. **CV:** Hypotension, bradycardia, complete heart block and other ECG abnormalities. **Respiratory:** Respiratory depression.

INTERACTIONS Drug: Milk of Magnesia decreases absorption of **chlordiazepoxide, dicumarol, digoxin, isoniazid,** QUINOLONES, TETRACYCLINES.

PHARMACOKINETICS Absorption: 15–30% of magnesium is absorbed. **Onset:** 3–6 h. **Distribution:** Small amounts distributed in saliva and breast milk. **Elimination:** In feces; some renal excretion.

NURSING IMPLICATIONS

Assessment & Drug Effects
- Evaluate the patient's continued need for drug. Prolonged and frequent use of laxative doses may lead to dependence. Additionally, even therapeutic doses can raise urinary pH and thereby predispose susceptible patients to urinary infection and urolithiasis.
- Lab tests: Monitor serum magnesium with signs of hypermagnesemia such as bradycardia (see Appendix F), especially with frequent use or any degree of renal impairment.

Patient & Family Education
- Investigate the cause of persistent or recurrent constipation or gastric distress with physician.

MAGNESIUM OXIDE

(mag-nes′i-um)

Mag-Ox, Maox, Par-Mag, Uro-Mag

Classifications: ANTACID; SALINE CATHARTIC

Therapeutic: ANTACID; MAGNESIUM SUPPLEMENT; LAXATIVE

Prototype: Magnesium hydroxide

Pregnancy Category: A

AVAILABILITY 400 mg, 420 mg, 500 mg tablets; 140 mg capsules

ACTION & *THERAPEUTIC EFFECT* Nonsystemic antacid with high neutralizing capacity and relatively long duration of action. *Acts as an antacid in low doses and a mild saline laxative at higher doses. Also effective as a magnesium supplement.*

USES Essentially the same as magnesium hydroxide. May also be used as magnesium supplement.

CONTRAINDICATIONS Abdominal pain, nausea, vomiting, diarrhea, severe kidney dysfunction, fecal impaction, intestinal obstruction or perforation, ileus; rectal bleeding, colostomy, ileostomy; AV block; hypermagnesia; children younger than 2 y.

CAUTIOUS USE Cardiac disease, renal disease, renal impairment; electrolyte imbalance; pregnancy (category A), lactation.

ROUTE & DOSAGE

Antacid

Adult: **PO** 280–1500 mg with water or milk q.i.d., p.c. and at bedtime

Laxative

Adult: **PO** 2–4 g with water or milk at bedtime

Magnesium Supplement

Adult: **PO** 400–1200 mg/day in divided doses

ADMINISTRATION

Oral

- Separate administration of this drug from other oral drugs by 1–2 h.
- Store at 15°–30° C (59°–86° F) in airtight containers. On exposure to air, magnesium oxide rapidly absorbs moisture and carbon dioxide.

ADVERSE EFFECTS (≥1%) **GI:** *Diarrhea,* abdominal cramps, nausea; hypermagnesemia, kidney stones (chronic use).

INTERACTIONS Drug: See magnesium hydroxide.

PHARMACOKINETICS Absorption: 30–50% from GI tract. **Elimination:** In urine.

NURSING IMPLICATIONS

Assessment & Drug Effects

- Monitor for dehydration, hypokalemia, and hyponatremia (see Appendix F) since drug may cause intense bowel evacuation.
- Lab tests: Check patients on prolonged therapy periodically for electrolyte imbalance (i.e., hypermagnesemia).

Patient & Family Education

- Liquid preparation is reportedly more effective than the tablet form, as with other antacids.

MAGNESIUM SALICYLATE

(mag-nes′i-um)

Doan's Pills, Magan, Mobidin

Classification: ANALGESIC, NONSTEROIDAL ANTI-INFLAMMATORY DRUG (NSAID)

Therapeutic: NONNARCOTIC ANALGESIC, NSAID; ANTIPYRETIC
Prototype: Aspirin
Pregnancy Category: C first and second trimester; D third trimester

AVAILABILITY 467 mg, 500 mg, 580 mg caplets; 545 mg, 600 mg tablets

ACTION & *THERAPEUTIC EFFECT* Sodium-free salicylate derivative that is a nonsteroidal anti-inflammatory drug (NSAID). It inhibits prostaglandin synthesis. Does not inhibit platelet aggregation or increase bleeding time. *In equal doses, less potent than aspirin as an analgesic and antipyretic. Has anti-inflammatory effects.*

M

USES Relief of pain and inflammation in rheumatoid arthritis, osteoarthritis, bursitis, and other musculoskeletal disorders.

CONTRAINDICATIONS Hypersensitivity to salicylates; erosive gastritis, peptic ulcer; advanced renal insufficiency, liver damage; thrombolytic therapy; bleeding disorders; before surgery; pregnancy (category D third trimester); children younger than 12 y.
CAUTIOUS USE Serious acid base imbalances; renal disease, history of GI bleeding, or peptic ulcers; SLE; history of acute bronchospasm; pregnancy (category C first and second trimester), lactation.

ROUTE & DOSAGE

Analgesic/Antipyretic
Adult: **PO** 650 mg t.i.d. or q.i.d.

Arthritic Conditions
Adult: **PO** Up to 9.6 g/day in divided doses

ADMINISTRATION

Oral
- Give with a full glass of water, food, or milk to minimize gastric irritation.

ADVERSE EFFECTS (≥1%) **Body as a Whole:** Salicylism [dizziness, drowsiness, tinnitus, hearing loss, nausea, vomiting, hypermagnesemia (with high doses in patients with renal insufficiency)].

INTERACTIONS Drug: Aminosalicylic acid increases risk of SALICYLATE toxicity; **ammonium chloride** and other ACIDIFYING AGENTS decrease renal elimination and increase risk of SALICYLATE toxicity; anticoagulants—added risk of bleeding with ANTICOAGULANTS; CARBONIC ANHYDRASE INHIBITORS enhance SALICYLATE toxicity; CORTICOSTEROIDS compound ulcerogenic effects; increases **methotrexate** toxicity; low doses of SALICYLATES may antagonize uricosuric effects of **probenecid, sulfinpyrazone.**

PHARMACOKINETICS Absorption: Well absorbed from the GI tract. **Peak:** 20 min. **Distribution:** Widely distributed with high levels of salicylic acid in liver and kidney, crosses placenta, excreted in breast milk. **Metabolism:** Salicylic acid is metabolized in liver. **Elimination:** In kidneys. **Half-Life:** 2–3 h with single dose, 15–30 h with chronic dosing.

NURSING IMPLICATIONS

Assessment & Drug Effects
- Lab tests: Monitor serum magnesium levels for hypermagnesemia if used in high dosages or in patients with any degree of renal impairment.

Patient & Family Education
- Report to physician promptly tinnitus, hearing loss, or dizziness.

- Do not to take aspirin-containing drugs without consent of physician.
- Check ingredients. Doan's pills may contain acetaminophen plus salicylamide.

MAGNESIUM SULFATE

(mag-nes'i-um)

Epsom Salt

Classifications: SALINE CATHARTIC; ELECTROLYTE REPLACEMENT; ANTICONVULSANT

Therapeutic: LAXATIVE; ELECTROLYTE REPLACEMENT; ANTICONVULSANT

Prototype: Magnesium hydroxide

Pregnancy Category: A

AVAILABILITY 0.8 mEq/mL, 1 mEq/mL, 4 mEq/mL injection

ACTION & *THERAPEUTIC EFFECT* **Orally:** Acts as a laxative by osmotic retention of fluid, which distends colon, increases water content of feces, and causes mechanical stimulation of bowel activity. **Parenterally:** Acts as a CNS depressant and also as a depressant of smooth, skeletal, and cardiac muscle function. Anticonvulsant properties thought to be produced by CNS depression by decreasing the amount of acetylcholine liberated from motor nerve terminals, producing peripheral neuromuscular blockade. *Effective parenterally as a CNS depressant, smooth muscle relaxant and anticonvulsant in labor and delivery, and in cardiac disorders. It is a laxative when taken orally.*

USES Orally to relieve acute constipation and to evacuate bowel in preparation for x-ray of intestines. Parenterally to control seizures in toxemia of pregnancy, epilepsy, and acute nephritis and for prophylaxis and treatment of hypomagnesemia. Topically to reduce edema, inflammation, and itching.

UNLABELED USES To inhibit premature labor (tocolytic action) and as adjunct in hyperalimentation, to alleviate bronchospasm of acute asthma, to reduce mortality post-MI.

CONTRAINDICATIONS Myocardial damage; AV heart block; cardiac arrest except for certain arrhythmias; hypermagnesemia; GI obstruction; IV administration during the 2 h preceding delivery; PO use in patients with abdominal pain, nausea, vomiting, fecal impaction, or intestinal irritation, obstruction, or perforation.

CAUTIOUS USE Renal disease; renal failure; renal impairment; acute MI; digitalized patients; neuromuscular blocking agents, or cardiac glycosides; pregnancy (category A), children.

ROUTE & DOSAGE

Laxative

Adult: **PO** 10–15 g once/day

Seizures

Adult: **IV** 1 g, may need to repeat dose

Preeclampsia, Eclampsia

Adult: **IM/IV** 4–5 g slowly; simultaneously, 5 g **IM** in alternate buttocks q4h

Hypomagnesemia

Adult: **IM/IV** *Mild,* 1 g q6h for 4 doses; *Severe,* 5 g infused over 3 h

Child: **IV** 25–50 mg/kg q4–6h prn (max single dose: 2000 mg)

Total Parenteral Nutrition

Adult: **IV** 0.5–3 g/day

M

ADMINISTRATION

Oral

- Give in the morning or mid-afternoon in a glass of water for laxative action. Disguise bitter, salty taste by chilling or flavoring with lemon or orange juice.

Intramuscular

- Give deep using the 50% concentration for adults and the 20% concentration for children.

Intravenous

Note: Verify correct IV concentration and rate of infusion for administration to infants, children with physician.

PREPARE: **Direct/IV Infusion:** Give solutions with concentrations of 20% or less undiluted. ▪ Dilute more concentrated solutions to 20% (200 mg/mL) or less with D5W or NS.

ADMINISTER: **Direct:** Give at a rate of 150 mg over at least 1 min. Note: 20% solution contains 200 mg/mL, 10% solution contains 100 mg/mL. **IV Infusion:** Give required dose over 4 h. Do not exceed the direct rate.

INCOMPATIBILITIES **Solution/additive:** **10% fat emulsion, amphotericin B, calcium, chlorpromazine, clindamycin, cyclosporine, dobutamine, hydralazine, polymyxin B, procaine, prochlorperazine, sodium bicarbonate.** **Y-site:** **Amiodarone, amphotericin B, cholesteryl, cefepime, ciprofloxacin, haloperidol, lansoprazole.**

ADVERSE EFFECTS (≥1%) **Body as a Whole:** Flushing, sweating, extreme thirst, sedation, confusion, depressed reflexes or no reflexes, muscle weakness, flaccid paralysis, hypothermia. **CV:** Hypotension, depressed cardiac function, complete heart block, circulatory collapse. **Respiratory:** Respiratory paralysis. **Metabolic:** Hypermagnesemia, hypocalcemia, dehydration, electrolyte imbalance including hypocalcemia with repeated laxative use.

INTERACTIONS Drug: NEUROMUSCULAR BLOCKING AGENTS add to respiratory depression and apnea.

PHARMACOKINETICS Onset: 1–2 h PO; 1 h IM. **Duration:** 30 min IV; 3–4 h PO. **Distribution:** Crosses placenta; distributed into breast milk. **Elimination:** In kidneys.

NURSING IMPLICATIONS

Assessment & Drug Effects

- Observe constantly when given IV. Check BP and pulse q10–15min or more often if indicated.
- Lab tests: Monitor plasma magnesium levels in patients receiving drug parenterally (normal: 1.8–3 mEq/L). Plasma levels in excess of 4 mEq/L are reflected in depressed deep tendon reflexes and other symptoms of magnesium intoxication (see ADVERSE EFFECTS). Cardiac arrest occurs at levels in excess of 25 mEq/L. Monitor calcium and phosphorus levels also.
- Early indicators of magnesium toxicity (hypermagnesemia) include cathartic effect, profound thirst, feeling of warmth, sedation, confusion, depressed deep tendon reflexes, and muscle weakness.
- Monitor respiratory rate closely. Report immediately if rate falls below 12.
- Check urinary output, especially in patients with impaired kidney function. Therapy is generally not continued if urinary output is less than 100 mL during the 4 h preceding each dose.

- Observe newborns of mothers who received parenteral magnesium sulfate within a few hours of delivery for signs of toxicity, including respiratory and neuromuscular depression.
- Observe patients receiving drug for hypomagnesemia for improvement in the following signs of deficiency: Irritability, choreiform movements, tremors, tetany, twitching, muscle cramps, tachycardia, hypertension, psychotic behavior.
- Have calcium gluconate readily available in case of magnesium sulfate toxicity.

Patient & Family Education
- Drink sufficient water during the day when drug is administered orally to prevent net loss of body water.

MANNITOL Pr
(man′ni-tole)
Osmitrol
Classifications: ELECTROLYTIC AND WATER BALANCE AGENT; OSMOTIC DIURETIC
Therapeutic: OSMOTIC DIURETIC
Pregnancy Category: B

AVAILABILITY 5%, 10%, 15%, 20%, 25% injection

ACTION & *THERAPEUTIC EFFECT* Increases rate of electrolyte excretion by the kidney, particularly sodium, chloride, and potassium. Induces diuresis by raising osmotic pressure of glomerular filtrate, thereby inhibiting tubular reabsorption of water and solutes. Reduces elevated intraocular and cerebrospinal pressures by increasing plasma osmolality, thus inducing diffusion of water from these fluids back into plasma and extravascular space. *Osmotic diuretic that reduces intracranial pressure, cerebral edema, intraocular pressure, and promotes diuresis, thus preventing or treating oliguria.*

USES To promote diuresis in prevention and treatment of oliguric phase of acute kidney failure following cardiovascular surgery, severe traumatic injury, surgery in presence of severe jaundice, hemolytic transfusion reaction. Also used to reduce elevated intraocular (IOP) and intracranial pressure (ICP), to measure glomerular filtration rate (GFR), to promote excretion of toxic substances, to relieve symptoms of pulmonary edema, and as irrigating solution in transurethral prostatic reaction to minimize hemolytic effects of water. Commercially available in combination with sorbitol for urogenital irrigation.

CONTRAINDICATIONS Anuria; severe renal failure with azotemia or increasing oliguria; marked pulmonary congestion or edema; severe CHF; metabolic edema; hypovolemia; organic CNS disease, intracranial bleeding; shock, severe dehydration; concomitantly with blood.
CAUTIOUS USE Older adult; electrolyte imbalance; pregnancy (category B), lactation.

ROUTE & DOSAGE

Acute Kidney Failure
Adult: **IV Test Dose** 0.2 g/kg over 3–5 min if partial response may repeat test dose 1 time. If still negative, do not use. **Treatment** 50–100 g as 15–20% solution over 90 min to several hours
Child: **IV Test Dose** 0.2 g/kg (max: 12.5 g) over 3–5 min **Positive Response** Urine flow of 1 mL/kg/h for 1–2 h **Maintenance** 0.25–0.5 g/kg q4–6h

M

Edema, Ascites

Adult: **IV** 100 g as a 10–20% solution over 2–6 h

Elevated IOP or ICP

Adult: **IV** 1.5–2 g/kg as a 15–25% solution over 30–60 min

Acute Chemical Toxicity

Adult: **IV** 100–200 g depending on urine output

Measurement of GFR

Adult: **IV** 100 mL of 20% solution diluted with 180 mL NaCl injection infused at a rate of 20 mL/min

ADMINISTRATION

Intravenous

Note: Verify correct IV concentration and rate of infusion for administration to infants, children with physician.

PREPARE: **IV Infusion:** Give undiluted.

ADMINISTER: **IV Infusion:** Give a single dose over 30–90 min. ***Oliguria:*** A test dose is given to patients with marked oliguria to check adequacy of kidney function. Response is considered satisfactory if urine flow of at least 30–50 mL/h is produced over 2–3 h after drug administration; then rate is adjusted to maintain urine flow at 30–50 mL/h with a single dose usually being infused over 90 min or longer. ▪ Concentrations higher than 15% have a greater tendency to crystallize. ▪ Use an administration set with a 5 micron in-line IV filter when infusing concentrations of 15% or above.

INCOMPATIBILITIES **Solution/additive:** **Furosemide, imipenem-cilastatin, meropenem, potassium chloride, sodium chloride, whole blood.** **Y-site:** **Cefepime, doxorubicin liposome, filgrastim, pantoprazole.**

▪ Store at 15°–30° C (59°–86° F) unless otherwise directed. Avoid freezing.

ADVERSE EFFECTS (≥1%) **CNS:** Headache, tremor, convulsions, dizziness, transient muscle rigidity. **CV:** Edema, CHF, angina-like pain, hypotension, hypertension, thrombophlebitis. **Eye:** Blurred vision. **GI:** Dry mouth, nausea, vomiting. **Urogenital:** Marked diuresis, urinary retention, nephrosis, uricosuria. **Metabolic:** *Fluid and electrolyte imbalance,* especially <u>hyponatremia</u>; dehydration, acidosis. **Other:** With extravasation (local edema, skin necrosis; chills, fever, allergic reactions).

INTERACTIONS Drug: Increases urinary excretion of **lithium,** SALICYLATES, BARBITURATES, **imipramine, potassium.**

PHARMACOKINETICS Onset: 1–3 h diuresis; 30–60 min IOP; 15 min ICP. **Duration:** 4–6 h IOP; 3–8 h ICP. **Distribution:** Confined to extracellular space; does not cross blood–brain barrier except with very high plasma levels in the presence of acidosis. **Metabolism:** Small quantity metabolized to glycogen in liver. **Elimination:** Rapidly excreted by kidneys. **Half-Life:** 100 min.

NURSING IMPLICATIONS

Assessment & Drug Effects

- Take care to avoid extravasation. Observe injection site for signs of inflammation or edema.
- Lab tests: Monitor closely serum and urine electrolytes and kidney function during therapy.
- Measure I&O accurately and record to achieve proper fluid balance.

- Monitor vital signs closely. Report significant changes in BP and signs of CHF.
- Monitor for possible indications of fluid and electrolyte imbalance (e.g., thirst, muscle cramps or weakness, paresthesias, and signs of CHF).
- Be alert to the possibility that a rebound increase in ICP sometimes occurs about 12 h after drug administration. Patient may complain of headache or confusion.
- Take accurate daily weight.

Patient & Family Education

- Report any of the following: Thirst, muscle cramps or weakness, paresthesia, dyspnea, or headache.
- Family members should immediately report any evidence of confusion.

MAPROTILINE HYDROCHLORIDE

(ma-proe′ti-leen)

Classification: TETRACYCLIC ANTIDEPRESSANT
Therapeutic: ANTIDEPRESSANT
Prototype: Mirtazapine
Pregnancy Category: B

AVAILABILITY 25 mg, 50 mg, 75 mg tablets

ACTION & *THERAPEUTIC EFFECT* It selectively inhibits reuptake of norepinephrine at central nervous system (CNS) adrenergic synapses; this appears to produce antidepressant as well as antianxiety effects of maprotiline. *Useful in depression associated with anxiety and sleep disturbances.*

USES Treatment of depressive neurosis (dysthymic disorder) and manic-depressive illness, depressed type (major depressive disorder).

UNLABELED USES Bulimia, pain, panic attack, enuresis.

CONTRAINDICATIONS Acute MI, AV block, cardiac arrhythmias, QT prolongation; MAOI therapy within 14 days; tricyclic antidepressant therapy; children younger than 18 y; history of alcoholism; suicidal ideation.

CAUTIOUS USE History of seizure activity; psychotic disorders; history of suicidal tendencies; diabetes mellitus; hepatic disease; GI disease; GERD; BPH; respiratory depression; labor and delivery; pregnancy (category B), lactation.

ROUTE & DOSAGE

Mild to Moderate Depression

Adult: **PO** Start at 75 mg/day and may increase q2wk up to 150 mg/day in single or divided doses

Geriatric: **PO** Start with 25 mg at bedtime may increase to 50–75 mg/day

Severe Depression

Adult: **PO** Start at 100–150 mg/day may increase up to 300 mg/day in single or divided doses if needed

Pharmacogenetic Dosage Adjustment

Poor CYP2D6 metabolizers: Start with 40% of dose

ADMINISTRATION

Oral

- Give as single dose or in divided doses. Initiate therapy with low dosages to reduce risk of seizures.
- Store at 15°–30° C (59°–86° F) unless otherwise specified.

ADVERSE EFFECTS (≥1%) **CNS:** Seizures, exacerbation of psychosis, hallucinations, tremors, excitement, confusion, dizziness, *drowsiness*. **CV:** *Orthostatic hypotension,* hypertension, tachycardia. **Special Senses:** Accommodation disturbances, blurred vision, mydriasis. **GI:** Nausea, vomiting, epigastric distress, *constipation, dry mouth*. **Urogenital:** *Urinary retention,* frequency. **Skin:** Hypersensitivity reactions (skin rash, urticaria, photosensitivity).

INTERACTIONS Drug: May decrease some response to ANTIHYPERTENSIVES; CNS DEPRESSANTS, **alcohol,** HYPNOTICS, BARBITURATES, SEDATIVES potentiate CNS depression; may increase hypoprothrombinemic effect of ORAL ANTICOAGULANTS; transient delirium with **ethchlorvynol;** with **levodopa,** SYMPATHOMIMETICS (e.g., **epinephrine, norepinephrine**) there is possibility of sympathetic hyperactivity with hypertension and **hyperpyrexia;** with MAO INHIBITORS or **linezolid** there is possibility of severe reactions, toxic psychosis, cardiovascular instability; **methylphenidate** increases plasma TCA levels; THYROID DRUGS increase possibility of arrhythmias; **cimetidine** may increase plasma TCA levels.

PHARMACOKINETICS Absorption: Slowly absorbed from GI tract. **Peak:** 12 h. **Distribution:** Distributed chiefly to brain, lungs, liver, and kidneys. **Metabolism:** In liver. **Elimination:** 70% in urine, 30% in feces. **Half-Life:** 51 h.

NURSING IMPLICATIONS

Assessment & Drug Effects

- Monitor for therapeutic effectiveness; 2–3 wk are usually necessary for full effect.
- Monitor for increased suicidality, unusual changes in behavior, or suicide attempt. Inform the physician immediately.
- Assess level of sedative effect. If recovering patient becomes too lethargic to care for personal hygiene or to maintain food intake and interactions with others, report to physician.
- Monitor bowel elimination pattern and I&O ratio. Severe constipation and urinary retention are potential problems, especially in the older adult. Advise increased fluid intake (at least 1500 mL/day).
- Observe seizure precautions; risk of seizures appears to be high in heavy drinkers.
- Bear in mind that if patient uses excessive amounts of alcohol, potentiated effects of maprotiline may increase the danger of overdosage or suicide attempt.

Patient & Family Education

- Report symptoms of stomatitis and dry mouth when taking high doses. Sore or dry mouth can lead to lack of compliance.
- Use caution with tasks that require alertness and skill; ability may be impaired during early therapy.
- Do not change dose or dose schedule without consulting physician.
- Do not use OTC drugs unless approved by physician.
- Avoid alcohol; the effects of maprotiline are potentiated when both are used together and for 2 wk after maprotiline is discontinued.

MARAVIROC

(mar-a-vir′ok)

Selzentry

Classifications: ANTIRETROVIRAL; FUSION INHBITOR

Therapeutic: ANTIRETROVIRAL

Pregnancy Category: B

AVAILABILITY 150 mg, 300 mg tablets

ACTION & *THERAPEUTIC EFFECT* Selectively binds to human chemokine coreceptor-5 (CCR-5) on cell membranes of helper T cell lymphocytes preventing interaction with the HIV-1 envelope protein necessary for the HIV virus to enter helper T cells. *Prevents infection of helper T cells by HIV-1 viruses with CCR-5 tropism.*

USES Treatment of human immunodeficiency virus (HIV-1) infection in combination with other antiretroviral agents in treatment-experienced patients who express CCR-5 and who have evidence of HIV-1 replication and HIV-1 strains resistant to multiple antiretroviral agents.

CONTRAINDICATIONS Patients with dual/mixed, or chemokine-related receptor (CCR-4)-tropic HIV-1 virus; treatment naïve adults or children with HIV-1; S&S of hepatitis, or allergic reaction to drug; lactation; children younger than 16 y.

CAUTIOUS USE Hepatic impairment, hepatitis B or C; renal impairment; CrCl less than 50 mL/min; cardiac disease or increased risk for cardiovascular events; older adults; pregnancy (category B).

ROUTE & DOSAGE

Regimen without CYP3A Inducers or Inhibitors

Adult: **PO** 300 mg b.i.d.

Regimen with CYP3A Inhibitor with/without CYP3A Inducer

Adult: **PO** 150 mg b.i.d.

Regimen with CYP3A Inducers without a Strong CYP3A Inhibitor

Adult: **PO** 600 mg b.i.d.

ADMINISTRATION

- **Must be** given in combination with other antiretroviral drugs.
- Store at 15°–30° C (59°–86° F).

ADVERSE EFFECTS (≥1%) **Body as a Whole:** Appetite disorders, herpes infection, pain and discomfort, *pyrexia*. **CNS:** Depression, disturbances in consciousness, *sleep disorders, dizziness,* paresthesias and dysesthesias, peripheral neuropathies, sensory abnormalities. **CV:** Vascular hypertension disorders. **GI:** *Abdominal pain,* constipation, dyspepsia, stomatitis, ulceration. **Hematologic:** Neutropenia. **Metabolic:** Elevated AST levels. **Musculoskeletal:** Joint-related signs and symptoms, muscle pains, *musculoskeletal symptoms.* **Respiratory:** Breathing abnormalities, bronchitis, bronchospasm, *cough,* influenza, paranasal sinus disorder, pneumonia, respiratory tract disorders, sinusitis, *upper respiratory tract infection*. **Skin:** Apocrine and eccrine gland disorders, benign neoplasms, dermatitis, eczema, folliculitis, lipodystrophies, pruritis, *rash*. **Urogenital:** Bladder and urethral symptoms, condyloma acuminatum, urinary tract signs and symptoms.

INTERACTIONS Drug: STRONG CYP3A4 INHIBITORS (HIV PROTEASE INHIBITORS with the exception of **tipranavir/ritonavir, delavirdine, ketoconazole, itrazonazole, clarithromycin**) increase maraviroc plasma level. CYP3A4 INDUCERS (**efavirenz, rifampin, carbamazepine, phenobarbital, phenytoin**) decrease maraviroc plasma level. **Food:** Coadministration with a high-fat meal decreases the plasma levels of maraviroc. **Herbal: St. John's wort** may decrease the plasma levels of maraviroc.

PHARMACOKINETICS Absorption: Bioavailability is 23–33%. **Peak:** 0.5–4 h (dose-dependent). **Distribution:** 75% protein bound. **Metabolism:** In liver via CYP3A4. **Elimination:** Primarily in stool. **Half-Life:** 14–18 h.

NURSING IMPLICATIONS

Assessment & Drug Effects

- Monitor for and report promptly S&S of hepatotoxicity, hepatitis or infection.
- Monitor BP especially in those on antihypertensive drugs and with a history of postural hypotension.
- Monitor CV status especially in those with preexisting conditions that cause myocardial ischemia.
- Lab tests: Baseline and periodic CD4+ cell count and HIV RNA viral load; periodic LFTs, WBC with differential.

Patient & Family Education

- Exercise caution when arising from a lying or sitting positing. Dizziness is a common adverse effect.
- Do not engage in dangerous activities until response to drug is known.
- Report promptly any of the following: Itchy rash, yellow skin or eyes, nausea or vomiting, upper abdominal pain, flu-like symptoms, unexplained fatigue.

M

MEBENDAZOLE Pr

(me-ben′da-zole)

Classification: ANTHELMINTIC
Therapeutic: ANTHELMINTIC
Pregnancy Category: C

AVAILABILITY 100 mg tablets

ACTION & *THERAPEUTIC EFFECT* Carbamate with unusually broad spectrum of anthelmintic activity. Inhibits formation of worm's microtubules and inhibits glucose and other nutrient uptake by susceptible helminths. *Effective against susceptible helminths (nematodes) by interfering with their survival.*

USES Treatment of *Trichuris trichiura* (whipworm), *Enterobius vermicularis* (pinworm), *Ascaris lumbricoides* (roundworm), *Ancylostoma duodenale* (common hookworm), *Necator americanus* (American hookworm) in single or mixed infections.

UNLABELED USES Beef, dwarf, and pork tapeworm and threadworm infections.

CONTRAINDICATIONS Safety in children younger than 2 y is not established.

CAUTIOUS USE Inflammatory bowel disease, ulcerative colitis, Crohn's disease; hepatic disease; pregnancy (category C), lactation.

ROUTE & DOSAGE

Enterobiasis

Adult: **PO** 100 mg as single dose
Child: **PO** 100 mg as single dose

Other Infestations

Adult: **PO** 100 mg b.i.d. × 3 days
Child: **PO** 100 mg b.i.d. × 3 days

ADMINISTRATION

Oral

- Allow tablets to be chewed and swallowed, or crushed and mixed with food if needed.

ADVERSE EFFECTS (≥1%) **GI:** Transient abdominal pain, diarrhea. **Body as a Whole:** Dizziness, fever (possibly due to tissue necrosis in cysts).

INTERACTIONS Drug: Carbamazepine, phenytoin can increase metabolism of mebendazole.

PHARMACOKINETICS Absorption: Minimal from GI tract (2–10% of dose). **Metabolism:** Metabolized to inactive metabolite. **Elimination:** Primarily in feces. **Half-Life:** 3–9 h.

NURSING IMPLICATIONS

Assessment & Drug Effects

- Initiate second course of treatment if cure does not occur within 3 wk.
- Examine and treat all family members simultaneously because pinworms are readily transmitted from person to person.

Patient & Family Education

- Practice thorough hand washing after touching any potentially contaminated item.
- Change underclothing, bedclothes, towels, and facecloths daily; bathe frequently, preferably by showering. Infected person should sleep alone.

MECAMYLAMINE HYDROCHLORIDE

(mek-a-mill'a-meen)

Inversine

Classification: CENTRAL ACTING ANTIHYPERTENSIVE

Therapeutic: ANTIHYPERTENSIVE

Prototype: Methyldopa

Pregnancy Category: C

AVAILABILITY 2.5 mg tablets

ACTION & *THERAPEUTIC EFFECT* Potent, long-acting nondepolarizing ganglionic blocking agent. Blocks neurotransmission at both sympathetic and parasympathetic ganglia by competing with acetylcholine (Ach) for cholinergic receptor sites on postsynaptic membranes. *Reduces BP in both normotensive and hypertensive individuals. Effective in treating the signs and symptoms of Tourette's syndrome.*

USES Moderately severe to severe hypertension and uncomplicated malignant hypertension.

CONTRAINDICATIONS Hypersensitivity to mecamylamine; coronary insufficiency, pyloric stenosis; glaucoma; uremia, chronic pyelonephritis; recent MI; mild, moderate, or labile hypertension; unreliable uncooperative patients; lactation. Safety and efficacy in children not established.

CAUTIOUS USE Rising or elevated BUN; renal, cerebral, or coronary vascular pathology; recent CVA; prostatic hypertrophy, bladder neck obstruction, urethral stricture; pregnancy (category C).

ROUTE & DOSAGE

Moderately Severe to Severe Hypertension

Adult: **PO** 2.5 mg b.i.d. p.c. for 2 days, increased by increments of 2.5 mg at intervals of 2 days or more until desired BP response is attained (2.5–25 mg/day in 2–4 divided doses)

ADMINISTRATION

Oral

- Give after meals for more gradual absorption and smoother control of BP. Schedule consistently relative to meals.
- Do not suddenly discontinue drug; may result in severe hypertensive rebound with CVA and acute CHF. Usually, other antihypertensive therapy **must be** substituted grad-

ually, and patient **must be** supervised daily during period of dosage adjustment.

- Store at 15°–30° C (59°–86° F) unless otherwise directed.

ADVERSE EFFECTS (≥1%) **CNS:** Weakness, fatigue, sedation, headache, paresthesias, confusion, depression, choreiform movements, tremor. **CV:** *Orthostatic hypotension,* changes in heart rate, dizziness, syncope, precipitation of angina. **Special Senses:** Mydriasis, *blurred vision,* cycloplegia, nasal congestion, *dry mouth* with dysphagia, glossitis. **GI:** *Anorexia, nausea, vomiting, constipation, diarrhea,* adynamic ileus. **Urogenital:** Decreased libido, impotence, *urinary retention.*

INTERACTIONS Drug: Alcohol, other ANTIHYPERTENSIVE AGENTS, **bethanechol,** THIAZIDE DIURETICS potentiate hypotensive effects; **acetazolamide, sodium bicarbonate** increase mecamylamine toxicity because they decrease its elimination.

PHARMACOKINETICS Absorption: Almost completely from GI tract. **Onset:** 30 min–2 h. **Peak:** 3–5 h. **Duration:** 6–12 h. **Distribution:** Crosses blood–brain barrier and placenta; distributed into breast milk. **Metabolism:** In liver. **Elimination:** Primarily in urine.

NURSING IMPLICATIONS

Assessment & Drug Effects

- Monitor therapeutic effectiveness by taking BP readings in standing position at time of maximal drug effect. Assess for symptoms of orthostatic hypotension (faintness, dizziness, lightheadedness). Also note any changes in pulse rate.
- Monitor BP closely. Partial tolerance may develop in some patients, necessitating dosage adjustment.
- Report promptly constipation, frequent loose stools with abdominal distention, or decreased bowel sounds; may be the first signs of paralytic ileus (relatively frequent). Paralytic ileus is sometimes preceded by small, frequent stools.

Patient & Family Education

- Make position changes slowly and in stages, particularly from recumbent to upright posture; sit on edge of bed and move ankles and feet before walking.
- Lie down immediately if feeling light-headed or dizzy. Report adverse reactions immediately because drug effects may last hours to days after drug is discontinued.
- Do not drive or engage in potentially hazardous activities until response to drug is known.
- Promptly report any of the following: Frequent loose stools with abdominal distention, difficult urination, tremors, or uncontrollable muscle movements.

M

MECHLORETHAMINE HYDROCHLORIDE

(me-klor-eth′a-meen)

Mustargen

Classifications: ANTINEOPLASTIC; ALKYLATING AGENT; NITROGEN MUSTARD

Therapeutic: ANTINEOPLASTIC

Prototype: Cyclophosphamide

Pregnancy Category: D

AVAILABILITY 10 mg powder for injection

ACTION & *THERAPEUTIC EFFECT* Analog of mustard gas that forms highly reactive carbonium ion that causes cross-linking and abnormal base-pairing in DNA, thereby interfering with DNA replication and RNA and protein synthesis. Cell-cycle nonspecific inhibitor of DNA and RNA synthesis. *Antineoplastic agent that simulates actions of x-ray therapy, but nitrogen mustards produce more acute tissue damage and more rapid recovery.*

USES Generally confined to nonterminal stages of neoplastic disease, as single agent or in combination with other agents in palliative treatment of Hodgkin's disease (stages III and IV), lymphosarcoma, mycosis fungoides, polycythemia vera, bronchogenic carcinoma, chronic myelocytic or chronic lymphocytic leukemia. Also for intrapleural, intrapericardial, and intraperitoneal palliative treatment of metastatic carcinoma resulting in effusion.

CONTRAINDICATIONS Myelosuppression; infectious granuloma; known infectious diseases, acute herpes zoster; intracavitary use with other systemic bone marrow suppressants; pregnancy (category D), lactation.

CAUTIOUS USE Bone marrow infiltration with malignant cells, chronic lymphocytic leukemia; men or women in childbearing age.

ROUTE & DOSAGE

Advanced Hodgkin's Disease

Adult: **IV** 6 mg/m^2 on day 1 and 8 of a 28-day cycle

Other Neoplasms

Adult: **IV** 0.4 mg/kg given as a single dose or in divided doses of 0.1–0.2 mg/kg/day, may repeat course in 3–6 wk

Obesity Dosage Adjustment

Dose based on IBW

ADMINISTRATION

Intravenous

Wear surgical gloves during preparation and administration of solution. ▪ Avoid inhalation of vapors and dust and contact of drug with eyes and skin. ▪ Flush contaminated area immediately if drug contacts the skin. Use copious amounts of water for at least 15 min, followed by 2% sodium thiosulfate solution. Irritation may appear after a latent period. ▪ Irrigate immediately if eye contact occurs. Use copious amounts of NS followed by ophthalmologic examination as soon as possible.

PREPARE: **Direct:** Reconstitute immediately before use by adding 10 mL sterile water for injection or NS injection to vial to yield 1 mg/mL. With needle still in stopper, shake vial several times to dissolve. ▪ Discard colored solution or contents of any vial with drops of moisture.

ADMINISTER: **Direct:** To reduce risk of severe infections from extravasation or high concentration of the drug, inject slowly over 3–5 min into tubing or sidearm of freely flowing IV infusion. Flush vein with running IV solution for 2–5 min to clear tubing of any remaining drug. ▪ Be alert for extravasation. Treat promptly with subcutaneous or intradermal injection with isotonic sodium thiosulfate solution (1/6 molar) and application of ice compresses intermittently for a 6–12 h period to reduce local tissue damage and discomfort. ▪ Tissue induration and tenderness may persist 4–6 wk, and tissue may slough.

INCOMPATIBILITIES **Solution/additive: D5W, methohexital, normal saline. Y-site: Allopurinol, cefepime.**

ADVERSE EFFECTS (≥1%) **CNS:** Neurotoxicity: Vertigo, tinnitus, headache, drowsiness, peripheral neuropathy, light-headedness, paresthesias, cerebral deterioration, coma. **GI:** Stomatitis, xerostomia, anorexia, *nausea, vomiting,* diarrhea. **Hematologic:** Leukopenia, *thrombocytopenia,* lymphocytopenia, agranulocytosis, *anemia,* hyperheparinemia. **Skin:** Pruritus, hyperpigmentation, herpes zoster, alopecia. **Urogenital:** Amenorrhea, azoospermia, chromosomal abnormalities, hyperuricemia. **Body as a Whole:** Weakness, hypersensitivity reactions. *With extravasation: Painful inflammatory reaction, tissue sloughing, thrombosis, thrombophlebitis.*

INTERACTIONS Drug: May reduce effectiveness of ANTIGOUT AGENTS by raising serum **uric acid** levels; dosage adjustments may be necessary; may prolong neuromuscular blocking effects of **succinylcholine;** may potentiate bleeding effects of ANTICOAGULANTS, SALICYLATES, NSAIDS, PLATELET INHIBITORS.

PHARMACOKINETICS Metabolism: Rapid hydrolysis and demethylation. **Elimination:** In urine. **Half-Life:** Less than 1 min.

NURSING IMPLICATIONS

Assessment & Drug Effects

- Establish baseline data for body weight, I&O ratio and pattern, and blood labs as reference for design of drug and care regimens.
- Lab tests: Monitor CBC with differential and platelet count. Periodic serum uric acid levels.
- Record daily weight. Alert physician to sudden or slow, steady weight gain.
- Monitor and record patient's fluid losses carefully. Prolonged vomiting and diarrhea can produce volume depletion.
- Report immediately petechiae, ecchymoses, or abnormal bleeding from intestinal and buccal membranes. Keep injections and other invasive procedures to a minimum during period of thrombocytopenia.
- Report symptoms of agranulocytosis (e.g., unexplained fever, chills, sore throat, tachycardia, and mucosal ulceration).
- Prevent exposure to people with infection, especially upper respiratory tract infections.
- Note and record state of hydration of oral mucosa, condition of gingiva, teeth, tongue, mucosa, and lips.

Patient & Family Education

- Report any signs of bleeding immediately.
- Use caution to prevent falls or other traumatic injuries, especially during periods of low platelet counts.
- Increase fluid intake up to 3000 mL/day if allowed to minimize risk of kidney stones. Report promptly all symptoms, including flank or joint pain, swelling of lower legs and feet, changes in voiding pattern.

MECLIZINE HYDROCHLORIDE (Pr)

(mek'li-zeen)

Antivert, Antrizine, Bonamine ♣, Bonine, Dizmiss, RuVert-M

Classifications: ANTIHISTAMINE; H_1-RECEPTOR ANTAGONIST; ANTI-VERTIGO

Common adverse effects in *italic*, life-threatening effects underlined; generic names in **bold**; classifications in SMALL CAPS; ♣ Canadian drug name; (Pr) Prototype drug

Therapeutic: ANTIHISTAMINE, ANTIVERTIGO
Pregnancy Category: B

AVAILABILITY 12.5 mg, 25 mg, 50 mg tablets; 25 mg, 30 mg capsules

ACTION & *THERAPEUTIC EFFECT* Long-acting antihistamine, with marked effect in blocking histamine-induced vasopressive response but only slight anticholinergic action. Marked depressant action on labyrinthine excitability and on conduction in vestibular-cerebellar pathways. *Exhibits antivertigo, and antiemetic effects.*

USES Management of nausea, vomiting, and dizziness associated with motion sickness and in vertigo associated with diseases affecting vestibular system.

CONTRAINDICATIONS Hypersensitivity to meclizine; GI obstruction, ileus.
CAUTIOUS USE Angle-closure glaucoma, older adults, asthma, prostatic hypertrophy, pregnancy (category B), lactation. Safety in children younger than 12 y is not established.

ROUTE & DOSAGE

Motion Sickness
Adult: **PO** 25–50 mg 1 h before travel, may repeat q24h if necessary for duration of journey

Vertigo
Adult: **PO** 25–100 mg/day in divided doses

ADMINISTRATION

Oral
- Give without regard to meals.
- Ensure that chewable tablets are chewed or crushed before being swallowed with a liquid.

ADVERSE EFFECTS (≥1%) **CNS:** *Drowsiness.* **GI:** Dry mouth. **Special Senses:** Blurred vision. **Body as a Whole:** Fatigue.

INTERACTIONS Drug: Alcohol, CNS DEPRESSANTS may potentiate sedative effects of meclizine.

PHARMACOKINETICS Absorption: Readily absorbed from GI tract. **Onset:** 1 h. **Duration:** 8–24 h. **Distribution:** Crosses placenta. **Elimination:** Primarily in feces. **Half-Life:** 6 h.

NURSING IMPLICATIONS

Assessment & Drug Effects
- Supervision of ambulation, particularly with the older adult, since drug may cause drowsiness.
- Assess effectiveness of drug and inform physician when prescribed for vertigo; dosage adjustment may be required.

Patient & Family Education
- Do not drive or engage in potentially hazardous activities until response to drug is known.
- Be aware that sedative action may add to that of alcohol, barbiturates, narcotic analgesics, or other CNS depressants.
- Take 1 h before departure when prescribed for motion sickness.

MECLOFENAMATE SODIUM

(me-kloe-fen-am′ate)
Classification: ANALGESIC, NONSTEROIDAL ANTI-INFLAMMATORY DRUG (NSAID)
Therapeutic: ANALGESIC, NSAID; ANTIPYRETIC; ANTIRHEUMATIC
Prototype: Ibuprofen
Pregnancy Category: C first and second trimester; D third trimester

AVAILABILITY 50 mg, 100 mg capsules

ACTION & *THERAPEUTIC EFFECT* Inhibits prostaglandin synthesis by inhibiting both the COX-1 and COX-2 enzymes necessary for its synthesis and competes for binding at prostaglandin receptor sites. Does not appear to alter course of arthritis. *Palliative anti-inflammatory and analgesic activity.*

USES Symptomatic treatment of acute or chronic rheumatoid arthritis and osteoarthritis. Also in combination with gold salts or corticosteroids in treatment of rheumatoid arthritis.

UNLABELED USES Management of psoriatic arthritis, mild to moderate postoperative pain, dysmenorrhea.

M

CONTRAINDICATIONS Hypersensitivity to aspirin or other NSAIDS; active peptic ulcer, ulcerative colitis; perioperative pain related to CABG surgery; renal disease; pregnancy (category D third trimester), children younger than 14 y, patient designated as functional class IV rheumatoid arthritis (incapacitated, bedridden, etc).

CAUTIOUS USE History of upper GI tract disease; coronary artery disease; acute MI, cardiac arrhythmias; CVA; diabetes mellitus; SLE; compromised cardiac and kidney function, or other conditions predisposing to fluid retention; pregnancy (category C first and second trimester), lactation.

ROUTE & DOSAGE

Inflammatory Disease

Adult: **PO** 200–400 mg/day in 3–4 divided doses (max: 400 mg/day)

ADMINISTRATION

Oral

- Give with food or milk if patient complains of GI distress. An aluminum and magnesium hydroxide antacid (Maalox) also may be prescribed. Consult physician if symptoms persist.
- Withhold dose and report to physician if significant diarrhea occurs.
- Store at 15°–30° C (59°–86° F) in airtight, light-resistant container.

ADVERSE EFFECTS (≥1%) **CNS:** *Dizziness,* vertigo, lack of concentration, confusion, *headache,* tinnitus. **CV:** Edema. **GI:** *Severe diarrhea (dose-related),* peptic ulceration, GI bleeding, dyspepsia, abdominal pain, *nausea,* vomiting (may be severe), flatulence, eructation, pyrosis, anorexia, constipation. **GI:** *Abnormal liver function tests,* cholestatic jaundice. **Special Senses:** Blurred vision. **Urogenital:** Elevated BUN and creatinine, kidney failure. **Skin:** Rash, pruritus, urticaria.

INTERACTIONS Drug: ORAL ANTICOAGULANTS, **heparin** may prolong bleeding time; may increase **lithium** toxicity; increases pharmacologic and toxic activity of **phenytoin,** SULFONYLUREAS, SULFONAMIDES, **warfarin** through protein-binding displacement. **Herbal: Feverfew, garlic, ginger, ginkgo** increase bleeding potential.

PHARMACOKINETICS Absorption: Rapidly and completely from GI tract. **Peak:** 1–2 h. **Duration:** 2–4 h. **Distribution:** Crosses placenta. **Metabolism:** In liver. **Elimination:** 60% in urine, 30% in feces. **Half-Life:** 2–3.3 h.

NURSING IMPLICATIONS

Assessment & Drug Effects

- Report diarrhea promptly. It is the most frequent adverse effect and usually dose related.
- Lab tests: Monitor kidney function where incidence of adverse reactions is potentially high because drug is excreted primarily by the kidneys. Monitor PT, PTT, and INR frequently with concurrent anticoagulant therapy.
- Monitor I&O ratio. Encourage fluid intake of at least 8 glasses of liquid a day.
- Consider sodium content of meclofenamate tablets if patient is on restricted sodium intake.

Patient & Family Education

- Stop taking drug and promptly notify the physician if nausea, vomiting, severe diarrhea, and abdominal pain occur. Generally dose reduction or temporary withdrawal will control symptoms.
- Report to physician without delay: Blurred vision, tinnitus, or taste disturbances.
- Schedule ophthalmic examinations before and periodically during treatment and whenever you experience visual disturbances.
- Notify physician if you become pregnant.
- Weigh under standard conditions (similar clothing, same time of day) twice weekly. Report weight gain of more than 2.5 to 3.5 kg (3–4 lb)/wk as well as signs of edema: Swollen ankles, tibiae, hands, feet.
- Dizziness, a troublesome early side effect, frequently disappears in time. Avoid driving a car or potentially hazardous activities until response to drug is known.
- Report immediately to physician any sign of bleeding (e.g., melena, epistaxis, ecchymosis) when taking concomitant oral anticoagulant.

MEDROXYPROGESTERONE ACETATE

(me-drox′ee-proe-jess′te-rone)

Depo-Provera, Depo-subQ Provera 104, Provera

Classification: PROGESTIN

Therapeutic: PROGESTIN

Prototype: Progesterone

Pregnancy Category: X

AVAILABILITY 2.5 mg, 5 mg, 10 mg tablets; 104 mg/0.65 mL, 150 mg/mL, 400 mg/mL injection

ACTION & *THERAPEUTIC EFFECT* Induces and maintains endometrium, preventing uterine bleeding; inhibits production of pituitary gonadotropin, thus preventing ovulation and producing thick cervical mucus resistant to passage of sperm. *Slows release of luteinizing hormone (LH) preventing follicular maturation and ovulation.*

USES Dysfunctional uterine bleeding; secondary amenorrhea; parenteral form (Depo-Provera) used in adjunctive, palliative treatment of inoperable, recurrent, and metastatic endometrial or renal carcinoma; contraception; endometriosis-associated pain.

UNLABELED USES Obstructive sleep apnea.

CONTRAINDICATIONS History of thromboembolic disorders; breast cancer, cervical cancer, uterine cancer, vaginal cancer; hepatic disease; abnormal vaginal bleeding, incomplete abortion; pregnancy (category X); lactation.

CAUTIOUS USE Asthma, seizure disorders, CVA; migraine, cardiac or kidney dysfunction, liver disease.

M

ROUTE & DOSAGE

Secondary Amenorrhea

Adult: **PO** 5–10 mg/day for 5–10 days beginning any time if endometrium is adequately estrogen primed (withdrawal bleeding occurs in 3–7 days after discontinuing therapy)

Abnormal Bleeding Due to Hormonal Imbalance

Adult: **PO** 5–10 mg/day for 5–10 days beginning on the assumed or calculated 16th or 21st day of menstrual cycle; if bleeding is controlled, administer 2 subsequent cycles

Carcinoma

Adult: **IM** 400–1000 mg/wk; continue at 400 mg/mo if improvement occurs and disease stabilizes

Contraceptive

Adult: **IM** 100 mg q3mo

Sleep Apnea

Adult: **PO** 20 mg t.i.d.

ADMINISTRATION

Oral

- Oral drug may be given with food to minimize GI distress.

Intramuscular

- Administer IM deep into a large muscle.
- Store both formulations at 15°–30° C (59°–86° F); protect from freezing.

ADVERSE EFFECTS (≥1%) **CNS:** Cerebral thrombosis or hemorrhage, depression. **CV:** Hypertension, pulmonary embolism, edema. **GI:** Vomiting, nausea, cholestatic jaundice, abdominal cramps. **Urogenital:** *Breakthrough bleeding,* changes in menstrual flow, dysmenorrhea, vaginal candidiasis. **Skin:** Angioneurotic edema. **Body as a Whole:** Weight changes; *breast tenderness,* enlargement or secretion. **Musculoskeletal:** Loss of bone mineral density.

INTERACTIONS Drug: Aminoglutethimide decreases serum concentrations of medroxyprogesterone; BARBITURATES, **carbamazepine, oxcarbazepine, phenytoin, primidone, rifampin, modafinil, rifabutin, topiramate** can increase metabolism and decrease serum levels of medroxyprogesterone. **Herbal:** Intermenstrual bleeding and loss of contraceptive efficacy may occur with **St. John's wort.**

PHARMACOKINETICS Peak: 2–4 h PO, 3 wk IM. **Distribution:** Greater than 90% protein bound. **Metabolism:** In liver. **Elimination:** Primarily in feces. **Half-Life:** 30 days PO, 50 days IM.

NURSING IMPLICATIONS

Assessment & Drug Effects

- See progesterone for numerous additional nursing implications.
- Be aware that IM injection may be painful. Monitor sites for evidence of sterile abscess. A residual lump and discoloration of tissue may develop.
- Monitor for S&S of thrombophlebitis (see Appendix F).
- Note: Planned menstrual cycling with medroxyprogesterone may benefit the patient with a history of recurrent episodes of abnormal uterine bleeding.

Patient & Family Education

- Be aware that after repeated IM injections, infertility and amenorrhea may persist as long as 18 mo.
- Learn breast self-examination.
- Review package insert to ensure complete understanding of progestin therapy.

MEFENAMIC ACID

(me-fe-nam′ik)

Ponstel

Classification: ANALGESIC, NONSTEROIDAL ANTI-INFLAMMATORY DRUG (NSAID)

Therapeutic: ANALGESIC, NSAID; ANTIPYRETIC

Prototype: Ibuprofen

Pregnancy Category: C

AVAILABILITY 250 mg tablets

ACTION & *THERAPEUTIC EFFECT* NSAID that inhibits COX-1 and COX-2 enzymes necessary for prostaglandin synthesis. It affects platelet function. *Analgesic and anti-inflammatory actions.*

USES Short-term relief of mild to moderate pain including primary dysmenorrhea.

CONTRAINDICATIONS Hypersensitivity to drug; GI inflammation, or ulceration. Safety in children younger than 14 y is not established.

CAUTIOUS USE Hypersensitivity to aspirin, history of kidney or liver disease; blood dyscrasias; asthma; cardiac arrhythmias; CHF; edema; diabetes mellitus; SLE; pregnancy (category C), lactation. Long term use increases risk of serious adverse events (see DRUG INTERACTIONS).

ROUTE & DOSAGE

Mild to Moderate Pain

Adult: **PO Loading Dose** 500 mg **PO Maintenance Dose** 250 mg q6h prn

ADMINISTRATION

Oral

- Give with meals, food, or milk to minimize GI adverse effects.
- Duration of therapy should not exceed 1 wk (manufacturer's warning).

ADVERSE EFFECTS (≥1%) **CNS:** Drowsiness, insomnia, dizziness, nervousness, confusion, headache. **GI:** *Severe diarrhea,* ulceration, and bleeding; *nausea, vomiting,* abdominal cramps, flatus, constipation, hepatic toxicity. **Hematologic:** Prolonged prothrombin time, severe autoimmune hemolytic anemia (long-term use), leukopenia, eosinophilia, agranulocytosis, thrombocytopenic purpura, megaloblastic anemia, pancytopenia, bone marrow hypoplasia. **Urogenital:** Nephrotoxicity, dysuria, albuminuria, hematuria, elevation of BUN. **Skin:** Urticaria, rash, facial edema. **Special Senses:** Eye irritation, loss of color vision (reversible), blurred vision, ear pain. **Body as a Whole:** Perspiration. **CV:** Palpitation. **Respiratory:** Dyspnea; acute exacerbation of asthma; bronchoconstriction (in patients sensitive to aspirin).

DIAGNOSTIC TEST INTERFERENCE False-positive reactions for ***urinary bilirubin*** (using ***diazo tablet test***).

INTERACTIONS Drug: Mefenamic acid may prolong bleeding time with ORAL ANTICOAGULANTS, **heparin;** may increase **lithium** toxicity; increases pharmacologic and toxic activity of **phenytoin,** SULFONYLUREAS, SULFONAMIDES, **warfarin** because of protein binding displacement. **Herbal: Feverfew, garlic, ginger, ginkgo** increase bleeding potential.

PHARMACOKINETICS Absorption: Rapidly and completely from GI tract. **Peak:** 2–4 h. **Duration:** 6 h. **Distribution:** Distributed in breast milk. **Metabolism:** Partially in liver. **Elimination:** 50% in urine, 50% in feces. **Half-Life:** 2 h.

NURSING IMPLICATIONS

Assessment & Drug Effects

- Assess patients who develop severe diarrhea and vomiting for dehydration and electrolyte imbalance.
- Lab tests: With long-term therapy (not recommended) obtain periodic complete blood counts, Hct and Hgb, and kidney function tests.

Patient & Family Education

- Discontinue drug promptly if diarrhea, dark stools, hematemesis, ecchymoses, epistaxis, or rash occur and do not use again. Contact physician.
- Notify physician if persistent GI discomfort, sore throat, fever, or malaise occur.
- Do not drive or engage in potentially hazardous activities until response to drug is known. It may cause dizziness and drowsiness.
- Monitor blood glucose for loss of glycemic control if diabetic.

M

MEFLOQUINE HYDROCHLORIDE

(me-flo′quine)

Classifications: ANTIPROTOZOAL; ANTIMALARIAL

Therapeutic: ANTIMALARIAL

Prototype: Chloroquine

Pregnancy Category: C

AVAILABILITY 250 mg tablets

ACTION & *THERAPEUTIC EFFECT* Antimalarial agent, structurally related to quinine. *Effective against all types of malaria, including chloroquine-resistant malaria.*

USES Treatment of mild to moderate acute malarial infections, prevention of chloroquine-resistant malaria caused by *Plasmodium falciparum* and *P. vivax*.

CONTRAINDICATIONS Hypersensitivity to mefloquine or a related compound; with a calcium channel blocking agent, severe heart arrhythmias, history of QT_c prolongation; aggressive behavior; active depression, or history of depression, suicidal ideation; generalized anxiety disorder, psychosis, schizophrenia, or other major psychiatric disorders; seizure disorders; lactation.

CAUTIOUS USE Persons piloting aircraft or operating heavy machinery; pregnancy (category C).

ROUTE & DOSAGE

Note: The U.S. Public Health Service does NOT recommend its use in children less than 15 kg or in pregnant women

Treatment of Malaria

Adult: PO 1250 mg (5 tablets) as single oral dose taken with at least 8 oz of water

Child: **PO** 20–25 mg/kg as single dose

Prophylaxis for Malaria

Adult: **PO** 250 mg once/wk × 4 wk (beginning 1 wk before travel), then 250 mg every other wk for duration of exposure and for 2 doses after leaving endemic area

Child: **PO** Given weekly: *Weight 15–19 kg,* 1/4 tablet; *weight 20–30 kg,* 1/2 tablet; *weight 31–45 kg,* 3/4 tablet

ADMINISTRATION

Oral

- Give with food and at least 8 oz water.

- Do not give concurrently with quinine or quinidine; wait at least 12 h beyond last dose of either drug before administering mefloquine.
- Store at 15°–30° C (59°–86° F).

ADVERSE EFFECTS (≥1%) **Body as a Whole:** Arthralgia, chills, fatigue, fever. **CNS:** Dizziness, nightmares, visual disturbances, headache, syncope, confusion, psychosis, aggression, suicide ideation (rare). **CV:** Bradycardia, ECG changes (including QT_c prolongation), first-degree AV block. **GI:** Nausea, vomiting, abdominal pain, anorexia, diarrhea. **Skin:** Rash, itching.

DIAGNOSTIC TEST INTERFERENCE Transient increase in ***liver transaminases***.

INTERACTIONS Drug: Mefloquine can prolong cardiac conduction in patients taking BETA-BLOCKERS, CALCIUM CHANNEL BLOCKERS, and possibly **digoxin. Quinine** may decrease plasma mefloquine concentrations. Mefloquine may decrease **valproic acid** serum concentrations by increasing its hepatic metabolism. Administration with **chloroquine** may increase risk of seizures. Increased risk of cardiac arrest and seizures with **quinidine.**

PHARMACOKINETICS Absorption: 85% absorbed, concentrates in red blood cells. **Onset:** 59 and 28 h for parasite and fever clearance times in patients with *P. vivax* infections, respectively; 166 and 93 h in patients with *P. malariae* infections. **Distribution:** Concentrated in red blood cells due to high-affinity binding to red blood cell membranes; 98% protein bound; distributed minimally into breast milk. **Metabolism:** In liver. **Elimination:** Primarily in bile and feces. **Half-Life:** 10–21 days (shorter in patients with acute malaria).

NURSING IMPLICATIONS

Assessment & Drug Effects

- Monitor carefully during prophylactic use for development of unexplained anxiety, depression, restlessness, or confusion; such manifestations may indicate a need to discontinue the drug.
- Evaluate cardiac and liver functions periodically with prolonged use.
- Lab tests: Monitor periodically CBC with differential during prolonged use.
- Monitor blood levels of anticonvulsants with concomitant therapy closely.

Patient & Family Education

- Take drug on the same day each week when used for malaria prophylaxis.
- Do not perform potentially hazardous activities until response to drug is known.
- Report any of the following immediately: Fever, sore throat, muscle aches, visual problems, anxiety, confusion, mental depression, hallucinations.

MEGESTROL ACETATE

(me-jess'trole)

Megace, Megace ES

Classifications: ANTINEOPLASTIC; PROGESTIN

Therapeutic: ANTINEOPLASTIC; APPETITE ENHANCER

Prototype: Progesterone

Pregnancy Category: X (oral suspension); D (tablets)

AVAILABILITY 40 mg/mL, 125 mg/mL suspension; 20 mg, 40 mg tablets

M

ACTION & *THERAPEUTIC EFFECT* Progestational hormone with antineoplastic properties for which an antiluteinizing effect mediated via the pituitary has been postulated. *Effective for treating breast, renal cell, or endometrial carcinoma. Also effective as an appetite enhancer. Has a local effect when instilled directly into the endometrial cavity.*

USES Palliative agent for treatment of advanced carcinoma of breast or endometrium. AIDS-related wasting or cachexia.

CONTRAINDICATIONS Diagnostic test for pregnancy; pregnancy (category X oral suspension; category D tablet); lactation.

CAUTIOUS USE Older adults; severe hepatic disease; diabetes mellitus; renal impairment; thromboembolic disease.

ROUTE & DOSAGE

Palliative Treatment for Advanced Breast Cancer

Adult: **PO** 40 mg q.i.d.

Palliative Treatment for Advanced Endometrial Cancer

Adult: **PO** 40–320 mg/day in divided doses

Appetite Stimulation

Adult: **PO** 200 mg q6h

HIV-Related Cachexia

Adult: **PO (suspension)** 800 mg daily or 625 mg of **Megace ES**

ADMINISTRATION

Oral

- Give with meals or food if GI distress occurs.
- Shake oral suspension well before use.
- Store at 15°–30° C (59°–86° F) in tightly closed container.

ADVERSE EFFECTS (≥1%) **Urogenital:** Vaginal bleeding. **Body as a Whole:** Breast tenderness, headache, increased appetite, weight gain, allergic-type reactions (including bronchial asthma). **GI:** Abdominal pain, nausea, vomiting. **Hematologic:** DVT.

INTERACTIONS Drug: May increase levels of **warfarin;** may decrease renal clearance of **dofetilide.**

PHARMACOKINETICS Absorption: Appears to be well absorbed from GI tract. **Onset:** Onset of objective response in breast cancer in 6–8 wk. **Peak:** 1–3 h. **Duration:** 3–12 mo. **Metabolism:** Completely metabolized in liver. **Elimination:** 57–78% of dose excreted in urine within 10 days.

NURSING IMPLICATIONS

Assessment & Drug Effects

- Monitor weight periodically.
- Notify physician if abdominal pain, headache, nausea, vomiting, or breast tenderness become pronounced.
- Monitor for allergic reactions, including breathing distress characteristic of asthma, rash, urticaria, anaphylaxis, tachypnea, anxiety. Stop medication if they appear and notify physician.

Patient & Family Education

- Use contraception measures during therapy for carcinoma.
- Learn breast self-examination.
- Learn S&S of thrombophlebitis (see Appendix F).
- Review package insert to ensure understanding of megestrol therapy.

MELOXICAM

(mel-ox′-i-cam)

Mobic

Classification: ANALGESIC, NONSTEROIDAL ANTI-INFLAMMATORY DRUG (NSAID)

Therapeutic: ANALGESIC, NSAID; ANTIPYRETIC; ANTIRHEUMATIC

Prototype: Ibuprofen

Pregnancy Category: C

AVAILABILITY 7.5 mg tablets

ACTION & *THERAPEUTIC EFFECT* Is a nonsteroidal anti-inflammatory drug (NSAID) that is less selective in inhibiting only COX-2 enzyme than celecoxib; meloxicam inhibits both COX-1 and COX-2 enzymes that are necessary for synthesis of prostaglandin. *Exhibits anti-inflammatory and analgesic actions.*

USES Relief of the signs and symptoms of osteoarthritis, rheumatoid arthritis.

CONTRAINDICATIONS Hypersensitivity to meloxicam, aspirin, salicylates, or NSAIDs; GI bleeding; peptic ulcer disease; severe renal or hepatic disease; perioperative pain with CABG surgery; lactation.

CAUTIOUS USE *Helicobacter pylori* infections; history of coagulation defects, liver dysfunction, gastrointestinal disease or ulceration, anemia; asthma; bone marrow suppression; dehydration, edema, older adults; females of childbearing age; GI bleeding, GI diseases, GI perforation; heart failure; hepatic disease, renal impairment; hypertension, hypovolemia, immunosuppression; jaundice, lactase deficiency, advanced renal dysfunction; hypertension or cardiac conditions aggravated by fluid retention and edema; pregnancy (category C).

ROUTE & DOSAGE

Osteoarthritis

Adult: **PO** 7.5–15 mg once daily

Rheumatoid Arthritis

Adult: **PO** 15 mg once daily

ADMINISTRATION

Oral

- Do not exceed the maximum recommended daily dose of 15 mg.
- Use the lowest effective dose for the shortest duration to minimize risk of serious adverse effects.
- Store at 15°–30° C (59°–86° F).

ADVERSE EFFECTS (≥1%) **Body as a Whole:** Edema, fall, flu-like syndrome, pain. **GI:** Abdominal pain, diarrhea, dyspepsia, flatulence, nausea, constipation, <u>ulceration, GI bleed</u>. **Hematologic:** Anemia. **Musculoskeletal:** Arthralgia. **CNS:** Dizziness, headache, insomnia. **Respiratory:** Pharyngitis, upper respiratory tract infection, cough. **Skin:** Rash, pruritus. **Urogenital:** Micturition frequency, urinary tract infection.

INTERACTIONS Drug: May decrease effectiveness of ACE INHIBITORS, DIURETICS; **aspirin, warfarin** may increase risk of bleed; may increase **lithium** levels and toxicity. **Herbal: Feverfew, garlic, ginger, ginkgo** may increase bleeding potential.

PHARMACOKINETICS Absorption: 89% bioavailable. **Peak:** 4–5 h. **Distribution:** Greater than 99% protein bound, distributes into synovial fluid. **Metabolism:** In liver

(CYP2C9). **Elimination:** Equally in urine and feces. **Half-Life:** 15–20 h.

NURSING IMPLICATIONS

Assessment & Drug Effects

- Monitor for and immediately report S&S of GI ulceration or bleeding, including black, tarry stool, abdominal or stomach pain; hepatotoxicity, including fatigue, lethargy, pruritus, jaundice, flu-like symptoms; skin rash; weight gain and edema.
- Withhold drug and notify physician if hepatotoxicity or GI bleeding is suspected.
- Monitor carefully patients with a history of CHF, HTN, or edema for fluid retention.
- Lab tests: Hgb and Hct, CBC with differential, liver function tests, serum electrolytes, BUN, and creatinine within 3 mo of initiating therapy and every 6–12 mo thereafter; with high-risk patients (e.g., older than 60 y, history of peptic ulcer disease, prolonged or high-dose NSAID therapy, concurrent use of corticosteroids or anticoagulants) monitor within first 3–4 wk and every 3–6 mo thereafter.
- Coadministered drugs: With warfarin, closely monitor INR when meloxicam is initiated or dose changed; monitor for lithium toxicity, especially during addition, withdrawal, or change in dose of meloxicam.

Patient & Family Education

- Report any of the following to the physician immediately: Nausea, black tarry stool, abdominal or stomach pain, unexplained fatigue or lethargy, itching, jaundice, flu-like symptoms, skin rash, weight gain, or edema.
- Discontinue drug if hepatotoxicity or GI bleeding is suspected. Note that GI bleeding may occur without forewarning and is more likely in older adults, in those with a history of ulcers or GI bleeding, and with alcohol consumption and cigarette smoking.
- Do not take aspirin or other NSAIDs while on this medication.

M

MELPHALAN

(mel'fa-lan)

Alkeran

Classifications: ANTINEOPLASTIC; ALKYLATING AGENT

Therapeutic: ANTINEOPLASTIC

Prototype: Cyclophosphamide

Pregnancy Category: D

AVAILABILITY 2 mg tablets; 50 mg/vial injection

ACTION & *THERAPEUTIC EFFECT* Forms a highly reactive carbonium ion that causes cross-linking and abnormal base-pairing in DNA, thereby interfering with DNA and RNA replication as well as protein synthesis. *Antineoplastic effects result from its activity against both resting and rapidly dividing tumor cells.*

USES Palliative treatment of multiple myeloma and other neoplasms, including Hodgkin's disease and carcinomas of breast and ovary.

UNLABELED USES Polycythemia vera.

CONTRAINDICATIONS Severe bone marrow suppression; hepatic disease; renal impairment, renal failure; severe electrolyte imbalance; pregnancy (category D), lactation; men and women of childbearing age.

CAUTIOUS USE Recent treatment with other chemotherapeutic agents;

severe anemia, neutropenia, or thrombocytopenia.

ROUTE & DOSAGE

Multiple Myeloma

Adult: **PO** 6 mg/day for 2–3 wk, drug then withdrawn for 4–5 wk, restart at 2 mg/day when WBC and platelet counts start to rise
IV 16 mg/m^2 over 15 min q2wk for 4 doses

Epithelial Ovarian Cancer

Adult: **PO** 0.2 mg/kg/day for 5 days as single course, may repeat course q4–5wk

ADMINISTRATION

Oral

- Give with meals to reduce nausea and vomiting. An antiemetic may be ordered.

Intravenous

PREPARE: **IV Infusion:** Reconstitute melphalan powder by **RAPIDLY** injecting 10 mL of the provided diluent into the vial to yield 5 mg/mL. Shake vigorously until clear. ▪ Immediately dilute further with NS to a concentration of 0.45 mg/mL or less. ▪ Note: 45 mg in 100 mL yields 0.45 mg/mL. ▪ Do not refrigerate reconstituted solution prior to infusion.

ADMINISTER: **IV Infusion:** Give over 15 min or longer. Administration **Must be** completed within 60 min of reconstitution of drug because both reconstituted and diluted solutions are unstable. ▪ Ensure patency of IV site prior to infusion.

INCOMPATIBILITIES **Solution/Additive: D5W, lactated Ringer's. Y-site: Amphotericin B, chlorpromazine.**

- Store at 15°–30° C (59°–86° F) in light-resistant, airtight containers.

ADVERSE EFFECTS (≥1%) **Hematologic:** Leukopenia, agranulocytosis, thrombocytopenia, anemia, acute nonlymphatic leukemia. **Body as a Whole:** Uremia, angioneurotic peripheral edema. **GI:** Nausea, vomiting, stomatitis. **Skin:** Temporary alopecia. **Respiratory:** Pulmonary fibrosis.

INTERACTIONS **Drug:** Increases risk of nephrotoxicity with **cyclosporine, cimetidine** may decrease efficacy. **Food:** Food decreases absorption.

PHARMACOKINETICS **Absorption:** Incompletely and variably absorbed from GI tract. **Peak:** 2 h. **Distribution:** Widely distributed to all tissues. **Metabolism:** By spontaneous hydrolysis in plasma. **Elimination:** 25–50% in feces; 25–30% in urine. **Half-Life:** 1.5 h.

NURSING IMPLICATIONS

Assessment & Drug Effects

- Lab tests: Monitor WBC and platelet counts 2–3 times/wk during dosage adjustment period; determine WBC each week for 6–8 wk during maintenance therapy. Monitor serum uric acid levels.
- Monitor laboratory reports to anticipate leukopenic and thrombocytopenic periods.
- A degree of myelosuppression is maintained during therapy so as to keep leukocyte count in range of 3000–3500/mm^3.
- Assess for flank and joint pains that may signal onset of hyperuricemia.

Patient & Family Education

- Be alert to onset of fever, profound weakness, chills, tachycardia, cough, sore throat, changes

M

in kidney function, or prolonged infections and report to physician.

- Understand that reversible hair loss is an expected adverse effect.

MEMANTINE

(me-man′teen)

Namenda

Classifications: N-METHYL-D-ASPARTATE (NMDA) RECEPTOR ANTAGONIST; ANTIDEMENTIA

Therapeutic: ANTIDEMENTIA; ANTI-ALZHEIMER'S

Pregnancy Category: B

AVAILABILITY 5 mg, 10 mg tablets; 2 mg/mL solution

M

ACTION & *THERAPEUTIC EFFECT* Excess glutamate may play a role in Alzheimer's disease by overstimulating NMDA receptors. Blockade of NMDA receptors may slow intracellular calcium accumulation, preventing nerve damage without interfering with actions of glutamate that are required for memory and learning. *Improves cognitive functioning in moderate to severe Alzheimer's disease (AD) and in mild to moderate vascular dementia.*

USES Treatment of symptoms of moderate to severe Alzheimer's disease.

UNLABELED USES Treatment of moderate to severe vascular dementia.

CONTRAINDICATIONS Known memantine hypersensitivity; renal failure. Safety and efficacy in children are unknown.

CAUTIOUS USE Moderate to severe renal impairment; severe hepatic impairment; history of seizure disorder; older adults; pregnancy (category B), lactation.

ROUTE & DOSAGE

Alzheimer's Disease

Adult: **PO** Initiate with 5 mg once daily, increase dose by 5 mg/wk over a 3-wk period to target dose of 10 mg b.i.d.

Severe Renal Impairment Dosage Adjustment

Decrease to 5 mg b.i.d.

ADMINISTRATION

Oral

- Note: The recommended interval between dose increases is 1 wk.
- Dose reductions should be considered with moderate renal impairment.
- Store between 15°–30° C (59°–86° F).

ADVERSE EFFECTS (≥1%) **Body as a Whole:** Fatigue, pain, flu-like symptoms, peripheral edema. **CNS:** Dizziness, headache, confusion, somnolence, hallucinations, agitation, insomnia, abnormal gait, depression, anxiety, syncope, TIA, vertigo, ataxia, hypokinesia, aggressive reaction. **CV:** Hypertension, cardiac failure. **GI:** Constipation, vomiting, diarrhea, nausea, anorexia. **Hematologic:** Anemia. **Metabolic:** Weight loss, increased alkaline phosphatase. **Musculoskeletal:** Back pain, arthralgia. **Respiratory:** Coughing, dyspnea, bronchitis, upper respiratory infections, pneumonia. **Skin:** Rash. **Special Senses:** Conjunctivitis. **Urogenital:** Urinary incontinence, UTI, frequent micturition.

INTERACTIONS Drug: Drugs that increase the pH of the urine (CARBONIC ANHYDRASE INIBITORS, **sodium bicar-**

bonate) may increase levels of memantine; may enhance the effects of **amantadine, dextromethorphan, ketamine, bromocriptine, pergolide, pramipexole,** and **ropinirole;** may enhance the adverse effects of **levodopa**-containing drugs.

PHARMACOKINETICS Absorption: 100% from GI tract. **Duration:** 4–6 h. **Distribution:** Easily crosses the blood–brain barrier. **Metabolism:** Minimal. **Elmination:** Primarily excreted unchanged in urine. Increases in urinary pH can decrease elimination of drug. **Half-Life:** 60–80 h.

NURSING IMPLICATIONS

Assessment & Drug Effects

- Monitor respiratory and CV status, especially with preexisting heart disease.
- Assess for and report S&S of focal neurologic deficits (e.g., TIA, ataxia, vertigo).
- Lab tests: Periodic Hct and Hgb, serum sodium, alkaline phosphatase, and blood glucose.
- Monitor diabetics for loss of glycemic control.

Patient & Family Education

- Report any of the following to the physician: Problems with vision, skin rash, shortness of breath, swelling in throat or tongue, agitation or restlessness, confusion, dizziness, or incontinence.
- Do not drive or engage in other hazardous activities until reaction to drug is known.

MEPERIDINE HYDROCHLORIDE

(me-per′i-deen)

Demerol, Pethadol ♣, Pethidine Hydrochloride ♣

Classification: NARCOTIC (OPIATE AGONIST) ANALGESIC
Therapeutic: NARCOTIC ANALGESIC
Prototype: Morphine
Pregnancy Category: B (D at term)
Controlled Substance: Schedule II

AVAILABILITY 50 mg, 100 mg tablets; 50 mg/5 mL syrup; 10 mg/mL, 25 mg/mL, 50 mg/mL, 75 mg/mL, 100 mg/mL injection

ACTION & *THERAPEUTIC EFFECT* Analgesia is mediated through changes in the perception of pain at the spinal cord (mu_2, delta, kappa receptors) and higher levels in the CNS (mu_1 and $kappa_3$ receptors). *Control of moderate to severe pain. Does not alter pain threshold.*

USES Relief of moderate to severe pain, for preoperative medication, for support of anesthesia, and for obstetric analgesia.

CONTRAINDICATIONS Hypersensitivity to meperidine; convulsive disorders; acute abdominal conditions prior to diagnosis; MAOI therapy; pregnancy (category D at term).
CAUTIOUS USE Head injuries, increased intracranial pressure; asthma and other respiratory conditions; supraventricular tachycardias; prostatic hypertrophy; urethral stricture; glaucoma; older adult or debilitated patients; impaired kidney or liver function, hypothyroidism, Addison's disease; pregnancy (category B).

ROUTE & DOSAGE

Moderate to Severe Pain
NOTE: Should be titrated to pain response

M

Adult: **PO/Subcutaneous/IM/IV** 50–150 mg q3–4h prn
Child: **PO/Subcutaneous/IM/IV** 1–1.8 mg/kg q3–4h (max: 100 mg q4h) prn

Preoperative

Adult: **IM/Subcutaneous** 50–100 mg 30–90 min before surgery
Child: **IM/Subcutaneous** 1.1–2.2 mg/kg 30–90 min before surgery

Obstetric Analgesia

Adult: **IM/Subcutaneous** 50–100 mg when pains become regular, may be repeated q1–3h

Hepatic/Renal Impairment Dosage Adjustment

Adjust based on patient response

ADMINISTRATION

Oral

- Give syrup formulation in half a glass of water. Undiluted syrup may cause topical anesthesia of mucous membranes.

Subcutaneous and Intramuscular Injections

- Be aware that subcutaneous route is painful and can cause local irritation. IM route is generally preferred when repeated doses are required.
- Aspirate carefully before giving IM injection to avoid inadvertent IV administration. IV injection of undiluted drug can cause a marked increase in heart rate and syncope.

Intravenous

Note: Verify correct IV concentration and rate of infusion/injection for administration to infants or children with physician.

PREPARE: **Direct:** Dilute 50 mg in at least 5 mL of NS or sterile water to yield 10 mg/mL. **IV Infusion:** Dilute to a concentration of 1–10 mg/mL in NS, D5W, or other compatible solution.

ADMINISTER: **Direct:** Give slowly over 3–5 min at a rate not to exceed 25 mg/min. Slower injection preferred. **IV Infusion:** Usually given through a controlled infusion device at a rate not to exceed 25 mg/min.

INCOMPATIBILITIES **Solution/additive: Aminophylline,** BARBITURATES, **furosemide, heparin, methicillin, morphine, phenytoin, sodium bicarbonate. Y-site: Allopurinol, amphotericin B cholesteryl complex, cefepime, cefoperazone, doxorubicin liposome, furosemide, idarubicin, imipenem/cilastatin, lansoprazole, mezlocillin, minocycline, tetracycline.**

- Store at 15°–30° C (59°–86° F) in tightly closed, light-resistant containers unless otherwise directed by manufacturer.

ADVERSE EFFECTS (≥1%) **Body as a Whole:** Allergic (*Pruritus,* urticaria, skin rashes, wheal and flare over IV site), profuse perspiration. **CNS:** *Dizziness,* weakness, euphoria, dysphoria, *sedation,* headache, uncoordinated muscle movements, disorientation, decreased cough reflex, miosis, corneal anesthesia, <u>respiratory depression</u>. Toxic doses: Muscle twitching, tremors, hyperactive reflexes, excitement, hypersensitivity to external stimuli, agitation, confusion, hallucinations, dilated pupils, <u>convulsions</u>. **CV:** Facial flushing, light-headedness, hypotension, syncope, palpitation, bradycardia, tachycardia, <u>cardiovascular collapse, cardiac arrest (toxic doses)</u>. **GI:** Dry mouth, *nausea,* vomiting, *constipation,* biliary tract spasm. **Urogenital:** Oliguria, urinary retention. **Respiratory:** <u>Respiratory depression in</u>

newborn, bronchoconstriction (large doses). **Skin:** Phlebitis (following IV use), pain, tissue irritation and induration, particularly following subcutaneous injection. **Metabolic:** Increased levels of serum amylase, BSP retention, bilirubin, AST, ALT.

DIAGNOSTIC TEST INTERFERENCE High doses of meperidine may interfere with ***gastric emptying studies*** by causing delay in gastric emptying.

INTERACTIONS Drug: Alcohol and other CNS DEPRESSANTS, **cimetidine** cause additive sedation and CNS depression; AMPHETAMINES may potentiate CNS stimulation; MAO INHIBITORS, **selegiline** may cause excessive and prolonged CNS depression, convulsions, cardiovascular collapse; **phenytoin** may increase toxic meperidine metabolites. **Herbal: St. John's wort** may increase sedation.

PHARMACOKINETICS Absorption: 50–60% from GI tract. **Onset:** 15 min PO; 10 min IM, Subcutaneous; 5 min IV. **Peak:** 1 h PO, IM, Subcutaneous. **Duration:** 2–4 h PO, IM, Subcutaneous; 2 h IV. **Distribution:** Crosses placenta; distributed into breast milk. **Metabolism:** In liver. **Elimination:** In urine. **Half-Life:** 3–5 h.

NURSING IMPLICATIONS

Assessment & Drug Effects

- Give narcotic analgesics in the smallest effective dose and for the least period of time compatible with patient's needs.
- Assess patient's need for prn medication. Record time of onset, duration, and quality of pain.
- Note respiratory rate, depth, and rhythm and size of pupils in patients receiving repeated doses. If respirations are 12/min or below and pupils are constricted or dilated (see ACTION and USES) or breathing is shallow, or if signs of CNS hyperactivity are present, consult physician before administering drug.
- Monitor vital signs closely. Heart rate may increase markedly, and hypotension may occur. Meperidine may cause severe hypotension in postoperative patients and those with depleted blood volume.
- Schedule deep breathing, coughing (unless contraindicated), and changes in position at intervals to help to overcome respiratory depressant effects.
- Chart patient's response to drug and evaluate continued need.
- Repeated use can lead to tolerance as well as psychic and physical dependence of the morphine type.
- Be aware that abrupt discontinuation following repeated use results in morphine-like withdrawal symptoms. Symptoms develop more rapidly (within 3 h, peaking in 8–12 h) and are of shorter duration than with morphine. Nausea, vomiting, diarrhea, and pupillary dilatation are less prominent, but muscle twitching, restlessness, and nervousness are greater than produced by morphine.

Patient & Family Education

- Exercise caution with ambulation and moving from a lying/sitting position to a standing position.
- Be aware nausea, vomiting, dizziness, and faintness associated with fall in BP are more pronounced when walking than when lying down (these symptoms may also occur in patients without pain who are given meperidine). Symptoms are aggravated by the head-up position.

M

- Do not drive or engage in potentially hazardous activities until any drowsiness and dizziness have passed.
- Do not take other CNS depressants or drink alcohol because of their additive effects.

MEPHOBARBITAL

(me-foe-bar'bi-tal)

Mebaral, Methylphenobarbital

Classifications: ANTICONVULSANT; BARBITURATE; SEDATIVE-HYPNOTIC

Therapeutic: ANTICONVULSANT; SEDATIVE-HYPNOTIC

Prototype: Phenobarbital

Pregnancy Category: D

Controlled Substance: Schedule IV

M

AVAILABILITY 32 mg, 50 mg, 100 mg tablets

ACTION & *THERAPEUTIC EFFECT* Long-acting barbiturate that limits the spread of seizure activity by increasing the threshold for motor cortex stimuli. Exerts strong sedative effect and mild hypnotic effect. *Reduces seizure activity by decreasing excitability in nerve cells. Depresses CNS producing drowiness, hypnosis, and sedation.*

USES To control grand mal and petit mal epilepsy, alone or in combination with other anticonvulsant agents, and for sedative effect in management of delirium tremens and other acute agitation and anxiety states.

CONTRAINDICATIONS Hypersensitivity to barbiturates; coma; ethanol intoxication, hepatic encephalopathy; porphyria; status epilepticus; pregnancy (category D).

CAUTIOUS USE Fever, hyperthyroidism, alcoholism; respiratory disorders, COPD, sleep apnea; mental status changes, major depression; suicidal ideation; liver, kidney, or cardiac dysfunction; lactation.

ROUTE & DOSAGE

Anticonvulsant

Adult: **PO** 400–600 mg/day in divided doses

Child: **PO** *Younger than 5 y,* 16–32 mg t.i.d. or q.i.d.; *5 y or older,* 32–64 mg t.i.d. or q.i.d.

Sedative

Adult: **PO** 32–100 mg t.i.d. or q.i.d.

Child: **PO** *Younger than 5 y,* 16–32 mg t.i.d. or q.i.d.; *5 y or older,* 32–64 mg t.i.d. or q.i.d.

Delirium Tremens

Adult: **PO** 200 mg t.i.d. or q.i.d.

ADMINISTRATION

Oral

- Change from other anticonvulsant by gradually tapering off the former as mephobarbital doses are increased to maintain seizure control.
- When prescribed concurrently with phenobarbital, dose should be about one-half the amount of each used alone. When prescribed concurrently with phenytoin, the dose of phenytoin is usually reduced.
- Reduce discontinued drug dosage gradually over 4 or 5 days to avoid precipitating seizures of status epilepticus.

ADVERSE EFFECTS (≥1%) **CNS:** *Drowsiness,* dizziness, unsteadiness, hangover, paradoxical excitement. **GI:** Nausea, vomiting, constipation. **Body as a Whole:** Hypersensitivity reactions, respiratory depression.

INTERACTIONS Drug: Alcohol, CNS DEPRESSANTS compound CNS depression; may decrease absorption and increase metabolism of ORAL ANTICOAGULANTS; increases metabolism of CORTICOSTEROIDS, ORAL CONTRACEPTIVES, ANTICONVULSANTS, **digitoxin,** possibly decreasing their effects; ANTIDEPRESSANTS potentiate adverse effects; **griseofulvin** decreases absorption of mephobarbitol. **Herbal: Kava, valerian** may potentiate sedation.

PHARMACOKINETICS Absorption: 50% from GI tract. **Onset:** 60 min. **Duration:** 10–12 h. **Metabolism:** In liver to phenobarbital. **Elimination:** In urine. Alkalinization of urine or increase of urinary flow significantly increases the rate of phenobarbital excretion. **Half-Life:** 34 h.

NURSING IMPLICATIONS

Assessment & Drug Effects

- Monitor respiratory status, especially with concurrent CNS therapy with other drugs.
- Be prepared for paradoxical response to barbiturate therapy (i.e., irritability, marked excitement, aggression in children, depression, confusion) in older adults, debilitated patients, or children.

Patient & Family Education

- Be aware that abrupt cessation after prolonged therapy may result in withdrawal symptoms (tremulousness, weakness, insomnia, delirium, convulsions).
- Avoid driving and potentially hazardous activities until response to drug has stabilized.
- Do not take alcohol in any amount with a barbiturate.

MEPROBAMATE Pr

(me-proe-ba′mate)

Classifications: CARBAMATE; ANXIOLYTIC; SEDATIVE-HYPNOTIC

Therapeutic: ANTIANXIETY; SEDATIVE-HYPNOTIC

Pregnancy Category: D

Controlled Substance: Schedule IV

AVAILABILITY 200 mg, 400 mg tablets

ACTION & *THERAPEUTIC EFFECT* Carbamate derivative and CNS depressant. Acts on multiple sites in CNS and appears to block corticothalamic impulses. *Antianxiety agent. Hypnotic doses suppress REM sleep.*

USES To relieve anxiety and tension of psychoneurotic states and as adjunct in disease states associated with anxiety and tension. Also used to promote sleep in anxious, tense patients.

CONTRAINDICATIONS History of hypersensitivity to meprobamate or related carbamates; history of acute intermittent porphyria; pregnancy (category D), lactation, children younger than 6 y.

CAUTIOUS USE Impaired kidney or liver function; convulsive disorders; history of alcoholism or drug abuse; patients with suicidal tendencies.

ROUTE & DOSAGE

Sedative

Adult: **PO** 1.2–1.6 g/day in 3–4 divided doses (max: 2.4 g/day)
Child (6 y or older): **PO** 100–200 mg b.i.d. or t.i.d.

Hypnotic

Adult: **PO** 400–800 mg
Geriatric: **PO** 200 mg
Child (6 y or older): **PO** 200 mg

ADMINISTRATION

Oral

- Give with food to minimize gastric distress.

- Treatment physical dependence by gradual drug withdrawal over 1–2 wk to prevent onset of withdrawal symptoms.
- Store at 15°–30° C (59°–86° F) unless otherwise specified by manufacturer.

ADVERSE EFFECTS (≥1%) **Body as a Whole:** Allergy or idiosyncratic reactions (itchy, urticarial, or erythematous maculopapular rash; exfoliative dermatitis, petechiae, purpura, ecchymoses, eosinophilia, peripheral edema, angioneurotic edema, adenopathy, fever, chills, proctitis, bronchospasm, oliguria, anuria, Stevens-Johnson syndrome); anaphylaxis. **CNS:** *Drowsiness* and *ataxia,* dizziness, vertigo, slurred speech, headache, weakness, paresthesias, impaired visual accommodation, paradoxic euphoria and rage reactions, seizures in epileptics, panic reaction, rapid EEG activity. **CV:** Hypotensive crisis, syncope, palpitation, tachycardia, arrhythmias, transient ECG changes, circulatory collapse (toxic doses). **GI:** Anorexia, nausea, vomiting, diarrhea. **Hematologic:** Aplastic anemia (rare): Leukopenia, agranulocytosis, thrombocytopenia, exacerbation of acute intermittent porphyria. **Respiratory:** Respiratory depression.

DIAGNOSTIC TEST INTERFERENCE Meprobamate may cause falsely high ***urinary steroid*** determinations. ***Phentolamine*** tests may be falsely positive; meprobamate should be withdrawn at least 24 h and preferably 48–72 h before the test.

INTERACTIONS Drug: Alcohol, entacapone, TRICYCLIC ANTIDEPRESSANTS, ANTIPSYCHOTICS, OPIATES, SEDATING ANTIHISTAMINES, **pentazocine, tramadol,** MAOIS, SEDATIVE-HYPNOTICS, ANXIOLYTICS may potentiate CNS depression. **Herbal: Kava, valerian** may potentiate sedation.

PHARMACOKINETICS Absorption: Well absorbed from GI tract. **Peak:** 1–3 h. **Onset:** 1 h. **Distribution:** Uniformly throughout body; crosses placenta. **Metabolism:** Rapidly in liver. **Elimination:** Renally excreted; excreted in breast milk. **Half-Life:** 10–11 h.

NURSING IMPLICATIONS

Assessment & Drug Effects

- Supervise ambulation, if necessary. Older adults and debilitated patients are prone to oversedation and to the hypotensive effects, especially during early therapy.
- Utilize safety precautions for hospitalized patients. Hypnotic doses may cause increased motor activity during sleep.
- Consult physician if daytime psychomotor function is impaired. A change in regimen or drug may be indicated.
- Withdraw gradually in physically dependent patients to prevent preexisting symptoms or withdrawal reactions within 12–48 h: Vomiting, ataxia, muscle twitching, mental confusion, hallucinations, convulsions, trembling, sleep disturbances, increased dreaming, nightmares, insomnia. Symptoms usually subside within 12–48 h.

Patient & Family Education

- Take drug as prescribed. Psychic or physical dependence may occur with long-term use of high doses.
- Be aware that tolerance to alcohol will be lowered.
- Make position changes slowly, especially from lying down to upright; dangle legs for a few minutes before standing.

- Avoid driving or engaging in hazardous activities until response to drug is known.
- Report immediately onset of skin rash, sore throat, fever, bruising, unexplained bleeding.

MEQUINOL/TRETINOIN

(me-qui′nol/tre-ti′noyn)

Solagé

Classification: RETINOID

Therapeutic: DEPIGMENTING AGENT RETINOID

Prototype: Isotretinoin

Pregnancy Category: X

AVAILABILITY 2%/0.01% solution

ACTION & *THERAPEUTIC EFFECT* Mequinol is a depigmenting agent and tretinoin is a retinoid used to improve dermatologic changes (e.g., fine wrinkling, mottled hyperpigmentation, roughness) associated with photo-damage and aging. Mequinol's mechanism of depigmentation is probably due to oxidation by tyrosine to cytotoxic products in melanocytes, and/or inhibition of melanin formation. Tretinoin, a retinoid, is used to improve photo-damage to the skin by acting via retinoic acid receptors (RARs). *Mequinol has depigmenting properties; tretinoin improves sun-damaged skin.*

USES Treatment of solar lentigines (age spots).

UNLABELED USES Facial wrinkles.

CONTRAINDICATIONS Hypersensitivity to mequinol or tretinoin; pregnancy (category X), lactation, children.

CAUTIOUS USE History of hypersensitivity to acitretin, isotretinoin, etretinate, or other vitamin A derivatives, or hydroquinone; patients with eczema, moderate to severe skin pigmentation, vitiligo; cold weather.

ROUTE & DOSAGE

Solar Lentigines

Adult: **Topical** Apply to solar lentigines b.i.d. at least 8 h apart

ADMINISTRATION

Topical

- Apply doses at least 8 h apart; avoid application to unaffected areas.
- Avoid contact with eyes, lips, mucous membranes, or paranasal creases.
- Protect from light.

ADVERSE EFFECTS (≥1%) **Skin:** *Erythema, burning, stinging, tingling, desquamation, pruritus,* skin irritation, temporary hypopigmentation, rash, dry skin, crusting, application site reaction.

INTERACTIONS Drug: THIAZIDE DIURETICS, TETRACYCLINES, FLUOROQUINOLONES, PHENOTHIAZINES, SULFONAMIDES may augment phototoxicity.

PHARMACOKINETICS Absorption: 4.4% through skin. **Peak:** 1–2 h.

NURSING IMPLICATIONS

Assessment & Drug Effects

- Monitor for and report peeling, erythema, or hypopigmentation.
- Monitor for signs of tretinoin toxicity: Headache, fever, weakness, and fatigue.

Patient & Family Education

- Do not apply larger than recommended amounts.
- Do not wash affected area for at least 6 h after drug application; do not apply cosmetics to af-

fected area for at least 30 min after drug application.

- Minimize exposure to sunlight or sunlamps. Use extra caution if also taking concurrently other drugs that are photosensitizing (e.g., thiazide diuretics, phenothiazines).
- Notify physician if vitiligo (hypopigmentation of skin) or S&S of tretinoin toxicity develop (see ASSESSMENT & DRUG EFFECTS).

MERCAPTOPURINE (6-MP, 6-MERCAPTOPURINE) Pr

(mer-kap-toe-pyoor'een)

Purinethol

Classifications: ANTINEOPLASTIC; ANTIMETABOLITE, PURINE ANTAGONIST

Therapeutic: ANTINEOPLASTIC; IMMUNOSUPPRESSANT

Pregnancy Category: D

AVAILABILITY 50 mg tablets

ACTION & *THERAPEUTIC EFFECT* Antimetabolite and purine antagonist that inhibits purine metabolism. Blocks conversion of inosinic acid to adenine and xanthine ribotides within sensitive tumor cells. Also inhibits adenine-containing coenzymes, suggesting an influence over multiple cellular reactions. *Delayed immunosuppressive properties and carcinogenic potential.*

USES Primarily for acute lymphocytic and myelogenous leukemia. Response in adults is less than in children, but mercaptopurine is initial drug of choice. In chronic granulocytic leukemia, produces temporary remission.

UNLABELED USES Prevention of transplant graft rejection; SLE; rheumatoid arthritis; Crohn's disease.

CONTRAINDICATIONS Prior resistance to mercaptopurine; infections; pregnancy (category D); lactation.

CAUTIOUS USE Impaired kidney or liver function.

ROUTE & DOSAGE

Leukemias

Adult/Child: **PO Loading Dose** 2.5 mg/kg/day, may increase up to 5 mg/kg/day after 4 wk if needed **PO Maintenance Dose** 1.25–2.5 mg/kg/day

ADMINISTRATION

Oral

- Give total daily dose at one time.
- Reduce dose of mercaptopurine usually by 1/3–1/4 when given concurrently with allopurinol.
- Store tablets in light- and air-resistant container.

ADVERSE EFFECTS (≥1%) **GI:** Stomatitis, esophagitis, anorexia, nausea, vomiting, diarrhea, intestinal ulcerations, impaired liver function, <u>hepatic necrosis</u>. **Hematologic:** <u>Leukopenia</u>, anemia, eosinophilia, pancytopenia, <u>thrombocytopenia</u>, abnormal bleeding, bone marrow hypoplasia. **Urogenital:** Hyperuricemia, oliguria, renal impairment. **Skin:** Rash. **Body as a Whole:** Drug fever.

INTERACTIONS Drug: Allopurinol may inhibit metabolism and thus increase toxicity of mercaptopurine; may potentiate or antagonize anticoagulant effects of **warfarin.**

PHARMACOKINETICS Absorption: Approximately 50% absorbed from GI tract. **Peak:** 2 h. **Distribution:** Distributes into total body water. **Metabolism:** Rapidly by xanthine oxidase in liver. **Elimination:** 11% in urine within 6 h. **Half-Life:** 20–50 min.

NURSING IMPLICATIONS

Assessment & Drug Effects

- Lab tests: Monitor CBC with differential, platelet count, Hgb, Hct, and liver functions closely.
- Monitor for S&S of liver damage. Hepatic toxicity occurs most often when dose exceeds 2.5 mg/kg/day. Jaundice signals onset of hepatic toxicity and may necessitate terminating use.
- Withhold drug and notify physician at the first sign of an abnormally large or rapid fall in platelet and leukocyte counts.
- Record baseline data related to I&O ratio and pattern and body weight.
- Check vital signs daily. Report febrile states promptly.
- Protect patient from exposure to trauma, infections, or other stresses (restrict visitors and personnel who have colds) during periods of leukopenia.
- Report nausea, vomiting, or diarrhea. These may signal excessive dosage, especially in adults.
- Watch for signs of abnormal bleeding (ecchymoses, petechiae, melena, bleeding gums) if thrombocytopenia develops; report immediately.

Patient & Family Education

- Report any signs of bleeding (e.g., hematuria, bruising, bleeding gums).
- Report signs of hepatic toxicity (see Appendix F).
- Increase hydration (10–12 glasses of fluid daily) to reduce risk of hyperuricemia. Consult physician about desirable volume.
- Notify physician of onset of chills, nausea, vomiting, flank or joint pain, swelling of legs or feet, or symptoms of anemia.

MEROPENEM

(mer-o′pe-nem)

Merrem

Classification: CARBAPENEM ANTIBIOTIC

Therapeutic: ANTIBIOTIC

Prototype: Imipenem

Pregnancy Category: B

AVAILABILITY 500 mg, 1 g injection

ACTION & *THERAPEUTIC EFFECT* Broad-spectrum carbapenem antibiotic that inhibits cell wall synthesis of gram-positive and gram-negative bacteria by its strong affinity for penicillin-binding proteins of bacterial cell wall. *Effective against both gram-positive and gram-negative bacteria.*

USES Complicated appendicitis and peritonitis, bacterial meningitis caused by susceptible bacteria, complicated skin infections, intra-abdominal infections, skin/soft tissue infections.

UNLABELED USES Febrile neutropenia.

CONTRAINDICATIONS Hypersensitivity to meropenem, other carbapenem antibiotics including imipenem, penicillins, cephalosporins, or other beta-lactams. Safety and effectiveness in infants younger than 3 mo not established.

CAUTIOUS USE History of asthma or allergies, renal impairment, renal disease; epileptics, history of neurologic disorders, older adult, pregnancy (category B), lacatation.

ROUTE & DOSAGE

Intra-abdominal Infections

Adult/Child (weight greater than 50 kg): **IV** 1 g q8h
Child (3 mo or older, weight less than 50 kg): **IV** 20 mg/kg q8h (max: 1 g q8h)

Bacterial Meningitis

Adult/Child (weight greater than 50 kg): **IV** 2 g q8h
Child (3 mo or older, weight less than 50 kg): **IV** 40 mg/kg q8h (max: 2 g q8h)

Complicated Skin Infection

Adult/Child (weight greater than 50 kg): **IV** 500 mg q8h
Child (older than 3 mo, weight less than 50 kg): **IV** 10 mg/kg q8h (max: 500 mg q8h)

M

Renal Impairment Dosage Adjustment

CrCl 26–50 mL/min: q12h; 10–25 mL/min: 1/2 dose q12h; less than 10 mL/min: 1/2 dose q24h

ADMINISTRATION

Intravenous

Note: Dosage reduction is recommended for older adults.

PREPARE: **Direct:** Reconstitute the 500-mg or 1-g vial, respectively, by adding 10 or 20 mL sterile water for injection to yield approximately 50 mg/mL. ▪ Shake to dissolve and let stand until clear.
IV Infusion: Further dilute reconstituted solution in 50–250 mL of D5W, NS, or D5/NS.

ADMINISTER: **Direct:** Give doses of 5–20 mL over 3–5 min. **IV Infusion:** Give over 15–30 min.

INCOMPATIBILITIES **Solution/additive: D5W, lactated Ringer's, mannitol, amphotericin B, metronidazole, multivitamins, sodium bicarbonate. Y-site: Amphotericin B, diazepam, doxycycline, metronidazole, ondansetron, zidovudine.**

▪ Store undiluted at 15°–30° C (59°–86° F), diluted IV solutions should generally be used within 1 h of preparation.

ADVERSE EFFECTS (≥1%) **GI:** Diarrhea, nausea, vomiting, constipation. **Other:** Inflammation at injection site, phlebitis, thrombophlebitis. **CNS:** Headache. **Skin:** Rash, pruritus, diaper rash. **Body as a Whole:** Apnea, oral moniliasis, sepsis, shock. **Hematologic:** Anemia.

INTERACTIONS Drug: Probenecid delays meropenem excretion; may decrease **valproic acid** serum levels.

PHARMACOKINETICS Distribution: Attains high concentrations in bile, bronchial secretions, cerebrospinal fluid. **Metabolism:** Renal and extrarenal metabolism via dipeptidases or nonspecific degradation. **Elimination:** In urine. **Half-Life:** 0.8–1 h.

NURSING IMPLICATIONS

Assessment & Drug Effects

- Lab tests: Perform C&S tests prior to therapy. Monitor periodically liver and kidney function.
- Determine history of hypersensitivity reactions to other beta-lactams, cephalosporins, penicillins, or other drugs.
- Discontinue drug and immediately report S&S of hypersensitivity (see Appendix F).
- Report S&S of superinfection or pseudomembranous colitis (see Appendix F).
- Monitor for seizures especially in older adults and those with renal insufficiency.

Patient & Family Education

- Learn S&S of hypersensitivity, superinfection, and pseudomembranous colitis; report any of these to physician promptly.

MESALAMINE Pr

(me-sal'a-meen)

Asacol, Canasa, Lialda, Pentasa, Rowasa, Salofalk ♣

Classifications: ANTI-INFLAMMATORY; PROSTAGLANDIN INHIBITOR

Therapeutic: GI; ANTI-INFLAMMATORY

Pregnancy Category: B

AVAILABILITY 250 mg controlled release capsule (Pentasa); 400 mg delayed release tablet (Asacol); 1.2 g delayed release tablet (Lialda); 500 mg suppository, 4 g/60 mL rectal suspension (Rowasa); 500 mg suppositories (Canasa)

ACTION & *THERAPEUTIC EFFECT* Thought to diminish inflammation by blocking cyclooxygenase and inhibiting prostaglandin synthesis in the colon. *Provides topical anti-inflammatory action in the colon of patients with ulcerative colitis.*

USES Indicated in active mild to moderate distal ulcerative colitis, proctosigmoiditis, or proctitis; maintenance of remission of ulcerative colitis.

UNLABELED USES Crohn's disease.

CONTRAINDICATIONS Hypersensitivity to mesalamine, aminosalicylates, or salicylates.

CAUTIOUS USE Sulfite hypersensitivity; sensitivity to sulfasalazine; renal disease, renal impairment; pregnancy (category B), lactation.

ROUTE & DOSAGE

Ulcerative Colitis

Adult: **Rectal** (Rowasa) 4 g once/day at bedtime, enema should be retained for about 8 h if possible or 1 suppository (500 mg) b.i.d.; (Canasa) 500 mg b.i.d., may increase up to 500 mg t.i.d. **PO** (Asacol) 800 mg t.i.d. × 6 wk; (Pentasa) 500 mg t.i.d. × 6 wk; (Lialda) 2.4 g daily or 4.8 mg daily **Maintenance Dose** (Asacol) 800 mg b.i.d. or 400 mg q.i.d.
Child: **PO** 50 mg/kg/day divided q6–12h

ADMINISTRATION

Oral

- Ensure that controlled-release and enteric forms of the drug are not crushed or chewed.
- Shake the bottle well to make sure the suspension is mixed.

Rectal

- Use rectal suspension at bedtime with the objective of retaining it all night.
- Store at 15°–30° C (59°–86° F) away from heat and light.

ADVERSE EFFECTS (≥1%) **CNS:** *Headache,* fatigue, asthenia, malaise, weakness, dizziness. **GI:** *Abdominal pain, cramps,* or *discomfort,* flatulence, nausea, diarrhea, constipation, hemorrhoids, rectal pain, hepatitis (rare). **Skin:** Sensitivity reactions, rash, pruritus, alopecia. **Body as a Whole:** Fever. **Hematologic:** Thrombocytopenia (rare), eosinophilia. **Urogenital:** Interstitial nephritis.

INTERACTIONS Drug: May decrease the absorption of **digoxin.**

PHARMACOKINETICS Absorption: Rectal 5–35% absorbed from colon depending on retention time of enema or suppository. PO Asacol, approximately 28% absorbed; 80% of drug is released in colon 12 h after ingestion. PO Pentasa, 50% of drug is released in colon at a pH less than 6. **Peak:** 3–6 h. **Distribution:** Rectal administration may reach as high as the ascending colon. Asacol is released in the ileum and colon; Pentasa is released in the jejunum, ileum, and colon. Low concentrations of mesalamine and higher concentrations of its metabolites are excreted in breast milk. **Metabolism:** Rapidly acetylated in the liver and colon wall. **Elimination:** Primarily in feces; absorbed drug excreted in urine. **Half-Life:** 2–15 h (depending on formulation).

NURSING IMPLICATIONS

Assessment & Drug Effects

- Lab tests: Monitor carefully urinalysis, BUN, and creatinine, especially in patients with preexisting kidney disease. The kidney is the major target organ for toxicity.
- Assess for S&S of allergic-type reactions (e.g., hives, itching, wheezing, anaphylaxis). Suspension contains a sulfite that may cause reactions in asthmatics and some nonasthmatic persons.
- Expect response to therapy within 3–21 days; however, the usual course of therapy is from 3–6 wk depending on symptoms and sigmoidoscopic examinations.

Patient & Family Education

- Report to physician promptly: Cramping, abdominal pain, bloody diarrhea, or other signs of rectal irritation.
- Check with physician before using any new medicine (prescription or OTC).
- Continue medication for full time of treatment even if you are feeling better.

MESNA

(mes′na)

Mesnex

Classifications: CHEMOPROTECTANT; DETOXIFYING AGENT

Therapeutic: DETOXIFYING AGENT

Pregnancy Category: B

AVAILABILITY 100 mg/mL injection; 400 mg tablet

ACTION & *THERAPEUTIC EFFECT* Detoxifying agent used to inhibit hemorrhagic cystitis induced by ifosfamide. *Reacts chemically with urotoxic ifosfamide metabolites, resulting in their detoxification, and thus significantly decreases the incidence of hematuria.*

USES Prophylaxis for ifosfamide-induced hemorrhagic cystitis. Not effective in preventing hematuria due to other pathologic conditions such as thrombocytopenia.

UNLABELED USES Reduces the incidence of cyclophosphamide-induced hemorrhagic cystitis.

CONTRAINDICATIONS Hypersensitivity to mesna or other thiol compounds; neonates.

CAUTIOUS USE Autoimmune diseases; infants (injection); pregnancy (category B), lactation.

ROUTE & DOSAGE

Ifosfamide-Induced Hemorrhagic Cystitis

Adult: **IV** Dose = 20% of ifosfamide dose given 15 min before ifosfamide administration and 4 and 8 h after ifosfamide dose **PO** 40% of ifosfamide dose 2 and 6 h after each ifosfamide dose

ADMINISTRATION

▪ Note: To be effective, mesna **must be** administered with each dose of ifosfamide.

Intravenous

PREPARE: **Direct:** Add 4 mL of D5W, NS, or LR for each 100 mg of mesna to yield 20 mg/mL.
ADMINISTER: **Direct:** Give a single dose by direct IV over 60 sec.
INCOMPATIBILITIES **Solution/additive:** **Carboplatin, cisplatin, ifosfamide with epirubicin.** **Y-site:** **Amphotericin B cholesteryl complex, lansoprazole.**
▪ Inspect parenteral drug products visually for particulate matter and discoloration prior to administration. ▪ Discard any unused portion of the ampul because drug oxidizes on contact with air.

▪ Refrigerate diluted solutions or use within 6 h of mixing even though diluted solutions are chemically and physically stable for 24 h at 25° C (77° F). ▪ Store unopened ampul at 15°–30° C (59°–86° F) unless otherwise specified.

ADVERSE EFFECTS (≥1%) **GI:** *Bad taste in mouth, soft stools,* nausea, vomiting.

DIAGNOSTIC TEST INTERFERENCE May produce a false-positive result in test for ***urinary ketones.***

INTERACTIONS Drug: May decrease the effect of **warfarin.**

PHARMACOKINETICS Bioavailability: 45%–79% **Metabolism:** Rapidly oxidized in liver to active metabolite dimesna; dimesna is further metabolized in kidney. **Elimination:** 65% in urine within 24 h. **Half-Life:** Mesna 0.36 h, dimesna 1.17 h.

NURSING IMPLICATIONS

Assessment & Drug Effects

- Monitor urine for hematuria.
- About 6% of patients treated with mesna along with ifosfamide still develop hematuria.

Patient & Family Education

- Mesna prevents ifosfamide-induced hemorrhagic cystitis; it will not prevent or alleviate other adverse reactions or toxicities associated with ifosfamide therapy.
- Report any unusual or allergic reactions to physician.
- Check with physician before using any new prescription or OTC medicine.

METAPROTERENOL SULFATE

(met-a-proe-ter′e-nole)
Alupent, Metaprel
Classifications: BETA-ADRENERGIC AGONIST; BRONCHODILATOR
Therapeutic: BRONCHODILATOR
Prototype: Albuterol
Pregnancy Category: C

AVAILABILITY 10 mg, 20 mg tablets; 10 mg/5 mL syrup; 75 mg, 150 mg metered dose inhaler; 0.4%, 0.6%, 5% solution for inhalation

ACTION & *THERAPEUTIC EFFECT* Potent synthetic beta-adrenergic agonist that acts selectively on $beta_2$-adrenergic receptors to relax smooth muscle of bronchi, uterus, and blood vessels supplying skeletal muscles. *Effective as a bronchodilator; also, it controls bronchospasm in asthmatics.*

USES Bronchodilator in symptomatic relief of asthma and reversible bronchospasm associated with bronchitis and emphysema.

UNLABELED USES Treatment and prophylaxis of heart block and to avert progress of premature labor (tocolytic action).

CONTRAINDICATIONS Sensitivity to metaproterenol or other sympathomimetic agents; seizure disorders, seizures; diabetes mellitus; hyperthyroidism. Safety in children younger than 12 y (for aerosol use) and children younger than 6 y (tablets) is not established.

CAUTIOUS USE Older adults; hypertension, cardiovascular disorders including coronary artery disease, cardiac arrhythmias, QT prolongation; MAOI therapy; pregnancy (category C), lactation.

ROUTE & DOSAGE

Bronchospasm

Adult: **PO** 20 mg q6–8h **Metered Dose Inhaler** 2–3 inhalations q3–4h (max: 12 inhalations/day) **Nebulizer** 5–10 inhalations of undiluted 5% solution **IPPB** 2.5 mL of 0.4–0.6% solution q4–6h
Geriatric: **PO** 10 mg 3–4 times/day, may increase to 20 mg 3–4 times/day
Child: **PO** *Younger than 2 y,* 0.4 mg/kg t.i.d.–q.i.d.; *2–6 y,* 1.2–2.6 mg/kg/day in 3–4 divided doses; *6–9 y,* 10 mg q6–8h; *older than 9 y,* 20 mg q6–8h

ADMINISTRATION

- Note: Patient may use tablets and aerosol concomitantly.

Oral

- Give with food to reduce GI distress.

Inhalation

- Instruct patient to shake metered dose aerosol container, exhale through nose as completely as possible, administer aerosol while inhaling deeply through mouth, and to hold breath about 10 sec before exhaling slowly. Administer second inhalation 10 min after first.
- Store all forms at 15°–30° C (59°–86° F); protect from light and heat.

ADVERSE EFFECTS (≥1%) **CNS:** Nervousness, weakness, drowsiness, *tremor (particularly after PO administration),* headache, fatigue. **CV:** *Tachycardia,* hypertension, cardiac arrest, palpitation. **GI:** Nausea, vomiting, bad taste. **Urogenital:** Occasional difficulty in micturition and muscle cramps. **Respiratory:** Throat irritation, cough, exacerbation of asthma.

INTERACTIONS Drug: Epinephrine, other SYMPATHOMIMETIC BRONCHODILATORS may compound effects of metaproterenol; MAO INHIBITORS, TRICYCLIC ANTIDEPRESSANTS potentiate action of metaproterenol on vascular system; the effects of both metaproterenol and BETA-ADRENERGIC BLOCKERS are antagonized.

PHARMACOKINETICS Absorption: 40% of PO doses reach systemic circulation. **Onset:** Inhaled: 1 min; PO 15 min. **Peak:** 1 h all routes. **Duration:** Inhaled: 1–5 h; PO 4 h. **Metabolism:** In liver. **Elimination:** In urine.

NURSING IMPLICATIONS

Assessment & Drug Effects

- Monitor respiratory status. Auscultate lungs before and after inhalation to determine efficacy of drug in decreasing airway resistance.
- Monitor cardiac status. Report tachycardia and hypotension.

Patient & Family Education

- Report failure to respond to usual dose. Drug may have shorter duration of action after long-term use.

- Do not increase dose or frequency unless ordered by physician; there is the possibility of serious adverse effects.
- Anticipate tremor as a possible adverse effect.

METFORMIN (Pr)

(met-for'min)

Fortamet, Glucophage, Glucophage XR, Glumetza, Riomet

Classifications: ANTIDIABETIC; BIGUANIDE

Therapeutic: ANTIHYPERGLYCEMIC

Pregnancy Category: B

AVAILABILITY 500 mg, 850 mg, 1000 mg tablets; 500 mg, 750 mg, 1000 mg sustained release tablets; 100 mg/mL oral solution

ACTION & *THERAPEUTIC EFFECT* Biguanide oral hypoglycemic agent thought to both increase the binding of insulin to its receptors and potentiate insulin action. Improves tissue sensitivity to insulin, increases glucose transport into skeletal muscles and fat, and suppresses gluconeogenesis and hepatic production of glucose. *Effective in suppressing hepatic production of glucose as well as increasing the binding of insulin to its receptors in muscle tissue, thus lowering glucose levels.*

USES Treatment of type 2 diabetes mellitus as adjunct to diet and exercise.

CONTRAINDICATIONS Hypersensitivity to metformin; hepatic or cardiopulmonary insufficiency; alcoholism; concurrent infection; acute MI, cardiogenic shock; diabetic ketoacidosis; hypoxemia, lactic acidosis; radiographic contrast administration; renal disease, renal failure, renal impairment; sepsis; surgery; children younger than 10 y.

CAUTIOUS USE Previous hypersensitivity to phenformin or buformin; anemia; coma; dehydration, diarrhea; older adults; ethanol intoxication; fever; gastroparesis, GI obstruction; heart failure; hyperthyroidism, pituitary insufficiency; polycystic ovary syndrome; trauma, emesis; pregnancy (category B), lactation.

ROUTE & DOSAGE

Type 2 Diabetes Mellitus

Adult: **PO** Start with 500 mg daily to t.i.d. or 850 mg daily to b.i.d. with meals, may increase by 500–850 mg/day q1–3wk (max: 2550 mg/day); or start with 500 mg sustained release with p.m. meal, may increase by 500 mg/day at p.m. meal qwk (max: 2000 mg/day)

Adolescent/Child (older than 10 y): **PO** Glucophage only; 500 mg b.i.d., may increase by 500 mg/day qwk (max: 2000 mg/day)

ADMINISTRATION

Oral

- Ensure that extended release tablets are not crushed or chewed. They **must be** swallowed whole.
- Use a calibrated oral syringe or container to measure the oral solution for accurate dosing.
- Give with or shortly after main meals.
- Withhold metformin 48 h before and 48 h after receiving IV contrast dye.
- Dose increments are usually made at 2- to 3-wk intervals.
- Store at 15°–30° C (59°–86° F).

ADVERSE EFFECTS (≥1%) **CNS:** Headache, dizziness, agitation, fatigue. **Metabolic:** Lactic acidosis. **GI:** *Nausea, vomiting, abdominal pain, bitter or metallic taste, diarrhea, bloatedness, anorexia;* malabsorption of amino acids, vitamin B_{12}, and folic acid possible.

INTERACTIONS Drug: Captopril, furosemide, nifedipine may increase risk of hypoglycemia. **Cimetidine** reduces clearance of metformin. Concomitant therapy with AZOLE ANTIFUNGAL AGENTS (**fluconazole, ketoconazole, itraconazole**) and ORAL HYPOGLYCEMIC DRUGS has been reported in severe hypoglycemia. IODINATED RADIOCONTRAST DYES can cause lactic acidosis and acute kidney failure. **Amiloride, cimetidine digoxin, dofetilide, midodrine, morphine, procainamide, quinidine, quinine, ranitidine, triamterene, trimethoprim,** or **vancomycin** may decrease metformin elimination by competing for common renal tubular transport systems. **Acarbose** may decrease metformin levels. **Iodinated contrast dyes** may cause lactic acidosis or acute kidney failure. **Herbal: Garlic, ginseng, glucomannan** may increase hypoglycemic effects. **Guar gum** decreases absorption.

PHARMACOKINETICS Absorption: 50–60% of dose reaches systemic circulation. **Peak:** 1–3 h. **Distribution:** Not bound to plasma proteins. **Metabolism:** Not metabolized. **Elimination:** In urine. **Half-Life:** 6.2–17.6 h.

NURSING IMPLICATIONS

Assessment & Drug Effects

- Monitor vital signs and fasting and postprandial blood glucose values.
- Report promptly any of the following signs of lactic acidosis: Malaise, myalgia, somnolence, respiratory depression, abdominal distress.
- Lab tests: Obtain baseline and periodic kidney and liver function tests; drug contraindicated in the presence of renal or hepatic insufficiency. Monitor blood glucose and HbA1C, and lipid profile periodically.
- Monitor known or suspected alcoholics carefully for decreased liver function.
- Monitor cardiopulmonary status throughout course of therapy; cardiopulmonary insufficiency may predispose to lactic acidosis.

Patient & Family Education

- Be aware that hypoglycemia is not a risk when drug is taken in recommended therapeutic doses unless combined with other drugs which lower blood glucose.
- Report to physician immediately S&S of infection, which increase the risk of lactic acidosis (e.g., abdominal pains, nausea, and vomiting, anorexia).
- Report promptly severe vomiting, diarrhea, fever, or any illness that causes limited fluid intake.
- Avoid drinking alcohol while taking this drug.

METHADONE HYDROCHLORIDE

(meth'a-done)

Dolophine, Methadose

Classifications: NARCOTIC (OPIATE AGONIST); ANALGESIC

Therapeutic: NARCOTIC ANALGESIC; TOXICOLOGY AGENT

Prototype: Morphine

Pregnancy Category: C

Controlled Substance: Schedule II

AVAILABILITY 5 mg, 10 mg, 40 mg tablets; 1 mg/mL, 2 mg/mL, 10 mg/mL oral solution; 10 mg/mL injection

ACTION & *THERAPEUTIC EFFECT* Synthetic narcotic that is a CNS depressant, which causes sedation and respiratory depression. Highly addictive, with abuse potential; abstinence syndrome develops more slowly, and withdrawal symptoms are less intense but more prolonged. *Relieves severe pain and manages withdrawal therapy from narcotics, especially heroin.*

USES To relieve severe pain; for detoxification and temporary maintenance treatment in hospital and in federally controlled maintenance programs for ambulatory patients with narcotic abstinence syndrome.

CONTRAINDICATIONS Severe pulmonary disease; COPD; obstetric analgesia; lactation.
CAUTIOUS USE History of QT prolongation; liver, kidney, or cardiac dysfunction; pregnancy (category C).

ROUTE & DOSAGE

Pain
Adult: **PO/Subcutaneous/IM** 2.5–10 mg q3–4h prn **IV** 2.5–10 mg q8–12h prn (opiate naïve patient)
Child: **PO/IV/Subcutaneous/IM** 0.1–0.2 mg/kg q4h × 2–3 doses, then q6–12h prn (max: 5–10 mg/dose)

Detoxification Treatment
Adult: **PO/Subcutaneous/IM** 15–40 mg once/day, usually maintained at 20–120 mg/day

Renal Impairment Dosage Adjustment
CrCl less than 10 mL/min: Use 50–75% of dose

ADMINISTRATION

Oral
- Give for analgesic effect in the smallest effective dose to minimize the possible tolerance and physical and psychic dependence.
- Dilute dispersible tablets in 120 mL of water or fruit juice and allow at least 1 min for dispersion.

Subcutaneous/Intramuscular
- Note: IM route is preferred over subcutaneous when repeated parenteral administration is required (subcutaneous injections may cause local irritation and induration). Rotate injection sites.

Intravenous

PREPARE: **Direct/IV Infusion:** May be given undiluted or diluted with 1–5 mL of NS.
ADMINISTER: **Direct/IV Infusion:** Give over 5 or more minutes.
INCOMPATIBILITIES **Y-site: Phenytoin.**

- Store at 15°–30° C (59°–86° F) in tight, light-resistant containers.

ADVERSE EFFECTS (≥1%) **CNS:** *Drowsiness,* light-headedness, dizziness, hallucinations. **GI:** Nausea, vomiting, dry mouth, *constipation.* **Body as a Whole:** Transient fall in BP, bone and muscle pain. **Urogenital:** Impotence. **Respiratory:** <u>Respiratory depression</u>.

INTERACTIONS Drug: Alcohol and other CNS DEPRESSANTS, **cimetidine** add to sedation and CNS depression; AMPHETAMINES may potentiate CNS stimulation; with MAO INHIBITORS, **selegiline, furazolidone**

causes excessive and prolonged CNS depression, convulsions, cardiovascular collapse. **Food: Grapefruit juice** may increase serum levels and adverse effects. **Herbal: St. John's wort** decreases plasma levels.

PHARMACOKINETICS Absorption: Well absorbed from GI tract, variable IM absorption. **Onset:** 30–60 min PO; 10–20 min IM/Subcutaneous. **Peak:** 1–2 h. **Duration:** 6–8 h PO, IM, Subcutaneous; may last 22–48 h with chronic dosing. **Distribution:** Crosses placenta; distributed into breast milk. **Metabolism:** In liver (CYP3A4). **Elimination:** In urine. **Half-Life:** 15–25 h.

NURSING IMPLICATIONS

Assessment & Drug Effects

- Evaluate patient's continued need for methadone for pain. Adjustment of dosage and lengthening of between-dose intervals may be possible.
- Monitor respiratory status. Principal danger of overdosage, as with morphine, is extreme respiratory depression.
- Be aware that because of the cumulative effects of methadone, abstinence symptoms may not appear for 36–72 h after last dose and may last 10–14 days. Symptoms are usually of mild intensity (e.g., anorexia, insomnia, anxiety, abdominal discomfort, weakness, headache, sweating, hot and cold flashes).
- Observe closely for recurrence of respiratory depression during use of narcotic antagonists such as naloxone.

Patient & Family Education

- Be aware that orthostatic hypotension, sweating, constipation, drowsiness, GI symptoms, and other transient adverse effects of therapeutic doses appear to be more prominent in ambulatory patients. Most adverse effects disappear over a period of several weeks.
- Make position changes slowly, particularly from lying down to upright position; sit or lie down if you feel dizzy or faint.
- Do not drive or engage in potentially hazardous activities until response to drug is known.

M

METHAMPHETAMINE HYDROCHLORIDE

(meth-am-fet'a-meen)

Desoxyephedrine, Desoxyn

Classifications: ADRENERGIC AGONIST; CEREBRAL STIMULANT; AMPHETAMINE

Therapeutic: CEREBRAL STIMULANT; ANOREXIANT

Prototype: Amphetamine sulfate

Pregnancy Category: C

Controlled Substance: Schedule II

AVAILABILITY 5 mg tablets; 5 mg, 10 mg, 15 mg long-acting tablets

ACTION & *THERAPEUTIC EFFECT* CNS stimulant actions approximately equal to those of amphetamine, but accompanied by less peripheral activity. *CNS stimulation results in increased motor activity, diminished sense of fatigue, alertness, increased focus, and mood elevation. Anorexigenic effect is due to direct inhibition of hypothalamic appetite center.*

USES Short-term adjunct in management of exogenous obesity, as adjunctive therapy in attention deficit disorder (ADD), narcolepsy, epilepsy, and postencephalitic parkinsonism, and in treatment of certain depressive reactions, especially when characterized by apathy and psychomotor retardation.

CONTRAINDICATIONS Children with structural cardiac abnormalities; as anorexiant in children younger than 12 y and ADHD treatment in children younger than 6 y; patients receiving MAO inhibitors; arteriosclerotic parkinsonism; lactation.
CAUTIOUS USE Mild hypertension; psychopathic personalities; hyperexcitability states; history of suicide attempts; older adult or debilitated patients; pregnancy (category C).

ROUTE & DOSAGE

Attention Deficit Disorder
Child (6 y or older): **PO** 2.5–5 mg 1–2 times/day, may increase by 5 mg at weekly intervals up to 20–25 mg/day

Obesity
Adult: **PO** 2.5–5 mg 1–3 times/day 30 min before meals or 5–15 mg of long-acting form once/day

ADMINISTRATION

Oral
- Give early in the day, if possible, to avoid insomnia.
- Ensure that long-acting tablets are not chewed or crushed; these need to be swallowed whole.
- Give 30 min before each meal when used for treatment of obesity. If insomnia results, advise patient to inform physician.
- Preserve in tight, light-resistant containers.

ADVERSE EFFECTS (≥1%) **CNS:** Restlessness, tremor, hyperreflexia, insomnia, headache, nervousness, anxiety, dizziness, euphoria or dysphoria. **CV:** Palpitation, arrhythmias, hypertension, hypotension, circulatory collapse. **GI:** Dry mouth, unpleasant taste, nausea, vomiting, diarrhea, constipation. **Special Senses:** Increased intraocular pressure.

INTERACTIONS Drug: Acetazolamide, sodium bicarbonate decreases methamphetamine elimination; **ammonium chloride, ascorbic acid** increases methamphetamine elimination; effects of both methamphetamine and BARBITURATES may be antagonized; **furazolidone** may increase BP effects of AMPHETAMINES—interaction may persist for several weeks after discontinuing **furazolidone;** antagonizes antihypertensive effects of **guanethidine;** MAO INHIBITORS, **selegiline** can cause hypertensive crisis (fatalities reported)—do not administer AMPHETAMINES during or within 14 days of administration of these drugs; PHENOTHIAZINES may inhibit mood elevating effects of AMPHETAMINES; TRICYCLIC ANTIDEPRESSANTS enhance methamphetamine effects because they increase norepinephrine release; BETA-ADRENERGIC AGONISTS increase adverse cardiovascular effects of AMPHETAMINES.

PHARMACOKINETICS Absorption: Readily absorbed from the GI tract. **Duration:** 6–12 h. **Distribution:** All tissues especially the CNS; excreted in breast milk. **Metabolism:** In liver. **Elimination:** Renal elimination.

NURSING IMPLICATIONS

Assessment & Drug Effects
- Monitor weight throughout period of therapy.
- Be alert for a paradoxical increase in depression or agitation in depressed patients. Report immediately; drug should be withdrawn.
- Do not exceed duration of a few weeks for treatment of obesity.

M

Patient & Family Education

- Be alert for development of tolerance; happens readily, and prolonged use may lead to drug dependence. Abuse potential is high.
- Withdrawal after prolonged use is frequently followed by lethargy that may persist for several weeks.
- Weigh every other day under standard conditions and maintain a record of weight loss.

METHAZOLAMIDE

(meth-a-zoe′la-mide)

Classifications: EYE PREPARATION; CARBONIC ANHYDRASE INHIBITOR; ANTIGLAUCOMA
Therapeutic: ANTIGLAUCOMA
Prototype: Acetazolamide
Pregnancy Category: C

AVAILABILITY 25 mg, 50 mg tablets

ACTION & *THERAPEUTIC EFFECT* Inhibits carbonic anhydrase activity in eye by reducing rate of aqueous humor formation with consequent lowering of intraocular pressure. *Effective in lowering intraocular pressure in glaucoma patients.*

USES Adjunctive treatment in chronic simple (open-angle) glaucoma and secondary glaucoma and preoperatively in acute angle-closure glaucoma when delay of surgery is desired in order to lower intraocular pressure. May be used concomitantly with miotic and osmotic agents.

CONTRAINDICATIONS Glaucoma due to severe peripheral anterior synechiae, severe or absolute glaucoma, hemorrhagic glaucoma; hypokalemia, hyponatremia; dialysis; hepatic disease; renal disease, anuria, renal failure.
CAUTIOUS USE Pulmonary disease, COPD; diabetes mellitus; renal impairment; pregnancy (category C), lactation.

ROUTE & DOSAGE

Glaucoma
Adult: **PO** 50–100 mg b.i.d. or t.i.d.

ADMINISTRATION

Oral

- Give with meals to minimize GI distress.

ADVERSE EFFECTS (≥1%) **Body as a Whole:** Malaise, drowsiness, fatigue, lethargy. **GI:** Mild GI disturbance, anorexia. **CNS:** Headache, vertigo, paresthesias, mental confusion, depression.

INTERACTIONS Drug: Renal excretion of AMPHETAMINES, **ephedrine, flecainide, quinidine, procainamide,** TRICYCLIC ANTIDEPRESSANTS may be decreased, thereby enhancing or prolonging their effects; increases renal excretion of **lithium;** excretion of **phenobarbital** may be increased; **amphotericin B,** CORTICOSTEROIDS may add to potassium loss; hypokalemia caused by methazolamide may predispose patients on DIGITALIS GLYCOSIDES to **digitalis** toxicity; patients on high doses of SALICYLATES are at higher risk for SALICYLATE toxicity.

PHARMACOKINETICS Absorption: Slowly from GI tract. **Onset:** 2–4 h. **Peak:** 6–8 h. **Duration:** 10–18 h. **Distribution:** Throughout body, concentrating in RBCs, plasma, and kidneys; crosses placenta. **Metabolism:** Partially in liver. **Elimination:** Primarily in urine.

NURSING IMPLICATIONS

Assessment & Drug Effects

- Supervise ambulation in older adult, since drug may cause vertigo.
- Assess patient's ability to perform ADL since drug may cause fatigue and lethargy.
- Lab tests: Obtain periodic serum electrolytes, especially in older adults. Monitor lithium levels with concurrent administration of lithium and methazolamide.

Patient & Family Education

- Be aware that drug may cause drowsiness. Advise caution with hazardous activities until response to drug is known.

METHENAMINE HIPPURATE

(meth-en'a-meen hip'yoo-rate)

Hiprex, Urex

METHENAMINE MANDELATE

Mandelamine

Classification: URINARY TRACT ANTI-INFECTIVE

Therapeutic: URINARY TRACT ANTI-INFECTIVE

Prototype: Trimethoprim

Pregnancy Category: C

AVAILABILITY Methenamine Hippurate: 1 g tablets; **Methenamine Mandelate:** 0.5 g, 1 g tablets; 0.5 g/5 mL suspension

ACTION & *THERAPEUTIC EFFECT* Tertiary amine liberates formaldehyde in an acid medium. Nonspecific antibiotic agent with bactericidal activity. *Most bacteria and fungi are susceptible to formaldehyde; however, bacteria that are urease-positive (e.g.,* Proteus *sp.) convert urea to ammonium hydroxide, which prevents the generation of formaldehyde from methenamine.*

USES Prophylactic treatment of recurrent urinary tract infections (UTIs). Also long-term prophylaxis when residual urine is present (e.g., neurogenic bladder).

CONTRAINDICATIONS Renal insufficiency; liver disease; gout; severe dehydration; combined therapy with sulfonamides. Safety during lactation is not established.

CAUTIOUS USE Oral suspension for patients susceptible to lipoid pneumonia (e.g., older adults, debilitated patients); gout; pregnancy (category C).

ROUTE & DOSAGE

UTI Prophylaxis

Adult: **PO** (Hippurate) 1 g b.i.d.; (Mandelate) 1 g q.i.d.
Child: **PO** 6 y or younger, (Mandelate) 18.4 mg/kg q.i.d.; 6–12 y, (Hippurate) 0.5–1 g b.i.d.; (Mandelate) 500 mg q.i.d. or 50 mg/kg/day in 3 divided doses

ADMINISTRATION

Oral

- Give after meals and at bedtime to minimize gastric distress.
- Give oral suspension with caution to older adult or debilitated patients because of the possibility of lipid (aspiration) pneumonia; it contains a vegetable oil base.
- Store at 15°–30° C (59°–86° F) in tightly closed container; protect from excessive heat.

ADVERSE EFFECTS (≥1%) **GI:** Nausea, vomiting, diarrhea, abdominal cramps, anorexia. **Renal:** Bladder irritation, dysuria, frequency, albuminuria, hematuria, crystalluria.

DIAGNOSTIC TEST INTERFERENCE Methenamine (formaldehyde) may produce falsely elevated values for ***urinary catecholamines*** and ***urinary steroids (17-hydroxycorticosteroids)*** (by ***Reddy method***). Possibility of false ***urine glucose determinations*** with ***Benedict's*** test. Methenamine interferes with ***urobilinogen*** and possibly ***urinary VMA*** determinations.

INTERACTIONS Drug: Sulfamethoxazole forms insoluble precipitate in acid urine; **acetazolamide, sodium bicarbonate** may prevent hydrolysis to formaldehyde.

PHARMACOKINETICS Absorption: Readily from GI tract, although 10–30% of dose is hydrolyzed to formaldehyde in stomach. **Peak:** 2 h. **Duration:** Up to 6 h or until patient voids. **Distribution:** Crosses placenta; distributed into breast milk. **Metabolism:** Hydrolyzed in acid pH to formaldehyde. **Elimination:** In urine. **Half-Life:** 4 h.

NURSING IMPLICATIONS

Assessment & Drug Effects

- Monitor urine pH; value of 5.5 or less is required for optimum drug action.
- Monitor I&O ratio and pattern; drug most effective when fluid intake is maintained at 1500 or 2000 mL/day.
- Consult physician about changing to enteric-coated tablet if patient complains of gastric distress.
- Supplemental acidification to maintain pH of 5.5 or below required for drug action may be necessary. Accomplish by drugs (ascorbic acid, ammonium chloride) or by foods.

Patient & Family Education

- Do not self-medicate with OTC antacids containing sodium bicarbonate or sodium carbonate (to prevent raising urine pH).
- Achieve supplementary acidification by limiting intake of foods that can increase urine pH [e.g., vegetables, fruits, and fruit juice (except cranberry, plum, prune)] and increasing intake of foods that can decrease urine pH (e.g., proteins, cranberry juice, plums, prunes).

METHIMAZOLE

(meth-im′a-zole)
Tapazole
Classification: ANTITHYROID HORMONE
Therapeutic: ANTITHYROID
Prototype: Propylthiouracil
Pregnancy Category: D

AVAILABILITY 5 mg, 10 mg, 15 mg, 20 mg tablets

ACTION & *THERAPEUTIC EFFECT* Inhibits synthesis of thyroid hormones as the drug accumulates in the thyroid gland. Does not affect existing T_3 or T_4 levels. *Corrects hyperthyroidism by inhibiting synthesis of the thyroid hormone.*

USES Hyperthyroidism and prior to surgery or radiotherapy of the thyroid; may be used cautiously to treat hyperthyroidism in pregnancy.

CONTRAINDICATIONS Pregnancy (category D).
CAUTIOUS USE Other drugs known to cause agranulocytosis; bone marrow suppression; older adults; hepatic disease.

ROUTE & DOSAGE

Hyperthyroidism
Adult: **PO** 5–15 mg q8h
Child: **PO** 0.2–0.4 mg/kg/day divided q8h

ADMINISTRATION

Oral

- Give at same time each day relative to meals.
- Store at 15°–30° C (59°–86° F) in light-resistant container.

ADVERSE EFFECTS (≥1%) **GI:** Hepatotoxicity (rare). **Endocrine:** Hypothyroidism. **Hematologic:** *Leukopenia,* agranulocytosis, granulocytopenia, thrombocytopenia, pancytopenia, and aplastic anemia. **Musculoskeletal:** Arthralgia. **CNS:** Peripheral neuropathy, drowsiness, neuritis, paresthesias, vertigo. **Skin:** Rash, alopecia, skin hyperpigmentation, urticaria, and pruritus. **Urogenital:** Nephrotic syndrome.

INTERACTIONS Drug: Can reduce anticoagulant effects of **warfarin;** may increase serum levels of **digoxin;** may alter **theophylline** levels; may need to decrease dose of BETA-BLOCKERS.

PHARMACOKINETICS Absorption: Readily absorbed from GI tract. **Onset:** 30–40 min. **Peak:** 1 h. **Duration:** 2–4 h. **Distribution:** Crosses placenta; distributed into breast milk. **Elimination:** 12% in urine within 24 h. **Half-Life:** 5–13 h.

NURSING IMPLICATIONS

Assessment & Drug Effects

- Lab tests: Baseline and periodic thyroid function tests; periodic prothrombin time and LFTs.
- Closely monitor PT and INR in patients on oral anticoagulants. Anticoagulant activity may be potentiated.

Patient & Family Education

- Be aware that skin rash or swelling of cervical lymph nodes may indicate need to discontinue drug and change to another antithyroid agent. Consult physician.
- Notify physician promptly if the following symptoms appear: Bruising, unexplained bleeding, sore throat, fever, jaundice.
- Methimazole does not induce hypothyroiditis.

METHOCARBAMOL

(meth-oh-kar'ba-mole)

Robaxin

Classifications: SKELETAL MUSCLE RELAXANT, CENTRAL-ACTING; CARBAMATE

Therapeutic: SKELETAL MUSCLE RELAXANT

Prototype: Cyclobenzaprine

Pregnancy Category: C

AVAILABILITY 500 mg, 750 mg tablet; 100 mg/mL injection

ACTION & *THERAPEUTIC EFFECT* Exerts skeletal muscle relaxant action by depressing multisynaptic pathways in the spinal cord and possibly by sedative effect. *No direct action on skeletal muscles; instead, acts on multisynaptic pathways in spinal cord that control muscular spasms.*

USES Adjunct to physical therapy and other measures in management of discomfort associated with acute musculoskeletal disorders. Also used intravenously as adjunct in management of neuromuscular manifestations of tetanus.

CONTRAINDICATIONS Comatose states; CNS depression; acidosis, older adults; kidney dysfunction (injectable methocarbamol contains polyethylene glycol 300 in vehicle, which may cause urea retention and acidotic problems).

CAUTIOUS USE Epilepsy; females of childbearing age; renal disease, renal failure, renal impairment, seizure disorder; pregnancy (category C), lactation, children younger than 16 y.

ROUTE & DOSAGE

Acute Musculoskeletal Disorders

Adult: **PO** 1.5 g q.i.d. for 2–3 days, then 4–4.5 g/day in 3–6 divided doses **IV/IM** 1 g q8h

Tetanus

Adult: **IV** 1–3 g may be repeated q6h

Child: **PO** 15 mg/kg repeated q6h as needed up to 1.8 g/m^2/day for 3 consecutive days if necessary

ADMINISTRATION

Oral

- Tablets may be crushed, suspended in water, and given through an NG tube.

Intramuscular

- Do not exceed IM dose of 5 mL (0.5 g) into each gluteal region. Insert needle deep and carefully aspirate. Inject drug slowly. Rotate injection sites and observe daily for evidence of irritation.

Intravenous

PREPARE: **Direct:** May be given undiluted or diluted in up to 250 mL of NS or D5W. **IV Infusion:** May dilute in up to 250 mL of NS or D5W.

ADMINISTER: **Direct:** Give at a rate of 300 mg or fraction thereof over 1 min or longer. **IV Infusion:** Infuse at a rate consistent with amount of fluid, but do not exceed direct rate. ▪ Keep patient recumbent during and for at least 15 min after IV injection in order to reduce possibility of orthostatic hypotension and other adverse reactions. ▪ Monitor vital signs and IV flow rate. ▪ Take care to avoid extravasation of IV solution, which may result in thrombophlebitis and sloughing.

INCOMPATIBILITIES **Y-site: Furosemide.**

- Store at 15°–30° C (59°–86° F).

ADVERSE EFFECTS (≥1%) **Body as a Whole:** Fever, <u>anaphylactic reaction</u>, flushing, syncope, convulsions. **Skin:** Urticaria, pruritus, rash, thrombophlebitis, pain, sloughing (with extravasation). **Special Senses:** Conjunctivitis, blurred vision, nasal congestion. **CNS:** *Drowsiness, dizziness, lightheadedness,* headache. **CV:** Hypotension, bradycardia. **GI:** Nausea, metallic taste. **Hematologic:** Slight reduction of white cell count with prolonged therapy. **Renal:** Polyethylene glycol in the injection may increase preexisting acidosis and urea retention in patients with renal impairment.

DIAGNOSTIC TEST INTERFERENCE Methocarbamol may cause false increases in ***urinary 5-HIAA*** (with ***nitrosonaphthol reagent***) and ***VMA (Gitlow method).***

INTERACTIONS Drug: Alcohol and other CNS DEPRESSANTS enhance CNS depression.

PHARMACOKINETICS Absorption: Readily absorbed from GI tract. **Onset:** 30 min. **Peak:** 1–2 h. **Metabolism:** In liver. **Elimination:** In urine. **Half-Life:** 1–2 h.

NURSING IMPLICATIONS

Assessment & Drug Effects

- Lab tests: Obtain periodic WBC counts during prolonged therapy.
- Monitor vital signs closely during IV infusion.
- Supervise ambulation following parenteral administration.

Patient & Family Education

- Make position changes slowly, particularly from lying down to upright position; dangle legs before standing.

- Be aware that adverse reactions after oral administration are usually mild and transient and subside with dosage reduction. Use caution regarding drowsiness and dizziness. Avoid activities requiring mental alertness and physical coordination until response to drug is known.
- Urine may darken to brown, black, or green on standing.

METHOHEXITAL SODIUM

(meth-oh-hex'i-tal)

Brevital Sodium

Classifications: GENERAL ANESTHETIC; BARBITURATE

Therapeutic: GENERAL ANESTHETIC

Prototype: Thiopental

Pregnancy Category: B

Controlled Substance: Schedule IV

AVAILABILITY 500 mg, 2.5 g, 5 g powder for injection

ACTION & *THERAPEUTIC EFFECT* Rapid, ultra-short-acting barbiturate anesthetic agent. More potent than thiopental but of shorter duration of action, and recovery is more rapid. *Induces brief general anesthesia by depression of the CNS without analgesia.*

USES Induction of anesthesia, as supplement for other anesthetics, and as general anesthetic for brief operative procedures.

CONTRAINDICATIONS Hypersensitivity to methohexital sodium; agranulocytosis; barbiturate hypersensitivity; hepatic encephalopathy; intra-arterial administration; shock, heart failure, PVD, severe hypo- and hypertension, respiratory depression, infants younger than 1 mo; neonates.

CAUTIOUS USE Adrenal insufficiency, anemia, carbamazepine or hydantoin hypersensitivity; cardiac disease, COPD; uncontrolled asthma, status asthmaticus, sleep apnea, respiratory insufficiency, CNS depression; depression, ethanol intoxication; exfoliative dermatitis; hepatic disease; older adult; neuromuscular disease; obesity; porphyria; pulmonary disease, renal disease, uremia, renal impairment; seizure disorders, status epilepticus; shock; pregnancy (category B), lactation.

ROUTE & DOSAGE

Induction of Anesthesia

Adult: **IV** 50–120 mg at a rate of 5 mg q5min, then 20–40 mg q4–7min prn

Child/Infant: **IM** 6.6–10 mg/kg of 5% solution **IV** 1–2 mg/kg **Rectal** 20–35 mg/kg (max: 500 mg/dose)

ADMINISTRATION

Intravenous

Give to recumbent patient. Fall in BP may occur in susceptible patients receiving drug in upright position.

- Note: Verify with physician correct IV or IM concentration for infants or children as well as rate of IV infusion for administration to children.

***PREPARE:* Direct:** Prepare a 1% solution (10 mg/mL) by diluting with sterile water for injection, D5W, or NS. Use only clear, colorless solutions. ▪ Do not allow contact with rubber stoppers or parts of syringes treated with silicone because solution is incompatible with acid solutions (see IMCOMPATIBILITIES).

ADMINISTER: **Direct:** Give 5 mg over 5–10 sec.

INCOMPATIBILITIES **Solution/additive:** **Atropine, chlorpromazine, glycopyrrolate, hydralazine, kanamycin, lidocaine, mechlorethamine, methyldopa, prochlorperazine, promazine, promethazine, streptomycin.** **Y-site:** **Fenoldopam.**

- Store drug in sterile water for injection at room temperature for at least 6 wk. Solutions prepared with isotonic NaCl injection or 5% dextrose injection are stable for **ONLY** about 24 h.

ADVERSE EFFECTS (≥1%) **CV:** Hypotension, cardiac arrhythmias, cardiac arrest. **Musculoskeletal:** Muscle spasm. **CNS:** Postoperative psychomotor impairment that persists for 24 hours, anxiety, drowsiness, emergence delirium, restlessness, and seizures. **Respiratory:** Bronchospasm, cough, hiccups, respiratory depression, apnea, dyspnea, <u>respiratory arrest</u>. **Skin:** Phlebitis and nerve injury adjacent to the injection site, local irritation, edema, ulceration, necrosis.

INTERACTIONS Drug: **Alcohol** and other CNS DEPRESSANTS enhance CNS depression.

PHARMACOKINETICS Absorption: 17% absorbed PR. **Distribution:** Crosses CNS, placenta and excreted in breast milk. **Metabolism:** Oxidized in liver. **Elimination:** Primarily excreted in urine.

NURSING IMPLICATIONS

Assessment & Drug Effects

- Hiccups are common, particularly with rapid injection; they sometimes persist after anesthesia.
- Keep facilities for assisting respiration and administration of oxygen readily available in the event of respiratory distress.

METHOTREXATE SODIUM

(meth-oh-trex′ate)

MTX

Classifications: ANTINEOPLASTIC; ANTIMETABOLITE; IMMUNOSUPPRESSANT; DISEASE-MODIFYING ANTIRHEUMATIC DRUG (DMARD)

Therapeutic: ANTINEOPLASTIC; ANTIFOLATE; ANTIRHEUMATIC; ANTIPSORIATIC

Pregnancy Category: X

AVAILABILITY 2.5 mg tablets; 2.5 mg/mL, 25 mg/mL injection

ACTION & *THERAPEUTIC EFFECT* Antimetabolite and folic acid antagonist. Blocks folic acid participation in nucleic acid synthesis, thereby interfering with mitotic cell process. Rapidly proliferating tissues (malignant cells, bone marrow) are sensitive to interference of the mitotic process by this drug. *In psoriasis, reproductive rate of epithelial cells is higher than in normal cells. Induces remission slowly; use often preceded by other antineoplastic therapies. Also has immunosuppressant effects, and antirheumatic effects.*

USES Principally in combination regimens to maintain induced remissions in neoplastic diseases. Effective in treatment of gestational choriocarcinoma and hydatidiform mole and as immunosuppressant in kidney transplantation, for acute and subacute leukemias and leukemic meningitis, especially in children. Used in lymphosarcoma, in certain inoperable tumors of head, neck, and pelvis, and in mycosis fungoides. Also used to treat severe psoriasis nonresponsive to other forms of therapy, rheumatoid arthritis.

UNLABELED USES Psoriatic arthritis, SLE, polymyositis.

CONTRAINDICATIONS Hepatic and renal insufficiency; concomitant administration of hepatotoxic drugs and hematopoietic depressants; alcohol; ultraviolet exposure to psoriatic lesions; preexisting blood dyscrasias; pregnancy (category X), men and women in childbearing age; lactation.

CAUTIOUS USE Infections; peptic ulcer, ulcerative colitis; very young or old patients; cancer patients with preexisting bone marrow impairment; poor nutritional status.

ROUTE & DOSAGE

Trophoblastic Neoplasm

Adult: **PO/IM** 15–30 mg/day for 5 days, repeat for 3–5 courses

Leukemia

Adult: **IM/IV Loading Dose** 3.3 $mg/m^2/day$ **PO/IM/IV Maintenance Dose** 30 mg/m^2 weekly in 2 doses

Meningeal Leukemia

Child: **Intrathecal** 10–15 mg/m^2

Lymphoma

Adult: **PO** 10–25 mg/kg for 4–8 days

Osteosarcoma

Adult: **IV** 12 g/m^2, dose repeated at weeks 4, 5, 6, 7, 11, 12, 15, 16, 29, 39, 44, 45

Psoriasis/Rheumatoid Arthritis

Adult: **PO** 2.5 mg q12h for 3 doses each wk or 7.5 mg once/wk

Child: **PO/IM** 5–15 $mg/m^2/wk$ as single dose or in 3 divided doses 12 h apart

Mycosis Fungoides

Adult: **PO/IM** 5–50 mg weekly

ADMINISTRATION

Oral

- May be taken without respect to meals.
- Avoid skin exposure and inhalation of drug particles.

Intramuscular

- Inject deeply into a large muscle.

Intravenous

Note: Verify correct IV concentration and rate of infusion for administration to children with physician.

PREPARE: **Direct:** Reconstitute powder vial by adding 2 mL of NS or D5W without preservatives to each 5 mg to yield 2.5 mg/mL. Reconstitute 1 g high-dose vial with 19.4 mL D5W or NS to yield 50 mg/mL. **IV Infusion:** Further dilute contents of the reconstituted 1 g high-dose vial in D5W or NS to a 25 mg/mL or less.

ADMINISTER: **Direct:** Give at rate of 10 mg or fraction thereof over 60 sec. **IV Infusion:** Give over 1–4 h or as prescribed.

INCOMPATIBILITIES **Solution/additive:** **Bleomycin, metoclopramide, prednisolone, ranitidine.** **Y-site:** **Chlorpromazine, droperidol, gemcitabine, idarubicin, ifosfamide, midazolam, nalbuphine, promethazine, propofol.**

- Preserve drug in tight, light-resistant container.

ADVERSE EFFECTS (≥1%) **CNS:** *Headache,* drowsiness, blurred vision, dizziness, aphasia, hemiparesis; arachnoiditis, convulsions (after intrathecal administration); mental confusion, tremors, ataxia, coma. **GI:** Hepatotoxicity, GI ulcerations and hemorrhage, *ulcerative stomatitis, glossitis, gingivitis,* pharyngitis, nausea, vomiting, diarrhea, hepatic cirrhosis. **Urogenital:** Defective oogenesis or spermatogenesis, nephropathy, hematuria, menstrual dysfunction, infertility, abortion, fetal defects. **Hematologic:** *Leukopenia, thrombocytopenia,* anemia, marked myelosuppression, aplastic bone marrow, telangiectasis, thrombophlebitis at intra-arterial catheter site, hypogammaglobulinemia, and hyperuricemia. **Skin:** Erythematous rashes, pruritus, urticaria, folliculitis, vasculitis, photosensitivity, depigmentation, hyperpigmentation, alopecia. **Body as a Whole:** Malaise, undue fatigue, systemic toxicity (after intrathecal and intra-arterial administration), chills, fever, decreased resistance to infection, septicemia, osteoporosis, metabolic changes precipitating diabetes and sudden death, pneumonitis, pulmonary fibrosis.

M

DIAGNOSTIC TEST INTERFERENCE Severe reactions may occur when ***live vaccines*** are administered because of immunosuppressive activity of methotrexate.

INTERACTIONS Drug: Acitretin, alcohol, azathioprine, sulfasalazine increase risk of hepatotoxicity; **chloramphenicol, etretinate,** SALICYLATES, NSAIDS, SULFONAMIDES, SULFONYLUREAS, **phenylbutazone, phenytoin,** TETRACYCLINES, **PABA, penicillin, probenecid** may increase methotrexate levels with increased toxicity; **folic acid** may alter response to methotrexate. May increase **theophylline** levels; **cholestyramine** enhances methotrexate clearance. **Herbal: Echinacea** may increase risk of hepatotoxicity. **Food: Caffeine** greater than 180 mg/day (3–4 cups) may decrease effectiveness for rheumatoid arthritis.

PHARMACOKINETICS Absorption: Readily absorbed from GI tract. **Peak:** 0.5–2 h IM/IV; 1–4 h PO. **Distribution:** Widely distributed with highest concentrations in kidneys, gallbladder, spleen, liver, and skin; minimal passage across blood–brain barrier; crosses placenta; distributed into breast milk. **Metabolism:** In liver. **Elimination:** Primarily in urine. **Half-Life:** 2–4 h.

NURSING IMPLICATIONS

Assessment & Drug Effects

- Lab tests: Obtain baseline liver and kidney function, CBC with differential, platelet count, and chest x-rays. Repeat weekly during therapy. Monitor blood glucose and HbA1C periodically in diabetics.
- Prolonged treatment with small frequent doses may lead to hepatotoxicity, which is best diagnosed by liver biopsy.
- Monitor for and report ulcerative stomatitis with glossitis and gingivitis, often the first signs of toxicity. Inspect mouth daily; report patchy necrotic areas, bleeding and discomfort, or overgrowth (black, furry tongue).
- Monitor I&O ratio and pattern. Keep patient well hydrated (about 2000 mL/24 h).
- Prevent exposure to infections or colds during periods of leukopenia. Be alert to onset of agranulocytosis (cough, extreme fatigue, sore throat, chills, fever) and report symptoms promptly.
- Be alert for and report symptoms of thrombocytopenia (e.g., ecchymoses, petechiae, epistaxis, melena, hematuria, vaginal bleeding, slow and protracted oozing following trauma).

Common adverse effects in *italic*, life-threatening effects underlined; generic names in **bold**; classifications in SMALL CAPS; ♣ Canadian drug name; ⓟ Prototype drug

Patient & Family Education

- Report promptly any of the following: Diarrhea, mouth sores, fever, dehydration, cough, bleeding, shortness of breath, any signs of infection, or a skin rash.
- Avoid or moderate alcohol ingestion, which increases the incidence and severity of methotrexate hepatotoxicity.
- Practice fastidious mouth care to prevent infection, provide comfort, and maintain adequate nutritional status.
- Do not self-medicate with vitamins. Some OTC compounds may include folic acid (or its derivatives), which alters methotrexate response.
- Use contraceptive measures during and for at least 3 mo following therapy.
- Avoid exposure to sunlight and ultraviolet light. Wear sunglasses and sunscreen.

METHOXSALEN (Pr)

(meth-ox'a-len)

8-MOP, Oxsoralen, Uvadex

Classifications: PSORALEN; PIGMENTING AGENT

Therapeutic: PIGMENTING AGENT; ANTIPSORIATIC

Pregnancy Category: C

AVAILABILITY 10 mg capsules, 20 mcg/mL solution; 1% lotion

ACTION & *THERAPEUTIC EFFECT* Plant derivative with strong photosensitizing effects: Used with ultraviolet-A light (UVA) in therapeutic regimens called PUVA (P-psoralen). After photoactivation by long wavelength, UVA, methoxsalen combines with epidermal cell DNA causing photodamage (cytotoxic action). *Photo-damage inhibits rapid and uncontrolled epidermal cell turnover characteristic of psoriasis. Results in an inflammatory reaction with erythema. Strongly melanogenic.*

USES With controlled exposure to UVA to repigment vitiliginous skin and for symptomatic treatment of severe disabling psoriasis that is refractory to other forms of therapy.

UNLABELED USES (PUVA therapy) mycosis fungoides.

CONTRAINDICATIONS Sunburn, sensitivity (or its history) to psoralens, diseases associated with photosensitivity (e.g., SLE, albinism, melanoma or its history); invasive squamous cell cancer; cataract; aphakia; previous exposure to arsenic or ionizing radiation. Safety **(oral)** in children is not established.

CAUTIOUS USE Hepatic insufficiency; GI disease; chronic infection; treatment with known photosensitizing agents; immunosuppressed patient; cardiovascular disease; pregnancy (category C), lactation. Safety (**lotion**) in children younger than 12 y is not established.

ROUTE & DOSAGE

Idiopathic Vitiligo

Adult: **Topical** Apply lotion 1–2 h before exposure to UV light once/wk

Psoriasis

Adult: **PO** Give 1.5–2 h before exposure to UV light 2–3 times/wk: *weight less than 30 kg,* 10 mg; *weight 30–50 kg,* 20 mg; *weight 51–65 kg,* 30 mg; *weight 66–80 kg,* 40 mg; *weight 81–90 kg,* 50 mg; *weight 91–115 kg,* 60 mg; *weight greater than 115 kg,* 70 mg

M

ADMINISTRATION

- Note: Methoxsalen therapy with UV light (PUVA therapy) should be done under the complete control of a physician with special competence and experience in photochemotherapy.

Oral

- Give with milk or food to prevent GI distress.
- Maintain consistent time relationship between food–drug ingestion. Food digestion and absorption appear to affect drug serum levels.

Topical

- Only small (less than 10 cm^2), well-defined areas are treated with lotion. Systemic treatment is used for large areas.
- Apply lotion with cotton swabs, allow to dry 1–2 min, then reapply. Protect borders of the lesion with petrolatum and sunscreen lotion to prevent hyperpigmentation.
- Use finger cots or gloves to apply lotion and prevent photosensitization and burned skin.
- Apply sunscreen lotion to the skin for about one third of the initial exposure time during PUVA therapy until there is sufficient tanning. Do not apply to psoriatic areas before treatment.
- Store lotion and capsules at 15°–30° C (59°–86° F) in light-resistant containers unless otherwise directed by manufacturer.

ADVERSE EFFECTS (≥1%) **CNS:** Nervousness, dizziness, headache, mental depression or excitation, vertigo, insomnia. **Special Senses:** Cataract formation, ocular damage. **GI:** Cheilitis, *nausea* and other GI disturbances, toxic hepatitis. **Skin:** Phototoxic effects: <u>Severe edema and erythema</u>, *pruritus,* painful blisters; <u>burning</u>, peeling, thinning, freckling, and accelerated aging of skin; hyper- or hypopigmentation; severe skin pain (lasting 1–2 mo), photoallergic contact dermatitis (with topical use), exacerbation of latent photosensitive dermatoses, <u>malignant melanoma</u> (rare). **Body as a Whole:** Transient loss of muscular coordination, edema, leg cramps, systemic immune effects, drug fever.

INTERACTIONS Drug: Anthralin, coal tar, griseofulvin, PHENOTHIAZINES, **nalidixic acid,** SULFONAMIDES, BACTERIOSTATIC SOAPS, TETRACYCLINES, THIAZIDES compound photosensitizing effects. **Food:** Food will increase peak and extent of absorption.

PHARMACOKINETICS Absorption: Variably from GI tract. **Peak:** 2 h. **Duration:** 8–10 h. **Distribution:** Preferentially taken up by epidermal cells; distributes into lens of eye. **Elimination:** 80–90% in urine within 8 h. **Half-Life:** 0.75–2.4 h.

NURSING IMPLICATIONS

Assessment & Drug Effects

- Schedule a pretreatment ophthalmologic exam to rule out cataracts; repeat periodically during treatment and at yearly intervals thereafter.
- Lab tests: Monitor CBC, kidney and liver function, and antinuclear antibody tests during oral therapy.
- Fair-skinned patients appear to be at greatest risk for phototoxicity from PUVA therapy (see ADVERSE EFFECTS).
- Be aware that repigmentation is more rapid on fleshy areas (i.e., face, abdomen, buttocks) than on hands or feet.

Patient & Family Education

- Expect that effective repigmentation may require 6–9 mo of treatment; periodic treatment usually is necessary to retain pigmentation. If, after 3 mo of treatment, there is no apparent response, drug is discontinued.

- Avoid additional exposure to UV light (direct or indirect) for at least 8 h after oral drug ingestion and UVA exposure.
- Understand intended treatment schedule: After topical application, the initial sunlight exposure is limited to 1 min, with subsequent gradual and incremental exposures by prescription.
- Avoid additional UV light for 24–48 h after topical application and UVA exposure.
- Wear sunscreen lotion (with SPF 15 or higher) and protective clothing (hat, gloves) to cover all exposed areas including lips, to prevent burning or blistering if sunlight cannot be avoided after the treatment.
- Do not sunbathe for at least 48 h after PUVA treatment. Sunburn and photochemotherapy are additive in the production of burning and erythema.
- Wear wraparound sunglasses with UVA-absorbing properties both indoors and outdoors during daylight hours for 24 h. Do not substitute prescription sunglasses or photosensitive darkening glasses; they may actually increase danger of cataract formation.
- Alert physician to appearance of new psoriatic areas, flares, or regressed cleared skin areas during treatment and maintenance periods.

METHSCOPOLAMINE BROMIDE

(meth-skoe-pol′a-meen)

Pamine

Classifications: ANTICHOLINERGIC; ANTIMUSCARINIC; ANTISPASMODIC

Therapeutic: ANTISPASMODIC; ANTISECRETORY

Prototype: Atropine

Pregnancy Category: C

AVAILABILITY 2.5 mg tablets

ACTION & *THERAPEUTIC EFFECT*
Decreases GI tone and amplitude as well as frequency of peristaltic contractions of the esophagus, stomach, duodenum, jejunum, ileum, and colon. *Its spasmolytic and antisecretory actions are quantitatively similar to those of atropine but they last longer.*

USES Adjunct in treatment of peptic ulcer, irritable bowel syndrome, and a variety of other GI conditions. Also may be used to control excessive sweating and salivation, migraine headaches, and premenstrual cramps.

CONTRAINDICATIONS Hypersensitivity to any of the drug's constituents; prostatic hypertrophy; pyloric obstruction; intestinal atony; tachycardia, cardiac disease; MS; pyloric stenosis; lactation.

CAUTIOUS USE Older adult and debilitated patients; chronic obstructive pulmonary diseases (COPD); pregnancy (category C).

ROUTE & DOSAGE

Irritable Bowel Syndrome

Adult: **PO** 2.5–5 mg 30 min a.c. and at bedtime

ADMINISTRATION

Oral

- Give 30 min before meals and at bedtime.
- Preserve in tight, light-resistant containers.

ADVERSE EFFECTS (≥1%) **GI** Dry mouth, constipation. **Special Senses**

M

Blurred vision. **CNS** Dizziness, drowsiness, flushing of skin. **Urogenital** Urinary hesitancy or retention.

INTERACTIONS Drug: Amantadine, TRICYCLIC ANTIDEPRESSANTS increase anticholinergic effects; may increase effects of **atenolol, digoxin;** may decrease effectiveness of PHENOTHIAZINES.

PHARMACOKINETICS Absorption: Erratic after PO administration. **Onset:** Approximately 1 h. **Duration:** 4–6 h. **Elimination:** Primarily in urine and bile; some unchanged drug excreted in feces.

NURSING IMPLICATIONS

Assessment & Drug Effects

- Incidence and severity of adverse effects are generally dose related. Dosage is usually maintained at a level that produces slight dryness of mouth.
- Report urinary retention promptly; may indicate need to discontinue drug.

Patient & Family Education

- Do not drive or engage in potentially hazardous activities until response to drug is known.
- Make position changes slowly and in stages.
- Learn measures to relieve dry mouth; rinse mouth frequently with water, suck hard candy.

M

METHYCLOTHIAZIDE

(meth-i-kloe-thye′a-zide)

Duretic ✤, Enduron

Classifications: THIAZIDE DIURETIC; ANTIHYPERTENSIVE

Therapeutic: THIAZIDE DIURETIC; ANTIHYPERTENSIVE

Prototype: Hydrochlorothiazide

Pregnancy Category: D first trimester; C second and third trimester

AVAILABILITY 2.5 mg, 5 mg tablets

ACTION & *THERAPEUTIC EFFECT* Diuretic effect results from inhibition of the renal tubular reabsorption of electrolytes. Excretion of sodium and chloride is enhanced, along with a loss of potassium ions via the kidney. BP is lowered, probably by the loss of sodium, chloride and water, and, consequently, blood volume. Edema is also decreased in CHF patients by the same mechanism. *Antihypertensive effect as well as enhanced excretion of sodium and water.*

USES Antihypertensive treatment and adjunctively in the management of edema associated with CHF, renal pathology, and hepatic cirrhosis.

CONTRAINDICATIONS Hypersensitivity to thiazides, and sulfonamide derivatives; anuria, hypokalemia, pregnancy (category D first trimester), lactation.

CAUTIOUS USE Renal disease; impaired kidney or liver function; older adults; gout; SLE; hypercalcemia; diabetes mellitus; pregnancy (category C second and third trimester); children.

ROUTE & DOSAGE

Edema

Adult: **PO** 2.5–10 mg once/day or 3–5 times/wk

Hypertension

Adult: **PO** 2.5–10 mg/day
Child: **PO** 0.05–0.2 mg/kg/day

ADMINISTRATION

Oral

- Give early in a.m. after eating (reduces gastric irritation) to prevent sleep interruption because of diuresis. If 2 doses are ordered, administer second dose no later than 3 p.m.
- Store at 15°–30° C (59°–86° F) unless otherwise instructed.

ADVERSE EFFECTS (≥1%) **Body as a Whole:** Postural hypotension, sialadenitis, unusual fatigue, dizziness, paresthesias. **Skin:** Photosensitivity. **Special Senses:** Yellow vision. **Metabolic:** *Hypokalemia*. **Hematologic:** <u>Agranulocytosis</u>.

INTERACTIONS Drug: Amphotericin B, CORTICOSTEROIDS increase hypokalemic effects; may antagonize hypoglycemic effects of **insulin,** SULFONYLUREAS; **cholestyramine, colestipol** decrease thiazide absorption; intensifies hypoglycemic and hypotensive effects of **diazoxide;** increased potassium and magnesium loss may cause **digoxin** toxicity; decreases **lithium** excretion, increasing its toxicity; NSAIDS may attenuate diuresis, and risk of NSAID-induced kidney failure increased.

PHARMACOKINETICS Absorption: Incompletely absorbed. **Onset:** 2 h. **Peak:** 6 h. **Duration:** Greater than 24 h. **Distribution:** Distributed throughout extracellular tissue; concentrates in kidney; crosses placenta; distributed in breast milk. **Metabolism:** Does not appear to be metabolized. **Elimination:** In urine.

NURSING IMPLICATIONS

Assessment & Drug Effects

- Expect antihypertensive effects in 3–4 days; maximal effects may require 3–4 wk.
- Monitor BP and I&O ratio during first phase of antihypertensive therapy. Report a sudden fall in BP, which may initiate severe postural hypotension and potentially dangerous perfusion problems, especially in the extremities.
- Lab tests: Periodic serum electrolytes and CBC with differential.
- Monitor patient for S&S of hypokalemia (see Appendix F). Report promptly. Physician may change dose and institute replacement therapy.

Patient & Family Education

- Eat a balanced diet to protect against hypokalemia; generally not severe even with long-term therapy. Prevent onset by eating potassium-rich foods including a banana (about 370 mg potassium) and at least 180 mL (6 oz) orange juice (about 330 mg potassium) every day.
- Watch carefully for loss of glycemic control (diabetics) and early signs of hyperglycemia (see Appendix F). Symptoms are slow to develop.
- Avoid OTC drugs unless the physician approves them. Many preparations contain both potassium and sodium, and may induce electrolyte imbalance adverse effects.
- Older adults are more responsive to excessive diuresis; orthostatic hypotension may be a problem.
- Change positions slowly and in stages from lying down to upright positions; avoid hot baths or showers, extended exposure to sunlight, and standing still. Accept assistance as necessary to prevent falling.
- Do not drive or engage in potentially hazardous activities until adjustment to the hypotensive effects of drug has been made.

M

METHYLDOPA (Pr)

(meth-ill-doe′pa)

Apo-Methyldopa ✦, Novomedopa ✦

METHYLDOPATE HYDROCHLORIDE

(meth-ill-doe′pate)

Classifications: CENTRAL-ACTING ANTIHYPERTENSIVE; ALPHA-ADRENERGIC AGONIST

Therapeutic: ANTIHYPERTENSIVE, CENTRAL-ACTING

Pregnancy Category: B

AVAILABILITY 125 mg, 250 mg, 500 mg tablets; 50 mg/mL injection

ACTION & *THERAPEUTIC EFFECT* Structurally related to catecholamines and their precursors. Inhibits decarboxylation of dopa, thereby reducing concentration of dopamine, a precursor of norepinephrine. It also inhibits the precursor of serotonin. Reduces renal vascular resistance; maintains cardiac output without acceleration, but may slow heart rate; tends to support sodium and water retention. *Lowers standing and supine BP.*

USES Treatment of sustained moderate to severe hypertension, particularly in patients with kidney dysfunction. Also used in selected patients with carcinoid disease. Parenteral form has been used for treatment of hypertensive crises but is not preferred because of its slow onset of action.

CONTRAINDICATIONS Active liver disease (hepatitis, cirrhosis); pheochromocytoma; blood dyscrasias.

CAUTIOUS USE History of impaired liver or kidney function or disease; renal failure; autoimmune disease; cardiac disease; angina pectoris; history of mental depression; Parkinson's disease; young or older adult patients; pregnancy (category B).

ROUTE & DOSAGE

Hypertension

Adult: **PO** 250 mg b.i.d. or t.i.d., may be increased up to 3 g/day in divided doses, usual range 250–1000 mg total per day **IV** 250–500 mg q6h, may be increased up to 1 g q6h

Geriatric: **PO** 125 mg b.i.d. or t.i.d., may increase gradually (max: 3 g/day)

Child: **PO** 10 mg/kg/day in 2–4 divided doses (max: 3 g/day) **IV** 2–4 mg/kg/day in divided doses (max: 3 g/day)

Renal Impairment Dosage Adjustment

CrCl greater than 50 mL/min: Dose q8h; 10–50 mL/min: Dose q8–12h; less than 10 mL/min: Dose q12–24h

ADMINISTRATION

Oral

- Make dosage increases in evening to minimize daytime sedation.

Intravenous

PREPARE: **Intermittent:** Dilute in 100–200 mL of D5W, as needed, to yield 10 mg/mL.

ADMINISTER: **Intermittent:** Give over 30–60 min.

INCOMPATIBILITIES **Solution/additive:** **Amphotericin B, hydrocortisone, methohexital, tetracycline.** **Y-site:** **Fat emulsion.**

ADVERSE EFFECTS (≥1%) **Body as a Whole:** Hypersensitivity (*fever*, skin eruptions, ulcerations of soles of feet, flu-like symptoms, lymphadenopathy, eosinophilia). **CNS:** *Sedation, drowsiness,* sluggishness, headache, weakness, fatigue, dizziness, vertigo, *decrease in mental acuity,* inability to concentrate, amnesia-like syndrome, parkinsonism, mild psychoses, depression, nightmares. **CV:** Orthostatic hypotension, syncope, bradycardia, myocarditis, edema, weight gain *(sodium and water retention),* paradoxic hypertensive reaction (especially with IV administration). **GI:** Diarrhea, constipation, abdominal distention, malabsorption syndrome, nausea, vomiting, dry mouth, sore or black tongue, sialadenitis, abnormal liver function tests, jaundice, hepatitis, hepatic necrosis (rare). **Hematologic:** *Positive direct Coombs' test* (common especially in African-Americans), granulocytopenia. **Special Senses:** *Nasal stuffiness.* **Endocrine:** Gynecomastia, lactation, *decreased libido, impotence,* hypothermia (large doses), positive tests for lupus and rheumatoid factors. **Skin:** Granulomatous skin lesions.

DIAGNOSTIC TEST INTERFERENCE Methyldopa may interfere with ***serum creatinine*** measurements using ***alkaline picrate method, AST*** by ***colorimetric methods,*** and ***uric acid*** measurements by ***phosphotungstate method*** (with high methyldopa blood levels); it may produce false elevations of ***urinary catecholamines*** and increase in ***serum amylase*** in methyldopa-induced sialadenitis.

INTERACTIONS Drug: AMPHETAMINES, TRICYCLIC ANTIDEPRESSANTS, PHENOTHIAZINES, BARBITUATES may attenuate antihypertensive response; methyldopa may inhibit effectiveness of **ephedrine; haloperidol** may exacerbate psychiatric symptoms; with **levodopa** additive hypotension, increased CNS toxicity, especially psychosis; increases risk of **lithium** toxicity; **methotrimeprazine** causes excessive hypotension; MAO INHIBITORS may cause hallucinations; **phenoxybenzamine** may cause urinary incontinence. **Herbal: Licorice** may affect electrolyte levels; **ephedra, yohimbe, ginseng** may decrease efficacy.

PHARMACOKINETICS Absorption: About 50% absorbed from GI tract. **Peak:** 4–6 h. **Duration:** 24 h PO; 10–16 h IV. **Distribution:** Crosses placenta, distributed into breast milk. **Metabolism:** In liver and GI tract. **Elimination:** Primarily in urine. **Half-Life:** 1.7 h.

NURSING IMPLICATIONS

Assessment & Drug Effects

- Check BP and pulse at least q30min until stabilized during IV infusion and observe for adequacy of urinary output.
- Take BP at regular intervals in lying, sitting, and standing positions during period of dosage adjustment.
- Supervision of ambulation in older adults and patients with impaired kidney function; both are particularly likely to manifest orthostatic hypotension with dizziness and light-headedness during period of dosage adjustment.
- Monitor fluid and electrolyte balance and I&O. Weigh patient daily, and check for edema because methyldopa favors sodium and water retention.
- Lab tests: Baseline and periodic blood counts and liver function tests especially during first 6–12 wk of therapy or if patient develops unexplained fever; periodic serum electrolytes.

- Be alert that rising BP indicating tolerance to drug effect may occur during week 2 or 3 of therapy.

Patient & Family Education

- Exercise caution with hot baths and showers, prolonged standing in one position, and strenuous exercise that may enhance orthostatic hypotension. Make position changes slowly, particularly from lying down to upright posture; dangle legs a few minutes before standing.
- Be aware that transient sedation, drowsiness, mental depression, weakness, and headache commonly occur during first 24–72 h of therapy or whenever dosage is increased. Symptoms tend to disappear with continuation of therapy or dosage reduction.
- Avoid potentially hazardous tasks such as driving until response to drug is known; drug may affect ability to perform activities requiring concentrated mental effort, especially during first few days of therapy or whenever dosage is increased.
- Do not to take OTC medications unless approved by physician.

M

METHYLERGONOVINE MALEATE

(meth-ill-er-goe-noe′veen)

Methergine

Classifications: ADRENERGIC ANTAGONIST; ERGOT ALKALOID; OXYTOCIC

Therapeutic: OXYTOCIC

Prototype: Ergotamine

Pregnancy Category: C

AVAILABILITY 0.2 mg tablets; 0.2 mg/mL injections

ACTION & *THERAPEUTIC EFFECT* Ergot alkaloid that induces rapid, sustained tetanic uterine contraction that shortens third stage of labor and reduces blood loss. *Administered after delivery of the placenta to minimize the risk of postpartal hemorrhage.*

USES Routine management after delivery of placenta and for postpartum atony, subinvolution, and hemorrhage. With full obstetric supervision, may be used during second stage of labor.

CONTRAINDICATIONS Hypersensitivity to ergot preparations; induction of labor; use prior to delivery of placenta; threatened spontaneous abortion; prolonged use; uterine sepsis; hypertension; toxemia; angina; arteriosclerosis; CAD; dysfunctional uterine bleeding; eclampsia; hypertension; MI; neonates; PVD; preeclampsia; Raynaud's disease; sepsis; stroke; thromboangiitis obliterans; thrombophlebitis.

CAUTIOUS USE Diabetes mellitus; hepatic disease; migraine headaches; renal failure, renal impairment; pulmonary disease; pregnancy (category C), lactation.

ROUTE & DOSAGE

Postpartum Hemorrhage

Adult: **PO** 0.2 q6–8h × 2–7 days **IM/IV** 0.2 mg q2–4h (max: 5 doses)

ADMINISTRATION

- Use parenteral routes only in emergencies.

Oral

- Note: Dosing should not exceed 1 wk.

Intramuscular

- Inject undiluted deep into a large muscle.

Intravenous

PREPARE: **Direct:** Give undiluted or diluted in 5 mL of NS.
ADMINISTER: **Direct:** Give 0.2 mg or fraction thereof over 60 sec.
- Do not use ampules containing discolored solution or visible particles.

- Store at 15°–30° C (59°–86° F) unless otherwise directed. Protect from light.

ADVERSE EFFECTS (≥1%) **GI:** *Nausea, vomiting* (especially with IV doses). **CV:** Severe hypertensive episodes, bradycardia. **Body as a Whole:** Allergic phenomena including shock, ergotism.

INTERACTIONS Drug: PARENTERAL SYMPATHOMIMETICS, other ERGOT ALKALOIDS, TRIPTANS add to pressor effects and carry risk of hypertension; PROTEASE INHIBITORS, **itraconazole** may increase the risk of toxicity.

PHARMACOKINETICS Absorption: Readily from GI tract. **Onset:** 5–15 min PO; 2–5 min IM; immediate IV. **Duration:** 3 or more h PO; 3 h IM; 45 min IV. **Distribution:** Distributed into breast milk. **Metabolism:** Slowly in liver. **Elimination:** Mainly in feces, small amount in urine. **Half-Life:** 0.5–2 h.

NURSING IMPLICATIONS

Assessment & Drug Effects

- Monitor vital signs (particularly BP) and uterine response during and after parenteral administration of methylergonovine until partum period is stabilized (about 1–2 h).
- Notify physician if BP suddenly increases or if there are frequent periods of uterine relaxation.

Patient & Family Education

- Report severe cramping or increased bleeding.
- Report any of the following: Cold or numb fingers or toes, nausea or vomiting, chest or muscle pain.

METHYLNALTREXONE BROMIDE

(meth-yl-nal-trex′own bro′mide)
Relistor
Classification: NARCOTIC (OPIATE ANTAGONIST)
Therapeutic: NARCOTIC ANTAGONIST
Prototype: Naloxone
Pregnancy Category: B

AVAILABILITY 12 mg/0.6 mL solution for injection

ACTION & *THERAPEUTIC EFFECT* A selective, peripherally acting antagonist of opioid binding to mu-opioid receptors in tissues such as the GI tract. *Decreases constipating effects of opioids without interfering with analgesic effect of opioids in the CNS.*

USES Treatment of opioid-induced constipation in patients with advanced illness who are receiving palliative care when response to laxative therapy has not been sufficient.

UNLABELED USES Management of nausea and vomiting related to morphine. Treatment of pruritus related to morphine. Management of urinary retention caused by opioids.

CONTRAINDICATIONS Known or suspected mechanical GI obstruction; severe or persistent diarrhea.

CAUTIOUS USE Severe renal impairment; pregnancy (category B); lactation. Safety and efficacy in children not established.

M

ROUTE & DOSAGE

Opioid-Induced Constipation

Adult: **Subcutaneous** Administer every other day based on weight: *weight less than 38 kg,* 0.15 mg/kg; *weight 38 to less than 62 kg,* 8 mg; *weight 62 to less than 114 kg,* 12 mg

Renal Impairment Dosage Adjustment

CrCl less than 30 mL/min: Reduce normal adult dose by 50%

ADMINISTRATION

Subcutaneous

- An 8 mg dose equals 0.4 mL and a 12 mg dose equals 0.6 mL.
- Insert needle at a 45-degree angle into a pinched fold of skin on the abdomen, thigh, or upper arm. Release skin and inject. Rotate injection sites.
- Store at 20°–25° C (68°–77° F) away from light. May store drawn up into syringe for 24 h at room temperature with ambient light.

ADVERSE EFFECTS (≥1%) **CNS:** Dizziness. **GI:** *Abdominal pain*, diarrhea, *flatulence, nausea*.

PHARMACOKINETICS Peak: 0.5 h. **Distribution:** 11–15% protein bound. **Metabolism:** Hepatic. **Elimination:** Primarily eliminated unchanged (85%) in urine and feces. **Half-Life:** 8 h.

NURSING IMPLICATIONS

Assessment & Drug Effects

- Monitor bowel pattern.
- Withhold drug and report promptly severe or persistent diarrhea.

Patient & Family Education

- Ensure that patient/caregiver knows how to correctly inject subcutaneous medication.
- Stop methylnaltrexone and notify physician if severe or persistent diarrhea develops.

METHYLPHENIDATE HYDROCHLORIDE

(meth-ill-fen′i-date)

Concerta, Daytrana, Metadate CD, Metadate ER, Methylin, Methylin ER, Ritalin, Ritalin LA, Ritalin SR

Classification: CEREBRAL STIMULANT
Therapeutic: CEREBRAL STIMULANT
Prototype: Amphetamine
Pregnancy Category: C
Controlled Substance: Schedule II

AVAILABILITY 5 mg, 10 mg, 20 mg tablets; 2.5 mg, 5 mg, 10 mg chewable tablets; 5 mg/5 mL, 10 mg/5 mL oral solution; 10 mg, 20 mg, 30 mg, 40 mg, 50 mg, 60 mg sustained release capsules; 10 mg, 18 mg, 20 mg, 27 mg, 36 mg, 54 mg sustained release tablets; 10 mg, 15 mg, 20 mg, 30 mg transdermal patch

ACTION & *THERAPEUTIC EFFECT* Acts mainly on cerebral cortex exerting a stimulant effect. Results in mild CNS and respiratory stimulation with potency intermediate between amphetamine and caffeine. *Effects are more prominent on mental rather than on motor activities. Also believed to have an anorexiant effect.*

USES Adjunctive therapy in hyperkinetic syndromes characterized by

attention deficit disorder, narcolepsy.
UNLABELED USES Depression.

CONTRAINDICATIONS Hypersensitivity to drug; history of marked anxiety, agitation; aortic stenosis; serious cardiac disorders including arrhythmias; valvular heart disease; ventricular dysfunction; motor tics or Tourette's disease; substance abuse; severe anxiety, psychosis, major depression, suicidal ideation; glaucoma; lactation, children younger than 6 y of age.
CAUTIOUS USE Alcoholic; emotionally unstable patient; abrupt discontinuation; recent MI, anxiety, cardiac arrhythmias, cardiac disease, dysphagia, older adults; esophageal stricture, GI obstruction, heart failure, hepatic disease, hyperthyroidism, history of paralytic ileus, cystic fibrosis, mania, radiographic contrast administration, seizure disorder, hypertension; history of seizures; pregnancy (category C).

ROUTE & DOSAGE

Narcolepsy
Adult: **PO** 10 mg b.i.d. or t.i.d. 30–45 min p.c. (range: 10–60 mg/day)
Adolescent/Child (older than 6 y): **PO** 5 mg b.i.d., may increase weekly (max dose: 60 mg/day)

Attention Deficit Disorder
Adult: **PO** Immediate release products: 20–30 mg daily in divided doses. Concerta extended release product: 18–36 mg daily
Child: **PO** 5–10 mg before breakfast and lunch, with a gradual increase of 5–10 mg/wk as needed (max: 60 mg/day) or 20–40 mg sustained release daily before breakfast (max dose: 72 mg daily). Concerta extended release product: 18 mg daily (max: 54 mg/day)
Transdermal patch 10 mg patch worn for 9 hours × 1 wk then taper as needed. Increase no more than once weekly. Apply 2 h before desired effect.

ADMINISTRATION

Oral
- Give 30–45 min before meals. To avoid insomnia, give last dose before 6 p.m.
- Ensure that sustained release form is not chewed or crushed. It **must be** swallowed whole.
- Can open Metadate CD capsules and sprinkle on food
- Store at 15°–30° C (59°–86° F).

Transdermal
- Apply patch to hip area 2 h before desired effect and remove not later than 9 h after application. Patch may be removed earlier than 9 h if a shorter duration of effect is desired.
- Alternate application site daily. Do not apply under tight clothing.

ADVERSE EFFECTS (≥1%) **CNS:** Dizziness, drowsiness, *nervousness, insomnia.* **CV:** Palpitations, changes in BP and pulse rate, angina, cardiac arrhythmias, exacerbation of underlying CV conditions. **Special Senses:** Difficulty with accommodation, blurred vision. **GI:** Dry throat, anorexia, nausea; hepatotoxicity; abdominal pain. **Body as a Whole:** Hypersensitivity reactions (rash, fever, arthralgia, urticaria, exfoliative dermatitis, erythema multiforme); long-term growth suppression.

INTERACTIONS Drug: MAO INHIBITORS may cause hypertensive crisis;

M

antagonizes hypotensive effects of **guanethidine, bretylium;** potentiates action of CNS STIMULANTS (e.g. **amphetamine, caffeine**); may inhibit metabolism and increase serum levels of **fosphenytoin, phenytoin, phenobarbital,** and **primidone, warfarin,** TRICYCLIC ANTIDEPRESSANTS.

PHARMACOKINETICS Absorption: Readily from GI tract. Transdermal absorption increased with heat or inflamed skin. **Peak:** 1.9 h; 4–7 h sustained release, 2 h transdermal. **Duration:** 3–6 h; 8 h sustained release. **Elimination:** In urine.

NURSING IMPLICATIONS

Assessment & Drug Effects

- Monitor BP and pulse at appropriate intervals.
- Lab tests: Obtain periodic CBC with differential and platelet counts during prolonged therapy.
- Monitor closely patient with a history of drug dependence or alcoholism. Chronic abusive use can lead to tolerance, psychic dependence, and psychoses.
- Assess patient's condition with periodic drug-free periods during prolonged therapy.
- Supervise drug withdrawal carefully following prolonged use. Abrupt withdrawal may result in severe depression and psychotic behavior.

Patient & Family Education

- Report adverse effects to physician, particularly nervousness and insomnia. These effects may diminish with time or require reduction of dosage or omission of afternoon or evening dose.
- Check weight at least 2 or 3 times weekly and report weight loss. Check height and weight in children; failure to gain in either should be reported to physician.
- Withhold patch from an ADHD child who exhibits anxiety, tension or agitation. Consult physician.
- Do not apply heat or heating pad over area where patch is located.

METHYLPREDNISOLONE

(meth-ill-pred-niss'oh-lone)
Medrol

METHYLPREDNISOLONE ACETATE

Depo-Medrol

METHYLPREDNISOLONE SODIUM SUCCINATE

A-Methapred, Solu-Medrol

Classifications: BIOLOGICAL RESPONSE MODIFIER; IMMUNOSUPPRESSANT; ADRENAL CORTICOSTEROID; ANTI-INFLAMMATORY
Therapeutic: ANTI-INFLAMMATORY
Prototype: Prednisone
Pregnancy Category: C

AVAILABILITY Methylprednisolone: 2 mg, 4 mg, 8 mg, 16 mg, 24 mg, 32 mg tablets; **Methylprednisolone Acetate:** 20 mg/mL, 40 mg/mL, 80 mg/mL injection; **Methylprednisolone Sodium Succinate:** 40 mg, 125 mg, 500 mg, 1 g, 2 g powder for injection

ACTION & *THERAPEUTIC EFFECT* Intermediate-acting synthetic adrenal corticosteroid with glucocorticoid activity. It inhibits phagocytosis, and release of allergic substances. It also modifies the immune response of the body to various stimuli. **Sodium succinate** form is characterized by rapid onset of action and is used for emergency therapy of short duration. *Has anti-inflammatory and immunosuppressive properties.*

USES An anti-inflammatory agent in the management of acute and chronic inflammatory diseases, for palliative management of neoplastic diseases, and for control of severe acute and chronic allergic processes. High-dose, short-term therapy: Management of acute bronchial asthma, prevention of fat embolism in patient with long-bone fracture. Short-term management of rheumatic disorders.

UNLABELED USES Acetate form used as a long-acting contraceptive and for spinal cord injury, lupus nephritis, multiple sclerosis.

CONTRAINDICATIONS Hypersensitivity to corticosteroid drugs; systemic fungal infections; use of solutions with benzyl alcohol preservative for premature infants or neonates.

CAUTIOUS USE Cushing's syndrome; GI disease, GI ulceration; hepatic disease; renal disease; hypertension; varicella, vaccinia; CHF; diabetes mellitus; glaucoma; coagulopathy; emotional instability or psychotic tendencies; pregnacy (category C), lactation.

ROUTE & DOSAGE

Inflammation

Adult: **PO** 2–60 mg/day in 1 or more divided doses **IM** (Acetate) 10–80 mg/wk weekly or every other week; (Succinate) 10–80 mg daily **IV** 10–40 mg prn or 30 mg/kg q4–6h × 48 h

Child: **PO/IM/IV** 0.5–1.7 mg/kg/day divided q6–12h

Status Asthmaticus

Adult/Child: **IV** 2 mg/kg then 1–5 mg/kg qh

Acute Spinal Cord Injury

Adult/Child: **IV** 30 mg/kg over 15 min, followed in 45 min by 5.4 mg/kg/h × 23 h

Obesity Dosage Adjustment

Dose based on IBW if lower than actual weight

ADMINISTRATION

Oral

- Crush tablet before and give with fluid of patient's choice.
- Note: Preparation less irritating if given with food.
- Use alternate day therapy when given over long period.

Intramuscular

- Give injection deep into large muscle (not deltoid).

Intravenous

Note: Do NOT use methylprednisolone acetate for IV.

PREPARE: **Direct/Intermittent:** Available in ACT-O-Vial from which the desired dose may be withdrawn after initial dilution with supplied diluent. ▪ May be further diluted according to physician's orders. Recommended dilution is 0.25 mg/mL.

ADMINISTER: **Direct:** Give each 500 mg or fraction thereof over 2–3 min. **Intermittent:** Give over 15–30 min.

INCOMPATIBILITIES **Solution/additive:** **Dextrose 5%/sodium chloride 0.45%, aminophylline, calcium gluconate, glycopyrrolate, metaraminol, nafcillin, penicillin G sodium.** **Y-site:** **Allopurinol, amsacrine, ciprofloxacin, cisatracurium** (2 mg/mL or greater concentration), **diltiazem, docetaxel, etoposide, filgrastim, fenoldopam, gemcitabine, ondansetron, pacli-**

taxel, potassium chloride, propofol, sargramostim, vinorelbine.

- Store at 15°–30° C (59°–86° F). Do not freeze.

ADVERSE EFFECTS (≥1%) **CNS:** Euphoria, headache, insomnia, confusion, psychosis. **CV:** CHF, edema. **GI:** Nausea, vomiting, peptic ulcer. **Musculoskeletal:** Muscle weakness, delayed wound healing, muscle wasting, osteoporosis, aseptic necrosis of bone, spontaneous fractures. **Endocrine:** Cushingoid features, growth suppression in children, carbohydrate intolerance, hyperglycemia. **Special Senses:** Cataracts. **Hematologic:** Leukocytosis. **Metabolic:** Hypokalemia.

INTERACTIONS Drug: Amphotericin B, furosemide, THIAZIDE DIURETICS increase potassium loss; with ATTENUATED VIRUS VACCINES, may enhance virus replication or increase vaccine adverse effects; **isoniazid, phenytoin, phenobarbital, rifampin** decrease effectiveness of methylprednisolone because they increase metabolism of STEROIDS.

PHARMACOKINETICS Absorption: Readily absorbed from GI tract. **Peak:** 1–2 h PO; 4–8 days IM. **Duration:** 1.25–1.5 days PO; 1–5 wk IM. **Metabolism:** In liver. **Half-Life:** Greater than 3.5 h; HPA suppression: 18–36 h.

NURSING IMPLICATIONS

Assessment & Drug Effects

- Lab tests: Monitor periodically kidney and liver function, thyroid function, CBC, serum electrolytes, weight, and total cholesterol.
- Monitor diabetics for loss of glycemic control.
- Monitor serum potassium and report S&S of hypokalemia (see Appendix F).
- Monitor for and report S&S of Cushing's syndrome (see Appendix F).

Patient & Family Education

- Consult physician for any of the following: Slow wound healing, significant insomnia or confusion, or unexplained bone pain.
- Do not alter established dosage regimen (i.e., not to increase, decrease, or omit doses or change dose intervals). Withdrawal symptoms (rebound inflammation, fever) can be induced with sudden discontinuation of therapy.
- Report onset of signs of hypocorticism adrenal insufficiency immediately: Fatigue, nausea, anorexia, joint pain, muscular weakness, dizziness, fever.

METHYLTESTOSTERONE

(meth-ill-tess-toss′te-rone)

Android, Metandren ✦, Testred, Virilon

Classification: ANDROGEN/ANABOLIC STEROID

Therapeutic: ANABOLIC STEROID

Prototype: Testosterone

Pregnancy Category: X

Controlled Substance: Schedule III

AVAILABILITY 10 mg, 25 mg tablets

ACTION & *THERAPEUTIC EFFECT* Short-acting steroid with androgen/anabolic activity ratio (1:1) similar to that of testosterone but less effective than its esters. *Androgen activity is similar to testosterone; used in replacement therapy, and palliative treatment of postmenopausal female breast cancer.*

USES Androgen replacement therapy, delayed puberty (male), palliation of female mammary cancer (1–

5 y postmenopausal), postpartum breast engorgement.

CONTRAINDICATIONS Liver dysfunction; prostate cancer; severe cardiac, renal, or hepatic disease; pregnancy (category X), lactation.
CAUTIOUS USE Mild or moderate liver, kidney, or cardiac dysfunction; heart failure, diabetes mellitus; prostatic hypertrophy.

ROUTE & DOSAGE

Replacement
Adult: **PO** 10–50 mg/day in divided doses

Breast Cancer
Adult: **PO** 50–200 mg/day in divided doses for duration of therapeutic response or no longer than 3 mo if no remission

Postpartum Breast Engorgement
Adult: **PO** 80 mg/day for 3–5 days

ADMINISTRATION

Oral
- Place buccal tablets between cheek and gum. Ensure that tablet is absorbed, not chewed or swallowed; and eating or drinking avoided until absorption is complete.
- Store at 15°–30° C (59°–86° F). Avoid freezing.

ADVERSE EFFECTS (≥1%) **GI:** Cholestatic hepatitis with jaundice, irritation of oral mucosa with buccal administration. **Urogenital:** Renal calculi (especially in immobilized patient), priapism. **Endocrine:** *Acne, gynecomastia, edema,* oligospermia, menstrual irregularities.

INTERACTIONS **Drug:** Increases risk of bleeding associated with ORAL ANTICOAGULANTS; possibly increases risk of **cyclosporine** toxicity; may decrease glucose level, making adjustment of doses of **insulin,** SULFONYLUREAS necessary. **Herbal: Echinacea** may increase risk of hepatotoxicity.

PHARMACOKINETICS Absorption: Readily from GI tract. **Metabolism:** In liver. **Elimination:** In urine.

NURSING IMPLICATIONS

Assessment & Drug Effects
- Lab tests: Monitor liver function periodically; report signs of hepatic toxicity (see Appendix F).
- Monitor for flank pain, abdominal pain radiating to groin, or other symptoms of renal calculi.

Patient & Family Education
- Be prepared for distressing and undesirable adverse effects of virilization (women) since dosage sufficient to produce remission in breast cancer is quantitatively similar to that used for androgen replacement in the male.
- Report signs of virilism promptly. Voice change and hirsutism may be irreversible, even after drug is withdrawn.
- Report priapism (men) or other signs of excess sexual stimulation. The physician will terminate therapy.
- Report symptoms of jaundice with or without pruritus to physician; appears to be dose related. If liver function tests are altered at the same time, this drug will be withdrawn.

METIPRANOLOL HYDROCHLORIDE

(me-ti-pran′ol-ol)
OptiPranolol
Pregnancy Category: C
See Appendix A-1.

M

METOCLOPRAMIDE HYDROCHLORIDE Pr

(met-oh-kloe-pra′mide)

Emex ✤, Maxeran ✤, Metozolv ODT, Octamide PFS, Reglan

Classification: PROKINETIC AGENT (GI STIMULANT)

Therapeutic: GI STIMULANT; ANTIEMETIC

Pregnancy Category: B

AVAILABILITY 5 mg, 10 mg tablets; 5 mg/5 mL solution; 5 mg/mL injection; 5 mg, 10 mg orally disintegrating tablet

ACTION & *THERAPEUTIC EFFECT* Potent central dopamine receptor antagonist that increases resting tone of esophageal sphincter, and tone and amplitude of upper GI contractions. Thus gastric emptying and intestinal transit are accelerated. Antiemetic action results from drug-induced elevation of CTZ threshold and enhanced gastric emptying. *Effective as an antiemetic agent as part of a chemotherapy regimen. In diabetic gastroparesis, it relieves anorexia, nausea, vomiting, or persistent fullness after meals.*

USES Management of diabetic gastric stasis (gastroparesis); to prevent nausea and vomiting associated with emetogenic cancer chemotherapy (e.g., cisplatin, dacarbazine) or surgery; to facilitate intubation of small bowel; symptomatic treatment of gastroesophageal reflux.

UNLABELED USES Tourette's syndrome, hiccups.

CONTRAINDICATIONS Sensitivity or intolerance to metoclopramide; uncontrolled seizures; allergy to sulfiting agents; concurrent use of drugs that can cause extrapyramidal symptoms; pheochromocytoma; mechanical GI obstruction or perforation; ileus; history of breast cancer.

CAUTIOUS USE CHF, cardiac disease; sulfite hypersensitivity, asthma, hypokalemia, hypertension; depression; hepatic disease, infertility, methemoglobin reductase deficiency, Parkinson's disease, kidney dysfunction; GI hemorrhage; G6PD deficiency, procainamide hypersensitivity, seizure disorder, seizures, tardive dyskinesia; history of intermittent porphyria; pregnancy (category B); lactation.

ROUTE & DOSAGE

Gastroesophageal Reflux

Adult: **PO** 10–15 mg q.i.d. a.c. and at bedtime
Child: **PO** 0.1–0.2 mg/kg q.i.d.

Diabetic Gastroparesis

Adult: **PO/IV/IM** 10 mg q.i.d. a.c. and at bedtime for 2–8 wk
Geriatric: **PO** 5 mg a.c and at bedtime

Small-Bowel Intubation, Radiologic Examination

Adult: **IM/IV** 10 mg administered over 1–2 min
Child: **IM/IV** *Younger than 6 y,* 0.1 mg/kg over 1–2 min; *6–14 y,* 2.5–5 mg over 1–2 min

Chemotherapy-Induced Emesis

Adult: **PO** 20–40 mg q4–6h, may repeat **IM/IV** 2 mg/kg 30 min before antineoplastic administration, may repeat q2h for 2 doses, then q3h for 3 doses if needed

Postoperative Nausea/Vomiting

Adult: **IM/IV** 10–20 mg near end of surgery

ADMINISTRATION

Oral

- Give 30 min before meals and at bedtime.

Intravenous

Note: Verify correct IV concentration and rate of infusion for administration to infants or children with physician.

PREPARE: **Direct:** Doses of 10 mg or less may be given undiluted. **IV Infusion:** Doses greater than 10 mg IV should be diluted in at least 50 mL of D5W, NS, D5/0.45% NaCl, LR or other compatible solution.

ADMINISTER: **Direct:** Give over 1–2 min (or longer in pediatric patients). **IV Infusion:** Give over not less than 15 min.

INCOMPATIBILITIES **Solution/additive:** **Calcium gluconate, chloramphenicol, cisplatin, dexamethasone, erythromycin, floxacillin, fluorouracil, furosemide, lorazepam, methotrexate, penicillin G potassium, sodium bicarbonate,** TETRACYCLINES. **Y-site:** **Allopurinol, amphotericin B cholesteryl complex, amsacrine, cefepime, doxorubicin liposome, furosemide, propofol, TPN.**

- Discard open ampules; do not store for future use.
- Store at 15°–30° C (59°–86° F) in light-resistant bottle. Tablets are stable for 3 y; solutions and injections, for 5 y.

ADVERSE EFFECTS (≥1%) **CNS:** *Mild sedation, fatigue, restlessness,* agitation, headache, insomnia, disorientation, *extrapyramidal symptoms* (acute dystonic type), tardive dyskinesia, neurologic malignant syndrome with injection. **GI:** Nausea, constipation, *diarrhea,* dry mouth, altered drug absorption. **Skin:** Urticarial or maculopapular rash. **Body as a Whole:** Glossal or periorbital edema. **Hematologic:** Methemoglobinemia. **Endocrine:** Galactorrhea, gynecomastia, amenorrhea, impotence. **CV:** <u>Hypertensive crisis</u> (rare).

DIAGNOSTIC TEST INTERFERENCE Metoclopramide may interfere with gonadorelin test by increasing ***serum prolactin*** levels.

INTERACTIONS Drug: Alcohol and other CNS DEPRESSANTS add to sedation; ANTICHOLINERGICS, OPIATE ANALGESICS may antagonize effect on GI motility; PHENOTHIAZINES may potentiate extrapyramidal symptoms; may decrease absorption of **acetaminophen, aspirin, atovaquone, diazepam, digoxin, lithium, tetracycline;** may antagonize the effects of **amantadine, bromocriptine, levodopa, pergolide, ropinirole, pramipexole;** may cause increase in extrapyramidal and dystonic reactions with PHENOTHIAZINES, THIOXANTHENES, **droperidol, haloperidol, loxapine, metyrosine;** may prolong neuromuscular blocking effects of **succinylcholine.**

PHARMACOKINETICS Absorption: Readily from GI tract. **Onset:** 30–60 min PO; 10–15 min IM; 1–3 min IV. **Peak:** 1–2 h. **Duration:** 1–3 h. **Distribution:** To most body tissues including CNS; crosses placenta; distributed into breast milk. **Metabolism:** Minimally in liver. **Elimination:** 95% in urine, 5% in feces. **Half-Life:** 2.5–6 h.

NURSING IMPLICATIONS

Assessment & Drug Effects

- Report immediately the onset of restlessness, involuntary movements, facial grimacing, rigidity, or tremors. Extrapyramidal symptoms are most likely to occur in children, young adults, and the older adult and with high-dose treatment of vomiting associated with cancer chemotherapy. Symptoms can take months to regress.

- Be aware that during early treatment period, serum aldosterone may be elevated; after prolonged administration periods, it returns to pretreatment level.
- Lab tests: Periodic serum electrolytes.
- Monitor for possible hypernatremia and hypokalemia (see Appendix F), especially if patient has HF or cirrhosis.
- Adverse reactions associated with increased serum prolactin concentration (galactorrhea, menstrual disorders, gynecomastia) usually disappear within a few weeks or months after drug treatment is stopped.

M

Patient & Family Education

- Avoid driving and other potentially hazardous activities for a few hours after drug administration.
- Avoid alcohol and other CNS depressants.
- Report S&S of acute dystonia, such as trembling hands and facial grimacing (see Appendix F), immediately.

METOLAZONE

(me-tole′a-zone)

Zaroxolyn ✤

Classifications: THIAZIDE DIURETIC; ANTIHYPERTENSIVE

Therapeutic: DIURETIC; ANTIHYPERTENSIVE

Prototype: Hydrochlorothiazide

Pregnancy Category: D

AVAILABILITY 2.5 mg, 5 mg, 10 mg tablets

ACTION & *THERAPEUTIC EFFECT* Diuretic action is associated with interference with transport of sodium ions across renal tubular epithelium. This enhances excretion of sodium, chloride, potassium, bicarbonate, and water. *Produces a decrease in the systolic and diastolic BPs, and reduces edema in CHF and kidney failure patients.*

USES Management of hypertension as sole agent or to enhance effectiveness of other antihypertensives in severe form of hypertension; also edema associated with CHF and kidney disease.

CONTRAINDICATIONS Anuria, hypokalemia; hepatic coma or precoma; hypersensitivity to metolazone and sulfonamides; SLE; pregnancy (category D), lactation.

CAUTIOUS USE History of gout; elderly; allergies; concomitant use of digitalis glycosides; kidney and liver dysfunction.

ROUTE & DOSAGE

Edema

Adult: **PO** 5–20 mg/day

Child: **PO** 0.2–0.4 mg/kg/day divided q12–24h

Hypertension

Adult: **PO** 2.5–5 mg/day

ADMINISTRATION

Oral

- Do not interchange slow availability tablets and rapid availability tablets. They are not equivalent.
- Schedule doses to avoid nocturia and interrupted sleep. Give early in a.m. after eating to prevent gastric irritation (if given in 2 doses,

schedule second dose no later than 3 p.m.).

- Store at 15°–30° C (59°–86° F) in tightly closed container.

ADVERSE EFFECTS (≥1%) **GI:** Cholestatic jaundice. **Body as a Whole:** Vertigo, orthostatic hypotension. **Hematologic:** Venous thrombosis, leukopenia. **Metabolic:** Dehydration, *hypokalemia, hyperuricemia, hyperglycemia*.

INTERACTIONS Drug: Amphotericin B, CORTICOSTEROIDS increase hypokalemic effects; may antagonize hypoglycemic effects of SULFONYLUREAS, **insulin; cholestyramine, colestipol** decrease thiazide absorption; intensifies hypoglycemic and hypotensive effects of **diazoxide;** because of increased potassium and magnesium loss, may cause **digoxin** toxicity; decreases **lithium** excretion, increasing its toxicity; NSAIDS may attenuate diuresis—increased risk of NSAID-induced kidney failure.

PHARMACOKINETICS Absorption: Incomplete. **Onset:** 1 h. **Peak:** 2–8 h. **Duration:** 12–24 h. **Distribution:** Distributed throughout extracellular tissue; concentrates in kidney; crosses placenta; distributed in breast milk. **Metabolism:** Does not appear to be metabolized. **Elimination:** In urine. **Half-Life:** 14 h.

NURSING IMPLICATIONS

Assessment & Drug Effects

- Anticipate overdosage and adverse reactions in geriatric patients; may be more sensitive to effects of usual adult dose.
- Terminate therapy when adverse reactions are moderate to severe.
- Expect possible antihypertensive effects in 3 or 4 days, but 3–4 wk are required for maximum effect.
- Lab tests: Determine serum potassium at regular intervals. Prolonged treatment and inadequate potassium intake increase potential for hypokalemia (see Appendix F). Periodic plasma glucose and urinalysis determinations.

Patient & Family Education

- Do not drink alcohol; it potentiates orthostatic hypotension.
- Antihypertensive therapy may require as adjunct a high-potassium, low-sodium, and low-calorie diet.
- Include potassium-rich foods in the diet.
- Be aware that if hypokalemia develops, dietary potassium supplement of 1000–2000 mg (25–50 mEq) is usually adequate treatment.

METOPROLOL TARTRATE

(me-toe′proe-lole)

Apo-Metoprolol ♣, Betaloc ♣, Lopressor, Toprol XL

Classifications: CARDIOSELECTIVE BETA-ADRENERGIC ANTAGONIST; ANTIHYPERTENSIVE; ANTIANGINAL

Therapeutic: ANTIHYPERTENSIVE; ANTIANGINAL

Prototype: Propranolol

Pregnancy Category: C

AVAILABILITY 25 mg, 50 mg, 100 mg tablets; 25 mg, 50 mg, 100 mg, 200 mg sustained release tablets; 1 mg/mL injection

ACTION & *THERAPEUTIC EFFECT* Beta-adrenergic antagonist with preferential effect on $beta_1$ receptors located primarily on cardiac muscle. Antihypertensive action may be due to competitive antagonism of catecholamines at cardiac adrenergic neuron sites, drug-induced reduction of sympathetic outflow to the periphery, and to suppression of renin activity. *Reduces heart rate and cardiac output at rest and during exercise; lowers both supine and standing BP, slows sinus rate and decreases myocardial automaticity. Antianginal effect is like that of propranolol.*

USES Management of mild to severe hypertension (monotherapy or in combination with a thiazide or vasodilator or both); long-term treatment of angina pectoris and prophylactic management of stable angina pectoris reduce the risk of mortality after an MI.

UNLABELED USES CHF, migraine prophylaxis, arrythmias.

CONTRAINDICATIONS Cardiogenic shock, sinus bradycardia, advanced AV block without a pacemaker, bradycardia, sick sinus syndrome; pheochromocytoma, hypotension, moderate to severe cardiac failure, right ventricular failure secondary to pulmonary hypertension; abrupt discontinuation. Safe use in children younger than 6 y is not known.

CAUTIOUS USE Impaired liver or kidney function; cardiomegaly, CHF controlled by digitalis and diuretics; major depression; bronchial asthma and other bronchospastic diseases; history of allergy; thyrotoxicosis; diabetes mellitus; peripheral vascular disease; myasthenia gravis; cerebrovascular insufficiency; pregnancy (category C), lactation.

ROUTE & DOSAGE

Hypertension

Adult: **PO** 50–100 mg/day in 1–2 divided doses, may increase weekly up to 100–450 mg/day

Geriatric: **PO** 25 mg/day (range: 25–300 mg/day)

Child (older than 6 y): **PO** 1 mg/kg daily (max: 200 mg)

Angina Pectoris

Adult: **PO** 100 mg/day in 2 divided doses, may increase weekly up to 100–400 mg/day

Myocardial Infarction

Adult: **IV** 5 mg q2min for 3 doses, followed by PO therapy **PO** 50 mg q6h for 48 h, then 100 mg b.i.d.

ADMINISTRATION

Oral

- Ensure that sustained-release form is not chewed or crushed. It **must be** swallowed whole.
- Give with food to slightly enhance absorption; however, administration with food not essential. It is important to give with or without food consistently to minimize possible variations in bioavailability.

Intravenous

PREPARE: **Direct:** Give undiluted.

ADMINISTER: **Direct:** Give at a rate of 5 mg over 60 sec. ▪ Note conditions which are contraindications to drug administration.

INCOMPATIBILITIES **Y-site:** **Amphotericin B cholesteryl complex.**

- Store at 15°–30° C (59°–86° F). Protect from heat, light, and moisture.

ADVERSE EFFECTS (≥1%) **Body as a Whole:** Hypersensitivity (erythematous rash, fever, headache, muscle aches, sore throat, laryngospasm, respiratory distress). **CNS:** *Dizziness, fatigue, insomnia,* increased dreaming, mental depression. **CV:** *Bradycardia,* palpitation, cold extremities, Raynaud's phenomenon, intermittent claudication, angina pectoris, CHF, intensification of AV block, AV dissociation, complete heart block, cardiac arrest. **GI:** Nausea, *heartburn,* gastric pain, diarrhea or constipation, flatulence. **Hematologic:** Eosinophilia, thrombocytopenic and nonthrombocytopenic purpura, agranulocytosis (rare). **Skin:** Dry skin, pruritus, skin eruptions. **Special Senses:** Dry mouth and mucous membranes. **Metabolic:** Hypoglycemia. **Respiratory:** Bronchospasm (with high doses), *shortness of breath.*

DIAGNOSTIC TEST INTERFERENCE In common with other beta-blockers, metoprolol may cause elevated ***BUN*** and ***serum creatinine levels*** (patients with severe heart disease), elevated ***serum transaminase, alkaline phosphatase, lactate dehydrogenase,*** and ***serum uric acid.***

INTERACTIONS Drug: BARBITURATES, **rifampin** may decrease effects of metoprolol; **cimetidine, methimazole, propylthiouracil,** ORAL CONTRACEPTIVES may increase effects of metoprolol; additive bradycardia with **digoxin;** effects of both metoprolol and **hydralazine** may be increased; **indomethacin** may attenuate hypotensive response; BETA AGONISTS and metoprolol mutually antagonistic; **verapamil** may increase risk of heart block and bradycardia; increases **terbutaline** serum levels.

PHARMACOKINETICS Absorption: Readily from GI tract; 50% of dose reaches systemic circulation. **Onset:** 15 min. **Peak:** 1.5 h; 20 min (IV). **Duration:** 13–19 h. **Distribution:** Crosses blood–brain barrier and placenta; distributed into breast milk. **Metabolism:** Extensively in liver (CYP2D6). **Elimination:** In urine. **Half-Life:** 3–4 h.

NURSING IMPLICATIONS

Assessment & Drug Effects

- Take apical pulse and BP before administering drug. Report to physician significant changes in rate, rhythm, or quality of pulse or variations in BP prior to administration.
- Monitor BP, HR, and ECG carefully during IV administration.
- Expect maximal effect on BP after 1 wk of therapy.
- Take several BP readings close to the end of a 12 h dosing interval to evaluate adequacy of dosage for patients with hypertension, particularly in patients on twice daily doses. Some patients require doses 3 times a day to maintain satisfactory control.
- Observe hypertensive patients with CHF closely for impending heart failure: Dyspnea on exertion, orthopnea, night cough, edema, distended neck veins.
- Lab tests: Obtain baseline and periodic evaluations of blood cell counts, blood glucose, liver and kidney function.
- Monitor I&O, daily weight; auscultate daily for pulmonary rales.
- Monitor for and report signs of mental depression.

Patient & Family Education

- Learn how to take radial pulse before each dose. Report to physician if pulse is slower than base rate (e.g., 60 bpm) or becomes irregular. Consult physician for parameters.
- Reduce insomnia or increased dreaming by avoiding late evening doses.
- Monitor blood glucose (diabetics) for loss of glycemic control. Drug may mask some symptoms of hypoglycemia (e.g., BP and HR changes) and prolong hypoglycemia. Be alert to other possible

M

signs of hypoglycemia not affected by metoprolol and report to physician if present: Sweating, fatigue, hunger, inability to concentrate.

- Protect extremities from cold and do not smoke. Report cold, painful, or tender feet or hands or other symptoms of Raynaud's disease (intermittent pallor, cyanosis or redness, paresthesias). Physician may prescribe a vasodilator.
- Report immediately to physician the onset of problems with vision.
- Learn measures to relieve dry mouth; rinse mouth frequently with water, increase noncalorie liquid intake if inadequate, chew sugarless gum or suck hard candy.
- Relieve eye dryness by using sterile artificial tears available OTC.
- Do not drive or engage in potentially hazardous activities until response to drug is known.
- Reduce dosage gradually over a period of 1–2 wk when drug is discontinued. Sudden withdrawal can result in increase in anginal attacks and MI in patients with angina pectoris and thyroid storm in patients with hyperthyroidism.

M

METRONIDAZOLE Pr

(me-troe-ni'da-zole)

Flagyl, Flagyl ER, Flagyl IV, MetroCream, MetroGel, MetroGel Vaginal, MetroLotion, Noritate, Vandazole

Classifications: ANTITRICHOMONAL; AMEBICIDE; ANTIBIOTIC

Therapeutic: AMEBICIDE

Pregnancy Category: B

AVAILABILITY 250 mg, 500 mg tablets; 375 mg capsules; 750 mg sustained release tablets; 500 mg vials; 0.75% lotion, emulsion; 0.75%, 1% cream; 0.75%, 1% gel

ACTION & *THERAPEUTIC EFFECT*

Synthetic compound with trichomonacidal and amebicidal activity as well as antibacterial activity. *Has direct trichomonacidal and amebicidal activity; exhibits antibacterial activity against obligate anaerobic bacteria, gram-negative anaerobic bacilli, and* Clostridia.

USES Asymptomatic and symptomatic trichomoniasis in females and males; acute intestinal amebiasis and amebic liver abscess; preoperative prophylaxis in colorectal surgery, elective hysterectomy or vaginal repair, and emergency appendectomy. IV metronidazole is used for the treatment of serious infections caused by susceptible anaerobic bacteria in intra-abdominal infections, skin infections, gynecologic infections, septicemia, and for both pre- and postoperative prophylaxis, bacterial vaginosis. *Topical:* Rosacea.

UNLABELED USES Treatment of pseudomembranous colitis, Crohn's disease, *H. pylori* eradication.

CONTRAINDICATIONS Blood dyscrasias; active CNS disease; lactation.

CAUTIOUS USE Coexistent candidiasis; seizure disorders; heart failure; older adults; severe hepatic disease; renal impairment/failure; pregnancy (category B); alcoholism; liver disease.

ROUTE & DOSAGE

Trichomoniasis

Adult: **PO** 2 g once or 250 mg t.i.d. × 7 days

Child/Infant: **PO** 15–30 mg/kg/day q8h × 7 days

Giardiasis, *Gardnerella*

Adult: **PO** 500 mg b.i.d. × 7 days OR 750 ER tablet daily × 7 days

Vaginal Once or twice daily × 5 days

Amebiasis

Adult: **PO** 500–750 mg t.i.d. × 5–10 days
Child: **PO** 35–50 mg/kg/day in 3 divided doses × 10 days

Anaerobic Infections

Adult: **PO** 7.5 mg/kg q6h (max: 4 g/day) **IV Loading Dose** 15 mg/kg **IV Maintenance Dose** 7.5 mg/kg q6h (max: 4 g/day)
Child: **PO** 15–35 mg/kg/day divided q8h (max: 4 g/day) **IV** 30 mg/kg/day divided q6h
Neonate: **IV** *Weight less than 1.2 kg,* 7.5 mg q48h; *younger than 7 days/weight 1.2 kg–2 kg,* 7.5 mg q24h; *younger than 7 days/weight greater than 2 kg,* 15 mg/kg q12h; *older than 7 days/weight 1.2 kg–2 kg,* 15 mg/kg q12h; *older than 7 days/weight greater than 2 kg,* 30 mg/kg q12h

Pseudomembranous Colitis

Adult: **PO** 250–500 mg 3–4 times daily × 10 days

Rosacea

Adult: **Topical** Apply 0.75% gel as a thin film to affected area b.i.d.; apply 1% gel as a thin film to affected area daily

ADMINISTRATION

Oral

- Crush tablets before ingestion if patient cannot swallow whole.
- Ensure that Flagyl ER (extend release form) is not chewed or crushed. It **must be** swallowed whole. Give on an empty stomach, 1 h before or 2 h after meals.
- Give immediately before, with, or immediately after meals or with food or milk to reduce GI distress.
- Give lower than normal doses in presence of liver disease.

Topical

- Apply a thin film to affected area only.

Intravenous

Note: Verify correct IV concentration and rate of infusion for administration to neonates, infants, or children with physician.

PREPARE: **Intermittent:** Single-dose flexible containers (500 mg/100 mL) are ready for use without further dilution. ▪ *Flagyl IV powder vial:* Sequence for preparing solution (important) consists of (1) reconstitution with 4.4 mL sterile water or NS, (2) dilution in IV solution to yield 8 mg/mL in NS, D5W, or LR, (3) pH neutralization with approximately 5 mEq sodium bicarbonate injection for each 500 mg of Flagyl IV used. ▪ Avoid use of aluminum-containing equipment when manipulating IV product (including syringes equipped with aluminum needles or hubs).

ADMINISTER: **Intermittent:** Give IV solution slowly at a rate of one dose per hour.

INCOMPATIBILITIES **Solution/additive: TPN, amoxicillin/clavulanate, aztreonam, dopamine. Y-site: Amphotericin B cholesteryl complex, aztreonam, filgrastim, meropenem, warfarin.**

- Note: Precipitation occurs if neutralized solution is refrigerated. ▪ Note: Use diluted and neutralized solution within 24 h of preparation.

- Store at 15°–30° C (59°–86° F); protect from light. ▪ Reconstituted Flagyl

M

IV is chemically stable for 96 h when stored below 30° C (86° F) in room light. ▪ Diluted and neutralized IV solutions containing Flagyl IV should be used within 24 h of mixing.

ADVERSE EFFECTS (≥1%) **Body as a Whole:** Hypersensitivity (rash, urticaria, pruritus, flushing), fever, fleeting joint pains, overgrowth of *Candida*. **CNS:** Vertigo, headache, ataxia, confusion, irritability, depression, restlessness, weakness, fatigue, drowsiness, insomnia, paresthesias, sensory neuropathy (rare). **GI:** *Nausea,* vomiting, anorexia, epigastric distress, abdominal cramps, diarrhea, constipation, dry mouth, metallic or bitter taste, proctitis. **Urogenital:** Polyuria, dysuria, pyuria, incontinence, cystitis, decreased libido, dyspareunia, dryness of vagina and vulva, sense of pelvic pressure. **Special Senses:** Nasal congestion. **CV:** ECG changes (flattening of T wave).

DIAGNOSTIC TEST INTERFERENCE **Metronidazole** may interfere with certain chemical analyses for ***AST,*** resulting in decreased values.

INTERACTIONS Drug: ORAL ANTICOAGULANTS potentiate hypoprothrombinemia; **alcohol** may elicit disulfiram reaction; oral solutions of **citalopram, ritonavir; lopinavir/ritonavir,** and IV formulations of **sulfamethoxazole; trimethoprim, nitroglycerin** may elicit disulfiram reaction due to the alcohol content of the dosage form; **disulfiram** causes acute psychosis; **phenobarbital** increases metronidazole metabolism; may increase **lithium** levels; **fluorouracil, azathioprine** may cause transient neutropenia.

PHARMACOKINETICS Absorption: 80% absorbed from GI tract. **Peak:** 1–3 h. **Distribution:** Widely distributed to most body tissues, including CSF, bone, cerebral and hepatic abscesses; crosses placenta; distributed in breast milk. **Metabolism:** 30–60% in liver. **Elimination:** 77% in urine; 14% in feces within 24 h. **Half-Life:** 6–8 h.

NURSING IMPLICATIONS

Assessment & Drug Effects

- Discontinue therapy immediately if symptoms of CNS toxicity (see Appendix F) develop. Monitor especially for seizures and peripheral neuropathy (e.g., numbness and paresthesia of extremities).
- Lab tests: Obtain total and differential WBC counts before, during, and after therapy, especially if a second course is necessary.
- Monitor for S&S of sodium retention, especially in patients on corticosteroid therapy or with a history of CHF.
- Monitor patients on lithium for elevated lithium levels.
- Report appearance of candidiasis or its becoming more prominent with therapy to physician promptly.
- Repeat feces examinations, usually up to 3 mo, to ensure that amebae have been eliminated.

Patient & Family Education

- Adhere closely to the established regimen without schedule interruption or changing the dose.
- Refrain from intercourse during therapy for trichomoniasis unless male partner wears a condom to prevent reinfection.
- Have sexual partners receive concurrent treatment. Asymptomatic trichomoniasis in the male is a frequent source of reinfection of the female.
- Do not drink alcohol during therapy; may induce a disulfiram-type

reaction (see Appendix F). Avoid alcohol or alcohol-containing medications for at least 48 h after treatment is completed.

- Urine may appear dark or reddish brown (especially with higher than recommended doses). This appears to have no clinical significance.
- Report symptoms of candidal overgrowth: Furry tongue, color changes of tongue, glossitis, stomatitis; vaginitis, curd-like, milky vaginal discharge; proctitis. Treatment with a candidacidal agent may be indicated.

METYROSINE

(me-tye'roe-seen)

Demser

Classification: ENZYME INHIBITOR

Therapeutic: PHEOCHROMOCYTOMA AGENT

Pregnancy Category: C

AVAILABILITY 250 mg capsules

ACTION & *THERAPEUTIC EFFECT* Blocks the enzyme tyrosine hydroxylase, thus inhibiting the conversion of tyrosine to DOPA, which is the initial and rate-setting step in synthesis of catecholamines (dopamine, epinephrine, norepinephrine). *In patients with pheochromocytoma, reduces catecholamine synthesis as much as 80%, ameliorating hypertensive attacks and associated symptoms.*

USES Short-term management of pheochromocytoma until surgery is performed, in long-term control when surgery is contraindicated, and in patients with malignant pheochromocytoma.

UNLABELED USES Has been used in selected patients with schizophrenia to potentiate antipsychotic effects of phenothiazines.

CONTRAINDICATIONS Control of essential hypertension; dehydration. Safe use in children younger than 12 y is not established.

CAUTIOUS USE Impaired liver or kidney function; Parkinson's disease; pregnancy (category C), lactation.

ROUTE & DOSAGE

Pheochromocytoma

Adult: **PO** 250 mg q.i.d., may increase to 2–3 g/day in divided doses (max: 4 g/day)

ADMINISTRATION

Oral

- Give each dose with a full glass of water and be consistent about time medication is to be taken.
- Store at 15°–30° C (59°–86° F).

ADVERSE EFFECTS (≥1%) **CNS:** *Sedation,* fatigue; *extrapyramidal signs: Drooling, difficulty in speaking (dysarthria), tremors,* jaw stiffness (trismus); frank parkinsonism, psychic disturbances (anxiety, depression, hallucinations, disorientation, confusion), headache, muscle spasms. **GI:** *Diarrhea,* nausea, vomiting, abdominal pain, dry mouth. **Skin:** Rash, urticaria. **Urogenital:** Transient dysuria, crystalluria, hematuria, impotence, failure of ejaculation. **Endocrine:** Breast swelling, galactorrhea. **Body as a Whole:** Peripheral edema, nasal stuffiness, shortness of breath. **Hematologic:** Eosinophilia.

DIAGNOSTIC TEST INTERFERENCE False increases in ***urinary catecholamines*** may occur because of catechol metabolites of metyrosine.

INTERACTIONS Drug: Alcohol and other CNS DEPRESSANTS add to sedation and CNS depression; **droperidol, haloperidol,** PHENOTHIAZINES potentiate extrapyramidal effects.

PHARMACOKINETICS Absorption: Readily absorbed from GI tract. **Peak:** 2–3 days. **Duration:** 3–4 days. **Distribution:** Crosses blood–brain barrier. **Elimination:** In urine. **Half-Life:** 3.4–7.2 h.

NURSING IMPLICATIONS

Assessment & Drug Effects

- Monitor therapeutic effectiveness with frequent assessment of vital signs.
- Monitor I&O ratio and pattern. Fluid intake **must be** enough (e.g., 10–12 glasses or more) to maintain urinary output of 2000 mL or more to minimize risk of crystalluria.
- Perform routine urinalysis; if crystals occur, increase fluid intake further. If crystalluria persists, decrease drug dosage or discontinued.
- Lab tests: Obtain baseline and periodic measurements of urinary catecholamines and their metabolites (metanephrines and VMA). Metabolite excretion should decrease in patients with pheochromocytoma. Other baseline and regular determinations include kidney and liver function tests (in patients with dysfunction), and blood and urine glucose tests.
- Supervise ambulation. Sedative effects occur commonly within the first 24 h after drug is started. Maximal sedative effects in 2 or 3 days.

Patient & Family Education

- Notify physician if following adverse effects occur: Diarrhea, particularly if it is severe or persists, painful urination, jaw stiffness, drooling, difficult speech, tremors, disorientation. Dosage reduction or discontinuation of drug may be indicated.
- Avoid driving and potentially hazardous activities until response to drug is known.
- Be aware that abrupt withdrawal of metyrosine may result in psychic stimulation, feeling of increased energy, temporary changes in sleep pattern (usually insomnia). Symptoms may last for 2 or 3 days.
- Carry medical identification at all times if on prolonged therapy and notify all physicians and dentists involved in care about drug regimen.

MEXILETINE

(mex-il′e-teen)

Mexitil

Classification: ANTIARRHYTHMIC, CLASS IB

Therapeutic: ANTIARRHYTHMIC, CLASS IB

Prototype: Lidocaine

Pregnancy Category: C

AVAILABILITY 150 mg, 200 mg, 250 mg capsules

ACTION & *THERAPEUTIC EFFECT* Analog of lidocaine with class IB antiarrhythmic properties. Shortens action potential refractory period duration and improves resting potential. Produces modest suppression of sinus node automatically and AV nodal conduction. Prolongs the His-to-ventricular interval only if patient has preexisting conduction disturbance. *Has antiarrhythmic properties for ventricular disturbances.*

USES Acute and chronic ventricular arrhythmias; prevention of recurrent cardiac arrests; suppression of PVCs due to ventricular tachyarrhythmias.

UNLABELED USES Wolff-Parkinson-White syndrome and supraventricular arrhythmias.

CONTRAINDICATIONS Severe left ventricular failure, cardiogenic shock, severe bradyarrhythmias. Preexisting second- or third-degree heart block without pacemaker; cardiogenic shock; concurrent administration of drugs which alter urinary pH; lactation.

CAUTIOUS USE Patients with sinus node conduction irregularities, intraventricular conduction abnormalities; hypotension; severe congestive heart failure; renal failure; liver dysfunction; pregnancy (category C).

ROUTE & DOSAGE

Ventricular Arrhythmias

Adult: **PO** 200–300 mg q8h (max: 1200 mg/day)
Child: **PO** 1.4–5 mg/kg q8h

ADMINISTRATION

Oral

- Give with food or milk to reduce gastric distress.

ADVERSE EFFECTS (≥1%) **CNS:** *Dizziness, tremor, nervousness, incoordination,* headache, blurred vision, paresthesias, numbness. **CV:** Exacerbated arrhythmias, palpitations, chest pain, syncope, hypotension. **GI:** *Nausea, vomiting, heartburn,* diarrhea, constipation, dry mouth, abdominal pain. **Skin:** Rash. **Body as a Whole:** Dyspnea, edema, arthralgia, fever, malaise, hiccups. **Urogenital:** Impotence, urinary retention.

INTERACTIONS Drug: Phenytoin, phenobarbital, rifampin may decrease mexiletine levels; **cimetidine, fluvoxamine** may increase mexiletine levels; may increase **theophylline** levels; may increase proarrhythmic effects of **dofetilide** (separate administration by at least 1 wk).

PHARMACOKINETICS Absorption: Readily from GI tract. **Peak:** 2–3 h. **Distribution:** Distributed into breast milk. **Metabolism:** In liver. **Elimination:** In urine; renal elimination increases with urinary acidification. **Half-Life:** 10–12 h.

NURSING IMPLICATIONS

Assessment & Drug Effects

- Check pulse and BP before administration; make sure both are stabilized.
- Effective serum concentration range is 0.5–2 mcg/mL.
- Lab tests: Baseline and periodic liver function tests.
- Supervise ambulation in the weak, debilitated patient or the older adult during drug stabilization period. CNS adverse reactions predominate (e.g., intention tremors, nystagmus, blurred vision, dizziness, ataxia, confusion, nausea).
- Encourage drug compliance; affected particularly by the distressing adverse effects of tremor, ataxia, and eye symptoms.
- Check frequently with patient about adherence to drug regimen. If adverse effects are increasing, consult physician. Dose adjustment or discontinuation may be needed.

Patient & Family Education

- Learn about pulse parameters to be reported: Changes in rhythm and rate (bradycardia = pulse below 60); symptomatic bradycardia (light-headedness, syncope, dizziness), and postural hypotension.

M

MICAFUNGIN

(my-ca-fun'gin)
Mycamine
Classification: ANTIFUNGAL, ECHINOCANDIN
Therapeutic: ANTIFUNGAL
Prototype: Caspofungin
Pregnancy Category: C

AVAILABILITY 50 mg vial

ACTION & *THERAPEUTIC EFFECT* Micafungin is an antifungal agent that inhibits the synthesis of glucan, an essential component of fungal cell walls. Micafungin does not allow *Candida* fungi to replicate. *Has antifungal effects against various species of* Candida.

USES Treatment of patients with esophageal candidiasis, and for prophylaxis of *Candida* infections in patients undergoing hematopoietic stem cell transplantation. Susceptible organisms include *C. albicans*, *C. glabrata*, *C. krusei*, *C. parapsilosis*, and *C. tropicalis*.

UNLABELED USES Treatment of pulmonary *Aspergillus* infection.

CONTRAINDICATIONS Hypersensitivity to any component in micafungin. Safety and efficacy in children younger than 18 y are unknown.

CAUTIOUS USE Hepatic and renal dysfunction; older adult; pregnancy (category C); lactation.

ROUTE & DOSAGE

Esophageal Candidiasis
Adult: **IV** 150 mg/day over 1 h × 14 days

Candidiasis Prophylaxis in Hematopoietic Stem Cell Transplantation Patients
Adult: **IV** 50 mg/day over 1 h × 18 days

ADMINISTRATION

Intravenous

***PREPARE:* IV Infusion:** Reconstitute the 50 or 100 mg vial with 5 mL NS (without a bacteriostatic agent) to yield 10 mg/mL or 20 mg/mL, respectively. ▪ Gently swirl, but do not shake, to dissolve. Solution should be clear. ▪ Add required dose to 100 mL NS.

***ADMINISTER:* IV Infusion:** Give slowly over 1 h. ▪ Flush existing IV line with NS before/after infusion. ▪ Protect IV solution from light.

INCOMPATIBILITIES Do not mix or infuse with any other medications.

▪ Store reconstituted vial and IV solution for up to 24 h at 25° C (77° F). ▪ Protect from light.

ADVERSE EFFECTS (≥1%) **CNS:** *Headache,* dizziness, somnolence. **CV:** Flushing, hypertension, phlebitis. **GI:** *Nausea, vomiting, diarrhea,* abdominal pain. **Hematologic/Lymphatic:** Anemia, hemolytic anemia, leukemia, neutropenia, thrombocytopenia. **Hepatic:** Elevated liver enzymes, jaundice. **Metabolic:** Hypocalcemia, hypokalemia, hypomagnesemia. **Skin:** Pruritus, rash. **Body as a Whole:** Injection site pain, pyrexia, rigors.

INTERACTIONS Drug: Micafungin increases levels of **sirolimus** and **nifedipine.**

PHARMACOKINETICS Distribution: 99% protein bound. **Metabolism:** Biotransformation primarily in the liver. **Elimination:** Fecal (major) and renal. **Half-Life:** 14–17 h.

NURSING IMPLICATIONS

Assessment & Drug Effects

- Monitor for S&S of hypersensitivity during IV infusion; frequently monitor IV site for thrombophlebitis.

Common adverse effects in *italic*, life-threatening effects <u>underlined</u>; generic names in **bold**; classifications in SMALL CAPS; ♣ Canadian drug name; ℗ Prototype drug

- Monitor for S&S of hemolytic anemia (i.e., jaundice).
- Lab tests: Periodic LFTs, kidney function tests, serum electrolytes, and CBC.
- Monitor blood levels of sirolimus or nifedipine with concurrent therapy. If sirolimus or nifedipine toxicity occurs, dosages of these drugs should be reduced.

Patient & Family Education

- Report immediately any of the following: Facial swelling, wheezing, difficulty breathing or swallowing, tightness in chest, rash, hives, itching, or sensation of warmth.

MICONAZOLE NITRATE

(mi-kon′a-zole)

Monistat-Derm, Monistat 3, Monistat 7, Femizol-M, M-Zole, Micatin, Tetterine, Fungoid, Lotrimin AF, Desenex

Classification: AZOLE ANTIFUNGAL
Therapeutic: ANTIFUNGAL
Prototype: Fluconazole
Pregnancy Category: C

AVAILABILITY 100 mg, 200 mg vaginal suppositories; 2% cream; 2% ointment; 2% powder; 2% spray; 2% solution

ACTION & *THERAPEUTIC EFFECT* Broad-spectrum agent with fungicidal activity. Appears to inhibit uptake of components essential for cell reproduction and growth as well as cell wall structure, thus promoting cell death of fungi. *Effective against* Candida albicans *and other species of this genus. Inhibits growth of common dermatophytes, and the organism responsible for tinea versicolor.*

USES Vulvovaginal candidiasis, tinea pedis (athlete's foot), tinea cruris, tinea corporis, and tinea versicolor caused by dermatophytes.

CONTRAINDICATIONS Hypersensitivity to miconazole; children younger than 2 y (**topical**); children younger than 12 y (**vaginal**).
CAUTIOUS USE Hypersensitivity to azole antifungals; diabetes mellitus; bone marrow suppression; pregnancy (category C), lactation.

ROUTE & DOSAGE

Fungal Infection

Adult: **Topical** Apply cream sparingly to affected areas twice a day, and once daily for tinea versicolor, for 2 wk (improvement expected in 2–3 days, tinea pedis is treated for 1 mo to prevent recurrence) **Intravaginal** Insert suppository or vaginal cream each night × 7 days (100 mg) or 3 days (200 mg)

ADMINISTRATION

Topical

- Apply cream sparingly to intertriginous areas (between skin folds) to avoid maceration of skin.
- Massage affected area gently until cream disappears.
- Store at 15°–30° C (59°–86° F) unless otherwise directed.

ADVERSE EFFECTS (≥1%) **Urogenital:** Vulvovaginal burning, itching, or irritation; maceration, allergic contact dermatitis.

INTERACTIONS Drug: May increase INR with **warfarin;** may inactivate **nonoxynol-9** spermicides.

PHARMACOKINETICS Absorption: Small amount absorbed from vagina. **Metabolism:** Rapidly metabolized in liver. **Elimination:** In urine and feces. **Half-Life:** 2.1–24 h.

NURSING IMPLICATIONS

Assessment & Drug Effects

- Expect clinical improvement from topical application in 1 or 2 wk. If no improvement in 4 wk, diagnosis is reevaluated. Treat tinea pedis infection for 1 mo to assure permanent recovery.

Patient & Family Education

- Complete full course of treatment to ensure recovery.
- Do not interrupt vaginal application during menstrual period.
- Avoid contact of drug with eyes.

M

MIDAZOLAM HYDROCHLORIDE

(mid'az-zoe-lam)

Classifications: ANESTHETIC; BENZODIAZEPINE; ANXIOLYTIC; SEDATIVE-HYPNOTIC
Therapeutic: ANESTHETIC; ANTIANXIETY; SEDATIVE-HYPNOTIC
Prototype: Lorazepam
Pregnancy Category: D
Controlled Substance: Schedule IV

AVAILABILITY 2 mg/mL syrup; 1 mg/mL, 5 mg/mL injection

ACTION & *THERAPEUTIC EFFECT* Short-acting benzodiazepine that intensifies activity of gamma-aminobenzoic acid (GABA), a major inhibitory neurotransmitter of the brain, interfering with its reuptake and promoting its accumulation at neuronal synapses. Calms the patient, relaxes skeletal muscles, and in high doses produces sleep. *Is a CNS depressant with muscle relaxant, sedative-hypnotic, anticonvulsant, and amnestic properties.*

USES Sedation before general anesthesia, induction of general anesthesia; to impair memory of perioperative events (anterograde amnesia); for conscious sedation prior to short diagnostic and endoscopic procedures; and as the hypnotic supplement to nitrous oxide and oxygen (balanced anesthesia) for short surgical procedures.

CONTRAINDICATIONS Intolerance to benzodiazepines; acute narrow-angle glaucoma; shock, coma; acute alcohol intoxication; intra-arterial injection; status asthmaticus; pregnancy (category D), obstetric delivery, lactation.

CAUTIOUS USE COPD; chronic kidney failure; cardiac disease; pulmonary insufficiency; dementia; electrolyte imbalance; neuromuscular disease; Parkinson's disease; psychosis; CHF; older adults; bipolar disorder.

ROUTE & DOSAGE

Conscious Sedation

Adult: **IM** 0.07–0.08 mg/kg 30–60 min before procedure **IV** 1–2.5 mg, may repeat in 2 min prn; Intubated Patients, 0.05–0.2 mg/kg/h by continuous infusion
Child: **IM** 0.08 mg/kg × 1 dose **PR** 0.3 mg/kg × 1 dose; *Intubated Patients,* 2 mcg/kg/min by continuous infusion, may increase by 1 mcg/kg/min q30min until light sleep is induced
Neonate: **IV** 0.5–1 mcg/kg/min

IV Induction for General Anesthesia

Adult: **IV** Premedicated, 0.15–0.25 mg/kg over 20–30 sec, allow 2 min for effect **IV** Non-premedicated, 0.3–0.35 mg/kg over 20–30 sec, allow 2 min for effect

Child: **IV** 0.15 mg/kg followed by 0.05 mg/kg q2min × 1–3 doses

Status Epilepticus

Child: **IV Loading Dose** Older than 2 mo, 0.15 mg/kg **IV Maintenance Dose** 1 mcg/kg/min infusion, may titrate upward as needed q5min

Preoperative Sedation

Child: **PO** *Younger than 5 y,* 0.5 mg/kg; *older than 5 y,* 0.4–0.5 mg/kg

ADMINISTRATION

Intramuscular

- Inject IM drug deep into a large muscle mass.

Intravenous

PREPARE: **Direct:** Dilute in D5W or NS to a concentration of 0.25 mg/mL (e.g., 1 mg in 4 mL or 5 mg in 20 mL). **IV Infusion:** Add 5 mL of the 5 mg/mL concentration to 45 mL of D5W or NS to yield 0.5 mg/mL.

ADMINISTER: **Direct for Conscious Sedation:** Give over 2 min or longer. **Direct for Induction of Anesthesia:** Give over 20–30 sec. **Direct for Neonate:** DO NOT give bolus dose; give over at least 2 min. **IV Infusion:** Give at a rate based on weight.

INCOMPATIBILITIES Solution/additive: **Lactated Ringer's, pentobarbital, perphenazine, prochlorperazine.** Y-site: **Albumin, amoxicillin, amoxicillin/clavulanate, amphotericin B cholesteryl complex, ampicillin, bumetanide, butorphanol, ceftazidime, cefuroxime, clonidine, dexamethasone, foscarnet, fosphenytoin, furosemide, hydrocortisone, imipenem/cilastatin, methotrexate, nafcillin, omeprazole, sodium bicarbonate, thiopental, TPN, trimethoprim/sulfamethoxazole.**

- Store at 15°–30° C (59°–86° F), therapeutic activity is retained for 2 y from date of manufacture.

ADVERSE EFFECTS (≥1%) **CNS:** *Retrograde amnesia,* headache, euphoria, drowsiness, excessive sedation, confusion. **CV:** Hypotension. **Special Senses:** Blurred vision, diplopia, nystagmus, pinpoint pupils. **GI:** Nausea, vomiting. **Respiratory:** Coughing, laryngospasm (rare), respiratory arrest. **Skin:** Hives, swelling, burning, pain, induration at injection site, tachypnea. **Body as a Whole:** Hiccups, chills, weakness.

INTERACTIONS Drug: Alcohol, CNS DEPRESSANTS, ANTICONVULSANTS potentiate CNS depression; **cimetidine** increases midazolam plasma levels, increasing its toxicity; may decrease antiparkinsonism effects of **levodopa;** may increase **phenytoin** levels; **smoking** decreases sedative and antianxiety effects. **Food: Grapefruit juice** (greater than 1 qt/day) may increase risk of myopathy and rhabdomyolysis. **Herbal: Kava, valerian** may potentiate sedation. **Echinacea, St. John's wort** may reduce efficacy.

PHARMACOKINETICS Onset: 1–5 min IV; 5–15 min IM, 20–30 min PO. **Peak:** 20–60 min. **Duration:** Less than 2 h IV; 1–6 h IM. **Distribution:** Crosses blood–brain barrier and placenta. **Metabolism:** In liver (CYP3A4). **Elimination:** In urine. **Half-Life:** 1–4 h.

NURSING IMPLICATIONS

Assessment & Drug Effects

- Inspect insertion site for redness, pain, swelling, and other signs of extravasation during IV infusion.

- Monitor closely for indications of impending respiratory arrest. Resuscitative drugs and equipment should be immediately available.
- Monitor for hypotension, especially if the patient is premedicated with a narcotic agonist analgesic.
- Monitor vital signs for entire recovery period. In obese patient, half-life is prolonged during IV infusion; therefore, duration of effects is prolonged (i.e., amnesia, postoperative recovery).
- Be aware that overdose symptoms include somnolence, confusion, sedation, diminished reflexes, coma, and untoward effects on vital signs.

Patient & Family Education

- Do not drive or engage in potentially hazardous activities until response to drug is known. You may feel drowsy, weak, or tired for 1–2 days after drug has been given.

M

MIDODRINE HYDROCHLORIDE

(mid'o-dreen)

Orvaten, ProAmatine

Classification: VASOPRESSOR

Therapeutic: ANTIHYPOTENSIVE

Prototype: Methoxamine

Pregnancy Category: C

AVAILABILITY 2.5 mg, 5 mg, 10 mg tablets

ACTION & *THERAPEUTIC EFFECT* Vasopressor and $alpha_1$ agonist that activates the alpha-adrenergic receptors of the arteries and veins, resulting in increased vascular tone and elevation in blood pressure. *Affects standing, sitting, and supine systolic and diastolic blood pressures. Indicated by an increase in 1-min standing systolic BP and subjective feelings of clinical improvement.*

USES Treatment of symptomatic orthostatic hypotension.

CONTRAINDICATIONS Severe organic heart disease; heart failure; kidney disease, renal failure; urinary retention; pheochromocytoma; thyrotoxicosis; MAOI therapy; persistent and excessive supine hypertension.

CAUTIOUS USE Renal impairment, hepatic impairment; history of visual problems; diabetes with hypotension or visual disorders; pregnancy (category C), lactation. Safety and efficacy in children are not established.

ROUTE & DOSAGE

Orthostatic Hypotension

Adult: **PO** 10 mg t.i.d. during the daytime hours, dosed not less than 3 h apart with last dose at least 4 h before bedtime (max: 20 mg/dose)

ADMINISTRATION

Oral

- Do not give at bedtime or before napping (within 4 h of lying supine for any length of time).
- Give with caution in persons with pretreatment, supine systolic BP 170 mm Hg or higher.
- Store at 15°–30° C (59°–86° F).

ADVERSE EFFECTS (≥1%) **Body as a Whole:** *Paresthesia,* chills, pain, facial flushing. **CNS:** Confusion, nervousness, anxiety. **CV:** *Hypertension.* **GI:** Dry mouth. **Skin:** *Pruritus, piloerection,* rash. **Urogenital:** *Dysuria, urinary retention, urinary frequency.*

INTERACTIONS Drug: May antagonize effects of **doxazosin, prazosin, terazosin;** may potentiate vasoconstrictive effects of **ephed-**

rine, phenylephrine, pseudoephedrine; may cause hypertensive crisis with MAOIS.

PHARMACOKINETICS Absorption: Rapidly from GI tract. **Peak:** Midodrine 0.5 h; desglymidodrine 1–2 h. **Metabolism:** Rapidly metabolized to desglymidodrine, the active metabolite. **Elimination:** In urine. **Half-Life:** Midodrine 25 min, desglymidodrine 3–4 h.

NURSING IMPLICATIONS

Assessment & Drug Effects

- Lab tests: Evaluate kidney and liver function prior to initiating therapy.
- Monitor supine and standing BP regularly. Withhold drug and notify physician if supine BP increases excessively; determine acceptable parameters.
- Monitor carefully effect of the drug in diabetics with orthostatic hypotension and those taking fludrocortisone acetate, which may increase intraocular pressure.

Patient & Family Education

- Take last daily dose 4 h before bedtime.
- Report immediately to physician sensations associated with supine hypertension (e.g., pounding in ears, headache, blurred vision, awareness of heart beating).
- Discontinue drug and report to physician if S&S of bradycardia develop (e.g., dizziness, pulse slowing, fainting).
- Do not take allergy drugs, cold preparations, or diet pills without consulting physician.

MIGLITOL

(mig'li-tol)

Glyset

Classifications: ANTIDIABETIC; ALPHA-GLUCOSIDASE INHIBITOR
Therapeutic: ANTIDIABETIC; GLYCEMIC CONTROL ENHANCER
Prototype: Acarbose
Pregnancy Category: B

AVAILABILITY 25 mg, 50 mg, 100 mg tablets

ACTION & *THERAPEUTIC EFFECT* Enzyme inhibition of intestinal glucosidases delaying the formation of glucose from saccharides in the small intestine. Miglitol does not enhance insulin secretion. *It delays the digestion of carbohydrates, lowers the postprandial hyperglycemia, and reduces the levels of glysylated hemoglobin (HbA1C) in type 2 diabetics.*

USES Adjunct to diet for control of type 2 diabetes; may be used alone or with a sulfonylurea.

CONTRAINDICATIONS Diabetic ketoacidosis; digestive or absorptive disorders; history of or partial intestinal obstruction, inflammatory bowel disease; hypersensitivity to miglitol; lactation.

CAUTIOUS USE Hypersensitivity to acarbose; creatinine clearance greater than 2 mg/dL; high stress conditions (i.e., surgery, trauma, etc.); pregnancy (category B). Safety and efficacy in children younger than 18 y unknown.

ROUTE & DOSAGE

Type 2 Diabetes Mellitis

Adult: **PO** 25 mg t.i.d. at the start of each meal, may increase after 4–8 wk to 50 mg t.i.d. (max: 100 mg t.i.d.)

ADMINISTRATION

Oral
- Give drug with first bite of each of the three main meals.
- Store at 15°–30° C (59°–86° F).

ADVERSE EFFECTS (≥1%) **GI:** *Abdominal pain, diarrhea, flatulence.* **Skin:** Rash. **Metabolic:** Hypoglycemia.

INTERACTIONS Drug: Miglitol may reduce bioavailability of **propranolol, ranitidine; charcoal, pancreatin, amylase, pancrelipase** may decrease effectiveness of miglitol. **Herbal: Garlic, ginseng** may potentiate hypoglycemic effects.

PHARMACOKINETICS Absorption: 25 mg dose is completely absorbed, amount absorbed decreases with increasing dose to where 100 mg dose is 50–70% absorbed. **Peak:** 2–3 h. **Distribution:** Minimal protein binding (less than 4%). **Metabolism:** Not metabolized. **Elimination:** Half-life 2 h; 95% excreted unchanged in urine, lower doses should be used in patients with renal impairment.

NURSING IMPLICATIONS

Assessment & Drug Effects
- Monitor for therapeutic effectiveness: Indicated by improved blood glucose levels and decreased HbA1C.
- Monitor for S&S of hypoglycemia when used in combination with sulfonylureas, insulin, other hypoglycemia agents.
- Lab tests: Monitor postprandial blood glucose values and HbA1C q3mo.
- Treat hypolgycemia with oral glucose (dextrose); miglitol interferes with the breakdown of sucrose (table sugar).

Patient & Family Education
- Keep a source of oral glucose available to treat low blood sugar; miglitol prevents digestive breakdown of table sugar.
- Abdominal discomfort, flatulence, and diarrhea tend to diminish with continued therapy.

MILNACIPRAN

(mil-na-see′pran)
Savella
Classifications: SEROTONIN NOREPHINEPHRINE REUPTAKE INHIBITOR (SNRI); ANALGESIC
Therapeutic: ANALGESIC; SNRI
Prototype: Venlafaxine
Pregnancy Category: C

AVAILABILITY 12.5 mg, 25 mg, 50 mg, 100 mg tablets

ACTION & *THERAPEUTIC EFFECT* Exact mechanism of central pain inhibition is unknown. Is a potent inhibitor of both neuronal norepinephrine and serotonin reuptake without affecting uptake of other neurotransmitters. *Effective in reducing the pain associated with fibromyalgia.*

USES Management of fibromyalgia.
UNLABELED USES Treatment of depression.

CONTRAINDICATIONS Within 14 days discontinued use of MAOIs; abrupt discontinuation of milnacipran; suicidal ideation; major depressive disorder; uncontrolled narrow-angle glaucoma; substantial alcohol use; chronic liver disease; ESRD; lactation; children younger than 17 y.
CAUTIOUS USE Suicidal tendencies; history of seizures or depression; history of cardiac disease or pre-ex-

isting tachyarrhythmias; male obstructive uropathies; history of GI bleeding; moderate and severe renal impairment; hepatic impairment; elderly; pregnancy (category C).

ROUTE & DOSAGE

Fibromyalgia

Adults/Adolescents (17 y or older): **PO** Initial dose of 12.5 mg once daily on day 1, increase to 12.5 mg b.i.d. on days 2 and 3, 25 mg b.i.d. on days 4–7, and then 50 mg b.i.d. Dose can be increased to 100 mg b.i.d. if needed.

Renal Impairment Dosage Adjustment

CrCl 5–29 mL/min: Decrease dose by 50% (i.e., 25–50 mg b.i.d.); less than 5 mL/min: Use not recommended

ADMINISTRATION

Oral

- Dose titration should occur over a period of 1 wk to the recommended dose.
- Give with food, if needed, to improve tolerability of drug.
- Do not give within 14 days of an MAOI.
- Store at 15°–30° C (59°–86° F).

ADVERSE EFFECTS (≥2%) **Body as a Whole:** Chest pain and discomfort, chills. **CNS:** Anxiety, *dizziness, headache,* hypoesthesia, *insomnia,* migraine, paresthesia, tension headache, tremor. **CV:** *Hot flush,* increased blood pressure, increased heart rate, palpitations, tachycardia. **GI:** Abdominal pain, *constipation,* dry mouth, *nausea,* vomiting. **Metabolic:** Decreased appetite. **Respiratory:** Dyspnea, upper respiratory tract infection. **Skin:** Hyperhidrosis, pruritus, rash. **Special Senses:** Blurred vision. **Urogenital:** Decreased urine flow, dysuria, ejaculation disorder, erectile dysfunction, libido decreased, prostatitis, scrotal pain, testicular pain and swelling, urinary hesitation and retention, urethral pain.

INTERACTIONS Drug: Lithium may increase risk of serotonin syndrome. Milnacipran may inhibit antihypertensive effect of **clonidine** and other ALPHA$_2$ AGONISTS. **Digoxin** may increase the risk of postural hypotension and tachycardia. Milnacipran may increase bleeding with **warfarin, aspirin**, and NSAIDS; concurrent use with **epinephrine** or **norepinephrine** may cause paroxysmal hypertension and arrhythmia; concurrent use with SELECTIVE SEROTONIN REUPTAKE INHIBITORS, SELECTIVE NOREPINEPHRINE REUPTAKE INHIBITORS, **tramadol**, OR 5-HT-2B/2D AGONISTS (TRIPTANS) may cause additive serotonergic effects, hypertension, and coronary vasoconstriction.

PHARMACOKINETICS Absorption: 85–90% bioavailability. **Distribution:** Minimal (13%) plasma protein binding. **Metabolism:** Less than 50% metabolized by liver. **Elimination:** Primarily renal. **Half-Life:** 6–8 h.

NURSING IMPLICATIONS

Assessment & Drug Effects

- Monitor for and report promptly unusual changes in behavior (e.g., depression, anxiety, panic attack, insomnia, aggressiveness, mania) or suicidal ideation. Monitor closely during initial few months of therapy and during periods of dosage adjustment.
- Monitor HR and BP closely and report promptly sustained BP elevations. Pre-existing hypertension should be controlled before initiating this drug.

- Monitor for orthostatic hypotension and tachycardia with concurrent digoxin use.
- Lab tests: Periodic serum sodium, especially with concurrent diuretic therapy.

Patient & Family Education

- Do not abruptly stop taking this drug. It should be tapered off gradually after extended use.
- Report prompt unusual changes in behavior or suicidal ideas.
- Do not engage in potentially hazardous activities until reaction to drug is known.
- Exercise care to take prescribed BP medications exactly as ordered.
- Concurrent use of aspirin or NSAIDs is not recommended due to increased risk of bleeding. Consult physician.
- Avoid consuming alcohol while taking this drug.

M

MILRINONE LACTATE

(mil′ri-none)

Primacor

Classifications: INOTROPIC AGENT; VASODILATOR

Therapeutic: INOTROPIC AGENT

Prototype: Inamrinone

Pregnancy Category: C

AVAILABILITY 200 mcg/mL, 1 mg/mL injection

ACTION & *THERAPEUTIC EFFECT* Has a positive inotropic action and is a vasodilator with little chronotropic activity. Inhibitory action against cyclic-AMP phosphodiesterase in cardiac and smooth vascular muscle. Increases cardiac contractility and myocardial contractility. *Therefore, increases cardiac output and decreases pulmonary wedge pressure and vascular resistance, without increasing myocardial oxygen demand or significantly increasing heart rate.*

USES Short-term management of CHF.

UNLABELED USES Short-term use to increase the cardiac index in patients with low cardiac output after surgery. To increase cardiac function prior to heart transplantation.

CONTRAINDICATIONS Hypersensitivity to milrinone; valvular heart disease; acute MI.

CAUTIOUS USE Older adult; atrial fibrillation, atrial flutter; renal disease; renal impairment, renal failure; pregnancy (category C), lactation. Safety and efficacy in children are not established.

ROUTE & DOSAGE

Heart Failure

Adult: **IV Loading Dose** 50 mcg/kg IV over 10 min **IV Maintenance Dose** 0.375–0.75 mcg/kg/min

ADMINISTRATION

Intravenous

Note: Correct preexisting hypokalemia before administering milrinone. ▪ See manufacturer's information for dosage reduction in the presence of renal impairment.

PREPARE: **IV Infusion Loading Dose:** Give undiluted or dilute each 1 mg in 1 mL NS or 0.45% NaCl. **IV Infusion Maintenance Dose:** Dilute 20 mg of milrinone in D5W, NS, or 0.45% NaCl to yield: 100 mcg/mL with 180 mL diluent; 150 mcg/mL with 113 mL diluent; 200 mcg/mL with 80 mL diluent.

ADMINISTER: **IV Infusion Loading Dose:** Give 50 mcg/kg over 10 min. **IV Infusion Maintenance Dose:** Give at a rate based on weight. Use a microdrip set and infusion pump.

INCOMPATIBILITIES **Solution/additive:** **Furosemide, procainamide.** **Y-site:** **Furosemide, imipenem/cilastatin, procainamide.**

- Store according to manufacturer's directions.

ADVERSE EFFECTS (≥1%) **CV:** Increased ectopic activity, PVCs, ventricular tachycardia, ventricular fibrillation, supraventricular arrhythmias; possible increase in angina symptoms, hypotension.

INTERACTIONS Drug: Disopyramide may cause excessive hypotension.

PHARMACOKINETICS Peak: 2 min. **Duration:** 2 h. **Distribution:** 70% protein bound. **Elimination:** 80–85% excreted unchanged in urine within 24 h. Active renal tubular secretion is primary elimination pathway. **Half-Life:** 1.7–2.7 h.

NURSING IMPLICATIONS

Assessment & Drug Effects

- Monitor cardiac status closely during and for several hours following infusion. Supraventricular and ventricular arrhythmias have occurred.
- Monitor BP and promptly slow or stop infusion in presence of significant hypotension. Closely monitor those with recent aggressive diuretic therapy for decreasing blood pressure.
- Monitor fluid and electrolyte status. Hypokalemia should be corrected whenever it occurs during administration.

Patient & Family Education

- Report immediately angina that occurs during infusion to physician.
- Be aware that drug may cause a headache, which can be treated with analgesics.

MINOCYCLINE HYDROCHLORIDE

(mi-noe-sye'kleen)

Arestin, Dynacin, Minocin

Classification: TETRACYCLINE ANTIBIOTIC

Therapeutic: ANTIBIOTIC

Prototype: Tetracycline

Pregnancy Category: D

AVAILABILITY 50 mg, 75 mg, 100 mg capsules; 50 mg, 75 mg, 100 mg tablets; 50 mg/5 mL suspension; 1 mg sustained release microspheres

ACTION & *THERAPEUTIC EFFECT* Semisynthetic tetracycline derivative which appears to be active against strains of *Staphylococci* resistant to other tetracyclines. Bacteriostatic action appears to be a result of reversible binding to ribosomal units of susceptible bacteria and inhibition of bacterial protein synthesis. *Effective against gram-positive and gram-negative bacteria, but usually used against gram-negative bacteria.*

USES Treatment of mucopurulent cervicitis, granuloma inguinale, lymphogranuloma venereum, proctitis, bronchitis, lower respiratory tract infections caused by *Mycoplasma pneumoniae,* Rickettsial infections, chlamydial infections, non-gonococcal urethritis, chlamydial conjunctivitis, plague, brucellosis, bartonellosis, tularemia, UTI, and prostatitis; acne vulgaris, gonorrhea, cholera, meningococcal carrier state.

M

CONTRAINDICATIONS Hypersensitivity to tetracyclines; oral administration in meningococcal infections; sunlight (UV) exposure; pregnancy (category D); children younger than 8 y.
CAUTIOUS USE Renal and hepatic impairment; older adults; lactation.

ROUTE & DOSAGE

Anti-infective
Adult: **PO** 200 mg followed by 100 mg q12h
Child (older than 8 y): **PO** 4.4 mg/kg followed by 2 mg/kg q12h

Acne
Adult: **PO** 50 mg 1–3 times/day

Meningococcal Carrier State
Adult: **PO** 100 mg q12h × 5 days
Child (older than 8 y): **PO** 4 mg/kg followed by 2 mg/kg q12h × 5 days (max: 100 mg/dose)

ADMINISTRATION

Oral
- Shake suspension well before administration.
- Ensure that sustained release tablets are swallowed whole.
- Check expiration date. Outdated tetracycline can cause severe adverse effects.

ADVERSE EFFECTS (≥1%) **CNS:** *Weakness, lightheadedness, ataxia, dizziness, or vertigo.* **GI:** Nausea, cramps, diarrhea, flatulence. **Hepatic:** Hepatitis, increased liver enzyme, hepatotoxicity.

INTERACTIONS Drug: ANTACIDS, **iron, calcium, magnesium, zinc, kaolin and pectin, sodium bicarbonate, bismuth subsalicylate** can significantly decrease minocycline absorption; effects of both **desmopressin** and minocycline antagonized; increases **digoxin** absorption, increasing risk of **digoxin** toxicity; **methoxyflurane** increases risk of kidney failure. **Food:** Dairy products significantly decrease minocycline absorption; food may also decrease its absorption.

PHARMACOKINETICS Absorption: 90–100% from GI tract. **Peak:** 2–3 h. **Distribution:** Tends to accumulate in adipose tissue; crosses placenta; distributed into breast milk. **Metabolism:** Partially metabolized. **Elimination:** 20–30% in feces; ~12% in urine. **Half-Life:** 11–26 h.

NURSING IMPLICATIONS

Assessment & Drug Effects
- Obtain history of hypersensitivity reactions prior to administration; drug is contraindicated with known tetracycline hypersensitivity.
- Lab: C&S should be drawn prior to initiation of therapy.
- Monitor carefully for signs of hypersensitivity response (see Appendix F), particularly in patients with history of allergies, especially to drugs.
- Monitor at-risk patients for S&S of superinfection (see Appendix F).
- Assess risk of toxic effects carefully; increases with renal and hepatic impairment.
- Supervise ambulation, since lightheadedness, dizziness, and vertigo occur frequently.

Patient & Family Education
- Avoid hazardous activities or those requiring alertness while taking minocycline.
- Use sunscreen when outdoors and otherwise protect yourself from direct sunlight since photosensitivity reaction may occur.

- Report vestibular adverse effects (e.g., dizziness), which usually occur during first week of therapy. Effects are reversible if drug is withdrawn.
- Report loose stools or diarrhea or other signs of superinfection promptly to physician.
- Use or add barrier contraceptive while taking this drug if using hormonal contraceptive.

MINOXIDIL

(mi-nox′i-dill)

Rogaine

Classifications: NONNITRATE VASODILATOR; ANTIHYPERTENSIVE

Therapeutic: ANTIHYPERTENSIVE

Prototype: Hydralazine

Pregnancy Category: C

AVAILABILITY 2.5 mg, 10 mg tablets; 2% solution

ACTION & *THERAPEUTIC EFFECT* Direct-acting vasodilator that appears to act by blocking calcium uptake through cell membranes. Reduces elevated systolic and diastolic blood pressures in supine and standing positions, by decreasing peripheral vascular resistance. *Effective as an antihypertensive agent. It increases heart rate and cardiac output. Topical minoxidil reverses balding to some degree.*

USES Treat severe hypertension that is symptomatic or associated with damage to target organs and is not manageable with maximum therapeutic doses of a diuretic plus two other antihypertensive drugs. Used with a diuretic to prevent fluid retention and a beta adrenergic blocking agent (e.g., propranolol) or an alpha-adrenergic agonist (e.g., clonidine or methyldopa) to prevent tachycardia. **Topical:** to treat alopecia areata and male pattern alopecia.

CONTRAINDICATIONS Pheochromocytoma; recent acute MI, dissecting aortic aneurysm, valvular dysfunction, heart failure; cardiac disease, angina, CAD, CVA; pulmonary hypertension; severe renal failure CrCl less than 10 mL/min; children younger than 12 y.

CAUTIOUS USE Severe renal impairment; recent MI (within preceding month); coronary artery disease, chronic CHF; pregnancy (category C), lactation.

ROUTE & DOSAGE

Hypertension

Adult: **PO** 5 mg/day, increased q3–5days up to 40 mg/day in single or divided doses as needed (max: 100 mg/day)
Child: **PO** 0.2 mg/kg/day (max: 5 mg/day) initially, gradually increased to 0.25–1 mg/kg/day in divided doses (max: 50 mg/day)

Alopecia

Adult: **Topical** Apply 1 mL of 2% solution to affected area b.i.d.

ADMINISTRATION

Oral

- Dose increments are usually made at 3–5 days intervals. If more rapid adjustment is necessary, adjustments can be made q6h with careful monitoring.

Topical

- Do not apply topical product to an irritated scalp (e.g., sunburn, psoriasis).
- Store at 15°–30° C (59°–86° F) in tightly covered container unless otherwise directed.

M

ADVERSE EFFECTS (≥1%) **CV:** *Tachycardia,* angina pectoris, *ECG changes,* pericardial effusion and tamponade, rebound hypertension (following drug withdrawal); *edema,* including pulmonary edema; *CHF (salt and water retention).* **Skin:** *Hypertrichosis,* transient pruritus, darkening of skin, hypersensitivity rash, Stevens-Johnson syndrome. With topical use: Itching, flushing, scaling, dermatitis, folliculitis. **Body as a Whole:** Fatigue.

DIAGNOSTIC TEST INTERFERENCE ***Hct, Hgb,*** and ***erythrocyte count*** usually decrease (about 7%) during early therapy; ***serum alkaline phosphatase, BUN,*** and ***creatinine*** may increase during early therapy.

INTERACTIONS Drug: Epinephrine, norepinephrine cause excessive cardiac stimulation; **guanethidine** causes profound orthostatic hypotension.

PHARMACOKINETICS Absorption: Readily absorbed from GI tract. **Onset:** 30 min PO; at least 4 mo topical. **Peak:** 2–8 h PO. **Duration:** 2–5 days PO; new hair growth will remain 3–4 mo after withdrawal of topical. **Distribution:** Widely distributed including into breast milk. **Metabolism:** In liver. **Elimination:** 97% in urine and feces. **Half-Life:** 4.2 h.

NURSING IMPLICATIONS

Assessment & Drug Effects

- Take BP and apical pulse before administering medication and report significant changes. Consult physician for parameters.
- Lab tests: Periodic serum electrolytes.
- Do not stop drug abruptly. Abrupt reduction in BP can result in CVA and MI. Keep physician informed.
- Monitor fluid and electrolyte balance closely throughout therapy. Sodium and water retention commonly occur. Consult physician regarding sodium restriction. Monitor potassium intake and serum potassium levels in patient on diuretic therapy.
- Monitor I&O and daily weight. Report unusual changes in I&O ratio or daily weight gain, greater than 1 kg (2 lb).
- Observe patient daily for edema and auscultate lungs for rales. Be alert to signs and symptoms of CHF (see Appendix F).
- Observe for symptoms of pericardial effusion or tamponade. Symptoms are similar to those of CHF, but additionally patient may have paradoxical pulse (normal inspiratory reduction in systolic BP may fall as much as 10–20 mm Hg).

Patient & Family Education

- Learn about usual pulse rate and count radial pulse for one full minute before taking drug. Report an increase of 20 or more bpm.
- Notify physician promptly if the following S&S appear: Increase of 20 or more bpm in resting pulse; breathing difficulty; dizziness; lightheadedness; fainting; edema (tight shoes or rings, puffiness, pitting); weight gain, chest pain, arm or shoulder pain; easy bruising or bleeding.
- Be aware of possibility of hypertrichosis: Elongation, thickening, and increased pigmentation of fine body hair, especially of face, arms, and back. Develops 3–9 wk after start of therapy and occurs in approximately 80% of patients; reversible within 1–6 mo after drug withdrawal.

MIRTAZAPINE Pr

(mir-taz′a-peen)

Remeron, Remeron SolTab

Classifications: ANTIDEPRESSANT, TETRACYCLIC; ANXIOLYTIC

Therapeutic: ANTIDEPRESSANT; ANTI-ANXIETY

Pregnancy Category: C

AVAILABILITY 15 mg, 30 mg, 45 mg tablets and orally disintegrating tablets

ACTION & *THERAPEUTIC EFFECT* Tetracyclic antidepressant pharmacologically and therapeutically similar to tricyclic antidepressants. Tetracyclics enhance central nonadrenergic and serotonergic activity; thought to be due to normalization of neurotransmission efficacy. Mirtazapine is a potent antagonist of 5-HT_2 and 5-HT_3 serotonin receptors. *Acts as antidepressant. Effectiveness is indicated by mood elevation.*

USES Treatment of depression.

CONTRAINDICATIONS Hypersensitivity to mirtazapine or mianserin; hypersensitivity to other antidepressants (e.g., tricyclic antidepressants and MAOI depressants), acute MI; fever, infection; agranulocytosis, neutropenia, hematologic disease; suicidal ideation; jaundice, ethanol intoxication; lactation.

CAUTIOUS USE History of cardiovascular or GI disorders; BPH, urinary retention; narrow-angle glaucoma, increased intraocular pressure; hepatic or renal impairment, renal failure; hypercholesterolemia, hypertriglyceridemia, thrombocytopenia; older adults; angina, cardiac arrhythmias, anticholinergic medications; bipolar disorder, mania, bone marrow suppression, PKU, history of MI; cerebrovascular disease, seizure disorder, seizures, stroke; depression; hypovolemia, surgery; closed-angle glaucoma; ileus, GI obstruction, dehydration; diabetes mellitus, diabetic ketoacidosis; pregnancy (category C). Safety and effectiveness in children are not established.

ROUTE & DOSAGE

Depression

Adult: **PO** 15 mg/day in single dose at bedtime, may increase q1–2wk (max: 45 mg/day)
Geriatric: **PO** Use lower doses

Renal or Hepatic Impairment Dosage Adjustment

Use lower doses

ADMINISTRATION

Oral

- Give preferably prior to sleep to minimize injury potential.
- Begin drug no sooner than 14 days after discontinuation of an MAO inhibitor.
- Reduce dosage as warranted with severe renal or hepatic impairment and in older adults.
- Store at 20°–25° C (68°–77° F) in tight, light-resistant container.

ADVERSE EFFECTS (≥1%) **Body as a Whole:** Asthenia, flu syndrome, back pain, general and peripheral edema, malaise. **CNS:** *Somnolence,* dizziness, abnormal dreams, abnormal thinking, tremor, confusion, depression, agitation, vertigo, twitching. **CV:** Hypertension, vasodilation. **GI:** Nausea, vomiting, abdominal pain, *increased appetite*/weight gain, *dry mouth, constipation,* anorexia, cholecystitis, stomatitis, colitis, abnormal liver function tests. **Respiratory:** Dyspnea, cough, sinusitis. **Skin:** Pruritus, rash. **Urogenital:** Urinary frequency.

M

INTERACTIONS Drug: Additive cognitive and motor impairment with **alcohol** or BENZODIAZEPINES; increase risk of hypertensive crisis with MAOIS. **Herbal: Kava, valerian** may potentiate sedative effects.

PHARMACOKINETICS Absorption: Rapidly absorbed from GI tract, 50% reaches systemic circulation. **Peak:** 2 h. **Distribution:** 85% protein bound. **Metabolism:** In liver by cytochrome P450 system (CYP2D6, CYP1A2, CYP3A4). **Elimination:** 75% in urine, 15% in feces. **Half-Life:** 20–40 h.

NURSING IMPLICATIONS

Assessment & Drug Effects

- Lab tests: Monitor WBC count with differential, lipid profile, and ALT/AST periodically.
- Monitor for worsening of depression or suicidal ideation.
- Assess for weight gain and excessive somnolence or dizziness.
- Monitor for orthostatic hypotension with a history of cardiovascular or cerebrovascular disease. Periodically monitor ECG especially in those with known cardiovascular disease.
- Monitor those with history of seizures for lowering of the seizure threshold.

Patient & Family Education

- Do not drive or engage in potentially hazardous activities until response to drug is known.
- Do not use alcohol while taking drug.
- Report immediately unexplained fever or S&S of infection, especially flu-like symptoms, to physician.
- Do not take other prescription or OTC drugs without consulting physician.
- Make position changes slowly especially from lying or sitting to standing. Report dizziness, palpitations, and fainting.
- Monitor weight periodically and report significant weight gains.

MISOPROSTOL

(my-so-prost'ole)
Cytotec
Classification: PROSTAGLANDIN
Therapeutic: PROSTAGLANDIN
Pregnancy Category: X

AVAILABILITY 100 mcg, 200 mcg tablets

ACTION & *THERAPEUTIC EFFECT* Synthetic prostaglandin E_1 analog, with both antisecretory (inhibiting gastric acid secretion) and mucosal protective properties. Increases bicarbonate and mucosal protective properties. Inhibits basal and nocturnal gastric acid secretion and acid secretion in response to a variety of stimuli, including meals, histamine, pentagastrin, and coffee. Produces uterine contractions that may endanger pregnancy and cause a miscarriage. *Inhibits basal and nocturanal gastric acid secretion.*

USES Prevention of NSAID (including aspirin-induced) gastric ulcers in patients at high risk of complications from a gastric ulcer (e.g., the older adult and patients with a concomitant debilitating disease or a history of ulcers). Drug is taken for the duration of NSAID therapy and does not interfere with the efficacy of the NSAID.

UNLABELED USES Short-term treatment of duodenal ulcers; cervical ripening and induction of labor.

CONTRAINDICATIONS History of allergies to prostaglandins; **topical:** Abnormal fetal position, caesarean

section, ectopic pregnancy; fetal disease, incomplete abortion; multiparity, placenta previa, vaginal bleeding; pregnancy (category X).
CAUTIOUS USE Renal impairment; inflammatory bowel disease; lactation. Safety in children younger than 18 y is not established.

ROUTE & DOSAGE

Prevention of NSAID-Induced Ulcers
Adult: **PO** 100–200 mcg q.i.d. p.c. and at bedtime or 200 mcg b.i.d. or t.i.d.

ADMINISTRATION

Oral
- Give with food to minimize GI adverse effects (manufacturer recommendation).
- Store away from heat, light, and moisture.

ADVERSE EFFECTS (≥1%) **CNS:** Headache. **GI:** *Diarrhea, abdominal pain,* nausea, flatulence, dyspepsia, vomiting, constipation. **Urogenital:** Spotting, cramps, dysmenorrhea, uterine contractions.

INTERACTIONS Drug: MAGNESIUM-CONTAINING ANTACIDS may increase diarrhea.

PHARMACOKINETICS Absorption: Readily from GI tract; extensive first pass metabolism. **Onset:** 30 min. **Peak:** 60–90 min. **Duration:** At least 3 h. **Metabolism:** In liver. **Elimination:** Primarily in urine; small amount in feces. **Half-Life:** 20–40 min.

NURSING IMPLICATIONS

Assessment & Drug Effects
- Monitor for diarrhea; may be minimized by giving drug after meals and at bedtime. Diarrhea is a common adverse effect that is dose related and usually self-limiting (often resolving in 8 days).

Patient & Family Education
- Avoid using concurrent magnesium-containing antacids because of increased incidence of diarrhea.
- Report postmenopausal bleeding to physician; it may be drug related.
- Avoid pregnancy during misoprostol therapy; use an effective contraception method while taking drug.
- Drug has abortifacient property. Contact physician and immediately discontinue drug if you become pregnant.

MITOMYCIN

(mye-toe-mye'sin)
Mutamycin, Mytozytrex
Classification: ANTINEOPLASTIC ANTIBIOTIC
Therapeutic: ANTINEOPLASTIC
Prototype: Doxorubicin
Pregnancy Category: D

AVAILABILITY 5 mg, 20 mg, 40 mg injection

ACTION & *THERAPEUTIC EFFECT* Potent antibiotic antineoplastic effective in certain tumors unresponsive to surgery, radiation, or other agents. It selectively inhibits synthesis of DNA. At high concentrations, cellular and enzymatic RNA as well as protein synthesis are suppressed. *Highly destructive to rapidly proliferating cells and slowly developing carcinomas.*

USES In combination with other chemotherapeutic agents in palliative, adjunctive treatment of disseminated adenocarcinoma of breast, pancreas, or stomach, squamous cell carcinoma of head, neck, lung, and cervix. Not recommended to replace surgery or radiotherapy or as a single primary therapeutic agent.

CONTRAINDICATIONS Hypersensitivity or idiosyncratic reaction; severe bone marrow suppression; thrombocytopenia; coagulation disorders or bleeding tendencies; overhydration; severe renal impairment with CrCl less than 30 mL/min; pregnancy (category D), lactation.

CAUTIOUS USE Renal impairment; myelosuppression; pulmonary disease or respiratory insufficiency; older adults.

ROUTE & DOSAGE

Cancer

Adult/Child: **IV** 10–20 mg/m²/day as a single dose q6–8wk, additional doses based on hematologic response

Renal Impairment Dosage Adjustment

CrCl less than 10 mL/min: Use 75% of dose

ADMINISTRATION

Intravenous

Note: Verify correct IV concentration and rate of infusion/injection for administration to children with physician.

PREPARE: **Direct:** Reconstitute each 5 mg vial with 10 mL sterile water for injection. Shake to dissolve. If product does not clear immediately, allow to stand at room temperature until solution is obtained. Reconstituted solution is purple. **IV Infusion:** Reconstituted solution may be further diluted to concentrations of 20–40 mcg in D5W, NS, or LR.

ADMINISTER: **Direct:** Give reconstituted solution over 5–10 min or longer. **IV Infusion:** Give over 10 min or longer as determined by total volume of solution. ▪ D5W IV solutions **must be** infused within 3 h of preparation (see storage, below). ▪ Monitor IV site closely. Avoid extravasation to prevent extreme tissue reaction (cellulitis) to the toxic drug.

INCOMPATIBILITIES **Solution/additive:** DEXTROSE-CONTAINING SOLUTIONS, **bleomycin. Y-site: Aztreonam, cefepime, etoposide, filgrastim, gemcitabine, piperacillin/tazobactam, sargramostim, topotecan, vinorelbine.**

▪ Store drug reconstituted with sterile water for injection (0.5 mg/mL) for 14 days refrigerated or 7 days at room temperature. ▪ Drug diluted in D5W (20–40 mcg/mL) is stable at room temperature for 3 h.

ADVERSE EFFECTS (≥1%) **CNS:** Paresthesias. **GI:** Stomatitis, *nausea, vomiting,* anorexia, hematemesis, diarrhea. **Hematologic:** Bone marrow toxicity (*thrombocytopenia, leukopenia* occurring 4–8 wk after treatment onset), thrombophlebitis, anemia. **Respiratory:** Acute bronchospasm, hemoptysis, dyspnea, nonproductive cough, pneumonia, interstitial pneumonitis. **Skin:** Desquamation; induration, pain, necrosis, cellulitis at injection site; reversible alopecia, purple discoloration of nail beds. **Body as a Whole:** Pain, headache, fatigue, edema. **Urogenital:** Hemolytic uremic syndrome, renal toxicity.

PHARMACOKINETICS Metabolism: Metabolized rapidly in liver. **Elimination:** In urine. **Half-Life:** 23–78 min.

NURSING IMPLICATIONS

Assessment & Drug Effects

- Lab tests: Perform WBC with differential, platelet count, PT, INR, aPTT, Hgb, Hct, and serum creatinine frequently during and for at least 7 wk after treatment.
- Do not administer if serum creatinine is greater than 1.7 mg/dL or if platelet count falls below 150,000/mm³ and WBC is down to 4000/mm³ or if prothrombin or bleeding times are prolonged.
- Monitor I&O ratio and pattern. Report any sign of impaired kidney function: Change in ratio, dysuria, hematuria, oliguria, frequency, urgency. Keep patient well hydrated (at least 2000–2500 mL orally daily if tolerated). Drug is nephrotoxic.
- Observe closely for signs of infection. Monitor body temperature frequently.
- Inspect oral cavity daily for signs of stomatitis or superinfection (see Appendix F).

Patient & Family Education

- Report respiratory distress to physician immediately.
- Report signs of common cold to physician immediately.
- Understand that hair loss is reversible after cessation of treatment.

MITOTANE

(mye'toe-tane)

Lysodren

Classification: ANTINEOPLASTIC

Therapeutic: ANTINEOPLASTIC

Pregnancy Category: C

AVAILABILITY 500 mg tablets

ACTION & *THERAPEUTIC EFFECT* Cytotoxic agent with suppressant action on the adrenal cortex. Modifies peripheral metabolism of steroids and reduces production of adrenal steroids. Extra-adrenal metabolism of cortisol is altered, leading to reduction in 17-hydroxycorticosteroids (17-OHCS); however, plasma levels of corticosteroids do not fall. *Cytotoxic agent with suppressant action on the adrenal cortex.*

USES Inoperable adrenal cortical carcinoma (functional and nonfunctional).

UNLABELED USES Cushing's syndrome secondary to pituitary disorders.

CONTRAINDICATIONS Shock, severe trauma; lactation; children.

CAUTIOUS USE Liver disease; infection; preexisting neurologic disease; pregnancy (category C).

ROUTE & DOSAGE

Adrenocortical Carcinoma

Adult: **PO** Initially 2–6 g/day in divided doses t.i.d. or q.i.d. then increased to 9–10 g/day in divided doses (tolerated dose range: 2–16 g/day)

ADMINISTRATION

Oral

- Withhold temporarily and consult physician if shock or trauma occurs, since adrenal suppression is its prime action. Exogenous steroids may be required until the already depressed adrenal starts secreting steroids.
- Store at 15°–30° C (59°–86° F) in tight, light-resistant containers.

ADVERSE EFFECTS (≥1%) **CNS:** Vertigo, dizziness, drowsiness, tiredness, depression, *lethargy, sedation,* headache, confusion, tremors. **CV:** Hypertension, hypotension, flushing **GI:** *Anorexia, nausea, vom-*

iting, diarrhea. **Urogenital:** Hematuria, hemorrhagic cystitis, albuminuria. **Endocrine:** Adrenocortical insufficiency. **Special Senses:** Blurred vision, diplopia, lens opacity, toxic retinopathy. **Body as a Whole:** Generalized aching, fever, muscle twitching, hypersensitivity reactions, hyperpyrexia. **Skin:** *Rash,* cutaneous eruptions and pigmentation. **Metabolic:** *Hypouricemia, hypercholesterolemia.*

DIAGNOSTIC TEST INTERFERENCE Mitotane decreases ***protein-bound iodine (PBI)*** and ***urinary 17-OHCS levels.***

INTERACTIONS Drug: Potentiates sedative effects of **alcohol** and other CNS DEPRESSANTS; may increase the metabolism of **phenytoin, phenobarbital, warfarin,** decreasing their effectiveness. POTASSIUM SPARING DIURETICS may decrease the effect.

PHARMACOKINETICS Absorption: Approximately 40% absorbed from GI tract. **Onset:** 2–4 wk. **Peak:** 3–5 h. **Distribution:** Deposits in most body tissues, especially adipose tissue. **Metabolism:** In liver. **Elimination:** 10% in urine, 1–17% in feces **Half-Life:** 18–159 days.

NURSING IMPLICATIONS

Assessment & Drug Effects

- Monitor pulse and BP for early signs of shock (adrenal insufficiency).
- Observe for symptoms of hepatotoxicity (see Appendix F). Report them promptly, since reduced hepatic capacity can increase toxicity of mitotane and because dose may have to be decreased.
- Notify physician if following persist and become more severe: Aching muscles, fever, flushing, and muscle twitching.
- Monitor obese patient for symptoms of adrenal hypofunction. Because a large portion of the drug deposits in fatty tissue, the obese are particularly susceptible to prolonged adverse effects.
- Make neurologic and behavioral assessments at regular intervals throughout therapy.

Patient & Family Education

- Be aware that mitotane does not cure but does reduce tumor mass, pain, weakness, anorexia, and steroid symptoms.
- Report symptoms of adrenal insufficiency (weakness, fatigue, orthostatic hypotension, pigmentation, weight loss, dehydration, anorexia, nausea, vomiting, and diarrhea) to physician.
- Exercise caution when driving or performing potentially hazardous tasks requiring alertness because of drug-induced drowsiness, tiredness, dizziness. Symptoms tend to recede with continuation in therapy.

MITOXANTRONE HYDROCHLORIDE

(mi-tox′an-trone)

Novantrone

Classification: ANTINEOPLASTIC
Therapeutic: ANTINEOPLASTIC; IMMUNOSUPPRESSANT
Prototype: Doxorubicin
Pregnancy Category: D

AVAILABILITY 2 mg/mL injection

ACTION & *THERAPEUTIC EFFECT* Non–cell-cycle specific antitumor agent with less cardiotoxicity than doxorubicin. Interferes with DNA synthesis by intercalating with the DNA double helix, blocking effective DNA and RNA transcription. *Highly destructive to rapidly proliferating cells in all stages of cell division.*

USES In combination with other drugs for the treatment of acute nonlymphocytic leukemia (ANLL) in adults, bone pain in advanced prostate cancer. Reducing neurologic disability and/or frequency of clinical relapses in multiple sclerosis.

UNLABELED USES Breast cancer, non-Hodgkin's lymphomas, autologous bone marrow transplant.

CONTRAINDICATIONS Hypersensitivity to mitoxantrone; myelosuppression; baseline LVEF less than 50%; multiple sclerosis patients; intrathecal administration; pregnancy (category D), lactation.

CAUTIOUS USE Impaired cardiac function; impaired liver and kidney function; systemic infections; previous treatment with daunorubicin or doxorubicin due to increased possibility of decreased cardiac function. Safe use in children has not been established.

ROUTE & DOSAGE

Combination Therapy (with Cytarabine) for ANLL

Adult: **IV Induction Therapy:** 12 mg/m²/day on days 1–3, may need to repeat induction course
IV Consolidation Therapy: 12 mg/m² on days 1 and 2 (max lifetime dose: 80–120 mg/m²)

Prostate Cancer

Adult: **IV** 12–14 mg/m² q21days

Multiple Sclerosis

Adult: **IV** 12 mg/m² over 5–15 min q3mo (max lifetime dose: 140 mg/m²). Discontinue drug in MS patients if LVEF drops below 50% or if there is a clinically significant reduction in LVEF.

ADMINISTRATION

Intravenous

If mitoxantrone touches skin, wash immediately with copious amounts of warm water.

PREPARE: **IV Infusion: Must be** diluted prior to use. Withdraw contents of vial and add to at least 50 mL of D5W or NS. ▪ May be diluted to larger volumes to extend infusion time. ▪ Use goggles, gloves, and protective gown during drug preparation and administration.

ADMINISTER: **IV Infusion:** Administer into the tubing of a freely running IV of D5W or NS and infused over at least 3 min or longer (i.e., 30–60 min) depending on the total volume of IV solution. ▪ If extravasation occurs, stop infusion and immediately restart in another vein.

INCOMPATIBILITIES **Solution/additive: Heparin, hydrocortisone, paclitaxel. Y-site: Amphotericin B cholesteryl complex, aztreonam, cefepime, doxorubicin liposome, paclitaxel, piperacillin/tazobactam, propofol, TPN.**

▪ Discard unused portions of diluted solution. ▪ Once opened, multiple-use vials may be stored refrigerated at 2°–8° C (35°–46° F) for 14 days.

ADVERSE EFFECTS (≥1%) **CV:** Arrhythmias, decreased left ventricular function, CHF, tachycardia, ECG changes, MI (occurs with cumulative doses of greater than 80–100 mg/m²), edema, increased risk of cardiotoxicity. **GI:** *Nausea, vomiting,* constipation, diarrhea, hepato-

M

toxicity. **Hematologic:** Leukopenia, thrombocytopenia. **Other:** Discolors urine and sclera a blue-green color. **Skin:** Mild phlebitis, blue skin discoloration, alopecia.

INTERACTIONS Drug: May impair immune response to VACCINES such as influenza and pneumococcal infections. May have increased risk of infection with **yellow fever vaccine.**

PHARMACOKINETICS Distribution: Rapidly taken up by tissues and slowly released into plasma, 95% protein bound. **Metabolism:** In liver. **Elimination:** Primarily in bile. **Half-Life:** 37 h.

NURSING IMPLICATIONS

Assessment & Drug Effects

- Monitor IV insertion site. Transient blue skin discoloration may occur at site if extravasation has occurred.
- Monitor cardiac functioning throughout course of therapy including LVEF; report signs and symptoms of CHF or cardiac arrhythmias.
- Lab tests: Perform liver function tests prior to and during course of treatment. Monitor serum uric acid levels and initiate hypouricemic therapy before antileukemic therapy. Monitor carefully CBC with differential prior to and during therapy.

Patient & Family Education

- Understand potential adverse effects of mitoxantrone therapy.
- Expect urine to turn blue-green for 24 h after drug administration; sclera may also take on a bluish color.
- Be aware that stomatitis/mucositis may occur within 1 wk of therapy.
- Do not to risk exposure to those with known infections during the periods of myelosuppression.

M

MIVACURIUM CHLORIDE

(miv-a-cur′i-um)

Mivacron

Classification: SKELETAL MUSCLE RELAXANT, NONDEPOLARIZING

Therpeutic: SKELETAL MUSCLE RELAXANT; NEUROMUSCULAR BLOCKER

Prototype: Atracurium

Pregnancy Category: C

AVAILABILITY 2 mg/mL injection

ACTION & *THERAPEUTIC EFFECT* Short-acting, skeletal muscle relaxant that combines competitively to cholinergic receptors on the motor neuron end-plate. Antagonizes action of acetylcholine, and blocks neuromuscular transmission. This blocking action is readily reversible with an anticholinesterase agent. *Blocks nerve impulse transmission, which results in skeletal muscle relaxation and paralysis.*

USES Adjunct to general anesthesia, to facilitate tracheal intubation, and to provide skeletal muscle relaxation during surgery or mechanical ventilation.

CONTRAINDICATIONS Allergic reactions to mivacurium or its ingredients; neonates; children younger than 2 y.

CAUTIOUS USE Kidney function impairment, liver function impairment; older adult patients; pulmonary disease, COPD; pregancy (category C), lactation.

ROUTE & DOSAGE

Tracheal Intubation and Mechanical Ventilation

Adult: **IV Loading Dose** 0.15–0.25 mg/kg given over 5–15 sec (over 60 sec in patients with cardiovascular disease) **IV Mainte-**

nance Dose 0.1 mg/kg generally q15min **IV Continuous Infusion** Initial infusion of 9–10 mcg/kg/min, then 6–7 mcg/kg/min
Child (2–12 y): **IV Loading Dose** 0.2 mg/kg given over 5–15 sec (range: 0.09–0.2 mg/kg) then 14 mcg/kg/min

Obesity Dosage Adjustment

Use IBW

Renal Impairment Dosage Adjustment

Decrease infusion rates by up to 50%

Hepatic Impairment Dosage Adjustment

May decrease infusion rate up to 50%

ADMINISTRATION

Intravenous

PREPARE: **Direct/Continuous:** Add 3 mL of D5W, NS, D5/NS, LR, or D5/LR to each 1 mL mivacurium to yield 0.5 mg/mL.

ADMINISTER: **Direct Loading Dose:** Give over 5–15 sec (60 sec for those with CV disease). **Continuous:** Give at the rate determined by weight. ▪ Refer to manufacturer's infusion rate tables.

▪ Store diluted solution at 5°–25° C (41°–77° F) for up to 24 h.

ADVERSE EFFECTS (≥1%) **CV:** Transient decrease in arterial BP, hypotension, increases and decreases in heart rate. **Skin:** *Transient flushing about the face, neck, and/or chest* (especially with rapid administration).

INTERACTIONS Drug: GENERAL ANESTHETICS may enhance the degree of neuromuscular blockade produced by mivacurium. AMINOGLYCOSIDES, TETRACYCLINES, **bacitracin,** POLYMYXINS, **lincomycin, clindamycin, colistin, magnesium salts, lithium,** LOCAL ANESTHETICS, **procainamide,** and **quinidine** may enhance the neuromuscular blockade.

PHARMACOKINETICS Peak: 2–6 min. **Duration:** 25–30 min in adults, 8–16 min in children. **Distribution:** Limited tissue distribution. **Metabolism:** Rapidly hydrolyzed by plasma cholinesterase.

NURSING IMPLICATIONS

Assessment & Drug Effects

- Assess patients with neuromuscular disease carefully and adjust drug dosage using a peripheral nerve stimulator when they experience prolonged neuromuscular blocks.
- Monitor hemodynamic status carefully in patients with significant cardiovascular disease or those with potentially greater sensitivity to release of histamine-type mediators (e.g., asthma).
- Monitor for significant drop in BP because overdose may increase the risk of hemodynamic adverse effects.

MODAFINIL

(mod-a′fi-nil)

Provigil, Alertec ♣

ARMODAFINIL

Nuvigil

Classification: CNS STIMULANT, ANALEPTIC

Therapeutic: CNS STIMULANT; ANTINARCOLEPTIC

Pregnancy Category: C

Controlled Substance: Schedule IV

AVAILABILITY 100 mg, 200 mg capsules; 50 mg, 150 mg, 200 mg tablets

ACTION & *THERAPEUTIC EFFECT* Primary sites of CNS stimulant activity of modafinil appear to be in the hippocampus, the centrolateral nucleus of the thalamus, and the central nucleus of the amygdala. Modafinil may increase excitatory transmission in the thalamus and hippocampus. *Modafinil causes wakefulness, increased locomotor activity, and psychoactive and euphoric effects.*

USES Improve wakefulness in patients with narcolepsy or excessive sleepiness associated with shift work sleep disorder, obstructive sleep apnea/hypopnea syndrome.

UNLABELED USES Fatigue related to organic brain syndrome or multiple sclerosis.

M

CONTRAINDICATIONS Hypersensitivity to modafinil; acute MI, valvular heart disease. Safety and efficacy in children younger than 16 y are unknown.

CAUTIOUS USE Cardiovascular disease including left ventricular hypertrophy; cardiac disease, ischemic ECG changes, chest pain, arrhythmias, mitral valve prolapse, recent MI, unstable angina; older adults; history of drug or alcohol abuse; psychosis or emotional instability, depression, mania; leukopenia, MI, neurologic disease, hypertension, severe hepatic disease, severe renal impairment, renal failure, seizure disorder, sleep apnea; pregnancy (category C), lactation.

ROUTE & DOSAGE

Narcolepsy, Fatigue

Adult: **PO** (Provigil) 200 mg/day as single dose in the morning; (Nuvigil) 150–250 mg qa.m.

Shift-Work Sleep Disorder

Adult: **PO** (Nuvigil) 150 mg 1 h prior to shift

Hepatic Impairment Dosage Adjustment

Reduce dose by 50%

ADMINISTRATION

Oral

- Give in the morning shortly after awakening.
- Store at 15°–30° C (59°–86° F).

ADVERSE EFFECTS (≥1%) **Body as a Whole:** Chest pain, neck pain, chills, eosinophilia. **CNS:** *Headache,* nervousness, dizziness, depression, anxiety, cataplexy, insomnia, paresthesia, dyskinesia, hypertonia. **CV:** Hypotension, hypertension, vasodilation, arrhythmia, syncope. **GI:** *Nausea,* diarrhea, dry mouth, anorexia, abnormal LFTs, vomiting, mouth ulcer, gingivitis, thirst. **Respiratory:** Rhinitis, pharyngitis, lung disorder, dyspnea. **Skin:** Dry skin. **Special Senses:** Amblyopia, abnormal vision.

INTERACTIONS Drug: Methylphenidate may delay absorption of modafinil; modafinil may decrease levels of **cyclosporine,** ORAL CONTRACEPTIVES; modafinil may increase levels of **clomipramine, phenytoin, warfarin,** TRICYCLIC ANTIDEPRESSANTS.

PHARMACOKINETICS Absorption: Rapidly absorbed. **Peak:** 2–4 h. **Distribution:** Approximately 60% protein bound. **Metabolism:** In liver to inactive metabolites. **Elimination:** In urine. **Half-Life:** 15 h.

NURSING IMPLICATIONS

Assessment & Drug Effects

- Therapeutic effectiveness: Indicated by improved daytime wakefulness.

- Monitor BP and cardiovascular status, especially with preexisting hypertension and mitral valve prolapse or other CV condition.
- Monitor for S&S of psychosis, especially when history of psychotic episodes exists.
- Lab tests: Periodic liver function tests.
- Coadministered drugs: Monitor INR with warfarin for first several months and when dosage is changed; monitor for toxicity with phenytoin.

Patient & Family Education

- Use barrier contraceptive instead of/in addition to hormonal contraceptive.
- Inform physician of all prescription or OTC drugs in/added to your regimen.
- Notify physician if any S&S of an allergic reaction appear.

MOEXIPRIL HYDROCHLORIDE

(mo-ex'i-pril)

Univasc

Classifications: ANGIOTENSIN-CONVERTING ENZYME (ACE) INHIBITOR; ANTIHYPERTENSIVE

Therapeutic: ANTIHYPERTENSIVE

Prototype: Enalapril

Pregnancy Category: C first trimester; D second and third trimester

AVAILABILITY 7.5 mg, 15 mg tablets

ACTION & *THERAPEUTIC EFFECT*
ACE inhibitor that results in decreased conversion of angiotensin I to angiotensin II. Results in decreased vasopressor activity and aldosterone secretion. Lowering angiotensin II plasma levels results in blood pressure decreases and plasma renin activity increases. *ACE inhibition and decreased aldosterone secretion are responsible for its antihypertensive effect.*

USES Hypertension.
UNLABELED USES CHF, left ventricular dysfunction.

CONTRAINDICATIONS Hypersensitivity to moexipril; history of angioedema related to an ACE inhibitor; pregnancy (category D second and third trimester).
CAUTIOUS USE Hypersensitivity to any other ACE inhibitor; renal impairment, renal artery stenosis, volume-depleted patients; hypertensive patient with CHF; history of autoimmune disease; severe liver dysfunction; immunosuppressed patients; hyperkalemia; patients undergoing surgery/anesthesia; preexisting neutropenia; concurrent lithium therapy; pregnancy (category C first trimester), lactation. Safety and efficacy in children are not established.

ROUTE & DOSAGE

Hypertension
Adult: **PO** 7.5 mg once/day, may increase up to 30 mg/day in divided doses

Renal Impairment Dosage Adjustment
CrCl 40 mL/min or less: Start with 3.75 mg daily (also if patient is volume depleted or on diuretics)

ADMINISTRATION

Oral

- Give 1 h before or 2 h after meals. Food greatly reduces absorption of moexipril.
- May need to reduce starting dose 50% in patients with possible volume depletion or a history of renal insufficiency.

- Store at 15°–30° C (59°–86° F).

ADVERSE EFFECTS (≥1%) **CNS:** Headache, *dizziness,* drowsiness, sleep disturbances, nervousness, anxiety, mood changes. **CV:** Hypotension, chest pain, angina, peripheral edema, MI, palpitations, arrhythmias. **Endocrine:** Hyperkalemia. **GI:** Diarrhea, nausea, dyspepsia, abdominal pain, taste disturbances, constipation, vomiting, dry mouth, pancreatitis. **Urogenital:** Urinary frequency, increased BUN and serum creatinine. **Hematologic:** Neutropenia, hemolytic anemia. **Respiratory:** Cough, pharyngitis, rhinitis, flu-like symptoms. **Skin:** Angioedema (rare), rash, flushing.

INTERACTIONS Drug: Capsaicin may exacerbate cough. NSAIDS may reduce antihypertensive effects. May increase **lithium** levels and toxicity. POTASSIUM SUPPLEMENTS and POTASSIUM-SPARING DIURETICS may increase risk of hyperkalemia. **Food:** Food greatly reduces absorption of moexipril.

PHARMACOKINETICS Absorption: Readily absorbed from GI tract; approximately 13% of active metabolite reaches systemic circulation; absorption greatly reduced by food. **Onset:** 1 h. **Duration:** 24 h. **Distribution:** Approximately 50% protein bound. **Metabolism:** In liver to moexiprilat (active metabolite). **Elimination:** 13% in urine, 53% in feces. **Half-Life:** 2–9 h.

NURSING IMPLICATIONS

Assessment & Drug Effects

- Monitor closely for systematic hypotension that may occur within 1–3 h of first dose, especially in those with high blood pressure, on a diuretic or restricted salt intake, or otherwise volume depleted.
- Monitor BP and HR frequently during initiation of therapy, whenever a diuretic is added, and periodically throughout therapy.
- Determine trough BP (just before next dose) before dose adjustments are made.
- Lab tests: Monitor serum electrolytes, WBC with differential, Hct and Hgb, urinalysis, and kidney and liver function tests periodically throughout therapy.
- Supervise therapeutic response closely in patients with CHF.

Patient & Family Education

- Report to physician immediately swelling around face or neck or in extremities.
- Report S&S of hypotension (e.g., dizziness, weakness, syncope); nonproductive cough; skin rash; flu-like symptoms; jaundice; irregular heartbeat or chest pains; and dehydration from vomiting, diarrhea, or diaphoresis.
- Consult physician before using potassium-containing salt substitutes.

MOLINDONE HYDROCHLORIDE

(moe-lin'done)

Moban

Classification: ANTIPSYCHOTIC, PHENOTHIAZINE

Therapeutic: ANTIPSYCHOTIC

Prototype: Chlorpromazine

Pregnancy Category: C

AVAILABILITY 5 mg, 10 mg, 25 mg, 50 mg tablets

ACTION & *THERAPEUTIC EFFECT* Phenothiazine antipsychotic thought to block postsynaptic dopamine receptors in the brain. EEG studies suggest ascending reticular system is chief site of action. *Produces tranquilization without compromising alertness. Antipsychotic effect includes reduction in bizarre behavior, and control of aggressiveness.*

USES Management of manifestations of psychotic disorders.

CONTRAINDICATIONS Known hypersensitivity to molindone or to phenothiazines, or sulfites; severe CNS depression; severe cardiovascular disease; comatose states; dementia-related psychosis; mental retardation; children younger than 12 y, lactation.

CAUTIOUS USE Those harmed by increase in physical activity; prostatic hypertrophy; cardiovascular disease; older adults; history of seizures; previously detected cancer of breast; pregnancy (category C).

ROUTE & DOSAGE

Psychotic Disorders

Adult: **PO** 50–75 mg/day in 3–4 divided doses, may be increased to 100 mg/day in 3–4 days or may be able to decrease to 15–60 mg/day in divided doses (max: 225 mg/day)

ADMINISTRATION

Oral

- Be certain patient swallows the medication.
- Store medication in tightly capped, light-resistant bottles. Protect from heat and moisture.

ADVERSE EFFECTS (≥1%) **CNS:** *Transient drowsiness,* insomnia, *extrapyramidal symptoms* (dose related), euphoria, <u>neuroleptic malignant syndrome</u>. **GI:** Dry mouth, constipation, <u>hepatotoxicity</u>. **Special Senses:** Tinnitus, blurred vision, nasal congestion. **Urogenital:** Urinary retention. **Skin:** Mild photosensitivity. **CV:** Tachycardia. **Body as a Whole:** Change in weight. **Endocrine:** SLE-like syndrome, heavy menses, amenorrhea, galactorrhea, gynecomastia, increased libido, premature ejaculation.

INTERACTIONS Drug: May potentiate CNS depression with CNS DEPRESSANTS, **alcohol. Herbal: Kava** may increase risk and severity of dystonic reactions.

PHARMACOKINETICS Absorption: Readily from GI tract. **Peak:** 1 h. **Duration:** 24–36 h. **Distribution:** Into breast milk. **Metabolism:** In liver. **Elimination:** In urine and feces. **Half-Life:** 1.5 h.

NURSING IMPLICATIONS

Assessment & Drug Effects

- Withhold dose and consult with physician if the following symptoms occur: Tremor, involuntary twitching, exaggerated restlessness, changes in vision, light-colored stools, sore throat, fever, rash.
- Monitor bowel pattern and urinary output. The depressed patient may not report constipation or urinary retention, both adverse effects of this medicine.
- Supervise ambulation and other ADL in the older adult or debilitated or patient with impaired vision to prevent injury or falling because drug increases motor activity.
- Be alert early during treatment to onset of parkinsonism (extrapyramidal) symptoms: Rigidity, immobility, reduction of voluntary movements, tremors, fine vermicular tongue movements. Withhold dose and report promptly to physician.

M

Patient & Family Education

- Take drug as prescribed: Do not alter dose regimen or stop medication without consulting physician.
- Dizziness during early therapy usually disappears as treatment continues.
- Do not drive or engage in potentially hazardous activities requiring mental or physical coordination until response to drug is known.
- Avoid alcohol and self-medication with other depressants during therapy. Get physician approval before using any OTC drug.
- Avoid overexertion (patient with angina) and report increase in frequency of precordial pain.
- Schedule periodic ophthalmic examinations when treatment is long term.

M

MOMETASONE FUROATE

(mo-met′a-sone)

Asmanex Twisthaler, Elocon, Nasonex

Pregnancy Category: C

See Appendix A-3.

MONTELUKAST

(mon-te-lu′cast)

Singulair

Classifications: BRONCHODILATOR (RESPIRATORY SMOOTH MUSCLE RELAXANT); LEUKOTRIENE RECEPTOR ANTAGONIST

Therapeutic: BRONCHODILATOR

Prototype: Zafirlukast

Pregnancy Category: B

AVAILABILITY 5 mg, 10 mg tablets; 4 mg chewable tablets; 4 mg oral granules

ACTION & *THERAPEUTIC EFFECT* Selective receptor antagonist of leukotriene, thus inhibiting bronchoconstriction. Leukotrienes—inflammatory agents—induce bronchoconstriction and mucus production. Elevated sputum and blood levels of leukotrienes are present during acute asthma attacks. Montelukast controls asthmatic attacks by inhibiting leukotriene release as well as inflammatory action associated with the attack. *Effectiveness is indicated by improved pulmonary functions and better controlled asthmatic symptoms.*

USES Prophylaxis and chronic treatment of asthma or allergic rhinitis; exercise-induced bronchoconstriction (EIB).

CONTRAINDICATIONS Hypersensitivity to montelukast; acute asthma attacks; bronchoconstriction due to acute asthma; status asthmaticus; concurrent use of aspirin or NSAIDs with known allergy to either; children younger than 6 mo with asthma or periennial allergic rhinitis.

CAUTIOUS USE Hypersensitivity to other leukotriene receptor antagonists (e.g., zafirlukast, zileuton); severe liver disease; jaundice, PKU; severe asthma; pregnancy (category B), lactation.

ROUTE & DOSAGE

Asthma

Adult: **PO** 10 mg daily in evening

Child: **PO** *12 mo–5 y,* 4 mg daily in evening; *6–14 y,* 5 mg chewable tablet daily in evening

EIB

Adult/Adolescent (older than 15 y): **PO** 10 mg 2 h before exercise (not more than 1 per day)

ADMINISTRATION

Oral

- Give in the evening for maximum effectiveness.
- Ensure chewable tablets for children are not swallowed whole.
- Store at 15°–30° C (59°–86° F) in a tightly closed container and protect from light.

ADVERSE EFFECTS (≥1%) **Body as a Whole:** Asthenia, fever, trauma. **CNS:** Dizziness, *headache*. **GI:** Abdominal pain, dyspepsia, gastroenteritis, dental pain, abnormal liver function tests (ALT, AST), diarrhea, nausea. **Respiratory:** Nasal congestion, cough, influenza, laryngitis, pharyngitis, sinusitis. **Skin:** Rash. **Urogenital:** Pyuria.

PHARMACOKINETICS Absorption: Rapidly absorbed from GI tract, bioavailability 64%. **Peak:** 3–4 h for oral tablet, 2–2.5 h for chewable tablet. **Distribution:** Greater than 99% protein bound. **Metabolism:** Extensively metabolized by CYP3A4 and 2C9. **Elimination:** In feces. **Half-Life:** 2.7–5.5 h.

NURSING IMPLICATIONS

Assessment & Drug Effects

- Monitor effectiveness carefully when used in combination with phenobarbital or other potent cytochrome P450 enzyme inducers.
- Lab test: Periodic liver function tests.

Patient & Family Education

- Do not use for reversal of an acute asthmatic attack.
- Inform physician if short-acting inhaled bronchodilators are needed more often than usual with montelukast.
- Use chewable tablets (contain phenylalanine) with caution with PKU.

MORPHINE SULFATE (Pr)

(mor′feen)

Astramorph PF, Avinza, Depo-Dur, Duramorph, Embeda, Epimorph ✦, Infumorph, Kadian, MS Contin, MSIR, Oramorph SR, RMS, Roxanol, Statex ✦

Classifications: ANALGESIC; NARCOTIC (OPIATE) AGONIST

Therapeutic: NARCOTIC ANALGESIC

Pregnancy Category: C (D in long-term use, high dose, or close to term)

Controlled Substance: Schedule II

AVAILABILITY 10 mg, 15 mg, 30 mg tablets/capsules; 10 mg, 15 mg, 20 mg, 30 mg, 50 mg, 60 mg, 90 mg, 100 mg, 120 mg, 200 mg controlled release tablets/capsules; 10 mg/2.5 mL, 10 mg/5 mL, 20 mg/mL, 20 mg/5 mL, 30 mg/1.5 mL, 100 mg/5 mL oral solution; 0.5 mg/mL, 1 mg/mL, 2 mg/mL, 4 mg/mL, 5 mg/mL, 8 mg/mL, 10 mg/mL, 15 mg/mL, 25 mg/mL, 50 mg/mL injection; 10 mg/mL extended release lysosomal injection; 5 mg, 10 mg, 20 mg, 30 mg suppositories

ACTION & *THERAPEUTIC EFFECT* Natural opium alkaloid with agonist activity by binding with the same receptors as endogenous opioid peptides. Narcotic agonist effects are identified with different locations of receptors: Analgesia at supraspinal level, euphoria, respiratory depression and physical dependence; analgesia at spinal level, sedation and miosis; and dysphoric, hallucinogenic, and cardiac stimulant effects. *Controls severe pain; also used as an adjunct to anesthesia.*

USES Symptomatic relief of severe acute and chronic pain after nonnarcotic analgesics have failed and as preanesthetic medication; also used to relieve dyspnea of acute left ventricular failure and pulmonary edema and pain of MI.

CONTRAINDICATIONS Hypersensitivity to opiate agonists; increased intracranial pressure; convulsive disorders; acute bronchial asthma, respiratory depression; chemical-irritant induced pulmonary edema; hypovolemia; prostatic hypertrophy; undiagnosed acute abdominal conditions; following biliary tract surgery and surgical anastomosis; pancreatitis, GI ileus; severe liver or renal insufficiency; Addison's disease; hypothyroidism; during labor for delivery of a premature infant, premature infants; pregnancy (category D in long-term use, when high dose is used, or close to term).

CAUTIOUS USE Head trauma; toxic psychosis; mild or moderate hepatic or renal impairment; cardiac arrhythmias, cardiovascular disease; ulcerative colitis; constipation; emphysema; kyphoscoliosis; cor pulmonale; severe obesity; reduced blood volume; BPH; renal disease; history of substance abuse or alcoholism; very old, very young, or debilitated patients; labor, pregnancy (category C for low doses, short-term use, and not close to term).

ROUTE & DOSAGE

Pain Relief

Adult: **PO** 10–30 mg q4h prn or 15–30 mg sustained release q8–12h; **(Kadian)** dose q12–24h, increase dose prn for pain relief; **(Avinza)** dose q24h **IV** 2.5–15 mg/70 kg q2–4h or 0.8–10 mg/h by continuous infusion, may increase prn to control pain or 5–10 mg given epidurally q24h **Epidural** (DepoDur only) 10–15 mg as single dose 30 min before surgery (max: 20 mg) **IM/Subcutaneous** 5–20 mg q4h **PR** 10–20 mg q4h prn
Child: **IV** 0.05–0.1 mg/kg q4h or 0.025–2.6 mg/kg/h by continuous infusion (max: 10 mg/dose) **IM/Subcutaneous** 0.1–0.2 mg/kg q4h (max: 15 mg/dose) **PO** 0.2–0.5 mg/kg q4–6h; 0.3–0.6 mg/kg sustained release q12h
Neonate: **IV/IM/Subcutaneous** 0.05 mg/kg q4–8h (max: 0.1 mg/kg/dose) or 0.01–0.02 mg/kg/h

Renal Impairment Dosage Adjustment

CrCl 10–50 mL/min: Use 75% of dose, if lower use 50% of dose

ADMINISTRATION

Oral

- A fixed, individualized schedule is recommended when narcotic analgesic therapy is started to provide effective management; blood levels can be maintained and peaks of pain can be prevented (usually a 4-h interval is adequate).
- Lower dosages are recommended for older adult or debilitated patients.
- Do not break in half, crush, or allow sustained release tablet to be chewed.
- Do not give patient sustained release tablet within 24 h of surgery.
- Dilute oral solution in approximately 30 mL or more of fluid or semisolid food. A calibrated dropper comes with the bottle. Read labels carefully when using liquid preparation; available solutions: 20 mg/mL; 100 mg/mL.

Intramuscular/Subcutaneous

▪ Give undiluted.

Intravenous

Note: Verify correct IV concentration and rate of infusion/injection for administration to neonates, infants, or children with physician.

PREPARE: **Direct:** Dilute 2–10 mg in at least 5 mL of sterile water for injection. **Continuous:** Typically diluted to a range of 0.1–1 mg/mL. ▪ More concentrated solutions may be required with fluid restriction.

ADMINISTER: **Direct:** Give a single dose over 4–5 min. Avoid rapid administration. **Continuous:** Infuse via a controlled infusion device at a rate determined by patient response as ordered.

INCOMPATIBILITIES **Solution/additive:** **Alteplase, aminophylline, amobarbital, chlorothiazide, floxacillin, fluorouracil, haloperidol, heparin, meperidine, nitrofurantoin, pentobarbital, phenobarbital, perphenazine, phenytoin, sodium bicarbonate, thiopental.** **Y-site:** **Amphotericin B cholesteryl complex, azithromycin, cefepime, doxorubicin liposome, gallium, minocycline, phenytoin, sargramostim, tetracycline.**

▪ Store at 15°–30° C (59°–86° F). Avoid freezing. Refrigerate suppositories. Protect all formulations from light.

ADVERSE EFFECTS (≥1%) **Body as a Whole:** Hypersensitivity [*pruritus,* rash, urticaria, edema, hemorrhagic urticaria (rare), anaphylactoid reaction (rare)], sweating, skeletal muscle flaccidity; cold, clammy skin, hypothermia. **CNS:** Euphoria, insomnia, disorientation, visual disturbances, dysphoria, paradoxic CNS stimulation (restlessness, tremor, delirium, insomnia), convulsions (infants and children); decreased cough reflex, drowsiness, dizziness, deep sleep, coma, continuous intrathecal infusion may cause granulomas leading to paralysis. **Special Senses:** Miosis. **CV:** Bradycardia, palpitations, syncope; flushing of face, neck, and upper thorax; orthostatic hypotension, cardiac arrest. **GI:** *Constipation,* anorexia, dry mouth, biliary colic, *nausea,* vomiting, elevated transaminase levels. **Urogenital:** Urinary retention or urgency, dysuria, oliguria, reduced libido or potency (prolonged use). **Other:** Prolonged labor and respiratory depression of newborn. **Hematologic:** Precipitation of porphyria. **Respiratory:** Severe respiratory depression (as low as 2–4/min) or arrest; pulmonary edema.

DIAGNOSTIC TEST INTERFERENCE False-positive ***urine glucose*** determinations may occur using ***Benedict's solution. Plasma amylase*** and ***lipase*** determinations may be falsely positive for 24 h after use of morphine; ***transaminase levels*** may be elevated.

INTERACTIONS Drug: CNS DEPRESSANTS, SEDATIVES, BARBITURATES, BENZODIAZEPINES, and TRICYCLIC ANTIDEPRESSANTS potentiate CNS depressant effects. Use MAO INHIBITORS cautiously; they may precipitate hypertensive crisis. PHENOTHIAZINES may antagonize analgesia. Use with **alcohol** may lead to potentially fatal overdoses. **Herbal: Kava, valerian, St. John's wort** may increase sedation.

PHARMACOKINETICS Absorption: Variably from GI tract. **Peak:** 60 min PO; 20–60 min PR; 50–90 min subcutaneous; 30–60 min IM; 20 min

IV. **Duration:** Up to 7 h. **Distribution:** Crosses blood–brain barrier and placenta; distributed in breast milk. **Metabolism:** In liver. **Elimination:** 90% in urine in 24 h; 7–10% in bile.

NURSING IMPLICATIONS

Assessment & Drug Effects

- Obtain baseline respiratory rate, depth, and rhythm and size of pupils before administering the drug. Respirations of 12/min or below and miosis are signs of toxicity. Withhold drug and report to physician.
- Observe patient closely to be certain pain relief is achieved. Record relief of pain and duration of analgesia.
- Differentiate among restlessness as a sign of pain and the need for medication, restlessness associated with hypoxia, and restlessness caused by morphine-induced CNS stimulation (a paradoxic reaction that is particularly common in women and older adult patients).
- Monitor carefully those at risk for severe respiratory depression after epidural or intrathecal injection: Older adult or debilitated patients or those with decreased respiratory reserve (e.g., emphysema, severe obesity, kyphoscoliosis).
- Continue monitoring for respiratory depression for at least 24 h after each epidural or intrathecal dose.
- Assess vital signs at regular intervals. Morphine-induced respiratory depression may occur even with small doses, and it increases progressively with higher doses (generally max: 90 min after subcutaneous, 30 min after IM, and 7 min after IV).
- Encourage changes in position, deep breathing, and coughing (unless contraindicated) at regularly scheduled intervals. Narcotic analgesics also depress cough and sigh reflexes and thus may induce atelectasis, especially in postoperative patients.
- Be alert for nausea and orthostatic hypotension (with light-headedness and dizziness) in ambulatory patients or when a supine patient assumes the head-up position or in patients not experiencing severe pain.
- Monitor I&O ratio and pattern. Report oliguria or urinary retention. Morphine may dull perception of bladder stimuli; therefore, encourage the patient to void at least q4h. Palpate lower abdomen to detect bladder distention.

Patient & Family Education

- Avoid alcohol and other CNS depressants while receiving morphine.
- Do not use of any OTC drug unless approved by physician.
- Do not ambulate without assistance after receiving drug.
- Use caution or avoid tasks requiring alertness (e.g., driving a car) until response to drug is known since morphine may cause drowsiness, dizziness, or blurred vision.

MOXIFLOXACIN HYDROCHLORIDE

(mox-i-flox'a-sin)

Avelox, Vigamox

Classifications: ANTIBIOTIC; QUINOLONE

Therapeutic: ANTIBIOTIC

Prototype: Ciprofloxacin

Pregnancy Category: C

AVAILABILITY 400 mg tablets; 0.5% ophth solution; 400 mg/250 mL infusion

ACTION & *THERAPEUTIC EFFECT* Moxifloxacin is a synthetic broad-spectrum fluoroquinolone antibiotic. It inhibits DNA gyrase, an enzyme required for DNA replication, transcription, repair, and recombination of bacterial DNA. *Broad spectrum antibiotic that is bactericidal against gram-positive and gram-negative organisms.*

USES Treatment of acute bacterial sinusitis, acute bacterial exacerbation of chronic bronchitis, community-acquired pneumonia, skin and skin structure infections, bacterial conjunctivitis, complicated skin infections.

CONTRAINDICATIONS Hypersensitivity to moxifloxacin or other quinolones; moderate to severe hepatic insufficiency; syphilis; patients with history of prolonged QT_c interval on ECG, history of ventricular arrhythmias, atrial fibrillation, hypokalemia, bradycardia, acute myocardial ischemia, acute MI, patients receiving Class IA or Class III antiarrhythmic drugs; tendon pain; viral infection; history of torsades de pointes; lactation. **Ocular preparation:** use in children younger than 1 y.

CAUTIOUS USE CNS disorders; cerebrovascular disease, colitis, diarrhea, GI disease; diabetes mellitus; mild or moderate heart insufficiency; myasthenia gravis; seizure disorder; sunlight (UV) exposure; pregnancy (category C).

ROUTE & DOSAGE

Acute Bacterial Sinusitis, Acute Bacterial Exacerbation of Chronic Bronchitis, Community-Acquired Pneumonia, Skin Infections

Adult: **PO/IV** 400 mg daily × 5–14 days

Complicated Skin Infection

Adult: **PO/IV** 400 mg daily × 7–21 days

Bacterial Conjunctivitis

Adult/Child (older than 1 y): **Ophthalmic** 1 drop in affected eye(s) t.i.d. × 7 days

ADMINISTRATION

Oral

- Administer 4 h before or 8 h after multivitamins (containing iron or zinc), antacids (containing magnesium, calcium, or aluminum), sucralfate, or didanosine.

Intravenous

PREPARE: **IV Infusion:** Avelox (400 mg) is supplied in ready-to-use 250 mL IV bags. No further dilution is necessary.

ADMINISTER: **IV Infusion:** Give over 60 min. AVOID RAPID OR BOLUS DOSE.

- Store at 15°–30° C (59°–86° F); protect from high humidity.

ADVERSE EFFECTS (≥1%) **CNS:** Dizziness, headache, peripheral neuropathy. **GI:** Nausea, diarrhea, abdominal pain, vomiting, taste perversion, abnormal liver function tests, dyspepsia. **Musculoskeletal:** Tendon rupture, cartilage erosion. **CV:** Arrythmia, QT prolongation

DIAGNOSTIC TEST INTERFERENCE May cause false positive on ***opiate screening tests.***

INTERACTIONS Drug: Iron, zinc, ANTACIDS, **aluminum, magnesium, calcium, sucralfate** decrease absorption; **atenolol, erythromycin,** ANTIPSYCHOTICS, TRICYCLIC ANTIDEPRESSANTS, **quinidine, procainamide,**

amiodarone, sotalol may cause prolonged QT_c interval.

PHARMACOKINETICS Absorption: 90% bioavailable. **Steady State:** 3 d. **Distribution:** 50% protein bound. **Metabolism:** In liver. **Elimination:** Unchanged drug: 20% in urine, 25% in feces; metabolites: 38% in feces, 14% in urine. **Half-Life:** 12 h.

NURSING IMPLICATIONS

Assessment & Drug Effects

- Monitor for and notify physician immediately of adverse CNS effects.
- Notify physician immediately for S&S of hypersensitivity (see Appendix F).
- Lab tests: C&S before initiation of therapy and baseline serum potassium with history of hypokalemia.

M

Patient & Family Education

- Exercise care in timing of consumption of vitamins and antacids (see ADMINISTRATION).
- Drink fluids liberally, unless directed otherwise.
- Increased seizure potential is possible, especially when history of seizure exists.
- Stop taking drug and notify physician if experiencing palpitations, fainting, skin rash, severe diarrhea, ankle/foot pain, agitation, insomnia.
- Avoid engaging in hazardous activities until reaction to drug is known.

MUPIROCIN

(mu-pi-ro′sin)

Bactroban, Bactroban Nasal

Classification: PSEUDOMONIC ACID ANTIBIOTIC

Therapeutic: ANTIBIOTIC

Pregnancy Category: B

AVAILABILITY 2% ointment; cream

ACTION & *THERAPEUTIC EFFECT* Topical antibacterial produced by fermentation of *Pseudomonas fluorescens*. Inhibits bacterial protein synthesis by binding with the bacterial transfer RNA. *Susceptible bacteria are* Staphylococcus aureus *[including methicillin-resistant (MRSA) and beta-lactamase-producing strains] and other* Staphylococcus *and* Streptococcus pyogenes.

USES Impetigo due to *Staphylococcus aureus*, beta-hemolytic *Streptococci*, and *Streptococcus pyogenes;* nasal carriage of *S. aureus*.

UNLABELED USES Superficial skin infections; burns.

CONTRAINDICATIONS Hypersensitivity to any of its components and for ophthalmic use; lactation (do not apply to breast); children younger than 12 y (intranasal form); moderate to severe renal impairment.

CAUTIOUS USE Pregnancy (category B), lactation.

ROUTE & DOSAGE

Impetigo

Adult/Child: **Topical** Apply to affected area t.i.d., if no response in 3–5 days, reevaluate (usually continue for 1–2 wk)

Elimination of Staphylococcal Nasal Carriage

Child: **Intranasal** Apply intranasally b.i.d. to q.i.d. for 5–14 days

ADMINISTRATION

Topical

- Apply thin layer of medication to affected area.

- Cover area being treated with a gauze dressing if desired.

ADVERSE EFFECTS (≥1%) **Skin:** Burning, stinging, pain, pruritus, rash, erythema, dry skin, tenderness, swelling. **Special Senses:** Intranasal, local stinging, soreness, dry skin, pruritus.

INTERACTIONS Drug: Incompatible with **salicylic acid 2%**; do not mix in HYDROPHILIC VEHICLES (e.g., **Aquaphor**) or COAL TAR SOLUTIONS; **chloramphenicol** may interfere with bactericidal action of mupirocin.

PHARMACOKINETICS Absorption: Not systemically absorbed.

NURSING IMPLICATIONS

Assessment & Drug Effects

- Watch for signs and symptoms of superinfection (see Appendix F). Prolonged or repeated therapy may result in superinfection by nonsusceptible organisms.
- Reevaluate drug use if patient does not show clinical response within 3–5 days.
- Discontinue the drug and notify physician if signs of contact dermatitis develop or if exudate production increases.

Patient & Family Education

- Discontinue drug and contact physician if a sensitivity reaction or chemical irritation occurs (e.g., increased redness, itching, burning).

MUROMONAB-CD3

(myoo-roe-moe′nab)

Orthoclone OKT3

Classifications: BIOLOGICAL RESPONSE MODIFIER; MONOCLONAL ANTIBODY; IMMUNOSUPPRESSANT

Therapeutic: IMMUNOSUPPRESSANT
Prototype: Cyclosporine
Pregnancy Category: C

AVAILABILITY 1 mg/mL injection

ACTION & *THERAPEUTIC EFFECT* Murine monoclonal antibody (purified IgG_2). Specifically targets the T_3 (CD_3) antigen site of the human T-cell membrane. CD_3-positive T-cells are rapidly removed from circulation, and T-lymphocyte action leading to renal inflammation and destruction is blocked. This reverses graft rejection. *CD_3-positive T-lymphocyte immunosuppressive activity results in reversing graft rejection of a transplanted kidney.*

USES Acute allograft rejection in kidney transplant patients.
UNLABELED USES Acute allograft rejection in heart and liver transplant patients.

CONTRAINDICATIONS Intolerance to any product of murine origin; fluid overload; uncompensated heart failure; weight gain of more than 3% within week prior to treatment; infection: Chickenpox (existing, recent, including recent exposure), seizure disorders; herpes zoster; lactation.
CAUTIOUS USE Recent MI; ischemic cardiac disease, CAD; pulmonary edema; repeated courses; pregnancy (category C).

ROUTE & DOSAGE

Transplant Rejection

Adult: **IV** 5 mg/day for 10–14 days
Child: **IV** *Weight 30 kg or less,* 2.5 mg daily; *weight greater than 30 kg,* 5 mg daily

M

ADMINISTRATION

Note: Only persons experienced with immunosuppressive therapy and management of kidney transplant patients should administer muromonab-CD3 and only in an area equipped with staff and facilities to deal with cardiac resuscitation.

Intravenous

Note: Verify correct rate of IV injection for administration to infants or children with physician. ▪ Administer IV methylprednisolone sodium succinate before and IV hydrocortisone sodium succinate 30 min after muromonab-CD3 to decrease incidence of first dose reaction. ▪ Be aware that concomitant maintenance immunosuppressive therapy is reduced or discontinued during drug therapy with muromonab-CD3 and resumed about 3 days prior to end of therapy.

PREPARE: **Direct:** Give undiluted. Do not shake ampule. ▪ Draw sterile solution into syringe through a low protein-binding 0.2- or 0.22-micron filter. ▪ Discard filter; attach syringe to an appropriate needle for IV bolus injection.

ADMINISTER: **Direct:** Give by rapid (bolus) injection. ▪ Do not give by IV infusion or in conjunction with other drug solutions.

▪ Store at 2°–8° C (36°–46° F) unless otherwise stipulated. Avoid freezing.

ADVERSE EFFECTS (≥1%) **All:** Especially during first 2 days of therapy. **GI:** *Nausea, vomiting, diarrhea.* **Respiratory:** <u>Severe pulmonary edema</u>, *dyspnea, chest pain, wheezing.* **Body as a Whole:** *Fever, chills,* malaise, *tremor, increased susceptibility to cytomegalovirus, herpes simplex,* Pneumocystis carinii, Legionella, Cryptococcus, Serratia *organisms, and gram-negative bacteria.* **CV:** Tachycardia.

PHARMACOKINETICS Onset: The number of circulating CD_3-positive T-cells decreases within minutes. **Peak:** 2–7 days. **Duration:** 7 days.

NURSING IMPLICATIONS

Assessment & Drug Effects

- Monitor patient's response closely for 48 h for first dose reaction (occurs within 45–60 min after first dose and lasts several hours). It may occur (less severe) after second dose; then usually does not occur with subsequent doses. Symptoms: Chills, dyspnea, malaise, high fever.
- Assess and monitor vital signs. If temperature rises above 37.8° C (100° F), suspect infection (commonly observed in first 45 days of therapy). Take temperature before treatment and several hours after drug administration to detect first signs of infection.
- Consult physician if patient has a fever exceeding 37.8° C (100° F) before treatment. Make immediate attempts to lower temperature to at least 37.8° C (100° F) with antipyretics before muromonab-CD3 is administered.
- Be alert to susceptibility of patient with pretreatment fluid over-load to acute pulmonary edema (may be fatal). Be prepared for prompt intubation, oxygenation, and corticosteroid drug administration should it occur.
- Lab tests: Periodic WBC with differential, CD_3 T cells, LFTs, kidney function tests.

Patient & Family Education

- Report any of the following to physician: Chest pain, difficulty breathing, wheezing, nausea and vomiting, significant weight gain, an infection, or fever.

- Use an effective method of birth control for 12 wk following the end of therapy.

MYCOPHENOLATE MOFETIL

(my-co-phen′o-late mo′fe-till)
CellCept

MYCOPHENOLATE ACID

Myfortic

Classifications: BIOLOGICAL RESPONSE MODIFIER; IMMUNOSUPPRESSANT
Therapeutic: IMMUNOSUPPRESSANT
Prototype: Cyclosporine
Pregnancy Category: D

AVAILABILITY 250 mg capsules; 500 mg tablets; 180 mg, 360 mg delayed release tablets; 500 mg injection; 200 mg/mL oral solution

ACTION & *THERAPEUTIC EFFECT* Prodrug of mycophenolic acid with immunosuppressant properties; inhibits T- and B-lymphocyte responses, thus it inhibits antibody formation and generation of cytotoxic T-cells. It may also inhibit recruitment of leukocytes into sites of inflammation and graft sites in transplant patients. *Antirejection effects attributed to decreased number of activated lymphocytes in the graft site. It is synergistic with cyclosporine.*

USES Prophylaxis of organ rejection in patients receiving allogenic kidney, liver, or heart transplants.

UNLABELED USES Treatment of rheumatoid arthritis and psoriasis.

CONTRAINDICATIONS Hypersensitivity to mycophenolate mofetil, mycophenolic acid, polysorbate 80; vaccination, varicella; severe neutropenia; pregnancy (category D), lactation. **PO form:** Infants younger than 3 mo. **IV form:** Safety and efficacy in children have not been established.

CAUTIOUS USE Viral or bacterial infections; presence or history of carcinoma; bone marrow suppression; active peptic ulcer disease; cholestasis; gallbladder disease; GI disease, severe diarrhea; malabsorption syndromes; hepatic encephalopathy, hepatic or renal impairment; renal failure, uremia; herpes infection, infection; hypoalbuminemia; PKU; lactase deficiency; females of childbearing age, older adults.

ROUTE & DOSAGE

Note: CellCept and Myfortic are not interchangeable.

Prophylaxis for Kidney Transplant Rejection

Adult: **PO/IV** Start within 24 h of transplant, 1 g (mofetil) or 720 mg (sodium) b.i.d. in combination with corticosteroids and cyclosporine

Child: **PO** 600 mg/m^2 (mofetil) or 400 mg/m^2 (sodium) b.i.d. (max: 2 g/day mofetil, 720 mg/day sodium)

Prophylaxis for Heart/Liver Transplant Rejection

Adult: **PO/IV** 1.5 g (mofetil) b.i.d. started within 24 h of transplant

Toxicity Dosage Adjusment

If neutropenia develops, stop or reduce dose

ADMINISTRATION

Oral

- Give oral drug on an empty stomach.
- Adjust dosage with severe chronic kidney failure.
- Do not open or crush capsules; avoid contact with powder in cap-

sules, and wash thoroughly with soap and water if contact occurs.

Intravenous

PREPARE: **IV Infusion:** Reconstitute each vial with 14 mL D5W. Further dilute each 500 mg in an additional 70 mL of D5W to yield 6 mg/mL.

ADMINISTER: **IV Infusion:** Slowly infuse over 2 h or longer. Avoid rapid injection.

INCOMPATIBILITIES **Solution/additive & Y-site:** Do not mix or infuse with other medications.

- Begin IV mycophenolate mofetil within 24 h of transplant and continue for up to 14 days. ▪ Switch patient to oral drug as soon as possible.

- Store at 15°–30° C (59°–86° F).

ADVERSE EFFECTS (≥1%) **CNS:** *Headache, tremor,* insomnia, dizziness, weakness. **CV:** *Hypertension.* **Endocrine:** Hyperglycemia, hypercholesterolemia, hypophosphatemia, hypokalemia, hyperkalemia, *peripheral edema,* increased risk of miscarriage. **GI:** *Diarrhea, constipation, nausea,* anorexia, vomiting, *abdominal pain, dyspepsia.* **Urogenital:** *UTI, hematuria,* renal tubular necrosis, burning, frequency, vaginal burning or itching, vaginal bleeding, kidney stones. **Hematologic:** *Leukopenia, anemia, thrombocytopenia,* hypochromic anemia, leukocytosis. **Respiratory:** *Respiratory infection, dyspnea,* increased cough, pharyngitis. **Skin:** Rash. **Body as a Whole:** Leg or hand cramps, bone pain, myalgias, *sepsis (bacterial, fungal, viral),* progressive multifocal leukoencephalopathy.

INTERACTIONS Drug: Acyclovir, ganciclovir may increase mycophenolate serum levels. ANTACIDS, **cholestyramine** decreases mycophenolate absorption. **Mycophenolate** may decrease protein binding of **phenytoin** or **theophylline,** causing increased serum levels. **Azathioprine** increases risk of adverse effects

PHARMACOKINETICS Absorption: Rapidly from GI tract; 94% reaches systemic circulation; absorption decreased by food. **Onset:** 4 wk. **Metabolism:** In liver to active form, mycophenolic acid. **Elimination:** 87% in urine. **Half-Life:** 11 h.

NURSING IMPLICATIONS

Assessment & Drug Effects

- Prior to initiating therapy: Baseline CBC with differential.
- Withhold dose and notify physician if neutropenia develps (ANC less than 1.3 × 10^3/mcL).
- Lab tests: Monitor CBC weekly for first month, biweekly for second and third months, then once per month for first year; periodic kidney function tests, LFTs, serum electrolytes, lipase, amylase, blood glucose, and routine urinalysis.
- Monitor for and report any S&S of sepsis or infection.

Patient & Family Education

- Comply exactly with dosing regimen and scheduled laboratory tests.
- Report to physician immediately S&S of infection, such as UTI or respiratory infection, or signs of bleeding (e.g., black tarry stools, blood in urine, easy bruising).
- Report all troubling adverse reactions (e.g., blood in urine and swelling in arms and legs) to physician as soon as possible.
- Avoid taking OTC antacids simultaneously with mycophenolate mofetil. Separate the two drugs by 2 h.
- Women should use effective contraception during and for 6 wk after treatment is completed.

NABILONE

(nab'i-lone)

Cesamet

Classifications: SYNTHETIC CANNABINOID; ANTIEMETIC

Therapeutic: ANTIEMETIC; CANNABINOID

Pregnancy Category: C

Controlled Substance: Schedule II

AVAILABILITY 1 mg capsules

ACTION & *THERAPEUTIC EFFECT* Nabilone is a synthetic cannabinoid with multiple effects on the CNS. It is thought that the antiemetic effect results from its interaction with the cannabinoid receptor system (CB 1 receptor) in neural tissues. In therapeutic doses, it produces relaxation, drowsiness, and euphoria. *It effectively controls emesis in patients receiving chemotherapy when other drugs have failed.*

USES Prevention and treatment of nausea and vomiting in adult patients induced by cancer chemotherapy refractory to standard antiemetic therapy.

CONTRAINDICATIONS Hypersensitivity to any cannabinoid; hypovolemia; lactation.

CAUTIOUS USE Children; older adults; history of psychosis; pregnancy (category C).

ROUTE & DOSAGE

Nausea and Vomiting

Adult: **PO** Initial dose of 1 or 2 mg b.i.d. 1–3 h before chemotherapy. May increase to max of 2 mg t.i.d. May continue for 48 h after last dose of chemotherapy.

ADMINISTRATION

Oral

- Give 1–3 h before chemotherapy is begun. A dose of 1–2 mg the night before chemotherapy may be helpful in relieving nausea.
- Store at 15°–30° C (59°–86° F).

ADVERSE EFFECTS (≥1%) **CNS:** Asthenia, *ataxia, confusion difficulties,* depersonalization, *depression,* disorientation, *drowsiness, dysphoria, euphoria,* headache, sedation, *sleep disturbance, vertigo.* **CV:** Hypotension. **GI:** Anorexia, *dry mouth,* increased appetite, nausea. **Special Senses:** *Visual disturbances.*

INTERACTIONS Drug: SEDATIVES, HYPNOTICS, and other psychoactive substances can potentiate the CNS effects of nabilone. Coadministration of cannabinoids with **amphetamine, cocaine,** TRICYCLIC ANTIDEPRESSANTS, and/or SYMPATHOMIMETIC AGENTS can produce additive hypertension and tachycardia. Coadministration of cannabinoids with ANTIHISTAMINES or ANTICHOLINERGIC AGENTS can produce additive tachycardia and drowsiness. Coadministration of cannabinoids with BARBITURATES, BENZODIAZEPINES, **buspirone, ethanol, lithium,** MUSCLE RELAXANTS, OPIOIDS, and other CNS DEPRESSANTS can produce additive drowsiness and CNS-depressant effects. **Food: Alcohol** can potentiate the CNS effects of nabilone.

PHARMACOKINETICS Absorption: Complete absorption from GI tract. **Peak:** 2 h. **Metabolism:** Extensive hepatic metabolism. **Elimination:** Fecal (major) and urine. **Half-Life:** 2 h.

NURSING IMPLICATIONS

Assessment & Drug Effects

- Monitor for and report S&S of adverse psychiatric reactions (e.g.,

N

disorientation, hallucinations, psychosis) for 48–72 h after last dose of nabilone.

- Monitor for S&S of tachycardia and postural hypotension, especially in the older adult and those with a history of heart disease or hypertension.
- Lab tests: Periodic CBC with Hgb and Hct.

Patient & Family Education

- Do not use alcohol or other CNS depressants while using this medication.
- Do not drive or engage in potentially hazardous activities until response to drug is known.
- Report any of the following to a health care provider: Confusion, disorientation, hallucinations, or other bizarre behavior.

N

NABUMETONE

(na-bu-me'tone)

Relafen

Classification: ANALGESIC, NONSTEROIDAL ANTI-INFLAMMATORY DRUG (NSAID)

Therapeutic: ANALGESIC, NSAID; ANTIRHEUMATIC; ANTIPYRETIC

Prototype: Ibuprofen

Pregnancy Category: C

AVAILABILITY 500 mg, 750 mg tablets

ACTION & *THERAPEUTIC EFFECT* Blocks prostaglandin synthesis by inhibiting cyclooxygenase, an enzyme that converts arachidonic acid to precursors of prostaglandins. *Anti-inflammatory, analgesic, and antipyretic effects. Inhibits platelet aggregation and prolongs bleeding time.*

USES Rheumatoid arthritis and osteoarthritis.

CONTRAINDICATIONS Patients in whom urticaria, severe rhinitis, bronchospasm, angioedema, or nasal polyps are precipitated by aspirin or other NSAIDS; salicylate hypersensitivity; active peptic ulcer; bleeding abnormalities; CABG perioperative pain; lactation. Safe use in children younger than 6 mo is not established.

CAUTIOUS USE Hypertension, fluid retention, heart failure; history of GI ulceration, impaired liver or kidney function, chronic kidney failure, cardiac decompensation, bone marrow suppression; patients with SLE; elderly; pregnancy (category C).

ROUTE & DOSAGE

Rheumatoid & Osteoarthritis

Adult: **PO** 1000 mg/day as a single dose, may increase (max: 2000 mg/day in 1–2 divided doses)

ADMINISTRATION

Oral

- Give with food, milk, or antacid (if prescribed) to reduce the possibility of GI upset.
- Store at 15°–30° C (59°–86° F).

ADVERSE EFFECTS (≥1%) **GI:** Diarrhea, abdominal pain, nausea, dyspepsia, flatulence, melena, ulcers, constipation, dry mouth, gastritis. **CNS:** Tinnitus, dizziness, headache, insomnia, vertigo, fatigue, diaphoresis, nervousness, somnolence. **Skin:** Rash, pruritus.

INTERACTIONS Drug: May attenuate the antihypertensive response to DIURETICS. NSAIDS increase the risk of **methotrexate** toxicity. **Food:** Food may increase the peak but not the overall absorption of nabumetone.

Herbal: Feverfew, garlic, ginger, ginkgo may increase bleeding potential.

PHARMACOKINETICS Absorption: Readily absorbed from GI tract; approximately 35% is converted to its active metabolite on first pass through the liver. **Onset:** 1–3 wk for antirheumatic action. **Peak:** 3–6 h. **Distribution:** 99% protein bound; distributes into synovial fluid. **Metabolism:** In liver to its active metabolite, 6-methoxy-2-naphthylacetic acid (6MNA). **Elimination:** 80% of dose is excreted in urine as 6MNA; 10% excreted in feces. **Half-Life:** 24 h (6MNA).

NURSING IMPLICATIONS

Assessment & Drug Effects

- Lab tests: Obtain baseline and periodic evaluation of Hgb and Hct levels with prolonged or high-dose therapy.
- Monitor for signs and symptoms of GI bleeding.

Patient & Family Education

- Use caution with hazardous activities since nabumetone may cause dizziness, drowsiness, and blurred vision.
- Report abdominal pain, nausea, dyspepsia, or black tarry stools.
- Be aware that alcohol and aspirin will increase the risk of GI ulceration and bleeding.
- Notify your physician if any of the following occur: Persistent headache, skin rash or itching, visual disturbances, weight gain, or edema.

NADOLOL

(nay-doe'lole)

Corgard

Classifications: BETA-ADRENERGIC ANTAGONIST (ADRENERGIC BLOCKING AGENT); ANTIHYPERTENSIVE

Therapeutic: ANTIHYPERTENSIVE
Prototype: Propranolol
Pregnancy Category: C

AVAILABILITY 20 mg, 40 mg, 80 mg, 120 mg, 160 mg tablets

ACTION & *THERAPEUTIC EFFECT* Nonselective beta-adrenergic blocking agent that inhibits response to adrenergic stimuli by competitively blocking these receptors within the heart. Reduces heart rate and cardiac output at rest and during exercise, and also decreases conduction velocity through AV node and myocardial automaticity. *Decreases both systolic and diastolic BP at rest and during exercise.*

USES Hypertension, either alone or in combination with a diuretic. Also long-term prophylactic management of angina pectoris.

CONTRAINDICATIONS Bronchial asthma, severe COPD, inadequate myocardial function, sinus bradycardia, greater than first-degree conduction block, overt cardiac failure, cardiogenic shock; abrupt withdrawal; lactation. Safe use in children younger than 18 y is not established. **CAUTIOUS USE** CHF; diabetes mellitus; hyperthyroidism; renal failure, renal impairment; pregnancy (category C).

ROUTE & DOSAGE

Hypertension, Angina
Adult: **PO** 40 mg once/day, may increase up to 240–320 mg/day in 1–2 divided doses

ADMINISTRATION

Note: Dose is usually titrated up in 40–80 mg increments until optimum dose is achieved.

Oral

- Do not discontinue abruptly; reduce dosage over a 1–2-wk period. Abrupt withdrawal can precipitate MI or thyroid storm in susceptible patients.
- Store at 15°–30° C (59°–86° F); protect drug from light.

ADVERSE EFFECTS (≥1%) **Body as a Whole:** Hypersensitivity (rash, pruritus, laryngospasm, respiratory disturbances). **CV:** *Bradycardia, peripheral vascular insufficiency (Raynaud's type),* palpitation, postural hypotension, conduction or rhythm disturbances, CHF. **GI:** Dry mouth. **CNS:** *Dizziness, fatigue,* sedation, headache, paresthesias, behavioral changes. **Special Senses:** Blurred vision, dry eyes. **Skin:** Dry skin. **Urogenital:** Impotence.

INTERACTIONS Drug: NSAIDS may decrease hypotensive effects; may mask symptoms of a hypoglycemic reaction to **insulin,** SULFONYLUREAS; **prazosin, terazosin** may increase severe hypotensive response to first dose.

PHARMACOKINETICS Absorption: 30–40% of PO dose absorbed. **Peak:** 2–4 h. **Duration:** 17–24 h. **Distribution:** Widely distributed; crosses placenta; distributed in breast milk. **Elimination:** 70% in urine; also in feces. **Half-Life:** 10–24 h.

NURSING IMPLICATIONS

Assessment & Drug Effects

- Assess heart rate and BP before administration of each dose. Withhold drug and notify physician if apical pulse drops below 60 bpm or systolic BP below 90 mm Hg.
- Monitor weight. Advise patient to report weight gain of 1–1.5 kg (2–3 lb) in a day and any other possible signs of CHF (e.g., cough, fatigue, dyspnea, rapid pulse, edema).
- Evaluate effectiveness for patients with angina by reduction in frequency of anginal attacks and improved exercise tolerance. Improvement should coincide with steady state serum concentration reached within 6–9 days. Keep physician informed of drug effect.
- Monitor patients with diabetes mellitus closely. Beta-adrenergic blockade produced by nadolol may prevent important clinical manifestations of hypoglycemia (e.g., tachycardia, BP changes).
- Monitor I&O ratio and creatinine clearance in patients with impaired kidney function or with cardiac problems. Dosage intervals will be lengthened with decreases in creatinine clearance.

Patient & Family Education

- Check pulse before taking each dose. Do not take your medication if pulse rate drops below 60 (or other parameter set by physician) or becomes irregular. Consult your physician right away.
- Do not stop taking your medication or alter dosage without consulting your physician.
- Do not drive or engage in potentially hazardous activities until response to drug is known.

NAFARELIN ACETATE

(na-fa're-lin)

Synarel

Classification: GONADOTROPIN-RELEASING HORMONE (GnRH) ANALOG

Therapeutic: GnRH ANALOG

Prototype: Leuprolide

Pregnancy Category: X

AVAILABILITY 0.2 mg/spray solution

ACTION & *THERAPEUTIC EFFECT* Potent agonist analog of gonadotropin-releasing hormone (GnRH). Inhibits pituitary gonadotropin secretion of LH and FSH. *Decrease in serum estradiol or testosterone concentrations results in the quiescence of tissues and functions that depend on LH and FSH.*

USES Endometriosis and precocious puberty.

UNLABELED USES Uterine leiomyomas, benign prostatic hypertrophy.

CONTRAINDICATIONS Hypersensitivity to GnRH or GnRH agonist analog; undiagnosed abnormal vaginal bleeding; pregnancy (category X), lactation.

CAUTIOUS USE Polycystic ovarian disease; osteoporosis.

ROUTE & DOSAGE

Endometriosis

Adult: **Inhalation** 2 inhalations/day (200 mcg/inhalation), one in each nostril, begin between days 2 and 4 of menstrual cycle; in patients with persistent regular menstruation after 2 mo of therapy, may increase to 800 mcg/day as 2 inhalations (one in each nostril) b.i.d.; do not exceed 6 mo of treatment

Precocious Puberty

Child: **Inhalation** 800–1200 mcg/day divided q8–12h

ADMINISTRATION

Inhalation

- Withhold any topical nasal decongestant, if being used, until at least 30 min after nafarelin administration.
- Store at 15°–30° C (59°–86° F); protect from light.

ADVERSE EFFECTS (≥1%) **GI:** *Bloating, abdominal cramps,* weight gain, nausea. **Endocrine:** *Hot flashes, anovulation, amenorrhea, vaginal dryness,* galactorrhea. **Metabolic:** Decreased bone mineral content (reversible). **CNS:** Transient headache, inertia, mild depression, moodiness, fatigue. **Respiratory:** Nasal irritation. **Urogenital:** *Impotence, decreased libido,* dyspareunia.

DIAGNOSTIC TEST INTERFERENCE Increased ***alkaline phosphatase;*** marked increase in ***estradiol*** in first 2 wk, then decrease to below baseline; decreased ***FSH*** and ***LH*** levels; decreased ***testosterone*** levels.

INTERACTIONS Drug: No clinically significant interactions established.

PHARMACOKINETICS Absorption: 21% absorbed from nasal mucosa. **Onset:** 4 wk. **Peak:** 12 wk. **Duration:** 30–50 days after discontinuing drug. **Distribution:** 78–84% bound to plasma proteins; crosses placenta. **Metabolism:** Hydrolyzed in kidney. **Elimination:** 44–55% in urine over 7 days, 19–44% in feces. **Half-Life:** 2.7 h.

NURSING IMPLICATIONS

Assessment & Drug Effects

- Make appropriate inquiries about breakthrough bleeding, which may indicate that patient has missed successive drug doses.

Patient & Family Education

- Read the information pamphlet provided with nafarelin.
- Inform physician if breakthrough bleeding occurs or menstruation persists.
- Use or add barrier contraceptive during treatment.

NAFCILLIN SODIUM

(naf-sill'in)

Classifications: BETA-LACTAM ANTIBIOTIC; PENICILLIN
Therapeutic: ANTISTAPHYLOCOCCAL PENICILLIN
Prototype: Penicillin G potassium
Pregnancy Category: B

AVAILABILITY 1 g, 2 g injection

ACTION & *THERAPEUTIC EFFECT* Semisynthetic, acid-stable, penicillinase-resistant penicillin. Interfering with synthesis of mucopeptides essential to formation and integrity of bacterial cell wall leading to bacterial cell lysis. *Effective against both penicillin-sensitive and penicillin-resistant strains of* Staphylococcus aureus. *Also active against pneumococci and group A beta-hemolytic streptococci.*

N

USES Primarily, infections caused by penicillinase-producing staphylococci. Serum concentrations are considerably enhanced by concurrent use of probenecid.

CONTRAINDICATIONS Hypersensitivity to penicillins, cephalosporins, and other allergens; use of oral drug in severe infections, gastric dilatation, cardiospasm, or intestinal hypermotility.

CAUTIOUS USE History of or suspected atopy or allergy (eczema, hives, hay fever, asthma); GI disease; hepatic disease; pregnancy (category B); lactation.

ROUTE & DOSAGE

Staphylococcal Infections
Adult: **IV** 500 mg–1 g q4h (max: 12 g/day) **IM** 500 mg q4–6h
Child: **IV** 50–200 mg/kg/day divided q4–6h (max: 12 g/day) **IM** *Weight greater than 40 kg,* 500 mg q4–6h; *weight less than 40 kg,* 25 mg/kg b.i.d.
Neonate: **IV** 50–100 mg/kg/day divided q6–12h **IM** 25–50 mg/kg b.i.d.

ADMINISTRATION

Intramuscular

- Reconstitute each 500 mg with 1.7 mL of sterile water for injection or NaCl injection to yield 250 mg/mL. Shake vigorously to dissolve.
- In adults: Make certain solution is clear. Select site carefully. Inject deeply into gluteal muscle. Rotate injection sites.
- In children: The preferred IM site in children younger than 3 y is the midlateral or anterolateral thigh. Check agency policy.
- Label and date vials of reconstituted solution. Remains stable for 7 days under refrigeration and for 3 days at 15°–30° C (59°–86° F).

Intravenous

Note: Verify correct IV concentration and rate of infusion in neonates, infants, children with physician.

PREPARE: **Direct:** Reconstitute as for IM injection. ▪ Further dilute with 15–30 mL of D5W, NS, or 0.45% NaCl. **Intermittent:** Dilute the required dose of reconstituted solution in 100–150 mL of compatible IV solution. **Continuous:** Add the required dose of reconstituted solution to a volume of IV solution that maintains concentration of drug between 2–40 mg/mL.

ADMINISTER: **Direct:** Give over at least 10 min. **Intermittent:** Give over 30–90 min. **Continuous:** Give at ordered rate.

INCOMPATIBILITIES **Solution/additive:** **Aminophylline, ascor-**

bic acid, aztreonam, bleomycin, cytarabine, gentamicin, hydrocortisone, methylprednisolone, promazine. Y-site: **Diltiazem, droperidol, insulin regular, labetalol, midazolam, nalbuphine, pentazocine, vancomycin, verapamil.**

- Note: Usually, limit IV therapy to 24–48 h because of the possibility of thrombophlebitis (see Appendix F), particularly in older adults.
- Discard unused portions 24 h after reconstitution.

ADVERSE EFFECTS (≥1%) **Body as a Whole:** Drug fever, anaphylaxis (particularly following parenteral therapy). **GI:** Nausea, vomiting, *diarrhea,* increase in serum transaminase activity (following IM). **Hematologic:** Eosinophilia, thrombophlebitis following IV; neutropenia (long-term therapy). **Metabolic:** Hypokalemia (with high IV doses). **Skin:** Urticaria, pruritus, rash, pain and tissue irritation. **Urogenital:** Allergic interstitial nephritis.

DIAGNOSTIC TEST INTERFERENCE Nafcillin in large doses can cause false-positive ***urine protein*** tests using ***sulfosalicylic acid method*** or serum protein tests.

INTERACTIONS Drug: May antagonize hypoprothrombinemic effects of **warfarin. Probenecid** increases serum concentrations.

PHARMACOKINETICS Peak: 30–120 min IM; 15 min IV. **Duration:** 4–6 h IM. **Distribution:** Distributes into CNS with inflamed meninges; crosses placenta; distributed into breast milk, 90% protein bound. **Metabolism:** Enters enterohepatic circulation. **Elimination:** Primarily in bile; 10–30% in urine. **Half-Life:** 1 h.

NURSING IMPLICATIONS

Assessment & Drug Effects

- Lab tests: Perform C&S prior to initiation of therapy and periodically thereafter.
- Obtain a careful history before therapy to determine any prior allergic reactions to penicillins, cephalosporins, and other allergens.
- Inspect IV site for inflammatory reaction. Also check IV site for leakage; in the older adult patient especially, loss of tissue elasticity with aging may promote extravasation around the needle.
- Note: Allergic reactions, principally rash, occur most commonly.
- Lab tests: Baseline and periodic WBC with differential; periodic LFTs, and kidney function tests with nafcillin therapy longer than 2 wk.
- Monitor neutrophil count. Nafcillin-induced neutropenia (agranulocytosis) occurs commonly during third week of therapy. It may be associated with malaise, fever, sore mouth, or throat. Perform periodic assessments of liver and kidney functions during prolonged therapy.
- Be alert for signs of bacterial or fungal superinfections (see Appendix F) in patients on prolonged therapy.
- Determine IV sodium intake for patients with sodium restriction. Nafcillin sodium contains approximately 3 mEq of sodium per gram.

Patient & Family Education

- Report promptly S&S of neutropenia (see Assessment & Drug Effects), superinfection, or hypokalemia (see Appendix F).

NAFTIFINE

(naf'ti-feen)

N

Naftin
Classifications: ANTIBIOTIC; ANTIFUNGAL
Therapeutic: ANTIFUNGAL
Prototype: Terbinafine
Pregnancy Category: B

AVAILABILITY 1% cream, gel

ACTION & *THERAPEUTIC EFFECT* Synthetic broad-spectrum antifungal agent that may be fungicidal depending on the organism. Interferes in the synthesis of ergosterol, the principal sterol in the fungus cell membrane. Ergosterol becomes depleted and membrane function is affected. *Effective against topical infections caused by fungal organisms.*

USES Tinea pedis, tinea cruris, and tinea corporis.

CONTRAINDICATIONS Hypersensitivity to naftifine; occlusive dressing.
CAUTIOUS USE Pregnancy (category B), lactation. Safety and efficacy in children are not established.

N

ROUTE & DOSAGE

Tinea Infections
Adult: **Topical** Apply cream daily, or apply gel twice daily, up to 4 wk

ADMINISTRATION

Topical
- Gently massage into affected area and surrounding skin. Wash hands before and after application.
- Do not apply occlusive dressing unless specifically directed to do so.
- Store at 15°–30° C (59°–86° F).

ADVERSE EFFECTS (≥1%) **Skin:** Burning or stinging, dryness, erythema, itching, local irritation.

INTERACTIONS No clinically significant interactions established.

PHARMACOKINETICS Absorption: 2.5–6% absorbed through intact skin. **Onset:** 7 days. **Metabolism:** In liver. **Elimination:** In urine and feces. **Half-Life:** 2–3 days.

NURSING IMPLICATIONS

Assessment & Drug Effects
- Assess for irritation or sensitivity to cream; these are indications to discontinue use.
- Reevaluate use of drug if no improvement is noted after 4 wk.

Patient & Family Education
- Learn correct application technique.
- Avoid contact with eyes or mucous membranes.

NALBUPHINE HYDROCHLORIDE

(nal'byoo-feen)
Nubain
Classifications: ANALGESIC; NARCOTIC (OPIATE) AGONIST-ANTAGONIST
Therapeutic: NARCOTIC ANALGESIC
Prototype: Pentazocine
Pregnancy Category: B; D in prolonged use or in high does at term

AVAILABILITY 10 mg/mL, 20 mg/mL injection

ACTION & *THERAPEUTIC EFFECT* Synthetic narcotic analgesic with agonist and weak antagonist properties that is a potent analgesic. *Analgesic action that relieves moderate to severe pain with apparently low potential for dependence.*

USES Symptomatic relief of moderate to severe pain. Also preoperative sedation analgesia and as a supplement to surgical anesthesia.

CONTRAINDICATIONS History of hypersensitivity to nalbuphine, opiate agonists; pregnancy (category D in prolonged use or in high doses at term).

CAUTIOUS USE History of emotional instability or drug abuse; head injury, increased intracranial pressure; cardiac disease; impaired respirations, COPD; GI disorders; impaired kidney or liver function; MI; biliary tract surgery; pregnancy (category B; see CONTRAINDICATIONS), lactation.

ROUTE & DOSAGE

Moderate to Severe Pain

Adult: **IV/IM/Subcutaneous** 10 mg/70 kg q3–6h prn (max: 160 mg/day)

Surgery Anesthesia Supplement

Adult: **IV** 0.3–3 mg/kg, then 0.25–0.5 mg/kg as required

ADMINISTRATION

Intramuscular/Subcutaneous

- Inject undiluted.

Intravenous

PREPARE: **Direct:** Give undiluted.
ADMINISTER: **Direct:** Give at a rate of 10 mg or fraction thereof over 3–5 min.
INCOMPATIBILITIES **Solution/additive:** **Diazepam, dimenhydrinate, ketorolac, pentobarbital, promethazine, thiethylperazine.** **Y-site:** **Allopurinol, amphotericin B cholesteryl, cefepime, docetaxel, methotrexate, nafcillin, pemetrexed, piperacillin/tazobactam, sargramostim, sodium bicarbonate.**

- Store at 15°–30° C (59°–86° F), avoid freezing.

ADVERSE EFFECTS (≥1%) **CV:** Hypertension, hypotension, bradycardia, tachycardia, flushing. **GI:** Abdominal cramps, bitter taste, *nausea, vomiting,* dry mouth. **CNS:** *Sedation, dizziness,* nervousness, depression, restlessness, crying, euphoria, dysphoria, distortion of body image, unusual dreams, confusion, hallucinations; numbness and tingling sensations, headache, vertigo. **Respiratory:** Dyspnea, asthma, <u>respiratory depression</u>. **Skin:** Pruritus, urticaria, burning sensation, *sweaty, clammy skin.* **Special Senses:** Miosis, blurred vision, speech difficulty. **Urogenital:** Urinary urgency.

INTERACTIONS Drug: Alcohol and other CNS DEPRESSANTS add to CNS depression.

PHARMACOKINETICS Onset: 2–3 min IV; 15 min IM. **Peak:** 30 min IV. **Duration:** 3–6 h. **Distribution:** Crosses placenta. **Metabolism:** In liver. **Elimination:** In urine. **Half-Life:** 5 h.

NURSING IMPLICATIONS

Assessment & Drug Effects

- Assess respiratory rate before drug administration. Withhold drug and notify physician if respiratory rate falls below 12.
- Watch for allergic response in persons with sulfite sensitivity.
- Administer with caution to patients with hepatic or renal impairment.
- Monitor ambulatory patients; nalbuphine may produce drowsiness.
- Watch for respiratory depression of newborn if drug is used during labor and delivery.
- Avoid abrupt termination of nalbuphine following prolonged use, which may result in symptoms

similar to narcotic withdrawal: Nausea, vomiting, abdominal cramps, lacrimation, nasal congestion, piloerection, fever, restlessness, anxiety.

Patient & Family Education

- Do not drive or engage in potentially hazardous activities until response to drug is known.
- Avoid alcohol and other CNS depressants.

NALIDIXIC ACID

(nal-i-dix′ik)

NegGram

Classifications: URINARY TRACT ANTIINFECTIVE; ANTIBIOTIC, QUINOLONE

Therapeutic: URINARY TRACT; ANTIBIOTIC

Prototype: Ciprofloxacin

Pregnancy Category: C

N

AVAILABILITY 250 mg, 500 mg, 1 g tablets

ACTION & *THERAPEUTIC EFFECT* Synthetic quinolone with intracellular action that inhibits microbial DNA replication and RNA synthesis. *Marked bactericidal activity against most gram-negative urinary tract pathogens with the exception of strains of* Pseudomonas.

USES Urinary tract infections caused by susceptible gram-negative organisms including most *Proteus* strains, *Klebsiella*, *Enterobacter*, and *Escherichia coli*.

UNLABELED USES GI tract infections caused by susceptible strains of *Shigella sonnei;* prophylaxis of bacteriuria and in bladder irrigation for low-grade cystitis.

CONTRAINDICATIONS History of convulsive disorders; first trimester of pregnancy; infants younger than 3 mo.

CAUTIOUS USE Prepubertal child; kidney or liver disease; epilepsy; cerebral arteriosclerosis; respiratory insufficiency; patients and breast-feeding infants with G6PD deficiency; pregnancy (category C), lactation.

ROUTE & DOSAGE

Urinary Tract Infections

Adult: **PO** Acute therapy: 1 g q.i.d.; Chronic therapy: 500 mg q.i.d.

Child (older than 3 mo): **PO** Acute therapy: 55 mg/kg/day in 4 divided doses; Chronic therapy: 33 mg/kg/day in 4 divided doses

ADMINISTRATION

Oral

- Give with food or milk if drug causes GI distress. Otherwise, give on an empty stomach 1 h before or 2 h after meals.
- Store at 15°–30° C (59°–86° F) in tight container and avoid freezing.

ADVERSE EFFECTS (≥1%) **Body as a Whole:** Angioedema, fever, chills, arthralgia, hypersensitivity pneumonitis, <u>anaphylaxis</u> (rare). **CNS:** Drowsiness, headache, malaise, dizziness, vertigo, syncope, weakness, myalgia, peripheral neuritis, confusion, excitement, mental depression, seizures, insomnia. **GI:** Abdominal pain, *nausea, vomiting,* diarrhea, cholestasis, transient increase in AST. **Hematologic:** Eosinophilia, hemolytic anemia (especially in G6PD deficiency). **Skin:** Photosensitivity, pruritus, urticaria, rash. **Other:** Cartilage erosion.

DIAGNOSTIC TEST INTERFERENCE False-positive urine tests for ***glucose*** with ***cupric sulfate reagent*** (e.g.,

Benedict's or ***Clinitest***) but not with ***glucose oxidase methods*** (e.g., ***Clinistix, TesTape***). May cause elevation of ***urinary 17-keto-steroids (Zimmerman method)*** and ***urine vanillylmandelic acid (VMA).***

INTERACTIONS Drug: ANTACIDS, **sucralfate, calcium, magnesium, didanosine,** MULTIVITAMINS (containing **iron** or **zinc**) may decrease absorption of nalidixic acid; may increase hypoprothrombinemic effects of **warfarin.**

PHARMACOKINETICS Absorption: Readily from GI tract. **Peak:** Urine: 3–4 h. **Distribution:** Crosses placenta; distributed into breast milk. **Metabolism:** Partially in liver; some in kidneys. **Elimination:** In urine. **Half-Life:** 1.1–2.5 h.

NURSING IMPLICATIONS

Assessment & Drug Effects

- Lab tests: Perform C&S tests prior to initiation of treatment and periodically thereafter. Obtain blood counts and kidney or liver function tests if therapy is continued longer than 2 wk.
- Watch for CNS reactions, which tend to occur 30 min after initiation of treatment or after second or third dose. Infants, children, and older adults are especially susceptible. Report immediately the onset of marked irritability, vomiting, bulging of anterior fontanelle, headache, excitement or drowsiness, papilledema, vertigo.

Patient & Family Education

- Use drug exactly as prescribed and do not change dosage. Omitted doses, especially in early days of therapy, may promote development of bacterial resistance. Take full amount of medication.
- Contact physician immediately for unexplained behavior changes or severe headaches.
- Maintain adequate hydration (2000–3000 mL/day if tolerated) during treatment period. Consult physician if you notice a change in your urination pattern.
- Avoid exposure to direct sunlight or ultraviolet light while receiving drug. Contact physician if photosensitivity occurs. You may be photosensitive up to 3 mo after termination of drug.
- Contact your physician if you notice visual disturbances during first few days of therapy. Symptoms usually disappear promptly with reduction of dosage or discontinuation of therapy.

NALOXONE HYDROCHLORIDE (Pr)

(nal-ox'one)

Narcan

Classification: NARCOTIC (OPIATE ANTAGONIST)

Therapeutic: NARCOTIC ANTAGONIST

Pregnancy Category: C

AVAILABILITY 0.02 mg/mL, 0.4 mg/mL, 1 mg/mL injection

ACTION & *THERAPEUTIC EFFECT* A "pure" narcotic antagonist, essentially free of agonistic (morphine-like) properties. It possesses potent narcotic antagonist action. *Reverses the effects of opiates, including respiratory depression, sedation, and hypotension.*

USES Narcotic overdosage; complete or partial reversal of narcotic depression. Drug of choice when nature of depressant drug is not known and for diagnosis of sus-

pected acute opioid overdosage. Challenge for opioid dependence.
UNLABELED USES Shock and to reverse alcohol-induced or clonidine-induced coma or respiratory depression.

CONTRAINDICATIONS Hypersensitivity to naloxone, naltrexone, nalmefene; respiratory depression due to nonopioid drugs; substance abuse.
CAUTIOUS USE Known or suspected narcotic dependence; brain tumor, head trauma, increased ICP; history of substance abuse; cardiac irritability; seizure disorders; pregnancy (category C), lactation.

ROUTE & DOSAGE

Opiate Overdose

Adult: **IV** 0.4–2 mg, may repeat q2–3min up to 10 mg if necessary
Child (5 y or older and weight at least 20 kg): **IV** 2 mg, may repeat q2–3min if needed
Child/Infant (weight less than 20 kg): **IV** 0.01–0.1 mg/kg, may repeat q2–3min up to 10 mg if necessary
Neonate: **IV/Subcutaneous/IM** 0.01 mg/kg, may repeat q2–3min

Postoperative Opiate Depression

Adult: **IV** 0.1–0.2 mg, may repeat q2–3min for up to 3 doses if necessary
Child: **IV** 0.005–0.01 mg/kg, may repeat q2–3min up to 3 doses if necessary

Challenge for Opioid Dependence

Adult: **IM** 0.2 mg, observe for 30 sec for signs/symptoms of withdrawal, if no signs/symptoms then 0.6 mg and observe for 20 min

ADMINISTRATION

Intramuscular/Subcutaneous

- Inject undiluted.

Intravenous

PREPARE: **Direct:** May be given undiluted. **IV Infusion:** Dilute 2 mg in 500 mL of D5W or NS to yield 4 mcg/mL (0.004 mg/mL).
ADMINISTER: **Direct:** Give bolus dose over 10–15 sec. **IV Infusion:** Adjust rate according to patient response.
INCOMPATIBILITIES **Y-site: Amphotericin B cholesteryl complex, lansoprazole.**

- Use IV solutions within 24 h.
- Store at 15°–30° C (59°–86° F), protect from excessive light.

ADVERSE EFFECTS (≥1%) **Body as a Whole:** Reversal of analgesia, tremors, hyperventilation, slight drowsiness, sweating. **CV:** Increased BP, tachycardia. **GI:** Nausea, vomiting. **Hematologic:** Elevated partial thromboplastin time.

INTERACTIONS Drug: Reverses analgesic effects of NARCOTIC (OPIATE) AGONISTS and NARCOTIC (OPIATE) AGONIST-ANTAGONISTS.

PHARMACOKINETICS Onset: 2 min. **Duration:** 45 min. **Distribution:** Crosses placenta. **Metabolism:** In liver. **Elimination:** In urine. **Half-Life:** 60–90 min.

NURSING IMPLICATIONS

Assessment & Drug Effects

- Observe patient closely; duration of action of some narcotics may exceed that of naloxone. Keep physician informed; repeat naloxone dose may be necessary.
- May precipitate opiate withdrawal if administered to a patient who is opiate dependent.

- Note: Effects of naloxone generally start to diminish 20–40 min after administration and usually disappear within 90 min.
- Monitor respirations and other vital signs.
- Monitor surgical and obstetric patients closely for bleeding. Naloxone has been associated with abnormal coagulation test results. Also observe for reversal of analgesia, which may be manifested by nausea, vomiting, sweating, tachycardia.

Patient & Family Education

- Report postoperative pain that emerges after administration of this drug to physician.

NALTREXONE HYDROCHLORIDE

(nal-trex′one)

ReVia, Vivitrol

METHYLNALTREXONE

Relistor

Classification: NARCOTIC (OPIATE ANTAGONIST)

Therapeutic: NARCOTIC ANTAGONIST

Prototype: Naloxone HCl

Pregnancy Category: C

AVAILABILITY 25 mg, 50 mg, 100 mg tablets; 380 mg injection; **Methylnaltrexone:** 12 mg/0.6 mL injection

ACTION & *THERAPEUTIC EFFECT* Pure opioid antagonist with a mechanism of action that appears to result from competitive binding at opioid receptor sites reduces euphoria and drug craving without supporting the addiction. *Weakens or completely and reversibly blocks the subjective effects (the "high") of IV opioids and analgesics possessing both agonist and antagonist activity.*

USES Adjunct to the maintenance of an opioid-free state in detoxified addicts who are and desire to remain narcotic free. Management of alcohol dependence as an adjunct to social and psychotherapeutic methods. Opioid-related constipation in patients nonresponsive to laxatives.

UNLABELED USES Obesity.

CONTRAINDICATIONS Patients receiving opioid analgesics; opiate agonist use within 7–10 days; acute opioid agonist withdrawal; opioid-dependent patient; acute hepatitis, liver failure, hepatic encephalopathy; suicidal ideation; any individual who (1) fails naloxone challenge, (2) has a positive urine screen for opioids, or (3) has a history of sensitivity to naltrexone; lactation. Safe use in children younger than 18 y is not established.

CAUTIOUS USE Mild to moderate hepatic impairment (Child-Pugh class A or B); history of suicidal tendencies; renal impairment; pregnancy (category C); **IM form:** Special at-risk patients: Thrombocytopenia, coagulopathy (e.g., hemophilia), severe hepatic impairment.

ROUTE & DOSAGE

Treatment of Opiate Cessation

Adult: **PO** 25 mg followed by another 25 mg in 1 h if no withdrawal response; maintenance regimen is individualized (max: 800 mg/day)

Alcohol Dependence

Adult: **PO** 50 mg once/day **IM** 380 mg qmo

N

Opioid-Related Constipation (Relistor)

Adult: **Subcutaneous** *Weight less than 38 kg or greater than 114 kg,* 0.15 mg/kg every other day (max: 0.15 mg/kg in 24 h); *weight 38–62 kg,* 8 mg every other day (max: 8 mg/24 h); *weight 62–114 kg,* 12 mg every other day (max: 12 mg/24 h)

Renal Impairment Dosage Adjustment (Relistor)

CrCl less than 30 mL/min: Reduce dose by 50%

ADMINISTRATION

Oral

- Give without regard to food.

Intramuscular

- Give IM into the gluteal muscle, alternating buttocks per injection. Aspirate before injection to ensure that drug is not injected IV.

Subcutaneous (Methylnaltrexone Only)

- Give subcutaneously into upper arm, abdomen, or thigh.

ADVERSE EFFECTS (≥1%) **GI:** Dry mouth, anorexia, *nausea, vomiting,* constipation, *abdominal cramps/pain,* hepatotoxicity. **Musculoskeletal:** *Muscle and joint pains.* **CNS:** *Difficulty sleeping, anxiety, headache, nervousness,* reduced or increased energy, irritability, dizziness, depression. **Skin:** Skin rash. **Hematologic: IM extended release form:** Hematoma formation at injection site. **Body as a Whole:** Chills.

INTERACTIONS Drug: Increased somnolence and lethargy with PHENOTHIAZINES; reverses analgesic effects of NARCOTIC (OPIATE) AGONISTS and NARCOTIC (OPIATE) AGONIST-ANTAGONISTS.

PHARMACOKINETICS Absorption: Rapidly from GI tract; 20% reaches systemic circulation (first pass effect). **Onset:** 15–30 min. **Peak:** 1 h; 30 min (Relistor). **Duration:** 24–72 h PO; 4 wk IM. **Metabolism:** In liver to active metabolite. **Elimination:** In urine. **Half-Life:** 10–13 h PO, 5–10 days IM.

NURSING IMPLICATIONS

Assessment & Drug Effects

- Lab tests: Check liver function before the treatment is started, at monthly intervals for 6 mo, and then periodically as indicated.

Patient & Family Education

- Note: Naltrexone therapy may put you in danger of overdosing if you use opiates. Small doses even at frequent intervals will give no desired effects; however, a dose large enough to produce a high is dangerous and may be fatal.
- It may be possible to transfer from methadone to naltrexone. This can be done after gradual withdrawal and final discontinuation of methadone.
- Report promptly onset of signs of hepatic toxicity (see Appendix F) to physician. The drug will be discontinued.
- Do not self-dose with OTC drugs for treatment of cough, colds, diarrhea, or analgesia. Many available preparations contain small doses of an opioid. Consult physician for safe drugs if they are needed.
- Tell a doctor or dentist before treatment that you are using naltrexone.
- Wear identification jewelry indicating naltrexone use.

NANDROLONE DECANOATE

(nan′droe-lone)

Classification: ANABOLIC/ANDROGEN STEROID
Therapeutic: ANABOLIC STEROID
Prototype: Testosterone
Pregnancy Category: X
Controlled Substance: Schedule III

AVAILABILITY 100 mg/mL, 200 mg/mL injection

ACTION & *THERAPEUTIC EFFECT* Synthetic steroid with high ratio of anabolic activity to androgenic activity. Actions last 3–4 wk. *Increases hemoglobin and red cell mass and increases lean body mass in patients with cachexia (muscle wasting).*

USES Control of metastatic breast cancer, management of anemia of renal insufficiency.

CONTRAINDICATIONS Males with prostate or breast cancer; severe cardiac disease; liver dysfunction, severe renal disease; nephrotic syndrome, hypercalcemia; children younger than 2 y; pregnancy (category X), lactation.

CAUTIOUS USE Benign prostatic hypertrophy, history of MI; CAD; diabetes mellitus; heart failure; BPH; children.

ROUTE & DOSAGE

Anemia (Decanoate)

Adult: **IM** 50–200 mg/wk
Child (2–13 y): **IM** 25–50 mg q3–4wk

Metastatic Breast Cancer

Adult: **IM** 50–100 mg/wk

ADMINISTRATION

Intramuscular

- Inject drug deep IM, preferably into gluteal muscle in adult. Follow agency policy regarding IM site in small child.
- Intermittent therapy is usually recommended (4-mo course of treatment followed by 6–8-wk rest period).

ADVERSE EFFECTS (≥1%) **Body as a Whole:** Muscle cramps. **GI:** *Nausea, vomiting,* diarrhea, anorexia, abdominal fullness, cholestatic jaundice, <u>hepatic necrosis, hepatocellular neoplasms</u>. **Hematologic:** Leukopenia. **Metabolic:** Sodium, chloride, water, potassium, phosphate, and calcium retention, ankle edema, glucose intolerance, increased cholesterol. **CNS:** Excitation, insomnia, chills, toxic confusion. **Endocrine:** *Acne, virilization.*

INTERACTIONS Drug: May increase hypoprothrombinemic effects of **warfarin;** may decrease **insulin** and SULFONYLUREA requirements; CORTICOSTEROIDS may increase edema. **Herbal: Echinacea** may increase risk of hepatotoxicity.

PHARMACOKINETICS Absorption: Slowly absorbed from IM injection site over 4 days. **Peak:** 3–6 days. **Metabolism:** In liver to active metabolite. **Half-Life:** 6–8 days.

NURSING IMPLICATIONS

Assessment & Drug Effects

- Lab tests: Obtain baseline and periodic liver function evaluations and electrolyte levels.
- Monitor for S&S of hepatic toxicity (see Appendix F) and electrolyte imbalance, especially hyperkalemia and hypercalcemia (see Appendix F).
- Monitor diabetics for loss of glycemic control.

Patient & Family Education

- Note: In women, the drug may cause virilization (e.g., increased facial and body hair, deepening of voice).

N

NAPHAZOLINE HYDROCHLORIDE

(naf-az′oh-leen)

Ak-Con, Albalon, Allerest, Clear Eyes, Comfort, Degest-2, Naf-azair, Naphcon, Privine, Vaso-Clear, Vasocon

Classifications: EYE AND EAR PREPARATION; VASOCONSTRICTOR; ALPHA-ADRENERGIC AGONIST; DECONGESTANT

Therapeutic: DECONGESTANT

Pregnancy Category: C

AVAILABILITY 0.012%, 0.02%, 0.03%, 0.1% ophth solution; 0.05% nasal solution

ACTION & *THERAPEUTIC EFFECT* Direct-acting alpha-adrenergic agonist that produces rapid and prolonged vasoconstriction of arterioles. *It decreases fluid exudation and mucosal engorgement.*

USES Nasal decongestant and ocular vasoconstrictor.

CONTRAINDICATIONS Narrow-angle glaucoma; concomitant use with MAO inhibitors or tricyclic antidepressants; lactation. Safe use in children younger than 6 y has not been established.

CAUTIOUS USE Hypertension, cardiac irregularities, advanced arteriosclerosis; diabetes; hyperthyroidism; older adult patients; pregnancy (category C).

ROUTE & DOSAGE

Congestion

Adult: **Intranasal** 2 drops or sprays of 0.05% solution in each nostril q3–6h for no more than 3–5 days **Ophthalmic** See Appendix A

Child: **Intranasal** 1–2 drops or sprays of 0.025% solution q3–6h for no more than 3–5 days

ADMINISTRATION

Instillation

- Instill nasal spray with patient in upright position. If administered in reclining position, a stream rather than a spray may be ejected, with possibility of systemic reaction.
- Minimize amount of drug swallowed by taking care not to direct the flow toward nasopharynx and by positioning patient properly with the head tilted slightly downward.
- Store at 15°–30° C (59°–86° F), protect from freezing.

ADVERSE EFFECTS (≥1%) **Body as a Whole:** Hypersensitivity reactions, headache, nausea, weakness, sweating, drowsiness, hypothermia, <u>coma</u>. **CV:** Hypertension, bradycardia, <u>shock-like hypotension</u>. **Special Senses:** Transient nasal stinging or burning, dryness of nasal mucosa, pupillary dilation, increased intraocular pressure, rebound redness of the eye.

INTERACTIONS Drug: TRICYCLIC ANTIDEPRESSANTS, **maprotiline** may potentiate pressor effects.

PHARMACOKINETICS Onset: Within 10 min. **Duration:** 2–6 h.

NURSING IMPLICATIONS

Assessment & Drug Effects

- Watch for rebound congestion and chemical rhinitis with frequent and continued use.
- Monitor BP periodically for development or worsening of hyper-

tension, especially with ophthalmic route.
- Overdose: Bradycardia and hypotension can result. Report promptly.

Patient & Family Education
- Do not exceed prescribed regimen. Systemic effects can result from swallowing excessive medication.
- Discontinue medication and contact physician if nasal congestion is not relieved after 5 days.
- Prevent contamination of eye solution by taking care not to touch eyelid or surrounding area with dropper tip.

NAPROXEN
(na-prox′en)

Apo-Naproxen ♣, EC-Naprosyn, Naprelan, Naprosyn, Naxen ♣, Novonaprox ♣

NAPROXEN SODIUM
Aleve, Anaprox, Anaprox DS

Classifications: ANALGESIC, NONSTEROIDAL ANTI-INFLAMMATORY DRUG (NSAID); ANTIPYRETIC

Therapeutic: ANALGESIC, NSAID

Prototype: Ibuprofen

Pregnancy Category: B first and second trimester; D third trimester

AVAILABILITY 200 mg, 250 mg, 375 mg, 500 mg tablets; 375 mg, 500 mg sustained release tablets

ACTION & *THERAPEUTIC EFFECT* Propionic acid derivative. An NSAID with properties similar to ibuprofen, fenoprofen, and ketoprofen. Mechanism of action is related to inhibition of prostaglandin synthesis by inhibiting COX-1 and COX-2 isoenzymes. *Analgesic, anti-inflammatory, and antipyretic effects; also inhibits platelet aggregation and prolongs bleeding time.*

USES Anti-inflammatory and analgesic effects in symptomatic treatment of acute and chronic rheumatoid arthritis, juvenile arthritis (naproxen only), and for treatment of primary dysmenorrhea. Also management of ankylosing spondylitis, osteoarthritis, and gout.

UNLABELED USES Paget's disease of bone, Bartter's syndrome.

CONTRAINDICATIONS Active peptic ulcer; patients in whom asthma, rhinitis, urticaria, bronchospasm, or shock is precipitated by aspirin or other NSAIDs; perioperative pain associated with CABG; hypersensitivity to any NSAID; cardiac disease; pregnancy (category D third trimester); lactation. Safety in children younger than 2 y is not established.

CAUTIOUS USE History of upper GI tract disorders; impaired kidney, liver, or cardiac function; patients on sodium restriction (**naproxen sodium**); low pretreatment Hgb concentration; fluid retention, hypertension, heart failure; older adults; coagulopathy; SLE; pregnancy (category B first and second trimester).

ROUTE & DOSAGE

Note: 275 mg naproxen sodium = 250 mg naproxen

Inflammatory Disease

Adult: **PO** 250–500 mg b.i.d. (max: 1000 mg/day naproxen, 1100 mg/day naproxen sodium); Naprelan is dosed daily

Child (older than 2 y): **PO** 10–15 mg/kg/day in 2 divided doses (max: 1000 mg/day)

Mild to Moderate Pain, Dysmenorrhea
Adult: **PO** 500 mg followed by 200–250 mg q6–8h prn up to 1250 mg/day
Child (older than 2 y): **PO** 5–7 mg/kg q8–12h

ADMINISTRATION

Oral

- Ensure that extended release or enteric-coated form is not chewed or crushed. It **must be** swallowed whole.
- Give with food or an antacid (if prescribed) to reduce incidence of GI upset.
- Store at 15°–30° C (59°–86° F) in tightly closed container; protect from freezing.

ADVERSE EFFECTS (≥1%) **CNS:** *Headache, drowsiness, dizziness,* lightheadedness, depression. **CV:** Palpitation, dyspnea, peripheral edema, CHF, tachycardia. **Special Senses:** Blurred vision, tinnitus, hearing loss. **GI:** *Anorexia, heartburn,* indigestion, *nausea,* vomiting, thirst, GI bleeding, elevated serum ALT, AST. **Hematologic:** Thrombocytopenia, leukopenia, eosinophilia, inhibited platelet aggregation, agranulocytosis (rare). **Skin:** Pruritus, rash, ecchymosis. **Urogenital:** Nephrotoxicity. **Respiratory:** Pulmonary edema.

DIAGNOSTIC TEST INTERFERENCE Transient elevations in ***BUN*** and serum ***alkaline phosphatase*** may occur. Naproxen may interfere with some urinary assays of ***5-HIAA*** and may cause falsely high ***urinary 17-KGS*** levels (using ***m-dinitrobenzene reagent***). Naproxen should be withdrawn 72 h before adrenal function tests.

INTERACTIONS Drug: Bleeding time effects of ORAL ANTICOAGULANTS, **heparin** may be prolonged; may increase **lithium** toxicity. **Herbal: Feverfew, garlic, ginger, ginkgo, evening primrose oil** may increase bleeding potential.

PHARMACOKINETICS Absorption: Almost completely from GI tract when taken on empty stomach. **Peak:** 2 h naproxen; 1 h naproxen sodium. **Duration:** 7 h. **Metabolism:** In liver. **Elimination:** Primarily in urine; some biliary excretion (less than 1%). **Half-Life:** 12–15 h.

NURSING IMPLICATIONS

Assessment & Drug Effects

- Take detailed drug history prior to initiation of therapy. Observe for signs of allergic response in those with aspirin or other NSAID sensitivity.
- Lab tests: Obtain baseline and periodic evaluations of Hgb and kidney and liver function in patients receiving prolonged or high dose therapy.
- Baseline and periodic auditory and ophthalmic examinations are recommended in patients receiving prolonged or high dose therapy.
- Monitor therapeutic effectiveness. Patients with arthritis may experience symptomatic relief (reduction in joint pain, swelling, stiffness) within 24–48 h with naproxen sodium therapy and in 2–4 wk with naproxen.

Patient & Family Education

- Be aware that the therapeutic effect of naproxen may not be experienced for 3–4 wk.
- Do not drive or engage in potentially hazardous activities until response to drug is known.
- Avoid alcohol and aspirin (as well as other NSAIDs) unless otherwise advised by a physician. Potential to increase risk of GI ulceration and bleeding.

- Tell your dentist or surgeon if you are taking naproxen before any treatment; it may prolong bleeding time.

NARATRIPTAN

(nar-a-trip'tan)
Amerge
Classification: SEROTONIN 5-HT_1 RECEPTOR AGONIST
Therapeutic: ANTIMIGRAINE
Prototype: Sumatriptan
Pregnancy Category: C

AVAILABILITY 1 mg, 2.5 mg tablets

ACTION & *THERAPEUTIC EFFECT* Binds to the serotonin receptors (5-HT_{1D} and 5-HT_{1B}) on intracranial blood vessels, resulting in selective vasoconstriction of dilated vessels in the carotid circulation. It also inhibits the release of inflammatory neuropeptides associated with a migraine attack. *Inhibits vasoconstriction of dilated vessels selectively. This results in the relief of acute migraine headache attacks.*

USES Acute migraine headaches with or without aura.

CONTRAINDICATIONS Hypersensitivity to naratriptan; severe renal impairment (creatinine clearance less than 15 mL/min); severe hepatic impairment; history of ischemic heart disease (i.e., angina pectoris, MI), arteriosclerosis, cardiac arrhythmias; cardiac disease, CAD, older adults, peripheral vascular disease; cerebrovascular syndromes (i.e., strokes or TIA); uncontrolled hypertension; patients with hemiplegic or basilar migraine; older adults.

CAUTIOUS USE Cardiovascular disease; renal or hepatic insufficiency; elderly; pregnancy (category C), lactation. Safety and efficacy in children younger than 18 y are not established.

ROUTE & DOSAGE

Acute Migraine

Adult: **PO** 1–2.5 mg; may repeat in 4 h if necessary (max: 5 mg/24 h); patients with mild or moderate renal or hepatic impairment should not exceed 2.5 mg/24 h

ADMINISTRATION

Oral

- Give any time after symptoms of migraine appear. If the first tablet was effective but symptoms return, a second tablet may be given, but no sooner than 4 h after the first. Do not exceed 5 mg in 24 h.
- If there is no response to the first tablet, contact physician before administering a second tablet.
- Do not give within 24 h of an ergot-containing drug or other 5-HT_1 agonist.
- Store at 2°–25° C (36°–77° F); protect from light.

ADVERSE EFFECTS (≥1%) **Body as a Whole:** Asthenia, fatigue, malaise, pain, pressure sensation, paresthesias, throat pressure, warm/cold sensations, hot flushes. **CNS:** Somnolence, dizziness, drowsiness, headache, hypesthesia, decreased mental acuity, euphoria, tremor. **CV:** Coronary artery vasospasm, transient myocardial ischemia, MI, ventricular tachycardia, ventricular fibrillation, chest pain/tightness/heaviness, palpitations. **GI:** Dry mouth, nausea, vomiting, diarrhea. **Respiratory:** Dyspnea. **Skin:** Flushing.

N

INTERACTIONS Drug: Dihydroergotamine, methysergide, and other 5-HT$_1$ AGONISTS may cause prolonged vasospastic reactions; SSRIS have rarely caused weakness, hyperreflexia, and incoordination; MAOIS should not be used with 5-HT$_1$ AGONISTS. **Herbal: Gingko, ginseng, echinacea, St. John's wort** may increase triptan toxicity.

PHARMACOKINETICS Absorption: Rapidly absorbed, 70% bioavailability. **Peak:** 2–4 h. **Distribution:** 28–31% protein bound. **Metabolism:** In liver. **Elimination:** Primarily in urine. **Half-Life:** 6 h.

NURSING IMPLICATIONS

Assessment & Drug Effects

- Monitor carefully cardiovascular status following first dose in patients at risk for CAD (e.g., postmenopausal women, men older than 40 y, persons with known CAD risk factors) or coronary artery vasospasms.
- Be aware that ECG is recommended following first administration of naratriptan to someone with known CAD risk factors and periodically with long-term use.
- Report immediately to the physician: Chest pain, nausea, or tightness in chest or throat that is severe or does not quickly resolve.
- Obtain periodic cardiovascular evaluation with continued use.

Patient & Family Education

- Carefully review patient information leaflet and guidelines for administration.
- Contact physician immediately for any of the following: Symptoms of angina (e.g., severe and/or persistent pain or tightness in chest or throat, severe nausea); hypersensitivity (e.g., wheezing, facial swelling, skin rash, or hives); or abdominal pain.
- Report any other adverse effects (e.g., tingling, flushing, dizziness) at next physician visit.

NATALIZUMAB

(na-tal′-i-zu-mab)

Tysabri

Classifications: BIOLOGICAL RESPONSE MODIFIER; MONOCLONAL ANTIBODY; INTEGRIN INHIBITOR

Therapeutic: IMMUNOMODULATOR; MONOCLONAL ANTIBODY (IgG)

Prototype: Basiliximab

Pregnancy Category: C

AVAILABILITY 300 mg/15 mL injection

ACTION & *THERAPEUTIC EFFECT* Natalizumab is a recombinant immunoglobulin-G4 (IgG4) monoclonal antibody thought to interfere with the migration of lymphocytes and monocytes into the CNS endothelium of patients with multiple sclerosis, thereby reducing inflammation and demyelination of CNS white matter. *Inhibition of T-cell infiltration into the brain is thought to impede the demyelinating process of multiple sclerosis. It reduces relapses and occurrence of brain lesions. Natalizumab is also thought to attenuate T-lymphocyte–mediated intestinal inflammation in Crohn's disease and possibly ulcerative colitis.*

USES Treatment of relapsing forms of multiple sclerosis, treatment of Crohn's disease.

CONTRAINDICATIONS Prior hypersensitivity to natalizumab; murine protein hypersensitivity; have or have had progressive multifocal leukoencephalopathy (PML); active infection; S&S of PML; females of childbearing age; lactation; children younger than 18 y. **CAUTIOUS USE** Diabetes mellitus, immunocompromised patients; exposure to infection or tuberculosis; hepatic dysfunction; pregnancy (category C).

ROUTE & DOSAGE

Multiple Sclerosis/Moderate to Severe Crohn's Disease

Adult: **IV** 300 mg infused over 1 h every 4 wk

ADMINISTRATION

Intravenous

PREPARE: **IV Infusion:** Before and after dilution, solution should be colorless and clear to slightly opaque. Do not use if the solution has visible particles, flakes, color, or is cloudy. ▪ Withdraw 300 mg (15 mL) from the vial and add to an IV bag with 100 mL of NS. Do not use with any other diluent. ▪ Gently invert the bag to mix; do not shake. ▪ The IV solution **must be** used within 8 h.

ADMINISTER: **IV Infusion:** Flush IV line before/after with NS. Infuse over 1 h. ▪ Do not give a bolus dose. ▪ Stop infusion immediately if S&S of hypersensitivity appear.

INCOMPATIBILITIES **Solution/additive/Y-site:** Do not mix or infuse with other drugs.

▪ Store IV solution for up to 8 h at 2°–8° C (36°–46° F). ▪ Allow solution to warm to room temperature before administration

ADVERSE EFFECTS (≥1%) **Body as a Whole:** <u>Anaphylaxis</u> (rare, usually within 2 h of infusion), infections, fatigue, rigors, <u>risk of progressive multifocal leukoencephalopathy</u>. **CNS:** Depression, headache, syncope, tremor. **CV:** Chest discomfort. **GI:** Abdominal discomfort, abnormal liver function tests. **Hematologic:** Local bleeding from infusion site. **Musculoskeletal:** Arthralgia. **Respiratory:** Pneumonia. **Skin:** Acute urticaria. **Urogenital:** Urinary frequency, irregular menstruation, amenorrhea, dysmenorrhea. **Other:** Infusion-related reactions (headache, dizziness, fatigue, hypersensitivity reactions, urticaria, pruritus, and rigors).

INTERACTIONS Drug: May reduce the effectiveness of VACCINES and TOXOIDS; may increase risk of infection with IMMUNOSUPPRESSANTS.

PHARMACOKINETICS Half-Life: 11 days.

NURSING IMPLICATIONS

Assessment & Drug Effects

- During IV infusion and for 1–2 h after, monitor closely for S&S of hypersensitivity (e.g., urticaria, dizziness, fever, rash, chills, pruritus, nausea, flushing, hypotension, dyspnea, and chest pain).
- Monitor neurologic status frequently. Report promptly any emerging S&S of dysfunction.
- Lab tests: Baseline and periodic CBC with differential.

Patient & Family Education

- Report immediately any of the following during/after IV infusion: Difficulty breathing, wheezing or shortness of breath, swelling or tightness about the neck and throat, chest pain, skin rash or hives.
- Report promptly S&S of infection (e.g., cough, fever, chills, or sore throat).

NATAMYCIN

(na-ta-mye′sin)
Natacyn
Classification: ANTIFUNGAL ANTIBIOTIC
Therapeutic: ANTIFUNGAL
Prototype: Amphotericin B
Pregnancy Category: C

AVAILABILITY 5% suspension

ACTION & *THERAPEUTIC EFFECT* Mechanism of action simulates that of amphotericin B by binding to sterols in the fungal cell membrane resulting in cell death of fungi. *Effective against many yeasts and filamentous fungi including* Candida, Aspergillus, Cephalosporium, Fusarium, *and* Penicillium.

USES Blepharitis, conjunctivitis, and keratitis caused by susceptible fungi. Drug of choice for *Fusarium solani* keratitis.

UNLABELED USES Oral, cutaneous, and vaginal candidiasis; intranasal treatment of pulmonary aspergillosis.

CONTRAINDICATIONS Concomitant administration of a corticosteroid.

CAUTIOUS USE Pregnancy (category C), lactation. Safety and efficacy in children are not established.

ROUTE & DOSAGE

Fungal Keratitis

Adult: **Ophthalmic** 1 drop in conjunctival sac of infected eye q1–2h for 3–4 days, then decrease to 1 drop q6–8h, then gradually decrease to 1 drop q4–7days

ADMINISTRATION

Instillation

- Wash hands thoroughly before and after treatment. Infection is easily transferred from infected to noninfected eye and to other individuals.
- Shake well before using.
- Store at 2°–24° C (36°–75° F).

ADVERSE EFFECTS (≥1%) **Special Senses:** Blurred vision, photophobia, eye pain. Uneven adherence of suspension to epithelial ulcerations or in fornices.

INTERACTIONS Drug: No clinically significant interactions established.

PHARMACOKINETICS Absorption: Drug adheres to ulcerated surface of the cornea and is retained in conjunctival fornices. Does not appear to be systemically absorbed.

NURSING IMPLICATIONS

Assessment & Drug Effects

- Inspect eye for response and tolerance at least twice weekly.
- Note: Lack of improvement in keratitis within 7–10 days suggests that causative organisms may not be susceptible to natamycin. Reevaluation is indicated and possibly a change in therapy.

Patient & Family Education

- Learn appropriate technique for application of eye drops.
- Expect temporary light sensitivity. Be prepared to wear sunglasses outdoors after drug administration and perhaps for a few hours indoors.
- Return to ophthalmologist for reevaluation of eye problem if you experience symptoms of conjunctivitis: Pain, discharge, itching, scratching “foreign body sensation,” changes in vision.
- Do not share facecloths and hand towels; this will help prevent transmission of the fungal infection.

NATEGLINIDE

(nat-e′gli-nide)

Starlix

Classifications: ANTIDIABETIC; MEGLITINIDE

Therapeutic: ANTIDIABETIC

Prototype: Repaglinide

Pregnancy Category: C

AVAILABILITY 60 mg, 120 mg tablets

ACTION & *THERAPEUTIC EFFECT* Lowers blood glucose levels by stimulating the release of insulin from the pancreatic cells of a type 2 diabetic. Significantly reduces postprandial blood glucose in type 2 diabetics and improves glycemic control when given before meals. *Effectiveness is indicated by preprandial blood glucose between 80 and 120 mg/dL and HbA1C 6.5% or less.*

USES Alone or in combination with metformin for the treatment of non-insulin-dependent diabetes mellitus.

CONTRAINDICATIONS Prior hypersensitivity to nateglinide. Type 1 (insulin-dependent) diabetes mellitus, diabetic ketoacidosis; hypoglycemia.

CAUTIOUS USE Renal impairment; liver dysfunction; adrenal or pituitary insufficiency; malnutrition; infection, trauma, surgery or unusual stress; surgery; trauma; pregnancy (category C), lactation.

ROUTE & DOSAGE

Diabetes Mellitus

Adult: **PO** 60–120 mg t.i.d. 1–30 min prior to meals

ADMINISTRATION

Oral

- Give, preferably, 1–30 min before meals. Omit the dose if the meal is skipped. Add a dose if an extra meal is eaten. Never double the dose.
- Store at 15°–30° C (59°–86° F).

ADVERSE EFFECTS (≥1%) **Body as a Whole:** Back pain, flu-like symptoms. **CV:** Dizziness. **GI:** Diarrhea. **Metabolic:** Hypoglycemia. **Musculoskeletal:** Arthropathy. **Respiratory:** Upper respiratory infection, bronchitis, cough.

INTERACTIONS Drug: NSAIDS, SALICYLATES, MAO INHIBITORS, BETA-ADRENERGIC BLOCKERS, may potentiate hypoglycemic effects; THIAZIDE DIURETICS, CORTICOSTEROIDS, THYROID PREPARATIONS, SYMPATHOMIMETIC AGENTS may attenuate hypoglycemic effects. **Herbal: Garlic, ginseng** may potentiate hypoglycemic effects.

PHARMACOKINETICS Absorption: Rapidly absorbed, 73% bioavailability. **Peak:** 1 h. **Distribution:** 98% protein bound. **Metabolism:** In liver by CYP2C9 (70%) and CYP3A4 (30%). **Elimination:** Primarily in urine. **Half-Life:** 1.5 h.

NURSING IMPLICATIONS

Assessment & Drug Effects

- Lab tests: Frequent 2 h postprandial BS monitoring, FBS monitoring and HbA1C q3mo.
- Monitor carefully for S&S of hypoglycemia especially during the 1-wk period following transfer from a longer acting sulfonylurea.

Patient & Family Education

- Take only before a meal to lessen the chance of hypoglycemia.

- When transferred to nateglinide from another oral hypoglycemia drug, start nateglinide the morning after the other agent is stopped, unless directed otherwise by physician.
- Watch for S&S of hyperglycemia or hypoglycemia (see Appendix F); report poor blood glucose control to physician.
- Report gastric upset or other bothersome GI symptoms to physician.

NEBIVOLOL HYDROCHLORIDE

(ne-bi-vol′ol)

Bystolic

Classifications: BETA-ADRENERGIC ANTAGONIST; ANTIHYPERTENSIVE
Therapeutic: ANTIHYPERTENSIVE
Prototype: Propranolol
Pregnancy Category: C

N

AVAILABILITY 2.5 mg, 5 mg, and 10 mg tablets

ACTION & *THERAPEUTIC EFFECT* A beta-adrenergic receptor blocker that is a beta-1 selective antagonist in majority of individuals and a nonselective beta-blocker in poor metabolizers. At higher doses nebivolol blocks both beta-1 and beta-2 receptors. *Effectiveness is measured by decreasing both systolic and diastolic pressures associated with hypertension.*

USES Management of hypertension either alone or in combination with other antihypertensive agents.
UNLABELED USES Management of heart failure.

CONTRAINDICATIONS Severe bradycardia; greater than first degree heart block; sick sinus syndrome without pacemaker; severe hepatic impairment (Child-Pugh greater than class B); decompensated HF; bronchospastic disease; lactation.
CAUTIOUS USE Compensated CHF; history of angina or recent MI; peripheral vascular disease; moderate hepatic and moderate to severe renal impairment; spontaneous hypoglycemia or DM; pregnancy (category C). Safety and efficacy in children not established.

ROUTE & DOSAGE

Hypertension
Adult: **PO** 5 mg PO daily; can increase q2wk up to 40 mg daily

Hepatic Impairment Dosage Adjustment
Moderate hepatic impairment (Child-Pugh class B): Decrease to 2.5 mg daily and increase cautiously as needed; severe hepatic impairment: Use is contraindicated

Renal Impairment Dosage Adjustment
CrCl less than 30 mL/min: Decrease to 2.5 mg PO daily and cautiously increase as needed

ADMINISTRATION

Oral

- May give without regard to meals.
- Store at 20°–25° C (68°–77° F) in a tight, light-resistant container.

ADVERSE EFFECTS (≥1%) **Body as a Whole:** Chest pain, peripheral edema. **CNS:** Asthenia, dizziness, fatigue, *headache*, insomnia, paresthesia. **CV:** Bradycardia. **GI:** Abdominal pain, diarrhea, nausea.

Metabolic: Decreased HDL levels, decreased platelet count, hypercholesterolemia, hypertriglyceridemia, hyperuricemia, increased blood urea nitrogen. **Respiratory:** Dyspnea. **Skin:** Rash.

INTERACTIONS Drug: Catecholamine-depleting agents (**reserpine, guanethidine**) may produce excessive reduction in sympathetic activity if used with nebivolol. Compounds that inhibit CYP2D6 (**fluoxetine, paroxetine, propafenone, quinidine**) may increase nebivolol levels. If used in combination with **clonidine,** simultaneous discontinuation of both drugs may cause life-threatening increases in blood pressure. Combination use with **digoxin** may increase the risk of bradycardia. **Cimetidine** increases the levels of nebivolol metabolites. **Verapamil** and **diltiazem** may increase the pharmacologic effects of nebivolol. Nebivolol may decrease the clearance of **disopyramide.** Nebivolol may decrease the AUC and C_{max} of **sildenafil.**

PHARMACOKINETICS Peak: 1.5–4 h. **Distribution:** 98% Plasma protein bound. **Metabolism:** Hepatic; extent depends on genetic profile. **Elimination:** In urine (38–67%) and feces (13–44%). **Half-Life:** 12–19 h depending on genetic differences in metabolism.

NURSING IMPLICATIONS

Assessment & Drug Effects

- Monitor closely BP and HR. Report promptly significant bradycardia or S&S of heart failure.
- Monitor closely during the perioperative period for depressed cardiac functioning.
- Monitor diabetics for loss of glycemia control.
- Monitor respiratory status in those at risk for bronchospasm.
- Lab tests: Periodic lipid profile and LFTs; frequent blood glucose monitoring with DM.

Patient & Family Education

- Use caution with dangerous activities until reaction to drug is known.
- Report promptly any of the following: Sudden weight gain, increasing shortness of breath, swelling in lower legs and feet; heart rate less than 60 beats per minute or other value established by physician.
- Diabetics may experience hypoglycemia without the usual signs and symptoms while on this drug.
- Do not abruptly stop taking this medication. It should be tapered off over 1–2 wk.

NEFAZODONE

(nef-a-zo′done)

Classifications: ANTIDEPRESSANT; SEROTONIN NOREPINEPHRINE REUPTAKE INHIBITOR (SNRI)
Therapeutic: ANTIDEPRESSANT; SNRI
Prototype: Fluoxetine HCl
Pregnancy Category: C

AVAILABILITY 50 mg, 100 mg, 150 mg, 200 mg, 250 mg tablets

ACTION & *THERAPEUTIC EFFECT* Antidepressant with a dual mechanism of action. Inhibits neuronal serotonin (5-HT_2) and norepinephrine reuptake. *Effective in treating major depression without major cardiovascular adverse effects.*

USES Treatment of depression.

CONTRAINDICATIONS Hypersensitivity to nefazodone or alcohol; active hepatic disease, hepatitis, jaundice; elevated hepatic transaminase levels; MAOI therapy; mania; severe restlessness, suicidal ideation; surgery.
CAUTIOUS USE Older adults, women of childbearing age; history of seizure disorders, seizures; renal impairment; recent MI, unstable cardiac disease; hypotension; angina, stroke, hypovolemia, dehydration, bipolar disorder; history of mania; ECT therapy; pregnancy (category C), lactation. Safety and efficacy in children younger than 18 y are not established.

ROUTE & DOSAGE

Depression
Adult: **PO** 50–100 mg b.i.d., may need to increase up to 300–600 mg/day in 2–3 divided doses
Geriatric: **PO** Start with 50 mg b.i.d.

N

ADMINISTRATION

Oral
- Do not give within 14 days of discontinuation of an MAO inhibitor.
- Store at 15°–30° C (59°–86° F).

ADVERSE EFFECTS (≥1%) **Body as a Whole:** Anaphylactic reactions, angioedema. **CNS:** *Headache, dizziness, drowsiness,* asthenia, tremor, insomnia, agitation, anxiety. **GI:** Dry mouth, constipation, nausea, liver toxicity, <u>liver failure</u>. **Special Senses:** Visual disturbances, blurred vision, scotomata. **Endocrine:** Galactorrhea, gynecomastia, serotonin syndrome. **Skin:** <u>Stevens-Johnson syndrome</u>.

INTERACTIONS Drug: May cause serotonin syndrome (see Appendix F) with MAOIS or SSRIS; may increase plasma levels of some BENZODIAZEPINES, including **alprazolam** and **triazolam.** May decrease plasma levels and effects of **propranolol.** May increase levels and toxicity of **buspirone, carbamazepine, cilostazol, digoxin;** reports of QT_c prolongation and ventricular arrhythmias with **pimozide;** increased risk of rhabdomyolysis with **lovastatin, simvastatin;** increased risk of **ergotamine** toxicity with **dihydroergotamine, ergotamine. Herbal: St. John's wort** may cause **serotonin** syndrome.

PHARMACOKINETICS Onset: 1 wk. **Peak:** 3–5 wk. **Metabolism:** In liver to at least two active metabolites. **Half-Life:** Nefazodone 3.5 h, metabolites 2–33 h.

NURSING IMPLICATIONS

Assessment & Drug Effects
- Monitor for worsening of depression or emergence of suicidal ideation.
- Evaluate concurrent drugs for possible interactions.
- Monitor patients with a history of seizures for increased activity.
- Assess safety, as dizziness and drowsiness are common adverse effects.
- Lab tests: Monitor periodically liver function and CBC during long-term therapy.

Patient & Family Education
- Be aware that significant improvement in mood may not occur for several weeks following initiation of therapy.
- Do not drive or engage in potentially hazardous activities until response to the drug is known.
- Report changes in visual acuity.
- Report signs of jaundice such as yellow coloration of the cornea of the eye or other S&S of liver dys-

function (anorexia, GI complaints, malaise, etc).

NELARABINE
Arranon
Classifications: ANTINEOPLASTIC; PYRIMIDINE, ANTIMETABOLITE
Therapeutic: ANTINEOPLASTIC
Prototype: 5-Fluorouracil
Pregnancy Category: D

AVAILABILITY 5 mg/mL solution

ACTION & *THERAPEUTIC EFFECT* Nelarabine inhibits DNA synthesis in lymphoblastic T-cells of acute leukemia and lymphoma. *The incorporation of a nelarabine metabolite in the leukemic blast cells halts DNA synthesis and causes cell death.*

USES Treatment of patients with T-cell acute lymphoblastic leukemia lymphoma.

CONTRAINDICATIONS Hepersensitivity to nelarabine; severe bone marrow suppression; older adults; pregnancy (category D); lactation.
CAUTIOUS USE Severe renal impairment, severe renal failure; hepatic impairment; risk of infection, bleeding.

ROUTE & DOSAGE

Adult T-Cell Leukemia/ Lymphoma

Adult: **IV** 1500 mg/m² on days 1, 3, and 5, repeated every 21 days
Child: **IV** 650 mg/m² over 1 h for 5 days, repeated every 21 days

Toxicity Dosage Adjustment

Grade 2 or higher neurologic toxicity: Discontinue therapy; hematologic toxicities: Delay therapy

ADMINISTRATION
- Standard IV hydration, urine alkalinization, and prophylaxis with allopurinol are advised to manage hyperuricemia in those at risk for tumor lysis syndrome.
- Use gloves and protective clothing to prevent skin contact.

Intravenous

PREPARE: **IV Infusion:** Do not dilute. Transfer the required dose to a PVC or glass container for infusion.

ADMINISTER: **IV Infusion for Adult:** Give over 2 h. **IV Infusion for Child:** Give over 1 h.
- Discontinue IV and notify physician for neurologic adverse events of NCI Common Toxicity Criteria grade 2 or greater.

- Store vials at 15°–30° C (59°–86° F). Nelarabine is stable in PVC bags or glass infusion containers for 8 h up to 30° C.

ADVERSE EFFECTS (≥1%) **Body as a Whole:** Abnormal gait, *fatigue, pyrexia,* rigors. **CNS:** *Asthenia,* ataxia, *dizziness, headache, hypoesthesia, neuropathy, paresthesia, somnolence,* tremor. **CV:** Chest pain, *edema,* hypotension, *petechiae,* sinus tachycardia. **GI:** Abdominal pain, *constipation, diarrhea, nausea, vomiting,* stomatitis. **Hematologic/Lymphatic:** *Anemia, neutropenia, thrombocytopenia,* increased risk of infection. **Hepatic:** AST levels increased. **Metabolic:** Anorexia, dehydration, hyperglycemia. **Musculoskeletal:** Arthralgia, back pain, muscular weakness, *myalgia,* pain in extremities. **Respiratory:** *Cough, dyspnea, pleural effusion,* epistaxis, wheezing.

PHARMACOKINETICS Distribution: Extensive. **Metabolism:** Bioactivation to ara-GTP, oxidized to uric

N

acid. **Elimination:** Renal. **Half-Life:** 3 h (active metabolite).

NURSING IMPLICATIONS

Assessment & Drug Effects

- Monitor for and report immediately S&S of adverse CNS effects, including altered mental status (e.g., confusion, severe somnolence), seizures, and peripheral neuropathy (e.g., numbness, paresthesias, motor weakness, ataxia, paralysis). Note: Previous or concurrent treatment with intrathecal chemotherapy or previous craniospinal irradiation may increase risk of CNS toxicity.
- Monitor for S&S of bleeding, especially with platelet counts less than 50,000/mm^3.
- Lab tests: Baseline and periodic CBC with differential and platelet count; periodic serum electrolytes, serum uric acid, LFTs, and renal function test.
- Monitor diabetics for loss of glycemic control.
- Note: Previous or concurrent treatment with intrathecal chemotherapy or previous craniospinal irradiation may increase risk of CNS toxicity.

Patient & Family Education

- Do not drive or engage in potentially hazardous activities until response to drug is known.
- Report any of the following to a health care provider: Seizures; tingling or numbness in hands and feet; problems with fine motor coordination; unsteady gait and increased weakness with ambulating; fever or other signs of infections; black tarry stools, blood tinged urine, or other signs of bleeding.
- Use effective contraceptive measures to avoid pregnancy while taking this drug.

N

NELFINAVIR MESYLATE

(nel-fin′a-vir)

Viracept

Classifications: ANTIRETROVIRAL; PROTEASE INHIBITOR

Therapeutic: PROTEASE INHIBITOR

Prototype: Saquinavir

Pregnancy Category: B

AVAILABILITY 250 mg, 625 mg tablets; 50 mg/g powder

ACTION & *THERAPEUTIC EFFECT* Inhibits HIV-1 protease, which is responsible for the production of HIV-1 viral particles in an infected individual. This prevents the cleavage of viral polypeptide, resulting in the production of an immature, noninfectious virus. *Effectiveness is indicated by decreased viral load.*

USES Treatment of HIV infection in combination with a nucleoside analog.

CONTRAINDICATIONS Hypersensitivity to nelfinavir; concurrent administration with amiodarone, quinidine, rifampin, triazolam, or midazolam; pancreatitis; lactation. Safety and effectiveness in children younger than 2 y are not established.

CAUTIOUS USE Liver function impairment, hemophilia; diabetes mellitus, hyperglycemia; pregnancy (category B).

ROUTE & DOSAGE

HIV Infection

Adult: **PO** 750 mg t.i.d. or 1250 mg (2 × 625 mg) b.i.d. with food

Child (2–13 y): **PO** 20–30 mg/kg t.i.d. with food (max: 750 mg/dose)

ADMINISTRATION

Oral

- Give with a meal or light snack.

- Oral powder may be mixed with a small amount of water, milk, soy milk, or dietary supplements; liquid should be consumed immediately. Do not mix oral powder in original container nor with acid food or juice (e.g., orange or apple juice, or applesauce).
- Store at 15°–30° C (59°–86° F).

ADVERSE EFFECTS (≥1%) **Body as a Whole:** Allergic reactions, back pain, fever, malaise, pain, asthenia, myalgia, arthralgia. **CNS:** Headache, anxiety, depression, dizziness, insomnia, seizures. **GI:** Abdominal pain, *diarrhea,* nausea, flatulence, anorexia, dyspepsia, GI bleeding, hepatitis, vomiting, pancreatitis, increased liver function tests. **Hematologic:** Anemia, leukopenia, thrombocytopenia. **Respiratory:** Dyspnea, pharyngitis, rhinitis. **Skin:** Rash, pruritus, sweating, urticaria. **Endocrine:** Lipodystrophy, insulin resistance, dyslipidemia.

INTERACTIONS Drug: Other PROTEASE INHIBITORS, **ketoconazole** may increase nelfinavir levels; **rifabutin, rifampin,** PROTON PUMP INHIBITORS may decrease nelfinavir levels; nelfinavir will decrease ORAL CONTRACEPTIVE levels; may increase levels of **amiodarone, atorvastatin, simvastatin, slidenafil,** PDE 5 INHIBITORS; increase risk of **ergotamine** toxicity with **dihydroergotamine, ergotamine,** HMG-COA REDUCTASE INHIBITORS may have increased risk of rhabdomyolysis. BENZODIAZEPINES may increase risk of sedation. **Herbal: St. John's wort, garlic** may decrease antiretroviral activity.

PHARMACOKINETICS Absorption: Food increases the amount of drug absorbed. **Distribution:** Greater than 98% protein bound. **Metabolism:** In the liver (CYP3A). **Elimination:** Primarily in feces. **Half-Life:** 3.5–5 h.

NURSING IMPLICATIONS

Assessment & Drug Effects

- Monitor hemophiliacs (type A or B) closely for spontaneous bleeding.
- Monitor carefully patients with hepatic impairment for toxic drug effects.

Patient & Family Education

- Drug **must be** taken exactly as prescribed. Do not alter dose or discontinue drug without consulting physician.
- Use a barrier contraceptive even if using hormonal contraceptives.
- Be aware that diarrhea is a common adverse effect that can usually be controlled by OTC medications.

NEOMYCIN SULFATE

(nee-oh-mye′sin)

Mycifradin, Myciguent, Neo-Tabs, Neo-fradin

Classification: AMINOGLYCOSIDE ANTIBIOTIC

Therapeutic: ANTIBIOTIC

Prototype: Gentamicin

Pregnancy Category: C

AVAILABILITY 500 mg tablet; 125 mg/5 mL oral solution; 3.5 mg/g ointment, cream

ACTION & *THERAPEUTIC EFFECT* Aminoglycoside antibiotic that inhibits bacterial protein synthesis through irreversible binding to the 30S ribosomal subunit within susceptible bacteria. Causes bacteria not to replicate. *Active against a wide variety of gram-negative bacteria. Effective against certain gram-positive organisms, particularly penicillin-sensitive and some methicillin-resistant strains of* Staphylococcus aureus *(MRSA).*

USES Severe diarrhea caused by enteropathogenic *Escherichia coli;* preoperative intestinal antisepsis; to inhibit nitrogen-forming bacteria of GI tract in patients with cirrhosis or hepatic coma and for urinary tract infections caused by susceptible organisms. Also topically for short-term treatment of eye, ear, and skin infections.

CONTRAINDICATIONS Use of oral drug in patients with intestinal obstruction; ulcerative bowel lesions; IBD: Topical applications over large skin areas; hypersensitivity to aminoglycosides.

CAUTIOUS USE Dehydration; renal disease, renal impairment; hearing impairment; myasthenia gravis, parkinsonism; children, pregnancy (category C), lactation. **Topical otic applications:** Patients with perforated eardrum.

N

ROUTE & DOSAGE

Intestinal Antisepsis

Adult: **PO** 1 g q1h × 4 doses, then 1 g q4h × 5 doses
Child: **PO** 10.3 mg/kg q4–6h for 3 days

Hepatic Coma

Adult: **PO** 4–12 g/day in 4 divided doses for 5–6 days
Child: **PO** 437.5–1225 mg/m^2 q6h for 5–6 days

Diarrhea

Adult: **PO** 50 mg/kg in 4 divided doses for 2–3 days
Child: **PO** 8.75 mg/kg q6h for 2–3 days

Cutaneous Infections

Adult: **Topical** Apply 1–3 times/day

ADMINISTRATION

Oral

- Preoperative bowel preparation: Saline laxative is generally given immediately before neomycin therapy is initiated.

Topical

- Consult physician about what to use for cleansing skin before each application.
- Make sure ear canal is clean and dry prior to instillation for topical therapy of external ear.

ADVERSE EFFECTS (≥1%) **Body as a Whole:** Neuromuscular blockade with muscular and respiratory paralysis; hypersensitivity reactions. **GI:** Mild laxative effect, diarrhea, nausea, vomiting; prolonged therapy: Malabsorption-like syndrome including cyanocobalamin (vitamin B_{12}) deficiency, low serum cholesterol. **Urogenital:** Nephrotoxicity. **Special Senses:** Ototoxicity. **Skin:** *Redness,* scaling, pruritus, dermatitis.

INTERACTIONS Drug: May decrease absorption of **cyanocobalamin.**

PHARMACOKINETICS Absorption: 3% absorbed from GI tract in adults; up to 10% absorbed in neonates. **Peak:** 1–4 h. **Elimination:** 97% excreted unchanged in feces. **Half-Life:** 3 h.

NURSING IMPLICATIONS

Assessment & Drug Effects

- Monitor closely for ototoxicity and nephrotoxicity. Risk is greatest in those with impaired renal function.
- Lab tests: Obtain baseline and daily urinalysis for albumin, casts, and cells; BUN every other day; baseline and daily creatinine clearance in elderly patients.
- Monitor I&O in patients receiving drug orally. Report oliguria or

changes in I&O ratio. Inadequate neomycin excretion results in high serum drug levels and risk of nephrotoxicity.

Patient & Family Education

- Stop treatment and consult your physician if irritation occurs when you are using topical neomycin. Allergic dermatitis is common.
- Report any unusual symptom related to ears or hearing (e.g., tinnitus, roaring sounds, loss of hearing acuity, dizziness).
- Do not exceed prescribed dosage or duration of therapy.

NEOSTIGMINE METHYLSULFATE (Pr)

(nee-oh-stig′meen)

Prostigmin

Classifications: CHOLINERGIC AGENT; CHOLINESTERASE INHIBITOR

Therapeutic: CHOLINESTERASE INHIBITOR

Pregnancy Category: C

AVAILABILITY 1:1000, 1:2000, 1:4000 injection

ACTION & *THERAPEUTIC EFFECT*

Produces reversible cholinesterase inhibition or inactivation with direct stimulant action on voluntary muscle fibers and possibly on autonomic ganglia and CNS neurons. Allows intensified and prolonged effect of acetylcholine at cholinergic synapses (basis for use in myasthenia gravis). *Produces generalized cholinergic response including miosis, increased tonus of intestinal and skeletal muscles, constriction of bronchi and ureters, slower pulse rate, and stimulation of salivary and sweat glands.*

USES To prevent and treat postoperative abdominal distention and urinary retention; for symptomatic control of and sometimes for differential diagnosis of myasthenia gravis; and to reverse the effects of nondepolarizing muscle relaxants (e.g., tubocurarine).

CONTRAINDICATIONS Hypersensitivity to neostigmine, cholinergics; bromides; cholinesterase inhibitor toxicity; GI obstruction; ileus; bradycardia, hypotension; mechanical obstruction of intestinal or urinary tract; peritonitis; administration with other cholinergic drugs; lactation.

CAUTIOUS USE Recent ileorectal anastomoses; epilepsy; bronchial asthma; hepatic disease; bradycardia, recent coronary occlusion; vagotonia; hyperthyroidism; cardiac arrhythmias; renal failure; renal impairment; renal disease; peptic ulcer; seizure disorder; pregnancy (category C).

ROUTE & DOSAGE

Diagnosis of Myasthenia Gravis

Adult: **IM** 0.02 mg/kg
Child: **IM** 0.04 mg/kg

Treatment of Myasthenia Gravis

Adult: **IM/Subcutaneous** 0.5–2.5 mg q1–3h (max: 10 mg/day)
Child: **IM/Subcutaneous** 0.01–0.04 mg/kg q2–4h

Reversal of Nondepolarizing Neuromuscular Blockade

Adult: **IV** 0.5–2.5 mg slowly (max dose: 5 mg); may repeat
Child: **IV** 0.025–0.08 mg/kg
Infant: **IV** 0.025–0.1 mg/kg

Postoperative Abdominal Distention and Urinary Retention

Adult: **IM/Subcutaneous** 0.25 mg q4–6h for 2–3 days

Myasthenia Gravis

Adult: **IV** 0.5–2 mg q1–3h

Child: **IV** 0.01–0.04 mg/kg q2–4h

Renal Impairment Dosage Adjustment

CrCl 10–50 mL/min: Use 50% of dose; less than 10 mL/min: Use 25% of dose

ADMINISTRATION

Intramuscular/Subcutaneous

- Note: 1 mg = 1 mL of the 1:1000 solution; 0.5 mg = 1 mL of the 1:2000 solution; 0.25 mg = 1 mL of the 1:4000 solution.
- Give undiluted.

Intravenous

PREPARE: **Direct:** Give undiluted.
ADMINISTER: **Direct:** Give at a rate of 0.5 mg or a fraction thereof over 1 min.

ADVERSE EFFECTS (≥1%) **Body as a Whole:** Muscle cramps, *fasciculations,* twitching, pallor, fatigability, generalized weakness, paralysis, agitation, fear, death. **CV:** Tightness in chest, bradycardia, hypotension, elevated BP. **GI:** *Nausea,* vomiting, eructation, epigastric discomfort, abdominal cramps, diarrhea, involuntary or difficult defecation. **CNS:** CNS stimulation. **Respiratory:** *Increased salivation* and bronchial secretions, sneezing, cough, dyspnea, diaphoresis, respiratory depression. **Special Senses:** Lacrimation, miosis, blurred vision. **Urogenital:** Difficult micturition.

INTERACTIONS Drug: Succinylcholine decamethonium may prolong phase I block or reverse phase II block; neostigmine antagonizes effects of **tubocurarine; atracurium, vecuronium, pancuronium; procainamide, quinidine, atropine** antagonize effects of neostigmine.

PHARMACOKINETICS Onset: 10–30 min IM or IV. **Peak:** 20–30 min IM or IV. **Distribution:** Not reported to cross placenta or appear in breast milk. **Metabolism:** In liver. **Elimination:** 80% of drug and metabolites excreted in urine within 24 h. **Half-Life:** 50–90 min.

NURSING IMPLICATIONS

Assessment & Drug Effects

- Check pulse before giving drug to bradycardic patients. If below 60/min or other established parameter, consult physician. Atropine will be ordered to restore heart rate.
- Monitor respiration, maintain airway or assisted ventilation, and give oxygen as indicated when used as antidote for tubocurarine or other nondepolarizing neuromuscular blocking agents (usually preceded by atropine).
- Monitor pulse, respiration, and BP during period of dosage adjustment in treatment of myasthenia gravis.
- Report promptly and record accurately the onset of myasthenic symptoms and drug adverse effects in relation to last dose.
- Note carefully time of muscular weakness onset. It may indicate whether patient is in cholinergic or myasthenic crisis: Weakness that appears approximately 1 h after drug administration suggests cholinergic crisis (overdose) and is treated by prompt withdrawal of neostigmine and immediate administration of atropine. Weakness that occurs 3 h or more after drug administration is more likely due to myasthenic crisis (underdose or drug resistance) and is treated by more intensive anticholinesterase therapy.

- Record drug effect and duration of action. S&S of myasthenia gravis relieved by neostigmine include lid ptosis; diplopia; drooping facies; difficulty in chewing, swallowing, breathing, or coughing; and weakness of neck, limbs, and trunk muscles.
- Manifestations of neostigmine overdosage often appear first in muscles of neck and those involved in chewing and swallowing, with muscles of shoulder girdle and upper extremities affected next.
- Report to physician if patient does not urinate within 1 h after first dose when used to relieve urinary retention.

Patient & Family Education

- Keep a diary of "peaks and valleys" of muscle strength.
- Keep an accurate record for physician of your response to drug. Learn how to recognize adverse effects, how to modify dosage regimen according to your changing needs, or how to administer atropine if necessary.
- Be aware that certain factors may require an increase in size or frequency of dose (e.g., physical or emotional stress, infection, menstruation, surgery), whereas remission requires a decrease in dosage.

NEPAFENAC

(nep'a-fe-nac)

Nevanac

Pregnancy Category: C

See Appendix A-1.

NESIRITIDE

(nes-ir'i-tide)

Natrecor

Classifications: CARDIOVASCULAR; ATRIAL NATRIURETIC PEPTIDE HORMONE

Therapeutic: ATRIAL NATRIURETIC HORMONE (ANH)

Pregnancy Category: C

AVAILABILITY 1.5 mg vial

ACTION & *THERAPEUTIC EFFECT* Nesiritide is a human B-type natriuretic peptide (hBNP), produced by recombinant DNA, which mimics the actions of human atrial natriuretic hormone (ANH). ANH is secreted by the right atrium when atrial blood pressure increases. Nesiritide, like ANH, inhibits antidiuretic hormone (ADH) by increasing urine sodium loss by the kidney and triggering the formation of a large volume of dilute urine. Nesiritide binds to a cyclic nucleic acid, which results in smooth muscle cell relaxation. *Effective in causing smooth muscle relaxation. The drug also causes dilation of veins and arteries. It is effective in managing dyspnea at rest in patients with acute CHF.*

USES Acute treatment of decompensated CHF in patients who have dyspnea at rest or with minimal activity.

CONTRAINDICATIONS Hypersensitivity to nesiritide, *Escherichia coli* protein, patients with a systolic blood pressure less than 90 mm Hg, cardiogenic shock, patients with low cardiac filling pressures, patients who should not receive vasodilators, such as those with significant valvular stenosis, restrictive or obstructive cardiomyopathy, pericardial perfusion; constrictive pericarditis, pericardial tamponade.

CAUTIOUS USE Pregnancy (category C), lactation. Safety and efficacy in pediatric patients have not been established.

ROUTE & DOSAGE

Acute Decompensated CHF

Adult: **IV** 2 mcg/kg bolus administered over 60 sec, followed by a continuous infusion of 0.01 mcg/kg/min (0.1 mL/kg/h) (max: 0.03 mcg/kg/min). Monitor blood pressure. If hypotension occurs, the dose should be reduced or discontinued. The infusion can subsequently be restarted at a dose that is reduced by 30% (with no bolus administration) after stabilization of hemodynamics.

ADMINISTRATION

Intravenous

N

PREPARE: **Direct and IV Infusion:** Reconstitute one 1.5 mg vial by adding 5 mL of IV solution removed from a 250 mL bag of selected diluent (i.e., D5W, NS, D5/0.45% NaCl, D5/0.2% NaCl). ▪ Rock the vial gently so that all surfaces, including the stopper, contact the diluent ensuring complete reconstitution. Do not shake the vial. ▪ Add the entire contents of the vial to the 250 mL IV bag to yield approximately 6 mcg/mL. Invert the bag several times to mix completely. ▪ Use within 24 h. ▪ Prime the IV tubing with 25 mL prior to connecting to the vascular access port.

ADMINISTER: **Direct:** Bolus dose **MUST BE** withdrawn from the prepared infusion bag. Determine dose as follows: Bolus volume (mL) = (0.33) × (patient weight in kg). ▪ Give the bolus dose over 60 sec through an IV port in the tubing. **IV Infusion:** Infuse remainder of IV infusion immediately following the bolus dose. ▪ Determine the infusion rate as follows: Flow rate (mL/h) = (0.1) × (patient weight in kg).

INCOMPATIBILITIES **Solution/additive: Promethazine. Y-site: Bumetanide, enalaprilat, ethacrynic acid, furosemide, heparin, hydralazine, regular insulin, micafungin.**

▪ Store at controlled room temperature at 20°–25° C (68°–77° F) or refrigerated.

ADVERSE EFFECTS (≥1%) **Body as a Whole:** Headache, back pain, catheter pain, fever, injection site pain, leg cramps. **CNS:** Insomnia, dizziness, anxiety, confusion, paresthesia, somnolence, tremor. **CV:** *Hypotension,* ventricular tachycardia, ventricular extrasystoles, angina, bradycardia, tachycardia, atrial fibrillation, AV node conduction abnormalities. **GI:** Abdominal pain, nausea, vomiting. **Respiratory:** Cough, hemoptysis, apnea. **Skin:** Sweating, pruritus, rash. **Special Senses:** Amblyopia. **Renal:** Renal failure in acutely decompensated heart failure patients.

INTERACTIONS Drug: Additive effects with ANTIHYPERTENSIVES.

PHARMACOKINETICS Onset: 15 min. **Duration:** Greater than 60 min depending on dose. **Metabolism:** Proteolytic cleavage, proteolysis. **Half-Life:** 18 min.

NURSING IMPLICATIONS

Assessment & Drug Effects

- Monitor hemodynamic parameters (e.g., BP, PCWP, HR, ECG) throughout therapy.

- Establish hypotension parameters prior to initiating therapy. Notify physician immediately if systolic BP falls below 90 mm Hg.
- Reduce the dose or withhold the drug if hypotension occurs during administration. Reinitiate therapy infusion only after hypotension is corrected. Subsequent doses following a hypotensive episode are usually reduced by 30% and given without a prior bolus dose.
- Lab tests: Baseline and periodic serum creatinine.

NEVIRAPINE

(ne-vir'a-peen)
Viramune
Classifications: ANTIRETROVIRAL; NONNUCLEOSIDE REVERSE TRANSCRIPTASE INHIBITOR (NNRTI)
Therapeutic: ANTIRETROVIRAL; NNRTI
Prototype: Efavirenz
Pregnancy Category: B

AVAILABILITY 200 mg tablets; 10 mg/mL suspension

ACTION & *THERAPEUTIC EFFECT* Nonnucleoside reverse transcriptase inhibitor (NNRTI) of HIV-1. Binds directly to reverse transcriptase and blocks RNA- and DNA-dependent polymerase activities, thus preventing replication of the virus. *Prevents replication of the HIV-1 virus. Resistant strains appear rapidly.*

USES In combination with nucleoside analogs for treatment of HIV.

CONTRAINDICATIONS Hypersensitivity to nevirapine; development of rash; severe skin reactions to the drug; hepatitis B or C: Increased transaminases combined with rash or sign of hepatotoxicity; hormonal contraceptives; neonates; lactation; Child-Pugh class B or C.

CAUTIOUS USE Renal disease; mild or moderate hepatic impairment, hemodialysis; CNS disorders; pregnant women with CD4+ lymphocyte counts greater than 250/mm³; pregnancy (category B).

ROUTE & DOSAGE

HIV

Adult/Adolescent: **PO** 200 mg once daily for 14 days, then increase to 200 mg b.i.d.
Child/Infant (older than 15 days): **PO** 150 mg/m² daily × 14 days, then 150 mg/m² twice daily (max: 400 mg) (max: 200 mg/dose)

ADMINISTRATION

Oral

- Reinitiate with 200 mg/day for 14 days, then increase to b.i.d. dosing, when dosing is interrupted for more than 7 days.
- Store at 15°–30° C (59°–86° F) in a tightly closed container.

ADVERSE EFFECTS (≥1%) **Body as a Whole:** Fever, paresthesia, myalgia. **CNS:** Headache. **GI:** Nausea, diarrhea, abdominal pain, hepatitis, increased liver function tests, hepatotoxicity (including fulminant and cholestatic hepatitis, hepatic necrosis, and hepatic failure, especially with long-term use). **Hematologic:** Anemia, neutropenia. **Skin:** *Rash*, Stevens-Johnson syndrome.

INTERACTIONS Drug: May decrease plasma concentrations of PROTEASE INHIBITORS, ORAL CONTRACEPTIVES; may decrease **methadone, dronedarone** levels. **Herbal: St. John's wort, garlic** may decrease antiretroviral activity.

PHARMACOKINETICS Absorption: Rapidly from GI tract. **Peak:** 4h. **Distribution:** 60% protein bound, crosses placenta, distributed into breast milk. **Metabolism:** In liver (CYP3A). **Elimination:** Primarily in urine. **Half-Life:** 25–40 h.

NURSING IMPLICATIONS

Assessment & Drug Effects

- Lab tests: Obtain baseline and periodic liver and kidney function tests, routine blood chemistry, and CBC.
- Monitor weight, temperature, respiratory status with chest x-ray throughout therapy.
- Monitor carefully, especially during first 6 wk of therapy, for severe rash (with or without fever, blistering, oral lesions, conjunctivitis, swelling, joint aches, or general malaise).
- Withhold drug and notify physician if rash develops or liver function tests are abnormal.

N

Patient & Family Education

- Learn about common adverse effects.
- Withhold drug and notify physician if severe rash appears.
- Do not drive or engage in potentially hazardous activities until response to drug is known. There is a high potential for drowsiness and fatigue.
- Use or add barrier contraceptive if using hormonal contraceptive.

NIACIN (VITAMIN B_3, NICOTINIC ACID)

(nye'a-sin)

Niacor, Niaspan, Nicobid, Nico-400, Nicotinex, Novoniacin ✤, Slo-Niacin, Tri-B3 ✤

NIACINAMIDE (NICOTINAMIDE)

Classifications: VITAMIN B_3; ANTILIPEMIC

Therapeutic: ANTILIPEMIC; LIPID-LOWERING AGENT

Pregnancy Category: C

AVAILABILITY 50 mg, 100 mg, 250 mg, 500 mg tablets; 125 mg, 250 mg, 400 mg, 500 mg, 750 mg, 1000 mg sustained release tablets, capsules

ACTION & *THERAPEUTIC EFFECT* Water-soluble, heat-stable, B-complex vitamin (B_3) that functions with riboflavin as a control agent in coenzyme system that converts protein, carbohydrate, and fat to energy through oxidation-reduction. Niacinamide, an amide of niacin, is used as an alternative in the prevention and treatment of pellagra. *Produces vasodilation by direct action on vascular smooth muscles. Inhibits hepatic synthesis of VLDL, cholesterol, and triglyceride, and, indirectly, LDL. Large doses effectively reduce elevated serum cholesterol and total lipid levels in hypercholesterolemia and hyperlipidemic states.*

USES In prophylaxis and treatment of pellagra, usually in combination with other B-complex vitamins, and in deficiency states accompanying carcinoid syndrome, isoniazid therapy, Hartnup's disease, and chronic alcoholism. Also in adjuvant treatment of hyperlipidemia (elevated cholesterol or triglycerides) in patients who do not respond adequately to diet or weight loss. Also as vasodilator in peripheral vascular disorders, Ménière's disease, and labyrinthine syndrome, as well as to counteract LSD toxicity and to distinguish between psychoses of dietary and nondietary origin.

CONTRAINDICATIONS Hypersensitivity to niacin; hepatic impairment; severe hypotension; hemorrhaging or arterial bleeding; active peptic ulcer; lactation, and children younger than 16 y.

CAUTIOUS USE History of gallbladder disease, liver disease, and peptic ulcer; severe renal impairment; glaucoma; angina; coronary artery disease; diabetes mellitus; predisposition to gout; allergy; thrombocytopenia; pregnancy (category C).

ROUTE & DOSAGE

Niacin Deficiency

Adult: **PO** 10–20 mg/day

Pellagra

Adult: **PO** 50–100 mg 3–4 times/day
Child: **PO** 50–100 mg t.i.d.

Hyperlipidemia

Adult: **PO** 1.5–3 g/day in divided doses, may increase up to 6 g/day if necessary
Child: **PO** 100–250 mg/day in 3 divided doses, may increase by 250 mg/day q2–3wk as tolerated

ADMINISTRATION

Oral

- Give with meals to decrease GI distress. Give with cold water (not hot beverage) to facilitate swallowing.
- Ensure that sustained release form is not chewed or crushed. It **must be** swallowed whole.
- Store at 15°–30° C (59°–86° F) in a light and moisture proof container.

ADVERSE EFFECTS (≥1%) **CNS:** *Transient headache, tingling of extremities,* syncope. With chronic use: Nervousness, panic, toxic amblyopia, proptosis, blurred vision, loss of central vision. **CV:** *Generalized flushing with sensation of warmth,* postural hypotension, vasovagal attacks, arrhythmias (rare). **GI:** *Abnormalities of liver function tests; jaundice, bloating, flatulence, nausea,* vomiting, GI disorders, activation of peptic ulcer, xerostomia. **Skin:** *Increased sebaceous gland activity,* dry skin, skin rash, *pruritus,* keratitis nigricans. **Metabolic:** Hyperuricemia, hyperglycemia, glycosuria, hypoprothrombinemia, hypoalbuminemia.

DIAGNOSTIC TEST INTERFERENCE Niacin causes elevated serum ***bilirubin, uric acid, alkaline phosphatase, AST, ALT, LDH*** levels and may cause ***glucose intolerance.*** Decreases ***serum cholesterol*** 15–30% and may cause false elevations with certain ***fluorometric methods*** of determining ***urinary catecholamines.*** Niacin may cause false-positive ***urine glucose*** tests using ***copper sulfate reagents*** (e.g., ***Benedict's*** solution).

INTERACTIONS Drug: Potentiates hypotensive effects of ANTIHYPERTENSIVE AGENTS.

PHARMACOKINETICS Absorption: Readily from GI tract. **Peak:** 20–70 min. **Distribution:** Into breast milk. **Metabolism:** In liver. **Elimination:** Primarily in urine. **Half-Life:** 45 min.

NURSING IMPLICATIONS

Assessment & Drug Effects

- Monitor therapeutic effectiveness and record effect of therapy on clinical manifestations of deficiency (fiery red tongue, excessive saliva secretion and infection of oral membranes, nausea, vomiting, diarrhea, confusion). Therapeutic response usually begins within 24 h.

N

- Lab tests: Obtain baseline and periodic tests of blood glucose and liver function in patients receiving prolonged high dose therapy.
- Monitor diabetics and patients on high doses for decreased glucose tolerance and loss of glycemic control.
- Observe patients closely for evidence of liver dysfunction (jaundice, dark urine, light-colored stools, pruritus) and hyperuricemia in patients predisposed to gout (flank, joint, or stomach pain; altered urine excretion pattern).

Patient & Family Education

- Be aware that you may feel warm and flushed in face, neck, and ears within first 2 h after oral ingestion and it may last several hours. Effects are usually transient and subside as therapy continues.
- Sit or lie down and avoid sudden posture changes if you feel weak or dizzy. Report these symptoms and persistent flushing to your physician.
- Be aware that alcohol and large doses of niacin cause increased flushing and sensation of warmth.
- Avoid exposure to direct sunlight until lesions have entirely cleared if you have skin manifestations.

N

NICARDIPINE HYDROCHLORIDE

(ni-car′di-peen)

Cardene, Cardene SR

Classifications: CALCIUM CHANNEL BLOCKER; ANTIHYPERTENSIVE

Therapeutic: ANTIHYPERTENSIVE; ANTIANGINAL

Prototype: Nifedipine

Pregnancy Category: C

AVAILABILITY 20 mg, 30 mg capsules; 30 mg, 45 mg, 60 mg sustained release capsules; 2.5 mg/mL injection

ACTION & *THERAPEUTIC EFFECT* Calcium channel entry blocker that inhibits the transmembrane influx of calcium ions into cardiac muscle and smooth muscle, thus affecting contractility. Selectively affects vascular smooth muscle more than cardiac muscle. *Significantly decreases systemic vascular resistance. It reduces BP at rest and during isometric and dynamic exercise.*

USES Either alone or with beta-blockers for chronic, stable (effort-associated) angina; either alone or with other antihypertensives for essential hypertension.

UNLABELED USES CHF, cerebral ischemia, migraine.

CONTRAINDICATIONS Hypersensitivity to nicardipine; advanced aortic stenosis; cardiogenic shock; hypotension; lactation.

CAUTIOUS USE CHF; renal and hepatic impairment; severe bradycardia; older adult; GERD; hiatal hernia; renal disease; renal impairment; acute stroke; acute myocardial infarction; pregnancy (category C).

ROUTE & DOSAGE

Hypertension, Angina

Adult: **PO** 20–40 mg t.i.d. or 30–60 mg SR b.i.d. **IV** Initiation of therapy in a drug-free patient: 5 mg/h initially, increase dose by 2.5 mg/h q15min (or faster) (max: 15 mg/h); for severe hypertension: 4–7.5 mg/h; for postop hypertension: 10–15 mg/h initially, then 1–3 mg/h

Substitute for Oral Nicardipine

Adult: **IV** 20 mg q8h **PO** 0.5 mg/h; 30 mg q8h **PO** 1.2 mg/h; 40 mg q8h **PO** 2.2 mg/h

Common adverse effects in *italic*, life-threatening effects underlined; generic names in **bold**; classifications in SMALL CAPS; ♣ Canadian drug name; ⓟ Prototype drug

ADMINISTRATION

Note: To prevent symptoms of withdrawal, do not abruptly discontinue drug.

Oral

- Give on empty stomach. High-fat meals may decrease blood levels.
- Ensure that sustained release form is not chewed or crushed. It **must be** swallowed whole.
- When converting from IV to oral dose, give first dose of t.i.d. regimen 1 h before discontinuing infusion.

Intravenous

PREPARE: **IV Infusion:** Dilute each 25 mg ampule with 240 mL of D5W or NS to yield 0.1 mg/mL.

ADMINISTER: **IV Infusion:** Usually initiated at 50 mL/h (5 mg/h) with rate increases of 25 mL/h (2.5 mg/h) q5–15min up to a maximum of 150 mL/h. ▪ Infusion is usually slowed to 30 mL/h once the target BP is reached. *Substitute for oral doses:* Oral 20 mg q8h, IV equivalent is 0.5 mg/h; oral 30 mg q8h, IV equivalent is 1.2 mg/h; oral 40 mg q8h, IV equivalent is 2.2 mg/h.

INCOMPATIBILITIES **Solution/additive: Sodium bicarbonate. Y-site: Ampicillin, ampicillin/sulbactam, cefoperazone, furosemide, heparin, thiopental.**

ADVERSE EFFECTS (≥1%) **CNS:** Dizziness or headache, fatigue, anxiety, depression, paresthesias, insomnia, somnolence, nervousness. **CV:** Pedal edema, hypotension, flushing, palpitations, tachycardia, increased angina. **GI:** Anorexia, nausea, vomiting, dry mouth, constipation, dyspepsia. **Skin:** Rash, pruritus. **Body as a Whole:** Arthralgia or arthritis.

INTERACTIONS Drug: Adenosine prolongs bradycardia. **Amiodarone** may cause sinus arrest and AV block. **Benazepril** blunts increase in heart rate and increase in plasma **norepinephrine** and **aldosterone** seen with nicardipine. BETA-BLOCKERS cause hypotension and bradycardia. **Cimetidine** increases levels of nicardipine, resulting in hypotension. Concomitant nicardipine and **cyclosporine** result in significant increase in **cyclosporine** serum concentrations 1–30 days after initiation of nicardipine therapy; following withdrawal of nicardipine, **cyclosporine** levels decrease. **Magnesium,** when used to retard premature labor, may cause severe hypotension and neuromuscular blockade. **Food: Grapefruit juice** (greater than 1 qt/day) may increase plasma concentrations and adverse effects.

PHARMACOKINETICS Absorption: Immediately 35% of oral dose reaches systemic circulation. **Onset:** 1 min IV; 20 min PO. **Peak:** 0.5–2 h. **Duration:** 3 h IV. **Distribution:** 95% protein bound; distributed in breast milk. **Metabolism:** Rapidly and extensively in liver (CYP3A4); active metabolite has less than 1% activity of parent compound. **Elimination:** 35% in feces, 60% in urine; not affected by hemodialysis. **Half-Life:** 8.6 h.

NURSING IMPLICATIONS

Assessment & Drug Effects

- Establish baseline data before treatment is started including BP and pulse.
- Monitor closely BP values during initiation and titration of dosage. Hypotension with or without an increase in heart rate may occur.
- Avoid too rapid reduction in either systolic or diastolic pressure during parenteral administration.

- Discontinue IV infusion if hypotension or tachycardia develop.
- Observe for large peak and trough differences in BP. Initially, measure BP at peak effect (1–2 h after dosing) and at trough effect (8 h after dosing).

Patient & Family Education

- Record and report any increase in frequency, duration, and severity of angina when initiating or increasing dosage. Keep a record of nitroglycerin use and promptly report any changes in previous anginal pattern.
- Do not change dosage regimen without consulting physician.
- Be aware that abrupt withdrawal may cause an increased frequency and duration of chest pain. This drug **must be** gradually tapered under medical supervision.
- Rise slowly from a recumbent position; avoid driving or operating potentially dangerous equipment until response to nicardipine is known.
- Notify physician if any of the following occur: Irregular heartbeat, shortness of breath, swelling of the feet, pronounced dizziness, nausea, or drop in BP.

NICOTINE (Pr)

(nik′o-teen)

Nicotrol NS, Nicotrol Inhaler, Commit

NICOTINE POLACRILEX

Nicorette Gum, Nicorette DS

NICOTINE TRANSDERMAL SYSTEM

Habitrol, Nicoderm, Nicotrol, ProStep

Classifications: SMOKING DETERRENT; CHOLINERGIC RECEPTOR ANTAGONIST

Therapeutic: SMOKING DETERRENT

Pregnancy Category: D (nasal spray, transdermal system); C (gum)

AVAILABILITY 2 mg, 4 mg gum; 2 mg, 4 mg lozenges; 0.5 mg spray; 4 mg inhaler; 7 mg/day, 14 mg/day, 21 mg/day, 5 mg/day, 10 mg/day, 15 mg/day, 11 mg/day, 22 mg/day transdermal patch

ACTION & *THERAPEUTIC EFFECT*

Ganglionic cholinergic receptor antagonist that has both adrenergic and cholinergic effects. Includes stimulant and depressant effects on the peripheral nervous system and CNS; respiratory stimulation; peripheral vasoconstriction; increased heart rate, cardiac output, and stroke volume; increased tone and motor activity of GI smooth muscles; increased bronchial secretions (initially); antidiuretic activity. Heavy smokers are tolerant of these effects. *Rationale for use is to reduce withdrawal symptoms accompanying cessation of smoking. Success rate appears to be greatest in smokers with high "physical" type of nicotine dependence.*

USES In conjunction with a medically supervised behavior modification program, as a temporary and alternate source of nicotine by the nicotine-dependent smoker who is withdrawing from cigarette smoking.

CONTRAINDICATIONS Nonsmokers, immediate post-MI period; life-threatening arrhythmias; active temporomandibular joint disease; severe angina pectoris; women with childbearing potential (unless effective contraception is used).

Nicotine Transdermal, Inhaler System: Pregnancy (category D). Safety in children and adolescents is not established.

CAUTIOUS USE Vasospastic disease (e.g., Buerger's disease, Prinzmetal's variant angina), cardiac arrhythmias, hyperthyroidism, type 1 diabetes, pheochromocytoma, esophagitis, oral and pharyngeal inflammation; denture use, denture caps, or partial bridges; hypertension and peptic ulcer disease (active or inactive); GERD. **Gum:** Pregnancy (category C). During lactation, only if benefit of a smoking cessation program outweighs risks.

ROUTE & DOSAGE

Smoking Cessation

Adult: **PO** Chew 1 piece of gum whenever have urge to smoke, may be repeated as needed (max: 30 pieces of gum/day) **Intranasal** 1 dose = 2 sprays, 1 in each nostril, start with 1–2 doses (2–4 sprays) each hour (max: 5 doses/h, 40 doses/day), may continue for 3 mo **Topical** Apply 1 transdermal patch q24h by the following schedule: ***Habitrol, Nicoderm:*** 21 mg/day × 6 wk, 14 mg/day × 2 wk, 7 mg/day × 2 wk; *weight less than 45 kg (100 lb), smoke less than 1/2 pack/day, or have cardiovascular disease,* 14 mg/day × 6 wk, 7 mg/day × 2–4 wk ***ProStep:*** 22 mg/day × 4–8 wk, 11 mg/day × 2–4 wk; *weight less than 45 kg (100 lb), smoke less than 1/2 pack/day, or have cardiovascular disease,* 11 mg/day × 4–8 wk. ***Nicotrol:*** Apply 1 transdermal patch 16 h/day by the following schedule: 15 mg/day × 4–12 wk, 10 mg/day × 2–4 wk, 5 mg/day × 2–4 wk

ADMINISTRATION

Oral

- Note: Most adverse local effects (irritation of tongue, mouth, and throat, jaw-muscle aches, dislike of taste) are transient and subside in a few days. Modification of the chewing technique may help.

Transdermal

- Remove the old patch before applying the next new patch.
- Apply patch to nonhairy, clean, dry skin site; immediately remove from protective container.
- Store at or below 30° C (86° F); patches are sensitive to heat.

ADVERSE EFFECTS (≥1%) **CNS:** *Headache, dizziness, lightheadedness,* insomnia, irritability, dependence on nicotine. **CV:** Arrhythmias, tachycardia, palpitations, hypertension. **GI:** Air swallowing, *jaw ache, nausea,* belching, salivation, anorexia, dry mouth, laxative effects, constipation, *indigestion,* diarrhea, dyspepsia, vomiting, sialorrhea, abdominal pain, diarrhea. **Respiratory:** *Sore mouth or throat, cough, hiccups,* hoarseness; injury to mouth, teeth, temporomandibular joint pain, *irritation/tingling of tongue.* **Skin:** *Erythema, pruritus, local edema, rash;* skin reactions may be delayed, occurring after 3 wk of patch use. **Special Senses:** *Runny nose, nasal irritation, throat irritation, watering eyes,* minor epistaxis, nasal ulceration. **Body as a Whole:** Acute overdose/nicotine intoxication (perspiration; severe headache; dizziness; disturbed hearing and vision; mental confusion; severe weakness; fainting; hypotension; dyspnea; weak, rapid, irregular pulse; sei-

N

zures); death (from respiratory failure secondary to drug-induced respiratory muscle paralysis).

INTERACTIONS Drug: May increase metabolism of **caffeine, theophylline, acetaminophen, insulin, oxazepam, pentazocine propranolol. Food:** Coffee, cola may decrease nicotine absorption from nicotine gum.

PHARMACOKINETICS Absorption: Approximately 90% of the nicotine in a piece of gum is released slowly over 15–30 min; rate of release is controlled by vigor and duration of chewing; readily absorbed from buccal mucosa; transdermal 75–90% absorbed through skin; 53–58% of nasal spray is absorbed. **Peak:** Transdermal 8–9 h; nasal spray 4–15 min. **Distribution:** Crosses placenta; distributed into breast milk. **Metabolism:** In liver, primarily to cotinine. **Elimination:** In urine. **Half-Life:** 30–120 min.

N

NURSING IMPLICATIONS

Assessment & Drug Effects

- Be aware that transient erythema, pruritus, or burning is common with transdermal patch and usually disappears 24 h after patch removal.
- Differentiate cutaneous hypersensitivity (contact sensitization) that does not resolve in 24 h from a transient local reaction. The former is an indication to discontinue the transdermal patch.

Patient & Family Education

- Chew a piece of gum for approximately 30 min to get the full dose of nicotine.
- Chew only one piece of gum at a time. Chewing gum too rapidly can cause excessive buccal absorption and lead to adverse effects: Nausea, hiccups, throat irritation.
- Gradually decrease number of pieces of gum chewed in 24 h. Usually, a period of 3 mo is allowed before tapering use of gum.
- Promptly discontinue use of transdermal patch and notify physician if a severe or persistent local or generalized skin reaction occurs.
- Smoking while using the transdermal nicotine patch increases the risk of adverse reactions.

NIFEDIPINE (Pr)

(nye-fed'i-peen)

Adalat CC, Procardia, Procardia XL

Classifications: CALCIUM CHANNEL BLOCKER; ANTIANGINAL, ANTIHYPERTENSIVE

Therapeutic: ANTIHYPERTENSIVE, ANTIANGINAL

Pregnancy Category: C

AVAILABILITY 10 mg, 20 mg capsules; 30 mg, 60 mg, 90 mg sustained release tablets

ACTION & *THERAPEUTIC EFFECT* Blocks calcium ion influx across cell membranes of cardiac muscle and vascular smooth muscle. Reduces myocardial oxygen utilization and supply and relaxes and prevents coronary artery spasm. Decreases peripheral vascular resistance and increases cardiac output. *The rise in peripheral blood flow is the basis for use in treatment of Raynaud's phenomenon as well as hypertension. Effective antianginal agent.*

USES Vasospastic "variant" or Prinzmetal's angina and chronic stable angina without vasospasm. Mild to moderate hypertension alone or in combination with a diuretic.

Common adverse effects in *italic*, life-threatening effects underlined; generic names in **bold**; classifications in SMALL CAPS; ♣ Canadian drug name; (Pr) Prototype drug

UNLABELED USES Esophageal disorders; vascular headaches; Raynaud's phenomenon; asthma; cardiomyopathy; primary pulmonary hypertension.

CONTRAINDICATIONS Known hypersensitivity to nifedipine; unstable angina; acute MI; cardiogenic shock; aortic stenosis; GI obstruction. Safety in children is not established.

CAUTIOUS USE GERD; CHF; pregnancy (category C), lactation.

ROUTE & DOSAGE

Angina
Adult: **PO** 10–20 mg t.i.d. up to 180 mg/day

Hypertension
Adult: **PO** 10–20 mg t.i.d. up to 180 mg/day or 30–90 mg sustained release once/day

ADMINISTRATION

Oral

- Do not give within the first 1–2 wk following an MI.
- Use only the sustained release form to treat chronic hypertension. Ensure that sustained release form is not chewed or crushed. It **must be** swallowed whole.
- Discontinue drug gradually, with close medical supervision to prevent severe hypertension and other adverse effects.
- Store at 15°–25° C (59°–77° F); protect from light and moisture.

ADVERSE EFFECTS (≥1%) **Body as a Whole:** Sore throat, weakness, fever, sweating, chills, febrile reaction. **CNS:** *Dizziness, lightheadedness,* nervousness, mood changes, weakness, jitteriness, sleep disturbances, blurred vision, retinal ischemia, difficulty in balance, *headache.* **CV:** Hypotension, *facial flushing, heat sensation,* palpitations, *peripheral edema,* MI (rare), prolonged systemic hypotension with overdose. **GI:** Nausea, heartburn, *diarrhea,* constipation, cramps, flatulence, gingival hyperplasia, hepatotoxicity. **Musculoskeletal:** Inflammation, joint stiffness, muscle cramps. **Respiratory:** Nasal congestion, dyspnea, cough, wheezing. **Skin:** Dermatitis, pruritus, urticaria. **Urogenital:** Sexual difficulties, possible male infertility.

DIAGNOSTIC TEST INTERFERENCE Nifedipine may cause mild to moderate increases of ***alkaline phosphatase, CPK, LDH, AST, ALT.***

INTERACTIONS Drug: BETA-BLOCKERS may increase likelihood of CHF; may increase risk of **phenytoin** toxicity. **Herbal: Melatonin** may increase blood pressure and heart rate. **Ginkgo, ginseng** may increase plasma concentrations. **St. John's wort** may decrease plasma concentrations. **Food: Grapefruit juice** (greater than 1 qt/day) may increase plasma concentrations and adverse effects.

PHARMACOKINETICS Absorption: Readily absorbed from GI tract; 45–75% reaches systemic circulation (first pass metabolism). **Onset:** 10–30 min. **Peak:** 30 min. **Distribution:** Distributed into breast milk. **Metabolism:** In liver. **Elimination:** 75–80% in urine, 15% in feces. **Half-Life:** 2–5 h.

NURSING IMPLICATIONS

Assessment & Drug Effects

- Monitor BP carefully during titration period. Patient may become severely hypotensive, especially if also taking other drugs known to lower BP. Withhold drug and notify physician if systolic BP less than 90.

- Monitor blood sugar in diabetic patients. Nifedipine has diabetogenic properties.
- Monitor for gingival hyperplasia and report promptly. This is a rare but serious adverse effect (similar to phenytoin-induced hyperplasia).

Patient & Family Education

- Keep a record of nitroglycerin use and promptly report any changes in previous pattern. Occasionally, people develop increased frequency, duration, and severity of angina when they start treatment with this drug or when dosage is increased.
- Be aware that withdrawal symptoms may occur with abrupt discontinuation of the drug (chest pain, increase in anginal episodes, MI, dysrhythmias).
- Inspect gums visually every day. Changes in gingivae may be gradual, and bleeding may be exhibited only with probing.
- Seek prompt treatment for symptoms of gingival hyperplasia (easy bleeding of gingivae and gradual enlarging of gingival mass, especially on buccal side of lower anterior teeth). Drug will be discontinued if gingival hyperplasia occurs.
- Research shows that smoking decreases the efficacy of nifedipine and has direct and adverse effects on the heart in the patient on nifedipine treatment.

N

NILOTINIB HYDROCHLORIDE

(ni-lot'i-nib hy-dro-chlor'ide)

Tasigna

Classifications: ANTINEOPLASTIC; TYROSINE KINASE INHIBITOR (TKI)

Therapeutic: ANTINEOPLASTIC; TKI

Prototype: Gefitinib

Pregnancy Category: D

AVAILABILITY 200 mg capsules

ACTION & *THERAPEUTIC EFFECT*

Nilotinib is a tyrosine kinase inhibitor designed to selectively inhibit the BCR-ABL tyrosine kinase on the Philadelphia chromosome found in chronic myelogenous leukemia (CML). It prevents tyrosine kinase enzyme from converting to its active conformation. Thus, it prevents proliferation of BCR-ABL cells and ultimately induces cell death in CML. Nilotinib enhances binding site affinity by offering alternate binding pathways for the ABL tyrosine kinases. *Increased kinase selectivity and binding site affinity makes nilotinib more potent than other similar drugs (imatinib) in preventing the proliferation of CML.*

USES Treatment of chronic and accelerated phase Philadelphia chromosome positive (Ph^+) chronic myelogenous leukemia (CML) in patients resistant to or intolerant to prior therapy that included imatinib.

CONTRAINDICATIONS Hypoglycemia; hypomagnesemia; long QT syndrome; concurrent use of strong CYP3A4 inhibitors/inducers; severe galactose or lactose intolerance; pregnancy (category D), lactation.

CAUTIOUS USE History of pancreatitis; history of cardiac disease; myelosuppression. Safety and efficacy in children not established.

ROUTE & DOSAGE

Chronic Myelogenous Leukemia

Adult: **PO** 400 mg b.i.d.

QT Prolongation Dosage Adjustment

If QT_c greater than 480 msec, withhold nilotinib

If QT_c returns to less than 450 msec and to within 20 msec of the baseline within 2 wk, resume at previous dose.
If QT_c is 450–480 msec after 2 wk, resume at 400 mg PO daily.
If QT_c is greater than 480 msec while taking 400 mg daily, discontinue nilotinib.

Myelosuppression Dosage Adjustment

If ANC less than 1×10^9/L or platelet count less than 50×10^9/L, withhold nilotinib.
If ANC greater than 1×10^9/L and platelet count greater than 50×10^9/L within 2 wk, resume previous dose.
If ANC less than 1×10^9/L or platelet count less than 50×10^9/L for more than 2 wk, resume at 400 mg PO daily

Nonhematologic Abnormalities Dosage Adjustment

For grade 3 or higher serum lipase, amylase, bilirubin, or hepatic transaminases: Withhold nilotinib and monitor abnormal level(s).
Resume nilotinib at 400 mg PO daily if toxicity resolves to grade 1 or lower. Other moderate/severe nonhematologic toxicities: Withhold nilotinib until toxicity resolves, then resume at 400 mg PO daily. May increase to 400 mg b.i.d.

ADMINISTRATION

Oral

- Give on an empty stomach, at least 2 h before or 1 h after eating.
- Ensure that capsules are swallowed whole with water.
- Note: Hypokalemia and hypomagnesemia should be corrected prior to drug administration.
- Store at 15°–30° C (59°–86° F)

ADVERSE EFFECTS (≥1%) **Body as a Whole:** *Peripheral edema, pyrexia.* **CNS:** *Asthenia*, dizziness, *fatigue, headache*, insomnia, paresthesia. **CV:** Flushing, hypertension, palpitations, <u>QT prolongation</u>. **GI:** *Abdominal pain, constipation, diarrhea*, dyspepsia, flatulence, *nausea.* **Hematologic:** *Anemia, neutropenia*, pancytopenia, *thrombocytopenia.* **Metabolic:** Decreased albumin, elevated alkaline phosphatase, elevated ALT, elevated AST, elevated bilirubin, *elevated lipase, hyperglycemia*, hyperkalemia, hypocalcemia, hypokalemia, hyponatremia, *hypophosphatemia.* **Musculoskeletal:** *Arthralgia, back pain, bone pain*, chest pain, *muscle spasms, myalgia, pain in extremity.* **Respiratory:** *Cough*, dysphonia, *dyspnea, nasopharyngitis.* **Skin:** Alopecia, dry skin, eczema, hyperhidrosis, night sweats, *pruritus, rash*, urticaria. **Special Senses:** Vertigo.

INTERACTIONS Drug: Inducers of CYP3A4 (**carbamazepine, dexamethasone, phenobarbital, phenytoin, rifabutin, rifampin, rifapentine**) decrease nilotinib levels. Inhibitors of CYP3A4 (**clarithromycin, indinavir, itraconazole, ketoconazole, nefazodone, nelfinavir, ritonavir, saquinavir, telithromycin, voriconazole**) increase nilotinib levels. P-glycoprotein inhibitors increase the levels of nilotinib. Nilotinib increases the levels of **midazolam, warfarin,** and P-glycoprotein substrates. **Food:** Food increases bioavailability. **Grapefruit** products may increase nilotinib levels. **Herbal: St. John's wort** decreases nilotinib levels.

N

PHARMACOKINETICS Peak: 3 h. **Distribution:** 98% plasma protein bound. **Metabolism:** Hepatic to inactive metabolites. **Elimination:** 93% fecal. **Half-Life:** 17 h.

NURSING IMPLICATIONS

Assessment & Drug Effects

- Obtain a baseline ECG, then again 7 days after first drug dose, and periodically thereafter. Withhold drug and report immediately QT prolongation.
- Monitor closely patients with hepatic impairment for QT interval prolongation.
- Lab tests: Baseline and periodic serum electrolytes; hepatic function tests; CBC q2wk first 2 mo then monthly thereafter; periodic serum lipase.
- Monitor diabetics for loss of glycemic control.

Patient & Family Education

- Nilotinib should not be taken with food (see Administration).
- Women of childbearing age should use reliable forms of contraception, including a barrier type.
- Avoid grapefruit products while on nilotinib.

N

NILUTAMIDE

(ni-lu′ta-mide)

Nilandron

Classifications: ANTINEOPLASTIC; ANTIANDROGEN

Therapeutic: ANTINEOPLASTIC; ANTIANDROGEN

Prototype: Flutamide

Pregnancy Category: C

AVAILABILITY 150 mg tablets

ACTION & *THERAPEUTIC EFFECT* Nonsteroidal with antiandrogen activity. Blocks the effects of testosterone at the androgen receptor sites, thus preventing the normal androgenic response. *Effective in blocking testosterone in treatment of metastatic prostate carcinoma.*

USES Use with surgical castration for metastatic prostate cancer.

CONTRAINDICATIONS Severe hepatic impairment; severe respiratory insufficiency; hypersensitivity to nilutamide; lactation.

CAUTIOUS USE Asian patients relative to causing interstitial pneumonitis; alcoholics; pregnancy (category C). Safety and effectiveness in children are not established.

ROUTE & DOSAGE

Metastatic Prostate Cancer

Adult: **PO** 300 mg daily × 30 days, then 150 mg daily

ADMINISTRATION

Oral

- Give first dose on the day of or day after surgical castration.
- Store below 15°–30° C (59°–86° F) and protect from light.

ADVERSE EFFECTS (≥1%) **Body as a Whole:** *Hot flushes, impotence, decreased libido, malaise,* edema, weight loss, arthritis. **CNS:** Nervousness, paresthesias. **CV:** Angina, heart failure, syncope. **GI:** Diarrhea, GI hemorrhage, melena, dry mouth. **Respiratory:** Cough, interstitial lung disease, rhinitis. **Skin:** Pruritus. **Other:** Alcohol intolerance. **Special Senses:** Cataracts, photophobia.

INTERACTIONS Drug: Carbamazepine, rifampin, phenytoin may decrease level; **fluconazole, gemfibrozil, omeprazole** may increase levels. **Herbal: St. John's wort** may decrease levels.

Common adverse effects in *italic*, life-threatening effects underlined; generic names in **bold**; classifications in SMALL CAPS; ♣ Canadian drug name; ⓟ Prototype drug

PHARMACOKINETICS Absorption: Rapidly from GI tract. **Metabolism:** In the liver (CYP2C19). **Elimination:** In urine. **Half-Life:** 38–50 h.

NURSING IMPLICATIONS

Assessment & Drug Effects

- Obtain baseline chest x-ray before treatment and periodically thereafter.
- Closely monitor for S&S of pneumonitis; at the first sign of adverse pulmonary effects, withhold drug and notify physician. Abnormal ABGs may indicate need to discontinue drug.
- Lab tests: Monitor liver function before beginning treatment and at 3-mo intervals; if serum transaminases increase greater than 2–3 × ULN, treatment is usually discontinued.
- Monitor patients taking phenytoin, theophylline, or warfarin closely for toxic levels of these drugs.

Patient & Family Education

- Report to physician immediately the following S&S of adverse effects on lungs: Development of chest pain, dyspnea, and cough with fever.
- Report S&S of liver injury to physician: Jaundice, dark urine, fatigue, or signs of GI distress including nausea, vomiting, abdominal pain.
- Use caution when moving from lighted to dark areas because the drug may slow visual adaptation to darkness. Tinted glasses may partially alleviate the problem.

NIMODIPINE

(ni-mo′di-peen)

Classifications: CALCIUM CHANNEL BLOCKER; CEREBRAL ANTISPASMODIC
Therapeutic: CEREBRAL ANTISPASMODIC

Prototype: Nifedipine
Pregnancy Category: C

AVAILABILITY 30 mg capsule

ACTION & *THERAPEUTIC EFFECT* Calcium channel blocking agent that is relatively selective for cerebral arteries compared with arteries elsewhere in the body. *Reduces vascular spasms in cerebral arteries during a stroke.*

USES To improve neurologic deficits due to spasm following subarachnoid hemorrhage from ruptured congenital intracranial aneurysms in patients who are in good neurologic condition posticus (e.g., Hunt and Hess Grades I–III).

UNLABELED USES Migraine headaches, ischemic seizures.

CONTRAINDICATIONS Near-fatal reaction to intravenous administration; hypotension; cardiogenic shock; lactation.

CAUTIOUS USE Hepatic impairment; acute MI; bradycardia, heart failure, ventricular dysfunction; elderly; pregnancy (category C). Safety and effectiveness in children are not established.

ROUTE & DOSAGE

Subarachnoid Hemorrhage

Adult: **PO** 60 mg q4h for 21 days, start therapy within 96 h of subarachnoid hemorrhage

Hepatic Impairment Dosage Adjustment

Decrease dose to 30 mg q4h

ADMINISTRATION

Oral

- Make a hole in both ends of the capsule with an 18-gauge needle and extract the contents into a sy-

ringe if patient is unable to swallow. Empty the contents into an enteral (if in use) tube and wash down with 30 mL of NS.
- Store below 40° C (104° F); protect from light.

ADVERSE EFFECTS (≥1%) **CNS:** Headache. **CV:** *Hypotension*. **GI:** Hemorrhage, mild, transient increase in liver function tests.

INTERACTIONS Drug: Hypotensive effects increased when combined with other CALCIUM CHANNEL BLOCKERS. **Food: Grapefruit juice** (greater than 1 qt/day) may increase plasma concentrations and adverse effects.

PHARMACOKINETICS Absorption: Readily from GI tract; approximately 13% reaches systemic circulation (first pass metabolism). **Peak:** 1 h. **Distribution:** Crosses blood–brain barrier; possibly crosses placenta; distributed into breast milk. **Metabolism:** 85% in liver; 15% in kidneys. **Elimination:** Greater than 50% in urine, 32% in feces. **Half-Life:** 8–9 h.

NURSING IMPLICATIONS

Assessment & Drug Effects

- Take apical pulse prior to administering drug and hold it if pulse is below 60. Notify the physician.
- Establish baseline data before treatment is started: BP, pulse, and laboratory evaluations of liver and kidney function.
- Monitor frequently for adverse drug effects, including hypotension, peripheral edema, tachycardia, or skin rash.
- Monitor frequently for dizziness or lightheadedness in older adult patients; risk of hypotension is increased.

Patient & Family Education

- Report gradual weight gain and evidence of edema (e.g., tight rings on fingers, ankle swelling).
- Keep follow-up appointments for monitoring of progress during therapy.

NISOLDIPINE

(ni-sol′di-peen)

Sular

Classifications: CALCIUM CHANNEL BLOCKER; ANTIHYPERTENSIVE

Therapeutic: ANTIHYPERTENSIVE; ANTIANGINAL

Prototype: Nifedipine

Pregnancy Category: C

AVAILABILITY 8.5 mg, 17 mg, 20 mg, 25.5 mg, 30 mg, 34 mg, 40 mg extended release tablets

ACTION & *THERAPEUTIC EFFECT* Inhibits calcium ion influx across cell membranes of cardiac muscle and vascular smooth muscle, which results in vasodilation, inotropism, and negative chronotropism. Inhibits vasoconstriction in the peripheral vasculature. *Significantly reduces total peripheral resistance, decreases blood pressure, and increases cardiac output. It is also a potent coronary vasodilator.*

USES Hypertension.

UNLABELED USES CHF, angina.

CONTRAINDICATIONS Hypersensitivity to nisoldipine or other calcium blockers; systolic BP less than 90 mm Hg, advanced aortic stenosis, cardiogenic shock, severe hypotension, acute MI, sick sinus syndrome; lactation. Safety and efficacy in children not established.

CAUTIOUS USE Liver dysfunction; severe obstructive coronary artery disease; class II to IV heart failure, especially with concurrent administration of a beta-blocker; paroxysmal atrial fibrillation; GERD; CHF; digital ischemia, ulceration, or gangrene; nonobstructive hypertrophic cardiomyopathy; Duchenne muscular dystrophy; older adult; pregnancy (category C).

ROUTE & DOSAGE

Hypertension

Adult: **PO** 17 mg daily may increase by 8.5 mg weekly as needed
Geriatric: **PO** 8.5 mg daily, may increase weekly as needed

ADMINISTRATION

Oral

- Give drug with food to decrease GI distress, but do not give with grapefruit juice or a high-fat meal.
- Ensure that extended release form is not chewed or crushed. It **must be** swallowed whole.
- Drug is usually discontinued gradually to prevent adverse effects.
- Store at 15°–30° C (59°–86° F).

ADVERSE EFFECTS (≥1%) **CNS:** Dizziness, anxiety, tremor, weakness, fatigue, *headache*. **CV:** Hypotension, peripheral edema, palpitations, orthostatic hypotension. **GI:** Abdominal pain, cramps, constipation, dry mouth, diarrhea, nausea. **Skin:** *Flushing,* rash, erythema, urticaria. **Urogenital:** Urinary frequency. **Respiratory:** Pulmonary edema (patients with CHF), wheezing, dyspnea. **Body as a Whole:** Myalgia.

INTERACTIONS Drug: May cause significant increase in **digoxin** level in patients with CHF. BETA-BLOCKERS may cause hypotension and bradycardia. **Phenytoin, carbamazepine, phenobarbital** may significantly decrease levels. Azole antifungals may affect metabolism; avoid combination. **Food:** High-fat food increases availability.

PHARMACOKINETICS Absorption: Rapidly from GI tract; 4–8% reaches systemic circulation. **Peak Effect:** 1–3 h. **Duration:** 8–12 h for hypertension, 7–8 h for angina. **Distribution:** 99% protein bound. **Metabolism:** Extensively in liver. **Elimination:** 70–75% in urine as metabolites. **Half-Life:** 2–14 h.

NURSING IMPLICATIONS

Assessment & Drug Effects

- Monitor blood pressure carefully during period of drug initiation and with dosage increments.
- Monitor cardiovascular status especially heart rate, frequency of angina attacks, or worsening heart failure.
- Assess for and report edematous weight gain.
- Monitor digoxin levels closely with concurrent use and watch for S&S of digoxin toxicity (see Appendix F).

Patient & Family Education

- Do not discontinue the drug abruptly.
- Report symptoms of orthostatic hypotension or other bothersome adverse effects to physician.
- Do not drive or engage in potentially hazardous activities until response to drug is known.

NITAZOXANIDE

(nit-a-zox′-a-nide)
Alinia
Classification: ANTIPROTOZOAL
Therapeutic: ANTIPROTOZOAL
Prototype: Metronidazole
Pregnancy Category: B

N

AVAILABILITY 100 mg/5 mL oral suspension; 500 mg tablets

ACTION & *THERAPEUTIC EFFECT* Antiprotozoal activity believed to be due to interference with an essential enzyme needed for anaerobic energy metabolism in protozoa. *Inhibits growth of sporozoites and oocysts of* Cryptosporidium parvum *and trophozoites of* Giardia lamblia.

USES Treatment of diarrhea caused by *Cryptosporidium parvum* and *Giardia lamblia*.

CONTRAINDICATIONS Prior hypersensitivity to nitazoxanide.
CAUTIOUS USE Hepatic and biliary disease, renal disease, renal impairment, renal failure, and combined renal and hepatic disease; pregnancy (category B); lactation. Safety and efficacy in children younger than 1 y have not been studied.

N

ROUTE & DOSAGE

Diarrhea
Adult: **PO** 500 mg q12h × 3 days
Child: **PO** *12–47 mo,* 100 mg q12h × 3 days; *4–11 y,* 200 mg q12h × 3 days

ADMINISTRATION

Oral
- Prepare suspension as follows: Tap bottle until powder loosens. Draw up 48 mL of water, add half to bottle, shake to suspend powder, then add remaining 24 mL of water and shake vigorously.
- Give required dose (5 or 10 mL) with food.
- Keep container tightly closed, and shake well before each administration.
- Suspension may be stored for 7 days at 15°–30° C (59°–86° F), after which any unused portion **must be** discarded.

ADVERSE EFFECTS (≥1%) **CNS:** Headache. **GI:** Abdominal pain, diarrhea, vomiting.

INTERACTIONS Food: Increases levels.

PHARMACOKINETICS Peak: 1–4 h. **Distribution:** 99% protein bound. **Metabolism:** Rapidly hydrolyzed in liver to an active metabolite, tizoxanide (desacetyl-nitazoxanide). **Elimination:** In urine, bile, and feces.

NURSING IMPLICATIONS

Assessment & Drug Effects
- Monitor for therapeutic effectiveness: No watery stools and 2 or less soft stools with no hematochezia within the past 24 h or no symptoms and no unformed stools within the past 48 h.
- Monitor closely patients with preexisting hepatic or biliary disease for adverse reactions.
- Assess appetite, level of abdominal discomfort and extent of bloating.
- Assess frequency and quantity of diarrhea and monitor total hydration status.
- Weigh daily to aid in assessment of possible fluid loss from diarrhea.

Patient & Family Education
- Note that 5 mL of the oral suspension contains approximately 1.5 g of sucrose.
- Report either no improvement in or worsening of diarrhea and abdominal discomfort.

NITROFURANTOIN
(nye-troe-fyoor'an-toyn)
Furadantin, Novo-Furan ♣

NITROFURANTOIN MACROCRYSTALS

Macrobid, Macrodantin

Classification: URINARY TRACT ANTI-INFECTIVE

Therapeutic: URINARY TRACT ANTIBIOTIC

Pregnancy Category: B

AVAILABILITY 25 mg/5 mL suspension; 25 mg, 50 mg, 100 mg capsules

ACTION & *THERAPEUTIC EFFECT* Synthetic nitrofuran derivative presumed to act by interfering with several bacterial enzyme systems. Highly soluble in urine and reportedly most active in acid urine. Antimicrobial concentrations in urine exceed those in blood. *Active against wide variety of gram-negative and gram-positive microorganisms.*

USES Uncomplicated urinary tract infection, including cystitis.

CONTRAINDICATIONS Hypersensitivity to nitrofurantoin including hepatic dysfunction; anuria, oliguria, significant impairment of kidney function (CrCl less than 60 mL/min); G6PD deficiency; history of cholestatic jaundice; infants younger than 1 mo; pregnancy at term (38–42 wk), labor, or obstetric delivery; lactation.

CAUTIOUS USE History of asthma, anemia, diabetes, vitamin B deficiency, hepatic disease; pulmonary disease; mild to moderate renal disease; electrolyte imbalance, debilitating disease; B_{12} deficiency; pregnancy (category B).

ROUTE & DOSAGE

UTI, Cystitis

Adult: **PO** 50–100 mg q.i.d. × 7 days, or 3 days after sterile urine sample
Child/Infant (1 mo–12 y): **PO** 1.25–1.75 mg/kg q6h (max: 400 mg/day)
Adult/Adolescent (Macrobid only): **PO** 100 mg q12h × 7 days

Chronic Suppressive Therapy for UTI

Adult: **PO** 50–100 mg at bedtime
Child (1 mo–12 y): **PO** 1–2 mg/kg/day in 1–2 divided doses (max: 100 mg/day)

Renal Impairment Dosage Adjustment

Avoid if CrCl less than 60 mL/min

ADMINISTRATION

Oral

- Give with food or milk to minimize gastric irritation.
- Avoid crushing tablets because of the possibility of tooth staining; dilute oral suspension in milk, water, or fruit juice, and rinse mouth thoroughly after taking drug.

ADVERSE EFFECTS (≥1%) **CNS:** Peripheral neuropathy, headache, nystagmus, drowsiness, vertigo. **GI:** *Anorexia, nausea, vomiting,* abdominal pain, diarrhea, cholestatic jaundice, hepatic necrosis. **Hematologic (rare):** Hemolytic or megaloblastic anemia (especially in patients with G6PD deficiency), granulocytosis, eosinophilia. **Body as a Whole:** Angioedema, anaphylaxis, drug fever, arthralgia. **Respiratory:** Allergic pneumonitis, asthmatic attack (patients with history of asthma), pulmonary sensitivity reactions (interstitial pneumonitis or fibrosis). **Skin:** Skin eruptions, pruritus, urticaria, exfoliative dermatitis, transient alopecia. **Urogenital:** Genitourinary superinfections (especially with *Pseudomonas*), crystalluria (older adult

N

patients), dark yellow or brown urine. **Other:** Tooth staining from direct contact with oral suspension and crushed tablets (infants).

DIAGNOSTIC TEST INTERFERENCE Nitrofurantoin metabolite may produce false-positive ***urine glucose*** test results with Benedict's reagent.

INTERACTIONS Drug: ANTACIDS may decrease absorption of nitrofurantoin; **nalidixic acid,** other QUINOLONES may antagonize antimicrobial effects; **probenecid, sulfinpyrazone** increase risk of nitrofurantoin toxicity.

PHARMACOKINETICS Absorption: Readily from GI tract. **Peak:** Urine: 30 min. **Distribution:** Crosses placenta; distributed into breast milk. **Metabolism:** Partially in liver. **Elimination:** Primarily in urine. **Half-Life:** 20 min.

N

NURSING IMPLICATIONS

Assessment & Drug Effects

- Lab tests: Perform C&S prior to therapy; recommended in patients with recurrent infections.
- Monitor I&O. Report oliguria and any change in I&O ratio.
- Be alert to signs of urinary tract superinfections (e.g., milky urine, foul-smelling urine, perineal irritation, dysuria).
- Assess for nausea (which occurs fairly frequently). May be relieved by using macrocrystalline preparation (Macrodantin).
- Watch for acute pulmonary sensitivity reaction, usually within first week of therapy and apparently more common in older adults. May be manifested by mild to severe flu-like syndrome.
- With prolonged therapy, monitor for subacute or chronic pulmonary sensitivity reaction, commonly manifested by insidious onset of malaise, cough, dyspnea on exertion, altered ABGs.
- Monitor for S&S of peripheral neuropathy, which can be severe and irreversible. Withhold drug and notify physician immediately.

Patient & Family Education

- Report promptly muscle weakness, tingling, numbness.
- Nitrofurantoin may impart a harmless brown color to urine.
- Consult physician regarding fluid intake. Generally, fluids are not forced; however, intake should be adequate.

NITROGLYCERIN ℗

(nye-troe-gli'ser-in)

Minitran, Nitrocap, Nitrodisc, Nitro-Dur, Nitrogard, Nitrogard-SR, Nitrong SR, Nitrospan, Nitrostat, Nitrostat I.V.

Classification: NITRATE VASODILATOR

Therapeutic: ANTIANGINAL; VASODILATOR

Pregnancy Category: C

AVAILABILITY 5 mg/mL injection; 0.3 mg, 0.4 mg, 0.6 mg sublingual tablets; 2.5 mg, 6.5 mg, 9 mg sustained release tablets, capsules; 0.1 mg/h, 0.2 mg/h, 0.3 mg/h, 0.4 mg/h, 0.6 mg/h, 0.8 mg/h transdermal patch; 2% ointment

ACTION & *THERAPEUTIC EFFECT* Organic nitrate and potent vasodilator that relaxes vascular smooth muscle. After conversion to nitric oxide, it leads to dose-related dilation of both venous and arterial blood vessels. Promotes peripheral pooling of blood, reduction of peripheral resistance, and decreased venous return to the heart. Both left ventricular preload and afterload are reduced and myocardial oxygen consumption or demand is decreased. *Produces antianginal, anti-ischemic, and antihypertensive effects.*

USES Prophylaxis, treatment, and management of angina pectoris. IV nitroglycerin is used to control BP in perioperative hypertension, CHF associated with acute MI; to produce controlled hypotension during surgical procedures, and to treat angina pectoris in patients who have not responded to nitrate or beta-blocker therapy.

UNLABELED USES Sublingual and topical to reduce cardiac workload in patients with acute MI and in CHF. Ointment for adjunctive treatment of Raynaud's disease.

CONTRAINDICATIONS Hypersensitivity, idiosyncrasy, or tolerance to nitrates; severe anemia; head trauma, increased ICP; glaucoma (sustained release forms). **IV form:** Hypotension, uncorrected hypovolemia, constrictive pericarditis, pericardial tamponade.

CAUTIOUS USE Severe liver or kidney disease, conditions that cause dry mouth, early MI; pregnancy (category C), lactation.

ROUTE & DOSAGE

Angina

Adult: **Sublingual** 1–2 sprays (0.4–0.8 mg) or a 0.3–0.6-mg tablet q3–5min as needed (max: 3 doses in 15 min) **PO** 1.3–9 mg q8–12h **IV** Start with 5 mcg/min and titrate q3–5min until desired response (up to 200 mcg/min) **Transdermal Unit** Apply once q24h or leave on for 10–12 h, then remove and have a 10–12 h nitrate free interval

Topical Apply 1.5–5 cm (1/2–2 in) of ointment q4–6h

Child: **IV** 0.25–0.5 mcg/kg/min, titrate by 0.5–1 mcg/kg/min q3–5min (max: 5 mg/kg/min)

ADMINISTRATION

Sublingual Tablet

- Give 1 tablet and if pain is not relieved, give additional tablets at 5-min intervals, but not more than 3 tablets in a 15-min period.
- Typically available for self-administration in their original container. Instruct in correct use. Request patient to report all attacks.
- Instruct to sit or lie down upon first indication of oncoming anginal pain and to place tablet under tongue or in buccal pouch (hypotensive effect of drug is intensified in the upright position).

Sustained Release Tablet or Capsule

- Give on an empty stomach (1 h before or 2 h after meals), with a full glass of water. Ensure it is swallowed whole.
- Be aware that sustained release form helps to prevent anginal attacks; it is not intended for immediate relief of angina.

Transdermal Ointment

- Using dose-determining applicator (paper application patch) supplied with package, squeeze prescribed dose onto this applicator. Using applicator, spread ointment in a thin, uniform layer to premarked 5.5 by 9 cm (2 1/4 by 3 1/2 in.) square. Place patch with ointment side down onto nonhairy skin surface (areas commonly used: Chest, abdomen, anterior thigh, forearm). Cover with transparent wrap and secure with tape. Avoid getting ointment on fingers.

- Rotate application sites to prevent dermal inflammation and sensitization. Remove ointment from previously used sites before reapplication.

Transdermal Unit

- Apply transdermal unit (transdermal patch) at the same time each day, preferably to skin site free of hair and not subject to excessive movement. Avoid abraded, irritated, or scarred skin. Clip hair if necessary.
- Change application site each time to prevent skin irritation and sensitization.

Intravenous

- Check to see if patient has transdermal patch or ointment in place before starting IV infusion. The patch (or ointment) is usually removed to prevent overdosage.

N

PREPARE: **IV Infusion:** Nitroglycerin is available undiluted and premixed in D5W IV solutions of varying concentrations. ▪ *IV Infusion from Concentrate:* Use only non-PVC plastic or glass bottles and manufacturer-supplied IV tubing. ▪ Withdraw contents of one vial (25 or 50 mg) into syringe and inject immediately into 500 mL of IV solution to minimize contact with plastic; yields 50 mcg/mL or 100 mcg/mL. ▪ If less fluid is desired, add 5 mg to 100 mL to yield 50 mcg/mL. Other concentrations within the range of 25–400 mcg/mL may be used. ▪ Do not exceed 400 mcg/mL.

ADMINISTER: **IV Infusion:** Give by continuous infusion regulated exactly by an infusion pump. ▪ IV dosage titration requires careful and continuous hemodynamic monitoring.

INCOMPATIBILITIES **Solution/additive:** **Caffeine, hydralazine, phenytoin. Y-site: Alteplase, levofloxacin.**

- Use only glass containers for storage of reconstituted IV solution. Polyvinyl chloride (PVC) plastic can absorb nitroglycerin and therefore should not be used.
- Non-polyvinyl-chloride (non-PVC) sets are recommended or provided by manufacturer.

ADVERSE EFFECTS (≥1%) **CNS:** *Headache,* apprehension, blurred vision, weakness, vertigo, dizziness, faintness. **CV:** *Postural hypotension,* palpitations, tachycardia (sometimes with paradoxical bradycardia), increase in angina, syncope, and circulatory collapse. **GI:** Nausea, vomiting, involuntary passing of urine and feces, abdominal pain, dry mouth. **Hematologic:** Methemoglobinemia (high doses). **Skin:** Cutaneous vasodilation with flushing, rash, exfoliative dermatitis, contact dermatitis with transdermal patch; topical allergic reactions with ointment: Pruritic eczematous eruptions, anaphylactoid reaction characterized by oral mucosal and conjunctival edema. **Body as a Whole:** Muscle twitching, pallor, perspiration, cold sweat; local sensation in oral cavity at point of dissolution of sublingual forms.

DIAGNOSTIC TEST INTERFERENCE Nitroglycerin may cause increases in determinations of ***urinary catecholamines*** and ***VMA;*** may interfere with the ***Zlatkis-Zak color reaction,*** causing a false report of decreased ***serum cholesterol.***

INTERACTIONS Drug: Alcohol, ANTIHYPERTENSIVE AGENTS compound hypotensive effects; IV nitroglycerin may antagonize **heparin** anticoagulation. Vasodilating effects may be enhanced by **sildenafil, vardenafil,** or **tadalafil,** so this combination should be avoided.

PHARMACOKINETICS Absorption: Significant loss to first pass metabolism after oral dosing. **Onset:** 2 min SL; 3 min PO; 30 min ointment. **Duration:** 30 min SL; 3–5 h PO; 3–6 h ointment. **Distribution:** Widely distributed; not known if distributes to breast milk. **Metabolism:** Extensively in liver. **Elimination:** Inactive metabolites in urine. **Half-Life:** 1–4 min.

NURSING IMPLICATIONS

Assessment & Drug Effects

- Administer IV nitroglycerin with extreme caution to patients with hypotension or hypovolemia since the IV drug may precipitate a severe hypotensive state.
- Monitor patient closely for change in levels of consciousness and for dysrhythmias.
- Be aware that moisture on sublingual tissue is required for dissolution of sublingual tablet. However, because chest pain typically leads to dry mouth, a patient may be unresponsive to sublingual nitroglycerin.
- Assess for headaches. Approximately 50% of all patients experience mild to severe headaches following nitroglycerin. Transient headache usually lasts about 5 min after sublingual administration and seldom longer than 20 min. Assess degree of severity and consult as needed with physician about analgesics and dosage adjustment.
- Supervise ambulation as needed, especially with older adult or debilitated patients. Postural hypotension may occur even with small doses of nitroglycerin. Patients may complain of dizziness or weakness due to postural hypotension.
- Take baseline BP and heart rate with patient in sitting position before initiation of treatment with transdermal preparations.
- One hour after transdermal (ointment or unit) medication has been applied, check BP and pulse again with patient in sitting position. Report measurements to physician.
- Assess for and report blurred vision or dry mouth.
- Assess for and report the following topical reactions: Contact dermatitis from the transdermal patch; pruritus and erythema from the ointment.

Patient & Family Education

- Store tablet form in its original container.
- Sit or lie down upon first indication of oncoming anginal pain.
- Relax for 15–20 min after taking tablet to prevent dizziness or faintness.
- Be aware that pain not relieved by 3 sublingual tablets over a 15-min period may indicate acute MI or severe coronary insufficiency. Contact physician immediately or go directly to emergency room.
- Note: Sublingual tablets may be taken prophylactically 5–10 min prior to exercise or other stimulus known to trigger angina (drug effect lasts 30–60 min).
- Keep record for physician of number of angina attacks, amount of medication required for relief of each attack, and possible precipitating factors.
- Remove transdermal unit or ointment immediately from skin and notify physician if faintness, dizziness, or flushing occurs following application.
- You can use a sublingual formulation while transdermal unit or ointment is in place.

- Report blurred vision or dry mouth. Both warrant withdrawal of drug.
- Change position slowly and avoid prolonged standing. Dizziness, lightheadedness, and syncope (due to postural hypotension) occur most frequently in older adults.
- Report any increase in frequency, duration, or severity of anginal attack.

NITROPRUSSIDE SODIUM

(nye-troe-pruss'ide)

Nitropress

Classifications: NONNITRATE VASODILATOR; ANTIHYPERTENSIVE

Therapeutic: ANTIHYPERTENSIVE; VASODILATOR

Prototype: Hydralazine

Pregnancy Category: C

N

AVAILABILITY 50 mg injection

ACTION & *THERAPEUTIC EFFECT*
Potent, rapid-acting hypotensive agent that acts directly on vascular smooth muscle to produce peripheral vasodilation, with consequently marked lowering of arterial BP, mild decrease in cardiac output, and moderate lowering of peripheral vascular resistance. *Effective antihypertensive agent used for rapid reduction of high blood pressure.*

USES Short-term, rapid reduction of BP in hypertensive crises and for producing controlled hypotension during anesthesia to reduce bleeding.

UNLABELED USES Refractory CHF or acute MI.

CONTRAINDICATIONS Compensatory hypertension, as in atriovenous shunt or coarctation of aorta, and for control of hypotension in patients with inadequate cerebral circulation; lactation.

CAUTIOUS USE Hepatic insufficiency, hypothyroidism, severe renal impairment, hyponatremia, older adult patients with low vitamin B_{12} plasma levels or with Leber's optic atrophy; pregnancy (category C).

ROUTE & DOSAGE

Hypertensive Crisis

Adult: **IV** 0.3–0.5 mcg/kg/min (average 3 mcg/kg/min)
Child: **IV** 1 mcg/kg/min (average 3 mcg/kg/min) (max: 5 mcg/kg/min)

ADMINISTRATION

Intravenous

PREPARE: **Continuous:** Dissolve each 50 mg in 2–3 mL of D5W. Further dilute in 250 mL D5W to yield 200 mcg/mL or 500 mL D5W to yield 100 mcg/mL. ▪ Lower concentrations may be desirable depending on patient weight. ▪ Following reconstitution, solutions usually have faint brownish tint; if solution is highly colored, do not use it. Promptly wrap container with aluminum foil or other opaque material to protect drug from light.

ADMINISTER: **Continuous:** Administer by infusion pump or similar device that will allow precise measurement of flow rate required to lower BP. ▪ Give at the rate required to lower BP, usually between 0.5–10 mcg/kg/min. ▪ DO NOT exceed the maximum dose of 10 mcg/kg/min nor give this dose for longer than 10 min.

INCOMPATIBILITIES **Solution/additive:** **Amiodarone, propafenone.** **Y-site:** **Cisatracurium, haloperidol, levofloxacin.**

- Store reconstituted solutions and IV solution at 15°–30° C (59°–86° F) protected from light; stable for 24 h.

ADVERSE EFFECTS (≥1%) **Body as a Whole:** Diaphoresis, apprehension, restlessness, muscle twitching, retrosternal discomfort. Thiocyanate toxicity (profound hypotension, tinnitus, blurred vision, fatigue, metabolic acidosis, pink skin color, absence of reflexes, faint heart sounds, loss of consciousness). **CV:** Profound hypotension, palpitation, increase or transient lowering of pulse rate, bradycardia, tachycardia, ECG changes. **GI:** Nausea, retching, abdominal pain. **Metabolic:** Increase in serum creatinine, fall or rise in total plasma cobalamins. **CNS:** Headache, dizziness. **Special Senses:** Nasal stuffiness. **Other:** Irritation at infusion site.

INTERACTIONS No clinically significant interactions established.

PHARMACOKINETICS Onset: Within 2 min. **Duration:** 1–10 min after infusion is terminated. **Metabolism:** Rapidly converted to cyanogen in erythrocytes and tissue, which is metabolized to thiocyanate in liver. **Elimination:** Excreted in urine primarily as thiocyanate. **Half-Life:** (Thiocyanate): 2.7–7 days.

NURSING IMPLICATIONS

Assessment & Drug Effects

- Monitor constantly to titrate IV infusion rate to BP response.
- Relieve adverse effects by slowing IV rate or by stopping drug; minimize them by keeping patient supine.
- Notify physician immediately if BP begins to rise after drug infusion rate is decreased or infusion is discontinued.
- Monitor I&O.
- Lab tests: Monitor blood thiocyanate level in patients receiving prolonged treatment or in patients with severe kidney dysfunction (levels usually are not allowed to exceed 10 mg/dL). Determine plasma cyanogen level following 1 or 2 days of therapy in patients with impaired liver function.

NIZATIDINE

(ni-za′ti-deen)

Axid, Axid AR

Classifications: H_2-RECEPTOR ANTAGONIST; ANTISECRETORY

Therapeutic: ANTIULCER; ANTISECRETORY

Prototype: Cimetidine

Pregnancy Category: B

AVAILABILITY 75 mg tablets; 150 mg, 300 mg capsules; 15 mg/mL oral solution

ACTION & *THERAPEUTIC EFFECT* Inhibits secretion of gastric acid by reversible, competitive blockage of histamine at the H_2 receptor, particularly those in the gastric parietal cells. *Significantly reduces nocturnal gastric acid secretion for up to 12 h.*

USES Active duodenal ulcers; maintenance therapy for duodenal ulcers.

CONTRAINDICATIONS Hypersensitivity to nizatidine; lactation; children 12 y or younger.

CAUTIOUS USE Hypersensitivity to other H_2-receptor antagonists; renal impairment or renal failure; older adults; pregnancy (category B).

ROUTE & DOSAGE

Active Duodenal Ulcer

Adult: **PO** 150 mg b.i.d. or 300 mg at bedtime

N

Maintenance Therapy
Adult: **PO** 150 mg at bedtime

ADMINISTRATION

Oral
- Give drug usually once daily at bedtime. Dose may be divided and given twice daily.
- Administer oral liquid drug using a calibrated measuring device.
- Be aware that antacids consisting of aluminum and magnesium hydroxides with simethicone decrease nizatidine absorption by about 10%. Administer the antacid 2 h after nizatidine.

ADVERSE EFFECTS (≥1%) **CNS:** Somnolence, fatigue. **Skin:** Pruritus, sweating. **Metabolic:** Hyperuricemia.

INTERACTIONS Drug: May decrease absorption of **delavirdine, didanosine, itraconazole, ketoconazole;** ANTACIDS may decrease absorption of nizatidine. May increase **alcohol** levels.

PHARMACOKINETICS Absorption: Greater than 90% from GI tract. **Peak:** 0.5–3 h. **Metabolism:** In liver. **Elimination:** 60% in urine unchanged. **Half-Life:** 1–2 h.

NURSING IMPLICATIONS

Assessment & Drug Effects
- Monitor patient for alleviation of symptoms. Most ulcers should heal within 4 wk.
- Monitor for persistence of ulcer symptoms in patients who continue to smoke during therapy.
- Lab tests: Periodic LFTs and kidney function tests with long-term therapy.

Patient & Family Education
- Take medications for the full course of therapy even though symptoms may be relieved.
- Do not take other prescription or OTC medications without consulting physician.
- Stop smoking; smoking adversely affects healing of ulcers and effectiveness of the drug.

NONOXYNOL-9

(noe-nox'ee-nole)
Conceptrol, Delfen, Emko, Gynol II, Koromex
Classification: SPERMICIDE CONTRACEPTIVE
Therapeutic: SPERMICIDE CONTRACEPTIVE
Pregnancy Category: C

AVAILABILITY 1%, 2%, 2.2%, 3.5%, 4%, 5% gel; 8%, 12.5% foam; 2.27%, 100 mg, 150 mg suppositories

ACTION & *THERAPEUTIC EFFECT* Nonionic surfactant spermicidal incorporated into foams, gels, jelly, or suppositories. Immobilizes sperm by cell membrane disruption. *Applied over the cervix, blocks entrance to uterus by sperm, traps and absorbs seminal fluid, then releases the immediately available spermicide.*

USES As barrier contraceptive alone or in conjunction with a vaginal diaphragm or with a condom.

CONTRAINDICATIONS Cystocele, prolapsed uterus, sensitivity or allergy to polyurethane or to nonoxynol-9; vaginitis; history of TSS; immediately after delivery or abortion; during menstruation.

CAUTIOUS USE HIV patients; pregnancy (category C); menstruation.

ROUTE & DOSAGE

Contraceptive
Adult: **Topical** Apply or insert 30–60 min before intercourse. Repeat before each intercourse.

ADMINISTRATION

Topical

- Apply foams, gels, jelly, cream: Fully load intravaginal applicator and insert about 2/3 of its length [7.5–10 cm (3–4 in.)] into vagina.
- Use with diaphragm: Place 1–3 tsp spermicide formulation in dome prior to insertion. After diaphragm is in place, additional spermicide is recommended. Leave spermicide and diaphragm in place 6 h after intercourse.

ADVERSE EFFECTS (≥1%) **Urogenital:** *Candidiasis;* vaginal irritation and dryness; increase in vaginal infections; menstrual and nonmenstrual toxic shock syndrome (TSS).

INTERACTIONS Drug: Intravaginal AZOLE ANTIFUNGALS may inactivate the spermicides.

PHARMACOKINETICS Onset: Spermicidal action is prompt upon contact with sperm; minimal systemic absorption.

NURSING IMPLICATIONS

Patient & Family Education

- Stop using nonoxynol-9 if pregnancy is suspected.
- Report symptoms of vaginal infection to physician: Burning, inflammation, intense vaginal and vulvar itching, cheesy, curd-like discharge, painful intercourse, dysuria. Nonoxynol-9 antifungal properties are weaker than its antibacterial potency, thus vulvovaginal candidiasis frequently occurs.
- Use spermicide before the first and every subsequent act of intercourse.

NOREPINEPHRINE BITARTRATE

(nor-ep-i-nef'rin)

Levarterenol, Levophed, Noradrenaline

Classifications: ADRENERGIC AGONIST; VASOCONSTRICTOR

Therapeutic: VASOPRESSOR; CARDIAC INOTROPIC

Prototype: Epinephrine

Pregnancy Category: C

AVAILABILITY 1 mg/mL injection

ACTION & *THERAPEUTIC EFFECT* Direct-acting sympathomimetic amine identical to natural catecholamine norepinephrine. Acts directly and predominantly on alpha-adrenergic receptors; little action on beta receptors except in heart ($beta_1$ receptors). Causes vasoconstriction and cardiac stimulation; also produces powerful constrictor action on resistance and capacitance blood vessels. *Peripheral vasoconstriction and moderate inotropic stimulation of heart result in increased systolic and diastolic blood pressure, myocardial oxygenation, coronary artery blood flow, and workload of the heart.*

USES To restore BP in certain acute hypotensive states such as shock, sympathectomy, pheochromocytomectomy, spinal anesthesia, poliomyelitis, MI, septicemia, blood transfusion, and drug reactions. Also as adjunct in treatment of cardiac arrest.

CONTRAINDICATIONS Use as sole therapy in hypovolemic states, except as temporary emergency measure; mesenteric or peripheral vascular thrombosis; profound hypoxia or hypercarbia; use during cyclopropane or halothane anesthesia; hypertension; hyperthyroidism; MAOI therapy.

CAUTIOUS USE Severe heart disease; older adult patients; within 14 days of MAOI therapy; patients receiving tricyclic antidepressants; pregnancy (category C), lactation.

ROUTE & DOSAGE

Hypotension
Adult: **IV** Initial 0.5–1 mcg/min, titrate to response; usual range 8–30 mcg/min
Child: **IV** 0.05–0.1 mcg/kg/min; titrate to response (max: 1–2 mcg/kg/min)

ADMINISTRATION

Intravenous

PREPARE: **IV Infusion:** Dilute a 4 mL ampule in 1000 mL of D5W or D5/NS. ▪ More concentrated solutions (e.g., 4 mg in 500 mL to yield 8 mcg/mL) may be used based on fluid requirements. ▪ Do not use solution if discoloration or precipitate is present. Protect from light.

ADMINISTER: **IV Infusion:** Initial rate of infusion is 2–3 mL/min (8–12 mcg/min), then titrated to maintain BP, usually 0.5–1 mL/min (2–4 mcg/min). ▪ An infusion pump is used. Usually give at the slowest rate possible required to maintain BP. Constantly monitor flow rate. ▪ Check infusion site frequently and immediately report any evidence of extravasation: Blanching along course of infused vein (may occur without obvious extravasation), cold, hard swelling around injection site. ▪ Antidote for extravasation ischemia: Phentolamine, 5–10 mg in 10–15 mL NS injection, is infiltrated throughout affected area (using syringe with fine hypodermic needle) as soon as possible. ▪ If therapy is to be prolonged, change infusion sites at intervals to allow effect of local vasoconstriction to subside. ▪ Avoid abrupt withdrawal; when therapy is discontinued, infusion rate is slowed gradually.

INCOMPATIBILITIES **Solution/additive:** **Aminophylline, amobarbital, ampicillin, whole blood, cephapirin, chlorothiazide, chlorpheniramine, diazepam, pentobarbital, phenobarbital, phenytoin, secobarbital, sodium bicarbonate, sodium iodide, streptomycin, thiopental, warfarin.** **Y-site:** **Insulin, thiopental.**

ADVERSE EFFECTS (≥1%) **Body as a Whole:** Restlessness, anxiety, *tremors,* dizziness, weakness, insomnia, pallor, plasma volume depletion, edema, hemorrhage, intestinal, <u>hepatic</u>, or renal <u>necrosis</u>, retrosternal and pharyngeal pain, profuse sweating. **CV:** Palpitation, hypertension, reflex bradycardia, <u>fatal arrhythmias</u> (large doses), severe hypertension. **GI:** Vomiting. **Metabolic:** Hyperglycemia. **CNS:** Headache, violent headache, <u>cerebral hemorrhage</u>, convulsions. **Respiratory:** Respiratory difficulty. **Skin:** Tissue necrosis at injection site (with extravasation). **Special Senses:** Blurred vision, photophobia.

INTERACTIONS Drug: ALPHA- and BETA-BLOCKERS antagonize pressor effects; ERGOT ALKALOIDS, **furazolidone, guanethidine, methyldopa,** TRICYCLIC ANTIDEPRESSANTS may potentiate pressor effects; **halothane, cyclopropane** increase risk of arrhythmias.

PHARMACOKINETICS Onset: Very rapid. **Duration:** 1–2 min after infusion. **Distribution:** Localizes in sympathetic nerve endings; crosses placenta. **Metabolism:** In liver and other tissues by catecholamine O-methyltransferase and monoamine oxidase. **Elimination:** In urine.

NURSING IMPLICATIONS

Assessment & Drug Effects

- Monitor constantly while patient is receiving norepinephrine. Take baseline BP and pulse before start of therapy, then q2min from initiation of drug until stabilization occurs at desired level, then every 5 min during drug administration.
- Adjust flow rate to maintain BP at low normal (usually 80–100 mm Hg systolic) in normotensive patients. In previously hypertensive patients, systolic is generally maintained no higher than 40 mm Hg below preexisting systolic level.
- Observe carefully and record mental status (index of cerebral circulation), skin temperature of extremities, and color (especially of earlobes, lips, nail beds) in addition to vital signs.
- Monitor I&O. Urinary retention and kidney shutdown are possibilities, especially in hypovolemic patients. Urinary output is a sensitive indicator of the degree of renal perfusion. Report decrease in urinary output or change in I&O ratio.
- Be alert to patient's complaints of headache, vomiting, palpitation, arrhythmias, chest pain, photophobia, and blurred vision as possible symptoms of overdosage. Reflex bradycardia may occur as a result of rise in BP.
- Continue to monitor vital signs and observe patient closely after cessation of therapy for clinical sign of circulatory inadequacy.

NORETHINDRONE (Pr)

(nor-eth-in′drone)

Micronor, Norlutin, Nor-Q.D.

NORETHINDRONE ACETATE

Aygestin ♣, Norlutate ♣

Classification: PROGESTIN
Therapeutic: PROGESTIN; CONTRACEPTIVE
Pregnancy Category: X

AVAILABILITY 0.35 mg, 5 mg tablets

ACTION & *THERAPEUTIC EFFECT* Synthetic progestational hormone with androgenic, anabolic, and estrogenic properties. Progestin-only contraceptives alter cervical mucus, exert progestational effect on endometrium, interfere with implantation, and, in some cases, suppress ovulation. *Contraceptive that suppresses the midcycle surge of luteinizing hormone (LH).*

USES Amenorrhea, abnormal uterine bleeding due to hormonal imbalance in absence of organic pathology; endometriosis. Also alone or in combination with an estrogen for birth control.

CONTRAINDICATIONS Thromboembolic disorders, cerebral vascular or coronary vascular disease; carcinoma of breast, endometrium, or liver; abnormal vaginal bleeding; known or suspected pregnancy (category X); children younger than 16 y.

CAUTIOUS USE Cardiac disease; history of depression, seizure disorders, migraine; diabetes mellitus; CHF; history of thrombophlebitis or thromboembolic disease; lactation.

ROUTE & DOSAGE

Amenorrhea

Adult: **PO Norethindrone** 5–20 mg on day 5 through day 25 of menstrual cycle; **Acetate** 2.5–10 mg on day 5 through day 25 of menstrual cycle

N

Endometriosis

Adult: **PO Norethindrone** 10 mg/day for 2 wk; increase by 5 mg/day q2wk up to 30 mg/day, dose may remain at this level for 6–9 mo or until breakthrough bleeding; **Acetate** 5 mg/day for 2 wk, increase by 2.5 mg/day q2wk up to 15 mg/day, dose may remain at this level for 6–9 mo or until breakthrough bleeding

Progestin-Only Contraception

Adult: **PO Norethindrone** 0.35 mg/day starting on day 1 of menstrual flow, then continuing indefinitely

ADMINISTRATION

Oral

- Note: Dosing schedule is based on a 28-day menstrual cycle.
- Use or add a barrier contraceptive when starting the minipill regimen (progestin-only contraception) for the first cycle or for 3 wk to ensure full protection.
- Protect drug from light and from freezing.

ADVERSE EFFECTS (≥1%) **CNS:** Cerebral thrombosis or hemorrhage, depression. **CV:** Hypertension, pulmonary embolism, edema. **GI:** Nausea, vomiting, cholestatic jaundice, abdominal cramps. **Urogenital:** *Breakthrough bleeding,* cervical erosion, changes in menstrual flow, dysmenorrhea, vaginal candidiasis. **Other:** *Weight changes; breast tenderness,* enlargement or secretion.

INTERACTIONS Drug: BARBITURATES, **carbamazepine, fosphenytoin, modafinil, phenytoin, primidone, pioglitazone, rifampin rifabutin, rifapentine, topiramate, troglitazone** can decrease contraceptive effectiveness.

PHARMACOKINETICS Absorption: Readily absorbed from GI tract. **Metabolism:** In liver. **Elimination:** In urine and feces as metabolites.

NURSING IMPLICATIONS

Assessment & Drug Effects

- Monitor for S&S of thrombophlebitis (see Appendix F).
- Withhold drug and notify physician if any of the following occur: Sudden, complete, or partial loss of vision, proptosis, diplopia, or migraine headache.

Patient & Family Education

- Wait at least 3 mo before becoming pregnant after stopping the minipill to prevent birth defects. Use a barrier or nonhormonal method of contraception until pregnancy is desired.
- If you have not taken all your pills and you miss a period, consider the possibility of pregnancy after 45 days from the last menstrual period; stop using this drug until pregnancy is ruled out.
- If you have taken all your pills and you miss 2 consecutive periods, rule out pregnancy and use a barrier or nonhormonal method of contraception before continuing the regimen.
- Promptly report prolonged vaginal bleeding or amenorrhea.
- Keep appointments for physical checkups (q6–12mo) while you are taking hormonal birth control.

NORFLOXACIN

(nor-flox'a-sin)

Noroxin

Classification: QUINOLONE ANTIBIOTIC

Therapeutic: ANTIBIOTIC

Prototype: Ciprofloxacin

Pregnancy Category: C

AVAILABILITY 400 mg tablets

ACTION & *THERAPEUTIC EFFECT* Potent broad-spectrum antibiotic activity. Alters structure of bacterial DNA gyrase, thus promoting double-stranded DNA breakage, thus interfering with synthesis of bacterial protein and blocking bacterial survival. *Active against many bacterial pathogens of the urinary tract.*

USES Complicated and uncomplicated urinary tract infection (UTI); gonorrhea, prostatitis.

UNLABELED USES Gastroenteritis and prevention of travelers' diarrhea.

CONTRAINDICATIONS Use in individual with known factors that predispose to seizures; history of hypersensitivity to norfloxacin and other quinolone antibiotics; history of QT prolongation; tendon pain; lactation; children younger than 18 y.

CAUTIOUS USE Impaired kidney function, adolescents if skeletal growth is complete; G6PD deficiency; GI disease; myasthenia gravis; pregnancy (category C).

ROUTE & DOSAGE

Urinary Tract Infection/Prostatitis

Adult: **PO** 400 mg b.i.d. × 3–21 days (depending on causative agent)

Gonorrhea or Gonococcal Urethritis (Not CDC Recommended)

Adult: **PO** 800 mg once/day

Renal Impairment Dosage Adjustment

CrCl 30 mL/min or less: 400 mg once daily

ADMINISTRATION

Oral

- Give 1 h before or 2 h after meals with a full glass of water.
- Administer concomitant antacid at least 2 h after norfloxacin to prevent interference with absorption. Aluminum or magnesium ions in the antacid may bind to and form insoluble complexes with the quinolone in GI tract.
- Store at 40° C (104° F) or lower in tightly closed container. Do not freeze.

ADVERSE EFFECTS (≥1%) **Musculoskeletal:** Joint swelling, cartilage erosion in weight-bearing joints, tendonitis. In immunosuppressed adult: Acute ankle and hip pain followed by acute pain, tenderness, and swelling of tendon sheath of middle finger of both hands after 4 wk of therapy. **CNS:** *Headache,* dizziness, lightheadedness, fatigue, drowsiness, somnolence, depression, insomnia, seizures, peripheral neuropathy. **GI:** *Nausea,* abdominal pain, diarrhea, vomiting, anorexia, dyspepsia, dysphagia, dry mouth, bitter taste, heartburn, flatulence, pruritus ani, increased serum AST, ALT, alkaline phosphatase. **Hematologic:** Leukopenia, neutropenia. **Urogenital:** With high doses: Crystalluria (not associated with renal toxicity), vulvar irritation.

DIAGNOSTIC TEST INTERFERENCE May cause false positive on ***opiate screening tests.***

INTERACTIONS Drug: ANTACIDS, **iron, sucralfate**, zinc decrease absorption; **nitrofurantoin** may antagonize antibacterial effects; may increase hypoprothrombinemic effects of **warfarin;** may cause slight increase in **theophylline** levels; concurrent administration with CLASS

N

IA and CLASS III ANTIARRHYTHMICS may result in development of QT prolongation as well as torsades de points.

PHARMACOKINETICS Absorption: 30–40% from GI tract. **Peak:** 1–2 h. **Distribution:** Renal parenchyma, gallbladder, liver, prostate; crosses placenta; distributed into breast milk. **Metabolism:** In liver. **Elimination:** In urine and feces. **Half-Life:** 3–4 h.

NURSING IMPLICATIONS

Assessment & Drug Effects

- Collect urine specimens for testing before initiating antibiotic.
- Monitor patient for tendon pain. Norfloxacin should be discontinued and physician informed.
- Lab tests: Periodic WBC with differential, liver enzymes, and alkaline phosphatase, especially with prolonged use.
- Report to the physician if patient is adequately hydrated, yet I&O ratio and pattern changes are noted, or if condition does not improve within a few days. Dosage may need to be modified.

Patient & Family Education

- Take drug at same time each day.
- Take drug exactly as prescribed. Erratic dosing can encourage emergence of resistant bacteria; underdosing or premature discontinuation of treatment can cause return of UTI symptoms.
- Keep fluid intake high (at least 2500–3000 mL/day if tolerated) to provide adequate urine output and hydration, important in the prevention of crystalluria (rare side effect).

NORMAL SERUM ALBUMIN, HUMAN (Pr)

(al-byoo'min)

Albuminar, Albutein, Buminate, Plasbumin

Classifications: PLASMA DERIVATIVE; PLASMA VOLUME EXPANDER

Therapeutic: PLASMA VOLUME EXPANDER

Pregnancy Category: C

AVAILABILITY 5%, 20%, 25% injection

ACTION & *THERAPEUTIC EFFECT* Obtained by fractionating pooled venous and placental human plasma, which is then sterilized by filtration and heated to minimize transmitting hepatitis B or HIV. Plasma volume expander that increases the osmotic pressure of plasma. *Expands volume of circulating blood by osmotically shifting tissue fluid into general circulation.*

USES To restore plasma volume and maintain cardiac output in hypovolemic shock; for prevention and treatment of cerebral edema; as adjunct in exchange transfusion for hyperbilirubinemia and erythroblastosis fetalis; to increase plasma protein level in treatment of hypoproteinemia; and to promote diuresis in refractory edema. Also used for blood dilution prior to or during cardiopulmonary bypass procedures. Has been used as adjunct in treatment of adult respiratory distress syndrome (ARDS).

CONTRAINDICATIONS Hypersensitivity to albumin; severe anemia; cardiac failure; within 24 h of severe burns; heart failure; patients with normal or increased intravascular volume.

CAUTIOUS USE Low cardiac reserve, pulmonary disease, absence of albumin deficiency; liver or kidney failure, dehydration, hypertension, hypernatremia; restricted sodium intake; pregnancy (category C).

ROUTE & DOSAGE

Emergency Volume Replacement

Adult: **IV** 25 g, may repeat in 15–30 min if necessary (max: 250 g)

Colloidal Volume Replacement (Nonemergency)

Child: **IV** 12.5 g, may repeat in 15–30 min if necessary

Hypoproteinemia

Adult: **IV** 50–75 g (max: 2 mL/min)
Child: **IV** 25 g (max: 2 mL/min)

ADMINISTRATION

Intravenous

PREPARE: **IV Infusion:** Normal serum albumin, 5%, is infused without further dilution. ▪ Normal serum albumin, 20% and 25%, may be infused undiluted or diluted in NS or D5W (with sodium restriction).

ADMINISTER: **IV Infusion for Hypovolemic Shock:** Give initially as rapidly as necessary to restore blood volume. As blood volume approaches normal, rate should be reduced to avoid circulatory overload and pulmonary edema. ▪ Give 5% albumin at rate not exceeding 2–4 mL/min. Give 20% and 25% albumin at a rate not to exceed 1 mL/min. **IV Infusion with Normal Blood Volume:** Give 5% albumin human at a rate not to exceed 5–10 mL/min; give 20% and 25% albumin at a rate not to exceed 2 or 3 mL/min. **IV Infusion for Children:** Usual rate is 25%–50% of the adult rate.

INCOMPATIBILITIES **Solution/additive:** **Amino acids, verapamil.** **Y-site:** **Fat emulsion, midazolam, vancomycin, verapamil.**

▪ Store at temperature not to exceed 37° C (98.6° F). ▪ Use solution within 4 h, once container is opened, because it contains no preservatives or antimicrobials. Discard unused portion.

ADVERSE EFFECTS (≥1%) **Body as a Whole:** Fever, chills, flushing, increased salivation, headache, back pain. **Skin:** Urticaria, rash. **CV:** Circulatory overload, pulmonary edema (with rapid infusion); hypotension, hypertension, dyspnea, tachycardia. **GI:** Nausea, vomiting.

DIAGNOSTIC TEST INTERFERENCE False rise in ***alkaline phosphatase*** when albumin is obtained partially from pooled placental plasma (levels reportedly decline over period of weeks).

NURSING IMPLICATIONS

Assessment & Drug Effects

- Monitor BP, pulse and respiration, and IV albumin flow rate. Adjust flow rate as needed to avoid too rapid a rise in BP.
- Lab tests: Monitor dosage of albumin using plasma albumin (normal): 3.5–5 g/dL; total serum protein (normal): 6–8.4 g/dL; Hgb; Hct; and serum electrolytes.
- Observe closely for S&S of circulatory overload and pulmonary edema (see Appendix F). If S&S appear, slow infusion rate just sufficiently to keep vein open, and report immediately to physician.
- Monitor I&O ratio and pattern. Report changes in urinary output. Increase in colloidal osmotic pressure usually causes diuresis, which may persist 3–20 h.
- Withhold fluids completely during succeeding 8 h, when albumin is given to patients with cerebral edema.

Patient & Family Education

- Report chills, nausea, headache, or back pain to physician immediately.

NORTRIPTYLINE HYDROCHLORIDE

(nor-trip'ti-leen)

Aventyl, Pamelor

Classification: TRICYCLIC ANTIDEPRESSANT

Therapeutic: TRICYCLIC ANTIDEPRESSANT

Prototype: Imipramine

Pregnancy Category: D

AVAILABILITY 10 mg, 25 mg, 50 mg, 75 mg capsules; 10 mg/5 mL solution

ACTION & *THERAPEUTIC EFFECT* Secondary amine derivative of amitriptyline that inhibits the action of many chemical agents including catecholamines. Mood elevation may be due to its inhibition of reuptake of serotonin or another neurotransmitter at the presynaptic membrane. *Effective in improving depressive moods.*

USES Endogenous depression. Similar in actions, uses, limitations, and interactions to imipramine.

UNLABELED USES Nocturnal enuresis in children.

CONTRAINDICATIONS Hypersensitivity to tricyclic antidepressants; acute recovery period after MI; AV block; history of QT prolongation; suicidal ideation; during or within 14 days of MAO inhibitor therapy; children younger than 6 y, pregnancy (category D), lactation.

CAUTIOUS USE Narrow-angle glaucoma, cardiac disease; history of suicidal tendencies; hyperthyroidism, concurrent administration of thyroid medications, concurrent use with electroshock therapy; history of suicides; Parkinson's disease; asthma; bipolar disorder; older adults.

ROUTE & DOSAGE

Antidepressant

Adult: **PO** 25 mg t.i.d. or q.i.d., gradually increased to 100–150 mg/day

Geriatric: **PO** Start with 10–25 mg at bedtime, increase by 25 mg q3days to 75 mg at bedtime (max: 150 mg/day)

Adolescent: **PO** 30–50 mg/day in divided doses

Child (6–12 y): **PO** 10–20 mg/day in 3–4 divided doses

Nocturnal Enuresis

Child: **PO** 6–7 y, 10 mg/day; 8–11 y, 10–20 mg/day; *older than 11 y*, 25–35 mg/day given 30 min before bedtime

Pharmacogenetic Dosage Adjustment

Poor CYP2D6 metabolizers: Start with 50% of dose

ADMINISTRATION

Oral

- Give with food to decrease gastric distress.
- In older adults, total daily dose may be given once a day at bedtime (preferred).
- Be aware that nortriptyline is a 4% alcohol solution.
- Supervise drug ingestion to be sure patient swallows medication.
- Store at 15°–30° C (59°–86° F) in tightly closed container.

ADVERSE EFFECTS (≥1%) **Body as a Whole:** Tremors, hyperhidrosis. **CV:** *Orthostatic hypotension*. **GI:** Paralytic ileus, *dry mouth*. **Hemato-**

Common adverse effects in *italic*, life-threatening effects underlined; generic names in **bold**; classifications in SMALL CAPS; ♣ Canadian drug name; ℗ Prototype drug

logic: Agranulocytosis (rare). **CNS:** Drowsiness, confusional state (especially in older adults and with high dosage). **Skin:** Photosensitivity reaction. **Special Senses:** Blurred vision. **Urogenital:** *Urinary retention.*

INTERACTIONS Drug: May decrease response to ANTIHYPERTENSIVES; CNS DEPRESSANTS, **alcohol,** HYPNOTICS, BARBITURATES, SEDATIVES potentiate CNS depression; may increase hypoprothrombinemic effect of ORAL ANTICOAGULANTS; **levodopa,** SYMPATHOMIMETICS (e.g., **epinephrine, norepinephrine**) pose possibility of sympathetic hyperactivity with hypertension and hyperpyrexia; MAO INHIBITORS pose possibility of severe reactions: Toxic psychosis, cardiovascular instability; **methylphenidate** increases plasma TCA levels; THYROID DRUGS may increase possibility of arrhythmias; **cimetidine** may increase plasma TCA levels. **Herbal: Ginkgo** may decrease seizure threshold. **St. John's wort** may cause serotonin syndrome (see Appendix F).

PHARMACOKINETICS Absorption: Rapidly from GI tract. **Peak:** 7–8.5 h. **Duration:** Crosses placenta; distributed in breast milk. **Metabolism:** In liver (CYP2D6). **Elimination:** Primarily in urine. **Half-Life:** 16–90 h.

NURSING IMPLICATIONS

Assessment & Drug Effects

- Be aware that nortriptyline has a narrow therapeutic plasma level range, or "therapeutic window." Drug levels above or below the therapeutic window are associated with decreased rate of response.
- Therapeutic response may not occur for 2 wk or more.
- Monitor carefully for signs and symptoms of suicidality in children and adults.
- Monitor BP and pulse rate during adjustment period of TCA therapy. If systolic BP falls more than 20 mm Hg or if there is a sudden increase in pulse rate, withhold medication and notify the physician.
- Notify physician if psychotic signs increase.
- Inspect oral membranes daily if patient is on high doses of TCA. Urge outpatient to report stomatitis or dry mouth. Sore mouth can be a major cause of poor nutrition and noncompliance. Consult physician about use of a saliva substitute (e.g., VA-Oralube, Moi-Stir).
- Monitor bowel elimination pattern and I&O ratio. Urinary retention and severe constipation are potential problems, especially in older adults. Advise increased fluid intake; consult physician about stool softener.
- Observe patient with history of glaucoma. Symptoms that may signal acute attack (severe headache, eye pain, dilated pupils, halos of light, nausea, vomiting) should be reported promptly.

Patient & Family Education

- Be aware that your ability to perform tasks requiring alertness and skill may be impaired. Do not engage in hazardous activities until response to drug is known.
- Do not use OTC drugs unless physician approves.
- Consult physician about safe amount of alcohol, if any, that can be ingested. Alcohol and nortriptyline both have increased effects when used together and for up to 2 wk after the TCA is discontinued.
- Nortriptyline enhances the effects of barbiturates and other CNS depressants are enhanced.

NYSTATIN

(nye-stat'in)

Mycostatin, Nadostine ♣, Nilstat, Nyaderm ♣, Nystex, O-V Statin

Classification: ANTIFUNGAL ANTIBIOTIC

Therapeutic: ANTIFUNGAL

Prototype: Amphotericin B

Pregnancy Category: C

AVAILABILITY 500,000 unit tablets; 100,000 units/mL oral suspension; 200,000 troches; 100,000 units vaginal tablets; 100,000 units/g cream, ointment, powder

ACTION & *THERAPEUTIC EFFECT* Nontoxic, nonsensitizing antifungal antibiotic that binds to sterols in fungal cell membrane, thereby changing membrane potential and allowing leakage of intracellular components that leads to fungi cell death. *Fungistatic and fungicidal activity against a variety of yeasts and fungi.*

USES Local infections of skin and mucous membranes caused by *Candida* sp. including *Candida albicans* (e.g., paronychia; cutaneous, oropharyngeal, vulvovaginal, and intestinal candidiasis).

CONTRAINDICATIONS Use of vaginal tablets during pregnancy (category C); vaginal infections caused by *Gardnerella vaginalis* or *Trichomonas* sp.

CAUTIOUS USE Diabetes mellitus; pregnancy (category C), lactation.

ROUTE & DOSAGE

Candida Infections

Adult: **PO** 500,000–1,000,000 units t.i.d.; 1–4 troches 4–5 times/day; Suspension: 400,000–600,000 units q.i.d. **Intravaginal** 1–2 tablets daily for 2 wk

Child: **PO** Suspension: 400,000–600,000 units q.i.d.

Infant: **PO** 100,000–200,000 units q.i.d.

ADMINISTRATION

Oral

- Give reconstituted powder for oral suspension immediately after mixing.
- Rinse mouth with 1–2 tsp oral suspension. Should be kept in mouth (swish) as long as possible (at least 2 min), then liquid should be spit out or swallowed (if "swish and swallow" is ordered).
- For children, infants: Apply drug with swab to each side of mouth. Avoid food or drink for 30 min after treatment.
- The troche dosage form should dissolve in mouth (about 30 min). Troches should not be chewed or swallowed. Food and drink should be avoided during period of dissolving and for 30 min after treatment.

Topical

- Do not apply occlusive dressings over topical applications unless specifically directed to do so.

Intravaginal

- Store vaginal tablets in refrigerator below 15° C (59° F).

ADVERSE EFFECTS (≥1%) **GI:** Nausea, vomiting, epigastric distress, diarrhea (especially with high oral doses).

PHARMACOKINETICS Absorption: Poorly absorbed from GI tract. **Elimination:** In feces.

NURSING IMPLICATIONS

Assessment & Drug Effects

- Monitor oral cavity, especially the tongue, for signs of improvement.

Patient & Family Education

- This drug may cause contact dermatitis. Stop using the drug and report to physician if redness, swelling, or irritation develops.
- Take for oral candidiasis (thrush) treatment after meals and at bedtime.
- Care of dentures: Remove dentures before each rinse with oral suspension and before use of troche. Remove dentures at night (infection occurs more frequently in person who wears dentures 24 h a day).
- Dust shoes and stockings, as well as feet, with nystatin dusting powder.
- Gently clean infected areas with tepid water before each application of topical preparation.
- Continue medication for vulvovaginal candidiasis during menstruation.
- Use vaginal tablets up to 6 wk before term to prevent thrush in the newborn.

OCTREOTIDE ACETATE Pr

(oc-tre′o-tide)

Sandostatin, Sandostatin LAR depot

Classification: SOMATOSTATIN ANALOG

Therapeutic: HORMONE SUPPRESSANT; ACROMEGALY AGENT; ANTIDIARRHEAL

Pregnancy Category: B

AVAILABILITY 0.05 mg/mL, 0.1 mg/mL, 0.2 mg/mL, 0.5 mg/mL, 1 mg/mL injection; 10 mg/5 mL, 20 mg/5 mL, 30 mg/5 mL depot injection

ACTION & *THERAPEUTIC EFFECT* A long-acting peptide that mimics natural hormone somatostatin. Suppresses secretion of serotonin, pancreatic peptides, gastrin, vasoactive intestinal peptide, insulin, glucagon, secretin, and motilin. *Stimulates fluid and electrolyte absorption from the GI tract and prolongs intestinal transit time; also inhibits the growth hormone.*

USES Symptomatic treatment of severe diarrhea and flushing episodes associated with metastatic carcinoid tumors. Also watery diarrhea associated with vasoactive intestinal peptide (VIP) tumors, acromegaly.

UNLABELED USES Acromegaly associated with pituitary tumors, fistula drainage, variceal bleeding.

CONTRAINDICATIONS Hypersensitivity to octreotide.

CAUTIOUS USE Cholelithiasis, renal impairment; dialysis; hepatic disease, liver cirrhosis; cardiac disease, CHF; diabetes, hypothyroidism; older adults; pregnancy (category B); lactation.

ROUTE & DOSAGE

Carcinoid Syndrome

Adult: **Subcutaneous/IV** 100–600 mcg/day in 2–4 divided doses, titrate to response **IM** May switch to depot injection after 2 wk at 20 mg q4wk × 3 mo

VIPoma

Adult: **Subcutaneous/IV** 200–300 mcg/day in 2–4 divided doses, titrate to response **IM** May switch to depot injection after 2 wk at 20 mg q4wk × 2 mo

Acromegaly

Adult: **Subcutaneous** 50 mcg t.i.d., titrate up to 100 mcg–500 mcg t.i.d. **IM** May switch to depot injection after 2 wk at 20 mg q4wk × at least 3 mo, then reassess

Renal Impairment Dosage Adjustment

Dialysis: Reduce dose

ADMINISTRATION

Subcutaneous/Intramuscular

- **Sandostatin LAR Depot** should be given IM. Reconstitute according to manufacturer's directions.
- **Sandostatin** may be given subcutaneously or IV.
- Minimize GI side effects by giving injections between meals and at bedtime.
- Avoid multiple injections into the same site. Rotate subcutaneous sites on abdomen, hip, and thigh.
- Give deep IM into a large muscle. To reduce local irritation, allow solution to reach room temperature before injection and administer slowly.

Intravenous

PREPARE: **Direct:** Give **Sandostatin** undiluted. **Intermittent:** Dilute in 50–200 mL D5W.

ADMINISTER: **Direct:** Give a single dose over 3–5 min. In emergency (eg, carcinoid crisis), give rapid IV bolus over 60 sec. **Intermittent:** Give over 15–30 min.

INCOMPATIBILITIES **Solution/additive:** **Fat emulsion, regular insulin.** **Y-site:** **Dantrolene, diazepam, micafungin, phenytoin, pantoprazole.**

ADVERSE EFFECTS (≥1%) **CNS:** Headache, fatigue, dizziness. **GI:** *Nausea, diarrhea, abdominal pain and discomfort.* **CV:** Bradycardia. **Metabolic:** Hypoglycemia, hyperglycemia, increased liver transaminases, hypothyroidism (after long-term use), cholelithiasis, pancreatitis. **Body as a Whole:** Flushing, edema, *injection site pain*, pruritus.

INTERACTIONS Drug: May decrease **cyclosporine** levels; may alter other drug and nutrient absorption because of alterations in GI motility.

PHARMACOKINETICS Absorption: Rapidly from subcutaneous injection. **Peak:** 0.4 h. **Duration:** Up to 12 h. **Metabolism:** In liver. **Elimination:** In urine. **Half-Life:** 1.5 h.

NURSING IMPLICATIONS

Assessment & Drug Effects

- Lab tests: Periodic blood glucose, LFTs, and serum electrolytes. As specific conditions indicate, periodic: Plasma serotonin levels with carcinoid tumors, plasma VIP levels with VIPoma, serum GH, serum IGF-1, and thyroid function tests.
- Monitor for hypoglycemia and hyperglycemia (see Appendix F), because octreotide may alter the balance between insulin, glucagon, and growth hormone.
- Monitor fluid and electrolyte balance, as octreotide stimulates fluid and electrolyte absorption from GI tract.
- Monitor vitals signs, especially BP.
- Monitor bowel function, including bowel sounds and stool consistency.

Patient & Family Education

- Learn proper technique for subcutaneous injection if self-medication is required.
- Note: Preferred sites for subcutaneous injections of octreotide are the hip, thigh, and abdomen.

Multiple injections at the same subcutaneous injection site within short periods of time are not recommended. This is to avoid irritating the area.

OFATUMUMAB

(o-fa-tu'mu-mab)

Arzerra

Classifications: BIOLOGICAL RESPONSE MODIFIER; MONOCLONAL ANTIBODY; ANTINEOPLASTIC

Therapeutic: ANTINEOPLASTIC

Prototype: Basiliximab

Pregnancy Category: C

AVAILABILITY 100 mg/5 mL solution for injection

ACTION & *THERAPEUTIC EFFECT* A CD20 cytolytic IgG1 kappa monoclonal antibody. The CD20 molecule is present on normal B lymphocytes, both mature and immature lymphocytes as well as on B-cell chronic lymphocytic leukemia (CLL). Ofatumumab causes B-cell lysis possibly by antibody-dependent, cell-mediated cytotoxicity. *Effectiveness in treatment of CLL refractory to the standard drug regimen is based on the clinical improvement in response to ofatumumab.*

USES Chronic lymphocytic leukemia refractory to fludarabine and alemtuzumab.

CONTRAINDICATIONS Serious infusion reaction; moderate to severe COPD; leukoencephalopathy; viral hepatitis; live vaccines. Safety and effectiveness in children are not established.

CAUTIOUS USE History of hepatitis B; elderly; pregnancy (category C); lactation.

ROUTE & DOSAGE

Chronic Lymphocytic Leukemia (CLL)

Adult: **IV** Initial dose of 300 mg followed 1 wk later by 2000 mg qwk for 7 doses, followed by 2000 mg q4wk for 4 doses

ADMINISTRATION

Intravenous

PREPARE: **Infusion:** Do not shake drug vials. ▪ Determine the volume of the required drug dose and withdraw an equal volume of NS from a 1000 mL polyolefin IV bag. Add ofatumumab to the IV bag and mix by gentle inversion.

ADMINISTER: **Infusion:** Infuse through an in-line filter and PVC administration set supplied with product. ▪ Do **NOT** give IV push or bolus. ▪ Do not mix or administer with any other drugs or solutions. *For doses 1 and 2:* Initiate infusion at 12 mL/h. If no infusion reaction occurs from 0–30 min, may increase rate q30min as follows: 31–60 min, 25 mL/h; 61–90 min, 50 mL/h; 91–120 min, 100 mL/h; after 120 min, 200 mL/h. ▪ *For doses 3–12:* Initiate infusion at 25 mL/h. If no infusion reaction occurs from 0–30 min, may increase rate q30min as follows: 31–60 min, 50 mL/h; 61–90 min, 100 mL/h; 91–120 min, 200 mL/h; after 120 min, 400 mL/h.

▪ Store diluted solution between 2°–8° C (36°–46° F). ▪ Use within 12 h of preparation. Discard solution after 24 h.

ADVERSE EFFECTS (≥1%) **Body as a Whole:** Chills, *fatigue,* herpes zoster infection, *infusion reactions,* peripheral edema, *pyrexia,* sepsis. **CNS:** Headache, insomnia. **CV:** Hy-

O

pertension, hypotension, tachycardia. **GI:** *Diarrhea, nausea.* **Hematologic:** *Anemia, neutropenia.* **Musculoskeletal:** Back pain, muscle spasms. **Respiratory:** *Bronchitis, cough, dyspnea,* nasopharyngitis, *pneumonia,* sinusitis, *upper respiratory tract infections.* **Skin:** Hyperhidrosis, *rash,* urticaria.

PHARMACOKINETICS Half-Life: 14 days.

NURSING IMPLICATIONS

Assessment & Drug Effects

- Monitor for infusion reactions and stop infusion for any of the following: Bronchospasm, dyspnea, angioedema, flushing, significant changes in BP, tachycardia, back or abdominal pain, fever, rash, or urticaria.
- Monitor for and report promptly S&S of changes in neurologic status or suspected intestinal obstruction.
- Lab tests: Baseline and periodic CBC with differential.

O

Patient & Family Education

- Report promptly any of the following: New or worsening abdominal pain or nausea, confusion, dizziness, loss of balance, difficulty talking or problems with vision, sore throat, fever, or other signs of infections.
- Avoid live vaccinations and close contact with those who have received live vaccines.

OFLOXACIN

(o-flox'a-cin)

Floxin, Ocuflox

Classification: ANTIBIOTIC, QUINOLONE

Therapeutic: ANTIBIOTIC

Prototype: Ciprofloxacin

Pregnancy Category: C

AVAILABILITY 200 mg, 300 mg, 400 mg tablets; 0.3% ophth solution; 0.3% otic solution

ACTION & *THERAPEUTIC EFFECT* A fluoroquinolone antibiotic that inhibits DNA gyrase, an enzyme necessary for bacterial DNA replication and some aspects of its transcription, repair, recombination, and transposition. *Has a broad spectrum of activity against gram-positive and gram-negative bacteria. Most effective against aerobic and anaerobic gram-negative bacteria.*

USES Uncomplicated gonorrhea, prostatitis, respiratory tract infections, skin and skin structure infections, urinary tract infections, superficial ocular infections, pelvic inflammatory disease. Otic: Otitis externa, otitis media with perforated tympanic membranes.

UNLABELED USES EENT infections, *Helicobacter pylori* infections, *Salmonella* gastroenteritis, anthrax.

CONTRAINDICATIONS Hypersensitivity to ofloxacin or other quinolone antibacterial agents; tendon pain; sunlight (UV) exposure; QT prolongation; viral infection; lactation.

CAUTIOUS USE Renal disease; patients with a history of epilepsy, psychosis, or increased intracranial pressure, cerebrovascular disease, CNS disorders such as seizures, epilepsy, myasthenia gravis; GI disease, colitis, dehydration; syphilis; atrial fibrillation; acute MI; CVA; children and adolescents younger than 18 y (except for otic preparation); pregnancy (category C).

ROUTE & DOSAGE

Uncomplicated Gonorrhea (Not CDC Recommended)

Adult: **PO** 400 mg for 1 dose

Respiratory Tract and Skin and Skin Structure Infections

Adult: **PO** 200–400 mg q12h × 10 days

Urinary Tract Infection

Adult: **PO** 200 mg q12h × 3–10 days

Pelvic Inflammatory Disease

Adult: **PO** 400 mg b.i.d. × 14 days

Prostatitis

Adult: **PO** 300 mg b.i.d. × 6 wk

Superficial Ocular Infections

Adult/Adolescent/Child: **Ophthalmic** Instill 1–2 drops q2–4h for first 2 days, then q.i.d. for up to 5 additional days

Otitis Media with Perforation

Adult: **Otic** 10 drops (0.5 mL) q12h for 14 days
Child (1 y or older): **Otic** 5 drops (0.25 mL) q12h for 14 days

Otitis Externa

Adult: **Otic** 10 drops (0.5 mL) q12h for 7 days
Child (6 mo–13 y): **Otic** 5 drops (0.25 mL) q12h for 7 days

Renal Impairment Dosage Adjustment

CrCl 20–50 mL/min: Dose should be given q24h; less than 20 mL/min: 1/2 the dose q24h

Hepatic Impairment Dosage Adjustment

Severe impairment: 400 mg daily

ADMINISTRATION

Oral

- Do not give with meals.
- Avoid administering mineral supplements or vitamins with iron or zinc within 2 h of drug.
- Do not give antacids with magnesium, aluminum, or sucralfate within 4 h before or 2 h after drug.

Instillation

- Do NOT allow tip of dropper for ocular preparation to contact any surface.

ADVERSE EFFECTS (≥1%) **CNS:** *Headache, dizziness, insomnia,* hallucinations. **GI:** Nausea, vomiting, diarrhea, GI discomfort. **Urogenital:** Pruritus, pain, irritation, burning, vaginitis, vaginal discharge, dysmenorrhea, menorrhagia, dysuria, urinary frequency. **Skin:** Pruritus, rash. **Other:** Cartilage erosion.

DIAGNOSTIC TEST INTERFERENCE May cause false positive on ***opiate screening tests.***

INTERACTIONS Drug: Ofloxacin absorption decreased when it is administered with MAGNESIUM- or ALUMINUM-CONTAINING ANTACIDS. Other CATIONS, including **calcium, iron,** and **zinc,** also appear to interfere with ofloxacin absorption. May have additive effect with ANTIDIABETICS.

PHARMACOKINETICS Absorption: 90–98% from GI tract. **Peak:** 1–2 h. **Distribution:** Distributes to most tissues; 50% crosses into CSF with inflamed meninges; 20–32% protein bound; crosses placenta; distributed into breast milk. **Metabolism:** Slightly in liver. **Elimination:** 72–98% in urine within 48 h. **Half-Life:** 5–7.5 h.

NURSING IMPLICATIONS

Assessment & Drug Effects

- Lab tests: Do C&S tests prior to initial dose. Treatment may be implemented pending results.
- Determine history of hypersensitivity reactions to quinolones or other drugs before therapy is started.
- Withhold ofloxacin and notify physician at first sign of tendon

O

pain, a skin rash, or other allergic reaction.

- Monitor for seizures, especially in patients with known or suspected CNS disorders. Discontinue ofloxacin and notify physician immediately if seizure occurs.
- Assess for signs and symptoms of superinfection (see Appendix F).

Patient & Family Education

- Drink fluids liberally unless contraindicated.
- Be aware that dizziness or lightheadedness may occur; use appropriate caution.
- Avoid excessive sunlight or artificial ultraviolet light because of the possibility of phototoxicity.

OLANZAPINE

(o-lan′za-peen)

Zyprexa, Zyprexa Zydis

Classification: ANTIPSYCHOTIC, ATYPICAL

Therapeutic: ANTIPSYCHOTIC, ANTIMANIC

Prototype: Clozapine

Pregnancy Category: C

AVAILABILITY 2.5 mg, 5 mg, 7.5 mg, 10 mg, 15 mg tablets; 10 mg, 15 mg, 20 mg orally disintegrating tablets; 10 mg powder for injection

ACTION & *THERAPEUTIC EFFECT* Antipsychotic activity is thought to be due to antagonism for both serotonin 5-$HT_{2A/2C}$ and dopamine D_{1-4} receptors. May inhibit the CNS presynaptic neuronal reuptake of serotonin and dopamine. *Has effective antipsychotic activity.*

USES Management of psychotic disorders, treatment of bipolar disorder, acute agitation (IM).

UNLABELED USES Alzheimer's dementia.

CONTRAINDICATIONS Hypersensitivity to olanzapine; abrupt discontinuation, coma, severe CNS depression; dementia-related psychosis in elderly. **IM form:** Tardive dyskinesia; infants; lactation.

CAUTIOUS USE Known cardiovascular disease, neurologic disease, stroke, cerebrovascular disease, Parkinson's disease; history of seizures, conditions that predispose to hypotension (i.e., dehydration, hypovolemia); history of syncope; history of breast cancer; Japanese; diabetes mellitus; prostatic hypertrophy; closed-angle glaucoma; paralytic ileus; urinary retention; hepatic or renal impairment, jaundice; predisposition to aspiration pneumonia; may increase risk of stroke in elderly patients with dementia; history of or high risk for suicide; pregnancy (category C). **IM form:** Elderly, debilitated or at risk for hypotension. Safety and effectiveness in children 6 y and younger are not established.

ROUTE & DOSAGE

Psychotic Disorders

Adult: **PO** Start with 5–10 mg once/day, may increase by 2.5–5 mg qwk until desired response (usual range 10–15 mg/day, max: 20 mg/day)

Geriatric: **PO** Start with 5 mg once/day

Bipolar Mania

Adult: **PO** Start with 10–15 mg once/day, may increase by 5 mg q24h if needed

Acute Agitation

Adult: **IM** 10 mg, do not repeat more frequently than q2h (max: 30 mg/24h)

Geriatric: **IM** 2.5–5 mg once

ADMINISTRATION

Oral

- Do not push orally disintegrating tablet through blister foil. Peel foil back and remove tablet. Tablet will disintegrate with/without liquid.

Intramuscular

- Reconstitute with 2.1 mL of sterile water for injection to yield 5 mg/mL. Use within 1 h of reconstitution.
- Give deep IM into the gluteal muscle. Do not inject more than 5 mL into one site.

ADVERSE EFFECTS (≥1%) **Body as a Whole:** *Weight gain,* fever, back and chest pain, peripheral and lower extremity edema, joint pain, twitching, premenstrual syndrome. **CNS:** *Somnolence, dizziness, headache, agitation, insomnia, nervousness, hostility,* anxiety, personality disorder, akathisia, hypertonia, tremor amnesia, euphoria, stuttering, extrapyramidal symptoms (dystonic events, *parkinsonism, akathisia*), tardive dyskinesia. **CV:** Postural hypotension, hypotension, tachycardia. **Special Senses:** Amblyopia, blepharitis. **GI:** Abdominal pain, constipation, dry mouth, increased appetite, increased salivation, nausea, vomiting, elevated liver function tests. **Metabolic:** Hyperglycemia, diabetes mellitus. **Urogenital:** Premenstrual syndrome, hematuria, urinary incontinence, metrorrhagia. **Respiratory:** Rhinitis, cough, pharyngitis, dyspnea. **Skin:** Rash.

INTERACTIONS Drug: May enhance hypotensive effects of ANTIHYPERTENSIVES. May enhance effects of other CNS ACTIVE DRUGS, **alcohol. Carbamazepine, omeprazole, rifampin** may increase metabolism and clearance of olanzapine. **Fluvoxamine** may inhibit metabolism and clearance of olanzapine.

PHARMACOKINETICS Absorption: Rapidly from GI tract; 60% reaches systemic circulation. **Onset:** 15 min IM. **Peak:** 6 h. **Distribution:** 93% protein bound, secreted into breast milk of animals (human secretion unknown). **Metabolism:** In liver (CYP1A2). **Elimination:** Approximately 57% in urine, 30% in feces. **Half-Life:** 21–54 h.

NURSING IMPLICATIONS

Assessment & Drug Effects

- Monitor closely cerebrovascular status in elderly patients with dementia-related psychosis.
- Monitor diabetics for loss of glycemic control.
- Withhold drug and immediately report S&S of neuroleptic malignant syndrome (see Appendix F); assess for and report S&S of tardive dyskinesia (see Appendix F).
- Lab tests: Periodically monitor ALT, especially in those with hepatic dysfunction or being treated with other potentially hepatotoxic drugs. Periodic blood glucose monitoring.
- Monitor BP and HR periodically. Monitor temperature, especially under conditions such as strenuous exercise, extreme heat, or treatment with other anticholinergic drugs.
- Monitor for and report orthostatic hypotension, especially during the initial dose-titration period.
- Monitor for seizures, especially in older adults and cognitively impaired persons.

Patient & Family Education

- Carefully monitor blood glucose levels if diabetic.

O

- Do not drive or engage in potentially hazardous activities until response to drug is known; drug increases risk of orthostatic hypotension and cognitive impairment.
- Learn common adverse effects and possible drug interactions.
- Avoid alcohol and do not take additional medications without informing physician.
- Do not become overheated; avoid conditions leading to dehydration.

OLMESARTAN MEDOXOMIL

(ol-me-sar′tan)

Benicar

Classification: ANGIOTENSIN II RECEPTOR (TYPE AT_1) ANTAGONIST, ANTIHYPERTENSIVE

Therapeutic: ANTIHYPERTENSIVE

Prototype: Losartan

Pregnancy Category: C first trimester; D second and third trimester

O

AVAILABILITY 5 mg, 20 mg, 40 mg tablets

ACTION & *THERAPEUTIC EFFECT* Angiotensin II receptor (type AT_1) antagonist acts as a potent vasodilator and primary vasoactive hormone of the renin-angiotensin-aldosterone system. Selectively blocks the binding of angiotensin II to the AT_1 receptors found in many tissues (e.g., vascular smooth muscle, adrenal glands). *Antihypertensive effect is due to its potent vasodilation effect.*

USES Treatment of hypertension.

CONTRAINDICATIONS Hypersensitivity to pimecrolimus or components in the cream; Netherton's syndrome; application to active cutaneous viral infection; pregnancy (category D second and third trimester); lactation, children.

CAUTIOUS USE Renal artery stenosis; heart failure; severe renal impairment; hypovolemia; pregnancy (category C first trimester).

ROUTE & DOSAGE

Hypertension

Adult: **PO** 20 mg daily, may increase to 40 mg daily. Start with 5–10 mg daily if volume depleted.

ADMINISTRATION

Oral

- Determine if patient is volume depleted (e.g., patients treated with diuretics) prior to first administration of drug. If volume depletion is suspected, a lower starting dose is recommended.
- Store at 20°–25° C (68°–77° F).

ADVERSE EFFECTS (≥1%) **Body as a Whole:** Back pain, flu-like symptoms. **CNS:** Headache. **CV:** Hypotension (especially if dehydrated). **GI:** Diarrhea. **Metabolic:** Increased CPK, hyperglycemia, hypertriglyceridemia. **Respiratory:** Bronchitis, pharyngitis, rhinitis, sinusitis, upper respiratory infection. **Urogenital:** Hematuria.

INTERACTIONS Drug: May increase hypotensive effect of other ANTIHYPERTENSIVES; may cause hyperkalemia with POTASSIUM-SPARING DIURETICS, POTASSIUM SUPPLEMENTS; increase risk of **lithium** toxicity. **Herbal: Ephedra, ma-huang** may antagonize antihypertensive effects.

PHARMACOKINETICS Absorption: Rapidly absorbed, 26% reaches systemic circulation. **Peak:** 1–2 h. **Distribution:** 99% protein bound. **Metabolism:** Not metabolized by CYP 450 system. **Elimination:** 50% in urine, 50% in feces. **Half-Life:** 13 h.

NURSING IMPLICATIONS

Assessment & Drug Effects

- Monitor closely any volume-depleted patient following initial drug doses. If serious hypotension occurs, place patient in supine position and notify physician immediately.
- Monitor BP and HR at drug trough (prior to a scheduled dose). Report hypotension or bradycardia.
- Monitor drug effectiveness, especially in African Americans, when olmesartan is used as monotherapy.
- Lab tests: Monitor baseline and periodic renal functions; monitor CBC, electrolytes, and liver function with long-term therapy.

Patient & Family Education

- Discontinue drug and notify physician if you experience swelling of the face, tongue, or throat, or if you believe you are pregnant.
- Notify physician of symptoms of hypotension (e.g., dizziness, fainting).

OLOPATADINE HYDROCHLORIDE

(o-lo-pa′ta-deen)

Patase, Patanol

Pregnancy Category: C

See Appendix A-1.

OLSALAZINE SODIUM

(ol-sal′a-zeen)

Dipentum

Classification: ANTI-INFLAMMATORY

Therapeutic: GI ANTI-INFLAMMATORY

Prototype: Mesalamine

Pregnancy Category: C

AVAILABILITY 250 mg capsules

ACTION & *THERAPEUTIC EFFECT* Converted to 5-aminosalicylic acid (5-ASA) by colonic bacteria. The 5-ASA is absorbed slowly, resulting in a very high local concentration in the colon. 5-ASA inhibits prostaglandin production in the colon, thus leading to its anti-inflammatory properties. *5-ASA has anti-inflammatory activity in ulcerative colitis.*

USES Maintenance therapy in patients with ulcerative colitis.

UNLABELED USES Acute flare-up of ulcerative colitis.

CONTRAINDICATIONS Hypersensitivity to salicylates or 5-ASA.

CAUTIOUS USE Patients with preexisting kidney disease; elderly; colitis; pregnancy (category C), lactation. Safety and effectiveness in children are not established.

ROUTE & DOSAGE

Ulcerative Colitis

Adult: **PO** 500 mg b.i.d., may increase up to 1.5–3 g/day in 2–4 divided doses

ADMINISTRATION

Oral

- Give with food in two evenly divided doses.

ADVERSE EFFECTS (≥1%) **CNS:** Headache. **GI:** *Diarrhea,* nausea, abdominal pain, indigestion, vomiting, bloating. **Skin:** Rash. **Body as a Whole:** Arthralgia.

PHARMACOKINETICS Absorption: 1–3% from GI tract; high colonic concentrations are associated with efficacy. **Metabolism:** Olsalazine, a prodrug, is composed of 2 molecules of 5-ASA; colonic bacterial azo-reductases break the azo bond, releasing 2 active molecules of 5-

O

ASA. **Elimination:** Primarily in feces as 5-ASA. **Half-Life:** At least 6 h.

NURSING IMPLICATIONS

Assessment & Drug Effects

- Monitor kidney function in patients with preexisting renal disease.
- Monitor for S&S of a hypersensitivity reaction (see Appendix F). Withhold olsalazine and notify physician at first sign of an allergic response.

Patient & Family Education

- Report diarrhea, a possible adverse effect, to the physician.

O

OMALIZUMAB

(o-mal-i-zoo'mab)

Xolair

Classifications: BIOLOGICAL RESPONSE MODIFIER; MONOCLONAL ANTIBODY; RESPIRATORY ANTI-INFLAMMATORY

Therapeutic: ANTIALLERGIC; ANTIASTHMATIC; ANTI-INFLAMMATORY

Pregnancy Category: B

AVAILABILITY 75 mg, 150 mg vial

ACTION & *THERAPEUTIC EFFECT* DNA recombinant monoclonal antibody that selectively binds to human IgE. It inhibits binding of IgE to high-affinity IgE receptors on the surface of mast cells and basophils, limiting the release of inflammatory mediators. *Inhibits release of mediators of the allergic response and has an anti-inflammatory action on the respiratory system.*

USES Control of moderate to severe allergic asthma.

UNLABELED USES Seasonal allergic rhinitis, food allergies.

CONTRAINDICATIONS Hypersensitivity to omalizumab; severe infections, including chicken pox and other viral infections; acute bronchospasm, acute asthma, status asthmaticus; malignancies; children younger than 12 y.

CAUTIOUS USE Live vaccines; pregnancy (category B), lactation.

ROUTE & DOSAGE

Allergic Asthma

Adult/Adolescent: **Subcutaneous** 150–375 mg q2–4wk. Dose is based on baseline IgE serum levels.

ADMINISTRATION

Subcutaneous

- Reconstitute as follows: (1) Draw 1.4 mL of sterile water for injection into a 3-mL syringe with a 1-inch, 18-gauge needle. (2) Place vial upright on flat surface and inject sterile water. Keep vial upright and gently swirl for about 1 min to wet powder. Do not shake. (3) Gently swirl vial for 5–10 sec q5min to dissolve remaining solids. Some vials may take longer than 20 min to dissolve. Do not use if not completely dissolved by 40 min. (4) Once dissolved, invert vial for 15 sec to allow solution to drain toward stopper. (5) Using a new 3-mL syringe with a 1-inch, 18-gauge needle, insert needle into inverted vial with tip at the very bottom of solution, then withdraw solution. Before removing needle from vial, pull the plunger to end of syringe barrel to remove all solution from inverted vial. (6) Replace 18-gauge needle with a 25-gauge needle for subcutaneous injection. (7) Expel air, large bubbles, and any excess solution to obtain the required 1.2 mL dose. A thin layer of small bubbles may remain at top of the solution in syringe.

- Give subcutaneously and rotate injection sites. Solution is viscous and takes 5–10 sec to inject.
- Use within 8 h of reconstitution when stored in the vial at 2°–8° C (36°–46° F), or within 4 h of reconstitution when stored at room temperature.

ADVERSE EFFECTS (≥1%) **Body as a Whole:** Anaphylaxis/anaphylactoid reactions, *injection site reactions (bruising, erythema, warmth, burning, stinging, pruritus, hive formation, pain, induration, inflammation),* fatigue, generalized pain. **CNS:** Headache, dizziness. **GI:** *Nausea, vomiting, diarrhea, abdominal pain.* **Hematologic:** Epistaxis, menorrhagia, hematoma, anemia. **Musculoskeletal:** Arthralgia. **Respiratory:** Upper respiratory tract infections, sinusitis, pharyngitis. **Skin:** Rash, pruritus, urticaria, dermatitis. **Special Senses:** Earache.

PHARMACOKINETICS Absorption: Slowly absorbed from subcutaneous site; 53–71% reaches systemic circulation. **Peak:** 7–8 days. **Half-Life:** 22 days.

NURSING IMPLICATIONS

Assessment & Drug Effects

- Monitor for injection site reactions including bruising, redness, warmth, burning, stinging, itching, hive formation, pain, indurations, mass, and inflammation.
- Lab test: Platelet counts if signs of increased tendency to bleed appear.

Patient & Family Education

- Do not use this drug for relief of acute bronchospasm or status asthmaticus.
- Promptly report any of the following: Bleeding or unusual bruising, difficulty breathing or shortness of breath, skin rash or hives.
- Do not accept a live virus vaccine without consulting physician.

OMEGA-3 FATTY ACIDS (EICOSAPENTAENOIC ACID AND DOCOSAHEXAENOIC ACID) EPA & DHA

(o-me'ga-3)

Dr. Sears OmegaRx, Eskimo-3, Fish Oil, Omega-3 Fatty Acids, ICAR Prenatal Essential Omega-3, Mega Twin EPA, Natrol DHA Neuromins, Natrol Omega-3, Natural Fish Oil, Oleomed Heart, Omacor, Omega-3 Fish Oil Concentrate, Sea Omega, ZonePerfect Omega 3

Classifications: NUTRITIONAL SUPPLEMENT; OMEGA-3 FATTY ACIDS

Therapeutic: OMEGA-3 FATTY ACIDS; ANTILIPEMIC

Pregnancy Category: C

AVAILABILITY 100 mg, 200 mg, 300 mg, 360 mg, 375 mg, 500 mg, 517 mg, 840 mg, 1000 mg, 1760 mg capsules; 900 mg/5 mL and 1800 mg/5 mL oil for oral ingestion

ACTION & *THERAPEUTIC EFFECT* Mechanism of action of omega-3-acid ethyl esters is not completely understood. May include inhibition of acetyl-CoA and increased peroxisomal beta-oxidation in the liver. *Triglyceride lowering is the most consistent effect observed.*

USES Adjunct to diet to reduce hypertriglyceridemia.

UNLABELED USES Adjunct nutritional supplementation for hypertriglyceridemia, rheumatoid arthritis, or for the general purpose of maintaining a healthy heart.

CONTRAINDICATIONS Hypersensitivity to any component of the medication; infants.

CAUTIOUS USE Known sensitivity or allergy to fish; concurrent use of anticoagulants or thrombolytics; pregnancy (catgory C), lactation.

ROUTE & DOSAGE

Hypertriglyceridemia
Adult: **PO** 4 g b.i.d. or daily

ADMINISTRATION

Oral
- The daily dose may be given as one dose or divided b.i.d.
- Store 15°–30° C (59°–86° F).

ADVERSE EFFECTS (≥1%) **Body as a Whole:** Back pain, flu syndrome, unspecified pain. **GI:** Diarrhea, dyspepsia, eructation, nausea, vomiting. **Metabolic/Nutritional:** Increased total cholesterol and/or LDL levels, weight gain. **Skin:** Rash. **Special Senses:** Halitosis, taste disturbances.

INTERACTIONS Drug: ANTICOAGULANTS and THROMBOLYTICS are affected by inhibition of platelet aggregation with omega-3 fatty acids.

PHARMACOKINETICS Metabolism: Extensive liver metabolism.

NURSING IMPLICATIONS

Assessment & Drug Effects
- Monitor for S&S of hypersensitivity in those with known allergy to fish.
- Monitor diabetics for loss of glycemic control.
- Lab tests: Baseline and periodic lipid profile.
- Note: Poor therapeutic response after 2 mo is an indication to discontinue drug.
- Monitor blood levels of anticoagulants with concurrent therapy.

Patient & Family Education
- Do not take omega-3 fatty acids without consulting physician if you have a chronic medical disorder.

O

OMEPRAZOLE (Pr)

(o-me′pra-zole)
Losec ♣, Prilosec, Prilosec OTC, Zegerid
Classification: PROTON PUMP INHIBITOR
Therapeutic: ANTIULCER
Pregnancy Category: C

AVAILABILITY 10 mg, 20 mg, 40 mg capsules; 2.5 mg, 10 mg powder for oral suspension; 20 mg delayed release tablet

ACTION & *THERAPEUTIC EFFECT* An antisecretory compound that is a gastric acid pump inhibitor. Suppresses gastric acid secretion by inhibiting the H^+, K^+-ATPase enzyme system [the acid (proton H^+) pump] in the parietal cells. *Suppresses gastric acid secretion relieving gastrointestinal distress and promoting ulcer healing.*

USES Duodenal and gastric ulcer. Gastroesophageal reflux disease including severe erosive esophagitis (4 to 8 wk treatment). Long-term treatment of pathologic hypersecretory conditions such as Zollinger-Ellison syndrome, multiple endocrine adenomas, and systemic mastocytosis. In combination with clarithromycin to treat duodenal ulcers associated with *Helicobacter pylori*. Dyspepsia occurring more than twice weekly.

UNLABELED USES Healing or prevention of NSAID-related ulcers.

CONTRAINDICATIONS Long-term use for gastroesophageal reflux disease (GERD), duodenal ulcers; proton pump inhibitors (PPIs), hypersensitivity; children younger than 2 y; use of OTC formulation in children younger than 18 y or GI bleeding; use of Zegerid in metabolic alkalosis, hypocalcemia, vomiting, GI bleeding; lactation.

CAUTIOUS USE Dysphagia; metabolic or respiratory alkalosis; hepatic disease; pregnancy (category C).

ROUTE & DOSAGE

Gastroesophageal Reflux, Erosive Esophagitis, Duodenal Ulcer

Adult/Adolescent: **PO** 20–40 mg once/day for 4–8 wk

Gastric Ulcer

Adult: **PO** 20 mg b.i.d. for 4–8 wk

Hypersecretory Disease

Adult: **PO** 60 mg once/day up to 120 mg t.i.d.

Duodenal Ulcer Associated with *H. pylori*

Adult: **PO** 40 mg once/day for 14 days, then 20 mg/day for 14 days, in combination with clarithromycin 500 mg t.i.d. for 14 days

Dyspepsia

Adult: **PO** 20 mg daily × 14 days

ADMINISTRATION

Oral

- Give before food, preferably breakfast; capsules **must be** swallowed whole (do not open, chew, or crush).
- Note: Antacids may be administered with omeprazole.
- *For NG tube administration:* Into a catheter-tipped syringe, empty a 2.5 mg packet of omeprazole spheres into 5 mL of water or a 10 mg packet into 15 mL of water. Immediately shake syringe then allow to thicken for 2–3 min. Shake syringe again, then inject into NG tube.

ADVERSE EFFECTS (≥1%) **CNS:** Headache, dizziness, fatigue. **GI:** Diarrhea, abdominal pain, nausea, mild transient increases in liver function tests. **Urogenital:** Hematuria, proteinuria. **Skin:** Rash.

DIAGNOSTIC TEST INTERFERENCE Omeprazole has been reported to significantly impair peak **cortisol** response to exogenous ACTH. This finding is undergoing further investigation. May result in false-negative 13C-urea breath test.

INTERACTIONS Drug: May increase **diazepam, phenytoin, warfarin** levels. May affect levels of ANTIRETROVIRAL AGENTS. **Herbal: Ginkgo, St. John's wort** may decrease plasma concentrations. **Food:** Food decreases absorption by up to 35%.

PHARMACOKINETICS Absorption: Poorly from GI tract; 30–40% reaches systemic circulation. **Onset:** 0.5–3.5 h. **Peak:** Peak inhibition of gastric acid secretion: 5 days. **Metabolism:** In liver (CYP2C19). **Elimination:** 80% in urine, 20% in feces. **Half-Life:** 0.5–1.5 h.

NURSING IMPLICATIONS

Assessment & Drug Effects

- Lab tests: Monitor urinalysis for hematuria and proteinuria. Periodic liver function tests with prolonged use.

Patient & Family Education

- Report any changes in urinary elimination such as pain or discomfort associated with urination, or blood in urine.
- Report severe diarrhea; drug may need to be discontinued.

ONDANSETRON HYDROCHLORIDE

(on-dan'si-tron)

Zofran, Zofran ODT

Classifications: 5-HT$_3$ ANTAGONIST; ANTIEMETIC

Therapeutic: ANTIEMETIC

Pregnancy Category: B

AVAILABILITY 4 mg, 8 mg, 16 mg, 24 mg tablets; 4 mg, 8 mg orally disintegrating tablets; 4 mg/5 mL oral solution; 2 mg/mL, 8 mg/50 mL, 32 mg/50 mL injection

ACTION & *THERAPEUTIC EFFECT* Selective serotonin (5-HT$_3$) receptor antagonist. Serotonin receptors are located centrally in the chemoreceptor trigger zone (CTZ) and peripherally on the vagal nerve terminals. Serotonin is released from the wall of the small intestine and stimulates the vagal efferent nerves through the serotonin receptors and initiates the vomiting reflex. *Prevents nausea and vomiting associated with cancer chemotherapy and anesthesia.*

USES Prevention of nausea and vomiting associated with initial and repeated courses of cancer chemotherapy, including high-dose cisplatin; postoperative nausea and vomiting.

UNLABELED USES Treatment of hyperemesis gravidarum

CONTRAINDICATIONS Hypersensitivity to ondansetron; **PO:** children younger than 4 y.

CAUTIOUS USE Hepatic disease; QT prolongation; PKU; pregnancy (category B), lactation.

O

ROUTE & DOSAGE

Prevention of Chemotherapy-Induced Nausea and Vomiting

Adult: **PO** 8–24 mg 30 min before chemotherapy, then q8h times 2 more doses **IV** 32 mg or three 0.15 mg/kg doses starting 30 min before chemotherapy, then 4 and 8 h after

Adult/Child/Infant (6 mo–18 y): **IV** 0.15 mg/kg infused over 15 min beginning 30 min before start of chemotherapy, then 4 and 8 h after first dose of ondansetron

Child (older than 4 y): **PO** 4 mg 30 min before chemotherapy, then q8h times 2 more doses

Nausea and Vomiting with Highly Emetogenic Chemotherapy

Adult: **PO** Single 24 mg dose 30 min before administration of single-day highly emetogenic chemotherapy

Postoperative Nausea and Vomiting

Adult: **PO** 8–16 mg 1 h preoperatively **IM/IV** 4 mg injected immediately prior to anesthesia induction or once postoperatively if patient experiences nausea/vomiting shortly after surgery

Child/Infant: **IV** *1 mo–12 y, weight less than 40 kg,* 0.1 mg/kg *1 mo–12 y, weight greater than 40 kg,* 4 mg dose

Hepatic Impairment Dosage Adjustment

Child-Pugh class C: Maximum dose 8 mg/day

ADMINISTRATION

Oral

- Give tablets 30 min prior to chemotherapy and 1–2 h prior to radiation therapy.
- Do NOT push orally disintegrating tablet through blister foil. Peel foil back and remove tablet. Tablets will disintegrate with/without liquid.

Intravenous

PREPARE: **Direct for Postoperative N&V:** May be given undiluted. **IV Infusion for Chemotherapy-Induced N&V:** Dilute a single dose in 50 mL of D5W or NS. ▪ May be further diluted in selected IV solution.

ADMINISTER: **Direct for Postoperative N&V:** Give over at least 30 sec, 2–5 min preferred. **IV Infusion for Chemotherapy-Induced N&V:** Give over 15 min. ▪ When three separate doses are administered, infuse each over 15 min.

INCOMPATIBILITIES **Solution/additive:** **Meropenem.** **Y-site:** **Acyclovir, allopurinol, aminophylline, amphotericin B, amphotericin B cholesteryl, ampicillin, ampicillin/sulbactam, amsacrine, cefepime, cefoperazone, fluorouracil, furosemide, ganciclovir, lansoprazole, lorazepam, meropenem, methylprednisolone, piperacillin, pemetrexed, sargramostim, sodium bicarbonate, TPN.**

ADVERSE EFFECTS (≥1%) **CNS:** Dizziness and light-headedness, *headache, sedation.* **GI:** *Diarrhea,* constipation, dry mouth, transient increases in liver aminotransferases and bilirubin. **Body as a Whole:** Hypersensitivity reactions.

INTERACTIONS Drug: Rifampin may decrease ondansetron levels.

PHARMACOKINETICS Peak: 1–1.5 h. **Metabolism:** In liver (CYP3A4). **Elimination:** 44–60% in urine within 24 h; ~25% in feces. **Half-Life:** 3 h.

NURSING IMPLICATIONS

Assessment & Drug Effects

- Monitor fluid and electrolyte status. Diarrhea, which may cause fluid and electrolyte imbalance, is a potential adverse effect of the drug.
- Monitor cardiovascular status, especially in patients with a history of coronary artery disease. Rare cases of tachycardia and angina have been reported.

Patient & Family Education

- Be aware that headache requiring an analgesic for relief is a common adverse effect.

O

OPIUM, POWDERED OPIUM TINCTURE (LAUDANUM)

(oh′pee-um)

Deodorized Opium Tincture

Classifications: NARCOTIC (OPIATE AGONIST) ANALGESIC; ANTIDIARRHEAL

Therapeutic: NARCOTIC ANALGESIC; ANTIDIARRHEAL

Prototype: Morphine

Pregnancy Category: C

Controlled Substance: Schedule II

AVAILABILITY 10%, 2 mg/5 mL liquid

ACTION & *THERAPEUTIC EFFECT* Contains several natural alkaloids including morphine, codeine, papaverine. Antidiarrheal due to inhibition of GI motility and propulsion; leads to prolonged transit of intestinal contents, desiccation of feces, and constipation. *Antidiarrheal activity due to inhibition of GI motility.*

USES Symptomatic treatment of acute diarrhea and to treat severe withdrawal symptoms in neonates born to women addicted to opiates.

CONTRAINDICATIONS Diarrhea caused by poisoning (until poison is completely eliminated).

CAUTIOUS USE History of opiate agonist dependence; asthma; severe prostatic hypertrophy; hepatic disease; pregnancy (category C), lactation.

ROUTE & DOSAGE

Acute Diarrhea

Adult: **PO** 0.6 mL q.i.d. up to 1 mL q.i.d. (max: 6 mL/day)

Child: **PO** 0.005–0.01 mL/kg q3–4h (max: 6 doses/24 h)

Neonatal Withdrawal

Child: **PO** Make a 1:25 aqueous dilution, then give 3–6 drops q3–6h as needed or 0.2 mL q3h, may increase by 0.05 mL q3h until withdrawal symptoms are controlled, then gradually decrease dose after withdrawal symptoms have stabilized

O

ADMINISTRATION

Oral

- Do not confuse this preparation with camphorated opium tincture (paregoric), which contains only 2 mg anhydrous morphine/5 mL, thus requiring a higher dose volume than that required for therapeutic dose of Deodorized Opium Tincture.
- Give drug diluted with about one third glass of water to ensure passage of entire dose into stomach.
- Store in tight, light-resistant containers.

ADVERSE EFFECTS (≥1%) **GI:** Nausea and other GI disturbances. **CNS:** Depression of CNS.

INTERACTIONS Drug: Alcohol and other CNS DEPRESSANTS add to CNS effects.

PHARMACOKINETICS Absorption: Variable absorption from GI tract. **Distribution:** Crosses placenta; distributed into breast milk. **Metabolism:** In liver. **Elimination:** In urine.

NURSING IMPLICATIONS

Assessment & Drug Effects

- Withhold medication and report to physician if respirations are 12/min or below or have changed in character and rate.
- Discontinue as soon as diarrhea is controlled; note character and frequency of stools.
- Offer small amounts of fluid frequently but attempt to maintain 3000–4000 mL fluid total in 24 h.
- Monitor body weight, I&O ratio and pattern, and temperature. If patient develops fever of 38.8° C (102° F) or above, electrolyte and hydration levels may need to be evaluated. Consult physician.

Patient & Family Education

- Be aware that constipation may be a consequence of antidiarrheal therapy but that normal habit pattern usually is reestablished with resumption of normal dietary intake.
- Note: Addiction is possible with prolonged use or with drug abuse.

OPRELVEKIN

(o-prel've-kin)

Neumega

Classifications: BLOOD FORMER; HEMATOPOIETIC GROWTH FACTOR

Therapeutic: HEMATOPOIETIC GROWTH FACTOR

Prototype: Epoetin alfa

Pregnancy Category: C

AVAILABILITY 5 mg injection

ACTION & *THERAPEUTIC EFFECT* Hematopoietic growth factor (interleukin-11) that is produced by recombinant DNA. *Effectiveness indicated by return of postnadir platelet count toward normal (50,000 or higher). Increases platelet count in a dose-dependent manner.*

USES Prevention of severe thrombocytopenia following myelosuppressive chemotherapy (not effective after myeloablative chemotherapy).

CONTRAINDICATIONS Hypersensitivity to oprelvekin; myeloablative chemotherapy; myeloid malignancies; lactation.

CAUTIOUS USE Patients with left ventricular dysfunction, cardiac disease, CHF, history of atrial arrhythmias, or other arrhythmias; electrolyte imbalance, hypokalemia; respiratory disease; papilledema; thromboembolic disorders; older adults; cerebrovascular disease, stroke, TIAs; pleural effusion, pericardial effusion, ascites; increased intracranial pressure, brain tumor, visual disturbances; hepatic or renal dysfunction; children; pregnancy (category C).

ROUTE & DOSAGE

Thrombocytopenia

Adult: **Subcutaneous** 50 mcg/kg once daily starting 6–24 h after completing chemotherapy and continuing until platelet count is 50,000 cells/mcL or higher or up to 21 days

Child/Infant (8 mo–17 y): **Subcutaneous** 75–100 mcg/kg once daily starting 6–24 h after completing chemotherapy and continuing until platelet count is 50,000 cells/mcL or higher or up to 21 days

ADMINISTRATION

- Note: Do not use if solution is discolored or if it contains particulate matter.

Subcutaneous

- Reconstitute solution by gently injecting 1 mL of sterile water for injection (without preservative) toward the sides of the vial. Keep needle in vial and gently swirl to dissolve but do not shake solution. Without removing needle, withdraw specified amount of oprelvekin for injection.
- Give as single dose into the abdomen, thigh, hip, or upper arm.
- Discard any unused portion of the vial. It contains no preservatives.
- Use reconstituted solution within 3 h; store at 2°–8° C (36°–46° F) until used.
- Store unopened vials at 2°–8° C (36°–46° F). Do not freeze.

ADVERSE EFFECTS (≥1%) **Body as a Whole:** *Edema, neutropenic fever, fever,* asthenia, pain, chills, myalgia, bone pain, dehydration. **CNS:** *Headache, dizziness, insomnia,* nervousness. **CV:** *Tachycardia,* vasodilation, palpitations, syncope, atrial fibrillation/flutter, peripheral edema, capillary leak syndrome. **GI:** *Nausea, vomiting, mucositis, diarrhea,* oral moniliasis, anorexia, constipation, dyspepsia. **Hematologic:** Ecchymosis. **Respiratory:** *Dyspnea, rhinitis, cough, pharyngitis,* pleural effusion, pulmonary edema, exacerbation of preexisting pleural effusion. **Skin:** Alopecia, *rash,* skin discoloration, exfoliative dermatitis. **Special Senses:** Conjunctival injection, amblyopia.

INTERACTIONS Drug: No clinically significant interactions established.

PHARMACOKINETICS Absorption: 80% from subcutaneous injection site. **Onset:** Days 5–9. **Duration:** 7 days after last dose. **Distribution:** Distributes to highly perfused organs. **Elimination:** In urine. **Half-Life:** 6.9 h.

NURSING IMPLICATIONS

Assessment & Drug Effects

- Lab tests: Monitor platelet counts until adequate recovery; periodically monitor CBC with differential and serum electrolytes.
- Monitor carefully for and immediately report S&S of fluid overload, hypokalemia, and cardiac arrhythmias.
- Monitor persons with preexisting fluid retention carefully (e.g., CHF, pleural effusion, ascites) for worsening of symptoms.

Patient & Family Education

- Review patient information leaflet with special attention to administration directions.
- Report any of the following to the physician: Shortness of breath, edema of arms and/or legs, chest pain, unusual fatigue or weakness, irregular heartbeat, blurred vision.

ORLISTAT

(or′li-stat)

Alli, Xenical

Classifications: ANORECTANT; NONSYSTEMIC LIPASE INHIBITOR

Therapeutic: ANORECTANT
Prototype: Diethylpropion
Pregnancy Category: B

AVAILABILITY 60 mg, 120 mg capsules

ACTION & *THERAPEUTIC EFFECT* Nonsystemic inhibitor of gastrointestinal lipase. Reduces intestinal absorption of dietary fat by forming inactive enzymes with pancreatic and gastric lipase in the GI tract. *Indicated by weight loss/decreased body mass index (BMI). Reduces the intestinal absorption of dietary fat because at least 95% of orlistat is eliminated in the feces; reduces caloric intake in obese individuals.*

USES Weight loss and weight maintenance in patients with BMI 30 kg/m^2 or greater or 27 kg/m^2 or greater in patients with other risk factors. Reduce risk for weight regain after prior weight loss.

CONTRAINDICATIONS Hypersensitivity to orlistat; malabsorption syndrome; cholestasis; gallbladder disease; hypothyroidism; organic causes of obesity; anorexia nervosa, bulimia nervosa. Safety and efficacy in children younger than 16 y are not established.

CAUTIOUS USE Gastrointestinal diseases including frequent diarrhea; known dietary deficiencies in fat soluble vitamins (i.e., A, D, E); history of calcium oxalate nephrolithiasis or hyperoxaluria; older adults; pregnancy (category B), lactation.

ROUTE & DOSAGE

Weight Loss

Adult/Adolescent (older than 16 y): **PO** 60–120 mg t.i.d. with each main meal containing fat

ADMINISTRATION

Oral

- Give during or up to 1 h after a meal containing fat.
- Omit dose with nonfat-containing meal or if meal is skipped.
- Store at 15°–30° C (59°–86° F). Keep bottle tightly closed; do **NOT** use after the printed expiration date.

ADVERSE EFFECTS (≥1%) **Body as a Whole:** Fatigue. **CNS:** *Headache,* dizziness, anxiety. **CV:** Hypertension, stroke. **GI:** *Oily spotting, flatus with discharge, fecal urgency, fatty/oily stool, oily evacuation, increased defecation,* fecal incontinence, *abdominal pain/discomfort,* nausea, infectious diarrhea, rectal pain/discomfort, tooth disorder, gingival disorder, vomiting. **Skin:** Rash. **Urogenital:** Menstrual irregularity.

DIAGNOSTIC TEST INTERFERENCE Monitor PT/INR in patients on chronic stable doses of **warfarin.**

INTERACTIONS Drug: Orlistat may increase absorption of **pravastatin;** may decrease absorption of fat soluble VITAMINS (A, D, E, K).

PHARMACOKINETICS Absorption: Minimal. **Metabolism:** In gastrointestinal wall. **Elimination:** In feces. **Half-Life:** 1–2 h.

NURSING IMPLICATIONS

Assessment & Drug Effects

- Monitor weight and BMI; closely monitor diabetics for hypoglycemia.
- Coadministered drugs: Monitor PT/INR with warfarin.
- Monitor BP frequently, especially with preexisting hypertension.

Patient & Family Education

- Take a daily multivitamin containing fat-soluble vitamins at least 2 h before/after orlistat.
- Remember common GI adverse effects typically resolve after 4 wk therapy.
- Avoid high fat meals to minimize adverse GI effects. Distribute fat calories over three main meals daily.
- Monitor weight several times weekly. Diabetics: Monitor blood glucose carefully following any weight loss.

ORPHENADRINE CITRATE

(or-fen′a-dreen)

Norflex

Classification: SKELETAL MUSCLE RELAXANT, CENTRAL ACTING

Therapeutic: SKELETAL MUSCLE RELAXANT

Prototype: Cyclobenzaprine

Pregnancy Category: C

AVAILABILITY 100 mg sustained release tablets; 30 mg/mL injection

ACTION & *THERAPEUTIC EFFECT* Tertiary amine anticholinergic agent and central-acting skeletal muscle relaxant. Relaxes tense skeletal muscles indirectly, possibly by analgesic action or by atropine-like central action. *Relieves skeletal muscle spasm.*

USES To relieve muscle spasm discomfort associated with acute musculoskeletal conditions.

CONTRAINDICATIONS Narrow-angle glaucoma; achalasia; pyloric or duodenal obstruction, stenosing peptic ulcers; prostatic hypertrophy or bladder neck obstruction, urinary tract obstruction; myasthenia gravis; cardiospasm (megaloesophagus); tachycardia. Safe use in the pediatric age group is not established.

CAUTIOUS USE History of cardiac disease, arrhythmias, coronary insufficiency; asthma; GERD; hepatic disease; renal disease; renal impairment; elderly; pregnancy (category C), lactation.

ROUTE & DOSAGE

Muscle Spasm

Adult: **PO** 100 mg b.i.d. **IM/IV** 60 mg, may repeat in 12 h if needed

ADMINISTRATION

Oral

- Ensure that sustained release form is not chewed or crushed. It **must be** swallowed whole.

Intramuscular

- Give undiluted deep into a large muscle.

O

Intravenous

PREPARE: **Direct:** Give undiluted. Protect from light.

ADMINISTER: **Direct:** Give at a rate of 60 mg (2 mL) over 5 min with patient in supine position. ▪ Keep supine for 5–10 min post-injection.

ADVERSE EFFECTS (≥1%) **CNS:** *Drowsiness,* weakness, headache, dizziness; mild CNS stimulation (high doses: restlessness, anxiety, tremors, confusion, hallucinations, agitation, tachycardia, palpitation, syncope). **Special Senses:** Increased ocular tension, dilated pupils, blurred vision. **GI:** *Dry mouth,* nausea, vomiting, abdominal cramps, constipation. **Urogenital:** *Urinary hesitancy* or *retention.* **Body as a Whole:** Hypersensitivity [pruritus, urticaria, rash, <u>anaphylactic reaction</u> (rare)].

INTERACTIONS Drug: Propoxyphene may cause increased confusion, anxiety, and tremors; may worsen schizophrenic symptoms, or increase risk of tardive dyskinesia with **haloperidol;** additive CNS depressant with ANXIOLYTICS, SEDATIVES, HYPNOTICS, **butorphanol, nalbuphine,** OPIATE AGONISTS, **pentazocine, tramadol, cyclobenzaprine** may increase anticholinergic effects. **Herbal: Valerian, kava** potentiate sedation.

PHARMACOKINETICS Absorption: Readily from GI tract. **Peak:** 2 h. **Duration:** 4–6 h. **Distribution:** Rapidly distributed in tissues; crosses placenta. **Metabolism:** In liver. **Elimination:** In urine. **Half-Life:** 14 h.

NURSING IMPLICATIONS

Assessment & Drug Effects

- Lab tests: Periodic blood, urine, and liver function studies with prolonged therapy.
- Report complaints of mouth dryness, urinary hesitancy or retention, headache, tremors, GI problems, palpitation, or rapid pulse to physician. Dosage reduction or drug withdrawal is indicated.
- Monitor elimination patterns. Older adults are particularly sensitive to anticholinergic effects (urinary hesitancy, constipation); closely observe.
- Monitor therapeutic drug effect. In the patient with parkinsonism, orphenadrine reduces muscular rigidity but has little effect on tremors. Some reduction in excessive salivation and perspiration may occur, and patient may appear mildly euphoric.

Patient & Family Education

- Relieve mouth dryness by frequent rinsing with clear tepid water, increasing noncaloric fluid

intake, sugarless gum, or lemon drops. If these measures fail, a saliva substitute may help.
- Do not drive or engage in potentially hazardous activities until response to drug is known.
- Avoid concomitant use of alcohol and other CNS depressants; these may potentiate depressant effects.

OSELTAMIVIR PHOSPHATE

(o-sel'tam-i-vir)
Tamiflu
Classification: ANTIVIRAL
Therapeutic: ANTIVIRAL
Pregnancy Category: C

AVAILABILITY 30 mg, 45 mg, 75 mg capsule; 12 mg/mL suspension

ACTION & *THERAPEUTIC EFFECT* Inhibits influenza A and B viral neuraminidase enzyme, preventing the release of newly formed virus from the surface of the infected cells. Inhibits replication of the influenza A and B virus. *Effectiveness indicated by relief of flu symptoms. Prevents viral spread across the mucous lining of the respiratory tract.*

USES Treatment of uncomplicated acute influenza in adults symptomatic for no more than 2 days; prophylaxis of influenza.

CONTRAINDICATIONS Hypersensitivity to oseltamivir; severe hepatic impairment or severe hepatic disease; viral infections other than flu; infants younger than 1 y or neonates. Safety in immunosuppression has not been established.

CAUTIOUS USE Hereditary fructose intolerance; cardiac disease; COPD, pediatric patients with asthma; mild or moderate hepatic impairment; psychiatric disorders; renal impairment; pregnancy (category C), lactation. Safety and efficacy in chronic cardiac/respiratory disease are not established.

ROUTE & DOSAGE

Influenza Treatment

Adult/Adolescent: **PO** 75 mg b.i.d. × 5 days
Child (1–12 y): **PO** *Weight greater than 40 kg,* 75 mg b.i.d. × 5 days; *weight 23–40 kg,* 60 mg b.i.d. × 5 days; *weight 15–22 kg,* 45 mg b.i.d. × 5 days; *weight less than 15 kg,* 30 mg b.i.d. × 5 days

Influenza Prevention

Adult/Adolescent/Child (older than 1 y): **PO** 75 mg daily × 10 days; begin within 2 days of contact with infected person

Renal Impairment Dosage Adjustment

CrCl less than 30 mL/min: (treatment) 75 mg daily (prophylaxis) 75 mg every other day or 30 mg daily

ADMINISTRATION

Oral
- Give with food to decrease the risk of GI upset.
- Start within 48 h of onset of flu symptoms.
- Take missed dose as soon as possible unless next dose is due within 2 h.
- Store at 15°–30° C (59°–86° F); protect from moisture, keep dry.

ADVERSE EFFECTS (≥1%) **Body as a Whole:** Fatigue. **CNS:** Dizziness,

O

headache, insomnia, vertigo. **GI:** Nausea, vomiting, diarrhea, abdominal pain. **Respiratory:** Bronchitis, cough.

PHARMACOKINETICS Absorption: Readily absorbed, 75% bioavailable. **Distribution:** 42% protein bound. **Metabolism:** Extensively metabolized to active metabolite oseltamivir carboxylate by liver esterases. **Elimination:** Primarily in urine. **Half-Life:** 1–2 h; oseltamivir carboxylate 6–10 h.

NURSING IMPLICATIONS

Assessment & Drug Effects

- Monitor ambulation in frail and older adult patients due to potential for dizziness and vertigo.
- Monitor children for abnormal behavior such as delirium or self-injury.

Patient & Family Education

- Contact your physician regarding the use of this drug in children.

O

OXACILLIN SODIUM

(ox-a-sill'in)

Bactocill

Classifications: ANTIBIOTIC, PENICILLIN; ANTISTAPHYLOCOCCAL PENICILLIN

Therapeutic: ANTIBIOTIC

Prototype: Penicillin G

Pregnancy Category: C

AVAILABILITY 250 mg, 500 mg capsules; 250 mg/5 mL suspension; 250 mg, 500 mg, 1 g, 2 g, 4 g injection

ACTION & *THERAPEUTIC EFFECT* Semisynthetic, acid-stable, penicillinase-resistant isoxazolyl penicillin. Oxacillin inhibits final stage of bacterial cell wall synthesis by preferentially binding to specific penicillin-binding proteins (PBPs) located within the bacterial cell wall, leading to destruction of the cell wall of the organism. *It is highly active against most penicillinase-producing staphylococci, and is generally ineffective against gram-negative bacteria and methicillin-resistant staphylococci (MRSA).*

USES Infections caused by staphylococci.

CONTRAINDICATIONS Infections caused by staphylococci. Hypersensitivity to penicillins or cephalosporins.

CAUTIOUS USE History of or suspected atopy or allergy (hives, eczema, hay fever, asthma); history of GI disease; hepatic disease; renal disease; premature infants, neonates, pregnancy (category C), lactation (may cause infant diarrhea).

ROUTE & DOSAGE

Staphylococcal Infections

Adult: **PO** 500 mg–1 g q4–6h **IM/IV** 250 mg–1 g q4–6h (max: 12 g/day)

Child: **PO** 50–100 mg/kg/day divided q4–6h **IM/IV** 100–200 mg/kg/day divided q4–6h (max: 12 g/day)

Neonate: **IV** 50–100 mg/kg/day divided q6–12h

ADMINISTRATION

Note: The total sodium content (including that contributed by buffer) in each gram of oxacillin is approximately 3.1 mEq or 71 mg.

Oral

- Give with a full glass of water on an empty stomach (either 1 h before meals or 2 h after meals). Food reduces absorption.

Intramuscular

- Reconstitute each 250 mg with 1.4 mL sterile water for injection to yield 250 mg/1.5 mL. Shake vial vigorously until drug is completely dissolved. Discard unused portions after 3 days at room temperature or 7 days under refrigeration.
- Administer deep IM to adults by deep intragluteal injection. Follow agency policy for IM site in young children and infants. Rotate injection sites.

Intravascular

Note: Verify correct IV concentration and rate of infusion/injection with physician before IV administration to neonates, infants, children.

PREPARE: **Direct:** Reconstitute each 500 mg or fraction thereof with 5 mL with sterile water for injection or NS to yield 250 mg/1.5 mL. **Intermittent:** Dilute required dose of reconstituted solution in 50–100 mL of D5W, NS, D5/NS, or LR. **Continuous:** Dilute required dose of reconstituted solution in up to 1000 mL of compatible IV solutions.

ADMINISTER: **Direct:** Give at a rate of 1 g or fraction thereof over 10 min. **Intermittent:** Give over 15–30 min. **Continuous:** Give over 6 h.

INCOMPATIBILITIES **Solution/additive:** **Caffeine citrate, cephalothin, cytarabine, erythromycin, hyaluronidase, hydrocortisone, nitrofurantoin, pentobarbital, phenobarbital,** TETRACYCLINES, **warfarin.** **Y-site:** **Caffeine citrate, sodium bicarbonate, verapamil.**

ADVERSE EFFECTS (≥1%) **Body as a Whole:** Thrombophlebitis (IV therapy), superinfections, wheezing, sneezing, fever, <u>anaphylaxis</u>. **GI:** Nausea, vomiting, flatulence, *diarrhea,* hepatocellular dysfunction (elevated AST, ALT, hepatitis). **Hematologic:** Eosinophilia, leukopenia, thrombocytopenia, granulocytopenia, <u>agranulocytosis</u>; neutropenia (reported in children). **Skin:** Pruritus, rash, urticaria. **Urogenital:** Interstitial nephritis, transient hematuria, albuminuria, azotemia (newborns and infants on high doses).

DIAGNOSTIC TEST INTERFERENCE Oxacillin in large doses can cause false-positive ***urine protein tests*** using sulfosalicylic acid methods.

PHARMACOKINETICS Absorption: Incompletely and erratically absorbed orally. **Peak:** 30–120 min IM; 15 min IV. **Duration:** 4 h PO; 4–6 h IM. **Distribution:** Distributes into CNS with inflamed meninges; crosses placenta; distributed into breast milk, 90% protein bound. **Metabolism:** Enters enterohepatic circulation. **Elimination:** Primarily in urine, some in bile. **Half-Life:** 0.5–1 h.

O

NURSING IMPLICATIONS

Assessment & Drug Effects

- Ask patient prior to first dose about hypersensitivity reactions to penicillins, cephalosporins, and other allergens.
- Lab tests: Periodic liver functions, CBC with differential, platelet count, and urinalysis.
- Hepatic dysfunction (possibly a hypersensitivity reaction) has been associated with IV oxacillin; it is reversible with discontinuation of drug. Symptoms may resemble viral hepatitis or general signs of hypersensitivity and should be reported promptly: Hives, rash, fever, nausea, vomiting, abdominal discomfort, anorexia, malaise, jaundice (with dark yellow to brown urine, light-colored or clay-colored stools, pruritus).

- Withhold next drug dose and report the onset of hypersensitivity reactions and superinfections (see Appendix F).

Patient & Family Education

- Take oral medication around the clock; do not miss a dose. Take all of the medication prescribed even if you feel better, unless otherwise directed by physician.

OXALIPLATIN

(ox-a-li-pla'tin)
Eloxatin
Classifications: ANTINEOPLASTIC; ALKYLATING AGENT
Therapeutic: ANTINEOPLASTIC
Prototype: Cyclophosphamide
Pregnancy Category: D

AVAILABILITY 5 mg/mL injection

ACTION & *THERAPEUTIC EFFECT* Oxaliplatin forms inter- and intrastrand DNA cross-links that inhibit DNA replication and transcription. The cytotoxicity of oxaliplatin is cell-cycle nonspecific. *Antitumor activity of oxaliplatin in combination with 5-fluorouracil (5-FU) has antiproliferative activity against colon carcinoma that is greater than either compound alone.*

USES Metastatic cancer of colon and rectum.
UNLABELED USES Non–small-cell lung cancer, non-Hodgkin's lymphoma, ovarian cancer.

CONTRAINDICATIONS History of known allergy to oxaliplatin or other platinum compounds; myelosuppression; pregnancy (category D); lactation. Safety and effectiveness in children are not established.

CAUTIOUS USE Renal impairment, because clearance of ultrafilterable platinum is decreased in mild, moderate, and severe renal impairment; older adults; hepatic impairment.

ROUTE & DOSAGE

Metastatic Colon or Rectal Cancer

Adult: **IV** 85 mg/m² infused over 120 min once every 2 wk × 6 mo; adjust for toxicities

Renal Impairment Dosage Adjustment

CrCl less than 19 mL/min: Omit dose or change therapy

ADMINISTRATION

Intravenous

Premedication with an antiemetic is recommended.

PREPARE: **IV Infusion:** NEVER reconstitute with NS or any solution containing chloride. ▪ Reconstitute the 50 mg vial or the 100 mg vial by adding 10 mL or 20 mL, respectively, of sterile water for injection or D5W. ▪ MUST further dilute in 250–500 mL of D5W for infusion.

ADMINISTER: **IV Infusion:** Do NOT use needles or infusion sets containing aluminum parts. ▪ Flush infusion line with D5W before and after administration of any other concomitant medication. ▪ Give over 120 min with frequent monitoring of the IV insertion site. ▪ Discontinue at the first sign of extravasation and restart IV in a different site.

INCOMPATIBILITIES **Solution/additive:** CHLORIDE-CONTAINING SOLUTIONS, ALKALINE SOLUTIONS, including **sodium bicarbonate, 5-fluorouracil (5-FU). Y-site:** ALKALINE SOLUTIONS, including **sodium bi-**

carbonate, diazepam, 5-fluorouracil (5-FU).

▪ Store reconstituted solution up to 24 h under refrigeration at 2°–8° C (36°–46° F). ▪ After final dilution, the IV solution may be stored for 6 h at room temperature [20°–25° C (68°–77° F)] or up to 24 h under refrigeration.

ADVERSE EFFECTS (≥1%) **Body as a Whole:** *Fever, edema, pain,* allergic reaction, arthralgia, rigors. **CNS:** *Fatigue, neuropathy, headache,* dizziness, insomnia. **CV:** Chest pain. **GI:** *Diarrhea, nausea, vomiting, anorexia, stomatitis, constipation, abdominal pain,* reflux, dyspepsia, taste perversion, mucositis, flatulence. **Hematologic:** *Anemia, leukopenia, thrombocytopenia,* neutropenia, thromboembolism. **Metabolic:** Hypokalemia, dehydration. **Respiratory:** *Dyspnea, cough,* rhinitis, pharyngitis, epistaxis, hiccup. **Skin:** Flushing, rash, alopecia, injection site reaction. **Urogenital:** Dysuria.

INTERACTIONS Drug: AMINOGLYCOSIDES, **amphotericin B, vancomycin,** and other **nephrotoxic drugs** may increase risk of renal failure.

PHARMACOKINETICS Distribution: Greater than 90% protein bound. **Metabolism:** Rapid and extensive nonenzymatic biotransformation. **Elimination:** Primarily in urine. **Half-Life:** 391 h.

NURSING IMPLICATIONS

Assessment & Drug Effects

- Monitor for S&S of hypersensitivity (e.g., rash, urticaria, erythema, pruritus; rarely, bronchospasm and hypotension). Discontinue drug and notify physician if any of these occur.
- Monitor insertion site. Extravasation may cause local pain and inflammation that may be severe and lead to complications, including necrosis.
- Monitor for S&S of coagulation disorders including GI bleeding, hematuria, and epistaxis.
- Monitor for S&S of peripheral neuropathy (e.g., paresthesia, dysesthesia, hypoesthesia in the hands, feet, perioral area, or throat, jaw spasm, abnormal tongue sensation, dysarthria, eye pain, and chest pressure). Symptoms may be precipitated or exacerbated by exposure to cold temperature or cold objects.
- Lab tests: Before each administration cycle, monitor WBC count with differential, hemoglobin, platelet count, and blood chemistries (including ALT, AST, bilirubin, and creatinine). Monitor baseline and periodic renal functions.
- Do not apply ice to oral mucous membranes (e.g., mucositis prophylaxis) during the infusion of oxaliplatin as cold temperature can exacerbate acute neurological symptoms.

Patient & Family Education

- Use effective methods of contraception while receiving this drug.
- Avoid cold drinks, use of ice, and cover exposed skin prior to exposure to cold temperature or cold objects.
- Do not drive or engage in potentially hazardous activities until response to drug is known.
- Report any of the following to a health care provider: Difficulty writing, buttoning, swallowing, walking; numbness, tingling or other unusual sensations in extremities; non-productive cough or shortness of breath; fever, particularly if associated with persistent diarrhea or other evidence of infection.

- Report promptly S&S of a bleeding disorder such as black tarry stool, coke-colored or frankly bloody urine, bleeding from the nose or mucous membranes.

OXANDROLONE

(ox-an′dro-lone)

Oxandrin

Classification: ANDROGEN/ANABOLIC STEROID

Therapeutic: ANABOLIC STEROID

Prototype: Testosterone

Pregnancy Category: X

Controlled Substance: Schedule III

AVAILABILITY 2.5 mg tablets

ACTION & *THERAPEUTIC EFFECT* Synthetic steroid with anabolic and androgenic activity. ***Androgenic activity:*** *Responsible for the growth spurt of the adolescent and for growth termination by epiphyseal closure. Increases erythropoiesis, possibly by stimulating production of erythropoietin, and promotes vascularization and darkening of skin. Antagonizes effects of estrogen excess on female breast and endometrium.* ***Anabolic activity:*** *Increases protein metabolism and decreases its catabolism. Large doses suppress spermatogenesis, thereby causing testicular atrophy. Controls development and maintenance of secondary sexual characteristics.*

USES Adjunctive therapy to promote weight gain, offset protein catabolism associated with prolonged administration of corticosteroids, relieve bone pain accompanying osteoporosis.

CONTRAINDICATIONS Hypersensitivity or toxic reactions to androgens; severe cardiac, hepatic, or renal disease; possibility of virilization of external genitalia of female fetus; polycythemia; hypercalcemia; known or suspected prostatic or breast cancer in males; benign prostatic hypertrophy with obstruction; patients easily stimulated sexually; asthenic males who may react adversely to androgenic overstimulation; conditions aggravated by fluid retention; hypertension; pregnancy (category X), lactation.

CAUTIOUS USE Cardiac, hepatic, and mild to moderate renal disease, hypercholesterolemia, heart failure, peripheral edema, arteriosclerosis, coronary artery disease, MI; cholestasis; diabetes mellitus; prostatic hypertrophy; prepubertal males, geriatric patients, acute intermittent porphyria; older adults.

ROUTE & DOSAGE

Weight Gain

Adult: **PO** 2.5 mg b.i.d. to q.i.d. (max: 20 mg/day) for 2–4 wk

Child: **PO** 0.1 mg/kg/day

ADMINISTRATION

Oral

- Individualize doses; great variations in response exist.
- Store at 15°–30° C (59°–86° F).

ADVERSE EFFECTS (≥1%) **CNS:** Habituation, excitation, insomnia, depression, changes in libido. **Urogenital:** *Males:* Phallic enlargement, increased frequency or persistence of erections, inhibition of testicular function, testicular atrophy, oligospermia, impotence, chronic priapism, epididymitis, bladder irritability; *Females:* Clitoral enlargement, menstrual irregularities. **Hepatic:** Cholestatic jaundice with or without hepatic necrosis and death, hepatocellular neoplasms, peliosis hepatitis (long-term use). **Skin:** Hirsutism and male pattern baldness in females, acne. **Endocrine:** Gynecomastia, deepening of voice in females, premature closure of epiphyses in children, edema, decreased glucose tolerance.

DIAGNOSTIC TEST INTERFERENCE May decrease levels of thyroxine-binding globulin (decreased total T_4 and increased T_3 RU and free T_4).

INTERACTIONS Drug: May increase INR with **warfarin.** May inhibit metabolism of ORAL HYPOGLYCEMIC AGENTS. Concomitant STEROIDS may increase edema. **Herbal: Echinacea** may increase risk of hepatotoxicity.

PHARMACOKINETICS Half-Life: 10–13 h (increased in elderly patients).

NURSING IMPLICATIONS

Assessment & Drug Effects

- Monitor weight closely throughout therapy.
- Assess for and report development of edema or S&S of jaundice (see Appendix F).
- Lab tests: Monitor periodically liver function, lipid profile, Hct and Hgb, PT and INR, serum electrolytes, and CPK.
- Withhold and notify physician if hypercalcemia develops in breast cancer patient.
- Monitor growth in children closely.

Patient & Family Education

- Women: Report signs of virilization, including acne and changes in menstrual periods.
- Men: Report too frequent or prolonged erections or appearance/worsening of acne.
- Report S&S of jaundice (see Appendix F) or edema.
- Monitor blood glucose for loss of glycemic control if diabetic.

OXAPROZIN

(ox-a-pro′zin)

Daypro

Classification: ANALGESIC, NONSTEROIDAL ANTI-INFLAMMATORY DRUG (NSAID)

Therapeutic: NONNARCOTIC ANALGESIC, NSAID; ANTIRHEUMATIC; ANTIPYRETIC

Prototype: Ibuprofen

Pregnancy Category: C first and second trimester; D third trimester

AVAILABILITY 600 mg tablets

ACTION & *THERAPEUTIC EFFECT* Long-acting NSAID agent, which is an effective prostaglandin synthetase inhibitor. It inhibits COX-1 and COX-2 enzymes needed for prostaglandin synthesis at the site of inflammation. *Has anti-inflammatory, antipyretic, and analgesic properties.*

USES Treatment of osteoarthritis and rheumatoid arthritis.

UNLABELED USES Ankylosing spondylitis, chronic pain, gout, oral surgery pain, temporal arteritis, tendinitis.

CONTRAINDICATIONS Hypersensitivity to oxaprozin or any other NSAID; complete or partial syndrome of nasal polyps; angioedema; CABG perioperative pain; pregnancy (category D third trimester); lactation.

CAUTIOUS USE History of GI bleeding, alcoholism, smoking; history of severe hepatic dysfunction, renal insufficiency; cardiac disease; coagulopathy; photosensitivity; older adults; pregnancy (category C first and second trimester). Safety and effectiveness in children younger than 6 y are not established.

ROUTE & DOSAGE

Osteoarthritis, Rheumatoid Arthritis

Adult: **PO** 600–1200 mg daily (max: 1800 mg/day or 25 mg/kg, whichever is lower)

ADMINISTRATION

Oral

- Give with meals or milk to decrease GI distress.
- Divide doses in those unable to tolerate once-daily dosing.
- Use lower starting doses for those with renal or hepatic dysfunction, advanced age, low body weight, or a predisposition to GI ulceration.

ADVERSE EFFECTS (≥1%) **CNS:** Tinnitus, headache, insomnia, somnolence. **GI:** Diarrhea, abdominal pain, nausea, dyspepsia, flatulence, melena, ulcers, constipation, dry mouth, gastritis. **Skin:** Rash, pruritus. **Urogenital:** Dysuria, urinary frequency.

O

DIAGNOSTIC TEST INTERFERENCE May cause false-positive reactions for BENZODIAZEPINES with ***urine drug-screening*** tests.

INTERACTIONS Drug: May attenuate the antihypertensive response to DIURETICS. NSAIDS increase the risk of **methotrexate** or **lithium** toxicity. May increase **aspirin** toxicity. **Herbal: Feverfew, garlic, ginger, ginkgo** may increase risk of bleeding.

PHARMACOKINETICS Absorption: Readily from GI tract. **Peak:** 125 min. **Onset:** 1–6 wk for maximum therapeutic effect. **Distribution:** 99% protein bound. Distributes into synovial fluid, crosses placenta. Distributed into breast milk. **Metabolism:** In the liver. **Elimination:** 60% in urine, 30–35% in feces. **Half-Life:** 40 h.

NURSING IMPLICATIONS

Assessment & Drug Effects

- Monitor for S&S of GI bleeding, especially in patients with a history of inflammation or ulceration of upper GI tract, or those treated chronically with NSAIDs.
- Monitor patients with CHF for increased fluid retention and edema. Report rapid weight increases accompanied by edema.
- Lab tests: Perform baseline and periodic evaluation of Hgb, kidney and liver function. Auditory and ophthalmologic exams are recommended with prolonged or high-dose therapy.

Patient & Family Education

- Report immediately dark tarry stools, "coffee ground" or bloody emesis, or other GI distress.
- Avoid aspirin or other NSAIDs without explicit permission of physician.
- Be aware of the possibility of photosensitivity, which results in a rash on sun-exposed skin.
- Report immediately to physician ringing in ears, decreased hearing, or blurred vision.
- Do not exceed ordered dose. The goal of therapy is lowest effective dose.

OXAZEPAM

(ox-a′ze-pam)

Ox-Pam ♣, Serax, Zapex ♣

Classifications: ANXIOLYTIC; SEDATIVE-HYPNOTIC; BENZODIAZEPINE

Therapeutic: ANTIANXIETY; SEDATIVE-HYPNOTIC

Prototype: Lorazepam

Pregnancy Category: D

Controlled Substance: Schedule IV

AVAILABILITY 10 mg, 15 mg, 30 mg capsules; 15 mg tablets

ACTION & *THERAPEUTIC EFFECT* Benzodiazepine derivative related to lorazepam. Effects are mediated by the inhibitory neurotransmitter GABA. Acts on the thalamic, hypothalamic, and limbic levels of CNS. *Has anxiolytic, sedative, hypnotic, and skeletal muscle relaxant effects.*

USES Management of anxiety and tension associated with a wide range of emotional disturbances. Also to control acute withdrawal symptoms in chronic alcoholism.

CONTRAINDICATIONS Hypersensitivity to oxazepam and other benzodiazepines; respiratory depression; psychoses, suicidal ideation; acute alcohol intoxication; acute-angle glaucoma; pregnancy (category D), lactation, children younger than 6 y.

CAUTIOUS USE Older adult and debilitated patients; impaired kidney and liver function; alcoholism; addiction-prone patients; COPD; history of seizures; history of suicide; mental depression; bipolar disorder.

ROUTE & DOSAGE

Anxiety
Adult: **PO** 10–30 mg t.i.d. or q.i.d.

Acute Alcohol Withdrawal
Adult: **PO** 15–30 mg t.i.d. or q.i.d.

ADMINISTRATION

Oral
- Give with food if GI upset occurs.
- Store in tightly closed container at 15°–30° C (59°–86° F) unless otherwise specified.

ADVERSE EFFECTS (≥1%) **CNS:** *Drowsiness,* dizziness, mental confusion, vertigo, ataxia, headache, lethargy, syncope, tremor, slurred speech, paradoxic reaction (euphoria, excitement). **GI:** Nausea, xerostomia, jaundice. **Skin:** Skin rash, edema. **CV:** Hypotension, edema. **Hematologic:** Leukopenia. **Urogenital:** Altered libido.

INTERACTIONS Drug: Alcohol, CNS DEPRESSANTS, ANTICONVULSANTS potentiate CNS depression; **cimetidine** increases oxazepam plasma levels, increasing its toxicity; may decrease antiparkinsonism effects of **levodopa;** may increase **phenytoin** levels; smoking decreases sedative and antianxiety effects. **Herbal: Kava, valerian** may potentiate sedation.

PHARMACOKINETICS Absorption: Readily absorbed from GI tract. **Peak:** 2–3 h. **Distribution:** Crosses placenta; distributed into breast milk. **Metabolism:** In liver. **Elimination:** Primarily in urine, some in feces. **Half-Life:** 2–8 h.

NURSING IMPLICATIONS

Assessment & Drug Effects
- Observe older adult patients closely for signs of overdosage. Report to physician if daytime psychomotor function is depressed.
- Monitor for increased signs and symptoms of suicidality.
- Lab tests: Perform liver function and white blood cell counts on a regular planned basis.
- Note: Excessive and prolonged use may cause physical dependence.

Patient & Family Education
- Report promptly any mild paradoxic stimulation of affect and excitement with sleep disturbances that may occur within the first 2 wk of therapy. Dosage reduction is indicated.

- Consult physician before self-medicating with OTC drugs.
- Do not drive or engage in potentially hazardous activities until response to drug is known.
- Do not drink alcoholic beverages while taking oxazepam. The CNS depressant effects of each agent may be intensified.
- Contact physician if you intend to or do become pregnant during therapy about discontinuing the drug.
- Withdraw drug slowly following prolonged therapy to avoid precipitating withdrawal symptoms (seizures, mental confusion, nausea, vomiting, muscle and abdominal cramps, tremulousness, sleep disturbances, unusual irritability, hyperhidrosis).

OXCARBAZEPINE

(ox-car'ba-ze-peen)
Trileptal
Classification: ANTICONVULSANT
Therapeutic: ANTICONVULSANT
Prototype: Carbamazepine
Pregnancy Category: C

AVAILABILITY 150 mg, 300 mg, 600 mg tablets; 300 mg/5 mL suspension

ACTION & *THERAPEUTIC EFFECT* Anticonvulsant properties may result from blockage of voltage-sensitive sodium channels, which results in stabilization of hyperexcited neural membranes. *Inhibits repetitive neuronal firing, and decreased propagation of neuronal impulses.*

USES Monotherapy or adjunctive therapy in the treatment of partial seizures in adults and children age 4–16 y.

CONTRAINDICATIONS Hypersensitivity to oxcarbazepine; children younger than 3 y.

CAUTIOUS USE Older adults; renal impairment; renal failure; infertility, hyponatremia, SIADH, and drugs associated with SIADH as an adverse effect; pregnancy (category C), lactation; children younger than 8 y.

ROUTE & DOSAGE

Partial Seizures

Adult: **PO** Start with 300 mg b.i.d. and increase by 600 mg/day qwk to 2400 mg/day in 2 divided doses for monotherapy or 1200 mg/day as adjunctive therapy
Child: **PO** *4–16 y,* Initiate with 8–10 mg/kg/day divided b.i.d. (max: 600 mg/day), gradually increase weekly to target dose (divided b.i.d.) based on weight: *Weight 20–29 kg,* 900 mg/day; *weight 29.1–39 kg,* 1200 mg/day; *weight greater than 39 kg,* 1800 mg/day

Renal Impairment Dosage Adjustment

CrCl less than 30 mL/min: Initiate at 1/2 usual starting dose (300 mg b.i.d.)

ADMINISTRATION

Oral

- Initiate therapy at one-half the usual starting dose (300 mg/day) if creatinine clearance less than 30 mL/min.
- Do not abruptly stop this medication; withdraw drug gradually when discontinued to minimize seizure potential.
- Store preferably at 25° C (77° F), but room temperature permitted. Keep container tightly closed.

ADVERSE EFFECTS (≥1%) **Body as a Whole:** *Fatigue,* asthenia, peripheral edema, generalized edema, chest pain, weight gain. **CV:** Hypotension. **GI:** *Nausea, vomiting, abdominal pain,* diarrhea, dyspepsia, constipation, gastritis, anorexia, dry mouth. **Hematologic:** Lymphadenopathy. **Metabolic:** Hyponatremia. **Musculoskeletal:** Muscle weakness. **CNS:** *Headache, dizziness, somnolence, ataxia, nystagmus, abnormal gait,* insomnia, tremor, nervousness, agitation, abnormal coordination, speech disorder, confusion, abnormal thinking, aggravate convulsions, emotional lability. **Respiratory:** Rhinitis, cough, bronchitis, pharyngitis. **Skin:** Acne, hot flushes, purpura, <u>Stevens-Johnson syndrome, toxic epidermal necrolysis</u>. **Special Senses:** *Diplopia, vertigo, abnormal vision,* abnormal accommodation, taste perversion, ear ache. **Urogenital:** Urinary tract infection, micturition frequency, vaginitis.

INTERACTIONS Drug: Carbamazepine, phenobarbital, phenytoin, valproic acid, verapamil, CALCIUM CHANNEL BLOCKERS may decrease oxcarbazepine levels; may increase levels of **phenobarbital, phenytoin;** may decrease levels of **felodipine,** ORAL CONTRACEPTIVES. **Herbal: Ginkgo** may decrease anticonvulsant effectiveness. **Evening primrose oil** may decrease the seizure threshold.

PHARMACOKINETICS Absorption: Rapidly and completely from GI tract. **Peak:** Steady-state levels reached in 2–3 days. **Distribution:** 40% protein bound. **Metabolism:** Extensively metabolized in liver to active 10-monohydroxy metabolite (MHD). **Elimination:** 95% in kidneys. **Half-Life:** 2 h, MHD 9 h.

NURSING IMPLICATIONS

Assessment & Drug Effects

- Monitor for and report S&S of: Hyponatremia (e.g., nausea, malaise, headache, lethargy, confusion); CNS impairment (e.g., somnolence, excessive fatigue, cognitive deficits, speech or language problems, incoordination, gait disturbances).
- Monitor phenytoin levels when administered concurrently.
- Lab tests: Periodic serum sodium, T_4 level; when oxcarbazepine is used as adjunctive therapy, closely monitor plasma level of the concomitant antiepileptic drug during titration of the oxcarbazepine dose.

Patient & Family Education

- Notify physician of the following: Dizziness, excess drowsiness, frequent headaches, malaise, double vision, lack of coordination, or persistent nausea.
- Exercise special caution with concurrent use of alcohol or CNS depressants.
- Use caution with potentially hazardous activities and driving until response to drug is known.
- Use or add barrier contraceptive since drug may render hormonal methods ineffective.

O

OXICONAZOLE NITRATE

(ox-i-con′a-zole)

Oxistat

Classification: AZOLE ANTIFUNGAL
Therapeutic: ANTIFUNGAL
Prototype: Fluconazole
Pregnancy Category: B

AVAILABILITY 1% cream, lotion

ACTION & *THERAPEUTIC EFFECT* Topical synthetic antifungal agent that presumably works by altering the cellular membrane of the fungi, resulting in increased membrane permeability, secondary metabolic effects, and growth inhibition. *Effective against fungi.*

USES Topical treatment of tinea pedis, tinea cruris, and tinea corporis due to *Trichophyton rubrum* and *Trichophyton mentagrophytes;* also used for cutaneous candidiasis caused by *Candida albicans* and *Candida tropicalis.*

CONTRAINDICATIONS Hypersensitivity to oxiconazole.
CAUTIOUS USE Hypersensitivity to other azole antifungals; pregnancy (category B), lactation.

ROUTE & DOSAGE

Tinea and Other Dermal Infections
Adult: **Topical** Apply to affected area once daily in the evening

ADMINISTRATION

Topical
- Apply cream to cover the affected areas once daily (in the evening).
- Treat tinea corporis and tinea cruris for 2 wk; tinea pedis for 1 mo to reduce the possibility of recurrence.
- Store at 15°–30° C (59°–86° F).

ADVERSE EFFECTS (≥1%) **Skin:** Transient burning and stinging, dryness, erythema, pruritus, and local irritation.

INTERACTIONS Drug: No clinically significant interactions established.

PHARMACOKINETICS Absorption: Less than 0.3% is absorbed systemically.

NURSING IMPLICATIONS

Patient & Family Education
- Use only externally. Do not use intravaginally.
- Discontinue drug and contact physician if irritation or sensitivity develops.
- Avoid contact with eyes.
- Contact physician if no improvement is noted after the prescribed treatment period.

OXTRIPHYLLINE

(ox-trye′fi-lin)
Choledyl SA
Classifications: BRONCHODILATOR (RESPIRATORY SMOOTH MUSCLE RELAXANT); XANTHINE
Therapeutic: BRONCHODILATOR
Prototype: Theophylline
Pregnancy Category: C

AVAILABILITY 400 mg, 600 mg sustained release tablets

ACTION & *THERAPEUTIC EFFECT* Relaxes smooth muscle by direct action, particularly of bronchi and pulmonary vessels, and stimulates medullary respiratory center with resulting increase in vital capacity. *Relaxes bronchi smooth muscle and stimulates respiratory center in the medulla of the brain.*

USES As bronchodilator to control asthma or COPD.

CONTRAINDICATIONS Hypersensitivity to xanthines; coronary artery disease; renal or hepatic impairment; lactation. Safe use in children younger than 1 y is not established.
CAUTIOUS USE Peptic ulcer; prostatic hypertrophy; diabetes mellitus; glaucoma; pregnancy (category C).

ROUTE & DOSAGE

Asthma, COPD

Adult: **PO** 4.7 mg/kg (usual dose 200 mg) q8h

Child: **PO** *1–9 y,* 6.2 mg/kg q6h; *9–16 y, adult smoker,* 4.7 mg/kg (usual dose 200 mg) q6h

ADMINISTRATION

Oral

- Give on an empty stomach (30 min to 1 h before or 2 h after meals); may be taken after meals and at bedtime to reduce GI distress. Sustained release tablet permits dosing q12h.
- Ensure that sustained release form is not chewed or crushed. It **must be** swallowed whole.
- Protect elixir from light.

ADVERSE EFFECTS (≥1%) **CNS:** Restlessness, dizziness, insomnia, convulsions, *muscle twitching.* **CV:** Palpitation, tachycardia, flushing, hypotension. **GI:** *Nausea,* vomiting, anorexia, epigastric pain, diarrhea, activation of peptic ulcer. **Urogenital:** Transient urinary frequency, kidney irritation. **Body as a Whole:** Urticaria, fever, dehydration.

INTERACTIONS Drug: Lowers lithium levels; **cimetidine,** high dose **allopurinol** (600 mg/day), **ciprofloxacin, erythromycin, troleandomycin** can significantly increase levels. **Herbal: St. John's wort** may decrease plasma levels.

PHARMACOKINETICS Absorption: Well absorbed from GI tract. **Duration:** 4–8 h; varies with age, smoking, and liver function. **Distribution:** Crosses placenta; distributed into breast milk. **Metabolism:** Extensively in liver. **Elimination:** Parent drug and metabolites excreted by kidneys. **Half-Life:** 4 h in adults.

NURSING IMPLICATIONS

Note: See theophylline for numerous additional nursing implications.

Assessment & Drug Effects

- Use safety precautions with older adults during early therapy; dizziness is a relatively common adverse effect.
- Monitor vital signs and I&O. Improvement in quality of pulse and respiration and diuresis are expected clinical effects.
- Observe and report early signs of possible toxicity: Anorexia, nausea, vomiting, dizziness, shakiness, restlessness, abdominal discomfort, irritability, palpitation, tachycardia, marked hypotension, cardiac arrhythmias, seizures.

Patient & Family Education

- Report gastric distress, palpitation, and CNS stimulation (irritability, restlessness, nervousness, insomnia) to physician. Reduction in dosage may be indicated.
- Limit caffeine intake; it may increase incidence of adverse effects.
- Do not take OTC medications, especially cough suppressants, which may cause retention of secretions and CNS depression, without consulting physician.
- Drink adequate fluids (at least 2000 mL/day) to decrease viscosity of airway secretions.

OXYBUTYNIN CHLORIDE Pr

(ox-i-byoo′ti-nin)

Ditropan, Ditropan XL, Gelnique, Oxytrol

Classifications: ANTICHOLINERGIC; ANTIMUSCARINIC; GU ANTISPASMODIC

Therapeutic: GU ANTISPASMODIC

Pregnancy Category: B

AVAILABILITY 5 mg tablets; 5 mg, 10 mg sustained release tablets; 5 mg/5 mL syrup; 3.9 mg/day transdermal patch; 10% topical gel

ACTION & *THERAPEUTIC EFFECT* Synthetic tertiary amine that exerts direct antispasmodic action and inhibits muscarinic effects of acetylcholine on smooth muscle of the urinary muscle. *Prominent antispasmodic activity of the urinary muscle.*

USES To relieve symptoms associated with voiding in patients with uninhibited neurogenic bladder and reflex neurogenic bladder. Also has been used to relieve pain of bladder spasm following transurethral surgical procedures.

CONTRAINDICATIONS Hypersensitivity of oxybutynin; narrow-angle glaucoma, myasthenia gravis, partial or complete GI obstruction, gastric retention, paralytic ileus, intestinal atony (especially older adult or debilitated patients), megacolon, severe colitis, GU obstruction, urinary retention, unstable cardiovascular status; extended release form with renal impairment; lactation, infants.
CAUTIOUS USE Older adults; autonomic neuropathy, hiatus hernia with reflex esophagitis; hepatic or renal dysfunction; urinary infection; hyperthyroidism; CHF, coronary artery disease, hypertension; prostatic hypertrophy; pregnancy (category B).

O

ROUTE & DOSAGE

Overactive Bladder

Adult/Adolescent: **PO** 5 mg 2–4 times/day (max: 20 mg/day) or 5 mg sustained release daily, may increase up to 30 mg/day
Topical Apply 1 patch twice weekly; or apply contents of 1 package once daily
Child (older than 6 y): **PO** 5 mg b.i.d., not more than three doses/day (immediate release) or 5 mg daily (sustained release)
Geriatric: **PO** 2.5–5 mg b.i.d. (max: 15 mg/day) or 5 mg sustained release daily, may increase up to 30 mg/day
Topical Apply 1 patch twice weekly
Child: **PO** *1–5 y,* 0.2 mg/kg b.i.d.–q.i.d.; *older than 5 y,* 5 mg b.i.d. (max: 15 mg/day)

ADMINISTRATION

Oral

- Ensure that sustained release form is not chewed or crushed. It **must be** swallowed whole.

Topical

- Ensure that old patch is removed prior to application of new patch.

ADVERSE EFFECTS (≥1%) **Body as a Whole:** Severe allergic reactions including urticaria, skin rashes, suppression of lactation, decreased sweating, fever. **CNS:** *Drowsiness,* dizziness, weakness, insomnia, restlessness, psychotic behavior (overdosage). **CV:** Palpitations, tachycardia, flushing. **Special Senses:** Mydriasis, *blurred vision,* cycloplegia, increased ocular tension. **GI:** *Dry mouth,* nausea, vomiting, *constipation,* bloated feeling. **Skin:** *Pruritus at application site,* rash, application site reactions, erythema. **Urogenital:** Urinary hesitancy or retention, impotence.

PHARMACOKINETICS Absorption: Diffuses across intact skin. **Onset:** 0.5–1 h. **Peak:** 3–6 h. **Duration:** 6–10 h. **PO:** 96 h transdermal. **Metabolism:** In liver. **Elimination:** Primarily in urine. **Half-Life:** 2–5 h

NURSING IMPLICATIONS

Assessment & Drug Effects

- Periodic interruptions of therapy are recommended to determine patient's need for continued treatment. Tolerance has occurred in some patients.
- Keep physician informed of expected responses to drug therapy (e.g., effect on urinary frequency, urgency, urge incontinence, nocturia, completeness of bladder emptying).
- Monitor patients with colostomy or ileostomy closely; abdominal distention and the onset of diarrhea in these patients may be early signs of intestinal obstruction or of toxic megacolon.

Patient & Family Education

- Do not drive or engage in potentially hazardous activities until response to drug is known.
- Exercise caution in hot environments. By suppressing sweating, oxybutynin can cause fever and heat stroke.

OXYCODONE HYDROCHLORIDE

(ox-i-koe′done)

OxyContin, Percolone, Endocodone, OxyFAST, Roxicodone

Classifications: NARCOTIC (OPIATE AGONIST); ANALGESIC

Therapeutic: NARCOTIC ANALGESIC

Prototype: Morphine

Pregnancy Category: B; D for prolonged use or use of high doses at term

Controlled Substance: Schedule II

AVAILABILITY 5 mg, 15 mg, 30 mg tablets; **OxyContin:** 10 mg, 20 mg, 40 mg, 80 mg, 160 mg sustained release tablets; 5 mg/5 mL, 20 mg/mL oral solution

ACTION & *THERAPEUTIC EFFECT* Semisynthetic derivative of an opium alkaloid with actions qualitatively similar to those of morphine. Binds with stereo-specific receptors in various sites of CNS to alter both perception of pain and emotional response to pain. *Active against moderate to moderately severe pain. Appears to be more effective in relief of acute than long-standing pain.*

USES Relief of moderate to moderately severe pain such as may occur with bursitis, dislocations, simple fractures and other injuries, and neuralgia. Relieves postoperative, postextractional, postpartum pain.

CONTRAINDICATIONS Hypersensitivity to oxycodone and principal drugs with which it is combined; bronchial asthma; pregnancy (category D for prolonged use or high doses at term); lactation, children younger than 6 y.

CAUTIOUS USE Alcoholism; renal or hepatic disease; viral infections; Addison's disease; cardiac arrhythmias; chronic ulcerative colitis; history of drug abuse or dependency; gallbladder disease, acute abdominal conditions; head injury, intracranial lesions; hypothyroidism; prostatic hypertrophy; respiratory disease; urethral stricture; older adult or debilitated patients; peptic ulcer or coagulation abnormalities (combination products containing aspirin); pregnancy (category B except for prolonged use).

ROUTE & DOSAGE

Moderate to Severe Pain

Adult: **PO** 5–10 mg q6h prn; OxyContin can be dosed q8h

Child: **PO** *6–12 y,* 1.25 mg q6h prn; *12 y or older,* 2.5 mg q6h prn

ADMINISTRATION

Oral

- Ensure that sustained release form is not chewed or crushed. It **must be** swallowed whole.
- Store at 15°–30° C (59°–86° F). Protect from light.

ADVERSE EFFECTS (≥1%) **CNS:** Euphoria, dysphoria, lightheadedness, dizziness, *sedation*. **GI:** Anorexia, nausea, vomiting, *constipation,* jaundice, hepatotoxicity (combinations containing acetaminophen). **Respiratory:** Shortness of breath, respiratory depression. **Skin:** Pruritus, skin rash. **CV:** Bradycardia. **Body as a Whole:** Unusual bleeding or bruising. **Urogenital:** Dysuria, frequency of urination, urinary retention.

O

DIAGNOSTIC TEST INTERFERENCE ***Serum amylase*** levels may be elevated because oxycodone causes spasm of sphincter of Oddi. ***Blood glucose determinations:*** False decrease (measured by ***glucose oxidase-peroxidase method***). ***5-HIAA determination:*** False positive with use of ***nitroisonaphthol reagent*** (quantitative test is unaffected).

INTERACTIONS Drug: Alcohol and other CNS DEPRESSANTS add to CNS depressant activity. **Herbal: St. John's wort** may increase sedation.

PHARMACOKINETICS Absorption: Readily from GI tract. **Onset:** 10–15 min. **Peak:** 30–60 min. **Duration:** 4–5 h. **Distribution:** Crosses placenta; distributed into breast milk. **Metabolism:** In liver. **Elimination:** Primarily in urine. **Half-Life:** 3–5 h.

NURSING IMPLICATIONS

Assessment & Drug Effects

- Monitor patient's response closely, especially to sustained-release preparations.
- Consult physician if nausea continues after first few days of therapy.
- Note: Light-headedness, dizziness, sedation, or fainting appear to be more prominent in ambulatory than in nonambulatory patients and may be alleviated if patient lies down.
- Evaluate patient's continued need for oxycodone preparations. Psychic and physical dependence and tolerance may develop with repeated use. The potential for drug abuse is high.
- Lab tests: Check hepatic function and hematologic status periodically in patients on high dosage.
- Be aware that serious overdosage of any oxycodone preparation presents problems associated with a narcotic overdose (respiratory depression, circulatory collapse, extreme somnolence progressing to stupor or coma).

Patient & Family Education

- Do not alter dosage regimen by increasing, decreasing, or shortening intervals between doses. Habit formation and liver damage may result.
- Avoid potentially hazardous activities such as driving a car or operating machinery while using oxycodone preparation.
- Do not drink large amounts of alcoholic beverages while using oxycodone preparations; risk of liver damage is increased.
- Check with physician before taking OTC drugs for colds, stomach distress, allergies, insomnia, or pain.
- Inform surgeon or dentist that you are taking an oxycodone prepara-

tion before any surgical procedure is undertaken.

OXYMETAZOLINE HYDROCHLORIDE

(ox-i-met-az'oh-leen)

Afrin, Dristan Long Lasting, Duramist Plus, Duration, Nafrine ✦, Neo-Synephrine 12 Hour, Nostrilla, Sinex Long Lasting

Classifications: NASAL PREPARATION; DECONGESTANT
Therapeutic: DECONGESTANT
Prototype: Naphazoline
Pregnancy Category: C

AVAILABILITY 0.025%, 0.05% solution

ACTION & *THERAPEUTIC EFFECT* Sympathomimetic agent that acts directly on alpha receptors of sympathetic nervous system resulting in relief of nasal congestion. *Constricts smaller arterioles in nasal passages and has prolonged decongestant effect.*

USES Relief of nasal congestion in a variety of allergic and infectious disorders of the upper respiratory tract; used as nasal tampon to facilitate intranasal examination or before nasal surgery. Also used as adjunct in treatment and prevention of middle ear infection by decreasing congestion of eustachian ostia.

CONTRAINDICATIONS Use in children younger than 2 y; closed-angle glaucoma; lactation.
CAUTIOUS USE Within 14 days of MAO inhibitors, coronary artery disease, hypertension, hyperthyroidism, diabetes mellitus; pregnancy (category C).

ROUTE & DOSAGE

Nasal Congestion
Adult: **Intranasal** 2–3 drops or 2–3 sprays of 0.05% solution into each nostril b.i.d. for up to 3–5 days
Child: **Intranasal** *2–5 y,* 2–3 drops or 2–3 sprays of 0.025% solution into each nostril b.i.d. for up to 3–5 days; *older than 6 y,* same as for adult

ADMINISTRATION

Instillation
- Place spray nozzle in nostril without occluding it and tilt head slightly forward prior to instillation of spray; instruct patient to sniff briskly during administration.
- Rinse dropper or spray tip in hot water after each use to prevent contamination of solution by nasal secretions.

ADVERSE EFFECTS (≥1%) **Special Senses:** *Burning,* stinging, dryness of nasal mucosa, *sneezing.* **Body as a Whole:** Headache, lightheadedness, drowsiness, insomnia, palpitations, *rebound congestion.*

INTERACTIONS Drug: No clinically significant interactions established.

PHARMACOKINETICS Onset: 5–10 min. **Duration:** 6–10 h.

NURSING IMPLICATIONS

Assessment & Drug Effects
- Monitor for S&S of excess use. If noted, discuss possibility of rebound congestion.

Patient & Family Education
- Wash hands carefully after handling oxymetazoline. Anisocoria (inequality of pupil size, blurred vision) can develop if eyes are rubbed with contaminated fingers.
- Do not to exceed recommended dosage. Rebound congestion

(chemical rhinitis) may occur with prolonged or excessive use.
- Systemic effects can result from swallowing excessive medication.

OXYMETHOLONE

(ox-i-meth'oh-lone)
Anadrol-50
Classification: ANDROGEN/ANABOLIC STEROID
Therapeutic: ANABOLIC STEROID
Prototype: Testosterone
Pregnancy Category: X
Controlled Substance: Schedule III

AVAILABILITY 50 mg tablets

ACTION & *THERAPEUTIC EFFECT* Mechanism of action in refractory anemias is unclear but may be due to direct stimulation of bone marrow, protein anabolic activity, or to androgenic stimulation of erythropoiesis. *Stimulates formation of red blood cells in the bone marrow. Stimulates bone growth, aids in bone matrix reconstitution.*

O

USES Aplastic anemia.
UNLABELED USES Osteoporosis, catabolic conditions.

CONTRAINDICATIONS Hypersensitivity to oxymetholone; prostatic hypertrophy with obstruction; prostatic or male breast cancer; carcinoma of the breast in women with hypercalcemia; cardiac, renal, hepatic decompensation; nephrosis or nephrotic stage of nephritis; premature infant; pregnancy (category X), lactation.
CAUTIOUS USE Prepubertal males; geriatric male patients; diabetes mellitus; coronary disease.

ROUTE & DOSAGE

Aplastic Anemia
Adult/Child: **PO** 1–5 mg/kg/day

ADMINISTRATION

Oral
- For treatment of anemias, a minimum trial period of 3–6 mo is recommended, since response tends to be slow.
- Store at 15°–30° C (59°–86° F). Protect from heat and light.

ADVERSE EFFECTS (≥1%) **Endocrine:** Androgenic in women: Suppression of ovulation, lactation, or menstruation; *hoarseness or deepening of voice* (often irreversible); *hirsutism; oily skin; acne;* clitoral enlargement; regression of breasts; male-pattern baldness (in disseminated breast cancer). Hypoestrogenic effects in women: Flushing, sweating; vaginitis with pruritus, drying, bleeding; menstrual irregularities. Males: Prepubertal: Premature epiphyseal closure, phallic enlargement, priapism. Postpubertal: Testicular atrophy, decreased ejaculatory volume, azoospermia, oligospermia (after prolonged administration or excessive dosage), impotence, epididymitis, gynecomastia. **CV:** *Edema,* skin flush. **GI:** *Nausea, vomiting, anorexia,* diarrhea, jaundice, <u>hepatotoxicity</u>. **Urogenital:** Bladder irritability. **Metabolic:** Hypercalcemia.

INTERACTIONS Drug: May enhance hypoprothrombinemic effects of **warfarin. Herbal: Echinacea** may increase risk of hepatotoxicity.

PHARMACOKINETICS Absorption: Readily from GI tract. **Metabolism:** In liver. **Elimination:** In urine. **Half-Life:** 9 h.

NURSING IMPLICATIONS

Assessment & Drug Effects
- Monitor patient with a history of seizures closely because an increase in their frequency may be noted.

- Monitor periodically for edema that may develop with or without CHF.
- Monitor for hypercalcemia (see Appendix F), especially in women with breast cancer.
- Lab tests: Periodic serum calcium; periodic liver function tests are especially important for the older adult patient. Drug should be stopped with first sign of liver toxicity (jaundice).

Patient & Family Education

- Monitor blood glucose for loss of glycemic control if diabetic.
- Women: Notify physician of signs of virilization.

OXYMORPHONE HYDROCHLORIDE

(ox-i-mor'fone)

Numorphan, Opana, Opana ER

Classifications: NARCOTIC (OPIATE AGONIST); ANALGESIC

Therapeutic: NARCOTIC ANALGESIC

Prototype: Morphine

Pregnancy Category: C

Controlled Substance: Schedule II

AVAILABILITY 1 mg/mL, 1.5 mg/mL injection; 5 mg suppositories; 10 mg extended release tablets; 10 mg tablets

ACTION & *THERAPEUTIC EFFECT* Structurally and pharmacologically related to morphine. Analgesic action for moderate to severe pain. Produces mild sedation and, unlike morphine, has little antitussive action. *Effective in relief of moderate to severe pain.*

USES Relief of moderate to severe pain, preoperative medication, obstetric analgesia, support of anesthesia, and relief of anxiety in patients with dyspnea associated with acute ventricular failure and pulmonary edema.

CONTRAINDICATIONS Pulmonary edema resulting from chemical respiratory irritants; ileus; status asthmaticus; children younger than 12 y.

CAUTIOUS USE Alcoholism; biliary tract disease; bladder obstruction; severe pulmonary disease, respiratory insufficiency, COPD; depression; older adults; pregnancy (category C), lactation.

ROUTE & DOSAGE

Moderate to Severe Pain

Adult: **PO** 10–20 mg q4–6h prn; extended release 5–10 mg q12h **Subcutaneous/IM** 1–1.5 mg q4–6h prn **IV** 0.5 mg q4–6h then switch to alternate route **PR** 5 mg q4–6h prn

Analgesia during Labor

Adult: **IM** 0.5–1 mg

ADMINISTRATION

Subcutaneous/Intramuscular

- Give undiluted.

Intravenous

PREPARE: **Direct:** May be given undiluted or diluted in 5 mL of sterile water or NS.

ADMINISTER: **Direct:** Give at a rate of 0.5 mg over 2–5 min.

- Protect drug from light. Store suppositories in refrigerator 2°–15° C (36°–59° F).

ADVERSE EFFECTS (≥1%) **GI:** *Nausea, vomiting, euphoria.* **CNS:** *Dizziness,* lightheadedness, sedation. **Respiratory:** Respiratory depression (see morphine), apnea, respiratory arrest. **Body as a Whole:** Sweating, coma, shock. **CV:** Cardiac arrest, circulatory depression.

INTERACTIONS Drug: Alcohol and other CNS DEPRESSANTS add to CNS depression; **propofol** increases risk of bradycardia.

PHARMACOKINETICS Onset: 5–10 min IV; 10–15 min IM; 15–30 min PR. **Peak:** 1–1.5 h. **Duration:** 3–6 h. **Distribution:** Crosses placenta. **Metabolism:** In liver. **Elimination:** In urine. **Half-Life:** PO 7–9 h; extended release 9–11 h.

NURSING IMPLICATIONS

Assessment & Drug Effects

- Monitor respiratory rate. Withhold drug and notify physician if rate falls below 12 breaths/min.
- Supervise ambulation and advise patient of possible light-headedness. Older adult and debilitated patients are most susceptible to CNS depressant effects of drug.
- Evaluate patient's continued need for narcotic analgesic. Prolonged use can lead to dependence of morphine type.
- Medication contains sulfite and may precipitate a hypersensitivity reaction in susceptible patient.

Patient & Family Education

- Use caution when walking because of potential for injury from dizziness.
- Do not consume alcohol while taking oxymorphone.

O

OXYTOCIN INJECTION (Pr)

(ox-i-toe'sin)

Pitocin

Classification: OXYTOCIC

Therapeutic: OXYTOCIC

Pregnancy Category: X

AVAILABILITY 10 units/mL injection

ACTION & *THERAPEUTIC EFFECT* Synthetic, water-soluble polypeptide identical pharmacologically to the natural oxytocin released by posterior pituitary. By direct action on myofibrils, produces phasic contractions characteristic of normal delivery. Uterine sensitivity to oxytocin increases during gestation period and peaks sharply before parturition. *Effective in initiating or improving uterine contractions at term.*

USES To initiate or improve uterine contraction at term, management of inevitable, incomplete, or missed abortion; stimulation of uterine contractions during third stage of labor; stimulation to overcome uterine inertia; control of postpartum hemorrhage and promotion of postpartum uterine involution. Also used to induce labor in cases of maternal diabetes, preeclampsia, eclampsia, and erythroblastosis fetalis.

CONTRAINDICATIONS Hypersensitivity to oxytocin; significant cephalopelvic disproportion, unfavorable fetal position or presentations that are undeliverable without conversion before delivery, obstetric emergencies that favor surgical intervention, fetal distress in which delivery is not imminent, prematurity, placenta previa, prolonged use in severe toxemia or uterine inertia, hypertonic uterine patterns, conditions predisposing to thromboplastin or amniotic fluid embolism (dead fetus, abruptio placentae), grand multiparity, invasive cervical carcinoma, primipara older than 35 y, past history of uterine sepsis or of traumatic delivery; pregnancy (category X); lactation.

CAUTIOUS USE Preeclampsia; history of seizures; history of mental hypertension.

ROUTE & DOSAGE

Labor Induction

Adult: **IV** 0.5–2 milliunits/min, may increase by 1–2 milliunits/min q15–60min (max: 20 milliunits/min); dose is decreased when labor is established. High dose regimen: 6 milliunits/min, may increase by 6 milliunits/min q15–60min until contraction pattern established.

Postpartum Bleeding

Adult: **IM** 10 units total dose **IV** Infuse a total of 10–40 units at a rate of 20–40 milliunits/min after delivery

Incomplete Abortion

Adult: **IV** 10–20 milliunits/min

ADMINISTRATION

Intramuscular

- Give 10 units IM after delivery of the placenta.

Intravenous

PREPARE: **IV Infusion:** When diluting oxytocin for IV infusion, rotate bottle gently to distribute medicine throughout solution. **IV Infusion for Inducing Labor:** Add 10 units (1 mL) to 1 L of D5W, NS, LR, or D5NS to yield 10 milliunits/mL. **IV Infusion for Postpartum Bleeding/Incomplete Abortion:** Add 10–40 units (1–4 mL) to 1 L of D5W, NS, LR, or D5NS to yield 10–40 milliunits/mL. ***ADMINISTER:*** **IV Infusion:** Use an infusion pump for accurate control of infusion rate. **IV Infusion for Inducing Labor:** Initially infuse 0.5–2 milliunits/min; increase by 1–2 milliunits/min at 30–60 min intervals. **IV Infusion for Postpartum Bleeding:** Initially infuse 10–40 milliunits/min, then adjust to control uterine atony. **IV Infusion for Incomplete Abortion:** Infuse 10–20 milliunits/min. Do not exceed 30 units in 12 h.

INCOMPATIBILITIES **Solution/additive:** **Fibrinolysin, norepinephrine, prochlorperazine, warfarin.**

ADVERSE EFFECTS (≥1%) **Body as a Whole:** Fetal trauma from too rapid propulsion through pelvis, fetal <u>death</u>, anaphylactic reactions, postpartum hemorrhage, precordial pain, edema, cyanosis or redness of skin. **CV:** Fetal bradycardia and arrhythmias, maternal cardiac arrhythmias, hypertensive episodes, <u>subarachnoid hemorrhage</u>, increased blood flow, <u>fatal afibrinogenemia</u>, ECG changes, PVCs, <u>cardiovascular spasm and collapse</u>. **GI:** Neonatal jaundice, maternal nausea, vomiting. **Endocrine:** ADH effects leading to severe water intoxication and hyponatremia, hypotension. **CNS:** Fetal <u>intracranial hemorrhage</u>, anxiety. **Respiratory:** Fetal hypoxia, maternal dyspnea. **Urogenital:** Uterine hypertonicity, tetanic contractions, <u>uterine rupture</u>, pelvic hematoma.

INTERACTIONS Drug: VASOCONSTRICTORS cause severe hypertension; **cyclopropane anesthesia** causes hypotension, maternal bradycardia, arrhythmias. **Herbal: Ephedra, ma huang** may cause hypertension.

PHARMACOKINETICS Duration: 1 h. **Distribution:** Distributed throughout extracellular fluid; small amount may cross placenta. **Metabolism:** Rapidly destroyed in liver and kidneys. **Elimination:** Small amounts excreted unchanged in urine. **Half-Life:** 3–5 min.

NURSING IMPLICATIONS

Assessment & Drug Effects

- Start flow charts to record maternal BP and other vital signs, I&O ratio, weight, strength, duration, and frequency of contractions, as well as fetal heart tone and rate, before instituting treatment.
- Monitor fetal heart rate and maternal BP and pulse at least q15min during infusion period; evaluate tonus of myometrium during and between contractions and record on flow chart. Report change in rate and rhythm immediately.
- Stop infusion to prevent fetal anoxia, turn patient on her side, and notify physician if contractions are prolonged (occurring at less than 2-min intervals) and if monitor records contractions about 50 mm Hg or if contractions last 90 sec or longer. Stimulation will wane rapidly within 2–3 min. Oxygen administration may be necessary.
- If local or regional (caudal, spinal) anesthesia is being given to the patient receiving oxytocin, be alert to the possibility of hypertensive crisis (sudden intense occipital headache, palpitation, marked hypertension, stiff neck, nausea, vomiting, sweating, fever, photophobia, dilated pupils, bradycardia or tachycardia, constricting chest pain).
- Monitor I&O during labor. If patient is receiving drug by prolonged IV infusion, watch for symptoms of water intoxication (drowsiness, listlessness, headache, confusion, anuria, weight gain). Report changes in alertness and orientation and changes in I&O ratio (i.e., marked decrease in output with excessive intake).
- Check fundus frequently during the first few postpartum hours and several times daily thereafter.

Patient & Family Education

- Be aware of purpose and anticipated effect of oxytocin.
- Report sudden, severe headache immediately to health care providers.

PACLITAXEL Pr

(pac-li-tax'el)

Abraxane, Taxol

Classifications: ANTINEOPLASTIC; TAXANE

Therapeutic: ANTINEOPLASTIC; ANTIMICROTUBULE

Pregnancy Category: D

AVAILABILITY 6 mg/mL injection; 100 mg powder for injection (with 900 mg human albumin)

ACTION & *THERAPEUTIC EFFECT* During cell division, paclitaxel is an antimicrotubular agent that interferes with the microtubule network essential for interphase and mitosis. This results in abnormal spindle formation and multiple asters during mitosis. *Interferes with growth of rapidly dividing cells including cancer cells, and eventually causes cell death. Additionally, the breakup of the cytoskeleton within nondividing cells interrupts intracellular transport and communications.*

USES Ovarian cancer, breast cancer, Kaposi's sarcoma, non–small-cell lung cancer (NSCLC).

UNLABELED USES Squamous cell head and neck cancer, small-cell lung cancer, endometrial cancer, esophageal cancer, gastric cancer, testicular cancer, germ cell tumors, and other solid tumors, leukemia, melanoma.

CONTRAINDICATIONS Taxol: Hypersensitivity to paclitaxel, or taxane; baseline neutrophil count less than 1500 cells/mm³; thrombocytopenia; with AIDS-related Kaposi's sarcoma baseline neutrophil count less than 1000 cells/mm³. For **Abraxane:** Baseline neutrophil count less than 1500 cells/mm³; pregnancy (category D), lactation.
CAUTIOUS USE Cardiac arrhythmias, cardiac disease; impaired liver function; alcoholism; older adults; peripheral neuropathy. Safety and efficacy in children are not established.

ROUTE & DOSAGE

Ovarian Cancer, NSCLC
Adult: **IV** 135 mg/m² 24-h infusion repeated q3wk

Breast Cancer
Adult: **IV** 175–250 mg/m² over 3 h q3wk
Abraxane: **IV** 260 mg/m² over 30 min q3wk

Kaposi's Sarcoma
Adult: **IV** 135 mg/m² infused over 3 h q3wk or 100 mg/m² infused over 3 h q2wk

ADMINISTRATION

Intravenous

Note: Premedication as follows (except with **Abraxane**) to avoid severe hypersensitivity: Dexamethasone 20 mg (10 mg with AIDS-related Kaposi's) PO/IV at 12 and 6 h prior to infusion; diphenhydramine 50 mg IV 30–60 min prior to infusion; and cimetidine 300 mg or ranitidine 50 mg IV 30 min before infusion.

- Do not administer to patients with AIDS-related Kaposi's unless neutrophil count is at least 1000/mm³; for all others, do not administer unless neutrophil count is at least 1500/mm³.
- Follow institutional or standard guidelines for preparation, handling, and disposal of cytotoxic agents.

PREPARE: **IV Infusion: Dilution of Conventional Paclitaxel:** Do not use equipment or devices containing polyvinyl chloride (PVC) in preparation of infusion. ▪ Dilute to a final concentration of 0.3–1.2 mg/mL in any of the following: D5W, NS, D5/NS, or D5W in Ringer's injection. The prepared solution may be hazy, but this does not indicate a loss of potency.
Abraxane Vial Reconstitution: Slowly inject 20 mL NS over at least 1 min onto the inside wall of the vial to yield 5 mg/mL. ▪ DO NOT inject directly into the cake powder. Allow vial to sit for at least 5 min, then gently swirl for at least 2 min to completely dissolve. If foaming occurs, let stand for at least 15 min until foam subsides. ▪ If particulates or settling are visible, gently invert vial to ensure complete resuspension prior to use. ▪ Remove the required dose and inject into an empty sterile, PVC or non-PVC type IV bag.

ADMINISTER: **IV Infusion:** Because tissue necrosis occurs with extravasation, frequently assess patency of a peripheral IV site. ▪ **Conventional Paclitaxel:** Infuse over 3 h through IV tubing containing an in-line (0.22 micron or less) filter. Do not use equipment containing PCV. ▪ **Abraxane:** DO NOT use an in-line filter. Infuse over 30 min.

P

INCOMPATIBILITIES **Solution/additive: PVC bags** and **infusion sets** should be avoided (except with Abraxane) due to leaching of DEHP (plasticizer). Do not mix with any other medications. **Y-site: Amphotericin B, amphotericin B cholesteryl sulfate complex, chlorpromazine, doxorubicin liposome, hydroxyzine, methylprednisolone, mitoxantrone.**

- **Conventional paclitaxel** solutions diluted for infusion are stable at room temperature (approximately 25° C/77° F) for up to 27 h. - Reconstituted **Abraxane** should be used immediately but may be kept refrigerated for up to 8 h if needed.

ADVERSE EFFECTS (≥1%) **CV:** Ventricular tachycardia, ventricular ectopy, *transient bradycardia,* chest pain. **CNS:** Fatigue, headaches, *peripheral neuropathy,* weakness, seizures. **GI:** *Nausea, vomiting,* diarrhea, taste changes, *mucositis,* elevations in serum triglycerides. **Hematologic:** Neutropenia, *anemia,* thrombocytopenia. **Body as a Whole:** *Hypersensitivity reactions (hypotension, dyspnea with* bronchospasm, *urticaria, abdominal and extremity pain, diaphoresis,* angioedema), *myalgias, arthralgias, alopecia.* **Skin:** *Alopecia,* tissue necrosis with extravasation. **Urogenital:** Minor elevations in kidney and liver function tests.

INTERACTIONS Drug: Increased myelosuppression if **cisplatin, doxorubicin** is given before paclitaxel; **ketoconazole** can inhibit metabolism of paclitaxel; additive bradycardia with BETA-BLOCKERS, **digoxin, verapamil;** additive risk of bleeding with ANTICOAGULANTS, NSAIDS, PLATELET INHIBITORS (including **aspirin**), THROMBOLYTIC AGENTS.

PHARMACOKINETICS Distribution: Greater than 90% protein bound; does not cross CSF. **Metabolism:** In liver (CYP3A4, 2C8). **Elimination:** Feces 70%, urine 14%. **Half-Life:** 1–9 h.

NURSING IMPLICATIONS

Assessment & Drug Effects

- Monitor for hypersensitivity reactions, especially during first and second administrations of the paclitaxel. S&S requiring treatment, but not necessarily discontinuation of the drug, include dyspnea, hypotension, and chest pain. Discontinue immediately and manage symptoms aggressively if angioedema and generalized urticaria develop.
- Monitor vital signs frequently, especially during the first hour of infusion. Bradycardia occurs in approximately 12% of patients, usually during infusion. It does not normally require treatment. Cardiac monitoring is indicated for those with severe conduction abnormalities.
- Lab tests: Monitor hematologic status throughout course of treatment. Severe neutropenia is common but usually of short duration (less than 500/mm³ for less than 7 days) with the nadir occurring about day 11. Thrombocytopenia occurs less often and is less severe with the nadir around day 8 or 9. The incidence and severity of anemia increase with exposure to paclitaxel.
- Monitor for peripheral neuropathy, the severity of which is dose dependent. Severe symptoms occur primarily with higher than recommended doses.

Patient & Family Education

- Immediately report to physician S&S of paclitaxel hypersensitivity: Difficulty breathing, chest pain, palpitations, angioedema (subcuta-

P

neous swelling usually around face and neck), and skin rashes or itching.
- Be sure to have periodic blood work as prescribed.
- Avoid aspirin, NSAIDS, and alcohol to minimize GI distress.
- Be aware of high probability of developing hair loss (greater than 80%).

PALIFERMIN

(pal-i-fur'men)

Kepivance

Classifications: BIOLOGICAL RESPONSE MODIFIER; KERATINOCYTE GROWTH FACTOR; CYTOKINE

Therapeutic: KERATINOCYTE GROWTH FACTOR (KGF)

Pregnancy Category: C

AVAILABILITY 6.25 mg powder for injection

ACTION & *THERAPEUTIC EFFECT* Naturally occurring keratinocyte growth factor (KGF) is produced and regulated in response to epithelial tissue injury. Binding of KGF to its receptors in epithelial cells results in proliferation, differentiation, and repair of injury to epithelial cells. Palifermin is a synthetic form of KCG; thus it enhances replacement of injured cells. *Palifermin reduces the incidence of severe oral mucositis that interferes with food consumption in the cancer patient.*

USES Reduction of the incidence and duration of severe oral mucositis in patients with hematologic malignancies who are receiving myelotoxic therapy requiring hematopoietic stem cell support.

CONTRAINDICATIONS Hypersensitivity to *Escherichia coli*–derived protein, palifermin; nonhematologic malignancies; within 24 h of chemotherapy. Safe use in children not established.

CAUTIOUS USE Use contraception for females of childbearing age; pregnancy (category C), lactation.

ROUTE & DOSAGE

Oral Mucositis

Adult: **IV** 60 mcg/kg/day for 3 days before and 3 days after myelotoxic therapy. **Premyelotoxic therapy:** Final dose should be given 24–48 h before therapy. **Postmyelotoxic therapy:** First dose should be given after but on the same day of hematopoietic stem cell infusion, and at least 4 days after the most recent administration of palifermin.

ADMINISTRATION

Intravenous

Do not give within 24 h before/after or during myelotoxic chemotherapy.

PREPARE: **Direct:** Reconstitute powder with 1.2 mL sterile water to yield 5 mg/mL. Gently swirl to dissolve but do not shake. ▪ Powder will dissolve in about 3 min. Should be used immediately.

ADMINISTER: **Direct:** Give as a bolus dose. ▪ If heparin is used to maintain the IV line, flush before/after with NS. ▪ If diluted solution was refrigerated, may warm to room temperature for up to 1 h but protect from light.

INCOMPATIBILITIES **Y-site: Heparin.**

- Store powder vial at 2°–8° C (36°–46° F). Protect from light.
- If needed, may store reconstituted solution refrigerated for up to 24 h.
- Discard any reconstituted solution left at room temperature for longer than 1 h.

ADVERSE EFFECTS (≥5%) **Body as a Whole:** *Edema, fever, pain.* **CNS:** *Dysesthesia.* **GI:** *Mouth/tongue thickness or discoloration, taste alterations.* **Metabolic:** *Elevated serum amylase, elevated serum lipase.* **Musculoskeletal:** *Arthralgia.* **Skin:** *Erythema, pruritus, rash.* **Urogenital:** Proteinuria.

INTERACTIONS Drug: Administration of palifermin within 24 h of **myelotoxic chemotherapy** increases the severity and duration of oral mucositis.

PHARMACOKINETICS Distribution: Extravascular distribution. **Half-Life:** 4.5 h.

NURSING IMPLICATIONS

Assessment & Drug Effects

- Monitor for improvement in mucositis.
- Monitor for S&S of oral toxicities and skin toxicities.

Patient & Family Education

- Report any of the following to a health care provider: Alteration of taste, discoloration or enlargement of the tongue, lack of sensation around the mouth, skin rash, itching, or edema.

P

PALIPERIDONE

(pa-li'per-i-done)

Invega

PALIPERIDONE PALMITATE

Invega Sustenna

Classification: ANTIPSYCHOTIC, ATYPICAL

Therapeutic: ATYPICAL ANTIPSYCHOTIC

Prototype: Clozapine

Pregnancy Category: C

AVAILABILITY 1.5 mg, 3 mg, 6 mg, 9 mg extended release tablets; extended release injection

ACTION & *THERAPEUTIC EFFECT* Interferes with binding of dopamine to dopamine type 2 (D_2) receptors, serotonin (5-HT_{2A}) receptors, and alpha-adrenergic receptors. *Effective in controlling symptoms of schizophrenia as well as other psychotic symptoms.*

USES Treatment of schizophrenia, schizoaffective disorder.

CONTRAINDICATIONS Hypersensitivity to paliperidone, risperidone; elderly with dementia-related psychosis; concurrent administration with drugs that produce QT_c prolongation including Class IA or Class III antiarrhythmic medications, antipsychotic medications, and antibiotics that prolong the QT interval; hyperglycemia, ketoacidosis; GI narrowing (pathologic or iatrogenic); lactation; children younger than 18 y.

CAUTIOUS USE History of cerebrovascular events; hypovolemia, dehydration; cardiovascular disease; renal impairment; older adults; history of hypotension; CNS pathology; systemic infection; diabetes mellitus, obesity, family history of diabetes mellitus; history of seizures; Parkinson's disease; disorders that may lead to aspiration pneumonia (e.g., severe Alzheimer's dementia); potential for suicidality; pregnancy (category C).

ROUTE & DOSAGE

Schizophrenia

Adult: **PO** Initially 6 mg/day; may adjust up/down in 3 mg increments; at least 5 day intervals needed for dosage increments (max: 12 mg/day) **IM** 234 mg on day 1, then 156 mg 1 wk later, then monthly dose of 117 mg (dose may vary based on patient response) **Converting PO to IM** 3 mg/day PO = 39–78 mg/mo IM; 60 mg/day PO = 117 mg/mo IM; 12 mg/day PO = 234 mg/mo IM

Schizoaffective Disorder

Adult: **PO** 6 mg daily, dose adjusted at intervals of more than 4 days (max: 12 mg/day)

Renal Impairment Dosage Adjustment

CrCl 50–79 mL/min: Max 6 mg/day; IM injection: Use 156 on day 1 and 117 mg 1 wk later, then monthly 78 mg injections
CrCl 10–49 mL/min: Max 3 mg/day; IM not recommended

ADMINISTRATION

- Extended release tablets **must be** swallowed whole. They should not be chewed or crushed.
- Give in the morning with or without food.
- Store at 15°–30° C (59°–86° F). Protect from moisture.

ADVERSE EFFECTS (≥1%) **Body as a Whole:** Back pain, cough, pain in extremity, pyrexia; injection site reaction. **CNS:** *Akathisia, anxiety,* asthenia, dizziness, dystonia, extrapyramidal disorder, fatigue, *headache,* hypertonia, parkinsonism, *somnolence,* tremor. **CV:** Atrioventricular block, bundle branch block, ECG T-wave abnormalities, hypertension, orthostatic hypotension, QT_c prolongation, sinus arrhythmia, tachycardia. **GI:** Abdominal pain, dry mouth, dyspepsia, nausea, salivary hypersecretion. **Metabolic:** Increased insulin levels. **Special Senses:** Blurred vision.

INTERACTIONS Drug: Enhanced CNS depression with **alcohol** or CNS DEPRESSANTS. Paliperidone may enhance the effects of ANTIHYPERTENSIVE AGENTS. Paliperidone can diminish the effects of DOPAMINE AGONISTS (**levodopa, bromocriptine, cabergoline, pergolide, pramipexole, ropinirole**). **Carbamazepine** decreases effectiveness. **Food:** High fat/high caloric meal increases paliperidone levels.

PHARMACOKINETICS Absorption: Bioavailability is 28%. **Peak:** 24 h. **Distribution:** 74% protein bound. **Metabolism:** In liver (26–41%). **Elimination:** Urine (major, 50–70% unchanged) and stool (minor). **Half-Life:** 23 h.

NURSING IMPLICATIONS

Assessment & Drug Effects

- Baseline ECG recommended to rule out congenital, long-QT syndrome.
- Prior to initiating therapy, hypokalemia and hypomagnesemia should be corrected.
- Monitor CV status and monitor BP especially in those prone to hypotension.
- Reassess patient periodically in order to maintain on the lowest effective drug dose.
- Monitor closely neurologic status of older adults.
- Supervise closely those with suicidal ideation.
- Monitor closely those at risk for seizures.
- Assess degree of cognitive and motor impairment, and assess for environmental hazards.
- Lab tests: Baseline and periodic serum electrolytes; periodic blood glucose, and complete blood counts.
- Monitor diabetics for loss of glycemic control.

Patient & Family Education

- Exercise caution with hazardous activities until response to drug is known.

- Carefully monitor blood glucose levels if diabetic.
- Do not engage in potentially hazardous activities until the response to drug is known.
- Be aware of the risk of orthostatic hypotension.
- The shell of the tablet may be eliminated in the stool whole, but this does not mean the drug was not absorbed.
- Monitor for signs and symptoms of suicidal ideation.
- Be aware of the possibility of seizure activity.

PALIVIZUMAB

(pal-i-viz′u-mab)

Synagis

Classifications: IMMUNOMODULATOR; MONOCLONAL ANTIBODY; IMMUNOGLOBULIN

Therapeutic: IMMUNOGLOBULIN (IgG)

Pregnancy Category: C

P

AVAILABILITY 100 mg vial

ACTION & *THERAPEUTIC EFFECT* Monoclonal antibody ($IgG1_k$) produced by recombinant DNA technology to the respiratory syncytial virus (RSV). *Provides passive immunity against respiratory syncytial virus. Indicated by prevention of lower respiratory tract infection.*

USES Prevention of serious lower respiratory tract infections in children susceptible to RSV.

CONTRAINDICATIONS Hypersensitivity to palivizumab; lactation.

CAUTIOUS USE Hypersensitivity to other immunoglobulin preparations, blood products, or other medications; kidney or liver dysfunction; acute RSV infection; pregnancy (category C).

ROUTE & DOSAGE

RSV

Child: **IM** 15 mg/kg qmo during RSV season

ADMINISTRATION

Intramuscular

- Reconstitute solution by gently injecting 1 mL of sterile water for injection (without preservative) toward the sides of the vial. Gently swirl for 30 sec to dissolve (do not shake solution). Allow to stand at room temperature for at least 20 min until solution clears.
- Give IM only into the anterolateral aspect of the thigh. Volumes greater than 1 mL should be divided and given in different sites.
- Use reconstituted solution within 6 h. Discard any unused portion of the vial. It contains no preservatives.

ADVERSE EFFECTS (≥1%) **Body as a Whole:** *Otitis media,* pain, hernia. **GI:** Increased AST, diarrhea, nausea, vomiting, gastroenteritis. **Respiratory:** *URI, rhinitis,* pharyngitis, cough, wheeze, bronchiolitis, asthma, croup, dyspnea, sinusitis, apnea. **Skin:** *Rash.*

PHARMACOKINETICS Half-Life: 20 days.

NURSING IMPLICATIONS

Assessment & Drug Effects

- Lab tests: Periodic monitoring of liver functions may be warranted.
- Monitor carefully for and immediately report S&S of respiratory illness including fever, cough, wheezing, and chest retractions.
- Assess for and report erythema or indurations at injection site.

Patient & Family Education

- Contact physician for S&S of respiratory illness, vomiting, diarrhea, or if redness develops at injection site.

PALONOSETRON

(pal-o-no′si-tron)
Aloxi
Classifications: SEROTONIN 5-HT_3 RECEPTOR ANTAGONIST; ANTIEMETIC
Therapeutic: ANTIEMETIC
Prototype: Ondansetron
Pregnancy Category: B

AVAILABILITY 0.25 mg/5 mL injection

ACTION & *THERAPEUTIC EFFECT* Selectively blocks serotonin 5-HT_3 receptors found centrally in the chemoreceptor trigger zone (CTZ) of the hypothalamus, and peripherally at vagal nerve endings in the intestines. *Prevents acute chemotherapy-induced nausea and vomiting associated with initial and repeat courses of moderately or highly emetogenic chemotherapy.*

USES Prevention of acute and delayed nausea and vomiting associated with highly emetogenic cancer chemotherapy.
UNLABELED USES Postoperative nausea/vomiting.

CONTRAINDICATIONS Hypersensitivity to palonosetron; lactation, children younger than 18 y.
CAUTIOUS USE Dehydration; cardiac arrhythmias, QT prolongation; electrolyte imbalance; pregnancy (category B).

ROUTE & DOSAGE

Prevention of Chemotherapy-Induced Nausea and Vomiting
Adult: **IV** 0.25 mg infused over 30 sec 30 min prior to chemotherapy; do not repeat for at least 7 days

Hepatic Impairment/Renal Impairment Dosage Adjustment
No adjustment necessary

ADMINISTRATION

Intravenous

PREPARE: **Direct:** Do not dilute and do not mix with other drugs.
ADMINISTER: **Direct:** Give over 30 sec. Flush IV line with NS before and after administration.
INCOMPATIBILITIES Do not mix with other drugs.

- Store at room temperature of 15°–30° C (59°–86° F). Protect from light.

ADVERSE EFFECTS (≥1%) **CNS:** Headache, anxiety, dizziness. **GI:** Constipation, diarrhea, abdominal pain. **Dermatologic:** Pruritus.

INTERACTIONS Drug: Can cause profound hypotension with **apomorphine.**

PHARMACOKINETICS Metabolism: In liver (CYP2D6, 1A2, 3A4). **Elimination:** Primarily renal. **Half-Life:** 40 h.

NURSING IMPLICATIONS

Assessment & Drug Effects

- Monitor closely cardiac status especially in those taking diuretics or otherwise at risk for hypokalemia or hypomagnesemia, with congenital QT syndrome, or patients taking antiarrhythmic or other drugs that lead to QT prolongation.

Patient & Family Education

- Report promptly any of the following: Difficulty breathing, wheezing, or shortness of breath; palpitations or chest tightness; skin rash or itching; swelling of the face, tongue, throat, hands, or feet.

PAMIDRONATE DISODIUM

(pa-mi'dro-nate)
Aredia
Classification: BISPHOSPHONATE (REGULATORY, BONE METABOLISM)
Therapeutic: BONE METABOLISM REGULATORY
Prototype: Etidronate
Pregnancy Category: D

AVAILABILITY 30 mg, 60 mg, 90 mg powder for injection; 3 mg, 6 mg, 9 mg solution for injection

ACTION & *THERAPEUTIC EFFECT* A bone-resorption inhibitor thought to absorb calcium phosphate crystals into bone. May also inhibit osteoclast activity, thus contributing to inhibition of bone resorption. Does not inhibit bone formation or mineralization. *Reduces bone turnover and, when used in combination with adequate hydration, it increases renal excretion of calcium, thus reducing serum calcium concentrations.*

P

USES Hypercalcemia of malignancy and Paget's disease, bone metastases in multiple myeloma or breast cancer.

UNLABELED USES Primary hyperparathyroidism, osteoporosis prophylaxis.

CONTRAINDICATIONS Hypersensitivity to pamidronate; breast cancer, severe renal disease, hypercalcemia, hypercholesterolemia, polycythemia, pregnancy (category D), prostatic cancer. Safety and effectiveness in children are not established.

CAUTIOUS USE Heart failure, nephrosis or nephrotic syndrome, moderate renal disease; hepatic disease, cholestasis; peripheral edema, prostate hypertrophy; chronic kidney failure; cancer patients with stomatitis; lactation.

ROUTE & DOSAGE

Moderate Hypercalcemia of Malignancy (corrected calcium 12–13.5 mg/dL)

Adult: **IV** 60–90 mg infused over 4–24 h, may repeat in 7 days

Severe Hypercalcemia of Malignancy (corrected calcium greater than 13.5 mg/dL)

Adult: **IV** 90 mg infused over 4–24 h, may repeat in 7 days

Paget's Disease

Adult: **IV** 30 mg once daily for 3 days (90 mg total)

Osteolytic Metastases

Adult: **IV** 90 mg once/mo

ADMINISTRATION

Intravenous

PREPARE: **IV Infusion:** Add 10 mL sterile water for injection to reconstitute the 30 or 90 mg vial to yield 3 or 9 mg/mL, respectively. Allow to completely dissolve. **IV Infusion for Hypercalcemia of Malignancy:** Withdraw the required dose and dilute in D5W, NS, or 1/2NS as follows: Use 1000 mL. **IV Infusion for Paget's Disease and Multiple Myeloma:** Withdraw the required dose and dilute in D5W, NS, or 1/2NS as follows: Use 500 mL. **IV Infusion for Breast Cancer Bone Metastases:** Withdraw the required dose and dilute in D5W, NS, or 1/2NS as follows: Use 250 mL.

ADMINISTER: **IV Infusion:** Regulate infusion rate carefully. Rapid infusion may cause renal damage. **IV Infusion for Hypercalcemia of Malignancy:** Infuse over 2–24 h. **IV Infusion for Paget's disease and Multiple Myeloma:** Infuse over 4 h. **IV Infusion for**

Breast Cancer Bone Metastases: Infuse over 2 h.

INCOMPATIBILITIES **Solution/additive:** CALCIUM-CONTAINING SOLUTIONS (including **lactated Ringer's**).

- Refrigerate reconstituted pamidronate solution at 2°–8° C (36°–46° F); the IV solution may be stored at room temperature. Both are stable for 24 h.

ADVERSE EFFECTS (≥1%) **Body as a Whole:** *Fever with or without rigors* generally occurs within 48 h and subsides within 48 h despite continued therapy; *thrombophlebitis at injection site;* general malaise lasting for several weeks; transient increase in bone pain; jaw osteonecrosis. **Metabolic:** *Hypocalcemia.* **GI:** Nausea, abdominal pain, *epigastric discomfort.* **CV:** Hypertension. **Skin:** Rash.

INTERACTIONS Drug: Concurrent use of **foscarnet** may further decrease serum levels of ionized calcium.

PHARMACOKINETICS Absorption: 50% of dose is retained in body. **Onset:** 24–48 h. **Peak:** 6 days. **Duration:** 2 wk–3 mo. **Distribution:** Accumulates in bone; once deposited, remains bound until bone is remodeled. **Metabolism:** Not metabolized. **Elimination:** 50% excreted in urine unchanged. **Half-Life:** 28 h.

NURSING IMPLICATIONS

Assessment & Drug Effects

- Assess IV injection site for thrombophlebitis.
- Lab tests: Monitor serum calcium, phosphate, magnesium, and potassium at frequent intervals; CBC with differential; Hct and Hgb; and kidney function tests throughout course of therapy.
- Monitor for S&S of hypocalcemia, hypokalemia, hypomagnesemia, and hypophosphatemia.
- Monitor for seizures especially in those with a preexisting seizure disorder.
- Monitor vital signs. Be aware that drug fever, which may occur with pamidronate use, is self-limiting, usually subsiding in 48 h even with continued therapy.
- Monitor I&O and hydration status. Patient should be adequately hydrated, without fluid overload.

Patient & Family Education

- Be aware that transient, self-limiting fever with/without chills may develop.
- Generalized malaise, which may last for several weeks following treatment, is an anticipated adverse effect.
- Report to physician immediately perioral tingling, numbness, and paresthesia. These are signs of hypocalcemia.

PANCRELIPASE (Pr)

(pan-kre-li'pase)

Cotazym, Cotazym-S, Festal II, Ilozyme, Ku-Zyme-Hp, Pancrease, Ultrase, Viokase

Classification: ENZYME REPLACEMENT THERAPY

Therapeutic: PANCREATIC ENZYME REPLACEMENT THERAPY

Pregnancy Category: C

AVAILABILITY Tablets or capsules containing lipase, protease, and amylase

ACTION & *THERAPEUTIC EFFECT* Pancreatic enzyme concentrate of porcine origin standardized for lipase content. Similar to pancreatin but on a weight basis has 12 times the lipolytic activity and at least 4 times the trypsin and amylase content of pancreatin. *Facilitates the hydrolysis of fats into glycerol and fatty acids, starches into dextrins and sugars, and proteins into peptides for easier absorption.*

USES Replacement therapy in symptomatic treatment of malabsorption syndrome due to cystic fibrosis and other conditions associated with exocrine pancreatic insufficiency.

CONTRAINDICATIONS History of allergy to porcine protein or enzymes; esophageal strictures; pancreatitis.
CAUTIOUS USE GI disease, Crohn's disease, short bowel syndrome; CF; pregnancy (category C), lactation.

ROUTE & DOSAGE

Pancreatic Insufficiency
Adult: **PO** 1–3 capsules or tablets or 1–2 packets of powder 1–2 h before, during, or 1 h after meals, with an extra dose taken with any food eaten between meals
Child: **PO** 1–2 capsules or tablets 1–2 h before, during, or 1 h after meals, with an extra dose taken with any food eaten between meals

ADMINISTRATION

Oral
- Ensure that enteric-coated preparations are not crushed or chewed.
- Note: For children, powder form may be sprinkled on food.
- Open capsule and sprinkled contents on soft food, which should be swallowed without chewing to prevent mucus membrane irritation. Follow with a full glass of water or juice. Cimetidine, ranitidine, or an antacid may be prescribed to be given before pancrelipase to prevent drug's destruction by gastric pepsin and acid pH.
- Determine dosage in relation to fat content in diet (suggested ratio: 300 mg pancrelipase for each 17 g dietary fat).

ADVERSE EFFECTS (≥1%) **GI:** Anorexia, nausea, vomiting, diarrhea. **Metabolic:** Hyperuricosuria.

INTERACTIONS Drug: Iron absorption may be decreased.

PHARMACOKINETICS Absorption: Not absorbed. **Distribution:** Acts locally in GI tract. **Elimination:** In feces.

NURSING IMPLICATIONS

Assessment & Drug Effects
- Monitor I&O and weight. Note appetite and quality of stools, weight loss, abdominal bloating, polyuria, thirst, hunger, itching. Pancreatic insufficiency is frequently associated with steatorrhea, bulky stools, and insulin-dependent diabetes.

Patient & Family Education
- Learn proper timing of medication in relation to meals.

PANCURONIUM BROMIDE
(pan-kyoo-roe'nee-um)
Classification: SKELETAL MUSCLE RELAXANT, NONDEPOLARIZING
Therapeutic: SKELETAL MUSCLE RELAXANT
Prototype: Atracurium
Pregnancy Category: C

AVAILABILITY 1 mg/mL, 2 mg/mL injection

ACTION & *THERAPEUTIC EFFECT* Synthetic curariform nondepolarizing neuromuscular blocking agent that produces skeletal muscle relaxation or paralysis by competing with acetylcholine at cholinergic receptor sites on skeletal muscle endplate and thus blocks nerve impulse transmission. *Induces skeletal muscle relaxation or paralysis.*

USES Adjunct to anesthesia to induce skeletal muscle relaxation. Also to facilitate management of patients undergoing mechanical ventilation.

CONTRAINDICATIONS Hypersensitivity to the drug or bromides; tachycardia.

CAUTIOUS USE Debilitated patients; dehydration; myasthenia gravis; neuromuscular disease; pulmonary, liver, or kidney disease; fluid or electrolyte imbalance; pregnancy (category C), lactation.

ROUTE & DOSAGE

Skeletal Muscle Relaxation

Adult/Child/Infant: **IV** 0.04–0.1 mg/kg initial dose, may give additional doses of 0.01 mg/kg at 30–60 min intervals
Neonate: **IV** 0.02 mg/kg test dose, then 0.03 mg/kg

Obesity Dosage Adjustment

Use IBW

Renal Impairment Dosage Adjustment

CrCl 10–50 mL/min: Use 50% of dose; less than 10 mL/min: Do not use

ADMINISTRATION

Intravenous

Plastic syringe may be used for administration, but drug may adsorb to plastic with prolonged storage.

PREPARE: **Direct:** Give undiluted.
ADMINISTER: **Direct:** Give over 30–90 sec.
INCOMPATIBILITIES **Solution/additive:** **Furosemide.**

- Refrigerate at 2°–8° C (36°–46° F). Do not freeze.

ADVERSE EFFECTS (≥1%) **CV:** *Increased pulse rate and BP,* ventricular extrasystoles. **Skin:** Transient acneiform rash, burning sensation along course of vein. **Body as a Whole:** Salivation, skeletal muscle weakness, <u>respiratory depression</u>.

DIAGNOSTIC TEST INTERFERENCE Pancuronium may decrease ***serum cholinesterase*** concentrations.

INTERACTIONS Drug: GENERAL ANESTHETICS increase neuromuscular blocking and duration of action; AMINOGLYCOSIDES, **bacitracin, polymyxin B, clindamycin, lidocaine,** parenteral **magnesium, quinidine, quinine, trimethaphan, verapamil** increase neuromuscular blockade; DIURETICS may increase or decrease neuromuscular blockade; **lithium** prolongs duration of neuromuscular blockade; NARCOTIC ANALGESICS possibly add to respiratory depression; **succinylcholine** increases onset and depth of neuromuscular blockade; **phenytoin** may cause resistance to or reversal of neuromuscular blockade.

PHARMACOKINETICS Onset: 30–45 sec. **Peak:** 2–3 min. **Duration:** 60 min. **Distribution:** Well distributed to tissues and extracellular fluids; crosses placenta in small amounts. **Metabolism:** Small amount in liver. **Elimination:** Primarily in urine. **Half-Life:** 2 h.

NURSING IMPLICATIONS

Assessment & Drug Effects

- Assess cardiovascular and respiratory status continuously.
- Observe patient closely for residual muscle weakness and signs of respiratory distress during recovery period. Monitor BP and vital signs. Peripheral nerve stimulator may be used to assess the effects of pancuronium and to monitor restoration of neuromuscular function.
- Note: Consciousness is not affected by pancuronium. Patient will be awake and alert but unable to speak.

PANITUMUMAB

(pan-i-tu-mu′mab)

Vectibix

Classifications: ANTINEOPLASTIC; BIOLOGICAL RESPONSE MODIFIER; MONOCLONAL ANTIBODY; EPIDERMAL GROWTH FACTOR RECEPTOR (EGFR) INHIBITOR

Therapeutic: ANTINEOPLASTIC

Prototype: Gefitinib

Pregnancy Category: C

P

AVAILABILITY 20 mg/mL solution for injection in 5 mL, 10 mL, and 20 mL vials

ACTION & *THERAPEUTIC EFFECT* Overexpression of epidermal growth factor receptors (EGFRs) occurs in many human cancers, including those of the colon and rectum. EGFRs control the activity of intracellular tyrosine kinases that regulate transcription of DNA molecules involved in cellular growth, survival, motility, proliferation, and transformation. *Panitumumab inhibits upregulation or overexpression of EGFR in cancer cells, decreasing their capacity for cell proliferation, cell survival, and decreasing their invasive capacity and metastases.*

USES Treatment of EGFR-expressing metastatic colorectal carcinoma in patients with disease progression on or following fluoropyrimidine-, oxaliplatin-, and irinotecan-containing chemotherapy regimens.

CONTRAINDICATIONS Pulmonary fibrosis; interstitial lung disease. Use contraception for females of childbearing age; lactation. Safe use in children not established.

CAUTIOUS USE Photosensitivity with drug use; electrolyte imbalances, especially hypomagnesemia, and hypocalcemia; lung disorders; pregnancy (category C).

ROUTE & DOSAGE

Metastatic Colorectal Carcinoma

Adult: **IV** 6 mg/kg q14days

Dosage Adjustments for Infusion Reactions and Dermatologic Reactions

Mild or moderate infusion reactions (Grade 1 or 2): Reduce infusion rate by 50%

Severe infusion reactions (Grade 3 or 4): Discontinue permanently

Intolerable or severe dermatologic toxicity (greater than Grade 3): Withhold drug. If toxicity does not improve to at least grade 2 within 1 mo, permanently discontinue. If toxicity improves to at least grade 2 and patient is symptomatically improved after withholding no more than 2 doses, resume at 50% of original dose. If toxicities recur, discontinue permanently. If toxicities do not recur, subsequent doses may be increased by increments of 25% of original dose until 6 mg/kg is reached.

ADMINISTRATION

Intravenous

PREPARE: **IV Infusion:** Dilute doses up to 1000 mg with NS to a total volume of 100 mL. ▪ Dilute higher doses with NS to a total volume of 150 mL. ▪ Final concentration should not exceed 10 mg/mL. ▪ Mix by gentle inversion and do not shake. Solution will contain small translucent particles that will be removed by filtration during infusion.

ADMINISTER: **IV Infusion:** Infuse doses less than 1000 mg over 60 min. ▪ Infuse doses greater than 1000 mg over 90 min. ▪ Use an infusion pump and a 0.2 or 0.22 micron in-line filter. ▪ Flush the line before/after infusion with NS. ▪ Discontinue infusion immediately if an anaphylactic reaction is suspected (i.e., bronchospasm, fever, chills, hypotension).

▪ Store unopened vials at 2°–8° C (36°–46° F). Protect vials from direct sunlight. ▪ Use diluted infusion solution within 6 h if stored at room temperature, or within 24 h if stored at 2°–8° C (36°– 46° F).

ADVERSE EFFECTS (≥1%) **Body as a Whole:** *Fatigue,* <u>infectious sequelae and septic death</u>, infusion reactions, peripheral edema. **GI:** *Abdominal pain, constipation, diarrhea,* mucosal inflammation, *nausea,* stomatitis, *vomiting*. **Metabolic:** *Hypomagnesemia*. **Respiratory:** *Cough,* pulmonary fibrosis. **Skin:** *Acneiform dermatitis, dry skin, erythema, pruritus, skin exfoliation, skin fissures, nail disorders, paronychia*. **Special Senses:** Conjunctivitis, eye/eyelid irritation, increased lacrimation, ocular hyperemia.

PHARMACOKINETICS Half-Life: 7.5 days.

NURSING IMPLICATIONS

Assessment & Drug Effects

- Monitor for S&S of a severe infusion reaction; check vital signs q30min during infusion and 30 min post-infusion.
- Monitor for and report S&S of dermatologic toxicity such as acne-like dermatitis, pruritus, erythema, rash, skin exfoliation, dry skin, and skin fissures; inflammatory or infectious sequelae in those who experience severe dermatologic toxicities.
- Withhold drug and notify physician for any signs of drug toxicity.
- Lab tests: Periodic serum electrolytes during and for 8 wk following completion of therapy.

Patient & Family Education

- Immediately report any discomfort experienced during and shortly after drug infusion.
- Wear sunscreen and limit sun exposure while receiving panitumumab.
- Report any of the following to a health care provider: Any signs of irritation, inflammation, or infection of the skin, nails, or eyes; shortness of breath or any other breathing difficulty.
- Women of childbearing age should use reliable means of contraception during and for 6 mo after the last dose of panitumumab.

PANTOPRAZOLE SODIUM

(pan-to'pra-zole)

Protonix, Protonix IV

Classifications: GASTRIC PROTON PUMP INHIBITOR; ANTISECRETORY

Therapeutic: ANTIULCER

Prototype: Omeprazole

Pregnancy Category: B

P

AVAILABILITY 20 mg, 40 mg enteric coated tablets; 40 mg injection; 40 mg delayed release oral suspension

ACTION & *THERAPEUTIC EFFECT* Gastric acid pump inhibitor; belongs to a class of antisecretory compounds. Gastric acid secretion is decreased by inhibiting the H^+, K^+-ATPase enzyme system responsible for acid production. *Specifically, suppresses gastric acid secretion by inhibiting the acid (proton H^+) pump in the parietal cells.*

USES Short-term treatment of erosive esophagitis associated with gastroesophageal reflux disease (GERD), hypersecretory disease.
UNLABELED USES Peptic ulcer disease.

CONTRAINDICATIONS Hypersensitivity to pantoprazole or other proton pump inhibitors (PPIs); lactation.
CAUTIOUS USE Mild to severe hepatic insufficiency, cirrhosis; concurrent administration of EDTA-containing products; pregnancy (category B). Safety and effectiveness in children younger than 18 y are not established.

ROUTE & DOSAGE

Erosive Esophagitis

Adult: **PO** 40 mg daily × 8–16 wks **IV** 40 mg daily × 7–10 days

Hypersecretory Disease

Adult: **PO** 40 mg b.i.d. (doses up to 240 mg/day have been used) **IV** 80 mg b.i.d.; adjust based on acid output

Renal Impairment/Hepatic Impairment Dosage Adjustment

Adjustment not needed
Hemodialysis Dosage Adjustment: Drug not removed

ADMINISTRATION

Oral

- Do not crush or break in half. **Must be** swallowed whole.
- Granules for oral suspension should be given 30 min before meals. Granules should be put into apple juice or applesauce, not water.
- *NG tube administration:* Add granules for suspension to a catheter tip syringe. Add 40 mL of apple juice in 10 mL increments to fully suspend granules and ensure that all of the drug is washed into the stomach.
- Store preferably at 20°–25° C (66°–77° F), but room temperature permitted.

Intravenous

PREPARE: **IV Infusion:** Reconstitute each 40 mg vial with 10 mL NS to yield 4 mg/mL. ▪ The required dose of 40 or 80 mg may be further diluted to a **total volume** of 100 mL in D5W, NS, or LR to yield 0.4 mg/mL or 0.8 mg/mL, respectively.

ADMINISTER: **IV Infusion:** Give through a dedicated line or flushed IV line before and after each dose with D5W, NS, or LR. ▪ Give the 4 mg/mL concentration over at least 2 min. ▪ Infuse the 0.4 or 0.8 mg/mL concentration over 15 min.

INCOMPATIBILITIES **Solution/additive:** Solutions containing **zinc.** **Y-site:** **Midazolam, zinc.**

▪ Reconstituted solution may be stored for up to 6 h at 15–30° C (59–86° F) before further dilution. ▪ The diluted 100 mL solution should be infused within 24 h or infused within 24 h of reconstitution.

ADVERSE EFFECTS (≥1%) **GI:** Diarrhea, flatulence, abdominal pain.

P

CNS: Headache, insomnia. **Skin:** Rash.

INTERACTIONS Drug: May decrease absorption of **ampicillin,** IRON SALTS, **itraconazole, ketoconazole;** increases INR with **warfarin. Herbal: Ginkgo** may decrease plasma levels. **Lab Test:** May cause false-positive urine tetrahydrocannabinol (THC) test.

PHARMACOKINETICS Absorption: Well absorbed with 77% bioavailability. **Peak:** 2.4 h. **Distribution:** 98% protein bound. **Metabolism:** In liver (CYP2C19). **Elimination:** 71% in urine, 18% in feces. **Half-Life:** 1 h.

NURSING IMPLICATIONS

Assessment & Drug Effects

- Monitor for and immediately report S&S of angioedema or a severe skin reaction.
- Lab tests: Urea breath test 4–6 wk after completion of therapy.

Patient & Family Education

- Contact physician promptly if any of the following occur: Peeling, blistering, or loosening of skin; skin rash, hives, or itching; swelling of the face, tongue, or lips; difficulty breathing or swallowing.

PAPAVERINE HYDROCHLORIDE

(pa-pav′er-een)

Classification: NONNITRATE VASODILATOR

Therapeutic: VASODILATOR; SMOOTH MUSCLE RELAXANT

Prototype: Hydralazine

Pregnancy Category: C

AVAILABILITY 150 mg sustained release capsule; 30 mg/mL injection

ACTION & *THERAPEUTIC EFFECT* Exerts nonspecific direct spasmolytic effect on smooth muscles unrelated to innervation. Acts directly on myocardium, depresses conduction and irritability, and prolongs refractory period. *Relaxes the smooth muscle of the heart as well as produces relaxation of the vascular smooth muscles.*

USES Primarily for relief of cerebral and peripheral ischemia associated with arterial spasm and MI complicated by arrhythmias. Also visceral spasm as in ureteral, biliary, and GI colic.

UNLABELED USES Impotence, cardiac bypass surgery.

CONTRAINDICATIONS Parenteral use in complete AV block.

CAUTIOUS USE Glaucoma; myocardial depression; glaucoma; QT prolongation, angina pectoris; recent stroke; pregnancy (category C); lactation.

ROUTE & DOSAGE

Cerebral and Peripheral Ischemia

Adult: **PO** 150–300 mg q8–12h
IM/IV 30–120 mg q3h as needed
Child: **IM/IV** 6 mg/kg/day divided into 4 doses

ADMINISTRATION

Oral

- Give with or following meals; give milk or prescribed antacid to reduce possibility of nausea.
- Ensure that sustained release form is not chewed or crushed. **Must be** swallowed whole.

Intramuscular

- Aspirate carefully before injecting IM to avoid inadvertent entry into blood vessel, and administer slowly.

Intravenous

- IV administration to children: Verify correct IV concentration and rate of infusion with physician.

PREPARE: **Direct:** Give undiluted or diluted in an equal volume of sterile water for injection.
ADMINISTER: **Direct:** Give slowly over 1–2 min. AVOID rapid injection.
INCOMPATIBILITIES **Solution/additive:** **Aminophylline, heparin, lactated Ringer's.**

ADVERSE EFFECTS (≥1%) **Body as a Whole:** General discomfort, facial flushing, sweating, weakness, coma. **CNS:** Dizziness, drowsiness, headache, sedation. **CV:** Slight rise in BP, paroxysmal tachycardia, transient ventricular ectopic rhythms, AV block, arrhythmias. **GI:** Nausea, anorexia, constipation, diarrhea, abdominal distress, dry mouth and throat, hepatotoxicity (jaundice, eosinophilia, abnormal liver function tests); with rapid IV administration. **Respiratory:** Increased depth of respiration, respiratory depression, fatal apnea. **Skin:** Pruritus, skin rash. **Special Senses:** Diplopia, nystagmus. **Urogenital:** Priapism.

P

INTERACTIONS Drug: May decrease **levodopa** effectiveness; **morphine** may antagonize smooth muscle relaxation effect of papaverine.

PHARMACOKINETICS Absorption: Readily from GI tract. **Peak:** 1–2 h. **Duration:** 12 h sustained release. **Metabolism:** In liver. **Elimination:** In urine chiefly as metabolites. **Half-Life:** 90 min.

NURSING IMPLICATIONS

Assessment & Drug Effects

- Monitor pulse, respiration, and BP in patients receiving drug parenterally. If significant changes are noted, withhold medication and report promptly to physician.
- Lab tests: Perform liver function and blood tests periodically. Hepatotoxicity (thought to be a hypersensitivity reaction) is reversible with prompt drug withdrawal.

Patient & Family Education

- Notify physician if any adverse effect persists or if GI symptoms, jaundice, or skin rash appear. Liver function tests may be indicated.
- Do not drive or engage in potentially hazardous activities until response to drug is known. Alcohol may increase drowsiness and dizziness.

PAREGORIC (CAMPHORATED OPIUM TINCTURE)

(par-e-gor'ik)

Classifications: ANTIDIARRHEAL; NARCOTIC (OPIATE AGONIST) ANALGESIC
Therapeutic: ANTIDIARRHEAL; NARCOTIC ANALGESIC
Prototype: Loperamide
Pregnancy Category: C
Controlled Substance: Schedule III

AVAILABILITY 2 mg/5 mL liquid

ACTION & *THERAPEUTIC EFFECT* Pharmacologic activity is due to morphine content. Increases smooth muscle tone of GI tract, decreases motility and effective propulsive peristalsis while diminishing digestive secretions. *Delayed transit of intestinal contents results in desiccation of feces and constipation.*

USES Short-term treatment for symptomatic relief of acute diarrhea and abdominal cramps.

CONTRAINDICATIONS Hypersensitivity to opium alkaloids; diarrhea caused by poisons (until eliminated); COPD.

CAUTIOUS USE Asthma; liver disease; GI disease; history of opiate agonist dependence; severe prostatic hypertrophy; pregnancy (category C), lactation.

ROUTE & DOSAGE

Acute Diarrhea

Adult: **PO** 5–10 mL after loose bowel movement, 1–4 times daily if needed
Child: **PO** 0.25–0.5 mL/kg 1–4 times/day

ADMINISTRATION

Oral

- Give paregoric in sufficient water (2 or 3 swallows) to ensure its passage into the stomach (mixture will appear milky).

ADVERSE EFFECTS (≥1%) **GI:** Anorexia, nausea, vomiting, *constipation,* abdominal pain. **Body as a Whole:** Dizziness, faintness, drowsiness, facial flushing, sweating, physical dependence.

INTERACTIONS Drug: Alcohol and other CNS DEPRESSANTS add to CNS effects.

PHARMACOKINETICS Absorption: Readily from GI tract. **Duration:** 4–5 h. **Distribution:** Crosses placenta; distributed into breast milk. **Metabolism:** In liver. **Elimination:** In urine. **Half-Life:** 2–3 h.

NURSING IMPLICATIONS

Assessment & Drug Effects

- Paregoric may worsen the course of infection-associated diarrhea by delaying the elimination of pathogens.
- Be aware that adverse effects are primarily due to morphine content. Paregoric abuse results because of the narcotic content of the drug.
- Assess for fluid and electrolyte imbalance until diarrhea has stopped.

Patient & Family Education

- Adhere strictly to prescribed dosage schedule.
- Maintain bed rest if diarrhea is severe with a high level of fluid loss.
- Replace fluids and electrolytes as needed for diarrhea. Drink warm clear liquids and avoid dairy products, concentrated sweets, and cold drinks until diarrhea stops.
- Observe character and frequency of stools. Discontinue drug as soon as diarrhea is controlled. Report promptly to physician if diarrhea persists more than 3 days, if fever is higher than 38.8° C (102° F), abdominal pain develops, or if mucus or blood is passed.
- Understand that constipation is often a consequence of antidiarrheal treatment and a normal elimination pattern is usually established as dietary intake increases.

PARICALCITOL

(par-i-cal′ci-tol)
Zemplar
Classification: VITAMIN D ANALOG
Therapeutic: VITAMIN D ANALOG
Prototype: Calcitriol
Pregnancy Category: C

AVAILABILITY 2 mcg/mL, 5 mcg/mL vial; 1 mcg, 2 mcg, 4 mcg capsules

ACTION & *THERAPEUTIC EFFECT* Synthetic vitamin D analog that reduces parathyroid hormone (PTH) activity levels in chronic kidney failure (CRF) patients. Lowers serum levels of calcium and phosphate. Decreases the parathyroid hormone as well as bone resorption in some patients. *Effectiveness indicated by iPTH levels less than 1.5–3 times the upper limit of normal.*

USES Prevention and treatment of secondary hyperparathyroidism associated with CRF.

CONTRAINDICATIONS Hypersensitivity to paricalcitol; hypercalcemia; evidence of vitamin D toxicity; concurrent administration of phosphate preparations and vitamin D; children younger than 5 y.

CAUTIOUS USE Severe liver disease; concurrent administration of digitalis; abnormally low levels of PTH; pregnancy (category C), lactation.

ROUTE & DOSAGE

CRF-Associated Secondary Hyperparathyroidism

Adult: **IV** 0.04 mcg/kg–0.1 mcg/kg (max: 0.24 mcg/kg), no more than every other day during dialysis **PO** iPTH less than 500 pg/mL, 1 mcg/day or 2 mcg 3 times/wk; iPTH greater than 500 pg/mL, 2 mcg/day or 4 mcg 3 times/wk

Child (5–17 y): **IV** 0.04 mcg/kg 3 times/wk during dialysis

ADMINISTRATION

Oral

- Give no more frequently than every other day when dosing 3 times/wk.
- Store at 15–30° C (59–86° F).

Intravenous

PREPARE: **Direct:** Give undiluted.

ADMINISTER: **Direct:** Give IV bolus dose anytime during dialysis.

- Store at 25° C (77° F). Discard unused portion of a single dose vial.

ADVERSE EFFECTS (≥1%) **Body as a Whole:** Chills, feeling unwell, fever, flu-like symptoms, sepsis, edema. **CNS:** Lightheadedness. **CV:** Palpitations. **GI:** Dry mouth, <u>GI bleeding</u>, *nausea*, vomiting. **Respiratory:** Pneumonia. **Metabolic:** Hypercalcemia.

INTERACTIONS Drug: Hypercalcemia may increase risk of **digoxin** toxicity; may increase **magnesium** absorption and toxicity in renal failure. **Herbal:** Be cautious of **vitamin D** content in herbal and OTC products.

PHARMACOKINETICS Distribution: Greater than 99% protein bound. **Metabolism:** Via CYP3A4. **Elimination:** Primarily in feces (74%). **Half-Life:** 15 h.

NURSING IMPLICATIONS

Assessment & Drug Effects

- Monitor for S&S of hypercalcemia (see Appendix F).
- Lab tests: Serum calcium and phosphate 2 times a wk during initiation of therapy; then monthly; serum PTH q3mo; periodic serum magnesium, alkaline phosphatase, 24-urinary calcium and phosphate. Increase frequency of lab tests during dosage adjustments.
- Withhold drug and notify physician if hypercalcemia occurs.
- Coadministered drugs: Monitor for digoxin toxicity if serum calcium level is elevated.

Patient & Family Education

- Report immediately any of the following to the physician: Weakness, anorexia, nausea, vomiting, abdominal cramps, diarrhea, muscle or bone pain, or excessive thirst.

- Adhere strictly to dietary regimen of calcium supplementation and phosphorus restriction to ensure successful therapy.
- Avoid excessive use of aluminum-containing compounds such as antacids/vitamins.

PAROMOMYCIN SULFATE (Pr)

(par-oh-moe-mye′sin)

Classifications: AMINOGLYCOSIDE ANTIBIOTIC; AMEBICIDE
Therapeutic: AMEBICIDE
Pregnancy Category: C

AVAILABILITY 250 mg capsules

ACTION & *THERAPEUTIC EFFECT* Aminoglycoside antibiotic with broad spectrum antibacterial activity. *Exerts direct bactericidal and amebicidal action, primarily in lumen of GI tract. Ineffective against extraintestinal amebiasis.*

USES Acute and chronic intestinal amebiasis and to rid bowel of nitrogen-forming bacteria in patients with hepatic coma; used preoperatively to suppress intestinal flora. Also tapeworm infestation.

CONTRAINDICATIONS Aminoglycoside hypersensitivity; intestinal obstruction; impaired kidney function. **CAUTIOUS USE** GI ulceration; renal failure, renal impairment; older adults; myasthenia gravis; parkinsonism; pregnancy (category C).

ROUTE & DOSAGE

Intestinal Amebiasis
Adult/Child: **PO** 25–35 mg/kg divided in 3 doses for 7–10 days

Hepatic Coma
Adult: **PO** 4 g/day in divided doses for 5–10 days

ADMINISTRATION

Oral

- Give after meals to prevent gastric distress.

ADVERSE EFFECTS (≥1%) **CNS:** Headache, vertigo. **GI:** *Diarrhea, abdominal cramps,* steatorrhea, *nausea, vomiting, heartburn,* secondary enterocolitis. **Skin:** Exanthema, rash, pruritus. **Special Senses:** Ototoxicity. **Urogenital:** Nephrotoxicity (in patients with GI inflammation or ulcerations). **Body as a Whole:** Eosinophilia, overgrowth of nonsusceptible organisms.

DIAGNOSTIC TEST INTERFERENCE Prolonged use of paromomycin may cause reduction in ***serum cholesterol.***

INTERACTIONS Drug: May decrease absorption of **cyanocobalamin.**

PHARMACOKINETICS Absorption: Poorly from intact GI tract. **Elimination:** In feces.

NURSING IMPLICATIONS

Assessment & Drug Effects

- Monitor therapeutic effectiveness. Criterion of cure is absence of amoebae in stool specimens examined at weekly intervals for 6 wk after completion of treatment, and thereafter at monthly intervals for 2 y.
- Monitor for appearance of a superinfection during therapy (see Appendix F).
- Lab test: Baseline WBC with differential. Repeat if superinfection is suspected.
- Monitor closely patients with history of GI ulceration for nephrotoxicity and ototoxicity (see Appendix

P

F). Drug absorption can take place through diseased mucosa.

Patient & Family Education

- Do not prepare, process, or serve food until treatment is complete when receiving drug for intestinal amebiasis. Isolation is not required.
- Practice strict personal hygiene, particularly hand washing after defecation and before eating food.

PAROXETINE

(par-ox′e-teen)

Pexeva, Paxil, Paxil CR

Classifications: ANTIDEPRESSANT; SELECTIVE SEROTONIN 5-HT REUPTAKE INHIBITOR (SSRI)

Therapeutic: ANTIDEPRESSANT; SSRI; ANTIANXIETY

Prototype: Fluoxetine

Pregnancy Category: D

AVAILABILITY 10 mg, 20 mg, 30 mg, 40 mg tablets; 12.5 mg, 25 mg, 37.5 mg sustained release tablets; 10 mg/5 mL suspension

P

ACTION & *THERAPEUTIC EFFECT* Antidepressant structurally unrelated to other serotonin 5-HT reuptake inhibitors. Potent and highly selective inhibitor of serotonin reuptake by neurons in CNS. *Efficacious in depression resistant to other antidepressants and in depression complicated by anxiety.*

USES Depression, obsessive-compulsive disorders, panic attacks, excessive social anxiety, generalized anxiety, post-traumatic stress disorder (PTSD), premenstrual dysphoric disorder (PMDD).

UNLABELED USES Diabetic neuropathy, myoclonus, bipolar depression in conjunction with lithium, chronic headache, premature ejaculation, fibromyalgia.

CONTRAINDICATIONS Hypersensitivity to paroxetine; suicidal ideation; concomitant use of MAO inhibitors, alcohol; pregnancy (category D); children or adolescents with major depressive disorder.

CAUTIOUS USE History of mania, suicidal tendencies; anorexia nervosa, ECT therapy; seizure disorder; renal/hepatic impairment, renal failure; history of metabolic disorders; volume-depleted patients, recent MI, unstable cardiac disease; lactation. Safety and efficacy have not been established in children younger than 18 y.

ROUTE & DOSAGE

Depression

Adult: **PO** 10–50 mg/day (max: 80 mg/day); 25 mg sustained release daily in morning, may increase by 12.5 mg (max: 62.5 mg/day); use lower starting doses for patients with renal or hepatic insufficiency and geriatric patients

Geriatric: **PO** Start with 10 mg/day (12.5 mg/day sustained release), [max: 40 mg/day (50 mg/day sustained release)]

Obsessive-Compulsive Disorder

Adult: **PO** 20–60 mg/day

Panic Attacks

Adult: **PO** 40 mg/day

Social Anxiety Disorder

Adult: **PO** 20–60 mg/day

Generalized Anxiety, PTSD

Adult: **PO** Start with 10 mg once daily, may increase by 10 mg/day at weekly intervals if needed to target dose of 40 mg once daily (max: 60 mg/day)

Geriatric: **PO** Start with 10 mg PO once daily, may increase by 10 mg/day at weekly intervals if needed (max: 40 mg/day)

Premenstrual Dysphoric Disorder
Adult: **PO** 12.5 mg once daily (up to 25 mg once daily) throughout the month or daily for 2 wk before menstrual period

Pharmacogenetic Dosage Adjustment
Poor CYP2D6 metabolizers: Start with 65% of dose

ADMINISTRATION

Oral

- Ensure that sustained release form is not chewed or crushed. **Must be** swallowed whole.
- Be aware that at least 14 days should elapse when switching a patient from/to an MAO inhibitor to/from paroxetine.

ADVERSE EFFECTS (≥1%) **CV:** Postural hypotension. **CNS:** *Headache,* tremor, agitation or nervousness, anxiety, paresthesias, dizziness, insomnia, *sedation.* **GI:** *Nausea,* constipation, vomiting, anorexia, diarrhea, dyspepsia, flatulence, increased appetite, taste aversion, *dry mouth.* **Urogenital:** Urinary hesitancy or frequency. **Hepatic:** Isolated reports of elevated liver enzymes. **Special Senses:** Blurred vision. **Skin:** Diaphoresis, rash, pruritus. **Metabolic:** Hyponatremia in older adult. **Body as a Whole:** Bone fracture (in older adults).

INTERACTIONS Drug: Activated charcoal reduces absorption of paroxetine. **Cimetidine** increases paroxetine levels. MAO INHIBITORS, **selegiline** may cause an increased vasopressor response leading to hypertensive crisis or death. **Phenytoin** can cause liver enzyme induction resulting in lower paroxetine levels and shorter half-life. **Warfarin** may increase risk of bleeding and **thioridazine** levels, and prolong QT_c interval leading to heart block; increase **ergotamine** toxicity with **dihydroergotamine, ergotamine.** May reduce the efficacy of **tamoxifen. Herbal: St. John's wort** may cause serotonin syndrome (headache, dizziness, sweating, agitation).

PHARMACOKINETICS Absorption: 99% from GI tract. **Onset:** 2 wk. **Peak:** 5–8 h. **Distribution:** Very lipophilic. 95% protein bound. Distributes into breast milk. **Metabolism:** Extensively in the liver to inactive metabolites via CYP2D6. **Elimination:** Less than 2% is excreted unchanged in urine. 65% of dose appears in urine as metabolites. Metabolites of paroxetine are also excreted in feces, presumably via bile. **Half-Life:** 24 h.

NURSING IMPLICATIONS

Assessment & Drug Effects

- Monitor for worsening of depression or emergence of suicidal ideation. Closely monitor those younger than 18 y for suicidal thinking and behavior.
- Monitor for adverse effects, which include headache, weakness, sedation, dizziness, insomnia; nausea, constipation, or diarrhea; dry mouth; sweating; male ejaculatory disturbance. These occur in more than 10% of all patients and may result in poor compliance with drug regimen.
- Monitor older adult for fluid and sodium imbalances.
- Monitor for significant weight loss.
- Monitor patients with history of mania for reactivation of condition.
- Monitor patients with preexisting cardiovascular disease carefully because paroxetine may adversely affect hemodynamic status.

Patient & Family Education

- Monitor children and adolescents for changes in behavior that may indicate suicidal ideation.
- Use caution when operating hazardous machinery or equipment until response to drug is known.
- Concurrent use of alcohol may increase risk of adverse CNS effects.
- Adaptation to some adverse effects (especially dizziness and nausea) may occur over a period of 4–6 wk.
- Do not stop drug therapy after improvement in emotional status occurs.
- Notify physician of any distressing adverse effects.

PAZOPANIB

(pas-o′pa-nib)
Votrient
Classifications: ANTINEOPLASTIC; TYROSINE KINASE INHIBITOR (TKI)
Therapeutic: ANTINEOPLASTIC; TKI
Prototype: Gefitinib
Pregnancy Category: D

AVAILABILITY 200 mg, 400 mg tablets

ACTION & *THERAPEUTIC EFFECT* A multi-tyrosine kinase inhibitor (TKI) of vascular endothelial growth factor receptor (VEGFR). Overexpression of VEGFR is present in many cancers. *Pazopanib inhibits growth of advanced renal cell carcinoma.*

USES Treatment of advanced renal cell carcinoma

CONTRAINDICATIONS Hepatotoxicity; severe hepatic impairment; ALT elevation greater than 3 × ULN concurrently with bilirubin elevation of greater than 2 × ULN; cerebral or GI bleeding within last 6 mo; uncontrolled hypertension; surgical procedures; pregnancy (category D); lactation. Safety and effectives in pediatric patients have not been established.

CAUTIOUS USE Risk for QT prolongation; risk for or history of thrombotic event; risk for or history of GI perforation or fistula; moderate hepatic impairment; elderly.

ROUTE & DOSAGE

Renal Cell Carcinoma

Adult: **PO** 800 mg once daily at least 1 h prior or 2 h after a meal; reduce to 400 mg once daily if larger dose isn't tolerated or if patient is taking a strong CYP3A4 inhibitor

Hepatic Impairment Dosage Adjustment

Moderate impairment: Reduce dose to 200 mg once daily
Severe impairment: Not recommended for use

ADMINISTRATION

Oral

- Give without food at least 1 h before or 2 h after a meal.
- Ensure that the tablets are swallowed whole. They should not be crushed or chewed.

ADVERSE EFFECTS (≥1%) **Body as a Whole:** Alopecia, *asthenia*, epistaxis, *fatigue*, *hair color changes*. **CNS:** *Headache*. **CV:** Chest pain, *hypertension*, <u>myocardial infarction</u>, QT elevation, <u>transient ischemic attack</u>. **GI:** *Abdominal pain*, *diarrhea*, dyspepsia, *nausea*, rectal hemorrhage, *vomiting*. **Hematologic:** *Leukopenia*, *lymphocytope-*

nia, neutropenia, thrombocytopenia. **Metabolic:** *Alterations in glucose, anorexia, AST and ALT elevation, decreased magnesium, decreased phosphorus, decreased sodium,* decreased weight, *elevated bilirubin,* hypothyroidism, lipase enzyme elevation, proteinuria. **Respiratory:** Hemoptysis. **Skin:** Facial edema, palmar-plantar erythrodysesthesia, rash, skin depigmentation. **Special Senses:** Dysgeusia. **Urogenital:** Hematuria.

INTERACTIONS Drug: Strong INHIBITORS OF CYP3A4 (e.g., **ketoconazole, ritonavir, clarithromycin**) may increase pazopanib levels. INDUCERS OF CYP3A4 (e.g., **rifampin**) may decrease pazopanib levels. Pazopanib may increase the levels of other drugs that require CYP3A4, CYP2D6, or CYP2C8 for their metabolism. **Food: Grapefruit juice** may increase pazopanib levels.

PHARMACOKINETICS Peak: 2–4 h. **Distribution:** Greater than 99% plasma protein bound. **Metabolism:** Hepatic oxidation by CYP3A4. **Elimination:** Primarily fecal. **Half-Life:** 30.9 h.

NURSING IMPLICATIONS

Assessment & Drug Effects

- Monitor BP closely. Consult physician for desired parameters and report promptly BP elevations above desired levels.
- Monitor cardiac status, especially in those at higher risk for QT interval prolongation. ECG monitoring as warranted.
- Lab tests: Baseline LFTs, then q4wk for 4 mo, and periodically thereafter; periodic thyroid function tests, urinalysis for proteinuria; baseline and periodic serum electrolytes.
- Withhold drug and notify physician immediately if ALT exceeds 3 × ULN and bilirubin exceeds 2 × ULN.

Patient & Family Education

- Report promptly any of the following: Unexplained signs of bleeding, jaundice, unusually dark urine, unusual tiredness, or pain the right upper abdomen.
- Do not take OTC drugs, herbs, vitamins or dietary supplements without consulting physician.
- Women of childbearing age should use adequate means of contraception to avoid pregnancy while on this drug.

PEGFILGRASTIM

(peg-fil-gras′tim)

Neulasta

Classifications: HEMATOPOIETIC GROWTH FACTOR; GRANULOCYTE COLONY-STIMULATING FACTOR (G-CSF)

Therapeutic: HEMATOPOIETIC GROWTH FACTOR; G-CSF

Prototype: Filgrastim

Pregnancy Category: C

AVAILABILITY 10 mg/mL injection

ACTION & *THERAPEUTIC EFFECT* Human granulocyte colony-stimulating factor (G-CSF) produced by recombinant DNA. Endogenous G-CSF regulates the production of neutrophils within the bone marrow; primarily affects neutrophil proliferation, differentiation, and selected end-cell functional activity (including enhanced phagocytic activity, antibody-dependent killing, and increased expression of some functions associated with cell-surface antigens). *Increases neutrophil proliferation and differentiation within the bone marrow.*

USES To decrease the incidence of infection, as manifested by febrile neutropenia, in patients with non-myeloid malignancies receiving myelosuppressive anticancer drugs associated with a significant incidence of severe neutropenia with fever; to decrease neutropenia associated with bone marrow transplant; to treat chronic neutropenia.

CONTRAINDICATIONS Hypersensitivity to *E. coli*–derived proteins, 14 days before or 24 h after administration of chemotherapy; myeloid cancers; splenomegaly; ARDS; children weighing less than 45 kg.

CAUTIOUS USE Sickle cell disorders. For use in peripheral blood stem cells (PBSC) mobilization; neutropenic patients with sepsis; leukemia; pregnancy (category C), lactation.

ROUTE & DOSAGE

Neutropenia

Adult (weight greater than 45 kg): **Subcutaneous** 6 mg once per chemotherapy cycle at least 24 h after chemotherapy

ADMINISTRATION

Subcutaneous

- Do not administer pegfilgrastim in the period 14 days before or 24 h after cytotoxic chemotherapy.
- Use only one dose per vial; do not reenter the vial.
- Prior to injection, pegfilgrastim may be allowed to reach room temperature for a maximum of 6 h. Discard any vial left at room temperature for longer than 6 h.
- Aspirate prior to injection to avoid injection into a blood vessel. Inject subcutaneously; do not inject intradermally. Recommended injection sites include outer area of upper arms, abdomen (excluding 2-in. area around navel), front of middle thighs, and upper outer areas of the buttocks.
- Store refrigerated at 2°–8° C (36°–46° F). Do not freeze. Avoid shaking.

ADVERSE EFFECTS (≥1%) **Body as a Whole:** *Bone pain,* hyperuricemia, *fever.* **Hematologic:** Anemia. **GI:** Nausea, anorexia, increased LFTs. **Body as a Whole:** *Bone pain,* hyperuricemia, *fever.*

INTERACTIONS Drug: Can interfere with activity of CYTOTOXIC AGENTS; do not use 14 days before or less than 24 h after CYTOTOXIC AGENTS; **lithium** may increase release of neutrophils.

PHARMACOKINETICS Absorption: Readily absorbed from subcutaneous site. **Half-Life:** 15–80 h.

NURSING IMPLICATIONS

Assessment & Drug Effects

- Lab tests: Obtain a baseline CBC with differential and platelet count prior to administering drug. Obtain CBC twice weekly during therapy to monitor neutrophil count and leukocytosis. Monitor Hct and platelet count regularly.
- Discontinue pegfilgrastim if absolute neutrophil count exceeds 10,000/mm^3 after the chemotherapy-induced nadir. Neutrophil counts should then return to normal.
- Monitor patients with preexisting cardiac conditions closely. MI and arrhythmias have been associated with a small percent of patients receiving pegfilgrastim.
- Monitor temperature q4h. Incidence of infection should be reduced after administration of pegfilgrastim.
- Assess degree of bone pain if present. Consult physician if non-

narcotic analgesics do not provide relief.

Patient & Family Education

- Report bone pain and, if necessary, request analgesics to control pain.
- Note: Proper drug administration and disposal is important. A puncture-resistant container for the disposal of used syringes and needles should be utilized.

PEGINTERFERON ALFA-2A (Pr)

(peg-in-ter-fer′on)

Pegasys

Classifications: BIOLOGICAL RESPONSE MODIFIER; IMMUNOMODULATOR; ALPHA INTERFERON

Therapeutic: ANTIVIRAL; ANTIHEPATITIS

Pregnancy Category: C

AVAILABILITY 180 mcg/mL vials; 180 mcg prefilled syringes

ACTION & *THERAPEUTIC EFFECT* Interferon-stimulated genes modulate processes leading to inhibition of viral replication in infected cells, inhibition of cell proliferation, and immunomodulation. Stimulates production of effector proteins that raise body temperature, and causes reversible decreases in leukocyte and platelet counts. *Induces antiviral effects by activation of macrophages, natural killer cells, and T-cells, thus boosting cellular immunity and suppressing hepatic inflammation and replication of hepatitis C virus.*

USES Chronic hepatitis C with or without **ribavirin** in patients coinfected with HIV; treatment of patients with BHeAg-positive or -negative chronic hepatitis B.

CONTRAINDICATIONS Hypersensitivity to peginterferon alfa-2a or any of its components; severe immunosuppression; autoimmune thyroid diseases (e.g., Graves' disease, thyroiditis); autoimmune hepatitis; dental work; sepsis; *E. coli* hypersensitivity, decompensated hepatic disease prior to or during treatment; in neonates and infants because it contains benzyl alcohol; females of childbearing age; lactation.

CAUTIOUS USE History of neuropsychiatric disorder; alcoholism, substance abuse, bipolar disorder, mania, psychosis; bone marrow suppression; cardiac arrhythmias, history of MI, cardiac disease, heart failure, uncontrolled hypertension; pulmonary disease, including COPD; thyroid dysfunction; diabetes mellitus; older adults; autoimmune disorders; autoimmune hepatitis; ulcerative and hemorrhagic colitis; pancreatitis; pulmonary disorders; HBV or HIV coinfection; retinal disease; renal impairment with creatinine clearance less than 50 mL/min; organ transplant recipients; pregnancy (category C); children younger than 18 y.

ROUTE & DOSAGE

Chronic Hepatitis C

Adult: **Subcutaneous** 180 mcg once weekly × 48 wk, may decrease to 135 mcg once weekly if not tolerated

Renal Impairment Dosage Adjustment

End stage renal disease: Reduce dose to 135 mcg once weekly

Hepatic Impairment Dosage Adjustment

Reduce dose to 90 mcg once weekly if LFTs progressively increase over baseline

P

ADMINISTRATION

Subcutaneous

- Give dose on the same day of each week. Administer subcutaneously in the abdomen or thigh and rotate injection sites.
- Warm refrigerated vial by rolling in hands for about 1 min. Do not use if particulate matter is visible in the vial or product is discolored. Discard any unused portion.
- Withhold drug and notify physician for any of the following: ANC less than 750/mm³ or platelet count less than 50, 000/mm³.
- Store in the refrigerator at 36°–46° F (2°–8° C), do not freeze or shake. Protect from light. Vials are for single use only.

ADVERSE EFFECTS (≥1%) **Body as a Whole:** *Musculoskeletal pain, myalgia, arthralgia, fatigue, inflammation at injection site, flu-like symptoms, rigors, fever,* pain, malaise, asthenia, exacerbation of autoimmune disease. **CNS:** *Headache, depression,* anxiety, *irritability, insomnia, dizziness,* impaired concentration, impaired memory, <u>suicidal ideation, suicide attempt</u>. **GI:** *Nausea, diarrhea, abdominal pain, anorexia,* dry mouth. **Hematologic:** Thrombocytopenia, *neutropenia.* **Skin:** *Alopecia, pruritus,* dermatitis, sweating, rash.

INTERACTIONS Drug: May increase **theophylline** levels; increased risk of fetal defects with **ribavirin;** additive myelosuppression with ANTINEOPLASTICS.

PHARMACOKINETICS Peak: 72–96 h. **Elimination:** 30% in urine. **Half-Life:** 80 h.

NURSING IMPLICATIONS

Assessment & Drug Effects

- Monitor for S&S of hypersensitivity (e.g., angioedema, bronchoconstriction) and, if noted, institute appropriate medical action immediately. Note that transient rashes are not an indication to discontinue treatment.
- Withhold drug and notify physician for any of the following: Severe neuropsychiatric events (e.g., psychosis, hallucinations, suicidal ideation, depression, bipolar disorders and mania), severe neutropenia or thrombocytopenia, abdominal pain accompanied by bloody diarrhea and fever, S&S of pancreatitis, new or worsening ophthalmologic disorders, or any other severe adverse event (see CAUTIOUS USE).
- Monitor respiratory and cardiovascular status; report dyspnea, chest pain, and hypotension immediately; perform baseline and periodic ECG and chest X-ray.
- Lab tests: Baseline and periodic creatinine clearance, uric acid, CBC with differential, platelet count, Hct and Hgb, TSH, ALT, AST, bilirubin, blood glucose; retest CBC with differential, platelet count, Hct and Hgb after 2 wk and other blood chemistries after 4 wk. Serum HCV RNA levels after 24 wk of treatment.
- Baseline and periodic ophthalmology exams are recommended.

Patient & Family Education

- If you miss a drug dose and remember within 2 days of the scheduled dose, take the dose and continue with your regular schedule. If more than 2 days have passed, contact physician for instructions.
- Notify physician immediately for any of the following: Severe depression or suicidal thoughts, severe chest pain, difficulty breathing, changes in vision, unusual bleeding or bruising, bloody diarrhea, high fever, severe stomach or

lower back pain, severe chest pain, development of a new or worsening of a preexisting skin condition.
- Follow up with lab tests; compliance with lab testing is extremely important while taking this drug.
- Do not drive or engage in other potentially hazardous activities until reaction to drug is known.
- Women should use reliable means of contraception while taking this drug and notify physician immediately if they become pregnant.

PEGINTERFERON ALFA-2B

(peg-in-ter-fer'on)
PEG-Intron
Classifications: BIOLOGICAL RESPONSE MODIFIER; IMMUNOMODULATOR; ALPHA INTERFERON
Therapeutic: ANTIVIRAL; ANTIHEPATITIS
Prototype: Peginterferon alfa-2a
Pregnancy Category: C

AVAILABILITY 100 mcg/mL, 160 mcg/mL, 240 mcg/mL, 300 mcg/mL powder for injection

ACTION & *THERAPEUTIC EFFECT* Binds to specific membrane receptors on the cell surface, thereby initiating suppression of cell proliferation, enhanced phagocytic activity of macrophages, augmentation of specific cytotoxic lymphocytes for target cells, and inhibition of viral replication in virus-infected cells. *Induces antiviral effects by activation of macrophages, natural killer cells, and T-cells, thus boosting cellular immunity and suppressing hepatic inflammation and replication of hepatitis C virus.*

USES Chronic hepatitis C.
UNLABELED USES Renal carcinoma.

CONTRAINDICATIONS Hypersensitivity to peginterferon; autoimmune hepatitis; decompensated liver disease; persistently severe or worsening S&S of life-threatening neuropsychiatric, autoimmune, ischemic, or infectious disorders.

CAUTIOUS USE History of neuropsychiatric disorder; bone marrow suppression; ulcerative and hemorrhagic colitis; pulmonary disorders; HBV or HIV coinfection; thyroid dysfunction; diabetes mellitus; cardiovascular disease; autoimmune disorders; pulmonary disease, COPD; retinal disease; renal impairment with creatinine clearance less than 50 mL/min; older adults; pregnancy (category C), lactation. Safety and efficacy in children younger than 18 y are not established.

ROUTE & DOSAGE

Chronic Hepatitis C

Adult: **Subcutaneous** Based on weight and injected once weekly × 1 y: *Weight 37–45 kg,* 40 mcg; *weight 46–56 kg,* 50 mcg; *weight 57–72 kg,* 64 mcg; *weight 73–88 kg,* 80 mcg; *weight 89–106 kg,* 96 mcg; *weight 107–136 kg,* 120 mcg; *weight 137–160 kg,* 150 mcg

ADMINISTRATION

Subcutaneous
- Give dose on the same day of each week.
- Be aware that two Safety Lok™ syringes are provided in the drug package: One for reconstitution and one for injection. Reconstitute with only 0.7 mL of supplied diluent and discard remaining diluent. Enter the vial only once as it does not contain a preservative. Swirl gently to produce a clear, colorless solution. Use solution immediately.

- Serious adverse reactions warrant reduction or discontinuation of dose.
- Store dry vial at 15°–30° C (59°–86° F). If necessary, store reconstituted solution up to 24 h at 2°–8° C (36°–46° F).

ADVERSE EFFECTS (≥1%) **Body as a Whole:** *Musculoskeletal pain, fatigue, inflammation at injection site, flu-like symptoms, rigors, fever, weight loss, viral infection,* pain, malaise, hypertonia. **CNS:** *Headache, depression, anxiety, emotional lability, irritability, insomnia, dizziness.* **GI:** *Nausea, anorexia, diarrhea, abdominal pain,* vomiting, dyspepsia, hepatomegaly. **Endocrine:** Hypothyroidism. **Hematologic:** Thrombocytopenia, neutropenia. **Respiratory:** *Pharyngitis,* sinusitis, cough. **Skin:** *Alopecia, pruritus, dry skin,* sweating, rash, flushing.

INTERACTIONS Drug: May increase **theophylline** levels; additive myelosuppression with ANTINEOPLASTICS; **zidovudine** may increase hematologic toxicity; increase **doxorubicin** toxicity, increase neurotoxicity with **vinblastine; aldesleukin (IL-2)** may potentiate the risk of kidney failure.

PHARMACOKINETICS Peak: 15–44 h. **Duration:** 48–72 h. **Elimination:** 30% in urine. **Half-Life:** 40 h (22–60 h).

NURSING IMPLICATIONS

Assessment & Drug Effects

- Monitor for S&S of hypersensitivity (e.g., angioedema, bronchoconstriction) and, if noted, institute appropriate medical action immediately. Note that transient rashes are not an indication to discontinue treatment.
- Monitor for and report immediately S&S of neuropsychiatric disorders (e.g., psychosis, hallucinations, suicidal ideation, depression).
- Monitor respiratory and cardiovascular status; report dyspnea, chest pain, and hypotension immediately; baseline and periodic ECG and chest X-ray.
- Lab tests: Baseline and periodic creatinine clearance, CBC with differential, platelet count, Hct and Hgb, TSH, ALT, AST, bilirubin, blood glucose; with diabetics or hypertensives. Serum HCV RNA levels are assessed after 24 wk of treatment.
- Withhold drug and notify physician for any of the following: Severe neuropsychiatric events, severe neutropenia or thrombocytopenia, abdominal pain accompanied by bloody diarrhea and fever, S&S of pancreatitis, or any other severe adverse event (see CAUTIOUS USE).
- Baseline and periodic ophthalmology exams are recommended.

Patient & Family Education

- Drink fluids liberally while taking this drug, especially during the initial stages of therapy.
- Learn reasons for withholding drug (see ASSESSMENT & DRUG EFFECTS).
- Use effective means of contraception while taking this drug. Women should not become pregnant.
- Follow up with lab tests; compliance with lab testing is extremely important while taking this drug.

PEGVISOMANT

(peg-vis′o-mant)

Somavert

Classifications: GROWTH HORMONE MODIFIER; GROWTH HORMONE RECEPTOR ANTAGONIST

Therapeutic: GROWTH HORMONE ANTAGONIST

Pregnancy Category: B

Common adverse effects in *italic*, life-threatening effects underlined; generic names in **bold**; classifications in SMALL CAPS; ♣ Canadian drug name; ⓟ Prototype drug

AVAILABILITY 10 mg, 15 mg, 20 mg powder for injection

ACTION & *THERAPEUTIC EFFECT* A growth hormone (GH) receptor antagonist that binds to GH receptors on cell surfaces where it blocks its action and ability to stimulate production of insulin-like growth factor I (IGF-I). *Produces a significant decrease in the level of serum insulin-like growth factor I (IGF-I), the primary mediator of GH effects on body tissues.*

USES Treatment of acromegaly when other treatments have failed or are inappropriate.

CONTRAINDICATIONS Hypersensitivity to pegvisomant or latex.
CAUTIOUS USE Pituitary tumors; diabetes mellitus; hepatic and/or renal impairment; neoplastic disease; elderly; pregnancy (category B); lactation; children.

ROUTE & DOSAGE

Acromegaly
Adult: **Subcutaneous** 40 mg loading dose, then 10 mg once daily. Adjust dose in 5 mg increments, up to 30 mg/day, based on serum IGF-I concentrations.

ADMINISTRATION

Subcutaneous
- Allow vials to reach room temperature, then reconstitute by adding 1 mL of supplied diluent (sterile water for injection) to the vial. Direct diluent against the glass wall of vial, then mix by gently rolling between palms of hands to dissolve. DO NOT SHAKE. ▪ Solution should be clear and colorless. ▪ Use within 6 h of reconstitution.
- Inject subcutaneously and exercise caution not to inject IV.
- Rotate injection sites and do not use any site more than once every 1–2 mo.
- Store vials of powder at 2°–8° C (36°–46° F).

ADVERSE EFFECTS (≥1%) **Body as a Whole:** Asthenia, flu-like syndrome, infection, injection site reactions, back pain, paresthesias, peripheral edema. **CNS:** Dizziness. **CV:** Angina, chest pain, hypertension, MI. **GI:** Elevated liver function tests, diarrhea, nausea, vomiting. **Metabolic:** Hypercholesterolemia, hypoglycemia, and low titer non-neutralizing antigrowth hormone antibodies. **Musculoskeletal:** Arthralgia. **Respiratory:** Sinusitis.

DIAGNOSTIC TEST INTERFERENCE Similar to growth hormone and may cross-react with ***growth hormone assays.*** Do not use these assays to monitor pegvisomant therapy.

INTERACTIONS Drug: OPIATE AGONISTS may lead to higher pegvisomant dosing requirements; may need to decrease doses of **insulin,** ORAL ANTIDIABETIC AGENTS; **octreotide** may affect response.

PHARMACOKINETICS Absorption: 57% from subcutaneous injection site. **Peak:** 33–77 h. **Half-Life:** 6 days.

NURSING IMPLICATIONS

Assessment & Drug Effects
- Montior CV status with baseline and periodic BP measurements.
- Monitor diabetics for loss of glycemic control.
- Withhold drug and notify physician for significant elevation in AST/ALT or S&S of hepatitis.
- Lab tests: IGF-I levels 4–6 wk after initiation of therapy or any

P

dose adjustment, then q6mo after IGF-I levels have normalized; periodic LFTs and lipid profile; frequent blood glucose monitoring, especially if diabetic.

Patient & Family Education

- Report promptly any of the following: Chest pain or tightness, signs of infection (e.g., fever, chills, flu-like symptoms).
- Discontinue drug and notify physician immediately if jaundice appears.
- Do not drive or engage in other hazardous activities until reaction to drug is known.

PEMETREXED

(pe-me-trex′ed)
Alimta
Classifications: ANTINEOPLASTIC; ANTIMETABOLITE, ANTIFOLATE
Therapeutic: ANTINEOPLASTIC
Prototype: Methotrexate
Pregnancy Category: D

P

AVAILABILITY 500 mg powder for injection

ACTION & *THERAPEUTIC EFFECT* Suppresses tumor growth by inhibiting both DNA synthesis and folate metabolism at multiple target enzymes. *Appears to arrest the cell cycle, thus inhibiting tumor growth.*

USES Treatment of malignant pleural mesothelioma that is unresectable or in patients that are not surgery candidates in combination with cisplatin; treatment of locally advanced or metastatic non-small cell lung cancer (NSCLC).

UNLABELED USES Solid tumors, including bladder, breast, colorectal, gastric, head and neck, pancreatic, and renal cell cancers.

CONTRAINDICATIONS Mannitol hypersensitivity; creatinine clearance is less than 45 mL/min, renal failure, moderate or severe renal impairment; active infection; vaccines; children younger than 18 y; pregnancy (category D); lactation.

CAUTIOUS USE Anemia, thrombocytopenia, neutropenia, dental disease; older adults; hepatic disease, hypoalbuminemia, hypovolemia, dehydration, ascites, pleural effusion.

ROUTE & DOSAGE

Malignant Mesothelioma, Non–Small-Cell Lung Cancer

Adult: **IV** 500 mg/m^2 on day 1 of each 21-day cycle

Renal Impairment Dosage Adjustment

Not recommended if CrCl less than 45 mL/min

ADMINISTRATION

Intravenous

Pre-/posttreatment with folic acid, vitamin B_{12}, and dexamethasone are needed to reduce hematologic and gastrointestinal toxicity, and the possibility of severe cutaneous reactions from pemetrexed.

PREPARE: **IV Infusion:** Reconstitute each 500 mg vial with 20 mL of preservative-free NS. ▪ Do not use any other diluent. Swirl gently to dissolve. Each vial will contain 25 mg/mL. ▪ Withdraw the needed amount of reconstituted solution and add to 100 mL of preservative-free NS. ▪ Discard any unused portion.

ADMINISTER: **IV Infusion:** Do NOT give a bolus dose. ▪ Infuse over 10 min.

INCOMPATIBILITIES **Solution/additive:** Solutions containing **cal-**

cium, lactated Ringer's.: Y-site: **Amphotericin B, calcium, cefazolin, cefotaxime, cefotetan, cefoxitin, ceftazidime, chlorpromazine, ciprofloxacin, dobutamine, doxorubicin, doxycycline, droperidol, gemcitabine, gentamicin, irinotecan, metronidazole, minocycline, mitoxantrone, nalbuphine, ondansetron, prochlorperazine, tobramycin, topotecan.**

▪ Store unopened single-use vials at room temperature between 15°–30° C (59°–86° F). ▪ The reconstituted drug is stable for up to 24 h at 2°–8° C (36°–46° F) or at 25° C (77° F).

ADVERSE EFFECTS (≥1%) **Body as a Whole:** *Fatigue, fever,* hypersensitivity reaction, edema, myalgia, arthralgia. **CNS:** Neuropathy, *mood alteration, depression.* **CV:** Chest pain, thromboembolism. **GI:** *Nausea, vomiting, constipation, anorexia, stomatitis, diarrhea,* dehydration, dysphagia, esophagitis, odynophagia, increased LFTs. **Hematologic:** *Neutropenia, leukopenia, anemia, thrombocytopenia.* **Respiratory:** *Dyspnea.* **Skin:** *Rash, desquamation,* alopecia. **Urogenital:** *Increases serum creatinine,* renal failure.

INTERACTIONS Drug: Increased risk of renal toxicity with other nephrotoxic drugs (**acyclovir, adefovir, amphotericin B,** AMINOGLYCOSIDES, **carboplatin, cidofovir, cisplatin, cyclosporine, foscarnet, ganciclovir, sirolimus, tacrolimus, vancomycin**); NSAIDS may increase risk of renal toxicity in patients with preexisting renal insufficiency; may cause additive risk of bleeding with ANTICOAGULANTS, PLATELET INHIBITORS, **aspirin,** THROMBOLYTIC AGENTS.

PHARMACOKINETICS Metabolism: Not extensively. **Elimination:** Primarily in urine. **Half-Life:** 3.5 h.

NURSING IMPLICATIONS

Assessment & Drug Effects

- Withhold drug and notify physician if the absolute neutrophil count (ANC) is less than 1500 cells/mm³ or the platelet count is less than at least 100,000 cells/mm³, or if the CrCl is less than 45 mL/min.
- Lab tests: Baseline and periodic CBC with differential; monitor for nadir and recovery before each dose (on day 8 and 15, respectively, of each cycle); periodic LFTs, serum creatinine and BUN.
- Notify physician for S&S of neuropathy (paresthesia) or thromboembolism.

Patient & Family Education

- Report promptly any of the following to physician: Symptoms of anemia (e.g., chest pain, unusual weakness or tiredness, fainting spells, lightheadedness, shortness of breath); symptoms of poor blood clotting (e.g., bruising; red spots on skin; black, tarry stools; blood in urine); symptoms of infection (e.g., fever or chills, cough, sore throat, pain or difficulty passing urine); symptoms of liver problems (e.g., yellowing of skin).
- Do not take nonsteroidal anti-inflammatory drugs (NSAIDs) without first consulting the physician.

PEMIROLAST POTASSIUM

(pem-ir′o-last po-tass′i-um)
Alamast
Pregnancy Category: C
See Appendix A-1.

P

PENBUTOLOL

(pen-bu'tol-ol)

Levatol

Classifications: BETA-ADRENERGIC ANTAGONIST; ANTIHYPERTENSIVE

Therapeutic: ANTIHYPERTENSIVE

Prototype: Propranolol

Pregnancy Category: C

AVAILABILITY 20 mg tablets

ACTION & *THERAPEUTIC EFFECT* Synthetic $beta_1$- and $beta_2$-adrenergic blocking agent that competes with epinephrine and norepinephrine for available beta receptor sites. Lowers both supine and standing BP in hypertensive patients. Hypotensive effect is associated with decreased cardiac output, suppressed renin activity as well as beta blockage. *Effective in lowering mild to moderate blood pressure.*

USES Mild to moderate hypertension alone or with other antihypertensive agents.

P

CONTRAINDICATIONS Hypersensitivity to penbutolol; clients with cardiogenic shock, acute CHF, sinus bradycardia, second and third degree AV block; bronchial asthma, acute bronchospasm; Raynaund's disease; COPD.

CAUTIOUS USE Cardiac failure; PVD; chronic bronchitis; diabetes; mental depression; myasthenia gravis, cerebrovascular insufficiency, stroke; renal disease; pregnancy (category C), lactation. Safety and effectiveness in children is not established.

ROUTE & DOSAGE

Hypertension

Adult: **PO** 10–20 mg daily, may increase to 40–80 mg/day

ADMINISTRATION

Oral

- Discontinue by reducing the dose gradually over 1 to 2 wk.

ADVERSE EFFECTS (≥1%) **CNS:** Dizziness, fatigue, *headache,* insomnia. **CV:** AV block, bradycardia. **GI:** Nausea, diarrhea, dyspepsia. **Respiratory:** Cough, dyspnea. **Urogenital:** Impotence.

INTERACTIONS Drug: DIURETICS and other HYPOTENSIVE AGENTS increase hypotensive effect; effects of **albuterol, metaproterenol, terbutaline, pirbuterol,** and **penbutolol** are antagonized; NSAIDS blunt hypotensive effect; decreases hypoglycemic effect of **glyburide; amiodarone** increases risk of bradycardia and sinus arrest.

PHARMACOKINETICS Absorption: Readily from GI tract. **Peak:** 2–3 h. **Duration:** 20 h. **Metabolism:** In liver. **Elimination:** In urine. **Half-Life:** 5 h.

NURSING IMPLICATIONS

Assessment & Drug Effects

- Take apical pulse before administering drug. If pulse is below 60, or other established parameter, hold the drug and contact physician.
- Take a BP reading before giving drug, if BP is not stabilized. If systolic pressure is 90 mm Hg or less, hold drug and contact physician.
- Check BP near end of dosage interval or before administration of next dose to evaluate effectiveness.
- Monitor therapeutic effectiveness. Full effectiveness of the drug may not be seen for 4–6 wk.
- Watch for S&S of bronchial constriction. Report promptly and withhold drug.

- Monitor diabetics for loss of glycemic control. Drug suppresses clinical signs of hypoglycemia (e.g., BP changes, increased pulse rate) and may prolong hypoglycemic state.
- Monitor carefully for exacerbation of angina during drug withdrawal.

Patient & Family Education

- Do not discontinue the drug without physician's advice because of the possible exacerbation of ischemic heart disease.
- If diabetic, report persistent S&S of hypoglycemia (see Appendix F) to physician (diabetics).
- Avoid driving or other potentially hazardous activities until response to drug is known.
- Make position changes slowly and avoid prolonged standing. Notify physician if dizziness and light-headedness persist.
- Comply with and do not alter established regimen (i.e., do not omit, increase, or decrease dosage or change dosage interval).
- Avoid prolonged exposure of extremities to cold.
- Avoid excesses of alcohol. Heavy alcohol consumption [i.e., greater than 60 mL (2 oz)/day] may elevate arterial pressure; therefore, to maintain treatment effectiveness, either avoid alcohol or drink moderately (less than 60 mL/day). Consult physician.

PENCICLOVIR

(pen-cy′clo-vir)

Denavir

Classification: ANTIVIRAL

Therapeutic: TOPICAL ANTIVIRAL

Prototype: Acyclovir

Pregnancy Category: B

AVAILABILITY 10 mg/g cream

ACTION & *THERAPEUTIC EFFECT*
Antiviral agent active against herpes simplex virus type 1 (HSV-1) and type 2 (HSV-2). HSV-1 and HSV-2 infected cells phosphorylate penciclovir utilizing viral thymidine kinase. Competes with viral DNA, thus inhibiting both viral DNA synthesis and replication. *Effectiveness is measured in decreased viral load.*

USES Treatment of recurrent herpes labialis (cold sores).

CONTRAINDICATIONS Hypersensitivity to penciclovir or famciclovir, lactation.

CAUTIOUS USE Acyclovir, or related antiviral hypersensitivity; pregnancy (category B). Safety and efficacy in children younger than 12 y have not been established. Safety in immunocompromised patients is not established.

ROUTE & DOSAGE

Cold Sores

Adult: **Topical** Apply q2h while awake × 4 days

ADMINISTRATION

Topical

- Apply as soon as possible after developing lesion.
- Do not apply to mucous membranes or near the eyes.
- Store at or below 30° C (86° F). Do not freeze.

ADVERSE EFFECTS (≥1%) **CNS:** Headache. **Skin:** Erythema.

PHARMACOKINETICS Absorption: Minimally absorbed from cold sore.

NURSING IMPLICATIONS

Assessment & Drug Effects

- Monitor the extent of lesions and treatment effectiveness.

P

Patient & Family Education

- Wash hands before and after application. Avoid contact of drug with eyes.
- Apply sunscreen to lips; may minimize recurrence of lesions.

PENICILLAMINE

(pen-i-sill'a-meen)

Cuprimine, Depen

Classifications: CHELATING AGENT; DISEASE-MODIFIYING ANTIRHEUMATIC DRUG (DMARD)

Therapeutic: CHELATING AGENT; ANTIRHEUMATIC (DMARD)

Pregnancy Category: D

AVAILABILITY 250 mg capsules

ACTION & *THERAPEUTIC EFFECT*
Combines chemically with cystine to form a soluble disulfide complex that prevents stone formation and may even dissolve existing cystic stones. Forms stable soluble chelate with copper, zinc, iron, lead, mercury, and possibly other heavy metals and promotes their excretion in urine. Mechanism of action in rheumatoid arthritis appears to be related to inhibition of collagen formation. *With Wilson's disease, therapeutic effectiveness is indicated by improvement in psychiatric and neurologic symptoms, visual symptoms, and liver function. With rheumatoid arthritis, therapeutic effectiveness is indicated by improvement in grip strength, decrease in stiffness following immobility, reduction of pain, decrease in sedimentation rate and rheumatoid factor.*

USES To promote renal excretion of excess copper in Wilson's disease (hepatolenticular degeneration); active rheumatoid arthritis in patients who have failed to respond to conventional therapy; cystinuria.

UNLABELED USES Scleroderma, primary biliary cirrhosis, porphyria cutanea tarda, lead poisoning.

CONTRAINDICATIONS Hypersensitivity to penicillamine or to any penicillin; history of penicillamine-related aplastic anemia or agranulocytosis; rheumatoid arthritis patients with renal insufficiency or who are pregnant; renal failure; concomitant administration with drugs that can cause severe hematologic or renal reactions (e.g., antimalarials, gold salts); pregnancy (category D), lactation.

CAUTIOUS USE Allergy-prone individuals; diabetes mellitus; renal disease, renal impairment; hepatic impairment, hepatic disease; history of hematologic disease.

ROUTE & DOSAGE

Wilson's Disease

Adult: **PO** 250 mg q.i.d., with 3 doses 1 h a.c. and the last dose at least 2 h after the last meal
Child: **PO** 20 mg/kg/day in 2–4 divided doses (max: 1 g/day)

Cystinuria

Adult: **PO** 250–500 mg q.i.d., with doses adjusted to limit urinary excretion of cystine to 100–200 mg/day
Child: **PO** 30 mg/kg/day in 4 divided doses with doses adjusted to limit urinary excretion of cystine to 100–200 mg/day

Rheumatoid Arthritis (RA)

Adult: **PO** 125–250 mg/day; may increase at 1–3 mo intervals up to 1–1.5 g/day
Child: **PO** 3 mg/kg/day (up to 250 mg/day) × 3 mo, then 6 mg/kg/day (up to 500 mg/day) in 2 divided doses × 3 mo [max:

10 mg/kg/day (up to 1.5 g/day) in 3–4 divided doses]

Lead Poisoning

Child: **PO** 30–40 mg/kg/day in 3–4 divided doses (max: 1.5 g/day); initiate at 25% target dose, gradually increase to full dose over 2–3 wk

Renal Impairment Dosage Adjustment

If CrCl less than 50 mL/min, avoid use

Hemodialysis Dosage Adjustment: In RA patients dose may be decreased from 250 mg daily to 250 mg 3 times/wk

ADMINISTRATION

Oral

- Give on empty stomach (60 min before or 2 h after meals) to avoid absorption of metals in foods by penicillamine.
- Give contents in 15–30 mL of chilled fruit juice or pureed fruit (e.g., applesauce) if patient cannot swallow capsules or tablets.

ADVERSE EFFECTS (≥1%) **Body as a Whole:** Fever, arthralgia, lymphadenopathy, thyroiditis, SLE-like syndrome, thrombophlebitis, hyperpyrexia, myasthenia gravis syndrome, tingling of feet, weakness. **GI:** *Anorexia, nausea, vomiting,* epigastric pain, diarrhea, oral lesions, *reduction or loss of taste perception (particularly salt and sweet), metallic taste,* activation of peptic ulcer, pancreatitis. **Urogenital:** Membranous glomerulopathy, *proteinuria,* hematuria. **Hematologic:** Thrombocytopenia, leukopenia, agranulocytosis, thrombotic thrombocytopenic purpura, hemolytic anemia, aplastic anemia. **Metabolic:** Pyridoxine deficiency. **Skin:** *Generalized pruritus, urticaria,* mammary hyperplasia, alveolitis, skin friability, excessive skin wrinkling, *early and late occurring rashes,* pemphigus-like rash, alopecia. **Special Senses:** Tinnitus, optic neuritis, ptosis.

INTERACTIONS Drug: ANTIMALARIALS, CYTOTOXICS, **gold** therapy may potentiate hematologic and renal adverse effects; **iron** may decrease penicillamine absorption.

PHARMACOKINETICS Absorption: Readily from GI tract. **Peak:** 1 h. **Distribution:** Crosses placenta. **Metabolism:** In liver. **Elimination:** In urine. **Half-Life:** 1–7 h.

NURSING IMPLICATIONS

Assessment & Drug Effects

- Lab tests: Check WBC with differential, direct platelet counts, Hgb, and urinalyses prior to initiation of therapy and every 3 days during the first month of therapy, then every 2 wk thereafter. Perform liver function tests and eye examinations before start of therapy and at least twice yearly thereafter.
- Withhold drug and contact physician if the patient with rheumatoid arthritis develops proteinuria greater than 1 g (some clinicians accept greater than 2 g) or if platelet count drops to less than 100,000/mm³, or platelet count falls below 3500–4000/mm³, or neutropenia occurs.

Patient & Family Education

- Note: Clinical evidence of therapeutic effectiveness may not be apparent until 1–3 mo of drug therapy.
- Take exactly as prescribed. Allergic reactions occur in about one third of patients receiving penicillamine. Temporary interruptions

P

of therapy increase possibility of sensitivity reactions.
- Take temperature nightly during first few months of therapy. Fever is a possible early sign of allergy.
- Observe skin over pressure sites: Knees, elbows, shoulder blades, toes, buttocks. Penicillamine increases risk of skin breakdown.
- Report unusual bruising or bleeding, sore mouth or throat, fever, skin rash, or any other unusual symptoms to physician.

PENICILLIN G BENZATHINE

(pen-i-sill'in)

Bicillin, Bicillin L-A, Permapen

Classifications: BETA-LACTAM ANTIBIOTIC; NATURAL PENICILLIN

Therapeutic: ANTIBIOTIC

Prototype: Penicillin G potassium

Pregnancy Category: B

AVAILABILITY 300,000 units/mL, 600,000 units/mL, 1,200,000 units/2 mL, 2,400,000 units/4 mL injection

ACTION & *THERAPEUTIC EFFECT* Acid-stable, penicillinase-sensitive, long-acting form of natural penicillin. Acts by interfering with synthesis of mucopeptides essential to formation and integrity of the bacterial cell wall. *Effective against many strains of* Staphylococcus aureus, *gram-positive cocci, gram-negative cocci. Also effective against gram-positive bacilli and gram-negative bacilli as well as some strains of* Salmonella, Shigella, *and spirochetes.*

USES Infections highly susceptible to penicillin G, such as streptococcal, pneumococcal, and staphylococcal infections, venereal disease such as syphilis (including early, late, and congenital forms), and nonvenereal diseases (e.g., yaws, bejel, and pinta). Also used in prophylaxis of rheumatic fever.

CONTRAINDICATIONS Hypersensitivity to penicillins; IV administration. **CAUTIOUS USE** History of or suspected allergy (eczema, hives, hay fever, asthma); hypersensitivity to cephalosporins or carbapenems; history of colitis; IBD; renal disease, renal impairment; GI disease; pregnancy (category B); lactation; infants, neonates.

ROUTE & DOSAGE

Mild to Moderate Infections

Adult: **IM** 1,200,000 units once/day

Child: **IM** *Weight greater than 27 kg,* 900,000 units once/day; *weight less than 27 kg,* 300,000–600,000 units once/day

Syphilis

Adult: **IM** Less than 1 y duration: 2,400,000 units as single dose; greater than 1 y duration: 2,400,000 units/wk for 3 wk

Child: **IM** Congenital: 50,000 units/kg as single dose

Prophylaxis for Rheumatic Fever

Adult: **IM** 1,200,000 units q4wk

Child: **IM** 1,200,000 units q3–4wk

ADMINISTRATION

Intramuscular
- Do not confuse penicillin G benzathine with preparations containing procaine penicillin G (e.g., Bicillin C-R).
- Make IM injection deep into upper outer quadrant of buttock. In infants and small children, the pre-

ferred site is the midlateral aspect of the thigh.

- Shake multiple-dose vial vigorously before withdrawing desired IM dose. Shake prepared cartridge unit vigorously before injecting drug.
- Select IM site with care. Injection into or near a major peripheral nerve can result in nerve damage.
- Inadvertent IV administration has resulted in arterial occlusion and cardiac arrest.
- Make injections at a slow steady rate to prevent needle blockage.
- Store at 15°–30° C (59°–86° F).

ADVERSE EFFECTS (≥1%) **Body as a Whole:** *Local pain,* tenderness, and fever associated with IM injection, chills, fever, wheezing, anaphylaxis, neuropathy, nephrotoxicity; superinfections, Jarisch-Herxheimer reaction in patients with syphilis. **Skin:** Pruritus, urticaria, and other skin eruptions. **Hematologic:** Eosinophilia, hemolytic anemia, and other blood abnormalities. Also see PENICILLIN G POTASSIUM.

INTERACTIONS Drug: Probenecid decreases renal elimination; may decrease efficacy of ORAL CONTRACEPTIVES.

PHARMACOKINETICS Absorption: Slowly absorbed from IM site. **Peak:** 12–24 h. **Duration:** 26 days. **Distribution:** Crosses placenta; distributed into breast milk. **Metabolism:** Hydrolyzed to penicillin in body. **Elimination:** Excreted slowly by kidneys.

NURSING IMPLICATIONS

Note: See penicillin G potassium for numerous additional clinical implications.

Assessment & Drug Effects

- Determine history of hypersensitivity reactions to penicillins, cephalosporins, or other allergens prior to initiation of drug therapy.
- Lab tests: Perform C&S tests prior to initiation of therapy and periodically thereafter. Perform periodic renal function tests.

Patient & Family Education

- Report immediately to physician the onset of an allergic reaction. There is great risk of severe and prolonged reactions because drug is absorbed so slowly.

PENICILLIN G POTASSIUM (Pr)

(pen-i-sill'in)

Megacillin ♣

PENICILLIN G SODIUM

Classifications: BETA-LACTAM ANTIBIOTIC; NATURAL PENICILLIN

Therapeutic: ANTIBIOTIC

Pregnancy Category: B

AVAILABILITY 1,000,000 units, 5,000,000 units, 10,000,000 units, 20,000,000 units vials; 1,000,000 units/50 mL, 2,000,000 units/50 mL 3,000,000 units/50 mL injection

ACTION & *THERAPEUTIC EFFECT* Acid-labile, penicillinase-sensitive, natural penicillin. Antimicrobial spectrum is narrow compared to that of semisynthetic penicillins. Acts by interfering with synthesis of mucopeptides essential to formation and integrity of bacterial cell wall. *Highly active against gram-positive cocci (e.g., non-penicillinase-producing* Staphylococcus, Streptococcus *groups) and gram-negative cocci. Also effective against gram-positive bacilli and gram-negative bacilli as well as some strains of* Salmonella *and* Shigella *and spirochetes.*

USES Moderate to severe systemic infections caused by penicillin-sensitive microorganisms. Certain staphylococcal infections; streptococcal infections. Also used as prophylaxis in patients with rheumatic or congenital heart disease. Since oral preparations are absorbed erratically and thus **must be** given in comparatively high doses, this route is generally used only for mild or stabilized infections or long-term prophylaxis.

CONTRAINDICATIONS Hypersensitivity to any of the penicillins or corn; administration of oral drug to patients with severe infections; nausea, vomiting, hypermotility, gastric dilatation; cardiospasm; viral infections; patients on sodium restriction.
CAUTIOUS USE History of or suspected allergy (asthma, eczema, hay fever, hives); history of allergy to cephalosporins; GI disorders; kidney or liver dysfunction, electrolyte imbalance; renal disease or renal impairment; myasthenia gravis, epilepsy, neonates, young infants; pregnancy (category B). Use during lactation may lead to sensitization of infants.

P

ROUTE & DOSAGE

Moderate to Severe Infections
Adult: **IV/IM** 2–24 million units divided q4h
Child: **IV/IM** 250,000–400,000 units/kg divided q4h

ADMINISTRATION

Note: Check whether physician has prescribed penicillin G potassium or sodium.

Intramuscular
- Do not use the 20,000,000 unit dosage form for IM injection.
- Reconstitute for IM: Loosen powder by shaking bottle before adding diluent (sterile water for injection or sterile NS). Keep the total volume to be injected small. Solutions containing up to 100,000 units/mL cause the least discomfort. Adding 10 mL diluent to the 1,000,000 unit vial = 100,000 units/mL. Shake well to dissolve.
- Select IM site carefully. IM injection is made deep into a large muscle mass. Inject slowly. Rotate injection sites.

Intravenous

PREPARE: **Intermittent/Continuous:** Reconstitute as for IM injection then withdraw the required dose and add to 100–1000 mL of D5W or NS IV solution, depending on length of each infusion.
ADMINISTER: **Intermittent:** *Adults:* Give over at least 1 h; *Infants and Children:* Give over 15–30 min. **Continuous:** Give at a rate required to infuse the daily dose in 24 h. ▪ With high doses, IV penicillin G should be administered slowly (usually over 24 h) to prevent electrolyte imbalance from potassium or sodium content. ▪ Physician will often prescribe specific flow rate.
INCOMPATIBILITIES **Solution/additive:** **Dextran 40, fat emulsion, aminophylline, amphotericin B, cephalothin, chlorpromazine, dopamine, hydroxyzine, metaraminol, metoclopramide, pentobarbital, prochlorperazine, promazine, sodium bicarbonate,** TETRACYCLINES, **thiopental.**

▪ Store dry powder (for parenteral use) at room temperature. After reconstitution (initial dilution), store solutions for 1 wk under refrigeration. ▪ Intravenous infusion solutions containing penicillin G are stable at room temperature for at least 24 h.

ADVERSE EFFECTS (≥1%) **Body as a Whole:** Coughing, sneezing, feeling of uneasiness; systemic anaphylaxis, fever, widespread increase in capillary permeability and vasodilation with resulting edema (mouth, tongue, pharynx, larynx), laryngospasm, malaise, serum sickness (fever, malaise, pruritus, urticaria, lymphadenopathy, arthralgia, angioedema of face and extremities, neuritis prostration, eosinophilia), SLE-like syndrome, Injection site reactions (pain, inflammation, abscess, phlebitis), superinfections (especially with *Candida* and gram-negative bacteria), neuromuscular irritability (twitching, lethargy, confusion, stupor, hyperreflexia, multifocal myoclonus, localized or generalized seizures, coma). **CV:** Hypotension, circulatory collapse, cardiac arrhythmias, cardiac arrest. **GI:** Vomiting, diarrhea, severe abdominal cramps, nausea, epigastric distress, diarrhea, flatulence, dark discoloration of tongue, sore mouth or tongue. **Urogenital:** Interstitial nephritis, Loeffler's syndrome, vasculitis. **Hematologic:** Hemolytic anemia, thrombocytopenia. **Metabolic:** Hyperkalemia (penicillin G potassium); hypokalemia, alkalosis, hypernatremia, CHF (penicillin G sodium). **Respiratory:** Bronchospasm, asthma. **Skin:** Itchy palms or axilla, pruritus, *urticaria,* flushed skin, *delayed skin rashes* ranging from urticaria to exfoliative dermatitis, Stevens-Johnson syndrome, fixed-drug eruptions, contact dermatitis.

DIAGNOSTIC TEST INTERFERENCE ***Blood grouping and compatibility tests:*** Possible interference associated with penicillin doses greater than 20 million units daily. ***Urine glucose:*** Massive doses of penicillin may cause false-positive test results with ***Benedict's solution*** and possibly ***Clinitest*** but not with ***glucose oxidase methods*** (e.g., ***Clinistix, Diastix, TesTape***). ***Urine protein:*** Massive doses of penicillin can produce false-positive results when turbidity measures are used (e.g., ***acetic acid*** and ***heat, sulfo-salicylic acid***); ***Ames reagent*** reportedly not affected. ***Urinary PSP excretion tests:*** False decrease in urinary excretion of PSP. ***Urinary steroids:*** Large IV doses of penicillin may interfere with accurate measurement of ***urinary 17-OHCS*** (***Glenn-Nelson technique*** not affected).

INTERACTIONS Drug: Probenecid decreases renal elimination; penicillin G may decrease efficacy of ORAL CONTRACEPTIVES; **colestipol** decreases penicillin absorption; POTASSIUM-SPARING DIURETICS may cause hyperkalemia with penicillin G potassium. **Food:** Food increases breakdown in stomach.

PHARMACOKINETICS Peak: 15–30 min IM. **Distribution:** Widely distributed; good CSF concentrations with inflamed meninges; crosses placenta; distributed in breast milk. **Metabolism:** 16–30% metabolized. **Elimination:** 60% in urine within 6 h. **Half-Life:** 0.4–0.9 h.

NURSING IMPLICATIONS

Assessment & Drug Effects

- Obtain an exact history of patient's previous exposure and sensitivity to penicillins and cephalosporins and other allergic reactions of any kind prior to treatment with penicillin.
- Hypersensitivity reactions are more likely to occur with parenteral penicillin than with the oral drug. Skin rash is the most common type al-

P

lergic reaction and should be reported promptly to physician.

- Lab tests: Perform C&S tests prior to initiation of therapy; treatment may be started before results are known. Evaluate renal, hepatic, and hematologic systems at regular intervals in patients on high-dose therapy. Additionally, check electrolyte balance periodically in patients receiving high parenteral doses.
- Observe all patients closely for at least 30 min following administration of parenteral penicillin. The rapid appearance of a red flare or wheal at the IM or IV injection site is a possible sign of sensitivity. Also suspect an allergic reaction if patient becomes irritable, has nausea and vomiting, breathing difficulty, or sudden fever. Report any of the foregoing to physician immediately.
- Be aware that reactions to penicillin may be rapid in onset or may not appear for days or weeks. Symptoms usually disappear fairly quickly once drug is stopped, but in some patients may persist for 5 days or more.
- Allergy to penicillin is unpredictable. It has occurred in patients with a negative history of penicillin allergy and also in patients with no known prior contact with penicillin (sensitization may have occurred from penicillin used commercially in foods and beverages).
- Be alert for neuromuscular irritability in patients receiving parenteral penicillin in excess of 20 million units/day who have renal insufficiency, hyponatremia, or underlying CNS disease, notably myasthenia gravis or epilepsy. Seizure precautions are indicated. Symptoms usually begin with twitching, especially of face and extremities.
- Monitor I&O, particularly in patients receiving high parenteral doses. Report oliguria, hematuria, and changes in I&O ratio. Consult physician regarding optimum fluid intake. Dehydration increases the concentration of drug in kidneys and can cause renal irritation and damage.
- Observe closely for signs of toxicity, especially in neonates, young infants, the older adult, and patients with impaired kidney function receiving high-dose penicillin therapy. Urinary excretion of penicillin is significantly delayed in these patients.
- Observe patients on high-dose therapy closely for evidence of bleeding, and bleeding time should be monitored. (In high doses, penicillin interferes with platelet aggregation.)

Patient & Family Education

- Understand that hypersensitivity reaction may be delayed. Report skin rashes, itching, fever, malaise, and other signs of a delayed reaction to physician immediately (see ADVERSE EFFECTS).
- Notify physician if following symptoms appear when taking penicillin for treatment of syphilis: Headache, chills, fever, myalgia, arthralgia, malaise, and worsening of syphilitic skin lesions. Reaction is usually self-limiting. Check with physician if symptoms do not improve within a few days or get worse.
- Report S&S of superinfection (see Appendix F).

PENICILLIN G PROCAINE

(pen-i-sill'in)

Classifications: BETA-LACTAM ANTIBIOTIC; NATURAL PENICILLIN
Therapeutic: ANTIBIOTIC
Prototype: Penicillin G potassium

Pregnancy Category: B

AVAILABILITY 600,000 units/mL, 300,000 units/mL

ACTION & *THERAPEUTIC EFFECT* Long-acting form of penicillin G. The procaine salt has low solubility and thus creates a tissue depot from which penicillin is slowly absorbed. Onset of action is slower and produces lower serum concentrations than penicillin G potassium, but has longer duration of action. It inhibits the final stage of bacterial cell wall synthesis by binding to specific penicillin-binding proteins (PBPs) located in the bacterial cell wall. This results in cell death of bacteria. *Same actions and antibacterial activity as for penicillin G potassium and is similarly inactivated by penicillinase and gastric acid.*

USES Moderately severe infections due to penicillin G-sensitive microorganisms that are susceptible to low but prolonged serum penicillin concentrations. Commonly, uncomplicated pneumococcal pneumonia, uncomplicated gonorrheal infections, and all stages of syphilis. May be used concomitantly with penicillin G or probenecid when more rapid action and higher blood levels are indicated.

CONTRAINDICATIONS History of hypersensitivity to any of the penicillins, or to procaine or any other "caine-type" local anesthetic; lactation.

CAUTIOUS USE History of or suspected allergy, hypersensitivity to cephalosporins, carbapenem; asthmatics; GI disease, renal disease; renal impairment; pregnancy (category B); infants, neonates.

ROUTE & DOSAGE

Moderate to Severe Infections

Adult: **IM** 600,000–1,200,000 units once/day
Child: **IM** 300,000 units once/day

Pneumococcal Pneumonia

Adult: **IM** 600,000 units q12h

Uncomplicated Gonorrhea

Adult: **IM** 4,800,000 units divided between 2 different injection sites at one visit preceded by 1 g of probenecid 30 min before injections

Syphilis

Adult: **IM** Primary, secondary, latent: 600,000 units/day for 8 days; late latent, tertiary, neurosyphilis: 600,000 units/day for 10–15 days
Child: **IM** 500,000–1,000,000 units/m^2 once/day

ADMINISTRATION

Intramuscular

- Shake multiple-dose vial thoroughly before withdrawing medication to ensure uniform suspension of drug.
- Use 20-gauge needle to avoid clogging.
- Give IM deep into upper outer quadrant of gluteus muscle; in infants and small children midlateral aspect of thigh is generally preferred. Select IM site carefully. Accidental injection into or near major peripheral nerves and blood vessels can cause neurovascular damage.
- Aspirate carefully before injecting drug to avoid entry into a blood vessel. Inadvertent IV administration reportedly has resulted in pulmonary infarcts and death.

P

- Inject drug at a slow, but steady rate to prevent needle blockage. Give in two sites if the dose is very large. Rotate injection sites.

ADVERSE EFFECTS (≥1%) **Body as a Whole:** Procaine toxicity [e.g., mental disturbances (anxiety, confusion, depression, combativeness, hallucinations), expressed fear of impending death, weakness, dizziness, headache, tinnitus, unusual tastes, palpitation, changes in pulse rate and BP, seizures]. Also see PENICILLIN G POTASSIUM.

INTERACTIONS Drug: Probenecid decreases renal elimination; may decrease efficacy of ORAL CONTRACEPTIVES.

PHARMACOKINETICS Absorption: Slowly from IM site. **Peak:** 1–3 h. **Duration:** 15–20 h. **Distribution:** Crosses placenta; distributed into breast milk. **Metabolism:** Hydrolyzed to penicillin in body. **Elimination:** By kidneys within 24–36 h.

P

NURSING IMPLICATIONS

Assessment & Drug Effects

- Obtain an exact history of patient's previous exposure and sensitivity to penicillins, cephalosporins, and to procaine, and other allergic reactions of any kind prior to treatment.
- Test patient by injecting 0.1 mL of 1–2% procaine hydrochloride intradermally if sensitivity is suspected. Appearance of a wheal, flare, or eruption indicates procaine sensitivity.
- Be alert to the possibility of a transient toxic reaction to procaine, particularly when large single doses are administered. The reaction manifested by mental disturbance and other symptoms (see ADVERSE EFFECTS) occurs almost immediately and usually subsides after 15–30 min.

Patient & Family Education

- Report any skin reaction at the site of injection.
- Report onset of rash, itching, fever, chills or other symptoms of an allergic reaction to physician.

PENICILLIN V

PENICILLIN V POTASSIUM

(pen-i-sill'in)

Apo-Pen-VK ✦, Beepen VK, Betapen-VK, Ledercillin VK, Nadopen-V ✦, Novopen-VK ✦, Penicillin VK, Pen-V, Pen-Vee K, Robicillin VK, V-Cillin K, Veetids

Classifications: BETA-LACTAM ANTIBIOTIC; NATURAL PENICILLIN
Therapeutic: ANTIBIOTIC
Prototype: Penicillin G potassium
Pregnancy Category: B

AVAILABILITY 250 mg, 500 mg tablets; 125 mg/5 mL, 250 mg/5 mL suspension

ACTION & *THERAPEUTIC EFFECT* Acid-stable analog of penicillin G with which it shares actions. It binds with the necessary penicillin-binding proteins (PBP) in cell wall of bacteria interfering with cell wall synthesis and resulting in cell lysis. *Penicillin V is bactericidal and is inactivated by penicillinase. Less active than penicillin G against gonococci and other gram-negative microorganisms.*

USES Mild to moderate infections caused by susceptible *Streptococci, Pneumococci,* and *Staphylococci*. Also Vincent's infection and as prophylaxis in rheumatic fever.

CONTRAINDICATIONS Hypersensitivity to any penicillin; lactation.
CAUTIOUS USE History of or suspected allergy (hay fever, asthma, hives, eczema) reactions; hypersensitivity to cephalosporins, beta-lactamase inhibitors, or carbapenem; GI disease; cystic fibrosis; renal impairment, hepatic impairment; pregnancy (category B).

ROUTE & DOSAGE

Mild to Moderate Infections
Adult: **PO** 125–500 mg q6h
Child (younger than 12 y): **PO** 15–50 mg/kg/day in 3–6 divided doses

Endocarditis Prophylaxis
Adult: **PO** 2 g 30–60 min before procedure, then 500 mg q6h for 8 doses
Child (weight less than 30 kg): **PO** 1 g 30–60 min before procedure, then 250 mg q6h for 8 doses

ADMINISTRATION

Oral
- Give after a meal rather than on an empty stomach; drug may be better absorbed and result in higher blood levels.
- Shake well before pouring. Following reconstitution, oral solution is stable for 14 days under refrigeration.

ADVERSE EFFECTS (≥1%) **Body as a Whole:** Nausea, vomiting, *diarrhea,* epigastric distress. *Hypersensitivity reactions* (e.g., flushing, pruritus, urticaria or other skin eruptions, eosinophilia, anaphylaxis; hemolytic anemia, leukopenia, thrombocytopenia, neuropathy, superinfections).

INTERACTIONS Drug: Probenecid decreases renal elimination; may decrease efficacy of ORAL CONTRACEPTIVES; **colestipol** decreases absorption. **Food:** Food increases breakdown in stomach.

PHARMACOKINETICS Absorption: 60–73% absorbed from GI tract. **Peak:** 30–60 min. **Duration:** 6 h. **Distribution:** Highest levels in kidneys; crosses placenta; distributed into breast milk. **Elimination:** In urine. **Half-Life:** 30 min.

NURSING IMPLICATIONS

Note: See penicillin G potassium for numerous additional nursing implications.

Assessment & Drug Effects
- Obtain careful history concerning hypersensitivity reactions to penicillins, cephalosporins, and other allergens before therapy begins.
- Lab tests: Perform C&S tests prior to initiation and at regular intervals throughout therapy. Evaluate renal, hepatic, and hematologic systems at regular intervals in patients receiving prolonged therapy.

Patient & Family Education
- Take penicillin V around the clock at specific intervals to maintain a constant blood level.
- Do not miss any doses and continue taking medication until it is all gone unless otherwise directed by the physician.
- Discontinue medication and promptly report to physician the onset of hypersensitivity reactions and superinfections (see Appendix F).
- Use specially marked measuring device to ensure accurate doses of oral liquid preparation.

PENTAMIDINE ISETHIONATE
(pen-tam'i-deen)

Nebupent, Pentacarinat ♣, Pentam 300
Classification: ANTIPROTOZOAL
Therapeutic: ANTIPROTOZOAL
Pregnancy Category: C

AVAILABILITY 300 mg injection; 300 mg aerosol

ACTION & *THERAPEUTIC EFFECT* Aromatic diamide antiprotozoal drug that appears to block parasite reproduction by interfering with nucleotide (DNA, RNA), phospholipid, and protein synthesis. *Effective against the protozoan parasite* Pneumocystis carinii *in AIDS patients.*

USES *P. carinii* pneumonia (PCP).
UNLABELED USES African trypanosomiasis and visceral leishmaniasis. (Drug supplied for the latter uses is through the Centers for Disease Control and Prevention, Atlanta, GA.)

CONTRAINDICATIONS QT prolongation, history of torsades de pointes; lactation.
CAUTIOUS USE Hypertension, hypotension; hyperglycemia; pancreatitis; hypoglycemia; hypocalcemia; blood dyscrasias; liver or kidney dysfunction; diabetes mellitus; pancreatitis; asthma; cardiac arrhythmias; pregnancy (category C).

P

ROUTE & DOSAGE

Treatment of *Pneumocystis carinii* Pneumonia

Adult/Child: **IM/IV** 4 mg/kg/day for 14–21 days; infuse IV over 60 min

Prophylaxis of *Pneumocystis carinii* Pneumonia

Adult: **Inhaled** 300 mg per nebulizer q3–4wk
Child: **IV/IM** 4 mg/kg monthly

ADMINISTRATION

Inhaled
- Reconstitute contents of one vial in 6 mL sterile water (not saline) and administer using nebulizer.
- Do not mix with any other drug.

Intramuscular
- Dissolve contents of 1 vial (300 mg) in 3 mL sterile water for injection.
- Give deep IM into a large muscle.
- The IM injection is painful and frequently causes local reactions (pain, indurations, swelling). Select alternate sites for daily doses and institute local treatment if indicated.

Intravenous

PREPARE: **IV Infusion:** Dissolve contents of 1 vial in 3–5 mL sterile water for injection or D5W. ▪ Further dilute in 50–250 mL of D5W.
ADMINISTER: **IV Infusion:** Give over 60 min.
INCOMPATIBILITIES **Y-site: Aldesleukin,** CEPHALOSPORINS, **fluconazole, foscarnet, linezolid.**

- Note: IV solutions are stable at room temperature for up to 24 h. Protect solution from light.

ADVERSE EFFECTS (≥1%) **CNS:** Confusion, hallucinations, neuralgia, dizziness, sweating. **CV:** Sudden, severe hypotension, cardiac arrhythmias, ventricular tachycardia, phlebitis. **GI:** Anorexia, nausea, vomiting, pancreatitis, unpleasant taste. **Urogenital:** Acute kidney failure. **Hematologic:** Leukopenia, thrombocytopenia, anemia. **Metabolic:** Hypoglycemia, hypocalcemia, *hyperkalemia.* **Respiratory:** *Cough, bronchospasm,* laryngitis, shortness of breath, chest pain, pneumothorax. **Skin:** Stevens-Johnson syndrome, facial flush (with IV injection), *local reactions at injection site.*

INTERACTIONS Drug: AMINOGLYCOSIDES, **amphotericin B, cidofovir, cisplatin, ganciclovir, cyclosporine, vancomycin,** other nephrotoxic drugs increase risk of nephrotoxicity.

PHARMACOKINETICS Absorption: Readily after IM injection. **Distribution:** Leaves bloodstream rapidly to bind extensively to body tissues. **Elimination:** 50–66% in urine within 6 h; small amounts found in urine for as long as 6–8 wk. **Half-Life:** 6.5–13.2 h.

NURSING IMPLICATIONS

Assessment & Drug Effects

- Monitor BP and HR continuously during the infusion, every half hour for 2 h thereafter, and then every 4 h until BP stablizes. Sudden severe hypotension may develop after a single dose. Place patient in supine position while receiving the drug.
- Lab tests: Monitor periodically serum electrolytes, renal function, CBC with differential, platelet count, and blood glucose.
- Measure and record I&O ratio and pattern.
- Be alert and report promptly S&S of impending kidney dysfunction (e.g., changed I&O ratio, oliguria, edema).
- Characteristics of pneumonia in the immunocompromised patient include constant fever, scanty (if any) sputum, dyspnea, tachypnea, and cyanosis.
- Monitor temperature changes and institute measures to lower the temperature as indicated. Fever is a constant symptom in *P. carinii* pneumonia, but may be rapidly elevated [as high as 40° C (104° F)] shortly after drug infusion.

Patient & Family Education

- Report promptly to physician increasing respiratory difficulty.
- Monitor blood glucose for loss of glycemic control if diabetic.
- Report any unusual bruising or bleeding. Avoid using aspirin or other NSAIDs.
- Increase fluid intake (if not contraindicated) to 2–3 qt (L) per day.

PENTAZOCINE HYDROCHLORIDE (Pr)

(pen-taz′oh-seen)

Talwin

Classifications: NARCOTIC (OPIATE AGONIST-ANTAGONIST); ANALGESIC

Therapeutic: NARCOTIC ANALGESIC

Pregnancy Category: C

Controlled Substance: Schedule IV

AVAILABILITY 30 mg/mL injection

ACTION & *THERAPEUTIC EFFECT* Synthetic analgesic with potency approximately one-third that of morphine. Opiates exert their effects by stimulating specific opiate receptors that produce analgesia, respiratory depression, and euphoria as well as physical dependence. *Effective for moderate to severe pain relief. Acts as weak narcotic antagonist and has sedative properties.*

USES Relief of moderate to severe pain; also used for preoperative analgesia or sedation, and as supplement to surgical anesthesia.

CONTRAINDICATIONS Hypersensitivity to sulfite; head injury, increased intracranial pressure; seizures; emotionally unstable patients, or history of drug abuse; pregnancy (other than labor). Safe use in children younger than 12 y is not established.

CAUTIOUS USE Impaired kidney or liver function; cardiac disease; COPD, asthmas, respiratory depression; GI obstruction; biliary surgery; patients with MI who have nausea and vomiting; pregnancy (category C), lactation.

ROUTE & DOSAGE

Moderate to Severe Pain (Excluding Patients in Labor)

Adult: **IM/IV/Subcutaneous** 30–60 mg q3–4h (max: 360 mg/day)
Child: **IM** 15–30 mg

Women in Labor

Adult: **IM** 20–30 mg; 20 mg may be repeated 1 or 2 times at 2–3 h intervals

Renal Impairment Dosage Adjustment

CrCl 10–50 mL/min: Give 75% of dose; less than 10 mL/min: Give 50% of dose

ADMINISTRATION

Subcutaneous/Intramuscular

- IM is preferred to subcutaneous route when frequent injections over an extended period are required.
- Observe injection sites daily for signs of irritation or inflammation.

Intravenous

PREPARE: **Direct:** Give undiluted or diluted with 1 mL sterile water for injection for each 5 mg.
ADMINISTER: **Direct:** Give slowly at a rate of 5 mg over 60 sec.
INCOMPATIBILITIES **Solution/additive:** **Aminophylline,** BARBITURATES, **sodium bicarbonate, glycopyrrolate, heparin, nafcillin. Y-site: Nafcillin.**

ADVERSE EFFECTS (≥1%) **Body as a Whole:** Flushing, allergic reactions, <u>shock</u>. **CNS:** *Drowsiness,* sweating, *dizziness, lightheadedness, euphoria,* psychotomimetic effects, confusion, anxiety, hallucinations, disturbed dreams, bizarre thoughts, euphoria and other mood alterations. **CV:** Hypertension, palpitation, tachycardia. **GI:** *Nausea, vomiting,* constipation, dry mouth, alterations of taste. **Urogenital:** Urinary retention. **Respiratory:** <u>Respiratory depression</u>. **Skin:** Injection-site reactions (induration, nodule formation, sloughing, sclerosis, cutaneous depression), rash, pruritus. **Special Senses:** Visual disturbances.

INTERACTIONS Drug: Alcohol and other CNS DEPRESSANTS add to CNS depression; NARCOTIC ANALGESICS may precipitate narcotic withdrawal syndrome.

PHARMACOKINETICS Onset: 15 min IM, Subcutaneous; 2–3 min IV. **Peak:** 1 h IM, 15 min IV. **Duration:** 3 h IM, 1 h IV. **Distribution:** Crosses placenta. **Metabolism:** Extensively in liver. **Elimination:** Primarily in urine; small amount in feces. **Half-Life:** 2–3 h.

NURSING IMPLICATIONS

Assessment & Drug Effects

- Monitor therapeutic effect. Tolerance to analgesic effect sometimes occurs. Psychologic and physical dependence have been reported in patients with history of drug abuse, but rarely in patients without such history. Addiction liability matches that of codeine.
- Monitor vital signs and assess for respiratory depression. Keep supine to minimize adverse efffects.

- Monitor drug-induced CNS depression.
- Be aware that pentazocine may produce acute withdrawal symptoms in some patients who have been receiving opioids on a regular basis.
- Monitor I&O as drug may cause urinary retention.

Patient & Family Education

- Avoid driving and other potentially hazardous activities until response to drug is known.
- Do not discontinue drug abruptly following extended use; may result in chills, abdominal and muscle cramps, yawning, runny nose, tearing, itching, restlessness, anxiety, drug-seeking behavior.

PENTOBARBITAL

(pen-toe-bar′bi-tal)

PENTOBARBITAL SODIUM

Nembutal Sodium, Novopentobarb ♣

Classifications: ANXIOLYTIC; SEDATIVE-HYPNOTIC; BARBITURATE; ANTICONVULSANT
Therapeutic: ANTIANXIETY; SEDATIVE-HYPNOTIC; ANTICONVULSANT
Prototype: Secobarbital
Pregnancy Category: D
Controlled Substance: Schedule II

AVAILABILITY 50 mg/mL injection

ACTION & *THERAPEUTIC EFFECT*
Short-acting barbiturate with anticonvulsant properties. Potent respiratory depressant. Initially, barbiturates suppress REM sleep, but with chronic therapy REM sleep returns to normal. *Effective as a sedative and hypnotic and anticonvulsant.*

USES Sedative or hypnotic for preanesthetic medication, induction of general anesthesia, adjunct in manipulative or diagnostic procedures, and emergency control of acute convulsions.

CONTRAINDICATIONS History of sensitivity to barbiturates; parturition, fetal immaturity, uncontrolled pain; ethanol intoxication; hepatic encephalopathy; porphyria; suicidal ideation; pregnancy (category D), lactation.
CAUTIOUS USE COPD, sleep apnea; heart failure; hypertension, hypotension, pulmonary disease; alcoholism; mental status changes, suicidality, major depression; neonates; renal impairment, renal failure; children.

ROUTE & DOSAGE

Preoperative Sedation
Adult: **IM** 150–200 mg in 2 divided doses
Child: **IV** 1–3 mg/kg (max: 100 mg)

Hypnotic
Adult: **IM** 150–200 mg **IV** 100 mg q1–3min up to 500 mg dose
Child: **IM** 2–6 mg/kg (max: 100 mg)

Status Epilepticus
Adult: **IV** 2–15 mg/kg loading, then 0.5–3 mg/kg/h
Child: **IM** 5–15 mg/kg loading, then 0.5–5 mg/kg/h

ADMINISTRATION

Note: Do not give within 14 days of starting/stopping an MAO inhibitor.

Intramuscular

- Do not use parenteral solutions that appear cloudy or in which a precipitate has formed.
- Make IM injections deep into large muscle mass, preferably upper

outer quadrant of buttock. Aspirate needle carefully before injecting it to prevent inadvertent entry into blood vessel. Inject no more than 5 mL (250 mg) in any one site because of possible tissue irritation.

Intravenous

PREPARE: **Direct:** Give undiluted or diluted (preferred) with sterile water, D5W, NS, or other compatible IV solutions.

ADMINISTER: **Direct:** Give slowly. Do not exceed rate of 50 mg/min.

INCOMPATIBILITIES **Solution/additive: Atropine, butorphanol, chlorpheniramine, chlorpromazine, cimetidine, codeine, dimenhydrinate, diphenhydramine, droperidol, ephedrine, fentanyl, glycopyrrolate, hydrocortisone, hydroxyzine, inulin, levorphanol, meperidine, methadone, midazolam, morphine, nalbuphine, norepinephrine,** TETRACYCLINES, **penicillin G, pentazocine, perphenazine, phenytoin, promazine, prochlorperazine, promethazine, ranitidine, sodium bicarbonate, streptomycin, succinylcholine, triflupromazine, vancomycin. Y-site: Amphotericin B cholesteryl, fenoldopam, TPN.**

▪ Take extreme care to avoid extravasation. Necrosis may result because parenteral solution is highly alkaline. ▪ Do not use cloudy or precipitated solution.

ADVERSE EFFECTS (≥1%) **Body as a Whole:** Drowsiness, lethargy, hangover, paradoxical excitement in the older adult patient. **CV:** Hypotension with rapid IV. **Respiratory:** With rapid IV (<u>respiratory depression, laryngospasm</u>, bronchospasm, <u>apnea</u>).

INTERACTIONS Drug: Phenmetrazine antagonizes effects of pentobarbital; CNS DEPRESSANTS, **alcohol,** SEDATIVES add to CNS depression; MAO INHIBITORS cause excessive CNS depression; **methoxyflurane** creates risk of nephrotoxicity. **Herbal: Kava, valerian** may potentiate sedation.

PHARMACOKINETICS Onset: 10–15 min IM; 1 min IV. **Duration:** 15 min IV. **Distribution:** Crosses placenta. **Metabolism:** Primarily in liver. **Elimination:** In urine. **Half-Life:** 4–50 h.

NURSING IMPLICATIONS

Assessment & Drug Effects

- Monitor BP, pulse, and respiration q3–5min during IV administration. Observe patient closely; maintain airway. Have equipment for artificial respiration immediately available.
- Observe patient closely for adverse effects for at least 30 min after IM administration of hypnotic dose.
- Monitor for hypersensitivity reactions (see Appendix F) especially with a history of asthma or angioedema.
- Monitor for adverse CNS effects including exacerbation of depression and suicide ideation.
- Monitor those in acute pain, children, the elderly, and debilitated patients for paradoxical excitement restlessness.
- Lab tests: Periodic pentobarbital levels. Note: Plasma levels greater than 30 mcg/mL may be toxic and 65 mcg/mL and above may be lethal.
- Concurrent drug: Monitor warfarin and phenytoin levels frequently to ensure therapeutic range.

Patient & Family Education

- Exercise caution when driving or operating machinery for the remainder of day after taking drug.

- Avoid alcohol and other CNS depressants for 24 h after receiving this drug.
- Women using oral contraceptives should use an additional, alternative form of contraception.

PENTOXIFYLLINE

(pen-tox-i'fi-leen)

Pentoxil, Trental

Classifications: HEMATOLOGIC; RED BLOOD CELL MODIFIER; BLOOD VISCOSITY REDUCER

Therapeutic: RED BLOOD CELL MODIFIER; BLOOD VISCOSITY IMPROVER

Pregnancy Category: C

AVAILABILITY 400 mg sustained release tablets

ACTION & *THERAPEUTIC EFFECT* Useful in restoration of blood flow through capillary microcirculation that has been compromised by structural and flow dynamic changes in cerebral and peripheral vascular disorders. Maintains the flexibility of RBCs, increasing erythrocyte cAMP activity, thus allowing erythrocyte membranes to maintain their integrity and become more resistant to deformity. Improvement in blood viscosity results in increased blood flow to the microcirculation and enhanced tissue oxygenation. *Results in increased blood flow to the extremities, reduced pain and paresthesia of intermittent claudication.*

USES Intermittent claudication associated with occlusive peripheral vascular disease; diabetic angiopathies.

UNLABELED USES To improve psychopathologic symptoms in patient with cerebrovascular insufficiency and to reduce incidence of stroke in the patient with recurrent TIAs.

CONTRAINDICATIONS Intolerance to pentoxifylline or to methylxanthines (caffeine and theophylline); intracranial bleeding; retinal bleeding; lactation. Safety in children younger than 18 y is not established.

CAUTIOUS USE Angina, hypotension, arrhythmias, cerebrovascular disease; peptic ulcer disease; renal failure; renal impairment; risk of bleeding; pregnancy (category C).

ROUTE & DOSAGE

Intermittent Claudication

Adult: **PO** 400 mg t.i.d. with meals

ADMINISTRATION

Oral

- Give on an empty stomach or with food; be consistent with time of day and relationship to food in establishing the daily regimen.
- Store tablets at 15°–30° C (59°–86° F).

ADVERSE EFFECTS (≥1%) **Body as a Whole:** Fever, flushing, convulsions, somnolence, loss of consciousness. **CNS:** Agitation, nervousness, *dizziness,* drowsiness, headache, insomnia, tremor, confusion. **CV:** Angina, chest pain, dyspnea, arrhythmias, palpitations, hypotension, edema, flushing. **Eye:** Blurred vision, conjunctivitis, scotomas. **GI:** Abdominal discomfort, belching, flatus, bloating, diarrhea, *dyspepsia, nausea, vomiting.* **Skin:** Brittle fingernails, pruritus, rash, urticaria. **Other:** Earache, unpleasant taste, excessive salivation, leukopenia, malaise, sore throat, swollen neck glands, weight change.

INTERACTIONS Drug: Ciprofloxacin, cimetidine may increase levels and toxicity, **warfarin** may have additive effects. **Herbal: Evening primrose oil, ginseng** may increase bleeding risk.

P

PHARMACOKINETICS Absorption: Readily from GI tract; 10–50% reaches systemic circulation (first pass metabolism). **Peak:** 2–4 h. **Distribution:** Distributed into breast milk. **Metabolism:** In liver and erythrocytes. **Elimination:** Primarily in urine. **Half-Life:** 0.4–0.8 h.

NURSING IMPLICATIONS

Assessment & Drug Effects

- Monitor therapeutic effectiveness which is indicated by relief from pain and cramping in calf muscles, buttocks, thighs, and feet during exercise and improves walking performance (time and duration).
- Monitor BP if patient is also on antihypertensive treatment. Drug may slightly decrease an already stabilized BP, necessitating a reduced dose of the hypotensive drug.

Patient & Family Education

- Consult physician to determine CV status and capacity before reestablishing walking as exercise.
- Pay particular attention to care of the feet because of arterial insufficiency (diminished perfusion to feet).
- Be aware that bleeding and prolonged PT/INR associated with this treatment have been reported. Report promptly unexplained bleeding, easy bruising, nose bleed, pinpoint rash to physician.
- Avoid driving or working with hazardous machinery until drug response has stabilized because of potential for tiredness, blurred vision, dizziness.

PERINDOPRIL ERBUMINE

(per-in'do-pril)
Aceon

Classifications: ANGIOTENSIN-CONVERTING ENZYME (ACE) INHIBITOR; ANTIHYPERTENSIVE
Therapeutic: ANTIHYPERTENSIVE
Prototype: Captopril
Pregnancy Category: D

AVAILABILITY 2 mg, 4 mg, 8 mg tablets

ACTION & *THERAPEUTIC EFFECT*
Angiotensin-converting enzyme (ACE) inhibitor. ACE catalyzes the conversion of angiotensin I to angiotensin II, a potent vasoconstrictor substance. Lowers BP by inhibition of ACE. Reduced aldosterone is associated with potassium-sparing effect. In addition, it decreases systemic vascular resistance (afterload) and pulmonary capillary wedge pressure (PCWP), a measure of preload, and improves cardiac output as well as activity tolerance. *Effective in lowering blood pressure by vasodilatation resulting from inhibition of ACE. Improves cardiac output as well as activity tolerance in coronary artery disease.*

USES Hypertension, myocardial infarction prophylaxis.
UNLABELED USES Heart failure.

CONTRAINDICATIONS Hypersensitivity to perindopril or any other ACE inhibitor; history of angioedema induced by an ACE inhibitor, pregnancy (category D); patients with hypertrophic cardiomyopathy, renal artery stenosis.
CAUTIOUS USE Renal insufficiency, volume-depleted patients, severe liver dysfunction; autoimmune diseases, immunosuppressant drug therapy; hyperkalemia or potassium-sparing diuretics; older adult; surgery; neutropenia; febrile illness; lactation.

ROUTE & DOSAGE

Hypertension, Stable Coronary Artery Disease

Adult: **PO** 2–4 mg once daily, may be increased to 8 mg daily in 1 or 2 divided doses (max: 16 mg/day)

Myocardial Infarction Prophylaxis

Adult: **PO** 4 mg daily × 2 wk, then 8 mg daily

Renal Impairment Dosage Adjustment

CrCl 30–59 mL/min: Start 2 mg daily; CrCl 16–29 mL/min: Start 2 mg every other day; CrCl less than 16 mL/min: Give 2 mg on dialysis days only

ADMINISTRATION

Oral

- Manufacturer recommends an initial dose of 2–4 mg in 1 or 2 divided doses if concurrently ordered diuretic cannot be discontinued 2–3 days before beginning perinodopril. Consult physician.
- Give on an empty stomach 1 h before meals.
- Dosage adjustments are generally made at intervals of at least 1 wk.
- Store at 20°–25° C (68°–77° F) and protect from moisture.

ADVERSE EFFECTS (≥1%) **CNS:** Dizziness, lightheadedness (in the absence of postural hypotension), headache, mood and sleep disorders, fatigue. **CV:** Palpitations. **Endocrine:** Hyperkalemia. **GI:** Nausea, vomiting, epigastric pain, diarrhea, taste disturbances, dyspepsia. **Urogenital:** Proteinuria, impotence, sexual dysfunction. **Special Senses:** Dry eyes, blurred vision. **Body as a Whole:** *Cough,* angioedema, pruritus, muscle cramps, sinusitis, hypertonia, fever. **Skin:** Rash.

INTERACTIONS Drug: POTASSIUM-SPARING DIURETICS (**amiloride, spironolactone, triamterene**) may increase the risk of hyperkalemia. POTASSIUM SUPPLEMENTS increase the risk of hyperkalemia; lithium levels can be increased. Use with **azathioprine** may cause anemia and leukopenia. **Pregabalin** may increase risk of angioedema. **Food:** Food can decrease drug absorption 35%.

PHARMACOKINETICS Absorption: Readily from GI tract, absorption significantly decreased when taken with food. **Peak: Perindopril:** 1 h; **perindoprilat:** 3–7 h. **Duration:** 24 h. **Metabolism:** Hydrolyzed in the liver to its active form, perindoprilat. **Elimination:** Primarily in urine. **Half-Life: Perindopril:** 0.8–1 h, **perindoprilat:** 30–120 h.

NURSING IMPLICATIONS

Assessment & Drug Effects

- Monitor BR and HR carefully following initial dose for several hours until stable, especially in patients using concurrent diuretics, on salt restriction, or volume depleted.
- Place patient immediately in a supine position if excess hypotension develops.
- Lab tests: Periodic serum potassium, serum sodium, BUN and creatinine, ALT, blood glucose, lipid profile, and WBC with differential.
- Monitor closely kidney function in patients with CHF.
- Monitor serum lithium levels and assess for S&S of lithium toxicity when used concurrently; increased caution is needed when diuretic therapy is also used.

P

Patient & Family Education

- Discontinue drug and immediately report S&S of angioedema (i.e., swelling) of face or extremities to physician. Seek emergency help for swelling of the tongue or any other signs of potential airway obstruction.
- Be aware that light-headedness can occur, especially during early therapy; excess fluid loss of any kind (e.g., vomiting, diarrhea) will increase risk of hypotension and fainting.
- Avoid using potassium supplements unless specifically directed to do so by physician.
- Report S&S of infection (e.g., sore throat, fever) promptly to physician.

PERMETHRIN (Pr)

(per-meth'rin)

Nix, Elimite, Acticin

Classifications: SCABICIDE; PEDICULICIDE

Therapeutic: SCABICIDE; PEDICULICIDE

Pregnancy Category: B

P

AVAILABILITY 5% cream; 1% liquid

ACTION & *THERAPEUTIC EFFECT* Pediculicidal and ovicidal activity against *Pediculus humanus* var. *capitis* (head louse). Inhibits sodium ion influx through nerve cell membrane channels, resulting in delayed repolarization of the action potential and paralysis of the pest. *It prevents burrowing into host's skin. Since lice are completely dependent on blood for survival, they die within 24–48 h. Also active against ticks, mites, and fleas.*

USES Pediculosis capitis.

CONTRAINDICATIONS Hypersensitivity to pyrethrins, chrysanthemums, sulfites, or other preservatives or dyes; acute inflammation of the scalp; lactation.

CAUTIOUS USE Children younger than 2 y (**liquid**), and less than 2 mo (**lotion**); asthma; pregnancy (category B).

ROUTE & DOSAGE

Head Lice

Adult/Child (older than 2 y): **Topical** Apply sufficient volume to clean wet hair to saturate the hair and scalp; leave on 10 min, then rinse hair thoroughly

ADMINISTRATION

Topical

- Saturate scalp as well as hair with the lotion; this is not a shampoo. Shake lotion well before application.
- Hair should be washed with regular shampoo before treatment with permethrin, thoroughly rinsed and dried.
- Rinse hair and scalp thoroughly and dry with a clean towel following 10 min exposure to the medication. Head lice are usually eliminated with one treatment.
- Store drug away from heat at 15°–25° C (59°–77° F) and direct light. Avoid freezing.

ADVERSE EFFECTS (≥1%) **Skin:** *Pruritus, transient tingling,* burning, stinging, numbness; erythema, edema, rash.

PHARMACOKINETICS Absorption: Less than 2% of amount applied is absorbed through intact skin. **Metabolism:** Rapidly hydrolyzed to inactive metabolites. **Elimination:** Primarily in urine.

NURSING IMPLICATIONS

Assessment & Drug Effects

- Do not attempt therapy if patient is known to be sensitive to any pyrethrin or pyrethroid. Stop treatment if a reaction occurs.

Patient & Family Education

- When hair is dry, comb with a fine-tooth comb (furnished with medication) to remove dead lice and remaining nits or nit shells.
- Be aware that drug remains on hair shaft up to 14 days; therefore, recurrence of infestation rarely occurs (less than 1%).
- Inspect hair shafts daily for at least 1 wk to determine drug effectiveness. Contact physician if live lice are observed after 7 days. Signs of inadequate treatment: Itching, redness of skin, skin abrasion, infected scalp areas.
- Resume regular shampooing after treatment; residual deposit of drug on hair is not reduced.
- Be aware that drug is usually irritating to the eyes and mucosa. Flush well with water if medicine accidentally gets into eyes.

PERPHENAZINE

(per-fen′a-zeen)

Classifications: PHENOTHIAZINE ANTIPSYCHOTIC; ANTIEMETIC

Therapeutic: ANTIPSYCHOTIC; ANTIEMETIC

Prototype: Chlorpromazine

Pregnancy Category: C

AVAILABILITY 2 mg, 4 mg, 6 mg, 8 mg, 16 mg tablets; 16 mg/5 mL liquid

ACTION & *THERAPEUTIC EFFECT* Affects all parts of CNS, particularly the hypothalamus. Antipsychotic effect is due to its ability to antagonize neurotransmitter dopamine by acting on its receptors in the brain. Antiemetic action results from direct blockade of dopamine in the chemoreceptor trigger zone (CTZ) in the medulla. *Has antipsychotic and antiemetic properties.*

USES Psychotic disorders, symptomatic control of severe nausea and vomiting.

CONTRAINDICATIONS Hypersensitivity to perphenazine and other phenothiazines; preexisting liver damage; suspected or established subcortical brain damage, comatose states, CNS depression; hepatic encephalopathy; QT prolongation; bone marrow depression; lactation.

CAUTIOUS USE Previously diagnosed breast cancer; liver or kidney dysfunction; cardiovascular disorders; alcohol withdrawal, epilepsy, psychic depression, patients with suicidal tendency; cardiac and pulmonary disease; glaucoma; history of intestinal or GU obstruction; geriatric or debilitated patients; patients who will be exposed to extremes of heat or cold, or to phosphorous insecticides; pregnancy (category C).

ROUTE & DOSAGE

Psychotic Disorders

Adult: **PO** 4–16 mg b.i.d. to q.i.d. (max: 64 mg/day)

Child: **PO** 4 mg b.i.d. to q.i.d. (max: 16 mg/day)

Nausea

Adult: **PO** 8–16 mg b.i.d. to q.i.d. (up to 24 mg/day)

Hemodialysis Dosage Adjustment: Not dialyzable

Pharmacogenetic Adjustment

Poor CYP2D6 metabolizers: Start with 30% of dose

ADMINISTRATION

Oral

- Ensure that sustained release form is not chewed or crushed. **Must be** swallowed whole.
- Dilute oral concentrate before administration: Dilute each 5 mL (16 mg) in 60 mL water, milk, saline solution, 7-Up, or other compatible carbonated beverages. Do not use liquids that cause color changes or precipitate.

ADVERSE EFFECTS (≥1%) **CNS:** *Extrapyramidal effects (dystonic reactions, akathisia, parkinsonian syndrome, tardive dyskinesia), sedation,* convulsions. **CV:** *Orthostatic hypotension,* tachycardia, bradycardia. **Special Senses:** Mydriasis, blurred vision, corneal and lenticular deposits. **GI:** Constipation, *dry mouth,* increased appetite, adynamic ileus, abnormal liver function tests, cholestatic jaundice. **Urogenital:** *Urinary retention,* gynecomastia, menstrual irregularities, inhibited ejaculation. **Hematologic:** Agranulocytosis, thrombocytopenic purpura, aplastic or hemolytic anemia. **Body as a Whole:** Photosensitivity, itching, erythema, urticaria, angioneurotic edema, drug fever, anaphylactoid reaction, sterile abscess. Nasal congestion, decreased sweating. **Metabolic:** Hyperprolactinemia, galactorrhea, weight gain.

DIAGNOSTIC TEST INTERFERENCE Perphenazine may cause falsely abnormal ***thyroid function*** tests because of elevations of ***thyroid globulin.***

INTERACTIONS Drug: Alcohol and other CNS DEPRESSANTS enhance CNS depression; ANTACIDS, ANTIDIARRHEALS may decrease absorption of phenothiazines; ANTICHOLINERGIC AGENTS add to anticholinergic effects including fecal impaction and paralytic ileus; BARBITURATES, ANESTHETICS increase hypotension and excitation. **Herbal: Kava** increased risk and severity of dystonic reactions.

PHARMACOKINETICS Absorption: Poorly absorbed from GI tract; 20% reaches systemic circulation. **Peak:** 4–8 h PO. **Duration:** 6–12 h. **Distribution:** Crosses placenta. **Metabolism:** In liver (CYP2D6) with some metabolism in GI tract. **Elimination:** In urine and feces. **Half-Life:** 9.5 h.

NURSING IMPLICATIONS

Assessment & Drug Effects

- Establish baseline BP before initiation of drug therapy and check it at regular intervals, especially during early therapy.
- Report restlessness, weakness of extremities, dystonic reactions (spasms of neck and shoulder muscles, rigidity of back, difficulty swallowing or talking); motor restlessness (akathisia: inability to be still); and parkinsonian syndrome (tremors, shuffling gait, drooling, slow speech). A high incidence of extrapyramidal effects accompanies use of perphenazine, particularly with high doses.
- Withhold medication and report IMMEDIATELY to physician S&S of tardive dyskinesia (i.e., fine, wormlike movements or rapid protrusions of the tongue, chewing motions, lip smacking). Patients on long-term therapy are at high risk. Teach patients and responsible family members about symptoms because early reporting is essential.
- Lab tests: Obtain CBC with differential, liver and kidney function studies.
- ECG and ophthalmologic examination are recommended prior to

initiation and periodically during therapy.
- Suspect hypersensitivity, withhold drug, and report to physician if jaundice appears between weeks 2 and 4.
- Monitor urine and bowel elimination pattern.

Patient & Family Education
- Make all position changes slowly and in stages, particularly from recumbent to upright posture, and to lie down or sit down if light-headedness or dizziness occurs.
- Do not drive or engage in potentially hazardous activities until response to drug is known.
- Discontinue drug and report to physician immediately if jaundice appears between weeks 2 and 4.
- Avoid long exposure to sunlight and to sunlamps. Photosensitivity results in skin color changes from brown to blue-gray.
- Adhere strictly to dosage regimen. Contact physician before changing it for any reason.
- Drug should be discontinued gradually over a period of several weeks following prolonged therapy.
- Avoid OTC drugs unless physician prescribes them.
- Be aware that perphenazine may discolor urine reddish brown.

PHENAZOPYRIDINE HYDROCHLORIDE

(fen-az-oh-peer′i-deen)

Azo-Standard, Baridium, Geridium, Phenazo ♣, Phenazodine, Pyridiate, Pyridium, Pyronium ♣, Urodine, Urogesic

Classification: URINARY TRACT ANALGESIC
Therapeutic: URINARY TRACT ANALGESIC
Pregnancy Category: B

AVAILABILITY 95 mg, 97.2 mg, 100 mg, 150 mg, 200 mg tablets

ACTION & *THERAPEUTIC EFFECT* Azo dye that has local anesthetic action on urinary tract mucosa, which imparts little or no antibacterial activity. *Effective as a urinary tract analgesic.*

USES Symptomatic relief of pain, burning, frequency, and urgency arising from irritation of urinary tract mucosa, as from infection, trauma, surgery, or instrumentation.

CONTRAINDICATIONS Renal insufficiency, renal disease including glomerulonephritis, pyelonephritis, renal failure, uremia; hepatic disease; glucose-6-phosphate dehydrogenase deficiency, severe hepatitis.

CAUTIOUS USE GI disturbances; older adults; pregnancy (category B), lactation.

ROUTE & DOSAGE

Cystitis
Adult: **PO** 200 mg t.i.d.
Child: **PO** 12 mg/kg/day in 3 divided doses

ADMINISTRATION

Oral
- Give with or after meals.

ADVERSE EFFECTS (≥1%) **Body as a Whole:** Headache, vertigo. **GI:** Mild GI disturbances. **Urogenital:** Kidney stones, transient acute kidney failure. **Metabolic:** Methemoglo-

P

binemia, hemolytic anemia. **Skin:** Skin pigmentation. **Special Senses:** May stain soft contact lenses.

DIAGNOSTIC TEST INTERFERENCE Phenazopyridine may interfere with any urinary test that is based on color reactions or spectrometry: ***Bromsulphalein*** and ***phenolsulfonphthalein*** excretion tests; urinary ***glucose*** test using ***Clinistix*** or ***TesTape*** (***copper-reduction methods*** such as ***Clinitest*** and ***Benedict's test*** reportedly not affected); ***bilirubin*** using "foam test" or ***Ictotest; ketones*** using ***nitroprusside*** (e.g., ***Acetest, Ketostix,*** or ***Gerhardt ferric chloride***); ***urinary protein*** using ***Albustix, Albutest,*** or ***nitric acid ring test;*** urinary ***steroids; urobilinogen; assays*** for ***porphyrins.***

INTERACTIONS Drug: No clinically significant interactions established.

PHARMACOKINETICS Absorption: Readily absorbed from GI tract. **Distribution:** Crosses placenta in trace amounts. **Metabolism:** In liver and other tissues. **Elimination:** Primarily in urine.

P

NURSING IMPLICATIONS

Assessment & Drug Effects

- Monitor for therapeutic effectiveness as indicated by relief from pain and burning upon urination.

Patient & Family Education

- Drug will impart an orange to red color to urine and may stain clothing.

PHENELZINE SULFATE Pr

(fen'el-zeen)

Nardil

Classifications: ANTIDEPRESSANT; MONOAMINE OXIDASE (MAO) INHIBITOR

Therapeutic: ANTIDEPRESSANT; MAO INHIBITOR

Pregnancy Category: C

AVAILABILITY 15 mg tablets

ACTION & *THERAPEUTIC EFFECT* Potent hydrazine monoamine oxidase (MAO) inhibitor. Antidepressant believed to be due to irreversible inhibition of MAO, thereby permitting increased concentrations of endogenous epinephrine, norepinephrine, serotonin, and dopamine within presynaptic neurons and at receptor sites. *Antidepressant utilization is limited to individuals who do not respond well to other classes of antidepressants.*

USES Management of endogenous depression, depressive phase of manic-depressive psychosis, and severe exogenous (reactive) depression not responsive to more commonly used therapy.

CONTRAINDICATIONS Hypersensitivity to MAO inhibitors; suicidal ideation; pheochromocytoma; hyperthyroidism; CHF, acute MI, cardiac arrhythmias, hypertension, history of angina pectoris; cardiovascular or cerebrovascular disease; increased intracranial pressure; intracranial bleeding; renal failure; severe renal impairment, hypernatremia; atonic colitis; glaucoma; history of frequent or severe headaches; history of liver disease, abnormal liver function tests; alcoholism; within 10 days of surgery; depression, accompanying alcoholism or drug addiction; older adult or debilitated patients; paranoid schizophrenia; lactation. Safety in children younger than 6 y is not established.
CAUTIOUS USE Epilepsy; pyloric stenosis; diabetes; manic-depressive states; agitated patients; schizophrenia or psychosis; seizures; suicidal

tendencies; chronic brain syndromes; pregnancy (category C).

ROUTE & DOSAGE

Depression

Adult: **PO** 15 mg t.i.d., rapidly increase to at least 60 mg/day, may need up to 90 mg/day

ADMINISTRATION

Oral

- Avoid rapid discontinuation, particularly after high dosage, since a rebound effect may occur (e.g., headache, excitability, hallucinations, and possibly depression).
- Store in tightly covered containers away from heat and light.

ADVERSE EFFECTS (≥1%) **Body as a Whole:** Dizziness or vertigo, headache, *orthostatic hypotension,* drowsiness or *insomnia,* weakness, fatigue, edema, tremors, twitching, akathisia, ataxia, hyperreflexia, faintness, hyperactivity, marked agitation, anxiety, seizures, trismus, opisthotonos, <u>respiratory depression, coma</u>. **CNS:** Mania, hypomania, confusion, memory impairment, delirium, hallucinations, euphoria, acute anxiety reaction, toxic precipitation of schizophrenia, convulsions, peripheral neuropathy. **CV:** <u>Hypertensive crisis</u> (intense occipital headache, palpitation, marked hypertension, stiff neck, nausea, vomiting, sweating, fever, photophobia, dilated pupils, bradycardia or tachycardia, constricting chest pain, intracranial bleeding), hypotension or hypertension, <u>circulatory collapse</u>. **GI:** *Constipation, dry mouth, nausea,* vomiting, *anorexia,* weight gain. **Hematologic:** Normocytic and normochromic anemia, leukopenia. **Skin:** Hyperhidrosis, skin rash, photosensitivity. **Special Senses:** Blurred vision.

DIAGNOSTIC TEST INTERFERENCE Phenelzine may cause a slight false increase in ***serum bilirubin.***

INTERACTIONS Drug: TRICYCLIC ANTIDEPRESSANTS may cause hyperpyrexia, seizures; **fluoxetine, sertraline, paroxetine** may cause serotonin syndrome (see Appendix F); SYMPATHOMIMETIC AGENTS (e.g., **amphetamine, phenylephrine, phenylpropanolamine**), **guanethidine** and **reserpine** may cause hypertensive crisis; CNS DEPRESSANTS have additive CNS depressive effects; OPIATE ANALGESICS (especially **meperidine**) may cause hypertensive crisis and circulatory collapse; **buspirone,** hypertension; GENERAL ANESTHETICS, prolonged hypotensive and CNS depressant effects; hypertension, headache, hyperexcitability reported with **dopamine, methyldopa, levodopa, tryptophan; metrizamide** may increase risk of seizures; HYPOTENSIVE AGENTS and DIURETICS have additive hypotensive effects. **Food:** Aged meats or aged cheeses, protein extracts, sour cream, alcohol, anchovies, liver, sausages, overripe figs, bananas, avocados, chocolate, soy sauce, bean curd, natural yogurt, fava beans—**tyramine**-containing foods—may precipitate hypertensive crisis. Avoid **chocolate** or **caffeine. Herbal: Ginseng, ephedra, ma huang, St. John's wort** may cause hypertensive crisis.

PHARMACOKINETICS Absorption: Readily absorbed from GI tract. **Onset:** 2 wk. **Metabolism:** Rapidly metabolized. **Elimination:** 79% of metabolites excreted in urine in 96 h.

NURSING IMPLICATIONS

Assessment & Drug Effects

- Prior to initiation of treatment, evaluate patient's BP in standing and recumbent positions.

P

- Monitor BP and pulse between doses when titrating initial dosages. Observe closely for evidence of adverse drug effects. Thereafter, monitor at regular intervals throughout therapy.
- Monitor children, adolescents, and adults for changes in behavior that may indicate suicidality.
- Lab tests: Baseline and periodic CBC and LFTs.
- Report immediately if hypomania (exaggeration of motility, feelings, and ideas) occurs as depression improves. This reaction may also appear at higher than recommended doses or with long-term therapy.
- Observe for and report therapeutic effectiveness of drug: Improvement in sleep pattern, appetite, physical activity, interest in self and surroundings, as well as lessening of anxiety and bodily complaints.
- Observe patient with diabetes closely for S&S of hypoglycemia (see Appendix F).
- Patients on prolonged therapy should be checked periodically for altered color perception, changes in fundi or visual fields. Changes in red-green vision may be the first indication of eye damage.

P

Patient & Family Education

- Maximum antidepressant effects generally appear in 2–6 wk and persist several weeks after drug withdrawal.
- Avoid self-medication. OTC preparations (e.g., cough, cold, and hay fever remedies, appetite suppressants) can precipitate severe hypertensive reactions if taken during therapy or within 2–3 wk after discontinuation of an MAO inhibitor.
- Report immediately to physician the onset of headache and palpitation, or any other unusual effects which may indicate need to discontinue therapy.
- Do not consume foods and beverages containing tyramine or tryptophan or drugs containing pressor agent. These can cause severe hypertensive reactions. Get a list from your care provider.
- Avoid drinking excessive caffeine and chocolate beverages (e.g., coffee, tea, cocoa, or cola).
- Make position changes slowly, especially from recumbent to upright posture, and dangle legs over bed a few minutes before rising to walk. Avoid standing still for prolonged periods. Also avoid hot showers and baths (resulting vasodilatation may potentiate hypotension); lie down immediately if feeling lightheaded or faint.
- Check weight 2 or 3 times per wk and report unusual gain.
- Report jaundice. Hepatotoxicity is believed to be a hypersensitivity reaction unrelated to dosage or duration of therapy.

PHENOBARBITAL Pr

(fee-noe-bar'bi-tal)
Solfoton

PHENOBARBITAL SODIUM

Luminal
Classifications: ANTICONVULSANT; SEDATIVE-HYPNOTIC; BARBITURATE
Therapeutic: ANTICONVULSANT; SEDATIVE-HYPNOTIC
Pregnancy Category: D
Controlled Substance: Schedule IV

AVAILABILITY 15 mg, 16 mg, 30 mg, 60 mg, 90 mg, 100 mg tablets; 16 mg capsules; 15 mg/5 mL, 20 mg/5 mL liquid; 30 mg/mL, 60 mg/mL, 65 mg/mL, 130 mg/mL injection

ACTION & *THERAPEUTIC EFFECT* Long-acting barbiturate, while the sodium form of phenobarbital is short acting; both forms have anticonvulsant properties. Sedative and hypnotic effects appear to be due primarily to interference with impulse transmission of cerebral cortex by inhibition of reticular activating system. Limits spread of seizure activity results by increasing the threshold for motor cortex stimulation. *Effective as a sedative, hypnotic, and an anticonvulsant with no analgesic effect.*

USES Long-term management of tonic-clonic (grand mal) seizures and partial seizures; status epilepticus, eclampsia, febrile convulsions in young children. Also used as a sedative in anxiety or tension states; in pediatrics as preoperative and postoperative sedation and to treat pylorospasm in infants.

UNLABELED USES Treatment and prevention of hyperbilirubinemia in neonates and in the management of chronic cholestasis; benzodiazepine withdrawal.

CONTRAINDICATIONS Hypersensitivity to barbiturates; manifest hepatic or familial history of porphyria; severe respiratory or kidney disease; history of previous addiction to sedative hypnotics; alcohol intoxication; uncontrolled pain; renal failure, anuria; pregnancy (category D).

CAUTIOUS USE Impaired liver, kidney, cardiac, or respiratory function; sleep apnea; COPD; history of allergies; older adult or debilitated patients; patients with fever; hyperthyroidism; diabetes mellitus or severe anemia; seizure disorders; during labor and delivery; patient with borderline hypoadrenal function; lactation, young children and neonates.

ROUTE & DOSAGE

Anticonvulsant

Adult: **PO/IV** 1–3 mg/kg/day in divided doses
Child: **PO/IV** 4–8 mg/kg/day in divided doses

Status Epilepticus

Adult: **IV** 300-800 mg, then 120–240 mg q20min (total max: 1–2 g)
Child: **IV** 10–20 mg/kg in single or divided doses, then 5 mg/kg/dose q15–30min (total max: 40 mg/kg)
Neonate: **IV** 15–20 mg/kg in single or divided doses

Sedative/Hypnotic

Adult: **PO** 30–120 mg/day **IV/IM** 100–320 mg/day
Child: **PO** 2 mg/kg/day in 3 divided doses **IV/IM** 3–5 mg/kg

Renal Impairment Dosage Adjustment

CrCl less than 10 mL/min: Dose q12–16h
Hemodialysis Dosage Adjustment: 20–50% dialyzed

ADMINISTRATION

Oral

- Give crushed and mixed with a fluid or with food if patient cannot swallow pill. Do not permit patient to swallow dry crushed drug.

Intramuscular

- Give IM deep into large muscle mass; do not exceed 5 mL at any one site.

P

Intravenous

Note: Verify correct IV concentration and rate of infusion for neonates, infants, children with physician. Use IV route ONLY if other routes are not feasible.

PREPARE: **Direct:** May be given undiluted or diluted in 10 mL of sterile water for injection.

ADMINISTER: **Direct:** Give 60 mg or fraction thereof over at least 60 sec. Give within 30 min after preparation.

INCOMPATIBILITIES **Solution/additive:** **Ampicillin, cephalothin, chlorpromazine, cimetidine, clindamycin, codeine phosphate, dexamethasone, diphenhydramine, erythromycin, ephedrine, hydralazine, hydrocortisone sodium succinate, hydroxyzine, insulin, kanamycin, levorphanol, meperidine, methadone, methylphenidate, morphine, nitrofurantoin, norepinephrine, pentazocine, pentobarbital, phytonadione, procaine, prochlorperazine, promazine, promethazine, sodium bicarbonate, streptomycin,** TETRACYCLINES, **vancomycin, warfarin.** **Y-site:** **Amphotericin B cholesteryl complex, hydromorphone, TPN with albumin.**

- Be aware that extravasation of IV phenobarbital may cause necrotic tissue changes that necessitate skin grafting. Check injection site frequently.

P

ADVERSE EFFECTS (≥1%) **Body as a Whole:** Myalgia, neuralgia, CNS depression, coma, and death. **CNS:** *Somnolence,* nightmares, insomnia, "hangover," headache, anxiety, thinking abnormalities, dizziness, nystagmus, irritability, paradoxic excitement and exacerbation of hyperkinetic behavior (in children); confusion or depression or marked excitement (older adult or debilitated patients); ataxia. **CV:** Bradycardia, syncope, hypotension. **GI:** Nausea, vomiting, constipation, diarrhea, epigastric pain, liver damage. **Hematologic:** Megaloblastic anemia, agranulocytosis, thrombocytopenia. **Metabolic:** Hypocalcemia, osteomalacia, rickets. **Musculoskeletal:** Folic acid deficiency, vitamin D deficiency. **Respiratory:** Respiratory depression. **Skin:** Mild maculopapular, morbilliform rash; erythema multiforme, Stevens-Johnson syndrome, exfoliative dermatitis (rare).

DIAGNOSTIC TEST INTERFERENCE BARBITURATES may affect ***bromsulphalein*** retention tests (by enhancing liver uptake and excretion of dye) and increase ***serum phosphatase.***

INTERACTIONS Drug: Alcohol, CNS DEPRESSANTS compound CNS depression; phenobarbital may decrease absorption and increase metabolism of ORAL ANTICOAGULANTS; increases metabolism of CORTICOSTEROIDS, ORAL CONTRACEPTIVES, ANTICONVULSANTS, **digitoxin,** possibly decreasing their effects; ANTIDEPRESSANTS potentiate adverse effects of phenobarbital; **griseofulvin** decreases absorption of phenobarbital; **quinine** increases plasma levels. **Herbal: Kava, valerian** may potentiate sedation.

PHARMACOKINETICS Absorption: 70–90% slowly from GI tract. **Peak:** 8–12 h PO; 30 min IV. **Duration:** 4–6 h IV. **Distribution:** 20–45% protein bound; crosses placenta; enters breast milk. **Metabolism:** In liver (CYP2C19). **Elimination:** In urine. **Half-Life:** 2–6 days.

NURSING IMPLICATIONS

Assessment & Drug Effects

- Observe patients receiving large doses for at least 30 min to ensure that sedation is not excessive.

- Chronic use in children or infants requires continuous assessment related to normal cognitive and behavioral functioning.
- Keep patient under constant observation when drug is administered IV, and record vital signs at least every hour or more often if indicated.
- Check IV injection site very frequently to prevent extravasation of phenobarbital. It could result in tissue damage requiring skin grafting.
- Lab tests: Periodic LFTs, CBC with differential, Hct and Hgb, serum folate, and vitamin D levels during prolonged therapy.
- Monitor serum drug levels. Serum concentrations greater than 50 mcg/mL may cause coma. Therapeutic serum concentrations of 15–40 mcg/mL produce anticonvulsant activity in most patients. These values are usually attained after 2 or 3 wk of therapy with a dose of 100–200 mg/day.
- Expect barbiturates to produce restlessness when given to patients in pain because these drugs do not have analgesic action.
- Be prepared for paradoxical responses and report promptly in older adult or debilitated patient and children [i.e., irritability, marked excitement (inappropriate tearfulness and aggression in children), depression, and confusion].
- Monitor for drug interactions. Barbiturates increase the metabolism of many drugs, leading to decreased pharmacologic effects of those drugs.
- Monitor for and report chronic toxicity symptoms (e.g., ataxia, slurred speech, irritability, poor judgment, slight dysarthria, nystagmus on vertical gaze, confusion, insomnia, somatic complaints).

Patient & Family Education

- Be aware that anticonvulsant therapy may cause drowsiness during first few weeks of treatment, but this usually diminishes with continued use.
- Avoid potentially hazardous activities requiring mental alertness until response to drug is known.
- Do not consume alcohol in any amount when taking a barbiturate; it may severely impair judgment and abilities.
- Increase vitamin D-fortified foods (e.g., milk products) because drug increases vitamin D metabolism. A vitamin D supplement may be prescribed.
- Maintain adequate dietary folate intake: Fresh vegetables (especially green leafy), fresh fruits, whole grains, liver. Long-term therapy may result in nutritional folate (B_9) deficiency. A supplement of folic acid may be prescribed.
- Adhere to drug regimen (i.e., do not change intervals between doses or increase or decrease doses) without contacting physician.
- Do not stop taking drug abruptly because of danger of withdrawal symptoms (8–12 h after last dose), which can be fatal.
- Report to physician the onset of fever, sore throat or mouth, malaise, easy bruising or bleeding, petechiae, jaundice, rash when on prolonged therapy.
- Avoid pregnancy when receiving barbiturates. Use or add barrier device to hormonal contraceptive when taking prolonged therapy.

PHENOXYBENZAMINE HYDROCHLORIDE

(fen-ox-ee-ben′za-meen)

Dibenzyline

Classifications: ALPHA-ADRENERGIC RECEPTOR ANTAGONIST; ANTIHYPERTENSIVE
Therapeutic: ALPHA-BLOCKER; ANTIHYPERTENSIVE
Prototype: Prazosin
Pregnancy Category: C

AVAILABILITY 10 mg capsules

ACTION & *THERAPEUTIC EFFECT* Long-acting alpha-adrenergic receptor antagonist that produces noncompetitive blockade of alpha-adrenergic receptor sites at postganglionic synapses. Alpha-receptor sites are thus unable to react to the endogenous or exogenous sympathomimetic agents epinephrine and norepinephrine. *Blocks excitatory effects of epinephrine, including vasoconstriction, but does not affect adrenergic cardiac inhibitory actions. It produces a "chemical sympathectomy" and it can maintain it.*

USES Management of pheochromocytoma.

UNLABELED USES To improve circulation in peripheral vasospastic conditions such as Raynaud's acrocyanosis and frostbite sequelae, for adjunctive treatment of shock, hypertensive crisis.

CONTRAINDICATIONS Instances when fall in BP would be dangerous; lactation.

CAUTIOUS USE Marked cerebral or coronary arteriosclerosis, compensated congestive heart failure, coronary artery disease; older adults; renal insufficiency; respiratory infections; pregnancy (category C).

ROUTE & DOSAGE

Management of Pheochromocytoma
Adult: **PO** 10 mg b.i.d., may increase by 10 mg/day at 4-day intervals to desired response (usual range: 20–40 mg/day in 2–3 divided doses)
Child: **PO** 0.2 mg/kg/day, may increase by 0.2 mg/kg/day to desired response (usual range: 0.4–1.2 mg/kg/q6–8h)

ADMINISTRATION

Oral
- Give with milk or in divided doses to reduce gastric irritation.
- Preserve in airtight containers protected from light.

ADVERSE EFFECTS (≥1%) **Body as a Whole:** *Dizziness,* fainting, drowsiness, sedation, tiredness, weakness, lethargy, confusion, headache, <u>shock</u>. **CNS:** CNS stimulation (large doses). **CV:** *Postural hypotension, tachycardia,* palpitation. **GI:** Dry mouth. **Urogenital:** Inhibition of ejaculation. **Respiratory:** *Nasal congestion.* **Skin:** Allergic contact dermatitis. **Special Senses:** *Miosis,* drooping of eyelids.

INTERACTIONS Drug: Inhibits effects of **methoxamine, norepinephrine, phenylephrine;** additive hypotensive effects with ANTIHYPERTENSIVES.

PHARMACOKINETICS Absorption: Variably (approximately 30%) from GI tract. **Onset:** 2 h. **Peak:** 4–6 h. **Duration:** 3–4 days. **Distribution:** Accumulates in adipose tissue. **Elimination:** 80% in urine and bile within 24 h. **Half-Life:** 24 h.

NURSING IMPLICATIONS

Assessment & Drug Effects

- Monitor BP and note pulse quality, rate, and rhythm in recumbent and standing positions during period of dosage adjustment. Observe patient closely for at least 4 days from one dosage increment to the next; hypotension and tachycardia are most likely to occur in standing position.

- Drug has cumulative action, thus onset of therapeutic effects may not occur until after 2 wk of therapy, and full therapeutic effects may not be apparent for several more weeks.

Patient & Family Education

- Make position changes slowly, particularly from reclining to upright posture, and dangle legs and exercise ankles and feet for a few minutes before standing.
- Be aware that light headedness, dizziness, and palpitations usually disappear with continued therapy but may reappear under conditions that promote vasodilation, such as strenuous exercise or ingestion of a large meal or alcohol.
- Pupil constriction, nasal stuffiness, and inhibition of ejaculation generally decrease with continued therapy.
- Do not take OTC medications for coughs, colds, or allergy without approval of physician. Many contain agents that cause BP elevation.

PHENTERMINE HYDROCHLORIDE

(phen-ter′meen)

Ionamin, Fastin, Zantryl, Adipex-P, Obe-Nix-30

Classification: ANOREXIANT
Therapeutic: APPETITE SUPPRESSANT
Prototype: Diethylpropion
Pregnancy Category: C
Controlled Substance: Schedule IV

AVAILABILITY 8 mg, 30 mg, 37.5 mg tablets; 15 mg, 18.75 mg, 30 mg, 37.5 mg capsules

ACTION & *THERAPEUTIC EFFECT* Sympathetic amine with actions that include CNS stimulation and blood pressure elevation. *Appetite suppression or metabolic effects along with diet adjustment result in weight loss in obese individuals.*

USES Short-term (8–12 wk) adjunct for weight loss.

CONTRAINDICATIONS History of hypertension, moderate to severe hypertension, advanced arteriosclerosis, cardiovascular disease, including cardiac arrhythmias and valvular heart disease; hyperthyroidism; known hypersensitivity to sympathetic amines; agitated states; psychosis; schizophrenia; history of drug abuse; during or within 14 days of administration of MAO inhibitor; concurrent administration of selective serotonin reuptake inhibitors (SSRIs); valvular heart disease; glaucoma; lactation, or children younger than 16 y.

CAUTIOUS USE Mild hypertension, diabetes mellitus; pregnancy (category C).

ROUTE & DOSAGE

Obesity

Adult: **PO** 8 mg t.i.d. 30 min before meals or 15–37.5 mg daily before breakfast or 10–14 h before retiring

ADMINISTRATION

Oral

- Ensure that at least 14 days have elapsed between the first dose of phentermine and the last dose of an MAO inhibitor.
- Give 30 min before meals.
- Do not administer if an SSRI is currently prescribed.
- Store in a tight container.

P

ADVERSE EFFECTS (≥1%) **Body as a Whole:** Hypersensitivity (urticaria, rash, erythema, burning sensation), chest pain, excessive sweating, clamminess, chills, flushing, fever, myalgia. **CV:** Palpitations, tachycardia, arrhythmias, hypertension or hypotension, syncope, precordial pain, pulmonary hypertension. **GI:** Dry mouth, altered taste, nausea, vomiting, abdominal pain, diarrhea, constipation, stomach pain. **Endocrine:** Gynecomastia. **Hematologic:** Bone marrow suppression, agranulocytosis, leukopenia. **Musculoskeletal:** Muscle pain. **CNS:** Overstimulation, nervousness, restlessness, dizziness, insomnia, weakness, fatigue, malaise, anxiety, euphoria, drowsiness, depression, agitation, dysphoria, tremor, dyskinesia, dysarthria, confusion, incoordination, headache, change in libido. **Skin:** Hair loss, ecchymosis. **Special Senses:** Mydriasis, blurred vision. **Urogenital:** Dysuria, polyuria, urinary frequency, impotence, menstrual upset.

P

INTERACTIONS Drug: MAO INHIBITORS, **furazolidone** may increase pressor response resulting in hypertensive crisis. TRICYCLIC ANTIDEPRESSANTS may decrease anorectic response. May decrease hypotensive effects of **guanethidine.**

PHARMACOKINETICS Absorption: Absorbed from the small intestine. **Duration:** 4–14 h. **Elimination:** Primarily in urine. **Half-Life:** 19–24 h.

NURSING IMPLICATIONS

Assessment & Drug Effects

- Assess for tolerance to the anorectic effect of the drug. Withhold drug and report to physician when this occurs.
- Lab tests: Periodic CBC with differential and blood glucose.
- Monitor periodic cardiovascular status, including BP, exercise tolerance, peripheral edema.
- Monitor weight at least 3 times/wk.

Patient & Family Education

- Do not take this drug late in the evening because it could cause insomnia.
- Report immediately any of the following: Shortness of breath, chest pains, dizziness or fainting, swelling of the extremities.
- Tolerance to the appetite suppression effects of the drug usually develops in a few weeks. Notify physician, but do not increase the drug dose.
- Weigh yourself at least 3 times/wk at the same time of day with the same amount of clothing.

PHENTOLAMINE MESYLATE

(fen-tole′a-meen)

Regitine, Rogitine ♣

Classifications: ALPHA-ADRENERGIC RECEPTOR ANTAGONIST; VASODILATOR

Therapeutic: VASODILATOR

Prototype: Prazosin

Pregnancy Category: C

AVAILABILITY 5 mg injection

ACTION & *THERAPEUTIC EFFECT* Alpha-adrenergic blocking agent that competitively blocks alpha-adrenergic receptors, but action is transient and incomplete. Causes vasodilation and decreases general vascular resistance as well as pulmonary arterial pressure, primarily by direct action on vascular smooth muscle. *Prevents hypertension resulting from elevated levels of circulating epinephrine or norepinephrine.*

USES Diagnosis of pheochromocytoma and to prevent or control hypertensive episodes prior to or during pheochromocytomectomy.

UNLABELED USES Prevention of dermal necrosis and sloughing following IV administration or extravasation of norepinephrine.

CONTRAINDICATIONS Hypersensitivity to phentolamine; MI (previous or present), coronary artery disease; peptic ulcer disease; lactation.
CAUTIOUS USE Gastritis; pregnancy (category C).

ROUTE & DOSAGE

To Prevent Hypertensive Episode during Surgery
Adult: **IV/IM** 5 mg 1–2 h before surgery, repeat as needed
Child: **IV/IM** 0.05–0.1 mg/kg/dose (max: 5 mg/dose)

To Test for Pheochromocytoma
Adult: **IV/IM** 5 mg
Child: **IV/IM** 0.05–0.1 mg/kg (max: 5 mg)

To Treat Extravasation
Adult: **Intradermal** 5–10 mg diluted in 10 mL of normal saline injected into affected area within 12 h of extravasation
Child: **Intradermal** 0.1–0.2 mg/kg diluted with normal saline injected into affected area within 12 h of extravasation

ADMINISTRATION

Note: Place patient in supine position when receiving drug parenterally. ▪ Monitor BP and pulse q2min until stabilized.

Intramuscular

- Reconstitute 5 mg vial with 1 mL of sterile water for injection.

Intravenous

PREPARE: **Direct:** Reconstitute as for IM. May be further diluted with up to 10 mL of sterile water. ▪ Use immediately.

ADMINISTER: **Direct:** Give a single dose over 60 sec.

ADVERSE EFFECTS (≥1%) **Body as a Whole:** Weakness, dizziness, flushing, *orthostatic hypotension*. **GI:** *Abdominal pain, nausea, vomiting, diarrhea, exacerbation of peptic ulcer.* **CV:** *Acute and prolonged hypotension, tachycardia, anginal pain,* cardiac arrhythmias, MI, cerebrovascular spasm, shock-like state. **Special Senses:** Nasal stuffiness, conjunctival infection.

INTERACTIONS Drug: May antagonize BP raising effects of **epinephrine, ephedrine.**

PHARMACOKINETICS Peak: 2 min IV; 15–20 min IM. **Duration:** 10–15 min IV; 3–4 h IM. **Elimination:** In urine. **Half-Life:** 19 min.

NURSING IMPLICATIONS

Assessment & Drug Effects

Test for pheochromocytoma:

- *IV administration:* Keep patient at rest in supine position throughout test, preferably in quiet darkened room. ▪ Prior to drug administration, take BP q10min for at least 30 min to establish that BP has stabilized before IV injection. ▪ Record BP immediately after injection and at 30-sec intervals for first 3 min; then at 1-min intervals for next 7 min.
- *IM administration:* Post-injection, BP determinations at 5-min intervals for 30–45 min.

Patient & Family Education

- Avoid sudden changes in position, particularly from reclining to upright posture and dangle legs and exercise ankles and toes for a few minutes before standing to walk.
- Lie down or sit down in head-low position immediately if lightheaded or dizzy.

P

PHENYLEPHRINE HYDROCHLORIDE

(fen-ill-ef′rin)

AK-Dilate Ophthalmic, Alconefrin, Isopto Frin, Mydfrin, Neo-Synephrine, Nostril, Rhinall, Sinarest Nasal, Sinex

Classifications: EYE AND NOSE PREPARATION; ALPHA-ADRENERGIC AGONIST; MYDRIATIC; VASOPRESSOR; DECONGESTANT

Therapeutic: VASOCONSTRICTOR; DECONGESTANT; MYDRIATIC

Prototype: Methoxamine

Pregnancy Category: C

AVAILABILITY 10 mg chewable tablet; 0.125%, 0.16%, 0.5%, 1% nasal solution; 0.12%, 2.5%, 10% ophth solution; 10 mg/mL injection

ACTION & *THERAPEUTIC EFFECT*
Potent, synthetic, direct-acting sympathomimetic with strong alpha-adrenergic cardiac stimulant actions. Elevates systolic and diastolic pressures through arteriolar constriction. Reduces intraocular pressure by increasing outflow and decreasing rate of aqueous humor secretion. *Topical applications to eye produce vasoconstriction and prompt mydriasis of short duration, usually without causing cycloplegia. Nasal decongestant action qualitatively similar to that of epinephrine but more potent and has longer duration of action. Effective antihypotensive agent.*

USES Parenterally to maintain BP during anesthesia, to treat vascular failure in shock, and to overcome paroxysmal supraventricular tachycardia. Used topically for rhinitis of common cold, allergic rhinitis, and sinusitis; in selected patients with wide-angle glaucoma; as mydriatic for ophthalmoscopic examination or surgery, and for relief of uveitis.

CONTRAINDICATIONS Severe coronary disease, severe hypertension, atrial fibrillation, atrial flutter, cardiac arrhythmias; severe organic cardiac disease, cardiomyopathy; uncontrolled hypertension; ventricular fibrillation or tachycardia; acute MI, angina; cerebral arteriosclerosis, MAOI; narrow-angle glaucoma (ophthalmic preparations); labor, delivery.

CAUTIOUS USE Hyperthyroidism; diabetes mellitus; older adult patients; 21 days before or following termination of MAO inhibitor therapy; pregnancy (category C), lactation.

ROUTE & DOSAGE

Hypotension
Adult: **IM/Subcutaneous** 1–10 mg (initial dose not to exceed 5 mg) q10–15min as needed **IV** 0.1–0.18 mg/min until BP stabilizes; then 0.04–0.06 mg/min for maintenance

Ophthalmoscopy
See Appendix A

Supraventricular Tachycardia
Adult: **IV** 0.25–0.5 mg bolus, then 0.1–0.2 mg doses (total max: 1 mg)

Vasoconstrictor
Adult: **Ophthalmic** See Appendix A-1 **Intranasal** Small amount of nasal jelly placed into each nostril q3–4h as needed or 2–3 drops or sprays of 0.25–0.5% solution q3–4h as needed
Child: **Intranasal** *Younger than 6 y,* 2–3 drops or sprays of 0.125% solution q3–4h as needed; *6–12 y,* 2–3 drops or sprays of 0.25% solution q3–4h as needed

ADMINISTRATION

Instillation

- Nasal preparations: Instruct patient to blow nose gently (with both nostrils open) to clear nasal passages before administration of medication.
- Instillation (drops): Tilt head back while sitting or standing up, or lie on bed and hang head over side. Stay in position a few minutes to permit medication to spread through nose. (Spray): With head upright, squeeze bottle quickly and firmly to produce 1 or 2 sprays into each nostril; wait 3–5 min, blow nose, and repeat dose. (Jelly): Place in each nostril and sniff it well back into nose.
- Clean tips and droppers of nasal solution dispensers with hot water after use to prevent contamination of solution. Droppers of ophthalmic solution bottles should not touch any surface including the eye.
- Ophthalmic preparations: To avoid excessive systemic absorption, apply pressure to lacrimal sac during and for 1–2 min after instillation of drops.

Subcutaneous/Intramuscular

- Give undiluted.

Intravenous

Note: Ensure patency of IV site prior to administration.

PREPARE: **Direct:** Dilute each 10 mg (1 mL) of 1% solution in 9 mL of sterile water. **IV Infusion:** Dilute each 10 mg in 500 mL D5W or NS (concentration: 0.02 mg/mL).

ADMINISTER: **Direct:** Give a single dose over 60 sec. **IV Infusion:** Titrate to maintain BP.

INCOMPATIBILITIES **Solution/additive:** **Phenytoin** **Y-site:** **Propofol, thiopental.**

- Protect from exposure to air, strong light, or heat, any of which can cause solutions to change color to brown, form a precipitate, and lose potency.

ADVERSE EFFECTS (≥1%) **Special Senses:** *Transient stinging,* lacrimation, brow ache, headache, blurred vision, allergy (pigmentary deposits on lids, conjunctiva, and cornea with prolonged use), increased sensitivity to light. *Rebound nasal congestion* (hyperemia and edema of mucosa), *nasal burning,* stinging, dryness, *sneezing.* **CV:** Palpitation, tachycardia, bradycardia (overdosage), extrasystoles, hypertension. **Body as a Whole:** Trembling, sweating, pallor, sense of fullness in head, tingling of extremities, sleeplessness, dizziness, light-headedness, weakness, restlessness, anxiety, precordial pain, *tremor,* <u>severe visceral or peripheral vasoconstriction</u>, necrosis if IV infiltrates.

INTERACTIONS Drug: ERGOT ALKALOIDS, **guanethidine, reserpine,** TRICYCLIC ANTIDEPRESSANTS increase pressor effects of phenylephrine; **halothane, digoxin** increase risk of arrhythmias; MAO INHIBITORS cause hypertensive crisis; **oxytocin** causes persistent hypertension; ALPHA-BLOCKERS, BETA-BLOCKERS antagonize effects of phenylephrine.

PHARMACOKINETICS Onset: Immediate IV; 10–15 min IM/Subcutaneous. **Duration:** 15–20 min IV; 30–120 min IM/Subcutaneous; 3–6 h topical. **Metabolism:** In liver and tissues by monoamine oxidase.

NURSING IMPLICATIONS

Assessment & Drug Effects

- Monitor infusion site closely as extravasation may cause tissue necrosis and gangrene. If extravasation does occur, area should be immediately injected with 5–10 mg of phentolamine (Regitine) diluted in 10–15 mL of NS.

- Monitor pulse, BP, and central venous pressure (q2–5min) during IV administration.
- Control flow rate and dosage to prevent excessive dosage. IV overdoses can induce ventricular dysrhythmias.
- Observe for congestion or rebound miosis after topical administration to eye.

Patient & Family Education

- Be aware that instillation of 2.5–10% strength ophthalmic solution can cause burning and stinging.
- Do not exceed recommended dosage regardless of formulation.
- Inform the physician if no relief is experienced from preparation in 5 days.
- Wear sunglasses in bright light because after instillation of ophthalmic drops, pupils will be large and eyes may be more sensitive to light than usual. Stop medication and notify physician if sensitivity persists beyond 12 h after drug has been discontinued.
- Be aware that some ophthalmic solutions may stain contact lenses.

P

PHENYTOIN Pr

(fen′i-toy-in)

Dilantin-125, Dilantin

PHENYTOIN SODIUM EXTENDED

Dilantin Kapseals, Phentek

PHENYTOIN SODIUM PROMPT

Dilantin

Classifications: ANTICONVULSANT; HYDANTOIN

Therapeutic: ANTICONVULSANT
Pregnancy Category: D

AVAILABILITY 100 mg capsule; 100 mg, 200 mg, 300 mg sustained release capsule; 50 mg chewable tablet; 125 mg/5 mL suspension; 50 mg/mL injection

ACTION & *THERAPEUTIC EFFECT*
Anticonvulsant action elevates the seizure threshold and/or limits the spread of seizure discharge. Phenytoin is accompanied by reduced voltage, frequency, and spread of electrical discharges within the motor cortex. *Inhibits seizure activity. Effective in treating arrhythmias associated with QT prolongation.*

USES To control tonic-clonic (grand mal) seizures, psychomotor and nonepileptic seizures (e.g., Reye's syndrome, after head trauma). Also used to prevent or treat seizures occurring during or after neurosurgery. Is not effective for absence seizures.
UNLABELED USES Antiarrhythmic agent (phenytoin IV) especially in treatment of digitalis-induced arrhythmias; treatment of trigeminal neuralgia (tic douloureux).

CONTRAINDICATIONS Hypersensitivity to hydantoin products; rash; seizures due to hypoglycemia; sinus bradycardia, complete or incomplete heart block; Adams-Stokes syndrome; pregnancy (category D).
CAUTIOUS USE Impaired liver or kidney function; alcoholism; blood dyscrasias; hypotension, severe myocardial insufficiency, impending or frank heart failure; older adult, debilitated, gravely ill patients; pancreatic adenoma; diabetes mellitus, hyperglycemia; respiratory depression; acute intermittent porphyria.

ROUTE & DOSAGE

Anticonvulsant

Adult: **PO** 15–20 mg/kg loading dose, then 300 mg/day in 1–3 divided doses, may be gradually increased by 100 mg/wk until seizures are controlled **IV** 10–15 mg/kg then 300 mg/day in divided doses

Child: **PO/IV** 15–20 mg/kg loading dose, then 5 mg/kg in 2 divided doses

ADMINISTRATION

Oral

- Ensure that sustained release form is not chewed or crushed. **Must be** swallowed whole.
- Do not give within 2–3 h of antacid ingestion.
- Shake suspension vigorously before pouring to ensure uniform distribution of drug.
- Note: Prompt release capsules and chewable tablets are not intended for once-a-day dosage since drug is too quickly bioavailable and can therefore lead to toxic serum levels.
- Use sustained release capsules ONLY for once-a-day dosage regimens.

Intravenous

Note: Verify correct rate of IV injection for administration to infants or children with physician.

- Inspect solution prior to use. May use a slightly yellowed injectable solution safely. Precipitation may be caused by refrigeration, but slow warming to room temperature restores clarity.

PREPARE: **Direct:** Give undiluted. Use only when clear without precipitate.

ADMINISTER: **Direct for Adult:** Give 50 mg or fraction thereof over 1 min (25 mg/min in older adult or when used as antiarrhythmic). ▪ Follow with an injection of sterile saline through the same in-place catheter or needle. DO NOT use solutions containing dextrose.

Direct for Child/Neonate: Give 1 mg/kg/min. ▪ Follow with an injection of sterile saline through the same in-place catheter or needle. DO NOT use solutions containing dextrose.

INCOMPATIBILITIES **Solution/additive:** **5% dextrose, lactated Ringer's, fat emulsion, sodium chloride, amikacin, aminophylline, bretylium, cephalothin, cephapirin, chloramphenicol, chlordiazepoxide, clindamycin, codeine phosphate, diphenhydramine, dobutamine, hydromorphone, insulin, levorphanol, lidocaine, lincomycin, meperidine, metaraminol, methadone, morphine, nitroglycerin, norepinephrine, penicillin G, pentobarbital, phenylephrine, phytonadione, procaine, prochlorperazine, secobarbital, streptomycin, warfarin.** **Y-site:** **Amikacin, amphotericin B cholesteryl complex, bretylium, cimetidine, ciprofloxacin, clarithromycin, clindamycin, diltiazem, dobutamine, enalaprilat, fenoldopam, gatifloxacin, heparin, hydromorphone, lidocaine, linezolid, methadone, morphine, ondansetron, potassium chloride, propofol, sufentanil, tacrolimus, theophylline, TPN, vitamin B complex with C.**

- Observe injection site frequently during administration to prevent infiltration. Local soft tis-

P

sue irritation may be serious, leading to erosion of tissues.

ADVERSE EFFECTS (≥1%) **CNS:** Usually dose-related: Nystagmus, *drowsiness,* ataxia, dizziness, mental confusion, tremors, insomnia, headache, seizures. **CV:** Bradycardia, hypotension, cardiovascular collapse, ventricular fibrillation, phlebitis. **Special Senses:** Photophobia, conjunctivitis, diplopia, blurred vision. **GI:** *Gingival hyperplasia,* nausea, vomiting, constipation, epigastric pain, dysphagia, loss of taste, weight loss, hepatitis, liver necrosis. **Hematologic:** Thrombocytopenia, leukopenia, leukocytosis, agranulocytosis, pancytopenia, eosinophilia; megaloblastic, hemolytic, or aplastic anemias. **Metabolic:** Fever, hyperglycemia, glycosuria, weight gain, edema, transient increase in serum thyrotropic (TSH) level, osteomalacia or rickets associated with hypocalcemia and elevated alkaline phosphatase activity. **Skin:** Alopecia, hirsutism (especially in young female); rash: scarlatiniform, maculopapular, urticaria, morbilliform; bullous, exfoliative, or purpuric dermatitis; Stevens-Johnson syndrome, toxic epidermal necrolysis, keratosis, neonatal hemorrhage. **Urogenital:** Acute renal failure, Peyronie's disease. **Respiratory:** Acute pneumonitis, pulmonary fibrosis. **Body as a Whole:** Periarteritis nodosum, acute systemic lupus erythematosus, craniofacial abnormalities (with enlargement of lips); lymphadenopathy.

DIAGNOSTIC TEST INTERFERENCE Phenytoin (HYDANTOINS) may produce lower than normal values for ***dexamethasone*** or ***metyrapone*** tests; may increase serum levels of ***glucose, BSP,*** and ***alkaline phosphatase*** and may decrease ***PBI*** and ***urinary steroid*** levels.

INTERACTIONS Drug: Alcohol decreases phenytoin effects; OTHER ANTICONVULSANTS may increase or decrease phenytoin levels; phenytoin may decrease absorption and increase metabolism of ORAL ANTICOAGULANTS; phenytoin increases metabolism of CORTICOSTEROIDS, ORAL CONTRACEPTIVES, and **nisoldipine,** decreasing their effectiveness; **amiodarone, chloramphenicol, omeprazole,** and **ticlopidine** increase phenytoin levels; ANTITUBERCULOSIS AGENTS decrease phenytoin levels. **Food: Folic acid, calcium,** and **vitamin D** absorption may be decreased by phenytoin; phenytoin absorption may be decreased by enteral nutrition supplements. **Herbal: Ginkgo** may decrease anticonvulsant effectiveness.

PHARMACOKINETICS Absorption: Completely from GI tract. **Peak:** 1.5–3 h prompt release; 4–12 h sustained release. **Distribution:** 95% protein bound; crosses placenta; small amount in breast milk. **Metabolism:** Oxidized in liver to inactive metabolites. **Elimination:** By kidneys. **Half-Life:** 22 h.

NURSING IMPLICATIONS

Assessment & Drug Effects

- Monitor infusion site closely as extravasation may cause tissue necrosis.
- Continuously monitor vital signs and symptoms during IV infusion and for an hour afterward. Watch for respiratory depression. Constant observation and a cardiac monitor are necessary with older adults or patients with cardiac disease. Margin between toxic and therapeutic IV doses is relatively small.
- Be aware of therapeutic serum concentration: 10–20 mcg/mL; toxic level: 30–50 mcg/mL; lethal

level: 100 mcg/mL. Steady-state therapeutic levels are not achieved for at least 7–10 days.

- Lab tests: Periodic serum phenytoin concentration; CBC with differential, platelet count, and Hct and Hgb; serum glucose, serum calcium, and serum magnesium; and liver funtion tests.
- Observe patient closely for neurologic adverse effects following IV administration.
- Monitor for gingival hyperplasia, which appears most commonly in children and adolescents and never occurs in patients without teeth.
- Make sure patients on prolonged therapy have adequate intake of vitamin D-containing foods and sufficient exposure to sunlight.
- Monitor diabetics for loss of glycemic control.
- Monitor for S&S of hypocalcemia (see Appendix F), especially in patients receiving other anticonvulsants concurrently, as well as those who are inactive, have limited exposure to sun, or whose dietary intake is inadequate.
- Observe for symptoms of folic acid deficiency: Neuropathy, mental dysfunction.
- Be alert to symptoms of hypomagnesemia (see Appendix F); neuromuscular symptoms: Tetany, positive Chvostek's and Trousseau's signs, seizures, tremors, ataxia, vertigo, nystagmus, muscular fasciculations.

Patient & Family Education

- Be aware that drug may make urine pink or red to red-brown.
- Report symptoms of fatigue, dry skin, deepening voice when receiving long-term therapy because phenytoin can unmask a low thyroid reserve.
- Do not alter prescribed drug regimen. Stopping drug abruptly may precipitate seizures and status epilepticus.
- Do not request/accept change in drug brand when refilling prescription without consulting physician.
- Understand the effects of alcohol: Alcohol intake may increase phenytoin serum levels, leading to phenytoin toxicity.
- Discontinue drug immediately if a measles-like skin rash or jaundice appears and notify physician.
- Be aware that influenza vaccine during phenytoin treatment may increase seizure activity. Consult physician.

PHYSOSTIGMINE SALICYLATE

(fi-zoe-stig′meen)

Antilirium

Classification: CHOLINESTERASE INHIBITOR

Therapeutic: ANTICHOLINERGIC ANTIDOTE, CHOLINESTERASE INHIBITOR

Prototype: Neostigmine

Pregnancy Category: C

AVAILABILITY 1 mg/mL injection

ACTION & *THERAPEUTIC EFFECT* Physostigmine competes with acetylcholine (ACE) for its binding site on acetylcholinesterase, thereby potentiating action of ACE on the skeletal muscle, GI tract and within the CNS. *Effective in reversing anticholingeric toxicity.*

USES To reverse anticholinergic toxicity.

CONTRAINDICATIONS Asthma; diabetes mellitus; gangrene, cardiovascular disease; mechanical obstruction of intestinal or urogenital tract; peptic ulcer disease; asthma; any vagotonic state; closed-angle glaucoma; secondary glaucoma; inflammatory disease of iris or ciliary body; lactation.

CAUTIOUS USE Epilepsy; parkinsonism; bradycardia; hyperthyroidism; seizure disorders; hypotension; pregnancy (category C).

ROUTE & DOSAGE

Reversal of Anticholinergic Effects

Adult: **IM/IV** 0.5–2 mg (IV not faster than 1 mg/min), repeat as needed
Child: **IV** 0.02 mg/kg/dose, may repeat q5–10min (max total dose: 2 mg)

ADMINISTRATION

- Use only clear, colorless solutions. Red-tinted solution indicates oxidation, and such solutions should be discarded.

Intramuscular

- Give undiluted.

Intravenous

Note: Verify correct rate of IV injection for infants or children with physician.

PREPARE: **Direct:** Give undiluted.
ADMINISTER: **Direct for Adult:** Give slowly at a rate of no more than 1 mg/min. ▪ Rapid administration and overdosage can cause a cholinergic crisis. **Direct for Child:** Give 0.5 mg or fraction thereof over at least 1 min. ▪ Rapid administration and overdosage can cause a cholinergic crisis.
INCOMPATIBILITIES **Solution/additive: Phenytoin, ranitidine. Y-site: Dobutamine.**

ADVERSE EFFECTS (≥1%) **Body as a Whole:** *Sweating,* cholinergic crisis (acute toxicity), hyperactivity, respiratory distress, convulsions. **CNS:** Restlessness, hallucinations, twitching, tremors, *sweating,* weakness, ataxia, convulsions, collapse. **GI:** *Nausea, vomiting, epigastric pain, diarrhea, salivation.* **Urogenital:** Involuntary urination or defecation. **Special Senses:** Miosis, *lacrimation,* rhinorrhea. **Respiratory:** Dyspnea, bronchospasm, respiratory paralysis, pulmonary edema. **Cardiovascular:** Irregular pulse, palpitations, bradycardia, rise in BP.

INTERACTIONS Drug: Antagonizes effects of **echothiophate, isoflurophate.**

PHARMACOKINETICS Absorption: Readily from mucous membranes, muscle, subcutaneous tissue; 10–12% absorbed from GI tract. **Onset:** 3–8 min IM/IV. **Duration:** 0.5–5 h IM/IV. **Distribution:** Crosses blood–brain barrier. **Metabolism:** In plasma by cholinesterase. **Elimination:** Small amounts in urine. **Half-Life:** 15–40 min.

NURSING IMPLICATIONS

Assessment & Drug Effects

- Monitor vital signs and state of consciousness closely in patients receiving drug for atropine poisoning. Since physostigmine is usually rapidly eliminated, patient can lapse into delirium and coma within 1 to 2 h; repeat doses may be required.
- Monitor closely for adverse effects related to CNS and for signs of sensitivity to physostigmine. Have atropine sulfate readily available for clinical emergency.
- Discontinue parenteral or oral drug if following symptoms arise: Excessive salivation, emesis, frequent urination, or diarrhea.
- Eliminate excessive sweating or nausea with dose reduction.

PHYTONADIONE (VITAMIN K$_1$)

(fye-toe-na-dye'one)

Mephyton

Classifications: VITAMIN K; ANTIDOTE

Therapeutic: VITAMIN K, ANTIDOTE

Pregnancy Category: C

AVAILABILITY 5 mg tablets; 2 mg/mL, 10 mg/mL injection

ACTION & *THERAPEUTIC EFFECT* Fat-soluble substance chemically identical to and with similar activity as naturally occurring vitamin K. Vitamin K is essential for hepatic biosynthesis of blood clotting Factors II, VII, IX, and X. *Promotes liver synthesis of clotting factors.*

USES Drug of choice as antidote for overdosage of coumarin and indandione oral anticoagulants. Also reverses hypoprothrombinemia secondary to administration of oral antibiotics, quinidine, quinine, salicylates, sulfonamides, excessive vitamin A, and secondary to inadequate absorption and synthesis of vitamin K (as in obstructive jaundice, biliary fistula, ulcerative colitis, intestinal resection, prolonged hyperalimentation). Also prophylaxis of and therapy for neonatal hemorrhagic disease.

CONTRAINDICATIONS Hypersensitivity to phytonadione, benzyl alcohol or castor oil; severe liver disease. **CAUTIOUS USE** Biliary tract disease, obstructive jaundice; elderly (IV use); pregnancy (category C).

ROUTE & DOSAGE

Anticoagulant Overdose

Adult: **PO/Subcutaneous/IM** 2.5–10 mg; rarely up to 50 mg/day, may repeat parenteral dose after 6–8 h if needed or PO dose after 12–24 h **IV** Emergency only: 10–15 mg at a rate of 1 mg/min or less, may be repeated in 4 h if bleeding continues

Hemorrhagic Disease of Newborns

Infant: **IM/Subcutaneous** 0.5–1 mg immediately after delivery, may repeat in 6–8 h if necessary

Other Prothrombin Deficiencies

Adult: **IM/Subcutaneous/IV** 2–25 mg

Child/Infant: **IM/Subcutaneous/IV** 0.5–5 mg

ADMINISTRATION

Oral

- Bile salts must be given with tablets if patient has deficient bile production.
- Store in tightly closed container and protect from light. Vitamin K is rapidly degraded by light.

Intramuscular/Subcutaneous

- Subcutaneous route is preferred. IM route has been associated with severe reactions.
- Apply gentle pressure to site following injection. Swelling (internal bleeding) and pain sometimes occur with injection.

Intravenous

Note: Reserve IV route only for emergencies.

PREPARE: **Direct:** Dilute a single dose in 10 mL D5W, NS, or D5/NS. ▪ Protect infusion solution from light.

ADMINISTER: **Direct:** Give solution immediately after dilution at a rate not to exceed 1 mg/min.

INCOMPATIBILITIES **Solution/additive: Ascorbic acid, cephalothin, dobutamine, doxycy-**

cline, magnesium sulfate, nitrofurantoin, phenobarbital, ranitidine, thiopental, vancomycin, warfarin. Y-site: Dobutamine.
▪ Protect infusion solution from light by wrapping container with aluminum foil or other opaque material. ▪ Discard unused solution and contents in open ampule.

ADVERSE EFFECTS (≥1%) **Body as a Whole:** Hypersensitivity or anaphylaxis-like reaction: Facial flushing, cramp-like pains, convulsive movements, chills, fever, diaphoresis, weakness, dizziness, shock, cardiac arrest. **CNS:** Headache (after oral dose), brain damage, death. **GI:** Gastric upset. **Hematologic:** Paradoxic hypoprothrombinemia (patients with severe liver disease), severe hemolytic anemia. **Metabolic:** Hyperbilirubinemia, kernicterus. **Respiratory:** Bronchospasm, dyspnea, sensation of chest constriction, respiratory arrest. **Skin:** Pain at injection site, hematoma, and nodule formation, erythematous skin eruptions (with repeated injections). **Special Senses:** Peculiar taste sensation.

P

DIAGNOSTIC TEST INTERFERENCE Falsely elevated ***urine steroids*** (by modifications of ***Reddy, Jenkins, Thorn procedure***).

INTERACTIONS Drug: Antagonizes effects of **warfarin; cholestyramine, colestipol, mineral oil** decrease absorption of oral phytonadione.

PHARMACOKINETICS Absorption: Readily from intestinal lymph if bile is present. **Onset:** 6–12 h PO; 1–2 h IM/Subcutaneous; 15 min IV. **Peak:** Hemorrhage usually controlled within 3–8 h; normal prothrombin time may be obtained in 12–14 h after administration. **Distribution:** Concentrates briefly in liver after absorption; crosses placenta; distributed into breast milk. **Metabolism:** Rapidly in liver. **Elimination:** In urine and bile.

NURSING IMPLICATIONS

Assessment & Drug Effects

- Monitor patient constantly. Severe reactions, including fatalities, have occurred during and immediately after IV and IM injection (see ADVERSE EFFECTS).
- Lab tests: Baseline and frequent PT/INR.
- Frequency, dose, and therapy duration are guided by PT/INR clinical response.
- Monitor therapeutic effectiveness which is indicated by shortened PT, INR, bleeding, and clotting times, as well as decreased hemorrhagic tendencies.
- Be aware that patients on large doses may develop temporary resistance to coumarin-type anticoagulants. If oral anticoagulant is reinstituted, larger than former doses may be needed. Some patients may require change to heparin.

Patient & Family Education

- Maintain consistency in diet and avoid significant increases in daily intake of vitamin K–rich foods when drug regimen is stabilized. Know sources rich in vitamin K: Asparagus, broccoli, cabbage, lettuce, turnip greens, pork or beef liver, green tea, spinach, watercress, and tomatoes.

PILOCARPINE HYDROCHLORIDE (Pr)

PILOCARPINE NITRATE

(pye-loe-kar′peen)

Adsorbocarpine, Isopto Carpine, Minims Pilocarpine ♣, Miocarpine ♣, Ocusert, Pilo, Pilocar, Salagen

Classifications: EYE PREPARATION; MIOTIC (ANTIGLAUCOMA); DIRECT-ACTING CHOLINERGIC

Therapeutic: ANTIGLAUCOMA

Pregnancy Category: C

AVAILABILITY 0.25%, 0.5%, 1%, 2%, 3%, 4%, 5%, 6%, 8%, 10% ophth solution; 4% ophth gel; 20 mcg/h, 40 mcg/h ocular insert; 5 mg tablets

ACTION & *THERAPEUTIC EFFECT* In open-angle glaucoma, pilocarpine causes contraction of the ciliary muscle, increasing the outflow of aqueous humor, which reduces intraocular pressure (IOP). In closed-angle glaucoma, it induces miosis by opening the angle of the anterior chamber of the eye, through which aqueous humor exits. *Decrease in IOP results from stimulation of ciliary and papillary sphincter muscles, thus facilitating outflow of aqueous humor.*

USES Open-angle and angle-closure glaucomas; to reduce IOP and to protect the lens during surgery and laser iridotomy; to counteract effects of mydriatics and cycloplegics following surgery or ophthalmoscopic examination; to treat xerostomia.

CONTRAINDICATIONS Secondary glaucoma, acute iritis, acute inflammatory disease of anterior segment of eye; uncontrolled asthma; lactation. **Ocular therapeutic system:** Not used in acute infectious conjunctivitis, keratitis, retinal detachment, or when intense miosis is required, contact lens use.

CAUTIOUS USE Bronchial asthma; biliary tract disease; COPD; hypertension; pregnancy (category C).

ROUTE & DOSAGE

Acute Glaucoma

Adult/Child: **Ophthalmic** 1 drop of 1–2% solution in affected eye q5–10min for 3–6 doses, then 1 drop q1–3h until IOP is reduced

Chronic Glaucoma

Adult/Child: **Ophthalmic** 1 drop of 0.5–4% solution in affected eye q4–12h or 1 ocular system (Ocusert) q7days

Miotic

Adult/Child: **Ophthalmic** 1 drop of 1% solution in affected eye

Xerostomia

Adult: **PO** 5 mg t.i.d., may increase up to 10 mg t.i.d.

ADMINISTRATION

Oral

- Give with a full glass of water, if not contraindicated.

Instillation

- Note: During acute phase, physician may prescribe instillation of drug into unaffected eye to prevent bilateral attack of acute glaucoma.
- Apply gentle digital pressure to periphery of nasolacrimal drainage system for 1–2 min immediately after instillation of drops to prevent delivery of drug to nasal mucosa and general circulation.

ADVERSE EFFECTS (≥1%) **CNS:** Oral (asthenia, headaches, dizziness, chills). **Special Senses:** Ciliary spasm with brow ache, twitching of eyelids, eye pain with change in eye focus, miosis, *diminished vision in poorly illuminated areas,* blurred vision, reduced visual acuity, sensitivity, contact allergy, lacrimation, follicular conjunctivitis, conjunctival irritation, cataract, retinal detachment. **GI:** *Nausea,* vomiting, abdominal cramps, diarrhea, epigastric distress, *salivation*. **Respiratory:** Bronchospasm, rhinitis. **CV:** Tachycardia. **Body as a Whole:** Tremors, *increased sweating,* urinary frequency.

INTERACTIONS Drug: The actions of pilocarpine and **carbachol** are additive when used concomitantly. Oral form may cause conduction disturbances with BETA-BLOCKERS. Antagonizes the effects of concurrent ANTICHOLINERGIC DRUGS (e.g., **atropine, ipratropium**). **Food:** High-fat meal decreases absorption of pilocarpine.

PHARMACOKINETICS Absorption: Topical penetrates cornea rapidly; readily absorbed from GI tract. **Onset:** Miosis 10–30 min; IOP reduction 60 min; salivary stimulation 20 min. **Peak:** Miosis 30 min; IOP reduction 75 min; salivary stimulation 60 min. **Duration:** Miosis 4–8 h; IOP reduction 4–14 h (7 days with Ocusert); salivary stimulation 3–5 h. **Metabolism:** Inactivated at neuronal synapses and in plasma. **Elimination:** In urine. **Half-Life:** 0.76–1.35 h.

P

NURSING IMPLICATIONS

Assessment & Drug Effects

- Be aware that hourly tonometric tests may be done during early treatment because drug may cause an initial transitory increase in IOP.
- Monitor changes in visual acuity.
- Monitor for adverse effects. Brow pain and myopia tend to be more prominent in younger patients and generally disappear with continued use of drug.

Patient & Family Education

- Understand that therapy for glaucoma is prolonged and that adherence to established regimen is crucial to prevent blindness.
- Do not drive or engage in potentially hazardous activities until vision clears. Drug causes blurred vision and difficulty in focusing.
- Discontinue medication if symptoms of irritation or sensitization persist and report to physician.

PIMECROLIMUS

(pim-e-cro-lim′us)

Elidel

Classifications: BIOLOGICAL RESPONSE MODIFIER; IMMUNOMODULATOR

Therapeutic: IMMUNOSUPPRESSANT; ANTI-INFLAMMATORY

Prototype: Cyclosporine

Pregnancy Category: C

AVAILABILITY 1% cream

ACTION & *THERAPEUTIC EFFECT* Pimecrolimus selectively inhibits inflammatory action of skin cells by blocking T-cell activation and cytokine release. It appears to inhibit the production of IL-2, IL-4, IL-10, and interferon gamma in T-cells. *Produces significant anti-inflammatory activity without evidence of skin atrophy.*

USES Short-term intermittent treatment of mild to moderate atopic dermatitis.

CONTRAINDICATIONS Hypersensitivity to pimecrolimus or components in the cream; Netherton's syndrome; application to active cutaneous viral infection; occlusive dressing; artificial or natural sunlight (UV) exposure; lactation; children younger than 2 y.

CAUTIOUS USE Infection at topical treatment sites; history of untoward effects with topical cyclosporine or tacrolimus; skin papillomas; immunocompromised patients; pregnancy (category C).

ROUTE & DOSAGE

Atopic Dermatitis
Adult: **Topical** Apply thin layer to affected skin b.i.d.

ADMINISTRATION

Topical
- Do not apply to any skin surface that appears to be infected.

ADVERSE EFFECTS (≥1%) **Body as a Whole:** Flu-like symptoms, infections, fever, increased risk of cancer. **CNS:** Headache. **GI:** Gastroenteritis, abdominal pain, nausea, vomiting, diarrhea, constipation. **Respiratory:** Sore throat, *upper respiratory infection, cough,* nasal congestion, asthma exacerbation, rhinitis, epistaxis. **Skin:** *Burning,* irritation, pruritus, skin infection, impetigo, folliculitis, skin papilloma, herpes simplex dermatitis, urticaria, acne. **Special Senses:** Ear infection, earache, conjunctivitis.

PHARMACOKINETICS Absorption: Minimal through intact skin. **Metabolism:** No evidence of skin-mediated metabolism, metabolized in liver by CYP3A4. **Elimination:** Primarily in feces.

NURSING IMPLICATIONS

Assessment & Drug Effects
- Assess for and report persistent skin irritation that develops following application of the cream and lasts for more than 1 wk.

Patient & Family Education
- Minimize exposure of treated area to natural or artificial sunlight.
- Immediately report a new or changed skin lesion to the physician.
- Stop topical application once signs of dermatitis have disappeared. Resume application at the first sign of recurrence.
- Wash hand thoroughly after application if hands are not the treatment sites.
- Report any significant skin irritation that results from application of the cream.

PIMOZIDE

(pi′moe-zide)
Orap
Classification: ANTIPSYCHOTIC
Therapeutic: ANTIPSYCHOTIC
Prototype: Haloperidol
Pregnancy Category: C

AVAILABILITY 1 mg, 2 mg tablets

ACTION & *THERAPEUTIC EFFECT* Potent central dopamine antagonist that alters release and turnover of central dopamine stores. Blockade of CNS dopaminergic receptors results in suppression of the motor and phonic tics that characterize Tourette's disorder. *Effective in suppressing motor and phonic tics associated with Tourette's disorder.*

USES To suppress severe motor and phonic tics in patient with Tourette's disorder who has failed to respond satisfactorily to standard treatment (e.g., haloperidol).
UNLABELED USES Schizophrenia.

CONTRAINDICATIONS Treatment of simple tics other than those associated with Tourette's disorder; drug-induced tics; history of cardiac dysrhythmias and conditions marked by prolonged QT syndrome, patient taking drugs that may prolong QT interval (e.g., quinidine); congenital heart defects, cardiac arrhythmias; electrolyte imbalance;

P

Parkinson's disease; severe toxic CNS depression; lactation.

CAUTIOUS USE Kidney and liver dysfunction; patients receiving anticonvulsant therapy; cardiac disease; glaucoma; BPH; urinary retention; pregnancy (category C). Safe use in children younger than 12 y is not known.

ROUTE & DOSAGE

Tourette's Disorder

Adult: **PO** 1–2 mg/day in divided doses, gradually increase dose every other day up to 0.2 mg/kg/day or 10 mg/day in divided doses, whichever is less (max: 0.2 mg/kg/day or 10 mg/day)
Adolescent: **PO** 0.05 mg/kg/day at bedtime, gradually increase as needed (max: 0.2 mg/kg/day or 10 mg, whichever is less)

ADMINISTRATION

Oral

- Increase drug dose gradually, usually over 1–3 wk, until maintenance dose is reached.
- Follow regimen prescribed by physician for withdrawal: Usually slow, gradual changes over a period of days or weeks (drug has a long half-life). Sudden withdrawal may cause reemergence of original symptoms (motor and phonic tics) and of neuromuscular adverse effects of the drug.

P

ADVERSE EFFECTS (≥1%) **Body as a Whole:** *Akathisia,* speech disorder, *torticollis, tremor,* handwriting changes, *akinesia,* fainting, hyperpyrexia, tardive dyskinesia, *rigidity, oculogyric crisis,* hyperreflexia; seizures, neuroleptic malignant syndrome; *extrapyramidal dysfunction,* hyperthermia, autonomic dysfunction; diaphoresis, weight changes, asthenia, chest pain, periorbital edema. **CNS:** Headache, *sedation, drowsiness,* insomnia, seizures, stupor. **CV:** Prolongation of QT interval, inverted or flattened T wave, appearance of U wave, labile blood pressure. **Urogenital:** Loss of libido, impotence, nocturia, urinary frequency, amenorrhea, dysmenorrhea, mild galactorrhea, urinary retention, acute renal failure. **Respiratory:** Dyspnea, respiratory failure. **Skin:** Sweating, skin irritation. **Special Senses:** Visual disturbances, photosensitivity, decreased accommodation, blurred vision, cataracts. **GI:** Increased salivation, nausea, vomiting, diarrhea, anorexia, abdominal cramps, constipation.

INTERACTIONS Drug: Alcohol and other CNS DEPRESSANTS increase CNS depression; ANTICHOLINERGIC AGENTS (e.g., TRICYCLIC ANTIDEPRESSANTS, **atropine**) increase anticholinergic effects; PHENOTHIAZINES, TRICYCLIC ANTIDEPRESSANTS, ANTIARRHYTHMICS, MACROLIDE ANTIBIOTICS, AZOLE ANTIFUNGALS, PROTEASE INHIBITORS, **nefazodone, sertraline, zileuton** increase risk of arrhythmias and heart block; pimozide antagonizes effects of ANTICONVULSANTS—there is loss of seizure control. **Food: Grapefruit juice** (greater than 1 qt/day) may increase plasma concentrations and adverse effects.

PHARMACOKINETICS Absorption: Slowly and variably from GI tract (40–50% absorbed). **Peak:** 6–8 h. **Metabolism:** In liver (by CYP3A4). **Elimination:** 80–85% in urine, 15–20% in feces. **Half-Life:** 55 h.

NURSING IMPLICATIONS

Note: See haloperidol for additional nursing implications.

Assessment & Drug Effects

- Obtain ECG baseline data at beginning of therapy and check pe-

riodically, especially during dosage adjustments.
- Notify physician immediately for widening or prolongation of the QT interval, which suggests developing cardiotoxicity.
- Risk of tardive dyskinesia appears to be greatest in women, older adults, and those on high-dose therapy.
- Be aware that extrapyramidal reactions often appear within the first few days of therapy, are dose-related, and usually occur when dose is high.
- Be aware that anticholinergic effects (dry mouth, constipation) may increase as dose is increased.

Patient & Family Education
- Adhere to established drug regimen (i.e., do not change dose or intervals and discontinue only with physician's guidance).
- Use measures to relieve dry mouth (frequent rinsing with water, saliva substitute, increased fluid intake) and constipation (increased dietary fiber, drink 6–8 glasses of water daily).
- Do not drive or engage in potentially hazardous activities because drug-caused hand tremors, drowsiness, and blurred vision may impair alertness and abilities.
- Pseudoparkinsonism symptoms are usually mild and reversible with dose adjustment.
- Be alert to the earliest symptom of tardive dyskinesia ("flycatching"—an involuntary movement of the tongue), and report promptly to the physician.
- Return to physician for periodic assessments of therapy benefit and cardiac status.
- Understand dangers of ingesting alcohol to prevent augmenting CNS depressant effects of pimozide.

PINDOLOL
(pin'doe-lole)
Visken
Classifications: BETA-ADRENERGIC RECEPTOR ANTAGONIST; ANTIHYPERTENSIVE; ANTIANGINAL
Therapeutic: ANTIHYPERTENSIVE; ANTIANGINAL
Prototype: Propranolol
Pregnancy Category: B

AVAILABILITY 5 mg, 10 mg tablets

ACTION & *THERAPEUTIC EFFECT* Hypotensive mechanism results from its competitively blocking beta-adrenergic receptors primarily in myocardium, and beta receptors within smooth muscle. *Lowers blood pressure by decreasing peripheral vascular resistance. Exerts vasodilation as well as hypotensive effects.*

USES Management of hypertension concurrently with a thiazide diuretic or as single agent. Used in patient who has failed to respond to diet, exercise, and weight reduction.
UNLABELED USES Stress and exercise-induced chronic stable angina pectoris.

CONTRAINDICATIONS Bronchospastic diseases, asthma; severe bradycardia, cardiogenic shock, AV block, sick sinus syndrome; cardiac failure; pulmonary failure; lactation. Safety in children is not established.
CAUTIOUS USE Nonallergic bronchospasm; COPD; CHF; diabetes mellitus; hyperthyroidism; myasthenia gravis; impaired liver and kidney function; pregnancy (category B).

ROUTE & DOSAGE

Hypertension
Adult: **PO** 5 mg b.i.d., may increase by 10 mg/day q2–3wk if needed up (max: 60 mg/day in 2–3 divided doses)
Geriatric: **PO** Start with 5 mg daily

Angina Pectoris
Adult: **PO** 15–40 mg/day in 3–4 divided doses

ADMINISTRATION

Oral
- Give drug at same time of day each day with respect to time of food intake for most predictable results.
- Withdraw or discontinue treatment gradually over a period of 1–2 wk.

ADVERSE EFFECTS (≥1%) **CNS:** *Fatigue,* dizziness, insomnia, drowsiness, confusion, fainting, decreased libido. **CV:** *Bradycardia,* hypotension, CHF. **GI:** Nausea, *diarrhea, constipation,* flatulence. **Respiratory:** <u>Bronchospasm</u>, pulmonary edema, dyspnea. **Body as a Whole:** Back or joint pain. Sensitivity reactions seen as antinuclear antibodies (ANA) (10–30% of patients). **Hematologic:** <u>Agranulocytosis</u>. **Urogenital:** Impotence. **Metabolic:** Hypoglycemia (may mask symptoms of a hypoglycemic reaction).

INTERACTIONS Drug: DIURETICS and other HYPOTENSIVE AGENTS increase hypotensive effect; effects of **albuterol, metaproterenol, terbutaline, pirbuterol** and **pindolol** antagonized; NSAIDS blunt hypotensive effect; decreases hypoglycemic effect of **glyburide; amiodarone** increases risk of bradycardia and sinus arrest.

PHARMACOKINETICS Absorption: Rapidly from GI tract; 50–95% reaches systemic circulation (first pass metabolism). **Onset:** 3 h. **Peak:** 1–2 h. **Duration:** 24 h. **Distribution:** Distributed into breast milk. **Metabolism:** 40–60% in liver. **Elimination:** In urine. **Half-Life:** 3–4 h.

NURSING IMPLICATIONS

Assessment & Drug Effects
- Monitor HR and BP. Report bradycardia and hypotension. Dosage adjustment may be indicated.
- Note: Hypotensive effect may begin within 7 days but is not at maximum therapeutically until about 2 wk after beginning of treatment.
- Lab test: Periodic CBC with differential, kidney function tests, and blood glucose.

Patient & Family Education
- Pindolol masks the dizziness and sweating symptoms of hypoglycemia. Monitor blood glucose for loss of glycemic control.
- Adhere to the prescribed drug regimen; if a change is desired, consult physician first. Abrupt withdrawal of drug might precipitate a thyroid crisis in a patient with hyperthyroidism, and angina in the patient with ischemic heart disease, leading to an MI.

PIOGLITAZONE HYDROCHLORIDE

(pi-o-glit′a-zone)
Actos
Classifications: ANTIDIABETIC; THIAZOLIDINEDIONE
Therapeutic: ANTIDIABETIC; INSULIN SENSITIZER
Prototype: Rosiglitazone maleate
Pregnancy Category: C

Common adverse effects in *italic*, life-threatening effects <u>underlined</u>; generic names in **bold**; classifications in SMALL CAPS; ♣ Canadian drug name; ⊕ Prototype drug

AVAILABILITY 15 mg, 30 mg, 45 mg tablets

ACTION & *THERAPEUTIC EFFECT* Decreases hepatic glucose output and increases insulin-dependent muscle glucose uptake in skeletal muscle and adipose tissue. Improves glycemic control in noninsulin-dependent diabetics (type 2) by enhancing insulin sensitivity of cells without stimulating pancreatic insulin secretion. *Improves glycemic control as indicated by improved blood glucose levels and decreased HbA1C to 6.5 or lower.*

USES Adjunct to diet in the treatment of type 2 diabetes mellitus.

CONTRAINDICATIONS Hypersensitivity to pioglitazone, troglitazone, rosiglitazone, englitazone; type 1 diabetes, or treatment of DKA; New York Heart Association (NYHA) Class III or IV heart failure; active liver disease or ALT levels greater than 2.5 times normal limit; jaundice; lactation.

CAUTIOUS USE Liver dysfunction; cardiovascular disease; hypertension, CHF, anemia, edema; renal impairment; older adults; pregnancy (category C). Safety and efficacy in children younger than 18 y are not established.

ROUTE & DOSAGE

Type 2 Diabetes Mellitus

Adult: **PO** 15–30 mg once daily (max: 45 mg daily)

ADMINISTRATION

Oral

- Give without regard to food.
- Do not initiate therapy if baseline serum ALT greater than 2.5 times normal.
- Store at 15°–30° C (59°–86° F) in tightly closed container; protect from humidity and moisture.

ADVERSE EFFECTS (≥1%) **Body as a Whole:** Headache, myalgia, edema. **CV:** Edema, fluid retention, exacerbation of heart failure. **GI:** Tooth disorder. **Respiratory:** *Upper respiratory tract infection,* sinusitis, pharyngitis. **Metabolic:** Hypoglycemia, mild anemia.

INTERACTIONS Drug: Pioglitazone may decrease serum levels of ORAL CONTRACEPTIVES; **ketoconazole, gemfibrozil** may increase serum levels of **pioglitazone. Herbal: Garlic, ginseng** may potentiate hypoglycemic effects.

PHARMACOKINETICS Absorption: Rapidly absorbed. **Peak:** 2 h; steady state concentrations within 7 days. **Duration:** 24 h. **Distribution:** Greater than 99% protein bound. **Metabolism:** In liver to active metabolites. **Elimination:** Primarily in bile and feces. **Half-Life:** 16–24 h.

P

NURSING IMPLICATIONS

Assessment & Drug Effects

- Monitor for S&S hypoglycemia (possible when insulin/sulfonylureas are coadministered).
- Monitor closely for S&S of CHF or exacerbation of symptoms with preexisting CHF.
- Lab tests: Baseline serum ALT, then q2mo for first year, then periodically (more often if elevated); periodic HbA1C, Hgb and Hct, and lipid profile.
- Discontinue drug if ALT greater than 3 × ULN or patient has jaundice.
- Monitor weight and notify physician of development of edema.

Patient & Family Education

- Be aware that resumed ovulation is possible in nonovulating premenopausal women.
- Use or add barrier contraceptive if using hormonal contraception.
- Report immediately to physician: Unexplained anorexia, nausea, vomiting, abdominal pain, fatigue, dark urine; or S&S of fluid retention such as weight gain, edema, or activity intolerance.
- Combination therapy: May need adjustment of other antidiabetic drugs to avoid hypoglycemia.
- Learn of and adhere strictly to guideliness for liver function tests. Be sure to have blood tests for liver function every 2 mo for first year; then periodically.

PIPERACILLIN SODIUM (Pr)

(pi-per′a-sill-in)

Classifications: BETA-LACTAM ANTIBIOTIC; PENICILLIN
Therapeutic: ANTIBIOTIC
Pregnancy Category: B

AVAILABILITY 2 g, 3 g, 4 g injection

ACTION & *THERAPEUTIC EFFECT* Piperacillin is a beta-lactam antibiotic that inhibits final stage of bacterial cell wall synthesis by preferentially binding to specific penicillin-binding proteins (PBPs) located inside the bacterial cell wall. This interferes with cell wall synthesis promoting cell death. *Extended-spectrum penicillin with antibiotic activity against most gram-negative and many gram-positive anaerobic and aerobic organisms.*

USES Susceptible organisms that cause gynecologic, skin and skin structure, gonococcal, and streptococcal infections; lower respiratory tract, intra-abdominal, and bone and joint infections; septicemia, urinary tract infections. Also used prophylactically prior to and during surgery and as empiric antiinfective therapy in granulocytopenic patients.

CONTRAINDICATIONS Hypersensitivity to penicillins.
CAUTIOUS USE Liver and kidney dysfunction; hypersensitivity to cephalosporins or carbapenem; cystic fibrosis; eczema, asthma; GI disease; pregnancy (category B); lactation.

ROUTE & DOSAGE

Uncomplicated Urinary Tract Infection
Adult: **IV/IM** 6–8 g/day divided q6–12h

Complicated UTIs
Adult: **IV** 8–16 g/day divided q6–8h

Mild to Moderate Infections
Child: **IV** 200–300 mg/kg/day divided q4–6h (max: 24 g/day)
Neonate: **IV** 150–200 mg/kg/day divided q6–8h

Moderate to Severe Infections
Adult: **IV/IM** 1–3 g q6–8h

Life-Threatening Infection, *Pseudomonas* Infections
Adult: **IV** 12–18 g/day divided q4–6h)

Uncomplicated Gonococcal Infections
Adult: **IM** 2 g with 1 g oral probenecid given 30 min before

Renal Impairment Dosage Adjustment
CrCl 20–40 mL/min: Use 3–4 g q8h; less than 20 mL/min: Give q12h

Hemodialysis Dosage Adjustment: 20–50% dialyzable

ADMINISTRATION

Note: Patients undergoing hemodialysis usually receive a maximum dosage of 2 g piperacillin q8h and an additional 1 g dose after each dialysis period. Doses and frequency are usually modified if creatinine clearance is less than 40 mL/min.

Intramuscular

- Limit IM injections to 2 g/site. Use the gluteal muscle, preferably. Use deltoid muscle only if well developed.
- Diluents for reconstitution include sterile or bacteriostatic water for injection, bacteriostatic NaCl injection, and sterile lidocaine HCl injection 0.5–1.0% without epinephrine for IM. When reconstituted, solution contains 1 g/2.5 mL.

Intravenous

Note: Verify correct IV concentration and rate of infusion for administration to neonates, infants, or children with physician.

PREPARE: **Direct:** Reconstitute by diluting each 1 g or fraction thereof with 5 mL sterile water or NS for injection. Shake well until dissolved. **Intermittent:** Further dilute reconstituted solution with 50–100 mL NS, D5W, D5NS, or LR. ▪ Note: Must administer within 2 h if diluted in LR.

ADMINISTER: **Direct:** Give over 3–5 min. Avoid rapid injection. **Intermittent:** Give over 30 min.

INCOMPATIBILITIES **Solution/additive:** AMINOGLYCOSIDES. **Y-site:** AMINOGLYCOSIDES, **amiodarone, amphotericin B cholesteryl complex, cisatracurium, filgrastim, fluconazole, gatifloxacin, gemcitabine, ondansetron, sargramostim, vancomycin, vinorelbine.**

ADVERSE EFFECTS (≥1%) **Body as a Whole:** Coughing, sneezing, feeling of uneasiness; systemic anaphylaxis, fever, widespread increase in capillary permeability and vasodilation with resulting edema (mouth, tongue, pharynx, larynx), laryngospasm, malaise, serum sickness (fever, malaise, pruritus, urticaria, lymphadenopathy, arthralgia, angioedema of face and extremities, neuritis prostration, eosinophilia), SLE-like syndrome, injection site reactions (pain, inflammation, abscess, phlebitis), superinfections (especially with *Candida* and gram-negative bacteria), neuromuscular irritability (twitching, lethargy, confusion, stupor, hyperreflexia, multifocal myoclonus, localized or generalized seizures, coma). **CV:** Hypotension, circulatory collapse, cardiac arrhythmias, cardiac arrest. **GI:** Vomiting, diarrhea, severe abdominal cramps, nausea, epigastric distress, diarrhea, flatulence, dark discoloration of tongue, sore mouth or tongue. **Urogenital:** Interstitial nephritis, Loeffler's syndrome, vasculitis. **Hematologic:** Hemolytic anemia, thrombocytopenia. **Metabolic:** Hyperkalemia (penicillin G potassium); hypokalemia, alkalosis, hypernatremia, CHF (penicillin G sodium). **Respiratory:** Bronchospasm, asthma. **Skin:** Itchy palms or axilla, pruritus, *urticaria*, flushed skin, *delayed skin rashes* ranging from urticaria to exfoliative dermatitis, Stevens-Johnson syndrome, fixed-drug eruptions, contact dermatitis.

INTERACTIONS Drug: May increase risk of bleeding with ANTICOAGULANTS; **probenecid** decreases elimination of piperacillin.

PHARMACOKINETICS Peak: 45 min IM; 5 min IV. **Distribution:** Widely distributed; highest concentrations in urine and bile; adequate CSF penetration with inflamed meninges; crosses placenta; distributed into breast milk. **Metabolism:** In liver. **Elimination:** Primarily in urine, partly in bile. **Half-Life:** 0.6–1.35 h.

NURSING IMPLICATIONS

Assessment & Drug Effects

- Obtain history of hypersensitivity to penicillins, cephalosporins, or other drugs prior to administration.
- Lab tests: C&S prior to first dose of the drug; start drug pending results. Periodic CBC with differential, platelet count, Hgb and Hct, and serum electrolytes.
- Monitor for hypersensitivity response; discontinue drug and notify physician if allergic response noted.
- Lab tests: Periodic CBC with differential, platelet count, Hgb and Hct, and serum electrolytes.
- Monitor for hemorrhagic manifestations because high doses may induce coagulation abnormalities.

Patient & Family Education

- Report significant, unexplained diarrhea.
- Withhold drug and report to physician if signs of an allergic reaction develop (e.g., itching, rash, hives).

P

PIPERACILLIN/TAZOBACTAM

(pi-per′a-cil-lin/taz-o-bac′tam)

Zosyn

Classifications: BETA-LACTAM ANTIBIOTIC; PENICILLIN

Therapeutic: ANTIBIOTIC

Prototype: Piperacillin sodium

Pregnancy Category: B

AVAILABILITY 2 g, 3 g, 4 g injection

ACTION & *THERAPEUTIC EFFECT* Antibacterial combination product consisting of the semisynthetic piperacillin and the beta-lactamase inhibitor tazobactam. Tazobactam has little antibacterial activity itself; however, in combination with piperacillin, it extends the spectrum of bacteria that are susceptible to piperacillin. *Two-drug combination has antibiotic activity against an extremely broad spectrum of gram-positive, gram-negative, and anaerobic bacteria.*

USES Treatment of moderate to severe appendicitis, uncomplicated and complicated skin and skin structure infections, endometritis, pelvic inflammatory disease, or nosocomial or community-acquired pneumonia caused by beta-lactamase-producing bacteria.

CONTRAINDICATIONS Hypersensitivity to piperacillin, tazobactam, penicillins; coagulopathy.

CAUTIOUS USE Hypersensitivity to cephalosporins, carbapenem or beta-lactamase inhibitors such as clavulanic acid and sulbactam; GI disease, colitis; cystic fibrosis; eczema; kidney failure; complicated urinary tract infections; pregnancy (category B), lactation.

ROUTE & DOSAGE

Moderate to Severe Infections

Adult: **IV** 3.375 g q6h, infused over 30 min, for 7–10 days

Child: **IV** *Younger than 6 mo,* 150–300 mg piperacillin/kg/day divided q6–8h; *6 mo or older,* 240 mg piperacillin component/kg/day divided q8h

Nosocomial Pneumonia

Adult: **IV** 4.5 g q6h, infused over 30 min, for 7–10 days

Renal Insufficiency Dosage Adjustment

CrCl 20–40 mL/min: 2.25 g q6h; less than 20 mL/min: 2.25 g q8h

Hemodialysis Dosage Adjustment: 2.25 g q12h (for nosocomial pneumonia dose q8h); give additional 0.75 g after dialysis session

ADMINISTRATION

Note: Verify correct IV concentration and rate of infusion for administration to infants or children with physician.

Intravenous

PREPARE: **Intermittent:** Reconstitute powder with 5 mL of diluent (e.g., D5W, NS) for each 1 g or fraction thereof; shake well until dissolved. ▪ Further dilute to a total of 50 mL or less in selected diluent [e.g., NS, sterile water for injection, D5W, dextran 6% in NS, and LR only with solution containing EDTA].

ADMINISTER: **Intermittent:** Give over at least 30 min. ▪ DO NOT administer through a line with another infusion.

INCOMPATIBILITIES **Solution/additive:** **Aminoglycosides, lactated Ringer's, albumin, blood products, solutions containing sodium bicarbonate.** **Y-site:** **Acyclovir, aminoglycosides, amiodarone, amphotericin B, amphotericin B cholesteryl complex, azithromycin, chlorpromazine, cisatracurium, cisplatin, dacarbazine, daunorubicin, dobutamine, doxorubicin, doxorubicin liposome, doxycycline, droperidol, famotidine, ganciclovir, gatifloxacin, gemcitabine, haloperidol, hydroxyzine, idarubicin, miconazole, minocycline, mitomycin, mitoxantrone, nalbuphine, prochlorperazine, promethazine, streptozocin, vancomycin.**

ADVERSE EFFECTS (≥1%) **CNS:** Headache, insomnia, fever. **GI:** Diarrhea, constipation, nausea, vomiting, dyspepsia, <u>pseudomembranous colitis</u>. **Skin:** Rash, pruritus, hypersensitivity reactions.

INTERACTIONS Drug: May increase risk of bleeding with ANTICOAGULANTS; **probenecid** decreases elimination of piperacillin.

PHARMACOKINETICS Distribution: Distributes into many tissues, including lung, blister fluid, and bile; crosses placenta; distributed into breast milk. **Metabolism:** In liver. **Elimination:** In urine. **Half-Life:** 0.7–1.2 h.

NURSING IMPLICATIONS

Assessment & Drug Effects

- Obtain history of hypersensitivity to penicillins, cephalosporins, or other drugs prior to administration.
- Lab tests: C&S prior to first dose of the drug; start drug pending results. Monitor hematologic status with prolonged therapy (Hct and Hgb, CBC with differential and platelet count).
- Monitor patient carefully during the first 30 min after initiation of the infusion for signs of hypersensitivity (see Appendix F).

Patient & Family Education

- Report rash, itching, or other signs of hypersensitivity immediately.

- Report loose stools or diarrhea as these may indicate pseudomembranous colitis.

PIRBUTEROL ACETATE

(pir-bu′ter-ol)

Maxair

Classifications: BETA-ADRENERGIC AGONIST; BRONCHODILATOR
Therapeutic: BRONCHODILATOR
Prototype: Albuterol
Pregnancy Category: C

AVAILABILITY 0.2 mg aerosol

ACTION & *THERAPEUTIC EFFECT* Selective agonist of beta$_2$-adrenergic receptors that relaxes bronchospasm and increases ciliary motion. Activates the enzyme that catalyzes the conversion of ATP to cyclic adenosine monophosphate (cAMP). Increased cAMP is associated with relaxation of bronchial smooth muscle and inhibition of the release of histamine and other mediators of hypersensitivity from mast cells. *Effective bronchodilator and decreases the release of mediators within the mast cell that cause a hypersensitivity reaction.*

USES Prevention and reversal of bronchospasm associated with asthma.

CONTRAINDICATIONS Hypersensitivity to pirbuterol or any other adrenergic agent such as epinephrine, albuterol, or isoproterenol; lactation, children younger than 12 y.

CAUTIOUS USE Heart disease, irregular heartbeat; QT prolongation, AV block; high blood pressure, history of stroke or seizures; diabetes; Parkinson's disease; thyroid disease; prostate disease; glaucoma; pregnancy (category C).

ROUTE & DOSAGE

Asthma
Adult/Child (older than 12 y): **Inhaled** 2 inhalations (0.4 mg) q6h (max: 12 inhalations/day)

ADMINISTRATION

Inhalation

- Shake inhaler canister well immediately before using.
- Direct patient to exhale deeply, loosely close lips around mouthpiece, then inhale slowly and deeply through mouthpiece while pressing top of canister.
- Store at 15°–30° C (59°–86° F).

ADVERSE EFFECTS (≥1%) **CNS:** Nervousness, headache, dizziness, tremor. **CV:** Palpitations, tachycardia. **GI:** Dry mouth, nausea, glossitis, abdominal pain, cramps, anorexia, diarrhea, stomatitis. **Other:** Cough, tolerance.

INTERACTIONS Drug: Epinephrine and other SYMPATHOMIMETIC BRONCHODILATORS may have additive effects. BETA-BLOCKERS may antagonize the effects.

PHARMACOKINETICS Onset: 5 min. **Peak:** 30 min. **Duration:** 3–4 h. **Metabolism:** In liver. **Elimination:** By kidneys. **Half-Life:** 2–3 h.

NURSING IMPLICATIONS

Assessment & Drug Effects

- Monitor arterial blood gases and pulmonary functions periodically.
- Monitor vital signs. Report tachycardia, palpitations, and hypertension or hypotension.

Patient & Family Education

- Learn proper technique for using the inhaler.
- Report palpitations, chest pain, nervousness, tremors, or other bother-

some adverse effects promptly to physician.

- Contact physician immediately if symptoms of asthma worsen or you do not respond to the usual dose.
- Adhere rigidly to dosing directions and contact physician if breathing difficulty persists.

PIROXICAM

(peer-ox'i-kam)

Feldene

Classification: ANALGESIC, NONSTEROIDAL ANTI-INFLAMMATORY DRUG (NSAID)

Therapeutic: ANALGESIC, NSAID; ANTIPYRETIC

Prototype: Ibuprofen

Pregnancy Category: C

AVAILABILITY 10 mg, 20 mg capsules

ACTION & *THERAPEUTIC EFFECT* Nonsteroidal anti-inflammatory agent that strongly inhibits enzyme cyclooxygenase, both COX1 and COX2, the catalyst of prostaglandin synthesis. Decreased prostaglandin results in anti-inflammatory properties, analgesic and antipyretic effects. *Decreases inflammatory processes in bone-joint disease, as well as has analgesic and antipyretic effects.*

USES Acute and long-term relief of mild to moderate pain and for symptomatic treatment of osteoarthritis and rheumatoid arthritis.

UNLABELED USES Acute and chronic relief of mild to moderate pain.

CONTRAINDICATIONS Hypersensitivity to NSAIDs or salicylates; hemophilia; active peptic ulcer, GI bleeding; CABG perioperative pain; ST-elevated MI; lactation. Safety in children is not established.

CAUTIOUS USE History of upper GI disease including ulcerative colitis; SLE; kidney dysfunction; hepatic disease; CHF; acute MI; compromised cardiac function; hypertension or other conditions predisposing to fluid retention; renal disease; alcoholism; coagulation disorders; elderly; pregnancy (category C).

ROUTE & DOSAGE

Arthritis, Pain

Adult: **PO** 10–20 mg 1–2 times/day

ADMINISTRATION

Oral

- Give at the same time every day.
- Give capsule with food or fluid to help reduce GI irritation.
- Dose adjustments should be made on basis of clinical response at intervals of weeks rather than days in order to prevent over dosage.
- Store in tightly closed container at 15°–30° C (59°–86° F) unless otherwise directed.

ADVERSE EFFECTS (≥1%) **CNS:** Somnolence, dizziness, vertigo, depression, insomnia, nervousness. **CV:** Peripheral edema, hypertension, worsening of CHF, exacerbation of angina. **Special Senses:** Tinnitus, hearing loss, blurred vision, reduced visual acuity, changes in color vision, scotomas, corneal deposits, retinal disturbances. **GI:** *Nausea, vomiting, dyspepsia,* <u>GI bleeding</u>, diarrhea, constipation, flatulence, dry mouth, <u>peptic ulceration</u>, anorexia, jaundice, hepatitis. **Hematologic:** Anemia, decreases in Hgb, Hct; leukopenia, eosinophilia, <u>aplastic anemia</u>; thrombocytopenia, *prolonged bleeding time.* **Skin:** Urticaria, erythema multiforme, maculopapular, vesiculobullous rash; photosensitivity, sweating, Stevens-Johnson syndrome, bruising, dermatitis. **Body as a Whole:** Allergic rhinitis, angioedema, fever, palpitations, syncope, muscle cramps, fever, hypersensitivity reactions. **Metabolic:** Hypoglycemia, hyperglycemia, hyperkalemia, weight gain. **Urogenital:** Dysuria, acute kidney failure, papillary necrosis, hematuria, proteinuria, nephrotic syndrome. **Respiratory:** Bronchospasm, dyspnea.

INTERACTIONS Drug: ORAL ANTICOAGULANTS, **heparin** may prolong bleeding time; may increase **lithium** toxicity; **alcohol, aspirin** increase risk of GI hemorrhage. **Herbal: Feverfew, garlic, ginger, ginkgo** may increase bleeding potential.

PHARMACOKINETICS Absorption: Extenstively from GI tract. **Onset:** 1 h analgesia; 7 days for rheumatoid arthritis. **Peak:** 3–5 h analgesia; 2–4 wk antirheumatic. **Duration:** 48–72 h analgesia. **Distribution:** Small amount distributed into breast milk. **Metabolism:** Extensively in liver. **Elimination:** Primarily in urine, some in bile (less than 5%). **Half-Life:** 30–86 h.

NURSING IMPLICATIONS

Assessment & Drug Effects

- Wait at least 7 days to evaluate antirheumatic effect.
- Clinical evidence of benefits from drug therapy include pain relief in motion and in rest, reduction in night pain, stiffness, and swelling; increased ROM (range of motion) in all joints.
- Be aware that adverse effects may not appear for 7–10 days after start of therapy (except for an allergic reaction).
- Lab tests: Periodic BUN, ALT, AST, CBC, Hgb and Hct in patient (especially the older adult) receiving drug for an extended period.

Patient & Family Education

- If a dose is missed, take drug when missed dose is discovered if it is 6–8 h before the next scheduled dose. Otherwise, omit dose and reestablish regimen at next scheduled hour.
- Do not self-dose with aspirin or other OTC drug without physician's advice.
- Do not increase dosage beyond prescribed regimen. Understand that long half-life of drug may cause delayed therapeutic effect. Higher than recommended doses are associated with increased incidence of GI irritation and peptic ulcer.
- Incidence of GI bleeding with this drug is relatively high. Report symptoms of GI bleeding (e.g., dark, tarry stools, coffee-colored emesis) or severe gastric pain promptly to physician.
- Be alert to symptoms of drug-induced anemia: Profound fatigue, skin and mucous membrane pallor, lethargy.
- Avoid alcohol since it may increase the risk of GI bleeding.
- Be alert to signs of hypoprothrombinemia including bruises, pinpoint rash, unexplained bleeding, nose bleed, blood in urine, when piroxicam is taken concomitantly with an anticoagulant.
- Do not drive or engage in potentially hazardous activities until response to drug is known.
- Drink at least 6–8 full glasses of water daily and report signs of renal insufficiency (see Appendix F) to physician because most of drug is excreted by kidneys and

impaired kidney function increases danger of toxicity.

PITAVASTATIN CALCIUM

(pit-a-vah-stat′in)

Livalo

Classifications: ANTIHYPERLIPIDEMIC; LIPID-LOWERING AGENT; HMG-COA REDUCTASE INHIBITOR (STATIN)

Therapeutic: ANTILIPEMIC; LIPID-LOWERING AGENT; STATIN

Prototype: Lovastatin

Pregnancy Category: X

AVAILABILITY 1 mg, 2 mg, 4 mg tablets

ACTION & *THERAPEUTIC EFFECT* Pitavastatin is a HMG-CoA reductase inhibitor that reduces plasma cholesterol levels by interfering with the production of cholesterol in the liver. It also promotes removal of LDL and VLDL from plasma. *Effectiveness is measured by decrease in blood level of total cholesterol, LDL cholesterol and triglycerides and an increase in HDL cholesterol.*

USES Treatment of hypercholesterolemia, hyperlipoproteinemia, and/or hypertriglyceridemia as an adjunct to dietary control. Pitavastatin reduces elevated total cholesterol, LDL cholesterol, apolipoprotein B, and triglyceride concentrations, and increases HDL cholesterol in patients with primary hypercholesterolemia or mixed dyslipidemia.

UNLABELED USES Regression of coronary atherosclerosis in patients with acute coronary syndrome (ACS).

CONTRAINDICATIONS Hypersensitivity to pitavastatin; myopathy and rhabdomyolysis; acute renal failure; ESRD not on hemodialysis; active liver disease; pregnancy (category X); lactation. Safety and effectiveness have not been established.

CAUTIOUS USE Moderate or mild renal impairment; elderly.

ROUTE & DOSAGE

Hypercholesterolemia, Hyperlipoproteinemia, and/or Hypertriglyceridemia

Adult: **PO** Initially 2 mg once daily; can be adjusted to 1–4 mg once daily.

Renal Impairment Dosage Adjustment

CrCl 30 to less than 60 mL/min: Initially, 1 mg once daily; do not exceed 2 mg once daily
CrCl less than 30 mL/min on hemodialysis: Initially, 1 mg once daily; do not exceed 2 mg once daily
CrCl less than 30 mL/min not on hemodialysis: Not recommended

ADMINISTRATION

Oral

- May give without regard to meals any time of day.
- Store at 15°–30° C (59°–86° F).

ADVERSE EFFECTS (≥1%) **Body as a Whole:** Pain in extremity, influenza. **CNS:** Headache. **GI:** Constipation, diarrhea. **Hematologic:** Elevated creatine phosphokinase (CPK), elevated transaminase (AST and ALT) levels. **Musculoskeletal:** Arthralgia, back pain, myalgia. **Respiratory:** Nasopharyngitis. **Skin:** Pruritus, rash, urticaria.

INTERACTIONS Drug: Cyclosporine, erythromycin, HIV PROTEASE INHIBITORS, and **rifampin** increase pi-

P

tavastatin levels. FIBRATES may increase the risk of myopathy and rhabdomyolysis. Combination use with **niacin** may increase the risk of skeletal muscle effects.

PHARMACOKINETICS Absorption: 51% bioavailable. **Peak:** 1 h. **Distribution:** Greater than 99% plasma protein bound. **Metabolism:** In liver. **Elimination:** Primarily fecal (79%) with minor renal (15%) elimination. **Half-Life:** 12 h.

NURSING IMPLICATIONS

Assessment & Drug Effects

- Monitor for and report muscle pain, tenderness, or weakness.
- Withhold drug and notify physician for ALT/AST greater than 3 × ULN.
- Lab tests: Lipid profile at baseline, at 4 wk, and periodically thereafter; LFTs at baseline, at 12 wk after initiation or elevation of dose, and periodically thereafter; creatine kinase levels if patient experiences muscle pain.

Patient & Family Education

- Report promptly unexplained muscle pain, tenderness, or weakness.
- Avoid or minimize alcohol consumption while on this drug.
- Use effective contraceptive measures to avoid pregnancy while taking this drug.

PLASMA PROTEIN FRACTION

(plas′ma)

Plasmanate, Plasma-Plex, Protenate

Classification: PLASMA VOLUME EXPANDER

Therapeutic: PLASMA VOLUME EXPANDER; ALBUMIN

Prototype: Normal serum albumin, human

Pregnancy Category: C

AVAILABILITY 5% injection

ACTION & *THERAPEUTIC EFFECT* Provides plasma proteins that increase colloidal osmotic pressure within the intravascular compartment equal to human plasma. It shifts water from the extravascular tissues back into the intravascular space, thus expanding plasma volume. *Used to maintain cardiac output by expanding plasma volume in the treatment of shock due to various causes.*

USES Emergency treatment of hypovolemic shock due to burns, trauma, surgery, infections; temporary measure in treatment of blood loss when whole blood is not available; to replenish plasma protein in patients with hypoproteinemia (if sodium restriction is not a problem).

CONTRAINDICATIONS Hypersensitivity to albumin; severe anemia; cardiac failure; patients undergoing cardiopulmonary bypass surgery.

CAUTIOUS USE Patients with low cardiac reserve; absence of albumin deficiency; liver or kidney failure; pregnancy (category C).

ROUTE & DOSAGE

Plasma Volume Expansion

Adult: **IV** 250–500 mL at a maximum rate of 10 mL/min
Child: **IV** 6.6–30 mL/kg at a rate of 5–10 mL/min

Hypoproteinemia

Adult: **IV** 1–1.5 L/day infused at a rate not to exceed 5–8 mL/min

ADMINISTRATION

Intravenous

Do not use solutions that show a sediment or appear turbid.

- Do not use solutions that have been frozen.

PREPARE: **IV Infusion:** Give undiluted. ▪ Once container is opened, solution should be used within 4 h because it contains no preservatives. ▪ Discard unused portions.

ADMINISTER: **IV Infusion:** Rate of infusion and volume of total dose will depend on patient's age, diagnosis, degree of venous and pulmonary congestion, Hct, and Hgb determinations. As with any oncotically active solution, infusion rate should be relatively slow. Range may vary from 1–10 mL/min.

INCOMPATIBILITIES PROTEIN HYDROLYSATES or solutions containing alcohol.

ADVERSE EFFECTS (≥1%) **GI:** Nausea, vomiting, hypersalivation, headache. **Body as a Whole:** Tingling, chills, fever, cyanosis, chest tightness, backache, urticaria, erythema, <u>shock (systemic anaphylaxis)</u>, circulatory overload, pulmonary edema.

NURSING IMPLICATIONS

Assessment & Drug Effects

- Monitor vital signs (BP and pulse). Frequency depends on patient's condition. Flow rate adjustments are made according to clinical response and BP. Slow or stop infusion if patient suddenly becomes hypotensive.
- Report a widening pulse pressure (difference between systolic and diastolic); it correlates with increase in cardiac output.
- Report changes in I&O ratio and pattern.
- Observe patient closely during and after infusion for signs of hypervolemia or circulatory overload (see Appendix F). Report these symptoms immediately to physician.
- Make careful observations of patient who has had either injury or surgery in order to detect bleeding points that failed to bleed at lower BP.

PODOPHYLLUM RESIN (PODOPHYLLIN)

(pode-oh-fill′um)

Podo-ben, Podofin

PODOFILOX

Condylox

Classification: KERATOLYTIC

Therapeutic: CYTOTOXIC; KERATOLYTIC

Pregnancy Category: C

AVAILABILITY Podophyllum: 25% liquid; **Podofilox:** 0.5% gel, solution

ACTION & *THERAPEUTIC EFFECT*

Potent cytotoxic and keratolytic agent that directly affects epithelial cell metabolism, causing degeneration and arrest of mitosis. *Slow disruption of cells and tissue erosion as a result of its caustic action. Selectively affects embryonic and tumor cells more than adult cells.*

USES Benign growths including external genital and perianal warts, papillomas, fibroids.

CONTRAINDICATIONS Birthmarks, moles, or warts with hair growth from them; cervical, urethral, oral warts; normal skin and mucous membranes peripheral to treated areas; diabetes mellitus; patient with poor circulation; irritated, or bleeding skin; application of drug over large area.

CAUTIOUS USE Pregnancy (category C), lactation. Safe use in children is not known.

P

ROUTE & DOSAGE

Condylomata Acuminata

Adult: **Topical** Use 10% solution and repeat 1–2 times/wk for up to 4 applications

Verruca Vulgaris (Common Wart)

Adult: **Topical** Apply 0.5% solution q12h for up to 4 wk

Multiple Superficial Epitheliomatosis, Keratoses

Adult: **Topical** Apply 0.5% solution or gel daily for several days

ADMINISTRATION

Note: Use 10–25% solution for areas less than 10 cm^2 or 5% solution for areas of 10–20 cm^2, anal, or genital warts; apply drug to dry surface, allowing area to dry between drops, wash off after 1–4 h.

Topical

- Avoid podophyllum resin contact with eyes or similar mucosal surfaces; if it occurs, flush thoroughly with lukewarm water for 15 min and remove film precipitated by the water.
- Avoid application of drug to normal tissue. If it occurs, remove with alcohol. Protect surfaces surrounding area to be treated with a layer of petrolatum or flexible collodion.
- Remove drug thoroughly with soap and water after each treatment of accessible tissue surface.
- Apply a protective coat of talcum powder after treatment and drying of anogenital area.
- Remove drug with alcohol, if application causes extreme pain, pruritus, or swelling.
- Store in a tight, light-resistant container; avoid exposure to excessive heat.

ADVERSE EFFECTS (≥1%) **Body as a Whole:** Severe systemic toxicity (sometimes fatal), sensorimotor neuropathy (reversible), symptomatic orthostatic hypotension, paresthesias and weakness of extremities, stocking-glove sensory loss, absent ankle reflexes, decreased response to painful stimuli. **CNS:** Lethargy, mental confusion, disorientation, delirium, agitation, seizures, progressive stupor, polyneuritis, pyrexia, coma, visual and auditory hallucinations, acute psychotic reaction, ataxia, hypotonia, areflexia, increased CSF protein, paralytic ileus. **CV:** Sinus tachycardia. **Hematologic:** Bone marrow suppression similar to that caused by antineoplastic drug toxicity, leukopenia, thrombocytopenia. **GI:** *Nausea, vomiting, diarrhea, abdominal pain,* hepatotoxicity, increased serum concentrations of LDH, AST, and alkaline phosphatase. **Urogenital:** Renal failure, urinary retention. **Respiratory:** Decreased respirations, apnea, hyperventilation.

NURSING IMPLICATIONS

Assessment & Drug Effects

- Warts become blanched, then necrotic within 24–48 h. Sloughing begins after about 72 h with no scarring. Frequently, a mild topical anti-infective agent, with or without a dressing, is applied until the healing is complete.
- Monitor neurologic status. Sensorimotor polyneuropathy, if it occurs, appears about 2 wk after application of drug, worsens for 3 mo, and may persist for up to 9 mo. Cerebral effects may persist for 7–10 days; ataxia, hypotonia,

Common adverse effects in *italic*, life-threatening effects underlined; generic names in **bold**; classifications in SMALL CAPS; ♣ Canadian drug name; Prototype drug

and areflexia improve more slowly than effects on sensorium.

Patient & Family Education

- Learn proper technique of treatment if self-administered as treatment of verruca vulgaris (common wart). Also be fully aware of the need to report treatment failure to physician.
- Be aware that as with any STD, the patient's sex partner should be examined.
- Systemic toxicity may be severe and serious and is associated with application of drug to large areas, to tissue that is friable, bleeding, or recently biopsied, or for prolonged time. Toxicity may occur within hours of application. There are significant dangers from overuse or misuse of this drug.
- Learn symptoms of toxicity and report any that appear promptly to physician (see ADVERSE EFFECTS).

POLYCARBOPHIL

(pol-i-kar'boe-fil)

Equalactin, FiberNorm

Classifications: BULK LAXATIVE; ANTIDIARRHEAL

Therapeutic: BULK LAXATIVE; ANTIDIARRHEAL

Prototype: Psyllium

Pregnancy Category: C

AVAILABILITY 500 mg, 625 mg tablets; 500 mg, 625 mg chewable tablets

ACTION & *THERAPEUTIC EFFECT* Hydrophilic agent that absorbs free water in intestinal tract and opposes dehydrating forces of bowel by forming a gelatinous mass. *Restores more normal moisture level and motility in the lower GI tract; produces well-formed stool and reduces diarrhea.*

USES Constipation or diarrhea associated with acute bowel syndrome, diverticulosis, irritable bowel and in patients who should not strain during defecation. Also choleretic diarrhea, diarrhea caused by small-bowel surgery or vagotomy, and disease of terminal ileum.

CONTRAINDICATIONS Partial or complete GI obstruction; fecal impaction; dysphagia; acute abdominal pain; rectal bleeding; undiagnosed abdominal pain, or other symptoms symptomatic of appendicitis; poisonings; before radiologic bowel examination; bowel surgery. Safety in children younger than 3 y is not established.

CAUTIOUS USE Renal failure, renal impairment; pregnancy (category C).

ROUTE & DOSAGE

Constipation or Diarrhea

Adult: **PO** 1 g q.i.d. prn (max: 6 g/day)

Child: **PO** *3–6 y,* 500 mg b.i.d. prn (max: 1.5 g/day); *6–12 y,* 500 mg t.i.d. prn (max: 3 g/day)

ADMINISTRATION

Oral

- Chewable tablets should be chewed well before swallowing.
- Give each dose with a full glass [240 mL (8 oz)] of water or other liquid.
- Repeat dose every 30 min up to the maximum dose in 24 h with severe diarrhea.
- Store at 15°–30° C (59°–86° F) in tightly closed container unless otherwise directed.

ADVERSE EFFECTS (≥1%) **GI:** Esophageal blockage, intestinal impaction, *abdominal fullness.* **Metabolic:** Low serum potassium, ele-

P

vated blood glucose levels (with extended use). **Respiratory:** Asthma. **Skin:** Skin rash.

INTERACTIONS Drug: May decrease absorption and clinical effects of ANTIBIOTICS, **warfarin, digoxin, nitrofurantoin,** SALICYLATES.

PHARMACOKINETICS Absorption: Not absorbed from GI tract. **Onset:** 12–24 h. **Peak:** 1–3 days.

NURSING IMPLICATIONS

Assessment & Drug Effects

- Determine duration and severity of diarrhea in order to anticipate signs of fluid-electrolyte losses.
- Monitor and record number and consistency of stools per day, presence and location of abdominal discomfort (i.e., tenderness, distention), and bowel sounds.
- Monitor and record I&O ratio and pattern. Dehydration is indicated if output is less than 30 mL/h.
- Inspect oral cavity for dryness, and be alert to systemic signs of dehydration (e.g., thirst and fever). Dehydration from an episode of diarrhea appears rapidly in young children and older adults.

P

Patient & Family Education

- Consult physician if sudden changes in bowel habit persist more than 1 wk, action is minimal or ineffective for 1 wk, or if there is no antidiarrheal action within 2 days.
- Be aware that extended use of this drug may cause dependence for normal bowel function.
- Do not discontinue polycarbophil unless physician advises if also taking an oral anticoagulant, digoxin, salicylates, or nitrofurantoin.

POLYMYXIN B SULFATE

(pol-i-mix′in)

Classifications: ANTIBIOTIC; PENICILLIN

Therapeutic: ANTIBIOTIC

Pregnancy Category: C (IV/IM form); B (topical form)

AVAILABILITY 500,000 unit injection

ACTION & *THERAPEUTIC EFFECT* Antibiotic that binds to lipid phosphates in bacterial membranes and changes permeability to permit leakage of cytoplasm from bacterial cells, resulting in cell death. *Bactericidal against susceptible gram-negative but not gram-positive organisms.*

USES Topically and in combination with other anti-infectives or corticosteroids for various superficial infections of eye, ear, mucous membrane, and skin. Concurrent systemic anti-infective therapy may be required for treatment of intraocular infection and severe progressive corneal ulcer. Used parenterally only in hospitalized patients for treatment of severe acute infections of urinary tract, bloodstream, and meninges; and in combination with Neosporin for continuous bladder irrigation to prevent bacteremia associated with use of indwelling catheter.

CONTRAINDICATIONS Hypersensitivity to polymyxin antibiotics; concurrent and sequential use of other nephrotoxic and neurotoxic drugs; respiratory insufficiency; concurrent use of products that inhibit peristalsis, skeletal muscle relaxants, ether, or sodium citrate. Safety in children younger than 1 mo is not established.

CAUTIOUS USE Impaired kidney function, renal failure; inflammatory bowel disease; myasthenia gravis;

pulmonary disease; **IV/IM form:** Pregnancy (category C), lactation; **topical form:** Pregnancy (category B).

ROUTE & DOSAGE

Infections

Adult/Child: **IV** 15,000–25,000 units/kg/day divided q12h **IM** 25,000–30,000 units/kg/day divided q4–6h **Intrathecal** 50,000 units × 3–4 days then every other day; *older than 2 y,* 20,000 units × 3–4 days, then 25,000 units every other day

Infant: **IV/IM** Up to 40,000 units/kg/day

Renal Impairment Dosage Adjustment

CrCl 5–20 mL/min: 7500–12,500 units/kg/day IV divided q12h; less than 5 mL/min: 2250–3750 units/kg/day IV divided q12h

ADMINISTRATION

Intramuscular

- Routine administration by IM routes not recommended because it causes intense discomfort, along the peripheral nerve distribution, 40–60 min after IM injection.
- Make IM injection in adults deep into upper outer quadrant of buttock. Select IM site carefully to avoid injection into nerves or blood vessels. Rotate injection sites. Follow agency policy for IM site used in children.

Intravenous

PREPARE: **Intermittent:** Reconstitute by dissolving 500,000 units in 5 mL sterile water for injection or NS to yield 100,000 units/mL. Withdraw a single dose and then further dilute in 300–500 mL of D5W.

ADMINISTER: **Intermittent:** Infuse over period of 60–90 min. ▪ Inspect injection site for signs of phlebitis and irritation.

INCOMPATIBILITIES **Solution/additive: Amphotericin B, cefazolin, cephalothin, cephapirin, chloramphenicol, heparin, nitrofurantoin, prednisolone, tetracycline.**

▪ Protect unreconstituted product and reconstituted solution from light and freezing. Store in refrigerator at 2°–8° C (36°–46° F). ▪ Parenteral solutions are stable for 1 wk when refrigerated. Discard unused portion after 72 h.

ADVERSE EFFECTS (≥1%) **Body as a Whole:** Irritability, facial flushing, ataxia, circumoral, lingual, and peripheral paresthesias (stocking-glove distribution); severe pain (IM site), thrombophlebitis (IV site), superinfections, electrolyte disturbances (prolonged use; also reported in patients with acute leukemia); local irritation and burning (topical use), <u>anaphylactoid reactions</u> (rare). **CNS:** Drowsiness, dizziness, vertigo, convulsions, coma; <u>neuromuscular blockade (generalized muscle weakness, respiratory depression or arrest)</u>; meningeal irritation, increased protein and cell count in cerebrospinal fluid, fever, headache, stiff neck (intrathecal use). **Special Senses:** Blurred vision, nystagmus, slurred speech, dysphagia, ototoxicity (vestibular and auditory) with high doses. **GI:** GI disturbances. **Urogenital:** Albuminuria, cylindruria, azotemia, hematuria; nephrotoxicity.

INTERACTIONS Drug: ANESTHETICS and NEUROMUSCULAR BLOCKING AGENTS may prolong skeletal muscle relaxation. AMINOGLYCOSIDES and **ampho-**

P

tericin B have additive nephrotoxic potential.

PHARMACOKINETICS Peak: 2 h IM. **Distribution:** Widely distributed except to CSF, synovial fluid, and eye; does not cross placenta. **Metabolism:** Unknown. **Elimination:** 60% excreted unchanged in urine. **Half-Life:** 4.3–6 h.

NURSING IMPLICATIONS

Assessment & Drug Effects

- Lab tests: Obtain C&S tests prior to first dose and periodically thereafter to determine continuing sensitivity of causative organisms. Perform baseline serum electrolytes and kidney function tests before parenteral therapy. Frequent monitoring of kidney function and serum drug levels is advised during therapy. Monitor electrolytes at regular intervals during prolonged therapy.
- Review electrolyte results. Patients with low serum calcium are particularly prone to develop neuromuscular blockade.
- Inspect tongue every day. Assess for S&S of superinfection (see Appendix F). Polymyxin therapy supports growth of opportunistic organisms. Report symptoms promptly.
- Monitor I&O. Maintain fluid intake sufficient to maintain daily urinary output of at least 1500 mL. Some degree of renal toxicity usually occurs within first 3 or 4 days of therapy even with therapeutic doses. Consult physician.
- Withhold drug and report findings to physician for any of the following: Decreases in urine output (change in I&O ratio), proteinuria, cellular casts, rising BUN, serum creatinine, or serum drug levels (not associated with dosage increase). All can be interpreted as signs of nephrotoxicity.
- Nephrotoxicity is generally reversible, but it may progress even after drug is discontinued. Therefore, close monitoring of kidney function is essential, even following termination of therapy.
- Be alert for respiratory arrest after the first dose and also as long as 45 days after initiation of therapy. It occurs most commonly in patients with kidney failure and high plasma drug levels and is often preceded by dyspnea and restlessness.

Patient & Family Education

- Report to physician immediately any muscle weakness, shortness of breath, dyspnea, depressed respiration. These symptoms are rapidly reversible if drug is withdrawn.
- Report promptly to physician transient neurologic disturbances (burning or prickling sensations, numbness, dizziness). All occur commonly and usually respond to dosage reduction.
- Report promptly to physician the onset of stiff neck and headache (possible symptoms of neurotoxic reactions, including neuromuscular blockade). This response is usually associated with high serum drug levels or nephrotoxicity.
- Report promptly S&S of superinfection (see Appendix F).
- Report any S&S of colitis for up to 2 mo following discontinuation of drug.

PORACTANT ALPHA

(por-ac′tant)

Curosurf

Classification: LUNG SURFACTANT

Therapeutic: LUNG SURFACTANT

Prototype: Beractant

AVAILABILITY 80 mg/mL suspension

ACTION & *THERAPEUTIC EFFECT* Endogenous pulmonary surfactant lowers the surface tension on alveoli surfaces during respiration, and stabilizes the alveoli against collapse at resting pressures. *Alleviates respiratory distress syndrome (RDS) in premature infants caused by deficiency of surfactant.*

USES Treatment (rescue) of respiratory distress syndrome in premature infants.

CONTRAINDICATIONS Hypersensitivity to porcine products or poractant alpha.

CAUTIOUS USE Infants born greater than 3 wk after ruptured membranes; intraventricular hemorrhage of grade III or IV; major congenital malformations; nosocomial infection; pretreatment of hypothermia or acidosis due to increased risk of intracranial hemorrhage; lactation.

ROUTE & DOSAGE

Respiratory Distress Syndrome

Neonate: **Intratracheal** 2.5 mL/kg birth weight, may repeat with 1.25 mL/kg q12h × 2 more doses if needed (max: 5 mL/kg)

ADMINISTRATION

Note: Correction of acidosis, hypotension, anemia, hypoglycemia, and hypothermia is recommended prior to administration of poractant alfa.

Intratracheal

- Warm vial slowly to room temperature; gently turn upside down to form uniform suspension, but do NOT shake.
- Withdraw slowly the entire contents of a vial (concentration equals 80 mg/mL) into a 3 or 5 mL syringe through a large gauge (greater than 20 gauge) needle.
- Attach a 5 French catheter, precut to 8 cm, to the syringe.
- Fill the catheter with poractant alfa and discard excess through the catheter so that only the total dose to be given remains in the syringe.
- Refer to specific instruction provided by manufacturer for proper dosing technique. Follow instructions carefully regarding installation of drug and ventilation of infant. Note that catheter tip should not extend beyond distal tip of endotracheal tube.
- Store refrigerated at 2°–8° C (36°–46° F) and protect from light. Do not shake vials. Do not warm to room temperature and return to refrigeration more than once.

ADVERSE EFFECTS (≥1%) **CV:** Bradycardia, hypotension. **Respiratory:** Intratracheal tube blockage, oxygen desaturation; pulmonary hemorrhage.

PHARMACOKINETICS Not studied.

NURSING IMPLICATIONS

Assessment & Drug Effects

- Stop administration of poractant alfa and take appropriate measures if any of the following occur: Transient episodes of bradycardia, decreased oxygen saturation, reflux of poractant alfa into endotracheal tube, or airway obstruction. Dosing may resume after stabilization.
- Do not suction airway for 1 h after poractant alfa instillation unless there is significant airway obstruction.

POSACONAZOLE

(pos-a-con′a-zole)

Noxafil
Classification: AZOLE ANTIFUNGAL
Therapeutic: ANTIFUNGAL
Prototype: Fluconazole
Pregnancy Category: C

AVAILABILITY 200 mg/5 mL oral suspension

ACTION & *THERAPEUTIC EFFECT* Azole antifungals inhibit ergosterol synthesis, the principal sterol in the fungal cell membrane, thus interfering with the functions of fungal cell membrane. This results in increased membrane permeability causing leakage of cellular contents. *Has a broad spectrum of antifungal activity against common fungal pathogens.*

USES Prophylactic treatment of invasive *Aspergillus* and *Candida* infections in patients 13 y of age and older who are at high risk due to immunosuppression (e.g., hematopoietic stem cell transplant recipients with graft versus host disease, or patients with hematologic malignancies with prolonged neutropenia from chemotherapy).

UNLABELED USES Treatment of febrile neutropenia or refractory invasive fungal infection; treatment of periorbital cellulitis due to *Rhizopus* sp.; treatment of refractory histoplasmosis; treatment of refractory coccidioidomycosis; treatment of fungal necrotizing fasciitis.

CONTRAINDICATIONS Hypersensitivity to posaconazole; coadministration with ergot alkaloids, or CYP3A4 substrates; history of QT prolongation; abnormal levels of potassium, magnesium, or calcium; lactation; children younger than 13 y.

CAUTIOUS USE Hypersensitivity to other azole antifungal antibiotics; hepatic disease or hepatitis; cardiac arrhythmias; history of proarrhythmic conditions; CHF, myocardial ischemia, atrial fibrillation; AIDS; pregnancy (category C).

ROUTE & DOSAGE

Prophylactic Treatment of Invasive *Aspergillus* and *Candida* Infections

Adult: **PO** 200 mg t.i.d.

ADMINISTRATION

Oral

- Shake well before use. Give with a full meal or liquid nutritional supplement.
- Store at 15°–30° C (59°–86° F).

ADVERSE EFFECTS (≥1%) **Body as a Whole:** Anxiety, *bacteremia, dizziness, edema, fatigue, fever, headache, infection, insomnia, rigors,* weakness. **CNS:** QT/QT_c prolongation, tremor. **CV:** *Hypertension, hypotension, tachycardia.* **GI:** *Abdominal pain, anorexia constipation, diarrhea, dyspepsia, mucositis, nausea,* vomiting. **Hematologic:** *Anemia, febrile neutropenia, neutropenia, petechiae, thrombocytopenia.* **Metabolic:** *Bilirubinemia,* creatinine levels increased, elevated liver enzymes, hypocalcemia, *hyperglycemia, hypokalemia, hypomagnesemia.* **Musculoskeletal:** *Arthralgia, back pain, musculoskeletal pain.* **Respiratory:** *Cough, dyspnea, epistaxis, pharyngitis,* upper respiratory tract infection. **Skin:** *Pruritus, rash.* **Special Senses:** Blurred vision, taste disturbances. **Urogenital:** *Vaginal hemorrhage.*

INTERACTIONS Drug: Rifabutin and **phenytoin** increase the metabolism of posaconazole resulting in decreased plasma levels. **Cimetidine** decreases the absorption of posaconazole. Posaconazole is known to increase the plasma levels of **cyclosporine, tacrolimus, rifabutin, midazolam,** and **phenytoin.** Coadministration with other drugs that cause QT prolongation (e.g., **quinidine**) can result in torsades de pointes. Posaconazole may increase the plasma levels of ERGOT ALKALOIDS, VINCA ALKALOIDS, HMG COA REDUCTASE INHIBITORS, and CALCIUM CHANNEL BLOCKERS. **Food:** Administration with food increases absorption of posaconazole.

PHARMACOKINETICS Peak: 3–5 h. **Distribution:** 98% protein bound. **Metabolism:** Conjugated to inactive metabolites. **Elimination:** Primarily fecal elimination (71%) with minor renal elimination. **Half-Life:** 35 h.

NURSING IMPLICATIONS

Assessment & Drug Effects

- Monitor for and report S&S of breakthrough fungal infections, especially in those with severe renal impairment, or experiencing vomiting and diarrhea, or who cannot tolerate a full meal or supplement along with posaconazole.
- Monitor and report degree of improvement of oropharyngeal candidiasis.
- Monitor those with proarrhythmic conditions for development of arrhythmias.
- Lab tests: Baseline and periodic LFTs; baseline serum electrolytes.
- Withhold drug and notify physician of abnormal serum potassium, magnesium, or calcium levels.
- Monitor blood levels of phenytoin, cyclosporine, tacrolimus, and sirolimus with concurrent therapy. Monitor for adverse effects of concurrently administered statins or calcium channel blockers.

Patient & Family Education

- Do not take any prescription or nonprescription drugs without informing your physician.
- Know parameters for withholding drug (i.e., inability to take with a full meal or nutritional supplement).
- Report immediately any of the following to your health care provider: Vomiting, diarrhea, inability to eat, jaundice of skin, yellowing of eyes, itching, or skin rash.

POTASSIUM CHLORIDE

(poe-tass′ee-um)

Apo-K ♣, K-10, Kalium Durules ♣, Kaochlor, Kaochlor-20 Concentrate, Kaon-Cl, KCl 5% and 20%, K-Long ♣, Klor, Klor-10%, Klor-Con, Kloride, Klorvess, Klotrix, K-Dur, K-Lyte/Cl, K-tab, Micro-K Extentabs, SK-Potassium Chloride, Slo-Pot ♣, Slow-K

POTASSIUM GLUCONATE

Kaon, Kaylixir

Classification: ELECTROLYTIC REPLACEMENT SOLUTION

Therapeutic: ELECTROLYTE REPLACEMENT

Pregnancy Category: C

AVAILABILITY Chloride: 6.7 mEq, 8 mEq, 10 mEq, 20 mEq sustained release tablets; 500 mg, 595 mg tablets; 20 mEq, 25 mEq, 50 mEq effervescent tablets; 20 mEq/15 mL, 40 mEq/15 mL, 45 mEq/15 mL liquid; 15 mEq, 20 mEq, 25 mEq powder; 2 mEq/mL injection; 10 mEq, 20 mEq, 30 mEq, 40 mEq, 60 mEq, 90 mEq vials; **Gluconate:** 20 mEq/15 mL liquid

ACTION & *THERAPEUTIC EFFECT* Principal intracellular cation that is essential for maintenance of intracellular isotonicity, transmission of nerve impulses, contraction of cardiac, skeletal, and smooth muscles, maintenance of normal kidney function, and for enzyme activity. *Effectiveness in hypokalemia is measured by serum potassium concentration greater than 3.5 mEq/liter.*

USES To prevent and treat potassium deficit secondary to diuretic or corticosteroid therapy. Also indicated when potassium is depleted by severe vomiting, diarrhea; intestinal drainage, fistulas, or malabsorption; prolonged diuresis, diabetic acidosis. Effective in the treatment of hypokalemic alkalosis (chloride, not the gluconate).

CONTRAINDICATIONS Severe renal impairment; severe hemolytic reactions; untreated Addison's disease; crush syndrome; early postoperative oliguria (except during GI drainage); adynamic ileus; acute dehydration; heat cramps, hyperkalemia, patients receiving potassium-sparing diuretics, digitalis intoxication with AV conduction disturbance.

CAUTIOUS USE Cardiac or kidney disease; systemic acidosis; slow-release potassium preparations in presence of delayed GI transit or Meckel's diverticulum; extensive tissue breakdown (such as severe burns); pregnancy (category C), lactation.

P

ROUTE & DOSAGE

Hypokalemia

Adult: **PO** 10–100 mEq/day in divided doses **IV** 10–60 mEq/h diluted to at least 10–20 mEq/100 mL of solution (max: 200–400 mEq/day, monitor higher doses carefully)

Child: **PO** 1–3 mEq/kg/day in divided doses; sustained release tablets not recommended
IV Up to 3 mEq/kg/24 h at a rate less than 0.02 mEq/kg/min

ADMINISTRATION

Oral

- Give while patient is sitting up or standing (never in recumbent position) to prevent drug–induced esophagitis. Some patients find it difficult to swallow the large sized KCl tablet.
- Do not crush or allow to chew any potassium salt tablets. Observe to make sure patient does not suck tablet (oral ulcerations have been reported if tablet is allowed to dissolve in mouth).
- Swallow whole tablet with a large glass of water or fruit juice (if allowed) to wash drug down and to start esophageal peristalsis.
- Follow exactly directions for diluting various liquid forms of KCl. In general, dilute each 20 mEq potassium in at least 90 mL water or juice and allowed to dissolve completely before administration.
- Dilute liquid forms as directed before giving it through nasogastric tube.

Intravenous

PREPARE: **IV Infusion:** Add desired amount to 100–1000 mL IV solution (compatible with all standard solutions). ▪ Usual maximum is 80 mEq/1000 mL, however, 40 mEq/L is preferred to lessen irritation to veins. Note: **NEVER** add KCl to an IV bag/bottle which is hanging. ▪ After adding KCl invert bag/bottle several times to ensure even distribution.
ADMINISTER: **IV Infusion for Adult/Child:** KCl is **never** given

direct IV or in concentrated amounts by any route. ▪ Too rapid infusion may cause fatal hyperkalemia. **IV Infusion for Adult:** Infuse at rate not to exceed 10 mEq/h; in emergency situations, may infuse very cautiously up to 40 mEq/h with continuous cardiac monitoring. **IV Infusion for Child:** Infuse at a rate not to exceed 0.5–1.0 mEq/kg/h.

INCOMPATIBILITIES **Solution/additive:** **Furosemide, pentobarbital, phenobarbital, succinylcholine.** **Y-site:** **Amphotericin B cholesteryl complex, azithromycin, chlordiazepoxide, chlorpromazine, diazepam, ergotamine, methylprednisolone, phenytoin.**

▪ Take extreme care to prevent extravasation and infiltration. At first sign, discontinue infusion and select another site.

ADVERSE EFFECTS (≥1%) **GI:** *Nausea, vomiting,* diarrhea, abdominal distention. **Body as a Whole:** Pain, mental confusion, irritability, listlessness, paresthesias of extremities, muscle weakness and heaviness of limbs, difficulty in swallowing, flaccid paralysis. **Urogenital:** Oliguria, anuria. **Hematologic:** Hyperkalemia. **Respiratory:** Respiratory distress. **CV:** Hypotension, bradycardia; cardiac depression, arrhythmias, or arrest; altered sensitivity to digitalis glycosides. *ECG changes in hyperkalemia:* Tenting (peaking) of T wave (especially in right precordial leads), lowering of R with deepening of S waves and depression of RST; prolonged P-R interval, widened QRS complex, decreased amplitude and disappearance of P waves, prolonged QT interval, signs of right and left bundle block, deterioration of QRS contour and finally ventricular fibrillation and death.

INTERACTIONS Drug: POTASSIUM-SPARING DIURETICS, ANGIOTENSIN-CONVERTING ENZYME (ACE) INHIBITORS may cause hyperkalemia.

PHARMACOKINETICS Absorption: Readily from upper GI tract. **Elimination:** 90% in urine, 10% in feces.

NURSING IMPLICATIONS

Assessment & Drug Effects

- Monitor I&O ratio and pattern in patients receiving the parenteral drug. If oliguria occurs, stop infusion promptly and notify physician.
- Lab test: Frequent serum electrolytes are warranted.
- Monitor for and report signs of GI ulceration (esophageal or epigastric pain or hematemesis).
- Monitor cardiac status of patients receiving parenteral potassium. Irregular heartbeat is usually the earliest clinical indication of hyperkalemia.
- Be alert for potassium intoxication (hyperkalemia, see S&S, Appendix F); may result from any therapeutic dosage, and the patient may be asymptomatic.
- The risk of hyperkalemia with potassium supplement increases (1) in older adults because of decremental changes in kidney function associated with aging, (2) when dietary intake of potassium suddenly increases, and (3) when kidney function is significantly compromised.

Patient & Family Education

- Do not be alarmed when the tablet carcass appears in your stool. The sustained release tablet (e.g., Slow-K) utilizes a wax matrix as carrier for KCl crystals that passes through the digestive system.
- Learn about sources of potassium with special reference to foods and OTC drugs.

P

- Do not use any salt substitute unless it is specifically ordered by the physician. These contain a substantial amount of potassium and electrolytes other than sodium.
- Do not self-prescribe laxatives. Chronic laxative use has been associated with diarrhea-induced potassium loss.
- Notify physician of persistent vomiting because losses of potassium can occur.
- Report continuing signs of potassium deficit to physician: Weakness, fatigue, polyuria, polydipsia.
- Advise dentist or new physician that a potassium drug has been prescribed as long-term maintenance therapy.
- Do not open foil-wrapped powders and tablets before use.

POTASSIUM IODIDE

(poe-tass′ee-um)

Pima, SSKI, Thyro-Block ♣

Classifications: ANTITHYROID; EXPECTORANT

Therapeutic: ANTITHYROID; EXPECTORANT

Prototype: Guaifenesin

Pregnancy Category: D

AVAILABILITY 325 mg/5 mL syrup; 1 g/mL solution

ACTION & *THERAPEUTIC EFFECT* Appears to increase secretion of respiratory fluids by direct action on bronchial tissue, thereby decreasing mucus viscosity. When the thyroid gland is hyperplastic, excess iodide ions temporarily inhibit secretion of thyroid hormone, foster accumulation in thyroid follicles, and decrease vascularity of gland. *Administration for hyperthyroidism is limited to short-term therapy. As an expectorant, the iodine ion increases mucous secretion formation in bronchi, and decreases viscosity of mucus.*

USES To facilitate bronchial drainage and cough in emphysema, asthma, chronic bronchitis, bronchiectasis, and respiratory tract allergies characterized by difficult-to-raise sputum. Also used alone for hyperthyroidism or in conjunction with antithyroid drugs and propranolol in treatment of thyrotoxic crisis; in immediate preoperative period for thyroidectomy to decrease vascularity, fragility, and size of thyroid gland and for treatment of persistent or recurring hyperthyroidism that occurs in Graves' disease patients. Used as a radiation protectant in patients receiving radioactive iodine and to shield the thyroid gland from radiation in the wake of a serious nuclear plant accident. (Use as an expectorant has been largely replaced by other agents.)

CONTRAINDICATIONS Hypersensitivity or idiosyncrasy to iodine; hyperthyroidism; hyperkalemia; acute bronchitis; pregnancy (category D), lactation.

CAUTIOUS USE Renal impairment; cardiac disease; pulmonary tuberculosis; Addison's disease.

ROUTE & DOSAGE

To Reduce Thyroid Vascularity

Adult/Child: **PO** 50–250 mg t.i.d. for 10–14 days before surgery

Expectorant

Adult: **PO** 300–650 mg p.c. b.i.d. or t.i.d.

Child: **PO** 60–250 mg p.c. b.i.d. or t.i.d.

Thyroid Blocking in Radiation Emergency

Adult: **PO** 130 mg/day for 10 days

Child: **PO** *Younger than 1 y,* 65 mg/day for 10 days; *older than 1 y,* 130 mg/day for 10 days

ADMINISTRATION

Oral

- Give with meals in a full glass (240 mL) of water or fruit juice and at bedtime with juice to disguise salty taste and minimize gastric distress.
- Avoid giving KI with milk; absorption of the drug may be decreased by dairy products.
- Adhere strictly to schedule and accurate dose measurements when iodide is administered to prepare thyroid gland for surgery, particularly at end of treatment period when possibility of "escape" (from iodide) effect on thyroid gland increases.
- Place container in warm water and gently agitate to dissolve if crystals are noted in the solution.
- Discard any solution that has turned a brownish yellow on standing, especially if exposed to light (caused by liberated trace of free iodine).
- Store in airtight, light-resistant container.

ADVERSE EFFECTS (≥1%) **GI:** Diarrhea, nausea, vomiting, stomach pain, nonspecific small bowel lesions (associated with enteric coated tablets). **Body as a Whole:** Angioneurotic edema, cutaneous and mucosal hemorrhage, fever, arthralgias, lymph node enlargement, eosinophilia, paresthesias, periorbital edema, weakness. *Iodine poisoning (iodism):* Metallic taste, stomatitis, salivation, coryza, sneezing; swollen and tender salivary glands (sialadenitis), frontal headache, vomiting (blue vomitus if stomach contained starches, otherwise yellow vomitus), bloody diarrhea. **Metabolic:** Hyperthyroid adenoma, goiter, hypothyroidism, collagen disease–like syndromes. **CV:** Irregular heartbeat. **CNS:** Mental confusion. **Skin:** Acneiform skin lesions (prolonged use), flare-up of adolescent acne. **Respiratory:** Productive cough, pulmonary edema.

DIAGNOSTIC TEST INTERFERENCE Potassium iodide may alter ***thyroid function*** test results and may interfere with ***urinary 17-OHCS*** determinations.

INTERACTIONS Drug: ANTITHYROID DRUGS, **lithium** may potentiate hypothyroid and goitrogenic actions; POTASSIUM-SPARING DIURETICS, POTASSIUM SUPPLEMENTS, ACE INHIBITORS increase risk of hyperkalemia.

PHARMACOKINETICS Absorption: Adequately absorbed from GI tract. **Distribution:** Crosses placenta. **Elimination:** Cleared from plasma by renal excretion or thyroid uptake.

NURSING IMPLICATIONS

Assessment & Drug Effects

- Lab tests: Determine serum potassium levels before and periodically during therapy.
- Keep physician informed about characteristics of sputum: Quantity, consistency, color.

Patient & Family Education

- Report to physician promptly the occurrence of abdominal pain, distension, nausea, or vomiting.
- Report clinical S&S of iodism (see ADVERSE EFFECTS). Usually, symptoms will subside with dose reduction and lengthened intervals between doses.
- Avoid foods rich in iodine if iodism develops: Seafood, fish liver oils, and iodized salt.

- Be aware that sudden withdrawal following prolonged use may precipitate thyroid storm.
- Do not use OTC drugs without consulting physician. Many preparations contain iodides and could augment prescribed dose [e.g., cough syrups, gargles, asthma medication, salt substitutes, cod liver oil, multiple vitamins (often suspended in iodide solutions)].
- Be aware that optimum hydration is the best expectorant when taking KI as an expectorant. Increase daily fluid intake.

PRALATREXATE

(pra-la-trex'ate)

Folotyn

Classifications: ANTINEOPLASTIC; ANTIMETABOLITE, ANTIFOLATE

Therapeutic: ANTINEOPLASTIC

Prototype: Methotrexate

Pregnancy Category: D

P

AVAILABILITY 20 mg/mL, 40 mg/2 mL solution for injection

ACTION & *THERAPEUTIC EFFECT* Antimetabolite and folic acid antagonist. Blocks folic acid participation in nucleic acid synthesis, thereby interfering with cell division (mitosis). Rapidly dividing cells, including cancer cells, are sensitive to this interference in the mitotic process. *Effective in treatment of relapsed or refractory peripheral T-cell lymphoma (PTCL).*

USES Treatment of relapsed or refractory peripheral T-cell lymphoma (PTCL).

CONTRAINDICATIONS Concomitant administration of hepatotoxity drugs; pregnancy (category D); lactation.

CAUTIOUS USE Thrombocytopenia, neutropenia, anemia; moderate to severe renal function impairment; liver function impairment; ulcerative colitis; poor nutritional status.

ROUTE & DOSAGE

Peripheral T-Cell Lymphoma

Adult: **IV** 30 mg/m² over 3–5 min. Repeat weekly for 6 wk in 7-wk cycles.

Adjustments Based on Drug Hematologic Toxicities

- Platelet count less than 50,000/mm³ for 1 wk: Omit dose, resume dose when platelet count is at least 50,000/mm³
- Platelet count less than 50,000/mm³ for 2 wk: Omit dose, resume at 20 mg/m² when platelet count is at least 50,000/mm³
- Platelet count less than 50,000/mm³ for 3 wk: Discontinue therapy.
- ANC 500–1,000/mm³ and no fever for 1 wk: Omit dose; resume dose when ANC is at least 1,000/mm³.
- ANC 500–1,000/mm³ and fever or ANC less than 500/mm³ for 1 wk: Omit dose; give G-CSF or GM-CSF support; resume dose and continue G-CSF or GM-CSF support when ANC is at least 1,000/mm³ and fever resolves.
- ANC 500–1,000/mm³ and fever or ANC less than 500/mm³ for 2 wks or recurrence of toxicity: Omit dose; give G-CSF or GM-CSF support; resume at 20 mg/m² and continue G-CSF or GM-CSF support when ANC is at least 1,000/mm³ and fever resolves.

- ANC 500–1,000/mm³ and fever or ANC less than 500/mm³ for 3 wk's duration or 2nd recurrence of toxicity: Discontinue therapy

Adjustments Based on Mucositis

- Grade 2 mucositis: Omit dose; resume dose when toxicity grade is 1 or less
- Grade 2 mucositis recurrence: Omit dose; resume at 20 mg/m² when toxicity grade is 1 or less
- Grade 3 mucositis: Omit dose; resume at 20 mg/m² when toxicity grade is 1 or less
- Grade 4 mucositis: Discontinue therapy

Adjustments for All Other Treatment-Related Toxicities

- Grade 3 toxicities: Omit dose and resume at 20 mg/m² when toxicity is grade 2 or less
- Grade 4 toxicities: Discontinue therapy

Hepatic Impairment Dosage Adjustment

Included above with general grade 3 and grade 4 treatment-related toxicities.

ADMINISTRATION

Intravenous

PREPARE: **Direct:** Withdraw from vial into syringe immediately before use. Do not dilute. Use gloves and other protective clothing during handling and preparation. ▪ Flush thoroughly if drug contacts skin or mucous membranes.

ADMINISTER: **Direct:** Give over 3–5 min via a side port of a free-flowing NS IV line. ▪ Withhold drug and notify physician for any of the following: Platelet count less than 100,000/mcL for first dose or less than 50,000/mcL for all subsequent doses, ANC less than 1000/mcL, or grade 2 or higher mucositis.

▪ Refrigerate at 2°–8° C (36°–46° F) until use and protect from light. ▪ Vials are stable at room temperature for up to 72 h if left in original carton.

ADVERSE EFFECTS (≥10%) **Body as a Whole:** Abdominal pain, asthenia, *edema, fatigue,* night sweats, pain in extremity, *pyrexia,* <u>sepsis</u>. **CV:** <u>Tachycardia</u>. **GI:** *Constipation, diarrhea, mucositis, nausea, vomiting.* **Hematologic:** *Anemia,* leukopenia, *neutropenia, thrombocytopenia.* **Metabolic:** Anorexia, elevated AST and ALT, hypokalemia. **Musculoskeletal:** Back pain. **Respiratory:** *Cough, dyspnea, epistaxis,* pharyngolaryngeal pain, upper respiratory tract infection. **Skin:** Pruritus, rash.

INTERACTIONS Drug: Probenecid may increase pralatrexate levels. Drugs that are subject to substantial renal clearance (e.g., NSAIDS, **trimethoprim/sulfamethoxazole**) may delay the clearance of pralatrexate.

PHARMACOKINETICS Distribution: 67% bound to plasma proteins. **Metabolism:** Not extensively metabolized. **Elimination:** Primarily excreted in the urine. **Half-Life:** 12–18 h.

NURSING IMPLICATIONS

Assessment & Drug Effects

- Monitor vitals signs. Report immediately S&S of infection, especially fever of 100.5° F or greater.
- Monitor status of mucus membranes because mucositis is a dose-limiting toxicity.
- Lab tests: Prior to each dose, CBC with differential and platelet count; baseline and periodic LFTs and kidney function tests.

Patient & Family Education

- Practice meticulous oral hygiene.
- Monitor for S&S of an infection. Contact the physician immediately if an infection is suspected or if your temperature is elevated.
- Report promptly unexplained bleeding or symptoms of anemia (e.g., excessive weakness, fatigue, intolerance to activity, pale skin).
- Folic acid and vitamin B_{12} supplementation are recommended to reduce the risk of drug-related toxicities. Consult with physician.
- Use effective means of contraception to avoid pregnancy while taking this drug. If a pregnancy does occur, notify physician immediately.
- Do not take aspirin or NSAIDs without consulting physician.

PRALIDOXIME CHLORIDE

(pra-li-dox'eem)

2-PAM, Protopam Chloride

Classifications: CHOLINESTERASE RECEPTOR AGONIST; DETOXIFICATION AGENT

Therapeutic: ANTIDOTE; CHOLINESTERASE ENHANCER

Pregnancy Category: C

AVAILABILITY 1 g injection

ACTION & *THERAPEUTIC EFFECT* Reactivates cholinesterase by displacing the enzyme from its receptor sites; the free enzyme then can resume its function of degrading accumulated acetylcholine, thereby restoring normal neuromuscular transmission. *More active against effects of anticholinesterases at skeletal neuromuscular junction than at autonomic effector sites or in CNS respiratory center; therefore, atropine* ***must be*** *given concomitantly to block effects of acetylcholine and its accumulation in these sites.*

USES Antidote in treatment of poisoning by organophosphate insecticides and pesticides with anticholinesterase activity (e.g., parathion, TEPP, sarin) and to control overdosage by anticholinesterase drugs used in treatment of myasthenia gravis (cholinergic crisis).

UNLABELED USES To reverse toxicity of echothiophate ophthalmic solution.

CONTRAINDICATIONS Hypersensitivity to pralidoxime; use in poisoning by insecticide of the carbonate class (Sevin), inorganic phosphates, or organophosphates having no anticholinesterase activity; patients receiving aminophylline, theophylline, morphine, succinylcholine, reserpine, or phenothiazines.

CAUTIOUS USE Myasthenia gravis; renal insufficiency; asthma; peptic ulcer; severe cardiac disease; concomitant use of barbiturates in organophosphorus poisoning; pregnancy (category C), lactation.

ROUTE & DOSAGE

Organophosphate Poisoning

Adult: **IV** 1–2 g in 100 mL NS infused over 15–30 min; or 1–2 g as 5% solution in sterile water over not less than 5 min, may repeat after 1 h if muscle weakness not relieved. **IM/Subcutaneous** 1–2 g if IV route is not feasible.
Child: **IV** 20–50 mg/kg. May repeat in 1–2 h if needed.

Anticholinesterase Overdose in Myasthenia Gravis

Adult: **IV** 1–2 g in 100 mL NS infused over 15–30 min, followed by increments of 250 mg q5min prn

ADMINISTRATION

Subcutaneous/Intramuscular

- Give only if unable to give IV; NOT preferred routes.
- Reconstitute as for direct IV injection (see below).

Intravenous

PREPARE: **Direct:** Reconstitute 1-g vial by adding 20 mL sterile water for injection to yield 50 mg/mL (a 5% solution). ▪ If pulmonary edema is present, give without further dilution. **IV Infusion (preferred):** Further dilute reconstituted solution in 100 mL NS.

ADMINISTER: **Direct:** In pulmonary edema, 1 g or fraction thereof over 5 min; do not exceed 200 mg/min. **IV Infusion (preferred):** Give over 15–30 min.

▪ Stop infusion or reduce rate if hypertension occurs.

ADVERSE EFFECTS (≥1%) **CNS:** Dizziness, headache, drowsiness. **GI:** Nausea. **Special Senses:** Blurred vision, diplopia, impaired accommodation. **CV:** Tachycardia, hypertension (dose-related). **Body as a Whole:** Hyperventilation, muscular weakness, laryngospasm, muscle rigidity.

INTERACTIONS Drug: May potentiate the effects of BARBITURATES.

PHARMACOKINETICS Peak: 5–15 min IV; 10–20 min IM. **Distribution:** Distributed throughout extracellular fluids; crosses blood–brain barrier slowly if at all. **Metabolism:** Probably in liver. **Elimination:** Rapidly in urine. **Half-Life:** 0.8–2.7 h.

NURSING IMPLICATIONS

Assessment & Drug Effects

- Monitor BP, vital signs, and I&O. Report oliguria or changes in I&O ratio.
- Monitor closely. It is difficult to differentiate toxic effects of organophosphates or atropine from toxic effects of pralidoxime.
- Be alert for and report immediately: Reduction in muscle strength, onset of muscle twitching, changes in respiratory pattern, altered level of consciousness, increases or changes in heart rate and rhythm.
- Observe necessary safety precautions with unconscious patient because excitement and manic behavior reportedly may occur following recovery of consciousness.
- Keep patient under close observation for 48–72 h, particularly when poison was ingested, because of likelihood of continued absorption of organophosphate from lower bowel.
- In patients with myasthenia gravis, overdosage with pralidoxime may convert cholinergic crisis into myasthenic crisis.

PRAMIPEXOLE DIHYDROCHLORIDE

(pra-mi-pex′ole)

Mirapex

Classifications: DOPAMINE RECEPTOR AGONIST; ANTIPARKINSON

Therapeutic: ANTIPARKINSON

Prototype: Levodopa

Pregnancy Category: C

AVAILABILITY 0.125 mg, 0.25 mg, 1 mg, 1.5 mg tablets

ACTION & *THERAPEUTIC EFFECT*

Nonergot dopamine receptor agonist for treatment of Parkinson's disease. Exhibits high affinity for the D_2 subfamily of dopamine receptors in the brain and higher binding affinity to D_3 than other dopamine receptor subtypes. *Effectiveness is indicated by improved*

P

control of neuromuscular functioning. Improves ADLs.

USES Treatment of idiopathic Parkinson's disease and moderate to severe primary restless legs syndrome (RLS).

CONTRAINDICATIONS Hypersensitivity to pramipexole or ropinirole; lactation.
CAUTIOUS USE Renal and liver function impairment; concomitant use of CNS depressants; impulse control symptoms; pregnancy (category C). Safety and efficacy in children are not established.

ROUTE & DOSAGE

Parkinson's Disease

Adult: **PO** Start with 0.125 mg t.i.d. × 1 wk, then 0.25 mg t.i.d. for 1 wk, continue to increase by 0.25 mg/dose t.i.d. qwk to a target dose of 1.5 mg t.i.d.

Restless Legs Syndrome

Adult: **PO** 0.125 mg taken 2–3 h before bed; dose can be increased every 4–7 days

Renal Impairment Dosage Adjustment

CrCl 35–60 mL/min: Same titration schedule dosed b.i.d. (max: 1.5 mg b.i.d.); 15–35 mL/min: Same titration schedule dosed daily (max: 1.5 mg daily)

ADMINISTRATION

Oral

- Titrate dose increments gradually with at least 4–7 days between increases.
- Reduce doses for creatinine clearance greater than 60 mL/min.
- Give with food if nausea develops.

ADVERSE EFFECTS (≥1%) **Body as a Whole:** *Asthenia,* general edema, malaise, fever, decreased weight. **CNS:** *Dizziness, somnolence, sudden sleep attacks, insomnia, hallucinations, dyskinesia, extrapyramidal syndrome,* headache, confusion, amnesia, hypesthesia, dystonia, akathisia, myoclonus, peripheral edema. **CV:** *Postural hypotension,* chest pain. **GI:** *Nausea, constipation,* anorexia, dysphagia, dry mouth. **Respiratory:** Dyspnea, rhinitis. **Urogenital:** Decreased libido, impotence, urinary frequency or incontinence. **Special Senses:** Vision abnormalities.

INTERACTIONS Drug: Cimetidine decreases clearance; BUTYROPHENONES, **metoclopramide**, PHENOTHIAZINES may antagonize effects.

PHARMACOKINETICS Absorption: Rapidly from GI tract, greater than 90% bioavailability. **Peak:** 2 h. **Distribution:** 15% protein bound. **Metabolism:** Minimally in the liver. **Elimination:** Primarily in urine. **Half-Life:** 8–12 h.

NURSING IMPLICATIONS

Assessment & Drug Effects

- Monitor for S&S of orthostatic hypotension, especially when the dosage is increased.
- Monitor cardiac status, especially in those with significant orthostatic hypotension.
- Lab tests: Monitor BUN and creatinine periodically; monitor CPK with complaints of muscle pain.
- Monitor for and report signs of tardive dyskinesia (see Appendix F).

Patient & Family Education

- Hallucinations are an adverse effect of this drug and occur more often in older adults.

- Make position changes slowly especially from a lying or sitting to standing.
- Use caution with potentially dangerous activities until response to drug is known; drowsiness is a common adverse effect.
- Avoid alcohol and use extra caution if taking other prescribed CNS depressants; both may exaggerate drowsiness, dizziness, and orthostatic hypotension.
- Do not abruptly stop taking this drug. It should be discontinued over a period of 1 wk.

PRAMLINTIDE

Symlin

Classifications: ANTIDIABETIC; AMYLIN ANALOG

Therapeutic: ANTIHYPERGLYCEMIC

Pregnancy Category: C

AVAILABILITY 0.6 mg/mL injection

ACTION & *THERAPEUTIC EFFECT* Pramlintide is a synthetic analog of human amylin, a hormone secreted by pancreatic beta cells. In type 2 diabetic patients using insulin and in type 1 diabetics, beta cells in the pancreas are either damaged or destroyed, resulting in reduced secretion of both insulin and amylin after meals. Amylin reduces postmeal glucagon levels, thus lowering serum glucose level. *Pramlintide is an antihyperglycemic drug that controls postprandial blood glucose levels.*

USES Adjunct treatment of diabetes mellitus type 1 and type 2 in patients who use mealtime insulin therapy and who have failed to achieve desired glucose control despite optimal insulin therapy.

CONTRAINDICATIONS Hypersensitivity to pramlintide, cresol; noncompliance with insulin regime or medical care; HbA1C greater than 9%; hypoglycemia; gastroparesis; concomitant use of drugs to stimulate GI motility; renal failure or dialysis. Safety and efficacy in children not established.

CAUTIOUS USE Osteoporosis; alcohol; thyroid disease; pregnancy (category C), lactation.

ROUTE & DOSAGE

Type 1 Diabetes Mellitus

Adult: **Subcutaneous** 15 mcg immediately before each major meal; may increase by 15 mcg increments if no clinically significant nausea for 3–7 days. If nausea or vomiting persists at 45 mcg or 60 mcg, reduce to 30 mcg.

Type 2 Diabetes Mellitus

Adult: **Subcutaneous** 60 mcg immediately before each major meal; may increase to 120 mcg if no clinically significant nausea for 3–7 days. If nausea or vomiting persists at 120 mcg, reduce to 60 mcg.

ADMINISTRATION

Subcutaneous

- Give subcutaneously into the abdomen or thigh (not the arm) immediately before each major meal. Rotate injection sites.
- Never mix pramlintide and insulin in the same syringe. Separate injection sites.
- Use a U100 insulin syringe to administer. One unit of pramlintide drawn from a 0.6 mg/mL vial contains 6 mcg of medication. Thus, a 30 mcg dose is equal to 5 units in a U100 syringe.
- Do not administer to patients with HbA1C greater than 9% or

those taking drugs to stimulate GI motility.

- Note: When initiating pramlintide therapy, insulin dose reduction is required.
- Store at 2°–8° C (36°–46° F), and protect from light. Do not freeze. Discard vials that have been frozen or overheated. Discard open vials after 28 days.

ADVERSE EFFECTS (≥1%) **CNS:** Dizziness, fatigue, *headache*. **GI:** Abdominal pain, *anorexia, nausea, vomiting*. **Musculoskeletal:** Arthralgia. **Respiratory:** *Coughing*, pharyngitis. **Body as a Whole:** *Allergic reaction, inflicted injury*.

INTERACTIONS Drugs: Pramlintide can decrease rate and/or extent of GI absorption of other oral drugs. Significant slowing of gastric motility with ANTIMUSCARINICS.

PHARMACOKINETICS Absorption: 30–40% bioavailability. **Peak:** 20 min. **Distribution:** 40% protein bound. **Metabolism:** Extensive renal metabolism. **Half-Life:** 48 min.

NURSING IMPLICATIONS

Assessment & Drug Effects

- Monitor for severe hypoglycemia, which usually occurs within 3 h of injection. Hypoglycemia is worse in type 1 diabetics.
- Monitor diabetics for loss of glycemic control.
- Lab tests: Baseline and periodic HbA1C; frequent pre/postmeal plasma glucose levels.
- Withhold drug and notify physician for clinically significant nausea or increased frequency or severity of hypoglycemia.

Patient & Family Education

- Follow directions for taking the drug (see Administration). Use a new needle for each injection.
- Note: Patients should reduce a.c. rapid-acting or short-acting insulin dosages by 50% when pramlintide is initiated. Check with physician.
- Do not drive or engage in potentially hazardous activities until response to drug is known.
- Report any of the following to physician: Persistent, significant nausea; episodes of hypoglycemia (e.g., hunger, headache, sweating, tremor, irritability, or difficulty concentrating).

PRAMOXINE HYDROCHLORIDE

(pra-mox′een)

Fleet Relief Anesthetic Hemorrhoidal, Prax, ProctoFoam, Tronolane, Tronothane ♣

Classifications: LOCAL ANESTHETIC (MUCOSAL); ANTIPRURITIC
Therapeutic: LOCAL ANESTHETIC; ANTIPRURITIC
Prototype: Procaine
Pregnancy Category: C

AVAILABILITY 1% cream, gel, lotion, spray

ACTION & *THERAPEUTIC EFFECT* Produces anesthesia by blocking conduction and propagation of sensory nerve impulses in skin and mucous membranes. *Provides temporary relief from pain and itching on skin or mucous membrane.*

USES To relieve pain caused by minor burns and wounds; for temporary relief of pruritus secondary to dermatoses, hemorrhoids, and anal fissures; and to facilitate sigmoidoscopic examination.

CONTRAINDICATIONS Application to large areas of skin; prolonged use; preparation for laryngopharyngeal examination, bronchoscopy,

or gastroscopy. Safety in children younger than 2 y is not established.
CAUTIOUS USE Extensive skin disorders; pregnancy (category C), lactation.

ROUTE & DOSAGE

Relief of Minor Pain and Itching
Adult/Child (older than 2 y): **Topical** Apply t.i.d. or q.i.d.

ADMINISTRATION

Topical
- Clean thoroughly and dry rectal area before use for temporary relief of hemorrhoidal pain and itching.
- Administer rectal preparations in the morning and evening and after bowel movement or as directed by physician.
- Apply lotion or cream to affected surfaces with a gloved hand. Wash hands thoroughly before and after treatment.
- Do not apply to eyes or nasal membranes.

ADVERSE EFFECTS (≥1%) **Skin:** Burning, stinging, sensitization.

INTERACTIONS No clinically significant interactions established.

PHARMACOKINETICS **Onset:** 3–5 min. **Duration:** Up to 5 h.

NURSING IMPLICATIONS

Assessment & Drug Effects
- Monitor for and report promptly significant tissue irritation or sloughing.

Patient & Family Education
- Drug is usually discontinued if condition being treated does not improve within 2–3 wk or if it worsens, or if rash or condition not present before treatment appears, or if treated area becomes inflamed or infected.
- Discontinue and consult physician if rectal bleeding and pain occur during hemorrhoid treatment.

PRASUGREL

(pra-soo′grel)
Effient
Classifications: ANTIPLATELET; PLATELET INHIBITOR; ADP RECEPTOR ANTAGONIST
Therapeutic: PLATELET INHIBITOR
Prototype: Clopidogrel
Pregnancy Category: B

AVAILABILITY 5 mg, 10 mg tablets

ACTION & *THERAPEUTIC EFFECT*
Prasugrel is an inhibitor of platelet activation and aggregation through irreversible binding to adenosine diphosphate (ADP) receptors on platelets. *Prasugrel prolongs bleeding time, thereby reducing atherosclerotic events in selected high risk patient managed with percutaneous coronary intervention (PCI).*

USES Prophylaxis of arterial thromboembolism in patients with acute coronary syndrome, including unstable angina, non–ST-elevation myocardial infarction (NSTEMI), or ST-elevation acute myocardial infarction (STEMI), who are being managed with percutaneous coronary intervention (PCI)

CONTRAINDICATIONS Active pathologic bleeding disorder; active bleeding; history of TIA or stroke; within 7 days of CABG surgery or any surgery; concomitant use of NSAIDs or other drugs that increase risk of bleeding.

CAUTIOUS USE Severe hepatic impairment (Child-Pugh class C, total score greater than 10); older adults over 75 y; pregnancy (category B); lactation.

ROUTE & DOSAGE

Thromboembolism Prophylaxis

Adult: **PO** *Younger than 75 y, weight 60 kg or greater;* 60 mg loading dose, then 10 mg once daily; *younger than 75 y, weight less than 60 kg;* 60 mg loading dose, then 5 mg once daily

ADMINISTRATION

Oral
- Give without regard to food.
- Daily aspirin is recommended with prasugrel.
- Do not administer to patient with active bleeding or who is likely to undergo urgent CABG.
- Store at 15°–30° C (59°–86° F).

ADVERSE EFFECTS (≥1%) **Body as a Whole:** Fatigue, non-cardiac chest pain, pain in extremity, peripheral edema, pyrexia. **CNS:** Dizziness, headache. **CV:** Artial fibrillation, bradycardia, hypertension, hypotension. **GI:** Diarrhea, gastrointestinal hemorrhage, nausea. **Hematologic:** *Epistaxis, increased bleeding tendency*. **Metabolic:** Hypercholesterolemia, hyperlipidemia, leukopenia. **Musculoskeletal:** Back pain. **Respiratory:** Cough, dyspnea.

INTERACTIONS Drug: Warfarin or NSAIDS may increase the risk of bleeding.

PHARMACOKINETICS Absorption: 79% or higher. **Peak:** 30 min. **Metabolism:** Hydrolysis and oxidation to active metabolite. **Elimination:** Urine (68%) and feces (27%). **Half-Life:** 7 h.

NURSING IMPLICATIONS

Assessment & Drug Effects
- Monitor vital signs. Suspect bleeding if patient is hypotensive and has recently undergone an invasive or surgical procedure.
- Monitor for and report promptly any S&S of active bleeding.
- Lab tests: Periodic lipid profile.

Patient & Family Education
- Report promptly unexplained prolonged or excessive bleeding, or blood in urine or stool.
- Report immediately any of the following: Weakness, extremely pale skin, purple skin patches, jaundice, or fever.
- Inform all medical providers that you are taking prasugrel.
- Do not take OTC anti-inflammatory or pain medications without consulting physician.

PRAVASTATIN

(pra-vah-stat′in)
Pravachol
Classifications: ANTILIPEMIC; HMG-COA REDUCTASE INHIBITOR (STATIN)
Therapeutic: ANTILIPEMIC; STATIN
Prototype: Lovastatin
Pregnancy Category: X

AVAILABILITY 10 mg, 20 mg, 40 mg, 80 mg tablets

ACTION & *THERAPEUTIC EFFECT* Competitively inhibits 3-hydroxy-3-methylglutaryl-coenzyme A (HMG-CoA) reductase, the enzyme that catalyzes cholesterol biosynthesis. HMG-CoA reductase inhibitors (statins) increase serum HDL cholesterol, decrease serum LDL cholesterol, VLDL cholesterol, and plasma triglyceride levels. *It is effective in reducing total and LDL* *cholesterol in various forms of hypercholesterolemia.*

USES Hypercholesterolemia (alone or in combination with bile acid sequestrants) and familial hypercholesterolemia.

CONTRAINDICATIONS Hypersensitivity to pravastatin; active liver disease or unexplained elevated liver function test; hepatic encephalopathy, hepatitis, jaundice, rhabdomyolysis; pregnancy (category X), lactation. Safety and efficacy in children younger than 8 y are not established.
CAUTIOUS USE Alcoholics, history of liver disease; renal impairment; renal disease; seizure disorders.

ROUTE & DOSAGE

Hyperlipidemia
Adult: **PO** 10–80 mg daily
Child (8–13 y): **PO** 20 mg daily

ADMINISTRATION

Oral
- Give without regard to meals.
- Give in the evening.

ADVERSE EFFECTS (≥1%) **GI:** Nausea, diarrhea, abdominal pain, vomiting, constipation, flatulence, heartburn, transient elevations in serum liver transaminase levels. **Other:** Fatigue, rhinitis, cough, transient elevations in CPK.

INTERACTIONS Drug: May increase PT when administered with **warfarin.**

PHARMACOKINETICS Absorption: Poorly from GI tract; 17% reaches systemic circulation. **Onset:** 2 wk. **Peak:** 4 wk. **Distribution:** 43–55% protein bound; does not cross blood–brain barrier; crosses placenta; distributed into breast milk. **Metabolism:** Extensive first-pass metabolism in liver; has no active metabolites. **Elimination:** 20% of dose excreted in urine, 71% in feces. **Half-Life:** 1.8–2.6 h.

NURSING IMPLICATIONS

Assessment & Drug Effects
- Lab tests: Baseline LFTs at start of therapy and then at 12 wk. If normal at 12 wk, may change to semiannual monitoring. Monitor cholesterol levels throughout therapy.
- Monitor coagulation studies with patients receiving concurrent warfarin therapy. PT may be prolonged.
- Monitor CPK levels if patient experiences unexplained muscle pain.

Patient & Family Education
- Report unexplained muscle pain, tenderness, or weakness, especially if accompanied by malaise or fever, to physician promptly.
- Report signs of bleeding to physician promptly when taking concomitant warfarin therapy.

P

PRAZIQUANTEL

(pray-zi-kwon'tel)
Biltricide
Classification: ANTHELMINTIC
Therapeutic: ANTHELMINTIC
Prototype: Mebendazole
Pregnancy Category: B

AVAILABILITY 600 mg tablets

ACTION & *THERAPEUTIC EFFECT* Synthetic agent with broad-spectrum anthelmintic activity against all developmental stages of schistosomes and other trematodes (flukes) and against cestodes (tapeworm). Increases permeability of parasite cell membrane to calcium. Leads to immobilization of their suckers and dislodgment from their residence in blood vessel walls. *Active against all developmental stages of schistosomes, including cercaria (free-swimming larvae). Also active against other trematodes (flukes) and cestodes (tapeworms).*

USES All stages of schistosomiasis (bilharziasis) caused by all *Schistosoma* species pathogenic to humans. Other trematode infections caused by Chinese liver fluke.
UNLABELED USES Lung, sheep liver, and intestinal flukes and tapeworm infections.

CONTRAINDICATIONS Hypersensitivity to praziquantel; ocular cysticercosis. Safety in children younger than 4 y is not established; women should not breast feed on day of praziquantel therapy or for 72 h after last dose of drug.
CAUTIOUS USE Hepatic disease; cardiac arrhythmias; pregnancy (category B).

P

ROUTE & DOSAGE

Schistosomiasis

Adult/Child (older than 4 y): **PO** 60 mg/kg in 3 equally divided doses at 4–6 h intervals on the same day, may repeat in 2–3 mo after exposure

Other Trematodes

Adult/Child (older than 4 y): **PO** 75 mg/kg in 3 equally divided doses at 4–6 h intervals on the same day

Cestodiasis (Adult or Intestinal Stage)

Adult: **PO** 10–20 mg/kg as single dose

Cestodiasis (Larval or Tissue Stage)

Adult: **PO** 50 mg/kg in 3 divided doses/day for 14 days

ADMINISTRATION

Oral
- Give dose with food and fluids. Tablets can be broken into quarters but should NOT be chewed.
- Advise patient to take sufficient fluid to wash down the medication. Tablets are soluble in water; gagging or vomiting because of bitter taste may result if tablets are retained in the mouth.
- Store tablets in tight containers at less than 30° C (86° F).

ADVERSE EFFECTS (≥1%) **CNS:** *Dizziness, headache, malaise,* drowsiness, lassitude, CSF reaction syndrome (exacerbation of neurologic signs and symptoms such as seizures, increased CSF protein concentration, increased anticysticercal IgG levels, hyperthermia, intracranial hypertension) in patient treated for cerebral cysticercosis. **GI:** *Abdominal pain or discomfort with or without nausea;* vomiting, anorexia, diarrhea. **Hepatic:** *Increased AST, ALT (slight).* **Skin:** Pruritus, urticaria. **Body as a Whole:** Fever, sweating, symptoms of host-mediated immunologic response to antigen release from worms (fever, eosinophilia).

DIAGNOSTIC TEST INTERFERENCE Be mindful that selected drugs may interfere with stool studies for ova and parasites: ***Iron, bismuth, oil (mineral*** or ***castor), Metamucil*** (if ingested within 1 wk of test), ***barium, antibiotics, antiamebic*** and ***antimalarial drugs,*** and ***gallbladder dye*** (if administered within 3 wk of test).

INTERACTIONS Drug: Phenytoin can lead to therapeutic failure. **Food: Grapefruit juice** (greater than 1 qt/day) may increase plasma concentrations and adverse effects.

PHARMACOKINETICS Absorption: Rapidly, 80% reaches systemic circulation. **Peak:** 1–3 h. **Distribution:** Enters cerebrospinal fluid. **Metabolism:** Extensively to inactive metabolites. **Elimination:** Primarily in urine. **Half-Life:** 0.8–1.5 h.

NURSING IMPLICATIONS

Assessment & Drug Effects

- Patient is reexamined in 2 or 3 mo to ensure complete eradication of the infections.

Patient & Family Education

- Do not drive or operate other hazardous machinery on day of treatment or the following day because of potential drug-induced dizziness and drowsiness.
- Usually, all schistosomal worms are dead 7 days following treatment.
- Contact physician if you develop a sustained headache or high fever.

PRAZOSIN HYDROCHLORIDE (Pr)

(pra′zoe-sin)

Minipress

Classifications: ALPHA-ADRENERGIC RECEPTOR ANTAGONIST; ANTIHYPERTENSIVE; VASODILATOR

Therapeutic: ANTIHYPERTENSIVE

Pregnancy Category: C

AVAILABILITY 1 mg, 2 mg, 5 mg capsules

ACTION & *THERAPEUTIC EFFECT* Selective inhibition of alpha$_1$-adrenoceptors that produces vasodilation in both resistance (arterioles) and capacitance (veins) vessels with the result that both peripheral vascular resistance and blood pressure are reduced. *Lowers blood pressure in supine and standing positions with most pronounced effect on diastolic pressure.*

USES Treatment of hypertension.

UNLABELED USES Severe refractory congestive heart failure, Raynaud's disease or phenomenon, ergotamine-induced peripheral ischemia, pheochromocytoma, benign prostatic hypertrophy.

CONTRAINDICATIONS Hypotension.

CAUTIOUS USE Renal impairment; chronic kidney failure; hypertensive patient with cerebral thrombosis; angina; men with sickle cell trait; elderly; pregnancy (category C); lactation.

ROUTE & DOSAGE

Hypertension

Adult: **PO** Start with 1 mg at bedtime, then 1 mg b.i.d. or t.i.d., may increase to 20 mg/day in divided doses

Child: **PO** Start with 5 mcg/kg q6h, gradually increase to 25 mcg/kg q6h (max: 15 mg or 0.4 mg/kg/day)

ADMINISTRATION

Oral

- Give initial dose at bedtime to reduce possibility of adverse effects such as postural hypotension and syncope. However, if first dose is taken during the day, advise patient not to drive a car for about 4 h after ingestion of drug.
- Give drug with food to reduce incidence of faintness and dizziness;

P

food may delay absorption but does not affect extent of absorption.

- Store in tightly closed container away from strong light. Do not freeze.

ADVERSE EFFECTS (≥1%) **CNS:** *Dizziness, headache, drowsiness,* nervousness, vertigo, depression, paresthesia, insomnia. **CV:** Edema, dyspnea, syncope *first-dose phenomenon,* postural hypotension, *palpitations,* tachycardia, angina. **Special Senses:** Blurred vision, tinnitus, reddened sclerae. **GI:** Dry mouth, *nausea,* vomiting, diarrhea, constipation, abdominal discomfort, pain. **Urogenital:** Urinary frequency, incontinence, priapism (especially in men with sickle cell anemia), impotence. **Skin:** Rash, pruritus, alopecia, lichen planus. **Body as a Whole:** Diaphoresis, epistaxis, nasal congestion, arthralgia, transient leukopenia, increased serum uric acid, and BUN.

INTERACTIONS Drug: DIURETICS, HYPOTENSIVE AGENTS and alcohol increase hypotensive effects. **Sildenafil, vardenafil,** and **tadalafil** may enhance hypotensive effects.

PHARMACOKINETICS Absorption: Approximately 60% of oral dose reaches the systemic circulation. **Onset:** 2 h. **Peak:** 2–4 h. **Duration:** Less than 24 h. **Distribution:** Widely distributed, including into breast milk. **Metabolism:** Extensively in liver. **Elimination:** 6–10% in urine, rest in bile and feces. **Half-Life:** 2–4 h.

NURSING IMPLICATIONS

Assessment & Drug Effects

- Be alert for first-dose phenomenon (rare adverse effect: 0.15% of patients); characterized by a precipitous decline in BP, bradycardia, and consciousness disturbances (syncope) within 90–120 min after the initial dose of prazosin. Recovery is usually within several hours. Preexisting low plasma volume (from diuretic therapy or salt restriction), beta-adrenergic therapy, and recent stroke appear to increase the risk of this phenomenon.
- Monitor blood pressure. If it falls precipitously with first dose, notify physician promptly.
- Full therapeutic effect may not be achieved until 4–6 wk of therapy.

Patient & Family Education

- Avoid situations that would result in injury if you should faint, particularly during early phase of treatment. In most cases, effect does not recur after initial period of therapy; however, it may occur during acute febrile episodes, when drug dose is increased, or when another antihypertensive drug is added to the medication regimen.
- Make position and direction changes slowly and in stages. Dangle legs and move ankles a minute or so before standing when arising in the morning or after a nap.
- Lie down immediately if you experience light-headedness, dizziness, a sense of impending loss of consciousness, or blurred vision. Attempting to stand or walk may result in a fall.
- Do not drive or engage in other potentially hazardous activities until response to drug is known.
- Take drug at same time(s) each day.
- Report priapism or impotence. A change in the drug regimen usually reverses these difficulties.
- Do not take OTC medications, especially remedies for coughs, colds, and allergy, without consulting physician.

- Be aware that adverse effects usually disappear with continuation of therapy, but dosage reduction may be necessary.

PREDNISOLONE

(pred-niss'oh-lone)

Prelone

PREDNISOLONE ACETATE

Flo-Pred, Pred Forte, Pred Mild

PREDNISOLONE SODIUM PHOSPHATE

AK-Pred, Inflamase Forte, Inflamase Mild

Classification: ADRENAL CORTICOSTEROID

Therapeutic: ANTI-INFLAMMATORY; IMMUNOSUPPRESSANT

Prototype: Prednisone

Pregnancy Category: C

AVAILABILITY Prednisolone: 1 mg, 2.5 mg, 5 mg tablet; 5 mg/5 mL, 15 mg/5 mL syrup; **Acetate:** 1% ophth suspension; **Sodium Phosphate:** 5 mg/5 mL liquid; 0.125%, 1%, 0.9%, 0.11% ophth solution

ACTION & *THERAPEUTIC EFFECT* Has glucocorticoid activity similar to the naturally occurring hormone. It prevents or suppresses inflammation and immune responses. Its actions include inhibition of leukocyte infiltration at the site of inflammation, interference in the function of inflammatory mediators, and suppression of humoral immune resonses. *Effective as an anti-inflammatory agent.*

USES Principally as an anti-inflammatory and immunosuppressant agent.

CONTRAINDICATIONS Fungal infections; GI bleeding.

CAUTIOUS USE Cataracts; coagulopathy; diabetes mellitus; seizure disorders; renal disease; psychosis; emotional instability; GI disorders; pregnancy (category C).

ROUTE & DOSAGE

Anti-inflammatory

Adult: **PO** 5–60 mg/day in single or divided doses **Ophthalmic** See Appendix A-1

Child: **PO** 0.1–2 mg/kg/day in divided doses

ADMINISTRATION

Oral

- Give with meals to reduce gastric irritation. If distress continues, consult physician about possible adjunctive antacid therapy.

Alternate-Day Therapy (ADT) for Patient on Long-Term Therapy

- With ADT, the 48-h requirement for steroids is administered as a single dose every other morning.
- Be aware that ADT minimizes adverse effects associated with long-term treatment while maintaining the desired therapeutic effect.
- See PREDNISONE for numerous additional nursing implications.

ADVERSE EFFECTS (≥1%) **Endocrine:** Hirsutism (occasional), adverse effects on growth and development of the individual and on sperm. **Special Senses:** Perforation of cornea (with topical drug). **Body as a Whole:** Sensitivity to heat; fat embolism, hypotension and shock-like reactions. **CNS:** Insomnia. **GI:** Gastric irritation or ulceration. **Skin:** Ecchymotic skin lesions; vasomotor symptoms. Also see PREDNISONE.

INTERACTIONS Drug: BARBITURATES, **phenytoin, rifampin** increase steroid metabolism, therefore may need increased doses of prednisolone; **amphotericin B,** DIURETICS add to **potassium** loss; **ambenonium, neostigmine, pyridostig-**

mine may cause severe muscle weakness in patients with myasthenia gravis; VACCINES, TOXOIDS may inhibit antibody response. **Food: Licorice** may elevate plasma levels and adverse effects.

PHARMACOKINETICS Absorption: Readily from GI tract. **Peak:** 1–2 h. **Duration:** 1–1.5 days. **Distribution:** Crosses placenta; distributed into breast milk. **Metabolism:** In liver. **Elimination:** HPA suppression: 24–36 h; in urine. **Half-Life:** 3.5 h.

NURSING IMPLICATIONS

Assessment & Drug Effects

- Be alert to subclinical signs of lack of improvement such as continued drainage, low-grade fever, and interrupted healing. In diseases caused by microorganisms, infection may be masked, activated, or enhanced by corticosteroids. Observe and report exacerbation of symptoms after short period of therapeutic response.
- Be aware that temporary local discomfort may follow injection of prednisolone into bursa or joint.

Patient & Family Education

- Adhere to established dosage regimen (i.e., do not increase, decrease, or omit doses or change dose intervals).
- Report gastric distress or any sign of peptic ulcer.

P

PREDNISONE (Pr)

(pred′ni-sone)

Apo-Prednisone ✦, Deltasone, Meticorten, Orasone, Panasol, Prednicen-M, Sterapred, Winpred ✦

Classification: ADRENAL CORTICOSTEROID

Therapeutic: IMMUNOSUPPRESSANT; ANTI-INFLAMMATORY

Pregnancy Category: C

AVAILABILITY 1 mg, 2.5 mg, 5 mg, 10 mg, 20 mg, 50 mg tablets; 5 mg/5 mL, 5 mg/mL solution

ACTION & *THERAPEUTIC EFFECT* Immediate-acting synthetic analog of hydrocortisone that is biotransformed in the liver into prednisolone. Sodium retention and potassium depletion can occur. *Has anti-inflammatory and immunosuppressant properties.*

USES May be used as a single agent or conjunctively with antineoplastics in cancer therapy; also used in treatment of myasthenia gravis and inflammatory conditions as an immunosuppressant; acute respiratory distress syndrome, Addison's disease, adrenal hyperplasic, gout, gouty arthritis, headache, hemolytic anemia, sarcoidosis, Stevens-Johnson syndrome.

UNLABELED USES Absence seizures.

CONTRAINDICATIONS Systemic fungal infections and known hypersensitivity; cataracts.

CAUTIOUS USE Patients with infections; nonspecific ulcerative colitis; diverticulitis; active or latent peptic ulcer; renal insufficiency; coagulopathy; psychosis; seizure disorders; thromboembolic disease; hypertension; osteoporosis; myasthenia gravis; pregnancy (category C).

ROUTE & DOSAGE

Anti-inflammatory

*Doses are highly individualized (ranges are provided)

Adult: **PO** 5–60 mg/day in single or divided doses

Child: **PO** 0.1–0.15 mg/kg/day in single or divided doses

Acute Asthma
Child: **PO** *Younger than 1 y,* 1–2 mg/kg/day × 3–5 days or 10 mg q12h; *1–4 y,* 20 mg q12h; *5–13 y,* 30 mg q12h; *older than 13 y,* 40 mg q12h × 3–5 days

ADMINISTRATION

Oral

- Crush tablet and give with fluid of patient's choice if unable to swallow whole.
- Give at mealtimes or with a snack to reduce gastric irritation.
- Dose adjustment may be required if patient is subjected to severe stress (serious infection, surgery, or injury) or if a remission or disease exacerbation occurs.
- Do not abruptly stop drug. Reduce dose gradually by scheduled decrements (various regimens) to prevent withdrawal symptoms and permit adrenals to recover from drug-induced partial atrophy.

Alternate-Day Therapy (ADT) for Patient on Long-Term Therapy

- With ADT, the 48-h requirement for steroids is administered as a single dose every other morning.
- Be aware that ADT minimizes adverse effects associated with long-term treatment while maintaining the desired therapeutic effect.

ADVERSE EFFECTS (≥1%) **CNS:** Euphoria, headache, insomnia, confusion, psychosis. **CV:** CHF, edema. **GI:** Nausea, vomiting, peptic ulcer. **Musculoskeletal:** Muscle weakness, delayed wound healing, muscle wasting, osteoporosis, aseptic necrosis of bone, spontaneous fractures. **Endocrine:** Cushingoid features, growth suppression in children, carbohydrate intolerance, hyperglycemia. **Special Senses:** Cataracts. **Hematologic:** Leukocytosis. **Metabolic:** Hypokalemia.

INTERACTIONS Drug: BARBITURATES, **phenytoin, rifampin** increase steroid metabolism—increased doses of prednisone may be needed; **amphotericin B,** DIURETICS increase **potassium** loss; **ambenonium, neostigmine, pyridostigmine** may cause severe muscle weakness in patients with myasthenia gravis; may inhibit antibody response to VACCINES, TOXOIDS.

PHARMACOKINETICS Absorption: Readily from GI tract. **Peak:** 1–2 h. **Duration:** 1–1.5 days. **Distribution:** Crosses placenta; distributed into breast milk. **Metabolism:** In liver. **Elimination:** Hypothalamus-pituitary axis suppression: 24–36 h; in urine. **Half-Life:** 3.5 h.

NURSING IMPLICATIONS

Assessment & Drug Effects

- Establish baseline and continuing data regarding BP, I&O ratio and pattern, weight, fasting blood glucose level, and sleep pattern. Start flow chart as reference for planning individualized pharmacotherapeutic patient care.
- Check and record BP during dose stabilization period at least 2 times daily. Report an ascending pattern.
- Monitor patient for evidence of HPA axis suppression during long-term therapy by determining plasma cortisol levels at weekly intervals.
- Lab tests: Obtain fasting blood glucose, serum electrolytes, and routine laboratory studies at regular intervals during long-term steroid therapy.
- Be aware that older adult patients and patients with low serum albumin are especially susceptible to adverse effects because of excess circulating free glucocorticoids.
- Be alert to signs of hypocalcemia (see Appendix F). Patients with

P

hypocalcemia have increased requirements for pyridoxine (vitamin B_6), vitamins C and D, and folates.
- Be alert to possibility of masked infection and delayed healing (anti-inflammatory and immunosuppressive actions). Prednisone suppresses early classic signs of inflammation. When patient is on an extended therapy regimen, incidence of oral *Candida* infection is high. Inspect mouth daily for symptoms: White patches, black furry tongue, painful membranes and tongue.
- Monitor bone density. Compression and spontaneous fractures of long bones and vertebrae present hazards, particularly in long-term corticosteroid treatment of rheumatoid arthritis or diabetes, in immobilized patients, and older adults.
- Be aware of previous history of psychotic tendencies. Watch for changes in mood and behavior, emotional stability, sleep pattern, or psychomotor activity, especially with long-term therapy, that may signal onset of recurrence. Report symptoms to physician.
- Monitor for withdrawal syndrome (e.g., myalgia, fever, arthralgia, malaise) and hypocorticism (e.g., anorexia, vomiting, nausea, fatigue, dizziness, hypotension, hypoglycemia, myalgia, arthralgia) with abrupt discontinuation of corticosteroids after long-term therapy.

Patient & Family Education

- Take drug as prescribed and do not alter dosing regimen or stop medication without consulting physician.
- Be aware that a slight weight gain with improved appetite is expected, but after dosage is stabilized, a sudden slow but steady weight increase [2 kg (5 lb)/wk] should be reported to physician.
- Avoid or minimize alcohol, which may contribute to steroid-ulcer development in long-term therapy.
- Report symptoms of GI distress to physician and do not self-medicate to find relief.
- Do not use aspirin or other OTC drugs unless they are prescribed specifically by the physician.
- Be fastidious about personal hygiene; give special attention to foot care, and be particularly cautious about bruising or abrading the skin.
- Report persistent backache or chest pain (possible symptoms of vertebral or rib fracture) that may occur with long-term therapy.
- Tell dentist or new physician about prednisone therapy.

PREGABALIN

Lyrica

Classifications: ANTICONVULSANT; GABA-ANALOG; ANALGESIC/MISCELLANEOUS; ANXIOLYTIC

Therapeutic: ANTICONVULSANT; ANALGESIC; ANTIANXIETY

Prototype: Gabapentin

Pregnancy Category: C

Controlled Substance: Schedule V

AVAILABILITY 25 mg, 50 mg, 75 mg, 100 mg, 150 mg, 200 mg, 225 mg, 300 mg capsules

ACTION & *THERAPEUTIC EFFECT*

Pregabalin is an analog of gamma-aminobutyric acid (GABA) that increases neuronal GABA levels and reduces calcium currents in the calcium channels of neurons; this may account for its control of pain and anxiety. Its affinity for voltage-gated calcium channels may account for its antiseizure activity. *Has analgesic, anti-anxiety, and anticonvulsant properties.*

USES Management of neuropathic pain associated with diabetic peripheral neuropathy, adjunctive therapy for adult patients with partial-onset seizures, management of postherpetic neuralgia, fibromyalgia.

UNLABELED USES Treatment of generalized anxiety disorders, treatment of social anxiety disorder, treatment of moderate pain.

CONTRAINDICATIONS Hypersensitivity to pregabalin or gabapentin; alcohol; lactation. Safety and efficacy in children younger than 18 y have not been established.

CAUTIOUS USE Renal impairment or failure, hemodialysis; elderly; congestive heart failure, NYHA (Class III or IV) cardiac status; pregnancy (category C).

ROUTE & DOSAGE

Neuropathic Pain (Diabetic Peripheral Neuropathy)

Adult: **PO** 50–100 mg t.i.d.

Partial-Onset Seizures

Adult: **PO** Initial dose 75 mg or less b.i.d or 50 mg t.i.d; may increase to 300 mg b.i.d. or 200 mg t.i.d.

Fibromyalgia

Adult: **PO** 75 mg b.i.d., may increase up to 150 b.i.d. within first week, then up to 225 b.i.d. (max dose: 450 mg/day)

Postherpetic Neuralgia

Adult: **PO** Initial dose 75 mg b.i.d. or 50 mg t.i.d; may increase to 150–300 mg b.i.d. or 100–200 mg t.i.d.

Renal Impairment Dosage Adjustment

CrCl 30–60 mL/min: 75–300 mg/day given in 2 or 3 divided doses; 15–30 mL/min: 25–150 mg/day given in 1 or 2 divided doses; less than 15 mL/min: 25–75 mg once daily

Hemodialysis Dosage Adjustment: Dose based on renal function, give supplemental dose

ADMINISTRATION

Oral

- Dosage reduction is required with renal dysfunction.
- Drug should not be abruptly stopped; discontinue by tapering over a minimum of 1 wk.
- Give a supplemental dose immediately following dialysis.
- Store at 15°–30° C (59°– 86° F).

ADVERSE EFFECTS (≥1%) **Body as a Whole:** *Accidental injury,* flu syndrome, pain. **CNS:** Abnormal gait, amnesia, *ataxia,* confusion, *dizziness,* euphoria, headache, incoordination, myoclonus, nervousness, neuropathy, *somnolence,* speech disorder, abnormal thinking, tremor, twitching, vertigo. **CV:** Chest pain. **GI:** Constipation, dry mouth, flatulence, increased appetite, vomiting. **GU:** Urinary incontinence. **Metabolic/Nutritional:** Edema, facial edema, hypoglycemia, *peripheral edema, weight gain.* **Musculoskeletal:** Back pain, myasthenia. **Respiratory:** Bronchitis, dyspnea. **Special Senses:** Abnormal vision, *blurry vision, diplopia.*

INTERACTIONS Drug: Concomitant use with THIAZOLIDINEDIONES may exacerbate weight gain and fluid retention.

PHARMACOKINETICS Absorption: 90% bioavailability. **Peak:** 1.5 h. **Metabolism:** Negligible. **Elimination:** Primarily in the urine. **Half-Life:** 6 h.

P

NURSING IMPLICATIONS

Assessment & Drug Effects

- Monitor for and report promptly mental status or behavior changes (e.g., anxiety, panic attacks, restlessness, irritability, depression, suicidal thoughts).
- Monitor for weight gain, peripheral edema, and S&S of heart failure, especially with concurrent thiazolidinedione (e.g., rosiglitazone) therapy.
- Lab tests: Baseline and periodic kidney function tests; periodic platelet counts.
- Monitor diabetics for increased incidences of hypoglycemia.
- Supervise ambulation especially when other CNS drugs are used concurrently.

Patient & Family Education

- Do not drive or engage in potentially hazardous activities until response to drug is known.
- Report any of the following to a health care provider: Changes in vision (i.e., blurred vision); dizziness and incoordination; weight gain and swelling of the extremities, behavior or mood changes, especially suicidal thoughts.
- Avoid alcohol consumption while taking this drug.
- Inform your physician if you plan to become pregnant or father a child.

PRIMAQUINE PHOSPHATE

(prim′a-kween)

Primaquine

Classification: ANTIMALARIAL

Therapeutic: ANTIMALARIAL

Prototype: Chloroquine

Pregnancy Category: C

AVAILABILITY 26.3 mg tablets; 5 g, 25 g, 100 g, 500 g powder

ACTION & *THERAPEUTIC EFFECT* Acts on primary exoerythrocytic forms of *Plasmodium vivax* and *Plasmodium falciparum*. Destroys late tissue forms of *P. vivax* and thus effects radical cure (prevents relapse). *Gametocidal activity against all species of Plasmodia that infect humans; interrupts transmission of malaria.*

USES To prevent relapse ("radical" or "clinical" cure) of *P. vivax* and *P. ovale* malarias and to prevent attacks after departure from areas where *P. vivax* and *P. ovale* malarias are endemic. With clindamycin for the treatment of *Pneumocystis carinii* pneumonia (PCP) in AIDS.

CONTRAINDICATIONS Hypersensitivity to primaquine or iodoquinol; rheumatoid arthritis; lupus erythematosus (SLE); hemolytic drugs, concomitant or recent use of agents capable of bone marrow depression (e.g., quinacrine; patients with G6PD deficiency).

CAUTIOUS USE Bone marrow depression; hematologic disease; methemoglobin reductase deficiency; pregnancy (category C), lactation.

ROUTE & DOSAGE

Malaria Treatment

Adult: **PO** 30 mg daily for 14 days concomitantly or consecutively with chloroquine or hydroxychloroquine on first 3 days of acute attack

Child: **PO** 0.5 mg/kg daily for 14 days concomitantly or consecutively with chloroquine or hydroxychloroquine on first 3 days of acute attack

Malaria Prophylaxis

Adult: **PO** 15 mg daily for 14 days beginning immediately after leaving malarious area

Child: **PO** 0.3 mg/kg daily for 14 days beginning immediately after leaving malarious area

ADMINISTRATION

Oral

- Give drug at mealtime or with an antacid (prescribed); may prevent or relieve gastric irritation. Notify physician if GI symptoms persist.
- Store in tight, light-resistant containers.

ADVERSE EFFECTS (≥1%) **Hematologic:** Hematologic reactions including granulocytopenia and acute hemolytic anemia in patients with G6PD deficiency, moderate leukocytosis or leukopenia, anemia, granulocytopenia, agranulocytosis. **GI:** Nausea, vomiting, epigastric distress, abdominal cramps. **Skin:** Pruritus. **Metabolic:** Methemoglobinemia (cyanosis). **Body as a Whole:** Headache, confusion, mental depression. **Special Senses:** Disturbances of visual accommodation. **CV:** Hypertension, arrhythmias (rare).

INTERACTIONS Drug: Toxicity of both **quinacrine** and primaquine increased.

PHARMACOKINETICS Absorption: Readily from GI tract. **Peak:** 6 h. **Metabolism:** Rapidly in liver to active metabolites. **Elimination:** In urine. **Half-Life:** 3.7–9.6 h.

NURSING IMPLICATIONS

Assessment & Drug Effects

- Be aware drug may precipitate acute hemolytic anemia in patients with G6PD deficiency, an inherited error of metabolism carried on the X chromosome, present in about 10% of American black males and certain white ethnic groups: Sardinians, Sephardic Jews, Greeks, and Iranians. Whites manifest more intense expression of hemolytic reaction than do blacks. Screen for prior to initiation of therapy.
- Lab tests: Perform repeated hematologic studies (particularly blood cell counts and Hgb) and urinalyses during therapy.

Patient & Family Education

- Examine urine after each voiding and to report to physician darkening of urine, red-tinged urine, and decrease in urine volume. Also report chills, fever, precordial pain, cyanosis (all suggest a hemolytic reaction). Sudden reductions in hemoglobin or erythrocyte count suggest an impending hemolytic reaction.

PRIMIDONE

(pri'mi-done)

Apo-Primidone ◆, Mysoline

Classifications: ANTICONVULSANT; BARBITURATE

Therapeutic: ANTICONVULSANT

Prototype: Phenobarbital

Pregnancy Category: D

AVAILABILITY 50 mg, 250 mg tablets; 250 mg/5 mL suspension

ACTION & *THERAPEUTIC EFFECT* Antiepileptic properties result from raising the seizure threshold and changing seizure patterns. *Effective as an anticonvulsant in all types of seizure disorders except absence seizures.*

USES Alone or concomitantly with other anticonvulsant agents in the prophylactic management of complex partial (psychomotor) and generalized tonic-clonic (grand mal) seizures.

UNLABELED USES Essential tremor.

CONTRAINDICATIONS Hypersensitivity to barbiturates, porphyria; ethanol intoxication, hepatic encephalopathy, suicidal ideation; pregnancy (category D).

CAUTIOUS USE Chronic lung disease, sleep apnea; liver or kidney disease, dialysis; hyperactive children; mental status changes, major depression, suicidal tendencies; lactation; children.

ROUTE & DOSAGE

Seizures

Adult/Child (8 y or older): **PO** 250 mg/day, increased by 250 mg/wk (max: 2 g in 2–4 divided doses)

Child (Younger than 8 y): **PO** 125 mg/day, increased by 125 mg/wk (max: 2 g/day in 2–4 divided doses)

ADMINISTRATION

Oral

- Give whole or crush with fluid of patient's choice.
- Give with food if drug causes GI distress.

ADVERSE EFFECTS (≥1%) **CNS:** *Drowsiness, sedation, vertigo, ataxia, headache,* excitement (children), confusion, unusual fatigue, hyperirritability, emotional disturbances, acute psychoses (usually patients with psychomotor epilepsy). **Special Senses:** Diplopia, nystagmus, swelling of eyelids. **GI:** *Nausea, vomiting, anorexia.* **Hematologic:** Leukopenia, thrombocytopenia, eosinophilia, decreased serum folate levels, megaloblastic anemia (rare). **Skin:** Alopecia, maculopapular or morbilliform rash, edema, lupus erythematosus-like syndrome. **Urogenital:** Impotence. **Body as a Whole:** Lymphadenopathy, osteomalacia.

INTERACTIONS Drug: Alcohol, CNS DEPRESSANTS compound CNS depression; **phenobarbital** may decrease absorption and increase metabolism of ORAL ANTICOAGULANTS; increases metabolism of CORTICOSTEROIDS, ORAL CONTRACEPTIVES, ANTICONVULSANTS, **digitoxin,** possibly decreasing their effects; ANTIDEPRESSANTS potentiate adverse effects of primidone; **griseofulvin** decreases absorption of primidone. **Herbal: Kava, valerian** may potentiate sedation.

PHARMACOKINETICS Absorption: Approximately 60–80% from GI tract. **Peak:** 4 h. **Distribution:** Distributed into breast milk. **Metabolism:** In liver to phenobarbital and PEMA. **Elimination:** In urine. **Half-Life:** Primidone 3–24 h, PEMA 24–48 h; phenobarbital 72–144 h.

NURSING IMPLICATIONS

Assessment & Drug Effects

- Lab tests: Perform baseline and periodic CBC, complete blood chemistry (q6mo), and primidone blood levels. (Therapeutic blood level for primidone: 5–10 mcg/mL.)
- Monitor primidone plasma levels (concentrations of primidone greater than 10 mcg/mL are usually associated with significant ataxia and lethargy).
- Therapeutic response may not be evident for several weeks.
- Observe for S&S of folic acid deficiency: Mental dysfunction, psychiatric disorders, neuropathy, megaloblastic anemia. Determine serum folate levels if indicated.

Patient & Family Education

- Avoid driving and other potentially hazardous activities during beginning of treatment because drowsiness, dizziness, and ataxia may be severe. Symptoms tend to disappear with continued therapy; if they persist, dosage reduction or drug withdrawal may be necessary.

- Avoid alcohol and other CNS depressants unless otherwise directed by physician.
- Do not take OTC medications unless approved by physician.
- Pregnant women should receive prophylactic vitamin K therapy for 1 mo prior to and during delivery to prevent neonatal hemorrhage.
- Withdraw primidone gradually to avoid precipitating status epilepticus.

PROBENECID (Pr)

(proe-ben′e-sid)

Benemid, Benuryl ✦, Probalan, SK-Probenecid

Classifications: URICOSURIC; ANTIGOUT

Therapeutic: ANTIGOUT

Pregnancy Category: B

AVAILABILITY 0.5 g tablet

ACTION & *THERAPEUTIC EFFECT* Competitively inhibits renal tubular reabsorption of uric acid, thereby promoting its excretion and reducing serum urate levels. *Prevents formation of new tophaceous deposits and uric acid buildup in the serum and tissues. As an additive to penicillin, it increases serum concentration of penicllins and prolongs their serum concentration.*

USES Hyperuricemia in chronic gouty arthritis and tophaceous gout.

UNLABELED USES Adjuvant to therapy with penicillin G and penicillin analogs to elevate and prolong plasma concentrations of these antibiotics; to promote uric acid excretion in hyperuricemia secondary to administration of thiazides and related diuretics, furosemide, ethacrynic acid, pyrazinamide.

CONTRAINDICATIONS Blood dyscrasias; uric acid kidney stones; during or within 2–3 wk of acute gouty attack; overexcretion of uric acid (greater than 1000 mg/day); patients with creatinine clearance less than 50 mg/min; use with penicillin in presence of known renal impairment; use for hyperuricemia secondary to cancer chemotherapy. Safe use as adjunct to penicillin or cephalosporin therapy in children younger than 2 y is not established.

CAUTIOUS USE History of peptic ulcer; pregnancy (category B), lactation.

ROUTE & DOSAGE

Gout

Adult: **PO** 250 mg b.i.d. for 1 wk, then 500 mg b.i.d. (max: 3 g/day)

Adjunct for Penicillin or Cephalosporin Therapy

Adult: **PO** 500 mg q.i.d. or 1 g with single dose therapy (e.g., gonorrhea)

Child (2–14 y or weight less than 50 kg): **PO** 25–40 mg/kg/day in 4 divided doses

ADMINISTRATION

Oral

- Therapy is usually not initiated during an acute gouty attack. Consult physician.
- Minimize GI adverse effects by giving after meals, with food, milk, or antacid (prescribed). If symptoms persist, dosage reduction may be required.
- Give with a full glass of water if not contraindicated.
- Be aware that physician may prescribe concurrent prophylactic doses of colchicine for first 3–6 mo

P

of therapy because frequency of acute gouty attacks may increase during first 6–12 mo of therapy.

ADVERSE EFFECTS (≥1%) **Body as a Whole:** Flushing, dizziness, fever, anaphylaxis. **CNS:** *Headache*. **GI:** *Nausea, vomiting, anorexia,* sore gums, hepatic necrosis (rare). **Urogenital:** Urinary frequency. **Hematologic:** Anemia, hemolytic anemia (possibly related to G6PD deficiency), aplastic anemia (rare). **Musculoskeletal:** Exacerbations of gout, uric acid kidney stones. **Skin:** Dermatitis, pruritus. **Respiratory:** Respiratory depression.

DIAGNOSTIC TEST INTERFERENCE False-positive ***urine glucose*** tests are possible with ***Benedict's solution*** or ***Clinitest*** [***glucose oxidase methods*** not affected (e.g., ***Clinistix, TesTape***)].

INTERACTIONS Drug: SALICYLATES may decrease uricosuric activity; may decrease **methotrexate** elimination, causing increased toxicity; decreases **nitrofurantoin** efficacy and increases its toxicity. Decreases clearance of PENICILLINS, CEPHALOSPORINS, and NSAIDS.

PHARMACOKINETICS Absorption: Readily from GI tract. **Onset:** 30 min. **Peak:** 2–4 h. **Duration:** 8 h. **Distribution:** Crosses placenta. **Metabolism:** In liver. **Elimination:** In urine. **Half-Life:** 4–17 h.

NURSING IMPLICATIONS

Assessment & Drug Effects

- Lab tests: Periodic serum urate levels, Hct and Hgb, and urinalysis. Determine acid–base balance periodically when urinary alkalinizers are used.
- Patients taking sulfonylureas may require dosage adjustment. Probenecid enhances hypoglycemic actions of these drugs (see DIAGNOSTIC TEST INTERFERENCES).
- Expect urate tophaceous deposits to decrease in size. Classic locations are in cartilage of ear pinna and big toe, but they can occur in bursae, tendons, skin, kidneys, and other tissues.

Patient & Family Education

- Drink fluid liberally (approximately 3000 mL/day) to maintain daily urinary output of at least 2000 mL or more. This is important because increased uric acid excretion promoted by drug predisposes to renal calculi.
- Physician may advise restriction of high-purine foods during early therapy until uric acid level stabilizes. Foods high in purine include organ meats (sweetbreads, liver, kidney), meat extracts, meat soups, gravy, anchovies, and sardines. Moderate amounts are present in other meats, fish, seafood, asparagus, spinach, peas, dried legumes, wild game.
- Avoid alcohol because it may increase serum urate levels.
- Do not stop taking drug without consulting physician. Irregular dosage schedule may sharply elevate serum urate level and precipitate acute gout.
- Report symptoms of hypersensitivity to physician. Discontinuation of drug is indicated.
- Do not take aspirin or other OTC medications without consulting physician. If a mild analgesic is required, acetaminophen is usually allowed.

PROCAINAMIDE HYDROCHLORIDE Pr

(proe-kane-a'mide)

Pronestyl, Pronestyl SR
Classification: ANTIARRHYTHMIC, CLASS IA
Therapeutic: ANTIARRHYTHMIC, CLASS IA
Pregnancy Category: C

AVAILABILITY 250 mg, 375 mg, 500 mg tablets, capsules; 250 mg, 500 mg, 750 mg, 1000 mg sustained release tablets; 100 mg/mL, 500 mg/mL injection

ACTION & *THERAPEUTIC EFFECT* Potent class IA antiarrhythmic that depresses excitability of myocardium to electrical stimulation, reduces conduction velocity in atria, ventricles, and His-Purkinje system. Produces peripheral vasodilation and hypotension, especially with IV use. *Effectively used for atrial arrhythmias; suppresses automaticity of His-Purkinje ventricular muscle.*

USES Prophylactically to maintain normal sinus rhythm following conversion of atrial flutter or fibrillation by other methods; to prevent recurrence of paroxysmal atrial fibrillation and tachycardia, paroxysmal AV junctional rhythm, ventricular tachycardia, ventricular and atrial premature contractions. Also cardiac arrhythmias associated with surgery and anesthesia.

UNLABELED USES Malignant hyperthermia.

CONTRAINDICATIONS Hypersensitivity to procainamide or procaine, yellow dye 5 (tartrazine); blood dyscrasias; bundle branch block; complete AV block, second and third degree AV block unassisted by pacemaker; QT prolongation, torsades de pointes; non-life-threatening ventricular arrhythmias; leukopenia or agranulocytosis; SLE; concurrent use with other antiarrhythmic agents; myasthenia gravis.

CAUTIOUS USE Patient who has undergone electrical conversion to sinus rhythm; first-degree heart block; bone marrow suppression or cytopenia; hypotension, cardiac enlargement, CHF, MI, ischemic heart disease; coronary occlusion, ventricular dysrhythmia from digitalis intoxication, ventricular arrhythmias; hepatic or renal insufficiency; electrolyte imbalance; bronchial asthma; aspirin hypersensitivity; cytopenia; pregnancy (category C), lactation.

ROUTE & DOSAGE

Arrhythmias

Adult: **PO** 50 mg/kg/day in divided doses (b.i.d. for Procanbid); max: 5 g/day **IM** 0.5–1 g q4–8h until able to take PO **IV** 100 mg q5min at a rate of 25–50 mg/min until arrhythmia is controlled or 1 g given, then 2–6 mg/min
Child: **PO** 15–50 mg/kg/day divided q3–6h **IM** 50 mg/kg/day divided q3–6 until PO tolerated **IV** 3–6 mg/kg q10–30min (max: 100 mg/dose), then 20–80 mcg/kg/min

Renal Impairment Dosage Adjustment

Oral doses CrCl 10–50 mL/min: Give q6–12h; less than 10 mL/min: Give q8–24h. **IV doses** Reduce loading dose to 12 mg/kg, then maintenance by 1/3 to 2/3.
Hemodialysis Dosage Adjustment: Give 200 mg supplemental dose post dialysis

ADMINISTRATION

Oral

- Give first PO dose at least 4 h after last IV dose

P

- Give oral preparation on empty stomach, 1 h before or 2 h after meals, with a full glass of water to enhance absorption. If drug causes gastric distress, give with food.
- Crush immediate release (but NOT sustained release) tablet if patient is unable to swallow it whole.
- Swallow sustained release tablet whole. It has a wax matrix that is not absorbed but appears in the stool.

Intramuscular

- IM route should be used only when IV route is not feasible.

Intravenous

Use IV route for emergency situations.

PREPARE: **Direct:** Dilute each 100 mg with 5–10 mL of D5W or sterile water for injection. **IV Infusion:** Add 1 g of procainamide to 250–500 mL of D5W solution to yield 4 mg/mL in 250 mL or 2 mg/mL in 500 mL.

ADMINISTER: **Direct:** Usual rate is 20 mg/min. Faster rates (up to 50 mg/min) should be used with caution. **IV Infusion for Adult:** 2–6 mg/min. **IV Infusion for Child:** 20–80 mcg/kg/min. ▪ Control IV administration over several hours by assessment of procainamide plasma levels. ▪ Use an infusion pump with constant monitoring. ▪ Keep patient in supine position. ▪ Be alert to signs of too rapid administration of drug (speed shock: Irregular pulse, tight feeling in chest, flushed face, headache, loss of consciousness, shock, cardiac arrest).

INCOMPATIBILITIES **Solution/additive:** **Bretylium, esmolol, ethacrynate, milrinone, phenytoin.** **Y-site:** **Inamrinone (amrinone), milrinone.**

- Store solution for up to 24 h at room temperature and for 7 days under refrigeration at 2°–8° C (36°–46° F). ▪ Slight yellowing does not alter drug potency, but discard solution if it is markedly discolored or precipitated.

ADVERSE EFFECTS (≥1%) **CNS:** Dizziness, psychosis. **CV:** Severe hypotension, pericarditis, <u>ventricular fibrillation</u>, AV block, tachycardia, flushing. **GI:** Bitter taste, nausea, vomiting, diarrhea, anorexia, (all mostly PO). **Hematologic:** <u>Agranulocytosis with repeated use</u>; thrombocytopenia. **Body as a Whole:** Fever, muscle and joint pain, angioneurotic edema, myalgia, *SLE-like syndrome (50% of patients on large doses for 1 y):* Polyarthralgias, pleuritic pain, pleural effusion. **Skin:** Maculopapular rash, pruritus. erythema, skin rash.

DIAGNOSTIC TEST INTERFERENCE Procainamide increases the plasma levels of ***alkaline phosphatase, bilirubin, lactic dehydrogenase*** and ***AST.*** It may also alter results of the ***edrophonium test.***

INTERACTIONS Drug: Other ANTIARRHYTHMICS add to therapeutic and toxic effects; ANTICHOLINERGIC AGENTS compound anticholinergic effects; ANTIHYPERTENSIVES add to hypotensive effects; **cimetidine** may increase levels with increase in toxicity.

PHARMACOKINETICS Absorption: 75–95% from GI tract. **Peak:** 15–60 min IM; 30–60 min PO. **Duration:** 3 h; 8 h with sustained release. **Distribution:** Distributed to CSF, liver, spleen, kidney, brain, and heart; crosses placenta; distributed into breast milk. **Metabolism:** In liver to *N*-acetylprocainamide (NAPA), an active metabolite (30–60% metabolized to NAPA). **Elimination:**

In urine. **Half-Life:** 3 h procainamide, 6 h NAPA.

NURSING IMPLICATIONS

Assessment & Drug Effects

- Check apical radial pulses before each dose during period of adjustment to the oral route.
- Patients with severe heart, liver, or kidney disease and hypotension are at particular risk for adverse effects.
- Monitor the patient's ECG and BP continuously during IV drug administration.
- Discontinue IV drug temporarily when (1) arrhythmia is interrupted, (2) severe toxic effects are present, (3) QRS complex is excessively widened (greater than 50%), (4) PR interval is prolonged, or (5) BP drops 15 mm Hg or more. Obtain rhythm strip and notify physician.
- Ventricular dysrhythmias are usually abolished within a few minutes after IV dose and within an hour after PO or IM administration.
- Report promptly complaints of chest pain, dyspnea, and anxiety. Digitalization may have preceded procainamide in patients with atrial arrhythmias. Cardiotonic glycosides may induce sufficient increase in atrial contraction to dislodge atrial mural emboli, with subsequent pulmonary embolism.
- Therapeutic procainamide blood levels are reached in approximately 24 h if kidney function is normal but are delayed in presence of renal impairment.

Patient & Family Education

- Keep a record of weekly weight. Notify physician if weight gain of 1 kg (2 lb) or more is accompanied by local edema.
- Record and report date, time, and duration of fibrillation episodes when taking maintenance doses: Light-headedness, giddiness, weakness, or faintness.
- Keep a record of pulse rates. Report to physician changes in rate or quality.
- Report to physician signs of reduced procainamide control: Weakness, irregular pulse, unexplained fatigability, anxiety.
- Do not double dose or change an interval because a previous dose was missed. Take procainamide at evenly spaced intervals around the clock unless otherwise prescribed.

PROCAINE HYDROCHLORIDE (Pr)

(proe'kane)

Novocain

Classification: LOCAL ANESTHETIC (ESTER-TYPE)

Therapeutic: LOCAL ANESTHETIC

Pregnancy Category: C

P

AVAILABILITY 1%, 10% injection

ACTION & *THERAPEUTIC EFFECT* Decreases sodium flux into nerve cell, thus depressing initial depolarization and preventing propagation and conduction of the nerve impulse. *Local anesthetic action produces loss of sensation and motor activity in circumscribed areas that are treated.*

USES Spinal anesthesia and epidural and peripheral nerve block by injection and infiltration methods.

CONTRAINDICATIONS Known hypersensitivity to procaine or to other drugs of similar chemical structure, to PABA, and to parabens; generalized septicemia, inflammation, or sepsis at proposed injection site; cerebrospinal diseases (e.g., meningitis, syphilis); heart block, hypotension, hypertension; bowel pathology, GI hemorrhage; coagulopathy, anticoagulants, thrombocytopenia. **CAUTIOUS USE** Debilitated, older adults, or acutely ill patients; obstetric delivery; increased intra-abdominal pressure; known drug allergies and sensitivities; impaired cardiac function, dysrhythmias; shock; pregnancy (category C), lactation.

ROUTE & DOSAGE

Spinal Anesthesia

Adult: **Intrathecal** 10% solution diluted with NS at 1 mL/5 sec

Infiltration Anesthesia/ Peripheral Nerve Block

Adult: **Regional** 0.25–0.5% solution

ADMINISTRATION

Subcutaneous

- Reconstitute solution: To prepare 60 mL of a 0.5% solution (5 mg/mL), dilute 30 mL of 1% solution with 30 mL sterile distilled water. Add 0.5–1 mL epinephrine 1:1000/100 mL anesthetic solution for vasoconstrictive effect (1:200,000–1:100,000).
- Do not use solutions that are cloudy, discolored, or that contain crystals. Discard unused portion of solutions not containing a preservative. Avoid use of solution with preservative for spinal, epidural, or caudal block.
- With subcutaneous administration, inject slowly with frequent aspirations to avoid inadvertent intravascular administration, which can lead to a systemic reaction.

INCOMPATIBILITIES **Solution/additive: Aminophylline, amobarbital, chlorothiazide, magnesium sulfate, phenobarbital, phenytoin, secobarbital, sodium bicarbonate.**

ADVERSE EFFECTS (≥1%) **CNS:** Anxiety, nervousness, dizziness, circumoral paresthesia, tremors, drowsiness, sedation, convulsions, <u>respiratory arrest</u>. With spinal anesthesia: postspinal headache, arachnoiditis, palsies, spinal nerve paralysis, meningism. **Special Senses:** Tinnitus, blurred vision. **CV:** Myocardial depression, arrhythmias including bradycardia (also fetal bradycardia); hypotension. **GI:** Nausea, vomiting. **Skin:** Cutaneous lesions of delayed onset, urticaria, pruritus, angioneurotic edema, sweating, syncope, <u>anaphylactoid reaction</u>. **Urogenital:** Urinary retention, fecal or urinary incontinence, loss of perineal sensation and sexual function, slowing of labor and increased incidence of forceps delivery (all with caudal or epidural anesthesia).

INTERACTIONS Drug: May antagonize effects of SULFONAMIDES; increased risk of hypotension with MAOIS, ANTIHYPERTENSIVES.

PHARMACOKINETICS Absorption: Rapidly from injection site. **Onset:** 2–5 min. **Duration:** 1 h. **Metabolism:** Hydrolyzed by plasma pseudocholinesterases. **Elimination:** 80% of metabolites excreted in urine. **Half-Life:** 7.7 min.

NURSING IMPLICATIONS

Assessment & Drug Effects

- Be aware that reactions during dental procedure are usually mild, transient, and produced by epinephrine added to local anesthetic (e.g., headache, palpitation, tachycardia, hypertension, dizziness).

- Use procaine with epinephrine with caution in body areas with limited blood supply (e.g., fingers, toes, ears, nose). If used, inspect particular area for evidence of reduced perfusion (vasospasm): Pale, cold, sensitive skin.
- Hypotension is the most important complication of spinal anesthesia. Risk period is during first 30 min after induction and is intensified by changes in position that promote decreased venous return, or by preexisting hypertension, pregnancy, old age, or hypovolemia.

Patient & Family Education

- Understand that there will be temporary loss of sensation in the area of the injection.
- Do not consume hot liquids or foods until sensation returns when drug used for dental procedure.

PROCARBAZINE HYDROCHLORIDE

(proe-kar'ba-zeen)

Matulane, Natulan ♣

Classifications: ANTINEOPLASTIC; ALKYLATING AGENT

Therapeutic: ANTINEOPLASTIC

Prototype: Cyclophosphamide

Pregnancy Category: D

AVAILABILITY 50 mg capsules

ACTION & *THERAPEUTIC EFFECT* Hydrazine derivative with antimetabolite properties that is cell cycle–specific for the S phase of cell division. Suppresses mitosis at interphase, and causes chromatin derangement. *Highly toxic to rapidly proliferating tissue.*

USES Adjunct in palliative treatment of Hodgkin's disease.

UNLABELED USES Solid tumors.

CONTRAINDICATIONS Severe myelosuppression; pheochromocytoma; alcohol ingestion; foods high in tyramine content; sympathomimetic drugs. MAO inhibitors should be discontinued 14 days prior to therapy; tricyclic antidepressants, 7 days before therapy; pregnancy (category D), lactation.

CAUTIOUS USE Concomitant administration with CNS depressants; hepatic or renal impairment; cardiac disease; bipolar disorder, mania, paranoid schizophrenia; G6PD deficiency; parkinsonism; following radiation or chemotherapy before at least 1 mo has elapsed; alcoholism; infection; diabetes mellitus.

ROUTE & DOSAGE

Adjunct for Hodgkin's Disease

Adult: **PO** 2–4 mg/kg/day in single or divided doses for 1 wk, then 4–6 mg/kg/day until WBC less than 4000/mm^3 or platelets are less than 100,000/mm^3 or maximum response obtained; drug is then discontinued until bone marrow recovery is satisfactory; treatment is started again at 1–2 mg/kg/day

Child: **PO** 50 mg/m^2/day in single or divided doses for 1 wk, then 100 mg/m^2/day until WBC is less than 4000/mm^3 or platelets are less than 100,000/mm^3 or maximum response obtained; drug is then discontinued until bone marrow recovery is satisfactory; treatment is started again at 50 mg/m^2/day

ADMINISTRATION

Oral

- Do not give if WBC count is less than 4000/mm^3 or platelet count is less than 100,000/mm³. Consult physician.

- Store at 15°–30° C (59°–86° F). Protect from freezing, moisture, and light.

ADVERSE EFFECTS (≥1%) **CNS:** Myalgia, arthralgia, paresthesias, weakness, fatigue, lethargy, drowsiness, neuropathies, mental depression, acute psychosis, hallucinations, dizziness, headache, ataxia, nervousness, insomnia, coma, confusion, seizures. **GI:** *Severe nausea and vomiting,* anorexia, stomatitis, dry mouth, dysphagia, diarrhea, constipation, jaundice, ascites. **Hematologic:** Bone marrow suppression (leukopenia, anemia, thrombocytopenia), hemolysis, bleeding tendencies. **Skin:** Dermatitis, pruritus, herpes, hyperpigmentation, flushing, alopecia. **Respiratory:** *Pleural effusion, cough,* hoarseness. **CV:** Hypotension, tachycardia. **Body as a Whole:** Chills, fever, sweating, photosensitivity; intercurrent infections. **Urogenital:** Gynecomastia, depressed spermatogenesis, atrophy of testes.

P

INTERACTIONS Drug: Alcohol, PHENOTHIAZINES, and other CNS DEPRESSANTS add to CNS depression; TRICYCLIC ANTIDEPRESSANTS, MAO INHIBITORS, SYMPATHOMIMETICS, **ephedrine, phenylpropanolamine** may precipitate hypertensive crisis, hyperpyrexia; seizures, or death. Procarbazine may enhance the effects of **CNS depressants.** A disulfiram-like reaction may occur following ingestion of **alcohol. Food: Tyramine**-containing foods may precipitate hypertensive crisis [see **phenelzine sulfate** (MAO INHIBITOR)].

PHARMACOKINETICS Absorption: Readily from GI tract. **Peak:** 1 h. **Distribution:** Widely distributed with high concentrations in liver, kidneys, intestinal wall, and skin. **Metabolism:** In liver. **Elimination:** In urine. **Half-Life:** 1 h.

NURSING IMPLICATIONS

Assessment & Drug Effects

- Monitor baseline and periodic BP, weight, temperature, pulse, and I&O ratio and pattern.
- Lab tests: Determine hematologic status (Hgb, Hct, WBC with differential, reticulocyte, and platelet counts) initially and at least q3–4days. Hepatic and renal studies (transaminase, alkaline phosphatase, BUN, urinalysis) are also indicated initially and at least weekly during therapy.
- Protect patient from exposure to infection and trauma when nadir of leukopenia is approached. Note and report changes in voiding pattern, hematuria, and dysuria (possible signs of urinary tract infection). Monitor I&O ratio and temperature closely.
- Withhold drug and notify physician of any of the following: CNS S&S (e.g., paresthesias, neuropathies, confusion); leukopenia [WBC count less than 4000/mm³; thrombocytopenia (platelet count less than 100,000/mm³)]; hypersensitivity reaction, the first small ulceration or persistent spot of soreness in oral cavity, diarrhea, and bleeding.
- Monitor for and report any of the following: Chills, fever, weakness, shortness of breath, productive cough. Drug will be discontinued.
- Assess for signs of liver dysfunction: Jaundice (yellow skin, sclerae, and soft palate), frothy or dark urine, clay-colored stools.
- Tolerance to nausea and vomiting (most common adverse effects) usually develops by end of first week of treatment. Doses are kept

at a minimum during this time. If vomiting persists, therapy will be interrupted.

Patient & Family Education

- Avoid OTC nose drops, cough medicines, and antiobesity preparations containing ephedrine, amphetamine, epinephrine, and tricyclic antidepressants because they may cause hypertensive crises. Do not to use OTC preparations without physician's approval.
- Report to physician any sign of impending infection.
- Do not eat foods high in tyramine content (e.g., aged cheese, beer, wine).
- Avoid alcohol; ingestion of any form of alcohol may precipitate a disulfiram-type reaction (see Appendix F).
- Report to physician immediately signs of hemorrhagic tendencies: Bleeding into skin and mucosa, easy bruising, nose bleeds, or blood in stool or urine. Bone marrow depression often occurs 2–8 wk after start of therapy.
- Avoid excessive exposure to the sun because of potential photosensitivity reaction: Cover as much skin area as possible with clothing, and use sunscreen lotion (SPF higher than 12) on all exposed skin surfaces.
- Use caution while driving or performing hazardous tasks until response to drug is known since drowsiness, dizziness, and blurred vision are possible adverse effects.
- Use contraceptive measures during procarbazine therapy.

PROCHLORPERAZINE Pr

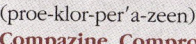

(proe-klor-per′a-zeen)

Compazine, Compro

PROCHLORPERAZINE EDISYLATE

Compazine

PROCHLORPERAZINE MALEATE

Compazine, Stemetil ♣

Classifications: ANTIPSYCHOTIC, PHENOTHIAZINE; ANTIEMETIC

Therapeutic: ANTIPSYCHOTIC; ANTIEMETIC

Pregnancy Category: C

AVAILABILITY 5 mg, 10 mg, 25 mg tablets; 10 mg, 15 mg, 30 mg sustained release capsule; 2.5 mg, 5 mg, 25 mg suppositories; 5 mg/mL injection; **Edisylate:** 5 mg/mL injection

ACTION & *THERAPEUTIC EFFECT* Strong antipsychotic effects thought to be due to blockade of postsynaptic dopamine receptors in the brain. Antiemetic effect is produced by suppression of the chemoreceptor trigger zone (CTZ). *Effective antipsychotic and antiemetic properties.*

USES Management of manifestations of psychotic disorders, of excessive anxiety, tension, and agitation, and to control severe nausea and vomiting.

UNLABELED USES Behavioral syndromes in dementia.

CONTRAINDICATIONS Hypersensitivity to phenothiazines; bone marrow depression; blood dyscrasias, jaundice; comatose or severely depressed states; dementia-related psychosis in elderly; children weighing less than 9 kg (20 lb) or younger than 2 y of age; pediatric surgery; short-term vomiting in children or vomiting of unknown etiology; Reye's syndrome or other encephalopathies; history of dyskinetic reactions or epilepsy; lactation.

CAUTIOUS USE Patient with previously diagnosed breast cancer, children with acute illness or dehydration; Parkinson's disease; GI obstruction; hepatic disease; seizure disorders; urinary retention, BPH; pregnancy (category C).

ROUTE & DOSAGE

Severe Nausea, Vomiting

Adult: **PO** 5–10 mg 3–4 times/day; sustained release: 10–15 mg q12h **IM** 5–10 mg q3–4h up to 40 mg/day **IV** 2.5–10 mg q3–4h (max: 40 mg/day) **PR** 25 mg b.i.d.

Child (weight greater than 9 kg): **PO/PR** 2.5 mg 1–3 times/day or 5 mg b.i.d. (max: 15 mg/day) **IM** 0.13 mg/kg q3–4h

Psychotic Disorders

Adult: **PO** 5–10 mg 3–4 times/day; titrate up q2–3days **IM** 10–20 mg; may repeat q1–4h to gain control, then q4–6h

Child (2–12 y): **PO/PR** 2.5 mg 2–3 times/day (max: 20 mg daily ages 2–5 and 25 mg daily ages 6–12)

ADMINISTRATION

Oral

- Dosages for older adults, emaciated patients and children should be increased slowly.
- Ensure that sustained release form is not chewed or crushed. **Must be** swallowed whole.
- Do not give oral concentrate to children.
- Avoid skin contact with oral concentrate or injection solution because of possibility of contact dermatitis.

Intramuscular

- Do not inject drug subcutaneously.
- Make injection deep into the upper outer quadrant of the buttock in adults. Follow agency policy regarding IM injection site for children.

Intravenous

PREPARE: **Direct:** May be given undiluted or diluted in small amounts of NS. **IV Infusion:** Dilute in 50–100 mL of D5W, NS, D5/0.45% NaCl, LR or other compatible solution.

ADMINISTER: **Direct:** DO NOT give a bolus dose. Give at a maximum rate of 5 mg/min. **IV Infusion:** Give over 15–30 min. Do not exceed direct IV rate.

INCOMPATIBILITIES Solution/additive: **Aminophylline, amphotericin B, ampicillin, calcium gluconate, cephalothin, chloramphenicol, chlorothiazide, dimenhydrinate, epinephrine, erythromycin, furosemide, hydrocortisone, hydromorphone, kanamycin, ketorolac, methohexital, midazolam, morphine, penicillin G sodium, pentobarbital, phenobarbital, tetracycline, thiopental, vancomycin, warfarin.** Y-site: **Aldesleukin, allopurinol, amifostine, amphotericin B cholesteryl complex, aztreonam, bivalirudin, cefepime, etoposide, fenoldopam, filgrastim, fludarabine, foscarnet, gemcitabine, piperacillin-tazobactam.**

- Discard markedly discolored solutions; slight yellowing does not appear to alter potency.

ADVERSE EFFECTS (≥1%) **CNS:** *Drowsiness,* dizziness, *extrapyramidal reactions (akathisia, dystonia, or parkinsonism),* <u>persistent tardive</u>

dyskinesia, acute catatonia. **CV:** Hypotension. **GI:** Cholestatic jaundice. **Skin:** Contact dermatitis, photosensitivity. **Endocrine:** Galactorrhea, amenorrhea. **Special Senses:** Blurred vision. **Hematologic:** Leukopenia, agranulocytosis.

INTERACTIONS Drug: Alcohol, CNS DEPRESSANTS increase CNS depression; ANTACIDS, ANTIDIARRHEALS decrease absorption, therefore, administer 2 h apart; **phenobarbital** increases metabolism of prochlorperazine; GENERAL ANESTHETICS increase excitation and hypotension; antagonizes antihypertensive action of **guanethidine; phenylpropanolamine** poses possibility of sudden death; TRICYCLIC ANTIDEPRESSANTS intensify hypotensive and anticholinergic effects; decreases seizure threshold—ANTICONVULSANT dosage may need to be increased. **Herbal: Kava** may increase risk and severity of dystonic reactions.

PHARMACOKINETICS Absorption: Readily from GI tract. **Onset:** 30–40 min PO; 60 min PR; 10–20 min IM. **Duration:** 3–4 h PO; 10–12 h sustained release PO; 3–4 h PR; up to 12 h IM. **Distribution:** Crosses placenta; distributed into breast milk. **Metabolism:** In liver. **Elimination:** In urine.

NURSING IMPLICATIONS

Assessment & Drug Effects

- Position carefully to prevent aspiration of vomitus; may have depressed cough reflex.
- Most older adult and emaciated patients and children, especially those with dehydration or acute illness, appear to be particularly susceptible to extrapyramidal effects. Be alert to onset of symptoms: Early in therapy watch for pseudoparkinson's and acute dyskinesia. After 1–2 mo, be alert to akathisia.
- Keep in mind that the antiemetic effect may mask toxicity of other drugs or make it difficult to diagnose conditions with a primary symptom of nausea.
- Lab tests: Periodic CBC with differential in long-term therapy.
- Be alert to signs of high core temperature: Red, dry, hot skin; full bounding pulse; dilated pupils; dyspnea; confusion; temperature over 40.6° C (105° F); elevated BP. Exposure to high environmental temperature places this patient at risk for heat stroke. Inform physician and institute measures to reduce body temperature rapidly.

Patient & Family Education

- Take drug only as prescribed and do not alter dose or schedule. Consult physician before stopping the medication.
- Avoid hazardous activities such as driving a car until response to drug is known because drug may impair mental and physical abilities, especially during first few days of therapy.
- Be aware that drug may color urine reddish brown. It also may cause the sun-exposed skin to turn gray-blue.
- Protect skin from direct sun's rays and use a sunscreen lotion (SPF higher than 12) to prevent photosensitivity reaction.
- Withhold dose and report to the physician if the following symptoms persist more than a few hours: Tremor, involuntary twitching, exaggerated restlessness. Other reportable symptoms include light-colored stools, changes in vision, sore throat, fever, rash.

PROGESTERONE Pr

(proe-jess'ter-one)

Crinone Gel, Endrometrin, Gesterol 50, Progestaject, Prometrium

Classification: PROGESTIN

Therapeutic: PROGESTIN

Pregnancy Category: X; B (vaginal gel in early pregnancy)

AVAILABILITY 100 mg capsules; 50 mg/mL injection; 4%, 8% gel; 100 mg vaginal insert

ACTION & *THERAPEUTIC EFFECT* Has estrogenic, anabolic, and androgenic activity. Transforms endometrium from proliferative to secretory state; suppresses pituitary gonadotropin secretion, thereby blocking follicular maturation and ovulation. *Relaxes estrogen-primed myometrium and prohibits spontaneous contraction of uterus. Sudden drop in blood levels of progestin (and estradiol) causes "withdrawal bleeding" from endometrium. Intrauterine placement of progesterone hypothetically inhibits sperm survival, and suppresses endometrial proliferation (antiestrogenic effect).*

USES Secondary amenorrhea, functional uterine bleeding, endometriosis, and premenstrual syndrome. Largely supplanted by new progestins, which have longer action and oral effectiveness. Treatment of infertile women with progesterone deficiency.

CONTRAINDICATIONS Hypersensitivity to progestins, known or suspected breast or genital malignancy; use as a pregnancy test; thrombophlebitis, thromboembolic disorders; ectopic pregnancy; cerebral apoplexy (or its history); severely impaired liver function or disease; undiagnosed vaginal bleeding, incomplete abortion; use during first 4 mo of pregnancy (category X) other than vaginal gel used for assisted reproductive technology (ART) in early pregnancy.

CAUTIOUS USE Anemia; diabetes mellitus; history of psychic depression; persons susceptible to acute intermittent porphyria or with conditions that may be aggravated by fluid retention (asthma, seizure disorders, cardiac or kidney function, migraine); impaired liver function; previous ectopic pregnancy; presence or history of salpingitis; venereal disease; unresolved abnormal Pap smear; genital bleeding of unknown etiology; previous pelvic surgery; **Vaginal gel:** in early first trimester (category B); lactation.

ROUTE & DOSAGE

Amenorrhea

Adult: **IM** 5–10 mg for 6–8 consecutive days **PO** 400 mg at bedtime × 10 days **Vaginal gel** 45 mg every other day (up to 6 doses)

Uterine Bleeding

Adult: **IM** 5–10 mg/day for 6 days

Premenstrual Syndrome

Adult: **PR** 200–400 mg/day

Assisted Reproductive Technology

Adult: **Vaginally** 90 mg gel daily or b.i.d. until placental autonomy OR 10–12 wk; 100 mg insert 2–3 times daily up to 10 wk

ADMINISTRATION

Oral

- Give at bedtime and advise caution with ambulation because drug may cause drowsiness or dizziness.

- Do not give oral capsules, which contain peanut oil, to patients allergic to peanuts.

Intramuscular

- Immerse vial in warm water momentarily to redissolve crystals (if present) and to facilitate aspiration of drug into syringe.
- Inject deeply IM. Injection site may be irritated. Inspect IM sites carefully and rotate areas systematically.

Vaginal

- When given using the supplied applicators, a measured dose of 4% vaginal gel contains 45 mg and a measured dose of 8% gel contains 90 mg. Dosage increases from 4% to 8% cannot be achieved by an increase in volume of 4% gel; the 8% gel must be used to supply a 90 mg dose.

- Store drug at 15°–30° C (59°–86° F) unless otherwise specified by manufacturer. Protect from freezing and light.

ADVERSE EFFECTS (≥1%) **CNS:** Migraine headache, *dizziness,* lethargy, mental depression, somnolence, insomnia. **CV:** <u>Thromboembolic disorder, pulmonary embolism</u>. **Special Senses:** Change in vision, proptosis, diplopia, papilledema, retinal vascular lesions. **GI:** Hepatic disease, cholestatic jaundice; *nausea,* vomiting, *abdominal cramps.* **Urogenital:** Vaginal candidiasis, chloasma, cervical erosion and changes in secretions, *breakthrough bleeding,* dysmenorrhea, amenorrhea, pruritus vulvae. **Metabolic:** Hyperglycemia, decreased libido, transient increase in sodium and chloride excretion, pyrexia. **Skin:** *Acne,* pruritus, allergic rash, photosensitivity, urticaria, hirsutism, alopecia. **Body as a Whole:** *Edema, weight changes;* pain at injection site; fatigue. **Endocrine:** Gynecomastia, galactorrhea.

DIAGNOSTIC TEST INTERFERENCE PROGESTINS may decrease levels of ***urinary pregnanediol*** and increase levels of ***serum alkaline phosphatase, plasma amino acids, urinary nitrogen,*** and ***coagulation factors VII, VIII, IX,*** and ***X.*** They also decrease ***glucose tolerance*** (may cause false-positive ***urine glucose tests***) and lower ***HDL*** (high-density lipoprotein) levels.

INTERACTIONS Drug: BARBITURATES, **carbamazepine, phenytoin, rifampin** may alter contraceptive effectiveness; **ketoconazole** may inhibit progesterone metabolism; may antagonize effects of **bromocriptine.**

PHARMACOKINETICS Absorption: Rapid from IM site; PO peaks at 3 h. **Metabolism:** Extensively in liver. **Elimination:** Primarily in urine; excreted in breast milk. **Half-Life:** 5 min.

NURSING IMPLICATIONS

Assessment & Drug Effects

- Record baseline data for comparative value about patient's weight, BP, and pulse at onset of progestin therapy. Report deviations promptly.
- Lab tests: Periodic liver function tests, blood glucose, and serum electrolytes.
- Monitor for and report immediately S&S of thrombophlebitis or thromboembolic disease.

Patient & Family Education

- Avoid exposure to UV light and prolonged periods of time in the sun. Photosensitivity severity is related to both time of exposure and dose. A phototoxic drug reaction usually looks like an exaggerated sunburn and occurs within

5–18 h after exposure to sun and is maximal by 36–72 h.

- Use sunscreen lotion (SPF higher than 12) on exposed skin surfaces whenever outdoors, even on dark days.
- Inform physician promptly if any of the following occur: Sudden severe headache or vomiting, dizziness or fainting, numbness in an arm or leg, pain in calves accompanied by swelling, warmth, and redness; acute chest pain or dyspnea.
- Report to physician promptly unexplained sudden or gradual, partial or complete loss of vision, ptosis, or diplopia.
- Monitor for loss of glycemic control if diabetic.
- Notify physician if you become or suspect pregnancy. Learn the potential risk to the fetus from exposure to progestin.

P

PROMETHAZINE HYDROCHLORIDE

(proe-meth'a-zeen)

Histantil ♣, Phenergan

Classifications: ANTIHISTAMINE; ANTIEMETIC; ANTIVERTIGO

Therapeutic: ANTIHISTAMINE; ANTIEMETIC; ANTIVERTIGO

Prototype: Prochlorperazine

Pregnancy Category: C

AVAILABILITY 12.5 mg, 25 mg, 50 mg tablets; 6.25 mg/5 mL syrup; 12.5 mg, 25 mg, 50 mg suppositories; 25 mg/mL, 50 mg/mL injection

ACTION & *THERAPEUTIC EFFECT* An antihistamine that exerts antiserotonin, anticholinergic, and local anesthetic action. Antiemetic action thought to be due to depression of CTZ in medulla. *Long-acting derivative of phenothiazine with marked antihistamine activity and prominent sedative, amnesic, antiemetic, and anti-motion sickness actions.*

USES Symptomatic relief of various allergic conditions, to ameliorate and prevent reactions to blood and plasma, and in prophylaxis and treatment of motion sickness, nausea, and vomiting. Preoperative, postoperative, and obstetric sedation and as adjunct to analgesics for control of pain.

CONTRAINDICATIONS Hypersensitivity to phenothiazines; acute MI; angina, atrial fibrillation, atrial flutter, cardiac arrhythmias, cardiomyopathy uncontrolled hypertension; MAOI therapy; comatose or severely depressed states; children with Reye's syndrome, hepatic encephalopathy, hepatic diseases; acutely ill or dehydrated children; children younger than 2 y; newborn or premature infants; lactation.

CAUTIOUS USE Impaired liver function; epilepsy; bone marrow depression; cardiovascular disease; peripheral vascular disease; asthma; acute or chronic respiratory impairment (particularly in children); hypertension; narrow angle glaucoma; stenosing peptic ulcer, pyloroduodenal obstruction; prostatic hypertrophy; bladder neck obstruction; older adult or debilitated patients; pregnancy (category C).

ROUTE & DOSAGE

Motion Sickness

Adult: **PO/PR** 25 mg q12h prn
Child (older than 2 y): **PO/PR** 10.5 mg/kg/dose q12h prn (max: 25 mg/dose)

Nausea

Adult: **PO/PR/IM/IV** 12.5–25 mg q4–6h prn

Child (older than 2 y): **PO/PR/IM/IV** 0.25–0.5 mg/kg q4–6h prn (max: 25 mg/dose)

Allergies

Adult: **PO/PR** 12.5 mg q.i.d. or 25 mg at bedtime **IM/IV** 25 mg, repeat in 2 h if necessary, switch to PO

Child (older than 2 y): **PO** 0.1 mg/kg q6h and 0.05 mg/kg at bedtime prn

Sedation

Adult: **PO/PR/IM/IV** 25–50 mg/dose

Child (older than 2 y): **PO/PR/IM/IV** 12.5–25 mg/dose (max: 50 mg)

ADMINISTRATION

Oral

- Give with food, milk, or a full glass of water may minimize GI distress.
- Tablets may be crushed and mixed with water or food before swallowing.
- Oral doses for allergy are generally prescribed before meals and on retiring or as single dose at bedtime.

Intramuscular

- Give IM injection deep into large muscle mass. Aspirate carefully before injecting drug. Intra-arterial injection can cause arterial or arteriolar spasm, with resultant gangrene.
- Subcutaneous injection (also contraindicated) can cause chemical irritation and necrosis. Rotate injection sites and observe daily.

Intravenous

PREPARE: **Direct:** The 25 mg/mL concentration may be given undiluted. ▪ Dilute the 50 mg/mL concentration in NS to yield no more than 25 mg/mL (e.g., diluting the 50 mg/mL concentration in 4 mL yields 10 mg/mL). ▪ Inspect parenteral drug before preparation. Discard if it is darkened or contains precipitate.

ADMINISTER: **Direct:** Give each 25 mg or fraction thereof over at least 1 min.

INCOMPATIBILITIES **Solution/additive:** **Aminophylline, ampicillin, carbenicillin, cefazolin, cefotetan, ceftizoxime, chloramphenicol, chlordiazepoxide, chlorothiazide, dexamethasone, dimenhydrinate. furosemide, heparin, hydrocortisone, ketorolac, methicillin, methohexital, nalbuphine, nitrofurantoin, penicillin G sodium, pentobarbital, phenobarbital, thiopental.** **Y-site:** **Aldesleukin, allopurinol, amphotericin B cholesteryl complex, cefepime, cefmetazole, cefoperazone, cefotetan, doxorubicin liposome, foscarnet, furosemide, heparin, methotrexate, piperacillin/tazobactam, TPN.**

- Store at 15°–30° C (59°–86° F) in tight, light-resistant container unless otherwise directed.

ADVERSE EFFECTS (≥1%) **Body as a Whole:** Deep sleep, coma, convulsions, cardiorespiratory symptoms, extrapyramidal reactions, nightmares (in children), CNS stimulation, abnormal movements. **Respiratory:** Irregular respirations, <u>respiratory depression, apnea</u>. **CNS:** Sedation *drowsiness,* confusion, dizziness, disturbed coordination, restlessness, tremors. **CV:** Transient mild hypotension or hypertension. **GI:** Anorexia, nausea, vomiting, constipation. **Hematologic:** Leuko-

P

penia, agranulocytosis. **Special Senses:** *Blurred vision, dry mouth,* nose, or throat. **Skin:** Photosensitivity. **Urogenital:** Urinary retention.

DIAGNOSTIC TEST INTERFERENCE May interfere with ***blood grouping in ABO system*** and may produce false results with ***urinary pregnancy tests*** (***Gravindex,*** false-positive; ***Prepurex*** and ***Dap tests,*** false-negative). Promethazine can cause significant alterations of ***flare response*** in ***intradermal allergen tests*** if performed within 4 days of patient receiving promethazine.

INTERACTIONS Drug: Alcohol and other CNS DEPRESSANTS add to CNS depression and anticholinergic effects.

PHARMACOKINETICS Absorption: Readily from GI tract. **Onset:** 20 min PO/PR/IM; 5 min IV. **Duration:** 2–8 h. **Distribution:** Crosses placenta. **Metabolism:** In liver (CYP2D6, 2B6). **Elimination:** Slowly in urine and feces.

P

NURSING IMPLICATIONS

Assessment & Drug Effects

- Supervise ambulation. Promethazine sometimes produces marked sedation and dizziness.
- Be aware that antiemetic action may mask symptoms of unrecognized disease and signs of drug overdosage as well as dizziness, vertigo, or tinnitus associated with toxic doses of aspirin or other ototoxic drugs.
- Patients in pain may develop involuntary (athetoid) movements of upper extremities following parenteral administration. These symptoms usually disappear after pain is controlled.
- Monitor respiratory function in patients with respiratory problems, particularly children. Drug may suppress cough reflex and cause thickening of bronchial secretions.

Patient & Family Education

- For motion sickness: Take initial dose 30–60 min before anticipated travel and repeat at 8–12 h intervals if necessary. For duration of journey, repeat dose on arising and again at evening meal.
- Do not drive or engage in other potentially hazardous activities requiring mental alertness and normal reaction time until response to drug is known.
- Avoid sunlamps or prolonged exposure to sunlight. Use sunscreen lotion during initial drug therapy.
- Do not take OTC medications without physician's approval.
- Avoid alcohol and other CNS depressants.
- Relieve dry mouth by frequent rinses with water or by increasing noncaloric fluid intake (if allowed), chewing sugarless gum, or sucking hard candy. If these measures fail, add a saliva substitute (e.g., Moi-Stir, Orex, Xero-Lube).

PROPAFENONE

(pro-pa'fen-one)

Rythmol

Classification: ANTIARRHYTHMIC CLASS IC

Therapeutic: ANTIARRHYTHMIC CLASS IC

Prototype: Flecainide

Pregnancy Category: C

AVAILABILITY 150 mg, 225 mg, 300 mg tablets

ACTION & *THERAPEUTIC EFFECT* Class IC antiarrhythmic drug with a direct stabilizing action on myocardial membranes. Reduces spontaneous automaticity. Exerts a negative inotropic effect on the myocardium. *Decreases rate of single and multiple PVCs and suppresses ventricular arrhythmias.*

USES Ventricular arrhythmias.
UNLABELED USES Atrial tachyarrhythmias, reentrant arrhythmias, Wolff-Parkinson-White syndrome.

CONTRAINDICATIONS Hypersensitivity to propafenone; uncontrolled CHF, cardiogenic shock, sinoatrial, AV or intraventricular disorders (e.g., sick sinus node syndrome, AV block) without a pacemaker; cardiogenic shock; bradycardia, QT prolongation; marked hypotension; bronchospastic disorders; electrolyte imbalances; non–life-threatening arrhythmias. Safety and efficacy in children are not established.
CAUTIOUS USE CHF, COPD, chronic bronchitis; AV block; hepatic/renal impairment; older adult patients; pregnancy (category C), lactation.

ROUTE & DOSAGE

Ventricular Arrhythmias
Adult: **PO** Initiate with 150 mg q8h, may be increased at 3–4 days intervals (max: 300 mg q8h)

ADMINISTRATION
- Dosage increments are usually made gradually with older adults or those with previous extensive myocardial damage.
- Significant dose reduction is warranted with severe liver dysfunction. Consult physician.
- Store at 15°–30° C (59°–86° F).

ADVERSE EFFECTS (≥1%) **CNS:** *Blurred vision, dizziness,* paresthesias, fatigue, somnolence, vertigo, headache. **CV:** Arrhythmias, ventricular tachycardia, hypotension, bundle branch block, AV block, complete heart block, sinus arrest, CHF. **Hematologic:** Leukopenia, granulocytopenia (both rare). **GI:** Nausea, abdominal discomfort, constipation, vomiting, dry mouth, *taste alterations,* cholestatic hepatitis. **Skin:** Rash.

INTERACTIONS Drug: Amiodarone, quinidine increases the levels and toxicity of propafenone. May increase levels and toxicity of TRICYCLIC ANTIDEPRESSANTS, **cyclosporine, digoxin,** BETA-BLOCKERS, **theophylline,** and **warfarin** may increase levels of both **propafenone** and **diltiazem. Phenobarbital** decreases levels of **propafenone.**

PHARMACOKINETICS Absorption: Readily from GI tract. **Peak:** 3.5 h. **Distribution:** 97% protein bound, highest concentrations in the lung. Crosses placenta, distributed into breast milk. **Metabolism:** Extensively metabolized in the liver. **Elimination:** 18.5–38% of dose excreted in urine as metabolites. **Half-Life:** 5–8 h.

NURSING IMPLICATIONS

Assessment & Drug Effects
- Monitor cardiovascular status frequently (e.g., ECG, Holter monitor) to determine effectiveness of drug and development of new or worsened arrhythmias.
- Monitor closely patients with preexisting CHF for worsening of this condition. Monitor for digoxin toxicity with concurrent use, because drug may increase serum digoxin levels.
- Report development of second- or third-degree AV block or significant widening of the QRS complex. Dosage adjustment may be warranted.

Patient & Family Education

- Report to physician any of following: Chest pain, palpitations, blurred or abnormal vision, dyspnea, or signs and symptoms of infection.
- Be aware when taking concurrent warfarin of possible increase in plasma levels that increase bleeding risk. Report unusual bleeding or bruising.
- Monitor radial pulse daily and report decreased heart rate or development of an abnormal heartbeat.
- Be aware of possibility of dizziness and need for caution with walking, especially in older adult or debilitated patients.

PROPANTHELINE BROMIDE

(proe-pan'the-leen)

Pro-Banthine, Propanthel ✦

Classifications: ANTICHOLINERGIC; ANTIMUSCARINIC; ANTISPASMODIC

Therapeutic: ANTISPASMODIC

Prototype: Atropine

Pregnancy Category: C

AVAILABILITY 7.5 mg, 15 mg tablets

ACTION & *THERAPEUTIC EFFECT* Has potent antimuscarinic activity and postganglionic nicotinic receptor blocking action. *Decreases motility (smooth muscle tone) in the GI, biliary, and urinary tracts, resulting in antispasmodic action.*

USES Adjunct in treatment of peptic ulcer, irritable bowel syndrome, pancreatitis, ureteral and urinary bladder spasm. Also used prior to radiologic diagnostic procedures to reduce duodenal motility.

CONTRAINDICATIONS Narrow-angle glaucoma; tachycardia, MI; paralytic ileus, GI obstructive disease; hemorrhagic shock; myasthenia gravis. Safety in children is not established.

CAUTIOUS USE CAD, CHF, cardiac arrhythmias; liver disease, ulcerative colitis, hiatus hernia, esophagitis; kidney disease; prostatic hypertrophy; glaucoma; debilitated patients; hyperthyroidism; autonomic neuropathy; brain damage; Down's syndrome; spastic disorders; pregnancy (category C), lactation.

ROUTE & DOSAGE

Irritable Bowel Syndrome

Adult: **PO** 15 mg 30 min a.c. and 30 mg at bedtime (max: 120 mg/day)

Geriatric: **PO** 7.5 mg 2–3 times/day a.c. (max: 90 mg/day)

ADMINISTRATION

Oral

- Give 30–60 min before meals and at bedtime. Advise not to chew tablet; drug is bitter.
- Give at least 1 h before or 1 h after an antacid (or antidiarrheal agent).
- Store dry powder and tablets at 15°–30° C (59°–86° F); protect from freezing and moisture.

ADVERSE EFFECTS (≥1%) **GI:** *Constipation, dry mouth.* **Special Senses:** Blurred vision, mydriasis, increased intraocular pressure. **CNS:** Drowsiness. **Urogenital:** Decreased sexual activity, difficult urination.

INTERACTIONS Drug: Decreased absorption of **ketoconazole;** ORAL POTASSIUM may increase risk of GI ulcers. **Food:** Food significantly decreases absorption.

PHARMACOKINETICS Absorption: Incompletely from GI tract. **Onset:** 30–45 min. **Duration:** 4–6 h. **Metab-**

olism: 50% in GI tract before absorption; 50% in liver. **Elimination:** Primarily in urine; some in bile. **Half-Life:** 9 h.

NURSING IMPLICATIONS

Assessment & Drug Effects

- Assess bowel sounds, especially in presence of ulcerative colitis, since paralytic ileus may develop, predisposing to toxic megacolon.
- Be aware that older adult or debilitated patients may respond to a usual dose with agitation, excitement, confusion, drowsiness. Stop drug and report to physician if these symptoms are observed.
- Check BP, heart sounds and rhythm periodically in patients with cardiac disease.

Patient & Family Education

- Void just prior to each dose to minimize risk of urinary hesitancy or retention. Record daily urinary volume and report problems to physician.
- Relieve dry mouth by rinsing with water frequently, chewing sugar-free gum or sucking hard candy.
- Maintain adequate fluid and high-fiber food intake to prevent constipation.
- Make all position changes slowly and lie down immediately if faintness, weakness, or palpitations occur. Report symptoms to physician.
- Do not drive or engage in potentially hazardous activities until response to drug is known.

PROPOFOL

(pro′po-fol)

Diprivan

FOSPROPOFOL

Lusendra

Classifications: GENERAL ANESTHESIA; SEDATIVE-HYPNOTIC
Therapeutic: SEDATIVE-HYPNOTIC; GENERAL ANESTHESIA
Prototype: Thiopental
Pregnancy Category: B

AVAILABILITY 10 mg/mL, 35 mg/mL injection

ACTION & *THERAPEUTIC EFFECT* Sedative-hypnotic used in the induction and maintenance of anesthesia or sedation. Rapid onset (40 sec) and minimal excitation during induction of anesthesia. *Effectively used for conscious sedation and maintenance of anesthesia.*

USES Induction or maintenance of anesthesia as part of a balanced anesthesia technique; conscious sedation in mechanically ventilated patients.

CONTRAINDICATIONS Hypersensitivity to propofol or propofol emulsion, which contain soybean oil and egg phosphatide; obstetrical procedures; patients with increased intracranial pressure or impaired cerebral circulation; lactation. **Propofol:** Do not use for induction of anesthesia in children younger than 3 y and for maintenance of anesthesia in infants younger than 2 mo. **Fospropofol:** Children younger than 18 y.

CAUTIOUS USE Patients with severe cardiac or respiratory disorders, respiratory depression, hypoxemia, hypertension; history of epilepsy or seizures; hypovolemia; elderly; pregnancy (category B).

ROUTE & DOSAGE

Induction of Anesthesia
Adult: **IV** 2–2.5 mg/kg q10sec until induction onset

Adult (older than 55 y): **IV** 1–1.5 mg/kg q10sec until induction onset
Adolescent/Child (3 y or older): **IV** 2.5–3.5 mg/kg over 20–30 sec

Maintenance of Anesthesia

Adult: **IV** 100–200 mcg/kg/min
Adult (older than 55 y): **IV** 50–100 mcg/kg/min
Child/Infant (older than 2 months): **IV** 125–150 mcg/kg/min

Conscious Sedation

Adult: **IV** 5 mcg/kg/min for at least 5 min, may increase by 5–10 mcg/kg/min q5–10min until desired level of sedation is achieved (may need maintenance rate of 5–80 mcg/kg/min)

Monitored Anesthesia Care or Sedation (Fospropofol)

Adult (healthy): **IV** *Weight greater than 90 kg,* 577.5 mg bolus, then may supplement no more than q4min to a max of 140 mg/dose; *weight 61–89 kg,* 6.5 mg/kg (max: 577.5 mg) bolus, then supplement doses up to 1.6 mg/kg no more than q4min; *weight less than 60 kg,* 385 mg bolus, supplement up to 105 mg/dose no more than q4min
Adult (severe systemic disease): **IV** *Weight greater than 90 kg,* 437.5 mg as bolus; give supplemental doses up to 105 mg per dose no more frequently than q4min; *weight 61–89 kg,* initially, give 75% of standard dosing regimen; give supplemental doses of 75% of standard dosing regimen; *weight less than 60 kg,* 297.5 mg bolus; give supplemental doses to a max of 70 mg per dose no more frequently than q4min

Elderly: Use decreased starting dose

ADMINISTRATION

- Use strict aseptic technique to prepare propofol for injection; drug emulsion supports rapid growth of microorganisms.
- Inspect for particulate matter and discoloration. Discard if either is noted.
- Shake well before use. Inspect for separation of the emulsion. Do not use if there is evidence of separation of phases of the emulsion.

Intravenous

PREPARE: **IV Infusion:** Give undiluted or diluted in D5W to a concentration not less than 2 mg/mL. Begin drug administration immediately after preparation and complete within 6 h.

ADMINISTER: **IV Infusion:** Use syringe or volumetric pump to control rate. ▪ Rate is determined by patient weight in kg. Depending on the form of the drug, indication, patient's health status and age, drug my be given by variable rate infusion or intermittent IV bolus (usually over 3–5 min). ▪ Administer immediately after spiking the vial. Complete infusion within 6 h.

INCOMPATIBILITIES **Y-site: Amikacin, amphotericin B, ascorbic acid, atracurium, atropine, bretylium, calcium chloride, ciprofloxacin, cisatracurium, diazepam, digoxin, doripenem, doxorubicin, hydroxocobalamine, gentamicin, levofloxacin, methotrexate, methylprednisolone, metoclopramide, minocycline, mitoxantrone, netilmicin, nimodipine, phenytoin,**

P

remifentanil, tobramycin, verapamil.

- Store unopened between 4° C (40° F) and 22° C (72° F). Refrigeration is not recommended. Protect from light.

ADVERSE EFFECTS (≥1%) **CNS:** Headache, dizziness, *twitching, bucking, jerking, thrashing, clonic/myoclonic movements.* **Special Senses:** Decreased intraocular pressure. **CV:** Hypotension, ventricular asystole (rare). **GI:** Vomiting, abdominal cramping. **Respiratory:** Cough, hiccups, apnea. **Other:** Pain at injection site.

DIAGNOSTIC TEST INTERFERENCE Propofol produces a temporary reduction in ***serum cortisol levels.*** However, propofol does not seem to inhibit adrenal responsiveness to ***ACTH.***

INTERACTIONS Drug: Concurrent continuous infusions of propofol and **alfentanil** produce higher plasma levels of **alfentanil** than expected. CNS DEPRESSANTS cause additive CNS depression.

PHARMACOKINETICS Onset: 9–36 sec. **Duration:** 6–10 min. **Distribution:** Highly lipophilic, crosses placenta, excreted in breast milk. **Metabolism:** Extensively in the liver (CYP2B6, 2C9). **Elimination:** Approximately 88% of the dose is recovered in the urine as metabolites. **Half-Life:** 5–12 h.

NURSING IMPLICATIONS

Assessment & Drug Effects

- Monitor hemodynamic status and assess for dose-related hypotension.
- Take seizure precautions. Tonic-clonic seizures have occurred following general anesthesia with propofol.
- Be alert to the potential for drug induced excitation (e.g., twitching, tremor, hyperclonus) and take appropriate safety measures.
- Provide comfort measures; pain at the injection site is quite common especially when small veins are used.

PROPOXYPHENE HYDROCHLORIDE

(proe-pox′i-feen)

Darvon 642 ✤, **Novopropoxyn** ✤

PROPOXYPHENE NAPSYLATE

Darvon-N

Classification: NARCOTIC (OPIATE AGONIST) ANALGESIC

Therapeutic: NARCOTIC ANALGESIC

Prototype: Morphine

Pregnancy Category: C; D for prolonged use or at term

Controlled Substance: Schedule IV

AVAILABILITY Napsylate: 100 mg tablets; **Hydrochloride:** 65 mg capsules

ACTION & *THERAPEUTIC EFFECT* Centrally acting opioid structurally related to methadone. Acts as a weak agonist at opiate receptors within the CNS. *Potent analgesic.*

USES Relief of mild to moderate pain.

CONTRAINDICATIONS Hypersensitivity to drug; suicidal individuals; alcoholism; concurrent use of selegiline or rasagiline; dependence on opiates; pregnancy (category D for prolonged use or at term), children.

CAUTIOUS USE Kidney or liver disease; cardiac disease; biliary tract disease; pulmonary insufficiency;

pregnancy (category C if not prolonged use or at term).

ROUTE & DOSAGE

Mild to Moderate Pain

Adult: **PO** 65 mg–100 mg q4h prn (max: 390 mg HCl/day, 600 mg napsylate/day)

ADMINISTRATION

- Empty capsules and mix contents with water or food if unable to swallow capsule whole.
- Be aware that absorption may be delayed by presence of food in stomach.
- Store at 15°–30° C (59°–86° F).

ADVERSE EFFECTS (≥1%) **CNS:** Dizziness, lightheadedness, *drowsiness,* sedation, unusual fatigue or weakness, restlessness, tremor, euphoria, dysphoria, headache, paradoxic excitement, mental confusion, toxic psychosis, coma, convulsions. **GI:** Nausea, vomiting, abdominal pain, constipation, liver dysfunction. **Special Senses:** Minor visual disturbances, pinpoint pupils (dilate with advancing hypoxia). **Skin:** Skin eruptions (hypersensitivity). **Metabolic:** Hypoglycemia (patients with impaired kidney function), acidosis, nephrogenic diabetes insipidus. **Respiratory:** Respiratory depression, pulmonary edema. **CV:** Circulatory collapse, ECG abnormalities.

INTERACTIONS Drug: Alcohol and other CNS DEPRESSANTS add to CNS depression, also fatalities reported with alcohol use; may increase hypoprothrombinemic effects of **warfarin;** may increase **carbamazepine** toxicity through decreased metabolism; **orphenadrine** increases CNS stimulation, anxiety, tremors, confusion. **Selegiline** or **rasagiline** use may cause coma, respiratory depression, or death.

PHARMACOKINETICS Absorption: Readily from upper part of small intestine. **Onset:** 15–60 min. **Peak:** 2–3 h. **Duration:** 4–6 h. **Distribution:** Crosses placenta; distributed into breast milk. **Metabolism:** In liver. **Elimination:** In urine. **Half-Life:** 6–12 h, 30–36 h for metabolite.

NURSING IMPLICATIONS

Assessment & Drug Effects

- Evaluate need for drug since abuse potential is high.
- Monitor CNS effects, respiratory status and therapeutic effectiveness.
- Overdose: Prompt action required; fatalities occur commonly within first hour following overdosage.

Patient & Family Education

- Do not drive or engage in potentially hazardous activities until response to drug is known.
- Do not exceed recommended dose; do not use alcohol and other CNS depressants with propoxyphene.
- Lie down if dizziness, lightheadedness, drowsiness, nausea, or vomiting occur while ambulating.
- Be aware that tolerance and physical or psychic dependence of the morphine type can occur with excessive use.

PROPRANOLOL HYDROCHLORIDE (Pr)

(proe-pran'oh-lole)

Apo-Propranolol ♣, Inderal, Inderal LA, InnoPran XL, Novo-pranol ♣

Common adverse effects in *italic*, life-threatening effects underlined; generic names in **bold**; classifications in SMALL CAPS; ♣ Canadian drug name; (Pr) Prototype drug

Classifications: BETA-ADRENERGIC RECEPTOR ANTAGONIST; ANTIHYPERTENSIVE; ANTIARRHYTHMIC, CLASS II
Therapeutic: ANTIHYPERTENSIVE; ANTIARRHYTHMIC, CLASS II; ANTIANGINAL
Pregnancy Category: C

AVAILABILITY 10 mg, 20 mg, 40 mg, 60 mg, 80 mg, 90 mg tablets; 60 mg, 80 mg, 120 mg, 160 mg sustained release capsules; 4 mg/mL, 8 mg/mL, 80 mg/mL solution; 1 mg/mL injection

ACTION & *THERAPEUTIC EFFECT* Nonselective beta-blocker of both cardiac and bronchial adrenoreceptors that competes with epinephrine and norepinephrine for available beta receptor sites. In higher doses, it depresses cardiac function including contractility and arrhythmias. Lowers both supine and standing blood pressures in hypertensive patients. *Reduces heart rate, myocardial irritability (Class II antiarrhythmic), and force of contraction, depresses automaticity of sinus node and ectopic pacemaker, and decreases AV and intraventricular conduction velocity. Hypotensive effect is associated with decreased cardiac output. Has migraine prophylactic effects.*

USES Management of cardiac arrhythmias, myocardial infarction, tachyarrhythmias associated with digitalis intoxication, anesthesia, and thyrotoxicosis, hypertrophic subaortic stenosis, angina pectoris due to coronary atherosclerosis, pheochromocytoma, hereditary essential tremor; also treatment of hypertension alone, but generally with a thiazide or other antihypertensives.

UNLABELED USES Anxiety states, migraine prophylaxis, essential tremors, schizophrenia, tardive dyskinesia, acute panic symptoms (e.g., stage fright), recurrent GI bleeding in cirrhotic patients, treatment of aggression and rage.

CONTRAINDICATIONS Greater than first-degree heart block; right ventricular failure secondary to pulmonary hypertension; ventricular dysfunction; sinus bradycardia, cardiogenic shock, significant aortic or mitral valvular disease; bronchial asthma or bronchospasm, severe COPD, pulmonary edema; abrupt discontinuation; major depression; PVD, Raynaud's disease.

CAUTIOUS USE Peripheral arterial insufficiency; history of systemic insect sting reaction; patients prone to nonallergenic bronchospasm (e.g., chronic bronchitis, emphysema); major surgery; cerebrovascular disease, stroke; renal or hepatic disease; pheochromocytoma, vasospastic angina; older adults; diabetes mellitus; patients prone to hypoglycemia; hyperthyroidism, thyrotoxicosis; surgery; myasthenia gravis; Wolff-Parkinson-White syndrome; pregnancy (category C), lactation.

ROUTE & DOSAGE

Hypertension

Adult: **PO** 40 mg b.i.d., usually need 160–480 mg/day in divided doses; **InnoPran XL** dose 80 mg each night, may increase to 120 mg at bedtime

Child: **PO** 0.5–1 mg/kg/day in 2 divided doses (max: 16 mg/kg/day)

Neonate: **PO** 0.25 mg/kg q6–8h (max: 5 mg/kg/day)

Angina

Adult: **PO** 80–320 mg mg/day in divided doses

Arrhythmias

Adult: **PO** 10–30 mg q6–8h **IV** 1–3 mg q4h
Child: **PO** 0.5–1 mg/kg/day in divided doses, titrate up to daily dose of 2–6 mg/kg/day (max: 16 mg/kg/day)

Acute MI

Adult: **PO** 180–240 mg/day in divided doses

Migraine Prophylaxis

Adult: **PO** 80 mg/day in divided doses, may need 160–240 mg/day
Hemodialysis Dosage Adjustment: No supplemental dose needed

ADMINISTRATION

- Take apical pulse and BP before administering drug. Withhold drug if heart rate less than 60 bpm or systolic BP less than 90 mm Hg. Consult physician for parameters.

Oral

- Do not give within 2 wk of an MAO inhibitor.
- Note that InnoPran XL should be given at bedtime.
- Be consistent with regard to giving with food or on an empty stomach to minimize variations in absorption.
- Ensure that sustained release form is not chewed or crushed. **Must be** swallowed whole.
- Reduce dosage gradually over a period of 1–2 wk and monitor patient closely when discontinued.

Intravenous

Note: Verify correct IV concentration and rate of infusion for neonates with physician.

- Take apical pulse and BP before administering drug. Withhold drug if heart rate less than 60 bpm or systolic BP less than 90 mm Hg. ▪ Consult physician for parameters.

PREPARE: **Direct:** May be given undiluted or dilute each 1 mg in 10 mL of D5W. **Intermittent:** Dilute a single dose in 50 mL of NS.

ADMINISTER: **Direct:** Give each 1 mg or fraction thereof over 1 min. **Intermittent:** Give each dose over 15–20 min.

INCOMPATIBILITIES **Y-site: Amphotericin B cholesteryl complex, diazoxide.**

- Store at 15°–30° C (59°–86° F) in tightly closed, light-resistant containers.

ADVERSE EFFECTS (≥1%) **Body as a Whole:** Fever; pharyngitis; respiratory distress, weight gain, LE-like reaction, cold extremities, leg fatigue, arthralgia, anaphylactic/anaphylactoid reactions. **Urogenital:** Impotence or decreased libido. **Skin:** Erythematous, psoriasis-like eruptions; pruritus, Stevens-Johnson syndrome, toxic epidermal necrolysis, erythema multiforme, exfoliative dermatitis, urticaria. Reversible alopecia, hyperkeratoses of scalp, palms, feet; nail changes, dry skin. **CNS:** Drug-induced psychosis, sleep disturbances, depression, *confusion,* agitation, giddiness, lightheadedness, *fatigue,* vertigo, syncope, weakness, *drowsiness,* insomnia, vivid dreams, visual hallucinations, delusions, reversible organic brain syndrome. **CV:** Palpitation, profound *bradycardia,* AV heart block, cardiac standstill, hypotension, angina pectoris, tachyarrhythmia, acute CHF, peripheral arterial insufficiency resembling Raynaud's disease, myotonia, paresthesia of *hands.* **Special Senses:** Dry eyes (gritty sensation), visual disturbances, conjunctivitis, tinnitus, hearing loss, nasal stuffiness. **GI:** Dry mouth, nausea, vomiting, heartburn, diarrhea, constipation, flatulence, abdominal cramps, mesenteric arterial thrombosis, ischemic colitis, pancreatitis. **Hematologic:** Transient eosinophilia, thrombocytopenic or nonthrombocytopenic purpura, agranulocytosis. **Metabolic:** Hypoglycemia, hyperglycemia, hypocalcemia (patients with hyperthyroidism). **Respiratory:** Dyspnea, laryngospasm, bronchospasm.

DIAGNOSTIC TEST INTERFERENCE BETA-ADRENERGIC BLOCKERS may produce false-negative test results in exercise tolerance ECG tests, and elevations in ***serum potassium, peripheral platelet count, serum uric acid, serum transaminase, alkaline phosphatase, lactate dehydrogenase, serum creatinine, BUN,*** and an increase or decrease in ***blood glucose*** levels in diabetic patients.

INTERACTIONS Drug: PHENOTHIAZINES have additive hypotensive effects. BETA-ADRENERGIC AGONISTS (e.g., **albuterol**) antagonize effects. **Atropine** and TRICYCLIC ANTIDEPRESSANTS block bradycardia. DIURETICS and other HYPOTENSIVE AGENTS increase hypotension. High doses of **tubocurarine** may potentiate neuromuscular blockade. **Cimetidine** decreases clearance, increases effects. ANTACIDS, **ascorbic acid** may decrease absorption. **Herbal: Black pepper** may increase plasma levels.

PHARMACOKINETICS Absorption: Completely from GI tract; undergoes extensive first-pass metabolism. **Peak:** 60–90 min immediate release; 6 h sustained release; 5 min IV. **Distribution:** Widely distributed including CNS, placenta, and breast milk. **Metabolism:** Almost completely in liver (CYP1A2, 2D6). **Elimination:** 90–95% in urine as metabolites; 1–4% in feces. **Half-Life:** 2.3 h.

NURSING IMPLICATIONS

Assessment & Drug Effects

- Obtain careful medical history to rule out allergies, asthma, and obstructive pulmonary disease. Propranolol can cause bronchiolar constriction even in normal subjects.
- Monitor apical pulse, respiration, BP, and circulation to extremities closely throughout period of dosage adjustment. Consult physician for acceptable parameters.
- Evaluate adequate control or dosage interval for patients being treated for hypertension by checking blood pressure near end of dosage interval or before administration of next dose.
- Be aware that adverse reactions occur most frequently following IV administration soon after therapy is initiated; however, incidence is also high following oral use in the older adult and in patients with impaired kidney function. Reactions may or may not be dose related.
- Lab tests: Obtain periodic hematologic, kidney, liver, and cardiac functions when propranolol is given for prolonged periods.
- Monitor I&O ratio and daily weight as significant indexes for detecting fluid retention and developing heart failure.
- Consult physician regarding allowable salt intake. Drug plasma volume may increase with consequent risk of CHF if dietary sodium is not restricted in patients not receiving concomitant diuretic therapy.
- Fasting for more than 12 h may induce hypoglycemic effects fostered by propranolol.
- If patient complains of cold, painful, or tender feet or hands, examine carefully for evidence of impaired circulation. Peripheral

P

pulses may still be present even though circulation is impaired. Caution patient to avoid prolonged exposure of extremities to cold.

Patient & Family Education

- Learn usual pulse rate and take radial pulse before each dose. Report to physician if pulse is below the established parameter or becomes irregular.
- Be aware that propranolol suppresses clinical signs of hypoglycemia (e.g., BP changes, increased pulse rate) and may prolong hypoglycemia.
- Understand importance of compliance. Do not alter established regimen (i.e., do not omit, increase, or decrease dosage or change dosage interval).
- Do not discontinue abruptly; can precipitate withdrawal syndrome (e.g., tremulousness, sweating, severe headache, malaise, palpitation, rebound hypertension, MI, and life-threatening arrhythmias in patients with angina pectoris).
- Be aware that drug may cause mild hypotension (experienced as dizziness or lightheadedness) in normotensive patients on prolonged therapy. Make position changes slowly and avoid prolonged standing. Notify physician if symptoms persist.
- Do not drive or engage in potentially hazardous activities until response to drug is known.
- Consult physician before self-medicating with OTC drugs.
- Inform dentist, surgeon, or ophthalmologist that you are taking propranolol (drug lowers normal and elevated intraocular pressure).

P

PROPYLTHIOURACIL (PTU) Pr

(proe-pill-thye-oh-yoor'a-sill)

Propyl-Thyracil ♣

Classification: ANTITHYROID

Therapeutic: ANTITHYROID

Pregnancy Category: D

AVAILABILITY 50 mg tablets

ACTION & *THERAPEUTIC EFFECT* Interferes with use of iodine and blocks synthesis of thyroxine (T_4) and triiodothyronine (T_3). Antithyroid action is delayed days and weeks until preformed T_3 and T_4 are degraded. *Effective as an antithyroid agent in various hyperthyroid conditions.*

USES Hyperthyroidism, iodine-induced thyrotoxicosis, and hyperthyroidism associated with thyroiditis; to establish euthyroidism prior to surgery or radioactive iodine treatment; palliative control of toxic nodular goiter.

CONTRAINDICATIONS Hypersensitivity to propylthiouracil; concurrent administration of sulfonamides or coal tar derivatives such as aminopyrine or antipyrine; pregnancy (category D), lacation.

CAUTIOUS USE Infection; concomitant administration of anticoagulants or other drugs known to cause agranulocytosis; bone marrow depression; impaired liver function.

ROUTE & DOSAGE

Hyperthyroidism

Adult: **PO** 300–450 mg/day divided q8h, may need 600–1200 mg/day initially

Geriatric: **PO** 150–300 mg/day divided q8h

Child: **PO** *6–10 y,* 50–150 mg/day; *older than 10 y,* 150–300 mg/day or 150 mg/m²/day

Neonates: **PO** 5–10 mg/kg/day

Thyrotoxic Crisis
Adult: **PO** 200 mg q4–6h until full control achieved

ADMINISTRATION

Oral

- Give at the same time each day with relation to meals. Food may alter drug response by changing absorption rate.
- If drug is being used to improve thyroid state before radioactive iodine (RAI) treatment, discontinued 3 or 4 days before treatment to prevent uptake interference. PTU therapy may be resumed if necessary 3–5 days after the RAI administration.
- Store drug at 15°–30° C (59°–86° F) in light-resistant container.

ADVERSE EFFECTS (≥1%) **CNS:** Paresthesias, headache, vertigo, drowsiness, neuritis. **GI:** Nausea, vomiting, diarrhea, dyspepsia, loss of taste, sialoadenitis, hepatitis. **Hematologic:** Myelosuppression, lymphadenopathy, periarteritis, hypoprothrombinemia, thrombocytopenia, leukopenia, agranulocytosis. **Metabolic:** Hypothyroidism (goitrogenic): Enlarged thyroid, reduced GI motility, periorbital edema, puffy hands and feet, bradycardia, cool and pale skin, worsening of ophthalmopathy, sleepiness, fatigue, mental depression, dizziness, vertigo, sensitivity to cold, paresthesias, nocturnal muscle cramps, changes in menstrual periods, unusual weight gain. **Skin:** Skin rash, urticaria, pruritus, hyperpigmentation, lightening of hair color, abnormal hair loss. **Body as a Whole:** Drug fever, lupus-like syndrome, arthralgia, myalgia, hypersensitivity vasculitis.

DIAGNOSTIC TEST INTERFERENCE Propylthiouracil may elevate ***prothrombin time*** and serum ***alkaline phosphatase, AST, ALT*** levels.

INTERACTIONS Drug: Amiodarone, potassium iodide, sodium iodide, THYROID HORMONES can reverse efficacy.

PHARMACOKINETICS Absorption: Rapidly from GI tract. **Peak:** 1–1.5 h. **Distribution:** Appears to concentrate in thyroid gland; crosses placenta; some distribution into breast milk. **Metabolism:** Rapidly to inactive metabolites. **Elimination:** 35% in urine within 24 h. **Half-Life:** 1–2 h.

NURSING IMPLICATIONS

Assessment & Drug Effects

- Be aware that about 10% of patients with hyperthyroidism have leukopenia less than 4000 cells/mm³ and relative granulocytopenia.
- Observe for signs of clinical response to PTU (usually within 2 or 3 wk): Significant weight gain, reduced pulse rate, reduced serum T_4.
- Lab tests: Baseline and periodic T_3 and T_4; periodic CBC with differential and platelet count.
- Satisfactory euthyroid state may be delayed for several months when thyroid gland is greatly enlarged.
- Be alert to signs of hypoprothrombinemia: Ecchymoses, purpura, petechiae, unexplained bleeding. Warn ambulatory patients to report these signs promptly.
- Be alert for important diagnostic signs of excess dosage: Contraction of a muscle bundle when pricked, mental depression, hard and nonpitting edema, and need for high thermostat setting and extra blankets in winter (cold intolerance).
- Monitor for urticaria (occurs in 3–7% of patients during weeks 2–8 of treatment). Report severe rash.

P

Patient & Family Education

- Note that PTU treatment may be reinstituted if surgery fails to produce normal thyroid gland function.
- Report severe skin rash or swelling of cervical lymph nodes. Therapy may be discontinued.
- Report to physician sore throat, fever, and rash immediately (most apt to occur in first few months of treatment). Drug will be discontinued and hematologic studies initiated.
- Avoid use of OTC drugs for asthma, or cough treatment without checking with the physician. Iodides sometimes included in such preparations are contraindicated.
- Learn how to take pulse accurately and check daily. Report to physician continued tachycardia.
- Report diarrhea, fever, irritability, listlessness, vomiting, weakness; these are signs of inadequate therapy or thyrotoxicosis.
- Chart weight 2 or 3 times weekly; clinical response is monitored through changes in weight and pulse.
- Do not alter drug regimen (e.g., increase, decrease, omit doses, change dosage intervals).
- Check with physician about use of iodized salt and inclusion of seafood in the diet.

PROTAMINE SULFATE

(proe'ta-meen)

Classifications: ANTIDOTE; HEPARIN ANTAGONIST

Therapeutic: ANTIHEMORRHAGIC

Pregnancy Category: C

AVAILABILITY 10 mg/mL injection

ACTION & *THERAPEUTIC EFFECT* Combines with heparin to produce a stable complex; thus it neutralizes the anticoagulant effect of heparin. *Effective antidote to heparin overdose.*

USES Antidote for heparin overdosage (after heparin has been discontinued).

UNLABELED USES Antidote for heparin administration during extracorporeal circulation.

CONTRAINDICATIONS Hemorrhage not induced by heparin overdosage; lactation.

CAUTIOUS USE Cardiovascular disease; history of allergy to fish; vasectomized or infertile males; diabetes mellitus; patients who have received protamine-containing insulin; pregnancy (category C).

ROUTE & DOSAGE

Antidote for Heparin Overdose

Adult/Child: **IV** 1 mg for every 100 units of heparin to be neutralized (max: 100 mg in a 2 h period), give the first 25–50 mg by slow direct IV and the rest over 2–3 h

ADMINISTRATION

Note: Titrate dose carefully to prevent excess anticoagulation because protamine has a longer half-life than heparin and also has some anticoagulant effect of its own.

Intravenous

Note: Verify correct IV concentration and rate of infusion for infants or children with physician.

PREPARE: **Direct:** May be given as supplied direct IV. **Continuous:** Dilute in 50 mL or more of NS or D5W.

ADMINISTER: **Direct:** Give each 50 mg or fraction thereof slowly over 10–15 min. ▪ NEVER give more than 50 mg in any 10 min period or 100 mg in any 2 h period.

Continuous: Do not exceed direct rate. Give over 2–3 h or longer as determined by coagulation studies.

INCOMPATIBILITIES **Solution/additive:** RADIOCONTRAST MATERIALS, **furosemide.**

- Store protamine sulfate injection at 15°–30° C (59°–86° F). ▪ Solutions do not contain preservatives and should not be stored.

ADVERSE EFFECTS (≥1%) **CV:** *Abrupt drop in BP* (with rapid IV infusion), bradycardia. **Body as a Whole:** Urticaria, angioedema, pulmonary edema, anaphylaxis, dyspnea, lassitude; transient flushing and feeling of warmth. **GI:** Nausea, vomiting. **Hematologic:** Protamine overdose or "heparin rebound" (hyperheparinemia).

INTERACTIONS No clinically significant interactions established.

PHARMACOKINETICS Onset: 5 min. **Duration:** 2 h.

NURSING IMPLICATIONS

Assessment & Drug Effects

- Do not use protamine if only minor bleeding occurs during heparin therapy because withdrawal of heparin will usually correct minor bleeding within a few hours.
- Monitor BP and pulse q15–30min, or more often if indicated. Continue for at least 2–3 h after each dose, or longer as dictated by patient's condition.
- Lab tests: Monitor aPTT or ACT values. Coagulation tests are usually performed 5–15 min after administration of protamine, and again in 2–8 h if desirable.
- Observe closely patients undergoing extracorporeal dialysis or patients who have had cardiac surgery for bleeding (heparin rebound). Even with apparent adequate neutralization of heparin by protamine, bleeding may occur 30 min to 18 h after surgery. Monitor vital signs closely. Additional protamine may be required in these patients.

PROTEIN C CONCENTRATE (HUMAN)

(pro′teen)

Ceprotin

Classifications: HEMATOLOGIC; THROMBOLYTIC; PROTEIN INHIBITOR

Therapeutic: PROTEIN C REPLACEMENT THERAPY

Pregnancy Category: C

AVAILABILITY 500 unit, 1000 unit vials of lyophilized powder

ACTION & *THERAPEUTIC EFFECT* Protein C is a critical element in a pathway that provides a natural mechanism for control of the coagulation system. This prevents excess procoagulant responses to activating stimuli. *Protein C is necessary to decrease thrombin generation and intravascular clot formation.*

USES Treatment of patients with severe congenital protein C deficiency; protein C replacement therapy for the prevention and treatment of venous thrombosis and purpura fulminans in children and adults.

CONTRAINDICATIONS Hypersensitivity to human protein C; concurrent administration with tissue plasminogen activator (tPA); hypernatremia; lactation.

CAUTIOUS USE Concurrent administration of anticoagulants; heparin induced thrombocytopenia (HIT); renal impairment; hepatic impairment; older adults; pregnancy (category C).

ROUTE & DOSAGE

Acute Episodes of Venous Thrombosis and Purpura Fulminans and Short-Term Prophylaxis

Adult: **IV** Initial dose 100–120 units/kg; then 60–80 units/kg q6h × 3. Maintenance dose: 45–60 units/kg q6–12h.

ADMINISTRATION

Intravenous

PREPARE: **Direct/IV Infusion:** Bring powder and supplied diluent to room temperature. Insert supplied double-ended transfer needle into diluent vial, then invert and rapidly insert into protein C powder vial. (If vacuum does not draw diluent into vial, discard.) ▪ Remove transfer needle and gently swirl to dissolve. ▪ Resulting solution concentration is 100 units/mL and it should be colorless to slightly yellowish, clear to slightly opalescent and free from visible particles. ▪ Withdraw required dose with the supplied filter needle.

ADMINISTER: **Direct/IV Infusion:** Infuse at 2 mL/min. **Direct/IV Infusion for Child weighing greater than 10 kg:** Infuse at 0.2 mL/kg/min.

▪ Store at room temperature for no more than 3 h after reconstitution. ▪ Prior to reconstitution, protect from light.

ADVERSE EFFECTS (≥1%) **Body as a Whole:** Fever, hyperhidrosis, hypersensitivity reactions (rash, pruritits), restlessness. **CNS:** Lightheadedness. **CV:** Hemothorax, hypotension.

INTERACTIONS Drug: Protein C concentrate can increase bleeding caused by **alteplase, reteplase,** or **tenecteplase.**

PHARMACOKINETICS Peak: 0.5–1 h. **Half-Life:** 9.9 h.

NURSING IMPLICATIONS

Assessment & Drug Effects

- Monitor for and promptly report S&S of bleeding or hypersensitivity reactions (see Appendix F).
- Monitor vital signs including BP and temperature.
- Lab tests: Baseline and periodic protein C activity, protein C trough level with acute thrombotic events; platelet counts; frequent serum sodium with renal function impairment.

Patient & Family Education

- Report immediately early signs of hypersensitivity reactions including hives, generalized itching, tightness in chest, wheezing, difficulty breathing.
- Report immediately any signs of bleeding including black tarry stools, pink/red-tinged urine, unusual bruising.

PROTRIPTYLINE HYDROCHLORIDE

(proe-trip'te-leen)

Triptil ♣, Vivactil

Classification: TRICYCLIC ANTIDEPRESSANT

Therapeutic: ANTIDEPRESSANT

Prototype: Imipramine

Pregnancy Category: C

AVAILABILITY 5 mg, 10 mg tablets

ACTION & *THERAPEUTIC EFFECT*

Tricyclic antidepressant (TCA) that is believed to enhance actions of norepinephrine and serotonin by blocking their reuptake at the neuronal membrane. *Effective in the treatment of depressed individuals, particularly those who are withdrawn.*

USES Symptomatic treatment of endogenous depression in patients under close medical supervision. Particularly effective for depression manifested by psychomotor retardation, apathy, and fatigue.

CONTRAINDICATIONS Hypersensitivity to TCAs; concurrent use of MAOIs; acute recovery phase following MI; QT prolongation, bundle branch block; within 14 days of MAOI therapy; cardiac conduction defects; suicidal ideation.

CAUTIOUS USE Hepatic, cardiovascular, or kidney dysfunction; diabetes mellitus; hyperthyroidism; history of alcoholism; patients with insomnia; asthma; bipolar disorder; suicidal tendencies; children and adolescents; pregnancy (category C), lactation.

ROUTE & DOSAGE

Antidepressant

Adult: **PO** 15–40 mg/day in 3–4 divided doses (max: 60 mg/day)
Adolescent: **PO** 15 mg/day in divided doses

ADMINISTRATION

Oral

- Give whole or crush and mix with fluid or food.
- Give dosage increases in the morning dose to prevent sleep interference and because this TCA has psychic energizing action.
- Give last dose of day no later than midafternoon; insomnia rather than drowsiness is a frequent adverse effect.
- Store at 15°–30° C (59°–86° F) in tightly closed container.

ADVERSE EFFECTS (≥1%) **Body as a Whole:** Photosensitivity, <u>edema</u> (general or of face and <u>tongue</u>). **GI:** *Xerostomia, constipation,* paralytic ileus. **Special Senses:** Blurred vision. **Urogenital:** *Urinary retention.* **CNS:** Insomnia, headache, confusion. **CV:** Change in heat or cold tolerance; *orthostatic hypotension, tachycardia.*

INTERACTIONS Drug: May decrease some response to ANTIHYPERTENSIVES; CNS DEPRESSANTS, **alcohol,** HYPNOTICS, BARBITURATES, SEDATIVES potentiate CNS depression; ORAL ANTICOAGULANTS may increase hypoprothrombinemic effects; **ethchlorvynol** causes transient delirium; **levodopa** SYMPATHOMIMETICS (e.g., **epinephrine, norepinephrine**) increases possibility of sympathetic hyperactivity with hypertension and hyperpyrexia; MAO INHIBITORS present possibility of severe reactions—toxic psychosis, cardiovascular instability; **methylphenidate** increases plasma TCA levels; THYROID DRUGS may increase possibility of arrhythmias; **cimetidine** may increase plasma TCA levels. **Herbal: Ginkgo** may decrease seizure threshold; **St. John's wort** may cause serotonin syndrome (headache, dizziness, sweating, agitation).

PHARMACOKINETICS Absorption: Rapidly from GI tract. **Peak levels:** 24–30 h. **Distribution:** Crosses placenta; distributed into breast milk. **Metabolism:** In liver. **Elimination:** Primarily in urine. **Half-Life:** 54–98 h.

NURSING IMPLICATIONS

Assessment & Drug Effects

- Monitor therapeutic effectiveness. Onset of initial effect characterized by increased activity and energy is fairly rapid, usually within 1 wk af-

P

ter therapy is initiated. Maximum effect may not occur for 2 wk or more.

- Monitor adolescents as well as adults for changes in behavior that may indicate suicidality. Suicide is an inherent risk with any depressed patient and may remain until there is significant improvement.
- Monitor vital signs closely and CV system responses during early therapy, particularly in patients with cardiovascular disorders and older adults receiving daily doses in excess of 20 mg. Withhold drug and inform physician if BP falls more than 20 mm Hg or if there is a sudden increase in pulse rate.
- Lab tests: Periodic LFTs.
- Monitor I&O ratio and bowel pattern during early therapy and when patient is on large doses.
- Assess and advise physician as indicated for prominent anticholinergic effects (xerostomia, blurred vision, constipation, paralytic ileus, urinary retention, delayed micturition).
- Assess condition of oral membranes frequently; institute symptomatic treatment if necessary. Xerostomia can interfere with appetite, fluid intake, and integrity of tooth surfaces.

Patient & Family Education

- Report promptly changes in mood or behavior indicative of suicidal thinking.
- Consult physician about safe amount of alcohol, if any, that can be taken. Actions of both alcohol and protriptyline are potentiated when used together for up to 2 wk after the TCA is discontinued.
- Consult physician before taking any OTC medications.
- Be aware that effects of barbiturates and other CNS depressants are enhanced by TCAs.
- Avoid potentially hazardous activities requiring alertness and skill until response to drug is known.
- Avoid exposure to the sun without protecting skin with sunscreen lotion (SPF higher than 12). Photosensitivity reactions may occur.

PSEUDOEPHEDRINE HYDROCHLORIDE

(soo-doe-e-fed′rin)

Cenafed, Decongestant Syrup, Dorcol Children's Decongestant, Eltor ✦, Eltor 120 ✦, Halofed, Novafed, PediaCare, Pseudofrin ✦, Robidrine ✦, Sudafed, Sudrin

Classifications: ALPHA- AND BETA-ADRENERGIC RECEPTOR AGONIST; DECONGESTANT

Therapeutic: NASAL DECONGESTANT

Prototype: Epinephrine

Pregnancy Category: C

AVAILABILITY 30 mg, 60 mg tablets; 120 mg, 240 mg sustained release tablets; 15 mg/5 mL, 30 mg/5 mL liquid; 7.5 mg/0.8 mL drops

ACTION & *THERAPEUTIC EFFECT* Sympathomimetic amine that produces decongestion of respiratory tract mucosa by stimulating the sympathetic nerve endings including alpha-, $beta_1$, and $beta_2$ receptors. *Effect is caused by vasoconstriction and thus increased nasal airway patency.*

USES Symptomatic relief of nasal congestion associated with rhinitis, coryza, and sinusitis and for eustachian tube congestion.

CONTRAINDICATIONS Hypersensitivity to sympathomimetic amines; severe hypertension; severe coronary artery disease; use within 14 days of MAOIS; hyperthyroidism; prostatic hypertrophy. Safe use in children younger than 2 y **(PO form)**, children younger than 12 y **(sustained release form)** is not established.

CAUTIOUS USE Hypertension, heart disease, renal impairment; acute MI, angina; closed-angle glaucoma; concurrent use of ACE INHIBITOR; pregnancy (category C), lactation.

ROUTE & DOSAGE

Nasal Congestion

Adult: **PO** 60 mg q4–6h or 120 mg sustained release q12h
Geriatric: **PO** 30–60 mg q6h prn
Child: **PO** *2–6 y*, 15 mg q4–6h (max: 60 mg/day); *6–11 y*, 30 mg q4–6h (max: 120 mg/day)

ADMINISTRATION

Oral

- Ensure that sustained release form is not chewed or crushed. **Must be** swallowed whole.

ADVERSE EFFECTS (≥1%) **Body as a Whole:** *Transient stimulation*, tremulousness, difficulty in voiding. **CV:** Arrhythmias, palpitation, *tachycardia*. **CNS:** *Nervousness*, dizziness, headache, sleeplessness, numbness of extremities. **GI:** Anorexia, dry mouth, nausea, vomiting.

INTERACTIONS Drug: Other SYMPATHOMIMETICS increase pressor effects and toxicity; MAO INHIBITORS may precipitate hypertensive crisis; BETA-BLOCKERS may increase pressor effects; may decrease antihypertensive effects of **guanethidine, methyldopa, reserpine.**

PHARMACOKINETICS Absorption: Readily from GI tract. **Onset:** 15–30 min. **Duration:** 4–6 h (8–12 h sustained release). **Distribution:** Crosses placenta; distributed into breast milk. **Metabolism:** Partially metabolized in liver. **Elimination:** In urine.

NURSING IMPLICATIONS

Assessment & Drug Effects

- Monitor HR and BP, especially in those with a history of cardiac disease. Report tachycardia or hypertension.

Patient & Family Education

- Do not take drug within 2 h of bedtime because drug may act as a stimulant.
- Discontinue medication and consult physician if extreme restlessness or signs of sensitivity occur.
- Consult physician before concomitant use of OTC medications; many contain ephedrine or other sympathomimetic amines and might intensify action of pseudoephedrine.

PSYLLIUM HYDROPHILIC MUCILLOID (Pr)

(sill′i-um)

Hydrocil, Instant, Karasil ♣, Konsyl, Metamucil, Modane Bulk, Perdiem Plain, Reguloid, Serutan, Siblin, Syllact, V-Lax

Classification: BULK LAXATIVE
Therapeutic: BULK LAXATIVE
Pregnancy Category: C

AVAILABILITY 3.4 g/dose powder; 2.5 g, 3.4 g, 4.03 g/teaspoon granules

ACTION & *THERAPEUTIC EFFECT* Bulk-producing laxative that absorbs liquid in the GI tract, facilitating peristalsis and bowel motility. *Bulk-producing laxative that promotes peristalsis and natural elimination.*

USES Chronic atonic or spastic constipation and constipation associated with rectal disorders or anorectal surgery.

CONTRAINDICATIONS Esophageal and intestinal obstruction, dysphagia; nausea, vomiting, fecal impaction, acute abdomen; undiagnosed abdominal pain, appendicitis; children younger than 6 y.
CAUTIOUS USE Diabetics; pregnancy (category C).

ROUTE & DOSAGE

Constipation or Diarrhea
Adult: **PO** 1–2 rounded tsp or 1 packet 1–3 times/day prn
Child (younger than 6 y): **PO** 1 tsp in water at bedtime

ADMINISTRATION

Oral
- Fill an 8-oz (240-mL) water glass with cool water, milk, fruit juice, or other liquid; sprinkle powder into liquid; stir briskly; and give immediately (if effervescent form is used, add liquid to powder). Granules should not be chewed.
- Follow each dose with an additional glass of liquid to obtain best results.
- Exercise caution with older adult patient who may aspirate the drug.

ADVERSE EFFECTS (≥1%) **Hematologic:** Eosinophilia. **GI:** Nausea and vomiting, diarrhea (with excessive use); GI tract strictures when drug used in dry form, abdominal cramps.

INTERACTIONS Drug: Psyllium may decrease absorption and clinical effects of ANTIBIOTICS, **warfarin, digoxin, nitrofurantoin,** SALICYLATES.

PHARMACOKINETICS Absorption: Not absorbed from GI tract. **Onset:** 12–24 h. **Peak:** 1–3 days.

NURSING IMPLICATIONS

Assessment & Drug Effects
- Report promptly to physician if patient complains of retrosternal pain after taking the drug. Drug may be lodged as a gelatinous mass (because of poor mixing) in the esophagus.
- Monitor therapeutic effectiveness. When psyllium is used as either a bulk laxative or to treat diarrhea, the expected effect is formed stools. Laxative effect usually occurs within 12–24 h. Administration for 2 or 3 days may be needed to establish regularity.
- Assess for complaints of abdominal fullness. Smaller, more frequent doses spaced throughout the day may be indicated to relieve discomfort of abdominal fullness.
- Monitor warfarin and digoxin levels closely if either is given concurrently.

Patient & Family Education
- Note sugar and sodium content of preparation if on low-sodium or low-calorie diet. Some preparations contain natural sugars, whereas others contain artificial sweeteners.
- Understand that drug works to relieve both diarrhea and constipation by restoring a more normal moisture level to stool.
- Be aware that drug may reduce appetite if it is taken before meals.

PYRANTEL PAMOATE
(pi-ran′tel)
Antiminth, Pin-Rid
Classification: ANTHELMINTIC
Therapeutic: ANTHELMINTIC
Prototype: Mebendazole
Pregnancy Category: C

AVAILABILITY 180 mg capsules; 50 mg/mL suspension

ACTION & *THERAPEUTIC EFFECT* Exerts selective depolarizing neuromuscular blocking action that results in spastic paralysis of worm. *Causes evacuation of worms from intestines.*

USES *Enterobius vermicularis* (pinworm) and *Ascaris lumbricoides* (roundworm) infestations.

UNLABELED USES Hookworm infestations; trichostrongylosis.

CONTRAINDICATIONS Hypersensitivity to pyrantel.

CAUTIOUS USE Liver dysfunction; malnutrition; dehydration; anemia; pregnancy (category C).

ROUTE & DOSAGE

Pinworm or Roundworm

Adult/Child: **PO** 11 mg/kg as a single dose (max: 1 g)

ADMINISTRATION

Oral

- Shake suspension well before pouring it to ensure accurate dosage.
- Give with milk or fruit juices and without regard to prior ingestion of food or time of day.
- Store below 30° C (86° F). Protect from light.

ADVERSE EFFECTS (≥1%) **CNS:** Dizziness, headache, drowsiness, insomnia. **GI:** Anorexia, *nausea,* vomiting, abdominal distention, diarrhea, *tenesmus,* transient elevation of AST. **Skin:** Skin rashes.

INTERACTIONS Drug: Piperazine and pyrantel may be mutually antagonistic.

PHARMACOKINETICS Absorption: Poorly from GI tract. **Peak:** 1–3 h. **Metabolism:** In liver. **Elimination:** Greater than 50% in feces, 7% in urine.

NURSING IMPLICATIONS

Assessment & Drug Effects

- Lab tests: Monitor baseline and periodic AST/ALT in individuals with known liver dysfunction.

Patient & Family Education

- Do not drive or engage in other potentially hazardous activities until response to drug is known.

PYRAZINAMIDE

(peer-a-zin′a-mide)

PZA, Tebrazid ♣

Classifications: ANTIBIOTIC; ANTITUBERCULOSIS

Therapeutic: ANTITUBERCULOSIS

Pregnancy Category: C

AVAILABILITY 500 mg tablets

ACTION & *THERAPEUTIC EFFECT* Pyrazinoic acid amide, analog of nicotinamide. *Bacteriostatic against* Mycobacterium tuberculosis. *Not used as sole agent against TB infection.*

USES Short-term therapy of advanced tuberculosis before surgery and to treat patients unresponsive to primary agents (e.g., isoniazid, streptomycin).

CONTRAINDICATIONS Severe liver damage, acute gout.

CAUTIOUS USE History of gout or diabetes mellitus; impaired kidney function; alcoholism; history of peptic ulcer; acute intermittent porphyria; pregnancy (category C), lactation.

ROUTE & DOSAGE

Tuberculosis
Adult: **PO** 15–35 mg/kg/day in 3–4 divided doses (max: 2 g/day)
Child: **PO** 20–40 mg/kg/day divided q12–24h (max: 2 g/day)

ADMINISTRATION

Oral

- Discontinue drug if hepatic reactions (jaundice, pruritus, icteric sclerae, yellow skin) or hyperuricemia with acute gout (severe pain in great toe and other joints) occurs.
- Store at 15°–30° C (59°–86° F) in tightly closed container.

ADVERSE EFFECTS (≥1%) **Body as a Whole:** *Active gout,* arthralgia, lymphadenopathy. **Urogenital:** Difficulty in urination. **CNS:** Headache. **Skin:** Urticaria. **Hematologic:** Hemolytic anemia, decreased plasma prothrombin. **GI:** Splenomegaly, fatal hemoptysis, aggravation of peptic ulcer, *hepatotoxicity, abnormal liver function tests.* **Metabolic:** *Rise in serum uric acid.*

DIAGNOSTIC TEST INTERFERENCE Pyrazinamide may produce a temporary decrease in ***17-ketosteroids*** and an increase in ***protein-bound iodine.***

INTERACTIONS Drug: Increase in liver toxicity (including fatal hepatoxicity in when treating latent TB) with **rifampin.**

PHARMACOKINETICS Absorption: Readily from GI tract. **Peak:** 2 h. **Distribution:** Crosses blood–brain barrier. **Metabolism:** In liver. **Elimination:** Slowly in urine. **Half-Life:** 9–10 h.

NURSING IMPLICATIONS

Assessment & Drug Effect

- Observe and supervise closely. Patients should receive at least one other effective antituberculosis agent concurrently.
- Examine patients at regular intervals and question about possible signs of toxicity: Liver enlargement or tenderness, jaundice, fever, anorexia, malaise, impaired vascular integrity (ecchymoses, petechiae, abnormal bleeding).
- Hepatic reactions appear to occur more frequently in patients receiving high doses.
- Lab tests: Baseline LFTs (especially AST, ALT, serum bilirubin) and at 2–4 wk intervals during therapy. Blood uric acid determinations are advised before, during, and following therapy.

Patient & Family Education

- Report to physician onset of difficulty in voiding. Keep fluid intake at 2000 mL/day if possible.
- Monitor blood glucose (diabetics) for possible loss of glycemic control.

PYRETHRINS

(peer'e-thrins)

A-200 Pyrinate, Barc, Blue, Pyrinate, Pyrinyl, R & C, RID, TISIT, Triple X

Classifications: ANTIPARASITIC; PEDICULICIDE
Therapeutic: SCABICIDE
Prototype: Permethrin
Pregnancy Category: C

AVAILABILITY 0.18%, 0.2%, 0.3% liquid; 0.3% gel; 0.3% shampoo

ACTION & *THERAPEUTIC EFFECT* Pediculicide solution that acts as a contact poison affecting the parasite's nervous system, causing paralysis and death. *Controls head lice, pubic (crab) lice, and body lice and their eggs (nits).*

USES External treatment of *Pediculus humanus* infestations.

CONTRAINDICATIONS Sensitivity to solution components; skin infections and abrasions.

CAUTIOUS USE Ragweed-sensitized patient; asthma; pregnancy (category C), lactation, infants, children.

ROUTE & DOSAGE

Pediculus humanus Infestations

Adult: **Topical** See Administration for appropriate application

ADMINISTRATION

Topical

- Apply enough solution to completely wet infested area, including hair. Allow to remain on area for 10 min.
- Wash and rinse with large amounts of warm water.
- Use fine-toothed comb to remove lice and eggs from hair.
- Shampoo hair to restore body and luster.
- Repeat treatment once in 24 h if necessary.
- Repeat treatment in 7–10 days to kill newly hatched lice.
- Do not apply to eyebrows or eyelashes without consulting physician.
- Flush eyes with copious amounts of warm water if accidental contact occurs.

ADVERSE EFFECTS (≥1%) **Body as a Whole:** Irritation with repeated use.

NURSING IMPLICATIONS

Patient & Family Education

- Do not swallow, inhale, or allow pyrethrins to contact mucosal surfaces or the eyes.
- Discontinue use and consult physician if treated area becomes irritated.
- Examine each family member carefully; if infested, treat immediately to prevent spread or reinfestation of previously treated patient.
- Dry clean, boil, or otherwise treat contaminated clothing. Sterilize (soak in pyrethrins) combs and brushes used by patient.
- Do not share combs, brushes, or other headgear with another person.

PYRIDOSTIGMINE BROMIDE

(peer-id-oh-stig′meen)

Mestinon, Regonol

Classifications: CHOLINERGIC; ANTICHOLINESTERASE

Therapeutic: CHOLINESTERASE INHIBITOR

Prototype: Neostigmine

Pregnancy Category: C

AVAILABILITY 60 mg/5 mL syrup; 60 mg tablet; 180 mg extended release tablet; 5 mg/mL injection

ACTION & *THERAPEUTIC EFFECT* Indirect-acting cholinergic that inhibits cholinesterase activity. Facilitates transmission of impulses across myoneural junctions by blocking destruction of acetylcholine. *Has direct stimulant action on voluntary muscle fibers and possibly on autonomic ganglia and CNS neurons. Produces increased tone in skeletal muscles.*

USES Myasthenia gravis and as an antagonist to nondepolarizing skeletal muscle relaxants (e.g., curariform drugs).

CONTRAINDICATIONS Hypersensitivity to anticholinesterase agents; mechanical obstruction of urinary or intestinal tract; hypotension; neonates.

CAUTIOUS USE Hypersensitivity to bromides; bronchial asthma; epilepsy; recent cardiac occlusion; renal impairment; vagotonia; hyperthyroidism; peptic ulcer; cardiac dysrhythmias; bradycardia; pregnancy (category C).

ROUTE & DOSAGE

Myasthenia Gravis

Adult: **PO** 60 mg–1.5 g/day spaced according to response of individual patient; sustained release: 180–540 mg 1–2 times/day at intervals of at least 6 h **IM/IV** Approximately 1/30 of PO dose

Child: **PO** 7 mg/kg/day divided into 5–6 doses

Neonates: **PO** 5 mg q4–6h **IM/IV** 0.05–0.15 mg/kg q4–6h

Reversal of Muscle Relaxants

Adult: **IV** 10–20 mg immediately preceded by IV atropine

P

ADMINISTRATION

Oral

- Give with food or fluid.
- Ensure that sustained release form is not chewed or crushed. **Must be** swallowed whole.
- Note: A syrup is available. Some patients may not like it because it is sweet; try to make it more palatable by giving it over ice chips. The syrup formulation contains 5% alcohol.

Intramuscular

- Note: Parenteral dose is about 1/30 the oral adult dose.
- Give deep IM into a large muscle.

Intravenous

PREPARE: **Direct:** Give undiluted. Do NOT add to IV solutions.

ADMINISTER: **Direct:** Give at a rate of 0.5 mg over 1 min for myasthenia gravis; 5 mg over 1 min for reversal of muscle relaxants.

- Store at 15°–30° C (59°–86° F). Protect from light and moisture.

ADVERSE EFFECTS (≥1%) **Skin:** Acneiform rash. **Hematologic:** Thrombophlebitis (following IV administration). **GI:** *Nausea, vomiting, diarrhea.* **Special Senses:** *Miosis.* **Body as a Whole:** *Excessive salivation and sweating,* weakness, fasciculation. **Respiratory:** Increased bronchial secretion, <u>bronchoconstriction</u>. **CV:** Bradycardia, hypotension.

INTERACTIONS Drug: Atropine NONDEPOLARIZING MUSCLE RELAXANTS antagonize effects of pyridostigmine.

PHARMACOKINETICS Absorption: Poorly from GI tract. **Onset:** 30–45 min PO; 15 min IM; 2–5 min IV. **Duration:** 3–6 h. **Distribution:** Crosses placenta. **Metabolism:** In liver and in serum and tissue by cholinesterases. **Elimination:** In urine.

NURSING IMPLICATIONS

Assessment & Drug Effects

- Report increasing muscular weakness, cramps, or fasciculations. Failure of patient to show improvement may reflect either underdosage or overdosage.
- Observe patient closely if atropine is used to abolish GI adverse effects or other muscarinic adverse effects because it may mask signs of overdosage (cholinergic crisis): Increasing muscle weakness, which through involvement of respiratory muscles can lead to death.
- Monitor vital signs frequently, especially respiratory rate.

- Observe for signs of cholinergic reactions (see Appendix F), particularly when drug is administered IV.
- Observe neonates of myasthenic mothers, who have received pyridostigmine, closely for difficulty in breathing, swallowing, or sucking.
- Observe patient continuously when used as muscle relaxant antagonist. Airway and respiratory assistance **must be** maintained until full recovery of voluntary respiration and neuromuscular transmission is assured. Complete recovery usually occurs within 30 min.

Patient & Family Education

- Be aware that duration of drug action may vary with physical and emotional stress, as well as with severity of disease.
- Report onset of rash to physician. Drug may be discontinued.
- Sustained release tablets may become mottled in appearance; this does not affect their potency.

PYRIDOXINE HYDROCHLORIDE (VITAMIN B_6)

(peer-i-dox'een)

Classification: VITAMIN
Therapeutic: VITAMIN B_6 REPLACEMENT
Pregnancy Category: A (C if greater than RDA)

AVAILABILITY 25 mg, 50 mg, 100 mg, 250 mg, 500 mg tablets; 100 mg/mL injection

ACTION & *THERAPEUTIC EFFECT* Water-soluble complex of three closely related compounds with B_6 activity. Converted in body to pyridoxal, a coenzyme that functions in protein, fat, and carbohydrate metabolism and in facilitating release of glycogen from liver and muscle. In protein metabolism, participates in enzymatic transformations of amino acids and conversion of tryptophan to niacin and serotonin. Aids in energy transformation in brain and nerve cells, and is thought to stimulate heme production. *Effectiveness is evaluated by improvement of B_6 deficiency manifestations: Nausea, vomiting, skin lesions resembling those of riboflavin and niacin deficiency, edema, CNS symptoms, hypochromic microcytic anemia.*

USES Prophylaxis and treatment of pyridoxine deficiency, as seen with inadequate dietary intake, drug-induced deficiency (e.g., isoniazid, oral contraceptives), and inborn errors of metabolism (vitamin B_6–dependent convulsions or anemia). Also to prevent chloramphenicol-induced optic neuritis, to treat acute toxicity caused by overdosage of cycloserine, hydralazine, isoniazid (INH); alcoholic polyneuritis; sideroblastic anemia associated with high serum iron concentration. Has been used for management of many other conditions ranging from nausea and vomiting in radiation sickness and pregnancy to suppression of postpartum lactation.

CONTRAINDICATIONS IV form: Cardiac disease.
CAUTIOUS USE Renal impairment; neonatal prematurity with renal impairment; cardiac disease; pregnancy [category A (C if greater than RDA)].

ROUTE & DOSAGE

Dietary Deficiency
Adult: **PO/IM/IV** 10–20 mg/day × 2–3 wk
Child: **PO** 5–25 mg/day × 3 wk, then 1.5–2.5 mg/day

Pyridoxine Deficiency Syndrome
Adult: **PO/IM/IV** Initial dose up to 600 mg/day may be required; then up to 50 mg/day

Isoniazid-Induced Deficiency

Adult: **PO/IM/IV** 100 mg/day × 3 wk, then 30 mg/day
Child: **PO** 10–50 mg/day × 3 wk, then 1–2 mg/kg/day

Pyridoxine-Dependent Seizures

Neonate/Infant: **PO/IM/IV** 50–100 mg/day

ADMINISTRATION

Oral

- Ensure that sustained release and enteric forms are not chewed or crushed. **Must be** swallowed whole.

Intramuscular

- Give deep IM into a large muscle.

Intravenous

PREPARE: **Direct:** Give undiluted. **Continuous:** May be added to most standard IV solutions.
ADMINISTER: **Direct:** Give at a rate of 50 mg or fraction thereof over 60 seconds. **Continuous:** Give according to ordered rate for infusion.

- Store at 15°–30° C (59°–86° F) in tight, light-resistant containers. Avoid freezing.

ADVERSE EFFECTS (≥1%) **Body as a Whole:** Paresthesias, slight flushing or feeling of warmth, temporary burning or stinging pain in injection site. **CNS:** Somnolence seizures (particularly following large parenteral doses). **Metabolic:** Low folic acid levels.

INTERACTIONS Drug: Isoniazid, cycloserine, penicillamine, hydralazine, and ORAL CONTRACEPTIVES may increase pyridoxine requirements; may reverse or antagonize therapeutic effects of **levodopa.**

PHARMACOKINETICS Absorption: Readily from GI tract. **Distribution:** Stored in liver; crosses placenta. **Metabolism:** In liver. **Elimination:** In urine.

NURSING IMPLICATIONS

Assessment & Drug Effects

- Monitor neurologic status to determine therapeutic effect in deficiency states.
- Record a complete dietary history so poor eating habits can be identified and corrected (a single vitamin deficiency is rare; patient can be expected to have multiple vitamin deficiencies).
- Lab tests: Periodic Hct and Hgb, and serum iron.

Patient & Family Education

- Learn rich dietary sources of vitamin B_6: Yeast, wheat germ, whole grain cereals, muscle and glandular meats (especially liver), legumes, green vegetables, bananas.
- Do not self-medicate with vitamin combinations (OTC) without first consulting physician.

PYRIMETHAMINE

(peer-i-meth'a-meen)

Daraprim

Classification: FOLIC ACID ANTAGONIST
Therapeutic: ANTIMALARIAL
Prototype: Chloroquine
Pregnancy Category: C

AVAILABILITY 25 mg tablets

ACTION & *THERAPEUTIC EFFECT* Long-acting folic acid antagonist. Selectively inhibits action of dehydrofolic reductase in parasites with resulting blockade of folic acid metabolism. *Prevents development of fertilized gametes in the mosquito and thus helps to prevent transmission of malaria.*

USES Prophylaxis of malaria due to susceptible strains of plasmodia. May be used conjointly with fast-acting antimalarial (e.g., chloroquine, quinacrine, quinine) to initiate transmission control and suppressive cure. Used with a sulfonamide to provide synergistic action in treatment of toxoplasmosis.

CONTRAINDICATIONS Chloroguanide-resistant malaria; hypersensitivity to sulfonamides; megaloblastic anemia caused by folate deficiency; children younger than 2 mo; lactation.

CAUTIOUS USE Convulsive disorders; asthma; bone marrow suppression; folate deficiency; hepatic disease; renal disease; seizure disorder; pregnancy (category C).

ROUTE & DOSAGE

Malaria Chemoprophylaxis
Adult: **PO** 25 mg once/wk
Child: **PO** *Younger than 4 y,* 6.25 mg once/wk; *4–10 y,* 12.5 mg once/wk; *older than 10 y,* 25 mg once/wk

Toxoplasmosis
Adult: **PO** 50–75 mg/day with a sulfonamide for 1–3 wk, then decrease dose by half and continue for 1 mo
Child: **PO** 1 mg/kg/day divided into 2 doses with a sulfonamide for 1–3 wk, then decrease to 0.5 mg/kg/day for 1 mo (max: 25 mg/day)

ADMINISTRATION

Oral

- Minimize GI distress by giving with meals. If symptoms persist, dosage reduction may be necessary.
- Give on same day each week for malaria prophylaxis. Begin when individual enters malarious area and continue for 10 wk after leaving the area.

ADVERSE EFFECTS (≥1%) **GI:** Anorexia, vomiting, atrophic glossitis, abdominal cramps, diarrhea. **Skin:** Skin rashes. **Hematologic:** *Folic acid deficiency* (*megaloblastic anemia, leukopenia, thrombocytopenia, pancytopenia,* diarrhea). **CNS:** CNS stimulation including convulsions, respiratory failure.

INTERACTIONS Drug: Folic acid, *para*-aminobenzoic acid (PABA) may decrease effectiveness against toxoplasmosis.

PHARMACOKINETICS Absorption: Readily from GI tract. **Peak:** 2 h. **Distribution:** Concentrates in kidneys, lungs, liver, and spleen; distributed into breast milk. **Elimination:** Slowly in urine; excretion may extend over 30 days or longer. **Half-Life:** 54–148 h.

NURSING IMPLICATIONS

Assessment & Drug Effects

- Monitor patient response closely. Dosages required for treatment of toxoplasmosis approach toxic levels.
- Lab tests: Perform blood counts, including platelets, twice weekly during therapy.
- Withhold drug and notify physician if hematologic abnormalities appear.

Patient & Family Education

- Be aware that folic acid deficiency may occur with long-term use of pyrimethamine. Report to physician weakness, and pallor (from anemia), ulcerations of oral mucosa, superinfections, glossitis; GI disturbances such as diarrhea and poor fat absorption, fever. Folate (folinic acid) replacement may be prescribed. Increase food sources of folates (if allowed) in diet.

P

QUAZEPAM

(qua′ze-pam)

Doral

Classifications: BENZODIAZEPINE; ANXIOLYTIC; SEDATIVE-HYPNOTIC

Therapeutic: ANTIANXIETY; SEDATIVE-HYPNOTIC

Prototype: Lorazepam

Pregnancy Category: X

Controlled Substance: Schedule IV

AVAILABILITY 15 mg tablets

ACTION & *THERAPEUTIC EFFECT* Believed to potentiate gamma-aminobutyric acid (GABA) neuronal inhibition in the limbic, neocortical, and mesencephalic reticular systems. *Significantly decreases total wake time and significantly increases sleep time. REM sleep is essentially unchanged.*

USES Insomnia characterized by difficulty in falling asleep, frequent nocturnal awakenings, or early morning awakenings.

CONTRAINDICATIONS Hypersensitivity to quazepam or benzodiazepines; sleep apnea; pregnancy (category X), lactation.

CAUTIOUS USE Impaired liver and kidney function; compromised respiratory function; history of seizures; elderly; debilitated clients. Safety and effectiveness in children younger than 18 y are not established.

ROUTE & DOSAGE

Insomnia

Adult: **PO** 7.5–15 mg at bedtime

ADMINISTRATION

Oral

- Initial dose is usually 15 mg but can often be effectively reduced after several nights of therapy.
- Use lowest effective dose in older adults as soon as possible.

ADVERSE EFFECTS (≥1%) **CNS:** *Drowsiness, headache*, fatigue, dizziness, dry mouth. **GI:** Dyspepsia.

INTERACTIONS Drug: Alcohol, CNS DEPRESSANTS, ANTICONVULSANTS potentiate CNS depression; **cimetidine** increases quazepam plasma levels, increasing its toxicity; may decrease antiparkinsonism effects of **levodopa;** may increase **phenytoin** levels; **smoking** decreases sedative effects of quazepam. **Herbal: Kava, valerian** may potentiate sedation.

PHARMACOKINETICS Absorption: Readily from GI tract. **Onset:** 30 min. **Peak:** 2 h. **Distribution:** Crosses placenta; distributed into breast milk. **Metabolism:** In liver to active metabolites. **Elimination:** In urine and feces. **Half-Life:** 39 h.

NURSING IMPLICATIONS

Assessment & Drug Effects

- Monitor for respiratory depression in patients with chronic respiratory insufficiency.
- Monitor for suicidal tendencies in previously depressed clients.
- Daytime drowsiness is more likely to occur in older adult clients.

Patient & Family Education

- Inform physician about any alcohol consumption and prescription or nonprescription medication that you take. Avoid alcohol use since it potentiates CNS depressant effects.
- Inform physician immediately if you become pregnant. This drug causes birth defects.
- Do not drive or engage in potentially hazardous activities until response to drug is known.
- Do not increase the dose of this drug; inform physician if the drug no longer works.

- This drug may cause daytime sedation, even for several days after drug is discontinued.

QUETIAPINE FUMARATE

(ke-ti-a′peen)

Seroquel, Seroquel XR

Classification: ATYPICAL ANTIPSYCHOTIC

Therapeutic: ANTIPSYCHOTIC

Prototype: Clozapine

Pregnancy Category: C

AVAILABILITY 25 mg, 100 mg, 200 mg tablets; 50 mg, 200 mg, 300 mg, 400 mg extended release tablets

ACTION & *THERAPEUTIC EFFECT* Antagonizes multiple neurotransmitter receptors in the brain including serotonin (5-HT_{1A} and 5-HT_2) as well as dopamine D_1 and D_2 receptors. *Effectiveness indicated by a reduction in psychotic behavior.*

USES Management of schizophrenia, maintenance of acute bipolar disorder, and add-on therapy for major depressive disorder.

UNLABELED USES Management of agitation and dementia.

CONTRAINDICATIONS Hypersensitivity to quetiapine; lactation; alcohol use; suicidal ideation; **extended release tablets:** Dementia-related psychosis. Safe use in children younger than 18 y is not established.

CAUTIOUS USE Liver function impairment, **immediate release tablets only for:** Older adults, or hepatic impairment; cardiovascular disease (history of MI or ischemic heart disease, heart failure, arrhythmias, CVA, hypotension, dehydration, treatment with antihypertensives); history of seizures or suicide; breast cancer; Alzheimer's, Parkinson's disease; patient at risk for aspiration pneumonia; debilitated patients; cerebrovascular disease; pregnancy (category C).

ROUTE & DOSAGE

Bipolar Depression

Adult: **PO** Day 1: 50 mg at bedtime, Day 2: 100 mg at bedtime, Day 3: 200 mg at bedtime, then 300 mg daily at bedtime

Schizophrenia

Adult: **PO** *(Immediate release)* Start 25 mg b.i.d., may increase by 25–50 mg b.i.d. to t.i.d. on the second or third day as tolerated to a target dose of 300–400 mg/day divided b.i.d. to t.i.d., may adjust dose by 25–50 mg b.i.d. daily as needed (max: 800 mg/day); *(Extended release)* 300 mg daily at bedtime, titrate up to 400–800 mg daily (max: 800 mg/day)

Manic Episodes in Bipolar Disorder Monotherapy or with Lithium/Divalproex (Immediate Release Only)

Adult: **PO** Start with total of 100 mg (in two doses) day 1, increase to 400 mg/day (in two doses) by day 4 OR extended release 300 mg on day 1, then 600 mg on day 2, may adjust by 400–800 mg/day based on response

Geriatric: Titrate more slowly due to risk of orthostatic hypotension

Bipolar I Disorder Maintenance

Adult: **PO** 200–400 mg b.i.d.

Hepatic Impairment Dosage Adjusment

Immediate release: Start with 25 mg dose and increase by 25–50 mg/day; Extended release: Start with 50 mg PO on day 1, then increase by 50 mg/day to the lowest effective and tolerable dose

Q

ADMINISTRATION

Oral

- Dose is usually retitrated over a period of several days when patient has been off the drug for longer than 1 wk.
- Follow recommended lower doses and slower titration for the older adults, the debilitated, and those with hepatic impairment or a predisposition to hypotension.
- Store at 15°–30° C (59°–86° F).

ADVERSE EFFECTS (≥1%) **Body as a Whole:** Asthenia, fever, hypertonia, dysarthria, flu syndrome, weight gain, peripheral edema, <u>increased risk of suicidal thinking</u>. **CNS:** *Dizziness, headache, somnolence*. **CV:** Postural hypotension, tachycardia, palpitations. **GI:** Dry mouth, dyspepsia, abdominal pain, constipation, anorexia. **Metabolic:** Hyperglycemia, diabetes mellitus. **Respiratory:** Rhinitis, pharyngitis, cough, dyspnea. **Skin:** Rash, sweating. **Hematologic:** Leukopenia.

INTERACTIONS Drug: BARBITURATES, **carbamazepine, phenytoin, rifampin, thioridazine** may increase clearance of quetiapine. Quetiapine may potentiate the cognitive and motor effects of **alcohol,** enhance the effects of ANTIHYPERTENSIVE AGENTS, antagonize the effects of **levodopa** and DOPAMINE AGONISTS. **Ketoconazole, itraconazole, fluconazole, erythromycin** may decrease clearance of quetiapine. Drugs that increase the QT interval (e.g., **amiodarone, clarithromycin,** ANTIARRHYTHMICS, **haloperidol**) increase risk of cardiac effects. Other ANTIPSYCHOTICS increase the risk of adverse effects. **Herbal: St. John's wort** may cause **serotonin** syndrome (see Appendix F).

PHARMACOKINETICS Absorption: Rapidly and completely absorbed from GI tract. **Peak:** 1.5 h. **Distribution:** 83% protein bound. **Metabolism:** In liver (CYP3A4). **Elimination:** 73% in urine, 20% in feces. **Half-Life:** 6 h.

NURSING IMPLICATIONS

Assessment & Drug Effects

- Monitor diabetics for loss of glycemic control.
- Monitor for changes in behavior that may indicate suicidality.
- Reassess need for continued treatment periodically.
- Withhold the drug and immediately report S&S of tardive dyskinesia or neuroleptic malignant syndrome (see Appendix F).
- Lab tests: Periodic LFTs, lipid profile, thyroid function, blood glucose, CBC with differential.
- Monitor ECG periodically, especially in those with known cardiovascular disease.
- Baseline cataract exam is recommended when therapy is started and at 6 mo intervals thereafter.
- Monitor patients with a history of seizures for lowering of the seizure threshold.

Patient & Family Education

- Carefully monitor blood glucose levels if diabetic.
- Exercise caution with potentially dangerous activities requiring alertness, especially during the first week of drug therapy or during dose increments.
- Make position changes slowly, especially when changing from lying or sitting to standing to avoid dizziness, palpitations, and fainting.
- Avoid alcohol consumption and activities that may cause overheating and dehydration.

QUINAPRIL HYDROCHLORIDE

(quin′a-pril)

Accupril

Classifications: ANGIOTENSIN-CONVERTING ENZYME (ACE) INHIBITOR; ANTIHYPERTENSIVE

Therapeutic: ANTIHYPERTENSIVE

Prototype: Enalapril

Pregnancy Category: D

AVAILABILITY 5 mg, 10 mg, 20 mg, 40 mg tablets

ACTION & *THERAPEUTIC EFFECT* Potent, long-acting ACE inhibitor that lowers BP by interrupting the conversion sequences initiated by renin to form angiotensin II, a vasoconstrictor. Also decreases circulating aldosterone, a secretory response to angiotensin II stimulation. Reduces pulmonary capillary wedge pressure, systemic vascular resistance, and mean arterial pressure, with concurrent increases in cardiac output, cardiac index, and stroke volume. *Lowers BP by producing vasodilation. Effective in the treatment of CHF because it improves cardiac indicators.*

USES Mild to moderate hypertension, CHF.

CONTRAINDICATIONS Hypersensitivity to quinapril or other ACE inhibitors; history of angioedema; pregnancy (category D), lactation, children.

CAUTIOUS USE Renal insufficiency; autoimmune disease, volume-depleted patients, aortic stenosis, hypertrophic cardiomyopathy; renal artery stenosis, neutropenia.

ROUTE & DOSAGE

Hypertension, CHF

Adult: **PO** 10–20 mg daily, may increase up to 80 mg/day in 1–2 divided doses

Geriatric: **PO** Start with 2.5–5 mg daily

Renal Impairment Dosage Adjustment

CrCl 30–60 mL/min: 5 mg daily initially; less than 10–30 mL/min: 2.5 mg/day initially

ADMINISTRATION

Oral

- When patient has been treated with a diuretic, the diuretic is usually discontinued 2–3 days before beginning quinapril. If the diuretic cannot be discontinued, initial quinapril dose is usually lowered to 5 mg.
- Store at 15°–30° C (59°–86° F) and protect from moisture.

ADVERSE EFFECTS (≥1%) **CV:** Edema, hypotension. **CNS:** Dizziness, fatigue, headache. **GI:** Nausea, vomiting, diarrhea. **Hematologic:** Eosinophilia, neutropenia. **Metabolic:** Hyperkalemia, proteinuria. **Respiratory:** Cough. **Body as a Whole:** <u>Angioedema</u>, myalgia.

DIAGNOSTIC TEST INTERFERENCE May increase ***BUN*** or ***serum creatinine.***

INTERACTIONS Drug: POTASSIUM-SPARING DIURETICS may increase risk of hyperkalemia. May elevate serum **lithium** levels, resulting in **lithium** toxicity.

PHARMACOKINETICS Absorption: Rapidly from GI tract. **Onset:** 1 h. **Peak:** 2–4 h. **Duration:** Up to 24 h. **Distribution:** 97% bound to plasma proteins; crosses placenta; not known if distributed into breast milk. **Metabolism:** Extensively metabolized in liver to its active metabolite, quinaprilat. **Elimination:** 50–60% in urine, primarily as quinaprilat; 30% in feces. **Half-Life:** 2 h.

Q

NURSING IMPLICATIONS

Assessment & Drug Effects

- Following initial dose, monitor for several hours for first-dose hypotension, especially in salt- or volume-depleted patients (e.g., those pretreated with a diuretic).
- Monitor BP at time of peak effectiveness, 2–4 h after dosing, and at end of dosing interval just before next dose.
- Report diminished antihypertensive effect toward end of dosing interval. Inadequate trough response may indicate need to divide daily dose.
- Lab tests: Baseline and periodic kidney function tests; periodic serum potassium; periodic WBC in those with collagen vascular disease or renal impairment.
- Observe for S&S of hyperkalemia (see Appendix F).

Patient & Family Education

- Discontinue quinapril and report S&S of angioedema (e.g., swelling of face or extremities, difficulty breathing or swallowing) to physician.
- Maintain adequate fluid intake and avoid potassium supplements or salt substitutes unless specifically prescribed by physician.
- Light-headedness and dizziness may occur, especially during the initial days of therapy. If fainting occurs, stop taking quinapril until the physician has been consulted.

QUINIDINE SULFATE

(kwin′i-deen sul-fate)

Apo-Quinidine ♣, Novoquinidin ♣

QUINIDINE GLUCONATE

Classification: ANTIARRHYTHMIC CLASS IA
Therapeutic: ANTIARRHYTHMIC CLASS IA
Prototype: Procainamide
Pregnancy Category: C

AVAILABILITY Quinidine sulfate: 200 mg, 300 mg tablets; 300 mg sustained release tablets; **Quinidine gluconate:** 324 mg sustained release tablets; 80 mg/mL injection

ACTION & *THERAPEUTIC EFFECT* Class IA antiarrhythmic that depresses myocardial excitability, contractility, automaticity, and conduction velocity as well as prolongs refractory period. *Depresses myocardial excitability, conduction velocity, and irregularity of nerve impulse conduction.*

USES Premature atrial, AV junctional, and ventricular contraction; paroxysmal atrial tachycardia, chronic ventricular tachycardia (when not associated with complete heart block); maintenance therapy after electrical conversion of atrial fibrillation or flutter; life-threatening malaria.

CONTRAINDICATIONS Hypersensitivity or idiosyncrasy to quinine or quinidine; thrombocytopenic purpura resulting from prior use of quinidine; intraventricular conduction defects, complete AV block, AV conduction disorders; left bundle branch block; marked QRS widening; thyrotoxicosis; extensive myocardial damage, frank CHF, hypotensive states; history of drug-induced torsades de pointes.
CAUTIOUS USE Incomplete heart block; impaired kidney or liver function; bronchial asthma or other respiratory disorders; myasthenia gravis; potassium imbalance; pregnancy (category C), lactation.

ROUTE & DOSAGE

Conversion to and/or Maintenance of Sinus Rhythm
Sulfate Immediate Release

Adult: **PO** 200–300 mg q6–8h until sinus rhythm restored or toxicity occurs (max: 3–4 g)

Sulfate Extended Release

Adult: **PO** 324–648 mg q8–12h

Gluconate

Adult: **IM** 600 mg salt, then 400 mg salt; can repeat q2h if needed **IV** 800 mg salt, monitor closely

Malaria

Adult/Adolescent/Child: **IV** 24 mg/kg loading dose, then 12 mg/kg q8h OR 10 mg/kg loading dose, then 0.02 mg/kg/min for 24 h

Renal Impairment Dosage Adjustment

CrCl less than 10 mL/min: Give 75% of dose

Hemodialysis Dosage Adjustment: 200 mg supplement dose postdialysis

ADMINISTRATION

Oral

- Give with a full glass of water on an empty stomach for optimum absorption (i.e., 1 h before or 2 h after meals). Administer drug with food if GI symptoms occur (nausea, vomiting, diarrhea are most common). Do not administer with grapefruit juice.
- Ensure that extended release tablets are swallowed whole. They should not be crushed or chewed.
- Store in tight, light-resistant containers away from excessive heat.

Intramuscular

- Aspirate carefully before injection to avoid inadvertent entry into blood vessel.

Intravenous

PREPARE: **IV Infusion:** Dilute 800 mg (10 mL) in at least 40 mL D5W to yield a maximum concentration of 16 mg/mL.

ADMINISTER: **IV Infusion:** Give via infusion pump at a rate not to exceed 16 mg (1 mL)/min.

INCOMPATIBILITIES Solution/additive: **Amiodarone, atracurium, furosemide.** Y-site: **Acyclovir, aminophylline, amphotericin B, ampicillin, aztreonam, bivalirudin, bretylium,** CEPHALOSPORINS, **clindamycin, dantrolene, daptomycin, dexamethasone, diazoxide, ertapenem, furosemide, ganciclovir, heparin in dextrose, hydrocortisone, indomethacin, insulin, ketorolac, methicillin, methylprednisolone, mezlocillin, minocycline, nafcillin, nitroprusside, oxacillin, pantoprazole, premetrexed, penicillin, pentobarbital, phenobarbital, phenytoin, piperacillin, sodium bicarbonate, SMP/TMX, ticarcillin.**

- Use supine position during drug administration; severe hypotension is most likely to occur in patients receiving drug via IV.
- Protect IV solutions from light and heat to prevent brownish discoloration and possibly precipitation.

ADVERSE EFFECTS (≥1%) **CNS:** Headache, fever, tremors, apprehension, delirium, syncope with sudden loss of consciousness, seizures. **CV:** Hypotension, CHF, <u>widened QRS complex</u>, bradycardia, <u>heart block</u>, atrial flutter, <u>ventricular flutter, fibril-</u>

lation or tachycardia; quinidine syncope, torsades de pointes. **Special Senses:** Mydriasis, blurred vision, disturbed color perception, reduced visual field, photophobia, diplopia, night blindness, scotomas, optic neuritis, disturbed hearing (tinnitus, auditory acuity). **GI:** *Nausea, vomiting, diarrhea, abdominal pain*, hepatic dysfunction. **Hematologic:** Acute hemolytic anemia (especially in patients with G6PD deficiency), hypoprothrombinemia, leukopenia. Thrombocytopenia, agranulocytosis (both rare). **Body as a Whole:** Cinchonism (nausea, vomiting, headache, dizziness, fever, tremors, vertigo, tinnitus, visual disturbances), angioedema, acute asthma, respiratory depression, vascular collapse. **Skin:** Rash, urticaria, cutaneous flushing with intense pruritus, photosensitivity. **Metabolic:** SLE, hypokalemia.

INTERACTIONS Drug: May increase **digoxin** levels by 50%; **amiodarone** may increase quinidine levels, increasing its risk of heart block; other ANTIARRHYTHMICS, PHENOTHIAZINES, **reserpine** add to cardiac depressant effects; ANTICHOLINERGIC AGENTS add to vagolytic effects; CHOLINERGIC AGENTS may antagonize cardiac effects; ANTICONVULSANTS, BARBITURATES, **rifampin** increase the metabolism of quinidine, thus decreasing its efficacy; CARBONIC ANHYDRASE INHIBITORS, **sodium bicarbonate,** CHRONIC ANTACIDS decrease renal elimination of quinidine, thus increasing its toxicity; **verapamil** causes significant hypotension; may increase hypoprothrombinemic effects of **warfarin. Diltiazem** may increase levels and decrease elimination of quinidine. **Food: Grapefruit juice** (greater than 1 qt/day) may decrease absorption.

PHARMACOKINETICS Absorption: Almost completely from GI tract. **Onset:** 1–3 h. **Peak:** 0.5–1 h. **Duration:** 6–8 h. **Distribution:** Widely distributed to most body tissues except the brain; crosses placenta; distributed into breast milk. **Metabolism:** In liver (CYP3A4). **Elimination:** Greater than 95% in urine, less than 5% in feces. **Half-Life:** 6–8 h.

NURSING IMPLICATIONS

Assessment & Drug Effects

- Observe cardiac monitor and report immediately the following indications for stopping quinidine: (1) Sinus rhythm, (2) widening QRS complex in excess of 25% (i.e., longer than 0.12 sec), (3) changes in QT interval or refractory period, (4) disappearance of P waves, (5) sudden onset of or increase in ectopic ventricular beats (extrasystoles, PVCs), (6) decrease in heart rate to 120 bpm. Also report immediately any worsening of minor side effects.
- Continuous monitoring of ECG and BP is required. Observe patient closely (check sensorium and be alert for any sign of toxicity); determine plasma quinidine concentrations frequently when large doses (more than 2 g/day) are used or when quinidine is given parenterally (i.e., quinidine gluconate).
- Observe patient closely following each parenteral dose. Amount of subsequent dose is gauged by response to preceding dose.
- Monitor vital signs q1–2h or more often as needed during acute treatment. Count apical pulse for a full minute. Report any change in pulse rate, rhythm, or quality or any fall in BP.
- Severe hypotension is most likely to occur in patients receiving high

oral doses or parenteral quinidine (i.e., quinidine gluconate).

- Lab tests: Periodic blood counts, serum electrolyte determinations, and kidney and liver function during long-term therapy. Periodic serum quinidine (target range 2–6 micrograms/mL or higher).
- Monitor I&O. Diarrhea occurs commonly during early therapy; most patients become tolerant to this side effect. Evaluate serum electrolytes, acid-base, and fluid balance when symptoms become severe; dosage adjustment may be required.

Patient & Family Education

- Report feeling of faintness to physician. "Quinidine syncope" is caused by quinidine-induced changes in ventricular rhythm resulting in decreased cardiac output and syncope.
- Do not self-medicate with OTC drugs without advice from physician.
- Do not increase, decrease, skip, or discontinue doses without consulting physician.
- Notify physician immediately of disturbances in vision, ringing in ears, sense of breathlessness, onset of palpitations, and unpleasant sensation in chest. Be sure to note the time of occurrence and duration of chest symptoms.

QUININE SULFATE

(kwye'nine)

Novoquinine ♣

Classification: ANTIMALARIAL

Therapeutic: ANTIMALARIAL

Prototype: Chloroquine

Pregnancy Category: X

AVAILABILITY 325 mg capsules

ACTION & *THERAPEUTIC EFFECT* Inhibits protein synthesis and depresses many enzyme systems in malaria parasite. *Effective against* Plasmodium vivax *and* Plasmodium malariae *but not* Plasmodium falciparum. *Generally replaced by less toxic and more effective agents in treatment of malaria.*

USES Chloroquine-resistant falciparum malaria and in combination with other antimalarials for radical cure of relapsing vivax malaria; also relief of nocturnal recumbency leg cramps.

CONTRAINDICATIONS Hypersensitivity to quinine; tinnitus, optic neuritis; myasthenia gravis; G6PD deficiency; pregnancy (category X).
CAUTIOUS USE Cardiac arrhythmias. Same precautions as for quinidine sulfate when used in patients with cardiovascular conditions; lactation.

ROUTE & DOSAGE

Acute Malaria

Adult: **PO** 650 mg q8h for 3 days
Child: **PO** 25 mg/kg/day in three divided doses q8h for 3 days

Malaria Chemoprophylaxis

Adult: **PO** 325 mg b.i.d. for 6 wk

Nocturnal Leg Cramps

Adult: **PO** 260–300 mg at bedtime

ADMINISTRATION

Oral

- Give with or after meals or a snack to minimize gastric irritation. Quinine has potent local irritant effect on gastric mucosa. Do not crush capsule; drug is not only irritating but also extremely bitter.
- Store in tight, light-resistant containers.

Q

ADVERSE EFFECTS (≥1%) **Body as a Whole:** Cinchonism (tinnitus, decreased auditory acuity, dizziness, vertigo, headache, visual impairment, *nausea, vomiting, diarrhea,* fever); hypersensitivity (cutaneous flushing, visual impairment, pruritus, skin rash, fever, gastric distress, dyspnea, tinnitus); hypothermia, coma. **CNS:** Confusion, excitement, apprehension, syncope, delirium, convulsions, blackwater fever (extensive intravascular hemolysis with renal failure), death. **CV:** Angina, hypotension, tachycardia, cardiovascular collapse. **Hematologic:** Leukopenia, thrombocytopenia, agranulocytosis, hypoprothrombinemia, hemolytic anemia. **Respiratory:** Decreased respiration.

DIAGNOSTIC TEST INTERFERENCE Quinine may interfere with determinations of ***urinary catecholamines*** (***Sobel*** and ***Henry modification procedure***) and ***urinary steroids (17-hydroxycorticosteroids)*** (modification of ***Reddy, Jenkins, Thorn*** method).

INTERACTIONS Drug: May increase **digoxin** levels; ANTICHOLINERGIC AGENTS add to vagolytic effects; CHOLINERGIC AGENTS may antagonize cardiac effects; ANTICONVULSANTS, BARBITURATES, **rifampin** increase the metabolism of quinine, thus decreasing its efficacy; CARBONIC ANHYDRASE INHIBITORS, **sodium bicarbonate,** CHRONIC ANTACIDS decrease renal elimination of quinine, thus increasing its toxicity; **warfarin** may increase hypoprothrombinemic effects. **Amantadine, carbamazepine, phenobarbital** levels may be increased. **Food: Grapefruit juice** (greater than 1 qt/day) may increase plasma concentrations and adverse effects.

PHARMACOKINETICS Absorption: Well from GI tract. **Peak:** 1–3 h. **Duration:** 6–8 h. **Distribution:** Widely distributed to most body tissues except the brain; crosses placenta; distributed into breast milk. **Metabolism:** In liver. **Elimination:** Greater than 95% in urine, less than 5% in feces. **Half-Life:** 8–21 h.

NURSING IMPLICATIONS

Assessment & Drug Effects

- Be alert for S&S of rising plasma concentration of quinine marked by tinnitus and hearing impairment, which usually do not occur until concentration is 10 mcg/mL or more.
- Follow the same precautions with quinine as are used with quinidine in patients with atrial fibrillation; quinine may produce cardiotoxicity in these patients.

Patient & Family Education

- Learn possible adverse reactions and report onset of any unusual symptom promptly to physician.

QUINUPRISTIN/ DALFOPRISTIN

(quin-u-pris′tin/dal′fo-pris-tin)

Synercid

Classifications: STREPTOGRAMIN ANTIBIOTIC; CYCLIC MACROLIDE
Therapeutic: ANTIBIOTIC
Pregnancy Category: B

AVAILABILITY 500 mg vial (150 mg quinupristin/350 mg dalfopristin)

ACTION & *THERAPEUTIC EFFECT* Dalfopristin inhibits the early phase of protein synthesis of bacteria, while quinupristin inhibits the late phase of protein synthesis of bacteria. Both actions lead to death of the bacteria organisms. *Effectiveness indicated by clinical improvement in S&S of life-threatening bacteria. Active against gram-positive pathogens including vancomycin-resistant* Enterococcus faecium *(VREF), as well as some gram-negative anaerobes.*

USES Serious or life-threatening infections associated with VREF bacteremia; complicated skin and skin structure infections caused by *Staphylococcus aureus* or *Streptococcus pyogenes.*

CONTRAINDICATIONS Hypersensitivity to quinupristin/dalfopristin, pristinamycin, other streptogramins; children younger than 16 y.

CAUTIOUS USE Renal or hepatic dysfunction; pregnancy (category B); lactation.

ROUTE & DOSAGE

Vancomycin-Resistant *Enterococcus faecium*

Adult: **IV** 7.5 mg/kg infused over 60 min q8h

Complicated Skin and Skin Structure Infections

Adult: **IV** 7.5 mg/kg infused over 60 min q12h × 7 days

ADMINISTRATION

Intravenous

PREPARE: **Intermittent:** Reconstitute a single 500 mg vial by adding 5 mL D5W or sterile water for injection to yield 100 mg/mL. ▪ Gently swirl to dissolve but do NOT shake. Allow solution to clear. ▪ Withdraw the required dose and further dilute by adding to 100 mL (central line) or 250–500 mL (peripheral site) of D5W.

ADMINISTER: **Intermittent:** Flush line before and after with D5W. Do NOT use saline. ▪ Administer over 1 h.

INCOMPATIBILITIES **Solution/additive:** **Saline solutions** and **lactated Ringer's** solution (flush lines with **D5W** before infusing other drugs). **Y-site:** Any drugs diluted in **saline.**

▪ Refrigerate unopened vials. After reconstitution solution is stable for 5 h at room temperature and 54 h refrigerated.

ADVERSE EFFECTS (≥1%) **Body as a Whole:** Headache, pain, *myalgia, arthralgia.* **GI:** Nausea, diarrhea, vomiting. **Skin:** Rash, pruritus. **Other:** *Inflammation, pain, or edema at infusion site, other infusion site reactions,* thrombophlebitis.

INTERACTIONS Drug: Inhibits CYP3A4 metabolism of **cyclosporine, midazolam, nifedipine,** PROTEASE INHIBITORS, **vincristine, vinblastine, docetaxel, paclitaxel, diazepam, tacrolimus, carbamazepine, quinidine, lidocaine, disopyramide.**

PHARMACOKINETICS Distribution: Moderately protein bound. **Metabolism:** Metabolized to several active metabolites. **Elimination:** Primarily in feces (75–77%). **Half-Life:** 3 h quinupristin, 1 h dalfopristin.

NURSING IMPLICATIONS

Assessment & Drug Effects

- Monitor for S&S of infusion site irritation; change infusion site if irritation is apparent.
- Monitor for cutaneous reaction (e.g., pruritus/erythema of neck, face, upper body).
- Lab tests: C&S from site of infection prior to initiating therapy; WBC with differential; and liver

function (especially with preexisting hepatic insufficiency).

Patient & Family Education

- Report burning, itching, or pain at infusion site to physician.
- Report any sensation of swelling of face and tongue; difficulty swallowing.

RABEPRAZOLE SODIUM

(rab-e-pra′zole)

AcipHex

Classification: PROTON PUMP INHIBITOR
Therapeutic: ANTIULCER
Prototype: Omeprazole
Pregnancy Category: B

AVAILABILITY 20 mg tablets

ACTION & *THERAPEUTIC EFFECT* Gastric proton pump inhibitor that specifically suppresses gastric acid secretion by inhibiting the H^+, K^+-ATPase enzyme system [the acid (proton H^+) pump] in the parietal cells of the stomach. Produces an antisecretory effect on the hydrogen ion (H^+) in the parietal cells. *Effectiveness indicated by a negative urea breath test for* H. pylori *with preexisting gastric ulcer; also by elimination of S&S of GERD or peptic ulcers.*

USES Healing and maintenance of healing of erosive or ulcerative gastroesophageal reflux disease (GERD); healing of duodenal ulcers; treatment of hypersecretory conditions.

CONTRAINDICATIONS Hypersensitivity to rabeprazole, lansoprazole, or omeprazole or proton pump inhibitors (PPIs); lactation.

CAUTIOUS USE Severe hepatic impairment; mild to moderate hepatic disease; Japanese; pregnancy (category B). Safety and efficacy in children younger than 16 y are not established.

ROUTE & DOSAGE

Healing of Erosive GERD
Adult: **PO** 20 mg daily × 48 wk, may continue up to 16 wk if needed
Adolescent: **PO** 20 mg daily for up to 8 wk

Maintenance Therapy for GERD
Adult: **PO** 20 mg daily

Healing Duodenal Ulcer
Adult: **PO** 20 mg daily × 4 wk

Hypersecretory Disease
Adult: **PO** 60 mg daily in 1–2 divided doses (max: 100 mg daily or 60 mg b.i.d.)

ADMINISTRATION

Oral

- Ensure that the tablet is swallowed whole. It should not be crushed or chewed.
- Store at 15°–30° C (59°–86° F).

ADVERSE EFFECTS (≥1%) **Body as a Whole:** Headache. **Skin:** (Rare) Stevens-Johnson syndrome, toxic epidermal necrolysis, erythema multiforme.

INTERACTIONS Drug: May decrease absorption of **ketoconazole;** may increase **digoxin** levels; may decrease **nelfinavir** levels. **Herbal: Ginkgo** may decrease plasma levels.

PHARMACOKINETICS Absorption: 52% bioavailability. **Distribution:** 96% protein bound. **Metabolism:** In liver by (CYP3A4, 2C19). **Elimination:** Primarily in urine. **Half-Life:** 1–2 h.

NURSING IMPLICATIONS

Assessment & Drug Effects

- Lab tests: Periodic LFTs.
- Coadministered drugs: Monitor for changes in digoxin blood level.

Patient & Family Education

- Report diarrhea, skin rash, other bothersome adverse effects to physician.

RALOXIFENE HYDROCHLORIDE

(ra-lox′i-feen)

Evista

Classification: SELECTIVE ESTROGEN RECEPTOR ANTAGONIST/AGONIST

Therapeutic: OSTEOPOROSIS PROPHYLACTIC

Prototype: Tamoxifen

Pregnancy Category: X

AVAILABILITY 60 mg tablets

ACTION & *THERAPEUTIC EFFECT* Tamoxifen analog that exhibits selective estrogen receptor antagonist activity on uterus and breast tissue. Prevents tissue proliferation in both sites. Decreases bone resorption and increases bone density. *Effectiveness indicated by increased bone mineral density. Reduces the risk of invasive breast cancer in high risk postmenopausal women (e.g., breast cancer in situ, or atypical hyperplasia).*

USES Prevention and treatment of osteoporosis in postmenopausal women; breast cancer prophylaxis.

CONTRAINDICATIONS Active thromboembolic event; hypersensitivity to raloxifene; pregnancy (category X), lactation, children.

CAUTIOUS USE Concurrent use of raloxifene and estrogen hormone replacement therapy and lipid-lowering agents; hyperlipidemia; hepatic impairment.

ROUTE & DOSAGE

Prevention/Treatment of Osteoporosis

Adult: **PO** 60 mg daily

Breast Cancer Prophylaxis

Postmenopausal Adult: **PO** 60 mg daily

ADMINISTRATION

Oral

- Calcium and vitamin D supplementation are recommended with raloxifene: 1500 mg/day of elemental calcium and 400–800 units/day of vitamin D.
- Store at 15°–30° C (59°–86° F) in a tightly closed container and protect from light.

ADVERSE EFFECTS (≥1%) **Body as a Whole:** Infection, flu-like syndrome, leg cramps, fever, arthralgia, myalgia, arthritis. **CNS:** Migraine headache, depression, insomnia. **CV:** *Hot flashes*, chest pain, peripheral edema, decreased serum cholesterol. **GI:** Nausea, dyspepsia, vomiting, flatulence, GI disorder, gastroenteritis, weight gain. **Respiratory:** Sinusitis, pharyngitis, cough, pneumonia, laryngitis. **Skin:** Rash, sweating. **Urogenital:** Vaginitis, UTI, cystitis, leukorrhea, endometrial disorder, breast pain, vaginal bleeding.

INTERACTIONS Drug: Use of ESTROGENS not recommended; absorption reduced by **cholestyramine;** use with **warfarin** or other coumarin derivatives may result in changes in prothrombin time (PT). **Herbal: Soy isoflavones** should be used with caution.

PHARMACOKINETICS Absorption: 60% absorbed, absolute bioavailability 2%. **Metabolism:** Extensive first-pass metabolism in liver. **Elimination:** Primarily in feces. **Half-Life:** 27.7–32.5 h.

NURSING IMPLICATIONS

Assessment & Drug Effects

- Lab tests: Periodically monitor LFTs; with concurrent oral anticoagulants, carefully monitor PT and INR.
- Monitor carefully for and immediately report S&S of thromboembolic events.
- Do not give drug concurrently with cholestyramine; however, if unavoidable, space the two drugs as widely as possible.

Patient & Family Education

- Contact physician immediately if unexplained calf pain or tenderness occurs.
- Avoid prolonged restriction of movement during travel.
- Drug does not prevent and may induce hot flashes.
- Do not take drug with other estrogen-containing drugs.
- Raloxifene is normally discontinued 72 h prior to prolonged immobilization (e.g., post-surgical recovery, prolonged bedrest). Consult physician.

R

RALTEGRAVIR

(ral-te-gra′vir)

Isentress

Classifications: ANTIRETROVIRAL; INTEGRASE INHIBITOR

Therapeutic: ANTIRETROVIRAL

Pregnancy Category: C

AVAILABILITY 400 mg tablets

ACTION & *THERAPEUTIC EFFECT* Inhibits HIV-1 integrase, an enzyme required for integration of proviral DNA into the helper T-cell genome, thus preventing formation of the HIV-1 provirus. *Inhibiting integration prevents replication and proliferation of the HIV-1 virus.*

USES In combination with other antiretroviral agents for the treatment of HIV-1 infection in treatment-experienced adult patients who have evidence of viral replication and HIV-1 strains resistant to multiple antiretroviral agents.

CONTRAINDICATIONS Treatment of naïve HIV-1 patients; lactation; children younger than 16 y. Safety and efficacy in patients with severe hepatic impairment are unknown.

CAUTIOUS USE Mild to moderate hepatic impairment; pregnancy (category C).

ROUTE & DOSAGE

HIV-1 Infection

Adult/Adolescent: **PO** 400 mg b.i.d.

HIV Infection (with Concurrent Rifampin)

Adult/Adolescent: **PO** 800 mg b.i.d.

ADMINISTRATION

- May be given without regard to food.
- Give before dialysis.
- Store at 15–30° C (59–86° F).

ADVERSE EFFECTS (≥1%) **Body as a Whole:** Asthenia, fatigue, pyrexia. **CNS:** Dizziness, headache. **GI:** Abdominal pain, *diarrhea*, nausea, vomiting. **Skin:** Lipodystrophy. **Hematologic:** Anemia, neutropenia.

INTERACTIONS Drug: Atazanavir may increase plasma levels of raltegravir; **rifampin** and **tipranavir/ritonavir** may decrease plasma levels of raltegravir.

PHARMACOKINETICS Peak: 3 h. **Distribution:** 83% protein bound.

Metabolism: In the liver. **Elimination:** Stool and urine. **Half-Life:** 9 h.

NURSING IMPLICATIONS

Assessment & Drug Effects

- Monitor for and report S&S of immune reconstitution syndrome (inflammatory response to residual opportunistic infections such as MAC, CMV, PCP, or reactivation of varicella zoster).
- Lab tests: Baseline and periodic CD4+ cell count and HIV RNA viral load; periodic CBC with differential, LFTs.
- Monitor diabetics for loss of glycemic control.

Patient & Family Education

- Inform physician immediately if you plan to become or become pregnant during therapy.
- Report promptly unexplained leg pain or muscle cramping.

RAMELTEON

(ra-mel'tee-on)

Rozerem

Classifications: MELATONIN RECEPTOR AGONIST; SEDATIVE-HYPNOTIC
Therapeutic: SEDATIVE-HYPNOTIC
Pregnancy Category: C

AVAILABILITY 8 mg tablets

ACTION & *THERAPEUTIC EFFECT* Ramelteon is a melatonin receptor agonist with high affinity for melatonin receptors in the brain. This activity is believed to promote sleep, as these receptors, in response to endogenous melatonin, are thought to be involved in maintaining the circadian rhythm underlying the normal sleep-wake cycle. *Effective in promoting onset of sleep.*

USES Treatment of insomnia characterized by difficulty with sleep onset.

CONTRAINDICATIONS Hypersensitivity to ramelteon; severe hepatic function impairment (Child-Pugh class C); severe sleep apnea or severe COPD; concurrent use of alcohol; severe depression; suicidal ideation; lactation.

CAUTIOUS USE Moderate hepatic function impairment (Child-Pugh class B); depression with suicidal tendencies; elderly; pregnancy (category C).

ROUTE & DOSAGE

Insomnia
Adult: **PO** 8 mg within 30 min of bedtime

ADMINISTRATION

Oral

- Give within 30 min of bedtime.
- Do not administer to anyone on concurrent fluvoxamine therapy without alerting physician. This combination causes a dramatic increase in ramelteon blood level.
- Store at 15°–30° C (59°– 86° F).

ADVERSE EFFECTS (≥1%) **CNS:** Depression, dizziness, fatigue, headache, insomnia, somnolence. **GI:** Diarrhea, unpleasant taste, nausea. **Musculoskeletal:** Arthralgia, myalgia. **Respiratory:** Upper respiratory tract infection.

INTERACTIONS Drug: Concurrent use with **ethanol** produces additive CNS depressant effects; **ketoconazole, itraconazole,** and **fluvoxamine** increase ramelteon levels; other CYP1A2 INHIBITORS (e.g., **ciprofloxacin, enoxacin, mexiletine, norfloxacin, tacrine**) may also increase ramelteon levels; **rifampin** decreases ramelteon levels. **Food:** High fat meal, **grapefruit** or **grapefruit juice** increase ramelteon level.

PHARMACOKINETICS Absorption: 84%. **Peak:** 45 min. **Distribution:**

R

82% protein bound. **Metabolism:** Rapid and extensive first pass hepatic metabolism; one metabolite, M-II, is active. **Elimination:** Primarily renal. **Half-Life:** 1–2.5 h.

NURSING IMPLICATIONS

Assessment & Drug Effects

- Monitor for and report worsening insomnia and cognitive or behavioral changes.
- Monitor for S&S of decreased testosterone levels (e.g., loss of libido) or increased prolactin levels (galactorrhea).
- Lab test: Baseline LFTs.

Patient & Family Education

- Do not take with or immediately after a high fat meal.
- Do not drive or engage in potentially hazardous activities until response to drug is known.
- Do not consume alcohol while taking this drug.
- Report any of the following to physician: Worsening insomnia, cognitive or behavioral changes, problem with reproductive function.

RAMIPRIL

(ram'i-pril)

Altace

Classifications: ANGIOTENSIN-CONVERTING ENZYME (ACE) INHIBITOR; ANTIHYPERTENSIVE

Therapeutic: ANTIHYPERTENSIVE

Prototype: Enalapril

Pregnancy Category: C first trimester; D second and third trimester

AVAILABILITY 1.25 mg, 2.5 mg, 5 mg, 10 mg capsules; 1.25 mg, 2.5 mg, 5 mg, 10 mg tablets

ACTION & *THERAPEUTIC EFFECT* Reduces peripheral vascular resistance by inhibiting the formation of angiotensin II, a potent vasoconstrictor. This also decreases serum aldosterone levels and reduces peripheral arterial resistance (afterload) as well as improves cardiac output and exercise tolerance. *Lowers BP, and improves cardiac output as well as exercise tolerance.*

USES Mild to moderate hypertension, CHF, stroke prophylaxis, myocardial infarction prophylaxis, post myocardial infarction.

UNLABELED USES Diabetic nephropathy, proteinuria.

CONTRAINDICATIONS Hypersensitivity to ramipril or any other ACE inhibitor, patients with history of angioneurotic edema; jaundice; hyperkalemia; pregnancy (category D second and third trimester), lactation.

CAUTIOUS USE Impaired kidney or liver function, surgery or anesthesia; CHF; pregnancy (category C first trimester). Safety and effectiveness in children are not established.

ROUTE & DOSAGE

Hypertension, CHF, Stroke Prophylaxis, Myocardial Infarction Prophylaxis

Adult: **PO** 2.5–5 mg daily, may increase up to 20 mg/day in 1–2 divided doses

Post Myocardial Infarction

Adult: **PO** 1.25–2.5 mg b.i.d. (may titrate up to 5 mg b.i.d.)

ADMINISTRATION

Oral

- When patient has been treated with a diuretic, the diuretic is usually discontinued 2–3 days before beginning ramipril. If the diuretic cannot be discontinued, initial ramipril dose is usually lowered to 1.25 mg.
- Store at 15°–30° C (59°–86° F) and protect from moisture.

ADVERSE EFFECTS (≥1%) **CNS:** Dizziness, fatigue, headache. **GI:** Nausea, vomiting, diarrhea, eructation. **Metabolic:** Hyperkalemia, hyponatremia. **Skin:** Erythema, pruritus. **Body as a Whole:** Angioedema. **Respiratory:** Cough.

INTERACTIONS Drug: POTASSIUM-SPARING DIURETICS may increase risk of hyperkalemia. May, elevate, serum **lithium** levels, resulting in lithium toxicity. NSAIDS may attenuate antihypertensive effects. Use with **azathioprine** increases risk of hematologic side effects. **Pregabalin** use increases the risk of angioedema.

PHARMACOKINETICS Absorption: 60% absorbed from GI tract. **Onset:** 2 h. **Peak:** 6–8 h. **Duration:** Up to 24 h. **Distribution:** Crosses placenta; not known if distributed into breast milk. **Metabolism:** Rapidly metabolized in liver to its active metabolite, ramiprilat. **Elimination:** 40–60% in urine, 40% in feces. **Half-Life:** 2–3 h.

NURSING IMPLICATIONS

Assessment & Drug Effects

- Monitor BP at time of peak effectiveness, 3–6 h after dosing and at end of dosing interval just before next dose.
- Report diminished antihypertensive effect.
- Monitor for first-dose hypotension, especially in salt- or volume-depleted persons.
- Lab tests: Monitor BUN and serum creatinine periodically. Increases may necessitate dose reduction or discontinuation of drug. Monitor serum potassium values.
- Observe for S&S of hyperkalemia (see Appendix F).

Patient & Family Education

- Discontinue drug and report S&S of angioedema to physician (e.g., swelling of face or extremities, difficulty breathing or swallowing).
- Maintain adequate fluid intake and avoid potassium supplements or salt substitutes unless specifically prescribed by the physician.
- Light-headedness and dizziness may occur, especially during the initial days of therapy. If fainting occurs, stop taking ramipril until the physician has been consulted.

RANITIDINE HYDROCHLORIDE

(ra-nye'te-deen)

Zantac, Zantac-75

Classification: ANTISECRETORY (H_2-RECEPTOR ANTAGONIST)

Therapeutic: ANTIULCER

Prototype: Cimetidine

Pregnancy Category: B

AVAILABILITY 75 mg, 150 mg, 300 mg tablets; 25 mg, 150 mg effervescent tablets; 150 mg, 300 mg capsules; 15 mg/mL syrup; 1 mg/mL, 25 mg/mL injection

ACTION & *THERAPEUTIC EFFECT* Potent anti-ulcer drug that competitively inhibits histamine action at H_2-receptor sites on parietal cells, blocking gastric acid secretion. Indirectly reduces pepsin secretion. *Blocks daytime and nocturnal basal gastric acid secretion stimulated by histamine and reduces gastric acid release in response to food, caffeine, pentagastrin, and insulin.*

USES Short-term treatment of active duodenal ulcer; maintenance therapy for duodenal ulcer patient after healing of acute ulcer; treatment of gastroesophageal reflux disease; short-term treatment of active, benign gastric ulcer; treatment of pathologic GI hypersecretory conditions (e.g., Zollinger-Ellison syndrome, systemic mastocytosis, and postoperative hypersecretion); heartburn.

CONTRAINDICATIONS Hypersensitivity to ranitidine; acute porphyria; **OTC form:** children younger than 12 y.

CAUTIOUS USE Hypersensitivity to H_2-blockers; hepatic and renal dysfunction; renal failure; elderly; PKU; pregnancy (category B), infants younger than 1 mo, lactation.

ROUTE & DOSAGE

Duodenal Ulcer, Gastric Ulcer, Gastroesophageal Reflux

Adult: **PO** 150 mg b.i.d. or 300 mg at bedtime **IV** 50 mg q6–8h; 150–300 mg/24 h by continuous infusion

Child: **PO** 4–5 mg/kg/day divided q8–12h (max: 300 mg/day) **IM/IV** 2–4 mg/kg/day divided q6–8h (max: 200 mg/day)

Infant (younger than 2 wk): **PO** 1.5–2 mg/kg/day divided q12h **IV** 1.5 mg/kg/day divided q12h or 0.04 mg/kg/h by continuous infusion

Duodenal Ulcer, Maintenance Therapy

Adult: **PO** 150 mg at bedtime

Pathologic Hypersecretory Conditions

Adult: **PO** 150 mg b.i.d. up to 6 g/day **IV** 1 mg/kg/h, adjusted for gastric output

Heartburn

Adult: **PO** 75–150 mg b.i.d.

Renal Impairment Dosage Adjustment

If CrCl less than 50 mL/min, use PO dose q24h, use IV dose q18–24h

Hemodialysis Dosage Adjustment: Time dose to administer at the end of dialysis

R

ADMINISTRATION

Oral

- May be given without regard to meals.
- Effervescent tablets should not be chewed, swallowed whole, or allowed to dissolve on tongue. Dissolve 25 mg tablet in at least 5 mL of water; dissolve 150 mg tablet in 6–8 oz water. Allow tablet to dissolve completely before administration.
- Store tablets in light-resistant, tightly capped container at 15°–30° C (59°–86° F) in a dry place.

Intramuscular

- Note: Does not need to be diluted.

Intravenous

Note: Verify correct IV concentration and rate of infusion for infants and children with physician.

PREPARE: **Direct:** Dilute 50 mg NS, D5W, LR, or other compatible IV solution to a total volume of 20 mL. **Intermittent:** Dilute 50 mg in 50–100 mL of NS, D5W, LR, or other compatible IV solution. **Continuous:** Dilute total daily dose in 250 mL of NS, D5W, LR, or other compatible IV solution. Final concentration should be 2.5 mg/mL or less.

ADMINISTER: **Direct:** Give at a rate of 4 mL/min or 20 mL over not less than 5 min. **Intermittent:** Give over 15–30 min. **Continuous:** Give over 24 h. Do not exceed 6.25 mg/h.

INCOMPATIBILITIES **Solution/additive:** **Amphotericin B, atracurium, cefazolin, cefoxitin, ceftazidime, cefuroxime, clindamycin, chlorpromazine, diazepam, ethacrynic acid,**

hydroxyzine, methotrimeprazine, midazolam, pentobarbital, phenobarbital, phytonadione. Y-site: **Amphotericin B cholesteryl complex, hetastarch in normal saline, insulin.**

- Schedule dose to coincide with end of treatment if patient is having hemodialysis.

ADVERSE EFFECTS (≥1%) **CNS:** Headache, malaise, dizziness, somnolence, insomnia, vertigo, mental confusion, agitation, depression, hallucinations in older adults. **CV:** Bradycardia (with rapid IV push). **GI:** Constipation, nausea, abdominal pain, diarrhea. **Skin:** Rash. **Hematologic:** Reversible decrease in WBC count, thrombocytopenia. **Body as a Whole:** Hypersensitivity reactions, anaphylaxis (rare).

DIAGNOSTIC TEST INTERFERENCE Ranitidine may produce slight elevations in ***serum creatinine*** (without concurrent increase in ***BUN***); (rare) increases in ***AST, ALT, alkaline phosphatase, LDH,*** and total ***bilirubin.*** Produces false-positive tests for ***urine protein*** with ***Multistix*** (use ***sulfosalicylic acid*** instead).

INTERACTIONS Drug: May reduce absorption of **cefpodoxime, cefuroxime, delavirdine, ketoconazole, itraconazole.**

PHARMACOKINETICS Absorption: Incompletely from GI tract (50% reaches systemic circulation). **Peak:** 2–3 h PO. **Duration:** 8–12 h. **Distribution:** Distributed into breast milk. **Metabolism:** In liver. **Elimination:** In urine, with some excreted in feces. **Half-Life:** 2–3 h.

NURSING IMPLICATIONS

Assessment & Drug Effects

- Potential toxicity results from decreased clearance (elimination), which causes prolonged action; greatest risk for toxicity is in older adult patients or those with hepatic or renal dysfunction.
- Lab tests: Periodic liver functions. Monitor creatinine clearance if renal dysfunction is present or suspected.
- Be alert for early signs of hepatotoxicity: Jaundice (dark urine, pruritus, yellow sclera and skin), elevated transaminases (especially ALT) and LDH.
- Long-term therapy may lead to vitamin B_{12} deficiency.

Patient & Family Education

- Note: Long duration of action provides ulcer pain relief that is maintained through the night as well as the day.
- Adhere to scheduled periodic laboratory checkups during ranitidine treatment.
- Do not supplement therapy with OTC remedies for gastric distress or pain without physician's advice.

RANOLAZINE

(ra-no′la-zeen)

Ranexa

Classifications: ANTIANGINAL; PARTIAL FATTY ACID OXIDATION (PFOX) INHIBITOR

Therapeutic: ANTIANGINAL

Pregnancy Category: C

AVAILABILITY 500 mg, 1000 mg extended release tablets

ACTION & *THERAPEUTIC EFFECT* Ranolazine is a partial fatty-acid oxidation inhibitor that shifts myocardial metabolism away from fatty acids to glucose. This shift requires less oxygen for oxidation and results in decreased oxygen demand. *Improves exercise tolerance and angina symptoms.*

R

USES Treatment of chronic stable angina in combination with calcium channel blockers, beta-blockers, or nitrates.

CONTRAINDICATIONS Severe hepatic impairment; severe renal impairment, renal failure, hypokalemia, hypomagnesemia; history of acute MI; lactation; children.
CAUTIOUS USE History of QT prolongation or torsades de pointes; renal impairment; older adult; pregnancy (category C).

ROUTE & DOSAGE

Chronic Stable Angina
Adult: **PO** 500 mg b.i.d. (max: 1000 mg b.i.d.) (patients taking concurrent CYP3A4 inhibitors have a max dose of 500 mg b.i.d.)

ADMINISTRATION

Oral
- **Must be** swallowed whole. Should not be crushed, broken, or chewed.
- Store at 15°–30° C (59°–86° F).

ADVERSE EFFECTS (≥1%) **Body as a Whole:** Peripheral edema. **CNS:** *Dizziness,* headache. **CV:** Palpitations. **GI:** Abdominal pain, *constipation,* dry mouth, nausea, vomiting. **Respiratory:** Dyspnea. **Special Senses:** Tinnitus, vertigo.

DIAGNOSTIC TEST INTERFERENCE Ranolazine is not known to interfere with any diagnostic laboratory test.

INTERACTIONS Drug: INHIBITORS OF P-GLYCOPROTEIN (e.g., **ritonavir, cyclosporine**) may increase ranolazine absorption. Ranolazine increases the plasma concentrations of **digoxin** and **simvastatin.** INHIBITORS OF CYP3A4 [e.g., **diltiazem, erythromycin, grapefruit juice,** HIV PROTEASE INHIBITORS, **ketoconazole,** MACROLIDE ANTIBIOTICS (especially **ketoconazole**), **verapamil**] can increase plasma levels and QT_c elevation. **Paroxetine,** a CYP2D6 INHIBITOR, increases the plasma levels of ranolazine. CLASS I or III ANTIARRHYTHMICS (e.g., **quinidine, dofetilide, sotalol**), **thioridazine,** and **ziprasidone** can cause additive increases in QT_c elevation. **Food: Grapefruit juice**.

PHARMACOKINETICS Absorption: 73% of PO dose absorbed. **Peak:** 2–5 h. **Distribution:** 62% protein bound. **Metabolism:** Extensive hepatic metabolism. **Elimination:** 75% in urine; 25% in feces. **Half-Life:** 7 h.

NURSING IMPLICATIONS

Assessment & Drug Effects
- Monitor ECG at baseline and periodically for prolongation of the QT_c interval.
- Lab tests: Baseline and periodic HbA1c in diabetics.
- Monitor blood levels of digoxin with concurrent therapy.
- When coadministered with simvastatin, monitor for and report unexplained muscle weakness or pain.

Patient & Family Education
- Do not engage in hazardous activities until response to drug is known.
- Contact physician if you experience fainting while taking ranolazine.
- Do not drink grapefruit juice or eat grapefruit while taking this drug.

RASAGILINE
(ras-a-gi'leen)
Azilect
Classifications: MONOAMINE OXIDASE-B (MAO-B) INHIBITOR; ANTIPARKINSON

Therapeutic: ANTIPARKINSON
Pregnancy Category: C

AVAILABILITY 0.5 mg, 1 mg tablets

ACTION & *THERAPEUTIC EFFECT* Rasagiline is a potent monoamine oxidase B (MAO-B) inhibitor that prevents the enzyme monoamine oxidase B from breaking down dopamine in the brain. Rasagiline also interferes with dopamine reuptake at synapses in the brain. *Rasagiline helps to overcome dopaminergic motor dysfunction in Parkinson's disease.*

USES Treatment of Parkinson's disease, either as monotherapy or as an adjunct to levodopa.

CONTRAINDICATIONS Moderate to severe hepatic impairment; alcoholism; biliary cirrhosis; pheocheomocytoma; elective surgery; increased intracranial pressure, cerebrovascular disease, intracranial bleeding, recent head trauma, stroke; controlled hypertension; concurrent use of MAOI therapy or antihypertensive drugs; elective surgery; children.

CAUTIOUS USE Mild hepatic dysfunction; cardiovascular disease; diabetes mellitus; asthma, bronchitis, hyperthyroidism; postural or orthostatic hypotension; migraine headaches; moderate to severe renal impairment, anuria; epilepsy or preexisting seizure disorders; pregnancy (category C), lactation.

ROUTE & DOSAGE

Parkinson's Disease
Adult: **PO** 1 mg/day as monotherapy; 0.5–1 mg/day if adjunctive therapy

Hepatic Impairment Dosage Adjustment
Mild Impairment: 0.5 mg/day

ADMINISTRATION

Oral

- May be given without regard to food.
- Store at 15°–30° C (59°–86° F).

ADVERSE EFFECTS (≥1%) **Body as a Whole:** Accidental injury, allergic reaction, alopecia, gingivitis, hernia, infection, neck pain, pruritus. **CNS:** Abnormal dreams, abnormal gait, amnesia, anxiety, asthenia, ataxia, confusion, depression, dizziness, *dyskinesia,* dystonia, *fall,* fever, flu syndrome, hallucinations, *headache,* hyperkinesias, hypertonia, malaise, neuropathy, neck pain, paresthesia, somnolence, syncope, tremor, vertigo. **CV:** Angina pectoris, <u>bundle branch block</u>, <u>cerebrovascular accident</u>, chest pain, postural hypotension. **GI:** Abdominal pain, anorexia, constipation, diarrhea, dry mouth, dyspepsia, dysphagia, gastroenteritis, GI hemorrhage, *nausea,* vomiting. **Hematologic:** Anemia, hemorrhage. **Metabolic:** Abnormal liver function tests, albuminuria, weight loss. **Musculoskeletal:** Arthralgia, arthritis, bursitis, leg cramps, myasthenia, tenosynovitis. **Respiratory:** Asthma, dyspnea, epistaxis, increased cough, rhinitis. **Skin:** Ecchymosis, eczema, skin carcinoma, skin ulcer, sweating, urticaria, vesiculobullous rash. **Special Senses:** Conjunctivitis. **Urogenital:** Decreased libido, hematuria, impotence, urinary incontinence.

INTERACTIONS Drug: INHIBITORS OF CYP1A2 (e.g., **atazanavir, ciprofloxacin, mexiletine, tacrine**) may increase rasagiline plasma levels. Rasagiline increases the plasma levels of ANESTHETICS; thus it **must be** discontinued 14 days prior to elective surgery. Rasagiline can cause severe CNS toxicity, including hyperpyrexia and death, with ANTIDE-

R

PRESSANTS, SELECTIVE SEROTONIN REUPTAKE INHIBITORS (SSRI), SEROTONIN-NOREPINEPHRINE REUPTAKE INHIBITORS (SNRI), NONSELECTIVE MAO INHIBITORS, or SELECTIVE MAO-B INHIBITORS. Rasagiline can increase the plasma levels of **cyclobenzaprine** and SYMPATHOMIMETIC AMINES. Rasagiline and **dextromethorphan** can cause brief episodes of psychosis and bizarre behavior. Rasagiline can potentiate the dopaminergic effects of **levodopa.** Rasagiline can increase the plasma levels of **meperidine, methadone, propoxyphene,** and **tramadol,** resulting in coma, severe hypertension or hypotension, severe respiratory depression, convulsions, and death. **Herbal:** Rasagiline increases the plasma levels of **St. John's wort.**

PHARMACOKINETICS Absorption: Rapidly absorbed with 36% bioavailability. **Peak:** 1 h. **Distribution:** 88–94% protein bound. **Metabolism:** Extensive hepatic metabolism. **Elimination:** Primarily renal (62%) with minor fecal elimination. **Half-Life:** 3 h.

NURSING IMPLICATIONS

Assessment & Drug Effects

- Monitor for and report S&S of dopaminergic side effects (e.g., dyskinesia, hallucinations, etc.) with concurrent levodopa.
- Monitor for and report suspicious skin changes suggestive of melanoma or other skin cancers.
- Lab tests: Baseline and periodic LTFs; periodic renal function tests, CBC with Hct and Hgb.
- Note all contraindicated drugs and drug groups and exercise caution not to administer a contraindicated substance.
- Note all drug interactions and monitor for the indicated effects.

Patient & Family Education

- Do not take any prescription or nonprescription drug without consulting physician.
- Periodic skin examinations should be scheduled with a dermatologist. If you notice changes in a skin mole or new skin lesion, contact the dermatologist.
- Avoid foods and beverages containing tyramine (e.g., aged cheeses and meats, tap beer, red wine, soybean products).
- Make position changes slowly, especially when standing from a lying or sitting position.
- Do not drive or engage in potentially hazardous activities until response to drug is known.
- Report immediately any of the following to a health care provider: Palpitations, severe headache, blurred vision, difficulty thinking, seizures, chest pain, unexplained nausea or vomiting, or any sudden weakness or paralysis.

RASBURICASE

(ras-bur'i-case)

Elitek, Fasturtec ♣

Classifications: ANTIGOUT; ANTIMETABOLITE

Therapeutic: ANTIGOUT

Pregnancy Category: C

AVAILABILITY 1.5 mg/vial powder for injection

ACTION & *THERAPEUTIC EFFECT* A recombinant urate-oxidase enzyme produced by DNA technology. In humans, uric acid is the final step in the catabolic pathway of purines. Rasburicase catalyzes enzymatic oxidation of uric acid; thus it is only active at the end of the purine catabolic pathway. *Used to manage plasma uric acid levels in pediatric* *patients with leukemia, lymphoma, and solid tumor malignancies who are receiving anticancer therapy that results in tumor lysis, and therefore elevates plasma uric acid.*

USES Initial management of increased uric acid levels secondary to tumor lysis.

CONTRAINDICATIONS Hypersensitivity to rasburicase; deficiency in glucose-6-phosphate dehydrogenase (G6PD); history of anaphylaxis; hemolytic reactions or methemoglobinemia reactions to rasburicase; lactation, children younger than 1 mo.
CAUTIOUS USE Patients at risk for G6PD deficiency (e.g., African or Mediterranean ancestry); asthma; bone marrow suppression, pregnancy (category C). Safety and efficacy in adults and elderly are unknown.

ROUTE & DOSAGE

Hyperuricemia
Child (older than 1 mo): **IV** 0.15–0.2 mg/kg/day × 5 days starting 4–24 h before chemotherapy

ADMINISTRATION

Intravenous

PREPARE: **IV Infusion:** Reconstitute each 1.5 mg vial with 1 mL of the provided diluent and mix by swirling very gently. **Do not shake.** Discard if particulate matter is visible or if product is discolored after reconstitution. ▪ Remove the predetermined dose from the reconstituted vials and inject into enough NS in an infusion bag to achieve a final total volume of 50 mL.

ADMINISTER: **IV Infusion:** Give over 30 min. **DO NOT GIVE BOLUS DOSE.** Infuse through an **unfiltered** line used for no other medications. ▪ If a separate line is not possible, flush the line with at least 15 mL of saline solution before/after infusion of rasburicase.

▪ Immediately discontinue IV infusion and institute emergency measures for S&S of anaphylaxis including chest pain, dyspnea, hypotension, and/or urticaria.

INCOMPATIBILITIES Do not mix or infuse with other drugs.

ADVERSE EFFECTS (≥1%) **Body as a Whole:** *Fever,* sepsis, severe hypersensitivity reactions including anaphylaxis at any time during treatment. **CNS:** *Headache.* **GI:** *Mucositis, vomiting, nausea, diarrhea, abdominal pain.* **Hematologic:** Neutropenia. **Skin:** *Rash.*

DIAGNOSTIC TEST INTERFERENCE May give false elevations for ***uric acid*** if blood sample is left at room temperature.

PHARMACOKINETICS Half-Life: 18 h.

NURSING IMPLICATIONS

Assessment & Drug Effects

- Lab tests: Patients at higher risk for G6PD deficiency (e.g., patients of African or Mediterranean ancestry) should be screened prior to starting therapy as this deficiency is a contraindication for this drug.
- Monitor closely for S&S of hypersensitivity and be prepared to institute emergency measures for anaphylaxis.
- Monitor cardiovascular, respiratory, neurologic, and renal status throughout therapy.

Patient & Family Education

- Report immediately any distressing S&S to physician.

R

REMIFENTANIL HYDROCHLORIDE

(rem-i-fent'a-nil)

Ultiva

Classifications: ANALGESIC, NARCOTIC (OPIATE AGONIST); GENERAL ANESTHESIA

Therapeutic: NARCOTIC ANALGESIC; GENERAL ANESTHESIA

Prototype: Morphine

Pregnancy Category: C

Controlled Substance: Schedule II

AVAILABILITY 1 mg/mL, 2 mg/mL, 5 mg/mL injection

ACTION & *THERAPEUTIC EFFECT* Synthetic, potent narcotic agonist analgesic that is rapidly metabolized; therefore respiratory depression is of shorter duration when discontinued. *Used as the analgesic component of an anesthesia regime.*

USES Analgesic during induction and maintenance of general anesthesia, as the analgesic component of monitored anesthesia care.

CONTRAINDICATIONS Hypersensitivity to fentanyl analogs, epidural or intrathecal administration.

CAUTIOUS USE Head injuries, increased intracranial pressure; older adults, debilitated, morbid obesity, poor-risk patients; COPD, other respiratory problems, bradyarrhythmia; pregnancy (category C), lactation. Safety in labor and delivery has not been demonstrated.

ROUTE & DOSAGE

Adjunct to Anesthesia

Adult: **IV** 0.5–1 mcg/kg/min or 1 mcg/kg bolus

Child: **IV** *Birth–2 mo,* 0.4–1 mcg/kg/min; *1–12 y,* 0.5–1 mcg/kg/min or 1 mcg/kg bolus

Obesity Dosage Adjustment

Dose based on IBW

ADMINISTRATION

Intravenous

IV administration to infants and children: Verify correct IV concentration and rate of infusion with physician.

PREPARE: **Direct/Continuous Infusion:** Reconstitute by adding 1 mL of sterile water for injection, D5W, NS, D5NS, 1/2NS, or D5LR to each 1 mg of remifentanil to yield 1 mg/mL. Shake well to dissolve. ▪ Further dilute to a final concentration of 20, 25, 50, or 250 mcg/mL by adding the required dose to the appropriate amount of IV solution.

ADMINISTER: **Direct/Continuous Infusion:** Give at the ordered rate according to patient's weight. ▪ Note that bolus doses should NOT be given during a continuous infusion of remifentanil. ▪ Flush IV tubing thoroughly following infusion.

INCOMPATIBILITIES **Solution/additive:** Unknown. **Y-site:** **Amphotericin B, amphotericin B cholesteryl, cefoperazone, chlorpromazine, diazepam.**

▪ Clear IV tubing completely of the drug following discontinuation of remifentanil infusion to ensure that inadvertent administration of the drug will not occur at a later time. ▪ Reconstituted solution is stable for 24 h at room temperature. Store vials of powder at 2°–25° C (36°–77° F).

ADVERSE EFFECTS (≥1%) **Body as a Whole:** Muscle rigidity, shivering. **CNS:** Dizziness, headache. **CV:** Hypotension, hypertension, bradycardia. **GI:** *Nausea*, vomiting. **Respira-**

tory: Respiratory depression, apnea. **Skin:** Pruritus.

INTERACTIONS Drug: Alcohol and other CNS DEPRESSANTS potentiate effects; MAO INHIBITORS may precipitate hypertensive crisis.

PHARMACOKINETICS Duration: 12 min. **Distribution:** 70% protein bound. **Metabolism:** Hydrolyzed by nonspecific esterases in the blood and tissues. **Elimination:** In urine. **Half-Life:** 3–10 min.

NURSING IMPLICATIONS

Assessment & Drug Effects

- Monitor vital signs during postoperative period; observe for and immediately report any S&S of respiratory distress or respiratory depression, or skeletal and thoracic muscle rigidity and weakness.
- Monitor for adequate postoperative analgesia.

REPAGLINIDE Pr

(rep-a-gli′nide)

Prandin, GlucoNorm ♣

Classifications: ANTIDIABETIC; MEGLITINIDE

Therapeutic: ANTIHYPERGLYCEMIC

Pregnancy Category: C

AVAILABILITY 0.5 mg, 1 mg, 2 mg tablets

ACTION & *THERAPEUTIC EFFECT* Hypoglycemic agent that lowers blood glucose levels by stimulating release of insulin from the pancreatic islets. *Significantly reduces postprandial blood glucose in type 2 diabetes [preprandial blood glucose between 80 and 120 mg/dL and HbA1C (glycosylated Hgb less than 6.5%)]. Minimal effects on fasting blood glucose.*

USES Adjunct to diet and exercise in type 2 diabetes. May also be used in combination with metformin.

CONTRAINDICATIONS Hypersensitivity to repaglinide; insulin-dependent diabetes, diabetic ketoacidosis, lactation; children.

CAUTIOUS USE Hypoglycemia; loss of glycemic control due to secondary failure; hepatic impairment; severe renal impairment; older adults, surgery, fever, systemic infection, trauma; pregnancy (category C).

ROUTE & DOSAGE

Type 2 Diabetes

Adult: **PO** Initial dose: 0.5 mg 15–30 min a.c.; initial dose for patients previously using glucose-lowering agents: 1–2 mg 15–30 min a.c. (2–4 doses/day depending on meal pattern; max: 16 mg/day); dosage range: 0.5–4 mg 15–30 min a.c.

ADMINISTRATION

Oral

- Give within 30 min of beginning a meal.
- Store at 15°–30° C (59°–86° F) in a tightly closed container and protect from moisture.

ADVERSE EFFECTS (≥1%) **Body as a Whole:** Arthralgia, back pain, paresthesia, allergy. **CNS:** Headache. **CV:** Chest pain, angina. **GI:** Nausea, diarrhea, constipation, vomiting, dyspepsia. **Respiratory:** URI, sinusitis, rhinitis, bronchitis. **Metabolic:** *Hypoglycemia.*

INTERACTIONS Drug: Erythromycin, ketoconazole may inhibit metabolism and potentiate hypoglycemia; BARBITURATES, **carbamazepine, rifabutin, rifampin,**

R

rifapentine, pioglitazone may induce metabolism and cause hyperglycemia; **gemfibrozil** may increase risk of hypoglycemia and duration of action. **Herbal: Ginseng, garlic** may increase hypoglycemic effects. **Food: Grapefruit juice** (greater than 1 qt/day) may increase plasma concentrations and adverse effects.

PHARMACOKINETICS Absorption: Rapidly from GI tract, 56% bioavailability. **Peak:** 1 h. **Distribution:** 98% protein bound. **Metabolism:** In liver (CYP3A4). **Elimination:** 90% in feces. **Half-Life:** 1 h.

NURSING IMPLICATIONS

Assessment & Drug Effects

- Lab tests: Frequent FBS and postprandial blood glucose monitoring and HbA1C q3mo to determine effective dose.
- Monitor carefully for S&S of hypoglycemia especially during the 1-wk period following transfer from a longer-acting sulfonylurea.

Patient & Family Education

- Take only with meals to lessen the chance of hypoglycemia. If a meal is skipped, skip a dose; if a meal is added, add a dose.
- Start repaglinide the morning after the other agent is stopped when changing from another oral hypoglycemia drug.
- Be alert for S&S of hyperglycemia or hypoglycemia (see Appendix F); report poor blood glucose control to physician.

RESERPINE Pr

(re-ser′peen)

Serpalan, Sk-Reserpine

Classifications: RAUWOLFIA ALKALOID; ANTIHYPERTENSIVE

Therapeutic: ANTIHYPERTENSIVE

Pregnancy Category: D

AVAILABILITY 0.1 mg, 0.25 mg tablets

ACTION & *THERAPEUTIC EFFECT* Interferes with binding of serotonin at receptor sites, decreases synthesis of norepinephrine by depleting dopamine (its precursor), and competitively inhibits their reuptake in storage granules. Depletes norepinephrine and serotonin in CNS, peripheral nervous system, heart, and other organs and tissues. *Sympathetic inhibition seen in small but persistent decrease in BP, frequently associated with bradycardia, and reduced cardiac output.*

USES Mild essential hypertension and as adjunctive therapy with other antihypertensive agents in the more severe forms of hypertension. Also used in agitated psychotic states, primarily in patients intolerant to phenothiazine or patients who also require antihypertensive medication.

UNLABELED USES Reduce vasospastic attacks in Raynaud's phenomenon and other peripheral vascular disorders, and for short-term symptomatic treatment of thyrotoxicosis.

CONTRAINDICATIONS Hypersensitivity to rauwolfia alkaloids; history of mental depression; acute peptic ulcer, ulcerative colitis; patients receiving electroconvulsive therapy; within 7–14 days of MAO inhibitor therapy; pregnancy (category D), lactation. Safe use in children is not established.

CAUTIOUS USE Renal insufficiency; cardiac arrhythmias; cardiac damage; cerebrovascular accident; history of peptic ulcers; epilepsy; bronchitis, asthma; older adults, de-

R

bilitated patients; gallstones; obesity; chronic sinusitis; parkinsonism; pheochromocytoma.

ROUTE & DOSAGE

Hypertension

Adult: **PO** 0.5 mg/day initially, reduced to 0.1–0.25 mg/day
Geriatric: **PO** Start with 0.05 mg daily, increase by 0.05 mg/wk

ADMINISTRATION

Oral

- Give with meals or with milk or other food to minimize possibility of gastric irritation (drug increases gastric secretions).
- Store in tight, light-resistant containers, preferably at 15°–30° C (59°–86° F), unless otherwise directed by manufacturer.

ADVERSE EFFECTS (≥1%) **CNS:** *Drowsiness,* sedation, *lethargy,* mental depression, nervousness, anxiety, nightmares, increased dreaming, headache, dizziness, increased appetite, dull sensorium; prolonged use of large doses: CNS stimulation (parkinsonian syndrome): Tremors, muscle rigidity; <u>respiratory depression</u>, convulsions, hypothermia. **CV:** Bradycardia, *edema,* orthostatic hypotension, increased AV conduction time (prolonged therapy); angina-like symptoms, arrhythmias, CHF (rare). **Special Senses:** *Nasal congestion,* epistaxis, lacrimation, blurred vision; miosis, ptosis, conjunctival congestion (acute toxicity). **GI:** Dry mouth or excessive salivation, nausea, vomiting, abdominal cramps, diarrhea, reactivation of peptic ulcer (hypersecretion), heartburn, biliary colic. **Hematologic:** Thrombocytopenic purpura, anemia, prolonged BT. **Body as a Whole:** Hypersensitivity (pruritus, rash, asthma), muscle aches, dysuria, fixed-drug eruptions. **Urogenital:** Menstrual irregularities, breast engorgement, galactorrhea, gynecomastia, feminization (males), impaired sexual function, impotence.

DIAGNOSTIC TEST INTERFERENCE Possibility of elevated ***blood glucose*** values; however, it is also reported that reserpine may decrease thiazide-induced hyperglycemia. Increase in ***serum prolactin*** with chronic administration of ***rauwolfia*** alkaloids; overdoses may cause initial increase in excretion of ***urinary catecholamines;*** decreases with chronic administration. Large doses may cause initial rise in ***urinary 5 HIAA*** excretion. Initial IM doses may increase ***urinary VMA*** excretion followed by decrease by end of third day of therapy (with oral or parenteral administration). Possible interference with ***urinary steroid*** colorimetric determinations: ***17-OHCS*** and ***17-KS.***

INTERACTIONS Drug: Diuretics, other HYPOTENSIVE AGENTS compound hypotensive effects; CARDIAC GLYCOSIDES (**digoxin**) may increase risk of arrhythmias; MAO INHIBITORS may cause excitation and hypertension; CNS DEPRESSANTS compound depression; may decrease response to **levodopa. Herbal: St. John's wort** may antagonize hypotensive effects.

PHARMACOKINETICS Peak: 2 h. **Distribution:** Widely distributed, especially to adipose tissue; crosses blood–brain barrier and placenta; distributed in breast milk. **Metabolism:** Extensively metabolized to inactive compounds. **Elimination:** Slowly excreted, 60% in feces within 96 h and 10% in urine. **Half-Life:** 4.5 and 11.3 h.

R

NURSING IMPLICATIONS

Assessment & Drug Effects

- Assess vital signs at frequent intervals. (Note: Drop in BP may be accompanied by bradycardia.)
- Lab tests: Periodic CBC with differential, platelet count, serum electrolytes, and plasma glucose.
- Supervise ambulation as indicated; postural hypotension occurs more frequently in elderly patients.
- Monitor I&O, especially in patients with impaired kidney function. Report changes in I&O ratio and pattern.
- Full therapeutic effect of oral drug for hypertension may not occur until 2–3 wk of therapy, and effects may persist for as long as 4–6 wk after drug is discontinued.
- Be aware that mental depression is a serious adverse effect and may be severe. It occurs most commonly in high dosage regimens (e.g., 0.5–1 mg/day or more) and may not appear until 2–8 mo of therapy and may last for several months after drug is withdrawn.

Patient & Family Education

- Take drug at the same time each day, do not skip or double doses, and do not stop therapy without advice of physician.
- Do not drive or engage in potentially hazardous activities until response to drug is known.
- Learn about possible adverse effects and report promptly to physician.
- Report the following possible beginning symptoms of depression: Early morning insomnia, anorexia, inability to concentrate, despondency, self-deprecation, attitude of detachment, mood swings, or impotence.
- Make position changes slowly, particularly from recumbent to upright posture, and lie down or sit down (head-low position) if patient feels faint. Do not take hot showers or hot tub baths, and do not to stand still for prolonged periods. Report symptoms of dizziness or lightheadedness to physician.
- Check for edema and record weight daily. Consult physician about gain of 1–2 kg (3–5 lb) in 1 wk.
- Do not take OTC medications without consulting physician or pharmacist (many preparations for coughs and colds contain agents that affect the actions of reserpine).

R

RESPIRATORY SYNCYTIAL VIRUS IMMUNE GLOBULIN (RSV-IVIG)

(res-pir'a-tory sin-cy'ti-al)

RespiGam

Classifications: BIOLOGICAL RESPONSE MODIFIER; IMMUNOGLOBULIN (IgG)

Therapeutic: IMMUNOGLOBULIN

Prototype: Immune globulin

Pregnancy Category: C

AVAILABILITY 2500 mg/50 mL vial

ACTION & *THERAPEUTIC EFFECT* Contains IgG immune globulin antibodies from human plasma. *The preparation contains large amounts of RSV-neutralizing antibodies.*

USES Prevention of serious lower respiratory tract infection caused by RSV in children younger than 24 mo with bronchopulmonary dysplasia or history of premature birth; hypervolemia.

CONTRAINDICATIONS Previous severe reaction to RespiGam or other human immunoglobulin preparation, selective IgA deficiency; congenital heart disease, fluid overload; hepatic disease; lactation.

CAUTIOUS USE Immunodeficiency, AIDS, pulmonary disease; CHF; renal failure; pregnancy (category C).

ROUTE & DOSAGE

RSV

Child/Infant/Neonate: **IV** 750 mg/kg, may repeat monthly as needed

ADMINISTRATION

Intravenous

PREPARE: **IV Infusion:** Give undiluted. Do not shake vial.

ADMINISTER: **IV Infusion:** Infuse at 1.5 mL/kg/h for first 15 min, then 3 mL/kg/h for next 15 min, then 6 mL/kg/h for rest of infusion. Infuse vial contents undiluted through a separate IV line if possible; if "piggyback" **must be** used, see manufacturer's directions. DO NOT EXCEED IV INFUSION RATES given in Route & Dosage table! ▪ Use a constant infusion pump.

INCOMPATIBILITIES **Solution/additive or Y-site:** Do not mix with other drugs.

- Store vials at 2°–8° C (35°–46° F). Begin infusion within 6 h after vial is entered and complete within 12 h.

ADVERSE EFFECTS (≥1%) **Body as a Whole:** Fever, pyrexia, fluid overload. **CV:** Tachycardia, hypertension. **GI:** Vomiting, diarrhea, gastroenteritis. **Respiratory:** Respiratory distress, wheezing, rales, hypoxia, hypoxemia, tachypnea. **Skin:** Injection site inflammation.

INTERACTIONS Drug: May interfere with immune response to LIVE VIRUS VACCINES (mumps, rubella, measles), may need to repeat vaccine if given within 10 mo of RespiGam.

PHARMACOKINETICS Half-Life: 22–28 days.

NURSING IMPLICATIONS

Assessment & Drug Effects

- Monitor closely during and after each IV rate change.
- Assess vital signs and respiratory status prior to infusion, during and after each rate change, and at 30-min intervals until 30 min after infusion is completed, and periodically thereafter for 24 h.
- Slow infusion immediately if S&S of fluid overload appear and report to physician.
- Lab tests: Monitor routine blood chemistry, serum electrolytes, blood gases, osmolality.
- Monitor for aseptic meningitis syndrome, which may begin up to 2 days after infusion.

Patient & Family Education

- Be aware of the possibility of aseptic meningitis syndrome; learn S&S to report (headache, drowsiness, fever, photophobia, painful eye movements, muscle rigidity, nausea, vomiting).

RETAPAMULIN

Altabax

Classifications: ANTIBIOTIC; PLEUROMUTILIN

Therapeutic: TOPICAL ANTIBIOTIC

Pregnancy Category: B

AVAILABILITY 1% (10 mg/g) topical ointment

ACTION & *THERAPEUTIC EFFECT* Selectively inhibits bacterial protein synthesis at a site on the 50S subunit of the bacterial ribosome. *Effective against* Staphylococcus *(MRSA) and* Streptococcus *organisms.*

USES Topical treatment of impetigo due to susceptible stains of *Staphylococcus aureus* (methicillin-sensitive strains only) or *Streptococcus*

R

pyogenes in patients 9 mo of age or older.

CONTRAINDICATIONS Hypersensitivity to retapamulin; children less than 9 mo.
CAUTIOUS USE Pregnancy (category B); lactation.

ROUTE & DOSAGE

Impetigo Infection
Adult/Child/Infant (9 mo or older): Apply in thin layer b.i.d. × 5 days

ADMINISTRATION

Topical
- Apply a thin layer to infected region. May cover with gauze dressing.
- Store at 15°–30° C (59°–86° F).

ADVERSE EFFECTS (≥1%) **Body as a Whole:** Application-site irritation, pyrexia. **CNS:** Headache. **GI:** Diarrhea, nausea. **Metabolic:** Creatinine phosphokinase increased. **Respiratory:** Nasopharyngitis. **Skin:** Eczema, pruritus.

PHARMACOKINETICS Absorption: Minimal systemic absorption. **Metabolism:** In liver.

R

NURSING IMPLICATIONS

Assessment & Drug Effects
- Monitor for excessive skin irritation. Report swelling, blistering, or oozing.

Patient & Family Education
- Report any of the following at application site: Redness, itching, burning, swelling, blistering, or oozing.

RETEPLASE RECOMBINANT

(re′te-plase)

Retavase
Classification: THROMBOLYTIC ENZYME, TISSUE PLASMINOGEN ACTIVATOR (t-PA)
Therapeutic: THROMBOLYTIC
Prototype: Alteplase
Pregnancy Category: C

AVAILABILITY 10.4 international unit vials

ACTION & *THERAPEUTIC EFFECT* DNA recombinant human tissue-type plasminogen activator (t-PA) that acts as a catalyst in the cleavage of plasminogen to plasmin. Responsible for degrading the fibrin matrix of a clot. *Has antithrombolytic properties.*

USES Thrombolysis management of acute MI to reduce the incidence of CHF and mortality.

CONTRAINDICATIONS Active internal bleeding, history of CVA, recent neurologic surgery or trauma, intercranial neoplasm, or aneurysm, bleeding disorders, severe uncontrolled hypertension.
CAUTIOUS USE Any condition in which bleeding constitutes a significant hazard (i.e., severe hepatic or renal disease, CVA, hypertension, acute pancreatitis, septic thrombophlebitis); pregnancy (category C), lactation. Safety and efficacy in children are not established.

ROUTE & DOSAGE

Thrombolysis during Acute MI
Adult: **IV** 10 units injected over 2 min. Repeat dose in 30 min (20 units total).

ADMINISTRATION

Intravenous

PREPARE: **Direct:** Reconstitute using only the diluent, syringe, needle, and dispensing pin provided with reteplase. ▪ Withdraw diluent with syringe provided. Remove needle from syringe, replace with dispensing pin and transfer diluent to vial of reteplase. Leave pin and syringe in place in vial and swirl to dissolve. Do NOT shake. ▪ When completely dissolved, remove 10 mL solution, replace dispensing pin with a 20-gauge needle.

ADMINISTER: **Direct:** Flush IV line before and after with 30 mL NS or D5W and do NOT give any other drug simultaneously through the same IV line. ▪ Give a single dose evenly over 2 min.

INCOMPATIBILITIES **Solution/additive: Heparin. Y-site: Bivalirudin, heparin.**

▪ Store drug kit unopened at 2°–25° C (36°–77° F).

ADVERSE EFFECTS (≥1%) **Hematologic:** *Hemorrhage* (including *intracranial*, GI, genitourinary), anemia. **CV:** Reperfusion arrhythmias.

DIAGNOSTIC TEST INTERFERENCE Causes decreases in plasminogen and fibrinogen, making ***coagulation*** and ***fibrinolytic*** tests unreliable.

INTERACTIONS Drug: Aspirin, abciximab, dipyridamole, heparin may increase risk of bleeding.

PHARMACOKINETICS Elimination: In urine. **Half-Life:** 13–16 min.

NURSING IMPLICATIONS

Assessment & Drug Effects

- Discontinue concomitant heparin immediately if serious bleeding not controllable by local pressure occurs and, if not already given, withhold the second reteplase bolus.
- Monitor carefully all potential bleeding sites; monitor for S&S of internal hemorrhage (e.g., GI, GU, intracranial, retroperitoneal, pulmonary).
- Monitor carefully cardiac status for arrhythmias associated with reperfusion.
- Avoid invasive procedures, arterial and venous punctures, IM injections, and nonessential handling of the patient during reteplase therapy.

Patient & Family Education

- Report changes in consciousness or signs of bleeding to physician immediately.

RH_0(D) IMMUNE GLOBULIN

(row)

RhoGAM, Rhophylac, WinRho SDF

RH_0(D) IMMUNE GLOBULIN MICRO-DOSE

BayRho-D Mini Dose, MICRhoGAM

Classifications: BIOLOGICAL RESPONSE MODIFIER; IMMUNOGLOBULIN (IgG)

Therapeutic: IMMUNOGLOBULIN

Prototype: Immune globulin

Pregnancy Category: C

AVAILABILITY RhoGAM, MICRhoGAM: 5% solution in prefilled syringes; **Rhophylac:** 300 mcg prefilled syringe; **WinRho SDF:** 120 mcg, 300 mcg, 1000 mcg vials

ACTION & *THERAPEUTIC EFFECT* Sterile nonpyrogenic gamma globulin solution containing immunoglobulins (IgG), which provides passive immunity by suppressing active antibody response and formation of anti-Rh_0(D) in Rh-negative [Rh_0(D)-negative] individuals previously exposed to Rh-positive

[$Rh_0(D)$-positive, D^u-positive] blood. *Effective for exposure in Rh-negative women when Rh-positive fetal RBCs enter maternal circulation during third stage of labor, fetal-maternal hemorrhage (as early as second trimester), amniocentesis, or other trauma during pregnancy, termination of pregnancy, and following transfusion with Rh-positive RBC, whole blood, or components (platelets, WBC) prepared from Rh-positive blood.*

USES To prevent isoimmunization in Rh-negative individuals exposed to Rh-positive RBC (see above). $Rh_0(D)$ immune globulin microdose is for use only after spontaneous or induced abortion or termination of ectopic pregnancy up to and including 12 wk of gestation. Treatment of idiopathic thrombocytopenia purpura.

CONTRAINDICATIONS $Rh_0(D)$-positive patient; person previously immunized against $Rh_0(D)$ factor, severe immune globulin hypersensitivity, bleeding disorders; neonates.

CAUTIOUS USE IgA deficiency; pregnancy (category C).

R

ROUTE & DOSAGE

Note: Only WinRho SDF and Rhophylac can be given IV. BayRho-D and RhoGAM are available in regular and mini-dose vials.

Antepartum Prophylaxis

Adult: **IM/IV** 300 mcg at approximately 28-wk gestation; followed by 1 vial of mini-dose or 120 mcg within 72 h of delivery if infant is Rh-positive

Postpartum Prophylaxis

Adult: **IM/IV** 300 mcg preferably within 72 h of delivery if infant is Rh-positive

Following Amniocentesis, Miscarriage, Abortion, Ectopic Pregnancy

Adult: **IM** If over 13-wk gestation, 300 mcg, preferably within 3 h but at least within 72 h; if less than 13 wk, give 50 mcg

Transfusion Accident

Adult: **IM/IV** 300 mcg for each volume of RBCs infused divided by 15, given within at least 72 h of accident
Child: **IV** Administer 600 mcg q8h until total dose given. Exposure to positive whole blood 9 mcg/mL, exposure to positive RBCs 18 mcg/mL. **IM** Administer 1200 mcg q12h until total dose given. Exposure to positive whole blood 12 mcg/mL, exposure to positive RBCs 24 mcg/mL.

Idiopathic Thrombocytopenia Purpura

Adult/Child: **IV** 50 mcg/kg, then 25–60 mcg/kg depending on response

ADMINISTRATION

- BayRho-D (HyperRHO S/D), MIC-RhoGam, and RhoGAM are administered by IM route only. NEVER give IV.
- WinRho SDF and Rhophylac may be given IM or IV depending on the indication.

Intramuscular

- Use the deltoid muscle. Give in divided doses at different sites, all at once or at intervals, as long as the entire dose is given within 72 h after delivery or termination of pregnancy.

- Reconstitute lyophilized powder with 1.25 mL of NS (using the same method to dissolve as for IV). Give immediately after reconstitution.
- Observe patient closely for at least 20 min after administration. Keep epinephrine immediately available; systemic allergic reactions sometimes occur.

Intravenous

PREPARE: **Direct:** No dilution is required for products supplied in liquid form. ▪ Reconstitute lyophilized powder vials according to specific manufacturer's directions. ▪ WinRho SDF: Remove entire contents of vial to obtain the labeled dosage. If partial vial is needed for dosage calculation, withdraw the entire contents to ensure accurate calculation of dosage requirement. ▪ Rhophylac: Bring to room temperature before use.

ADMINISTER: **Direct:** Rhophylac: Give at a rate of 2 mL per 15–60 sec for ITP. ▪ WinRho SDF: Give over 3–5 min.

▪ Refrigerate commercially prepared solutions, although it may remain stable up to 30 days at room temperature according to manufacturer. ▪ Discard solutions that have been frozen. ▪ Store powder at 2°–8° C (36°–46° F) unless otherwise directed; avoid freezing.

ADVERSE EFFECTS (≥1%) **Body as a Whole:** Injection site irritation, slight fever, myalgia, lethargy.

INTERACTIONS Drug: May interfere with immune response to LIVE VIRUS VACCINE; should delay use of LIVE VIRUS VACCINES for 3 mo after administration of $Rh_0(D)$ immune globulin.

PHARMACOKINETICS Peak: 2 h IV, 5–10 days IM. **Half-Life:** 25 days.

NURSING IMPLICATIONS

Assessment & Drug Effects

- Obtain history of systemic allergic reactions to human immune globulin preparations prior to drug administration.
- Send sample of newborn's cord blood to laboratory for cross-match and typing immediately after delivery and before administration of $Rh_0(D)$ immune globulin. Confirm that mother is $Rh_0(D)$ and D^u-negative. Infant **must be** Rh-positive.

Patient & Family Education

- Be aware that administration of $Rh_0(D)$ immune globulin (antibody) prevents hemolytic disease of the newborn in a subsequent pregnancy.

RIBAVIRIN

(rye-ba-vye′rin)

Virazole, Rebetol, Copegus, Ribasphere

Classification: ANTIVIRAL
Therapeutic: ANTIVIRAL
Prototype: Acyclovir
Pregnancy Category: X

AVAILABILITY 6 g vial for nebulizer; 200 mg tablets; 200 mg capsules; 40 mg/mL oral solution

ACTION & *THERAPEUTIC EFFECT* Synthetic nucleoside with broad-spectrum antiviral activity against DNA and RNA viruses. Mode is believed to involve multiple mechanisms including selective interference with viral ribonucleic protein synthesis. *Active against many RNA and DNA viruses, including respira-*

R

tory syncytial virus (RSV), influenza A and B, parainfluenza, measles, mumps, Lassa fever, enterovirus 72 (formerly called hepatitis A), yellow fever, HIV, herpes simplex virus (HSV-1 and HSV-2), and vaccinia.

USES Aerosol product used for selected infants and young children with respiratory syncytial virus (RSV). Oral product used in combination with interferon-alfa-2b to treat hepatitis C or in combination with peginterferon alpha for treatment of hepatitis C.

UNLABELED USES Prophylaxis and treatment of influenza A and B, pneumonia caused by adenovirus; Lassa fever, measles, HSV-1, HSV-2, hepatitis A, SARS, cytomegalovirus.

CONTRAINDICATIONS Mild RSV infections of lower respiratory tract; infants requiring simultaneous assisted ventilation; pancreatitis; autoimmune hepatitis; renal failure; hemoglobinopathy; pregnancy (category X), lactation.

CAUTIOUS USE COPD, asthma; anemia; history of MI, cardiac arrhythmias, cardiac disease; older adults, decreased renal, hepatic, or cardiac function; respiratory depression; history of depression or suicidal tendencies.

R

ROUTE & DOSAGE

RSV

Child: **Inhalation** 20 mg via SPAG-2 nebulizer administered over 12–18 h/day for 3–7 days

Hepatitis C

(in combination with interferon-alfa)

Adult: **PO** *Weight greater than 75 kg,* 600 mg b.i.d. for 24–48 wk; *weight less than 75 kg,* 400 mg in a.m., 600 mg in p.m. for 24–48 wk

Child/Adolescent: **PO** *Weight greater than 73 kg,* 15 mg/kg/day or 1200 mg/day in divided doses; *weight 60–73 kg,* 15 mg/kg/day or 1000 mg/day in divided doses; *weight 47–59 kg,* 15 mg/kg/day or 800 mg/day in divided doses; *older than 3 y, weight less than 47 kg,* 15 mg/kg/day in divided doses

Chronic Hepatitis C (with Peginterferon Alfa-2b)

Adult: **PO** 800–1400 mg daily in divided doses

Adolescent/Child (older than 3 y): **PO** *Weight greater than 73 kg,* 15 mg/kg/day or 1200 mg/day in divided doses; *weight 60–73 kg,* 15 mg/kg/day or 1000 mg/day in divided doses; *weight 47–59 kg,* 15 mg/kg/day or 800 mg/day in divided doses; *weight less than 47 kg,* 15 mg/kg/day in divided doses

Renal Impairment Dosage Adjustment

CrCl less than 50 mL/min: Oral ribavirin should not be used

ADMINISTRATION

- Give tablets with food. Ensure that tablets and capsules are swallowed whole. They should not be opened, crushed, or chewed.

Inhalation

- Administer only by SPAG-2 aerosol generator, following manufacturer's directions.
- Caution: Ribavirin has demonstrated teratogenicity in animals. Advise pregnant health care personnel of the potential teratogenic risks associated with exposure during ribavirin administration to patients.

- Do not give other aerosol medication concomitantly with ribavirin.
- Discard solution in the SPAG-2 reservoir at least q24h and whenever liquid level is low before fresh reconstituted solution is added.
- Store unopened vial in a dry place at 15°–25° C (59°–78° F) unless otherwise directed.
- Following reconstitution, store solution at 20°–30° C (68°–86° F) for 24 h.

ADVERSE EFFECTS (≥1%) **CV:** Hypotension (faintness, lightheadedness, unusual fatigue), MI, cardiac arrest. **Special Senses:** Conjunctivitis, erythema of eyelids. **Hematologic:** Reticulocytosis, hemolytic anemia (especially in combination with interferon alpha). **Respiratory:** Deterioration of respiratory function, dyspnea, apnea, chest soreness, bacterial pneumonia, ventilator dependence. **GI:** Transient increases in AST, ALT, bilirubin; abdominal cramps, jaundice.

INTERACTIONS Drug: Ribavirin may antagonize the antiviral effects of **zidovudine** against HIV; increased risk of fetal defects with **peginterferon.**

PHARMACOKINETICS Absorption: Rapidly absorbed orally (44%) and systemically from lungs. **Peak:** Inhaled 60–90 min. PO 1.7–3 h. **Distribution:** Crosses placenta; distributed into breast milk. **Metabolism:** In cells to an active metabolite. **Elimination:** 85% in urine, 15% in feces. **Half-Life:** 24 h in plasma, 16–40 days in RBCs.

NURSING IMPLICATIONS

Assessment & Drug Effects

- Obtain specimens for rapid diagnosis of RSV infection before therapy is initiated or at least during the first 24 h of ribavirin therapy. Do not continue therapy without laboratory confirmation of RSV infection.
- Lab tests: Baseline CBC with differential and platelet count, repeat at 2 and 4 wk, and periodically thereafter; baseline and periodic serum electrolytes, LFTs, and TSH.
- Monitor respiratory function and fluid status closely during therapy. Note baseline rate and character of respirations and pulse. Observe for signs of labored breathing: Dyspnea, apnea; rapid, shallow respirations, intercostal and substernal retraction, nasal flaring, limited excursion of lungs, cyanosis. Auscultate lungs for abnormal breath sounds.
- Observe patients requiring simultaneous assisted ventilation closely for S&S of worsening pulmonary function. Check equipment carefully every 2 h, including endotracheal tube, for malfunction. Precipitation of ribavirin and accumulation of fluid in tubing can obstruct the apparatus and cause inadequate ventilation and gas exchange.
- Monitor cardiac status, including ECG, especially in those with preexisiting cardiac dysfunction.

Patient & Family Education

- Both male and female patients should take every precaution to prevent pregnancy during treatment and for 6 mo following the end of therapy.
- Inform physician immediately if a pregnancy occurs within 6 mo of completing therapy.
- Drink fluids liberally unless otherwise advised by physician.
- Use caution with hazardous activities until response to drug is known.

RIBOFLAVIN (VITAMIN B_2)

(rye'bo-flay-vin)

Riboflavin (Vitamin B_2)

Classification: VITAMIN
Therapeutic: VITAMIN REPLACEMENT
Pregnancy Category: A (C if greater than RDA)

AVAILABILITY 50 mg, 100 mg tablets

ACTION & *THERAPEUTIC EFFECT* Water-soluble vitamin and component of the flavoprotein enzymes, which work together with a wide variety of proteins to catalyze many cellular respiratory reactions by which the body derives its energy. *Evaluated by improvement of clinical manifestations of deficiency: Digestive disturbances, headache, burning sensation of skin (especially "burning" feet), cracking at corners of mouth (cheilosis), glossitis, seborrheic dermatitis (and other skin lesions), mental depression, corneal vascularization (with photophobia, burning and itchy eyes, lacrimation, roughness of eyelids), anemia, neuropathy.*

USES To prevent riboflavin deficiency and to treat ariboflavinosis; also to treat microcytic anemia and as a supplement to other B vitamins in treatment of pellagra and beri-beri.

R

CAUTIOUS USE Pregnancy (category A; category C if greater than RDA).

ROUTE & DOSAGE

Nutritional Supplement
Adult: **PO** 5–10 mg/day
Child: **PO** 1–4 mg/day

Nutritional Deficiency
Adult: **PO** 5–30 mg/day in divided doses
Child: **PO** 3–10 mg/day

ADMINISTRATION

Oral

- Give with food to enhance absorption.
- Store in airtight containers protected from light.

ADVERSE EFFECTS (≥1%) **Urogenital:** May discolor urine bright yellow.

DIAGNOSTIC TEST INTERFERENCE In large doses, riboflavin may produce yellow-green fluorescence in ***urine*** and thus cause false elevations in certain ***fluorometric determinations*** of ***urinary catecholamines.***

INTERACTIONS Drug: No clinically significant interactions established.

PHARMACOKINETICS Absorption: Readily absorbed from GI tract. **Distribution:** Little is stored; excess amounts are excreted in urine. **Elimination:** In urine. **Half-Life:** 66–84 min.

NURSING IMPLICATIONS

Assessment & Drug Effects

- Collaborate with physician, dietitian, patient, and responsible family member in planning for diet. A complete dietary history is an essential part of vitamin replacement so that poor eating habits can be identified and corrected. Deficiency in one vitamin is usually associated with other vitamin deficiencies.

Patient & Family Education

- Be aware that large doses may cause an intense yellow discoloration of urine.
- Note: Rich dietary sources of riboflavin are found in liver, kidney, beef, pork, heart, eggs, milk and milk products, yeast, whole-grain cereals, vitamin B–enriched breakfast cereals, green vegetables, and mushrooms.

RIFABUTIN

(rif-a-bu′tin)
Ansamycin, Mycobutin

Classifications: ANTIBIOTIC; ANTI-TUBERCULOSIS
Therapeutic: ANTITUBERCULOSIS
Prototype: Rifampin
Pregnancy Category: B

AVAILABILITY 150 mg capsules

ACTION & *THERAPEUTIC EFFECT* Semisynthetic bacteriostatic antibiotic. Mode of action may be to inhibit DNA-dependent RNA polymerase in susceptible bacterial cells but not in human cells. *Effective against* Mycobacterium avium *complex (MAC) (or* M. avium-intracellulare*) and many strains of* M. tuberculosis.

USES The prevention of disseminated *Mycobacterium avium* complex (MAC) disease in patients with advanced HIV infection.

CONTRAINDICATIONS Hypersensitivity to rifabutin or any other rifamycins; lactation.
CAUTIOUS USE Older adults, pregnancy (category B).

ROUTE & DOSAGE

Prevention of MAC
Adult: **PO** 300 mg daily, may give 150 mg b.i.d. if nausea is a problem
Child: **PO** 75 mg daily

ADMINISTRATION

Oral
- Give the usual dose of 300 mg/day or in two divided doses of 150 mg with food if needed to reduce GI upset.
- Store at room temperature, 15°–30° C (59°–86° F), unless otherwise directed.

ADVERSE EFFECTS (≥1%) **CNS:** *Headache.* **GI:** *Abdominal pain, dyspepsia, nausea, taste perversion, increased liver enzymes.* **Hematologic:** Thrombocytopenia, eosinophilia, leukopenia, neutropenia. **Skin:** Rash. **Other:** *Turns urine, feces, saliva, sputum, perspiration, and tears orange. Soft contact lenses may be permanently discolored.*

INTERACTIONS Drug: May decrease levels of BENZODIAZEPINES, BETA-BLOCKERS, **clofibrate, dapsone,** NARCOTICS, ANTICOAGULANTS, CORTICOSTEROIDS, **cyclosporine, quinidine,** ORAL CONTRACEPTIVES, PROGESTINS, SULFONYLUREAS, **ketoconazole, fluconazole,** BARBITURATES, **theophylline,** and ANTICONVULSANTS, resulting in therapeutic failure.

PHARMACOKINETICS Absorption: 12–20% of oral dose reaches the systemic circulation. **Peak:** 2–3 h. **Distribution:** 85% protein bound. Widely distributed, high concentrations in the lungs, liver, spleen, eyes, and kidney. Crosses placenta, distributed into breast milk. **Metabolism:** In the liver. Causes induction of hepatic enzymes. **Elimination:** Approximately 53% of dose is excreted in urine as metabolites, 30% is excreted in feces. **Half-Life:** 16–96 h (average 45 h).

NURSING IMPLICATIONS

Assessment & Drug Effects
- Monitor patients for S&S of active TB. Report immediately.
- Lab tests: Monitor periodic blood work for neutropenia and thrombocytopenia.
- Evaluate patients on concurrent oral hypoglycemic therapy for loss of glycemic control.
- Review patient's complete drug regimen because dosage adjustment of a significant number of drugs may be needed when rifabutin is added to regimen.

Patient & Family Education

- Learn S&S of TB and MAC (e.g., persistent fever, progressive weight loss, anorexia, night sweats, diarrhea) and notify physician if any of these develop.
- Notify physician of following: Muscle or joint pain, eye pain or other discomfort, chest pain with dyspnea, rash, or a flu-like syndrome.
- Be aware that urine, feces, saliva, sputum, perspiration, tears, and skin may be colored brown-orange. Soft contact lens may be permanently discolored.
- Rifabutin may reduce the activity of a wide variety of drugs. Provide a complete and accurate list of concurrent drugs to the physician for evaluation.

RIFAMPIN (Pr)

(rif'am-pin)

Rifadin, Rimactane, Rofact ♣

Classifications: ANTIBIOTIC; ANTITUBERCULOSIS

Therapeutic: ANTITUBERCULOSIS

Pregnancy Category: C

AVAILABILITY 150 mg, 300 mg capsules; 600 mg injection

ACTION & *THERAPEUTIC EFFECT* Semisynthetic derivative of rifamycin B that inhibits DNA-dependent RNA polymerase activity in susceptible bacterial cells, thereby suppressing RNA synthesis. *Active against* Mycobacterium tuberculosis, M. leprae, Neisseria meningitidis, *and a wide range of gram-negative and gram-positive organisms.*

USES Primarily as adjuvant with other antituberculosis agents in initial treatment and retreatment of clinical tuberculosis; as short-term therapy to eliminate meningococci from nasopharynx of asymptomatic carriers of *N. meningitidis* when risk of meningococcal meningitis is high.

UNLABELED USES Chemoprophylaxis in contacts of patients with *Haemophilus influenzae* type B infection; alone or in combination with dapsone and other anti-infectives in treatment of leprosy (especially dapsone-resistant leprosy). Also infections caused by susceptible gram-negative and gram-positive bacteria that fail to respond to other anti-infectives; in combination with erythromycin or tetracycline for treatment of Legionnaire's disease.

CONTRAINDICATIONS Hypersensitivity to rifampin; obstructive biliary disease; meningococcal disease; intermittent rifampin therapy. Safe use in children younger than 5 y is not established.

CAUTIOUS USE Hepatic disease; history of alcoholism; concomitant use of other hepatotoxic agents; pregnancy (category C).

ROUTE & DOSAGE

Pulmonary Tuberculosis

Adult: **PO/IV** 600 mg daily in conjunction with other antituberculosis agents

Child: **PO/IV** 10–20 mg/kg/day (max: 600 mg/day)

Meningococcal Carriers

Adult: **PO** 600 mg q12h for 2 consecutive days

Child: **PO** 10–20 mg/kg q12h for 2 consecutive days (max: 600 mg/day)

Prophylaxis for *H. influenzae* Type B

Adult: **PO** 600 mg/day for 4 days

Child: **PO** 20 mg/kg/day for 4 days (max: 600 mg/day)

Dapsone-Sensitive Multibacillary Leprosy
Adult: **PO** 600 mg once/mo with clofazimine and dapsone for a minimum of 2 y

ADMINISTRATION

Oral

- Give 1 h before or 2 h after a meal. Peak serum levels are delayed and may be slightly lower when given with food; capsule contents may be emptied into fluid or mixed with food.
- Note: An oral suspension can be prepared from capsules for use with pediatric patients. Consult pharmacist for directions.
- Keep a desiccant in bottle containing capsules to prevent moisture causing instability.

Intravenous

***PREPARE:* IV Infusion:** Reconstitute vial by adding 10 mL of sterile water for injection to each 600-mg to yield 60 mg/mL. Swirl to dissolve. ▪ Withdraw the ordered dose and further dilute in 500 mL of D5W (preferred) or NS. ▪ If absolutely necessary, 100 mL of D5W or NS may be used.
***ADMINISTER:* IV Infusion:** Infuse 500 mL solution over 3 h and 100 mL solution over 30 min. ▪ Note: A less concentrated solution infused over a longer period is preferred.
INCOMPATIBILITIES Solution/additive: **Minocycline.** Y-site: **Diltiazem.**

- Use NS solutions within 24 h and D5W solutions within 4 h of preparation.

ADVERSE EFFECTS (≥1%) **CNS:** Fatigue, drowsiness, headache, ataxia, confusion, dizziness, inability to concentrate, generalized numbness, pain in extremities, muscular weakness. **Special Senses:** Visual disturbances, transient low-frequency hearing loss, conjunctivitis. **GI:** *Heartburn, epigastric distress, nausea, vomiting, anorexia, flatulence, cramps, diarrhea,* <u>pseudomembranous colitis</u>, *transient elevations in liver function tests* (bilirubin, BSP, alkaline phosphatase, ALT, AST), pancreatitis. **Hematologic:** Thrombocytopenia, transient leukopenia, anemia, including hemolytic anemia. **Body as a Whole:** Hypersensitivity (fever, pruritus, urticaria, skin eruptions, soreness of mouth and tongue, eosinophilia, hemolysis), flu-like syndrome. **Urogenital:** Hemoglobinuria, hematuria, <u>acute renal failure</u>, light-chain proteinuria, menstrual disorders, <u>hepatorenal syndrome</u>, (with intermittent therapy). **Respiratory:** Hemoptysis. **Other:** Increasing lethargy, liver enlargement and tenderness, jaundice, brownish-red or orange discoloration of skin, sweat, saliva, tears, and feces; unconsciousness.

DIAGNOSTIC TEST INTERFERENCE Rifampin interferes with contrast media used for ***gallbladder study;*** therefore, test should precede daily dose of rifampin. May also cause retention of ***BSP.*** Inhibits standard assays for ***serum folate*** and ***vitamin*** B_{12}.

INTERACTIONS Drug: Alcohol, isoniazid, pyrazinamide, ritonavir, saquinavir increase risk of drug-induced hepatotoxicity (including fatal hepatotoxicity when used for latent TB); ***p*-aminosalicylic acid (PAS)** decreases concentrations of rifampin; decreases concentrations of **alfentanil, alosetron, alprazolam, amprenavir,** BARBITURATES, BENZODIAZEPINES, **carbamazepine, atovaquone, cevimeline, chloramphenicol, clofibrate,** CORTICOSTEROIDS, **cyclosporine, dapsone,**

delavirdine, diazepam, digoxin, diltiazem, disopyramide, estazolam, estramustine, fentanyl, fosphenytoin, fluconazole galantamine, indinavir, itraconazole, ketoconazole, lamotrigine, levobupivacaine, lopinavir, methadone, metoprolol, mexiletine, midazolam, nelfinavir, ORAL SULFONYLUREAS, ORAL CONTRACEPTIVES, **phenytoin,** PROGESTINS, **propafenone, propranolol, quinidine, quinine, ritonavir, sirolimus, theophylline,** THYROID HORMONES, **tocainide, tramadol, verapamil, warfarin, zaleplon,** and **zonisamide,** leading to potential therapeutic failure. Do not use with **simvastatin.**

PHARMACOKINETICS Absorption: Readily from GI tract. **Peak:** 2–4 h. **Distribution:** Widely distributed, including CSF; crosses placenta; distributed into breast milk. **Metabolism:** In liver to active and inactive metabolites; is enterohepatically cycled. **Elimination:** Up to 30% in urine, 60–65% in feces. **Half-Life:** 3 h.

NURSING IMPLICATIONS

Assessment & Drug Effects

- Lab tests: Periodic liver function tests are advised. Closely monitor patients with hepatic disease.
- Check prothrombin time daily or as necessary to establish and maintain required anticoagulant activity when patient is also receiving an anticoagulant.

Patient & Family Education

- Do not interrupt prescribed dosage regimen. Hepatorenal reaction with flu-like syndrome has occurred when therapy has been resumed following interruption.
- Be aware that drug may impart a harmless red-orange color to urine, feces, sputum, sweat, and tears. Soft contact lenses may be permanently stained.
- Report onset of jaundice, hypersensitivity reactions, and persistence of GI adverse effects to physician.
- Use or add barrier contraceptive if using hormonal contraception. Concomitant use of rifampin and oral contraceptives leads to decreased effectiveness of the contraceptive and to menstrual disturbances (spotting, breakthrough bleeding).
- Keep drug out of reach of children.

RIFAPENTINE

(rif'a-pen-teen)

Priftin

Classifications: ANTIBIOTIC; ANTITUBERCULOSIS; MYCOBACTERIUM

Therapeutic: ANTITUBERCULOSIS

Prototype: Rifampin

Pregnancy Category: C

AVAILABILITY 150 mg tablets

ACTION & *THERAPEUTIC EFFECT* Rifamycin derivative that inhibits DNA-dependent RNA polymerase activity in susceptible bacterial cells, thereby suppressing RNA synthesis. *Effective against* Mycobacterium tuberculosis, *indicated by improvement in clinical S&S (e.g., fever, cough, pleuritic pain, fatigue) and on chest x-ray.*

USES Pulmonary tuberculosis in conjunction with at least one other antitubercular agent.

CONTRAINDICATIONS Hypersensitivity to any rifamycins (e.g., rifampin, rifabutin, rifapentine); porphyria; lactation.

CAUTIOUS USE Patients with abnormal liver function tests or hepatic disease; older adults; HIV disease;

pregnancy (category C). Safe use in children younger than 12 y not established.

ROUTE & DOSAGE

Tuberculosis: Short-Course Therapy
Adult: **PO** 600 mg twice weekly (at least 72 h apart) × 2 mo, then 600 mg once weekly × 4 mo

ADMINISTRATION

Oral
- Give with an interval of NO LESS than 72 h between doses.
- Give with food to minimize GI upset.
- Store at 15°–30° C (59°–86° F) in a tightly closed container and protect from excess moisture.

ADVERSE EFFECTS (≥1%) **CNS:** Headache, dizziness. **CV:** Hypertension. **GI:** Increased liver function tests (ALT, AST), anorexia, nausea, vomiting, dyspepsia, diarrhea. **GU:** *Hyperuricemia*, pyuria, proteinuria, hematuria, urinary casts. **Hematologic:** Neutropenia, lymphopenia, anemia, leukopenia, thrombocytosis. **Respiratory:** Hemoptysis. **Skin:** Rash, pruritus, acne. **Body as a Whole:** Arthralgia, pain.

INTERACTIONS Drug: Decreased levels of **indinavir** and possibly other PROTEASE INHIBITORS; increased metabolism and decreased activity of ORAL CONTRACEPTIVES, **phenytoin, disopyramide, mexiletine, quinidine, tocainide, warfarin, fluconazole, itraconazole, ketoconazole, diazepam,** BETA-BLOCKERS, CALCIUM CHANNEL BLOCKERS, CORTICOSTEROIDS, **haloperidol,** SULFONYLUREAS, **cyclosporine, tacrolimus, levothyroxine,** NARCOTIC ANALGESICS, **quinine,** REVERSE TRANSCRIPTASE INHIBITORS, TRICYCLIC ANTIDEPRESSANTS, **sildenafil, theophylline.**

PHARMACOKINETICS Absorption: Approximately 70% absorbed. **Peak:** 5–6 h. **Distribution:** 97.7% protein bound. **Metabolism:** Hydrolyzed by esterase enzyme to active metabolite in liver; inducer of cytochromes P450 3A4 and 2C8/9. **Elimination:** 70% in feces, 17% in urine. **Half-Life:** 13.3 h.

NURSING IMPLICATIONS

Assessment & Drug Effects
- Lab tests: Sputum smear and culture, CBC, baseline liver functions (especially serum transaminases) to rule out preexisting hepatic disease and serum creatinine and BUN.
- Monitor carefully for S&S of toxicity with concurrent use of oral anticoagulants, digitalis preparations, or anticonvulsants.

Patient & Family Education
- Follow strict adherence to the prescribed dosing schedule to prevent emergence of resistant strains of tuberculosis.
- Be aware that food may be useful in preventing GI upset.
- Report immediately any of the following to the physician: Fever, weakness, nausea or vomiting, loss of appetite, dark urine or yellowing of eyes or skin, pain or swelling of the joints, severe or persistent diarrhea.
- Use or add barrier contraceptive if using hormonal contraception.

RIFAXIMIN

(ri-fax′i-min)
Xifaxan
Classifications: RIFAMYCIN ANTIBIOTIC; MYCOBACTERIUM

R

Therapeutic: MYCOBACTERIUM
Prototype: Rifampin
Pregnancy Category: C

AVAILABILITY 200 mg tablets

ACTION & *THERAPEUTIC EFFECT* A rifamycin antibiotic that inhibits bacterial RNA synthesis by binding to DNA-dependent RNA polymerase, thereby blocking RNA transcription. *Its spectrum of activity includes gram-positive and gram-negative aerobes and anaerobes.*

USES Treatment of traveler's diarrhea caused by noninvasive strains of *E. coli*.

CONTRAINDICATIONS Hypersensitivity to rifaximin, other rifamycin antimicrobial agents or to any of its components; dysentery; children younger than 12 y; lactation.
CAUTIOUS USE Diarrhea with fever and/or blood in the stool, or diarrhea due to organisms other than *E. coli;* IBD, worsening diarrhea or diarrhea persisting for longer than 24–48 h; pregnancy (category C).

ROUTE & DOSAGE

Traveler's Diarrhea
Adult: **PO** 200 mg t.i.d. for 3 days

ADMINISTRATION

Oral
- May be given without regard to food.
- Store at 15°–30° C (59°–86° F).

ADVERSE EFFECTS (≥1%) **Body as a Whole:** Fever. **CNS:** Headache. **GI:** *Flatulence,* abdominal pain, rectal tenesmus, defecation urgency, nausea, constipation, vomiting.

PHARMACOKINETICS Absorption: Less than 0.4% absorbed orally. **Peak:** 1.21 h. **Elimination:** In feces. **Half-Life:** 5.85 h.

NURSING IMPLICATIONS

Assessment & Drug Effects
- Withhold drug and notify physician if diarrhea worsens or lasts longer than 48 h after starting drug; an alternative treatment should be considered.
- Report promptly the appearance of blood in the stool.

Patient & Family Education
- Report promptly any of the following: Fever; difficulty breathing; skin rash, itching, or hives; worsening diarrhea during or after treatment or blood in the stool.

RILUZOLE

(ri-lu'zole)
Rilutek
Classifications: AMYOTROPHIC LATERAL SCLEROSIS (ALS) AGENT; GLUTAMATE ANTAGONIST
Therapeutic: ALS AGENT
Pregnancy Category: C

AVAILABILITY 50 mg tablets

ACTION & *THERAPEUTIC EFFECT* Glutamate antagonist that inhibits the presynaptic release of glutamic acid in the CNS. Effectiveness based on theory that pathogenesis of amyotrophic lateral sclerosis (ALS) is related to injury of motor neurons by glutamate. *Believed to reduce the degeneration of neurons in ALS.*

USES Treatment of ALS, may extend survival or time to tracheostomy.

CONTRAINDICATIONS Hypersensitivity to riluzole; lactation.
CAUTIOUS USE Hepatic dysfunction, renal impairment; hyperten-

sion, history of other CNS disorders; pregnancy (category C). Safe use in children younger than 12 y is not established.

ROUTE & DOSAGE

ALS

Adult: **PO** 50 mg q12h at least 1 h before or 2 h after meals

ADMINISTRATION

Oral

- Give at same time daily and at least 1 h before or 2 h after a meal. Do not give before/after a high-fat meal.
- Store at room temperature; protect from bright light.

ADVERSE EFFECTS (≥1%) **Body as a Whole:** *Asthenia,* headache, back pain, malaise, arthralgia, weight loss, peripheral edema, flu-like syndrome. **CNS:** Hypertonia, depression, dizziness, dry mouth, insomnia, somnolence, circumoral paresthesia. **CV:** Hypertension, tachycardia, phlebitis, palpitation. **GI:** Abdominal pain, *nausea,* vomiting, dyspepsia, anorexia, diarrhea, flatulence, stomatitis. **Respiratory:** *Decreased lung function,* rhinitis, increased cough, apnea, bronchitis, dysphagia, dyspnea. **Skin:** Pruritus, eczema, alopecia, exfoliative dermatitis (rare). **Urogenital:** UTI.

INTERACTIONS Drug: BARBITURATES, **carbamazepine** may increase risk of hepatotoxicity.

PHARMACOKINETICS Absorption: Well absorbed from GI tract, 60% reaches systemic circulation. **Peak:** Steady-state levels by day 5. **Distribution:** 96% protein bound. **Metabolism:** In liver by CYP1A2. **Elimination:** 90% in urine. **Half-Life:** 12 h.

NURSING IMPLICATIONS

Assessment & Drug Effects

- Lab tests: Monitor periodically Hct and Hgb, routine blood chemistries, and alkaline phosphatase. If febrile illness develops, monitor WBC count. Baseline LFTs, then monthly for 3 mo, then q3mo for remainder of first year, and periodically thereafter.
- Withhold drug and notify physician if liver enzymes are elevated.

Patient & Family Education

- Report any febrile illness to physician.
- Do not engage in potentially hazardous activities until response to drug is known.
- Learn common adverse effects and possible adverse interaction with alcohol.

RIMANTADINE

(ri-man'ta-deen)

Flumadine

Classifications: ANTIVIRAL; ADMANTANE

Therapeutic: ANTIVIRAL

Prototype: Amantadine

Pregnancy Category: C

AVAILABILITY 100 mg tablets

ACTION & *THERAPEUTIC EFFECT* Antiviral agent thought to exert an inhibitory effect early in the viral replication cycle, probably by interfering with the viral uncoating procedure of the influenza A virus. Inhibits synthesis of both viral RNA and viral protein, thus causing viral destruction. *Prevents or interrupts influenza A infections.*

USES Prophylaxis and treatment of influenza A.

R

CONTRAINDICATIONS Hypersensitivity to rimantadine and amantadine; lactation, children younger than 1 y.
CAUTIOUS USE History of seizures; renal or hepatic impairment; elderly; pregnancy (category C).

ROUTE & DOSAGE

Prophylaxis of Influenza A
Adult/Child (10 y or older): **PO** 100 mg b.i.d.
Child (1–9 y): **PO** 5 mg/kg daily (max: 150 mg/day) in divided doses
Geriatric: **PO** 100 mg daily

Treatment of Influenza A
Adult/Adolescent (older than 14 y): **PO** 100 mg b.i.d. started within 48 h of symptoms and continued for 5–7 days from initial symptoms
Geriatric: **PO** 100 mg daily started within 48 h of symptoms and continued for 5–7 days from initial symptoms

Hepatic Impairment Dosage Adjustment
100 mg daily with severe liver disease

Renal Impairment Dosage Adjustment
CrCl less than 10 mL/min: Extend dosing interval to 24 h

ADMINISTRATION

Oral
- Store at 15°–30° C (59°–86° F).

ADVERSE EFFECTS (≥1%) **CNS:** Nervousness, dizziness, headache, sleep disturbances, fatigue or malaise, drowsiness, anticholinergic effects. **GI:** Nausea, vomiting, diarrhea, dyspepsia, dry mouth, anorexia, abdominal pain.

INTERACTIONS Drug: Intranasal influenza vaccine should not be used within 48 h.

PHARMACOKINETICS Absorption: Readily absorbed from GI tract. **Peak:** Serum levels 3.2–4.3 h. **Distribution:** Concentrates in respiratory secretions. **Metabolism:** Extensively in liver. **Elimination:** By kidneys. **Half-Life:** 20–36 h.

NURSING IMPLICATIONS

Assessment & Drug Effects
- Monitor carefully for seizure activity in patients with a history of seizures. Seizures are an indication to discontinue the drug.
- Monitor cardiac, respiratory, and neurologic status while on drug. Report palpitations, hypertension, dyspnea, or pedal edema.

Patient & Family Education
- Report bothersome adverse effects to physician; especially hallucinations, palpitations, difficulty breathing, and swelling of legs.
- Use caution with hazardous activities until reaction to drug is known.

RIMEXOLONE
(rim-ex′o-lone)
Vexol
Pregnancy Category: C
See Appendix A-1.

RISEDRONATE SODIUM
(ri-se-dron′ate)
Actonel
Classifications: BISPHOSPHONATE; BONE METABOLISM REGULATOR
Therapeutic: BONE RESORPTION INHIBITOR; OSTEOPOROSIS TREATMENT
Prototype: Etidronate disodium
Pregnancy Category: C

AVAILABILITY 5 mg, 30 mg, 35 mg, 75 mg, 150 mg tablets

ACTION & *THERAPEUTIC EFFECT* Diphosphate preparation with primary action on bone. Lowers serum alkaline phosphatase, presumably by decreasing release of phosphate from bone and increasing excretion of parathyroid hormone. Slows rate of bone resorption and new bone formation in pagetic bone lesions and in normal remodeling process. *Effectiveness indicated by decreased bone and joint pain and improved bone density.*

USES Paget's disease, prevention and treatment of osteoporosis.

UNLABELED USE Osteolytic metastases.

CONTRAINDICATIONS Hypersensitivity to risedronate or other bisphosphonates; hypocalcemia, vitamin D deficiency; severe renal impairment (CrCl less than 30 mL/min); lactation.

CAUTIOUS USE Renal impairment; CHF; hyperphosphatemia; hepatic disease; fever related to infection or other causes; pregnancy (category C). Safety and efficacy in children younger than 18 y are not established.

ROUTE & DOSAGE

Paget's Disease

Adult: **PO** 30 mg daily for 2 mo, may repeat after 2 mo rest if necessary

Prevention and Treatment of Osteoporosis

Adult (female): **PO** 5 mg daily OR 35 mg once weekly OR 75 mg daily for 2 consecutive days each month OR 150 mg once monthly
Adult (men): **PO** 35 mg weekly
Adult (with chronic systemic glucocorticoid): **PO** 5 mg daily

Renal Impairment Dosage Adjustment

CrCl less than 30 mL/min: Use not recommended

ADMINISTRATION

Oral

- Give on an empty stomach (at least 30 min before first food or drink of the day) with at least 6–8 oz plain water. Ensure that tablet is swallowed whole. It should not be crushed or chewed.
- Note: Patient should be upright. Maintain upright position and empty stomach for at least 30 min after administration.
- Space calcium supplements and antacids as far as possible from risedronate.
- Store at 15°–30° C (59°–86° F) in a tightly closed container and protect from light.

ADVERSE EFFECTS (≥1%) **Body as a Whole:** Flu-like syndrome, asthenia, arthralgia, bone pain, leg cramps, myasthenia. **CNS:** Headache, dizziness. **CV:** Chest pain, peripheral edema. **GI:** *Diarrhea,* abdominal pain, nausea, constipation, belching, colitis. **Respiratory:** Bronchitis, sinusitis. **Skin:** Rash. **Special Senses:** Amblyopia, tinnitus, dry eyes.

DIAGNOSTIC TEST INTERFERENCE May interfere with the use of ***bone-imaging agents.***

INTERACTIONS Drug: Calcium, ANTACIDS significantly decrease absorption, use with NONSTEROIDAL ANTIINFLAMMATORIES may increase risk of gastric ulcer.

PHARMACOKINETICS Absorption: Minimally absorbed from GI tract, bioavailability 0.63%. **Peak:** 1 h. **Distribution:** Approximately 60% of

R

dose is distributed to bone. **Metabolism:** Not metabolized. **Elimination:** In urine; unabsorbed drug excreted in feces. **Half-Life:** 220 h.

NURSING IMPLICATIONS

Assessment & Drug Effects

- Lab tests: Baseline and periodic serum calcium, phosphorus, and alkaline phosphatase.
- Monitor carefully for and immediately report S&S of GI bleeding and hypocalcemia.

Patient & Family Education

- Administration guidelines regarding upright position, empty stomach, and spacing relative to calcium supplements and antacids **must be** strictly followed.
- Report any of the following to physician: Eye irritation, significant GI upset, or flu-like symptoms.

RISPERIDONE

(ris-per′i-done)

Risperdal, Risperdal M-TAB, Risperdal Consta

Classification: ATYPICAL ANTIPSYCHOTIC

Therapeutic: ANTIPSYCHOTIC

Prototype: Clozapine

Pregnancy Category: C

R

AVAILABILITY 0.25 mg, 0.5 mg, 1 mg, 2 mg, 3 mg, 4 mg tablets; 0.5 mg, 1 mg, 2 mg, 3 mg, 4 mg quick-dissolving tablets; 1 mg/mL solution; 12.5 mg, 25 mg, 37.5 mg, 50 mg injection

ACTION & *THERAPEUTIC EFFECT* Interferes with binding of dopamine to D_2-interlimbic region of the brain, serotonin (5-HT_2) receptors, and alpha-adrenergic receptors in the occipital cortex. It has low to moderate affinity for the other serotonin (5-HT) receptors. *Effective in controlling symptoms of schizophrenia as well as other psychotic symptoms.*

USES Treatment of schizophrenia; treatment of bipolar disorder; irritability associated with autism.

UNLABELED USES Management of patients with dementia-related psychotic symptoms. Adjunctive treatment of behavioral disturbances in patients with mental retardation.

CONTRAINDICATIONS Hypersensitivity to risperidone; elderly with dementia-related psychosis; QT prolongation, Reye's syndrome, brain tumor, severe CNS depression, head trauma; tardive dyskinesia; sunlight (UV) exposure, tanning beds; lactation, children younger than 13 y for schizophrenia; children younger than 10 y for bipolar disease; children younger than 5 y for autism.

CAUTIOUS USE Older adults; arrhythmias, hypotension, breast cancer, blood dyscrasia, cardiac disorders, cerebrovascular disease, hypotension, dehydration, diabetes mellitus, diabetic ketoacidosis, hyperglycemia, hypokalemia, hypomagnesemia, hyponatremia, MI, obesity, orthostatic hypotension, mild or moderate CNS depression, coma; GI obstruction, dysphagia; electrolyte imbalance, ethanol intoxication, heart failure, renal or hepatic dysfunction; seizure disorder, seizures, suicidal ideation; stroke, Parkinson's disease; pregnancy (category C).

ROUTE & DOSAGE

Schizophrenia

Adult/Adolescent (older than 13 y): **PO** 1–2 mg/day in 1 or 2 doses, then titrate up (max: 8 mg/day) **IM** 25 mg once q2wk (max: 50 mg)

Geriatric: **PO** Start 0.5 mg b.i.d. and increase by 0.5 mg b.i.d. daily to an initial target of 1.5 mg b.i.d. (max: 4 mg/day) **IM** 25 mg once q2wk (max: 25 mg)

Bipolar Disorder

Adult/Adolescent (older than 10 y): **PO** 2–3 mg once daily for up to 3 wk (max: 6 mg/day)

Geriatric: **PO** Start with 0.5 mg b.i.d. and increase by 0.5 mg b.i.d. daily to an initial target of 1.5 mg b.i.d. (max: 4 mg/day). May convert to once daily dosing after stabilized in b.i.d. 2–3 days.

Irritability Associated with Autism

Adolescent/Child (5 y or older, weight 20 kg or greater): **PO** 0.5 mg daily; after 4 days, increase to 1 mg daily; can increase by 0.5 mg q2wk

Child (5 y or older, weight less than 20 kg): **PO** 0.25 mg daily; after 4 days, increase to 0.5 mg daily; can increase by 0.25 mg q2wk

Renal Impairment Dosage Adjustment

CrCl less than 30 mL/min: Start with 0.5 mg b.i.d., increase by 0.5 mg b.i.d. daily to an initial target of 1.5 mg b.i.d., may increase by 0.5 mg b.i.d. at weekly intervals (max: 6 mg/day); lower IM dose may be required

Hepatic Impairment Dosage Adjustment

Start with dose of 0.5 mg b.i.d.

ADMINISTRATION

Oral

- The oral solution may be mixed with water, orange juice, low-fat milk, or coffee. It is not compatible with cola or tea.
- Orally disintegrating tablets should not be removed from the blister until immediately before administration. Tablets disintegrate immediately and may be swallowed with/without liquid.
- Store at 15°–30° C (59°–86° F).

Intramuscular

- Reconstitute the 25, 37.5, or 50 mg vial using the supplied 2 mL prefilled syringe. Shake vigorously for at least 10 sec to produce a uniform, thick, milky suspension. If 2 min or more pass before injection, shake vial again.
- Give deep IM into the upper-outer quadrant of the gluteal muscle with the supplied needle; do not substitute. Follow the manufacturer's instructions for use of the SmartSite Needle-Free Vial Access Device and Needle-Pro device.
- Store unopened vials at 2°–8° C (36°–46° F). Protect from light.

ADVERSE EFFECTS (≥1%) **Body as a Whole:** Orthostatic hypotension with initial doses, sweating, weakness, fatigue. **CNS:** *Sedation, drowsiness, headache,* transient blurred vision, *insomnia,* disinhibition, *agitation,* anxiety, increased dream activity, dizziness, catatonia, *extrapyramidal symptoms* (akathisia, dystonia, pseudoparkinsonism), especially with doses greater than 10 mg/day, neuroleptic malignant syndrome (rare), increased risk of stroke in elderly. **CV:** Prolonged QT_c interval, tachycardia. **GI:** Dry mouth, dyspepsia, nausea, vomiting, diarrhea, constipation, abdominal pain, elevated liver function tests (AST, ALT). **Endocrine:** Galactorrhea. **Metabolic:** Hyperglycemia, diabetes mellitus. **Respiratory:** Rhinitis, cough, dyspnea. **Skin:** Photosensitivity. **Urogenital:** Urinary retention, menorrhagia, decreased sexual desire, erectile dysfunction, sexual dysfunction male and female.

R

DIAGNOSTIC TEST INTERFERENCE ***Liver function tests (AST, ALT)*** are elevated.

INTERACTIONS Drug: Risperidone may enhance the effects of certain ANTIHYPERTENSIVE AGENTS. May antagonize the antiparkinson effects of **bromocriptine, cabergoline, levodopa, pergolide, pramipexole, ropinirole. Carbamazepine, phenytoin, phenobarbital, rifampin** may decrease risperidone levels. **Clozapine** may increase risperidone levels.

PHARMACOKINETICS Absorption: Rapidly; not affected by food. **Onset:** Therapeutic effect 1–2 wk. **Peak:** 1–2 h. **Distribution:** 0.7 L/kg; in animal studies, risperidone has been found in breast milk. **Metabolism:** Primarily in liver by cytochrome P450 with an active metabolite, 9-hydroxyrisperidone. **Elimination:** 70% in urine; 14% in feces. **Half-Life:** 20 h for slow metabolizers, 30 h for fast metabolizers.

NURSING IMPLICATIONS

Assessment & Drug Effects

- Monitor diabetics for loss of glycemic control.
- Reassess patients periodically and maintain on the lowest effective drug dose.
- Monitor closely neurologic status of older adults.
- Monitor cardiovascular status closely; assess for orthostatic hypotension, especially during initial dosage titration.
- Monitor closely those at risk for seizures.
- Assess degree of cognitive and motor impairment, and assess for environmental hazards.
- Lab tests: Monitor periodically blood glucose, serum electrolytes, liver function, and complete blood counts.

Patient & Family Education

- Carefully monitor blood glucose levels if diabetic.
- Do not engage in potentially hazardous activities until the response to drug is known.
- Be aware of the risk of orthostatic hypotension.
- Avoid alcohol while taking this drug.

RITONAVIR

(ri-ton′a-vir)

Norvir

Classifications: ANTIRETROVIRAL; PROTEASE INHIBITOR

Therapeutic: PROTEASE INHIBITOR

Prototype: Saquinavir

Pregnancy Category: B

AVAILABILITY 100 mg capsules; 80 mg/mL solution

ACTION & *THERAPEUTIC EFFECT* HIV protease is an enzyme required to produce the polyprotein procurers of functional proteins in infectious HIV. Prevent cleavage of the viral polyproteins, resulting in the formation of immature noninfectious virus particles. *Protease inhibitor of both HIV-1 and HIV-2 resulting in the formation of noninfectious viral particles.*

USES Alone or in combination with other antiretroviral agents or protease inhibitors for treatment of HIV infection. Often used to increase the effect of other antiretrovirals.

CONTRAINDICATIONS Hypersensitivity to ritonavir; antimicrobial resistance to protease inhibitors; pancreatitis; lactation. Safe use in children younger than 1 mo has not been established.

CAUTIOUS USE Hepatic diseases, liver enzyme abnormalities, or hepatitis, jaundice; diabetes mellitus, diabetic ketoacidosis, hyperlipidemia, hypertriglyceridemia; hemophilia A or B, renal insufficiency; pregnancy (category B).

ROUTE & DOSAGE

HIV

Adult: **PO** 600 mg b.i.d. 1 h before or 2 h after meal (may take with a light snack)
Child (older than 1 mo): **PO** 300–400 mg/m² b.i.d. (max: 600 mg b.i.d.), start with 250 mg/m² b.i.d., increase by 50 mg/m² q2–3days

ADMINISTRATION

Oral

- Give preferably with food; oral solution may be mixed with chocolate milk or nutritional therapy liquids within 1 h of dosing to improve taste.
- Store refrigerated at 2°–8° C (36°–46° F). Protect from light in tightly closed container.

ADVERSE EFFECTS (≥1%) **Body as a Whole:** Myalgia, allergic reaction, bronchitis, cough, rhinitis, taste alterations, visual disturbances, dysuria, hyperglycemia, diabetes. **CNS:** *Asthenia,* fatigue, headache, fever, malaise, circumoral or peripheral paresthesia, insomnia, dizziness, somnolence, abnormal thinking, amnesia, agitation, anxiety, confusion, convulsions, aphasia, ataxia, diplopia, emotional lability, euphoria, hallucinations, decreased libido, nervousness, neuralgia, neuropathy, peripheral neuropathy, paralysis, tremor, vertigo. **CV:** Palpitations, vasodilation, hypotension, postural hypotension, syncope, tachycardia, <u>prolonged QT interval</u>. **Hematologic:** Anemia, thrombocytopenia, lymphadenopathy. **GI:** *Nausea, diarrhea, vomiting,* abdominal pain, dyspepsia, stomatitis, anorexia, dry mouth, constipation, flatulence, cholecystitis, cholestasis, abnormal liver function tests, hepatitis. **Skin:** Rash, sweating, acne, contact dermatitis, pruritus, urticaria, skin ulceration, dry skin.

INTERACTIONS Drug: Carbamazepine, dexamethasone, phenobarbital, phenytoin, rifabutin, rifampin, smoking can decrease ritonavir levels. **Ritonavir** may increase serum levels and toxicity of **clarithromycin,** especially in patients with renal insufficiency (reduce **clarithromycin** dose in patients with CrCl less than 60 mL/min); **desipramine; saquinavir, amiodarone, bepridil, bupropion, clozapine, dihydroergotamine, flecainide, meperidine, pimozide, piroxicam, propoxyphene, quinidine, rifabutin, trazodone, alfuzosin, fluticasone.** Ritonavir decreases levels of ORAL CONTRACEPTIVES, **theophylline;** may increase **ergotamine** toxicity with **dihydroergotamine, ergotamine;** may increase systemic steroid exposure with **fluticasone.** Liquid formulation may cause disulfiram-like reaction with **alcohol** or **metronidazole.** See the complete prescribing information for a comprehensive table of potential, but not studied, drug interactions. Use with **darunavir** may increase risk of hepatoxicity. **Herbal: St. John's wort, garlic** may decrease antiretroviral activity.

PHARMACOKINETICS Absorption: Rapidly from GI tract. **Peak:** 2–4 h. **Distribution:** 98–99% protein bound. **Metabolism:** In liver (CYP3A4).

Elimination: Primarily in feces (greater than 80%).

NURSING IMPLICATIONS

Assessment & Drug Effects

- Lab tests: Monitor periodically CBC with differential and platelet count, liver function, kidney function, serum albumin, lipid profile, CPK, serum amylase, electrolytes, blood glucose HbA1C, and alkaline phosphatase.
- Withhold drug and notify physician in the presence of abnormal liver function.
- Assess for S&S of GI distress, peripheral neuropathy, and other potential adverse effects.

Patient & Family Education

- Learn potential adverse reactions and drug interactions; report to physician use of any OTC or prescription drugs.
- Take this drug exactly as prescribed. Do not skip doses. Take at same time each day.
- Do not take ritonavir with any of the following drugs as fatal reactions may occur: Amiodarone, astemizole, alfuzosin, bepridil, dihydroergotamine, ergotamine, ergonovine, flecainide, methylergonovine, midazolam, pimozide, propafenone, quinidine, triazolam, voriconazole.

R

RITUXIMAB

(rit-ux′i-mab)

Rituxan

Classifications: ANTINEOPLASTIC; IMMUNOMODULATOR; DISEASE-MODIFYING ANTIRHEUMATIC DRUG (DMARD)

Therapeutic: ANTINEOPLASTIC; ANTI-RHEUMATIC; DMARD

Pregnancy Category: C

AVAILABILITY 10 mg/mL injection

ACTION & *THERAPEUTIC EFFECT* Monoclonal antibody that binds with the CD20 antigen on the surface of normal and malignant B lymphocytes. B-cells are believed to play a role in the pathogenesis of rheumatoid arthritis and associated chronic synovitis. B-cells may be acting at multiple sites in the autoimmune/inflammatory process including rheumatoid factor and other autoantibody production, antigen presentation, T-cell activation, and/or proinflammatory cytokine production. Rituximab-induced depletion of peripheral B-lymphocytes in patients with rheumatoid arthritis (RA) and in non-Hodgkin's lymphoma results in a rapid and sustained depletion of circulating and tissue-based (e.g., thymus, spleen) B-lymphocytes. *Rituximab effectiveness in both rheumatoid arthritis and non-Hodgkin's lymphoma is measured by induced depletion of peripheral B-lymphocytes.*

USES Relapsed or refractory CD20 positive, B-cell non-Hodgkin's lymphoma, treatment of rheumatoid arthritis (with methotrexate).

UNLABELED USES RA in patients not responding to MTX therapy.

CONTRAINDICATIONS Hypersensitivity to murine proteins, rituximab, or abciximab; angina, cardiac arrhythmias, cardiac disease; pulmonary disease, chronic lymphocytic leukemia (CLL), lymphoma, severe hypotension; oliguria, rising serum creatinine; viral hepatitis B (HBV), vaccination; lactation.

CAUTIOUS USE Prior exposure to murine-based monoclonal antibodies; history of allergies; asthma and other pulmonary disease (increased risk of bronchospasm); respiratory insufficiency; older adults; CAD; thrombocytopenia; history of cardiac arrhythmias; hypertension, renal impairment; pregnancy (category C). Safety and efficacy in children are not established.

ROUTE & DOSAGE

Non-Hodgkin's Lymphoma

Adult: **IV** 375 mg/m² infused at 50 mg/h, may increase infusion rate q30min (max: 400 mg/h if tolerated), repeat dose on days 8, 15, and 22 (total of 4 doses)

Rheumatoid Arthritis

Adult: **IV** 1000 mg on days 1 and 15 (with methotrexate)

ADMINISTRATION

Intravenous

PREPARE: **IV Infusion:** Dilute ordered dose to 1–4 mg/mL by adding to an infusion bag of NS or D5W. ▪ Examples: 500 mg in 400 mL yields 1 mg/mL; 500 mg in 75 mL yields 4 mg/mL. ▪ Gently invert bag to mix. Discard unused portion left in vial.

ADMINISTER: **IV Infusion:** Infuse first dose at a rate of 50 mg/h; may increase rate at 50 mg/h increments q30min to maximum rate of 400 mg/h. ▪ For subsequent doses, infuse at a rate of 100 mg/h and increase by 100 mg/h increments q30min up to maximum rate of 400 mg/h. ▪ Slow or stop infusion if S&S of hypersensitivity appear (see Appendix F).

▪ Store unopened vials at 2°–8° C (36°–46° F) and protect from light.

ADVERSE EFFECTS (≥1%) **Body as a Whole:** Angioedema, *fatigue,* asthenia, night sweats, *fever, chills,* myalgia. **CNS:** Headache, dizziness, depression. **CV:** Hypotension, tachycardia, peripheral edema. **GI:** *Nausea,* vomiting, throat irritation, anorexia, abdominal pain, hepatitis B reactivation with <u>fulminant hepatitis, hepatic failure,</u> and <u>death</u>. **Hematologic:** <u>Leukopenia, thrombocytopenia, anemia, neutropenia</u>. **Respiratory:** Bronchospasm, dyspnea, rhinitis. **Skin:** Pruritus, rash urticaria. **Other:** Infusion-related reactions: *Fever, chills, rigors, pruritus, urticaria, pain, flushing,* chest pain, hypotension, hypertension, dyspnea; <u>fatal infusion-related reactions</u> have been reported.

INTERACTIONS Drug: ANTIHYPERTENSIVE AGENTS should be stopped 12 h prior to avoid excessive hypotension; **cisplatin** may cause additive nephrotoxicity.

PHARMACOKINETICS Duration: 6–12 mo. **Half-Life:** 60–174 h (increases with multiple infusions).

NURSING IMPLICATIONS

Assessment & Drug Effects

- Lab tests: Baseline and periodic CBC with differential, LFTs, and renal function tests. CBC with differential, peripheral CD20+ B lymphocytes.
- Monitor carefully BP and ECG status during infusion and immediately report S&S of hypersensitivity (e.g., fever, chills, urticaria, pruritus, hypotension, bronchospasms; see Appendix F for others).

Patient & Family Education

- Do not take antihypertensive medication within 12 h of rituximab infusions.
- Note: Use effective contraception during and for up to 12 mo following rituximab therapy.

R

- Report any of the following experienced during infusion: Itching, difficulty breathing, tightness in throat, dizziness, headache, or nausea.

RIVASTIGMINE TARTRATE

(ri-vas′tig-meen)
Exelon
Classifications: CHOLINESTERASE INHIBITOR; ANTIDEMENTIA
Therapeutic: ANTIALZHEIMER'S
Pregnancy Category: B

AVAILABILITY 2 mg/mL oral solution; 1.5 mg, 3 mg, 4.5 mg, 6 mg capsules

ACTION & *THERAPEUTIC EFFECT* Inhibits acetylcholinesterase G_1 form of this enzyme in the cerebral cortex and the hippocampus. The G_1 form of acetylcholinesterase is found in higher levels in the brains of patients with Alzheimer's disease. *Inhibits acetylcholinesterase more specifically in the brain (hippocampus and cortex) than in the heart or skeletal muscle in Alzheimer's disease.*

R

USES Treatment of mild to moderate dementia of the Alzheimer's type.

CONTRAINDICATIONS Hypersensitivity to rivastigmine or carbamate derivatives; lactation.
CAUTIOUS USE History of toxicity to cholinesterase inhibitors (e.g., tacrine); diabetes mellitus, cardiovascular/pulmonary disease; GI disorders including intestinal obstruction/peptic ulcer disease; concurrent use of other cholinergic agents, or anticholinergic agents; urogenital tract obstruction; Parkinson's disease; history of seizures; hepatic or renal insufficiency; pregnancy (category B).

ROUTE & DOSAGE

Alzheimer's Dementia
Adult/Geriatric: **PO** Start with 1.5 mg b.i.d with food, may increase by 1.5 mg b.i.d. q2wk if tolerated, target dose 3–6 mg b.i.d. (max: 12 mg b.i.d.) (if discontinued for a few doses, restart at last dose or lower; if treatment is interrupted for several days, reinitiate with 1.5 mg b.i.d. and titrate q2wk as above)

ADMINISTRATION

Oral
- Give both capsules and liquid with food.
- Give liquid form undiluted or mixed with water, juice, or soda (do not mix with other liquids). Stir completely to dissolve. Ensure that entire mixture is swallowed.
- Withhold drug and notify physician if significant anorexia, nausea, or vomiting occur.
- Store capsules and oral solution below 25° C (77° F). Ensure that bottle of liquid is in an UPRIGHT position.

ADVERSE EFFECTS (≥1%) **Body as a Whole:** Asthenia, increased sweating, syncope, fatigue, malaise, flu-like syndrome. **CV:** Hypertension. **GI:** *Nausea, vomiting, anorexia,* dyspepsia, *diarrhea, abdominal pain,* constipation, flatulence, eructation. **Metabolic:** Weight loss. **CNS:** *Dizziness, headache,* somnolence, tremor, insomnia, confusion, depression, anxiety, hallucination, aggressive reaction. **Respiratory:** Rhinitis.

INTERACTIONS Drug: May exaggerate muscle relations with **succinyl-**

choline and other NEUROMUSCULAR BLOCKING AGENTS, may attenuate effects of ANTICHOLINERGIC AGENTS.

PHARMACOKINETICS Absorption: Well absorbed, 40% reaches systemic circulation. **Peak:** 1 h. **Duration:** 10 h. **Distribution:** Crosses blood–brain barrier with CSF peak concentrations in 1.4–2.6 h, 40% protein bound. **Metabolism:** By cholinesterase-mediated hydrolysis. **Elimination:** In urine. **Half-Life:** 1.5 h.

NURSING IMPLICATIONS

Assessment & Drug Effects

- Monitor cognitive function and ability to perform ADLs.
- Monitor for and report S&S of GI distress: Anorexia, weight loss, nausea and vomiting.
- Lab tests: Periodic serum electrolytes, Hgb and Hct, urinalysis, blood glucose HbA1C, especially with long-term therapy.
- Monitor ambulation as dizziness is a common adverse effect.
- Monitor diabetics for loss of glycemic control.

Patient & Family Education

- Review instruction sheet provided with liquid form of the drug.
- Monitor weight at least weekly.
- Report any of the following to the physician: Loss of appetite, weight loss, significant nausea and/or vomiting.
- Supervise activity since there is a high potential for dizziness.

RIZATRIPTAN BENZOATE

(ri-za-trip'tan ben'zo-ate)

Maxalt, Maxalt-MLT

Classification: SEROTONIN 5-HT_1 RECEPTOR AGONIST

Therapeutic: ANTIMIGRAINE

Prototype: Sumatriptan
Pregnancy Category: C

AVAILABILITY 5 mg, 10 mg tablets; 5 mg, 10 mg disintegrating tablets

ACTION & *THERAPEUTIC EFFECT* Selective (5-$HT_{1B/1D}$) receptor agonist that reverses the vasodilation of cranial blood vessels associated with a migraine. *Activation of the 5-$HT_{1B/1D}$ receptors reduces the pain pathways associated with the migraine headache as well as reversing vasodilation of cranial blood vessels.*

USES Acute migraine headaches with or without aura.

CONTRAINDICATIONS Hypersensitivity to rizatriptan; CAD; Prinzmetal's angina (potential for vasospasm); ischemic heart disease; risk factors for CAD such as hypertension, hypercholesterolemia, obesity, diabetes, smoking, and strong family history; concurrent administration with ergotamine drugs or sumatriptan; concurrent administration with MAOIS; basilar or hemiplegic migraine.
CAUTIOUS USE Hypersensitivity to sumatriptan; renal or hepatic impairment; hypertension; asthmatic patients; pregnancy (category C), lactation. Safety and effectiveness in children younger than 18 y are not established.

ROUTE & DOSAGE

Acute Migraine

Adult: **PO** 5–10 mg, may repeat in 2 h if necessary (max: 30 mg/24 h); 5 mg with concurrent propranolol (max: 15 mg/24 h)

R

ADMINISTRATION

Oral

- Give any time after symptoms of migraine appear. If symptoms return, a second tablet may be given but no sooner than 2 h after the first.
- Do not exceed 30 mg (three doses) in any 24 h period.
- Do not give within 24 h of an ergot-containing drug or another 5-HT_1 agonist.
- Store at 15°–30° C (59°–86° F) and protect from light and moisture.

ADVERSE EFFECTS (≥1%) **Body as a Whole:** Asthenia, fatigue, pain, pressure sensation, paresthesias, throat pressure, warm/cold sensations. **CNS:** Somnolence, dizziness, headache, hypesthesia, decreased mental acuity, euphoria, tremor. **CV:** Coronary artery vasospasm, transient myocardial ischemia, MI, ventricular tachycardia, ventricular fibrillation, chest pain/tightness/heaviness, palpitations. **GI:** Dry mouth, nausea, vomiting, diarrhea. **Respiratory:** Dyspnea. **Skin:** Flushing. **Endocrine:** Hot flashes.

R

INTERACTIONS Drug: Propranolol may increase concentrations of rizatriptan, use smaller rizatriptan doses; **dihydroergotamine, methysergide,** other 5-HT_1 AGONISTS may cause prolonged vasospastic reactions; SSRIS have rarely caused weakness, hyperreflexia, and incoordination; MAOIS should not be used with 5-HT_1 AGONISTS. **Herbal: St. John's wort** may increase triptan toxicity.

PHARMACOKINETICS Absorption: 45% of oral dose reaches systemic circulation. **Peak:** 1–1.5 h for oral tabs; 1.6–2.5 h for orally disintegrating tablets. **Metabolism:** Via oxidative deamination by monoamine oxidase A. **Elimination:** Primarily in urine (82%). **Half-Life:** 2–3 h.

NURSING IMPLICATIONS

Assessment & Drug Effects

- Monitor cardiovascular status carefully following first dose in patients at risk for CAD (e.g., postmenopausal women, men older than 40 y, persons with known CAD risk factors) or coronary artery vasospasms.
- ECG is recommended following first administration of rizatriptan to someone with known CAD risk factors.
- Report immediately to physician: Chest pain or tightness in chest or throat that is severe or does not quickly resolve.
- Monitor periodically cardiovascular status with continued rizatriptan use.

Patient & Family Education

- Do not exceed 30 mg (three doses) in 24 h.
- Allow orally disintegrating tablets to dissolve on tongue; no liquid is needed.
- Contact physician immediately if any of the following develop following rizatriptan use: Symptoms of angina (e.g., severe and/or persistent pain or tightness in chest or throat), hypersensitivity (e.g., wheezing, facial swelling, skin rash, or hives), abdominal pain.
- Report any other adverse effects (e.g., tingling, flushing, dizziness) at next physician visit.

ROPINIROLE HYDROCHLORIDE

(ro-pi'ni-role)

Requip, Requip XL

Classifications: DOPAMINE RECEPTOR AGONIST; ANTIPARKINSON

Therapeutic: ANTIPARKINSON
Prototype: Levodopa
Pregnancy Category: C

AVAILABILITY 0.25 mg, 0.5 mg, 1 mg, 2 mg, 3 mg, 4 mg, 5 mg tablets; 2 mg, 4 mg, 6 mg, 8 mg, 12 mg extended release tablets

ACTION & *THERAPEUTIC EFFECT* Nonergot dopamine receptor agonist that has high affinity for the D_2 and D_3 subfamily of dopamine receptors. *Effectiveness indicated by improvement in idiopathic Parkinson's disease.*

USES Idiopathic Parkinson's disease, restless legs syndrome.

CONTRAINDICATIONS Hypersensitivity to ropinirole or pramipexole.
CAUTIOUS USE Hepatic impairment; severe renal impairment; mental instability; concomitant use of CNS depressants; pregnancy (category C), lactation. Safety and efficacy in children are not established.

ROUTE & DOSAGE

Parkinson's Disease
Adult: **PO** (Immediate release) Start with 0.25 mg t.i.d., titrate up by 0.25 mg/dose t.i.d. qwk to a target dose of 1 mg t.i.d.; if response is still not satisfactory, may continue to increase by 1.5 mg/day qwk to a dose of 9 mg/day, and then by 3 mg/day or less weekly (max: 24 mg/day) (Extended release) 2 mg daily for 1–2 wk then increase by 2 mg/day at one week intervals (max: 24 mg/day)

Restless Legs Syndrome
Adult: **PO** Take 0.25 mg 1–3 h before bed × 2 days, increase to 0.5 mg for the first wk, then increase by 0.5 mg qwk to a maximum of 4 mg

ADMINISTRATION

Oral
- Give with food to reduce occurrence of nausea.
- Do not crush extended release tablets. Ensure that they are swallowed whole.
- Drug should not be abruptly discontinued. Dose should be tapered over a period of days.
- Store at 15°–30° C (59°–86° F).

ADVERSE EFFECTS (≥1%) **Body as a Whole:** Increased sweating, dry mouth, flushing, asthenia, *fatigue,* pain, edema, malaise, *viral infection,* UTI, impotence. **CNS:** *Dizziness, somnolence, sudden sleep attacks,* hallucinations, confusion, amnesia, hypesthesia, yawning, hyperkinesia, impaired concentration, vertigo, hallucinations. **CV:** *Syncope,* chest pain, orthostatic symptoms, hypertension, palpitations, atrial fibrillation, extrasystoles, hypotension, tachycardia, peripheral edema, peripheral ischemia. **GI:** *Nausea, vomiting, dyspepsia,* abdominal pain, anorexia, flatulence. **Respiratory:** Pharyngitis, rhinitis, sinusitis, bronchitis, dyspnea. **Special Senses:** Abnormal vision, xerophthalmia, eye abnormality.

INTERACTIONS Drug: Ropinirole levels may be increased by ESTROGENS, QUINOLONE ANTIBIOTICS, **cimetidine, diltiazem, erythromycin, fluvoxamine, mexiletine, tacrine;** effects may be antagonized by PHENOTHIAZINES, BUTYROPHENONES, **metoclopramide zileuton** may increase ropinerole levels.

PHARMACOKINETICS Absorption: Rapidly from GI tract; 55% bioavailability. **Peak:** 1–2 h. **Distribution:** 30–40% protein bound. **Metabolism:** In liver (CYP1A2). **Elimination:** Primarily in urine. **Half-Life:** 6 h.

NURSING IMPLICATIONS

Assessment & Drug Effects

- Lab test: Periodically monitor BUN and creatinine, hepatic function.
- Monitor cardiac status. Report increases in BP and HR to physician.
- Monitor carefully for orthostatic hypotension, especially during dose escalation.
- Monitor level of alertness. Institute appropriate precautions to prevent injury due to dizziness or drowsiness.

Patient & Family Education

- Be aware that hallucinations are a possible adverse effect and occur more often in older adults.
- Make position changes slowly, especially after long periods of lying or sitting. Postural hypotension is common, especially during early treatment.
- Exercise caution with hazardous activities requiring alertness since drowsiness and sedation are common adverse effects. Effects are additive with alcohol or other CNS depressants.
- Report behavioral changes (e.g., impulsive behavior) to physician.

R

ROPIVACAINE HYDROCHLORIDE

(ro-piv′i-cane)

Naropin

Classification: LOCAL ANESTHETIC (ESTER-TYPE)

Therapeutic: LOCAL ANESTHETIC

Prototype: Procaine HCl

Pregnancy Category: B

AVAILABILITY 2 mg/mL, 5 mg/mL, 7.5 mg/mL, 10 mg/mL injection

ACTION & *THERAPEUTIC EFFECT* Blocks the generation and conduction of nerve impulses, probably by increasing the threshold for electrical excitability. *Local anesthetic action produces loss of sensation and motor activity in areas of the body close to the injection site.*

USES Local and regional anesthesia, postoperative pain management, anesthesia/pain management for obstetric procedures.

CONTRAINDICATIONS Hypersensitivity to ropivacaine or any local anesthetic of the amide type; generalized septicemia, inflammation or sepsis at the proposed injection site; cerebral spinal diseases (e.g., meningitis); heart block, hypotension, hypertension, GI hemorrhage. **CAUTIOUS USE** Debilitated, older adult, or acutely ill patients; arrhythmias, shock; pregnancy (category B), lactation.

ROUTE & DOSAGE

Surgical Anesthesia

Adult: **Epidural** 25–200 mg (0.5–1% solution) **Nerve block** 5–250 mg (0.5%, 0.75% solution)

Labor Pain

Adult: **Epidural** 20–40 mg (0.2% solution)

Postoperative Pain Management

Adult: **Epidural** 12–20 mg/h (0.2% solution) **Infiltration** 2–200 mg (0.2–0.5% solution)

ADMINISTRATION

Intrathecal

- Avoid rapid injection of large volumes of ropivacaine. Incremental doses should always be used to achieve the smallest effective dose and concentration.

- Use an infusion concentration of 2 mg/mL (0.2%) for postoperative analgesia.
- Do not use disinfecting agents containing heavy metal ions (e.g., mercury, copper, zinc, etc.) on skin insertion site or to clean the ropivacaine container top.
- Discard continuous infusions solution after 24 h; it contains no preservatives.
- Store unopened at 20°–25° C (68°–77° F).

ADVERSE EFFECTS (≥1%) **Body as a Whole:** Pain, fever, rigors, hypoesthesia. **CNS:** Paresthesia, headache, dizziness, anxiety. **CV:** *Hypotension,* bradycardia, hypertension, tachycardia, chest pain, fetal bradycardia. **GI:** Nausea. **Skin:** Pruritus. **Urogenital:** Urinary retention, oliguria. **Hematologic:** Anemia.

INTERACTIONS Drug: Additive adverse effects with other LOCAL ANESTHETICS.

PHARMACOKINETICS Onset: 1–30 min (average 10–20 min) depending on dose/route of administration. **Duration:** 0.5–8 h depending on dose/route of administration. **Distribution:** 94% protein bound. **Metabolism:** In the liver by CYP1A. **Elimination:** In urine. **Half-Life:** 1.8–4.2 h.

NURSING IMPLICATIONS

Assessment & Drug Effects

- Monitor carefully cardiovascular and respiratory status throughout treatment period. Assess for hypotension and bradycardia.
- Report immediately S&S of CNS stimulation or CNS depression.

Patient & Family Education

- Report any of the following to physician immediately: Restlessness, anxiety, tinnitus, blurred vision, tremors.

ROSIGLITAZONE MALEATE Pr

(ros-i-glit'a-zone)

Avandia

Classifications: ANTIDIABETIC; THIAZOLIDINEDIONES

Therapeutic: ANTIHYPERGLYCEMIC

Pregnancy Category: C

AVAILABILITY 2 mg, 4 mg, 8 mg tablets

ACTION & *THERAPEUTIC EFFECT* Antidiabetic agent that lowers blood sugar levels by improving target cell response to insulin in Type 2 diabetics. It reduces cellular insulin resistance and decreases hepatic glucose output (gluconeogenesis). *Reduces hyperglycemia and hyperlipidemia, thus improving hyperinsulinemia without stimulating pancreatic insulin secretion. Effectiveness indicated by decreased HbA1C.*

USES Adjunct to diet in the treatment of type 2 diabetes. May also be used in combination with metformin.

CONTRAINDICATIONS Hypersensitivity to rosiglitazone; cardiovascular disease, particularly hypertensive patients with New York Heart Association Class III and IV cardiac status (e.g., CHF); active hepatic disease; lactation.

CAUTIOUS USE As monotherapy in Type 1 diabetes mellitus or diabetic ketoacidosis; CHF or risk for CHF; hepatic impairment; pregnancy (category C). Safety and efficacy in children younger than 18 y are not established.

ROUTE & DOSAGE

Type 2 Diabetes Mellitus

Adult: **PO** Start at 4 mg daily or 2 mg b.i.d., may increase after 12

R

wk (max: 8 mg/day in 1–2 divided doses)

Hepatic Impairment Dosage Adjustment

Do not use if ALT greater than 2.5 × ULN

ADMINISTRATION

Oral

- May be given without regard to meals.
- Store at 15°–30° C (59°–86° F) in tight, light-resistant container.

ADVERSE EFFECTS (≥1%) **Body as a Whole:** Edema, anemia, headache, back pain, fatigue. **CV:** Edema, fluid retention, exacerbation of heart failure, increased risk of heart attack. **GI:** Diarrhea. **Respiratory:** Upper respiratory tract infection, sinusitis. **Special Senses:** Macular edema. **Other:** Hyperglycemia.

INTERACTIONS Drug: Insulin may increase risk of heart failure or edema; enhance hypoglycemia with ORAL ANTIDIABETIC AGENTS, **ketoconazole, gemfibrozil** may increase effect. **Bosentan** may reduce effect. **Herbal: Garlic, ginseng, green tea** may potentiate hypoglycemic effects.

PHARMACOKINETICS Absorption: 99% from GI tract. **Peak:** 1 h, food delays time to peak by 1.75 h. **Duration:** Greater than 24 h. **Distribution:** Greater than 99% protein bound. **Metabolism:** In liver (CYP2C8) to inactive metabolites. **Elimination:** 64% urine, 23% feces. **Half-Life:** 3–4 h. Liver disease increases serum concentrations and increases half-life by 2 h.

NURSING IMPLICATIONS

Assessment & Drug Effects

- Monitor for S&S of hypoglycemia (possible when insulin/sulfonylureas are coadministered).
- Monitor for S&S of CHF or exacerbation of symptoms with preexisting CHF.
- Lab tests: Baseline LFTs, then q2mo for first year; then periodically (more often when elevated); periodic HbA1C, Hgb and Hct, and lipid profile.
- Withhold drug and notify physician if ALT greater than 2.5 times normal or patient jaundiced.
- Monitor weight and notify physician of development of edema.

Patient & Family Education

- Report promptly any of the following: Rapid weight gain, edema, shortness of breath, or exercise intolerance.
- Be aware that resumed ovulation is possible in nonovulating premenopausal women.
- Use or add barrier contraceptive if using hormonal contraception.
- Report immediately to physician: S&S of liver dysfunction such as unexplained anorexia, nausea, vomiting, abdominal pain, fatigue, dark urine; or S&S of fluid retention such as weight gain, edema, or activity intolerance.
- Combination therapy: May need adjustment of other antidiabetic drugs to avoid hypoglycemia.

ROSUVASTATIN

(ro-su-va-sta′ten)

Crestor

Classifications: HMG-COA REDUCTASE INHIBITOR (STATIN); ANTILIPEMIC

Therapeutic: ANTIHYPERLIPEMIC; STATIN

Prototype: Lovastatin

Pregnancy Category: X

AVAILABILITY 5 mg, 10 mg, 20 mg, 40 mg tablets

ACTION & *THERAPEUTIC EFFECT*
Rosuvastatin is a potent inhibitor

of HMG-CoA reductase, an enzyme that catalyzes the conversion of HMG-CoA to mevalonic acid, an early and rate-limiting step in cholesterol biosynthesis. This results in reducing the amount of mevalonic acid, a precursor of cholesterol. *Reduces total cholesterol and LDL cholesterol; additionally, lowers plasma triglycerides and apolipoprotein B while increasing HDL.*

USES Adjunct to diet for the reduction of LDL cholesterol and triglycerides in patients with primary hypercholesterolemia, hypertriglyceridemia, and mixed dyslipidemia.

CONTRAINDICATIONS Hypersensitivity to any component of the product, active liver disease, pregnancy (category X), women of childbearing potential not using appropriate contraceptive measures, lactation.

CAUTIOUS USE Concomitant use of cyclosporine and gemfibrozil; excessive alcohol use or history of liver disease; renal impairment; advanced age; hypothyroidism.

ROUTE & DOSAGE

Hyperlipidemia

Adult/Adolescent/Child (older than 10 y): **PO** 10 mg once daily (5–40 mg/day), max dose 40 mg/day; If taking cyclosporine, gemfibrozil, lopinavir/ritonavir, start with 5 mg/day
Geriatric: Initial dose of 5 mg/day

Renal Impairment Dosage Adjustment

CrCl less than 30 mL/min: 5 mg once daily (max: 10 mg/day)

ADMINISTRATION

Oral

- Persons of Asian descent may be slow metabolizers and may require half the normal dose.
- May give any time of day without regard to food.
- Do not give within 2 h of an antacid.
- Store at or below 30° C (86° F).

ADVERSE EFFECTS (≥1%) **Body as a Whole:** Asthenia, back pain, flu syndrome, chest pain, infection, pain, peripheral edema. **CNS:** Headache, dizziness, insomnia, hypertonia, paresthesia, depression, anxiety, vertigo, neuralgia. **CV:** Hypertension, angina, vasodilatation, palpitations. **GI:** Diarrhea, dyspepsia, nausea, abdominal pain, constipation, gastroenteritis, vomiting, flatulence, gastritis. **Endocrine:** Diabetes. **Hematologic:** Anemia, ecchymosis. **Musculoskeletal:** Myalgia, arthritis, arthralgia, rhabdomyolysis (especially with dose greater than 40 mg). **Respiratory:** Pharyngitis, rhinitis, sinusitis, bronchitis, increased cough, dyspnea, pneumonia, asthma. **Skin:** Rash, pruritus. **Urogenital:** UTI.

INTERACTIONS Drug: Atazanavir, cyclosporine, gemfibrozil, niacin may increase risk of rhabdomyolysis; ANTACIDS may decrease rosuvastatin absorption; may cause increase in INR with **warfarin. Herbal: Red-yeast rice** increases rhabdomyolysis risk.

PHARMACOKINETICS Absorption: Well absorbed. **Peak:** 3–5 h. **Metabolism:** Limited metabolism in the liver (not CYP3A4). **Elimination:** Primarily in feces (90%). **Half-Life:** 20 h.

NURSING IMPLICATIONS

Assessment & Drug Effects

- Monitor for and report promptly S&S of myopathy (e.g., skeletal

R

muscle pain, tenderness or weakness).
- Withhold drug and notify physician if CPK levels are markedly elevated (10 or more × ULN) or if myopathy is diagnosed or suspected.
- Lab tests: CPK levels for S&S of myopathy; periodic LFTs; more frequent INR values with concomitant warfarin therapy.
- Monitor CV status, especially with a known history of hypertension or heart disease.
- Monitor diabetics for loss of glycemic control.

Patient & Family Education
- Do not take antacids within 2 h of taking this drug.
- Women should use reliable means of contraception to prevent pregnancy while taking this drug.

SALMETEROL XINAFOATE
(sal-me′ter-ol xin′a-fo-ate)
Serevent
Classifications: BETA$_2$-ADRENERGIC AGONIST; RESPIRATORY SMOOTH MUSCLE RELAXANT; BRONCHODILATOR
Therapeutic: BRONCHODILATOR
Prototype: Albuterol
Pregnancy Category: C

AVAILABILITY 50 mcg powder diskus for inhalation

ACTION & *THERAPEUTIC EFFECT* Long-acting beta$_2$-adrenoreceptor agonist that stimulates beta$_2$-adrenoreceptors, relaxes bronchospasm, and increases ciliary motility, thus facilitating expectoration. *Relaxes bronchospasm and increases ciliary motility, thus facilitating expectoration of pulmonary secretions.*

USES Maintenance therapy for asthma or bronchospasm. Prevention of exercise-induced bronchospasm. Do not use to treat acute bronchospasm.

CONTRAINDICATIONS Hypersensitivity to salmeterol; other long-acting beta$_2$-adrenergic agonists; primary treatment of status asthmaticus; acute bronchospasm; MAOI therapy; safety and efficacy in children younger than 4 y not established.
CAUTIOUS USE Cardiovascular disorders, cardiac arrhythmias, hypertension; history of seizures or thyrotoxicosis; liver and renal impairment, older adults, diabetes mellitus, sensitivity to other beta-adrenergic agonists; women in labor; pregnancy (category C), lactation.

ROUTE & DOSAGE

Asthma or Bronchospasm
Adult/Child (4 y or older): **Inhalation** 2 inhalations of aerosol (42 mcg) or 1 powder diskus (50 mcg) b.i.d. approximately 12 h apart

Prevention of Exercise-Induced Bronchospasm
Adult/Child (4 y or older): **Inhalation** 2 inhalations of aerosol (42 mcg) or 1 powder diskus (50 mcg) 30–60 min before exercise

ADMINISTRATION

Inhalation
- Do not use to relieve symptoms of acute asthma.
- Activate diskus by moving lever until it clicks. Patient should exhale fully (not into diskus), place diskus in mouth, and inhale quickly and deeply through the diskus. Diskus should be removed and breath held for 10 sec.
- Store at room temperature, 15°–30° C (59°–86° F).

ADVERSE EFFECTS (≥1%) **CNS:** Dizziness, headache, tremor. **CV:** Palpitations, sinus tachycardia. **Res-**

piratory: Respiratory arrest (rare). **Skin:** Rash. **Body as a Whole:** Tolerance (tachyphylaxis).

INTERACTIONS Drug: Effects antagonized by BETA-BLOCKERS.

PHARMACOKINETICS Onset: 10–20 min. **Peak:** Effect 2 h. **Duration:** Up to 12 h. **Distribution:** 94–95% protein bound. **Metabolism:** Dissociates in solution; salmeterol base and xinafoate salt are metabolized, absorbed, distributed, and excreted independently; salmeterol is extensively metabolized by hydroxylation. **Elimination:** Primarily in feces. **Half-Life:** 3–4 h.

NURSING IMPLICATIONS

Assessment & Drug Effects

- Withhold drug and notify physician immediately if bronchospasms occur following its use.
- Monitor cardiovascular status; report tachycardia.
- Lab tests: Monitor liver enzymes periodically with long-term therapy.

Patient & Family Education

- Never use a spacer device with the drug.
- Do not use this drug to treat an acute asthma attack.
- Notify physician immediately of worsening asthma or failure to respond to the usual dose of salmeterol.
- Do not use an additional dose prior to exercise if taking twice-daily doses of salmeterol.
- Take the preexercise dose 30–60 min before exercise and wait 12 h before an additional dose.

SALSALATE

(sal′sal-ate)

Artha-G, Mono-Gesic, Salflex, Salsitab

Classifications: ANALGESIC (SALICYLATE); NONSTEROIDAL ANTI-INFLAMMATORY DRUG (NSAID)
Therapeutic: NONNARCOTIC ANALGESIC, NSAID; DISEASE-MODIFYING ANTIRHEUMATIC DRUG (DMARD)
Prototype: Aspirin
Pregnancy Category: C

AVAILABILITY 500 mg, 750 mg tablets

ACTION & *THERAPEUTIC EFFECT* Anti-inflammatory and analgesic activity of salsalate may be mediated through inhibition of the prostaglandin synthetase enzyme complex. *Has analgesic, anti-inflammatory, and antirheumatic effects.*

USES Symptomatic treatment, rheumatoid arthritis, osteoarthritis, and related rheumatic disorders.

CONTRAINDICATIONS Hypersensitivity to salicylates or NSAIDs; chronic renal insufficiency; peptic ulcer; children younger than 12 y; hemophilia; chickenpox, influenza, tinnitus. Safety in children not established.
CAUTIOUS USE Liver function impairment; older adults; pregnancy (category C), lactation.

ROUTE & DOSAGE

Arthritis
Adult: **PO** 325–3000 mg/day in divided doses (max: 4 g/day)

ADMINISTRATION

Oral

- Give with a full glass of water or food or milk to reduce GI adverse effects.

ADVERSE EFFECTS (≥1%) **GI:** Nausea, dyspepsia, heartburn, vomiting, diarrhea, risk of GI bleed. **Spe-**

S

cial Senses: Tinnitus, hearing loss (reversible). **Body as a Whole:** Vertigo, flushing, headache, confusion, hyperventilation, sweating. **CNS:** Drowsiness.

DIAGNOSTIC TEST INTERFERENCE False-negative results for ***Clinistix;*** false-positives for ***Clinitest.***

INTERACTIONS Drug: Aminosalicylic acid increases risk of salicylate toxicity. **Ammonium chloride** and other ACIDIFYING AGENTS decrease renal elimination and increase risk of salicylate toxicity. ANTICOAGULANTS increase risk of bleeding. ORAL HYPOGLYCEMIC AGENTS increase hypoglycemic activity with salsalate doses greater than 2 g/day. CARBONIC ANHYDRASE INHIBITORS enhance salicylate toxicity. CORTICOSTEROIDS add to ulcerogenic effects. **Methotrexate** toxicity is increased. Low doses of salicylates may antagonize uricosuric effects of **probenecid** and **sulfinpyrazone. Herbal: Feverfew, garlic, ginger, ginkgo** may increase bleeding potential.

PHARMACOKINETICS Absorption: Readily absorbed from small intestine. **Peak:** 1.5–4 h. **Metabolism:** Hydrolyzed in liver, GI mucosa, plasma, whole blood, and other tissues. **Elimination:** In urine. **Half-Life:** 1 h.

S

NURSING IMPLICATIONS

Assessment & Drug Effects

- Symptom relief is gradual (may require 3–4 days to establish steady-state salicylate level).
- Monitor for adverse GI effects, especially in patient with a history of peptic ulcer disease.

Patient & Family Education

- Do not to take another salicylate (e.g., aspirin) while on salsalate therapy.
- Monitor blood glucose for loss of glycemic control in diabetes; drug may induce hypoglycemia when used with sulfonylureas.
- Report tinnitus, hearing loss, vertigo, rash, or nausea.

SAQUINAVIR MESYLATE (Pr)

(sa-quin′a-vir mes′y-late)

Invirase

Classifications: ANTIRETROVIRAL; PROTEASE INHIBITOR

Therapeutic: PROTEASE INHIBITOR

Pregnancy Category: B

AVAILABILITY 200 mg gelatin capsules; 500 mg tablets

ACTION & *THERAPEUTIC EFFECT* Synthetic peptide that inhibits the activity of HIV protease and prevents the cleavage of viral polyproteins essential for the maturation of HIV. *Effectiveness indicated by reduced viral load (decreased number of RNA copies), and increased number of T helper CD4 cells.*

USES Advanced HIV infection, usually in combination with zidovudine or zalcitabine.

CONTRAINDICATIONS Significant hypersensitivity to saquinavir; severe hepatic impairment; antimicrobial resistance to other protease inhibitors, monotherapy, lactation.

CAUTIOUS USE Mild to moderate hepatic insufficiency; severe renal impairment; hepatitis B or C; diabetes mellitus, diabetic ketoacidosis; older adults; hemophilia A or B, pregnancy (category B). Safety and efficacy in HIV-infected children younger than 12 y are not established.

ROUTE & DOSAGE

HIV

Adult/Adolescent: **PO** 1000 mg b.i.d. with ritonavir 100 mg b.i.d.

ADMINISTRATION

Oral

- Give with or up to 2 h after a full meal to ensure adequate absorption and bioavailability. Give with ritonavir.
- Do not administer to anyone taking rifampin or rifabutin because these drugs significantly decrease the plasma level of saquinavir.
- Store at 15°–30° C (59°–86° F) in tightly closed bottle.

ADVERSE EFFECTS (≥1%) **CNS:** Headache, paresthesia, numbness, dizziness, peripheral neuropathy, ataxia, confusion, convulsions, hyperreflexia, hyporeflexia, tremor, agitation, amnesia, anxiety, depression, excessive dreaming, hallucinations, euphoria, irritability, lethargy, somnolence. **CV:** Chest pain, hypertension, hypotension, syncope. **Endocrine:** Dehydration, hyperglycemia, diabetes, weight changes. **Hematologic:** Anemia, splenomegaly, thrombocytopenia, pancytopenia. **GI:** *Nausea, diarrhea, abdominal discomfort,* dyspepsia, mucosal damage, change in appetite, dry mouth. **Skin:** Rash, pruritus, acne, erythema, seborrhea, hair changes, photosensitivity, skin ulceration, dry skin. **Body as a Whole:** Myalgia, allergic reaction. **Respiratory:** Bronchitis, cough, dyspnea, epistaxis, hemoptysis, laryngitis, rhinitis. **Special Senses:** Xerophthalmia, earache, taste alterations, tinnitus, visual disturbances.

INTERACTIONS Drug: Rifampin, rifabutin significantly decrease saquinavir levels. **Phenobarbital, phenytoin, dexamethasone, carbamazepine** may also reduce saquinavir levels. Saquinavir levels may be increased by **delavirdine, ketoconazole, ritonavir, clarithromycin, indinavir.** May increase serum levels of **triazolam, midazolam,** ERGOT DERIVATIVES, **nelfinavir, sildenafil.** May significantly increase **simvastatin** levels and toxicity; may increase risk of **ergotamine** toxicity of **dihydroergotamine, ergotamine. Herbal: St. John's wort, garlic** may decrease antiretroviral activity. **Food: Grapefruit juice** (greater than 1 qt/day) may increase plasma concentrations and adverse effects.

PHARMACOKINETICS Absorption: Rapidly from GI tract; only 4% reaches systemic circulation; food significantly increases bioavailability. **Distribution:** 98% protein bound. **Metabolism:** In liver (CYP3A4), first-pass metabolism. **Elimination:** Primarily in feces (greater than 80%). **Half-Life:** 13 h.

NURSING IMPLICATIONS

Assessment & Drug Effects

- Lab tests: Monitor serum electrolytes, CBC with differential, liver function, blood glucose and HbA1C, CPK, and serum amylase prior to initiating therapy and periodically thereafter.
- Monitor for and report S&S of peripheral neuropathy.
- Assess for buccal mucosa ulceration or other distressing GI S&S.
- Monitor weight periodically.
- Monitor for toxicity if any of the following drugs is used concomitantly: Calcium channel blockers, clindamycin, dapsone, quinidine, triazolam, or simvastatin.

Patient & Family Education

- Take drug within 2 h of a full meal.
- Be aware of all drugs which should not be taken concurrently with saquinavir.
- Be aware that saquinavir is not a cure for HIV infection and that its long-term effects are unknown.
- Report any distressing adverse effects to physician.

SARGRAMOSTIM (GM-CSF)

(sar-gra′mos-tim)

Leukine

Classifications: HEMATOPOIETIC GROWTH FACTOR; GRANULOCYTE MACROPAHGE COLONY STIMULATING FACTOR (GM-CSF)

Therapeutic: HEMATPOIETIC GROWTH FACTOR; GM-CSF

Prototype: Filgrastim

Pregnancy Category: C

AVAILABILITY 250 mcg, 500 mcg injection

ACTION & *THERAPEUTIC EFFECT* Recombinant human granulocyte macrophage colony stimulating factor (GM-CSF) is produced by recombinant DNA technology. GM-CSF is a hematopoietic growth factor that stimulates proliferation and differentiation of progenitor cells in the granulocyte-macrophage pathways. *Effectiveness is measured by an increase in the number of mature white blood cells (i.e., neutrophil count).*

USES Febrile neutropenia, neutropenia caused by chemotherapy, peripheral blood stem cell (PBSC) mobilization.

UNLABELED USES Neutropenia secondary to other diseases; aplastic anemia, Crohn's disease, malignant melanoma.

S

CONTRAINDICATIONS Hypersensitivity to GM-CSF, yeast-derived products; excessive leukemic myeloid blasts in bone marrow or blood greater than or equal to 10%; within 24 h of chemotherapy or radiation treatment; if ANC exceeds 20,000 cells/mm^3 discontinue drug or use half the dose; increased growth of tumor size; lactation; neonates.

CAUTIOUS USE Hypersensitivity to benzl alcohol; history of cardiac arrhythmias, preexisting cardiac disease, renal or hepatic dysfunction, CHF, hypoxia, myelodysplastic syndromes; pulmonary infiltrates; fluid retention; kidney and liver dysfunction; use in AML for adults younger than 55 y; pregnancy (category C). Safety and efficacy in children are not established.

ROUTE & DOSAGE

Neutropenia following Stem Cell Transplantation

Adult: **IV** 250 mcg/m^2/day infused over 2 h for 21 days, begin 2–4 h after bone marrow transfusion and not less than 24 h after last dose of chemotherapy or 12 h after last radiation therapy

Following PBSC

Adult: **IV/Subcutaneous** 250 mg/m^2/day

Neutropenia following Chemotherapy/Febrile Neutropenia

Adult: **IV/Subcutaneous** 250 mcg/m^2/day starting ~day 11 or 4 days following induction chemotherapy

ADMINISTRATION

- Note: Do not give within 24 h preceding or following chemotherapy or within 12 h preceding or following radiotherapy.

Subcutaneous

- Reconstitute each 250 mcg vial with 1 mL of sterile water for injection (without preservative). Direct sterile water against side of vial and swirl gently. Avoid excessive or vigorous agitation. Do not shake. Use without further dilution for subcutaneous injection.

Intravenous

Note: Verify correct IV concentration and rate of infusion administration in infants and children with physician.

PREPARE: **IV Infusion:** Reconstitute as for subcutaneous, then further dilute reconstituted solution with NS. If the final concentration is less than 1 mcg/mL, add albumin (human) to NS before addition of sargramostim. ▪ Use 1 mg albumin per 1 mL of NS to give a final concentration of 0.1% albumin. ▪ Administer as soon as possible and within 6 h of reconstitution or dilution for IV infusion. ▪ Discard after 6 h. ▪ Sargramostim vials are single-dose vials, do not reenter or reuse. Discard unused portion.

ADMINISTER: **IV Infusion:** Give over 2, 4, or 24 h as ordered. ▪ Do not use an in-line membrane filter. ▪ Interrupt administration and reduce the dose by 50% if absolute neutrophil count exceeds 20,000/mm^3 or if platelet count exceeds 500,000/mm^3. Notify physician. ▪ Reduce the IV rate 50% if patient experiences dyspnea during administration. ▪ Discontinue infusion if respiratory symptoms worsen. Notify physician.

INCOMPATIBILITIES **Y-site: Acyclovir, amphotericin B, ampicillin, ampicillin/sulbactam, amsacrine, cefonicid, cefoperazone, ceftazidime, chlorpromazine, ganciclovir, haloperidol, hydrocortisone, hydromorphone, hydroxyzine, imipenem/cilastatin, lorazepam, methylprednisolone, mitomycin, morphine, nalbuphine, ondansetron, piperacillin, sodium bicarbonate, tobramycin.**

▪ Refrigerate the sterile powder, the reconstituted solution, and store diluted solution at 2°–8° C (36°–46° F). ▪ Do not freeze or shake.

ADVERSE EFFECTS (≥1%) **CNS:** Lethargy, malaise, headache, fatigue. **CV:** Abnormal ST segment depression, supraventricular arrhythmias, edema, *hypotension, tachycardia,* pericardial effusion, pericarditis. **Hematologic:** Anemia, *thrombocytopenia.* **GI:** Nausea, vomiting, diarrhea, anorexia. **Body as a Whole:** *Bone pain, myalgia, arthralgias,* weight gain, hyperuricemia, *fever.* **Respiratory:** Pleural effusion. **Skin:** *Rash, pruritus.* **Other:** *First-dose reaction* (some or all of the following symptoms: hypotension, tachycardia, fever, rigors, flushing, nausea, vomiting, diaphoresis, back pain, leg spasms, and dyspnea).

INTERACTIONS Drug: CORTICOSTEROIDS and **lithium** should be used with caution because it may potentiate the myeloproliferative effects.

PHARMACOKINETICS Absorption: Readily from subcutaneous site. **Onset:** 3–6h. **Peak:** 1–2 h. **Duration:** 5–10 days Subcutaneous. **Elimination:** Probably in urine. **Half-Life:** 80–150 min.

NURSING IMPLICATIONS

Assessment & Drug Effects

- Lab tests: Baseline and biweekly CBC with differential and platelet count; biweekly LFTs and kidney function tests in patients with established kidney or liver dysfunction.
- Discontinue treatment if WBC 50,000/mm^3. Notify the physician.
- Monitor cardiac status. Occasional transient supraventricular arrhythmias have occurred during administration, particularly in those with a history of cardiac arrhyth-

mias. Arrhythmias are reversed with discontinuation of drug.

- Give special attention to respiratory symptoms (dyspnea) during and immediately following IV infusion, especially in patients with preexisting pulmonary disease.
- Use drug with caution in patients with preexisting fluid retention, pulmonary infiltrates, or CHF. Peripheral edema, pleural or pericardial effusion has occurred after administration. It is reversible with dose reduction.
- Notify physician of any severe adverse reaction immediately.

Patient & Family Education

- Notify nurse or physician immediately of any adverse effect (e.g., dyspnea, palpitations, peripheral edema, bone or muscle pain) during or after drug administration.

SAXAGLIPTIN

(sax-a-glip'tin)

Onglyza

Classifications: HORMONE MODIFIER; ANTIDIABETIC; INCRETIN MODIFIER; DIPEPTIDYL PEPTIDASE-4 (DPP-4) INHIBITOR

Therapeutic: ANTIDIABETIC; DDP-4 INHIBITOR

Prototype: Sitagliptin

Pregnancy Category: B

S

AVAILABILITY 2.5 mg, 5 mg tablets

ACTION & *THERAPEUTIC EFFECT* Saxagliptin slows inactivation of incretin hormones [e.g. glucagon-like peptide-1 (GLP-1) and glucose-dependent insulinotropic polypeptide (GIP)]. As plasma glucose rises, incretin hormones stimulate release of insulin from the pancreas and GLP-1 also lowers glucagon secretion, resulting in reduced hepatic glucose production. *In type 2 diabetics, saxagliptin elevates the level of incretin hormones, thus increasing insulin secretion and reducing glucagon secretion. It lowers both fasting and postprandial plasma glucose levels.*

USES Treatment of type 2 diabetes mellitus in combination with exercise and diet.

CONTRAINDICATIONS Hypersensitivity to saxagliptin; type 1 diabetes mellitus, ketoacidosis; concurrent administration with insulin. Safety and effectiveness in children younger than 18 y have not been established.

CAUTIOUS USE Mild renal impairment (CrCl greater than 50 mL/min); elderly; pregnancy (category B); lactation.

ROUTE & DOSAGE

Type 2 Diabetes Mellitus

Adult: **PO** 2.5–5 mg once daily. Dose is limited to 2.5 mg once daily when co-administered with a strong CYP3A4/5 inhibitor.

Renal Impairment Dosage Adjustment

CrCl less than or equal to 50 mL/min: 2.5 mg PO once daily

ADMINISTRATION

Oral

- May be taken without regard to meals.
- Dosing in the older adults should be based on creatinine clearance.
- Store at 15°–30° C (59°–86° F).

ADVERSE EFFECTS (≥1%) **Body as a Whole:** Peripheral edema. **CNS:** *Headache.* **GI:** Abdominal pain, gasteroenteritis, vomiting. **Metabolic:** Hypoglycemia. **Respiratory:**

Nasopharyngitis, upper respiratory tract infection. **Skin:** Facial edema, urticaria. **Special Senses:** Sinusitis. **Urogenital:** *Urinary tract infection.*

DIAGNOSTIC TEST INTERFERENCE Dose-related decrease in ***absolute lymphocyte*** count.

INTERACTIONS Drug: Rifampin and other INDUCERS OF CYP3A4/5 enzymes decrease saxagliptin levels. Moderate (e.g., **amprenavir, aprepitant, erythromycin, fluconazole, fosamprenavir, verapamil**) and strong (e.g., **atazanavir, clarithromycin, indinavir, itraconazole, nefazodone, nelfinavir, ritonavir, saquinavir, telithromycin**) INHIBITORS OF CYP3A4/5 increase saxagliptin levels. **Food: Grapefruit juice** increases saxagliptin levels.

PHARMACOKINETICS Peak: 2 h. **Distribution:** Negligible plasma protein binding. **Metabolism:** Hepatic metabolism to active and inactive compounds. **Elimination:** Renal (75%) and fecal (22%). **Half-Life:** 2.5–3.1 h.

NURSING IMPLICATIONS

Assessment & Drug Effects

- Monitor for and report S&S of significant GI distress including NV&D.
- Monitor for S&S of hypoglycemia when used in combination with a sulfonylurea or insulin.
- Lab tests: Baseline and periodic creatinine clearance; periodic fasting and postprandial plasma glucose and HbA1C; lymphocyte count during periods of infection.

Patient & Family Education

- Carry out blood glucose monitoring as directed by physician.
- Consult physician during periods of stress and illness as dosage adjustments may be required.
- When taken alone to control diabetes, saxagliptin is unlikely to cause hypoglycemia because it only works when the blood sugar is rising after food intake.

SCOPOLAMINE

(skoe-pol'a-meen)

Transderm Scōp, Transderm-V ♣

SCOPOLAMINE HYDROBROMIDE

Hyoscine, Isopto-Hyoscine, Scopace, Murocoll, Triptone

Classifications: ANTICHOLINERGIC; ANTIMUSCARINIC; ANTISPASMODIC; ANTIVERTIGO

Therapeutic: ANTISPASMODIC; ANTI-EMETIC; ANTIVERTIGO

Prototype: Atropine

Pregnancy Category: C

AVAILABILITY Scopolamine: 1.5 mg transdermal patch; **Scopolamine HBr:** 0.4 mg tablets; 0.3 mg/mL, 0.4 mg/mL, 0.86 mg/mL, 1 mg/mL injection; 0.25% ophth solution

ACTION & *THERAPEUTIC EFFECT* Antimuscarinic agent that inhibits the action on acetylcholine (ACh) on postganglionic cholinergic nerves as well as on smooth muscles that lack cholinergic innervation. *Produces CNS depression with marked sedative and tranquilizing effects for use in anesthesia. Effective as a preanesthetic agent to control bronchial, nasal, pharyngeal, and salivary secretions. Additionally, it prevents nausea and vomiting associated with motion sickness.*

USES In obstetrics with morphine to produce amnesia and sedation ("twilight sleep") and as preanes-

S

thetic medication. To control spasticity (and drooling) in postencephalitic parkinsonism, paralysis agitans, and other spastic states, as prophylactic agent for motion sickness and as mydriatic and cycloplegic in ophthalmology. Therapeutic system: (**Transderm Scōp**) is used to prevent nausea and vomiting associated with motion sickness.

CONTRAINDICATIONS Hypersensitivity to anticholinergic drugs; hypersensitive to belladonna or barbiturates; asthma; hepatitis; closed-angle glaucoma or open-angle glaucoma; severe ulcerative colitis, GI obstruction; urinary tract obstruction diseases, BPH; myasthenia gravis, autonomic neuropathy; coronary heart disease, CHF, cardiac arrhythmias; toxemia of pregnancy.
CAUTIOUS USE Hypertension; patients older than 40 y, pyloric obstruction, autonomic neuropathy; thyrotoxicosis, liver disease; paralytic ileus; hiatal hernia, mild or moderate ulcerative colitis, gastric ulcer, GERD; renal impairment; parkinsonism; COPD, asthma or allergies; hyperthyroidism; brain damage, spastic paralysis; tartrazine or sulfite sensitivity; Down syndrome; older adults; pregnancy (category C); children, infants.

S

ROUTE & DOSAGE

Preanesthetic

Adult: **PO** 0.4–0.8 mg **IM/Subcutaneous/IV** 0.3–0.6 mg q4–6h
Child: **PO/IM/Subcutaneous/IV** 6 mcg/kg q6–8h (max: 0.3 mg/dose)

Motion Sickness

Adult: **Topical** 1 patch q72h starting 12 h before anticipated travel
Child: **PO** 6 mcg/kg 1 h before anticipated travel

Refraction

Adult: **Ophthalmic** 1–2 drops in eye 1 h before refraction

Uveitis

Adult: **Ophthalmic** 1–2 drops in eye up to q.i.d.

ADMINISTRATION

Instillation

- Minimize possibility of systemic absorption by applying pressure against lacrimal sac during and for 1 or 2 min following instillation of eye drops.

Transdermal

- Apply transdermal disc system (Transderm Scōp, a controlled-release system) to dry surface behind the ear.
- Replace with another disc on another site behind the ear if disc system becomes dislodged.

Subcutaneous or Intramuscular

- Give undiluted.

Intravenous

PREPARE: **Direct:** Dilute required dose with an equal volume of sterile water for injection.
ADMINISTER: **Direct:** Give a single dose slowly over 2–3 min.

- Preserve in tight, light-resistant containers.

ADVERSE EFFECTS (≥1%) **Body as a Whole:** Fatigue, dizziness, *drowsiness,* disorientation, restlessness, hallucinations, toxic psychosis. **GI:** *Dry mouth and throat, constipation.* **Urogenital:** Urinary retention. **CV:** Decreased heart rate. **Special Senses:** Dilated pupils, photophobia, blurred vision, *local irritation,* follicular conjunctivitis. **Respiratory:** <u>Depressed respiration</u>. **Skin:** Local irritation from patch adhesive, rash.

INTERACTIONS Drug: Amantadine, ANTIHISTAMINES, TRICYCLIC ANTIDEPRESSANTS, **quinidine, disopyramide, procainamide** add to anticholinergic effects; decreases **levodopa** effects; **methotrimeprazine** may precipitate extrapyramidal effects; decreases antipsychotic effects (decreased absorption) of PHENOTHIAZINES. **Food: Grapefruit juice** (greater than 1 qt/day) may increase plasma concentrations and adverse effects.

DIAGNOSTIC TEST INTERFERENCE Lab Test: Interferes with ***gastric secretion test.***

PHARMACOKINETICS Absorption: Readily from GI tract and percutaneously. **Peak:** 20–60 min. **Duration:** 5–7 days. **Distribution:** Crosses placenta; distributed to CNS. **Metabolism:** In liver. **Elimination:** In urine.

NURSING IMPLICATIONS

Assessment & Drug Effects

- Observe patient closely; some patients manifest excitement, delirium, and disorientation shortly after drug is administered until sedative effect takes hold.
- Use of side rails is advisable, particularly for older adults, because of amnesic effect of scopolamine.
- In the presence of pain, scopolamine may cause delirium, restlessness, and excitement unless given with an analgesic.
- Be aware that tolerance may develop with prolonged use.
- Terminate ophthalmic use if local irritation, edema, or conjunctivitis occur.

Patient & Family Education

- Vision may blur when used as mydriatic or cycloplegic; do not drive or engage in potentially hazardous activities until vision clears.
- Place disc on skin site the night before an expected trip or anticipated motion for best therapeutic effect.
- Wash hands carefully after handling scopolamine. Anisocoria (unequal size of pupils, blurred vision can develop by rubbing eye with drug-contaminated finger).

SECOBARBITAL SODIUM (Pr)

(see-koe-bar'bi-tal)

Seconal Sodium

Classifications: SEDATIVE-HYPNOTIC; BARBITURATE; ANXIOLYTIC
Therapeutic: SEDATIVE-HYPNOTIC
Pregnancy Category: D
Controlled Substance: Schedule II

AVAILABILITY 50 mg, 100 mg capsules

ACTION & *THERAPEUTIC EFFECT* Short-acting barbiturate with CNS depressant effects as well as mood alteration from excitation to mild sedation, hypnosis, and deep coma. Depresses the sensory cortex, decreases motor activity, alters cerebellar function and produces drowsiness, sedation, and hypnosis. *Alters cerebellar function and produces drowsiness, sedation, and hypnosis.*

USES Hypnotic for simple insomnia and preoperatively to provide basal hypnosis for general, spinal, or regional anesthesia.

CONTRAINDICATIONS History of sensitivity to barbiturates; porphyria; severe liver function; renal function impairment; severe respiratory disease; nephritic syndrome; parturition, fetal immaturity; uncontrolled pain. Use of sterile injection containing polyethylene glycol vehicle in patients with renal insufficiency; pregnancy (category D); children younger than 6 y.

CAUTIOUS USE Pregnant women with toxemia or history of bleeding;

labor and delivery; seizure disorders; aspirin hypersensitivity; liver function impairment; hyperthyroidism; diabetes mellitus; severe anemia; older adults, debilitated individuals; lactation.

ROUTE & DOSAGE

Sedative
Adult: **PO** 100–300 mg/day in 3 divided doses
Child: **PO** 4–6 mg/kg/day in 3 divided doses

Preoperative Sedative
Adult: **PO** 100–300 mg 1–2 h before surgery
Child: **PO** 50–100 mg 1–2 h before surgery

Hypnotic
Adult: **PO** 100–200 mg

ADMINISTRATION

Oral

- Give hypnotic dose only after patient retires for the evening.
- Crush and mix with a fluid or with food if patient cannot swallow pill.

ADVERSE EFFECTS (≥1%) **CNS:** Drowsiness, lethargy, hangover, paradoxical excitement in older adults. **Respiratory:** Respiratory depression, laryngospasm.

INTERACTIONS Drug: Phenmetrazine antagonizes effects of secobarbital; CNS DEPRESSANTS, **alcohol,** SEDATIVES compound CNS depression; MAO INHIBITORS cause excessive CNS depression; **methoxyflurane** increases risk of nephrotoxicity. **Herbal: Kava, valerian** may potentiate sedation.

PHARMACOKINETICS Absorption: 90% from GI tract. **Onset:** 15–30 min. **Duration:** 1–4 h. **Distribution:** Crosses placenta; distributed into breast milk. **Metabolism:** In liver. **Elimination:** In urine. **Half-Life:** 30 h.

NURSING IMPLICATIONS

Assessment & Drug Effects

- Be alert to unexpected responses and report promptly. Older adults or debilitated patients and children sometimes have paradoxical response to barbiturate therapy (i.e., irritability, marked excitement as inappropriate tearfulness and aggression in children, depression, and confusion).
- Be aware that barbiturates do not have analgesic action, and may produce restlessness when given to patients in pain.
- Lab tests: Obtain liver function and hematology tests, serum folate and vitamin D levels during prolonged therapy.
- Be alert for acute toxicity (intoxication) characterized by profound CNS depression, respiratory depression, hypoventilation, cyanosis, cold clammy skin, hypothermia, constricted pupils (but may be dilated in severe intoxication), shock, oliguria, tachycardia, hypotension, respiration arrest, circulatory collapse, and death.

Patient & Family Education

- Do not drive or engage in potentially hazardous activities until response to drug is established.
- Store barbiturates in a safe place; not on the bedside table or other readily accessible places. It is possible to forget having taken the drug, and in half-wakened conditions take more and accidentally overdose.
- Do not become pregnant. Use or add barrier contraception if using hormonal contraceptives.
- Report onset of fever, sore throat or mouth, malaise, easy bruising or bleeding, petechiae, jaundice,

rash to physician during prolonged therapy.

- Do not consume alcohol in any amount when taking a barbiturate. It may severely impair judgment and abilities.

SELEGILINE HYDROCHLORIDE (L-DEPRENYL)

(se-leg′i-leen)

Carbex, Eldepryl, Emsam, Zelapar

Classifications: ANTIPARKINSON; ANTIDEPRESSANT (MAOI)

Therapeutic: ANTIPARKINSON; ANTIDEPRESSANT

Pregnancy Category: C

AVAILABILITY 5 mg tablets, capsules; 1.25 mg orally disintegrating tab; 6 mg, 9 mg, 12 mg transdermal patch

ACTION & *THERAPEUTIC EFFECT* Increase in dopaminergic activity is thought to be primarily due to selective inhibition of MAO type B activity. Ability of selegiline to control parkinsonism is thought to be due to increased dopaminergic activity. It interferes with dopamine reuptake at the synapse of neurons as well as its inhibition of MAO type B dopaminergic activity in the brain. Interference with dopamine reuptake at the MAO type A dopaminergic receptors in the brain is thought to be the mechanism for antidepression. *Effectiveness is measured in decreased tremors, reduced akinesia, improved speech and motor abilities as well as improved walking. At slightly higher doses it is an effective antidepressant.*

USES Adjunctive therapy of Parkinson's disease for patients being treated with levodopa and carbidopa who exhibit deterioration in the quality of their response to therapy, major depressive disorder.

UNLABELED USES Attention deficit/hyperactivity disorder, extrapyramidal symptoms.

CONTRAINDICATIONS Hypersensitivity to selegiline; uncontrolled hypertension; concomitant use with meperidine and other opioids; suidical ideation; lactation.

CAUTIOUS USE Hypertension; history of suicide, bipolar disorder; psychosis; pregnancy (category C). Safety and efficacy in adolescents and children are not established.

ROUTE & DOSAGE

Parkinson's Disease

Adult: **PO** 5 mg b.i.d. with breakfast and lunch (doses greater than 10 mg/day are associated with increased risk of toxicity due to MAO inhibition) **PO (Zelapar)** 1.25 mg daily × 6 weeks (max: 2.5 mg daily)

Geriatric: **PO** Start with 5 mg qa.m.

Depression

Adult: **Transdermal** 6 mg/day, may increase by 3 mg/day q2wk up to 12 mg/day

ADMINISTRATION

Oral

- Do not give daily doses exceeding 10 mg/day.
- Note: Concurrent levodopa and carbidopa doses are usually reduced 10–30% after 2–3 days of selegiline therapy.
- Do not use concurrently with opioids (especially meperidine).
- Store at 15°–30° C (59°–86° F).

Transdermal

- Do not cut or trim patch.
- Before application wash the area with soap and warm water. Dry thoroughly.
- Apply to upper torso, upper thigh, or outer surface of upper arm. Do not apply to hairy, oily, irritated, broken, or calloused skin.
- Rotate sites.
- Wash hands after application.

ADVERSE EFFECTS (≥1%) **CNS:** Sleep disturbances, psychosis, agitation, confusion, dyskinesia, dizziness, hallucinations, dystonia, akathisia. **CV:** Hypotension. **GI:** Anorexia, *nausea,* vomiting, abdominal pain, constipation, diarrhea.

INTERACTIONS Drug: TRICYCLIC ANTIDEPRESSANTS may cause hyperpyrexia, seizures; **fluoxetine, sertraline, paroxetine** may cause hyperthermia, diaphoresis, tremors, seizures, delirium; SYMPATHOMIMETIC AGENTS (e.g., **amphetamine, phenylephrine, phenylpropanolamine**), **guanethidine,** and **reserpine** may cause hypertensive crisis; CNS DEPRESSANTS have additive CNS depressive effects; OPIATE ANALGESICS (especially **meperidine**) may cause hypertensive crisis and circulatory collapse; **buspirone,** hypertension; GENERAL ANESTHETICS—prolonged hypotensive and CNS depressant effects; hypertension, headache, hyperexcitability reported with **dopamine, methyldopa, levodopa, tryptophan; metrizamide** may increase risk of seizures; HYPOTENSIVE AGENTS and DIURETICS have additive hypotensive effects. **Food:** Aged meats or aged cheeses, protein extracts, sour cream, alcohol, anchovies, liver, sausages, overripe figs, bananas, avocados, chocolate, soy sauce, bean curd, natural yogurt, fava beans—**tyramine**-containing foods—may precipitate hypertensive crisis (less frequent with usual doses of **selegiline** than with other MAOIS). **Herbal: Ginseng, ephedra, ma huang, St. John's wort** may cause hypertensive crisis.

PHARMACOKINETICS Absorption: Rapid; 73% reaches systemic circulation. **Onset:** 1 h. **Duration:** 1–3 days. **Distribution:** Crosses placenta; not known if distributed into breast milk. **Metabolism:** In liver to *N*-desmethyldeprenyl-amphetamine and methamphetamine. **Elimination:** In urine. **Half-Life:** 15 min (metabolites 2–20 h).

NURSING IMPLICATIONS

Assessment & Drug Effects

- Monitor vital signs, particularly during period of dosage adjustment. Report alterations in BP or pulse. Indications for discontinuation of the drug include orthostatic hypotension, hypertension, and arrhythmias.
- Monitor for changes in behavior that may indicate increase suicidality, especially in adolescents or children being treated for depression.
- Monitor all patients closely for behavior changes (e.g., hallucinations, confusion, depression, delusions).

Patient & Family Education

- Do not exceed the prescribed drug dose.
- Report symptoms of MAO inhibitor-induced hypertension (e.g., severe headache, palpitations, neck stiffness, nausea, vomiting) immediately to physician.
- Do not drive or engage in potentially hazardous activities until response to drug is known.

- Make positional changes slowly and in stages. Orthostatic hypotension is possible as well as dizziness, light-headedness, and fainting.
- If the transdermal patch falls off, apply a new patch to a new area, and resume previous schedule.
- Only one should be worn at a given time. Remove the old transdermal patch.

SELENIUM SULFIDE

(se-lee′nee-um)

Exsel, Selsun, Selsun Blue

Classifications: ANTIBIOTIC, TOPICAL; ANTIFUNGAL

Therapeutic: TOPICAL ANTIFUNGAL; ANTISEBORRHEIC

Pregnancy Category: C

AVAILABILITY 1% lotion, shampoo

ACTION & *THERAPEUTIC EFFECT* Absorption of selenium sulfide into epithelial tissue cells is followed by degradation of compound to selenium and sulfide ions. Selenium ions block enzyme systems involved in epithelial cell growth. As a result, cell turnover rate is reduced. *Active against* Pityrosporum ovale*, a yeast-like fungus found in the normal flora of the scalp. Also decreases rate of growth of the epithelial cells of the scalp and other epithelial layers of cells in the body.*

USES Itching and flaking of the scalp associated with dandruff, seborrheic dermatitis of the scalp, and tinea versicolor.

CONTRAINDICATIONS Kidney failure or biliary tract obstruction, GI malfunction; Wilson's disease; application to damaged or inflamed skin surfaces; children younger than 2 y.

CAUTIOUS USE Prolonged skin contact; use in genital area or skin folds; pregnancy (category C); lactation.

ROUTE & DOSAGE

Dandruff Control, Seborrheic Dermatitis

Adult/Child: **Topical** Massage 5–10 mL of a 1–2.5% solution into wet scalp and leave on for 2–3 min, rinse thoroughly, then repeat application and rinse well again (initially, shampoo 2 times/wk for 2 wk, then decrease to once q1–4wk prn)

Tinea Versicolor

Adult/Child: **Topical** Apply a 2.5% solution to affected area with a small amount of water to form a lather, leave on for 10 min, then rinse thoroughly, repeat once/day for 7 days

ADMINISTRATION

Topical

- Wash hands thoroughly after application of selenium sulfide to affected areas. Remove jewelry before treatment; drug will damage it.
- Rinse genital areas and skin folds well with water and dry thoroughly after treatment for tinea versicolor to prevent irritation.
- Store at 15°–30° C (59°–86° F) in tight container; protected from heat. Avoid freezing.

ADVERSE EFFECTS (≥1%) **Skin:** *Skin irritation (stinging),* rebound oiliness of scalp, hair discoloration, diffuse hair loss (reversible), systemic toxicity (if applied to abraded, infected skin).

S

PHARMACOKINETICS Absorption: No percutaneous absorption if skin is intact.

NURSING IMPLICATIONS

Assessment & Drug Effects

- Monitor therapeutic effectiveness.

Patient & Family Education

- Rinse thoroughly with water if lotion contacts eyes in order to prevent chemical conjunctivitis.
- Do not use drug more frequently than required to maintain control of dandruff.
- Hair loss is reversible, usually within 2–3 wk after treatment is discontinued.
- Discontinue use if skin is irritated or treatment fails. Systemic toxicity may result from application of lotion to damaged skin (percutaneous absorption) or from prolonged use (overdosage). Toxicity symptoms include tremors, anorexia, occasional vomiting, lethargy, weakness, severe perspiration, garlicky breath, lower abdominal pain. Symptoms disappear 10–12 days after treatment is stopped.

S

SENNA (SENNOSIDES)

(sen′na)

Black-Draught, Gentlax B, Senexon, Senokot, Senolax

Classification: STIMULANT LAXATIVE

Therapeutic: STIMULANT LAXATIVE

Prototype: Bisacodyl

Pregnancy Category: C

AVAILABILITY 8.6 mg, 15 mg, 25 mg tablets; 8.6 mg/5 mL, 15 mg/5 mL syrup

ACTION & *THERAPEUTIC EFFECT* Senna glycosides are converted in colon to active aglycone, which stimulates peristalsis. Concentrate is purified and standardized for uniform action and is claimed to produce less colic than crude form. *Peristalsis stimulated by conversion of drug to active chemical.*

USES Acute constipation and preoperative and preradiographic bowel evacuation.

CONTRAINDICATIONS Hypersensitivity; appendicitis, fecal impaction; fluid and electrolyte imbalances; irritable colon, nausea, vomiting, undiagnosed abdominal pain, intestinal obstruction; children younger than 6 y.

CAUTIOUS USE Diabetes mellitus; children older than 6 y; fluid and electrolyte imbalances; pregnancy (category C).

ROUTE & DOSAGE

Constipation

Adult: **PO Standard Senna Concentrate** 1–2 tablets or 1/2–1 tsp at bedtime (max: 4 tablets or 2 tsp b.i.d.); **Syrup, Liquid** 10–15 mL at bedtime

Child: **PO Standard Senna Concentrate** *Weight greater than 27 kg,* 1 tablet or 1/2 tsp at bedtime; **Syrup, Liquid** *1 mo–1 y,* 1.25–2.5 mL at bedtime; *1–5 y,* 2.5–5 mL at bedtime; *5–15 y,* 5–10 mL at bedtime

ADMINISTRATION

Oral

- Give at bedtime, generally.
- Avoid exposing drug to excessive heat; protect fluid extracts from light.

ADVERSE EFFECTS (≥1%) **GI:** Abdominal cramps, flatulence, nausea, watery diarrhea, excessive loss of water and electrolytes, weight loss, melanotic segmentation of colonic mucosa (reversible).

PHARMACOKINETICS Onset: 6–10 h; may take up to 24 h. **Metabolism:** In liver. **Elimination:** In feces.

NURSING IMPLICATIONS

Assessment & Drug Effects

- Reduce dose in patients who experience considerable abdominal cramping.

Patient & Family Education

- Be aware that drug may alter urine and feces color; yellowish brown (acid), reddish brown (alkaline).
- Continued use may lead to dependence. Consult physician if constipation persists.
- See bisacodyl for additional nursing implications.

SERTACONAZOLE NITRATE

(ser-ta-con′a-zole)

Ertaczo

Classifications: ANTIBIOTIC; AZOLE ANTIFUNGAL

Therapeutic: ANTIFUNGAL

Prototype: Fluconazole

Pregnancy Category: C

AVAILABILITY 2% cream

ACTION & *THERAPEUTIC EFFECT* It is believed that azole antifungals act primarily by inhibiting cytochrome P450–dependent synthesis of ergosterol, a key component of the cell membrane of fungi resulting in fungal cell injury. *Has a broad spectrum of activity against common fungal pathogens.*

USES Treatment of tinea pedis in immunocompetent patients.

CONTRAINDICATIONS Onychomycosis; children younger than 12 y.

CAUTIOUS USE History of hypersensitivity to azole antifungals; pregnancy (category C), lactation.

ROUTE & DOSAGE

Tinea Pedis

Adult/Child (older than 12 y): **Topical** Apply thin layer to affected area twice daily for 4 wk

ADMINISTRATION

Topical

- Cleanse the affected area and dry thoroughly before application.
- Apply a thin layer of the cream to affected area between the toes and the immediately surrounding healthy skin. Gently rub into the skin.
- Store at 15°–30° C (57°–86° F).

ADVERSE EFFECTS (≥1%) **Skin:** Contact dermatitis, dry skin, burning, application site reaction, skin tenderness.

PHARMACOKINETICS Absorption: Negligible through intact skin.

NURSING IMPLICATIONS

Assessment & Drug Effects

- Monitor for clinical improvement, which should be seen about 2 wk after initiating treatment.

Patient & Family Education

- Report any of the following: Severe skin irritation, redness, burning, blistering, or itching.
- Do not stop using this medication prematurely. Athlete's foot takes about 4 wk to clear completely.
- Nursing mothers should ensure that this topical cream does not accidentally get on the breast.

SERTRALINE HYDROCHLORIDE

(ser′tra-leen)

Zoloft

Classifications: ANTIDEPRESSANT; SELECTIVE SEROTONIN REUPTAKE INHIBITOR (SSRI)

Therapeutic: ANTIDEPRESSANT; SSRI

Prototype: Fluoxetine

Pregnancy Category: C

AVAILABILITY 25 mg, 50 mg, 100 mg tablets; 20 mg/mL liquid

ACTION & *THERAPEUTIC EFFECT* Potent inhibitor of serotonin (5-HT) reuptake in the brain. Chronic administration results in downregulation of norepinephrine, a reaction found with other effective antidepressants. *Effective in controlling depression, obsessive-compulsive disorder, anxiety, and panic disorder.*

USES Major depression, obsessive-compulsive disorder, panic disorder, social anxiety disorder, premenstrual dysphoric disorder, generalized anxiety, post-traumatic stress disorder.

UNLABELED USES Eating disorders, generalized anxiety disorder.

S

CONTRAINDICATIONS Patients taking MAO inhibitors or within 14 days of discontinuing MAO inhibitor; concurrent use of Antabuse; suicidal ideation, hyponatremia; mania or hypomania. Safety and effectiveness in children younger than 6 y are not established.

CAUTIOUS USE Seizure disorders, major affective disorders, bipolar disorder, history of suicide; liver dysfunction, renal impairment; abrupt discontinuation; anorexia nervosa, recent history of MI or unstable cardiac disease, dehydration; diabetes mellitus; older adults; ECT therapy, seizure disorder, seizures; pregnancy (category C), lactation.

ROUTE & DOSAGE

Depression, Anxiety

Adult: **PO** Begin with 50 mg/day, gradually increase every few weeks according to response (range: 50–200 mg)

Geriatric: **PO** Start with 25 mg/day

Premenstrual Dysphoric Disorder

Adult: **PO** Begin with 50 mg/day for first cycle, may titrate up to 150 mg/day

Obsessive-Compulsive Disorder

Adult: **PO** Begin with 50 mg/day, may titrate at weekly intervals up to 200 mg/day

Child (6–12 y): **PO** Begin with 25 mg/day, may increase by 50 mg/wk, as tolerated and needed, up to 200 mg/day

ADMINISTRATION

Oral

- Give in the morning or evening.
- Do not give concurrently with an MAO inhibitor or within 14 days of discontinuing an MAO inhibitor.
- Dilute concentrate before use with 4 oz of water, ginger ale, lemon/lime soda, lemonade, or orange juice ONLY. Give immediately after mixing. Caution with latex sensitivity, as the dropper contains dry natural rubber.

ADVERSE EFFECTS (≥1%) **CV:** Palpitations, chest pain, hypertension, hypotension, edema, syncope, tachycardia. **CNS:** *Agitation, insomnia, headache, dizziness, somnolence, fatigue,* ataxia, incoordination, vertigo, abnormal dreams, aggressive behavior, delusions, hallucinations, emotional lability, paranoia, suicidal ideation, depersonalization. **Endocrine:** Gynecomastia, male sexual dysfunction. **GI:** Nausea, vomiting, diarrhea, constipation, indigestion, anorexia, flatulence, abdominal pain, dry mouth. **Special Senses:** Exophthalmos, blurred vision, dry eyes, diplopia, photophobia, tearing, conjunctivitis, mydriasis. **Skin:** Rash, urticaria, acne, alopecia. **Respiratory:** Rhinitis, pharyngitis, cough, dyspnea, bronchospasm. **Body as a Whole:** Myalgia, arthralgia, muscle weakness, bone fracture (older adults). **Metabolic:** Hyponatremia in older adults.

DIAGNOSTIC TEST INTERFERENCE May cause asymptomatic elevations in ***liver function tests.*** Slight decrease in ***uric acid.***

INTERACTIONS Drug: MAOIS (e.g., **selegiline, phenelzine**) should be stopped 14 days before sertraline is started because of serious problems with other SEROTONIN REUPTAKE INHIBITORS (shivering, nausea, diplopia, confusion, anxiety). **Sertraline** may increase levels and toxicity of **diazepam, pimozide, tolbutamide.** Use cautiously with other centrally acting CNS drugs; increase risk of **ergotamine** toxicity with **dihydroergotamine, ergotamine.** Concentrate interacts with **disulfiram. Herbal: St. John's wort** may cause **serotonin** syndrome (headache, dizziness, sweating, agitation). **Food: Grapefruit juice** (greater than 1 qt/day) may increase plasma concentrations and adverse effects.

PHARMACOKINETICS Absorption: Slowly from GI tract. **Onset:** 2–4 wk. **Distribution:** 99% protein bound; distribution into breast milk unknown. **Metabolism:** Extensive first-pass metabolism in liver to inactive metabolites. **Elimination:** 40–45% in urine, 40–45% in feces. **Half-Life:** 24 h.

NURSING IMPLICATIONS

Assessment & Drug Effects

- Supervise patients at risk for suicide closely during initial therapy.
- Monitor for worsening of depression or emergence of suicidal ideation.
- Monitor older adults for fluid and sodium imbalances.
- Monitor patients with a history of a seizure disorder closely.
- Lab tests: Monitor PT and INR with patients receiving concurrent warfarin therapy.

Patient & Family Education

- Report diarrhea, nausea, dyspepsia, insomnia, drowsiness, dizziness, or persistent headache to physician.
- Report emergence of agitation, irritability, hostility or aggression, mania.
- Report signs of bleeding promptly to physician when taking concomitant warfarin.

SEVELAMER HYDROCHLORIDE (Pr)

(se-vel'a-mer)

Renagel

Classifications: ELECTROLYTE AND WATER BALANCE AGENT; PHOSPHATE BINDER

Therapeutic: PHOSPHATE BINDER

Pregnancy Category: C

AVAILABILITY 400 mg, 800 mg tablets; oral powder for suspension

ACTION & *THERAPEUTIC EFFECT* Polymer that binds intestinal phos-

S

phate; interacts with phosphate by way of ion-exchange and hydrogen binding. Advantageously, does not contain aluminum or calcium in treating hyperphosphatemia in end-stage kidney failure. *Effectiveness indicated by a serum phosphate level 6.0 mg/dL or less.*

USES Reduction of serum phosphorus in patients with end-stage kidney disease.

CONTRAINDICATIONS Hypophosphatemia; hypersensitivity to sevelamer HCl; fecal impaction; bowel obstruction; hypophosphatemia; appendicitis; dysphagia, GI bleeding, major GI surgery; lactation. Safety and efficacy in children younger than 18 y are not established.
CAUTIOUS USE GI motility disorders; vitamin deficiencies (especially vitamins D, E, and K and folic acid); pregnancy (category C).

ROUTE & DOSAGE

Hyperphosphatemia
Adult: **PO** 800–1600 mg t.i.d. based on severity of hyperphosphatemia

S

ADMINISTRATION

Oral
- Give with meals; do not open or chew capsule.
- Give other oral medications 1 h before or 3 h after Renagel.
- Discard capsules after printed expiration date.
- Store at 15°–30° C (59°–86° F); protect from moisture.

ADVERSE EFFECTS (≥1%) **Body as a Whole:** Headache, infection, pain. **CV:** Hypertension, hypotension, thrombosis. **GI:** Diarrhea, dyspepsia, vomiting, nausea, constipation, flatulence. **Respiratory:** Increased cough.

NURSING IMPLICATIONS

Assessment & Drug Effects
- Lab tests: Obtain frequent serum phosphate levels.

Patient & Family Education
- Do not use capsules after printed expiration date.
- Take daily multivitamin supplement approved by physician.

SIBUTRAMINE HYDROCHLORIDE MONOHYDRATE
(si-bu′tra-meen)
Meridia
Classification: CNS STIMULANT, ANOREXIANT
Therapeutic: APPETITE SUPPRESSANT
Pregnancy Category: C
Controlled Substance: Schedule IV

AVAILABILITY 5 mg, 10 mg, 15 mg capsules

ACTION & *THERAPEUTIC EFFECT* Inhibits central reuptake of serotonin (5-HT_3), monoamine reuptake, as well as norepinephrine and dopamine reuptake by blocking their receptors. *Appetite suppression occurs by enhancing satiety and raising the metabolic rate. Effectiveness indicated by a loss of at least 4 lb during the first 4 wk of therapy.*

USES Management of obesity in patients with BMI of at least 30 kg/m^2 or BMI of at least 27 kg/m^2 and other risk factors (hypertension, diabetes, dyslipidemia).

CONTRAINDICATIONS Major eating disorders; anorexia nervosa, bulimia; arrhythmias; concurrent administration with other serotonin reuptake inhibitors (e.g., fluoxetine), MAOIs within 14 days, lithium, tryptophan; severe hepatic or renal impairment; ESRD, dialysis; CHF, stroke, CAD; uncontrolled or poorly controlled hypertension; seizures; lactation.

CAUTIOUS USE History of hypertension; older adults; narrow-angle glaucoma; mild or moderate hepatic disease; renal impairment; pregnancy (category C). Safety and efficacy in patients younger than 16 y are not established.

ROUTE & DOSAGE

Weight Loss

Adult/Adolescent: **PO** 10 mg once daily, preferably in morning, may be increased to 15 mg if inadequate weight loss (less than 4 lb) in 4 wk

ADMINISTRATION

Oral

- Note: Doses above 15 mg/day are not recommended.
- Allow at least 2 wk to elapse between discontinuing an MAOI and starting sibutramine.
- Store at 15°–30° C (59°–86° F) in a tightly closed container; protect from light.

ADVERSE EFFECTS (≥1%) **Body as a Whole:** Back pain, flu-like syndrome, asthenia, arthralgia. **CNS:** *Headache,* insomnia, migraine headache, dizziness, nervousness, anxiety, depression, paresthesias, seizures (rare). **CV:** Increase in BP, tachycardia, vasodilation, palpitations. **GI:** *Dry mouth,* anorexia, constipation, abdominal pain, increased appetite, nausea, dyspepsia, taste perversion. **Respiratory:** Rhinitis, pharyngitis, sinusitis, cough. **Skin:** Rash, sweating. **Urogenital:** Dysmenorrhea, UTI.

INTERACTIONS Drug: DECONGESTANTS, COUGH AND ALLERGY MEDICATIONS may cause additional increase in BP; MAOIS, ERGOT DERIVATIVES, **sumatriptan, naratriptan, rizatriptan, zolmitriptan, dextromethorphan, meperidine, pentazocine, fentanyl, lithium;** SSRIS may predispose to **serotonin** syndrome (see Appendix F); **ketoconazole, erythromycin** may inhibit metabolism of sibutramine. **Herbal: St. John's wort** may cause **serotonin** syndrome (see Appendix F).

PHARMACOKINETICS Absorption: Rapidly from GI tract. **Peak:** 1.2 h. **Distribution:** 97% protein bound; concentrates in liver and kidneys. **Metabolism:** In liver (CYP3A4) to active metabolites. **Elimination:** In urine. **Half-Life:** 14–16 h.

NURSING IMPLICATIONS

Assessment & Drug Effects

- Monitor weight changes carefully to determine therapeutic effect.
- Lab tests: Periodic liver function, bilirubin, alkaline phosphatases, lipid profile.
- Monitor BR and HR regularly; report sustained increases in BP or HR immediately.
- Monitor for and immediately report S&S of serotonin syndrome (see Appendix F).
- Monitor persons with narrow-angle glaucoma closely for worsening intraocular pressure.

Patient & Family Education

- Notify physician if any of the following develop: Rash, hives, or

other S&S of an allergic reaction; signs of hyperstimulation such as restlessness, shivering, profuse sweating, irritability, and tremor.
- Take in the morning; causes less interference with sleep.
- Check with physician before taking any OTC cough, cold, allergy, or weight-loss drugs.
- Maintain strict adherence to prescribed antihypertensives.
- Inform physician of all drugs being taken. Serious adverse effects may be experienced with concomitant use of some drugs used to treat depression.

SILDENAFIL CITRATE (Pr)

(sil-den′a-fil ci′trate)

Revatio, Viagra

Classifications: PHOSPHODIESTERASE (PDE) INHIBITOR; IMPOTENCE; PULMONARY ANTIHYPERTENSIVE

Therapeutic: PULMONARY ANTIHYPERTENSIVE; IMPOTENCE

Pregnancy Category: B

AVAILABILITY 20 mg, 25 mg, 50 mg, 100 mg tablets; 10 mg/12.5 mL injection

ACTION & *THERAPEUTIC EFFECT* Enhances vasodilation effect of nitric oxide in the corpus cavernosus of the penis, thus sustaining an erection. PDE-5 inhibitors reduce pulmonary vasodilation by sustaining levels of cyclic guanosine monophosphate (cGMP). Additionally, sildenafil produces a reduction in the pulmonary to systemic vascular resistance ratio. *Effective for treatment of erectile dysfunction, whether organic or psychogenic in origin. Sildenafil produces a significant improvement in arterial oxygenation in pulmonary arterial hypertension (PAH).*

USES Erectile dysfunction, pulmonary arterial hypertension.

UNLABELED USES Altitude sickness, Raynaud's phenomenon, sexual dysfunction.

CONTRAINDICATIONS Hypersensitivity to sildenafil; lactation, children, infants.

CAUTIOUS USE CAD, heart failure, MI, cardiac arrhythmias, stroke within 6 mo of starting drug; nitrate therapy; hypotension and hypertension; risk factors for CVA; aortic stenosis; anatomic deformity of the penis; sickle cell anemia, polycythemia; multiple myeloma; leukemia; active bleeding or a peptic ulcer, GERD, hiatal hernia; coagulopathy; retinitis pigmentosa; hepatic disease, hepatitis, cirrhosis; severe renal impairment (CrCl less than 30 mL/min); older adults; pregnancy (category B).

ROUTE & DOSAGE

Erectile Dysfunction

Adult: **PO** 50 mg 0.5–4 h before sexual activity (dose range: 25 to 100 mg once/day); max dose: 25 mg/day with itraconazole or ketoconazole; max dose: 25 mg/48 h with ritonavir

Geriatric: **PO** 25 mg approximately 1 h before sexual activity

Pulmonary Arterial Hypertension

Adult: **PO** 20 mg t.i.d. (4–6 h apart) **IV** 10 mg t.i.d.

Hepatic Impairment Dosage Adjustment

Child-Pugh class A or B: Starting dose of 25 mg

Renal Impairment Dosage Adjustment

CrCl less than 30 mL/min: Starting dose of 25 mg

S

ADMINISTRATION

Oral

- For erectile dysfunction: Dose 1 h prior to sexual activity (effective range is 0.5–4 h).
- Do not give within 24 h of taking any medication with nitrates (i.e., nitroglycerin).

Intravenous

PREPARE: **Direct:** Give undiluted. ***ADMINISTER:*** **Direct:** Give as a bolus dose.

- Store at 15°–30° C (59°–86° F) in a tightly closed container; protect from light.

ADVERSE EFFECTS (≥1%) **Body as a Whole:** Face edema, photosensitivity, shock, asthenia, pain, chills, fall, allergic reaction, arthritis, myalgia. **CNS:** *Headache,* dizziness, migraine, syncope, cerebral thrombosis, ataxia, neuralgia, paresthesias, tremor, vertigo, depression, insomnia, somnolence, abnormal dreams. **CV:** Flushing, chest pain, <u>MI</u>, angina, AV block, tachycardia, palpitation, hypotension, postural hypotension, <u>cardiac arrest</u>, <u>sudden cardiac death</u>, heart failure, cardiomyopathy, abnormal ECG, edema. **GI:** Dyspepsia, diarrhea, abdominal pain, vomiting, colitis, dysphagia, gastritis, gastroenteritis, esophagitis, stomatitis, dry mouth, abnormal liver function tests, thirst. **Respiratory:** Nasal congestion, asthma, dyspnea, laryngitis, pharyngitis, sinusitis, bronchitis, cough. **Skin:** Rash, urticaria, pruritus, sweating, <u>exfoliative dermatitis</u>. **Urogenital:** UTI. **Special Senses:** Abnormal vision (color changes, photosensitivity, blurred vision, sudden vision loss). **Hematologic:** Anemia, leukopenia. **Metabolic:** Gout, hyperglycemia, hyperuricemia, hypoglycemia, hypernatremia.

INTERACTIONS Drug: NITRATES increase risk of serious hypotension; if used within 4 h of **doxazosin, prazosin, terazosin, tamsulosin; cimetidine, erythromycin, ketoconazole, itraconazole,** PROTEASE INHIBITORS increase sildenafil levels; **rifampin** can decrease sildenafil levels. **Food: Grapefruit juice** (greater than 1 qt/day) may increase plasma concentrations and adverse effects.

PHARMACOKINETICS Absorption: Rapidly from GI tract. **Peak:** 30–120 min. **Distribution:** 96% protein bound. **Metabolism:** In liver (CYP3A4 and 2C9). **Elimination:** 80% in feces, 12% in urine. **Half-Life:** 4 h.

NURSING IMPLICATIONS

Assessment & Drug Effects

- Monitor carefully for and immediately report S&S of cardiac distress.

Patient & Family Education

- Do not take sildenafil within 4 h of taking doxazosin, prazosin, terazosin, or tamsulosin.
- Consuming a high-fat meal before taking drug may cause delay in drug action.
- Report to physician: Headaches, flushing, chest pain, indigestion, blurred vision, sensitivity to light, changes in color vision.

S

SILODOSIN

(sil′o-do-sin)

Rapaflo

Classifications: ALPHA-1 ADRENERGIC RECEPTOR ANTAGONIST; GENITOURINARY SMOOTH MUSCLE RELAXANT

Therapeutic: GENITOURINARY SMOOTH MUSCLE RELAXANT

Prototype: Tamsulosin

Pregnancy Category: B

AVAILABILITY 4 mg, 8 mg capsules

ACTION & *THERAPEUTIC EFFECT* Selective antagonist of post-synaptic alpha-1 adrenoreceptors located in the prostate, bladder base, bladder neck, prostatic capsule, and prostatic urethra. *Blockade of these alpha-1 adrenoreceptors causes the smooth muscle in these tissues to relax, resulting in improvement in urine flow and reduction in signs and symptoms of benign prostatic hyperplasia (BPH).*

USES Treatment of the signs and symptoms of BPH

CONTRAINDICATIONS Severe renal impairment (CrCl less than 30 mL/min); severe hepatic impairment (Child-Pugh score greater than or equal to 10); concomitant administration with strong CYP3A4 inhibitor drugs. Safety and efficacy in children have not been established.

CAUTIOUS USE Moderate renal impairment; cataract surgery; elderly; pregnancy (category B).

ROUTE & DOSAGE

Benign Prostatic Hyperplasia

Adult: **PO** 8 mg once daily with a meal

Renal Impairment Dosage Adjustment

CrCl 30–49 mL/min: Reduce dose to 4 mg once daily; less than 30 mL/min: Not recommended

ADMINISTRATION

Oral

- Give with meals.
- Store at 15°–30° C (59°–86° F). Protect from light and moisture.

ADVERSE EFFECTS (≥1%) **Body as a Whole:** Abdominal pain, asthenia. **CNS:** Dizziness, headache, insomnia. **CV:** Orthostatic hypotension. **GI:** Diarrhea. **Respiratory:** Nasal congestion, nasopharyngitis, rhinorrhea, sinusitis. **Urogenital:** *Retrograde ejaculation.*

DIAGNOSTIC TEST INTERFERENCE Increased ***prostate specific antigen (PSA).***

INTERACTIONS Drug: Strong CYP3A4 INHIBITORS (e.g., **itraconazole, ritonavir**) or strong P-GLYCOPROTEIN INHIBITORS (e.g., **ketoconazole**) greatly increases silodosin levels. Moderate CYP3A4 INHIBITORS (e.g., **diltiazem, erythromycin, verapamil**) may increase silodosin levels. Other ALPHA-BLOCKERS can cause additive pharmacodynamic effects. INHIBITORS OF UDP-GLUCURONOSYLTRANSFERASE 2B7 (e.g., **probenecid, valproic acid, fluconazole**) may increase silodosin levels.

PHARMACOKINETICS Absorption: 32% bioavailable. **Distribution:** Approximately 97% plasma protein bound. **Metabolism:** Hepatic oxidation and conjugation. **Elimination:** Renal and fecal. **Half-Life:** 13.3 h.

NURSING IMPLICATIONS

Assessment & Drug Effects

- Monitor I&O and ease of voiding.
- Monitor orthostatic vital signs (lying and then standing) at the beginning of therapy. Report a systolic pressure drop of 15 mm Hg or greater and HR increase of 15 beats or greater upon standing.
- Monitor for orthostatic hypotension, especially at the beginning of therapy and in those taking concurrent antihypertensive drugs.

Patient & Family Education

- Make position changes slowly and in stages to minimize risk of dizziness and fainting.
- Avoid hazardous activities until reaction to drug is known.
- Report unexplained skin eruptions or purple skin patches.

- If cataract surgery is planned, inform ophthalmologist that you are taking silodosin.

SILVER SULFADIAZINE

(sul-fa-dye'a-zeen)

Silvadene

Classification: SULFONAMIDE

Therapeutic: TOPICAL ANTIINFECTIVE

Prototype: Sulfisoxazole

Pregnancy Category: B

AVAILABILITY 1%/50 g cream

ACTION & *THERAPEUTIC EFFECT* Silver salt is released slowly and exerts bactericidal effect only on bacterial cell membrane and wall, rather than by inhibiting folic acid synthesis. *Broad antimicrobial activity including many gram-negative and gram-positive bacteria and yeast.*

USES Prevention and treatment of sepsis in second- and third-degree burns.

CONTRAINDICATIONS Hypersensitivity to other sulfonamides; pregnant women at term, premature infants and neonates younger than 1 mo.

CAUTIOUS USE Impaired kidney or liver function; porphyria; impaired respiratory function; G6PD deficiency; thrombocytopenia, leukopenia, hematological disease; pregnancy (category B), lactation.

ROUTE & DOSAGE

Burn Wound Treatment

Adult/Child: **Topical** Apply 1% cream 1–2 times/day to thickness of approximately 1.5 mm (1/16 in.)

ADMINISTRATION

Topical

- Do not use if cream darkens; it is water soluble and white.
- Apply with sterile, gloved hands to cleansed, debrided burned areas. Reapply cream to areas where it has been removed by patient activity; cover burn wounds with medication at all times.
- Bathe patient daily (in whirlpool or shower or in bed) as aid to debridement. Reapply drug.
- Note: Dressings are not required but may be used if necessary. Drug does not stain clothing.
- Store at room temperature away from heat.

ADVERSE EFFECTS (≥1%) **Body as a Whole:** Pain (occasionally), burning, itching, rash, reversible leukopenia. Potential for toxicity as for other sulfonamides if applied to extensive areas of the body surface.

INTERACTIONS Drug: PROTEOLYTIC ENZYMES are inactivated by silver in cream.

PHARMACOKINETICS Absorption: Not absorbed through intact skin, however, approximately 10% could be absorbed when applied to second- or third-degree burns. **Distribution:** Distributed into most body tissues. **Metabolism:** In the liver. **Elimination:** In urine.

NURSING IMPLICATIONS

Assessment & Drug Effects

- Observe for and report hypersensitivity reaction: Rash, itching, or burning sensation in unburned areas.
- Lab tests: Obtain serum sulfa concentrations, urinalysis, and kidney function tests when drug is applied to extensive areas. Significant quantities of drug may be absorbed.

S

- Observe patient for reactions attributed to sulfonamides.
- Note: Analgesic may be required. Occasionally, pain is experienced on application; intensity and duration depend on depth of burn.
- Continue treatment until satisfactory healing or burn site is ready for grafting, unless adverse reactions occur.

SIMVASTATIN

(sim-vah-sta′-tin)

Zocor

Classifications: HMG-COA REDUCTASE INHIBITOR (STATIN); ANTILIPEMIC
Therapeutic: ANTIHYPERLIPEMIC; STATIN
Prototype: Lovastatin
Pregnancy Category: X

AVAILABILITY 5 mg, 10 mg, 20 mg, 40 mg, 80 mg tablets

ACTION & *THERAPEUTIC EFFECT* Inhibitor of 3-hydroxy-3-methylglutaryl coenzyme A (HMG-CoA) reductase. HMG-CoA reductase inhibitors increase HDL cholesterol, and decrease LDL cholesterol, and total cholesterol synthesis. *Effectiveness indicated by decreased serum triglycerides, decreased LDL, cholesterol, and modest increases in HDL cholesterol.*

S

USES Hypercholesterolemia (alone or in combination with bile acid sequestrants), familial hypercholesterolemia. Reduces risk of coronary death and nonfatal MI.

CONTRAINDICATIONS Hypersensitivity to simvastatin; active liver disease or unexplained elevation of transaminase, hepatic encephalopathy, hepatitis, jaundice, AST or ALT of 3 × ULN; rhabdomyolysis, acute renal failure; cholestasis; myopathy; MS; pregnancy (category X), lactation; children younger than 10 y.

CAUTIOUS USE Homozygous familial hypercholesterolemia, history of liver disease, alcoholics; renal disease, renal impairment; DM; seizure disorder.

ROUTE & DOSAGE

Hypercholesterolemia

Adult: **PO** 5–40 mg daily (max: 80 mg daily). Patients taking danazol or cyclosporine should not exceed 10 mg daily. Patients taking verapamil or amiodarone should not exceed 20 mg daily.
Adolescent/Child (older than 10 y and in females at least 1 y postmenarche): **PO** 10 mg each night (may dose up to 40 mg each night)

Renal Impairment Dosage Adjustment

CrCl less than 20 mL/min: Start with 5 mg each night

ADMINISTRATION

Oral

- Adjust dosage usually at 4-wk intervals.
- Give in the evening.
- Store at 15°–30° C (59°–86° F).

ADVERSE EFFECTS (≥1%) **CV:** Angina. **CNS:** Dizziness, headache, vertigo, asthenia, fatigue, insomnia. **GI:** Nausea, diarrhea, vomiting, abdominal pain, constipation, flatulence, heartburn, transient elevations in liver transaminases, transient elevations in CPK. **Body as a Whole:** Fatigue. **Respiratory:** Rhinitis, cough.

INTERACTIONS Drug: May increase PT when administered with **warfarin; cyclosporine, gemfibro-**

zil, fenofibrate, clofibrate, antilipemic doses of **niacin, fluconazole, itraconazole, ketoconazole, miconazole, nefazodone, nelfinavir, ritonavir, saquinavir, sildenafil, tacrolimus, clarithromycin, erythromycin, telithromycin** may increase serum levels and increase risk of myopathy, rhabdomyolysis and acute kidney failure. Avoid use with **rifampin.** Use with **amiodarone** increases risk of rhabdomyolysis. **Food: Grapefruit juice** (greater than 1 qt/day) may increase risk of myopathy, rhabdomyolysis. **Herbal: Peppermint oil** may increase plasma concentrations. **St. John's wort** may decrease efficacy.

PHARMACOKINETICS Absorption: Rapidly from GI tract. **Onset:** 2 wk. **Peak:** 4–6 wk. **Distribution:** 95% protein bound; achieves high liver concentrations; crosses placenta. **Metabolism:** Extensive first-pass metabolism in liver to its active metabolite. **Elimination:** 13% in urine, 60% in bile and feces.

NURSING IMPLICATIONS

Assessment & Drug Effects

- Assess for and report unexplained muscle pain. Determine CPK level at onset of muscle pain.
- Lab tests: Obtain baseline and periodic (q6mo) liver function during the first year and yearly thereafter. Monitor cholesterol levels throughout therapy.
- Monitor coagulation studies with patients receiving concurrent warfarin therapy. PT may be prolonged.

Patient & Family Education

- Report unexplained muscle pain, tenderness, or weakness, especially if accompanied by malaise or fever, to physician.
- Report signs of bleeding to physician promptly when taking concurrent warfarin.
- Moderate intake of grapefruit juice while taking this medication.

SIROLIMUS

(sir-o-li′mus)

Rapamune

Classifications: IMMUNOMODULATOR; IMMUNOSUPPRESSANT

Therapeutic: IMMUNOSUPPRESSANT

Prototype: Cyclosporine

Pregnancy Category: C

AVAILABILITY 1 mg, 2 mg tablets; 1 mg/mL oral solution

ACTION & *THERAPEUTIC EFFECT* Immunomodulator structurally related to tacrolimus with immunosuppressive activity. Active in reducing a transplant rejection by inhibiting the response of helper T-lymphocytes and B-lymphocytes to cytokinesis [(interleukin) IL-2, IL-4, and IL-5]. *Inhibits antibody production and acute transplant rejection reaction in autoimmune disorders [e.g., systemic lupus erythematosus (SLE)]. Indicated by nonrejection of transplanted organ.*

USES Prophylaxis of kidney transplant rejection.

UNLABELED USES Treatment of psoriasis.

CONTRAINDICATIONS Hypersensitivity to sirolimus; lung or liver transplant patients; soya lecithin (soy fatty acids) hypersensitivity; lymphoma, neoplastic disease; children younger than 13 y; females of childbearing age; lactation.

CAUTIOUS USE Hypersensitivity to or concurrent administration with tacrolimus; impaired renal function;

S

concurrent use of aminoglycosides, and amphotericin B; renal transplant patients; dialysis patients, UV exposure, retransplant patients, multiorgan transplant recipients, African American transplant patients; viral or bacterial infection; hypertriglyceridemia, hyperlipidemia, diabetic patients, atrial fibrillation, CHF, hypervolemia, palpitations; mild to moderate hepatic disease; coronary artery disease; myelosuppression; liver disease; pregnancy (category C).

ROUTE & DOSAGE

Kidney Transplant

Adult/Adolescent (over 40 kg): **PO** 6 mg loading dose immediately after transplant, then 2 mg/day. Doses will need to be much higher (up to 40 mg/day) if using cyclosporine or corticosteroids.

Adolescent (13 y or older, weight less than 40 kg): **PO** 3 mg/m^2 loading dose immediately after transplant, then 1 $mg/m^2/day$. Doses will need to be much higher (up to 40 mg/day) if not on cyclosporine.

Hepatic Impairment Dosage Adjustment

Loading dose does not need to be modified. Reduce maintenance dose by 33% in moderate or mild impairment. In severe impairment, reduce by 50%.

S

ADMINISTRATION

Oral

- Give 4 h after oral cyclosporine.
- Tablets should be swallowed whole. They should not be crushed or chewed.
- Add prescribed amount of sirolimus oral solution to a glass containing 2 oz (60 mL) or more of water or orange juice (do not use any other type of liquid). Stir vigorously and administer immediately. Refill glass with 4 oz (120 mL) or more of water or orange juice. Stir vigorously and administer immediately.
- Give consistently with respect to amount and type of food.
- Refrigerate; protect from light; use multidose bottles within 1 mo of opening.

ADVERSE EFFECTS (≥1%) **Body as a Whole:** *Asthenia, back pain, chest pain, fever, pain, arthralgia;* flu-like syndrome; generalized edema; infection; lymphocele; malaise; sepsis, arthrosis, bone necrosis, leg cramps, myalgia, osteoporosis, tetany, abscess, ascites, cellulitis, chills, face edema, hernia, pelvic pain, peritonitis. **CNS:** *Insomnia, tremor, headache,* anxiety, confusion, depression, dizziness, emotional lability, hypertonia, hyperesthesia, hypotonia, neuropathy, paresthesia, somnolence. **CV:** *Hypertension,* atrial fibrillation, CHF, hypervolemia, hypotension, palpitation, peripheral vascular disorder, postural hypotension, syncope, tachycardia, thrombophlebitis, thrombosis, vasodilation. **GI:** *Constipation, diarrhea, dyspepsia, nausea, vomiting, abdominal pain,* anorexia, dysphagia, eructation, esophagitis, flatulence, gastritis, gastroenteritis, gingivitis, gum hyperplasia, ileus, mouth ulceration, oral moniliasis, stomatitis, abnormal liver function tests. **Hematologic:** *Anemia, thrombocytopenia,* leukopenia, hemorrhage, ecchymosis, leukocytosis, lymphadenopathy, polycythemia, thrombotic, thrombocytopenic purpura. **Metabolic:** *Edema, hypercholesterolemia, hyperkalemia, hyperlipidemia, hypokalemia, hypophosphatemia, peripheral edema, weight gain,* Cushing's syndrome, diabetes, acidosis, hypercalcemia, hyperglycemia, hyperphosphatemia, hypocalcemia, hypoglycemia, hypomagnesemia, hyponatremia; increased LDH, alkaline phosphatase, BUN, creatine phosphokinase, ALT, or AST; weight loss. **Respiratory:** *Dyspnea, pharyngitis, upper respiratory tract infection,* asthma, atelectasis, bronchitis, cough, epistaxis, hypoxia, lung edema, pleural effusion, pneumonia, rhinitis, sinusitis. **Skin:** *Acne, rash,* fungal dermatitis, hirsutism, pruritus, skin hypertrophy, skin ulcer, sweating. **Urogenital:** *UTI,* albuminuria, bladder pain, dysuria, hematuria, hydronephrosis, impotence, kidney pain, nocturia, renal tubular necrosis, oliguria, pyuria, scrotal edema, incontinence, urinary retention, glycosuria. **Special Senses:** Abnormal vision, cataract, conjunctivitis, deafness, ear pain, otitis media, tinnitus.

INTERACTIONS Drug: Sirolimus concentrations increased by **clarithromycin, cyclosporine, diltiazem, erythromycin, ketoconazole, itraconazole, telithromycin;** sirolimus concentrations decreased by **rifabutin, rifampin;** VACCINES may be less effective with sirolimus; **tacrolimus** increases mortality, hepatic artery thrombosis, and graft loss. **Food: Grapefruit juice** significantly increases plasma levels. High fat meals increase levels. **Herbal: St. John's wort** decreases efficacy.

PHARMACOKINETICS Absorption: Rapidly with 14% bioavailability. **Peak:** 2 h. **Distribution:** 92% protein bound, distributes in high concentrations to heart, intestines, kidneys, liver, lungs, muscle, spleen, and testes. **Metabolism:** In liver (CYP3A4). **Elimination:** 91% in feces, 2.2% in urine. **Half-Life:** 62 h.

NURSING IMPLICATIONS

Assessment & Drug Effects

- Monitor for S&S of graft rejection.
- Control hyperlipidemia prior to initiating drug.
- Lab tests: Draw trough whole-blood sirolimus levels 1 h before a scheduled dose. Obtain periodic lipid profile, CBC with differential, fasting plasma glucose, blood chemistry, BUN, and creatinine (especially with other drugs known to cause renal impairment).

Patient & Family Education

- Avoid grapefruit juice within 2 h of taking sirolimus.
- Limit exposure to sunlight (UV exposure).
- Note: Decreased effectiveness possible for vaccines during therapy.
- Use or add barrier contraceptive before, during, and for 12 wk after discontinuing therapy.

SITAGLIPTIN (Pr)

(sit-a-glip′tin)

Januvia

Classifications: HORMONE MODIFIER; ANTIDIABETIC; INCRETIN MODIFIER; DIPEPTIDYL PEPTIDASE-4 (DPP-4) INHIBITOR

Therapeutic: ANTIDIABETIC; DDP-4 INHIBITOR

Pregnancy Category: C

AVAILABILITY 25 mg, 50 mg, and 100 mg tablets

ACTION & *THERAPEUTIC EFFECT* Sitagliptin slows inactivation of incretin hormones [e.g., glucagon-like peptide-1 (GLP-1) and glucose-dependent insulinotropic polypeptide (GIP)] that are released by the intestine. As plasma glucose rises, incretin hormones stimulate release of insulin from the pancreas, and GLP-1 also lowers glucagon secretion, resulting in reduced hepatic glucose production. *Sitagliptin* *lowers both fasting and postprandial plasma glucose levels.*

USES Adjunct treatment of type 2 diabetes mellitus in combination with exercise and diet.

CONTRAINDICATIONS Type I diabetes mellitus, diabetic ketoacidosis. Safety and efficacy in children younger than 18 y are not known.
CAUTIOUS USE Moderate to severe renal impairment, renal failure, hemodialysis; older adults; pregnancy (category C), lactation.

ROUTE & DOSAGE

Type 2 Diabetes Mellitus
Adult: **PO** 100 mg/day

Renal Impairment Dosage Adjustment
CrCl between 30 mL/min and 50 mL/min: 50 mg/day; less than 30 mL/min: 25 mg/day

ADMINISTRATION

Oral
- May be given without regard to meals.
- Note that dosage adjustment is recommended for moderate to severe renal impairment.
- Store at 20°–25° C (68°–77° F).

S

ADVERSE EFFECTS (≥1%) **CNS:** Headache. **Respiratory:** Nasopharyngitis, upper respiratory tract infection. **Endocrine:** Acute pancreatitis.

INTERACTIONS Drug: Sitagliptin may increase **digoxin** levels. QUINOLONES may increase blood glucose.

PHARMACOKINETICS Absorption: 87% absorbed. **Peak:** 1–4 h. **Distribution:** 38% protein bound. **Metabolism:** 20% metabolized in the liver. **Elimination:** Primarily renal (87%) with minor elimination in the kidneys. **Half-Life:** 12.4 h.

NURSING IMPLICATIONS

Assessment & Drug Effects
- Monitor for and report S&S of significant GI distress, including NV&D.
- Monitor for S&S of hypoglycemia when used in combination with a sulfonylurea drug or insulin.
- Lab tests: Baseline and periodic CrCl; periodic fasting and postprandial plasma glucose and HbA1C.
- Monitor blood levels of digoxin with concurrent therapy.

Patient & Family Education
- Follow directions for taking the drug (see Administration).
- Note: When taken alone to control diabetes, sitagliptin is unlikely to cause hypoglycemia because it only works when your blood sugar is rising.

SODIUM BICARBONATE NA(HCO_3)

(sod'i-um bi-car'bon-ate)
Sodium Bicarbonate
Classifications: FLUID AND ELECTROLYTE BALANCE AGENT; ANTACID
Therapeutic: ANTACID
Pregnancy Category: C

AVAILABILITY 325 mg, 520 mg, 650 mg tablets; 4.2%, 5%, 7.5%, 8.4% injection

ACTION & *THERAPEUTIC EFFECT*
Rapidly neutralizes gastric acid to form sodium chloride, carbon dioxide, and water. After absorption of sodium bicarbonate, plasma alkali reserve is increased and excess sodium and bicarbonate ions are excreted in urine, thus rendering urine less acid. *Short-acting, potent systemic antacid; rapidly neutralizes gastric acid or systemic acidosis.*

USES Systemic alkalinizer to correct metabolic acidosis (as occurs in diabetes mellitus, shock, cardiac arrest, or vascular collapse), to minimize uric acid crystallization associated with uricosuric agents, to increase the solubility of sulfonamides, and to enhance renal excretion of barbiturate and salicylate overdosage. Commonly used as home remedy for relief of occasional heartburn, indigestion, or sour stomach. Used topically as paste, bath, or soak to relieve itching and minor skin irritations such as sunburn, insect bites, prickly heat, poison ivy, sumac, or oak. Sterile solutions are used to buffer acidic parenteral solutions to prevent acidosis. Also as a buffering agent in many commercial products (e.g., mouthwashes, douches, enemas, ophthalmic solutions).

CONTRAINDICATIONS Prolonged therapy with sodium bicarbonate; patients losing chloride (as from vomiting, GI suction, diuresis); hypocalcemia; metabolic alkalosis; respiratory alkalosis; peptic ulcer.

CAUTIOUS USE Edema, sodium-retaining disorders; heart disease, hypertension; preexisting respiratory acidosis; renal disease, renal insufficiency; hyperkalemia, hypokalemia; older adults; pregnancy (category C).

ROUTE & DOSAGE

Antacid

Adult: **PO** 0.3–2 g 1–4 times/day or 1/2 tsp of powder in glass of water

Urinary Alkalinizer

Adult: **PO** 4 g initially, then 1–2 g q4h
Child: **PO** 84–840 mg/kg/day in divided doses

Cardiac Arrest

Adult: **IV** 1 mEq/kg initially, then 0.5 mEq/kg q10min depending on arterial blood gas determinations (8.4% solutions contain 50 mEq/50 mL), give over 1–2 min
Child: **IV** 0.5–1 mEq/kg q10min depending on arterial blood gas determinations, give over 1–2 min

Metabolic Acidosis

Adult/Child: **IV** Dose adjusted according to pH, base deficit, $Paco_2$, fluid limits, and patient response

ADMINISTRATION

Oral

- Do not add oral preparation to calcium-containing solutions.

Intravenous

PREPARE: **Direct/IV Infusion:** May give 4.2% (0.5 mEq/mL) and 5% (0.595 mEq/mL) $NaHCO_3$ solutions undiluted. ▪ Dilute 7.5% (0.892 mEq/mL) and 8.4% (1 mEq/mL) solutions with compatible IV solutions to a maximum concentration of 0.5 mEq/mL. ▪ For infants and children, dilute to at least 4.2%.

ADMINISTER: **Direct:** Give a bolus dose over 1–2 min only in emergency situations. ▪ For neonates or infants younger than 2 y, use only 4.2% solution for direct IV injection. **IV Infusion:** Usual rate is 2–5 mEq/kg over 4–8 h; do not exceed 50 mEq/h. ▪ Flush line before/after with NS. ▪ Stop infusion immediately if extravasation occurs. Severe tissue damage has followed tissue infiltration.

INCOMPATIBILITIES **Solution/additive:** **Alcohol 5%, lactated Ringer's, amoxicillin, ascorbic**

S

acid, bupivacaine, carboplatin, carmustine, ciprofloxacin, cisplatin, codeine, corticotropin, dobutamine, dopamine, epinephrine, glycopyrrolate, hydromorphone, imipenem-cilastatin, insulin, isoproterenol, labetalol, levorphanol, magnesium sulfate, meperidine, meropenem, methadone, metoclopramide, morphine, norepinephrine, oxytetracycline, penicillin G, pentazocine, pentobarbital, phenobarbital, procaine, promazine, streptomycin, succinylcholine, tetracycline, thiopental, vancomycin, vitamin B complex with C. Y-site: **Allopurinol, amiodarone, amphotericin B cholesteryl complex, calcium chloride, ciprofloxacin, cisatracurium, diltiazem, doxorubicin liposome, fenoldopam, hetastarch, idarubicin, imipenem/cilastatin, inamrinone, leucovorin, lidocaine, midazolam, nalbuphine, ondansetron, oxacillin, sargramostim, verapamil, vincristine, vindesine, vinorelbine.**

▪ Store in airtight containers. ▪ Note expiration date.

S

ADVERSE EFFECTS (≥1%) **GI:** *Belching, gastric distention,* flatulence. **Metabolic:** Metabolic alkalosis; electrolyte imbalance: Sodium overload (pulmonary edema), hypocalcemia (tetany), hypokalemia, milk-alkali syndrome, dehydration. **Other:** Rapid IV in neonates (hypernatremia, reduction in CSF pressure, <u>intracranial hemorrhage</u>). **Skin:** Severe tissue damage following extravasation of IV solution. **Urogenital:** Renal calculi or crystals, impaired kidney function.

DIAGNOSTIC TEST INTERFERENCE Small increase in ***blood lactate*** levels (following IV infusion of sodium bicarbonate); false-positive ***urinary protein*** determinations (using ***ames reagent, sulfacetic acid,*** heat and ***acetic acid*** or ***nitric acid ring method***); elevated ***urinary urobilinogen*** levels (***urobilinogen*** excretion increases in alkaline urine).

INTERACTIONS Drug: May decrease absorption of **ketoconazole;** may decrease elimination of **dextroamphetamine, ephedrine, pseudoephedrine, quinidine;** may increase elimination of **chlorpropamide, lithium,** SALICYLATES, TETRACYCLINES.

PHARMACOKINETICS Absorption: Readily from GI tract. **Onset:** 15 min. **Duration:** 1–2 h. **Elimination:** In urine within 3–4 h.

NURSING IMPLICATIONS

Assessment & Drug Effects

- Be aware that long-term use of oral preparation with milk or calcium can cause milk-alkali syndrome: Anorexia, nausea, vomiting, headache, mental confusion, hypercalcemia, hypophosphatemia, soft tissue calcification, renal and ureteral calculi, renal insufficiency, metabolic alkalosis.
- Lab tests: Urinary alkalinization: Monitor urinary pH as a guide to dosage (pH testing with nitrazine paper may be done at intervals throughout the day and dosage adjustments made accordingly).
- Lab tests: Metabolic acidosis: Monitor patient closely by observations of clinical condition; measurements of acid-base status (blood pH, Po_2, Pco_2, HCO_3^-, and other electrolytes, are usually made several times daily during acute period). Observe for signs of alkalosis (over treatment) (see Appendix F).

- Observe for and report S&S of improvement or reversal of metabolic acidosis (see Appendix F).

Patient & Family Education

- Do not use sodium bicarbonate as antacid. A nonabsorbable OTC alternative for repeated use is safer.
- Do not take antacids longer than 2 wk except under advice and supervision of a physician. Self-medication with routine doses of sodium bicarbonate or soda mints may cause sodium retention and alkalosis, especially when kidney function is impaired.
- Be aware that commonly used OTC antacid products contain sodium bicarbonate: Alka-Seltzer, Bromo-Seltzer, Gaviscon.

SODIUM FERRIC GLUCONATE COMPLEX

(so'di-um fer'ric glu'co-nate)

Ferrlecit

Classifications: NUTRITIONAL SUPPLEMENT; IRON PREPARATION

Therapeutic: ANTIANEMIC; IRON REPLACEMENT

Prototype: Ferrous sulfate

Pregnancy Category: B

AVAILABILITY 62.5 mg elemental iron/5 mL ampule

ACTION & *THERAPEUTIC EFFECT* Stable iron complex used to restore iron loss in chronic kidney failure patients. The use of erythropoietin therapy and blood loss through hemodialysis require iron replacement. The ferric ion combines with transferrin and is transported to bone marrow where it is incorporated into hemoglobin. *Effectiveness indicated by improved Hgb and Hct, iron saturation, and serum ferritin levels.*

USES Treatment of iron deficiency in patients on chronic hemodialysis and receiving erythropoietin therapy.

CONTRAINDICATIONS Any anemia not related to iron deficiency; hypersensitivity to sodium ferric gluconate complex; hemochromatosis, hemosiderosis; hemolytic anemia; thalassemia; neonates.

CAUTIOUS USE Hypersensitivity to benzyl alcohol; active or suspected infection; cardiac disease; hepatic disease; older adults; pregnancy (category B), lactation. Safety and efficacy in children younger than 6 y are not established.

ROUTE & DOSAGE

Iron Deficiency in Dialysis Patients

Adult: **IV** 125 mg infused over 1 h
Child (older than 6 y): **IV** 1.5 mg/kg infused over 1 h (max: 125 mg/dose)

ADMINISTRATION

Intravenous

PREPARE: **Direct for Adult:** May be given undiluted. **Direct for Child:** Dilute required doses in 25 mL NS. **IV Infusion for Adult/Child:** Dilute 125 mg in 100 mL of NS. ▪ Use immediately after dilution.

ADMINISTER: **Direct for Adult:** Give no faster than 12.5 mg/min. **IV Infusion for Adult/Child:** Give over NOT less than 60 min.

INCOMPATIBILITIES **Solution/additive:** Do not mix with any other medications or add to parenteral nutrition solutions.

- Store unopened ampules at 20°–25° C (68°–77° F).

ADVERSE EFFECTS (≥1%) **Body as a Whole:** Hypersensitivity reaction (cardiovascular collapse, cardiac arrest, bronchospasm, oral/pharyngeal edema, dyspnea, angioedema, urticaria, pruritus). **CV:** Flushing, hypotension.

PHARMACOKINETICS Not studied.

NURSING IMPLICATIONS

Assessment & Drug Effects

- Monitor closely for S&S of severe hypersensitivity (see Appendix F) during IV administration.
- Monitor vital signs periodically during IV administration (transient hypotension possible especially during dialysis).
- Stop infusion immediately and notify physician if hypersensitivity is suspected.
- Lab tests: Periodic Hgb, Hct, Fe saturation, serum ferritin.

Patient & Family Education

- Report to physician immediately: Difficulty breathing, itching, flushing, rash, weakness, light-headedness, pain, or any other discomfort during infusion.

S

SODIUM FLUORIDE

(sod'i-um)

Fluorinse, Fluoritab, Flura-Drops, Karidium, Pediaflor, Point-Two, Thera-Flur-N

Classifications: ELECTROLYTE REPLACEMENT DENTAL PROPHYLACTIC
Therapeutic: DENTAL PROPHYLACTIC
Pregnancy Category: B (topical); C (oral)

AVAILABILITY 0.25 mg, 0.5 mg, 1 mg tablets; 0.125 mg, 0.25 mg, 0.5 mg drops; 0.2 mg/mL solution; 0.02%, 0.04%, 0.09%, 2% rinse; 0.5%, 1.2% gel

ACTION & *THERAPEUTIC EFFECT* Source of the fluorine ion, a trace element. Incorporates into developing tooth enamel, hardens surfaces, and increases resistance to cariogenic microbial processes. Topical application reduces acid production by bacteria in dental plaque and promotes remineralization of acid-damaged enamel. Application to exposed root surfaces supports formation of insoluble materials within dentinal tubules, thereby blocking transport of offending stimuli. *Oral form stimulates osteoblastic activity leading to increased bone mass. Topical application reduces acid production by bacteria in dental plaque and promotes remineralization of enamel.*

USES When fluoride ion concentration in drinking water is 0.7 ppm or less, to prevent periodontal disease and dental caries, to treat dental cervical hypersensitivity, and to control dental caries associated with xerostomia.

UNLABELED USES Adjunctive treatment of osteoporosis; management of bone lesions in multiple myeloma; to reduce bone pain in patient with metastatic prostatic carcinoma; to stabilize progression of hearing loss in a limited number of patients with otosclerosis.

CONTRAINDICATIONS When daily intake of fluoride from drinking water exceeds 0.7 ppm; low-sodium or sodium-free diets; rheumatoid arthritis; hypersensitivity to fluoride; gels or dental rinses by children younger than 6 y, 1 mg tablet or rinse in children younger than 3 y, or 1 mg rinse in children younger than 6 y; GI disease.

CAUTIOUS USE Renal dysfunction; rheumatoid arthritis; arthralgia; **topical:** pregnancy (category B); **oral:** pregnancy (category C), lactation.

ROUTE & DOSAGE

Prevent Periodontal Disease (Drinking Water Concentration Less Than 0.3 ppm)

Child: **PO** *Birth–2 y,* 0.25 mg/day; *2–3 y,* 0.5 mg/day; *3–13 y,* 1 mg/day

Prevent Periodontal Disease (Drinking Water Concentration 0.3–0.7 ppm)

Child: **PO** *Birth–2 y,* 0.125 mg/day; *2–3 y,* 0.25 mg/day; *3–13 y,* 0.5 mg/day

Prevent Dental Caries

Child: **Topical** *6–12 y,* 5 mL of 0.2% solution daily; *older than 12 y,* 10 mL of 0.2% solution daily

Desensitization of Exposed Root Surfaces

Child: **Topical** 0.2% rinsing solution once nightly after brushing and flossing

ADMINISTRATION

Oral

- Avoid giving sodium fluoride with milk or dairy products. Calcium from these products combines with fluorine, decreasing its absorption.
- Give drops preferably after meals. Give undiluted or mixed with fluids or foods.
- Dissolve tablets in the mouth or chew before swallowing. Administer at bedtime (after brushing the teeth).

Topical

- Apply all fluorine preparations after thoroughly brushing and flossing; preferably at bedtime.
- Do not swallow topical or rinse preparations.
- If patient's mouth is sore, the neutral preparation (Thera-Flur N) is better tolerated.
- Use as treatment for dental hypersensitivity: Thoroughly brush teeth; then swish PO solution around and between teeth for 1 min; expectorate. If gel is used, apply a few drops to toothbrush and brush gently onto affected surfaces.
- Apply Gel-drops with applicators supplied by the dentist. Spread gel on inner surfaces of applicators, which are placed over lower and upper teeth at the same time. User bites down lightly for 6 min, then removes applicators and rinses mouth thoroughly. Applicators are cleaned with cold water.
- Store all forms in tight plastic or paraffin-lined glass containers (sodium fluoride reacts with ordinary glass at a slow but appreciable rate) at 15°–30° C (59°–86° F). Avoid freezing.

ADVERSE EFFECTS (≥1%) **Skin:** Rash, atopic dermatitis, urticaria, stomatitis. **Body as a Whole:** GI and respiratory allergic reactions, salty or soapy taste, dehydration, thirst, excessive salivation, muscle weakness, tremors, <u>shock, death from cardiac and respiratory failure</u>. **Musculoskeletal:** Dental fluorosis (brown or white mottling of tooth enamel), osseous fluorosis (patchy mineralization and possible decrease in bone strength).

INTERACTIONS Drug: Aluminum, calcium, magnesium-containing products may decrease **fluoride** absorption.

PHARMACOKINETICS Absorption: Readily from GI tract. **Distribution:** Fluoride is stored in bones and teeth; crosses placenta; distributed into breast milk. **Elimination:** Rapidly excreted, primarily in urine with small amounts in feces.

S

NURSING IMPLICATIONS

Assessment & Drug Effect

- Monitor therapeutic effectiveness.

Patient & Family Education

- Do not eat, drink, or rinse mouth for at least 30 min after using the rinsing solution.
- Do not exceed recommended dosage. If mottling of teeth occurs, notify dentist.
- Apply sodium fluoride gel or solution used in orthodontic treatment regimen immediately before attachment or reattachment of the tooth-encircling bands.
- To be effective, fluoride supplementation **must be** consistent and continuous from infancy until 12–14 y.
- Consult dentist about continuing fluoride therapy if you move or there is a change in water supply (mottling may occur if drinking water has fluoride content greater than 1.5 ppm).

SODIUM OXYBATE (GHB)

(sod'i-um ox'y-bate)

Xyrem

Classification: CENTRAL NERVOUS SYSTEM (CNS) DEPRESSANT

Therapeutic: CNS DEPRESSANT

Pregnancy Category: C

Controlled Substance: Schedule III

S

AVAILABILITY 500 mg/mL solution

ACTION & *THERAPEUTIC EFFECT* CNS depressant; the precise mechanism by which sodium oxybate produces anticataplexy in narcolepsy is unknown. Sodium oxybate is GHB, a known drug of abuse. *Produces anticataplectic effects in narcolepsy and decreases the number of cataplexy events in individuals with narcolepsy. Also has sedative and amnestic properties.*

USES Treatment of cataplexy in patients with narcolepsy.

CONTRAINDICATIONS Alcohol or sedative-hypnotics or other CNS depressants; psychosis; coma; eclampsia; patients with succinic semialdehyde dehydrogenase deficiency; compromised respiratory drive, severe depression, or suicidal tendencies; children younger than 16 y.
CAUTIOUS USE Hepatic dysfunction; compromised respiratory function; sleep disorders; history of seizures; heart failure, hypertension, impaired renal function; previous history of depressive illness or suicide attempt; elderly; sleepwalking; pregnancy (category C).

ROUTE & DOSAGE

Cataplexy

Adult: **PO** Start with 2.25 g given at bedtime while in bed and repeated 2.5–4 h later. Dose may be increased by 1.5 g/day every 2 wk to a max of 9 g/day in 2 divided doses.

Hepatic Impairment Dosage Adjustment

Reduce dose by 50% in patients with hepatic impairment

ADMINISTRATION

Oral

- Give at bedtime at least 2–3 h after the evening meal.
- Dilute each dose with 2 oz (60 mL) of water in the dosing cups provided.
- Instruct patient to remain in bed after taking sodium oxybate.
- Discard any diluted dose that has not been used within 24 h.
- Store at 15°–30° C (59°–86° F).

ADVERSE EFFECTS (≥1%) **Body as a Whole:** *Pain, infection,* flu-like syndrome, asthenia, allergic reactions, chills. **CNS:** Confusion, depression, sleepwalking, *headache, dizziness, somnolence,* nervousness, abnormal dreams, insomnia, agitation, ataxia, convulsion, stupor, tremor. **CV:** Hypertension. **GI:** *Nausea,* diarrhea, vomiting, dyspepsia, abdominal pain, anorexia, constipation. **Metabolic:** Increased alkaline phosphatase, edema, hypercholesteremia, hypocalcemia, weight gain. **Respiratory:** *Pharyngitis,* rhinitis, sinusitis **Skin:** Increased sweating, acne, alopecia, rash. **Special Senses:** Amblyopia, tinnitus. **Urogenital:** Urinary incontinence, dysmenorrhea, albuminuria, cystitis, hematuria, metrorrhagia, urinary frequency.

INTERACTIONS Drug: Alcohol, SEDATIVE-HYPNOTICS, other CNS DEPRESSANTS may increase CNS depressant effects. **Food:** High-fat meal will significantly reduce absorption.

PHARMACOKINETICS Absorption: Incompletely absorbed, 25% reaches systemic circulation. **Peak:** 0.05–1.25 h. **Metabolism:** Oxidized in the Krebs' cycle to carbon dioxide and water. **Elimination:** Primarily eliminated as carbon dioxide in respiration. **Half-Life:** 0.5–1 h.

NURSING IMPLICATIONS

Assessment & Drug Effects

- Monitor for and report immediately any of the following: Seizure, respiratory depression, or decreased level of consciousness.
- Monitor closely patients with hepatic insufficiency for adverse events.
- Monitor for and report excessive weight gain and development of edema.
- Lab tests: Perform baseline LFTs; monitor periodically serum electrolytes and lipid profile.

Patient & Family Education

- Do not take sodium oxybate at any time other than at night, immediately before bedtime.
- Be consistent with timing of the evening meal and take this drug at least 2–3 h after eating.
- Prepare both doses prior to bedtime. After ingesting each dose remain in bed.
- Do not consume alcohol or use other sedative hypnotic drugs with sodium oxybate.
- Do not drive or engage in potentially hazardous activities until reaction to drug is known.

SODIUM POLYSTYRENE SULFONATE

(pol-ee-stye′reen)

Kayexalate, SPS Suspension

Classifications: ELECTROLYTE AND WATER BALANCE; CATION EXCHANGE

Therapeutic: CATION EXCHANGE

Pregnancy Category: C

AVAILABILITY 15 g/60 mL suspension; 100 mg/g powder

ACTION & *THERAPEUTIC EFFECT* Sulfonic cation-exchange resin that removes potassium by exchanging sodium ion for potassium, particularly in large intestine; potassium-containing resin is then excreted through the bowel. *Removes potassium by exchanging sodium ion for potassium through the large intestine.*

USES Hyperkalemia.

CONTRAINDICATIONS Patients with hypokalemia; hypersensitivity to

S

Kayexalate; GI obstruction; hypocalcemia, hypokalemia; lactation.
CAUTIOUS USE Older adults; acute or chronic kidney failure; low birth weight infants; neonates with reduced gut; patients receiving digitalis preparations; patients who cannot tolerate even a small increase in sodium load (e.g., CHF, severe hypertension, and marked edema); pregnancy (category C).

ROUTE & DOSAGE

Hyperkalemia

Adult: **PO** 15 g suspended in 70% sorbitol or 20–100 mL of other fluid 1–4 times/day **Rectal** 30–50 g/100 mL 70% sorbitol q6h as warm emulsion high into sigmoid colon
Child: **PO** Calculate appropriate amount on exchange rate of 1 mEq of potassium per gram of resin and suspend in 70% sorbitol or other appropriate solution (usual dose: 1 g/kg q6h) **Rectal** 1 g/kg q2–6h

ADMINISTRATION

Oral

- Give as a suspension in a small quantity of water or in syrup. Usual amount of fluid ranges from 20–100 mL or approximately 3–4 mL/g of drug.

Rectal

- Use warm fluid (as prescribed) to prepare the emulsion for enema.
- Administer at body temperature and introduce by gravity, keeping suspension particles in solution by stirring. Flush suspension with 50–100 mL of fluid; then clamp tube and leave it in place.
- Urge patient to retain enema at least 30–60 min but as long as several hours if possible.
- Irrigate colon (after enema solution has been expelled) with 1 or 2 qt flushing solution (non-sodium containing). Drain returns constantly through a Y-tube connection.
- Store remainder of prepared solution for 24 h; then discard.

ADVERSE EFFECTS (≥1%) **GI:** *Constipation, fecal impaction (in older adults);* anorexia, gastric irritation, nausea, vomiting, diarrhea (with sorbitol emulsions). **Metabolic:** Sodium retention, hypocalcemia, hypokalemia, hypomagnesemia.

INTERACTIONS Drug: ANTACIDS, LAXATIVES containing **calcium** or **magnesium** may decrease potassium exchange capability of the resin.

PHARMACOKINETICS Absorption: Not absorbed systemically. **Onset:** Several hours to days. **Metabolism:** Not metabolized. **Elimination:** In feces.

NURSING IMPLICATIONS

Assessment & Drug Effects

- Lab tests: Determine serum potassium levels daily throughout therapy. Monitor acid–base balance, electrolytes, and minerals in patients receiving repeated doses.
- Serum potassium levels do not always reflect intracellular potassium deficiency. Observe patient closely for early clinical signs of severe hypokalemia (see Appendix F). ECGs are also recommended.
- Consult physician about restricting sodium content from dietary and other sources since drug contains approximately 100 mg (4.1 mEq) of sodium per g (1 tsp, 15 mEq sodium).

Patient & Family Education

- Check bowel function daily. Usually, a mild laxative is prescribed to prevent constipation (common

S

adverse effect). Older adult patients are particularly prone to fecal impaction.

SOLIFENACIN SUCCINATE

(sol-i-fen′a-sin)

VESIcare

Classifications: ANTICHOLINERGIC; ANTIMUSCARINIC; ANTISPASMODIC

Therapeutic: ANTISPASMODIC

Prototype: Oxybutynin

Pregnancy Category: C

AVAILABILITY 5 mg, 10 mg tablets

ACTION & *THERAPEUTIC EFFECT* Solifenacin is a selective muscarinic antagonist that depresses both voluntary and involuntary bladder contractions caused by detrusor overactivity. *Solifenacin improves the volume of urine per void and reduces the frequency of incontinent and urgency episodes.*

USES Treatment of overactive bladder (OAB) with symptoms of urinary incontinence, urgency, and frequency.

CONTRAINDICATIONS Hypersensitivity to solifenacin; severe hepatic impairment; gastric retention; uncontrolled narrow-angle glaucoma; urinary retention; toxic megacolon; GI obstruction; ileus; GERD; lactation.

CAUTIOUS USE Bladder outflow obstruction; concurrent use of ketoconazole or other potent CYP3A4 inhibitors; obstructive disorders; decreased GI motility; hepatic impairment; history of QT prolongation or concurrent use of medications known to prolong the QT interval; controlled narrow-angle glaucoma; renal impairment; renal disease; renal failure; mild to moderate hepatic impairment; older adults; pregnancy (category C).

ROUTE & DOSAGE

Overactive Bladder

Adult: **PO** 5 mg once daily; may be increased to 10 mg once daily if tolerated (max: 5 mg/day if taking drugs that inhibit CYP3A4—see Interactions, Drug)

Hepatic Impairment Dosage Adjustment

If moderate hepatic impairment, do not exceed 5 mg/day. If severe hepatic impairment, do not use.

Renal Impairment Dosage Adjustment

CrCl less than 30 mL/min: Max dose 5 mg/day

ADMINISTRATION

Oral

- Tablets should be swallowed whole.
- Store at 15–30° C (59–86° F).

ADVERSE EFFECTS (≥1%) **Body as a Whole:** Edema, fatigue. **CNS:** Dizziness, depression. **CV:** Hypertension. **GI:** *Dry mouth, constipation,* nausea, vomiting, dyspepsia, upper abdominal pain. **Respiratory:** Cough. **Special Senses:** Blurred vision, dry eyes. **Urogenital:** Urinary tract infection, urinary retention.

INTERACTIONS Drug: CYP3A4 INHIBITORS (e.g., **clarithromycin, delavirdine, diltiazem, efavirenz, erythromycin, fluconazole, fluvoxamine, itraconazole, nefazodone, norfloxacin, omeprazole,** PROTEASE INHIBITORS, **quinine, verapamil, troleandomycin, voriconazole, zafirlukast**) may in-

S

crease levels and toxicity (max dose: 5 mg/day); **amantadine, amoxapine, bupropion, clozapine, cyclobenzaprine, diphenhydramine, disopyramide, maprotiline, olanzapine, orphenadrine,** PHENOTHIAZINES, TRICYCLIC ANTIDEPRESSANTS have additive anticholinergic adverse effects. **Food: Grapefruit juice** may increase solifenacin levels and toxicity.

PHARMACOKINETICS Absorption: 90% absorbed from GI tract. **Peak:** 3–8 h. **Metabolism:** Extensively metabolized in the liver by CYP3A4. **Elimination:** Primarily in urine, 22% in feces. **Half-Life:** 45–68 h.

NURSING IMPLICATIONS

Assessment & Drug Effects

- Monitor bladder function and report promptly urinary retention.
- Monitor ECG in patients with a known history of QT prolongation or patients taking medications that prolong the QT interval.

Patient & Family Education

- Stop taking this drug and report to physician if urinary retention occurs.
- Report promptly any of the following: Blurred vision or difficulty focusing vision, palpitations, confusion, or severe dizziness.
- Report to physician problems with bowel elimination, especially constipation lasting 3 days or longer.
- Exercise caution in hot environments, as the risk of heat prostration increases with this drug.

S

SOMATROPIN Pr

(soe-ma-troe′pin)

Accretropin, Genotropin, Miniquick, Humatrope, Norditropin, Nutropin, Nutropin AQ, Omnitrope, Serostim, Serostim LQ, Saizen, Zorbtive

Classification: GROWTH HORMONE

Therapeutic: GROWTH HORMONE

Pregnancy Category: B or C (depending on the brand)

AVAILABILITY 1.5 mg, 4 mg, 5 mg, 5.8 mg, 6 mg, 8 mg, 10 mg injection; 5 mg/1.5 mL, 15 mg/1.5 mL prefilled syringe

ACTION & *THERAPEUTIC EFFECT* Recombinant growth hormone with the natural sequence of 191 amino acids characteristic of endogenous growth hormone (GH), of pituitary origin. *Induces growth responses in children.*

USES Growth failure due to GH deficiency; replacement therapy prior to epiphyseal closure in patients with idiopathic GH deficiency; GH deficiency secondary to intracranial tumors or panhypopituitarism; inadequate GH secretion; short stature in girls with Turner's syndrome; AIDS wasting syndrome; short bowel syndrome.

UNLABELED USES Growth deficiency in children with rheumatoid arthitis.

CONTRAINDICATIONS Hypersensitivity to somatropin, growth hormone or any ingredient; patient with closed epiphyses; underlying progressive intracranial tumor, acute critical illness including open heart surgery, abdominal surgery, respiratory failure; diabetic retinopathy; respiratory insufficiency; during chemotherapy, radiation therapy, active neoplastic disease; selective cases or Prader-Willi syndrome; children with an intracranial tumor; intracranial hypertension; untreated hypothyroidism, obesity; neonates with benzyl alcohol hypersensitivity, and certain brands.

CAUTIOUS USE Diabetes mellitus or family history of the disease; concurrent use of insulin or antihypertensive agents; Prader-Willi syndrome; skeletal abnormalities; history of upper airway obstruction, sleep apnea, or unidentified URI; concomitant or prior use of thyroid or androgens in prepubertal male; hypothyroidism; chronic renal failure; pregnancy (category B or category C depending on the brand), lactation.

ROUTE & DOSAGE

Note: Dosing will vary with specific products

Growth Hormone Deficiency

Adult: **Subcutaneous Humatrope** 0.006 mg/kg (0.018 international unit/kg) daily, may increase [max: 0.0125 mg/kg/day (0.0375 international unit/kg/day)]; **Nutropin, Nutropin AQ** 0.006 mg/kg daily (max: *younger than 35 y,* 0.025 mg/kg/day; *older than 35 y,* 0.0125 mg/kg/day) **Genotropin, Omnitrope** 0.04 mg/kg qwk divided into daily doses (max: 0.08 mg/kg/wk) **Norditropin** Initially 0.004 mg/kg/day (max: 0.016 mg/kg)
Child: **Subcutaneous Genotropin** 0.16–0.24 mg/kg/wk divided into 6–7 daily doses; **Humatrope** 0.18 mg/kg/wk (0.54 international unit/kg/wk) divided into equal doses given on either 3 alternate days or 6 times/wk; **Norditropin** 0.024–0.034 mg/kg/day 6–7 times/wk; **Nutropin, Nutropin AQ** 0.3 mg/kg/wk (0.9 international unit/kg/wk) divided into 6–7 daily doses

Inadequate Growth Hormone Secretion

Child: **Subcutaneous Nutropin, Nutropin AQ** 0.3 mg/kg every week **Accretropin** 0.18–0.3 mg/kg/wk divided into daily doses **Genotropin** 0.16–0.24 mg/kg/wk divided into daily doses **Subcutanous or IM Humatrop, Saizen** 0.18 mg/kg/wk in divided doses

AIDS Wasting or Cachexia

Adult: **SC Serostim** *Weight greater than 55 kg,* 6 mg each night; *weight 45–55 kg,* 5 mg each night; *weight 35–45 kg,* 4 mg each night; *weight less than 35 kg,* 0.1 mg/kg each night
Child (6–17 y): **SC** 0.04–0.07 mg/kg/day

Short Bowel Syndrome

Adult: **SC Zorbtive** 0.1 mg/kg once daily for 4 wk (max: 8 mg/day)

ADMINISTRATION

Subcutaneous

- Reconstitute each brand following its manufacturer's instructions (vary from brand to brand).
- Read and carefully follow directions for use supplied with the Nutropin AQ Pen™ cartridge if this is the product being used.
- Rotate injection sites; abdomen and thighs are preferred sites. Do not use buttocks until the child has been walking for a year or more and the muscle is adequately developed.
- Store lyophilized powder at 2°–8° C (36°–46° F). After reconstitution, most preparations are stable for at least 14 days under refrigeration. DO NOT FREEZE.

S

ADVERSE EFFECTS (≥1%) **Body as a Whole:** Pain, swelling at injection site; myalgia. Fatalities reported in patients with Prader-Willi syndrome and one or more of the following: Severe obesity, history of respiratory impairment or sleep apnea, or unidentified respiratory infection, especially male patients. **Metabolic:** *Hypercalciuria;* oversaturation of bile with cholesterol, hyperglycemia, ketosis. **Endocrine:** High circulating GH antibodies with resulting treatment failure, accelerated growth of intracranial tumor.

INTERACTIONS Drug: ANABOLIC STEROIDS, **thyroid hormone,** ANDROGENS, ESTROGENS may accelerate epiphyseal closure; **ACTH,** CORTICOSTEROIDS may inhibit growth response to somatropin.

PHARMACOKINETICS Metabolism: In liver. **Elimination:** In urine. **Half-Life:** 15–50 min.

NURSING IMPLICATIONS

Assessment & Drug Effects

- Monitor growth at designated intervals.
- Lab test: Periodic serum and urine calcium and plasma glucose. Test for circulating GH antibodies (antisomatropin antibodies) in patients who respond initially but later fail to respond to therapy.
- Hypercalciuria, a frequent adverse effect in the first 2–3 mo of therapy, may be symptomless; however, it may be accompanied by renal calculi, with these reportable symptoms: Flank pain and colic, GI symptoms, urinary frequency, chills, fever, hematuria.
- Observe diabetics or those with family history of diabetes closely. Obtain regular fasting blood glucose and HbA1C.
- Examine patients with GH deficiency secondary to intracranial lesion frequently for progression or recurrence of underlying disease.

Patient & Family Education

- Be aware that during first 6 mo of successful treatment, linear growth rates may be increased 8–16 cm or more per year (average about 7 cm/y or approximately 3 in.). Additionally, subcutaneous fat diminishes but returns to pretreatment value later.
- Record accurate height measurements at regular intervals and report to physician if rate is less than expected.
- In general, growth response to somatropin is inversely proportional to duration of treatment.
- Bone age is typically assessed annually in all patients and especially those also receiving concurrent thyroid or androgen treatment, since these drugs may precipitate early epiphyseal closure. Take child for bone age assessment on appointed annual dates.

S

SORAFENIB

(sor-a-fe′nib)

Nexavar

Classifications: ANTINEOPLASTIC; TYROSINE KINASE INHIBITOR (TKI); MULTI-KINASE INHIBITOR

Therapeutic: ANTINEOPLASTIC

Prototype: Gefitinib

Pregnancy Category: D

AVAILABILITY 200 mg tablets

ACTION & *THERAPEUTIC EFFECT*

Sorafenib is a multi-kinase inhibitor targeting enzyme systems in both tumor cells and tumor vasculature. It appears to be cytostatic, requiring continued drug exposure for tumor growth inhibition. *Sorafenib inhibits enzymes respon-*

sible for uncontrolled tumor cellular proliferation and angiogenesis.

USES Treatment of advanced renal cell cancer.

UNLABELED USES Treatment of advanced malignant melanoma. Treatment of metastatic hepatocellular cancer.

CONTRAINDICATIONS Active infection; severe renal impairment (less than 30 mL/min), or hemodialysis; pregnancy (category D), lactation. Safe use in children younger than 18 y is not established.

CAUTIOUS USE Previous myelosuppressive therapy, either radiation or chemotherapy; mild or moderate renal disease; hepatic disease; heart failure, ventricular dysfunction, cardiac disease, peripheral edema; females of childbearing age.

ROUTE & DOSAGE

Renal Cell Cancer

Adult: **PO** 400 mg b.i.d.

Dosage Adjustments for Skin Toxicity

Grade 2 (1st episode): Continue therapy and treat symptoms. If no improvement in 7 days, discontinue until toxicity resolves to at least grade 1, then resume with 400 mg/day or 400 mg every other day

Grade 2 (2nd or 3rd episode): Discontinue until toxicity resolves to at least grade 1, then resume with 400 mg/day or 400 mg every other day

Grade 2 (4th episode): Discontinue therapy

Grade 3 (1st or 2nd episode): Discontinue until toxicity resolves to at least grade 1, then resume with 400 mg/day or 400 mg every other day

Grade 3 (3rd episode): Discontinue therapy

ADMINISTRATION

Oral

- Tablets **must be** swallowed whole. They should not be crushed, broken, or chewed.
- Give on an empty stomach 1 h before or 2 h after eating.
- Store at 15°–30° C (59°–86° F). Protect from moisture.

ADVERSE EFFECTS (≥1%) **Body as a Whole:** Asthenia, bone pain, decreased appetite, *fatigue,* influenza-like illness, *joint pain,* mouth pain, muscle pain, pyrexia. **CNS:** Depression, *headache, sensory neuropathy.* **CV:** *Hypertension.* **GI:** *Abdominal pain, anorexia, constipation, diarrhea,* dyspepsia, dysphagia, mucositis, *nausea,* stomatitis, *vomiting.* **Hematologic:** *Anemia,* <u>hemorrhage</u>, *leukopenia, lymphopenia, neutropenia, thrombocytopenia.* **Metabolic:** *Amylase elevation, hypophosphatemia, lipase elevation, weight loss.* **Musculoskeletal:** Arthralgia, myalgia. **Respiratory:** *Cough, dyspnea,* hoarseness. **Skin:** Acne, *alopecia, desquamation, dry skin,* erythema, exfoliative dermatitis, flushing, *hand-foot skin reaction, rash.* **Urogenital:** Erectile dysfunction.

INTERACTIONS Drug: Sorafenib may increase levels of drugs requiring glucuronidation by the UGT1A1 and UGT1A9 pathways (e.g., **irinotecan**). Due to thrombocytopenic effects, sorafenib can contribute to increased bleeding from NONSTEROIDAL ANTI-INFLAMMATORY DRUGS, PLATELET INHIBITORS (e.g., **aspirin, clopidogrel**), THROMBOLYTIC AGENTS, and **warfarin.** INDUCERS OF CYP3A4 (e.g., **carbamazepine, phenobarbital, phenytoin, rifampin**) may de-

S

crease the levels of sorafenib. **Food:** Food decreases the absorption of sorafenib. **Herbal: St. John's wort** may decrease the levels of sorafenib.

PHARMACOKINETICS Absorption: 38–49% absorbed. **Peak:** 3 h. **Distribution:** 99.5% protein bound. **Metabolism:** In the liver. **Elimination:** Primarily fecal (77%) with minor elimination in the urine (19%). **Half-Life:** 25–48 h.

NURSING IMPLICATIONS

Assessment & Drug Effects

- Monitor for and report S&S of skin toxicity (e.g., rash, erythema, dermatitis, paresthesia, swelling, or pain in hands or feet). Severe reactions may require temporary suspension of therapy or dose reduction.
- Monitor for S&S of bleeding, especially in those on anticoagulation therapy.
- Monitor BP weekly for the first 6 wk of therapy and periodically thereafter. New-onset hypertension has been associated with sorafenib.
- Lab tests: Periodic CBC with differential and platelet count, serum electrolytes, LFTs, lipase, amylase, and alkaline phosphatase.
- Monitor blood levels of warfarin with concurrent therapy.

S

Patient & Family Education

- Report any of the following to a health care provider: Skin rash; redness, blisters, pain or swelling of the palms or hands or soles of feet; signs of bleeding; unexplained chest, shoulder, neck and jaw, or back pain.
- Do not take any prescription or nonprescription drugs without consulting the physician.
- Male and female patients should use effective birth control during treatment and for at least 2 wk following completion of treatment.

SOTALOL

(so-ta'lol)

Betapace, Betapace AF

Classifications: BETA-ADRENERGIC ANTAGONIST; ANTIARRHYTHMIC CLASS II AND III

Therapeutic: ANTIARRHYTHMIC CLASS II AND III

Prototype: Amiodarone

Pregnancy Category: B

AVAILABILITY Betapace 80 mg, 120 mg, 160 mg, 240 mg tablets; **Betapace AF** 80 mg, 120 mg, 160 mg tablets

ACTION & *THERAPEUTIC EFFECT* Has both class II and class III antiarrhythmic properties. Slows heart rate, decreases AV nodal conduction, and increases AV nodal refractoriness. Produces significant reduction in both systolic and diastolic blood pressure. *Antiarrhythmic properties are effective in controlling ventricular arrhythmias as well as atrial fibrillation/flutter. Regulates blood pressure values.*

USES Treatment of life-threatening ventricular arrhythmias (sustained ventricular tachycardia) and maintenance of normal sinus rhythm in patients with atrial fibrillation/flutter.

UNLABELED USES Hypertension, angina.

CONTRAINDICATIONS Hypersensitivity to sotalol; bronchial asthma, acute bronchospasm; sinus bradycardia, sick sinus syndrome; second and third degree heart block, long QT syndrome, cardiogenic shock, uncontrolled CHF; chronic bronchitis, emphysema; hypokalemia less than 4 mEq/L; creatinine clearance of less than 40 mL/min.

CAUTIOUS USE CHF, electrolyte disturbances, recent MI, diabetes, sick sinus rhythm, renal impairment; excessive diarrhea, or profuse sweating; pregnancy (category B), lactation.

ROUTE & DOSAGE

Ventricular Arrhythmias (Betapace)

Adult: **PO** Initial dose of 80 mg b.i.d. or 160 mg daily taken prior to meals, may increase every 3–4 days in 40–160 mg increments (most patients respond to 240–320 mg/day in 2 or 3 divided doses, doses greater than 640 mg/day have not been studied)

Renal Impairment Dosage Adjustment

CrCl greater than 60 mL/min: q12h; 30–60 mL/min: q24h; 10–30 mL/min: q36–48h; less than 10 mL/min: Individualize carefully

Atrial Fibrillation/Flutter (Betapace AF)

Adult: **PO** Initial dose of 80 mg b.i.d., may increase every 3–4 days (max: 240 mg/day in 1–2 divided doses)

Renal Impairment Dosage Adjustment

CrCl greater than 60 mL/min: q12h; 40–60 mL/min: q24h; less than 40 mL/min contraindicated

ADMINISTRATION

Oral

- Give on an empty stomach 1 h before or 2 h after meals. Do not give with milk or milk products.
- Drug should be initiated and doses increased only under close supervision, preferably in a hospital with cardiac rhythm monitoring and frequent assessment.
- Use smallest effective dose for patients with nonallergic bronchospasms.
- Do not discontinue drug abruptly. Gradually reduce dose over 1–2 wk.
- Store at room temperature, 15°–30° C (59°–86° F).

ADVERSE EFFECTS (≥1%) **CV:** AV block, hypotension, aggravation of CHF, although the incidence of heart failure may be lower than for other beta-blockers, <u>life-threatening ventricular arrhythmias, including polymorphous ventricular tachycardia or torsades de pointes</u>, *bradycardia, dyspnea, chest pain, palpitation,* bleeding (less than 2%). **CNS:** Headache, *fatigue, dizziness,* weakness, lethargy, depression, lassitude. **GI:** Nausea, vomiting, diarrhea, dyspepsia, dry mouth. **Urogenital:** Impotence, decreased libido. **Metabolic:** Hyperglycemia. **Special Senses:** Visual disturbances. **Respiratory:** Respiratory complaints. **Skin:** Rash.

INTERACTIONS Drug: Antagonizes the effects of BETA AGONISTS. **Amiodarone** may lead to symptomatic bradycardia and sinus arrest. The hypoglycemic effects of ORAL HYPOGLYCEMIC AGENTS may be potentiated. May cause resistance to **epinephrine** in anaphylactic reactions. Should be used with caution with other ANTIARRHYTHMIC AGENTS. **Food:** Absorption may be reduced by food, especially **milk** and MILK PRODUCTS.

PHARMACOKINETICS Absorption: Slowly and completely from GI tract. Negligible first-pass metabolism. Reduced by food, especially milk and milk products. **Peak:** 2–3 h. **Duration:** 24 h. **Distribution:** Drug

S

is hydrophilic and will enter the CSF slowly (about 10%). Crosses placental barrier. Distributed in breast milk. Not appreciably protein bound. **Metabolism:** Does not undergo significant hepatic enzyme metabolism and no active metabolites have been identified. **Elimination:** In urine with 75% of the drug excreted unchanged within 72 h. **Half-Life:** 7–18 h.

NURSING IMPLICATIONS

Assessment & Drug Effects

- Monitor ECG at baseline and periodically thereafter (especially when doses are increased) because proarrhythmic events most often occur within 7 days of initiating therapy or increasing dose.
- Lab test: Baseline serum electrolytes. Correct electrolyte imbalances of hypokalemia or hypomagnesemia prior to initiating therapy.
- Monitor cardiac status throughout therapy. Exercise special caution when sotalol is used concurrently with other antiarrhythmics, digoxin, or calcium channel blockers.
- Monitor patients with bronchospastic disease (e.g., bronchitis, emphysema) carefully for inhibition of bronchodilation.
- Monitor diabetics for loss of glycemic control. Beta blockage reduces the release of endogenous insulin in response to hyperglycemia and may blunt symptoms of acute hypoglycemia (e.g., tachycardia, BP changes).

Patient & Family Education

- Be aware of risk for hypotension and syncope, especially with concurrent treatment with catecholamine-depleting drugs (e.g., reserpine, guanethidine).
- Take radial pulse daily and report marked bradycardia (pulse below 60 or other established parameter) to physician.
- Type 2 diabetics are at increased risk for hyperglycemia. All diabetics are at risk of possible masking of symptoms of hypoglycemia.
- Do not abruptly discontinue drug because of the risk of exacerbation of angina, arrhythmias, and possible myocardial infarction.

S

SPIRONOLACTONE (Pr)

(speer-on-oh-lak'tone)

Aldactone, Novospiroton ♣

Classifications: ELECTROLYTIC AND WATER BALANCE; ALDOSTERONE ANTAGONIST; POTASSIUM-SPARING DIURETIC

Therapeutic: POTASSIUM-SPARING DIURETIC; ANTIHYPERTENSIVE; ALDOSTERONE ANTAGONIST

Pregnancy Category: D

AVAILABILITY 25 mg, 50 mg, 100 mg tablets

ACTION & *THERAPEUTIC EFFECT* Steroidal compound and specific pharmacologic antagonist of aldosterone. Competes with aldosterone for cellular receptor sites in distal renal tubules. Promotes sodium and chloride excretion without loss of potassium. *A diuretic agent that promotes sodium and chloride excretion without concomitant loss of potassium. Lowers systolic and diastolic pressures in hypertensive patients. Effective in treatment of primary aldosteronism.*

USES Essential hypertension, refractory edema due to CHF, hepatic cirrhosis, nephrotic syndrome, hypokalemia, and idiopathic edema.

May be used to potentiate actions of other diuretics and antihypertensive agents or for its potassium-sparing effect. Also used for treatment of (and as presumptive test for) primary aldosteronism.

UNLABELED USES Hirsutism in women with polycystic ovary syndrome or idiopathic hirsutism; adjunct in treatment of myasthenia gravis and familial periodic paralysis.

CONTRAINDICATIONS Anuria, severe renal insufficiency; renal failure; diabetic nephropathy; progressing impairment of kidney function, hyperkalemia; pregnancy (category D).

CAUTIOUS USE BUN of 40 mg/dL or greater, mild or moderate renal impairment; liver disease.

ROUTE & DOSAGE

Edema

Adult: **PO** 25–200 mg/day in divided doses, continued for at least 5 days (dose adjusted to optimal response; if no response, a thiazide or loop diuretic may be added)
Child: **PO** 3.3 mg/kg/day in single or divided doses, continued for at least 5 days (dose adjusted to optimal response)
Neonate: **PO** 1–3 mg/kg/day divided q12–24h

Hypertension

Adult: **PO** 25–100 mg/day in single or divided doses, continued for at least 2 wk (dose adjusted to optimal response)

Primary Aldosteronism: Diagnosis

Adult: **PO** Short Test: 400 mg/day for 4 days; long test: 400 mg/day for 3–4 wk

Primary Aldosteronism

Adult: **PO** 100–400 mg/day in divided doses

Hypokalemia

Adult: **PO** 25–100 mg daily

ADMINISTRATION

Oral

- Give with food to enhance absorption.
- Crush tablets and give with fluid of patient's choice if unable to swallow whole.
- Store in tight, light-resistant containers. Suspension is stable for 1 mo under refrigeration.

ADVERSE EFFECTS (≥1%) **CNS:** Lethargy, mental confusion, fatigue (with rapid weight loss), headache, drowsiness, ataxia. **Endocrine:** Gynecomastia (both sexes), inability to achieve or maintain erection, androgenic effects (hirsutism, irregular menses, deepening of voice); parathyroid changes, decreased glucose tolerance, SLE. **GI:** Abdominal cramps, nausea, vomiting, anorexia, diarrhea. **Skin:** Maculopapular or erythematous rash, urticaria. **Metabolic:** Fluid and electrolyte imbalance (particularly hyperkalemia and hyponatremia); elevated BUN, mild acidosis, hyperuricemia, gout. **Body as a Whole:** Drug fever. **Hematologic:** Agranulocytosis. **CV:** Hypertension (post-sympathectomy patient).

DIAGNOSTIC TEST INTERFERENCE May produce marked increases in ***plasma cortisol*** determinations by ***Mattingly fluorometric*** method; these may persist for several days after termination of drug (spironolactone metabolite produces fluorescence). There is the possibility of false elevations in measurements of ***digoxin serum levels*** by ***RIA*** procedures.

S

INTERACTIONS Drug: Combinations of spironolactone and acidifying doses of **ammonium chloride** may produce systemic acidosis; use these combinations with caution. Diuretic effect of spironolactone may be antagonized by **aspirin** and other SALICYLATES. **Digoxin** should be monitored for decreased effect of CARDIAC GLYCOSIDES. Hyperkalemia may result with POTASSIUM SUPPLEMENTS, ACE INHIBITORS, ARBS, **heparin** may decrease **lithium** clearance resulting in increased tenacity; may alter anticoagulant response in **warfarin. Food:** Salt substitutes may increase risk of hyperkalemia.

PHARMACOKINETICS Absorption: ~73% from GI tract. **Onset:** Gradual. **Peak:** 2–3 days; maximum effect may take up to 2 wk. **Duration:** 2–3 days or longer. **Distribution:** Crosses placenta, distributed into breast milk. **Metabolism:** In liver and kidneys to active metabolites. **Elimination:** 40–57% in urine, 35–40% in bile. **Half-Life:** 1.3–2.4 h parent compound, 18–23 h metabolites.

NURSING IMPLICATIONS

Assessment & Drug Effects

- Check blood pressure before initiation of therapy and at regular intervals throughout therapy.
- Lab tests: Monitor serum electrolytes (sodium and potassium) especially during early therapy; monitor digoxin level when used concurrently.
- Assess for signs of fluid and electrolyte imbalance, and signs of digoxin toxicity.
- Monitor daily I&O and check for edema. Report lack of diuretic response or development of edema; both may indicate tolerance to drug.
- Weigh patient under standard conditions before therapy begins and daily throughout therapy. Weight is a useful index of need for dosage adjustment. For patients with ascites, physician may want measurements of abdominal girth.
- Observe for and report immediately the onset of mental changes, lethargy, or stupor in patients with liver disease.
- Adverse reactions are generally reversible with discontinuation of drug. Gynecomastia appears to be related to dosage level and duration of therapy; it may persist in some after drug is stopped.

Patient & Family Education

- Be aware that the maximal diuretic effect may not occur until third day of therapy and that diuresis may continue for 2–3 days after drug is withdrawn.
- Report signs of hyponatremia or hyperkalemia (see Appendix F), most likely to occur in patients with severe cirrhosis.
- Avoid replacing fluid losses with large amounts of free water (can result in dilutional hyponatremia).
- Weigh 2–3 times each wk. Report gains/loss of 5 lb or more.
- Do not drive or engage in potentially hazardous activities until response to the drug is known.
- Avoid excessive intake of high-potassium foods and salt substitutes.

STAVUDINE (D4T)

(sta′vu-deen)

Zerit

Classifications: ANTIRETROVIRAL; NUCLEOSIDE REVERSE TRANSCRIPTASE INHIBITOR (NRTI)

Therapeutic: ANTIRETROVIRAL; NRTI

Prototype: Lamivudine

Pregnancy Category: C

AVAILABILITY 15 mg, 20 mg, 30 mg, 40 mg capsules; 1 mg/mL oral solution

ACTION & *THERAPEUTIC EFFECT* Synthetic analog of thymidine (a nucleoside in DNA) with antiviral action against HIV. Appears to act by being incorporated into growing DNA chains by viral transcriptase, thus terminating viral replication. *Inhibits the replication of HIV in human cells and decreases viral load.*

USES Treatment of adults with HIV infection in combination with other antiretroviral agents.

CONTRAINDICATIONS Hypersensitivity to stavudine; lactic acidosis; lactation.

CAUTIOUS USE Previous hypersensitivity to zidovudine, didanosine, or zalcitabine; folic acid or B_{12} deficiency; liver and renal insufficiency; alcoholism; peripheral neuropathy; history of pancreatitis; pregnancy (category C).

ROUTE & DOSAGE

HIV Infection

Adult/Adolescent: **PO** *Weight less than 60 kg,* 30 mg q12h; *weight 60 kg or greater,* 40 mg q12h
Child: **PO** *Weight greater than 60 kg,* 40 mg q12h; *weight 30–60 kg,* 30 mg q12h
Child/Infant/Neonate (older than 14 days): **PO** *Weight less than 30 kg,* 1 mg/kg q12h
Neonate (younger than 13 days): **PO** 0.5 mg/kg q12h

Renal Impairment Dosage Adjustment

CrCl 25–50 mL/min: Reduce dose by 50%; less than 25 mL/min: Reduce dose by 50% and extend interval to q24h

Toxicity Dosage Adjustment

Adult/Adolescent: Weight greater than 60 kg, 20 mg q12h; *weight less than 60 kg,* 15 mg q12h
Child: Reduce dose by 50%

ADMINISTRATION

Oral

- Adhere strictly to 12-h interval between doses.
- Reconstitute powder by adding 202 mL of water to the container. Shake vigorously. Yields 200 mL of 1 mg/mL solution.
- Store at room temperature, 15°–30° C (59°–86° F).

ADVERSE EFFECTS (≥1%) **CNS:** *Peripheral neuropathy,* paresthesias. **GI:** *Anorexia, nausea, vomiting, diarrhea,* cramping, pancreatitis, abdominal pain, elevated liver function tests, abdominal pain. **Body as a Whole:** *Headache,* chills/fever, *myalgia*. **Hematologic:** Anemia, neutropenia. **Skin:** *Rash*. **Metabolic:** Lactic acidosis in pregnant women; hyperglycemia.

INTERACTIONS Drug: Didanosine may increase risk of pancreatitis and hepatotoxicity; **probenecid** can decrease elimination; **zalcitabine** increases risk of neuropathy; **zidovudine** may impact metabolism, avoid concurrent use. Use INTERFERONS, **ribavirin** cautiously.

PHARMACOKINETICS Absorption: Readily absorbed from GI tract; 82% reaches systemic circulation. **Peak:** Effect 6 wk. **Distribution:** Distributes into CSF; excreted in breast milk of animals. **Metabolism:** Unknown. **Elimination:** In urine. **Half-Life:** 1–1.6 h.

S

NURSING IMPLICATIONS

Assessment & Drug Effects

- Monitor for peripheral neuropathy and report numbness, tingling, or pain, which may indicate a need to interrupt stavudine.
- Lab tests: Monitor liver enzymes, CBC with differential, PT and INR, and kidney function periodically.
- Monitor for development of opportunistic infection.

Patient & Family Education

- Take drug exactly as prescribed.
- Report to physician any adverse drug effects that are bothersome.
- Report symptoms of peripheral neuropathy to physician immediately.

STREPTOMYCIN SULFATE

(strep-toe-mye'sin)

Classifications: AMINOGLYCOSIDE ANTIBIOTIC; ANTITUBERCULOSIS
Therapeutic: ANTIBIOTIC; ANTITUBERCULOSIS
Prototype: Gentamicin
Pregnancy Category: D

AVAILABILITY 400 mg/mL, 1 g injection

ACTION & *THERAPEUTIC EFFECT* Aminoglycoside antibiotic that works by inhibiting bacterial protein synthesis through irreversible binding to the 30S ribosomal subunit of susceptible bacteria. *Active against a variety of gram-positive, gram-negative, and acid-fast organisms.*

USES Only in combination with other antitubercular drugs in treatment of all forms of active tuberculosis caused by susceptible organisms. Used alone or in conjunction with tetracycline for tularemia, plague, and brucellosis. Also used with other antibiotics in treatment of subacute bacterial endocarditis due to *Enterococci* and *Streptococci* (viridans group) and *Haemophilus influenzae* and in treatment of peritonitis, respiratory tract infections, granuloma inguinale, and chancroid when other drugs have failed.

CONTRAINDICATIONS History of toxic reaction or hypersensitivity to aminoglycosides; labyrinthine disease; myasthenia gravis; pregnancy (category D).

CAUTIOUS USE Impaired kidney function (given in reduced dosages); use in older adults and in prematures, neonates, and children.

ROUTE & DOSAGE

Tuberculosis
Adult: **IM** 15 mg/kg up to 1 g/day as single dose
Geriatric: **IM** 10 mg/kg (max: 750 mg/day)
Child: **IM** 20–40 mg/kg/day up to 1 g/day as single dose
Infant: **IM** 10–15 mg/kg q12h
Neonate: **IM** 10–20 mg/kg q24h

Tularemia
Adult: **IM** 1–2 g/day in 1–2 divided doses for 7–10 days
Child: **IM** 20–40 mg/kg/day divided q6–12h

Plague
Adult: **IM** 2 g/day in 2–4 divided doses
Child: **IM** 30 mg/kg/day divided q8–12h

ADMINISTRATION

Intramuscular

- Give IM deep into large muscle mass to minimize possibility of irritation. Injections are painful.
- Avoid direct contact with drug; sensitization can occur. Use gloves during preparation of drug.

- Use commercially prepared IM solution undiluted; intended only for IM injection (contains a preservative, and therefore is not suitable for other routes).
- Store ampules at room temperature. Protect from light; exposure to light may slightly darken solution, with no apparent loss of potency.

ADVERSE EFFECTS (≥1%) **CNS:** Paresthesias (peripheral, facial). **Body as a Whole:** Hypersensitivity angioedema, drug fever, enlarged lymph nodes, anaphylactic shock, headache, inability to concentrate, lassitude, muscular weakness, *pain and irritation at IM site,* superinfections, neuromuscular blockade, arachnoiditis. **GI:** Stomatitis, hepatotoxicity. **Hematologic:** Blood dyscrasias (leukopenia, neutropenia, pancytopenia, hemolytic or aplastic anemia, eosinophilia). **Special Senses:** *Labyrinthine damage,* auditory damage, optic nerve toxicity (scotomas). **Urogenital:** Nephrotoxicity. **CNS:** Encephalopathy, CNS depression syndrome in infants (stupor, flaccidity, coma, paralysis, cardiac arrest). **Respiratory:** Respiratory depression. **Skin:** Skin rashes, pruritus, exfoliative dermatitis.

DIAGNOSTIC TEST INTERFERENCE Streptomycin reportedly produces false-positive ***urinary glucose*** tests using ***copper sulfate methods (Benedict's solution, Clinitest)*** but not with ***glucose oxidase methods*** (e.g., ***Clinistix, TesTape***). False increases in protein content in ***urine*** and ***CSF*** using ***Folin-Ciocalteau reaction*** and decreased ***BUN*** readings with ***Berthelot reaction*** may occur from test interferences. ***C&S*** tests may be affected if patient is taking salts such as sodium and potassium chloride, sodium sulfate and tartrate, ammonium acetate, calcium and magnesium ions.

INTERACTIONS Drug: May potentiate anticoagulant effects of **warfarin;** additive nephrotoxicity with **acyclovir, amphotericin B,** AMINOGLYCOSIDES, **carboplatin, cidofovir, cisplatin, cyclosporine, foscarnet, ganciclovir,** SALICYLATES, **tacrolimus, vancomycin.**

PHARMACOKINETICS Peak: 1–2 h. **Distribution:** Diffuses into most body tissues and extracellular fluids; crosses placenta; distributed into breast milk. **Elimination:** In urine. **Half-Life:** 2–3 h adults, 4–10 h newborns.

NURSING IMPLICATIONS

Assessment & Drug Effects

- Lab tests: Obtain C&S tests prior to and periodically during course of therapy. In patients with impaired kidney function, frequent determinations of serum drug concentrations and periodic kidney and liver function tests are advised (serum concentrations should not exceed 25 mcg/mL in these patients).
- Be alert for and report immediately symptoms of ototoxicity (see Appendix F). Symptoms are most likely to occur in patients with impaired kidney function, patients receiving high doses (1.8–2 g/day) or other ototoxic or neurotoxic drugs, and older adults. Irreversible damage may occur if drug is not discontinued promptly.
- Early damage to vestibular portion of eighth cranial nerve (higher incidence than auditory toxicity) is initially manifested by moderately severe headache, nausea, vomiting, vertigo in upright position, difficulty in reading, unsteadiness, and positive Romberg sign.

S

- Be aware that auditory nerve damage is usually preceded by vestibular symptoms and high-pitched tinnitus, roaring noises, impaired hearing (especially to high-pitched sounds), sense of fullness in ears. Audiometric test should be done if these symptoms appear, and drug should be discontinued. Hearing loss can be permanent if damage is extensive. Tinnitus may persist several days to weeks after drug is stopped.
- Monitor I&O. Report oliguria or changes in I&O ratio (possible signs of diminishing kidney function). Sufficient fluids to maintain urinary output of 1500 mL/24 h are generally advised. Consult physician.

Patient & Family Education

- Report any unusual symptoms. Review adverse reactions with physician periodically, especially with prolonged therapy.
- Be aware of possibility of ototoxicity and its symptoms (see Appendix F).
- Report to physician immediately any of the following: Nausea, vomiting, vertigo, incoordination, tinnitus, fullness in ears, impaired hearing.

S

STREPTOZOCIN

(strep-toe-zoe′sin)
Zanosar
Classification: ANTINEOPLASTIC, ALKYLATING
Therapeutic: ANTINEOPLASTIC
Prototype: Cyclophosphamide
Pregnancy Category: D

AVAILABILITY 1 g injection

ACTION & *THERAPEUTIC EFFECT* Streptozocin inhibits DNA synthesis in cells and prevents progression of cells into mitosis, affecting all phases of the cell cycle (cell-cycle nonspecific). *Successful therapy with streptozocin (alone or in combination) produces a biochemical response evidenced by decreased secretion of hormones as well as measurable tumor regression. Thus, serial fasting insulin levels during treatment indicate response to this drug.*

USES Metastatic functional and nonfunctional islet cell carcinoma of pancreas, as single agent or in combination with fluorouracil.

UNLABELED USES A variety of other malignant neoplasms including metastatic carcinoid tumor or carcinoid syndrome, refractory advanced Hodgkin's disease, and metastatic colorectal cancer.

CONTRAINDICATIONS Pregnancy (category D), lactation. Safety in children is not established.

CAUTIOUS USE Renal impairment; hepatic disease, hepatic impairment; patients with history of hypoglycemia; diabetes mellitus.

ROUTE & DOSAGE

Islet Cell Carcinoma of Pancreas

Adult: **IV** 500 mg/m²/day for 5 consecutive days q6wk or 1 g/m²/wk for 2 wk, then increase to 1.5 g/m²/wk, infuse dose over 15 min to 6 h

Renal Impairment Dosage Adjustment

If CrCl 10–50 mL/min, use 75% of dose; if less, use 50% of dose

ADMINISTRATION

Intravenous

Use only under constant supervision by physician experienced in therapy with cytotoxic agents and only when the benefit to risk ratio is fully and thoroughly understood by patient and family.

- Wear gloves to protect against topical exposure, which may pose a carcinogen hazard, when handling streptozocin. ▪ If solution or powder comes in contact with skin or mucosa, promptly flush the area thoroughly with soap and water.

PREPARE: **IV Infusion:** Reconstitute with 9.5 mL D5W or NS, to yield 100 mg/mL. Solution will be pale gold. ▪ May be further diluted with up to 250 mL of the original diluent. ▪ Protect reconstituted solution and vials of drug from light.

ADMINISTER: **IV Infusion:** Give over 15–60 min. ▪ Inspect injection site frequently for signs of extravasation (patient complaints of stinging or burning at site, swelling around site, no blood return or questionable blood return). ▪ If extravasation occurs, area requires immediate attention to prevent necrosis. Remove needle, apply ice, and contact physician regarding further treatment to infiltrated tissue.

INCOMPATIBILITIES **Y-site:** **Allopurinol, aztreonam, cefepime, piperacillin/tazobactam.**

▪ Note: An antiemetic given routinely every 4 or 6 h and prophylactically 30 min before a treatment may provide sufficient control to maintain the treatment regimen (even if it reduces but does not completely eliminate nausea and vomiting).

▪ Discard reconstituted solutions after 12 h (contains no preservative and not intended for multidose use).

ADVERSE EFFECTS (≥1%) **CNS:** Confusion, lethargy, depression. **GI:** *Nausea, vomiting,* diarrhea, transient increase in AST, ALT, or alkaline phosphatase; hypoalbuminemia. **Hematologic:** *Mild* to moderate myelosuppression *(leukopenia, thrombocytopenia, anemia).* **Metabolic:** Glucose tolerance abnormalities (moderate and reversible); glycosuria without hyperglycemia, <u>insulin shock</u> (rare). **Urogenital:** <u>Nephrotoxicity: Azotemia, anuria, proteinuria, hypophosphatemia, hyperchloremia</u>; *Fanconi-like syndrome* (proximal renal tubular reabsorption defects, alkaline pH of urine, glucosuria, acetonuria, aminoaciduria); hypokalemia, hypocalcemia. **Other:** Local necrosis following extravasation.

INTERACTIONS Drug: MYELOSUPPRESSIVE AGENTS add to hematologic toxicity; nephrotoxic agents (e.g., AMINOGLYCOSIDES, **vancomycin, amphotericin B, cisplatin**) increase risk of nephrotoxicity; **phenytoin** may reduce cytotoxic effect on pancreatic beta cells.

PHARMACOKINETICS Absorption: Undetectable in plasma within 3 h. **Distribution:** Metabolite enters CSF. **Metabolism:** In liver and kidneys. **Elimination:** 70–80% of dose in urine, 1% in feces, and 5% in expired air. **Half-Life:** 35–40 min.

NURSING IMPLICATIONS

Assessment & Drug Effects

- Lab tests: Weekly CBC; LFTs prior to each course of therapy; serial urinalyses and kidney function tests; baseline and weekly serum electrolytes, then for 4 wk after termination of therapy.
- Ensure that repeat courses of streptozocin treatment are not given un-

S

til patient's liver, kidney, and hematologic functions are within acceptable limits.

- Be alert to and report promptly early laboratory evidence of kidney dysfunction: Hypophosphatemia, mild proteinuria, and changes in I&O ratio and pattern.
- Mild adverse renal effects may be reversible following discontinuation of streptozocin, but nephrotoxicity may be irreversible, severe, or fatal.
- Be alert to symptoms of sepsis and superinfections or increased tendency to bleed (thrombocytopenia). Myelosuppression is severe in 10–20% of patients and may be cumulative and more severe if patient has had prior exposure to radiation or to other antineoplastics.
- Monitor and record temperature pattern to promptly recognize impending sepsis.

Patient & Family Education

- Inspect site at weekly intervals and report changes in tissue appearance if extravasation occurred during IV infusion.
- Report symptoms of hypoglycemia (see Appendix F) even though this drug has minimal, if any, diabetogenic action.
- Drink fluids liberally (2000–3000 mL/day). Hydration may protect against drug toxicity effects.
- Report S&S of nephrotoxicity (see Appendix F).
- Do not take aspirin or NSAIDs without consulting physician.
- Report to physician promptly any signs of bleeding: Hematuria, epistaxis, ecchymoses, petechial.
- Report symptoms that suggest anemia: Shortness of breath, pale mucous membranes and nail beds, exhaustion, rapid pulse.

S

SUCCINYLCHOLINE CHLORIDE (Pr)

(suk-sin-ill-koe'leen)

Anectine, Quelicin

Classification: DEPOLARIZING SKELETAL MUSCLE RELAXANT

Therapeutic: SKELETAL MUSCLE RELAXANT

Pregnancy Category: C

AVAILABILITY 20 mg/mL, 50 mg/mL, 100 mg/mL injection

ACTION & *THERAPEUTIC EFFECT* Synthetic, ultrashort-acting depolarizing neuromuscular blocking agent with high affinity for acetylcholine (ACh) receptor sites. *Initial transient contractions and fasciculations are followed by sustained flaccid skeletal muscle paralysis produced by state of accommodation that develops in adjacent excitable muscle membranes.*

USES To produce skeletal muscle relaxation as adjunct to anesthesia; to facilitate intubation and endoscopy, to increase pulmonary compliance in assisted or controlled respiration, and to reduce intensity of muscle contractions in pharmacologically induced or electroshock convulsions.

CONTRAINDICATIONS Hypersensitivity to succinylcholine; family history of malignant hyperthermia; burns; trauma.

CAUTIOUS USE During delivery by cesarean section; kidney, liver, pulmonary, metabolic, or cardiovascular disorders; myasthenia gravis; dehydration, electrolyte imbalance, patients taking digitalis, severe burns or trauma, fractures, spinal cord injuries, degenerative or dystrophic neuromuscular diseases, low plasma pseudocholinesterase levels (recessive genetic trait, but often associated with severe liver disease, severe anemia, dehydration, marked changes in body temperature, exposure to neurotoxic insecticides, certain drugs); collagen diseases, porphyria, intraocular surgery, glaucoma; pregnancy (category C), lactation.

ROUTE & DOSAGE

Surgical and Anesthetic Procedures

Adult: **IV** 0.3–1.1 mg/kg administered over 10–30 sec, may give additional doses prn **IM** 2.5–4 mg/kg up to 150 mg
Child: **IV** 1–2 mg/kg administered over 10–30 sec, may give additional doses prn **IM** 2.5–4 mg/kg up to 150 mg

Prolonged Muscle Relaxation

Adult: **IV** 0.5–10 mg/min by continuous infusion

Obesity Dosage Adjustment

Dose based on IBW

ADMINISTRATION

Intramuscular

- Give IM injections deeply, preferably high into deltoid muscle.

Intravenous

Use only freshly prepared solutions; succinylcholine hydrolyzes rapidly with consequent loss of potency.

- Give initial small test dose (0.1 mg/kg) to determine individual drug sensitivity and recovery time.

PREPARE: **Direct:** Give undiluted. **Intermittent/Continuous:** Dilute 1 g in 500–1000 mL of D5W or NS.
ADMINISTER: **Direct:** Give a bolus dose over 10–30 sec. **Intermittent/Continuous (Preferred):** Give at a rate of 0.5–10 mg/min. Do not exceed 10 mg/min.
INCOMPATIBILITIES **Solution/additive:** **Aminophylline, ampicillin, cephalothin, diazepam, epinephrine, hydrocortisone, methicillin, methohexital, nitrofurantoin, oxacillin, oxytetracycline, sodium bicarbonate, thiopental, warfarin.** **Y-site:** **Thiopental.**

- Note: Expiration date and storage before and after reconstitution; varies with the manufacturer.

ADVERSE EFFECTS (≥1%) **CNS:** *Muscle fasciculations,* profound and prolonged muscle relaxation, muscle pain. **CV:** *Bradycardia,* tachycardia, hypotension, hypertension, arrhythmias, sinus arrest. **Respiratory:** <u>*Respiratory depression*</u>, bronchospasm, hypoxia, <u>apnea</u>. **Body as a Whole:** <u>Malignant hyperthermia</u>, increased IOP, excessive salivation, enlarged salivary glands. **Metabolic:** Myoglobinemia, hyperkalemia. **GI:** Decreased tone and motility of GI tract (large doses).

INTERACTIONS **Drug:** **Aminoglycosides, colistin, cyclophosphamide, cyclopropane, echothiophate iodide, halothane, lidocaine,** MAGNESIUM SALTS, **methotrimeprazine,** NARCOTIC ANALGESICS, ORGANOPHOSPHAMIDE INSECTICIDES, MAO INHIBITORS, PHENOTHIAZINES, **procaine, procainamide, quinidine, quinine, propranolol** may prolong neuromuscular blockade; DIGITALIS GLYCOSIDES may increase risk of cardiac arrhythmias.

PHARMACOKINETICS **Onset:** 0.5–1 min IV; 2–3 min IM. **Duration:** 2–3 min IV; 10–30 min IM. **Distribution:** Crosses placenta in small amounts. **Metabolism:** In plasma by pseudocholinesterases. **Elimination:** In urine.

S

NURSING IMPLICATIONS

Assessment & Drug Effects

- Lab tests: Obtain baseline serum electrolytes. Electrolyte imbalance (particularly potassium, calcium, magnesium) can potentiate effects of neuromuscular blocking agents.
- Be aware that transient apnea usually occurs at time of maximal drug effect (1–2 min); spontaneous respiration should return in a few seconds or, at most, 3 or 4 min.
- Have immediately available: Facilities for emergency endotracheal intubation, artificial respiration, and assisted or controlled respiration with oxygen.
- Monitor vital signs and keep airway clear of secretions.

Patient & Family Education

- Patient may experience postprocedural muscle stiffness and pain (caused by initial fasciculations following injection) for as long as 24–30 h.
- Be aware that hoarseness and sore throat are common even when pharyngeal airway has not been used.
- Report residual muscle weakness to physician.

S

SUCRALFATE

(soo-kral′fate)

Carafate, Sulcrate ♣

Classifications: ANTIULCER; GASTRO-ADHESIVE

Therapeutic: ANTIULCER; GASTRO-PROTECTANT

Pregnancy Category: B

AVAILABILITY 1 g tablets; 1 g/10 mL suspension

ACTION & *THERAPEUTIC EFFECT* Sucralfate and gastric acid react to form a viscous, adhesive, paste-like substance that resists further reaction with gastric acid. This "paste" adheres to the GI mucosa with a major portion binding electrostatically to the positively charged protein molecules in the damaged mucosa of an ulcer crater or an acute gastric erosion. *Absorbs bile, inhibits the enzyme pepsin, and blocks back diffusion of H^+ ions. These actions plus adherence of the paste-like complex protect damaged mucosa against further destruction from ulcerogenic secretions and drugs.*

USES Short-term (up to 8 wk) treatment of duodenal ulcer.

UNLABELED USES Short-term treatment of gastric ulcer, aspirin-induced erosions, suspension for chemotherapy-induced mucositis.

CONTRAINDICATIONS Safety and efficacy in children are not established.

CAUTIOUS USE Chronic kidney failure or dialysis due to aluminum accumulation; renal impairment; pregnancy (category B).

ROUTE & DOSAGE

Duodenal Ulcer

Adult: **PO** 1 g q.i.d. 1 h a.c. and at bedtime **PO Maintenance** 1 g b.i.d.

ADMINISTRATION

Oral

- Use drug solubilized in an appropriate diluent by a pharmacist when given through nasogastric tube.
- Administer antacids prescribed for pain relief 30 min before or after sucralfate.
- Separate administration of quinolones, digoxin, phenytoin, tetracycline from that of sucralfate by 2 h to prevent sucralfate from bind-

ing to these compounds in the intestinal tract and reducing their bioavailability.

- Store in tight container at room temperature, 15°–30° C (59°–86° F). Stable for 2 y after manufacture.

ADVERSE EFFECTS (≥1%) **GI:** Nausea, gastric discomfort, *constipation,* diarrhea.

INTERACTIONS Drug: May decrease absorption of QUINOLONES (e.g., **ciprofloxacin, norfloxacin**), **digoxin, phenytoin, tetracycline.**

PHARMACOKINETICS Absorption: Minimally absorbed from GI tract (less than 5%). **Duration:** Up to 6 h (depends on contact time with ulcer crater). **Elimination:** 90% in feces.

NURSING IMPLICATIONS

Assessment & Drug Effects

- Be aware of drug interactions and schedule other medications accordingly.

Patient & Family Education

- Although healing has occurred within the first 2 wk of therapy, treatment is usually continued 4–8 wk.
- Be aware that constipation is a drug-related problem. Follow these measures unless contraindicated: Increase water intake to 8–10 glasses per day; increase physical exercise, increase dietary bulk. Consult physician: A suppository or bulk laxative (e.g., Metamucil) may be prescribed.

SUFENTANIL CITRATE

(soo-fen′ta-nil)

Sufenta

Classifications: NARCOTIC (OPIATE AGONIST) ANALGESIC; GENERAL ANESTHETIC

Therapeutic: NARCOTIC ANALGESIC; GENERAL ANESTHETIC
Prototype: Morphine
Pregnancy Category: C
Controlled Substance: Schedule II

AVAILABILITY 50 mcg/mL injection

ACTION & *THERAPEUTIC EFFECT* Synthetic opioid related to fentanyl. Onset of action and recovery from anesthesia occur more rapidly with sufentanil than with fentanyl. *Effective agent for analgesia as a supplement or as a primary anesthesia.*

USES Analgesic supplement in maintenance of balanced general anesthesia and also as a primary anesthetic.

CONTRAINDICATIONS Hypersensitivity to sufentanil or opiate agonists. **CAUTIOUS USE** Pulmonary disease, reduced respiratory reserve; COPD; cardiac disease; increased intracranial pressure; seizure disorders; impaired liver or kidney function; GI disease; pregnancy (category C), lactation.

ROUTE & DOSAGE

Adjunct to General Anesthesia

Adult: **IV** 1–8 mcg/kg, depending on duration of surgery, may give additional doses of 10–50 mcg if needed

As Primary Anesthetic

Adult: **IV** 1–30 mcg/kg administered with 100% oxygen and a muscle relaxant, may give additional doses of 10–50 mcg if needed

Child (younger than 12 y): **IV** 10–25 mcg/kg administered with 100% oxygen and a muscle relaxant, may give additional

S

doses of 25–50 mcg up to 1–2 mcg/kg/dose if needed

Obesity Dosage Adjustment

Use lean body weight

ADMINISTRATION

Intravenous

Administer only by qualified personnel, specifically trained in the use of IV anesthesia and in the management of respiratory depression.

- Have available a narcotic antagonist (e.g., naloxone) to reverse respiratory depression.

PREPARE: **Direct:** Examine solution for particulate matter and discoloration (solution should be clear) before administration. Give undiluted.

ADMINISTER: **Direct:** Give a bolus dose over 3–5 sec.

INCOMPATIBILITIES **Solution/additive:** **Diazepam, lorazepam, phenobarbital, phenytoin, sodium bicarbonate, sodium chloride.** **Y-site:** **Lorazepam, phenytoin, thiopental.**

- Store at 15°–30° C (59°–86° F) unless otherwise directed; protect from light.

ADVERSE EFFECTS (≥1%) **CV:** Bradycardia, tachycardia, hypotension, hypertension, arrhythmias. **GI:** Nausea, vomiting, constipation. **Respiratory:** Bronchospasm, respiratory depression, apnea. **Body as a Whole:** *Skeletal muscle rigidity (especially of trunk)*, chills, *itching*, spasms of sphincter of Oddi, urinary retention.

INTERACTIONS Drug: BETA-ADRENERGIC ANTAGONISTS increase incidence of bradycardia; **alcohol** and other CNS DEPRESSANTS such as BARBITURATES, TRANQUILIZERS, OPIATES, and INHALATION GENERAL ANESTHETICS add to CNS depression; **cimetidine** increases risk of respiratory depression.

PHARMACOKINETICS Onset: 1.5–3 min. **Duration:** 40 min. **Distribution:** Crosses blood–brain barrier. **Metabolism:** In liver (CYP3A4) and small intestine. **Elimination:** In urine and feces. **Half-Life:** 2–3 h.

NURSING IMPLICATIONS

Assessment & Drug Effects

- Monitor vital signs. Observe for skeletal muscle rigidity, especially of chest wall, and respiratory depression, particularly in older adults, and in patients who are obese, debilitated, or who have received high doses.
- Bear in mind that if naloxone is given to reverse respiratory depression, the duration of sufentanil-induced respiratory depression may exceed the duration of naloxone.

Patient & Family Education

- Avoid activities that require mental alertness for at least 24 h after receiving this drug.

SULFACETAMIDE SODIUM

(sul-fa-see'ta-mide)

AK-Sulf, Bleph 10, Cetamide, Isopto Cetamide, Ophthacet, Sebizon, Sodium Sulamyd, Sulf-10

SULFACETAMIDE SODIUM/ SULFUR

Sulfacet, Rosula

Classification: SULFONAMIDE ANTIBIOTIC

Therapeutic: ANTIBIOTIC

Prototype: Sulfisoxazole

Pregnancy Category: C; D near term

AVAILABILITY Sulfacetamide: 10% lotion; 1%, 10%, 15%, 30% solution; 10% ointment; **Sulfacetamide/Sulfur:** 10%/5% gel, lotion

ACTION & *THERAPEUTIC EFFECT* Highly soluble sulfonamide that exerts bacteriostatic effect by interfering with bacterial utilization of PABA, thereby inhibiting folic acid biosynthesis required for bacterial growth. *Effective against a wide range of gram-positive and gram-negative microorganisms.*

USES Ophthalmic preparations are used for conjunctivitis, corneal ulcers, and other superficial ocular infections and as adjunct to systemic sulfonamide therapy for trachoma. The topical lotion is used for scaly dermatoses, seborrheic dermatitis, seborrhea sicca, and other bacterial skin infections.

CONTRAINDICATIONS Hypersensitivity to sulfonamides; neonates, pregnancy (category D near term). Safe use in children not known.

CAUTIOUS USE Application of lotion to denuded or debrided skin; pregnancy (category C except near term), lactation.

ROUTE & DOSAGE

Conjunctivitis

Adult: **Ophthalmic** 1–3 drops of 10%, 15%, or 30% solution into lower conjunctival sac q2–3h, may increase interval as patient responds or use 1.5–2.5 cm (1/2–1 in.) of 10% ointment q6h and at bedtime

Seborrhea, Rosacea

Adult: **Topical** Apply thin film to affected area 1–3 times/day

ADMINISTRATION

Instillation

- Be aware that ophthalmic preparations and skin lotion are not interchangeable.
- Check strength of medication prescribed.
- See patient instructions for instilling eye drops.
- Discard darkened solutions; results when left standing for a long time.
- Store at 8°–15° C (46°–59° F) in tightly closed containers unless otherwise directed.

ADVERSE EFFECTS (≥1%) **Special Senses:** *Temporary stinging or burning sensation,* retardation of corneal healing associated with long-term use of ophthalmic ointment. **Body as a Whole:** Hypersensitivity reactions (Stevens-Johnson syndrome, lupus-like syndrome), superinfections with nonsusceptible organisms.

INTERACTIONS Drug: Tetracaine and other LOCAL ANESTHETICS DERIVED FROM PABA may antagonize the antibacterial effects of sulfonamides; SILVER PREPARATIONS may precipitate sulfacetamide from solution.

PHARMACOKINETICS Absorption: Minimal systemic absorption, but may be enough to cause sensitization. **Metabolism:** In liver to inactive metabolites. **Elimination:** In urine.

NURSING IMPLICATIONS

Assessment & Drug Effects

- Discontinue if symptoms of hypersensitivity appear (erythema, skin rash, pruritus, urticaria).

Patient & Family Education

- Wash hands thoroughly with soap and running water (before and after instillation).
- Examine eye medication; discard if cloudy or dark in color.

- Avoid contaminating any part of eye dropper that is inserted in bottle.
- Tilt head back, pull down lower lid. At the same time, look up while drop is being instilled into conjunctival sac. Immediately apply gentle pressure just below the eyelid and next to nose for 1 min. Close eyes gently, so as not to squeeze out medication.
- Report purulent eye discharge to physician. Sulfacetamide sodium is inactivated by purulent exudates.

SULFADIAZINE

(sul-fa-dye′a-zeen)

Microsulfon

Classification: SULFONAMIDE ANTIBIOTIC

Therapeutic: ANTIBIOTIC

Prototype: Sulfisoxazole

Pregnancy Category: C; D near term

AVAILABILITY 500 mg tablets

ACTION & *THERAPEUTIC EFFECT* Short-acting sulfonamide that exerts bacteriostatic effect by interfering with bacterial utilization of PABA, thereby inhibiting folic acid biosynthesis required for bacterial growth. *Effective against a wide range of gram-positive and gram-negative microorganisms.*

USES Used in combination with pyrimethamine for treatment of cerebral toxoplasmosis and chloroquine-resistant malaria.

CONTRAINDICATIONS Hypersensitivity to sulfonamides or to any ingredients in the formulation; porphyria; pregnancy (category D near term), lactation.

CAUTIOUS USE Application of lotion to denuded or debrided skin; dehydration; hepatic disease; impaired renal function; pregnancy (category C except near term).

ROUTE & DOSAGE

Mild to Moderate Infections

Adult: **PO Loading Dose** 2–4 g loading dose **PO Maintenance Dose** 2–4 g/day in 4–6 divided doses

Child (older than 2 mo): **PO Loading Dose** 75 mg/kg **PO Maintenance Dose** 150 mg/kg/day in 4–6 divided doses (max: 6 g/day)

Rheumatic Fever Prophylaxis

Adult: **PO** *Weight less than 30 kg,* 500 mg/day; *weight greater than 30 kg,* 1 g/day

Toxoplasmosis

Adult: **PO** 2–8 g/day divided q6h

Child (older than 2 mo): **PO** 100–200 mg/kg/day divided q6h

Neonate: **PO** 50 mg/kg q12h × 12 mo

ADMINISTRATION

Oral

- Maintain sufficient fluid intake to produce urinary output of at least 1500 mL/24 h for children between 3000 and 4000 mL/24 h for adults. Concomitant administration of urinary alkalinizer may be prescribed to reduce possibility of crystalluria and stone formation.
- Store in tight, light-resistant containers.

ADVERSE EFFECTS (≥1%) **CNS:** Headache, peripheral neuritis, peripheral neuropathy, tinnitus, hearing loss, vertigo, insomnia, drowsiness, mental depression, acute psychosis, ataxia, convulsions, kernicterus (newborns). **GI:** *Nausea, vomiting, diarrhea,* abdominal pains, hepatitis, jaundice, pancreatitis, stomatitis. **Hematologic:** Acute hemolytic anemia (especially in patients with G6PD deficiency), aplastic anemia, methemoglobinemia, agranulocytosis, thrombocytopenia, leukopenia, eosinophilia, hypoprothrombinemia. **Body as a Whole:** Headache, *fever,* chills, arthralgia, malaise, allergic myocarditis, serum sickness, anaphylactoid reactions, lymphadenopathy, local reaction following IM injection, fixed drug eruptions, diuresis, overgrowth of nonsusceptible organisms, LE phenomenon. **Skin:** Pruritus, urticaria, rash, erythema multiforme including *Stevens-Johnson syndrome, exfoliative dermatitis,* alopecia, photosensitivity, vascular lesions. **Urogenital:** *Crystalluria,* hematuria, proteinuria, anuria, toxic nephrosis, reduction in sperm count. **Metabolic:** Goiter, hypoglycemia. **Special Senses:** Conjunctivitis, conjunctival or scleral infection, retardation of corneal healing (ophthalmic ointment).

INTERACTIONS Drug: PABA-CONTAINING LOCAL ANESTHETICS may antagonize sulfa's effects; ORAL ANTICOAGULANTS potentiate hypoprothrombinemia; may potentiate SULFONYLUREA-induced hypoglycemia. May decrease concentrations of **cyclosporine;** may increase levels of **phenytoin.**

PHARMACOKINETICS Absorption: Readily absorbed from GI tract. **Peak:** 3–6 h. **Distribution:** Distributed to most tissues, including CSF; crosses placenta. **Metabolism:** In liver. **Elimination:** In urine.

NURSING IMPLICATIONS

Assessment & Drug Effects

- Lab tests: Baseline and periodic urine C&S to determine drug effectiveness; with long-term therapy, CBC, Hct, and Hgb.
- Monitor hydration status.

Patient & Family Education

- Take drug exactly as prescribed. Do not alter schedule or dose; take total amount prescribed unless physician changes the regimen.
- Drink fluids liberally unless otherwise directed.
- Report early signs of blood dyscrasias (sore throat, pallor, fever) promptly to the physician.

SULFAMETHOXAZOLE-TRIMETHOPRIM (SMZ-TMP)

(sul-fa-meth′ox-a-zole-tri-meth′o-prim)

Bactrim, Bactrim DS, Co-Trim, Septra, Septra DS

Classifications: URINARY TRACT AGENT; SULFONAMIDE

Therapeutic: URINARY TRACT ANTI-INFECTIVE

Prototype: Trimethoprim

Pregnancy Category: C; D near term

AVAILABILITY 400 mg SMZ/80 mg TMP, 800 mg SMZ/160 mg TMP tablets; 200 mg SMZ/40 mg TMP suspension; 80 mg SMZ/16 mg TMP injection

ACTION & *THERAPEUTIC EFFECT* Fixed combination of sulfamethoxazole (SMZ), an intermediate-acting anti-infective sulfonamide, and trimethoprim (TMP), a synthetic anti-infective. Both components of the combination are synthetic folate antagonist anti-infectives. Principal action is by enzyme inhibition that prevents bacterial synthesis of essential nucleic acids and proteins. *Effective against* Pneumocystis jiroveci *pneumonitis (formerly PCP),* Shigellosis *enteritis, and severely complicated UTIs due to most strains of the Enterobacteriaceae.*

USES *Pneumocystis jiroveci* pneumonitis (formerly PCP), shigellosis enteritis, and severe complicated UTIs. Also children with acute otitis media due to susceptible strains of *Haemophilus influenzae,* and acute episodes of chronic bronchitis in adults.

UNLABELED USES Isosporiasis; prevention of traveler's diarrhea; cholera; genital ulcers caused by *Haemophilus ducreyi;* prophylaxis for *P. jiroveci* pneumonia (formerly PCP) in neutropenic patients.

CONTRAINDICATIONS Hypersensitivity to SMZ, TMP, sulfonamides, or bisulfites, carbonic anhydrase inhibitors; group A beta-hemolytic streptococcal pharyngitis; megaloblastic anemia due to folate deficiency; creatinine clearance less than 15 mL/min; G6PD deficiency; hyperkalemia; porphyria; pregnancy (category D near term), lactation. Not recommended for infants younger than 2 mo.

CAUTIOUS USE Impaired kidney or liver function; bone marrow depression; possible folate deficiency; severe allergy or bronchial asthma; hypersensitivity to sulfonamide derivative drugs (e.g., acetazolamide, thiazides, tolbutamide); pregnancy (category C except near term).

S

ROUTE & DOSAGE

(Weight-based doses are calculated on TMP component)

Systemic Infections

Adult: **PO** 160 mg TMP/800 mg SMZ q12h **IV** 8–10 mg/kg/day TMP divided q6–12h

Child: **PO** *Older than 2 mo, weight less than 40 kg,* 4 mg/kg/day TMP q12h; *weight greater than 40 kg,* 160 mg TMP/800 mg SMZ q12h

Child/Infant (older than 2 mo): **IV** 6–10 mg/kg/day TMP divided q6–12h

***Pneumocystis jiroveci* Pneumonia (formerly PCP)**

Adult: **PO** 15–20 mg/kg/day TMP divided q6h

Adult/Adolescent/Child: **IV** 15–20 mg/kg/day TMP divided q6h

Prophylaxis for *Pneumocystis jiroveci* Pneumonia (formerly PCP)

Adult: **PO** 160 mg TMP/800 mg SMZ q24h

Child: **PO** 150 mg/m^2 TMP/750 mg/m^2 SMZ b.i.d. 3 consecutive days/wk (max: 320 mg TMP/day)

Renal Impairment Dosage Adjustment

CrCl 10–30 mL/min: Reduce dose by 50%; less than 10 mL/min: Reduce dose by 50–75%

ADMINISTRATION

Oral

- Give with a full glass of desired fluid.
- Maintain adequate fluid intake (at least 1500 mL/day) during therapy.
- Store at 15°–30° C (59°–86° F) in dry place protected from light. Avoid freezing.

Intravenous

PREPARE: **Intermittent:** Add contents of the 5 mL ampule to 125 mL D5W. ▪Use within 6 h. ▪If less fluid is desired, dilute in 75 of 100 mL and use within 2 or 4 h, respectively.

ADMINISTER: **Intermittent:** Infuse over 60–90 min. ▪ Avoid rapid infusion.

INCOMPATIBILITIES **Solution/additive:** Stability in **dextrose** and **normal saline** is concentration dependent, **fluconazole, linezolid, verapamil.** **Y-site: Amikacin, aminophylline, cisatracurium, fluconazole, foscarnet, midazolam, vinorelbine.**

- Store unopened ampule at 15–30° C (50–86° F)

ADVERSE EFFECTS (≥1%) **Skin:** *Mild to moderate rashes (including fixed drug eruptions),* <u>toxic epidermal necrolysis</u>. **GI:** *Nausea, vomiting,* diarrhea, *anorexia,* hepatitis, <u>pseudomembranous enterocolitis</u>, stomatitis, glossitis, abdominal pain. **Urogenital:** Kidney failure, oliguria, anuria, crystalluria. **Hematologic:** <u>Agranulocytosis</u> (rare), <u>aplastic anemia</u> (rare), megaloblastic anemia, hypoprothrombinemia, thrombocytopenia (rare). **Body as a Whole:** Weakness, arthralgia, myalgia, photosensitivity, <u>allergic myocarditis</u>.

DIAGNOSTIC TEST INTERFERENCE May elevate levels of serum creatinine, transaminase, bilirubin, alkaline phosphatase.

INTERACTIONS Drug: May enhance hypoprothrombinemic effects of ORAL ANTICOAGULANTS; may increase **methotrexate** toxicity. **Alcohol** may cause disulfiram reaction.

PHARMACOKINETICS Absorption: Readily from GI tract. **Peak:** 1–4 h (oral). **Distribution:** Widely distributed, including CNS; crosses placenta; distributed into breast milk. **Metabolism:** In liver. **Elimination:** In urine. **Half-Life:** 8–10 h TMP, 10–13 h SMZ.

NURSING IMPLICATIONS

Assessment & Drug Effects

- Be aware that IV Septra contains sodium metabisulfite, which produces allergic-type reactions in susceptible patients: Hives, itching, wheezing, anaphylaxis. Susceptibility (low in general population) is seen most frequently in asthmatics or atopic nonasthmatic persons.
- Lab tests: Baseline and follow-up urinalysis; CBC with differential, platelet count, BUN and creatinine clearance with prolonged therapy.
- Monitor coagulation tests and prothrombin times in patient also receiving warfarin. Change in warfarin dosage may be indicated.
- Monitor I&O volume and pattern. Report significant changes to forestall renal calculi formation. Also report failure of treatment (i.e., continued UTI symptoms).
- Older adult patients are at risk for severe adverse reactions, especially if liver or kidney function is compromised or if certain other drugs are given. Most frequently observed: Thrombocytopenia (with concurrent thiazide diuretics); severe decrease in platelets (with or without purpura); bone marrow suppression; severe skin reactions.
- Be alert for overdose symptoms (no extensive experience has been reported): Nausea, vomiting, anorexia, headache, dizziness, mental depression, confusion, and bone marrow depression.

Patient & Family Education

- Report immediately to physician if rash appears. Other reportable symptoms are sore throat, fever, purpura, jaundice; all are early signs of serious reactions.

- Monitor for and report fixed eruptions to physician. This drug can cause fixed eruptions at the same sites each time the drug is administered. Every contact with drug may not result in eruptions; therefore, patient may overlook the relationship.
- Drink 2.5–3 L (1 L is approximately equal to 1 qt) daily, unless otherwise directed.

SULFASALAZINE

(sul-fa-sal′a-zeen)

Azulfidine, PMS Sulfasalazine ♣, PMS Sulfasalazine E.C. ♣, Salazopyrin ♣, SAS Enteric-500 ♣, S.A.S.-500 ♣

Classifications: ANTI-INFLAMMATORY; SULFONAMIDE

Therapeutic: GI ANTI-INFLAMMATORY; IMMUNOMODULATOR; DISEASE-MODIFYING ANTIRHEUMATIC DRUG (DMARD)

Prototype: Mesalamine

Pregnancy Category: C; D near term

AVAILABILITY 500 mg tablets; 500 mg sustained release tablets

ACTION & *THERAPEUTIC EFFECT* Locally acting sulfonamide, believed to be converted by intestinal microflora to sulfapyridine (provides antibacterial action) and 5-aminosalicylic acid (5-ASA) or mesalamine, which may exert an anti-inflammatory effect. Inhibits prostaglandins known to cause diarrhea and affect mucosal transport as well as interference with absorption of fluids and electrolytes from colon. *Reduces* Clostridium *and* Escherichia coli *in the stools. Anti-inflammatory and immunomodulatory properties are effective in controlling the S&S of ulcerative colitis and rheumatoid arthritis.*

USES Ulcerative colitis and relatively mild regional enteritis; rheumatoid arthritis.

UNLABELED USES Granulomatous colitis, Crohn's disease, scleroderma.

CONTRAINDICATIONS Sensitivity to sulfasalazine, other sulfonamides and salicylates, trimethoprim; folate deficiency; megaloblastic anemia; renal failure, renal impairment; agranulocytosis; intestinal and urinary tract obstruction; porphyria; pregnancy (category D near term), lactation. Safety and efficacy in children younger than 2 y are unknown.

CAUTIOUS USE Severe allergy, or bronchial asthma; blood dyscrasias; hepatic or renal impairment; G6PD deficiency; older adults; pregnancy (category C except near term); children younger than 6 y.

ROUTE & DOSAGE

Ulcerative Colitis, Rheumatoid Arthritis

Adult: **PO** 1–2 g/day in 4 divided doses, may increase up to 8 g/day if needed

Child: **PO** 40–50 mg/kg/day in 4 divided doses (max: 75 mg/kg/day)

Juvenile Rheumatoid Arthritis

Child: **PO** 10 mg/kg/day, increase weekly by 10 mg/kg/day [usual dose: 15–25 mg/kg q12h (max: 2 g/day)]

ADMINISTRATION

Oral

- Give after eating to provide longer intestine transit time.
- Do not crush or chew sustained release tablets; **must be** swallowed whole.
- Use evenly divided doses over each 24-h period; do not exceed 8-h intervals between doses.

- Consult physician if GI intolerance occurs after first few doses. Symptoms are probably due to irritation of stomach mucosa and may be relieved by spacing total daily dose more evenly over 24 h or by administration of enteric-coated tablets.
- Store at 15°–30° C (59°–86° F) in tight, light-resistant containers.

ADVERSE EFFECTS (≥1%) **Body as a Whole:** *Nausea, vomiting, bloody diarrhea; anorexia,* arthralgia, rash, anemia, oligospermia (reversible), blood dyscrasias, liver injury, infectious mononucleosis–like reaction, *allergic reactions.*

INTERACTIONS Drug: Iron, ANTIBIOTICS may alter absorption of sulfasalazine.

PHARMACOKINETICS Absorption: 10–15% from GI tract unchanged; remaining drug is hydrolyzed in colon to sulfapyridine (most of which is absorbed) and 5-aminosalicylic acid (30% of which is absorbed). **Peak:** 1.5–6 h sulfasalazine; 6–24 h sulfapyridine. **Distribution:** Crosses placenta; distributed into breast milk. **Metabolism:** In intestines and liver. **Elimination:** All metabolites are excreted in urine. **Half-Life:** 5–10 h.

NURSING IMPLICATIONS

Assessment & Drug Effects

- Monitor for GI distress. GI symptoms that develop after a few days of therapy may indicate need for dosage adjustment. If symptoms persist, physician may withhold drug for 5–7 days and restart it at a lower dosage level.
- Be aware that adverse reactions generally occur within a few days to 12 wk after start of therapy; most likely to occur in patients receiving high doses (4 g or more).
- Lab tests: Measure RBC folate in patients on high doses (more than 2 g/day); a daily supplement may be prescribed.

Patient & Family Education

- Examine stools and report to physician if enteric-coated tablets have passed intact in feces. Some patients lack enzymes capable of dissolving coating; conventional tablet will be ordered.
- Be aware that drug may color alkaline urine and skin orange-yellow.
- Remain under close medical supervision. Relapses occur in about 40% of patients after initial satisfactory response. Response to therapy and duration of treatment are governed by endoscopic examinations.

SULFINPYRAZONE

(sul-fin-peer'a-zone)

Antazone ♣, Anturan ♣, Anturane, Apo-Sulfinpyrazone ♣, Novopyrazone ♣

Classifications: ANTIGOUT; URICOSURIC

Therapeutic: ANTIGOUT

Prototype: Probenecid

Pregnancy Category: C

AVAILABILITY 100 mg tablets; 200 mg capsules

ACTION & *THERAPEUTIC EFFECT* Potent renal tubular blocking agent of uric acid in the kidney that lowers its serum blood level. Inhibits release of adenosine diphosphate and 5-hydroxytryptophan, and thus decreases platelet adhesiveness and increases platelet survival time. *Promotes urinary excretion of uric acid and reduces serum urate* *levels by competitively inhibiting tubular reabsorption of uric acid in the kidney.*

USES Maintenance therapy in chronic gouty arthritis and tophaceous gout.

UNLABELED USES Drug-induced hyperuricemia, to decrease platelet aggregation and increase their survival in prevention of TIAs and stroke.

CONTRAINDICATIONS Known hypersensitivity to phenylbutazone, or pyrazoline derivatives or salicylates; active peptic ulcer; concurrent administration of salicylates; blood dyscrasias; patients with creatinine clearance less than 50 mg/min, treatment of hyperuricemia secondary to neoplastic disease or cancer chemotherapy; bone marrow suppression; hematologic disease; nephrolithiasis.

CAUTIOUS USE NSAID hypersensitivity; impaired kidney function; severe hepatic disease; history of healed peptic ulcer; concurrent use of anticoagulant therapy; thrombocytopenia; use in conjunction with sulfonamides and sulfonylureas; pregnancy (category C).

ROUTE & DOSAGE

Gout

Adult: **PO** 100–200 mg b.i.d. for 1 wk, then increase to 200–400 mg b.i.d., may reduce to 200 mg/d after serum urate levels are controlled (max: 800 mg/day)

Inhibition of Platelet Aggregation

Adult: **PO** 200 mg t.i.d. or q.i.d.

ADMINISTRATION

Oral

- Give with meals, milk, or antacid (prescribed) to prevent local drug irritant effect. Severity and frequency of symptoms increase with dosage. Persistence of GI symptoms may require discontinuation of drug.
- Ensure fluid intake sufficient to support urinary output of at least 2000–3000 mL/day during early therapy (consult physician). Also alkalinize urine (e.g., with large doses vitamin C) to increase solubility of uric acid and minimize risk of uric acid stones.

ADVERSE EFFECTS (≥1%) **GI:** *Nausea,* vomiting, diarrhea, *epigastric pain, blood loss, reactivation or aggravation of peptic ulcer,* jaundice. **CNS:** Ataxia, dizziness, vertigo, convulsions, coma. **Special Senses:** Tinnitus. **Body as a Whole:** Edema, labored respirations, hypersensitivity, reactions (skin rashes, fever). **Urogenital:** Precipitation of acute gout, urolithiasis, renal colic.

DIAGNOSTIC TEST INTERFERENCE Sulfinpyrazone decreases urinary excretion of ***aminohippuric acid*** and ***phenolsulfonphthalein.***

INTERACTIONS Drug: May decrease efficacy of **nitrofurantoin** for UTI and increase its systemic toxicity. May displace SULFONYLUREAS from protein binding and increase risk of hypoglycemia; may augment prothrombin time increased by **warfarin; cholestyramine** decreases absorption of sulfinpyrazone; **aspirin** may inhibit uricosuric effects of sulfinpyrazone.

PHARMACOKINETICS Absorption: Readily absorbed from GI tract. **Peak:** 1–2 h. **Duration:** 4–6 h; may persist up to 10 h. **Metabolism:** In liver to active and inactive metabolites. **Elimination:** Slowly in urine; 5% in feces. **Half-Life:** 3 h.

NURSING IMPLICATIONS

Assessment & Drug Effects

- Monitor frequency of acute attacks.
- Lab tests: Periodic serum urate levels; periodic CBC during prolonged therapy; periodic kidney function tests, particularly with renal impairment; PT and INR with concurrent warfarin use.
- Frequency of acute gouty attacks may increase during first 6–12 mo of therapy, even when serum urate levels appear to be controlled. Concurrent prophylactic doses of colchicine may be prescribed during first 3–6 mo of treatment to prevent or lessen severity of attacks.

Patient & Family Education

- Remain under close medical supervision; therapy is continued indefinitely.
- Do not experiment with dosage; subtherapeutic doses may enhance urate retention and large doses may increase risk of toxicity.
- Continue medication without interruption even during acute gouty attack. Contact physician for concomitant treatment with full therapeutic doses of colchicine or other anti-inflammatory agent.
- Avoid aspirin-containing medications. If an analgesic is required (in patients with normal kidney function), acetaminophen is generally recommended.

SULFISOXAZOLE (Pr)

(sul-fi-sox′a-zole)

Classification: SULFONAMIDE ANTIBIOTIC
Therapeutic: ANTIBIOTIC
Pregnancy Category: C; D near term

AVAILABILITY 500 mg tablets

ACTION & *THERAPEUTIC EFFECT* Short-acting derivative of sulfanilamide. Bacteriostatic action believed to be by competitive inhibition of *p*-aminobenzoic acid (PABA), thereby interfering with folic acid biosynthesis required for bacterial growth. *Exhibits broad antimicrobial spectrum against both gram-positive and gram-negative organisms.*

USES Acute, recurrent, and chronic urinary tract infections and chancroid; adjunctive therapy in trachoma, chloroquine-resistant strains of malaria, acute otitis media due to *Haemophilus influenzae,* and meningococcal and *H. influenzae* meningitis. Ophthalmic preparations used in treatment of conjunctivitis, corneal ulcer, and other superficial eye infections and as adjunct to systemic sulfonamide therapy for trachoma. Topical vaginal preparation used for *H. vaginalis* vaginitis.

CONTRAINDICATIONS History of hypersensitivity to sulfonamides, salicylates, or chemically related drugs; use in treatment of group A beta-hemolytic streptococcal infections; neonates; porphyria; G6PD deficiency; advanced kidney or liver disease; intestinal and urinary obstruction; pregnancy (category D if near term); infants less than 2 mo except for treatment of congenital toxoplasmosis.
CAUTIOUS USE Impaired kidney or liver function; severe allergy; bronchial asthma; blood dyscrasias; pregnancy (category C except near term).

ROUTE & DOSAGE

Infection

Adult: **PO** 2–4 g initially, followed by 4–8 g/day in 4–6 divided doses

Child (older than 2 mo): **PO** 75 mg/kg initially, followed by 150 mg/kg/day in 4–6 divided doses (max: 6 g/day)

ADMINISTRATION

Oral

- Give with full glass of water or other fluid; tablet may be crushed.
- Store at 15°–30° C (59°–86° F) in tight, light-resistant containers.

ADVERSE EFFECTS (≥1%) **CNS:** Headache, peripheral neuritis, peripheral neuropathy, tinnitus, hearing loss, vertigo, insomnia, drowsiness, mental depression, acute psychosis, ataxia, convulsions, kernicterus (newborns). **GI:** *Nausea, vomiting, diarrhea,* abdominal pains, hepatitis, jaundice, pancreatitis, stomatitis. **Hematologic:** Acute hemolytic anemia (especially in patients with G6PD deficiency), aplastic anemia, methemoglobinemia, agranulocytosis, thrombocytopenia, leukopenia, eosinophilia, hypoprothrombinemia. **Body as a Whole:** Headache, *fever,* chills, arthralgia, malaise, allergic myocarditis, serum sickness, anaphylactoid reactions, lymphadenopathy, local reaction following IM injection, fixed drug eruptions, diuresis, overgrowth of nonsusceptible organisms, LE phenomenon. **Skin:** Pruritus, urticaria, rash, erythema multiforme including *Stevens-Johnson syndrome exfoliative, dermatitis,* alopecia, photosensitivity, vascular lesions. **Urogenital:** *Crystalluria,* hematuria, proteinuria, anuria, toxic nephrosis, reduction in sperm count. **Metabolic:** Goiter, hypoglycemia. **Special Senses:** Conjunctivitis, conjunctival or scleral infection, retardation of corneal healing (ophthalmic ointment).

DIAGNOSTIC TEST INTERFERENCE Sulfonamides may interfere with ***BSP*** retention and ***PSP*** excretion tests and may affect results of ***thyroid function*** tests (***I-131*** may be decreased for about 7 days). Large doses of sulfonamides reportedly may produce false-positive ***urine glucose*** determinations with ***copper reduction methods*** (e.g., ***Benedict's*** and ***Clinitest***). SULFONAMIDES may produce false-positive results for ***urinary protein*** (with ***sulfosalicylic acid test***) and may interfere with ***urine urobilinogen*** determinations using ***Ehrlich's reagent*** or ***Urobilistix.*** Follow-up cultures are unreliable unless PABA is added to culture medium.

INTERACTIONS Drug: PABA-CONTAINING LOCAL ANESTHETICS may antagonize sulfa's effects; ORAL ANTICOAGULANTS potentiate hypoprothrombinemia; may potentiate SULFONYLUREA-induced hypoglycemia; may decrease concentrations of **cyclosporine;** may increase levels of **phenytoin.**

PHARMACOKINETICS Absorption: Readily from GI tract. **Peak:** 2–4 h. **Distribution:** Distributed in extracellular space; crosses blood–brain barrier and placenta; detected in breast milk. **Metabolism:** In liver. **Elimination:** 95% in urine in 24 h. **Half-Life:** 4.6–7.8 h.

NURSING IMPLICATIONS

Assessment & Drug Effects

- Lab tests: C&S prior to initiation of therapy; frequent kidney function tests and urinalyses; frequent CBC and LFTs, especially during regimens longer than 2 wk. Monitor sulfisoxazole blood levels, especially with high-dose therapy

S

(max levels should not exceed 200 mcg/mL).

- Monitor I&O. Report oliguria and changes in I&O ratio. Fluid intake should be adequate to support urinary output of at least 1500 mL/day to prevent crystalluria and stone formation.
- Report early manifestations of blood dyscrasias or hypersensitivity reactions immediately (fever with sore throat, malaise, unusual fatigue, joint pains, pallor, bleeding tendencies, rash, jaundice).
- Be alert for skin lesions, papular or vesiculobullous lesions, especially on sun-exposed areas, Stevens-Johnson syndrome (severe erythema multiforme) may be preceded by high fever, severe headache, stomatitis, conjunctivitis, rhinitis, urticaria, balanitis (inflammation of penis or clitoris). Termination of drug therapy is indicated.
- Observe diabetic patients receiving oral hypoglycemic agents closely for hypoglycemic reactions. Obtain blood glucose and HbA1C levels before and shortly after initiation of therapy.

Patient & Family Education

- Do not take OTC medications without consulting physician.
- Use or add barrier contraceptives if using hormonal contraceptives, which may be unreliable while taking this drug.
- Avoid exposure to ultraviolet light and excessive sunlight to prevent photosensitivity reaction during therapy and for several months after treatment is discontinued.
- Inform dentist or new physician that you are taking a sulfonamide.

SULINDAC

(sul-in′dak)

Clinoril

Classifications: ANALGESIC, NONSTEROIDAL ANTI-INFLAMMATORY DRUG (NSAID); ANTIPYRETIC

Therapeutic: NONNARCOTIC ANALGESIC, NSAID

Prototype: Ibuprofen

Pregnancy Category: C; D third trimester

AVAILABILITY 150 mg, 200 mg tablets

ACTION & *THERAPEUTIC EFFECT*
Anti-inflammatory action thought to result from inhibition of prostaglandin synthesis. *Exhibits anti-inflammatory, analgesic, and antipyretic properties.*

USES Acute and long-term symptomatic treatment of osteoarthritis, rheumatoid arthritis, ankylosing spondylitis; acute painful shoulder (acute subacromial bursitis or supraspinatus tendinitis); acute gouty arthritis.

CONTRAINDICATIONS Hypersensitivity to sulindac; hypersensitivity to aspirin (patients with "aspirin triad": Acute asthma, rhinitis, nasal polyps), other NSAIDs, or salicylates; significant kidney or liver dysfunction; CABG perioperative pain; pregnancy (category D third trimester), lactation. Safety in children is not established.

CAUTIOUS USE History of upper GI tract disorders; anticoagulant therapy; CHF; moderate or mild renal impairment; compromised cardiac function, hypertension, hemophilia or other bleeding tendencies; pregnancy (category C first and second trimesters).

S

ROUTE & DOSAGE

Arthritis, Ankylosing Spondylitis, Acute Gouty Arthritis

Adult: **PO** 150–200 mg b.i.d. (max: 400 mg/day)

ADMINISTRATION

Oral

- Crush and give mixed with liquid or food if patient cannot swallow tablet.
- Administer with food, milk, or antacid (if prescribed) to reduce possibility of GI upset. Note: Food retards absorption and delays and lowers peak concentrations.

ADVERSE EFFECTS (≥1%) **CNS:** Drowsiness, *dizziness, headache,* anxiety, nervousness. **CV:** Palpitation, peripheral edema, CHF, (patients with marginal cardiac function). **Special Senses:** Blurred vision, amblyopia, vertigo, tinnitus, decreased hearing. **GI:** *Abdominal pain, dyspepsia, nausea, vomiting, constipation,* diarrhea, ulceration, flatulence, anorexia; stomatitis, sore or dry mucous membranes, dry mouth; GI bleeding, gastritis. **Hematologic:** Prolonged bleeding time, aplastic anemia, thrombocytopenia, leukopenia, eosinophilia. **Body as a Whole:** Angioneurotic edema, fever, chills, anaphylaxis. **Skin:** Stevens-Johnson syndrome, toxic epidermal necrolysis syndrome, rash, pruritus. **Urogenital:** Renal impairment.

DIAGNOSTIC TEST INTERFERENCE Abnormalities in ***liver function tests*** may occur.

INTERACTIONS Drug: Heparin, ORAL ANTICOAGULANTS may prolong bleeding time; may increase **lithium** toxicity; **aspirin,** other NSAIDS add to ulcerogenic effects; may increase **methotrexate** toxicity; **dimethylsulfoxide (DMSO)** may decrease effects of sulindac. **Herbal: Feverfew, garlic, ginger, ginkgo** may increase bleeding potential.

PHARMACOKINETICS Absorption: 90% from GI tract. **Peak:** 2 h without food, 3–4 h with food. **Duration:** 10–12 h. **Distribution:** Minimal passage across placenta; distributed into breast milk. **Metabolism:** In liver to active sulfide metabolite. **Elimination:** 75% in urine, 25% in feces. **Half-Life:** 7.8 h sulindac, 16.4 h sulfide metabolite.

NURSING IMPLICATIONS

Assessment & Drug Effects

- Assess for and report promptly unexplained GI distress.
- Lab tests: Obtain baseline and periodic evaluations of Hgb, kidney and liver function.
- Schedule auditory and ophthalmic examinations in patients receiving prolonged or high-dose therapy.

Patient & Family Education

- Do not drive or engage in potentially hazardous activities until response to drug is known.
- Report any incidence of unexplained bleeding or bruising immediately to physician (e.g., bleeding gums, black and tarry stools, coffee-colored emesis).
- Report onset of skin rash, itching, hives, jaundice, swelling of feet or hands, sore throat or mouth, shortness of breath, or night cough to physician.
- Be aware that adverse GI effects are relatively common. Report abdominal pain, nausea, dyspepsia, diarrhea, or constipation.
- Avoid alcohol and aspirin as they may increase risk of GI ulceration and bleeding tendencies.

S

- Inform dentist or surgeon of drug regimen because bleeding time may be prolonged.

SUMATRIPTAN

(sum-a-trip′tan)
Imitrex
Classification: SEROTONIN 5-HT_1 RECEPTOR AGONIST
Therapeutic: ANTIMIGRAINE
Pregnancy Category: C

AVAILABILITY 25 mg, 50 mg tablets; 12 mg/mL injection; 5 mg, 20 mg nasal spray

ACTION & *THERAPEUTIC EFFECT* Selective agonist for a serotonin receptor (probably 5-HT_{1D}) that causes vasoconstriction of cranial carotid arteries. *Relieves migraine headache. Also relieves photophobia, phonophobia, nausea and vomiting associated with migraine attacks.*

USES Treatment of acute migraine attacks with or without aura, cluster headache.

CONTRAINDICATIONS Hypersensitivity to sumatriptan; IV use; coronary artery disease (CAD); acute MI, angina, arteriosclerosis; cerebrovascular disease; colitis; older adults; concurrent use with MAO inhibitors; uncontrolled hypertension; intracranial bleeding; PVD; Raynaud's disease; stroke; severe hepatic disease; Wolff-Parkinson-White syndrome; basilar or hemiplegic migraine.
CAUTIOUS USE Impaired liver or kidney function; pregnancy (category C); MAO inhibitors. Safety and effectiveness in children are not established.

ROUTE & DOSAGE

Migraine or Cluster Headache
Adult: **Subcutaneous** 6 mg any time after onset of migraine. If headache returns, may repeat with 6 mg subcutaneously at least 1 h after first injection (max: 12 mg/24 h). **PO** 25 mg × 1 dose, if headache returns may repeat once after 2 h (max: 100 mg). **Intranasal** 5, 10, or 20 mg in one nostril. If headache returns, may repeat once after 2 h (max: 40 mg/24 h).

ADMINISTRATION

Note: Do not give within 24 h of an ergot-containing drug.

Oral
- Give any time after symptoms of migraine appear.
- A second tablet may be given if symptoms return but no sooner than 2 h after the first tablet.
- Do not exceed 100 mg in a single oral dose or 300 mg/day.

Intranasal
- Note: A single dose is one spray into ONE nostril.

Subcutaneous
- A second injection may be given 1 h or longer following first injection if initial relief is not obtained or if migraine returns.
- Be aware that if adverse effects are dose limiting, a lower dose may be effective.
- Store all forms at room temperature, 15°–30° C (59°–86° F). Protect from light.

ADVERSE EFFECTS (≥1%) **CV:** Chest pressure and tightness, hypotension or hypertension, hypertensive crisis, syncope, peripheral cyanosis, thromboembolism, heart

S

block, sinus bradycardia, atrial fibrillation, ventricular fibrillation, ventricular tachycardia, coronary artery vasospasm, angina, transient myocardial ischemia, MI, cardiac arrest. **CNS:** *Tingling, warming sensation, pressure, numbness,* headache, *dizziness, vertigo,* drowsiness, sedation, seizure, CNS hemorrhage, subarachnoid hemorrhage, stroke. **Body as a Whole:** Dizziness, lightheadedness, myalgia, or muscle cramps, *pain on injection,* weakness, flushing and a sensation of warmth or burning after injection. **GI:** Abdominal pain, cramping, diarrhea, nausea, vomiting.

INTERACTIONS Drug: Dihydroergotamine, ERGOT ALKALOIDS may cause vasospasm and a slight elevation in blood pressure. MAO INHIBITORS increase sumatriptan levels and toxicity (especially the oral form); do not use concurrently or within 2 wk of stopping MAO INHIBITORS; use with other serotonin altering drugs increases risk of serotonin syndrome (see Appendix F). **Herbal: St. John's wort** may increase triptan toxicity.

PHARMACOKINETICS Onset: 10–30 min after subcutaneous administration. **Duration:** 1–2 h. **Distribution:** Widely distributed, 10–20% protein bound. May be excreted in breast milk. **Metabolism:** Hepatically to inactive metabolite. **Elimination:** 57% in urine, 38% in feces. **Half-Life:** 2 h.

S

NURSING IMPLICATIONS

Assessment & Drug Effects

- Monitor cardiovascular status carefully following first dose in patients at relatively high risk for coronary artery disease (e.g., postmenopausal women, men over 40 years old, persons with known CAD risk factors) or who have coronary artery vasospasms.
- Report to physician immediately chest pain or tightness in chest or throat that is severe or does not quickly resolve following a dose of sumatriptan.
- Monitor therapeutic effectiveness. Pain relief usually begins within 10 min of injection, with complete relief in approximately 65% of all patients within 2 h.

Patient & Family Education

- Review patient information leaflet provided by the manufacturer carefully.
- Learn correct use of autoinjector for self-administration of subcutaneous dose.
- Pain or redness at injection site is common but usually disappears in less than 1 h.
- Notify physician immediately if symptoms of severe angina (e.g., severe or persistent pain or tightness in chest, back, neck, or throat) or hypersensitivity (e.g., wheezing, facial swelling, skin rash, or hives) occur.
- Do not take any other serotonin receptor agonist (Axert, Maxalt, Zomig, Amerge) within 24 h of taking sumatriptan.
- Check with physician before taking any new OTC or prescription drugs.
- Report any other adverse effects (e.g., tingling, flushing, dizziness) at next physician visit.

SUNITINIB

(sun-i-ti′nib)

Sutent

Classifications: ANTINEOPLASTIC; PROTEIN-TYROSINE KINASE INHIBITOR

Therapeutic: ANTINEOPLASTIC
Prototype: Gefitinib
Pregnancy Category: D

AVAILABILITY 12.5 mg, 25 mg, 50 mg capsules

ACTION & *THERAPEUTIC EFFECT* An antineoplastic agent that is a selective inhibitor of receptor tyrosine kinases (RTKs) in solid tumors. Carcinogenic activity within these tumors is a result of tumor angiogenesis and proliferation. *Sunitinib causes tumor regression and decreased tumor growth.*

USES Treatment of advanced renal cell cancer; treatment of gastrointestinal stromal tumors (GIST) after disease progression on or intolerance to imatinib.

CONTRAINDICATIONS Hypersensitivity to sunitinib; uncontrolled hypertension, acute MI; fever, abnormal bleeding, sore throat; children, pregnancy (category D), lactation.
CAUTIOUS USE Cardiac disease, CHF, history of hypertension, history of MI; CVA; females of childbearing age.

ROUTE & DOSAGE

Advanced Renal Cell Cancer

Adult: **PO** 50 mg/day for 4 wk, followed by 2 wk off treatment; repeat 6-wk cycle as needed.

Dosage Adjustments with Concurrent Hepatic CYP3A4 Modifiers

CYP3A4 Inducers: Increase to maximum of 87.5 mg/day
CYP3A4 Inhibitors: Decrease to minimum of 37.5 mg/day

ADMINISTRATION

Oral

- Incremental dosage changes of 12.5 mg are recommended.
- Store at 15°–30° C (59°–86° F).

ADVERSE EFFECTS (≥1%) **Body as a Whole:** *Alopecia, asthenia, dizziness, fatigue, fever,* hair color change, *headache, peripheral edema.* **CV:** *Hypertension,* myocardial ischemia. **GI:** *Abdominal pain, altered taste, anorexia, constipation, diarrhea, dyspepsia, flatulence, glossodynia, nausea, mucositis, stomatitis, vomiting.* **Hematologic:** *Anemia, bleeding, neutropenia, lymphopenia, thrombocytopenia.* **Metabolic:** *Dehydration, elevated hepatic enzymes (AST/ALT, alkaline phosphatase, pancreatic enzymes, amylasemia, lipasemia),* hypothyroidism, *hyperbilirubinemia.* **Musculoskeletal:** *Arthralgia, back pain, myalgia/limb pain.* **Respiratory:** *Cough, dyspnea.* **Skin:** *Dry skin, hand-foot syndrome, rash, skin discoloration.*

INTERACTIONS Drug: Coadministration of CYP3A4 INDUCERS (e.g., **carbamazepine, dexamethasone, phenobarbital, phenytoin, rifabutin, rifampin, rifapentine**) may decrease plasma levels of sunitinib. Coadministration of CYP3A4 INHIBITORS (e.g., **atazanavir, clarithromycin, erythromycin, indinavir, itraconazole, ketoconazole, nefazodone, nelfinavir, ritonavir, saquinavir, telithromycin, voriconazole**) may increase plasma levels of sunitinib. **Food: Grapefruit** and **grapefruit juice** may increase the plasma levels of sunitinib. **Herbal: St. John's wort** may decrease the plasma levels of sunitinib.

PHARMACOKINETICS Peak: 6–12 h. **Distribution:** 95–98% protein bound. **Metabolism:** Extensive hepatic metabolism. **Elimination:** Primarily fecal elimination (61%) with minor renal elimination. **Half-Life:** 40–60 h.

S

NURSING IMPLICATIONS

Assessment & Drug Effects

- Monitor for and report S&S of bleeding (e.g., GI, GU, gingival, etc.).
- Monitor BP regularly and assess regularly for S&S of congestive heart failure. Withhold drug and notify physician if severe hypertension or signs of heart failure develop.
- Lab tests: At the beginning of each treatment cycle, CBC with differential and platelet count; periodic serum electrolytes; thyroid function tests with symptoms suggestive of hypothyroidism.

Patient & Family Education

- Do not use any prescription or nonprescription drugs without consulting a physician.
- Skin discoloration (yellow color) and/or loss of skin and hair pigmentation may occur with this drug.
- Report any of the following to a health care provider: Painful redness of palms and soles of feet; severe abdominal pain, vomiting, and diarrhea; signs of bleeding; chest pain or discomfort; shortness of breath; swelling of feet, legs, or hands; rapid weight gain.
- Women of childbearing age are advised not to become pregnant while taking sunitinib.

TACRINE

(tac'rine)

Cognex

Classifications: CHOLINESTERASE INHIBITOR; ANTIDEMENTIA

Therapeutic: ALZHEIMER'S

Pregnancy Category: C

AVAILABILITY 10 mg, 20 mg, 30 mg, 40 mg capsules

ACTION & *THERAPEUTIC EFFECT* Cholinesterase inhibitor that elevates acetylcholine in the cerebral cortex by slowing degradation of acetylcholine release by the remaining intact neurons. Balances pathologic changes in neurons that result in deficiency of acetylcholine in early stages of Alzheimer's disease. *Slows manifestations of Alzheimer's disease.*

USES Improvement of memory in mild to moderate Alzheimer's dementia.

UNLABELED USES HIV infection (severe dementia), tardive dyskinesia, acute anticholinergic syndrome with possible advantage over physostigmine.

CONTRAINDICATIONS Hypersensitivity to tacrine; patients who develop jaundice while taking tacrine.

CAUTIOUS USE Anesthesia, sick sinus rhythm, bradycardia; history of ulcers, GI bleeding, abnormal liver function; patients with asthma, hypotension, COPD, hyperthyroidism, seizure disorders; urinary tract obstruction, intestinal obstruction; pregnancy (category C), lactation. Safety and efficacy in children are not established.

ROUTE & DOSAGE

Alzheimer's Disease

Adult: **PO** 10 mg q.i.d. (taken between meals if tolerated), increase in 40 mg/day increments not sooner than q6wk (max: 160 mg/day)

Hepatic Impairment Dosage Adjustment

Dose-related hepatotoxic effects have been observed; use with caution or not at all in patients with history of past or current liver disease

ADMINISTRATION

Oral

- Give at least 1 h before meals; bioavailability reduced 30–40% when taken with food. Effectiveness depends on administration at regular intervals.
- Withhold drug and notify physician if ALT exceeds 3 × ULN. Note: Drug usually discontinued if ALT exceeds 5 × ULN.
- Store at room temperature, 15°–30° C (59°–86° F), away from moisture.

ADVERSE EFFECTS (≥1%) **CNS:** Agitation, dizziness and confusion, ataxia, insomnia, somnolence, hallucinations. **GI:** Nausea, *vomiting,* belching, *diarrhea,* abdominal discomfort, anorexia, *hepatotoxicity.* **Skin:** Purpura. **Urogenital:** Excessive micturition and incontinence with UTI infections. **Body as a Whole:** Diaphoresis.

INTERACTIONS Drug: Prolongs action of **succinylcholine** and possibly other NEUROMUSCULAR BLOCKING AGENTS due to inhibition of plasma pseudocholinesterase. Increases **theophylline** concentrations two-fold. **Cimetidine** increases concentration of tacrine by 64%. **Herbal: Echinacea** may increase risk of hepatotoxicity.

PHARMACOKINETICS Absorption: Approximately 17% absorbed from GI tract. Food decreases rate and extent of absorption by 30–40%. **Onset:** 30–90 min. **Peak:** 2 h. Steady state in 24–36 h. **Distribution:** Penetrates blood–brain barrier. Protein binding is 55%. **Metabolism:** Metabolized in the liver by cytochrome P450 system. At least three hydroxylated metabolites have been identified that may be biologically active. Females have lower activity in cytochrome P450 isoenzymes so plasma levels are approximately 50% higher than men with same dose. **Elimination:** Less than 3% of dose recovered in urine in 24 h. **Half-Life:** 3.5 h.

NURSING IMPLICATIONS

Assessment & Drug Effects

- Monitor for clinical improvement (defined as a 4-point improvement in Alzheimer's Disease Assessment Scale/Cognitive Subscale). Improvement has been observed after 1–4 wk; may take 6 mo for maximum benefit.
- Lab tests: Monitor serum transaminase (ALT) levels according to following schedule: Every 2 wk for first 16 wk, then monthly for 2 mo, then every 3 mo thereafter; resume weekly monitoring for 6 wk with each dose increase; continue weekly monitoring if ALT remains more than 2 times normal; if therapy is interrupted more than 4 wk then restarted, resume full ALT monitoring schedule.
- Monitor I&O because tacrine may cause bladder outflow obstruction.
- Monitor for seizure activity and take appropriate precautions.
- Monitor patients with history of angle-closure glaucoma for a worsening of this condition.
- Monitor for GI distress and bleeding, especially in patients with a history of peptic ulcer disease or on concurrent NSAID therapy.
- Supervise ambulation because dizziness occurs in more than 10% of patients.
- Monitor cardiovascular status including periodic ECG monitor-

ing. Assess for fluid retention and worsening of CHF.
- Monitor periodically for development of drug-induced diabetes.

Patient & Family Education
- Be aware of adverse effects related to initiation of therapy or dosage increases (e.g., nausea, vomiting, diarrhea) as well as delayed effects (e.g., rash, GI bleeding, jaundice). Report adverse effects to the physician.
- Do not discontinue or reduce dosage of 80 mg/day or more abruptly because it may precipitate acute deterioration of cognitive function.
- Make sure to have regular follow-up and liver function tests.
- Tacrine may induce seizures, vertigo, and syncope. Use appropriate precautions.
- Understand that tacrine therapy is not a cure and will become ineffective at some point as the disease progresses.

TACROLIMUS
(tac-rol'i-mus)
Prograf, Protopic
Classifications: BIOLOGICAL RESPONSE MODIFIER; IMMUNOSUPPRESSANT
Therapeutic: IMMUNOSUPPRESSANT
Prototype: Cyclosporine
Pregnancy Category: C

AVAILABILITY 0.5 mg, 1 mg, 5 mg capsules; 5 mg/mL injection; 0.1%, 0.03% ointment

ACTION & *THERAPEUTIC EFFECT* Inhibits helper T-lymphocytes by selectively inhibiting secretion of interleukin-2, interleukin-3, and interleukin-gamma, thus reducing transplant rejection. *Inhibits antibody production (thus subduing immune response) by creating an imbalance in favor of suppressor T-lymphocytes.*

USES Prophylaxis for organ transplant rejection, moderate to severe atopic dermatitis (e.g., eczema).
UNLABELED USES Acute organ transplant rejection, severe plaque-type psoriasis, ulcerative colitis, nephrotic syndrome.

CONTRAINDICATIONS Hypersensitivity to tacrolimus or castor oil; postoperative oliguria or renal failure with CrCl greater than or equal to 4 mg/dL; potassium sparing diretics; lactation, infants, neonates; **tacrolimus ointment:** children younger than 2 y.
CAUTIOUS USE Renal or hepatic insufficiency, hyperkalemia, QT prolongation; CHF; diabetes mellitus, gout, history of seizures, hypertension; cardiomyopathy, left ventricular dysfunction (e.g., heart failure); neoplastic disease, especially lymphoproliferative disorders; pregnancy (category C).

ROUTE & DOSAGE

Rejection Prophylaxis (Dose Varies Based on Organ)
Adult: **PO** 0.075–0.2 mg/kg/day in divided doses q12h, start no sooner than 6 h after transplant; give first oral dose 8–12 h after discontinuing IV therapy **IV** 0.01–0.05 mg/kg/day as continuous IV infusion, start no sooner than 6 h after transplant, continue until patient can take oral therapy
Child: **PO** 0.15–0.2 mg/kg/day **IV** 0.03–0.05 mg/kg/day

Atopic Dermatitis
Adult: **Topical** Apply thin layer to affected area b.i.d., continue until clearing of symptoms

Child (2–15 y): **Topical** Apply thin layer of 0.03% ointment to affected area b.i.d., continue until clearing of symptoms

Renal Impairment Dosage Adjustment

Start with lower dose

Hemodialysis Dosage Adjustment: Supplementation not necessary

ADMINISTRATION

Oral

- Patient should be converted from IV to oral therapy as soon as possible.
- Give first oral dose 8–12 h after discontinuing IV infusion.

Topical

- Ensure that skin is clean and completely dry before application.
- Apply a thin layer to the affected area and rub in gently and completely.
- Do not apply occlusive dressing over the site.

Intravenous

PREPARE: **IV Infusion:** Dilute 5 mg/mL ampules with NS or D5W to a concentration of 0.004–0.02 mg/mL (4–20 mcg/mL). ▪ Lower concentrations are preferred for children.

ADMINISTER: **IV Infusion:** Give as continuous IV. ▪ PVC-free tubing is recommended, especially at lower concentrations.

INCOMPATIBILITIES **Y-site:** **Acyclovir, allopurinol, azathioprine, cefoperazone, dantrolene, diazepam, diazoxide, esomeprazole, ganciclovir, lansoprazole, levothyroxine, omeprazole, phenytoin, thiopental.**

- Store ampules between 5° and 25° C (41° and 77° F); store capsules at room temperature, 15°–30° C (59°–86° F). ▪ Store the diluted infusion in glass or polyethylene containers and discard after 24 h.

ADVERSE EFFECTS (≥1%) **CNS:** *Headache, tremors, insomnia, paresthesia, hyperesthesia* and/or sensations of warmth, circumoral numbness. **CV:** *Mild to moderate hypertension.* **Endocrine:** Hirsutism, *hyperglycemia, hyperkalemia, hypokalemia, hypomagnesemia,* hyperuricemia, decreased serum cholesterol. **GI:** *Nausea, abdominal pain, gas,* appetite changes, *vomiting, anorexia, constipation,* diarrhea, ascites. **Hematologic:** *Anemia, leukocytosis, thrombocytopenia purpura.* **Urogenital:** UTI, oliguria, nephrotoxicity, nephropathy. **Respiratory:** *Pleural effusion, atelectasis, dyspnea.* **Special Senses:** Blurred vision, photophobia. **Skin:** *Flushing, rash, pruritus, skin irritation,* alopecia, erythema, folliculitis, hyperesthesia, <u>exfoliative dermatitis</u>, hirsutism, photosensitivity, skin discoloration, skin ulcer, sweating. **Body as a Whole:** *Pain, fever, peripheral edema, increased risk of cancer.*

INTERACTIONS Drug: Use with **cyclosporine** increases risk of nephrotoxicity. **Metoclopramide, lansoprazole,** CALCIUM CHANNEL BLOCKER, ANTIFUNGAL AGENTS, MACROLIDE ANTIBIOTICS, **bromocriptine, cimetidine, cyclosporine, methylprednisolone, omeprazole** may increase levels; **caspofungin, rifampin** may decrease levels. NSAIDS may lead to oliguria or anuria. **Herbal: St. John's wort** decreases efficacy. **Food: Grapefruit juice** (greater than 1 qt/day) may increase plasma concentrations and adverse effects.

PHARMACOKINETICS Absorption: Erratic and incompletely from GI tract; absolute bioavailability approximately 14–25%; absorption reduced by food. **Peak:** PO 1–4 h. **Duration:** IV 12 h. **Distribution:** Within plasma, tacrolimus is found primarily in lipoprotein-deficient fraction; 75–97% protein bound; distributed into red blood cells; blood:plasma ratio reported greater than 4; animal studies have demonstrated high concentrations of tacrolimus in lung, kidney, heart, and spleen; distributed into breast milk. **Metabolism:** Extensively in liver (CYP3A4). **Elimination:** Metabolites primarily in bile. **Half-Life:** 8.7–11.3 h.

NURSING IMPLICATIONS

Assessment & Drug Effects

- Lab tests: Monitor serum tacrolimus, serum electrolytes, blood glucose, LFTs, uric acid, BUN, and creatinine clearance periodically.
- Monitor kidney function closely; report elevated serum creatinine or decreased urinary output.
- Monitor for neurotoxicity, and report tremors, changes in mental status, or other signs of toxicity.
- Monitor cardiovascular status and report hypertension.

Patient & Family Education

- Report promptly unexplained hunger, thirst, and frequent urination.
- Be aware of potential adverse effects.
- Minimize exposure to natural or artificial sunlight while using the ointment.
- Notify physician of S&S of neurotoxicity.

TADALAFIL

(ta-dal′a-fil)
Cialis

Classifications: IMPOTENCE; PHOSPHODIESTERASE (PDE) INHIBITOR; VASODILATOR
Therapeutic: IMPOTENCE; PULMONARY ANTIHYPERTENSIVE
Prototype: Sildenafil
Pregnancy Category: B

AVAILABILITY 2.5 mg, 5 mg, 10 mg, 20 mg tablets

ACTION & *THERAPEUTIC EFFECT* Tadalafil is a selective phosphodiesterase (PDE) inhibitor. PDE is responsible for degradation of cyclic GMP in the corpus cavernosum of the penis. Cyclic GMP causes smooth muscle relaxation in lung tissue and the corpus cavernosum, thereby allowing inflow of blood into the penis. PDE-5 inhibitors reduce pulmonary vasodilation by sustaining levels of cyclic guanosine monophosphate (cGMP). *Additionally, tadalafil produces a reduction in the pulmonary to systemic vascular resistance ratio. Tadalafil promotes sustained erection only in the presence of sexual stimulation. Tadalafil produces a significant improvement in arterial oxygenation in pulmonary hypertension.*

USES Treatment of erectile dysfunction, pulmonary hypertension.

CONTRAINDICATIONS Hypersensitivity to tadalafil, vardenafil, or sildenafil; MI within last 90 days; Class 2 or greater heart failure within last 6 mo; unstable angina or angina during intercourse; uncontrolled cardiac arrhythmias; nitrate/nitrite therapy; hypotension, uncontrolled hypertension; retinitis pigmentosa; CVA within last 6 mo; left ventricular outflow obstruction, aortic stenosis; severe (Child-Pugh class C) hepatic failure; not recommended for women, lactation, or children younger than 18 y.

CAUTIOUS USE CAD, risk factors for CVA; renal insufficiency; mild to moderate (Child-Pugh class A or B) hepatic impairment, hepatic disease; anatomic deformity of the penis; sickle cell anemia; multiple myeloma; leukemia; active bleeding or a peptic ulcer; hiatal hernia, GERD; sickle cell disease; retinitis pigmentosa; hepatitis, cirrhosis; severe renal impairment; older adults; concurrent use with other medicines for penile dysfunction; pregnancy (category B).

ROUTE & DOSAGE

Erectile Dysfunction

Adult: **PO** 2.5 mg daily *OR* 10 mg prior to anticipated sexual activity. May increase to max dose 20 mg/day or reduce to 5 mg/day if needed. If taking ritonavir, itraconazole, ketoconazole, or voriconazole, max dose 10 mg q72h.

Pulmonary Hypertension

Adult: **PO** 40 mg

Hepatic Impairment Dosage Adjustment

Mild to moderate impairment (Child-Pugh class A and B): Max 10 mg/day; not recommended with severe hepatic impairment

Renal Impairment Dosage Adjustment

CrCl 30–50 mL/min: Start at 5 mg once daily (max: 10 mg q48h); less than 30 mL/min: Max dose 5 mg and once daily dosing is not recommended

Hemodialysis Dosage Adjustment: Once daily dosing is not recommended

ADMINISTRATION

Oral

- If not on the daily dose regimen, tadalafil is taken approximately 1 h before expected intercourse, but preferably not after a heavy or high-fat meal.
- Store at 15°–30° C (59°–86° F).

ADVERSE EFFECTS (≥1%) **Body as a Whole:** Flushing, back pain, asthenia, facial edema, fatigue, pain, transient global amnesia. **CNS:** *Headache,* dizziness, insomnia, somnolence, vertigo, hypesthesia, paresthesia. **CV:** Angina, chest pain, hypertension, hypotension, MI, orthostatic hypotension, palpitations, syncope, sinus tachycardia. **GI:** Dyspepsia, nausea, vomiting, abdominal pain, abnormal liver function tests, diarrhea, loose stools, dysphagia, esophagitis, gastritis, GERD, xerostomia. **Metabolic:** Increased GGTP. **Musculoskeletal:** Arthralgia, myalgia, neck pain. **Respiratory:** Nasal congestion, dyspnea, epistaxis, pharyngitis. **Skin:** Rash, pruritus, sweating. **Special Senses:** Blurred vision, changes in color vision, conjunctivitis, eye pain, lacrimation, swelling of eyelids, sudden vision loss. **Urogenital:** Spontaneous penile erection.

INTERACTIONS Drug: May potentiate hypotensive effects of ETHANOL, NITRATES, **alfuzosin, doxazosin, prazosin, tamsulosin** (doses greater than 0.4 mg/day), **terazosin; erythromycin** (and other MACROLIDES), **indinavir, itraconazole, ketoconazole,** PROTEASE INHIBITORS, **ritonavir, saquinavir, voriconazole** may increase levels and toxicity of tadalafil; **barbiturates, bosentan, carbamazepine, dexamethasone, fosphenytoin, nevirapine, rifampin phenytoin, rifabutin, troglitazone** may reduce level and effectiveness of tadalafil. **Food: Grapefruit juice** may increase levels and toxicity of tadalafil.

PHARMACOKINETICS Absorption: Rapidly absorbed, 15% reaches systemic circulation. **Onset:** 30–45 min. **Peak:** 2 h. **Duration:** Up to 36 h. **Metabolism:** In liver by CYP3A4. **Elimination:** In feces (61%) and urine (39%). **Half-Life:** 17.5 h.

NURSING IMPLICATIONS

Assessment & Drug Effects

- Monitor CV status and report angina or other S&S of cardiac dysfunction.
- Lab tests: Baseline and periodic LFTs.

Patient & Family Education

- Do not take more than once per day.
- Note: With moderate renal insufficiency, the maximum recommended dose is 10 mg not more than once in every 48 h.
- Moderate use of alcohol when taking this drug.
- Do not take this drug without consulting physician if you are taking drugs called "alpha-blockers" or "nitrates" or any other drugs for high blood pressure, chest pain, or enlarged prostate.
- Report promptly any of the following: Palpitations, chest pain, back pain, difficulty breathing, or shortness of breath; dizziness or fainting; changes in vision; swollen eyelids; muscle aches; painful or prolonged erection (lasting longer than 4 h); skin rash, or itching.

T

TAMOXIFEN CITRATE Pr

(ta-mox′i-fen)

Nolvadex, Nolvadex-D ♣, Tamofen ♣

Classifications: ANTINEOPLASTIC; SELECTIVE ESTROGEN RECEPTOR MODIFIER (SERM)

Therapeutic: ANTINEOPLASTIC; ANTI-ESTROGEN

Pregnancy Category: D

AVAILABILITY 10 mg, 20 mg tablets

ACTION & *THERAPEUTIC EFFECT* Nonsteroidal gonad-stimulating drug with potent antiestrogenic as well as estrogenic activity on various tissues. Competes with estradiol at estrogen receptor (ER-positive) sites in target tissues such as breast, uterus, vagina, anterior pituitary. Estrogen is thought to increase breast cancer in ER-positive tumors. Tamoxifen has no effect on the development of ER-negative breast cancer disease. *Has effects on tumor with high concentration of estrogen receptors. Tamoxifen-receptor complexes move into the cell nucleus, decreasing DNA synthesis and estrogen responses.*

USES Palliative treatment of advanced with metastatic estrogen receptors (ER)-positive breast cancer in postmenopausal women, adjunctively with surgery in the treatment of breast carcinoma with positive lymph nodes.

UNLABELED USES Investigationally to stimulate ovulation in selected anovulatory women desiring pregnancy.

CONTRAINDICATIONS Anticoagulant therapy including coumadin; preexisting endometrial hyperplasia; intramuscular injections if platelets less than 50,000/mm^3; history of thromboembolic disease; pregnancy (category D), especially during first trimester, lactation; children.

CAUTIOUS USE Vision disturbances; cataracts, visual disturbance; leukopenia, bone marrow suppression; thrombocytopenia; hypercalcemia; hypercholesterolemia, lipid protein abnormalities; women with ductal cardinoma in situ (DCIS).

ROUTE & DOSAGE

Breast Carcinoma

Adult: **PO** 10–20 mg 1–2 times/day (morning and evening)

Stimulation of Ovulation

Adult: **PO** 5–40 mg b.i.d. for 4 days

ADMINISTRATION

Oral

- Doses greater than 20 mg/day should be given in divided doses a.m. and p.m.
- Store at 20°–25° C (68°–77° F); protect from light. Oral solution should be used within 3 mo of opening.

ADVERSE EFFECTS (≥1%) **Body as a Whole:** Increased bone pain, and transient local disease flair; loss of hair, weight gain, shortness of breath, photosensitivity, *hot flashes.* **CNS:** Depression, lightheadedness, dizziness, headache, mental confusion, sleepiness. **CV:** Thrombosis, pulmonary embolism, increased risk of stroke. **GI:** *Nausea and vomiting (about 25% of patients),* distaste for food, anorexia. **Hematologic:** Leukopenia, thrombocytopenia. **Metabolic:** Hypercalcemia. **Skin:** Skin rash or dryness. **Special Senses:** Retinopathy, decreased visual acuity, blurred vision. **Urogenital:** Changes in menstrual period, milk production and leaking from breasts, vaginal discharge and bleeding, pruritus vulvae, risk of uterine malignancies.

DIAGNOSTIC TEST INTERFERENCE Tamoxifen may produce transient increase in ***serum calcium.***

INTERACTIONS Drug: May enhance hypoprothrombinemic effects of **warfarin;** may increase risk of thromboembolic events with CYTOTOXIC AGENTS; **bromocriptine** may elevate tamoxifen levels, SSRI ANTIDEPRESSANTS may decrease effectiveness of tamoxifen.

PHARMACOKINETICS Absorption: Slowly from GI tract. **Peak:** 3–6 h. **Metabolism:** In liver (CYP2D6), enterohepatically cycled. **Elimination:** Primarily in feces. **Half-Life:** 7 days.

NURSING IMPLICATIONS

Assessment & Drug Effects

- Administer analgesics for pain relief as necessitated by bone and tumor pain or local disease flair.
- Be aware that local swelling and marked erythema over preexisting lesions or the development of new lesions may signal soft-tissue disease response to tamoxifen. These symptoms rapidly subside.
- Lab tests: Assess CBC, including platelet counts, periodically. Transient leukopenia and thrombocytopenia (50,000–100,000/mm^3) without hemorrhagic tendency have been reported. Monitor serum calcium periodically.

Patient & Family Education

- Do not change established dose schedule.
- Report to physician any of the following: Marked weakness or numbness in face or leg, especially on one side of the body; difficulty walking or loss of balance; unexplained sleepiness or mental confusion; edema; shortness of breath; or blurred vision.
- Understand the possibility of drug-induced menstrual irregularities before starting treatment.
- Report promptly any unexpected vaginal discharge or pain or pressure in your pelvis.
- Avoid prolonged sun exposure, especially if skin is unprotected.

T

Apply sunscreen lotions (SPF 12 or greater) to all exposed skin surfaces.
- Avoid OTC drugs unless specifically prescribed by the physician; particularly OTC pain medicines.
- Report onset of tenderness or redness in an extremity.

TAMSULOSIN HYDROCHLORIDE (Pr)

(tam′su-lo-sin)

Flomax

Classification: ALPHA-ADRENERGIC RECEPTOR ANTAGONIST

Therapeutic: SMOOTH MUSCLE RELAXANT OF BLADDER OUTLET & PROSTATE GLAND

Pregnancy Category: B

AVAILABILITY 0.4 mg capsules

ACTION & *THERAPEUTIC EFFECT* Antagonist of the alpha$_{1A}$-adrenergic receptors located in the prostate. This blockage can cause smooth muscles in the bladder outlet and the prostate gland to relax, resulting in improvement in urinary blood flow and a reduction in symptoms of BPH. *Effectiveness is indicated by improved voiding. Improves symptoms related to benign prostatic hypertrophy (BPH) related to bladder outlet obstruction.*

USES Benign prostatic hypertrophy.

CONTRAINDICATIONS Hypersensitivity to tamsulosin; women; lactation, pediatric patients.

CAUTIOUS USE History of syncope, hypersensitivity to sulfonamides; hypotension; older adults; renal impairment, renal failure, renal disease; pregnancy (category B).

ROUTE & DOSAGE

Benign Prostatic Hypertrophy
Adult: **PO** 0.4 mg daily 30 min after a meal, may increase up to 0.8 mg daily

ADMINISTRATION

Oral
- Give 30 min after the same meal each day.
- Instruct to swallow capsules whole; not to crush, chew, or open.
- If dose is interrupted for several days, reinitiate at the lowest dose, 0.4 mg.
- Store at 20°–25° C (68°–77° F).

ADVERSE EFFECTS (≥1%) **Body as a Whole:** Asthenia, back or chest pain. **CNS:** *Headache, dizziness,* insomnia. **CV:** *Orthostatic hypotension (especially with first dose).* **GI:** Diarrhea, nausea. **Respiratory:** *Rhinitis,* pharyngitis, increased cough, sinusitis. **Urogenital:** Decreased libido, *abnormal ejaculation.* **Special Senses:** Amblyopia.

INTERACTIONS Drug: Cimetidine may decrease clearance of tamsulosin. **Sildenafil, vardenafil,** and **tadalafil,** and alcohol may enhance hypotensive effects.

PHARMACOKINETICS Absorption: Rapidly from GI tract. Greater than 90% bioavailability. **Peak:** 4–5 h fasting, 6–7 h fed. **Distribution:** Widely distributed in body tissues, including kidney and prostate. **Metabolism:** In the liver. **Elimination:** 76% in urine. **Half-Life:** 14–15 h.

NURSING IMPLICATIONS

Assessment & Drug Effects
- Monitor for signs of orthostatic hypotension; take BP lying down, then upon standing. Report a sys-

tolic pressure drop of 15 mm Hg or more or a HR 15 beats or more upon standing.

- Monitor patients on warfarin therapy closely.

Patient & Family Education

- Make position changes slowly to minimize orthostatic hypotension.
- Report dizziness, vertigo, or fainting to physician. Exercise caution with hazardous activities until response to drug is known.
- Be aware that concurrent use of cimetidine may increase the orthostatic hypotension adverse effect.

TAPENTADOL

(ta-pent'a-dol)

Nucynta

Classifications: CENTRALLY ACTING NARCOTIC ANALGESIC; MU-OPIOID RECEPTOR AGONIST; INHIBITOR OF NOREPINEPHRINE REUPTAKE

Therapeutic: CENTRALLY ACTING NARCOTIC ANALGESIC

Pregnancy Category: C

Controlled Substance: Schedule II

AVAILABILITY 50 mg, 75 mg, 100 mg tablets

ACTION & *THERAPEUTIC EFFECT* Tapentadol is a centrally acting synthetic analgesic that is a mu-opioid agonist and also thought to inhibit norepinephrine reuptake. *Effective in treatment of moderate to severe acute pain.*

USES Relief of acute moderate to severe pain.

CONTRAINDICATIONS Impaired pulmonary function (e.g., significant respiratory depression, acute or severe bronchial asthma, hypercapnia without monitoring or the absence of resuscitative equipment); paralytic ileus; concomitant use of MAOI or use within 14 days; head injury, intracranial pressure (ICP), concurrent use with other centrally acting drugs; severe hepatic or renal impairment; labor and delivery, lactation. Safety and effectiveness in children younger than 18 y are not established.

CAUTIOUS USE Elderly; debilitated patients; upper airway obstruction; cranial lesions without increased ICP; history of drug or alcohol abuse; history of seizures; mild or moderate renal or hepatic impairment; pregnancy (category C).

ROUTE & DOSAGE

Acute Moderate to Severe Pain

Adult: **PO** 50–100 mg q 4–6 h. On first day of dosing only may give a second dose 1 h later if initial dose ineffective (may titrate to max total daily dose: 700 mg day 1 and 600 mg thereafter).

Hepatic Impairment Dosage Adjustment

Moderate impairment: Reduce initial dose to 50 mg q 8 h. Severe impairment (Child-Pugh class C): Not recommended for use.

ADMINISTRATION

Oral

- On day 1 of therapy, a second dose may be given as soon as 1 h after the initial dose if pain relief is inadequate. All subsequent doses should be at 4–6 h intervals.
- Do not exceed a total daily dose of 700 mg on day 1 or 600 mg on subsequent days.
- Do not administer if a paralytic ileus is suspected.

- Do not give within 14 days of an MAOI.
- Store at 15°–30° C (59°–86° F).

ADVERSE EFFECTS (≥1%) **Body as a Whole:** Fatigue. **CNS:** Abnormal dreams, anxiety, confusional state, *dizziness,* insomnia, lethargy, *somnolence,* tremor. **CV:** Hot flush. **GI:** Constipation, dry mouth, dyspepsia, *nausea, vomiting.* **Metabolic:** Decrease appetite. **Musculoskeletal:** Arthralgia. **Respiratory:** Nasopharyngitis, <u>respiratory depression</u>, upper respiratory tract infection. **Skin:** Hyperhidrosis, pruritus, rash. **Urogenital:** Urinary tract infection.

INTERACTIONS Drug: Other OPIOID AGONISTS, GENERAL ANESTHETICS, PHENOTHIAZINES, ANTIEMETICS, other TRANQUILIZERS, SEDATIVES, HYPNOTICS, or other CNS DEPRESSANTS may cause additive CNS depression. MAO INHIBITORS can raise **norepinephrine** levels resulting in adverse cardiovascular events.

PHARMACOKINETICS Absorption: 32% bioavailability. **Peak:** 1.25 h. **Metabolism:** In liver. **Elimination:** Primarily renal. **Half-Life:** 4 h.

NURSING IMPLICATIONS

Assessment & Drug Effects

- Monitor degree of pain relief, mental status, and level of alertness.
- Monitor vital signs. Withhold drug and notify physician for a respiratory rate of 12/min or less.
- If an opioid antagonist is required to reverse the action of tapentadol, continue to monitor respiratory status since respiratory depression may outlast duration of action of the opioid antagonists.
- Withhold drug and report promptly S&S of serotonin syndrome (see Appendix F).
- Monitor ambulation. Fall precautions may be warranted.

Patient & Family Education

- Avoid engaging in hazardous activities until reaction to drug is known.
- Avoid alcohol while taking this drug.
- Consult physician before taking OTC drugs.

TAZAROTENE

(ta-zar′o-teen)

Avage, Tazorac

Classifications: RETINOID; ANTIACNE

Therapeutic: ANTIACNE

Prototype: Isotretinoin

Pregnancy Category: X

AVAILABILITY 0.05%, 0.1% gel, cream

ACTION & *THERAPEUTIC EFFECT* Retinoid prodrug that blocks epidermal cell proliferation and hyperplasia. Suppresses inflammation present in the epidermis of psoriasis. *Effectiveness indicated by improvement in acne or psoriasis.*

USES Topical treatment of plaque psoriasis on up to 20% of the body, mild to moderate acne, facial fine wrinkling, mottled hypo- and hyperpigmentation (blotchy skin discoloration), and benign facial lentigines.

CONTRAINDICATIONS Hypersensitivity to tazarotene; pregnancy (category X), women who are or may become pregnant; lactation.

CAUTIOUS USE Concurrent administration with drugs that are photosensitizers (e.g., thiazide diuretics, tetracyclines); retinoid hypersensitivity. Safety and efficacy in children younger than 12 y are not established.

ROUTE & DOSAGE

Plaque Psoriasis
Adult: **Topical** Apply thin film to affected area once daily in evening

Acne
Adult: **Topical** After cleansing and drying face, apply thin film to acne lesions once daily in evening

Fine Wrinkles
Adult: **Topical** Apply thin film of cream to affected area once daily

ADMINISTRATION

Topical

- Dry skin completely before application of a thin film of medication.
- Apply medication to no more than 20% of body surface in those with psoriasis.
- Apply only to affected areas; avoid contact with eyes and mucous membranes.

ADVERSE EFFECTS (≥1%) **Skin:** *Pruritus, burning/stinging, erythema, worsening of psoriasis, irritation, skin pain,* rash, desquamation of skin, irritant contact dermatitis, inflammation, fissuring, bleeding, dry skin, sunburn.

INTERACTIONS Drug: Increased risk of photosensitivity reactions with QUINOLONES (especially **sparfloxacin**), PHENOTHIAZINES, SULFONAMIDES, SULFONYLUREAS, TETRACYCLINES, THIAZIDE DIURETICS.

PHARMACOKINETICS Absorption: Rapidly absorbed through skin. **Distribution:** Active metabolite greater than 99% protein bound; crosses placenta, distributed into breast milk. **Metabolism:** Undergoes esterase hydrolysis to active metabolite AGN 190299. **Elimination:** In both urine and feces. **Half-Life:** 18 h.

NURSING IMPLICATIONS

Assessment & Drug Effects

- Monitor for photosensitivity in those concurrently using any of the following: Thiazides, tetracyclines, fluoroquinolones, phenothiazines, sulfonamides.

Patient & Family Education

- Understand fully the risk of serious fetal harm. Use reliable forms of effective contraception. Discontinue treatment and notify physician if pregnancy occurs.
- Alert: Immediately rinse thoroughly with water if contact with eyes occurs.
- Avoid all unnecessary exposure to sunlight or artificial UV light. If brief exposure is necessary, cover as much skin surface as possible and use sunscreens (minimum SPF 15).
- Do not apply to sunburned skin.
- Discontinue medication and notify physician if any of the following occur: Pruritus, burning, skin redness, excessive peeling, worsening of psoriasis.
- Limit application of topicals with strong skin-drying effects to skin areas being treated with tazarotene.

TELAVANCIN HYDROCHLORIDE

(tel-a-van'sin)
Vibativ
Classifications: ANTIBIOTIC; LIPOGLYCOPROTEIN
Therapeutic: ANTIBIOTIC
Pregnancy Category: C

AVAILABILITY 250 mg, 750 mg lyophilized powder for reconstitution and injection

ACTION & *THERAPEUTIC EFFECT* Telavancin is a lipoglycoprotein antibiotic derived from vancomycin with a mechanism of action related to inhibiting cell wall synthesis of bacteria. It binds to the bacterial membrane and disrupts the barrier function of the cell membrane of gram-positive bacteria. *Effective against a broad range of gram-positive bacteria.*

USES Treatment of complicated skin and skin structure infections caused by susceptible gram-positive bacteria.

UNLABELED USES Treatment of hospital-acquired nosocomial pneumonia caused by susceptible gram-positive bacteria.

CONTRAINDICATIONS End-stage renal disease or hemodialysis; QT prolongation. Safety and effectiveness in children younger than 18 y are not known.

CAUTIOUS USE Moderate or severe renal impairment; renal disease; elderly; ulcerative colitis; women of childbearing potential; pregnancy (category C), lactation.

ROUTE & DOSAGE

Complicated Skin and Skin Structure Infections

Adult: **IV** 10 mg/kg over 60 min q24h for 7–14 days

Renal Impairment Dosage Adjustment

CrCl 30–50 mL/min: Decrease to 7.5 mg/kg q 24 h; 10–29 mL/min: Decrease to 10 mg/kg q 48 h

ADMINISTRATION

Intravenous

PREPARE: **Infusion:** Reconstitute each 250 mg with 15 mL of D5W or NS to yield 15 mg/mL. Mix thoroughly to dissolve. For doses of 150–800 mg, must further dilute in 100–250 mL of IV solution. For doses less than 100 mg or greater than 800 mg, should be further diluted in D5W, NS, or LR to a final concentration in the range of 0.6–8 mg/mL.

ADMINISTER: **Infusion:** Infuse over 60 min or longer to minimize infusion-related reactions. Do not infuse through the same line with any other drugs or additives.

- Storage: Reconstituted vials or infusion solution should be used within 4 h if at room temperature or 72 h if refrigerated. **Important note:** The total time holding time for reconstituted vials plus infusion solution cannot exceed 4 h at room temperature or 72 h refrigerated.

ADVERSE EFFECTS (≥1%) **Body as a Whole:** Generalized pruritus, rigors, infusion site erythema and pain. **CNS:** Dizziness, *taste disturbance.* **GI:** Abdominal pain, *Clostridium difficile*-associated diarrhea, diarrhea, *nausea, vomiting.* **Metabolic:** Decreased appetite, *increased serum creatinine.* **Skin:** Pruritus, rash. **Urogenital:** *Foamy urine.*

DIAGNOSTIC TEST INTERFERENCE Telavancin may cause increases in ***PT, INR, aPTT,*** and ***ACT.*** Telavancin interferes with ***urine qualitative dipstick protein assays,*** as well as quantitative ***dye methods*** (e.g., ***pyrogallol red-molybdate***).

PHARMACOKINETICS Distribution: 93% bound to albumin. **Metabolism:** Metabolized to 3-hydroxylated metabolites. **Elimination:** Primarily via the urine. **Half-Life:** 8–9 h.

NURSING IMPLICATIONS

Assessment & Drug Effects

- Lab tests: Baseline culture and sensitivity test before initiation of therapy. Baseline and frequent (q48–72h) kidney function tests throughout therapy.

- Monitor for red man syndrome (i.e., flushing of upper body, urticaria, pruritus, or rash) during infusion. If syndrome develops, slow infusion immediately. If reaction does not cease, stop infusion and notify physician.
- Withhold drug and notify physician for CrCl of 50 mL/min or less.
- Monitor for and report promptly the onset of watery diarrhea with or without fever, passage of tarry or bloody stools, pus, or mucus.
- Monitor ECG with concurrent use of drugs known to prolong the QT interval.

Patient & Family Education

- Report promptly appearance of rash or itching during drug infusion.
- Report promptly loose stools or diarrhea even after completion of drug.
- Women should use effective means of contraception while on this drug. Notify physician if pregnancy occurs during treatment.

TELBIVUDINE

(tel-bi'vu-deen)

Tyzeka

Classifications: ANTIRETROVIRAL; NUCLEOSIDE REVERSE TRANSCRIPTASE INHIBITOR (NRTI)

Therapeutic: ANTIRETROVIRAL; NRTI

Prototype: Lamivudine

Pregnancy Category: B

AVAILABILITY 600 mg tablets; 100 mg/5mL oral solution

ACTION & *THERAPEUTIC EFFECT*

Telbivudine is a nucleoside analog with activity against hepatitis B virus (HBV) DNA polymerase. Its metabolite inhibits HBV DNA polymerase (reverse transcriptase) by competing with the natural nucleoside substrate. Incorporation into HBV viral DNA causes DNA chain termination, resulting in inhibition of HBV replication. *Effectiveness is measured by reducing the viral load and preventing infection of new hepatocytes.*

USES Treatment of chronic hepatitis B in patients with evidence of either histologically active disease or evidence of persistent elevations in serum aminotransferases (ALT or AST).

CONTRAINDICATIONS Hypersensitivity to telbivudine; lactation. Safe use in children younger than 16 y not established.

CAUTIOUS USE Moderate to severe renal impairment, hemodialysis; alcoholism; obesity in females; risk of hepatic disease; individuals with organ transplants; older adults; pregnancy (category B).

ROUTE & DOSAGE

Chronic Hepatitis B

Adults/Adolescents (16 y or older): **PO** 600 mg/day

Renal Impairment Dosage Adjustment

CrCl 50 mL/min or greater: No dosage adjustment
CrCl 30–49 mL/min: 600 mg q48h
CrCl less than 30 mL/min (not requiring dialysis): 600 mg q72h
CrCl less than 5–10 mL/min (ESRD): 600 mg q96h

ADMINISTRATION

Oral

- May be given without regard to food.
- Store at 15°–30° C (59°–86° F).

ADVERSE EFFECTS (≥1%) **Body as a Whole:** *Fatigue and malaise, headache, influenza-like syndrome, post-procedural pain,* pyrexia. **CNS:** Dizziness, insomnia. **GI:** *Abdominal pain, diarrhea and loose stools,* dyspepsia, *nausea, vomiting.* **Metabolic:** *Increased CPK levels,* lactic acidosis and severe hepatomegaly with steatosis. **Musculoskeletal:** Arthralgia, back pain, myalgia. **Respiratory:** *Cough, nasopharyngitis,* pharyngolaryngeal pain, *upper respiratory tract infection.* **Skin:** Rash.

INTERACTIONS Drug: Coadministration with drugs that alter renal function may alter plasma concentrations of telbivudine. Anti-HBV activity of telbivudine is additive with **adefovir** and is not antagonized by the HIV NRTIS **didanosine** and **stavudine.** Telbivudine is not antagonistic to anti-HIV activity of **abacavir, didanosine, emtricitabine, lamivudine, stavudine, tenofovir,** or **zidovudine.**

PHARMACOKINETICS Peak: 1–4 h. **Distribution:** Minimal protein binding; widely distributed in tissues. **Elimination:** Primarily unchanged in urine. **Half-Life:** 40–49 h.

T

NURSING IMPLICATIONS

Assessment & Drug Effects

- Monitor for and report S&S of lactic acidosis (e.g., anorexia, nausea, vomiting, bloating, abdominal pain, malaise, tachycardia or other arrhythmia, and difficulty in breathing).
- Withhold drug and notify physician of any of the following: Suspected lactic acidosis, steatosis, or markedly elevated liver enzymes.
- Lab tests: LFTs during and for several months after discontinuation of telbivudine; periodic serum bicarbonate.

Patient & Family Education

- Avoid all alcohol consumption while taking this drug.
- Report any of the following to a health care provider: Loss of appetite, nausea and vomiting, abdominal pain, palpitations, or difficulty breathing.

TELITHROMYCIN

(tel-i-thro-my′sin)

Ketek

Classifications: ANTIBIOTIC; KETOLIDE

Therapeutic: ANTIBIOTIC

Prototype: Erythromycin

Pregnancy Category: C

AVAILABILITY 400 mg tablets

ACTION & *THERAPEUTIC EFFECT* Telithromycin binds to bacterial ribosomal RNA site of the 50S subunit; this action results in inhibition of RNA-dependent protein synthesis of bacteria, thus resulting in cell death. Telithromycin concentrates in phagocytes where it works against intracellular respiratory pathogens. *Its broad spectrum of activity is effective against respiratory pathogens, including erythromycin- and penicillin-resistant pneumococci.*

USES Treatment of mild to moderate community-acquired pneumonia.

CONTRAINDICATIONS Macrolide antibiotic hypersensitivity; QT prolongation; ongoing proarrhythmic conditions such as hypokalemia, hypomagnesemia, significant bradycardia, myasthenia gravis unless no other therapeutic option is available; severe renal impairment or renal failure; viral infections. Safety and efficacy in children younger than 18 y are not established.

CAUTIOUS USE History of GI disease; hepatic disease; history of hepatitis or jaundice; pregnancy (category C), lactation.

ROUTE & DOSAGE

Community-Acquired Pneumonia
Adult: **PO** 800 mg once daily for 7–10 days

ADMINISTRATION

Oral

- Do not administer concurrently with simvastatin, lovastatin, atorvastatin, Class 1A (e.g., quinidine, procainamide) or Class III (e.g., dofetilide) antiarrhythmic agents.
- Store at 15°–30° C (59°–86° F). Keep container tightly closed. Protect from light.

ADVERSE EFFECTS (≥1%) **CNS:** Headache, dizziness. **CV:** Potential to cause QT_c prolongation. **GI:** *Diarrhea,* nausea, vomiting, loose stools, dysgeusia. **Metabolic:** Elevated LFTs, liver failure. **Musculoskeletal:** May exacerbate myasthenia gravis. **Special Senses:** Blurred vision, diplopia, difficulty focusing.

INTERACTIONS Drug: Pimozide or CLASS IA or CLASS III ANTIARRHYTHMICS may cause life-threatening arrhythmias; may increase concentrations of **atorvastatin, lovastatin, simvastatin,** BENZODIAZEPINES; **rifampin** decreases telithromycin levels; ERGOT DERIVATIVES (**ergotamine, dihydroergotamine**) may cause severe peripheral vasospasm; **theophylline** may exacerbate adverse GI effects. **Food: Grapefruit juice** (greater than 1 qt/day) may increase plasma concentrations and adverse effects.

PHARMACOKINETICS Absorption: 57% bioavailable. **Peak:** 1 h. **Metabolism:** 50% in liver (CYP3A4), 50% by CYP-independent mechanisms. **Elimination:** In urine and feces. **Half-Life:** 10 h.

NURSING IMPLICATIONS

Assessment & Drug Effects

- Monitor ECG in patients at risk for QT_c interval prolongation (i.e., bradycardia).
- Withhold drug and notify physician for S&S of QT_c interval prolongation such as dizziness or fainting.
- Monitor for and report promptly S&S of liver dysfunction: Fatigue, anorexia, nausea, clay-colored stools, etc.
- Lab tests: Baseline LFTs, BUN and creatinine, serum potassium.

Patient & Family Education

- Stop taking drug and notify physician for episodes of dizziness or fainting; report signs of jaundice (yellow color of the skin and/or eyes), unexplained fatigue, loss of appetite, nausea, dark urine, or clay-colored stool.
- Exercise caution when engaging in potentially hazardous activities; visual disturbances (e.g., blurred vision, difficulty focusing, double vision) are potential side effects of this drug. If visual problems occur, avoid quick changes in viewing between close and distant objects.

TELMISARTAN

(tel-mi-sar′tan)

Micardis

Classifications: ANGIOTENSIN II RECEPTOR ANTAGONIST; ANTIHYPERTENSIVE

Therapeutic: ANTIHYPERTENSIVE

Prototype: Losartan potassium

Pregnancy Category: C first trimester; D second and third trimester

AVAILABILITY 40 mg, 80 mg tablets

ACTION & *THERAPEUTIC EFFECT* Angiotensin II receptor (type AT_1) antagonist. Selectively blocks the binding of angiotensin II to the AT_1 receptors in many tissues (e.g., vascular smooth muscles, adrenal glands). Blocks the vasoconstricting and aldosterone-secreting effects of angiotensin II, thus resulting in an antihypertensive effect. *Effectiveness is indicated by a reduction in BP.*

USES Treatment of hypertension.

CONTRAINDICATIONS Hypersensitivity to telmisartan or other angiotensin receptor antagonists (e.g., losartan, eprosartan, etc.); pregnancy (category D second and third trimester), lactation.

CAUTIOUS USE Coronary artery disease (CAD); hypertropic cardiomyopathy; CHF; oliguria; hypotension; renal artery stenosis; older adult patients; biliary obstruction; liver dysfunction; renal impairment; pregnancy (category C first trimester). Safety and efficacy in children younger than 18 y are not established.

ROUTE & DOSAGE

Hypertension

Adult: **PO** 40 mg daily, may increase to 80 mg/day

ADMINISTRATION

Oral

- Do not remove tablets from blister pack until immediately before administration.
- Correct volume depletion prior to initial dose.
- Store at 15°–30° C (59°–86° F).

ADVERSE EFFECTS (≥1%) **Body as a Whole:** Back pain, flu-like syndrome, myalgia, headache, fatigue. **CNS:** Dizziness. **CV:** Hypotension, hypertension, chest pain, peripheral edema. **GI:** Diarrhea, dyspepsia, abdominal pain, nausea. **Respiratory:** Sinusitis, pharyngitis.

INTERACTIONS Drug: Telmisartan may increase **digoxin** levels.

PHARMACOKINETICS Absorption: Absorption is dose dependent, 42% of 40 mg dose is absorbed. **Peak:** 0.5–1 h. **Distribution:** Greater than 99% protein bound. **Metabolism:** Minimally metabolized. **Elimination:** Primarily in feces as unchanged drug. **Half-Life:** 24 h.

NURSING IMPLICATIONS

Assessment & Drug Effects

- Monitor BP carefully after initial dose; and periodically thereafter. Monitor more frequently with preexisting biliary obstructive disorders or hepatic insufficiency.
- Monitor dialysis patients closely for orthostatic hypotension.
- Lab tests: Periodic Hgb, creatinine clearance, liver enzymes.
- Monitor concomitant digoxin levels throughout therapy.

Patient & Family Education

- Report pregnancy to physician immediately.
- Allow between 2–4 wk for maximum therapeutic response.

TEMAZEPAM

(te-maz′e-pam)

Restoril

Classifications: BENZODIAZEPINE; ANXIOLYTIC; SEDATIVE-HYPNOTIC

Therapeutic: ANTIANXIETY; SEDATIVE-HYPNOTIC

Prototype: Lorazepam

Pregnancy Category: X

Controlled Substance: Schedule IV

AVAILABILITY 7.5 mg, 15 mg, 30 mg capsules

ACTION & *THERAPEUTIC EFFECT* Benzodiazepine derivative with hypnotic, anxiolytic, sedative effects. Principal effect is significant improvement in sleep parameters. Minimal change in REM sleep. *Reduces night awakenings and early morning awakenings; increases total sleep times, absence of rebound effects.*

USES To relieve insomnia associated with frequent nocturnal awakenings or early morning awakenings.

CONTRAINDICATIONS Benzodiazepine hypersensitivity; ethanol intoxication; narrow-angle glaucoma; psychoses; pregnancy (category X), lactation; safety in children younger than 18 y is not established.

CAUTIOUS USE Severely depressed patient or one with suicidal ideation; history of drug abuse or dependence, acute intoxication; alcoholism; COPD; liver or kidney dysfunction; older adults; sleep apnea.

ROUTE & DOSAGE

Insomnia

Adult: **PO** 7.5–30 mg at bedtime
Geriatric: **PO** 7.5 mg at bedtime

ADMINISTRATION

Oral

- Give 20–30 min before patient retires.
- Store at 15°–30° C (59°–86° F) in tight container unless otherwise specified by manufacturer.

ADVERSE EFFECTS (≥1%) **CNS:** *Drowsiness,* dizziness, lethargy, confusion, headache, euphoria, relaxed feeling, weakness. **GI:** Anorexia, diarrhea. **CV:** Palpitations.

INTERACTIONS Drug: Alcohol, CNS DEPRESSANTS, ANTICONVULSANTS potentiate CNS depression; **cimetidine** increases temazepam plasma levels, thus increasing its toxicity; may decrease antiparkinsonism effects of **levodopa;** may increase **phenytoin** levels; smoking decreases sedative effects. **Herbal: Kava, valerian** may potentiate sedation.

PHARMACOKINETICS Absorption: Readily from GI tract. **Onset:** 30–50 min. **Peak:** 2–3 h. **Duration:** 10–12 h. **Distribution:** Crosses placenta; distributed into breast milk. **Metabolism:** In liver to oxazepam. **Elimination:** In urine. **Half-Life:** 8–24 h.

NURSING IMPLICATIONS

Assessment & Drug Effects

- Be alert to signs of paradoxical reaction (excitement, hyperactivity, and disorientation) in older adults. Psychoactive drugs are the most frequent cause of acute confusion in this age group.
- CNS adverse effects are more apt to occur in the patient with hypoalbuminemia, liver disease, and in older adults. Report promptly incidence of bradycardia, drowsiness, dizziness, clumsiness, lack of coordination. Supervise ambulation, especially at night.

T

- Lab tests: Obtain liver and kidney function tests during long-term use.
- Be alert to S&S of overdose: Weakness, bradycardia, somnolence, confusion, slurred speech, ataxia, coma with reduced or absent reflexes, hypertension, and respiratory depression.

Patient & Family Education

- Be aware that improvement in sleep will not occur until after 2–3 doses of drug.
- Notify physician if dreams or nightmares interfere with rest. An alternate drug or reduced dose may be prescribed.
- Be aware that difficulty getting to sleep may continue. Drug effect is evidenced by the increased amount of rest once asleep.
- Consult physician if insomnia continues in spite of medication.
- Do not smoke after medication is taken.
- Do not use OTC drugs (especially for insomnia) without advice of physician.
- Consult physician before discontinuing drug especially after long-term use. Gradual reduction of dose may be necessary to avoid withdrawal symptoms.
- Avoid use of alcohol and other CNS depressants.
- Do not drive or engage in other potentially hazardous activities until response to drug is known. This drug may depress psychomotor skills and cause sedation.

T

TEMOZOLOMIDE

(tem-o-zol′o-mide)

Temodar

Classifications: ANTINEOPLASTIC; ALKYLATING AGENT

Therapeutic: ANTINEOPLASTIC

Prototype: Cyclophosphamide

Pregnancy Category: D

AVAILABILITY 5 mg, 20 mg, 100 mg, 140 mg, 180 mg, 250 mg capsules; 100 mg solution for injection

ACTION & *THERAPEUTIC EFFECT* Cytotoxic agent with alkylating properties that are cell cycle nonspecific. Interferes with purine (e.g., guanine) metabolism and thus protein synthesis in rapidly proliferating cells. *Effectiveness is indicated by objective evidence of tumor regression.*

USES Adult patients with refractory anaplastic astrocytoma, glioblastoma multiforme with radiotherapy.

CONTRAINDICATIONS Hypersensitivity to temozolomide, DTIC, or dacarbazine; severe bone marrow suppression; children younger than 3 y; pregnancy (category D), lactation.

CAUTIOUS USE Bacterial or viral infection; older adults; severe hepatic or renal impairment; myelosuppression; prior radiotherapy or chemotherapy.

ROUTE & DOSAGE

Astrocytoma

Adult: **PO/IV** 150 mg/m² daily days 1–5 per 28-day treatment cycle (may increase to 200 mg/m²/day); subsequent doses are based on absolute neutrophil count on day 21 or at least 48 h before next scheduled cycle (see prescribing information for dosage adjustments based on neutrophil count)

Glioblastoma Multiforme

Adult: **PO** 75 mg/m² daily for 42 days with focal radiotherapy; after

4 wk, maintenance phase of 150–200 mg/m² on days 1–5 of 28-day cycle

ADMINISTRATION

Oral

- Give consistently with regard to food.
- Do not administer unless absolute neutrophil count greater than 1500 per microliter and platelet count greater than 100,000 per microliter.
- Do not open capsules. Avoid inhalation or contact with skin or mucous membranes, if accidentally opened/damaged.
- Store at room temperature, 15°–30° C (59°–86° F).

ADVERSE EFFECTS (≥1%) **Body as a Whole:** *Headache, fatigue, asthenia, fever,* back pain, myalgia, weight gain; viral infection. **CNS:** *Convulsions, hemiparesis, dizziness, abnormal coordination, amnesia, insomnia,* paresthesia, somnolence, paresis, ataxia, dysphasia, abnormal gait, confusion, anxiety, depression. **CV:** *Peripheral edema.* **GI:** *Nausea, vomiting, constipation, diarrhea,* abdominal pain, anorexia. **Hematologic:** Anemia, neutropenia, thrombocytopenia, leukopenia, lymphopenia. **Respiratory:** Upper respiratory tract infection, pharyngitis, sinusitis, cough. **Skin:** Rash, pruritus. **Metabolic:** Adrenal hypercorticism. **Urogenital:** Urinary incontinence. **Special Senses:** Diplopia, abnormal vision.

INTERACTIONS Drug: Valproic acid may decrease **temozolomide** levels.

PHARMACOKINETICS Absorption: Rapidly. **Peak:** 1 h. **Metabolism:** Spontaneously metabolized to active metabolite MTIC. **Elimination:** Primarily in urine. **Half-Life:** 1.8 h.

NURSING IMPLICATIONS

Assessment & Drug Effects

- Monitor for S&S of toxicity: Infection, bleeding episodes, jaundice, rash, CNS disturbances.
- Lab tests: CBC with differential on day 22 and weekly until absolute neutrophil count (ANC) greater than 1500 per microliter and platelet count greater than 100,000 per microliter; periodic LFT and routine serum chemistry, including serum calcium.

Patient & Family Education

- Take consistently with respect to meals.
- Report to physician signs of infection, bleeding, discoloration of skin or skin rash, dizziness, lack of balance, or other bothersome side effects promptly.
- Exercise caution with hazardous activities until response to drug is known.
- Use effective methods of contraception; avoid pregnancy.

TEMSIROLIMUS

(tem-si-ro-li′mus)

Torisel

Classifications: BIOLOGICAL RESPONSE MODIFIER; ANTINEOPLASTIC; PROTEIN-TYROSINE KINASE INHIBITOR (TKI)

Therapeutic: ANTINEOPLASTIC

Prototype: Gefitinib

Pregnancy Category: D

AVAILABILITY 25 mg/mL concentrated solution

ACTION & *THERAPEUTIC EFFECT* Inhibits an intracellular protein that controls cell division in renal carcinoma and other tumor cells. *Results in arrest of growth in tumor cells.*

USES Treatment of advanced renal cell carcinoma.
UNLABELED USES Astrocytoma, mantle cell lymphoma (MCL).

CONTRAINDICATIONS Live vaccines; pregnancy (category D); lactation. Safe use in children has not been established.
CAUTIOUS USE Hypersensitivity to temsirolimus, sirolimus, polysorbate 80, or antihistamines; diabetes mellitus; history of hyperlipemia; respiratory disorders; perioperative period due to potential for abnormal wound healing; CNS tumors (primary or by metastasis); hepatic impairment.

ROUTE & DOSAGE

Renal Cell Carcinoma
Adult: **IV** 25 mg qwk

Dosage Adjustment
Regimen with a strong CYP3A4 inhibitor: 12.5 mg/wk
Regimen with a strong CYP3A4 inducer: 50 mg based on tolerability

ADMINISTRATION

Intravenous
Patients should receive prophylactic IV diphenhydramine 25 to 50 mg (or similar antihistamine) 30 min before each dose.

PREPARE: **IV Infusion:** Inject 1.8 mL of supplied diluent into the 25 mg/mL vial to yield 10 mg/mL. ▪ Withdraw the required dose and inject rapidly into a 250 mL DEHP-free container of NS. Invert to mix.
ADMINISTER: **IV Infusion:** Use DEHP-free infusion line with a 5 micron or less in-line filter. ▪ Infuse over 30–60 min. ▪ Complete infusion within 6 h of preparation.

INCOMPATIBILITIES **Solution/additive:** Do not add other drugs or agents to temsirolimus IV solutions.

▪ Store at 2°–8° C (36°–46° F). Protect from light. The 10 mg/mL drug solution is stable for up to 24 h at 15°–30° C (59°–86° F).

ADVERSE EFFECTS (≥1%) **Body as a Whole:** Allergic/hypersensitivity reactions, *asthenia,* chest pain, chills, *edema,* impaired wound healing, infections, pain, pyrexia. **CNS:** Depression, dysgeusia, headache, insomnia. **CV:** Hypertension, thrombophlebitis, venous thromboembolism. **GI:** Abdominal pain, *anorexia,* constipation, diarrhea, fatal bowel perforation, *mucositis, nausea,* vomiting. **Hematologic:** Decrease hemoglobin, *leukocytopenia, lymphopenia,* neutropenia, *thrombocytopenia.* **Metabolic:** *Elevated alkaline phosphatase, elevated AST, elevated serum creatinine,* hypokalemia, *hypophosphatemia,* hyperbilirubinemia, *hypercholesterolemia, hyperglycemia, hypertriglyceridemia,* weight loss. **Musculoskeletal:** Arthralgia, back pain, myalgia. **Respiratory:** Cough, dyspnea, epistaxis, interstitial lung disease, pharyngitis, pneumonia, rhinitis, upper respiratory tract infection. **Skin:** Acne, dry skin, nail disorder, pruritus, *rash.* **Special Senses:** Conjunctivitis. **Urogenital:** Urinary tract infection.

INTERACTIONS Drug: AZOLE ANTIFUNGAL AGENTS **(fluconazole, itraconazole, ketoconazole, posaconazole, voriconazole), cyclosporine,** INHIBITORS OF CYP3A4 (HIV PROTEASE INHIBITORS, **clarithromycin, diltiazem**), **mycophenolate mofetil,** and **sunitinib** increase the plasma levels of **temsirolimus.** INDUCERS OF CYP3A4 (**dexamethasone, rifampin, rifabutin, phenytoin**)

T

decrease the plasma level of temsirolimus. **Food: Grapefruit** and **grapefruit juice** increase the plasma level of temsirolimus. **Herbal: St. John's wort** decreases the plasma level of temsirolimus.

PHARMACOKINETICS Peak: 0.5–2 h. **Metabolism:** In liver. **Elimination:** Primarily in stool. **Half-Life:** 17.3 h.

NURSING IMPLICATIONS

Assessment & Drug Effects

- Withhold drug and notify physician for absolute neutrophil count less than 1000/mm³ or platelet count less than 75,000/mm³.
- Monitor for infusion-related reactions during and for at least 1 h after completion of infusion.
- Slow or stop infusion for infusion-related reactions. If infusion is restarted after 30–60 min of observation, slow rate to up to 60 min and continue observation.
- Monitor respiratory status and report promptly dyspnea, cough, S&S of hypoxia, fever.
- Lab tests: Baseline and periodic CBC with differential and platelet count, lipid profile, LFTs, alkaline phosphatase, kidney function tests, serum electrolytes, plasma glucose, ABGs.
- Monitor diabetics for loss of glycemic control.

Patient & Family Education

- Avoid live vaccines and close contact with those who have received live vaccines.
- Use effective contraceptive measures to prevent pregnancy.
- Men with partners of childbearing age should use reliable contraception throughout treatment and for 3 mo after the last dose of temsirolimus.
- Report promptly any of the following: S&S of infection, difficulty breathing, abdominal pain, blood in stools, abnormal wound healing, S&S of hypersensitivity (see Appendix F).

TENECTEPLASE RECOMBINANT

(ten-ect′e-plase)

TNKase

Classification: THROMBOLYTIC ENZYME, TISSUE PLASMINOGEN ACTIVATOR (t-PA)

Therapeutic: THROMBOLYTIC ENZYME

Prototype: Alteplase

Pregnancy Category: C

AVAILABILITY 50 mg vial

ACTION & *THERAPEUTIC EFFECT* Tenecteplase is a thrombolytic agent that activates plasminogen, a substance created by endothelial cells in response to arterial wall injury that contributes to clot formation. Plasminogen is converted to plasmin which breaks down the fibrin mesh that binds the clot together, thus dissolving the clot. *Effective in producing thrombolysis of a clot involved in a myocardial infarction.*

USES Reduction of mortality associated with acute myocardial infarction (AMI).

CONTRAINDICATIONS Active internal bleeding; history of CVA; intracranial or intraspinal surgery with 2 mo; intracranial neoplasm; arteriovenous malformation, or aneurysm; known bleeding diathesis; brain tumor; increased intracranial pressure; coagulopathy; head trauma; stroke; surgery; severe uncontrolled hypertension; lactation.

CAUTIOUS USE Recent major surgery, previous puncture of compressible vessels, CVA, recent GI or GU bleeding, recent trauma; hypertension, mitral valve stenosis, acute pericarditis, bacterial endocarditis; severe liver or kidney disease; hemorrhagic ophthalmic conditions; septic thrombophlebitis or occluded, infected AV cannula; advanced age; pregnancy (category C). Safety and efficacy in children are not established.

ROUTE & DOSAGE

Acute Myocardial Infarction

Adult: **IV** Infuse dose over 5 sec, *weight less than 60 kg,* 30 mg; *weight 60–70 kg,* 35 mg; *weight 70–80 kg,* 40 mg; *weight 80–90 kg,* 45 mg; *weight greater than 90 kg,* 50 mg

ADMINISTRATION

Intravenous

PREPARE: **Direct:** Read and follow instructions supplied with TwinPak™ Dual Cannula Device. ▪ Withdraw 10 mL of sterile water for injection from the supplied vial; inject entire contents into the TNKase vial directing the diluent stream into the powder. ▪ Gently swirl until dissolved but do not shake. The resulting solution contains 5 mg/mL. ▪ Withdraw the appropriate dose and discard any unused solution. ▪ Follow directions supplied with TwinPak™ for proper handling of syringe.

ADMINISTER: **Direct:** Dextrose-containing IV line **must be** flushed before and after bolus with NS. ▪ Give as a single bolus dose over 5 sec. ▪ The total dose given should not exceed 50 mg.

INCOMPATIBILITIES **Solution/additive: Dextrose** solutions.

▪ Store unopened TwinPak™ at or below 30° C (86° F) or under refrigeration at 2°–8° C (36°–46° F).

ADVERSE EFFECTS (≥1%) **Hematologic:** Major bleeding, *hematoma,* GI bleed, bleeding at puncture site, hematuria, pharyngeal, epistaxis.

DIAGNOSTIC TEST INTERFERENCE Unreliable results for ***coagulation test I*** and measures of ***fibrinolytic activity.***

PHARMACOKINETICS Metabolism: In liver. **Half-Life:** 90–130 min.

NURSING IMPLICATIONS

Assessment & Drug Effects

- Avoid IM injections and unnecessary handling or invasive procedures for the first few hours after treatment.
- Monitor for S&S of bleeding. Should bleeding occur, withhold concomitant heparin and antiplatelet therapy; notify physician.
- Monitor cardiovascular and neurologic status closely. Persons at increased risk for life-threatening cardiac events include those with: A high potential for bleeding, recent surgery, severe hypertension, mitral stenosis and atrial fibrillation, anticoagulant therapy, and advanced age.
- Lab tests: Baseline and 1 h after administration of drug determine cardiac enzymes, circulating myoglobin, cardiac troponin-1, creatine kinase-MB; Hgb and Hct post-infusion; frequent aPTT, PT, and thrombin time.
- Coagulation parameters may not predict bleeding episodes.

Patient & Family Education

- Notify physician of the following immediately: A sudden, severe headache; any sign of bleeding; signs or symptoms of hypersensitivity (see Appendix F).

- Stay as still as possible and do not attempt to get out of bed until directed to do so.

TENOFOVIR DISOPROXIL FUMARATE

(ten-o-fo'vir di-so-prox'il fum'a-rate)

Viread

Classifications: ANTIRETROVIRAL; NUCLEOSIDE REVERSE TRANSCRIPTASE INHIBITOR (NRTI)

Therapeutic: ANTIRETROVIRAL; NRTI

Prototype: Zidovudine

Pregnancy Category: B

AVAILABILITY 300 mg tablets

ACTION & *THERAPEUTIC EFFECT* Tenofovir is a potent inhibitor of retroviruses, including HIV-1. The active form of tenofovir persists in HIV-infected cells for prolonged periods, thus, it results in sustained inhibition of HIV replication. *It reduces the viral load (plasma HIV-RNA), and CD4 counts.*

USES In combination with other antiretrovirals for the treatment of HIV; chronic hepatitis B infection.

CONTRAINDICATIONS Hypersensitivity to tenofovir; lactic acidosis, severe hepatomegaly, concurrent administration of nephrotoxic agents, acute renal failure; lactation.

CAUTIOUS USE Hepatic dysfunction, alcoholism, know risks for hepatic dysfunction; renal impairment; obesity; pathologic bone fractures; older adults; children, pregnancy (category B).

ROUTE & DOSAGE

HIV Infection

Adult: **PO** 300 mg once daily with meal

Chronic Hepatitis B

Adult: **PO** 300 mg daily

Renal Impairment Dosage Adjustment

CrCl 30–49 mL/min: Dose q48h; 10–29 mL/min: Dose twice weekly

Hemodialysis Dosage Adjustment: Dose weekly or after 12 h of dialysis

ADMINISTRATION

Oral

- Give at the same time each day with a meal.
- Give 2 h before or 1 h after didanosine (if ordered concurrently).
- Store at room temperature; excursions to 15°–30° C (59°–80° F) are permitted.

ADVERSE EFFECTS (≥1%) **Body as a Whole:** Asthenia. **CNS:** Headache. **GI:** *Nausea,* vomiting, diarrhea, flatulence, abdominal pain, anorexia. **Hematologic:** Neutropenia. **Metabolic:** Increased *creatine kinase,* AST, ALT, serum amylase, triglycerides, serum glucose.

INTERACTIONS Drug: May increase **didanosine** toxicity; **acyclovir, amphotericin B, cidofovir, foscarnet, ganciclovir, probenecid, valacyclovir, valganciclovir** may increase tenofovir toxicity by decreasing its renal elimination. **Food:** Food increases absorption.

PHARMACOKINETICS Absorption: Bioavailability 25% fasting, 40% with high fat meal. **Peak:** 1 h. **Distribution:** Less than 7% protein bound. **Metabolism:** Not metabolized by CYP450 enzyme system. **Elimination:** Renally eliminated. **Half-Life:** 11–14 h.

T

NURSING IMPLICATIONS

Assessment & Drug Effects

- Lab tests: Monitor baseline and periodic renal function and LFTs; monitor periodically serum electrolytes, and ABGs if lactic acidosis is suspected.
- Monitor for S&S of bone abnormalities (e.g., bone pain, stress fractures).
- Monitor closely patients receiving other nephrotoxic agents for changes in serum creatinine and phosphorus. Withhold drug and notify physician for creatinine clearance less than 60 mL/min.
- Withhold drug and notify physician if patient develops clinical or lab findings suggestive of lactic acidosis or pronounced hepatotoxicity (e.g., hepatomegaly and steatosis even in the absence of marked transaminase elevations).

Patient & Family Education

- Take this drug exactly as prescribed. Do not miss any doses. If you miss a dose, take it as soon as possible and then take your next dose at its regular time. If it is almost time for your next dose, do not take the missed dose. Wait and take the next dose at the regular time. Do not double the next dose.
- Report any of the following to physician: Unexplained anorexia, nausea, vomiting, abdominal pain, fatigue, dark urine.

T

TERAZOSIN

(ter-ay′zoe-sin)

Hytrin

Classifications: ALPHA-ADRENERGIC RECEPTOR ANTAGONIST; ANTIHYPERTENSIVE

Therapeutic: ANTIHYPERTENSIVE BPH AGENT

Prototype: Prazosin

Pregnancy Category: C

AVAILABILITY 1 mg, 2 mg, 5 mg, 10 mg capsules

ACTION & *THERAPEUTIC EFFECT* Selectively blocks alpha$_1$-adrenergic receptors in vascular smooth muscle in many tissues, including vascular smooth muscle, the bladder neck, and the prostate. Promotes vasodilation, thus producing relaxation that leads to reduction of peripheral vascular resistance and lowered BP as well as increased urine flow. *Effectiveness is measured in lowering of blood pressure values and controlling the symptoms of benign prostate hypertrophy.*

USES To treat hypertension alone or in combination with other antihypertensive agents (beta-adrenergic blocking agents, diuretics). To treat benign prostatic hypertrophy (BPH) and urinary flow obstruction.

CONTRAINDICATIONS Hypersensitivity to terazosin. Safe use in children is not established.

CAUTIOUS USE Patients with BPH; prostate cancer; history of hypotensive episodes; angina; renal impairment, renal disease, renal failure; elderly; pregnancy (category C), lactation.

ROUTE & DOSAGE

Hypertension, Benign Prostatic Hypertrophy

Adult: **PO** Start with 1 mg at bedtime, then 1–5 mg/day (max: 20 mg/day)

ADMINISTRATION

Oral

- Give initial dose at bedtime to reduce the potential for severe hypotensive effect. After the initial dose, give any time of day.

- Store at 15°–30° C (59°–86° F) in tightly closed container away from heat and strong light. Do not freeze.

ADVERSE EFFECTS (≥1%) **CNS:** *Asthenia (weakness), dizziness, headache,* drowsiness, weakness. **CV:** Postural hypotension, palpitation, *first-dose phenomenon (syncope).* **Special Senses:** Blurred vision. **GI:** Nausea. **Body as a Whole:** Weight gain, pain in extremities, peripheral edema. **Respiratory:** Nasal congestion, sinusitis, dyspnea. **Urogenital:** Impotence.

INTERACTIONS Drug: Antihypertensive effects may be attenuated by NSAIDS. **Sildenafil, vardenafil,** and **tadalafil** may enhance hypotensive effects.

PHARMACOKINETICS Absorption: Readily from GI tract. **Peak:** 1–2 h. **Metabolism:** In liver. **Elimination:** 60% in feces, 40% in urine. **Half-Life:** 9–12 h.

NURSING IMPLICATIONS

Assessment & Drug Effects

- Be alert for possible first-dose phenomenon (precipitous decline in BP with consciousness disturbance). This is rare; occurs within 90–120 min of initial dose.
- Monitor BP at end of dosing interval (just before next dose) to determine level of antihypertensive control.
- Be aware that drug-induced decrease in BP appears to be more position dependent (i.e., greater in the erect position) during the first few hours after dosing than at end of 24 h.
- A greatly diminished hypotensive response at end of 24 h indicates need for change in dosage (increased dose or twice daily regimen). Report to physician.

Patient & Family Education

- Avoid situations that would result in injury should syncope (loss of consciousness) occur after first dose. If faintness develops, lie down promptly.
- Make position changes slowly (i.e., change in direction or from recumbent to upright posture). Dangle legs and move ankles a minute or so before standing when arising. Orthostatic hypotension (greatest shortly after dosing) can pose a problem with ambulation.
- Do not drive or engage in potentially hazardous activities for at least 12 h after first dose, after dosage increase, or when treatment is resumed after interruption of therapy.
- Monitor weight: Report sudden gain of more than 0.5–1 kg (1–2 lb) accompanied by edema in extremities to physician. Dose adjustment may be indicated.
- Do not alter established drug regimen. Consult physician if drug is omitted for several days. Drug will be started with the initial dosing regimen.
- Keep scheduled appointments for assessment of BP control and other clinically significant tests.
- Do not take OTC medications, particularly those that may contain an adrenergic agent (e.g., remedies for coughs, colds, allergy) without first consulting physician.

TERBINAFINE HYDROCHLORIDE (Pr)

(ter-bin'a-feen)

Lamisil, Lamisil DermaGel

Classifications: ANTIBIOTIC; ANTIFUNGAL

Therapeutic: ANTIFUNGAL

Pregnancy Category: B

AVAILABILITY 250 mg tablets; 1% cream; 1.12% gel

ACTION & *THERAPEUTIC EFFECT* Synthetic antifungal agent that inhibits its sterol biosynthesis in fungi and ultimately causes fungal cell death. *Effective as a topical antifungal treatment as well as in oral form.*

USES Topical treatment of superficial mycoses such as interdigital tinea pedis, tinea cruris, and tinea corporis due to *Epidermophyton floccosum, Trichophyton mentagrophytes,* or *T. rubrum;* oral treatment of onychomycosis due to tinea unguium.

CONTRAINDICATIONS Hypersensitivity to terbinafine; alcoholism; hepatic disease; hepatitis; jaundice; renal impairment; renal failure; lactation.
CAUTIOUS USE Pregnancy (category B). Safety and efficacy in children younger than 12 y are not established.

ROUTE & DOSAGE

Tinea Pedis, Tinea Cruris, or Tinea Corporis
Adult: **Topical** Apply daily or b.i.d. to affected and immediately surrounding areas until clinical signs and symptoms are significantly improved (1–7 wk)

Onychomycosis
Adult: **PO** 250 mg daily × 6 wk for fingernails or × 12 wk for toenails

ADMINISTRATION

Topical
- Apply externally. Avoid application to mucous membranes and avoid contact with eyes.
- Do not use occlusive dressings unless specifically directed to do so by physician.
- Store at 15°–30° C (59°–86° F).

ADVERSE EFFECTS (≥1%) **Skin:** Pruritus, local burning, dryness, rash, vesiculation, redness, contact dermatitis at application site. **CNS:** *Headache.* **GI:** Diarrhea, dyspepsia, abdominal pain, liver test abnormalities, liver failure (rare). **Hematologic:** Neutropenia (rare). **Special Senses:** Taste disturbances.

INTERACTIONS Drug: May increase **theophylline** levels; may decrease **cyclosporine** levels; **rifampin** may decrease **terbinafine** levels.

PHARMACOKINETICS Absorption: 70% PO; approximately 3.5% of topical dose is absorbed systemically. **Elimination:** In urine. **Half-Life:** 36 h.

NURSING IMPLICATIONS

Assessment & Drug Effects
- Monitor for and report increased skin irritation.

Patient & Family Education
- Learn correct technique for application of cream.
- Notify physician if drug causes increased skin irritation or sensitivity.
- Be aware that medication **must be** used for full treatment time to be effective.

TERBUTALINE SULFATE

(ter-byoo′te-leen)
Classifications: BETA-ADRENERGIC RECEPTOR AGONIST; BRONCHODILATOR
Therapeutic: RESPIRATORY SMOOTH MUSCLE RELAXANT; BRONCHODILATOR
Prototype: Albuterol
Pregnancy Category: B

AVAILABILITY 2.5 mg, 5 mg tablets; 0.2 mg aerosol; 1 mg/mL injection

ACTION & *THERAPEUTIC EFFECT* Synthetic adrenergic stimulant with selective $beta_2$-receptor activity in bronchial smooth muscles, inhibits histamine release from mast cells, and increases ciliary motility. *Relieves bronchospasm in chronic obstructive pulmonary disease (COPD) and significantly increases vital capacity. Increases uterine relaxation (thereby preventing or abolishing high intrauterine pressure).*

USES Orally or subcutaneously as a bronchodilator in bronchial asthma and for reversible airway obstruction associated with bronchitis and emphysema.

UNLABELED USES To delay delivery in preterm labor.

CONTRAINDICATIONS Known hypersensitivity to sympathomimetic amines; severe hypertension and coronary artery disease; tachycardia with digitalis intoxication; within 14 days of MAO inhibitor therapy; angle-closure glaucoma.

CAUTIOUS USE Angina, stroke, hypertension; diabetes mellitus; thyrotoxicosis; history of seizure disorders; MAOI therapy; cardiac arrhythmias; QT prolongation; thyroid disease; older adults; kidney and liver dysfunction; pregnancy (category B). Use further caution in second and third trimester (may inhibit uterine contractions and labor).

ROUTE & DOSAGE

Bronchodilator

Adult: **PO** 2.5–5 mg t.i.d. at 6 h intervals (max: 15 mg/day) **Subcutaneous** 0.25 mg q15–30min up to 0.5 mg in 4 h **Inhaled** 2 inhalations separated by 60 sec q4–6h

Adolescent (12–15 y): **PO** 2.5 mg t.i.d. at 6 h intervals (max: 7.5 mg/day) **Subcutaneous** 0.25 mg q15–30min up to 0.5 mg in 4 h **Inhaled** 2 inhalations separated by 60 sec q4–6h

Child (Younger than 12 y): **PO** 0.05 mg/kg q8h, gradually increase up to 0.15 mg/kg q8h (max: 5 mg/day) **Subcutaneous** 0.005–0.01 mg/kg (max: 0.4 mg) q15–20min × 2 doses

Premature Labor

Adult: **PO** 2.5 mg q4–6h

ADMINISTRATION

Oral

- Give with fluid of patient's choice; tablets may be crushed.
- Be certain about recommended doses: PO preparation, 2.5 mg; subcutaneous, 0.25 mg. A decimal point error can be fatal.
- Give with food if GI symptoms occur.

Subcutaneous

- Give subcutaneous injection into lateral deltoid area.
- Store all forms at 15°–30° C (59°–86° F); protect from light. Do not freeze.

ADVERSE EFFECTS (≥1%) **CNS:** *Nervousness, tremor,* headache, *lightheadedness,* drowsiness, fatigue, seizures. **CV:** *Tachycardia,* hypotension or hypertension, *palpitation,* maternal and fetal tachycardia. **GI:** Nausea, vomiting. **Body as a Whole:** Sweating, muscle cramps.

DIAGNOSTIC TEST INTERFERENCE Terbutaline may increase ***blood glucose*** and free ***fatty acids.***

INTERACTIONS Drug: Epinephrine, other SYMPATHOMIMETIC BRONCHODILATORS may add to effects; MAO INHIBITORS, TRICYCLIC ANTIDEPRESSANTS potentiate action on vascular sys-

T

tem; effects of both BETA-ADRENERGIC BLOCKERS and terbutaline antagonized.

PHARMACOKINETICS Absorption: 33–50% from GI tract. **Onset:** 30 min PO; less than 15 min Subcutaneous; 5–30 min inhaled. **Peak:** 2–3 h PO; 30–60 min Subcutaneous; 1–2 h inhaled. **Duration:** 4–8 h PO; 1.5–4 h Subcutaneous; 3–4 h inhaled. **Distribution:** Into breast milk. **Metabolism:** In liver. **Elimination:** Primarily in urine, 3% in feces. **Half-Life:** 3–4 h.

NURSING IMPLICATIONS

Assessment & Drug Effects

- Assess vital signs: Baseline pulse and BP and before each dose. If significantly altered from baseline level, consult physician. Cardiovascular adverse effects are more apt to occur when drug is given by subcutaneous route or it is used by a patient with cardiac arrhythmia.
- Most adverse effects are transient, however, rapid heart rate may persist for a relatively long time.
- Aerosolized drug produces minimal cardiac stimulation or tremors.
- Be aware that muscle tremor is a fairly common adverse effect that appears to subside with continued use.
- Monitor patient being treated for premature labor for CV S&S for 12 h after drug is discontinued. Report tachycardia promptly.
- Monitor I&O ratio. Fluid restriction may be necessary. Consult physician.

Patient & Family Education

- Inhalator therapy: Review instructions for use of inhalator (included in the package).
- Learn how to take your own pulse and the limits of change that indicate need to notify the physician.
- Consult physician if breathing difficulty is not relieved or if it becomes worse within 30 min after an oral dose.
- Consult physician if symptomatic relief wanes; tolerance can develop with chronic use.
- Do not self-dose this drug, particularly during long-term therapy. In the face of waning response, increasing the dose will not improve the clinical condition and may cause overdosage. Understand that decreasing relief with continued treatment indicates need for another bronchodilator, not an increase in dose.
- Do not puncture container, use or store it near heat or open flame, or expose to temperatures above 49° C (120° F), which may cause bursting. Contents of the aerosol (inhalator) are under pressure.
- Do not use any other aerosol bronchodilator while being treated with aerosol terbutaline. Do not self-medicate with an OTC aerosol.
- Do not use OTC drugs without physician approval. Many cold and allergy remedies, for example, contain a sympathomimetic agent that when combined with terbutaline may cause harmful adverse effects.

TERCONAZOLE

(ter-con′a-zole)
Terazol 7, Terazol 3
Classification: AZOLE ANTIFUNGAL
Therapeutic: VAGINAL ANTIFUNGAL
Prototype: Fluconazole
Pregnancy Category: C

AVAILABILITY 0.4%, 0.8% vaginal cream; 80 mg vaginal suppositories

ACTION & *THERAPEUTIC EFFECT* Terconazole is thought to exert an-

T

tifungal activity by disruption of normal fungal cell membrane permeability. *Exhibits fungicidal activity against* Candida albicans.

USES Local treatment of vulvovaginal candidiasis.

CONTRAINDICATIONS Hypersensitivity to terconazole or azole antifungals; use of tampons; lactation.
CAUTIOUS USE Pregnancy (category C). Safety and efficacy in children younger than 18 y are not established.

ROUTE & DOSAGE

Candidiasis
Adult: **Intravaginal** One suppository (2.5 g) each night × 3 days; one applicator full of 0.4% cream each night × 7 days; one applicator full of 0.8% cream each night × 3 days

ADMINISTRATION

Intravaginal

- Insert applicator high into the vagina (except during pregnancy).
- Wash applicator before and after each use.
- Store away from direct heat and light.

ADVERSE EFFECTS (≥1%) **CNS:** *Headache.* **Urogenital:** Vaginal itching, burning, irritation. **Body as a Whole:** Rash, flu-like syndrome (fever, chills, headache, hypotension).

INTERACTIONS Drug: May inactivate **nonoxynol-9** spermicides.

PHARMACOKINETICS Absorption: Slow minimal absorption from vagina. **Onset:** Within 3 days. **Metabolism:** In liver. **Elimination:** Half in urine, half in feces. **Half-Life:** 4–11 h.

NURSING IMPLICATIONS

Assessment & Drug Effects

- Do not use if patient has a history of allergic reaction to other antifungal agents, such as miconazole.
- Monitor for sensitization and irritation; these may indicate need to discontinue drug.

Patient & Family Education

- Use correct application technique.
- Do not use tampons concurrently with terconazole.
- Learn potential adverse reactions, including sensitization and allergic response.
- Be aware that terconazole may interact with diaphragms and latex condoms; avoid concurrent use within 72 h.
- Refrain from sexual intercourse while using terconazole.
- Wear only cotton underwear; change daily.

TERIPARATIDE

(ter-i-par′a-tide)
Forteo
Classification: PARATHYROID HORMONE AGONIST
Therapeutic: PARATHYROID HORMONE AGONIST
Pregnancy Category: C

AVAILABILITY 750 mcg/3 mL injection

ACTION & *THERAPEUTIC EFFECT* Parathyroid hormone (PTH) is the primary regulator of calcium and phosphate metabolism in bone and kidney. Biological actions of PTH and teriparatide are similar in bone and kidneys. *Stimulates new bone formation by preferential stimulation of osteoblastic activity over osteoclastic activity; improves bone microarchitecture, and increases* *bone mass and strength by stimulating new bone formation.*

USES Treatment of osteoporosis in postmenopausal women at high risk for fracture; increase bone mass in men with primary or hypogonadal osteoporosis who are at high risk for fracture.

CONTRAINDICATIONS Hypersensitivity to teriparatide; osteosarcoma; Paget's disease; unexplained elevations of alkaline phosphatase; bone metastases or a history of skeletal malignancies; metabolic bone diseases other than osteoporosis; preexisting hypercalcemia; prior history of radiation therapy involving the skeleton; pediatric patients or young adults with open epiphyses; lactation; children 18 y and younger.
CAUTIOUS USE Active or recent urolithiasis, hypercalciuria; hypotension; concurrent use of digitalis; hepatic, renal, and cardiac disease; pregnancy (category C).

ROUTE & DOSAGE

Osteoporosis
Adult: **Subcutaneous** 20 mcg daily

ADMINISTRATION

Subcutaneous
- Do not administer to anyone with hypercalcemia. Consult physician.
- Rotate subcutaneous injection sites.

ADVERSE EFFECTS (≥1%) **Body as a Whole:** *Pain,* asthenia, neck pain. **CNS:** Headache, dizziness, depression, insomnia, vertigo. **CV:** Hypertension, angina, syncope. **GI:** Nausea, constipation, dyspepsia, vomiting. **Metabolic:** *Transient increase in calcium levels,* increase in serum uric acid, antibodies to teriparatide after 12 mo therapy. **Musculoskeletal:** *Arthralgia,* leg cramps. **Respiratory:** Rhinitis, cough, pharyngitis, dyspnea, pneumonia. **Skin:** Rash, sweating.

INTERACTIONS Drug: May increase risk of **digoxin** toxicity.

PHARMACOKINETICS Absorption: Extensively absorbed from subcutaneous site. **Onset:** 2 h for calcium concentration increase. **Peak:** Max calcium concentrations 4–6 h. **Duration:** 16–24 h. **Metabolism:** Parathyroid hormone is metabolized by nonspecific enzymes. **Elimination:** Primarily in urine. **Half-Life:** 1 h Subcutaneous.

NURSING IMPLICATIONS

Assessment & Drug Effects
- Monitor cardiovascular status including BP and subjective reports of angina.
- Lab tests: Monitor periodically serum calcium, alkaline phosphatase, uric acid and bone density levels.
- Concurrent drugs: Monitor closely for digoxin toxicity with concurrent use.

Patient & Family Education
- Report unexplained leg cramps and bone pain.
- Learn correct technique for subcutaneous injection.

T

TESTOSTERONE (Pr)
(tess-toss'ter-one)
Androderm, AndroGel, Striant, Testim

TESTOSTERONE CYPIONATE
Andro-Cyp, Depo-Testosterone, Depotest

TESTOSTERONE ENANTHATE
Delatest, Delatestryl, Malogex ♣

Classifications: ANDROGEN/ANABOLIC STEROID; ANTINEOPLASTIC
Therapeutic: ANTINEOPLASTIC; ANABOLIC STEROID
Pregnancy Category: X
Controlled Substance: Schedule III

AVAILABILITY Testosterone: 75 mg implantable pellets; 2.5 mg/24 h, 4 mg/24 h, 5 mg/24 h, 6 mg/24 h, transdermal patch; 1% gel; 2.5 g, 5 g gel packets; 30 mg buccal patch; **Testosterone Cypionate:** 100 mg/mL, 200 mg/mL injection; **Testosterone Enanthate:** 100 mg/mL, 200 mg/mL injection

ACTION & *THERAPEUTIC EFFECT* Synthetic steroid compound with both androgenic and anabolic activity. Controls development and maintenance of secondary sexual characteristics. **Androgenic activity:** Responsible for the growth spurt of the adolescent, onset of puberty, and for growth termination by epiphyseal closure. **Anabolic activity:** Increases protein metabolism and decreases its catabolism. Large doses suppress spermatogenesis, thereby causing testicular atrophy. *Antagonizes effects of estrogen excess on female breast and endometrium. Responsible for the growth spurt of the adolescent male and onset of puberty.*

USES Androgen replacement therapy, delayed puberty (male), palliation of female mammary cancer (1–5 y postmenopausal), and to treat postpartum breast engorgement. Available in fixed combination with estrogens in many preparations.

CONTRAINDICATIONS Hypersensitivity or toxic reactions to androgens; serious cardiac, liver, or kidney disease; hypercalcemia; known or suspected prostatic or breast cancer in male; benign prostatic hypertrophy with obstruction; patients easily stimulated sexually; older adults; asthenic males who may react adversely to androgenic overstimulation; conditions aggravated by fluid retention; hypertension; pregnancy (category X), possibility of virilization of external genitalia of female fetus, lactation.

CAUTIOUS USE Cardiac, liver, and kidney disease; prepubertal males; diabetes mellitus; history of MI; CAD; BPH; geriatric patients, acute intermittent porphyria.

ROUTE & DOSAGE

Male Hypogonadism

Adult: **IM Cypionate, Enanthate** 50–400 mg q2–4wk **Topical** Start with 6 mg/day system applied daily, if scrotal area inadequate, use 4 mg/day system; **Androderm** Apply to torso; **AndroGel** Apply one packet to upper arms, shoulders, or abdomen once daily; **Striant** Apply one patch to the gum region just above the incisor tooth q12h

Delayed Puberty

Adult: **IM Cypionate, Enanthate** 50–200 mg q2–4wk

Metastatic Breast Cancer

Adult: **IM Cypionate, Enanthate** 200–400 mg q2–4wk

ADMINISTRATION

Buccal

- Apply buccal patch to gum just above the incisor tooth.

Transdermal

- Apply transdermal system on clean, dry scrotal skin. Dry shave scrotal hair for optimal skin contact. Do not use chemical depilatories. Wear patch for 22–24 h.

- Apply Androderm patches to abdomen, back, thigh, or upper arm. Alternate application site q24h with 7 days or longer between same site.
- Store at 15°–30° C (59°–86° F).

Intramuscular

- Give IM injections deep into gluteal musculature.
- Store IM formulations prepared in oil at room temperature. Warming and shaking vial will redisperse precipitated crystals.

ADVERSE EFFECTS (≥1%) **CNS:** Excitation, insomnia. **CV:** Skin flushing and vascularization. **GI:** Nausea, vomiting, anorexia, diarrhea, gastric pain, jaundice. **Hematologic:** Leukopenia. **Metabolic:** Hypercalcemia, hypercholesterolemia, *sodium and water retention (especially in older adults) with edema*. **Renal:** Renal calculi (especially in the immobilized patient), bladder irritability. **Urogenital:** *Increased libido.* **Skin:** *Acne,* injection site irritation and sloughing. **Body as a Whole:** Hypersensitivity to testosterone, <u>anaphylactoid reactions</u> (rare). **Hematologic:** Precipitation of acute intermittent porphyria. **Endocrine:** Female—suppression of ovulation, lactation, or menstruation; hoarseness or deepening of voice (often irreversible); hirsutism; oily skin; clitoral enlargement; regression of breasts; male-pattern baldness (in disseminated breast cancer); flushing, sweating; vaginitis with pruritus, drying, bleeding; menstrual irregularities. Male—prepubertal-premature epiphyseal closure, phallic enlargement, priapism. Postpubertal—testicular atrophy, decreased ejaculatory volume, azoospermia, oligospermia (after prolonged administration or excessive dosage), impotence, epididymitis, priapism, *gynecomastia*.

DIAGNOSTIC TEST INTERFERENCE Testosterone alters ***glucose tolerance*** tests; decreases ***thyroxine-binding globulin concentration*** (resulting in decreased ***total*** T_4 serum levels and increased ***resin of*** T_3 and T_4). Increases ***creatinine*** and ***creatinine*** excretion (lasting up to 2 wk after therapy is discontinued) and alters response to ***metyrapone test.*** It suppresses ***clotting factors II, V, VII, X*** and decreases excretion of ***17-ketosteroids.*** May increase or decrease ***serum cholesterol.***

INTERACTIONS Drug: ORAL ANTICOAGULANTS may potentiate hypoprothrombinemia. May decrease **insulin** requirements.

PHARMACOKINETICS Absorption: **Cypionate** and **enanthate** are slowly absorbed from lipid tissue. **Duration:** 2–4 wk **cypionate** and **enanthate. Distribution:** 98% bound to sex hormone-binding globulin. **Metabolism:** Primarily in liver. **Elimination:** 90% in urine, 6% in feces. **Half-Life:** 10–100 min.

NURSING IMPLICATIONS

Assessment & Drug Effects

- Check I&O and weigh patient daily during dose adjustment period. Weight gain (due to sodium and water retention) suggests need for decreased dosage. When dosage is stabilized, urge patient to check weight at least twice weekly and to report increases, particularly if accompanied by edema in dependent areas. Dose adjustment and diuretic therapy may be started.
- Lab tests: Periodic serum cholesterol, serum electrolytes as well as liver function tests throughout therapy.
- Monitor serum calcium closely. Androgenic therapy is usually ter-

T

minated if serum calcium rises above 14 mg/dL.

- Report S&S of hypercalcemia (see Appendix F) promptly. The immobilized patient is particularly prone to develop hypercalcemia, which indicates progression of bone metastasis in patients with metastatic breast cancer. Treatment includes withdrawing testosterone and checking calcium, phosphate, and BUN levels daily.
- Instruct diabetic to report sweating, tremor, anxiety, vertigo. Testosterone-induced anabolic action enhances hypoglycemia (hyperinsulinism). Dosage adjustment of antidiabetic agent may be required.
- Observe patients on concomitant anticoagulant treatment for signs of overdosage (e.g., ecchymoses, petechiae). Report promptly to physician; anticoagulant dose may need to be reduced.
- Monitor prepubertal or adolescent males throughout therapy to avoid precocious sexual development and premature epiphyseal closure. Skeletal stimulation may continue 6 mo beyond termination of therapy.

Patient & Family Education

- Review directions for application of transdermal patches.
- Report soreness at injection site, because a postinjection site boil may be an associated adverse reaction.
- Report priapism (sustained and often painful erections occurring especially in early replacement therapy), reduced ejaculatory volume, and gynecomastia to physician. Symptoms indicate necessity for temporary withdrawal or discontinuation of testosterone therapy.
- Notify physician promptly if pregnancy is suspected or planned. Masculinization of the fetus is most likely to occur if testosterone (androgen) therapy is provided during first trimester of pregnancy.
- Androgens may cause virilism in women at dosage required to treat carcinoma. Report increase in libido (early sign of toxicity), growth of facial hair, deepening of voice, male-pattern baldness. The onset of hoarseness can easily be overlooked unless its significance as an early and possibly irreversible sign of virilism is appreciated. Reevaluation of treatment plan is indicated.

TETRACAINE HYDROCHLORIDE

(tet′ra-kane)

Pontocaine

Classification: LOCAL ANESTHETIC (ESTER TYPE)

Therapeutic: LOCAL ANESTHETIC

Prototype: Procaine HCl

Pregnancy Category: C

AVAILABILITY 0.2%, 0.3%, 1% injection; 20 mg powder; 2% solution; 1%, 2% cream; 2% gel; 1% ointment; 0.5% ophth solution

ACTION & *THERAPEUTIC EFFECT*
A potent and toxic local anesthetic that depresses initial depolarization phase of the action potential, thus preventing propagation and conduction of the nerve impulse. *Effectiveness indicated by loss of sensation and motor activity in circumscribed body areas close to injection or application site.*

USES Spinal anesthesia (high, low, saddle block) and topically to produce surface anesthesia. **Eye:** To anesthetize conjunctiva and cornea prior to superficial procedures (including tonometry, gonioscopy,

T

removal of foreign bodies or sutures, corneal scraping). **Nose and Throat:** To abolish laryngeal and esophageal reflexes prior to bronchoscopy, esophagoscopy. **Skin:** To relieve pruritus, pain, burning.

CONTRAINDICATIONS Older adult and debilitated patients; prolonged use of ophthalmic preparations; known hypersensitivity to tetracaine or other local anesthetics of ester type (e.g., procaine, chloroprocaine, cocaine), sulfite, or to PABA or its derivatives; coagulopathy; anticoagulant therapy; thrombocytopenia; increased bleeding time; infection at application or injection site.

CAUTIOUS USE Shock; cachexia, cardiac decompensation; QT prolongation; elderly; pregnancy (category C), lactation; children younger than 16 y.

ROUTE & DOSAGE

Local Anesthesia

Adult: **Topical** Before procedure, 1–2 drops of 0.5% solution or 1.25–2.5 cm of ointment in lower conjunctival fornix or 0.5% solution or ointment to nose or throat
Spinal 1% solution diluted with equal volume of 10% dextrose injected in subarachnoid space

T

ADMINISTRATION

Topical

- Avoid use of solutions that are cloudy, discolored, or crystallized.
- When tetracaine is used on mucosa of larynx, trachea, or esophagus, the manufacturer recommends adding 0.06 mL of a 0.1% epinephrine solution to each mL tetracaine solution to slow absorption of the anesthetic.
- Store ophthalmic solution and ointment at 15°–30° C (59°–86° F); refrigerate topical. Avoid freezing. Use tight, light-resistant containers.

ADVERSE EFFECTS (≥1%) **Body as a Whole:** Anaphylactic reactions, convulsions, faintness, syncope. **CNS:** Postspinal headache, headache, spinal nerve paralysis, anxiety, nervousness, seizures. **CV:** Bradycardia, arrhythmias, hypotension. **Special Senses:** Stinging; corneal erosion, retardation or prevention of healing of corneal abrasion, transient pitting and sloughing of corneal surface, dry corneal epithelium; dry mucous membranes, prolonged depression of cough reflex.

INTERACTIONS Drug: May antagonize effects of SULFONAMIDES.

PHARMACOKINETICS Onset: 1 min eye; 3 min mucosal surface; 3 min spinal. **Duration:** Up to 15 min eye; 30–60 min mucosal surface; 1.5–3 h spinal. **Metabolism:** In liver and plasma. **Elimination:** In urine.

NURSING IMPLICATIONS

Assessment & Drug Effects

- Recovery from anesthesia to the pharyngeal area is complete when patient has feeling in the hard and soft palates and when muscles in the faucial (tonsillar) pillars contract with stimulation.
- Do not give food or liquids until these normal pharyngeal responses are present (usually about 1 h after anesthetic administration). The first small amount of liquid (water) should be given under supervision of care provider.
- Be aware that increased blood concentration of the drug may result from excess application of tetracaine to the skin (to relieve pruritus or burning), application to debrided or infected skin surfaces, or too rapid injection rate.

- High blood concentrations of tetracaine can lead to adverse systemic effects involving CNS and CV systems: Convulsions, respiratory arrest, dysrhythmias, cardiac arrest.

Patient & Family Education

- Do not use ophthalmic drug longer than prescribed period. Prolonged use to eye surface may cause corneal epithelial erosions and retard healing of corneal surface.
- Natural barriers to eye infection and injury are removed by the anesthesia. Do not rub eye after drug instillation until anesthetic effect has dissipated (evidenced by return of blink reflex). Patching for temporary protection of the corneal epithelium may be ordered.
- Wash or disinfect hands before and after self-administration of solutions or ointment.

TETRACYCLINE HYDROCHLORIDE (Pr)

(tet-ra-sye'kleen)

Novotetra ♣, Sumycin

Classifications: ANTIBIOTIC; TETRACYCLINE

Therapeutic: ANTIBIOTIC

Pregnancy Category: D

AVAILABILITY 100 mg, 125 mg, 250 mg, 500 mg capsules; 125 mg/5 mL suspension

ACTION & *THERAPEUTIC EFFECT* Tetracyclines exert antiacne action by suppressing growth of *Propionibacterium acnes* within sebaceous follicles. *Effective against a variety of gram-positive and gram-negative bacteria and against most chlamydiae, mycoplasmas, rickettsiae, and certain protozoa (e.g., amebae). Exerts antiacne action by suppressing growth of* Propionibacterium acnes *within sebaceous follicles.*

USES Chlamydial infections (e.g., lymphogranuloma venereum, psittacosis, trachoma, inclusion conjunctivitis, nongonococcal urethritis); mycoplasmal infections (e.g., *Mycoplasma pneumoniae*); rickettsial infections (e.g., Q fever, Rocky Mountain spotted fever, typhus); spirochetal infections: Relapsing fever *(Borrelia)*, leptospirosis, syphilis (penicillin-hypersensitive patients); amebiases; uncommon gram-negative bacterial infections [e.g., brucellosis, shigellosis, cholera, gonorrhea (penicillin-hypersensitive patients), granuloma inguinale, tularemia]; gram-positive infections (e.g., tetanus). Also used orally (solution) for inflammatory acne vulgaris.

UNLABELED USES Actinomycosis, acute exacerbations of chronic bronchitis; Lyme disease; pericardial effusion (metastatic); acute PID; sexually transmitted epididymoorchitis; with quinine for multidrug-resistant strains of *Plasmodium falciparum* malaria; anti-infective prophylaxis for rape victims; recurrent cystic thyroid nodules; melioidosis; and as fluorescence test for malignancy.

CONTRAINDICATIONS Hypersensitivity to tetracyclines or to any ingredient in the formulation; severe renal or hepatic impairment, common bile duct obstruction; UV exposure; pregnancy (category D), infancy, children younger than 8 y.

CAUTIOUS USE History of kidney or liver dysfunction; myasthenia gravis; history of allergy, asthma, hay fever, urticaria; undernourished patients.

T

ROUTE & DOSAGE

Systemic Infection

Adult: **PO** 250–500 mg b.i.d.–q.i.d. (1–2 g/day)
Child (older than 8 y): **PO** 25–50 mg/kg/day in 2–4 divided doses

Acne

Adult/Child (older than 8 y): **PO** 500–1000 mg/day in 4 divided doses

ADMINISTRATION

Oral

- Give with a full glass of water on an empty stomach at least 1 h before or 2 h after meals (food, milk, and milk products can reduce absorption by 50% or more).
- Do not give immediately before bed.
- Give with food if patient is having GI symptoms (e.g., nausea, vomiting, anorexia); do not give with foods high in calcium such as milk or milk products.
- Shake suspension well before pouring to ensure uniform distribution of drug. Use calibrated liquid measure to dispense.
- Check expiration date for all tetracyclines. Fanconi-like syndrome (renal tubular dysfunction) and also an LE-like syndrome have been attributed to outdated tetracycline preparations.
- Tetracycline decomposes with age, exposure to light, and when improperly stored under conditions of extreme humidity, heat, or cold. The resultant product may be toxic.
- Store at 15°–30° C (59°–86° F) in tightly covered container in dry place. Protect from light.

ADVERSE EFFECTS (≥1%) **CNS:** Headache, intracranial hypertension (rare). **Special Senses:** Pigmentation of conjunctiva due to drug deposit. **GI:** Reported mostly for oral administration, but also may occur with parenteral tetracycline (*nausea, vomiting,* epigastric distress, heartburn, *diarrhea,* bulky loose stools, steatorrhea, *abdominal discomfort, flatulence,* dry mouth); dysphagia, retrosternal pain, esophagitis, esophageal ulceration with oral administration, abnormally high liver function test values, decrease in serum cholesterol, <u>fatty degeneration of liver [jaundice, increasing nitrogen retention (azotemia), hyperphosphatemia, acidosis, irreversible shock]</u>; foul-smelling stools or vaginal discharge, stomatitis, glossitis; black hairy tongue (lingua nigra), diarrhea: Staphylococcal enterocolitis. **Body as a Whole:** Drug fever, angioedema, serum sickness, <u>anaphylaxis</u>. **Urogenital:** Particularly in patients with kidney disease; increase in BUN/serum creatinine, renal impairment even with therapeutic doses; <u>Fanconi-like syndrome (outdated tetracycline)</u> (characterized by polyuria, polydipsia, nausea, vomiting, glycosuria, proteinuria acidosis, aminoaciduria); vulvovaginitis, pruritus vulvae or ani (possibly hypersensitivity). **Skin:** Dermatitis, *phototoxicity:* Discoloration of nails, onycholysis (loosening of nails); cheilosis; fixed drug eruptions particularly on genitalia; thrombocytopenic purpura; urticaria, rash, <u>exfoliative dermatitis</u>; with topical applications: Skin irritation, dry scaly skin, transient stinging or burning sensation, slight yellowing of skin at application site, acute contact dermatitis. **Other:** Pancreatitis, local reactions: Pain and irritation (IM site), Jarisch-Herxheimer reaction.

DIAGNOSTIC TEST INTERFERENCE

TETRACYCLINES may cause false increases in ***urinary catecholamines***

Common adverse effects in *italic*, life-threatening effects <u>underlined</u>; generic names in **bold**; classifications in SMALL CAPS; ♣ Canadian drug name; ⓟ Prototype drug

(by ***fluorometric methods***), and false decreases in ***urinary urobilinogen.*** Parenteral TETRACYCLINES containing ***ascorbic acid*** reportedly may produce false-positive ***urinary glucose*** determinations by ***copper reduction methods*** (e.g., ***Benedict's reagent, Clinitest***); TETRACYCLINES may cause false-negative results with ***glucose oxidase methods*** (e.g., ***Clinistix, TesTape***).

INTERACTIONS Drug: ANTACIDS, **calcium**, and **magnesium** bind tetracycline in gut and decrease absorption. ORAL ANTICOAGULANTS potentiate hypoprothrombinemia. ANTIDIARRHEAL AGENTS with **kaolin** and pectin may decrease absorption. Effectiveness of ORAL CONTRACEPTIVES decreased. **Methoxyflurane** may produce fatal nephrotoxicity. **Food:** Dairy products and **iron, zinc** supplements decrease tetracycline absorption.

PHARMACOKINETICS Absorption: 75–80% of dose absorbed. **Peak:** 2–4 h. **Distribution:** Widely distributed, preferentially binds to rapid growing tissues; crosses placenta; enters breast milk. **Metabolism:** Not metabolized; enterohepatic cycling. **Elimination:** 50–60% in urine within 72 h. **Half-Life:** 6–12 h.

NURSING IMPLICATIONS

Assessment & Drug Effects

- Lab tests: Baseline and periodic C&S, kidney function tests, LFTs, and hematopoietic function tests, particularly during high-dose, long-term therapy. Determine serum tetracycline levels in patients at-risk for hepatotoxicity (occurs most frequently in patients receiving other hepatotoxic drugs or with history of renal or hepatic impairment).
- Report GI symptoms (e.g., nausea, vomiting, diarrhea) to physician. These are generally dose-dependent, occurring mostly in patients receiving 2 g/day or more and during prolonged therapy. Frequently, symptoms are controlled by reducing dosage or administering with compatible foods.
- Be alert to evidence of superinfections (see Appendix F). Regularly inspect tongue and mucous membrane of mouth for candidiasis (thrush). Suspect superinfection if patient complains of irritation or soreness of mouth, tongue, throat, vagina, or anus, or persistent itching of any area, diarrhea, or foul-smelling excreta or discharge.
- Withhold drug and notify physician if superinfection develops. Superinfections occur most frequently in patients receiving prolonged therapy, the debilitated, or those who have diabetes.
- Monitor I&O in patients receiving parenteral tetracycline. Report oliguria or any changes in appearance of urine or in I&O.

Patient & Family Education

- Report onset of diarrhea to physician. It is important to determine whether diarrhea is due to irritating drug effect or superinfections or pseudomembranous colitis (caused by overgrowth of toxin-producing bacteria: *Clostridium difficile*) (see Appendix F). The latter two conditions can be life threatening and require immediate withdrawal of tetracycline and prompt initiation of symptomatic and supportive therapy.
- Reduce incidence of superinfection (see Appendix F) by meticulous care of mouth, skin, and perineal area. Rinse mouth of food debris after eating; floss daily and use a soft-bristled toothbrush.
- Avoid direct exposure to sunlight during and for several days after therapy is terminated to reduce

possibility of photosensitivity reaction (appearing like an exaggerated sunburn).

- Exercise caution with potentially hazardous activities until reaction to drug is known.
- Report immediately sudden onset of painful or difficult swallowing (dysphagia) to physician. Esophagitis and esophageal ulceration have been associated with bedtime administration of tetracycline capsules or tablets with insufficient fluid, particularly to patients with hiatal hernia or esophageal problems.
- Response to acne therapy usually requires 2–8 wk, maximal results may not be apparent for up to 12 wk.

TETRAHYDROZOLINE HYDROCHLORIDE

(tet-ra-hye-drozz'a-leen)

Collyrium, Mallazine, Murine Plus, Optigene, Soothe, Tyzine, Visine

Classifications: EYE AND NOSE PREPARATION; VASOCONSTRICTOR; DECONGESTANT

Therapeutic: NASAL DECONGESTANT; OCULAR VASOCONSTRICTOR

Prototype: Naphazoline

Pregnancy Category: C

AVAILABILITY 0.05% ophth solution; 0.05%, 0.1% nasal solution

ACTION & *THERAPEUTIC EFFECT* Alpha-adrenergic agonist that causes intense vasoconstriction when applied topically to mucous membranes, and when applied as eyedrops. *Ophthalmic solution is effective for allergic reactions of the eye; nasal solution is anti-inflammatory and also decreases allergic congestion.*

USES Symptomatic relief of minor eye irritation and allergies and for nasopharyngeal congestion of allergic or inflammatory origin.

CONTRAINDICATIONS Hypersensitivity to tetrahydrozoline or any component; use of ophthalmic preparation in glaucoma or other serious eye diseases; use within 14 days of MAO inhibitor therapy. Use in children younger than 2 y; use of 0.1% or higher strengths in children younger than 6 y.

CAUTIOUS USE Hypertension; cardiovascular disease; hyperthyroidism; diabetes mellitus; young children; pregnancy (category C), lactation.

ROUTE & DOSAGE

Decongestant

Adult: **Ophthalmic** See Appendix A-1 **Nasal** 2–4 drops of 0.1% solution or spray in each nostril q3h prn

Child: **Nasal** *2–6 y,* 2–4 drops of 0.05% solution or spray in each nostril q3h prn; *6 y or older,* same as adult

ADMINISTRATION

Instillation

- Make sure interval between doses is at least 4–6 h since drug action lasts 4–8 h.
- Place patient in upright position when using nasal spray. (If patient is reclining, a stream rather than a spray may be ejected, with consequent overdosage.)
- Use lateral, head-low position to administer nasal drops.

ADVERSE EFFECTS (≥1%) **Special Senses:** *Transient stinging,* irritation, *sneezing,* dryness, headache, tremors, drowsiness, lightheadedness, insomnia, palpitation. **Body as a Whole:** With overdose: Marked drowsiness, sweating, coma, hypotension, shock, bradycardia.

PHARMACOKINETICS Absorption: May be absorbed from nasal mucosa. **Duration:** 4–8 h.

NURSING IMPLICATIONS

Patient & Family Education

- Discontinue medication and consult physician if relief is not obtained within 48 h or if symptoms persist or increase.
- Do not exceed recommended dosage. Rebound congestion and rhinitis may occur with frequent or prolonged use of nasal preparation.

THALIDOMIDE

(tha-lid'o-mide)

Thalomid

Classifications: IMMUNOMODULATOR; TUMOR NECROSIS FACTOR (TNF) MODIFIER

Therapeutic: IMMUNOSUPPRESSIVE; TNF MODIFIER

Pregnancy Category: X

AVAILABILITY 50 mg capsules

ACTION & *THERAPEUTIC EFFECT* Anti-inflammatory effects may be due to its inhibition of neutrophil chemotaxis and decrease of monocyte phagocytosis. Immunosuppressive effect may result from suppression of excessive tumor necrosis factor-alpha (TNF-alpha) production. Also, reduces helper T cells and increases suppressor T cells. *Effectiveness indicated by control of cutaneous manifestations of erythema nodosum leprosum and/or improvement in Crohn's disease.*

USES Acute and maintenance treatment of cutaneous manifestations of moderate to severe erythema nodosum leprosum. Refractory Crohn's disease.

UNLABELED USES Stimulate appetite in patients with HIV-associated cachexia, lupus, multiple myeloma.

CONTRAINDICATIONS Hypersensitivity to thalidomide; peripheral neuropathy; pregnancy (category X), lactation, children younger than 11 y.

CAUTIOUS USE Liver and kidney disease; CHF or hypertension; constipation or other GI disorders; neurologic disorders or history of neuritis.

ROUTE & DOSAGE

Erythema Nodosum Leprosum

Adult: **PO** 100–300 mg daily (max: 400 mg/day) × at least 2 wk

Child (11–17 y): **PO** 100 mg daily

Refractory Crohn's Disease

Adult: **PO** 50–100 mg daily (doses up to 300 mg studied)

ADMINISTRATION

Oral

- Give at bedtime and at least 1 h after the evening meal.
- Give this drug only to persons who understand and have signed the required consent form.
- Verify, prior to administration, that this drug was prescribed and dispensed only by persons registered by the STEPS (System for Thalidomide Education and Prescribing Safety) program.

- Store at 15°–30° C (59°–86° F); protect from light.

ADVERSE EFFECTS (≥1%) **Body as a Whole:** Asthenia, back pain, chills, facial edema, *fever,* malaise, pain. **CNS:** Drowsiness, *somnolence,* peripheral neuropathy (possibly irreversible), *dizziness,* orthostatic hypotension, headache, agitation, insomnia, nervousness, paresthesia, tremor, vertigo, seizures. **CV:** Bradycardia, peripheral edema, hyperlipidemia. **GI:** Abdominal pain, anorexia, constipation, *diarrhea,* dry mouth, flatulence, abnormal liver function tests, nausea, oral moniliasis. **Hematologic:** Neutropenia, anemia, *leukopenia,* lymphadenopathy. **Respiratory:** Pharyngitis, rhinitis, sinusitis. **Skin:** *Rash,* acne, nail disorder, fungal dermatitis, pruritus, sweating, <u>toxic epidermal necrolysis</u>. **Body as a Whole:** Hypersensitivity reaction (rash, fever, tachycardia, hypotension), HIV viral load increase, infection. **Urogenital:** Teratogenicity, albuminuria, hematuria, impotence.

INTERACTIONS Drug: Enhances sedation associated with BARBITURATES, **alcohol, chlorpromazine, reserpine.**

PHARMACOKINETICS Absorption: Slowly absorbed from GI tract. **Peak:** 2.9–5.7 h. **Distribution:** Crosses placenta; present in ejaculate in males. **Metabolism:** Does not appear to be hepatically metabolized. **Half-Life:** 6–7.5 h.

T

NURSING IMPLICATIONS

Assessment & Drug Effects

- Lab tests: Monitor WBC with differential prior to therapy and periodically thereafter.
- Monitor carefully for and immediately report S&S of peripheral neuropathy. Discontinue drug and notify prescriber if peripheral neuropathy is suspected.

Patient & Family Education

- Do not share this medication with anyone else under any circumstances.
- Use effective methods of birth control (both women and men); starting 1 mo before, during, and 1 mo following discontinuation of thalidomide therapy. Men **MUST** use condoms when engaging in sexual activity to prevent birth defects.
- Exercise caution while driving or engaging in potentially hazardous activities because drug may cause dizziness.
- Report pain, numbness, or tingling in the hands or feet to physician immediately.

THEOPHYLLINE (Pr)

(thee-off'i-lin)

Elixophyllin, Lanophyllin, PMS Theophylline ♣, Pulmophylline ♣, Theo-24, Theolair, Theophylline Ethylenediamine, Theospan-SR, Uniphyl

Classifications: BRONCHODILATOR (RESPIRATORY SMOOTH MUSCLE RELAXANT); XANTHINE

Therapeutic: BRONCHODILATOR

Pregnancy Category: C

AVAILABILITY 100 mg, 125 mg, 200 mg, 250 mg, 300 mg tablets; 100 mg, 200 mg capsules; 80 mg/15 mL, 150 mg/15 mL liquid; 100 mg, 200 mg, 250 mg, 300 mg, 450 mg, 500 mg, 600 mg sustained release tablets; 50 mg, 75 mg, 100 mg, 125 mg, 200 mg, 250 mg, 260 mg, 300 mg sustained release capsules; 200 mg, 400 mg, 800 mg injection

ACTION & *THERAPEUTIC EFFECT* Xanthine derivative that relaxes smooth muscle by direct action, particularly of bronchi and pulmonary vessels, and stimulates medullary respiratory center with resulting increase in vital capacity. *Effective for relief of bronchospasm in asthmatics, chronic bronchitis, and emphysema.*

USES Prophylaxis and symptomatic relief of bronchial asthma, as well as bronchospasm associated with chronic bronchitis and emphysema. Also used for emergency treatment of paroxysmal cardiac dyspnea and edema of CHF.

UNLABELED USES Treatment of apnea and bradycardia of premature infants and to reduce severe bronchospasm associated with cystic fibrosis and acute descending respiratory infection.

CONTRAINDICATIONS Hypersensitivity to xanthines; coronary artery disease or angina pectoris when myocardial stimulation might be harmful; severe renal or liver impairment.

CAUTIOUS USE Compromised cardiac or circulatory function, hypertension; acute pulmonary edema; multiple organ failure; CHF; hyperthyroidism; peptic ulcer; prostatic hypertrophy; glaucoma; diabetes mellitus; older adults; pregnancy (category C), lactation; children, and neonates.

ROUTE & DOSAGE

Bronchospasm

Adult/Child: **PO/IV Loading Dose** 5 mg/kg
Adult: **PO/IV Maintenance Dose*** *Nonsmoker,* 0.4 mg/kg/h; *Smoker,* 0.6 mg/kg/h; *with CHF or cirrhosis,* 0.2 mg/kg/h
Child: **PO/IV Maintenance Dose*** *1–9 y,* 0.8 mg/kg/h; *10–12 y,* 0.6 mg/kg/h
Infant: **PO/IV Maintenance Dose*** 0.5–0.7 mg/kg/h
Neonate: **PO/IV Maintenance Dose*** 0.13 mg/kg/h
*IV by continuous infusion, PO divided q6h (immediate release) or q8–12h (sustained release)

Obesity Dosage Adjustment

Dose based on IBW.

ADMINISTRATION

Note: All doses based on ideal body weight.

Oral

- Wait 4–6 h after the last IV dose, when switching from IV to oral dosing.
- Give with a full glass of water and after meals to minimize gastric irritation.
- Give sustained release forms and enteric-coated tablets whole. Chewable tablets **must be** chewed thoroughly before swallowing. Sustained release granules from capsules can be taken on an empty stomach or mixed with applesauce or water.
- Note: Timing of dose is critical. Be certain patient understands necessity to adhere to the correct intervals between doses.

Intravenous

PREPARE: **Direct/Intermittent:** Dilute, as needed, to a maximum concentration of 20 mg/mL. **IV Infusion:** Typically diluted to 0.8 mg/mL with D5W.

ADMINISTER: **Direct/Intermittent:** Typically infused over 20–30 min. DO NOT EXCEED 20 mg/min. **IV Infusion:** Infuse at a rate based on patient's weight.

INCOMPATIBILITIES **Solution/additive:** **Ascorbic acid, ceftriaxone, cimetidine, hetastarch. Y-site: Hetastarch, phenytoin.**

T

ADVERSE EFFECTS (≥1%) **CNS:** Stimulation (irritability, restlessness, insomnia, dizziness, headache, tremor, hyperexcitability, muscle twitching, drug-induced seizures). **CV:** Palpitation, *tachycardia,* extrasystoles, flushing, marked hypotension, circulatory failure. **GI:** *Nausea,* vomiting, anorexia, epigastric or abdominal pain, diarrhea, activation of peptic ulcer. **Urogenital:** Transient urinary frequency, albuminuria, kidney irritation. **Respiratory:** Tachypnea, respiratory arrest. **Body as a Whole:** Fever, dehydration.

DIAGNOSTIC TEST INTERFERENCE False-positive elevations of ***serum uric acid*** (***Bittner*** or ***colorimetric*** methods). ***Probenecid*** may cause false high ***serum theophylline*** readings, and spectrophotometric methods of determining ***serum theophylline*** are affected by a furosemide, sulfathiazole, phenylbutazone, probenecid, theobromine.

INTERACTIONS Drug: Increases **lithium** excretion, lowering lithium levels; **cimetidine,** high-dose **allopurinol** (600 mg/day), **tacrine,** QUINOLONES, MACROLIDE ANTIBIOTICS, and **zileuton** can significantly increase theophylline levels; **tobacco** use significantly decreases levels. **Herbal: St. John's wort** may decrease theophylline efficacy. **Daidzein** (in soy), **black pepper** increase serum concentrations and adverse effects.

T

PHARMACOKINETICS Absorption: Most products are 100% absorbed from GI tract. **Peak:** IV 30 min; uncoated tablet 1 h; sustained release 4–6 h. **Duration:** 4–8 h; varies with age, smoking, and liver function. **Distribution:** Crosses placenta. **Metabolism:** Extensively in liver. **Elimination:** Parent drug and metabolites excreted by kidneys; excreted in breast milk.

NURSING IMPLICATIONS

Assessment & Drug Effects

- Monitor vital signs. Improvement in respiratory status is the expected outcome.
- Observe and report early signs of possible toxicity: Anorexia, nausea, vomiting, dizziness, shakiness, restlessness, abdominal discomfort, irritability, palpitation, tachycardia, marked hypotension, cardiac arrhythmias, seizures.
- Monitor for tachycardia, which may be worse in patients with severe cardiac disease. Conversely, theophylline toxicity may be masked in patients with tachycardia.
- Lab tests: Monitor plasma level of theophylline. Be aware that therapeutic plasma level ranges from 10–20 mcg/mL (a narrow therapeutic range). Levels exceeding 20 mcg/mL are associated with toxicity.
- Monitor drug levels closely in heavy smokers. Cigarette smoking induces hepatic microsomal enzyme activity, decreasing serum half-life and increasing body clearance of theophylline. An increase of dosage from 50–100% is usual in heavy smokers.
- Monitor plasma drug level closely in patients with heart failure, kidney or liver dysfunction, alcoholism, high fever. Plasma clearance of xanthines may be reduced.
- Take necessary safety precautions and forewarn older adult patients of possible dizziness during early therapy.
- Monitor patients on sustained release preparations for S&S of overdosage. Continued slow absorption leads to high plasma concentrations for a prolonged period.

- Note: Neonates of mothers using this drug have exhibited slight tachycardia, jitteriness, and apnea.
- Monitor **CLOSELY** for adverse effects in infants younger than 6 mo and prematures; theophylline metabolism is prolonged as is the half-life in this age group.

Patient & Family Education

- Take medication at the same time every day.
- Avoid charcoal-broiled foods (high in polycyclic carbon content); may increase theophylline elimination and reduce the half-life as much as 50%.
- Limit caffeine intake because it may increase incidence of adverse effects.
- Cigarette smoking may significantly lower theophylline plasma concentration.
- Be aware that a low-carbohydrate, high-protein diet increases theophylline elimination, and a high-carbohydrate, low-protein diet decreases it.
- Drink fluids liberally (2000–3000 mL/day) if not contraindicated to decrease viscosity of airway secretions.
- Avoid self-dosing with OTC medications, especially cough suppressants, which may cause retention of secretions and CNS depression.

THIAMINE HYDROCHLORIDE (VITAMIN B_1)

(thye′a-min)

Classification: VITAMIN B_1
Therapeutic: VITAMIN B_1 REPLACEMENT THERAPY
Pregnancy Category: A; C if dose is above RDA

AVAILABILITY 50 mg, 100 mg, 250 mg tablets; 20 mg enteric-coated tablet; 100 mg/mL injection

ACTION & *THERAPEUTIC EFFECT* Water-soluble B_1 vitamin and member of B-complex group used for thiamine replacement therapy. Functions as an essential coenzyme in carbohydrate metabolism and has a role in conversion of tryptophan to nicotinamide. *Effectiveness is evidenced by improvement of clinical manifestations of thiamine deficiency (e.g., anorexia, depression, loss of memory, etc.).*

USES Treatment and prophylaxis of beriberi, to correct anorexia due to thiamine deficiency states, and in treatment of neuritis associated with pregnancy, pellagra, and alcoholism, including Wernicke-Korsakoff syndrome. Therapy generally includes other members of vitamin B complex, since thiamine deficiency rarely occurs alone. Severe deficiency is characterized by ophthalmoplegia, polyneuropathy, muscle wasting ("dry" beriberi), edema, serous effusions, and CHF ("wet" beriberi).

CAUTIOUS USE Pregnancy (category A; category C if above RDA).

ROUTE & DOSAGE

Thiamine Deficiency

Adult: **IV/IM** 50–100 mg t.i.d., then 5–10 mg PO for 1 mo
Child: **IV/IM** 10–25 mg t.i.d. then, 5–10 mg PO for 1 mo

Alcohol Withdrawal

Adult: **IV/IM** 100 mg/day until PO 50–100 mg/day as tolerated

Wernicke's Encephalopathy

Adult: **IV/IM** 100 mg/day then 50–100 mg/day until on normal diet

T

Dietary Supplement
Adult: **PO** 15–30 mg/day
Child: **PO** 10–50 mg/day

ADMINISTRATION

Oral

- Do not crush or chew enteric-coated tablets. These **must be** swallowed whole.

Intramuscular

- Give deep IM into a large muscle; may be painful. Rotate sites and apply cold compresses to area if necessary for relief of discomfort.

Intravenous

Note: Intradermal test dose is recommended prior to administration in suspected thiamine sensitivity. Deaths have occurred following IV use.

PREPARE: **Direct:** Give undiluted. **IV Infusion:** Diluted in 1000 mL of most IV solutions.

ADMINISTER: **Direct:** Give at a rate of 100 mg over 5 min. **IV Infusion:** Give at the ordered rate.

INCOMPATIBILITIES **Solution/additive: Amobarbital, diazepam, furosemide, phenobarbital.**

- Preserve in tight, light-resistant, nonmetallic containers. Thiamine is unstable in alkaline solutions (e.g., solutions of acetates, barbiturates, bicarbonates, carbonates, citrates) and neutral solutions.

ADVERSE EFFECTS (≥1%) **Body as a Whole:** Feeling of warmth, weakness, sweating, restlessness, tightness of throat, angioneurotic edema, <u>anaphylaxis</u>. **Respiratory:** Cyanosis, pulmonary edema. **CV:** <u>Cardiovascular collapse</u>, slight fall in BP following rapid IV administration. **GI:** GI hemorrhage, nausea. **Skin:** Urticaria, pruritus.

INTERACTIONS Drug: No clinically significant interactions established.

PHARMACOKINETICS Absorption: Limited from GI tract. **Distribution:** Widely distributed, including into breast milk. **Elimination:** In urine.

NURSING IMPLICATIONS

Assessment & Drug Effects

- Record patient's dietary history carefully as an essential part of vitamin replacement therapy. Collaborate with physician, dietitian, patient, and responsible family member in developing a diet teaching plan that can be sustained by patient.

Patient & Family Education

- Food–drug relationships: Learn about rich dietary sources of thiamine (e.g., yeast, pork, beef, liver, wheat and other whole grains, nutrient-added breakfast cereals, fresh vegetables, especially peas and dried beans).
- Body requirement of thiamine is directly proportional to carbohydrate intake and metabolic rate; requirement increases when diet consists predominantly of carbohydrates.

THIOGUANINE (TG, 6-THIOGUANINE)

(thye-oh-gwah′neen)
Lanvis ✦, Tabloid
Classifications: ANTINEOPLASTIC; ANTIMETABOLITE; PURINE ANTAGONIST
Therapeutic: ANTINEOPLASTIC
Prototype: Mercaptopurine
Pregnancy Category: D

AVAILABILITY 40 mg tablets

ACTION & *THERAPEUTIC EFFECT* Antimetabolite and purine antagonist with immunosuppressive activity. Drug is incorporated into the DNA and RNA of human bone marrow cells. *Delays myelosuppression; has potential mutagenic and carcinogenic properties.*

USES In combination with other antineoplastics for remission induction in acute myelogenous leukemia and as treatment of chronic myelogenous leukemia. Has little advantage over mercaptopurine.

CONTRAINDICATIONS Patients with prior resistance to this drug; severe bone marrow depression; pregnancy (category D), lactation.
CAUTIOUS USE Hepatic disease.

ROUTE & DOSAGE

Leukemia
Adult: **PO** 2 mg/kg/day, may increase to 3 mg/kg/day if no response after 4 wk

ADMINISTRATION

Oral
- Withhold drug and notify physician if toxicity develops. There is no known antagonist; prompt discontinuation of the drug is essential to avoid irreversible myelosuppression from toxicity.
- Store at 15°–30° C (59°–86° F) in airtight container.

ADVERSE EFFECTS (≥1%) **Hematologic:** Leukopenia, thrombocytopenia, anemia. **GI:** Jaundice, nausea, vomiting, anorexia, stomatitis, diarrhea. **Urogenital:** *Hyperuricemia.* **Other:** Hepatotoxicity (risk increased with long-term use).

INTERACTIONS Drug: Severe hepatotoxicity with **busulfan;** may decrease immune response to VACCINES; increase risk of bleeding with ANTICOAGULANTS; NSAIDS, SALICYLATES; PLATELET INHIBITORS, THROMBOLYTIC AGENTS; effects may be reversed by **filgrastim, sargramostim.**

PHARMACOKINETICS Absorption: Variable and incomplete absorption from GI tract. **Peak:** 8 h. **Distribution:** Crosses placenta. **Metabolism:** In liver. **Elimination:** In urine. **Half-Life:** 11 h.

NURSING IMPLICATIONS

Assessment & Drug Effects
- Lab tests: Monitor blood counts weekly (CBC with differential and platelet count); periodic LFTs with long-term use.
- Determine hematologic parameters for withholding drug.
- Monitor I&O ratio and report oliguria.
- Observe patient's skin and sclera for jaundice. It should be reported promptly as a symptom of toxicity; drug will be discontinued promptly.
- Expect that the drop in leukocyte count may be slow over a period of 2–4 wk. Treatment is interrupted if there is a rapid fall within a few days.

Patient & Family Education
- Maintenance doses are continued throughout remissions.

THIOPENTAL SODIUM (Pr)
(thye-oh-pen'tal)
Pentothal
Classifications: GENERAL ANESTHETIC; BARBITURATE; SEDATIVE-HYPNOTIC
Therapeutic: GENERAL ANESTHETIC; SEDATIVE-HYPNOTIC; ANTICONVULSIVE
Pregnancy Category: C
Controlled Substance: Schedule III

AVAILABILITY 20 mg/mL, 25 mg/mL injection

ACTION & *THERAPEUTIC EFFECT* Ultrashort-acting barbiturate that induces brief general anesthesia and hyposis without analgesia by depression of neuronal activity in the CNS. Rapid redistribution of agent out of brain reduces anesthesia level and increases reflex airway hyperactivity to mechanical stimulation. *Muscle relaxation is slight, and reflexes are poorly controlled. Since analgesia is slight, thiopental is seldom used alone except for brief minor procedures. Effective in controlling seizure activity as well as increased intracranial pressure (ICP).*

USES To induce hypnosis and anesthesia prior to or as supplement to other anesthetic agents or as sole agent for brief (15-min) operative procedures. Also used as an anticonvulsant and sedative-hypnotic and for narcoanalysis and narcosynthesis in psychiatric disorders.

CONTRAINDICATIONS Hypersensitivity to barbiturates; history of paradoxic excitation; status asthmaticus; acute intermittent or other hepatic porphyrias.

CAUTIOUS USE Coronary artery disease, hypotension, shock; conditions that may potentiate or prolong hypnotic effect including excessive premedication, liver or kidney dysfunction, myxedema, Addison's disease, severe anemia, increased BUN; increased intracranial pressure; myasthenia gravis; asthma and other respiratory diseases; pregnancy (category C).

ROUTE & DOSAGE

Induction

Adult: **IV Test Dose** 25–75 mg, then 50–75 mg at 20–40 sec intervals, an additional 50 mg may be given if needed

Child: **IV** 5–6 mg/kg initially, followed by 1 mg/kg if needed

Infant: **IV** 5–8 mg/kg

Convulsions

Adult: **IV** 75–250 mg, repeat as needed

Child: **IV** 2–3 mg/kg/dose, repeat as needed

Narcoanalysis

Adult: **IV** 100 mg/min until confusion occurs

Renal Impairment Dosage Adjustment

If CrCl less than 10 mL/min, give 75% of dose.

ADMINISTRATION

Intravenous

Note: Verify correct IV concentration and rate of infusion to neonates, infants, children with physician.

- *Test dose:* May be given to assess unusual sensitivity to drug. Following administration, observe patient for at least 1 min for unexpected deep anesthesia or respiratory depression.

PREPARE: **Direct:** Reconstitute each 500 mg of powder by adding at least 20 mL of sterile water for injection to yield a 2.5% solution (25 mg/1 mL). **Continuous:** May be further diluted for infusion by adding 20 mL of reconstituted solution to at least 100 mL of NS or D5W. ▪ Prepare solution freshly and use promptly. If a precipitate is present, discard solution. ▪ Unused portions should be discarded within 24 h.

ADMINISTER: **Direct:** Infuse each 25 mg over 1 min or more. **Continuous:** Titrate to achieve desired result.

T

INCOMPATIBILITIES Solution/additive: **Dextrose lactated Ringer's, 10% dextrose, fructose 10%, lactated Ringer's injection, amikacin, calcium chloride, calcium gluconate, cephalothin, cephapirin, chloramphenicol, chlorpromazine, cimetidine, clindamycin, codeine phosphate, dimenhydrinate, diphenhydramine, doxapram, ephedrine, fibrinolysin, glycopyrrolate, heparin, hydromorphone, insulin, levorphanol, meperidine, metaraminol, methadone, methicillin, morphine, norepinephrine, penicillin G, prochlorperazine, promazine, promethazine, sodium bicarbonate, succinylcholine, tetracycline, vancomycin.** Y-site: **Alfentanil, ascorbic acid, atracurium, atropine, cisatracurium, diltiazem, dobutamine, dopamine, ephedrine, epinephrine, fenoldopam, furosemide, hydromorphone, labetalol, lidocaine, lorazepam, midazolam, morphine, nicardipine, norepinephrine, pancuronium, phenylephrine, succinylcholine, sufentanil, vecuronium.**

▪ Consult physician if intra-arterial injection or extravasation occurs. The extravasation site will require particular attention to prevent arteritis, neuritis, and skin slough. ▪ An intra-arterial injection usually causes extreme pain before patient loses consciousness.

▪ Store at 15°–30° C (59°–86° F). Avoid excessive heat; protect from freezing.

ADVERSE EFFECTS (≥1%) **CNS:** Headache, retrograde amnesia, emergence delirium, prolonged somnolence and recovery. **CV:** Myocardial depression, arrhythmias, circulatory depression. **GI:** Nausea, vomiting, regurgitation of gastric contents, rectal irritation, cramping, rectal bleeding, diarrhea. **Respiratory:** Respiratory depression with apnea; hiccups, sneezing, coughing, bronchospasm, laryngospasm. **Body as a Whole:** Hypersensitivity reactions, anaphylaxis (rare), hypothermia, thrombosis and sloughing (with extravasation); salivation, shivering, skeletal muscle hyperactivity.

DIAGNOSTIC TEST INTERFERENCE ***Thiopental*** may cause decrease in ***I^{123} and I^{131} thyroidal uptake*** test results.

INTERACTIONS Drug: CNS DEPRESSANTS, **alcohol** potentiate CNS and respiratory depression. PHENOTHIAZINES increase risk of hypotension. **Probenecid** may prolong anesthesia. **Herbal: Kava, valerian** may potentiate sedation.

PHARMACOKINETICS Onset: 30–60 sec. **Duration:** 10–30 min. **Distribution:** Distributed into muscle and liver; crosses placenta. **Metabolism:** In liver. **Elimination:** In urine. **Half-Life:** 12 min.

NURSING IMPLICATIONS

Assessment & Drug Effects

- Monitor vital signs q3–5min before, during, and after anesthetic administration until recovery and into postoperative period, if necessary.
- Report increases in pulse rate or drop in blood pressure. Hypovolemia, cranial trauma, or premedication with opioids increases potential for apnea and symptoms of myocardial depression (decreased cardiac output and arterial pressure).

T

- Shivering, excitement, muscle twitching may develop during recovery period if patient is in pain.

Patient & Family Education

- Onset of drug effect is rapid, with loss of consciousness within 30–60 sec.

THIORIDAZINE HYDROCHLORIDE

(thye-o-rid'a-zeen)

Novoridazine ♣

Classification: PHENOTHIAZINE ANTIPSYCHOTIC

Therapeutic: ANTIPSYCHOTIC

Prototype: Chlorpromazine

Pregnancy Category: C

AVAILABILITY 10 mg, 15 mg, 25 mg, 50 mg, 100 mg, 150 mg, 200 mg tablets; 30 mg/mL, 100 mg/mL solution; 25 mg/5 mL suspension

ACTION & *THERAPEUTIC EFFECT* Thioridazine blocks postsynaptic dopamine receptors in the mesolimbic system of the brain. The decrease in dopamine neurotransmission has been found to correlate to antipsychotic effects. *Effective in reducing excitement, hypermotility, abnormal initiative, affective tension, and agitation by inhibiting psychomotor functions. Also effective as an antipsychotic agent, and for behavioral disorders in children.*

USES Management of nonpsychotic behavioral disturbances of senility, manifestations of psychotic disorders, alcohol withdrawal; symptomatic treatment of organic brain disease. Short-term treatment of moderate to marked depression and for management of hyperkinetic behavior syndrome (attention deficit disorder).

CONTRAINDICATIONS Hypersensitivity to phenothiazines. Severe CNS depression; CV disease; family history of QT prolongation; suicidal ideation; children younger than 2 y; lactation.

CAUTIOUS USE Premature ventricular contractions; previously diagnosed breast cancer; patients exposed to extremes in heat or to organophosphorus insecticides; history of suicidal ideation; Parkinson's disease; seizure disorders; closed-angle glaucoma; respiratory disorders; pregnancy (category C).

ROUTE & DOSAGE

Psychotic Disorders

Adult: **PO** 50–100 mg t.i.d., may increase up to 800 mg/day as needed or tolerated
Geriatric: **PO** 10 mg t.i.d., may increase up to 200 mg/day
Child (older than 2 y): **PO** 0.5–3 mg/kg/day in divided doses; if hospitalized, may start at 25 mg t.i.d.

Moderate to Marked Depression

Adult: **PO** 25 mg t.i.d., may increase up to 200 mg/day in divided doses

Dementia Behavior

Geriatric: **PO** 10–25 mg 1–2 times/day, may increase q4–7days (max: 400 mg/day in divided doses)

Pharmacogenetic Dosage Adjustment

Poor CYP2D6 metabolizers: Start with 40% of dose

ADMINISTRATION

Oral

- Give with fluid of patient's choice; tablet may be crushed.

- Schedule phenothiazine at least 1 h before or 1 h after an antacid or antidiarrheal medication.
- Dilute liquid concentrate just prior to administration with 1/2 glass of fruit juice, milk, water, carbonated beverage, or soup.
- Add increases in dose to the first dose of the day to prevent sleep disturbance.
- Store at 15°–30° C (59°–86° F) in tightly covered, light-resistant containers unless otherwise indicated.

ADVERSE EFFECTS (≥1%) **CNS:** *Sedation,* dizziness, drowsiness, lethargy, extrapyramidal syndrome, nocturnal confusion, hyperactivity. **Special Senses:** Nasal congestion, blurred vision, pigmentary retinopathy. **GI:** Xerostomia, *constipation,* paralytic ileus. **Urogenital:** Amenorrhea, breast engorgement, gynecomastia, galactorrhea, *urinary retention.* **CV:** Ventricular dysrhythmias, hypotension, prolonged QT_c interval.

INTERACTIONS Drug: Alcohol, ANXIOLYTICS, SEDATIVE-HYPNOTICS, other CNS DEPRESSANTS add to CNS depression; additive adverse effects with other PHENOTHIAZINES; **amiodarone, amoxapine, arsenic trioxide, bepridil, clarithromycin, daunorubicin, diltiazem, disopyramide, dofetilide, dolasetron, doxorubicin, encainide, erythromycin, flecainide, fluoxetine, fluvoxamine gatifloxacin, grepafloxacin, haloperidol, ibutilide, indapamide, local anesthetics, maprotiline, moxifloxacin, octreotide, paroxetine, pentamidine, pimozide, procainamide, probucol, quinidine, risperidone, sotalol, sertraline, sparfloxacin, terodiline, tocainide, tricyclic antidepressants, venlafaxine, verapamil, ziprasidone** can prolong QT_c interval resulting in arrhythmias. **Herbal: Kava** may increase risk and severity of dystonic reactions.

PHARMACOKINETICS Absorption: Well absorbed from GI tract. **Onset:** Days to weeks. **Distribution:** Crosses placenta; distributed into breast milk. **Metabolism:** In liver (CYP-2D6). **Elimination:** In urine. **Half-Life:** 26–36 h.

NURSING IMPLICATIONS

Assessment & Drug Effects

- Monitor for changes in behavior that may indicate increased possibility of suicide ideation.
- Orthostatic hypotension may occur in early therapy. Female patients appear to be more susceptible than males.
- Be aware that patients may be unable to adjust to extremes of temperature because drug effects heat regulatory center in the hypothalamus. Patient may complain of being cold even at average room temperature; older adults are particularly susceptible.
- Monitor I&O ratio and bowel elimination pattern. Check for abdominal distention and pain. Encourage adequate fluid intake as prophylaxis for constipation and xerostomia. The depressed patient may not seek help for either symptom or for urinary retention.
- Lab tests: Obtain periodic CBC and liver function tests during therapy.

Patient & Family Education

- Exercise care not to spill drug on skin because of danger of contact dermatitis. Wash skin well in soap and water if liquid drug is spilled.
- Take drug as prescribed and do not alter dosing regimen or stop medication without consulting physician.

- Avoid alcohol during phenothiazine therapy. Concomitant use enhances CNS depression effects.
- Be aware that marked drowsiness generally subsides with continued therapy or reduction in dosage.
- Do not drive or engage in potentially hazardous activities until response to drug is known.
- Make position changes slowly, particularly from lying down to upright posture; dangle legs a few minutes before standing.
- Vasodilation produced by hot showers or baths or by long exposure to environmental heat may accentuate hypotensive effect.
- Report the onset of any change in visual acuity, brownish coloring of vision, or impairment of night vision to physician. An ophthalmic consultation may be indicated.
- Note: Thioridazine may color urine pink-red to reddish brown.
- Do not use any OTC drugs unless approved by the physician.

THIOTEPA

(thye-oh-tep′a)

Classifications: ANTINEOPLASTIC; ALKYLATING AGENT
Therapeutic: ANTINEOPLASTIC
Prototype: Cyclophosphamide
Pregnancy Category: D

T

AVAILABILITY 15 mg, 30 mg injection

ACTION & *THERAPEUTIC EFFECT* Cell-cycle nonspecific alkylating agent that selectively reacts with DNA phosphate groups to produce chromosome cross-linkage and consequent blocking of nucleoprotein synthesis. Highly toxic hematopoietic agent. *Myelosuppression is cumulative and unpredictable and may be delayed.*

USES To produce remissions in malignant lymphomas, including Hodgkin's disease, and adenocarcinoma of breast and ovary. Also in chronic granulocytic and lymphocytic leukemia, superficial papillary carcinoma of urinary bladder, bronchogenic carcinoma, and in malignant effusions secondary to neoplastic disease of serosal cavities.
UNLABELED USES Prevention of pterygium recurrences following postoperative beta-irradiation; leukemia, malignant meningeal neoplasms.

CONTRAINDICATIONS Hypersensitivity to drug; acute leukemia; acute infection; pregnancy (category D), lactation.
CAUTIOUS USE Chronic lymphocytic leukemia; myelosuppression produced by radiation; bone marrow invasion by tumor cells; impaired kidney or liver function.

ROUTE & DOSAGE

Malignant Lymphomas

Adult: **IV** 0.3–0.4 mg/kg q1–4wk **Intracavitary** 0.6–0.8 mg/kg instilled through same tubing used for paracentesis at intervals of at least 1 wk **Intravesicular** 60 mg in 30–60 mL of distilled water instilled into bladder to be retained for 2 h once/wk for 4 wk **Intrathecal** 1–11.5 mg/m^2 1–2 times/wk
Child: **IV** 25–65 mg/m^2/dose every 21 days

ADMINISTRATION

Intravenous

Use only under constant supervision by physicians experienced in therapy with cytotoxic agents.

- Avoid exposure of skin and respiratory tract to particles of thiotepa during solution preparation.

PREPARE: **Direct:** Reconstitute each 15 mg vial with 1.5 mL sterile water for injection (supplied) to yield 10 mg/mL. ▪ Filter solution through a 0.22 micron filter to eliminate haze. Use immediately.

ADMINISTER: **Direct:** Give 60 mg or fraction thereof over 1 min.

INCOMPATIBILITIES **Solution/additive: Cisplatin. Y-site: Cisplatin, filgrastim, minocycline, vinorelbine.**

- Store powder for injection and reconstituted solutions at 2°–8° C (35°–46° F); protect from light. ▪ Solutions reconstituted with sterile water only are stable for 8 h under refrigeration.

ADVERSE EFFECTS (≥1%) **GI:** Anorexia, nausea, vomiting, stomatitis, ulceration of intestinal mucosa. **Hematologic:** Leukopenia, thrombocytopenia, anemia, pancytopenia. **Skin:** Hives, rash, pruritus. **Urogenital:** Amenorrhea, interference with spermatogenesis. **Body as a Whole:** Headache, febrile reactions, pain and weeping of injection site, hyperuricemia, slowed or lessened response in heavily irradiated area, sensation of throat tightness. **Other:** Reported with intravesical administration (lower abdominal pain, hematuria, hemorrhagic chemical cystitis, vesical irritability).

INTERACTIONS Drug: May prolong muscle paralysis with **mivacurium;** ANTICOAGULANTS, NSAIDS, SALICYLATES, ANTIPLATELET AGENTS may increase risk of bleeding.

PHARMACOKINETICS Absorption: Rapidly cleared from plasma. **Onset:** Gradual response over several wk. **Metabolism:** In liver. **Elimination:** 60% in urine within 24–72 h.

NURSING IMPLICATIONS

Assessment & Drug Effects

- Monitor closely because most patients will manifest some evidence of toxicity.
- Be aware that because of cumulative effects, maximum myelosuppression may be delayed 3–4 wk after termination of therapy.
- Withhold drug and notify physician if leukocyte count falls to 3000/mm^3 or below or if platelet count falls below 150,000/mm^3.
- Lab tests: Determine Hgb level, WBC with differential, and thrombocyte (i.e., platelet) counts at least weekly during therapy and for at least 3 wk after therapy is discontinued; periodic LFTs, kidney function tests, and serum uric acid.

Patient & Family Education

- Be aware of possibility of amenorrhea (usually reversible in 6–8 mo).
- Report onset of fever, bleeding, a cold or illness, no matter how mild to physician; medical supervision may be necessary.

THIOTHIXENE HYDROCHLORIDE

(thye-oh-thix′een)

Navane

Classification: PHENOTHIAZINE ANTIPSYCHOTIC

Therapeutic: ANTIPSYCHOTIC

Prototype: Chlorpromazine

Pregnancy Category: C

AVAILABILITY 1 mg, 2 mg, 5 mg, 10 mg, 20 mg capsules; 5 mg/mL solution

ACTION & *THERAPEUTIC EFFECT* Mechanism is related to blockade of postsynaptic dopamine receptors in the mesolimbic region of the brain. Additionally, blockade of alpha$_1$-adrenergic receptors in the CNS produces sedation and muscle relaxation. *Possesses antipsychotic, sedative, adrenolytic, and antiemetic activity.*

USES Manifestations of psychotic disorders.

UNLABELED USES Antidepressant.

CONTRAINDICATIONS Hypersensitivity to thioxanthenes and phenothiazines; comatose states; CNS depression; circulatory collapse; blood dyscrasias; lactation; children younger than 12 y.

CAUTIOUS USE History of convulsive disorders; alcohol withdrawal; glaucoma; prostatic hypertrophy; cardiovascular disease; patients who might be exposed to organophosphorus insecticides or to extreme heat; previously diagnosed breast cancer; pregnancy (category C).

ROUTE & DOSAGE

Psychotic Disorders

Adult: **PO** 2 mg t.i.d., may increase up to 15 mg/day as needed or tolerated (max: 60 mg/day) **IM** 4 mg b.i.d. to q.i.d. (max: 30 mg/day)

Dementia Behavior

Geriatric: **PO** 1–2 mg 1–2 times/day, may increase q4–7days (max: 30 mg/day in divided doses)

ADMINISTRATION

Oral

- Avoid contact between oral concentrate and skin or clothing to prevent contact dermatitis. If concentrate spills, wash skin promptly with water.
- Give oral concentrate (contains 7% alcohol) diluted in a cupful of water, fruit juice, carbonated beverage, milk, or soup.
- Capsules may be opened and mixed with food or water for ease of administration.

Intramuscular

- Give IM injection deep into upper outer quadrant of buttock. Aspirate carefully before injection. Rotate injection sites.
- Store at 15°–30° C (59°–86° F) in light-resistant containers unless otherwise indicated.

ADVERSE EFFECTS (≥1%) **CNS:** *Drowsiness,* insomnia, dizziness, cerebral edema, convulsions, *extrapyramidal symptoms (dose related),* paradoxical exaggeration of psychotic symptoms; sudden death, neuroleptic malignant syndrome, tardive dyskinesia, depressed cough reflex. **GI:** Xerostomia, constipation. **CV:** Tachycardia, *orthostatic hypotension* (especially with IM). **Urogenital:** Impotence, gynecomastia, galactorrhea, amenorrhea. **Skin:** Rash, contact dermatitis, photosensitivity. **Special Senses:** Blurred vision, pigmentary retinopathy. **Metabolic:** Decreased serum uric acid levels.

INTERACTIONS Drug: Alcohol, ANXIOLYTICS, SEDATIVE-HYPNOTICS, other CNS DEPRESSANTS add to CNS depression; additive adverse effects with other PHENOTHIAZINES; **Herbal: Kava** may increase risk and severity of dystonic reactions.

PHARMACOKINETICS Absorption: Slowly absorbed from GI tract. **Onset:** Days to weeks PO; 1–6 h IM. **Duration:** Up to 12 h. **Distribution:** May remain in body for several weeks; crosses placenta. **Metabolism:** In liver. **Elimination:** In bile and feces. **Half-Life:** 34 h.

NURSING IMPLICATIONS

Assessment & Drug Effects

- Monitor for therapeutic response. Although therapeutic response can be observed 1–6 h following IM injection, it may be days or several weeks before there is a response with oral drug.

- Keep patient recumbent for at least 1 h following IM because of possibility of orthostatic hypotension. Check BP periodically.
- Monitor BP for excessive hypotensive response when thiothixene is added to drug regimen of patient on hypertensive treatment until therapy is stabilized.
- Monitor response when patient is changed from IM to PO forms (capsules, concentrate). Dosage adjustment may be necessary.
- Lab tests: Periodic blood chemistry and LFTs with prolonged therapy.
- Report extrapyramidal effects (pseudoparkinsonism, akathisia, dystonia) to physician; dose adjustment or short-term therapy with an antiparkinsonism agent may provide relief.
- Be alert to first symptoms of tardive dyskinesia (see Appendix F). Withhold drug and notify physician.

Patient & Family Education

- Make position changes slowly, particularly from lying down to upright because of danger of lightheadedness; sit a few minutes before walking.
- Do not drive or engage in potentially hazardous activities until response to drug is known.
- Avoid alcohol and other depressants during therapy.
- Take drug as prescribed; do not alter dosing regimen or stop medication without consulting physician. Abrupt discontinuation can cause delirium.
- Do not use any OTC drugs without approval of physician.
- Avoid excessive exposure to sunlight to prevent a photosensitivity reaction. If sun exposure is expected, protect skin with sunscreen lotion (SPF 12 or above).
- Schedule periodic eye exams and report blurred vision to physician.

THROMBIN

(throm′bin)

Recothrom, Thrombinar, Thrombostat

Classification: COAGULATOR; TOPICAL HEMOSTATIC

Therapeutic: COAGULATOR; HEMOSTATIC

Pregnancy Category: C

AVAILABILITY 1000, 5000, 10,000, 20,000, 50,000 unit vials

ACTION & *THERAPEUTIC EFFECT* Plasma protein prepared from prothrombin of bovine origin. Induces clotting of whole blood or fibrinogen solution without addition of other substances. *Facilitates conversion of fibrinogen to fibrin resulting in clotting of whole blood.*

USES When oozing of blood from capillaries and small venules is accessible, as in dental extraction, plastic surgery, grafting procedures, and epistaxis; also to shorten bleeding time at puncture sites in heparinized patient (i.e., following hemodialysis).

CONTRAINDICATIONS Known hypersensitivity to any of drug components or to material of bovine origin; parenteral use; entry or infiltration into large blood vessels.

CAUTIOUS USE Pregnancy (category C). Safety and efficacy in children and infants are not established.

ROUTE & DOSAGE

Oozing Blood

Adult: **Topical** 100–2000 NIH units/mL, depending on extent of bleeding, may be used as solution, in dry form, by mixing thrombin with blood plasma to form a fibrin "glue," or in conjunction with absorbable gelatin sponge

ADMINISTRATION

Topical

- Ensure that sponge recipient area is free of blood before applying thrombin.
- Prepare solutions in sterile distilled water or isotonic saline.
- Use solutions within a few hours of preparation. If several hours are to elapse between time of preparation and use, solution should be refrigerated, or preferably frozen, and used within 48 h.
- Store lyophilized preparation at 2°–8° C (36°–46° F).

ADVERSE EFFECTS (≥1%) **Body as a Whole:** Sensitivity, allergic and febrile reactions, intravascular clotting and death when thrombin is allowed to enter large blood vessels.

THYROID

(thye'roid)

Armour Thyroid, Thyrar

Classification: THYROID HORMONE

Therapeutic: THYROID HORMONE REPLACEMENT

Prototype: Levothyroxine sodium

Pregnancy Category: A

AVAILABILITY 15 mg (1/4 grain), 30 mg (1/2 grain), 60 mg (1 grain), 90 mg (1 1/2 grain), 120 mg (2 grain), 180 mg (3 grain), 240 mg (4 grain), 300 mg (5 grain) tablets

ACTION & *THERAPEUTIC EFFECT* Animal thyroid gland containing active thyroid hormones, *l*-thyroxine (T_4) and *l*-triiodothyronine (T_3). T_4 is largely converted to T_3, which exerts the principal effects. Influences growth and maturation of various tissues (including skeletal and CNS) at critical periods. Promotes a generalized increase in metabolic rate of body tissues. *Effectiveness indicated by diuresis, followed by sense of well-being, increased pulse rate, increased pulse pressure, increased appetite, increased psychomotor activity, loss of constipation, normalization of skin texture and hair, and increased T_3 and T_4 serum levels.*

USES Replacement or substitution therapy in primary hypothyroidism (cretinism, myxedema, simple goiter, deficiency states in pregnancy and older adults) and secondary hypothyroidism caused by surgery, excess radiation, or antithyroid drug therapy. May be given as adjunct to antithyroid agents when it is desirable to limit release of thyrotropic hormones and to prevent goitrogenesis and hypothyroidism.

CONTRAINDICATIONS Thyrotoxicosis; acute MI not associated with hypothyroidism, cardiovascular disease; morphologic hypogonadism; nephrosis; uncorrected hypoadrenalism.

CAUTIOUS USE Angina pectoris, hypertension, older adults who may have occult cardiac disease; renal insufficiency; concomitant administration of catecholamines; diabetes mellitus; hyperthyroidism (history of); malabsorption states; pregnancy (category A).

ROUTE & DOSAGE

Mild to Moderate Hypothyroidism

Adult: **PO** 60 mg/day, may increase q30days to 60–180 mg/day

Severe Hypothyroidism
Adult: **PO** 15 mg/day, increased q2wk to 60 mg/day, then may increase q30days if needed
Child: **PO** 15 mg/day, may increase by 15 mg q2wk if needed

ADMINISTRATION

Oral

- Give preferably on an empty stomach.
- Initiate dosage generally at low level and systematically increase in small increments to desired maintenance dose.
- Store in dark bottle to minimize spontaneous deiodination. Keep desiccated thyroid dry.

ADVERSE EFFECTS (≥1%) **Endocrine:** Hyperthyroidism, thyroid storm [high temperature (as high as 41° C [106° F])], tachycardia, vomiting, shock, coma. **Special Senses:** Staring expression in eyes. **CV:** CHF, angina, cardiac arrhythmias, palpitation, tachycardia. **Body as a Whole:** Weight loss, tremors, headache, nervousness, fever, insomnia, warm and moist skin, heat intolerance, leg cramps, menstrual irregularities, shock, changes in appetite. **GI:** Diarrhea or abdominal cramps. **Metabolic:** Hyperglycemia (usually offset by increased tissue oxidation of sugar).

DIAGNOSTIC TEST INTERFERENCE Thyroid increases ***basal metabolic rate;*** may increase ***blood glucose levels, creatine phosphokinase, AST, LDH, PBI.*** It may decrease ***serum uric acid, cholesterol, thyroid-stimulating hormone (TSH), iodine 131*** uptake. Many medications may produce false results in ***thyroid function tests.***

INTERACTIONS Drug: ORAL ANTICOAGULANTS potentiate hypoprothrombinemia; may increase requirements for **insulin,** SULFONYLUREAS; **epinephrine** may precipitate coronary insufficiency; **cholestyramine** may decrease thyroid absorption.

PHARMACOKINETICS Absorption: Variably absorbed from GI tract. **Peak:** 1–3 wk. **Distribution:** Does not readily cross placenta; minimal amounts in breast milk. **Metabolism:** Deiodination in thyroid gland. **Elimination:** In urine and feces. **Half-Life:** T_3, 1–2 days; T_4, 6–7 days.

NURSING IMPLICATIONS

Assessment & Drug Effects

- Observe patient carefully during initial treatment for untoward reactions such as angina, palpitations, cardiac pain.
- Be alert for symptoms of overdosage (see ADVERSE EFFECTS) that may occur 1–3 wk after therapy is started.
- Monitor response until regimen is stabilized to prevent iatrogenic hyperthyroidism. In drug-induced hyperthyroidism, there may also be increased bone loss. Such a patient is vulnerable to pathologic fractures.
- Monitor vital signs: Assess pulse before each dose during period of dosage adjustment. Consult physician if rate is 100 or more or if there has been a marked change in rate or rhythm.
- Lab tests: Monitor thyroid function q3mo during dose adjustment period. Monitor prothrombin time if patient is receiving concurrent anticoagulant therapy. A decrease in requirement usually develops within 1–4 wk after starting treatment with thyroid.

Patient & Family Education

- Be aware that replacement therapy for hypothyroidism is lifelong; continued follow-up care is important.
- Monitor pulse rate and report increases greater than parameter set by physician.
- Report to physician onset of chest pain or other signs of aggravated CV disease (dyspnea, tachycardia).
- Report evidence of any unexplained bleeding to physician when taking concomitant anticoagulant.
- Use monthly height and weight measurement to monitor growth in juvenile undergoing treatment.

TIAGABINE HYDROCHLORIDE

(ti-a′ga-been)

Gabitril Filmtabs

Classifications: ANTICONVULSANT; GABA INHIBITOR

Therapeutic: ANTICONVULSANT

Prototype: Valproic acid sodium (sodium valproate)

Pregnancy Category: C

AVAILABILITY 2 mg, 4 mg, 12 mg, 16 mg, 20 mg tablets

ACTION & *THERAPEUTIC EFFECT* Potent and selective inhibitor of GABA uptake into presynaptic neurons; allows more GABA to bind to the surfaces of postsynaptic neurons in the CNS. *Effectiveness indicated by reduction in seizure activity.*

USES Adjunctive therapy for partial seizures.

CONTRAINDICATIONS Hypersensitivity to tiagabine; lactation; children younger than 12 y.

CAUTIOUS USE Liver function impairment; history of spike and wave discharge on EEG; status epilepticus; pregnancy (category C).

ROUTE & DOSAGE

Seizures

Adult: **PO** Start with 4 mg daily, may increase dose by 4–8 mg/day qwk (max: 56 mg/day in 2–4 divided doses)

Adolescent (12–18 y): **PO** Start with 4 mg daily, after 2 wk may increase dose by 4–8 mg/day qwk (max: 32 mg/day in 2–4 divided doses)

ADMINISTRATION

Oral

- Give with food.
- Make dosage increases, when needed, at weekly intervals.
- Store at 15°–30° C (59°–86° F) in a tightly closed container and protect from light.

ADVERSE EFFECTS (≥1%) **Body as a Whole:** Infection, flu-like syndrome, pain, myasthenia, allergic reactions, chills, malaise, arthralgia. **CNS:** *Dizziness, asthenia, tremor, somnolence, nervousness,* difficulty concentrating, ataxia, depression, insomnia, abnormal gait, hostility, confusion, speech disorder, difficulty with memory, paresthesias, emotional lability, agitation, dysarthria, euphoria, hallucinations, hyperkinesia, hypertonia, hypotonia, myoclonus, twitching, vertigo. Risk of new-onset seizures. **CV:** Vasodilation, hypertension, palpitations, tachycardia, syncope, edema, peripheral edema. **GI:** Abdominal pain, diarrhea, nausea, vomiting, increased appetite, mouth ulcers. **Respiratory:** Pharyngitis, cough, bronchitis, dyspnea, epistaxis, pneumonia. **Skin:** Rash, pruritus, alopecia, dry skin, sweating, ecchymoses. **Special Senses:** Am-

T

blyopia, nystagmus, tinnitus. **Urogenital:** Dysmenorrhea, dysuria, metrorrhagia, incontinence, vaginitis, UTI.

INTERACTIONS Drug: Carbamazepine, phenytoin, phenobarbital decrease levels of tiagabine. Use with ANTIDEPRESSANTS, ANTIPSYCHOTICS, STIMULANTS, and NARCOTICS may increase seizure risk. **Herbal: Ginkgo** may decrease anticonvulsant effectiveness. **Evening primrose oil** may affect seizure threshold.

PHARMACOKINETICS Absorption: Rapidly absorbed; 90% bioavailability. **Peak:** 45 min. **Distribution:** 96% protein bound. **Metabolism:** In liver, probably by cytochrome P450 3A isoform. **Elimination:** 25% in urine, 63% in feces. **Half-Life:** 7–9 h (4–7 h with other enzyme-inducing drugs).

NURSING IMPLICATIONS

Assessment & Drug Effects

- Lab tests: Measure plasma levels of tiagabine before and after changes are made in the drug regimen.
- Be aware that concurrent use of other anticonvulsants may decrease effectiveness of tiagabine or increase the potential for adverse effects.
- Monitor carefully for S&S of CNS depression.

Patient & Family Education

- Do not stop taking drug abruptly; may cause sudden onset of seizures.
- Exercise caution while engaging in potentially hazardous activities because drug may cause dizziness.
- Use caution when taking other prescription or OTC drugs that can cause drowsiness.
- Report any of the following to the physician: Rash or hives; red, peeling skin; dizziness; drowsiness; depression; GI distress; nervousness or tremors; difficulty concentrating or talking.

TICARCILLIN DISODIUM/ CLAVULANATE POTASSIUM

(tye-kar-sill'in/clav-yoo'la-nate)
Timentin
Classifications: ANTIBIOTIC; ANTIPSEUDOMONAL PENICILLIN
Therapeutic: ANTIBIOTIC
Prototype: Piperacillin
Pregnancy Category: B

AVAILABILITY 3.1 g injection

ACTION & *THERAPEUTIC EFFECT* Extended-spectrum penicillin and fixed combination of ticarcillin disodium with the potassium salt of clavulanic acid, a beta-lactamase inhibitor. Used alone, clavulanic acid antibacterial activity is weak, but in combination with ticarcillin prevents degradation by beta-lactamase and extends ticarcillin spectrum of activity. *Combination drug extends ticarcillin spectrum of activity against many strains of beta-lactamase–producing bacteria (synergistic effect).*

USES Infections of lower respiratory tract and urinary tract and skin and skin structures, infections of bone and joint, and septicemia caused by susceptible organisms. Also mixed infections and as presumptive therapy before identification of causative organism.

CONTRAINDICATIONS Hypersensitivity to penicillins or to cephalosporins, coagulopathy.
CAUTIOUS USE Diabetes mellitus; GI disease; asthma; history of allergies; renal impairment; pregnancy (category B), lactation.

ROUTE & DOSAGE

Moderate to Severe Infections
Adult (weight greater than 60 kg): **IV** 3.1 g q4–6h
Child (older than 3 mo): **IV** 200–300 mg/kg/day divided q4–6h (based on ticarcillin)
Infant (younger than 3 mo): **IV** 200–300 mg/kg/day divided q6–8h (based on ticarcillin)

Renal Impairment Dosage Adjustment
CrCl 30–60 mL/min: Give 2 g q4h or 3.1 g q8h; 10–30 mL/min: Give 2 g q8h or 3.1 g q12h; less than 10 mL/min: Give 2 g q12h
Hemodialysis Dosage Adjustment: 2 g q12h, supplement with 3.1 g after dialysis

ADMINISTRATION

Intravenous
Note: Verify correct IV concentration and rate of infusion for administration to infants and children with physician.

PREPARE: **Intermittent:** Reconstitute by adding 13 mL sterile water for injection or NS injection to the 3.1 g vial to yield 200 mg/mL ticarcillin with 6.7 mg/mL clavulanic acid. Shake until dissolved. ▪Further dilute the required does in NS, D5W, or LR to concentrations between 10–100 mg/mL. ▪DO NOT use if discoloration or particulate matter is present.

ADMINISTER: **Intermittent:** Give over 30 min.

INCOMPATIBILITIES **Solution/additive:** AMINOGLYCOSIDES, **sodium bicarbonate.** **Y-site:** AMINOGLYCOSIDES, **amphotericin B cholesteryl complex, azithromycin, vancomycin.**

▪Store vial with sterile powder at 21°–24° C (69°–75° F) or colder. ▪If exposed to higher temperature, powder will darken, indicating degradation of clavulanate potassium and loss of potency. Discard vial. ▪See package insert for information about storage and stability of reconstituted and diluted IV solutions of drug.

ADVERSE EFFECTS (≥1%) **Body as a Whole:** Hypersensitivity reactions, pain, burning, swelling at injection site; phlebitis, thrombophlebitis; superinfections. **CNS:** Headache, blurred vision, mental deterioration, convulsions, hallucinations, seizures, giddiness, neuromuscular hyperirritability. **GI:** *Diarrhea, nausea,* vomiting, disturbances of taste or smell, stomatitis, flatulence. **Hematologic:** Eosinophilia, thrombocytopenia, leukopenia, neutropenia, hemolytic anemia. **Metabolic:** Hypernatremia, transient increases in serum AST, ALT, BUN, and alkaline phosphatase; increases in serum LDH, bilirubin, and creatinine and decreased serum uric acid.

DIAGNOSTIC TEST INTERFERENCE May interfere with test methods used to determine ***urinary proteins*** except for tests for urinary protein that use ***bromphenol blue. Positive direct antiglobulin (Coombs') test*** results, apparently caused by clavulanic acid, have been reported. This test may interfere with ***transfusion cross-matching procedures.***

INTERACTIONS Drugs: May increase risk of bleeding with ANTICOAGULANTS; **probenecid** decreases elimination of ticarcillin.

PHARMACOKINETICS Distribution: Widely distributed with highest concentrations in urine and bile; crosses

T

placenta; distributed into breast milk. **Metabolism:** In liver. **Elimination:** In urine. **Half-Life:** 1.1–1.2 h ticarcillin, 1.1–1.5 h clavulanate.

NURSING IMPLICATIONS

Assessment & Drug Effects

- Lab tests: Obtain baseline C&S tests before initiating therapy; drug may be started pending results. Monitor kidney and liver functions, CBC, platelet count, and serum electrolytes during prolonged treatment.
- Be aware that serious and sometimes fatal anaphylactoid reactions have been reported in patients with penicillin hypersensitivity or history of sensitivity to multiple allergens. Reported incidence is low with this combination drug.
- Monitor cardiac status because of high sodium content of drug.
- Overdose symptoms: This drug may cause neuromuscular hyperirritability or seizures.

Patient & Family Education

- Report urticaria, rashes, or pruritus to physician immediately.
- Report frequent loose stools, diarrhea, or other possible signs of pseudomembranous colitis (see Appendix F) to physician.

TICLOPIDINE

(ti-clo′pi-deen)

Ticlid

Classifications: ANTICOAGULANT; PLATELET AGGREGATION INHIBITOR; ADP RECEPTOR ANTAGONIST

Therapeutic: PLATELET AGGREGATION INHIBITOR

Prototype: Clopidogrel

Pregnancy Category: B

AVAILABILITY 250 mg tablets

ACTION & *THERAPEUTIC EFFECT*
Platelet aggregation inhibitor that interferes with platelet membrane functioning and therefore platelet interactions. *Ticlopidine interferes with ADP-induced binding of fibrinogen to the platelet membrane at specific receptor sites. Platelet adhesion and platelet aggregation are therefore inhibited. Prevents release of platelet constituents and prolongs bleeding time.*

USES Reduction of the risk of thrombotic stroke in patients intolerant to aspirin.

UNLABELED USES Prevention of venous thromboembolic disorders; maintenance of bypass graft patency and of vascular access sites in hemodialysis patients; improvement of exercise performance in patients with ischemic heart disease and intermittent claudication; prevention of postoperative deep venous thrombosis (DVT).

CONTRAINDICATIONS Hypersensitivity to ticlopidine; hematopoietic disease, coagulopathy; leukemia; pathologic bleeding; severe liver impairment; lactation.

CAUTIOUS USE Hepatic function impairment, renal impairment; patients at risk for bleeding from trauma, surgery, or a bleeding disorder; GI bleeding; pregnancy (category B). Safe use in children younger than 18 y not established.

ROUTE & DOSAGE

Stroke Prevention

Adult: **PO** 250 mg b.i.d. with food

ADMINISTRATION

Oral

- Give with food or just after eating to minimize GI irritation.
- Do not give within 2 h of an antacid.
- Store at 15°–30° C (59°–86° F).

T

ADVERSE EFFECTS (≥1%) **CNS:** Dizziness. **GI:** Nausea, vomiting, abdominal cramps; dyspepsia, flatulence, anorexia; abnormal liver function tests (few cases of hepatotoxicity reported). **Hematologic:** Neutropenia (resolves in 1–3 wk), thrombocytopenia, leukopenia, agranulocytosis (usually within first 3 mo), and pancytopenia; hemorrhage (ecchymosis, epistaxis, menorrhagia, GI bleeding), thrombotic thrombocytopenia purpura (usually within first month). **Skin:** Urticaria, maculopapular rash, erythema nodosum (generally occur within the first 3 mo of therapy, with most occurring within the first 3–6 wk).

DIAGNOSTIC TEST INTERFERENCE Increases ***total serum cholesterol*** by 8–10% within 4 wk of beginning therapy. ***Lipoprotein ratios*** remain unchanged. Elevates ***alkaline phosphatase*** and ***serum transaminases.***

INTERACTIONS Drug: ANTACIDS decrease bioavailability of ticlopidine. ANTICOAGULANTS increase risk of bleeding. **Cimetidine** decreases clearance of ticlopidine. CORTICOSTEROIDS counteract increased bleeding time associated with ticlopidine. May decrease **cyclosporine** levels (one case report). Increases **theophylline** half-life by 42%, possibly increasing **theophylline** serum levels. May increase **phenytoin** levels. **Food:** Food may increase bioavailability of ticlopidine. **Herbal:** Evening primrose oil increases bleeding risk.

PHARMACOKINETICS Absorption: 90% absorbed from GI tract; increased absorption when taken with food. **Onset:** Antiplatelet activity, 24–48 h; maximal effect at 3–5 days. **Peak:** Peak serum levels at 2 h. **Duration:** Bleeding times return to baseline within 4–10 days. **Distribution:** 90% bound to plasma proteins. **Metabolism:** Rapidly and extensively metabolized in liver. **Elimination:** Only 1% excreted unchanged; 60% of metabolites excreted in urine, 23% in feces. **Half-Life:** 12.6 h; terminal half-life is 4–5 days with repeated dosing.

NURSING IMPLICATIONS

Assessment & Drug Effects

- Lab tests: Periodic platelet count and bleeding time. Monitor CBC with differentials q2wk from second week to end of third month of therapy and thereafter if S&S of infection develop.
- Report promptly laboratory values indicative of neutropenia, thrombocytopenia, or agranulocytosis.
- Monitor for signs of bleeding (e.g., ecchymosis, epistaxis, hematuria, GI bleeding).

Patient & Family Education

- Report promptly to physician any of the following: Nausea, diarrhea, rash, sore throat, or other signs of infection, signs of bleeding, or signs of cholestasis (e.g., yellow skin or sclera, dark urine or clay-colored stools).
- Understand risk of GI bleeding; do not take aspirin along with ticlopidine.
- Do not take antacids within 2 h of ticlopidine.
- Keep appointments for regularly scheduled blood tests.

TIGECYCLINE

(ti-ge-cy′cline)

Tygacil

Classifications: ANTIBIOTIC; GLYCYLCYCLINE

Therapeutic: ANTIBIOTIC

Prototype: Tetracycline

Pregnancy Category: D

AVAILABILITY 50 mg injection

ACTION & *THERAPEUTIC EFFECT* Tigecycline inhibits protein production in bacteria by binding to the 30S ribosomal subunit and blocking entry of transfer RNA molecules into the ribosome of the bacteria. This prevents formation of peptide chains within the bacteria, thus interfering with their growth. *Tigecycline is active against a broad spectrum of bacterial pathogens and is bacteriostatic.*

USES Treatment of complicated skin and skin structure infections, community acquired pneumonia, and complicated intra-abdominal infections.

CONTRAINDICATIONS Hypersensitivity to tigecycline; pregnancy (category D) and during tooth development of the fetus; viral infections.

CAUTIOUS USE Severe hepatic impairment (Child-Pugh class C); hypersensitivity to tetracycline, intestinal perforations, intra-abdominal infections; GI disorders; lactation; children younger than 18 y.

ROUTE & DOSAGE

Community Acquired Pneumonia, Complicated Skin/Intra-abdominal Infections

Adult: **IV** 100 mg initially, followed by 50 mg q12h over 30–60 min × 5–14 days

Hepatic Impairment Dosage Adjustment

Child-Pugh class C: Initial dose 100 mg, followed by 25 mg q12h

ADMINISTRATION

- Note that dosage adjustment is required with severe hepatic impairment.

Intravenous

PREPARE: **Intermittent:** Reconstitute each 50 mg with 5.3 mL of NS or D5W to yield 10 mg/mL. ▪ Swirl gently to dissolve; reconstituted solution should be yellow to orange in color. ▪ After reconstitution, immediately withdraw exactly 5 mL from each vial and add to 100 mL of NS or D5W for infusion. ▪ The maximum concentration in the IV bag should be 1 mg/mL (two 50 mg doses).

ADMINISTER: **Intermittent:** Give over 30–60 min; when using Y-site, flush IV line with NS or D5W before/after infusion.

INCOMPATIBILITIES **Y-site: Amphotericin B, chlorpromazine, methylprednisolone, voriconazole.**

- Store in the IV bag at room temperature for up to 6 h, or refrigerated at 2°–8° C (36°–46° F) for up to 24 h.

ADVERSE EFFECTS (≥1%) **CNS:** Asthenia, dizziness, headache, insomnia. **CV:** Hypertension, hypotension, peripheral edema, phlebitis. **GI:** Abdominal pain, constipation, diarrhea, dyspepsia, *nausea, vomiting*. **Hematologic/Lymphatic:** Abnormal healing, anemia, infection, leukocytosis, thrombocythemia. **Metabolic/Nutritional:** Alkaline phosphatase increased, ALT increased, amylase increased, AST increased, bilirubinemia, BUN increased, hyperglycemia, hypokalemia, hypoproteinemia, lactic dehydrogenase increased. **Musculoskeletal:** Back pain. **Respiratory:** Dyspnea, increased cough, pulmonary physical findings. **Skin:** Pruritus, rash, sweating. **Body as a Whole:** Abscess, fever, local reaction to injection, pain.

INTERACTIONS Drug: Increased concentrations of **warfarin** required close monitoring of INR. Efficacy of ORAL CONTRACEPTIVES may be decreased when used in combination with tigecycline.

T

PHARMACOKINETICS Distribution: 71–89% protein bound. **Metabolism:** Negligible. **Elimination:** Fecal (major) and renal. **Half-Life:** 27 h (single dose); 42 h (multiple doses).

NURSING IMPLICATIONS

Assessment & Drug Effects

- Monitor for hypersensitivity reaction in those with reported tetracycline allergy.
- Monitor for and report S&S of superinfection (see Appendix F) or pseudomembranous enterocolitis (see Appendix F).
- Lab tests: C&S prior to initiation of therapy; periodic serum electrolytes, LFTs and kidney function tests; PT and INR with concurrent anticoagulant therapy.
- Monitor diabetics for loss of glycemic control.

Patient & Family Education

- Avoid direct exposure to sunlight during and for several days after therapy is terminated to reduce risk of photosensitivity reaction.
- Report to physician loose stools or diarrhea either during or shortly after termination of therapy.
- Use a barrier contraceptive in addition to oral contraceptives if trying to avoid pregnancy.

T

TILUDRONATE DISODIUM

(til-u′dro-nate)

Skelid

Classification: REGULATOR, BONE METABOLISM (BISPHOSPHONATE)

Therapeutic: BONE METABOLISM REGULATOR

Prototype: Etidronate disodium

Pregnancy Category: C

AVAILABILITY 240 mg tablets

ACTION & *THERAPEUTIC EFFECT* This diphosphate inhibits osteoclastic activity that leads to resorption of the bone matrix. Acts primarily by inhibiting normal or abnormal bone resorption, thus reducing bone formation. *Effectiveness indicated by decreasing levels of alkaline phosphatase.*

USES Treatment of Paget's disease.

CONTRAINDICATIONS Hypersensitivity to diphosphonates (e.g., alendronate, etidronate, pamidronate, tiludronate); severe kidney failure (Clcr less than 30 mL/min); lactation. **CAUTIOUS USE** Hypocalcemia, renal impairment; active UGI problems (e.g., gastritis, dysphagia, ulcer, esophageal disease); vitamin D deficiency; CHF; pregnancy (category C). Safety and efficacy in children are not established.

ROUTE & DOSAGE

Paget's Disease

Adult: **PO** 400 mg/day with 6–8 oz of water × 3 mo

ADMINISTRATION

Oral

- Give with 6–8 oz of plain water 2 h before or after food.
- Do not give within 2 h of drugs containing calcium, aspirin, or indomethacin. Give aluminum- or magnesium-containing antacids no sooner than 2 h after tiludronate.
- Store in manufacturer's packaging at 15°–30° C (59°–86° F).

ADVERSE EFFECTS (≥1%) **Body as a Whole:** *Pain,* flu-like syndrome, edema. **CNS:** Headache, dizziness, paresthesias. **CV:** Chest pain. **GI:** *Nausea, diarrhea,* dyspepsia, vomiting, flatulence. **Special Senses:** Cataract, conjunctivitis, glaucoma. **Respiratory:** Rhinitis, sinusitis, coughing, pharyngitis. **Skin:** Rash. **Metabolic:** Hyperparathyroidism, vitamin D deficiency, **Musculoskeletal:** Arthralgia, arthrosis.

INTERACTIONS Drug: Absorption decreased by CALCIUM-, ALUMINUM- OR MAGNESIUM-CONTAINING ANTACIDS, **aspirin.** Absorption increased by **indomethacin.**

PHARMACOKINETICS Absorption: Poorly absorbed from GI tract. **Steady-State:** 30 days. **Metabolism:** Not metabolized. **Elimination:** Primarily in urine. **Half-Life:** 150 h.

NURSING IMPLICATIONS

Assessment & Drug Effects

- Monitor for S&S of upper GI dysfunction or ulceration.
- Lab tests: Periodic serum calcium and serum phosphate.

Patient & Family Education

- Do not remove tablets from foil strips until time to be taken.
- Wait at least 2 h after taking tiludronate to take aluminum- and magnesium-containing antacids.
- Consult physician to determine appropriate daily intake of vitamin D and calcium.

TIMOLOL MALEATE

(tye′moe-lole)

Betimol, Blocadren, Istalol, Timoptic, Timoptic XE

Classifications: BETA-ADRENERGIC ANTAGONIST; EYE PREPARATION; MIOTIC; ANTIHYPERTENSIVE; ANTIANGINAL

Therapeutic: MIOTIC; ANTIHYPERTENSIVE; ANTIANGINAL

Prototype: Propranolol

Pregnancy Category: C

AVAILABILITY 5 mg, 10 mg, 20 mg tablets; 0.25%, 0.5% ophth solution or gel

ACTION & *THERAPEUTIC EFFECT* Nonselective beta-adrenergic antagonist that demonstrates antihypertensive, antiarrhythmic, and antianginal properties, and suppresses plasma renin activity. When applied topically, lowers elevated and normal intraocular pressure (IOP) by reducing formation of aqueous humor and possibly by increasing outflow. *Topically, lowers elevated and normal intraocular pressure (IOP). Orally, therapeutically useful for mild hypertension, angina, and migraine headaches.*

USES Topically (ophthalmic solution) to reduce elevated IOP in chronic, open-angle glaucoma, aphakic glaucoma, secondary glaucoma, and ocular hypertension. May be used alone or in conjunction with epinephrine, pilocarpine, or a carbonic anhydrase inhibitor such as acetazolamide. Oral preparation is used as monotherapy or in combination with a thiazide diuretic to prevent reinfarction after MI and to treat mild hypertension.

UNLABELED USES Prophylactic management of stable, uncomplicated angina pectoris and migraine headaches.

CONTRAINDICATIONS Bronchospasm; severe COPD; bronchial asthma; heart failure; abrupt discontinuation, acute bronchospasm, AV block, bradycardia, cardiogenic shock, acute pulmonary edema, compromised left ventricular dysfunction, Raynaud's disease. Safety in children is not established.

CAUTIOUS USE Bronchitis, patients subject to bronchospasm, asthma; sinus bradycardia, greater than first-degree heart block, heart failure; re-

T

nal impairment; hepatic disease; vasospastic angina, peripheral vascular disease; pheochromocytoma; thyrotoxicosis, hyperthyroidism; right ventricular failure secondary to pulmonary hypertension, COPD; stroke, cerebrovascular disease; depression; older adults; psoriasis; myasthenia gravis; pregnancy (category C).

ROUTE & DOSAGE

Glaucoma
See Appendix A-1.

Hypertension, Post-MI Reinfarction
Adult: **PO** 10 mg b.i.d., may increase to 60 mg/day in 2 divided doses

Angina
Adult: **PO** 15–45 mg in 3 divided doses

ADMINISTRATION

Oral
- Give with fluid of patient's choice; tablet may be crushed.
- Dosage increases for hypertension should be made at weekly intervals.

ADVERSE EFFECTS (≥1%) **CNS:** Fatigue, lethargy, weakness, somnolence, anxiety, headache, dizziness, confusion, psychic dissociation, depression. **CV:** Palpitation, bradycardia, hypotension, syncope, AV conduction disturbances, CHF, aggravation of peripheral vascular insufficiency. **Special Senses:** *Eye irritation* including conjunctivitis, blepharitis, keratitis, superficial punctate keratopathy. **GI:** Anorexia, dyspepsia, nausea. **Skin:** Rash, urticaria. **Respiratory:** Difficulty in breathing, bronchospasm. **Body as a Whole:** Fever. **Metabolic:** Hypoglycemia, hypokalemia.

INTERACTIONS Drug: ANTIHYPERTENSIVE AGENTS, DIURETICS, SELECTIVE SEROTONIN REUPTAKE INHIBITORS potentiate hypotensive effects; NSAIDS may antagonize hypotensive effects.

PHARMACOKINETICS Absorption: 90% absorbed from GI tract; 50% reaches systemic circulation; some systemic absorption from topical application. **Peak:** 1–2 h PO; 1–5 h topical. **Distribution:** Distributed into breast milk. **Metabolism:** 80% metabolized in liver to inactive metabolites. **Elimination:** In urine.

NURSING IMPLICATIONS

Assessment & Drug Effects
- Check pulse before administering timolol, topical or oral. If there are extremes (rate or rhythm), withhold medication and notify physician.
- Assess pulse rate and BP at regular intervals and more aften in patients with severe heart disease.
- Note: Some patients develop tolerance during long-term therapy.

Patient & Family Education
- Be aware that drug may cause slight reduction in resting heart rate. Learn how to assess pulse rate and report significant changes. Consult physician for parameters.
- Do not stop drug abruptly; angina may be exacerbated. Dosage is reduced over a period of 1–2 wk.
- Report promptly to physician difficulty breathing. Drug withdrawal may be indicated.

TINIDAZOLE
(tin′i-da-zole)
Tindamax
Classification: AZOLE ANTIBIOTIC
Therapeutic: AZOLE ANTIBIOTIC; ANTIPROTOZOAL; AMEBICIDE

Prototype: Metronidazole
Pregnancy Category: X first trimester; C second and third trimester

AVAILABILITY 250 mg, 500 mg tablets

ACTION & *THERAPEUTIC EFFECT* Tinidazole is effective against dividing and nondividing cells of targeted bacteria and protozoa. It inhibits formation of their DNA helix and thus inhibits DNA synthesis of these organisms. This leads to bacterial and protozoal cell death. *Demonstrates activity against infections caused by protozoa and anaerobic bacteria.*

USES Treatment of trichomoniasis, giardiasis, amebiasis, bacterial vaginosis, and amebic liver abscess.

CONTRAINDICATIONS Hypersensitivity to tinidazole or other azole antibiotics; pregnancy (category X first trimester), lactation within 72 h of tinidazole use; children younger than 3 y.
CAUTIOUS USE CNS diseases, liver dysfunction, alcoholism, ethanol intoxication; hematologic disease; neurologic disease; bone marrow depression; dialysis; candidiasis; pregnancy (category C second and third trimester).

ROUTE & DOSAGE

Giardiasis

Adult: **PO** 2 g as single dose
Child (3 y or older): **PO** 50 mg/kg (up to 2 g) as single dose

Intestinal Amebiasis

Adult: **PO** 2 g once daily for 3 days
Child (3 y or older): **PO** 50 mg/kg/day (up to 2 g/day) once daily for 3 days

Amebic Liver Abscess

Adult: **PO** 2 g once daily for 3–5 days
Child (3 y or older): **PO** 50 mg/kg/day (up to 2 g/day) once daily for 3–5 days

Trichomoniasis

Adult: **PO** 2 g as single dose

Bacterial Vaginosis

Adult: **PO** 2 g daily × 2 days OR 1 g daily × 5 days
Hemodialysis Dosage Adjustment: If dose given on dialysis day, give supplemental dose (1/2 regular dose) post-dialysis

ADMINISTRATION

Oral
- Give with food to minimize GI distress; may be crushed in artificial cherry syrup if tablets cannot be swallowed whole.
- If given on a dialysis day, add a 50% dose of tinidazole at the end of hemodialysis.
- Separate the dosing of cholestyramine and tinidazole by 2–4 h when used concurrently.
- Do not give within 2 wk of the last dose of disulfiram.
- Store at 15°–30° C (59°–86° F). Protect from light.

ADVERSE EFFECTS (≥1%) **Body as a Whole:** Weakness, fatigue, malaise. **CNS:** Dizziness, headache. **GI:** Metallic/bitter taste, nausea, anorexia, dyspepsia, cramps, epigastric discomfort, vomiting, constipation.

INTERACTIONS Drug: May increase INR with **warfarin; alcohol** may cause **disulfiram**-like reaction; may increase the half-life of **fosphenytoin, phenytoin;** may increase levels and toxicity of **lith-**

ium, fluorouracil, cyclosporine, tacrolimus; cholestyramine may decrease absorption of tinidazole; **cimetidine** or **ketoconazole** may increase levels.

PHARMACOKINETICS Peak: 2 h. **Distribution:** Crosses blood–brain barrier and placenta and is excreted in breast milk. **Metabolism:** In the liver by CYP3A4. **Elimination:** Primarily in urine. **Half-Life:** 12–14 h.

NURSING IMPLICATIONS

Assessment & Drug Effects

- Withhold drug and notify physician for S&S of CNS dysfunction (e.g., seizures, numbness or paresthesia of extremities). Drug should be discontinued if abnormal neurologic signs appear.
- Lab tests: Baseline LTFs; CBC with differential, if retreatment is required.
- Monitor INR/PT frequently with concomitant oral anticoagulants. Continue monitoring for at least 8 days after discontinuation of tinidazole.
- Monitor serum lithium levels with concurrent use.
- Monitor for phenytoin toxicity with concurrent IV phenytoin.

Patient & Family Education

- Stop taking the drug and report promptly: Convulsions, numbness, tingling, pain, or weakness in the hands or feet; dizziness or unsteadiness; fever.
- Harmless urine discoloration may occur while taking this drug.

T

TINZAPARIN SODIUM

(tinz′a-par-in)

Innohep

Pregnancy Category: B

See Appendix A-2.

TIOCONAZOLE

(ti-o-con′a-zole)

Vagistat-1

Classifications: ANTIBIOTIC; AZOLE ANTIFUNGAL

Therapeutic: AZOLE ANTIFUNGAL

Prototype: Fluconazole

Pregnancy Category: C

AVAILABILITY 6.5% vaginal ointment

ACTION & *THERAPEUTIC EFFECT* Broad-spectrum antifungal agent that inhibits growth of human pathogenic yeasts by disrupting normal fungal cell membrane permeability. *Effective against* Candida albicans, *other species of* Candida, *and* Torulopsis glabrata.

USES Local treatment of vulvovaginal candidiasis.

CONTRAINDICATIONS Hypersensitivity to tioconazole or other imidazole antifungal agents; children younger than 12 y; lactation.

CAUTIOUS USE Diabetes mellitus; HIV infections; immunosuppression; pregnancy (category C).

ROUTE & DOSAGE

Candidiasis

Adult: **Intravaginal** One applicator full at bedtime × 1 day

ADMINISTRATION

Instillation

- Insert applicator high into the vagina (except during pregnancy).
- Wash applicator before and after each use.
- Store away from direct heat and light.

ADVERSE EFFECTS (≥1%) **Urogenital:** Mild erythema, burning, discomfort, rash, itching.

INTERACTIONS Drug: May inactivate spermicidal effects of **nonoxynol-9.**

PHARMACOKINETICS Absorption: Minimal absorption from vagina.

NURSING IMPLICATIONS

Assessment & Drug Effects

- Do not use for patient with a history of allergic reaction to other antifungal agents, such as miconazole.
- Monitor for sensitization and irritation; these may be an indication to discontinue drug.

Patient & Family Education

- Learn correct application technique.
- Understand potential adverse reactions, including sensitization and allergic response.
- Tioconazole may interact with diaphragms and latex condoms; avoid concurrent use within 72 h.
- Refrain from sexual intercourse while using tioconazole.
- Wear only cotton underwear; change daily.

TIOTROPIUM BROMIDE

(ti-o-tro′pi-um)

Spiriva

Classifications: ANTICHOLINERGIC; ANTIMUSCARINIC; ANTISPASMODIC; BRONCHODILATOR

Therapeutic: BRONCHODILATOR; ANTISPASMODIC

Prototype: Atropine

Pregnancy Category: C

AVAILABILITY 18 mcg capsules with powder for inhalation

ACTION & *THERAPEUTIC EFFECT* A long-acting, antispasmodic agent. In the bronchial airways, it exhibits inhibition of muscarinic receptors of the smooth muscle resulting in bronchodilation. *Bronchodilation after inhalation of tiotropium is predominantly a site-specific effect.*

USES Maintenance treatment of bronchospasm associated with chronic obstructive pulmonary disease (COPD); reducing COPD exacerbations.

CONTRAINDICATIONS Hypersensitivity to tiotropium, atropine, or ipratropium; acute bronchospasm; children younger than 18 y.

CAUTIOUS USE Decreased renal function; BPH, urinary bladder neck obstruction; narrow-angle glaucoma; older adults; pregnancy (category C), lactation.

ROUTE & DOSAGE

COPD

Adult: **Inhaled** Inhale 18 mcg once daily using hand inhaler device provided.

ADMINISTRATION

Inhalation

- Place capsule in HandiHaler® and press button to puncture. Instruct patient to exhale deeply then put the mouthpiece to the lips and breathe in the dose deeply and slowly; remove HandiHaler® and hold breath for at least 10 sec, and then exhale slowly; rinse mouth with water to minimize dry mouth.
- Ensure that drug does not contact the eyes.
- Store at 15°–30° C (59°–86° F).

ADVERSE EFFECTS (≥1%) **Body as a Whole:** Nonspecific chest pain, dependent edema, infection, moniliasis, flu-like syndrome, cough, allergic reactions. **CNS:** Dysphonia, paresthesia, depression. **GI:** Abdominal pain, constipation, *dry mouth, dyspepsia,* vomiting, reflux, stomati-

T

tis. **Metabolic:** Hypercholesterolemia, hyperglycemia. **Musculoskeletal:** Myalgia, skeletal pain. **Respiratory:** Epistaxis, *pharyngitis, rhinitis,* laryngitis, *sinusitis, upper respiratory tract infection.* **Skin:** Rash. **Special Senses:** Cataract. **Urogenital:** Urinary tract infection.

INTERACTIONS Drug: May cause additive anticholinergic effects with other ANTICHOLINERGIC AGENTS.

PHARMACOKINETICS Absorption: 19.5% absorbed from the lungs. **Peak:** 5 min. **Metabolism:** Less than 25% of dose is metabolized in liver by CYP2D6 and 3A4. **Elimination:** 14% of dose excreted in urine; remaining is excreted in feces as nonabsorbed drug. **Half-Life:** 5–6 days.

NURSING IMPLICATIONS

Assessment & Drug Effects

- Withhold drug and notify physician if S&S of angioedema occurs.
- Monitor for anticholinergic effects (e.g., tachycardia, urinary retention).

Patient & Family Education

- Do not allow powdered medication to contact the eyes, as this may cause blurring of vision and pupil dilation.
- Tiotropium bromide is intended as a once-daily maintenance treatment. It is not useful for treatment of acute episodes of bronchospasm (i.e., rescue therapy).
- Withhold drug and notify physician if swelling around the face, mouth, or neck occurs.
- Report any of the following: Constipation, increased heart rate, blurred vision, urinary difficulty.

T

TIPRANAVIR

(ti-pra′na-vir)

Aptivus

Classifications: ANTIRETROVIRAL; PROTEASE INHIBITOR
Therapeutic: ANTIRETROVIRAL; PROTEASE INHIBITOR
Prototype: Saquinavir
Pregnancy Category: C

AVAILABILITY 250 mg capsules; 100 mg/mL oral solution

ACTION & *THERAPEUTIC EFFECT*
A non-peptide protease inhibitor that inhibits virus-specific processing of the viral polyproteins in HIV-1 infected cells, thus preventing the formation of mature viral particles. *Helps decrease viral load of HIV-1 strains resistant to other protease inhibitors.*

USES Treatment of HIV-1 infection in adults with evidence of viral replication who are highly treatment-experienced or have HIV-1 strains resistant to multiple protease inhibitors. Tipranavir should be used in combination with ritonavir 200 mg and other antiretroviral agents.

CONTRAINDICATIONS Known hypersensitivity to tipranavir; moderate to severe (Child-Pugh class B and C, respectively) hepatic insufficiency; pancreatitis; lactation.
CAUTIOUS USE Hypersensitivity to sulfonamides; patients with chronic hepatitis B or hepatitis C coinfection; hemophilia; coagulopathy; elevated liver enzymes; diabetes mellitus or hyperglycemia; hyperlipidemia; pregnancy (category C); children.

ROUTE & DOSAGE

HIV-1 Infection
Adult: **PO** 500 mg (with 200 mg ritonavir) b.i.d.

Adolescent/Child: **PO** 14 mg/kg OR 375 mg/m^2 OR 500 mg b.i.d. (depending on ritonavir dose)

ADMINISTRATION

Oral

- Coadminister with ritonavir. Give with food.
- Store at 15°–30° C (59°–86° F). Once opened, use contents of bottle within 60 days.

ADVERSE EFFECTS (≥1%) **Body as a Whole:** Fatigue, pyrexia. **CNS:** Asthenia, depression, headache, insomnia. **GI:** Abdominal pain, *diarrhea,* nausea, vomiting. **Hematologic:** Decreased white blood cell levels, risk of hemorrhage. **Hepatic:** *Elevated liver enzymes (amylase, ALT, AST).* **Metabolic:** *Increased cholesterol, increased triglycerides.* **Respiratory:** Bronchitis, cough. **Skin:** Rash.

INTERACTIONS Drug: Aluminum- and **magnesium-**based ANTACIDS may decrease tipranavir absorption. AZOLE ANTIFUNGAL AGENTS, **clarithromycin, erythromycin,** and other inhibitors of CYP3A4 may increase tipranavir levels. **Efavirenz, loperamide,** NRTIS, and RIFAMYCINS (e.g., **rifampin**) may decrease tipranavir levels. Tipranavir increases **rifabutin** levels. Coadministration of tipranavir and **tenofovir** decreases the levels of both compounds. Tipranavir increases the concentration of BENZODIAZEPINES, **desipramine,** ERGOT ALKALOIDS, and numerous ANTIARRHYTHMIC AGENTS **(amiodarone, flecainide, propafenone, quinidine).** Tipranavir may decrease **ethinyl estradiol** levels by 50%. Combination use of tipranavir and HMG COA REDUCTASE INHIBITORS increases the risk of myopathy. Tipranavir capsules contain **alcohol** that can produce disulfiram-like reactions with **metronidazole** and **disulfiram.** Adjust **midazolam** dose. **Food:** Food enhances the bioavailability of tipranavir, avoid large doses of vitamin E. **Herbal: St. John's wort** decreases the levels of tipranavir.

PHARMACOKINETICS Peak: 3 h. **Distribution:** Greater than 99.9% protein bound. **Metabolism:** Extensive hepatic oxidation to inactive metabolites (when given alone); minimal metabolism (when given with ritonavir). **Elimination:** Fecal (primary) and renal (minimal). **Half-Life:** 6 h.

NURSING IMPLICATIONS

Assessment & Drug Effects

- Monitor for and report immediately S&S of liver toxicity.
- Monitor for S&S of adverse drug reactions and toxicity from concurrently administered drugs. Many drugs interact with tipranavir.
- Monitor diabetics for loss of glycemic control.
- Use barrier contraceptive if using hormonal contraceptive.
- Lab tests: Baseline and frequent LFTs, especially in those with hepatitis B or C; periodic lipid profile and fasting plasma glucose.
- Monitor blood levels of anticoagulants with concurrent therapy.

Patient & Family Education

- Follow directions for taking the drug (see Administration). If a dose is missed, take it as soon as possible and then return to the normal schedule. Never double a dose.
- Inform physician of all medications and herbal products you are taking.
- Protect against sunlight exposure to minimize risk of photosensitivity.
- Report any of the following to physician: Fatigue, weakness, loss of appetite, nausea, jaundice, dark urine, or clay colored stools.

TIROFIBAN HYDROCHLORIDE

(tir-o-fi′ban)
Aggrastat
Classifications: ANTICOAGULANT; ANTIPLATELET; GLYCOPROTEIN (GP) IIB/IIIA RECEPTOR INHIBITOR
Therapeutic: ANTIPLATELET
Prototype: Abciximab
Pregnancy Category: B

AVAILABILITY 250 mcg/mL, 50 mcg/mL injection

ACTION & *THERAPEUTIC EFFECT* Antiplatelet agent that binds to the glycoprotein IIb/IIIa receptor of platelets inhibiting platelet aggregation. *Effectiveness indicated by minimizing thrombotic events during treatment of acute coronary syndrome.*

USES Acute coronary syndromes (unstable angina, MI).

CONTRAINDICATIONS Hypersensitivity to tirofiban; active internal bleeding within 30 days; acute pericarditis; aortic dissection; intracranial aneurysm, intracranial mass, coagulopathy; history of aneurysm or AV malformation; history of intracranial hemorrhage or neoplasm; active abnormal bleeding; retinal bleeding; hemorrhagic retinopathy; major surgery or trauma within 3 days; stroke within 30 days; history of hemorrhagic stroke; thrombocytopenia following administration of tirofiban; within 4 h of PCI; lactation.

CAUTIOUS USE Platelet count less than 150,000 mm^3; severe renal insufficiency; pregnancy (category B). Safety and efficacy in children younger than 18 y are unknown.

ROUTE & DOSAGE

Acute Coronary Syndromes
Adult: **IV** 0.4 mcg/kg/min for 30 min, then 0.1 mcg/kg/min for 12–24 h after angioplasty or arteriectomy

Renal Impairment Dosage Adjustment
CrCl less than 30 mL/min: Reduce rate of infusion 50%

ADMINISTRATION

Intravenous

PREPARE: **IV Infusion:** *Dilution of 250 mcg/mL concentrate to 50 mcg/mL:* Withdraw 100 mL from a 500-mL bag of NS or D5W and replace with 100 mL of tirofiban HCl injection. ▪ If a 250-mL IV bag is used, withdraw 50 mL of IV solution and replace with 50 mL of tirofiban injection. ▪ Either preparation yields 50 mcg/mL. ▪ Mix well before infusing. ▪ Note: Commercially premixed IV tirofiban solutions are available.

ADMINISTER: **IV Infusion:** An initial loading dose of 0.4 mcg/kg/min for 30 min is usually followed by a maintenance infusion of 0.1 mcg/kg/min.

INCOMPATIBILITIES **Y-site: Diazepam, tenecteplase.**

▪ Discard unused IV solution 24 h following start of infusion. ▪ Store unopened containers at 15°–30° C (59°–86° F). ▪ Do not freeze and protect from light.

ADVERSE EFFECTS (≥1%) **Body as a Whole:** Edema, swelling, pelvic pain, vasovagal reaction, leg pain. **CNS:** Dizziness. **CV:** Bradycardia, <u>coronary artery dissection</u>. **GI:** GI bleeding. **Hematologic:** *Bleeding* (<u>major bleeding</u>), anemia, thrombocytopenia. **Skin:** Sweating.

INTERACTIONS Drug: Increased risk of bleeding with ANTICOAGULANTS, NSAIDS, SALICYLATES, ANTIPLATELET AGENTS. **Herbal: Feverfew, garlic, ginger, ginkgo, horse chestnut** may increase risk of bleeding.

PHARMACOKINETICS Duration: 4–8 h after stopping infusion. **Distribution:** 65% protein bound. **Metabolism:** Minimally metabolized. **Elimination:** 65% in urine, 25% in feces. **Half-Life:** 2 h.

NURSING IMPLICATIONS

Assessment & Drug Effects

- Lab tests: Monitor platelet count, Hgb and Hct before treatment, (within 6 h of infusing loading dose), and frequently throughout treatment; monitor aPTT and ACT.
- Withhold drug and notify physician if thrombocytopenia (platelets less than 100,000) is confirmed.
- Monitor carefully for and immediately report S&S of internal or external bleeding.
- Minimize unnecessary invasive procedures and devices to reduce the risk of bleeding.

Patient & Family Education

- Report unexplained pelvic or abdominal pain.

TIZANIDINE HYDROCHLORIDE

(ti-zan′i-deen)

Zanaflex

Classification: SKELETAL MUSCLE RELAXANT, CENTRAL-ACTING

Therapeutic: SKELETAL MUSCLE RELAXANT; ANTISPASMODIC

Prototype: Cyclobenzaprine

Pregnancy Category: C

AVAILABILITY 4 mg tablets; 2 mg, 4 mg, 6 mg capsules

ACTION & *THERAPEUTIC EFFECT* Centrally acting alpha-adrenergic agonist that reduces spasticity by increasing presynaptic inhibition of motor neurons. Greatest effect on polysynaptic afferent reflex activity at the spinal cord level. *Site of action is the spinal cord; reduces skeletal muscle spasms. Effectiveness indicated by decreased muscle tone.*

USES Acute and intermittent management of increased muscle tone associated with spasticity.

CONTRAINDICATIONS Hypersensitivity to tizanidine. Safety in labor and delivery is unknown.

CAUTIOUS USE Patients with hepatic impairment, hepatic disease; renal insufficiency (CrCl less than 25 mL/min), or renal failure; psychosis; women taking oral contraceptives; older adults because of renal impairment; pregnancy (category C), lactation. Safety and efficacy in children are not established.

ROUTE & DOSAGE

Spasticity

Adult: **PO** Start with 4 mg and gradually increase to 8 mg q6–8h prn (max: 3 doses or 36 mg/24 h)

Renal Impairment Dosage Adjustment

CrCl less than 25 mL/min: Use lower dose

ADMINISTRATION

Oral

- Dose increases are usually made gradually in 2- to 4-mg increments.
- Store at 15°–30° C (59°–86° F).

ADVERSE EFFECTS (≥1%) **Body as a Whole:** *Asthenia (tiredness),* flu-like syndrome, fever, myasthenia, back pain, infection. **CNS:** *Somnolence, dizziness,* dyskinesia, nervousness, depression, anxiety, paresthesia. **CV:** *Hypotension, bradycardia.* **GI:** *Dry mouth,* constipation, abnormal liver function tests, vomiting, abdominal pain, diarrhea, dyspepsia. **Respiratory:** Pharyngitis, rhinitis. **Skin:** Rash, sweating, skin ulcer. **Urogenital:** *UTI,* urinary frequency. **Special Senses:** Speech disorder, blurred vision.

INTERACTIONS Drug: ORAL CONTRACEPTIVES decrease clearance of **tizanidine. Alcohol** and other CNS DEPRESSANTS increase CNS depression. **Fluvoxamine, ciprofloxacin** increase tizanidine levels and toxicity. **Herbal: Kava, valerian** may potentiate sedation.

PHARMACOKINETICS Absorption: Rapidly absorbed from GI tract; 40% bioavailability. **Peak:** 1–2 h. **Duration:** 3–6 h. **Distribution:** Crosses placenta, distributed into breast milk. **Metabolism:** In the liver. **Elimination:** 60% in urine, 20% in feces. **Half-Life:** 2.5 h.

NURSING IMPLICATIONS

Assessment & Drug Effects

- Lab tests: Monitor LFTs during the first 6 mo of treatment (baseline, 1, 3, and 6 mo) and periodically thereafter.
- Monitor cardiovascular status and report orthostatic hypotension or bradycardia.
- Monitor closely older adults, those with renal impairment, and women taking oral contraceptives for adverse effects because drug clearance is reduced.

Patient & Family Education

- Exercise caution with potentially hazardous activities requiring alertness since sedation is a common adverse effect. Effects are additive with alcohol or other CNS depressants.
- Make position changes slowly because of the risk of orthostatic hypotension.
- Report unusual sensory experiences; hallucinations and delusions have occurred with tizanidine use.

TOBRAMYCIN SULFATE

(toe-bra-mye'sin)

AKTob, TobraDex, Tobrex, TOBI

Classification: AMINOGLYCOSIDE ANTIBIOTIC

Therapeutic: ANTIBIOTIC

Prototype: Gentamicin sulfate

Pregnancy Category: D

AVAILABILITY 10 mg/mL, 40 mg/mL injection; 300 mg/5 mL inhalation solution; 0.1%, 0.3% ophth solution; 0.1%, 0.3% ophth ointment

ACTION & *THERAPEUTIC EFFECT* Broad-spectrum, aminoglycoside antibiotic that binds irreversibly to one of two aminoglycoside binding sites on the 30S ribosomal subunit of the bacteria, thus inhibiting protein synthesis, resulting in bacterial cell death. *Effective in treatment of gram-negative bacteria. Exhibits greater antibiotic activity against* Pseudomonas aeruginosa *than other aminoglycosides.*

USES Treatment of severe infections caused by susceptible organisms.

CONTRAINDICATIONS History of hypersensitivity to tobramycin and other aminoglycoside antibiotics; pregnancy (category D).

CAUTIOUS USE Impaired kidney function; renal disease; dehydration; hearing impairment; myasthenia gravis; parkinsonism; premature and neonatal infants; older adults; lactation.

ROUTE & DOSAGE

Moderate to Severe Infections

Adult: **IV/IM** 3 mg/kg/day divided q8h up to 5 mg/kg/day OR 4–7 mg/kg/day single dose **Topical** 1–2 drops in affected eye q1–4h

Child: **IM/IV** *Younger than 5 y,* 2.5 mg/kg q8h **IV/IM** *5 y or older,* 2–2.5 mg/kg/day divided q8h

Neonate: **IM/IV** 2.5 mg/kg q12–24h

Cystic Fibrosis

Adult/Child: **IM/IV** 2.5–3.5 mg/kg q6–8h **Nebulized** 300 mg inhaled b.i.d. × 28 days, may repeat after 28-day drug-free period

Renal Impairment Dosage Adjustment

Increase interval.

Hemodialysis Dosage Adjustment: Administer dose after dialysis and monitor levels

Obesity Dosage Adjustment

Dose based on IBW; in morbid obesity, use dosing weight of IBW + 0.4 (Weight – IBW)

ADMINISTRATION

Note: All doses should be based on ideal body weight.

Inhalation

- Administer over 10–15 min using a handheld reusable nebulizer with a compressor (use only those supplied). Patient should sit upright and breathe normally through the nebulizer mouthpiece.

Intramuscular

- Give deep IM into a large muscle. Rotate injection sites.

Intravenous

Note: Verify correct IV concentration and rate of infusion to neonates, infants, or children with physician.

PREPARE: **Intermittent:** Dilute each dose in 50–100 mL or more of D5W, NS or D5/NS. ▪ Final concentration should not exceed 1 mg/mL.

ADMINISTER: **Intermittent:** Infuse diluted solution over 20–60 min. ▪ Avoid rapid infusion.

INCOMPATIBILITIES Solution/additive: **Alcohol 5% in dextrose, cefamandole, cefepime, cefoperazone, cefoxitin, clindamycin, heparin.** Y-site: **Allopurinol, amphotericin B cholesteryl complex, azithromycin, cefoperazone, heparin, hetastarch, indomethacin, propofol, sargramostim.**

- Store at 15°–30° C (59°–86° F) prior to reconstitution. After reconstitution, solution may be refrigerated and used within 96 h. ▪ If kept at room temperature, use within 24 h.

T

ADVERSE EFFECTS (≥1%) **CNS:** Neurotoxicity (including ototoxicity), *nephrotoxicity,* increased AST, ALT, LDH, serum bilirubin; anemia, fever, rash, pruritus, urticaria, nausea, vomiting, headache, lethargy, superinfections; hypersensitivity. **Special Senses:** *Burning, stinging of eye after drug instillation;* lid itching and edema.

INTERACTIONS Drug: ANESTHETICS, SKELETAL MUSCLE RELAXANTS add to neuromuscular blocking effects; **acyclovir, amphotericin B, bacitracin, capreomycin,** CEPHALOSPORINS, **colistin, cisplatin, carboplatin, methoxyflurane, polymyxin B, vancomycin, furosemide, ethacrynic acid** increased risk of ototoxicity, nephrotoxicity.

PHARMACOKINETICS Peak: 30–90 min IM. **Duration:** Up to 8 h. **Distribution:** Crosses placenta; accumulates in renal cortex. **Elimination:** In urine. **Half-Life:** 2–3 h in adults.

NURSING IMPLICATIONS

Assessment & Drug Effects

- Weigh patient before treatment for calculation of dosage.
- Obtain bacterial C&S tests prior to and during therapy.
- Observe patient receiving tobramycin closely because of the high potential for toxicity, even in conventional doses.
- Lab tests: Baseline and periodic kidney function; monitor serum drug concentrations to minimize rise of toxicity. Prolonged peak serum concentrations greater than 10 mcg/mL or trough concentrations greater than 2 mcg/mL are not recommended.
- Monitor auditory, and vestibular functions closely, particularly in patients with known or suspected renal impairment and patients receiving high doses.
- Be aware that drug-induced auditory changes are irreversible (partial or total); usually bilateral. Partial or bilateral deafness may continue to develop even after therapy discontinued.
- Monitor I&O. Report oliguria, changes in I&O ratio, and cloudy or frothy urine (may indicate proteinuria). Keep patient well hydrated to prevent chemical irritation in renal tubules; older adults are especially susceptible to renal toxicity.
- Be aware that prolonged use of ophthalmic solution may encourage superinfection with nonsusceptible organisms including fungi.
- Report overdose symptoms for eye medication: Increased lacrimation, keratitis, edema and itching of eyelids.

Patient & Family Education

- Report symptoms of superinfections (see Appendix F) to physician. Prompt treatment with an antibiotic or antifungal medication may be necessary.
- Report S&S of hearing loss, tinnitus, or vertigo to physician.

TOLAZAMIDE

(tole-az′a-mide)

Tolinase

Classifications: SULFONYLUREA ANTIDIABETIC

Therapeutic: ANTIDIABETIC

Prototype: Glyburide

Pregnancy Category: C

AVAILABILITY 100 mg, 250 mg, 500 mg tablets

ACTION & *THERAPEUTIC EFFECT* Sulfonylurea hypoglycemic that lowers blood glucose primarily by stimulating pancreatic beta cells to secrete insulin. Antidiabetic action is a result of stimulation of the pancreas to secrete more insulin in the presence of blood sugar; it requires functioning beta cells. *Effectiveness is measured in decreasing the serum blood level to within normal limits and decreasing HbA1C value to 6.5 or lower.*

USES Mild to moderately severe type 2 diabetes mellitus that cannot be controlled by diet and weight reduction and that is uncompli-

T

cated by acidosis, ketosis, coma. Effective in primary or secondary failures to other sulfonylurea

CONTRAINDICATIONS Known sensitivity to sulfonylureas and to sulfonamides; type 1 diabetes complicated by ketoacidosis; infection; trauma. Safety in lactation or children is not established.

CAUTIOUS USE Older adults; renal disease; renal failure, renal impairment; pregnancy (category C).

ROUTE & DOSAGE

Type 2 Diabetes Mellitus
Adult: **PO** 100 mg–1 g daily to b.i.d. a.c., may adjust dose by 100–250 mg/day at weekly intervals (max: 1 g/day)

ADMINISTRATION

Oral

- Give in the morning with or before meals.
- Divide dose of more than 500 mg and give b.i.d.
- Store at 15°–30° C (59°–86° F) in a tightly closed container unless otherwise directed. Keep drug out of the reach of children.

ADVERSE EFFECTS (≥1%) **GI:** Nausea, vomiting, cholestatic jaundice. **Metabolic:** Hypoglycemia. **CNS:** Vertigo. **Skin:** Photosensitivity. **Hematologic:** Agranulocytosis.

INTERACTIONS Drug: Alcohol elicits disulfiram-type reaction in some patients; ORAL ANTICOAGULANTS, **chloramphenicol, clofibrate, phenylbutazone,** MAO INHIBITORS, SALICYLATES, **probenecid,** SULFONAMIDES may potentiate hypoglycemic actions; THIAZIDES may antagonize hypoglycemic effects; **cimetidine** may increase tolazamide levels, causing hypoglycemia. **Herbal: Ginseng, karela** may potentiate hypoglycemic effects.

PHARMACOKINETICS Absorption: Slowly from GI tract. **Onset:** 60 min. **Peak:** 4–6 h. **Duration:** 10–15 h (up to 20 h in some patients). **Distribution:** Distributed in highest concentrations in liver, kidneys, and intestines; crosses placenta; distributed into breast milk. **Metabolism:** Extensively in liver. **Elimination:** 85% in urine, 15% in feces. **Half-Life:** 7 h.

NURSING IMPLICATIONS

Assessment & Drug Effects

- Monitor closely for daytime and nighttime hypoglycemia since tolazamide is long acting.
- Lab tests: Periodic HbA1C and frequent FBS; periodic CBC.
- Monitor for and report signs of an allergic reaction (e.g., rash, urticaria, pruritus).

Patient & Family Education

- Check blood glucose daily or as ordered by physician. Important to continue close medical supervision for first 6 wk of treatment.
- Learn the S&S of hypoglycemia and hyperglycemia and check blood glucose level when either is suspected.
- Report to physician if you experience frequent and/or severe episodes of hypoglycemia.
- Do not take OTC preparations unless approved or prescribed by physician.
- Understand that alcohol can precipitate a disulfiram-type reaction.
- Many drugs interact with tolazamide. Monitor blood glucose more frequently whenever a new drug is added to your regimen.

TOLBUTAMIDE

(tole-byoo'ta-mide)

T

Mobenol ♣, Novobutamide ♣, Orinase

TOLBUTAMIDE SODIUM

Orinase Diagnostic

Classification: SULFONYLUREA ANTIDIABETIC
Therapeutic: ANTIDIABETIC
Prototype: Glyburide
Pregnancy Category: C

AVAILABILITY 500 mg tablets; 1 g vial

ACTION & *THERAPEUTIC EFFECT* Short-acting sulfonylurea that lowers blood glucose concentration by stimulating pancreatic beta cells to synthesize and release insulin. No action demonstrated if functional beta cells are absent. *Lowers blood glucose concentration by stimulating pancreatic beta cells to synthesize and release insulin.*

USES Management of mild to moderately severe, stable type 2 diabetes that is not controlled by diet and weight reduction alone. Also used in treatment of patients who are unresponsive to other sulfonylureas and adjunctively with insulin to stabilize certain cases of labile diabetes. Used as diagnostic agent to rule out pancreatic islet cell adenoma or diabetes.

T

CONTRAINDICATIONS Hypersensitivity to sulfonylureas or to sulfonamides; history of repeated episodes of diabetic ketoacidosis (with or without coma); type 1 diabetes as sole therapy; diabetic coma; severe stress, infection, trauma, or major surgery; severe renal insufficiency, liver or endocrine disease. Safe use in children is not established.

CAUTIOUS USE Cardiac, thyroid, pituitary, or adrenal dysfunction; severe hepatic disease, renal disease, renal impairment, renal failure; history of peptic ulcer; alcoholism; infection; older adults, debilitated, malnourished, or uncooperative patient; pregnancy (category C), lactation.

ROUTE & DOSAGE

Type 2 Diabetes
Adult: **PO** 250 mg to 3 g/day in 1–2 divided doses

Diagnosis of Functioning Insulinoma
Adult: **IV** 1 g over 2–3 min

ADMINISTRATION

Oral

- Tablets may be crushed and given with full glass of water if patient desires.
- Do not give at bedtime because of danger of nocturnal hypoglycemia, unless specifically prescribed.
- Store below 40° C (104° F), preferably between 15°–30° C (59°–86° F) in well-closed container. Avoid freezing.

ADVERSE EFFECTS (≥1%) **GI:** Nausea, epigastric fullness, heartburn, anorexia, constipation, diarrhea, cholestatic jaundice (rare). **Hematologic:** <u>Agranulocytosis</u>, thrombocytopenia, leukopenia, hemolytic anemia, <u>aplastic anemia</u>, pancytopenia. **Metabolic:** Hepatic porphyria, disulfiram-like reactions, SIADH, hypoglycemia without loss of consciousness or neurologic symptoms (unusual fatigue, tremulousness, hunger, drowsiness, GI distress, sweating, anxiety, headache) severe hypoglycemia (visual disturbances, ataxia, paresthesias, confusion, tachycardia, seizures, <u>coma</u>). **Skin:** Allergic skin reactions: Pruritus, erythema, urticaria, morbilliform or maculopapular eruptions; porphyria cutanea tarda, photosensitivity. **Special Senses:** Taste alterations. **CNS:** Headache.

DIAGNOSTIC TEST INTERFERENCE The SULFONYLUREAS may produce abnormal ***thyroid function test*** results and reduced ***RAI uptake*** (after long-term administration). A tolbutamide metabolite may cause false-positive ***urinary protein*** values when turbidity procedures are used (such as heat and ***acetic acid*** or ***sulfosalicylic acid***); ***Ames reagent*** strips reportedly not affected.

INTERACTIONS Drug: Phenylbutazone increases hypoglycemic effects; THIAZIDE DIURETICS may attenuate hypoglycemic effects; **alcohol** may produce disulfiram reaction; BETA-BLOCKERS may mask symptoms of a hypoglycemic reaction. **Herbal: Ginseng, karela** may potentiate hypoglycemic effects.

PHARMACOKINETICS Absorption: Readily from GI tract. **Peak:** 3–5 h. **Distribution:** Into extracellular fluids. **Metabolism:** Principally in liver. **Elimination:** 75–85% in urine; some in feces. **Half-Life:** 7 h.

NURSING IMPLICATIONS

Assessment & Drug Effects

- Supervise closely during initial period of therapy until dosage is established. One or 2 wk of therapy may be required before full therapeutic effect is achieved.
- Monitor closely during adjustment period, watching for S&S of impending hypoglycemia (see Appendix F). Detection of a hypoglycemic reaction in a diabetic patient also receiving a beta-blocker, especially older adults, is difficult.
- Evaluate nondefinitive vague complaints; hypoglycemic symptoms may be especially vague in older adults. Observe patient carefully, especially 2–3 h after eating, check urine for sugar and ketone bodies and capillary blood glucose.
- Lab tests: Baseline liver and kidney function tests; periodic HbA1C, serum electrolytes, CBC with differential, and platelet counts.
- Report repetitive complaints of headache and weakness a few hours after eating; may signal incipient hypoglycemia.
- Be aware that pruritus and rash, frequently reported adverse effects, may clear spontaneously; if these persist, drug will be discontinued.

Patient & Family Education

- Learn the S&S of hyperglycemia (see Appendix A) and check blood glucose level when hyperglycemia is suspected.
- Hypoglycemia is frequently caused by overdosage of hypoglycemic drug, inadequate or irregular food intake, nausea, vomiting, diarrhea, and added exercise without caloric supplement or dose adjustment. Learn the S&S of hypoglycemia (see Appendix F) and check blood glucose level whenever hypoglycemia is suspected.
- Report any illness promptly. Physician may want to evaluate need for insulin.
- Do not self-medicate with OTC drugs unless approved or prescribed by physician.
- Be aware that alcohol, even in moderate amounts, can precipitate a disulfiram-type reaction (see Appendix F). A hypoglycemic response after ingesting alcohol requires emergency treatment.
- Protect exposed skin areas from the sun with a sunscreen lotion (SPF 12–15) because of potential

T

photosensitivity (especially in the alcoholic).

- Monitor blood glucose daily or as directed by physician.
- Be alert to added danger of loss of control (hyperglycemia) when a drug that affects the hypoglycemic action of sulfonylureas (see DRUG INTERACTIONS) is withdrawn or added to the tolbutamide regimen. Monitor blood glucose carefully.
- Use or add barrier contraceptive if using hormonal contraceptives.

TOLCAPONE (Pr)

(tol′ca-pone)

Tasmar

Classifications: ANTICHOLINERGIC; CATECHOLAMINE-O-METHYLTRANSFERASE (COMT) INHIBITOR

Therapeutic: ANTIPARKINSON

Pregnancy Category: C

AVAILABILITY 100 mg, 200 mg tablets

ACTION & *THERAPEUTIC EFFECT* Selective and reversible inhibitor of catecholamine-O-methyltransferase (COMT). COMT is the enzyme responsible for metabolizing catecholamines and, therefore, levodopa. *Concurrent administration of tolcapone and levodopa increases the amount of levodopa available to control Parkinson's disease by increasing dopaminergic brain stimulation.*

USES Idiopathic Parkinson's disease as adjunct to levodopa/carbidopa.

CONTRAINDICATIONS Hypersensitivity to tolcapone; liver disease; MAOI therapy.

CAUTIOUS USE History of hypersensitivity to other COMT inhibitors (e.g., entacapone, nitecapone); anorexia nervosa; hematuria; hypotension; syncopy; renal disease; renal impairment; pregnancy (category C), lactation.

ROUTE & DOSAGE

Parkinson's Disease

Adult: **PO** 100 mg t.i.d. (max: 200 mg t.i.d.)

ADMINISTRATION

Oral

- Give with food if GI upset occurs.
- Give only in conjunction with levodopa/carbidopa therapy.
- Therapy with tolcapone should NOT be initiated if patient has ALT/AST greater than 2 × ULN or has known liver disease.
- Store at 20°–25° C (68°–77° F) in a tightly closed container.

ADVERSE EFFECTS (≥1%) **Body as a Whole:** Muscle cramps, orthostatic complaints, fatigue, falling, balance difficulties, hyperkinesia, stiffness, arthritis, hypokinesia. **CNS:** *Dyskinesia, sleep disorder, dystonia, excessive dreaming,* somnolence, confusion, dizziness, headache, hallucination, syncope, paresthesias. **CV:** Chest pain, hypotension. **GI:** *Nausea,* anorexia, diarrhea, vomiting, constipation, <u>fulminant liver failure, severe hepatocellular injury</u>, dry mouth, abdominal pain, dyspepsia, flatulence. **Respiratory:** URI, dyspnea, sinus congestion. **Skin:** Sweating. **Urogenital:** UTI, urine discoloration, micturition disorder.

INTERACTIONS Drug: Will increase **levodopa** levels when taken simultaneously; CNS DEPRESSANTS may cause additive sedation; do not give with non-selective MAOIS **(isocarboxazid, phenelzine, or tranylcypromine furazolidone, linezolid, procarbazine). Food:** Decreases levels.

PHARMACOKINETICS Absorption: Rapidly from GI tract, bioavailability 65%. **Peak:** 2 h. **Distribution:** Over 99% protein bound. **Metabolism:** Extensively metabolized by COMT and glucuronidation. **Elimination:** 60% in urine, 40% in feces; clearance reduced by 50% in patients with liver disease. **Half-Life:** 2–3 h.

NURSING IMPLICATIONS

Assessment & Drug Effects

- Lab tests: Monitor LFTs monthly for first 3 mo, every 6 wk for the next 3 mo, and periodically thereafter.
- Withhold drug and notify physician if liver dysfunction is suspected.
- Monitor PT and INR carefully when given concurrently with warfarin.
- Monitor carefully for and immediately report S&S of hepatic impairment (e.g., jaundice, dark urine).

Patient & Family Education

- Do not engage in hazardous activities until response to drug is known. Avoid use of alcohol or sedative drugs while on tolcapone.
- Rise slowly from a sitting or lying position to avoid a rapid drop in BP with possible weakness or fainting.
- Nausea is a common possible adverse effect especially at the beginning of therapy.
- Do not suddenly stop taking this drug. Doses **must be** gradually reduced over time.
- Notify physician promptly about any of following: Increased loss of muscle control, fainting, yellowing of skin or eyes, darkening of urine, severe diarrhea, hallucinations.

TOLMETIN SODIUM

(tole′met-in)

Tolectin, Tolectin DS

Classifications: ANALGESIC, NONSTEROIDAL ANTI-INFLAMMATORY (NSAID); ANTIPYRETIC

Therapeutic: NONNARCOTIC ANALGESIC, NSAID; DISEASE-MODIFYING ANTIRHEUMATIC DRUG (DMARD)

Prototype: Ibuprofen

Pregnancy Category: C first and second trimester; D third trimester

AVAILABILITY 200 mg, 600 mg tablets; 400 mg capsules

ACTION & *THERAPEUTIC EFFECT* Nonsteroidal anti-inflammatory analgesic that competitively inhibits both cyclooxygenase (COX) isoenzymes, COX-1 and COX-2, by blocking arachidonate binding to prostaglandin sites, and thus inhibits prostaglandin synthesis. *Possesses analgesic, anti-inflammatory, and antipyretic and antirheumatic activity.*

USES In acute flares and management of chronic rheumatoid arthritis. May be used alone or in combination with gold or corticosteroids.

CONTRAINDICATIONS History of intolerance or hypersensitivity to tolmetin, aspirin, and other NSAIDs; active peptic ulcer, CABG perioperative pain; in patients with functional class IV rheumatoid arthritis (severely incapacitated, bedridden, or confined to a wheelchair). Safety during pregnancy (category D third trimester), lactation, or children younger than 2 y is not established.

T

CAUTIOUS USE History of upper GI tract disease; impaired kidney function; SLE; compromised cardiac function; pregnancy (category C first and second trimester).

ROUTE & DOSAGE

Arthritis

Adult: **PO** 400 mg t.i.d. (max: 2 g/day)
Child (2 y or older): **PO** 20 mg/kg/day in 3–4 divided doses (max: 30 mg/kg/day)

ADMINISTRATION

Oral

- Schedule to include a morning dose (on arising) and a bedtime dose.
- Give with fluid of patient's choice; crush tablet or empty capsule to mix with water or food if patient cannot swallow tablet/capsule.
- Store at 15°–30° C (59°–86° F) in tightly capped and light-resistant container unless otherwise instructed.

ADVERSE EFFECTS (≥1%) **CNS:** *Headache, dizziness, vertigo, lightheadedness,* mood elevation or depression, tension, nervousness, weakness, drowsiness, insomnia, tinnitus. **CV:** Mild edema (about 7% patients), sodium and water retention, mild to moderate hypertension. **GI:** Epigastric or abdominal pain, dyspepsia, *nausea,* vomiting, heartburn, constipation, peptic ulcer, GI bleeding. **Hematologic:** Transient and small decreases in hemoglobin and hematocrit, purpura, petechiae, granulocytopenia, leukopenia. **Urogenital:** Hematuria, proteinuria, increased BUN. **Skin:** Toxic epidermal necrolysis, morbilliform eruptions, urticaria, pruritus. **Body as a Whole:** Anaphylaxis (especially after drug is discontinued and then reinstituted).

DIAGNOSTIC TEST INTERFERENCE Tolmetin prolongs ***bleeding time,*** inhibits ***platelet aggregation,*** elevates ***BUN, alkaline phosphatase,*** and ***AST*** levels; may decrease ***hemoglobin*** and ***hematocrit*** values. Metabolites may produce false-positive results for ***proteinuria*** [with tests that rely on acid precipitation (e.g., ***sulfosalicylic acid***)].

INTERACTIONS Drug: ORAL ANTICOAGULANTS, **heparin** may prolong bleeding time; may increase **lithium** toxicity; **aspirin,** other NSAIDS add to ulcerogenic effects; may increase **methotrexate** toxicity. **Herbal: Feverfew, garlic, ginger, ginkgo** may increase bleeding potential.

PHARMACOKINETICS Absorption: Rapidly from GI tract. **Peak:** 30–60 min. **Distribution:** Crosses blood–brain barrier and placenta; distributed into breast milk. **Metabolism:** In liver. **Elimination:** In urine. **Half-Life:** 60–90 min.

NURSING IMPLICATIONS

Assessment & Drug Effects

- Monitor patients with kidney damage closely. Evaluate I&O ratio and encourage patient to increase fluid intake to at least 8 full glasses per day.
- Lab tests: Obtain periodic kidney function tests (routine urinalysis, creatinine clearance, and serum creatinine) for patient on long-term therapy.
- Check self-medicating habits of the patient. Sodium bicarbonate alkalinizes the urine, which increases urinary excretion of tolmetin and may reduce degree and duration of effectiveness.

Patient & Family Education

- Take drug with meals or milk if GI disturbances occur. Notify physician if symptoms persist;

dosage reduction may be necessary, or antacid added.

- Monitor weight and report an increase greater than 2 kg (4 lb)/wk with impaired kidney or cardiac function; check for swelling in ankles, tibiae, hands, and feet.
- Inform surgeon or dentist before treatment if you are taking tolmetin because of possible enhanced bleeding.
- Report promptly signs of abnormal bleeding (ecchymosis, epistaxis, melena, petechiae), itching, skin rash, persistent headache, edema.
- Avoid potentially hazardous activities until response to drug is known because dizziness and drowsiness are common adverse effects.

TOLNAFTATE

(tole-naf′tate)

Aftate, Pitrex ♣, Tinactin

Classification: ANTIFUNGAL ANTIBIOTIC

Therapeutic: ANTIFUNGAL

Pregnancy Category: C

AVAILABILITY 1% cream, solution, gel, powder, spray

ACTION & *THERAPEUTIC EFFECT* Synthetic topical antifungal agent. Tolnaftate distorts hyphae and stunts mycelial growth on susceptible fungi. *Fungistatic or fungicidal as well as anti-infective against bacteria, protozoa, and viruses.*

USES Tinea pedis (athlete's foot), tinea cruris (jock itch), tinea corporis (body ringworm); also tinea capitis and tinea unguium if infection is superficial, plantar or palmar lesions adjunctively with keratolytic agents, and tinea versicolor (caused by *Malassezia furfur*).

CONTRAINDICATIONS Skin irritations prior to therapy, nail and scalp infections; immunosuppressed patients, diabetes mellitus, peripheral vascular disease. Safe use in children younger than 2 y is not established.

CAUTIOUS USE Excoriated skin; pregnancy (category C), lactation.

ROUTE & DOSAGE

Tinea Infestations

Adult/Child: **Topical** Apply 0.5–1 cm (1/4–1/2 in.) of cream or 3 drops of solution b.i.d. in morning and evening; powder may be used prophylactically in normally moist areas

ADMINISTRATION

Topical

- Cleanse site thoroughly with water and dry completely before applying. Massage thin layer gently into skin. Make sure area is not wet from excess drug after application.
- Shake aerosol powder container well before use.
- Note: Cream and powder are not recommended for nail or scalp infection.
- Use liquids (solutions) for scalp infection or to treat hairy areas.
- Store cream, gel, powder, and topical solution in light-resistant containers at 15°–30° C (59°–86° F); store aerosol container at 2°–30° C (38°–86° F). Avoid freezing and exposure to light.

ADVERSE EFFECTS (≥1%) **Skin:** Local irritation, stinging of skin from aerosol formulation.

T

NURSING IMPLICATIONS

Patient & Family Education

- Expect relief from pruritus, soreness, and burning within 24–72 h after start of treatment.
- Continue treatment for 2–3 wk after disappearance of all symptoms to prevent recurrence.
- Return to physician for reevaluation in absence of improvement within 4 wk.
- Note: If skin has thickened as a result of the infection, desired clinical response may be delayed for 4–6 wk.
- Avoid contact with eyes of all drug forms.
- Place container in warm water to liquify contents if solution solidifies. Potency is unaffected.

TOLTERODINE TARTRATE

(tol-ter′o-deen tar′trate)

Detrol, Detrol LA

Classifications: ANTICHOLINERGIC; MUSCARINIC RECEPTOR ANTAGONIST

Therapeutic: ANTIMUSCARINIC; BLADDER ANTISPASMODIC

Prototype: Oxybutynin

Pregnancy Category: C

AVAILABILITY 1 mg, 2 mg tablets; 2 mg, 4 mg sustained release

ACTION & *THERAPEUTIC EFFECT* Selective muscarinic urinary bladder receptor antagonist. Reduces urinary incontinence, urgency, and frequency. *Controls urinary bladder incontinence by controlling contractions.*

USES Overactive bladder, urinary incontinence, urinary urgency.

CONTRAINDICATIONS Hypersensitivity to tolterodine; uncontrolled narrow-angle glaucoma; gastric retention; urinary retention; lactation.

CAUTIOUS USE Cardiovascular disease; liver disease; controlled narrow-angle glaucoma; urinary retention; severe hepatic impairment; obstructive GI disease; obstructive uropathy; paralytic ileus or intestinal atony; renal impairment; ulcerative colitis; pregnancy (category C).

ROUTE & DOSAGE

Overactive Bladder

Adult: **PO** 2 mg b.i.d. or 4 mg (sustained release) daily

Hepatic Impairment Dosage Adjustment

Reduce dose by 50%

Renal Impairment Dosage Adjustment

CrCl less than 30 mL/min: Reduce dose 50%

ADMINISTRATION

Oral

- Do not crush or chew sustained release tablets. These **must be** swallowed whole.
- Doses greater than 1 mg b.i.d. are not recommended for those with significantly reduced liver function or kidney function or concurrently receiving macrolide antibiotics, azole antifungal agents, or other cytochrome P450 3A4 inhibitors.
- Store at 20°–25° C (68°–77° F) in a tightly closed container.

ADVERSE EFFECTS (≥1%) **Body as a Whole:** Back pain, fatigue, flu-like syndrome, falls, arthralgia, weight gain. **CNS:** Headache, paresthesias, vertigo, dizziness, nervousness, somnolence. **CV:** Chest pain, hypertension. **GI:** *Dry mouth,* dyspepsia, constipation, abdominal pain, diarrhea, flatulence, nausea, vomiting. **Urogenital:** Dysuria, micturition frequency, urinary retention, UTI. **Respiratory:** Bronchitis, cough, pharyngitis, rhinitis, sinusitis, URI. **Skin:** Pruritus, rash, erythema, dry skin. **Special Senses:** Dry eyes, vision abnormalities.

INTERACTIONS Drug: Additive anticholinergic effects with **amantadine, amoxapine, bupropion, clozapine, cyclobenzaprine, disopyramide, maprotiline, olanzapine, orphenadrine,** SEDATING H_1-BLOCKERS, PHENOTHIAZINES, TRICYCLIC ANTIDEPRESSANTS. Increased effects with **clarithromycin, cyclosporine, erythromycin, itraconazole,** or **ketoconazole. Food: Grapefruit juice** may increase **tolterodine** levels in some patients.

PHARMACOKINETICS Absorption: 77% absorbed, decreased with food. **Peak:** 1–2 h. **Distribution:** 96% protein bound. **Metabolism:** In liver by CYP2D6 active metabolite. **Elimination:** 77% in urine, 17% in feces. **Half-Life:** 1.9–3.7 h.

NURSING IMPLICATIONS

Assessment & Drug Effects

- Monitor voiding pattern and report promptly urinary retention.
- Monitor vital signs carefully (HR and BP), especially in those with cardiovascular disease.

Patient & Family Education

- Notify physician promptly if you experience eye pain, rapid heartbeat, difficulty breathing, skin rash or hives, confusion, or incoordination.
- Report blurred vision, sensitivity to light, and dry mouth (all common adverse effects) to physician if bothersome.
- Avoid the use of alcohol or OTC antihistamines.

TOLVAPTAN

(tol-vap'tan)

Samsca

Classifications: ELECTROLYTE & WATER BALANCE AGENT; DIURETIC; VASOPRESSIN ANTAGONIST

Therapeutic: VASOPRESSIN ANTAGONIST; DIURETIC

Prototype: Conivaptan

Pregnancy Category: C

AVAILABILITY 15 mg, 30 mg tablets

ACTION & *THERAPEUTIC EFFECT* Tolvaptan is a selective vasopressin V_2-receptor antagonist, thus antagonizing the effect of vasopressin and causing an increase in urine water excretion, decrease in urine osmolality, and increase in serum sodium concentrations. *Effectiveness is measured by increase in serum sodium level toward lower limit of normal, and/or decrease in sign and symptoms of hyponatremia.*

USES Treatment of hypervolemic and euvolemic hyponatremia including patients with heart failure, cirrhosis, and syndrome of inappropriate antidiuretic hormone (SIADH).

CONTRAINDICATIONS Rapid correction of serum sodium (e.g. greater than12 mEq/L/24 h); cognitively impaired; serious neurologic symptoms; hypovolemic hyponatremia; hypertonic saline; concurrent administration with strong CYP3A inhibitors; lactation. Safety and effectiveness in children younger than 18 y are not established.

T

CAUTIOUS USE Must be initiated or reinitiated in a hospital setting; cirrhosis; pregnancy (category C).

ROUTE & DOSAGE

Hyponatremia

Adult: **PO** Initially 15 mg once daily; may be adjusted up to 60 mg once daily

ADMINISTRATION

Oral

- Doses may be increased at 24 h intervals or greater.
- Do not administer if patient is unable to sense or respond to thirst.
- Store at 15°–30°C (59°–86°F).

ADVERSE EFFECTS (≥2%) **Body as a Whole:** *Asthenia,* pyrexia, *thirst.* **GI:** *Constipation, dry mouth, nausea.* **Metabolic:** Anorexia, *hyperglycemia.* **Urogenital:** *Pollakiuria, polyuria.*

INTERACTIONS Drug: Strong CYP3A INHIBITORS (e.g., **clarithromycin, ketoconazole, itraconazole, telithromycin, saquinavir, nelfinavir, ritonavir, nefazodone**) may increase tolvaptan levels. Moderate CYP3A INHIBITORS (e.g., **erythromycin, fluconazole, aprepitant, diltiazem, verapamil**) may increase tolvaptan levels. P-GLYCOPROTEIN INHIBITORS (e.g., **cyclosporine**) may require tolvaptan dosage reduction. CYP3A INDUCERS (e.g., **rifabutin, rifapentine, rifampin, barbiturates, phenytoin, carbamazepine**) decrease the levels of tolvaptan. Tolvaptan increases the levels of **digoxin**. BETA-BLOCKERS, ANGIOTENSIN RECEPTOR BLOCKERS, ANGIOTENSIN-CONVERTING ENZYME INHIBITORS and POTASSIUM-SPARING DIURETICS may cause hyperkalemia. **Food:** Administration with **grapefruit juice** may increase tolvaptan levels. **Herbal: St. John's Wort** may decrease the levels of tolvaptan.

PHARMACOKINETICS Absorption: Approximately 40% absorbed. **Peak:** 2–4 h. **Distribution:** 99% plasma protein bound. **Metabolism:** In liver through CYP3A4. **Elimination:** Eliminated entirely by non-renal routes. **Half-Life:** 12 h.

NURSING IMPLICATIONS

Assessment & Drug Effects

- Monitor vital signs frequently throughout therapy. Monitor ECG as warranted
- Monitor weight and I&O closely as copious diuresis is expected.
- Fluid restriction should be avoided during the first 24 h of therapy.
- Lab tests: Baseline and frequent serum electrolytes and volume status; periodic blood glucose.
- Monitor mental status throughout treatment. Report promptly changes in mental status (e.g., lethargy, confusion, disorientation, hallucinations, seizures).
- Report promptly symptoms of osmotic demyelination syndrome (ODS): Dysarthria, mutism, dysphagia, lethargy, affective changes, spasticity, seizures, or coma.
- Monitor digoxin levels closely with concurrent administration.

Patient & Family Education

- Continue to drink fluid in response to thirst until otherwise directed. Fluid restrictions are usually required after the first 24 h of therapy.
- Report promptly any of the following: Trouble speaking or swallowing, drowsiness, mood changes, confusion, involuntary body movements, or muscle weakness in arms or legs.

TOPIRAMATE

(to-pir'a-mate)

Topamax

Classifications: GAMMA-AMINOBUTYRATE (GABA) ENHANCER; ANTICONVULSANT

Therapeutic: ANTICONVULSANT; ANTIEPILEPTIC

Pregnancy Category: C

AVAILABILITY 25 mg, 100 mg, 200 mg tablets; 15 mg, 25 mg, 50 mg capsules

ACTION & *THERAPEUTIC EFFECT* Sulfamate-substituted monosaccharide with a broad spectrum of anticonvulsant activity. Exhibits sodium channel-blocking action, as well as enhancing the ability of GABA to induce a flux of chloride ions into the neurons, thus potentiating the activity of this inhibitory neurotransmitter (GABA). *Effectiveness indicated by a decrease in seizure activity.*

USES Adjunctive therapy for partial-onset seizures in adults and children age 2–16 y; generalized tonic-clonic seizures; migraine prophylaxis.

UNLABELED USES Cluster headache, bulimia nervosa, neuropathic pain, infantile spasms, weight loss.

CONTRAINDICATIONS Hypersensitivity to topiramate; children younger than 2 y. Effect on labor and delivery is unknown.

CAUTIOUS USE Moderate and severe renal impairment, hepatic impairment; COPD; severe pulmonary disease; pregnancy (category C), lactation.

ROUTE & DOSAGE

Partial-Onset Seizures

Adult: **PO** Initiate with 25 mg b.i.d., increase by 50 mg/wk to efficacy **PO Maintenance Dose** 200–400 mg/day divided b.i.d. (max: 1600 mg/day)

Child (2–16 y): **PO** Initiate with 1–3 mg/kg at bedtime × 1 wk, then increase by 1–3 mg/kg/day in 2 divided doses q1–2wk to a target range of 5–9 mg/kg/day

Generalized Tonic-Clonic

Child: **PO** Initiate with 1–3 mg/kg at bedtime; titrate to 6 mg/kg/day by the end of 8 wk

Migraine Prophylaxis

Adult: **PO** Initiate with 25 mg b.i.d., increase by 25 mg/wk to 200 mg/day or max tolerated dose

Renal Impairment Dosage Adjustment

CrCl less than 70 mL/min: Decrease dose by 50%

ADMINISTRATION

Oral

- Make dosage increments of 50 mg at weekly intervals to the recommended dose, usually 400 mg/day.
- Do not break tablets unless absolutely necessary because of bitter taste.
- Store at 15°–30° C (59°–86° F) in a tightly closed container. Protect from light and moisture.

ADVERSE EFFECTS (≥1%) **Body as a Whole:** *Fatigue, speech problems,* weight loss; decreased sweating and hyperthermia in children; metabolic acidosis. **CNS:** *Somnolence, dizziness, ataxia, psychomotor slowing, confusion, nystagmus, paresthesia, memory difficulty, difficulty concentrating, nervousness,* depression, anxiety, tremor. **GI:** Anorexia. **Special Senses:** Angle closure glaucoma (rare).

INTERACTIONS Drug: Increased CNS depression with **alcohol** and other CNS DEPRESSANTS; may increase **phenytoin** concentrations; may decrease ORAL CONTRACEPTIVE, **valproate** concentrations; may increase risk of kidney stone formation with other CARBONIC ANHYDRASE INHIBITORS. **Carbamazepine, phenytoin, valproate** may decrease topiramate concentrations. **Herbal: Ginkgo** may decrease anticonvulsant effectiveness.

PHARMACOKINETICS Absorption: Rapidly absorbed from GI tract; 80% bioavailability. **Peak:** 2 h. **Distribution:** 13–17% protein bound. **Metabolism:** Minimally metabolized in the liver. **Elimination:** Primarily in urine. **Half-Life:** 21 h.

NURSING IMPLICATIONS

Assessment & Drug Effects

- Monitor mental status and report significant cognitive impairment.
- Lab tests: Periodically monitor CBC with Hgb and Hct.

Patient & Family Education

- Do not stop drug abruptly; discontinue gradually to minimize seizures.
- To minimize risk of kidney stones, drink at least 6–8 full glasses of water each day.
- Exercise caution with potentially hazardous activities. Sedation is common, especially with concurrent use of alcohol or other CNS depressants.
- Use or add barrier contraceptive if using hormonal contraceptives.
- Be aware that psychomotor slowing and speech/language problems may develop while on topiramate therapy.
- Report adverse effects that interfere with activities of daily living.

T

TOPOTECAN HYDROCHLORIDE (Pr)

(toe-po-tee'can)

Hycamtin

Classifications: ANTINEOPLASTIC; CAMPTOTHECIN; DNA TOPOISOMERASE I INHIBITOR

Therapeutic: ANTINEOPLASTIC

Pregnancy Category: D

AVAILABILITY 4 mg injection

ACTION & *THERAPEUTIC EFFECT* Antitumor mechanism is related to inhibition of the activity of topoisomerase I, an enzyme required for DNA replication. Topoisomerase I is essential for the relaxation of supercoiled double-stranded DNA that enables replication and transcription to proceed. *Topotecan permits uncoiling of DNA stands but prevents recoiling of the two strands of DNA, resulting in a permanent break in the DNA strands.*

USES Metastatic ovarian cancer, small cell lung cancer.

CONTRAINDICATIONS Previous hypersensitivity to topotecan, irinotecan, or other camptothecin analogs; acute infection; severe bone marrow depression; severe thrombocytopenia; pregnancy (category D), lactation.

CAUTIOUS USE Myelosuppression; severe renal impairment or renal failure; history of bleeding disorders; previous cytotoxic or radiation therapy.

ROUTE & DOSAGE

Metastatic Ovarian Cancer and Small Cell Lung Cancer

Adult: **IV** 1.5 mg/m² daily for 5 days starting on day 1 of a 21-

day course. Four courses of therapy recommended. Subsequent doses can be adjusted by 0.25 mg/m² depending on toxicity.

Renal Impairment Dosage Adjustment

CrCl 20–39 mL/min: Use 0.75 mg/m²
Hemodialysis Dosage Adjustment: Supplementation not needed

ADMINISTRATION

Intravenous

Initiate therapy only if baseline neutrophil count 1500/mm³ or higher and platelet count 100,000/mm³ or higher. ▪ Do not give subsequent doses until neutrophils 1000/mm³ or higher, platelets 100,000/mm³ or higher, and Hgb greater than 9.0 mg/dL.

- Note: Dosage adjustments to 0.75 mg/m² are recommended with moderate renal impairment.

PREPARE: **IV Infusion:** Reconstitute each 4-mg vial with 4 mL sterile water for injection to yield 1 mg/mL. ▪ Withdraw the required dose and inject into 50–100 mL of NS or D5W. ▪ If skin contacts drug during preparation, wash immediately with soap and water.

ADMINISTER: **IV Infusion:** Give over 30 min immediately after preparation.

INCOMPATIBILITIES **Y-site: Dexamethasone, fluorouracil, mitomycin.**

- Store vials at 20°–25° C (68°–77° F); protect from light. Reconstituted vials are stable for 24 h.

ADVERSE EFFECTS (≥1%) **Body as a Whole:** *Asthenia, fever, fatigue.* **GI:** *Nausea, vomiting, diarrhea, constipation, abdominal pain, stomatitis, anorexia,* transient elevations in liver function tests. **Hematologic:** *Leukopenia, neutropenia, anemia, thrombocytopenia.* **Respiratory:** *Dyspnea.* **Skin:** *Alopecia.*

INTERACTIONS Drug: Increased risk of bleeding with ANTICOAGULANTS, NSAIDS, SALICYLATES, ANTIPLATELET AGENTS.

PHARMACOKINETICS Distribution: 35% bound to plasma proteins. **Metabolism:** Undergoes pH-dependent hydrolysis. **Elimination:** ~30% in urine. **Half-Life:** 2–3 h.

NURSING IMPLICATIONS

Assessment & Drug Effects

- Lab tests: Obtain CBC counts with differential frequently; periodically monitor ALT.
- Assess for GI distress, respiratory distress, neurosensory symptoms, and S&S of infection throughout therapy.

Patient & Family Education

- Learn common adverse effects and measures to control or minimize when possible. Immediately report any distressing adverse effects to physician.
- Avoid pregnancy during therapy.

TOREMIFENE CITRATE

(tor-em'i-feen ci'trate)

Fareston

Classifications: ANTINEOPLASTIC; SELECTIVE ESTROGEN RECEPTOR MODIFIER (SERM)

Therapeutic: ANTINEOPLASTIC, ANTI-ESTROGEN

Prototype: Tamoxifen

Pregnancy Category: D

AVAILABILITY 60 mg tablets

T

ACTION & *THERAPEUTIC EFFECT* Nonsteroidal antiestrogen chemical derivative of tamoxifen. Antitumor activity thought to be due to ability to compete with estrogen for binding sites in cancer cells. *Depresses growth in estrogen receptor–positive tumors in postmenopausal women.*

USES Metastatic breast cancer in postmenopausal women who are estrogen receptor positive.

CONTRAINDICATIONS Hypersensitivity to toremifene; history of thromboembolic disease; pregnancy (category D); lactation.
CAUTIOUS USE Preexisting endometrial hyperplasia; bone metastases (may result in hypercalcemia); geriatric patients; leukopenia and thrombocytopenia; liver disease; history of thrombolytic disease.

ROUTE & DOSAGE

Breast Cancer
Adult: **PO** 60 mg daily

ADMINISTRATION

Oral
- Withhold drug and notify physician if severe hypercalcemia develops.
- Store at 15°–30° C (59°–86° F) in a tightly closed container and protect from light.

T

ADVERSE EFFECTS (≥1%) **Body as a Whole:** *Hot flashes, sweating,* edema. **CNS:** Dizziness. **GI:** *Nausea,* vomiting, abnormal liver function tests. **Respiratory:** Pulmonary embolism. **Urogenital:** *Vaginal discharge,* vaginal bleeding. **Special Senses:** Cataracts, dry eyes, corneal keratopathy.

INTERACTIONS Drug: THIAZIDE DIURETICS increase risk of hypercalcemia; increased PT on **warfarin; carbamazepine, phenobarbital, phenytoin** may increase toremifene metabolism.

PHARMACOKINETICS Absorption: Rapidly absorbed from GI tract. **Peak:** 3 h. **Distribution:** Greater than 99% protein bound; crosses placenta. **Metabolism:** In liver by cytochrome P450 3A4. **Elimination:** Primarily in feces. **Half-Life:** 5 days.

NURSING IMPLICATIONS

Assessment & Drug Effects
- Lab tests: Periodically monitor CBC with differential, serum calcium, liver and kidney functions.
- Monitor patients carefully with bone metastases or those on drugs that decrease calcium excretion (e.g., thiazide diuretics) for S&S of hypercalcemia (see Appendix F).
- Monitor PT and INR carefully when given concurrently with warfarin.

Patient & Family Education
- Report to physician promptly any of the following: Unexplained weakness or fatigue, musculoskeletal pain or calf pain and tenderness, sudden chest pain, vaginal bleeding.
- Schedule periodic eye exams with long-term therapy.

TORSEMIDE

(tor′se-mide)
Demadex
Classifications: ELECTROLYTE AND WATER BALANCE; LOOP DIURETIC
Therapeutic: DIURETIC; ANTIHYPERTENSIVE
Prototype: Furosemide
Pregnancy Category: B

AVAILABILITY 5 mg, 10 mg, 20 mg, 100 mg tablets; 10 mg/mL injection

ACTION & *THERAPEUTIC EFFECT* Long-acting potent sulfonamide "loop" diuretic that inhibits reabsorption of sodium and chloride primarily in the loop of Henle and renal tubules. Binds to the sodium/potassium/chloride carrier in the loop of Henle and in the renal tubules. *Long-acting potent "loop" diuretic and antihypertensive agent.*

USES Management of edema associated with CHF, chronic kidney failure, hepatic cirrhosis; hypertension.

CONTRAINDICATIONS Hypersensitivity to torsemide or sulfonamides; anuria, fluid and electrolyte depletion states; anuria; acute MI; hepatic coma.

CAUTIOUS USE Renal impairment; ventricular arrhythmias; gout or hyperuricemia; diabetes mellitus or history of pancreatitis; liver disease; hearing impairment; pregnancy (category B); lactation.

ROUTE & DOSAGE

Edema of CHF, Chronic Kidney Failure

Adult: **PO/IV** 10–20 mg once daily, may increase up to 200 mg/day as needed

Hepatic Cirrhosis

Adult: **PO/IV** 5–10 mg once daily administered with an aldosterone antagonist or potassium-sparing diuretic, may increase up to 40 mg/day as needed

Hypertension

Adult: **PO** 2.5–5 mg once daily, may increase to 10 mg/day if no response after 4–6 wk

ADMINISTRATION

- Note: With hepatic cirrhosis, use an aldosterone antagonist concomitantly to prevent hypokalemia and metabolic alkalosis.

Oral

- Be aware that oral and IV doses are therapeutically equivalent; patients may be switched between the two forms with no change in dosage.

Intravenous

PREPARE: **Direct:** Given undiluted.
ADMINISTER: **Direct:** Give slowly over 2 min.
INCOMPATIBILITIES **Solution/additive: Dobutamine.**

- Store at 15°–30° C (59°–86° F).

ADVERSE EFFECTS (≥1%) **CNS:** Headache, dizziness, fatigue, insomnia. **CV:** Orthostatic hypotension. **Endocrine:** *Hypokalemia,* hyponatremia, hyperuricemia. **GI:** Nausea, diarrhea. **Skin:** Rash, pruritus. **Body as a Whole:** Muscle cramps, rhinitis.

INTERACTIONS Drug: NSAIDS may reduce diuretic effects. Also see furosemide for potential drug interactions such as increased risk of **digoxin** toxicity due to hypokalemia, prolonged neuromuscular blockade with NEUROMUSCULAR BLOCKING AGENTS, and decreased **lithium** elimination with increased toxicity. **Herbal: Ginseng** may decrease efficacy.

PHARMACOKINETICS Absorption: Readily from GI tract. **Onset:** IV 10 min; PO 60 min. **Peak:** IV within 60 min; PO 60–120 min. **Duration:** 6–8 h. **Metabolism:** In liver (CYP system). **Elimination:** 80% in bile; 20% in urine. **Half-Life:** 210 min.

NURSING IMPLICATIONS

Assessment & Drug Effects

- Monitor BP often and assess for orthostatic hypotension; assess respiratory status for S&S of pulmonary edema.

T

- Monitor ECG, as electrolyte imbalances predispose to cardiac arrhythmias.
- Lab tests: Monitor serum electrolytes, uric acid, blood glucose, BUN, and creatinine periodically throughout the course of therapy.
- Monitor I&O with daily weights. Assess for improvement in edema.
- Monitor diabetics for loss of glycemic control.
- Monitor coagulation parameters and lithium levels in patients on concurrent anticoagulant and/or lithium therapy.

Patient & Family Education

- Check weight at least weekly and report abrupt gains or losses to physician.
- Understand the risk of orthostatic hypotension.
- Report symptoms of hypokalemia (see Appendix F) or hearing loss immediately to physician.
- Monitor blood glucose for loss of glycemic control if diabetic.

TRAMADOL HYDROCHLORIDE

(tra′ma-dol)

Ultram, Zydol ♣

Classifications: ANALGESIC; NARCOTIC (OPIATE AGONIST)

Therapeutic: NARCOTIC ANALGESIC

Prototype: Morphine sulfate

Pregnancy Category: C

Controlled Substance: Schedule IV

AVAILABILITY 50 mg tablets; 50 mg orally disintegrating tablets

ACTION & *THERAPEUTIC EFFECT* Centrally acting opiate receptor agonist that inhibits the uptake of norepinephrine and serotonin, suggesting both opioid and nonopioid mechanisms of pain relief. May produce opioid-like effects, but causes less respiratory depression than morphine. *Effective agent for control of moderate to moderately severe pain.*

USES Management of moderate to moderately severe pain.

CONTRAINDICATIONS Hypersensitivity to tramadol or other opioid analgesics; severe respiratory depression; severe or acute asthmas; patients on MAO inhibitors; substance abuse; alcohol intoxication; lactation; children younger than 16 y.
CAUTIOUS USE Debilitated patients; chronic respiratory disorders; respiratory depression; older adults; liver disease; renal impairment; myxedema, hypothyroidism, or hypoadrenalism; GI disease; acute abdominal conditions; increased ICP or head injury, increased intracranial pressure; history of seizures; patients older than 75 y; pregnancy (category C).

ROUTE & DOSAGE

Pain

Adult: **PO** 50–100 mg q4–6h prn (max: 400 mg/day), may start with 25 mg/day if not well tolerated, and increase by 25 mg q3days up to 200 mg/day

Geriatric: **PO** 50–100 mg q4–6h prn (max: 300 mg/day), may start with 25 mg/day if not well tolerated, and increase by 25 mg q3days up to 200 mg/day

Renal Impairment Dosage Adjustment

CrCl less than 30 mL/min: Decrease to 50–100 mg q12h

Hepatic Impairment Dosage Adjustment

Cirrhosis: Decrease to 50–100 mg q12h

ADMINISTRATION

Oral

- Extended release tablets should be swallowed whole. They should not be crushed or chewed.
- Store at 15°–30° C (59°–86° F).

ADVERSE EFFECTS (≥1%) **CNS:** Drowsiness, *dizziness, vertigo, fatigue, headache, somnolence,* restlessness, euphoria, confusion, anxiety, coordination disturbance, sleep disturbances, seizures. **CV:** Palpitations, vasodilation. **GI:** *Nausea, constipation,* vomiting, xerostomia, dyspepsia, diarrhea, abdominal pain, anorexia, flatulence. **Body as a Whole:** Sweating, anaphylactic reaction (even with first dose), withdrawal syndrome (anxiety, sweating, nausea, tremors, diarrhea, piloerection, panic attacks, paresthesia, hallucinations) with abrupt discontinuation. **Skin:** Rash. **Special Senses:** Visual disturbances. **Urogenital:** Urinary retention/frequency, menopausal symptoms.

DIAGNOSTIC TEST INTERFERENCE Increased ***creatinine, liver enzymes;*** decreased ***hemoglobin; proteinuria.***

INTERACTIONS Drug: Carbamazepine significantly decreases tramadol levels (may need up to twice usual dose). Tramadol may increase adverse effects of MAO INHIBITORS. TRICYCLIC ANTIDEPRESSANTS, **cyclobenzaprine,** PHENOTHIAZINES, SELECTIVE SEROTONIN-REUPTAKE INHIBITORS (SSRIS), MAO INHIBITORS may enhance seizure risk with tramadol. May increase CNS adverse effects when used with other CNS DEPRESSANTS. **Herbal: St. John's wort** may increase sedation.

PHARMACOKINETICS Absorption: Rapidly absorbed from GI tract; 75% reaches systemic circulation. **Onset:** 30–60 min. **Peak:** 2 h. **Duration:** 3–7 h. **Distribution:** Approximately 20% bound to plasma proteins; probably crosses blood–brain barrier; crosses placenta; 0.1% excreted into breast milk. **Metabolism:** Extensively in liver by cytochrome P450 system. **Elimination:** Primarily in urine. **Half-Life:** 6–7 h.

NURSING IMPLICATIONS

Assessment & Drug Effects

- Assess for level of pain relief and administer prn dose as needed but not to exceed the recommended total daily dose.
- Monitor vital signs and assess for orthostatic hypotension or signs of CNS depression.
- Withhold drug and notify physician if S&S of hypersensitivity occur.
- Assess bowel and bladder function; report urinary frequency or retention.
- Use seizure precautions for patients who have a history of seizures or who are concurrently using drugs that lower the seizure threshold.
- Monitor ambulation and take appropriate safety precautions.

Patient & Family Education

- Exercise caution with potentially hazardous activities until response to drug is known.
- Do not exceed the total number of mg prescribed for a 24 h period.
- Understand potential adverse effects and report problems with bowel and bladder function, CNS impairment, and any other bothersome adverse effects to physician.

TRANDOLAPRIL

(tran-do′la-pril)

Mavik
Classifications: ANGIOTENSIN-CONVERTING ENZYME (ACE) INHIBITOR; ANTIHYPERTENSIVE
Therapeutic: ANTIHYPERTENSIVE; ACE INHIBITOR
Prototype: Enalapril
Pregnancy Category: D

AVAILABILITY 1 mg, 2 mg, 4 mg tablets

ACTION & *THERAPEUTIC EFFECT* Inhibits ACE and interrupts conversion by renin which leads to the formation of angiotensin II from angiotensin I. Inhibition of ACE leads to vasodilation as well as to decreased aldosterone. Decreased aldosterone leads to diuresis and a slight increase in serum potassium. *Lowers blood pressure by specific inhibition of ACE. Unlike other ACE inhibitors, all racial groups respond to trandolapril, including low-renin hypertensives.*

USES Treatment of hypertension, alone or in combination with other antihypertensive agents.
UNLABELED USES CHF.

CONTRAINDICATIONS Hypersensitivity to trandolapril or ACE inhibitors; history of angioedema related to previous treatment with an ACE inhibitor; pregnancy (category D), lactation.
CAUTIOUS USE Renal impairment, hepatic insufficiency; patients prone to hypotension (e.g., CHF, ischemic heart disease, aortic stenosis, CVA, dehydration); SLE, scleroderma. Safety and effectiveness in children younger than 18 y are not established.

ROUTE & DOSAGE

Note: Discontinue diuretics 2–3 days before starting trandolapril.

Hypertension
Adult: **PO** 1 mg in nonblack patients, 2 mg in black patients once daily, may increase weekly to 2–4 mg once daily (max: 8 mg/day)

Renal Impairment Dosage Adjustment
CrCl less than 30 mL/min: Start with 0.5 mg once daily

Hepatic Impairment Dosage Adjustment
Hepatic cirrhosis: Start with 0.5 mg once daily

ADMINISTRATION

Oral
- Note: If concurrently ordered diuretic cannot be discontinued 2–3 days before beginning trandolapril therapy, initial dose is usually reduced to 0.5 mg.
- Dosage adjustments are typically made at intervals of at least 1 wk.
- Store at 15°–30° C (59°–86° F).

ADVERSE EFFECTS (≥1%) **Body as a Whole:** Fatigue, angioedema. **CNS:** Dizziness, headache. **CV:** Hypotension. **GI:** Diarrhea. **Respiratory:** Cough. **Skin:** Rash, pruritus. **Metabolic:** Hyperkalemia.

INTERACTIONS Drug: DIURETICS may enhance hypotensive effects. POTASSIUM-SPARING DIURETICS (**amiloride, spironolactone, triamterene**), POTASSIUM SUPPLEMENTS, POTASSIUM-CONTAINING SALT SUBSTITUTES may increase risk of hyperkalemia. May increase serum levels and toxicity of **lithium.**

PHARMACOKINETICS Absorption: Rapidly absorbed from GI tract and converted to active form, trandolaprilat, in liver; 70% of dose reaches systemic circulation as trandolaprilat. **Peak:** 4–10 h. **Distribution:** 80% protein bound; crosses placenta, secreted into breast milk of animals (human secretion unknown). **Metabolism:** In liver to active metabolite, trandolaprilat. **Elimination:** 33% in urine, 66% in feces. **Half-Life:** 6 h trandolapril, 10 h trandolaprilat.

NURSING IMPLICATIONS

Assessment & Drug Effects

- Monitor BP carefully for 1–3 h following initial dose, especially in patients using concurrent diuretics, on salt restriction, or volume depleted.
- Lab tests: Baseline LFTs and kidney function tests; periodic serum potassium and sodium.
- Monitor serum lithium levels frequently with concurrent lithium therapy and assess for S&S of lithium toxicity; increase caution when diuretic therapy is also used.

Patient & Family Education

- Discontinue drug and immediately report S&S of angioedema of face or extremities to physician. Seek emergency help for swelling of the tongue or any other sign of potential airway obstruction.
- Be aware that lightheadedness can occur, especially during early therapy. Excess fluid loss of any kind will increase risk of hypotension and syncope.

TRANYLCYPROMINE SULFATE

(tran-ill-sip′roe-meen)

Parnate

Classifications: ANTIDEPRESSANT; MONOAMINE OXIDASE INHIBITOR (MAOI)

Therapeutic: ANTIDEPRESSANT; MAOI

Prototype: Phenelzine

Pregnancy Category: C

AVAILABILITY 10 mg tablets

ACTION & *THERAPEUTIC EFFECT* Potent MAO with a antidepressant activity that arises from the increased availability of monoamines resulting from the inhibition of the enzyme MAO. This leads to increased concentration of neurotransmitters, such as epinephrine, norepinephrine, and dopamine in the CNS. *Drug of last choice for severe depression unresponsive to other MAO inhibitors.*

USES Severe depression.

CONTRAINDICATIONS Confirmed or suspected cerebrovascular defect, cardiovascular disease, CHF; hepatic disease; hypertension, pheochromocytoma, history of severe or recurrent headaches; acute MI; angina; renal failure; suicidal ideation; anuria; lactation; children.

CAUTIOUS USE Bipolar disorder; Parkinson's disease; psychosis; schizophrenia; seizure disorders; history of suicidal attempts; renal impairment; pregnancy (category C).

ROUTE & DOSAGE

Severe Depression

Adult: **PO** 30 mg/day in 2 divided doses (20 mg in a.m., 10 mg in p.m.), may increase by 10 mg/day at 3 wk intervals (max: 60 mg/day)

ADMINISTRATION

Oral

- Crush tablet and give with fluid or mix with food if patient cannot swallow pill.
- Note: Doses given in the late evening may cause insomnia.

ADVERSE EFFECTS (≥1%) **CNS:** Vertigo, dizziness, tremors, muscle

T

twitching, headache, blurred vision. **CV:** *Orthostatic hypotension,* arrhythmias, hypertensive crisis. **GI:** Dry mouth, anorexia, constipation, diarrhea, abdominal discomfort. **Skin:** Rash. **Urogenital:** Impotence. **Body as a Whole:** Peripheral edema, sweating.

INTERACTIONS Drug: TRICYCLIC ANTIDEPRESSANTS, **fluoxetine,** AMPHETAMINES, **ephedrine, reserpine, guanethidine, buspirone, methyldopa, dopamine, levodopa, tryptophan** may precipitate hypertensive crisis, headache, or hyperexcitability; **alcohol** and other CNS DEPRESSANTS add to CNS depressant effects; **meperidine** can cause fatal cardiovascular collapse; ANESTHETICS exaggerate hypotensive and CNS depressant effects; **metrizamide** increases risk of seizures; DIURETICS and other ANTIHYPERTENSIVE AGENTS add to hypotensive effects. **Food: Tyramine**-containing foods may precipitate hypertensive crisis (e.g., aged cheeses, processed cheeses, sour cream, wine, champagne, beer, pickled herring, anchovies, caviar, shrimp, liver, dry sausage, figs, raisins, overripe bananas or avocados, chocolate, soy sauce, bean curd, yeast extracts, yogurt, papaya products, meat tenderizers, broad beans). **Herbal: Ginseng, ephedra, ma huang, St. John's wort** may lead to hypertensive crisis; **ginseng** may lead to manic episodes.

PHARMACOKINETICS Absorption: Completely absorbed from GI tract. **Onset:** 10 days. **Metabolism:** Rapidly metabolized in liver to active metabolite. **Elimination:** Primarily in urine. **Half-Life:** 2.5 h (but may take 120 h for urinary tryptamine levels to return to normal).

NURSING IMPLICATIONS

Assessment & Drug Effects

- Monitor BP closely. Severe hypertensive reactions are known to occur with MAO inhibitors.
- Monitor for changes in behavior that could indicate increased suicidality.
- Expect therapeutic response within 3 days, but full antidepressant effects may not be obtained until 2–3 wk of drug therapy.

Patient & Family Education

- Do not eat tyramine-containing foods (see FOOD–DRUG INTERACTIONS).
- Be aware that excessive use of caffeine-containing beverages (chocolate, coffee, tea, cola) can contribute to development of rapid heartbeat, arrhythmias, and hypertension.
- Make position changes slowly, particularly from recumbent to upright posture.
- Avoid potentially hazardous activities until response to drug is known.
- Avoid alcohol or other CNS depressants because of their possible additive effects.

TRASTUZUMAB

(tra-stu′zu-mab)

Herceptin

Classifications: IMMUNOMODULATOR; MONOCLONAL ANTIBODY; ANTINEOPLASTIC; ANTI-HUMAN EPIDERMAL GROWTH FACTOR (ANTI-HER)

Therapeutic: ANTINEOPLASTIC; IMMUNOMODULATOR; ANTI-HER

Pregnancy Category: D

AVAILABILITY 21 mg/mL injection

T

ACTION & *THERAPEUTIC EFFECT* Recombinant DNA monoclonal antibody (I_gG_1 kappa) that selectively binds to the human epidermal growth factor receptor-2 protein (HER_2). *Inhibits growth of human tumor cells that overexpress HER_2 proteins.*

USES Metastatic breast cancer in those whose tumors overexpress the HER_2 protein. HER_2-positive breast cancer after surgery.

CONTRAINDICATIONS Concurrent administration of anthracycline or radiation; pregnancy (category D); lactation during and for 6 mo following administration of trastuzumab.

CAUTIOUS USE Preexisting cardiac dysfunction; pulmonary disease; previous administration of cardiotoxic therapy (e.g., anthracycline or radiation); older adults; hypersensitivity to benzyl alcohol (preservative in bacteriostatic water).

ROUTE & DOSAGE

Metastatic Breast Cancer

Adult: **IV** 4 mg/kg, then 2 mg/kg qwk

ADMINISTRATION

Intravenous

PREPARE: **IV Infusion:** Reconstitute each vial with 20 mL of supplied diluent (bacteriostatic water) to produce a multidose vial containing 21 mg/mL. ▪ Note: For patients with a hypersensitivity to benzyl alcohol, reconstitute with sterile water for injection; this solution **must be** used immediately with any unused portion discarded. ▪ Withdraw the ordered dose and add to a 250 mL of NS and invert bag to mix. ▪ Do not give or mix with dextrose solutions.

ADMINISTER: **IV Infusion:** Infuse loading dose (4 mg/kg) over 90 min; infuse subsequent doses (2 mg/kg) over 30 min. ▪ Do not give IV push or as a bolus dose.

INCOMPATIBILITIES **Solution/additive:** **Dextrose** solution; do not mix or coadminister with other drugs.

▪ Store unopened vials and reconstituted vials at 2°–8° C (36°–46° F). ▪ Discard reconstituted vials 28 days after reconstitution.

ADVERSE EFFECTS (≥1%) **Body as a Whole:** *Pain, asthenia, fever, chills,* flu syndrome, allergic reaction, bone pain, arthralgia, hypersensitivity (anaphylaxis, urticaria, bronchospasm, angioedema, or hypotension), increased incidence of infections, infusion reaction (*chills, fever,* nausea, vomiting, pain, rigors, headache, dizziness, dyspnea, hypotension, rash). **CNS:** *Headache, insomnia, dizziness, paresthesias,* depression, peripheral neuritis, neuropathy. **CV:** CHF, cardiac dysfunction (dyspnea, cough, paroxysmal nocturnal dyspnea, peripheral edema, S3 gallop, reduced ejection fraction), tachycardia, edema, cardiotoxicity. **GI:** *Diarrhea, abdominal pain, nausea, vomiting,* anorexia. **Hematologic:** *Anemia, leukopenia.* **Respiratory:** *Cough, dyspnea,* rhinitis, pharyngitis, sinusitis. **Skin:** *Rash,* herpes simplex, acne.

INTERACTIONS Drug: Paclitaxel may increase trastuzumab levels and toxicity.

PHARMACOKINETICS Half-Life: 5.8 days.

NURSING IMPLICATIONS

Assessment & Drug Effects

- Lab tests: Periodically monitor CBC with differential, platelet count, and Hgb and Hct.

T

- Monitor for chills and fever during the first IV infusion; these adverse events usually respond to prompt treatment without the need to discontinue the infusion. Notify physician immediately.
- Monitor carefully cardiovascular status at baseline and throughout course of therapy, assessing for S&S of heart failure (e.g., dyspnea, increased cough, PND, edema, S3 gallop). Those with preexisting cardiac dysfunction are at high risk for cardiotoxicity.

Patient & Family Education

- Report promptly any unusual symptoms (e.g., chills, nausea, fever) during infusion.
- Report promptly any of the following: Shortness of breath, swelling of feet or legs, persistent cough, difficulty sleeping, loss of appetite, abdominal bloating.

TRAVOPROST

(tra′-vo-prost)

Travatan

Pregnancy Category: C

See Appendix A-1.

TRAZODONE HYDROCHLORIDE

(tray′zoe-done)

Classification: ANTIDEPRESSANT

Therapeutic: ANTIDEPRESSANT

Prototype: Imipramine

Pregnancy Category: C

AVAILABILITY 50 mg, 100 mg, 150 mg, 300 mg tablets

ACTION & *THERAPEUTIC EFFECT* Centrally acting antidepressant that potentiates serotonin effects by selectively blocking its reuptake at presynaptic membranes in CNS. Produces varying degrees of sedation in normal and mentally depressed patient. *Increases total sleep time, decreases number and duration of awakenings in depressed patient, and decreases REM sleep. Has antianxiety effect in severely depressed patient.*

USES Both inpatient and outpatient with major depression with or without prominent anxiety.

UNLABELED USES Adjunctive treatment of alcohol dependence, anxiety neuroses, drug-induced dyskinesias, insomnia.

CONTRAINDICATIONS Initial recovery phase of MI; ventricular ectopy; electroshock therapy; suicidal ideation. Safe use in children younger than 6 y is not established.

CAUTIOUS USE Bipolar disorder, older adults; history of suicidal tendencies; cardiac arrhythmias or disease; hepatic disease, renal impairment; pregnancy (category C), lactation.

ROUTE & DOSAGE

Depression

Adult: **PO** 150 mg/day in divided doses, may increase by 50 mg/day q3–4days (max: 400–600 mg/day)

Geriatric: **PO** 25–50 mg at bedtime, may increase q3–7days to usual range of 75–150 mg/day

Child (6–18 y): **PO** 1.5–2 mg/kg/day in divided doses, increase q3–4days prn (max: 6 mg/kg/day)

Pharmacogenetic Dosage Adjustment

Poor CYP2D6 metabolizer: Start with 80% of normal dose

ADMINISTRATION

Oral

- Give drug with food; increases amount of absorption by 20% and appears to decrease incidence of dizziness or light-headedness. Maintain the same schedule for food-drug intake throughout treatment period to prevent variations in serum concentration.
- Store in tightly closed, light-resistant container at 15°–30° C (59°–86° F).

ADVERSE EFFECTS (≥1%) **CNS:** *Drowsiness,* light-headedness, tiredness, dizziness, insomnia, headache, agitation, impaired memory and speech, disorientation. **CV:** *Hypotension (including orthostatic hypotension),* hypertension, syncope, shortness of breath, chest pain, tachycardia, palpitations, bradycardia, PVCs, ventricular tachycardia (short episodes of 3–4 beats). **Special Senses:** Nasal and sinus congestion, blurred vision, eye irritation, sweating or clamminess, tinnitus. **GI:** *Dry mouth,* anorexia, constipation, abdominal distress, nausea, vomiting, dysgeusia, flatulence, diarrhea. **Urogenital:** Hematuria, increased frequency, delayed urine flow, early or absent menses, male priapism, ejaculation inhibition. **Hematologic:** Anemia. **Musculoskeletal:** Skeletal aches and pains, muscle twitches. **Skin:** Skin eruptions, rash, pruritus, acne, photosensitivity. **Body as a Whole:** Weight gain or loss.

INTERACTIONS Drug: ANTIHYPERTENSIVE AGENTS may potentiate hypotensive effects; **alcohol** and other CNS DEPRESSANTS add to depressant effects; may increase **digoxin** or **phenytoin** levels; MAO INHIBITORS may precipitate hypertensive crisis; **ketoconazole, indinavir, ritonavir** may increase levels and toxicity. **Herbal: Ginkgo** may increase sedation.

PHARMACOKINETICS Absorption: Readily from GI tract. **Onset:** 1–2 wk. **Peak:** 1–2 h. **Distribution:** Distributed into breast milk. **Metabolism:** In liver (CYP2D6). **Elimination:** 75% in urine, 25% in feces. **Half-Life:** 5–9 h.

NURSING IMPLICATIONS

Assessment & Drug Effects

- Monitor BP and heart rate and rhythm. Report to physician development of tachycardia, bradycardia, or palpitations.
- Monitor for orthostatic hypotension, especially in the elderly or those taking concurrent antihypertensive drugs.
- Monitor children and adolescents for changes in behavior that indicate increased suicidality.
- Observe patient's level of activity. If it appears to be increasing toward sleeplessness and agitation with changes in reality orientation, report to physician. Manic episodes have been reported.
- Be aware that overdose is characterized by an extension of common adverse effects: Vomiting, lethargy, drowsiness, and exaggerated anticholinergic effects.

Patient & Family Education

- Expect therapeutic response to begin in 1 wk; may require 2–4 wk to reach maximum levels. Adhere to regimen.
- Do not alter dose or intervals between doses.
- Consult physician if drowsiness becomes a distressing adverse effect. Dose regimen may be changed so that largest dose is at bedtime.
- Limit or abstain from alcohol use. The depressant effects of CNS de-

pressants and alcohol may be potentiated by this drug.

- Do not self-medicate with OTC drugs for colds, allergy, or insomnia treatment without advice of physician. Many of these drugs contain CNS depressants.
- Male patient should report inappropriate or prolonged penile erections. The drug may be discontinued.

TREPROSTINIL SODIUM

(tre-pros′tin-il)

Remodulin

Classifications: PROSTAGLANDIN; PULMONARY ANTIHYPERTENSIVE; VASODILATOR

Therapeutic: PULMONARY ANTIHYPERTENSIVE

Prototype: Epoprostenol

Pregnancy Category: B

AVAILABILITY 1 mg/mL, 2.5 mg/mL, 5 mg/mL, 10 mg/mL injection; 1.74 mg/2.9 mL solution for inhalation

ACTION & *THERAPEUTIC EFFECT* Causes direct vasodilation of the pulmonary and systemic arterial vascular beds, and inhibition of platelet aggregation. The vasodilatory effects reduce right and left ventricular afterload, and increase cardiac output and stroke volume. Also improves dyspnea, fatigue, and signs and symptoms of pulmonary arterial hypertension (PAH). *Vasodilation of the arteries in the pulmonary system results in lowering of pulmonary arterial hypertension (PAH).*

USES Treatment of pulmonary arterial hypertension (PAH).

UNLABELED USES Severe intermittent claudication.

CONTRAINDICATIONS Severe hepatic insufficiency; hypersensitivity to treprostinil.

CAUTIOUS USE Mild or moderate hepatic insufficiency; bleeding disorders; elderly; renal disease, renal impairment, renal failure; pregnancy (category B), lactation. Safety and efficacy in children younger than 16 y are not established.

ROUTE & DOSAGE

Pulmonary Arterial Hypertension

Adult/Adolescent: **Subcutaneous/IV** 1.25 ng/kg/min. If dose is not tolerated, reduce to 0.625 ng/kg/min. Then increase rate by no more than 1.25 ng/kg/min/wk for first 4 wk, then by 2.5 ng/kg/min/wk until achieve desired response. There is little experience with doses greater than 40 ng/kg/min. See package insert for cross taper schedule switching from epoprostenol to treprostenil.

Adult: **Inhalation** 3 breaths (18 mcg) via inhalation system 4 times/day, may increase by 3 breaths at 1–2 wk intervals.

ADMINISTRATION

Subcutaneous

- Administer Remodulin undiluted by continuous infusion through a subcutaneous catheter. Use an infusion pump designed for subcutaneous delivery.
- Avoid abrupt withdrawal or sudden large reductions in dosage as these may lead to worsening of PAH symptom.

Intravenous

May be given as IV infusion via a central line when the subcutaneous route is not feasible.

PREPARE: **Infusion:** Dilute with sterile water for injection or NS.

▪ Follow specific directions for preparation provided by the manufacturer.

ADMINISTER: **Infusion:** Given by continuous infusion via a central venous catheter. Interruptions in drug delivery MUST be avoided. ▪ Have backup delivery system readily available.

▪ Store at 15°–25° C (59°–77° F).

ADVERSE EFFECTS (≥1%) **Body as a Whole:** *Jaw pain,* flushing, syncope. **CNS:** *Headache,* dizziness. **CV:** *Vasodilation,* edema, hypotension. **GI:** *Diarrhea, nausea, vomiting.* **Skin:** *Rash,* pruritus. **Other:** *Infusion site reactions (erythema, hematoma, induration, pruritus, rash, injection site pain).*

INTERACTIONS Drug: NSAIDS, ANTICOAGULANTS may increase risk of bleeding; ANTIHYPERTENSIVE AGENTS, DIURETICS, VASODILATORS may exacerbate hypotension; **ephedrine, pseudoephedrine** may antagonize antihypertensive effects. **Herbal: Ephedra, ma huang** may antagonize antihypertensive effects.

PHARMACOKINETICS Absorption: Completely absorbed from subcutaneous site. **Onset:** Steady state reached in 10 h. **Metabolism:** Extensively in liver by unknown enzyme system. **Elimination:** 79% in urine, 13% in feces. **Half-Life:** 2–4 h.

NURSING IMPLICATIONS

Assessment & Drug Effects

- Monitor for therapeutic effectiveness indicated by less dyspnea and fatigue, increased activity tolerance, and improved hemodynamic parameters.
- Monitor for and report symptoms of excessive response to the drug including: Headache, nausea, emesis, restlessness, anxiety and infusion site pain or reaction (e.g., erythema, induration or rash). If these occur, the rate of subcutaneous infusion should be slowed.
- Monitor BP closely, especially if taking concurrent antihypertensive drugs (e.g., diuretics, vasodilators).
- Lab tests: Baseline and periodic LFTs and renal function tests. Monitor periodically coagulation parameters (more often if on concurrent anticoagulation therapy).

Patient & Family Education

- Note: Therapy with this drug may be needed for prolonged periods, possibly years.
- Report any of the following: Headache, nausea, vomiting, restlessness, anxiety, and infusion site pain.

TRETINOIN

(tret'i-noyn)

Avita, Renova, Retin-A, Retin-A Micro, Retinoic Acid, Vesanoid, Vitamin A Acid

Classifications: ANTINEOPLASTIC; ANTIACNE (RETINOID); ANTIPSORIATIC

Therapeutic: ANTINEOPLASTIC; ANTIACNE; ANTIPSORIATIC

Prototype: Isotretinoin

Pregnancy Category: D (oral form); C (topical form)

AVAILABILITY 0.025%, 0.05%, 0.1% cream; 0.025%, 0.01% gel; 0.05% liquid; 10 mg capsules

ACTION & *THERAPEUTIC EFFECT*

Antiacne activity: Contact irritant containing retinoic acid and vitamin A acid. Reverses retention hyperkeratosis and comedo formation, primary events in acne pathology. Suggests that keratinocytes in the sebaceous follicle become less adherent and turnover of follicular epithelial cells is increased; two processes that promote easy extrusion of the comedo and prevent it from reformation. **Antineoplastic activity:** Tretinoin induces cellular differentiation in malignant cells. As vitamin A (retinol) derivatives, retinoids are important regulators of cell reproduction, and cell proliferation and differentiation. Tretinoin represents a new class of anticancer drugs, differentiating agents. It is used in the treatment of acute promyelotic leukemia (APL). Tretinoin offers a less toxic means to induce complete remission than conventional chemotherapy. APL results from changes in the alpha-retinoic acid receptor (RAR) found on the long arm of chromosome 17. *Effective in early treatment and control of acne vulgaris grades I–III. Effective in treatment of APL.*

USES Topical treatment of acne vulgaris grades I–III, especially during early stages when number of comedones is greatest; adjunctively in management of associated comedones and in treatment of flat warts; oral for remission induction treatment of acute promyelocytic leukemia; cream as adjunctive therapy for mitigation of fine wrinkles.

UNLABELED USES Psoriasis, senile keratosis, ichthyosis vulgaris, keratosis palmaris and plantaris, basal cell carcinoma, photodamaged skin (photoaging), and other skin conditions. **Orphan drug:** For squamous metaplasia of conjunctiva or cornea with mucous deficiency and keratinization.

CONTRAINDICATIONS Hypersensitivity to retinoid; eczema; exposure to sunlight or ultraviolet rays, sunburn; pregnancy (**oral:** category D); lactation; children younger than 12 y.

CAUTIOUS USE Patient in an occupation necessitating considerable sun exposure or weather extremes; hepatic disease; pregnancy (**topical:** category C).

ROUTE & DOSAGE

Acne

Adult: **Topical** Apply once/day at bedtime

Acute Promyelocytic Leukemia

Adult: **PO** 45 mg/m²/day

Antiwrinkle Cream

Adult: **Topical** (0.05% cream) Apply to face once daily at bedtime

ADMINISTRATION

Topical

- Cleanse using a mild bland soap, and thoroughly dry areas being treated before applying drug. Avoid use of medicated, drying, or abrasive soaps and cleansers.
- Wash hands before and after treatment. Apply lightly over affected areas. Do not apply to nonaffected skin area.
- Avoid contact of drug with eyes, mouth, angles of nose, open wounds, mucous membranes.
- Store gel and liquid formulations below 30° C (86° F) and solution below 27° C (80° F).

ADVERSE EFFECTS (≥1%) **Body as a Whole: Note:** Listed adverse effects occur primarily with oral administration; only skin effects with topical administration. *Bone pain, malaise, shivering, hemorrhage, peripheral edema, pain, chest discomfort, weight gain or loss,* <u>DIC</u>. **CNS:** *Dizziness, paresthesias, anxiety, insomnia, depression, headache, fever, weakness, fatigue,* cerebral hemorrhage, intracranial hypertension, hallucinations. **CV:** *Arrhythmias, flushing, hypotension, hypertension,* CHF. **Special Senses:** Visual disturbances, ocular disturbances, change in visual acuity, earache. **GI:** *Nausea, vomiting, abdominal pain, diarrhea, constipation, dyspepsia,* <u>GI</u>

T

<u>hemorrhage</u>. **Respiratory:** *Dyspnea, respiratory insufficiency, pneumonia, rales, pleural effusion, wheezing.* **Skin:** Local inflammatory reactions, transient stinging or warmth on site, *redness, scaling, severe erythema,* blistering, crusting and peeling, temporary hypopigmentation or hyperpigmentation, *increased sweating.* **Urogenital:** Renal insufficiency, dysuria, acute kidney failure.

INTERACTIONS Drug: TOPICAL ACNE MEDICATIONS (including **sulfur, resorcinol, benzoyl peroxide,** and **salicylic acid**) may increase inflammation and peeling; topical products containing **alcohol** or **menthol** may cause stinging.

PHARMACOKINETICS Absorption: Minimally absorbed from intact skin, Topical; 60% absorbed, PO. **Elimination:** About 0.1% of topical dose is excreted in urine within 24 h; 63% excreted in urine and 31% in feces, PO. **Half-Life:** 45 min, Topical; 2–2.5 h, PO.

NURSING IMPLICATIONS

Assessment & Drug Effects

- Be aware that treatment to dark-skinned individuals may cause unsightly postinflammatory hyperpigmentation; that is reversible with termination of drug treatment.
- Clinical response should be evident in 2–3 wk; complete and satisfactory response (in 75% of the patients) may require 3–4 mo.
- Be aware that erythema and desquamation during the first 1–3 wk of treatment do not represent exacerbation of the skin problem but a probable response to the drug from deep previously unseen lesions.

Patient & Family Education

- As treatment is continued, lesions gradually disappear, leaving an inflammatory background; scaling and redness decrease after 8–10 wk of therapy.
- Wash face no more often than 2–3 times daily.
- Be aware that drug is not curative; relapses commonly occur within 3–6 wk after treatment has been discontinued.
- Avoid exposure to sun; when cannot be avoided, use a SPF 15 or higher sunscreen.
- Do not self-medicate with additional acne treatment because of danger of drug interactions.

TRIAMCINOLONE

(trye-am-sin'oh-lone)

Atolone, Kenacort, Kenalog-E

TRIAMCINOLONE ACETONIDE

Azmacort, Cenocort A_2, Kenalog, Nasacort HFA, Triam-A, Triamonide, Tri-kort, Trilog, Tri-Nasal

TRIAMCINOLONE DIACETATE

Kenacort

TRIAMCINOLONE HEXACETONIDE

Aristospan

Classifications: ADRENAL CORTICOSTEROID; GLUCOCORTICOID

Therapeutic: ANTI-INFLAMMATORY; IMMUNOSUPPRESSANT

Prototype: Prednisone

Pregnancy Category: C

AVAILABILITY Triamcinolone: 4 mg, 8 mg tablets; 4 mg/5 mL syrup; **Triamcinolone acetonide:** 3 mg/mL, 10 mg/mL, 40 mg/mL injection; 100 mcg aerosol; 55 mcg inhaler; 55 mcg spray; 0.5 mg/mL nasal spray; 0.025%, 0.1%, 0.5% cream, ointment, lotion; 10.3% topical spray; **Triamcinolone diacetate:** 4 mg tablet; **Triamcinolone hexacetonide:** 5 mg/mL, 20 mg/mL injection

ACTION & *THERAPEUTIC EFFECT* Immediate-acting synthetic fluorinated adrenal corticosteroid with glucocorticoid properties. Possesses minimal sodium and water retention properties in therapeutic doses. *Anti-inflammatory and immunosuppressant drug that is effective in the treatment of bronchial asthma.*

USES An anti-inflammatory or immunosuppressant agent. Orally inhaled: Bronchial asthma in patient who has not responded to conventional inhalation treatment. Therapeutic doses do not appear to suppress HPA (hypothalamic-pituitary-adrenal) axis.

CONTRAINDICATIONS Hypersensitivity to corticosteroids or benzyl alcohol; kidney dysfunction; glaucoma; acute bronchospasm; fungal infection; children younger than 6 y. **CAUTIOUS USE** Coagulopathy, hemophilia, diabetes mellitus, GI disease; congestive heart failure; herpes infection; infection; inflammatory bowel disease; myasthenia gravis; MI; ocular exposure, ocular infection; osteoporosis; peptic ulcer disease; PVD; skin abrasion; pregnancy (category C), lactation.

T

ROUTE & DOSAGE

Inflammation, Immunosuppression

Adult: **IM/Subcutaneous** 4–48 mg/day in divided doses **Intra-articular/Intradermal** 4–48 mg/day **Inhaled** 2–4 inhalations q.i.d. **Topical** See Appendix A
Child: **IM/Subcutaneous** 3.3–50 mg/m²/day in divided doses **Intra-articular/Intradermal** 3.3–50 mg/m²/day

Acetonide

Adult: **IM** 60 mg, may repeat with 20–100 mg q6wk **Intradermal** 1 mg per injection site (max: 30 mg total) **Intra-articular** 2.5–4.0 mg **Inhalation** See Appendix A
Child: **IM** *6–12 y*, 0.03–0.2 mg q1–7days **Inhalation** See Appendix A

Hexacetonide

Adult: **Intralesional** Up to 0.5 mg/in² of skin **Intra-articular** 2–20 mg q3–4wk

ADMINISTRATION

Inhalation

- Follow manufacturer's directions for specific oral or nasal inhaler and instruct patient on proper administration technique.

Subcutaneous/Intramuscular

- Do not give triamcinolone injection IV.
- IM injections should only be given into a large, well developed muscle such as the gluteal muscle.
- Store at 15°–30° C (59°–86° F). Protect from light.

ADVERSE EFFECTS (≥1%) **CNS:** Euphoria, headache, insomnia, confusion, psychosis. **CV:** CHF, edema. **GI:** Nausea, vomiting, peptic ulcer. **Musculoskeletal:** Muscle weakness, delayed wound healing, muscle wasting, osteoporosis, aseptic necrosis of bone, spontaneous fractures. **Endocrine:** Cushingoid features, growth suppression in children, carbohydrate intolerance, hyperglycemia. **Special Senses:** Cataracts. **Hematologic:** Leukocytosis. **Metabolic:** Hypokalemia. **Skin:** Burning, itching, folliculitis, hypertrichosis, hypopigmentation.

INTERACTIONS Drug: BARBITURATES, **phenytoin, rifampin** increase steroid metabolism—may need increased doses of triamcinolone; **amphotericin B,** DIURETICS add to potassium loss; **ambenonium, neostigmine, pyridostigmine** may cause severe muscle weakness in patients with myasthenia gravis; may inhibit antibody response to VACCINES, TOXOIDS.

PHARMACOKINETICS Absorption: Readily absorbed from all routes. **Onset:** 24–48 h PO, IM. **Peak:** 1–2 h PO; 8–10 h IM. **Duration:** 2.25 days PO; 1–6 wk IM. **Metabolism:** In liver. **Elimination:** In urine. **Half-Life:** 2–5 h; HPA suppression, 18–36 h.

NURSING IMPLICATIONS

Assessment & Drug Effects

- Notify physician if wheezing occurs immediately following a dose of inhaled triamcinolone.
- Do not use occlusive dressing over topical application unless specifically ordered to do so.
- Monitor growth in children receiving prolonged, systemic triamcinolone therapy.
- Monitor for signs of negative nitrogen balance (e.g., muscle atrophy), especially in older or debilitated patients receiving prolonged therapy.
- Lab tests: Periodic serum electrolytes and blood glucose.
- Report to physician immediately if a local infection develops at site of topical application.
- Report symptoms of hypercortisolism or Cushing's syndrome (see Appendix F), hyperglycemia (see Appendix F), and glucosuria (e.g., polyuria). These may arise from systemic absorption after topical application, especially in children and if used over extensive areas for prolonged periods or if occlusive dressings are used.

Patient & Family Education

- Report promptly any of the following: Sore throat, fever, swelling of feet or ankles, or muscle weakness.
- Adhere to drug regimen; do not increase or decrease established regimen and do not discontinue abruptly.
- Asthmatics should report promptly worsening of asthma symptoms following oral inhalation.

TRIAMTERENE

(trye-am′ter-een)

Dyrenium

Classifications: ELECTROLYTE AND WATER BALANCE AGENT; POTASSIUM-SPARING DIURETIC

Therapeutic: POTASSIUM-SPARING DIURETIC

Prototype: Spironolactone

Pregnancy Category: D

AVAILABILITY 50 mg, 100 mg capsules

ACTION & *THERAPEUTIC EFFECT* Has weak diuretic action with a potassium-sparing effect. Promotes excretion of sodium, chloride, and carbonate. Blocks potassium excretion by direct action on distal renal tubule rather than by inhibiting aldosterone. *Has a diuretic action and a potassium-sparing effect.*

USES Adjunct in the management of edema associated with CHF, hepatic cirrhosis, nephrotic syndrome, idiopathic edema, steroid-induced edema, and edema due to secondary hyperaldosteronism. Also alone or in conjunction with a thiazide or loop diuretic in patients with hypertension because of its potassium-sparing activity.

CONTRAINDICATIONS Hypersensitivity to drug; anuria, severe or progressive kidney disease or dysfunc-

T

tion; severe liver disease; diabetic neuropathy; elevated serum potassium; severe electrolyte or acid-base imbalance; pregnancy (category D).
CAUTIOUS USE Impaired kidney or liver function; gout; history of gouty arthritis; diabetes mellitus, older adults; history of kidney stones; lactation.

ROUTE & DOSAGE

Edema

Adult: **PO** 100 mg b.i.d. (max: 300 mg/day), may be able to decrease to 100 mg/day or every other day
Geriatric: **PO** 50 mg/day (max: 100 mg/day in 1–2 divided doses)
Child: **PO** 2–4 mg/kg/day in divided doses or every other day (max: 300 mg/day)

ADMINISTRATION

Oral

- Empty capsule and give with fluid or mix with food, if patient cannot swallow capsule.
- Give drug with or after meals to prevent or minimize nausea.
- Schedule doses to prevent interruption of sleep from diuresis (e.g., with or after breakfast if a single dose is taken, or no later than 6 p.m. if more than one dose is prescribed). Consult physician.
- Withdraw drug gradually in patients on prolonged or high-dose therapy in order to prevent rebound increased urinary excretion of potassium.
- Store in tight, light-resistant containers at 15°–30° C (59°–86° F) unless otherwise directed.

ADVERSE EFFECTS (≥1%) **GI:** Diarrhea, nausea, vomiting, and other GI disturbances. **CNS:** Dizziness, headache, dry mouth, anaphylaxis, weakness, muscle cramps. **Skin:** Pruritus, rash, photosensitivity. **CV:** Hypotension (large doses). **Metabolic:** *Hyperkalemia* and other electrolyte imbalances, elevated BUN, elevated uric acid (patients predisposed to gouty arthritis), hyperchloremic acidosis. **Hematologic:** Blood dyscrasias: Granulocytopenia, eosinophilia, megaloblastic anemia in patients with reduced folic acid stores (e.g., hepatic cirrhosis).

DIAGNOSTIC TEST INTERFERENCE Pale blue fluorescence in urine interferes with ***fluorometric assay*** of ***quinidine*** and ***lactic dehydrogenase activity.*** Triamterene may cause increases in ***blood glucose*** levels (diabetic patients), ***BUN, serum potassium, magnesium,*** and ***uric acid*** and ***urinary calcium excretion.***

INTERACTIONS Drug: May increase **lithium** levels, thus increasing its toxicity; **indomethacin** may decrease renal elimination of triamterene; ANGIOTENSIN-CONVERTING ENZYME (ACE) INHIBITORS, other POTASSIUM-SPARING DIURETICS may cause hyperkalemia. **Food:** High potassium foods may increase risk of hyperkalemia.

PHARMACOKINETICS Absorption: Rapidly but variably from GI tract. **Onset:** 2–4 h. **Duration:** 7–9 h. **Metabolism:** In liver to active and inactive metabolites. **Elimination:** In urine. **Half-Life:** 100–150 min.

NURSING IMPLICATIONS

Assessment & Drug Effects

- Monitor BP during periods of dosage adjustment. Hypotensive reactions, although rare, have been reported. Take care with ambulation, particularly for older adults.

- Weigh patient under standard conditions, prior to drug initiation and daily during therapy.
- Diuretic response usually occurs on first day of therapy; maximum effect may not occur for several days.
- Monitor and report oliguria and unusual changes in I&O ratio. Consult physician regarding allowable fluid intake.
- Be alert for S&S of kidney stone formation; reported in patients taking high doses or who have low urine volume and increased urine acidity.
- Lab tests: Baseline and periodic serum potassium and other electrolytes; periodic kidney function tests with known or suspected renal insufficiency; periodic blood studies with prolonged therapy or with cirrhosis to monitor for megaloblastic anemia.
- Observe for S&S of hyperkalemia (see Appendix F), particularly in patients with renal insufficiency, on high-dose or prolonged therapy, older adults, and those with diabetes.
- Monitor diabetics closely for loss of glycemic control.

Patient & Family Education

- Do not use salt substitutes; unlike most diuretics, triamterene promotes potassium retention.
- Do not restrict salt; there is a possibility of low-salt syndrome (hyponatremia). Consult physician.
- Report significant fatigue or weakness, malaise, fever, sore throat, or mouth and unusual bleeding or bruising to physician.
- Be aware that drug may cause photosensitivity; avoid exposure to sun and sunlamps.
- Drug may impart a harmless pale blue fluorescence to urine.

TRIAZOLAM

(trye-ay′zoe-lam)

Halcion

Classifications: BENZODIAZEPINE; ANXIOLYTIC; SEDATIVE-HYPNOTIC

Therapeutic: SEDATIVE-HYPNOTIC; ANTIANXIETY

Prototype: Lorazepam

Pregnancy Category: X

Controlled Substance: Schedule IV

AVAILABILITY 0.125 mg, 0.25 mg tablets

ACTION & *THERAPEUTIC EFFECT* Blockade of cortical and limbic arousal results in hypnotic activity. *Decreases sleep latency and number of nocturnal awakenings, decreases total nocturnal wake time, and increases duration of sleep.*

USES Short-term management of insomnia characterized by difficulty in falling asleep, frequent wakeful periods. Following long-term use, tolerance or adaptation may develop.

CONTRAINDICATIONS Hypersensitivity to triazolam and benzodiazepines; ethanol intoxication; suicidal ideations; pregnancy (category X), lactation.

CAUTIOUS USE Depression; bipolar disorder; dementia; psychosis; myasthenia gravis; Parkinson's disease; older adults and debilitated patients; patients with suicidal tendency; impaired kidney or liver function; chronic pulmonary insufficiency; sleep apnea.

ROUTE & DOSAGE

Insomnia

Adult: **PO** 0.125–0.25 mg at bedtime (max: 0.5 mg/day)
Geriatric: **PO** 0.0625–0.125 mg at bedtime

T

ADMINISTRATION

Oral

- Give immediately before bed; onset of drug action is rapid.
- Do not exceed recommended doses.
- Store at 15°–30° C (59°–86° F).

ADVERSE EFFECTS (≥1%) **CNS:** *Drowsiness,* lightheadedness, headache, dizziness, ataxia, visual disturbances, confusional states, *memory impairment, "rebound insomnia," anterograde amnesia,* paradoxical reactions, minor changes in EEG patterns. **GI:** Nausea, vomiting, constipation.

INTERACTIONS Drug: Alcohol, CNS DEPRESSANTS, ANTICONVULSANTS, **nefazodone,** BENZODIAZEPINES potentiate CNS depression; **cimetidine** increases triazolam plasma levels, thus increasing its toxicity; may decrease antiparkinsonism effects of **levodopa. Herbal: Kava, valerian** may potentiate sedation. **St. John's wort** may decrease efficacy. **Food: Grapefruit juice** (greater than 1 qt/day) may increase plasma concentrations and adverse effects.

PHARMACOKINETICS Absorption: Readily from GI tract. **Onset:** 15–30 min. **Peak:** 1–2 h. **Duration:** 6–8 h. **Distribution:** Crosses placenta; distributed into breast milk. **Elimination:** In urine. **Half-Life:** 2–3 h.

T

NURSING IMPLICATIONS

Assessment & Drug Effects

- Be aware that signs of developing tolerance or adaptation (with long-term use) include increased daytime anxiety, increased wakefulness during last one third of the night.
- Lab tests: Obtain periodic blood counts, urinalysis, and blood chemistries during long-term use.
- Evaluate smoking habit. As with other benzodiazepines, smoking may decrease hypnotic effects.
- Monitor for symptoms of overdosage: Slurred speech, somnolence, confusion, impaired coordination, and coma.

Patient & Family Education

- Do not drive or engage in potentially hazardous activities until response to drug is known.
- Avoid use of alcohol or other CNS depressants while on this drug; they may increase sedative effects.
- Do not stop taking drug suddenly, especially if you are subject to seizures. Withdrawal symptoms may occur and range from mild dysphoria to more serious symptoms (e.g., tremors, abdominal and muscle cramps, convulsions). Consult physician for schedule to discontinue therapy.
- Do not increase dose without physician's advice because of toxic potential of drug.

TRIFLUOPERAZINE HYDROCHLORIDE

(trye-floo-oh-per'a-zeen)

Novoflurazine ♣, Solazine ♣, Stelazine, Terfluzine ♣

Classification: ANTIPSYCHOTIC, PHENOTHIAZIDE

Therapeutic: ANTIPSYCHOTIC

Prototype: Chlorpromazine

Pregnancy Category: C

AVAILABILITY 1 mg, 2 mg, 5 mg, 10 mg tablets; 10 mg/mL liquid; 2 mg/mL injection

ACTION & *THERAPEUTIC EFFECT* Phenothiazine with antipsychotic effects thought to be related to blockade of postsynaptic dopamine receptors in the brain. *Effectiveness indicated by increase in mental and physical activity.*

USES Management of manifestations of psychotic disorders; "possibly effective" control of excessive anxiety and tension associated with neuroses or somatic conditions.

CONTRAINDICATIONS Hypersensitivity to phenothiazines or sulfites; comatose states; CNS depression; ethanol intoxication; blood dyscrasias; children younger than 6 y; hematologic disease, bone marrow depression; dementia in elderly; preexisting liver disease; lactation.
CAUTIOUS USE Previously detected breast cancer; history of QT prolongation; significant cardiac disease or pulmonary disease; compromised respiratory function; seizure disorders; impaired liver function; pregnancy (category C).

ROUTE & DOSAGE

Psychotic Disorders
Adult: **PO** 1–2 mg b.i.d., may increase up to 20 mg/day in hospitalized patients
Child (6–12 y): **PO** 1 mg 1–2 times/day, may increase up to 15 mg/day in hospitalized patients

Dementia Behavior
Geriatric: **PO** 0.5–1 mg 1–2 times/day, may increase q4-7days (max: 40 mg in divided doses)

ADMINISTRATION

Oral

- Dilute oral concentrate just before administration with about 60–120 mL suitable diluent (e.g., water, fruit juices, carbonated beverage, milk, soups, puddings).
- Crush tablet and give with fluid or mix with food if patient will not or cannot swallow pill.
- Store in light-resistant container at 15°–30° C (59°–86° F) unless otherwise directed.

ADVERSE EFFECTS (≥1%) **CNS:** *Drowsiness,* insomnia, dizziness, agitation, *extrapyramidal effects,* <u>neuroleptic malignant syndrome</u>. **Special Senses:** Nasal congestion, *dry mouth,* blurred vision, pigmentary retinopathy. **Hematologic:** <u>Agranulocytosis</u>. **Skin:** Photosensitivity, skin rash, sweating. **GI:** Constipation. **CV:** Tachycardia, *hypotension.* **Respiratory:** Depressed cough reflex. **Endocrine:** Gynecomastia, galactorrhea.

INTERACTIONS Drug: Alcohol and other CNS DEPRESSANTS add to CNS depression. **Herbal: Kava** may increase risk and severity of dystonic reactions.

PHARMACOKINETICS Absorption: Well absorbed from GI tract. **Onset:** Rapid onset. **Peak:** 2–3 h. **Duration:** Up to 12 h. **Metabolism:** In liver. **Elimination:** In bile and feces.

NURSING IMPLICATIONS

Assessment & Drug Effects

- Monitor HR and BP. Hypotension is a common adverse effect.
- Hypotension and extrapyramidal effects (especially akathisia and dystonia) are most likely to occur in patients receiving high doses or in older adults. Withhold drug and notify physician if patient has dysphagia, neck muscle spasm, or if tongue protrusion occurs.
- Monitor I&O ratio and bowel elimination pattern. Check for abdominal distention and pain. Encourage adequate fluid intake as prophylaxis for constipation and xerostomia.

T

- Lab tests: Periodic CBC and serum prolactin, especially with prolonged therapy.
- Agitation, jitteriness, and sometimes insomnia may simulate original psychotic symptoms. These adverse effects may disappear spontaneously.
- Expect maximum therapeutic response within 2–3 wk after initiation of therapy.

Patient & Family Education

- Take drug as prescribed; do not alter dosing regimen or stop medication without consulting physician.
- Consult physician about use of any OTC drugs during therapy.
- Do not take alcohol and other depressants during therapy.
- Avoid potentially hazardous activities such as driving or operating machinery, until response to drug is known.
- Cover as much skin surface as possible with clothing when you **must be** in direct sunlight. Use an SPF higher than 12 sunscreen on exposed skin.
- Urine may be discolored or reddish brown and this is harmless.

TRIFLURIDINE

(trye-flure'i-deen)

Viroptic

Classification: ANTIVIRAL

Therapeutic: ANTIVIRAL

Pregnancy Category: C

AVAILABILITY 1% ophth solution

ACTION & *THERAPEUTIC EFFECT* Pyrimidine nucleoside that appears to inhibit viral DNA synthesis and viral replication. *Active against herpes simplex virus (HSV) types 1 and 2, vaccinia virus, and certain strains of adenovirus.*

USES Topically to eyes for treatment of primary keratoconjunctivitis and recurring epithelial keratitis caused by herpes simplex virus types 1 and 2. Also for other herpetic ophthalmic infections including stromal keratitis, uveitis, and for infections caused by vaccinia and *Adenovirus,* but clinical effectiveness has not been established.

CONTRAINDICATIONS Lactation; children younger than 6 y.

CAUTIOUS USE Dry eye syndrome; pregnancy (category C).

ROUTE & DOSAGE

Viral Infections of Eye

Adult: **Ophthalmic** 1 drop 1% ophthalmic solution into affected eye q2h during waking hours until healing (reepithelialization) has occurred (max: 9 drops/day); when healing appears to be complete, dosage reduced to 1 drop q4h during waking hours for an additional 7 days (max: 5 drops/day); continuous administration beyond 21 days not recommended

ADMINISTRATION

Instillation

- Wait several minutes between applications when used concurrently with other eye drops.
- Store refrigerated at 2°–8° C (36°–46° F) unless otherwise directed.

ADVERSE EFFECTS (≥1%) **Special Senses:** Mild transient burning or stinging, mild irritation of conjunctiva or cornea, photophobia, edema of eyelids and cornea, punctal occlusion, superficial punctate keratopathy, epithelial keratopathy, stromal edema, keratitis sicca, hyperemia, increased intraocular pressure.

INTERACTIONS Drug: No clinically significant interactions established.

PHARMACOKINETICS Absorption: Following topical application to eye, trifluridine penetrates cornea and aqueous humor (inflammation enhances penetration). Systemic absorption does not appear to be significant.

NURSING IMPLICATIONS

Assessment & Drug Effects

- Expect epithelial eye infections to respond to therapy within 2–7 days, with complete healing occurring in 1–2 wk.

Patient & Family Education

- Inform physician of progress and keep follow-up appointments. Herpetic eye infections have a tendency to recur and can lead to corneal damage if not adequately treated.

TRIHEXYPHENIDYL HYDROCHLORIDE

(trye-hex-ee-fen′i-dill)

Aparkane ♣, Apo-Trihex ♣, Novohexidyl ♣

Classifications: CENTRALLY ACTING CHOLINERGIC RECEPTOR ANTAGONIST; ANTIPARKINSON AGENT; ANTISPASMODIC

Therapeutic: ANTIPARKINSON; ANTISPASMODIC

Prototype: Benztropine

Pregnancy Category: C

AVAILABILITY 2 mg, 5 mg tablets; 2 mg/5 mL elixir

ACTION & *THERAPEUTIC EFFECT* Thought to act by blocking excess of acetylcholine at certain cerebral synaptic sites. Relaxes smooth muscle by direct effect and by atropinelike blocking action on the parasympathetic nervous system. *Diminishes the characteristic tremor of Parkinson's disease.*

USES Symptomatic treatment of all forms of parkinsonism (arteriosclerotic, idiopathic, postencephalitic). Also to prevent or control drug-induced extrapyramidal disorders.

UNLABELED USES Huntington's chorea, spasmodic torticollis.

CONTRAINDICATIONS Narrow-angle glaucoma; tardive dyskinesia; lactation. Safe use in children is not established.

CAUTIOUS USE History of drug hypersensitivities; arteriosclerosis; hypertension; cardiac disease, kidney or liver disorders; myasthenia gravis; alcoholism; obstructive diseases of GI or genitourinary tracts; older adults with prostatic hypertrophy; pregnancy (category C).

ROUTE & DOSAGE

Parkinsonism

Adult: **PO** 1 mg day 1, 2 mg day 2, then increase by 2 mg q3–5days up to 6–10 mg/day in 3 or more divided doses (max: 15 mg/day)

Extrapyramidal Effects

Adult: **PO** 5–15 mg/day in divided doses

ADMINISTRATION

Oral

- Give before or after meals, depending on how patient reacts. Older adults and patients prone to excessive salivation (e.g., postencephalitic parkinsonism) may prefer to take drug after meals. If drug causes excessive mouth dryness, it may be better given before meals, unless it causes nausea.

- Do not crush or chew sustained release capsules. These **must be** swallowed whole.
- Store at 15°–30° C (59°–86° F) in tight container unless otherwise directed.

ADVERSE EFFECTS (≥1%) **GI:** *Dry mouth, nausea,* constipation. **Special Senses:** *Blurred vision,* mydriasis, photophobia, angle-closure glaucoma. **Urogenital:** Urinary hesitancy or retention. **CNS:** *Dizziness, nervousness,* insomnia, drowsiness, confusion, agitation, delirium, psychotic manifestations, euphoria. **CV:** Tachycardia, palpitations, hypotension, orthostatic hypotension. **Body as a Whole:** Hypersensitivity reactions.

INTERACTIONS Drug: Reduces therapeutic effects of **chlorpromazine, haloperidol,** PHENOTHIAZINES; increases bioavailability of **digoxin;** MAO INHIBITORS potentiate actions of trihexyphenidyl. **Herbal: Betel nut** may increase risk of extrapyramidal symptoms.

PHARMACOKINETICS Absorption: Readily from GI tract. **Onset:** Within 1 h. **Peak:** 2–3 h. **Duration:** 6–12 h. **Elimination:** In urine.

T

NURSING IMPLICATIONS

Assessment & Drug Effects

- Be aware that incidence and severity of adverse effects are usually dose related and may be minimized by dosage reduction. Older adults appear more sensitive to usual adult doses.
- Monitor vital signs. Pulse is a particularly sensitive indicator of response to drug. Report tachycardia, palpitations, paradoxical bradycardia, or fall in BP.
- Assess for and report severe CNS stimulation (see ADVERSE EFFECTS) that occurs with high doses, and in patients with arteriosclerosis, or those with history of hypersensitivity to other drugs.
- In patients with severe rigidity, tremors may appear to be accentuated during therapy as rigidity diminishes.
- Monitor daily I&O if patient develops urinary hesitancy or retention. Voiding before taking drug may relieve problem.
- Check for abdominal distention and bowel sounds if constipation is a problem.

Patient & Family Education

- Learn measures to relieve drug-induced dry mouth; rinse mouth frequently with water and suck ice chips, sugarless gum, or hard candy. Maintain adequate total daily fluid intake.
- Avoid excessive heat because drug suppresses perspiration and, therefore, heat loss.
- Do not to engage in potentially hazardous activities requiring alertness and skill. Drug causes dizziness, drowsiness, and blurred vision. Help walking may be indicated.

TRIMETHOBENZAMIDE HYDROCHLORIDE

(trye-meth-oh-ben′za-mide)

Tigan

Classification: ANTIEMETIC
Therapeutic: ANTIEMETIC
Prototype: Prochlorperazine
Pregnancy Category: C

AVAILABILITY 300 mg capsules; 100 mg/mL injection

ACTION & *THERAPEUTIC EFFECT* Primary locus of action is thought to be the chemoreceptor trigger zone (CTZ) in medulla. *Less effective than phenothiazine antiemetics but produces fewer adverse effects.*

USES Control of nausea and vomiting.

CONTRAINDICATIONS Uncomplicated vomiting in viral illness; parenteral use in children or infants; rectal administration in prematures and newborns; known sensitivity to benzocaine (in suppository) or to similar local anesthetics.

CAUTIOUS USE In presence of high fever, dehydration, electrolyte imbalance; children; pregnancy (category C), lactation.

ROUTE & DOSAGE

Nausea and Vomiting

Adult: **PO** 300 mg t.i.d. or q.i.d.
IM 200 mg t.i.d. or q.i.d. prn
Geriatric: May require dose reduction or changes in interval.

ADMINISTRATION

Oral

- Empty capsule and give with water or mix with food if patient cannot swallow capsule.

Intramuscular

- Give IM deep into upper outer quadrant of buttock.
- Minimize possibility of irritation and pain by avoiding escape of solution along needle track. Use Z-track technique. Rotate injection sites.

ADVERSE EFFECTS (≥1%) **Body as a Whole:** Hypersensitivity reactions (including allergic skin eruptions), muscle cramps, pain, stinging, burning, redness, irritation at IM site; local irritation following rectal administration. **CNS:** Pseudoparkinsonism. **CV:** Hypotension. **GI:** Diarrhea, exaggeration of nausea, acute hepatitis, jaundice.

INTERACTIONS Drug: Alcohol and other CNS DEPRESSANTS add to depressant activity; BELLADONNA ALKALOIDS may intensify anticholinergic effects; PHENOTHIAZINES may precipitate extrapyramidal syndrome.

PHARMACOKINETICS Onset: 10–40 min PO; 15 min IM. **Duration:** 3–4 h PO; 2–3 h IM. **Elimination:** 30–50% of dose excreted unchanged in urine within 48–72 h.

NURSING IMPLICATIONS

Assessment & Drug Effects

- Monitor BP. Hypotension may occur particularly in surgical patients receiving drug parenterally.
- Report promptly and stop drug therapy if an acute febrile illness accompanies or begins during therapy.
- Antiemetic effect of drug may obscure diagnoses of GI or other pathologic conditions or signs of toxicity from other drugs.

Patient & Family Education

- Report promptly to physician onset of rash or other signs of hypersensitivity (see Appendix F). Discontinue drug immediately.
- Do not drive or engage in potentially hazardous activities until response to drug is known.
- Do not drink alcohol or alcoholic beverages during therapy with this drug.

TRIMETHOPRIM Pr

(trye-meth'oh-prim)

Primsol, Proloprim

Classification: ANTI-INFECTIVE, URINARY TRACT

Therapeutic: URINARY TRACT ANTI-INFECTIVE

Pregnancy Category: C

AVAILABILITY 100 mg, 200 mg tablets; 50 mg/5 mL liquid

ACTION & *THERAPEUTIC EFFECT* Anti-infective and folic acid antagonist with slow bactericidal action. Binds and interferes with bacterial cell growth. *Effective against most common UTI pathogens. Most pathogens causing UTI are in normal vaginal and fecal flora. Effective in treatment of acute otitis media.*

USES Initial episodes of acute uncomplicated UTIs, acute otitis media in children.

UNLABELED USES Treatment and prophylaxis of chronic and recurrent UTI in both men and women; treatment in conjunction with dapsone of initial episodes of *Pneumocystis carinii* pneumonia; treatment of travelers' diarrhea.

CONTRAINDICATIONS Megaloblastic anemia secondary to folate deficiency; creatinine clearance less than 15 mL/min, impaired kidney or liver function; possible folate deficiency; children with fragile X chromosome associated with mental retardation; children younger than 6 mo.

CAUTIOUS USE Renal disease; mild or moderate renal impairment; pregnancy (category C), lactation.

ROUTE & DOSAGE

Urinary Tract Infection

Adult: **PO** 100 mg b.i.d. or 200 mg once/day

Child: **PO** 2–3 mg/kg q12h × 10 days

Acute Otitis Media

Child (older than 6 mo): **PO** 10 mg/kg divided q12h × 10 days

Travelers' Diarrhea

Adult: **PO** 200 mg b.i.d.

ADMINISTRATION

Oral

- Give with 240 mL (8 oz) of fluid if not contraindicated.
- Store at 15°–30° C (59°–86° F) in dry, light-protected place.

ADVERSE EFFECTS (≥1%) **GI:** Epigastric discomfort, nausea, vomiting, glossitis, abnormal taste sensation. **Hematologic:** Neutropenia, *megaloblastic anemia,* methemoglobinemia, leukopenia, thrombocytopenia (rare). **Skin:** *Rash, pruritus,* exfoliative dermatitis, photosensitivity. **Body as a Whole:** Fever. **Metabolic:** Increased serum transaminases (ALT, AST), bilirubin, creatinine, BUN.

DIAGNOSTIC TEST INTERFERENCE Interferes with serum ***methotrexate assays*** that use a competitive binding protein technique with a bacterial dihydrofolate reductase as the binding protein. May cause falsely elevated ***creatinine*** values when ***Jaffe reaction*** is used.

INTERACTIONS Drug: May inhibit **phenytoin** metabolism causing increased levels.

PHARMACOKINETICS Absorption: Almost completely absorbed from GI tract. **Peak:** 1–4 h. **Distribution:** Widely distributed, including lung, saliva, middle ear fluid, bile, bone, CSF; crosses placenta; appears in

T

breast milk. **Metabolism:** In liver. **Elimination:** 80% in urine unchanged. **Half-Life:** 8–11 h.

NURSING IMPLICATIONS

Assessment & Drug Effects

- Lab tests: Obtain C&S tests before trimethoprim therapy is initiated. Obtain periodic urine cultures, BUN, creatinine clearance, CBC, Hgb, and Hct.
- Reinforce necessity to adhere to established drug regimen. Recurrent infection after terminating prophylactic treatment of UTI may occur even after 6 mo of therapy.
- Assess urinary pattern during treatment. Altered pattern (frequency, urgency, nocturia, retention, polyuria) may reflect emerging drug resistance, necessitating change of drug regimen. Periodically check for bladder distention.
- Be alert for toxic effects on bone marrow, particularly in older adults, malnourished, alcoholic, pregnant, or debilitated patients. Recognize and report signs of infection or anemia.
- Drug-induced rash, a common adverse effect, is usually maculopapular, pruritic, or morbilliform and appears 7–14 days after start of therapy with daily doses of 200 mg or less.

Patient & Family Education

- Drink fluids liberally (2000–3000 mL/day, if not contraindicated) to help flush out urinary bacteria.
- Report pain and hematuria to physician immediately.
- Do not postpone voiding even though increases in fluid intake may cause more frequent urination.
- Do not use douches or sprays during treatment periods; practice careful perineal hygiene to prevent reinfection.
- Report to physician promptly any symptoms of a blood disorder (fever, sore throat, pallor, purpura, ecchymosis).
- Consult physician if severe traveler's diarrhea does not respond to 3–5 days therapy (i.e., persistence of symptoms of severe nausea, abdominal pain, diarrhea with mucus or blood, and dehydration).
- Drug-induced rash, a common adverse effect, may appear 7–14 days after start of therapy. Report rash to physician for evaluation.

TRIMIPRAMINE MALEATE

(tri-mip′ra-meen)

Surmontil

Classification: TRICYCLIC ANTIDEPRESSANT

Therapeutic: TRICYCLIC ANTIDEPRESSANT (TCA)

Prototype: Imipramine

Pregnancy Category: C

AVAILABILITY 25 mg, 50 mg, 100 mg capsules

ACTION & *THERAPEUTIC EFFECT* Tricyclic antidepressant (TCA) useful in depression associated with anxiety and sleep disturbances. Recent studies suggest strong, active H_2-receptor antagonism is a characteristic of TCAs. *More effective in alleviation of endogenous depression than other depressive states.*

USES Treatment of major depression.

UNLABELED USES Peptic ulcer disease.

CONTRAINDICATIONS Hypersensitivity to tricyclic antidepressants; prostatic hypertrophy; during recovery period after MI; AV block; QT prolongation; bundle-branch block; ileus; MAOI therapy; suicide ideation. Safety and efficacy in children are not established.

CAUTIOUS USE Schizophrenia, electroshock therapy, psychosis, bipolar disease; Parkinson's disease; seizure disorders; increased intraocular pressure; history of urinary retention; history of narrow-angle glaucoma; hyperthyroidism, suicidal tendency; cardiovascular, liver, thyroid, kidney disease; pregnancy (category C), lactation.

ROUTE & DOSAGE

Depression

Adult: **PO** 75–100 mg/day in divided doses, may increase gradually up to 300 mg/day if needed **PO Maintenance Dose** Usually 50–150 mg/day
Geriatric: **PO** 25 mg at bedtime, may increase q3days (max: 100 mg/day)

Pharmacogenetic Dosage Adjustment

Poor CYP2D6 metabolizer: Start with 30% of dose

T

ADMINISTRATION

Oral

- Give with food to decrease gastric distress.
- Store in tightly closed container at 15°–30° C (59°–86° F) unless otherwise specified.

ADVERSE EFFECTS (≥1%) **CNS:** Seizures, tremor, confusion, *sedation.* **Special Senses:** Blurred vision. **CV:** Tachycardia, *orthostatic hypotension,* hypertension. **GI:** *Xerostomia, constipation,* paralytic ileus. **Urogenital:** *Urinary retention.* **Skin:** Photosensitivity, sweating.

INTERACTIONS Drug: May decrease some antihypertensive response to ANTIHYPERTENSIVES; CNS DEPRESSANTS, **alcohol,** HYPNOTICS, BARBITURATES, SEDATIVES potentiate CNS depression; may increase hypoprothrombinemic effect of ORAL ANTICOAGULANTS; **ethchlorvynol** may cause transient delirium; with **levodopa**, SYMPATHOMIMETICS (e.g., **epinephrine, norepinephrine**), possibility of sympathetic hyperactivity with hypertension and hyperpyrexia; with MAO INHIBITORS, possibility of severe reactions, toxic psychosis, cardiovascular instability; **methylphenidate** increases plasma TCA levels; THYROID AGENTS may increase possibility of arrhythmias; **cimetidine** may increase plasma TCA levels. **Herbal: Ginkgo** may decrease seizure threshold; **St. John's wort** may cause **serotonin** syndrome.

PHARMACOKINETICS Absorption: Rapidly absorbed from GI tract. **Peak:** 2 h. **Metabolism:** In liver (CYP2D6). **Elimination:** In urine and feces. **Half-Life:** 9.1 h.

NURSING IMPLICATIONS

Assessment & Drug Effects

- Assess vital signs (BP and pulse rate) during adjustment period of tricyclic antidepressant (TCA) therapy. If BP falls more than 20 mm Hg or if there is a sudden increase in pulse rate, withhold medication and notify physician.
- Orthostatic hypotension may be sufficiently severe to require protective assistance when patient is ambulating. Instruct patient to change position from recum-

bency to standing slowly and in stages.
- Monitor for changes in behavior that may indicate increased incidence of suicidality.
- Report fine tremors, a distressing extrapyramidal adverse effect, to physician.
- Monitor bowel elimination pattern and I&O ratio. Severe constipation and urinary retention are potential problems, especially in older adults. Advise increased fluid intake to at least 1500 mL/day (if allowed).
- Inspect oral membranes daily with high-dose therapy. Urge outpatient to report symptoms of stomatitis or xerostomia.
- Regulate environmental temperature and patient's clothing carefully; drug may cause intolerance to heat or cold.

Patient & Family Education
- Be aware that your ability to perform tasks requiring alertness and skill may be impaired.
- Do not use OTC drugs unless approved by physician.
- Understand that the actions of both alcohol and trimipramine are increased when used together during therapy and for up to 2 wk after the TCA is discontinued. Consult physician about safe amounts of alcohol, if any, that can be taken.
- Be aware that the effects of barbiturates and other CNS depressants may also be enhanced by trimipramine.
- Expect that therapeutic response will be delayed because TCAs have a "lag period" of 2–4 wk. Increased dosage does not shorten period but rather increases incidence of adverse reactions. Keep physician advised and do not interrupt therapy.

TRIPELENNAMINE HYDROCHLORIDE

(tri-pel-enn′a-meen)

PBZ-SR, Pelamine, Pyribenzamine ♣

Classifications: ANTIHISTAMINE; H_1-RECEPTOR ANTAGONIST

Therapeutic: ANTIHISTAMINE

Prototype: Diphenhydramine

Pregnancy Category: B

AVAILABILITY 25 mg, 50 mg tablets; 100 mg sustained release tablets

ACTION & *THERAPEUTIC EFFECT*
Antagonizes histamine action (i.e., increased capillary permeability, edema formation, itching, and constriction of respiratory, GI, and vascular smooth muscle). *Has antihistamine, antitussive, anticholinergic, and local anesthetic action.*

USES To relieve symptoms of various allergic conditions, to ameliorate reactions to blood or plasma, and in anaphylaxis as adjunct to epinephrine and other standard measures after acute symptoms have been controlled. Also to provide oral mucous membrane analgesia in young children with herpetic gingivastomatitis.

CONTRAINDICATIONS Narrow-angle glaucoma; symptomatic prostatic hypertrophy; bladder neck obstruction; GI obstruction or stenosis; lower respiratory tract symptoms, including asthma; within 14 days of MAO inhibitor therapy. Safe use in neonates and premature infants is not established.

CAUTIOUS USE History of asthma; convulsive disorders; increased intraocular pressure; hyperthyroidism; cardiovascular disease; hypertension; diabetes mellitus; pregnancy (category B), lactation.

ROUTE & DOSAGE

Allergic Conditions

Adult: **PO** 25–50 mg q4–6h or 100 mg sustained release q8–12h (max: 600 mg/day)
Child: **PO** 5 mg/kg/day in 4–6 divided doses (max: 300 mg/day)

ADMINISTRATION

Oral

- Give with or immediately after meals or food or with a glass of milk or water to lessen GI adverse effects.
- Do not use sustained release formulation (100 mg) with children of any age.
- Do not crush, break, or chew sustained release tablets. These **must be** swallowed whole.
- Store in tight, light-resistant containers.

ADVERSE EFFECTS (≥1%) **Respiratory:** Thickened bronchial secretions, wheezing, sensation of chest tightness. **Special Senses:** Blurred vision, diplopia. **Urogenital:** Urinary hesitancy or retention; dysuria. **CV:** Palpitation, tachycardia, mild hypotension or hypertension, <u>cardiovascular collapse</u>. **CNS:** *Drowsiness,* dizziness, tinnitus, vertigo, fatigue, headache; disturbed coordination, tingling, tremors, euphoria, nervousness, restlessness, insomnia, hallucinations, excitement. **GI:** *Epigastric distress, anorexia, nausea, vomiting, constipation* or diarrhea, *dry mouth, nose,* and *throat.* **Hematologic:** Leukopenia, hemolytic anemia. **Skin:** Skin rash, urticaria, photosensitivity. **Body as a Whole:** <u>Anaphylactic shock</u>, fever, ataxia, athetosis, convulsions, <u>coma</u>.

INTERACTIONS Drug: Alcohol and other CNS DEPRESSANTS add to CNS depression; MAO INHIBITORS may intensify anticholinergic effects.

PHARMACOKINETICS Absorption: Readily from GI tract. **Onset:** 15–30 min. **Peak:** 2–3 h. **Duration:** 4–6 h (up to 8 h with sustained release). **Distribution:** Crosses placenta; distributed into breast milk. **Metabolism:** In liver. **Elimination:** In urine.

NURSING IMPLICATIONS

Assessment & Drug Effects

- Assist older adults during ambulation; dizziness, sedation, and hypotension are more likely to occur in this age group.
- Lab tests: Obtain periodic blood cell counts during long-term therapy with antihistamines.

Patient & Family Education

- Void just before taking drug if urinary hesitancy is a problem.
- Do not drive or engage in potentially hazardous activities until response to drug is known. Mild to moderate drowsiness, blurred vision, and dizziness occur in some patients.
- Be aware that the effects of antihistamines may be augmented by concomitant use of alcohol or other CNS depressants.
- Do not take OTC preparations without consulting physician.

TRIPTORELIN PAMOATE

(trip-tor'e-lyn)

Trelstar Depot

Classification: GONADOTROPIN-RELEASING HORMONE (GnRH) AGONIST ANALOG
Therapeutic: GnRH AGONIST ANALOG
Prototype: Leuprolide acetate
Pregnancy Category: X

AVAILABILITY 3.75 mg injection

ACTION & *THERAPEUTIC EFFECT* Synthetic luteinizing releasing hormone agonist (LHRH or GnRH) with greater potency than naturally occurring luteinizing hormone. Potent inhibitor of gonadotropin secretion that causes decreased formation of testosterone. *In men, the level of serum testosterone is equivalent to a surgically castrated man.*

USES Palliative treatment of advanced prostate cancer.

CONTRAINDICATIONS Hypersensitivity to triptorelin, other LHRH agonists, or LHRH; dysfunctional uterine bleeding; pregnancy (category X), lactation; children.
CAUTIOUS USE Prostatic carcinoma; hepatic or renal dysfunction; patients with impending spinal cord compression or severe urogenital disorder; premenstrual syndrome; renal insufficiency.

ROUTE & DOSAGE

Prostate Cancer
Adult: **IM** 3.75 mg qmo

ADMINISTRATION

Intramuscular
- Give deep into a large muscle.

ADVERSE EFFECTS (≥1%) **Body as a Whole:** *Hot flushes,* pain, leg pain, fatigue. **CV:** Hypertension. **GI:** Diarrhea, vomiting. **Hematologic:** Anemia. **Musculoskeletal:** Skeletal pain. **CNS:** Headache, dizziness, insomnia, impotence, emotional lability. **Skin:** Pruritus. **Urogenital:** Urinary retention, UTI. **Other:** Pain at injection site.

DIAGNOSTIC TEST INTERFERENCE May interfere with tests for ***pituitary-gonadal function.***

PHARMACOKINETICS Peak: 1–3 h. **Duration:** 1 mo. **Metabolism:** Unknown. **Elimination:** Eliminated by liver and kidneys. **Half-Life:** 3 h.

NURSING IMPLICATIONS

Assessment & Drug Effects
- Monitor for S&S of disease flare, especially during the first 1–2 wk of therapy: Increased bone pain, blood in urine, urinary obstruction, or symptoms of spinal compression.
- Lab tests: Periodic serum testosterone, PSA, acid phosphatase levels; urinary and serum calcium; urinary calcium/creatinine ratio; lipid profile in those at risk for atherosclerosis.

Patient & Family Education
- Disease flare (see ASSESSMENT & DRUG EFFECTS) is a common, temporary adverse effect of therapy; however, symptoms may become serious enough to report to the physician.
- Notify physician promptly of the following: S&S of an allergic reaction (itching, hives, swelling of face, arms, or legs; tingling in mouth or throat, tightness in chest or trouble breathing); weakness or loss of muscle control; rapid weight gain.

TROPICAMIDE

(troe-pik'a-mide)

Pregnancy Category: C

See Appendix A-1.

TROSPIUM CHLORIDE

(tro-spi'um)

Sanctura, Sanctura XR

Classifications: ANTICHOLINERGIC; ANTIMUSCARINIC; ANTISPASMODIC

Therapeutic: URINARY SMOOTH MUSCLE RELAXANT

Prototype: Oxybutynin

Pregnancy Category: C

AVAILABILITY 20 mg tablets; 60 mg extended release capsule

ACTION & *THERAPEUTIC EFFECT* Antagonizes the effect of acetylcholine on muscarinic receptors in smooth muscle. Its parasympatholytic action reduces the tonus of the smooth muscle of the bladder. *Decreases urinary frequency, urgency, and urge incontinence in patients with overactive bladders.*

USES Treatment of overactive (neurogenic) bladder, urinary incontinence.

T

CONTRAINDICATIONS Hypersensitivity to trospium; patients with or at risk for urinary retention; uncontrolled narrow-angle glaucoma; gastric tension, GI obstruction, ileus, pyloric stenosis, toxic megacolon, severe ulcerative colitis. Safety and effectiveness in children have not been established.

CAUTIOUS USE Significant bladder obstruction, closed-angle glaucoma; BPH; ulcerative colitis, GERD, intestinal atony; myasthenia gravis, autonomic neuropathy; moderate or severe hepatic dysfunction; severe renal insufficiency, renal failure; glaucoma; older adults; pregnancy (category C), lactation.

ROUTE & DOSAGE

Overactive Bladder

Adult: **PO** 20 mg twice daily OR 60 mg (extended release) daily

Geriatric (75 y or older): **PO** 20 mg once daily at bedtime if anticholinergic adverse effects are intolerable

Renal Impairment Dosage Adjustment

CrCl less than 30 mL/min: 20 mg once daily at bedtime

ADMINISTRATION

Oral

- Give at least 1 h before meals or on an empty stomach.
- Store at 20°–25° C (66°–77° F).

ADVERSE EFFECTS (≥1%) **Body as a Whole:** Fatigue. **CNS:** Headache. **GI:** *Dry mouth, constipation,* abdominal pain, dyspepsia, flatulence. **Special Senses:** Dry eyes. **Urogenital:** Urinary retention.

INTERACTIONS Drug: Increased anticholinergic adverse effects with ANTICHOLINERGIC AGENTS.

PHARMACOKINETICS Absorption: Less than 10% absorbed orally. **Peak:** 5–6 h. **Elimination:** Primarily in feces (unabsorbed dose), renal tubular secretion of absorbed dose. **Half-Life:** 20 h.

NURSING IMPLICATIONS

Assessment & Drug Effects

- Monitor bowel and bladder function. Report urinary hesitancy or significant constipation.

- Withhold drug and notify physician if urinary retention develops.
- Monitor for and report worsening of GI symptoms in those with GERD.

Patient & Family Education

- Report promptly any of the following: Signs of an allergic reaction, (e.g., itching or hives), blurred vision or difficulty focusing, confusion, dizziness, difficulty passing urine.
- Moderate intake of tea, coffee, caffeinated sodas, and alcohol to minimize side effects of this drug.
- Avoid situations in which overheating is likely, as drug may impair sweating, which is a normal cooling mechanism.
- Do not engage in hazardous activities until response to the drug is known.

VACCINIA IMMUNE GLOBULIN (VIG-IV)

(vac-cin′i-a)

Classifications: BIOLOGICAL RESPONSE MODIFIER; IMMUNOGLOBULIN
Therapeutic: IMMUNOGLOBULIN
Prototype: Immune globulin
Pregnancy Category: C

AVAILABILITY 50 mg/mL injection

ACTION & *THERAPEUTIC EFFECT* Vaccinia immune globulin, VIG (VIG-IV) is a purified human immunoglobulin G (IgG). It is derived from adult human plasma collected from donors who received booster immunizations with the smallpox vaccine. VIG (VIG-IV) contains high titers of antivaccinia antibodies. *VIG is effective in the treatment of smallpox vaccine adverse reactions secondary to continued vaccinia virus replication after vaccination.*

USES Prevention of serious complications of smallpox vaccine; treatment of progressive vaccinia; severe generalized vaccinia; eczema vaccinatum; vaccinia infection in patients with skin conditions (e.g., burns, impetigo, varicella-zoster, poison ivy, or eczematous skin lesions); treatment or modification of aberrant infections induced by vaccinia virus.

CONTRAINDICATIONS Predisposition to acute renal failure (i.e., preexisting renal insufficiency, diabetes mellitus, volume depletion, sepsis proteinemia, patients older than 65 y); AIDS; chronic skin conditions; bone marrow suppression; chemotherapy; radiation therapy; corticosteroid therapy, eczema; hematologic disease, thrombosis; hypotension; herpes infection; postvaccinal encephalitis; aseptic meningitis syndrome (AMS); pulmonary edema; lactation. Safety and efficacy in children are not established.
CAUTIOUS USE Renal impairment; autoimmune disease; cardiomyopathy, impaired cardiac output, cardiac disease, history of hypercoagulation; pregnancy (category C).

ROUTE & DOSAGE

Vaccinia
Adults: **IV** 100–500 mg/kg

Renal Impairment Dosage Adjustment
Maximum dose: 400 mg/kg

ADMINISTRATION

Intravenous

PREPARE: **IV Infusion:** No dilution required. Use solution as supplied.

ADMINISTER: **IV Infusion:** Begin infusion within 6 h of entering the vial. Complete infusion within 12 h of entering the vial. ▪ Use in-line filter (0.22 microns), infusion pump, and dedicated IV line [may infuse into a preexisting catheter if it contains NS, D2.5W, D5W, D10W, or D20W (or any combination of these)]. ▪ Infuse at 1 mL/kg/h the first 30 min, increase to 2 mL/kg/h the next 30 min, and then increase to 3 mL/kg/h until infused.

ADVERSE EFFECTS (≥1%) **Body as a Whole:** Injection site reaction. **CNS:** Dizziness, *headache*. **GI:** Abdominal pain, nausea, vomiting. **Musculoskeletal:** Arthralgia, back pain. **Respiratory:** Upper respiratory infection. **Skin:** Erythema, flushing.

INTERACTIONS Drug: May interfere with the immune response to LIVE VIRUS VACCINES. Vaccination with LIVE VIRUS VACCINES should be deferred until approximately 6 mo after administration of VIG-IV.

PHARMACOKINETICS Half-Life: 22 days.

NURSING IMPLICATIONS

Assessment & Drug Effects

- Monitor vital signs continuously during infusion, especially after infusion rate changes.
- Slow infusion rate for any of the following: Flushing, chills, muscle cramps, back pain, fever, nausea, vomiting, arthralgia, and wheezing.
- Discontinue infusion, institute supportive measures, and notify physician for any of the following: Increase in heart rate, increase in respiratory rate, shortness of breath, rales or other signs of anaphylaxis.
- Have loop diuretic available for management of fluid overload.

Patient & Family Education

- Promptly report any discomfort that develops while drug is being infused.

VALACYCLOVIR HYDROCHLORIDE

(val-a-cy′clo-vir)

Valtrex

Classification: ANTIVIRAL

Therapeutic: ANTIVIRAL

Prototype: Acyclovir

Pregnancy Category: B

AVAILABILITY 500 mg, 1 g tablets

ACTION & *THERAPEUTIC EFFECT* An antiviral agent hydrolyzed in the intestinal wall or liver to acyclovir; interferes with viral DNA synthesis. *Active against herpes simplex virus types 1 (HSV-1) and 2 (HSV-2), varicella zoster virus, and cytomegalovirus. Inhibits viral replication.*

USES Herpes zoster (shingles) in immunocompetent adults. Treatment and suppression of recurrent genital herpes; suppression of recurrent herpes in HIV-positive patients; treatment of cold sores.

CONTRAINDICATIONS Hypersensitivity to or intolerance of valacyclovir or acyclovir; children younger than 2 y.

CAUTIOUS USE Renal impairment, patients receiving nephrotoxic drugs, advanced HIV disease, allogeneic bone marrow transplant and renal transplant recipients, treatment of disseminated herpes zoster, immunocompromised patients, pregnancy (category B); lactation.

ROUTE & DOSAGE

Herpes Zoster

Adult: **PO** 1 g (2 × 500 mg) t.i.d. for 7 days, start within 48 h of onset of zoster rash

Renal Impairment Dosage Adjustment

CrCl 30–49 mL/min: 1 g q12h; 10–29 mL/min: 1 g q24h; less than 10 mL/min: 500 mg q24h

Treatment of Recurrent Genital Herpes

Adult: **PO** 500 mg b.i.d. × 3 days

Renal Impairment Dosage Adjustment

CrCl 29 mL/min or less: 500 mg daily

Suppression of Recurrent Genital Herpes

Adult: **PO** 1 g daily; concurrent HIV infection 500 mg b.i.d.

Treatment of Cold Sores

Adult/Child: **PO** 2 g 12 h × 2 doses

Chickenpox

Adolescent/Child (older than 2 y): **PO** 20 mg/kg t.i.d. × 5 days (max: 1 g t.i.d.)

ADMINISTRATION

Oral

- Start drug as soon as possible after diagnosis of herpes zoster, preferably within 48 h of onset of rash.
- Note: Dosage reduction is recommended for patients with renal impairment.
- Give valacyclovir after hemodialysis.
- Store at 15°–30° C (59°–86° F).

ADVERSE EFFECTS (≥1%) **CNS:** *Headache,* weakness, somnolence, dizziness, fatigue, lethargy, confusion. **GI:** *Nausea, vomiting, diarrhea,* abdominal pain, dyspepsia, flatulence. **Urogenital:** Glomerulonephritis, renal tubular damage, acute renal failure. **Skin:** Rash, urticaria, pruritus.

INTERACTIONS Drug: Probenecid, cimetidine decrease valacyclovir elimination. **Zidovudine** may cause increased drowsiness and lethargy.

PHARMACOKINETICS Absorption: Rapidly absorbed from GI tract; 54% reaches systemic circulation as acyclovir. **Peak:** 1.5 h. **Distribution:** 13.5–17.9% bound to plasma proteins; distributes into plasma, cerebrospinal fluid, saliva, and major body organs; crosses placenta; excreted in breast milk. **Metabolism:** Rapidly converted to acyclovir during first pass through intestine and liver. **Elimination:** 40–50% in urine. **Half-Life:** 2.5–3.3 h.

NURSING IMPLICATIONS

Assessment & Drug Effects

- Monitor kidney function in patients with kidney impairment or those receiving potentially nephrotoxic drugs.
- Monitor for S&S of hypersensitivity; if present, withhold drug and notify physician.

Patient & Family Education

- Be aware of potential adverse effects and do not discontinue drug until full course is completed.
- Note: Post-herpes pain is likely to be present for several months after completion of therapy.

VALGANCICLOVIR HYDROCHLORIDE

(val-gan-ci′clo-vir)

Valcyte
Classification: ANTIVIRAL
Therapeutic: ANTIVIRAL
Prototype: Acyclovir
Pregnancy Category: C

AVAILABILITY 450 mg tablets

ACTION & *THERAPEUTIC EFFECT* Rapidly converted to ganciclovir by intestinal and hepatic enzymes. In cells infected with cytomegalovirus (CMV), ganciclovir is converted to ganciclovir triphosphate that inhibits viral DNA synthesis. *Antiviral drug that prevents replication of viral CMV DNA.*

USES Treatment of CMV retinitis; prevention of CMV disease in high-risk kidney, kidney-pancreas, and heart transplant patients (not effective in liver transplants).

CONTRAINDICATIONS Hypersensitivity to valganciclovir, ganciclovir, or acyclovir; renal failure; dental work; antimicrobial resistance; neutropenia, thrombocytopenia; females of childbearing age; lactation.
CAUTIOUS USE Impaired kidney function; older adults; dental disease; anemia; leukopenia; bone marrow depression; concomitant use of myelosuppressive drugs; irradiation; pregnancy (category C). Safety and efficacy in children are not established.

ROUTE & DOSAGE

Cytomegalovirus Prophylaxis
Adult: **PO** 900 mg once daily with food, starting within 10 days of transplantation until 100 days post-transplantation

Cytomegalovirus Retinitis Induction
Adult: **PO** 900 mg b.i.d. with food × 21 days

Cytomegalovirus Retinitis Maintenance
Adult: **PO** 900 mg daily with food

Renal Impairment Dosage Adjustment
CrCl 40–59 mL/min: 450 mg b.i.d. (induction) or daily (maintenance); 25–39 mL/min: 450 mg daily (induction) or q2days (maintenance); 10–24 mL/min: 450 mg q2days (induction) or twice weekly (maintenance)

ADMINISTRATION

Oral
- Exercise caution in handling tablets. Do not crush or break tablets. Avoid direct contact of crushed or broken tablets with skin or mucous membranes.
- Give with food.
- Do not give to patients on hemodialysis.
- Store at 25°–30° C (77°–86° F).

ADVERSE EFFECTS (≥1%) **Body as a Whole:** *Fever,* local and systemic infections, hypersensitivity reactions. **CNS:** *Headache, insomnia,* peripheral neuropathy, paresthesia, convulsions, psychosis, confusion, hallucinations, agitation. **GI:** *Diarrhea, nausea, vomiting, abdominal pain.* **Hematologic:** *Neutropenia, anemia,* thrombocytopenia, pancytopenia, bone marrow suppression, aplastic anemia. **Special Senses:** *Retinal detachment.*

INTERACTIONS Drug: ANTINEOPLASTIC AGENTS, **amphotericin B, didanosine, trimethoprim-sulfamethoxazole (TMP-SMZ), dapsone, pentamidine, probenecid, zidovudine** may increase bone marrow suppression and other toxic effects of valganciclovir; may increase risk of nephrotoxicity from

cyclosporine; ANTIRETROVIRAL AGENTS may decrease valganciclovir levels; valganciclovir may increase levels and toxicity of ANTIRETROVIRAL AGENTS; may increase risk of seizures due to **imipenem-cilastatin.**

PHARMACOKINETICS Absorption: Well absorbed from GI tract, 60% reaches systemic circulation as ganciclovir. **Onset:** 3–8 days. **Peak:** 1–3 h. **Duration:** Clinical relapse can occur 14 days to 3.5 mo after stopping therapy; positive blood and urine cultures recur 12–60 days after therapy. **Distribution:** Distributes throughout body including CSF, eye, lungs, liver, and kidneys; crosses placenta in animals; not known if distributed into breast milk. **Metabolism:** Metabolized in intestinal wall to ganciclovir, ganciclovir is not metabolized. **Elimination:** 94–99% of dose is excreted unchanged in urine. **Half-Life:** 4 h.

NURSING IMPLICATIONS

Assessment & Drug Effects

- Withhold drug and notify physician for any of the following: Absolute neutrophil count less than 500 cells/mm³, platelet count less than 25,000/mm³, hemoglobin less than 8 g/dL, declining creatinine clearance.
- Monitor for S&S of bronchospasm in asthma patients; notify physician immediately.
- Lab tests: Baseline and frequent serum creatinine or creatinine clearance, CBC with differential, platelet count, Hct and Hgb.

Patient & Family Education

- Schedule ophthalmologic follow-up examinations at least every 4–6 wk while being treated with valganciclovir.
- Keep all scheduled appointments for laboratory tests.
- Do not drive or engage in potentially hazardous activities until response to drug is known.
- Report any of the following immediately: Unexpected bleeding, infection.
- Use effective methods of contraception (barrier and other types) during and for at least 90 days following treatment.
- Discontinue drug and notify physician immediately in the event of pregnancy.

VALPROIC ACID (DIVALPROEX SODIUM, SODIUM VALPROATE) Pr

(val-proe′ic)

Depacon, Depakene, Depakote, Depakote ER, Depakote Sprinkle, Epival ✦, Stavzor

Classifications: ANTICONVULSANT; GAMMA-AMINOBUTYRIC ACID (GABA) INHIBITOR

Therapeutic: ANTICONVULSANT

Pregnancy Category: D

AVAILABILITY 250 mg capsules; 125 mg sprinkle capsules; 125 mg, 250 mg, 500 mg delayed release tablets; 500 mg sustained release tablets; 250 mg/5 mL syrup; 100 mg/mL injection

ACTION & *THERAPEUTIC EFFECT* Anticonvulsant with increased bioavailability of the inhibitory neurotransmitter gamma-aminobutyric acid (GABA) to brain neurons. It may also suppress repetitive neuronal firing through inhibition of voltage-sensitive sodium channels. *Depresses abnormal neuron discharges in the CNS, thus decreasing seizure activity.*

USES Alone or with other anticonvulsants in management of absence

(petit mal) and mixed seizures; mania; migraine headache prophylaxis.
UNLABELED USES Status epilepticus refractory to IV diazepam, petit mal variant seizures, febrile seizures in children, other types of seizures including psychomotor (temporal lobe), myoclonic, akinetic and tonic-clonic seizures, photosensitivity seizures, and those refractory to other anticonvulsants.

CONTRAINDICATIONS Hypersensitivity to valproate sodium; urea cycle disorders (UCD), hyperammonemia, encephalopathy; suicidal ideations; thrombocytopenia, patient with bleeding disorders or liver dysfunction or disease, cirrhosis, hepatitis; pancreatitis; congenital metabolic disorders, those with severe seizures, or on multiple anticonvulsant drugs; encephalopathy; AIDS; fluid restriction or decreased food intake; pregnancy (category D); lactation; children younger than 10 y.
CAUTIOUS USE History of suicidal tendencies; history of kidney disease, renal impairment or failure; history of liver disease; adjunctive treatment with other anticonvulsants; congenital metabolic disorders, those with severe epilepsy, use as sole anticonvulsant drug; HIV; hypoalbuminemia; organic brain syndrome; older adults.

ROUTE & DOSAGE

Note: May need to increase dose when converting from immediate release to extended release products

Management of Seizures

Adult/Child (10 y or older): **PO/IV** 10–15 mg/kg/day in divided doses when total daily dose greater than 250 mg, increase at 1 wk intervals by 5–10 mg/kg/day until seizures are controlled or adverse effects develop (max: 60 mg/kg/day)
Conversion of PO to IV: Give normal dose in divided doses q6h

Migraine Headache Prophylaxis

Adult: **PO** 250 mg b.i.d. (max: 1000 mg/day) or **Depakote ER** 500 mg daily × 1 wk, may increase to 1000 mg daily

Mania

Adult: **PO** 750 mg/day administered in divided doses OR 25 mg/kg/day using extended release tabs

Hepatic Impairment Dosage Adjustment

Dose reduction recommended

Renal Impairment Dosage Adjustment

Severe impairment may require close monitoring

ADMINISTRATION

Oral

- Give tablets and capsules whole; instruct patient to swallow whole and not to chew. Instruct to swallow sprinkle capsules whole or sprinkle entire contents on teaspoonful of soft food, and instruct to not chew food.
- Avoid using a carbonated drink as diluent for the syrup because it will release drug from delivery vehicle; free drug painfully irritates oral and pharyngeal membranes.
- Reduce gastric irritation by administering drug with food.

Intravenous

PREPARE: **IV Infusion:** Dilute each dose in 50 mL or more of D5W, NS, or LR.

V

ADMINISTER: **IV Infusion:** Give a single dose over at least 60 min (20 mg/min or less). Avoid rapid infusion.

INCOMPATIBILITIES **Solution/additive:** Should avoid mixing with other drugs.

ADVERSE EFFECTS (≥1%) **CNS:** Breakthrough seizures, *sedation, drowsiness,* dizziness, increased alertness, hallucinations, emotional upset, aggression; deep coma, death (with overdose). **GI:** *Nausea, vomiting, indigestion (transient),* hypersalivation, anorexia with weight loss, increased appetite with weight gain, abdominal cramps, diarrhea, constipation, liver failure, pancreatitis. **Hematologic:** *Prolonged bleeding time,* leukopenia, lymphocytosis, thrombocytopenia, hypofibrinogenemia, bone marrow depression, anemia. **Skin:** Skin rash, photosensitivity, transient hair loss, curliness or waviness of hair. **Endocrine:** Irregular menses, secondary amenorrhea. **Metabolic:** Hyperammonemia (usually asymptomatic) hyperammonemic encephalopathy in patients with urea cycle disorders. **Respiratory:** Pulmonary edema (with overdose).

DIAGNOSTIC TEST INTERFERENCE Valproic acid produces false-positive results for ***urine ketones,*** elevated ***AST, ALT, LDH,*** and ***serum alkaline phosphatase,*** prolonged ***bleeding time,*** altered ***thyroid function tests.***

INTERACTIONS Drug: Alcohol and other CNS DEPRESSANTS potentiate depressant effects; other ANTICONVULSANTS, BARBITURATES increase or decrease anticonvulsant and BARBITURATE levels; **haloperidol, loxapine, maprotiline,** MAOIS, PHENOTHIAZINES, THIOXANTHENES, TRICYCLIC ANTIDEPRESSANTS can increase CNS depression or lower seizure threshold; **aspirin, dipyridamole, warfarin** increase risk of spontaneous bleeding; **clonazepam** may precipitate absence seizures; SALICYLATES, **cimetidine, isoniazid** may increase valproic acid levels and toxicity. **Mefloquine** can decrease valproic acid levels; **meropenem** may decrease valproic acid levels; **cholestyramine** may decrease absorption. **Herbal: Ginkgo** may decrease anticonvulsant effectiveness.

PHARMACOKINETICS Absorption: Readily from GI tract. **Peak:** 1–4 h valproic acid; 3–5 h divalproex. **Therapeutic Range:** 50–100 mcg/mL. **Distribution:** Crosses placenta; distributed into breast milk. **Metabolism:** In liver. **Elimination:** Primarily in urine; small amount in feces and expired air. **Half-Life:** 5–20 h.

NURSING IMPLICATIONS

Assessment & Drug Effects

- Monitor for therapeutic effectiveness achieved with serum levels of valproic acid at 50–100 mcg/mL.
- Monitor patient alertness especially with multiple drug therapy for seizure control.
- Monitor patient carefully during dose adjustments and promptly report presence of adverse effects. Increased dosage is associated with frequency of adverse effects.
- Lab tests: Baseline platelet count, bleeding time, and serum ammonia, then repeat at least q2mo, especially during the first 6 mo of therapy.
- Multiple drugs for seizure control increase the risk of hyperammonemia, marked by lethargy, anorexia, asterixis, increased seizure frequency, and vomiting. Report such symptoms promptly to physician. If they persist with decreased dosage, the drug will be discontinued.

Patient & Family Education

- Do not discontinue therapy abruptly; such action could result in loss of seizure control. Consult physician before you stop or alter dosage regimen.
- Note to diabetic patients: Drug may cause a false-positive test for urine ketones. Notify physician if this occurs.
- Notify physician promptly if spontaneous bleeding or bruising occurs (e.g., petechiae, ecchymotic areas, otorrhagia, epistaxis, melena).
- Withhold dose and notify physician for following symptoms: Visual disturbances, rash, jaundice, light-colored stools, protracted vomiting, diarrhea. Fatal liver failure has occurred in patients receiving this drug.
- Avoid alcohol and self-medication with other depressants during therapy.
- Consult physician before using any OTC drugs during anticonvulsant therapy, especially drugs containing aspirin or sedatives and medications for hay fever or other allergies.
- Do not drive or engage in potentially hazardous activities until response to drug is known.

VALRUBICIN

(val-roo′bi-sin)

Valstar

Classification: ANTINEOPLASTIC ANTHRACYCLINE

Therapeutic: ANTINEOPLASTIC

Prototype: Doxorubicin hydrochloride

Pregnancy Category: C

AVAILABILITY 40 mg/mL solution

ACTION & *THERAPEUTIC EFFECT*

A cytotoxic agent that inhibits the incorporation of nucleosides in DNA and RNA, resulting in extensive chromosomal damage. Valrubicin interferes with DNA topoisomerase II, which is responsible for the normal DNA separation of strands and the resealing of those DNA strands. *Valrubicin has higher antitumor efficacy and lower toxicity than doxorubicin.*

USES Intravesical therapy of BCG-refractory carcinoma *in situ* of the urinary bladder.

CONTRAINDICATIONS Hypersensitivity to valrubicin, doxorubicin, anthracyclines, or castor oil; patients with a perforated bladder, concurrent UTI, active infection; severe irritable bladder symptoms; severe myelosuppression; lactation.

CAUTIOUS USE Within 2 wk of a transureteral resection; compromised bladder mucosa; mild to moderate myelosuppression; history of bleeding disorders; GI disorders, renal impairment; pregnancy (category C).

ROUTE & DOSAGE

BCG-Refractory Bladder Carcinoma *in situ*

Adult: **Intravesically** 800 mg once/wk × 6 wk

ADMINISTRATION

Instillation

Avoid skin reactions by using gloves during preparation/administration.

- Use only glass, polypropylene, or polyolefin containers and tubing.

PREPARE: Slowly warm 4 vials (5 mL each) to room temperature. ▪ When a precipitate is initially present, warm vials in hands until solution clears. ▪ Add contents of 4 vials to 55 mL of 0.9% NaCl injection to yield 75 mL of diluted solution.

ADMINISTER: Aseptically insert a urethral catheter and drain the bladder. ▪ Use gravity drainage to instill valrubicin slowly over several min. ▪ Withdraw catheter; instruct patient not to void for 2 h. ▪ Note: Do not leave a clamped catheter in place.

▪ Refrigerate. Do not freeze.

ADVERSE EFFECTS (≥1%) **Body as a Whole:** Abdominal pain, asthenia, back pain, fever, headache, malaise, myalgia. **CNS:** Dizziness. **CV:** Vasodilation. **GI:** Diarrhea, flatulence, nausea, vomiting. **Urogenital:** *Urinary frequency, urgency, dysuria, bladder spasm, hematuria, bladder pain, incontinence, cystitis, UTI,* nocturia, local burning, urethral pain, pelvic pain, gross hematuria, urinary retention. **Respiratory:** Pneumonia. **Skin:** Rash. **Other:** Anemia, hyperglycemia, peripheral edema.

PHARMACOKINETICS Absorption: Not absorbed. **Distribution:** Penetrates bladder wall. **Metabolism:** Not metabolized. **Elimination:** Almost completely excreted by voiding the instillate.

NURSING IMPLICATIONS

Assessment & Drug Effects

- Therapeutic effectiveness: Indicated by regression of the bladder tumor.
- Notify physician if bladder spasms with spontaneous discharge of valrubicin occur during/shortly after instillation.

Patient & Family Education

- Expect red-tinged urine during the first 24 h after administration.
- Report prolonged passage of red-colored urine or prolonged bladder irritation.
- Drink plenty of fluids during 48 h period following administration.
- Use reliable contraception during therapy period (approximately 6 wk).

VALSARTAN

(val-sar′tan)

Diovan

Classifications: ANGIOTENSIN II RECEPTOR ANTAGONIST; ANTIHYPERTENSIVE

Therapeutic: ANTIHYPERTENSIVE; ANGIOTENSIN RECEPTOR (AT_1) ANTAGONIST

Prototype: Losartan

Pregnancy Category: D

AVAILABILITY 40 mg, 80 mg, 160 mg capsules

ACTION & *THERAPEUTIC EFFECT* An angiotensin II receptor (type AT_1 receptor subtype) antagonist that blocks the angiotensin converting enzyme (ACE). It inhibits the binding of angiotensin II to the AT_1 subtype receptors found in many tissues (e.g., vascular smooth muscle, adrenal glands). Angiotensin II is a potent vasoconstrictor and primary vasoactive hormone of the renin–angiotensin–aldosterone system (RAAS). *Blocking angiotensin II receptors results in vasodilation as well as decreasing the aldosterone-secreting effects of angiotensin II. These actions result in the antihypertensive effect of valsartan.*

USES Treatment of hypertension, heart failure.

CONTRAINDICATIONS Hypersensitivity to valsartan or losartan; severe heart failure with compromised renal function; volume depletion; history of ACE inhibitor–induced angioedema; pregnancy (category D), lactation; children younger than 6 y or with CrCl of 30 mL/min per 1.73 mm³.

CAUTIOUS USE Severe renal impairment; mild to moderate hepatic impairment; biliary stenosis; renal artery stenosis; hypovolemia; hyperkalemia; transient hypotension; use prior to surgery; history of angioedema; congestive heart failure.

ROUTE & DOSAGE

Hypertension

Adult: **PO** 80 mg daily (max: 320 mg daily)
Adolescent/Child (6–16 y): **PO** 1.3 mg/kg (up to 40 mg/day)

Heart Failure

Adult: **PO** Start with 40 mg b.i.d. and titrate up to 160 mg b.i.d.
Hemodialysis Dosage Adjustment: Adjustment not needed

ADMINISTRATION

Oral

- Give on an empty stomach.
- Correct volume depletion prior to initiation of therapy to prevent hypotension.
- Reduce dosage with severe hepatic or renal impairment.
- Note: Daily dose may be titrated up to 320 mg.
- Store at 15°–30° C (59°–86° F).

ADVERSE EFFECTS (≥1%) **Body as a Whole:** Arthralgia. **CNS:** Headache, dizziness. **GI:** Diarrhea, nausea. **Respiratory:** Cough, sinusitis. **Metabolic:** Hyperkalemia.

V

PHARMACOKINETICS Absorption: Rapidly from GI tract, 25% bioavailability. **Onset:** Blood pressure decreased in 2 wk. **Peak:** Plasma levels, 2–4 h; blood pressure effect 4 wk. **Distribution:** 99% protein bound. **Metabolism:** In the liver. **Elimination:** Primarily in feces. **Half-Life:** 6 h.

NURSING IMPLICATIONS

Assessment & Drug Effects

- Monitor BP periodically; take trough readings, just prior to the next scheduled dose, when possible.
- Lab tests: Periodic LFTs, BUN and creatinine, serum potassium, and CBC with differential.

Patient & Family Education

- Inform physician immediately if you become pregnant.
- Note: Maximum pressure lowering effect is usually evident between 2 and 4 wk after initiation of therapy.
- Notify physician of episodes of dizziness, especially those that occur when making position changes.
- Do not use potassium supplements or salt substitutes containing potassium without consulting the prescribing physician.

VANCOMYCIN HYDROCHLORIDE

(van-koe-mye'sin)

Vancocin

Classifications: ANTIBIOTIC; GLYCOPEPTIDE
Therapeutic: ANTIBIOTIC
Pregnancy Category: B

AVAILABILITY 125 mg, 250 mg capsules; 500 mg, 1 g, 5 g, 10 g injection

ACTION & *THERAPEUTIC EFFECT* Bactericidal action is due to inhibition of cell-wall biosynthesis and alteration of bacterial cell-membrane permeability and ribonucleic acid (RNA) synthesis. *Active against many gram-positive organisms.*

USES Parenterally for potentially life-threatening infections in patients allergic, nonsensitive, or resistant to other less toxic antimicrobial drugs. Used orally only in *Clostridium difficile* colitis (not effective by oral route for treatment of systemic infections).

CONTRAINDICATIONS Hypersensitivity to vancomycin, allergy to corn or corn products, previous hearing loss.

CAUTIOUS USE Older adults; impaired kidney function, renal failure, renal impairment, hearing impairment; colitis, inflammatory disorders of the intestine; pregnancy (category B), lactation; children, neonates.

ROUTE & DOSAGE

Systemic Infections

Adult/Adolescent: **IV** 500 mg q6h or 1 g q12h or 15 mg/kg q12h
Child/Infant (older than 1 mo): **IV** 30–40 mg/kg/day divided q6–8h
Neonate: **IV** 10–15 mg/kg q8–24h

***Clostridium difficile* Colitis**

Adult: **PO** 125–500 mg q6h
Child: **PO** 40 mg/kg/day divided q6h (max: 2 g/day)
Neonate: **PO** 10 mg/kg/day in divided doses

Surgical Prophylaxis (in Patients Allergic to Beta-Lactams)

Adult/Adolescent/Child (weight at least 27 kg): **IV** 10–15 mg/kg starting 1 h before surgery
Child (weight less than 27 kg): **IV** 20 mg/kg starting 1 h before surgery

Renal Impairment Dosage Adjustment

CrCl 40–60 mL/min: Dose q24h; less than 40 mL/min: Extend interval based on monitoring levels

Hemodialysis Dosage Adjustment: Not dialyzed

ADMINISTRATION

Oral

- May be given with or without food.
- Note: Some parenteral products may be administered orally; check manufacturer's package insert.

Intravenous

PREPARE: **Intermittent:** Reconstitute 500 mg vial or 1 g vial with 10 mL or 20 mL, respectively, of sterile water for injection to yield 50 mg/mL. ▪ Further dilute each 500 mg with at least 100 mL and each 1 g with at least 200 mL of D5W, NS, or LR.

ADMINISTER: **Intermittent:** Give a single dose at a rate of 10 mg/min or over NOT LESS than 60 min (whichever is longer). ▪ Avoid rapid infusion, which may cause sudden hypotension. ▪ Monitor IV site closely; necrosis and tissue sloughing will result from extravasation.

INCOMPATIBILITIES **Solution/additive:** **Aminophylline,** BARBITURATES, **aztreonam** (high concentration), **calcium chloride, chloramphenicol, chlorothiazide, dexamethasone, erythromycin, heparin, methicillin, sodium bicarbonate, warfarin.** **Y-site:** **Albumin, amphotericin B cholesteryl, aztreonam, bivalirudin, cefazolin, cefepime, cefotaxime, cefotetan, cefoxitin, ceftazidime, ceftriaxone, cefuroxime, drotrecogin, foscarnet, heparin, idarubicin, lansoprazole, nafcillin, omeprazole, piperacillin/tazobactam, sargramostim, ticarcillin, ticarcillin/clavulanate, warfarin.**

- Store oral and parenteral solutions in refrigerator for up to 14 days; after further dilution, parenteral solution is stable 24 h at room temperature.

ADVERSE EFFECTS (≥1%) **Special Senses:** Ototoxicity (auditory portion of eighth cranial nerve). **Urogenital:** Nephrotoxicity leading to uremia. **Body as a Whole:** Hypersensitivity reactions (chills, fever, skin rash, urticaria, shock-like state), anaphylactoid reaction with vascular collapse, superinfections, severe pain, thrombophlebitis at injection site, generalized tingling following rapid IV infusion. **Hematologic:** Transient leukopenia, eosinophilia. **GI:** Nausea, warmth. **Other:** Injection reaction that includes *hypotension accompanied by flushing and erythematous rash on face and upper body* ("red-neck syndrome") following rapid IV infusion.

INTERACTIONS Drug: Adds to toxicity of ototoxic and nephrotoxic drugs (AMINOGLYCOSIDES, **amphotericin B, colistin, capreomycin; cidofovir; cisplatin; cyclosporine; foscarnet; ganciclovir; IV pentamidine; polymyxin B; streptozocin; tacrolimus**). **Cholestyramine, colestipol** can decrease absorption of oral vancomycin; may increase risk of lactic acidosis with **metformin.**

V

PHARMACOKINETICS Absorption: Not absorbed. **Peak:** 30 min after end of infusion. **Distribution:** Diffuses into pleural, ascitic, pericardial, and synovial fluids; small amount penetrates CSF if meninges are inflamed; crosses placenta. **Elimination:** 80–90% of IV dose in urine within 24 h; PO dose excreted in feces. **Half-Life:** 4–8 h.

NURSING IMPLICATIONS

Assessment & Drug Effects

- Monitor BP and heart rate continuously through period of drug administration.
- Lab tests: Periodic urinalysis, kidney and liver functions, and hematologic studies. Monitor serial tests of vancomycin blood levels (peak and trough) in patients with borderline kidney function, in infants and neonates, and in patients older than 60 y.
- Assess hearing. Drug may cause damage to auditory branch (not vestibular branch) of eighth cranial nerve, with consequent deafness, which may be permanent.
- Be aware that serum levels of 60–80 mcg/mL are associated with ototoxicity. Tinnitus and high-tone hearing loss may precede deafness, which may progress even after drug is withdrawn. Older adults and those on high doses are especially susceptible.
- Monitor I&O: Report changes in I&O ratio and pattern. Oliguria or cloudy or pink urine may be a sign of nephrotoxicity (also manifested by transient elevations in BUN, albumin, and hyaline and granular casts in urine).

Patient & Family Education

- Notify physician promptly of ringing in ears.
- Adhere to drug regimen (i.e., do not increase, decrease, or interrupt dosage. The full course of prescribed drug therapy **must be** completed).

VARDENAFIL HYDROCHLORIDE

(var-den'a-fil hy-dro-chlo'ride)

Levitra

Classifications: IMPOTENCE AGENT; PHOSPHODIESTERASE (PDE) INHIBITOR; VASODILATOR
Therapeutic: IMPOTENCE; PDE INHIBITOR
Prototype: Sildenafil
Pregnancy Category: B

AVAILABILITY 2.5 mg, 5 mg, 10 mg, 20 mg tablets

ACTION & *THERAPEUTIC EFFECT* Phosphodiesterases-5 (PDE5) is an enzyme that speeds up the degradation of cyclic guanosine monophosphate (cGMP), an enzyme needed to cause and maintain increased blood flow into the penis necessary for an erection. Vardenafil is a PDE5 inhibitor. *It enhances erectile function by increasing the amount of cGMP in the penis.*

USES Treatment of erectile dysfunction.

CONTRAINDICATIONS Hypersensitivity to vardenafil or sildenafil; QT prolongation, renal failure, severe renal impairment; retinitis pigmentosa; lactation.

CAUTIOUS USE CAD, MI, or stroke within 6 mo; hypotension, or hypertension; risk factors for CVA; anatomic deformity of the penis; subaortic stenosis; sickle cell anemia, leukemia; multiple myeloma; leukemia; coagulopathy; active bleeding or a peptic ulcer; coagulopathy; GERD; hepatitis, cirrhosis; older adults; pregnancy (category B).

ROUTE & DOSAGE

Erectile Dysfunction

Adult: **PO** 10 mg approximately 60 min before sexual activity. May increase to max 20 mg/day if needed. If taking ritonavir, max dose is 2.5 mg/72 h. If taking erythromycin, indinavir, itraconazole, ketoconazole, max dose is 2.5–5 mg/24 h.

Geriatric: **PO** Start with 5 mg 60 min before sexual activity (max: 20 mg/day)

Hepatic Impairment Dosage Adjustment

Moderate impairment: Reduce dose to 5 mg (max: 10 mg/day)

ADMINISTRATION

Oral

- Take approximately 1 h before expected intercourse, but preferably not after a heavy or high-fat meal.
- Store at 15°–30° C (59°–86° F).

ADVERSE EFFECTS (≥1%) **Body as a Whole:** *Flushing,* flu-like syndrome, back pain, anaphylactoid reactions, asthenia, facial edema, pain, paresthesias. **CNS:** *Headache,* dizziness, insomnia, somnolence, vertigo. **CV:** Angina, hypertension, hypotension, MI, orthostatic hypotension, palpitations, syncope, sinus tachycardia. **GI:** Dyspepsia, nausea, vomiting, abdominal pain, abnormal liver function tests, diarrhea, dysphagia, esophagitis, gastritis, GERD, xerostomia. **Metabolic:** Increased creatine kinase. **Musculoskeletal:** Arthralgia, myalgia, hypertonia, hyperesthesia. **Respiratory:** Rhinitis, sinusitis, dyspnea, epistaxis, pharyngitis. **Skin:** Photosensitivity, rash, pruritus, sweating. **Special Senses:** Tinnitus, sudden vision loss, blurred vision, changes in color vision. **Urogenital:** Ejaculation dysfunction.

INTERACTIONS Drug: May potentiate hypotensive effects of NITRATES, **alfuzosin, doxazosin, prazosin, tamsulosin, terazosin; amiodarone, dofetilide, procainamide, quinidine, sotalol** may in-

V

crease QT_c interval leading to arrhythmias; **erythromycin** (and other MACROLIDES), **indinavir, itraconazole, ketoconazole,** PROTEASE INHIBITORS, **ritonavir, voriconazole** may increase level and toxicity of vardenafil.

PHARMACOKINETICS Absorption: Rapidly absorbed, 15% reaches systemic circulation. **Onset:** Within 1 h. **Peak:** 0.5–2 h. **Metabolism:** In liver by CYP3A4. **Elimination:** Primarily in feces (90–95%). **Half-Life:** 4–5 h.

NURSING IMPLICATIONS

Assessment & Drug Effects

- Monitor CV status and report angina or other S&S of cardiac dysfunction.
- Lab tests: Baseline and periodic LFTs.

Patient & Family Education

- Do not take more than once a day and never take more than the prescribed dose.
- Do not take this drug without consulting physician if you are taking drugs called "alpha-blockers" or "nitrates" or any other drugs for high blood pressure, chest pain, or enlarged prostate.
- Report promptly any of the following: Palpitations, chest pain, back pain, difficulty breathing, or shortness of breath; dizziness or fainting; changes in vision; dizziness; swollen eyelids; muscle aches; painful or prolonged erection (lasting longer than 4 h); skin rash, or itching.

V

VARENICLINE

(var-en′i-cline)

Chantix

Classifications: SMOKING DETERRENT; NICOTINIC RECEPTOR AGONIST

Therapeutic: SMOKING CESSATION

Prototype: Nicotine

Pregnancy Category: C

AVAILABILITY 0.5 mg, 1 mg capsules

ACTION & *THERAPEUTIC EFFECT* Nicotine increases dopamine release in the brain and cravings for nicotine are stimulated by low levels of dopamine during periods of abstinence. Varenicline is a partial agonist at nicotinic acetylcholine receptors (nAChRs), the sites responsible for the dopamine effects of nicotine. It partially stimulates these receptors to produce a modest level of dopamine but blocks nicotine from binding to many of the nicotinic receptor sites. *By blocking nicotinic receptors, it reduces effects of nicotine in cases where patient relapses and uses tobacco.*

USES Adjunct for smoking cessation in patients experiencing nicotine withdrawal.

CONTRAINDICATIONS Suicidal ideation; chronic depression; serious psychiatric disease; lactation. Safe use in children or adolescents younger than 18 y is not known.

CAUTIOUS USE History of suicidal tendencies, depression; renal disease, older adults; pregnancy (category C).

ROUTE & DOSAGE

Smoking Cessation

Adult: **PO** Begin with 0.5 mg/day for 3 days, increase to 0.5 mg b.i.d. for 4 days, then increase to 1 mg b.i.d. on day 8. Treat for 12 wk and may repeat an additional 12 wk.

Renal Impairment Dosage Adjustment

CrCl 50 mL/min or less: Titrate to 0.5 mg b.i.d. (max)

ADMINISTRATION

Oral

- Give after a meal with a full glass of water.
- Dose titration over 8 days (from 0.5 mg to 2 mg daily) is recommended to minimize adverse effects.
- Store at 15°–30° C (59°–86° F).

ADVERSE EFFECTS (≥1%) **Body as a Whole:** Fatigue, flushing, gingivitis, headache, influenza-like symptoms, lethargy, malaise, thirst. **CNS:** *Abnormal dreams,* anorexia, anxiety, asthenia, disturbance in attention, depression, dizziness, drowsiness, emotional lability, *insomnia,* irritability, *nightmares,* restlessness, sensory disturbance, *sleep disorder, suicidality.* **CV:** Chest pain, hypertension. **GI:** Abdominal pain, *constipation,* diarrhea, dyspepsia, *flatulence,* gastroesophageal reflux, *nausea, vomiting.* **Metabolic:** Abnormal liver function test, appetite stimulation, weight gain. **Musculoskeletal:** Arthralgia, back pain, muscle cramps, musculoskeletal pain, myalgia. **Respiratory:** Dyspnea, epistaxis, respiratory disorder, rhinorrhea. **Skin:** Hyperhidrosis, pruritus, rash. **Special Senses:** Dysgeusia, xerostomia. **Urogenital:** Menstrual irregularity, polyuria.

INTERACTIONS Drug: Cimetidine increases systemic exposure to varenicline by 29%.

PHARMACOKINETICS Absorption: Complete absorption from GI tract. **Peak:** 3–4 h. **Distribution:** Less than 20% protein bound. **Metabolism:** Minimal. **Elimination:** Primarily eliminated unchanged in the urine. **Half-Life:** 24 h.

NURSING IMPLICATIONS

Assessment & Drug Effects

- Monitor smoking cessation behavior and adverse effects.
- Monitor BP for new-onset hypertension.
- Monitor diabetics for loss of glycemic control.
- Monitor for increased suicidality, or increase in agitation or aggression.

Patient & Family Education

- Report persistent nausea, vomiting, or insomnia to a health care provider.
- Report new-onset of depressed mood, suicidal ideation, or changes in emotion and behavior resulting from the use of varenicline.

VARICELLA VACCINE

(var-i-cel′la)

Varivax

Classification: VACCINE

Therapeutic: VIRAL VACCINE

Prototype: Hepatitis B

Pregnancy Category: C

AVAILABILITY 1350 PFU/vial

ACTION & *THERAPEUTIC EFFECT* A live attenuated vaccine that acts against both chickenpox and shingles, both of which are caused by varicella zoster infection. *Effective in protecting healthy children and adults from varicella.*

USES Vaccination against varicella in individuals 12 mo or older.

CONTRAINDICATIONS Hypersensitivity to any component of the vaccine; history of anaphylactoid reaction to neomycin; individuals with blood dyscrasia, leukemia, lymphomas, bone marrow or lymphatic system malignancies, individuals with primary or acquired immunodeficient states; active untreated tuberculosis; any febrile respiratory illness or other febrile infections; children younger than 1 y.

V

CAUTIOUS USE Acute lymphoblastic leukemia in remission; IgA deficiency; pregnancy (category C), lactation.

ROUTE & DOSAGE

Varicella Protection

Adult: **Subcutaneous** Primary immunization of 0.5 mL followed by 0.5 mL 4–8 wk after first dose, may need to revaccinate 3 mo after initial series if patient fails to seroconvert

Child (12 mo–12 y): **Subcutaneous** Single dose of 0.5 mL

ADMINISTRATION

Subcutaneous

- Reconstitute vaccine with 0.7 mL of supplied diluent; gently agitate the vial to mix. Withdraw entire contents of vial (0.5 mL) into syringe for injection. Change needle on syringe and administer immediately or within 30 min of reconstitution.
- Give subcutaneously into the outer aspect of the deltoid. Exercise caution not to inject IV.
- Store powder vaccine in frost-free freezer at –15° C (+5° F) or colder. Store diluent separately at room temperature or in the refrigerator.

ADVERSE EFFECTS (≥1%) **CNS:** Headache, fever. **Hematologic:** Mild thrombocytopenia. **Skin:** *Redness, swelling, or rash at injection site.* **Other:** Herpes zoster infection (rare).

INTERACTIONS Drug: Acyclovir decreases vaccine's effectiveness. It is recommended that **yellow fever vaccine** be given at least 1 mo apart from varicella or any other LIVE VIRUS VACCINE. Avoid **salicylates** for 6 wk after vaccination to decrease risk of developing Reye's syndrome.

PHARMACOKINETICS Onset: Seroconversion approximately 42 days after vaccination. **Duration:** Older than 5–10 y in healthy children. **Distribution:** Crosses placenta; distributed into breast milk.

NURSING IMPLICATIONS

Assessment & Drug Effects

- Withhold vaccine and notify physician if patient has a history of hypersensitivity to neomycin or a current febrile infection.
- Monitor for signs and symptoms of hypersensitivity (see Appendix F) and administer epinephrine if an anaphylactoid reaction occurs.

Patient & Family Education

- Avoid use of salicylates (e.g., acetylsalicylic acid) for 6 wk after vaccination, especially with children and adolescents.
- Notify physician about all adverse reactions (i.e., fever, rash, respiratory illness).

VASOPRESSIN INJECTION Pr

(vay-soe-press'in)

Classifications: PITUITARY HORMONE; ANTIDIURETIC HORMONE (ADH)

Therapeutic: ADH REPLACEMENT

Pregnancy Category: C

AVAILABILITY 20 pressor units/mL injection

ACTION & *THERAPEUTIC EFFECT* Polypeptide hormone extracted from animal posterior pituitaries, and possesses pressor and antidiuretic (ADH) properties. Produces concentrated urine by increasing tubular reabsorption of water (ADH activity), thus reabsorbing up to 90% of water in renal tubules. Causes contraction of smooth muscles of the GI tract as well as the vascular system, especially capillaries, arterioles and venules. *Effective in reversing diuresis caused by diabetes insipidus. When given intravenously, it is effective as an adjunct in treating massive GI bleeding.*

USES Antidiuretic to treat diabetes insipidus, to dispel gas shadows in abdominal roentgenography, and as prevention and treatment of postoperative abdominal distention.

UNLABELED USES Test for differential diagnosis of nephrogenic, psychogenic, and neurohypophyseal diabetes insipidus; test to elevate ability of kidney to concentrate urine, and provocative test for pituitary release of corticotropin and growth hormone; emergency and adjunct pressor agent in the control of massive GI hemorrhage (e.g., esophageal varices).

CONTRAINDICATIONS Chronic nephritis accompanied by nitrogen retention; ischemic heart disease, PVCs, advanced arteriosclerosis; lactation.

CAUTIOUS USE Epilepsy; migraine; asthma; heart failure, angina pectoris; any state in which rapid addition to extracellular fluid may be hazardous; vascular disease; preoperative and postoperative polyuric patients, kidney disease; goiter with cardiac complications; older adult patients, labor and delivery, pregnancy (category C), children.

ROUTE & DOSAGE

Diabetes Insipidus

Adult: **IM/Subcutaneous** 5–10 units aqueous solution 2–4 times/day (5–60 units/day) or 1.25–2.5 units in oil q2–3days **Intranasal** Apply to cotton pledget or intranasal spray

Child: **IM/Subcutaneous** 2.5–10 units aqueous solution 2–4 times/day

Abdominal Distention, Abdominal Radiographic Procedures

Adult: **IM/Subcutaneous** 5 units with 5–10 units q3–4h prn or 5–15 units 2 h and 30 min prior to procedure

GI Hemorrhage

Adult: **IV** 20 units bolus then 0.2–0.4 units/min up to 0.9 units/min

ADMINISTRATION

Intramuscular/Subcutaneous

- Give 1–2 glasses of water with vasopressin to reduce adverse effects such as skin blanching, abdominal cramps and nausea.
- Give IM injection deeply into a large muscle.
- With subcutaneous injection, exercise caution not to inject intradermally.

Intravenous

PREPARE: **Direct/IV Infusion:** Dilute with NS or D5W to a concentration of 0.1–1 units/mL.

ADMINISTER: **Direct:** Give rapid bolus dose. **IV Infusion:** Titrate dose and rate to patient's response. ▪ Ensure patency prior to injection or infusion as extravasation may cause severe vasoconstriction with tissue necrosis and gangrene.

ADVERSE EFFECTS (≥1%) **Skin:** Rash, urticaria. **Body as a Whole:** Anaphylaxis; *tremor,* sweating, bronchoconstriction, *circumoral and facial pallor,* angioneurotic edema, *pounding in head, water intoxication* (especially with tannate), gangrene at injection site with intraarterial infusion. **GI:** *Eructations, passage of gas, nausea, vomiting,* heartburn, abdominal cramps, increased bowel movements secondary to excessive use. **CV:** Angina (in patient with coronary vascular disease); cardiac arrest, hypertension, bradycardia, minor arrhythmias, premature atrial contraction, heart block, peripheral vascular collapse, coronary insufficiency, MI; cardiac arrhythmia, pulmonary edema, bradycardia (with intra-arterial infusion). **Urogenital:** Uterine cramps. **Respiratory:** Congestion, rhinorrhea, irritation, mucosal ulceration and pruritus, postnasal drip. **Special Senses:** Conjunctivitis.

DIAGNOSTIC TEST INTERFERENCE Vasopressin increases ***plasma cortisol*** levels.

INTERACTIONS Drug: Alcohol, demeclocycline, epinephrine, heparin, lithium, phenytoin may decrease antidiuretic effects of vasopressin; **guanethidine, neostigmine** increase vasopressor actions; **chlorpropamide, clofibrate, carbamazepine,** THIAZIDE DIURETICS may increase antidiuretic activity.

PHARMACOKINETICS Duration: 2–8 h in aqueous solution, 48–72 h in oil, 30–60 min IV infusion. **Distribution:** Extracellular fluid. **Metabolism:** In liver and kidneys. **Elimination:** In urine. **Half-Life:** 10–20 min.

NURSING IMPLICATIONS

Assessment & Drug Effects

- Monitor infants and children closely. They are more susceptible to volume disturbances (such as sudden reversal of polyuria) than adults.
- Establish baseline data of BP, weight, I&O pattern and ratio. Monitor BP and weight throughout therapy. (Dose used to stimulate diuresis has little effect on BP.) Report sudden changes in pattern to physician.
- Be alert to the fact that even small doses of vasopressin may precipitate MI or coronary insufficiency, especially in older adult patients. Keep emergency equipment and drugs (antiarrhythmics) readily available.
- Check patient's alertness and orientation frequently during therapy. Lethargy and confusion associated with headache may signal onset of water intoxication, which, although insidious in rate of development, can lead to convulsions and terminal coma.
- Monitor urine output, specific gravity, and serum osmolality while patient is hospitalized.
- Withhold vasopressin, restrict fluid intake, and notify physician if urine-specific gravity is less than 1.015.

Patient & Family Education

- Be prepared for possibility of anginal attack and have coronary vasodilator available (e.g., nitroglycerin) if there is a history of coronary artery disease. Report to physician.
- With diabetes insipidus, measure and record data related to polydipsia and polyuria. Keep an accurate record of output. Understand that treatment should diminish intense thirst and restore undisturbed normal sleep.
- Avoid concentrated fluids (e.g., undiluted syrups), since these increase urine volume.

VECURONIUM

(vek-yoo-roe'nee-um)

Classifications: ACETYLCHOLINE RECEPTOR ANTAGONIST; NONDEPOLARIZING SKELETAL MUSCLE RELAXANT
Therapeutic: SKELETAL MUSCLE RELAXANT
Prototype: Atracurium
Pregnancy Category: C

V

AVAILABILITY 4 mg, 10 mg, 20 mg vials

ACTION & *THERAPEUTIC EFFECT* Intermediate-acting nondepolarizing skeletal muscle relaxant that inhibits neuromuscular transmission by competitively binding with acetylcholine at receptors located on motor endplate receptors. *Effective as a skeletal muscle relaxant.*

USES Adjunct for general anesthesia to produce skeletal muscle relaxation during surgery. Especially useful for patients with severe kidney disease, limited cardiac reserve, and history of asthma or allergy. Also to facilitate endotracheal intubation.

UNLABELED USES Continuous infusion for facilitation of mechanical ventilation.

CONTRAINDICATIONS Hypersensitivity to bromide; malignant hyperthermia.

CAUTIOUS USE Severe liver disease; impaired acid–base, fluid and electrolyte balance; severe obesity; adrenal or neuromuscular disease (myasthenia gravis, Eaton-Lambert syndrome); patients with slow circulation time (cardiovascular disease, old age, edematous states); obesity, children younger than 1 y and older than 7 wk; pregnancy (category C), lactation.

ROUTE & DOSAGE

Skeletal Muscle Relaxation

Adult/Child (10 y or older): **IV** 0.04–0.1 mg/kg initially, then after 25–40 min, 0.01–0.15 mg/kg q12–15min or 0.001 mg/kg/min by continuous infusion for prolonged procedures

Child (1–10 y)/Infant: **IV** Varies greatly; may require higher initial dose

Obesity Dosage Adjustment

Dose based on IBW

ADMINISTRATION

Note: Vecuronium is administered only by qualified clinicians.

Intravenous

PREPARE: **Direct:** Reconstitute the 10 or 20 mg vial with 10 or 20 mL, respectively, of sterile water for injection (supplied). **Continuous:** Further dilute the reconsituted solution in up to 100 mL D5W, NS, or LR to yield 0.1–0.2 mg/mL.

ADMINISTER: **Direct:** Give a bolus dose over 30 sec. **Continuous:** Give at the required rate.

INCOMPATIBILITIES **Y-site:** **Amphotericin B cholesteryl complex, diazepam, etomidate, furosemide, thiopental.**

- Refrigerate after reconstitution below 30° C (86° F), unless otherwise directed. Discard solution after 24 h.

ADVERSE EFFECTS (≥1%) **Body as a Whole:** Skeletal muscle weakness, malignant hyperthermia. **Respiratory:** Respiratory depression.

INTERACTIONS **Drug:** GENERAL ANESTHETICS increase neuromuscular blockade and duration of action; AMINOGLYCOSIDES, **bacitracin, polymyxin B, clindamycin, lidocaine, parenteral magnesium, quinidine, quinine, trimethaphan, verapamil** increase neuromuscular blockade; DIURETICS may increase or decrease neuromuscular blockade; **lithium** prolongs duration of neuromuscular blockade; NARCOTIC ANALGESICS increase possibility of additive respiratory depression; **succinyl-**

choline increases onset and depth of neuromuscular blockade; **phenytoin** may cause resistance to or reversal of neuromuscular blockade.

PHARMACOKINETICS Onset: Less than 1 min. **Peak:** 3–5 min. **Duration:** 25–40 min. **Distribution:** Well distributed to tissues and extracellular fluids; crosses placenta; distribution into breast milk unknown. **Metabolism:** Rapid nonenzymatic degradation in bloodstream. **Elimination:** 30–35% in urine, 30–35% in bile. **Half-Life:** 30–80 min.

NURSING IMPLICATIONS

Assessment & Drug Effects

- Lab tests: Baseline serum electrolytes, acid–base balance, and kidney and liver functions.
- Use peripheral nerve stimulator during and following drug administration to avoid risk of overdosage and to identify residual paralysis during recovery period. This is especially indicated when cautious use of drug is specified.
- Monitor vital signs at least q15min until stable, then q30min for the next 2 h. Also monitor airway patency until assured that patient has fully recovered from drug effects. Note rate, depth, and pattern of respirations. Obese patients and patients with myasthenia gravis or other neuromuscular disease may have ventilation problems.
- Evaluate patients for recovery from neuromuscular blocking (curare-like) effects as evidenced by ability to breathe naturally or take deep breaths and cough, to keep eyes open, and to lift head keeping mouth closed and by adequacy of hand grip strength. Notify physician if recovery is delayed.
- Note: Recovery time may be delayed in patients with cardiovascular disease, edematous states, and in older adults.

V

VENLAFAXINE Pr

(ven-la-fax′een)

Effexor, Effexor XR

DESVENLAFAXINE

Pristiq

Classifications: ANTIDEPRESSANT; SEROTONIN NOREPINEPHRINE REUPTAKE INHIBITOR (SNRI)

Therapeutic: ANTIDEPRESSANT; SNRI

Pregnancy Category: C

AVAILABILITY 25 mg, 37.5 mg, 50 mg, 75 mg, 100 mg tablets; 37.5 mg, 75 mg, 150 mg sustained release capsules; **Desvenlafaxine:** 50 mg, 100 mg extended release tablet

ACTION & *THERAPEUTIC EFFECT*

Potent inhibitor of neuronal serotonin and norepinephrine reuptake. *Antidepressant effect presumed to be due to potentiation of neurotransmitter activity in the CNS.*

USES Depression, generalized anxiety disorder; social anxiety disorder.

UNLABELED USES Obsessive-compulsive disorder.

CONTRAINDICATIONS Hypersensitivity to venlafaxine, or other SNRI drugs; concurrent administration with MAO inhibitors; abrupt discontinuation; suicide ideation; lactation, neonates.

CAUTIOUS USE Renal and hepatic impairment, renal failure; anorexia nervosa, history of mania, history of suicidal tendencies, especially in individuals younger than 24 y; elevated intraocular pressure, acute closed-angle glaucoma; cardiac disorders, recent MI, heart failure; hypertension; hyperthyroidism; CNS depression; history of seizures or seizure disorders; older adults; pregnancy (category C). Safety in children younger than 18 y is not established.

ROUTE & DOSAGE

Depression

Adult: **PO** 25–125 mg t.i.d. **Desvenlafaxine:** 50 mg daily, may increase dose (max: 400 mg/day)
Geriatric: **PO (venlafaxine and desvenlafaxine)** Start with lower doses in older adults

Anxiety

Adult: **PO** Start with 37.5 mg sustained release daily and increase to 75–225 mg sustained release per day

Renal Impairment Dosage Adjustment

Venlafaxine: CrCl 10–70 mL/min: Reduce total daily dose by 25–50%; less than 10 mL/min: Reduce total daily dose by 50%
Desvenlafaxine: CrCl 3–50 mL/min: Max dose is 50 mg/day; less than 30 mL/min: 50 mg every other day

Pharmacogenetic Dosage Adjustment

Poor CYP2D6 metabolizer: Start with 70% of dose

ADMINISTRATION

Oral

- Give with food. Sustained release capsules **must be** swallowed whole, must not be opened or chewed.
- Dosage increments of up to 75 mg/day are usually made at 4 days or longer intervals.
- Allow 14 days interval after discontinuing an MAO inhibitor before starting venlafaxine or desvenlafaxine.
- Do not abruptly withdraw drug after 1 wk or more of therapy.
- Store at room temperature, 15°–30° C (59°–86° F).

ADVERSE EFFECTS (≥1%) **CV:** *Increased blood pressure and heart rate,* palpitations. **CNS:** *Dizziness,* fatigue, headache, anxiety, insomnia, *somnolence,* <u>suicidality</u>. **Endocrine:** Small but statistically significant increase in serum cholesterol, weight loss (approximately 3 lb). **GI:** *Nausea, vomiting, dry mouth,* constipation. **Urogenital:** Sexual dysfunction, erectile failure, delayed orgasm, anorgasmia, impotence, abnormal ejaculation. **Special Senses:** Blurred vision. **Body as a Whole:** *Sweating,* asthenia.

INTERACTIONS Drug: Cimetidine, MAO INHIBITORS, **desipramine, haloperidol** may increase levels and toxicity. Should not use in combination with MAO INHIBITORS: Do not start until greater than 14 days after stopping MAO INHIBITOR; do not start MAO INHIBITOR until 7 days after stopping venlafaxine/desvenlafaxine. **Trazodone** may lead to **serotonin** syndrome. **Herbal: St. John's wort, sour date nut** may cause **serotonin** syndrome.

PHARMACOKINETICS Absorption: Well absorbed from GI tract. **Onset:** 2 wk. **Peak:** Venlafaxine 1–2 h; metabolite 3–4 h. **Duration:** Approximately 30% protein bound, but extensively tissue bound. **Metabolism:** Undergoes substantial first-pass metabolism to its major active metabolite, *O*-desmethylvenlafaxine, with similar activity to venlafaxine. **Elimination:** ~60% in urine as parent compound and metabolites. **Half-Life:** Venlafaxine 3–4 h, *O*-desmethylvenlafaxine 10 h, desvenlafaxine ~11 h.

V

NURSING IMPLICATIONS

Assessment & Drug Effects

- Monitor for worsening of depression or emergence of suicidal ideation.
- Monitor cardiovascular status periodically with measurements of HR and BP.
- Lab tests: Periodic lipid profile.
- Monitor neurologic status and report excessive anxiety, nervousness, and insomnia.
- Monitor weight periodically and report excess weight loss.
- Assess safety, as dizziness and sedation are common.

Patient & Family Education

- Be aware of potential adverse effects and notify physician of those that are bothersome.
- Report promptly worsening mental status, especially thoughts of suicide.
- Do not drive or engage in potentially hazardous activities until response to drug is known.
- Avoid using alcohol while on venlafaxine.
- Do not use herbal medications without consulting physician.

VERAPAMIL HYDROCHLORIDE (Pr)

(ver-ap′a-mill)

Calan, Calan SR, Covera-HS, Isoptin, Isoptin SR, Verelan, Verelan PM

Classifications: CALCIUM CHANNEL BLOCKER; ANTIHYPERTENSIVE; ANTIARRHYTHMIC CLASS IV

Therapeutic: ANTIARRHYTHMIC; ANTIHYPERTENSIVE; ANTIANGINAL

Pregnancy Category: C

AVAILABILITY 40 mg, 80 mg, 120 mg tablets; 120 mg, 180 mg, 240 mg sustained release tablets; 100 mg, 120 mg, 180 mg, 200 mg, 240 mg, 300 mg sustained release capsules; 5 mg/2 mL injection

ACTION & *THERAPEUTIC EFFECT* Inhibits calcium ion influx through slow channels into cells of myocardial and arterial smooth muscle. Dilates coronary arteries and arterioles and inhibits coronary artery spasm. Decreases and slows SA and AV node conduction without affecting normal arterial action potential or intraventricular conduction. Dilates peripheral arterioles, causing decreased total peripheral resistance, and this results in lowering the BP. *Decreases angina attacks by dilating coronary arteries and inhibiting coronary vasospasms. Decreases nodal conduction, resulting in an antiarrhythmic effect. Decreased total peripheral vascular resistance; and therefore, reduction in BP.*

USES Supraventricular tachyarrhythmias; Prinzmetal's (variant) angina, chronic stable angina; unstable, crescendo or preinfarctive angina and essential hypertension.

UNLABELED USES Paroxysmal supraventricular tachycardia, atrial fibrillation; prophylaxis of migraine headache; and as alternate therapy in manic depression.

CONTRAINDICATIONS Severe hypotension (systolic less than 90 mm Hg), cardiogenic shock, cardiomegaly, digitalis toxicity, second- or third-degree AV block; Wolff-Parkinson-White syndrome including atrial flutter and fibrillation; accessory AV pathway, left ventricular dysfunction, severe CHF, sinus node disease, sick sinus syndrome (except in patients with functioning ventricular pacemaker); lactation; **extended release tablets:** children younger than 18 y.

CAUTIOUS USE Duchenne's muscular dystrophy; hepatic and renal impairment; MI followed by coronary occlusion, aortic stenosis; GI obstruction, GERD, hiatal hernia, ileus; pregnancy (category C).

ROUTE & DOSAGE

Angina

Adult: **PO** 80 mg q6–8h, may increase up to 320–480 mg/day in divided doses (Note: Covera-HS **must be** given once daily at bedtime)

Hypertension

Adult: **PO** 80 mg t.i.d. or 90–240 mg sustained release 1–2 times/day up to 480 mg/day (Note: Covera-HS **must be** given once daily at bedtime)

Supraventricular Tachycardia, Atrial Fibrillation

Adult/Adolescent (older than 15 y): **IV** 5–10 mg after 30 min may give 10 mg (max total dose: 20 mg)
Child/Adolescent (up to 15 y): **IV** 0.1–0.3 mg/kg (do not exceed 5 mg)
Infant: **IV** 0.1–0.2 mg/kg may repeat after 30 min

Renal Impairment Dosage Adjustment

CrCl less than 10 mL/min: Give 50–75% of dose
Hemodialysis Dosage Adjustment: Supplemental dose not necessary

Hepatic Impairment Dosage Adjustment

In cirrhosis, use 20–50% of normal dose

ADMINISTRATION

Oral

- Give with food to reduce gastric irritation.
- Capsules can be opened and contents sprinkled on food. Do NOT dissolve or chew capsule contents.
- Do not withdraw abruptly; may increase and extend duration of pain in the angina patient.

Intravenous

PREPARE: **IV Direct:** Given undiluted or diluted in 5 mL of sterile water for injection. ▪ Inspect parenteral drug preparation before administration. Make sure solution is clear and colorless.

ADMINISTER: **Direct:** Give a single dose over 2–3 min.

INCOMPATIBILITIES **Solution/additive:** **Albumin, aminophylline, amphotericin B, hydralazine, trimethoprim/sulfamethoxazole.** **Y-site:** **Albumin, amphotericin B cholesteryl complex, ampicillin, lansoprazole, mezlocillin, nafcillin, oxacillin, propofol, sodium bicarbonate.**

- Store at 15°–30° C (59°–86° F) and protect from light.

ADVERSE EFFECTS (≥1%) **CNS:** Dizziness, vertigo, *headache,* fatigue, sleep disturbances, depression, syncope. **CV:** *Hypotension,* congestive heart failure, bradycardia, severe tachycardia, peripheral edema, <u>AV block</u>. **GI:** Nausea, abdominal discomfort, *constipation,* elevated liver enzymes. **Body as a Whole:** Flushing, pulmonary edema, muscle fatigue, diaphoresis. **Skin:** Pruritus.

DIAGNOSTIC TEST INTERFERENCE Verapamil may cause elevations of serum ***AST, ALT, alkaline phosphatase.***

INTERACTIONS Drug: BETA-BLOCKERS increase risk of CHF, bradycardia, or heart block; significantly increased levels of **digoxin** and **carbamazepine** and toxicity; potentiates hypotensive effects of HYPOTENSIVE AGENTS; levels of **lithium** and **cyclosporine** may be increased, increasing their toxicity; **calcium salts** (IV) may antagonize verapamil effects. **Food: Grapefruit juice** may increase verapamil levels. **Herbal: Hawthorne** may have additive hypotensive effects. **St. John's wort** may decrease efficacy.

PHARMACOKINETICS Absorption: 90% absorbed, but only 25–30% reaches systemic circulation (first pass metabolism). **Peak:** 1–2 h PO; 4–8 h sustained release; 5 min IV. **Distribution:** Widely distributed, including CNS; crosses placenta; present in breast milk. **Metabolism:** In liver (CYP3A4). **Elimination:** 70% in urine; 16% in feces. **Half-Life:** 2–8 h.

NURSING IMPLICATIONS

Assessment & Drug Effects

- Establish baseline data and periodically monitor BP and pulse with oral administration.
- Lab tests: Baseline and periodic LFTs and kidney functions.
- Following IV infusion, instruct patient to remain in recumbent position for at least 1 h after dose is given to diminish subjective effects of transient asymptomatic hypotension that may accompany infusion.
- Monitor for AV block or excessive bradycardia when IV infusion is given concurrently with digitalis.
- Monitor I&O ratio during IV and early oral maintenance therapy. Renal impairment prolongs duration of action, increasing potential for toxicity and incidence of adverse effects. Advise patient to report gradual weight gain and evidence of edema.
- Monitor ECG continuously during IV administration. Essential because drug action may be prolonged and incidence of adverse reactions is highest during IV administration in older adults, patients with impaired kidney function, and patients of small stature.
- Check BP shortly before administration of next dose to evaluate degree of control during early treatment for hypertension.

Patient & Family Education

- Monitor radial pulse before each dose, notify physician of an irregular pulse or one slower than established guideline.
- Do not drive or engage in potentially hazardous activities until response to drug is known.
- Decrease intake of caffeine-containing beverage (i.e., coffee, tea, chocolate).
- Change positions slowly from lying down to standing to prevent falls because of drug-related vertigo until tolerance to reduced BP is established.
- Notify physician of easy bruising, petechiae, unexplained bleeding.
- Do not use OTC drugs, especially aspirin, unless they are specifically prescribed by physician.

VINBLASTINE SULFATE

(vin-blast'een)

Classifications: ANTINEOPLASTIC; MITOTIC INHIBITOR

Therapeutic: ANTINEOPLASTIC

Prototype: Vincristine

Pregnancy Category: D

AVAILABILITY 10 mg powder for injection; 1 mg/mL vial

ACTION & *THERAPEUTIC EFFECT* Cell cycle–specific drug that interferes with microtubules that form the mitotic spindle fibers required to complete the process of mitosis. Has an effect on cell energy production needed for mitosis and interferes with nucleic acid synthesis. *Interrupts the cell cycle in metaphase, thus preventing cell replication.*

USES Palliative treatment of Hodgkin's disease and non-Hodgkin's lymphomas, choriocarcinoma, lymphosarcoma, neuroblastoma, mycosis fungoides, advanced testicular germinal cell cancer, histiocytosis, and other malignancies resistant to other chemotherapy. Used singly or in combination with other chemotherapeutic drugs.

CONTRAINDICATIONS Severe bone marrow suppression, leukopenia, bacterial infection, adynamic ileus; older adult patients with cachexia or skin ulcers; men and women of childbearing potential; pregnancy (category D), lactation.

CAUTIOUS USE Malignant cell infiltration of bone marrow; obstructive jaundice, hepatic impairment; history of gout; use of small amount of drug for long periods; use in eyes.

ROUTE & DOSAGE

Antineoplastic

Adult: **IV** 7–10 mg/m^2 once weekly, dose varies based on protocol and may increase incrementally up to 18.5 mg/m^2 if tolerated

Child: **IV** 2.5 mg/m^2 may increase up to 12.5 mg/m^2 if tolerated

Hepatic Impairment Dosage Adjustment

Bilirubin 1.5–3 mg/dL: Reduce dose 50%; bilirubin over 3 mg/dL: Reduce dose 75%

ADMINISTRATION

Intravenous

PREPARE: **Direct:** Add 10 mL NS to 10 mg of drug to yield 1 mg/mL. Do not use other diluents. ▪ Avoid contact with eyes. Severe irritation and persisting corneal changes may occur. Flush immediately and thoroughly with copious amounts of water. Wash both eyes; do not assume one eye escaped contamination.

ADMINISTER: **Direct:** Drug is usually injected into tubing of running IV infusion of NS or D5W over period of 1 min. ▪ Stop injection promptly if extravasation occurs. Use applications of moderate heat and local injection of hyaluronidase to help disperse extravasated drug. ▪ Observe injection site for sloughing. ▪ Restart infusion in another vein.

INCOMPATIBILITIES **Solution/additive:** **Furosemide, heparin.** **Y-site:** **Cefepime, furosemide, lansoprazole.**

▪ Refrigerate reconstituted solution in tight, light-resistant containers up to 30 days without loss of potency.

ADVERSE EFFECTS (≥1%) **Body as a Whole:** Fever, weight loss, muscular pains, weakness, parotid gland pain and tenderness, tumor site pain, Raynaud's phenomenon. **CNS:** Mental depression, peripheral neuritis, numbness and paresthesias of tongue and extremities, loss of deep tendon reflexes, headache, convulsions. **GI:** Vesiculation of mouth, stomatitis, pharyngitis, anorexia, *nausea, vomiting,* diarrhea, ileus, abdominal pain, constipation, rectal bleeding, <u>hemorrhagic enterocolitis</u>, bleeding of old peptic ulcer. **Hematologic:** <u>Leukopenia</u>, thrombocytopenia, and anemia. **Skin:** *Alo-*

V

pecia (reversible), vesiculation, photosensitivity, phlebitis, cellulitis, and sloughing following extravasation (at injection site). **Urogenital:** Urinary retention, *hyperuricemia,* aspermia. **Respiratory:** Bronchospasm.

INTERACTIONS Drug: Mitomycin may cause acute shortness of breath and severe bronchospasm; may decrease **phenytoin** levels; ALFA INTERFERONS, **erythromycin, itraconazole** may increase vinblastine toxicity.

PHARMACOKINETICS Distribution: Concentrates in liver, platelets, and leukocytes; poor penetration of blood–brain barrier. **Metabolism:** Partially in liver. **Elimination:** In feces and urine. **Half-Life:** 24 h.

NURSING IMPLICATIONS

Assessment & Drug Effects

- Lab tests: Monitor WBC count. Recovery from leukopenic nadir occurs usually within 7–14 days. With high doses, total leukocyte count may not return to normal for 3 wk.
- Do not administer drug unless WBC count has returned to at least 4000/mm^3, even if 7 days have passed.
- Monitor for unexplained bruising or bleeding, which should be promptly reported, even though thrombocyte reduction seldom occurs unless patient has had prior treatment with other antineoplastics.
- Adverse reactions seldom persist beyond 24 h with exception of epilation, leukopenia, and neurological adverse effects.
- Monitor bowel elimination pattern and bowel sounds to recognize severe constipation or paralytic ileus. A stool softener may be necessary.
- Inspect skin surfaces over pressure areas daily if patient is not ambulating. Note condition of skin of older adults especially.
- Report promptly if oral mucosa tissue breakdown is noted.

Patient & Family Education

- Be aware that temporary mental depression sometimes occurs on second or third day after treatment begins.
- Avoid exposure to infection, injury to skin or mucous membranes, and excessive physical stress, especially during leukocyte nadir period.
- Notify physician promptly about onset of symptoms of agranulocytosis (see Appendix F). Do not delay seeking appropriate treatment.
- Avoid exposure to sunlight unless protected with sunscreen lotion (SPF greater than 12) and clothing.

V

VINCRISTINE SULFATE (Pr)

(vin-kris′teen)

Classifications: ANTINEOPLASTIC; MITOTIC INHIBITOR

Therapeutic: ANTINEOPLASTIC

Pregnancy Category: D

AVAILABILITY 1 mg/mL injection

ACTION & *THERAPEUTIC EFFECT* Cell cycle–specific vinca alkaloid arrests mitosis at metaphase by inhibition of mitotic spindle function, thereby inhibiting cell division. *Induction of metaphase arrest in 50% of cells results in inhibition of cancer cell proliferation.*

USES Acute lymphoblastic and other leukemias, Hodgkin's disease, lymphosarcoma, neuroblastoma, Wilms' tumor, lung and breast cancer, reticular cell carcinoma, and osteogenic and other sarcomas.

UNLABELED USES Idiopathic thrombocytopenic purpura, alone or adjunctively with other antineoplastics.

CONTRAINDICATIONS Obstructive jaundice; active infection; adynamic ileus; radiation of the liver; patient with demyelinating form of Charcot-Marie-Tooth syndrome; men and women of childbearing potential; pregnancy (category D), lactation.

CAUTIOUS USE Leukopenia; preexisting neuromuscular or neurologic disease; hypertension; hepatic or biliary tract disease; elderly.

ROUTE & DOSAGE

Antineoplastic

Adult: **IV** 1.4 mg/m² (max: 2 mg/m²) at weekly intervals
Child: **IV** *Weight greater than 10 kg,* 1–2 mg/m² at weekly intervals; *weight less than 10 kg,* 0.05 mg/kg initial weekly dose, then titrate

Hepatic Impairment Dosage Adjustment

Bilirubin 1.5–3 mg/dL: Use 50% of dose; 3–5 mg/dL: Use 25% of dose; greater than 5 mg/dL: Skip dose

ADMINISTRATION

Intravenous

PREPARE: **Direct:** No dilution is required. Administer as supplied. ▪ Avoid contact with eyes. Severe irritation and persisting corneal changes may occur. Flush immediately and thoroughly with copious amounts of water. Wash both eyes; do not assume one eye escaped contamination.

ADMINISTER: **Direct:** Drug is usually injected into tubing of running infusion over a 1 min period. ▪ Stop injection promptly if extravasation occurs. Use applications of moderate heat and local injection of hyaluronidase to help disperse extravasated drug. ▪ Restart infusion in another vein. Observe injection site for sloughing.

INCOMPATIBILITIES **Solution/additive:** **Furosemide.** **Y-site:** **Cefepime, furosemide, idarubicin, lansoprazole, sodium bicarbonate.**

▪ Store solution in the refrigerator.

ADVERSE EFFECTS (≥1%) **CNS:** *Peripheral neuropathy,* neuritic pain, *paresthesias, especially of hands and feet;* foot and hand drop, sensory loss, athetosis, ataxia, loss of deep tendon reflexes, muscle atrophy, dysphagia, weakness in larynx and extrinsic eye muscles, ptosis, diplopia, mental depression. **Special Senses:** Optic atrophy with blindness; transient cortical blindness, ptosis, diplopia, photophobia. **GI:** Stomatitis, pharyngitis, anorexia, nausea, vomiting, diarrhea, abdominal cramps, *severe constipation (upper-colon impaction), paralytic ileus (especially in children),* rectal bleeding; <u>hepatotoxicity</u>. **Urogenital:** Urinary retention, polyuria, dysuria, SIADH (high urinary sodium excretion, hyponatremia, dehydration, hypotension); uric acid nephropathy. **Skin:** Urticaria, rash, *alopecia,* cellulitis and phlebitis following extravasation (at injection site). **Body as a Whole:** Convulsions with hypertension, malaise, fever, headache, pain in parotid gland area, weight loss. **Metabolic:** Hyperuricemia, hyperkalemia. **CV:** Hypertension, hypotension. **Respiratory:** Bronchospasm.

INTERACTIONS Drug: Mitomycin may cause acute shortness of breath and severe bronchospasm; may decrease **digoxin, phenytoin** levels.

PHARMACOKINETICS Distribution: Concentrates in liver, platelets, and leukocytes; poor penetration of blood–brain barrier. **Metabolism:** Partially in liver (CYP3A4). **Elimination:** Primarily in feces. **Half-Life:** 10–155 h.

NURSING IMPLICATIONS

Assessment & Drug Effects

- Monitor I&O ratio and pattern, BP, and temperature daily.
- Monitor for and report steady weight gain.
- Lab tests: Monitor serum electrolytes and CBC with differential. Complete bone marrow remission in leukemia varies widely and may not occur for as long as 100 days after therapy is started.
- Be aware that neuromuscular adverse effects, most apt to appear in the patient with preexisting neuromuscular disease, usually disappear after 6 wk of treatment. Children are especially susceptible to neuromuscular adverse effects.
- Assess for hand muscular weakness, and check deep tendon reflexes (depression of Achilles reflex is the earliest sign of neuropathy). Also observe for and report promptly: Mental depression, ptosis, double vision, hoarseness, paresthesias, neuritic pain, and motor difficulties.
- Provide special protection against infection or injury during leukopenic days. Leukopenia occurs in a significant number of patients; leukocyte count in children usually reaches nadir on fourth day and begins to rise on fifth day after drug administration.
- Avoid use of rectal thermometer or intrusive tubing to prevent injury to rectal mucosa.
- Monitor ability to ambulate and supply support as needed.
- Start a prophylactic regimen against constipation and paralytic ileus at beginning of treatment (paralytic ileus is most likely to occur in young children).

Patient & Family Education

- Notify physician promptly of stomach, bone, or joint pain, and swelling of lower legs and ankles.
- Report changes in bowel habit as soon as manifested.
- Report a steady gain or sudden weight change to physician.

VINORELBINE TARTRATE

(vin-o-rel′been)

Navelbine

Classifications: ANTINEOPLASTIC; MITOTIC INHIBITOR

Therapeutic: ANTINEOPLASTIC

Prototype: Vincristine

Pregnancy Category: D

AVAILABILITY 10 mg/mL injection

ACTION & *THERAPEUTIC EFFECT* A semisynthetic vinca alkaloid with antineoplastic activity. Inhibits polymerization of tubules into microtubules, which disrupts mitotic spindle formation. *Arrests mitosis at metaphase, thereby inhibiting cell division in cancer cells.*

USES Non–small-cell lung cancer.

UNLABELED USES Breast cancer, ovarian cancer, Hodgkin's disease.

CONTRAINDICATIONS Hypersensitivity to vinorelbine, infection; severe bone marrow suppression; granylocyte counts greater than or equal to 1000 cells/mm^3; pulmo-

V

nary toxicity to drug; constipation, ileus; pregnancy (category D), lactation.

CAUTIOUS USE Hypersensitivity to vincristine or vinblastine; leukopenia or other indicator(s) of bone marrow suppression; chickenpox or herpes zoster infection; hepatic insufficiency, severe liver disease; pulmonary disease; preexisting neurologic or neuromuscular disorders; older adults. Safety and efficacy in children are not established.

ROUTE & DOSAGE

Non–Small-Cell Lung Cancer

Adult: **IV** 25–30 mg/m² weekly; may require toxicity adjustment

Hepatic Impairment Dosage Adjustment

Bilirubin 2.1–3 mg/dL: Use 50% of dose; greater than 3 mg/dL: Use 25% of dose

ADMINISTRATION

Intravenous

Use caution to prevent contact with skin, mucous membranes, or eyes during preparation.

PREPARE: **Direct:** Dilute each 10 mg in a syringe with either 2 or 5 mL of D5W or NS to yield 3 mg/mL or 1.5 mg/L, respectively. **IV Infusion:** Dilute the required dose in an IV bag with D5W, NS, or LR to a final concentration of 0.5–2 mg/mL (example: 10 mg diluted in 19 mL yields 0.5 mg/mL).

ADMINISTER: **IV Infusion:** Give diluted solution over 6–10 min into the side port closest to an IV bag with free-flowing IV solution; follow by flushing with at least 75–125 mL of IV solution over 10 min. ▪ Take every precaution to avoid extravasation. If suspected, discontinue IV immediately and begin in a different site.

INCOMPATIBILITIES **Solution/additive:** **Acyclovir, aminophylline, amphotericin B, ampicillin, cefazolin, cefoperazone, ceforanide, cefotaxime, cefotetan, ceftazidime, ceftriaxone, cefuroxime, fluorouracil, furosemide, ganciclovir, methylprednisolone, mitomycin, piperacillin, sodium bicarbonate, thiotepa, trimethoprim–sulfamethoxazole.** **Y-site:** **Acyclovir, allopurinol, aminophylline, amphotericin B, amphotericin B cholesteryl complex, ampicillin, cefazolin, cefoperazone, cefotetan, ceftriaxone, cefuroxime, fluorouracil, furosemide, ganciclovir, heparin, lansoprazole, methylprednisolone, mitomycin, piperacillin, sodium bicarbonate, thiotepa, trimethoprim-sulfamethoxazole.**

- Store at 2°–8° C (36°–46° F).

ADVERSE EFFECTS (≥1%) **CNS:** *Decreased deep tendon reflexes, paresthesia, fatigue, asthenia, peripheral neuropathy,* myalgia, jaw pain. **Hematologic:** *Anemia,* *<u>neutropenia, granulocytopenia</u>*, thrombocytopenia. **GI:** Paralytic ileus, *constipation, nausea, vomiting, diarrhea,* stomatitis, mucositis, hepatotoxicity *(elevated LFT).* **Body as a Whole:** *Pain on injection,* venous pain, thrombophlebitis, *alopecia,* myalgia, muscle weakness.

INTERACTIONS Drug: Increased severity of granulocytopenia in combination with **cisplatin;** increased risk of acute pulmonary reactions in combination with **mitomycin; paclitaxel** may increase neuropathy.

PHARMACOKINETICS Distribution: 60–80% bound to plasma proteins

V

(including platelets and lymphocytes); sequestered in tissues, especially lung, spleen, liver, and kidney, and released slowly. **Metabolism:** In liver (CYP3A4). **Elimination:** Primarily in bile and feces (50%), 10% in urine. **Half-Life:** 42–45 h.

NURSING IMPLICATIONS

Assessment & Drug Effects

- Withhold drug and notify physician if the granulocyte count is less than 1000 cells/mm^3.
- Monitor for neurologic dysfunction including paresthesia, decreased deep tendon reflexes, weakness, constipation, and paralytic ileus.
- Lab tests: Monitor CBC with differential throughout therapy and on the day of treatment prior to each infusion. Monitor kidney and liver functions, and serum electrolytes periodically.
- Monitor for S&S of infection, especially during period of granulocyte nadir 7–10 days after dosing.

Patient & Family Education

- Be aware of potential and inevitable adverse effects.
- Women should use reliable forms of contraception to prevent pregnancy.
- Notify physician of distressing adverse effects, especially symptoms of leukopenia (e.g., chills, fever, cough) and peripheral neuropathy (e.g., pain, numbness, tingling in extremities).
- Report changes in bowel habits as soon as manifested.

V

VITAMIN A

(vye′ta-min A)

Aquasol A, Del-Vi-A

Classification: VITAMIN SUPPLEMENT
Therapeutic: VITAMIN A REPLACEMENT

Pregnancy Category: A (X if greater than RDA)

AVAILABILITY 5000 international unit tablets; 10,000 international unit, 15,000 international unit, 25,000 international unit capsules; 50,000 international units/mL injection

ACTION & *THERAPEUTIC EFFECT* Vitamin A, a fat-soluble vitamin, acts as a cofactor in mucopolysaccharide synthesis, cholesterol synthesis, and the metabolism of hydroxysteroids. *Essential for normal growth and development of bones and teeth, for integrity of epithelial and mucosal surfaces, and for synthesis of visual purple necessary for visual adaptation to the dark. Has antioxidant properties.*

USES Vitamin A deficiency and as dietary supplement during periods of increased requirements, such as pregnancy, lactation, infancy, and infections. Used as replacement therapy in conditions that affect absorption, mobilization, or storage of vitamin A (e.g., steatorrhea, severe biliary obstruction, liver cirrhosis, total gastrectomy). Used in skin disorders [e.g., folliculosis keratosis (Darier's disease), psoriasis]; however, other retinoids are being preferentially selected. Also used as a screening test for fat malabsorption.

CONTRAINDICATIONS History of sensitivity to vitamin A, hypervitaminosis A, oral administration to patients with malabsorption syndrome. Safe use in amounts exceeding 6000 international units during pregnancy (category X if greater than RDA) is not established.

CAUTIOUS USE Women on oral contraceptives, children, hepatic disease, hepatic dysfunction, hepatitis; low-birth-weight infants; renal disease;

pregnancy (category A within RDA limit), lactation.

ROUTE & DOSAGE

Severe Deficiency

Adult/Child (older than 8 y): **PO** 500,000 international units/day for 3 days followed by 50,000 international units/day for 2 wk, then 10,000–20,000 international units/day for 2 mo **IM** 100,000 international units/day for 3 days followed by 50,000 international units/day for 2 wk

Child: **PO/IM** *Younger than 1 y,* 10,000 international units/kg/day for 3 days followed by 7500–15,000 international units/day for 10 days; *1–8 y,* 10,000 international units/kg/day for 3 days followed by 17,000–35,000 international units/day for 2 wk

Dietary Supplement

Child: **PO** *Younger than 4 y,* 10,000 international units/day; *4–8 y,* 15,000 international units/day

ADMINISTRATION

Oral

- Give on an empty stomach or following food or milk if GI upset occurs.
- Store in tight, light-resistant containers.

Intramuscular

- Use IM route only if oral route not feasible.
- Inject deeply into a large muscle.

ADVERSE EFFECTS (≥1%) **CNS:** Irritability, headache, intracranial hypertension (pseudotumor cerebri), increased intracranial pressure, bulging fontanelles, papilledema, exophthalmos, miosis, nystagmus. **Metabolic:** Hypervitaminosis A syndrome (malaise, lethargy, abdominal discomfort, anorexia, vomiting), hypercalcemia. **Musculoskeletal:** Slow growth; deep, tender, hard lumps (subperiosteal thickening) over radius, tibia, occiput; migratory arthralgia; retarded growth; premature closure of epiphyses. **Skin:** Gingivitis, lip fissures, excessive sweating, drying or cracking of skin, pruritus, increase in skin pigmentation, massive desquamation, brittle nails, alopecia. **Urogenital:** Hypomenorrhea. **GI:** Hepatosplenomegaly, jaundice. **Endocrine:** Polydipsia, polyurea. **Hematologic:** Leukopenia, hypoplastic anemias, vitamin A plasma levels greater than 1200 international units/dL, elevations of sedimentation rate and prothrombin time. **Body as a Whole:** Anaphylaxis, death (after IV use).

DIAGNOSTIC TEST INTERFERENCE Vitamin A may falsely increase ***serum cholesterol*** determinations ***(Zlatkis-Zak reaction);*** may falsely elevate ***bilirubin*** determination (with ***Ehrlich's reagent***).

INTERACTIONS Drug: Mineral oil, cholestyramine may decrease absorption of vitamin A.

PHARMACOKINETICS Absorption: Readily absorbed from GI tract in presence of bile salts, pancreatic lipase, and dietary fat. **Distribution:** Stored mainly in liver; small amounts also found in kidney and body fat; distributed into breast milk. **Metabolism:** In liver. **Elimination:** In feces and urine.

NURSING IMPLICATIONS

Assessment & Drug Effects

- Take dietary and drug history (e.g., intake of fortified foods, dietary supplements, self-administration or

V

prescription drug sources). Women taking oral contraceptives tend to have significantly higher plasma vitamin A levels.

- Monitor therapeutic effectiveness. Vitamin A deficiency is often associated with protein malnutrition as well as other vitamin deficiencies. It may manifest as night blindness, restriction of growth and development, epithelial alterations, susceptibility to infection, abnormal dryness of skin, mouth, and eyes (xerophthalmia) progressing to keratomalacia (ulceration and necrosis of cornea and conjunctiva), and urinary tract calculi.

Patient & Family Education

- Avoid use of mineral oil while on vitamin A therapy.
- Notify physician of symptoms of overdosage (e.g., nausea, vomiting, anorexia, drying and cracking of skin or lips, headache, loss of hair).

VITAMIN B_1

See Thiamine HCl.

VITAMIN B_2

See Riboflavin.

VITAMIN B_3

See Niacin.

VITAMIN B_6

See Pyridoxine.

VITAMIN B_9

See Folic acid.

VITAMIN B_{12}

See Cyanocobalamin.

VITAMIN B_{12A}

See Hydroxocobalamin.

VITAMIN C

See Ascorbic acid.

VITAMIN D

See Calcitriol, Ergocalciferol.

VITAMIN E (TOCOPHEROL)

(vit′a-min E)

Aquasol E, Vita-Plus E, Vitec

Classification: VITAMIN SUPPLEMENT

Therapeutic: VITAMIN E SUPPLEMENT

Pregnancy Category: A within RDA

AVAILABILITY 100 international unit, 200 international unit, 400 international unit, 500 international unit, 800 international unit tablets; 100 international unit, 200 international unit, 400 international unit, 1000 international unit capsules; 15 international units/0.3 mL, 15 international units/30 mL liquid

ACTION & *THERAPEUTIC EFFECT* A group of naturally occurring fat-soluble substances known as tocopherols. Alpha tocopherol, comprising 90% of the tocopherols, is the most biologically potent. An antioxidant, it prevents peroxidation, a process that gives rise to free radicals (highly reactive chemical structures that damage cell membranes and alter nuclear proteins). *Prevents cell membrane and protein damage, protects against blood clot formation by decreasing platelet aggregation, enhances vitamin A utilization, and promotes normal growth, development, and tone of muscles.*

USES To treat and prevent hemolytic anemia due to vitamin E deficiency in premature neonates; to prevent retrolental fibroplasia secondary to oxygen treatment in neonates, and in treatment of diseases with secondary erythrocyte membrane abnormalities (e.g., sickle cell anemia, and G6PD deficiency and as supplement in malabsorption syndromes). Used in patients on diets containing large amounts of polyunsaturated fats for long periods and in the patient who abruptly discontinues such a diet. Also used topically for dry or chapped skin and minor skin disorders.

UNLABELED USES Muscular dystrophy and a number of other conditions with no conclusive evidence of value. A component of many multivitamin formulations and of topical deodorant preparations as an antioxidant.

CONTRAINDICATIONS Bleeding disorders; thrombocytopenia.

CAUTIOUS USE Large doses may exacerbate iron deficiency anemia; pregnancy (category A within RDA).

ROUTE & DOSAGE

Vitamin E Deficiency

Adult: **PO** 60–75 international units/day

Child: **PO** 1 international units/kg/day

Prophylaxis for Vitamin E Deficiency

Adult: **PO** 12–15 international units/day

Child: **PO** 7–10 international units/day

Neonate: **PO** 5 international units/day

ADMINISTRATION

Oral

- Give on an empty stomach or following food or milk if GI upset occurs.
- Ensure that capsules are swallowed whole. They should not be crushed or chewed.
- Store in tight containers protected from light.

ADVERSE EFFECTS (≥1%) **Body as a Whole:** Skeletal muscle weakness, headache, fatigue (with excessive doses). **GI:** Nausea, diarrhea, intestinal cramps. **Urogenital:** Gonadal dysfunction. **Metabolic:** Increased serum creatine kinase, cholesterol, triglycerides; decreased serum thyroxine and triiodothyronine; increased urinary estrogens, androgens; creatinuria. **Skin:** Sterile abscess, thrombophlebitis, contact dermatitis. **Special Senses:** Blurred vision.

INTERACTIONS Herbal: Mineral oil, cholestyramine may decrease absorption of vitamin E; may enhance anticoagulant activity of **warfarin.**

PHARMACOKINETICS Absorption: 20–60% absorbed from GI tract if fat absorption is normal; enters blood via lymph. **Distribution:** Stored mainly in adipose tissue; crosses placenta. **Metabolism:** In liver. **Elimination:** Primarily in bile.

NURSING IMPLICATIONS

Patient & Family Education

- Natural sources of vitamin E are found in wheat germ (the richest source) as well as in vegetable oils (sunflower, corn, soybean, cottonseed), green leafy vegetables, nuts, dairy products, eggs, cereals, meat, and liver.

VORICONAZOLE

(vor-i-con′a-zole)

Vfend

Classifications: ANTIBIOTIC; AZOLE ANTIFUNGAL

Therapeutic: ANTIFUNGAL
Prototype: Fluconazole
Pregnancy Category: D

AVAILABILITY 50 mg, 200 mg tablets; 200 mg injection

ACTION & *THERAPEUTIC EFFECT* Inhibits fungal cytochrome P450 enzymes used for an essential step in fungal ergosterol biosynthesis. The subsequent loss of ergosterol in the fungal cell wall is thought to be responsible for the antifungal activity. *Voriconazole is active against* Aspergillus *and* Candida.

USES Treatment of invasive aspergillosis, esophageal candidiasis, candidemia in nonneutropenic patients and disseminated skin infections, and abdomen, kidney, bladder wall, and wound infections due to *Candida.*

CONTRAINDICATIONS Known hypersensitivity to voriconazole; **IV form:** Should be avoided in moderate or severe renal impairment (CrCl less than 50 mL/min) and severe Child-Pugh class C hepatic impairment. History of galactose intolerance; Lapp lactase deficiency or glucose-galactose malabsorption; sunlight (UV) exposure; pregnancy (category D); lactation.

CAUTIOUS USE Mild to moderate hepatic cirrhosis, hepatitis, Child-Pugh class A and B hepatic disease; renal disease. **PO & IV form:** Mild or moderate renal impairment; ocular disease; hypersensitivity to other azole antifungal agents such as fluconazole. Safety and efficacy have not been established in children younger than 12 y.

V

ROUTE & DOSAGE

Aspergillosis

Adult: **IV** 6 mg/kg q12h day 1, then 3–4 mg/kg q12h. Treatment continues until 7–14 days after symptom resolution. **PO** *Weight greater than 40 kg,* 400 mg q12h day 1, then 200 mg q12h. May increase to 300 mg q12h if inadequate response. *Weight less than 40 kg,* 400 mg q12h day 1, then 100 mg q12h. May increase to 150 mg q12h if inadequate response.

Esophageal Candidiasis

Adult: **PO** *Weight greater than 40 kg,* 200 mg q12h for a minimum of 14 days and for at least 7 days after resolution of symptoms; *weight less than 40 kg,* 100 mg q12h for a minimum of 14 days and for at least 7 days after resolution of symptoms

Dose Adjustment for Concomitant Fosphenytoin or Phenytoin

Adult: **IV** 6 mg/kg q12h day 1, then 5 mg/kg q12h. **PO** *Weight greater than 40 kg,* 400 mg q12h day 1, then 400 mg q12h; *weight less than 40 kg,* 400 mg q12h day 1, then 200 mg q12h

Renal Impairment Dosage Adjustment

CrCl less than 50 mL/min: Switch to PO therapy after loading dose; hemodialysis does not require supplemental dose

Hepatic Impairment Dosage Adjustment

Child-Pugh class A or B: Reduce maintenance dose by 50%; Child-Pugh class C: Avoid drug use

ADMINISTRATION

Oral

- Give at least 1 h before or 1 h following a meal.
- Store tablets at 15°–30° C (59°–86° F).

Intravenous

PREPARE: **Intermittent:** Use a 20 mL syringe to reconstitute each 200 mg powder vial with exactly 19 mL of sterile water for injection to yield 10 mg/mL. Discard vial if a vacuum does not pull the diluent into vial. Shake until completely dissolved. ▪ Calculate the required dose of voriconazole based on patient's weight. ▪ From an IV infusion bag of NS, D5W, D5/NS, D5/.45NS, LR or other suitable solution, withdraw and discard a volume of IV solution equal to the required dose. ▪ Inject the required dose of voriconazole into the IV bag. The IV solution should have a final voriconazole concentration of 0.5–5 mg/mL. ▪ Infuse immediately.

ADMINISTER: **Intermittent:** Infuse over 1–2 h at a maximum rate of 3 mg/kg/h. ▪ DO NOT give a bolus dose.

INCOMPATIBILITIES **Solution/additive:** Do not dilute with **sodium bicarbonate;** do not mix with any other drugs. **Y-site:** Do not infuse with other drugs.

▪ Store unreconstituted vials at 15°–30° C (59°–86° F).

ADVERSE EFFECTS (≥1%) **Body as a Whole:** Peripheral edema, fever, chills. **CNS:** Headache, hallucinations, dizziness. **CV:** Tachycardia, hypotension, hypertension, vasodilation. **GI:** Nausea, vomiting, abdominal pain, abnormal LFTs, diarrhea, cholestatic jaundice, dry mouth. **Metabolic:** Increased alkaline phosphatase, AST, ALT, hypokalemia, hypomagnesemia. **Skin:** Rash, pruritus. **Special Senses:** *Abnormal vision (enhanced brightness, blurred vision, or color vision changes),* photophobia.

INTERACTIONS Drug: Due to significant increased toxicity or decreased activity, the following drugs are contraindicated with voriconazole: BARBITURATES, **carbamazepine, efavirenz,** ERGOT ALKALOIDS, **pimozide, quinidine, rifabutin, sirolimus; fosphenytoin, phenytoin, rifampin, ritonavir** may significantly decrease voriconazole levels. PROTEASE INHIBITORS (except **indinavir**) may increase voriconazole toxicity; voriconazole may increase the toxicity of BENZODIAZEPINES, **cyclosporine,** PROTEASE INHIBITORS (except **indinavir**), NONNUCLEOSIDE REVERSE TRANSCRIPTASE INHIBITORS, **omeprazole, tacrolimus, vinblastine, vincristine, warfarin;** NONNUCLEOSIDE REVERSE TRANSCRIPTASE INHIBITORS may increase or decrease voriconazole levels. **Food:** Absorption reduced with high-fat meals. **Herbal: St. John's wort** may decrease efficacy.

PHARMACOKINETICS Absorption: 96% absorbed. Has a nonlinear pharmacokinetic profile, a small change in dose may cause a large change in serum levels. Steady state not achieved until day 5–6 if no loading dose is given. **Peak:** 1–2 h. **Metabolism:** In liver by (and inhibits) CYP3A4, 2C9 and 2C19. **Elimination:** Primarily in urine. **Half-Life:** 6 h–6 days depending on dose.

NURSING IMPLICATIONS

Assessment & Drug Effects

- Visual acuity, visual field, and color perception should be monitored if treatment continues beyond 28 days.
- Withhold drug and notify physician if skin rash develops.
- Monitor cardiovascular status especially with preexisting CV disease.
- Lab tests: Monitor baseline and periodic LFTs including bilirubin; patients who develop abnormal LFTs during therapy should be moni-

V

tored for the development of more severe hepatic injury. Monitor frequently renal function tests, especially serum creatinine. Monitor periodic CBC with platelet count, Hct and Hgb, serum electrolytes, alkaline phosphatase, blood glucose, and lipid profile.

- Concurrent drugs: Monitor PT/INR closely with warfarin as dose adjustments of warfarin may be needed. Monitor frequently blood glucose levels with sulfonylurea drugs as reduction in the sulfonylurea dosage may be needed. Monitor for and report any of the following: S&S of rhabdomyolysis in patient receiving a statin drug; prolonged sedation in patient receiving a benzodiazepine; S&S of heart block, bradycardia, or CHF in patient receiving a calcium channel blocker.

Patient & Family Education

- Use reliable means of birth control to prevent pregnancy. If you suspect you are pregnant, contact physician immediately.
- Do not drive at night while taking voriconazole as the drug may cause blurred vision and photophobia.
- Do not drive or engage in other potentially hazardous activities until reaction to drug is known.
- Avoid strong, direct sunlight while taking voriconazole.

WARFARIN SODIUM

(war′far-in)

Coumadin Sodium, Warfilone ♣

Classification: ANTICOAGULANT

Therapeutic: ANTICOAGULANT

Pregnancy Category: X

AVAILABILITY 1 mg, 2 mg, 2.5 mg, 3 mg, 4 mg, 5 mg, 6 mg, 7.5 mg, 10 mg tablets; 2.5 mg/mL injection

ACTION & *THERAPEUTIC EFFECT* Indirectly interferes with blood clotting by depressing hepatic synthesis of vitamin K-dependent coagulation factors: II, VII, IX, and X. *Deters further extension of existing thrombi and prevents new clots from forming.*

USES Prophylaxis and treatment of deep vein thrombosis and its extension, pulmonary embolism; treatment of atrial fibrillation with embolization. Also used as adjunct in treatment of coronary occlusion, cerebral transient ischemic attacks (TIAs), and as a prophylactic in patients with prosthetic cardiac valves. Used extensively as rodenticide.

CONTRAINDICATIONS Hemorrhagic tendencies, vitamin C or K deficiency, hemophilia, coagulation factor deficiencies, dyscrasias; active bleeding; open wounds, active peptic ulcer, visceral carcinoma, esophageal varices, malabsorption syndrome; uncontrolled hypertension, cerebral vascular disease; heparin-induced thrombocytopenia (HIT); pericarditis with acute MI; severe hepatic or renal disease; continuous tube drainage of any orifice; subacute bacterial endocarditis; recent surgery of brain, spinal cord, or eye; regional or lumbar block anesthesia; threatened abortion; unreliable patients; pregnancy (category X).

CAUTIOUS USE Alcoholism, allergic disorders, during menstruation, older adults, senility, psychosis; debilitated patients. Endogenous factors that may increase prothrombin time response (enhance anticoagulant effect): Carcinoma, CHF, collagen diseases, hepatic and renal insufficiency, diarrhea, fever, pancreatic disorders, malnutrition, vitamin K deficiency. Endogenous factors that may decrease prothrombin time response (decrease anticoagulant response): Edema, hypothyroidism, hyperlipidemia, hypercholesterolemia, chronic alcoholism, hereditary resistance to coumarin therapy.

ROUTE & DOSAGE

Anticoagulant
Adult: **PO/IV** Usual dose 2–10 mg daily with dose adjusted to maintain a PT 1.2–2 × control or INR of 2–3
Child: **PO** 0.1–0.3 mg/kg/day, adjust to maintain INR of 2–3

Pharmacogenetic Dosage Adjustment
Variations in CYP2C9 or VKORC1 may require dose adjustments

ADMINISTRATION

Note: Antidote for bleeding—anticoagulant effect usually is reversed by omitting 1 or more doses of warfarin and by administration of specific antidote phytonadione (vitamin K_1) 2.5–10 mg orally. Physician may advise patient to carry vitamin K_1 at all times, but not to take it until after consultation. If bleeding persists or progresses to a severe level, vitamin K 15–25 mg IV is given, or a fresh whole blood transfusion may be necessary.

Oral

- Give tablet whole or crushed with fluid of patient's choice.

Intravenous

PREPARE: **Direct:** Add 2.7 mL of sterile water for injection to the 5 mg vial.

ADMINISTER: **Direct:** Give required dose over 1–2 min.

INCOMPATIBILITIES **Solution/additive:** **Ammonium chloride, 5% dextrose, lactated Ringer's, atropine, calcium chloride, calcium gluconate, chloramphenicol, chlorothiazide, chlortetracycline, erythromycin, methicillin, nitrofurantoin, oxacillin, oxytetracycline, penicillin, pentobarbital, phenobarbital, promethazine, sodium bicarbonate, succinyl chloride, vitamin B with C.** **Y-site:** **Aminophylline, ammonium chloride, bretylium, ceftazidime, cephalothin, cimetidine, ciprofloxacin, dobutamine, esmolol, gentamicin, labetalol, metronidazole, promazine, lactated Ringer's, vancomycin.**

- Store at 15°–30° C (59°–86° F). Discard discolored or precipitated solutions. Protect all preparations from light and moisture.

ADVERSE EFFECTS (≥1%) **Body as a Whole:** Major or minor hemorrhage from any tissue or organ; hypersensitivity (dermatitis, urticaria, pruritus, fever). **GI:** Anorexia, nausea, vomiting, abdominal cramps, diarrhea, steatorrhea, stomatitis. **Other:** Increased serum transaminase levels, hepatitis, jaundice, burning sensation of feet, transient hair loss. **Overdosage:** Internal or external bleeding, paralytic ileus; skin necrosis of toes (purple toes syndrome), tip of nose, buttocks, thighs, calves, female breast, abdomen, and other fat-rich areas.

DIAGNOSTIC TEST INTERFERENCE
Warfarin (coumarins) may cause alkaline urine to be red-orange; may enhance ***uric acid*** excretion, cause elevation of ***serum transaminases,*** and may increase ***lactic dehydrogenase*** activity.

INTERACTIONS Drug: In addition to the drugs listed below, many other drugs have been reported to alter the expected response to warfarin; however, clinical importance of

W

these reports has not been substantiated. The addition or withdrawal of any drug to an established drug regimen should be made cautiously, with more frequent INR determinations than usual and with careful observation of the patient and dose adjustment as indicated. The following may enhance the anticoagulant effects of warfarin: **Acetohexamide, acetaminophen,** ALKYLATING AGENTS, **allopurinol,** AMINOGLYCOSIDES, **aminosalicylic acid, amiodarone,** ANABOLIC STEROIDS, ANTIBIOTICS (ORAL), ANTIMETABOLITES, ANTIPLATELET DRUGS, **aspirin, asparaginase, capecitabine, celecoxib, chloramphenicol, chlorpropamide, chymotrypsin, cimetidine, clofibrate, co-trimoxazole, danazol, dextran, dextrothyroxine, diazoxide, disulfiram, erythromycin, ethacrynic acid, fluconazole, glucagons, guanethidine,** HEPATOTOXIC DRUGS, **influenza vaccine, isoniazid, itraconazole, ketoconazole,** MAO INHIBITORS, **meclofenamate, mefenamic acid, methyldopa, methylphenidate, metronidazole, miconazole, mineral oil, nalidixic acid, neomycin (oral),** NONSTEROIDAL ANTI-INFLAMMATORY DRUGS, **oxandrolone, plicamycin,** POTASSIUM PRODUCTS, **propoxyphene, propylthiouracil, quinidine, quinine, rofecoxib, salicylates, streptokinase, sulindac,** SULFONAMIDES, SULFONYLUREAS, TETRACYCLINES, THIAZIDES, THYROID DRUGS, **tolbutamide,** TRICYCLIC ANTIDEPRESSANTS, **urokinase, vitamin E, zileuton.** The following may increase or decrease the anticoagulant effects of warfarin: **Alcohol** (acute intoxication may increase, chronic alcoholism may decrease effects), **chloral hydrate,** DIURETICS. The following may decrease the anticoagulant effects of warfarin: BARBITURATES, **carbamazepine, cholestyramine,** CORTICOSTEROIDS, **corticotropin, ethchlorvynol, glutethimide, griseofulvin,** LAXATIVES, **mercaptopurine,** ORAL CONTRACEPTIVES, **rifampin, spironolactone, vitamin C, vitamin K.** **Herbal: Boldo, capsicum, celery, chamomile, chondroitin, clove, coenzyme Q10, danshen, devil's claw, dong quai, echinacea, evening primrose oil, fenugreek, feverfew, fish oil, garlic, ginger, ginkgo, glucosamine, horse chestnut, licorice root, passionflower herb, turmeric, willow bark** may increase risk of bleeding; **ginseng, green tea, seaweed, soy, St. John's wort** may decrease effectiveness of warfarin. **Food: Cranberry juice** may increase INR. Green leafy vegetables may affect efficacy. **Avocado** may decrease effectiveness of warfarin.

PHARMACOKINETICS Absorption: Well absorbed from GI tract. **Onset:** 2–7 days. **Peak:** 0.5–3 days. **Distribution:** 97% protein bound; crosses placenta. **Metabolism:** In liver (CYP2C9). **Elimination:** In urine and bile. **Half-Life:** 0.5–3 days.

NURSING IMPLICATIONS

Assessment & Drug Effects

- Determine PT/INP prior to initiation of therapy and then daily until maintenance dosage is established.
- Obtain a COMPLETE medication history prior to start of therapy and whenever altered responses to therapy require interpretation; extremely IMPORTANT since many drugs interfere with the activity of anticoagulant drugs (see INTERACTIONS).
- Dose is typically adjusted to maintain PT at $1^{1}/_{2}$–$2^{1}/_{2}$ times the control (12–15 sec), or 15–35% of normal prothrombin activity, or

an INR of 2–4 depending on diagnosis.

- Lab tests: For maintenance dosage, PT/INR determinations at 1–4-wk intervals depending on patient's response; periodic urinalyses, stool guaiac, and LFTs. Blood samples for PT/INR should be drawn at 12–18 h after last dose (optimum).
- Note: Patients at greatest risk of hemorrhage include those whose PT/INR are difficult to regulate, who have an aortic valve prosthesis, who are receiving long-term anticoagulant therapy, and older adult and debilitated patients.

Patient & Family Education

- Understand that bleeding can occur even though PT/INR are within therapeutic range. Stop drug and notify physician immediately if bleeding or signs of bleeding appear: Blood in urine, bright red or black tarry stools, vomiting of blood, bleeding with tooth brushing, blue or purple spots on skin or mucous membrane, round pinpoint purplish red spots (often occur in ankle areas), nosebleed, bloody sputum; chest pain; abdominal or lumbar pain or swelling, profuse menstrual bleeding, pelvic pain; severe or continuous headache, faintness or dizziness; prolonged oozing from any minor injury (e.g., nicks from shaving).
- Stop drug and report immediately any symptoms of hepatitis (dark urine, itchy skin, jaundice, abdominal pain, light stools) or hypersensitivity reaction (see Appendix F).
- Take drug at same time each day, and do NOT alter dose.
- Risk of bleeding is increased for up to 1 mo after receiving the influenza vaccine.
- Fever, prolonged hot weather, malnutrition, and diarrhea lengthen PT/INR (enhanced anticoagulant effect).
- A high-fat diet, sudden increase in vitamin K–rich foods (cabbage, cauliflower, broccoli, asparagus, lettuce, turnip greens, onions, spinach, kale, fish, liver), coffee or green tea (caffeine), or by tube feedings with high vitamin K content shorten PT/INR.
- Avoid excess intake of alcohol.
- Use a soft toothbrush and floss teeth gently with waxed floss.
- Use barrier contraceptive measures; if you become pregnant while on anticoagulant therapy the fetus is at great potential risk of congenital malformations.
- Do not take any other prescription or OTC drug unless specifically approved by physician or pharmacist.

XYLOMETAZOLINE HYDROCHLORIDE

(zye-loe-met-az′oh-leen)

Otrivin

Classifications: NASAL DECONGESTANT; VASOCONSTRICTOR

Therapeutic: NASAL DECONGESTANT

Prototype: Naphazoline

Pregnancy Category: C

AVAILABILITY 0.05%, 0.1% nasal solution

ACTION & *THERAPEUTIC EFFECT* Markedly constricts dilated arterioles of nasal membrane. *Decreases fluid exudate and mucosal engorgement associated with rhinitis and may open up obstructed eustachian tubes.*

USES Temporary relief of nasal congestion associated with common cold, sinusitis, acute and chronic rhinitis, and hay fever and other allergies.

X

CONTRAINDICATIONS Sensitivity to adrenergic substances; angle-closure glaucoma; concurrent therapy with MAO inhibitors or tricyclic antidepressants; lactation, **PO:** children younger than 12 y, **Nasal:** children younger than 2 y and infants.
CAUTIOUS USE Hypertension; hyperthyroidism; heart disease, including angina; advanced arteriosclerosis, older adults, pregnancy (category C).

ROUTE & DOSAGE

Nasal Congestion
Adult/Child (12 y or older): **Nasal** 1–2 sprays or 1–2 drops of 0.1% solution in each nostril q8–10h (max: 3 doses/day)
Child (2 –12 y): **Nasal** 1 spray or 2–3 drops of 0.05% solution in each nostril q8–10h (max: 3 doses/day)

ADMINISTRATION

Instillation

- Have patient clear each nostril gently before administering spray or drops.
- Store at 15°–30° C (59°–86° F) in a tight, light-resistant container.

ADVERSE EFFECTS (≥1%) **All:** Usually mild and infrequent; local stinging, burning, dryness and ulceration, sneezing, headache, insomnia, drowsiness. **With Excessive Use:** *Rebound nasal congestion* and vasodilation, tremulousness, hypertension, palpitations, tachycardia, arrhythmia, somnolence, sedation, <u>coma</u>.

INTERACTIONS Drug: May cause increase BP with **guanethidine, methyldopa,** MAO INHIBITORS; PHENOTHIAZINES may decrease effectiveness of nasal decongestant.

PHARMACOKINETICS Onset: 5–10 min. **Duration:** 5–6 h.

NURSING IMPLICATIONS

Assessment & Drug Effects

- Evaluate for development of rebound congestion (see ADVERSE EFFECTS).

Patient & Family Education

- Prevent contamination of nasal solution and spread of infection by rinsing dropper and tip of nasal spray in hot water after each use; restrict use to the individual patient.
- Note: Prolonged use can cause rebound congestion and chemical rhinitis. Do NOT exceed prescribed dosage and report to physician if drug fails to provide relief within 3–4 days.
- Do NOT self-medicate with OTC drugs, sprays, or drops without physician's approval.
- Note: Excessive use by a child may lead to CNS depression.

ZAFIRLUKAST (Pr)

(za-fir-lu'kast)
Accolate
Classifications: RESPIRATORY SMOOTH MUSCLE RELAXANT; LEUKOTRIENE RECEPTOR ANTAGONIST (LTRA); BRONCHODILATOR
Therapeutic: BRONCHODILATOR; LTRA
Pregnancy Category: B

AVAILABILITY 10 mg, 20 mg tablets

ACTION & *THERAPEUTIC EFFECT* Selective leukotriene receptor antagonist (LTRA) that inhibits binding of leukotriene D_4 and E_4, thus inhibiting inflammation and bronchoconstriction. Leukotriene production and receptor affinity have been correlated with the pathogenesis of asthma. *Zafirlukast helps to prevent the signs and symptoms of asthma, including airway edema, smooth muscle con-*

striction, and altered cellular activity due to inflammation.

USES Prophylaxis and chronic treatment of asthma in adults and children older than 5 y (not for acute bronchospasm).

CONTRAINDICATIONS Hypersensitivity to zafirlukast; acute asthma attacks, including status asthmaticus, acute bronchospasm; lactation, children younger than 5 y.

CAUTIOUS USE Hepatic impairment, hepatic disease; corticosteroid withdrawal or reduction in dose; patients 65 y or older, pregnancy (category B).

ROUTE & DOSAGE

Asthma

Adult: **PO** 20 mg b.i.d. 1 h before or 2 h after meals
Child (older than 5 y): **PO** 10 mg b.i.d.

ADMINISTRATION

Oral

- Give 1 h before or 2 h after meals.
- Store at 20°–25° C (68°–77° F); protect from light and moisture.

ADVERSE EFFECTS (≥1%) **Body as a Whole:** Generalized pain, asthenia, myalgia, fever, back pain. **CNS:** *Headache,* dizziness. **GI:** Nausea, diarrhea, abdominal pain, vomiting, dyspepsia; liver dysfunction, increased liver function tests, hepatic failure. **Other:** Churg-Strauss syndrome (fever, muscle aches and pains, weight loss).

INTERACTIONS Drug: May increase prothrombin time (PT) in patients on **warfarin. Erythromycin** decreases bioavailability of zafirlukast.

PHARMACOKINETICS Absorption: Rapidly from GI tract, bioavailability significantly reduced by food. **Onset:** 1 wk. **Peak:** 3 h. **Distribution:** Greater than 99% protein bound; secreted into breast milk. **Metabolism:** In liver (CYP2C9). **Elimination:** 90% in feces, 10% in urine. **Half-Life:** 10 h.

NURSING IMPLICATIONS

Assessment & Drug Effects

- Assess respiratory status and airway function regularly.
- Lab tests: Periodic LFTs.
- Monitor closely PT and INR with concurrent warfarin therapy.
- Monitor closely phenytoin level with concurrent phenytoin therapy.

Patient & Family Education

- Taking medication regularly, even during symptom-free periods.
- Note: Drug is not intended to treat acute episodes of asthma.
- Report S&S of hepatic toxicity (see Appendix F) or flu-like symptoms to physician. Follow-up lab work is very important.
- Notify physician immediately if condition worsens while using prescribed doses of all antiasthmatic medications.

ZALEPLON

(zal′ep-lon)
Sonata
Classifications: ANXIOLYTIC; SEDATIVE-HYPNOTIC; NONBENZODIAZEPINE
Therapeutic: SEDATIVE-HYPNOTIC; ANTIANXIETY
Prototype: Zolpidem
Pregnancy Category: C
Controlled Substance: Schedule IV

AVAILABILITY 5 mg, 10 mg capsules

ACTION & *THERAPEUTIC EFFECT* Short-acting nonbenzodiazepine

Z

with sedative-hypnotic, muscle relaxant, and anticonvulsant activity. *Reduces difficulty in initially falling asleep. Preserves deep sleep (stage 3 through stage 4) at hypnotic dose with minimal-to-absent rebound insomnia when discontinued.*

USES Short-term treatment of insomnia.

CONTRAINDICATIONS Hypersensitivity to zaleplon, or tartrazine dye (Yellow 5); suicidal ideation; lactation. Safe use in children is not established.
CAUTIOUS USE Hypersensitivity to salicylates; concurrent use of other CNS depressants (e.g., benzodiazepines, alcohol); chronic depression; history of drug abuse; COPD; respiratory insufficiency; hepatic or renal impairment; pulmonary disease; pregnancy (category C).

ROUTE & DOSAGE

Insomnia
Adult: **PO** 10 mg at bedtime (max: 20 mg at bedtime)
Geriatric: **PO** 5 mg at bedtime (max: 10 mg at bedtime)

ADMINISTRATION

Oral
- Give immediately before bedtime; not while patient is still ambulating.
- Store at 20°–25° C (68°–77° F).

ADVERSE EFFECTS (≥1%) **Body as a Whole:** Asthenia, fever, *headache,* migraine, myalgia, back pain. **CNS:** Amnesia, dizziness, paresthesia, somnolence, tremor, vertigo, depression, hypertonia, nervousness, difficulty concentrating. **GI:** Abdominal pain, dyspepsia, nausea, constipation, dry mouth. **Respiratory:** Bronchitis. **Skin:** Pruritus, rash. **Special Senses:** Eye pain, hyperacusis, conjunctivitis. **Urogenital:** Dysmenorrhea.

INTERACTIONS Drug: Alcohol, imipramine, thioridazine may cause additive CNS impairment; **rifampin** increases metabolism of **zaleplon; cimetidine** increases serum levels of **zaleplon. Herbal: Valerian, melatonin** may produce additive sedative effects. **Food:** High-fat meals may delay absorption.

PHARMACOKINETICS Absorption: Rapidly and completely absorbed, 30% reaches systemic circulation. **Onset:** 15–20 min. **Peak:** 1 h. **Duration:** 3–4 h. **Distribution:** 60% protein bound. **Metabolism:** Extensively in liver (CYP3A4) to inactive metabolites. **Elimination:** 70% in urine, 17% in feces. **Half-Life:** 1 h.

NURSING IMPLICATIONS

Assessment & Drug Effects
- Monitor behavior and notify physician for significant changes. Use extra caution with preexisting clinical depression.
- Provide safe environment and monitor ambulation after drug is ingested.
- Monitor respiratory status with preexisting compromised pulmonary function.

Patient & Family Education
- Exercise caution when walking; avoid all hazardous activities after taking zaleplon.
- Do not take in combination with alcohol or any other sleep medication.
- Note: Exhibits altered effectiveness if taken with/immediately after high-fat meal.
- Do not use longer than 2–3 wk.
- Expect possible mild/brief rebound insomnia after discontinuing regimen.
- Report use of OTC medications to physician (e.g., cimetidine).
- Report pregnancy to physician immediately.

ZANAMIVIR

(zan'a-mi-vir)

Relenza

Classification: ANTIVIRAL

Therapeutic: ANTIINFLUENZA

Pregnancy Category: C

AVAILABILITY 5 mg/Rotadisk blister

ACTION & *THERAPEUTIC EFFECT* Inhibitor of influenza A and B viral enzyme; does not permit the release of newly formed viruses from the surface of the infected cells. *Prevents viral spread across the mucus lining of the respiratory tract, and inhibits the replication of influenza A and B virus. Relieves flu-like symptoms.*

USES Uncomplicated acute influenza in patients symptomatic less than 2 days; prophylaxis for influenza.

CONTRAINDICATIONS Hypersensitivity to zanamivir or milk protein; severe renal impairment, renal failure; COPD; severe asthma.

CAUTIOUS USE Renal impairment; cardiac disease; older adults; severe metabolic disease; pregnancy (category C), lactation. **Acute influenza:** Safety and efficacy in children younger than 7 y are unknown. **Influenza prophylaxis:** Safe use in children younger than 5 y is unknown.

ROUTE & DOSAGE

Acute Influenza

Adult/Child (older than 7 y): **Inhaled** 2 inhalations (one 5 mg blister/inhalation) b.i.d. (approximately 12 h apart) × 5 days

Influenza Prophylaxis

Adult/Child (older than 5 y): **Inhaled** 2 inhalations daily for 10 days (household prophylaxis) or 2 inhalations daily for 28 days (community outbreak)

ADMINISTRATION

Inhalation

- Most effective if initiated within 48 h of onset of flu-like symptoms.
- Give any scheduled inhaled bronchodilator before zanamivir.
- Store at 25° C (77° F).

ADVERSE EFFECTS (≥1%) **Body as a Whole:** Headache, abnormal behavior. **CNS:** Dizziness. **GI:** Nausea, diarrhea, vomiting. **Respiratory:** Nasal symptoms, bronchitis, cough, sinusitis; ear, nose, throat infection.

INTERACTIONS Drug: Do not use with LIVE VACCINES.

PHARMACOKINETICS Absorption: 4–17% of inhaled dose is systemically absorbed. **Peak:** 1–2 h. **Distribution:** Less than 10% protein bound. **Metabolism:** Not metabolized. **Elimination:** In urine. **Half-Life:** 2.5–5.1 h.

NURSING IMPLICATIONS

Patient & Family Education

- Start within 48 h of onset of flu-like symptoms for most effective response.
- Use any scheduled inhaled bronchodilator first; then use zanamivir.

ZICONOTIDE

(zi-con'o-tide)

Prialt

Classifications: NONNARCOTIC ANALGESIC; N-TYPE CALCIUM CHANNEL BLOCKER

Z

Therapeutic: NONNARCOTIC ANALGESIC
Pregnancy Category: C

AVAILABILITY 25 mcg/mL, 100 mcg/mL injection

ACTION & *THERAPEUTIC EFFECT* Ziconotide binds to N-type calcium channels located on the afferent nerves in the dorsal horn in the spinal cord. It is thought that these binding blocks of N-type calcium channels lead to a blockade of excitatory neurotransmitter release in the afferent nerve endings. *Ziconotide is effective in controlling severe chronic pain that is intractable to other analgesics.*

USES Management of severe chronic pain in patients for whom intrathecal (IT) therapy is warranted.

UNLABELED USES Spasticity associated with spinal cord trauma.

CONTRAINDICATIONS Hypersensitivity to ziconotide; epidural or intravenous administration; preexisting history of psychosis; sepsis; depression with suicidal ideation; cognitive impairment; bipolar disorder; schizophrenia; dementia; presence of infection at the injection site, uncontrolled bleeding, or spinal canal obstruction that impairs circulation of CSF; coagulopathy; seizures; lactation. Safety and efficacy in children or infants are not established.

CAUTIOUS USE Elderly; renal, hepatic, and cardiac impairment; older adults; pregnancy (category C).

ROUTE & DOSAGE

Severe Chronic Pain

Adult: **Intrathecal** Initial 0.1 mcg/h; may titrate up 0.1 mcg/h q2–3days to 0.8 mcg/h (19.2 mcg/day)

ADMINISTRATION

Intrathecal

- May be administered undiluted (25 mcg/mL in 20 mL vial) or diluted using the 100 mcg/mL vials. Diluted ziconotide is prepared with NS without preservatives.
- Administer using an implanted variable-rate microinfusion device or an external microinfusion device and catheter.
- Note: Due to serious adverse events, 19.2 mcg/day (0.8 mcg/h) is the maximum recommended dose.
- Doses should normally be titrated upward by no more than 2.4 mcg/day (0.1 mcg/h) at intervals of 2–3 times/wk.
- Refrigerate all ziconotide solutions after preparation and begin infusion within 24 h. Discard any unused portion left in a vial.

ADVERSE EFFECTS (≥1%) **Body as a Whole:** Accidental injury, back pain, catheter complication, catheter-site pain, cellulitis, chest pain, chills, *fever,* flu syndrome, infection, malaise, neck pain, neck rigidity, *pain,* pump-site complication, pump-site mass, pump-site pain, viral infection. **CNS:** Abnormal dreams, *abnormal gait,* agitation, *anxiety, aphasia, asthenia, ataxia,* CSF abnormal, *confusion,* depression, difficulty concentrating, *dizziness,* dry mouth, *dysesthesia,* emotional lability, *headache,* hostility, hyperesthesia, *hypertonia,* incoordination, insomnia, *memory impairment,* mental slowing, meningitis, *nervousness,* neuralgia, paranoid reaction, *paresthesia,* reflexes decreased, *somnolence, speech disorder,* stupor, abnormal thinking, tremor, twitching, *vertigo.* **CV:** Hypertension, hypotension, postural hypotension, syncope, tachycardia, vasodilation. **GI:** Abdominal pain, *anorexia,* constipation, *diar-*

Common adverse effects in *italic*, life-threatening effects underlined; generic names in **bold**; classifications in SMALL CAPS; ♣ Canadian drug name; ⓟ Prototype drug

rhea, dyspepsia, gastrointestinal disorder, *nausea, vomiting.* **GU:** Dysuria, urinary incontinence, *urinary retention,* urinary tract infection, impaired urination. **Hematologic:** Anemia, ecchymosis. **Metabolic/Nutritional:** Creatinine phosphokinase increased, dehydration, edema, hypokalemia, peripheral edema, weight loss. **Musculoskeletal:** Arthralgia, arthritis, leg cramps, myalgia, myasthenia. **Respiratory:** Bronchitis, cough increased, dyspnea, lung disorder, pharyngitis, pneumonia, rhinitis, sinusitis. **Skin:** Cutaneous surgical complication, dry skin, pruritus, rash, skin disorder, sweating. **Special Senses:** *Abnormal vision,* diplopia, *nystagmus,* photophobia, taste perversion, tinnitus.

INTERACTIONS Drug: Ethanol and other CNS DEPRESSANTS may increase drowsiness, dizziness, and confusion.

PHARMACOKINETICS Distribution: 50% protein bound. **Metabolism:** Hydrolyzed by peptidases. **Half-Life:** 4.6 h.

NURSING IMPLICATIONS

Assessment & Drug Effects

- Monitor for and report S&S of meningitis, cognitive impairment, hallucinations, changes in mood or consciousness, or other psychiatric symptoms.
- Lab tests: Serum creatine kinase every other week for first month and monthly thereafter.

Patient & Family Education

- Report any of the following to physician: Muscle pain, soreness, or weakness, confusion, unusual behavior, symptoms of depression or suicidal thoughts, fever, headache, stiff neck, nausea or vomiting, seizures.
- Note: Taking this drug with other depressants (e.g., alcohol, sedatives, tranquilizers) will increase the risk of side effects.

ZIDOVUDINE (FORMERLY AZIDOTHYMIDINE, AZT)

(zye-doe′vyoo-deen)

Retrovir

Classifications: ANTIVIRAL; NUCLEOSIDE REVERSE TRANSCRIPTASE INHIBITOR

Therapeutic: ANTIVIRAL; NRTI

Prototype: Lamivudine

Pregnancy Category: C

AVAILABILITY 300 mg tablets; 100 mg capsules; 50 mg/5 mL syrup; 10 mg/mL injection

ACTION & *THERAPEUTIC EFFECT* Appears to act by being incorporated into growing DNA chains by viral reverse transcriptase, thereby terminating viral replication. *Zidovudine has antiviral action against HIV, LAV (lymphadenopathy-associated virus), and ARV (AIDS-associated retrovirus).*

USES Patients who are HIV positive and have a CD4 count 500/mm^3 or less, asymptomatic HIV infection, early and late symptomatic HIV disease, prevention of perinatal transfer of HIV during pregnancy.

UNLABELED USES Pediatric patients, postexposure chemoprophylaxis.

CONTRAINDICATIONS Life-threatening allergic reactions to any of the components of the drug; lactic acidosis; lactation.

CAUTIOUS USE Impaired renal or hepatic function, alcoholism; anemia; chemotherapy; radiation therapy; bone marrow depression; pregnancy (category C).

ROUTE & DOSAGE

Symptomatic HIV Infection
Adult: **PO** 300 mg b.i.d. OR 200 mg t.i.d. **IV** 1–2 mg/kg q4h (1200 mg/day)
Child (3 mo–13 y): **PO** 160 mg/m^2 q8h

Prevention of Maternal-Fetal Transmission
Neonate: **PO** *Greater than 34 wk:* 2 mg/kg q6h for 6 wk beginning within 12 h after birth; *30–35 wk gestation:* 2 mg/kg q12h for 2 wk, then q8h for 4 wk; *less than 30 wk gestation:* 2 mg/kg q12h for 4 wk, then q8h for 2 wk **IV** *Full term:* 1.5 mg/kg q6h × 6 wk
Maternal: **PO** 100 mg 5 times daily OR 300 mg b.i.d. from 14 wk gestation until delivery **IV** During labor, 2 mg/kg loading dose, then 1 mg/kg/h until clamping umbilical cord

Toxicity Dosage Adjustment
Hemoglobin falls below 7.5 g/dL or falls 25% from baseline: Interrupt therapy. *ANC falls below 750 cells/mm3 or decreases 50% from baseline:* Interrupt therapy.

ADMINISTRATION

Oral
- Do not expose capsules and syrup to light during drug preparation.

Intravenous

PREPARE: **Intermittent:** Withdraw required dose from vial and dilute with D5W to a concentration not to exceed 4 mg/mL.
ADMINISTER: **Intermittent for HIV infection:** Give calculated dose at a constant rate over 60 min; avoid rapid infusion. **IV Infusions for Prevention of Maternal-Fetal Transmission:** Give maternal loading dose over 1 h, then continuous infusion at 1 mg/kg/h. **Intermittent Infusion for Prevention of Maternal Transmission of HIV to Neonate:** Give calculated dose at a constant rate over 30 min.
INCOMPATIBILITIES **Solution/additive: Meropenem. Y-site: Lansoprazole, meropenem.**

- Store at 15°–25° C (59°–77° F) and protect from light. Store diluted IV solutions refrigerated for 24 h.

ADVERSE EFFECTS (≥1%) **Body as a Whole:** *Fever,* dyspnea, *malaise,* weakness, *myalgia,* myopathy. **CNS:** *Headache,* insomnia, dizziness, paresthesias, mild confusion, anxiety, restlessness, agitation. **GI:** *Nausea,* diarrhea, *vomiting, anorexia,* GI pain. **Hematologic:** *Bone marrow depression, granulocytopenia, anemia.* **Respiratory:** *Cough, wheezing.* **Skin:** *Rash,* itching, diaphoresis.

INTERACTIONS Drug: Acetaminophen ganciclovir, interferon-alfa may enhance bone marrow suppression; **atovaquone, amphotericin B, aspirin, dapsone, doxorubicin, fluconazole, flucytosine, indomethacin, interferon alfa, methadone, pentamidine, vincristine, valproic acid** may increase risk of AZT toxicity; **probenecid** will decrease AZT elimination, resulting in increased serum levels and thus toxicity. **Nelfinavir, rifampin, ritonavir** may decrease zidovudine (AZT) concentrations; other ANTIRETROVIRAL AGENTS may cause lactic acidosis and severe hepatomegaly with steatosis; **stavudine, doxorubicin** may antagonize AZT effects.

PHARMACOKINETICS Absorption: Readily from GI tract; 60–70% reaches systemic circulation (first-pass metabolism). **Peak:** 0.5–1.5 h.

Distribution: Crosses blood–brain barrier and placenta. **Metabolism:** In liver. **Elimination:** 63–95% in urine. **Half-Life:** 1 h.

NURSING IMPLICATIONS

Assessment & Drug Effects

- Evaluate patient at least weekly during the first month of therapy.
- Lab tests: Baseline and frequent (at least q2wk) blood counts, CD4 (T_4) lymphocyte count, Hgb, and granulocyte count to detect hematologic toxicity.
- Myelosuppression results in anemia, which commonly occurs after 4–6 wk of therapy, and granulocytopenia in 6–8 wk. Frequently, both respond to dosage adjustment. Significant anemia (Hgb less than 7.5 g/dL or reduction greater than 25% of baseline value), or granulocyte count less than 750/mm^3 (or reduction greater than 50% of baseline) may require temporary interruption of therapy and transfusions.
- Monitor for common adverse effects, especially severe headache, nausea, insomnia, and myalgia.

Patient & Family Education

- Contact physician promptly if health status worsens or any unusual symptoms develop.
- Understand that this drug is not a cure for HIV infection; you will continue to be at risk for opportunistic infections.
- Do not share drug with others; take drug exactly as prescribed.
- Drug does NOT reduce the risk of transmission of HIV infection through body fluids.

ZILEUTON

(zi-leu′ton)

Zyflo, Zyflo CR

Classifications: RESPIRATORY SMOOTH MUSCLE RELAXANT; BRONCHODILATOR; LEUKOTRIENE RECEPTOR ANTAGONIST (LTRA)
Therapeutic: BRONCHODILATOR; LTRA
Prototype: Zafirlukast
Pregnancy Category: C

AVAILABILITY 600 mg immediate release and controlled release tablets

ACTION & *THERAPEUTIC EFFECT* Inhibits 5-lipoxygenase, the enzyme needed to start the conversion of arachidonic acid to leukotrienes, which are important inflammatory agents that induce bronchoconstriction and mucus production. *Zileuton helps to prevent the signs and symptoms of asthma including airway edema, smooth muscle constriction, and altered cellular activity due to inflammation.*

USES Prophylaxis and chronic treatment of asthma in adults and children younger than 12 y.

CONTRAINDICATIONS Hypersensitivity to zileuton or zafirlukast, active liver disease, status asthmaticus; QT prolongation; lactation.
CAUTIOUS USE Hepatic insufficiency; alcoholism; older adults; older females; fever; infection; history of QT prolongation; pregnancy (category C). Safety and effectiveness in children younger than 12 y are not established.

ROUTE & DOSAGE

Asthma

Adult/Child (older than 12 y): **PO** 1200 mg controlled release tablets b.i.d. or 600 mg immediate release tablets q.i.d.

ADMINISTRATION

Oral

- Ensure that controlled release tablets are swallowed whole. They should not be crushed or chewed.
- Store at room temperature, 15°–30° C (59°–86° F); protect from light.

ADVERSE EFFECTS (≥1%) **Body as a Whole:** Pain, asthenia, myalgia, arthralgia, fever, malaise, neck pain/rigidity. **CNS:** *Headache,* dizziness, insomnia, nervousness, somnolence. **CV:** Chest pain. **GI:** Abdominal pain, *dyspepsia,* nausea, constipation, flatulence, vomiting, elevated liver function tests, asymptomatic hepatitis. **Skin:** Pruritus. **Other:** Conjunctivitis, hypertonia, lymphadenopathy, vaginitis, UTI, leukopenia.

INTERACTIONS Drug: May double **theophylline** levels and increase toxicity. Increases hypoprothrombinemic effects of **warfarin.** May increase levels of BETA-BLOCKERS (especially **propranolol**), leading to hypotension and bradycardia.

PHARMACOKINETICS Absorption: Rapidly from GI tract. **Peak:** 1.7 h. **Duration:** 5–8 h. **Distribution:** 93% protein bound; secreted in the breast milk of rats. **Metabolism:** In liver primarily via glucuronide conjugation. **Elimination:** Primarily in urine (94%). **Half-Life:** 2.5 h.

NURSING IMPLICATIONS

Assessment & Drug Effects

- Assess respiratory status and airway function regularly.
- Lab tests: Periodic CBC and routine blood chemistry; monthly LFTs for 3 mo, then every 2–3 mo for rest of first year, then periodically.
- Instructions for CONCURRENT THERAPIES: Monitor closely each of the following with concurrent drug therapy: With theophylline, theophylline levels; with warfarin, PT and INR; with phenytoin, phenytoin level; with propranolol, HR and BP for excessive beta blockade.

Patient & Family Education

- Take medication regularly even during symptom-free periods.
- Drug is not intended to treat acute episodes of asthma.
- Report to physician promptly S&S of hepatic toxicity (see Appendix F) or flu-like symptoms. Follow-up lab work is very important.
- Notify physician if condition worsens while using prescribed doses of all antiasthmatic medications.

ZIPRASIDONE HYDROCHLORIDE

(zip-ra-si′done)

Geodon

Classification: ANTIPSYCHOTIC, ATYPICAL

Therapeutic: ATYPICAL ANTIPSYCHOTIC

Prototype: Clozapine

Pregnancy Category: C

AVAILABILITY 20 mg, 40 mg, 60 mg, 80 mg capsules; 20 mg/mL injection

ACTION & *THERAPEUTIC EFFECT* Exerts antischizophrenic effects through dopamine (D_2) and serotonin (5-HT_{2A}) receptor antagonist. Exerts antidepressant effects through 5-HT_{1A} agonism, 5-HT_{1D} antagonism, and serotonin/norepinephrine reuptake inhibition. *Improves symptoms of schizophrenia, schizoaffective disorder, and psychotic depression.*

USES Treatment of schizophrenia, acute bipolar mania, acute psychosis, agitation.

UNLABELED USES Tourette's syndrome.

CONTRAINDICATIONS Hypersensitivity to ziprasidone; history of QT prolongation including congenital long QT syndrome or with other drugs known to prolong the QT interval; AV block, bundle branch block, cardiac arrhythmias, congenital heart disease, recent MI or uncompensated heart failure; bradycardia, hypokalemia or hypomagnesemia; neuroleptic malignant syndrome and tardive dyskinesia; dehydration or hypovolemia; UV exposure and tanning beds; lactation. Safety and efficacy in children or adolescents (except for treatment of Tourette's syndrome) are not established.

CAUTIOUS USE History of seizures, CVA, dementia, Parkinson's disease, or Alzheimer disease; known cardiovascular disease, conduction abnormalities, cerebrovascular disease; hepatic impairment; seizure disorder, seizures; breast cancer; risk factors for elevated core body temperature; esophageal motility disorders and risk of aspiration pneumonia; schizophrenia; suicide potential; pregnancy (category C); children older than 7 y for use in Tourette's syndrome only.

ROUTE & DOSAGE

Schizophrenia
Adult: **PO** Start with 20 mg b.i.d. with food, may increase q2days up to 80 mg b.i.d. if needed

Acute Episodes of Agitation/Acute Psychosis
Adult: **IM** 10 mg q2h or 20 mg q4h up to max of 40 mg/day

Acute Mania/Bipolar Disorder
Adult: **PO** Start with 40 mg b.i.d. with food; may increase q2days up to 80 mg b.i.d. if needed

ADMINISTRATION

Note: CONTRAINDICATIONS for this drug. Do NOT administer to anyone with a history of cardiac arrhythmias or other cardiac disease, hypokalemia, hypomagnesemia, prolonged QT/QT_c interval, or to anyone on other drugs known to prolong the QT_c interval.

- Withhold drug and consult physician if any of the foregoing conditions are present.

Oral

- Give with food.
- Make dosage adjustments at intervals of 2 days or more.

Intramuscular

- Give deep IM into a large muscle.
- Store at 15°–30° C (59°–86° F).

ADVERSE EFFECTS (≥1%) **Body as a Whole:** Asthenia, myalgia, weight gain, flu-like syndrome, face edema, chills, hypothermia. **CNS:** *Somnolence,* akathisia, dizziness, extrapyramidal effects, dystonia, hypertonia, agitation, tremor, dyskinesias, hostility, paresthesia, confusion, vertigo, hypokinesia, hyperkinesias, abnormal gait, oculogyric crisis, hypesthesia, ataxia, amnesia, cogwheel rigidity, delirium, hypotonia, akinesia, dysarthria, withdrawal syndrome, buccoglossal syndrome, choreoathetosis, diplopia, incoordination, neuropathy. **CV:** Tachycardia, postural hypotension, prolonged QT_c interval, hypertension. **GI:** *Nausea,* constipation, dyspepsia, diarrhea, dry mouth, anorexia, abdominal pain, vomiting. **Metabolic:** Hyperglycemia, diabetes mellitus. **Respiratory:** Rhinitis, increased cough, dyspnea. **Skin:** Rash, fungal dermatitis, photosensitivity. **Special Senses:** Abnormal vision.

INTERACTIONS Drug: Carbamazepine may decrease **ziprasidone**

levels; **ketoconazole** may increase **ziprasidone** levels; may enhance hypotensive effects of ANTIHYPERTENSIVE AGENTS; may antagonize effects of **levodopa;** increased risk of arrhythmias and heart block due to prolonged QT_c interval with ANTIARRHYTHMIC AGENTS, **amoxapine, arsenic trioxide, chlorpromazine, clarithromycin, daunorubicin, diltiazem, dolasetron, doxorubicin, droperidol, erythromycin, halofantrine, indapamide, levomethadyl,** LOCAL ANESTHETICS, **maprotiline, mefloquine, mesoridazine, octreotide, pentamidine, pimozide, probucol, gatifloxacin, grepafloxacin, levofloxacin, moxifloxacin, sparfloxacin,** TRICYCLIC ANTIDEPRESSANTS, **tacrolimus, thioridazine, troleandomycin;** additive CNS depression with SEDATIVE-HYPNOTICS, ANXIOLYTICS, **ethanol,** OPIATE AGONISTS.

PHARMACOKINETICS Absorption: Well absorbed with 60% reaching systemic circulation. **Peak:** 6–8 h. **Metabolism:** In liver (CYP3A4). **Elimination:** Feces and urine. **Half-Life:** 7 h.

NURSING IMPLICATIONS

Assessment & Drug Effects

- Lab tests: Baseline and periodic ECG, serum potassium and serum magnesium, especially with concomitant diuretic therapy. Periodically monitor blood glucose.
- Monitor diabetics for loss of glycemic control.
- Monitor for S&S of torsade de pointes (e.g., dizziness, palpitations, syncope), tardive dyskinesia (see Appendix F) especially in older adult women and with prolonged therapy, and the appearance of an unexplained rash. Withhold drug and report to physician immediately if any of these develop.
- Monitor for signs and symptoms of suicidality.
- Monitor I&O ratio and pattern: Notify physician if diarrhea, vomiting or any other conditions develops which may cause electrolyte imbalance.
- Monitor BP lying, sitting, and standing. Report orthostatic hypotension to physician.
- Monitor cognitive status and take appropriate precautions.
- Monitor for loss of seizure control, especially with a history of seizures or dementia.

Patient & Family Education

- Carefully monitor blood glucose levels if diabetic.
- Be aware that therapeutic effect may not be evident for several weeks.
- Report any of the following to a health care provider immediately: Palpitations, faintness or loss of consciousness, rash, abnormal muscle movements, vomiting or diarrhea.
- Do not drive or engage in potentially hazardous activities until response to drug is known.
- Make position changes slowly and in stages to prevent dizziness upon arising.
- Avoid strenuous exercise, exposure to extreme heat, or other activities that may cause dehydration.

ZOLEDRONIC ACID

(zo-le-dron'ic)

Aclasta ♦, Reclast, Zometa

Classifications: BISPHOSPHONATE; REGULATOR, BONE METABOLISM

Therapeutic: BONE METABOLISM REGULATOR

Prototype: Etidronate disodium

Pregnancy Category: D

Z

AVAILABILITY 4 mg/5 mL, 5 mg/100 mL injection

ACTION & *THERAPEUTIC EFFECT* Zoledronic acid inhibits various stimulatory factors of osteoclastic activity produced by bone tumors. It also induces osteoclast apoptosis. *Zoledronic acid blocks osteoclastic resorption of bone, thus reducing the amount of calcium released from bone.*

USES Treatment of hypercalcemia of malignancy, multiple myeloma, and bony metastases from solid tumors, Paget's disease (Reclast), postmenopausal or glucocorticoid-induced osteoporosis (Reclast).

CONTRAINDICATIONS Hypersensitivity to zoledronic acid or other bisphosphonates; preexisting hypocalcemia; serum creatinine of 0.5 mg/dL; pregnancy (category D); lactation.

CAUTIOUS USE Aspirin-sensitive asthma; cancer chemotherapy; renal and/or hepatic impairment; dental work; multiple myeloma; older adults. Safety and effectiveness of zoledronic acid in children have not been established.

ROUTE & DOSAGE

Hypercalcemia of Malignancy (Zometa)

Adult: **IV** 4 mg over a minimum of 15 min. May consider retreatment if serum calcium has not returned to normal, may repeat after 7 days

Multiple Myeloma and Bony Metastases from Solid Tumors (Zometa)

Adult: **IV** 4 mg over a minimum of 15 min q3–4wk

Osteoporosis (Reclast)

Adult: **IV** 5 mg infusion once per year

Osteoporosis Prophylaxis in Postmenopausal Women

Adult: **IV** 5 mg every other year

Paget's Disease (Reclast)

Adult: **IV** 5 mg dose, retreatment may be necessary

Renal Impairment Dosage Adjustment (Zometa)

CrCl 50–60 mL/min: 3.5 mg; 40–49 mL/min: 3.3 mg; 30–39 mL/min: 3 mg; less than 30 mL/min: Do not use

Renal Impairment Dosage Adjustment (Reclast)

Do not use if CrCl less than 35 mL/min

ADMINISTRATION

Intravenous

Do not administer to anyone who is dehydrated or suspected of being dehydrated. Consult physician.

- Do not administer zoledronic acid unless patient is adequately rehydrated.
- Do not administer until serum creatinine values have been evaluated by the physician.

PREPARE: **IV Infusion:** *Injection Concentrate:* Withdraw required dose from the 4 mg/5 mL vial and dilute in 100 mL of D5W or NS. DO NOT use lactated Ringer's solution. ▪ If not used immediately, refrigerate. The total time between reconstitution and end of infusion must not exceed 24 h.

ADMINISTER: **IV Infusion:** Infuse a single dose over NO LESS than 15 min.

INCOMPATIBILITIES **Solution/additive and Y-site:** Do not mix or infuse with **calcium**-containing solutions (e.g., **lactated Ringer's**).

Z

▪ Store at 2°–8° C (36°–46° F) following dilution. ▪ **Must be** completely infused within 24 h of reconstitution.

ADVERSE EFFECTS (≥1%) **Body as a Whole:** *Fever,* flu-like syndrome, redness and swelling at injection site, asthenia, chest pain, leg edema, mucositis, rigors. **CNS:** *Insomnia, anxiety, confusion, agitation,* headache, somnolence. **CV:** *Hypotension.* **GI:** *Nausea, vomiting, constipation, abdominal pain, anorexia,* dysphagia. **Hematologic:** *Anemia,* granulocytopenia, thrombocytopenia, pancytopenia. **Metabolic:** *Hypophosphatemia, hypokalemia, hypomagnesemia,* hypocalcemia, dehydration. **Musculoskeletal:** Skeletal pain, arthralgias, osteonecrosis of the jaw in cancer patients. **Respiratory:** *Dyspnea, cough,* pleural effusion. **Skin:** Alopecia, dermatitis. **Urogenital:** Renal deterioration (increase in S_{cr}).

INTERACTIONS Drug: LOOP DIURETICS may increase risk of hypocalcemia; **thalidomide** and other NEPHROTOXIC DRUGS may increase risk of renal toxicity.

PHARMACOKINETICS Onset: 4–10 days. **Duration:** 3–4 wk. **Metabolism:** Not metabolized. **Elimination:** In urine. **Half-Life:** 146 h.

NURSING IMPLICATIONS

Assessment & Drug Effects

- Lab tests: Baseline renal function tests prior to each dose and periodically thereafter; periodic ionized calcium or corrected serum calcium levels, serum phosphate and magnesium, electrolytes, CBC with differential, Hct and Hgb.
- Notify physician immediately of deteriorating renal function as indicated by rising serum creatinine levels over baseline value.
- Withhold zoledronic acid and notify physician if serum creatinine is not within 10% of the baseline value.
- Monitor closely patient's hydration status. Note that loop diuretics should be used with caution due to the risk of hypocalcemia.
- Monitor for S&S of bronchospasm in aspirin-sensitive asthma patients; notify physician immediately.

Patient & Family Education

- Maintain adequate daily fluid intake. Consult with physician for guidelines.
- Report unexplained weakness, tiredness, irritation, muscle pain, insomnia, or flu-like symptoms.
- Use reliable means of birth control to prevent pregnancy. If you suspect you are pregnant, contact physician immediately.

ZOLMITRIPTAN

(zol-mi-trip'tan)

Zomig, Zomig ZMT, Zomig Nasal Spray

Classifications: SEROTONIN $5\text{-}HT_1$ RECEPTOR AGONIST; ERGOT ALKALOID

Therapeutic: ANTIMIGRAINE

Prototype: Sumatriptan

Pregnancy Category: C

AVAILABILITY 2.5 mg, 5 mg tablets orally disintegrating tablets; 5 mg nasal spray

ACTION & *THERAPEUTIC EFFECT* Selective serotonin ($5\text{-}HT_{1B/1D}$) receptor agonist. The agonist effects at $5\text{-}HT_{1B/1D}$ reverse the vasodilation of cranial blood vessels and inhibit release of pro-inflammatory neuropeptides. *Vasoconstricts dilated cranial blood vessels and decreased*

Z

neuropeptide release relieve the pain of a migraine headache.

USES Acute migraine headaches with or without aura.

CONTRAINDICATIONS Hypersensitivity to zolmitriptan; ischemic heart disease (angina pectoris, arteriosclerosis, ECG changes, history of MI or Prinzmetal's angina); cardiac arrhythmias, symptomatic Wolff-Parkinson-White syndrome, uncontrolled hypertension; hemiplegia or basilar migraine; concurrent administration of ergotamine or sumatriptan; PKU; children younger than 18 y.

CAUTIOUS USE Men older than 40 y; postmenopausal women; patients with other cardiac risk factors, such as diabetes, obesity, cigarette smoking, high cholesterol levels, strong family history of CAD; concurrent administration of MAOIs; GI disease, PVD, ischemic colitis, Raynaud's disease, cerebrovascular disease, stroke, intracranial bleeding; renal failure or renal disease; adults older than 65 y; pregnancy (category C), lactation.

ROUTE & DOSAGE

Acute Migraine

Adult: **PO** 2.5–5 mg, may repeat in 2 h if necessary (max: 10 mg/24 h) **Nasal Spray** One spray into one nostril

ADMINISTRATION

Oral

- Give any time after symptoms of migraine appear. Give 2.5 mg or less by breaking a 5 mg tablet in half. If headache returns, may repeat q2h up to 10 mg in 24 h.
- Do NOT give zolmitriptan within 24 h of an ergot-containing drug or other 5-HT_1 agonist.
- Discard unused tablets that have been removed from the packaging.

Intranasal

- Unit-dose spray device delivers a 5 mg dose. Do not exceed the maximum dose of 10 mg in 24 h.
- Store at 2°–25° C (36°–77° F) and protect from light.

ADVERSE EFFECTS (≥1%) **Body as a Whole:** Asthenia, fatigue, malaise, pain, pressure sensation, paresthesia, throat pressure, warm/cold sensations, hypesthesia. **CNS:** Somnolence, dizziness, drowsiness, headache, hypesthesia, decreased mental acuity, euphoria, tremor. **CV:** Coronary artery vasospasm, transient myocardial ischemia, MI, ventricular tachycardia, ventricular fibrillation, chest pain/tightness/heaviness, palpitations. **GI:** Dry mouth, nausea, vomiting. **Respiratory:** Dyspnea. **Skin:** Flushing. **Other:** Hot flushes.

INTERACTIONS Drug: Dihydroergotamine, methysergide, other 5-HT_1 AGONISTS may cause prolonged vasospastic reactions; SSRIS have rarely caused weakness, hyperreflexia, and incoordination; MAOIS should not be used with 5-HT_1 AGONISTS; **cimetidine** increases half-life of zolmitriptan. **Herbal: St. John's wort** may increase triptan toxicity.

PHARMACOKINETICS Absorption: Rapidly absorbed, 40% bioavailability. **Peak:** 2–3 h. **Distribution:** 25% protein bound. **Metabolism:** In liver to active metabolite. **Elimination:** Primarily in urine (65%), 30% in feces. **Half-Life:** 3 h.

NURSING IMPLICATIONS

Assessment & Drug Effects

- Monitor for therapeutic effectiveness: Relief or reduction of migraine pain within 1–4 h.

- Monitor cardiovascular status carefully following first dose in patients at risk for CAD (e.g., postmenopausal women, men older than 40 y, persons with known CAD risk factors) or coronary artery vasospasms.
- Periodic cardiovascular evaluation is recommended with long-term use.
- Report to physician immediately chest pain, nausea, or tightness in chest or throat that is severe or does not quickly resolve.

Patient & Family Education

- Carefully review patient information insert and guidelines for taking drug.
- Do NOT take zolmitriptan during the aura phase, but as early as possible after onset of migraine.
- Do not remove orally disintegrating tablet from blister until just prior to dosing.
- Concurrent oral contraceptive use may increase incidence of adverse effects.
- Contact physician immediately if any of the following occur after zolmitriptan use: Symptoms of angina (e.g., severe or persistent pain or tightness in chest or throat, sudden nausea), hypersensitivity (e.g., wheezing, facial swelling, skin rash, hives), fainting, or abdominal pain.
- Report any other adverse effects (e.g., tingling, flushing, dizziness) at next physician visit.

ZOLPIDEM Pr

(zol′-pi-dem)

Ambien, Ambien CR, Edluar, Tovalt ODT, Zolpimist

Classifications: ANXIOLYTIC; SEDATIVE-HYPNOTIC, NON-BENZODIAZEPINE

Therapeutic: SEDATIVE-HYPNOTIC; ANTIANXIETY

Pregnancy Category: C

Controlled Substance: Schedule IV

AVAILABILITY 5 mg, 10 mg tablets; 6.25 mg, 12.5 mg extended release tablets; 5 mg, 10 mg orally disintegrating tablets; lingual spray

ACTION & *THERAPEUTIC EFFECT* An agonist that binds the gamma-aminobutyric acid (GABA)-A receptor chloride channel, thus inhibiting its action potential in the cortical region of the brain. *Sedative, anticonvulsant, and antianxiety effects thought to be due to GABA-A agonism.*

USES Short-term treatment of insomnia.

CONTRAINDICATIONS Suicidal ideation; labor or obstetric delivery, children younger than 18 y.

CAUTIOUS USE Depressed patients, hepatic/renal impairment, older adults, alcohol or drug abuse; patients with compromised respiratory status, COPD, sleep apnea; chronic depression; pregnancy (category C).

ROUTE & DOSAGE

Short-Term Treatment of Insomnia

Adult: **PO** 10 mg (immediate release/ODT) OR 12.5 mg (extended release) at bedtime **Spray** 1–2 sprays before bedtime

Geriatric: **PO** 5 mg (immediate release) or 6.25 mg (extended release) at bedtime **Spray** 1 spray before bedtime (max: 2 sprays)

Hepatic Impairment Dosage Adjustment

5 mg (immediate release) or 6.25 mg (extended release) at bedtime

ADMINISTRATION

Oral

- Give immediately before bedtime; for more rapid sleep onset, do NOT give with or immediately after a meal.
- Extended release tablets should be swallowed whole. Ensure that they are not crushed or chewed.
- Store at room temperature, 15°–30° C (59°–86° F).

ADVERSE EFFECTS (≥1%) **CNS:** Headache on awakening, drowsiness or fatigue, lethargy, drugged feeling, depression, anxiety, irritability, dizziness, double vision. Confusion and falls reported in elderly. Doses greater than 10 mg may be associated with anterograde amnesia or memory impairment. **GI:** Dyspepsia, nausea, vomiting. **Other:** Myalgia.

INTERACTIONS Drug: CNS DEPRESSANTS, **alcohol,** PHENOTHIAZINES by augmenting CNS depression. **Food:** Extent and rate of absorption of zolpidem are significantly decreased.

PHARMACOKINETICS Absorption: Readily from GI tract. 70% reaches systemic circulation. **Onset:** 7–27 min. **Peak:** 0.5–2.3 h. **Duration:** 6–8 h. **Distribution:** Highly protein bound. Lowest concentrations in CNS, highest concentrations in glandular tissue and fat. Crosses placenta. **Metabolism:** In the liver to 3 inactive metabolites. **Elimination:** 79–96% in the bile, urine, and feces. **Half-Life:** 1.7–2.5 h.

NURSING IMPLICATIONS

Assessment & Drug Effects

- Assess respiratory function in patients with compromised respiratory status. Report immediately to physician significantly depressed respiratory rate (less than 12/min).
- Monitor patients for S&S of depression (see Appendix F); zolpidem may increase level of depression.
- Monitor closely older adult or debilitated patients for impaired cognitive or motor function and unusual sensitivity to the drug's effects.

Patient & Family Education

- Avoid taking alcohol or other CNS depressants while on zolpidem.
- Do not drive or engage in other potentially hazardous activities until response to drug is known.
- Report vision changes to physician.
- Note: Onset of drug is more rapid when taken on an empty stomach.

ZONISAMIDE Pr

(zon-i'sa-mide)

Zonegran

Classifications: ANTICONVULSANT; SULFONAMIDE

Therapeutic: ANTICONVULSANT

Pregnancy Category: C

AVAILABILITY 25 mg, 50 mg, 100 mg capsules

ACTION & *THERAPEUTIC EFFECT* A broad-spectrum anticonvulsant that facilitates dopaminergic and serotonergic neurotransmission but does not potentiate the activity of gamma-aminobutyric acid (GABA) in the synapses of the CNS neurons. *Suppresses focal spike discharges and electroshock seizures. Effective against a variety of seizure types.*

USES Adjunctive therapy for partial seizures in adults.

UNLABELED USES Bipolar disorder.

CONTRAINDICATIONS Hypersensitivity to sulfonamides or zonisamide; lactation; children younger than 16 y.

CAUTIOUS USE Renal or hepatic insufficiency, dehydration, hypovolemia; renal impairment; older adults; pregnancy (category C).

ROUTE & DOSAGE

Partial Seizures
Adult: **PO** Start at 100 mg daily, may increase after 2 wk to 200 mg/day, may then increase q2wk, if necessary (max: 400 mg/day in 1–2 divided doses)

ADMINISTRATION

Oral
- Do not crush or break capsules; ensure capsules are swallowed whole with adequate fluid.
- Withdraw drug gradually when discontinued to minimize seizure potential.
- Store at 25° C (77° F); room temperature permitted. Protect from light and moisture.

ADVERSE EFFECTS (≥1%) **Body as a Whole:** Flu-like syndrome, weight loss. **CNS:** Agitation, irritability, anxiety, ataxia, confusion, depression, difficulty concentrating, difficulty with memory, *dizziness,* fatigue, *headache,* insomnia, mental slowing, nervousness, nystagmus, paresthesia, schizophrenic behavior, *somnolence,* tiredness, tremor, convulsion, abnormal gait, hyperesthesia, incoordination. **GI:** Abdominal pain, *anorexia,* constipation, diarrhea, dyspepsia, nausea, dry mouth, flatulence, gingivitis, gum hyperplasia, gastritis, stomatitis, cholelithiasis, glossitis, melena, rectal hemorrhage, ulcerative stomatitis, ulcer, dysphagia. **Metabolic:** Oligohidrosis, sometimes resulting in heat stroke and hyperthermia in children. **Respiratory:** Rhinitis, pharyngitis, cough. **Skin:** Ecchymosis, rash, pruritus. **Special Senses:** Difficulties in verbal expression, diplopia, speech abnormalities, taste perversion, amblyopia, tinnitus. **Urogenital:** Kidney stones.

INTERACTIONS Drug: Phenytoin, carbamazepine, phenobarbital, valproic acid may decrease half-life of zonisamide.

PHARMACOKINETICS Peak: 2–6 h. **Distribution:** 40% protein bound, extensively binds to erythrocytes. **Metabolism:** Acetylated in liver by CYP3A4. **Elimination:** Primarily in urine. **Half-Life:** 63–105 h.

NURSING IMPLICATIONS

Assessment & Drug Effects
- Withhold drug and notify physician if an unexplained rash or S&S of hypersensitivity appear (see Appendix F).
- Monitor for and report S&S of CNS impairment (somnolence, excessive fatigue, cognitive deficits, speech or language problems, incoordination, gait disturbances); oligohidrosis (lack of sweating) and hyperthermia in pediatric patients.
- Lab tests: Periodic BUN and serum creatinine, and CBC with differential.

Patient & Family Education
- Do not abruptly stop taking this medication.
- Increase daily fluid intake to minimize risk of renal stones. Notify physician immediately of S&S of renal stones: Sudden back or abdominal pain, and blood in urine.
- Report any of the following: Dizziness, excess drowsiness, frequent headaches, malaise, double vision, lack of coordination, persistent nausea, sore throat, fever, mouth ulcers, or easy bruising.
- Exercise special caution with concurrent use of alcohol or CNS depressants.
- Do not drive or engage in other potentially hazardous activities until response to drug is known.

Appendixes

◆ APPENDIX A

(Generic names are in **bold**)

APPENDIX A-1

OCULAR MEDICATIONS:

BETA-ADRENERGIC BLOCKERS Prototype for classification: Propranolol HCl Use: Intraocular hypertension and chronic open-angle glaucoma.

Betaxolol HCl Betoptic, Betoptic S, 0.25%, 0.5% solution	*Adult:* **Topical** 1 drop of 0.5% solution or 0.25% suspension in affected eye twice daily.
Carteolol HCl Ocupress, 1% solution	*Adult:* **Topical** 1 drop b.i.d.
Levobetaxolol Betaxon, 0.5% suspension	*Adult:* **Topical** 1 drop b.i.d.
Levobunolol Betagan, 0.25%, 0.5% solution	*Adult:* **Topical** 1–2 drops 1–2 times/day.
Metipranolol HCl OptiPranolol, 0.3% solution	*Adult:* **Topical** 1 drop b.i.d.
Timolol maleate Betimol, Timoptic, Timoptic XE, Istalol, 0.25%, 0.5% solution	*Adult:* **Topical** 1 drop of 0.25–0.5% solution b.i.d.; may decrease to daily. Apply gel daily. Apply Istalol solution once daily.

Adverse Effects/Clinical Implications: May cause *mild ocular stinging* and discomfort; tearing; may also have the adverse effects of systemic beta-blockers. May mask symptoms of acute hypoglycemia in diabetic patients (tachycardia, tremor, but not sweating). May precipitate thyroid storm in patients with hyperthyroidism. Patients with impaired cardiac function and the elderly should report to physician signs and symptoms of CHF (see Appendix G). Monitor BP for hypotension and heart rate for bradycardia.

MIOTICS Prototype for classification: Pilocarpine HCl Use: Open-angle and angle-closure glaucomas; to reduce IOP and to protect the lens during surgery and laser iridotomy; to counteract effects of mydriatics and cycloplegics following surgery or ophthalmoscopic examination.

Apraclonidine HCl Iopidine, 0.5%, 1% solution	**Intraoperative and Postsurgical Increase in IOP:** *Adult:* **Topical** 1 drop of 1% solution in affected eye 1 h before surgery and 1 drop in same eye immediately after surgery. **Open-Angle Glaucoma:** *Adult:* **Topical** 1 drop of 0.5% solution in affected eye q12h.

Brimonidine tartrate Alphagan P, 0.1%, 0.15% solution	**Glaucoma:** *Adult:* **Topical** 1 drop in affected eye(s) t.i.d. approximately 8 h apart.
Brinzolamide Azopt, 1% suspension	**Ocular Hypertension or Open-Angle Glaucoma:** *Adult:* **Topical** 1 drop in affected eye(s) t.i.d.
Carbachol Carbastat, Miostat, 0.01% solution	*Adult:* **Intraocular** 0.5 ml of 0.01% solution injected into anterior chamber of eye.
Dorzolamide Trusopt, 2% solution	**Ocular Hypertension or Open-Angle Glaucoma:** *Adult, Child:* **Topical** 1 drop in affected eye(s) t.i.d.
Echothiophate iodide Phospholine Iodide, 0.125% solution	**Glaucoma:** *Adult:* **Topical** 1 drop of 0.03–0.25% solution in conjunctival sac 1–2 times/day. **Accommodative Esotropia:** *Adult:* **Topical** ***Diagnosis:*** 1 drop of 0.125% solution in both eyes once/day at bedtime for 2–3 wk. ***Treatment:*** 1 drop of 0.125% solution every other day or 1 drop of 0.06% solution daily (max: 1 drop 0.125% solution daily).
Pilocarpine HCl Isopto Carpine, Miocarpine, Pilopine HS, 0.5%, 1%, 2%, 3%, 4%, 6% solution	**Acute Glaucoma:** *Adult:* **Topical** 1 drop of 1–2% solution in affected eye q5–10min for 3–6 doses, then 1 drop q1–3h until IOP is reduced. **Chronic Glaucoma:** *Adult:* **Topical** 1 drop of 0.5–4% solution in affected eye q4–12h or 1 ocular system (Ocusert) q7days **Miotic:** *Adult:* **Topical** 1 drop of 1% solution in affected eye.

Adverse Effects/Clinical Implications: Ocular: Ciliary spasm with brow ache, twitching of eyelids, eye pain with change in eye focus, miosis, *diminished vision in poorly illuminated areas,* blurred vision, reduced visual acuity, sensitivity, contact allergy, lacrimation, follicular conjunctivitis, conjunctival irritation, cataract, retinal detachment. **CNS:** *Headache, drowsiness,* depression, syncope. **GI:** Abnormal taste, dry mouth. **Clinical Implications:** Wait 15 min after instillation before inserting soft contact lenses to avoid staining the lenses. Use with MAO inhibitors may have increased risk of hypertensive emergency. May increase the effects of beta-blockers and other antihypertensives on blood pressure and heart rate. TCAs may reduce the effects of **brimonidine. Brinzolamide** is a carbonic anhydrase inhibitor (prototype: Acetazolamide) and is a sulfonamide. It should not be used by patients with sulfa allergies. Reconstituted solutions of **echothiophate** remain stable for 1 mo at room temperature. Expiration date should appear on label. The length of time solutions remain stable under refrigeration varies with manufacturer. **Echothiophate** therapy is generally discontinued 2–6 wk before surgery. If necessary, alternate miotic therapy is substituted. Medication should be given in the evening. Give at least 5 min apart from other topical ophthalmic drugs. The patient with brown or hazel eyes may require a stronger ophthalmic solution or more frequent instillation of **physostigmine** for desired effects than the patient with blue eyes.

PROSTAGLANDINS Prototype for classification: Latanoprost
Use: Open-angle glaucoma and intraocular hypertension.

Bimatoprost Lumigan, 0.03% solution	*Adult:* **Topical** 1 drop in affected eye(s) once daily in the evening.
Latanoprost Xalatan, 0.005% solution	*Adult:* **Topical** 1 drop (1.5 mcg) in affected eye(s) once daily in the evening.
Travoprost Travatan, 0.004% solution	*Adult:* **Topical** 1 drop in affected eye(s) once daily in the evening.

Adverse Effects: Ocular: *Conjunctival hyperemia, growth of eyelashes, ocular pruritus,* ocular dryness, visual disturbance, ocular burning, foreign body sensation, eye pain, pigmentation of the periocular skin, blepharitis, cataract, superficial punctate keratitis, eyelid erythema, ocular irritation, eyelash darkening, eye discharge, tearing, photophobia, allergic conjunctivitis, increases in iris pigmentation (brown pigment), conjunctival edema. **Body as a Whole:** Headaches, abnormal liver function tests, asthenia, and hirsutism. **Clinical Implications:** Should instill in the evening. Wait 15 min after instillation before inserting soft contact lenses to avoid staining the lenses. Give at least 5 min apart from other topical ophthalmic drugs.

MYDRIATIC Prototype for classification: Homatropine HBr
Use: Mydriatic for ocular examination and as cycloplegic to measure errors of refraction. Also inflammatory conditions of uveal tract, ciliary spasm, as a cycloplegic and mydriatic in preoperative and postoperative conditions, and as an optical aid in select patients with axial lens opacities.

Cyclopentolate HCl AK-Pentolate, Cyclogyl, 0.5%, 1%, 2% solution	**Cycloplegic Refraction:** *Adult:* **Topical** 1 drop of 1% solution in eye 40–50 min before procedure, followed by 1 drop in 5 min; may need 2% solution in patients with darkly pigmented eyes. *Child:* **Topical** 1 drop of 0.5–1% solution in eye 40–50 min before procedure, followed by 1 drop in 5 min; may need 2% solution in patients with darkly pigmented eyes.
Dipivefrin HCl Propine, 0.1% solution	**Glaucoma:** *Adult:* **Topical** 1 drop in eye q12h.

Homatropine HBr AK-Homatropine, Homatrine, Isopto Homatropine, 2%, 5% solution	**Cycloplegic Refraction:** *Adult:* **Topical** 1–2 drops of 2% or 5% solution in eye repeated in 5–10 min if necessary. **Ocular Inflammation:** *Adult:* **Topical** 1–2 drops of 2% or 5% solution in eye up to q3–4h.
Hydroxyamphetamine HBr/ Tropicamide Paremyd, 0.25%, 1% solution	**Dilation of pupil:** *Adult:* **Topical** 1–2 drops in conjunctival sac.
Phenylephrine HCl AK-Dilate Ophthalmic, Alconefrin, Mydfrin, Neo-Synephrine, 0.12%, 0.125%, 0.16%, 0.25%, 0.5%, 1%, 1.5%, 10% solution	**Ophthalmoscopy:** *Adult:* **Topical** 1 drop of 2.5% or 10% solution before examination. *Child:* **Topical** 1 drop of 2.5% solution before examination. **Vasoconstrictor:** *Adult:* **Topical** 2 drops of 0.12–0.15% solution q3–4h as necessary.
Tropicamide Mydriacyl, Tropicacyl, 0.5%, 1% solution	**Refraction:** *Adult:* **Topical** 1–2 drops of 1% solution in each eye, repeat in 5 min; if patient is not seen within 20–30 min, an additional drop may be instilled. **Examination of Fundus:** *Adult:* **Topical** 1–2 drops of 0.5% solution in each eye 15–20 min prior to examination; may repeat q30min if necessary.

Contraindicated in: Primary (narrow-angle) glaucoma or predisposition to glaucoma; children younger than 6 y. **Cautious Use in:** Increased IOP, infants, children, pregnancy (category C), the elderly or debilitated; hypertension; hyperthyroidism; diabetes; cardiac disease. **Adverse Effects:** Increased IOP, *blurred vision, photophobia*. **Prolonged Use:** Local irritation, congestion, edema, eczema, follicular conjunctivitis. **Excessive Dosage/Systemic Absorption:** Symptoms of atropine poisoning (flushing, dry skin, mouth, nose; decreased sweating; fever, rash, rapid/irregular pulse; abdominal and bladder distention; hallucinations, confusion). **CNS:** Psychotic reaction, behavior disturbances, ataxia, incoherent speech, restlessness, hallucinations, somnolence, disorientation, failure to recognize people, grand mal seizures. **Clinical Implications:** Carefully monitor **cyclopentolate** patients with seizure disorders, since systemic absorption may precipitate a seizure. Photophobia associated with mydriasis may require patient to wear dark glasses. Since drug causes blurred vision, supervision of activity may be indicated.

VASOCONSTRICTOR; DECONGESTANT **Prototype for classification: Naphazoline HCl** **Use:** Ocular vasoconstrictor.

Naphazoline HCl AK-Con, Albalon, Allerest, Clear Eyes, Comfort, Degest-2, Nafazair, Naphcon, Privine, VasoClear, Vasocon, 0.012%, 0.02%, 0.03%, 0.1% solution	*Adult:* **Topical** 1–3 drops of 0.1% solution q3–4h prn or 1–2 drops of a 0.01–0.03% solution q4h prn.
Tetrahydrozoline HCl Collyrium, Mallazine, Murine Plus, Optigene, Soothe, Tyzine, Visine, 0.05% solution	*Adult:* **Topical** 1–2 drops of 0.05% solution in eye b.i.d. or t.i.d.

Contraindicated in: Narrow-angle glaucoma; concomitant use with MAO INHIBITORS or TRICYCLIC ANTIDEPRESSANTS **Cautious Use in:** Hypertension, cardiac irregularities, advanced arteriosclerosis; diabetes; hyperthyroidism; elderly patients. **Adverse Effects:** Pupillary dilation, increased intraocular pressure, rebound redness of the eye, headache, hypertension, nausea, weakness, sweating. **Overdosage:** Drowsiness, hypothermia, bradycardia, shocklike hypotension, coma.

CORTICOSTEROID, ANTI-INFLAMMATORY **Prototype for classification: Hydrocortisone** **Use:** Inflammation. **Unlabeled Use:** Anterior uveitis.

Dexamethasone sodium phosphate Maxidex Ophthalmic, 0.1% suspension	*Adult:* **Topical** 1–2 drops in conjunctival sac up to 4–6 times/day; may instill hourly for severe disease.
Difluprednate Durezol, 0.05% suspension	*Adult:* **Topical** 1 drop in conjunctival sac q.i.d. for the first 24 h; q.i.d. for 2 wk then b.i.d. for 2 wk.
Fluorometholone Fluor-Op, FML Forte, FML Liquifilm, FML S.O.P., 0.1%, 0.25% suspension; 0.1% ointment	*Adult/Child (older than 2 y):* **Topical** 1–2 drops of suspension in conjunctival sac q.h. for the first 24–48 h; then b.i.d. to q.i.d.; or a thin strip of ointment q4h for the first 24–48 h; then 1–3 times/day.
Loteprednol etabonate Alrex, Lotemax, 0.2%, 0.5% suspension	*Adult:* **Topical** 1–2 drops in conjunctival sac q.i.d. during initial treatment, may increase to q1h if necessary.

Prednisolone sodium phosphate Inflamase Mild, Pred Mild, Prednisol, Inflamase Forte, 0.11%, 0.12%, 0.9% suspension	*Adult:* **Topical** 1–2 drops in conjunctival sac q.h. during the day; then q2h at night; may decrease to 1 drop t.i.d. or q.i.d.
Rimexolone Vexol, 1% solution	**Postoperative Ocular Inflammation:** *Adult:* **Topical** 1–2 drops q.i.d. beginning 24 h after surgery, continue through first 2 wk postoperatively. **Anterior Uveitis:** *Adult:* **Topical** 1–2 drops in affected eye every hour while awake for first week, then q2h for second week, then taper frequency until uveitis resolves.

Contraindicated in: Ocular fungal diseases, *herpes simplex* keratitis, ocular infections, ocular mycobacterial infections, viral disease of cornea or conjunctiva such as vaccinia, varicella. **Adverse Effects: Ocular:** Blurred vision, photophobia, conjunctival edema, corneal edema, erosion, eye discharge, dryness, irritation, pain; prolonged use: Glaucoma, ocular hypertension, damage to optic nerve, defects in visual acuity and visual fields, posterior subcapsular cataract formation, secondary ocular infections. **Other:** Headache, taste perversion. **Clinical Implications:** Shake all products well before use.

OCULAR ANTIHISTAMINES Prototype for classification: Emedastine
Use: Relief of signs and symptoms of allergic conjunctivitis.

Azelastine HCl OPTIVAR, 0.05% solution	*Adult/Child (older than 3 y):* **Topical** 1 drop in affected eye(s) b.i.d.
Bepotastine Bepreve, 1.5% solution	*Adult:* **Topical** 1 drop in affected eye(s) b.i.d.
Cromolyn sodium Crolom, Opticrom, 4% solution	*Adult:* **Topical** 1–2 drops in each eye 4–6 times/day.
Emedastine difumarate Emadine, 0.05% solution	*Adult/Child (older than 3 y):* **Topical** 1 drop in affected eye(s) up to q.i.d.
Epinastine hydrochloride Elestat, 0.05% solution	*Adult/Child (older than 3 y):* **Topical** 1 drop in affected eye(s) up to b.i.d.
Ketotifen fumarate Zaditor, 0.025% solution	*Adult:* **Topical** 1 drop in affected eye(s) q8–12h.
Lodoxamide Alomide, 0.1% solution	*Adult/Child (older than 2 mo):* **Topical** 1–2 drop in affected eye(s) q.i.d. for up to 3 mo.
Nedocromil sodium Alocril, 2% solution	*Adult/Child (older than 3 y):* **Topical** 1–2 drops in affected eye(s) b.i.d.
Olopatadine HCl Patanol, 0.1% solution Pataday, 0.2% solution Patanase, 665 mcg nasal spray	*Adult/Child (older than 3 y):* **Topical** 1–2 drops in affected eye(s) b.i.d. at least 6–8 h apart. *Adult/Adolescent:* **Intranasal** 1 spray in each nostril b.i.d.

Pemirolast potassium Alamast, 0.1% solution	*Adult:* **Topical** 1–2 drops in affected eye(s) q.i.d.

Adverse Effects: Ocular: Allergic reactions, *burning, stinging,* discharge, dry eyes, eye pain, eyelid disorder, itching, keratitis, lacrimation disorder, mydriasis, photophobia, rash. **CNS:** Drowsiness, fatigue, headache. **Other:** Dry mouth, cold syndrome, pharyngitis, rhinitis, sinusitis, taste perversion. **Clinical Implications:** Wait 10 min after instilling **emedastine** before inserting soft contact lenses; do not use **olopatadine** with soft contact lenses.

OCULAR NONSTEROIDAL ANTI-INFLAMMATORY DRUGS:
Prototype for classification: Ibuprofen **Use:** Treatment of ocular pain and inflammation associated with cataract surgery.

Bromfenac Xibrom, 0.09% solution	*Adult:* **Topical** 1 drop into affected eye(s) b.i.d. beginning 24 h after cataract surgery and continuing for 14 days.
Ketorolac Acular, Acuvail, 0.45%, 0.5% solution	*Adult:* **Topical** 1 drop to affected eye(s) 4 times/day beginning 24 h after surgery and continuing for 14 days.
Nepafenac Nevanac, 0.1% suspension	*Adult/Child (older than 10 y):* **Topical** 1 drop into affected eye(s) t.i.d. beginning 24 h after cataract surgery and continuing for 14 days.

Adverse Effects: Ocular: Conjunctival hyperemia, ocular hypertension, foreign body sensation, decreased visual acuity, headache, iritis, ocular inflammation (e.g., edema, erythema), ocular irritation (burning/stinging), ocular pruritus, ocular pain, photophobia, lacrimation, abnormal sensation in the eye, delayed wound healing, keratitis, lid margin crusting, corneal erosion, corneal perforation, corneal thinning, and epithelial breakdown. Continued use can lead to ulceration or perforation. **Clinical Implications: Nepafenac** suspension **must be** shaken well prior to use.

OCULAR ANTIBIOTIC, QUINOLONE
Prototype for classification: Ciprofloxacin **Use:** Treatment of ocular infection.

Besifloxacin Besivance, 0.6% suspension	*Adult/Adolescent/Child:* **Topical** 1 drop in affected eye(s) t.i.d. × 7 days
Ciprofloxacin Ciloxin, 0.3% solution	*Adult/Adolescent/Child (older than 1 y):* **Topical** 1–2 drops in affected eye(s) q2h × 2 days then q4h × 5 days.
Gatifloxacin Zymar, 0.3% solution	*Adult/Adolescent/Child (older than 1 y):* **Topical** 1 drop in affected eye(s) q2h × 2 days then 1 drop in affected eye(s) up to 4 times/day.
Moxifloxacin Vigamox, 0.5% solution	*Adult/Child (older than 1 y):* **Topical** 1 drop in affected eye(s) t.i.d. × 7 days.

Adverse Effects: Ocular: Conjunctival redness, blurred vision, irritation, pain, pruritus. **CNS:** Headache.

APPENDIX A-2

LOW MOLECULAR WEIGHT HEPARINS:

ANTICOAGULANT, LOW MOLECULAR WEIGHT HEPARIN Prototype for classification: Enoxaparin Use: Prevention and treatment of DVT following hip or knee replacement or abdominal surgery, unstable angina, acute coronary syndromes.

Dalteparin sodium Fragmin, 10,000 international units/mL, 25,000 international units/mL	**DVT Prophylaxis, Abdominal Surgery:** *Adult:* **Subcutaneous** 2500 international units daily starting 1–2 h prior to surgery and continuing for 5–10 days postoperatively. **DVT Prophylaxis, Total Hip Arthroplasty:** *Adult:* **Subcutaneous** 2500–5000 international units daily starting 1–2 h prior to surgery and continuing for 5–14 days postoperatively. **Acute Thromboembolism:** *Adult:* **Subcutaneous** 120 international units/kg b.i.d. for at least 5 days. **Recurrent Thromboembolism:** *Adult:* **Subcutaneous** 5000 international units b.i.d. for 3–6 mo. **Unstable Angina/Non–Q-Wave MI:** *Adult:* **Subcutaneous** 120 international units/kg (max: 10,000 international units) q12h. **DVT Prophylaxis with risk of PE:** *Adult:* **Subcutaneous** 5000 international units once daily for 12–14 days. **Extended Treatment of VTE or Proximal DVT:** *Adult:* **Subcutaneous** 200 international units/kg daily for 1 mo then 150 international units/kg daily for 2-6 mo.
Enoxaparin Lovenox, 100 mg/mL	**Prevention of DVT after Hip or Knee Surgery:** *Adult:* **Subcutaneous** 30 mg subcutaneously b.i.d. for 10–14 days starting 12–24 h post-surgery. **Prevention of DVT after Abdominal Surgery:** *Adult:* **Subcutaneous** 40 mg daily starting 2 h before surgery and continuing for 7–10 days (max: 12 days). **Treatment of DVT and Pulmonary Embolus:** *Adult:* **Subcutaneous** 1 mg/kg b.i.d.; monitor anti-Xa activity to determine appropriate dose. **Acute Coronary Syndrome:** *Adult:* **Subcutaneous** 1 mg/kg q12h × 2–8 days. Give concurrently with aspirin 100–325 mg/day.
Tinzaparin sodium Innohep, 20,000 international units/mL	**Treatment of DVT:** *Adult:* **Subcutaneous** 175 anti-Xa international units/kg daily × at least 6 days.

Contraindicated in: Hypersensitivity to ardeparin, other low molecular weight heparins, pork products, or parabens; active major bleeding, thrombocytopenia that is positive for antiplatelet antibodies with ardeparin; uncontrolled hypertension; nursing mothers. **Cautious Use in:** Hypersensitivity to heparin; history of heparin-induced thrombocytopenia; bacterial endocarditis; severe and uncontrolled hypertension, cerebral aneurysm or hemorrhagic stroke, bleeding disorders, recent GI bleeding or associated GI disorders (e.g., ulcerative colitis), thrombocytopenia, or platelet disorders; severe liver or renal disease, diabetic retinopathy, hypertensive retinopathy, invasive procedures; pregnancy (category C). **Adverse Effects: Body as a Whole:** Allergic reactions (rash, urticaria), arthralgia, pain and inflammation at injection site, peripheral edema, fever. **CNS:** *CVA,* dizziness, headache, insomnia. **CV:** Chest pain. **GI:** Nausea, vomiting. **Hematologic:** *Hemorrhage,* thrombocytopenia, ecchymoses, anemia. **Respiratory:** Dyspnea. **Skin:** Rash, pruritus. **Drug Interactions: Aspirin,** NSAIDS, **warfarin** can increase risk of hemorrhage **Clinical Implications:** Alternate injection sites using the abdomen, anterior thigh, or outer aspect of upper arms. **Lab Tests:** CBC with platelet count, urinalysis, and stool for occult blood should be tested throughout therapy. Routine coagulation tests are not required. Carefully monitor for and immediately report S&S of excessive anticoagulation (e.g., bleeding at venipuncture sites or surgical site) or hemorrhage (e.g., drop in BP or Hct). Patients on oral anticoagulants, platelet inhibitors, or with impaired renal function **must be** very carefully monitored for hemorrhage. Patient should be sitting or lying supine for injection. Inject deep subcutaneously with entire length of needle inserted into skin fold. Hold skin fold gently throughout injection and do not rub site after injection.

APPENDIX A-3

INHALED CORTICOSTEROIDS (ORAL AND NASAL INHALATIONS):

CORTICOSTEROID, ANTIINFLAMMATORY Prototype for classification: Hydrocortisone Use: Oral inhalation to treat steroid-dependent asthma, nasal inhalation for the management of the symptoms of seasonal or perennial rhinitis.

Beclomethasone dipropionate Beconase AQ, QVAR, Vancenase AQ	**Asthma:** *Adult:* **Oral Inhaler** 2 inhalations t.i.d. or q.i.d. up to 20 inhalations/day; may try to reduce systemic steroids after 1 wk of concomitant therapy; QVAR 40–80 mcg b.i.d. (max: 320 mcg/day). *Child (6–12 y):* **Oral Inhaler** 1–2 inhalations t.i.d. or q.i.d. up to 10 inhalations/day; QVAR 5–11 y, 40–80 mcg b.i.d. (max: 160 mcg/day). **Allergic Rhinitis:** *Adult:* **Nasal Inhaler** 1 spray per nostril b.i.d. to q.i.d. *Child (older than 6 y):* 1–2 sprays daily.

Budesonide Pulmicort, Turbuhaler, Pulmicort, Respules, Rhinocort, Rhinocort Aqua, Rhinocort, Turbuhaler	**Asthma, Maintenance Therapy:** *Adult:* **Oral Inhalation** 1 or 2 inhalations (200 mcg/inhalation) daily–b.i.d. (max: 800 mcg b.i.d.). *Child (6 y or older):* **Oral Inhalation** 1 inhalation (200 mcg/inhalation) daily–b.i.d. (max: 400 mcg b.i.d.). *Child (12 mo–8 y):* **Nebulization** 0.5 mg/day in 1–2 divided doses. **Rhinitis:** *Adult/Child (6 y or older):* **Intranasal** 2 sprays per nostril in the morning and evening or 4 sprays per nostril in the morning. Each actuation releases 32 mcg from the nasal adapter.
Ciclesonide Omnaris, 50 mcg/spray 80 mcg, 160 mcg inhaled solution	**Rhinitis:** *Adult/Child (older than 6 y):* **Intranasal** 1–2 sprays per nostril once daily (200 mcg/day). **Asthma:** *Adult/Child (older than 12 y):* **Inhaled** 80 mcg b.i.d.; may increase to 160 mcg b.i.d.
Dexamethasone Decadron, Decaspray, 0.04% solution	*Adult:* **Oral Inhalation** Up to 3 inhalations t.i.d. or q.i.d. (max: 12 inhalations/day). **Intranasal** 2 sprays per nostril b.i.d. or t.i.d. (max: 12 sprays/day). *Child:* **Oral Inhalation** Up to 2 inhalations q.i.d. (max: 8 inhalations/day). **Intranasal** 1 or 2 sprays per nostril b.i.d. (max: 8 sprays/day).
Flunisolide AeroBid, Nasalide, Nasarel, 250 mcg/spray	**Allergic Rhinitis:** *Adult:* **Inhaled/Intranasal** 2 sprays orally, or intranasally per nostril, b.i.d.; may increase to t.i.d., if needed. *Child:* **Inhaled/Intranasal** 6–14 y, 1 spray orally, or intranasally per nostril t.i.d. or 2 sprays b.i.d.
Fluticasone Flonase, Flovent, Flovent HFA, 44 mcg, 110 mcg, 220 mcg aerosol, Veramyst, 27.5 mcg/actuation	**Seasonal Allergic Rhinitis:** *Adult:* **Intranasal** 100 mcg (1 inhalation) per nostril 1–2 times daily (max: 4 times daily). **Inhalation** 1–2 inhalations b.i.d. *Child (4 y or older):* **Intranasal** 1 spray per nostril once daily. May increase to 2 sprays per nostril once daily if inadequate response, then decrease to 1 spray per nostril once daily when control is achieved. *Adult/Adolescent/Child (12 y or older):* **Intranasal (Veramyst)** 2 sprays per nostril daily then reduce to 1 spray daily. *Child (2–11 y):* **Intranasal (Veramyst)** 1 spray per nostril daily, may increase to 2 sprays per nostril daily if necessary. *Adult/Adolescent:* **Inhaled (Advair)** 1–2 inhalations q12h
Mometasone furoate Asmanex, Nasonex, Twisthaler, 220 mcg/inhalation, 50 mcg/inhalation	*Adult:* **Intranasal** 2 sprays (50 mcg each) in each nostril once daily. *Child (2 y or older):* **Intranasal** 1 spray in each nostril once daily. *Adult/Child (older than 12 y):* **Powder for Inhalation** 1 inhalation (220 mcg) once daily (max: 1 inhalation b.i.d.). *Child (4–11 y):* **Powder for Inhalation** 100 mcg daily.

Triamcinolone acetonide Azmacort, 100 mcg/ inhalation	*Adult:* **Inhalation** 2 puffs 3–4 times/day (max: 16 puffs/day) or 4 puffs b.i.d. **Nasal Spray** 2 sprays/nostril once daily (max: 8 sprays/day). *Child (6–12 y):* **Inhalation** 1–2 sprays t.i.d. or q.i.d. (max: 12 sprays/day) or 2–4 sprays b.i.d.

Contraindicated in: Nonasthmatic bronchitis, primary treatment of status asthmaticus, acute attack of asthma. **Cautious Use in:** Patients receiving systemic corticosteroids; use with extreme caution if at all in respiratory tuberculosis, untreated fungal, bacterial, or viral infections, and ocular herpes simplex; nasal inhalation therapy for nasal septal ulcers, nasal trauma, or surgery. **Adverse Effects: Oral Inhalation:** *Candidal infection of oropharynx* and occasionally larynx, hoarseness, dry mouth, sore throat, sore mouth. **Nasal (Inhaler):** *Transient nasal irritation, burning, sneezing,* epistaxis, bloody mucous, nasopharyngeal itching, dryness, crusting, and ulceration; headache, nausea, vomiting. **Other:** With excessive doses, symptoms of hypercorticism. Increase risk of adverse effects if Advair is used with other long-acting beta-agonists. **Clinical Implications:** Note that oral inhalation and nasal inhalation products are not to be used interchangeably. **Oral Inhaler:** Emphasize the following: (1) Shake inhaler well before using. (2) After exhaling fully, place mouthpiece well into mouth with lips closed firmly around it. (3) Inhale slowly through mouth while activating the inhaler. (4) Hold breath 5–10 sec, if possible, then exhale slowly. (5) Wait 1 min between puffs. Clean inhaler daily. Separate parts as directed in package insert, rinse them with warm water, and dry them thoroughly. Rinsing mouth and gargling with warm water after each oral inhalation removes residual medication from oropharyngeal area. Mouth care may also delay or prevent onset of oral dryness, hoarseness, and candidiasis. **Nasal Inhaler:** Directions for use of nasal inhaler provided by manufacturer should be carefully reviewed with patient. Emphasize the following points: (1) Gently blow nose to clear nostrils. (2) Shake inhaler well before using. (3) If 2 sprays in each nostril are prescribed, direct one spray toward upper, and the other toward lower part of nostril. (4) Wash cap and plastic nosepiece daily with warm water; dry thoroughly. Inhaled steroids do not provide immediate symptomatic relief and are not prescribed for this purpose.

APPENDIX A-4

TOPICAL CORTICOSTEROIDS:

CORTICOSTEROID, ANTI-INFLAMMATORY Prototype for classification: Hydrocortisone Use: As a topical corticosteroid, the drug is used for the relief of the inflammatory and pruritic manifestations of corticosteroid-responsive dermatoses.

Contraindicated in: Topical steroids contraindicated in presence of varicella, vaccinia, on surfaces with compromised circulation, and in children younger than 2 y. **Cautious Use in:** Children; diabetes mellitus; stromal *herpes simplex;* glaucoma, tuberculosis of eye; osteoporosis; untreated fungal, bacterial, or viral infections **Adverse Effects: Skin:** Skin thinning and atrophy, *acne, impaired wound healing;* petechiae, ecchymosis, easy bruising; suppression of skin test reaction; hypopigmentation

Hydrocortisone Aeroseb-HC, Alphaderm, Cetacort, Cortaid, Cortenema, Dermolate, Hytone, Rectacort, Synacort, Caldecort, 0.5%, 1%, 2.5% cream, lotion, ointment, spray **Hydrocortisone acetate** Anusol HC, Carmol HC, Coli foam, Cortaid, Cort-Dome, Corticaine, Cortifoam, Epifoam, 0.5%, 1% ointment, cream	*Adult:* **Topical** Apply a small amount to the affected area 1–4 times/day. **PR** Insert 1% cream, 10% foam, 10–25 mg suppository, or 100 mg enema nightly.
Alclometasone dipropionate Aclovate, 0.05% cream, ointment	*Adult:* **Topical** 0.05% cream or ointment applied sparingly b.i.d. or t.i.d.; may use occlusive dressing for resistant dermatoses.
Amcinonide Cyclocort, 0.1% cream, lotion, ointment	*Adult:* **Topical** Apply thin film b.i.d. or t.i.d.
Betamethasone dipropionate Diprolene, Diprolene AF, Diprosone, Maxivate, 0.05% cream, gel, lotion, ointment	*Adult:* **Topical** Apply thin film b.i.d.
Betamethasone valerate Luxiq, Valisone, Psorion, Beta-Val, 0.1% cream, ointment, lotion; 0.12% aerosol foam	*Adult:* **Topical** Apply sparingly b.i.d.
Clobetasol propionate Clobex, Cormax, Embeline, Olux, Temovate, 0.05% cream, gel, ointment, lotion, aerosol foam	*Adult:* **Topical** Apply sparingly b.i.d. (max: 50 g/wk), or b.i.d. 3 day/wk or 1–2 times/wk for up to 6 mo.
Clocortolone pivalate Cloderm, 0.1% cream	*Adult:* **Topical** Apply thin layer 1–4 times/day.
Desonide DesOwen, Tridesilon, 0.05% cream, ointment, lotion	*Adult:* **Topical** Apply thin layer b.i.d. to q.i.d.
Desoximetasone Topicort, Topicort-LP, 0.05% cream, ointment	*Adult:* **Topical** Apply thin layer b.i.d.

Diclofenac Flector, Pennsaid, 1.3% topical patch; 1% topical gel	*Adult:* **Topical** Up to 4 g 4 times/day on affected joint (max: 16 g).
Diflorasone diacetate Florone, Florone E, Maxiflor, Psorcon E, Psorcon, 0.05% cream, ointment	*Adult:* **Topical** Apply thin layer of ointment 1–3 times/day or cream 2–4 times/day.
Fluocinolone acetonide Fluoderm, Synalar, 0.025% ointment, cream 0.2% cream; 0.01% cream, solution, shampoo, oil; 0.59 mg ophthalmic insert	*Adult:* **Topical** Apply thin layer b.i.d. to q.i.d.
Fluocinonide Lidemol, Lidex, Lidex-E, Lyderm, Topsyn, Vanos, 0.05% cream, ointment, solution, gel; 0.1% cream	*Adult:* **Topical** Apply thin layer b.i.d. to q.i.d.
Flurandrenolide Cordran, Cordran SP, Drenison, 0.025% ointment, cream; 0.05% ointment, cream, lotion	*Adult:* **Topical** Apply thin layer b.i.d. or t.i.d.; apply tape 1–2 times/day at 12 h intervals. *Child:* **Topical** Apply thin layer 1–2 times/day; apply tape once/day.
Fluticasone Cutivate, 0.005%, 0.05% cream; 0.005% ointment	*Adult/Child (older than 3 mo):* **Topical** Apply a thin film of cream or ointment to affected area once or twice daily.
Halcinonide Halog, 0.1% cream, ointment, solution	*Adult:* **Topical** Apply thin layer b.i.d. or t.i.d. *Child:* **Topical** Apply thin layer once/day.
Halobetasol Ultravate, 0.05% cream, ointment	*Adult:* **Topical** Apply sparingly b.i.d.
Mometasone furoate Elocon, 0.1% cream, lotion, ointment	*Adult:* **Topical** Apply a thin film of cream or ointment or a few drops of lotion to affected area once/day.
Triamcinolone Aristocort, Kenacort, Kenalog, Triderm, 0.025%, 0.5%, 0.1% cream; 0.025%, 0.5%, 0.1% ointment; 0.025%, 0.1% lotion	*Adult:* **Topical** Apply sparingly b.i.d. or t.i.d.

or hyperpigmentation, hirsutism, acneiform eruptions, subcutaneous fat atrophy; allergic dermatitis, urticaria, angioneurotic edema, increased sweating. **Clinical Implications:** Administer retention enema preferably after a bowel movement. The enema should be retained at least 1 h or all night if possible. If an occlusive dressing is to be used, apply medication sparingly, rub until it disappears, and then reapply, leaving a thin coat over lesion. Completely cover area with transparent plastic or other occlusive device or vehicle. Avoid covering a weeping or exudative lesion. Usually, occlusive dressings are not applied to face, scalp, scrotum, axilla, and groin. Inspect skin carefully between applications for ecchymotic, petechial, and purpuric signs, maceration, secondary infection, skin atrophy, striae or miliaria; if present, stop medication and notify physician. Warn patient not to self-dose with OTC topical preparations of a corticosteroid more than 7 days. They should not be used for children younger than 2 y. If symptoms do not abate, consult physician. Usually, topical preparations are applied after a shower or bath when skin is damp or wet. Cleansing and application of prescribed preparation should be done with extreme gentleness because of fragility, easy bruisability, and poor-healing skin. Hazard of systemic toxicity is higher in small children because of the greater ratio of skin surface area to body weight. Apply sparingly. Urge patient on long-term therapy with topical corticosterone to check expiration date.

Schedule I

High potential for abuse and of no currently accepted medical use. Examples: heroin, LSD, marijuana, mescaline, peyote. Not obtainable by prescription but may be legally procured for research, study, or instructional use.

Schedule II

High abuse potential and high liability for severe psychological or physical dependence. Prescription required and cannot be renewed.[a] Includes opium derivatives, other opioids, and short-acting barbiturates. Examples: amphetamine, cocaine, meperidine, morphine, secobarbital.

Schedule III

Potential for abuse is less than that for drugs in Schedules I and II. Moderate to low physical dependence and high psychological dependence. Includes certain stimulants and depressants not included in the above schedules and preparations containing limited quantities of certain opioids. Examples: chlorphentermine, glutethimide, mazindol, paregoric, phendimetrazine. Prescription required.[b]

Schedule IV

Lower potential for abuse than Schedule III drugs. Examples: certain psychotropics (tranquilizers), chloral hydrate, chlordiazepoxide, diazepam, meprobamate, phenobarbital. Prescription required.[a]

Schedule V

Abuse potential less than that for Schedule IV drugs. Preparations contain limited quantities of certain narcotic drugs; generally intended for antitussive and antidiarrheal purposes and may be distributed without a prescription provided that:

1. Such distribution is made only by a pharmacist.
2. Not more than 240 mL or not more than 48 solid dosage units of any substance containing opium, nor more than 120 mL or not more than 24 solid dosage units of any other controlled substance may be distributed at retail to the same purchaser in any given 48-hour period without a valid prescription order.
3. The purchaser is at least 18 years old.
4. The pharmacist knows the purchaser or requests suitable identification.
5. The pharmacist keeps an official written record of: name and address of purchaser, name and quantity of controlled substance purchased, date of sale, initials of dispensing pharmacist. This record is to be made available for inspection and copying by U.S. officers authorized by the Attorney General.

6. Other federal, state, or local law does not require a prescription order.

Under jurisdiction of the Federal Controlled Substances Act:
[a]Except when dispensed directly by a practitioner, other than a pharmacist, to an ultimate user, no controlled substance in Schedule II may be dispensed without a *written* prescription, except that in emergency situations such drug may be dispensed upon oral prescription and a written prescription must be obtained within the time frame prescribed by law. No prescription for a controlled substance in Schedule II may be refilled.
[b]Refillable up to 5 times within 6 mo, but only if so indicated by physician.

◆ APPENDIX C FDA PREGNANCY CATEGORIES

The FDA requires that all prescription drugs absorbed systemically or known to be potentially harmful to the fetus be classified according to one of five pregnancy categories (A, B, C, D, X). The identifying letter signifies the level of risk to the fetus and is to appear in the precautions section of the package insert. The categories described by the FDA are as follows:

Category A

Controlled studies in women fail to demonstrate a risk to the fetus in the first trimester (and there is no evidence of risk in later trimesters), and the possibility of fetal harm appears remote.

Category B

Either animal-reproduction studies have not demonstrated a fetal risk but there are no controlled studies in pregnant women, or animal-reproduction studies have shown an adverse effect (other than a decrease in fertility) that was not confirmed in controlled studies in women in the first trimester (and there is no evidence of a risk in later trimesters).

Category C

Either studies in animals have revealed adverse effects on the fetus (teratogenic or embryocidal effects or other) and there are no controlled studies in women, or studies in women and animals are not available. Drugs should be given only if the potential benefit justifies the potential risk to the fetus.

Category D

There is positive evidence of human fetal risk, but the benefits from use in pregnant women may be acceptable despite the risk (e.g., if the drug is needed in a life-threatening situation or for a serious disease for which safer drugs cannot be used or are ineffective). There will be an appropriate statement in the "warnings" section of the labeling.

Category X

Studies in animals or human beings have demonstrated fetal abnormalities or there is evidence of fetal risk based on human experience, or both, and the risk of the use of the drug in pregnant women clearly outweighs any possible benefit. The drug is contraindicated in women who are or may become pregnant. There will be an appropriate statement in the "contraindications" section of the labeling.

◆ APPENDIX D ORAL DOSAGE FORMS THAT SHOULD NOT BE CRUSHED

Some oral dosage forms should not be crushed or chewed. These dosage forms have been specially designed to release the drug slowly over several hours, to protect the drug from the low pH of the stomach, and/or to protect the stomach from the irritating effects of the drug.

Drugs may have an **enteric coating** which is designed to allow the drug to pass through the stomach intact with the drug being released in the intestines. This protects the stomach from the irritating effects of the drug, protects the drug from being destroyed by the acid pH of the stomach, and can delay the onset of action.

Extended release (slow release, SR) formulations are designed to release the drug over an extended period of time. These formulations can include multiple-layer compressed tablets where drug is released as each layer dissolves, mixed-release pellets that dissolve at different time intervals, and special tablets that are themselves inert but are designed to release drug slowly from the formulation. Some extended release dosage forms are scored and may be broken in half without affecting the release mechanism but still should not be crushed or chewed. Some mixed-release capsule formulations can be opened and the contents sprinkled on food. However, the pellets should not be crushed or chewed. Some extended release formulations can be identified by common abbreviations used in their brand names. These abbreviations include: CR (controlled release), CRT (controlled release tablet), LA (long acting), SR (sustained release), TR (time release), SA (sustained action), and XL or XR (extended release).

Occasionally, drugs should not be crushed because they are oral mucosa irritants, are extremely bitter, or contain dyes that may stain teeth or mucosal tissue. Many medications that are combinations (containing multiple ingredients) should not be split.

The table contains a list of drugs found in the Guide that should not be crushed or chewed. A liquid dosage form may be available for many of these drugs. However, the dose or frequency of administration may be different from the slow-release product. Check with your pharmacist for liquid availability and dosing conversions.

	Generic Name	Comments
Accutane	isotretinoin	mucous membrane irritant
AcipHex	rabeprazole	slow release
Actiq Oralet	fentanyl citrate	lozenge product
Adalat CC	nifedipine	slow release
Adderall XR	amphetamine	slow release
Advicor	niacin/lovastatin	slow release

	Generic Name	Comments
Aggrenox	aspirin/dipyridamole	slow release; may be opened and contents taken without crushing
Allegra D	fexofenadine/ pseudoephedrine	slow release
Aptivus	tipranavir	taste
Arthrotec	diclofenac/misoprostol	enteric coated
Asacol	mesalamine	slow release
Augmentin XR	amoxicillin/clavulanic acid	slow release; may be scored and broken
Avinza	morphine	slow release; capsule may be opened
Avodart	dutasteride	skin contact may cause tumor production
Azor	amlodipine/olmesartan	combination product
Azulfidine En-tabs	sulfasalazine	enteric coated
Bayer Extra Strength Enteric 500	aspirin, enteric coated	enteric coated; slow release
Bayer Low Adult 81 mg	aspirin, enteric coated	enteric coated
Bayer Caplet	aspirin, enteric coated	enteric coated
Biaxin XL	clarithromycin	slow release
Bisacodyl	bisacodyl	enteric coated
Bisco-Lax	bisacodyl	enteric coated
Boniva	ibandronate	irritant
Calan SR	verapamil	slow release; may break tablet
Cama Arthritis Strength	aspirin, magnesium oxide, aluminum hydroxide	special tablet formulation
Cardizem, Cardizem CD, Cardizem SR, Cardizem LA	diltiazem	slow release; capsules may be opened and contents taken without chewing or crushing
Ceftin	cefuroxime	taste; use liquid formulation
Cellcept	mycophenolate	teratogenic potential
Chloral Hydrate	chloral hydrate	liquid-filled capsule
Chlor-Trimeton Repetab	chlorpheniramine	slow release
Choledyl SA	oxtriphylline	slow release

	Generic Name	Comments
Cipro	ciprofloxacin	taste
Compazine Spansule	prochlorperazine	slow release; capsules may be opened and contents taken without chewing or crushing
Concerta	methylphenidate	slow release
Constant T	theophylline	slow release; capsules may be opened and contents taken without chewing or crushing
Cotazym S	pancrelipase	enteric coated; capsules may be opened and contents taken without chewing or crushing
Covera-HS	verapamil	slow release
Cymbalta	duloxetine	enteric coated
Deconamine SR	chlorpheniramine, pseudoephedrine	slow release
Depakene	valproic acid	slow release; mucous membrane irritant
Depakote	valproate disodium	enteric coated
Desoxyn Gradumets	methamphetamine	slow release
Detrol LA	tolterodine	slow release
Dexedrine Spansule	dextroamphetamine	slow release
Diamox Sequels	acetazolamide	slow release
Dilacor XR	diltiazem	slow release
Dilatrate-SR	isosorbide dinitrate	slow release
Disophrol Chronotab	dexbrompheniramine, pseudoephedrine	slow release
Donnatal Extentab	atropine, scopolamine, hyoscyamine, phenobarbital	slow release
Donnazyme	pancreatin, pepsin, bile salts, atropine, scopolamine, hyoscyamine, phenobarbital	slow release
Drixoral	dexbrompheniramine, pseudoephedrine	slow release
Dulcolax	bisacodyl	enteric coated
Duratuss	phenylephedrine, guaifenesin	slow release

	Generic Name	Comments
Easprin	aspirin	enteric coated
Ecotrin	aspirin	enteric coated
E.E.S. 400	erythromycin ethyl-succinate	enteric coated
Effexor XR	venlafaxine	slow release
Elixophyllin SR	theophylline	slow release; capsules may be opened and contents taken without chewing or crushing
E-Mycin	erythromycin	enteric coated
Ergostat	ergotamine	sublingual tablet
Eryc	erythromycin	enteric coated; capsules may be opened and contents taken without chewing or crushing
Ery-Tab	erythromycin	enteric coated
Erythrocin Stearate	erythromycin	enteric coated
Erythromycin Base	erythromycin	enteric coated
Eskalith CR	lithium	slow release
Fedahist Timecaps	chlorpheniramine, pseudoephedrine	slow release
Feldene	piroxicam	mucous membrane irritant
Feosol	ferrous sulfate	enteric coated
Feosol Spansule	ferrous sulfate	slow release; capsules may be opened and contents taken without chewing or crushing
Fergon	ferrous gluconate	slow release; capsules may be opened and contents taken without chewing or crushing
Ferro-Sequels	ferrous fumarate, docusate	slow release
Fero-Gradumet	ferrous sulfate	slow release
Festal II	pancrelipase	enteric coated
Glucophage XR	metformin	slow release
Glucotrol XL	glipizide	slow release
Gris-Peg	griseofulvin ultramicrosize	crushing may result in precipitation of drug as larger particles
Ilotycin	erythromycin	enteric coated

	Generic Name	Comments
Imdur	isosorbide mononitrate	slow release
Inderal LA	propranolol	slow release
Indocin SR	indomethacin	slow release; capsules may be opened and contents taken without chewing or crushing
Intelence	etravirine	*may be dissolved in water
Isoptin SR	verapamil	slow release
Iso-Bid	isosorbide dinitrate	slow release
Isosorbide Dinitrate SR	isosorbide dinitrate	slow release
Isuprel Glossets	isoproterenol	sublingual
Janumet	sitagliptin/metformin	combination product
Kadian	morphine	slow release
Kaon CL 10	potassium chloride	slow release
Klor-Con	potassium chloride	slow release
Klotrix	potassium chloride	slow release
K-Tab	potassium chloride	slow release
Levsinex Timecaps	hyoscyamine	slow release
Lithobid	lithium	slow release
Meprospan	meprobamate	slow release; capsules may be opened and contents taken without chewing or crushing
Mestinon Timespan	pyridostigmine	slow release
Micro K	potassium chloride	slow release
MS Contin	morphine	slow release
Mucinex	guaifenesin	slow release
Nico-400	niacin	slow release
Nicobid	niacin	slow release
Nitro Bid	nitroglycerin	slow release; capsules may be opened and contents taken without chewing or crushing
Nitroglyn	nitroglycerin	slow release; capsules may be opened and contents taken without chewing or crushing
Nitrong SR	nitroglycerin	slow release

	Generic Name	Comments
Norflex	orphenadrine	slow release
Norpace CR	disopyramide	slow release
Novafed A	pseudoephedrine, chlorpheniramine	slow release
Oramorph SR	morphine	slow release
Pancrease	pancrelipase	enteric coated
Papaverine Sustained Action	papaverine	slow release
PBZ-SR	tripelennamine hydrochloride	slow release
Perdiem	psyllium hydrophilic mucilloid	wax coated
Peritrate SA	pentaerythritol tetranitrate	slow release
Permitil Chronotab	fluphenazine	slow release
Phazyme, Phazyme 95	simethicone	slow release
Phyllocontin	aminophylline	slow release
Plendil	felodipine	slow release
Polaramine Repetabs	dexchlorpheniramine	slow release
Prevacid	lansoprazole	slow release; capsules may be opened and contents taken without chewing or crushing
Prilosec	omeprazole	slow release
Procainamide HCl SR	procainamide	slow release
Procan SR	procainamide	slow release
Procardia XL	nifedipine	slow release
Pronestyl SR	procainamide	slow release
Proventil Repetabs	albuterol	slow release
Quibron-T SR	theophylline	slow release
Quinaglute Dura Tabs	quinidine gluconate	slow release
Quinidex Extentabs	quinidine sulfate	slow release
Respid	theophylline	slow release

	Generic Name	Comments
Ritalin SR	methylphenidate	slow release
Robimycin Robitab	erythromycin	enteric coated
Rondec TR	pseudoephedrine, carbinoxamine	slow release
Roxanol SR	morphine	slow release
Sinemet CR	levodopa, carbidopa	slow release; tablet is scored and may be broken in half
Slo-Bid Gyrocaps	theophylline	slow release; capsules may be opened and contents taken without chewing or crushing
Slo-Phyllin Gyrocaps	theophylline	slow release; capsules may be opened and contents taken without chewing or crushing
Slow-Fe	ferrous sulfate	slow release
Slow-K	potassium chloride	slow release
Sorbitrate SA	isosorbide dinitrate	slow release
Strattera	atomoxetine	slow release
Sudafed 12 hour	pseudoephedrine	slow release
Tarka	trandolapril, verapamil	slow release
Teldrin	chlorpheniramine	slow release; capsules may be opened and contents taken without chewing or crushing
Tepanil Ten-Tab	diethylpropion	slow release
Tessalon Perles	benzonatate	slow release
Theo-24	theophylline	slow release
Thorazine Spansule	chlorpromazine	slow release
Toprol XL	metoprolol	slow release
Trental	pentoxifylline	slow release
Trilafon Repetabs	perphenazine	slow release
Triptone Caplets	scopolamine	slow release
Uniphyl	theophylline	slow release
Valrelease	diazepam	slow release
Verelan	verapamil	slow release; capsules may be opened and contents taken without chewing or crushing
Volmax	albuterol	slow release

	Generic Name	Comments
Wellbutrin SR, Wellbutrin XL	bupropion	slow release; mucous membrane irritant
ZORprin	aspirin	slow release
Zyban	bupropion	slow release

Note: This listing is not comprehensive. Please check with your pharmacist for additional questions.

Information from The Institute for Safe Medication Practices available at: http://www.ismp.org/tools/DoNotCrush.pdf

◆ APPENDIX E PRESCRIPTION COMBINATION DRUGS*

Acanya (ANTIACNE) *gel:* benzoyl peroxide 2.5%/clindamycin (see p. 348) 1.2%.

Accuretic (ANTIHYPERTENSIVE) *tablet:* quinapril (see p. 1325) 10 mg/hydrochlorothiazide (see p. 749) 12.5 mg; 20 mg quinapril (see p. 1325)/12.5 mg hydrochlorothiazide; 20 mg quinapril/25 mg hydrochlorothiazide.

Activella (HORMONE REPLACEMENT THERAPY) *tablet:* estradiol (see p. 587) 1 mg/norethindrone acetate (see p. 1107) 0.5 mg.

Actonel with Calcium (BISPHOSPHONATE) *tablet:* risedronate (see p. 1364) 35 mg/1250 calcium carbonate (see p. 224).

ACTOplus Met (ANTIDIABETIC) *tablet:* pioglitazone (see p. 1236) 15 mg/metformin (see p. 969) 500 mg; pioglitazone 15 mg/metformin 850 mg.

Advair Diskus (BRONCHODILATOR) *Inhalation powder:* fluticasone propionate (see p. 671) 100 mcg/salmeterol (see p. 1380) 50 mcg; fluticasone propionate 250 mcg/salmeterol 50 mcg; fluticasone propionate 115 mcg/salmeterol 21 mcg; fluticasone propionate 230 mcg/salmeterol 21 mcg; fluticasone propionate 45 mcg/salmeterol 21 mcg.

Advicor (ANTILIPEMIC) *tablets, sustained release:* niacin (see p. 1082) 500 mg/lovastatin (see p. 918) 20 mg; niacin 1000 mg/lovastatin 20 mg.

Aggrenox (ANTIPLATELET) *extended release capsule:* dipyridamole (see p. 488) 200 mg/aspirin (see p. 120) 25 mg.

Aldactazide 25/25 (DIURETIC) *tablet:* spironolactone (see p. 1424) 25 mg/hydrochlorothiazide (see p. 749) 25 mg.

Aldactazide 50/50 (DIURETIC) *tablet:* spironolactone (see p. 1424) 50 mg/hydrochlorothiazide (see p. 749) 50 mg.

Allegra D 12 hour (ANTIHISTAMINE, DECONGESTANT) *tablet, extended release:* fexofenadine (see p. 643) 60 mg/pseudoephedrine (see p. 1312) 120 mg.

Allegra D 24 hour (ANTIHISTAMINE, DECONGESTANT) *tablet, extended release:* fexofenadine (see p. 643) 180 mg/pseudoephedrine (see p. 1312) 240 mg.

Anexsia (NARCOTIC ANALGESIC [schedule III]) *tablet:* hydrocodone (see p. 751) 5 mg/acetaminophen (see p. 9) 500 mg.

Anexsia 5/325 (NARCOTIC ANALGESIC [schedule III]) *tablet:* hydrocodone (see p. 751) 5 mg/acetaminophen (see p. 9) 325 mg.

Anexsia 7.5/325 (NARCOTIC ANALGESIC [schedule III]) *tablet:* hydrocodone (see p. 751) 7.5 mg/acetaminophen (see p. 9) 325 mg.

Anexsia 7.5/650 (NARCOTIC ANALGESIC [schedule III]) *tablet:* hydrocodone (see p. 751) 7.5 mg/acetaminophen (see p. 9) 650 mg.

Angeliq (HORMONE) *tablet:* drospirenone 0.5 mg/estradiol (see p. 587) 1 mg.

Apresazide 25/25 (ANTIHYPERTENSIVE) *capsule:* hydralazine hydrochloride (see p. 747) 25 mg/hydrochlorothiazide (see p. 749) 25 mg.

Apresazide 50/50 (ANTIHYPERTENSIVE) *capsule:* hydralazine hydrochloride (see p. 747) 50 mg/hydrochlorothiazide (see p. 749) 50 mg.

Apresodex (ANTIHYPERTENSIVE) *tablet:* hydralazine hydrochloride (see p. 747) 25 mg/hydrochlorothiazide (see p. 749) 15 mg.

*For a complete list that includes non-prescription drugs, please see our companion website at www.prenhall.com

Aralen Phosphate with Primaquine Phosphate (ANTIMALARIAL) *tablet:* chloroquine phosphate (see p. 309) 500 mg (300 mg base)/primaquine phosphate (see p. 1278) 79 mg (45 mg base).

Arthrotec 50 (NSAID) *tablet:* diclofenac sodium (see p. 466) 50 mg/misoprostol (see p. 1024) 200 mcg.

Arthrotec 75 (NSAID) *tablet:* diclofenac sodium (see p. 466) 75 mg/misoprostol (see p. 1024) 200 mcg.

Atacand HCT (ANTIHYPERTENSIVE) *tablet:* candesartan (see p. 232) 32 mg/hydrochlorothiazide (see p. 749) 12.5 mg; candesartan 16 mg/hydrochlorothiazide 12.5 mg.

Atripla (ANTIRETROVIRAL) *tablet:* 600 mg efavirenz (see p. 537)/200 mg emtricitabine (see p. 543)/300 mg tenofovir (see p. 1475).

Augmentin (ANTIBIOTIC) *tablet:* amoxicillin (see p. 83) 250 mg/clavulanic acid 125 mg; amoxicillin 500 mg/clavulanic acid 125 mg; amoxicillin 875 mg/clavulanic acid 125 mg; amoxicillin 1000 mg/clavulanic acid 125 mg; *chewable tablet:* amoxicillin 125 mg/clavulanic acid 31.25 mg; amoxicillin 200 mg/clavulanic acid 28.5 mg; amoxicillin 250 mg/clavulanic acid 62.5 mg; amoxicillin 400 mg/clavulanic acid 57 mg; *suspension (per 5 mL):* amoxicillin 125 mg/clavulanic acid 31.25 mg; amoxicillin 200 mg/clavulanic acid 28.5 mg; amoxicillin 250 mg/clavulanic acid 62.5 mg; amoxicillin 400 mg/clavulanic acid 57 mg; amoxicillin 600 mg/clavulanic acid 42.9 mg.

Auralgan Otic (OTIC PREPARATION: DECONGESTANT, ANALGESIC) *solution:* acetic acid 0.1%, antipyrine 5.4%, benzocaine (see p. 164) 1.4%, u-polycosanol 410 0.01%.

Avalide (ANTIHYPERTENSIVE) *tablet:* irbesartan (see p. 820) 150 mg/hydrochlorothiazide (see p. 749) 12.5 mg; irbesartan 300 mg/hydrochlorothiazide 12.5 mg; irbesartan 300 mg/hydrochlorothiazide 25 mg.

Avandamet (HYPOGLYCEMIC AGENT) *tablet:* 1 mg rosiglitazone maleate (see p. 1377)/500 mg metformin HCl (see p. 969); 2 mg rosiglitazone/500 mg metformin; 4 mg rosiglitazone/500 mg metformin; 2 mg rosiglitazone/1000 mg metformin; 4 mg rosiglitazone/1000 mg metformin.

Avandaryl (HYPOGLYCEMIC AGENT) *tablet:* rosiglitazone (see p. 1377) 4 mg/glimepiride (see p. 712) 1 mg; rosiglitazone 4 mg/glimepiride 2 mg; rosiglitazone 4 mg/glimepiride 4 mg.

Azo Gantanol (URINARY ANTI-INFECTIVE, ANALGESIC) *tablet:* sulfamethoxazole (see p. 1439) 500 mg, phenazopyridine hydrochloride (see p. 1211) 100 mg.

Azo Gantrisin (URINARY ANTI-INFECTIVE, ANALGESIC) *tablet:* sulfisoxazole (see p. 1445) 500 mg/phenazopyridine hydrochloride (see p. 1211) 50 mg.

Azor (ANTIHYPERTENSIVE) *tablet:* amlodipine (see p. 79) 10 mg/olmesartan (see p. 1122) 20 mg; amlodipine 10 mg/olmesartan 40 mg; amlodipine 5 mg/olmesartan 20 mg; amlodipine 5 mg/olmesartan 40 mg.

B-A-C (ANALGESIC) acetaminophen (see p. 9) 650 mg/caffeine (see p. 218) 40 mg/butalbital 50 mg.

Bacticort Ophthalmic (ANTI-INFLAMMATORY) *suspension:* hydrocortisone (see p. 752) 1%/neomycin sulfate (see p. 1075) 0.35%/polymyxin B (see p. 1250) 10,000 units.

Bactrim (URINARY TRACT AGENT) *tablet:* sulfamethoxazole (see p.

1439) 400 mg/trimethoprim (see p. 1564) 80 mg.

Bactrim DS (URINARY TRACT AGENT) *tablet:* sulfamethoxazole (see p. 1439) 800 mg/trimethoprim (see p. 1564) 160 mg.

Benicar HCT (ANTIHYPERTENSIVE) *tablet:* 20 mg olmesartan medoxomil (see p. 1122)/12.5 mg hydrochlorothiazide (see p. 749); 40 mg olmesartan medoxomil/12.5 mg hydrochlorothiazide; 40 mg olmesartan medoxomil/25 mg hydrochlorothiazide.

Betoptic Pilo Suspension (ANTIGLAUCOMA) *suspension:* betaxolol (see p. 173) 0.25%/pilocarpine (see p. 1230) 1.75%.

BiDil (ANTIHYPERTENSIVE) *tablet:* isosorbide dinitrate (see p. 833) 20 mg/hydralazine (see p. 747) 37.5 mg.

Blephamide (OPHTHALMIC STEROID, SULFONAMIDE) *suspension:* prednisolone acetate (see p. 1273 0.2%/sulfacetamide sodium (see p. 1436) 10%.

Blephamide S.O.P. (OPHTHALMIC STEROID, SULFONAMIDE) *ointment:* prednisolone acetate (see p. 1273) 0.2%/sulfacetamide sodium (see p. 1436) 10%.

Brevicon (MONOPHASIC ORAL CONTRACEPTIVE [ESTROGEN, PROGESTIN]) *tablet:* ethinyl estradiol (see p. 608) 35 mcg/norethindrone (see p. 1107) 0.5 mg.

Bromfed (DECONGESTANT, ANTIHISTAMINE) *sustained release capsule:* pseudoephedrine hydrochloride (see p. 1312) 120 mg/brompheniramine maleate (see p. 197) 12 mg.

Bromfed-PD (DECONGESTANT, ANTIHISTAMINE) *sustained release capsule:* pseudoephedrine hydrochloride (see p. 1312) 60 mg/brompheniramine maleate (see p. 197) 6 mg.

Bronchial Capsules (ANTIASTHMATIC) *capsule:* theophylline (see p. 1492) 150 mg/guaifenesin (see p. 728) 90 mg.

Caduet (ANTIHYPERTENSIVE/ANTILIPEMIC) *tablet:* 2.5 mg amlodipine (see p. 79)/10 mg atorvastatin (see p. 129); 2.5 mg amlodipine/20 mg atorvastatin; 2.5 mg amlodipine/40 mg atorvastatin; 5 mg amlodipine/10 mg atorvastatin; 10 mg amlodipine/10 mg atorvastatin; 5 mg amlodipine/20 mg atorvastatin; 10 mg amlodipine/20 mg atorvastatin; 5 mg amlodipine/40 mg atorvastatin; 10 mg amlodipine/40 mg atorvastatin; 5 mg amlodipine/80 mg atorvastatin; 10 mg amlodipine/80 mg atorvastatin.

Cafergot Suppositories (ANTIMIGRAINE) *suppository:* ergotamine tartrate (see p. 571) 2 mg/caffeine (see p. 218) 100 mg.

Cam-ap-es (ANTIHYPERTENSIVE) *suspension, tablet:* hydrochlorothiazide (see p. 749) 15 mg/reserpine (see p. 1346) 0.1 mg/hydralazine hydrochloride (see p. 747) 25 mg.

Capital with Codeine (NARCOTIC ANALGESIC [schedule V]) *suspension (per 5 mL):* codeine phosphate (see p. 370) 12 mg/acetaminophen (see p. 9) 120 mg.

Capozide 25/15 (ANTIHYPERTENSIVE) *tablet:* captopril (see p. 237) 25 mg, hydrochlorothiazide (see p. 749) 15 mg.

Capozide 25/25 (ANTIHYPERTENSIVE) *tablet:* captopril (see p. 237) 25 mg/hydrochlorothiazide (see p. 749) 25 mg.

Capozide 50/15 (ANTIHYPERTENSIVE) *tablet:* captopril (see p. 237) 50 mg/hydrochlorothiazide (see p. 749) 15 mg.

Capozide 50/25 (ANTIHYPERTENSIVE) *tablet:* captopril (see p. 237) 50 mg/hydrochlorothiazide (see p. 749) 25 mg.

Carisoprodol Compound (SKELETAL MUSCLE RELAXANT, ANALGESIC) *tablet:* carisoprodol (see p. 248) 200 mg/aspirin (see p. 120) 325 mg.

Carmol HC (ANTI-INFLAMMATORY) *cream:* hydrocortisone acetate (see p. 752) 1%/urea 10%.

Celestone-Soluspan (GLUCOCORTICOID) *injection (suspension) (per mL):* betamethasone acetate (see p. 171) 3 mg/betamethasone sodium phosphate (see p. 171) 3 mg.

Cetacaine (TOPICAL ANESTHETIC) *gel, liquid, ointment, aerosol:* benzocaine (see p. 164) 14%/tetracaine hydrochloride (see p. 1485) 2%/butamben 2%/benzalkonium chloride (see p. 163) 0.5%.

Cheracol Syrup (NARCOTIC ANTITUSSIVE, EXPECTORANT [schedule V]) *syrup (per 5 mL):* codeine phosphate (see p. 370) 10 mg/guaifenesin (see p. 728) 100 mg/alcohol 4.75%.

Cipro HC Otic (ANTI-INFECTIVE/ANTI-INFLAMMATORY) *topical:* ciprofloxacin (see p. 335) 2 mg/dexamethasone (see p. 442) 10 mg otic suspension.

Ciprodex Otic (ANTI-INFECTIVE/ANTI-INFLAMMATORY) *topical:* ciprofloxacin (see p. 335) 0.3%/dexamethasone (see p. 442) 0.1% otic suspension.

Claritin D (ANTIHISTAMINE, DECONGESTANT) loratadine (see p. 913), 5 mg/pseudoephedrine (see p. 1312) 120 mg; loratadine 10 mg/pseudoephedrine 240 mg.

Clarinex D 24 hr (ANTIHISTAMINE, DECONGESTANT) *tablet:* desloratadine (see p. 438) 5 mg/pseudoephedrine (see p. 1312) 240 mg.

Climara Pro (HORMONE REPLACEMENT THERAPY) *transdermal patch:* estradiol (see p. 587) 0.045 mg/levonorgestrel acetate 0.015 mg.

Codiclear DH Syrup (ANTITUSSIVE [schedule III]) *syrup (per 5 mL):* hydrocodone (see p. 751) 5 mg/guaifenesin (see p. 728) 100 mg/alcohol 10%.

Codimal DH (ANTITUSSIVE [schedule III]) *syrup (per 5 mL):* phenylephrine hydrochloride (see p. 1222) 5 mg/pyrilamine maleate 8.33 mg/hydrocodone bitartrate (see p. 751) 1.66 mg.

Codimal PH (ANTITUSSIVE [schedule III]) *syrup (per 5 mL):* codeine (see p. 370) 10 mg/pyrilamine maleate 8.33 mg/phenylephrine (see p. 1222) 5 mg.

Co-Gesic (NARCOTIC ANALGESIC [schedule V]) *tablet:* hydrocodone (see p. 751) 5 mg/acetaminophen (see p. 9) 500 mg.

Coly-Mycin S Otic (OTIC: STEROID, ANTIBIOTIC) *suspension (per mL):* hydrocortisone acetate (see p. 752) 1%/neomycin sulfate (see p. 1075) 3.3 mg/colistin sulfate 3 mg/thonzonium bromide 0.05%.

Combigan (GLAUCOMA) *ophthalmic solution:* brimonidine (see p. 195) 0.2%/timolol (see p. 1515) 0.5%.

CombiPatch (HORMONE REPLACEMENT THERAPY) *transdermal patch:* estradiol (see p. 587) 0.05 mg/norethindrone acetate (see p. 1107) 0.14 mg; estradiol 0.05 mg/norethindrone acetate 0.25 mg.

Combivir (ANTIVIRAL) *tablet:* zidovudine (see p. 1615) 300 mg/lamivudine (see p. 860) 150 mg.

Cortisporin (OPHTHALMIC STEROID, ANTIBIOTIC) *suspension (per mL):* hydrocortisone (see p. 751) 1%/neomycin sulfate (see p. 1075) (equivalent to 0.35% neomycin base)/polymyxin B sulfate (see p. 1250) 10,000 units.

Cortisporin Ointment (OPHTHALMIC STEROID, ANTIBIOTIC) *oint-*

ment: hydrocortisone (see p. 751) 1%/neomycin sulfate (see p. 1075) (equivalent to 0.35% neomycin base)/bacitracin zinc (see p. 150) 400 units, polymyxin B sulfate (see p. 1250) 10,000 units/g.

Corzide 40/5 (ANTIHYPERTENSIVE) *tablet:* nadolol (see p. 1049) 40 mg/bendroflumethiazide 5 mg.

Corzide 80/5 (ANTIHYPERTENSIVE) *tablet:* nadolol (see p. 1049) 80 mg/bendroflumethiazide 5 mg.

Cosopt (OPHTHALMIC, GLAUCOMA) *ophthalmic solution:* dorzolamide (see p. 507) 2%/timolol (see p. 1515) 0.5%.

Cotrim (ANTI-INFECTIVE) *tablet:* trimethoprim (see p. 1564) 80 mg/sulfamethoxazole (see p. 1439) 400 mg.

Cotrim DS (Double Strength) (ANTI-INFECTIVE) *tablet:* trimethoprim (see p. 1564) 160 mg/sulfamethoxazole (see p. 1439) 800 mg.

Cotrim Pediatric (ANTI-INFECTIVE) *suspension:* trimethoprim (see p. 1564) 40 mg/sulfamethoxazole (see p. 1439) 200 mg/5 mL.

Cyclomydril (OPHTHALMIC DECONGESTANT) *ophthalmic solution:* cyclopentolate hydrochloride (see p. 390) 0.2%/phenylephrine hydrochloride (see p. 1222) 1%.

Darvocet-A 500 (NARCOTIC AGONIST ANALGESIC [schedule IV]) *tablet:* propoxyphene napsylate (see p. 1301) 100 mg/acetaminophen (see p. 9) 500 mg.

Darvocet-N 50 (NARCOTIC AGONIST ANALGESIC [schedule IV]) *tablet:* propoxyphene napsylate (see p. 1301) 50 mg/acetaminophen (see p. 9) 325 mg.

Darvocet-N 100 (NARCOTIC AGONIST ANALGESIC [schedule IV]) *tablet:* propoxyphene napsylate (see p. 1301) 100 mg/acetaminophen (see p. 9) 650 mg.

Decadron with Xylocaine (GLUCOCORTICOID) *injection (per mL):* dexamethasone sodium phosphate (see p. 442) 4 mg/lidocaine hydrochloride (see p. 891) 10 mg.

Deconamine (DECONGESTANT, ANTIHISTAMINE) *syrup (per 5 mL):* pseudoephedrine hydrochloride (see p. 1312) 30 mg/chlorpheniramine maleate (see p. 313) 2 mg; *tablet:* pseudoephedrine hydrochloride 60 mg/chlorpheniramine maleate 4 mg.

Deconamine SR (DECONGESTANT, ANTIHISTAMINE) *sustained release capsule:* pseudoephedrine hydrochloride (see p. 1312) 120 mg/chlorpheniramine maleate (see p. 313) 8 mg.

Demulen 1/50 (ORAL CONTRACEPTIVE) *tablet:* ethinyl estradiol (see p. 608) 50 mcg/norethindrone (see p. 1107) 1 mg.

Depo-Testadiol (ESTROGEN, ANDROGEN) *injection (per mL):* estradiol cypionate (see p. 587) 2 mg/testosterone cypionate (see p. 1482) 50 mg.

Dilaudid Cough Syrup (NARCOTIC ANTITUSSIVE [schedule II]) *syrup:* hydromorphone (see p. 756) 1 mg/guaifenesin (see p. 728) 100 mg/alcohol 5%.

Dilor G (ANTIASTHMATIC) *liquid (per 5 mL):* dyphylline (see p. 530) 100 mg/guaifenesin (see p. 728) 100 mg.

Diovan HCT (ANTIHYPERTENSIVE) *tablet:* hydrochlorothiazide (see p. 749) 12.5 mg/valsartan (see p. 1579) 80 mg; hydrochlorothiazide 12.5 mg/valsartan 160 mg; hydrochlorothiazide 25 mg/valsartan 160 mg; hydrochlorothiazide 12.5 mg/valsartan 320 mg; hydrochlorothiazide 25 mg/valsartan 320 mg.

Donnatal (GASTROINTESTINAL ANTICHOLINERGIC, SEDATIVE) *cap-*

sule, tablet, elixir: atropine sulfate (see p. 135) 0.0194 mg/scopolamine hydrobromide (see p. 1387) 0.0065 mg/hyoscyamine hydrobromide or sulfate (see p. 765) 0.1037 mg/phenobarbital (see p. 1214) 16.2 mg. The elixir contains alcohol 23%/5 mL.

Donnatal Extentab (GASTROINTESTINAL ANTICHOLINERGIC, SEDATIVE) *tablet:* atropine sulfate (see p. 135) 0.0582 mg/scopolamine hydrobromide (see p. 1387) 0.0195 mg/hyoscyamine sulfate (see p. 765) 0.3111 mg/phenobarbital (see p. 1214) 48.6 mg.

Donnatal No. 2 (GASTROINTESTINAL ANTICHOLINERGIC, SEDATIVE) *tablet:* atropine sulfate (see p. 135) 0.0194 mg/scopolamine hydrobromide (see p. 1387) 0.0065 mg/hyoscyamine hydrobromide or sulfate (see p. 765) 0.1037 mg/phenobarbital (see p. 1214) 32.4 mg.

Duac (ANTIACNE) *gel:* clindamycin (see p. 348) 1%/benzoyl peroxide 5%.

Duetact (ANTIDIABETIC) *tablet:* pioglitazone (see p. 1236) 30 mg/glimepiride (see p. 712) 2 mg; pioglitazone 30 mg/glimepiride 4 mg.

DuoNeb (BETA-AGONIST/ANTICHOLINERGIC BRONCHODILATOR) *inhalation solution:* 3 mg albuterol sulfate (see p. 29)/0.5 mg ipratropium bromide (see p. 819) per 3 mL.

Dyazide (DIURETIC) *capsule:* triamterene (see p. 1555) 37.5 mg/hydrochlorothiazide (see p. 749) 25 mg.

Embeda (ANALGESIC [schedule II]) *tablet:* morphine (see p. 1037) 20 mg/naltrexone (see p. 1059) 0.8 mg; morphine 30 mg/naltrexone 1.2 mg; morphine 50 mg/naltrexone 2 mg; morphine 60 mg/naltrexone 2.4 mg; morphine 80 mg/naltrexone 3.2 mg; morphine 100 mg/naltrexone 4 mg.

Endocet (NARCOTIC ANALGESIC [schedule II]) *tablet:* oxycodone (see p. 1149) 7.5 mg/acetaminophen (see p. 9) 325 mg; oxycodone 7.5 mg/acetaminophen 500 mg; oxycodone 10 mg/acetaminophen 325 mg; oxycodone 10 mg/acetaminophen 650 mg.

Epiduo (ANTIACNE) *gel:* adapalene (see p. 23) 0.1%/benzoyl peroxide 2.5%.

Epzicom (ANTIRETROVIRAL AGENT) *tablet:* abacavir (see p. 1) 600 mg/lamivudine (see p. 860) 300 mg.

Estratest (ESTROGEN, ANDROGEN) *tablet:* esterified estrogens (see p. 597) 1.25 mg/methyltestosterone (see p. 996) 2.5 mg.

Estratest H.S. (ESTROGEN, ANDROGEN) *tablet:* esterified estrogens (see p. 597) 0.625 mg/methyltestosterone (see p. 996) 1.25 mg.

Exforge (ANTIHYPERTENSIVE) *tablet:* amlodipine (see p. 79) 5 mg/valsartan (see p. 1579) 160 mg; amlodipine 10 mg/valsartan 160 mg; amlodipine 5 mg/valsartan 320 mg; amlodipine 10 mg/valsartan 320 mg.

Exforge HCT (ANTIHYPERTENSIVE) *tablet:* amlodipine (see p. 79) 5 mg/valsartan (see p. 1579) 160 mg/hydrochlorothiazide (see p. 749) 12.5 mg; amlodipine 5 mg/valsartan 160 mg/hydrochlorothiazide 25 mg; amlodipine 10 mg/valsartan 160 mg/hydrochlorothiazide 12.5 mg; amlodipine 10 mg/valsartan 160 mg/hydrochlorothiazide 25 mg.

Femhrt (HORMONES) *tablet:* ethinyl estradiol (see p. 608) 5 mcg/norethindrone acetate (see p. 1107) 1 mg; ethinyl estradiol 2.5 mcg/norethindrone acetate 0.5 mg.

Fioricet (NONNARCOTIC AGONIST ANALGESIC) *tablet:* acetaminophen (see p. 9) 325 mg/butalbital 50 mg/caffeine (see p. 218) 40 mg.

Fiorinal (NONNARCOTIC AGONIST ANALGESIC [schedule III]) *capsule, tablet:* aspirin (see p. 120) 325 mg/butalbital 50 mg/caffeine (see p. 218) 40 mg.

Fiorinal with Codeine (NARCOTIC AGONIST ANALGESIC [schedule III]) *capsule:* codeine phosphate (see p. 370) 30 mg/aspirin (see p. 120) 325 mg/caffeine (see p. 218) 40 mg/butalbital 50 mg.

Fluress (OPHTHALMIC ANESTHETIC) *ophthalmic solution:* benoxinate hydrochloride 0.4%/fluorescein sodium (see p. 658) 0.25%.

Fosamax Plus D (BISPHOSPHONATE) *tablet:* alendronate (see p. 35) 70 mg/vitamin D (see p. 1602) 2800 international units.

Glucovance (ANTIDIABETIC) *tablet:* glyburide (see p. 716) 1.25 mg/metformin (see p. 969) 250 mg; glyburide 2.5 mg/metformin 500 mg; glyburide 5 mg/metformin 500 mg.

Helidac (ANTIULCER, ANTIBIOTIC) *tablet:* bismuth subsalicylate (see p. 183) 262.4 mg/metronidazole (see p. 1004) 250 mg/tetracycline (see p. 1487) 500 mg.

Hycodan (ANTITUSSIVE [schedule III]) *tablet, syrup:* hydrocodone bitartrate (see p. 751) 5 mg/homatropine methylbromide 1.5 mg.

Hycotuss Expectorant (ANTITUSSIVE [schedule III]) guaifenesin (see p. 728) 100 mg/hydrocodone (see p. 751) 5 mg.

Hydrocet (NARCOTIC ANALGESIC [schedule III]) *capsule:* hydrocodone (see p. 751) 5 mg/acetaminophen (see p. 9) 500 mg.

Hyzaar (ANTIHYPERTENSIVE) *tablet:* losartan (see p. 916) 50 mg/hydrochlorothiazide (see p. 749) 12.5 mg/losartan 100 mg/hydrochlorothiazide 12.5 mg/losartan 100 mg/hydrochlorothiazide 25 mg.

Inderide 40/25 (ANTIHYPERTENSIVE) *tablet:* propranolol hydrochloride (see p. 1302) 40 mg/hydrochlorothiazide (see p. 749) 25 mg.

Janumet (ANTIDIABETIC) *tablet:* sitagliptin (see p. 1407) 50 mg/metformin (see p. 969 500 mg; sitagliptin 50 mg/metformin 1000 mg.

Levlen (ORAL CONTRACEPTIVE) *tablet:* ethinyl estradiol (see p. 608) 30 mcg/levonorgestrel 0.15 mg.

LidoSite (LOCAL ANESTHETIC) *transdermal patch:* lidocaine (see p. 891) 100 mg/epinephrine (see p. 555) 1.05 mg.

Limbitrol (PSYCHOTHERAPEUTIC [schedule IV]) *tablet:* chlordiazepoxide (see p. 305) 5 mg/amitriptyline (see p. 76) 12.5 mg.

Limbitrol DS (PSYCHOTHERAPEUTIC [schedule IV]) *tablet:* chlordiazepoxide (see p. 305) 10 mg/amitriptyline (see p. 76) 25 mg.

Loestrin 1/20 (ORAL CONTRACEPTIVE) *tablet:* ethinyl estradiol (see p. 608) 20 mcg/norethindrone acetate (see p. 1107) 1 mg.

Loestrin 1/20 Fe (ORAL CONTRACEPTIVE) *tablet:* ethinyl estradiol (see p. 608) 20 mcg/norethindrone acetate (see p. 1107) 1 mg/ferrous fumarate 75 mg in last 7 tablets.

Loestrin 1.5/30 (ORAL CONTRACEPTIVE) *tablet:* ethinyl estradiol (see p. 608) 30 mcg/norethindrone acetate (see p. 1107) 1.5 mg.

Loestrin 1.5/30 Fe (ORAL CONTRACEPTIVE) *tablet:* ethinyl estradiol (see p. 608) 30 mcg/norethindrone acetate (see p. 1107) 1.5 mg/ferrous fumarate 75 mg in last 7 tablets.

Lomotil (ANTIDIARRHEAL) *tablet:* diphenoxylate (see p. 486) 2.5 mg/atropine (see p. 135) 0.025 mg.

Lo/Ovral (ORAL CONTRACEPTIVE) *tablet:* ethinyl estradiol (see p. 608) 30 mcg/norgestrel 0.3 mg.

Lopressor HCT 50/25 (ANTIHYPERTENSIVE) *tablet:* metoprolol tartrate (see p. 1001) 50 mg/hydrochlorothiazide (see p. 749) 25 mg.

Lopressor HCT 100/25 (ANTIHYPERTENSIVE) *tablet:* metoprolol tartrate (see p. 1001) 100 mg/hydrochlorothiazide (see p. 749) 25 mg.

Lopressor HCT 100/50 (ANTIHYPERTENSIVE) *tablet:* metoprolol tartrate (see p. 1001) 100 mg/hydrochlorothiazide (see p. 749) 50 mg.

Lorcet (NARCOTIC ANALGESIC [schedule III]) *tablet:* hydrocodone (see p. 751) 5 mg/acetaminophen (see p. 9) 500 mg.

Lorcet 10/650 (NARCOTIC ANALGESIC [schedule III]) *tablet:* hydrocodone (see p. 751) 10 mg/acetaminophen (see p. 9) 650 mg.

Lorcet-HD (NARCOTIC ANALGESIC [schedule III]) *tablet:* hydrocodone (see p. 751) 5 mg/acetaminophen (see p. 9) 500 mg.

Lortab 5 (NARCOTIC ANALGESIC [schedule III]) *tablet:* hydrocodone (see p. 751) 5 mg/acetaminophen (see p. 9) 500 mg.

Lortab 7.5/500 (NARCOTIC ANALGESIC [schedule III]) *tablet:* hydrocodone (see p. 751) 7.5 mg/acetaminophen (see p. 9) 500 mg.

LoSeasonique (ORAL CONTRACEPTIVE) *tablet:* ethinyl estradiol (see p. 608) 0.01 mg/ethinyl estradiol 0.02 mg/levonorgestrol (see p. 887) 0.1 mg.

Lotensin HCT 20/25 (ANTIHYPERTENSIVE) *tablet:* hydrochlorothiazide (see p. 749) 25 mg/benazepril (see p. 160) 20 mg.

Lotensin HCT 20/12.5 (ANTIHYPERTENSIVE) *tablet:* hydrochlorothiazide (see p. 749) 12.5/benazepril (see p. 160) 20 mg.

Lotensin HCT 10/12.5 (ANTIHYPERTENSIVE) *tablet:* hydrochlorothiazide (see p. 749) 12.5 mg/benazepril (see p. 160 10 mg.

Lotrel (ANTIHYPERTENSIVE) *tablet:* amlodipine (see p. 79) 2.5 mg/benazepril (see p. 160) 10 mg; amlodipine 5 mg/benazepril 10 mg; amlodipine 5 mg/benazepril 20 mg; amlodipine 10 mg/benazepril 20 mg.

Lotrisone (CORTICOSTEROID, ANTIFUNGAL) *cream:* betamethasone (see p. 171) (as dipropionate) 0.05%/clotrimazole (see p. 364) 1%.

Malarone (ANTIMALARIAL) *tablet:* atovaquone (see p. 132) 250 mg/proguanil HCl (see p. 132) 100 mg; atovaquone 62.5 mg/proguanil HCl 25 mg.

Maxitrol (OPHTHALMIC STEROID, ANTIBIOTIC) *ophthalmic ointment, ophthalmic suspension:* dexamethasone (see p. 442) 0.1%/neomycin sulfate (see p. 175) (equivalent to 0.35% neomycin base)/polymyxin B sulfate (see p. 1250) 10,000 units.

Maxzide (DIURETIC) *tablet:* triamterene (see p. 1555) 75 mg/hydrochlorothiazide (see p. 749) 50 mg.

Maxzide 25 (DIURETIC) *tablet:* triamterene (see p. 1555) 37.5 mg/hydrochlorothiazide (see p. 749) 25 mg.

Metaglip (HYPOGLYCEMIC AGENT) *tablet:* glipizide (see p. 713) 2.5 mg/metformin HCl (see p. 969) 250 mg; glipizide 2.5 mg/metformin 500 mg; glipizide 5 mg/metformin 500 mg.

Micardis HCT (ANTIHYPERTENSIVE) *tablet:* telmisartan (see p. 1468) 40 mg/hydrochlorothiazide (see p. 749) 12.5 mg; telmisartan 80 mg/hydrochlorothiazide 12.5 mg; telmisartan 80 mg/hydrochlorothiazide 25 mg.

Minizide (ANTIHYPERTENSIVE) *capsule:* polythiazide 0.5 mg/prazosin hydrochloride (see p. 1271) 1 mg; polythiazide 0.5 mg/prazosin hydrochloride 2 mg; polythiazide 0.5 mg/prazosin hydrochloride 5 mg.

Modicon (ORAL CONTRACEPTIVE) *tablet:* ethinyl estradiol (see p. 608) 35 mcg/norethindrone (see p. 1107) 0.5 mg.

Moduretic (DIURETIC) *tablet:* amiloride hydrochloride (see p. 65) 5 mg/hydrochlorothiazide (see p. 749) 50 mg.

Mycitracin (OPHTHALMIC ANTIBIOTIC) *ophthalmic ointment:* polymyxin B sulfate (see p. 1250) 10,000 units/neomycin sulfate (see p. 1075) 3.5 mg/bacitracin (see p. 150) 500 units/g.

Mycodone (NARCOTIC ANALGESIC [schedule III]) *syrup (per 5 mL):* homatropine methylbromide 1.5 mg/hydrocodone (see p. 751) 5 mg.

Mycolog II (CORTICOSTEROID, ANTIFUNGAL) *cream, ointment:* triamcinolone acetonide (see p. 1553) 0.1%/nystatin (see p. 1114) 100,000 units/g.

Neo-Cortef (CORTICOSTEROID ANTIBIOTIC) *water-soluble cream, topical ointment:* hydrocortisone acetate (see p. 752) 1%/neomycin sulfate (see p. 1075) 0.5%.

Neosporin (OPHTHALMIC ANTIBIOTIC) *ophthalmic drops:* polymyxin B sulfate (see p. 1250) 10,000 units/neomycin sulfate (see p. 1075) 1.75 mg/gramicidin 0.025 mg/mL; *ophthalmic ointment:* polymyxin B sulfate 10,000 units/neomycin sulfate 3.5 mg/bacitracin zinc (see p. 150) 400 units/g.

Neosporin G.U. Irrigant (ANTIBIOTIC) *solution:* neomycin sulfate (see p. 1075) 40 mg/polymyxin B sulfate (see p. 1250) 200,000 units/mL.

Neutra-Phos (PHOSPHORUS REPLACEMENT) *capsule, powder:* phosphorus 250 mg/potassium (see p. 1258) 278 mg/sodium (see p. 1408) 164 mg/combination of monobasic, dibasic, sodium, and potassium phosphate.

Norco (NARCOTIC AGONIST ANALGESIC [schedule III]) *tablet:* hydrocodone bitartrate (see p. 751) 10 mg/acetaminophen (see p. 9) 325 mg; hydrocodone bitartrate 7.5 mg/acetaminophen 325 mg.

Nordette (ORAL CONTRACEPTIVE) *tablet:* ethinyl estradiol (see p. 608) 30 mcg/levonorgestrel (see p. 887) 0.15 mg.

Norethin 1/35 E (ORAL CONTRACEPTIVE) *tablet:* ethinyl estradiol (see p. 608) 35 mcg/norethindrone (see p. 1107) 1 mg.

Norethin 1/50 M (ORAL CONTRACEPTIVE) *tablet:* mestranol 50 mcg/norethindrone (see p. 1107) 1 mg.

Norgesic (SKELETAL MUSCLE RELAXANT) *tablet:* orphenadrine citrate (see p. 1133) 25 mg/aspirin (see p. 120) 385 mg/caffeine (see p. 218) 30 mg.

Norgesic Forte (SKELETAL MUSCLE RELAXANT, ANALGESIC) *tablet:* orphenadrine citrate (see p. 1133) 50 mg/aspirin (see p. 120) 770 mg/caffeine (see p. 218) 60 mg.

Norinyl 1+35 (ORAL CONTRACEPTIVE) *tablet:* ethinyl estradiol (see p. 608) 35 mcg/norethindrone (see p. 1107) 1 mg.

Norinyl 1+50 (ORAL CONTRACEPTIVE) *tablet:* mestranol 50 mcg/norethindrone (see p. 1107) 1 mg.

Ortho Evra (CONTRACEPTIVE) *transdermal patch:* norelgestromin 0.15 mg/ethinyl estradiol (see p. 608) 0.02 mg.

Paremyd (MYDRIATIC) *ophthalmic solution:* 1% hydroxyamphetamine hydrobromide, 0.25% tropicamide (see p. 1570).

Percocet (NARCOTIC ANALGESIC [schedule II]) *tablet:* oxycodone (see p. 1149) 2.5 mg/acetaminophen (see p. 9) 325 mg; oxycodone 7.5 mg/acetaminophen 325 mg; oxycodone 10 mg/acetaminophen 325 mg; oxycodone 10 mg/acetaminophen 650 mg.

Percodan (NARCOTIC ANALGESIC [schedule II]) *tablet:* oxycodone hydrochloride (see p. 1149) 4.5 mg/oxycodone terephthalate 0.38 mg/aspirin (see p. 120) 325 mg.

Phrenilin (NONNARCOTIC AGONIST ANALGESIC) *tablet:* acetaminophen (see p. 9) 325 mg/butalbital 50 mg.

Phrenilin Forte (NONNARCOTIC AGONIST ANALGESIC) *capsule:* acetaminophen (see p. 9) 650 mg/butalbital 50 mg.

Polysporin Ointment (ANTI-INFECTIVE [OPHTHALMIC]) *ophthalmic ointment:* polymyxin B sulfate (see p. 1250) 10,000 units/bacitracin zinc (see p. 150) 500 units/g.

Prandimet (HYPOGLYCEMIC AGENT) *tablet:* repaglinide (see p. 1345) 1 mg/metformin (see p. 969) 500 mg; repaglinide 2 mg/metformin 500 mg.

Pravigard Pac (LIPID-LOWERING AGENT) *tablet:* pravastatin (see p. 1268) 20 mg/buffered aspirin (see p. 120) 81 mg; pravastatin 20 mg/buffered aspirin 325 mg; pravastatin 40 mg/aspirin 81 mg; pravastatin 40 mg/buffered aspirin 325 mg; pravastatin 80 mg/buffered aspirin 81 mg; pravastatin 80 mg/buffered aspirin 325 mg.

Premarin with Methyltestosterone (ESTROGEN, ANDROGEN) *tablet:* conjugated estrogens (see p. 596) 0.625 mg/methyltestosterone (see p. 996) 5 mg.

Premphase (ESTROGEN, PROGESTERONE) *tablet:* conjugated estrogens (see p. 596) 0.625 mg/medroxyprogesterone acetate (see p. 945) 5 mg.

Prempro (ESTROGEN, PROGESTIN) *tablet:* conjugated estrogens (see p. 596) 0.3 mg/medroxyprogesterone (see p. 945) 1.5 mg; conjugated estrogen 0.45 mg/medroxyprogesterone 1.5 mg; conjugated estrogen 0.625 mg/medroxyprogesterone 2.5 mg; conjugated estrogen 0.625 mg/medroxyprogesterone 5 mg.

Prevacid NapraPAC (PROTON PUMP INHIBITOR/ANTI-INFLAMMATORY) *capsules and tablets:* lansoprazole (see p. 865) 15 mg capsule/naproxen sodium (see p. 1063) 375 mg table; lansoprazole 15 mg capsule/naproxen sodium 500 mg tablet.

Prevpac (ANTIBIOTIC/ANTISECRETORY) *capsules and tablets:* amoxicillin (see p. 83) 500 mg capsules, clarithromycin (see p. 344) 500 mg tablets, lansoprazole (see p. 865) 30 mg capsules.

Prinzide (ANTIHYPERTENSIVE) *tablet:* hydrochlorothiazide (see p. 749) 12.5 mg/lisinopril (see p. 903) 10 mg; hydrochlorothiazide 12.5 mg/lisinopril 20 mg; hydrochlorothiazide 25 mg/lisinopril 20 mg.

Probenecid and Colchicine (ANTIGOUT) *tablet:* probenecid (see p. 1281) 500 mg/colchicine (see p. 371) 0.5 mg.

Pyridium Plus (ANALGESIC) *tablet:* phenazopyridine hydrochloride (see p. 1211) 150 mg/hyoscyamine hydrobromide (see p. 765) 0.3 mg/butalbital 15 mg.

Rebetron (INTERFERON, ANTIVIRAL) ribavirin (see p. 1353) tablet polythiazide 2 mg/reserpine (see p. 1346) 0.25 mg.

Rifamate (ANTITUBERCULOSIS) *capsule:* isoniazid (see p. 829) 150 mg/rifampin (see p. 1358) 300 mg.

Rifater (ANTITUBERCULOSIS) *tablet:* rifampin (see p. 1358) 120 mg/isoniazid (see p. 829) 50 mg/pyrazinamide (see p. 1315) 300 mg.

Rimactane/INH Dual Pack (ANTITUBERCULOSIS) *pack:* thirty isoniazid (see p. 829) 300 mg tablets, sixty rifampin (see p. 1358) 300 mg capsules.

Robitussin A-C (ANTITUSSIVE, EXPECTORANT [schedule V]) *syrup (per 5 mL):* codeine phosphate (see p. 370) 10 mg/guaifenesin (see p. 728) 100 mg/alcohol 3.5%.

Rondec (DECONGESTANT, ANTIHISTAMINE) *tablet:* pseudoephedrine hydrochloride (see p. 1312) 60 mg/carbinoxamine maleate 4 mg; *drops (per mL):* pseudoephedrine hydrochloride 25 mg/carbinoxamine maleate 2 mg; *syrup (per mL):* pseudoephedrine hydrochloride 60 mg/carbinoxamine maleate 4 mg.

Roxicet (NARCOTIC ANALGESIC [schedule II]) *tablet:* oxycodone (see p. 1149) 5 mg/acetaminophen (see p. 9) 325 mg; *syrup (per 5 mL):* oxycodone 5 mg/acetaminophen 325 mg.

Simcor (ANTILIPIDEMIC) *extended release tablet:* niacin (see p. 1082) 1000 mg/simvastatin (see p. 1408) 20 mg; niacin 500 mg/simvastatin 20 mg; niacin 750 mg/simvastatin 20 mg.

Soma Compound (SKELETAL MUSCLE RELAXANT) *tablet:* carisoprodol (see p. 248) 200 mg/aspirin (see p. 120) 325 mg.

Soma Compound with Codeine (SKELETAL MUSCLE RELAXANT [schedule III]) *tablet:* carisoprodol (see p. 248) 200 mg, aspirin (see p. 120) 325 mg/codeine phosphate (see p. 370) 16 mg.

Stalevo (ANTIPARKINSON AGENT) *tablet:* carbidopa (see p. 242) 12.5 mg/levodopa (see p. 882) 50 mg/entacapone (see p. 551) 200 mg; carbidopa 18.75 mg/levodopa 75 mg/entacapone 200 mg; carbidopa 25 mg/levodopa 100 mg/entacapone 200 mg; carbidopa 31.25 mg/levodopa 125 mg/entacapone 200 mg; carbidopa 37.5 mg/levodopa 150 mg/entacapone 200 mg.

Suboxone (ANALGESIC) *sublingual tablet:* buprenorphine (see p. 204) 2 mg/naloxone (see p. 1057) 0.5 mg; buprenorphine 8 mg/naloxone 2 mg.

Symbicort (MINERALOCORTICOID/BRONCHODILATOR) *inhaler:* budesonide (see p. 199) 0.08 mg/formoterol (see p. 678) 0.045 mg; budesonide 0.16 mg/formoterol 0.045 mg.

Symbyax (ATYPICAL ANTIPSYCHOTIC/SSRI) *capsule:* olanzapine (see p. 1120) 6 mg/fluoxetine (see p. 661) 25 mg; olanzapine 6 mg/fluoxetine 50 mg; olanzapine 12 mg/fluoxetine 25 mg; olanzapine 12 mg/fluoxetine 50 mg.

Synalgos-DC (NARCOTIC AGONIST ANALGESIC [schedule III]) *capsule:* dihydrocodeine bitartrate 16 mg/aspirin (see p. 120) 356.4 mg/caffeine (see p. 218) 30 mg.

Synera (LOCAL ANESTHETIC) *transdermal patch:* lidocaine (see p. 891) 70 mg/tetracycline (see p. 1487) 70 mg.

Syntest D.S. (ESTROGEN, ANDROGEN) *tablet:* esterified estrogens (see p. 597) 1.25 mg/methyltestosterone (see p. 996) 2.5 mg.

Syntest H.S. (ESTROGEN, ANDROGEN) *tablet:* esterified estrogens (see p. 597) 0.625 mg/methyltestosterone (see p. 996) 1.25 mg.

Taclonex Scalp (NSAID) *topical suspension:* betamethasone (see p. 171) 0.064%/calcipotriene (see p. 219) 0.005%.

Talacen (NARCOTIC AGONIST-ANTAGONIST ANALGESIC [schedule IV]) *tablet:* pentazocine hydrochloride (see p. 1201) 25 mg/acetaminophen (see p. 9) 625 mg.

Talwin NX (NARCOTIC ANALGESIC [schedule IV]) *tablet:* pentazocine (see p. 1201) 50 mg/naloxone (see p. 1057) 0.5 mg.

Tanafed DP (DECONGESTANT, ANTIHISTAMINE) *suspension:* pseudoephedrine (see p. 1312) 75 mg/chlorpheniramine tannate 4.5 mg.

Tarka (ANTIHYPERTENSIVE) *tablet:* trandolapril (see p. 1543) 2 mg/verapamil HCl (see p. 1592) 180 mg; trandolapril 4 mg/verapamil HCl 240 mg; trandolapril 1 mg/verapamil HCl 240 mg, trandolapril 2 mg/verapamil HCl 240 mg.

Tecturna HCT (ANTIHYPERTENSIVE) *tablet:* aliskiren (see p. 39) 150 mg/hydrochlorothiazide (see p. 749) 12.5 mg.

Tenoretic 50 (ANTIHYPERTENSIVE) *tablet:* chlorthalidone (see p. 320) 25 mg/atenolol (see p. 126) 50 mg.

Tenoretic 100 (ANTIHYPERTENSIVE) *tablet:* chlorthalidone (see p. 320) 25 mg/atenolol (see p. 126) 100 mg.

Terra-Cortril Suspension (OCULAR STEROID AND ANTIBIOTIC) *suspension:* hydrocortisone acetate (see p. 752) 1.5%/oxytetracycline 0.5%.

Teveten HCT (ANTIHYPERTENSIVE) *tablet:* eprosartan mesylate (see p. 566) 600 mg/hydrochlorothiazide (see p. 749) 12.5 mg; eprosartan 600 mg/hydrochlorothiazide 25 mg.

Timolide (ANTIHYPERTENSIVE) *tablet:* hydrochlorothiazide (see p. 749) 25 mg/timolol maleate (see p. 1515) 10 mg.

Tobradex (ANTI-INFECTIVE) *ophthalmic suspension:* dexamethasone (see p. 442) 0.1%/tobramycin (see p. 1524) 0.3%; *ophthalmic ointment:* dexamethasone 0.1%/tobramycin 0.3%.

Treximet (ANALGESIC) *tablet:* naproxen (see p. 1063) 500 mg/sumatriptan (see p. 1449) 85 mg.

Triacin-C Cough Syrup (ANTITUSSIVE [schedule V]) *syrup:* pseudoephedrine (see p. 1312) 30 mg/triprolidine 1.25 mg/codeine (see p. 370) 10 mg.

Tri-Hydroserpine (ANTIHYPERTENSIVE) *tablet:* hydrochlorothiazide (see p. 749) 15 mg/reserpine (see p. 1346) 0.1 mg/hydralazine hydrochloride (see p. 747) 25 mg.

Tri-Levlen (ORAL CONTRACEPTIVE) *tablet:* ethinyl estradiol (see p. 608) 30 mcg/levonorgestrel (see p. 887) 0.05 mg × 6 days, ethinyl estradiol 40 mcg/levonorgestrel 0.075 mg × 5 days, ethinyl estradiol 30 mcg/levonorgestrel 0.125 mg × 10 days.

Tri-Luma Cream (STEROID) *cream:* 4% hydroquinone (see p. 758)/0.05% tretinoin (see p. 1551)/0.01% fluocinolone acetonide (see p. 658).

Tri-Norinyl (ORAL CONTRACEPTIVE) *tablet:* ethinyl estradiol (see p. 608) 35 mcg/norethindrone (see p. 1107) 0.5 mg × 7 d, ethinyl estradiol 35 mcg/norethindrone 1 mg × 9 d, ethinyl estradiol 35 mcg/norethindrone 0.5 mg × 5 d.

Triphasil (ORAL CONTRACEPTIVE) *tablet:* ethinyl estradiol (see p. 608) 30 mcg/levonorgestrel (see p. 887) 0.05 mg × 6 days, ethinyl estradiol 40 mcg/levonorgestrel 0.075 mg × 5 days, ethinyl estradiol 30 mcg/levonorgestrel 0.125 mg × 10 days.

Triple Antibiotic (OPHTHALMIC ANTIBIOTIC) *ophthalmic ointment:* hydrocortisone (see p. 752) 1%/neomycin sulfate (see p. 1075) 0.5%/bacitracin zinc (see p. 148) 400 units/polymyxin B sulfate (see p. 1250) 10,000 units/g.

Trizivir (REVERSE TRANSCRIPTASE INHIBITOR) *tablet:* abacavir (see p. 1) 300 mg/lamivudine (see p. 860) 150 mg/zidovudine (see p. 1615) 300 mg.

Truvada (NUCLEOSIDE REVERSE TRANSCRIPTASE INHIBITOR) *tablet:* emtricitabine (see p. 543) 200 mg/tenofovir disoproxil fumarate (see p. 1475) 300 mg.

Tussicap (ANTITUSSIVE [schedule III]) *extended release capsule:* chlorpheniramine (see p. 313) 8 mg/hydrocodone (see p. 751) 10 mg.

Tussigon (ANTITUSSIVE [schedule III]) *tablet:* homatropine methylbromide 1.5 mg/hydrocodone (see p. 751) 5 mg.

Tussionex (ANTITUSSIVE [schedule III]) *tablet:* chlorpheniramine (see p. 313) 8 mg/hydrocodone (see p. 751) 10 mg.

Twinrix (VACCINE) *injection:* hepatitis A vaccine (see p. 741) 720 ELU/hepatitis B recombinant vaccine (see p. 743) 20 mcg per single dose vial.

Tylenol with Codeine Elixir (NARCOTIC AGONIST ANALGESIC [schedule V]) *elixir (per 5 mL)* acetaminophen (see p. 9) 120 mg/codeine phosphate (see p. 370) 12 mg/alcohol 7%.

Tylenol with Codeine No. 1 (NARCOTIC AGONIST ANALGESIC [schedule III]) *tablet:* acetaminophen (see p. 9) 300 mg/codeine phosphate (see p. 370) 7.5 mg.

Tylenol with Codeine No. 2 (NARCOTIC AGONIST ANALGESIC [schedule III]) *tablet:* acetaminophen (see p. 9) 300 mg/codeine phosphate (see p. 370) 15 mg.

Tylenol with Codeine No. 3 (NARCOTIC AGONIST ANALGESIC [schedule III]) *tablet:* acetaminophen (see p. 9) 300 mg/codeine phosphate (see p. 370) 30 mg.

Tylenol with Codeine No. 4 (NARCOTIC AGONIST ANALGESIC [schedule III]) *tablet:* acetaminophen (see p. 9) 300 mg/codeine phosphate (see p. 370) 60 mg.

Tylox (NARCOTIC AGONIST ANALGESIC [schedule II]) *capsule:* oxycodone hydrochloride (see p. 1149) 5 mg/acetaminophen (see p. 9) 500 mg.

Ultracet (ANALGESIC/ANTIPYRETIC) *tablet:* tramadol (see p. 1542) 37.5 mg/acetaminophen (see p. 9) 325 mg.

Uniretic (ANTIHYPERTENSIVE) *tablet:* moexipril (see p. 1033) 7.5 mg/hydrochlorothiazide (see p. 749) 12.5 mg; moexipril 15 mg/hydrochlorothiazide 12.5 mg, moexipril 15 mg/hydrochlorothiazide 25 mg.

Urised (URINARY ANTI-INFECTIVE) *tablet:* methenamine (see p. 975) 40.8 mg/phenyl salicylate 18.1 mg/atropine sulfate (see p. 135) 0.03 mg/hyoscyamine (see p. 765) 0.03 mg/benzoic acid 4.5 mg/methylene blue 5.4 mg.

Valturna (ANTIHYPERTENSIVE) *tablet:* aliskiren (see p. 39) 150 mg/valsartan (see p. 1579) 160 mg; aliskiren 300 mg/valsartan 320 mg.

Vaseretic (ANTIHYPERTENSIVE) *tablet:* enalapril maleate (see p. 545)

10 mg/hydrochlorothiazide (see p. 749) 25 mg.

Vasocidin (OPHTHALMIC CORTICOSTEROID, ANTI-INFECTIVE) *ophthalmic solution:* prednisolone sodium phosphate (see p. 1273) 0.23%/sulfacetamide sodium (see p. 1436) 10%.

Vasocon-A (OPHTHALMIC DECONGESTANT) *ophthalmic solution:* naphazoline hydrochloride (see p. 1062) 0.05%/antazoline phosphate 0.5%.

Vicodin (NARCOTIC AGONIST ANALGESIC [schedule III]) *tablet:* hydrocodone bitartrate (see p. 751) 5 mg/acetaminophen (see p. 9) 500 mg.

Vicodin ES (NARCOTIC AGONIST ANALGESIC [schedule III]) *tablet:* hydrocodone (see p. 751) 7.5 mg/acetaminophen (see p. 9) 750 mg.

Vicodin HP (NARCOTIC AGONIST ANALGESIC [schedule III]) *tablet:* hydrocodone (see p. 751) 10 mg/acetaminophen (see p. 9) 660 mg.

Vicoprofen (NARCOTIC AGONIST ANALGESIC [schedule III]) *tablet:* hydrocodone bitartrate (see p. 751) 7.5 mg/ibuprofen (see p. 768) 200 mg.

Vytorin (ANTILIPEMIC AGENT) *tablet:* ezetimibe (see p. 622) 10 mg/simvastatin (see p. 1404) 10 mg; ezetimibe 10 mg/simvastatin 20 mg; ezetimibe 10 mg/simvastatin 40 mg; ezetimibe 10 mg/simvastatin 80 mg.

Wygesic (NARCOTIC AGONIST ANALGESIC [schedule IV]) *tablet:* propoxyphene hydrochloride (see p. 1301) 65 mg/acetaminophen (see p. 9) 650 mg.

Yasmin (ORAL CONTRACEPTIVE) *tablet:* ethinyl estradiol (see p. 608) 30 mcg/drospirenone 3 mg.

Zestoretic (ANTIHYPERTENSIVE) *tablet:* hydrochlorothiazide (see p. 749) 12.5 mg/lisinopril (see p. 903) 10 mg; hydrochlorothiazide 12.5 mg/lisinopril 20 mg; hydrochlorothiazide 25 mg/lisinopril 20 mg.

Ziac (ANTIHYPERTENSIVE) *tablet:* bisoprolol (see p. 184) 2.5 mg/hydrochlorothiazide (see p. 749) 6.25 mg; bisoprolol 5 mg/hydrochlorothiazide 6.25 mg; bisoprolol 10 mg/hydrochlorothiazide 6.25 mg.

Zylet (OPHTHALMIC ANTIBIOTIC) *solution:* loteprednol etabonate (see p. 917) 0.5%/tobramycin (see p. 1524) 0.3%.

Zyrtec-D (ANTIHISTAMINE/DECONGESTANT) *tablet, sustained release:* cetirizine (see p. 294) 5 mg/pseudoephedrine (see p. 1312) 120 mg.

◆ APPENDIX F GLOSSARY OF KEY TERMS, CLINICAL CONDITIONS, AND ASSOCIATED SIGNS AND SYMPTOMS

acute coronary syndrome an acute ischemic event with or without marked ST segment elevation.

acute dystonia extrapyramidal symptom manifested by abnormal posturing, grimacing, spastic torticollis (neck torsion), and oculogyric (eyeball movement) crisis.

adverse effect unintended, unpredictable, and nontherapeutic response to drug action. Adverse effects occur at doses used therapeutically or for prophylaxis or diagnosis. They generally result from drug toxicity, idiosyncrasies, or hypersensitivity reactions caused by the drug itself or by ingredients added during manufacture (e.g., preservatives, dyes, or vehicles).

afterload resistance that ventricles must work against to eject blood into the aorta during systole.

agranulocytosis sudden drop in leukocyte count; often followed by a severe infection manifested by high fever, chills, prostration, and ulcerations of mucous membrane such as in the mouth, rectum, or vagina.

akathisia extrapyramidal symptom manifested by a compelling need to move or pace, without specific pattern, and an inability to be still.

analeptic restorative medication that enhances excitation of the CNS without affecting inhibitory impulses.

anaphylactoid reaction excessive allergic response manifested by wheezing, chills, generalized pruritic urticaria, diaphoresis, sense of uneasiness, agitation, flushing, palpitations, coughing, difficulty breathing, and cardiovascular collapse.

anticholinergic actions inhibition of parasympathetic response manifested by dry mouth, decreased peristalsis, constipation, blurred vision, and urinary retention.

bioavailability fraction of active drug that reaches its action sites after administration by any route. Following an IV dose, bioavailability is 100%; however, such factors as first-pass effect, enterohepatic cycling, and biotransformation reduce bioavailability of an orally administered drug.

blood dyscrasia pathological condition manifested by fever, sore mouth or throat, unexplained fatigue, easy bruising or bleeding.

cardiotoxicity impairment of cardiac function manifested by one or more of the following: hypotension, arrhythmias, precordial pain, dyspnea, electrocardiogram (ECG) abnormalities, cardiac dilation, congestive failure.

cholinergic response stimulation of the parasympathetic response manifested by lacrimation, diaphoresis, salivation, abdominal cramps, diarrhea, nausea, and vomiting.

circulatory overload excessive vascular volume manifested by increased central venous pressure (CVP), elevated blood pressure, tachycardia, distended neck veins, peripheral edema, dyspnea, cough, and pulmonary rales.

CNS stimulation excitement of the CNS manifested by hyperactivity, excitement, nervousness, insomnia, and tachycardia.

CNS toxicity impairment of CNS function manifested by ataxia, tremor, incoordination, paresthesias, numbness, impairment of pain or touch sensation, drowsiness, confusion, headache, anxiety, tremors, and behavior changes.

congestive heart failure (CHF) impaired pumping ability of the heart manifested by paroxysmal nocturnal dyspnea, cough, fatigue or dyspnea on exertion, tachycardia, peripheral or pulmonary edema, and weight gain.

Cushing's syndrome fatty swellings in the interscapular area (buffalo hump) and in the facial area (moon face), distention of the abdomen, ecchymoses following even minor trauma, impotence, amenorrhea, high blood pressure, general weakness, loss of muscle mass, osteoporosis, and psychosis.

dehydration decreased intracellular or extracellular fluid manifested by elevated temperature, dry skin and mucous membranes, decrease tissue turgor, sunken eyes, furrowed tongue, low blood pressure, diminished or irregular pulse, muscle or abdominal cramps, thick secretions, hard feces and impaction, scant urinary output, urine specific gravity above 1.030, an elevated hemoglobin.

disulfiram-type reaction Antabuse-type reaction manifested by facial flushing, pounding headache, sweating, slurred speech, abdominal cramps, nausea, vomiting, tachycardia, fever, palpitations, drop in blood pressure, dyspnea, and sense of chest constriction. Symptoms may last up to 24 hours.

enzyme induction stimulation of microsomal enzymes by a drug resulting in its accelerated metabolism and decreased activity. If reactive intermediates are formed, drug-mediated toxicity may be exacerbated.

first-pass effect reduced bioavailability of an orally administered drug due to metabolism in GI epithelial cells and liver or to biliary excretion. Effect may be avoided by use of sublingual tablets or rectal suppositories.

fixed drug eruption drug-induced circumscribed skin lesion that persists or recurs in the same site. Residual pigmentation may remain following drug withdrawal.

half-life ($t_{1/2}$) time required for concentration of a drug in the body to decrease by 50%. Half-life also represents the time necessary to reach steady state or to decline from steady state after a change (i.e., starting or stopping) in the dosing regimen. Half-life may be affected by a disease state and age of the drug user.

heart failure left- and/or right-sided failure associated with systolic and/or diastolic dysfunction.

heat stroke a life-threatening condition manifested by absence of sweating; red, dry, hot skin; dilated pupils; dyspnea; full bounding pulse; temperature above 40° C (105° F); and mental confusion.

hepatic toxicity impairment of liver function manifested by jaundice, dark urine, pruritus, light-colored stools, eosinophilia, itchy skin or rash, and persistently high elevations of alanine amino-transferase (ALT) and aspartate aminotransferase (AST).

hyperammonemia elevated level of ammonia or ammonium in the blood manifested by lethargy, decreased appetite, vomiting, asterixis (flapping tremor), weak pulse, irritability, decreased responsiveness, and seizures.

hypercalcemia elevated serum calcium manifested by deep bone and flank pain, renal calculi, anorexia, nausea, vomiting, thirst, constipation, muscle hypotonicity, pathologic fracture, bradycardia, lethargy, and psychosis.

hyperglycemia elevated blood glucose manifested by flushed, dry skin, low blood pressure and elevated pulse, tachypnea, Kussmaul's respirations, polyuria, polydipsia; polyphagia, lethargy, and drowsiness.

hyperkalemia excessive potassium in blood, which may produce life-threatening cardiac arrhythmias, including bradycardia and heart block, unusual fatigue, weakness or heaviness of limbs, general muscle weakness, muscle cramps, paresthesias, flaccid paralysis of extremities, shortness of breath, nervousness, confusion, diarrhea, and GI distress.

hypermagnesemia excessive magnesium in blood, which may produce cathartic effect, profound thirst, flushing, sedation, confusion, depressed deep tendon reflexes (DTRs), muscle weakness, hypotension, and depressed respirations.

hypernatremia excessive sodium in blood, which may produce confusion, neuromuscular excitability, muscle weakness, seizures, thirst, dry and flushed skin, dry mucous membranes, pyrexia, agitation, and oliguria or anuria.

hypersensitivity reactions excessive and abnormal sensitivity to given agent manifested by urticaria, pruritus, wheezing, edema, redness, and anaphylaxis.

hyperthyroidism excessive secretion by the thyroid glands, which increases basal metabolic rate, resulting in warm, flushed, moist skin; tachycardia, exophthalmos; infrequent lid blinking; lid edema; weight loss despite increased appetite; frequent urination; menstrual irregularity; breathlessness; hypoventilation; congestive heart failure; excessive sweating.

hyperuricemia excessive uric acid in blood, resulting in pain in flank; stomach, or joints, and changes in intake and output ratio and pattern.

hypocalcemia abnormally low calcium level in blood, which may result in depression; psychosis; hyperreflexia; diarrhea; cardiac arrhythmias; hypotension; muscle spasms; paresthesias of feet, fingers, tongue; positive Chvostek's sign. Severe deficiency (tetany) may result in carpopedal spasms, spasms of face muscle, laryngospasm, and generalized convulsions.

hypoglycemia abnormally low glucose level in the blood, which may result in acute fatigue, restlessness, malaise, marked irritability and weakness, cold sweats, excessive hunger, headache, dizziness, confusion, slurred speech, loss of consciousness, and death.

hypokalemia abnormally low level of potassium in blood, which may result in malaise, fatigue, paresthesias, depressed reflexes, muscle weakness and cramps, rapid, irregular pulse, arrhythmias, hypotension, vomiting, paralytic ileus, mental confusion, depression, delayed thought process, abdominal distention, polyuria, shallow breathing, and shortness of breath.

hypomagnesemia abnormally low level of magnesium in blood, resulting in nausea, vomiting, cardiac arrhythmias, and neuromuscular symptoms (tetany, positive Chvostek's and Trousseau's signs, seizures, tremors, ataxia, vertigo, nystagmus, muscular fasciculations).

hyponatremia a decreased serum concentration (less than 125 mEq) of sodium that results in intracellular swelling. The resulting signs and symptoms include nausea, malaise, headache, lethargy, obtundation, seizures, and coma. There is significant variability in the symptomatology of hyponatremia manifested in patients.

hypophosphatemia abnormally low level of phosphates in blood, resulting in muscle weakness, anorexia, malaise, absent deep tendon reflexes, bone pain, paresthesias, tremors, negative calcium balance, osteomalacia, osteoporosis.

hypothyroidism condition caused by thyroid hormone deficiency that lowers basal metabolic rate and may result in periorbital edema, lethargy, puffy hands and feet, cool, pale skin, vertigo, nocturnal cramps, decreased GI motility, constipation, hypotension, slow pulse, depressed muscular activity, and enlarged thyroid gland.

hypoxia insufficient oxygenation in the blood manifested by dyspnea, tachypnea, headache, restlessness, cyanosis, tachycardia, dysrhythmias, confusion, decreased level of consciousness, and euphoria or delirium.

international normalizing ratio measurement that normalizes for the differences obtained from various laboratory readings in the value for thromboplastin blood level.

leukopenia abnormal decrease in number of white blood cells, usually below 5000 per cubic millimeter, resulting in fever, chills, sore mouth or throat, and unexplained fatigue.

liver toxicity manifested by anorexia, nausea, fatigue, lethargy, itching, jaundice, abdominal pain, dark-colored urine, and flu-like symptoms.

metabolic acidosis decrease in pH value of the extracellular fluid caused by either an increase in hydrogen ions or a decrease in bicarbonate ions. It may result in one or more of the following: lethargy, headache, weakness, abdominal pain, nausea, vomiting, dyspnea, hyperpnea progressing to Kussmaul breathing, dehydration, thirst, weakness, flushed face, full bounding pulse, progressive drowsiness, mental confusion, combativeness.

metabolic alkalosis increase in pH value of the extracellular fluid caused by either a loss of acid from the body (e.g., through vomiting) or an increased level of bicarbonate ions (e.g., through ingestion of sodium bicarbonate). It may result in muscle weakness, irritability, confusion, muscle twitching, slow and shallow respirations, and convulsive seizures.

microsomal enzymes drug-metabolizing enzymes located in the endoplasmic reticulum of the liver and other tissues chiefly responsible for oxidative drug metabolism (e.g., cytochrome P450).

myopathy any disease or abnormal condition of striated muscles manifested by muscle weakness, myalgia, diaphoresis, fever, and reddish-brown urine (myoglobinuria) or oliguria.

nephrotoxicity impairment of the nephrons of the kidney manifested by one or more of the following: oliguria, urinary frequency, hematuria, cloudy urine, rising BUN and serum creatinine, fever, graft tenderness or enlargement.

neuroleptic malignant syndrome (NMS) potentially fatal complication associated with antipsychotic drugs manifested by hyperpyrexia, altered mental status, muscle rigidity, irregular pulse, fluctuating BP, diaphoresis, and tachycardia.

orphan drug (as defined by the Orphan Drug Act, an amendment of the Federal Food, Drug, and Cosmetic Act which took effect in January 1983): drug or biological product used in the treatment, diagnosis, or prevention of a rare disease. A rare disease or condition is one that affects fewer than 200,000 persons in the United States, or affects more than 200,000 persons but for which there is no reasonable expectation that drug research and development costs can be recovered from sales within the United States.

ototoxicity impairment of the ear manifested by one or more of the following: headache, dizziness or vertigo, nausea and vomiting with motion, ataxia, nystagmus.

pharmacogenetic genetic variation affecting response to different drugs.

prodrug inactive drug form that becomes pharmacologically active through biotransformation.

protein binding reversible interaction between protein and drug resulting in a drug-protein complex (bound drug) which is in equilibrium with free (active) drug in plasma and tissues. Since only free drug can diffuse to action sites, factors that influence drug-binding (e.g., displacement of bound drug by another drug, or decreased albumin concentration) may potentiate pharmacologic effect.

pseudomembranous enterocolitis life-threatening superinfection characterized by severe diarrhea and fever.

pseudoparkinsonism extrapyramidal symptom manifested by slowing of volitional movement (akinesia), mask facies, rigidity and tremor at rest (especially of upper extremities); and pill rolling motion.

pulmonary edema excessive fluid in the lung tissue manifested by one or more of the following: shortness of breath, cyanosis, persistent productive cough (frothy sputum may be blood tinged), expiratory rales, restlessness, anxiety, increased heart rate, sense of chest pressure.

renal insufficiency reduced capacity of the kidney to perform its functions as manifested by one or more of the following: dysuria, oliguria, hematuria, swelling of lower legs and feet.

serotonin syndrome manifested by restlessness, myoclonus, mental status changes, hyperreflexia, diaphoresis, shivering, and tremor.

Somogyi effect rebound phenomenon clinically manifested by fasting hyperglycemia and worsening of diabetic control due to unnecessarily large p.m. insulin doses. Hormonal response to unrecognized hypoglycemia (i.e., release of epinephrine, glucagon, growth hormone, cortisol) causes insensitivity to insulin. Increasing the amount of insulin required to treat the hyperglycemia intensifies the hypoglycemia.

superinfection new infection by an organism different from the initial infection being treated by antimicrobial therapy manifested by one or more of the following: black, hairy tongue; glossitis, stomatitis; anal itching; loose, foul-smelling stools; vaginal itching or discharge; sudden fever; cough.

tachyphylaxis rapid decrease in response to a drug after administration of a few doses. Initial drug response cannot be restored by an increase in dose.

tardive dyskinesia extrapyramidal symptom manifested by involuntary rhythmic, bizarre movements of face, jaw, mouth, tongue, and sometimes extremities.

vasovagal symptoms transient vascular and neurogenic reaction marked by pallor, nausea, vomiting, bradycardia, and rapid fall in arterial blood pressure.

water intoxication (dilutional hyponatremia) less than normal concentration of sodium in the blood resulting from excess extracellular and intracellular fluid and producing one or more of the following: lethargy, confusion, headache, decreased skin turgor, tremors, convulsions, coma, anorexia, nausea, vomiting, diarrhea, sternal fingerprinting, weight gain, edema, full bounding pulse, jugular vein distention, rales, signs and symptoms of pulmonary edema.

◆ APPENDIX G ABBREVIATIONS

ABGs	arterial blood gases
a.c.	before meals (*ante cibum*)
ACD	acid–citrate–dextrose
ACE	angiotensin-converting enzyme
ACh	acetylcholine
ACIP	Advisory Committee on Immunization Practices
ACLS	advanced cardiac life support
ACS	acute coronary syndrome
ACT	activated clotting time
ACTH	adrenocorticotropic hormone
AD	Alzheimer's disease
ADD	attention deficit disorder
ADH	antidiuretic hormone
ADLs	activities of daily living
ad lib	as desired (*ad libitum*)
ADP	adenosine diphosphate
ADT	alternate-day drug (administration)
AF	atrial fibrillation
AFL	atrial flutter
AIDS	acquired immunodeficiency syndrome
alpha1-PI	alpha1-proteinase inhibitor
ALS	amyotrophic lateral sclerosis
ALT	alanine aminotransferase (formerly SGPT)
AMI	acute myocardial infarction
AML	acute myelogenous leukemia
AMP	adenosine monophosphate
ANA	antinuclear antibody(ies)
ANC	absolute neutrophil count
ANH	atrial natriuretic hormone
ANLL	acute nonlymphocytic leukemia
aPTT	activated partial thromboplastin time
ARC	AIDS-related complex
ARDS	adult respiratory distress syndrome
ASHD	arteriosclerotic heart disease
AST	aspartate aminotransferase (formerly SGOT)
AT_1	angiotensin II receptor subtype I
AT_2	angiotensin II receptor subtype II
ATP	adenosine triphosphate
AV	atrioventricular
b.i.d.	two times a day
BMD	bone mineral density
BMI	body mass index
BMR	basal metabolic rate
BP	blood pressure
BPH	benign prostatic hypertrophy
bpm	beats per minute
BSA	body surface area

BSE	breast self-exam
BSP	bromsulphalein
BT	bleeding time
BUN	blood urea nitrogen
C	centigrade, Celsius
CAD	coronary artery disease
cAMP	cyclic adenosine monophosphate
CBC	complete blood count
CCR5	cellular chemokine coreceptor-5
CDC	Centers for Disease Control and Prevention
CF	cystic fibrosis
cGMP	cyclic guanosine monophosphate
CHF	congestive heart failure
CKD	chronic kidney disease
CLL	chronic lymphocytic leukemia
cm	centimeter
CML	chronic myeloid leukemia
CMV	cytomegalovirus-I
CNS	central nervous system
Coll	collyrium (eye wash)
COMT	catecholamine-*O*-methyl transferase
COPD	chronic obstructive pulmonary disease
COX-2	cyclooxygenase-2
CPK	creatinine phosphokinase
CPR	cardiopulmonary resuscitation
CrCl	creatinine clearance
CRF	chronic renal failure
CRFD	chronic renal failure disease
C&S	culture and sensitivity
CSF	cerebrospinal fluid
CSP	cellulose sodium phosphate
CSSSI	complicated skin and skin structure infections
CT	clotting time
CTZ	chemoreceptor trigger zone
CV	cardiovascular
CVA	cerebrovascular accident
CVP	central venous pressure
CYP	cytochrome P450 system of enzymes
CYP3A4	cytochrome 3A4
CYP3A	cytochrome 3A
D5W	5% dextrose in water
D&C	dilation and curettage
DIC	disseminated intravascular coagulation
DKA	diabetic ketoacidosis
dL	deciliter (100 mL or 0.1 liter)
DM	diabetes mellitus
DMARD	disease-modifying antirheumatic drug
DNA	deoxyribonucleic acid
DPD	dihydropyrimidine dehydrogenase
DTRs	deep tendon reflexes

DVT	deep venous thrombosis
ECG, EKG	electrocardiogram
ECT	electroconvulsive therapy
EEG	electroencephalogram
EENT	eye, ear, nose, throat
e.g.	for example (*exempli gratia*)
EGFR	epidermal growth factor receptor
EIB	exercise-induced bronchoconstriction
ENT	ear, nose, throat
EPS	extrapyramidal symptoms (or syndrome)
ER	estrogen receptor
ESRF	end-stage renal failure
F	Fahrenheit
FBS	fasting blood sugar
FDA	Food and Drug Administration
FSH	follicle-stimulating hormone
FTI	free thyroxine index
5-FU	5-fluorouracil
FUO	fever of unknown origin
g	gram
G6PD	glucose-6-phosphate dehydrogenase
GABA	gamma-aminobutyric acid
GERD	gastroesophageal reflux disease
GFR	glomerular filtration rate
GH	growth hormone
GI	gastrointestinal
GIST	gastrointestinal stomal tumor
GM-CSF	granulocyte-macrophage colony-stimulating factor
GnRH	gonadotropic releasing hormone
GPIIb/IIIa	glycoprotein IIb/IIIa
GU	genitourinary
h	hour
HACA	human antichimeric antibody
HbA1C	glycosylated hemoglobin
hBNP	human B-type natriuretic peptide
HBV	viral hepatitis B
HCG	human chorionic gonadotropin
Hct	hematocrit
HDD-CKD	hemodialysis-dependant chronic kidney disease
HDL-C	high-density-lipoprotein cholesterol
HER	human epidermal growth factor
HF	heart failure
Hgb	hemoglobin
5-HIAA	5-hydroxyindoleacetic acid
HIT	heparin-induced thrombocytopenia
HIV	human immunodeficiency virus
HMG-CoA	3-hydroxy-3-methyl-glutaryl coenzyme A
HPA	hypothalamic–pituitary–adrenocortical (axis)
HPV	human papillomavirus
HR	heart rate

HSV-1	herpes simplex virus type 1
HSV-2	herpes simplex virus type 2
5-HT	5-hydroxytryptamine (serotonin receptor)
IBD	inflammatory bowel disease
IBW	ideal body weight
IC	intracoronary
ICP	intracranial pressure
ICU	intensive care unit
ID	intradermal
IFN	interferon
Ig	immunoglobulin
IGF-1	insulin-like growth factor 1
IL	interleukin
IM	intramuscular
INR	international normalized ratio
IOP	intraocular pressure
IPPB	intermittent positive pressure breathing
iPTH	idiopathic parathyroid hormone
IT	intrathecal
ITP	idiopathic thrombocytopenic purpura
IV	intravenous
JRA	juvenile rheumatoid arthritis
kg	kilogram
KGF	keratinocyte growth factor
17-KGS	17-ketogenic steroids
17-KS	17-ketosteroids
KVO	keep vein open
L	liter
LDH	lactic dehydrogenase
LDL	low density lipoprotein
LDL-C	low-density-lipoprotein cholesterol
LE	lupus erythematosus
LFT	liver function test
LH	luteinizing hormone
LR	lactated Ringer's
LSD	lysergic acid diethylamide
LTRA	leukotriene receptor antagonist
LVEDP	left ventricular end diastolic pressure
LVEF	left ventricular ejection fraction
M	molar (strength of a solution)
m^2	square meter (of body surface area)
MAO	monoamine oxidase
MAOI	monoamine oxidase inhibitor
MBD	minimal brain dysfunction
MCH	mean corpuscular hemoglobin
MCHC	mean corpuscular hemoglobin concentration
mCi	millicurie
mcg	microgram (1/1000 of a milligram)
MDI	metered dose inhaler
MDR	minimum daily requirements

MDS	muscular dystrophy syndrome
mEq	milliequivalent
mg	milligram
min	minute
MI	myocardial infarction
MIC	minimum inhibitory concentration
mL	milliliter (0.001 liter)
mm	millimeter
mo	month
MPS I	mucopolysaccharidosis I
MRSA	methicillin-resistant *Staphylococcus aureus*
MS	multiple sclerosis
mu-m	micrometer
N	normal (strength of a solution)
NADH	reduced form of nicotine adenine dinucleotide
NAPA	*N*-acetyl procainamide
nb	note well (*nota bene*)
NDD	non-hemodialysis dependent
NDD-CKD	non–hemodialysis-dependent chronic kidney disease
ng	nanogram (1/1000 of a microgram)
NMS	neuroleptic malignant syndrome
NNRTI	nonnucleoside reverse transcriptase inhibitor
NON-PVC	nonpolyvinyl chloride IV bag or tubing
NPN	nonprotein nitrogen
NPO	nothing by mouth
NRTI	nucleoside reverse transcriptase inhibitor
NS	normal saline
NSAID	nonsteroidal anti-inflammatory drug
NSCLC	non–small-cell lung cancer
NSR	normal sinus rhythm
NYHA Class I, II, III, IV	New York Heart Association classes of heart failure
OAB	overactive bladder
OC	oral contraceptive
ODT	oral disintegrating tablet
17-OHCS	17-hydroxycorticosteroids
OTC	over the counter (nonprescription)
P450	cytochrome P450 system of enzymes
PABA	*para*-aminobenzoic acid
PAS	*para*-aminosalicylic acid
PAWP	pulmonary artery wedge pressure
PBI	protein-bound iodine
PBP	penicillin-binding protein
p.c.	after meals (*post cibum*)
PCI	percutaneous coronary intervention
PCP	*Pneumocystis carinii* pneumonia
PCWP	pulmonary capillary wedge pressure
PDD	peritoneal dialysis dependent
PDD-CKD	peritoneal dialysis–dependent chronic kidney disease

PDE	phosphodiesterase
PDE5	phosphodiesterase type-5
PE	pulmonary embolism
PERLA	pupils equal, react to light and accommodation
PG	prostaglandin
PGE_2	prostaglandin E_2
pH	hydrogen ion concentration
Ph	Philadelphia (chromosome)
PID	pelvic inflammatory disease
PJP	*Pneumocystis jirovecii* pneumonia
PKU	phenylketonuria
PMDD	premenstrual dysphoric disorder
PML	progressive multifocal leukoencephalopathy
PND	paroxysmal nocturnal dyspnea
PO	by mouth or orally (*per os*)
PPI	proton pump inhibitor
PPM	parts per million
PR	rectally (*per rectum*)
prn	when required (*pro re nata*)
PSA	prostate-specific antigen
PSP	phenolsulfonphthalein
PSVT	paroxysmal supraventricular tachycardia
PT	prothrombin time
PTCL	peripheral T-cell lymphocyte
PTH	parathyroid hormone
PTT	partial thromboplastin time
PUD	peptic ulcer disease
PVC	polyvinyl chloride IV bag or tubing
PVC	premature ventricular contraction
PVD	peripheral vascular disease
PZI	protamine zinc insulin
q.i.d.	four times daily
RA	rheumatoid arthritis
RAI	radioactive iodine
RAR	retinoic acid receptor
RAST	radioallergosorbent test
RBC	red blood (cell) count
RDA	recommended (daily) dietary allowance
RDS	respiratory distress syndrome
REM	rapid eye movement
rem	radiation equivalent man
RES	reticuloendothelial system
RIA	radioimmunoassay
RNA	ribonucleic acid
ROM	range of motion
RSV	respiratory syncytial virus
RT	reverse transcriptase
RT_3U	total serum thyroxine concentration
S&S	signs and symptoms
SA	sinoatrial

SBE	subacute bacterial endocarditis
SC	subcutaneous
S_{cr}	serum creatinine
sec	second
SERMs	selective estrogen receptor modulators
SGGT	serum gamma-glutamyl transferase
SGOT	serum glutamic–oxaloacetic transaminase (*see* AST)
SGPT	serum glutamic–pyruvic transaminase (*see* ALT)
SIADH	syndrome of inappropriate antidiuretic hormone
SI Units	International System of Units
SK	streptokinase
SL	sublingual
SLE	systemic lupus erythematosus
SMA	sequential multiple analysis
SNRI	serotonin norepinephrine reuptake inhibitor
SOS	if necessary (*si opus cit*)
sp	species
SPF	sun protection factor
sq	square
SR	sedimentation rate
SRS-A	slow-reactive substance of anaphylaxis
SSRI	selective serotonin reuptake inhibitor
stat	immediately
STD	sexually transmitted disease
SVT	supraventricular tachyarrhythmias
$t_{1/2}$	half-life
T_3	triiodothyronine
T_4	thyroxine
TCA	tricyclic antidepressant
TG	total triglycerides
TIA	transient ischemic attack
t.i.d.	three times a day (*ter in die*)
TKI	tyrosine kinase inhibitor
TNF	tumor necrosis factor
tPA	tissue plasminogen activator
TPN	total parenteral nutrition
TPR	temperature, pulse, respirations
TSH	thyroid-stimulating hormone
TSS	toxic shock syndrome
TT	thrombin time
UA	urinary analysis
ULN	upper limit of normal
URI	upper respiratory infection
USP	United States Pharmacopeia
USPHS	United States Public Health Service
UTI	urinary tract infection
UV-A, UVA	ultraviolet A wave
VDRL	Venereal Disease Research Laboratory
VEGF	vascular endothelial growth factor
VLDL	very low density lipoprotein

VMA	vanillylmandelic acid
VREF	vancomycin-resistant *Enterococcus faecium*
VRSA	vancomycin-resistant *Staphylococcus aureus*
VS	vital signs
wk	week
WBC	white blood (cell) count
WBCT	whole blood clotting time
y	year

◆ APPENDIX H HERBAL AND DIETARY SUPPLEMENT TABLE

As patient interest in dietary supplements and other natural products increases, there continues to be an elevated need for information on this topic. These products are not standardized or regulated by FDA guidelines; therefore, caution should be used when discussing these products. Consumers should note that since rigid quality control standards are not required for these products, substantial variability can occur in both potency and purity of a given product, especially between different commercial companies.

Many of these products have limited research on safety; thus, side effects and potential drug interactions are not well understood. Dietary supplements may either increase or decrease the level of a drug in the patient's body.

This table provides basic information on some of the most commonly sold dietary supplements. For additional information, a specialty resource on herbal and/or dietary supplements should be consulted.

Name	Most Common Use	Significant Safety Concerns
Bilberry	Eye health	Long-term, high-dose use can cause liver problems
Black cohosh	Menopausal symptoms	Should be avoided in pregnant patients
Cranberry	Urinary tract infections	Considered safe at usual doses; high dose may increase bleeding risk
Echinacea	Infections	May cause allergic reactions; should be used only short-term
Eleuthera (Siberian ginseng)	Energy	Avoid use with digoxin
Evening primrose	Menopausal symptoms	May affect seizure threshold
Garlic	Cholesterol	Significant drug interactions with drugs metabolized by CYP system
Ginkgo	Memory enhancement	Potential increased bleeding risk
Ginger	Nausea	Overdoses may cause cardiac arrhythmias
Ginseng (American ginseng)	Energy	Should not be used with MAO inhibitors; may affect anticoagulants

Name	Most Common Use	Significant Safety Concerns
Glucosamine	Osteoarthritis	Considered safe at usual doses; at higher doses, possible interaction with warfarin and other coumarin anticoagulants
Green tea	Energy, weight loss	High doses may cause cardiovascular side effects
Horny goat weed	Sexual function	Should be avoided in pregnant/lactating women
Horse chestnut	Congestive heart failure	Potential hepatotoxicity
Milk thistle	Liver function	May affect CYP metabolism and interact with drugs metabolized by this system
Saw palmetto	Benign prostatic hyperplasia	Adverse effects appear mild
Soy	Menopausal symptoms	GI-related side effects may be significant for some patients
St. John's wort	Depression	Significant drug interactions with several drugs metabolized by CYP system
Valerian	Sleep disorder	Potentially hepatotoxic
Yohimbe	Sexual function	Do not use with drugs affecting serotonin system

◆ APPENDIX I LOOK-ALIKE, SOUND-ALIKE MEDICATIONS

There are a number of medications whose names look or sound similar when pronounced. The Institute of Safe Medication Practices, the Food and Drug Administration, the Joint Commission, and other patient safety groups have reported multiple medication errors related to these medications. The list below comes from the FDA approved list of established drug names that require use of Tall Man Letters (capitalized letters to more easily distinguish between similar medication names). More extensive lists of drugs and medications are available at http://www.ismp.org.

acetoHEXAMIDE	acetaZOLAMIDE	
buPROPion	busPIRone	
chlorproMAZINE	chlorproPAMIDE	
clomiPHENE	clomiPRAMINE	
cycloSPORINE	cycloSERINE	
DAUNOrubicin	DOXOrubicin	
dimenhyDRINATE	diphenhydrAMINE	
DOBUTamine	DOPamine	
glipiZIDE	glyBURIDE	
hydrALAZINE	hydrOXYzine	
medoxyPROGESTERone	methylPREDNISolone	methylTESTOSTERone
niCARdipine	NIFEdipine	
predniSONE	prednisoLONE	
sulfADIAZINE	sulfiSOXAZOLE	
TOLAZamide	TOLBUTamide	
vinBLAStine	vinCRIStine	

Bibliography

American Academy of Pediatrics Committee on Drugs. The transfer of drugs and other chemicals into human milk. *Pediatrics*. 2001;108:776–89.

American Hospital Formulary Service (AHFS) Drug Information. 09. Bethesda, MD: American Society of Health-System Pharmacists. 2009.

Bindler R, Howry L. *Prentice Hall Pediatric Drug Guide with Nursing Implications*. Upper Saddle River, NJ: Prentice Hall Health. 2005.

Clinical Pharmacology. http://www.gsm.com. Gold Standard Media. 2009.

Drug Facts and Comparisons. http://factsandcomparisons.com. Version 4.0 online. St. Louis: Wolters Kluwer Health, Inc. 2009.

Food and Drug Administration. http://www.fda.gov. 2009.

King Guide to Parenteral Admixtures. 35th ed. Napa, CA: King Guide Publications, Inc. 2006.

Kirschheiner J, Nickchen K, Bauer M, et al. Pharmacogenetics of antidepressants and antipsychotics: the contribution of allelic variations to the phenotype of drug response. Preview. *Mol Psychiatry*. 2004;9:442–73.

Lacy CF, Armstrong LL, Goldman MP, Lance LL. *Drug Information Handbook*. 15th ed. Hudson, OH: Lexi-Comp. 2008.

Phelps SJ, Hak EB, Crill CM. *Pediatric Injectable Drugs (Teddy Bear Book)*. 8th ed. American Society of Health-System Pharmacists (ASHP). 2007.

Physicians' Desk Reference. 63rd ed. Montvale, NJ: Thompson Healthcare. 2009.

Semla TP, Beizer JL, Higbee MD. *Geriatric Dosage Handbook*. 10th ed. Hudson, OH: Lexi-Comp. 2005.

Tatro DS. *Drug Interaction Facts: Herbal Supplements and Food*. 1st ed (Paperback). Facts and Comparisons. 2004.

Trissel LA. *Handbook of Injectable Drugs*. 14th ed. Bethesda, MD: American Society of Health-System Pharmacists. 2007.

USP DI: Advice to Patients. Rockville, MD: US Pharmacopeial Convention. 2008.

USP DI: Drug Information for the Health Care Professional. Rockville, MD: US Pharmacopeial Convention. 2008.

Index

A

Drug categories are in SMALL CAPS. Prototypes in **bold.**
Generic drug names are given in parentheses.

Drug categories are in SMALL CAPS. Prototypes in **bold.**
Generic drug names are given in parentheses.

Drug categories are in SMALL CAPS. Prototypes in **bold.**
Generic drug names are given in parentheses.

Drug categories are in SMALL CAPS. Prototypes in **bold.**
Generic drug names are given in parentheses.

Drug categories are in SMALL CAPS. Prototypes in **bold.**
Generic drug names are given in parentheses.

Drug categories are in SMALL CAPS. Prototypes in **bold.**
Generic drug names are given in parentheses.

Drug categories are in SMALL CAPS. Prototypes in **bold.**
Generic drug names are given in parentheses.

Drug categories are in SMALL CAPS. Prototypes in **bold.**
Generic drug names are given in parentheses.

C

Drug categories are in SMALL CAPS. Prototypes in **bold.**
Generic drug names are given in parentheses.

Drug categories are in SMALL CAPS. Prototypes in **bold.**
Generic drug names are given in parentheses.

Drug categories are in SMALL CAPS. Prototypes in **bold.**
Generic drug names are given in parentheses.

Drug categories are in SMALL CAPS. Prototypes in **bold**.
Generic drug names are given in parentheses.

E

Drug categories are in SMALL CAPS. Prototypes in **bold.**
Generic drug names are given in parentheses.

F

Drug categories are in SMALL CAPS. Prototypes in **bold.**
Generic drug names are given in parentheses.

G

Drug categories are in SMALL CAPS. Prototypes in **bold.**
Generic drug names are given in parentheses.

Drug categories are in SMALL CAPS. Prototypes in **bold.**
Generic drug names are given in parentheses.

I

J

K

L

Drug categories are in SMALL CAPS. Prototypes in **bold.**
Generic drug names are given in parentheses.

M

Drug categories are in SMALL CAPS. Prototypes in **bold.**
Generic drug names are given in parentheses.

Drug categories are in SMALL CAPS. Prototypes in **bold.**
Generic drug names are given in parentheses.

N

Drug categories are in SMALL CAPS. Prototypes in **bold.**
Generic drug names are given in parentheses.

Drug categories are in SMALL CAPS. Prototypes in **bold.**
Generic drug names are given in parentheses.

Drug categories are in SMALL CAPS. Prototypes in **bold.**
Generic drug names are given in parentheses.

P

Drug categories are in SMALL CAPS. Prototypes in **bold.**
Generic drug names are given in parentheses.

Drug categories are in SMALL CAPS. Prototypes in **bold.**
Generic drug names are given in parentheses.

Drug categories are in SMALL CAPS. Prototypes in **bold.**
Generic drug names are given in parentheses.

Q

R

Drug categories are in SMALL CAPS. Prototypes in **bold.**
Generic drug names are given in parentheses.

Drug categories are in SMALL CAPS. Prototypes in **bold.**
Generic drug names are given in parentheses.

Drug categories are in SMALL CAPS. Prototypes in **bold.**
Generic drug names are given in parentheses.

Drug categories are in SMALL CAPS. Prototypes in **bold.**
Generic drug names are given in parentheses.

T

Drug categories are in SMALL CAPS. Prototypes in **bold.**
Generic drug names are given in parentheses.

Drug categories are in SMALL CAPS. Prototypes in **bold.**
Generic drug names are given in parentheses.

U

Drug categories are in SMALL CAPS. Prototypes in **bold.**
Generic drug names are given in parentheses.

W

Drug categories are in SMALL CAPS. Prototypes in **bold.**
Generic drug names are given in parentheses.

X

Y

Z

COMMON DRUG IV-SITE COMPATIBILITY CHART

	AMINOPHYLLINE	DOBUTAMINE	DOPAMINE	HEPARIN	MEPERIDINE	MORPHINE	NITROGLYCERIN	ONDANSETRON	POTASSIUM CL
digoxin	C	C	C	C	C	C	C	C	C
diltiazem	I/C	C	C	I/C	C	C	C		C
diphenydramine	I	C	C	I/C	C	C	C	C	C
dobutamine	I	C	C	I/C	C	C	C	C	C
dopamine	C	C	C	C	C	C	C	C	C
doxycycline	C	C	C	I	C	C	C	C	C
enalapril/enalaprilat	C	C	C	C	C	C	C	C	C
epinephrine	I	C	C	C	C	C	C	C	C
eptifibatide	C	C		C	C	C	C	C	C
erythromycin	C	C	C	I/C	C	C	C	C	I/C
esmolol	C	C	C	I/C	C	C	C	C	C
famotidine	C	C	C	C	C	C	C	C	C
filgrastim	C			I	C	C		C	C
fluconazole	C	C	C	C	C	C	C	C	C
foscarnet	C	I	C	C		C			
furosemide	C	I/C	I/C	C	I/C	I/C	I/C	I	C
ganciclovir	I	I	I	C	I	I		I	C
gentamicin	C	C	I/C	I	C	C	C	C	C
heparin	C	I/C	I/C	C	I/C	C	C	C	C
hydrocortisone	C	I	C	C	I/C	C	C	C	C
hydromorphone	C	C	C	C		C	C	C	C
imipenem/cilastatin			C	C	I/C	C	C	C	C
inamrinone	C	C	I/C	I	I/C	I	I/C	I	I/C
insulin	C	I/C		C	C	I/C	C	I/C	C
isoproterenol	I	C	C	C	C		C	C	C
labetolol	C	C	C	I/C	C	C	C	C	C
lidocaine	C	C	C	C	C	C	C	C	C
lorazepam	C	C	C	C	I	C	C	I	C

COMMON DRUG IV-SITE COMPATIBILITY CHART

	AMINOPHYLLINE	DOBUTAMINE	DOPAMINE	HEPARIN	MEPERIDINE	MORPHINE	NITROGLYCERIN	ONDANSETRON	POTASSIUM CL
acyclovir	C	I	I	C	I/C	I/C	C	I	C
alteplase		I	I	I			I		
amikacin	C	C	C	I	C	C	C	C	C
amino acids (TPN)	I/C	C	C	C	C	C			C
aminophylline	C	I	I/C	C	C	C	C	I	C
amiodarone	I	C	C	I	C	C	C		C
ampicillin	I	I	I	I/C	I/C	I/C	I/C	I	I/C
ampicillin/sulbactam	I/C	I		I/C	I/C	I/C	I/C	I	I/C
aztreonam	C	C	C	C	C	C	C	C	C
bretylium	C	I/C	C	C	C	C	C	C	C
bumetanide		I/C	C	C	C	C	C	C	C
calcium chloride	C	C	C	C	C	C	C	C	C
cefazolin	C	I	I	C	C	C	C	C	C
cefoperazone	C	I	I	C	I	I/C	C	I	C
cefotaxime	C		C	C	C	C	C	C	C
cefotetan	C	I	C	C	I/C	C	C	I/C	C
cefoxitin		I	C	C	C	C	C	C	C
ceftazidime	C	I/C	C	C	C	C	C	I/C	C
ceftizoxime	C		C	C	C	C	C	C	C
ceftriaxone	C	I	C	C	C	C	C	I/C	C
cefuroxime	C	I	C	C	C	C	C	C	C
chloramphenicol	C	I	C	C	I/C	C	C	I	C
cimetidine	C	C	C	C	C	C	C	C	C
ciprofloxacin	I	C	C	I	C			C	C
clindamycin	I/C		C	C	C	C	C	C	C
dexamethasone	C	I	C	C	C	C	C	C	C
diazepam	I	I/C	I	I	I	I/C	I	I/C	I